The New York School of Regional Anesthesia

HADZIC'S TEXTBOOK OF REGIONAL ANESTHESIA AND ACUTE PAIN MANAGEMENT

NOTICE

Medicine is an ever-changing science. As new research and clinical experience broaden our knowledge, changes in treatment and drug therapy are required. The authors and the publisher of this work have checked with sources believed to be reliable in their efforts to provide information that is complete and generally in accord with the standards accepted at the time of publication. However, in view of the possibility of human error or changes in medical sciences, neither the authors nor the publisher nor any other party who has been involved in the preparation or publication of this work warrants that the information contained herein is in every respect accurate or complete, and they disclaim all responsibility for any errors or omissions or for the results obtained from use of the information contained in this work. Readers are encouraged to confirm the information contained herein with other sources. For example and in particular, readers are advised to check the product information sheet included in the package of each drug they plan to administer to be certain that the information contained in this work is accurate and that changes have not been made in the recommended dose or in the contraindications for administration. This recommendation is of particular importance in connection with new or infrequently used drugs.

The New York School of Regional Anesthesia

HADZIC'S TEXTBOOK OF REGIONAL ANESTHESIA AND ACUTE PAIN MANAGEMENT

SECOND EDITION

Editor

Admir Hadzic, MD, PhD
Professor of Anesthesiology
Director, New York School of Regional Anesthesia
New York, New York
Consultant, Anesthesiology, Intensive Care, Emergency Medicine and Pain Therapy
Ziekenhuis Oost-Limburg
Genk, Belgium

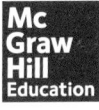

New York   Chicago   San Francisco   Athens   London   Madrid   Mexico City
Milan   New Delhi   Singapore   Sydney   Toronto

2 3 4 5 6 7 8 9   DSS   22 21 20 19 18 17

ISBN 978-0-07-171759-5
MHID 0-07-171759-5

This book was set in Minion by Adobe Garamond Pro by Cenveo® Publisher Services.
The editors were Brian Belval and Christie Naglieri.
The production supervisor was Catherine H. Saggese.
The cover designer was Randomatrix.
Production management was provided by Sonam Arora, Cenveo Publisher Services.

This book is printed on acid-free paper.

Library of Congress Cataloging-in-Publication Data

Names: Hadzic, Admir, editor. | New York School of Regional Anesthesia.
Title: Textbook of regional anesthesia and acute pain management / editor,
    Admir Hadzic.
Description: Second edition. | New York : McGraw-Hill Education, [2017] |
    Includes bibliographical references and index.
Identifiers: LCCN 2016008484| ISBN 9780071717595 (hardcover) |
    ISBN 0071717595 (hardcover)
Subjects: | MESH: Anesthesia, Conduction—methods | Pain Management
Classification: LCC RD84 | NLM WO 300 | DDC 617.9/64—dc23 LC record available at
    http://lccn.loc.gov/2016008484

McGraw-Hill are available at special quantity discounts to use as premiums and sales promotions,
or for use in corporate training programs. To contact a representative please visit the Contact Us pages at
www.mhprofessional.com.

This book is dedicated to Dr. Steven Dewaele (1974–2016), for he, the Ironman and essential marine of NYSORA's team, has inspired many by his zeal for life and the dedication with which he pursued everything he aimed at.

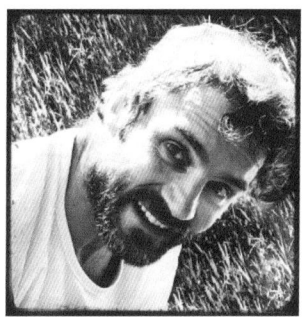

"The most dangerous risk of all is the risk of spending your life not doing what you want on the bet that you can buy yourself the freedom to do it later."

CONTENTS

PART 1

HISTORY

PART 2

FOUNDATIONS OF LOCAL AND REGIONAL ANESTHESIA

PART 3

CLINICAL PRACTICE OF REGIONAL ANESTHESIA

PART 4

ULTRASOUND IMAGING OF NEURAXIAL AND PERIVERTEBRAL SPACE

PART 5

OBSTETRIC ANESTHESIA

PART 6

PEDIATRIC ANESTHESIA

PART 7

ANESTHESIA IN PATIENTS WITH SPECIFIC CONSIDERATIONS

PART 8

REGIONAL ANESTHESIA IN THE EMERGENCY DEPARTMENT

PART 9

COMPLICATIONS OF LOCAL AND REGIONAL ANESTHESIA

PART 10

LAST: LOCAL ANESTHETIC SYSTEMIC TOXICITY

PART 11

PERIOPERATIVE OUTCOME AND ECONOMICS OF REGIONAL ANESTHESIA

PART 12

ACUTE PAIN MANAGEMENT

PART 13

EDUCATION IN REGIONAL ANESTHESIA

PART 14

STATISTICS AND PRINCIPLES OF RESEARCH DESIGN IN REGIONAL ANESTHESIA AND ACUTE PAIN MEDICINE

PART 15

NERVE STIMULATOR AND SURFACE ANATOMY-BASED NERVE BLOCKS

APPENDICES

CONTRIBUTORS

Sherif Abbas, MD
Anesthesiology Assistant
Catholic University of Leuven
Leuven, Belgium

Jolaade Adebayo, MD, D.ABA
Staff Anesthesiologist
Tanner Health System
Department of Surgery
Carrollton, Georgia

José Aguirre, MD
Team Leader Anesthesia Education and Research
Study Coordination UCAR
Consultant Anesthetist
Balgrist University Hospital
Zurich, Switzerland

Imran Ahmad, FRCA
Honorary Senior Lecturer, King's College
Consultant Anaesthetist
Clinical Lead for Airway Management
Guy's Hospital
Guy's and St. Thomas' NHS Foundation Trust
London, United Kingdom

Omar Ahmed, MD
Anesthesiologist
Premier Care Anesthesia
New York Medical College
Orange County, California

Michael H. Andreae, MD
Department of Anesthesiology
Montefiore Medical Center
Albert Einstein College of Medicine
New York, New York

Riánsares Arriazu, PharmD, PhD
Histology Laboratory
Institute of Applied Molecular Medicine
Department of Basic Medical Sciences
School of Medicine, CEU-San Pablo University
Madrid, Spain

Arthur Atchabahian, MD
Professor of Clinical Anesthesiology
Department of Anesthesiology, Perioperative Care, and Pain
    Medicine
NYU School of Medicine
New York, New York

Michael J. Barrington, MB, BS, FANZCA, PhD
Associate Professor
University of Melbourne
Senior Staff Anaesthetist
Department of Anaesthesia and Acute Pain Medicine
St. Vincent's Hospital Melbourne, Fitzroy
Victoria, Australia

David Beausang, MD
Assistant Professor
Department of Anesthesiology
Sidney Kimmel Medical College
Thomas Jefferson University and Hospitals
Philadelphia, Pennsylvania

Thomas Fichtner Bendtsen, MD, PhD
Associate Professor of Anesthesiology
Consultant, Anesthesiology
Aarhus University Hospital
Aarhus, Denmark

Honorio T. Benzon, MD
Professor of Anesthesiology
Northwestern University Feinberg School of Medicine
Chicago, Illinois

David J. Birnbach, MD, MPH
Professor of Anesthesiology and Obstetrics and Gynecology
Chief of Women's Anesthesia
Jackson Memorial Hospital
University of Miami
Miami, Florida

Rafael Blanco, MD, BS, FRCA, DEAA
Senior Consultant Anaesthetist
Corniche Hospital
Abu Dhabi
United Arab Emirates

Stephan Blumenthal, MD
Assistant Professor
Head of Institute of Anesthesiology
Bulach Hospital
Bulach, Switzerland

Alain Borgeat, MD
Professor of Anesthesiology
Director, University of Balgrist
Zurich, Switzerland

Herve Bouaziz, MD
Professor of Anesthesiology
Department of Anaesthesiology and Critical Care.
Nancy University Hospital,
Nancy, France

Cedric Bouts, MD
Anaesthesia Resident
Katholieke Universiteit Leuven (KUL)
Ziekenhuis Oost-Limburg, ZOL
Genk, Belgium

Richard Brull, MD, FRCPC
Professor of Anesthesia
University of Toronto
Chief, Department of Anesthesia
Women's College Hospital
Toronto, Ontario, Canada

Robbert Buck, MD
Anaesthesia Resident
University of Antwerp
Ziekenhuis Oost-Limburg, ZOL
Genk, Belgium

Chester "Trip" Buckenmaier III, MD
Professor of Anesthesiology
Director, Defense and Veterans Center for Integrative Pain
    Management
Uniformed Services University
Rockville, Maryland

Christiana C. Burts, BA, MB, FRCA
Consultant Anesthetist
Papworth Hospital NHS Foundation Trust
Cambridge, United Kingdom

John Butterworth IV, MD
Professor and Chairman
Department of Anesthesiology
Virginia Commonwealth University School of Medicine
Richmond, Virginia

Asokumar Buvanendran, MD
Professor, Department of Anesthesiology
William Gottschalk, Endowed Chair of Anesthesiology
Vice Chair Research and Director of Orthopedic Anesthesia
Rush University Medical Center
Chicago, Illinois

Bram Byloos, MD
Anaesthesia Resident
Katholieke Universiteit Leuven (KUL)
Ziekenhuis Oost-Limburg, ZOL
Genk, Belgium

Kenneth D. Candido, MD
Professor of Clinical Anesthesiology
Clinical Professor of Surgery
University of Illinois Chicago
Chairman, Department of Anesthesiology
Advocate Illinois Masonic Medical Center
Chicago, Illinois

Xavier Capdevila, MD, PhD
Professor or Anesthesiology and
    Critical Care Medicine
Head, Department of Anesthesiology
    and Critical Care Medicine
Lapeyronie University Hospital
NeuroScience Institute
Montpellier University
Montpellier, France

Anna Carrera, MD, PhD
Professor of Human Anatomy
NEOMA Research Group
Medical Science Department
Faculty of Medicine, University of Girona
Girona, Spain

Gregory M. Casey, DDS, MD
Cosmetic Facial Surgery Private Practice
Associate Clinical Professor
University of Florida
Oral and Maxillofacial Surgery
Naples, Florida

Tessy Castermans, MD
Anaesthesia Resident
University of Antwerp
Ziekenhuis Oost-Limburg, ZOL
Genk, Belgium

Vincent Chan, MD, FRCPC, FRCA
Professor
Department of Anesthesia
University of Toronto
Toronto, Ontario, Canada

Adrian Chin, MBBS, FANZCA
Department of Anesthesiology
Royal Brisbane and Women's Hospital
Brisbane, Queensland, Australia

Ki Jinn Chin, MBBS, MMed, FRCPC
Associate Professor
Department of Anesthesia,
Toronto Western Hospital
University of Toronto
Toronto, Ontario, Canada

Jason Choi, MD
Attending Anesthesiologist
White Plains Hospital
White Plains, New York

Lynn Choi, MD
Assistant Clinical Professor
Department of Anesthesiology and Perioperative Medicine
University of California, Los Angeles
Los Angeles, California

Stephen Choi, MD, FRCPC, MSc
Assistant Professor of Anesthesiology
Sunnybrook Health Sciences Centre
University of Toronto
Toronto, Ontario, Canada

Olivier Choquet, MD, MSc
Consultant, Associate Professor
Department of Anesthesia and Critical Care Unit
Lapeyronie University Hospital
Montpellier France

Alwin Chuan, MBBS, PhD, PGCertCU, FANZCA
Senior Clinical Lecturer
University of New South Wales
Consultant, Anaesthesiology
Liverpool Hospital
Sydney, Australia

Laura Clark, MD
Professor
Residency Program Director
Director of Regional Anesthesia and Acute Pain
University of Louisville
Louisville, Kentucky

Thomas B. Clark, DC, RVT, RMSK
Professor of Radiology
Logan University
St. Louis, Missouri

Stacy A. Coffin, MD
Anesthesiologist
St. Luke's Hospital of Duluth
Duluth, Minnesota

Kathleen Colfer, MSN, RN-BC
Clinical Nurse Specialist and Manager
Acute Pain Management Service
Department of Anesthesiology
Thomas Jefferson University Hospital
Philadelphia, Pennsylvania

Erika Cvetko, DD, PhD
Professor of Anatomy
Head of the Institute of Anatomy
Faculty of Medicine
University of Ljubljana
Ljubljana, Slovenia

Christophe Dadure, MD, PhD
Professor of Anesthesiology and
    Critical Care Medicine
Head of Department of Anesthesiology
Lapeyronie University Hospital
Montpellier, France

Elyad Davidson, MD
Anesthesiologist
Miami, Florida

Jose A de Andrés, MD, PhD, FIPP, EDRA
Professor of Anesthesia
Valencia School of Medicine
Chairman Anesthesia, Critical Care and Pain Management
    Department
General University Hospital
Valencia, Spain

Belen De Jose Maria, MD, PhD, ECFMG
Consultant in Pediatric Anesthesia
Hospital Sant Joan de Deu, University of Barcelona
Barcelona, Spain

Rick Delmonte, DPM, FACFAS
Foot and Ankle Surgeon
NYU Langone Medical Center
New York, New York

Gildasio S. De Oliveira Jr, MD, MSCI
Assistant Professor of Anesthesiology
Associate Chair for Research
Department of Anesthesiology
Northwestern University
Feinberg School of Medicine
Chicago, Illinois

Steven Dewaele, MD
Consultant, Anesthesiology
Intensive Care Medicine
Emergency Medicine
Ziekenhuis Oost-Limburg
Genk, Belgium

Franklin Dexter, MD, PhD
Professor, Department of Anesthesia
Director, Division of Management Consulting
University of Iowa
Iowa City, Iowa

Rishi M. Diwan, FRCA, MD, MBBS
Consultant Paediatric Anaesthetist and
    Acute Pain Lead
Deputy Clinical Director
Jackson Rees Department of Anaesthetics
Alder Hey Children's NHS Foundation Trust
Liverpool, United Kingdom

Lisa Doan, MD
Assistant Professor
Department of Anesthesiology, Perioperative Care and
    Pain Medicine
New York University School of Medicine
New York, New York

Jennifer E. Dominguez, MD, MHS
Anesthesiologist
Duke University Hospital
Durham, North Carolina

Joris Duerinckx, MD
Consultant, Orthopaedic and Hand Surgery
Ziekenhuis Oost-Limburg, ZOL
Genk, Belgium

Dimitri Dylst, MD
Consultant, Anesthesiology
Intensive Care Medicine
Emergency Medicine
Ziekenhuis Oost-Limburg
Genk, Belgium

Hesham Elsharkawy, MD, MSc
Staff, Anesthesiology Institute
Cleveland Clinic
Assistant Professor of Anesthesiology
CCLCM of Case Western Reserve
University of Cleveland
Cleveland, Ohio

Trent Emerick, MD
Assistant Clinical Professor
Department of Anesthesiology and Division of Chronic Pain
University of Pittsburgh
Pittsburgh, Pennsylvania

Hillenn Cruz Eng, MD
Assistant Professor
Department of Anesthesiology and Perioperative Medicine
Penn State Health
Hershey, Pennsylvania

Holly Evans, MD
Assistant Professor, University of Ottawa
Anesthesiologist, The Ottawa Hospital
Ottawa, Ontario, Canada

Paul Fettes, MBChB, BSc
Consultant Anaesthetist and
    Honorary Senior Lecturer
Department of Anaesthesia
Ninewells Hospital and Medical School
Dundee, Scotland, United Kingdom

Michael Fettiplace, MD
PhD Student at University of Illinois
College of Medicine
Chicago, Illinois

Peter Foldes, MD
Anesthesiologist
Department of Anesthesiology
Tulane University Medical Center
New Orleans, Louisiana

Elisabeth Fouché, MD
Digital Editor, Designer
Paris, France

Carlo D. Franco, MD
Professor Anesthesiology and Anatomy
Chairman Regional Anesthesia
JHS Hospital of Cook County
Chicago, Illinois

Jeff Gadsden, MD, FRCPC, FANZCA
Associate Professor
Duke University School of Medicine
Chief, Division of Orthopaedic, Plastic and Regional Anesthesiology
Duke University Medical Center
Durham, North Carolina

Elizabeth Gaertner, MD
Department of Anesthesiology
Hautepierre Hospital
Strasbourg, France

Tong J. Gan, MD, MHS, FRCA
Professor and Chairman
Department of Anesthesiology
Stony Brook University
Stony Brook, New York

Zoe S. Gan, BA
Medical Student
University of North Carolina School of Medicine
Chapel Hill, North Carolina

Philippe E. Gautier, MD
Head of Department
Director of Obstetric and Regional Anesthesia
Clinique Ste-Anne St.-Remi
Brussels, Belgium

Andrew J. Gentilin, MD
Anesthesiologist
CAMC Health System
Charleston, West Virginia

Liane Germond, MD
Anesthesiologist
Ochsner Medical Center
New Orleans, Lousiana

Christopher Gharibo, MD
Associate Professor of Anesthesiology and Pain Medicine
Associate Professor of Orthopedics
NYU School of Medicine
New York, New York

Marina Gitman, MD
Assistant Professor of Anesthesiology
University of Illinois Hospital
Chicago, Illinois

Michael S. Gold, PhD
Professor of Anesthesiology
Center for Pain Research
University of Pittsburgh
Pittsburgh, Pennsylvania

Monika Golebiewski, MD
Research Associate
NYSORA Europe
Munich, Germany

Paul M. Greenberg, DPM, FACFAS
Fellow, American College of Foot and Ankle Surgeons
Diplomate, American Board of Foot and Ankle Surgery
NYU Faculty Group Practice-Podiatry Associates Upper West Side
NYU Langone Medical Center
New York, New York

Roy A. Greengrass, MD, FRCP
Professor of Anesthesiology
Fellowship Director Acute Pain and Regional Anesthesia
Mayo Clinic Jacksonville Florida

Yavuz Gürkan, MD
Professor of Anaesthesiology
Kocaeli University Hospital
Kocaeli, Turkey

Patrick J. Hackett, MD
Department of Anesthesiology
Spectrum Medical Group
Maine Medical Center
Portland, Maine

Admir Hadzic, MD, PhD
Professor of Anesthesiology
Director of NYSORA
New York, New York
Consultant, Anesthesiology, Intensive Care, Emergency Medicine
    and Pain Therapy
Ziekenhuis Oost-Limburg
Genk, Belgium

Thomas M. Halaszynski, DMD, MD, MBA
Associate Professor of Anesthesiology
Senior Director of Regional Anesthesiology/Acute Pain Medicine
Yale University School of Medicine
New Haven, Connecticut

Sarah Hall, MD
Department of Anesthesiology and Critical Care Medicine
Johns Hopkins Hospital
Baltimore, Maryland

Marie N. Hanna, MD
Associate Professor, Anesthesia and Critical Care Medicine
Chief, Division of Regional Anesthesia and Acute Pain Management
Johns Hopkins Hospital
Baltimore, Maryland

Brian E. Harrington, MD
Anesthesiology/Pain Medicine
Billings Clinic Hospital
Billings, Montana

William Harrop-Griffiths, MD
Consultant Anaesthetist
Imperial College Healthcare NHS Trust
London, England

Ilvana Hasanbegovic, MD, PhD
Professor at Department of Anatomy
Faculty of Medicine
University of Sarajevo
Sarajevo, Bosnia and Herzegovina

James R. Hebl, MD
Professor of Anesthesiology
Regional Vice-President
Mayo Clinic
Rochester, Minnesota

Andrew A. Herring, MD
Assistant Clinical Professor
Department of Emergency Medicine
University of California, San Francisco
Director Emergency Pain and Addiction Treatment
Highland Hospital, Alameda Health System
Oakland, California

Adam T. Hershkin, DMD
Department of Oral and Maxillofacial Surgery
Mount Sinai St. Luke's Hospital
New York, New York

Loreen A. Herwaldt, MD
Department of Internal Medicine
Carver College of Medicine
Program of Hospital Epidemiology
University of Iowa Hospitals and Clinics
Iowa City, Iowa

Anthony M.-H. Ho, MD, FRCPC, FCCP
Professor
Department of Anesthesiology and Perioperative Medicine
Director, Pediatric Anesthesia
Queen's University
Kingston, Ontario, Canada

Paul Hobeika, MD
Assistant Professor of Orthopedic Surgery
Staff Orthopedic Surgeon
St. Luke's–Roosevelt Hospital
College of Physicians and Surgeons
Columbia University
New York, New York

Brian M. Ilfeld, MD, MS
Professor of Anesthesiology
University of California
San Diego, California

Vivian H. Y. Ip, MBChB, MRCP, FRCA
Clinical Assistant Professor
Director, Ambulatory Regional Anesthesia
Staff Anesthesiologist
University of Alberta Hospital
Edmonton, Alberta, Canada

Rasha S. Jabri, MD
Chief, Section of Pain Medicine
Tawam Hospital
Abu Dhabi, United Arab Emirates
Adjunct Assistant Professor of Anesthesiology
Johns Hopkins Hospital
Baltimore, Maryland

Adam K. Jacob, MD
Assistant Professor of Anesthesiology
Mayo Clinic, Indiana
University School of Medicine
Rochester, Minnesota

Hassanin Jalil, MD
Consultant Anesthesiologist
Intensive Care Specialist
Hospital Hasselt
Hasselt, Belgium

Eldan Kapur, MD
Associate Professor of Anatomy
Department of Anatomy
Medicine School
University of Sarajevo
Sarajevo, Bosnia and Herzegovina

Manoj K. Karmakar, MD
Associate Professor
Department of Anaesthesia and Intensive Care
The Chinese University of Hong Kong
Prince of Wales Hospital
Shatin, New Territories
Hong Kong

Joseph Kay, MD
Assistant Professor of Anesthesiology
Department of Anesthesia
Sunnybrook and Women's College Health Sciences Centre
University of Toronto
Toronto, Ontario, Canada

Paul Kessler, MD, PhD
Professor of Anesthesiology
Head of Department of Anesthesiology
Intensive Care and Pain Medicine
Orthopedic University Hospital Frankfurt
Frankfurt, Germany

Kyle R. Kirkham, MD, FRCPC
Lecturer, Department of Anesthesia
University of Toronto
Staff Anesthesiologist-Women's College Hospital
    and University Health Network-Toronto Western Hospital
Toronto, Canada

Sandra Kopp, MD
Associate Professor of Anesthesiology
Vice Chair, Integration and Convergence, Department of
    Anesthesiology
Chair, Division of Community Anesthesia
Consultant, Anesthesiology
Mayo Clinic College of Medicine
Rochester, Minnesota

Zbigniew J. Koscielniak-Nielsen, MD, PhD, FRCA
Assistant Professor
Orthopedic Anesthesia Research
Rigshospitalet
Copenhagen, Denmark

Maxine M. Kuroda, PhD, MPH
Epidemiologist/Biostatistician
Clinical Research Manager
NYSORA-SciMedBE
Ziekenhuis Oost-Limburg
Genk, Belgium

Joseph Largi, MD
Anesthesiologist
NYU Langone Medical Center
New York, New York

Malikah Latmore, MD
Assistant Professor of Anesthesiology
Mount Sinai St. Luke's and
    Mount Sinai West Hospitals
New York, New York

John Laur, MD, MS
Clinical Associate Professor
Chief of Anesthesiology
William S Middleton VA Hospital
University of Wisconsin-Madison
Madison, Wisconsin

Suzanne Lenart, RNC
Acute Pain Nurse
Department of Anesthesiology
Thomas Jefferson University Hospital
Philadelphia, Pennsylvania

Ine Leunen, MD
Regional Anesthesia Fellow
NYSORA Europe
Ziekenhuis Oost-Limburg
Genk, Belgium

Matthew Levine, MBChB, FANZCA
Specialist Anaesthetist
Capital and Coast District Health Board
Wellington, New Zealand

Jinlei Li, MD, PhD
Director of Education
Regional Anesthesia and Acute Pain Medicine Fellowship
Director of Regional Anesthesiology for YNHH Saint Raphael
    Campus and Center for Musculoskeletal Disease
Department of Anesthesia
Yale University
New Haven, Connecticut

Pulsar Li, DO
Instructor, Department of Anesthesiology
Pediatric Division
Loyola University Medical Center
Chicago, Illinois

Emily Lin, MD, MS
Assistant Anesthesiologist
Department of Anesthesiology and Critical Care Medicine
Memorial Sloan Kettering Cancer Center
New York, New York

Jui-An Lin, MD, PhD
Assistant Professor of Anesthesiology
College of Medicine, Taipei Medical University
Staff Physician, Department of Anesthesiology
Wan Fang Hospital
Taipei, Taiwan

Sanford Littwin, MD
Associate Professor of Anesthesiology
Clinical Director Operating Rooms
UPP Department of Anesthesiology
UPMC Presbyterian and Montefiore Hospitals
Pittsburgh, Pennsylvania

Qing Liu, MD, PhD
Assistant Professor
Department of Anesthesiology
University of Pittsburgh Medical Center
Pittsburgh, Pennsylvania

Ana M. López, MD, PhD, DESA
Associate Professor of Anesthesiology
Consultant, Department of Anesthesiology
Hospital Clinic de Barcelona
Barcelona, Spain

Andrés López, MD
Head, Department of Anesthesiology
HM Hospitales
Madrid, Spain

Sofie Louage, MD
Regional Anesthesia Fellow
NYSORA Europe
Ziekenhuis Oost-Limburg
Genk, Belgium

Amanda Lukof, MD
Department of Anesthesiology
Thomas Jefferson University Hospital
Philadelphia, Pennsylvania

Fabiola Machés, MD
Anesthesiologist
HM Hospitales
Madrid, Spain

Navin A. Mallavaram, MD
Founder, Medical Director
California Pain
Multidisciplinary Pain Management Clinic
Pleasanton, California

Colin J. L. McCartney, MBChB, PhD, FRCA, FCARCSI, FRCPC
Chair of Anesthesiology and Pain Medicine
University of Ottawa
Head of Anesthesiology and Pain Medicine
The Ottawa Hospital
Ottawa, Ontario, Canada

Patrick M. McQuillan, MD
Professor, Anesthesiology and Pediatrics
Department of Anesthesiology and
    Perioperative Medicine
Penn State Health
Hershey, Philadelphia

Shaun De Meirsman, MD
Anaesthesia Resident
Katholieke Universiteit Leuven (KUL)
Ziekenhuis Oost-Limburg, ZOL
Genk, Belgium

M. Steve Melton, MD
Assistant Professor
Department of Anesthesiology
Duke University Medical Center
Durham, North Carolina

Stavros G. Memtsoudis, MD, PhD, FCCP
Clinical Professor of Anesthesiology and Healthcare Policy and
    Research
Weill Cornell Medical College
Senior Scientist and Attending Anesthesiologist
Director, Critical Care Services
Hospital for Special Surgery
New York, New York

Marija Meznaric, MD, PhD
Assistant Professor of Anatomy
Institute of Anatomy
Faculty of Medicine
University of Ljubljana
Ljubljana, Slovenia

Andres Missair, MD, EDRA
Associate Professor
University of Miami
Section Chief, Associate Director Fellowship Program, Acute Pain
    Medicine
Department of Anesthesiology
VA Hospital
Miami, Florida

Amanda M. Monahan, MD
Assistant Clinical Professor
Department of Anesthesiology
University of California
San Diego, California

Hiroaki Murata, MD, PhD
Associate Professor
Department of Anesthesiology
Nagasaki University Graduate School of Biomedical Sciences
Nagasaki, Japan

Tatsuo Nakamoto, MD, PhD
Professor of Regional Anesthesia and Pain Medicine
Department of Anesthesiology
Kansai Medical University
Hirakata, Japan

Joseph M. Neal, MD
Anesthesiology Faculty
Virginia Mason Medical Center
Clinical Professor of Anesthesiology
University of Washington
Seattle, Washington

Andrew Neice, MD
Assistant Professor
Department of Anesthesia and Perioperative Medicine
Oregon Health and Science University
Portland, Oregon

Ariana Nelson, MD
Assistant Professor of Anesthesiology and Pain Medicine
University of California
Irvine Orange, California

Ahtsham U. Niazi, MBBS, FCARCSI, FRCPC
Associate Professor of Anesthesia
University of Toronto
Staff Anesthetist
Toronto Western Hospital
University Health Network
Toronto, Ontario, Canada

Karen C. Nielsen, MD
Associate Professor of Anesthesiology
Duke University Medical Center
Durham, North Carolina

Steven L. Orebaugh, MD
Professor of Anesthesiology
University of Pittsburgh School of Medicine
Pittsburgh, Pennsylvania

Tatjana Stopar Pintaric, MD, PhD, DEAA
Associate Professor
Consultant Anaesthesiologist
Clinical Department of Anaesthesiology and Intensive Therapy
University Medical Centre Ljubljana
Ljubljana, Slovenia

Jean M. Pottinger, RN, MA
Program of Hospital Epidemiology
University of Iowa Hospitals and Clinics
Iowa City, Iowa

John-Paul J. Pozek, MD
Assistant Professor
Department of Anesthesiology
Sidney Kimmel Medical College
Thomas Jefferson University and Hospitals
Philadelphia, Pennsylvania

Alberto Prats-Galino, MD, PhD
Professor of Human Anatomy and Embryology
Director, Laboratory of Surgical NeuroAnatomy (LSNA)
Department of Surgery and Medical-Surgical Specialities
Faculty of Medicine, University of Barcelona
Barcelona, Spain

Benaifer D. Preziosi, DMD
Diplomate of the American Board of Oral and
    Maxillofacial Surgery
Department Chair of Oral and Maxillofacial Surgery
AtlantiCare Regional Medical Center
Linwood, New Jersey

Stavros Prineas, BSc(Med), MBBS, FRCA, FANZCA
Consultant Anaesthetist
Sydney Eye Hospital
Nepean Hospital
Sydney, Australia

John Rae, MBChB
Specialty Trainee in Anaesthesia
Department of Anaesthesia
Ninewells Hospital and Medical School
Dundee, Scotland, United Kingdom

Johan Raeder, MD, PhD
Professor
Faculty of Medicine, University of Oslo
Senior Consultant
Department of Anaesthesiology
Oslo University Hospital
Oslo, Norway

Jayanthie S. Ranasinghe, MD
Professor of Clinical Anesthesiology
University of Miami Health System
Miami, Florida

Miguel A. Reina, MD, PhD
Professor of Anesthesiology
School of Medicine
CEU San Pablo University, Madrid
Senior Associate in Department of Anesthesiology
Madrid-Montepríncipe University Hospital
Madrid, Spain

Steve Roberts, MBChB, FRCA
Consultant Paediatric Anaesthetist
Jackson Rees Department of Anaesthesia
Alder Hey Children's Foundation Trust
Liverpool, United Kingdom

Xavier Sala-Blanch, MD
Associate Professor of Anatomy
Head of Orthopedic Anesthesia
Hospital Clinic de Barcelona
Barcelona, Spain

Alan C. Santos, MD, MPH
Professor of Anesthesiology
Executive Vice-Chairman
Texas Tech University Health Sciences Center
Lubbock, Texas

Leslie Schechter, PharmD
Advanced Practice Pharmacist
Thomas Jefferson University Hospital
Philadelphia, Pennsylvania

Ruben Schreurs, MD
Anaesthesia Resident
Katholieke Universiteit Leuven (KUL)
Ziekenhuis Oost-Limburg, ZOL
Genk, Belgium

Sebastian Schulz-Stübner, MD, PhD
Professor of Anesthesiology
Chief Physician
German Consulting Center for Infection Control and Prevention
    (BZH GmbH)
Freiburg, Germany

Kara G. Segna, MD
Assistant Professor of Anesthesiology and Critical Care Medicine
Johns Hopkins Hospital
Baltimore, Maryland

Paul J. Seider, MD
Oral and Maxillofacial Surgeon
Fort Lauderdale, Florida

Ann-Sofie Smeets, MD
Resident of Anaesthesiology, KUL
Ziekenhuis Oost-Limburg, ZOL
Genk, Belgium

Chrystelle Sola, MD, MSc
Associate Professor
Pediatric Anesthesia Unit
Department of Anesthesia and Critical Care Medicine
Lapeyronie University Hospital
Montpellier, France

Christina M. Spofford, MD, PhD
Associate Professor of Anesthesiology
Director, Regional Anesthesia and Acute Pain Fellowship
Medical College of Wisconsin
Milwaukee, Wisconsin

Ulrich J. Spreng, MD, PhD
Head of the Department in Anesthesiology, Critical Care and
    Emergencies
Baerum Hospital
Vestre Viken HF, Norway

Susan M. Steele, MD
Anesthesiologist
American Anesthesiology of North Carolina
Raleigh, North Carolina

Ottokar Stundner, MD
Assistant Professor of Anesthesiology and Intensive Care Medicine
Lecturer, Department of Anesthesiology
Perioperative Medicine and Intensive Care Medicine
Paracelsus Medical University
Salzburg, Austria

Yanxia Sun, MD, PHD
Staff Anesthesiologist
Department of Anesthesiology
Beijing Tongren Hospital
Capital Medical University
Beijing, China

Suzuko Suzuki, MD
Anesthesiology
Brigham and Women's Hospital
Boston, Massachusetts

Anthony R. Tharian, MD
Director of Regional Anesthesia and Acute Pain Management
Advocate Illinois Masonic Medical Center
Clinical Assistant Professor
University of Illinois
Chicago, Illinois

Daniel M. Thys, MD
Professor Emeritus
Columbia University
Chairman Emeritus
St. Luke's–Roosevelt Hospital Center
New York, New York

Luc Tielens, MD
Pediatric Anesthesiologist
Radboud University Medical Center
Nijmegen, The Netherlands

Knox H. Todd, MD, MPH, FACEP
Founding Chair
Department of Emergency Medicine
MD Anderson Cancer Center
Director, EMLine.org
Mendoza, Argentina

Roulhac D. Toledano, MD, PhD
Director, Obstetric Anesthesia
NYU Lutheran Medical Center
New York, New York
Assistant Professor of Anesthesiology
SUNY Downstate Medical Center
Brooklyn, New York

Tony Tsai, MD
Assistant Professor of Anesthesiology
Regional Anesthesiologist
St. Luke's–Roosevelt Hospital
College of Physicians and Surgeons
Columbia University
New York, New York

Ban C. H. Tsui, BPharm, MSc, MD, FRCP(C), PG Dip Echo
Professor of Anesthesiology
Adult and Pediatric Anesthesiologist
Department of Anesthesiology, Perioperative and Pain Medicine
Stanford University School of Medicine
Stanford, California

Sam Van Boxstael, MD
Emergency Physician
Resident in Anesthesiology, KUL
Ziekenhuis Oost-Limburg, ZOL
Genk, Belgium

Catherine Vandepitte, MD
Consultant, Anesthesiology
Ziekenhuis Oost-Limburg
Genk, Belgium

Marc Van de Velde, MD, PhD, EDRA
Professor of Anesthesiology
Chair, Department of Anesthesiology
Department of Cardiovascular Sciences, KUL
Department of Anesthesiology, UZ Leuven
Leuven, Belgium

Pascal Vanelderen, MD, PhD
Consultant, Anesthesiology
Intensive Care Medicine
Emergency Medicine
Pain Medicine
Ziekenhuis Oost-Limburg
Genk, Belgium

Luc Van Keer, MD
Staff Physician, Department of Anesthesiology
Ziekenhuis Oost Limburg, ZOL
Genk, Belgium

André Van Zundert, MD, PhD, FRCA, EDRA, FANZCA
Professor and Chair, Anaesthesiology
The University of Queensland
Royal Brisbane and Women's Hospital
Brisbane, Queensland, Australia

Tom C. Van Zundert, MD, PhD, EDRA
Department of Anaesthesia and Pain Medicine
Fiona Stanley Hospital
Murdoch, Western Australia

Alexandru Visan, MD, MBA
CEO
Executive Cortex Consulting, LLC
Miami, Florida

Eugene R. Viscusi, MD
Professor of Anesthesiology
Director, Acute Pain Management Service
Department of Anesthesiology
Thomas Jefferson University
Philadelphia, Pennsylvania

Jerry D. Vloka, MD
Associate Professor of Anesthesiology
St. Luke's–Roosevelt Hospital Center
College of Physicians and Surgeons
Columbia University
New York, New York

E. Gina Votta-Velis, MD, PhD
Associate Professor of Anesthesiology
Program Director, Acute Pain, Chronic Pain and Regional
    Anesthesia Fellowship
Department of Anesthesiology
University of Illinois at Chicago College of Medicine
Chicago, Illinois

Alicia L. Warlick, MD
Assistant Professor Anesthesiology
Regional Anesthesia Division
Duke University Medical Center
Durham, North Carolina

James C. Watson, MD
Associate Professor of Neurology
Vice Chair, Department of Neurology—Practice Analytics
Consultant, Departments of Neurology and Anesthesiology,
    Pain Division
Mayo Clinic
Rochester, Minnesota

Guy Weinberg, MD
Professor
University of Illinois at Chicago, College of Medicine
Staff Physician, Jesse Brown VA Medical Center
Chicago, Illinois

Paul F. White, MD, PhD, FANZCA
Director of Research and Education
Department of Anesthesia
Cedars-Sinai Medical Center in Los Angeles
The Sea Ranch, California

Brian A. Williams, MD, MBA
Professor of Anesthesiology
University of Pittsburgh
Director of Ambulatory/Regional Anesthesia
Acute Pain Medicine and Preoperative Optimization
VA Pittsburgh Healthcare System
Pittsburgh, Pennsylvania

Alon P. Winnie, MD
Professor Emeritus
Department of Anesthesiology
Northwestern University
Feinberg School of Medicine
Chicago, Illinois

Thomas Witkowski, MD
Assistant Professor of Anesthesiology
Sidney Kimmel Medical College
Thomas Jefferson University
Medical Director, Preop Testing Center
Philadelphia, Pennsylvania

Daquan Xu, MB, MSc, MPH
Research Associate
NYSORA
New York, New York

Takayuki Yoshida, MD, PhD
Assistant Professor
Department of Anesthesiology
Kansai Medical University Hospital
Hirakata, Osaka, Japan

Adam C. Young, MD
Assistant Professor
Rush University Medical Center
Chicago, Illinois

Associate Editors

Michael J. Barrington

Thomas F. Bendtsen

Honorio T. Benzon

Jose A de Andrés

Jeff Gadsden

Maxine Kuroda

Ana M. Lopez

Steven L. Orebaugh

Miguel Anguel Reina

Steve Roberts

Xavier Sala-Blanch

Catherine Vandepitte

Marc Van de Velde

PREFACE

The first edition of *NYSORA's Textbook of Regional Anesthesia and Acute Pain Management* (McGraw-Hill, 2007) was a compendium of knowledge in regional anesthesia and acute pain medicine that quickly became a gold standard for students, practitioners, and test-takers alike. Yet, clinical practice marches on, and over 200 key opinion leaders and the worldwide community of NYSORA's educators worked diligently over the past 4 years to update the first edition. It is now my privilege to present the second edition of the textbook.

The material in this edition has been organized into thematic sections. Writings on history of local and regional anesthesia is often unjustly limited to its very beginnings in the late 1800s and early 1900s. However, a great deal of innovative and pioneering work has taken place in more recent history, that is now featured in the current edition. We have added numerous new anatomical dissections, diagrams, and functional anatomy illustrations developed by the NYSORA team for practitioners of regional anesthesia and pain medicine. NYSORA's teaching of these techniques is based on the principles of injecting local anesthetics within connective tissue sheaths; consequently, significant effort was invested in functional regional anesthesia anatomy and in illustrations that demonstrate the importance of this concept. Sections on connective tissues and the ultrastructural anatomy of the neuraxial meninges were contributed by a group of Spanish collaborators, led by Dr Miguel Angel Reina. Their sections represent a collection of uniquely educational electron microscopic images that offer insights into the mechanisms of neural blockade, causes of failures and the anatomical basis for vulnerability of neural structures to anesthesiology interventions. I believe that these sections and their timeless images will be remain relevant for generations of students to come.

The section on pharmacology features exciting information that is emerging on controlled-release local anesthetics that extend the analgesic benefits of neural blockade. New knowledge on this topic is being published as this textbook is being printed; the reader is suggested to check the latest relevant literature to complement the information that was available at the time of publication.

The section on equipment for peripheral nerve blocks features an expanded chapter on new equipment, such as the development of needles and catheters and novel equipment for needle-nerve and injection monitoring. For instance, Chapter 14 gives an overview of the role of peripheral nerve stimulation in modern practice of ultrasound-guided peripheral nerve blocks and step-by-step algorithms to facilitate understanding of this often-confusing topic.

New to the second edition is an entire section on patient management considerations and regional anesthesia pathways. In Chapter 15, Dr Barrington's team contributes a didactic outline of the steps and processes toward evidence-based clinical pathways that incorporate big data, such as building pathways for specific surgical populations. The section also features two chapters on the effect of local anesthetics and regional anesthesia on cancer recurrence. The immune system and how it can be influenced by surgery and anesthesia are evaluated for possible mechanisms by which regional anesthesia could confer benefits in patients with cancer in Chapters 17 and 18.

Part 3B discusses the clinical practice of regional anesthesia, starting with local and infiltration anesthesia. Dr Raeder's team describes the use of local anesthetics for intra-articular and periarticular infiltration (Chapter 19), and Dr Imran Ahmad shares a wealth of clinical and teaching experience on the use of local anesthetics and ultrasound technology for airway management (Chapter 20).

Intravenous regional (Bier) blocks are still practiced worldwide. A revised chapter on intravenous regional anesthesia for upper and lower extremity surgery was contributed by Dr Alon Winnie and his former students. The chapter features an updated reference list and step-by-step guidance for clinical practice.

In Part 3C, the chapters on neuraxial and epidural anesthesia have been thoroughly updated and feature a wealth of anatomical, practical, and clinical considerations, including complications and their management. A new chapter on the etiology and management of failed spinal anesthesia is highly practical and will be of interest to both students and practitioners of anesthesiology (Chapter 23A). The chapter on epidural anesthesia contributed by Drs Toledano and Van de Velde features vast amount of physiologic, pharmacologic, and practical management information, and it is a good example of the efforts invested in making this edition of the textbook up-to-date.

Chapter 27 on postdural puncture headache now includes a number of electron microscopic images that facilitate understanding of the underlying pathophysiology and instructional diagrams that guide treatment.

Part 3D focuses on the latest techniques and information pertaining to ultrasound-guided nerve blocks. Beginning with equipment and the physics behind image optimization and artifact reduction, the chapters progress to the practical aspects of ultrasound-guided techniques for peripheral nerve blocks of the upper and lower extremities (Chapters 33A–33H) and for truncal blocks (Chapters 34 and 35). The techniques of locoregional anesthesia for maxillofacial and eye surgery have also been updated with highly illustrative, all-new NYSORA illustrations that we developed over the past 3 years. Chapters 39 and 40 focus on ultrasound imaging of the paravertebral and neuraxial space.

The sections on pediatric regional anesthesia and the utility of ultrasound have been greatly expanded by some of most respected practitioners and educators in pediatric anesthesiology and perioperative care.

Part seven features updated and much expanded chapters on the practice of regional anesthesia in patients with specific considerations and comorbidities.

The etiology of and avoiding complications of regional anesthesia are topics of great interest for practitioners of regional anesthesia. Part 9 discusses the mechanisms of and evidence-based recommendations on how to improve the management of patients with neurologic complications, including sections on advances in monitoring and medicolegal documentation.

Medical care is increasingly driven by evidence-based and cost-effectiveness considerations. Consequently, several chapters address the principles of pharmacoeconomics as they relate to regional anesthesia, rehabilitation, and postoperative outcome.

Part 12 of the book discusses the principles and practice of acute pain management, organization of the acute pain service, the role of intravenous patient-controlled analgesia and perineural catheters, and the epidemiology of pain. Special consideration was given to multimodal analgesia and pharmacologic interventions that increase patient's experience of anesthesia and surgery may have a role in preventing persistent postoperative pain (Chapter 75).

Part 13 focuses on education in regional anesthesia and the development of regional anesthesia fellowship programs in the United States.

Although the current trend toward ultrasound guidance is likely to become the most prevalent method of delivering most regional anesthesia techniques in the developed world, surface-based and electrical nerve stimulation techniques will likely continue to be practiced in many geographic areas without expertise ultrasound equipment. Because this edition was envisioned as a standardized text for global education in regional

anesthesia and acute pain medicine, for completeness we opted to include principles of peripheral nerve blockade without ultrasound guidance (Part 15). These sections have been thoroughly updated from the previous edition, many practice updates being adopted from what we have learned utilizing ultrasound guidance. These chapters also include fascinating historical perspectives on the development of peripheral nerve block techniques throughout decades passed and how advances in anatomical, pharmacologic, and equipment influenced the their developments. The chapters also contain a wealth of anatomical information, teaching diagrams, and illustrations that add meaningful value to this textbook regardless of the needle guidance and techniques methods.

Finally, the book features two practical appendices. Appendix 1 contains a pragmatic guide for the use of regional anesthesia in the anticoagulated patient adopted for practices in Europe. The Appendix 2 illustrates the principles of disposition of injectates in tissue sheaths in common regional anesthesia techniques, contributed by a true pioneer in this area, Dr Philippe Gautier (BE).

No book is complete or without unavoidable errors regardless of the efforts invested. However, I believe that we have put together one of the most comprehensive texts on regional anesthesia and pain medicine to date and have spared no efforts to accomplish this. I thank and sincerely congratulate all collaborators and cordially invite readers to send along any discrepancies or suggestions to ana.lopez.517@gmail.com. As with the first edition, we will do our best to use the feedback to improve the textbook in a future edition to come a few years from now.

Respectfully,
Prof. Admir Hadzic

ACKNOWLEDGMENTS

Writing a textbook is an overwhelming endeavor; only those who have undertaken the work on a book can understand the efforts and the sacrifice that it entails. Throughout the couple of years it took to compile the new information and collaborate with such a large group of opinion leaders, researchers, and educators, a number of outstanding individuals were crucial to its successful completion.

Sincerest appreciation to my wife, life and work partner, Dr Catherine Vandepitte, without whose wisdom, advice, and esthetic guidance this book would not see the light of the day.

Huge thanks go to NYSORA's incredible illustrator, Vali Lancea. Thank you to Dr Monika Golebiewski's impeccable organizational skills, eye for detail, and beyond-describable work ethics, Monika was truly instrumental in tying the loose ends in the final push to complete this project.

A big thank you to the entire NYSORA support team: NYSORA-Europe, NYSORA's new CREER (Center for Research, Education, and Enhanced Recovery); our top surgeons and nurses at ZOL Anesthesiology; and more. Many thanks to Dr Alex Visan for his advice on the economics of regional anesthesia as well. Thank you to all current and former NYSORA fellows who have inspired much of the work.

The current NYSORA-Europe research team deserves a resounding thank you: Ingrid Meex, Gulhan Ozyurek, Aysu Emine Salviz, Marijke Cipers, Max Kuroda, and Greet Van Meir. You really rock!

Finally, thank you to the amazing managing editor, Brian Belval; your professionalism, common sense, and experience have provided the crucial guidance for this book to come together. Combined with co-managing editor Christie Naglieri, the production supervisor Catherine H. Saggese, and production manager Sonam Arora, we had the best team possible to make this book the gold standard it inspires to be.

Prof. Admir Hadzic

HISTORY

The History of Local Anesthesia

Alwin Chuan and William Harrop-Griffiths

INTRODUCTION

The history of local anesthesia lacks a distinct *Eureka moment.* It can be argued that regional anesthesia does not have in its history a pivotal day that signified the wholesale change from an era before local anesthesia to the dawn of a new and wonderful age that included parts of the body being rendered insensate for therapeutic reasons. We do not have the equivalent of October 16, 1846, and the trembling hands of William Thomas Green Morton. What we have is a remarkably slow concatenation of the three elements necessary for the administration of the vast majority of local anesthetics: a syringe, a needle, and a local anesthetic drug. Many, however, would argue that to these three need be added several other factors: a detailed knowledge of anatomy and an appreciation of the body's pain mechanisms and more objective methods to localize peripheral nerves and monitor administration of local anesthetics. We make no excuse for concentrating in this chapter on the early history of local anesthesia to dissect the development of these three vital components.

BEFORE COCAINE

The origins of the first attempts at some form of local analgesia or anesthesia are lost in the mists of time. Direct nerve compression and the direct application of ice to peripheries before surgery have distant origins but were certainly in regular use from the latter half of the eighteenth century. The first detailed appreciation of the benefits of local anesthesia was written by James Young Simpson and published in 1848, decades before local anesthesia became a practical possibility (Figure 1–1). In this paper, he also described his own unsuccessful experiments with the topical application of a variety of liquids and vapors in an attempt to produce local anesthesia. The paper was published less than 2 years after Oliver Wendell Holmes had coined the term *anesthesia,* and it therefore almost certainly represents the first use of the term *local anesthesia,* although Simpson would have used the (arguably more correct) English spelling *anaesthesia.* However, Simpson was well aware that his were far from the first attempts to produce peripheral insensibility, for he refers to some ancient methods, which he considered "apocryphal," and also to Moore's method of nerve compression (Figure 1–2).[1]

Another distinguished British physician and president of the Medical Society of London in 1868 was Sir Benjamin Ward Richardson. He spent many years in the attempt to alleviate pain by modifying substances capable of producing general or local anesthesia. He brought into use no fewer than 14 anesthetics and invented the first double-valved mouthpiece for the administration of chloroform. He initially experimented with electricity before turning to the effects of cold as an anesthetic. Cold was known to produce a numbing effect and was used as far back as Napoleon's time when his surgeon, Baron Larrey, used its effects to alleviate pain. He introduced a method of producing local insensibility by freezing the part with an *ether spray,* which became the most practical method of using local anesthesia until cocaine's actions became apparent. The ether spray was utilized as a local agent until it was replaced in 1880 by ethyl chloride[2] (Figure 1–3).

COCAINE ANESTHESIA

The Origins

If local anesthesia has a Eureka moment, then it may have happened in the forests of South America. Centuries ago, an unnamed inhabitant of these climates may have been experimenting by putting leaves of various plants into his mouth and giving them a good chew. We can imagine that this would be a largely unrewarding hobby, but let us focus on the moment when he first placed a coca leaf into his mouth and masticated

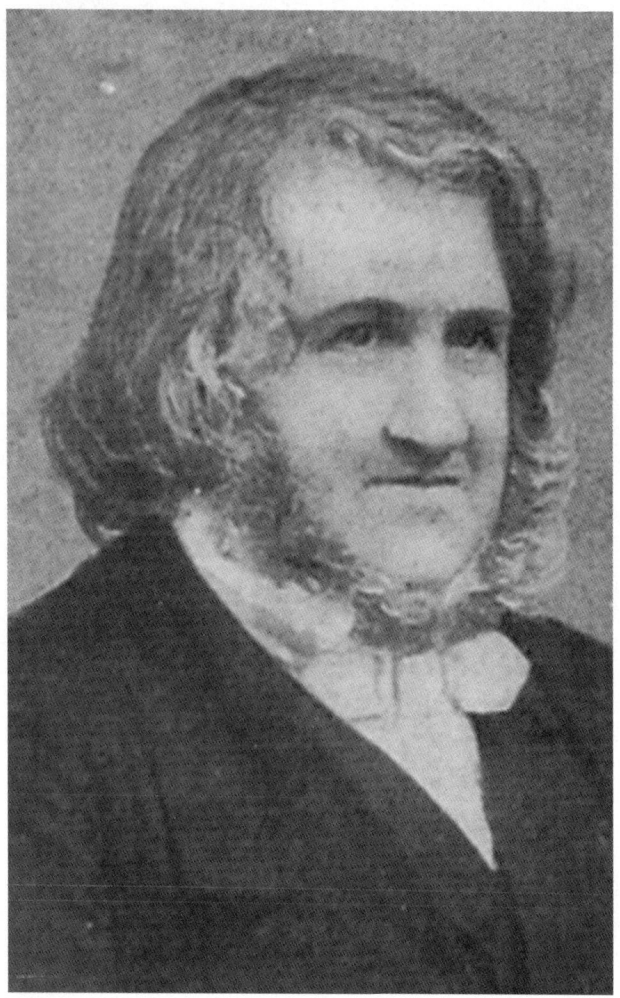

FIGURE 1–1. James Young Simpson.

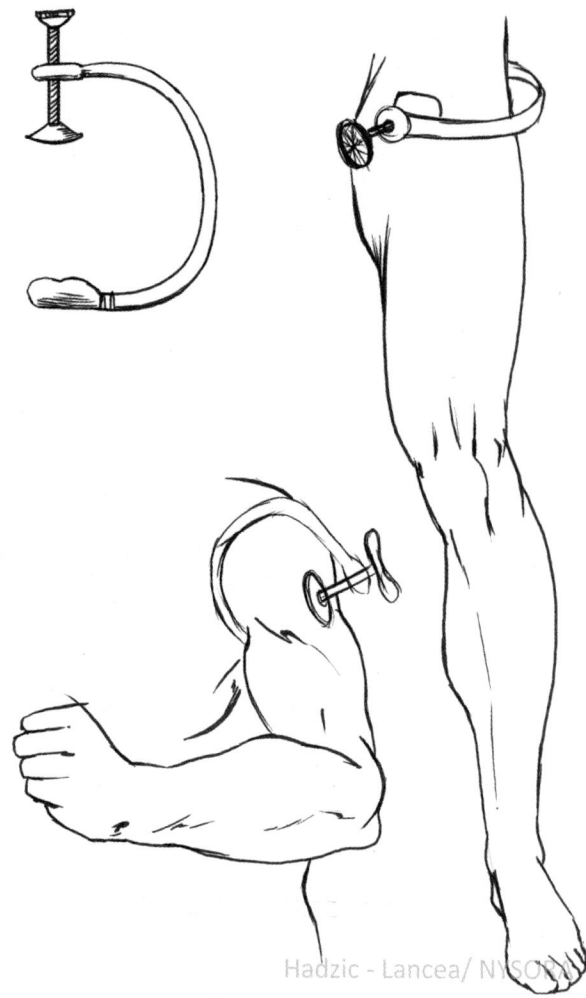

FIGURE 1–2. Nerve compression technique.

vigorously. Did he fall to his knees and shout in wonderment: "My lips have gone numb—surely this is the dawn of a new age of painless surgery!"? Almost certainly not—although he might have later told his friends that he felt somewhat excited, energetic, and euphoric while he chewed the leaves.

For thousands of years, South American peoples have chewed the coca leaf. It is a remarkable plant in that it contains vital nutrients as well as numerous alkaloids, most notably cocaine. The coca leaves are taken from a shrub of the genus *Erythroxylon coca*, named by Patrico Browne because of the reddish hue of the wood of the main species.[3] Many species of this genus have been grown in Nicaragua, Venezuela, Bolivia, and Peru since pre-Columbian times. *Erythroxylon coca* contains the highest concentration of the alkaloid known as cocaine in its leaves[3,4] (Figure 1–4).

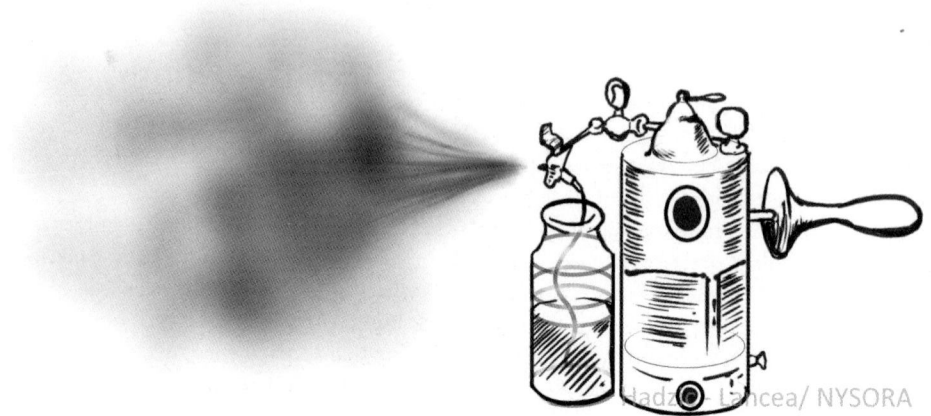

FIGURE 1–3. Ether spray.

Erythroxylon Coca Lam

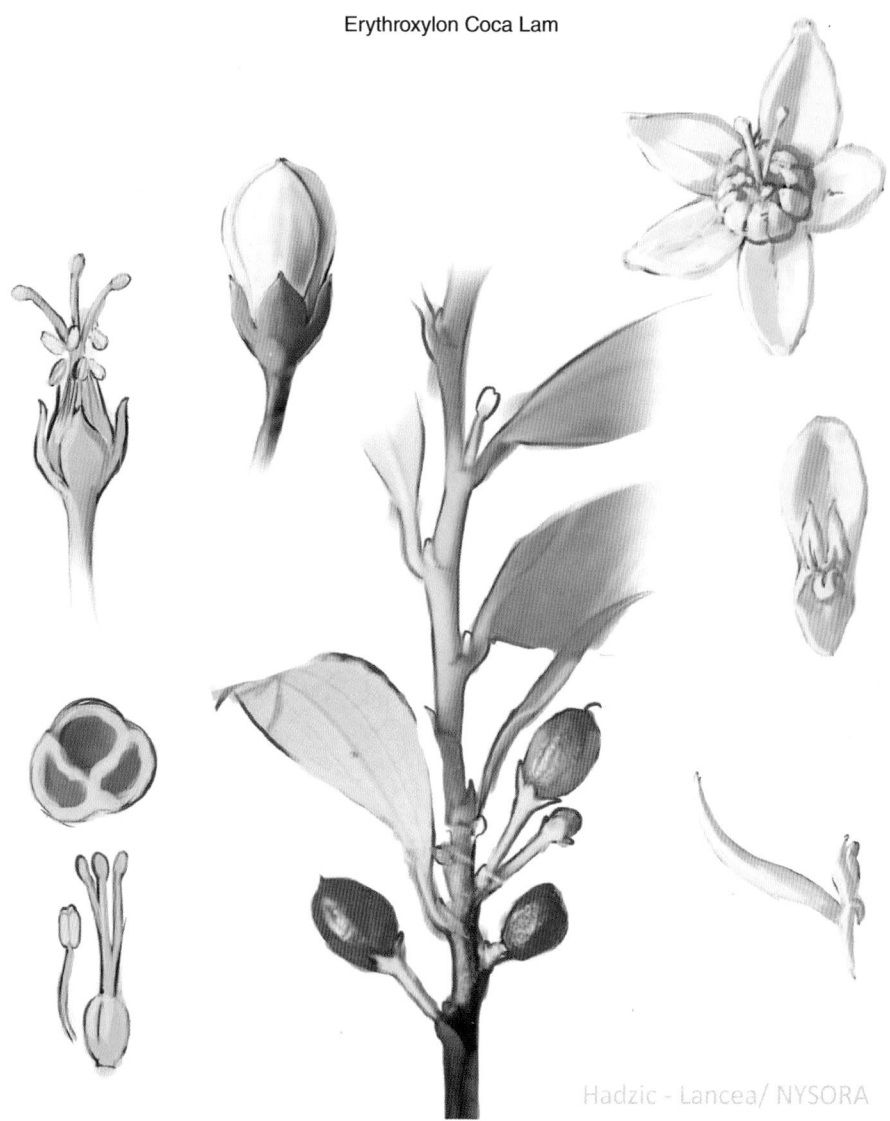

Hadzic - Lancea/ NYSORA

FIGURE 1−4. Coca leaf.

Traditionally, the leaves were chewed for social, mystical, medicinal, and religious purposes. The Florentine cartographer Amerigo Vespucci (1451–1512) was arguably the first European to document the human use of the coca leaf.[5,6] In his account of his voyage to America on the second expedition of Alonso de Ojeda and Juan de la Cosa from 1499 to 1500, he reported that the inhabitants of the Island of Margarita chewed certain herbs containing a white powder.[7] Among sixteenth-century Spanish chroniclers, the appearance of coca is associated with Francisco Pizarro's (1475–1541) conquest of the Inca or Tawantinsuyo Empire in 1532. Pedro Pizarro (1515–1571), Francisco Pizarro's cousin, who played a leading role in the capture of the last king of the Incas, described coca consumption by the nobles and high officials of the Inca Empire.[8] After the fall of the Inca Empire in the early 1500s, coca consumption spread to the population at large, creating a drastic change in the entire social system.

When the Spaniards conquered South America, they initially ignored the aboriginal claims that the leaf gave them vigor and liveliness. They self-righteously declared the practice of chewing the leaf the "work of the Devil."[5] But, once they found that the claims of the natives were true, they not only legalized the leaf but also taxed it—taking 10% of the value of each crop. The taxes were then used to support the Roman Catholic Church—the main source of revenue for the church to thrive. In 1609, Padre Blas Valera wrote: "Coca protects the body from many ailments, and our doctors use it in powdered form to reduce the swelling of wounds, to strengthen broken bones, to expel cold from the body or prevent it from entering, and to cure rotten wounds or sores that are full of maggots. And if it does so much for outward ailments, will not its singular virtue have even greater effect in the entrails of those who eat it?"[9] If the padre had been blessed with the ability to foresee the future, perhaps his enthusiasm would have been redirected toward limiting the use of the leaf, and the field of anesthesia might have taken a different turn.

Another member of the clergy, Bernabé Cobo, who spent his life bringing Christianity to the Incas, was the first to describe the anesthetic effects of coca. In a 1653 manuscript, he mentioned that toothaches could be alleviated by chewing the coca leaves. In 1859, an Italian physician by the name of Paolo Mantegazza had witnessed the use of coca by the natives in Peru. He wrote a paper describing the medicinal use in the treatment of "a furred tongue in the morning, flatulence and whitening of the teeth."[10]

Needles and Syringes

If local anesthetic drugs are the bullets used when fighting pain, the gun needed to fire these bullets is made up of a syringe and a needle. Without the bullets, the gun is useless, and just as certainly, without the gun, the bullets will have little effect. The development of the hypodermic syringe and needle was therefore an important prerequisite for the use of cocaine for anything but topical application. A thorough sifting of the available historical evidence and independent reexamination of the sources support the following outline of the facts: In 1845, Francis Rynd described the idea of introducing a solution of morphine hypodermically in the neighborhood of a peripheral nerve to alleviate neuralgic pain.[11] He introduced the solution by means of gravity, passively through a cannula once the trocar had been removed.

Several centuries passed before the development of a syringe to deliver medicine was described by Alexander Wood (Figure 1–5). Wood, a contemporary of James Young Simpson, in 1855 was the first to combine needle and syringe for hypodermic medication. He used the equipment manufactured by a gentleman by the name of Ferguson, who had developed the graduated glass syringe and hollow needle for the purpose of treating aneurysms by injecting ferric perchloride into the aneurysm to form a coagulated mass. Wood, a physician interested in the treatment of neuralgia, reasoned that morphine might be more effective if it were injected close to the nerve supplying the affected area. Although morphine may have some peripheral actions, and the effect of Wood's morphine was almost certainly central, he was nevertheless the first to think of the possibility of producing nerve blockade by direct drug injection. Thus, he has been called the "father-in-law" of local anesthesia—all he lacked was an agent that worked locally. Wood's contribution was therefore his procedure of subcutaneous injection. This technique was subsequently adopted by C. Hunter and renamed hypodermic injection, presumably because Hunter's purpose was to provide systemic absorption of medications injected.[12,13]

The Introduction of Cocaine

The growth in Western science and technology exploded during the nineteenth century. Six years after Charles Darwin's controversial book, *On the Origin of Species by Means of Natural Selection,* Joseph Lister was an important figure in changing the

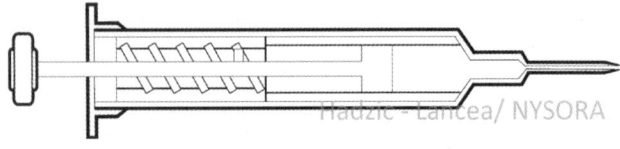

FIGURE 1–5. Early syringe.

face of surgery. He applied Pasteur's principles of bacterial growth in eliminating sepsis in the operating theatre. Other prominent figures contributed to the understanding of human physiology, such as Sydney Ringer's discovery of the need for calcium and potassium to maintain cardiac excitability, significantly advancing medical care. And then—there was cocaine.

Although the stimulant and hunger-suppressant effects of coca had been known for years, the isolation of the cocaine alkaloid was not achieved until 1855. Scientists attempted to isolate cocaine, but no one was successful for two reasons: Coca did not grow in the colder environment of Europe, and the chemistry involved was unknown at that time. Finally, in 1855, the German chemist Friedrich Gaedcke was able to isolate the cocaine alkaloid and publish the description in the journal *Archiv der Pharmacie.* In 1856, Friedrich Wöhler asked a colleague to bring him a large amount of coca leaves from South America. Wöhler then gave the leaves to Albert Niemann, a PhD student at the University of Göttingen in Germany, who then developed an improved purification process. His dissertation, *On a New Organic Base in the Coca Leaves,* published in 1860, earned him his doctoral degree. Of interest, he described cocaine as having "a bitter taste, promotes the flow of saliva, and leaves a peculiar numbness, followed by a sense of cold when applied to the tongue."[14,15]

Following Niemann, the first experimental study on cocaine was conducted by a former naval surgeon from Peru, Thomas Moreno y Maiz. He discovered that the injection of cocaine solutions caused insensitivity in rats, guinea pigs, and frogs. But, it was not until 1880, when Basil Von Anrep experimented on himself, that the application of cocaine for surgery was appreciated. Von Anrep injected a small amount of cocaine under the skin on his arm and noted that the area became insensitive to pinpricks. He did the same to his tongue with the same effect. He published his findings with the caveat "the animal experiments have no practical application; nevertheless I would recommend trying cocaine as a local anesthetic in persons of melancholy disposition."[16]

The groundwork was in place, but the final step toward the clinical use of cocaine had yet to be taken. Viennese ophthalmologist Karl Koller (1857–1944) rose to the challenge (Figure 1–6). Koller was an intern working in the Viennese General Hospital, where he was befriended by Sigmund Freud[17] (Figure 1–7). Freud wanted to know more about the stimulating action of cocaine, which he hoped might prove useful in curing one of his close friends of morphine addiction. This friend was a pathologist and had developed an agonizingly painful thenar neuroma secondarily to cutting himself during the performance of an autopsy. Freud was able to obtain a supply of cocaine from the pharmaceutical firm Merck. He shared it with Koller, who during the spring of 1884 helped him investigate its effects on the nervous system.[18]

Koller had dreams of achieving an appointment to assistant and knew his chances would be greatly enhanced by the creation of a respectable piece of research. The research he produced proved worthy enough, but interpersonal animosity intervened, and he was not awarded the position. Deeply disappointed, he moved first to the Netherlands, then to the United States.[19] In July 1884, Freud published a review of

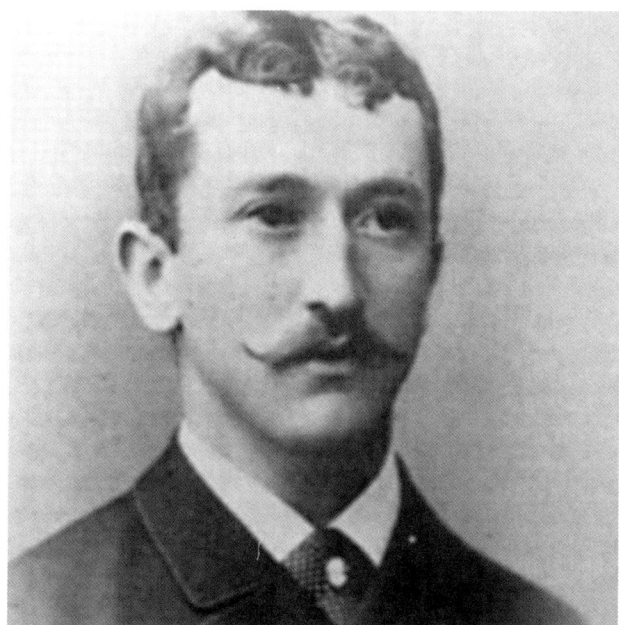

FIGURE 1–6. Carl Koller.

cocaine and his experiments with the drug, again noting, but without lending any particular attention to, the alkaloid's anesthetic effect on mucous membranes.[20] It was Koller who grasped the importance of this observation. His discovery was no accident, for he was keenly aware of the limitations of general anesthesia in ophthalmic surgery. Because of his past experience in the field of ophthalmology, Koller understood what others had failed to recognize. Many eye surgeries at that time were still being performed without anesthesia. Almost four decades after the discovery of ether, general anesthesia by mask had a number of limitations for ophthalmic surgery (eg, the anesthetized patient could not cooperate with the surgeon, the

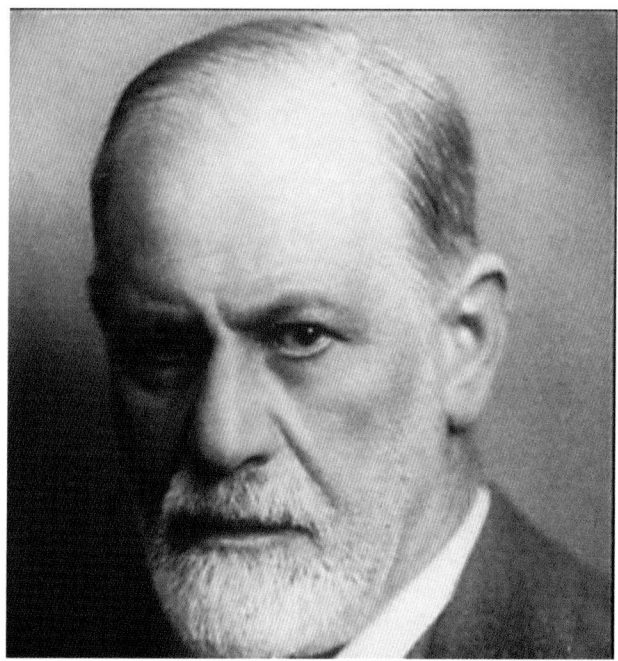

FIGURE 1–7. Sigmund Freud.

anesthesiologist's apparatus interfered with surgical access). At that time, many surgical incisions in the eye were not closed, as fine sutures were not yet available. Vomiting from chloroform or ether threatened to cause extrusion of the internal contents of the globe, markedly increasing the risk of permanent blindness. As a medical student, Koller had worked in a laboratory searching for a topical ophthalmic anesthetic to overcome the restrictions posed by general anesthesia. The medications available at that time had proved to be ineffective.

One day, Freud gave Koller a small sample of cocaine in an envelope, which he slipped into his pocket (an everyday occurrence in many American and European cities to this day). When the envelope leaked, a few grains of cocaine stuck to Koller's finger, which he casually licked with his tongue. His tongue became numb—if he had been able to mouth the word *Eureka* with a numb tongue, he may well have done so at this precise instant. At that moment, Koller realized that he had found what he had been searching for. He immediately created a suspension of cocaine crystals in his laboratory.[2] Koller realized that this had been noted by all who had worked with cocaine and that "in the moment it flashed upon me that I was carrying in my pocket the local anesthetic for which I had searched some years earlier."[1] In Freud's absence, he and another colleague, Joseph Gartner, dissolved a trace of the white powder in distilled water and instilled the solution into the conjunctival sac of a frog. After a minute or so, "the frog allowed his cornea to be touched and he also bore injury to the cornea without a trace of reflex action or defense." Koller wrote: "One more step had yet to be taken. We trickled the solution under each other's lifted eyelids. Then we placed a mirror before us, took pins, and with the head tried to touch the cornea. Almost simultaneously we were able to state 'I can't feel anything.'"[21,22] Then, he experimented with dog and guinea pig corneas with 2% to 5% cocaine solutions.[23]

Koller soon achieved the extraordinary notoriety he had longed for when in September 1884 he performed the first ophthalmologic surgical procedure using local anesthesia on a patient with glaucoma. The German Ophthalmologist Society Congress was to meet in Heidelberg in September 1884 and Koller was going to present his findings. Unfortunately, he was unable to attend. He asked Dr. Joseph Brettauer, an ophthalmologist from Trieste, to present his paper at the Congress. The effect of his work was immediate. Koller was able to present his findings in October of that year to the Viennese Medical Society. In late 1884, he published his findings.[21]

Physicians in the United States soon heard about Koller's amazing work. Dr. Henry Noyes of New York, an attendee of the Heidelberg Congress, published a summary of Koller's work in the *New York Medical Record*.[24] Another American physician, Dr. Bloom, translated Koller's article into English and published it in *The Lancet* in December of that same year. Koller's work was the trigger for the development of regional/local anesthesia. In the subsequent year, more than 60 publications on local anesthesia with cocaine appeared in the United States and Canada.

One of the most significant publications was that of N. J. Hepburn, an ophthalmologist from New York.[15] Self-experimentation was the standard for drug trials in those days.

To determine whether a drug was safe or effective, the researcher or physician commonly tried the drug personally. It takes courage to try a new drug on a patient, but it takes a particular and much greater form of courage to try that drug on yourself. Hepburn was no different from his colleagues. He gave himself a succession of subcutaneous injections of 0.4 mL (8 mg) of cocaine at 5-min intervals. By the eighth injection, the stimulating effects of the drug were strong enough that he decided it was best to stop. Unfortunately, Hepburn did not stop with those initial injections. He repeated the "experiment" 2 days later and 4 days after that, each time increasing the total amount of cocaine injected. Most likely by this time, he was hopelessly addicted.

By November 1884, the ophthalmologist C. S. Bull reported that he had been able to use cocaine to produce anesthesia of the cornea and conjunctiva in more than 150 cases.[25] He was enthusiastic about the advantages of the drug in that he saved time required for complete anesthesia with ether; patients were less nauseated, the engorgement of the ocular blood vessels (caused by ether) was eliminated, and he was less hampered by the anesthesia equipment required for inhalation anesthesia. Cocaine revolutionized eye, nose, and mouth surgery. Operations that had been exceedingly difficult or painful became routine when topical or injectable cocaine was used. Koller did not forget the contribution of his friend, Freud. He gave him the credit as his muse. Despite his disillusionment at not being foremost with the discovery, Freud is considered by many to be the founder of psychopharmacology because of his initial use of cocaine. He is considered the predecessor in the discovery and experimentation with mescaline, LSD, and amphetamines to modify behavior and to attempt to cure mental illness.[20]

Dangers of Cocaine

The "wonder drug" cocaine was soon sold everywhere and in almost everything. Following its isolation from the coca leaf, cocaine emerged as an ingredient in wine both in the United States and in Europe in amounts up to 7 mg/oz. In the original recipe for Coca-Cola (1866), coca leaves were included in the ingredients. It was not until 1906 when the Pure Food and Drug Act was passed that the Coca-Cola company began using decocainized leaves.[14] Until 1916, cocaine could be purchased over the counter at Harrods in London. It was found in tonics, toothache cures, and medicines (Figure 1–8). Coca cigarettes were sold with the promise of lifting depression. Those who purchased cocaine were promised in ads by the pharmaceutical firm Parke-Davis that it could "make the coward brave, the silent eloquent, and render the sufferer insensitive to pain." In the operatic world, it became commonplace to use cocaine to ease the pain of sore throats and to shrink nasal mucous membranes to enable the singers to improve the resonation of their voices.

Had cocaine's use been restricted to enhancing opera singing and local anesthesia, it would have become the achievement of nineteenth-century medicine. As had happened earlier with brandy, tobacco, morphine, and other drugs, cocaine was administered in too high concentrations and with too few precautions. In 1886, William Hammond, a former US Army Surgeon General, assured an audience of physicians that cocaine addiction did not exist. Based on self-experimentation, he concluded that regular use of cocaine was as easy to stop as quitting coffee. It did not have the addictive qualities of drugs like opium. But, when Hammond finished his lecture, an addiction specialist named Jansen Mattison offered a rebuttal. He related incidences of fierce addictions in patients under his care. He described cocaine's damaging effect on nerves and its ability to produce hallucinations, delusions, and emaciation. Many other practitioners began to encounter serious side effects.[26,27]

Mattison knew what he was talking about. Over the next several years, medical journals published hundreds of case reports of "cocainism." Unfortunately, many of the addicts were medical practitioners who had experimented on themselves, most notably Freud and William Stewart Halsted.[28,29] The opiate

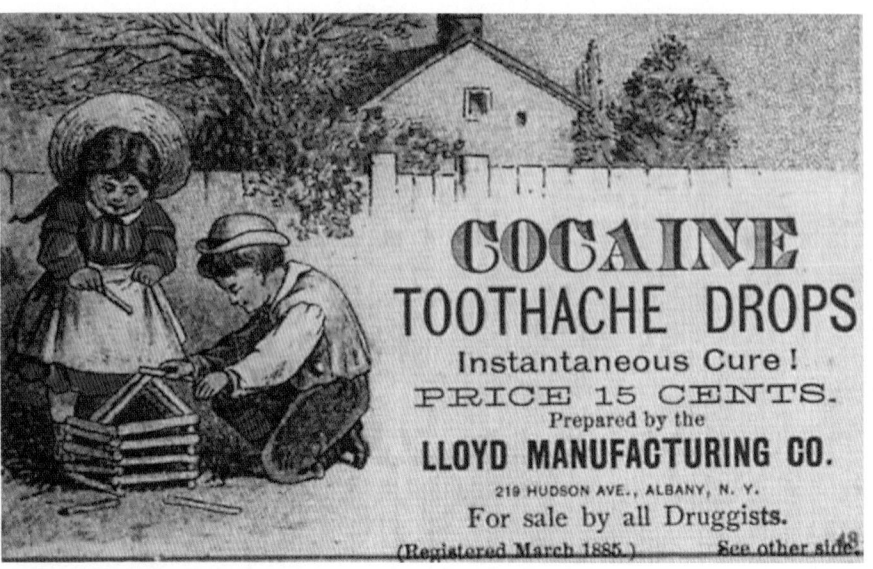

FIGURE 1–8. Cocaine toothache drops.

addicts, promised a cure for their addiction, switched to cocaine, but continued to use both drugs, further compromising their health.

Several researchers deserve the credit for making the infiltration of cocaine safer. Maximillian Oberst, Ludwig Per-nice, and Carl Ludwig Schleich, all from Germany, described the use of low concentrations of cocaine as effective means of local anesthesia.[30] The Parisian surgeon Paul Reclus described the use of very low concentrations of cocaine as effective anesthesia without harmful side effects for tooth extractions and pulpotomies.[31]

About the same time, Halsted was experimenting with low concentrations of cocaine applied by compression devices. Unfortunately, he also became addicted to both cocaine and morphine and could not publish his results.[12,17,29] Over time, the maximum "safe" cocaine dosage for infiltration anesthesia was established at 50 mg.

AFTER COCAINE

As the undesirable effects of cocaine, most notably addiction and toxicity, gradually became known, new anesthetic drugs were sought to replace it. Local methods to provide anesthesia had to await the development of less-toxic drugs. Once the clinical usefulness of cocaine became evident, efforts were made by various researchers to identify the active portion of the cocaine molecule and to create new substances that possessed local anesthetic activity without the adverse side effects. Most of the chemical work involving the creation of local anesthetics took place in Germany from 1900 to 1930.[32]

Niemann, as part of his pioneering work on purifying cocaine, had hydrolyzed benzoic acid from cocaine. In the search for other benzoic acid esters with local anesthetic properties, amylocaine (stovaine) was introduced in 1903. It became popular for spinal anesthesia until it was shown to be an irritant. But, it was the development of procaine in 1904 by the German chemist Alfred Einhorn that revolutionized local anesthetics.[33] On November 27, 1904, Einhorn (1856–1917) patented 18 *para*-aminobenzoic acid derivatives that had been developed in the Meister Lucius and Brüning plants at Höchst, in Hesse, Germany. His compound Number Two was to bring about a radical change in local anesthetic practice. He named the new anesthetic Novocain.[11] Procaine (Novocain) was introduced into clinical practice by Professor Heinrich Braun in 1905. Braun published a study comparing this new anesthetic to stovaine and alypine, two other promising local anesthetics.[34] Procaine was found to be safe and quickly became the standard local anesthetic drug. Within a short time, procaine completely replaced cocaine as the most commonly used local anesthetic. But, because of the short duration of action and prominent allergic potential limiting its clinical effectiveness, the search for longer-lasting compounds continued.[11,18,26,35]

In the years that followed, several local anesthetics were synthesized and used in clinical practice until side effects or other unfavorable characteristics were noted. In 1925, Karl Meischer synthesized dibucaine, and in 1928 Otto Eisleb synthesized tetracaine. Both were effective local anesthetics and had the desirable qualities of longer duration and potency, but systemic toxic effects limited their usefulness for regional techniques other than for spinal anesthesia. Most of the compounds developed during this time were amino ester derivatives, similar to cocaine, with similar allergic potential.

A major breakthrough came in the mid-1940s when the Swedish chemists Nils Löfgren and Bengt Lundquist developed a new local anesthetic they called lidocaine. Lidocaine was an amino amide derivative, a stable compound not influenced by exposure to high temperatures and, most importantly, one that did not have the allergic potential of the ester-type local anesthetics. With the development of this amide-type anesthetic drug, a whole new class of local anesthetics was synthesized. In 1957, Af Ekenstam developed mepivacaine and bupivacaine, and in 1969 Löfgren and Claes Tegnér developed prilocaine. Prilocaine's synthesis began because of a desire to produce a local anesthetic with a potency similar to that of lidocaine but without lidocaine's systemic toxic effects. Unfortunately, it was soon discovered that large doses of prilocaine produced a metabolite that caused methemoglobinemia. Although probably not clinically significant, this discovery severely limited its use in clinical practice.[36] In 1972, etidocaine was introduced to the clinical scene but was soon discovered to lack a differential sensory—motor blockade. Its clinical usefulness was therefore limited.

The only new ester local anesthetic developed in more recent times is chloroprocaine. Its rapid hydrolysis reduced the possibility of systemic toxicity, but its usefulness was restricted to procedures of short duration that did not produce a high degree of postoperative pain. In modern regional practices, it has been used both in spinal anesthesia and in nerve blocks for short, relatively painless procedures.

Two goals of modern pharmaceutical research have been development of amide anesthetics with lower toxicity and modification in the delivery of local anesthetics. Levobupivacaine and ropivacaine were both introduced commercially in 1996 as purified S-enantiomers rather than racemic solutions, with less risk of cardiac and central nervous system toxicity. More recently, liposomal delivery systems that allow slow release of commonly used local anesthetics have extended the duration of effect beyond 48 hours.

LOCAL ANESTHESIA TECHNIQUES

Infiltration Anesthesia

In 1895, a then-novel approach, termed *infiltration anesthesia,* had been promoted by Karl Ludwig Schleich (1859–1922).[35] Schleich applied the principle that pure water has a weak anesthetic effect but is painful on injection, whereas physiologic saline is not. In 1869, Pierre Carl Edouard Potain first observed that the subcutaneous injection of water produced local anesthesia. Halsted, a surgeon at Roosevelt Hospital in New York City, in a frank letter to the editor of the *New York Medical Journal* in 1885, declared that the "skin can be completely anesthetized to any extent by cutaneous injections of water."[37] In his own practice, Halsted had begun using water instead of cocaine in skin incisions, noting that the anesthesia did not subside completely when hyperemia reappeared.

In the belief that there was a solution capable of performing as a useful anesthetic that would not cause pain on injection, Schleich mixed 0.2% sodium chloride with 0.02% cocaine.

He used the mixture to produce cutaneous anesthesia for sebaceous cystectomy, hemorrhoidectomies, and small abscesses. Although Braun dismissed Schleich's solutions as "nonphysiologic," Schleich's work was important in advancing the application of small quantities of local anesthetics for surgical procedures. Because of the reported serious toxic reactions and fatalities reported with cocaine, enthusiasm for the utilization of local anesthesia had waned considerably. Paul Reclus undoubtedly understood that the cause of death from local anesthetics was related to overdose. He was able to demonstrate that absorption could be limited with lower concentrations of cocaine, a fact that Schleich obviously supported and implemented.[31] Schleich's approach still seems to be relevant, particularly with the recent European enthusiasm for *tumescent anesthesia,* in which sometimes-huge volumes of very dilute local anesthetic are used for surface surgery.

Conduction Anesthesia

With the excitement generated by Koller's report of cocaine anesthesia in 1884, several US surgeons concurrently entertained the idea of injecting cocaine directly into tissues to render them insensitive. William Burke injected five drops of 2% cocaine solution close to a metacarpal branch of the ulnar nerve and then painlessly removed a bullet from the base of his patient's little finger.[38] However, it was William Stewart Halsted (1852–1922; Figure 1–9) and his associate John Hall at Roosevelt Hospital in New York City who most clearly saw the great possibilities of conduction block.[39] Hall experimented on

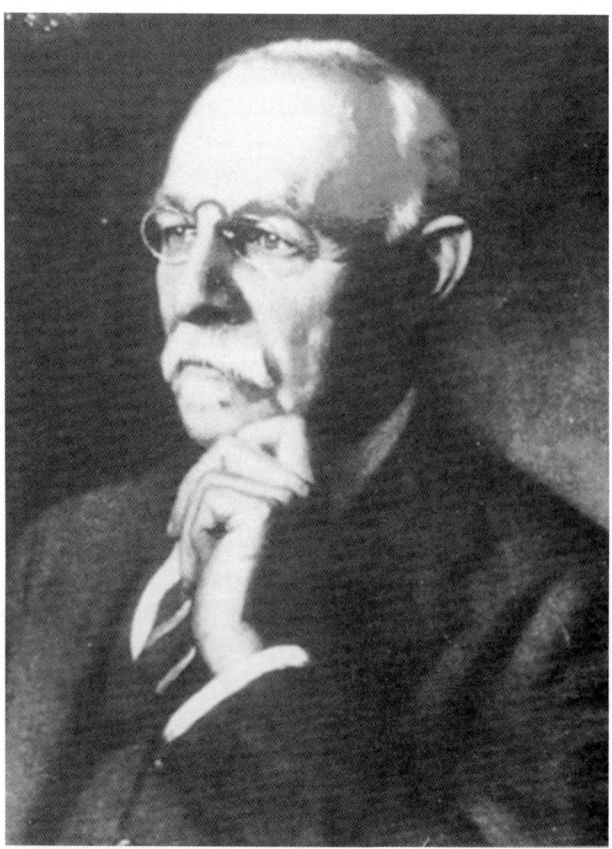

FIGURE 1–9. William Stewart Halsted.

himself by blocking a cutaneous branch of the ulnar nerve in his own forearm.[41] He and Halsted did not stop with upper extremity injections; they also successfully injected the musculocutaneous (superficial peroneal) nerve of the leg. Hall described the manifestation of systemic symptoms such as giddiness, severe nausea, cold perspiration, and dilated pupils, but these symptoms did not stop these daring scientists from further self-experimentation. Halsted blocked Hall's supratrochlear nerve to remove a congenital cystic tumor. One can assume that both Halsted and Hall had run out of minor surgical ailments in themselves and therefore had to look to others on whom they could experiment. In the days long before ethics committees and informed consent, one is tempted to speculate about the true "volunteer" status of the poor, and most likely unsuspecting, medical students. Hall's report was unequivocal in predicting that this mode of administration of cocaine would find wide application in outpatient surgery once the limits of safety had been determined—remarkably prescient of him.[40]

Although the conduction blocks were successful, unfortunately, several members of their group became addicted to cocaine. No further publications about the usefulness of cocaine anesthesia for surgical procedures were presented. It is one of the great sadnesses of the development of analgesic drugs in the history of humankind that two of the most effective agents, morphine and cocaine, are wickedly addictive. They deprived medicine of many of the potential discoveries of its most gifted sons and daughters. However, that Hall and Halsted were the true progenitors of conduction anesthesia can scarcely be doubted.[17,26]

In 1891, François-Franck was the first to apply the term *blocking* to the infiltration of a nerve trunk in any part.[41] He correctly discovered that the effect of the blocking drug was not limited to sensory fibers, but provided blockade of all nerves, both motor and sensory. He noted that sensory anesthesia became apparent more rapidly than the motor paralysis, a fact confirmed by von Anrep's 1880 observations.[16] François-Franck described the action of cocaine as transitory and noninjurious, "physiologic and segmental" anesthesia. He may well have borrowed part of it from J. Leonard Corning, who in 1886 wrote that "the thought of producing anaesthesia by abolishing conduction in sensory nerves, by suitable means, should have been rife in the minds of progressive physicians."[42] Corning most likely got the idea from Halsted because he had frequently observed Halsted and Hall's work at Roosevelt Hospital in New York.

The advantage of utilizing cocaine as a local anesthetic was that it anesthetized only the section of the body where surgery was to be performed, the goal of regional techniques in modern practice. But, the price to be paid was in the duration of action and toxicity, not to mention the more commonly recognized problem of addiction. The dose of cocaine was limited to 30 mg because of rapid absorption. Unfortunately, the duration of anesthesia was therefore no more than 15 minutes. Corning, in 1885, began researching means of prolonging the local anesthetic action of cocaine for surgery. He believed that once cocaine was injected beneath the skin, capillary circulation was responsible for distributing, diluting, and removing the anesthetic substance. In one experiment, he injected 0.3 mL of a 4% solution of cocaine into a cutaneous nerve of the arm and produced immediate anesthesia of the skin of the forearm. By compressing the extremity proximal to the site of injection with an Esmarch bandage, he was able to intensify and prolong the anesthesia to the forearm.[43]

Corning's successes with prolonging the action of local anesthetic with a physical tourniquet inspired Heinrich F. W. Braun to substitute epinephrine, a "chemical tourniquet," for the Esmarch tourniquet.[44] John Jacob Abel had isolated the pure form from the suprarenal medulla in 1897, and it had been subsequently used in ophthalmology to limit hemorrhage and in the treatment of glaucoma.[45] During its use in ophthalmology and subsequently in ear, nose, and throat surgeries, it was discovered that epinephrine prolonged the effect of cocaine, thereby allowing a reduction in dose and limiting side effects. Braun determined the optimal solution of epinephrine with cocaine by once again experimenting on himself. He discovered that the maximal dose that he could tolerate without side effects was 0.5 mg (0.5 mL of a 1:1000 solution of epinephrine). He coined the term *conduction anesthesia* when publishing the results of his experimentation.[46]

Intravenous Regional Anesthesia

The first reported use of intravenous regional anesthesia (IVRA) can be traced back to August Karl Gustav Bier (Figure 1–10), the originator of the infamous **Bier block**. Bier,

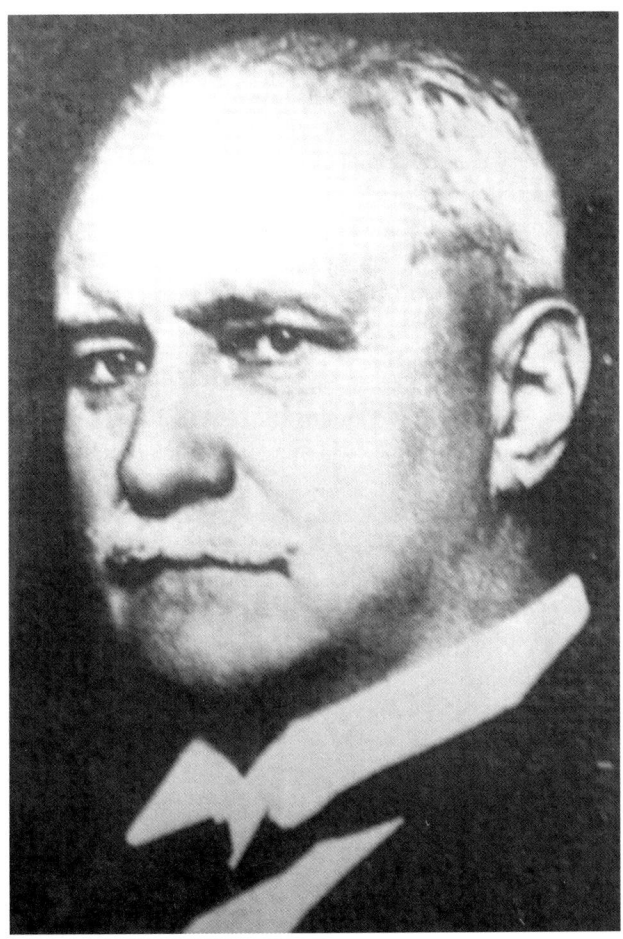

FIGURE 1–10. August Bier.

a German surgeon (1861–1949), influenced surgery, anesthesia, and general medicine with his contributions through the decades. IVRA was first described by Bier in 1908. His method consisted of occluding the circulation in a segment of the arm with two tourniquets. He then injected a solution of dilute procaine through a venous cutdown in the isolated segment. The injected solution diffused through the entire section of the limb quickly, producing **direct vein anesthesia** in just a few minutes.[47] The anesthesia lasted as long as the upper tourniquet was in place. Recovery of sensation was rapid after the tourniquet was removed.[48] Despite his successes, IVRA was not widely used until the technique was reintroduced in the 1960s by C. M. Holmes.[49]

Spinal Anesthesia

Soon after its introduction in 1884, local anesthesia became popular with surgeons, particularly those in France, Germany, and the United States.[18] This was in large part due to concerns about the safety of inhalational anesthesia, which, increased by the introduction of chloroform, had given rise to significant worries about toxicity. General anesthetic mortality was high at this time, and there was a distinct shortage of personnel trained to administer general anesthesia.[50] In a bizarre twist, the first spinal anesthetic was given some 5 years before the first lumbar puncture. The term *spinal anesthesia* was introduced by Corning, a neurologist, in his famous paper of 1885: "Spinal Anaesthesia and Local Medication of the Cord With Cocaine."[42] He theorized that interspinal blood vessels would carry the local anesthetic (cocaine) via communicating vessels into the spinal cord. He did not mention anything about cerebrospinal fluid or the depth of the needle insertion into the spinal space. It is speculated that he was aiming directly at the spinal cord as he introduced a needle between the 11th and 12th vertebrae. In his paper, he wrote: "I reasoned that it was highly probably that, if the anesthetic was placed between the spinous processes of the vertebrae, it would be rapidly transported by the blood to the substance of the cord and would give rise to anaesthesia of the sensory and perhaps also of the motor tracts of the same. To be more explicit, I hoped to produce artificially a temporary condition of things analogous in its physiological consequences to the effects observed in transverse myelitis or after total section of the cord."[42]

Corning's report was based on a series of two injections: one human and one animal (a dog). After first assessing its action in a dog, producing a blockade of rapid onset that was confined to the animal's rear legs, he administered cocaine to a man who was "addicted to masturbation." It may be that many anesthesiologists have spent much time wondering whether masturbation played any role in local anesthesia—this question can now be answered in the affirmative. Corning administered one dose without effect, and then, after a second dose had been given, the patient's legs "felt sleepy." The man had impaired sensibility in his lower extremity after about 20 minutes. He left Corning's office "none the worse for the experience"—although this experience itself may well have put him off his penchant for onanism. Corning had injected a total of 120 mg of cocaine, about four times the potentially lethal dose, in a period of 8 minutes.

What he achieved in this patient was probably what is now called *epidural,* or *extradural,* anesthesia. The dog probably received a spinal anesthetic with approximately 13 mg of cocaine, as judged by the rate of onset described.

Although Corning most assuredly had an innovative idea, his results were not more than a lucky accident because he injected a fatal dose of cocaine into the man. A direct communication between the extradural capillaries and the spinal cord does not exist. Based on the education that Corning received at the time, he was probably unaware of the existence of the subarachnoid space and cerebrospinal fluid.

Lumbar Puncture/Spinal Anesthesia

Heinrich Irenaeus Quincke (Figure 1–11) is credited with the introduction and popularization of the lumbar puncture. It was developed as a treatment for hydrocephalus in children with tubercular meningitis, then later as a diagnostic method for certain central nervous system diseases.[51] He based his approach on sound anatomic knowledge of the subarachnoid space and spinal cord. He used needles with an internal diameter of 0.5 to 1.2 mm and entered the subarachnoid space via a paravertebral approach. Interestingly, he prescribed bed rest for 24 hours following the puncture.

Despite the strides made by Quincke, utilizing his technique for spinal anesthesia did not occur for 8 years after Quincke's first publication. Bier published his renowned paper on spinal anesthesia in 1899. Bier had the good fortune to work at the

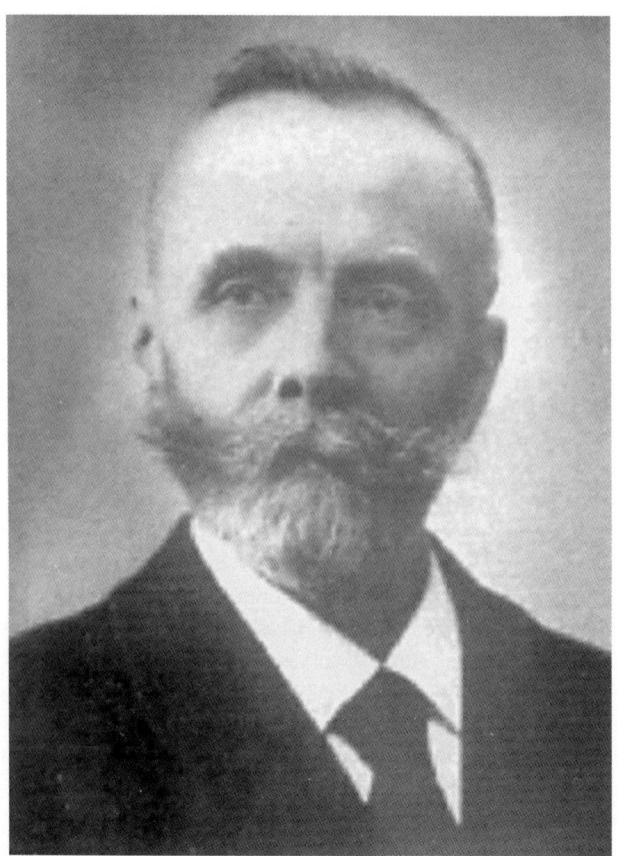

FIGURE 1–11. Heinrich Irenaeus Quincke.

same institution as Quincke and was most likely familiar with his work. His intention was to use spinal anesthesia with cocaine for major operations. He realized that he could produce a profound block with a minimum amount of the drug, thereby eliminating the majority of the adverse side effects noted by his colleagues. In his experiments, he noted that the extent of anesthesia produced was not always predictable. As was popular with his colleagues, he experimented on himself. He had his assistant, August Hildebrandt, perform lumbar punctures on him. In the first attempt, Hildebrandt was unable to administer an appreciable amount of cocaine before a large volume of cerebrospinal fluid leaked out of Bier. Because of the poor response, they were close to abandoning the experiment. Hildebrandt then offered to be the next "guinea pig" instead. Bier successfully placed the spinal anesthetic and proceeded to "punish" Hildebrandt with blows to the tibia, pulling on his testicle, and even putting out a cigar on Hildebrandt's thigh.[52,53] Unfortunately, both men developed violent headaches that lasted for days, leading Bier to recommend the following practices that are still being followed today: preventing the excessive loss of cerebrospinal fluid, using very fine (small) needles, and following strict bed rest if significant loss of cerebrospinal fluid cannot be avoided.[54] Intelligent prescience was at work again.

Bier was able to demonstrate that small amounts of local anesthetic (cocaine) injected into the subarachnoid space could provide surgical anesthesia for over 67% of the body. The anesthetic condition lasted approximately 45 minutes, an adequate time for many surgical procedures. His work provided the basis of spinal anesthesia as we practice it in modern medicine. Coincidentally, the practice of wearing rubber gloves emerged as a part of aseptic technique prior to Bier's work on spinal anesthesia, thus preventing many of the serious complications that could have occurred without this prophylactic measure.[55]

So, who deserves the laurels for the first spinal anesthetic? The history of anesthesiology is similar to that of other medical branches in that it has had its share of quarrels concerning priority. International disputes between the surgeon August Bier and his former colleague August Hildebrandt regarding the question of who was the actual inventor of spinal anesthesia are well documented. Although Hildebrandt and other colleagues frequently give credit to Corning, Bier insisted that he administered and described the technique of spinal anesthesia. In an extensive review (in the original language) of Corning's publication and those of Bier of Germany, Bier compared key factors, that is, the mention of cerebrospinal fluid, dose of injected cocaine, onset of action, and height of sensory analgesia. He noted that Corning's dose of local anesthetic was eight times higher than the dose given by Bier, yet the onset of analgesia was slower with a lower sensory block. Cerebrospinal fluid was not mentioned in Corning's paper. Bier concluded that Corning's injection was extradural, and that he (Bier) deserved to be acknowledged for introducing spinal anesthesia.[53,56–58]

After Bier's work in spinal anesthesia (published in 1899), interest in spinal anesthesia spread rapidly. Within 2 years of Bier's work, it has been estimated that more than 1000 papers were published relating to spinal anesthesia. Frederick Dudley Tait and Guido Caglieri in San Francisco were the first Americans to use true spinal anesthesia clinically.[59]

Rudoph Matas, head of the Department of Surgery at the University of Louisiana (later known as Tulane University), was the first American to report on spinal anesthesia. In his description of spinal anesthesia, Matas initially dissolved cocaine in water, creating a hypobaric solution. Later, he changed his "standard" mixture to cocaine with morphine, making him a pioneer in the use of spinal opioids to enhance central neuraxial anesthesia.[59]

With the vast interest in spinal anesthesia, serious complications from its application were soon observed. F. Gumprecht published a report of 15 cases of sudden death after spinal anesthesia.[60] Multiple cases of respiratory arrest and hypotension, following Harvey Cushing's introduction of blood pressure measurement, were also reported, leading to spinal anesthesia falling into disfavor.[61,62] Several pioneers sought to determine the causes of the variations in blood pressure from spinal anesthesia. Several theories emerged that have shaped our understanding of physiology today.

An extensive study was undertaken by L. G. Gray and H. T. Parsons of England to evaluate the causes for the changes in blood pressure after spinal anesthesia. They concluded that the decrease in arterial blood pressure was attributed to the diminished negative intrathoracic pressure during inspiration. High spinal anesthesia paralyzed the abdominal and thoracic muscles necessary to maintain that negative pressure.[63] With the understanding that hypotension was a primary danger with spinal anesthesia, G. Smith and W. Porter determined in 1915 that the fall in blood pressure was related to paralysis of the vasomotor fibers in the splanchnic area that regulated the tone of the blood vessels. They concluded that for spinal anesthesia to be effective without serious drops in blood pressure, cephalad diffusion of the local anesthetic should be avoided.[64] Gaston Labat contended that the serious adverse effects of spinal anesthesia were related to cerebral ischemia, not hypotension. He recommended that the patient should be placed in the Trendelenburg position after the spinal injection to keep the brain supplied with blood, therefore avoiding respiratory embarrassment.[65] Rather than looking at the position of the patient during injection, Arthur E. Barker promoted the idea that the baricity of the solution was instrumental in determining the cephalad spread. He made the injected solution stovaine, less toxic than cocaine but more irritating, hyperbaric with 5% glucose.[66] Barker was also a strong advocate for using sterile equipment and medication for spinal techniques. In 1934, Pitkin and Etherington-Wilson experimented with hypobaric solutions and changes in patient position to maintain control of the spread of the anesthetic.[32] Although there were other proponents of hypobaric spinal anesthesia, most had to deal with serious adverse effects, such as respiratory impairment and profound blood pressure changes requiring resuscitative maneuvers. It was not until 1920 that W. G. Hepburn and Lincoln Sise revived Barker's methods. Sise, an anesthesiologist at the Lahey Clinic in Boston, used hyperbaric tetracaine rather than stovaine.

Because of the irritating qualities of stovaine, Sise was interested in finding other local anesthetics that would provide sufficient length of anesthesia with limited side effects—something modern anesthesiologists can relate to in our daily practice. He was frustrated by the short duration of action of novocaine:

"The ending of a spinal anesthesia in the midst of an operation is always disturbing and annoying, but when this takes place in the midst of an abdominal operation, with the belly open, it may be dangerous as well."[67] He began using tetracaine because of its longer duration of action but was concerned about controlling the height of the block. Following Barker's recommendations regarding hyperbaric solutions, he added 10% glucose with success. He applied the same technique in 1935 to tetracaine.[67,68]

The most negative consequence of spinal anesthesia came from a trial in 1953. Two healthy young men had received spinal anesthesia on the same day in a hospital in England. Both developed *permanent* painful spastic paresis. Although the exact cause of the neurologic injury was never proven, it was suspected to be caused by contamination of the local anesthetic solution.[69,70] Several other cases of paralysis after spinal anesthesia followed, casting a dark shadow on the future application of this anesthetic technique. Fortunately, a follow-up analysis of over 10,000 spinal anesthetics was published by L. D. Vandam and R. D. Dripps. "The most gratifying result was the failure to discover persistent, progressive major neurological disease," providing the way for the spinal route to again emerge as a safe, effective means of providing anesthesia.[71]

The recurring problem of the inadequate duration of single-injection spinal anesthesia led a Philadelphia surgeon, William Lemmon, to report the development of an apparatus for continuous spinal anesthesia in 1940.[72] Lemmon began with the patient in the lateral position. The spinal tap was performed with a malleable silver needle that was left in position. As the patient was turned supine, the needle was positioned through a hole in the mattress and table. Additional injections of local anesthetic could be administered as required. Malleable silver needles also found a less-cumbersome and more common application in 1942 when Waldo Edwards and Robert Hingson encouraged the use of Lemmon's needles for continuous caudal anesthesia in obstetrics. In 1944, Edward Tuohy of the Mayo Clinic introduced important modifications of the continuous spinal techniques. He developed the now-familiar Tuohy needle as a means of improving the ease of passage of lacquered silk ureteral catheters through which he injected incremental doses of local anesthetic.[73]

Obstetric and Epidural Anesthesia

The origin of epidural analgesia began with Jean Enthuse Sicard, a neurologist, who introduced cocaine through the sacral hiatus for the treatment of sciatica and tabes. Independently, Fernand Cathelin used the same technique for surgical anesthesia.[74,75] In 1921, the Spanish surgeon Fidel Pagés-Miravé used a lumbar approach to the epidural space for surgical patients. His greatest contribution to the field of anesthesia was the introduction of *segmental anesthesia,* thereby eliminating some of the serious side effects of complete neuraxial blocks. Unfortunately, he died in an automobile accident before his methods could be shared by the students he worked with at the time. In 1931, Achille Dogliotti published a report on epidural injection of local anesthetics without knowledge of Pagés-Miravé's work. One of the most important features of

Dogliotti's work was his identification of the epidural space. He produced a textbook of his technique, which was both reproducible and easy to learn.[76] The limitation of epidural anesthesia was similar to that of spinal anesthesia—the duration of anesthesia provided. In 1947, Manuel Martinez Curbelo of Cuba is credited with using the Tuohy needle and a small ureteral catheter to provide continuous lumbar epidural analgesia.[77]

In the practice of obstetrics, religious beliefs obstructed the progress of pain relief for women in labor. It was commonly believed that providing anesthesia for the woman in labor went against God's will. James Young Simpson is credited with providing the first ether anesthetic for a complex obstetric delivery in 1847. He was severely criticized by both his peers and the clergy, but many women, most conspicuously Queen Victoria, began requesting anesthesia for the delivery of their children. There was not much progress in the field of obstetric analgesia/anesthesia from 1860 to 1940 until John Bonica, chief of anesthesia at the University of Washington, took over the management of his wife's anesthesia (and probably saved her life) during labor in 1943. She had a near-fatal complication during open drop ether anesthesia. From the time that he intervened in his wife's care, he devoted his career to the advancement of anesthetic care of the mother and fetus.[78]

When Bonica was chief of anesthesia, caudal anesthesia was the primary means used for providing labor analgesia. This followed a report by W. B. Edwards and R. A. Hingson that analgesia for labor and delivery could be satisfactorily achieved with caudal injections of tetracaine through a needle left in place within the sacral canal.[79] When commercially available catheters became available in the 1970s, continuous epidural analgesia gained popularity. In the years following Bonica's contributions, epidural anesthesia for obstetrics has become the norm. Modifications of the techniques and the introduction of either spinal or epidural opioids have made labor and delivery a more pleasant experience for expecting mothers.

A FEW THOUGHTS ON PAIN

Fundamental to modern neural blockade is the concept that pain is a sensory warning conveyed by specific nerve fibers, amenable, at least in principle, to modulation or interruption anywhere in the nerve's pathway. This outlook may be traced back to developments in the study of physiology that finally supplanted the view, first expressed by Plato and Aristotle, that pain, like pleasure, is a passion of the soul, that is, an emotion and not one of the senses. Philosophical changes growing out of the great revolutions of the eighteenth century and the birth of biology as a science gradually, although not entirely, effaced the religious connotations of pain in Western civilization. The doctrine of specific energies of the senses was first promulgated in 1826 by Johannes P. Müller (1801–1858).[80] This doctrine, although not specific for the conduction of pain, initiated the movement of scientific thought toward analysis and classification of the specific characters of different nerves. The theory that pain was a separate and distinct sense was first definitively developed by Moritz S. Schiff (1823–1896) in 1858. By examining the effect of incisions in the spinal cord, Schiff was able

to demonstrate that touch and pain were independent sensations. On animals, he demonstrated that injury to specific sections of the spinal cord resulted in loss of one modality without affecting the other.[81] Müller's theories led Erasmus Darwin (grandfather of Charles Darwin) to suggest the *intensive theory of pain*. Darwin felt that the sensation of pain was not a separate modality, but resulted from "whenever the sensorial motions are stronger than usual," theorizing that sensory overload leads to pain.[82] The theories of pain remained controversial throughout the early twentieth century, but by the middle of the twentieth century, the specificity theory (each sensory modality is transmitted along an independent pathway) became universally accepted as the most credible.

Applying drugs to transmitting nerves to alleviate neuralgic pain was first introduced by Francis Rynd in the early 1800s. Rynd's ideas possibly influenced the later development of both nerve blocks and opioid regional anesthesia.[81] When Carl Koller discovered the utility of cocaine as a surgical local anesthetic, a vast new world of local and regional analgesic therapy began. Corning is credited with the concept of direct application of an analgesic to the spinal cord for alleviation of pain, but it was not until the mechanism of pain was more fully understood that pain therapy could be focused on interrupting pain pathways. Unfortunately, by believing that pain pathway interruption was the complete answer to blocking pain, researchers focused only on that aspect, closing their minds to other related aspects of pain development. When Jean Joseph Emile Letievant described specific neurectomy techniques in the late nineteenth century, myriad surgical interventions, such as rhizotomy, cordotomy, and tractotomy, emerged to treat pain.[83] Unfortunately, most of these techniques were atrocious failures that often created more intense pain than was present prior to the procedure. Ronald Melzack and Patrick Wall's hypothesis that a spinal gate controls the cephalad transmission of nociception led to the modern introduction of electrical stimulation as a method of treating chronic pain. The concept proposed in the theory, that pain perception could be lessened by increasing activity in neural structures not associated with pain, led to chronic stimulation of the deep brain and spinal cord as a modality for the management of chronic pain. Consequently, both the brain and spinal structures emerged as targets for neuroaugmentation.[84,85] Although great strides have been made in our understanding of pain development and treatment, it is only through continued research that our understanding of preemptive pain control, such as those methods used in regional anesthesia, can be complete.

TWENTIETH-CENTURY REGIONAL ANESTHESIA

Orthopedic surgery has always lent itself to regional anesthesia techniques because of the ability to isolate anesthesia to the extremity being operated on. Initially, general anesthesia and nerve blocks were combined (still a somewhat common practice today). Harvey Cushing is credited with coining the name *regional anesthesia* for his method of blocking a nerve plexus under direct vision during general anesthesia. His goal was to decrease the anesthetic requirements and to provide postoperative pain relief. It is amazing to consider that he developed this technique in 1902, more than 100 years ago. A similar approach had been proposed by George Crile, 15 years earlier, to decrease the stress of surgery. Upper extremity anesthesia by blocking the brachial plexus percutaneously was achieved by many of our early colleagues. G. Hirschel is credited with developing the "blind" axillary brachial plexus block and D. Kulenkampff the supraclavicular technique, both in 1911. Because the risk of pneumothorax was high with the technique described by Kulenkampff, it was subsequently modified by A. Mulley using a lateral paravertebral approach. Mulley's approach is most likely the precursor of what is now commonly referred to as the "Winnie block" for the brachial plexus.

The spread of regional anesthesia in the United States was greatly facilitated by the work of Gaston Labat (Figure 1–12). Recruited to work at the Mayo Clinic in Rochester, Minnesota, Labat published his influential textbook, *Regional Anesthesia,* in which he described his techniques to the next generation of physicians, most notably Hippolite Wertheim, John Lundy, Ralph Waters, and Emery Rovenstine. Labat worked at the Mayo Clinic, then moved to Bellevue Hospital in New York City, where he worked with Wertheim. Together, they formed the first American Society of Regional Anesthesia. Labat's successor, Emery A. Rovenstine, was recruited to Bellevue to continue Labat's work. It was Rovenstine who was responsible for creating the specialty of anesthesiology in the 1920s and 1930s. He also is responsible for the creation of the first American clinic for the treatment of chronic pain, where he and his associates refined techniques of both lytic and therapeutic injections. Rovenstine and his successors used the American Society of Regional Anesthesia to educate physicians about pain management throughout the United States.[86]

The development of the multidisciplinary pain clinic was one of many contributions to anesthesiology made by John J. Bonica, a renowned teacher of regional techniques. During his periods of military, civilian, and university service at the University of Washington, John Bonica formulated a series of improvements in the management of chronic pain. His text, *The Management of Pain,* is regarded as a classic of the literature.[87,88]

THE POPULARITY AND USE OF LOCAL ANESTHESIA

Ever since Koller's original work, the popularity of local anaesthesia has waxed and waned, like that of many other medical developments. The announcement of his work produced a massive wave of enthusiasm, which was tempered as the problems of cocaine became increasingly appreciated. The first resurgence of interest came with the introduction of safer drugs at the beginning of the twentieth century and the second as a result of the efforts of Labat, Lundy, Maxson, Odom, and Pitkin in the United States in the years between the two world wars.

In Britain, general anesthesia has traditionally been administered by qualified doctors (although not always by specialists who practiced anesthesia exclusively). Standards have usually been high because the conduct of general anesthesia has been their entire responsibility. By contrast, local and regional techniques, if they were used at all, were performed by the surgeon, whose interest and attention were divided between anesthetic and operation. Regional anesthesia was not seen always to be to the patient's best advantage under such circumstances. Nevertheless, when the examination for the diploma in anaesthesia was instituted in 1935, the curriculum included local anesthesia. This, together with the establishment of anesthesia as an independent specialty within the UK National Health Service in 1948, did much to encourage local anesthetic techniques. Unfortunately, the years between 1950 and 1955 saw a sharp decrease in the use of local, and particularly spinal, anesthesia in the United Kingdom and in the United States. The many advances in general anesthesia then taking place were partly responsible because they encouraged the belief that a local technique was unnecessary. More important, though, was the fear of severe neurologic damage. The report, "The Grave Spinal Cord Paralyses Caused by Spinal Anesthesia," written in 1950 in New York by a British-trained neurologist, Foster Kennedy, was followed by the Woolley and Roe case and led to a virtual extinction of the use of regional techniques (see discussion in the section on spinal anesthesia).[70] After a number of reports of the safe use of local anesthetics for surgical procedures emerged, regional anesthesia techniques once again began to slowly emerge.

Local anesthetic techniques are of value in blocking afferent stimuli even in major surgery because of the reduction in the pain and stress suffered by the patient. This approach is now extending even to cardiac surgery, but the concept is far from new. As early as 1902, Harvey Cushing was advocating the combination of local with general anesthesia to decrease

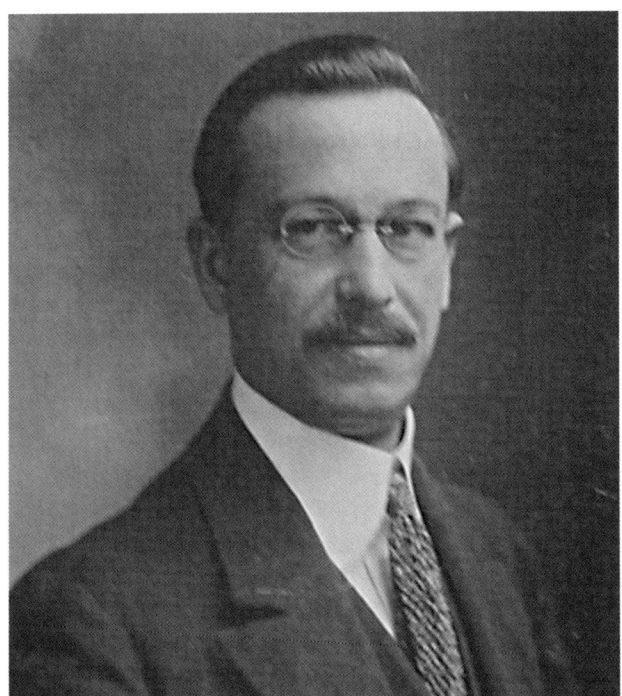

FIGURE 1–12. Gaston Labat.

"surgical shock," a concept that was further developed by Crile. The term *balanced anaesthesia* is common today and implies a triad of sleep produced by either inhalational or intravenous route, profound analgesia with opioid drugs, and muscle relaxation by neuromuscular block. But, interestingly, when Lundy first used the term in 1926, he intended that the second and third parts of the triad would be produced by a local anesthetic block, something proponents of regional anesthesia are implementing in modern anesthesia practice.

Other advances, although more difficult to quantify, have directly or indirectly helped the cause of regional anesthesia. For example, developments in the field of medical plastics have resulted in safe and reliable syringes, catheters, and filters, and the anesthesiologist can select from a wide variety of sedative and anxiolytic drugs that, when carefully used, can greatly improve the patient's acceptance of a nerve block. Of great importance has been the understanding of the effects and treatment of sympathetic block. Ephedrine became available in 1924 and was first used to treat hypotension during spinal anesthesia in 1927, but readily available intravenous fluids and equipment for their administration are more recent developments.

Most currently used techniques of regional anesthesia were devised during that first decade of the twentieth century: brachial plexus block, axillary and supraclavicular approaches; IVRA; celiac plexus block; caudal anesthesia; hyperbaric and hypobaric techniques of spinal anesthesia; and all the presently employed nerve blocks for the head and neck as applied in dentistry and plastic surgery. Thereafter, aside from technical innovation and understanding of some of the physiologic and toxicologic responses to local anesthetics, the great impetus to regional anesthesia came from the synthesis of the amide local anesthetics and an understanding of their pharmacodynamic and especially pharmacokinetic properties.[32]

In present-day practice, more advanced techniques of regional anesthesia (eg, continuous catheters, combination blocks, deep plexus blocks) have evolved because of the groundwork put in place by those earlier pioneers. With the advent of the Internet providing easier access to current medical practice, patients are better educated and are becoming advocates for regional anesthetic techniques.

It is appropriate to conclude by mentioning the organizations that seek to promote education and training in the use of regional anesthetic techniques. The American Society of Regional Anesthesia was reborn in 1975 and became firmly established. Its European counterpart (the European Society of Regional Anaesthesia and Pain Medicine) is younger but is now equally well established, and similar societies are flourishing in many other parts of the world. (founded in 1994 by Drs. Hadzic and Vloka), have been developed to continue to promote the safe and effective practice of regional anesthesia.

THE TWENTY-FIRST CENTURY AND BEYOND

The history of local and regional anesthesia did not end in the first half of the twentieth century. In fact, it is often said, "We are making history every day." For instance, important techniques developed in the last few decades have refined our ability to identify peripheral nerves accurately. With the increasingly enthusiastic introduction of the use of ultrasound for nerve location, the rate of development in this area of regional anesthetic practice will increase at a greater pace. Other technological advances have included needles optimized for visualization under ultrasound.

As detailed in other chapters of this textbook, there are current and exciting threads of enquiry on the morphology of nerves, combining insights on nerve electrical stimulation and pressure monitoring and a better understanding of the risks leading to nerve injury. Research continues on better agents and additives that can be used in regional anesthesia.

Perhaps the most important role for the regional anesthesiologists who will make history in the next few decades will be to document the clinical advantages and benefits of local and regional anesthesia. This endeavor will not only manifest itself as enthusiasm and skill but also will be based on the generation of convincing data through careful clinical research and academic cooperation within the regional anesthesia community. Books such as this are a vital part of building the future of regional anesthesia and in themselves will form a part of the history of local and regional anesthesia.

ACKNOWLEDGMENTS

We thank Bonnie Farrell, MD, Christopher Robards, MD, and Lakshmanasamy Somasundaram, MD, for their work on this chapter in the previous edition.

REFERENCES

1. Vandam L: Early American anesthetists: The origins of professionalism in anesthesia. Anesthesiology 1973;38:264–274.
2. Greene N: A consideration of factors in the discovery of anesthesia and their effects on its development. Anesthesiology 1971;38:264–274.
3. Cadwell J, Sever P: The biochemical pharmacology of abused drugs: I. Amphetamines, cocaine, and LSD. Clin Pharmacol Ther 1974;16:625–638.
4. Loza-Balsa G: *Monografia sobre la Coca.* Edita Sociedad Geografica de la Paz, 1991, pp 9–15.
5. Van Dyke C, Byck R: Cocaine. Sci Am 1982;246:128–141.
6. Guerra F: *The Pre-Columbian Mind.* Seminar Press 1971;1:47, 52, 126, 191.
7. Vespucci A: Cartas de viaje. Introduccion y notas de Luciano Formisano. Alianza Editorial SA 1986;48:102–137.
8. Romero C: Descubrimiento y conquista del Peru por Pedro Pizarro conquistador y poblador de este reino. Biografia de Pedro Pizarro 1917;6:1–187.
9. Ruetsch Y, Boni T, Borgeat A: From cocaine to ropivacaine: The history of local anesthetic drugs. Curr Topics Med Chem 2001;1:175–182.
10. Lossen W: Über das cocain. Ann Chem Pharmacol 1865;133:351–371.
11. Link W, Einhorn A: Inventor of novocaine. Dent Radiogr Photogr 1959;32:20.
12. Fink B: Leaves and needles: The introduction of surgical local anesthesia. Anesthesiology 1985;63:77.
13. Howard-Jones N: A critical study of the origins and early development of hypodermic medications. J Hist Med 1947;2:201.
14. Blejer-Prieto H: Coca leaf and cocaine addiction—some historical notes. Can Med Assoc J 1965;93:700–704.
15. Niemann A: Über eine neue organische Base in den Cocablattern. Arch Pharmacol 1860;153:129–155, 291–308.
16. von Anrep B: Über die physiologische Wirkung des Cocain. Pflugers Arch 1880;21:38.
17. Matas R: Local and regional anesthesia: A retrospect and prospect. Am J Surg 1934;25:189–196.

18. Koller K: Historical notes on the beginning of local anesthesia. JAMA 1928;90:1742–1743.

19. Buess H: Über die Anwendung der Koka und des Kokains in der Medizin. Ciba Z 1944;8:3362–3365.

20. Freud S: Über Coca. Centralbl Gesamte Ther 1884:289–314.

21. Koller C: On the use of cocaine for producing anaesthesia on the eye. Lancet 1884;2:990.

22. Becker H: Carl Koller and cocaine. Psychoanal Q 1963;32:309.

23. Koller K: Über die Verwendung des Cocain zur Aanasthesirung am Auge. Wien Med Wochenschr 1884;34:1276–1278.

24. Willstatter R, Wolfes D, Mader H: Synthese des naturlichen Cocains. Justus Liebigs Ann Chem 1923;434:111–139.

25. Hurtado P: *Indianos cacerenos. Notas biograficas de los hijos de la Alta Extremadura que sirvieron en America durante el primer siglo de su conquista.* Tipografia Luis Tasso, 1892, pp 38–39.

26. McAuley J: The early development of local anaesthesia. Br Dent J 1966;121:139–142.

27. Pernice L: Über Cocain anasthesie. Dtsch Med Wochenschr 1890;16:287–289.

28. Liljestrand G: Carl Koller and the development of local anesthesia. Acta Physiol Scand Suppl 1967;299:3–30.

29. Olch P, William S: Halsted and local anesthesia: Contributions and complications. Anesthesiology 1975;42:479–486.

30. Schleich C: Infiltration anasthesie (locale anasthesie) und ihr Verhaltniss zur allgemeinen Narcose (inhalation anasthesie). Verh Dtsch Ges Chiropractic 1892;21:121–127.

31. Reclus P: Analgesie locale par la cocaine. Rev Chiropr 1889;9:913.

32. Covino B: One hundred years plus two of regional anesthesia. Reg Anesth 1986;11:105.

33. Link W: Alfred Einhorn, Sc.D: Inventor of novocaine. Dent Radiogr Photogr 1959;32:1, 20.

34. Braun H: Über einige neue ortliche anaesthetica. Dtsch Med Wochenschr 1905;31:1667–1671.

35. Benedict H, Clark S, Freeman C: Studies in local anesthesia. J Am Dent Assoc 1932;19:2087–2105.

36. Ritchie J, Ritchie B, Greengard P: The active structure of local anesthetics. J Pharmacol Exp Ther 1965;150:152–159.

37. Halsted W: Water as a local anesthetic. N Y Med J 1885;42:327.

38. Burke W: Hydrochlorate of cocaine in minor surgery. N Y Med J 1884;40:616.

39. Halsted W: Practical comments on the use and abuse of cocaine; suggested by its invariably successful employment in more than a thousand minor surgical operations. N Y Med J 1885;42:327.

40. Hall R: Hydrochlorate of cocaine. N Y Med J 1884;40:643.

41. Francois-Frank C: Action patalysant locale de la cocaine sur les nerfs et les centres nerveux: Applications a la technique experimentale. Arch Physiol 1900;24:562.

42. Corning J: Spinal anaesthesia and local medication of the cord with cocaine. N Y Med J 1885;42:483.

43. Esmarch F: Über kunsstliche Blutleere. Arch Klin Chiropractic 1874;17:292.

44. Braun H: Über den Einfluss der Vitalitat der Gewebe auf die ortlichen und allgemeinen Giftwirkungen localanasthesirender Mittel und über die Bedeutung des Adrenalins für die Localanasthesie. Arch Klin Chiropr 1903;69:541.

45. Abel J: On the blood pressure raising constituent of the suprarenal capsule. Johns Hopkins Hosp Bull 1897;8:151.

46. Braun H: *Local Anesthesia: Its Scientific Basis and Practical Use,* 3rd ed. Lea & Febiger, 1914, p 541.

47. Rodola F, Vagnoni S, Ingletti S: An update on intravenous regional anaesthesia of the arm. Eur Rev Med Pharmacol Sci 2003;7:131–138.

48. Brill S, Middleton W, Brill G, et al: Bier's block; 100 years old and still going strong! Acta Anaesthesiol Scand 2004;48:117–122.

49. Holmes G: Intravenous regional anesthesia: A useful method of producing analgesia of the limbs. Lancet 1963;1:245–247.

50. Greene N: Anesthesia and the development of surgery (1846–1896). Anesth Analg 1979;58:5–12.

51. Quincke H: Die Lumbalpunction des Hydrocephalus. Ber Klin Wochenschr 1891;28:929.

52. Bier A: Versuche über Cocainisirung des Ruckenmarkes. Dtsch Z Chir 1899;51:361.

53. Marx G: The first spinal anesthesia. Who deserves the laurels? Reg Anesth 1994;19:429–430.

54. Bier A: Über einen neuen Weg Localanasgthesie an den Gliedmassen zu erzeugen. Arch Klin Chiropr 1908;86:1007.

55. Halsted W: *Surgical Papers by William Steward Halsted.* Johns Hopkins Press, 1924, pp 37–39.

56. Goerig M, Beck H: Priority conflict concerning the discovery of lumbar anesthesia between August Bier and August Hildebrandt. Anasthesiol Intensivemed Notfallmed Schmerzther 1996;31:111–119.

57. Goerig G, Esch J: In memory of August Bier (1861–1949). Anasthesiol Intensivemed Notfallmed Schmerzther 1999;34:463–474.

58. Goerig M, Agarwal K, Schulte-Steinberg O, et al: The versatile August Bier (1861–1949), father of spinal anesthesia. J Clin Anesth 2000;12:561–569.

59. Matas R: Local and regional anesthesia with cocaine and other analgesic drugs, including the subarachnoid method, as applied in general surgical practice. Phila Med J 1900;6:820–843.

60. Gumprecht F: Gefahren der Lumbalpunktion: Plotzliche Todesfalle danach. Dtsch Med Wochenschr 1900;27:386–389.

61. Cushing H: On routine determinations of arterial tension in operating room and clinic. Boston Med Surg J 1903;148:250–256.

62. Thorsen G: Neurologic complications after spinal anesthesia and results from 2493 follow-up cases. Acta Chir Scand 1950;(Suppl)121:385–398.

63. Gray H, Parsons L: Blood pressure variations associated with lumbar puncture and the induction of spinal anesthesia. Q J Med 1912;5:339.

64. Smith G, Porter W: Spinal anesthesia in the cat. Am J Physiol 1915;38:108.

65. Labat G: Circulatory disturbances associated with subarachnoid nerve block. Long Island Med J 1927;21:573.

66. Barker A: Clinical experiences with spinal analgesia in 100 cases and some reflections on the procedure. BMJ 1907;I:665.

67. Sise L: Pontocain-Glucose solution for spinal anesthesia. In Faulconer A, Keys T (eds): *Foundations of Anesthesiology.* Thomas, 1965, pp 874–882.

68. Sise L: Spinal anesthesia for upper and lower abdominal operations. New Engl J Med 1928;199:61.

69. Cope R: The Wooley and Roe case. Anaesthesia 1954;9:249–270.

70. Kennedy F, Effron A, Perry G: The grave spinal cord paralysis caused by spinal anesthesia. Surg Gynecol Obstet 1950;91:385–398.

71. Vandam L, Dripps R: Long-term follow-up of patients who received 10,098 spinal anesthetics. In Faulconer A, Keys T (eds): *Foundations of Anesthesiology.* Thomas, 1965, pp 901–913.

72. Lemmon W: A method for continuous spinal anesthesia, a preliminary report. In Faulconer A, Keys T (eds): *Foundations of Anesthesiology.* Thomas, 1965, pp 883–900.

73. Tuohy E: Continuous spinal anesthesia: Its usefulness and technic involved. Anesthesiology 1944;5:142.

74. Sicard M: Les injections medicamenteuses extradurales par voie sacro-coccygienne. C R Soc Dev Biol 1901;53:396–398.

75. Cathelin M: Une nouvelle voie d'injection rachidienne. Methodes des injections epidurales par le precede du canal sacre. C R Soc Dev Biol 1901;53:452–453.

76. Dogliotti A: Eine neue Methode der regionaren Anasthesie: Die peridurale segmentaire Anasthesie. Zentralbl Chir 1931;58:3141–3145.

77. Curbelo M: Continuous peridural segemental anesthesia by means of a ureteral catheter. Anesth Analg 1949;28:13–23.

78. Chadwick H: Obstetric anesthesia—then and now. Minerva Anestesiol 2005;71:517–520.

79. Edwards W, Hingson R: Continuous caudal anesthesia in obstetrics. Am J Surg 1942;57:459–464.

80. Wade N: *Muller's Elements of Physiology,* Thoemmes Continuum: The History of Ideas, 2003, pp 1–11.

81. Bonica J: Evolution of pain concepts and pain clinics. Clin Anesthesiol 1985;3:1.

82. Darwin E: *Zoonomia, or the Laws of Organic Life.* Johnson, 1794.

83. Spicher C, Kohut G: Jean Joseph Emile Letievant: A review of his contributions to surgery and rehabilitation. J Reconstr Microsurg 2001;17:169–177.

84. Gildenberg P: History of neuroaugmentative procedures. Neurosurg Clin North Am 2003;14:327–337.

85. Stanton-Hicks M, Salamon J: Stimulation of the central and peripheral nervous system for the control of pain. J Clin Neurophysiol 1997;14:46–62.

86. Bacon D: Gaston Labat, John Lundy, Emery Rovenstine, and the Mayo Clinic: The spread of regional anesthesia in American between the World Wars. J Clin Anesth 2002;14:315–320.

87. Bonica J: *The Management of Pain,* 2nd ed. Lea and Febiger, 1953.

88. Benedetti C, Chapman C: John J. Bonica. A biography. Minerva Anestesiol 2005;71:391–396.

FOUNDATIONS OF LOCAL AND REGIONAL ANESTHESIA

Embryology

Patrick M. McQuillan

INTRODUCTION

A thorough understanding of the underlying anatomy is fundamental to a logical approach to the techniques used in regional anesthesia. An appreciation for the embryologic development of tissues and structures can significantly add to the understanding of functional anatomy as it relates to regional anesthesia. In this chapter, I emphasize the embryologic development of the brain, spinal cord, peripheral and autonomic nervous systems, as well as the musculoskeletal system as it pertains to regional anesthesia. Many excellent comprehensive texts on embryology are available. For this chapter, I have relied heavily on information from primary texts and refer the reader to them for a complete discussion of all embryologic development. The first two, *Langman's Medical Embryology*[1] and *Basic Concepts in Embryology,*[2] are valuable for their ease of readability, clarity of figures, and clinical correlations. *Human Embryology and Developmental Biology*[3] is a good contemporary, comprehensive explanation of the molecular genetics of embryologic development. *The Developing Human: Clinically Oriented Embryology*[4] is the time-tested standard text of embryology.

GENERAL EMBRYOLOGY

The prenatal period is divided into two major periods: the embryonic period, from fertilization through 2 months, and the fetal period, from the third month through birth.

Embryonic Period

The embryonic period is the time when all tissues are formed and, particularly during the second month, all organs are formed. The fetal period is a time of organ growth.[2] Embryologic development begins with fertilization, the process by which the male and female gametes unite to give rise to a zygote. Approximately 3 days after fertilization, cells of the compacted embryo divide to form a **morula,** which is composed of an inner and outer cell mass. The inner cell mass gives rise to the tissues of the **embryoblast,** and the outer cell mass forms the **trophoblast,** which later contributes to the placenta. After a period of cell division, during which time the morula enters the uterine cavity, the **blastocoele** forms, and the embryo is known as a **blastocyst** (Figure 2–1).

By the eighth day of development, the blastocyst is partially embedded in the endometrium. At this time, the trophoblast differentiates into an inner and an outer layer. Lacunae develop in the outer layer, maternal sinusoids are eroded, and by the end of the second week a primitive uteroplacental circulation begins to develop.

The inner cell mass, or embryoblast, differentiates into two layers, the **epiblast** and the **hypoblast,** which together form the bilaminar germ disk.

The most characteristic event occurring during the third week of gestation is **gastrulation.** This is the process that establishes all three germ layers: **endoderm, ectoderm,** and **mesoderm** in the embryo (Figure 2–2). Gastrulation begins

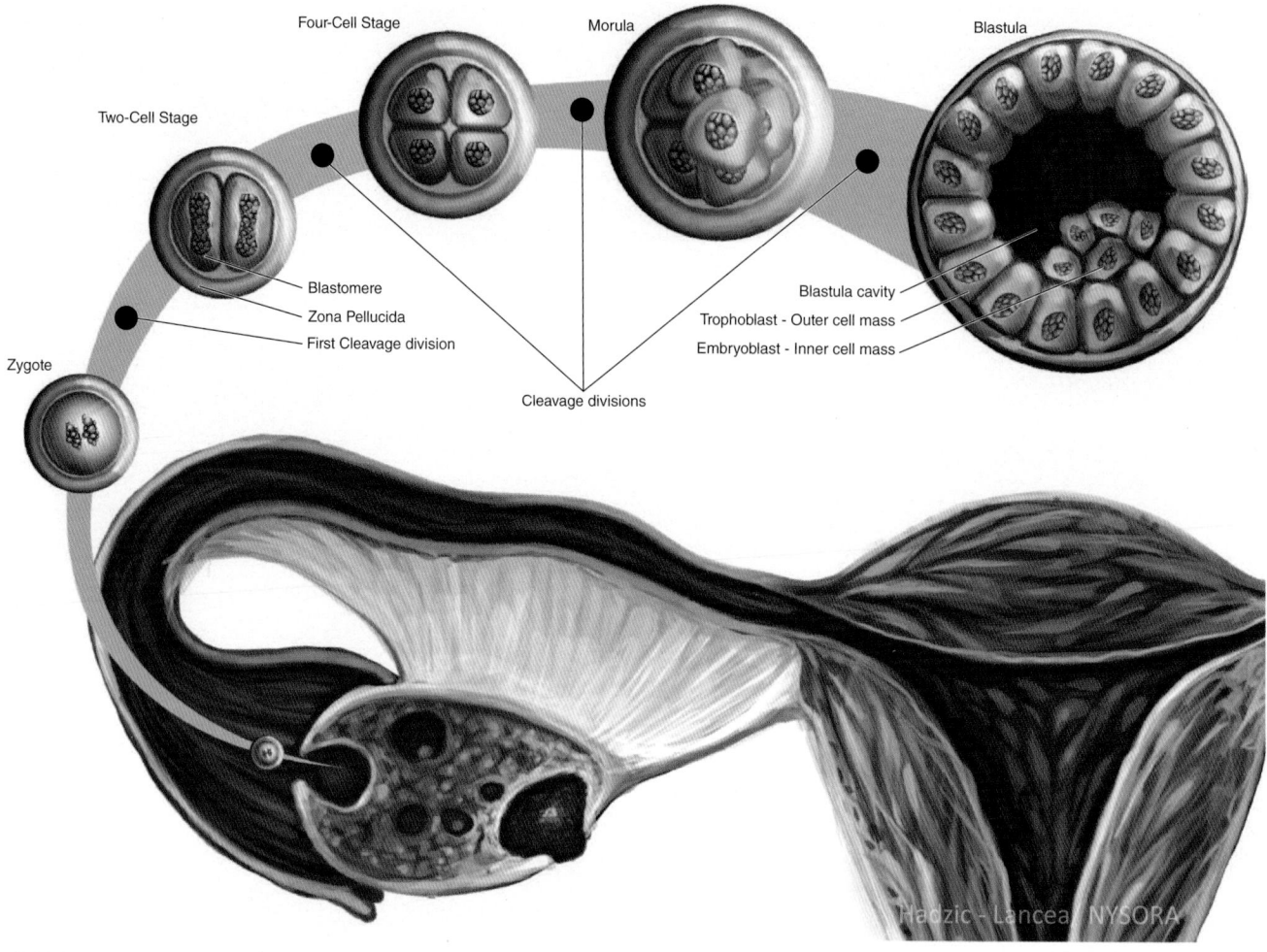

FIGURE 2–1. Formation of the blastocyst.

with the formation of the **primitive streak** on the surface of the epiblast portion of the bilaminar germ disk. Cells migrate toward the primitive streak, detach from the epiblast, and slip beneath it. This inward movement is known as **invagination.** Once the cells have invaginated, some displace the hypoblast, creating the new embryonic endoderm. Other cells come to lie between the epiblast and the newly created endoderm to form the mesoderm. Cells remaining in the epiblast then form the ectoderm. Through the process of gastrulation, the epiblast therefore becomes the source of all the germ layers in the embryo.[1] Developments during the first 3 weeks of the embryonic period produce an embryo with one germ layer (week 1), two germ layers (week 2), and three germ layers with a recognizable three-dimensional body form (week 3)[2] (Figure 2–3).

In general terms, the **ectoderm** germ layer gives rise to organs and structures that allow us to maintain contact with the outside world.[4] It gives rise to the central and peripheral nervous systems; the sensory epithelium of the eye, ear, and nose; the epidermis and its appendages; hair and nails, mammary glands; the hypophysis, subcutaneous glands; and the enamel of the teeth.

The **mesoderm** gives rise to supporting structures of the body, such as cartilage, bone, and connective tissue; striated and smooth muscle; the heart, blood, lymph vessels, and cells; and

the kidneys, gonads, and serous membranes lining the body cavities, spleen, and the cortex of the adrenal gland.

The **endoderm** produces the epithelial lining of the gastrointestinal and respiratory tracts, as well as the epithelial lining of the bladder and urethra, tympanic cavity, antrum, and auditory tube. It also engenders the parenchyma of the tonsils, thyroid, parathyroid thymus, liver, and pancreas.

As the embryo forms, it rapidly develops along several axes,[2] the first of which is the craniocaudal axis. It is established while the embryo is still a flat disk or sheet of cells. This axis runs from the future head to the future tail of the body form. The dorsoventral axis is the next to be established. This occurs as the body folds and defines the future front and back sides of the body form.

Establishment of the body axes takes place prior to and during the period of gastrulation. Cells at the posterior margin of the embryonic disk signal the craniocaudal axis. The dorsoventral orientation of tissue is controlled by a complex interaction of proteins and growth factors.

This early orientation of cells in the body is a result of the expression of *Hox* genes. There are four *Hox* gene complexes in vertebrates: *Hox a, b, c,* and *d.* Each consists of a group of between 9 and 11 genes arranged sequentially along a particular chromosome. A cascade of genes producing signaling factors

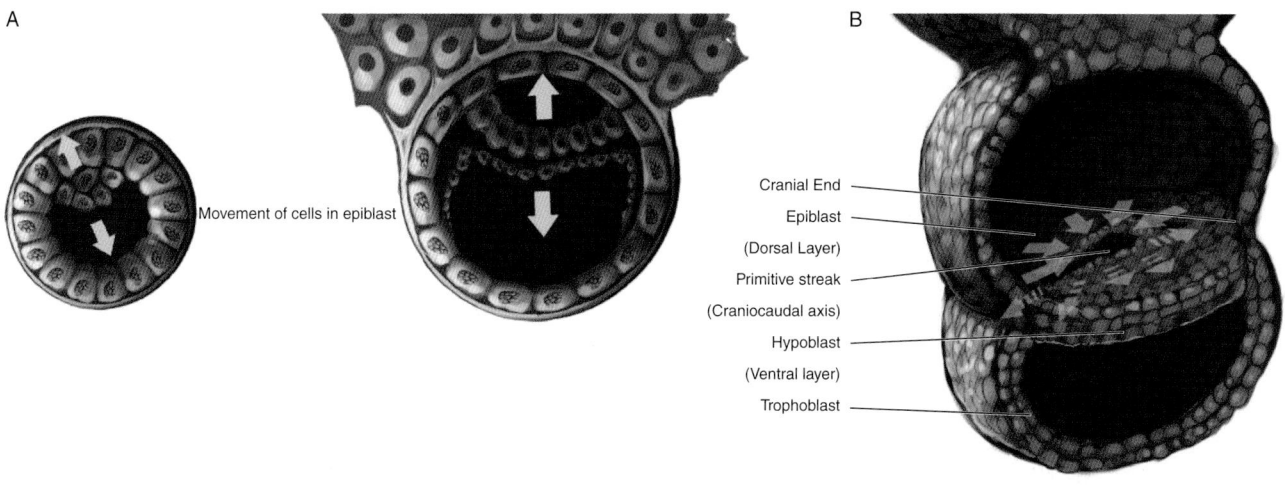

A

Movement of cells in epiblast

B

Cranial End
Epiblast
(Dorsal Layer)
Primitive streak
(Craniocaudal axis)
Hypoblast
(Ventral layer)
Trophoblast

Movement of gastrulating cells below epiblast

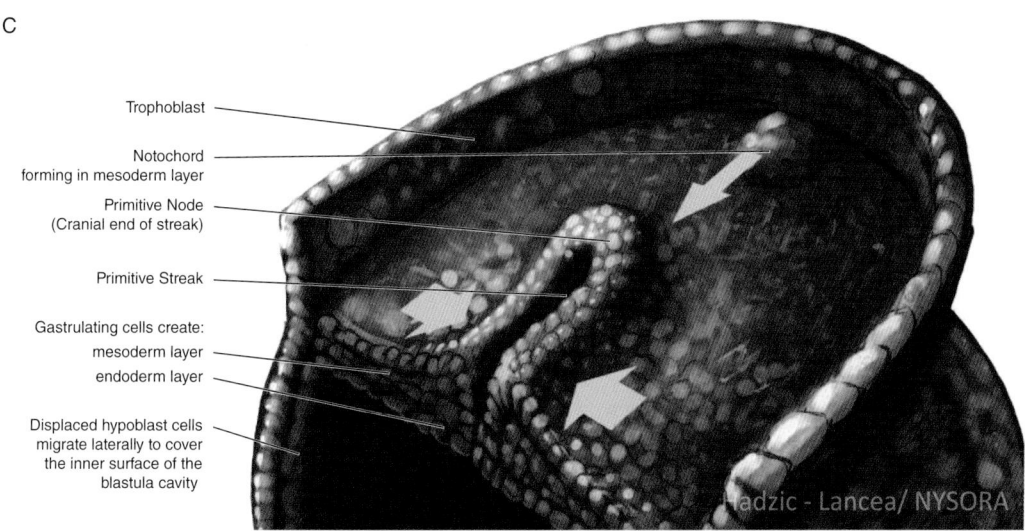

C

Trophoblast
Notochord
forming in mesoderm layer
Primitive Node
(Cranial end of streak)
Primitive Streak
Gastrulating cells create:
mesoderm layer
endoderm layer
Displaced hypoblast cells
migrate laterally to cover
the inner surface of the
blastula cavity

Hadzic - Lancea/ NYSORA

FIGURE 2–2. Establishment of the three basic germ layers in the embryo: endoderm, ectoderm, and mesoderm. **A:** Trophoblast with the shell removed. **B:** Gastrulation viewed from the dorsal surface. Solid arrows show movement of cells in epiblast; dashed arrows show movement of gastrulating cells below the epiblast. **C:** Differentiation of the basic germ layers.

also orchestrates left-right asymmetry, which is established early in development. As a result of complex interactions, for example, the heart and spleen lie on the left side of the body and the main lobe of the liver lies on the right.

Regions of the epiblast that migrate and ingress through the primitive streak have been mapped and their ultimate fates determined. Mesoderm cells that ingress through the cranial region of the primitive node become the notochord; those migrating at the lateral edges of the primitive node and from the cranial end of the primitive streak become the paraxial mesoderm. Cells migrating through the midstreak region become the intermediate mesoderm, and those migrating through the caudal part of the streak form the lateral plate mesoderm. This orientation of the mesoderm is important in understanding limb development.

The embryonic disk, initially flat and almost round, gradually becomes elongated, with a broad cephalic and a narrow caudal end. Expansion of the embryonic disk occurs mainly in the cephalic region. This growth in elongation is caused by continuous migration of cells from the primitive streak region

in a cephalad direction. Invagination and migration forward and laterally of surface cells in the primitive streak continue until the end of the fourth week. Germ cell layers in the cephalic region begin their specific differentiation by the middle of the third week, whereas those in the caudal part differentiate beginning by the end of the fourth week. This causes the embryo to develop in a cephalocaudal direction (Figure 2–4).

At the beginning of the third week of development, the ectodermal germ layer has the shape of the disk. The ectoderm gives rise to two subdivisions: neuroectoderm, which forms all neural tissue, and the epidermal covering of the body.[2] Appearance of the notochord and prechordal mesoderm induces the overlying ectoderm to thicken and form the neural plate (Figure 2–5). Cells of the neural plate make up the neuroectoderm, and their induction represents the initial event in the process of **neurulation.** By the end of the third week, the lateral edges of the neural plate become elevated to form neural folds, and the depressed midregion forms the neural groove. Gradually, the neural folds approach each other in the midline, where they fuse, resulting in formation of the neural tube. Neurulation is then complete, and the central nervous

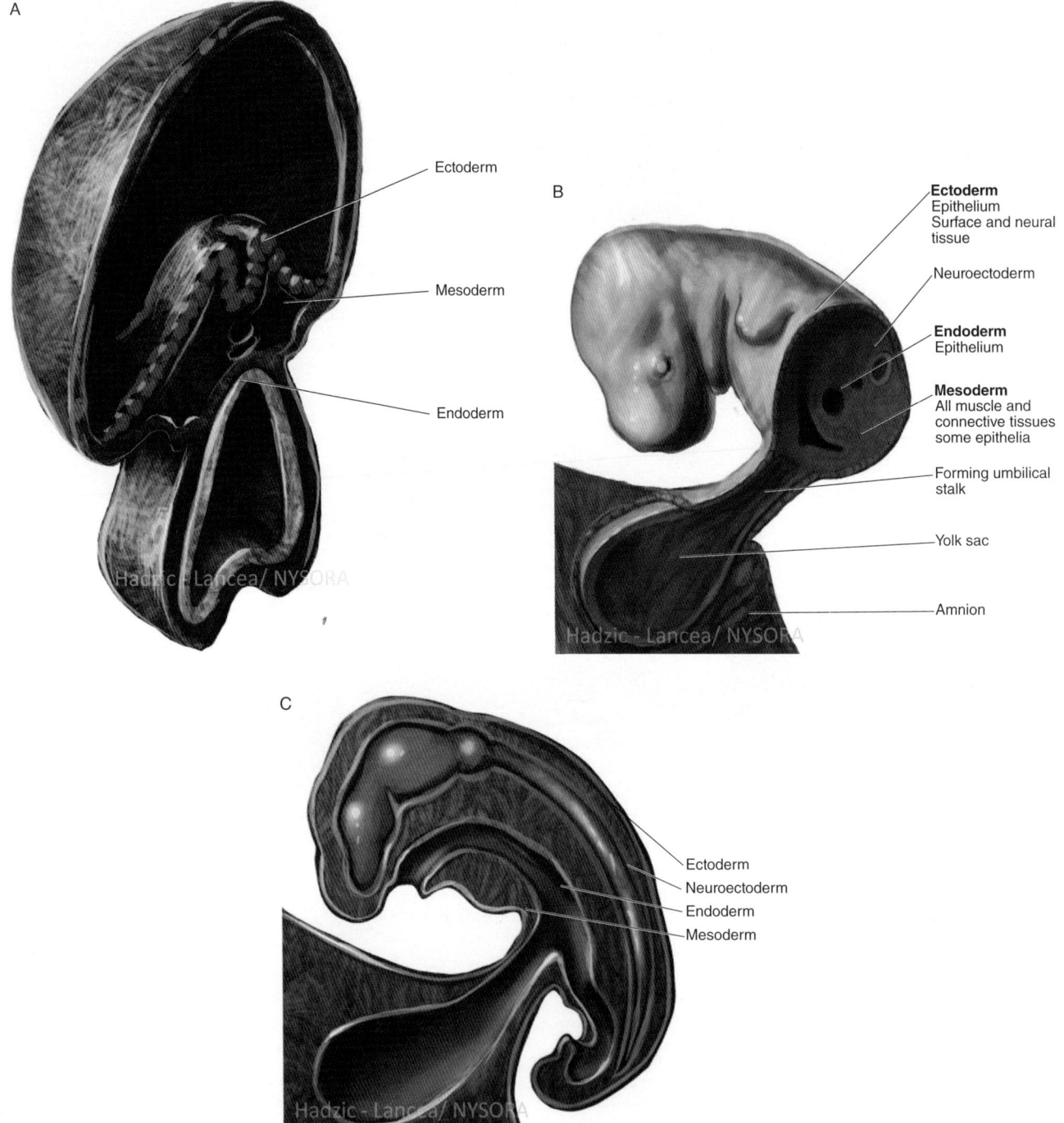

A

Ectoderm

Mesoderm

Endoderm

B

Ectoderm
Epithelium
Surface and neural
tissue

Neuroectoderm

Endoderm
Epithelium

Mesoderm
All muscle and
connective tissues
some epithelia

Forming umbilical
stalk

Yolk sac

Amnion

C

Ectoderm
Neuroectoderm
Endoderm
Mesoderm

FIGURE 2–3. Cross section of germ layers as they appear during embryonic folding. **A:** Cross section. **B:** Cross section of germ layers after folding is completed. **C:** Longitudinal section.

system (CNS) is represented by a closed tubular structure with a narrow caudal portion, the spinal cord, and a much broader cephalic portion characterized by a number of dilations, the brain vesicles. As the neural folds elevate and fuse, cells at the lateral border begin to dissociate from their neighbors. This cell population, called the **neural crest,** will undergo a transition as they leave the neuroectoderm to enter the underlying mesoderm.

During the body-folding process, the endoderm is formed into an epithelial tube, which runs the length of the body. The derivatives of the endoderm tube are all epithelial tissues (Figure 2–6).

Initially, cells of the mesoderm germ layer form a thin sheet of tissue on each side of the midline.[1] These cells proliferate and form a thick end plate of tissue known as paraxial mesoderm (Figure 2–7). More laterally, the mesoderm remains thin and is known as the lateral plate. This lateral plate divides into two layers: a somatic, or parietal, mesoderm layer and a splanchnic, or visceral, mesoderm layer. Together, these layers form the intraembryonic cavity. Intermediate mesoderm connects the paraxial and lateral plate mesoderm.

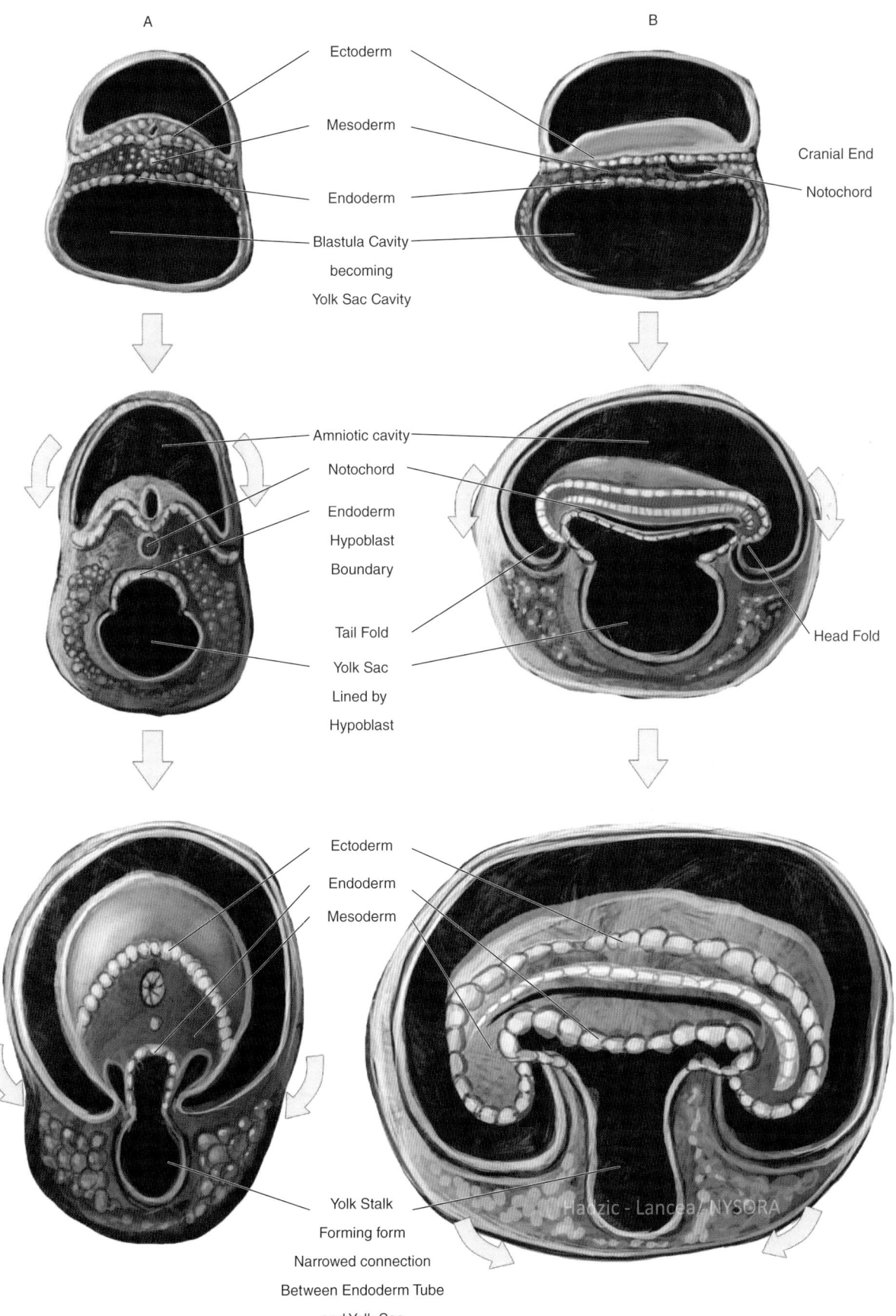

A
Ectoderm
Mesoderm
Endoderm
Blastula Cavity
becoming
Yolk Sac Cavity

B
Cranial End
Notochord

Amniotic cavity
Notochord
Endoderm
Hypoblast
Boundary
Tail Fold
Yolk Sac
Lined by
Hypoblast

Head Fold

Ectoderm
Endoderm
Mesoderm

Yolk Stalk
Forming form
Narrowed connection
Between Endoderm Tube
and Yolk Sac

FIGURE 2–4. Development of the embryo in a cephalocaudal direction. **A:** Lateral body folds, cross-sectional views. **B:** Craniocaudal body folds, longitudinal views.

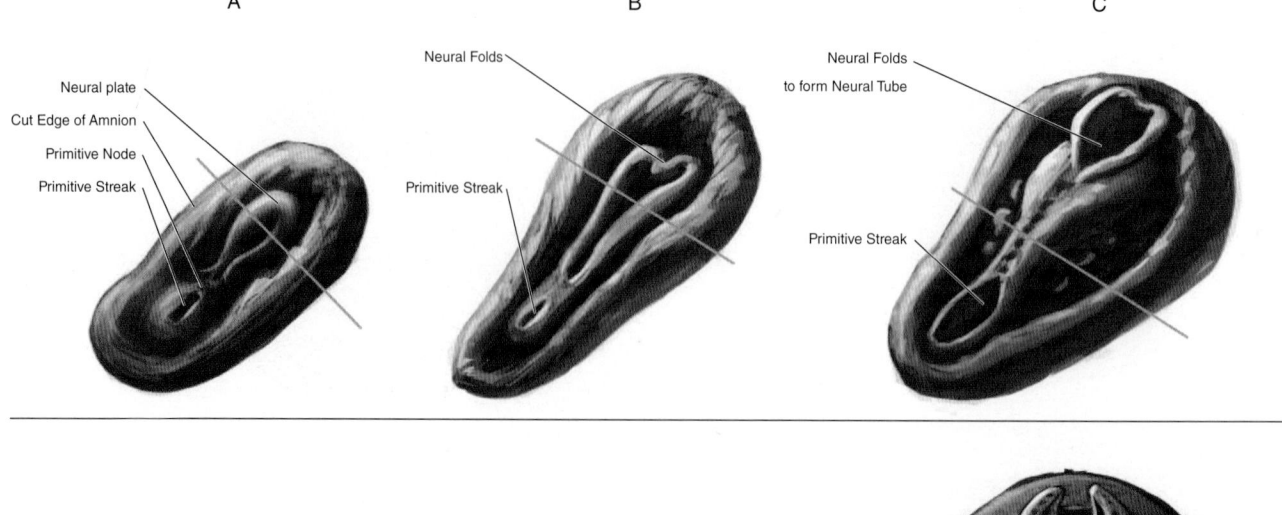

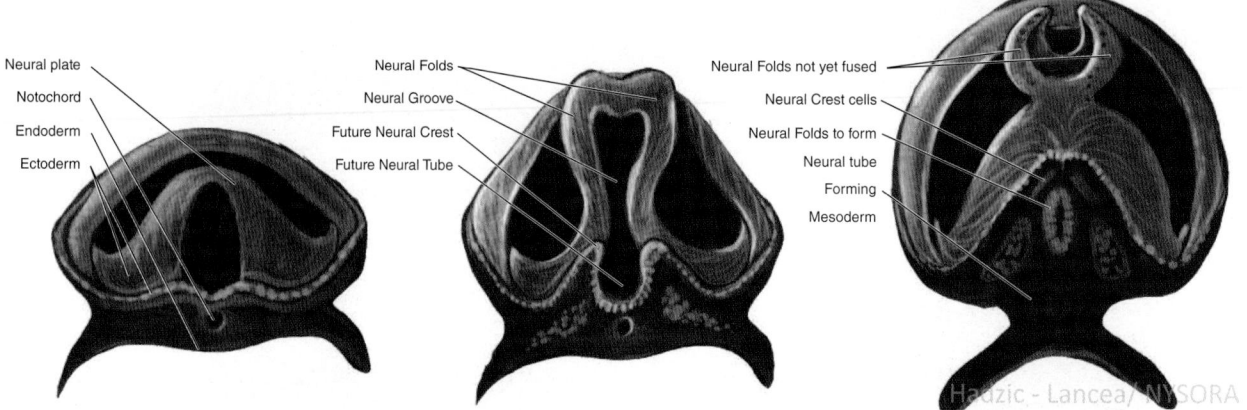

FIGURE 2–5. Formation of the neural plate. **A:** Formation of the neural plate. **B:** Formation of the neural folds and neural groove. **C:** Completion of neurulation, the creation of the neural tube.

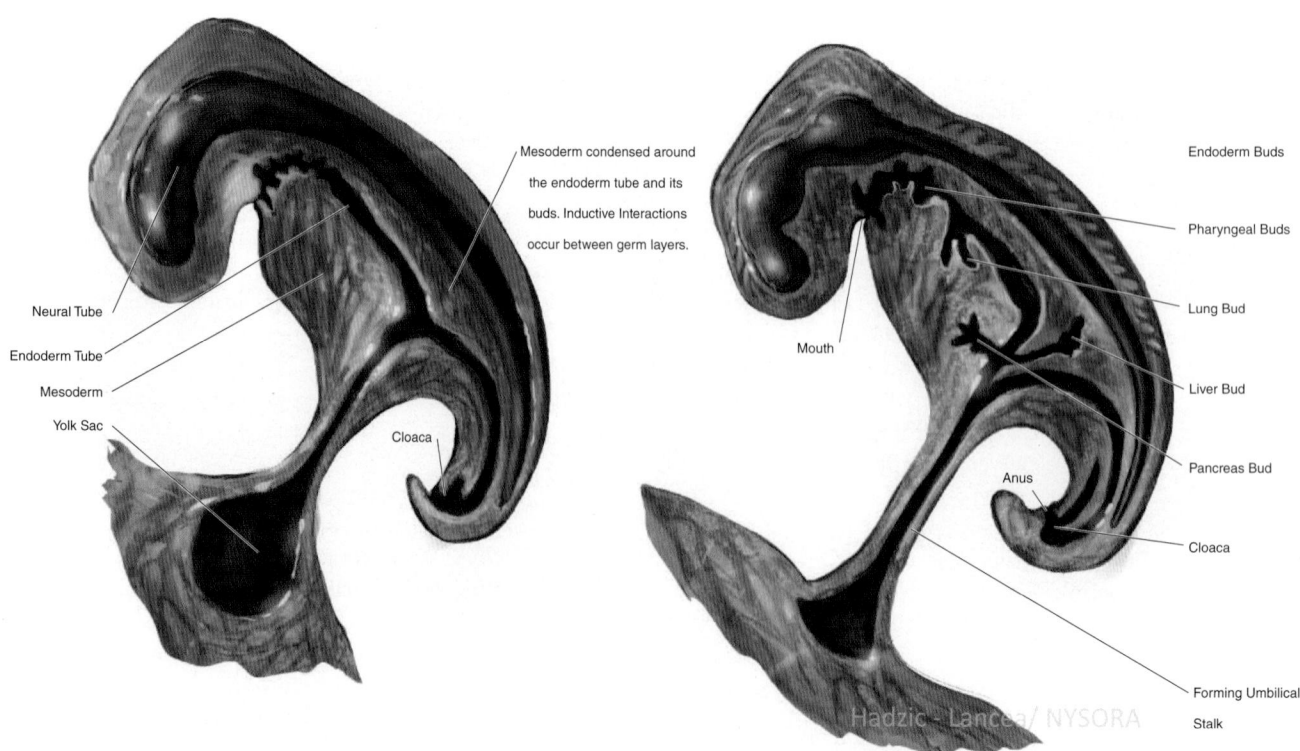

FIGURE 2–6. Formation of the endoderm.

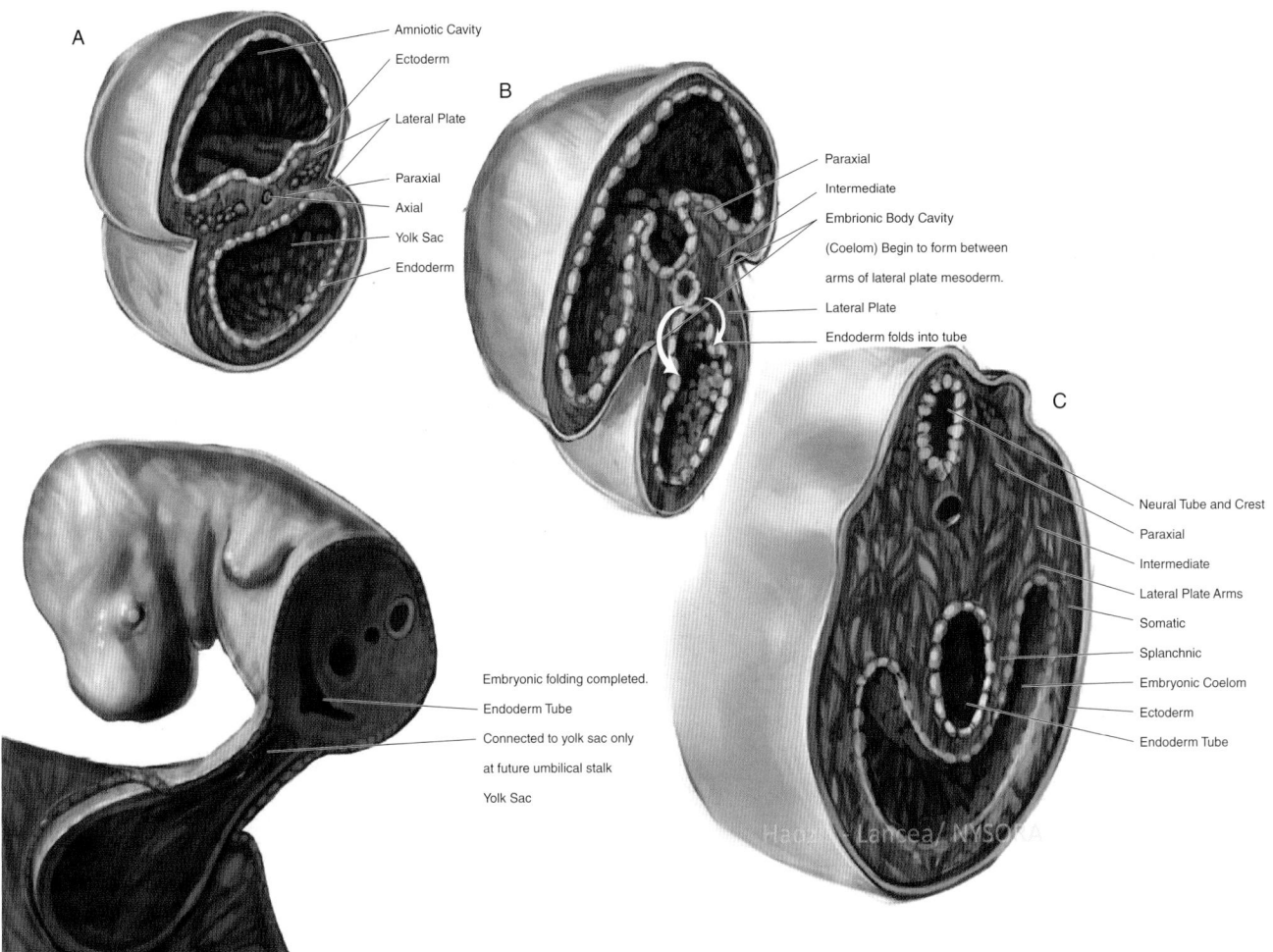

FIGURE 2–7. Formation of paraxial mesoderm (**A**), embryonic cavity (**B**), and embryonic folding (**C**).

By the beginning of the third week, paraxial mesoderm is organized into segments. These segments are known as **somitomeres.** They first appear in the cephalic region of the embryo, and their formation proceeds in a craniocaudal direction. In the head region, somitomeres transition, in association with segmentation of the neural plate, into neuromeres. From the occipital region caudally, somitomeres further organize into **somites.** Somites give rise to the **myotome** (ultimately muscle tissue), **sclerotome** (ultimately cartilage and bone), and **dermatome** (ultimately subcutaneous tissue of the skin). Collectively, these are all supporting tissues of the body (Figure 2–8).

Signaling for this somite differentiation arises from surrounding structures, including the notochord, neural tube, epidermis, and lateral plate mesoderm. By the beginning of the fourth week, cells forming the ventral and medial walls of the somite lose their compact organization and shift their position to surround the notochord (the dense cord of mesoderm that induces neuroectoderm). These cells, collectively known as the sclerotome, form a loosely woven tissue called the mesenchyme. They will surround the spinal cord and notochord to form the vertebral column. Cells at the dorsolateral portion of the somite also migrate as precursors of limb and body wall structures. Following migration of these muscle cells and cells of the sclerotome, cells at the dorsomedial portion of the somite

proliferate and migrate down the ventral side of the remaining dorsal epithelium of the somite to form a new layer, the myotome. The remaining dorsal epithelium forms the dermatome, and together these layers constitute the dermomyotome. Each segmentally arranged myotome contributes to muscles of the back, whereas the dermatomes disperse to form the dermis and subcutaneous tissue of the skin. Each myotome and dermatome retains its innervation from the segment of origin, no matter where the cells migrate. Therefore, each somite forms its own sclerotome, the cartilage and bone component; its own myotome, providing the segmental muscle component; and its own dermatome, the segmental skin component. Each myotome and dermatome also has its owns segmental nerve component (Figure 2–9).

During the second month, the external appearance of the embryo is changed greatly by the enormous size of the head and formation of the limbs, face, ears, nose, and eyes.[1] By the beginning of the fifth week, forelimbs and hind limbs appear as paddle-shaped buds (Figure 2–10). The forelimbs are located dorsal to the pericardial swelling at the level of the fourth cervical to first thoracic somites, which explains their innervation by the brachial plexus. Hind-limb buds appear slightly later just caudal to the attachment of the umbilical stock at the level of the lumbar and uppers sacral somites. With further growth, the

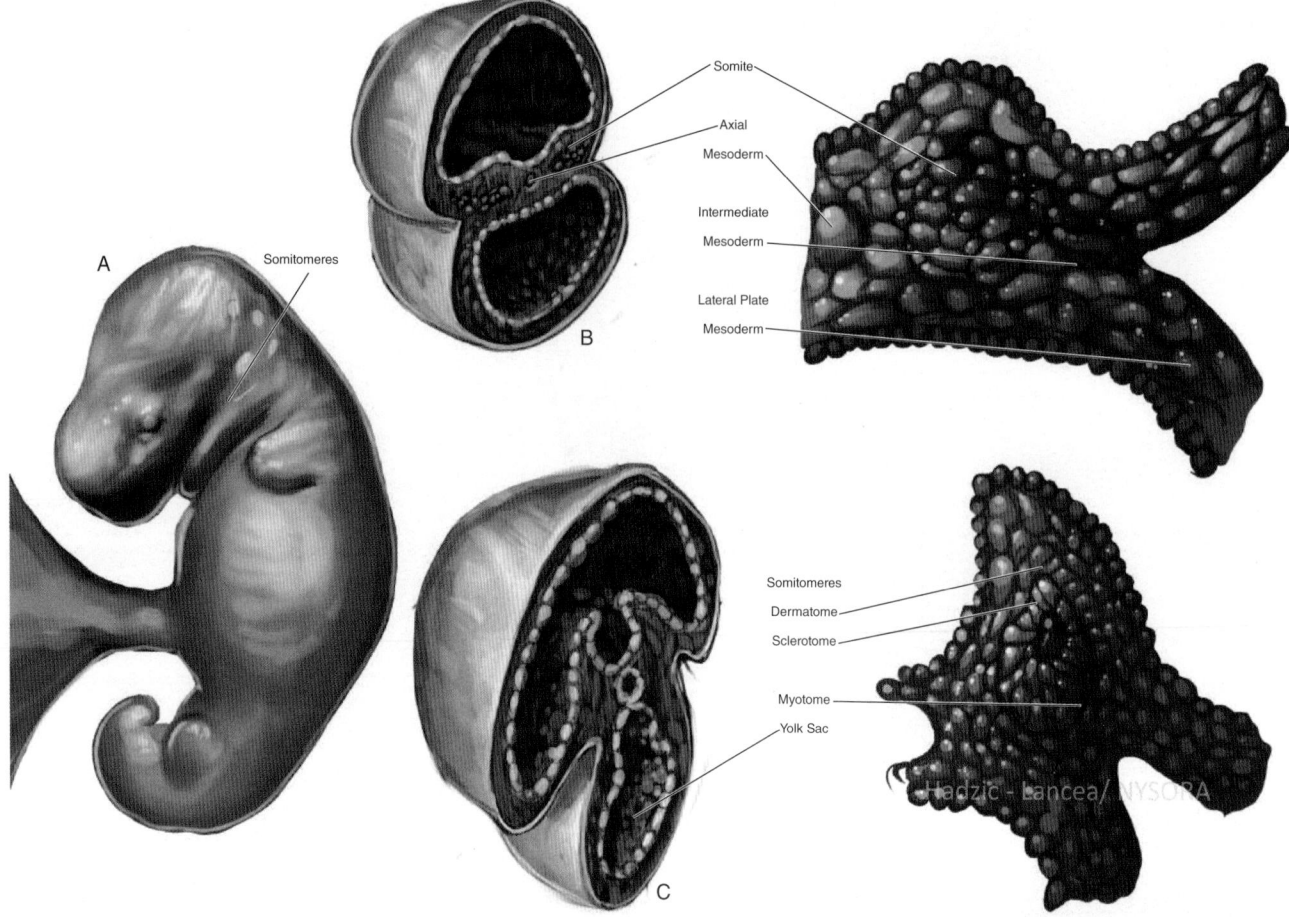

FIGURE 2–8. Development of the supporting tissues of the body myotome (muscle tissue), sclerotome (cartilage and bone), and dermatome (subcutaneous tissue). **A:** Paraxial mesoderm condenses to form the somite. **B:** Somite forms three regions. **C:** Somitomeres develop into somites.

terminal portions of the buds flatten, and a circular constriction separates them from the proximal, more cylindrical segment. Soon, four radial grooves separating five slightly thicker areas appear on the distal portion of the buds. This development foreshadows formation of the digits. These grooves, known as rays, appear in the hand region first and, shortly afterward, in the foot because the upper limb is slightly more advanced in development than the lower limb. While fingers and toes are being formed, a second constriction divides the proximal portion of the buds into two segments, and the three parts characteristic of the adult extremities can be recognized.

Fetal Period

The period from the beginning of the ninth week to the end of the intrauterine life is known as the fetal period.[1] It is characterized by maturation of tissues and organs and rapid growth of the body in length. This is particularly striking during the third, fourth, and fifth months, and increasing weight is most striking during the last 2 months of gestation. During the third month, the face becomes more human looking, and the limbs reach their relative length in comparison with the rest of the body, although the lower limbs are still a little shorter and less well developed than the upper

extremities. Primary ossification centers are present in the long bones and the skull by the 12th week.

Skeletal System: Limb Growth and Development

The skeletal system develops from paraxial and lateral plate mesoderm as well as neural crest tissue.[1] The somites (as previously described) differentiate into a ventromedial component called the sclerotome and a dorsolateral component called the dermomyotome. This organization of cells forms a loosely woven tissue called the mesenchyme. The mesenchyme migrates and differentiates into fibroblasts, chondroblasts, and osteoblasts.

At the end of the fourth week of development, limb buds become visible as outpocketings of the ventrolateral body wall.[1] Initially, they consist of a mesenchymal core derived from the somatic layer of lateral plate mesoderm that will form the bones and connective tissue of the limb, covered by a layer of ectoderm. Ectoderm at the distal border of the limb thickens and forms a specialized inducing tissue known as the **apical ectodermal ridge (AER).** The AER exerts an inductive influence on the adjacent mesenchyme, causing it to remain as a population of undifferentiated, rapidly proliferating cells

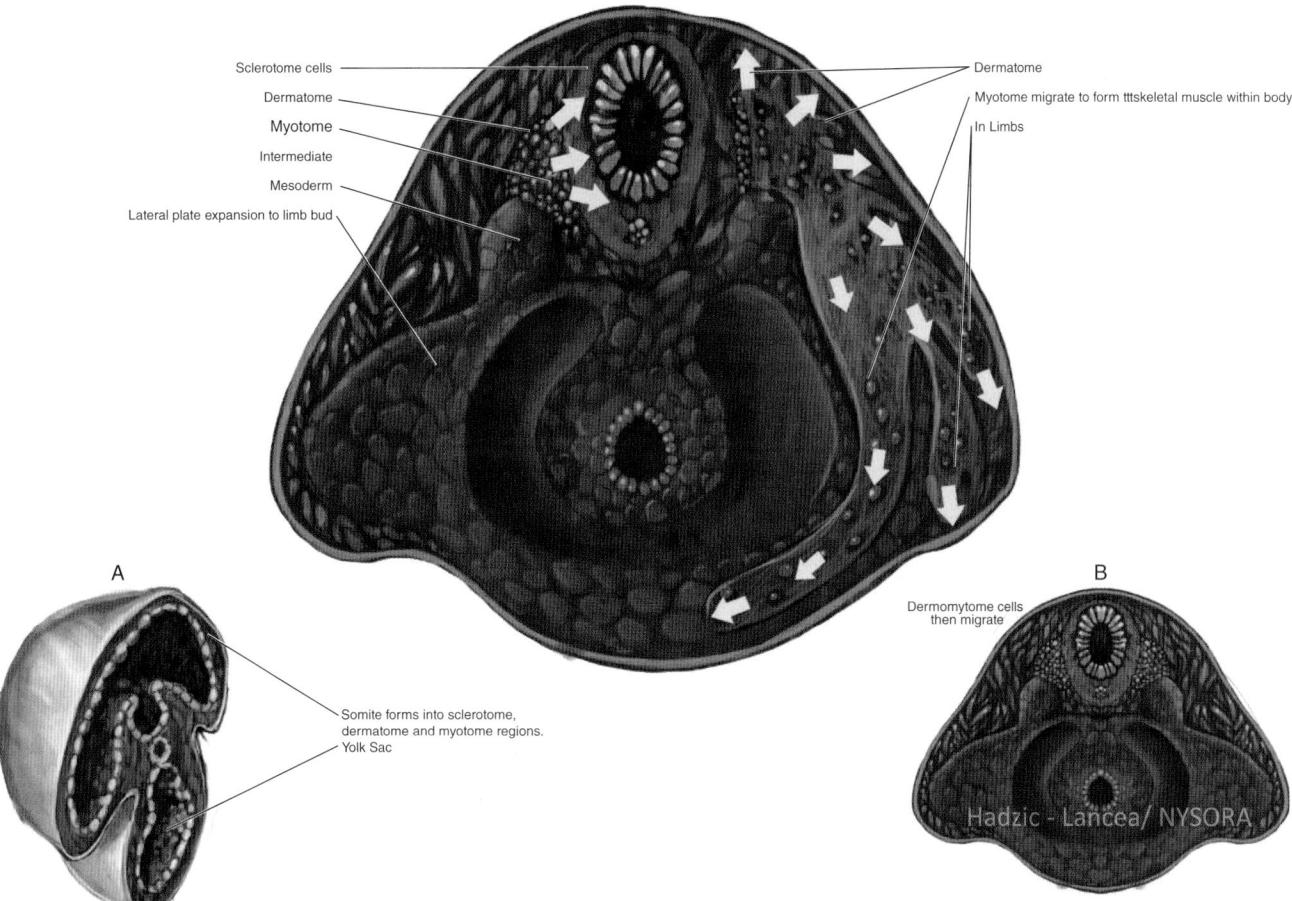

FIGURE 2–9. Cells of each somite region migrate separately to target destinations before forming specific tissues. Each somite forms its own sclerotome, myotome, and dermatome. **A:** Sclerotome cells migrate medially to form bones (vertebrae and ribs). **B:** Dermatome cells then migrate under ectoderm to form connective tissue of skin (dermis).

called the **progress zone.** As the limb grows, cells farther from the influence of the AER begin to differentiate into cartilage and muscle. In this manner of development, the limb proceeds proximodistally. In 6-week-old embryos, the terminal portion of the limb buds becomes flattened to form hand and footplates and is separated from the proximal segment by a circular constriction. Later, a second constriction divides the proximal portions into two segments, and the main parts of the extremities can be recognized.[1] Fingers and toes are formed when programmed cell death in the AER separates this ridge into five parts. Further formation of the digits depends on their continued outgrowth under the influence of the five remaining segments of ridge ectoderm. This results in condensation of the mesenchyme to form cartilaginous digital rays. Development of the upper and lower limbs is similar except that morphogenesis of the lower limb is approximately 1–2 days behind that of the upper limb.

During the seventh week of gestation, a key event occurs that is critical in understanding the final orientation and innervation of the limbs. The limbs rotate in opposite directions. The upper limb rotates 90° **laterally** so that the extensor muscles lie on the lateral and posterior surface and the thumbs lie laterally. The lower limb rotates approximately 90° **medially,** placing the extensor muscles on the anterior surface and the

great toe medially.[1] This explains why *homologous joints* of the upper and lower extremities (knees and elbows) *point in opposite directions.* This limb rotation results in the following[2]:

1. The final orientation of the limbs.
2. The final location and orientation of muscle groups (because the muscles are connected to the limb bones prior to rotation).
3. The patterns of sensory innervation of the skin (also because nerve fibers are connected with the dermis layer of the skin prior to rotation and are pulled along).

While the external shape is being established, mesenchyme in the buds begins to condense, and by the sixth week of development, the first hyaline cartilage models can be recognized. Ossification of the bones of the extremities begins by the end of the embryonic period. Primary ossification centers are present in all long bones of the limbs by the 12th week of development.

Molecular Regulation of Limb Development

Positioning of the limbs along the craniocaudal axis in the flank regions of the embryo is regulated by the *Hox* genes expressed

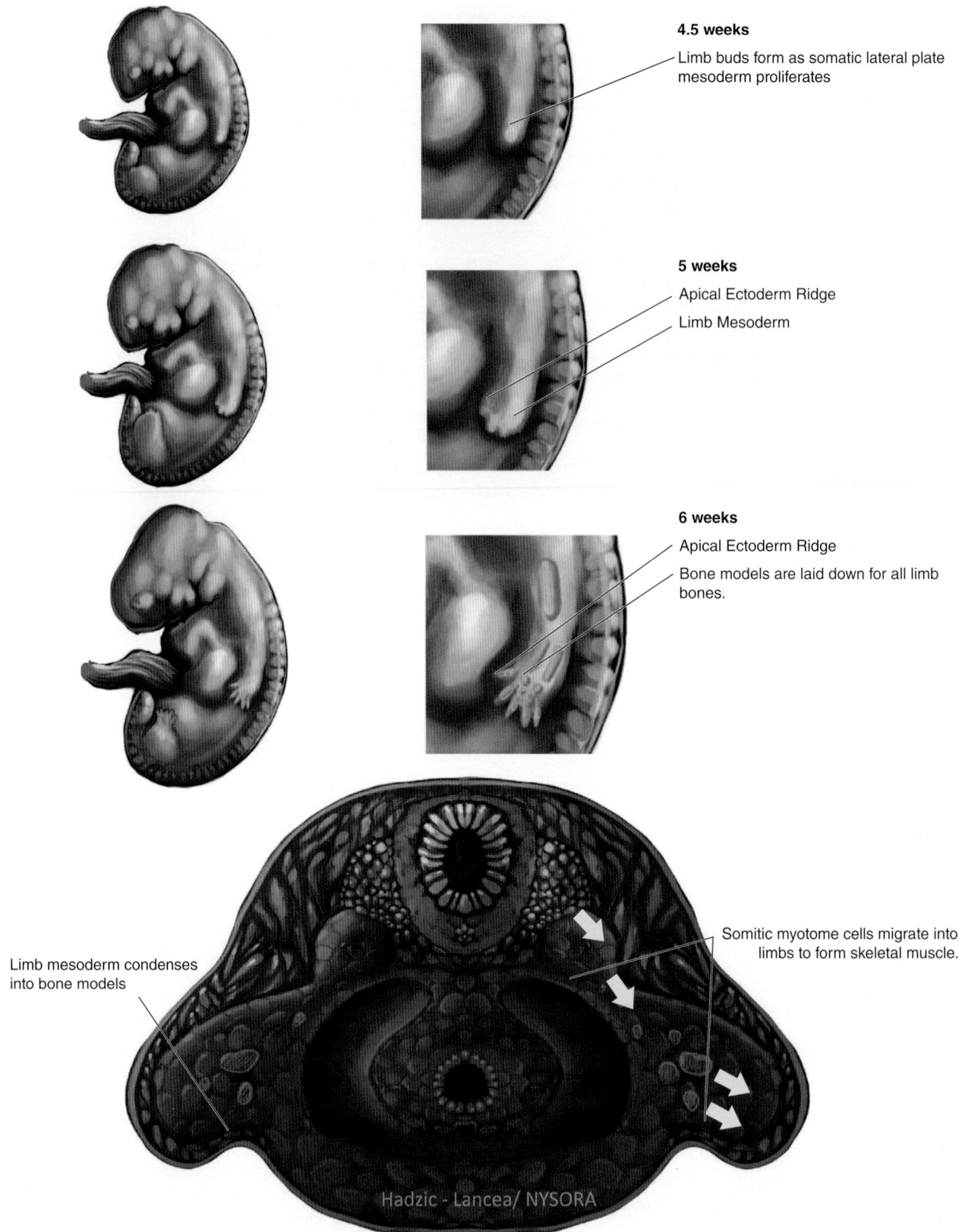

4.5 weeks

Limb buds form as somatic lateral plate mesoderm proliferates

5 weeks

Apical Ectoderm Ridge

Limb Mesoderm

6 weeks

Apical Ectoderm Ridge

Bone models are laid down for all limb bones.

Somitic myotome cells migrate into limbs to form skeletal muscle.

Limb mesoderm condenses into bone models

Hadzic - Lancea/ NYSORA

FIGURE 2–10. During the second month of development, the external appearance of the embryo greatly changes by rapid appearance of the large size of the head and formation of the limbs, face, ears, nose, and eyes. By the beginning of the fifth week, forelimbs and hind limbs appear as paddle-shaped buds. The arrows in the figure indicate direction of buds.

along this axis.[1] Once positioning along this axis is determined, growth must also be regulated along the proximodistal, anteroposterior, and dorsoventral axes. Patterning of the anteroposterior axis of the limb is regulated by the **zone of polarizing activity (ZPA),** a cluster of cells at the posterior border of the limb near the flank. These cells produce retinoic acid, which initiates expression of **sonic hedgehog (Shh),** a secreted factor that regulates development along this axis.[1] This regulation results in digits appearing in the proper order, with the thumb on the radial (anterior) side. As the limb grows, the ZPA moves distally to remain in proximity to the posterior border of the AER. The dorsoventral axis is patterned in a similar fashion by the dorsal ectoderm of the limb.

Although patterning genes for the limb axes have been predetermined, it is the *Hox* genes that regulate the types and shapes of the bones of the limbs. These *Hox* genes are nested in overlapping patterns of expression that somehow regulate patterning.[1] As a result, variations in their combinations create patterns of expression that may account for differences in fore- and hind-limb structures.

Vertebral Column

During the fourth week of development, cells of the sclerotome shift their position to surround both the spinal cord and the notochord.[1] During further development, the caudal portion of each sclerotome segment proliferates extensively and condenses. This proliferation is so extensive that it proceeds into the subjacent intersegmental tissue and binds the caudal half of one sclerotome to the cephalic half of the adjacent sclerotome. By incorporation of this intersegmental tissue into the precartilaginous vertebral body, the body of the vertebrae becomes intersegmental (Figure 2–11). *Hox* genes also control this patterning. Mesenchymal cells between cephalic and caudal parts of the original sclerotome form the intervertebral disk. Although the notochord regresses entirely in the region of the vertebral bodies, it persists and enlarges in the region of the intervertebral disk. Here, it contributes to the nucleus pulposus, which is later surrounded by circular fibers of the anulus fibrosus. Together, these structures form the intervertebral disk.[1]

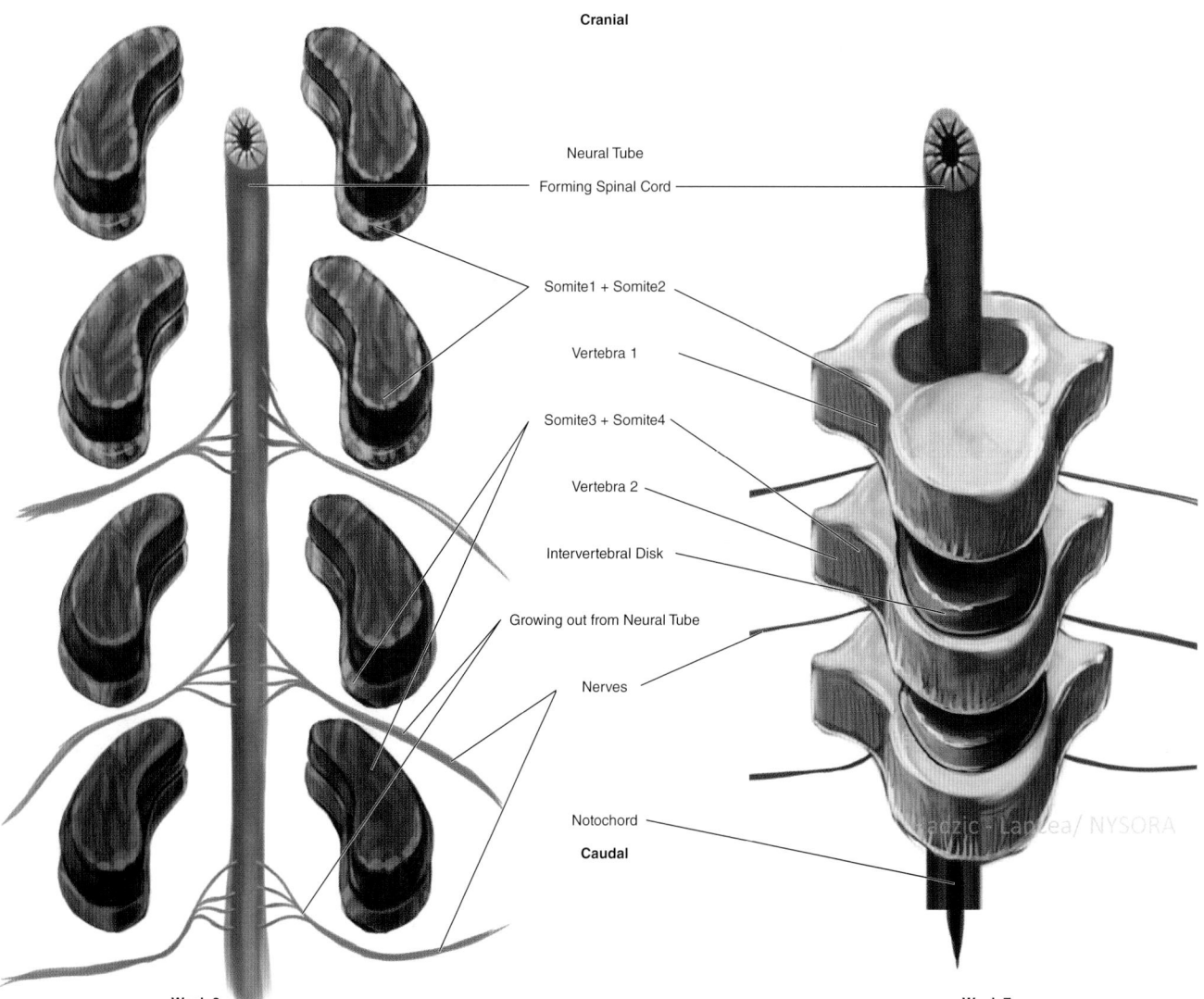

FIGURE 2–11. Formation of the vertebrae by fusion of sclerotome cells from two different somite levels.

Muscular and Peripheral Nervous Systems

With the exception of some smooth muscle tissue, the muscular system develops from the mesoderm germ layer.[1] Skeletal muscle is derived from paraxial mesoderm, which forms somites from the occipital to sacral regions and somitomeres in the head. The somites and somitomeres form the musculature of the axial skeleton body wall, limbs, and head. From the occipital region caudally, somites form and differentiate into this sclerotome, dermatome, and two muscle-forming regions. One of these is in the dorsolateral region of the somite and provides progenitor cells (myoblasts) for the limb and body wall musculature. The other region lies dorsomedially, migrates ventrally to cells that form the dermatome, and forms the myotome. Patterns of muscle formation are under the influence of the surrounding connective tissue into which myoblasts migrate. In the head region, this connective tissue is derived from neural crest cells. In cervical and occipital regions, muscles differentiate from somitic mesoderm, whereas in the body wall and limbs, they originate from the somatic mesoderm. By the end of the fifth week, prospective muscle cells are collected into two parts: a small dorsal portion, the **epimere,** and a larger ventral part called the **hypomere.**[1] Nerves innervating segmental muscles are also divided into a dorsal primary ramus for the epimere and a ventral primary ramus for the hypomere. These nerves remain with their original muscle segment throughout its migration. Myoblasts of the epimere form extensor muscles of the vertebral column, and those of the hypomere give rise to the muscles of the limbs and body wall. The first indication of limb musculature is observed in the seventh week of development as a condensation of mesenchyme near the base of the limb buds. This mesenchyme is derived from dorsolateral cells of the somites that migrate into the limb bud to form the muscles. This connective tissue dictates the pattern of muscle formation and is derived from somatic mesoderm, which also gives rise to the bones of the limb.[1]

With elongation of the limb buds, the muscle tissue splits into flexor and extensor components. The upper limb bud lies opposite the lower five cervical and upper two thoracic segments. The lower limb buds lie opposite the lower four lumbar and upper two sacral segments. As soon as the buds form, ventral primary rami from the appropriate spinal nerves penetrate into the mesenchyme (Figure 2–12). At first, each ventral ramus enters with isolated dorsal and ventral branches, but soon these branches unite to form large dorsal and ventral nerves. Thus, in the upper extremity, the radial nerve supplies all the extensor musculature and is formed by a combination of dorsal segmental branches. The ulnar and median nerves, which supply all the flexor muscles, are formed by a combination of the ventral branches[1] (Figure 2–13). Immediately after the nerves have entered the limb buds, they establish contact

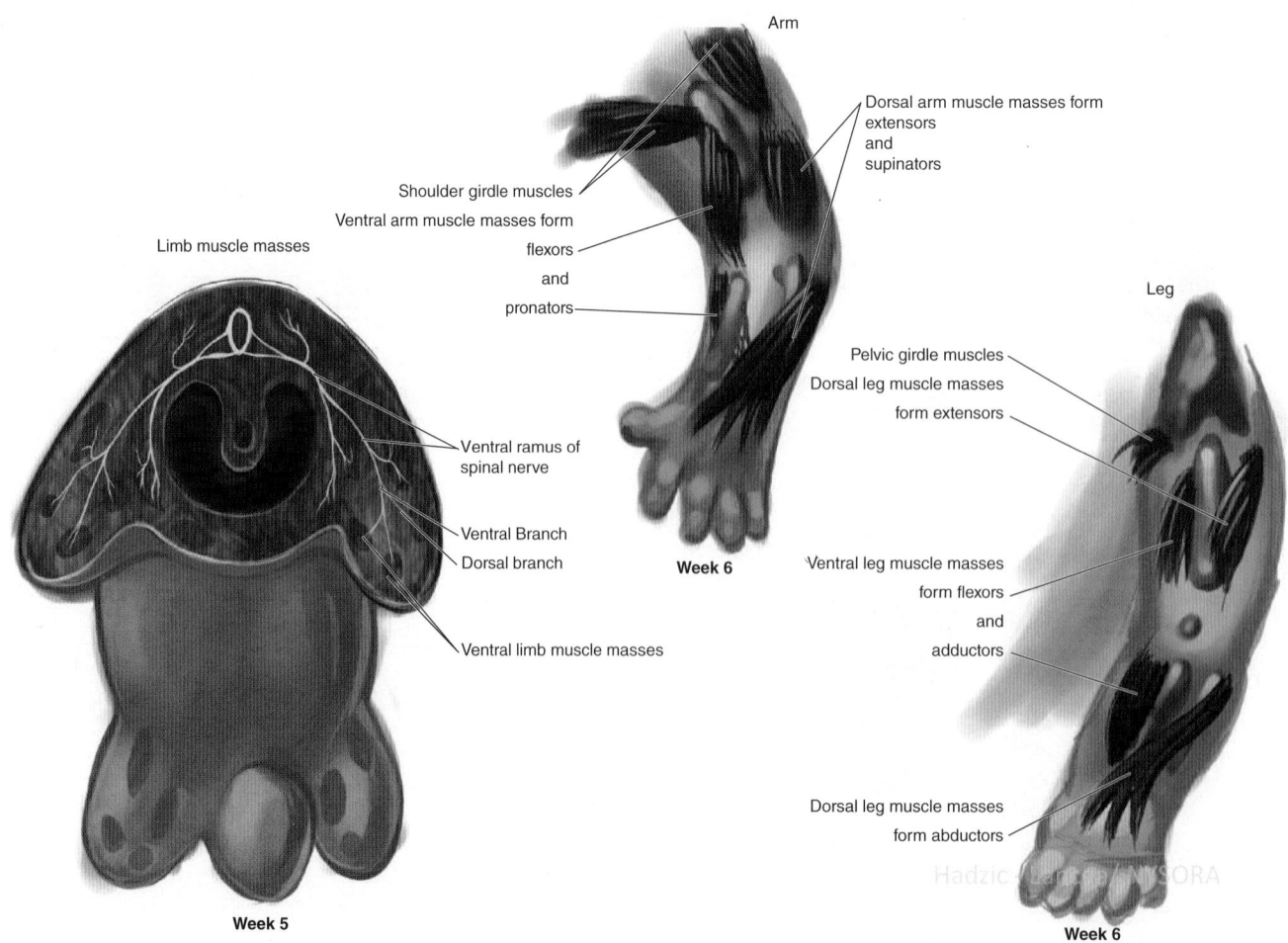

FIGURE 2–12. Formation of the spinal nerves.

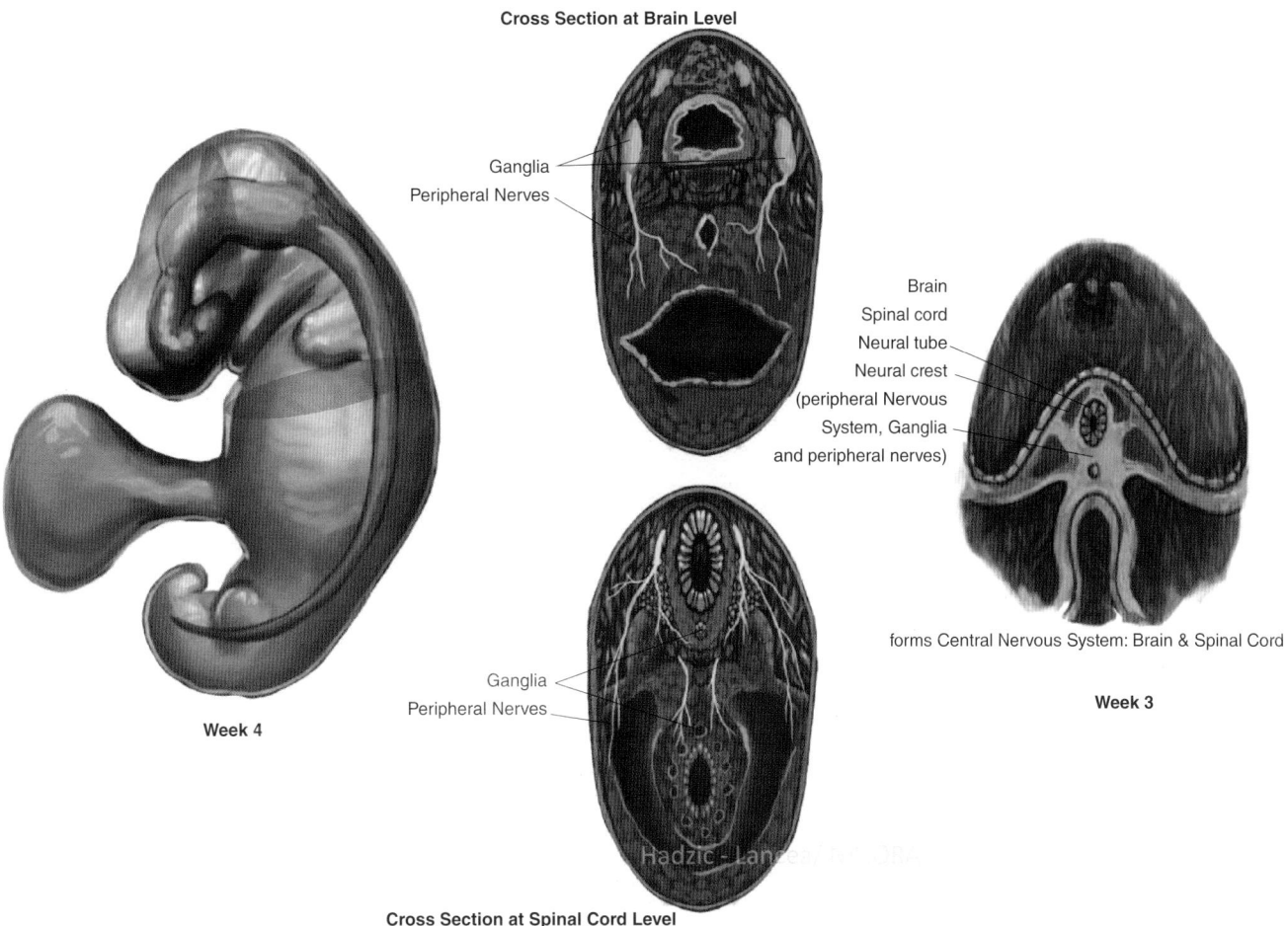

Cross Section at Brain Level

Ganglia
Peripheral Nerves

Brain
Spinal cord
Neural tube
Neural crest
(peripheral Nervous
System, Ganglia
and peripheral nerves)

forms Central Nervous System: Brain & Spinal Cord

Week 3

Ganglia
Peripheral Nerves

Week 4

Cross Section at Spinal Cord Level

FIGURE 2–13. Development of the peripheral nervous system.

with the differentiating mesoderm condensations. This early contact is a prerequisite for their complete functional differentiation. Spinal nerves therefore play an important role in differentiation and motor innervation of the limb musculature, as well as providing sensory innervation for the dermatomes. Although the original dermatomal pattern changes with growth of the extremities, an orderly sequence can still be recognized in the adult.

Central Nervous System

The CNS originates in the ectoderm and appears as the **neural plate** at the middle of the third week[1] (Figure 2–14). After the edges of the plate fold, the **neural folds** approach each other in the midline to fuse, forming the **neural tube.** The CNS then forms as a tubular structure with a broad cephalic portion (the brain) and a long caudal portion (the spinal cord). A basal plate, containing the motor neurons, and an alar plate, containing the sensory neurons, characterize the spinal cord, which forms the caudal end of the CNS.

The walls of the recently closed neural tube consist of neuroepithelial cells. These cells give rise to another type of cell, the **neuroblasts,** which are primitive nerve cells. They form a **mantle layer** around the neuroepithelial layer. This mantle layer later forms the gray matter of the spinal cord. The outermost layer of the spinal cord, called the **marginal layer,** contains nerve fibers emerging from neuroblasts in the mantle layer. As a result of myelination, this layer takes on a white appearance and is called the white matter of the spinal cord.[1] Because of the continuous addition of neuroblasts to the mantle layer, each side of the neural tube shows ventral and dorsal thickening. The ventral thickening (the basal plates) contains ventral motor horn cells. The dorsal thickening (the alar plates) forms the sensory areas. A group of neurons accumulate between these two areas, forming a small intermediate horn, which contains neurons of the sympathetic portion of the autonomic nervous system and is present only at thoracic and upper lumbar levels of the spinal cord[1] (Figure 2–15).

Spinal Nerves

Motor nerve fibers begin to appear in the fourth week, arising from nerve cells in the basal plates of the spinal cord.[4] They collect into bundles known as ventral nerve roots. Likewise, dorsal nerve roots form as collections of fibers originating from cells in dorsal root ganglia. Central processes from these ganglia form processes that grow into the spinal cord opposite the dorsal horns, and distal processes join the ventral nerve roots to form a spinal nerve. Spinal nerves divide into dorsal and ventral primary rami. Dorsal rami innervate dorsal axial musculature, vertebral joints, and the skin of the back. Ventral primary rami

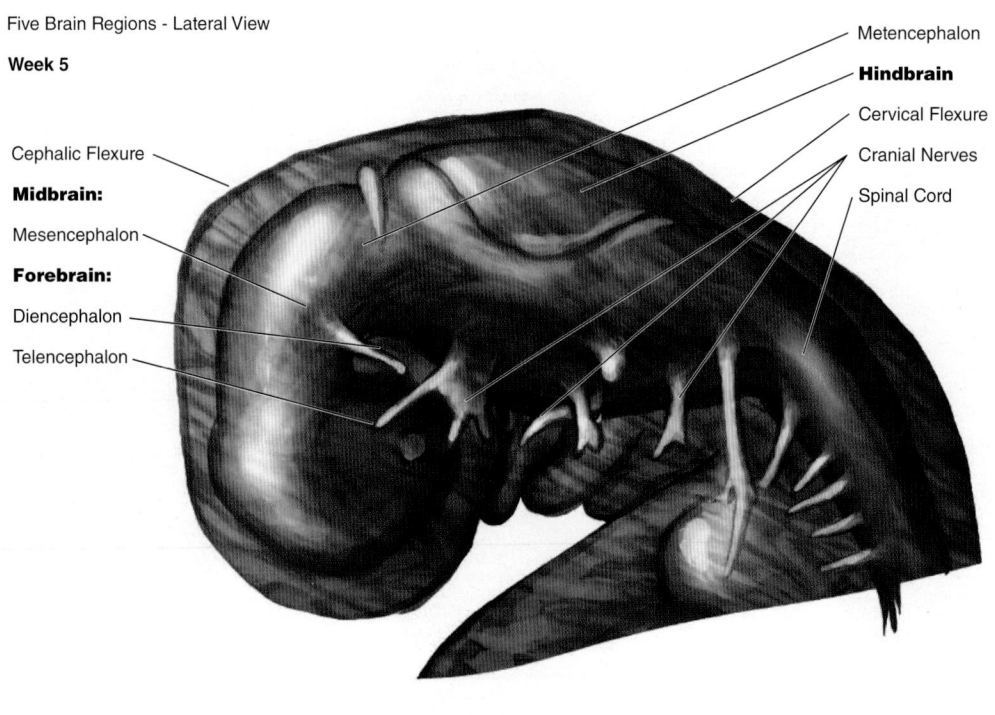

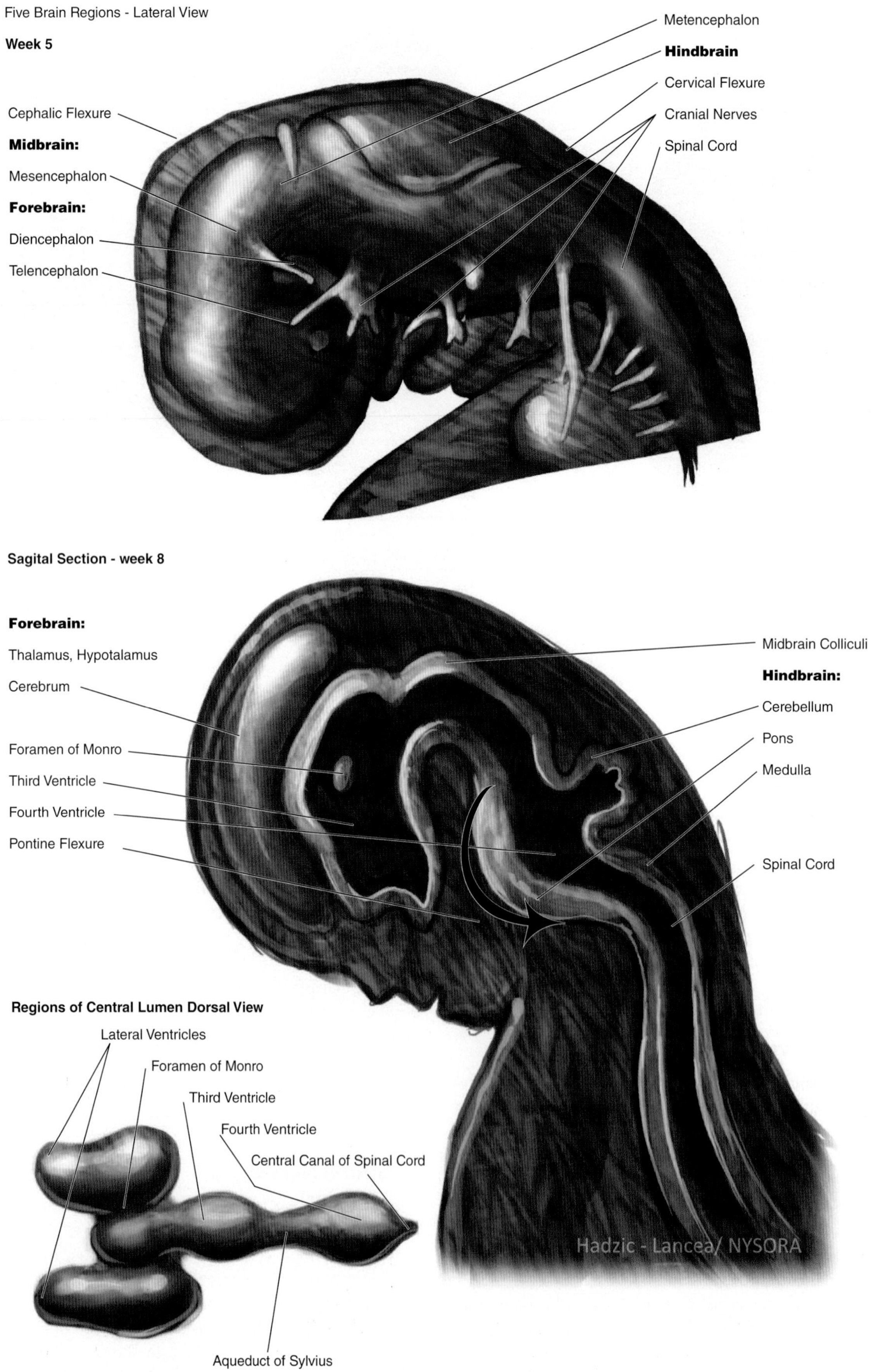

Five Brain Regions - Lateral View

Week 5

Cephalic Flexure

Midbrain:

Mesencephalon

Forebrain:

Diencephalon

Telencephalon

Metencephalon

Hindbrain

Cervical Flexure

Cranial Nerves

Spinal Cord

Sagital Section - week 8

Forebrain:

Thalamus, Hypotalamus

Cerebrum

Foramen of Monro

Third Ventricle

Fourth Ventricle

Pontine Flexure

Midbrain Colliculi

Hindbrain:

Cerebellum

Pons

Medulla

Spinal Cord

Regions of Central Lumen Dorsal View

Lateral Ventricles

Foramen of Monro

Third Ventricle

Fourth Ventricle

Central Canal of Spinal Cord

Aqueduct of Sylvius

Hadzic - Lancea/ NYSORA

FIGURE 2–14. Development of the central nervous system.

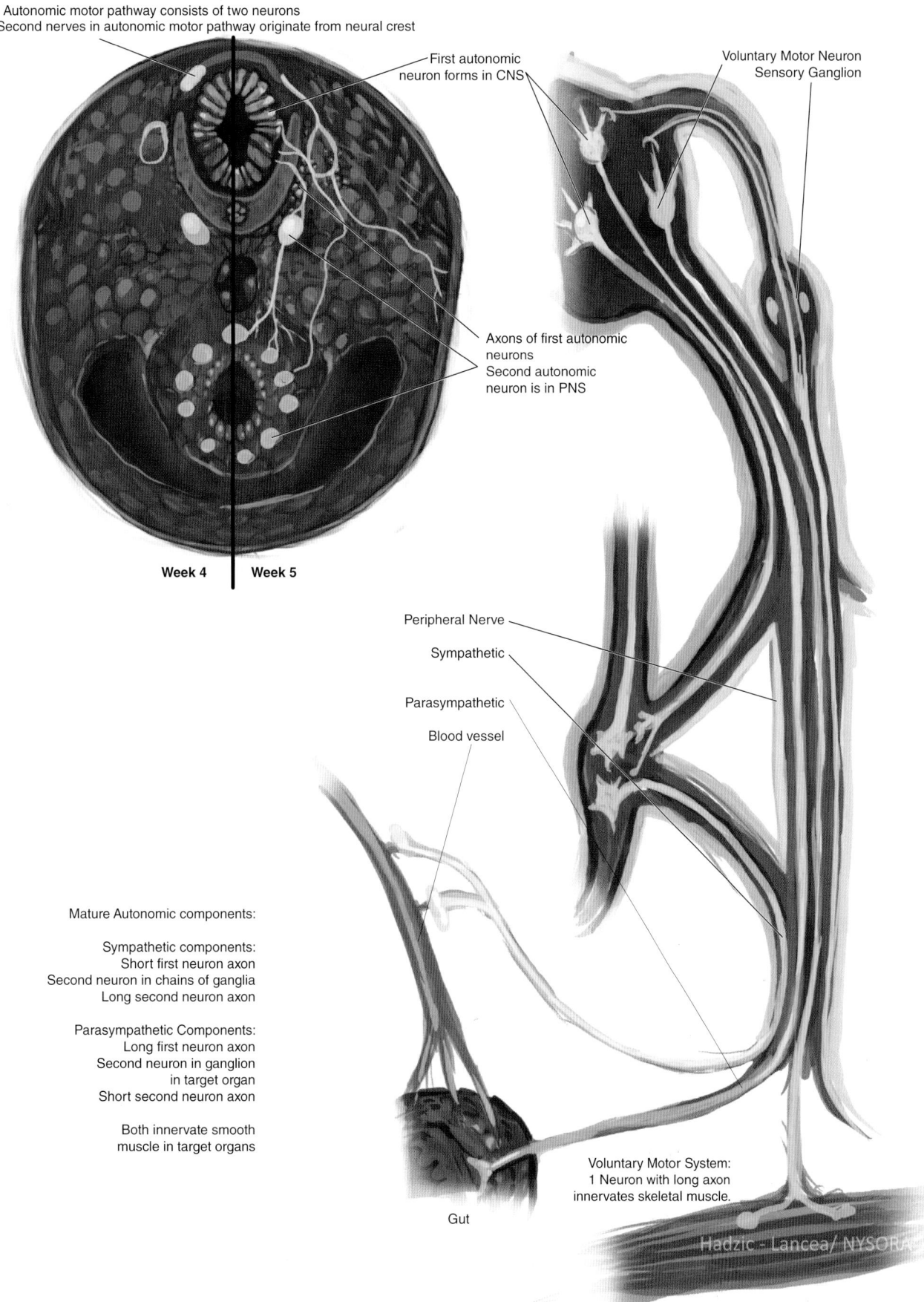

Autonomic motor pathway consists of two neurons
Second nerves in autonomic motor pathway originate from neural crest

First autonomic
neuron forms in CNS

Voluntary Motor Neuron
Sensory Ganglion

Axons of first autonomic
neurons
Second autonomic
neuron is in PNS

Week 4   **Week 5**

Peripheral Nerve

Sympathetic

Parasympathetic

Blood vessel

Mature Autonomic components:

Sympathetic components:
Short first neuron axon
Second neuron in chains of ganglia
Long second neuron axon

Parasympathetic Components:
Long first neuron axon
Second neuron in ganglion
in target organ
Short second neuron axon

Both innervate smooth
muscle in target organs

Voluntary Motor System:
1 Neuron with long axon
innervates skeletal muscle.

Gut

Hadzic - Lancea/ NYSORA

FIGURE 2–15. Development of autonomic nervous system.

innervate the limbs and ventral body wall and form the major nerve plexuses.[1]

In the third month of development, the spinal cord extends the entire length of the embryo, and spinal nerves pass through the intervertebral foramina at their level of origin. With increasing age, the vertebral column and dura lengthen more rapidly than the neural tube, resulting in the terminal end of the spinal cord gradually shifting to a higher level. At birth, this level is at the third lumbar vertebra. In the adult, the spinal cord terminates at the level of L2 to L3, whereas the dural sac and subarachnoid space extend to S2. As a result of this disproportionate growth, spinal nerves run obliquely from their segment of origin in the spinal cord to the corresponding level of the vertebral column. Below L2 to L3, a thread-like extension of the pia mater forms the filum terminale, which is attached to the periosteum of the first coccygeal vertebra and marks the tract of regression of the spinal cord.[1]

The Brain

The brain consists originally of three vesicles: the **rhombencephalon** (hindbrain), **mesencephalon** (midbrain), and **prosencephalon** (forebrain). The rhombencephalon will ultimately form the medulla oblongata, pons, and cerebellum. The mesencephalon resembles the spinal cord with its basal and alar plates. It will contain the anterior and posterior colliculi, forming the relay stations for visual and auditory reflex centers. The prosencephalon will ultimately give rise to the thalamus and hypothalamus as well as the cerebral hemispheres.[1]

Autonomic Nervous System

Functionally, the autonomic nervous system can be divided into two parts: a sympathetic portion in the thoracolumbar region and a parasympathetic portion in the cephalic and sacral regions. Both components of the autonomic nervous system consist of two tiers of neurons: pre- and postganglionic (Figure 2–16).

Sympathetic Nervous System

Preganglionic neurons of the sympathetic nervous system arise from the intermediate horn of the gray matter in the spinal cord.[3] At levels from T1 to L2, their myelinated axons grow from the cord *through* the ventral roots, paralleling the motor axons that supply the skeletal musculature. Shortly after the dorsal and ventral roots of the spinal nerve join, the preganglionic sympathetic axons, derived from the neuroepithelium of the neural tube, leave the spinal nerve via a **white communicating ramus.** They soon enter one of a series of sympathetic ganglia to synapse with neural crest-derived postganglionic neurons. The sympathetic ganglia, the bulk of which are organized as two chains running ventrolateral to the vertebral bodies, are laid down by neural crest cells that migrate from the closing neural tube along a special pathway. Once the migrating sympathetic neuroblasts have reached the site at which the sympathetic chain ganglia form, they spread both cranially and caudally until the extent of the chains approximates that seen in the adult. Some of the sympathetic neuroblasts migrate farther ventrally than the level of the chain ganglion to form a variety of other collateral ganglia. The adrenal medulla can be broadly viewed as a highly modified sympathetic ganglion. The outgrowing preganglionic sympathetic neurons either terminate within the chain ganglia or pass through on their way to more distant sympathetic ganglia to form synapses with the cell bodies of the second-order, or postganglionic, sympathetic neuroblasts. Axons of some postganglionic neuroblasts, which are unmyelinated, leave the chain ganglion as a parallel group and reenter the nearest spinal nerve through the **gray communicating ramus.** Once in the spinal nerve, these axons continue to grow until they reach their peripheral targets.

During the fifth week of development, cells originating in the neural crest of the thoracic region migrate on each side of the spinal cord toward the region immediately behind the dorsal aorta.[1] Here, they form a bilateral chain of segmentally arranged sympathetic ganglia interconnected by longitudinal nerve fibers. Together, they form the sympathetic chains on each side of the vertebral column. From their position in the thorax, neuroblasts migrate toward the cervical and lumbosacral regions, extending the sympathetic chains to their full length. Some sympathetic neuroblasts migrate in front of the aorta to form preaortic ganglia, such as the celiac and mesenteric ganglia. Other sympathetic cells migrate to the heart, lungs, and gastrointestinal tract, where they give rise to sympathetic organ plexuses. Once the sympathetic chains have been established, nerve fibers originating in the intermediate horn of the thoracolumbar segments of the spinal cord penetrate the ganglia of the chain. They are known as preganglionic fibers, have a myelin sheath, and stimulate sympathetic ganglion cells. Passing from spinal nerves to the sympathetic ganglia, they form the **white communicating rami.** Axons of the sympathetic ganglion cells, the postganglionic fibers, have no myelin sheath. They either pass to other levels of the sympathetic chain or extend to the heart, lungs, and intestinal tract. Other fibers, the gray communicating rami, which are found at all levels of the spinal cord, pass from the sympathetic chain to spinal nerves and from there to peripheral blood vessels, hair, and sweat glands.

Parasympathetic Nervous System

Neurons in the brainstem and the sacral region of the spinal cord give rise to preganglionic parasympathetic fibers.[1] Although also organized on a preganglionic and postganglionic basis, the parasympathetic nervous system has a distribution quite different from that of the sympathetic system. Like those of the sympathetic nervous system, preganglionic parasympathetic neurons originate in the intermediate column of the CNS. However, the levels of origin of these neuroblasts are the mid- and hindbrain and in the second to fourth sacral segments of the developing spinal cord. Axons from these preganglionic neuroblasts grow long distances before they meet the neural crest–derived postganglionic neurons. These are typically embedded in small, scattered ganglia or plexuses in the walls of the organs they innervate.

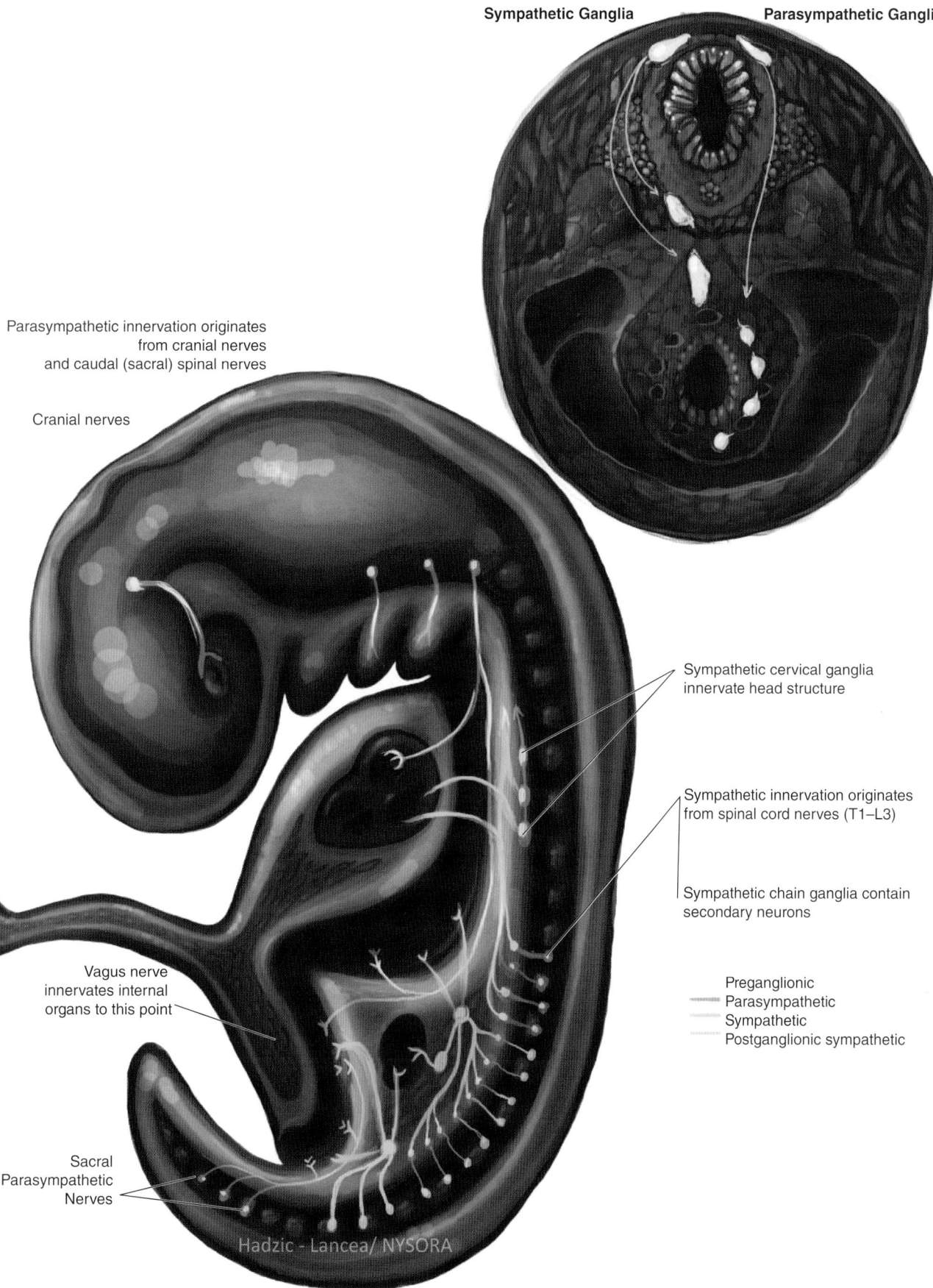

Sympathetic Ganglia   **Parasympathetic Ganglia**

Parasympathetic innervation originates
from cranial nerves
and caudal (sacral) spinal nerves

Cranial nerves

Sympathetic cervical ganglia
innervate head structure

Sympathetic innervation originates
from spinal cord nerves (T1–L3)

Sympathetic chain ganglia contain
secondary neurons

Preganglionic
Parasympathetic
Sympathetic
Postganglionic sympathetic

Vagus nerve
innervates internal
organs to this point

Sacral
Parasympathetic
Nerves

Hadzic - Lancea/ NYSORA

FIGURE 2–16. Development of autonomic nervous system: pre- and postganglionic neurons.

CLINICAL RELEVANCE

Functional Analysis of the Brachial Plexus

The separation of the trunks of the brachial plexus into anterior and posterior divisions places the nerves into relation with muscles formed from primitive anterior and posterior mesoderm masses during the development of the limbs. Once these relationships are established, they are never reversed, and the same fundamental correlation exists in the adult.[5,6] The anterior divisions of the trunks unite to form the lateral and medial chords of the brachial plexus, and the posterior divisions join to form the single posterior cord. Thus, all branches of the lateral and medial chords carry nerve bundles derived from the anterior divisions of the trunks, and the branches of the posterior cord conduct exclusively fibers from the posterior divisions. The discrete compartments of the upper extremity contain muscle groups of similar and related functions as well as the blood vessels and nerves that supply them. This concept is emphasized in the word *preaxial* to designate the component and structures anterior to the bone and fascial plane or axis of the limb and the word *postaxial* to designate structures behind the bony and fascial axis. With the limb in the anatomical position, those parts anterior to the bony axis are all in a continuous plane down the front of the limb, with the ventral axial line extending along the anterior surface of the arm and forearm. The postaxial parts are positioned continuously down the back of the limb.

The branches of the lateral and medial chords are all preaxial and innervate the preaxial muscles of the limb, whereas the posterior cord branches are postaxial and innervate the postaxial musculature. The radial nerve, being the only postaxial nerve below the shoulder, supplies all the postaxial muscles in the remainder of the limb. The median, musculocutaneous, and ulnar nerves share preaxial innervation.

The musculocutaneous nerve is muscular in the arm and cutaneous in the forearm, and it is the sole preaxial muscular nerve in the arm. The preaxial median and ulnar nerves are nerves of passage in the arm, but in the forearm and hand, each contributes to innervation, the median nerve more heavily in the forearm, the ulnar nerve more heavily in the hand.

In the shoulder region, many of the supra- and infraclavicular branches of the brachial plexus arise from recognizable pre- and postaxial cords or divisions. Their origins have the same significance as the major anterior and posterior divisions of the trunks. An example of this is the clavicle and the scapula. The clavicle is an anterior and the scapula a posterior bone. An exception to this designation involves the scapula because its coracoid process has a phylogenetic history as a separate bone and fuses with the scapula. Therefore, all muscles arising from the scapula, exclusive of the coracoid process (pectoralis minor, coracobrachialis, and short head of biceps), belong to a postaxial group at the shoulder, and those from the clavicle and coracoid belong to a preaxial group. The nerve-muscle correlation is maintained in that all muscles of scapular origin are supplied by postaxial branches of the brachial plexus, and all muscles derived from the clavicle and coracoid are supplied by preaxial branches.

Functional Analysis of the Lumbosacral Plexus

The innervation of the lower extremity follows the same pattern of pre- and postaxial orientation as described for the upper extremity. The primordial dermatomal pattern has disappeared, but an orderly sequence of dermatomes can still be recognized. Most of the original ventral surface of the lower limb lies on the back of the adult limb. The ventral axial line extends along the medial side of the thigh and knee to the posteromedial aspect of the leg to the heel.

As previously described, this results from the medial rotation of the lower limb at the end of the embryonic period. The lumbar plexuses are formed by the ventral rami of the first three lumbar nerves and part of the fourth lumbar nerve. The primary preaxial components are the genitofemoral nerve, which derives from L1 and L2, and obturator and accessory obturator nerves, which are derived from L2 and L3, respectively. The primary postaxial components are the lateral femoral cutaneous nerve, derived from L2 and L3, and the femoral nerve, derived from L2 through L4. The sacral plexus combines the ventral rami of part of L4 and L5 and S1 through S3, as well as part of S4. All these nerves, except S4, divide into anterior and posterior branches. Like the brachial plexus, the anterior branches form preaxial nerves related to preaxial muscle masses in skin areas, and the posterior branches form similarly related postaxial nerves. The principal nerve of the sacral plexus is the sciatic, which is composed of a preaxial nerve (the tibial nerve) and a postaxial nerve (the common peroneal), which is enclosed within a single sheath.

SUMMARY

In summary, regional anesthesia may be considered a practice of applied anatomy. Successful neuraxial and peripheral nerve blockade alike require a logical approach to the anatomic principles. Knowledge of the embryologic development of tissues and neural structures can significantly add to the understanding of functional anatomy as it relates to regional anesthesia.

REFERENCES

1. Sadler TW: *Langman's Medical Embryology*, 9th ed. Lippincott Williams & Wilkins, 2003.
2. Sweeney LJ: *Basic Concepts in Embryology: A Student's Survival Guide.* McGraw-Hill, 1998.
3. Carlson B: *Human Embryology and Developmental Biology*, 3rd ed. Mosby, 2004.
4. Moore KL: *The Developing Human: Clinically Oriented Embryology*, 7th ed. Saunders, 2003.
5. Woodburne RT: *Essentials of Human Anatomy*, 6th ed. Oxford University Press, 1978.
6. Larsen WJ: *Human Embryology*, 2nd ed. Churchill Livingstone, 1997.

Functional Regional Anesthesia Anatomy

Anna Carrera, Ana M. Lopez, Xavier Sala-Blanch, Eldan Kapur,
Ilvana Hasanbegovic, and Admir Hadzic

INTRODUCTION

The practice of regional anesthesia is inconceivable without sound knowledge of the functional regional anesthesia anatomy. Just as surgical technique relies on surgical anatomy or pathology leans on pathologic anatomy, the anatomic information necessary for the practice of regional anesthesia must be specific to this application. In the past, many nerve block techniques and approaches were devised by academicians merely relying on idealized anatomic diagrams and schematics, rather than on functional anatomy. However, once the anatomic layers and tissue sheets are dissected, the anatomy of nerve structures without the tissue sheaths around them is of little relevance to the clinical practice of regional anesthesia. This is because accurate placement of the needle and the spread of the local anesthetic after an injection depend on the interplay between neurologic structures and the neighboring tissues where local anesthetic pools and accumulates, rather than on the mere anatomic organization of the nerves and plexuses. Much research on functional regional anesthesia, a term introduced by Dr. Jerry Vloka in the 1990s, has contributed to better understanding of the anatomy of regional nerve blockade. Moreover, the introduction of ultrasound in the practice of regional anesthesia has further clarified the relationship of the needle and the nerve and the dynamics of local anesthetic spread.

The goal of this chapter is to provide a generalized and rather concise overview of anatomy relevant to the practice of regional anesthesia; more specific anatomic discussions pertaining to individual regional anesthesia techniques are detailed in their respective chapters. The reader is referred to Figure 3–1 for an easier orientation of the body planes discussed throughout the book.

ANATOMY OF PERIPHERAL NERVES

All peripheral nerves are similar in structure. The **neuron** is the basic functional neuronal unit responsible for the conduction of nerve impulses. Neurons are the longest cells in the body, many reaching a meter in length. Most neurons are incapable of dividing under normal circumstances and have limited ability to repair themselves after injury. A typical neuron consists of a cell body (soma) that contains a large nucleus. The cell body is attached to several branching processes, called dendrites, and a single axon. Dendrites receive incoming messages; axons conduct outgoing messages. Axons vary in length, and there is one only per neuron. In peripheral nerves, axons are long and slender. They are also called nerve fibers. The peripheral nerve is composed of three parts: (1) somatosensory or afferent neurons, (2) motor or efferent neurons, and (3) autonomic neurons.

Individual nerve fibers bind together, somewhat like individual wires in an electric cable (Figure 3–2). In the peripheral nerve, individual axons are eveloped by the endoneurium, which is a delicate layer of loose connective tissue around each axon. Groups of axons are closely associated within a bundle called a nerve fascicle that is surrounded by the perineurium, which imparts mechanical strength to the peripheral nerve. In surgical procedures, the perineurium holds sutures without tearing. In addition to its mechanical strength, the perineurium functions as a diffusion barrier to the fascicle, isolating the endoneural space around the axon from the surrounding tissue.[1] This barrier helps to preserve the ionic milieu of the axon and functions as a blood–nerve barrier. The **perineurium** surrounds each fasciculus and splits with it at each branching point. The fascicular bundles in turn are embedded in loose connective tissue called the **interfascicular epineurium,** which

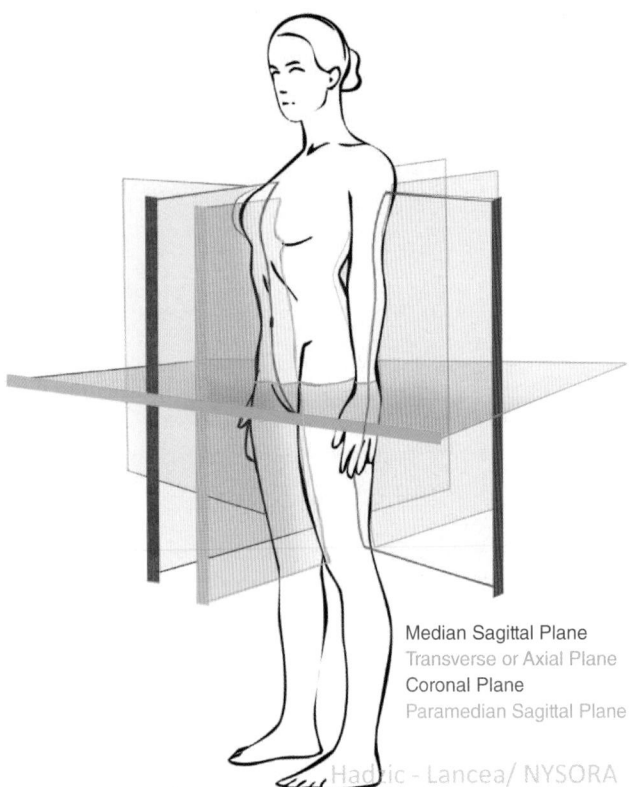

Median Sagittal Plane
Transverse or Axial Plane
Coronal Plane
Paramedian Sagittal Plane

Hadzic - Lancea/ NYSORA

FIGURE 3–1. Conventional body planes.

contains adipose tissue, fibroblasts, mastocytes, blood vessels (with small nerve fibers innervating these vessels), and lymphatics. In contrast, a more dense collagenous tissue forms the **epineurium** that surrounds the entire nerve and holds it loosely to the connective tissue through which it travels.

Of note, the fascicular bundles are not continuous throughout the peripheral nerve. They divide and anastomose with one another as frequently as every few millimeters.[1] However, the axons within a small set of adjacent bundles redistribute themselves so that the axons remain in approximately the same quadrant of the nerve for several centimeters. This arrangement is a practical concern to the surgeons trying to repair a severed nerve. If the cut is clean, it may be possible to suture individual fascicular bundles together. In such a scenario, there is a greater chance that the distal segment of nerves synapsing with the muscles will be sutured to the central stump of motor or sensory axons. In such cases, good functional recovery is more likely. If a short segment of the nerve is missing, however, the fascicles in the various quadrants of the stump may no longer correspond with one another, good axial alignment may not be possible, and functional recovery is greatly compromised or improbable.[1] This arrangement of the peripheral nerve helps explain why intraneural injections may result in disastrous consequences.

The connective tissue of a nerve is tougher, compared to the nerve fibers themselves, and allows a certain amount of "stretch" without damage to the nerve fibers. For instance, the axons are somewhat "wavy," and when stretched, the connective tissue around them is also stretched—giving it some protection. This feature plays a "safety" role in nerve blockade by allowing the nerves to be "pushed" rather than pierced by the advancing needle, as often seen on ultrasound. For this reason, it is prudent to avoid stretching the nerves and nerve plexuses during nerve blockade (eg, in axillary brachial plexus blocks and some approaches to the sciatic block).

The **paraneurium** consists of loose connective tissue that holds a stable relationship between adjacent structures filling the space in between them, such as the neurovascular bundles of intermuscular septae. This tissue contributes to functional mobility of nerves during joint and muscular movement.

Nerves receive blood from the adjacent blood vessels running along their course. These feeding branches to larger nerves are macroscopic in size and irregularly arranged, forming anastomoses to become longitudinally running vessel(s) that supply the nerve and give off subsidiary branches. Although the connective tissue sheath enveloping nerves serves to protect the nerves from stretching, it is also believed that neuronal injury after nerve blockade may be due, at least partly, to the pressure or stretch within connective sheaths that do not stretch well and the consequent interference with the vascular supply to the nerve.

Communication Between the Central and Peripheral Nervous Systems

The functional boundary between the central nervous system (CNS) and the peripheral nervous system (PNS) lies at the junction where oligodendrocytes meet Schwann cells along the axons that form the cranial and spinal nerve. The CNS communicates with the body through spinal nerves. Spinal nerves have both sensory and motor components (Figure 3–3). The **sensory fibers** arise from neurons in the dorsal root ganglia. Fibers enter the dorsolateral aspect of the spinal cord to form the dorsal root. The **motor fibers** arise from neurons in the ventral horn of the spinal cord. The fibers pass through the ventrolateral aspect of the spinal cord and form the ventral root. The dorsal and ventral roots converge in the intervertebral foramen to form a spinal nerve. After passing through the intervertebral foramen, the spinal nerve divides into dorsal and ventral rami. The dorsal ramus innervates muscle, bones, joints, and the skin of the back. The ventral ramus innervates muscle, bones, joints, and the skin of the anterior neck, thorax, abdomen, pelvis, and the extremities.

Spinal Nerves

There are 31 pairs of spinal nerves (Figure 3-4). The spinal nerves are enumerated by region: 8 cervical, 12 thoracic, 5 lumbar, 5 sacral, and 1 coccygeal. Spinal nerves pass through the vertebral column at the intervertebral foramina. The first cervical nerve (C1) passes superior to the C1 vertebra (atlas). The second cervical nerve (C2) passes between the C1 (atlas) and C2 (axis) vertebrae. This pattern continues down the cervical spine. A shift in pattern occurs at the C8 nerve because there is no C8 vertebra. The C8 nerve passes between the C7 and T1 vertebrae. The T1 nerve passes between the T1 and T2 vertebrae. This pattern continues down the remainder of the spine. The vertebral arch of the fifth sacral and first coccygeal

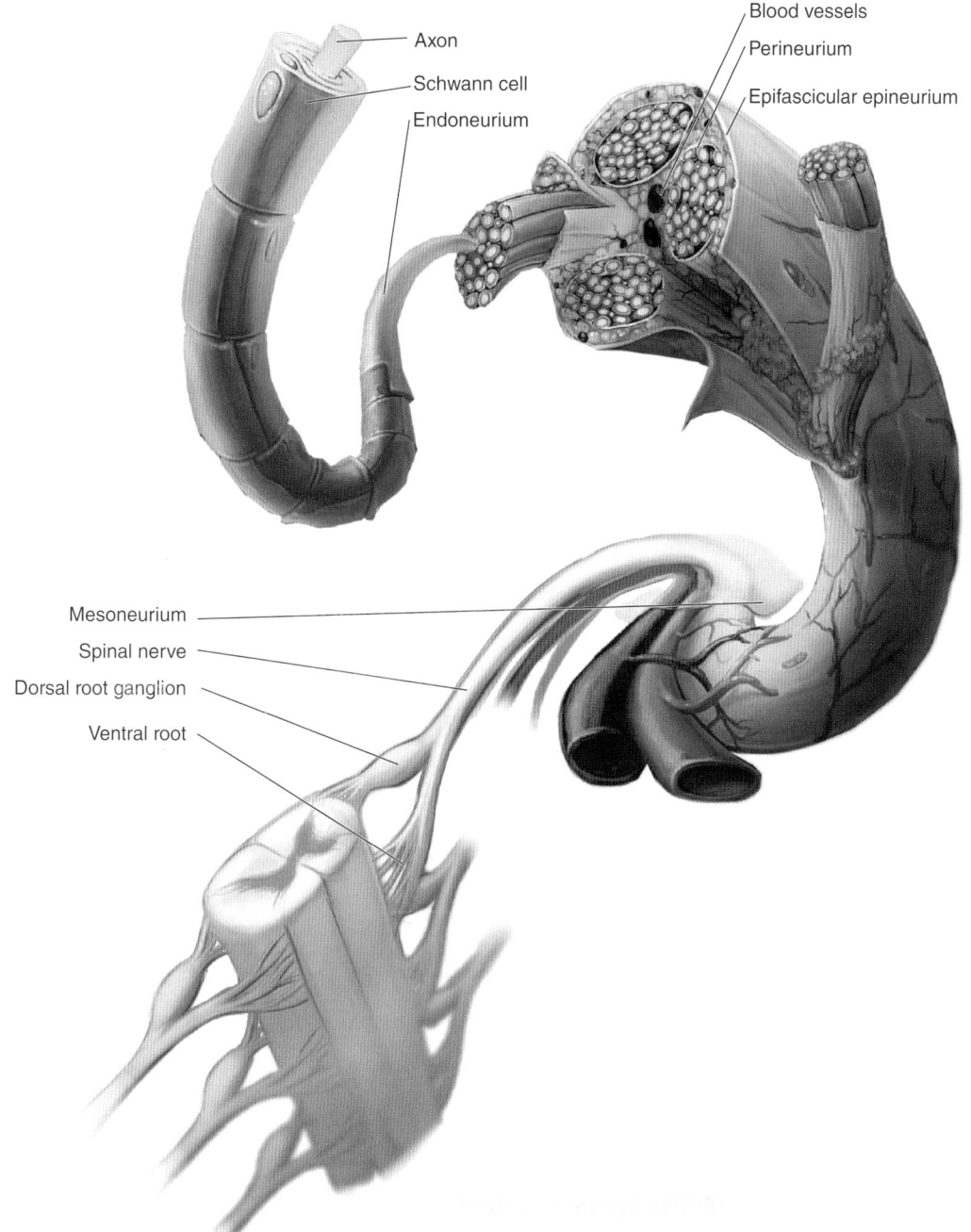

FIGURE 3–2. Organization of the peripheral nerve.

vertebrae is rudimentary. Because of this, the vertebral canal opens inferiorly at the sacral hiatus. The fifth sacral and first coccygeal nerves pass through the sacral hiatus. Because the inferior end of the spinal cord (conus medullaris) in adults is located at the L1 to L2 vertebral level, roots of spinal nerves must descend through the vertebral canal before exiting the vertebral column through the appropriate intervertebral foramen. Collectively, these roots are called the cauda equina.

Outside the vertebral column, ventral rami from different spinal levels coalesce to form intricate networks called plexuses. From the plexuses, nerves extend into the neck, the arms, and the legs.[1,2]

DERMATOMES, MYOTOMES, AND OSTEOTOMES

Dermatomal, myotomal, and osteotomal innervations are often emphasized in regional anesthesiology texts as important for the application of nerve blocks. In clinical practice of regional anesthesia, however, it is more practical to think in terms of which block techniques provide adequate analgesia and anesthesia for specific surgical procedures, rather than attempt to match nerves and spinal segments to the relevant dermatomal, myotomal, and osteotomal territory. Nevertheless, the description of dermatomal, myotomal, and osteotomal innervation is

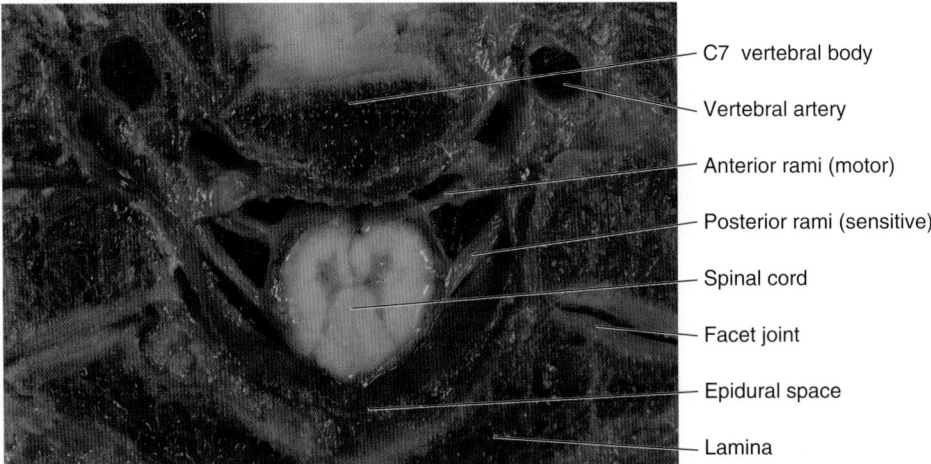

C7 vertebral body

Vertebral artery

Anterior rami (motor)

Posterior rami (sensitive)

Spinal cord

Facet joint

Epidural space

Lamina

FIGURE 3–3. Transverse section of cervical spine showing the spine with the origin of spinal nerves.

of didactic importance in regional anesthesia and is briefly presented here.

A **dermatome** is an area of the skin supplied by the dorsal (sensory) root of the spinal nerve (Figures 3–5a, 3–5b, and 3–6). In the trunk, each segment is horizontally disposed, except C1, which does not have a sensory component. The dermatomes of the limbs from the fifth cervical to the first thoracic nerve and from the third lumbar to the second sacral vertebrae extend as a series of bands from the midline of the trunk posteriorly into the limbs. It should be noted that considerable overlapping occurs between adjacent dermatomes; that is, each segmental nerve overlaps the territories of its neighbors.[3]

A **myotome** is the segmental innervation of skeletal muscle by the ventral (motor) root(s) of the spinal nerve(s). Major myotomes, their function, and corresponding spinal levels are represented in Figure 3–7. The innervation of the bones and

joints (**osteotome**) often does not follow the same segmental pattern as the innervation of the muscles and other soft tissues (Figure 3–8).

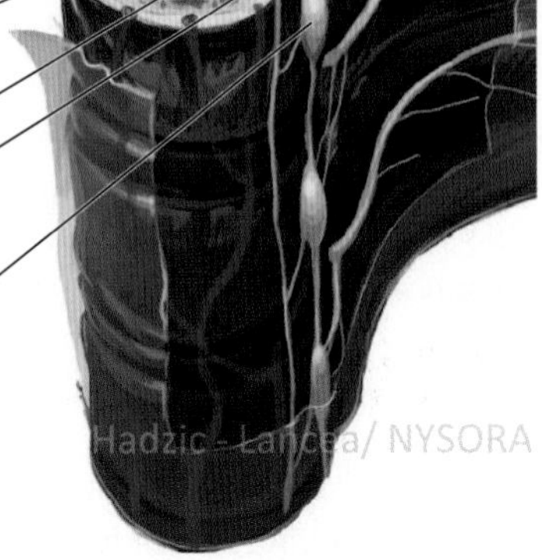

ANATOMY OF PLEXUSES AND PERIPHERAL NERVES

Cervical Plexus

The cervical plexus innervates muscles, joints, and skin in the anterior neck (Table 3–1). It is formed by the ventral rami of C1 through C4 (Figures 3–9 and 3–10). The rami form a loop called the ansa cervicalis that sends branches to the infrahyoid muscles. In addition, the rami form nerves that pass directly to several structures in the neck and thorax, including the scalene muscles, diaphragm, clavicular joints, and skin covering the anterior neck.

Ansa Cervicalis

The ventral ramus of C1 attaches to the ventral rami of C2 to C3. The attachment forms a loop called the ansa cervicalis, which sends branches to the infrahyoid muscles. The infrahyoid muscles consist of the omohyoid, sternohyoid, and sternothyroid muscles. They attach to the anterior surface of the hyoid bone or to the thyroid cartilage. Contraction of these muscles moves the hyoid bone or thyroid cartilage downward, effectively opening the laryngeal aditus, promoting inspiration. The C1 component also sends fibers to the thyrohyoid and geniohyoid muscles. Contraction of these muscles moves the anterior hyoid bone superiorly, closing the laryngeal aditus. Closure of the laryngeal aditus is necessary for swallowing to occur safely. This is one of the reasons why high levels of spinal anesthesia result in airway compromise and the risk of aspiration.

Nerves to Scalene Muscles

The ventral rami of C2 to C4 send branches directly to the scalene muscles, which attach between the cervical spine and ribs. When the cervical spine is stabilized, contraction elevates the ribs. This promotes inspiration. Interscalene block may result in block of the scalene muscles in addition to the phrenic block.

Lateral ramus

Medial ramus

of

dorsal ramus (posterior)

Dorsal root
(Sensory root)

Ventral root
(Motor root)

Spinal ganglion

Meningeal ramus

Spinal nerve

Ramus communicans

Ventral ramus

Sympathetic ganglion

Hadzic - Lancea / NYSORA

FIGURE 3–4. Anatomy of a spinal nerve (intercostal nerve).

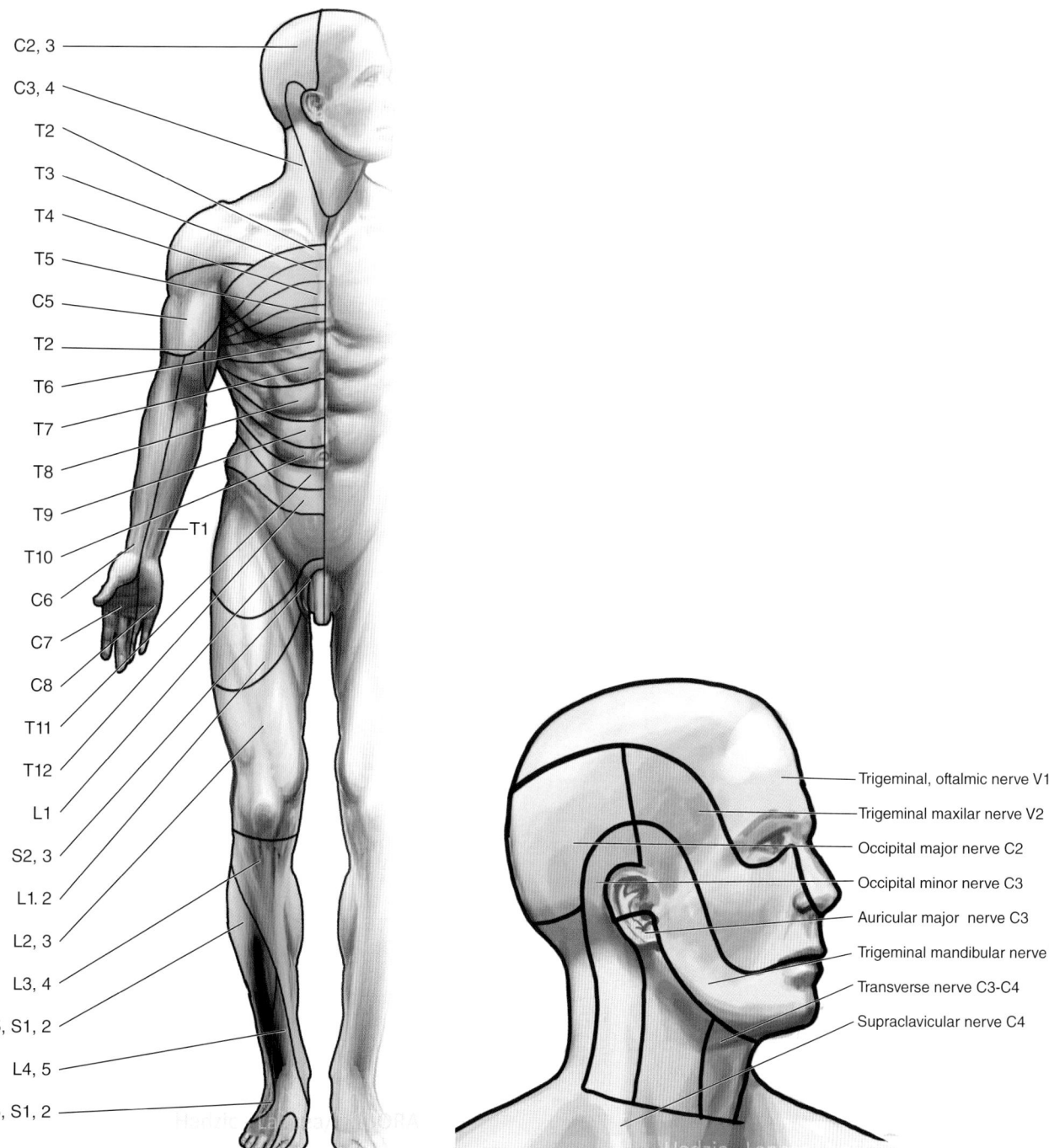

FIGURE 3–5. a, b: Dermatomes, anterior.

This is typically asymptomatic in healthy patients but may result in acute respiratory insufficiency in patients with borderline pulmonary function or in those with an exacerbation of asthma or chronic obstructive bronchitis. It is recommended that more distal approaches to a brachial plexus block and smaller injection volumes be used to limit the cephalad extension of the block, as well as shorter-acting local anesthetics to avoid prolonged blockade in case of respiratory insufficiency.

Phrenic Nerve

The phrenic nerve is formed by junction of fibers from C3 to C5, (Figure 3-10) and it innervates the diaphragm. The

phrenic nerve descends through the neck on the anterior surface of the anterior scalene muscle, passing through the superior thoracic aperture and descending on the walls of the mediastinum to the diaphragm. In addition to muscular fibers, the phrenic nerve transmits sensory fibers to the superior and inferior surfaces of the diaphragm. All approaches to the block of the brachial plexus above the clavicle with high volumes result in phrenic blockade (Figure 3-12).

Cutaneous Nerves of the Anterior Neck

Cutaneous sensory nerves arise from the cervical plexus, pass around the posterior margin of sternocleidomastoid, and

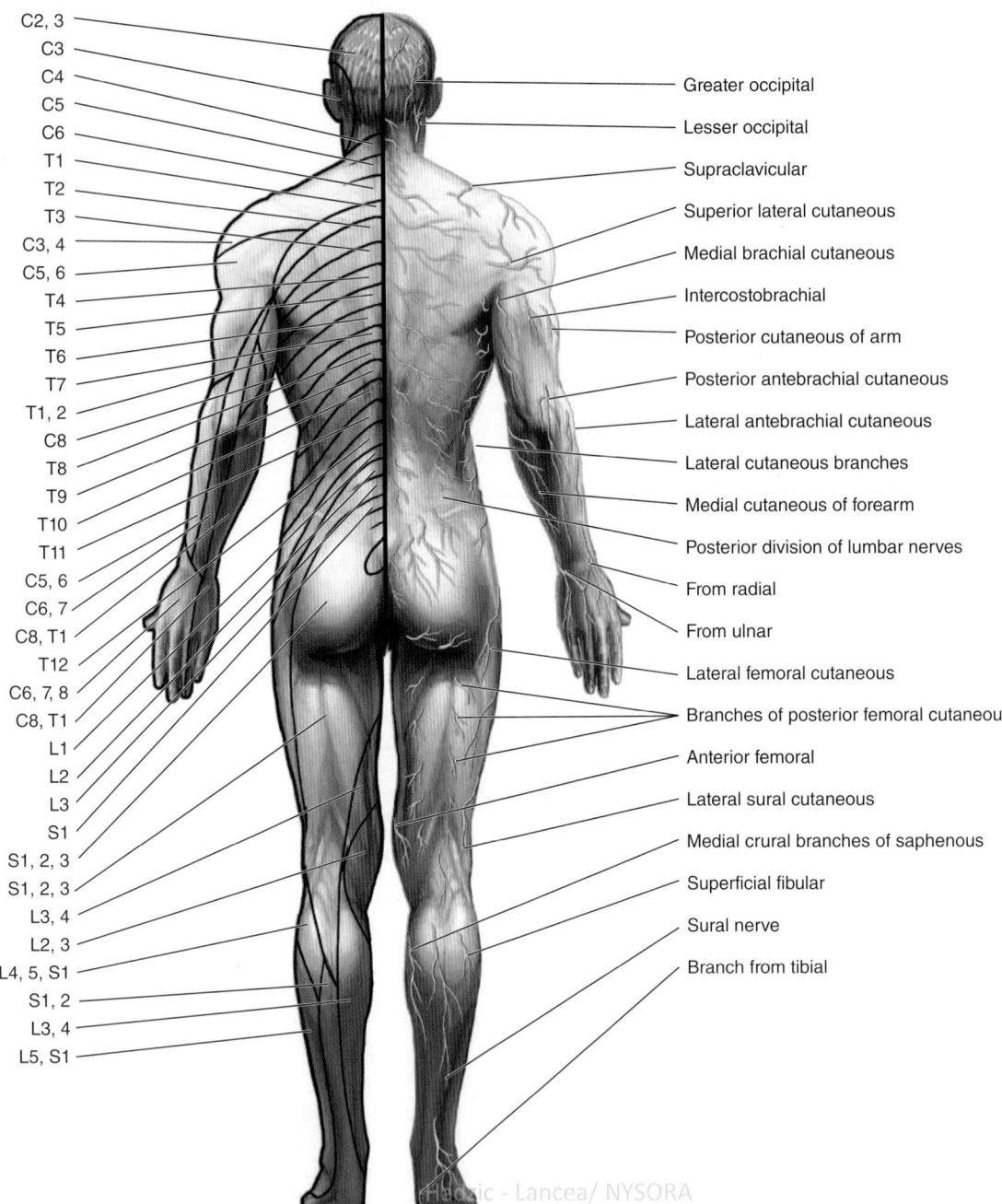

C2, 3
C3
C4
C5
C6
T1
T2
T3
C3, 4
C5, 6
T4
T5
T6
T7
T1, 2
C8
T8
T9
T10
T11
C5, 6
C6, 7
C8, T1
T12
C6, 7, 8
C8, T1
L1
L2
L3
S1
S1, 2, 3
S1, 2, 3
L3, 4
L2, 3
L4, 5, S1
S1, 2
L3, 4
L5, S1

Greater occipital
Lesser occipital
Supraclavicular
Superior lateral cutaneous
Medial brachial cutaneous
Intercostobrachial
Posterior cutaneous of arm
Posterior antebrachial cutaneous
Lateral antebrachial cutaneous
Lateral cutaneous branches
Medial cutaneous of forearm
Posterior division of lumbar nerves
From radial
From ulnar
Lateral femoral cutaneous
Branches of posterior femoral cutaneous
Anterior femoral
Lateral sural cutaneous
Medial crural branches of saphenous
Superficial fibular
Sural nerve
Branch from tibial

FIGURE 3–6. Dermatomes, posterior.

terminate in the scalp and anterior neck. The minor occipital nerve passes to the posterior auricular region of the scalp. The major auricular nerve passes to the auricle of the ear and to the region of the face anterior to the tragus. The transverse cervical nerve supplies the anterior neck. A series of supraclavicular nerves innervates the region covering the clavicle. Furthermore, the supraclavicular nerves may provide articular branches to the sternoclavicular and acromioclavicular joints.[4]

Brachial Plexus

The brachial plexus innervates bones, joints, muscles, and the skin of the upper extremity (Table 3–2). It is formed by ventral rami of C5 to T1 (Figures 3–11 and 3–12). In the posterior cervical triangle between the anterior and middle scalene muscles, the ventral rami join to form trunks. C5 and C6 join to form the superior trunk. C7 forms the middle trunk. C8 and T1 join to form the inferior trunk. All trunks branch into anterior and posterior divisions. All the posterior divisions join to form the posterior cord. The anterior divisions of the superior and middle trunks join to form the lateral cord. The anterior division of the inferior trunk forms the medial cord. Several terminal nerves arise within the posterior cervical triangle. Because they arise superior to the clavicle, they are called supraclavicular branches. The supraclavicular branches include the dorsal scapular nerve, the long thoracic nerve, the suprascapular nerve, and the nerve to the subclavius.[5–7]

A
B
C
D
C5
C6, 7, 8
C5-C6
C6, 7, 8
C7-T1
C6-C7
C8-T1
C6, 7
C5, 6
L5, S1
L5, S1
L2-L4
C5-C7
C5-C7
L4, 5
L2, 3
L5, S1
L3, 4

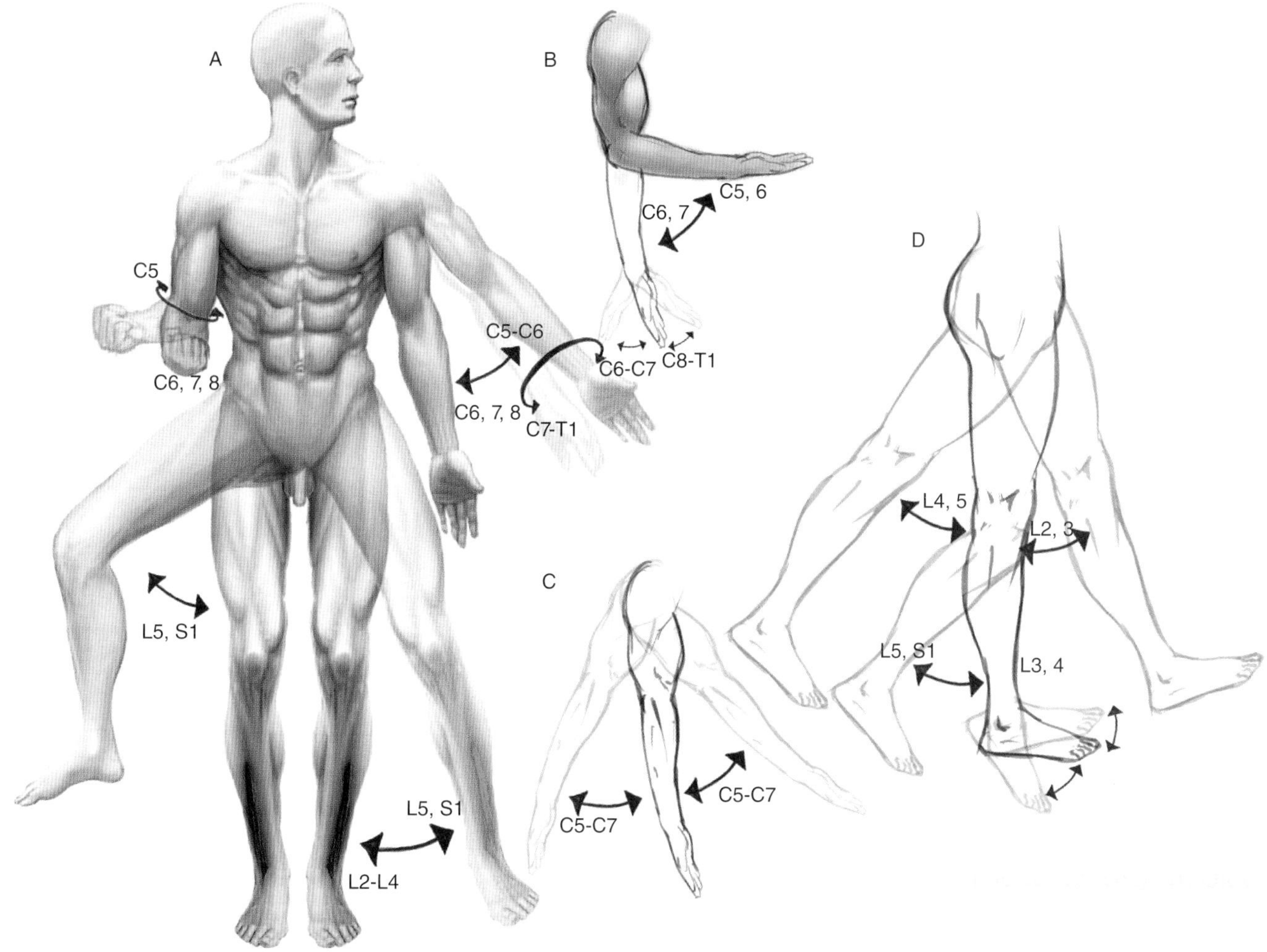

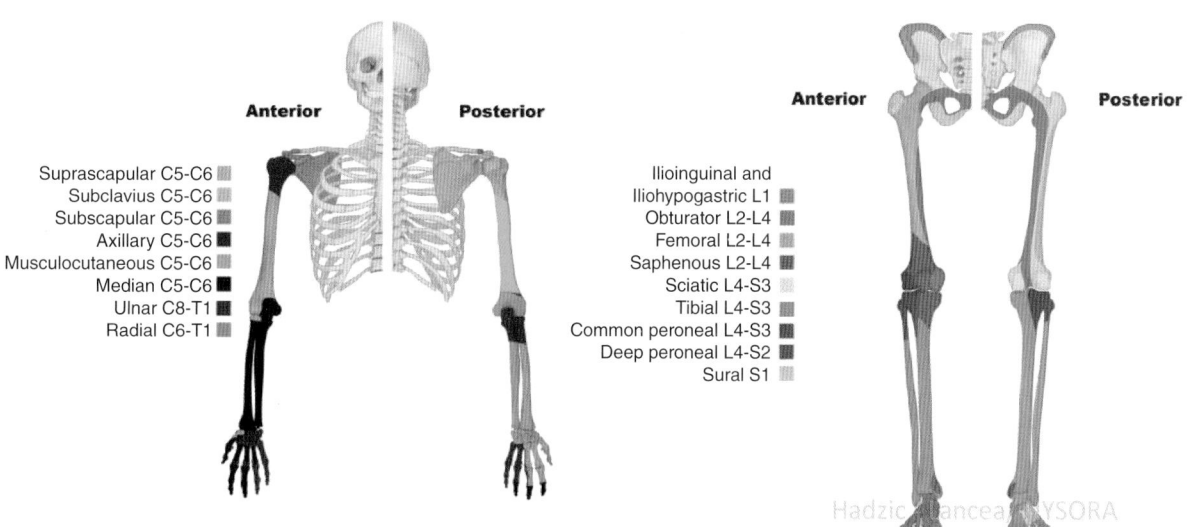

FIGURE 3–7. Functional innervation of the muscles (myotomes): **A:** Medial and lateral rotation of shoulder and hip, pronation and supination of wrist and forearm. Abduction and adduction of shoulder and hip. **B:** Flexion and extension of elbow and wrist. **C:** Flexion and extension of shoulder. **D:** Flexion and extension of hip, and knee. Dorsiflexion and plantar flexion of ankle, lateral views.

Anterior
Posterior
Suprascapular C5-C6
Subclavius C5-C6
Subscapular C5-C6
Axillary C5-C6
Musculocutaneous C5-C6
Median C5-C6
Ulnar C8-T1
Radial C6-T1
Anterior
Posterior
Ilioinguinal and
Iliohypogastric L1
Obturator L2-L4
Femoral L2-L4
Saphenous L2-L4
Sciatic L4-S3
Tibial L4-S3
Common peroneal L4-S3
Deep peroneal L4-S2
Sural S1
Hadzic Vancea NYSORA

FIGURE 3–8. Innervation of the major bones (osteotomes).

TABLE 3–1. Organization and distribution of the cervical plexus.

Nerves	Spinal Segments	Distribution
Ansa cervicalis (superior and inferior branches)	C1 to C4	Five of the extrinsic laryngeal muscles (sternothyroid, sternohyoid, omohyoid, geniohyoid, and thyrohyoid) by way of CN XII
Lesser occipital, transverse cervical, supraclavicular, and greater auricular nerves	C2 to C3	Skin of upper chest, shoulder, neck, and ear
Phrenic nerve	C3 to C5	Diaphragm
Cervical nerves	C1 to C5	Levator scapulae, scalenes, sternocleidomastoid, and trapezius muscles (with CN XI)

CN = cranial nerve.

Supraclavicular Branches
Dorsal Scapular Nerve

The dorsal scapular nerve arises from the ventral ramus of C5. It follows the levator scapula muscle to the scapula and descends the medial border of the scapula on the deep surface of the rhomboid muscles. In its route, the dorsal scapular nerve innervates the levator scapula and rhomboid muscles.

Long Thoracic Nerve

The long thoracic nerve arises from the ventral rami of C5 to C7. It descends along the anterior surface of the middle scalene to

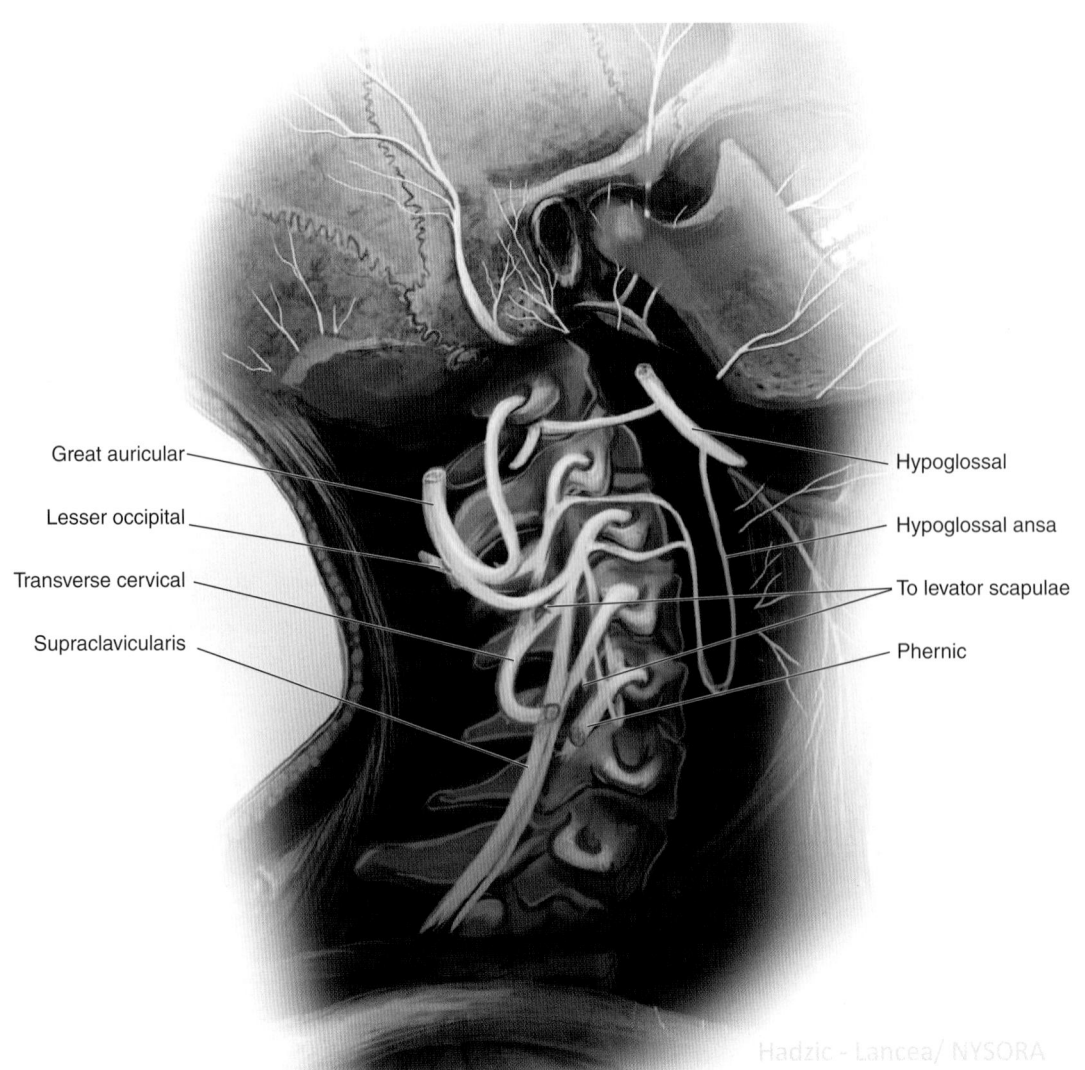

Great auricular
Lesser occipital
Transverse cervical
Supraclavicularis

Hypoglossal
Hypoglossal ansa
To levator scapulae
Phernic

FIGURE 3–9. Cervical plexus.

PART 2

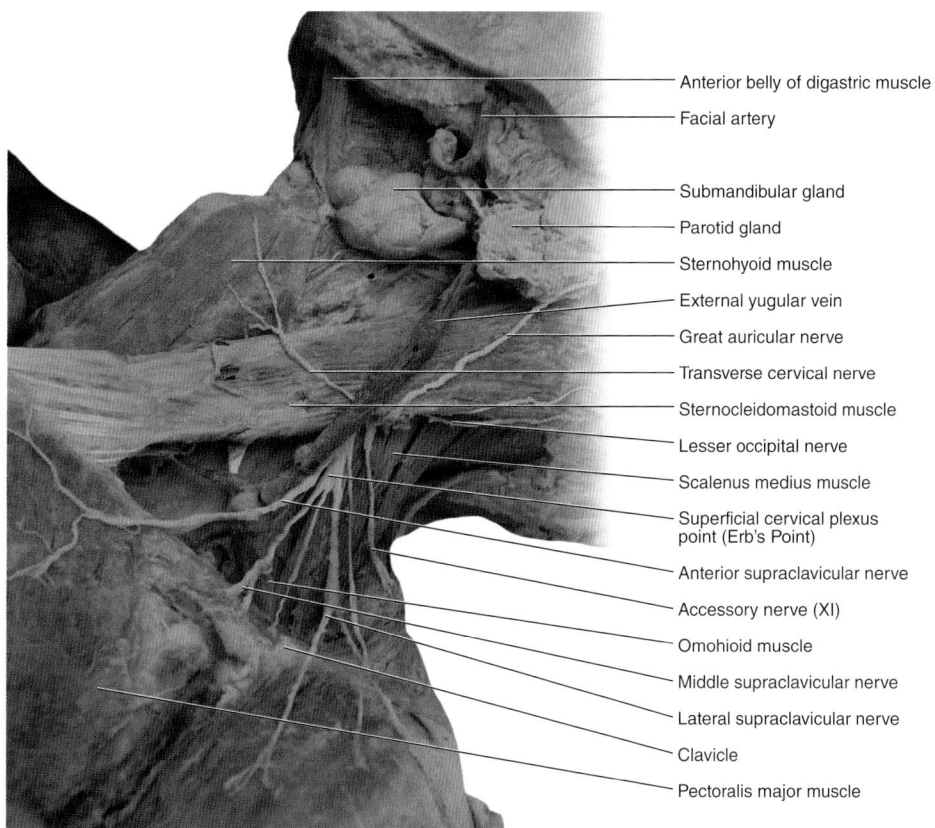

Anterior belly of digastric muscle
Facial artery
Submandibular gland
Parotid gland
Sternohyoid muscle
External yugular vein
Great auricular nerve
Transverse cervical nerve
Sternocleidomastoid muscle
Lesser occipital nerve
Scalenus medius muscle
Superficial cervical plexus point (Erb's Point)
Anterior supraclavicular nerve
Accessory nerve (XI)
Omohioid muscle
Middle supraclavicular nerve
Lateral supraclavicular nerve
Clavicle
Pectoralis major muscle

FIGURE 3–10. Dissection of cervical plexus.

TABLE 3–2. Organization and distribution of the brachial plexus.

Nerves(s)	Spinal Segments	Distribution
Nerves to subclavius	C4 to C6	Subclavius muscle
Dorsal scapular nerve	C5	Rhomboid muscles and levator scapulae muscle
Long thoracic nerve	C5 to C7	Serratus anterior muscle
Suprascapular nerve	C5, C6	Supraspinatus and infraspinatus muscles
Pectoralis nerve (median and lateral)	C5 to T1	Pectoralis muscles
Subscapular nerves	C5, C6	Subscapularis and teres major muscles
Thoracodorsal nerve	C6 to C8	Latissimus dorsi muscle
Axillary nerve	C5, C6	Deltoid and teres minor muscles; skin of shoulder
Radial nerve	C5 to T1	Extensor muscle of the arm and forearm (triceps brachii, extensor carpi radialis, supinator and anconeus muscles, and extensor carpi ulnaris muscles) and brachioradialis muscle; digital extensors and abductor pollicis muscle; skin over the posterolateral surface of the arm
Musculocutaneous nerve	C5 to C7	Flexor muscles on the arm (biceps brachii, brachialis, and coracobrachialis muscles); skin over lateral surface of forearm
Median nerve	C6 to T1	Flexor muscles on the forearm (flexor carpi radialis and palmaris longus muscles); pronator quadratus and pronator teres muscles; digital flexors (through the palmar interosseous nerve); skin over anterolateral surface of hand
Ulnar nerve	C8, T1	Flexor carpi ulnaris muscle, adductor pollicis muscle, and small digital muscles; medial part of flexor digitorum profundus muscle; skin over medial surface of the hand

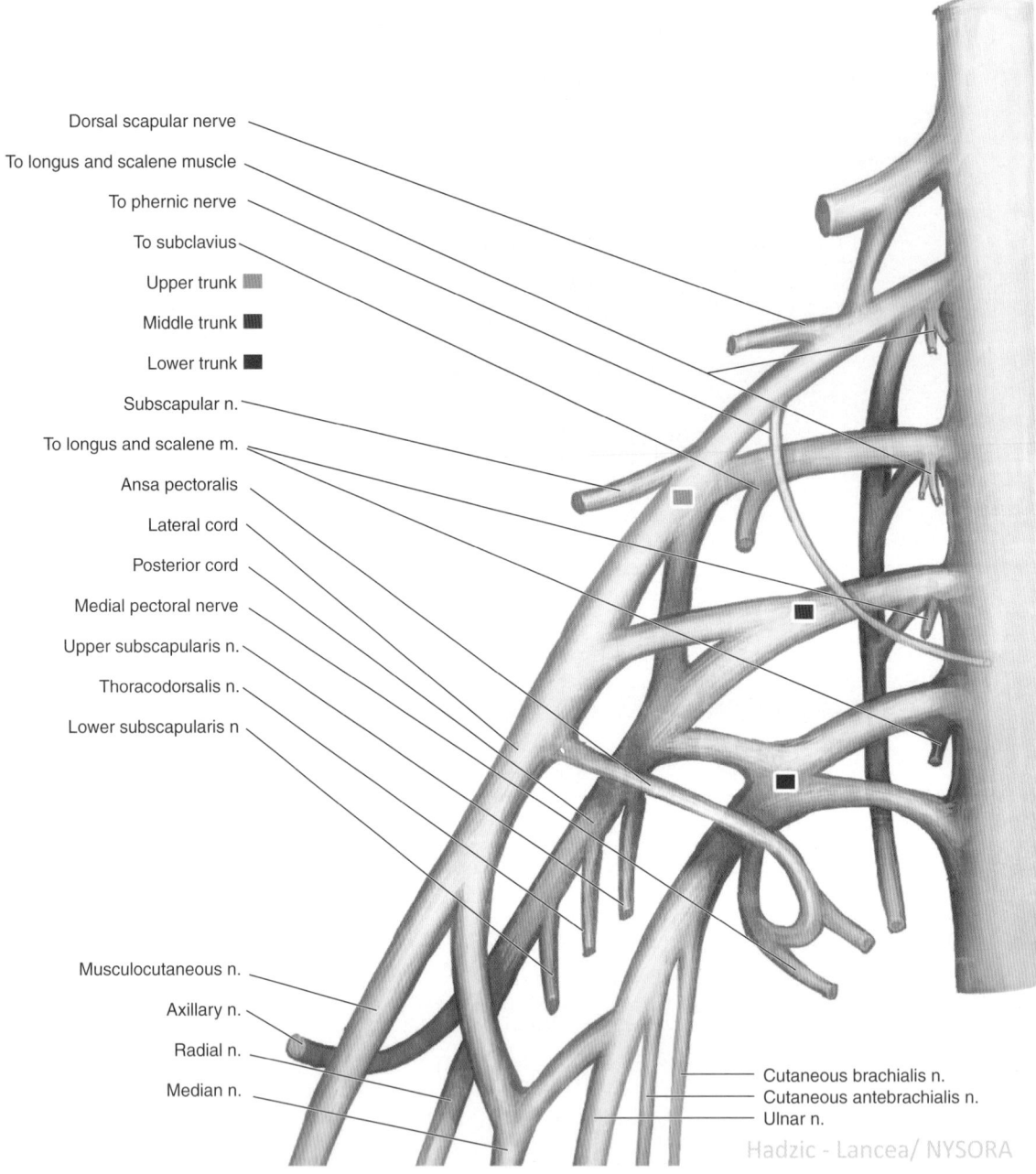

Dorsal scapular nerve
To longus and scalene muscle
To phernic nerve
To subclavius
Upper trunk
Middle trunk
Lower trunk
Subscapular n.
To longus and scalene m.
Ansa pectoralis
Lateral cord
Posterior cord
Medial pectoral nerve
Upper subscapularis n.
Thoracodorsalis n.
Lower subscapularis n
Musculocutaneous n.
Axillary n.
Radial n.
Median n.

Cutaneous brachialis n.
Cutaneous antebrachialis n.
Ulnar n.

Hadzic - Lancea/ NYSORA

FIGURE 3-11. Scheme of organization of the brachial plexus.

the first rib and then transfers onto the serratus anterior muscle, which it innervates.

Suprascapular Nerve

The suprascapular nerve arises from the superior trunk. It follows the inferior belly of the omohyoid muscle to the scapula; passes through the superior notch into the supraspinatus fossa, where it innervates the supraspinatus muscle; and continues around the scapular notch (lateral margin of the scapular spine) to the infraspinatus fossa, where it innervates the infraspinatus muscle. In addition to muscle, the suprascapular nerve innervates the posterior aspect of the glenohumeral joint, subacromial bursa, and acromioclavicular joint.

Nerve to Subclavius

The nerve to subclavius arises from the superior trunk. It passes anteriorly a short distance to innervate the subclavius muscle and the sternoclavicular joint.

The cords of the brachial plexus leave the posterior cervical triangle and enter the axilla through the axillary inlet. The remainder of the terminal branches arise within the axilla from the cords (Figure 3-12).

Posterior Cord Branches

The posterior cord forms the upper and lower subscapular nerves, thoracodorsal nerve, axillary nerve, and radial nerve.

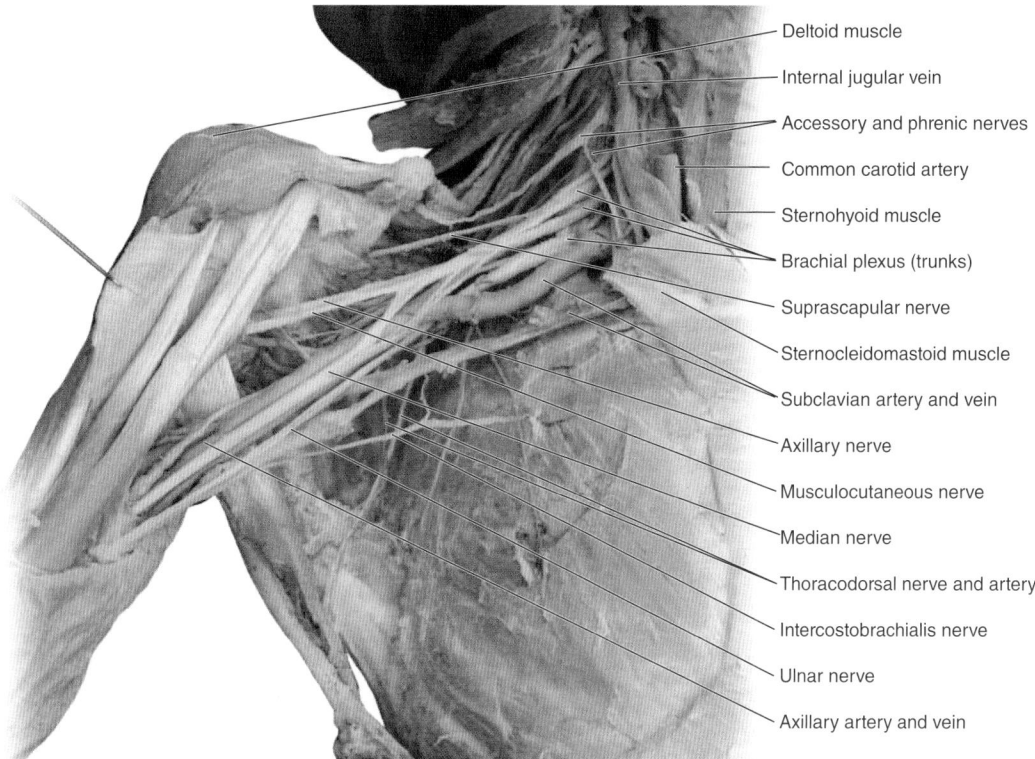

- Deltoid muscle
- Internal jugular vein
- Accessory and phrenic nerves
- Common carotid artery
- Sternohyoid muscle
- Brachial plexus (trunks)
- Suprascapular nerve
- Sternocleidomastoid muscle
- Subclavian artery and vein
- Axillary nerve
- Musculocutaneous nerve
- Median nerve
- Thoracodorsal nerve and artery
- Intercostobrachialis nerve
- Ulnar nerve
- Axillary artery and vein

FIGURE 3–12. Dissection of the brachial plexus.

Subscapular Nerves

The subscapular nerves are formed by fibers from C5 to C6. The upper subscapular nerve is the first nerve to arise from the posterior cord. It passes onto the anterior surface of the subscapularis muscle, which it innervates. The lower subscapular nerve arises more distally. It descends across the anterior surface of the subscapularis muscle to the teres major muscle and innervates both the subscapularis and teres major muscles.

Thoracodorsal Nerve

The thoracodorsal nerve is formed by fibers from C5 to C7. It arises from the posterior cord, usually between the subscapular nerves, and descends across the subscapularis and teres major muscle to the latissimus dorsi muscle. It innervates the latissimus dorsi.

Axillary Nerve

The axillary nerve is formed by fibers from C5 to C6 (Box 3–1). It passes from the axilla into the shoulder between the teres major and minor muscles, the long head of triceps and humerus quadrangular space of Velpeau. It innervates the teres minor. The nerve continues posterior to the surgical neck of the humerus to innervate the deltoid muscle. The superior lateral brachial cutaneous branch of the axillary nerve passes around the posterior margin of the deltoid to innervate the skin covering the deltoid. In addition to muscle and skin, the axillary nerve innervates the glenohumeral and acromioclavicular joints. Throughout its course, the nerve is associated with the posterior circumflex humeral artery and its branches.

Radial Nerve

The radial nerve is formed by fibers from C5 to T1 (Box 3–2). It passes from the axilla into the arm through the triangular space. The triangular space is located inferior to the teres major between the long head of the triceps brachii and the humerus. The radial nerve innervates the long head of the triceps muscle and sends a posterior brachial cutaneous branch to the skin covering this muscle. It descends along the shaft of the humerus in the spiral groove in association with the deep radial artery. In the spiral groove, the radial nerve innervates the medial and lateral heads of the triceps brachii as well as the anconeus muscles. In addition to innervating these muscles, it sends an inferior lateral brachial cutaneous nerve to the skin covering the posterior arm and a posterior antebrachial cutaneous branch to the skin

---

BOX 3–1. Axillary nerve (C5 to C6).

Muscular branches
- Abduction, flexion, or extension of shoulder
  - Deltoid
- Lateral rotation the shoulder; stabilization of glenohumeral joint
  - Teres minor

Articular branches
- Acromioclavicular joint
- Anterior aspect of glenohumeral joint

Cutaneous branch
- Superior lateral brachial cutaneous nerve

BOX 3–2. Radial nerve.

Muscular branches
- Extension of shoulder
  - Triceps brachii—long head
- Extension of elbow
  - Triceps brachii—long, lateral, medial heads
  - Anconeus
- Supination of forearm
  - Supinator
- Extension of wrist
  - Extensor carpi radialis—longus and brevis
  - Extensor carpi ulnaris
  - Extensor muscles of fingers and thumb listed next
- Extension of fingers (metacarpophalangeal and interphalangeal joints)
  - Extensor digitorum communis (index, middle, ring, little fingers)
  - Extensor indicis (index finger)
  - Extensor digiti minimi (little finger)
- Extension of thumb
  - Extensor pollicis longus (metacarpophlangeal and interphalangeal)
  - Extensor pollicis brevis (metacarpophalangeal joint)
- Abduction of thumb
  - Abductor pollicis longus

Articular branches
- Elbow (humeroradial and humeroulnar joints)
- Radioulnar joints—proximal and distal
- Radiocarpal joint

Cutaneous branches
- Posterior brachial cutaneous nerve
- Inferior lateral brachial cutaneous nerve
- Posterior antebrachial cutaneous nerve
- Superficial branch of the radial nerve

BOX 3–3. Musculocutaneous nerve (C5 to C7).

Muscular branches
- Flexion of the shoulder
  - Biceps brachii—long head
  - Coracobrachialis
- Flexion of elbow
  - Brachialis (humeroulnar joint)
  - Biceps brachii—long and short heads (humeroradial joint)
- Supination of forearm
  - Biceps brachii—long and short heads

Articular branches
- Elbow (humeroulnar and humeroradial joints)
- Proximal radioulnar joint

Cutaneous branch
- Lateral antebrachial cutaneous nerve

---

covering the posterior surface of the forearm. The radial nerve pierces the lateral intermuscular septum and crosses the elbow anterior to the lateral epicondyle between the brachialis and brachioradialis muscles. Here, it divides into a superficial and deep branch. The superficial branch descends the forearm on the deep surface of the brachioradialis. Proximal to the wrist, it enters the skin, providing innervation over the dorsum of the hand onto the thumb, index, middle, and ring fingers to the level of the distal interphalangeal joint. The deep branch pierces the supinator muscle and descends the forearm along the interosseous membrane as the posterior interosseous nerve. En route, it innervates the brachioradialis, extensor carpi radialis longus and brevis, supinator, extensor digitorum communis, extensor digiti minimi, extensor carpi ulnaris, extensor indicis, extensor pollicis longus and brevis, and abductor pollicis muscles. In addition, it innervates the humerus, elbow, radioulnar, and wrist joints.[8]

Branches From the Lateral Cord

The lateral cord forms the lateral pectoral nerve, musculocutaneous nerve, and part of the median nerve.

Lateral Pectoral Nerve

The lateral pectoral nerve is formed by fibers from C5 to C7. It crosses the axilla deep to the pectoralis minor muscle and penetrates the deep surface of pectoralis major muscle, which it innervates. In addition, it innervates the acromioclavicular joint.

Musculocutaneous Nerve

The musculocutaneous nerve is formed by fibers from C5 to C7 (Box 3–3). It pierces the coracobrachialis muscle and descends between the brachialis and biceps brachii muscles (see Figure 3–12). En route, it innervates all of these muscles. At the elbow, the musculocutaneous nerve becomes the lateral antebrachial cutaneous nerve and descends along the superficial surface of the brachioradialis muscle, innervating the skin covering that muscle. In addition to muscle and skin, the musculocutaneous nerve innervates the humerus elbow and proximal radioulnar joints.

Median Nerve

The median nerve is formed by junction of branches from the lateral and medial cords (Box 3–4). It descends the arm in association with the brachial artery and crosses the cubital fossa medial to the artery (see Figure 3–12). At the elbow, it innervates the pronator teres, flexor carpi radialis, and palmaris longus muscles. It passes into the forearm between the humeral and radial heads of the pronator teres muscle and descends in the space between the flexor digitorum superficialis and profundus muscles. En route, it innervates the flexor digitorum superficialis, the lateral part of the flexor digitorum profundus (fibers to the index and middle fingers), the flexor pollicis longus, and the pronator quadratus muscles. In addition, the median nerve sends a palmar cutaneous branch to the skin covering the thenar eminence. At the wrist, the median nerve passes through the carpal tunnel deep to the flexor retinaculum. In the hand, the median nerve sends branches to the thenar muscles, which are the abductor pollicis brevis, flexor pollicis brevis, and opponens pollicis. The median nerve divides into three common palmar digital

BOX 3–4. Median nerve.

Muscular branches
- Flexion of the elbow
  - Flexor carpi radialis
  - Pronator teres
- Pronation of forearm
  - Pronator teres
  - Pronator quadratus
- Flexion of wrist
  - Flexor carpi radialis
  - Palmaris longus
  - Flexor digitorum superficialis and profundus
  - Flexor pollicis longus
- Flexion of fingers
  - Flexor digitorum superficialis (index, middle, ring, little fingers)
  - Flexor digitorum profundus (index, middle fingers)
- Flexion of metacarpophalangeal and extension of interphalangeal joints
  - Lumbricals (index, middle finger)
- Flexion of thumb
  - Flexor pollicis longus
  - Flexor pollicis brevis
- Abduction of thumb
  - Abductor pollicis brevis
- Opposition of thumb
  - Opponens pollicis

Articular branches
- Elbow (humeroulnar and humeroradial joints)
- Radioulnar joints—proximal and distal
- All joints of the wrist and hand

Cutaneous branches
- Palmar branch of median nerve
- Proper palmar digital nerves

branches, which innerve the lateral two lumbrical muscles. The common palmar branches divide into proper palmar branches that innervate the skin of the thumb, index, middle, and ring (lateral half) fingers. The innervation covers the palmar surface and the nail beds. In addition to muscle and skin, the median nerve innervates the diaphysis of the radius and ulna, and the anterior elbow and all joints distal to it.[9,10]

Medial Cord Branches

The medial cord forms the medial pectoral nerve, medial brachial cutaneous nerve, medial antebrachial cutaneous nerve, and ulnar nerve and sends fibers to the median nerve.

Medial Pectoral Nerve

The medial pectoral is formed by fibers from C8 to T1. It pierces the pectoralis minor and ends by branching on the deep surface of the pectoralis major, innervating both muscles. Contraction of the pectoralis minor in conjunction with the serratus anterior and rhomboid muscles pulls the pectoral girdle

(clavicle and scapula) against the chest wall when load is applied to the upper extremity. Without this stabilization of the proximal joints, movement of the distal joint in the upper extremity would collapse.

Medial Brachial and Antebrachial Cutaneous Nerves

Both medial brachial and antebrachial cutaneous nerves descend in the arm associated with the brachial artery. The medial brachial cutaneous nerve distributes fibers to the skin covering the medial surface of the arm. Occasionally, the medial brachial nerve joins the lateral cutaneous branch of the second intercostal nerve to form the intercostobrachial nerve. The medial antebrachial cutaneous nerve crosses the cubital fossa and enters the skin to innervate the medial aspect of the forearm.[4]

Ulnar Nerve

The ulnar nerve is formed by fibers from C8 to T1 (Box 3–5). It descends the arm in association with the brachial artery (see

BOX 3–5. Ulnar nerve (C8 to T1).

Muscular branches
- Flexion of wrist
  - Flexor carpi ulnaris
  - Flexor digitorum profundus
- Flexion of fingers
  - Flexor digitorum profundus (ring, little finger)
  - Flexor digiti minimi (little finger)
- Flexion of knuckles and extension of fingers
  - Lumbricals (ring, little finger)
  - Interosseous muscles (index, middle, ring, little fingers)
- Adduction of fingers (metacarpophalangeal joint)
  - Palmar interosseous muscles (index, middle, ring, little finger)
- Abduction of fingers
  - Dorsal interosseous muscles (index, middle, ring finger)
  - Abductor digiti minimi (little finger)
- Opposition of little finger
  - Opponens digiti minimi
  - Palmaris brevis
- Adduction of thumb
  - Adductor pollicis
- Flexion of thumb
  - Flexor pollicis brevis

Articular branches
- Ulnocarpal joint
- All joints of the hand except interphalangeal joint of the thumb

Cutaneous branches
- Dorsal branch of the ulnar nerve
- Palmar branch of the ulnar nerve
- Proper palmar digital branches

Figures 3-11 and 3-12), pierces the medial intermuscular septum, and crosses the elbow posterior to the medial epicondyle. After crossing the elbow, the ulnar nerve descends the forearm between the flexor carpi ulnaris and flexor digitorum profundus, innervating both muscles. The ulnar innervation of the flexor digitorum is limited to fibers affecting the ring and little fingers. Proximal to the wrist, the ulnar nerve sends a palmar branch to the skin covering the hypothenar eminence and a dorsal branch to the skin covering the dorsal and medial surface of the hand and the skin covering the dorsal surface of the ring and little fingers. The ulnar nerve passes through Guyon's canal (deep to the transverse carpal ligament) to enter the hand. It divides into a superficial and a deep branch. The superficial branch sends branches to all muscles of the hypothenar eminence, including the abductor digiti minimi, flexor digiti minimi, and opponens digiti minimi. Then, it divides into common palmar digital branches, which in turn divide into proper palmar digital branches. These branches innervate the skin covering the palmar surface of the ring and little fingers. The innervation continues on to the nail beds of these fingers. The deep branch of the ulnar nerve passes beneath the adductor pollicis muscle, which it innervates. The ulnar nerve sends fibers to all interosseous muscles in the hand and to the lumbrical muscles affecting the ring and little fingers. The ulnar nerve ends by innervating the deep head of the flexor pollicis brevis muscle.[9,10]

Along its course, the ulnar nerve supplies the medial aspect of the elbow joint, the ulna and all joints of the medial aspect of the wrist, hand, and ring and little fingers.

Thoracic Spinal Nerves

Thoracic spinal nerves innervate the muscles, joints, skin, and pleuroperitoneal lining of the thoracic and abdominal walls. Because the nerves travel within the intercostal spaces, they are called intercostal nerves. The intercostal nerves comprise the anterior rami of the upper 11 thoracic spinal nerves. Each intercostal nerve enters the neurovascular plane posteriorly and gives a collateral branch that supplies the intercostal muscles of the space. Except for the first, each intercostal nerve gives off a lateral cutaneous branch that pierces the overlying muscle near the midaxillary line. This cutaneous nerve divides into anterior and posterior branches, which supply the adjacent skin (Figure 3–13). The intercostal nerves of the second to the sixth spaces enter the superficial fascia near the lateral border of the sternum and divide into medial and lateral cutaneous branches. Most of the fibers of the anterior ramus of the first thoracic spinal nerve join the brachial plexus for distribution to the upper limb. The small first intercostal nerve is the collateral branch and supplies only the muscles of the intercostal space, not the overlying skin.

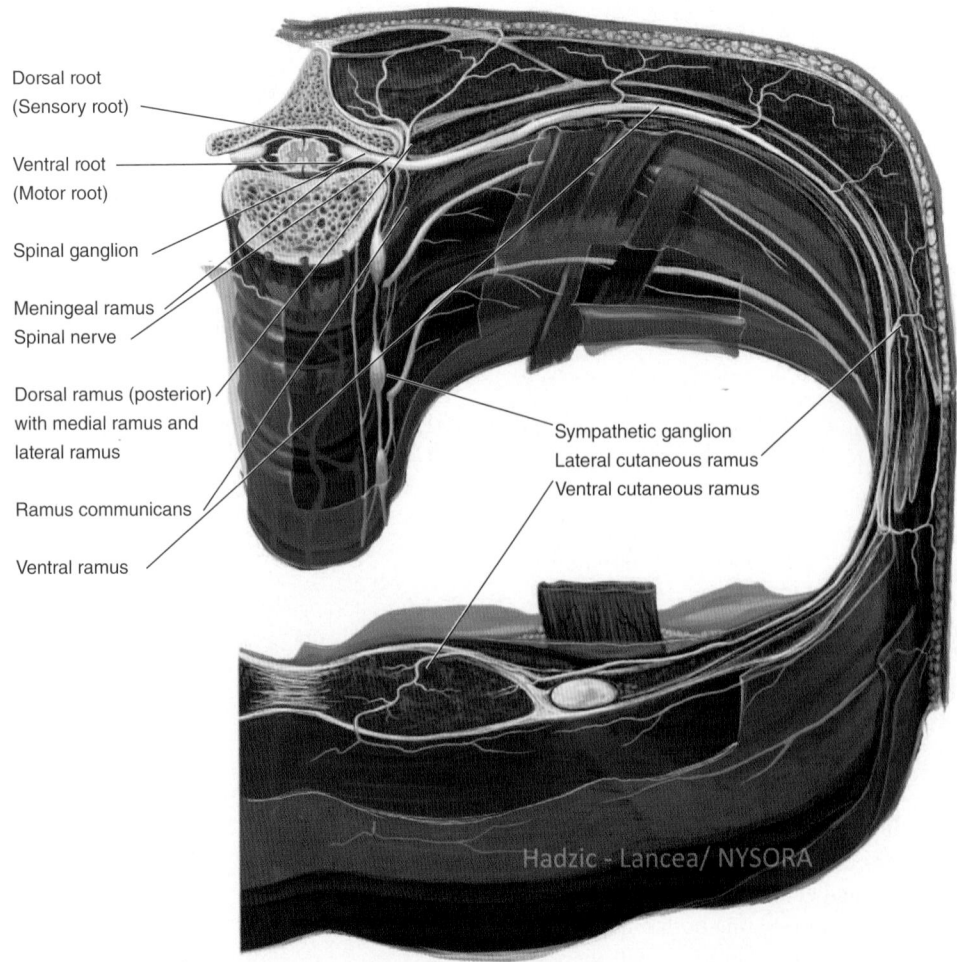

Dorsal root
(Sensory root)

Ventral root
(Motor root)

Spinal ganglion

Meningeal ramus
Spinal nerve

Dorsal ramus (posterior)
with medial ramus and
lateral ramus

Ramus communicans

Ventral ramus

Sympathetic ganglion
Lateral cutaneous ramus
Ventral cutaneous ramus

Hadzic - Lancea/ NYSORA

FIGURE 3–13. Organization and distribution of the spinal nerves at the thoracic level.

The intercostal nerves can be divided into two groups. One group is formed by nerves arising from T1 through T5. These nerves remain in the intercostal spaces throughout their course. The second group is formed by nerves arising from T6 to T12. These nerves initially travel in the intercostal spaces, but then cross the costal margin and terminate in the abdominal wall. This subgroup of intercostal nerves is called the thoracoabdominal nerves. The ventral ramus of T12 forms the subcostal nerve. This nerve travels entirely in the abdominal wall.

Intercostal Nerves

The intercostal nerves arise from the ventral rami of T1 through T11. They travel along the inferior margin of the rib of the corresponding number (eg, T1 nerve travels along the inferior margin of rib 1). En route, the nerve is located between the deepest (transverse thoracis muscle) and intermediate layer (internal intercostals muscle) of muscle. It is associated with the intercostal arteries and veins. From the top to the bottom, the neurovascular bundle is arranged as vein, artery, and nerve (mnemonic VAN). The intercostal nerves send branches to the transverse thoracis, internal intercostals, and external intercostal muscles. They innervate the costal joints. Through lateral and anterior cutaneous branches, they innervate the skin covering the respective intercostal spaces as well as the parietal pleura lining the intercostal spaces.

Thoracoabdominal (Intercostals T6 to T11) Nerves

The T6 through T11 intercostal (thoracoabdominal) nerves begin as typical intercostal nerves but then send branches across the costal margin into the muscles of the anterior abdominal wall. These branches innervate the transverse abdominis, internal abdominal oblique, external abdominal oblique, and rectus abdominis muscles. In addition, they innervate the skin of the anterior wall in a metameric manner from the xiphoid process to the umbilicus.

Subcostal Nerve

The T12, or subcostal, nerve never enters an intercostal space. It travels through the abdominal wall, terminating between the umbilicus and the pubic symphysis. It innervates muscle and skin along its course.

Lumbosacral Plexus

The lumbosacral plexus innervates the muscles, joints, skin, and peritoneal lining of the abdominopelvic wall[11,12] (Tables 3–3 and 3–4). It also innervates the inferior extremities. It is formed by the ventral rami of L1 to S5 (Figures 3–14 and 3–15). The ventral rami join to form the terminal nerves. Between the L2 and S3 levels, the plexus is more complex. The ventral rami divide into anterior and posterior divisions that join to form the terminal nerves. The plexus is located in the posterior abdominal wall between the psoas major and quadratus lumborum muscles (see Figure 3-15).

Iliohypogastric Nerve

The iliohypogastric nerve arises from the ventral ramus of L1 and travels in the abdominal wall to the level of the pubic symphysis (see Figures 3-15 and 3-16). It innervates the muscle, skin, and parietal peritoneum along its course.

Ilioinguinal Nerve

The ilioinguinal nerve (see Figures 3-15 and 3-16) arises from the ventral rami of L1, travels in the abdominal wall, pierces in the posterior wall of the inguinal canal, passes through the superficial inguinal ring, and terminates on the anterior scrotum or labia majora. It innervates the muscle, skin, and parietal peritoneum along its course.

TABLE 3–3. Organization and distribution of the lumbar plexus.

Nerves(s)	Spinal Segments	Distribution
Iliohypogastric nerve	T12 to L1	Abdominal muscles (external and internal oblique muscles, transverse abdominis muscles); skin over inferior abdomen and buttocks
Ilioinguinal nerve	L1	Abdominal muscles (with iliohypogastric nerve); skin over superior, medial thigh and portions of external genitalia
Genitofemoral nerve	L1, L2	Skin over anteromedial surface of thigh and portions over genitalia
Lateral femoral cutaneous nerve	L2, L3	Skin over anterior, lateral, and posterior surfaces of thigh
Femoral nerve	L2 to L4	Anterior muscles of thigh (sartorius muscle and quadriceps group); adductor of thigh (pectineus and iliopsoas muscles); skin over anteromedial surface of thigh, medial surface of leg, and foot
Obturator nerve	L2 to L4	Adductors of thigh (adductors magnus, brevis, and longus); gracilis muscle; skin over medial surface of thigh
Saphenous nerve	L2 to L4	Skin over medial surface of leg

TABLE 3–4. Organization and distribution of the sacral plexus.

Nerves(s)	Spinal Segments	Distribution
Gluteal nerves:		
Superior inferior	L4 to S2	Abductors of thigh (gluteus minimus, gluteus medius, and tensor fasciae latae); extensor of thigh (gluteus maximus)
Posterior femoral cutaneous nerve	S1 to S3	Skin of perineum and posterior surface of thigh and leg
Sciatic nerve:	L4 to S3	Three of the hamstrings (semitendinosus and semimembranosus long head of biceps femoris); adductor magnus (with obturator nerve)
Tibial nerve		Flexor of knee and plantar flexors of ankle (popliteus, gastrocnemius, soleus plantaris, and tibialis posterior muscles and long head of biceps femoris muscle); flexors of toes; skin over posterior surface of leg, plantar surface of foot
Common peroneal nerve		Biceps femoris muscle (short head); fibularis (brevis and longus) and tibialis anterior muscles; extensors of toes, skin over anterior surface of leg and dorsal surface of foot; skin over lateral portion of foot (through the sural nerve)
Pudendal nerve	S2 to S4	Muscles of perineum, including urogenital diaphragm and external anal and urethral sphincter muscles; skin of external genitalia and related skeletal muscles (bulbospongiosus, ischiocavernosus muscles)

Genitofemoral Nerve

The genitofemoral nerve arises from the ventral rami from L1 and L2 (see Figure 3–15). It travels in the abdominal wall and passes through the deep inguinal ring into the inguinal canal. A femoral branch pierces the anterior wall of the canal and innervates the skin covering the femoral hiatus in the crural fascia. The genital branch passes through the superficial inguinal ring to innervate the skin on the scrotum or labia majora. En route, it innervates the cremaster muscle. Contraction of the cremaster elevates the scrotum.

Nerve to the Coccygeus and Levator Ani

The nerve to the coccygeus and levator ani muscles arises from the posterior division of the ventral rami at S3 to S4. It travels anteriorly onto the superior surface of the coccygeus and levator ani.

Pudendal Nerve

The pudendal nerve arises from the anterior division of the ventral rami from S2 to S4. It passes from the pelvis through the greater sciatic foramen into the gluteal region. It enters the gluteal region inferior to the piriformis muscle, passes posterior to the ischial spine, then enters the perineum by passing through the lesser sciatic foramen. It innervates the muscle and skin of the perineum, anal canal and external anal sphincter.

Superior Gluteal Nerve

The superior gluteal nerve arises from the posterior division of the ventral rami at L4 to S1. It passes from the pelvis through the greater sciatic foramen to the gluteal region. It enters the gluteal region superior to the piriformis muscle, passes in the plane between gluteal medius and minimus muscles,

and terminates in the tensor fascia lata muscle. En route, it innervates the gluteus medius and minimus muscles as well as the tensor fascia lata.

Inferior Gluteal Nerve

The inferior gluteal nerve arises from the posterior division of the ventral rami at L5 to S2. It passes from the pelvis through the greater sciatic foramen into the gluteal region. It enters the gluteal region inferior to the piriformis muscle and terminates on the deep surface of the gluteal maximus muscle, which it innervates.

Nerve to Piriformis

The nerve to piriformis arises from the posterior division of the ventral rami at S1 to S2 and passes onto the deep surface of the piriformis muscle, which it innervates.

Nerve to Obturator Internus and Superior Gemellus

The nerve to the obturator internus and superior gemellus muscles arises from the anterior division of the ventral rami at L5 and S1. It passes from the pelvis through the greater sciatic foramen into the gluteal region. In enters the gluteal region inferior to the piriformis muscle and passes along the deep surface of the superior gemellus to the obturator internus, innervating these last two muscles.

Nerve to the Quadratus Femoris and Inferior Gemellus

The nerve to the quadratus femoris and inferior gemellus muscles arises from the anterior division of the ventral rami at L4 to L5. It passes from the pelvis through the greater sciatic foramen to the gluteal region and enters the gluteal region

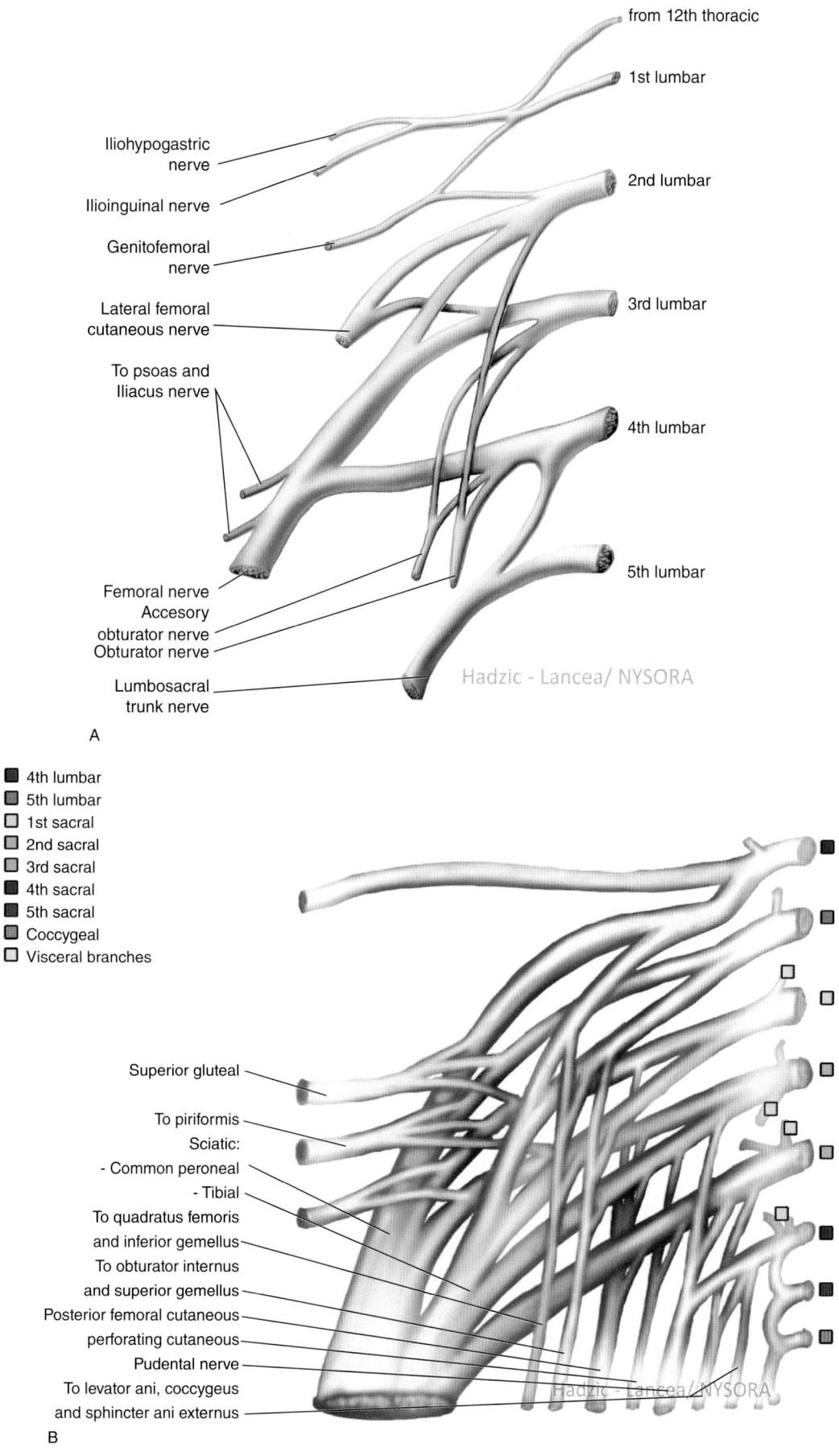

from 12th thoracic

1st lumbar

Iliohypogastric
nerve

2nd lumbar

Ilioinguinal nerve

Genitofemoral
nerve

3rd lumbar

Lateral femoral
cutaneous nerve

To psoas and
Iliacus nerve

4th lumbar

5th lumbar

Femoral nerve
Accesory
obturator nerve
Obturator nerve

Lumbosacral
trunk nerve

Hadzic - Lancea/ NYSORA

A

◼ 4th lumbar
◼ 5th lumbar
☐ 1st sacral
◻ 2nd sacral
◻ 3rd sacral
◼ 4th sacral
▦ 5th sacral
▦ Coccygeal
☐ Visceral branches

Superior gluteal

To piriformis
Sciatic:
- Common peroneal
- Tibial
To quadratus femoris
and inferior gemellus
To obturator internus
and superior gemellus
Posterior femoral cutaneous
perforating cutaneous
Pudental nerve
To levator ani, coccygeus
and sphincter ani externus

Hadzic - Lancea/ NYSORA

B

FIGURE 3–14. A, B: Organization schema of the lumbar and sacral plexuses.

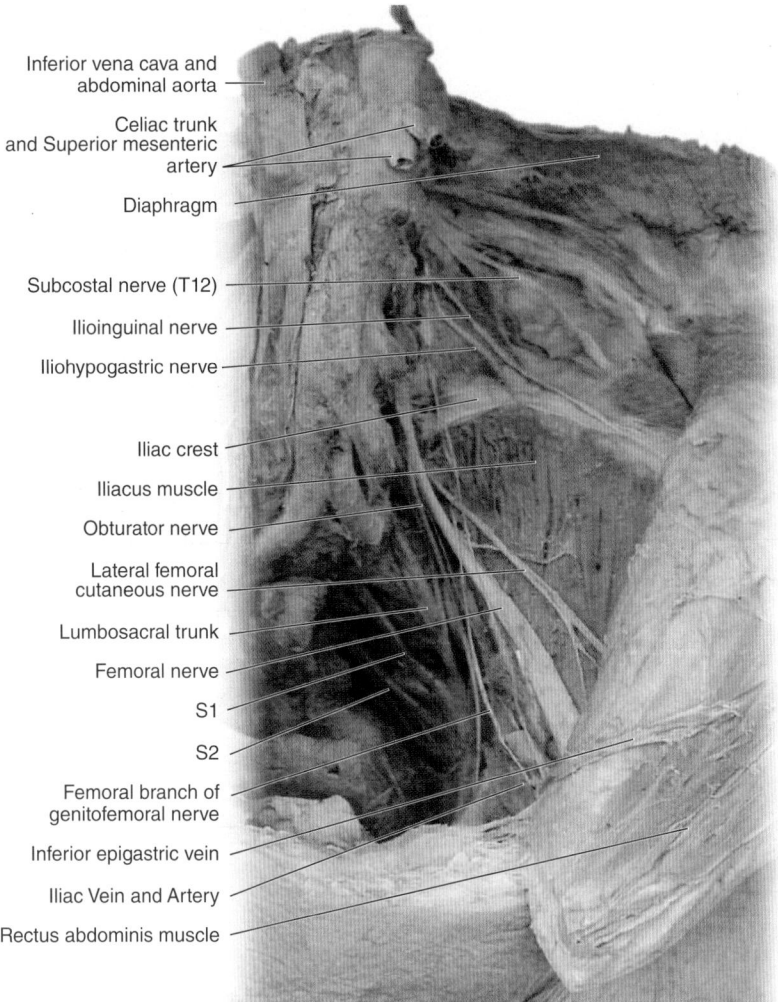

Inferior vena cava and abdominal aorta

Celiac trunk and Superior mesenteric artery

Diaphragm

Subcostal nerve (T12)

Ilioinguinal nerve

Iliohypogastric nerve

Iliac crest

Iliacus muscle

Obturator nerve

Lateral femoral cutaneous nerve

Lumbosacral trunk

Femoral nerve

S1

S2

Femoral branch of genitofemoral nerve

Inferior epigastric vein

Iliac Vein and Artery

Rectus abdominis muscle

FIGURE 3–15. Dissection of the lumbosacral plexus.

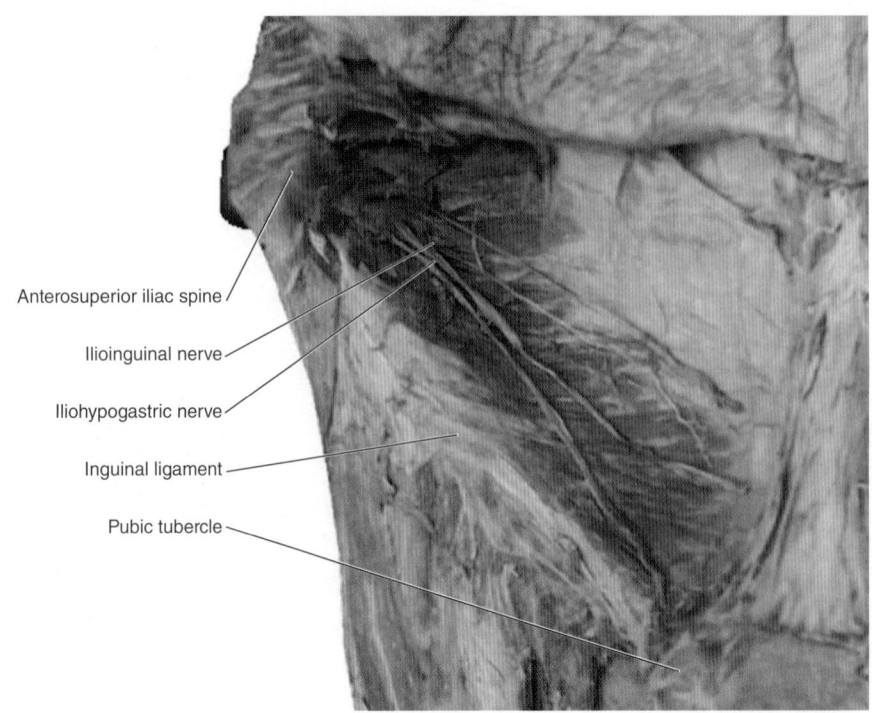

Anterosuperior iliac spine

Ilioinguinal nerve

Iliohypogastric nerve

Inguinal ligament

Pubic tubercle

FIGURE 3–16. Dissection of Ilioinguinal and iliohypogastric nerves.

inferior to piriformis, passing deep to the obturator internus to terminate innervating the inferior gemellus and quadratus femoris, as indicated by its name.

Lateral Femoral Cutaneous Nerve

The lateral femoral cutaneous nerve arises from the posterior divisions of the ventral rami at L2 to L3. It descends the posterior abdominal wall and crosses the iliac crest into the pelvis, where it descends on the iliacus muscle, passes deep to the inguinal ligament at the anterior iliac spine, and distributes cutaneous innervation on the lateral aspect of the thigh to the level of the knee (Figure 3–17).

Posterior Femoral Cutaneous Nerve

The posterior femoral cutaneous nerve arises from the anterior and posterior divisions of the ventral rami at S1 to S3. It passes from the pelvis through the greater sciatic foramen into the gluteal region. It enters the gluteal region inferior to the piriformis muscle, descends in the muscle plane between the gluteus maximus posteriorly and oburator internus anteriorly, and passes into the posterior thigh, where it supplies cutaneous innervation from the hip to the midcalf.[4]

Obturator Nerve

The obturator nerve (Box 3–6) arises from the anterior division of the ventral rami at L2 to L4 (Figure 3–18). It descends through the pelvis medial to the psoas major muscle, crosses the superior pubic ramus inferiorly, and passes through the obturator foramen into the medial compartment of the thigh, where it divides into posterior and anterior branches (see Figure 3–18). The posterior branch descends superficial to the adductor magnus muscle, which it innervates. The anterior branch passes superficial to the obturator externus muscle, descends the thigh in the muscle plane between the adductor brevis and adductor longus, and terminates in the gracilis muscle. En route, it innervates all of these muscles. Furthermore, it provides articular branches to the hip and cutaneous branches to the skin covering the medial thigh.

Femoral Nerve

The femoral nerve arises from the posterior division of the ventral rami at L2 to L4 (Box 3–7). It descends through the pelvis lateral to the psoas major muscle, passes deep to the inguinal ligament, and enters the anterior compartment of the thigh, where it divides into multiple branches supplying the muscle,

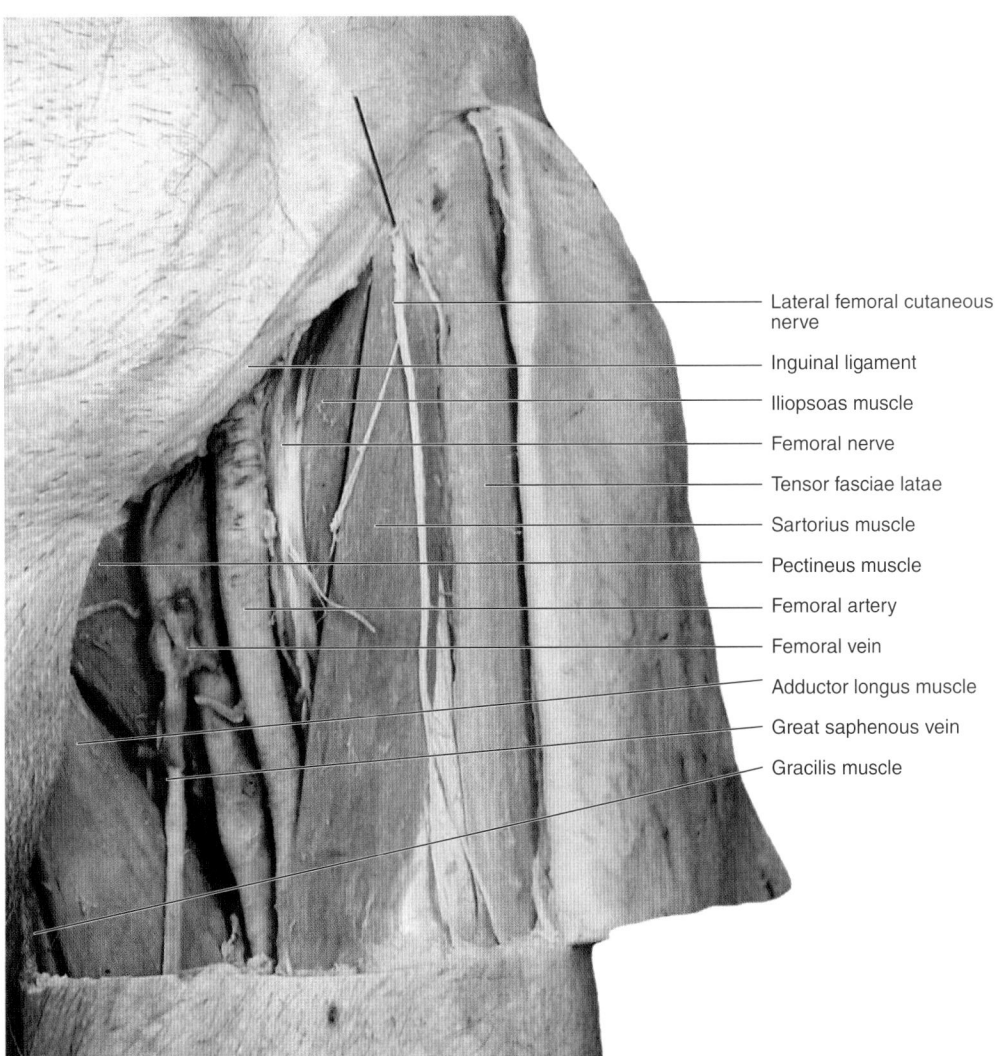

- Lateral femoral cutaneous nerve
- Inguinal ligament
- Iliopsoas muscle
- Femoral nerve
- Tensor fasciae latae
- Sartorius muscle
- Pectineus muscle
- Femoral artery
- Femoral vein
- Adductor longus muscle
- Great saphenous vein
- Gracilis muscle

FIGURE 3–17. Dissection of femoral triangle and laterofemoral cutaneous nerve.

BOX 3–6. Obturator nerve.

Muscular branches
- Adduction of hip
  - Adductor magnus, longus, and brevis
  - Gracilis
- Flexion of hip
  - Adductor magnus (anterior fibers)
  - Adductor longus and brevis
- Extension of hip
  - Adductor magnus (posterior fibers)

Articular branches
- Hip

Cutaneous branches
- Medial femoral cutaneous branches

joints, and skin in that region. In the femoral triangle–inguinal crease, the nerve is positioned lateral to the femoral artery and vein (mnemonic: NAVEL) (Figure 3–19). Muscular branches innervate the iliacus, psoas major, pectineus, rectus femoris, vastus lateralis, vastus intermedius, vastus medialis, and sartorius muscles. Articular branches innervate the hip and knee.[13]

Of note, the femoral nerve below the inguinal ligament consists of an anterior and a posterior part. The anterior part contains branches to the sartorius muscle and cutaneous branches of the anterior thigh, and the posterior contains the saphenous nerve (most medial part) and branches to the individual heads of the quadriceps muscle.[14]

Saphenous Nerve and Other Cutaneous Branches of the Femoral Nerve

The superficial branches of the femoral nerve supply the skin covering the anterior thigh. One cutaneous branch follows the deep surface of the sartorius muscle to its attachment on the tibia. Here, it passes onto the skin, providing innervation of the medial leg from the knee to the arch of the foot. En route, the nerve is accompanied by the saphenous vein, so it is called the saphenous branch of the femoral nerve (see Figure 3–19). As previously mentioned, the saphenous nerve is the most medial part of the femoral nerve at the inguinal (femoral) crease.[14]

Sciatic Nerve

The sciatic nerve is formed by the junction of the tibial and common peroneal nerves (Box 3–8). The tibial nerve arises from the anterior division of the ventral rami at L4 to S3 (see

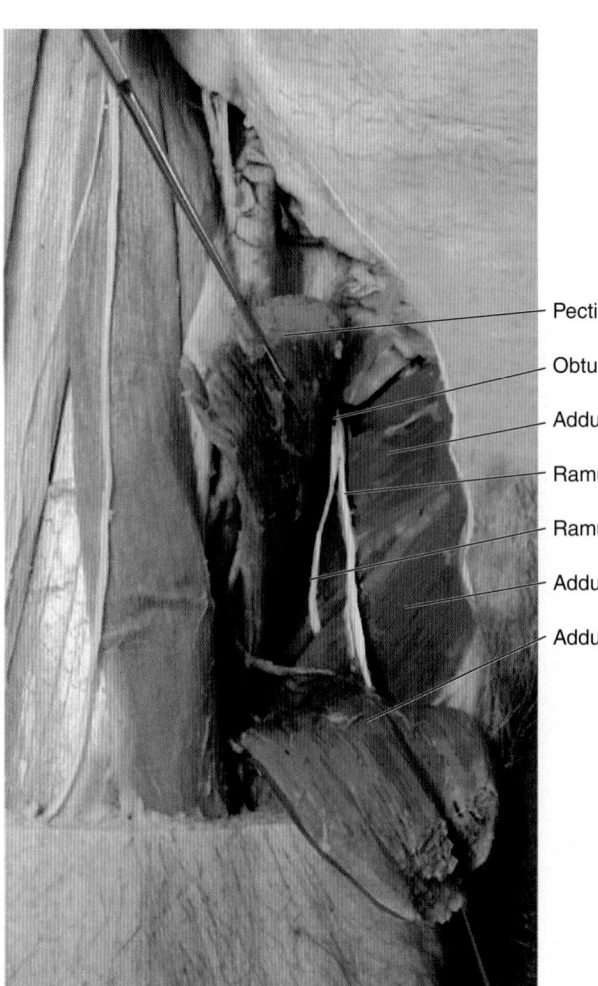

— Pectineus muscle
— Obturator nerve
— Adductor magnus muscle
— Ramus anterior
— Ramus posterior
— Adductor brevis muscle
— Adductor longus muscle

FIGURE 3–18. Anatomy of the obturator nerve.

BOX 3–7. Femoral nerve.

Muscular branches

- Flexion of hip
  - Iliacus
  - Psoas major
  - Pectineus
  - Rectus femoris
  - Sartorius
- Lateral rotation of hip
  - Sartorius
- Extension of knee
  - Rectus femoris
  - Vastus lateralis
  - Vastus intermedius
  - Vastus medialis
- Flexion of knee
  - Sartorius

Articular branches

- Hip
- Knee

Cutaneous branches

- Anterior femoral cutaneous nerves
- Saphenous branch of the femoral nerve

Figure 3–14). The common peroneal nerve arises from the posterior division of the ventral rami at L4 to S2. The sciatic nerve passes from the pelvis through the greater sciatic foramen into the gluteal region. It enters the gluteal region inferior to the piriformis muscle, descends in the muscle plane between the gluteus maximus posteriorly and the obturator internus anteriorly, and passes lateral to the ischial tuberosity to enter the posterior thigh (Figure 3–20). In the posterior thigh, it passes between the adductor magnus and the long head of the biceps femoris. It descends in the groove between the biceps femoris medially and the semitendinosus and semimembranosus laterally. En route, it innervates the adductor magnus, biceps femoris, semitendinosus, and semimembranosus muscles.[15] Posterior to the knee, the sciatic nerve descends into the popliteal fossa, where it diverges into the tibial and common peroneal nerves (Figure 3–21).[16]

Of note, these two branches are distinct from the onset and travel together enveloped in the same tissue sheath.[17] The tibial nerves exits the popliteal fossa passing between the heads of the gastrocnemius muscle into the superficial posterior compartment of the leg. Here, it descends deep to the plantaris and superficial to popliteus muscles. It passes between the tibial and fibular heads of the soleus muscle to enter the deep posterior compartment. The nerve passes posterior to the medial malleolus, where it enters the foot and divides into medial and lateral plantar

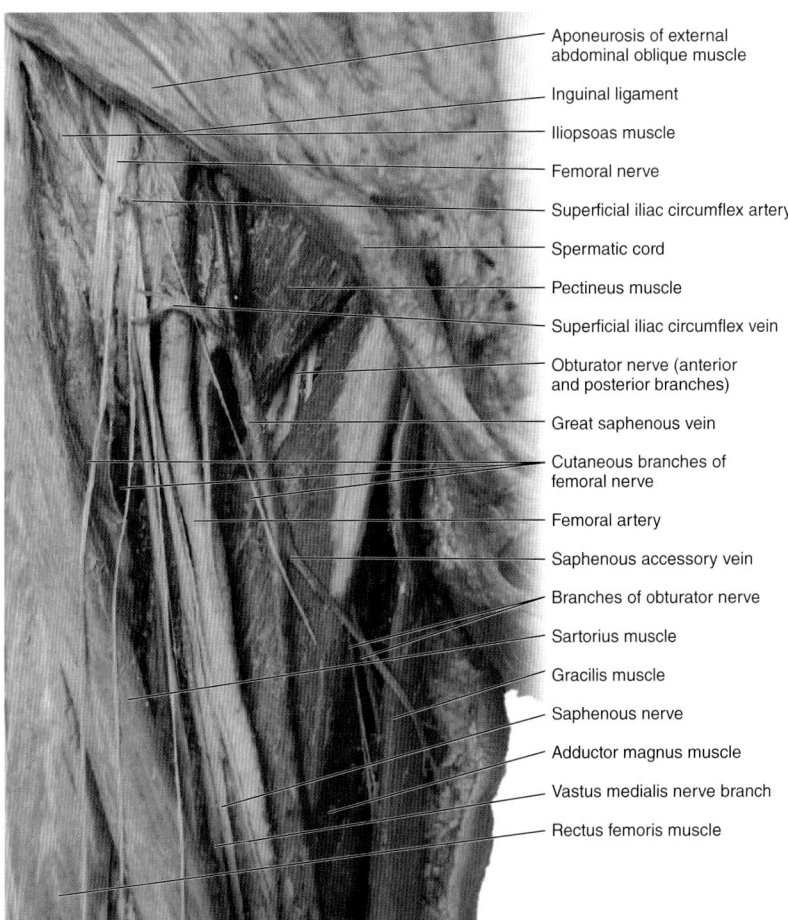

Aponeurosis of external abdominal oblique muscle

Inguinal ligament

Iliopsoas muscle

Femoral nerve

Superficial iliac circumflex artery

Spermatic cord

Pectineus muscle

Superficial iliac circumflex vein

Obturator nerve (anterior and posterior branches)

Great saphenous vein

Cutaneous branches of femoral nerve

Femoral artery

Saphenous accessory vein

Branches of obturator nerve

Sartorius muscle

Gracilis muscle

Saphenous nerve

Adductor magnus muscle

Vastus medialis nerve branch

Rectus femoris muscle

FIGURE 3–19. Anatomy of the femoral triangle.

BOX 3–8. Sciatic nerve.

Muscular branches
- Extension of hip—sciatic nerve
  - Biceps femoris—long head
- Flexion of knee—sciatic nerve
  - Biceps femoris—long and short heads
  - Semimembranosus
  - Semitendinosus
  - Popliteus—tibial division only
  - Gastrocnemius—tibial division only
- Plantar flexion of ankle—tibial nerve
  - Soleus
  - Gastrocnemius
  - Tibialis posterior
  - Flexor digitorum longus
  - Flexor hallucis longus
  - Peroneus longus and brevis—superficial peroneal nerve
- Dorsiflexion of ankle—deep peroneal nerve
  - Tibialis anterior
  - Extensor digitorum longus
  - Extensor hallucis longus
- Inversion of ankle—deep peroneal nerve
  - Tibialis anterior
- Eversion of ankle—superficial peroneal nerve
  - Peroneus longus and brevis

- Adduction of toes—tibial nerve
  - Plantar interosseus muscles
- Abduction of toes—tibial nerve
  - Dorsal interosseous muscles
  - Abductor hallucis
  - Abductor digiti minimi
- Flexion of toes—tibial nerve
  - Flexor digitorum longus and brevis
  - Flexor hallucis longus and brevis
- Extension of toes—deep peroneal nerve
  - Extensor digitorum longus and brevis
  - Extensor hallucis longus and brevis

Articular branches
- Knee
- Ankle
- Foot—all joints

Cutaneous branches
- Superficial peroneal
- Sural
- Calcaneal branches—medial and lateral
- Plantar nerves—medial and lateral

nerves that innervate the muscle and skin on the plantar surface of the foot. The common peroneal nerve follows the tendon of the biceps femoris to its attachment on the fibula. The nerve passes inferior to the neck of the fibula and divides into superficial and deep branches. The superficial branch enters the lateral compartment of the leg, where it innervates the peroneus longus and brevis muscles. The nerve terminates as cutaneous fibers on the dorsal and lateral surfaces of the foot. The deep peroneal nerve enters the anterior compartment of the leg, where it innervates the tibialis anterior, extensor digitorum longus, and extensor hallucis longus muscles. It crosses the anterior surface of the ankle into the foot, where it innervates the extensor digitorum brevis and extensor hallucis brevis muscles. It terminates as cutaneous fibers supplying skin between the hallux and second toe.[18]

SENSORY INNERVATION OF THE MAJOR JOINTS

Much of the practice of peripheral nerve blocks involves orthopedic and other joint surgery. Consequently, knowledge of the sensory innervation of the major joints is important for better understanding the neuronal components that need to be anesthetized to achieve anesthesia for, or analgesia, after joint surgery. Tables 3–5 and 3–6 summarize the sensory innervation of the major joints of the upper and lower extremities, respectively. Tables 3–7 and 3–8 summarize the innervation and kinetic function of the major muscle groups of the upper and lower extremities respectively.

Shoulder Joint

Innervation to the shoulder joints stems mostly from the axillary and suprascapular nerves (C5–C7). The skin over most medial parts of the shoulder receives nerves from the cervical plexus (see Figure 3-10). Such an arrangement explains why a brachial plexus block at the interscalene level is the most appropriate technique to achieve anesthesia to the shoulder (Figure 3–22).

Elbow Joint

Nerve supply to the elbow joint includes branches of all major nerves of the brachial plexus that cross the joint: musculocutaneous, radial, median, and ulnar nerves (Figure 3–23).

Wrist Joint

The wrist joint is supplied by the radial, ulnar, and median nerves (Figure 3–24), including interosseous branches of the radial and median nerves diverging at the proximal forearm. The cutaneous branches of these nerves, in addition to the antebrachial medial cutaneous and lateral cutaneous nerves, display frequent variations and connections among them at different levels, resulting in overlapping innervation areas.

Hip Joint

Nerves to the hip joint include the nerve to the rectus femoris from the femoral nerve, branches from the anterior division of the obturator nerve, and the nerve to the quadratus femoris from the sacral plexus (Figure 3–25).

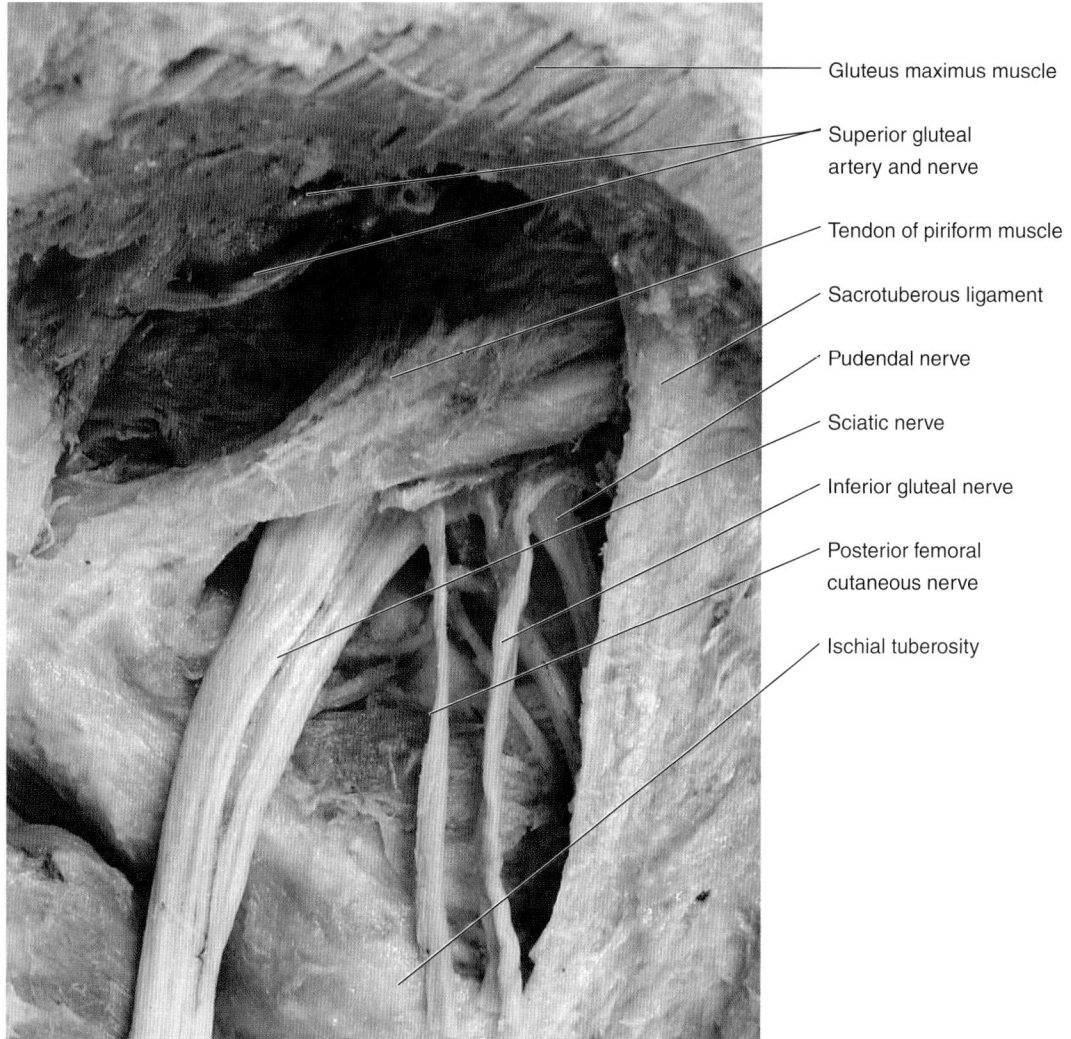

Gluteus maximus muscle

Superior gluteal artery and nerve

Tendon of piriform muscle

Sacrotuberous ligament

Pudendal nerve

Sciatic nerve

Inferior gluteal nerve

Posterior femoral cutaneous nerve

Ischial tuberosity

FIGURE 3–20. Anatomy of the sciatic nerve at gluteal level.

Knee Joint

Knee innervation is obtained from branches from the femoral, obturator, and sciatic nerves (Figure 3–26). The femoral nerve suplies the anterior aspect of the joint. Articular branches from the tibial and common peroneal divisions of the sciatic nerve innervate the posterior aspect, while fibers from the posterior division of the obturator nerve may contribute to the innervation of the medial aspect of the joint, together with fibers from the posterior division of the obturator nerve, may also contribute to the innervation of the joint.

Ankle Joint

The innervation of the ankle joint is complex and involves the terminal branches of the peroneal (deep and superficial peroneal nerves), tibial (posterior tibial nerve), and femoral nerves (saphenous nerve). A more simplistic view is that the entire innervation of the ankle joint stems from the sciatic nerve, with the exception of the skin on the medial aspect around the medial malleolus (saphenous nerve, a branch of the femoral nerve; Figure 3–27).

AUTONOMIC COMPONENT OF SPINAL NERVES

All spinal nerves transmit autonomic fibers to glands and smooth muscle in the region they innervate. The autonomic fibers are sympathetic. There are no parasympathetic fibers in spinal nerves. Sympathetic fibers originate in the spinal cord between T1 and L2. They pass from the spinal cord through the ventral roots of the T1 to L2 spinal nerves. They depart from the spinal nerve through white rami communicans to enter the sympathetic trunk. The sympathetic trunk is formed by a series of interconnected paravertebral ganglia, which are adjacent to the vertebral bodies and extend from the axis (C2 vertebra) to the sacrum. The preganglionic fibers synapse on cell bodies of neurons forming the paravertebral ganglia. The axons of the paravertebral ganglia (postganglionic fibers) can remain at the same level or they can change level by ascending or descending the trunk. The fibers pass from the trunk through gray rami communicans to spinal nerves. The sympathetic trunk sends a gray ramus to every spinal nerve. The sympathetic nerves travel along branches of the spinal nerve to the target destination[19] (Figure 3–28).

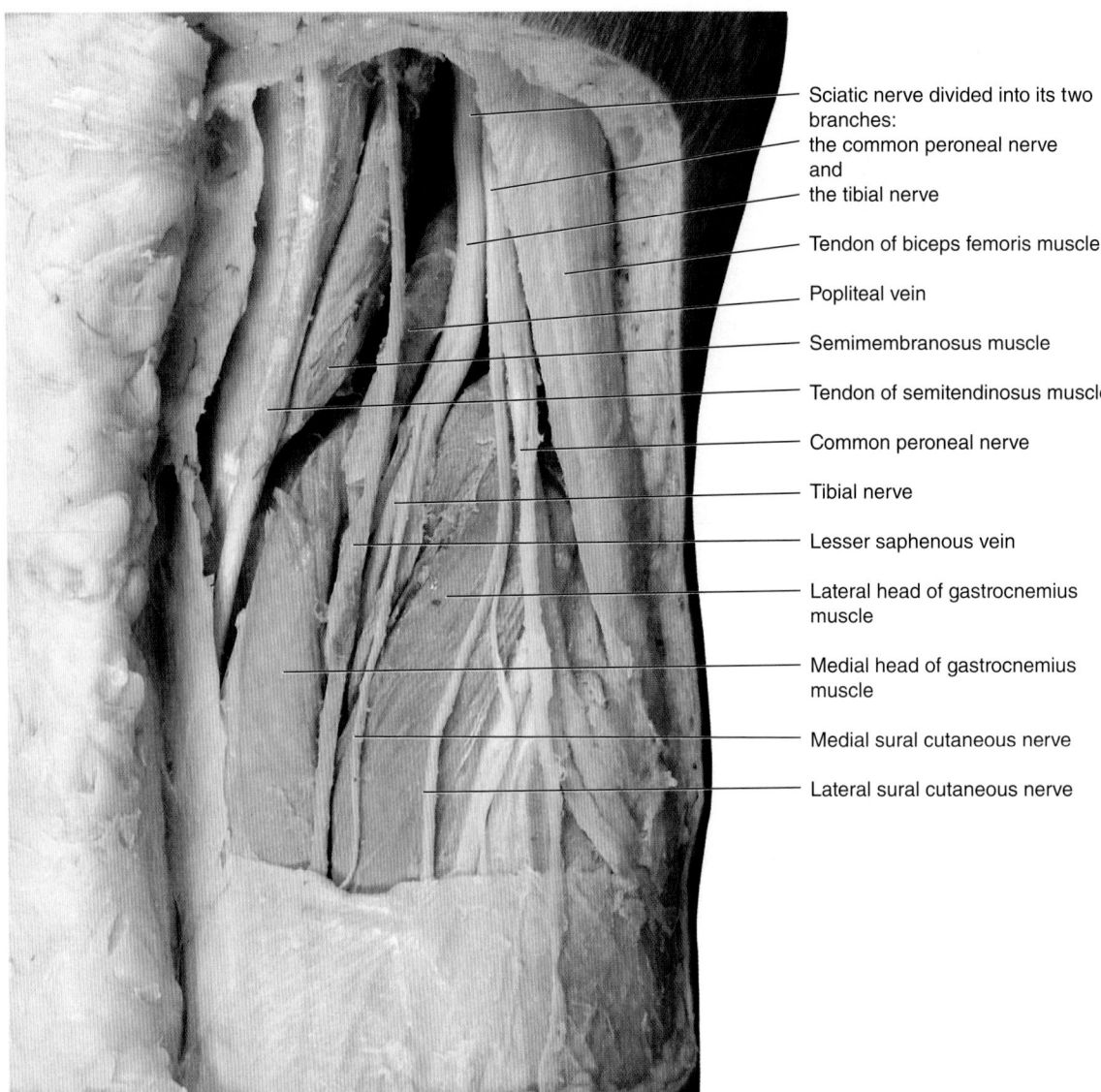

- Sciatic nerve divided into its two branches:
- the common peroneal nerve
- and
- the tibial nerve
- Tendon of biceps femoris muscle
- Popliteal vein
- Semimembranosus muscle
- Tendon of semitendinosus muscle
- Common peroneal nerve
- Tibial nerve
- Lesser saphenous vein
- Lateral head of gastrocnemius muscle
- Medial head of gastrocnemius muscle
- Medial sural cutaneous nerve
- Lateral sural cutaneous nerve

FIGURE 3–21. Anatomy of the sciatic nerve at the popliteal fossa.

TABLE 3–5. Innervation of joints in the superior extremity.

Joint	Innervation
Sternoclavicular	Medial supraclavicular, nerve to subclavius
Acromioclavicular	Axillary, lateral pectoral, lateral supraclavicular
Shoulder (glenohumeral)	Axillary, suprascapular, lateral pectoral
Elbow (humeroulnar, humeroradial)	Radial, musculocutaneous, ulnar
Radioulnar—proximal and distal	Median, radial, musculocutaneous
Wrist (radiocarpal, ulnocarpal)	Median, ulnar, radial
Intercarpal	Median, ulnar
Carpometacarpal	Median, ulnar, radial
Knuckle (metacarpophalangeal)	Median, ulnar
Interphalangeal—proximal and distal	Median, ulnar
Interphalangeal joint of the thumb	Median

TABLE 3–6. Innervation of joints of the inferior extremity.

Joint	Innervation
Hip (acetabulofemoral)	Femoral, obturator, superior gluteal, nerve to quadratus femoris and inferior gemellus
Knee (tibiofemoral)	Sciatic, femoral, obturator
Ankle (tibiotalar, talocalcaneal)	Tibial, deep peroneal
Metatarsophalangeal	Tibial
Interphalangeal	Tibial

TABLE 3–7. Summary of movement by joint—upper extremity.

Shoulder (Glenohumeral) Joint

Flexion	Biceps brachii—long head	Musculocutaneous nerve
	Coracobrachialis	
	Deltoid	Axillary nerve
	Pectoralis major	Medial and lateral pectoral nerve
Extension	Triceps brachii—long head	Radial nerve
	Latissimus dorsi	Thoracodorsal nerve
	Deltoid	Axillary nerve
Adduction	Latissimus dorsi	Thoracodorsal nerve
	Pectoralis major	Medial and lateral pectoral nerves
	Teres major	Lower subscapular nerve
	Subscapularis	Upper and lower subscapular nerve
Abduction	Supraspinatus	Suprascapular nerve
	Deltoid	Axillary nerve
Medial rotation	Pectoralis major	Medial and lateral pectoral nerve
	Latissimus dorsi	Thoracodorsal nerve
	Teres major	Lower subscapular nerve
	Subscapularis	Upper and lower subscapular nerves
Lateral rotation	Teres minor	Axillary nerve
	Infraspinatus	Suprascapular nerve

Elbow (Humeroulnar, Humeroradial) Joint

Flexion	Brachialis	Musculocutaneous
	Biceps brachii—long and short heads	
	Flexor carpi radialis	Median nerve
Extension	Triceps brachii—long lateral, medial head anconeus	Radial nerve

Radioulnar Joints

Supination	Biceps brachii—long and short head	Musculocutaneous
	Supinator	Radial nerve

(continued)

TABLE 3-7. Summary of movement by joint—upper extremity. *(Continued)*

Pronation	Pronator teres	Median nerve
	Pronator quadratus	

Wrist (Radiocarpal, Ulnocarpal) Joint

Flexion	Flexor carpi radialis	Median nerve
	Palmaris longus	
	Flexors of fingers listed below	
	Flexor carpi ulnaris	Ulnar nerve
Extension	Extensor carpi radialis longus and brevis	Radial nerve
	Extensors of fingers listed next	
	Extensor carpi ulnaris	

Carpometacarpal Joints

Opposition	Opponen pollicis	Median nerve
	Opponens digiti minimi	Ulnar nerve

Metacarpophalangeal Joints

Flexion	Flexor digitorum superficialis	Median nerve
	Flexor digitorum profundus	Median and ulnar nerves
	Flexor pollicis longus and brevis	Median nerve
	Interosseus	Ulnar nerve
	Lumbricals	Median and ulnar nerves
Extension	Extensor digitorum communis	Radial nerve
	Extensor indicis	
	Extensor digiti minimi	
Adduction	Palmar interosseous	Ulnar nerve
	Abductor pollicis	
Abduction	Dorsal interosseous	Ulnar nerve
	Abductor digiti minimi	
	Abductor pollicis longus	Radial nerve
	Abductor pollicis brevis	Median nerve

Interphalangeal Joints

Flexion	Flexor digitorum superficialis	Median nerve
	Flexor digitorum profundus	Median and ulnar nerves
	Flexor pollicis longus and brevis	Median nerve
Extension	Extensor digitorum communis	Radial nerve
	Extensor indicis	
	Extensor digiti minimi	
	Lumbricals (index, middle fingers)	Median nerve
	Lumbricals (ring, little fingers)	Ulnar nerve
	Interosseous muscles	

TABLE 3–8. Summary of movement by joints—lower extremity.

Hip (Acetabulofemoral) Joint

Flexion	Iliacus/psoas major	Femoral nerve
	Pectineus	
	Rectus femoris	
	Sartorius	
	Adductor magnus	Obturator nerve
	Adductor longus and brevis	
	Tensor fascia lata	Superior gluteal nerve
Extension	Biceps femoris—long head	Sciatic nerve
	Semimembranosis	
	Semitendinosis	
	Gluteus maximus	Inferior gluteal nerve
	Adductor magnus	Obturator nerve
Adduction	Adduct magnus, longus, brevis	Obturator nerve
	Gracilis	
	Pectineus	Femoral nerve
Abduction	Gluteus minimus	Superior gluteal nerve
	Gluteus medius	
	Tensor fascia lata	
Medial rotation	Gluteus minimus	Superior gluteal nerve
	Gluteus medius	
	Tensor fascia lata	
Lateral rotation	Piriformis	Nerve to piriformis
	Obturator internus	Nerve to obturator internus
	Superior gemelli	Nerve to obturator internus
	Inferior gemelli	Nerve to quadratus femoris
	Quadratus femoris	Nerve to quadratus femoris
	Sartorius	Femoral nerve

Knee (Tibiofemoral) Joint

Flexion	Bicep femoris—long and short heads	Sciatic nerve
	Semitendinosis	
	Semimembranosis	
	Popliteus	Tibial nerve
	Gastrocnemius	
	Sartorius	Femoral nerve
Extension	Rectus femoris	Femoral nerve
	Vastus lateralis	
	Vastus intermedius	
	Vastus medialis	

(continued)

TABLE 3–8. Summary of movement by joints—lower extremity. (*Continued*)

Medial rotation	Popliteus	Tibial nerve
	Semimembranosis	Sciatic nerve
	Semitendinosis	
Lateral rotation	Biceps femoris	Sciatic nerve
Ankle (Talocrural) Joint		
Plantarflexion	Soleus	Tibial nerve
	Gastronemius	
	Tibialis posterior	
	Flexor digitorum longus	
	Flexor hallucis longus	
	Peroneus longus and brevis	Superficial peroneal nerve
Dorsiflexion	Tibialis anterior	Deep peroneal nerve
	Extensor digitorum	
	Extensor hallucis longus	
Subtalar Joint		
Inversion	Tibialis anterior	Deep peroneal nerve
Eversion	Peroneus longus and brevis	Superficial peroneal nerve
Metatarsophalangeal Joints		
Flexion	Flexor digitorum longus and brevis	Tibial nerve
	Flexor hallucis longus and brevis	
	Flexor digiti minimi	
	Lumbricals	
	Interosseous muscles	
Extension	Extensor digitorum longus and brevis	Deep peroneal nerve
	Extensor hallucis longus and brevis	
Adduction	Plantar interosseous muscles	Tibial nerve
	Adductor hallucis	
Abduction	Dorsal interosseous	Tibial nerve
	Abductor hallucis	
	Abductor digiti minimi	
Interphalangeal Joints		
Flexion	Flexor digitorum longus and brevis	Tibial nerve
	Flexor hallucis longus and brevis	
Extension	Extensor digitorum longus and brevis	Deep peroneal nerve
	Extensor hallucis longus and brevis	
	Lumbricals	Tibial nerve
	Interosseous muscles	

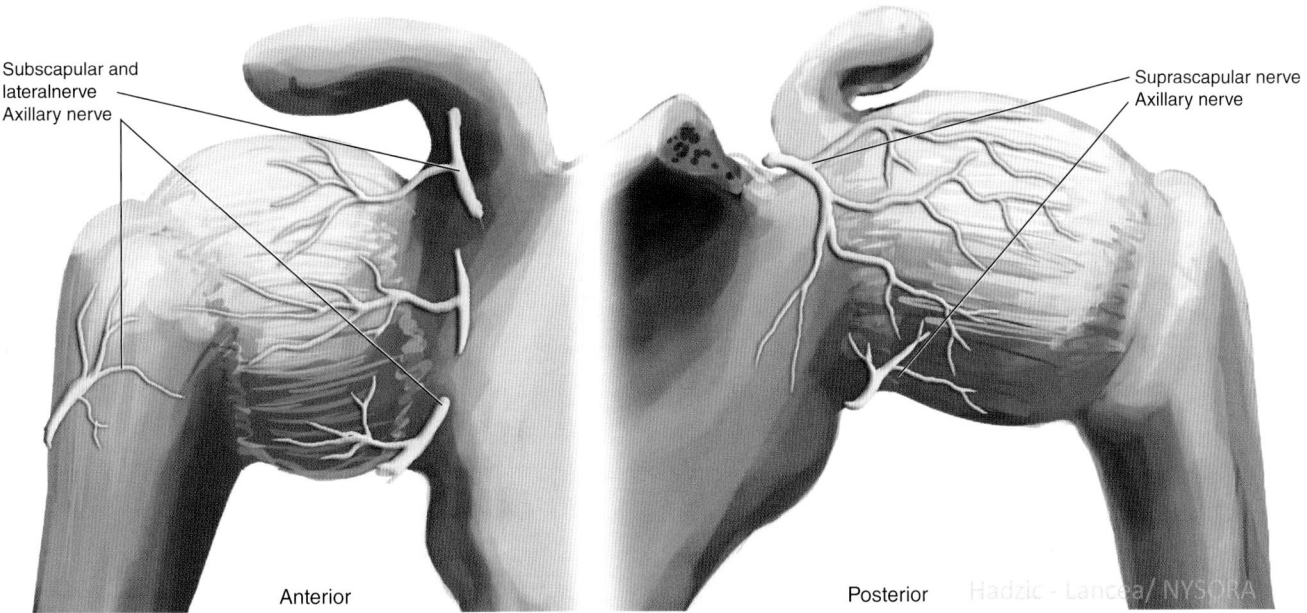

FIGURE 3-22. Shoulder joint: sensory innervation.

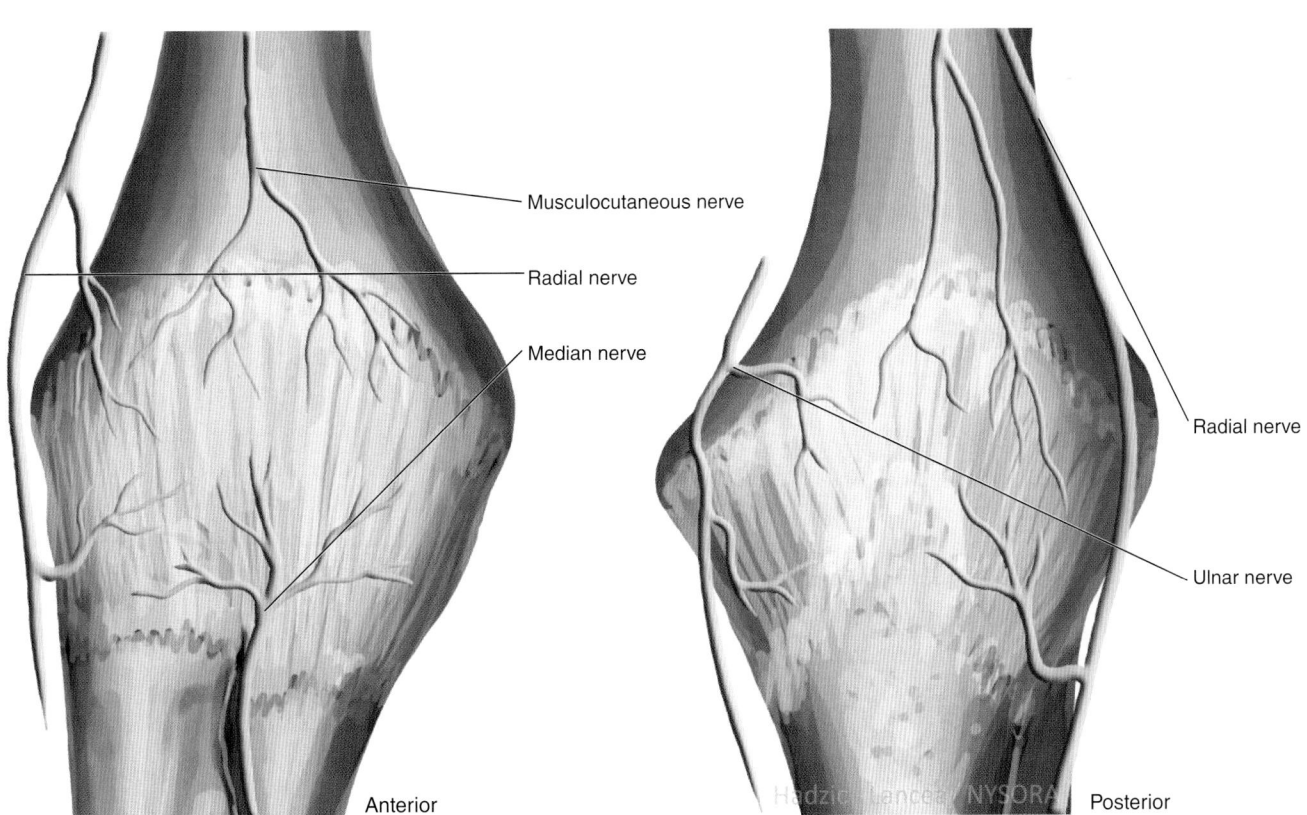

FIGURE 3-23. Elbow joint: sensory innervation.

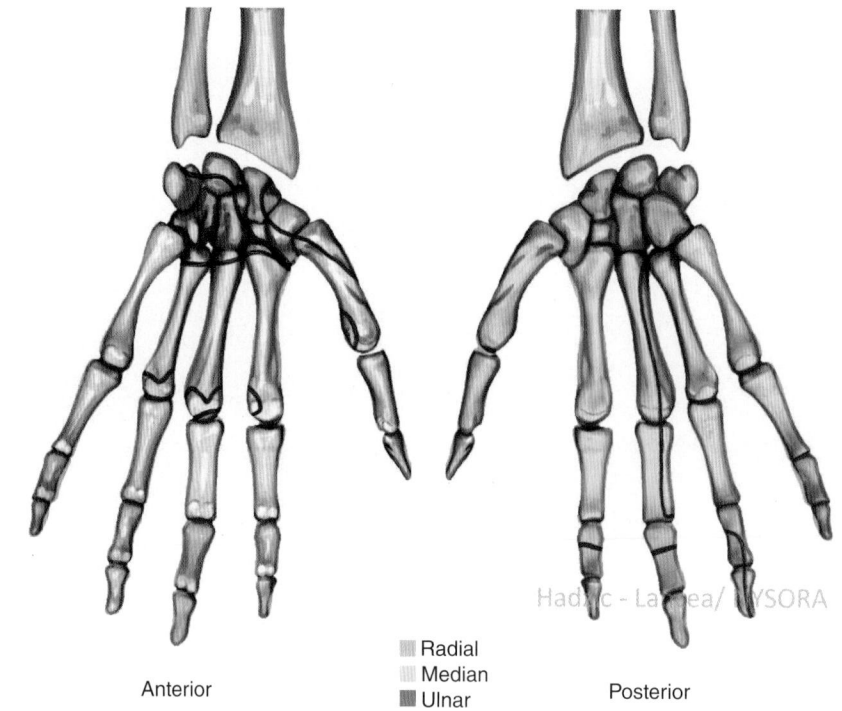

Radial
Median
Ulnar

Anterior   Posterior

FIGURE 3-24. Innervation of the wrist joint.

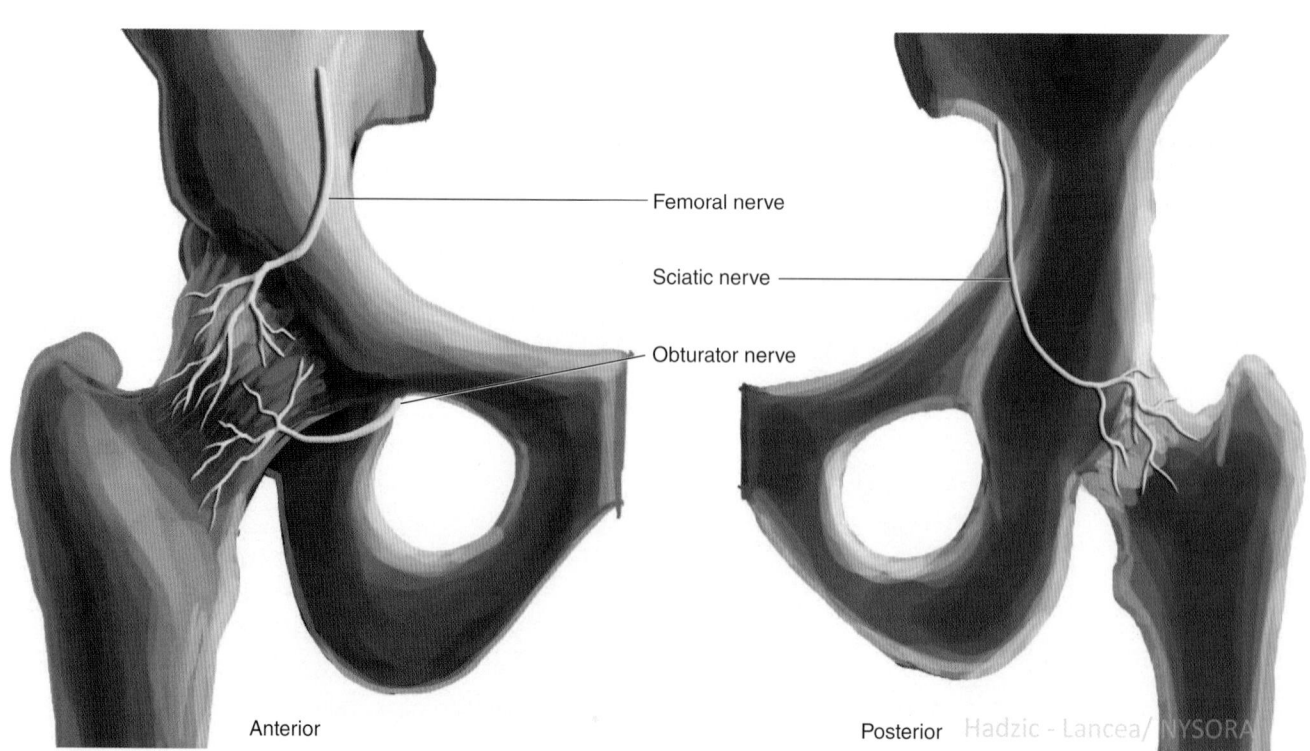

Femoral nerve

Sciatic nerve

Obturator nerve

Anterior   Posterior

FIGURE 3-25. Hip joint: sensory innervation.

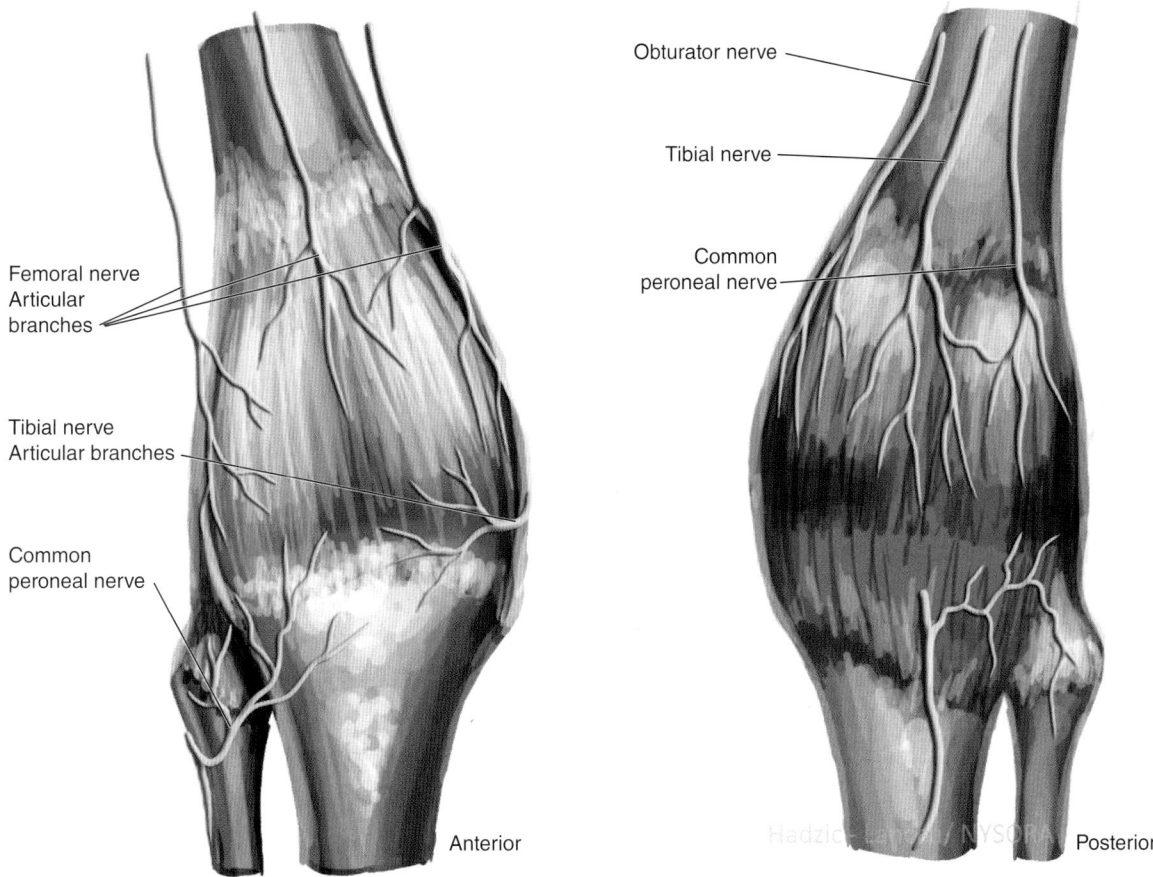

FIGURE 3–26. Knee joint: sensory innervation.

Parasympathetic fibers arise from the lumbosacral plexus. They originate in the spinal cord between S2 and S4, pass through the ventral roots, and enter the ventral rami of the S2 to S4 spinal nerves. The parasympathetic fibers separate from the ventral rami and form the pelvic splanchnic nerve. This nerve travels across the pelvic diaphragm (formed by levator ani and coccygeus muscles) to synapse on intramural ganglia in the wall of the pelvic viscera.[20,21]

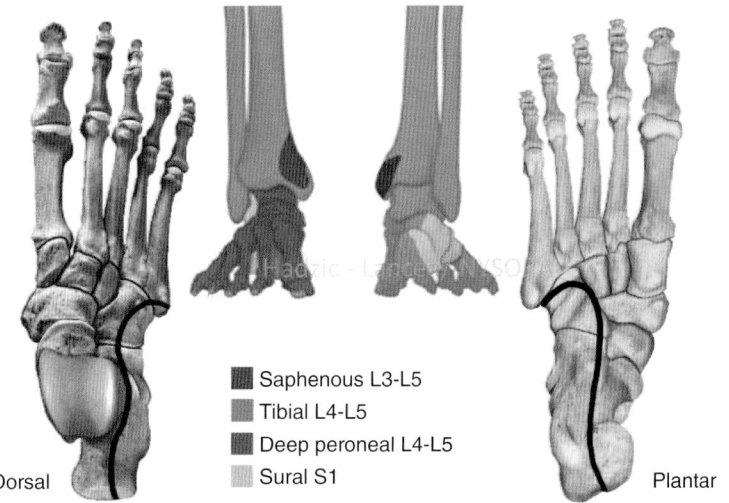

Saphenous L3-L5
Tibial L4-L5
Deep peroneal L4-L5
Sural S1

FIGURE 3–27. Innervation of joints in ankle and foot.

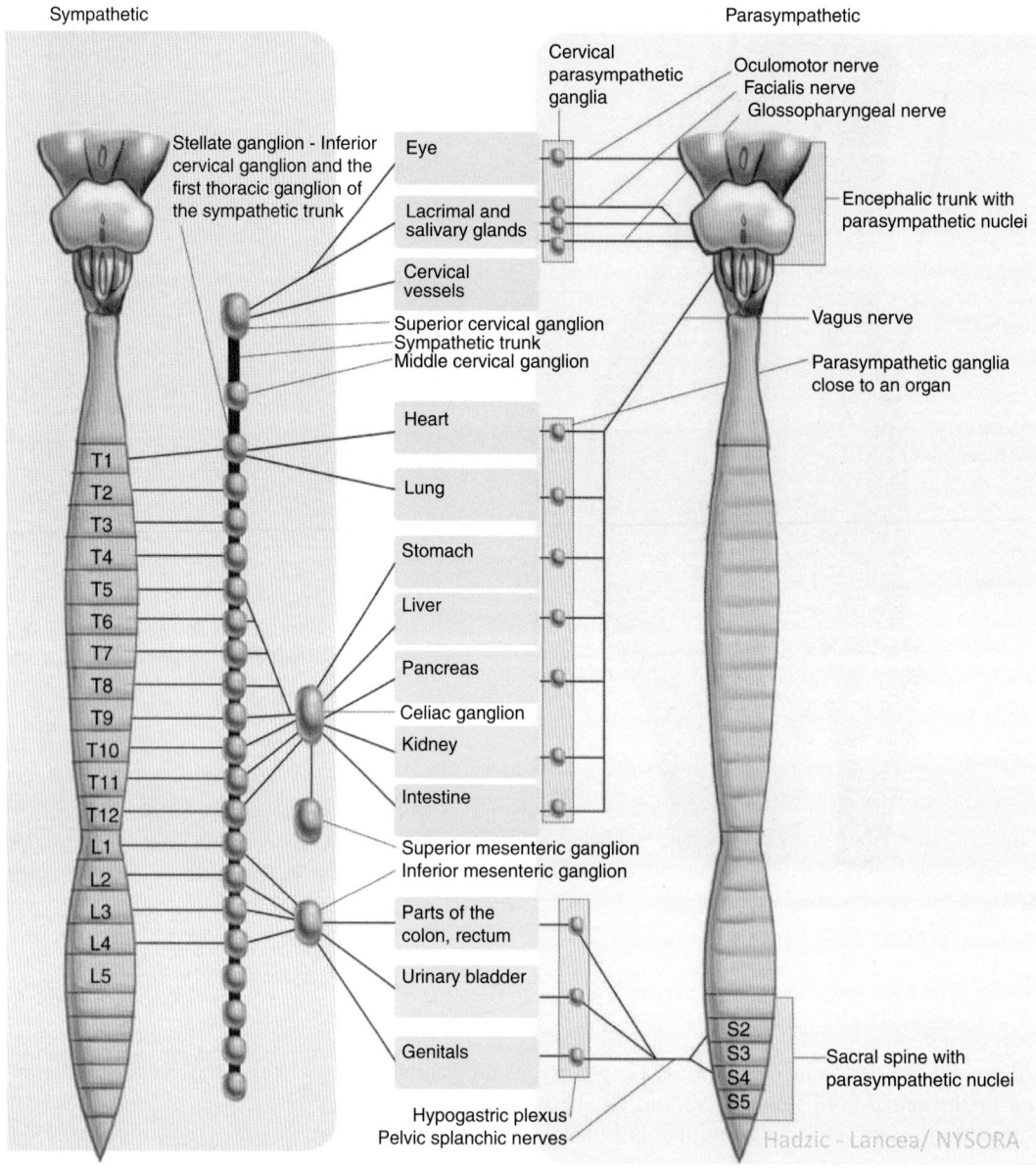

FIGURE 3–28. Organization of the autonomic nervous system.

REFERENCES

1. Kingsley R (ed): *The Gross Structure of the Nervous System, Concise Text of Neuroscience.* Lippincott Williams & Wilkins, 2000, pp 1–90.
2. Moore K, Dalley A: *Introduction to Clinically Oriented Anatomy.* Lippincott Williams & Wilkins, 1999, p 42.
3. Fix J: Neurohistology. In Baltimore KS (ed): *Neuroanatomy.* Williams & Wilkins, 1992, pp 59–69.
4. Gardner E, Bunge R: Gross anatomy of the peripheral nervous system. In Dyck P, Thomas P (eds): *Peripheral Neuropathy.* Elsevier Saunders, 2005, pp 11–34.
5. Spinal nerves. In Williams P, Bannister L, Berry M, et al (eds): *Gray's Anatomy: The Anatomical Basis of Medicine and Surgery,* 38th ed. Churchill-Livingstone, 1995, pp 1258–1292.
6. Foerster O: The dermatomes in man. Brain 1933:1–8.
7. Fix J: Spinal cord. In Baltimore KS (ed): *Neuroanatomy.* Williams & Wilkins, 1992, pp 59–69.
8. Moore K: Neck. In Moore K, Dalley A: *Introduction to Clinically Oriented Anatomy.* Lippincott Williams & Wilkins, 1999, p 42.
9. Harris W: The true form of the brachial plexus and its motor distribution. J Anat 1904;38:399.
10. Harris W: *The Morphology of the Brachial Plexus.* Humprey-Milford, 1939.
11. Kerr A: The brachial plexus of nerves in man, the variations in its formation and branches. Am J Anat 1918;23:285.
12. Sunderland S: The metrical and non-metrical features of the muscular branches of the radial nerve. J Comp Neurol 1946;85:93.
13. Sunderland S, Ray L: Metrical and nonmetrical features of the muscular branches of the median nerve. J Comp Neurol 1946;85:191.
14. Sunderland S, Hughes E: Metrical and nonmetrical features of the muscular branches of the ulnar nerve. J Comp Neurol 1946;85:113.
15. Moore K: Thorax and abdomen. In Moore K, Dalley A: *Introduction to Clinically Oriented Anatomy.* Lippincott Williams & Wilkins, 1999, p 85.
16. Horwitz M: The anatomy of the lumbosacral nerve plexus—Its relationship to vertebral segmentation and the posterior sacral nerve plexus. Anat Rec 1939;74:91.
17. Webber R: Some variations in the lumbar plexus of nerves in man. Acta Anat 1961;44:336–345.
18. Chung K: Abdomen. In Chung K (ed): *Gross Anatomy,* 3rd ed. Williams & Wilkins, 1995, pp 177–178.
19. Alast R: Innervation of the limbs. J Bone Joint Surg [Br] 1949;31:452.
20. Keegan J, Garrett F: The segmental distribution of the cutaneous nerves in the limbs of man. Anat Rec 1948;102:409.
21. Langley J: *The Autonomic Nervous System.* Heffer, 1926.

CHAPTER 4

Histology of the Peripheral Nerves and Light Microscopy

Erika Cvetko, Marija Meznarič, and Tatjana Stopar Pintaric

INTRODUCTION

Microscopic anatomy that emphasizes structure-function relations is important to the clinical practice of regional anesthesia. This chapter provides basis for understanding of the structure, classification, and organization of the peripheral nerves and insight into how the characteristics of the peripheral nerves (Figure 4–1) relate to the clinical practice of regional anesthesia.

ORGANIZATION OF THE PERIPHERAL NERVOUS SYSTEM

The nervous system enables the body to respond to continuous changes in its external and internal environments. It controls and integrates the functional activities of the organs and organ systems.

Nervous system cells consist of neurons and neuroglia. Neurons transmit nerve impulses to and from the central nervous system (CNS), thereby integrating motor and sensory functions. Neuroglial cells support and protect the neurons. In the CNS, myelin is produced by oligodendrocytes and in the peripheral nervous system (PNS) by the Schwann cells. Although both Schwann cells and oligodendrocytes are in charge of axon myelination, they have distinct morphological and molecular properties and different embryonic origins, the neural crest and the neural tube, respectively.[1]

The PNS consists of peripheral nerves (craniospinal, somatic, autonomic) with their associated ganglia and connective tissue investments. All lie peripheral to the pial covering of the CNS.[2–6]

Peripheral nerves contain fascicles of nerve fibers consisting of axons. In peripheral nerve fibers, axons are ensheathed by Schwann cells, which may or may not form myelin around the axons, depending on their diameter. Nerve fibers are grouped into fascicles of variable numbers. The size, number, and pattern of fascicles vary in different nerves and at different levels along their paths. Generally, their number increases and their size decreases at some distance proximal to the branching point.

NEURONS

A neuron is the structural and functional unit of the nervous system. It includes the cell body, dendrites, and axon.

The cell body (*perykarion*) is the dilated region of the neuron that contains a large, euchromatic nucleus with a prominent nucleolus and surrounding perinuclear cytoplasm (Figure 4–2). The perinuclear cytoplasm contains abundant rough-surfaced endoplasmic reticulum and free ribosomes. On light microscopy, the rough endoplasmic reticulum with rosettes of free ribosomes appears as small bodies, called Nissl bodies. The perinuclear cytoplasm contains numerous mitochondria, a large perinuclear Golgi apparatus, liposomes, microtubules, neurofilaments, transport vesicles, and inclusions. The presence of the euchromatic nucleus, large nucleolus, prominent Golgi apparatus, and Nissl bodies indicates the high level of anabolic activity needed to maintain these large cells.

Dendrites are elaborations of the receptive plasma membrane of the neuron. Most neurons possess multiple dendrites that typically arise from the cell body as single short trunks that ramify into smaller branches that taper at the ends. Dendrite-branching patterns are characteristic of each kind of neuron. The base of the dendrite contains the same organelles as the cell body, except the Golgi apparatus. Many organelles become sparse or absent toward the distal end of the dendrite. Dendrite branching results in several synaptic terminals and allows a neuron to receive and integrate multiple impulses.

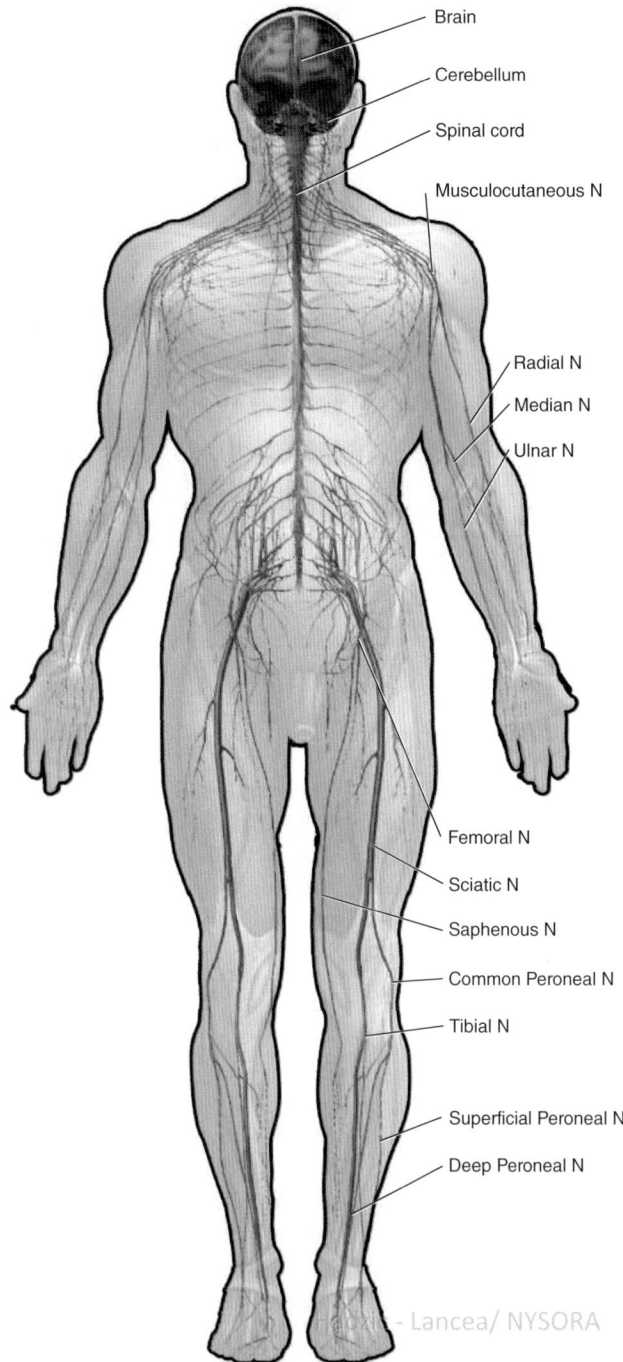

FIGURE 4–1. Peripheral and central nervous system. N = nerve.

The axon arises from the cell body as a single thin process, much longer than the dendrites. Its thickness is directly related to conduction velocity, which increases with axonal diameter. Some axons possess collateral branches. The portion of the axon between the cell body and the beginning of the myelin sheath is the initial segment.[7] At the end of the axon, the ramifications may form many small branches. The axonal cytoplasm is called *axoplasm.*

Almost all of the structural and functional protein molecules are synthesized in the cell body and are transported to distant locations within a neuron in a process known as axonal transport. Crucial to the trophic relations within the axon, axonal transport serves as a mode of intracellular communication carrying molecules and information along microtubules and intermediate filaments from the neuronal cell body to the axon terminal (anterograde transport) or from the axon terminal to the neuronal cell body (retrograde transport). Neurons communicate with other neurons and with effector cells by *synapses.* These special junctions between neurons and effector cells facilitate the transmission of nerve impulses from one (presynaptic) neuron to another (postsynaptic) neuron or from axons to effector (target) cells, such as muscle and gland cells.

Neurons have greater variation in size and shape than any other group of cells in the body. They are classified morphologically into three major types according to their shape and the arrangement of their processes. The most common neuron type, multipolar, possesses a single axon with various arrangements of multiple dendrites emanating from the cell body. The majority of multipolar neurons (Figure 4–2 and Figure 4–3) are motor neurons. A second type of neuron, unipolar or pseudounipolar (Figure 4–3), possesses only one process, the axon emanating from the cell body and opening up into the peripheral and central branches shortly after leaving the cell body. The central branch enters the CNS, while the peripheral branch proceeds to its corresponding receptor in the body. Each of the two branches is morphologically axonal and can propagate nerve impulses, although the very distal part of the peripheral branch arborizes, indicating its receptor function. The majority of unipolar neurons are sensory neurons, whose cell bodies are situated in the dorsal root ganglia of spinal nerves and in the sensory ganglia of cranial nerves. The third type of neuron, bipolar, possesses two processes emanating from the cell body: a single dendrite and a single axon. They can only be found in some cranial nerves.

Functionally, the nervous system has *somatic* and *autonomic* components. Nerve fibers innervating tissues derived from somites (muscles and skin) are described as somatic; nerve fibers innervating endodermal or other mesodermal derivatives (internal organs) are visceral. The somatic nervous system controls functions that are under conscious voluntary control with the exception of the reflex arch. It provides sensory and motor innervation to all parts of the body except the viscera, smooth muscles, cardiac muscle, and glands. The autonomic nervous system provides efferent involuntary innervation to smooth and cardiac muscles and glands. It also provides the afferent sensory innervation of the viscera (pain and autonomic reflexes).

Efferent Axons

Efferent axons arise from either the somatic or the autonomic nervous system. Somatic efferent (motor) neurons innervate skeletal muscle and have cell bodies located in somatic motor nuclei of the brainstem (cranial nerves) or in the ventral horns of the spinal cord (spinal nerves).

Preganglionic visceral efferent neurons of the sympathetic part of the autonomic nervous system arise from the intermediolateral column of the spinal cord between levels T1 and L2 and synapse on *paravertebral* or *prevertebral* (preaortic) ganglia. Peripheral nerves thus contain both preganglionic and postganglionic sympathetic fibers. Preganglionic visceral efferent neurons of the parasympathetic part of the autonomic nervous

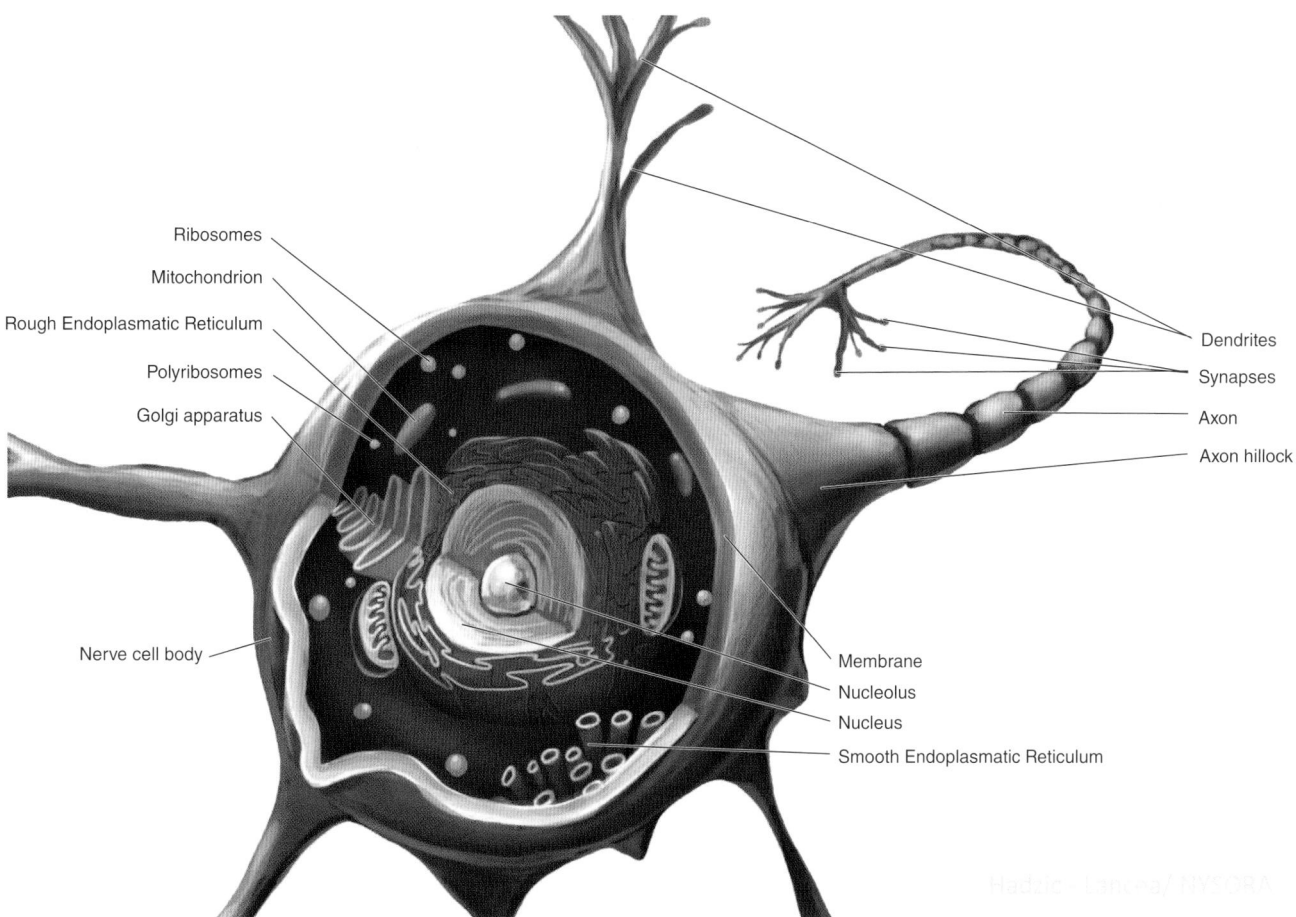

FIGURE 4–2. Diagram of a multipolar neuron. The nerve cell body, dendrites, and proximal part of the axon are within the CNS. The axons exiting the CNS distal to intervertebral foramina or foramina of the skull constitute the main part of the PNS.

system arise from the parasympathetic nuclei within the brainstem (cranial part of parasympathetic nervous system) or sacral spinal cord between the S2 and S4 segments (sacral part of the parasympathetic nervous system). Only preganglionic parasympathetic fibers travel along peripheral nerves to synapse on intramural ganglia in the wall of target organs.

Afferent Axons

Afferent axons are either somatic or visceral and have cell bodies either in the dorsal root ganglia of the spinal nerves or in the sensory ganglia of the cranial nerves. Somatic afferent (sensory) neurons transmit impulses from the receptors for touch, temperature, or pain (nociceptors) located in the body wall (skin) and from the proprioceptors in the skeletal muscles and joints. Visceral afferent neurons transmit information from viscera (interoceptors and nociceptors). The visceral afferent axons travel along the visceral efferent fibers and pass through the communicating branches and dorsal roots of the spinal nerves or along the vagus nerve to enter the CNS.

SCHWANN CELLS

Axons of peripheral nerves are ensheathed by Schwann cells. Their myelin sheath (modified plasmalemma) separates the axons from the endoneurium. Schwann cells are distributed

along the axons in longitudinal chains depending on myelination along the axon. The coordinated differentiation of the axons and their myelinating cells requires close communication between neurons and glia.[8] Signals provided by the axons regulate the proliferation, survival, and differentiation of glial cells.[9,10] On the other hand, reciprocal glial signals affect axonal cytoskeleton and transport[11] and are required for axonal survival[12,13] and regeneration.[14] Schwann cells also have a guiding function for growing axons,[15] indicating that glia do more than provide support to the axon.

Schwann cell phenotypes are characterized by distinct morphologies[5] and differential expression of myelin proteins, cell adhesion molecules, receptors, enzymes, intermediate filament proteins, ion channels, and extracellular matrix proteins.[6] All Schwann cells are surrounded by basal lamina, whose extracellular matrix molecules, such as laminin, regulate key aspects of Schwann cell development (for review, see Reference 16).

CLASSIFICATION OF NERVE FIBERS

Nerve fibers are classified according to axonal diameter, conduction velocity, type of receptor, and myelin sheath thickness (Table 4–1).[17] Conduction velocity is related to axonal diameter; that is, the larger the fiber is, the faster the conduction will be.

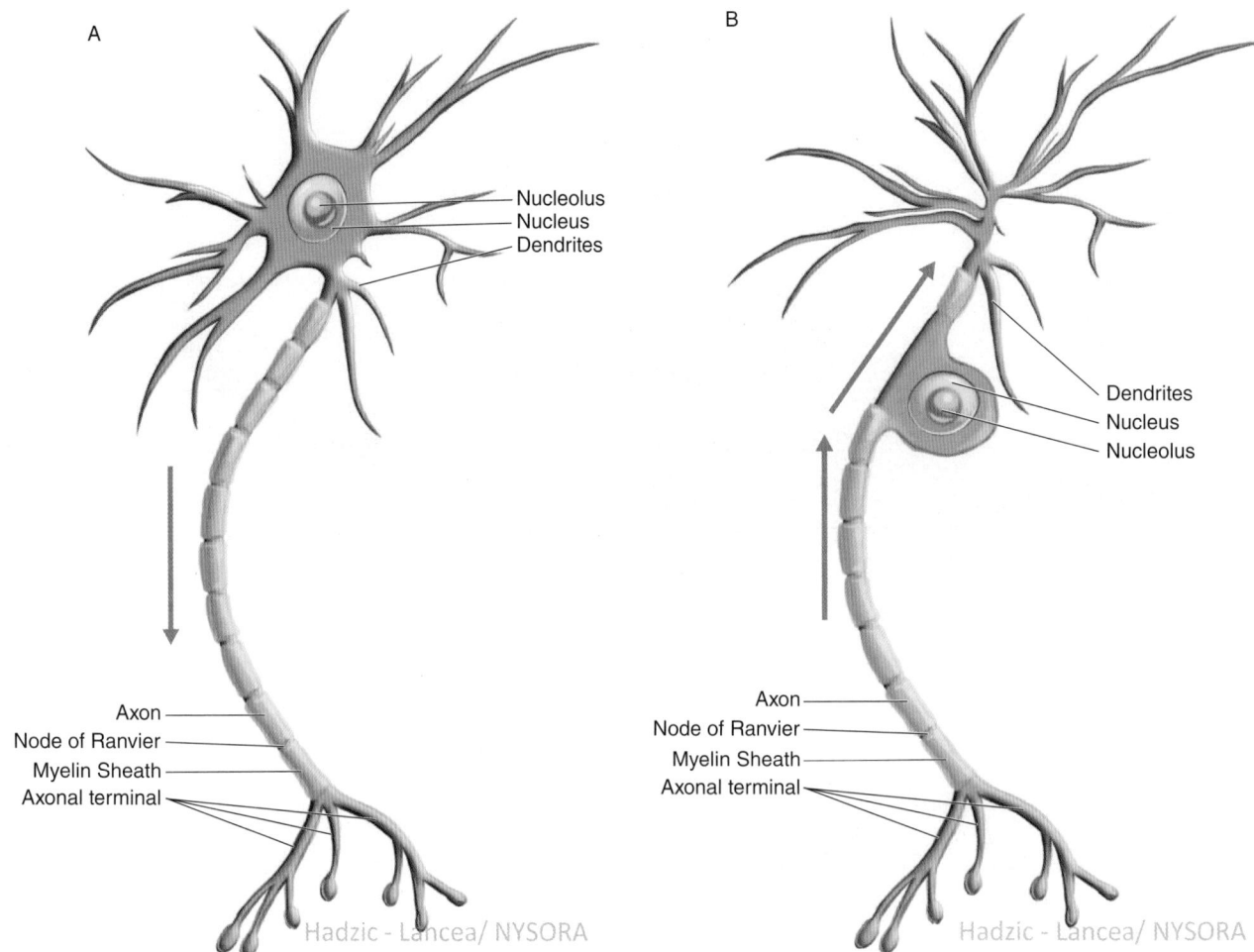

FIGURE 4–3. Diagram illustrating a multipolar (**A**) and unipolar or pseudounipolar (**B**) neuron. Arrows indicate the direction of nerve impulse propagation.

Clinical Pearl

- The larger the fiber, the more concentrated the local anesthetic must be to effect neural blockade.

MYELINATED NERVE FIBERS

Myelinated nerve fibers are ensheathed by myelin, greatly extended and modified plasmalemma of the Schwann cells (Figures 4–4 and 4–5). Myelin formation begins with extension of the Schwann cell cytoplasm and development of the inner mesaxon, which wraps around the axon several times. During the wrapping process, the cytoplasm is nearly extruded between the plasmalemma. Apposing extracellular faces of plasmalemma become "the major dense line," and apposing cytoplasmic faces form an "intraperiod line" of myelin. The proposed molecular structure of myelin fits the concept of plasmalemma as a lipid bilayer with integral and peripheral membrane proteins attached to the extracellular or to the cytoplasmic side of plasmalemma. In contrast to most biological membranes, myelin has a high ratio of lipid to protein (70%–85% lipid, 15%–30% protein), where the latter serve as structural proteins, enzymes, voltage channels, and signal transducers.[18]

Myelin sheath wraps the axon in segments. Areas of the axon covered by concentric lamellae of myelin and a single myelin-producing Schwann cell are called *internodes* and range in length from 200 to 1000 μm. Interruptions, which occur in the myelin sheath at regular intervals along the length of axons and expose the axon, are called nodes of Ranvier (Figure 4–6). Each node indicates an interface between the myelin sheaths of two different Schwann cells located along the axon.

The nodal region and its surroundings can be further subdivided into several domains (Figure 4–6) that contain a unique set of ion channels, cell adhesion molecules, and cytoplasmic adaptor proteins (for review, see Reference 8). In the PNS, the node is in contact with Schwann cell microvilli and covered by its basal lamina (Figure 4–6). An important characteristic of the *nodal* axolemma is its high density of voltage-gated Na$^+$ channels[19] as compared to the *juxtaparanodal* axolemma, which typically contains a high density of K$^+$ channels.[20] Na$^+$ channels potentiate the nerve impulse in a saltatory manner (Figure 4–7) along the myelinated fibers.[21,22] When the membrane at the node is excited, the local circuit that is generated cannot flow through the high-resistance myelin sheath. It therefore flows out and depolarizes the membrane at the next node, which may

TABLE 4–1. Classification of peripheral nerve fibers according to axonal diameter, conduction velocity, type of receptor, and myelin sheath thickness (myelination).

Axonal Diameter (μm)	Conduction Velocity (m/s)	Efferent Fibers	Afferent Fibers[a] (From Cutaneous Receptors)	Afferent Fibers From Skeletal Muscles, Tendons, and Joints	Myelination
12–20	60–120 30–70	Aα (to extrafusal muscle fibers)	Aα (from rapidly adapting mechanoreceptors)	Ia (from muscle spindles) Ib (from Golgi tendon organs)	Heavily myelinated
6–12	25–70		Aβ (from slowly adapting mechanoreceptors)	II (from joint proprioceptors)	Myelinated
3–8	15–30	Aγ (to intrafusal muscle fibers)			Myelinated
1–6	12–30		Aδ (from thermal and mechanical nociceptors and thermoreceptors—cold only)	III (from joint proprioceptors and joint nociceptors)	Thinly myelinated
1–3	3–15	B (preganglionic visceral)			Myelinated
0.2–1.5	0.5–2	C (postganglionic visceral)	C (from mechanical nociceptors and thermoreceptors—cold and warm, polymodal nociceptors)	IV (from joint nociceptors)	Unmyelinated

[a] Visceral afferent fibers (from interoceptors) are classified as Aδ and C fibers.

Source: Modified with permission from Cramer GD, Darby S: *Basic and Clinical Anatomy of the Spine, Spinal Cord, and ANS,* 2nd ed. Philadelphia: Elsevier/Mosby; 2005.

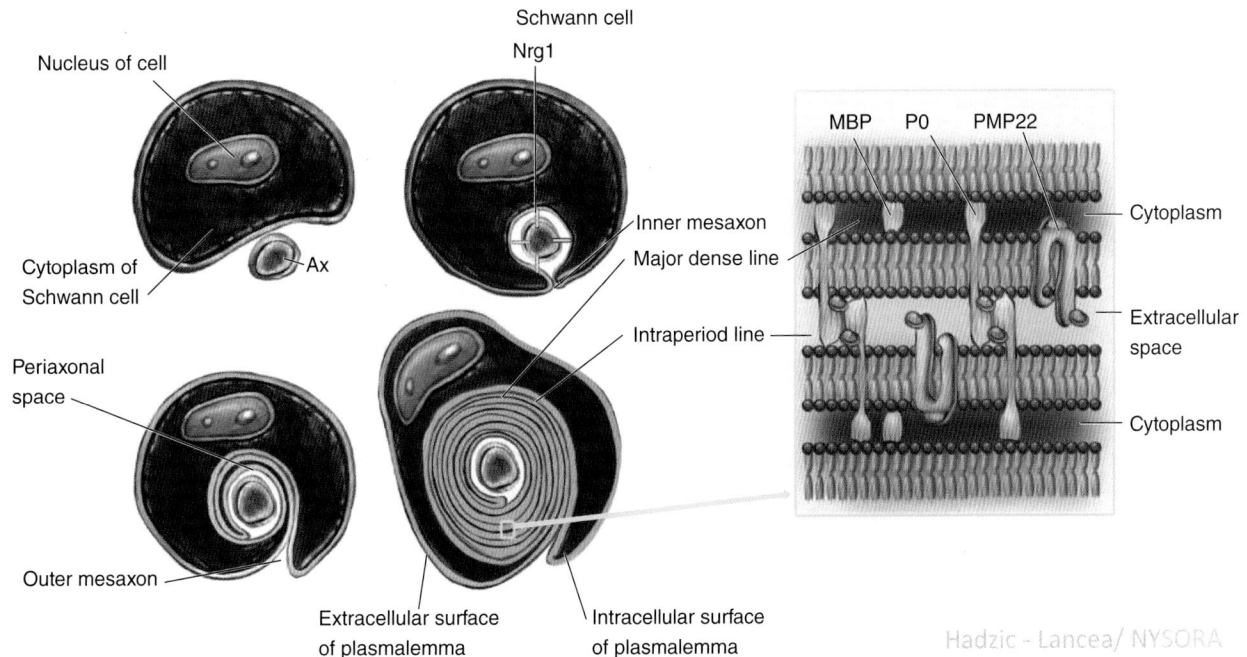

FIGURE 4–4. Schematic presentation of myelin formation and simplified scheme of its molecular organization. For simplification, the basal lamina of Schwann cells is not drawn. Nrg1 = neuregulin; MPB = myelin basic protein; P0 = protein zero; PMP22 = peripheral membrane protein of 22 kDa; Ax = axon. (Modified with permission from Ross M, Pawlina W: Histology: *A Text and Atlas With Correlated Cell and Molecular Biology,* 6th ed. Philadelphia: Wolters Kluwer; Lippincott Williams & Wilkins; 2011.)

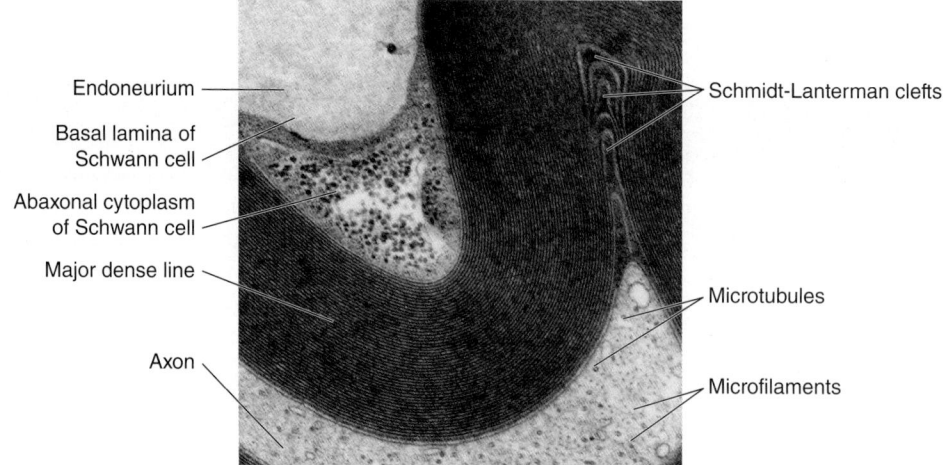

FIGURE 4–5. Electron micrograph of the myelinated fiber. Myelin is visualized as a series of alternating dark and less-dark lines. Biopsy of human sural nerve.

be 1 mm or farther away. The low capacitance of the sheath means that little energy is required to depolarize the remaining membrane between the nodes, resulting in increased speed of local circuit spreading.[18]

Myelination is an example of cell-to-cell communication in which axons interact with Schwann cells. The number of myelin layers is determined by the axon and not by the Schwann cell. Myelin sheath thickness is regulated by a growth factor called neuregulin 1 (Nrg1). The compaction of myelin sheath is associated with the expression of transmembrane myelin-specific proteins such as protein 0 (P0), a peripheral myelin protein of 22 kilodaltons (PMP22), and a myelin basic protein (MBP). The absence of proteins that regulate myelin sheath formation might result in severe hypomyelination or dismyelination in humans and experimental animals.[18]

UNMYELINATED NERVE FIBERS

Unmyelinated axons are also enveloped by Schwann cells and their basal lamina. An individual Schwann cell can ensheath a single or several unmyelinated axons (Figures 4–8 and 4–9). Unmyelinated fibers predominate in human cutaneous spinal nerves, where the average ratio of unmyelinated to myelinated fiber density is 3.7:1.[23] In unmyelinated fibers, conduction velocity is proportional to the square root of fiber diameter and is much slower compared to saltatory conduction in myelinated fibers (Table 4–1).

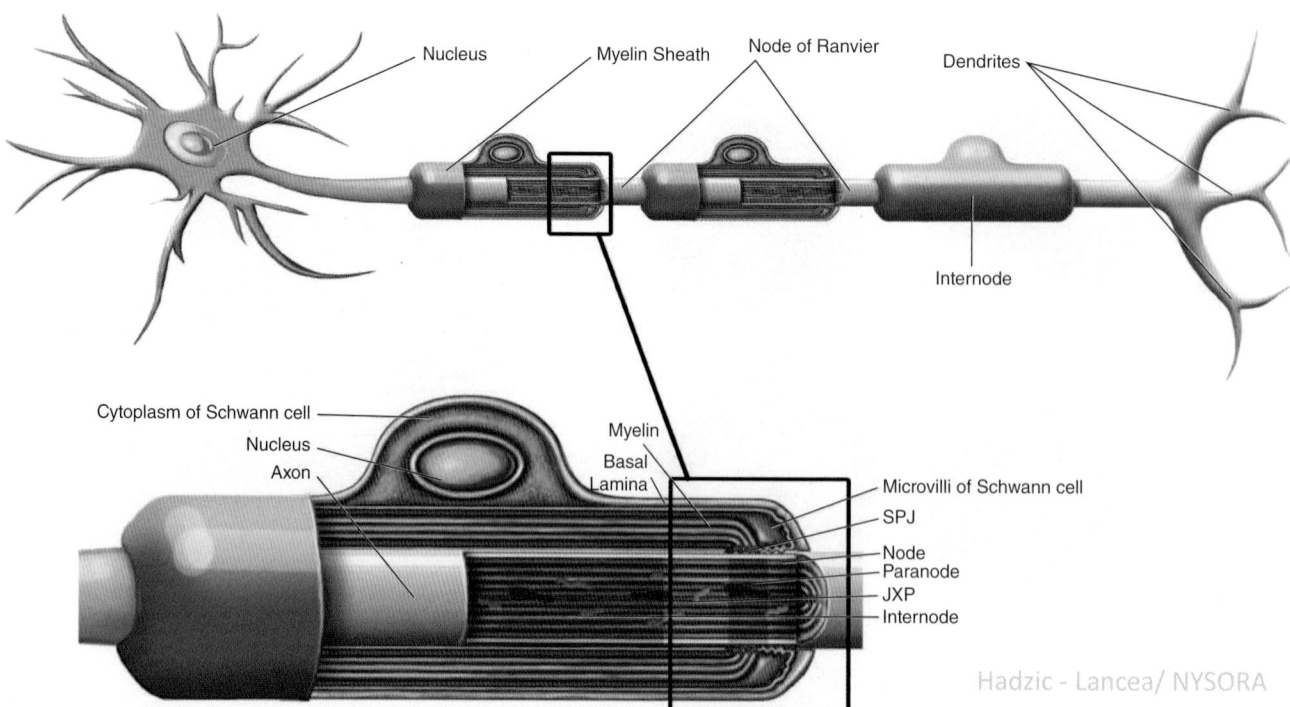

FIGURE 4–6. Distinct domains of the nodal region. The region occupied by distinct proteins located in the nodal axolemma is schematically depicted in black over axon. SPJ = septate like junctions; JXP = juxtaparanode. (Modified with permission from Poliak S, Peles E. The local differentiation of myelinated axons at nodes of Ranvier. *Nat Rev Neurosci.* 2003 Dec;4(12):968-980.)

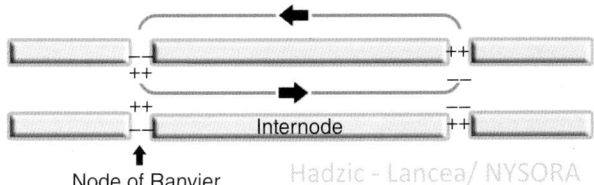

FIGURE 4–7. Saltatory conduction in myelinated nerve fiber. Na⁺ channels, located at nodal axolemma, potentiate the nerve impulse in a saltatory manner along myelinated nerve fiber.

CONNECTIVE TISSUE INVESTMENTS OF PERIPHERAL NERVES

In a peripheral nerve, nerve fibers and their supporting Schwann cells are held together by connective tissue organized into three distinctive components that have specific morphological and functional characteristics. The epineurium forms the outermost connective tissue of the peripheral nerve, the perineurium surrounds each nerve fascicle separately, while the individual nerve fibers are embedded in the endoneurium[2] (Figures 4–10 to 4–13).

Epineurium

The epineurium is a condensation of a loose areolar connective tissue that surrounds a peripheral nerve and binds its fascicles into a common bundle (Figure 4–10 and Figure 4–11).

Epineurium that extends between the fascicles is the interfascicular or inner epineurium, while epineurium that surrounds the entire nerve trunk is the epifascicular or external epineurium[24,25] called the epineurium comprises 30%–75% of the nerve cross-sectional area[26] but varies along the nerve. It is the thickest where continuous with the dura covering the CNS and more abundant in nerves adjacent to the joints, where nerves are subject to pressure.[27] Susceptibility to compression injury is therefore likely to be greater in unifascicular than in multifascicular nerves because the latter have greater amount of epineurium. As the peripheral nerve divides and the number of fascicles is reduced, the epineurium becomes progressively thinner and eventually disappears around monofascicular nerves.

The epineurium contains collagen, fibroblasts, mast cells, and fat cells. Collagen bundles have a predominant longitudinal orientation; however, an electron microscopy study found epineural collagen in bundles 10–20 μm in width are arrayed obliquely around the circumference of the nerve.[28] Elastic fibers are also present, particularly adjacent to the perineurium,[29,30] which are mainly oriented longitudinally. Collagen and elastic fibers are aligned and oriented to prevent damage by overstretching of the nerve bundle, suggesting that the epineurium is designed to accommodate the stretch.

Human epineurium is constructed predominantly of type I and type III collagen, with the type I predominating.[31] The diameter of the collagen fibrils averages 60–110 nm.[2]

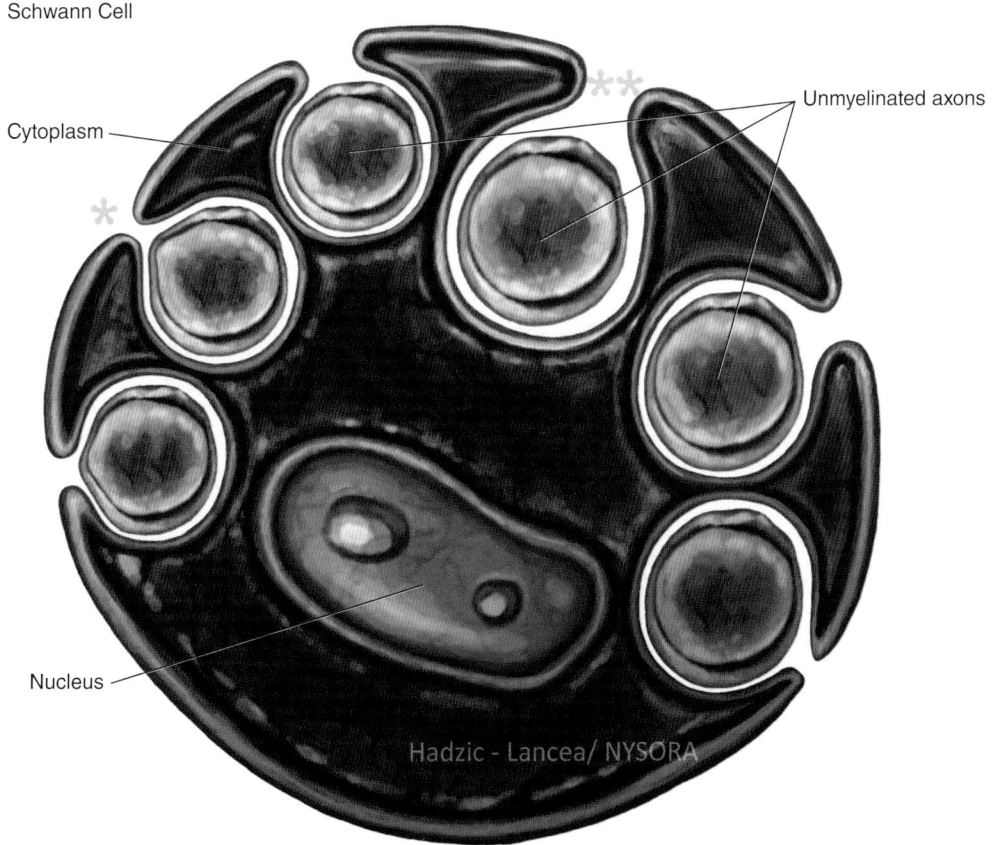

FIGURE 4–8. Schwann cell that engulfs several unmyelinated axons. The lips of the groove of cytoplasm can be closed (*), forming the mesaxon, or may be opened (**). Basal lamina of the Schwann cell is not drawn.

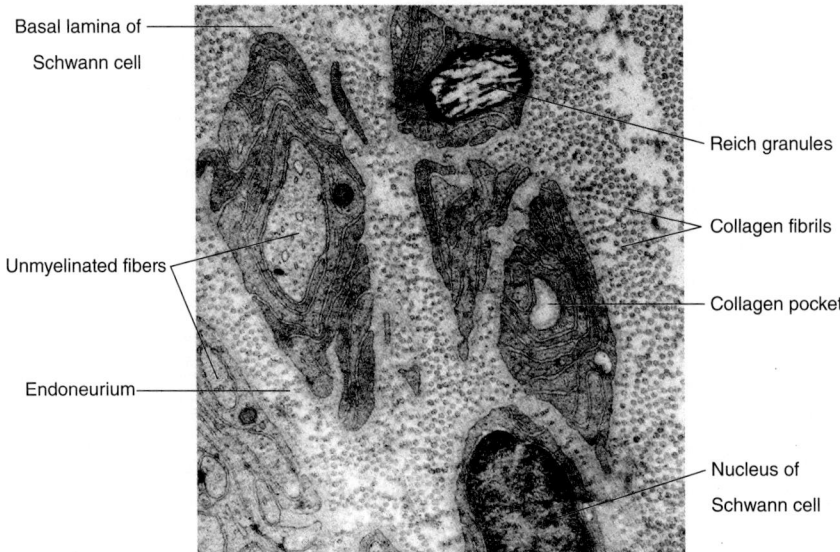

FIGURE 4–9. Electron micrograph of unmyelinated axons. Biopsy of human sural nerve.

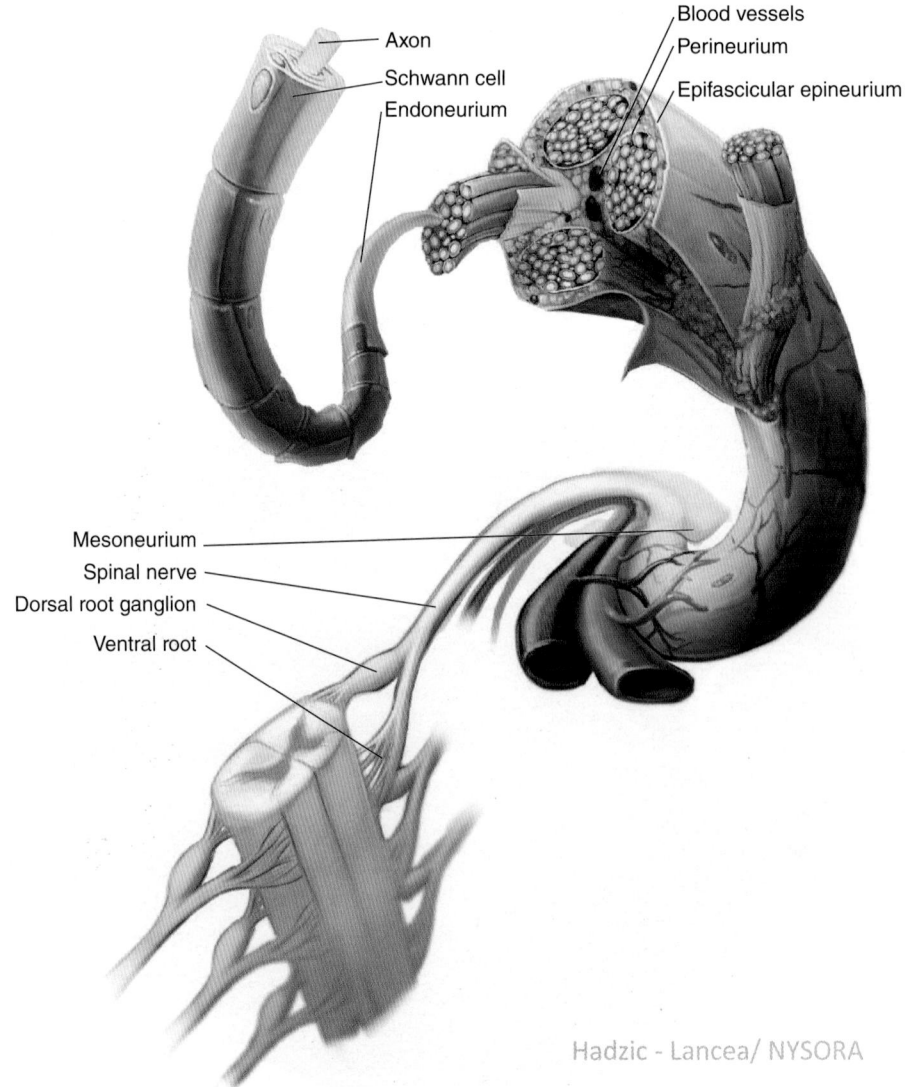

Hadzic - Lancea/ NYSORA

FIGURE 4–10. Connective tissue investments of peripheral nerve. The diagram demonstrates the arrangement of the peripheral nerve. A segment of the spinal nerve is enlarged to show the relation of the nerve fibers to the surrounding connective tissue (endoneurium, perineurium, and epineurium).

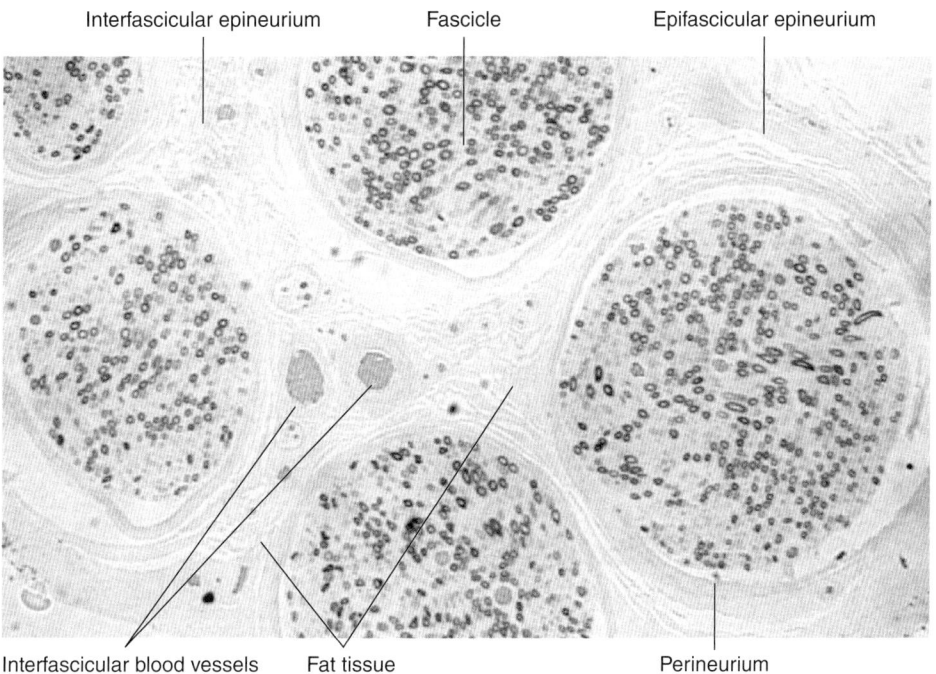

Interfascicular epineurium   Fascicle   Epifascicular epineurium

Interfascicular blood vessels   Fat tissue   Perineurium

FIGURE 4–11. Semithin section of human sural nerve fixed in osmium tetroxide. The myelin sheaths are preserved and stained black. Perineurium surrounds the nerve fascicle. Streaks of connective tissue originate from epifascicular epineurium inside the nerve as interfascicular epineurium. Fat tissue and blood vessels are localized in interfascicular epineurium.

Adipose tissue inside a nerve surrounds the fascicles and forms adipose sheaths that separate the fascicles from each other. The thickness of adipose sheaths varies from one fascicle to another and is greater in larger nerve trunks, highlighting its protective function in cushioning the fascicles against damage by compression.[27] Loss of epineural fat may present a risk factor for pressure-caused palsies in emaciated, bedridden patients.[2] In contrast, excessive adipose tissue can also delay the diffusion of local anesthetic injected near a nerve, thus interfering with the anesthetic blockade.[32] Epineurium is continuous with the connective tissue called adventitia or mesoneurium that surrounds the nerve when passing through, underneath, or between the muscle fascia, serving as (1) a conduit for the injected local anesthetic, (2) a path allowing for nerve gliding, and (3) a layer of protection against nerve trauma.[25] Because their attachment is loose, nerves are relatively mobile except where tethered by entering vessels or exiting nerve branches.[24]

Perineurium

The perineurium is a specialized connective tissue surrounding individual nerve fascicles (Figures 4–10 and 4–12). This protective cellular layer is thinner than the epineurium and separates the endoneurium from the epineurium.[2] The perineurium consists of alternating layers of flattened polygonal cells, which are thought to be derived from fibroblasts, and collagenous connective tissue,[29] the formation of which is controlled by the

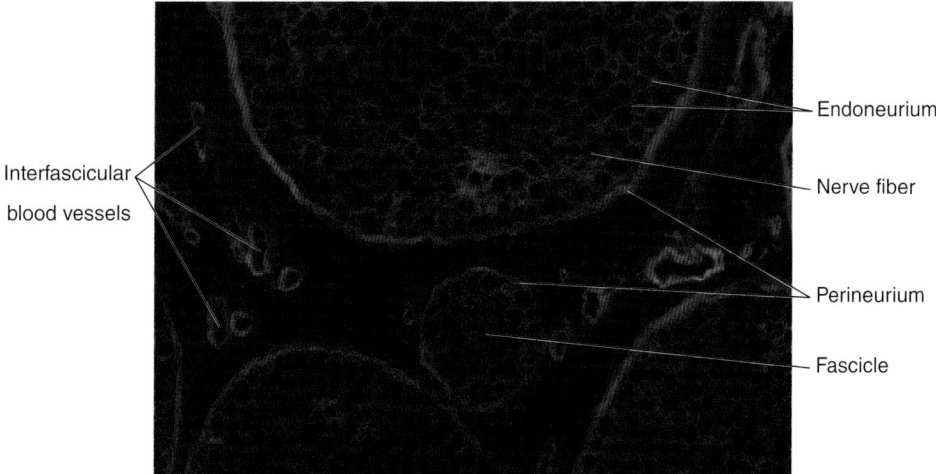

Interfascicular blood vessels

Endoneurium

Nerve fiber

Perineurium

Fascicle

FIGURE 4–12. Transverse section of pig sciatic nerve. Immunohistochemical staining for collagen. Blood vessels course through the interfascicular epineurium, which fills the space around the perineurium and fascicles.

PART 2

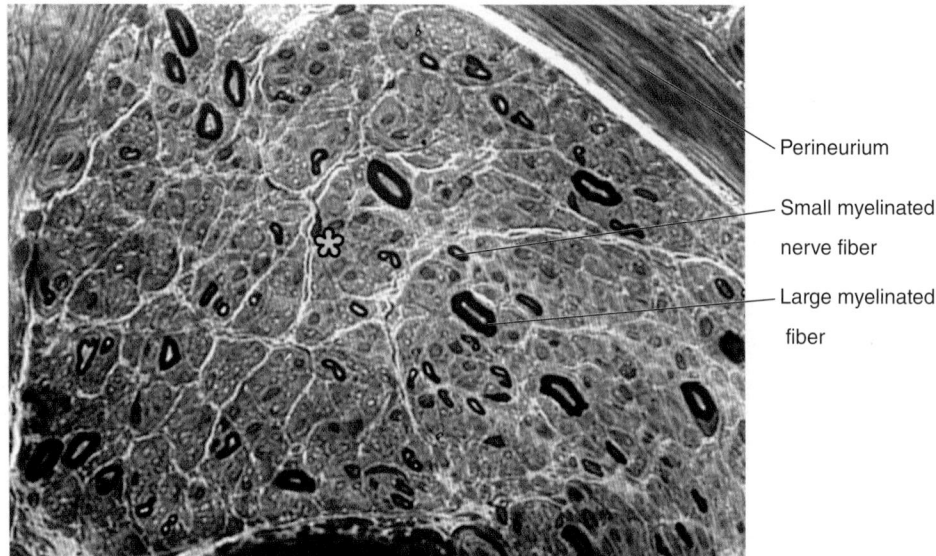

FIGURE 4–13. Semithin section of human sural nerve stained by cresyl violet. Axonal neuropathy with the predominant loss of large myelinated fibers. * Intrafascicular space between myelinated fibers (occupied by endoneurium, Schwann cell nuclei, and unmyelinated fibers).

Schwann cells.[33] The flattened polygonal cells, which constitute the lamellae, are specialized to function as a diffusion barrier.[34] The number of lamellae varies, depending mainly on the diameter of the fascicle; the larger the fascicle is, the greater the number of lamellae.[35] In mammalian nerve trunks, the perineurium contains 15–20 cell layers.[5] Contiguous cells in each layer interdigitate along extensive tight junctions.[30] The cells may branch and give rise to processes and contribute to the adjacent lamellae. Each layer of cells, enclosed by basal lamina, can reach a thickness of up to 0.5 μm in human nerves.[2,5]

Collagen fibers originate in a lattice-like arrangement, in which bundles are circular, longitudinal, and obliquely arranged. The innermost perineural cell layer adheres to a distinct boundary layer of densely woven collagen fibers and subperineurial fibroblasts that mechanically links the perineurium to the endoneurial contents.[28] Collagen fibers are predominantly type III, although type I collagen fibers are also present.[31] The diameter of the collagen fibrils is substantially smaller than that of the epineural fibrils, with an average of 52 nm in the rat sural nerve.[30] The basal lamina of polygonal cells is composed of collagens IV and V, fibronectin, heparan sulfate proteoglycan,[36] and laminin.[37] The ubiquitous presence of pinocytotic vesicles rich in phosphorylating enzymes underlie the assumption that the perineurium functions as a metabolically active diffusion barrier, playing an essential role in maintaining the osmotic milieu and fluid pressure within the endoneurium.[34] For instance, in one of our studies, inflammatory cells accumulated between the nerve fascicles in piglets after exposure of the nerve to ultrasound gel did not penetrate the perineurium.[38] Because of its tightly adherent cellular structure and more longitudinally oriented collagen, the perineurium is less tolerant to elongation than the epineurium. In the rabbit, mechanical failure during elongation coincided with a disruption of the perineurium while the epineurium remained intact.[39] The integrity of the diffusion barrier was maintained after 2 hours of 15%

elongation, while 27% elongation caused acute perineural disruption.[39]

Endoneurium

The endoneurium comprises loose intrafascicular connective tissue that does not include the perineural partitions that subdivide the fascicles and surrounds Schwann cells (Figure 4–12). Approximately 40%–50% of the intrafascicular space is occupied by nonneural elements (ie, other than axon and Schwann cells), of which the endoneurial fluid and connective tissue matrix occupy 20%–30%.[40] There are substantial variations among nerves in different species[5] and age groups.[41]

The endoneurium is composed of collagen fibers (produced by the underlying Schwann cells and fibroblasts); cellular components are bathed in endoneurial fluid, contained in substantial intrafascicular spaces. The nerve fibers tend to be grouped into small bundles with intervening clefts. Endoneurial fluid pressure is slightly higher than that of the surrounding epineurium. It is believed that this pressure gradient minimizes endoneurial contamination by toxic substances external to the nerve bundle.[42]

Endoneurial collagen fibrils are smaller than those in the epineurium and range between 30 and 65 nm in diameter in humans.[43] The fibrils run parallel to and around the nerve fibers, binding them into fascicles or bundles. They show condensations around capillaries and nerve fibers. Near the distal terminus of the axon, the endoneurium is reduced to a few reticular fibers surrounding the basal lamina of the Schwann cells. Types I, II, and III collagen are present in endoneurium.[44]

Cellular constituents of endoneurium are fibroblasts, endothelial cells of capillaries, mast cells, and macrophages. Mast cells occur in varying numbers, being especially numerous along blood vessels. Macrophages account for 2%–4% of the intrafascicular nuclei in rat peripheral nerve[45] and are the primary antigen-presenting cells of peripheral nerve. They scavenge extracellular proteins and present them to T cells emerging from circulation. The macrophages mediate immunologic surveillance and participate in nerve tissue repair. Following nerve injury, they proliferate and actively phagocytose myelin debris.

The extracellular matrix is rich in glycoproteins, glycosaminoglycans, and proteoglycans. The best characterized of these include the glycoprotein fibronectin, tenascin C, trombospondin, and the chondroitin sulfate proteoglycans versican and decorin.[46] Expression of these molecules changes after nerve injury, so they are potentially relevant during nerve regeneration.[46]

From a hydrodynamic point of view, the various tissues that comprise a peripheral nerve can be divided into the loose, high-compliance, expansible connective tissue of the epineurium and the low-compliance, disruptable fascicles and fascicular bundles, densely packed within the perineurium. These anatomical differences between connective tissues and fascicles or their bundles explain why an injection into fascicles requires more force (pressure) than injection into the loose connective tissue of the epineurium.[25,47]

Clinical Pearls

- The perineurium is a tough and resistant tissue, that tends to escape slowly advancing a blunt, short-bevel needle during nerve block procedure.[48]
- Higher force (pressure) is required for an injection into a low-compliant fascicle as opposed to the high-compliant epineurium.[49]
- In the interscalene and supraclavicular regions of the brachial plexus, the nerves are more densely packed and oligofascicular, while more distally, they are polyfascicular with a larger amount of stromal tissue.[50]
- Multifascicular nerves are less susceptible to injury as compared to unifascicular due to a reduced fascicular diameter and an increased epineurial protection.
- The abundance of loose epineurial tissue offers an explanation as to why most intraneural injections (intraneural, but extrafascicular) do not result in overt nerve injury.[51]

THE CENTRAL-PERIPHERAL TRANSITION REGION

The transition between the CNS and the PNS in cranial and spinal nerve roots is referred to as the *central-peripheral transition region* or *CNS-PNS border* (Figure 4–14). It represents an abrupt change in the type of myelin, supporting elements, and vascularization. The main glial components in the CNS are astrocytes and oligodendrocytes, while in the PNS the main components are the Schwann cells.[52] The nerve roots of spinal nerves are bathed in cerebrospinal fluid. The *transition region* is the length of the rootlet that contains both central and peripheral nervous tissue. Transition details distinguishing ensheathment of the spinal roots with the meninges and connective

tissue investments of the peripheral nerves have not been fully clarified.[5] Their structural arrangements however, are well documented in electron microscopic studies.[53–57]

The cellular components of the endoneurium in the spinal roots resemble those of peripheral nerves. The quantity of collagen is substantially less and is not organized in sheaths around the nerve fibers.[43] The region in which the spinal roots attach to the spinal cord is characterized by an irregularly designed transition from the peripheral nerve to the CNS, the Obersteiner-Redlich zone where Schwann cells are replaced by oligodendrocytes. The central portion of the root is limited at its periphery by marginal glia, composed of astrocytes covered by basal lamina.[5]

The spinal roots traverse the subarachnoid space covered by a multicellular root sheath and penetrate the dura at the subarachnoid angle (Figure 4–14). External to the subarachnoid angle, the nerve roots possess epineurium, perineurium, and endoneurium as in the peripheral nerve trunks. The epineurium is the continuation of the spinal dura, while the endoneurium is developed distal to the junction of the roots with the central nervous tissue. Perineurium ensheaths the spinal ganglia and is proximal to it. It is divided in the outer layers that pass between the dura and the arachnoid to form the "dural mesothelium,"[58] while the inner layers of perineurium continue over the roots as the "inner layer of the root sheath."[5,54]

The root sheath is composed of cellular and fibrous lamellae divided into two layers.[54] The outer layer consists of loosely associated cells bordering on the subarachnoid space. Where the roots become attached to the spinal cord, the cells of the outer layer of the root sheath become continuous with the pia.[59] At the subarachnoid angle, the outer layer becomes reflected to the external meningeal investments of the spinal cord (arachnoidea attached to the inner layer of spinal dura).[56] The inner layer of the root sheath consists of flattened cells that are closely associated with each other, are intermittently invested with a basal lamina, and resemble the perineurium but are not classifiable as perineural cells. It becomes continuous with the perineurium peripherally.

The subarachnoid space opens into a lateral recess that extends between the ventral and dorsal roots and may constitute a *communication* between the subarachnoid and endoneurial spaces.[54] This communication is clinically relevant because it allows inflammation to spread from the subarachnoid space to the endoneurium in the case of polyradiculoneuritides.

Clinical Pearls

- Local anesthetic injection within the epineurial cuff during performance of interscalene or lumbar plexus blocks may lead to spinal anesthesia due to dural cuff extension beyond the intervertebral foramen.[60]
- During performance of lumbar plexus block, epidural spread of local anesthetic is observed particularly when high injection pressure (force) is used during the injection process.[61]

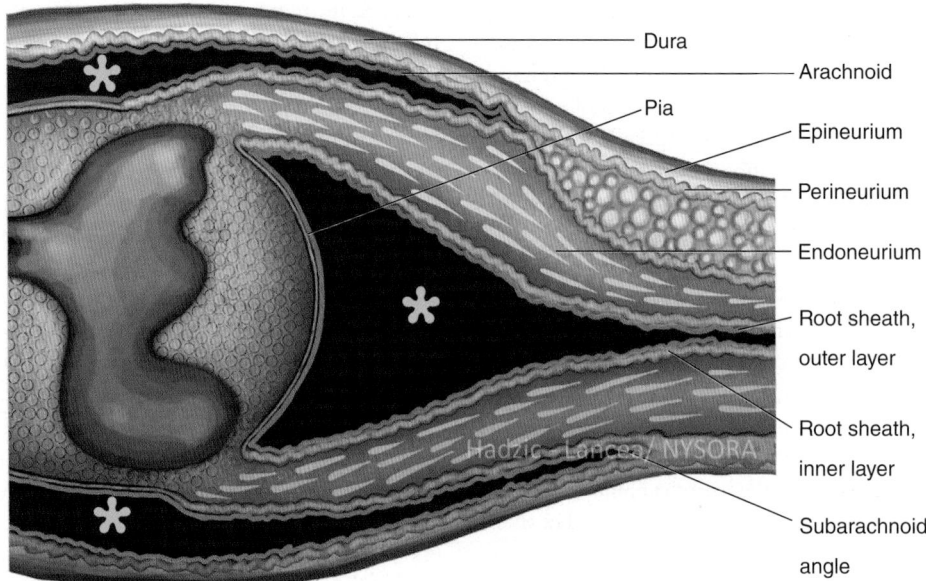

FIGURE 4–14. Central-peripheral transition region. The epineurium becomes continuous with the dura mater. The arachnoid is reflected over the roots at the subarachnoid angle and becomes continuous with the outer layer of the root sheath. At the junction with the spinal cord, the outer layer becomes continuous with the pia mater. The perineurium divides in two layers at the subarachnoid angle: The outer layer separates from the nerve root and runs between the dura and the arachnoid; the inner layer is adherent with spinal roots and constitutes the inner layer of the root sheath. Spinal ganglion is embedded in the perineurium. * Subarachnoid space. (Reproduced with permission from Haller FR, Low FN. The fine structure of the peripheral nerve root sheath in the subarachnoid space in the rat and other laboratory animals. *Am J Anat.* 1971 May;131(1):1-19.)

VASCULAR SUPPLY OF PERIPHERAL NERVES

The peripheral nerve is a well-vascularized structure,[62] supplied by vessels that originate from the nearby large arteries and veins as well as from smaller adjacent muscular and periostal blood vessels (Figure 4–12). Peripheral nerves have two separate, functionally independent, vascular systems: an extrinsic system (regional nutritive vessels and epineural vessels) and an intrinsic system (microvessels in the endoneurium).[63] There are rich anastomoses between the two systems, resulting in considerable overlap between the territories of the segmental arteries.

The epineurium is characterized by a predominantly longitudinal vascular plexus. Transperineural arterioles, 10–25 μm in diameter, pass from the epineurium to the endoneurium through sleeves of perineural tissue.[64] Their course through the perineurium is oblique, rendering them potentially susceptible to changes in intra- or extrafascicular pressure.[62] Epineurial and perineurial vessels have a rich perivascular plexus of peptidergic, serotoninergic, and adrenergic nerves that play an important role in the neurogenic control of endoneurial blood flow.[64]

The endoneurial vasculature is noted for its anatomical dissimilarities from a conventional capillary bed, although, physiologically, it serves similar metabolic functions. Transperineurial arterioles gradually lose their continuous muscle coat and become postarteriolar capillaries. Endoneurial capillaries have atypically greater diameter and intercapillary distances than those in many other tissues.[65] Such angioarchitecture suggests a lower exchange capacity.[66] Endoneurial arterioles have a poorly developed smooth muscle layer and thus limited capacity for autoregulation.[63] The density of endoneurial microvessels varies

significantly throughout peripheral nerves; these variations correlate with susceptibility to ischemic neuropathy.[67] This unique pattern of vessels, together with the high basal blood flow relative to metabolic requirements of the nerve, confer a high degree of resistance to ischemia so that nerve dysfunction does not occur during acute ischemia until blood flow is almost zero. The outstanding characteristic of the peripheral neurovascular system is its flexibility. Peripheral nerves may be surgically mobilized, severing their nutrition vessels without clinical consequences, to a surprising degree. However, the distribution of the circulation within the endoneurium is exquisitely sensitive to physical and chemical manipulation.[62]

Clinical Pearls

- Peripheral nerves are relatively resistant to ischemia because nerve dysfunction can only occur when the blood flow is almost zero.
- Local anesthetics have the ability to constrict vasculature and decrease the blood flow to the nerves.[68]

AGE-RELATED CHANGES IN PERIPHERAL NERVES

An intact aged PNS is characterized by several extensive structural, functional, and biochemical changes, which have been documented in both myelinated and unmyelinated fibers.[5,69] In the elderly, myelinated fiber density decreases.[23,41,70–72] A regular relation between internodal length and fiber diameter becomes less precise with aging.[41,73] This is associated with segmental demyelination and remyelination and the axonal degeneration and regeneration clinically evident as mild peripheral neuropathy.[5]

In unmyelinated fibers, regressive changes attributed to aging have been reported.[74,75] In unmyelinated fiber complexes of aging nerves, the proportion of Schwann cell bands devoid of axons increases (so-called collagen pockets; see Figure 4–9). An early age-related change appears to be the budding of Schwann cell processes into numerous flattened tongues, which usually occur in groups.[5] The perineurial index (ratio of perineurium thickness to fascicle diameter) shows a tendency to increase with age,[72] most probably reflecting age-related loss of nerve fibers.

Aging is associated with a decreased number of endoneurial capillaries and an increase in the thickness of capillary walls and the perineurium.[70] The rate of axonal regeneration becomes slower as density and number of regenerating axons decreases. Aging also impairs terminal sprouting of regenerated axons and collateral sprouting of intact adjacent axons, further limiting target reinnervation and functional recovery.[76]

The cause of changes related to aging is uncertain. It is not yet established whether they are the result of neuronal aging, giving rise to distal axonal degeneration and secondary demyelination, or local factors in the nerves, such as ischemia or the consequences of repeated minor trauma. Nevertheless, age-related changes in peripheral nerves probably result from the cumulative, lifelong effect of various pathogenic factors modified by genetic determinants and by a gradual decrease in regenerative capacity.[70]

Clinical Pearls

- Due to age-related nerve degeneration, less local anesthetic at lower concentration may be needed for nerve blockade.
- Age-related changes of the peripheral nerve may be responsible for the typically poorer ultrasonographic images of the peripheral nerves in the elderly as compared to younger subjects.[77]

RESPONSE OF PERIPHERAL NERVE TO INJURY

Injuries to the peripheral nerves result in loss of motor, sensory, and autonomic functions in the denervated segments of the body due to the interruption of axons, degeneration of distal nerve fibers, and eventual death of axotomized neurons.[78] Functional deficits caused by nerve injuries can be compensated by reinnervation of denervated targets by regenerating injured axons or by collateral branching of undamaged axons and remodeling of nervous system circuitry related to the lost functions. Nerve regeneration is possible if the cut ends remain near each other[76] otherwise, regeneration may not be complete or successful.

After an injury, the neuron attempts to repair the damage, regenerate the process, and restore function by initiating a series of structural and metabolic events called *axon reaction*. The reactions to the trauma are localized in three regions of the neuron: at the site of damage (local changes), distal to the site of damage (anterograde changes), and proximal to the site of damage (retrograde changes). Local reaction to injury involves removal of debris by neuroglial cells. The portion of the axon distal to an injury undergoes degeneration and is phagocytosed. The proximal portion of the injured axon undergoes degeneration followed by sprouting of a new axon whose growth is directed by Schwann cells.

Clinical Pearls

- The electrical stimulation threshold for a motor response of the sciatic nerve is increased in patients with diabetic foot gangrene, which may affect nerve identification.[79]
- Many postprocedure nerve injuries occur in nerves with preexisting pathology.[80]

SUMMARY

The knowledge that neural anatomy is unique at different anatomical sites is essential for a safe and effective practice of regional anesthesia. Understanding the peripheral nerve structure and its implication while using state-of-the-art monitors, including ultrasonography, nerve stimulation, and injection pressure monitoring, is helpful in minimizing the potential for patient injury.

REFERENCES

1. Jessen KR, Mirsky R: The origin and development of glial cells in peripheral nerves. Nat Rev Neurosci 2005;6(9):671–682.
2. Williams P: *Gray s Anatomy*, 38th ed. Churchill Livingstone, 1995.
3. Gartner L, Hiatt J: *Color Textbook of Histology*, 2nd ed. Saunders, 2001.
4. Ross M, Pawlina W: *Histology: A Text and Atlas With Correlated Cell and Molecular Biology*, 6th ed. Wolters Kluwer Lippincott Williams & Wilkins, 2011.
5. Thomas P, Berthold C, Ochoa J: Microscopic anatomy of the peripheral nervous system. In Dyck P, Thomas P (eds): *Peripheral Neuropathy*, 3rd ed. Saunders, 1993, pp 28–91.
6. Brushart T: *Nerve Repair*. Oxford University Press, 2011.
7. Palay SL, Sotelo C, Peters A, Orkand PM: The axon hillock and the initial segment. J Cell Biol 1968;38(1):193–201.
8. Poliak S, Peles E: The local differentiation of myelinated axons at nodes of Ranvier. Nat Rev Neurosci 2003;4(12):968–980.
9. Colognato H, Baron W, Avellana-Adalid V, et al: CNS integrins switch growth factor signalling to promote target-dependent survival. Nat Cell Biol 2002;4(11):833–841.
10. Fernandez PA, Tang DG, Cheng L, Prochiantz A, Mudge AW, Raff MC: Evidence that axon-derived neuregulin promotes oligodendrocyte survival in the developing rat optic nerve. Neuron 2000;28(1):81–90.
11. de Waegh SM, Lee VM, Brady ST. Local modulation of neurofilament phosphorylation, axonal caliber, and slow axonal transport by myelinating Schwann cells. Cell 1992;68(3):451–463.
12. Griffiths I, Klugmann M, Anderson T, et al: Axonal swellings and degeneration in mice lacking the major proteolipid of myelin. Science 1998;280(5369):1610–1613.
13. Lappe-Siefke C, Goebbels S, Gravel M, et al: Disruption of Cnp1 uncouples oligodendroglial functions in axonal support and myelination. Nat Genet 2003;33(3):366–374.

14. Nadim W, Anderson PN, Turmaine M: The role of Schwann cells and basal lamina tubes in the regeneration of axons through long lengths of freeze-killed nerve grafts. Neuropathol Appl Neurobiol 1990;16(5):411–421.

15. Noakes PG, Bennett MR: Growth of axons into developing muscles of the chick forelimb is preceded by cells that stain with Schwann cell antibodies. J Comp Neurol 1987;259(3):330–347.

16. Court FA, Wrabetz L, Feltri ML: Basal lamina: Schwann cells wrap to the rhythm of space-time. Curr Opin Neurobiol 2006;16(5):501–507.

17. Darby S, Frysztak R: Neuroanatomy of the spinal cord. In Cramer GD, Darby S (eds): *Basic and Clinical Anatomy of the Spine, Spinal Cord, and ANS*, 2nd ed. Elsevier Mosby, 2005, pp 339–410.

18. Morell P, Quarles R: Molecular architecture of myelin. In Siegel G, Agranoff B, Albers R (eds): *Basic Neurochemistry: Molecular, Cellular and Medical Aspects*, 6th ed. Lippincott-Raven, 1999, pp 51–71.

19. Ritchie JM, Rogart RB: Density of sodium channels in mammalian myelinated nerve fibers and nature of the axonal membrane under the myelin sheath. Proc Natl Acad Sci U S A 1977;74(1):211–215.

20. Wang H, Kunkel DD, Martin TM, Schwartzkroin PA, Tempel BL: Heteromultimeric K+ channels in terminal and juxtaparanodal regions of neurons. Nature 1993;365(6441):75–79.

21. Thaxton C, Pillai AM, Pribisko AL, Dupree JL, Bhat MA: Nodes of Ranvier act as barriers to restrict invasion of flanking paranodal domains in myelinated axons. Neuron 2011;69(2):244–257.

22. Waxman SG, Ritchie JM: Molecular dissection of the myelinated axon. Ann Neurol 1993;33(2):121–136.

23. Ochoa J, Mair WG: The normal sural nerve in man. I. Ultrastructure and numbers of fibres and cells. Acta Neuropathol 1969;13(3):197–216.

24. Millesi H, Terzis J: Nomenclature in peripheral nerve surgery. In Terzis J (ed): *Microreconstruction of Nerve Injuries*. Saunders, 1987, pp 3–13.

25. Sala-Blanch X, Vandepitte C, Laur JJ, et al: A practical review of perineural versus intraneural injections: A call for standard nomenclature. Int Anesthesiol Clin 2011;49(4):1–12.

26. Sunderland S, Bradley KC: The perineurium of peripheral nerves. Anat Rec 1952;113(2):125–141.

27. Sunderland S: The connective tissues of peripheral nerves. Brain 1965;88(4):841–854.

28. Ushiki T, Ide C: Three-dimensional organization of the collagen fibrils in the rat sciatic nerve as revealed by transmission- and scanning electron microscopy. Cell Tissue Res 1990;260(1):175–184.

29. Thomas PK. The connective tissue of peripheral nerve: an electron microscope study. J Anat 1963;97:35–44.

30. Thomas PK, Bhagat S: The effect of extraction of the intrafascicular contents of peripheral nerve trunks on perineurial structure. Acta Neuropathol 1978;43(1–2):135–141.

31. Lorimier P, Mezin P, Labat Moleur F, Pinel N, Peyrol S, Stoebner P: Ultrastructural localization of the major components of the extracellular matrix in normal rat nerve. J Histochem Cytochem 1992;40(6):859–868.

32. Reina MA, Lopez A, De Andres JA: [Adipose tissue within peripheral nerves. Study of the human sciatic nerve]. Rev Esp Anestesiol Reanim 2002;49(8):397–402.

33. Mirsky R, Parmantier E, McMahon AP, Jessen KR: Schwann cell-derived desert hedgehog signals nerve sheath formation. Ann N Y Acad Sci 1999;883:196–202.

34. Shanthaveerappa TR, Bourne GH: Perineural epithelium: A new concept of its role in the integrity of the peripheral nervous system. Science 1966;154(3755):1464–1467.

35. Lehmann HJ: [Structure and function of the perineural diffusion barrier]. Z Zellforsch Mikrosk Anat 1957;46(2):232–241.

36. Eldridge CF, Sanes JR, Chiu AY, Bunge RP, Cornbrooks CJ: Basal lamina-associated heparan sulphate proteoglycan in the rat PNS: Characterization and localization using monoclonal antibodies. J Neurocytol 1986;15(1):37–51.

37. Paetau A, Mellstrom K, Vaheri A, Haltia M: Distribution of a major connective tissue protein, fibronectin, in normal and neoplastic human nervous tissue. Acta Neuropathol 1980;51(1):47–51.

38. Stopar-Pintaric T, Cvetko E, Strbec M, et al: Intraneural and perineural inflammatory changes in piglets after injection of ultrasound gel, endotoxin, 0.9% NaCl or needle insertion without injection. Anaesth Analg 2014;115:1–6.

39. Rydevik BL, Kwan MK, Myers RR, et al: An in vitro mechanical and histological study of acute stretching on rabbit tibial nerve. J Orthop Res 1990;8(5):694–701.

40. Olsson Y: Microenvironment of the peripheral nervous system under normal and pathological conditions. Crit Rev Neurobiol 1990;5(3):265–311.

41. Jacobs JM, Love S: Qualitative and quantitative morphology of human sural nerve at different ages. Brain 1985;108(Pt 4):897–924.

42. Powell HC, Myers RR, Costello ML, Lampert PW: Endoneurial fluid pressure in wallerian degeneration. Ann Neurol 1979;5(6):550–557.

43. Gamble HJ, Eames RA. An electron microscope study of the connective tissues of human peripheral nerve. J Anat 1964;98:655–663.

44. Salonen V, Roytta M, Peltonen J: The effects of nerve transection on the endoneurial collagen fibril sheaths. Acta Neuropathol 1987;74(1):13–21.

45. Oldfors A: Macrophages in peripheral nerves. An ultrastructural and enzyme histochemical study on rats. Acta Neuropathol 1980;49(1):43–49.

46. Braunewell KH, Martini R, LeBaron R, et al: Up-regulation of a chondroitin sulphate epitope during regeneration of mouse sciatic nerve: Evidence that the immunoreactive molecules are related to the chondroitin sulphate proteoglycans decorin and versican. Eur J Neurosci 1995;7(4):792–804.

47. Kapur E, Vuckovic I, Dilberovic F, et al: Neurologic and histologic outcome after intraneural injections of lidocaine in canine sciatic nerves. Acta Anaesthesiol Scand 2007;51(1):101–107.

48. Jeng CL, Rosenblatt MA: Intraneural injections and regional anesthesia: The known and the unknown. Minerva Anestesiol 2011;77(1):54–58.

49. Orebaugh SL, Mukalel JJ, Krediet AC, et al: Brachial plexus root injection in a human cadaver model: Injectate distribution and effects on the neuraxis. Reg Anesth Pain Med 2012;37(5):525–529.

50. Moayeri N, Bigeleisen PE, Groen GJ: Quantitative architecture of the brachial plexus and surrounding compartments, and their possible significance for plexus blocks. Anesthesiology 2008;108(2):299–304.

51. Sala Blanch X, Lopez AM, Carazo J, et al: Intraneural injection during nerve stimulator-guided sciatic nerve block at the popliteal fossa. Br J Anaesth 2009;102(6):855–861.

52. Berthold CH, Carlstedt T. Observations on the morphology at the transition between the peripheral and the central nervous system in the cat. III. Myelinated fibres in S1 dorsal rootlets. Acta Physiol Scand Suppl 1977;446:43–60.

53. Andres KH: [The fine structure of the olfactory region of macrosmatic animals]. Z Zellforsch Mikrosk Anat 1966;69:140–154.

54. Haller FR, Low FN: The fine structure of the peripheral nerve root sheath in the subarachnoid space in the rat and other laboratory animals. Am J Anat 1971;131(1):11–19.

55. Himango WA, Low FN: The fine structure of a lateral recess of the subarachnoid space in the rat. Anat Rec 1971;171(1):1–19.

56. McCabe JS, Low FN: The subarachnoid angle: an area of transition in peripheral nerve. Anat Rec 1969;164(1):15–33.

57. Waggener JD, Beggs J: The membranous coverings of neural tissues: An electron microscopy study. J Neuropathol Exp Neurol 1967;26(3):412–426.

58. Pease DC, Schultz RL: Electron microscopy of rat cranial meninges. Am J Anat 1958;102(2):301–321.

59. Nabeshima S, Reese TS, Landis DM, Brightman MW: Junctions in the meninges and marginal glia. J Comp Neurol 1975;164(2):127–169.

60. Evans PJ, Lloyd JW, Wood GJ: Accidental intrathecal injection of bupivacaine and dextran. Anaesthesia 1981;36(7):685–687.

61. Gadsden JC, Lindenmuth DM, Hadzic A, Xu D, Somasundarum L, Flisinski KA: Lumbar plexus block using high-pressure injection leads to contralateral and epidural spread. Anesthesiology 2008;109(4):683–688.

62. Lundborg G. Intraneural microcirculation. Orthop Clin North Am 1988;19(1):1–12.

63. McManis PG, Schmelzer JD, Zollman PJ, Low PA: Blood flow and autoregulation in somatic and autonomic ganglia. Comparison with sciatic nerve. Brain 1997;120(Pt 3):445–449.

64. Beggs J, Johnson PC, Olafsen A, Watkins CJ, Cleary C: Transperineurial arterioles in human sural nerve. J Neuropathol Exp Neurol 1991;50(6):704–718.

65. Bell MA, Weddell AG: A morphometric study of intrafascicular vessels of mammalian sciatic nerve. Muscle Nerve 1984;7(7):524–534.

66. Smith DR, Kobrine AI, Rizzoli HV: Blood flow in peripheral nerves. Normal and post severance flow rates. J Neurol Sci 1977;33(3):341–346.

67. Kozu H, Tamura E, Parry GJ: Endoneurial blood supply to peripheral nerves is not uniform. J Neurol Sci 1992;111(2):204–208.

68. Perez-Castro R, Patel S, Garavito-Aguilar ZV, et al: Cytotoxicity of local anesthetics in human neuronal cells. Anesth Analg 2009;108(3):997–1007.

69. Drac H, Babiuch M, Wisniewska W: Morphological and biochemical changes in peripheral nerves with aging. Neuropatol Pol 1991;29(1–2):49–67.

70. Lehmann J: [Age-related changes in peripheral nerves]. Zentralbl Allg Pathol 1986;131(3):219–227.

71. Arnold N, Harriman DG: The incidence of abnormality in control human peripheral nerves studied by single axon dissection. J Neurol Neurosurg Psychiatry 1970;33(1):55–61.

72. Tohgi H, Tsukagoshi H, Toyokura Y: Quantitative changes with age in normal sural nerves. Acta Neuropathol 1977;38(3):213–220.

73. Vizoso AD: The relationship between internodal length and growth in human nerves. J Anat 1950;84(4):342–353.

74. Ochoa J, Mair WG: The normal sural nerve in man. II. Changes in the axons and Schwann cells due to ageing. Acta Neuropathol 1969;13(3): 217–239.

75. Ochoa J: Recognition of unmyelinated fiber disease: morphologic criteria. Muscle Nerve 1978;1(5):375–387.

76. Kovacic U, Sketelj J, Bajrovic FF: Chapter 26: Age-related differences in the reinnervation after peripheral nerve injury. Int Rev Neurobiol 2009;87:465–482.

77. Li X, Karmakar MK, Lee A, Kwok WH, Critchley LA, Gin T: Quantitative evaluation of the echo intensity of the median nerve and flexor muscles of the forearm in the young and the elderly. Br J Radiol 2012;85(1014):e140–e145.

78. Navarro X, Vivo M, Valero-Cabre A: Neural plasticity after peripheral nerve injury and regeneration. Prog Neurobiol 2007;82(4):163–201.

79. Keyl C, Held T, Albiez G, Schmack A, Wiesenack C: Increased electrical nerve stimulation threshold of the sciatic nerve in patients with diabetic foot gangrene: A prospective parallel cohort study. Eur J Anaesthesiol 2013;30(7):435–440.

80. Borgeat A, Ekatodramis G, Kalberer F, Benz C: Acute and nonacute complications associated with interscalene block and shoulder surgery: A prospective study. Anesthesiology 2001;95(4):875–880.

Connective Tissues of Peripheral Nerves

Miguel A. Reina, Xavier Sala-Blanch, Fabiola Machés, Riánsares Arriazu, and Alberto Prats-Galino

INTRODUCTION

A better understanding of some features of the fine structure of peripheral nerves may provide us with essential information that can be helpful in anesthetic clinical practice. This chapter reviews the ultrastructure of connective tissues of peripheral nerves to facilitate understanding of its role as the perineurial diffusion barrier and implication in regional anesthesia.

FASCICLES

Nerves and their principal branches (Figures 5–1 to 5–3) consist of parallel bundles of nerve fibers (nerve fascicles, fasciculi). The size, number, and pattern of fasciculi vary among nerves and at different distances from their origin. When the connective tissue of the peripheral nerve is removed, 20 or more tubular structures or fascicles are typically seen.

Inside each nerve, the axons form an intraneural plexus in such a fashion that one axon can contribute to different fascicles along the nerve length (Figure 5–4). In other words, an axon can travel from a peripheral position to a more central position as well as swap the fascicles altogether along its descent more peripherally.[1–4] Indeed, cross-sectional anatomy of nerves at close distance from each other demonstrates that the location and number of fascicles within nerves are highly variable (see Figure 5–3) with the presence of intraneural plexuses (Figures 5–5 and 5–6). The number, size, and location of fascicles in peripheral nerves are also variable even within a single nerve and can vary as much as 23 times along a 4- to 5-cm length of nerve.[5–8]

Clinical Pearl

- Inside each nerve, the axons form an intraneural plexus in such way that an axon can occupy different fascicles.

In a cross section of a sciatic nerve, fascicles comprise 25%–75% of the cross-sectional area (see Figures 5–1 and 5–3). This proportion varies in different nerves and at different levels of the same nerve. Up to 50% of the cross-sectional area is made up of non-neural tissue, including endoneural fluid and connective stroma. The number of fascicles increases at the level of nerve branching. In the proximity of joints, the fascicles are thinner, more numerous and have a thicker perineurium, which may confer better protection against pressure and stretching.[8]

CONNECTIVE TISSUE SHEATHS OF PERIPHERAL NERVES

The connective tissue inside nerves functions to support and protect nerves blood and lymphatic vessels (see Figure 5–1 and 5–2). The connective tissue of peripheral nerves takes different names according to its location.[1–3] On the outside of each peripheral nerve, there is collagenous tissue: *epineurium*. Surrounding every fascicle within the nerve is the *perineurium*. Individual nerve fibers within the fascicles are embedded in *endoneurium*, which fills the space bound by the perineurium. As the peripheral nerve divides and the number of fascicles decreases, the connective tissue sheaths become progressively thinner. For instance, in monofascicular nerves the epineurium is absent, distributed irregularly, or appears integrated with the perineurium. Connective tissue that connect nerves to the surrounding structures are thinner and disperse, often losing any distinguishable feature from that of general connective tissue.[9]

ENDONEURIUM

The endoneurium (Figures 5–7 and 5–8) intimately surrounds Schwann cells and fills the space bounded externally by the perineurium. Endoneurium contains collagen fibers,

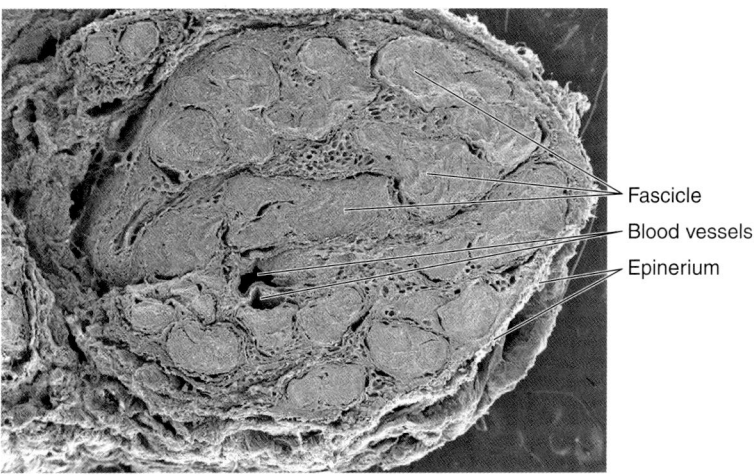

FIGURE 5-1. Sciatic nerve at the level of popliteal fossa. Scanning electron microscopy. Magnification ×25. (Reproduced with permission from Reina MA, Arriazu R, Collier CB, et al: Electron microscopy of human peripheral nerves of clinical relevance to the practice of nerve blocks. A structural and ultrastructural review based on original experimental and laboratory data, *Rev Esp Anestesiol Reanim*. Dec 2013;60(10):552-562.)

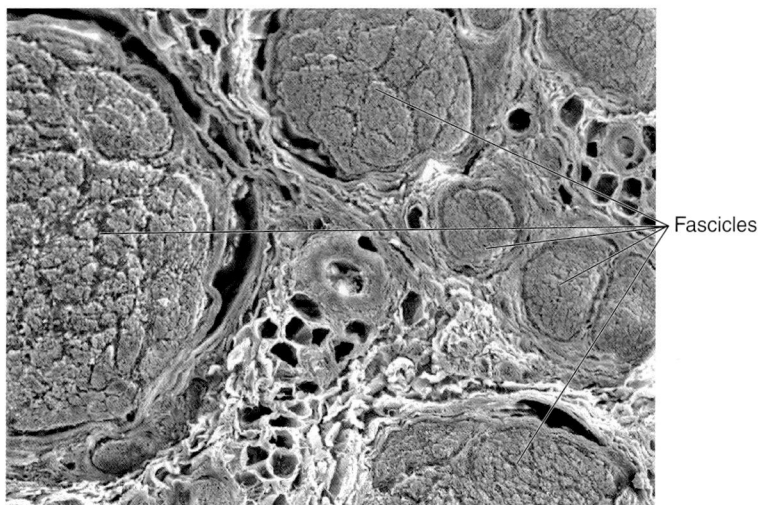

FIGURE 5-2. Scanning electron microscopy image of the human tibial nerve fascicles and adipose tissue that between fascicles. Magnification ×75. (Reproduced with permission from Wikinski J, Reina MA, Bollini C, et al: *Diagnóstico, prevención y tratamiento de las complicaciones neurológicas asociadas con la anestesia regional periférica y central*. Buenos Aires: Panamericana Ed; 2011.)

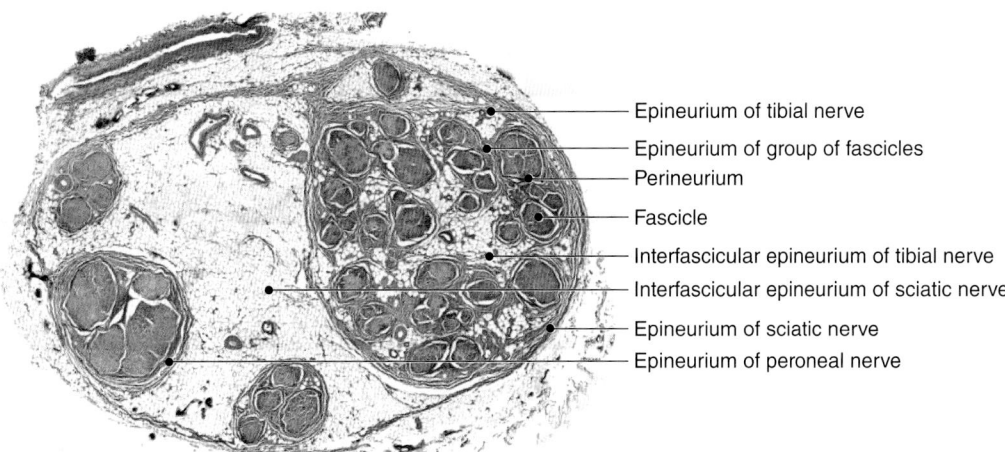

FIGURE 5-3. Sciatic nerve at the level of popliteal fossa. Hematoxylin-eosin. (Reproduced with permission from Reina MA, De Andres JA, Hernández JM, et al: Successive changes in extraneural structures from the subarachnoid nerve roots to the peripheral nerve, influencing anesthetic block, and treatment of acute postoperative pain. *Eur J Pain*. Suppl 2011;5(2):377-385.)

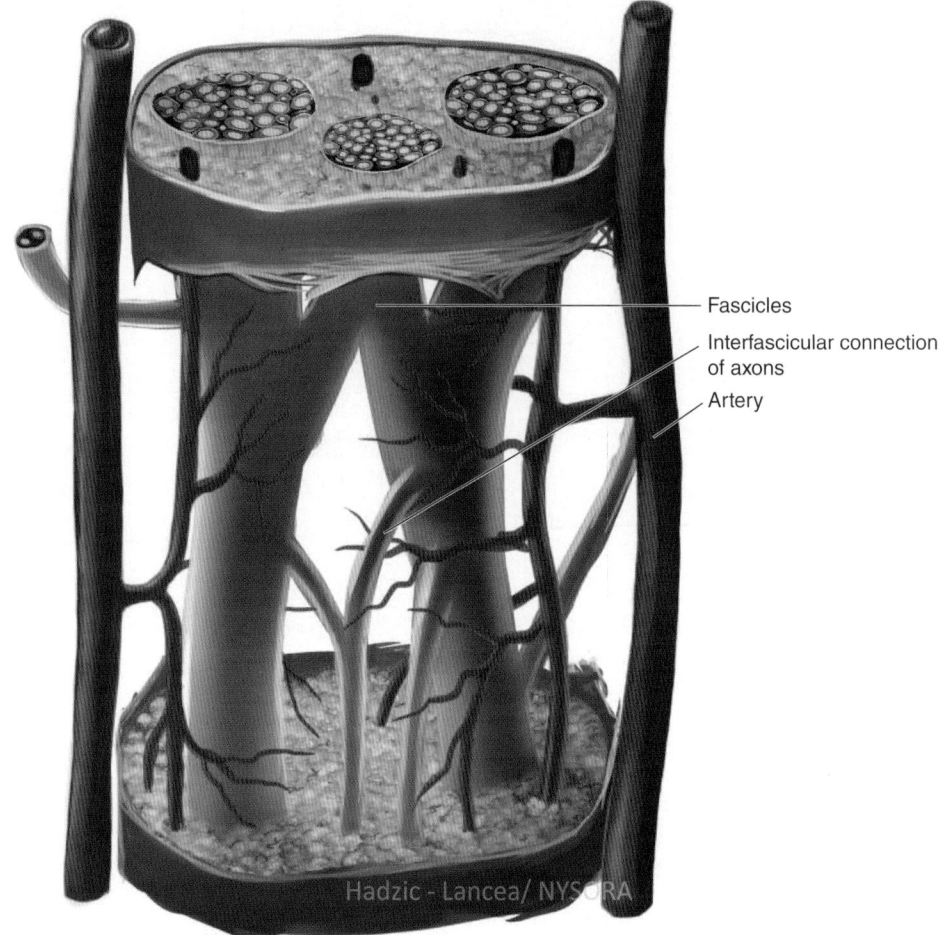

Fascicles

Interfascicular connection of axons

Artery

Hadzic - Lancea/ NYSORA

FIGURE 5–4. Diagram of intraneural plexus enclosed in a peripheral nerve. (Reproduced with permission from De Andrés JA, Reina MA, López A, et al: *Blocs nerveux périphériques, paresthésies et injections intraneurales*, Le Practicien en Anesthésie Réanimation 2010;14:213-221.)

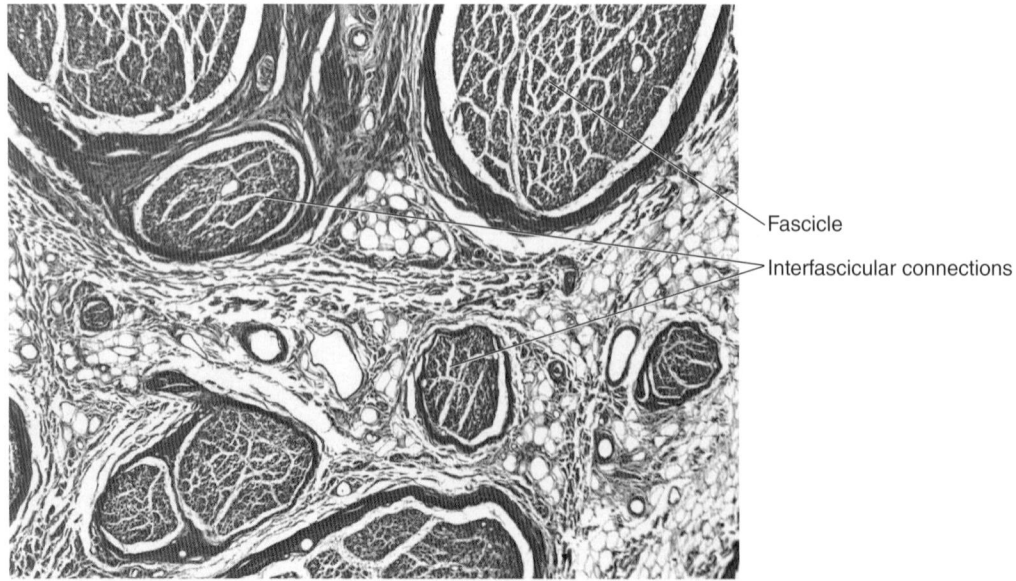

Fascicle

Interfascicular connections

FIGURE 5–5. Intraneural plexus within a peripheral nerve, from the brachial plexus. Hematoxylin-eosin. (Reproduced with permission from Reina MA, Arriazu R, Collier CB, et al: Electron microscopy of human peripheral nerves of clinical relevance to the practice of nerve blocks. A structural and ultrastructural review based on original experimental and laboratory data, *Rev Esp Anestesiol Reanim*. 2013 Dec;60(10):552-562.)

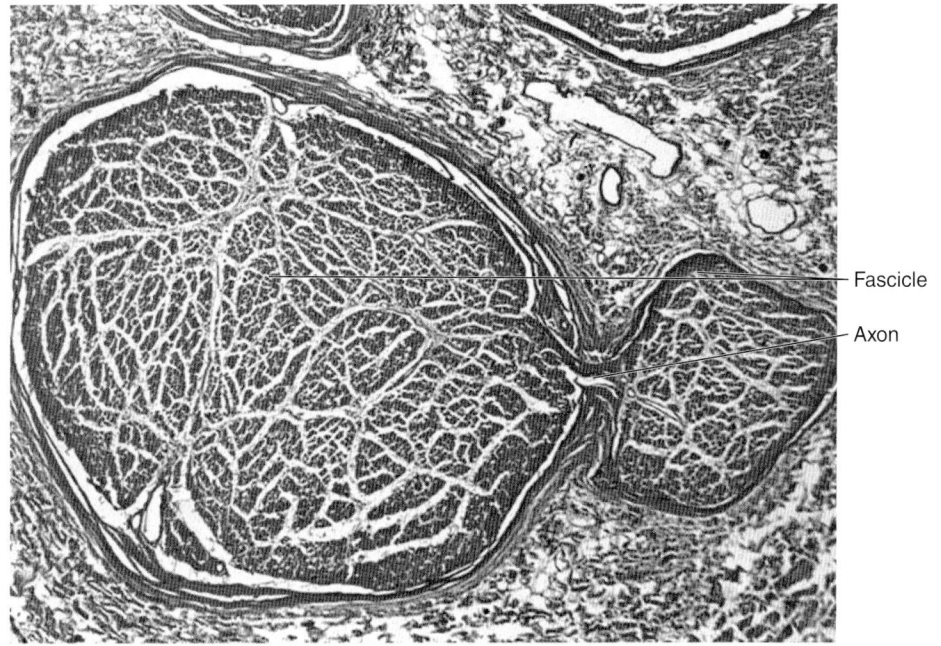

— Fascicle

— Axon

FIGURE 5–6. Intraneural plexus inside a peripheral nerve. Interfascicular connection from axons between two fascicles, obtained from the brachial plexus. Hematoxylin-eosin. (Reproduced with permission from Reina MA, Arriazu R, Collier CB, et al: Electron microscopy of human peripheral nerves of clinical relevance to the practice of nerve blocks. A structural and ultrastructural review based on original experimental and laboratory data. *Rev Esp Anestesiol Reanim*. 2013 Dec;60(10):552-562.)

fibroblasts, capillaries, and a few mast cells and macrophages. Collagen fibers are permeable and concentrated in a zone beneath the perineurium and around nerve fibers and blood vessels. The collagen fibers surround both myelinated and unmyelinated nerve fibers. However, the endoneurial sheaths around smaller myelinated fibers and around some unmyelinated axons are less well organized (Figure 5–9).

Fibroblasts are among the most abundant cell types of the endoneurium. They are responsible for fiber formation and production of ground substance. When sectioned transversely,

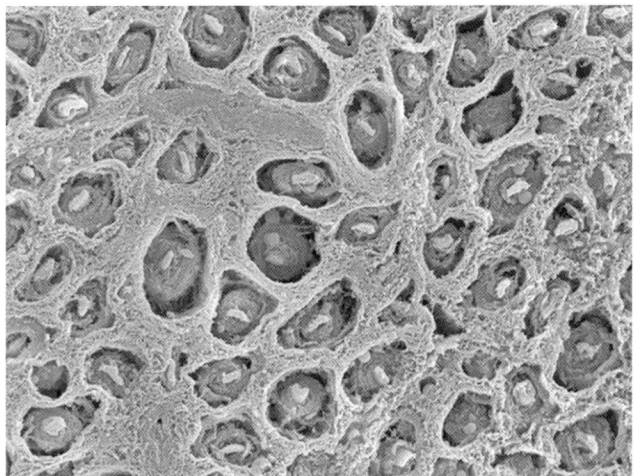

FIGURE 5–7. Endoneurium shaped as multiple canaliculi, enclosing fascicles of tibial nerve. Scanning electron microscopy. Magnification ×900. (Reproduced with permission from Reina MA: *Atlas of Functional Anatomy for Regional Anesthesia and Pain Medicine*. New York: Springer; 2015.)

endoneurial fibroblasts have triangular or rectangular perikaria. The appearance of fibroblasts varies depending on their functional activity. When the cell is metabolically active, as is the case with growth and in tissue regeneration after injury, the nucleus is larger and nucleoli are more prominent. The cytoplasm also stains more deeply and is basophilic in contrast with the lightly staining, slightly acidophilic cytoplasm of a relatively inactive cell. Like those in the epineurium, fibroblasts in the endoneurium lack a basal lamina.

Mast cells are especially numerous along the course of blood vessels. Mast cell granules are soluble in water and are therefore not easily revealed in sections routinely prepared with hematoxylin and eosin stain. After adequate fixation, the granules stain with most basic dyes and become metachromatic after certain dyes, such as toluidine blue. Electron microphotographs show that the secretory granules are membrane bound, and the granule matrices have varying densities and characteristic helical-type patterns (Figure 5–10). Macrophages are also found frequently around perivascular endoneurium (Figure 5–11). The endoneurium contributes to the stability of the internal medium where the Schwann cells and axons are located.[10] The endoneurium of cutaneous nerves contains more collagen fibers than deep nerves; this probably is related to its protective role. The endoneural collagen is believed to originate from the Schwann cells, which are 9:1 more prominent than fibroblasts. Schwann cells represent 90% of intrafascicular cells, whereas fibroblasts account for less than 5% of the remaining number. The endoneurium along with the epineurium and perineurium contribute to nerve protection against elongation under strain. The sinuous trajectories of axons confer additional protection on nerves. Endoneurial sheaths around axons is demonstrated in

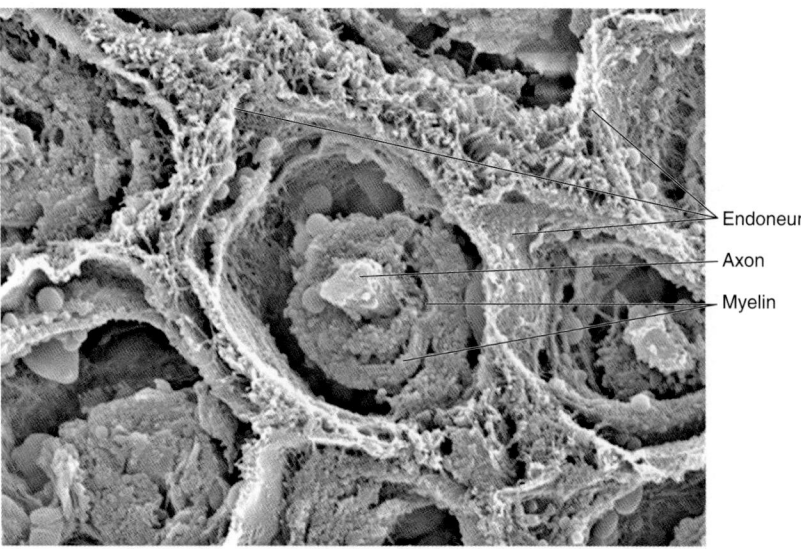

Endoneurium
Axon
Myelin

FIGURE 5–8. Endoneurium envelops myelinated axons in fascicles in a peripheral nerve. Scanning electron microscopy. Magnification ×3300. (Reproduced with permission from Reina MA, Arriazu R, Collier CB, et al: Electron microscopy of human peripheral nerves of clinical relevance to the practice of nerve blocks. A structural and ultrastructural review based on original experimental and laboratory data. *Rev Esp Anestesiol Reanim.* 2013 Dec;60(10):552-562.)

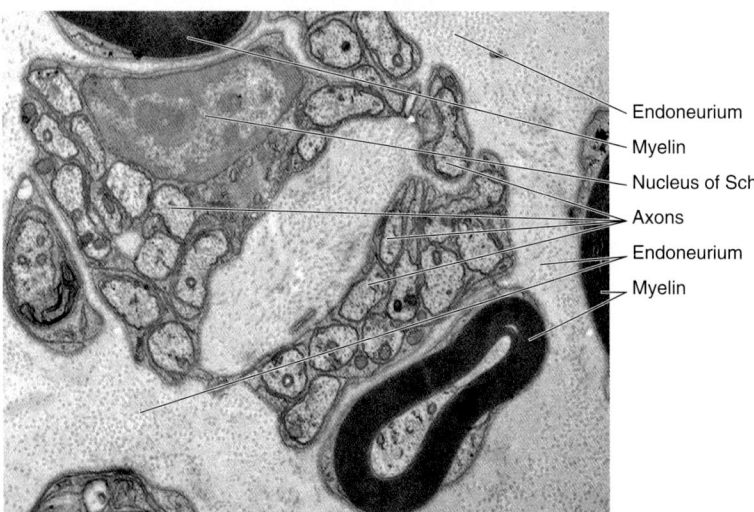

Endoneurium
Myelin
Nucleus of Schwann cell
Axons
Endoneurium
Myelin

FIGURE 5–9. Unmyelinated and myelinated axons enclosed by endoneurium. Transmission electron microscopy. Magnification ×20000. (Reproduced with permission from Reina MA, Arriazu R, Collier CB, et al: Electron microscopy of human peripheral nerves of clinical relevance to the practice of nerve blocks. A structural and ultrastructural review based on original experimental and laboratory data. *Rev Esp Anestesiol Reanim.* 2013 Dec;60(10):552-562.)

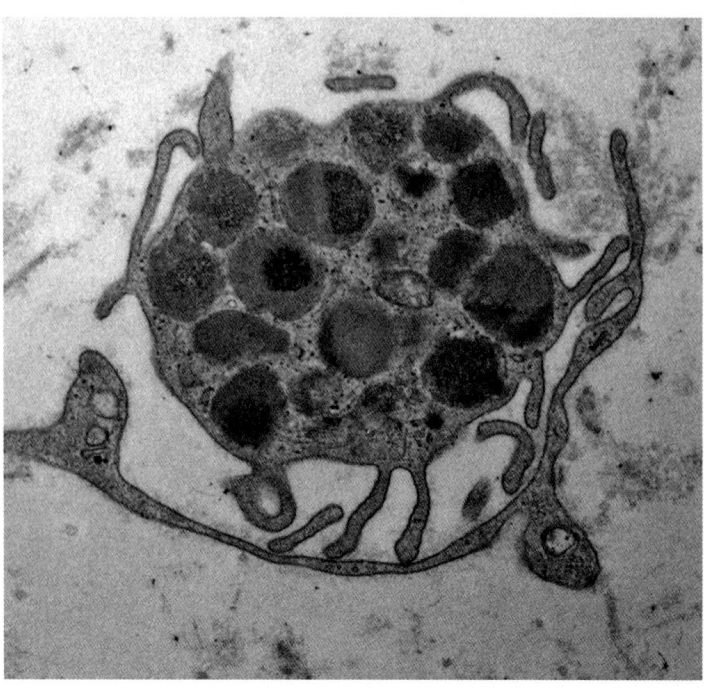

FIGURE 5–10. Mastocyte inside fascicles from tibial nerve. Transmission electron microscopy. Magnification ×7000. (Reproduced with permission from Reina MA: *Atlas of Functional Anatomy for Regional Anesthesia and Pain Medicine.* New York: Springer; 2015.)

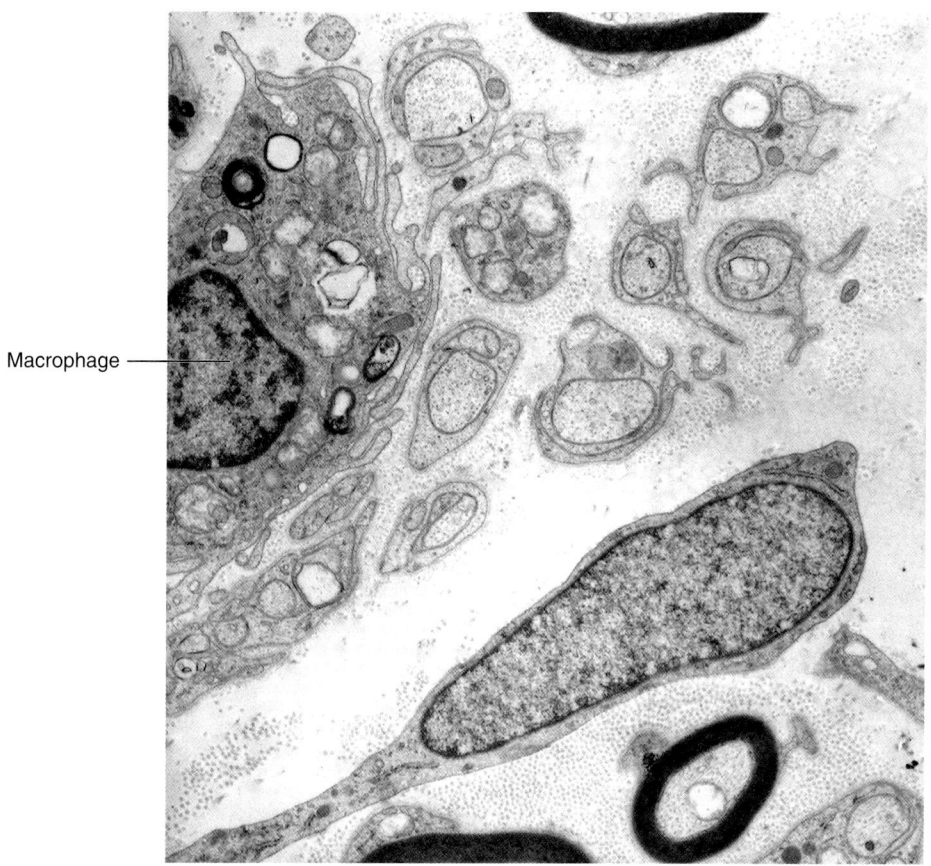

Macrophage —

FIGURE 5–11. Macrophage within fascicles as seen on Transmission electron microscopy. Magnification ×7000.

figures 5-7, 5-8 and 5-9. Instead of individually shaped endo-neurial layers, the endoneurium appears rather as a contin-uum, forming several canaliculi into which axons are embedded.

PERINEURIUM

Each fascicle is surrounded by a connective tissue sheath, the perineurium.[1–3,11–14] The perineurium consists of concentric layers of flattened cells separated by layers of collagen (Figures 5–12 to 5–16). The number of perineurial cell layers depends on the size of the fascicle. As many as 8–16 concentric layers may be present around large nerve fascicles, but a single layer of perineurial cells surrounds small distal fascicles. In larger peripheral nerves, concentric cell layers alternate with layers of collagen fibers arranged longitudinally, similar to those of the epineurium. Collagen fibers are thinner than those of the epineurium, and only a few elastic fibers are scattered among

them. Perineurial cells have a basal lamina on each side that may be considerably dense. At sites known as hemidesmo-somes, the perineurial cell plasma membrane strongly adheres to the basal lamina.[3,11]

With electron microscopy, perineurial cells are seen as thin sheets of cytoplasm containing small amounts of endoplasmic reticulum, filaments, and numerous endocytic vesicles. Tight junctions and gap junctions between adjacent cells within the same layer of perineurium are also observed.[3,11] Similar tight junctions may also appear between successive layers of the peri-neurium when their cells are in close proximity. Tight junctions in the inner layers of the perineurium and tight junctions in endoneurial capillaries form a blood-nerve barrier structure[14–16] (Figures 5–17 and 5–18). The *blood-nerve barrier* is not equiva-lent to the *blood-brain barrier*[11] as the blood-brain barrier astro-cytes help regulate the flow of compounds between blood and the brain. The perineural cells are metabolically active, and their cytoplasms contain enzymes like ATPase (adenosine triphosphatase), 5-nucleotidase, and so on. These cells probably play a role in maintaining electrolyte and glucose balance around the nerve cells.[17]

The perineurium forms a tubular wrapping that allows some axonal movement inside the fascicles. The thickness of the epineurium varies between 1 and 100 μm. As the number of fascicles within a nerve increases, the thickness of the perineu-rium generally decreases. For instance, along the trajectory of

92   FOUNDATIONS OF LOCAL AND REGIONAL ANESTHESIA

PART 2

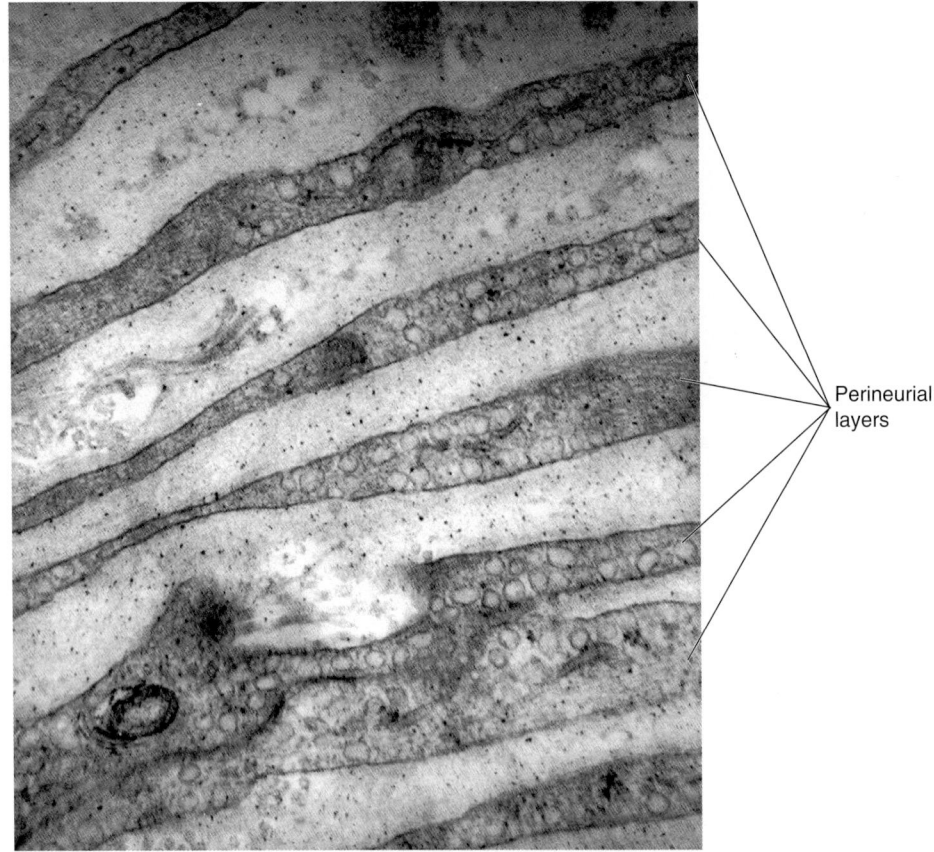

FIGURE 5–12. Concentric perineurial layers. Transmission electron microscopy. Magnification ×30,000. (Reproduced with permission from Reina MA, Arriazu R, Collier CB, et al: Electron microscopy of human peripheral nerves of clinical relevance to the practice of nerve blocks. A structural and ultrastructural review based on original experimental and laboratory data. *Rev Esp Anestesiol Reanim.* 2013 Dec;60(10):552-562.)

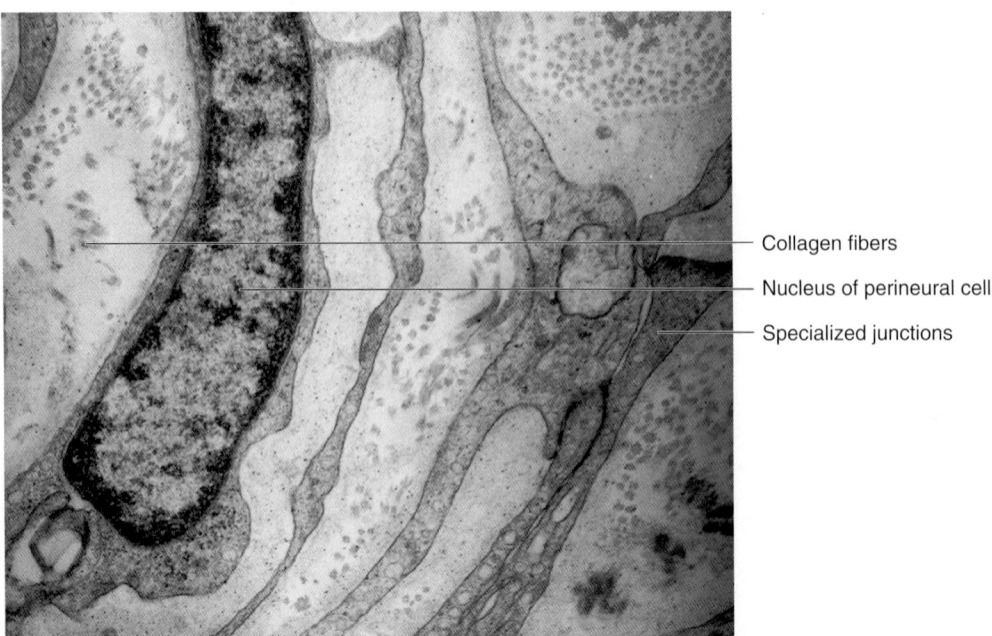

FIGURE 5–13. Perineurial layers and specialized junctions. Transmission electron microscopy. Magnification ×20,000. (Reproduced with permission from Reina MA, Arriazu R, Collier CB, et al: Electron microscopy of human peripheral nerves of clinical relevance to the practice of nerve blocks. A structural and ultrastructural review based on original experimental and laboratory data. *Rev Esp Anestesiol Reanim.* 2013 Dec;60(10):552-562.)

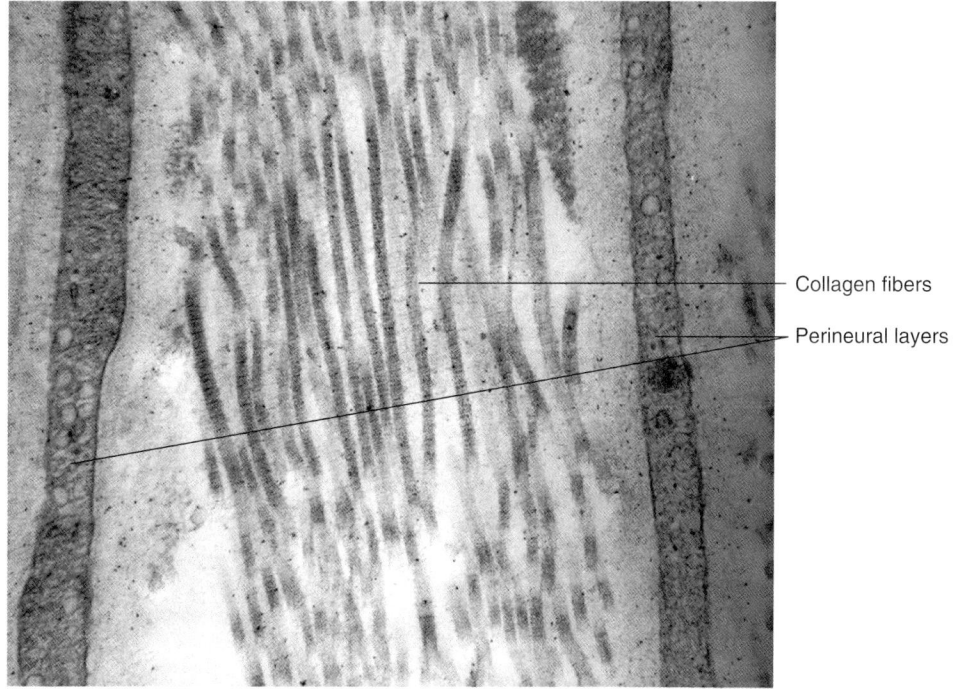

FIGURE 5–14. Collagen fibers among perineurial layers. Transmission electron microscopy. Magnification ×30,000. (Reproduced with permission from Reina MA: *Atlas of Functional Anatomy for Regional Anesthesia and Pain Medicine*. New York: Springer; 2015.)

the median nerve, the epineurium appears proportionally thicker in the wrist than in the axilla. There are three areas where the perineurium is absent and the epineurium becomes in contact with the endoneurium:nerve endings, around blood vessels, and in areas where reticular fibers penetrate the perineurium.

The role of the perineurium is to maintain intrafascicular pressure and to contribute to the barrier effect.[13,16,18] Pressure

exerted on the perineurium is transmitted to the endoneurium and ultimately the nerve fibers (axons).[19] The perineurium increases in thickness around points of nerve branching to provide additional protection.[20]

The perineurium may be also protective in limiting the extension of infection and inflammatory reactions. For instance, when a nerve with intact perineurium crosses an infected area, the nerve responds generally by thickening of its perineurial

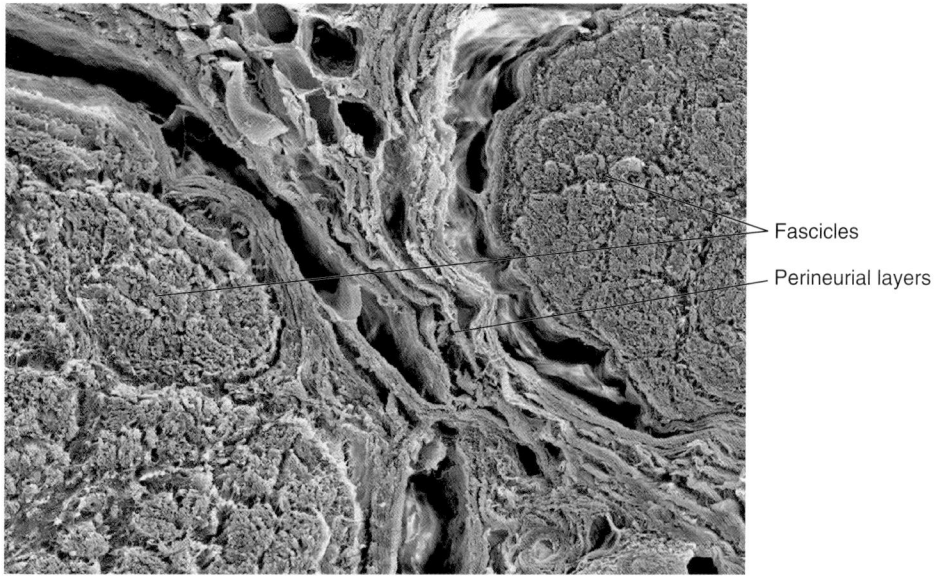

FIGURE 5–15. Perineurium and fascicles: three-dimensional features of perineural layers. Scanning electron microscopy. Magnification ×150. (Reproduced with permission from Reina MA, Arriazu R, Collier CB, et al: Electron microscopy of human peripheral nerves of clinical relevance to the practice of nerve blocks. A structural and ultrastructural review based on original experimental and laboratory data. *Rev Esp Anestesiol Reanim*. 2013 Dec;60(10):552-562.)

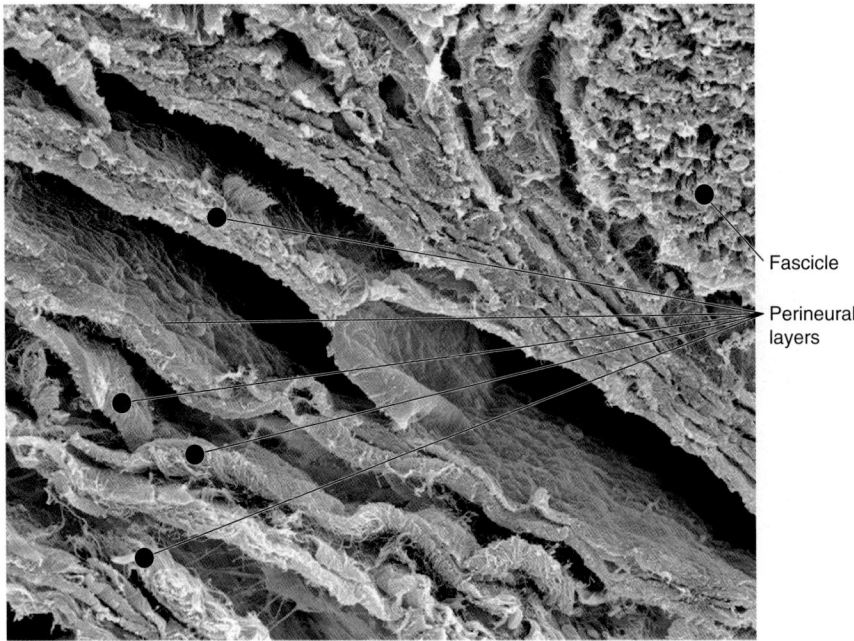

FIGURE 5–16. Three-dimensional image of perineural layers. Scanning electron microscopy. Magnification ×500. (Reproduced with permission from Reina MA, Arriazu R, Collier CB, et al: Electron microscopy of human peripheral nerves of clinical relevance to the practice of nerve blocks. A structural and ultrastructural review based on original experimental and laboratory data. *Rev Esp Anestesiol Reanim.* 2013 Dec;60(10):552-562.)

layer. Conversely, when perineurium is not intact, the infection easily spreads across nerve fascicles.[19] Injury to the epineurium, however, does not compromise the axonal safety to the same extent. Söderfelt demonstrated that the barrier effect of the epineurium is preserved for up to 22 hours postmortem in conditions of ischemia.[16] Olsson has studied the loss of the nerve barrier effect in vivo after nerve lesion. He also has demonstrated recovery of the effect between 2 and 30 days postinjury.[13]

Clinical Pearls

- Fascicles within the nerve are surrounded by perineurium which confers structural protection against penetration and over-stretching injury.
- A blood-nerve barrier is formed by tight junctions in the inner layers of the perineurium and tight junctions in endoneurial capillaries.

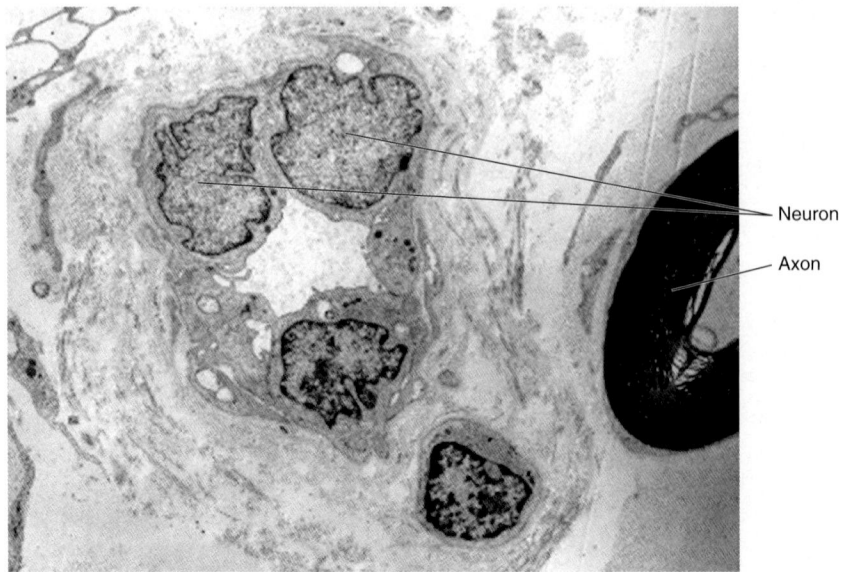

FIGURE 5–17. Endoneurium and capillaries inside fascicles of peripheral nerves. Transmission electron microscopy. Magnification ×3000. (Reproduced with permission from Reina MA, Arriazu R, Collier CB, et al: Electron microscopy of human peripheral nerves of clinical relevance to the practice of nerve blocks. A structural and ultrastructural review based on original experimental and laboratory data. *Rev Esp Anestesiol Reanim.* 2013 Dec;60(10):552-562.)

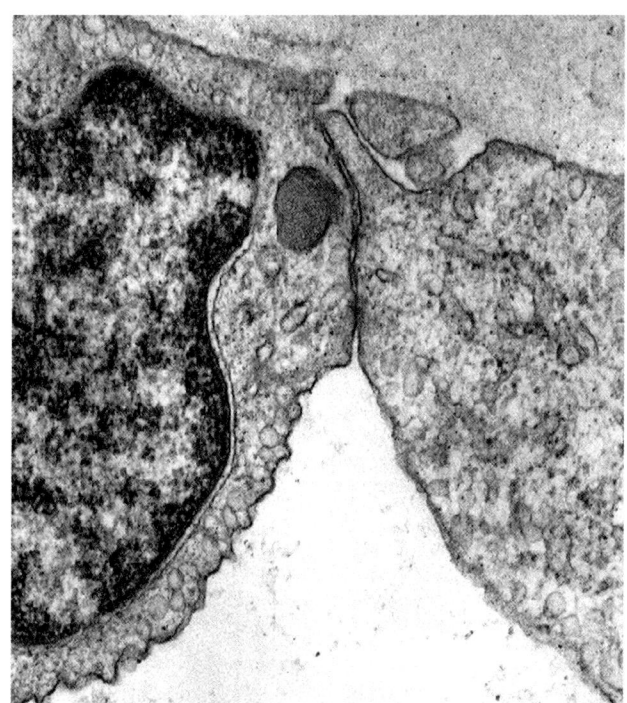

FIGURE 5–18. Endothelial cell from intrafascicular capillary. Transmission electron microscopy. Magnification ×20,000. (Reproduced with permission from Reina MA, López A, Villanueva MC, et al: The blood-nerve barrier in peripheral nerves. *Rev Esp Anestesiol Reanim.* 2003 Feb;50(2):80-86.)

EPINEURIUM

The outermost sheath of the epineurium consists of moderately dense connective tissue that binds nerve fascicles (Figures 5–3, 5–19, and 5–20). Epineurium merges with adipose tissue surrounding peripheral nerves, particularly in subcutaneous tissue. The amount of epineurial tissue varies along a nerve and is more abundant around joints. The thickness of the epineurium varies in different nerves and in different locations of the same nerve. For instance, the average thickness of the epineurium is 22% of the ulnar nerve at the level of the elbow and 88% of the sciatic nerve at the gluteal level. In general, the epineurium represents between 30% and 75% of the cross-sectional area of a nerve.[8,20,21] The proportion of epineurium is higher in larger nerves with increasing numbers of nerve fascicles. However, the epineurium is absent around monofascicular nerves and at nerve endings.

The epineurium contains adipocytes, fibroblasts, connective tissue fibers, mast cells, small blood and lymph vessels, and small nerve fibers innervating the vessels.[20] Epineurium is a permeable structure,[20,21] and its fibroblasts are ultrastructurally identical to fibroblasts elsewhere in the body. Scattered throughout the epineurium, fibroblasts form the epineurial collagen, the most prominent component of this layer. As collagen is a protein stained by most acid dyes, collagen fibers turn weak pink wiht eosin in preparations stained with hematoxylin-eosin. Under the electron microscope, fibers of mature collagen have frecuent cross bandings. Elastic fibers are also present, and these are considerably more compact than collagen fibers. They stain weak pink in sections stained with hematoxylin and eosin, brown with orcein, and blue-purple with resorcin-fuchsin. In electron micrographs, elastin fibers typically appear more stained (darker) at the periphery and are embedded in a substance containing thinner elastin filaments.

The epineurium of some nerves contains a considerable amount of fat, as is the case with the sciatic nerve. The common peroneal and tibial nerves, however, contain less fat than the sciatic nerve, and usually the former contains less fat than the latter.[8]

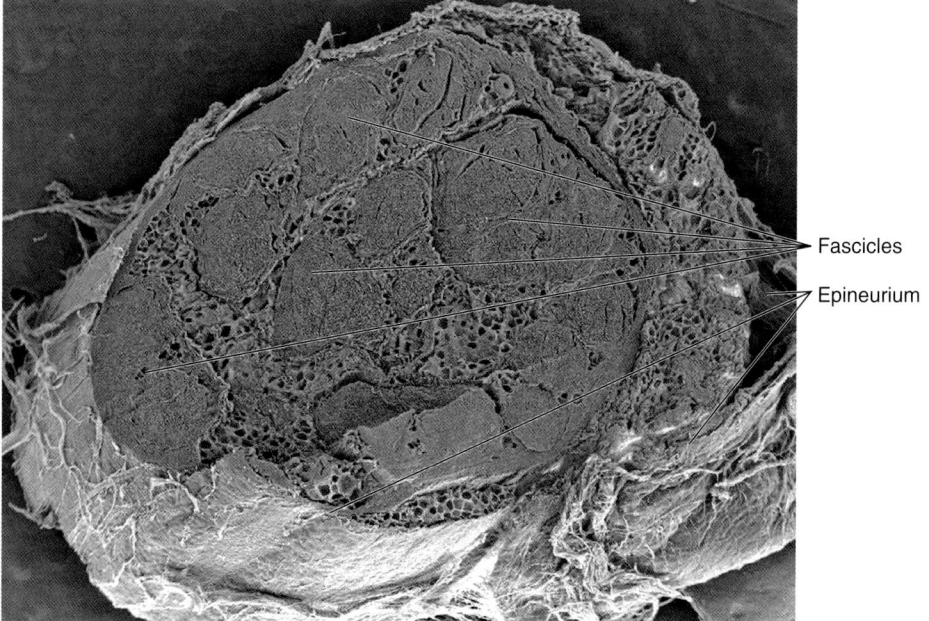

Fascicles

Epineurium

FIGURE 5–19. Epineurium in human tibial nerve. Scanning electron microscopy. Magnification ×20. (Reproduced with permission from Reina MA, Arriazu R, Collier CB, et al: Electron microscopy of human peripheral nerves of clinical relevance to the practice of nerve blocks. A structural and ultrastructural review based on original experimental and laboratory data. *Rev Esp Anestesiol Reanim.* 2013 Dec;60(10):552-562.)

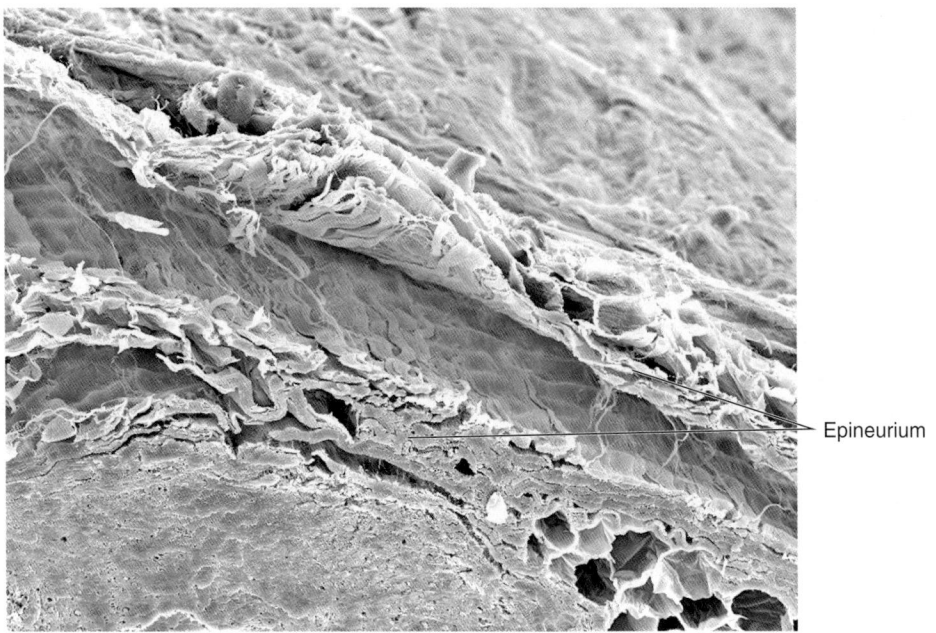

FIGURE 5–20. Epineurium in human tibial nerve. Scanning electron microscopy. Magnification ×180. (Reproduced with permission from Reina MA, Arriazu R, Collier CB, et al: Electron microscopy of human peripheral nerves of clinical relevance to the practice of nerve blocks. A structural and ultrastructural review based on original experimental and laboratory data. *Rev Esp Anestesiol Reanim.* 2013 Dec;60(10):552-562.)

Seen under the microscope, intraneural adipose cells resemble honeycombs, with empty vacuoles due to fat dissolution, during the fixation process[22] (Figure 5–21).

Mast cells are distributed throughout connective tissue and are often located in the proximity of small blood vessels.

Vasa nervorum supplying peripheral nerves arise from branches of regional arteries. Branches from these arteries enter the epineurium to form an vascular plexus (Figures 5–22 and 5–23). From the plexus, vessels penetrate the perineurium and enter the endoneurium as arterioles and capillaries. In nerves consisting of several fascicles, arteries, veins, and lymphatics run longitudinally and parallel to nerve fascicles.

Epineurium also projects longitudinal "ondulations" along its trajectory, providing elasticity especially in nerves supplying innervation to the extremities.

Clinical Pearls

- Epineurium is the outermost sheath of peripheral nerves.
- Epineurium is permeable and consists of moderately dense connective tissue that binds nerve fascicles.
- The epineurium contains adipocytes, fibroblasts, connective tissue fibers, mast cells, small lymphatics, as well as blood vessels and small nerve fibers innervating the vessels.

PARANEURAL SHEATHS AND COMMON EPINEURAL SHEATH

Whereas gross anatomy descriptions of distal peripheral nerves accurately identify each connective layer enclosing axons (endoneurium), nerve fascicles or bundles of axons (perineurium), and single peripheral nerves (epineurium), this becomes more complex where the connective tissue binds more than one nerve. An example of this is the sciatic nerve at the popliteal fossa. Various terms, such as paraneurium, paraneural sheaths,[23,24] common epineural sheath,[25] conjuctiva nervorum,[26] or adventitia,[27] are interchangeably used to refer to the same connective tissue.

Small nerves formed by a single group of fascicles feature a layer of perineurium enclosing each fascicle along with scarce amounts of adipose tissue. A connective tissue known as epineurium composed of collagenous fibers encloses the nerve.[3] Specific

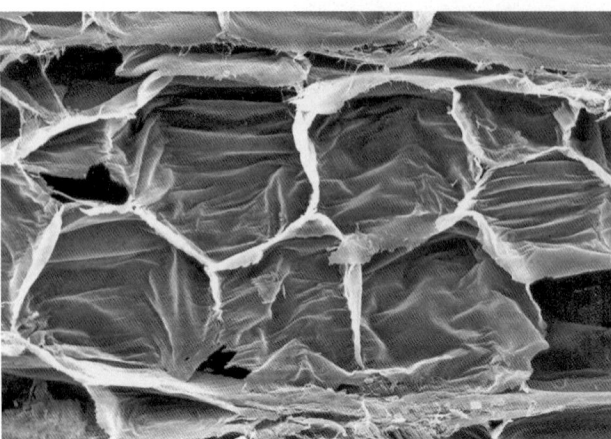

FIGURE 5–21. Adipocytes in interfascicular tissue of sciatic nerve. Scanning electron microscopy. Magnification ×400. (Reproduced with permission from Reina MA, López A, De Andrés JA: Adipose tissue within peripheral nerves. Study of the human sciatic nerve. *Rev Esp Anestesiol Reanim.* 2002 Oct;49(8):397-402.)

CHAPTER 5

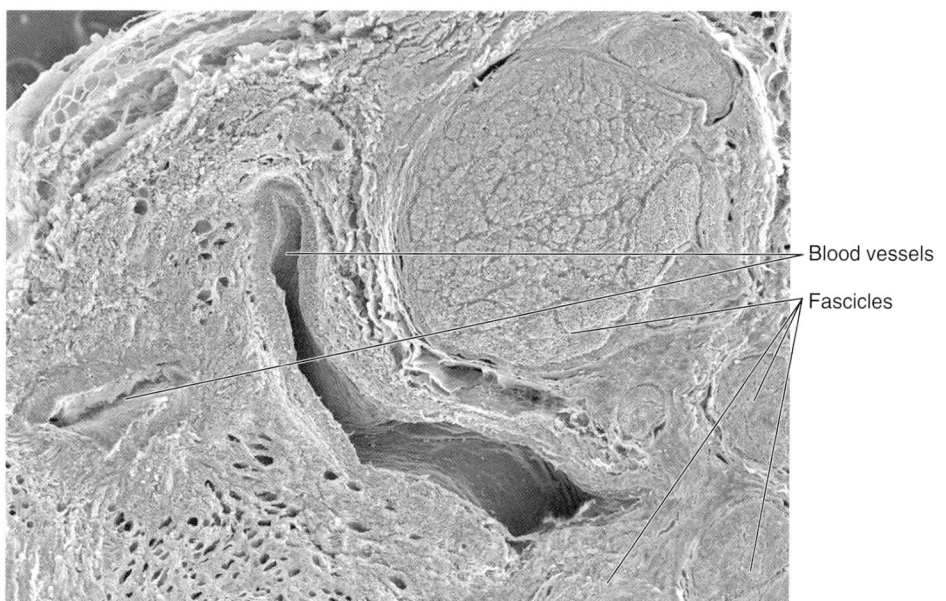

FIGURE 5–22. Interfascicular tissue and vessels in sciatic nerve. Scanning electron microscopy. Magnification ×50. (Reproduced with permission from Reina MA, López A, De Andrés JA: Adipose tissue within peripheral nerves. Study of the human sciatic nerve. *Rev Esp Anestesiol Reanim.* 2002 Oct;49(8):397-402.)

techniques enable identification of perineurium using staining methods positive for EMA (epithelial membrane antigen) and of collagen with Masson trichrome and EMA-negative stain.[3]

Similarly, staining techniques aid in the identification of structures in more complex nerves, such as the sciatic nerve, where groups of variable numbers of fascicles are present. In these types of nerves, EMA staining reveals that perineurium encloses each nerve fascicle, as opposed to connective tissue made up by collagen fibers typically present in epineurium that encloses groups of fascicles (detected with Masson trichromic stain).[3] Microscopic analysis of complex nerve structures such as the sciatic nerve at increasingly proximal locations shows that nerve branches within these nerve structures appear divided by their respective epineurial layers even before physical branch division materializes.

Each peripheral nerve at both plexus and terminal sites is encircled by concentric clusters of fat tissue, which appear just

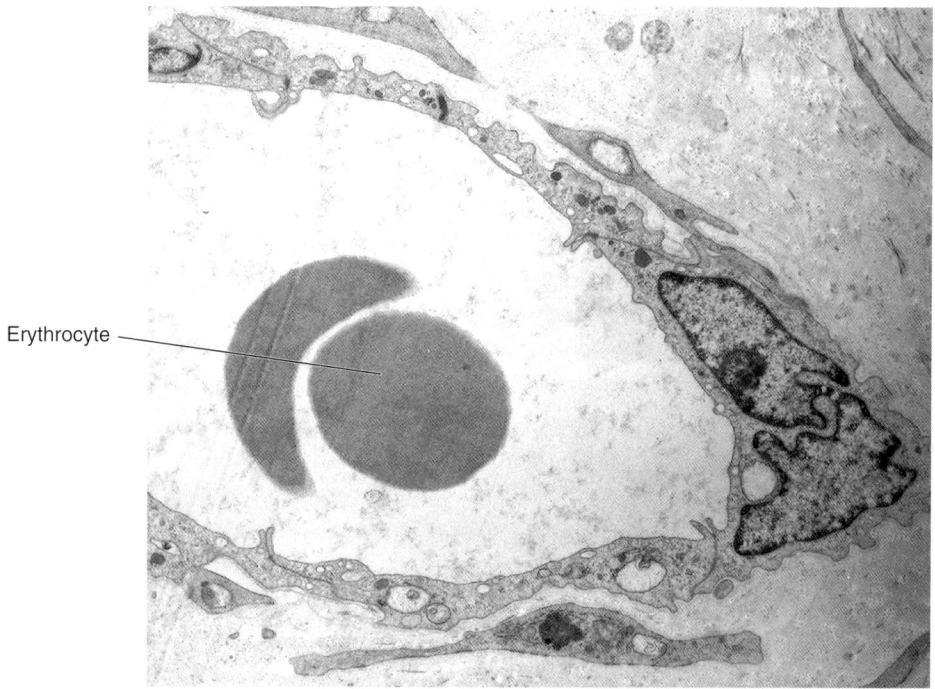

FIGURE 5–23. Blood vessel inside interfascicular tissue of sciatic nerve. Transmission electron microscopy. Magnification ×7000. (Used with permission from Miguel Angel Reina, MD.)

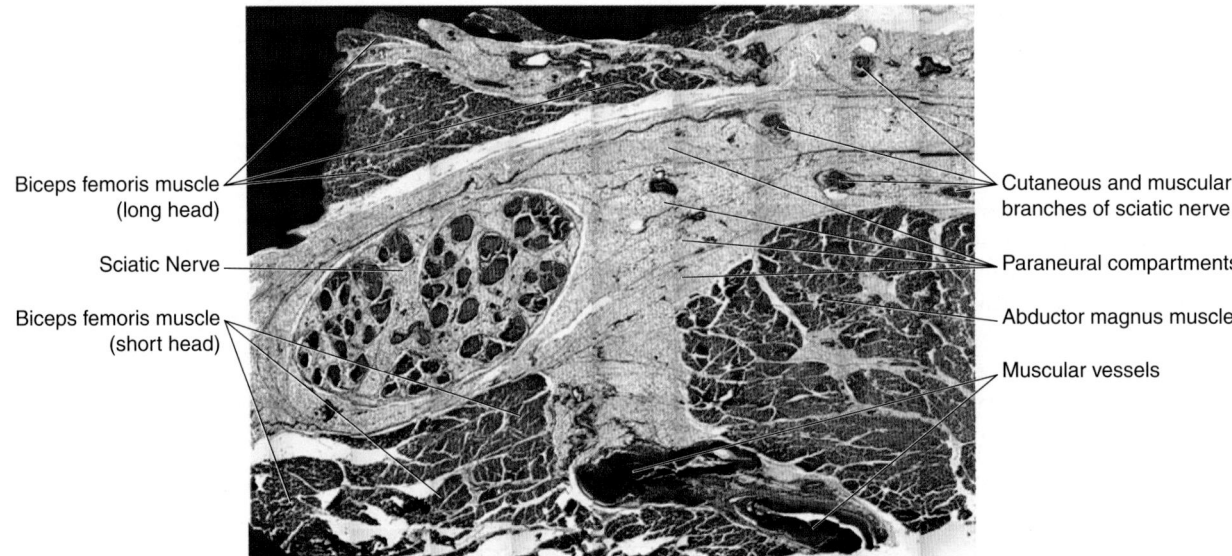

Biceps femoris muscle
(long head)

Sciatic Nerve

Biceps femoris muscle
(short head)

Cutaneous and muscular
branches of sciatic nerve

Paraneural compartments

Abductor magnus muscle

Muscular vessels

FIGURE 5–24. Sciatic nerve and its surrounding paraneurium at the level of the popliteal fossa. Hematoxylin-eosin. (Reproduced with permission from Reina MA: *Atlas of Functional Anatomy for Regional Anesthesia and Pain Medicine.* New York: Springer; 2015.)

prior to the division of the nerve (Figure 5–24 and 5–25). The adipose tissue extends alongside its collateral or terminal branches. The amount and shape of fat tissue vary along the nerve, progressively losing their concentric contour and becoming unevenly distributed. The collagen layer, similar to the epineurium, that wraps together the nerve components and the adipose tissue in between has been refered to as paraneurium, paraneural sheath, common epineural sheath, conjuctiva nervorum or adventitia by different authors.

In clinical practice, ultrasound-guided injection of local anesthetics enables the indirect identification of paraneurium as

the space between this layer and the nerve expands displaying a concentric shape. Neural layers surrounding fascicles, groups of fascicles, nerves, as well as more complex nerve structures have similar morphology, and they are mainly composed of collagen fibers. Therefore, it may seem reasonable to unify terminology noting that present denominations based on the anatomic location of each neural fascia seems rather confusing.[28,29] However, epineurium and paraneurium may best to avitted terms to avoid the present confusion. Both epineurium and paraneurium have similar functions, which include insulation and protection of nerves from injury. Paraneural compartments

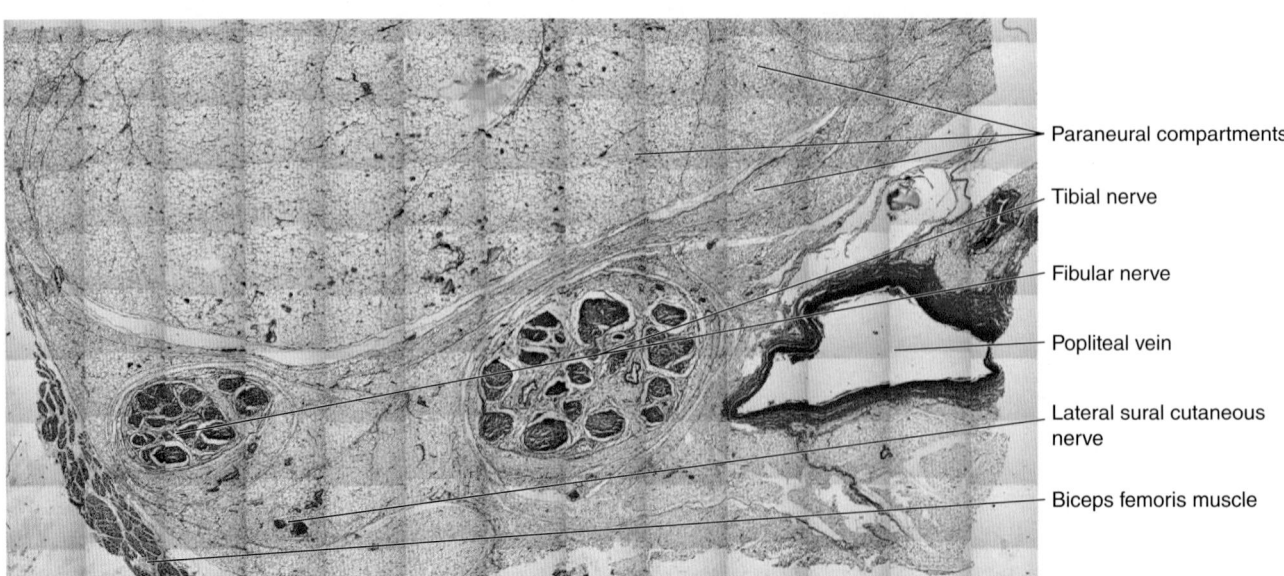

Paraneural compartments

Tibial nerve

Fibular nerve

Popliteal vein

Lateral sural cutaneous
nerve

Biceps femoris muscle

FIGURE 5–25. Tibial nerve, fibular nerve and its paraneurium at popliteal fossa. Hematoxylin-eosin. (Reproduced with permission from Reina MA: *Atlas of Functional Anatomy for Regional Anesthesia and Pain Medicine.* New York: Springer; 2015.)

facilitate longitudinal displacement of nerves controlling body movement. This movement is necessary to neutralize lateral compression by changing their shape.[30] If the tissue is exposed to external irritation, it reacts, leading to interfascicular fibrosis.[30]

In relation to the anatomic features of the sciatic nerves, Andersen et al[24] found the sheath surrounding the sciatic nerve to be a thin transparent structure that was clearly distinctive, both macroscopically and microscopically different from the epineurium. The sheath facilitated the spread of the injectate along the nerve. However, its projections did not completely encircle the nerve. The internal layers of the paraneurium around the sciatic nerve[31] had a similar structure of that sheath. Vloka et al[25] used the term *common epineural sheath*. Tran et al[32] compared the effectiveness of the sciatic nerve block in relation to what they called "subepineural" injection at the "bifurcation," which fills a common paraneural compartment shared by tibial and peroneal nerves close to their macroscopic division.

Orebaugh et al[33] reported that needle-tip placement in the interscalene region and injection of anesthetic solution took place frequently inside the epineurium. This occurred in approximately 50% of the nerve blocks without evidence of fascicular or axonal damage and no trace of dye within fascicles to suggest that the needle had traversed them.[33]

Spinner et al[34] demonstrated that intraepineurial injection of dye results in its dissection along paths of least resistance, suggesting the presence of anatomic constraints among epineurial compartments. When Spinner injected the inner epineurium, the dye expanded within the same compartment but did not cross over or extend to the common external epineurial space. Therefore, the concept of "intraneural injection" should be revised for each nerve examined, avoiding extrapolations based on studies of a single nerve[35,36,37] due to the considerable anatomic variability among peripheral nerves.

Clinical Pearl

- A peripheral nerve at both plexus and terminal sites is encircled by concentric clusters of adipose tissue. This explains why perineural injections result in low opening injection pressure.

PERIPHERAL NERVE BLOCKS

Diffusion of anesthetic into the axons is influenced by the presence and characteristics of the connective tissue sheaths (eg, perineurium, myelin) and the size and location of the axons inside fascicles. During intravenous peripheral anesthesia (Bier block), the local anesthetic most likely reaches the peripheral nerve endings through the intraneural capillary network.

Perineurium and endoneural capillary endothelium protect the axons from foreign substances thanks to their tight junctions between endothelial cells and among perineural cells.

Local anesthetic injected outside the epineurium of a nerve must traverse both the epineurium and perineurium to reach the axons. Subsequently, only a small proportion of the injected

anesthetic comes in direct contact with axons leading to delayed onset, incomplete or failed neural blockade. For instance, Popitz and collaborators[38] injected 1% lidocaine into the sciatic nerve of rats and found that when the block was complete, the intraneural amount of local anesthetic was around 1.6% of the injected dose.

SUMMARY

The composition and arrangement of the connective tissue of peripheral nerves play a major role in protection of the peripheral nerves and in the practice of regional anesthesia. Characteristics and variability of the connective tissue may substantially influence the spread of the local anesthetic during nerve block injection and therefore the dynamics and quality of the neural blockade.

REFERENCES

1. Reina MA, López A, Villanueva MC, De Andrés JA, León GI: Morphology of peripheral nerves, their sheaths, and their vascularization. Rev Esp Anestesiol Reanim 2000;47:464–475.
2. Reina MA, Wikinski J, Prats-Galino A, Machés F: Morfologia del nervio periférico. In: Wikinski J, Reina MA, Bollini C, et al (eds): *Diagnóstico, prevención y tratamiento de las complicaciones neurológicas asociadas con la anestesia regional periférica y central.* Panamericana Ed, 2011, pp 71–86.
3. Reina MA, Arriazu R, Collier CB, Sala-Blanch X: Histology and electron microscopy of human peripheral nerves of clinical relevance to the practice of nerve blocks. Rerv Esp Anestesiol Reanim 2013;60:552–562.
4. Reina MA, De Andres JA, Hernández JM, et al: Successive changes in extraneural structures from the subarachnoid nerve roots to the peripheral nerve, influencing anesthetic block, and treatment of acute postoperative pain. Eur J Pain Suppl 2011;5:377–385.
5. Sunderland S, Marshall RD, Swaney WE: The intraneural topography of the circumflex musculocutaneous and obturador nerves. Brain 1959;82:116–129.
6. Sunderland S, Ray LJ: The intraneural topography of the sciatic nerve and its popliteal divisions in man. Brain 1948;71:242–258.
7. Sunderland S: The intraneural topography of the radial, median and ulnar nerves. Brain 1945;68:243–255.
8. Sunderland S: *Troncos nerviosos periféricos.* Salvat Ed, 1985, pp 31–60.
9. Boyd IA, Davey MR: *Composition of Peripheral Nerves.* Churchill Livingstone, 1968.
10. Friede RL, Bischhausen R: The organization of endoneurial collagen in peripheral nerves as revealed with the scanning electron microscopy. J Neurol Sci 1978;38:83–89.
11. Reina MA, López A, De Andrés JA: The blood-nerve barrier in peripheral nerves. Rev Esp Anestesiol Reanim 2003;50:80–86.
12. De Andrés JA, Reina MA, López A, Sala-Blanch X, Prats A. Blocs nerveux périphériques, paresthésies et injections intraneurales. Prat Anesth Reanim 2010;14:213–221.
13. Olsson Y, Kristensson K: The perineurium as a diffusion barrier to protein tracers following trauma to nerves. Acta Neuropath 1973;23:105–111.
14. Sunderland S, Bradley KC: The perineurium of the peripheral nerves. Anat Rec 1952;113:125–142.
15. Olsson Y, Resse TS: Permeability of vas nervorum and perineurium in mouse sciatic nerve studied by fluorescence and electron microscopy. J Neuropathol Exp Neurol 1971;30:105–119.
16. Soderfeldt B, Olsson Y, Kristensson K: The perineurium as a diffusion barrier to protein tracers in human peripheral nerve. Acta Neuropath 1973;25:120–126.
17. Llewelyn JG, Thomas PK: Perineurial sodium-potasium ATPase activity in streptozotocin-diabetic rats. Exp Neurol 1987;97:375–382.
18. Lundborg G: Structure and function of the intraneural microvessels as related to trauma, edema formation and nerve function. J Bone Joint Surg 1975;57:938–948.
19. Sunderland S. The effect of rupture of the perineurium on the contained nerve fibres. Brain 1946;69:149–152.
20. Sunderland S: The connective tissues of peripheral nerves. Brain 1965;88:841–854.

21. Sunderland S: The adipose tissue of peripheral nerves. Brain 1945;68: 118–122.
22. Reina MA, López A, De Andrés JA: Adipose tissue within peripheral nerves. Study of the human sciatic nerve. Rev Esp Anestesiol Reanim 2002;49:397–402.
23. Krstic R. *Die Gewebe des Menschen und der Seaugetiere.* Springer, 1978.
24. Andersen HL, Andersen SL, Tranum-Jensen J. Injection inside the paraneural sheath of the sciatic nerve: Direct comparison among ultrasound imaging, macroscopic anatomy, and histologic analysis. Reg Anesth Pain Med. 2012;37:410–414.
25. Vloka JD, Hadzic A, Lesser JB, et al: A common epineural sheath for the nerves in the popliteal fossa and its possible implications for sciatic nerve block. Anesth Analg 1997;84:387–390; The division of the sciatic nerve in the popliteal fossa: anatomical implications for popliteal nerve blockade. Vloka JD, Hadzić A, April E, Thys DM. Anesth Analg. 2001 Jan;92(1):215-217.
26. Lang J. On connective tissue and blood vessels of the nerves. Z Anat Entwicklungsgesch 1962;123:61–79.
27. Van Beek A, Kleinert HE: Practical neurorrhaphy. Orthopedic Clin North Am 1977;8:377–386.
28. Sala-Blanch X, Reina MA, Ribalta T, Prats-Galino A. Sciatic nerve structure and nomenclature: Epineurium to paraneurium. Is this a new paradigm? Reg Anesth Pain Med 2013;38:463–465.
29. Sala-Blanch X, Vandepitte C, Laur J, et al: Practical review of perineural versus intraneural injections: a call for standard nomenclature. Int Anesth Clin 2011;49:1–12.
30. Millesi H, Hausner T, Schmidhammer R, Trattnig S, Tschabitscher M: Anatomical structures to provide passive motility of peripheral nerve trunks and fascicles. Acta Neurochir Suppl 2007;100:133–135.
31. Reina MA (ed): *Atlas of Functional Anatomy for Regional Anesthesia and Pain Medicine: Human Structure, Ultrastructure and 3D Reconstruction Images.* Springer, 2015.
32. Tran de QH, Dugani S, Pham K, Al-Shaafi A, Finlayson RJ: A randomized comparison between subepineural and conventional ultrasound-guided popliteal sciatic nerve block. Reg Anesth Pain Med 2011;36:548–552.
33. Orebaugh SL, McFadden K, Skorupan H, Bigeleisen PE: Subepineurial injection in ultrasound-guided interscalene needle tip placement. Reg Anesth Pain Med 2010;35:450–454.
34. Spinner RJ, Wang H, Carmichael SW, Amrami KK, Scheithauer BW: Epineurial compartments and their role in intraneural ganglion cyst propagation: An experimental study. Clin Anat 2007;20:826–833.
35. Ip V, Tsui B. Injection through the paraneural sheath rather than circumferential spread facilitates safe, effective sciatic nerve block. Reg Anesth Pain Med 2013;38:373.
36. Ip VH, Tsui BC. Kill 2 birds with 1 stone: Injection at the bifurcation during popliteal sciatic nerve block. Reg Anesth Pain Med 2011;36: 633–634.
37. Sala-Blanch X, López A, Prats-Galino A. Vloka sciatic nerve sheath: a tribute to a visionary. Reg Anesth Pain Med. 2015 Mar-Apr;40(2):174.
38. Popitz-Bergez S, Lee-Soon S, Strichartz GR, Thalhammer JG: Relation between functional deficit and intraneural local anesthetic during peripheral nerve block. A study in the rat sciatic nerve. Anesthesiology 1995;83:583–592.

Ultrastructural Anatomy of the Spinal Meninges and Related Structures

Miguel A. Reina, Carlo D. Franco, Alberto Prats-Galino, Fabiola Machés, Andrés López, and Jose A de Andrés

INTRODUCTION

Recent research on the ultrastructure of the human spinal dural sac and its contents has enhanced our understanding of the microstructure of the dura mater, arachnoid layer, trabecular arachnoid, pia mater, and nerve root cuffs. This chapter reviews new and traditional concepts regarding these structures and discusses their possible clinical implications. The distribution of epidural fat and its possible role in disposition and kinetics of neuraxial injections are also discussed.

DURAL SAC

The dural sac surrounds the spinal cord inside the vertebral column. It separates the epidural space from the subarachnoid space, ending at the second sacral vertebra. In an idealized shape, the dural sac is cylindrical with its thickness varying from about 1 mm in the cervical region and becoming gradually thinner as it descends (Figures 6–1 and 6–2). In the lumbar region, the thickness of the dural sac reaches 0.3 mm,[1] although measurements taken from anteroposterior or lateral may vary somewhat even at the same vertebral level. The dura mater is the most external layer of the dural sac and is responsible for 90% of its total thickness. This fibrous structure, although permeable, somewhat provides mechanical protection to the spinal cord and its neural elements. The internal 10% of the dural sac is formed by the arachnoid layer, which is a cellular lamina that adds little extra mechanical resistance.[2]

DURA MATER

Dura mater comprises approximately 80 concentric laminas[3–5] (Figure 6–3). Each dural lamina has a thickness of approximately 5 μm and consists of thinner laminas containing mostly collagen fibers (Figures 6–4 and 6–5). The collagen fibers are oriented in different directions but always within the concentric plane of the dural lamina; hence, they do not cross between the laminas. Each collagen fiber has a smooth surface and measures approximately 0.1 μm (Figure 6–6). The elastic fibers are fewer, measuring 2 μm in diameter, and have a rougher surface than that of the collagen fibers[6] (Figure 6–7).

Contrary to the classic description of fibers inside dural laminas being arranged longitudinally and parallel to the long axis of the vertebral column, the fibers are actually distributed multidirectionally at random inside each of the concentric dural laminas (Figures 6–8 to 6–10). Mastocytes and macrophages are also present within the dura mater (Figures 6–11 and 6–12).

ARACHNOID LAYER

Conventionally, the arachnoid layer is described as a fine membrane in close contact with but not adhering to the internal surface of the dura mater. Recent research, however, determined that there is no space between the dura mater and the arachnoid layer (see subdural space). The arachnoid layer is semipermeable and serves as a barrier to limit the passage of substances through the dural sac (Figures 6–13 and 6–14). Its thickness is about 50-60 μm[7] (Figures 6–15 and 6–16). In its interior, arachnoid cells strongly bond by specific membrane junctions with a thickness of about 10–15 μm. Collagen fibers at the center of the arachnoid layer give strength to the lamina and improve its mechanical resistance. Flat, elongated neurothelial cells occupy the outer portion of the layer. Tearing off the arachnoid layer exposes the subdural space. Neurothelial cells can be found attached either to the internal surface of the dura or to the external surface of the arachnoid layer[8,9] (Figure 6–17).

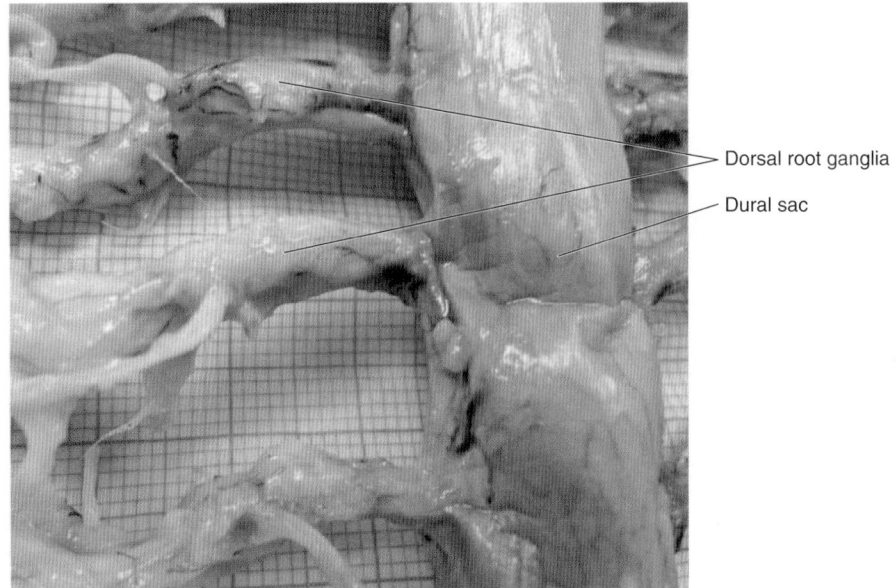

Dorsal root ganglia

Dural sac

FIGURE 6–1. Human dural sac. (Reproduced with permission from Reina MA, López García A, de Andrés JA, et al: Thickness variation of the dural sac. *Rev Esp Anestesiol Reanim.* 1999 Oct;46(8):344-349.)

NEURAXIAL BLOCKADE AND DURAL LESIONS

Piercing the dural sac during a subarachnoid block causes mechanical disruption of both the dura mater and the arachnoid layer. The cross-sectional area of the puncture site produced by a 25-gauge needle is similar regardless of whether the needle has a pencil point or a cutting end. However, the morphology of the lesion varies depending on the design of the needle tip. Pencil-point needles produce a greater and rougher-appearing injury to the dural fibers, while cutting needles produce a U-shaped lesion or flap resembling the open lid of a tin can[10–12] (Figures 6–18 to 6–31).

When using cutting (long bevel) needles, bevel orientation (eg, parallel or perpendicular to the main axis of the cord) does not significantly affect the size or morphology of the lesions in the dura and arachnoid lamina[10–12] (see Figure 6–24). The lesion that the needle produces in the dural sac has two components, dural and arachnoid. It is believed that the arachnoid component is vital in limiting cerebrospinal

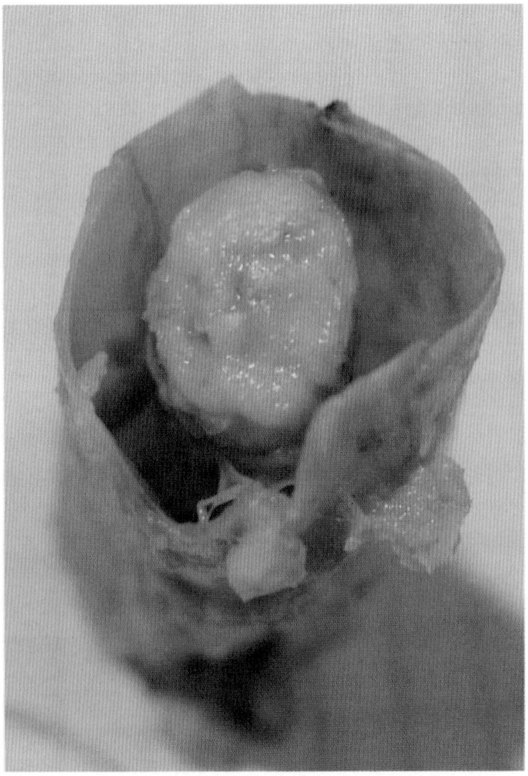

FIGURE 6–2. Human dural sac and end spinal cord. (Reproduced with permission from Reina MA, Pulido P, López A. El saco dural humano: *Rev Arg Anestesiol.* 2007; 65:167-184.)

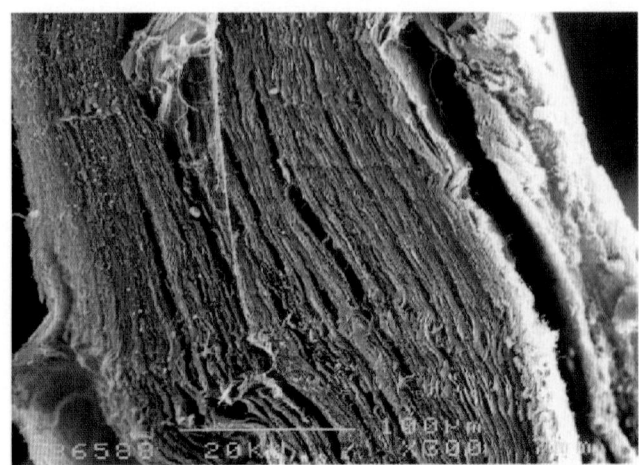

FIGURE 6–3. Thickness of the dural sac. Scanning electron microscopy. Magnification ×300. (Reproduced with permission from Reina MA, Dittmann M, López A, et al: New perspectives in the microscopic structure of human dura mater in the dorso lumbar region. *Reg Anesth.* 1997 Mar-Apr;22(2):161-166.)

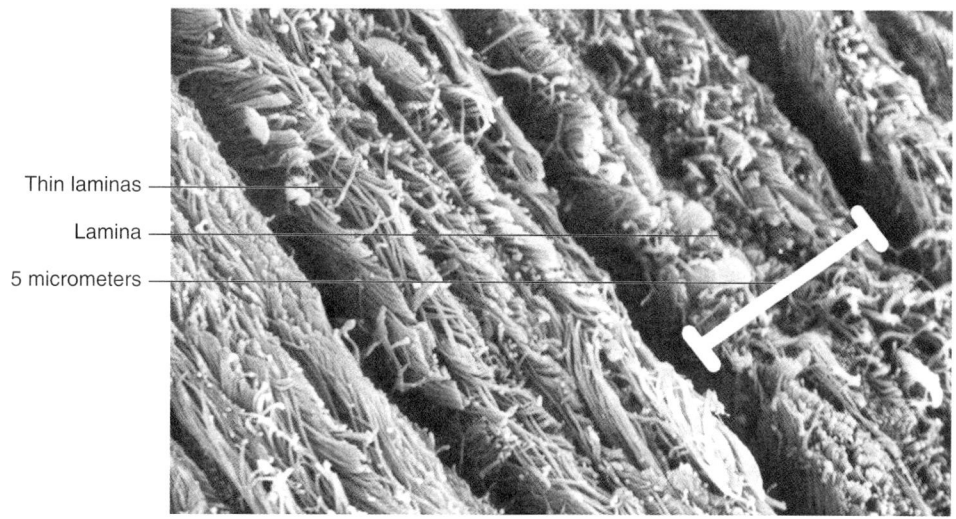

Thin laminas ——
Lamina ——
5 micrometers ——

FIGURE 6–4. Partial thickness of the dural sac. Details of dural laminas. Scanning electron microscopy. Magnification ×4,000. (Reproduced with permission from Reina MA, López A, Dittmann M, et al: Structure of human dura mater thickness by scanning electron microscopy. *Rev Esp Anestesiol Reanim.* 1996 Apr;43(4):135-137.)

fluid leakage from the subarachnoid space to the epidural space. Therefore, the size and morphology of arachnoid lesions seem to be more important for laminar sealing and cerebrospinal leakage than the size and morphology of dural lacerations.

The incidence of postdural puncture headache (PDPH) has been thought that is affected by the type of needle used (pencil point versus cutting) and of the bevel.

The traditional belief that cutting needles result in larger dural lesions (tears) was established in the 1940s and may have been the consequence of the imperfections in the needle design of that era. Modern needles, however, produce clean, U-shaped lesion or flap resembling the open lid of a tin can (see Figure 6–24).

After needle withdrawal, the U-shaped flap tends to return to its original position due to cerebrospinal fluid pressure and the elastic properties of the dura mater. The dural orifice is almost completely occluded after approximately 15 minutes. On the other hand, lesions produced by pencil-point needles involve a more complex lesion with fiber tearing, sectioning, and separation. The extent of the dural lesion caused by a needle depends on several factors, including the external diameter of the needle, dural and arachnoid sealing mechanisms, needle-tip design, and the quality of needle manufacturing. Needles having the same tip design but different manufacturing methods may not have the same surface quality and may contain microfractures or imperfections, resulting in more or less extensive dural fiber tearing and residual lesions.[13–15]

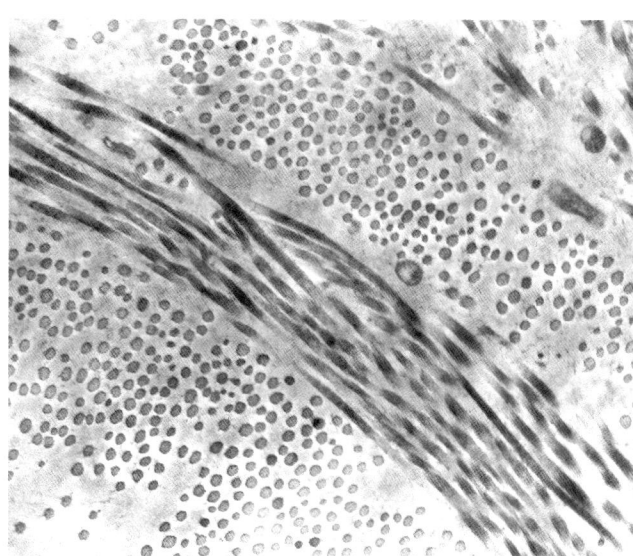

FIGURE 6–5. Partial thickness of the dural sac. Details of dural laminas. Transmission electron microscopy. Magnification ×20,000. (Reproduced with permission from Raj P: *Textbook of Regional Anesthesia.* Philadelphia: Churchill Livingstone; 2002.)

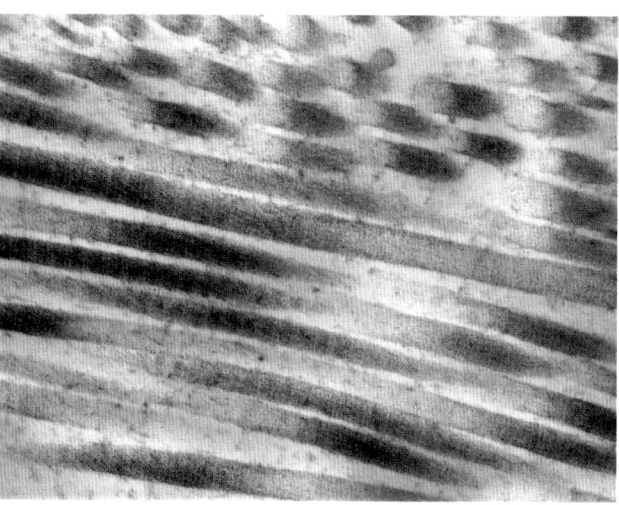

FIGURE 6–6. Collagen fibers in the thickness of the dural sac. Transmission electron microscopy. Magnification ×50,000. (Reproduced with permission from Raj P: *Textbook of Regional Anesthesia.* Philadelphia: Churchill Livingstone; 2002.)

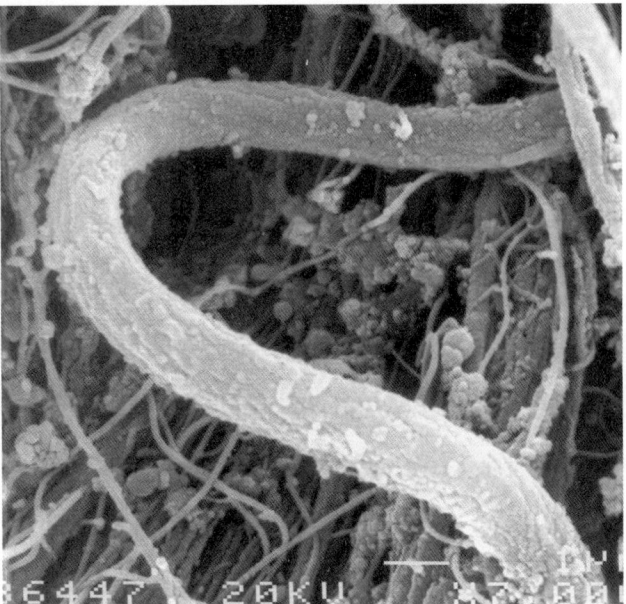

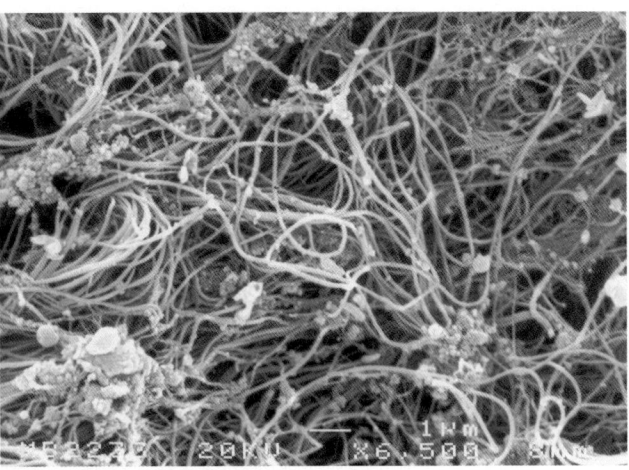

FIGURE 6–8. Detail of epidural surface of the dural sac. Scanning electron microscopy. Magnification ×6500. (Reproduced with permission from Dittmann M, Reina MA, López A: Neue ergebnisse bei der darstellung der dura mater spinalis mittles rasterelektronenmikroskopie. *Anaesthesist*. 1998 May;47(5):409-413.)

FIGURE 6–7. Elastic fibers of the dural sac. Scanning electron microscopy. Magnification ×7000. (Reproduced with permission from Reina MA, López A, Dittmann M, et al: External and internal surface of human dura mater by scanning electron microscopy. *Rev Esp Anestesiol Reanim*. 1996 Apr;43(4):130-4.)

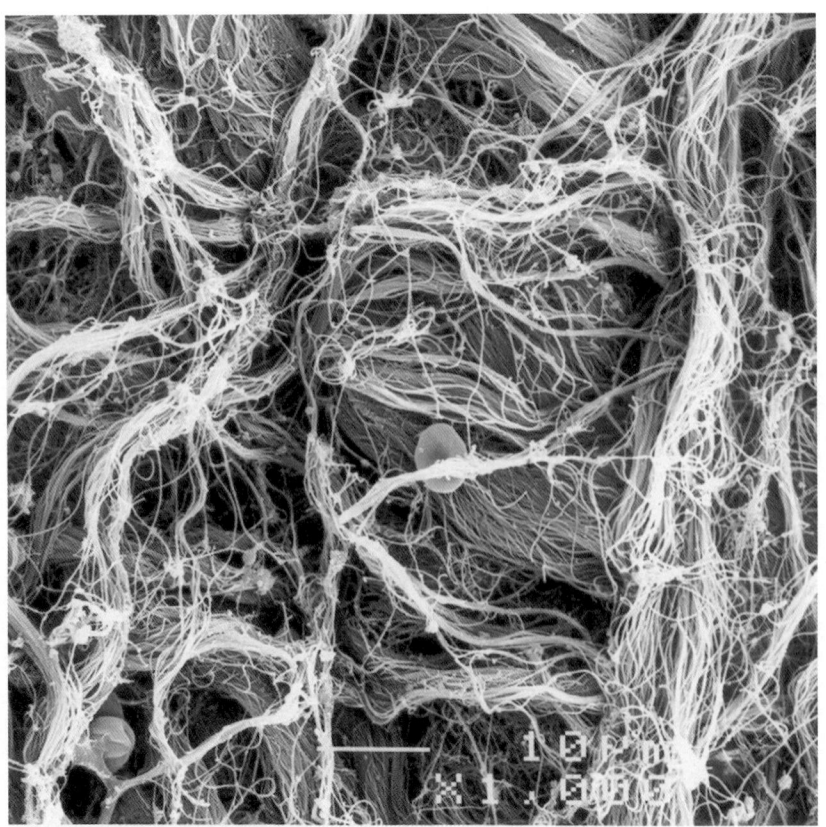

FIGURE 6–9. Detail of epidural surface of the dural sac. Scanning electron microscopy. Magnification ×1000. (Reproduced with permission from Reina MA, López A, Dittmann M, et al: External and internal surface of human dura mater by scanning electron microscopy. *Rev Esp Anestesiol Reanim*. 1996 Apr;43(4):130-4.)

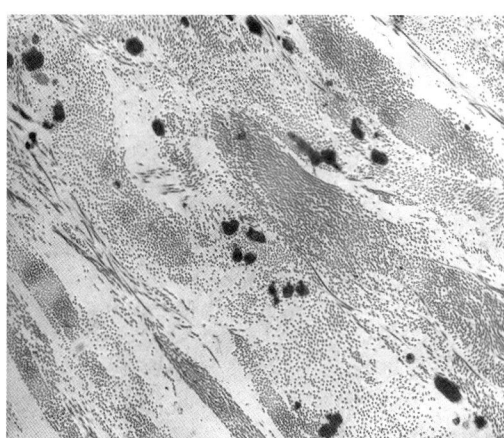

FIGURE 6–10. Collagen and elastic fibers in the thickness of the dural sac. Transmission electron microscopy. Magnification ×7,000. (Reproduced with permission from Raj P: *Textbook of Regional Anesthesia*. Philadelphia: Churchill Livingstone; 2002.)

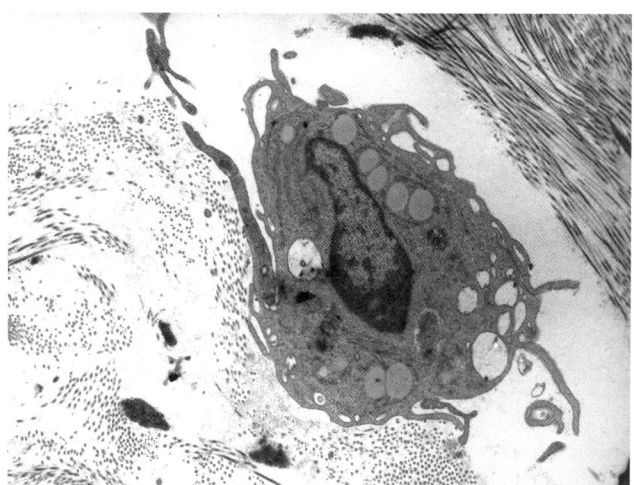

FIGURE 6–12. Macrophage in the thickness of the dura mater. Transmission electron microscopy. Magnification ×7000. (Reproduced with permission from Raj P: *Textbook of Regional Anesthesia*. Philadelphia: Churchill Livingstone; 2002.)

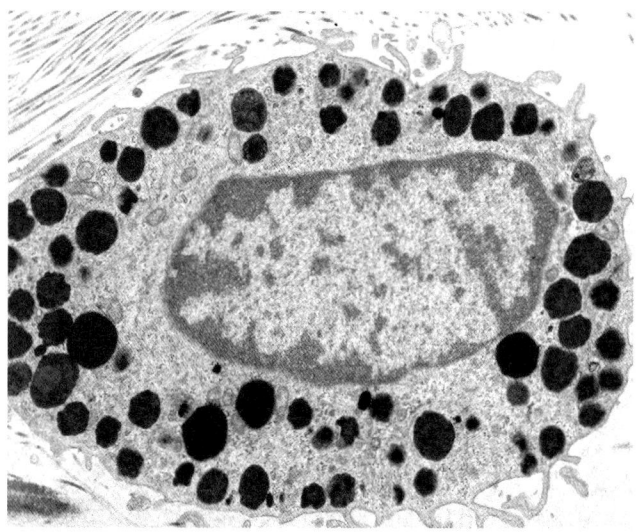

FIGURE 6–11. Mastocyte in the thickness of the dura mater. Transmission electron microscopy. Magnification ×15,000. (Reproduced with permission from Reina MA, Pulido P, López A. El saco dural humano: *Rev Arg Anestesiol*. 2007;65:167-184.)

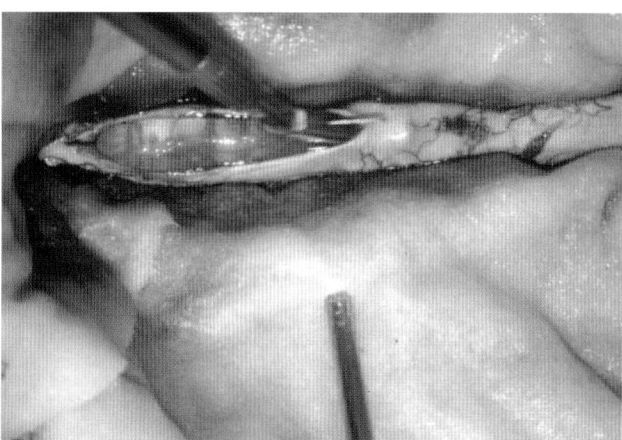

FIGURE 6–13. Dissection of human dural sac. (Reproduced with permission from Reina MA, Pulido P, López A. El saco dural humano. *Rev Arg Anestesiol*. 2007; 65:167-184.)

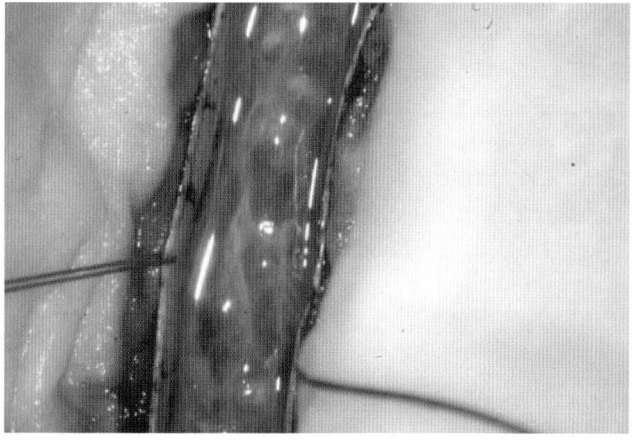

FIGURE 6–14. Dissection of human dural sac. Dura mater is open; arachnoid layer is closed. (Reproduced with permission from Reina MA, Pulido P, López A. El saco dural humano. *Rev Arg Anestesiol*. 2007; 65:167-184.)

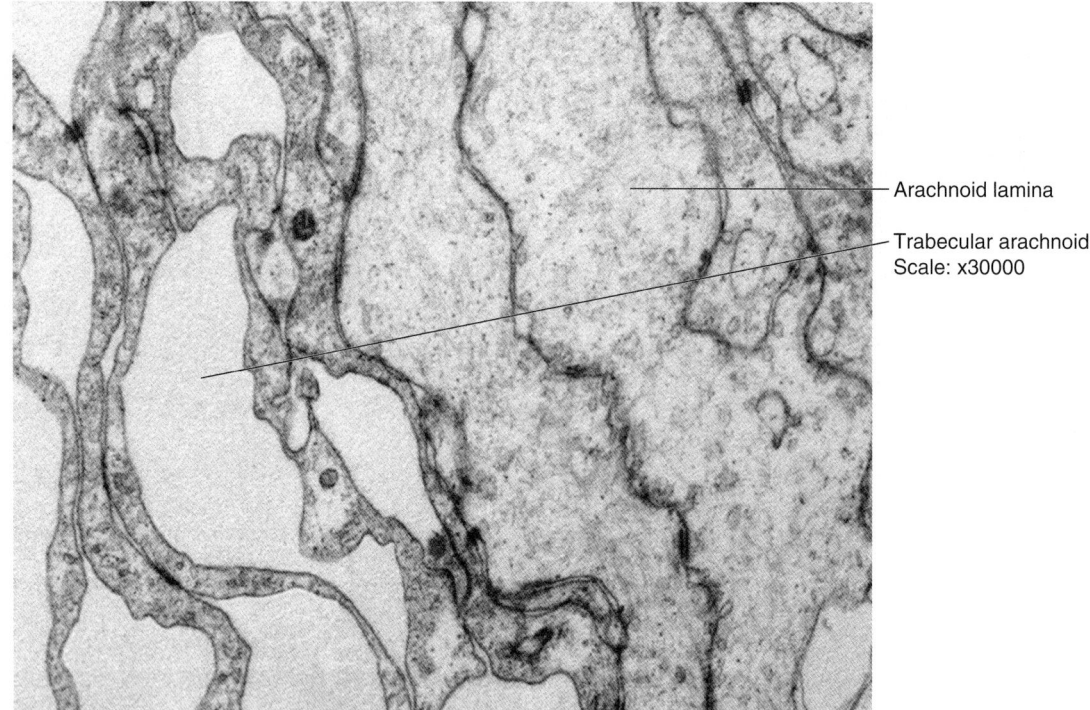

Arachnoid lamina

Trabecular arachnoid
Scale: x30000

FIGURE 6–15. Arachnoid cells in the thickness of arachnoid layer. Transmission electron microscopy. Magnification ×40,000.

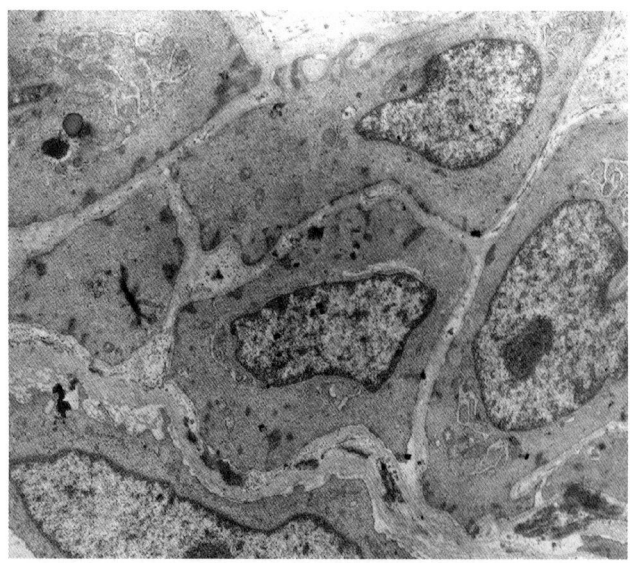

FIGURE 6–16. Arachnoid cells in the thickness of arachnoid layer. Transmission electron microscopy. Magnification ×4400. (Reproduced with permission from Raj P: *Textbook of Regional Anesthesia*. Philadelphia: Churchill Livingstone; 2002.)

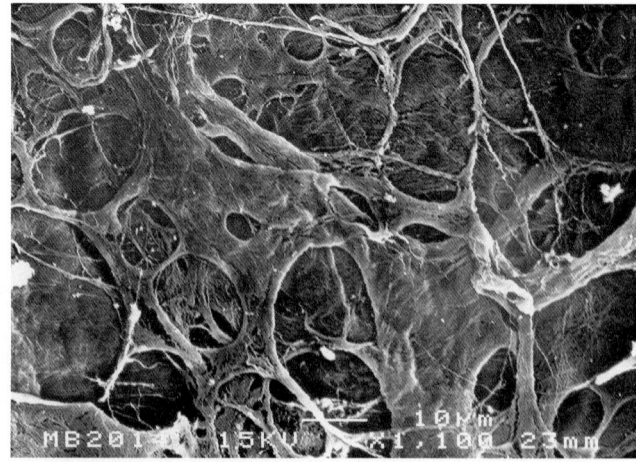

FIGURE 6–17. Internal surface of dura mater. Scanning electron microscopy. Magnification ×1100. (Reproduced with permission from Reina MA, Dittmann M, López A, et al: New perspectives in the microscopic structure of human dura mater in the dorso lumbar region. *Reg Anesth*. 1997 Mar-Apr;22(2):161-166.)

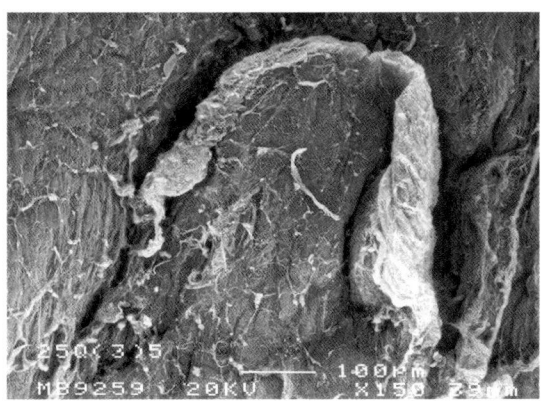

FIGURE 6–18. Dura-arachnoid lesion produced with 25-G Quincke needle. Epidural surface. Scanning electron microscopy. Magnification ×150. (Reproduced with permission from Reina MA, Castedo J, López A. Cefalea pospunción dural: Ultraestructura de las lesiones durales y agujas espinales usadas en las punciones lumbares. *Rev Arg Anestesiol.* 2008 Jan-Mar 66(1):6-26.)

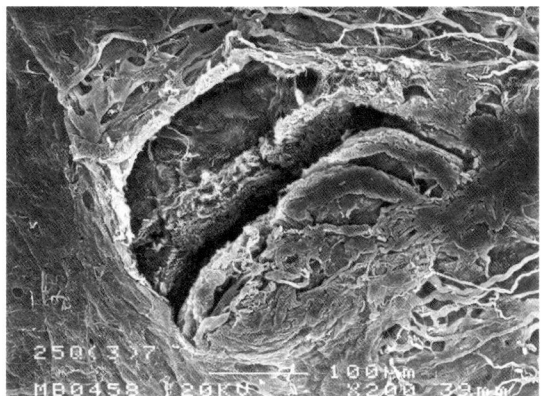

FIGURE 6–19. Dura-arachnoid lesion produced with 25-G Quincke needle. Arachnoid surface. Scanning electron microscopy. Magnification ×200. (Reproduced with permission from Reina MA, Castedo J, López A. Cefalea pospunción dural: Ultraestructura de las lesiones durales y agujas espinales usadas en las punciones lumbares. *Rev Arg Anestesiol.* 2008 Jan-Mar 66(1):6-26.)

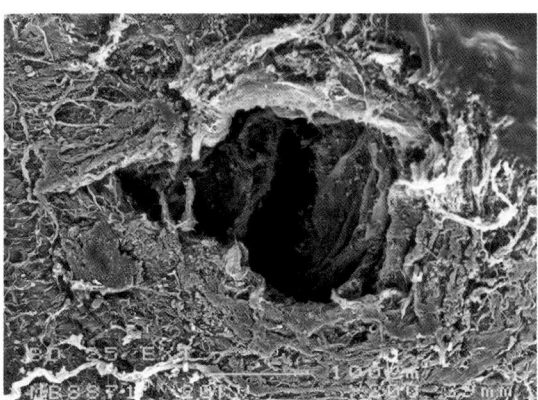

FIGURE 6–20. Dura-arachnoid lesion produced with 25-G Whitacre needle. Epidural surface. Scanning electron microscopy. Magnification ×200. (Reproduced with permission from Reina MA, López-García A, de Andrés-Ibáñez JA, et al: Electron microscopy of the lesions produced in the human dura mater by Quincke beveled and Whitacre needles. *Rev Esp Anestesiol Reanim.* 1997 Feb;44(2):56-61.)

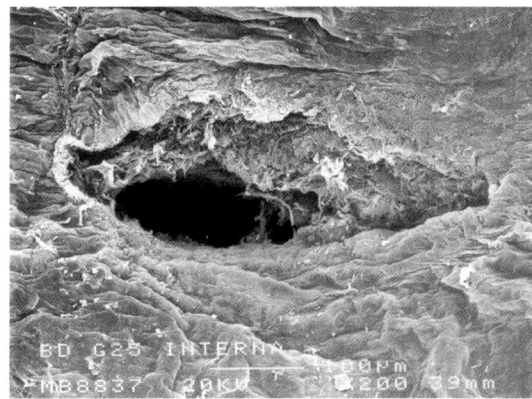

FIGURE 6–21. Dura-arachnoid lesion produced with 25-G Whitacre needle. Arachnoid surface. Scanning electron microscopy. Magnification ×200. (Reproduced with permission from Reina MA, López-García A, de Andrés-Ibáñez JA, et al: Electron microscopy of the lesions produced in the human dura mater by Quincke beveled and Whitacre needles. *Rev Esp Anestesiol Reanim.* 1997 Feb;44(2):56-61.)

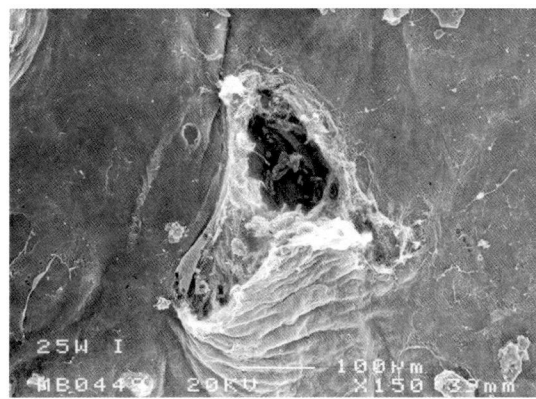

FIGURE 6–22. Dura-arachnoid lesion produced with 25-G Whitacre needle. Arachnoid surface. Scanning electron microscopy. Magnification ×150. (Reproduced with permission from Reina MA, De León Casasola OA, et al: An in vitro study of dural lesions produced by 25 Gauge Quincke and Whitacre needles evaluated by scanning electron microscopy. *Reg Anesth Pain Med.* 2000 Jul-Aug;25(4):393-402.)

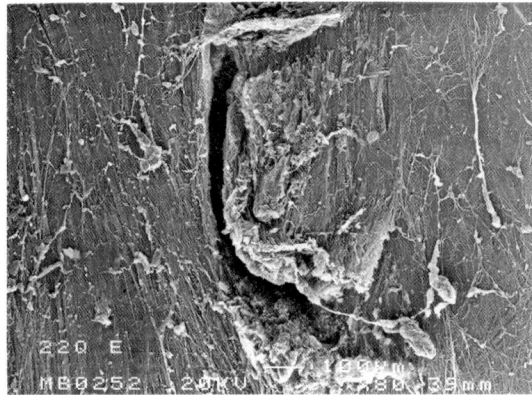

FIGURE 6–23. Dura-arachnoid lesion produced with 22-G Quincke needle. Epidural surface. Scanning electron microscopy. Magnification ×80. (Reproduced with permission from Reina MA, Castedo J, López A. Cefalea pospunción dural: Ultraestructura de las lesiones durales y agujas espinales usadas en las punciones lumbares. *Rev Arg Anestesiol.* 2008 Jan-Mar 66(1):6-26.)

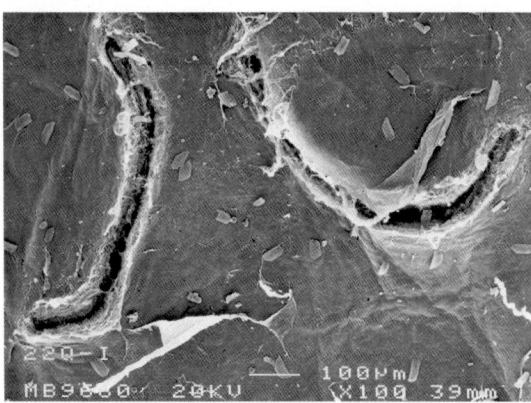

FIGURE 6–24. Dura-arachnoid lesion produced with 22-G Quincke needle. Arachnoid surface. Scanning electron microscopy. Magnification ×100. (Reproduced with permission from Raj P: *Textbook of Regional Anesthesia*. Philadelphia: Churchill Livingstone; 2002.)

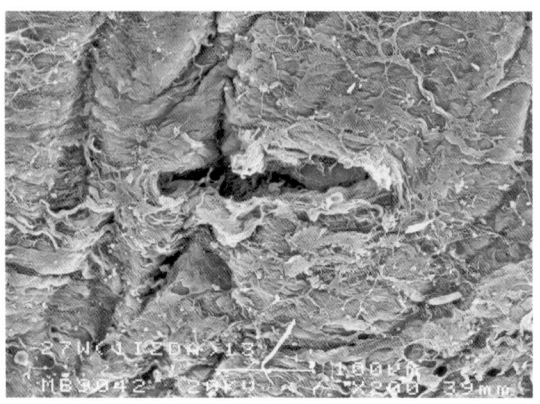

FIGURE 6–25. Dura-arachnoid lesion produced with 27-G Whitacre needle. Epidural surface. Scanning electron microscopy. Magnification ×200. (Reproduced with permission from Reina MA, Castedo J, López A. Cefalea pospunción dural: Ultraestructura de las lesiones durales y agujas espinales usadas en las punciones lumbares. *Rev Arg Anestesiol.* 2008 Jan-Mar 66(1):6-26.)

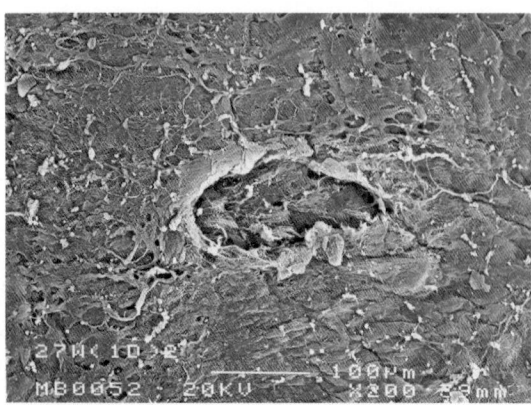

FIGURE 6–26. Dura-arachnoid lesion produced with 27-G Whitacre needle. Epidural surface. Scanning electron microscopy. Magnification ×200. (Reproduced with permission from Reina MA, Castedo J, López A. Cefalea pospunción dural: Ultraestructura de las lesiones durales y agujas espinales usadas en las punciones lumbares. *Rev Arg Anestesiol.* 2008 Jan-Mar 66(1):6-26.)

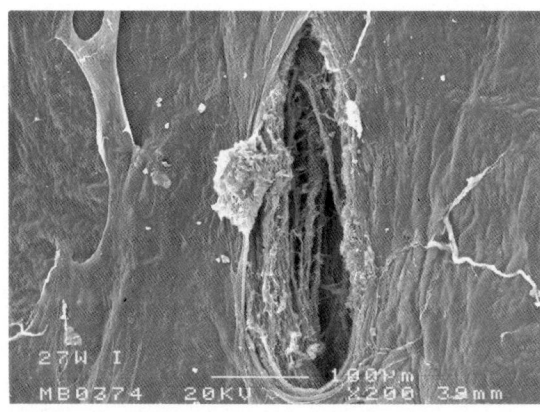

FIGURE 6–27. Dura-arachnoid lesion produced with 27-G Whitacre needle. Arachnoid surface. Scanning electron microscopy. Magnification ×200. (Reproduced with permission from Reina MA, Castedo J, López A. Cefalea pospunción dural: Ultraestructura de las lesiones durales y agujas espinales usadas en las punciones lumbares. *Rev Arg Anestesiol.* 2008 Jan-Mar 66(1):6-26.)

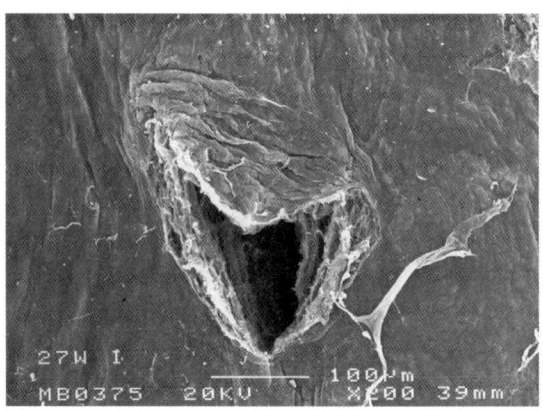

FIGURE 6–28. Dura-arachnoid lesion produced with 27-G Whitacre needle. Arachnoid surface. Scanning electron microscopy. Magnification ×200. (Reproduced with permission from Reina MA, Castedo J, López A. Cefalea pospunción dural: Ultraestructura de las lesiones durales y agujas espinales usadas en las punciones lumbares. *Rev Arg Anestesiol.* 2008 Jan-Mar 66(1):6-26.)

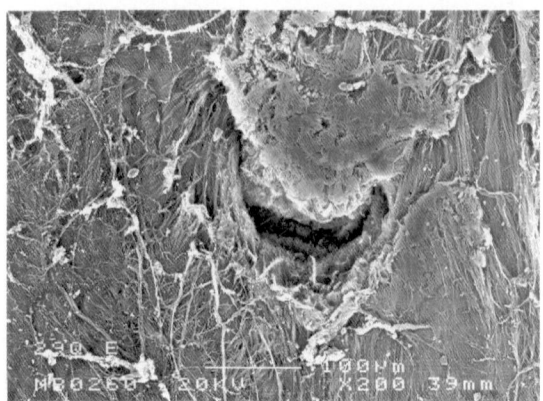

FIGURE 6–29. Dura-arachnoid lesion produced with 29-G Quincke needle. Epidural surface. Scanning electron microscopy. Magnification ×200. (Reproduced with permission from Reina MA, Castedo J, López A. Cefalea pospunción dural: Ultraestructura de las lesiones durales y agujas espinales usadas en las punciones lumbares. *Rev Arg Anestesiol.* 2008 Jan-Mar 66(1):6-26.)

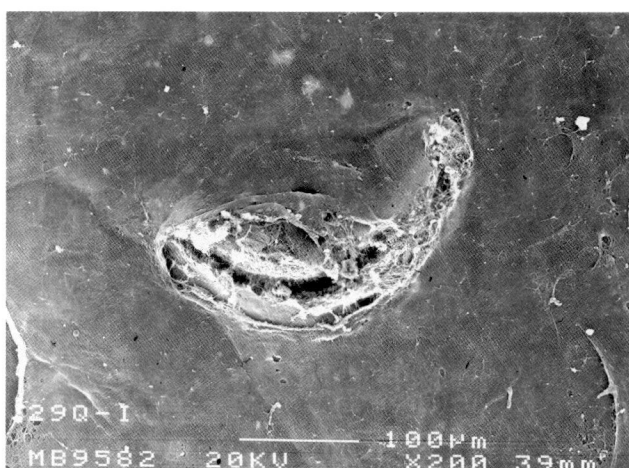

FIGURE 6–30. Dura-arachnoid lesion produced with 29-G Quincke needle. Arachnoid surface. Scanning electron microscopy. Magnification ×200. (Reproduced with permission from Reina MA, Castedo J, López A. Cefalea pospunción dural: Ultraestructura de las lesiones durales y agujas espinales usadas en las punciones lumbares. *Rev Arg Anestesiol.* 2008 Jan-Mar 66(1):6-26.)

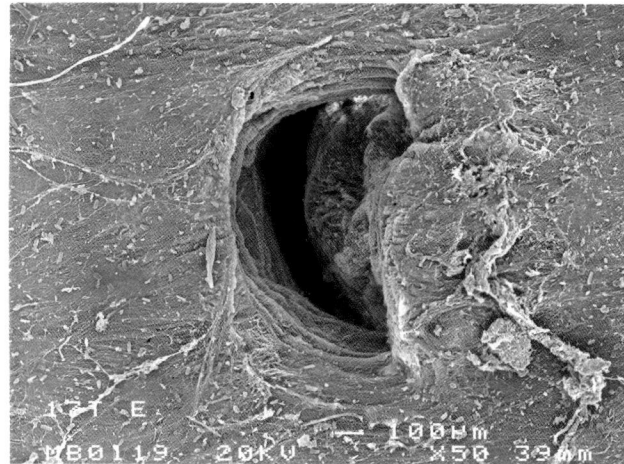

FIGURE 6–31. Dura-arachnoid lesion produced with 17-G Tuohy needle. Arachnoid surface. Scanning electron microscopy. Magnification ×50. (Reproduced with permission from Reina MA, Castedo J, López A. Cefalea pospunción dural: Ultraestructura de las lesiones durales y agujas espinales usadas en las punciones lumbares. *Rev Arg Anestesiol.* 2008 Jan-Mar 66(1):6-26.)

Deformation of the spinal needle caused by contacts with vertebral bones or other resistant structures during the neuraxial procedure can also increase the size of the dural lesion. Iatrogenic introduction of skin fragments into the subarachnoid space can also occur.[16–18]

POSTDURAL PUNCTURE HEADACHE AND TYPE OF NEEDLES

The etiology of PDPH is multifactorial. While the specific chapter on PDPH focuses on pathophysiology, prevention, and treatment, this section focuses on anatomical and equipment-related factors that may influence the occurrence and severity of PDPH. Initially, it was thought that pencil-point needles resulted in less-traumatic perforations of the dural sac. As the morphology of dural lesions became better known, other explanations have been proposed. Microscopic studies of lesions produced by spinal needles showed that the pencil-point needles produce a "burst"-type lesion with extensive fiber damage. However, the increased fiber tearing produced by pencil-point needles may promote greater inflammatory response at the edges of the lesion that paradoxically results in earlier occlusion and lower incidence of PDPH. Cutting needles, on the other hand, produce a "cleaner" tear of the dura with less inflammatory response that results in delayed puncture sealing, which could increase the incidence of spinal headache.

A needle tip blunted after colliding against bone can cause more damage to the fibers. Tip deformation depends on the collision angle and force applied. Cutting needles are especially susceptible to deformation of the needle tip after colliding against bone, contrary to pencil-point needles. However, because PDPH studies generally involve many anesthetists and different techniques, the definitive impact of the needle deformation on PDPH is difficult to study and at this time remains only hypothetical.

As mentioned, the dural lesion produced by the spinal needle has two components, a dura mater lesion and an arachnoid-layer lesion.[19] While the external or dural component of the sac provides mechanical resistance, it is not elastic enough to prevent cerebrospinal fluid leakage. In contrast, the internal or arachnoid lesion can retract to close the defect created by introduction of the needle into the subarachnoidal space and prevent the leakage of cerebrospinal fluid. Because the arachnoid component is probably more important in pathophysiology of PDPH than the dural itself, these lesions should be referred to as "dura-arachnoid" lesions.

TRABECULAR ARACHNOID

Arachnoid mater consists of two layers, the *trabecular* arachnoid and *arachnoid* layers. The trabecular arachnoid merges with the cellular plane of the pia mater and emits projections to all the structures that cross the subarachnoid space, including blood vessels and nerve roots. The projections that cover the nerve roots are called arachnoid sheaths[20,21] (Figures 6–32 to 6–40).

During movement, these sheaths stabilize and prevent excessive movements of the nerve roots within the dural sac. However, the sheaths confer little mechanical protection against trauma. Characteristics of the arachnoid sheaths in the cauda equina are variable; some are lax, while others are formed by superimposed planes of the same components with a more compact appearance. The thickness of an arachnoid sheath ranges from 10 to 60 μm. In some cases, one or more nerve roots are enveloped by a single arachnoid sheath, and in others, the nerve root has no sheath at all.[20,21]

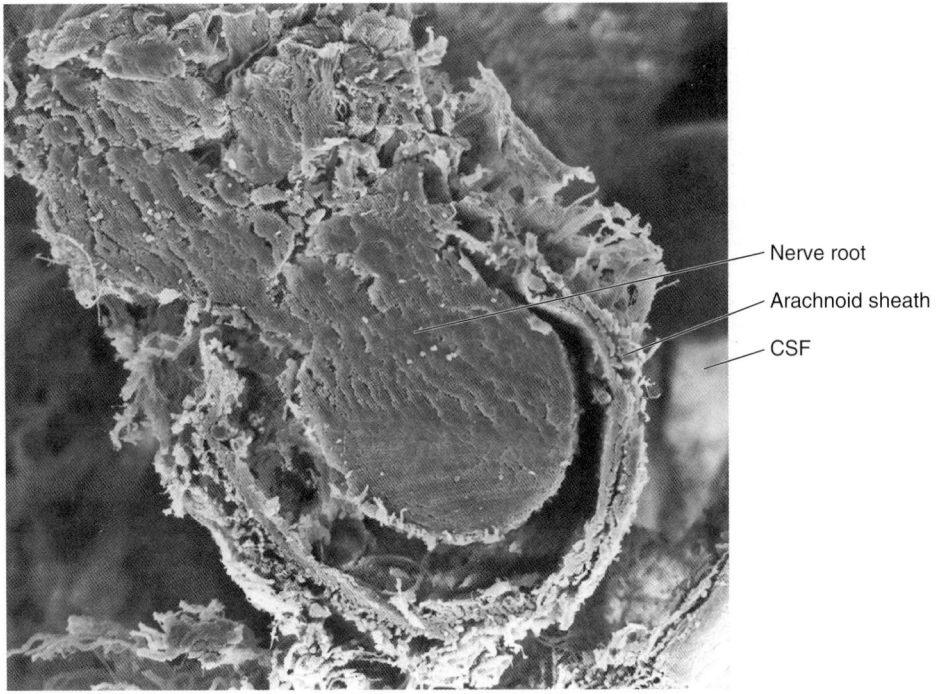

Nerve root
Arachnoid sheath
CSF

FIGURE 6–32. Trabecular arachnoid layer. The projections of trabecular arachnoid that cover nerve roots are called arachnoid sheaths. CSF = cerebrospinal fluid. Scanning electron microscopy. Magnification ×100. (Reproduced with permission from Reina MA, López A, De Andrés JA: Hypothesis concerning the anatomical basis of cauda equina syndrome and transient nerve root irritation after spinal anesthesia. *Rev Esp Anestesiol Reanim.* 1999 Mar;46(3):99-105.)

ARACHNOID SHEATHS OF NERVE ROOTS AND THEIR POTENTIAL ROLE IN NERVE LESIONS

Some cases of cauda equina syndrome and transient neurological syndrome could be explained by the existence of arachnoid sheaths surrounding nerve roots within the dural sac and the fact that needles or (micro)catheters can be inserted into them. An anesthetic solution accidentally injected into the arachnoid sheath of a spinal nerve may not be diluted by surrounding cerebrospinal fluid, thus exposing the nerve root to a higher anesthetic concentration than expected. Consequently, the concentration of the local anesthetic could be magnitudes higher (eg, 20–25 times) in comparison to the concentration of the anesthetic in the rest of the dural sac.[20,21] Such high local anesthetic concentration inside the arachnoid sheath could have deleterious effects on nerve roots, as opposed to a typical injection of the same anesthetic solution inside the dural sac

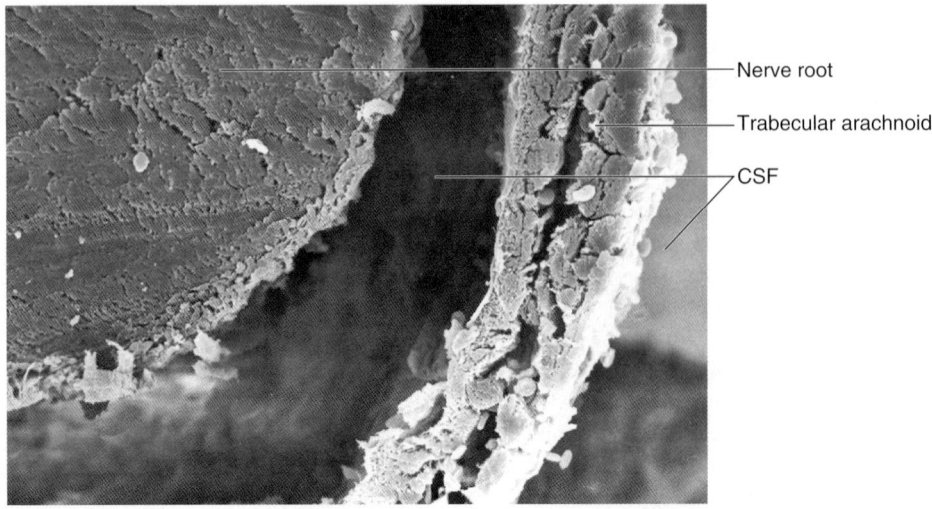

Nerve root
Trabecular arachnoid
CSF

FIGURE 6–33. Trabecular arachnoid layer. Detail of arachnoid sheaths. CSF = cerebrospinal fluid. Scanning electron microscopy. Magnification ×500. (Reproduced with permission from Raj P: *Textbook of Regional Anesthesia.* Philadelphia: Churchill Livingstone; 2002.)

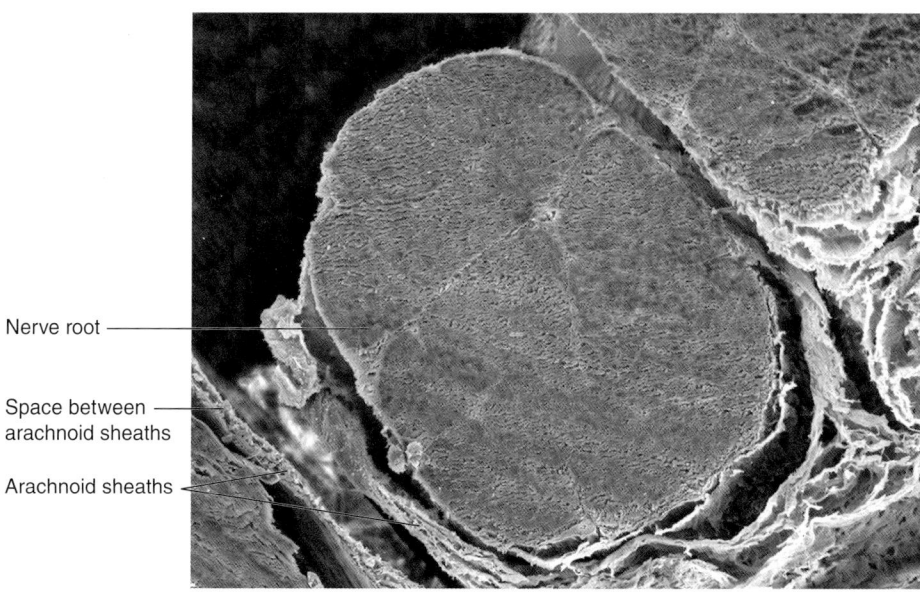

Nerve root

Space between arachnoid sheaths

Arachnoid sheaths

FIGURE 6–34. Nerve root and arachnoid sheath. Scanning electron microscopy. Magnification ×60. (Reproduced with permission from Torres LM: *Textbook of Anesthesia and Pain Management.* Aran Ed; 2001.)

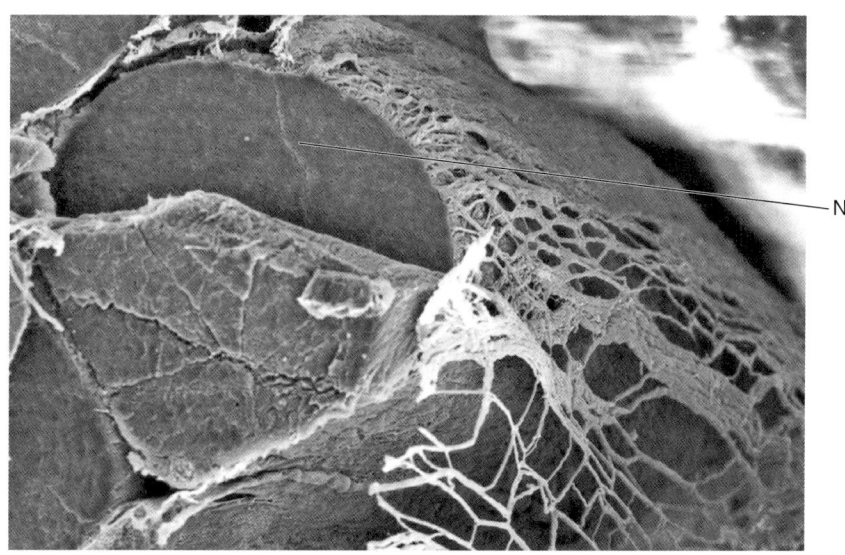

Nerve root

FIGURE 6–35. Nerve root and arachnoid sheath. Scanning electron microscopy. Magnification ×80. (Reproduced with permission from Reina MA, Villanueva MC, López A: Aracnoides trabecular, piamadre espinal humana y anestesia subaracnoidea, *Rev Arg Anestesiol* 2008;66: 111–133.)

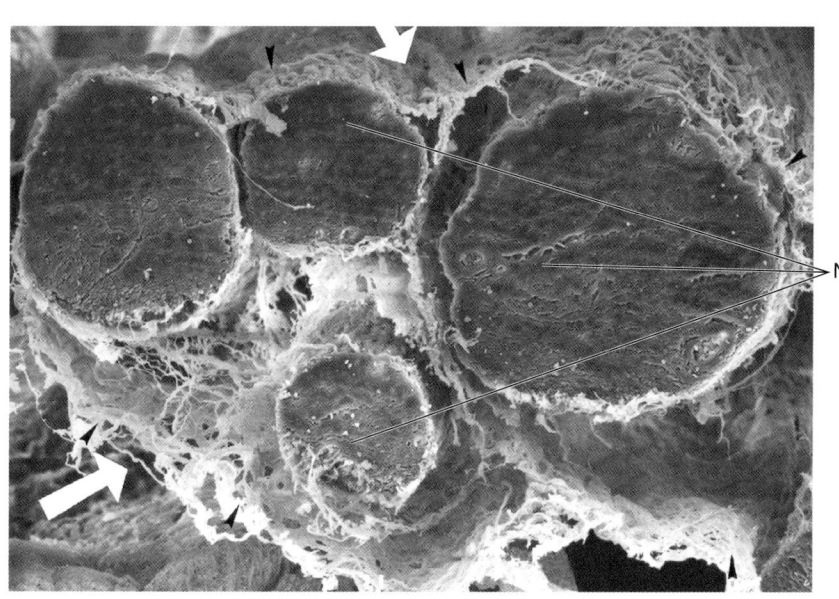

Nerve root

FIGURE 6–36. Four-nerve root and its arachnoid sheaths. Scanning electron microscopy. Magnification ×100. (Reproduced with permission from Reina MA, López A, De Andrés JA: Hypothesis concerning the anatomical basis of cauda equina syndrome and transient nerve root irritation after spinal anesthesia. *Rev Esp Anestesiol Reanim.* 1999 Mar;46(3):99-105.)

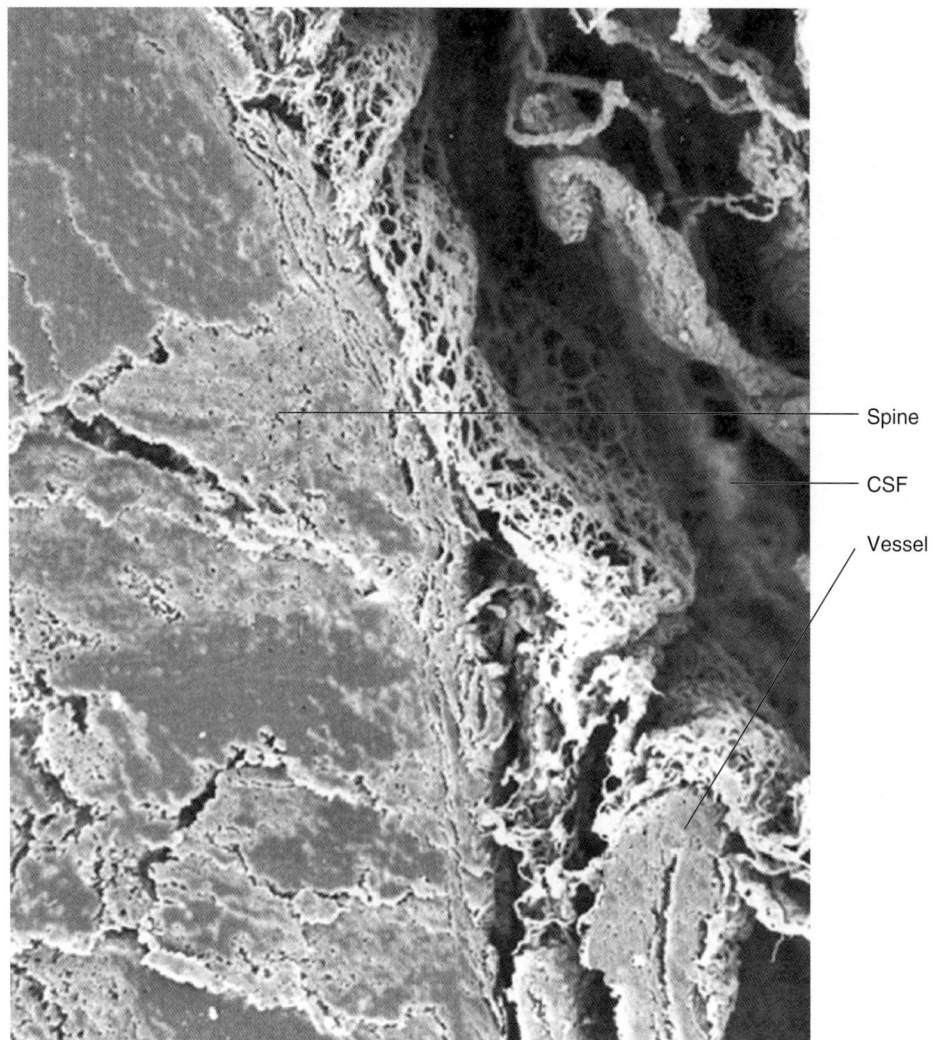

FIGURE 6–37. Human spinal cord and trabecular arachnoid layer. CSF = cerebrospinal fluid. Scanning electron microscopy. Magnification ×40. (Reproduced with permission from Reina MA, Machés F, López A, et al: The ultrastructure of the spinal arachnoid in humans and its impact on spinal anesthesia, cauda equina syndrome, and transient neurological syndrome. *Tech Reg Anesth Pain Management*. 2008 July;12(3):153-160.)

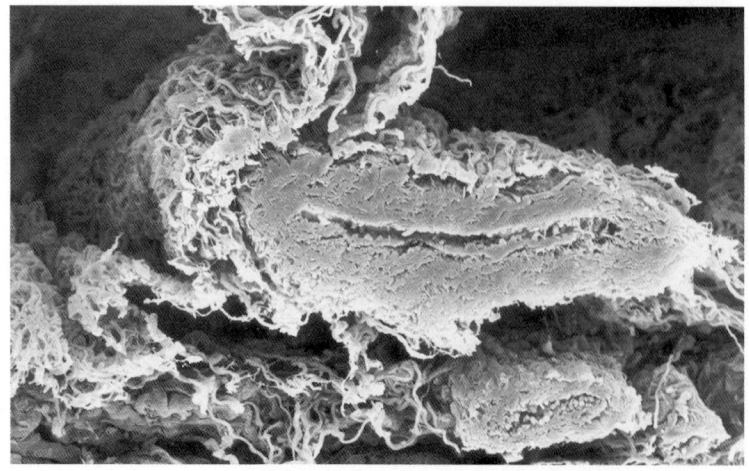

FIGURE 6–38. Subarachnoid vessel and trabecular arachnoid layer. Scanning electron microscopy. Magnification ×120. (Reproduced with permission from Raj P: *Textbook of Regional Anesthesia*. Philadelphia: Churchill Livingstone; 2002.)

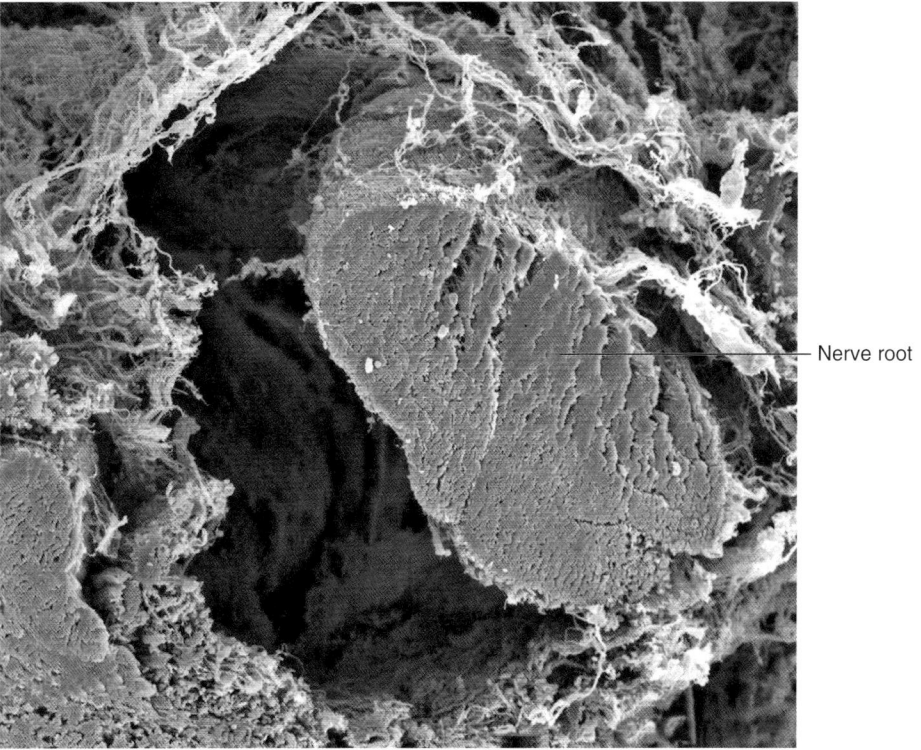

FIGURE 6–39. Nerve root and arachnoid sheath. Scanning electron microscopy. Magnification ×100. (Reproduced with permission from Torres LM: *Textbook of Anesthesia and Pain Management.* Aran Ed; 2001.)

but outside the arachnoid sheath. Because it takes time to establish equilibrium inside and outside the sheath, a nerve lesion could develop without direct needle trauma.

Injections of local anesthetic through a microcatheter into these arachnoid sheaths could be more devastating than a single injection. This is because the injection of a single large volume would eventually be diluted by leakage outside the sheath, whereas repeated doses of small volumes may be more likely to lead to neurotoxicity due to the continuous or repeated exposure to a high concentration of local anesthetics. Transient root

irritation syndrome and cauda equina syndrome may reflect different degrees of nerve damage related to local anesthetic concentration and duration of exposure. Injection of local anesthetic inside arachnoid sheaths in areas close to the spinal cord or to the conus medullaris could affect several nerve roots, while injection in more distal areas may affect single nerve roots.[20,21]

PIA MATER

The structure of the pia mater includes a cellular layer and a subpial compartment (Figures 6–41 and 6–42). The cellular layer consists of flat, overlapping pial cells with a smooth and bright appearance (Figure 6–43). Its thickness is 3 to 5 pial cells (10–15 μm) at the medullary level (Figures 6–44 to 6–46) and 2 to 3 cells (3–4 μm) at the nerve root level. Amorphous fundamental substance is found around the pial cells, and the cells measure on average 0.5–1 μm.[22-25]

The subpial compartment has large amounts of collagen fibers, amorphous fundamental substance, fibroblasts, and a small number of macrophages and blood vessels. The subpial compartment is enclosed between the pial cellular layer and a basal membrane in contact with neuroglial cells.

The subpial compartment from the low thoracic vertebrae has a thickness of 130–200 μm; here, variations in measurements are more significant than in the pial cellular layer (see Figures 6–41 and 6–42). At the level of the medullary cone, the thickness of the pia mater is reduced to 80–100 μm; its thickness continues to decrease to merely 50–60 μm in the origins

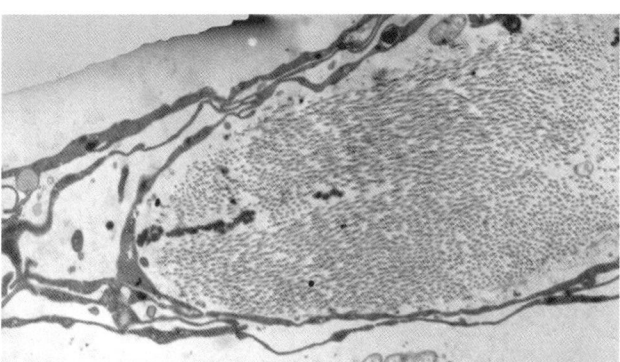

FIGURE 6–40. Detail of trabecular arachnoid layer. Transmission electron microscopy. Magnification ×5000. (Reproduced with permission from Reina MA, Villanueva MC, López A: Aracnoides trabecular, piamadre espinal humana y anestesia subaracnoidea. *Rev Arg Anestesiol.* 2008;66:111–133.)

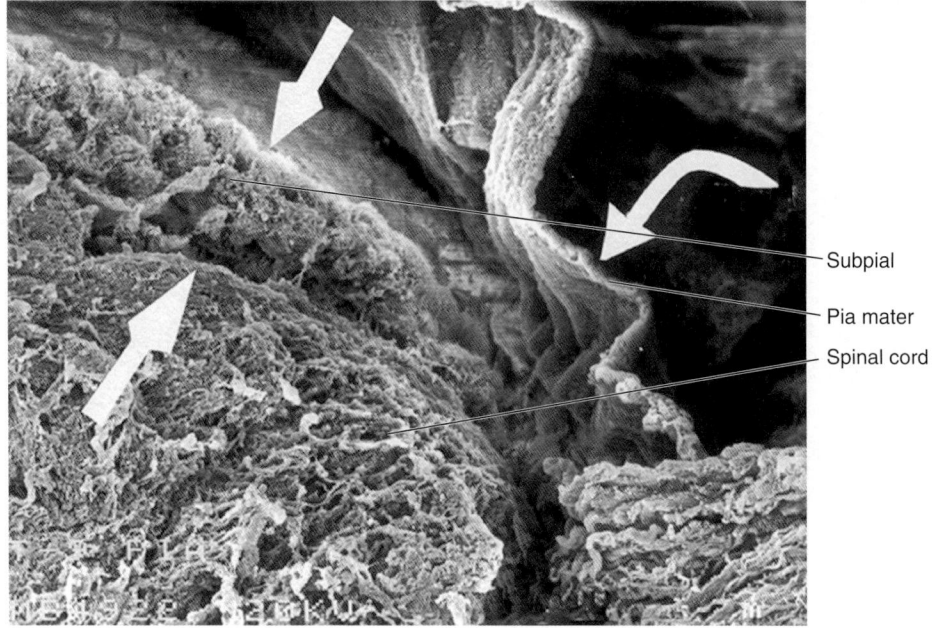

FIGURE 6–41. Human pia mater and spinal cord. Scanning electron microscopy. Magnification ×70. (Reproduced with permission from Reina MA, De Leon Casasola O, et al: Ultrastructural findings in human spinal pia mater in relation to subarachnoid anesthesia. *Anesth Analg.* 2004 May;98(5):1479-1485.)

of the cauda equina. At the nerve root level, the thickness of the subpial compartment is 10–12 μm.

At the level of the medullary cone, there are perforations or circular, ovoid, or elliptical fenestrations over the entire surface of the cellular layer of the pia mater (Figures 6–47 to 6–49). While the size of these fenestrations varies, most measure 12–15 μm in length and 4–8 μm in width. At the nerve root level, the pia mater shows similar fenestrations but smaller size (1–4 μm)[7,22,23] (Figure 6–50).

Numerous macrophages surround the pial cells. The macrophages differ from pial cells in that they lack long cytoplasmic processes, containing membrane-bound inclusions and a varying number of vacuoles, especially in the peripheral areas of their cytoplasm. The macrophages and other inflammatory

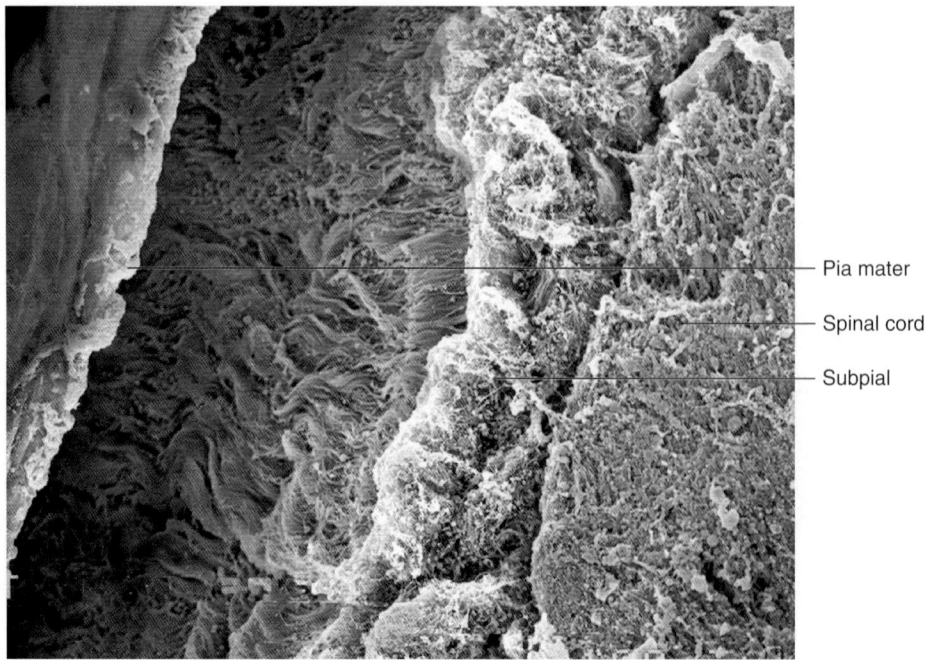

FIGURE 6–42. Human pia mater and subpial compartment. Scanning electron microscopy. Magnification ×100. (Reproduced with permission from Raj P: *Textbook of Regional Anesthesia.* Philadelphia: Churchill Livingstone; 2002.)

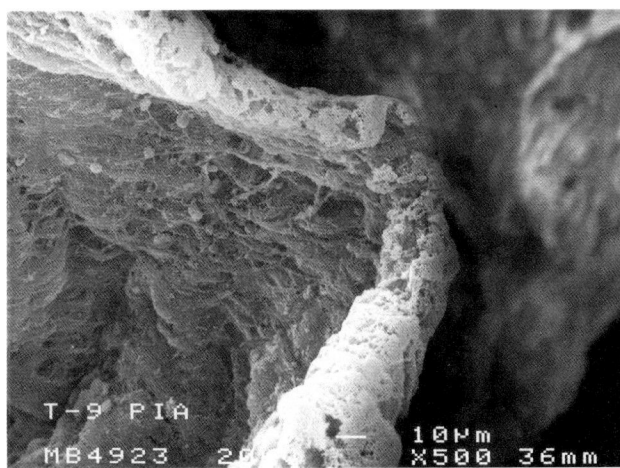

FIGURE 6–43. Detail of pia mater. Scanning electron microscopy. Magnification ×500. (Reproduced with permission from Reina MA, Wikinski J, De Andrés JA: Una rara complicación de la anestesia epidural y subaracnoidea. Tumores epidermoideos espinales iatrogénicos. *Rev Arg Anestesiol.* 2008;66:319-336.)

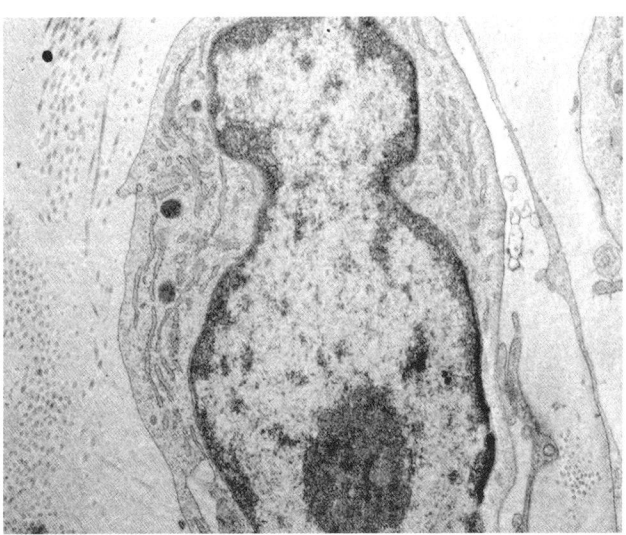

FIGURE 6–45. Detail of pial cells. Transmission electron microscopy. Magnification ×12,000. (Reproduced with permission from Reina MA, Wikinski J, De Andrés JA: Una rara complicación de la anestesia epidural y subaracnoidea. Tumores epidermoideos espinales iatrogénicos. *Rev Arg Anestesiol.* 2008;66:319-336.)

cells seen within the pia mater could originate from subpial and subarachnoid blood vessels or from immature pial cells as a result of an unknown stimulus. The fenestrations found in the pia mater appear to be associated with the migration of some immature pial cells as part of an inflammatory response.[23]

DURAL SAC LIGAMENTS

The epidural space contains fibrous formations that cross and anchor the dural sac to the vertebral canal. These connective tissue formations are referred to as the anterior, lateral, and posterior meningo-vertebral ligaments (Figures 6–51 and 6–52). The anterior meningo-vertebral ligament, which connects the dural sac with the posterior longitudinal ligament of the spine, is more compact. In some patients, fibrous flaps that fix the dural sac to the posterior longitudinal ligament may incompletely divide the anterior epidural space. Anterior ligaments extend from C7 to L5 with a craniocaudal orientation and acquire a transverse orientation at thoracic level T8–9. The length of these ligaments varies from about 0.5 to 29 mm. In

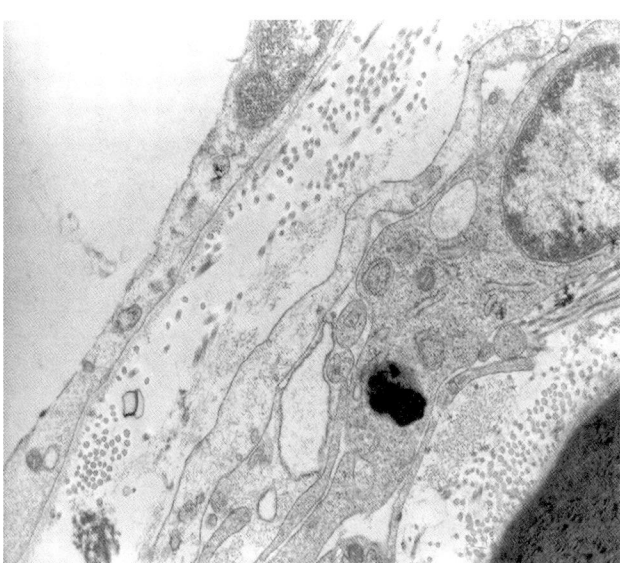

FIGURE 6–44. Human pia mater. Detail of pial cells. Transmission electron microscopy. Magnification ×12,000. (Reproduced with permission from Reina MA, Wikinski J, De Andrés JA: Una rara complicación de la anestesia epidural y subaracnoidea. Tumores epidermoideos espinales iatrogénicos. *Rev Arg Anestesiol.* 2008;66:319-336.)

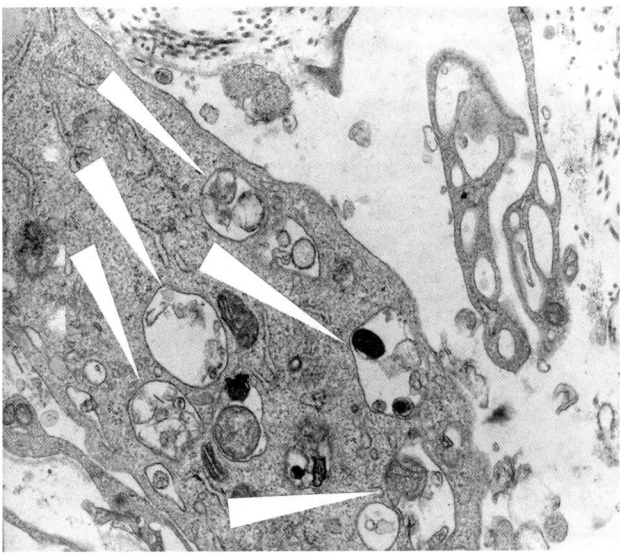

FIGURE 6–46. Detail of macrophagic cells in spinal pia mater. Transmission electron microscopy. Magnification ×12,000. (Reproduced with permission from Reina MA, Wikinski J, De Andrés JA: Una rara complicación de la anestesia epidural y subaracnoidea. Tumores epidermoideos espinales iatrogénicos. *Rev Arg Anestesiol.* 2008;66:319-336.)

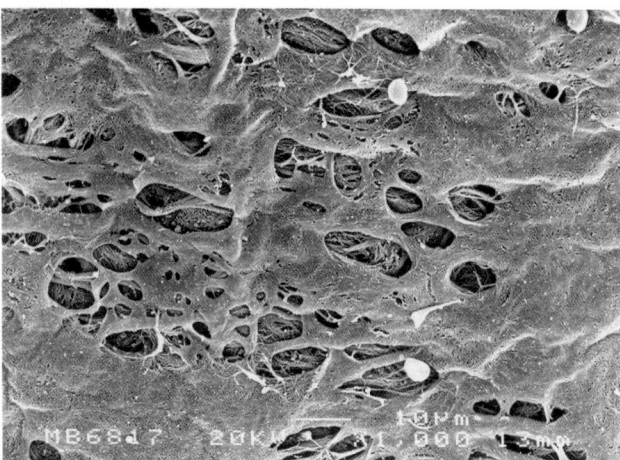

FIGURE 6–47. Fenestrations in human pia mater of conus medullaris. Scanning electron microscopy. Magnification ×1000. (Reproduced with permission from Reina MA, López García A, de Andrés JA: Anatomical description of a natural perforation present in the human lumbar pia mater. *Rev Esp Anestesiol Reanim.* 1998;45:4-7.)

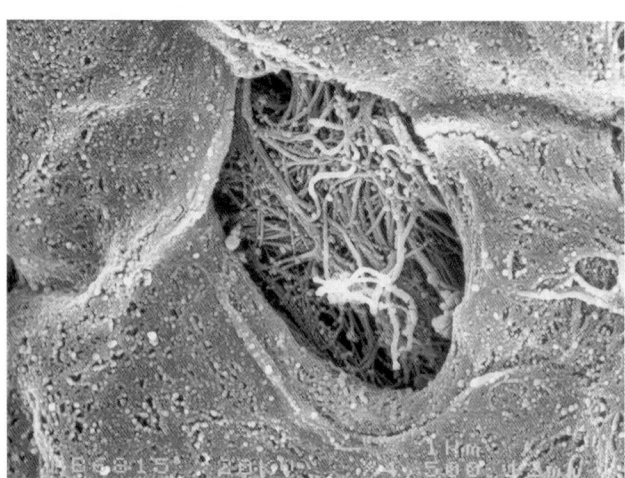

FIGURE 6–49. Detail of fenestration in human pia mater. Scanning electron microscopy. Magnification ×1500. (Reproduced with permission from Reina MA, López García A, de Andrés JA: Anatomical description of a natural perforation present in the human lumbar pia mater. *Rev Esp Anestesiol Reanim.* 1998;45:4-7.)

the sacral canal, the ligaments thicken to form a perforated medial septum, the "anterior sacral ligament of Trolard." The lateral meningo-vertebral ligament and the posterior ("Giordalengo") meningo-vertebral ligament are thinner and do not affect the circulation of fluids injected in the epidural space.

The "plica mediana dorsalis" is a longitudinal and discontinuous fibrous structure that can be found in the midsagittal region along the posterior epidural space, particularly in the lumbar region.[24,25]

EPIDURAL FAT

Epidural fat extends laterally toward the site where articular facets and ligamentum flavum meet. Located between the vertebral arches and the intervertebral foramina, fat wraps around

nerve roots within the dural sleeves but without adhering to them. This allows displacement of the dura within the vertebral canal during flexion/extension.

Epidural fat does adhere in the midline posteriorly by a vascular pedicle at a point where the right and left portions of the ligamentum flavum meet.[26] The amount of posterior epidural fat increases caudally, from L1–2 to L4–5, and can reach 16–25 mm. Its width also increases in the craniocaudal direction from 6 mm at the L1–2 interspace to 13 mm in the L4–5 interspace. The pedicle of the posterior epidural fat corresponds topographically with the plica mediana dorsalis.

Epidural fat deposits are in contact with the posterior surface of the dural sac and the vertebral lamina but adhere only to the vascular pedicle.[26] Regarding the posterior, epidural fat is

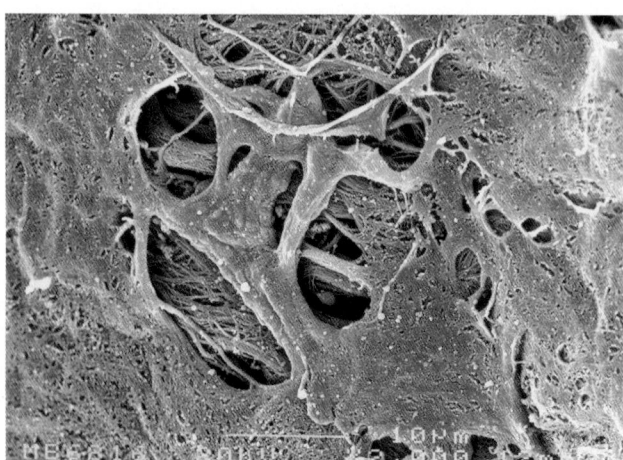

FIGURE 6–48. Fenestrations in human pia mater of conus medullaris. Scanning electron microscopy. Magnification ×2000. (Reproduced with permission from Reina MA, López García A, de Andrés JA: Anatomical description of a natural perforation present in the human lumbar pia mater. *Rev Esp Anestesiol Reanim.* 1998;45:4-7.)

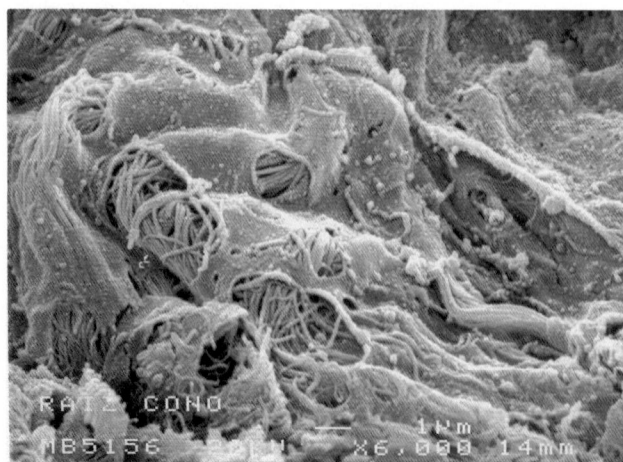

FIGURE 6–50. Fenestrations in human pia mater of nerve root. Scanning electron microscopy. Magnification ×6000. (Reproduced with permission from Reina MA, Villanueva MC, López A: Aracnoides trabecular, piamadre espinal humana y anestesia subaracnoidea. *Rev Arg Anestesiol.* 2008;66:111–133.)

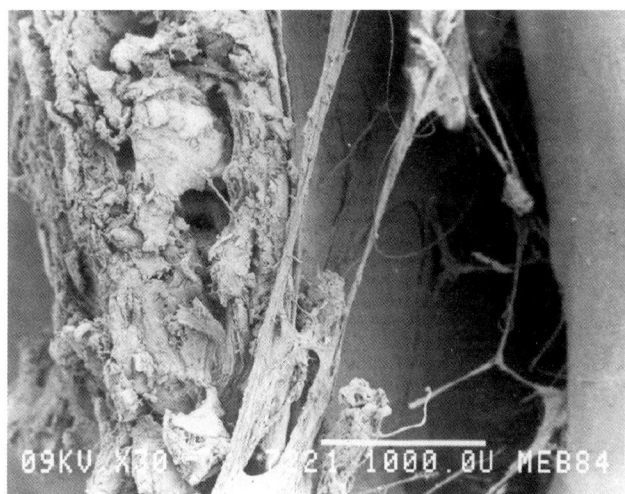

FIGURE 6–51. Epidural space. Fibrous formations that cross the epidural space. Scanning electron microscopy. Magnification ×30. (Reproduced with permission from Reina MA, Pulido P, López A. El saco dural humano. *Rev Arg Anestesiol.* 2007;65:167-184.)

homogeneous and is not separated by fibrous septae; laterally, epidural fat appears divided. Sometimes, a septal plane extends between the nerve root exit at the vertebral lamina and the posterior longitudinal ligament. Looking at the anterior, dura mater joins the vertebral canal at the height of the disks. It is in this anterior epidural region where the anterior venous vessels are found.

CHARACTERISTICS OF THE EPIDURAL FAT IN THE CERVICAL, THORACIC, LUMBAR, AND SACRAL REGIONS

The distribution of epidural fat is variable along the spinal canal, but it tends to be more consistent at different vertebral levels. For example, at the *cervical* level, adipose tissue is absent or almost nonexistent and sometimes forms a small posterior deposit seen

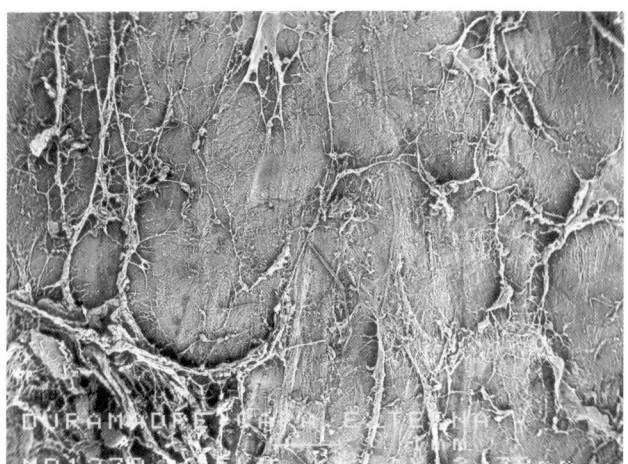

FIGURE 6–52. Epidural surface of the dural sac. Scanning electron microscopy. Magnification ×12. (Reproduced with permission from Reina MA, Dittmann M, López A, et al: New perspectives in the microscopic structure of human dura mater in the dorso lumbar region. *Reg Anesth.* 1997 Mar-Apr;22(2):161-166.)

with magnetic resonance imaging axial sections (C7 to T1), with increased signal intensity on T1-weighted sequences. Epidural fat is not generally found in the anterior and lateral regions.

At the *thoracic* level, epidural fat forms a broad posterior band with "indentations."[26] This band is thicker around the intervertebral space and around the intervertebral disk, becoming thinner at the level of the vertebral bodies and close to the base of the spinal processes of each vertebra. In the middle-upper thoracic region (T1–7), epidural fat follows a continuous pattern with more evident indentations, while in the lower thoracic region (T8–12) epidural fat becomes discontinuous.

At the lumbar level, epidural fat in the anterior and posterior epidural spaces remains separate. The posterior epidural fat is more prominent around the disks of L3–4 and L4–5. In some patients, the posterior epidural fat is cone shaped, with the apex located at the posterior. The thickness of the epidural fat in the lower lumbar zone occupies about 32% of the cross-sectional diameter of the vertebral canal.

Below L4–5, the dural sac ends and the sacral canal begins. Here, nerve roots are enveloped by dural sleeves, and epidural fat is the main component within the sleeves.[26]

The morphology and distribution of epidural fat can be altered in pathological conditions. Epidural lipomatosis, for example, is characterized by an increase in epidural fat volume.[27] Excessive fat deposits around the dural sac can cause spinal cord or nerve root compression, leading to neurological symptoms. In kyphoscoliosis, epidural fat is distributed asymmetrically and adipose tissue predominates in the concave portion of the curvature, while the spinal cord is displaced against the vertebral arch.[27] In patients with spinal canal stenosis, epidural fat is characteristically absent or markedly reduced around the stenotic zone.[27]

EPIDURAL FAT AND PHARMACOKINETICS OF EPDIURAL INJECTATES

The distribution of epidural fat in the lumbar vertebral canal is uneven, being more abundant in the dorsal region than in the ventral and lateral regions. The total amount, distribution, and morphology of fat in the epidural space and nerve root cuffs affect the diffusion of substances across these compartments.

Changes in the amount of epidural fat during pathological processes may alter absorption of drugs during epidural blockade. However, even in the absence of pathological processes, local variations in the amount of fat within the lumbar spinal canal could alter drug kinetics. It is possible that variations in the distance between fat and neighboring nerve tissues affect the disposition of drugs injected and kinetics of the lipophilic drugs. At present, however, the impact of the ultrastructure of epidural and nerve root cuffs on drug kinetics during epidural injection remains unclear.

SUBDURAL SPACE

In contrast to the classical description of a "subdural space" between the dura mater and the arachnoid dorsalis, studies have shown the presence of a solid but delicate tissue composed of specialized neurothelial cells[8,9] (Figure 6–53). Neurothelial cells

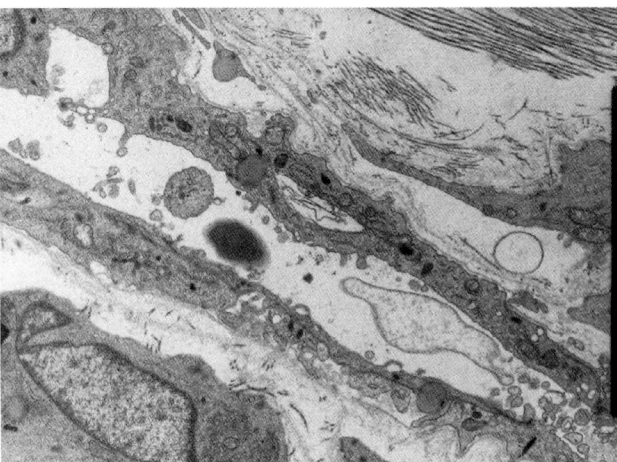

FIGURE 6–53. Neurothelial cells in the subdural compartment. Transmission electron microscopy. Magnification ×5000. (Reproduced with permission from Reina MA, De León Casasola OA, et al: The origin of the spinal subdural space. Ultrastructure finding. *Anesth Analg.* 2002 Apr;94(4):991-995.)

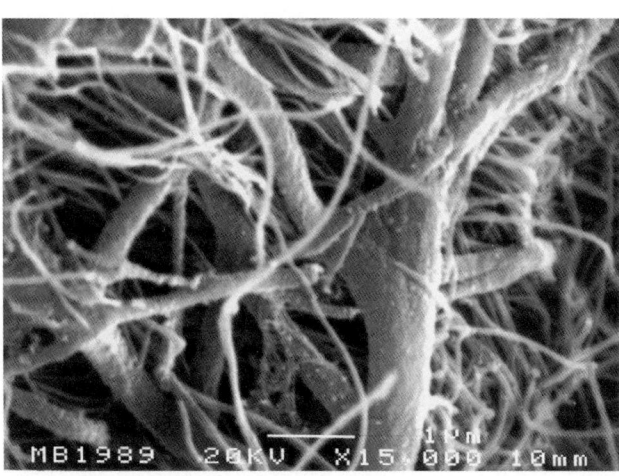

FIGURE 6–55. Neurothelial cells in the subdural compartment. Scanning electron microscopy. Magnification ×15,000. (Reproduced with permission from Reina MA, López A, De Andrés JA, Villanueva MC, Cortés L: Does the subdural space exist? *Rev Esp Anestesiol Reanim.* 1998 Nov;45(9):367-376.)

are also referred to as dural border cells. These elongated, fusiform cells with branched extensions are fragile and scantly cohesive to each other (Figures 6–54 and 6–55). Intercellular junctions between neurothelial cells are most susceptible to tearing, and cellular fragments may be seen next to torn neurothelial cells (Figures 6–56 and 6–57). When tearing occurs along the subdural compartment, small fissures merge into larger ones. Weak cohesive forces between neurothelial cells and lack of collagen fibers facilitate the widening of a fissure, producing the impression of a subdural space. Thus, the classic subdural space appears to be an iatrogenic artifact.[2]

Studying the structure of the subdural compartment may shed light on the origin of cranial and spinal subdural hematomas associated with cerebrospinal fluid hypotension.[28,29]

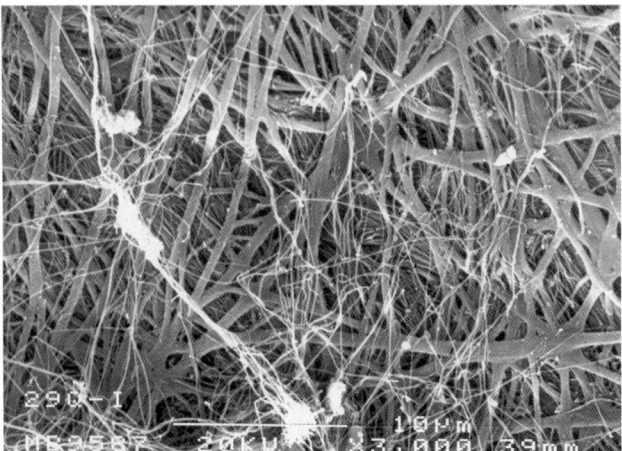

FIGURE 6–54. Neurothelial cells in the subdural compartment. Scanning electron microscopy. Magnification ×3000. (Reproduced with permission from Reina MA, De León Casasola OA, et al: The origin of the spinal subdural space. Ultrastructure finding. *Anesth Analg.* 2002 Apr;94(4):991-995.)

Subdural anesthetic blockade, caused by inadvertent injection of local anesthetic partially or entirely between the dura and arachnoid, results in highly unpredictable spinal or epidural anesthesia and complications due to an unanticipated high-level blockade. Dissection of the weak intercellular junctions between neurothelial cells may allow injected fluids to accumulate in the subdural space. Extent of the subdural block is unpredictable as it depends on the volume of local anesthetic injected and the nature of the dissection (cephalic or circumferential). If the dissection is mainly cephalad, only a few milliliters of anesthetic solution can block cardiorespiratory symptoms.

NERVE ROOT CUFFS

Bilateral projections of the dural sac (matter) onto the nerve roots form the nerve root cuffs or dural sleeves (Figure 6–58). Lateral extensions of the dura mater and the arachnoid layer surround the nerve roots as they exit the vertebral canal. The dural sac may contain a certain amount of cerebrospinal fluid around the nerve root. Nerve root cuffs (sleeves) have internal cellular and external fibrillar components[30] (Figure 6–59). Leptomeningeal cells, similar in nature to arachnoid or pial cells, form the cellular component of root cuffs. These cells are elongated, wider around the nucleus, stratified and oriented longitudinal to the nerve root axis (Figure 6–60).

At the *preganglion level*, the cellular component of a root cuff is 5.8–13 μm thick. These cells have cytoplasmic prolongations that encroach on neighboring cells, leaving little extracellular space. Unions between cell membranes are of the type desmosome and have tight junctions (Figure 6–61). Cells contain mitochondria in their cytoplasm and rough endoplasmic reticulum. Each cell is about 0.15–0.8 μm thick at both ends and 2.2–4.9 μm at the nucleus. The cellular component is arranged in two concentric layers held apart by collagen fibers.[31]

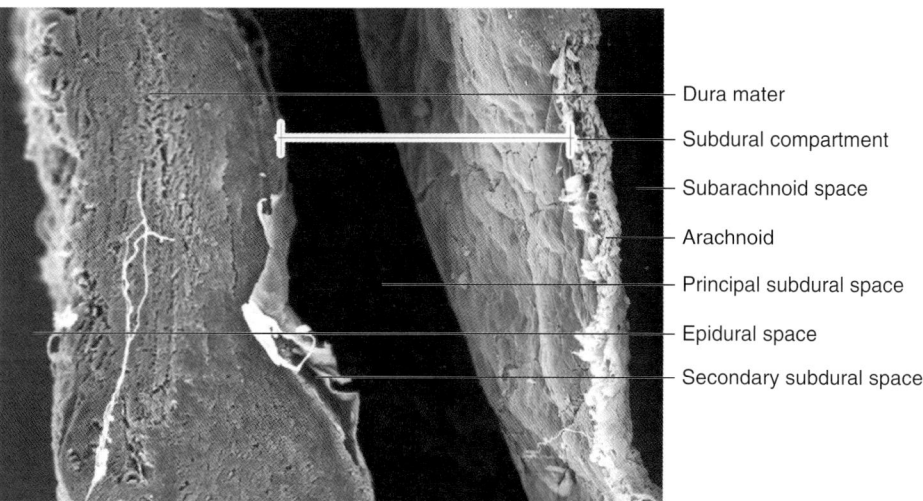

FIGURE 6-56. Human subdural space in the lumbar meninges. Scanning electron microscopy. Magnification ×180. (Reproduced with permission from Reina MA, López A, De Andrés JA, Villanueva MC, Cortés L: Does the subdural space exist? *Rev Esp Anestesiol Reanim.* 1998 Nov;45(9):367-376.)

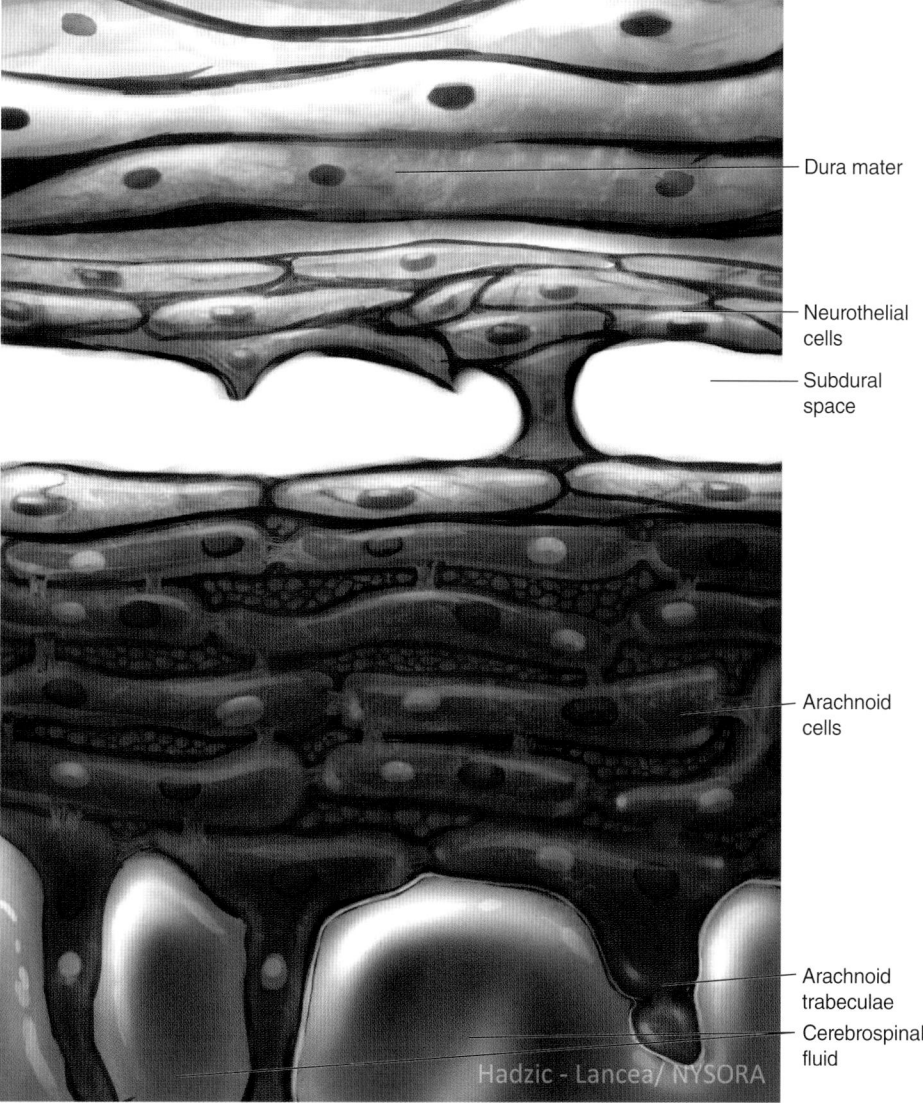

FIGURE 6-57. Diagram of origin of the subdural space.

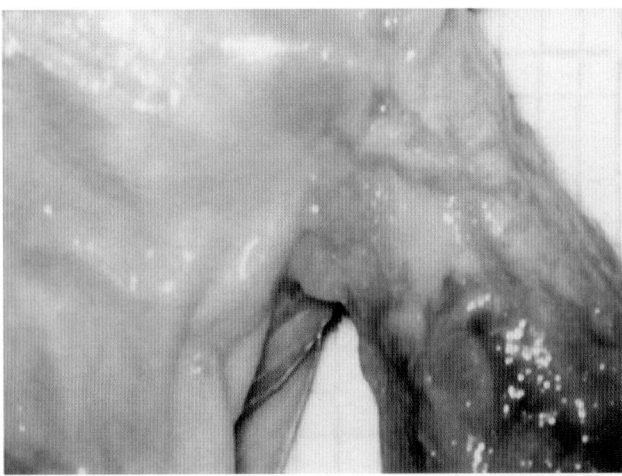

FIGURE 6–58. Human nerve root cuff. (Reproduced with permission from Reina MA, Villanueva MC, López A, et al: Fat inside the dural sheath of lumbar nerve roots in humans. *Rev Esp Anestesiol Reanim.* 2007 May;54(5):297-301.)

At the *postganglion level*, the cellular component has 9–14 single-cell concentric layers and measures 18–50 μm. Their unions are of the desmosome type.[31] The morphology of the cellular component at the ganglion level shows transitional changes while retaining many of the characteristics shown at the postganglion level. The cellular component consists of 25–30 concentric single-cell laminas and has a thickness of 55–60 μm.[31] Ultrastructural aspects of the cellular component at the pre-, post-, and ganglion levels are similar. The cells have rough endoplasmic reticulum widely distributed, and some also contain large vacuoles (0.1 μm) that occupy almost half of the cytoplasmic space. A membranous-like structure found in their cytoplasm may be involved in the production of vesicles (0.05–0.07 μm) needed for pinocytosis. Collagen fibers together with myelinated and unmyelinated axons are seen in the inner side of the cellular plane and are part of the endoneurial fibrillar structure. Specialized membrane unions among cells at the pre-, post-, and ganglion levels ensure a barrier effect, limiting the passage of substances from the epidural space to the nerve axons.

The fibrillar component[32] resides in the outer portion of the root cuff and has a thickness of 100–150 μm (Figure 6–62). It consists mostly of collagen fibers arranged in concentric laminas with scarce elastic fibers.[32] Large numbers of adipocytes separate dural laminas in groups of three to five concentric layers (Figure 6–63). Scanning electron microscopy shows adipocytes (Figure 6–63) extending from the dural sac to the dorsal root ganglia. Adipocytes can be found protruding from inside the wall built by the fibrillar component, out of the external epidural surface of the root cuff (Figures 6–64 and 6–65).

The fibrillar portion in the dural sac contains about 80 dural laminas with collagen fibers oriented in different directions and few elastic fibers. Its thickness varies between 270 and 350 μm at the lumbar level. Adipocytes are not found within the

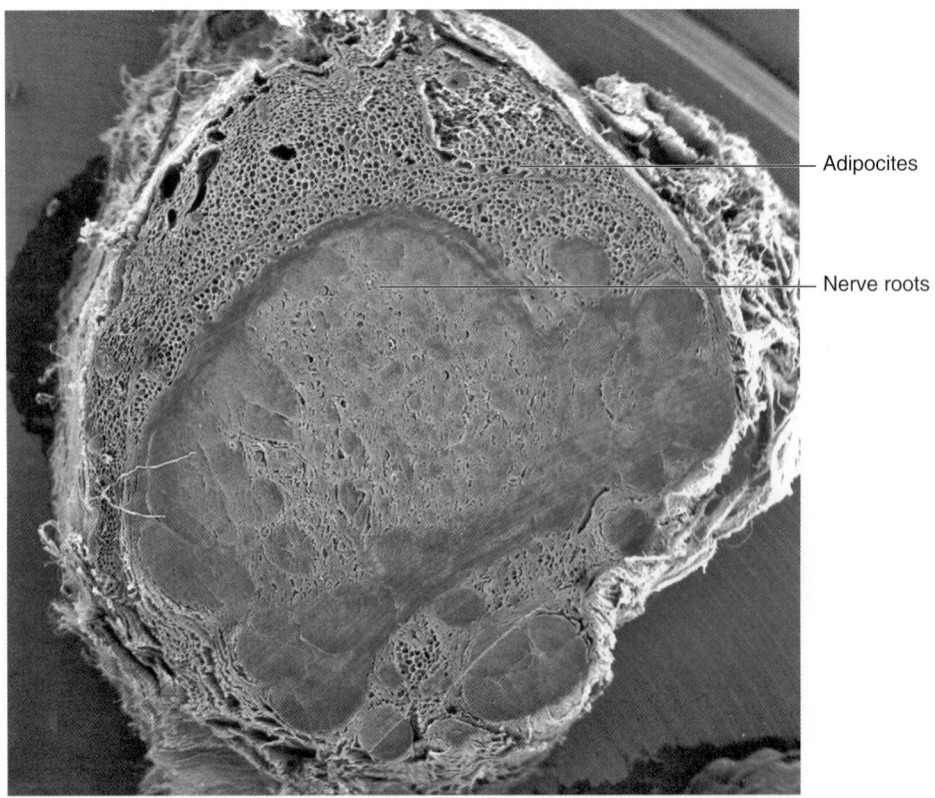

FIGURE 6–59. Human nerve root cuff. Scanning electron microscopy. Magnification ×12. (Reproduced with permission from Reina MA, Villanueva MC, Machés F, et al: Ultrastructure of human spinal nerve root cuff in lumbar spine. *Anesth Analg.* 2008 Jan;106(1): 339-344.)

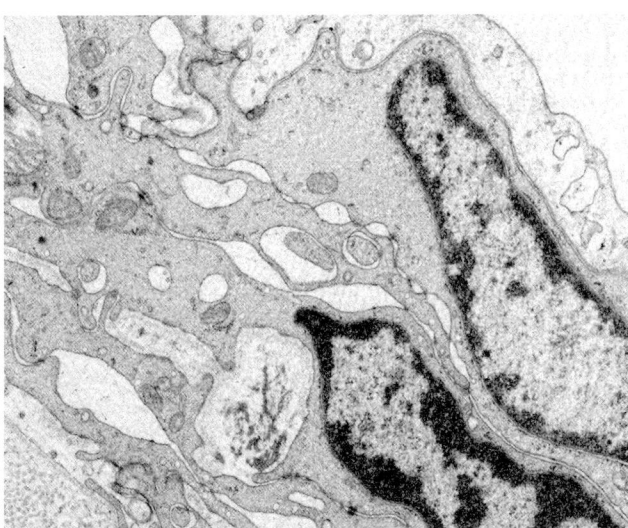

FIGURE 6–60. Human nerve root cuff. Detail of transition cellular barrier. Transmission electron microscopy. Magnification ×20,000. (Reproduced with permission from Reina MA, Villanueva MC, Machés F, et al: Ultrastructure of human spinal nerve root cuff in lumbar spine. *Anesth Analg.* 2008 Jan;106(1):339-344.)

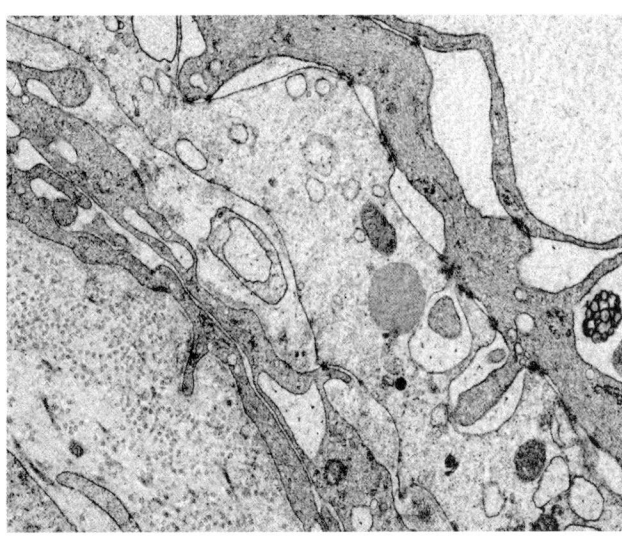

FIGURE 6–61. Human nerve root cuff. Detail of transition cellular barrier. Transmission electron microscopy. Magnification ×3000. (Reproduced with permission from Reina MA, Machés F, Pulido P, López A, De Andrés JA. Ultrastructure of Human Spinal Meninges. In: Aldrete A. *Arachnoiditis, Mexico*: Alfil Ed; 2010. pp. 29-46.)

thickness of the dural sac. Variations in dural thickness along the dural sac and differences related to the external fibrillar component do not alter the barrier effect, which is the exclusive responsibility of the cellular component.[33–37]

Scanning electron microscopy has shown that adipocytes measure 50–70 μm and are similar to those found in peripheral nerve samples of the sciatic nerve.[33] The fact that adipocytes appear smaller and lack a spherical shape is most likely due to loss of fat from their vacuoles during sample preparation. Fat in root cuffs covers groups of root axons, although adipocytes are not seen enclosing axons individually. This fat either partially or totally occupies the thickness of the root cuffs' fibrillar component.

ADIPOSE TISSUE IN ROOT CUFFS AND DRUG KINETICS

Adipose tissue can be found in the epidural space and inside the nerve root cuffs. Fat in nerve cuffs is in direct contact with nerve root axons and may play a role in the kinetics of

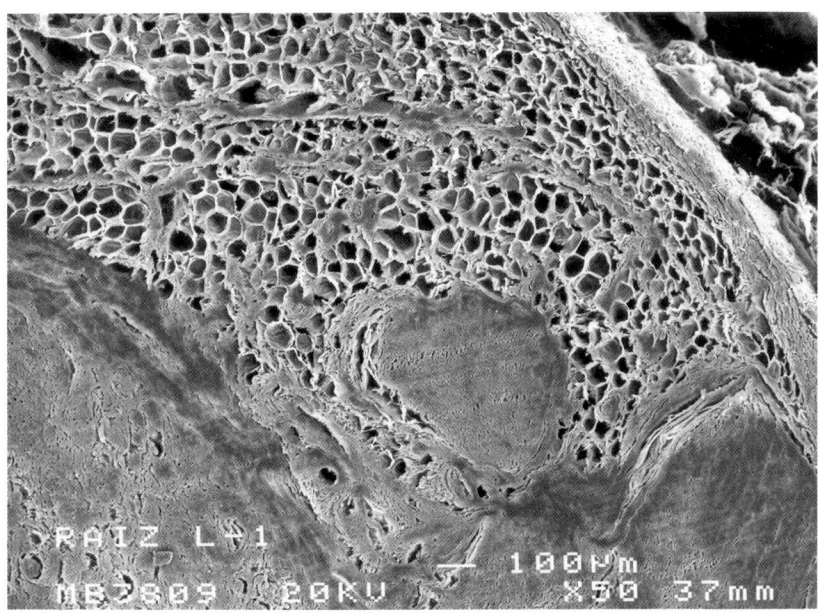

FIGURE 6–62. Human nerve root cuff. Detail of fat tissue in thickness of nerve root cuff. Scanning electron microscopy. Magnification ×50. (Reproduced with permission from Reina MA, Villanueva MC, López A, et al: Fat inside the dural sheath of lumbar nerve roots in humans. *Rev Esp Anestesiol Reanim.* 2007 May;54(5):297-301.)

PART 2

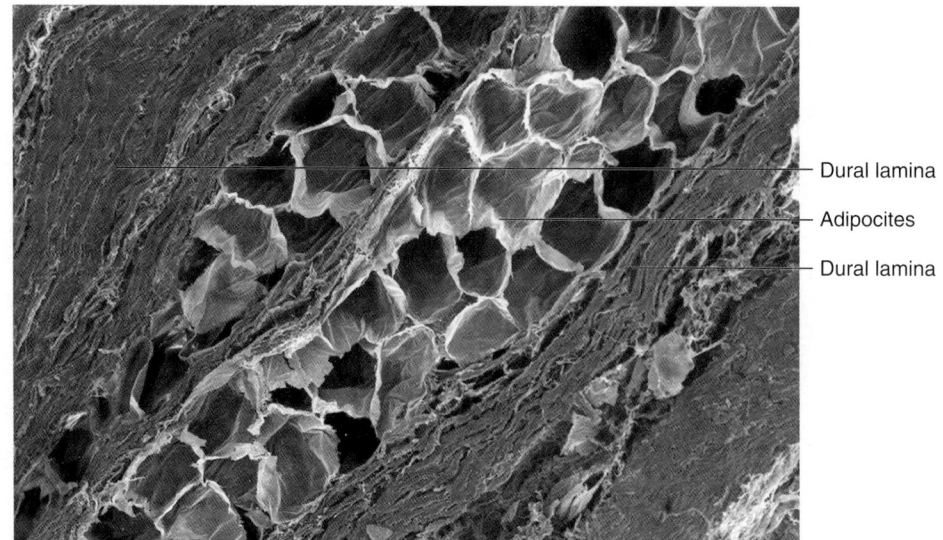

FIGURE 6–63. Human nerve root cuff. Detail of dural laminas in thickness of nerve root cuff. Scanning electron microscopy. Magnification ×150. (Reproduced with permission from Reina MA, Villanueva MC, Machés F, et al: Ultrastructure of human spinal nerve root cuff in lumbar spine. *Anesth Analg.* 2008 Jan;106(1):339-344.)

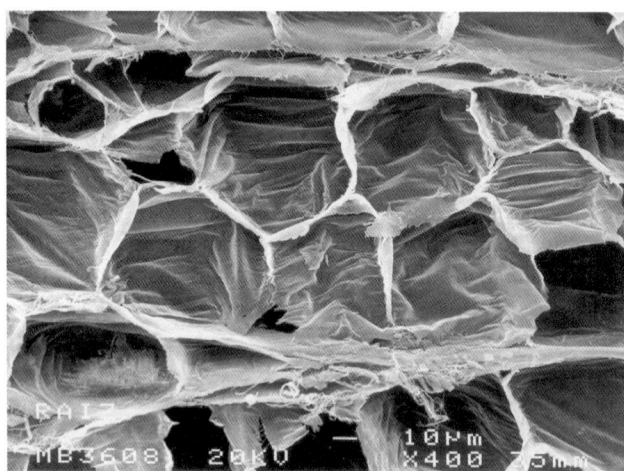

FIGURE 6–64. Human nerve root cuff. Adipocytes in nerve root cuff. Scanning electron microscopy. Magnification ×400. (Reproduced with permission from Reina MA, Villanueva MC, Machés F, et al: Ultrastructure of human spinal nerve root cuff in lumbar spine. *Anesth Analg.* 2008 Jan;106(1):339-344.)

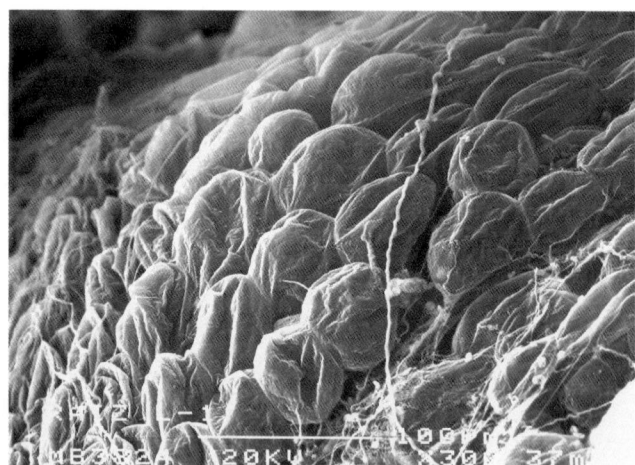

FIGURE 6–65. Adipocytes on epidural surface of nerve root cuff. Scanning electron microscopy. Magnification ×300. (Reproduced with permission from Reina MA, Villanueva MC, López A, et al: Fat inside the dural sheath of lumbar nerve roots in humans. *Rev Esp Anestesiol Reanim.* 2007 May;54(5):297-301.)

lipophilic substances injected near the nerve roots. The small space within the root cuffs and the large amount of drugs available in case of an injection into the cuff may expose the neural elements to a high concentration of local anesthetic as well as a retrograde spread toward the subarachnoidal space.[38]

SUMMARY

This chapter outlined the anatomical characteristics of the neuraxial meninges and related structures and discussed their potential clinical implications.

REFERENCES

1. Reina MA, López A, De Andrés JA: Variation of human dura mater thickness [in Spanish]. Rev Esp Anestesiol Reanim 1999;46:344–349.
2. Reina MA, Pulido P, López A: El saco dural humano. Rev Arg Anestesiol 2007; 65:167–184.
3. Reina MA, López A, Dittmann M, De Andrés JA: Structure of human dura mater thickness by scanning electron microscopy [in Spanish]. Rev Esp Anestesiol Reanim 1996;43:135–137.
4. Reina MA, Dittmann M, López A, van Zundert A: New perspectives in the microscopic structure of human dura mater in the dorso lumbar region. Reg Anesth 1997;22:161–166.
5. Dittmann M, Reina MA, López A: Neue ergebnisse bei der darstellung der dura mater spinalis mittles rasterelektronenmikroskopie. Anaesthesist 1998;47:409–413.

6. Reina MA, López A, Dittmann M, De Andrés JA: External and internal surface of human dura mater by scanning electron microscopy [in Spanish]. Rev Esp Anestesiol Reanim 1996;43:130–134.

7. Reina MA, Villanueva MC, López A: Aracnoides trabecular, piamadre espinal humana y anestesia subaracnoidea. Rev Arg Anestesiol 2008;66:111–133.

8. Reina MA, De León Casasola OA, López A, De Andrés JA, Mora M, Fernández A: The origin of the spinal subdural space. Ultrastructure finding. Anesth Analg 2002;94:991–995.

9. Reina MA, López A, De Andrés JA, Villanueva MC, Cortés L: ¿Subdural space exists? [in Spanish]. Rev Esp Anestesiol Reanim 1998;45:367–376.

10. Reina MA, De León Casasola OA, López A, De Andrés JA, Martín S, Mora M: An in vitro study of dural lesions produced by 25 gauge Quincke and Whitacre needles evaluated by scanning electron microscopy. Reg Anesth Pain Med 2000;25:393–402.

11. Reina MA, López A, Badorrey V, De Andrés JA, Martín S: Dura-arachnoids lesions produced by 22G Quincke spinal needles during a lumbar puncture. J Neurol Neurosurg Psychiatry 2004;75:893–897.

12. Reina MA, López-García A, de Andrés-Ibáñez JA, et al: Electron microscopy of the lesions produced in the human dura mater by Quincke beveled and Whitacre needles [in Spanish]. Rev Esp Anestesiol Reanim 1997;44:56–61.

13. Jokinen MJ, Pitkänen MT, Lehtonen E: Deformed spinal needle tips and associated dural perforations examined by scanning electrón microscopy. Acta Anaesthesiol Scand 1996;40:687–690.

14. Puolakka R, Andersson LC, Rosenberg PH: Microscopic analysis of three different spinal needle tips after experimental subarachnoid puncture. Reg Anesth Pain Med 2000;25:163–169.

15. Benham M: Spinal needle damage during routine clinical practice. Anaesthesia 1996;51:843–845.

16. Reina MA, López A, Manzarbeitia F, Amador V, Goxencia I, Olmedilla MC: Skin fragments carried by spinal needles in cadavers [in Spanish]. Rev Esp Anestesiol Reanim 1995;42:383–385.

17. Reina MA, López-García A, Dittmann M, de Andrés JA, Blázquez MG: Iatrogenic spinal epidermoid tumors. A late complication of spinal puncture [in Spanish]. Rev Esp Anestesiol Reanim 1996;43:142–146.

18. Reina MA, Wikinski J, De Andrés JA: Una rara complicación de la anestesia epidural y subaracnoidea. Tumores epidermoideos espinales iatrogénicos. Rev Arg Anestesiol 2008; 66:319–336.

19. Reina MA, Castedo J, López A: Cefalea pospunción dural: Ultraestructura de las lesiones durales y agujas espinales usadas en las punciones lumbares. Rev Arg Anestesiol 2008;66:6–26.

20. Reina MA, López A, De Andrés JA: Hypothesis on the anatomical bases of cauda equine syndrome and transitory radicular irritation syndrome post spinal anesthesia [in Spanish]. Rev Esp Anestesiol Reanim 1999;46:99–105.

21. Reina MA, Machés F, López A, De Andrés JA: The ultrastructure of the spinal arachnoid in humans and its impact on spinal anesthesia, cauda equina syndrome and transient neurological síndrome. Tech Reg Anesth Pain Management 2008;12:153–160.

22. Reina MA, De Leon Casasola O, Villanueva MC, López A, Maches F, De Andrés JA: Ultrastructural findings in human spinal pia mater in relation to subarachnoid anesthesia. Anesth Analg 2004;98:1479–1485.

23. Reina MA, López García A, de Andrés JA: Anatomical description of a natural perforation present in the human lumbar pia mater [in Spanish]. Rev Esp Anestesiol Reanim 1998;45:4–7.

24. Luyendijk W: The plica mediana dorsalis of the dura mater and its relation to lumbar peridurography. Neuroradiology 1976;11:147–149.

25. Blomberg R: The dorsomedian connective tissue band in the lumbar epidural space of humans: An anatomical study using epiduroscopy in autopsy cases. Anesth Analg 1986;65:747–752.

26. Reina MA, Pulido P, Castedo J, Villanueva MC, López A, De Sola R: Characteristics and distribution of the epidural fat [in Spanish]. Rev Esp Anestesiol Reanim 2006;53: 315–324.

27. Reina MA, Pulido P, Castedo J, Villanueva MC, López A, De Andrés JA: The epidural fat in different diseases. Contributions of magnetic resonance imaging and possible implications in the epidural and spinal anesthesia [in Spanish]. Rev Esp Anestesiol Reanim 2007;54:173–178.

28. Reina MA, López A, Benito-Leon J, Pulido P, María F: Intracraneal and spinal hematoma, a rare complication of epidural and spinal anesthesia [in Spanish]. Rev Esp Anestesiol Reanim 2004;51:28–39.

29. Reina MA, López A, Maches F, De Andrés JA: Origin of spinal subdural hematoma [in Spanish]. Rev Esp Anestesiol Reanim 2004;51:240–246.

30. Reina MA, Villanueva MC, Machés F, Carrera A, López A, De Andrés JA: Ultrastructure of human spinal nerve root cuff in lumbar spine. Anesth Analg 2008;106:339–344.

31. Reina MA, De Andrés J, Machés F, López A: New insights of human spinal root cuffs. In van Zundert A: *Highlights in Pain, Therapy and Regional Anaesthesia*, 16th ed. Permanyer, 2007, pp 163–173.

32. Reina MA, Villanueva MC, López A, De Andrés JA: Fat inside the dural sheath of lumbar nerve roots in human [in Spanish]. Rev Esp Anestesiol Reanim 2007;54:169–172.

33. Reina MA, López A, De Andrés JA: Adipose tissue within peripheral nerves. Study of the human sciatic nerve [in Spanish]. Rev Esp Anestesiol Reanim 2002;49:397–402.

34. Reina MA, Machés F, Pulido P, López A, De Andrés JA: Ultrastructure of human spinal meninges. In Aldrete A: *Arachnoiditis*. Alfil Ed, 2010, pp 29–246.

35. Reina MA. *Atlas of Functional Anatomy for Regional Anesthesia and Pain Medicine. Human Structure, Ultrastructure and 3D Reconstruction Images.* Springer, 2015, pp 705–748.

36. Reina MA, De Andrés JA, López A: Subarachnoid and epidural anesthesia. In Raj P: *Textbook of Regional Anesthesia.* Churchill Livingston, 2002, pp 307–324.

37. Reina MA, De Andrés JA, López García A: Anatomy in spinal blockade [in Spanish]. In Torres LM (ed). *Textbook of Anesthesia and Pain Management.* Aran Ed, 2001, pp 1135–1155.

38. Selander D, Sjöstrand J: Longitudinal spread of intraneurally injected local anesthetics. An experimental study of the initial neural distribution following intraneural injections. Acta Anaesthesiol Scand 1978;22:622–634.

Clinical Pearls

- The shape of the dural sac is cylindrical, and its thickness is variable.
- The dura mater is permeable and occupies 90% of the thickness of the dural sac.
- The arachnoid layer is semipermeable and governs the passage of substances.
- Dura-arachnoid lesions can differ depending on the type of spinal needle.
- Pencil-point needles produce a more destructive lesion, while cutting needles produce a U-shaped lesion, although the sizes of both are similar.
- The trabecular arachnoid covers the nerve roots and forms arachnoid sheaths.
- Pia mater has fenestrations at the level of the medullary cone.
- Epidural fat distribution is variable along the spinal canal but is consistent at different vertebral levels.
- Epidural fat volume is increased in epidural lipomatosis, distributed asymmetrically in kyphoscoliosis, and absent in stenosis.
- The "subdural space" is in fact occupied by delicate tissue composed of specialized neurothelial cells. The tearing of the subdural compartment gives origin to what we know as the subdural space.
- In root cuffs, there is a cellular component that governs the diffusion of substances. Root cuffs also contain large numbers of adipocytes in their thickness.

CHAPTER 7

Clinical Pharmacology of Local Anesthetics

John Butterworth IV

INTRODUCTION

Local and regional anesthesia and analgesia appear to be undergoing a renaissance, as judged by attendance at specialty meetings and substantial increase in research activity, as evidenced by growing number of scientific publications. In contrast to general anesthesia, in which the molecular mechanism remains the subject of speculation, the site at which local anesthetic (LA) drugs bind to produce nerve blocks has been cloned and mutated. This chapter focuses on mechanisms of anesthesia and toxicity, especially as knowledge of these mechanisms will assist the clinician in conducting safer and more effective regional anesthesia.

PREHISTORY AND HISTORY

The Incas regarded coca as a gift from the son of the sun God and limited its use to the "upper crust" of society.[1] They recognized and used the medicinal properties of cocaine long before the compound was brought to Europe for its properties to be "discovered." The Incas sometimes treated persistent headaches with trepanation, and coca was occasionally used to facilitate this procedure. Local anesthesia was accomplished by having the operator chew coca leaves and apply the macerated pulp to the skin and wound edges while using a tumi knife to bore through the bone.

By the sixteenth century, having disrupted Incan society, the conquistadors began paying laborers with cocaine paste. The laborers generally rolled the cocaine leaves into balls (called cocadas), bound together by guano or cornstarch.[1,2] These cocadas released the free-base cocaine as a consequence of the alkalinity of the guano and of the practice of chewing the cocadas with ash or lime (such alkaline compounds increase pH, favoring the free-base cocaine form over the positively charged hydrochloride salt). This practice probably marks the birth of "free-basing" cocaine and is the historic antecedent of the "rock" or "crack" cocaine so often abused in Western societies.

Cocaine was brought back to Vienna by an explorer/physician named Scherzer.[1] In Vienna, the chemist Albert Niemann isolated and crystallized pure cocaine hydrochloride in 1860. The Merck Company distributed batches of this agent to physicians for investigational purposes. Sigmund Freud was the most prominent of these cocaine experimenters. Freud reviewed his experimental work in a monograph devoted to cocaine, *Über Coca*. Freud and Carl Koller (an ophthalmology trainee) took cocaine orally and noticed that the drug rendered their tongues insensible.

Koller and Joseph Gartner began a series of experiments using cocaine to produce topical anesthesia of the conjunctiva. The birth of local and regional anesthesia dates from 1884, when Koller and Gartner reported their success at producing topical cocaine anesthesia of the eye in the frog, rabbit, dog, and human.[2-4]

The use of local anesthesia quickly spread around the world. The American surgeon William Halsted at Roosevelt Hospital in New York reported using cocaine to produce mandibular nerve block in 1884 and to produce brachial plexus block less than a year later.[5] These blocks were accomplished by surgically exposing the nerves, then injecting them under direct vision. Leonard Corning injected cocaine near the spine of dogs, producing what was likely the first epidural in 1885. Spinal

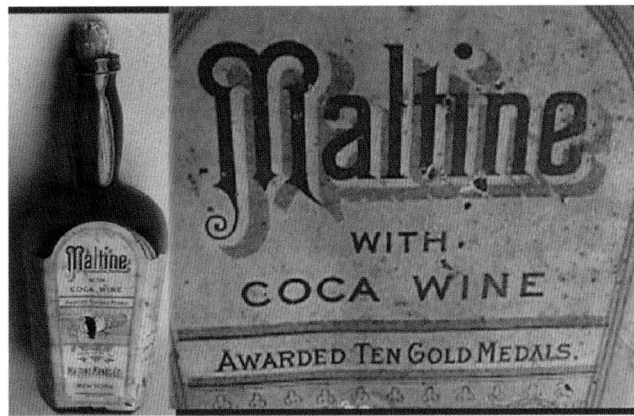

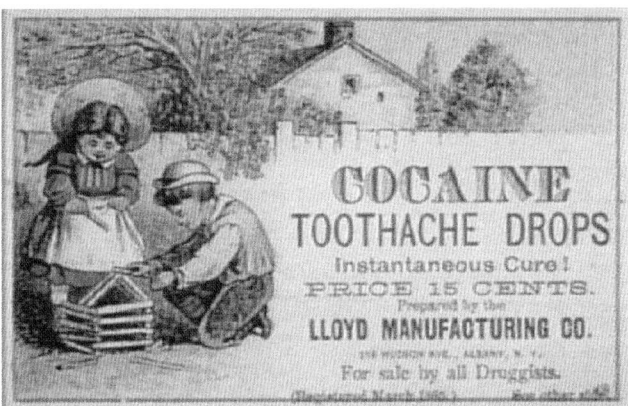

FIGURE 7–1. Examples of products that incorporated cocaine during the time before it became a controlled substance. Wines fortified with cocaine were particularly popular as "tonics." (Used with permission from Addiction Research Unit, University of Buffalo.)

Drug Brand name	Chemical structure	Class
Cocaine		Ester
Procaine Novocaine		Ester
Benzocaine		Ester
Tetracaine Pentocaine		Ester
2-Cloroprocaine Nescaine		Ester
Lidocaine Xylocaine		Amide
Prilocaine Citanest		Amide
Etidocaine Duranest		Amide
Mepivacaine Carbocaine		Amide
Ropivacaine Naropin		Amide
Bupivacaine Marcaine/Sensorcaine/ Levobupivacaine/ Chirocaine		Amide

FIGURE 7–2. Structures of commonly used local anesthetics.

anesthesia with cocaine was first accomplished in 1898 by August Bier. Cocaine spinal anesthesia was used to treat cancer pain in 1898. Caudal epidural anesthesia was introduced in 1902 by Sicard and Cathelin.[5] Bier described intravenous regional anesthesia in 1909. In 1911, Hirschel reported the first three percutaneous brachial plexus anesthesias. Fidel Pages reported using epidural anesthesia for abdominal surgery in 1921.

Cocaine was soon incorporated into many other products, including the original formulation of Coca-Cola devised by Pemberton in 1886. Wine tonics and other "patent" medicines of the day commonly contained cocaine (Figure 7–1). This practice ended when cocaine became regulated by the forerunner of the Food and Drug Administration (FDA) in the early 1900s.

MEDICINAL CHEMISTRY

Cocaine and all other LAs contain an aromatic ring and an amine at opposite ends of the molecule, separated by a hydrocarbon chain, and either an ester or an amide bond (Figure 7–2).[3,4,6,7] Cocaine, the archetypical ester, is the only naturally occurring LA. Procaine, the first synthetic ester LA,

was introduced in 1904 by Einhorn.[2] The introduction of the amide LA lidocaine in 1948 was transformative. Lidocaine quickly became used for all forms of regional anesthesia. Other amide LAs based on the lidocaine structure (prilocaine, etidocaine) subsequently appeared. A related series of amide LAs based on 2',6'-pipecoloxylidide was introduced (mepivacaine, bupivacaine, ropivacaine, and levobupivacaine). Ropivacaine and levobupivacaine are the only commercially available single-enantiomer (single-optical-isomer) LAs. Both are S(–)-enantiomers, avoiding the increased cardiac toxicity associated with racemic mixtures and the R(+)-isomers (this is discussed in a subsequent section). All other LAs either exist as racemates or have no asymmetric carbons.

Clinical Pearl

- All LAs contain an aromatic ring and an amine at opposite ends of the molecule, separated by a hydrocarbon chain, and either an ester or an amide bond.

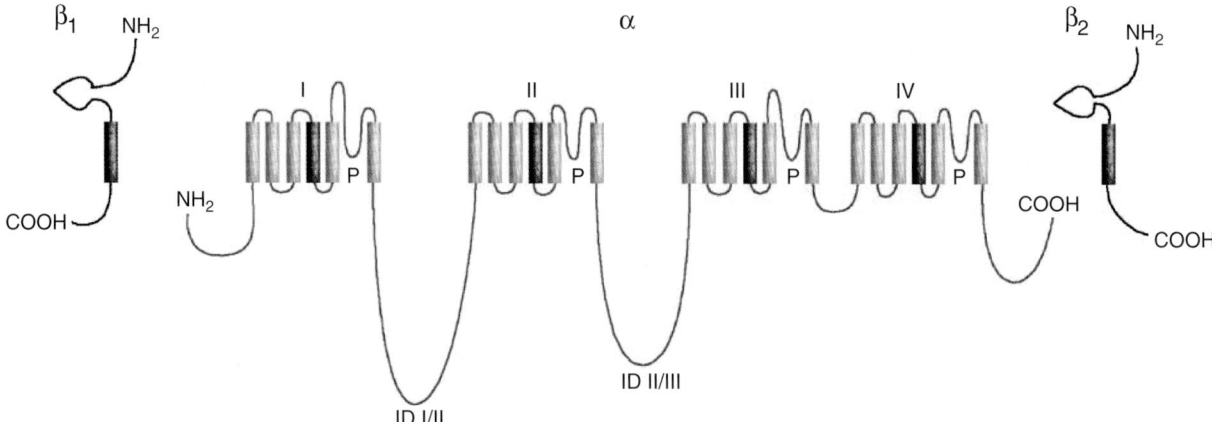

FIGURE 7–3. "Cartoon" structure of Na channel subunits. Note that the α-subunit has four domains that each contain six membrane-spanning segments. (Reproduced with permission from Plummer NW, Meisler MH: Evolution and diversity of mammalian sodium channel genes. *Genomics*. 1999 Apr 15;57(2):323-331.)

BIOPHYSICS OF VOLTAGE-GATED SODIUM CHANNELS AND LOCAL ANESTHETICS

Studies of the mechanisms of LA action on peripheral nerves are studies of interactions between LAs and voltage-gated Na channels because Na channels contain the LA-binding site. Na channels are integral membrane proteins that initiate and propagate action potentials in axons, dendrites, and muscle tissue; initiate and maintain membrane potential oscillations in specialized heart and brain cells; and shape and filter synaptic inputs.[8,9] Na channels share structural features with other similar voltage-gated ion channels that exist as tetramers, each with

six transmembrane helical segments (eg, voltage-gated Ca and K channels). Na channels contain one larger α-subunit and one or two smaller β-subunits, depending on the species and the tissue of origin. The α-subunit, the site of ion conduction and LA binding, has four homologous domains, each with six α-helical membrane-spanning segments (Figure 7–3).[8,9] The external surface of the α-subunit is heavily glycosylated, which serves to orient the channel properly within the plasma membrane (Figure 7–4).

Invertebrates have only one or two Na channel α-subunit genes, and the normal physiologic role of these channels is unclear (animals survive when the channels are not present).

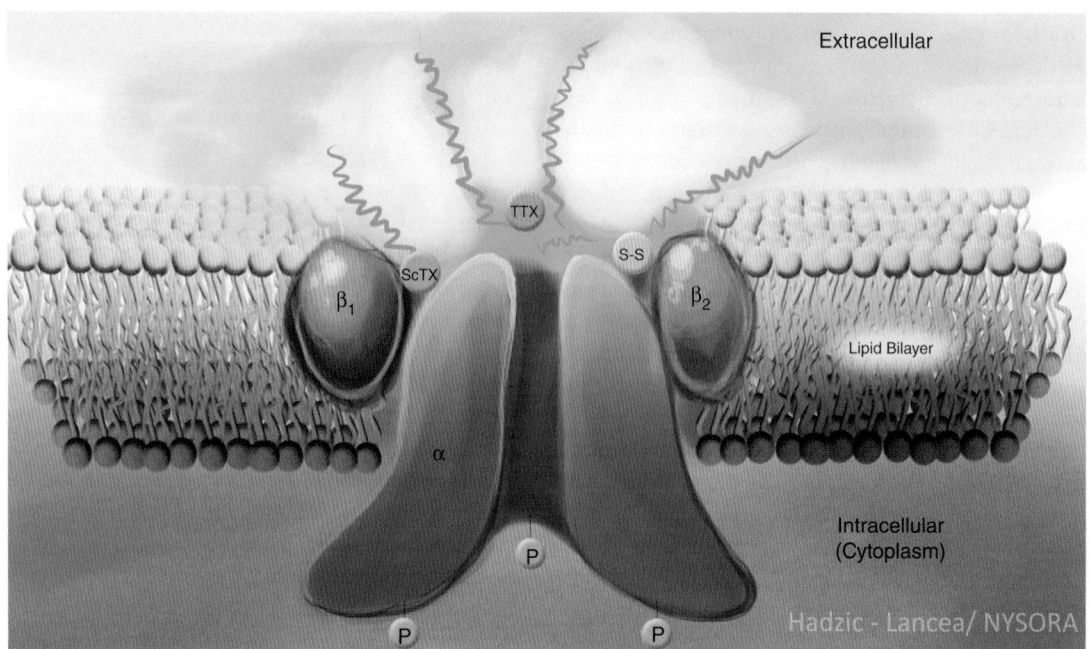

FIGURE 7–4. Cartoon of a Na channel in the plasma membrane. Note that all three subunits are heavily glycosylated on the extracellular side (see "squiggly" lines). In contrast to local anesthetics, note that both scorpion toxins (ScTX) and tetrodotoxin (TTX) have binding sites on the external surface of the channel. Note also that the cytoplasmic side of the channel is phosphorylated. (Reproduced with permission from Catterall WA: Cellular and molecular biology of voltage-gated sodium channels. *Physiol Rev.* 1992 Oct;72(4 Suppl):S15-S48.)

TABLE 7–1. Voltage-gated Na channel—neural isoforms.

	Na$_v$1.1	Na$_v$1.2	Na$_v$1.3	Na$_v$1.6	Na$_v$1.7	Na$_v$1.8	Na$_v$1.9
Chromosome	2	2	2	12	2	3	3
Where identified	CNS, DRG	CNS	CNS upregulated, after injury	DRG (large and small), CNS, Ranvier	DRG (large and small)	DRG (small)	DRG (small)
Inactivation	Fast	Fast	Fast	Fast	Fast	Slow	Slow
TTX	Sensitive	Sensitive	Sensitive	Sensitive	Sensitive	Insensitive	Insensitive

CNS = central nervous system; DRG = dorsal root gamglion; TTX = tetrodotoxin.

Source: Adapted with permission from Novakovic SD, Eglen RM, Hunter JC: Regulation of Na+ channel distribution in the nervous system. *Trends Neurosci.* 2001 Aug;24(8):473-478.

Humans, in contrast, have nine active Na channel α-subunit genes on four chromosomes, with cell-specific expression and localization of gene products.[10] The Na$_v$1.4 gene (by convention, geneticists refer to voltage-gated Na channel isoforms as Na$_v$1.x) supplies channels to skeletal muscle, and the Na$_v$1.5 gene supplies channels to cardiac muscle, leaving seven Na$_v$ isoforms in neural tissue (Table 7–1). Defined genes contribute specific Na channel forms to each of the unmyelinated axons, nodes of Ranvier in motor axons, and small dorsal root ganglion nociceptors.[10] Whereas all Na channel α-subunits will bind LAs similarly, their affinity for binding neurotoxins varies.

Na channel α- and β-subunit mutations lead to muscle, cardiac, and neural diseases.[11] For example, inherited mutations in Na$_v$1.5 have been associated with congenital long QT syndrome, Bruguda syndrome, and other conduction system diseases.[11] It has been shown that certain Na$_v$ isoforms proliferate in animal models of chronic pain. The existence of specific Na$_v$ gene α-subunit products offers the enticing possibility that inhibitors may someday be developed for each specific Na$_v$ α-subunit form. Such developments, already underway for some Na$_v$ isoforms, could revolutionize the treatment of chronic pain.

Blocking of impulses in a nerve fiber requires that a defined length of nerve become inexcitable (to prevent the impulse from "jumping over" the blocked segment). Thus, as the LA concentration increases, it must be applied along a shorter length of nerve to prevent impulse conduction, as is shown in Figure 7–5. Both normal conduction and the way in which LAs inhibit conduction differ between myelinated and unmyelinated nerve fibers. Conduction in myelinated fibers proceeds in jumps from one Ranvier node to the next, a process termed *saltatory conduction*. To block impulses in myelinated nerve fibers, it is generally necessary for LAs to inhibit channels in three successive Ranvier nodes (Figure 7–6). Unmyelinated fibers, lacking the saltatory mechanism, conduct much more slowly than myelinated fibers. Unmyelinated fibers are relatively resistant to LAs, despite their smaller diameter, due to dispersal of Na channels throughout their plasma membranes. These differences among nerve fibers arise during development when Na channels begin to cluster at Ranvier nodes in

myelinated axons. Nodal clustering of channels, essential for high-speed signal transmission, is initiated by Schwann cells in the peripheral nervous system and by oligodendrocytes in the central nervous system (CNS).[12]

Na channels may exist in at least three native conformations: "resting," "open," and "inactivated," first described by Hodgkin and Huxley.[13] During an action potential, neuronal Na channels open briefly, allowing extracellular Na ions to flow into the cell, depolarizing the plasma membrane. After only a few milliseconds, Na channels inactivate (whereupon the Na current ceases). Na channels return to the resting conformation with membrane repolarization. The process by which channels go from conducting to nonconducting forms is termed *gating*. Gating is assumed to result from movements of dipoles in response to changes in potential. The process by which voltage-gated channels operate likely involves movements of paddle-shaped voltage sensors within the channel's outer perimeter (Figure 7–7).[14,15] The speed of gating processes differs among

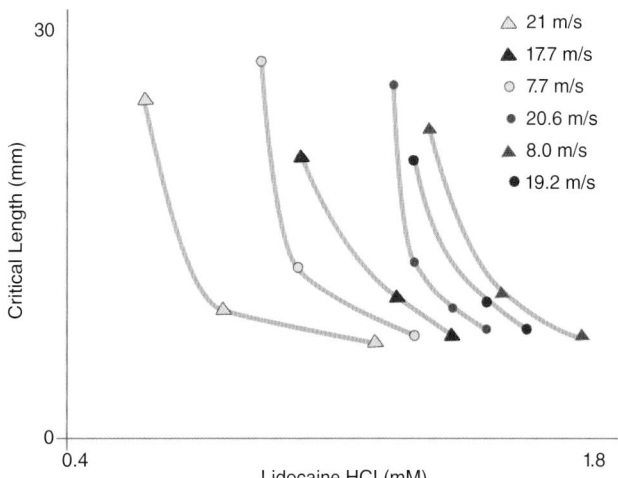

FIGURE 7–5. Note that the concentration of local anesthetic required to produce nerve block declines as the length of nerve exposed to the local anesthetic increases. (Reproduced with permission from Raymond SA, Steffensen SC, Gugino LD, et al: The role of length of nerve exposed to local anesthetics in impulse blocking action. *Anesth Analg.* 1989 May;68(5):563-570.)

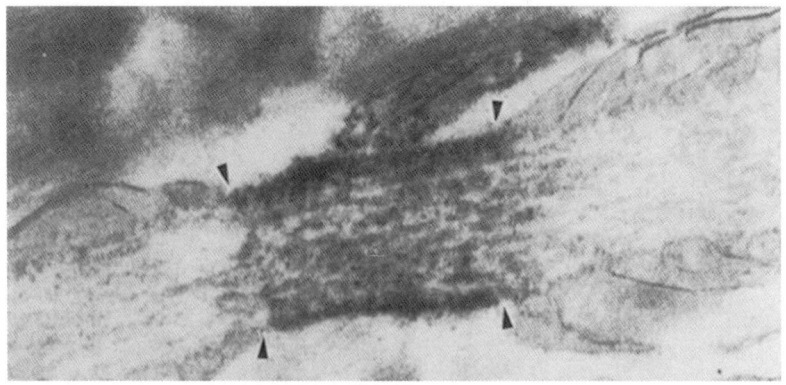

FIGURE 7–6. Electron micrograph of a node of Ranvier. Na channels have been immunolabeled and appear as dense granules within the four arrows. The paranodal region is indicated by "pn," and an astrocyte is indicated by "as." (Reproduced with permission from from Black JA, Friedman B, Waxman SG, et al: Immunoultrastructural localization of sodium channels at nodes of Ranvier and perinodal astro-cytes in rat optic nerve. *Proc R Soc Lond B Biol Sci.* 1989 Oct 23;238(1290):39-51.)

Na$_v$ α-subunit forms: Skeletal muscle and nerve forms gate quicker than cardiac forms.

Anesthesia results when LAs bind Na channels and inhibit the Na permeability that underlies action potentials.[6,8,9,13] Our understanding of LA mechanisms has been refined by several key observations. Taylor confirmed that LAs selectively inhibit Na channels in nerves.[16] Strichartz first observed use-dependent block with LAs, showing the importance of channel opening for LA binding.[17] *Use* (or *frequency*) *dependence* describes how LA inhibition of Na currents increases with repetitive depolarizations ("use").[13,17] Repetitive trains of depolarizations increase the likelihood that an LA will encounter an Na channel that is open or inactivated, with both forms having greater LA affinity than

do resting channels (Figure 7–8).[6,13,17] Thus, membrane potential influences both Na channel conformation and Na channel affinity for LAs. Use-dependent block appears important for the functioning of LAs as antiarrhythmics and may also underlie the effectiveness of reduced LA concentrations in managing pain.[6,8] Finally, using site-directed mutagenesis, Ragsdale and Wang[18,19] localized LA binding to specific amino acids in D4S6 of Na$_v$ 1.2 and Na$_v$ 1.4.

Some LA optical isomers confer greater apparent safety than their opposite enantiomer. For example, under voltage clamp, the R(+)-bupivacaine isomer more potently inhibits cardiac Na currents than the S(–)-bupivacaine (levobupivacaine) isomer (Figure 7–9).

Conventional Model

Paddle Model

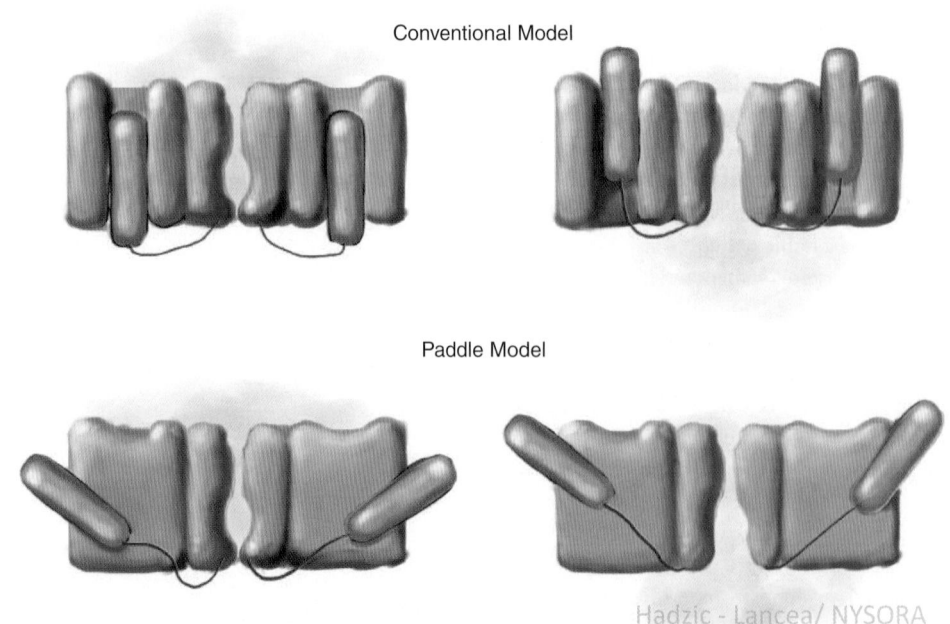

Hadzic - Lancea/ NYSORA

FIGURE 7–7. In the conventional model for voltage gating, the voltage-sensing part of the channel slides "in and out" of the membrane. More recent x-ray diffraction studies of the K channel suggest that a more appropriate mechanism is that of paddle-like structures sliding diagonally through the plasma membrane. (Reproduced with permission from Arhem P: Voltage sensing in ion channels: a 50-year-old mystery resolved? *Lancet.* 2004 Apr 10;363(9416):1221-1223.)

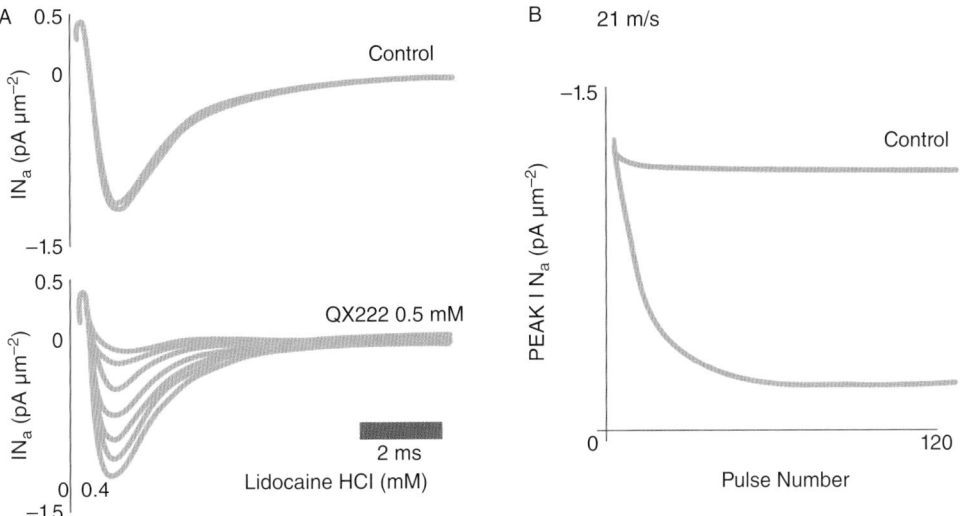

FIGURE 7-8. Use-dependent block of Na currents in Purkinje fibers. Under control conditions, each of a train of impulses results in identical current tracings. In the presence of the local anesthetic QX222, the first impulse is nearly the same size amplitude as under control conditions. Each succeeding impulse is smaller (reduced peak I_{Na}), reflecting an accumulating block of Na channels, until a nadir is reached. (Reproduced with permission from Hanck DA, Makielski JC, Sheets MF: Kinetic effects of quaternary lidocaine block of cardiac sodium channels: a gating current study. *J Gen Physiol.* 1994 Jan;103(1):19-43.)

Many other types of chemicals will also bind and inhibit Na channels, including general anesthetics, substance P inhibitors, α_2-adrenergic agonists, tricyclic antidepressants, and nerve toxins.[6,20-22] Nerve toxins are currently undergoing animal and human testing as possible replacements for LAs.

LOCAL ANESTHETIC PHARMACODYNAMICS

In clinical practice, LAs are typically described by their potency, duration of action, speed of onset, and tendency for differential sensory nerve block. These properties do not sort independently.

Potency and Duration

Nerve-blocking potency of LAs increases with increasing molecular weight and increasing lipid solubility.[23,24] Larger, more lipophilic LAs permeate nerve membranes more readily and bind Na channels with greater affinity. For example, etidocaine and bupivacaine have greater lipid solubility and potency than lidocaine and mepivacaine, to which they are closely related chemically.

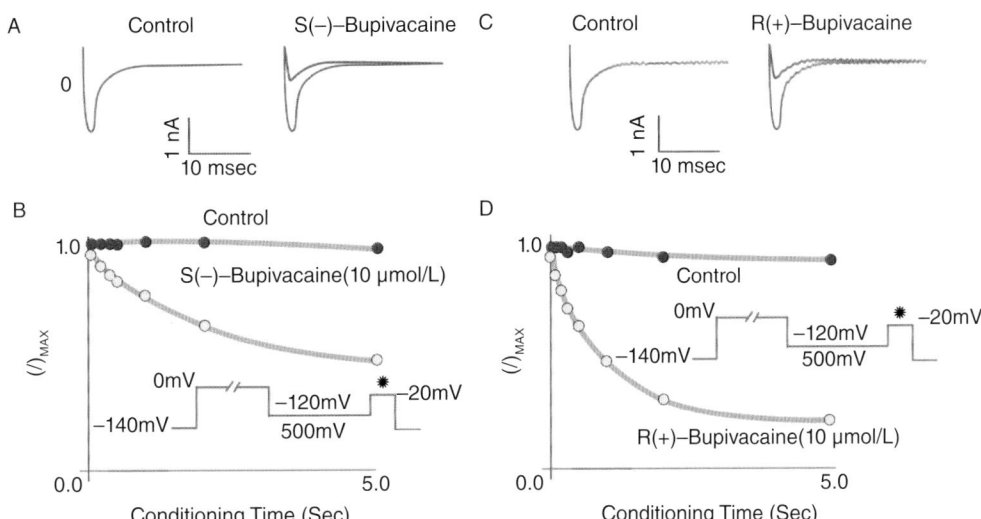

FIGURE 7-9. Reduced potency of *S*(−) bupivacaine relative to *R*(+)-bupivacaine at inhibiting cardiac Na currents under voltage clamp. After a standard "conditioning" depolarization of varying lengths, the *S*(−) isomer produces less reduction of VI_{max} than the *R*(+) isomer. (Reproduced with permission from Valenzuela C, Snyders DJ, Bennett PB, et al: Stereoselective block of cardiac sodium channels by bupivacaine in guinea pig ventricular myocytes. *Circulation.* 1995 Nov 15;92(10):3014-3024.)

Clinical Pearl

- Nerve-blocking potency of LAs increases with increasing molecular weight and increasing lipid solubility.

More lipid-soluble LAs are relatively water insoluble, highly protein bound in blood, less readily removed by the bloodstream from nerve membranes, and more slowly "washed out" from isolated nerves in vitro. Thus, increased lipid solubility is associated with increased protein binding in blood, increased potency, and longer duration of action. Extent and duration of anesthesia can be correlated with LA content of nerves in animal experiments.[25,26] In animals, blocks of greater depth and longer duration arise from smaller volumes of more concentrated LA, compared with larger volumes of less-concentrated LA.[27]

Speed of Onset

Many textbooks and review articles assert that the onset of anesthesia in isolated nerves slows with increasing LA lipid solubility and increasing pK_a (Table 7–2). At any pH, the percentage of LA molecules present in the uncharged form, largely responsible for membrane permeability, decreases with increasing pK_a.[23,24] However, of the two LAs with the fastest onset, etidocaine is highly lipid soluble and chloroprocaine has a pK_a greater than that of other LAs. Finally, the LA rate of onset is associated with the aqueous diffusion rate, which declines with increasing molecular weight.[28]

Differential Sensory Nerve Block

Regional anesthesia and pain management would be transformed by a LA that would selectively inhibit pain transmission while leaving other functions intact. However, sensory anesthesia sufficient for skin incision usually cannot be obtained without motor impairment.[3,4,6] As was first demonstrated by Gasser and Erlanger in 1929, all LAs will block smaller (diameter) fibers at lower concentrations than are required to block larger fibers of the same type.[29,30] As a group, unmyelinated fibers are resistant to LAs compared with larger myelinated A-δ fibers.[29,30] Bupivacaine and ropivacaine are relatively selective for sensory fibers. Bupivacaine produces

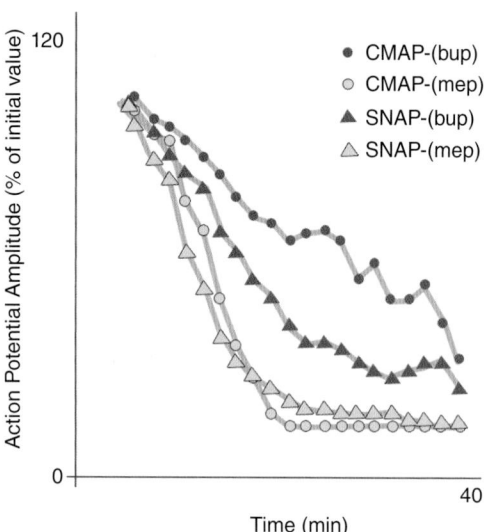

FIGURE 7–10. Differential onset of median nerve block with bupivacaine 0.3% (bup), but not with mepivacaine 1% (mep). Note that the compound motor action potential (CMAP) is inhibited less than the sensory nerve action potential (SNAP) during onset of bupivacaine block in these normal volunteer subjects. At steady state (20 min), CMAP and SNAP are comparably inhibited. On the other hand, mepivacaine produced faster inhibition of both CMAP and SNAP, and there was no differential onset of block. (Reproduced with permission from Butterworth J, Ririe DG, Thompson RB, et al: Differential onset of median nerve block: randomized, double-blind comparison of mepivacaine and bupivacaine in healthy volunteers. *Br J Anaesth.* 1998 Oct;81(4):515-521.)

more rapid onset of sensory than motor block, whereas the closely related chemical mepivacaine demonstrates no differential onset during median nerve blocks (Figure 7–10).[31] True differential anesthesia may be possible when Na_v isoform-selective antagonists become available. Certain Na_v isoforms have been found to be prevalent in dorsal root ganglia, and (as previously noted) the relative populations of various Na_v isoforms can change in response to various pain states.

Other Factors Influencing Local Anesthetic Activity

Many factors influence the ability of a given LA to produce adequate regional anesthesia, including the dose, site of administration, additives, temperature, and pregnancy. As the LA dose increases, the likelihood of success and the duration of anesthesia increase, while the delay of onset and tendency for differential block decrease. In general, the fastest onset and shortest duration of anesthesia occur with spinal or subcutaneous injections; a slower onset and longer duration are obtained with plexus blocks.[33]

Clinical Pearl

- The effectiveness of a given LA is influenced by the dose, site of administration, additives, temperature, and changes in neural susceptibility, as seen during pregnancy.

TABLE 7–2. Local anesthetic characteristics that tend to sort together.

Physical and Chemical
   Increasing lipid solubility
   Increased protein binding

Pharmacologic and Toxicologic
   Increasing potency
   Increasing onset time
   Increasing duration of action
   Increasing tendency for severe systemic toxicity
   In general, all tend to sort together

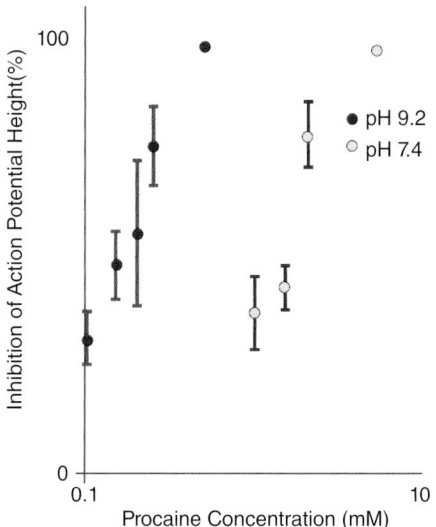

FIGURE 7–11. The potency of procaine at inhibiting compound action potentials in isolated frog sciatic nerves is dramatically increased at pH 9.2 as compared with pH 7.4. (Reproduced with permission from Butterworth JF, Lief PA, Strichartz GR: The pH-dependent local anesthetic activity of diethylaminoethanol, a procaine metabolite. *Anesthesiology.* 1988 Apr;68(4):501-506.)

Epinephrine is frequently added to LA solutions to cause vasoconstriction and to serve as a marker for intravascular injection.[4,7] Epinephrine and other α_1-agonists increase LA duration largely by prolonging and increasing intraneural concentrations of LAs. Blood flow is decreased only briefly, and the block will persist long after the α_1-adrenergic effect on blood flow has dissipated. Other popular LA additions include clonidine, $NaHCO_3$, opioids, dexamethasone, and hyaluronidase.

Uncharged local anesthetics have greater apparent potency at basic pH, where an increased fraction of LA molecules is uncharged, than at more acidic pH (Figure 7–11).[35] Uncharged LA bases diffuse across nerve sheaths and membranes more readily than charged LAs, hastening onset of anesthesia. Some clinical studies showed that the addition of sodium bicarbonate had an inconsistent action during clinical nerve block; however, not all studies demonstrated a faster onset of anesthesia. One might anticipate that bicarbonate would have its greatest effect when added to LA solutions to which epinephrine was added by the manufacturer. Such solutions are more acidic than "plain" (epinephrine-free) LA solutions to increase shelf life. Bicarbonate shortens the duration of lidocaine in animals.[27] Curiously, once LAs gain access to the cytoplasmic side of the Na channel, H+ ions potentiate use-dependent block.[6,13] Marked prolongation of local anesthesia can be achieved by incorporating LAs into liposomes, as has been done with bupivacaine in the some formulation.

Clinical Pearl

- Pregnancy increases neural susceptibility to LAs.

Pregnant women and pregnant animals demonstrate increased neural susceptibility to LAs.[36–38] In addition, spread of neuraxial anesthesia likely increases during pregnancy due to decreases in thoracolumbar cerebrospinal fluid volume.

BLOOD CONCENTRATIONS AND PHARMACOKINETICS

Peak LA concentrations vary by the site of injection (Figure 7–12). With the same LA dose, intercostal blocks consistently produce greater peak LA concentrations than epidural or plexus blocks.[4,7,33,39] As has been recently discussed by others, it makes little sense to speak of "maximal" doses of LAs except in reference to a specific nerve block procedure, since peak blood levels vary widely by block site.[40]

In blood, all LAs are partially protein bound, primarily to α_1-acid glycoprotein and secondarily to albumin.[3,4,7] Affinity for α_1-acid glycoprotein correlates with LA hydrophobicity and decreases with protonation (acidity).[41] Extent of protein binding is influenced by the concentration of α_1-acid glycoprotein. Both protein binding and protein concentration decline during pregnancy.[42] During longer-term infusion of LA and LA-opioid combinations, concentrations of LA-binding proteins progressively increase.[43] There is considerable first-pass uptake of LAs by the lungs,[44] and animal studies suggest that patients with right-to-left cardiac shunting may be expected to demonstrate LA toxicity after smaller intravenous bolus doses.[45]

Clinical Pearls

- Recommendations on maximal doses of LAs commonly found in pharmacology texts are not terribly useful in the practice of clinical regional anesthesia.
- The serum concentrations of LAs depend on the injection technique, place of injection, and addition of additives to the LA.
- Any recommendation on the maximal safe LA dose can be valid only in reference to a specific nerve block procedure.

Esters undergo rapid hydrolysis in blood, catalyzed by nonspecific esterases.[3,4,7] Procaine and benzocaine are metabolized to para-aminobenzoic acid (PABA), the species underlying anaphylaxis to these agents.[4] Higher doses of benzocaine, typically for topical anesthesia for endoscopy, can lead to life threatening levels of methemoglobinemia. The amides undergo metabolism in the liver. Lidocaine undergoes oxidative N-dealkylation (by the cytochromes CYP 1A2 and CYP 3A4 to monoethyl glycine xylidide and glycine xylidide).[3,4,7] Bupivacaine, ropivacaine, mepivacaine, and etidocaine also undergo N-dealkylation and hydroxylation.[3,4,7] Prilocaine is hydrolyzed to *o*-toluidine, the agent that causes methemoglobinemia.[4,24] Prilocaine doses of as little as 400 mg in fit adults may be expected to produce methemoglobinemia concentrations great enough to cause clinical cyanosis. Amide LA clearance is highly dependent on hepatic blood flow, hepatic extraction, and enzyme function; therefore, amide LA clearance is reduced by factors that decrease hepatic blood flow, such as β-adrenergic

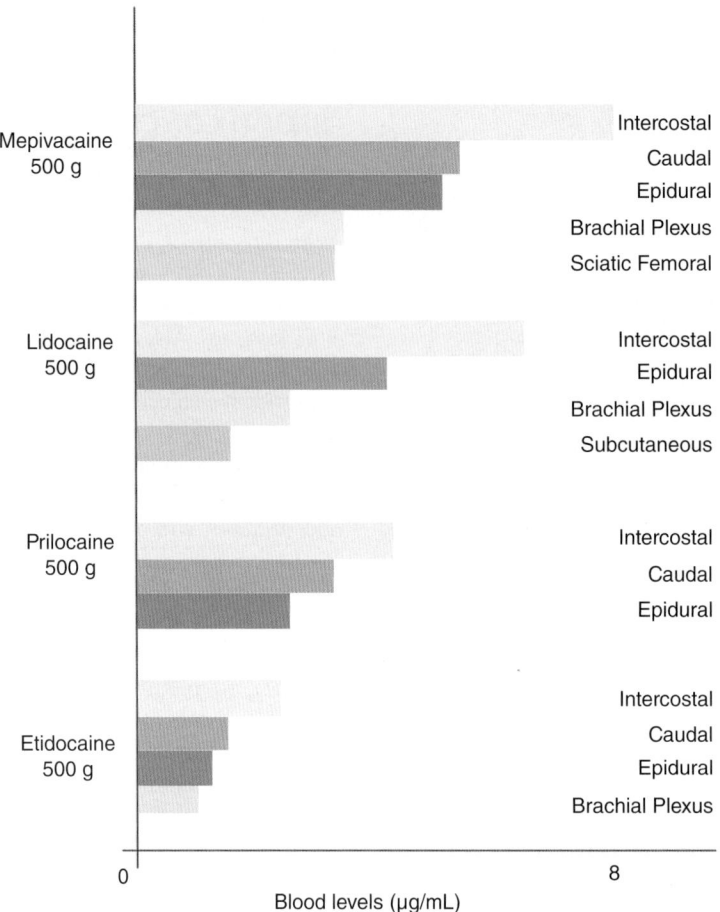

FIGURE 7–12. Peak blood concentrations of local anesthetics after various forms of regional anesthesia. Note that intercostal blocks consistently result in the greatest local anesthetic concentrations in blood, that plexus blocks result in the least local anesthetic concentrations in blood, and that epidural/caudal techniques are in between. (Reproduced with permission from Covino BG, Vassallo HG: *Local Anesthetics: Mechanisms of Action and Clinical Use.* Grune & Stratton; 1976.)

receptor or H_2-receptor blockers, and by heart or liver failure.[3,4,7]

Disposition of amide LAs is altered in pregnancy due to increased cardiac output, hepatic blood flow, and clearance, as well as the previously mentioned decline in protein binding. Renal failure tends to increase volume of distribution of amide LAs and to increase the accumulation of metabolic by-products of ester and amide LAs.

Theoretically, cholinesterase deficiency and cholinesterase inhibitors should increase the risk of systemic toxicity from ester LAs; however, there are no confirmatory clinical reports.

Some drugs inhibit various cytochromes responsible for LA metabolism; however, the importance of cytochrome inhibitors varies depending on the specific LA species. β-Blockers and H_2-receptor blockers inhibit CYP 2D6, which may contribute to reduced amide LA metabolism. Itraconazole has no effect on hepatic blood flow, but inhibits CYP 3A4 and bupivacaine elimination by 20%–25%.[46] Ropivacaine is hydroxylated by CYP 1A2 and metabolized to 2′,6′-pipecoloxylidide by CYP 3A4.[47,48] Fluvoxamine inhibition of CYP 1A2 reduces ropivacaine clearance by 70%. On the other hand, coadministration with strong inhibitors of CYP 3A4 (ketoconazole, itraconazole) has only a small effect on ropivacaine clearance.

DIRECT TOXIC SIDE EFFECTS

It is a common, but misguided, assumption that all LA actions, including toxic side effects, arise from interaction with voltage-gated Na channels. There is abundant evidence that LAs will bind many other targets aside from Na channels, including voltage-gated K and Ca channels, K_{ATP} channels, enzymes, *N*-methyl-D-aspartate receptors, β-adrenergic receptors, G-protein-mediated modulation of K and Ca channels, and nicotinic acetylcholine receptors.[6,49,50] LA binding to any one or all of these other sites could underlie LA production of spinal or epidural analgesia and could contribute to toxic side effects.[6,13,51]

Central Nervous System Side Effects

Local anesthetic CNS toxicity arises from selectively blocking the inhibition of excitatory pathways in the CNS, producing a stereotypical sequence of signs and symptoms as the LA concentration in blood gradually increases (Table 7–3).[3,4,7,33] With increased LA doses, seizures may arise in the amygdala.[3,4] With further LA dosing, CNS excitation progresses to CNS depression and eventual respiratory arrest. More potent (at nerve block) LAs produce seizures at lower blood concentrations and at lower doses than less-potent LAs. In animal studies, both

TABLE 7–3. Progression of signs and symptoms of toxicity as the local anesthetic dose (or concentration) gradually increases.

Vertigo

Tinnitus

Ominous feelings

Circumoral numbness

Garrulousness

Tremors

Myoclonic jerks

Convulsions

Coma

Cardiovascular collapse

metabolic and respiratory acidosis decreased the convulsive dose of lidocaine.[52]

Cardiovascular Toxicity

In laboratory experiments, most LAs will not produce cardiovascular (CV) toxicity until the blood concentration exceeds three times that necessary to produce seizures; however, there are clinical reports of simultaneous CNS and CV toxicity with bupivacaine (Table 7–4).[3,4,7] In dogs, supraconvulsant doses of bupivacaine more commonly produce arrhythmias than supraconvulsant doses of ropivacaine and lidocaine.[53] LAs produce CV signs of CNS excitation (increased heart rate, arterial blood pressure, and cardiac output) at lower concentrations than those associated with cardiac depression. Hypocapnia reduces ropivacaine-induced changes in ST segments and left ventricular contractility.[54]

Clinical Pearl

- In laboratory experiments, most LAs will not produce CV toxicity until the blood concentration exceeds three times that necessary to produce seizures.

TABLE 7–4. Convulsive versus lethal doses of local anesthetics in dogs.

	Lidocaine	Bupivacaine	Tetracaine
Dose producing convulsions in all animals (mg/kg)	22	5	4
Dose producing lethality in all animals (mg/kg)	76	20	27

Local anesthetics bind and inhibit cardiac Na channels (Na_v 1.5 isoform).[3,13] Bupivacaine binds more avidly and longer than lidocaine to cardiac Na channels.[55] As previously noted, certain R(+) optical isomers bind cardiac Na channels more avidly than S(–) optical isomers. These laboratory observations led to the clinical development of levobupivacaine and ropivacaine. Local anesthetics inhibit conduction in the heart with the same rank order of potency as for nerve block.[56,57]

Local anesthetics produce dose-dependent myocardial depression, possibly from interference with Ca signaling mechanisms within cardiac muscle.[56,58] These anesthetics bind and inhibit cardiac voltage-gated Ca and K channels at concentrations greater than those at which binding to Na channels is maximal.[6,13,58] The LAs bind β-adrenergic receptors and inhibit epinephrine-stimulated cyclic adenosine monophosphate (AMP) formation.[59,60] In rats, the rank order for cardiac toxicity appears to be bupivacaine > levobupivacaine > ropivacaine.[61–63] In dogs, lidocaine was the least potent, and bupivacaine and levobupivacaine were more potent than ropivacaine at inhibiting left ventricular function as assessed by echocardiography (Table 7–5). In dogs, both programmed electrical stimulation and epinephrine resuscitation elicited more arrhythmias after bupivacaine and levobupivacaine than after lidocaine or ropivacaine administration.[64–66]

The mechanism by which CV toxicity is produced may depend on which LA has been administered. When LAs were given to the point of extreme hypotension, dogs receiving lidocaine could be resuscitated but required continuing infusion of epinephrine to counteract LA-induced myocardial depression. Conversely, many dogs receiving bupivacaine or levobupivacaine to the point of extreme hypotension could not be resuscitated. After bupivacaine, levobupivacaine, or ropivacaine, dogs that could be defibrillated often required no additional therapy.[64–66] Similarly, in pigs, comparing lidocaine with bupivacaine, the ratio of potency for myocardial depression was 1:4, whereas it was 1:16 for arrhythmogenesis.[67] The LAs produce dilation of vascular smooth muscle at clinical concentrations.[68] Cocaine is the only LA that consistently produces local vasoconstriction.

Allergic Reactions

Clinical Pearls

- True immunologic reactions to LAs are rare.
- True anaphylaxis appears more common with ester LAs that are metabolized directly to PABA than other LAs.
- Accidental intravenous injections of LAs are sometimes misdiagnosed as allergic reactions.
- Some patients may react to preservatives, such as methylparaben, included with LAs.

True immunologic reactions to LAs are rare.[69] Accidental intravenous injections of LAs are sometimes misdiagnosed as allergic reactions. True anaphylaxis appears more common with ester LAs that are metabolized directly to PABA than to other

TABLE 7–5. Effects of local anesthetics on indices of myocardial function measured in dogs.

Local Anesthetic	LVEDP (EC$_{50}$ for 125% base) (mcg/mL)	dP/dt$_{max}$ (EC$_{50}$ for 65% base) (mcg/mL)	%FS (EC$_{50}$ for 65% base)(mcg/mL)
Bupivacaine	2.2 (1.2–4.4)	2.3 (1.7–3.1)	2.1 (1.47–3.08)
Levobupivacaine	1.7 (0.9–3.1)	2.4 (1.9–3.1)	1.3 (0.9–1.8)
Ropivacaine	4.0 (2.1–7.5)[a]	4.0 (3.1–5.2)[b]	3.0 (2.1–4.2)[a]
Lidocaine	6.8 (3.0–15.4)[c]	8.0 (5.7–11.0)[d]	5.5 (3.5–8.7)[d]

Note: Data provided are 50% effective concentrations (EC50s) and 95% confidence intervals.

[a]Ropivacaine > levobupivacaine, $p < .05$.

[b]Ropivacaine > bupivacaine, levobupivacaine, $p < .05$.

[c]Lidocaine > bupivacaine, levobupivacaine, $p < .01$.

[d]Lidocaine > bupivacaine, levobupivacaine, ropivacaine, $p < .01$.

EC$_{50}$, effective concentration for 50% of population; base, baseline; LVEDP = left ventricular end-diastolic pressure; dP/dt$_{max}$ = maximal rate of change of developed pressure (inotropy); %FS = percentage fractional shortening.

Source: Adapted with permission from Groban L, Dolinski SY: Differences in cardiac toxicity among ropivacaine, levobupivacaine, bupivacaine, and lidocaine. *Tech Reg Anesth Pain Manage.* 2001;April;5(2):48–55.

LAs. Some patients may react to preservatives, such as methyl-paraben, included with LAs. Several studies have shown that patients referred for evaluation of apparent LA allergy, even after exhibiting signs or symptoms of anaphylaxis, almost never demonstrate true allergy to the LA that was administered.[69,70] On the other hand, LA skin testing has an excellent negative predictive value. In other words, 97% of patients who fail to respond to LA skin testing will also not have an allergic reaction to the LA in a clinical setting.

Neurotoxic Effects

During the 1980s, 2-chloroprocaine (at that time formulated with sodium metabisulfite at a relatively acidic pH) occasionally produced cauda equina syndrome following accidental large-dose intrathecal injection during attempted epidural administration. Whether the "toxin" is 2-chloroprocaine or sodium metabisulfite remains unsettled: 2-chloroprocaine is now being tested as a substitute for lidocaine in human spinal anesthesia,[74] and a series of publications suggest that it may be safe and effective. At the same time, other investigators have linked neurotoxic reactions in animals to large doses of 2-chloroprocaine rather than to metabisulfite.[75] There is also controversy about transient neurologic symptoms and persistent sacral deficits after lidocaine spinal anesthesia. The reports and the controversy have persuaded many physicians to abandon lidocaine spinal anesthesia. Unlike other spinal LA solutions, lidocaine 5% permanently interrupts conduction when applied to isolated nerves or to isolated neurons.[76] This may be the result of lidocaine-induced increases in intracellular calcium and does not appear to involve Na channel blockade.[77] While it is impossible to "prove safety," multiple studies suggest that chloroprocaine or mepivacaine can be substituted for lidocaine for brief spinal anesthesias.

Treatment of Local Anesthetic Toxicity

Treatment of adverse LA reactions depends on their severity. Minor reactions can be allowed to terminate spontaneously. Seizures induced by LAs should be managed by maintaining a patent airway and by providing oxygen. Seizures may be terminated with intravenous midazolam (0.05–0.10 mg/kg) or propofol (0.5–1.5 mg/kg) or a paralytic dose of succinylcholine (0.5–1 mg/kg), followed by ventilation with bag and mask (or tracheal intubation).[4] LA CV depression manifested by moderate hypotension, may be treated by infusion of intravenous fluids and vasopressors (phenylephrine 0.5–5 μg/kg/min, norepinephrine 0.02–0.2 μg/kg/min, or vasopressin 40 μg IV). If myocardial failure is present, epinephrine (1–5 μg/kg IV bolus) may be required. When toxicity progresses to cardiac arrest, the guidelines for treatment of LA toxicity as developed by the American Society of Regional Anesthesia and Pain Medicine (ASRA) are reasonable,.[78] and certainly preferable to the chaotic resuscitation schemes identified in a national survey prior to publication of the guideline.[79] It makes sense that amiodarone be substituted for lidocaine and, based on multiple animal experiments, that smaller, incremental doses of epinephrine be used initially rather than 1-mg boluses.[80-82] Animal experiments and clinical reports demonstrate the remarkable ability of lipid infusion to resuscitate from bupivacaine-induced cardiac arrest (Figure 7–13).[83-85] Given the nearly nontoxic status of lipid infusion, one cannot make a convincing argument to withhold this therapy from a patient requiring resuscitation from LA intoxication. With unresponsive bupivacaine cardiac toxicity cardiopulmonary bypass should be considered.[86]

It appears that the threat from severe local anesthetic systemic toxicity may be on the decline, whether from better treatment or from changes in techniques.[87] A minority would argue

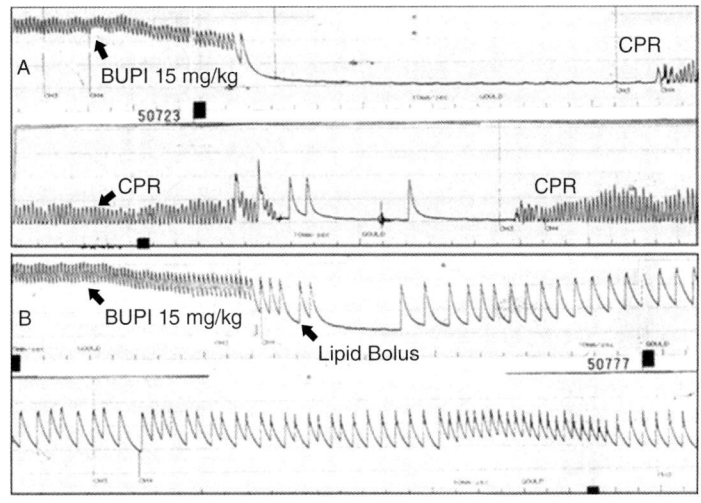

FIGURE 7–13. A: An anesthetized rat is given bupivacaine 15 mg/kg as indicated. The arterial blood pressure rapidly declines to cardiac arrest. Cardiopulmonary resuscitation (CPR) is given, but no arterial pressure is observed when CPR is discontinued. **B:** The same experiment is conducted, but a bolus of lipid is given; note that the arterial pressure is never lost (despite the same dose of bupivacaine being used), and that cardiac arrest does not ensue. (Reproduced with permission from Weinberg G: Current concepts in resuscitation of patients with local anesthetic cardiac toxicity. *Reg Anesth Pain Med.* 2002 Nov-Dec;27(6):568-575.)

that the risk was overstated from the start, at least in experienced hands.[88] Many practitioners believe that ultrasound guidance during peripheral nerve blocks has led to safer practices and less risk. While this view remains controversial, there are studies that support this belief.[89,90]

SUMMARY

After more than a century of use in Western medicine, LAs remain important tools for the twenty-first-century physician. Peripheral nerve blocks are almost certainly the result of LA inhibition of voltage-gated Na channels in neuronal membranes. The mechanisms of spinal and epidural anesthesia remain incompletely defined. The appropriate and safe dose of LAs varies with specific nerve block procedure. The mechanisms by which differing LAs produce CV toxicity likely vary: The more potent agents (eg, bupivacaine) may produce arrhythmias through a Na channel action, whereas the less-potent agents (eg, lidocaine) may produce myocardial depression through other pathways. Fears about LA systemic toxicity have abated with safer LAs, safer regional anesthesia practices, and improved treatments. There is renewed effort to produce clinically applicable delayed-release local anesthetic formulations to extend the duration of the currently available LAs.

REFERENCES

1. Vandam LD: Some aspects of the history of local anesthesia. In Strichartz GR (ed): *Local Anesthetics: Handbook of Experimental Pharmacology.* Springer-Verlag, 1987, pp 1–19.
2. Calatayud J, Gonzalez A: History of the development and evolution of local anesthesia since the coca leaf. Anesthesiology 2003;98:1503–1508.
3. Strichartz GR: *Local Anesthetics: Handbook of Experimental Pharmacology.* Springer-Verlag, 1987.
4. de Jong RH: *Local Anesthetics.* Mosby-Year Book, 1994.
5. Keys TE: *The History of Surgical Anesthesia.* Wood Library, Museum of Anesthesiology, 1996.
6. Butterworth JF IV, Strichartz GR: Molecular mechanisms of local anesthesia: A review. Anesthesiology 1990;72:711–734.
7. Tetzlaff J: *Clinical Pharmacology of Local Anesthetics.* Butterworth-Heinemann, 2000.
8. Ahern CA, Payandeh J, Bosmans F, Chanda B. The hitchhiker's guide to the voltage-gated sodium channel galaxy. J Gen Physiol. 2016;147:1–24.
9. de Lera Ruiz M, Kraus RL. Voltage-Gated Sodium Channels: Structure, Function, Pharmacology, and Clinical Indications. J Med Chem. 2015;58:7093–7118.
10. Lopreato GF, Lu Y, Southwell A, et al: Evolution and divergence of sodium channel genes in vertebrates. Proc Natl Acad Sci U S A 2001; 98:7588–7592.
11. Savio-Galmiberti E. Gollob MH, Darbar D: Voltage-gated sodium channels: Biophysics, pharmacology, and related channelopathies. Front Pharmacol 2012;3:1–19
12. Chen-Izu Y, Shaw RM, Pitt GS, et al. Na⁺ channel function, regulation, structure, trafficking and sequestration. J Physiol. 2015;593:1347–1360
13. Hille B: *Ionic Channels of Excitable Membranes*, 3rd ed. Sinauer, 2001.
14. Jiang Y, Lee A, Chen J, et al: X-ray structure of a voltage-dependent K⁺ channel. Nature 2003;423:33–41.
15. Freites JA, Tobias DJ. Voltage Sensing in Membranes: From Macroscopic Currents to Molecular Motions. J Membr Biol. 2015;248:419–430.
16. Taylor RE. Effect of procaine on electrical properties of squid axon membrane. Am J Physiol 1959;196:1070–1078.
17. Strichartz GR. The inhibition of sodium currents in myelinated nerve by quaternary derivatives of lidocaine. J Gen Physiol. 1973;62:37–57.
18. Ragsdale DS, McPhee JC, Scheuer T, et al: Molecular determinants of state-dependent block of Na⁺ channels by local anesthetics. Science 1994;265:1724–1728.
19. Wang GK, Quan C, Wang S: A common local anesthetic receptor for benzocaine and etidocaine in voltage-gated mu1 Na⁺ channels. Pflugers Arch 1998;435:293–302.
20. Sudoh Y, Cahoon EE, Gerner P, et al: Tricyclic antidepressants as long-acting local anesthetics. Pain 2003;103:49–55.
21. Kohane DS, Lu NT, Gokgol-Kline AC, et al: The local anesthetic properties and toxicity of saxitonin homologues for rat sciatic nerve block in vivo. Reg Anesth Pain Med 2000;25:52–59.
22. Butterworth JF IV, Strichartz GR: The alpha 2-adrenergic agonists clonidine and guanfacine produce tonic and phasic block of conduction in rat sciatic nerve fibers. Anesth Analg 1993;76:295–301.
23. Sanchez V, Arthur GR, Strichartz GR: Fundamental properties of local anesthetics. I. The dependence of lidocaine's ionization and octanol:buffer partitioning on solvent and temperature. Anesth Analg 1987;66: 159–165.

24. Strichartz GR, Sanchez V, Arthur GR, et al: Fundamental properties of local anesthetics. II. Measured octanol:buffer partition coefficients and pK$_a$ values of clinically used drugs. Anesth Analg 1990;71:158–170.

25. Popitz-Bergez FA, Leeson S, Strichartz GR, et al: Relation between functional deficit and intraneural local anesthetic during peripheral nerve block. A study in the rat sciatic nerve. Anesthesiology 1995;83:583–592.

26. Sinnott CJ, Cogswell LP III, Johnson A, et al: On the mechanism by which epinephrine potentiates lidocaine's peripheral nerve block. Anesthesiology 2003;98:181–188.

27. Nakamura T, Popitz-Bergez F, Birknes J, et al: The critical role of concentration for lidocaine block of peripheral nerve in vivo: Studies of function and drug uptake in the rat. Anesthesiology 2003;99: 1189–1197.

28. Brouneus F, Karami K, Beronius P, et al: Diffusive transport properties of some local anesthetics applicable for iontophoretic formulation of the drugs. Int J Pharm 2001;218:57–62.

29. Gissen AJ, Covino BG, Gregus J: Differential sensitivities of mammalian nerve fibers to local anesthetic agents. Anesthesiology 1980;53:467–474.

30. Raymond SA, Gissen AJ: Mechanisms of differential nerve block. In Strichartz GR (ed): Handbook of Experimental Pharmacology: Local Anesthetics. Springer-Verlag, 1987, pp 95–164.

31. Butterworth J, Ririe DG, Thompson RB, et al: Differential onset of median nerve block: Randomized, double-blind comparison of mepivacaine and bupivacaine in healthy volunteers. Br J Anaesth 1998; 81:515–521.

32. Novakovic SD, Eglen RM, Hunter JC: Regulation of Na$^+$ channel distribution in the nervous system. Trends Neurosci 2001;24:473–478.

33. Covino BG, Vasallo HG: Local Anesthetics. Grune & Stratton, 1976.

34. Kohane DS, Lu NT, Cairns BE, et al: Effects of adrenergic agonists and antagonists on tetrodotoxin-induced nerve block. Reg Anesth Pain Med 2001;26:239–245.

35. Butterworth JF IV, Lief PA, Strichartz GR: The pH-dependent local anesthetic activity of diethylaminoethanol, a procaine metabolite. Anesthesiology 1988;68:501–506.

36. Fagraeus L, Urban BJ, Bromage PR: Spread of epidural analgesia in early pregnancy. Anesthesiology 1983;58:184–187.

37. Butterworth JF IV, Walker FO, Lysak SZ: Pregnancy increases median nerve susceptibility to lidocaine. Anesthesiology 1990;72:962–965.

38. Popitz-Bergez FA, Leeson S, Thalhammer JG, et al: Intraneural lidocaine uptake compared with analgesic differences between pregnant and nonpregnant rats. Reg Anesth 1997;22:363–371.

39. Scott DB, Jebson PJ, Braid DP, et al: Factors affecting plasma levels of lignocaine and prilocaine. Br J Anaesth 1972;44:1040–1049.

40. Rosenberg PH, Veering BTh, Urmey WF: Maximum recommended doses of local anesthetics: A multifactorial concept. Reg Anesth Pain Med 2004;29:564–575.

41. Taheri S, Cogswell LP III, Gent A, et al: Hydrophobic and ionic factors in the binding of local anesthetics to the major variant of human alpha$_1$-acid glycoprotein. J Pharmacol Exp Ther 2003;304:71–80.

42. Fragneto RY, Bader AM, Rosinia F, et al: Measurements of protein binding of lidocaine throughout pregnancy. Anesth Analg 1994;79: 295–297.

43. Thomas JM, Schug SA: Recent advances in the pharmacokinetics of local anaesthetics. Long-acting amide enantiomers and continuous infusions. Clin Pharmacokinet 1999;36:67–83.

44. Rothstein P, Arthur GR, Feldman HS, et al: Bupivacaine for intercostal nerve blocks in children: Blood concentrations and pharmacokinetics. Anesth Analg 1986;65:625–632.

45. Bokesch PM, Castaneda AR, Ziemer G, et al: The influence of a right-to-left cardiac shunt on lidocaine pharmacokinetics. Anesthesiology 1987; 67:739–744.

46. Palkama VJ, Neuvonen PJ, Olkkola KT: Effect of itraconazole on the pharmacokinetics of bupivacaine enantiomers in healthy volunteers. Br J Anaesth 1999;83:659–661.

47. Oda Y, Furuichi K, Tanaka K, et al: Metabolism of a new local anesthetic, ropivacaine, by human hepatic cytochrome P450. Anesthesiology 1995; 82:214–220.

48. Ekstrom G, Gunnarsson UB: Ropivacaine, a new amide-type local anesthetic agent, is metabolized by cytochromes P450 1A and 3A in human liver microsomes. Drug Metab Dispos 1996;24:955–961.

49. Hirota K, Browne T, Appadu BL, et al: Do local anaesthetics interact with dihydropyridine binding sites on neuronal L-type Ca^{2+} channels? Br J Anaesth 1997;78:185–188.

50. Olschewski A, Olschewski H, Brau ME, et al: Effect of bupivacaine on ATP-dependent potassium channels in rat cardiomyocytes. Br J Anaesth 1999;82:435–438.

51. Sugimoto M, Uchida I, Fukami S, et al: The alpha and gamma subunit-dependent effects of local anesthetics on recombinant GABA(A) receptors. Eur J Pharmacol 2000;401:329–337.

52. Englesson S, Grevsten S: The influence of acid–base changes on central nervous system toxicity of local anaesthetic agents. II. Acta Anaesthesiol Scand 1974;18:88–103.

53. Feldman HS, Arthur GR, Covino BG: Comparative systemic toxicity of convulsant and supraconvulsant doses of intravenous ropivacaine, bupivacaine, and lidocaine in the conscious dog. Anesth Analg 1989;69: 794–801.

54. Porter JM, Markos F, Snow HM, et al: Effects of respiratory and metabolic pH changes and hypoxia on ropivacaine-induced cardiotoxicity in dogs. Br J Anaesth 2000;84:92–94.

55. Chernoff DM: Kinetic analysis of phasic inhibition of neuronal sodium currents by lidocaine and bupivacaine. Biophys J 1990;58:53–68.

56. Feldman HS, Covino BM, Sage DJ: Direct chronotropic and inotropic effects of local anesthetic agents in isolated guinea pig atria. Reg Anesth 1982;7:149–156.

57. Reiz S, Nath S: Cardiotoxicity of local anaesthetic agents. Br J Anaesth 1986;58:736–746.

58. McCaslin PP, Butterworth J: Bupivacaine suppresses [Ca(2+)](i) oscillations in neonatal rat cardiomyocytes with increased extracellular K$^+$ and is reversed with increased extracellular Mg(2+). Anesth Analg 2000;91:82–88.

59. Butterworth JF IV, Brownlow RC, Leith JP, et al: Bupivacaine inhibits cyclic-3′,5′-adenosine monophosphate production. A possible contributing factor to cardiovascular toxicity. Anesthesiology 1993;79:88–95.

60. Butterworth J, James RL, Grimes J: Structure-affinity relationships and stereospecificity of several homologous series of local anesthetics for the beta$_2$-adrenergic receptor. Anesth Analg 1997;85:336–342.

61. Ohmura S, Kawada M, Ohta T, et al: Systemic toxicity and resuscitation in bupivacaine-, levobupivacaine-, or ropivacaine-infused rats. Anesth Analg 2001;93:743–748.

62. Dony P, Dewinde V, Vanderick B, et al: The comparative toxicity of ropivacaine and bupivacaine at equipotent doses in rats. Anesth Analg 2000;91:1489–1492.

63. Chang DH, Ladd LA, Copeland S, et al: Direct cardiac effects of intracoronary bupivacaine, levobupivacaine and ropivacaine in the sheep. Br J Pharmacol 2001;132:649–658.

64. Groban L, Deal DD, Vernon JC, et al: Ventricular arrhythmias with or without programmed electrical stimulation after incremental overdosage with lidocaine, bupivacaine, levobupivacaine, and ropivacaine. Anesth Analg 2000;91:1103–1111.

65. Groban L, Deal DD, Vernon JC, et al: Cardiac resuscitation after incremental overdosage with lidocaine, bupivacaine, levobupivacaine, and ropivacaine in anesthetized dogs. Anesth Analg 2001;92:37–43.

66. Groban L, Deal DD, Vernon JC, et al: Does local anesthetic stereoselectivity or structure predict myocardial depression in anesthetized canines? Reg Anesth Pain Med 2002;27:460–468.

67. Nath S, Haggmark S, Johansson G, et al: Differential depressant and electrophysiologic cardiotoxicity of local anesthetics: An experimental study with special reference to lidocaine and bupivacaine. Anesth Analg 1986;65:1263–1270.

68. Carpenter RL, Kopacz DJ, Mackey DC: Accuracy of laser Doppler capillary flow measurements for predicting blood loss from skin incisions in pigs. Anesth Analg 1989;68:308–311.

69. deShazo RD, Nelson HS: An approach to the patient with a history of local anesthetic hypersensitivity: Experience with 90 patients. J Allergy Clin Immunol 1979;63:387–394.

70. Berkun Y, Ben-Zvi A, Levy Y, et al: Evaluation of adverse reactions to local anesthetics: Experience with 236 patients. Ann Allergy Asthma Immunol 2003;91:342–345.

71. Gissen AJ, Datta S, Lambert D: The chloroprocaine controversy. I. A hypothesis to explain the neural complications of chloroprocaine epidural. Reg Anesth 1984;9:124–134.

72. Gissen AJ, Datta S, Lambert D: The chloroprocaine controversy. II. Is chloroprocaine neurotoxic? Reg Anesth 1984;9:135–145.

73. Winnie AP, Nader AM: Santayana's prophecy fulfilled. Reg Anesth Pain Med 2001;26:558–564.

74. Kouri ME, Kopacz DJ: Spinal 2-chloroprocaine: A comparison with lidocaine in volunteers. Anesth Analg 2004;98:75–80.

75. Taniguchi M, Bollen AW, Drasner K: Sodium bisulfite: Scapegoat for chloroprocaine neurotoxicity? Anesthesiology 2004;100:85–91.

76. Lambert LA, Lambert DH, Strichartz GR: Irreversible conduction block in isolated nerve by high concentrations of local anesthetics. Anesthesiology 1994;80:1082–1093.

77. Gold MS, Reichling DB, Hampl KF, et al: Lidocaine toxicity in primary afferent neurons from the rat. J Pharmacol Exp Ther 1998;285:413–421.

78. Neal JM, Bernards CM, Butterworth JF 4th, et al. ASRA practice advisory on local anesthetic systemic toxicity. Reg Anesth Pain Med. 2010;35:152–61

79. Corcoran W, Butterworth J, Weller RS, et al. Local anesthetic-induced cardiac toxicity: a survey of contemporary practice strategies among academic anesthesiology departments. Anesth Analg. 2006;103:1322–6

80. El-Boghdadly K, Chin KJ. Local anesthetic systemic toxicity: Continuing Professional Development. Can J Anaesth. 2016;63:330–349

81. Krismer AC, Hogan QH, Wenzel V, et al: The efficacy of epinephrine or vasopressin for resuscitation during epidural anesthesia. Anesth Analg 2001;93:734–742.

82. Mayr VD, Raedler C, Wenzel V, et al: A comparison of epinephrine and vasopressin in a porcine model of cardiac arrest after rapid intravenous injection of bupivacaine. Anesth Analg 2004;98:1426–1431.

83. Weinberg GL, VadeBoncouer T, Ramaraju GA, et al: Pretreatment or resuscitation with a lipid infusion shifts the dose-response to bupivacaine-induced asystole in rats. Anesthesiology 1998;88:1071–1075.

84. Weinberg G, Ripper R, Feinstein DL, et al: Lipid emulsion infusion rescues dogs from bupivacaine-induced cardiac toxicity. Reg Anesth Pain Med 2003;28:198–202.

85. Fettiplace MR, Weinberg G. Past, Present, and Future of Lipid Resuscitation Therapy. JPEN J Parenter Enteral Nutr. 2015;39(1 Suppl):72S-83S.

86. Soltesz EG, van Pelt F, Byrne JG: Emergent cardiopulmonary bypass for bupivacaine cardiotoxicity. J Cardiothorac Vasc Anesth 2003;17:357–358.

87. Vasques F, Behr AU, Weinberg G, et al. A Review of Local Anesthetic Systemic Toxicity Cases Since Publication of the American Society of Regional Anesthesia Recommendations: To Whom It May Concern. Reg Anesth Pain Med. 2015;40:698–705.

88. Liu SS, Ortolan S, Sandoval MV, Curren J, Fields KG, Memtsoudis SG, YaDeau JT. Cardiac Arrest and Seizures Caused by Local Anesthetic Systemic Toxicity After Peripheral Nerve Blocks: Should We Still Fear the Reaper? Reg Anesth Pain Med. 2016;4:5–21.

89. Barrington MJ, Kluger R. Ultrasound guidance reduces the risk of local anesthetic systemic toxicity following peripheral nerve blockade. Reg Anesth Pain Med. 2013;38:289–299.

90. Neal JM, Brull R, Horn JL, et al. The Second American Society of Regional Anesthesia and Pain Medicine Evidence-Based Medicine Assessment of Ultrasound-Guided Regional Anesthesia: Executive Summary. Reg Anesth Pain Med. 2016;41:181–194.

CHAPTER 8

Controlled-Release Local Anesthetics

John-Paul J. Pozek, David Beausang, Kara G. Segna, and Eugene R. Viscusi

INTRODUCTION

Local anesthetics (LAs) are among the most useful drugs in anesthesiology practice and pain management. They are cornerstones in postoperative pain management within a multimodal analgesic pathway to reduce or eliminate opioids and their resulting adverse events. However, currently available LAs display a considerable range of onset and duration as well as tolerability across a wide range of uses, including infiltration, peripheral blocks, and epidural and spinal anesthesia. Their main limitation is duration of action, which in the treatment of postoperative pain may prevent adequate therapy of sufficient duration. For that reason, continuous catheter infusion systems are widely used but introduce challenges, such as catheter placement, catheter migration and maintenance, and the burden of the external pump. Therefore, long-acting LAs with predictable onset, delivery, and duration of action would be a near-ideal solution.

Local anesthetics can have considerably different properties depending on the body compartment where they are placed. Controlled-release LAs must be well studied for clinical efficacy and reliability in the various sites and modes of application. At this time, only one controlled-release drug is approved by the Food and Drug Administration (FDA) and is commercially available, although there are several others in development. In this chapter, we summarize the currently available information.

LOCAL ANESTHETIC CARRIERS

Since the 1970s, drug delivery systems for LAs have been the subject of considerable research efforts.[1-3] Development strategies are typically based on interdisciplinary approaches that combine polymer science, pharmaceutics, bioconjugate chemistry, and molecular biology.[4] The goals of these carriers are to provide a LA depot at the target site to prolong the drug effect and to decrease local and systemic toxicity by reducing the LA concentration and increasing LA permeability and absorption. These factors determine the concentration and the effect of the LA on the nervous tissue, influencing the latency, spread, intensity of the blockade, and the duration of action.[1]

Formulation approaches to systemically deliver LA have included the encapsulation in liposomes, complexation in cyclodextrins, association with biopolymers, transdermal nonliposomal carriers, and other carrier systems. Topical delivery systems for LA comprise of a wide spectrum of adjuvants, including viscosity-inducing agents, preservatives, permeation enhancers, and emollients. The physical state of these carriers varies from semisolid (gel, cream, ointment); liquid (emulsion, dispersion); to solid (patch) pharmaceutical forms.[1]

Liposome-Based Local Anesthetic Formulations

Liposomes, widely investigated as drug carriers for improving the delivery of therapeutic agents to specific sites in the body, are nonimmunogenic, biodegradable, nontoxic and work by encapsulating both hydrophilic and hydrophobic materials to deliver drugs.[4] The structural versatility combined with the ability to encapsulate different compounds, such as LAs, is due to microscopic mono- or bi-layer phospholipid vesicles.[1] The polar core of the liposphere allows hydrophilic drug molecules to become encapsulated. Amphiphilic and lipophilic molecules are solubilized within the phospholipid bilayer according to their affinity.[4]

Channel proteins can be incorporated into the liposome without a loss of activity within the hydrophobic domain of vesicle membranes, acting as a selective filter. Thus, drugs that are encapsulated with channel proteins are effectively protected from premature degradation by proteolytic enzymes and are able to diffuse through the channel driven by concentration gradients between the interior and exterior "nanocage."[4] Various types of liposomes can be prepared, depending on the number of lipid layers, size, surface charge, lipid composition, and methods of vesicle formation. In the case of liposomes and micro- or nanoparticle-based systems, the improved pharmacological action is generated by the slow rate of release of the encapsulated drug from these lipid bilayers.[1]

Benefits

Liposomes, composed of naturally occurring substances, offer the advantage of being nontoxic and biodegradable. The ability to entrap drugs in the aqueous or lipid form enables carrying of both hydrophilic and hydrophobic drugs.[4] The advantages of encapsulating LA in liposomes is controlled delivery via slow drug release to prolong anesthetic effect and reduce the risk of cardiovascular and central nervous system toxicity.[1]

Clinical Pearl

- Liposomes are microscopic spheres containing an aqueous core surrounded by a phospholipid bilayer.

Risks/Limitations

Although liposomes are the carrier of choice in many technologies, their use for LAs has not often been adequately explored. This could be because liposomes are considered unstable colloidal systems, either physically due to their size or chemically, as lipids are prone to oxidation.[4]

DepoFoam®

DepoFoam® consists of microscopic, spherical, lipid-based particles (Figure 8–1A).[5] The particles are composed of numerous polyhedral, nonconcentric, aqueous chambers containing the drug in solution. Each chamber in this multivesicular liposome is separated from adjacent chambers by lipid membranes

(Figure 8–1B). DepoFoam particles are distinguished structurally from unilamellar vesicles, multilamellar vesicles, and neosomes (Figure 8–2) by these closely packed, nonconcentric vesicles. The particles are tens of micrometers in diameter and have a large trapped volume. This allows delivery of relatively large quantities of medications in the encapsulated form with only a small volume of the formulation. Importantly, the liposomal platform that encapsulates the drug does so without altering the molecular structure. Therefore, a number of methods based on a manipulation of the lipid and aqueous composition may be used to control the rate of sustained release over a desired period from 1 to 30 days via erosion or reorganization of the lipid membranes.[6] DepoFoam has been used in to-date, two FDA-approved commercial products, including DepoCyt(e)® (cytarabine liposome injection), as well as EXPAREL® (bupivacaine liposome injectable suspension). DepoFoam can be released into the bloodstream via the interstitial space subcutaneously or intramuscularly or it can be delivered locally to a body compartment or joint via intrathecal, intraperitoneal, subcutaneous, epidural, or intraocular methods.[7,8]

Clinical Pearl

- DepoFoam technology consists of lipid-based particles with polyhedral, nonconcentric, aqueous chambers that contain the medication. This technology can be used with a number of different medications.

Benefits

DepoFoam is a ready-to-use product and can be administered with small-gauge needles and pen systems. With a flexible delivery system, it is designed to offer an immediate-release dose, followed by sustained delivery. DepoFoam is less than 3%

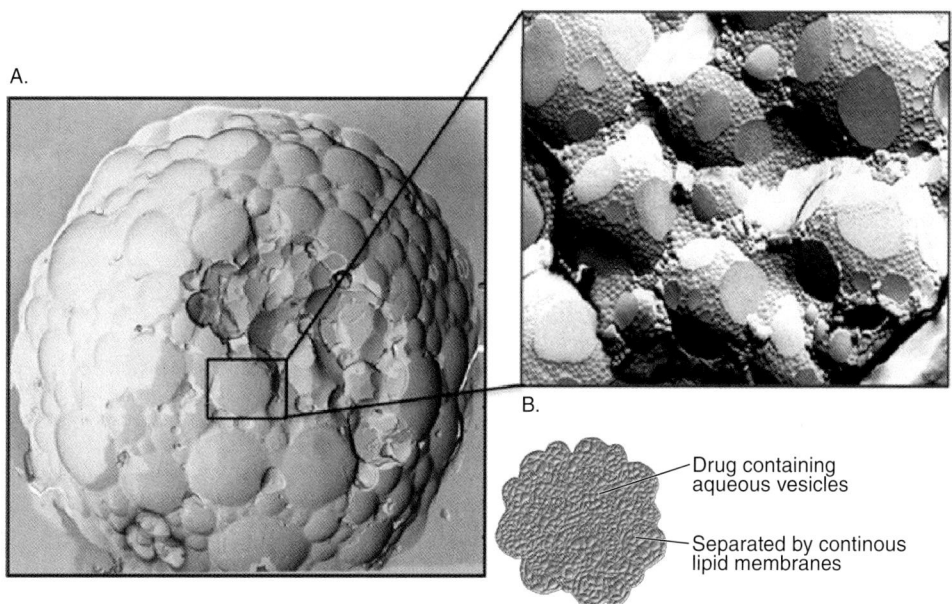

FIGURE 8–1. A: Scanning electron micrographic image of DepoFoam® with bupivacaine. **B:** Diagram representing the polyhedral, nonconcentric aqueous chambers filled with medication. (Used with permission from Pacira Pharmaceuticals, Inc.)

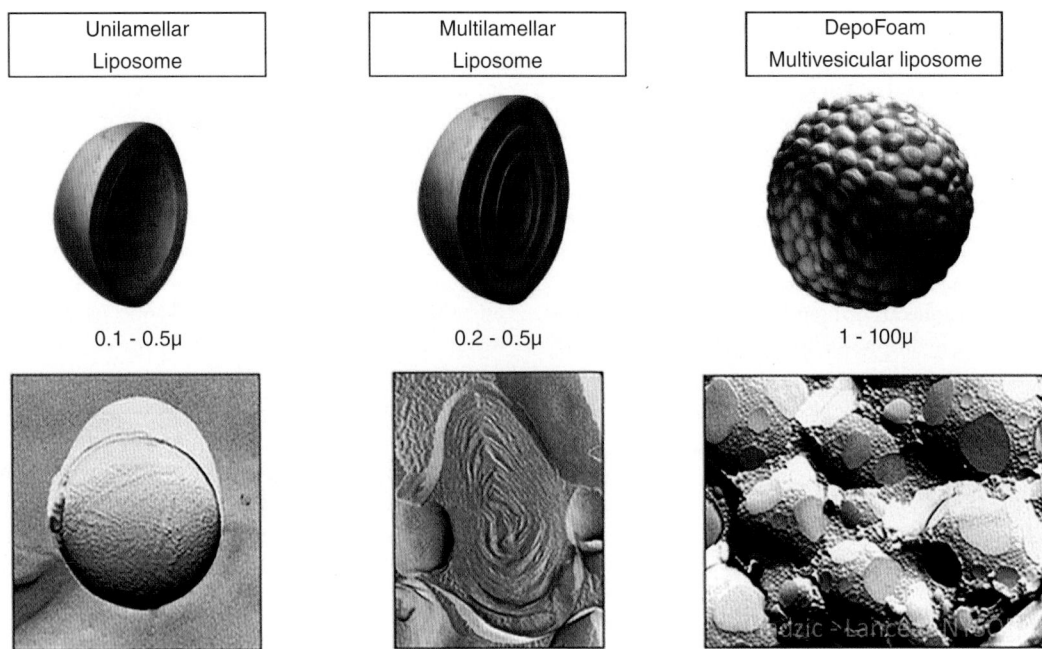

Unilamellar Liposome	Multilamellar Liposome	DepoFoam Multivesicular liposome
0.1 - 0.5μ	0.2 - 0.5μ	1 - 100μ

FIGURE 8–2. Comparison of unilamellar, multilamellar, and polylamellar formulations of liposomes.

lipid that is naturally occurring or a synthetic analogue of common lipids, including phospholipids, cholesterol, and triglycerides; therefore, it is biodegradable and biocompatible.[6]

Clinical trials have demonstrated limited to no adverse effects of DepoFoam. There is already considerable clinical experience with the delivery system as the formulation has been in use in products approved by the FDA and European Medicine Agency. Furthermore, at similar doses, this formulation can reduce systemic exposure and toxicity by reducing peak serum levels of a drug.[7,8]

Polymeric Micro- and Nanoparticle Formulations

Polymeric micro- or nanoparticles represent drug delivery systems made of natural or artificial polymer spheres or capsules, which must be biocompatible and biodegradable for drug delivery purposes.[1] Nanoparticles act as potential carriers for several classes of drugs, such as anticancer agents, antihypertensive agents, immunomodulators, and hormones, and for macromolecules such as nucleic acids, proteins, peptides, and antibodies. Nanoparticles can be designed for the site-specific delivery of drugs. The targeting and release capability of nanoparticles is influenced by particle size, surface charge, surface modification, and hydrophobicity. The performance of nanoparticles in vivo is influenced by morphological characteristics, surface chemistry, and molecular weight.[9] Polymer (micro- or nanoparticle) technologies are claimed to be applicable to all commercially available LA compounds.[1]

A variety of natural and synthetic polymers have been explored for the preparation of nanoparticles, of which poly(lactic acid) (PLA) and poly(glycolic acid) (PGA) and their copolymer poly(lactic-co-glycolic acid) (PLGA) have been extensively investigated for their biocompatibility and biodegradability. PLGA, one of the most successfully developed

biodegradable polymers,[9] attracted considerable attention due to the FDA and European Medicine Agency giving approval for parenteral administration. Other properties include well-described formulations and methods of production adapted to various types of drugs (eg, hydrophilic or hydrophobic small molecules or macromolecules) and protection of the drug from degradation.

Use of PLGA allows for the possibility of sustained release, the possibility to modify surface properties to provide better interaction with biological materials, and even a possibility toward targeting nanoparticles to specific organs or cells. Of note, after systemic administration, PLGA-based drug delivery systems are preferentially taken up by the reticuloendothelial system (RES) and present a high and selective uptake in inflamed areas. One of the reasons for the success of the carrier is that hydrolysis leads to the metabolite monomers lactic acid and glycolic acid, which are endogenous and easily metabolized by the body via the Krebs cycle. The PLGA delivery system is associated with a nearly negligible potential for toxicity.[10]

Benefits

Biodegradable nanoparticles have been used frequently as drug delivery vehicles due to their improved bioavailability, better encapsulation, and controlled release.[11] The literature describes that micro- or nanoencapsulation of LA greatly prolongs the duration of block and reduces systemic toxicity.[1]

Risks/Limitations

Despite the existing research on biodegradable microparticles containing macromolecular drugs, the effects of critical parameters influencing drug encapsulation are not sufficiently investigated for nanoscale carriers.[12] However, many novel techniques for preparation of drug-loaded nanoparticles are being developed and refined. The crux of the problem is the stability of nanoparticles after preparation, which is being addressed by freeze-drying using different classes of lyoprotectants.[9]

Another issue is that precise determination of the drug content is not easy because nanoparticles are colloidal systems. Encapsulation efficiency of drugs varies from 6% to 90% for dexamethasone and paclitaxel, respectively, while mean encapsulation efficiency is around 60% to 70% for various drugs, such as estradiol or xanthones. Another major pitfall of PLGA-based nanoparticles is that although PLGA-based nanoparticles often can present with high encapsulation efficiencies, the drug loading is generally poor (around 1%, which means that nanoparticles contain 1 mg active ingredient per 100 mg polymers of nanoparticles).

Yet another important pitfall is the consideration of high burst release of drug from nanoparticles. This phenomenon is described for most PLGA-based nanoparticles. Consequently, the drug might not be able to reach the target tissue or cells, leading to a loss of efficacy. Drug release mechanisms depend on the polymer used and on the loading efficiency. Generally, the rapid initial release is attributed to drug adsorbed to the nanoparticles' surface. Work is still being conducted to address these issues.[10]

LIPOSOMAL BUPIVACAINE

In October 2011, the FDA approved the use of single-injection liposomal bupivacaine for surgical site infiltration. To date, this is the only FDA-approved controlled-release LA.[4] Liposomal bupivacaine produces reliable plasma levels of bupivacaine up to 72 hours following infiltration. By comparison, traditional bupivacaine HCl has a duration of action of roughly 7 hours following tissue infiltration.[13] Liposomal bupivacaine encapsulates bupivacaine HCl within the carrier, DepoFoam. Prior to this development, extending the duration of action of an LA relied on indwelling catheters and infusion pumps. Infusion technology with an indwelling catheter carries a risk of infection, drug-filling errors, labeling errors, and variable infusion rates, particularly with elastometric pumps.[14] Replacement of elastomeric bags and targeted catheters with LA encapsulated in a liposome is a novel approach for providing analgesia. To date, liposomal bupivacaine has been studied in patients undergoing soft tissue surgery (hemorrhoidectomy, inguinal hernia repair, augmentation mammoplasty) or orthopedic surgery (bunionectomy and total knee arthroplasty).[5] Currently, it is approved for tissue infiltration.

> ## Clinical Pearl
>
> - Liposomal bupivacaine is a controlled-release LA that is FDA approved for wound (surgical site) infiltration.

Formulation

DepoFoam serves as the lipid-based carrier of bupivacaine HCl. When compared with other carriers, such as DepoDur® and DepoCyt, the major difference is the incorporation of dierucoylphosphatidylcholine into the DepoFoam.[15] It is comprised of nonemetogenic, naturally occurring or synthetic analogues of common lipids, making it generally well tolerated, although a tissue infiltration with DepoFoam bupivacaine in rabbits and dogs resulted in granulomatous inflammation, considered a natural reaction against the liposomes.[16]

Pharmacology

Liposomal bupivacaine is currently packaged in a 20-mL vial at a 1.3% concentration.[5] Single-dose administration is recommended, not exceeding 266 mg (one vial). Approximately 3% of the LA in liposomal bupivacaine is present in the free form. Because of this, the drug exhibits two peaks in plasma concentration T_{max} following tissue infiltration (Table 8–1).[17] This was observed by Langford et al in their study of patients receiving infiltration of liposomal bupivacaine for inguinal hernia repair. The first T_{max} occurs within the first hour, followed by a second T_{max} within 12 hours.[17] Systemic absorption depends on the total dose of drug administered, administration route, and vascularity of the administration site.[13] Liposomal bupivacaine has a 24-hour duration of action.[18]

As with traditional bupivacaine, liposomal bupivacaine is metabolized by the liver following its release from the drug delivery system.[13] Caution is recommended when using liposomal bupivacaine for patients with severe hepatic dysfunction. In phase 1, trial patients with moderate hepatic impairment

TABLE 8–1. Pharmacokinetics of controlled-release local anesthetics.

Drug	Carrier	T_{max} (h)	C_{max} (ng/mL)
Liposomal bupivacaine	DepoFoam	1–12[a]	365[b]
SABER-bupivacaine	SAIB	24–48[c]	625–989[c]
Bupivacaine-collagen implant	Bioidegradeable collagen matrix	0.5–20[d]	200[d]

[a]Reference 17.

[b]Reference 43.

[c]Reference 39.

[d]Reference 42.

SAIB = sucrose acetate isobutyrate.

had a 1.5-fold increase in the maximum plasma concentration C_{max} compared with healthy controls following single 300-mg infiltration of liposomal bupivacaine.[19] However, this is likely not of great clinical significance with single administration of liposomal bupivacaine. Significant accumulation of bupivacaine or its metabolites is not expected despite impaired liver function. Approximately 6% of bupivacaine is excreted unchanged in urine.[13]

Dosing and Administration

Dilution is recommended with sterile saline up to a maximum total volume of 300 mL.[20] Hypobaric solutions, such as sterile water, may disrupt the liposomal carrier, potentially leading to loss of sustained efficacy and high system drug levels.[18] Diluting liposomal bupivacaine with other drugs, such as lidocaine or bupivacaine HCl, may cause disruption of the carrier, accelerated release of bound bupivacaine and toxicity.[18] Additional LA, of any kind, is not recommended for 24 hours following liposomal bupivacaine administration. The liposomal carrier will maintain its integrity with injection through as small as 30-gauge needles.[18]

Clinical Pearl

- Diluting liposomal bupivacaine with other LA may cause disruption of the lipid carrier, possibly unbinding bupivacaine.

Clinical Evidence

In a phase 3 trial, an infiltration of 266 mg liposomal bupivacaine was compared with placebo in patients receiving hemorrhoidectomy. This randomized, double-blind study of 189 patients found that patients receiving liposomal bupivacaine had significantly less pain and fewer patients required opiate rescue.[21] A significant difference was also observed with regard to 72-hour opioid consumption, which was 45% lower compared with placebo.[21] Following this study, Onel and colleagues compared liposomal bupivacaine to bupivacaine HCl in a similar cohort of patients. This double-blind, randomized, controlled study examined 100 patients for hemorrhoidectomy. Patients had significantly less pain (47%) and required significantly less opioid (66%) over the first 72 hours with liposomal bupivacaine.[22]

Clinical Pearl

- Patients receiving wound infiltration with liposomal bupivacaine had significantly less pain and opioid usage than those who received bupivacaine HCl for hemorrhoidectomy and bunionectomy.

In a double-blind, randomized trial of 193 patients receiving bunionectomy with first-metatarsal osteotomy, liposomal bupivacaine showed significantly reduced pain at 24 and 36 hours when compared with placebo.[23] Although there was no statistically significant difference in pain scores, a liposomal bupivacaine dose-finding study of patients having unilateral inguinal hernia repair demonstrated benefits for secondary endpoints. The liposomal bupivacaine group trended toward lower opioid requirements in patients at all doses (155, 200, 266, 310 mg) compared with 100 mg bupivacaine HCl.[17]

In a randomized trial of women having bilateral breast augmentation surgery, subjects were randomized to injection of either 133 or 266 mg liposomal bupivacaine in one breast and 75 mg bupivacaine HCl in the contralateral breast.[24] In both groups, the subjects complained of more pain in the breast receiving bupivacaine HCl. The difference in opioid consumption between the two groups only reached significance after 48 hours which is commensurate with the delayed release of bupivacaine from liposome carriers.[24]

Use of liposomal bupivacaine in patients after implant-based breast reconstruction demonstrated significantly decreased visual analog scale (VAS) pain scores at 4–24 hours postoperatively when compared to bupivacaine HCl and placebo.[25] There was no difference in opioid and antiemetic usage between the three treatment groups.[25]

Multiple studies investigating analgesic efficacy of liposomal bupivacaine in wound infiltration after total knee arthroplasty have been performed. A study by Bagsby et al[26] compared periarticular injection with 2.6% liposomal bupivacaine versus 0.5% ropivacaine. Patients reported similar mean pain scores at 24 hours, but for the remainder of the hospitalization, pain scores were significantly increased in the liposomal bupivacaine group. Half of the ropivacaine group reported their pain as mild, compared with only 17% of patients receiving liposomal bupivacaine.[26]

A recent, large, randomized, controlled trial compared periarticular injection of liposomal bupivacaine versus bupivacaine HCl. All patients concurrently received multimodal analgesia. The two groups had no significant difference in terms of least, worst, and average daily pain at all time points.[27] Furthermore, there was no difference in consumption of opioids.[27]

A recent randomized prospective study compared local infiltration of liposomal bupivacaine with a single-injection femoral nerve block of ropivacaine and tetracaine. The nerve block group had significantly less pain in the first 24 hours postoperatively, but total opioid consumption was unchanged between the two groups.[28] Interestingly, the nerve block group had less opioid during the first day postoperatively, while the liposomal bupivacaine group consumed less on the second day.[28] The two treatments demonstrated no effect on total ambulation, but a greater percentage of patients ambulating and greater total distance was seen in the liposomal bupivacaine group.[28]

Safety

It is recommended that the dose of liposomal bupivacaine should not exceed the single 266-mg vial. Repeat LA administration is not recommended within 72 hours following infiltration. To ensure the liposomal carrier's integrity, liposomal bupivacaine should be diluted only with normal saline and administered through a needle that is 25 gauge or larger.[18] To avoid possible toxic levels of lidocaine and bupivacaine, liposomal bupivacaine infiltration should follow lidocaine infiltration by at least 20 minutes.[16] Overall, however, in over 1 million patient exposures, liposomal bupivacaine demonstrated a remarkable safety systemic toxicity profile.[29] Safety of liposomal bupivacaine in peripheral nerve blocks (PNBs) is discussed further in the chapter.[30]

Clinical Pearl

- Injection of liposomal bupivacaine should occur at least 20 minutes after infiltration of lidocaine to avoid potential toxicity.

Experimental Applications
Peripheral Nerve Blocks

The use of liposomal bupivacaine in PNBs has generated significant interest as a possible FDA-approved method to prolong nerve blockade without indwelling catheters. At the time of publication, liposomal bupivacaine has not been approved by the FDA for this indication.

Data from preclinical toxicology studies demonstrated no signs of neurotoxicity in animal models.[16,31,32] Similarly, a phase 1 study in healthy volunteers demonstrated no nerve injury with single-injection PNB.[33]

Efficacy of higher-dose liposomal bupivacaine was seen in femoral nerve blocks for patients receiving tricompartment knee arthroplasty. Patients receiving 133 and 266 mg had significantly decreased resting pain at 24 hours when compared with patients receiving 67 mg of liposomal bupivacaine or saline. A study by Ilfeld et al with variable doses of liposomal bupivacaine (0–80 mg) demonstrated prolonged motor and sensory block with higher doses of the medication.[33] All patients had motor and sensory blockade more than 24 hours in the 40-mg treatment group and more than 90% in the 80-mg treatment group.[33]

A recent review of literature examined the safety of liposomal bupivacaine over six studies with healthy volunteers and patients undergoing various surgical procedures. The most common side effects of perineural liposomal bupivacaine injection were nausea, pyrexia, constipation, vomiting, and pruritus.[34] There was no difference in adverse effects between liposomal bupivacaine and placebo. Treatment-related adverse events had lower incidence in the liposomal bupivacaine versus bupivacaine HCL groups, with the most common adverse event being hypesthesia.[34]

Potential deterrents for widespread use of liposomal bupivacaine in PNBs are a possible inability to achieve surgical anesthesia,[33] inferior analgesia compared to bupivacaine HCl over the first 12 postoperative hours, and inability to titrate the LA to effect. Prolonged sensory and motor blockade may affect early rehabilitation and increase fall risks.[35]

If approved for use in PNBs, single-injection liposomal bupivacaine may present a long-acting alternative to continuous PNB. There is potential for increased procedure efficiency and more widespread use of PNBs without the placement and fixation of a perineurial catheter, and the patient would avoid possible adverse events related to catheter placement.[35]

Epidural Anesthesia

Liposomal bupivacaine is currently not approved for epidural administration, although its pharmacologic profile following a single epidural injection has been studied. Viscusi, Candiotti, and colleagues performed a phase 1 randomized, double-blind, active-control, dose-escalating pilot study evaluating a single dose of liposomal bupivacaine at 89, 155, or 266 mg compared with bupivacaine HCl 50 mg in healthy volunteers. Their study concluded that epidural liposomal bupivacaine at 266 mg resulted in a longer duration of sensory block than liposomal bupivacaine 89 or 155 mg or bupivacaine HCl 50 mg.[36]

Interestingly, incidence of some degree of motor blockade was less with liposomal bupivacaine 266 mg versus bupivacaine HCl 50 mg.[36] The liposomal bupivacaine group had fewer patients who were unable to ambulate after 4 hours and a quicker resolution of complete motor blockade.[36] The high sensorimotor block ratio suggests significant utility for liposomal bupivacaine in epidural anesthesia, but further study is needed to document safety and efficacy.

EXPERIMENTAL MEDICATIONS
SABER-Bupivacaine

SABER (sucrose acetate isobutyrate extended release) technology (Durect Corporation) has been developed as a bioerodable injectable depot system with the potential of delivering a drug over a period of days to 3 months.[37]

Formulation

The SABER delivery system consists of sucrose acetate isobutyrate (SAIB), additives, and a solvent. SAIB is a hydrophobic, esterified sucrose derivative that exists as a viscous liquid (Figure 8–3). The SABER system can be mixed with a drug and injected subcutaneously or intramuscularly with up to a 25-gauge needle.[37]

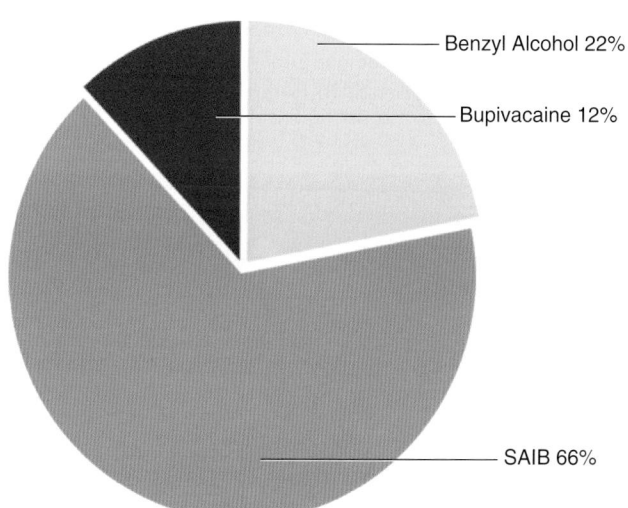

FIGURE 8–3. Formulation of SABER-bupivacaine. (Compiled from data in References 33–36.)

> **Clinical Pearl**
>
> - SABER-bupivacaine consists of a SAIB delivery system that is mixed with LA. After infiltration, the delivery system dissolves within tissues.

SABER-bupivacaine (Posidur™), developed by the Durect Corporation, awaits FDA approval.

Pharmacology

Solvent type and amount, drug loading, and other additives are possible variables to customize the duration of drug delivery. SABER formulations can carry a drug payload as high as 30%. On injection, the drug forms a depot in subcutaneous tissue, and its release begins immediately. The delivery system dissolves in situ, eliminating the need for removal.[38]

In a study comparing differing doses of SABER-bupivacaine (12% bupivacaine), the dose concentration response exhibited linear pharmacokinetics.[37] A large review of 11 clinical trials with both healthy subjects and those undergoing varied surgical procedures demonstrated a varied T_{max} at 24–48 hours (Table 8–1).[39] This seems to differ with surgical procedure, as T_{max} with administration after shoulder surgery was shorter when compared with abdominal surgery.[40] This is possibly due to rapid absorption of the drug when confined to a smaller surgical area.[40]

Clinical Evidence

In a 2012 double-blinded, randomized, controlled trial of 124 patients receiving open hernia repair, SABER-bupivacaine outperformed placebo after surgical site administration. A dose of 5 mL of SABER-bupivacaine (12% bupivacaine) had a significantly lower area under the curve (AUC) for mean pain intensity from 1 to 72 hours, compared to placebo (2.47 vs. 3.61; $p = .0036$). The 5-mL group achieved significantly reduced pain with movement and opioid consumption and increased time to first opioid when compared to placebo.[37]

Notably, the 2.5-mL formulation of SABER-bupivacaine did not reach the same levels of significance. A 2014 multicenter, randomized, double-blind study of 98 patients undergoing abdominal surgery showed clinically and statistically significant decreased pain for 3 days in patients given SABER-bupivacaine.[41]

Safety

Due to incomplete evidence of clinical safety, the FDA did not approve SABER-bupivacaine's new drug application in 2013. In 2012, Hadj et al reported no adverse events resulting from SABER-bupivacaine.[37] Wound healing was unchanged among the groups. Gan et al failed to identify any evidence of bupivacaine toxicity through evaluation of vital signs, physical exam, laboratory results, and Holter monitoring.[41]

▐ Bupivacaine-Collagen Implant

A collagen-based implant with LA that is currently waiting for phase 3 testing is a bupivacaine-collagen implant (XaraColl®). This medication is being developed by Innocoll Pharmaceuticals for implantation in sites of surgical trauma to provide postsurgical analgesia.[42]

Formulation

XaraColl is composed of a biodegradable and fully resorbable collagen matrix that is impregnated with bupivacaine (Figure 8–4). The matrix is implanted during surgery and is purported to begin releasing LA immediately.[42]

> **Clinical Pearl**
>
> - A bupivacaine-collagen implant is composed of a collagen matrix that is impregnated with LA. While the collagen matrix is resorbed, LA is released.

Pharmacology

Collagen implants have been studied with varying concentrations of bupivacaine. With slow resorption of the collagen matrix, controlled release of LA occurs. Systemic bupivacaine levels were demonstrated to be well below the toxicity threshold with a mean C_{max} of 0.22 µg/mL (Table 8–1).[43] Similar to liposomal bupivacaine, this medication demonstrated a biphasic peak of increased concentration.[43] In a study by Cusack, T_{max} ranged from 30 minutes to 20 hours, depending on which peak predominated.[43]

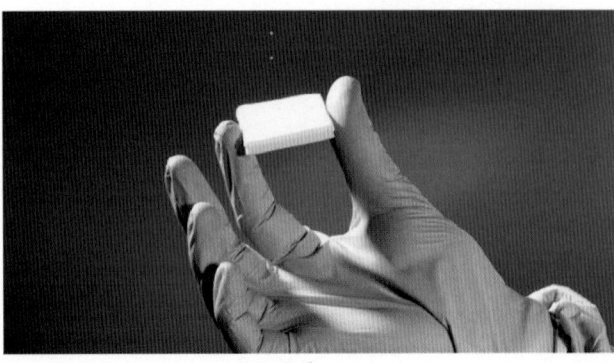

CollaRx® sponge

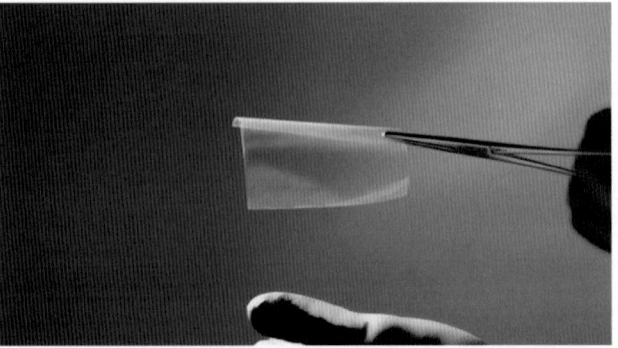

Collafilm® membrane

FIGURE 8–4. Delivery system of bupivacaine-collagen implant. (Used with permission from Innocoll Inc. Website. Accessed November 2015.)

Clinical Evidence

Two independent studies in men after unilateral inguinal hernia repair indicated a significant treatment effect for bupivacaine-collagen implants when compared to placebo. In one study, pain scores were significantly decreased in patients treated with implants versus placebo at both 24 and 48 hours with no significant change in opioid usage. In the second study, pain scores did not differ, but opioid usage decreased significantly in patients with bupivacaine-collagen implants. Pooled analysis of these studies suggested that this treatment effect extended over 72 hours postoperatively.[42]

Safety

Most common adverse events after implantation of bupivacaine-collagen implants were constipation, nausea, and headache.[41] One study demonstrated elevated liver enzymes and abnormal phosphorous levels after implantation, although none of these were clinically significant and resolved spontaneously. Visual disturbances possibly indicating bupivacaine toxicity were found in one patient, but serum sampling showed a low systemic concentration of bupivacaine.[43]

Phase 3 trials show a statistically significant decrease in pain scores 48 hours postoperatively in inguinal hernia repair when compared to placebo.[44]

SUMMARY

The clinical practice need for longer duration of analgesia and avoidance of the time-inefficient and procedurally more complex indwelling catheters has spurred interest in controlled-release LAs. Every technology to date has inherent compromises. Evidence to date suggests a clear utility for single-injection extended-released LAs but a continued role for delivery of LA by catheter and indwelling pump. Currently, the only medication in this class with FDA approval is liposomal bupivacaine, which is approved for wound infiltration. The search for new indications has inspired research in multiple modalities. Of particular interest to regional anesthesia and acute pain medicine are its potential use in PNBs and epidural anesthesia. FDA approval for use in these areas has the potential to positively affect the practice of regional anesthesia and quality of postoperative pain management. Controlled-release LAs are likely to become an important inherent part of a multimodal analgesia regimen. Controlled-release LAs, along with other analgesics, may further reduce the reliance on opioids as the primary postoperative analgesia consistent with all current published acute pain guidelines.

REFERENCES

1. Samad A, et al: Liposomal drug delivery systems: An update review. Curr Drug Deliv 2007;4(4):297–305.
2. Minkowitz HS, Singla NK, Evashenk MA, et al: Pharmacokinetics of sublingual sufentanil tablets and efficacy and safety in the management of postoperative pain. Reg Anesth Pain Med 2013;38:131–139.
3. Volltexte, et al: Cyclodextrins as drug carrier molecule: A review. Sci Pharm 2008;76:567–598.
4. Kulkarni PR, et al: Liposomes: A novel drug delivery system. Int J Curr Pharm Res 2011;3(2):10–18.
5. Formulary: Liposomal bupivacaine: A long acting local anesthetic for postsurgical analgesia.
6. Lambert WJ: DepoFoam multivesicular liposomes for the sustained release of macromolecules. In Rathbone MJ, Hadgraft J, Roberts MS, Lane ME (eds): *Modified Release Drug Delivery Technology*, 2nd ed. Informa Healthcare, 2008:207–214.
7. Angst MS, Drover DR: Pharmacology of drugs formulated with Depofoam: A sustained drug delivery system for parenteral administration using multivesicular liposome technologoy. Clin Pharmacokinet 2006;45(12):1153–1176.
8. Howell SB: Clinical applications of a novel sustained-release injectable drug delivery system: Depofoam technology. Cancer J 2001;7 (3): 219–227.
9. Bala I, et al: PLGA nanoparticles in drug delivery: the state of the art. Crit Rev Ther Drug Carrier Syst 2004;21(5):387–422.
10. Danhier F, et al: PLGA-based nanoparticles: An overview of biomedical applications. J Control Release 2012;161(2):505–522.
11. Pathak P, Nagarsenker M: Formulation and evaluation of lidocaine lipid nanosystems for dermal delivery. AAPS PharmSciTech 2009;10(3): 985–992.
12. Mundargi RC, et al: Nano/micro technologies for delivering macromolecular therapeutics using poly (D,L-lactide-co-glycolide) and its derivatives. J Control Release 2008;125(3):193–209.
13. *Marcaine (Bupivacaine HCl)* [US prescribing information]. Hospira Inc., 2009.
14. ISMP: *ISMP Calls for Safety Improvements in Use of Elastomeric Pain Relief Pumps*. Institute for Safe Medication Practices, 2009.
15. Richard BM, et al: Safety evaluation of EXPAREL (DepoFoam Bupivacaine) administered by repeated subcutaneous injection in rabbits and dogs: Species comparison. J Drug Deliv 2011;2011:467429.
16. Richard BM, Ott, LR, et al: The safety and tolerability evaluation of DepoFoam bupivacaine administered by incision wound infiltration in rabbits and dogs. Expert Opin Investig Drugs 2011;20(10):1327–1341.
17. Langford RM, et al: A single administration of depobupivacaine intraoperatively results in prolonged detectable plasma bupivacaine and analgesia in patients undergoing inguinal hernia repair. Presented at 62nd Postgraduate Assembly in Anesthesiology, December 12–16, 2008, New York, Poster 9088.
18. *Exparel (Bupivacaine Liposome Extended-Release Injectable Suspension)* [prescribing information]. Pacira Pharmaceuticals Inc., 2011.
19. Clinical Trial no SKY0402-C-110. An open-label, phase I study to assess the pharmacokinetics and safety of SKY0402 in subjects with impaired hepatic function. Pacira Pharmaceuticals Inc. (date on file).
20. Hadzic A, Abikhaled JA, Harmon WJ: Impact of volume expansion on the efficacy and pharmacokinetics of liposome bupivacaine. Local Reg Anesth 2015;8:105–111.
21. Gorfine SR, et al: Bupivacaine extended-release liposome injection for prolonged postsurgical analgesia in patients undergoing hemorrhoidectomy: A multicenter, randomized, double-blind, placebo-controlled trial. Dis Colon Rectum 2011;54(12)1552–1559.
22. Onel E, et al: Exparel, a liposomal bupivacaine local analgesic, extends pain relief and decreases opioid use. Presented at Annual Meeting of the American Society of Anesthesiologists, October 16–20, 2010, San Diego, CA.
23. Golf M, et al: A phase 3, randomized, placebo-controlled trial of DepoFoam® bupivacaine (extended-release bupivacaine local analgesic) in bunionectomy. Adv Ther 2011;28(9):776–788.
24. Clinical Trial no. SKY0402-C-210. A randomized, double-blind, active-control study to evaluate the safety and efficacy of a single local administration of SKY0402 for prolonged postoperative analgesia in subjects undergoing augmentation mammoplasty. Pacira Pharmaceuticals Inc. (date on file)
25. Butz DR, Shenaq DS, Rundell VL, et al: Postoperative pain and length of stay lowered by use of exparel in immediate, implant-based breast reconstruction. Plast Reconstr Surg Glob Open 2015;3(5):e391.
26. Bagsby DT, Ireland PH, Meneghini RM: Liposomal bupivacaine versus traditional periarticular injection for pain control after total knee arthroplasty. J Arthroplasty 2014;29(8):1687–1690.
27. Alijanipour et al: Peri-articular injection of liposomal bupivacaine offers no benefit over standard bupivacaine injection in total knee arthroplasty: a prospective, randomized, controlled trial. Presented at 2016 Annual Meeting of the American Academy of Orthopedic Surgeons, March 1, 2016. Orlando, FL.
28. Surdam JW, et al: The use of Exparel (liposomal bupivacaine) to manage postoperative pain in unilateral total knee arthroplasty patients. J Arthroplasty 2015;30:325–329.
29. Viscusi ER: The safety of liposome bupivacaine 2 years post-launch: A look back and a look forward. Expert Opin Drug Saf 2015;14(12): 1801–1803.

30. Ilfeld BM, Viscusi ER, Hadzic A, et al: Safety and side effect profile of liposome bupivacaine (Exparel) in peripheral nerve blocks. Reg Anesth Pain Med 2015;40(5):572–582.

31. McAlvin JB, et al: Multivesicular liposomal bupivacaine at the sciatic nerve. Biomaterials 2014;35:4557–4564.

32. Damjanovska M, Cvetko E, Hadzic A, et al: Neurotoxicity of perineural vs intraneural-extrafascicular injection of liposomal bupivacaine in the porcine model of sciatic nerve block. Anaesthesia 2015;70(12):1418–1426.

33. Ilfeld BM, et al: Liposomal bupivacaine as a single-injection peripheral nerve block: A dose-response study. Anesth Analg 2013;117:1248–1256.

34. Ilfeld BM, et al: Safety and side effect profile of liposome bupivacaine (Exparel) in peripheral nerve blocks. Reg Anesth Pain Med 2015;40:572–582.

35. Ilfeld BM, et al: A 4-day peripheral nerve block? Liposome bupivacaine: An introduction and update. ASA Newsletter 2014;78(8).

36. Viscusi ER, Candiotti KA, Onel E, Morren M, Ludbrook GL: The pharmacokinetics and pharmacodynamics of liposome bupivacaine administered via a single epidural injection to healthy volunteers. Reg Anesth Pain Med 2012;37(6):616–622.

37. Hadj A, et al: Safety and efficacy of extended-release bupivacaine local anesthetic in open hernia: A randomized controlled trial. ANZ J Surg 2012;82:251-257.

38. Sekar M, et al: Drug delivery of biologics: A controlled release strategy. Presented at IBC's 17th Annual TIDES Conference, May 3–6, 2015, San Diego, CA.

39. Shah J, et al: The PK profile of SABER-bupivacaine in humans across surgical models demonstrates sustained 72-hour drug delivery. Presented at 2014 Annual Meeting of the American Society of Anesthesiologists, October 15, 2014, New Orleans, LA.

40. Gan T, et al: SABER-bupivacaine reduced pain intensity for 72 hours following abdominal surgery relative to bupivacaine HCl. Presented at 2014 Annual Meeting of the American Society of Anesthesiologists, October 15, 2014, New Orleans, LA.

41. Cusack SL, et al: Clinical evaluation of XaraColl, a bupivacaine-collagen implant, for postoperative analgesia in two multicenter, randomized, double-blind, placebo-controlled pilot studies. J Pain Res 2012;5:217–225.

42. Cusack SL, et al: The pharmacokinetics and safety of an intraoperative bupivacaine-collagen implant (XaraColl®) for postoperative analgesia in women following total abdominal hysterectomy. J Pain Res 2013;6:151–159.

43. Hu D, et al: Pharmacokinetic profile of liposome bupivacaine injection following a single administration at the surgical site. Clin Drug Investig 2013;33:109–115.

44. Clinical Trial NCT02523599. A Phase 3, Randomized, Double-blind, Placebo-controlled Study to Investigate the Efficacy and Safety of the Xaracoll® Bupivacaine Implant (300mg Bupivacaine Hydrochloride) After Open Laparotomy Hernioplasty. Innocoll. (date on file)

Analgesic Adjuvants in the Peripheral Nervous System

Colin J. L. McCartney and Stephen Choi

NB: Several studies authored by Dr. S. Reuben that have since been retracted were referenced in the previous edition of this text. These references have been removed. All references remaining in which Dr. Reuben was involved that have not been retracted are still referenced.

INTRODUCTION

Peripheral nerve blocks provide many benefits for patients, including superior pain control and reduction in general anesthesia-related side effects. To optimize pain relief while reducing the total dose of local anesthetic, it would be of use to add a drug that both speeds onset and prolongs sensory blockade or analgesic effect. Improvements in our knowledge of peripheral nervous system (PNS) pain mechanisms allow us to develop methods of prolonging analgesia while reducing central and peripherally mediated adverse effects.

In the last 20 years, a number of drugs have been tested, and several have proven clinically useful when added to local anesthetic for peripheral nerve block or when used for local infiltration or intra-articular analgesia. These drugs are known as analgesic adjuvants.

This chapter examines the rationale and current evidence base for use of analgesic adjuvants and summarizes the best strategies for optimizing pain control and reducing adverse effects after surgery under peripheral nerve block, local infiltration, or injection of drugs in the intra-articular space.

RATIONALE FOR USE

Pain transmission in the CNS and PNS involves a complex array of neurotransmitters and pathways that are not easily blocked by one drug type or technique alone. Involvement of several classes of neurotransmitter at the injury site, peripheral nerve, dorsal horn of the spinal cord, and supraspinal sites is responsible for the transmission of nociception. Use of agonists at inhibitory receptors and antagonists at excitatory receptors allows a "multimodal" approach with optimization of pain control and reduction of adverse effects.[1]

In 1645, Descartes proposed a mechanism for pain transmission, suggesting that a peripheral pain impulse was transmitted directly from the periphery to the brain by a "hardwired" system without any intermediate modulation (Figure 9–1). This theory of pain transmission was widely held as true until as recently as 40 years ago.

In 1965, Melzack and Wall proposed their groundbreaking gate control theory of pain that suggested that pain could be modulated or "gated" at a number of points in the pain pathway. Subsequent research identified the dorsal horn (lamina II) of the spinal cord as an important site of potential modulation, and subsequent treatments for acute and chronic pain have utilized this knowledge to good effect. Treatments such as the use of spinal opioids and transcutaneous electrical nerve stimulation (TENS) have been developed in the light of this knowledge. The gate theory also changed many (often unsuccessful) pain management strategies from techniques where we tried to ablate pain pathways either chemically or surgically to more recent modulation techniques by which we attempt to inhibit excitatory influences and enhance inhibitory influences within the pain pathway.

In the last few decades, important advances have also occurred in our knowledge of how pain is generated and transmitted from the PNS to the central nervous system (CNS). Modulation of pain in the PNS also involves numerous transmitters and mechanisms that both excite and inhibit nociceptive pathways.

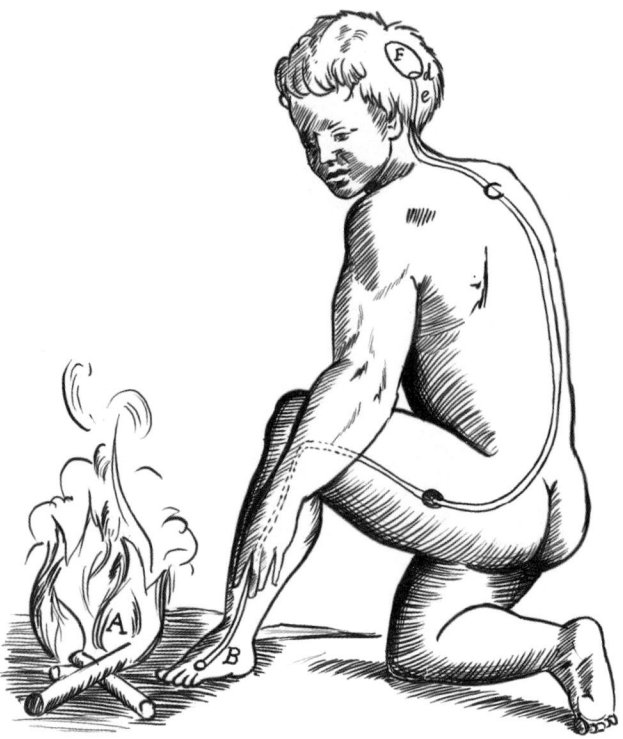

FIGURE 9–1. Descartes model of pain transmission in the peripheral nervous system.

In the PNS, under normal physiologic conditions nociceptive signals are produced when A-α and C fibers are stimulated by heat, pressure, or several chemicals produced by tissue damage and inflammation (potassium, histamine, bradykinin, prostaglandins, adenosine triphosphate [ATP]).[2] Nociceptive signals are transmitted to the superficial layers of lamina II of the dorsal horn in the spinal cord, where they are modulated at both the presynaptic and postsynaptic level and also by excitatory and inhibitory descending control pathways form the brainstem (Figure 9–2).[3] Signals that are successful in crossing this gate travel on to the brainstem and thalamus before reaching the cerebral cortex to produce a pain stimulus.

Chemical mediators in a wide array are produced in the PNS and have both excitatory and inhibitory influences on peripheral sensory nerve transmission[4] in both the acute and the chronic phase of injury (Figure 9–3).[5] These can directly activate the nerve (ATP, glutamate, 5-hydroxytryptamine [5-HT], histamine, bradykinin); enhance depolarization by sensitizing the nerve to other stimuli (prostaglandins, prostacyclin, and cytokines such as interleukins); or provide a regulatory role on the sensory neuron, inflammatory cells, and sympathetic fibers (bradykinin, tachykinin, and nerve growth factor).

RATIONALE FOR USE OF ANALGESIC ADJUVANTS

As previously noted, pain transmission in the CNS and PNS involves a complex array of neurotransmitters and pathways that are not easily blocked by one drug type or technique alone. A number of drugs in the anesthesiologist's armamentarium, including opioids, nonsteroidal anti-inflammatory drugs (NSAIDs), α_2-agonists, dexamethasone, and N-methyl-D-aspartate (NMDA) antagonists, have activity at these sites of action and may have benefit if applied in the PNS. Importantly, none has demonstrated neurotoxicity at clinically relevant concentrations.[6]

This knowledge can aid the regional anesthesiologist in a number of ways:

1. In the selection of adjuvants to local anesthetics to speed onset, prolong effect, and reduce total required dose.

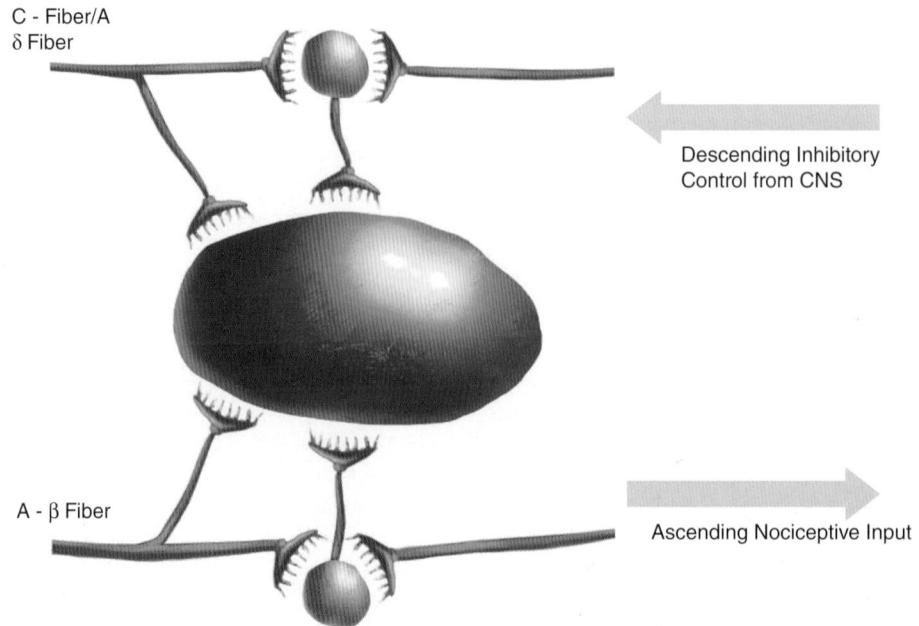

FIGURE 9–2. The gate theory proposed that small (C) fibers activated excitatory systems (black neuron) that subsequently excited output cells; these latter cells had their activity controlled by the balance of large fiber (A-β)-mediated inhibitions (mediated by endogenous opioids) and also by descending control systems from the central nervous system (mediated by norepinephrine and serotonin).

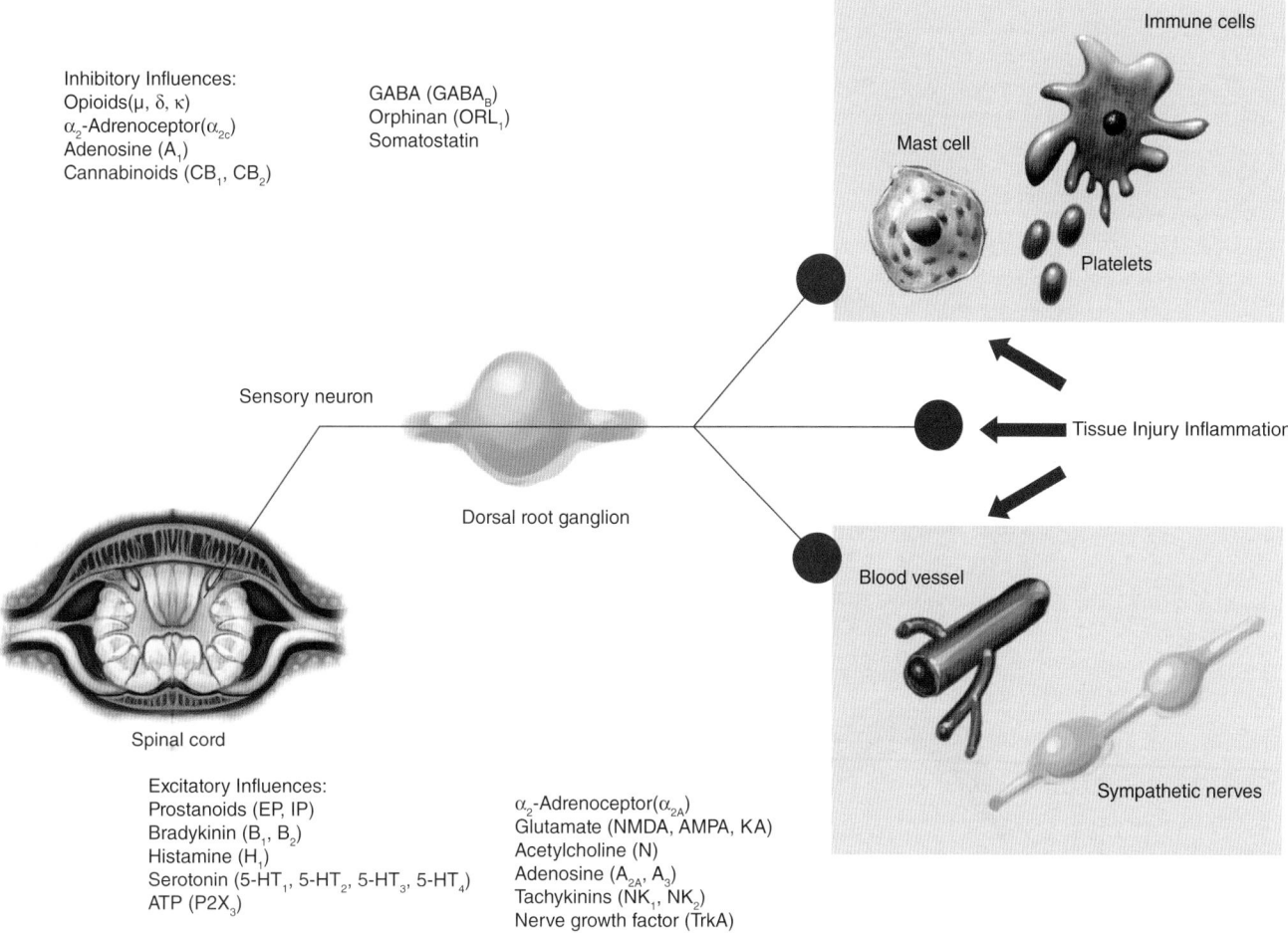

Inhibitory Influences:
Opioids(μ, δ, κ)
α_2-Adrenoceptor(α_{2c})
Adenosine (A_1)
Cannabinoids (CB_1, CB_2)

GABA ($GABA_B$)
Orphinan (ORL_1)
Somatostatin

Immune cells

Mast cell

Platelets

Sensory neuron

Tissue Injury Inflammation

Dorsal root ganglion

Blood vessel

Spinal cord

Sympathetic nerves

Excitatory Influences:
Prostanoids (EP, IP)
Bradykinin (B_1, B_2)
Histamine (H_1)
Serotonin (5-HT_1, 5-HT_2, 5-HT_3, 5-HT_4)
ATP ($P2X_3$)

α_2-Adrenoceptor(α_{2A})
Glutamate (NMDA, AMPA, KA)
Acetylcholine (N)
Adenosine (A_{2A}, A_3)
Tachykinins (NK_1, NK_2)
Nerve growth factor (TrkA)

FIGURE 9–3. Excitatory and inhibitory influences on peripheral nerve activity by mediators released by tissue injury and inflammation and by a variety of agents acting on neuroreceptors. AMPA = α-amino-3-hydroxy-5-methylisoxazole-4-propionic acid; KA = kainic acid; NMDA = N-methyl-D-aspartate; NK = neurokinin; TrkA = Tropomyosin receptor kinase A.

2. Suggest agents that can enhance postoperative analgesia without prolonging adverse effects of local anesthetics.

3. Suggest agents that predominantly act at peripheral sites without central effects, thereby optimizing analgesia while minimizing CNS side effects.

OPIOID ANALGESICS

During inflammation, opioid receptors are expressed in peripheral sensory fibers and immune cells[7]; moreover, endogenous opioids are released from these cells and balance the increased nociceptive state produced by inflammation.[8] An increasing body of work suggests an intimate relationship between endogenous opioids and the immune system. Christoph Stein and colleagues in Berlin have performed a number of pioneering studies[9,10] that described the ability of the immune system to deliver endogenous opioids and the ability of inflammation to stimulate movement of opioid receptors to the site of injury, thereby allowing antinociception to occur. However, these changes do not occur immediately after injury and can take up to 96 hours to occur.[11]

Opioid receptors and neuropeptides (eg, substance P) are synthesized in the dorsal root ganglion and transported along intra-axonal microtubules into central and peripheral processes of the primary afferent neuron (Figure 9–4). At the terminals, opioid receptors are incorporated into the neuronal membrane and become functional receptors. On activation by exogenous or endogenous opioids (released by immune cells), opioid receptors couple to inhibitory G proteins. This leads to direct or indirect (through decrease of cyclic adenosine monophosphate) suppression of Ca^{2+} or Na^+ currents and subsequent attenuation of substance P release. The permeability of the perineurium is increased within inflamed tissue, enhancing the ability of opioids to reach target receptors.

Numerous studies have applied opioids in the PNS to either peripheral nerves or the intra-articular space. Although many studies claimed an analgesic benefit of peripherally applied opioids, few studies incorporated a control group with a systemically applied opioid for comparison. Without inclusion of a control, it is impossible to interpret whether the peripheral opioid is having a true peripheral effect or is instead being carried to the CNS to induce analgesia. True peripherally mediated opioid analgesia may be beneficial if this is associated with improved analgesia or reduced adverse effects compared with systemic administration. If the effect is mediated centrally, then there is no clear benefit over systemic administration.

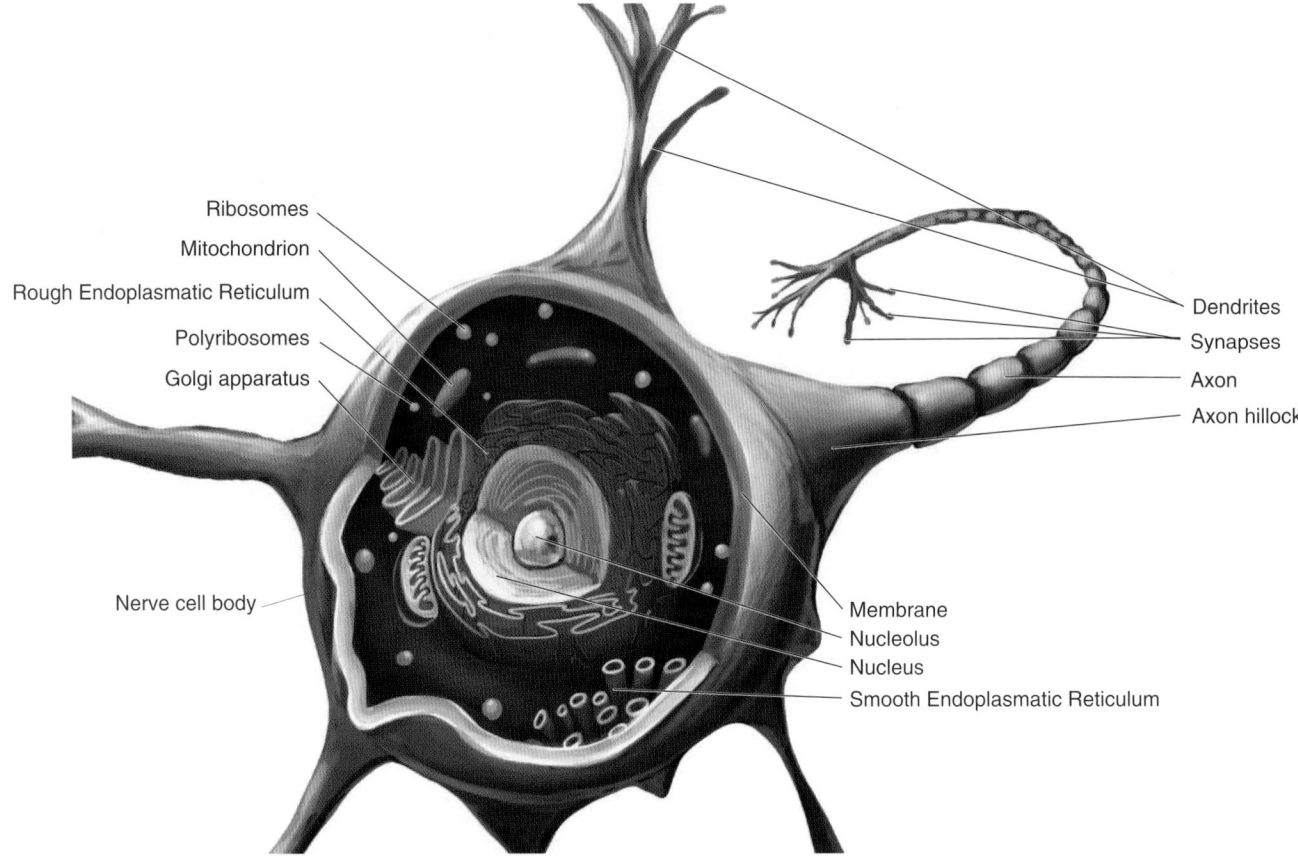

FIGURE 9–4. Opioid receptor transport and signaling in primary afferent neurons.

Perineural Opioids

Opioid receptors identified on primary afferent fibers are transported from the dorsal root ganglion to the site of inflammation; however, while they are undergoing axonal transport, they may not be easily reached by opioid agonists. This may explain the reason that two recent systematic reviews[12,13] published in 1997 and 2000 found little evidence for the benefit of adding opioids to local anesthetics in peripheral nerve blockade. An updated table of studies examining perineuronal administration of opioids[13–17] (excluding buprenorphine and tramadol) shows that analgesic benefit remains equivocal (Table 9–1). In addition, Peng and Choyce[18] reviewed the use of opioids in intravenous regional anesthesia (IVRA) with similar disappointing conclusions.

TABLE 9–1. Outcomes of studies examining the effect of perineuronal/perineural opioids (excluding tramadol and buprenorphine).

Total Studies	Overall Outcomes	Systemic Control Outcomes
19 studies	10 supportive	7 systemic control: 5 supportive; 2 negative
	9 negative	12 no systemic control: 5 supportive; 7 negative.

Despite these disappointing results, the two opioid agonists that have demonstrated analgesic efficacy when administered perineuronally are buprenorphine and tramadol. Buprenorphine is a partial μ-receptor agonist with a very high receptor affinity compared with fentanyl (24-fold) or morphine (50-fold). In addition, it has intermediate lipid solubility, which allows it to cross the neural membrane.[19,20] Candido and colleagues[21] added 0.3 mg buprenorphine (a partial opioid agonist) to a combination of mepivacaine and tetracaine in axillary block and found an almost 100% increase in the duration of analgesia compared with the administration of axillary block plus the same dose of intramuscular buprenorphine with no significant increase in adverse effects. This supports the peripheral analgesic effect of buprenorphine and the earlier findings of two studies that examined buprenorphine without a systemic control group.[22,23] Studies examining buprenorphine are presented in greater detail in Table 9–2.

Tramadol is a weak opioid agonist with some selectivity for the μ-receptor that also inhibits norepinephrine reuptake and stimulates serotonin release in the intrathecal space. Norepinephrine and serotonin are transmitters for the descending control pathway in the spinal cord and enhance analgesia.[24,25] Kapral and coworkers[26] used a 100-mg dose of tramadol as an adjuvant to mepivacaine in axillary brachial plexus block. They divided 60 patients into three groups: One group received mepivacaine 1% with 2 mL saline, the second group received mepivacaine 1% with 100 mg tramadol, and the third group received mepivacaine 1% with 2 mL saline and 100 mg

TABLE 9–2. Studies examining buprenorphine as an analgesic adjuvant with local anesthetics.

Author/ Date	Patients/ Groups	Block Type	Dose	Local Anesthetic	Systemic Control	Results
Viel[23] 1989	20/2	Supraclavicular	3 mcg/kg	Bupivacaine 0.5% 40 mL	No	Prolonged analgesia compared to morphine group (35 vs. 18.25 h); no difference in sensory block.
Bazin[24] 1997	89/4	Supraclavicular	3 µg/kg	Bupivacaine 0.5% Lidocaine 1%	No	Prolonged analgesia compared to control group (20 vs. 11.5 h)
Candido[22] 2001	40/2	Supraclavicular	0.3 mg	Mepivacaine 1% Tetracaine 0.2%	No	Prolonged analgesia compared to control group (17.4 vs. 5.3 h)
Candido[21] 2002	60/3	Axillary	0.3 mg	Mepivacaine 1% Tetracaine 0.2%	Yes IM	The mean duration of postoperative analgesia was 22.3 h in axillary group vs. 12.5 h in IM group and 6.6 h in placebo group.

IM = intramuscular

tramadol intravenously. This study demonstrated an increased duration of motor and sensory blockade in the axillary tramadol group that significantly ($p < .01$) outlasted both an intravenous and a placebo group. Robaux and colleagues[27] subsequently performed a dose-response study with placebo and 40-, 100-, and 200-mg doses of tramadol added to a fixed dose of mepivacaine 1.5% in axillary block and found that the 200-mg dose provided the best analgesia with no increased adverse effects. Alemanno and colleagues used a 1.5-mg/kg dose of tramadol as an adjuvant to 0.5% levobupivacaine (0.5 mL/kg) for interscalene block.[28] Here, 120 patients were divided into three groups: One group received local anesthetic alone, the second group received local anesthetic with systemic tramadol, and the third group received local anesthetic with perineural tramadol. While both groups receiving tramadol experienced prolonged analgesia compared to placebo, the group receiving perineural tramadol experienced prolonged analgesia compared to systemic tramadol (14.5 vs. 10.1 hours; $p < .001$).[28]

Intra-articular Opioids and Other Peripheral Routes of Administration

Opioid agonists administered into inflamed tissue will bind to opioid receptors on sensory terminals and induce analgesia. Animal studies indicated that these peripheral opioid receptors are expressed 96 hours after the initial inflammatory injury.[11] Intra-articular administration of opioids will therefore only produce analgesia in patients with preexisting inflammation. Kalso and coworkers[29] systematically examined the role of intra-articular opioids in 1997 and established that there existed evidence for a prolonged benefit from intra-articular

morphine without significant adverse effects at doses of 1 to 5 mg. No dose response was detected. Recent articles supported this finding and showed the benefit of intra-articular morphine,[30,31] tramadol,[32] buprenorphine,[33] and sufentanil.[34] However, a systematic review of the effects of intra-articular morphine demonstrated only a mild analgesic effect [visual analogue scale for pain (VAS) 12–17 mm reduction] but could not exclude that the effect was mediated by systemic absorption.[35]

ALPHA$_2$-AGONISTS AND CLONIDINE

Clonidine is an α_2-agonist with some α_1-stimulatory effects. It has traditionally been used as an antihypertensive agent and has been noted to have sedative and analgesic effects for many years. More recently, it was determined that α_2-receptors exist in the dorsal horn of the spinal cord, and stimulation of these receptors produces analgesic effects by inhibiting the presynaptic release of excitatory transmitters, including substance P and glutamate.[36-38] Intrathecal clonidine mediates analgesia by increasing acetylcholine levels, which in turn stimulates muscarinic receptors. Muscarinic excitation increases γ-amino butyric acid levels onto the primary afferent fiber, inhibiting the release of the excitatory neurotransmitter glutamate.[39]

Clonidine injected close to peripheral nerves with or without local anesthetic drugs appears to mediate analgesia in a number of ways. Clonidine has local anesthetic properties[40] and tonically inhibited compound action potentials of C fibers greater then A-α fibers in rat sciatic nerve and was comparable to lidocaine in its ability to inhibit C fibers in rabbit vagus nerve.[40,41] Clonidine also has a pharmacokinetic effect on local anesthetic redistribution mediated by a vasoconstrictor effect at the α_1-receptor.[42] Recent animal models have demonstrated and supported earlier work that clonidine predominantly facilitates peripheral nerve block through hyperpolarization-activated cationic current and that this effect is independent of any vasoconstrictor effect.[43]

A more recent addition to the selection of α_2-agonists is dexmedetomidine, which is selective for the α_2-receptor and which at present is mainly studied as a sedative agent in intensive care units. Dexmedetomidine may be expected to produce not only more profound analgesia but also greater adverse effects because of the selectivity of action.

Stimulation of the α_2-receptor produces hypotension, bradycardia, and sedation at higher doses, and these effects may outweigh any analgesic benefits produced by the use of these agents.

Perineuronal Application

Over 30 studies in humans have now examined the effect of clonidine on local anesthetics in peripheral nerve block. There is good evidence from these studies that clonidine in doses up to 1.5 µg/kg prolongs sensory block and analgesia when administered with local anesthetics for peripheral nerve block. This supports the early opinion of Murphy and colleagues[13] that clonidine is a beneficial adjuvant when added to peripheral nerve block and that the effect is most likely mediated in the PNS.

Although a number of studies have examined the effect of clonidine added to peripheral nerve block, only a few have controlled for a systemic effect. Singelyn and coworkers[44] evaluated 30 patients receiving an axillary brachial plexus block with 40 mL of 1% mepivacaine plus epinephrine 5 µg/mL. Patients were randomized to three groups and received (1) local anesthetic alone, (2) local anesthetic plus 150 µg of clonidine administered subcutaneously, or (3) 150 µg of clonidine in the brachial plexus block with local anesthetic. Clonidine added to the axillary brachial plexus block delayed the onset of pain twofold, without adverse effects when compared with systemic control.

Hutschala and coworkers[45] have recently demonstrated the peripheral analgesic effect of clonidine in volunteers when added to brachial plexus block with 0.25% bupivacaine. However, other recent studies demonstrated no overall benefit of adding clonidine to long-acting local anesthetics such as bupivacaine and ropivacaine.[46]

More recently, a meta-analysis by Popping and colleagues estimated that clonidine prolonged postoperative analgesia, sensory block, and motor block by 122, 74, and 141 minutes, respectively.[47] Clonidine, however, also increased the probability of hypotension (odds ratio [OR] 3.61), fainting (OR 5.07), sedation (OR 2.28), and bradycardia (OR 3.09). There was no observed dose response between a range of 30 and 300 µg, with the majority receiving 150 µg.

The addition of clonidine to continuous peripheral nerve blocks is not beneficial. Ilfeld and colleagues[48,49] have demonstrated in two studies that both 0.1 and 0.2 µg/mL of clonidine added to a continuous infusion of ropivacaine 0.2% failed to reduce pain scores or oral analgesic use after upper extremity surgery.

Dexmedetomidine, as previously postulated, does indeed produce a more profound effect on analgesia when applied perineurally in conjunction with local anesthetics. Four studies have recently examined this, and a meta-analysis suggested that dexmedetomidine prolongs the analgesic effects of brachial plexus blocks by 284 minutes. Interestingly, despite initial concerns that dexmedetomidine may have greater hemodynamic effects than clonidine, this does not appear to be the case.[50]

Intravenous Regional Anesthesia

Intravenous regional anesthesia is a useful, simple regional anesthetic technique especially for minor peripheral upper limb procedures that is limited by tourniquet tolerance and poor postoperative analgesia. Clonidine has been demonstrated in a number of studies to improve onset time[51] and intraoperative tourniquet tolerance.[52–54]

Only one study has demonstrated improved postoperative analgesia in the early postoperative period compared with placebo. Reuben and coworkers[49] randomized 45 patients to 40 mL 0.5% lidocaine with clonidine 1 µg/kg, lidocaine alone with intravenous clonidine, and lidocaine alone with intravenous saline. Patients who were given clonidine with lidocaine experienced significantly less pain and requested fewer analgesics then patients in the other two groups. Higher doses of clonidine (150 µg) produced significantly more sedation and incidence of hypotension.[52]

To date only one study has used dexmedetomidine in IVRA. Memis and colleagues[55] added 0.5 µg/kg of dexmedetomidine to 0.5% lidocaine and demonstrated reduction in onset time and improvement in postoperative analgesia compared with placebo with no significant adverse effects.

Intra-articular Techniques

The intra-articular effect of clonidine has been examined when administered with[56] and without local anesthetic[57–59] and been found to have beneficial effects on postoperative analgesia. The addition of morphine and clonidine may be expected to have additive effects. Two studies have examined this question, with one demonstrating improved analgesia[57] and the other no difference.[59]

Preclinical trials have demonstrated that, similar to opioids, clonidine-mediated analgesia is enhanced by inflammation, although at the present time the mechanism is not evident.[60]

DEXAMETHASONE

Dexamethasone is a potent synthetic corticosteroid with approximately seven times the anti-inflammatory potency of prednisolone[61] and very little mineralocorticoid activity. The half-life is approximately 36 to 54 hours in the perioperative setting. The effectiveness of dexamethasone as a postoperative antiemetic (4 to 10 mg intravenously) has been confirmed by over 60 randomized controlled trials, with a recent meta-analysis estimating on OR of 0.31 and a 3.7 number needed to treat (NNT).[62] Given its systemic anti-inflammatory properties, the analgesic effects of a single preoperative intravenous dose of dexamethasone have been investigated in over 24 randomized trials with modest effects up to 24 hours.[63] This meta-analysis, published in 2011, included 2751 patients and estimated that verbal rating scale for pain (VRS) scores were reduced to a maximum of 0.64 points up to 24 hours after dexamethasone administration.

Prior to these reviews, in vitro and murine studies of the specific pharmacologic action of dexamethasone yielded several novel applications in addition to systemic administration.

Perineural Application

Perineural corticosteroids are thought to exert their effect by several mechanisms, including attenuating the release of inflammatory mediators, reducing ectopic neuronal discharge, and inhibiting potassium channel–mediated discharge of nociceptive C fibers.[64–66] It is widely believed that dexamethasone improves the quality and duration of peripheral nerve blockade when administered in conjunction with local anesthetics. The US Food and Drug Administration (FDA) (or any other regulatory body), however, does not approve dexamethasone for perineural administration.

Nonetheless, multiple studies have assessed the effects of combining dexamethasone (4 to 10 mg) with local anesthetic for peripheral nerve blocks.[67–73] Upper and lower extremity peripheral nerve blocks performed with dexamethasone demonstrated prolongation of analgesia or sensory/motor block ranging from approximately 50% to 75% beyond that performed with local anesthetic alone.

Only one study to date has compared perineural to systemic dexamethasone in the context of peripheral nerve blocks.[73] This study randomized patients to interscalene brachial plexus block with placebo or 8 mg of perineural or systemic dexamethasone. The authors demonstrated block prolongation in both dexamethasone groups from 12 hours to approximately 20 and 22 hours for systemic and perineural administration, respectively, and concluded that systemic and perineural dexamethasone administration were equivalent. Further study is required comparing the effects of perineural and systemic dexamethasone before final conclusions can be drawn.

Concerns over complications related to dexamethasone, such as effects on blood glucose and neurotoxicity from the preservative used in multidose vials, have not been apparent in practice. In particular, a single dose of dexamethasone, whether administered perineurally or systemically, did not increase blood glucose to a clinically significant degree.[73–75] Murine studies of sodium bisulfite demonstrated no neurotoxicity with intrathecal administration.[76]

Intravenous Regional Anesthesia

Bigat and colleagues investigated the effects of adding dexamethasone to lidocaine IVRA in a randomized trial.[77] Seventy-five patients were randomized to lidocaine with placebo, 8 mg of dexamethasone with lidocaine, or 8 mg of systemic dexamethasone. In this study, systemic dexamethasone exerted no effect on the efficacy of IVRA, while lidocaine plus dexamethasone demonstrated improved block characteristics.

N-METHYL-D-ASPARTATE RECEPTOR ANTAGONISTS

Within the dorsal horn of the spinal cord both ionotropic [N-methyl-D-aspartate (NMDA)], α-amino-3-hydroxy-5-methylisoxazole-4-propionic acid (AMPA), kainic acid (KA), and metabotropic glutamate receptors are involved in nociceptive signaling and central sensitization in conditions of chronic pain.[78–90] Recently, multiple glutamate receptors have been found in peripheral nerve terminals and may contribute to peripheral pain signaling.[81] Injection of the NMDA receptor agonist glutamate into masseter muscle produces pain in both rats and humans.[82,83] Subsequent injection of NMDA receptor antagonists such as ketamine and dextromethorphan attenuates the pain.[84]

A number of studies have examined the effect of NMDA antagonists in producing peripherally mediated analgesia in patients. Tverskoy and colleagues[85] infiltrated bupivacaine with 0.3% ketamine or placebo for patients having inguinal herniorraphy and found that ketamine significantly enhanced the anesthetic and analgesic actions of a local anesthetic administered for infiltration anesthesia. Ketamine has been used as the sole anesthetic in IVRA, but patients suffered excessive adverse effects on tourniquet deflation.[86] Other workers have added ketamine (0.1 mg/mL) or clonidine (1 µg/kg) to lidocaine for IVRA.[87] Patients in the ketamine group had the best pain control, although both clonidine and ketamine significantly reduced analgesic consumption compared with lidocaine alone, with mild psychomimetic side effects in the ketamine group.

Two studies have examined the use of intra-articular ketamine. Dal and coworkers[88] randomized patients to intra-articular ketamine (0.5 mg/kg), neostigmine, bupivacaine, or placebo. Patients receiving all three drugs had similar improvements in analgesia with knee flexion compared with placebo; however, the ketamine group had the longest duration of analgesia. Brill and colleagues[89] performed a dose-response study using up to 1 mg/kg intra-articular ketamine after knee arthroscopy and found that the analgesic benefit only occurred in the first hour after surgery compared with placebo.

Magnesium has NMDA-blocking effects and blocks the ion channel on the NMDA receptor during normal physiologic states. Persistent nociceptive input in the dorsal horn of the spinal cord removes magnesium, allowing calcium influx and intracellular changes leading to persistent pain states.[80]

Turan et al[90] exploited this analgesic potential in the PNS by adding 1.5 g magnesium to lidocaine 0.5% for IVRA. Magnesium reduced onset time and significantly prolonged analgesic effect up to 6 hours after surgery with no difference in adverse effects.

Overall, NMDA antagonists may have significant potential for producing peripherally mediated analgesia in the future, although currently available agents (except magnesium in IVRA) have limited effects and at higher doses produce excessive adverse effects.

CYCLOOXYGENASE INHIBITION

Prostaglandins sensitize peripheral nerve endings to the effects of endogenous chemical mediators released during tissue injury. NSAIDs inhibit the production of prostaglandins through their well-known effect of inhibiting cyclooxygenase (COX). Application of NSAIDs directly in the PNS would therefore appear to make sense as a means of reducing pain by peripheral mechanism.

Intravenous Regional Anesthesia

A number of authors have added ketorolac to IVRA in doses from 5 to 60 mg, producing an improvement in intraoperative tourniquet tolerance and postoperative analgesia.[90] Steinberg and colleagues[91] performed a dose-response study with ketorolac in IVRA using placebo, 5-, 10-, 15-, 20-, 30-, and 60-mg doses of ketorolac. It was found that 20 mg was the ideal dose, with lower doses producing less analgesia and higher doses being no more effective.

Lysine acetylsalicylic acid 90 mg (equivalent to 50 mg acetylsalicylic acid) has been added to prilocaine for IVRA with prolongation of postoperative analgesia.[92]

Intra-articular Administration

The use of ketorolac alone, with local anesthetic or local anesthetic and morphine, is no more effective then local anesthetic alone when administered in the intra-articular space.

Infiltration

Ketorolac has been successfully infiltrated in a dose of 30 to 60 mg following hernia repair, giving an effect similar to infiltration with bupivacaine. However, local infiltration was found to be no more effective than systemic administration.[93–97]

CHOLINERGIC ANALGESIA

Muscarinic receptors mediate analgesia in the dorsal horn of the spinal cord, and neostigmine has produced analgesia when administered to both the intrathecal and epidural space.

Neostigmine has also been applied in the PNS in a number of studies, with generally disappointing results. Van Elstraete and coworkers[98] and Bone and colleagues[99] added neostigmine 500 μg to local anesthetic in axillary brachial plexus block. One study demonstrated no difference,[97] and the other found only significant reduction in pain at 24 hours, with no difference at other time points.[98]

Neostigmine added to local anesthetic for IVRA has also been disappointing. Turan and coworkers[100] added 500 μg neostigmine to prilocaine 0.5% and found improvement in sensory and motor block onset and offset with prolonged time to first analgesic request. However, McCartney and colleagues[101] performed a similar study using neostigmine 1 mg added to lidocaine 0.5%, with no differences found between groups. Overall, neostigmine appears disappointing as an analgesic adjuvant for peripheral nerve block or IVRA.

Neostigmine, however, has been used successfully as an analgesic adjuvant for intra-articular use after knee arthroscopy.[88,101–103] Yang and coworkers[102] performed a dose-response study and found 500 μg to be most effective, which was more effective than 2 mg of intra-articular morphine.

The effectiveness of the intra-articular cholinergic analgesic pathway compared with the poor results with perineuronal

TABLE 9–3. Best analgesic adjuvants in the peripheral nervous system by route of administration.

Route	Agent and Dose
Perineuronal/ perineural	Dexamethasone 4–10 mg; buprenorphine 0.3 mg; clonidine 1–2 μg/kg; tramadol 200 mg
IVRA	Dexmedetomidine 0.5 μg/kg; magnesium 1.5 g
Intra-articular	Clonidine 150 μg; morphine 5 mg
Local infiltration	Ketamine 3 mg/mL

application may be related to the presence of the inflammatory response in the intra-articular space, increasing the analgesic efficacy of acetylcholine by a mechanism that is yet to be defined.

SUMMARY

Peripheral nerve blocks provide significant anesthetic and analgesic benefits for our patients. Analgesic adjuvants such as opioids, α_2-agonists, NMDA receptor antagonists, and other agents can be added to local anesthetics both to facilitate onset and to prolong anesthetic and analgesic effects by mechanisms existing in the PNS. Several agents are effective when administered in the perineuronal or intra-articular space and when given in IVRA or local infiltration (Table 9–3). The effect size of each particular adjuvant is variable, with dexamethasone producing the largest effect size.

Our evolving knowledge of nociceptive mechanisms in the PNS will allow novel techniques to be developed in the future to further improve pain management.

REFERENCES

1. Kehlet H, Dahl JB: The value of "multimodal" or "balanced analgesia" in postoperative pain treatment. Anesth Analg 1993;77:1048–1056.
2. Raja SN, Meyer RA, Ringkamp M, et al: Peripheral neural mechanisms of nociception. In Wall PD, Melzack R (eds): *Textbook of Pain,* 4th ed. Churchill-Livingstone, 1999, pp 11–57.
3. Dickenson AH: Gate control theory of pain stands the test of time. Br J Anaesth 2002;88:755–757.
4. Millan MJ: The induction of pain: An integrative review. Prog Neurobiol 1999;57:1–164.
5. Sawynok J: Topical and peripherally acting analgesics. Pharmacol Rev 2003;55:1–20.
6. Williams BA, Hough KA, Tsui BY, Ibinson JW, Gold MS, Gebhart GF: Neurotoxicity of adjuvants used in perineural anesthesia and analgesia in comparison with ropivacaine. Reg Anesth Pain Med 2011; 36(3): 225–230.
7. Likar R, Mousa SA, Philippitsch G, et al: Increased numbers of opioid expressing inflammatory cells do not affect intraarticular morphine analgesia. Br J Anaesth 2004;93:375–380.
8. Brack A, Rittner HL, Machelska H, et al: Control of inflammatory pain by chemokine-mediated recruitment of opioid-containing polymorphonuclear cells. Pain 2004;112:229–238.
9. Machelska H, Cabot PJ, Mousa SA, et al: Pain control in inflammation governed by selectins. Nat Med 1998;4:1425–1428.
10. Stein C, Schafer M, Machelska H: Attacking pain at its source: New perspectives on opioids. Nat Med 2003;9:1003–1008.

11. Mousa SA, Zhang Q, Sitte N, et al: beta-Endorphin-containing memory-cells and mu-opioid receptors undergo transport to peripheral inflamed tissue. J Neuroimmunol 200;115:71–78.

12. Picard PR, Tramer MR, McQuay HJ, et al: Analgesic efficacy of peripheral opioids (all except intra-articular): A qualitative systematic review of randomised controlled trials. Pain 1997;72:309–318.

13. Murphy DB, McCartney CJ, Chan VW: Novel analgesic adjuncts for brachial plexus block: A systematic review. Anesth Analg 2000;90:1122–1128.

14. Fanelli G, Casati A, Magistris L, et al: Fentanyl does not improve the nerve block characteristics of axillary brachial plexus anaesthesia performed with ropivacaine. Acta Anaesthesiol Scand 2001;45:590–594.

15. Karakaya D, Buyukgoz F, Baris S, et al: Addition of fentanyl to bupivacaine prolongs anesthesia and analgesia in axillary brachial plexus block. Reg Anesth Pain Med 2001;26:434–438.

16. Likar R, Koppert W, Blatnig H, et al: Efficacy of peripheral morphine analgesia in inflamed, non-inflamed and perineural tissue of dental surgery patients. J Pain Symptom Manage 2001;21:330–337.

17. Nishikawa K, Kanaya N, Nakayama M, et al: Fentanyl improves analgesia but prolongs the onset of axillary brachial plexus block by peripheral mechanism. Anesth Analg 2000;91:384–387.

18. Choyce A, Peng P: A systematic review of adjuncts for intravenous regional anesthesia for surgical procedures. Can J Anaesth 2002;49:32–45.

19. Gutstein H, Akil H: Opioid analgesics. In Hardman J, Limbird L (eds): *Goodman & Gilman's The Pharmacologic Basis of Therapeutics,* 10th ed. McGraw-Hill, 2001, p 601.

20. Lanz E, Simko G, Theiss D, et al: Epidural buprenorphine—A double-blind study of postoperative analgesia and side effects. Anesth Analg 1984;63:593–598.

21. Candido KD, Winnie AP, Ghaleb AH, et al: Buprenorphine added to the local anesthetic for axillary brachial plexus block prolongs postoperative analgesia. Reg Anesth Pain Med 2002;27:162–167.

22. Candido KD, Franco CD, Khan MA, et al: Buprenorphine added to the local anesthetic for brachial plexus block to provide postoperative analgesia in outpatients. Reg Anesth Pain Med 2001;26:352–356.

23. Viel EJ, Eledjam JJ, De La Coussaye JE, et al: Brachial plexus block with opioids for postoperative pain relief: Comparison between buprenorphine and morphine. Reg Anesth 1989;14:274–278.

24. Bazin JE, Massoni C, Bruelle P, et al: The addition of opioids to local anaesthetics in brachial plexus block: The comparative effects of morphine, buprenorphine and sufentanil. Anaesthesia 1997;52:858–862.

25. Alhashemi JA, Kaki AM: Effect of intrathecal tramadol administration on postoperative pain after transurethral resection of prostate. Br J Anaesth 2003;91:536–540.

26. Kapral S, Gollmann G, Waltl B, et al: Tramadol added to mepivacaine prolongs the duration of an axillary brachial plexus blockade. Anesth Analg 1999;88:853–856.

27. Robaux S, Blunt C, Viel E, et al: Tramadol added to 1.5% mepivacaine for axillary brachial plexus block improves postoperative analgesia dose-dependently. Anesth Analg 2004;98:1172–1177.

28. Alemmano F, Ghisi D, Fanelli A, et al: Tramodol and 0.5% levobupivacaine for single shot interscalene block. Minerva Anestesiol 2013;78(3): 291–296.

29. Kalso E, Tramer MR, Carroll D, et al: Pain relief from intra-articular morphine after knee surgery: A qualitative systematic review. Pain 1997;71:127–134.

30. Brandsson S, Karlsson J, Morberg P, et al: Intraarticular morphine after arthroscopic ACL reconstruction: A double-blind placebo-controlled study of 40 patients. Acta Orthop Scand 2000;71:280–285.

31. Rasmussen S, Larsen AS, Thomsen ST, et al: Intra-articular glucocorticoid, bupivacaine and morphine reduces pain, inflammatory response and convalescence after arthroscopic meniscectomy. Pain 1998;78:131–134.

32. Alagol A, Calpur OU, Kaya G, et al: The use of intraarticular tramadol for postoperative analgesia after arthroscopic knee surgery: A comparison of different intraarticular and intravenous doses. Knee Surg Sports Traumatol Arthrosc 2004;12:184–188.

33. Varrassi G, Marinangeli F, Ciccozzi A, et al: Intra-articular buprenorphine after knee arthroscopy. A randomised, prospective, double-blind study. Acta Anaesthesiol Scand 1999;43:51–55.

34. Vranken JH, Vissers KC, de Jongh R, et al: Intraarticular sufentanil administration facilitates recovery after day-case knee arthroscopy. Anesth Analg 2001;92:625–628.

35. Gupta A, Bodin L, Holmstrom B, Berggren: A systematic review of the peripheral analgesic effects of intraarticular morphine. Anesth Analg 2001;93(3):761–770.

36. Unnerstall JR, Kopajtic TA, Kuhar MJ: Distribution of alpha 2 agonist binding sites in the rat and human central nervous system: Analysis of some functional, anatomic correlates of the pharmacologic effects of clonidine and related adrenergic agents. Brain Res 1984;319:69–101.

37. Kuraishi Y, Hirota N, Sato Y, et al: Noradrenergic inhibition of the release of substance P from the primary afferents in the rabbit spinal dorsal horn. Brain Res 1985;359:177–182.

38. Fleetwood-Walker SM, Mitchell R, Hope PJ, et al: An alpha 2 receptor mediates the selective inhibition by noradrenaline of nociceptive responses of identified dorsal horn neurones. Brain Res 1985;334:243–254.

39. Baba H, Kohno T, Okamoto M, et al: Muscarinic facilitation of GABA release in substantia gelatinosa of the rat spinal dorsal horn. J Physiol 1998;508:83–93.

40. Butterworth JF 5th, Strichartz GR: The alpha 2-adrenergic agonists clonidine and guanfacine produce tonic and phasic block of conduction in rat sciatic nerve fibers. Anesth Analg 1993;76:295–301.

41. Gaumann DM, Brunet PC, Jirounek P: Clonidine enhances the effects of lidocaine on C-fiber action potential. Anesth Analg 1992;74:719–725.

42. Eisenach JC, Gebhart GF: Intrathecal amitriptyline. Antinociceptive interactions with intravenous morphine and intrathecal clonidine, neostigmine, and carbamylcholine in rats. Anesthesiology 1995;83:1036–1045.

43. Kroin JS, Buvanendran A, Beck DR, et al: Clonidine prolongation of lidocaine analgesia after sciatic nerve block in rats is mediated via the hyperpolarization-activated cation current, not by alpha-adrenoreceptors. Anesthesiology 2004;101:488–494.

44. Singelyn FJ, Dangoisse M, Bartholomee S, et al: Adding clonidine to mepivacaine prolongs the duration of anesthesia and analgesia after axillary brachial plexus block. Reg Anesth 1992;17:148–150.

45. Hutschala D, Mascher H, Schmetterer L, et al: Clonidine added to bupivacaine enhances and prolongs analgesia after brachial plexus block via a local mechanism in healthy volunteers. Eur J Anaesthesiol 2004;21:198–204.

46. Culebras X, Van Gessel E, Hoffmeyer P, et al: Clonidine combined with a long acting local anesthetic does not prolong postoperative analgesia after brachial plexus block but does induce hemodynamic changes. Anesth Analg 2001;92:199–204.

47. Popping DM, Elia N, Marret E, Wenk M, Tramer MR. Clonidine as an adjuvant to local anesthetics for peripheral nerve and plexus blocks: A meta-analysis of randomized trials. Anesthesiology 2009;111(2):406–415.

48. Ilfeld BM, Morey TE, Enneking FK: Continuous infraclavicular perineural infusion with clonidine and ropivacaine compared with ropivacaine alone: A randomized, double-blinded, controlled study. Anesth Analg 2003;97:706–712.

49. Ilfeld BM, Morey TE, Thannikary LJ, et al: Clonidine added to a continuous interscalene ropivacaine perineural infusion to improve postoperative analgesia: A randomized, double-blind, controlled study. Anesth Analg 2005;100:1172–1178.

50. Abdallah FW, Brull R: Facilitatory effects of perineural dexmedetomidine on neuraxial and peripheral nerve block: a systematic review and meta-analysis. Br J Anaesth 2013;110(6):915–925.

51. Alayurt S, Memis D, Pamukcu Z: The addition of sufentanil, tramadol or clonidine to lignocaine for intravenous regional anaesthesia. Anaesth Intensive Care 2004;32:22–27.

52. Gentili M, Bernard JM, Bonnet F: Adding clonidine to lidocaine for intravenous regional anesthesia prevents tourniquet pain. Anesth Analg 1999;88:1327–1330.

53. Reuben SS, Steinberg RB, Klatt JL, et al: Intravenous regional anesthesia using lidocaine and clonidine. Anesthesiology 1999;91:654–658.

54. Lurie SD, Reuben SS, Gibson CS, et al: Effect of clonidine on upper extremity tourniquet pain in healthy volunteers. Reg Anesth Pain Med 2000;25:502–505.

55. Memis D, Turan A, Karamanlioglu B, et al: Adding dexmedetomidine to lidocaine for intravenous regional anesthesia. Anesth Analg 2004;98:835–840.

56. Joshi W, Reuben SS, Kilaru PR, et al: Postoperative analgesia for outpatient arthroscopic knee surgery with intraarticular clonidine and/or morphine. Anesth Analg 2000;90:1102–1106.

57. Tan PH, Buerkle H, Cheng JT, et al: Double-blind parallel comparison of multiple doses of apraclonidine, clonidine, and placebo administered intra-articularly to patients undergoing arthroscopic knee surgery. Clin J Pain 2004;20:256–260.

58. Gentili M, Juhel A, Bonnet F: Peripheral analgesic effect of intraarticular clonidine. Pain 1996;64:593–596.

59. Gentili M, Houssel P, Osman M, et al: Intra-articular morphine and clonidine produce comparable analgesia but the combination is not more effective. Br J Anaesth 1997;79:660–661.

60. Buerkle H, Schapsmeier M, Bantel C, et al: Thermal and mechanical antinociceptive action of spinal vs peripherally administered clonidine in the rat inflamed knee joint model. Br J Anaesth 1999;83:436–441.

61. Adrenal cortical steroids. In *Drug Facts and Comparisons*, 5th ed. Facts and Comparisons, 1997, pp 122–128.

62. De Oliveira GS Jr, Castro-Alves LJ, Ahmad S, Kendall MC, McCarthy RJ: Dexamethasone to prevent postoperative nausea and vomiting: An updated meta-analysis of randomized controlled trials. Anesth Analg 2013;116(1):58–74.

63. De Oliveira GS Jr, Almeida MD, Benzon HT, McCarthy RJ: Perioperative single dose systemic dexamethasone for postoperative pain: A meta-analysis of randomized controlled trials. Anesthesiology 2011;115(3): 575–588.

64. Attardi B, Takimoto K, Gealy R, Severns C, Levitan ES: Glucocorticoid induced up-regulation of a pituitary K⁺ channel mRNA in vitro and in vivo. Receptors Channels 1993;1:287–293.

65. Eker HE, Cok OY, Aribogan A, Arslan G: Management of neuropathic pain with methylprednisolone at the site of nerve injury. Pain Med 2012;13:443–451.

66. Johansson A, Hao J, Sjolund B: Local corticosteroid application blocks transmission in normal nociceptive C-fibres. Acta Anaesthesiol Scand 1990;34:335–338.

67. Cummings KC 3rd, Napierkowski DE, Parra-Sanchez I, et al: Effect of dexamethasone on the duration of interscalene nerve blocks with ropivacaine or bupivacaine. Br J Anaesth 2011;107:446–453.

68. Fredrickson MJ, Danesh-Clough TK, White R: Adjuvant dexamethasone for bupivacaine sciatic and ankle blocks: Results from 2 randomized placebo-controlled trials. Reg Anesth Pain Med 2013;38(4):300–307.

69. Movafegh A, Razazian M, Hajimaohamadi F, Meysamie A: Dexamethasone added to lidocaine prolongs axillary brachial plexus blockade. Anesth Analg 2006;102:263–267.

70. Parrington SJ, O'Donnell D, Chan VW, et al: Dexamethasone added to mepivacaine prolongs the duration of analgesia after supraclavicular brachial plexus blockade. Reg Anesth Pain Med 2010;35:422–426.

71. Tandoc MN, Fan L, Kolesnikov S, Kruglov A, Nader ND: Adjuvant dexamethasone with bupivacaine prolongs the duration of interscalene block: A prospective randomized trial. J Anesth 2011;25:704–709.

72. Vieira PA, Pulai I, Tsao GC, Manikantan P, Keller B, Connelly NR. Dexamethasone with bupivacaine increases duration of analgesia in ultrasound-guided interscalene brachial plexus blockade. Eur J Anaesthesiol 2010;27:285–288.

73. Desmet M, Braems H, Reynvoet M, et al: I.V. and perineural dexamethasone are equivalent in increasing the analgesic duration of a single-shot interscalene block with ropivacaine for shoulder surgery: A prospective, randomized, placebo-controlled study. Br J Anaesth 2013; 111(3):445–452. Epub ahead of print.

74. Thangaswamy CR, Rewari V, Trikha A, Dehran M, Chandralekha: Dexamethasone before total laparoscopic hysterectomy: A randomized controlled dose-response study. J Anesth 2010;24:24–30.

75. Worni M, Schudel HH, Seifert E, et al: Randomized controlled trial on single dose steroid before thyroidectomy for benign disease to improve postoperative nausea, pain, and vocal function. Ann Surg 2008;248: 1060–1066.

76. Taniguchi M, Bollen AW, Drasner K. Sodium bisulfite: Scapegoat for chloroprocaine neurotoxicity? Anesthesiology 2004;100(1):85–91.

77. Bigat Z, Boztug N, Hadimioglu N, Cete N, Coskunfirat N, Ertok E: Does dexamethasone improve the quality of intravenous regional anesthesia and analgesia? A randomized, controlled clinical study. Anesth Analg 2006;102(2):605–609.

78. Coderre TJ, Katz J, Vaccarino AL, et al: Contribution of central neuroplasticity to pathological pain: Review of clinical and experimental evidence. Pain 1993;52:259–285.

79. Price DD, Mao J, Mayer DJ: Central neural mechanisms of normal and abnormal pain states. In Fields HL, Liebskind JC (eds): *Progress in Pain Research and Management.* IASP Press, 1994;61–84.

80. Dickenson AH, Chapman V, Green GM: The pharmacology of excitatory and inhibitory amino acid-mediated events in the transmission and modulation of pain in the spinal cord. Gen Pharmacol 1997;28: 633–638.

81. Alfredson H, Forsgren S, Thorsen K, et al: Glutamate NMDAR1 receptors localised to nerves in human Achilles tendons. Implications for treatment? Knee Surg Sports Traumatol Arthrosc 2001;9:123–126.

82. Cairns BE, Hu JW, Arendt-Nielsen L, et al: Sex-related differences in human pain and rat afferent discharge evoked by injection of glutamate into the masseter muscle. J Neurophysiol 2001;86:782–791.

83. Svensson P, Cairns BE, Wang K, et al: Injection of nerve growth factor into human masseter muscle evokes long-lasting mechanical allodynia and hyperalgesia. Pain 2003;104:241–247.

84. Cairns BE, Svensson P, Wang K, et al: Activation of peripheral NMDA receptors contributes to human pain and rat afferent discharges evoked by injection of glutamate into the masseter muscle. J Neurophysiol 2003;90:2098–2105.

85. Tverskoy M, Oren M, Vaskovich M, et al: Ketamine enhances local anesthetic and analgesic effects of bupivacaine by peripheral mechanism: A study in postoperative patients. Neurosci Lett 1996;215:5–8.

86. Amiot JF, Bouju P, Palacci JH, et al: Intravenous regional anaesthesia with ketamine. Anaesthesia 1985;40:899–901.

87. Gorgias NK, Maidatsi PG, Kyriakidis AM, et al: Clonidine versus ketamine to prevent tourniquet pain during intravenous regional anesthesia with lidocaine. Reg Anesth Pain Med 2001;26:512–517.

88. Dal D, Tetik O, Altunkaya H, et al: The efficacy of intra-articular ketamine for postoperative analgesia in outpatient arthroscopic surgery. Arthroscopy 2004;20:300–305.

89. Brill S, McCartney CJ, Sawyer R, et al: Intra-articular ketamine analgesia following knee arthroscopy: A dose finding study. Pain Clin 2005;17: 25–29.

90. Turan A, Memis D, Karamanlioglu B, et al: Intravenous regional anesthesia using lidocaine and magnesium. Anesth Analg 2005;100: 1189–1192.

91. Reuben SS, Steinberg RB, Kreitzer JM, et al: Intravenous regional anesthesia using lidocaine and ketorolac. Anesth Analg 1995;81: 110–113.

92. Steinberg RB, Reuben SS, Gardner G: The dose-response relationship of ketorolac as a component of intravenous regional anesthesia with lidocaine. Anesth Analg 1998;86:791–793.

93. Corpataux JB, Van Gessel EF, Donald FA, et al: Effect on postoperative analgesia of small-dose lysine acetylsalicylate added to prilocaine during intravenous regional anesthesia. Anesth Analg 1997;84:1081–1085.

94. Reuben SS, Duprat KM: Comparison of wound infiltration with ketorolac versus intravenous regional anesthesia with ketorolac for postoperative analgesia following ambulatory hand surgery. Reg Anesth 1996;21:565–568.

95. Ben-David B, Katz E, Gaitini L, et al: Comparison of IM and local infiltration of ketorolac with and without local anaesthetic. Br J Anaesth 1995;75:409–412.

96. Connelly NR, Reuben SS, Albert M, et al: Use of preincisional ketorolac in hernia patients: Intravenous versus surgical site. Reg Anesth 1997; 22:229–232.

97. Bosek V, Cox CE: Comparison of analgesic effect of locally and systemically administered ketorolac in mastectomy patients. Ann Surg Oncol 1996;3:62–66.

98. Van Elstraete AC, Pastureau F, Lebrun T, et al: Neostigmine added to lidocaine axillary plexus block for postoperative analgesia. Eur J Anaesthesiol 2001;18:257–260.

99. Bone HG, Van Aken H, Booke M, et al: Enhancement of axillary brachial plexus block anesthesia by coadministration of neostigmine. Reg Anesth Pain Med 1999;24:405–410.

100. Turan A, Karamanlyoglu B, Memis D, et al: Intravenous regional anesthesia using prilocaine and neostigmine. Anesth Analg 2002;95(5): 1419–1422.

101. McCartney CJ, Brill S, Rawson R, et al: No anesthetic or analgesic benefit of neostigmine 1 mg added to intravenous regional anesthesia with lidocaine 0.5% for hand surgery. Reg Anesth Pain Med 2003;28: 414–417.

102. Yang LC, Chen LM, Wang CJ, et al: Postoperative analgesia by intra-articular neostigmine in patients undergoing knee arthroscopy. Anesthesiology 1998;88:334–339.

103. Gentili M, Enel D, Szymskiewicz O, et al: Postoperative analgesia by intraarticular clonidine and neostigmine in patients undergoing knee arthroscopy. Reg Anesth Pain Med 2001;26:342–347.

CHAPTER 10

Local Anesthetic Mixtures for Peripheral Nerve Blocks

Jason Choi and Jeff Gadsden

INTRODUCTION

Peripheral nerve blocks (PNBs) provide numerous advantages for surgical patients when used either as an analgesic supplement or as an alternative to general anesthesia. These advantages include superior pain control and avoidance of adverse effects associated with volatile anesthetics and opioids.[1] However, the benefits of PNBs are limited by the pharmacodynamics of the local anesthetic agents injected. Analgesia provided by PNBs lasts only as long as the duration of action of the local anesthetic at specific tissue sites. Typically, local anesthetics are characterized according to their latency ("onset time") and duration of action. For practical clinical purposes, local anesthetics can be grouped into one of three categories: (1) rapid onset and short duration (eg, chloroprocaine, procaine); (2) rapid onset and intermediate duration (eg, lidocaine, mepivacaine); and (3) slower onset and long duration (eg, bupivacaine, ropivacaine, tetracaine).[2]

An ideal local anesthetic for a PNB would have a fast onset coupled with a long duration and low toxicity.[3] At present, no such drug exists. In an attempt to achieve a single-injection PNB with characteristics close to ideal, mixtures of local anesthetics (most commonly, faster-onset, intermediate-duration local anesthetic and slower-onset, long-duration local anesthetic) for PNBs have been used clinically and have remained a common practice for over a century.[3–6] While compounding two drugs to obtain the "best" features of each is compelling, few studies have objectively examined the pharmacodynamics of mixtures of local anesthetics. Moreover, because many of the existing studies were conducted before the era of ultrasound guidance, it is difficult to extrapolate those data to current practice given the reduced volumes and doses of local anesthetic ultrasound guidance affords. This chapter examines the evidence base for utilizing local anesthetic mixtures for PNBs and summarizes the advantages and disadvantages of mixing local anesthetics. This chapter does not address the eutectic mixture of lidocaine and prilocaine used for topical analgesia.

PHARMACODYNAMICS OF LOCAL ANESTHETICS

In clinical practice, local anesthetics are described according to their clinical properties: potency, duration, latency, and toxicity. These clinical properties are not independent and are determined by each local anesthetic's structural, stereochemical, and physicochemical properties, such as pK_a, lipid solubility, and molecular weight (Table 10–1).

Latency is largely determined by pK_a and lipid solubility. The more nonionized drug present at the lipid membrane of the nerve, the more of the drug that can permeate to the sodium channel inside the axon. As such, drugs with lower pK_a's tend to have shorter latencies—for example, lidocaine (pK_a 7.8) has a faster onset than bupivacaine (pK_a 8.1). Local anesthetics with lower lipid solubilities tend to also have a prolonged latency (eg, bupivacaine and ropivacaine are far more lipid soluble than lidocaine). It may be difficult to predict latency based on a sole factor, as the individual factors combine to provide an overall latency. For example, two of the fastest local anesthetics are exceptions to the rules, as chloroprocaine has a high pK_a and etidocaine is highly lipid soluble. Molecular weight is often referred to as an important factor affecting latency, as smaller molecules have faster aqueous diffusion rates. Practically, however, local anesthetics have roughly similar molecular weights.

Duration of action is associated with the lipid solubility of the local anesthetic. This is due to a greater affinity of the drug to lipid membranes and, therefore, greater proximity to its sites

TABLE 10–1. Physicochemical properties of commonly used local anesthetics.

	Molecular Weight (Da)	pK$_a$ (at 25°C)	Nonionized at pH 7.4 (%)	Octanol/Buffer Partition Coefficient (Lipid Solubility)	Protein Binding (%)
Chloroprocaine	271	9.0	5	810	[a]
Tetracaine	264	8.5	7	5822	94
Lidocaine	234	7.8	24	366	64
Mepivacaine	246	7.7	39	130	77
Ropivacaine	262	8.2	17	775	94
Bupivacaine	288	8.1	17	3420	95

[a]The percentage protein binding of chloroprocaine is unknown.

of action. The longer the drug remains in the vicinity of the membrane, rather than being absorbed, the longer the effect on the Na$^+$ channel in the membrane. Greater lipid solubility also increases potency and therefore toxicity, decreasing the therapeutic index for highly lipophilic drugs. At standard pH and body temperature, bupivacaine has an aqueous solubility of 0.83 mg HCl salt/mL, compared to 15 mg HCl salt/mL for mepivacaine and 24 mg HCl salt/mL for lidocaine, and is therefore much more lipophilic than these two drugs with intermediate duration.[7]

Clinical Pearl

- A common misconception is that block duration is related to protein binding. In fact, dissociation times of local anesthetics from Na$^+$ channels are measured in seconds and do not have a bearing on the speed of recovery from the block. More important is the extent to which local anesthetic remains in the vicinity of the nerve. This is determined largely by three factors: lipid solubility, the degree of vascularity of the tissue, and the presence of vasoconstrictors that prevent vascular uptake.

LATENCY AND DURATION OF MIXTURES OF LOCAL ANESTHETICS

Early Investigations and Landmark-Based Techniques

Despite decades of clinical use of various local anesthetic combinations for PNBs, little has been published about the clinical properties of local anesthetic mixtures, with surprisingly few randomized controlled trials comparing specific local anesthetic mixtures versus single agents. As a resultant, substantial controversy still exists regarding advantages and disadvantages of various mixtures, and there are few available data to guide clinical practice.

In 1972, Moore et al reported on the safety and efficacy of a combination of tetracaine with several intermediate-duration local anesthetics, such as lidocaine, mepivacaine, and chloroprocaine, in a retrospective analysis of over 10,000 regional anesthetic procedures.[3] Compared to rapid-onset local anesthetics

alone, the onset of action of the local anesthetic mixture was unchanged by the addition of tetracaine, whereas the duration of action of the intermediate-duration local anesthetic was prolonged with the addition of tetracaine. In this report, however, the duration of the mixture was shorter than that of tetracaine alone. The authors suggested that the mixing of local anesthetics confers the optimal characteristics of each component for a single-dose technique. However, this retrospective study was limited both by the large variability of techniques and surgical procedures that were included and by the focus on epidural and spinal techniques. PNBs made up only a small minority of the data and consisted of a heterogeneous mix of PNBs.

Bromage and Gertel combined carbonated lidocaine 1% with bupivacaine 0.25% with epinephrine to perform supraclavicular brachial plexus blocks and compared the combination to single agents.[8] Again, latency of the mixture compared to bupivacaine alone was reduced but duration of action was compromised by up to 100 minutes, resulting in rapid block onset but moderate duration. However, the inconsistency in methodology between the two groups limits the interpretation of the data and its applicability to current practice. Although 60 mL total volume was used in the mixture group, only 25 to 50 mL of volume was used in the groups with a single local anesthetic.

Most of the earlier studies of local anesthetic mixtures involved epidural analgesia. Yet, there are few data, and much of these data are difficult to interpret due to methodological inconsistencies. Defalque et al in 1966 reported that, for mixtures of local anesthetics for epidurals in dogs, the mixture properties depended on the ratios of each component.[9] Latency was determined by the faster-acting component, while duration tended to reflect but did not equal the longer-acting component. The authors concluded that shorter latency comes at the expense of shorter duration than a single long-acting agent alone. Moreover, duration of the local anesthetic mixture varied and was less predictable.

Cohen et al compared epidural chloroprocaine 3% versus bupivacaine 0.5% versus an equal mixture of chloroprocaine 1.5% and bupivacaine 0.375% for labor analgesia and observed the latency and duration.[10] All three groups had similar onset times and block quality, although the bupivacaine 0.5% group had an extended time to two-segment regression compared to the other groups. In a separate study, Raj et al compared a mixture of chloroprocaine and bupivacaine to lidocaine and bupivacaine in both epidural and brachial plexus block models and found that latency was similar, although the authors pointed out that the plasma concentrations of chloroprocaine were significantly less, which may offer a safety advantage.[11] However, duration of action for either group was not measured. The authors suggested that chloroprocaine and bupivacaine act independently of each other, providing analgesia with rapid onset and long duration, but no reference or data were cited to substantiate this claim.

Seow et al randomized patients undergoing abdominal surgery to receive various ratios of lidocaine 2% and bupivacaine 0.5% (eg, ratios of 3:1, 2:2, 1:3), as well as each drug alone, by epidural administration.[12] Somewhat surprisingly, no difference in either latency or duration of action was observed when mixing bupivacaine 0.5% or lidocaine 2% versus either alone, although there was a slight trend toward prolonged duration in the bupivacaine alone group.

In the first randomized trial comparing a local anesthetic mixture with an individual agent, bupivacaine 0.5% was compared to a mixture of chloroprocaine 3% and bupivacaine 0.5% for axillary brachial plexus blocks in 25 subjects undergoing arm surgery.[13] In this case, the authors reported latency reductions of almost 50% with addition of chloroprocaine compared to bupivacaine alone. In addition, bupivacaine's latency was less predictable and with greater variation. Surprisingly, there was no difference in sensory duration between the two groups. However, the study was limited by its small sample size and the lack of a control group of chloroprocaine alone. It is important to note that unequal volumes of the compounded agents were used (10 mL of chloroprocaine and 20 mL of bupivacaine). This may limit the comparison of these results to other studies where 1:1 mixtures are used.

More recently, a double-blind, randomized, controlled trial involving equal volume mixtures of bupivacaine 0.5% or ropivacaine 0.75% with lidocaine 2% versus long-acting agents alone for both femoral and sciatic nerve blocks in patients undergoing lower extremity surgery reported significantly shorter latency by 33% to 50% with mixtures containing lidocaine.[14] Consistent with the majority of prior studies, equal-volume mixtures of lidocaine 2% with bupivacaine or ropivacaine resulted in significantly shorter duration than bupivacaine or ropivacaine alone by up to 4 to 9 hours. Interestingly, no significant decrease in postoperative analgesic requirements was found when comparing the three groups.

Although not considered a PNB, retrobulbar block performed using 2% lidocaine, 0.5% bupivacaine, or a 1:1 mixture of both resulted in identical latency of analgesia and eyeball akinesia, as well as first report of pain postoperatively following vitreoretinal surgery.[15]

The Age of Ultrasound

The use of ultrasound has a significant effect on PNB pharmacodynamics, with the majority of studies demonstrating decreased time to block onset and improved block success rates compared to landmark-based techniques.[16] The first randomized controlled trial to evaluate combinations of short- and long-acting local anesthetic with ultrasound-guided PNBs compared a mixture of 15 mL of mepivacaine 1.5% with 15 mL

bupivacaine 0.5% compared to equal volumes (30 mL) of bupivacaine 0.5% or mepivacaine 1.5% alone for interscalene block.[17] All three groups demonstrated similar onset times, whereas duration was variable: Mepivacaine alone had the shortest duration, bupivacaine alone had the longest duration, and the mixture group had an intermediate duration. The authors concluded that there is no tangible benefit to mixing these two local anesthetics for ultrasound-guided interscalene block, and that individual agents should be chosen on the basis of desired duration. For example, at our institution we typically use mepivacaine 1.5% alone for arteriovenous (AV) fistula creation, a procedure with limited postoperative pain intensity; bupivacaine 0.5% is frequently used for rotator cuff repair, where a prolonged duration of quality analgesia is required. The authors did note that 30 mL is a volume larger than normally given for interscalene brachial plexus block (ISBPB) and may account for the lack of difference in onset of block. Another potential factor in a lack of difference in onset is the possibility that the local anesthetic was more precisely placed in the interscalene sheath with ultrasound guidance compared to landmark techniques, effectively reducing any previously observed differences in time for the local anesthetic to diffuse across fascial planes and exert its effect. Of note, the mepivacaine group did have significantly greater predilection for block of the inferior trunk, which landmark-based interscalene brachial plexus block is known to variably cover.[18] The authors hypothesized that the hydrophilic nature of mepivacaine may have resulted in greater spread and thus more complete coverage of the brachial plexus.

The same group of investigators followed this study by comparing sequencing rather than mixing of local anesthetic to see if any differences were detectable by administering short-acting local anesthetic (mepivacaine 1.5%) before long-acting local anesthetic (bupivacaine 0.5%) during interscalene brachial plexus block or vice versa.[19] The rationale for this frequently used clinical sequencing seems logical, if unsubstantiated: Exposing roots and trunks of brachial plexus first to a solution of mepivacaine before injecting bupivacaine could result in the faster onset of interscalene block (ISB) (characteristics of the intermediate-acting drug), while the long-acting local anesthetic would provide a longer duration of action than the intermediate-acting drug alone. As reported by these authors, the onset times and duration for both groups were identical, showing that, if a mixture *is* administered, it does not matter which drug is injected first or last (Figures 10–1 and 10–2).

In the only other study using ultrasound guidance of PNB to investigate properties of local anesthetic mixtures, Laur et al compared 40 mL of bupivacaine 0.5% and 40 mL of mepivacaine 1.5% with an equivalent volume combination of each (total 40 mL) during ultrasound-guided infraclavicular block.[20] They reported that latencies were equal for the mepivacaine and mixed group and longer for the bupivacaine group. Similar to the studies by Gadsden et al, duration of action of the mixed group was shorter than bupivacaine alone, but longer than mepivacaine alone. The duration of sensory and motor block in the mixture group seemed unpredictable, with a wide range among subjects, echoing previous studies[9]. Another interesting finding was the substantially higher failure of blocks in the bupivacaine group, despite the same practitioners

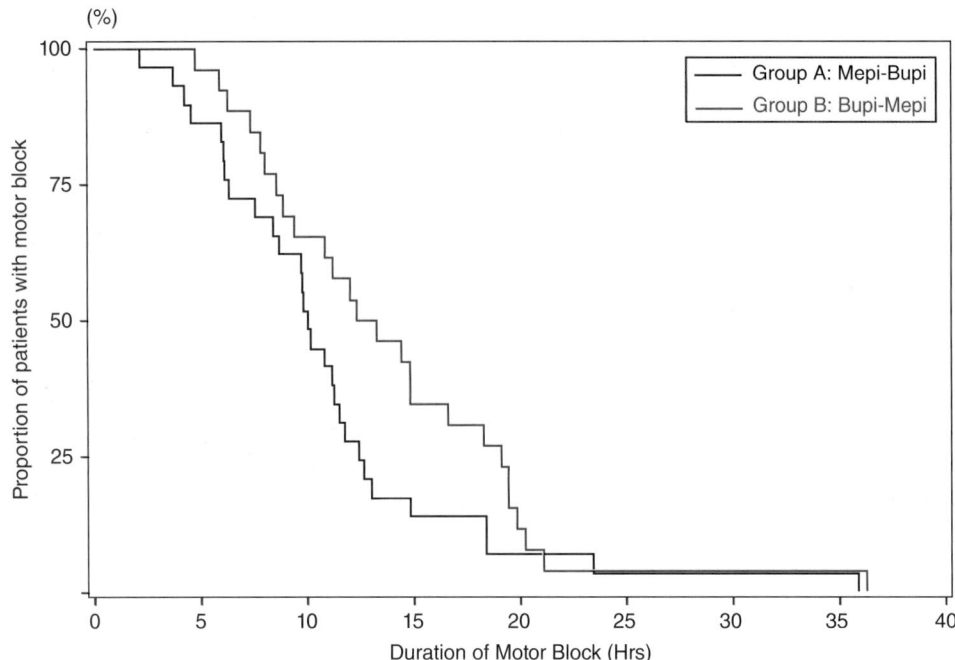

FIGURE 10-1. Decay curve showing proportion of patients with a motor block following administration of mepivacaine followed by bupivacaine (Group A: Mepi-Bupi) versus bupivacaine followed by mepivacaine (Group B: Bupi-Mepi).

and technique. With the use of ultrasound, onset time of PNBs appeared to be significantly less than observed in prior studies. While Laur et al demonstrated a significant difference in onset time of roughly 30%–50%, sensory onset was achieved by 12 minutes versus 6 minutes in 75% of subjects in the bupivacaine versus other groups. The controversy remains if this is a clinically relevant difference. Moreover, the question must be asked if an advantage of less than 10 minutes in latency justifies a roughly 50% reduction in duration.

Clinical Pearl

- For ultrasound-guided brachial plexus blocks, mixing short- and long-acting local anesthetics appears to have little influence on speed of onset. However, blocks performed with such a mixture will not last as long as a similar volume block performed with long-acting local anesthetic alone.

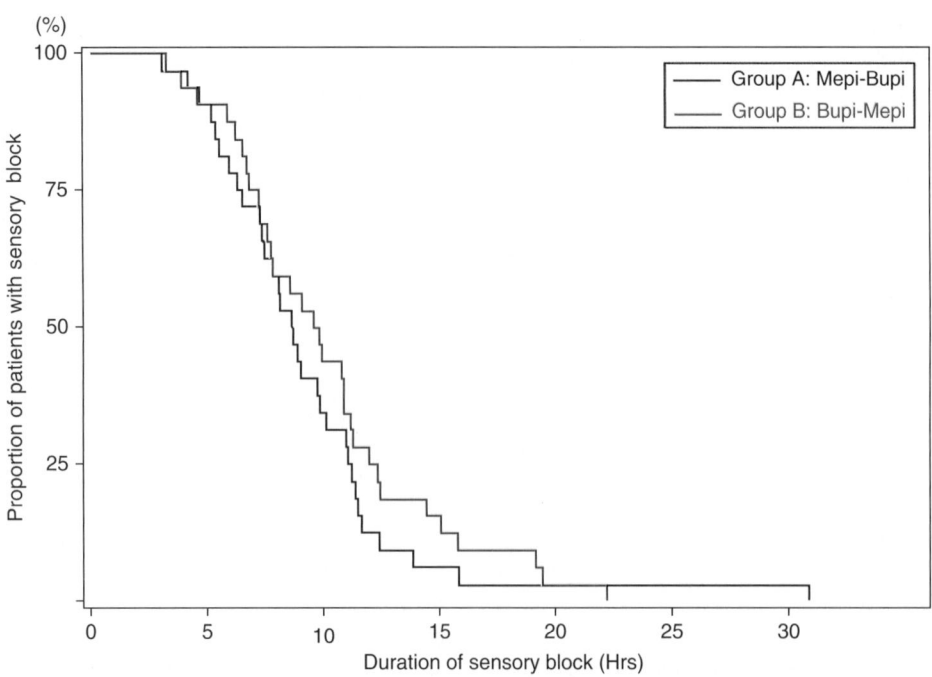

FIGURE 10-2. Decay curve showing proportion of patients with a sensory block following administration of mepivacaine followed by bupivacaine (Group A: Mepi-Bupi) versus bupivacaine followed by mepivacaine (Group B: Bupi-Mepi).

Overall, the evidence, with different methodologies, lack of standardization of technique, and various volumes, is difficult to extrapolate and apply clinically. While these more recent ultrasound-guided studies offer the most insight regarding current clinical practice, additional randomized trials of specific PNBs are needed to draw any conclusions.

Local Anesthetic Systemic Toxicity and Mixtures

Concern over systemic toxicity of local anesthetics grew primarily due to increasing numbers of toxic complications from bupivacaine used in regional anesthesia. Bupivacaine's elevated cardiac toxic potential highlighted a need for safer local anesthetic practices. Therapeutic and toxic windows are different for each local anesthetic. In particular, bupivacaine exhibits a narrow therapeutic window that has all too often led to local anesthetic systemic toxicity (LAST) and devastating consequences.

One of the theoretical advantages of compounding local anesthetics was decreased toxicity. By reducing the dose of each local anesthetic used, toxic levels of any individual drug should be decreased compared with a larger dose of each alone, which appears to be the case.[21] In a report of over 10,000 interventions, most of which involved neuraxial techniques, Moore et al showed mixtures of local anesthetics to be safe, and without increased risk of toxicity versus single agents alone, supporting the safety of admixing local anesthetic agents.[3]

However, toxicity of local anesthetic is additive,[22] and the calculation of the dose of each drug in a mixture required to avoid toxicity is unclear. Daos et al used a small-animal model to compare local anesthetic mixtures on the incidence of cardiotoxicity. These authors found that the addition of tetracaine to procaine, chloroprocaine, mepivacaine, or lidocaine reduced the time to cardiac arrest significantly, in some cases by 75%.[23] Another study investigated the possible synergistic or antagonistic role of amide-amide and amide-ester local anesthetic combinations in rats and determined that there was no evidence of either—the use of admixed local anesthetics resulted in the same additive toxic risk as if either parent drug had been administered sequentially.[24]

While cardiovascular adverse events are uncommon and ropivacaine and lidocaine are both considered to be relatively safe local anesthetics with clinically appropriate dosages, Reinikainen et al reported sudden cardiac arrest in a 97-kg young patient immediately following a landmark-based interscalene brachial plexus block.[25] The local anesthetic mixture used consisted of ropivacaine (150 mg) and lidocaine with epinephrine (360 mg), which represent 52% and 53% of the maximum recommended weight-based doses (3 mg/kg and 7 mg/kg), respectively. This highlights that, although each drug was under the maximum recommended limits, the total combined delivered dose was 105% of the recommended maximum. It is noteworthy that the use of epinephrine did not prevent this complication, neither in its role as an intravascular marker nor as a means to truncate the peak plasma concentration, further highlighting the need to carefully monitor dosages.

> ## Clinical Pearl
>
> - Local anesthetic toxicity is additive. When mixing local anesthetics, individual fractional contributions to overall maximum recommended dose limits should be considered.

To what extent these reports apply to the modern practice of regional anesthesia is unclear. In current clinical practice with ultrasound-guided regional anesthesia, much smaller volumes and doses are being used compared to the practice a decade ago. For instance, interscalene brachial plexus blocks can be achieved with as little as 5–7 mL compared to 40 mL historically.[26] Although the reality of most clinical practices lies somewhere in between, local anesthetic doses have dramatically decreased and are well under the recommended maximum limits, and there is now evidence that ultrasound guidance significantly reduces LAST compared to landmark-based techniques.[27]

Anatomical Considerations

Anatomical considerations must be considered in the examination of the latency and duration of PNBs, as it can have a significant effect on characteristics of individual PNBs. The popliteal sciatic nerve block is one particular instance for which anatomy and location of local anesthetic deposition significantly determine nerve block characteristics, as the components of the sciatic nerve in this location are surrounded by a tough connective tissue paraneural sheath. Recently, ultrasound-guided popliteal nerve blocks performed within the paraneural sheath have been shown to result in a more rapid onset compared to techniques where local anesthetic is placed outside the sheath, probably due to an increased exposure of the nerve's surface area to local anesthetic.[28,29] For this reason, latency for nerve blocks that rely on placement of local anesthetic within a sheath may have more to do with technique than choice of local anesthetics.[17,19] However, more studies are needed to corroborate these findings. No study to date has compared latency of various local anesthetics and their mixtures using ultrasound-guided intraneural injections at the popliteal sciatic nerve.

SUMMARY

The ideal local anesthetic for single-dose PNB with short latency and long duration has yet to be developed. Local anesthetic mixtures have long been used for PNBs in an attempt to create improved pharmacodynamics. However, interpreting the literature on this topic is difficult because (1) the literature is relatively scant and spread out over six decades; (2) the methodology is heterogeneous, with varying combinations of block locations, drug combinations, and evaluative methods; and (3) the results are somewhat conflicting. However, in considering the more recent, and especially the ultrasound-guided, PNB studies, a pattern emerges that suggests that latency is not significantly affected when high-potency, long-acting agents are admixed with low-potency, short-acting agents. At the same time, duration of neural blockade appears to suffer when bupivacaine alone is mixed with a shorter-acting agent.

With the precision of ultrasound-guided PNBs, latency of block onset is less an obstacle than duration. Duration of block is the most important determining characteristic in choosing local anesthetics. Due to the current shortcomings of local anesthetics, specifically duration, when utilized for single-injection PNBs, alternative solutions have been investigated. Adjuvants to local anesthetics have been used and are discussed in Chapter 9. Continuous methods have been developed and consist of a large portion of modern regional anesthesia practice today. Finally, recent advances in encapsulation of local anesthetic in liposomes offer promise, as these could extend the analgesic profile well beyond the usual 16–24 hours typically seen with our longest-acting agents.

REFERENCES

1. Kessler J, Marhofer P, Hopkins PM, Hollmann MW: Peripheral regional anaesthesia and outcome: Lessons learned from the last 10 years. Br J Anaesth 2015;114:728–745.
2. Tucker GT, Mather LE: Clinical pharmacokinetics of local anaesthetics. Clin Pharmacokinet 1979;4:241–278.
3. Moore DC, Bridenbaugh LD, Bridenbaugh PO, Thompson GE, Tucker GT: Does compounding of local anesthetic agents increase their toxicity in humans? Anesth Analg 1972;51:579–585.
4. Jafari S, Kalstein AI, Nasrullah HM, Hedayatnia M, Yarmush JM, SchianodiCola J: A randomized, prospective, double-blind trial comparing 3% chloroprocaine followed by 0.5% bupivacaine to 2% lidocaine followed by 0.5% bupivacaine for interscalene brachial plexus block. Anesth Analg 2008;107:1746–1750.
5. Duggan E, El Beheiry H, Perlas A, et al: Minimum effective volume of local anesthetic for ultrasound-guided supraclavicular brachial plexus block. Reg Anesth Pain Med 2009;34:215–218.
6. Cohen S: The rational use of local anesthetic mixtures. Reg Anesth 1979;4:11–12.
7. Cousins MJ, Bridenbaugh PO, Carr DB, Horlocker TT: *Cousins and Bridenbaugh's Neural Blockade in Clinical Anesthesia and Pain Medicine,* 4th ed. Lippincott Williams & Wilkins, 2008.
8. Bromage PR, Gertel M: Improved brachial plexus blockade with bupivacaine hydrochloride and carbonated lidocaine. Anesthesiology 1972;36:479–487.
9. Defalque RJ, Stoelting VK: Latency and duration of action of some local anesthetic mixtures. Anesth Analg 1966;45:106–116.
10. Cohen SE, Thurlow A: Comparison of a chloroprocaine—bupivacaine mixture with chloroprocaine and bupivacaine used individually for obstetric epidural analgesia. Anesthesiology 1979;51:288–292.
11. Raj PP, Rosenblatt R, Miller J, Katz RL, Carden E: Dynamics of local-anesthetic compounds in regional anesthesia. Anesth Analg. 1977;56:110–117.
12. Seow LT, Lips FJ, Cousins MJ, Mather LE: Lidocaine and bupivacaine mixtures for epidural blockade. Anesthesiology 1982;56:177–183.
13. Cunningham NL, Kaplan JA: A rapid-onset, long-acting regional anesthetic technique. Anesthesiology 1974;41:509–511.
14. Cuvillon P, Nouvellon E, Ripart J, et al: A comparison of the pharmacodynamics and pharmacokinetics of bupivacaine, ropivacaine (with epinephrine) and their equal volume mixtures with lidocaine used for femoral and sciatic nerve blocks: a double-blind randomized study. Anesth Analg 2009;108:641–649.
15. Jaichandran VV, Raman R, Gella L, Sharma T: Local anesthetic agents for vitreoretinal surgery: No advantage to mixing solutions. Ophthalmology 2015;122:1030–1033.
16. Salinas FV, Hanson NA: Evidence-based medicine for ultrasound-guided regional anesthesia. Anesthesiol Clin 2014;32:771–787.
17. Gadsden J, Hadzic A, Gandhi K, et al: The effect of mixing 1.5% mepivacaine and 0.5% bupivacaine on duration of analgesia and latency of block onset in ultrasound-guided interscalene block. Anesth Analg 2011;112:471–476.
18. Gadsden JC, Tsai T, Iwata T, Somasundarum L, Robards C, Hadzic A: Low interscalene block provides reliable anesthesia for surgery at or about the elbow. J Clin Anesth 2009;21:98–102.
19. Gadsden J, Shariat A, Hadzic A, Xu D, Patel V, Maliakal T: The sequence of administration of 1.5% mepivacaine and 0.5% bupivacaine does not affect latency of block onset or duration of analgesia in ultrasound-guided interscalene block. Anesth Analg. 2012;115:963–967.
20. Laur JJ, Bayman EO, Foldes PJ, Rosenquist RW: Triple-blind randomized clinical trial of time until sensory change using 1.5% mepivacaine with epinephrine, 0.5% bupivacaine, or an equal mixture of both for infraclavicular block. Reg Anesth Pain Med 2012;37:28–33.
21. Hashizume Y, Yamaguchi S, Mishio M, Takiguchi T, Okuda Y, Kitajima T: Pediatric caudal block with mepivacaine, bupivacaine or a mixture of both drugs: requirement for postoperative analgesia and plasma concentration of local anesthetics. J Clin Anesth 2001;13:30–34
22. Jong RH de, Bonin JD: Mixtures of local anesthetics are no more toxic than the parent drugs. Anesthesiology 1981;54:177–181.
23. Daos FG, Lopez L, Virtue RW: Local anesthetic toxicity modified by oxygen and by combination of agents. Anesthesiology 1962;23:755–761.
24. Spiegel DA, Dexter F, Warner DS, Baker MT, Todd MM: Central nervous system toxicity of local anesthetic mixtures in the rat. Anesth Analg 1992;75:922–928.
25. Reinikainen M, Hedman A, Pelkonen O, Ruokonen E: Cardiac arrest after interscalene brachial plexus block with ropivacaine and lidocaine. Acta Anaesthesiol Scand 2003;47:904–906.
26. Vandepitte C, Gautier P, Xu D, Salviz EA, Hadzic A: Effective volume of ropivacaine 0.75% through a catheter required for interscalene brachial plexus blockade. Anesthesiology 2013;118:863–867.
27. Barrington MJ, Kluger R: Ultrasound guidance reduces the risk of local anesthetic systemic toxicity following peripheral nerve blockade. Reg Anesth Pain Med 2013;38:289–297.
28. Perlas A, Wong P, Abdallah F, Hazrati L-N, Tse C, Chan V: Ultrasound-guided popliteal block through a common paraneural sheath versus conventional injection: a prospective, randomized, double-blind study. Reg Anesth Pain Med 2013;38:218–225.
29. Tran DQH, Dugani S, Pham K, Al-Shaafi A, Finlayson RJ: A randomized comparison between subepineural and conventional ultrasound-guided popliteal sciatic nerve block. Reg Anesth Pain Med 2011;36:548–552.

CHAPTER 11

Continuous Peripheral Nerve Blocks: Local Anesthetic Solutions and Infusion Strategies

Amanda M. Monahan and Brian M. Ilfeld

INTRODUCTION

Continuous peripheral nerve blocks are accomplished by infusion or intermittent boluses of local anesthetic solutions. Overwhelming plethora of options are available for nearly every aspect of continuous infusion administration, from the choice of infusate to choice of infusion rate and bolus regimen, to infusion pump selection.[1] An ideal perineural local anesthetic solution would provide analgesia while minimizing sensory, motor, and proprioception deficits. In addition, desirable attributes include a favorable toxicity profile and cost-efficacy. The optimal infusion strategy may be modified for the large number of clinical scenarios that the regional anesthesiologist will encounter in daily practice. Considerations include the indication for perineural catheter placement, the number and location of catheters, patient weight, and ambulatory versus inpatient status.

INFUSATES AND LOCAL ANESTHETIC CONCENTRATION

Local anesthetics were described[2] in continuous perineural infusions as early as 1946. Intermediate-duration local anesthetics such as mepivacaine have been used,[3] but long-acting local anesthetics such as ropivacaine, bupivacaine, and levobupivacaine are most frequently described.[1] These long-acting agents provide a favorable differential sensory-to-motor block. At the termination of an infusion, it is desirable for sensory and motor block to resolve quickly and predictably. Studies have suggested that sensory-and-motor block regresses faster with ropivacaine than with bupivacaine.[4]

It is currently unclear if local anesthetic concentration—or simply the total delivered dose—influences continuous block effects.[5,6] While the evidence suggests that for infusions involving the femoral nerve, local anesthetic concentration is of minimal importance compared with total dose, data for the sciatic nerve are lacking, and the brachial plexus information is conflicting.[7-9] Therefore, at this time it remains unknown if there is an "optimal" concentration of local anesthetic. Commonly described concentrations include ropivacaine 0.1%–0.4%,[4,6,10-13] bupivacaine 0.125%–0.15%,[4,14] and levobupivacaine 0.1%–0.125%.[15,16]

Clinical Pearl

- An infusion with ropivacaine 0.1%–0.2% is easier to titrate due to faster resolution of an insensate extremity but bupivacaine 0.1%–0.125% provides the same degree of analgesia and costs less in most regions and hospitals.

LOCAL ANESTHETIC DELIVERY STRATEGIES

Infusates are typically delivered using an infusion pump with a basal infusion, bolus dose, or combination of the two modalities. Regimens are often reported as basal rate (mL/hour)/bolus volume (mL)/bolus lockout time (minutes). The delivery regimen should minimize total local anesthetic consumption, supplemental opioid requirements, and disturbance of daily functioning/sleep. No single delivery regimen has proven ideal for all anatomic locations and clinical situations. In many cases, providing a basal infusion minimizes breakthrough pain and supplemental analgesic requirements.[1] Adding a patient-controlled bolus usually decreases the required basal infusion rate,[4,17,18] incidence of an insensate extremity,[19] and local anesthetic consumption, the last allowing for a longer infusion duration in the ambulatory setting.[20,21] For example, in the upper extremity, an interscalene infusion that includes a basal infusion has been found superior to a bolus-only regimen.[22]

Regarding specific basal infusion rates, the evidence is mixed, with many studies reporting few differences among various rates.[1] One study involving interscalene catheters suggested that a relatively large basal rate with small-volume bolus doses (8 mL/h basal, 2-mL bolus, 60-minute lockout) provides improved analgesia and functioning, but with higher overall local anesthetic consumption compared with a slower basal rate and larger bolus doses.[23] At the infraclavicular location, utilizing a basal infusion with bolus (in comparison to basal only or bolus only) also has been found to provide improved analgesia with decreased severity and incidence of breakthrough pain, sleep disturbances, as well as higher patient satisfaction.[24] Studies of axillary catheters are mixed.

In the lower extremity, some differences in dosing effects have been found in randomized controlled trials (RCTs) examining femoral versus popliteal sciatic locations. Findings of RCTs at the femoral or fascia iliaca location have not demonstrated an overwhelming preference for a specific regimen.[25–27] Sensory and motor effects are similar when comparing repeated, scheduled hourly bolus doses to a continuous basal infusion of the same hourly volume and dose.[17] Nearly all studies reported the total local anesthetic dose reduced with bolus-only dosing.[1]

Clinical Pearl

- Analgesia is optimized with an infusion pump that delivers both an adjustable basal rate and patient-controlled bolus doses.

INFUSATE ADDITIVES AND ADJUVANTS

Adjuvant pharmaceuticals have been added to the local anesthetic infusate in an attempt to improve analgesia quality, spare local anesthetic consumption, and minimize motor block. Many substances have been described with single-injection regional techniques. However, no analogous, clinically relevant benefits have been demonstrated for continuous peripheral nerve blocks.[28–31] In addition, no additive medications are currently approved for continuous perineural administration, and some additives that have been reported in clinical trials have unacceptable side effects.[32,33]

Clinical Pearl

- At this time, there are few data to support adding additives (adjuvants) to local anesthetic for perineural infusions.

INFUSION PUMPS

While intermittent clinician-administered boluses are theoretically possible, simply logistical considerations explain why most local anesthetic is administered using an infusion pump. The device used for administering a continuous infusion should be accurate, reliable, portable, and programmable. It is desirable for the pump to be quiet, inexpensive, and easy to refill.[34] In the ambulatory setting, the local anesthetic reservoir should accommodate enough infusate for 2 to 3 days.[34] Pumps can be arbitrarily categorized as nonelectronic and electronic (Figure 11–1). Examples of nonelectronic mechanisms include spring- and vacuum-powered devices, as well as elastomeric pumps. Due to issues with accuracy/consistency and reservoir volume,[35,36] spring- and vacuum-powered models are not typically used for the purposes of continuous peripheral nerve blocks.

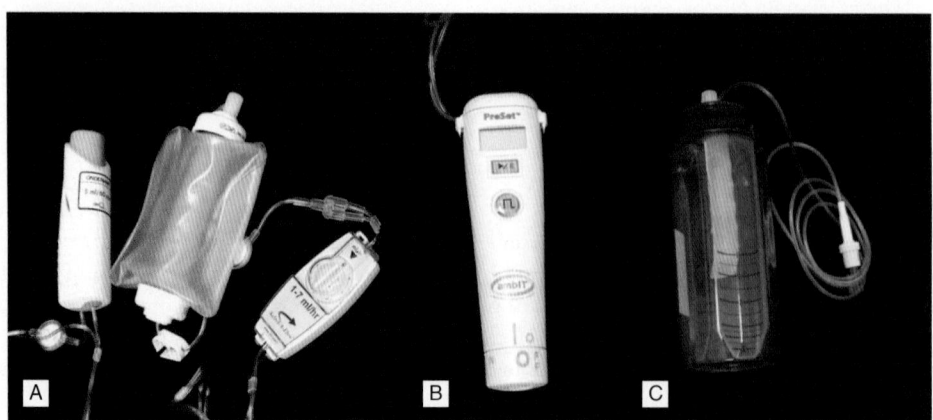

FIGURE 11–1. Examples of three infusion pumps designed for perineural local anesthetic infusion. **A:** An elastomeric device with adjustable basal infusion rate and 5-mL patient-controlled bolus function (ON-Q* C-bloc with ONDEMAND* and Select-A-Flow*, I-Flow/Kimberly-Clark, Lake Forest, CA). **B:** an electronic device with programmable basal infusion rate, patient-controlled bolus, lockout duration, and maximum total infused volume (ambIT Preset, Summit Medical Products, Sandy, UT). **C:** An elastomeric device with a manufacturer-determined/fixed basal infusion rate without a patient-controlled bolus function (LV5 Infusor, Baxter Healthcare International, Deerfield, IL).

Elastomeric pumps have been studied in depth for the purpose of continuous regional anesthesia. The acoustic silence of this modality may be desirable to many patients to minimize sleep disturbances. With regard to accuracy, these devices will infuse 110%–130% of the set basal rate in the first 3–8 hours and repeat this high rate in the final hours before pump emptying.[35–38] Some models allow for an adjustable basal rate as well as patient-controlled bolus dosing. The physics of the internal reservoir of the elastomeric devices limit ability to refill the pump, and even when technically possible,[39] it is neither recommended by manufacturers nor approved by regulatory bodies.[40]

Electronic pumps are reported to be the most accurate and consistent over the length of an infusion, usually within 5% of the programmed basal rate.[35–38] There are multiple models that are highly programmable, with various basal, patient controlled regional analgesia (PCRA) bolus, and lockout options. These pumps may emit noise during regular basal infusion and if/when an alarm is triggered. For models with an external reservoir, replacing the local anesthetic reservoir is easy to provide prolonged infusions. National pharmacologic guidelines have been developed for the preparing of regional anesthesia local anesthetic solutions. These guidelines require that the pump reservoir must be filled in an "ISO (International Organization for Standardization) class 5" environment. This entails compounding by a pharmacy using a "clean room" laminar flow workbench.[40]

Regardless of equipment type, it is important to educate patients both preoperatively and postoperatively regarding appropriate use of the pump functions. Preoperative counseling is desirable before any sedation is administered, and ideally a caretaker should be present in addition to the patient. Education should include the basic details and duration of the perineural infusion. Instructions should be given regarding when and how to use a patient-controlled bolus function. Patients are shown where the bolus button is located and how to deploy the button. They are counseled to use the bolus button whenever they have breakthrough pain and to expect a lag between bolus and local anesthetic effect. There is a risk for patients to have confusion about the roles of continuous perineural infusions and opioids as part of their multimodal analgesic plan. Patients may be instructed to use their bolus button, and if their pain is not at an acceptable level after 20 minutes, to add an oral opioid (or increase the basal infusion rate, depending on the pump capabilities). For ambulatory patients, written instructions are given with on-call contact information, as well as instructions for using the bolus button for pain, pausing the infusion in the event of an insensate extremity, or increasing/decreasing the basal rate, if necessary.

Clinical Pearl

- Electronic pumps provide a more stable basal infusion rate over the course of the infusion relative to elastomeric devices.

POSTOPERATIVE MANAGEMENT AND INFUSION STRATEGIES

As described in other chapters, the local anesthetic infusion strategy may be modified to manage common postoperative issues, such as breakthrough pain or an insensate extremity. To tailor the infusion strategy to a specific patient, the overall analgesic goals must be addressed. For example, a patient having major orthopedic surgery may require steady, around-the-clock analgesia, best provided with a continuous basal infusion in addition to patient-controlled bolus doses. In contrast, a patient following surgery for burns may primarily require the benefits of a larger bolus dose for daily bedside dressing changes and very low—if any—basal infusion. Because local anesthetics are bacteriostatic or -toxic, a continuous basal infusion rate is theoretically beneficial in reducing the risk of infection. Duration of local anesthetic infusion is an important postoperative consideration. While numerous infusion benefits have been demonstrated by RCT, longer duration of infusion (greater than 48 hours) has been associated with increased infection risk.[41] However, case reports of prolonged infusions have been described (34–85 days) without identified infection.[42,43]

Clinical Pearl

- An adjustable basal infusion rate allows an increase in the case of inadequate analgesia and a decrease in the case of an insensate extremity.

SUMMARY

An ideal continuous regional anesthesia infusate and administration strategy should provide reliable analgesia with minimal adverse effects. At this time, long-acting local anesthetics are favored due to the desire to minimize motor block. No pharmacologic additives or adjuvants have demonstrated additional benefits. Numerous administration strategies have been described, most combining a basal infusion with a patient-controlled bolus option. Both electronic and nonelectronic pumps are capable of providing these regimens. Optimal patient use of the infusion and pump bolus function requires appropriate perioperative counseling and support. Finally, infusion duration must balance analgesic and functional benefits with the risk of infection.

REFERENCES

1. Ilfeld BM: Continuous peripheral nerve blocks: A review of the published evidence. Anesth Analg 2011;113:904–925.
2. Ansbro FP: A method of continuous brachial plexus block. Am J Surg 1946;71:716–722.
3. Buettner J, Klose R, Hoppe U, Wresch P: Serum levels of mepivacaine-HCl during continuous axillary brachial plexus block. Reg Anesth 1989;14:124–127.
4. Borgeat A, Kalberer F, Jacob H, Ruetsch YA, Gerber C: Patient-controlled interscalene analgesia with ropivacaine 0.2% versus bupivacaine 0.15% after major open shoulder surgery: The effects on hand motor function. Anesth Analg 2001;92:218–223.

5. Ilfeld BM, Moeller LK, Mariano ER, et al: Continuous peripheral nerve blocks: Is local anesthetic dose the only factor, or do concentration and volume influence infusion effects as well? Anesthesiology 2010;112:347–354.

6. Bauer M, Wang L, Onibonoje OK, et al: Continuous femoral nerve blocks: Decreasing local anesthetic concentration to minimize quadriceps femoris weakness. Anesthesiology 2012;116:665–672.

7. Ilfeld BM, Loland VJ, Gerancher JC, et al: The effects of varying local anesthetic concentration and volume on continuous popliteal sciatic nerve blocks: A dual-center, randomized, controlled study. Anesth Analg 2008;107:701–707.

8. Le LT, Loland VJ, Mariano ER, et al: Effects of local anesthetic concentration and dose on continuous interscalene nerve blocks: A dual-center, randomized, observer-masked, controlled study. Reg Anesth Pain Med 2008;33:518–525.

9. Ilfeld BM, Le LT, Ramjohn J, et al: The effects of local anesthetic concentration and dose on continuous infraclavicular nerve blocks: A multicenter, randomized, observer-masked, controlled study. Anesth Analg 2009;108:345–350.

10. Ilfeld BM, Loland VJ, Sandhu NS, et al: Continuous femoral nerve blocks: the impact of catheter tip location relative to the femoral nerve (anterior versus posterior) on quadriceps weakness and cutaneous sensory block. Anesth Analg 2012;115:721–727.

11. Mariano ER, Sandhu NS, Loland VJ, et al: A randomized comparison of infraclavicular and supraclavicular continuous peripheral nerve blocks for postoperative analgesia. Reg Anesth Pain Med 2011;36:26–31.

12. Fredrickson MJ, Ball CM, Dalgleish AJ: Posterior versus anterolateral approach interscalene catheter placement: a prospective randomized trial. Reg Anesth Pain Med 2011;36:125–133.

13. Blumenthal S, Borgeat A, Neudorfer C, Bertolini R, Espinosa N, Aguirre J: Additional femoral catheter in combination with popliteal catheter for analgesia after major ankle surgery. Br J Anaesth 2011;106:387–393.

14. Ganesh A, Rose JB, Wells L, et al: Continuous peripheral nerve blockade for inpatient and outpatient postoperative analgesia in children. Anesth Analg 2007;105:1234–1242.

15. Watson MW, Mitra D, McLintock TC, Grant SA: Continuous versus single-injection lumbar plexus blocks: comparison of the effects on morphine use and early recovery after total knee arthroplasty. Reg Anesth Pain Med 2005;30:541–547.

16. Taboada M, Rodriguez J, Bermudez M, et al: Comparison of continuous infusion versus automated bolus for postoperative patient-controlled analgesia with popliteal sciatic nerve catheters. Anesthesiology 2009;110:150–154.

17. Charous MT, Madison SJ, Suresh PJ, et al: Continuous femoral nerve blocks: Varying local anesthetic delivery method (bolus versus basal) to minimize quadriceps motor block while maintaining sensory block. Anesthesiology 2011;115:774781.

18. Ilfeld BM, Duke KB, Donohue MC: The association between lower extremity continuous peripheral nerve blocks and patient falls after knee and hip arthroplasty. Anesth Analg 2010;111:1552–1554.

19. Ilfeld BM, Morey TE, Wang RD, Enneking FK: Continuous popliteal sciatic nerve block for postoperative pain control at home: A randomized, double-blinded, placebo-controlled study. Anesthesiology 2002;97:959–965.

20. Ilfeld BM, Thannikary LJ, Morey TE, Vander Griend RA, Enneking FK: Popliteal sciatic perineural local anesthetic infusion: A comparison of three dosing regimens for postoperative analgesia. Anesthesiology 2004;101:970–977.

21. Ilfeld BM, Enneking FK: A portable mechanical pump providing over four days of patient-controlled analgesia by perineural infusion at home. Reg Anesth Pain Med 2002;27:100–104.

22. Singelyn FJ, Seguy S, Gouverneur JM: Interscalene brachial plexus analgesia after open shoulder surgery: Continuous versus patient-controlled infusion. Anesth Analg 1999;89:1216–1220.

23. Ilfeld BM, Morey TE, Wright TW, Chidgey LK, Enneking FK: Interscalene perineural ropivacaine infusion: a comparison of two dosing regimens for postoperative analgesia. Reg Anesth Pain Med 2004;29:9–16.

24. Ilfeld BM, Morey TE, Enneking FK: Infraclavicular perineural local anesthetic infusion: A comparison of three dosing regimens for postoperative analgesia. Anesthesiology 2004;100:395–402.

25. Singelyn FJ, Vanderelst PE, Gouverneur JM: Extended femoral nerve sheath block after total hip arthroplasty: Continuous versus patient-controlled techniques. Anesth Analg 2001;92:455–459.

26. Singelyn FJ, Gouverneur JM: Extended "three-in-one" block after total knee arthroplasty: Continuous versus patient-controlled techniques. Anesth Analg 2000;91:176–180.

27. Eledjam JJ, Cuvillon P, Capdevila X, et al: Postoperative analgesia by femoral nerve block with ropivacaine 0.2% after major knee surgery: continuous versus patient-controlled techniques. Reg Anesth Pain Med 2002;27:604–611.

28. Ilfeld BM, Morey TE, Enneking FK: Continuous infraclavicular perineural infusion with clonidine and ropivacaine compared with ropivacaine alone: A randomized, double-blinded, controlled study. Anesth Analg 2003;97:706–712.

29. Ilfeld BM, Morey TE, Thannikary LJ, Wright TW, Enneking FK: Clonidine added to a continuous interscalene ropivacaine perineural infusion to improve postoperative analgesia: A randomized, double-blind, controlled study. Anesth Analg 2005;100:1172–1178.

30. Casati A, Vinciguerra F, Cappelleri G, et al: Adding clonidine to the induction bolus and postoperative infusion during continuous femoral nerve block delays recovery of motor function after total knee arthroplasty. Anesth Analg 2005;100:866–872.

31. Weber A, Fournier R, Van Gessel E, Riand N, Gamulin Z: Epinephrine does not prolong the analgesia of 20 mL ropivacaine 0.5% or 0.2% in a femoral three-in-one block. Anesth Analg 2001;93:1327–1331.

32. Brummett CM, Norat MA, Palmisano JM, Lydic R: Perineural administration of dexmedetomidine in combination with bupivacaine enhances sensory and motor blockade in sciatic nerve block without inducing neurotoxicity in rat. Anesthesiology 2008;109:502–511.

33. Esmaoglu A, Yegenoglu F, Akin A, Turk CY: Dexmedetomidine added to levobupivacaine prolongs axillary brachial plexus block. Anesth Analg 2010;111:1548–1551.

34. Ilfeld BM, Wright TW, Enneking FK, et al: Total shoulder arthroplasty as an outpatient procedure using ambulatory perineural local anesthetic infusion: A pilot feasibility study. Anesth Analg 2005;101:1319–1322.

35. Ilfeld BM, Morey TE, Enneking FK: The delivery rate accuracy of portable infusion pumps used for continuous regional analgesia. Anesth Analg 2002;95:1331–1336.

36. Ilfeld BM, Morey TE, Enneking FK: Portable infusion pumps used for continuous regional analgesia: Delivery rate accuracy and consistency. Reg Anesth Pain Med 2003;28:424–432.

37. Ilfeld BM, Morey TE, Enneking FK: New portable infusion pumps: Real advantages or just more of the same in a different package? Reg Anesth Pain Med 2004;29:371–376.

38. Valente M, Aldrete JA: Comparison of accuracy and cost of disposable, nonmechanical pumps used for epidural infusions. Reg Anesth 1997;22:260–266.

39. Grant CR, Fredrickson MJ: Regional anaesthesia elastomeric pump performance after a single use and subsequent refill: A laboratory study. Anaesthesia 2009;64:770–775.

40. Head S, Enneking FK: Infusate contamination in regional anesthesia: what every anesthesiologist should know. Anesth Analg 2008;107:1412–1418.

41. Capdevila X, Pirat P, Bringuier S, et al: Continuous peripheral nerve blocks in hospital wards after orthopedic surgery: A multicenter prospective analysis of the quality of postoperative analgesia and complications in 1,416 patients. Anesthesiology 2005;103:1035–1045.

42. Stojadinovic A, Auton A, Peoples GE, et al: Responding to challenges in modern combat casualty care: innovative use of advanced regional anesthesia. Pain Med 2006;7:330–338.

43. Borghi B, D'Addabbo M, White PF, et al: The use of prolonged peripheral neural blockade after lower extremity amputation: the effect on symptoms associated with phantom limb syndrome. Anesth Analg 2010;111:1308–1315.

SECTION 3 Equipment for Peripheral Nerve Blocks

CHAPTER 12

Equipment for Regional Anesthesia

Vivian H. Y. Ip and Ban C. H. Tsui

INTRODUCTION

Regional anesthesia has become commonplace in many practices worldwide due to the increasing evidence of patient benefit, such as reduction in pulmonary[1] and thromboembolic[2] complications, reduction in opioid consumption,[3] as well as reduced pain and time to discharge and better quality of life in the immediate postoperative period.[4] The increased popularity of regional anesthesia has resulted in advancement in techniques and equipment. The practice has evolved from using paresthesia for nerve localization to electrical nerve stimulation and, currently, to ultrasound. This chapter gives an overview of the equipment available in the practice of peripheral nerve blocks. It also outlines the equipment needed at various stages of the regional anesthesia procedure to ensure that it proceeds in an efficient and safe manner. The practice of regional anesthesia comprises equipment, protocols, and skills necessary to ensure that the block proceeds as smoothly and safely as possible—before, during, and after the block is administered.

REGIONAL BLOCKADE PREPARATION AND SETUP

Area and Monitoring

A quiet environment with all equipment necessary to perform regional anesthesia, together with resuscitation drugs and equipment within reach, is of paramount importance. An ideal location is an induction room where the patient can be monitored, premedicated and the regional block performed before transferring to the operating theater. A designated block area can be used to provide suitable, monitored procedure environment while optimizing operating room efficiency.

When performing the block, an assistant trained in regional anesthesia should be present to prepare and handle equipment and help with the injectate. The assistant should also be trained in performing resuscitation if it becomes necessary.

Regardless of where the block is performed, it is essential to have all equipment, drugs, and monitoring readily available. The best way to gather all the necessary equipment and drugs is the setup of a storage cart (Figure 12–1), which should be well labeled with the supplies readily identifiable.

Clinical Pearl

- An equipment cart should contain all of the drugs, needles, and catheters necessary for regional anesthesia as well as resuscitation medications and equipment.

Block Area General Equipment

Commonly used items should be stocked in the storage cart and refilled when necessary. The storage cart should contain the following:

- Sterile skin preparation solution, sponges/gauze, drape, marking pen, ruler for landmark identification, ultrasound gel, hypodermic needles for skin infiltration and drawing up 5% dextrose (5% dextrose in water, D5W).

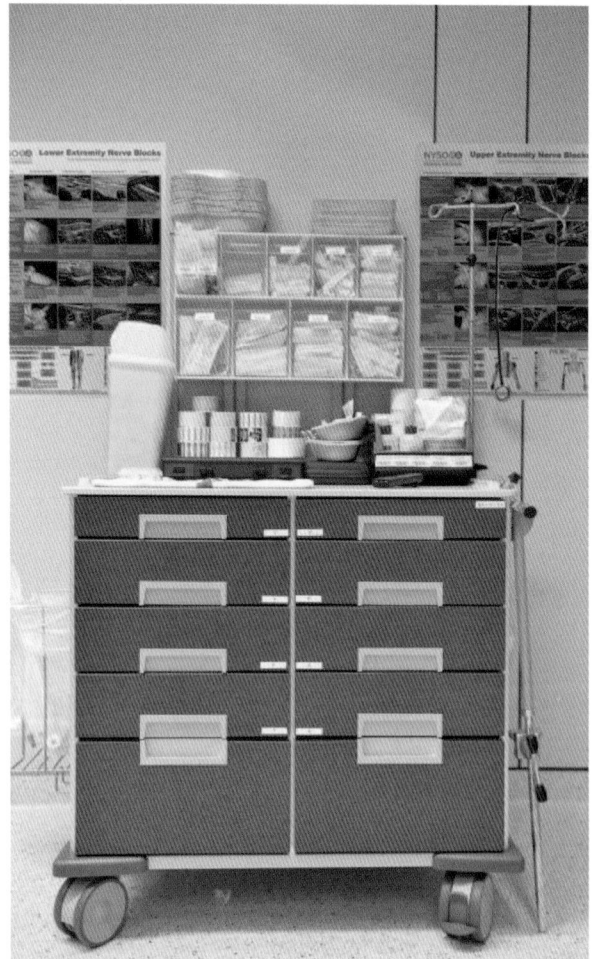

FIGURE 12–1. Equipment storage cart with clear identification of supplies and medication.

- A selection of sedatives, for example, midazolam (0.5–3 mg IV), and short-acting opioids such as fentanyl (50–100 μg IV), and propofol (20–100 mg IV) for nerve blocks that are more uncomfortable and require deeper sedation (eg, ankle block).
- Local anesthetics and normal saline for drug dilution if necessary. Local anesthetics are ideally stored in a separate compartment from intravenous drugs to avoid drug error.
- Intravenous cannulas. All patients should have an intravenous cannula inserted in case of local anesthetic toxicity.
- Dressings for intravenous cannulas, clear dressings for covering the ultrasound transducer used in single-shot nerve blocks, transducer cover, gel, and dressings for nerve block catheter insertion.

Emergency Drugs and Resuscitation Equipment

The use of ultrasound allows the visualization of the injectate and therefore, it has significantly reduced, but not eliminated, the risk of severe local anesthetic systemic toxicity (LAST). However, resuscitation equipment and medications should always be immediately available in the block area.[5]

Resuscitation Equipment

- Oxygen supply, nasal airway, and O_2 masks
- Oral airways of different sizes, laryngeal masks, and endotracheal tubes
- Laryngoscopes (Macintosh and Miller blades)
- Bag-mask ventilation device
- Suction
- Selection of various size intravenous cannulas
- Defibrillator

Resuscitation Drugs and Suggested Doses Intravenously

- Atropine (300–600 μg).
- Epinephrine (10–100 μg).
- Suxamethonium (40–100 mg).
- Ephedrine (5–15 mg).
- Phenylephrine (100–200 μg).
- Glycopyrrolate (200–400 μg).
- Intralipid® 20% (1.5 mL/kg over 1–2 minutes as an initial bolus, which can be repeated two to three times for persistent asystole. After the bolus, an infusion can be started at 0.25 mL/kg/min for 30 to 60 minutes; increase the infusion rate for refractory hypotension).[6–8] Ideally, Intralipid should be kept in a container with a protocol for use and equipment to draw up the drug.

Clinical Pearl

- During ultrasound-guided peripheral nerve block, visualization of injectate spread can minimize the risk of intravascular injection. The entire dose of local anesthetic should never be injected without seeing the spread of injectate on ultrasound, as this is suggestive of an intravenous injection

Documentation

A preblock checklist is paramount to ensure correct block performance at the appropriate site on the patient's body and includes documenting preoperative conditions (eg, relevant neurological deficits and comorbidities) and discussing risks and benefits and obtaining proper consent. In most countries, standardized medical documentation protocols have been established for induction and maintenance of general anesthesia. This documentation includes information about arterial blood pressure, heart rate, oxygenation, and details of common procedures such as maintaining airway status and providing endotracheal intubation. Likewise, there are similar standard guidelines for documenting neuraxial anesthesia, including information about block level; sterility provisions; equipment and technique used; incidence of cerebrospinal fluid, blood, or paresthesia; and local anesthetic injection. In contrast, no such guidelines exist for documenting peripheral nerve blocks, even though they are used routinely in clinical practice and possess the same medicolegal implications as general and neuraxial

Nerve Block(s)			

	Consent ☐	Coagulation OK ☐	Ultrasound ☐
Premedication	Left Right ☐ ☐	☐ Midazolam iv ......mg ☐ Ketamine iv ......mg ☐ Other: ....mg	
Sterility		☐ Sterile gloves, disinfection, drape, probe cover,	
Monitoring		☐ Full ASA monitoring ☐ In plane ☐ Out of plane ☐ Injection(s) made extraneural ☐ Number of injections .... ☐ OIP ≤ 15psi (Opening Injection Pressure) ☐ Nerve Stimulation (NS) ☐ No EMR ≤ 0.5 mA ☐ Not used	
Equipment		Needle:☐Stimuplex 22G Length.........mm ☐Other .....G Length.........mm ☐ Catheter:	
Local anesthetic		☐ Ropivacaine: ......% ......ml ☐ Bupivacaine: ......% ......ml ☐ Lidocaine: ......% ......ml ☐ Additives	☐ Adrenaline 1/.............. ☐ Other ....
Doctors		................................Hadzic Lancea/ NYSORA.	

FIGURE 12–2. An example of block documentation as used at NYSORA-Europe CREER (Center for Research, Education and Enhanced Recovery) at ZOL (Ziekenhuis Oost-Limburg, Genk, Belgium).

anesthesia. One limitation of the lack of a documentation protocol for peripheral nerve blocks is the relative dearth of information available for those who wish to retrospectively review a regional procedure for quality assurance, research, or legal reasons. An example of block documentation is seen Figure 12–2.

More information about monitoring and documenting of PNBs is addressed in Chapter 63.

EQUIPMENT FOR INDUCTION OF REGIONAL ANESTHESIA

Needles for Single-Shot Nerve Blocks

Currently, there are many different types of peripheral nerve block needles on the market. Insulated needles are commonly used with nerve stimulation. With the introduction of ultrasound, echogenic needles have been used widely for better visualization.[9] Commercially available needles for single-shot nerve blocks usually come with preattached extension tubing to facilitate aspiration and injection of D5W or local anesthetics and feature a female attachment for connection to a nerve stimulator. One should note that the Luer lock for the attached tubing may occasionally be loose, which can lead to leakage of injected local anesthetic as well as air on aspiration.

Needle-Tip Design

Nerve injury can be caused by direct nerve penetration or forceful needle-nerve contact. The bevel of the needle can have an impact on the extent of damage on needle insertion close to a nerve. Short-beveled needles (Figure 12–3) may have the advantage of reducing nerve damage caused by cutting or penetration of the nerve, whereas long-beveled (14°) needles have been shown to be more likely to penetrate perineurium and cause fascicular injury than a short-beveled (45°) needle, especially when oriented transversely to the nerve fibers.[10–12] On the

other hand, short-beveled needles can cause greater injury in case of nerve or fascicular penetration.[13] Blunt, noncutting needles and Tuohy needles provide better feedback and enhanced feel for the "pop" that occurs when puncturing through fascia. However, a needle that is too blunt may hinder fascial puncture, resulting in higher applied pressure and potentially "overshooting" after puncturing the fascia. Pencil-point and Tuohy needles can also cause greater post-traumatic inflammation, myelin damage, and intraneural hematoma.[14,15]

Neuraxial blocks can be performed with needles of different tip styles. Despite their description as atraumatic, Whitacre or Sprotte needles (Figure 12–4) can be traumatic to the tissues on entry, with tearing and severe disruption of collagen fibers (see Chapter 6). This contrasts with the Quincke needle, a so-called cutting needle[16] (Figure 12–4), also used for neuraxial blocks. Nevertheless, the overall consensus is that neuraxial blocks performed with an atraumatic needle is associated with less risk of postdural puncture headache.[17,18]

Needle Length

The choice of the needle length depends on the specific block. For instance, deeper blocks, such as sciatic nerve block, will require longer needles (eg, 100–120 mm). The use of ultrasound can help determine the distance of the trajectory toward

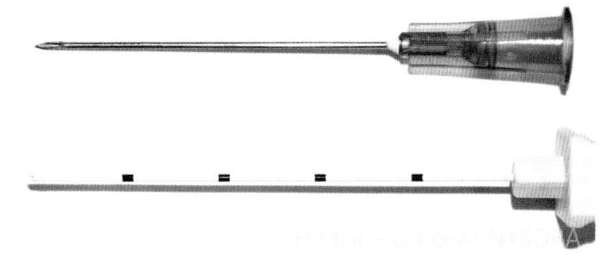

FIGURE 12–3. Short- (top) versus long-beveled needle (bottom).

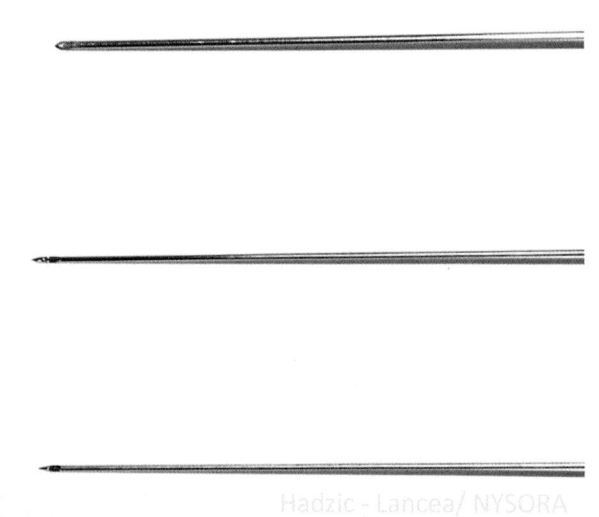

FIGURE 12–4. Different needles for spinal anesthesia: Whitacre (top), Sprotte (middle), and Quincke (bottom).

the target nerve. A needle that is too short will not reach the target site, while a long needle may be difficult to maneuver and may be advanced too deeply. Needles should have depth markings (Figure 12–5) for monitoring of the depth of penetration into the tissue. The correct needle length (shortest possible) will allow for better handling and manipulation.

Needle Gauge

In general, 22-gauge insulated needles are probably used most commonly for single-shot peripheral nerve blocks. With needle size, a balance must be sought between patient comfort and bending of the needle as it punctures through the skin. Because longer needles tend to bend more easily during advancement and are more difficult to steer during deep blocks, a larger-gauge needle may be required, as smaller-gauge needles lack rigidity and bend more readily. Larger-gauge needles should be used with caution, as they are associated with increased severity of tissue injury and hematoma, while smaller-gauge needles carry the more serious risk of the tip being inserted intrafascicularly.[15] Also, resistance tends to be increased on injection with smaller-gauge needles, and it also takes longer for blood to be aspirated back should the tip be intravascular.

Echogenic Needles

Since the introduction of ultrasound-guided peripheral nerve blocks, there has been an effort to manufacture needles with improved visibility on ultrasound. Echogenic needles reflect ultrasound beams through a variety of mechanisms, including a special coating that traps micro–air bubbles, grooves near the

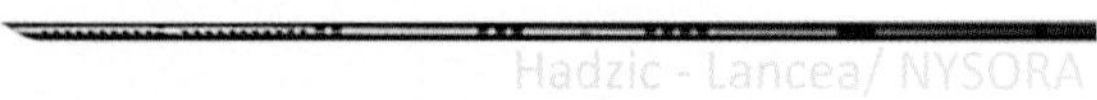

FIGURE 12–5. Nerve block needle showing centimeter markings that can be used as an example to monitor depth of penetration. Cornerstone reflectors to aid in visualization under ultrasound can also be seen at the distal end.

needle tip, or echogenic "dots" made by "cornerstone" reflectors (see distal end of needle in Figure 12–5). Needles with enhanced echogenicity may reduce visualization time during ultrasound-guided procedures.[9] An echogenic needle, with or without ultrasound beam steering, is better visualized compared to a nonechogenic needle at 60°–70° angles of insertion. In contrast, the nonechogenic needle with beam steering was more visible at a 40° insertion angle compared with the echogenic needle.[19]

Continuous Catheter Assemblies

Continuous infusion of local anesthetic has proved effective in providing long-term postoperative analgesia in a variety of settings. Peripheral nerve block catheters also enable titration of medication in small-dose aliquots. Equipment for continuous peripheral nerve blocks is discussed in detail in Chapter 13. Catheter-over-needle assemblies have been gaining popularity for delivering continuous regional anesthesia and analgesia and are discussed briefly in this chapter.

Historically, it has been well recognized that perineural catheters are associated with leakage and migration. However, the catheter-over-needle system design may reduce these obstacles and has renewed interest in continuous regional techniques.[20,21] The difference between this assembly and traditional catheter-through-needle assemblies is also the position of the needle in relation to the catheter, whether within or surrounding the catheter (Figure 12–6). With catheter-through-needle assemblies, a gap is left between the skin and the catheter on removal of the needle. In contrast, withdrawal of the needle in the catheter-over-needle assembly does not affect the snug fit of the catheter in the skin because the needle is housed inside the catheter.[22]

There are a few variations on this design that are marketed by different brands. For example, Contiplex (B-Braun Medical, Melsungen, Germany) design features the catheter-over-needle as a single unit (Figure 12–7).

Another variation is the recently introduced E-Cath (Pajunk MEDIZINTECHNOLOGIE GmbH, Geisingen, Germany kit with a "catheter-within-catheter" design, which features two components, the outer catheter sheath and the flexible inner catheter, that create a nonkinkable unit (Figure 12–8). The initial device resembles an intravenous cannula, with a needle within the outer catheter, which is inserted proximal to the target nerve under ultrasound guidance. The distal end of the needle protrudes for its electrical conductive property. Once in place, the needle is withdrawn from the unit, leaving the outer catheter in situ, and an inner catheter is inserted *into* the outer catheter to replace the needle and is Luer locked in place for injection (Figure 12–8). The inner catheter literally replaces the needle, and the inner catheter tip is essentially at the exact location where the needle tip was before needle withdrawal.

Several advantages of the catheter-over-needle design include potential:

- Simple to use with an insertion technique compared to that of a single-shot nerve block
- Less leakage from the catheter insertion site, for example, during shoulder surgery when the patient is in a

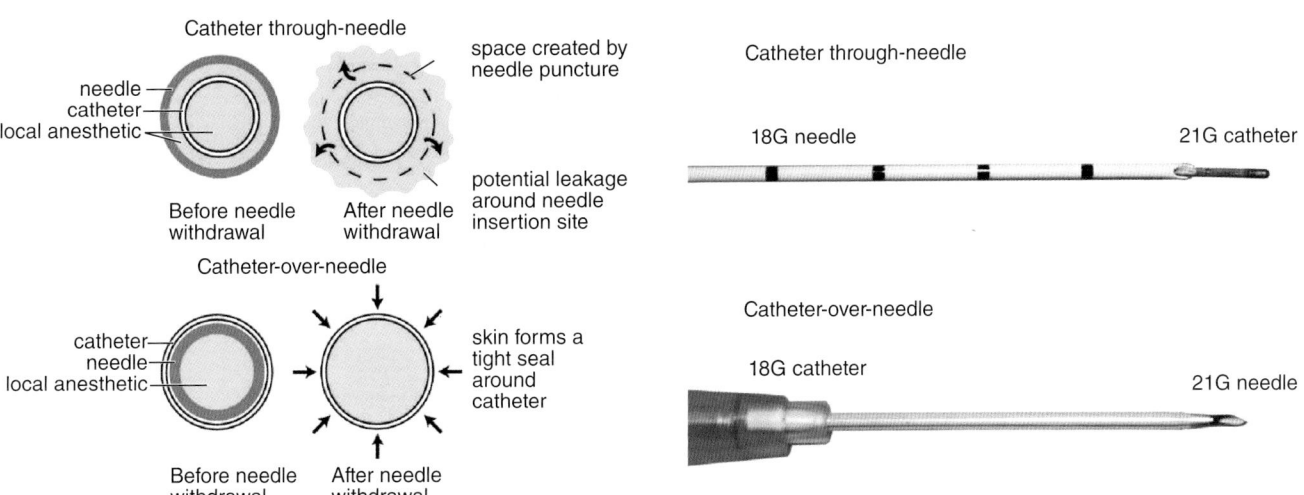

FIGURE 12–6. Left, schematic showing the difference between traditional catheter-through-needle (top) and catheter-over-needle (bottom) designs with respect to risk of leakage from the skin puncture site. In the former, the needle hole diameter is larger than the catheter diameter, leaving space for local anesthetic to leak when injected. In the latter, the puncture hole is smaller than the catheter diameter, allowing the catheter to be held tightly by the surrounding skin. Right, differing distal ends of catheter-though-needle (top) and catheter-over-needle (bottom) assemblies.

sitting position with a potential for surgical field contamination[23]
- Less risk of dressing adhesive disruption
- Fewer steps and less risk of dislodgement[24]
- Easy visualization of the catheter, especially the catheter tip[25]

Nerve-Locating Devices
Peripheral Nerve Stimulators

Peripheral nerve stimulators were the primary nerve-seeking device in the decades preceding widespread use of ultrasound guidance. The combined use of ultrasound and nerve stimulation creates a more objective method of achieving accurate and safe blocks while allowing monitoring and visualization of the block needle and targets in real time. With the introduction of ultrasound, the role of nerve stimulators has changed from nerve seeking to monitoring for needle-nerve contact or intraneural needle tip placement. In addition, nerve stimulation can be used as a confirmation technique and guide in placing

epidural catheters using the electrical epidural stimulation (Tsui) test.[26] Details of the physical properties underlying nerve stimulation are discussed in Chapter 18; key properties of commercially available nerve stimulators are briefly highlighted next (Figure 12–9).

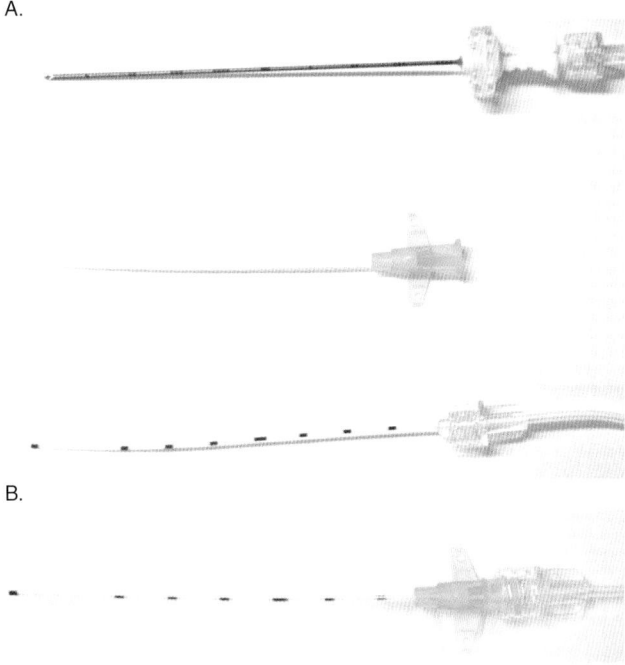

A.

B.

FIGURE 12–8. Detail of E-Cath (Pajunk MEDIZINTECHNOLOGIE GmbH, Geisingen, Germany catheter-over-needle components. **A:** Top, needle with extension tubing for nerve stimulator and a fluid giving set; middle, the catheter is placed over the needle to create a single unit that is inserted near the target nerve; bottom, the inner catheter is inserted into the outer catheter following needle withdrawal once the catheter-over-needle unit is at the desired position. **B:** Luer lock holding together the inner and outer catheters.

A.

B.

FIGURE 12–7. A: The Contiplex (B-Braun Medical, Melsungen, Germany) catheter-over-needle assembly, which features a long needle covered by the catheter and a clip that can be moved along the needle length for easy manipulation of the unit. **B:** B. Braun catheter-over-needle components: needle with extensions for nerve stimulation and injection (top) and catheter with centimeter marks (bottom).

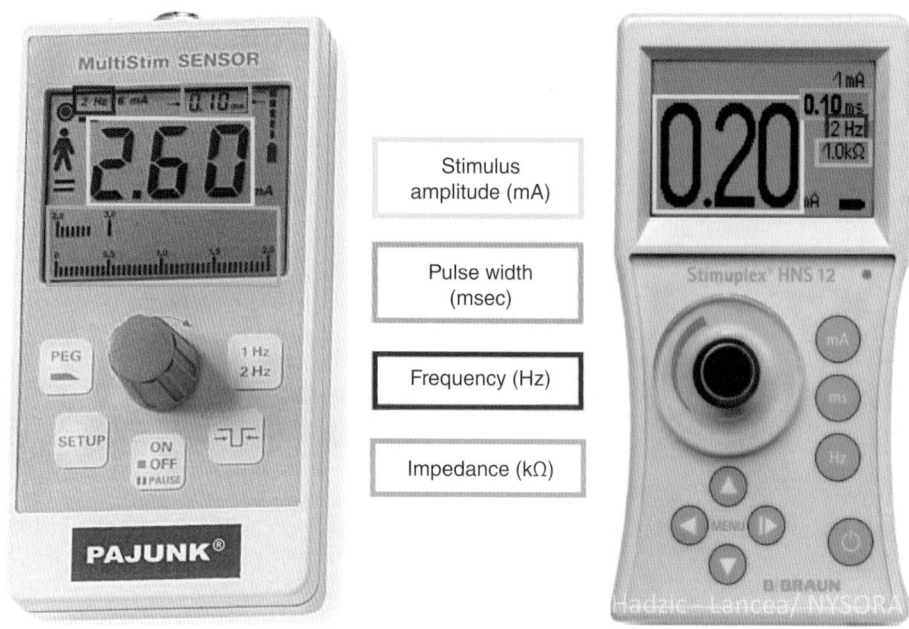

FIGURE 12–9. Peripheral nerve stimulators allowing measurement of stimulus amplitude, pulse width, frequency, and electrical impedance.

Constant Current Output and Display Most modern models now deliver constant current, and current output can be set in frequency, pulse width, and current milliamperes (mA). The primary advantage of a constant current output nerve stimulator is its ability to deliver a stable current output in the presence of varied resistances.

Display A clear digital display with accuracy to two decimal places is an important feature of the electrical nerve stimulator. This display must indicate the actual current delivered to the patient and not simply the target current setting. Some nerve stimulators are equipped with low- (up to 6 mA) and high-output (up to 80 mA) ranges. The lower range is used primarily to alert for potential intraneural needle placement, while the higher range is mainly used for the epidural stimulation test (1–10 mA).

Variable Pulse Width Short pulse widths (ie, 0.04 ms) are a better indicator of the distance between the needle and the nerve, based on changes in current. In contrast, with long pulse widths (ie, 1 ms), there is little difference in the current required to stimulate the nerve, regardless of whether the stimulating needle is in direct contact with the nerve or 1 cm away. At a pulse width of 0.04 ms, there is a large difference in the stimulating current required when comparing direct contact with the nerve versus a distance of 1 cm away.

Pulse width also has a role in successful use of the electrical epidural stimulation test. The proper pulse width must be used for different applications of the test, be it a peripheral or neuraxial block. Table 12–1 summarizes the appropriate pulse width for different applications.

Clearly Marked Polarity of the Electrodes The polarity of the needle will affect its ability to stimulate the nerve at a given current and should be clearly marked. The cathode (black) is selected as the stimulating electrode because it is three to four times more effective than the anode at depolarizing the nerve membrane.

Variable Pulse Frequency Most new stimulators have an option to change the frequency at which the electrical pulse is delivered. Although some commercially available peripheral nerve stimulators can allow adjustment of frequency up to 5 Hz, the optimal frequency of the electrical pulse is between 0.5 and 4 Hz. Most users select a frequency of 2 Hz. When using a lower frequency, such as 1 Hz (one stimulus per second), the needle must be advanced slowly to avoid missing the nerve between stimulations.

Disconnect and Malfunction Indicators The disconnection and malfunction of nerve stimulators should be easily detectable, and an indication of battery power is essential. Most

TABLE 12–1. Pulse widths for different applications during peripheral nerve block and neuraxial block.

Pulse Width	Application	Typical Threshold Range
0.1 ms	Motor peripheral nerve	Avoid < 0.3 mA
0.2 ms	Epidural space Intrathecal space	1–15 mA <1 mA
1 ms	Epidural space	6 mA

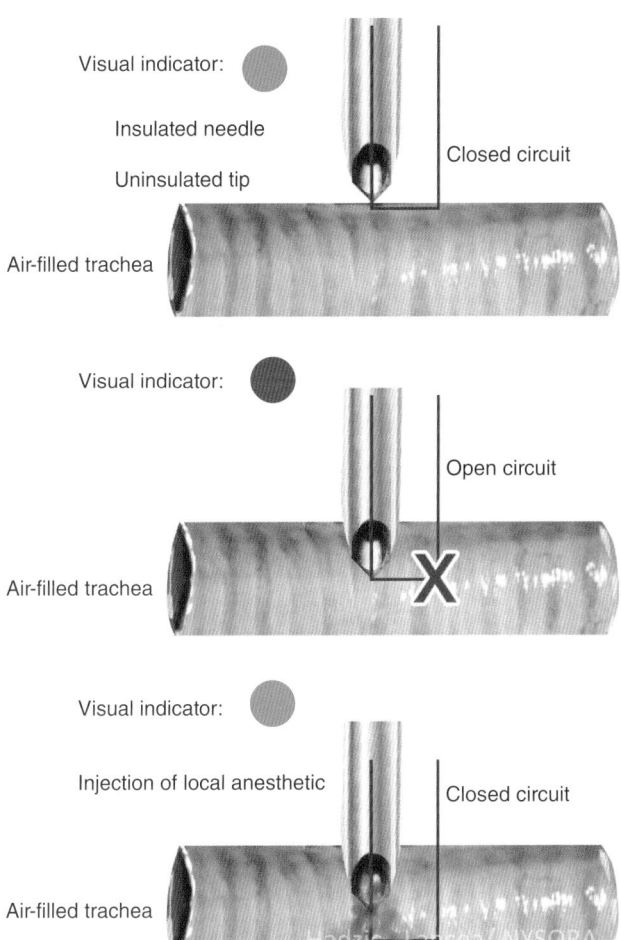

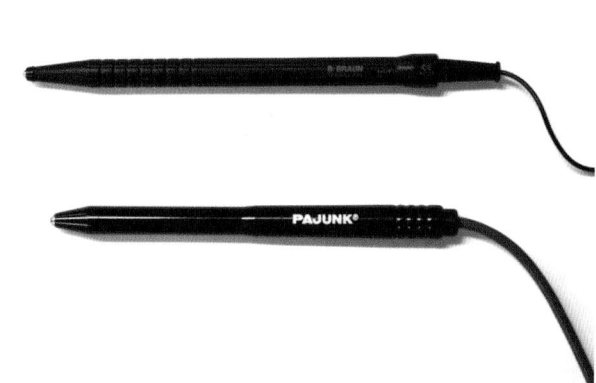

FIGURE 12–11. Surface nerve mapping probe for percutaneous electrode guidance.

FIGURE 12–10. Change in peripheral nerve stimulator light and tone signal on entry of uninsulated needle tip into tracheal lumen during airway topicalization (top and middle). With injection of local anesthetic, electrical current is closed, causing another light/tone signal change (bottom).

nerve stimulators use a change in tone or light to warn when the circuit is not complete and if the pulse current cannot be delivered. The value of the tone/light change on disconnection of the circuit was demonstrated recently with a novel use for a peripheral nerve stimulator in guiding an insulated needle with an uninsulated tip into the tracheal lumen for airway topicalization.[27] The change in tone/light indicated whether the tip was in contact with tissue (closed circuit) or suspended in the air-filled trachea (open circuit) (Figure 12–10).

Electrical Impedance Some modern nerve stimulators display the total impedance between the needle tip and ground electrode. The significance of this property in monitoring intraneural needle-tip placement is discussed in the section on monitoring devices in this chapter.

Other Accessories A probe may be used for performing percutaneous electrode guidance during surface nerve mapping (Figure 12–11). A small remote hand control or foot pedal allows a single operator to adjust the current output of a nerve

stimulator without an assistant, although this is seldom used clinically (Figure 12–12).

Ultrasound

The introduction of ultrasound technology has revolutionized the field of regional anesthesia, allowing nerve structures, needles, and other subcutaneous objects to be visualized in real time. Ultrasound undoubtedly can improve the safety and ease of performing nerve blocks; however, this is largely operator dependent.

There are a number of commercially available portable ultrasound machines that are suitable for regional anesthesia (Figure 12–13). These machines can be transported easily, and image quality and resolution are equivalent or similar to those of stationary ultrasound machines. The transducer (or probe) is the most important element of the ultrasound machine; transducers of various footprints and beam planes are available, allowing the user to scan most surfaces on individuals of various body habitus. The quality of ultrasound machines is constantly improving, with better ergonomic options and ease of use, higher resolution with improved transducers, improved portability, and reduction in cost. A more thorough discussion of ultrasound technology and application in regional anesthesia can be found in Chapters 28-30.

Monitoring Devices
Monitoring for the Patient

It is important to apply routine monitoring for patients undergoing regional anesthesia with or without sedation. Toxicity from local anesthetic overdose and intravascular injection and oversedation are potential complications of regional anesthesia. Therefore, one should be vigilant with regard to patient monitoring. One should also be aware that toxicity from local anesthetic can occur within the first half hour after injection of medication due to the peak in plasma concentration (typically 20–30 minutes).[28] Local anesthetic systemic toxicity is discussed in detail elsewhere.

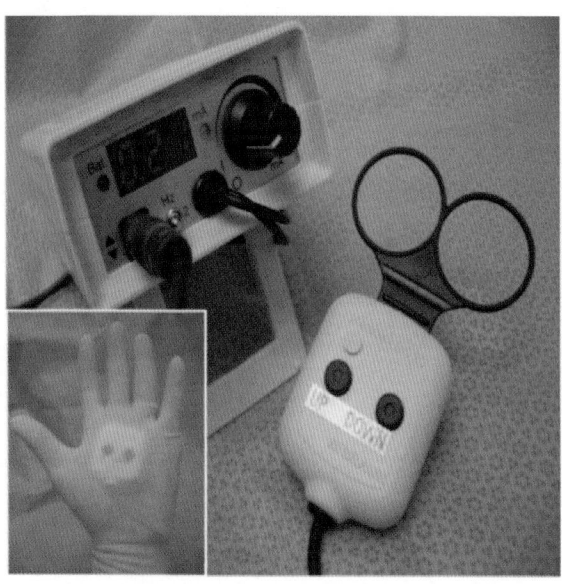
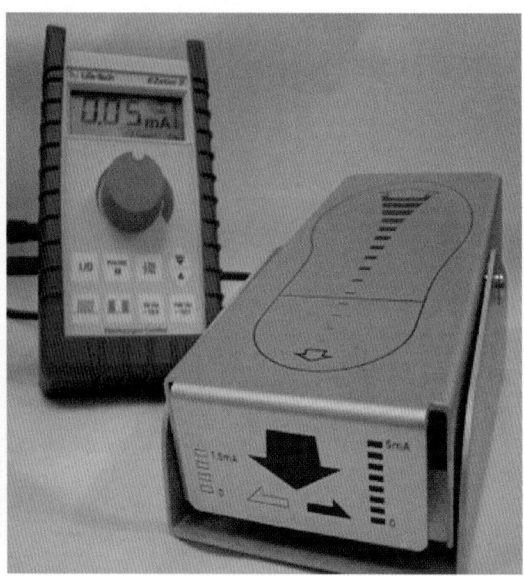

FIGURE 12–12. Remote hand-controlled (left) and foot-controlled (right) devices for adjusting nerve stimulator current output.

General monitoring for the patient includes examining the following:

- Electrocardiogram.
- Noninvasive blood pressure.
- Pulse oximetry.

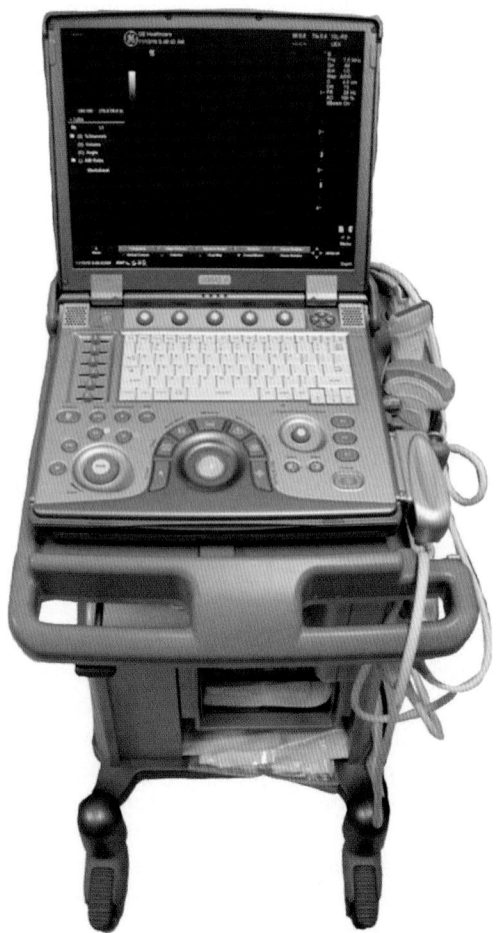

FIGURE 12–13. Portable ultrasound machine.

- For ventilation: The adequacy of ventilation for regional anesthesia without sedation can be performed by qualitative clinical monitoring. However, for patients who require sedation, capnography should be used unless it is precluded by the patient, procedure, or equipment.

Monitoring for Intraneural Injection

Paresthesia Prior to the introduction of nerve stimulation technology, paresthesia was the only means of nerve localization. However, there has been emerging evidence suggesting painful paresthesia can lead to persistent neurological symptoms and neuropathy. Thus, most clinicians are not only abandoning seeking paresthesia but also, with awake or lightly sedated patients, are using paresthesia as a signal to warn of needle-nerve proximity.

Electrical Nerve Stimulation The role of the nerve stimulator has shifted since the introduction of ultrasound. In most cases, nerve stimulation is no longer used as a primary tool for nerve localization but is instead used for monitoring to minimize intraneural injection. Nerve stimulators allow the user to monitor two electrophysiological properties during nerve block performance: the nerve stimulation threshold and electrical impedance.

Nerve stimulation threshold: A nerve stimulation threshold of less than 0.2 mA may suggest intraneural needle-tip location or needle-nerve contact.[29,30] When used alone, nerve stimulation lacks sensitivity[31] and should therefore be used in conjunction with other monitoring as described in this section. Observation of a motor response signifies needle-nerve proximity with a low threshold current; however, a lack of motor response at a 0.2 mA or less threshold with a pulse width of 0.1 ms does not always rule out intraneural needle placement.

Electrical impedance: Many modern nerve stimulators are capable of measuring impedance. In an electrical circuit, direct current (DC) is the flow of electric charge in only one direction, whereas alternating current (AC) describes flow of electric charge that reverses direction periodically. In nerve stimulation, pulsating DC is used. Because pulsating DC shares characteristics of both AC and DC waveforms, the electrical resistance of the nerve stimulation circuit is often referred to as impedance. Impedance is highly sensitive to tissue composition and varies depending on the water content of the tissue.[32] Because there is variation in water and lipid content between intraneural and extraneural spaces, with the former having a considerably greater amount of nonconduction lipid and lower water content, a significant difference in intraneural and extraneural impedance has been demonstrated.[33] A recent study in adult patients also showed that an increase in impedance greater than 4.3% may indicate intraneural needle placement.[34] Furthermore, discrimination between nerve tissue and other tissue types has been improved by combining several impedance variables at multiple measurement frequencies to increase precision.[35] Electrical impedance also changes on intravascular and perineural injection of D5W.[36] A change in impedance may therefore warn against injection in a location that could potentially cause nerve damage or other sequelae.

Clinical Pearl

- A sudden change in impedance may indicate that the needle is entering different tissues.

Ultrasound Imaging With the rising popularity of ultrasound guidance for peripheral nerve blocks, there has been a common misunderstanding that ultrasound can help avoid intraneural injection. To improve the safety margin, the needle tip should be visualized at all times during advancement of the needle during an in-plane approach; however, this can be challenging, even in experienced hands. In addition, there is a significant learning curve associated with using ultrasound in regional anesthesia, both with in-plane and out-of-plane approaches. When an out-of-plane approach is used, the needle shaft could be mistaken for the tip, which would be further downstream of the ultrasound beam. During injection, nerve swelling as a result of intraneural injection can also be difficult to note in real time. Moreover, by the time nerve swelling is noticed, it may be too late to prevent nerve injury as it takes only a miniscule volume of local anesthetic to rupture the perineurium when the needle is placed intrafascicularly. Finally, current ultrasound resolution is not high enough to recognize intrafascicular injection, the most severe event in terms of nerve damage. As such, nerve injury with peripheral nerve blocks despite the use of ultrasound continues to be reported.[37–39] The rate of residual paresthesia or numbness after ultrasound-guided peripheral nerve block is estimated to be 0.18% up to 16%.[40–43] Therefore, ultrasound should not be used as the sole guidance device but, rather, should be used in conjunction with other monitoring modalities to minimize the risk of intraneural injection.[44,45]

Injection Pressure Monitoring Monitoring injection pressure can help distinguish needle-tip location in the perineural tissue versus the needle-nerve contact or intrafascicular needle placement (ie, perineural vs. intraneural-intrafascicular).[46,47] Results of several studies suggest that high-pressure injection into the intraneural space, even with small volumes, can be a major contributor to mechanical injury of neurological tissue during peripheral nerve blocks.[48,49] The rationale and basis for nerve damage from high-pressure injection are likely a combination of mechanical injury from breaching the perineurium, leading to interference with endoneural microcirculation, and chemical injury from neurotoxicity of local anesthetics.[49–53]

Using canine models, it was shown that high injection pressure (>20 psi) can result in persistent neurological damage indicative of intrafascicular injection.[48] However, not all intraneural injection results in high injection pressure and subsequent neurological deficit.[31,54] This could be due to an intraneural extrafascicular injection or the beveled needle tip not being completely within the nerve. In these cases, the injectate may push the nerve out of the way, avoiding a high-pressure injection. Nevertheless, intraneural injection is generally not recommended. Forceful needle-nerve contact and displacement have also been shown to cause inflammatory changes to nerves.[55,56] Since a recent study demonstrated that high opening injection pressure (≥15 psi)—the pressure that must be overcome before injection can commence—may be indicative of intraneural needle placement, it is important to monitor injection pressure carefully during local anesthetic injection.[47] Furthermore, high injection pressure can also cause undesired neuraxial spread during certain regional blocks close to the neuraxis, for example, lumbar plexus block or brachial plexus block.[57,58]

Clinical Pearl

- It has been suggested that opening injection pressure should be kept below 15 psi to improve safety. Opening pressure is not dependent on needle size, needle type, injection speed, and syringe size.[47]

Methods of monitoring injection pressure include the following: syringe feel, in-line pressure manometer, and compressed air injection technique (CAIT).

Syringe feel. Traditionally in clinical practice, a subjective "syringe feel" technique has been used to assess resistance to injection of local anesthetic and is performed by the anesthesiologist or assistant while the anesthesiologist

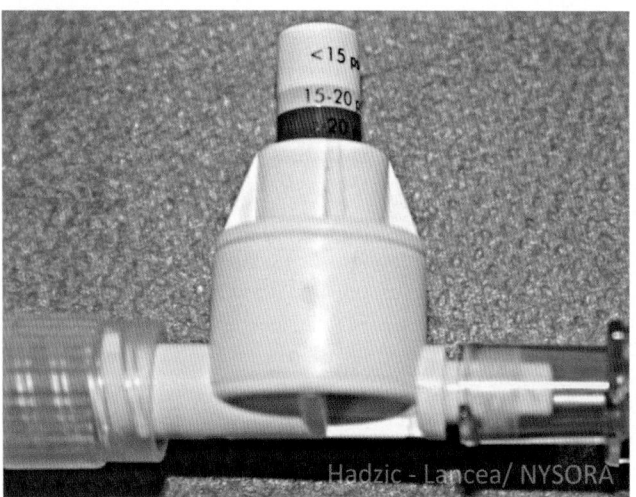

FIGURE 12–14. Commercially available disposable in-line pressure-monitoring device for monitoring injection pressure during peripheral nerve block (BSmart, BBraun Medical, Melsungen, GE).

maintains the correct needle position. Needless to say, this subjective approach is not reliable and is operator dependent.[59,60] Different needle lengths, diameter, and syringe types also affect the feel.

In-line pressure manometer. Commercially available objective disposable devices to measure injection pressure, such as BSmart™ (B-Braun Medical, Melsungen, Germany) (Figure 12–14), continuously displays the pressure during injection, allowing clinicians to quantify the injection

pressure information, which can be documented. The manometer is color coded such that when the pressure is 20 psi or greater, the indicator will be red to warn the operator. The in-line pressure monitor is placed proximal to the needle and in line with the nondistensible tubing. The other end of the pressure monitor is attached directly to the syringe. The principle is the same as in-line pressure sensors in devices such as syringe pumps for continuous pressure monitoring. The main principle behind the use of an injection pressure monitor is that a certain amount of injection pressure (opening pressure) must be reached before the injection (the flow of the anesthetic) can commence. The critical opening pressure necessary to inject local anesthetic when the needle is in contact with the nerve or is intrafascicular has been estimated in several studies to be more than 15 psi.[46,47] Therefore, if the injection is halted before the opening pressure is reached and flow of anesthetic is initiated, injection in vulnerable needle-nerve interaction can be avoided.

Compressed air injection technique. This is the clinical application of Boyle's law (Pressure × Volume = Constant). At a constant temperature, a set volume of gas (air) varies inversely with the pressure; for instance, if the volume of the gas is reduced by 50%, the pressure will be increased from 1 atmosphere to 2 atmospheres. This technique, designed by Tsui, involves aspirating a set amount of air above a volume of injectate within a syringe.[61] During injection, the volume of air is compressed and maintained at a certain percentage (Figure 12–15).

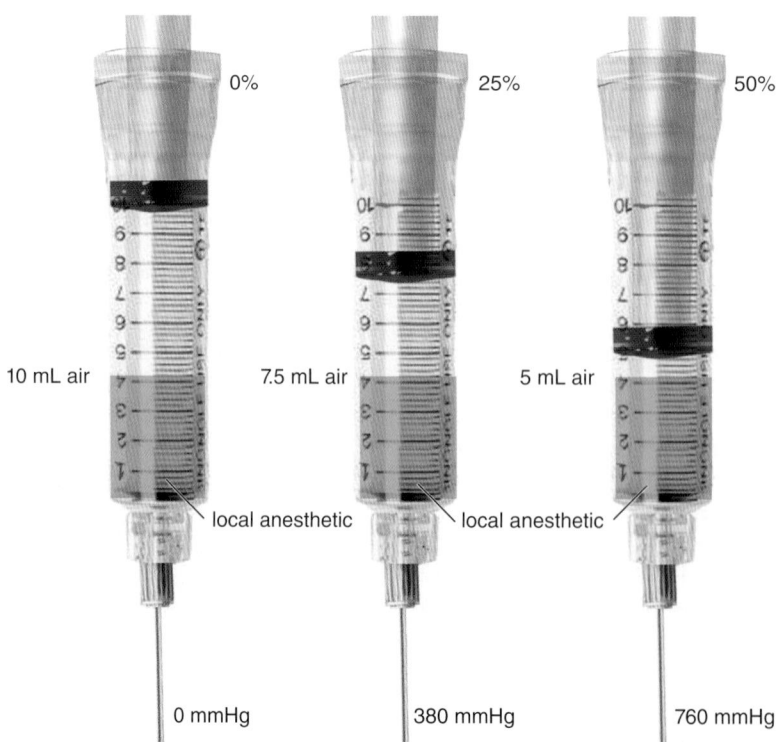

FIGURE 12–15. Compressed air injection technique (CAIT) to prevent high injection pressure; 50% compression of air volume in the syringe corresponds to an injection pressure of 760 mm Hg.

At 50% air compression, the injection pressure was 760 mm Hg or less, well below the threshold of less than 25 psi (1293 mm Hg).[61] CAIT is a simple and practical way to standardize the local anesthetic injection pressures in real time, ensuring the injection pressure is constantly below the threshold and minimizing the risk of clinically significant nerve injury. This method also inevitably reduces the speed of injection, which in turns decreases the risk of intrafascicular injection or siphoning the local anesthetic to unwanted tissue planes. The pressures generated by CAIT also remain consistently stable throughout the injection period, unlike the syringe feel technique, which produces high peak pressures. This is likely due to the "cushioning" effect from the volume of air, which dampens the initial high pressure.

Clinical Pearls

- In the era of ultrasound-guided peripheral nerve blocks, it is important not to dismiss the value of nerve stimulator and injection pressure monitoring to minimize the potential for nerve injury.
- It is important to use a combination of monitors to minimize the risk of intraneural, intrafascicular injection and needle-nerve trauma.

EQUIPMENT FOR POSTBLOCKADE MANAGEMENT

Block Assessment Tools

Various tools and techniques are available to monitor the progress of a regional block (Figure 12–16). Ideally, the monitoring tool or device should be as objective as possible, but due to physiological differences among individuals receiving a block, this is rarely the case. To date, there is no consensus on which is the most effective method. Nevertheless, most block-monitoring tools generally offer an acceptable interpretation of when surgical anesthesia is achieved. Similarly, tools and scales used to assess sensory and motor blockade vary greatly and offer subjective feedback on the degree to which a nerve block is achieving its desired goal. Commonly, pain scales or scores are used to indicate a patient's comfort level; as with block-monitoring tools, these scales and scores provide a more objective and reproducible means to assess the severity of pain.

Sensory (Dermatome) Testing

Regional block assessment tools are based on the assumption that the patient will not be able to perceive a stimulus on the area being blocked. These stimuli are usually temperature based (ice, alcohol swab), but a graded filament can also be used to measure diminishing and returning cutaneous sensation. In the case of trunk/neuraxial blocks, these methods can help

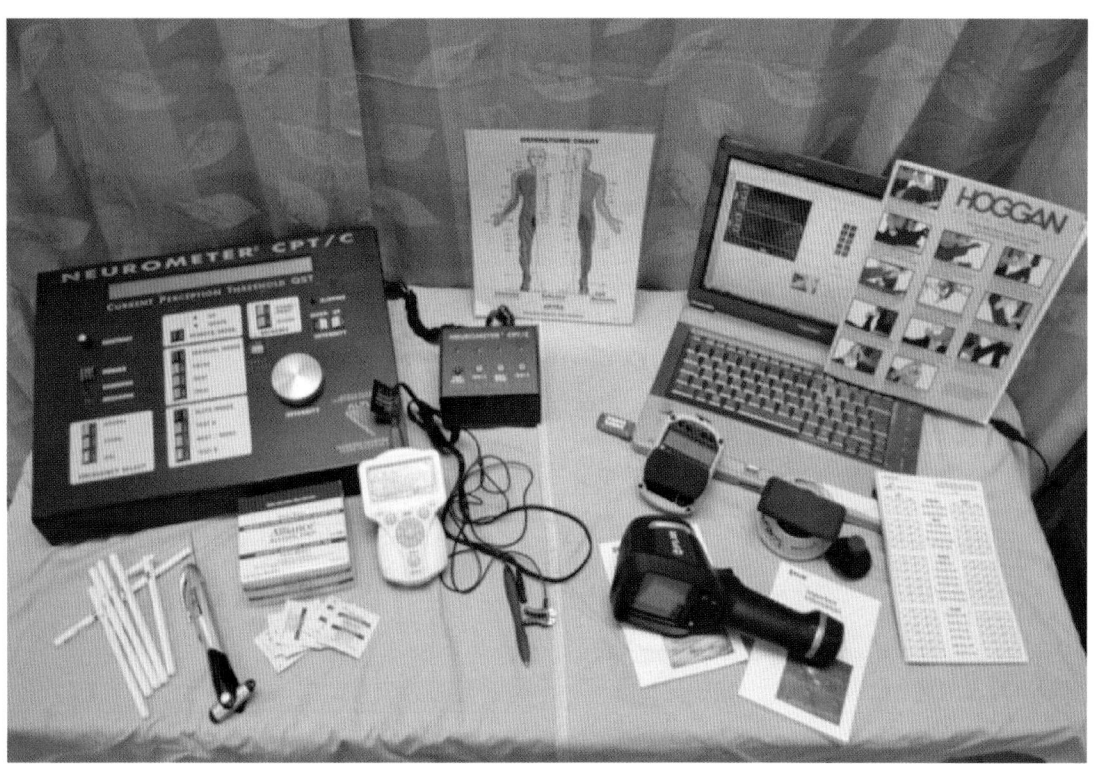

FIGURE 12–16. Selection of nerve block–monitoring equipment, including devices to measure current perception threshold (upper left), monofilaments and alcohol swabs for sensory perception (lower left), infrared scanning device (lower right), and force transducers with wireless data collection capability (upper right).

determine and follow block spread by observing which dermatomes are responsive to the stimulus.

Temperature/Infrared Recording

Recently, infrared thermal imaging has also been tested as a means to monitor block progression.[62,63] This test is based on the knowledge that skin temperature in the digits increases following brachial plexus block. The studies showed that infrared thermography of the digits had high positive predictive value for block success following brachial plexus anesthesia.

Current Perception Threshold

Current perception threshold (CPT) is a means of applying electrical current via a percutaneous electrode connected to a specialized current generator (eg, Neurometer[64]) to test sensory level. This method has been used to quantify degrees of neuropathy in conditions such as diabetes mellitus.[65,66] Recently, the reproducibility of this method has been tested in volunteers with acceptable results using a common peripheral nerve stimulator.[67] In this study, a peripheral nerve stimulator (see previous discussion) was used to apply an electrical stimulus to the blocked area; if the current required to elicit a sensory response was greater over time than the baseline (preblock or unblocked region) current, this was an indicator of block progression. Indeed, a subsequent study demonstrated that CPT can be an objective, reliable tool to monitor block onset in clinical scenarios.[68]

Pain Assessment

Numerous validated pain rating scales exist, with the most popular being variations on the 0–10 scale, where 0 indicates "no pain at all," and 10 indicates "worst pain ever." The numeric rating scale (NRS) and visual analog scale (VAS)[69] are two examples of this type. Other pain rating scales, such as the Defense and Veterans Pain Rating Scale (DVPRS),[70] feature notes on how the pain affects everyday living that can be used to more precisely define the severity of the pain. The DVPRS also features facial cartoons that can be used to obtain feedback on pain severity from individuals with limited communication ability. For elderly patients, the Pain Assessment Checklist for Seniors With Limited Ability to Communicate (PACSLAC)[71] can be used to assess pain in individuals with dementia or cognitive impairment and who have trouble communicating. For children, a variety of pain scales are available that can be used for different age groups and communication abilities.

Motor Block Assessment

The most common motor assessment tool is the Bromage score,[72] a 4-point scale ranging from 0 (full movement) to 3 (complete block/no movement). The original Bromage score was applied for cases of lower extremity block but can also be adapted to assessment of upper extremity block. Another more objective method that can assess onset of and recovery from a nerve block is strength testing. This can be performed with a portable force transducer: The patient is asked to exert force against the transducer with the limb or body part that has been blocked (eg, elbow extension to assess radial nerve function).

Some modern force transducers come equipped with a universal serial bus (USB) stick that, along with a portable computer, allows force data to be collected wirelessly in real time (Figure 12–16).

Maintenance of Regional Anesthesia

Regional anesthesia practice has relied on infusion pumps to provide continuous delivery of local anesthetic through a perineural catheter. This method remains the most popular method of continuous regional anesthesia, but new developments in technology and practice have allowed for flexibility in postoperative analgesia. Conventional methods for continuous nerve blocks are discussed in more detail in Chapters 11 and 13; new developments are covered here briefly.

Intermittent Bolus

In addition to the traditional continuous infusion regimen, it has become increasingly popular to use intermittent bolusing for continuous peripheral nerve block management. With its ability to target nerve structures with precision, catheter-over-needle technology (see previous discussion) greatly reduces the risk of catheter migration or dislodgement. An advantage of intermittent boluses is that the risk of local anesthetic toxicity is also reduced because constant delivery of local anesthetic is avoided and total dose is generally reduced.[73-75] An intermittent bolus regimen can be achieved by either a patient-controlled or preprogrammed approach.

Clinical Pearls

- One should consider and select pumps that allow delivery of intermittent boluses as well as continuous infusion.
- Because infusion pumps will be maintained and transported by the patient if they are mobile, the pump should be portable and easy to use.

Future Advances

Recently, the exciting prospect of controlling local anesthetic infusion by remote control was described.[76] In this system, pumps were set to adjust to patient need based on responses to questions about their pain control, and, in the event that settings needed to be changed, the practitioners were able to access the pump information via a secure server remotely, avoiding the need for a nurse or physician to be physically present.

CONCLUSION

With improvements in technology and equipment, regional anesthesia has progressed from an "art" practiced by few to a "science" that, with adequate training and experience, can be practiced by many. Regardless of who is performing the block or where it is being performed, there are several key guidelines that should be followed to ensure safe and effective regional anesthesia. It is essential that there be a designated area for performing nerve blocks and that all drugs and equipment are readily available. Careful documentation of the block procedure should be every institution's standard. Adequate patient monitoring is essential and should include standard ASA monitoring as well as objective ultrasound–nerve stimulator and injection pressure monitoring to help prevent nerve injury. The use of proper equipment, including appropriate needle length and gauge, will result in easier and more accurate needling. If a continuous block is desired, new catheter-over-needle assemblies can help mitigate the problems of traditional catheter-through-needle designs, and recent developments in long-term local anesthetic delivery methods, including intermittent bolus and remote control, represent valuable options.

In summary, current regional anesthesia practice depends on numerous tools, methods, and monitoring equipment. Although time is needed to gain adequate competency with some of these methods and tools, they are critical for ensuring that the regional block is performed in the safest and most effective manner possible during every stage of the procedure.

REFERENCES

1. van Lier F, van der Geest PJ, Hoeks SE, et al: Epidural analgesia is associated with improved health outcomes of surgical patients with chronic obstructive pulmonary disease. Anesthesiology 2011;115:315–3121.
2. Davies J, Fernando R: Effect of ropivacaine on platelet function. Anaesthesia 2001;56:709–710.
3. Richman JM, Liu SS, Courpas G, et al: Does continuous peripheral nerve block provide superior pain control to opioids? A meta-analysis. Anesth Analg 2006;102:248–257.
4. Salviz EA, Xu D, Frulla A, et al: Continuous interscalene block in patients having outpatient rotator cuff repair surgery: A prospective randomized trial. Anesth Analg 2013;117:1485–1492.
5. Sites BD, Taenzer AH, Herrick MD, et al: Incidence of local anesthetic systemic toxicity and postoperative neurologic symptoms associated with 12,668 ultrasound-guided nerve blocks: An analysis from a prospective clinical registry. Reg Anesth Pain Med 2012;37(5):478–482.
6. Cave G, Harvey M: Intravenous lipid emulsion as antidote beyond local anesthetic toxicity: A systematic review. Acad Emerg Med 2009;16:815–824.
7. Weinberg G, Ripper R, Feinstein DL, Hoffman W: Lipid emulsion infusion rescues dogs from bupivacaine-induced cardiac toxicity. Reg Anesth Pain Med 2003;28:198–202.
8. Weinberg, G: Treatment regimes. 2015. http://www.lipidrescue.org/.
9. Abbal B, Choquet O, Gourari A, et al: Enhanced visual acuity with echogenic needles in ultrasound-guided axillary brachial plexus block: A randomized, comparative, observer-blinded study. Minerva Anestesiol 2015;81:369–378.
10. Selander D, Dhuner KG, Lundborg G: Peripheral nerve injury due to injection needles used for regional anesthesia. An experimental study of the acute effects of needle point trauma. Acta Anaesthesiol Scand 1977;21:182–188.
11. Selander D: Peripheral nerve injury caused by injection needles. Br J Anaesth 1993;71:323–325.
12. Selander DE: Labat lecture 2006. Regional anesthesia: Aspects, thoughts, and some honest ethics; about needle bevels and nerve lesions, and back pain after spinal anesthesia. Reg Anesth Pain Med 2007;32:341–350.
13. Mackinnon SE, Hudson AR, Llamas F, et al: Peripheral nerve injury by chymopapain injection. J Neurosurg 1984;61:1–8.
14. Steinfeldt T, Graf J, Schneider J, et al: Histological consequences of needle-nerve contact following nerve stimulation in a pig model. Anesthesiol Res Pract 2011;2011:591851.
15. Steinfeldt T, Werner T, Nimphius W, et al: Histological analysis after peripheral nerve puncture with pencil-point or Tuohy needletip. Anesth Analg 2011;112:465–470.
16. Reina MA, de Leon-Casasola OA, Lopez A, et al: An in vitro study of dural lesions produced by 25-gauge Quincke and Whitacre needles evaluated by scanning electron microscopy. Reg Anesth Pain Med 2000;25:393–402.
17. Castrillo A, Tabernero C, Garcia-Olmos LM, et al: Postdural puncture headache: impact of needle type, a randomized trial. Spine J 2015;15:1571–1576.
18. Hammond ER, Wang Z, Bhulani N, et al: Needle type and the risk of post-lumbar puncture headache in the outpatient neurology clinic. J Neurol Sci 2011;306:24–28.
19. Uppal V, Sondekoppam RV, Ganapathy S: Effect of beam steering on the visibility of echogenic and non-echogenic needles: A laboratory study. Can J Anaesth 2014;61:909–915.
20. Ip VH, Tsui BC: The catheter-over-needle assembly facilitates delivery of a second local anesthetic bolus to prolong supraclavicular brachial plexus block without time-consuming catheterization steps: a randomized controlled study. Can J Anaesth 2013;60:692–699.
21. Tsui BC, Tsui J: Less leakage and dislodgement with a catheter-over-needle versus a catheter-through-needle approach for peripheral nerve block: An ex vivo study. Can J Anaesth 2012;59:655–661.
22. Ip VH, Rockley MC, Tsui BC: The catheter-over-needle assembly offers greater stability and less leakage compared with the traditional counterpart in continuous interscalene nerve blocks: A randomized patient-blinded study. Can J Anaesth 2013;60:1272–1273.
23. Ip V, Bouliane M, Tsui B: Potential contamination of the surgical site caused by leakage from an interscalene catheter with the patient in a seated position: A case report. Can J Anaesth 2012;59:1125–1129.
24. Tsui BC, Ip VH: Catheter-over-needle method reduces risk of perineural catheter dislocation. Br J Anaesth 2014;112:759–760.
25. Ip V, Tsui B. The safety of an interscalene catheter-over-needle technique. Anaesthesia 2013;68:774–775.
26. Tsui BC, Gupta S, Finucane B: Confirmation of epidural catheter placement using nerve stimulation. Can J Anaesth 1998;45:640–644.
27. Green JS, Tsui BC: Use of a nerve stimulator to assist cricothyroid membrane puncture during difficult airway topicalization. Can J Anaesth 2015;62:1126–1127.
28. Becker DE, Reed KL: Essentials of local anesthetic pharmacology. Anesth Prog 2006;53:98–108.
29. Bigeleisen PE, Moayeri N, Groen GJ: Extraneural versus intraneural stimulation thresholds during ultrasound-guided supraclavicular block. Anesthesiology 2009;110:1235–1243.
30. Robards C, Hadzic A, Somasundaram L, et al: Intraneural injection with low-current stimulation during popliteal sciatic nerve block. Anesth Analg 2009;109:673-677.
31. Chan VW, Brull R, McCartney CJ, et al: An ultrasonographic and histological study of intraneural injection and electrical stimulation in pigs. Anesth Analg 2007;104:1281–1284, tables.
32. Byrne K, Tsui BC: Practical concepts in nerve stimulation: Impedance and other recent advances. Int Anesthesiol Clin 2011;49:81–90.
33. Tsui BC, Pillay JJ, Chu KT, Dillane D: Electrical impedance to distinguish intraneural from extraneural needle placement in porcine nerves during direct exposure and ultrasound guidance. Anesthesiology 2008;109:479–483.
34. Bardou P, Merle JC, Woillard JB, et al: Electrical impedance to detect accidental nerve puncture during ultrasound-guided peripheral nerve blocks. Can J Anaesth 2013;60:253–258.
35. Kalvoy H, Sauter AR: Detection of intraneural needle-placement with multiple frequency bioimpedance monitoring: a novel method. J Clin Monit Comput 2106;30(2):185–192.
36. Chin J, Tsui BC: No change in impedance upon intravascular injection of D5W. Can J Anaesth 2010;57:559–564.
37. Cohen JM, Gray AT: Functional deficits after intraneural injection during interscalene block. Reg Anesth Pain Med 2010;35:397–399.
38. Reiss W, Kurapati S, Shariat A, Hadzic A: Nerve injury complicating ultrasound/electrostimulation-guided supraclavicular brachial plexus block. Reg Anesth Pain Med 2010;35:400–401.
39. Hara K, Sakura S, Yokokawa N, Tadenuma S: Incidence and effects of unintentional intraneural injection during ultrasound-guided subgluteal sciatic nerve block. Reg Anesth Pain Med 2012;37:289–293.
40. Sites BD, Taenzer AH, Herrick MD, et al: Incidence of local anesthetic systemic toxicity and postoperative neurologic symptoms associated with 12,668 ultrasound-guided nerve blocks: An analysis from a prospective clinical registry. Reg Anesth Pain Med 2012;37:478–482.
41. Liu SS, YaDeau JT, Shaw PM, et al: Incidence of unintentional intraneural injection and postoperative neurological complications with ultrasound-guided interscalene and supraclavicular nerve blocks. Anaesthesia 2011;66:168–174.

42. Widmer B, Lustig S, Scholes CJ, et al: Incidence and severity of complications due to femoral nerve blocks performed for knee surgery. Knee 2013;20:181–185.

43. Bilbao Ares A, Sabate A, Porteiro L, et al: [Neurological complications associated with ultrasound-guided interscalene and supraclavicular block in elective surgery of the shoulder and arm]. Prospective observational study in a university hospital]. Rev Esp Anestesiol Reanim 2013;60:384–391.

44. Brull R, Hadzic A, Reina MA, Barrington MJ: Pathophysiology and etiology of nerve injury following peripheral nerve blockade. Reg Anesth Pain Med 2015;40(5):479–490.

45. Neal JM, Barrington MJ, Brull R, et al: The second ASRA practice advisory on neurologic complications associated with regional anesthesia and pain medicine: Executive summary 2015. Reg Anesth Pain Med 2015;40(5):401–430.

46. Gadsden J, Latmore M, Levine DM, Robinson A: High opening injection pressure is associated with needle-nerve and needle-fascia contact during femoral nerve block. Reg Anesth Pain Med 2016;41(1):50–55.

47. Gadsden JC, Choi JJ, Lin E, Robinson A: Opening injection pressure consistently detects needle-nerve contact during ultrasound-guided interscalene brachial plexus block. Anesthesiology 2014;120(5):1246–1253.

48. Hadzic A, Dilberovic F, Shah S, et al: Combination of intraneural injection and high injection pressure leads to fascicular injury and neurologic deficits in dogs. Reg Anesth Pain Med 2004;29:417–423.

49. Kapur E, Vuckovic I, Dilberovic F, et al: Neurologic and histologic outcome after intraneural injections of lidocaine in canine sciatic nerves. Acta Anaesthesiol Scand 2007;51:101–107.

50. Gentili F, Hudson A, Kline DG, Hunter D: Peripheral nerve injection injury: An experimental study. Neurosurgery 1979;4:244–253.

51. Gentili F, Hudson AR, Hunter D, Kline DG: Nerve injection injury with local anesthetic agents: A light and electron microscopic, fluorescent microscopic, and horseradish peroxidase study. Neurosurgery 1980;6:263–272.

52. Myers RR, Kalichman MW, Reisner LS, Powell HC. Neurotoxicity of local anesthetics: Altered perineurial permeability, edema, and nerve fiber injury. Anesthesiology 1986;64:29–35.

53. Selander D, Brattsand R, Lundborg G, et al: Local anesthetics: importance of mode of application, concentration and adrenaline for the appearance of nerve lesions. An experimental study of axonal degeneration and barrier damage after intrafascicular injection or topical application of bupivacaine (Marcain). Acta Anaesthesiol Scand 1979;23:127–136.

54. Bigeleisen PE: Nerve puncture and apparent intraneural injection during ultrasound-guided axillary block does not invariably result in neurologic injury. Anesthesiology 2006;105:779–783.

55. Steinfeldt T, Wiesmann T, Nimphius W, et al: Perineural hematoma may result in nerve inflammation and myelin damage. Reg Anesth Pain Med 2014;39(6):513–519.

56. Steinfeldt T, Poeschl S, Nimphius W, et al: Forced needle advancement during needle-nerve contact in a porcine model: histological outcome. Anesth Analg 2011;113(2):417–420.

57. Gadsden JC, Lindenmuth DM, Hadzic A, et al: Lumbar plexus block using high-pressure injection leads to contralateral and epidural spread. Anesthesiology 2008;109:683–688.

58. Orebaugh SL, Mukalel JJ, Krediet AC, et al: Brachial plexus root injection in a human cadaver model: injectate distribution and effects on the neuraxis. Reg Anesth Pain Med 2012;37:525–529.

59. Claudio R, Hadzic A, Shih H, et al: Injection pressures by anesthesiologists during simulated peripheral nerve block. Reg Anesth Pain Med 2004;29(3):201–205.

60. Theron PS1, Mackay Z, Gonzalez JG, Donaldson N, Blanco R. An animal model of "syringe feel" during peripheral nerve block. Reg Anesth Pain Med 2009;34(4):330–332.

61. Tsui BC, Li LX, Pillay JJ: Compressed air injection technique to standardize block injection pressures. Can J Anaesth 2006;53: 1098–1102.

62. Asghar S, Bjerregaard LS, Lundstrom LH, et al: Distal infrared thermography and skin temperature after ultrasound-guided interscalene brachial plexus block: a prospective observational study. Eur J Anaesthesiol 2014;31:626–634.

63. Asghar S, Lundstrom LH, Bjerregaard LS, Lange KH: Ultrasound-guided lateral infraclavicular block evaluated by infrared thermography and distal skin temperature. Acta Anaesthesiol Scand 2014;58:867–874.

64. Masson EA, Veves A, Fernando D, Boulton AJ: Current perception thresholds: A new, quick, and reproducible method for the assessment of peripheral neuropathy in diabetes mellitus. Diabetologia 1989;32:724–728.

65. Matsutomo R, Takebayashi K, Aso Y: Assessment of peripheral neuropathy using measurement of the current perception threshold with the neurometer in patients with type 2 diabetes mellitus. J Int Med Res 2005; 33:442–453.

66. Nather A, Keng LW, Aziz Z, et al: Assessment of sensory neuropathy in patients with diabetic foot problems. Diabet Foot Ankle 2011;2:6367. doi:10.3402/dfa.v2i0.6367

67. Tsui BC, Shakespeare TJ, Leung DH, et al: Reproducibility of current perception threshold with the Neurometer((R)) vs the Stimpod NMS450 peripheral nerve stimulator in healthy volunteers: an observational study. Can J Anaesth 2013;60:753–760.

68. Gaudreault F, Drolet P, Fallaha M, Varin F: The reliability of the current perception threshold in volunteers and its applicability in a clinical setting. Anesth Analg 2015;120:678–683.

69. Huskisson EC: Visual analogue scales. In Melczak R (ed): *Pain Measurement and Assessment*. Raven Press, 1983, pp 33–37.

70. Buckenmaier CC III, Galloway KT, Polomano RC, et al: Preliminary validation of the Defense and Veterans Pain Rating Scale (DVPRS) in a military population. Pain Med 2013;14:110–123.

71. Fuchs-Lacelle S, Hadjistavropoulos T: Development and preliminary validation of the pain assessment checklist for seniors with limited ability to communicate (PACSLAC). Pain Manag Nurs 2004;5:37–49.

72. Bromage PR. *Epidural Analgesia*. Saunders, 1978.

73. Byeon GJ, Shin SW, Yoon JU, et al: Infusion methods for continuous interscalene brachial plexus block for postoperative pain control after arthroscopic rotator cuff repair. Korean J Pain 2015;28:210–216.

74. Patkar CS, Vora K, Patel H, et al: A comparison of continuous infusion and intermittent bolus administration of 0.1% ropivacaine with 0.0002% fentanyl for epidural labor analgesia. J Anaesthesiol Clin Pharmacol 2015;31:234–238.

75. Spencer AO, Tsui BC: Intermittent bolus via infraclavicular nerve catheter using a catheter-over-needle technique in a pediatric patient. Can J Anaesth 2014;61:684–685.

76. Macaire P, Nadhari M, Greiss H, et al: Internet remote control of pump settings for postoperative continuous peripheral nerve blocks: A feasibility study in 59 patients. Ann Fr Anesth Reanim 2014;33:e1–e7.

Equipment for Continuous Peripheral Nerve Blocks

Holly Evans, Karen C. Nielsen, M. Steve Melton, Roy A. Greengrass, and Susan M. Steele

INTRODUCTION

Continuous peripheral nerve blocks (CPNBs) provide a number of advantages in the perioperative period. These techniques provide the flexibility to prolong intraoperative anesthesia while avoiding the risks and side effects of general anesthesia. Following surgery, CPNBs offer extended postoperative analgesia. When compared to parenteral opioid analgesia, CPNBs are associated with superior analgesia, reduced opioid consumption, and decreased opioid-related side effects such as postoperative nausea and vomiting, sedation, and respiratory depression.[1–11] Analgesia of similar quality to epidural anesthesia is the result; however, less hypotension, urinary retention, pruritus, and mobility restrictions occur with CPNBs.[7,12–14] There is also evidence supporting the beneficial effect of CPNBs on postoperative sleep patterns and cognitive function[15,16] as well as early rehabilitation.[7,8] Concurrent sympathectomy is ideal following microvascular, reimplantation, and free-flap surgery,[17,18] as well as for treatment of accidental intra-arterial drug injection.[19–21] Extended analgesia can also be provided for patients with chronic pain[22] and those requiring palliation of terminal illness.[23] Finally, preoperative use can reduce phantom limb sensation in patients undergoing amputation.[24]

Despite these benefits, CPNBs have historically been relatively underused. This early lack of popularity was multifactorial; however, inadequate CPNB equipment likely contributed. The development of CPNB needles, catheters, and nerve localization technology has been essential for the safe use and advancement of these regional anesthesia techniques. This chapter summarizes the equipment required for continuous plexus anesthesia and will review the chronology of the development of modern-day CPNB equipment.

PRE-BLOCK CONSIDERATIONS

Block Room

A perineural catheter can be placed in a block room just as the preceding patient's procedure is finishing. This enhances operating room efficiency and flow. A block room allows the supplies and monitors discussed next to be stocked and stored in one location. The block room should be a clean, semi-sterile room in close proximity to the operating room suite.

Block Cart

Table 13–1 outlines block cart supplies necessary for the performance of CPNBs. Supplies are sterile where applicable.

Monitoring

Patients receiving a perineural catheter often receive sedation and large doses of local anesthetic. They should have standard American Society of Anesthesiologists (ASA) monitors applied. Furthermore, these patients should be monitored by an individual with Advanced Cardiac Life Support (ACLS) resuscitation knowledge and skills.

Resuscitative Medication and Equipment

A number of life-threatening complications can occur during placement of a CPNB. Table 13–2 lists the resuscitative medications and equipment that should be readily available.

Premedication and Sedation

Table 13–3 lists various agents that can be used to provide sedation and analgesia for perineural catheter placement.

TABLE 13–1. Block cart supplies necessary for continuous peripheral nerve blocks.

Sterile gloves ± gown for anesthesiologist
Disinfecting solution (2% chlorhexidine gluconate with 70% isopropyl alcohol)
Clear drapes
Needles for subcutaneous local anesthetic infiltration (ie, 25-gauge 1½ inch)
Syringes for subcutaneous local anesthetic infiltration (ie, 3 mL)
2 × 2 in. gauze
Selection of block needles and catheter sets of appropriate diameter and length
Nerve stimulator and electrodes
Ultrasound machine
Selection of ultrasound probes of appropriate frequency, shape, and size
Sterile ultrasound probe covers
Sterile gel for ultrasound imaging
Dextrose 5% in water
Local anesthetics and adjuvants (see below)
Occlusive dressing, Epi-Guard, tape, Mastisol, Dermabond®
Connectors for proximal tip of catheter
Oxygen source
Oxygen masks
Suction

Most advocate the use of light sedation, thus allowing communication with the patient regarding potential side effects.

Local Anesthetic Solutions and Adjuvants
Block Initiation

A variety of local anesthetics should be available on the block cart to initiate the nerve block. Short-acting agents such as lidocaine or mepivacaine allow for rapid onset yet early recovery of the sensorimotor block. This facilitates prompt assessment of neurological function following surgery and prior to starting a continuous perineural infusion. Block initiation with long-acting agents such as bupivacaine or ropivacaine extend the duration of dense anesthesia and analgesia. Ropivacaine is often selected instead of bupivacaine for its more favorable safety profile. Concentrated solutions provide effective intraoperative anesthesia and analgesia. Dilute local anesthetic solutions can provide selective sensory anesthesia while minimizing motor block after surgery.

TABLE 13–2. Necessary resuscitative medications and equipment.

ACLS drugs (ie, epinephrine, vasopressin, atropine)
Cardioverter/defibrillator
Intralipid® 20% (1.5-mL/kg bolus over 1 minute and every 3–5 minutes up to 3 mL/kg, 0.25 mL/kg/min infusion, maximum total dose 8 mL/kg)

TABLE 13–3. Agents for sedation and analgesia for perineural catheter placement.

Benzodiazepines (ie, midazolam)
Opiates (ie, fentanyl)
N-Methyl-ᴅ-aspartate antagonists (ie, ketamine)
Alpha-2 antagonists (ie, clonidine, dexmedetomidine)
Anesthetics (ie, propofol, etomidate)

When appropriate, epinephrine 1:200,000 or 1:400,000 is added to the local anesthetic solution. The epinephrine serves as a marker of intravascular injection and can limit the systemic absorption of perineurally placed local anesthetic.

Further adjuvants such as clonidine and dexamethasone have been used to enhance the duration and quality of analgesia.

Continuous Infusion

The nerve block is typically maintained with a continuous infusion of dilute, long-acting local anesthetic. Patient-controlled boluses are often added to the continuous infusion to enhance analgesia. The local anesthetic solution should be prepared in a clean environment, such as in a pharmacy using a laminar flow workbench. Minimizing bacterial contamination is critical to reducing the likelihood of infectious neurological complications.

Clinical Pearl

- Safe practice of regional anesthesia requires the immediate availability of monitors, resuscitation drugs, and equipment as well as a health care practitioner familiar with ACLS protocols.

NEEDLE-AND-CATHETER SYSTEMS

Historical Perspective

The earliest report of CPNB is attributed to Ansbro's 1946 work[25] (Figure 13–1). He attached a malleable blunt needle to injection tubing and a syringe. The needle was placed blindly in the supraclavicular area lateral to the pulsations of the subclavian artery and approximately 1 cm cephalad to the midpoint of the clavicle. A cork stopper from a can of ether was used to secure the needle in place. Intermittent injections of procaine were given to 27 patients to extend the duration of intraoperative anesthesia for up to 4 hours and 20 minutes.

Almost a quarter century later, continuous subclavian perivascular, interscalene, and axillary brachial plexus blocks were reported by DeKrey et al,[26] Winnie,[27] and Selander[28] (Figure 13–2), respectively. In all reports, the authors used an intravenous-type needle-and-cannula set. The brachial plexus was identified with a paresthesia or fascial pop technique, the inner needle was removed, and the outer plastic cannula was advanced into a perineural location.

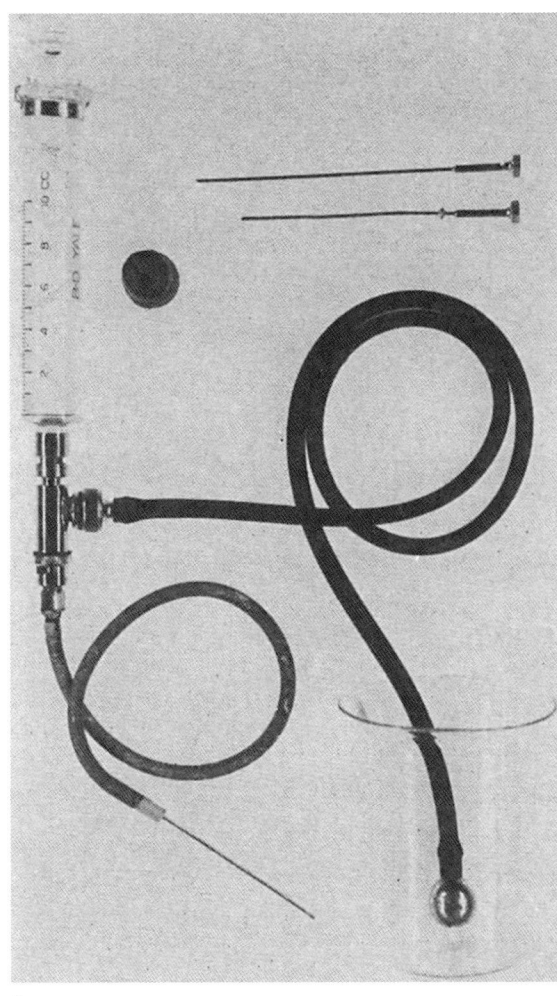

A

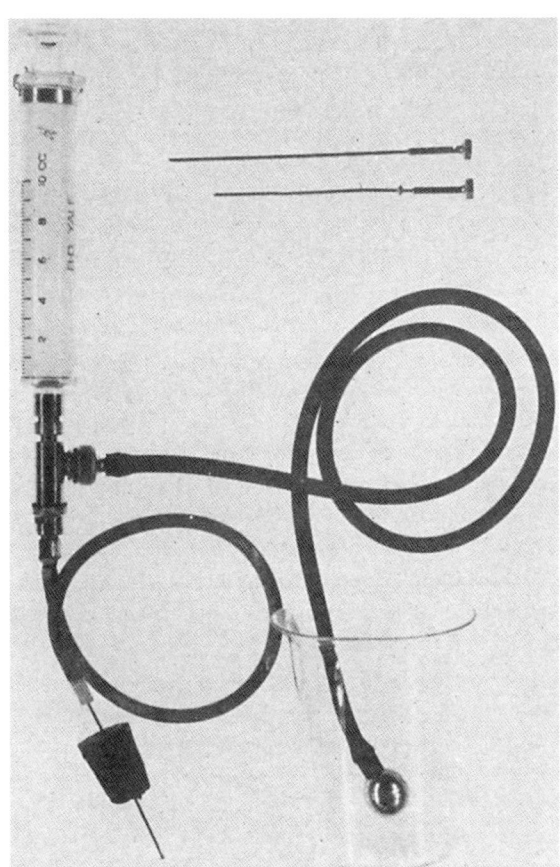

B

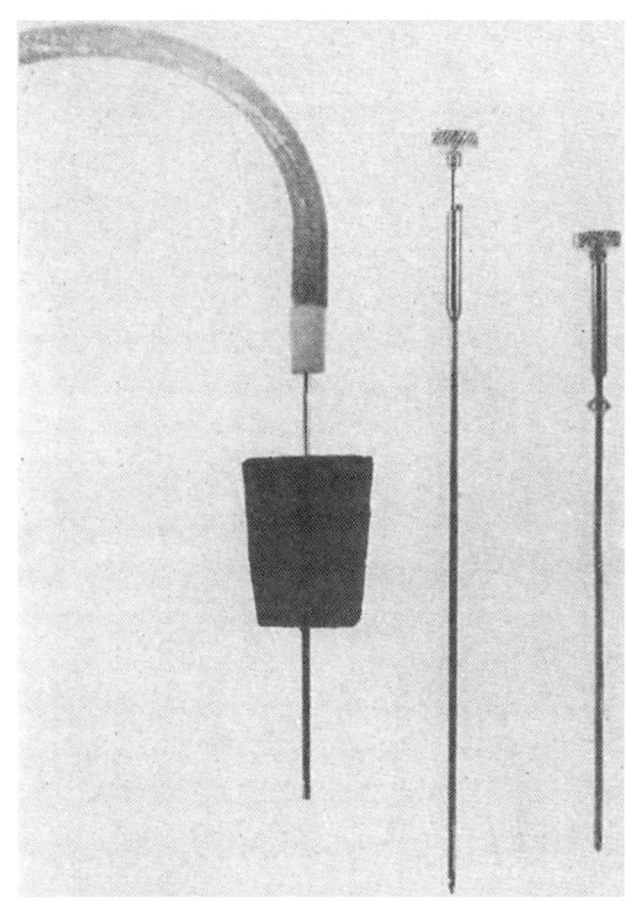

C

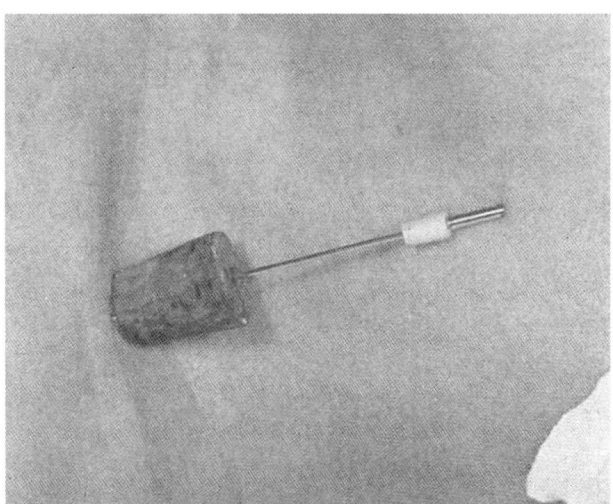

D

FIGURE 13–1. A: Apparatus consists of a 10-mL Luer lock syringe and the two-way valve as used in the Hingson-Edwards continuous caudal method. The tubing can be of any desired length (18 inches is sufficient). A malleable needle (Becton-Dickinson & Company) that has been filed to a blunt end to prevent perforation of blood vessels is used. A cork stopper from an ether can completes the apparatus. **B:** Apparatus with needle through the cork, usually 4 to 6 cm. **C:** Close view of blunted needle through the cork guard. The cork, when placed flush with the skin in the supraclavicular area, prevents the needle from going in deeper. **D:** Needle in place in the supraclavicular area. The cork prevents displacement inward and holds it upright.

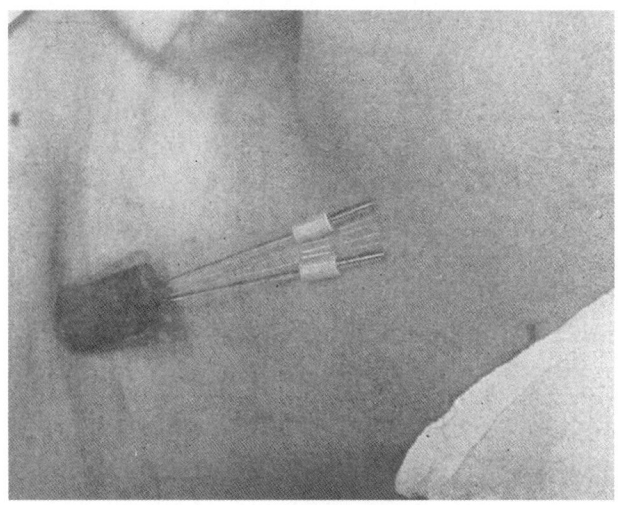

E

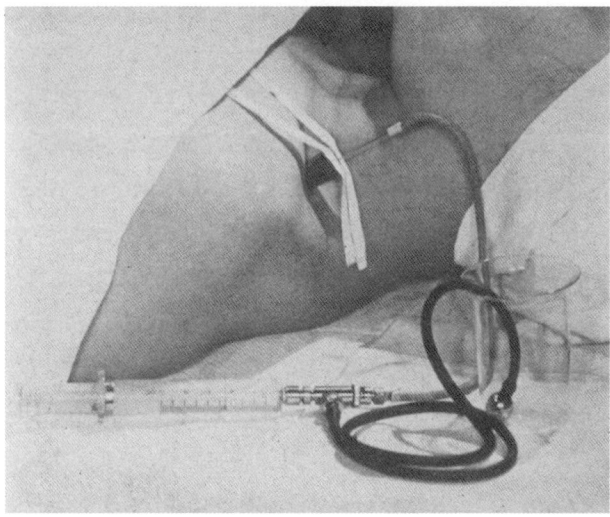

F

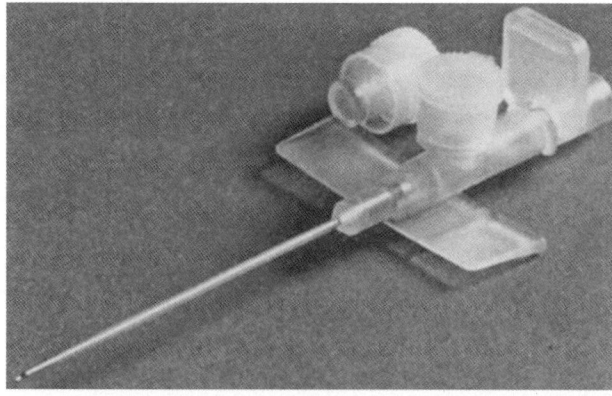

A

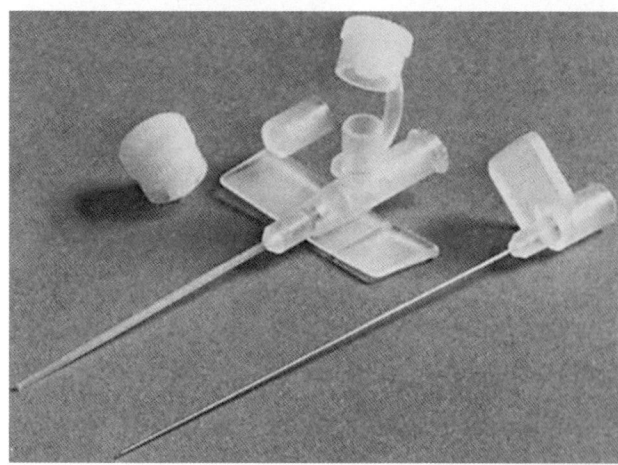

B

FIGURE 13–2. A, B: The Venflon cannula. (Reproduced with permission from Selander D: Catheter technique in axillary plexus block. Presentation of a new method. *Acta Anaesthesiol Scand.* 1977;21(4):324-329.)

FIGURE 13–1. (*Continued*) **E:** Pulsation of the needle indicating its close apposition to the subclavian artery. If the needle is placed lateral to the artery and on top of the first rib, of necessity it is in close proximity to the plexus. Injection of 30 to 40 mL of 1% procaine will induce anesthesia within 15 minutes. **F:** Apparatus in place and ready for fractional injections. The adhesive strapping over the cork keeps the needle in place and prevents its outward displacement. The cork firmly holding the needle prevents its inward displacement. (Reproduced with permission from Ansbro FP: A method of continuous brachial plexus block. *Am J Surg.* 1946 Jun;71:716-722.)

While these early accounts primarily involved "cannula-over-needle" devices, subsequent descriptions also included "catheter-through-needle" equipment. In the earliest report of a continuous lower extremity block, Brands and Callahan[29] performed continuous lumbar plexus blocks that lasted 72 to 96 hours for patients who sustained femoral neck fractures. The authors used an 18-gauge, 15 cm long needle and the loss-of-resistance method to identify the lumbar plexus psoas compartment and subsequently threaded an epidural catheter through the needle.

The identification of important neuroanatomical features occurred concurrently with the description of these early CPNBs. This knowledge was instrumental to the further understanding of plexus anatomy and to the development of continuous regional anesthesia techniques. Landmark papers were published by Winnie[27] as well as Thompson and Rorie[30] outlining the existence of a brachial plexus sheath and suggesting the potential for continuous plexus anesthesia. Tuominen et al[31] provided early evidence for the safety of continuous plexus infusions of local anesthetic when they studied blood levels of bupivacaine during continuous axillary brachial plexus infusion.

Reflecting the popularity of the paresthesia, fascial pop, and loss-of-resistance techniques from the 1970s through the early 1990s, the majority of subsequent reports of CPNBs also involved the use of intravenous-type needles and cannula (cannula-over-needle devices)[31–36] as well as epidural-type needles and catheters (catheter-through-needle equipment).[23,37–40]

Development of Insulated Systems

In the late 1970s, concern surfaced in the regional anesthesia literature over the potential for long-bevel needles and the paresthesia technique to cause neurologic complications.[41,42] The introduction of nerve stimulator techniques[43] led to a decline in the popularity of the paresthesia, fascial pop, and loss-or-resistance methods in favor of identification of neural structures by electrolocation. Uninsulated, short-bevel needles could be used with nerve stimulators; however, insulated needles were found to provide more focused current output and consequently more accurate localization of neural structures.[44] As nerve stimulator techniques came into more widespread use in the 1990s, commercially insulated single-injection needles became available, but the design of CPNB needles and catheters initially failed to keep pace. For many years, regional anesthesia practitioners assembled intravenous access, spinal, and epidural equipment to create their own insulated CPNB apparatus.

Numerous reports described connecting an intravenous needle and cannula to a current source to enable nerve stimulation. For example, Anker-Moller et al[45] adapted a 14-gauge intravenous needle and cannula set (Viggo, Sweden) to provide a continuous femoral nerve block. The nerve stimulator was attached inside the hub of the metal needle. The femoral nerve was identified with nerve stimulator assistance, the inner needle was removed, and a 16-gauge epidural catheter (Portex, UK) was inserted through the intravenous cannula (Figure 13–3).

Ben-David et al[46] inserted the metal needle of a 20-gauge intravenous catheter (Venflon, Viggo, Sweden) inside the proximal end of a 16-gauge central venous pressure needle (Secalon, Viggo, Sweden). They attached the negative electrode of the nerve stimulator to the exposed metal needle of the 20-gauge intravenous catheter and obtained appropriate stimulation during lumbar plexus block. The over-the-needle central venous cannula was then advanced beyond the tip of the needle and used for continuous lumbar plexus block (Figure 13–4).

Concepcion[47] wrapped the stylet of a 26-gauge spinal needle around the metal introducer of a typical intravenous over-the-needle cannula. An alligator clip was then attached to the stylet to allow electrical stimulation using a nerve stimulator.

Prosser[48] devised yet another method to provide nerve stimulation during CPNBs for pediatric patients. This author connected a jackplug electrode into the hub of an intravenous cannula (Abbocath-T Venisystems, Abbott, Ireland) to make an electrical contact between the nerve stimulator and the central metal needle of the intravenous set (Figure 13–5). The surrounding Teflon®-coated sheath insulated all but the tip of the cannula. This adaptation was successful with 20-, 22-, and 24-gauge intravenous catheters and consequently was ideal for the pediatric population.

Further advancing pediatric regional anesthesia, Tan et al[49] used a radial artery catheterization set (#RA-04120; Arrow, Reading, PA) with a 20-gauge cannula over a 22-gauge, thin-walled, short-beveled needle for continuous axillary brachial plexus block. The set had a 0.018-inch integral spring wire that this group connected via an alligator clip to the negative pole of a nerve stimulator to enable electrolocation of the brachial plexus. Using a Seldinger technique, the guidewire was then advanced and used to direct the cannula into the brachial plexus sheath.

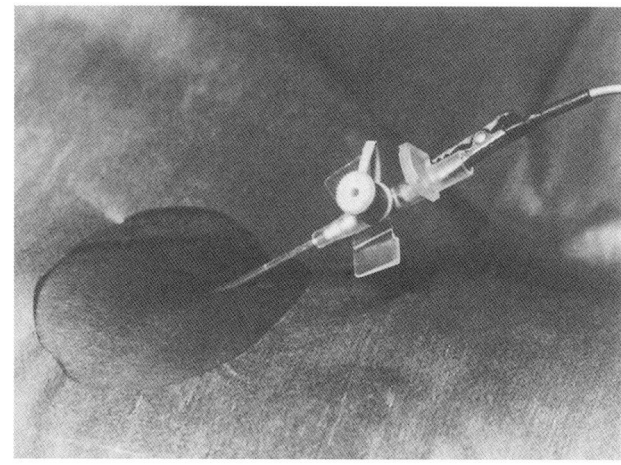

A

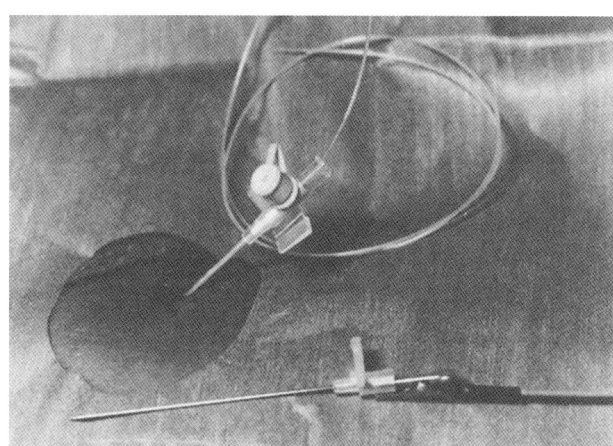

B

FIGURE 13–3. A: Placement of the infusion cannula. Nerve stimulator attached to the trocar (lateral view). **B:** The catheter is inserted through the infusion cannula (lateral view). (Reproduced with permission from Anker-Møller E1, Spangsberg N, Dahl JB, et al: Continuous blockade of the lumbar plexus after knee surgery: a comparison of the plasma concentrations and analgesic effect of bupivacaine 0.250% and 0.125%. *Acta Anaesthesiol Scand.* 1990 Aug;34(6):468-472.)

Spinal and epidural equipment has similarly been adapted for CPNBs performed with nerve stimulators. Several groups[1,50] have placed an 18-gauge intravenous cannula over a 22-gauge spinal needle to provide insulation to the distal part of the needle. A current source was then attached to the bare proximal metal needle, and local anesthetic was injected on identification of neural structures. The cannula was then threaded off the spinal needle into the perineural space and used for continuous infusion of local anesthetic for up to 2 days.

Alternatively, spinal needles and microcatheters have been used. The spinal microcatheters, however, were of such small size that injection was difficult, and they were prone to kinking. This equipment was eventually withdrawn from the market due to neurotoxicity associated with continuous spinal anesthesia.

While these designs allowed nerve stimulation through an insulated needle, a number of drawbacks still existed. Many

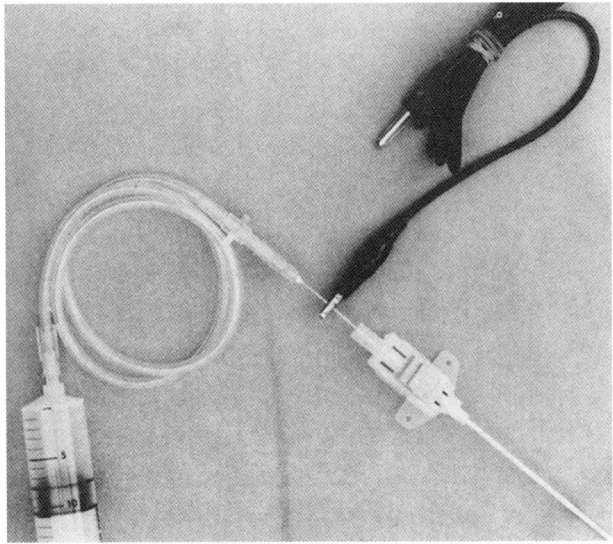

FIGURE 13–4. Assembly shows a 21-gauge needle inserted into the proximal end of the 16-gauge Secalon (Viggo, Sweden) central venous pressure catheter. Metal contact of the smaller needle inside the larger needle allows an electrical impulse to be conveyed to the Secalon needle tip. An alligator clip from the electrical stimulator is attached to the shaft of the 21-gauge needle. Intravenous extension tubing inserts into the hub of the 21-gauge needle. (Reproduced with permission from Ben-David B1, Lee E, Croitoru M: Psoas block for surgical repair of hip fracture: a case report and description of a catheter technique. *Anesth Analg.* 1990 Sep;71(3):298-301.)

steps were required between identification of the nerve and threading the catheter. This increased the risk of catheter misplacement and the likelihood of committing a breach in sterility. Despite the insulation provided by an intravenous-type cannula over a metal needle, the uninsulated area of the distal

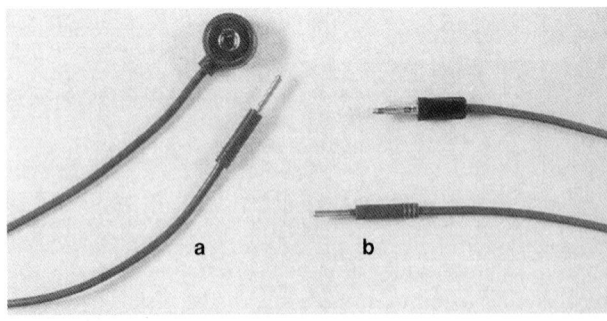

FIGURE 13–5. A: Peripheral nerve stimulator lead fitted with (a) standard press stud and jackplug connectors; (b) modified connectors, press stud replaced with second jackplug. **B:** Electrical contact between the Abbocath's central metal cannula and original jackplug from the lead. (Reproduced with permission from Prosser DP: Adaptation of an intravenous cannula for paediatric regional anaesthesia. *Anaesthesia.* 1996 May;51(5):510.)

needle tip was of significant size and could adversely affect the accuracy of nerve location. Unfortunately, in these self-assembled systems, the cannula rarely provided a snug fit over the needle. In addition, there was continued concern about the risk of neurologic complications from long-beveled intravenous-type needles. Finally, the shape of the needle tip did not facilitate catheter threading in directions other than parallel to the course of the needle.

Increased effort into the development of CPNB equipment and the introduction of the safer long-acting local anesthetic ropivacaine (Astra, Westborough, MA) in the 1990s further stimulated the expansion of CPNB techniques.

Commercially available cannula-over-needle systems were developed and marketed by various companies. B. Braun introduced a set that consisted of a cannula over a short-bevel needle with an accompanying catheter. The advantage was that the components were designed to fit snugly together (Figure 13–6). Both Pajunk (Geisengen, Germany) and B. Braun subsequently developed systems that involved a short-bevel needle with an integrated wire for nerve stimulation and with connection tubing for concurrent aspiration and injection (Figure 13–7). There was an accompanying catheter that could be threaded through the cannula. Some manufacturers offered the option of a Sprotte or Facet needle tip and a variety of sizes, some suitable for pediatric patients. Early Arrow equipment involved a bullet-tip needle for enhanced sensation of fascial penetration and a theoretical reduction in neurology injury (Figure 13–8).

Clinical Pearls

- Short-bevel block needles were used with the paresthesia technique to minimize nerve injury.
- Insulated needles are used with nerve stimulation to locate the nerve or plexus.
- The design of CPNB needles and catheters initially lagged behind the development of single-injection PNB equipment.

Modern Insulated Systems

The next advance in the development of insulated CPNB equipment involved catheter-through-needle systems (ie, Contiplex® Tuohy,[51] B. Braun Medical, Bethlehem, PA, and Plexolong®, Pajunk). A Tuohy needle was insulated along its length with the exception of a pinpoint area at its most distal tip. A stimulating wire was attached to the needle. Early prototypes involved a detachable wire with an alligator clip on one end and a plug for a nerve stimulator on the other end (Figure 13–9). In subsequent models, the stimulating wire was permanently affixed to the metal needle (Figures 13–10 and 13–11). This wire also served as a marker for the open face of the needle bevel distally. A 20-gauge, multiorifice epidural catheter and connector were included. The curved distal tip of the Tuohy needle facilitated advancement of the catheter parallel to the nerve(s) in question. Various needle lengths were

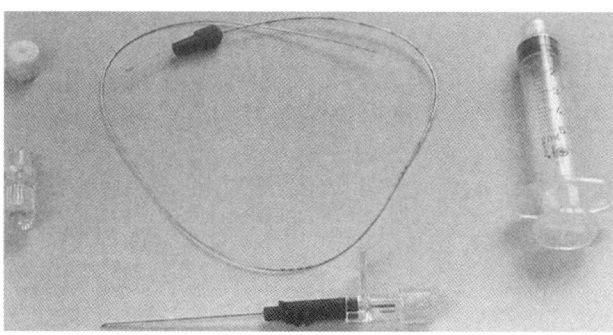

FIGURE 13–6. Brachial plexus infusion kit as used in this study (Contiplex®, B. Braun Australia Pty. Ltd.). The introducing cannula is 18 gauge, with a 0.85-mm diameter catheter, which is threaded into the axillary brachial plexus sheath. The needle within the cannula is a short-bevel type (30°). (Reproduced with permission from Mezzatesta JP, Scott DA, Schweitzer SA, et al: Continuous axillary brachial plexus block for postoperative pain relief. Intermittent bolus versus continuous infusion. *Reg Anesth.* 1997 Jul-Aug;22(4):357-362.)

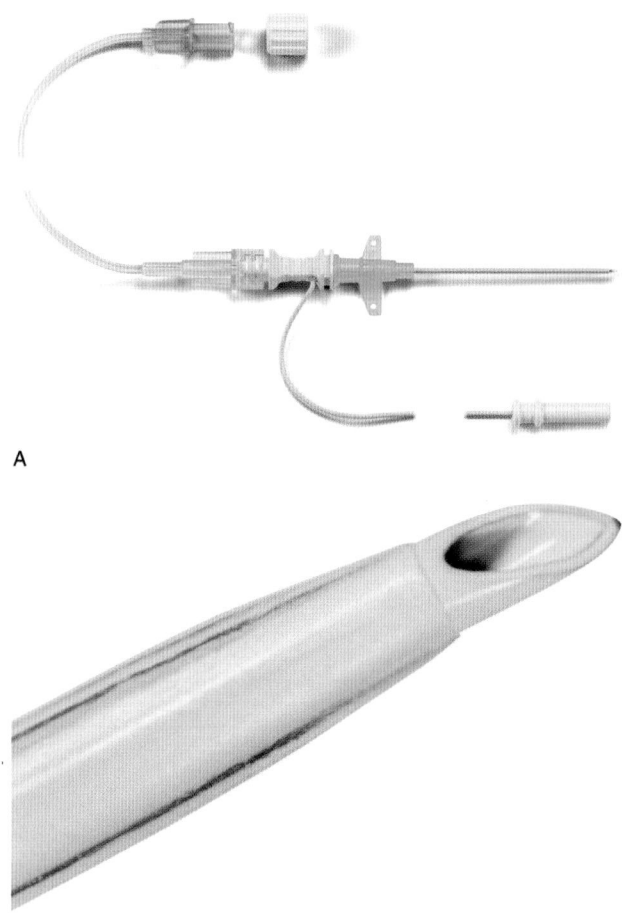

A

B

FIGURE 13–7. A: Pajunk MiniSet® consisting of a cannula-over-needle design and integrated stimulating cable and extension tubing. **B:** Pajunk MiniSet distal short-bevel needle tip and cannula. (Used with permission from Pajunk, Geisengen, Germany.)

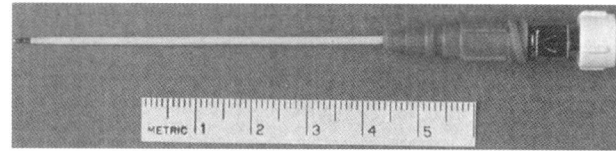

FIGURE 13–8. Arrow single-shot or continuous brachial plexus catheter. (Reproduced with permission from Longo SR, Williams DP: Bilateral fascia iliaca catheters for postoperative pain control after bilateral total knee arthroplasty: a case report and description of a catheter technique. *Reg Anesth.* 1997 Jul-Aug;22(4):372-377.)

manufactured, allowing CPNB of nerves of varying depths. Sprotte and Facet needle tips were also manufactured to enable catheter threading at various needle angle approaches.

Some CPNB equipment (Contiplex Tuohy[51]) incorporates an adapter with a Luer lock head and a hemostatic valve that can be fitted to the proximal end of the needle (Figure 13–10). The adapter has a central diaphragm that allows passage of a catheter through a port separate from where aspiration and injection occur. This eliminates the need for equipment disconnection and minimizes the likelihood of needle movement, catheter misplacement, and secondary block failure. This adapter also has a side arm connected to extension tubing that allows for continuous aspiration for blood and injection of solution by an assistant.

Catheters initially manufactured for epidural use have been adapted for CPNBs. They are well suited for this application as they are nonirritating and flexible and generate minimal friction on passage through needles. Graduated markings provide an indicator of insertion depth and radiopacity provides an additional method to confirm placement location. Some advocate the use of styletted catheters, believing that they are easier to advance; however, these may result in greater tissue or blood vessel trauma. Multiorifice catheters have a closed distal tip and

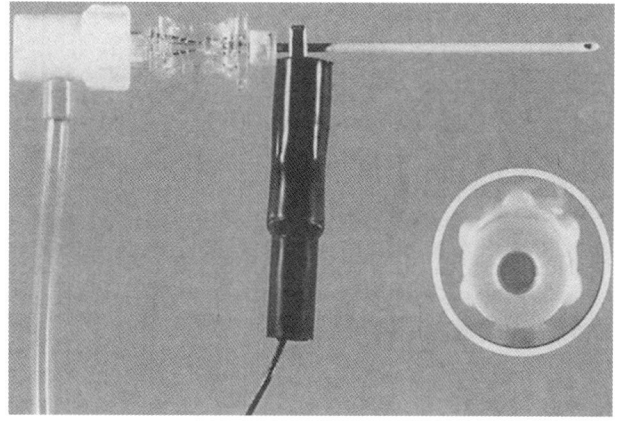

FIGURE 13–9. An 18-gauge, insulated Tuohy system (Braun, Contiplex®, B. Braun Medical, Bethlehem, PA). Inset shows a Luer lock head with central diaphragm at the proximal end of the needle. (Reproduced with permission from Klein SM, Grant SA, Greengrass RA, et al. Interscalene brachial plexus block with a continuous catheter insertion system and a disposable infusion pump. *Anesthesia & Analgesia.* Dec 2000;91(6):1473-1478.)

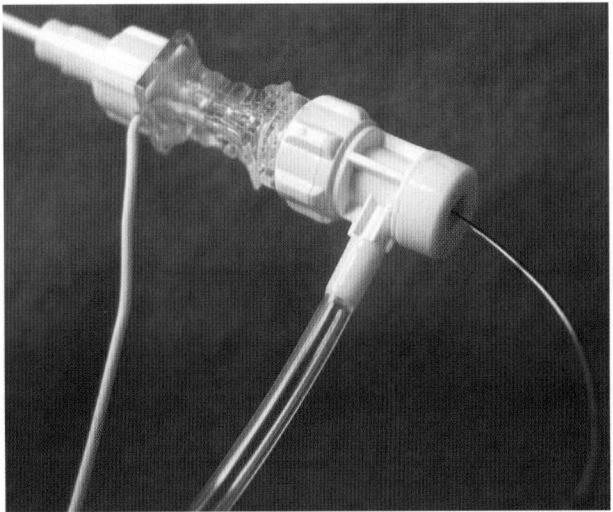

FIGURE 13–10. The Contiplex® Tuohy (B. Braun, Melsungen AG, Germany) consists of an insulated Tuohy needle with a pinpoint uninsulated tip, an integrated stimulating wire, extension tubing, and a connector with a hemostatic valve allowing the insertion of a catheter. This design enables simultaneous nerve stimulation, aspiration, and injection and allows for an immobile needle during catheter insertion. (Used with permission from Holly Evans, MD.)

three distal openings (0.5, 1.0, and 1.5 cm from the tip). Single-orifice catheters have a single opening at the distal end of the catheter (Figure 13–12). Multiorifice catheters provide better spread of local anesthetic solution that is administered by bolus; consequently, they are associated with improved analgesia compared to single-orifice catheters.[52]

Clinical Pearls

Continuous peripheral nerve block equipment typically includes the following:

- An insulated, large-bore needle (ie, Tuohy tip) with an integrated wire to allow nerve stimulation
- A flexible, atraumatic catheter that is threaded through the needle into a perineural location
- Clear, flexible tubing that can be attached to needle or catheter for injection and aspiration

Stimulating Catheters

Stimulating catheters provide the ability to conduct current to their distal end. They were developed as a tool to assess the proximity of the catheter's distal tip to the neural structures and in an attempt to reduce the likelihood of secondary block failure. In one of the first published reports, Sutherland[53] used a 1.0-mm outer-diameter ureteral catheter (Portex-Boots, Kent, UK) with a metal stylet. This author adapted the catheter by removing 50 mm from its distal tip and by rethreading the metal stylet so that it just protruded from the distal end

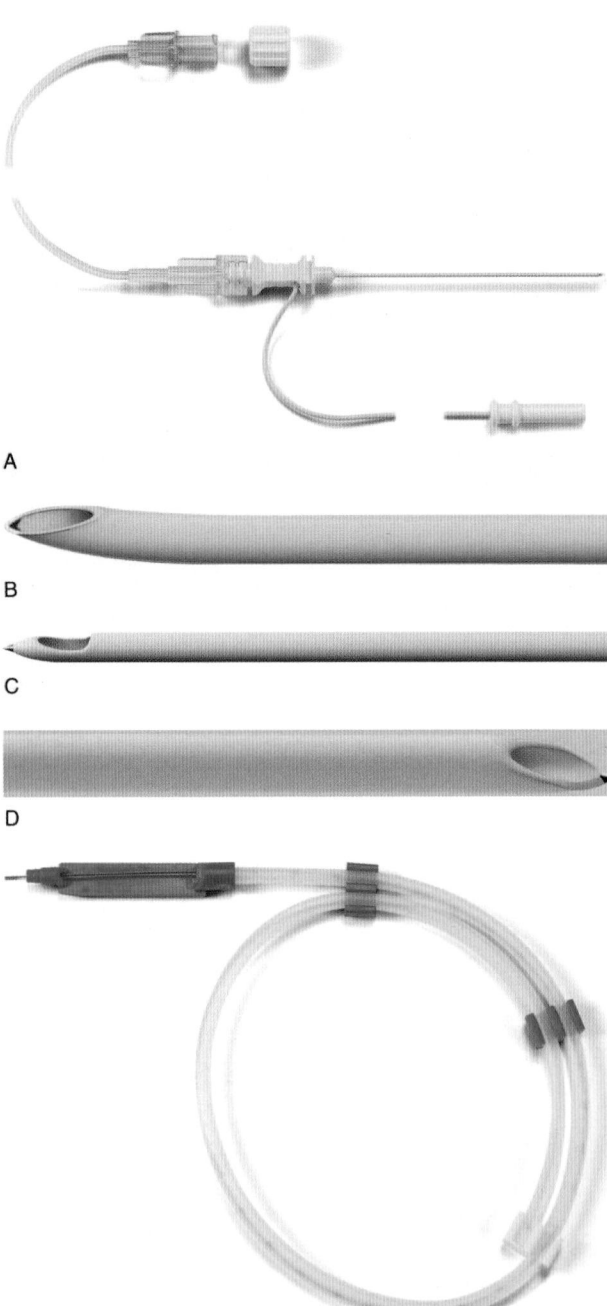

FIGURE 13–11. A: The Plexolong® system (Pajunk, Geisengen, Germany) incorporates an insulated needle, integrated stimulating wire, and extension tubing. **B:** The Plexolong Tuohy tip. **C:** The Plexolong Sprotte tip. **D:** The Plexolong Facet (or short-bevel) tip. **E:** The Plexolong catheter with thread-assist device. (Used with permission from Pajunk, Geisengen, Germany.)

(Figure 13–12). The proximal part of the stylet was folded over the proximal end of the catheter to maintain the correct length and to facilitate an electrical connection to the nerve stimulator. This equipment was used successfully for continuous sciatic nerve block following foot surgery.

Boezaart et al[54] subsequently described their adaptation of a wire-reinforced epidural catheter for use as a stimulating catheter. They used a polyurethane (Tecothane®) thermoplastic catheter

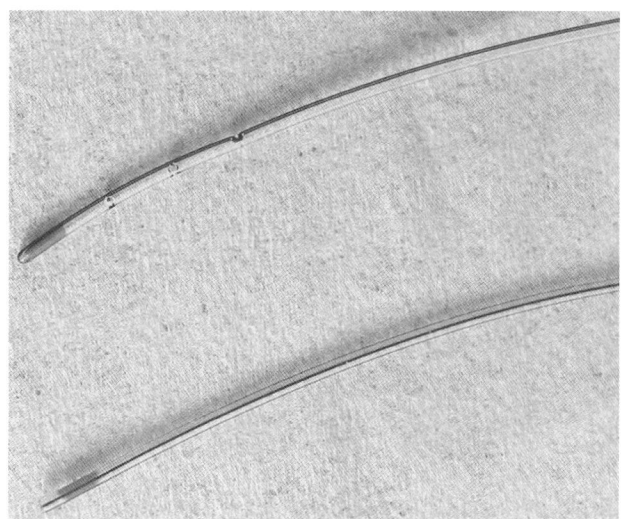

FIGURE 13–12. A closed-tip multiorifice catheter (top) and an open-tip single-orifice catheter (bottom). (Used with permission from Holly Evans, MD.)

with an inner steel spring reinforcement and a nonferromagnetic stainless steel stylet (Arrow Theracath®) and removed part of the outer catheter to provide a 5-mm unsheathed metal tip. These authors described removing the inner stylet from an uninsulated 17-gauge Tuohy needle and advancing the epidural catheter through the needle such that the metal tip of the catheter did not make contact with the metal needle. This effectively allowed electrolocation during needle and catheter placement for continuous interscalene brachial plexus block. A later modification involved the addition of an insulated needle with an inner metal stylet to the set (StimuCath®, Arrow International).[55,56] Further revisions resulted in the addition of an alligator clip to allow direct connection to a nerve stimulator (Figure 13–13)

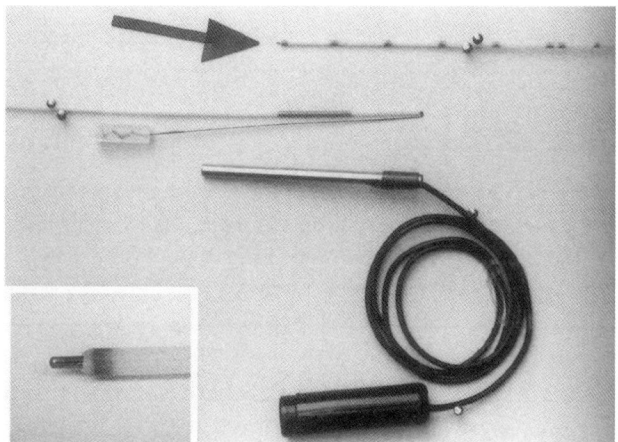

FIGURE 13–13. Shortened catheter with stylet just protruding from the distal end (inset) and folded over to maintain the position at the proximal end. Electrical connection is made by sliding a firmly fitting metal tube over the proximal end of the catheter. (Reproduced with permission from Sutherland ID: Continuous sciatic nerve infusion: expanded case report describing a new approach. *Reg Anesth Pain Med*. 1998 Sep-Oct;23(5):496-501.)

and, more recently, the addition of an integrated stimulating wire attached to the needle.

While this stimulating catheter was a significant advancement, several limitations existed. The needle bevel was sharper relative to other manufacturers' equipment and was associated with concern about neural injury. The opacity of the blue 20-gauge and white 19-gauge catheters made identification of aspirated blood challenging. The relatively large uninsulated segment at the distal tip of the needle could decrease the accuracy of nerve identification. And, there was a risk that the area of exposed wire at the distal tip of the catheter could uncoil in vivo if cut or traumatized.

In an attempt to address some of these shortcomings, Kick et al[57] developed another stimulating catheter (Stimulong® Catheter Set, Pajunk) and reported its reliability in a series of 10 supraclavicular brachial plexus blocks (Figures 13–14A and 13–14B). It consisted of a 20-gauge, single-hole, 400-mm polyamide catheter with a 405-mm indwelling removable conducting stylet. The metal wire stylet was insulated with Teflon coating along its length with the exception of the distal 0.3 mm. The proximal end had a plug to allow connection to a nerve stimulator. Subsequent modification involved incorporation of an integrated wire within the catheter (Stimulong Plus®, Pajunk)[58] (Figure 13–15).

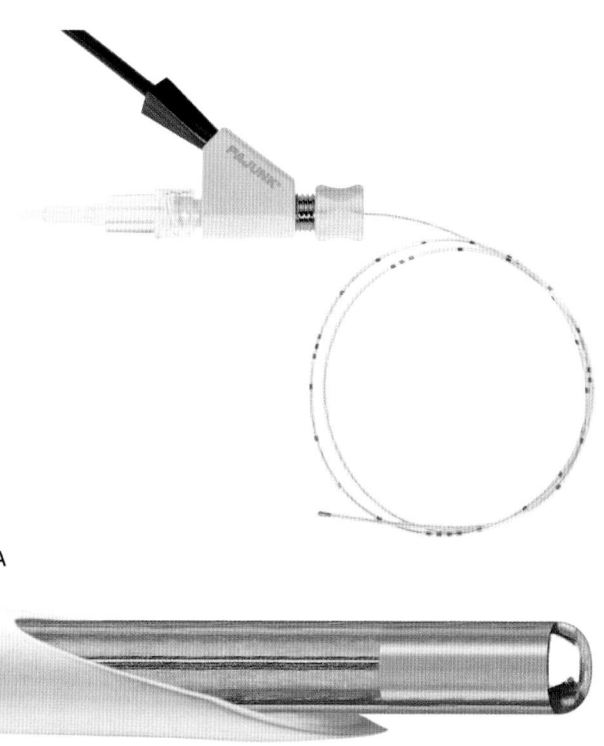

A

B

FIGURE 13–14. A: The stimulating catheter with integrated wire, Stimulong Plus® (Pajunk, Geisengen, Germany), is shown with its screw connector. The connector accepts an electric cable and extension tubing. **B:** The tip of the Stimulong Plus stimulating catheter is shown with its conductive golden tip. (Used with permission from Pajunk, Geisengen, Germany.)

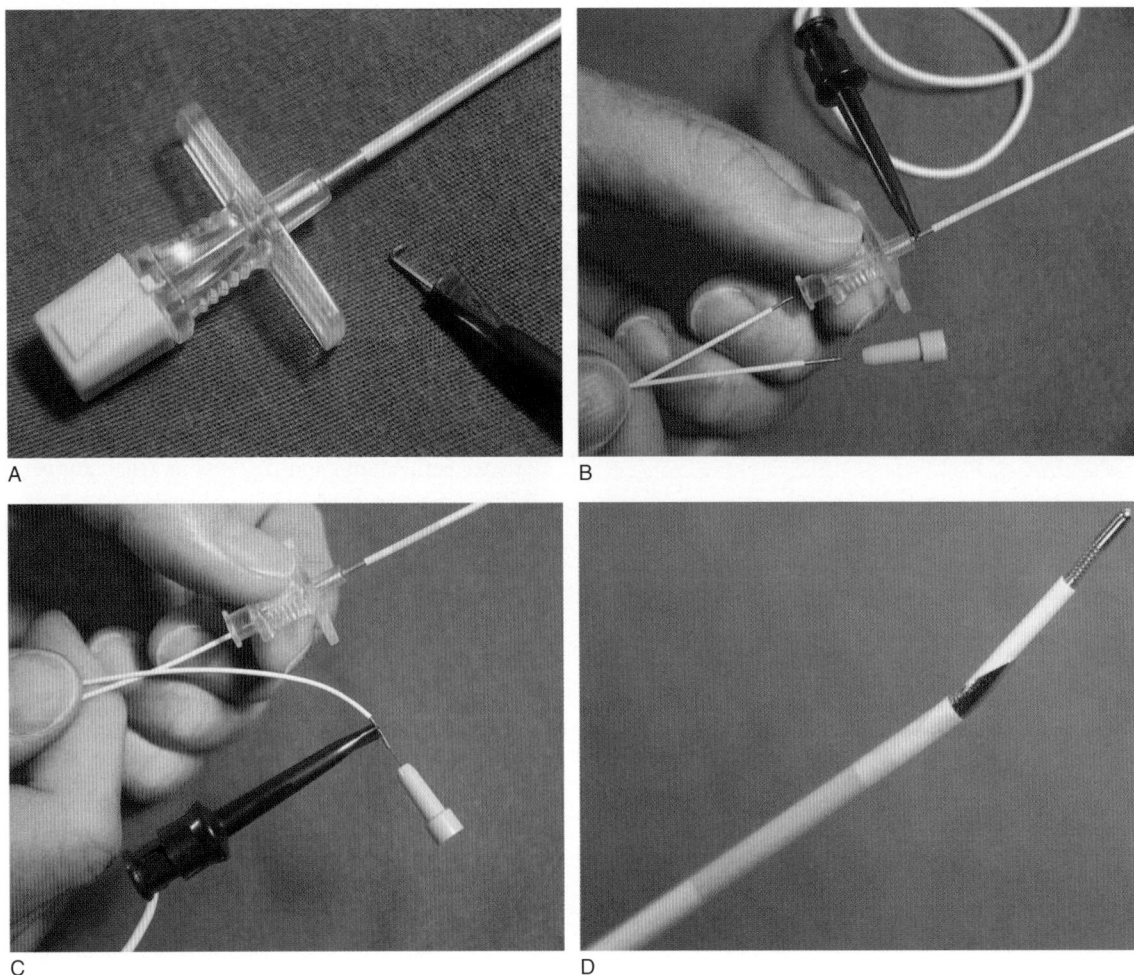

FIGURE 13–15. **A:** An alligator clip connects to an uninsulated segment on the proximal needle shaft of the StimuCath® system (Arrow International, Reading, PA). **B:** The StimuCath system consists of an insulated Tuohy tip needle, a stimulating catheter, and an alligator clip connector. **C:** The alligator clip is removed from the needle and attached to the catheter's proximal end. This provides current output to the catheter's distal tip. **D:** The Tuohy needle tip with a 5-mm long uninsulated segment is seen with the distal tip of the StimuCath stimulating catheter. (Used with permission from Holly Evans, MD.)

Stimulating catheters have been compared to nonstimulating catheters for CPNB. A stimulating catheter is associated with lower local anesthetic consumption and reduced requirement for additional opioid analgesia,[59–61]; however, it may be more technically challenging to place under ultrasound guidance.[62,63]

Clinical Pearl

- A stimulating catheter can confirm perineural location and may reduce the requirement for supplemental analgesia.

Echogenic Systems

The use of ultrasound to assist in the placement of CPNBs is now routine. Consequently, many manufacturers have incorporated echogenic features into their CPNB equipment. B. Braun incorporates laser reflectors into the needle of their Contiplex

Ultra series. Pajunk catheters are wire reinforced and contain radiocontrast strips at their distal end.

Clinical Pearl

- Echogenic needles and catheters improve visualization of equipment inserted under ultrasound guidance.

NERVE LOCALIZATION SYSTEMS

Nerve Stimulator

Nerve stimulators generate an electrical current that passes through to the tip of an insulated needle or stimulating catheter to stimulate a nerve/plexus. A motor twitch appropriate for the nerve in question is sought. The limits of this technique must be appreciated. Studies of nerve blocks performed with both nerve stimulation and ultrasound guidance have shown that a needle tip can contact a nerve without resulting in a motor twitch. Furthermore, a needle tip can be within a nerve even when there is no motor twitch at relatively low current.[64]

Ultrasound

Neural and perineural anatomy can be viewed with ultrasound imaging. Anatomical variants can be seen. The precise location and depth to neural structures can be estimated. Surrounding structures and vasculature can be identified and avoided. An image of the nerve block needle, catheter, and local anesthetic injection can be seen in relation to the nerve/plexus in real time. Though associated with the need for additional operator training and greater equipment expense, potential advantages of ultrasound include enhanced block success and reduced complications. Further details are provided in the relevant chapters.

Global Positioning System (Ultrasonix)

One of the newest nerve localization techniques involves the use of a global positioning system (ie, SonixGPS, Ultrasonix, Richmond, BC, Canada). Both the needle and the ultrasound probe contain sensors. As a result, the ultrasound screen displays the predicted needle trajectory and the location where the needle will intersect with the ultrasound beam.

Other: Fluoroscopy, Paresthesia, Fascial Click

There are additional nerve localization techniques. Fluoroscopy uses continuous x-ray imaging to localize a nearby bony structure. When appropriate, injection of contrast dye can be used to outline the location of perineural structures.

The paresthesia technique involves advancing the nerve block needle to contact a nerve/plexus. While sensory paresthesia may result, it is not guaranteed. Consequently, the paresthesia technique may be inaccurate and potentially harmful.

The fascial click technique involves a tactile "pop" sensation as a nerve block needle penetrates fascial layers. While this technique may be used for field blocks (i.e., fascia iliaca), its accuracy for nerve localization is limited.

Clinical Pearls

- Nerve stimulation can assist with identification of neural structures; however, limitations exist.
- Ultrasound guidance allows identification of important neural and perineural structures and allows confirmation of appropriate perineural injection of solute.

POSTBLOCK CONSIDERATIONS

Catheter Fixation Systems

One of the most common etiologies of secondary CPNB failure involves catheter displacement. Various techniques can be used to reduce the chance of catheter dislodgement. Subcutaneous tunneling of the catheter can be used in suitable locations.

A liquid adhesive can be applied where the catheter exits the skin and under the clear occlusive dressing. There are adhesive dressings that have been specifically designed to fix a catheter to the skin (i.e., Epi-Guard, Copenhagen MedLab, Glostrup, Denmark).

Infusion Pumps

The infusion pump selected should be reliable and accurate. It should contain an appropriate volume of local anesthetic solution for the anticipated duration of infusion. The pump should be adjustable and have the ability to provide a continuous infusion as well as patient-controlled boluses at specifically timed intervals. These features enable the CPNB to be tailored to changing patient requirements.

Outpatient perineural infusion pumps must be reliable, accurate, and compact in size. Electronic or elastomeric pumps are available for outpatient use. Some are disposable, whereas others are reusable and must be returned by the patient to the hospital.

Patient Follow-up

Patients with perineural catheters must be followed daily. The catheter site is inspected for cleanliness, integrity, and possible dislodgement. The catheter site is evaluated for signs of infection, such as redness, warmth, or purulent discharge. Adequacy of analgesia is assessed, and modifications to the pain management plan are made. The patient is educated about the care of the numb extremity and fall prevention strategies if applicable. Symptoms of local anesthetic toxicity are sought. Pump function is reviewed.

Outpatient Perineural Catheters

Outpatients are contacted daily by telephone, at which time the follow-up outlined previously is performed. The procedure for catheter removal is discussed and performed by the patient and the patient's caregiver at home. Disposable pumps are placed in the trash, while nondisposable pumps are returned in person or mailed to the hospital.

Clinical Pearl

- The safety and efficacy of CPNBs relies on properly securing the catheter to prevent dislodgement, appropriate follow-up by a knowledgeable health care worker, and adequate patient education regarding the care of the numb extremity, potential complications, and local anesthetic pump function.

CONCLUSION

This chapter highlights the equipment required for safe and effective perineural infusion of local anesthetic solutions. The development of specialized needle-and-catheter systems for this purpose was initially slow; however, currently available systems are reliable and applicable to most clinical situations.

When considering deterrents to the more widespread adoption of CPNBs, lack of operator training has frequently been cited in the past. Currently, there are numerous learning opportunities available, including hands-on courses, preceptorships, virtual reality, and simulation training. There has also been improvement in patient and surgeon education regarding the potential benefits of CPNBs. Nevertheless, some concern persists about potential side effects, including nerve injury and falls. While ongoing research has enhanced our understanding of the mechanism of nerve injury related to regional anesthesia, further information is required. Other factors limiting the clinical application of CPNBs may be institutional and should be addressed at a local level. These include time pressure in busy operating rooms, lack of qualified assistants for block performance, lack of funds for equipment, or lack of support for postoperative care.

REFERENCES

1. Serpell MG, Millar FA, Thomson MF: Comparison of lumbar plexus block versus conventional opioid analgesia after total knee replacement. Anaesthesia 1991;46(4):275–277.
2. Edwards ND, Wright EM: Continuous low-dose 3-in-1 nerve blockade for postoperative pain relief after total knee replacement. Anesth Analg 1992;75(2):265–267.
3. Matheny JM, Hanks GA, Rung GW, Blanda JB, Kalenak A: A comparison of patient-controlled analgesia and continuous lumbar plexus block after anterior cruciate ligament reconstruction. Arthroscopy 1993;9(1):87–90.
4. Borgeat A, Schappi B, Biasca N, Gerber C: Patient-controlled analgesia after major shoulder surgery: Patient-controlled interscalene analgesia versus patient-controlled analgesia. Anesthesiology 1997;87(6):1343–1347.
5. Singelyn FJ, Aye F, Gouverneur JM: Continuous popliteal sciatic nerve block: An original technique to provide postoperative analgesia after foot surgery. Anesth Analg 1997;84(2):383–386.
6. Borgeat A, Tewes E, Biasca N, Gerber C: Patient-controlled interscalene analgesia with ropivacaine after major shoulder surgery: PCIA vs PCA. Br J Anaesth 1998;81(4):603–605.
7. Singelyn FJ, Deyaert M, Joris D, Pendeville E, Gouverneur JM. Effects of intravenous patient-controlled analgesia with morphine, continuous epidural analgesia, and continuous three-in-one block on postoperative pain and knee rehabilitation after unilateral total knee arthroplasty. Anesth Analg 1998;87(1):88–92.
8. Capdevila X, Barthelet Y, Biboulet P, Ryckwaert Y, Rubenovitch J, d'Athis F. Effects of perioperative analgesic technique on the surgical outcome and duration of rehabilitation after major knee surgery. Anesthesiology 1999;91(1):8–15.
9. Lehtipalo S, Koskinen LO, Johansson G, Kolmodin J, Biber B. Continuous interscalene brachial plexus block for postoperative analgesia following shoulder surgery. Acta Anaesthesiol Scand 1999;43(3):258–264.
10. Chelly JE, Greger J, Gebhard R, et al. Continuous femoral blocks improve recovery and outcome of patients undergoing total knee arthroplasty. J Arthroplasty 2001;16(4):436–445.
11. White PF, Issioui T, Skrivanek GD, Early JS, Wakefield C: The use of a continuous popliteal sciatic nerve block after surgery involving the foot and ankle: Does it improve the quality of recovery? Anesth Analg 2003;97(5):1303–1309.
12. Matthews PJ, Govenden V: Comparison of continuous paravertebral and extradural infusions of bupivacaine for pain relief after thoracotomy. Br J Anaesth 1989;62(2):204–205.
13. Schultz P, Anker-Moller E, Dahl JB, Christensen EF, Spangsberg N, Fauno P: Postoperative pain treatment after open knee surgery: Continuous lumbar plexus block with bupivacaine versus epidural morphine. Reg Anesth 1991;16(1):34–37.
14. Turker G, Uckunkaya N, Yavascaoglu B, Yilmazlar A, Ozcelik S: Comparison of the catheter-technique psoas compartment block and the epidural block for analgesia in partial hip replacement surgery. Acta Anaesthesiol Scand 2003;47(1):30–36.
15. Nielsen KC, Greengrass RA, Pietrobon R, Klein SM, Steele SM: Continuous interscalene brachial plexus blockade provides good analgesia at home after major shoulder surgery-report of four cases. Can J Anaesth 2003;50(1):57–61.
16. Zaric D, Boysen K, Christiansen J, Haastrup U, Kofoed H, Rawal N:. Continuous popliteal sciatic nerve block for outpatient foot surgery—A randomized, controlled trial. Acta Anaesthesiol Scand 2004;48(3):337–341.
17. Buettner J, Klose R, Hoppe U, Wresch P: Serum levels of mepivacaine-HCl during continuous axillary brachial plexus block. Reg Anesth 1989;14(3):124–127.
18. van den Berg B, Berger A, van den Berg E, Zenz M, Brehmeier G, Tizian C: Continuous plexus anesthesia to improve circulation in peripheral microvascular interventions. Handchir Mikrochir Plast Chir 1983;15(2):101–104.
19. Camprubi Sociats I, Garcia Huete L, Sabate Pes A, Bartolome Sarvise C, Cochs Cristia J. Use of axillary perivascular blockage of the brachial plexus with a catheter as treatment in accidental intra-arterial injection of drugs. Rev Esp Anestesiol Reanim 1989;36(3):167–170.
20. Haynsworth RF, Heavner JE, Racz GB: Continuous brachial plexus blockade using an axillary catheter for treatment of accidental intra-arterial injections. Reg Anaesth 1985;10:187.
21. Berger JL, Nimier M, Desmonts JM: Continuous axillary plexus block in the treatment of accidental intraarterial injection of cocaine. N Engl J Med 1988;318(14):930.
22. Aguilar JL, Domingo V, Samper D, Roca G, Vidal F: Long-term brachial plexus anesthesia using a subcutaneous implantable injection system. Case report. Reg Anesth 1995;20(3):242–245.
23. Fischer HB, Peters TM, Fleming IM, Else TA: Peripheral nerve catheterization in the management of terminal cancer pain. Reg Anesth 1996;21(5):482–485.
24. Smith BE, Fischer HB, Scott PV. Continuous sciatic nerve block. Anaesthesia 1984;39(2):155–157.
25. Ansbro FP: A method of continuous brachial plexus block. Am J Surg 1946;71:716–722.
26. DeKrey JA, Schroeder CF, Buechel DR: Continuous brachial plexus block. Anesthesiology 1969;30(3):332.
27. Winnie AP: Interscalene brachial plexus block. Anesth Analg 1970;49(3):455–466.
28. Selander D: Catheter technique in axillary plexus block. Presentation of a new method. Acta Anaesthesiol Scand 1977;21(4):324–329.
29. Brands E, Callanan VI: Continuous lumbar plexus block--analgesia for femoral neck fractures. Anaesth Intensive Care 1978;6(3):256–258.
30. Thompson GE, Rorie DK: Functional anatomy of the brachial plexus sheaths. Anesthesiology 1983;59(2):117–122.
31. Tuominen M, Rosenberg PH, Kalso E: Blood levels of bupivacaine after single dose, supplementary dose, and during continuous infusion in axillary plexus block. Acta Anaesthesiol Scand 1983;27(4):303–306.
32. Manriquez RG, Pallares V: Continuous brachial plexus block for prolonged sympathectomy and control of pain. Anesth Analg 1978;57(1):128–130.
33. Economacos G, Skountzos V: Nerve blocking of the sciatic and femoral nerves. Continual block with vein catheter on 44 patients. Acta Anaesthesiol Belg 1980;31 Suppl:223–228.
34. Vatashsky E, Aronson HB: Continuous interscalene brachial plexus block for surgical operations on the hand. Anesthesiology 1980;53(4):356.
35. Sada T, Kobayashi T, Murakami S: Continuous axillary brachial plexus block. Can Anaesth Soc J 1983;30(2):201–205.
36. Neimkin RJ, May JW Jr, Roberts J, Sunder N: Continuous axillary block through an indwelling Teflon catheter. J Hand Surg Am 1984;9(6):830–833.
37. Conacher ID, Kokri M. Postoperative paravertebral blocks for thoracic surgery. A radiological appraisal. Br J Anaesth 1987;59(2):155–161.
38. Lonnqvist PA: Continuous paravertebral block in children. Initial experience. Anaesthesia 1992;47(7):607–609.
39. Vaghadia H, Kapnoudhis P, Jenkins LC, Taylor D: Continuous lumbosacral block using a Tuohy needle and catheter technique. Can J Anaesth 1992;39(1):75–78.
40. Chan V, Ferrante FM: Continuous thoracic paravertebral block. In Ferrante FM, VadeBoncoeur TR (eds): *Postoperative Pain Management.* Churchill Livingstone, 1993:403–414.
41. Selander D, Dhuner KG, Lundborg G: Peripheral nerve injury due to injection needles used for regional anesthesia. An experimental study of the acute effects of needle point trauma. Acta Anaesthesiol Scand 1977;21(3):182–188.
42. Selander D, Edshage S, Wolff T: Paresthesiae or no paresthesiae? Nerve lesions after axillary blocks. Acta Anaesthesiol Scand 1979;23(1):27–33.

43. Montgomery SJ, Raj PP, Nettles D, Jenkins MT: The use of the nerve stimulator with standard unsheathed needles in nerve blockade. Anesth Analg 1973;52(5):827–831.
44. Ford DJ, Pither C, Raj PP: Comparison of insulated and uninsulated needles for locating peripheral nerves with a peripheral nerve stimulator. Anesth Analg 1984;63(10):925–928.
45. Anker-Moller E, Spangsberg N, Dahl JB, Christensen EF, Schultz P, Carlsson P: Continuous blockade of the lumbar plexus after knee surgery: A comparison of the plasma concentrations and analgesic effect of bupivacaine 0.25% and 0.125%. Acta Anaesthesiol Scand 1990;34(6):468–472.
46. Ben-David B, Lee E, Croitoru M: Psoas block for surgical repair of hip fracture: A case report and description of a catheter technique. Anesth Analg 1990;71(3):298–301.
47. Conception M: Continuous brachial plexus techniques. In Ferrante FM, VadeBoncoeur TR (eds): *Postoperative Pain Management*. Churchill Livingstone, 1993:359–402.
48. Prosser DP: Adaptation of an intravenous cannula for paediatric regional anaesthesia. Anaesthesia 1996;51(5):510.
49. Tan TS, Watcha MF, Safavi F, McCulloch D, Payne CT, Tuefel A: Cannulation of the axillary brachial sheath in children. Anesth Analg 1995;80(3):640–641.
50. Rosenblatt R, Pepitone-Rockwell F, McKillop MJ: Continuous axillary analgesia for traumatic hand injury. Anesthesiology 1979;51(6):565–566.
51. Steele SM, Klein SM, D'Ercole FJ, Greengrass RA, Gleason D: A new continuous catheter delivery system. Anesth Analg 1998;87(1):228.
52. Fredrickson MJ, Ball CM, Dalgleish AJ: Catheter orifice configuration influences the effectiveness of continuous peripheral nerve blockade. Reg Anesth Pain Med 2011;36(5):470–475.
53. Sutherland ID: Continuous sciatic nerve infusion: Expanded case report describing a new approach. Reg Anesth Pain Med 1998;23(5):496–501.
54. Boezaart AP, de Beer JF, du Toit C, van Rooyen K: A new technique of continuous interscalene nerve block. Can J Anaesth 1999;46(3):275–281.
55. Boezaart AP, De Beer JF, Nell ML: Early experience with continuous cervical paravertebral block using a stimulating catheter. Reg Anesth Pain Med 2003;28(5):406–413.
56. Borene SC, Rosenquist RW, Koorn R, Haider N, Boezaart AP: An indication for continuous cervical paravertebral block (posterior approach to the interscalene space). Anesth Analg 2003;97(3):898–900.
57. Kick O, Blanche E, Pham-Dang C, Pinaud M, Estebe JP: A new stimulating stylet for immediate control of catheter tip position in continuous peripheral nerve blocks. Anesth Analg 1999;89(2):533–534.
58. Pham-Dang C, Kick O, Collet T, Gouin F, Pinaud M: Continuous peripheral nerve blocks with stimulating catheters. Reg Anesth Pain Med 2003;28(2):83–88.
59. Casati A, Fanelli G, Koscielniak-Nielsen Z, et al: Using stimulating catheters for continuous sciatic nerve block shortens onset time of surgical block and minimizes postoperative consumption of pain medication after halux valgus repair as compared with conventional nonstimulating catheters. Anesth Analg 2005;101(4):1192–1197.
60. de Tran QH, Munoz L, Russo G, Finlayson RJ: Ultrasonography and stimulating perineural catheters for nerve blocks: a review of the evidence. Can J Anaesth 2008;55(7):447–457.
61. Morin AM, Kranke P, Wulf H, Stienstra R, Eberhart LH: The effect of stimulating versus nonstimulating catheter techniques for continuous regional anesthesia: a semiquantitative systematic review. Reg Anesth Pain Med 2010;35(2):194–199.
62. Mariano ER, Loland VJ, Sandhu NS, et al: Comparative efficacy of ultrasound-guided and stimulating popliteal-sciatic perineural catheters for postoperative analgesia. Can J Anaesth 2010;57(10):919–926.
63. Gandhi K, Lindenmuth DM, Hadzic A, et al: The effect of stimulating versus conventional perineural catheters on postoperative analgesia following ultrasound-guided femoral nerve localization. J Clin Anesth 2011;23(8):626–631.
64. Robards C, Hadzic A, Somasundaram L, et al: Intraneural injection with low-current stimulation during popliteal sciatic nerve block. Anesth Analg 2009;109(2):673–677.

CHAPTER 14

Electrical Nerve Stimulators and Localization of Peripheral Nerves

André van Zundert and Admir Hadzic

INTRODUCTION

Peripheral nerve stimulation (PNS), an important tool to aid administration of peripheral nerve blocks. Improvements in electrical nerve localization technology have led to a number of commercially available nerve stimulators that are superior and more advanced compared to older devices. With the introduction of ultrasound-guided nerve blocks, however, there has been confusion on the role of nerve stimulation in the setting of ultrasound-guided nerve blocks. This review focuses on the foundation of nerve stimulation with a short historical background, the latest developments in the technology, and the role of nerve stimulation with ultrasound-guided peripheral nerve blocks.

HISTORY

Quick Facts

- 1780: Luigi Galvani[1] was the first to describe the effect of electrical neuromuscular stimulation in a frog experiment.
- 1912: Perthes[2] developed and described an electrical nerve stimulator.
- 1955: Pearson[3] introduced the concept of insulated needles for nerve location.
- 1962: Greenblatt and Denson[4] introduced a portable solid-state nerve stimulator with variable current output and described its use for nerve location.
- 1973: Montgomery et al[5] demonstrated that noninsulated needles require significantly higher current amplitudes than the insulated needles.
- 1984: Ford et al[6] reported a lack of accuracy with noninsulated needles once the needle tip passed the target nerve.
- Ford et al suggested the use of nerve stimulators with a constant current source, based on the comparison of the electrical characteristics of peripheral nerve stimulators.[7,8]

- In 2004, Hadzic & Vloka defined the electrical characteristics and suggested manufacturing standard for modern nerve stimulators.[9]

It took nearly 100 years from the concept of nerve stimulation to adoption of electrolocalization during peripheral nerve blockade in the 1990s. The more widespread introduction of nerve stimulation in the practice of peripheral nerve blockade led to research on the needle-nerve relationship and the effect of stimulus duration.[10,11] More recently, the principles of electrical nerve stimulation were applied to surface mapping of peripheral nerves using percutaneous electrode guidance[12–15] for confirmation and epidural catheter placement[16–18] and peripheral catheter placement.[19] This chapter discusses the electrophysiology of nerve stimulation, electrical nerve stimulators, various modes of localization of peripheral nerves, and integration of the technology into the realm of ultrasound-guided regional anesthesia.

What Is Electrical Peripheral Nerve Stimulation?

Electrical nerve stimulation in regional anesthesia is a method of using a low-intensity (up to 5 mA) and short-duration (0.05 to 1 ms) electrical stimulus (at 1- to 2-Hz repetition rate) to obtain a defined response (muscle twitch or sensation) to locate a peripheral nerve or nerve plexus with an (insulated) needle before injecting local anesthetic in close proximity to the nerve to block nerve conduction for surgery or acute pain management. The use of nerve stimulation can recognize an intraneural or intrafascicular needle placement injection, prevent further needle advancement intraneurally and help reduce the risk of nerve injury.

Electrical nerve stimulation can be used for a single-injection technique, as well as for guidance during the insertion of continuous nerve block catheters. More recently, ultrasound guidance in

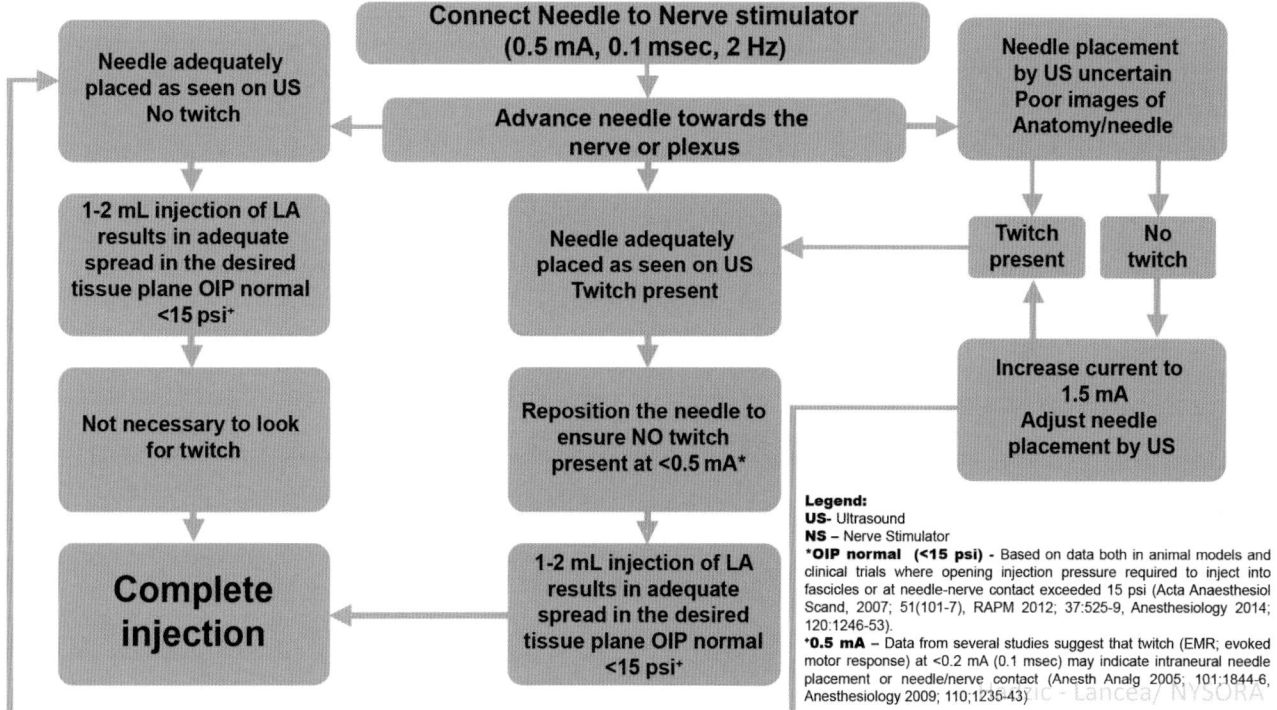

FIGURE 14–1. An algorithm for use of nerve stimulation with ultrasound-guided nerve blocks. Please note that the nerve stimulator here is used primarily as a safety-monitoring tool, rather than a nerve localization tool. The stimulator is set at 0.5 mA (0.1 ms), and the current is rarely manipulated. Instead, a motor response is obtained; extra caution is exercised as this indicates an intimate needle-nerve relationship. Instead of adjusting the current intensity to determine at which current the motor response extinguishes, the needle is slightly withdrawn to abolish the response and distance the needle tip from the nerve. A small amount of local anesthetic is then injected to determine the needle tip location while avoiding an opening pressure greater than 15 psi. LA, local anesthetic; OIP, opening injection pressure.

combination with nerve stimulation ("dual monitoring") has become a common practice to guide needle placement and robust medicolegal documentation of nerve block procedures.

Indications for the Use of PNS

In principle, almost all plexuses or other large peripheral nerves can be located using PNS.[20] When used with ultrasound guidance, PNS becomes primarily a safety tool. The goal of nerve stimulation is to place the tip of the needle (more specifically, its orifice for injection) in close proximity to the target nerve to inject the local anesthetic within the tissue space that contains the nerve. When used with ultrasound guidance, PNS becomes primarily a safety tool. An unexpected motor response during needle advancement may alert the operator that the needle is in immediate vicinity to the nerve and therefore, prevent further needle advancement when the needle tip position is not well seen on ultrasound. The motor response (twitch) to PNS is objective, reliable and independent from the patient's (subjective) response. Even with ultrasound guidance, nerve stimulation is often helpful to confirm that the structure imaged is actually the nerve that is sought. Likewise, the needle-nerve relationship may not always be visualized on ultrasound; an unexpected motor response can occur, alerting the operator that the needle is already in close proximity to the nerve. The occurrence of a motor response at a current intensity of less than 0.5 mA can serve as an indicator of a needle-nerve contact or intraneural needle placement.[21,22] Although this response may not be present even with an intraneural needle position

(low sensitivity), its presence is essentially always indicative of intraneural placement (high specificity). An algorithm for using nerve stimulation as a monitoring tool during ultrasound-guided blocks is provided in Figure 14–1.

The disadvantages of PNS include the need for additional equipment (nerve stimulator and insulated needles), the greater cost of insulated needles, and exceptional cases for which it may be difficult to elicit a motor response.

Clinical Pearls

- Occurrence of a motor response at 0.5 mA (0.1 ms) indicate needle-nerve contact or intraneural needle placement.
- Occurrence of the motor response at 0.5 mA should prompt caution. The practitioner should stop advancing the needle, withdraw the needle by 1 mm, and inject 1 mL of local anesthetic (assuming the opening pressure is less than 15 psi) to determine the needle tip position and adjust the needle and injection process accordingly.
- PNS should not be relied on in a patient receiving muscle relaxants.
- The presence of spinal or epidural anesthesia does not negatively affect the reliability of PNS.
- Multiple injection techniques may decrease PNS sensitivity due to the partial nerve blockade that occurs between injections.

BASICS OF NEUROPHYSIOLOGY AND ELECTROPHYSIOLOGY

Membrane Potential, Resting Potential, Depolarization, Action Potential, and Impulse Propagation

All living cells have a **membrane potential** (a voltage potential across their membrane, measured from the outside to the inside), which varies (depending on the species and the cell type) from about –60 to –100 mV. Nerve and muscle cells in mammals typically have a membrane potential (resting potential) of about –90 mV.

Only nerve and muscle cells have the capability of producing uniform electrical pulses, called **action potentials** (sometimes called spikes), which are propagated along their membranes, especially along the long extensions of nerve cells (nerve fibers, axons). A decrease in the electric potential difference (eg, from –90 to –55 mV, or **depolarization**) elicits an action potential. If the depolarization exceeds a certain *threshold*, an action potential or a series of action potentials is generated by the nerve membrane (also called firing) according to the all-or-nothing rule, resulting in propagation of the action potential along the nerve fiber (axon). To **depolarize** the nerve membrane from outside the cell (extracellular stimulation), the negative **polarity** of the electrical stimulus is more effective in removing the positive charge from the outside of the membrane. This in turn decreases the potential across the membrane toward the threshold level.

There are various types of nerve fibers. Each fiber type can be distinguished anatomically by its diameter and degree of myelination. Myelination is formed by an insulating layer of Schwann cells wrapped around the nerve fibers. These characteristics largely determine the electrophysiologic behavior of different nerve fibers, that is, the speed of impulse propagation of action potentials and the threshold of excitability. Most commonly, the distinguishing features are motor fibers (eg, Aα, Aβ) and pain fibers (C). The Aα motor fibers have the largest diameter and highest degree of myelination and therefore the highest speed of impulse propagation and a relatively low threshold for external stimulation. The C fibers (which transmit severe, dull pain) have little to no myelination and are of smaller diameter. Consequently, the speed of propagation in these fibers is relatively low, and the threshold levels to external stimulation, in general, are higher.

There are several other efferent fibers, which transmit responses from various skin receptors or muscle spindles (Aδ). These are thinner than Aα fibers and have less myelination. Some of these (afferent) sensory fibers, having a relatively low threshold level, transmit the typical tingling sensation associated with a lower level of pain sensation when electrically stimulated (similar to the sensation when hitting the "funny bone"). Such sensation can occur during transcutaneous stimulation before a motor response is elicited.

The basic anatomic structure of myelinated Aα fibers (motor) and nonmyelinated C fibers (pain) is shown schematically in Figure 14–2. The relationship between different stimuli and the triggering of the action potential in motor and

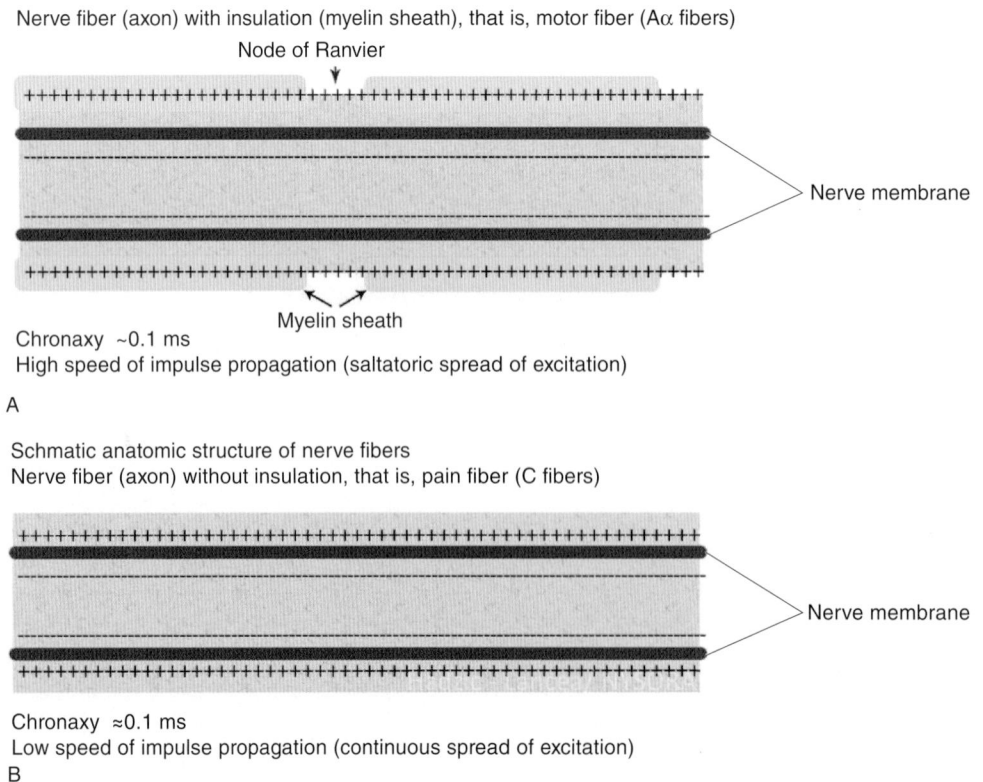

FIGURE 14–2. Schematic anatomic structures of nerve fibers. **A:** Nerve fiber (axon) with insulation (myelin sheath), (Aα fibers). **B:** Nerve fiber (axon) without insulation (C fiber).

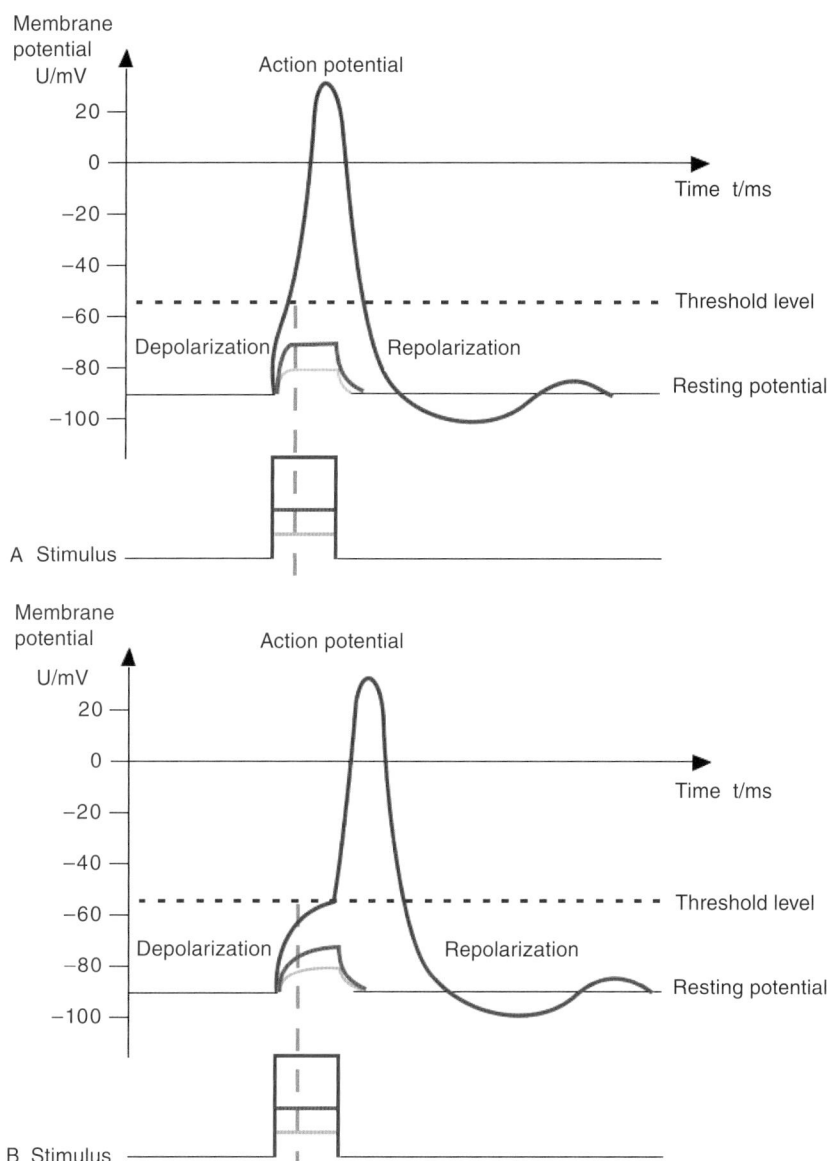

FIGURE 14–3. A: Action potential, threshold level, and stimulus. Motor fibers have a short chronaxy because of the relatively low capacitance of their myelinated membrane (only the area of the nodes of Ranvier count; see Figure 14–1); therefore, it takes only a short time to depolarize the membrane up to the threshold level. **B:** Action potential, threshold level, and stimulus. Pain fibers have a long chronaxy because of the higher capacitance of their nonmyelinated membrane (the entire area of the membrane counts); therefore, it takes a longer time to depolarize the membrane up to the threshold level. Short impulses (as indicated by the vertical dotted line) would not be able to depolarize the membrane below the threshold level.

pain fibers is illustrated in Figures 14–3A and 14–3B, respectively.

Threshold Level, Rheobase, Chronaxy

A certain minimum current intensity is necessary at a given pulse duration to reach the **threshold level** of excitation. The lowest threshold current (at infinitely long pulse durations) is called **rheobase**. The pulse duration (pulse width) at double the rheobase current is called **chronaxy**. Electrical pulses with the duration of the chronaxy are most effective (at relatively low amplitudes) to elicit action potentials. This is the reason why

motor response can be elicited at such short pulse duration (eg., 0.1 ms) at relatively low current amplitudes while avoiding the stimulation of C-type pain fibers. Typical chronaxy figures are 50–100 µs (Aα fibers), 170 µs (Aδ fibers), and 400 µs or greater (C fibers). The relationship of the rheobase to chronaxy for motor fibers versus pain nerve fibers is illustrated in Figure 14–4.

Impedance, Impulse Duration, and Constant Current

The electrical circuit is formed by the nerve stimulator, the nerve block needle and its tip design, the tissue characteristics

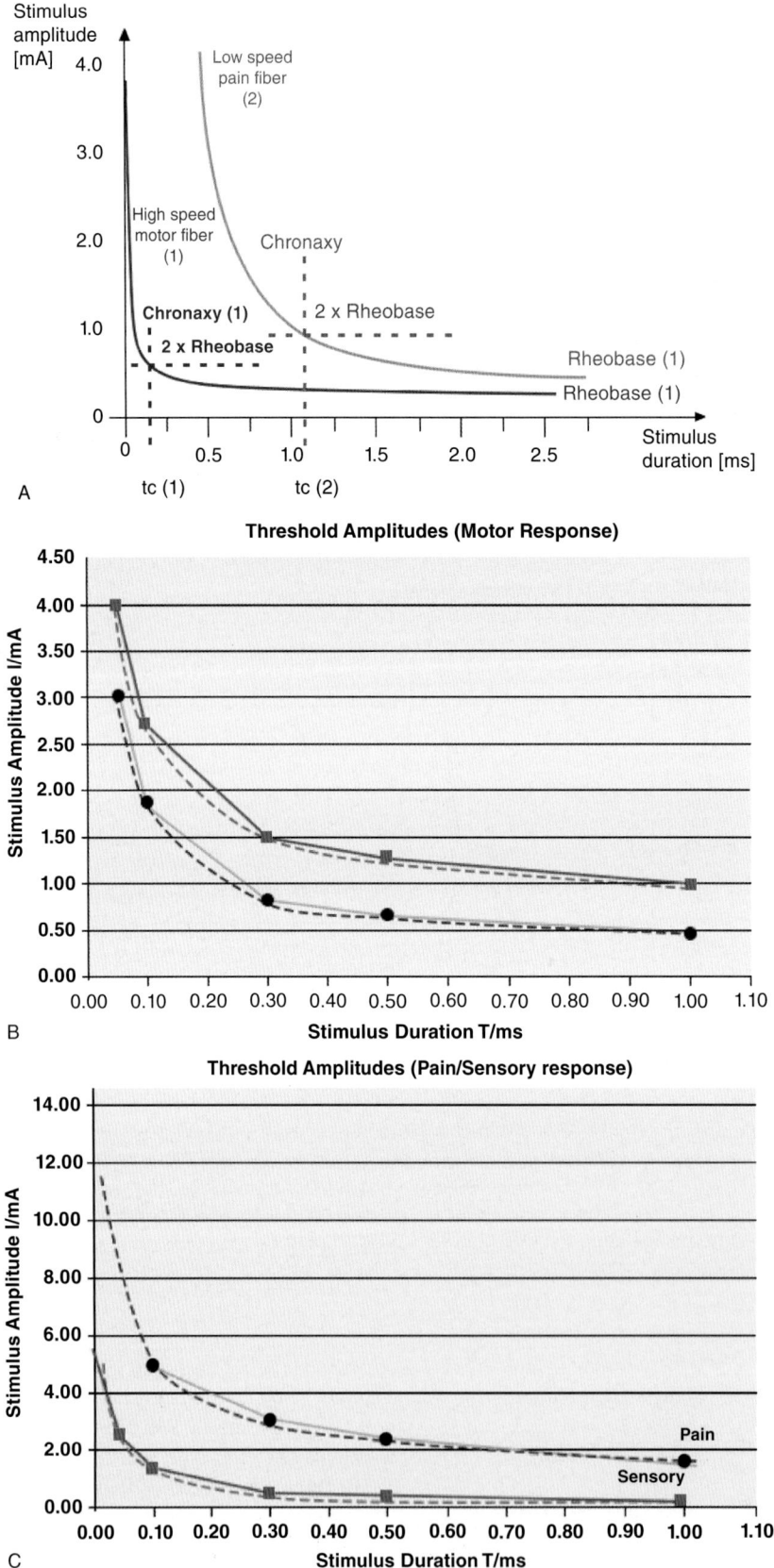

FIGURE 14–4. A: Comparison of threshold curves, chronaxy, and rheobase level of motor (high-speed) and pain (low-speed) fibers. **B:** Experimental data, threshold amplitudes obtained with percutaneous stimulation (Stimuplex Pen and Stimuplex HNS 12). Stimulation obtained with percutaneous stimulation of the median nerve near the wrist looking for motor response of the thumb. **C:** Threshold amplitudes obtained with percutaneous stimulation (Stimuplex Pen and Stimuplex HNS 12). Stimulation of the median and radial nerves near the wrist and at the midforearm looking for electric paresthesia (tingling sensation) in the middle and ring fingers (median nerve) or superficial pain sensation near the wrist (radial nerve), respectively.

of the patient, the skin, the skin electrode (grounding electrode), and the cables connecting all the elements. The resistance of this circuit is not just a simple Ohm's resistor equation because of the specific capacitances of the tissue, the electrocardiographic (ECG) electrode-to-skin interface, and the needle tip, which influence the overall resistance. The capacitance in the described circuit varies with the frequency content of the stimulation current, and it is called *impedance* or a *complex resistance,* which is dependent on the frequency content of the stimulus. In general, the shorter the impulse, the higher its frequency content is and, consequently, the lower the impedance of a circuit with a given capacitance. Conversely, a longer pulse duration has a lower frequency content. As an example, for a 0.1-ms stimulus, the main frequency content is 10 kHz plus its harmonics, whereas for a 1.0-ms impulse, the main frequency content is 1 kHz plus harmonics). In reality, the impedance of the needle tip and the electrode-to-skin impedance have the highest impact. The impedance of the needle tip largely depends on the geometry and insulation (conductive area). The electrode-to-skin impedance can vary considerably between individuals (eg, type of skin, hydration status) and can be influenced by the quality of the ECG electrode used.

Because of the variable impedance in the circuit, created primarily by the needle tip and electrode-to-skin interface, a nerve stimulator with a constant current source and sufficient (voltage) output power is necessary to compensate for the wide range of impedances encountered clinically.

CLINICAL USE OF PERIPHERAL NERVE STIMULATION

Setup and Checking the Equipment

The following are a few important aspects for successful electrolocalization of the peripheral nerves using PNS:

- Use only a nerve stimulator specifically manufactured for nerve blocks.
- Use insulated nerve stimulation needles (Table 14–1).
- Use high-quality skin electrodes with a low impedance.
  - Some lower-priced ECG electrodes can have too high an impedance/resistance.
- Before starting the procedure, check for the proper functioning of the nerve stimulator and the connecting cables.
- During the procedure, check frequently to assure that the current is being delivered and leads disconnect does not occur.

TABLE 14–1. Stimulation needle sizes recommended for various nerve blocks.

Nerve Block	Single-Shot Technique		Catheter Technique (Introducer Needle)	
	Length (mm)	Size, OD (mm/G)	Length (mm)	Size, OD (mm/G)
Anterior interscalene	25–50	0.5–0.7/25–22	33–55	1.1–1.3/20–18
Posterior interscalene	80–100	0.7/22	80–110	1.3/18
Vertical infraclavicular (VIB)	50	0.7/22	50–55	1.3/18
Axillary blockade	35–50	0.5–0.7/25–22	40–55	1.3/18
Suprascapular	35–50	0.5–0.7/25–22	40–55	1.3/18
Psoas compartment	80–120	0.7–0.8/22–21	80–150	1.3/18
Femoral nerve	50	0.7/22	50–55	1.3/18
Saphenous nerve	50–80	0.7/22	55–80	1.3/18
Obturator	80	0.7/22	80	1.3/18
Parasacral sciatic	80–120	0.7–0.8/22–21	80–110	1.3/18
Transgluteal sciatic	80–100	0.7–0.8/22–21	80–110	1.3/18
Anterior sciatic	100–150	0.7–0.9/22–20	100–150	1.3/18
Subtrochanteric sciatic	80–100	0.7–0.8/22–21	80–110	1.3/18
Lateral distal sciatic	50–80	0.7/22	55–80	1.3/18
Popliteal sciatic	50	0.7/22	55	1.3/18

OD = outside diameter; ON = Obturator nerve

Note: The nerve localization needle sizes given are only estimates; depending on the patient's size, a slightly shorter or longer size needle may be needed. Some manufacturers also offer smaller needle sizes for pediatric use.

Needles that longer than necessary for a given block procedure should not be used because the risk of complications may increase when inserting the needle too deeply.

- The design of the connectors should prevent a faulty polarity connection.
- Connect the nerve stimulation needle to the nerve stimulator (which should be turned on) and set the current amplitude and duration to the desired levels.
  - For superficial blocks, select 1.0 mA as a starting current intensity.
  - For deep blocks, select 1.5 mA as a starting current intensity.
  - Select between 0.1 and 0.3 ms of current duration for most purposes.
- With ultrasound guidance, select the current as 0.5 mA; it is rarely necessary to change the current as motor response with ultrasound guidance is not sought. However, when unexpectedly elicited, it warns the operator that the needle is in the immediate vicinity of the nerve or intraneurally placed.

Transcutaneous (Surface) Nerve Mapping

When ultrasound guidance is not used, a nerve-mapping pen can be used to locate superficial nerves (up to a maximum depth of approximately 3 cm) with transcutaneous nerve stimulation before the nerve block needle is inserted. Transcutaneous nerve mapping is particularly useful when identifying the best site for needle insertion in patients with difficult anatomy or when the landmarks prove difficult to identify. Figure 14–5 shows several available nerve-mapping pens.

Nerve mapping is also useful when teaching surface anatomy. It should be noted that longer stimulus duration (eg, 1 ms) is needed to accomplish transcutaneous nerve stimulation, as larger energy is required to elicit a motor response from the neural structures transcutaneously. The electrode tip of the pen should have an atraumatic, ball-shaped tip. The conductive tip diameter should not be larger than approximately 3 mm to provide sufficient current density and spatial discrimination, which may not be the case with larger tip diameters. Be aware that many nerve stimulators do not provide the required impulse duration of 1 ms

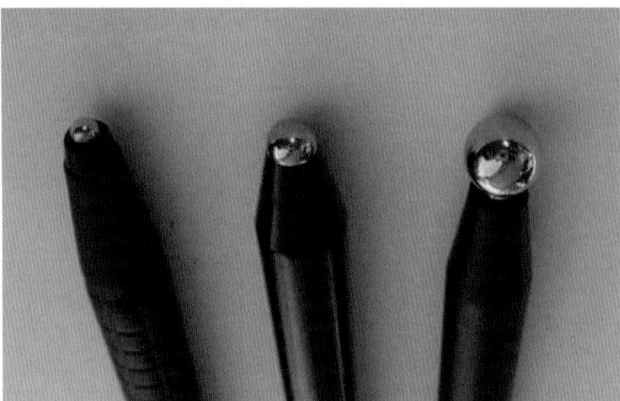

FIGURE 14–5. Tip configuration of several commercially available nerve-mapping PNS. From left to right: Stimuplex Pen (B. Braun, Melsungen (Germany); nerve-mapping pen (Pajunk, Germany); NeuroMap (HDC, USA).

or a strong enough constant current source (5 mA at minimum, 12 kΩ output load) to reliably use a nerve-mapping pen. Therefore, it is recommended that the mapping pen and the nerve stimulator be paired, ideally, by acquiring them from the same manufacturer.

The transcutaneous stimulation from a nerve-mapping pen can cause several kinds of sensation due to the stimulation of various sensory cells in the skin. This may be felt as tingling, a pinprick, or even a slight burning sensation. The perception varies greatly between individuals. Most patients tolerate transcutaneous stimulation with a nerve-mapping pen well; however, some individuals describe it as uncomfortable or even painful (depending on the stimulus amplitude and duration). However, the amount of energy delivered by nerve stimulators with a maximum output of 5 mA at 1-ms pulse duration is far too low to create any injury of the skin or the nerves. Moderate premedication is usually sufficient to make the procedure well tolerated by patients. Surface mapping was suggested as a useful tool in residents' training and particularly became popular in pediatric regional anesthesia in the 2000s. However, its use has been infrequent with the advent of ultrasound guidance.

Percutaneous Electrode Guidance

Percutaneous electrode guidance[10,11] combines transcutaneous nerve stimulation (nerve mapping) with nerve block needle guidance. In essence, a small aiming device is mounted and locked onto a conventional nerve block needle, which allows the conductive needle tip to make contact with the skin without scratching or penetrating the skin. Once the best response is obtained, the needle is advanced through the skin in the usual fashion, and the remainder of the apparatus continues to stabilize the needle and guide it toward the target. The device also allows the operator to make indentations in the skin and tissue so that the initial distance between the needle tip at the skin level and the target nerve is reduced, and the nerve block needle has less distance to travel through tissue. The technique allows for prelocation of the target nerve(s) prior to skin puncture (Figure 14–6).

Operating the Nerve Stimulator

The starting amplitude used for nerve stimulation depends on the local practice and the projected skin-nerve depth. For superficial nerves, an amplitude of 1 mA to start is chosen in most cases. For deeper nerves, it may be necessary to increase the initial current amplitude between 1.5 and 3 mA until motor response is elicited at a safe distance from the nerve. Too high current intensity, however, can lead to direct muscle stimulation or discomfort for the patient, both of which are undesirable.

Once the sought-after muscle response is obtained, the current intensity amplitude is gradually reduced, and the needle is slowly advanced farther. The needle must be advanced slowly to avoid too rapid advancement between the stimuli. Advancement of the needle and current reduction are continued until the desired motor response is achieved with a current of 0.2–0.5 mA

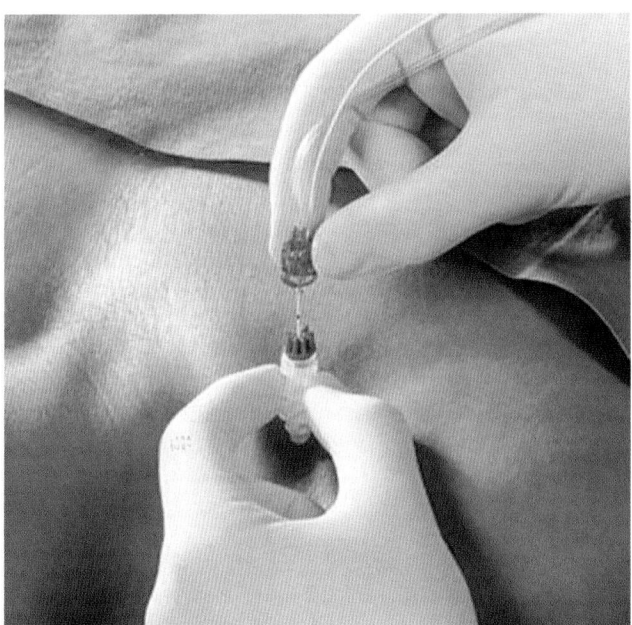

FIGURE 14–6. Percutaneous electrode guidance technique using Stimuplex Guide (B. Braun, Melsungen, Germany) during a vertical infraclavicular block procedure.

at 0.1-ms stimulus duration. The threshold level and duration of the stimulus are interdependent; in general, a short pulse duration is a better discriminator of the distance between the needle and the nerve.[20] When the motor twitch is lost during needle advancement, the stimulus intensity first should be increased to regain the muscle twitch rather than move the needle blindly. Once the needle is positioned properly, close enough to the nerve at around 0.3-mA current amplitude and 0.1-ms pulse duration, 1–2 mL of local anesthetic is injected as a test dose using low opening injection pressure, which abolishes the muscle twitch. The highly conductive injectate (eg, local anesthetic or normal saline solution) short-circuits the current to the surrounding tissue, effectively abolishing the motor response. In such situations, increasing the amplitude may not bring back the muscle twitch. Tsui and Kropelin[23] demonstrated that injection of dextrose 5% in water (D5W; which has low conductivity) does not lead to loss of the muscle twitch if the needle position is not changed. Then, the total amount of local anesthetic appropriate for the desired nerve block is injected.

It should be remembered that the absence of the motor response with a stimulating current of up to 1.5 mA does not rule out intraneural needle placement (low sensitivity). However, the presence of a motor response with a low-intensity current (≤0.2 mA, 0.1 ms) occurs only with intraneural and, possibly, intrafascicular needle placement. For this reason, if the motor response is still present at 0.2 mA or less (0.1 ms), the needle should be slightly withdrawn to avoid the risk of intrafascicular injection. The principle of the needle-to-nerve approach and its relation to the stimulation is depicted in Figures 14–7A, 14–7B, and 14–7C.

To avoid or minimize discomfort for the patient during the nerve location procedure, it is recommended that too high stimulating current be avoided. Again, the needle should not be advanced too fast because this can increase the risk of injury. Also, the best needle position, producing a good near-threshold motor response, may be missed.

The Role of Impedance Measurement

Measurement of the impedance can provide additional information if the electrical circuit is optimal. Theoretically, impedance can identify intraneural or intravascular placement of the needle tip. Tsui and colleagues[24] reported that the electrical impedance nearly doubles (12.1 to 23.2 kΩ), which is significant, when the needle is advanced from an extraneural to intraneural position in a porcine sciatic nerve. Likewise, injection of a small amount of D5W, which has a high impedance, results in a significantly higher increase of impedance in the perineural tissue than it does within the intravascular space.[25] Thus, measurement of the impedance before and after dextrose injection can potentially detect intravascular placement of the needle tip, thus identifying the placement prior to the injection of local anesthetic. In this report, the perineural baseline impedance (25.3 ± 2.0 kΩ) was significantly higher than the intravascular (17.2 ± 1.8 kΩ). On injection of 3 mL of D5W, the perineural impedance increased by 22.1 ± 6.7 kΩ to reach a peak of 50.2 ± 7.6 kΩ and remained almost constant at about 42 kΩ during the 30-s injection time. By contrast, intravascular impedance increased only by 2.5 ± 0.9 kΩ, which is significantly less compared to the perineural needle position. At present, however, more data are needed before these findings can be incorporated as an additional safety-monitoring method in clinical practice, although there have been significant recent advances in this regard.

Sequential Electrical Nerve Stimulation

Current nerve stimulation uses stimuli of identical duration (typically 0.1 ms), usually at 1- or 2-Hz repetition frequency. A common problem during nerve stimulation is that the evoked motor response is often lost while moving the needle to optimize its position. In such cases, it its recommended that the operator either increase the stimulus amplitude (mA) or increase the impulse duration (ms), the latter of which may not be possible. Alternatively, the operator can take a couple of steps, depending on the type of nerve stimulator used. The SENSe (sequential electrical nerve stimulation) technique incorporates an additional stimulus with a longer pulse duration after two regular impulses at 0.1-ms duration, creating a 3-Hz stimulation frequency.[26] The third longer impulse delivers more charge than the first two and therefore has a longer reach into the tissue. Consequently, an evoked motor response often is elicited at 1 Hz, even when the needle is distant from the nerve. Once the needle tip is positioned closer to the nerve, muscle twitches are seen at 3 Hz. The advantage of the SENSe technique is that a motor response (at 1/s) is maintained even when the twitches previously elicited by the first two impulses are lost due to slight needle movement. This feature prevents the operator from moving the needle "blindly."[26]

Figure 14–8 shows examples of the particular SENSe impulse patterns at different stimulus amplitudes. Eventually,

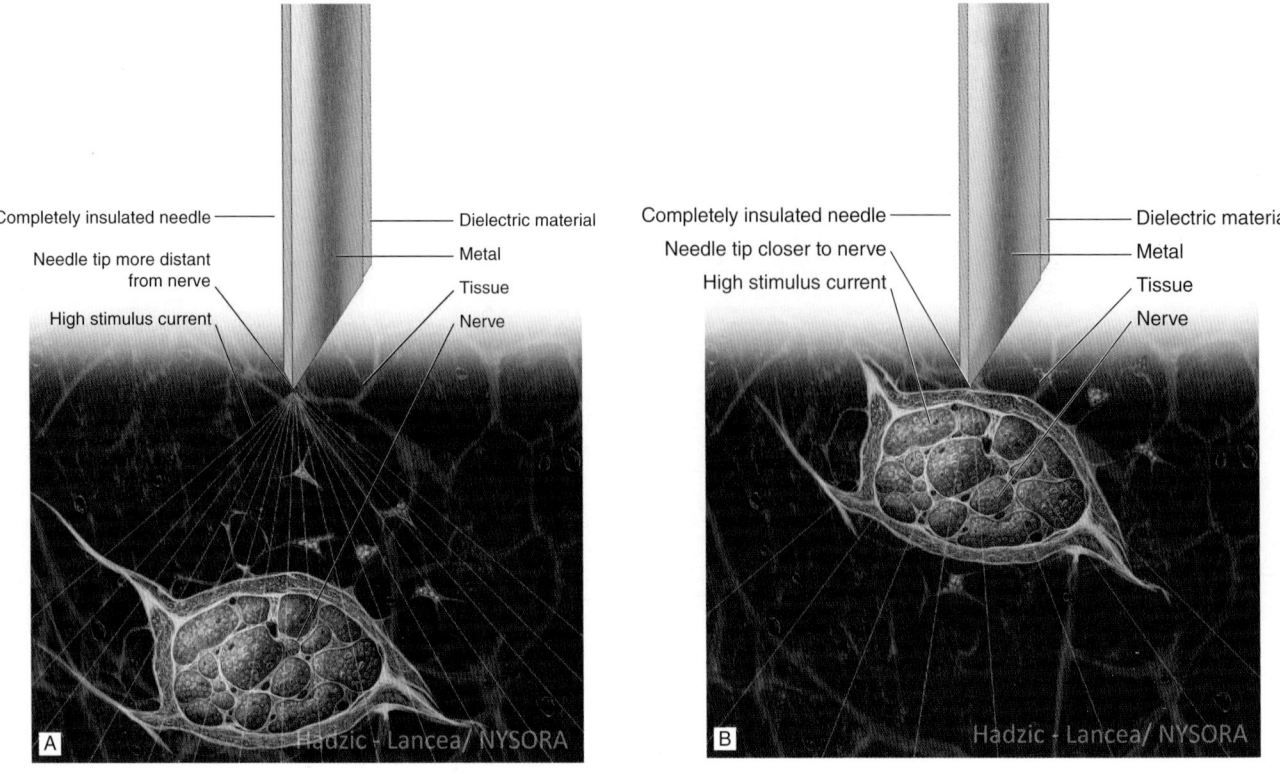

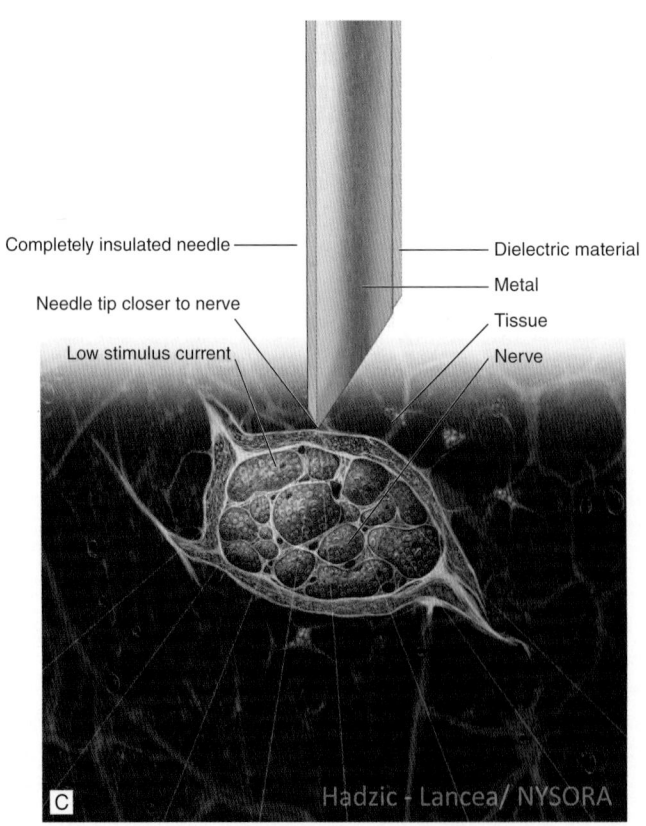

FIGURE 14–7. A: Stimulation needle at a distance to the nerve and high stimulus current eliciting a weak motor response. **B:** Stimulation needle close to the nerve and high stimulus current eliciting a strong motor response. **C:** Stimulation needle close to the nerve and low (near-threshold) stimulus current eliciting a weak motor response.

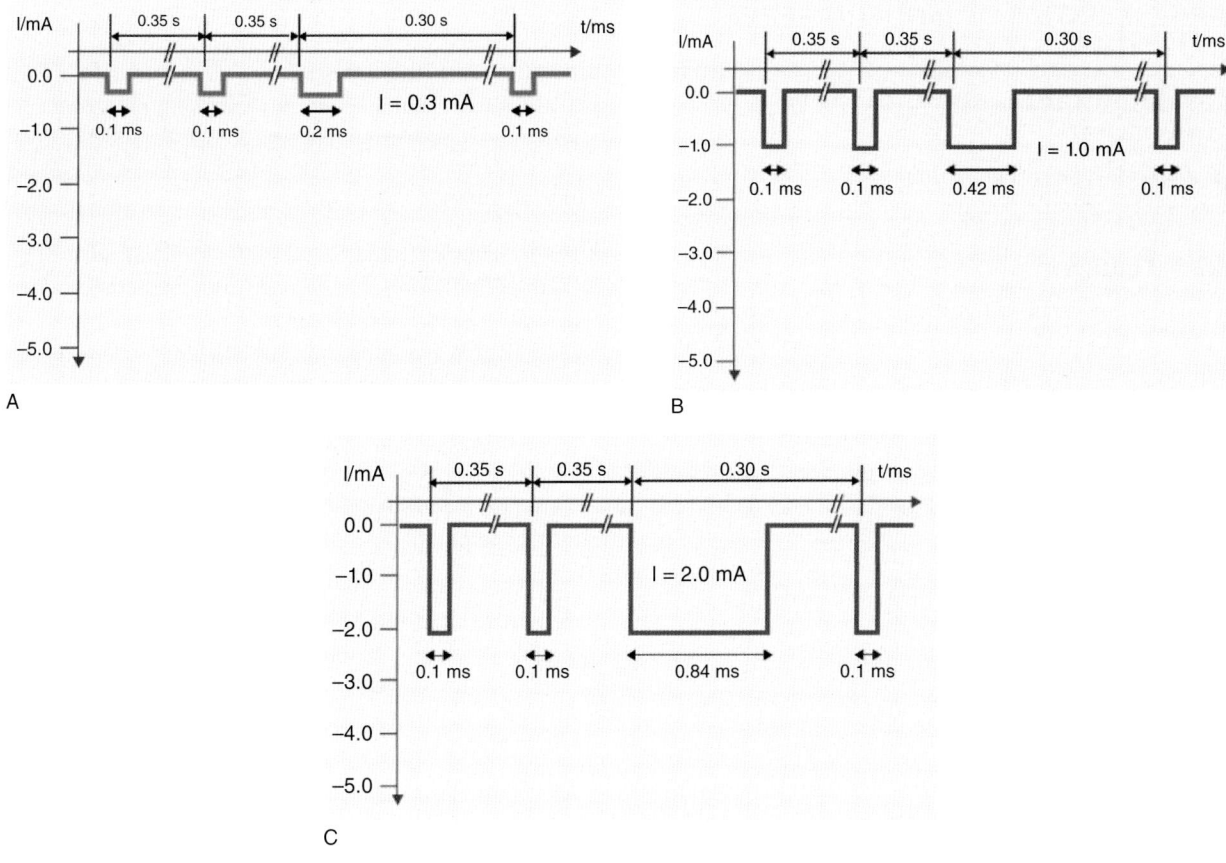

FIGURE 14–8. Sequential Electrical Nerve Stimulation (SENSe) impulse pattern of the Stimuplex HNS 12 nerve stimulator (B. Braun, Melsungen, Germany) depending on the actual stimulus amplitude. The impulse duration of the third impulse decreases with the stimulus amplitude below 2.5 mA from 1.0 ms to a minimum of 0.2 ms compared to the constant impulse duration of 0.1 ms of the first two impulses. **A:** Impulse pattern at 0.3 mA (threshold level). **B:** Impulse pattern at 1.0 mA. **C:** Impulse pattern at 2.0 mA.

the target threshold amplitude remains the same as usual (about 0.3 mA) but at 3 stimuli per second. With the SENSe technique, a motor response at only 1/s indicates that the needle is not yet placed correctly. Similar to the surface mapping, the utility of this technology has substantially decreased.

Troubleshooting During Nerve Stimulation

Table 14–2 lists the most common problems encountered during electrolocalization of the peripheral nerves and the corrective action.

TABLE 14–2. Common problems encountered during electrolocalization of peripheral nerves and corrective action.

Problem	Solution
Nerve stimulator does not work at all.	Check and replace battery; refer to stimulator operator's manual.
Nerve stimulator suddenly stops working.	Check and replace battery.
No motor response is achieved despite the appropriate needle placement.	Check connectors, skin electrode, cables, and stimulation needle for an interrupted circuit or too high impedance.
	Check and make sure that current is flowing—no disconnect indicator on the stimulator.
	Check the setting of amplitude (mA) and impulse duration.
	Check stimulator setting (some stimulators have a test mode or pause mode, which prevents current delivery).
Motor response disappears and cannot be regained even after increasing stimulus amplitude and duration.	Check for the causes listed previously. Can be caused by injection of local anesthetic.

CHARACTERISTICS OF MODERN NERVE STIMULATORS FOR NERVE BLOCKS

Most Important Features of Nerve Stimulators

This section addresses the most important features of nerve stimulators for monitoring during nerve block procedures.[20,27]

Electrical Features

- An adjustable constant current source with an operating range of 10 kΩ, minimally, output load (impedance), and ideally at 15 kΩ or greater.
- Adjustable stimulus amplitude (0–5 mA).
- A large and easy-to-read digital display of actual current delivered.
- A selectable pulse duration (width), at least between 0.1 and 1.0 ms (motor fibers are stimulated more easily with currents of shorter duration [0.1 ms] whereas sensory fibers require a longer stimulus duration [1.0 ms]).
- A stimulus frequency between 1 and 3 Hz (meaning 1 to 3 pulses per second). The best compromise is 2 Hz, which should be the default.
- A monophasic rectangular output pulse to provide reproducible stimuli.
- Configurable startup parameters so that the machine will comply with the hospital protocol and to avoid mistakes when multiple users are working with the same device (0.5 mA on startup, 0.1-ms pulse duration, 2-Hz stimulating frequency).
- A display of the circuit impedance (kΩ) is recommended to allow the operator to check the integrity of the electrical circuit and to detect a potential intraneural or intravascular placement of the needle tip.
- An automatic self-check process of the internal functioning of the unit with a warning message if something is wrong with the circuit.

Safety Features

- Easy and intuitive use.
- A large and easy-to-read display.
- Limited current range (0–5 mA) because an amplitude that is too high may be painful or uncomfortable for the patient.
- A display of all relevant parameters, such as amplitude (mA) (alternatively stimulus charge [nC]), stimulus duration (ms), stimulus frequency (Hz), impedance (kΩ), and battery status.
- Clear identification of output polarity (negative polarity at the needle).
- Meaningful instructions for use, with lists of operating ranges and allowed tolerances.
- Battery operation of the nerve stimulator, as opposed to electrical operation, provides intrinsic safety; there is no risk of serious electric shock or burns caused by a short circuit to the main supply of electricity.
- The maximum energy delivered by a nerve stimulator with 5 mA and 95-V output signal at 1-ms impulse duration is only 0.475 mWs.

- Combined units for *peripheral* (for peripheral nerve blockade) and *transcutaneous* (for muscle relaxation measurement) electrical nerve stimulation should not to be used because the transcutaneous function produced an unwanted high energy charge.

Alarms/warnings:

- Open circuit/disconnection alarm (optical and acoustic).
- Warning/indication if impedance is too high, that is, the desired current is not delivered.
- Displaying actual impedance is advisable.
- Near-threshold amplitude indication or alarm.
- Low-battery alarm.
- Internal malfunction alarm.

Table 14–3 provides a comparison of the most important features of commonly used nerve stimulators.

Stimulating Needles

Needles

A modern stimulating needle should have the following characteristics:

- A fully insulated needle hub and shaft to avoid current leakage
- Depth markings for easy identification and documentation of the needle insertion depth

Figures 14–9A and 14–9B show a comparison of the electrical characteristics of noninsulated and insulated needles with uncoated bevel (Figure 14–9A) and fully coated needles with a pinpoint electrode (Figure 14–9B). Even though a noninsulated needle provides for some discrimination (change in threshold amplitude) while approaching the nerve, there is virtually no ability to discriminate once the needle tip has passed the nerve. Therefore, spatial discrimination near the nerve is more precise in needles with a pinpoint electrode tip (Figure 14–9B) compared to needles with an uncoated bevel (Figure 14–9A).

Connectors

Connectors and cables should be fully insulated and include a safety connector to prevent current leakage as well as the risk of electric charge if the needle is not connected to the stimulator. Extension tubing with a Luer lock connector should be present for immobile needle technique.

Visualization of the Needle Under Ultrasound Imaging

Because ultrasound imaging is used more frequently (in particular with the use of the "dual-guidance" technique), the importance of good visualization of the nerve block needle is becoming an additional important feature. The visibility (distinct reflection signal) of the needle tip certainly is the most important aspect because this is the part of the needle that is placed in the target area next to the nerve. However, in

TABLE 14-3. Comparison of most relevant features of modern nerve stimulators.

Product/company Feature	Stimuplex HNS 12 (w/ SENSe) B. Braun	Stimuplex HNS 11 (replaced by HNS 12) B. Braun	Stimuplex DIG RC B. Braun	Multistim Sensor Pajunk	Multistim Vario Pajunk	Multistim Plex Pajunk	Plexygon Vygon	Polystim II Polymedic	Tracer III Life-Tech	NeuroTrace III / NMS 300 HDC/Xavant technology
Amplitude setting	Digital dial, 1 or 2 turns for full scale	Analog dial	Analog dial	Digital dial	Up/down keys	Up/down keys	Digital dial up/down keys	Analog dial	Analog dial	Up/down keys
Display size [WxH, mm] / type	62 × 41 graphic LCD	50 × 20 standard LCD	21 × 8 red LED	47 × 36 custom LCD	47 × 18 custom LCD	47 × 18 custom LCD	47.5 × 33.5 custom LCD	50 × 20 standard LCD	50 × 20 custom LCD	41 × 22 graphic LCD
Current range [mA]	0-1 0-5	0-1 0-5	0.2-5	0-6 0-60 (for nerve mapping only, max. 1 kOhm)	0-6 0-60 (for TENS only, max. 1.3 kOhm)	0-6	0-6 (at 0.05 ms) 0-5 (at 0.15 ms) 0-4 (at 0.3 ms)	0-1 0-5	0.05-5 0.05-1.5 (w/ foot pedal)	0.1-5 0-20 (nerve mapping) 0-80 (TENS)
Max. output voltage [V]	95	61	32	65	80	80	48	72	60	400 (for TENS)
Max. output load (impedance) nominal/max.	12/17 kOhm (5 mA) 90 kOhm (1 mA)	12/12 kOhm (mA) 60 kOhm (mA)	6/6 kOhm (5 mA) 30 kOhm (mA)	12/13 kOhm (5 mA) 65 kOhm (1 mA)	12/15 kOhm (5 mA) 80 kOhm (1 mA)	12/15 kOhm (5 mA) 80 kOhm (1 mA)	9/9 kOhm (5 mA) 48 kOhm (1 mA)	10/13 (5 mA) kOhm 72 kOhm (1 mA)	12/11 kOhm (5 mA)	80 kOhm (5 mA) (for TENS)
Impulse duration [ms]	0.05, 0.1, 0.3, 0.5, 1.0	0.1, 0.3, 1.0	0.1	0.05, 0.1, 0.2, 0.3, 0.5, 1.0	0.1, 0.3, 0.5, 1.0	0.1	0.05, 0.15, 0.3	0.1, 0.3, 1.0	0.05, 0.1, 0.3, 0.5, 1.0	0.04-0.200
Stimulus frequency [Hz]	1, 2, 3 (SENSe)	1, 2	1, 2	1, 2	1, 2, TOF, 50 Hz, 100 Hz	1, 2	1, 2, 4	1, 2, 3, 4, 5	1, 2	1, 2 TOF, DB, 50 Hz, 100 Hz
Display of patient current	YES	YES activated by key	NO	YES	YES activated by key	NO	YES	YES	NO	NO
Display of set current	YES if patient current is lower	YES activated by key	YES flashes if patient current is lower	YES if PAUSE key is pressed, or dial is turned	YES activated by key	YES (permanent)	YES if dial is turnd	YES activated by key	YES	YES; no indication if patient current deviates from displayed value
Display of impulse duration (ms)	YES	YES key LED	-	YES	YES	-	YES	YES key LED	YES	NO
Display of impedance	0-90 kOhm	NO	NO	NO	NO	NO	NO	NO	NO	NO

TABLE 14–3. Comparison of most relevant features of modern nerve stimulators. (*Continued*)

Product/company Feature	Stimuplex HNS 12 (w/ SENSe) B. Braun	Stimuplex HNS 11 (replaced by HNS 12) B. Braun	Stimuplex DIG RC B. Braun	Multistim Sensor Pajunk	Multistim Vario Pajunk	Multistim Plex Pajunk	Plexygon Vygon	Polystim II Polymedic	Tracer III Life-Tech	NeuroTrace III / NMS 300 HDC/Xavant technology
Display of charge (nC)	Optional, in addition to display of mA	NO	NO	NO	NO	NO	Alternative to mA	NO	NO	NO
Alarm signals	Special alarm and warning sounds; LED (red/yellow/green), display of respective text messages	Change of beep tone and LED stops flashing when no current, display icon	No tone and no yellow LED flash if no current; blinking display if current is lower than set	Change of beep tone if no current, display icon	Change of beep tone, display symbol, LED stops flashing if no current	Change of beep tone, display symbol, LED stops flashing if no current	Constant tone if open circuit, flashing display if current is lower than set	Click tone changes, LEDs stops flashing when current is lower than set	Flashing display and chirp sounds on open circuit	Chirp tone and display symbol for open circuit; no indication if current is lower than set
Threshold amplitude warning	Acoustic, LED yellow and display of text message	NO	NO	NO	NO	NO	NO	NO	NO	NO
Menu for setup and features	YES, full text menu, 26 languages	NO	NO	NO (setup w/o menu)	NO	NO	NO	NO	NO	YES, limited text
Percutaneous nerve mapping	YES stimuplex pen	YES stimuplex pen	NO	YES Pen + bipolar probe	NO	NO	NO	NO	NO	YES NeuroMap pen
Remote control	Handheld RC	NO	Hand held RC	NO	NO	NO	NO	NO	Foot pedal RC	NO
Power consumption at 5 mA output [mA]	3.6	3.6 (key LEDs off)	6.0	4.8	4.2	5.0	15.5	11.8 (key LEDs off)	No data	5.7
Size H × W × D [mm]	157 × 81 × 35	145 × 80 × 39	126 × 77 × 38	120 × 65 × 22	121 × 65 × 22	122 × 65 × 22	200 × 94 × 40	245 × 80 × 39	153 × 83 × 57	125 × 80 × 37
Weight w/ battery [g]	277	266	210	167	168	169	251	247	275	235

Note: Nerve stimulator models, features, and availability, July 2008.

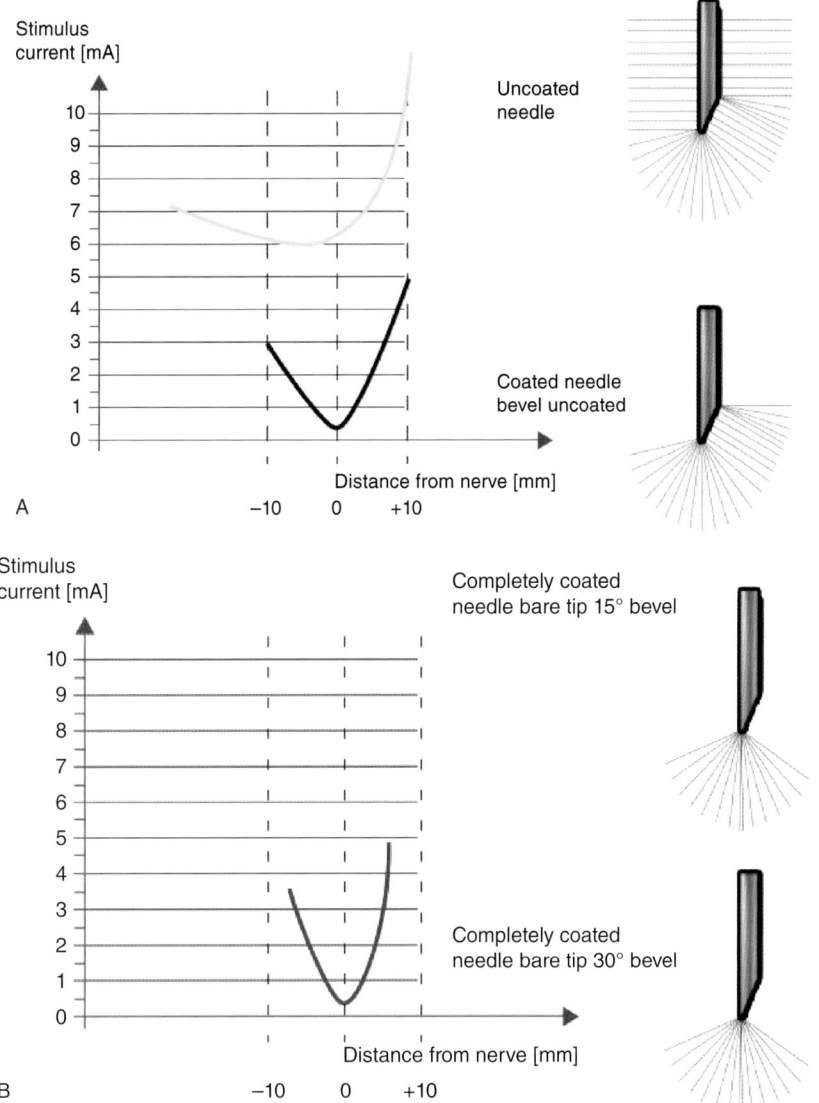

FIGURE 14–9. A: Threshold amplitude achieved with an uncoated needle and a coated needle with an uncoated bevel. **B:** Threshold amplitude achieved with a fully coated needle and a pinpoint electrode.

particular when using the in-plane approach, the visibility of the needle shaft is of interest as well because it helps to align the needle properly with the ultrasound beam to visualize the entire length to the target nerve.

Stimulating Catheters

In principle, stimulating catheters function like insulated needles.[28] The catheter body is made from insulating plastic material and usually contains a metallic wire inside, which conducts the current to its exposed tip electrode. Usually, such stimulating catheters are placed using a continuous nerve block needle, which is placed by first using nerve stimulation as described. It acts as an introducer needle for the catheter. Once this needle is placed close to the nerve or plexus to be blocked, the stimulating catheter is introduced through it, and the nerve stimulator is connected to the catheter. Stimulation through the catheter should reconfirm that the catheter tip is positioned in

close proximity to the target nerve(s). However, it must be noted that the threshold currents with stimulating catheters may be considerably higher. Injection of local anesthetic or saline (which is frequently used to widen the space for threading the catheter more easily) should be avoided because this may increase the threshold current considerably and can even prevent a motor response. D5W can be used to avoid losing a motor response.[23] Since the introduction of ultrasound monitoring of the distribution of the local anesthetic after needle or catheter placement, stimulating catheters have become nearly obsolete. This is because the ultimate test of the placement of the catheter tip in the therapeutic position is the distribution of the injectate in the tissue plane that contains the nerve or the plexus. Because the stimulating catheter can be placed in the proper position without obtaining the motor response, using the stimulation through the catheter will often lead to unnecessary needle and catheter manipulation. Nerve stimulation monitoring of the single-injection or continuous needle

208   FOUNDATIONS OF LOCAL AND REGIONAL ANESTHESIA

PART 2

placement is useful to avoid needle-nerve contact or intraneural placement and help decrease the risk of nerve inflammation or intraneural injection and consequent injury. In contrast, catheters are pliable and highly unlikely to cause nerve trauma or be inserted into a fascicle.[21]

Clinical Pearls

- Use low-intensity current nerve stimulation (0.5 mA) with ultrasound-guided nerve blocks and do not change the current intensity during the procedure.
- For nerve stimulator–guided nerve blocks, adjust the stimulus current amplitude: 1 mA (superficial blocks), 2 mA (deeper blocks) (eg, psoas compartment and deep sciatic blocks), 0.1 ms.
- Do not inject if the threshold current is 0.2–0.3 mA or less (0.1 ms) or opening injection pressure.

REFERENCES

1. Luigi Galvani (1737–1798). n.d. http://en.wikipedia.org/wiki/Galvani.
2. von Perthes G: Überleitungsanästhesie unter Zuhilfenahme elektrischer Reizung. Munch Med Wochenschr 1912;47:2545–2548.
3. Pearson RB: Nerve block in rehabilitation: A technique of needle localization. Arch Phys Med Rehabil 1955;26:631–633.
4. Greenblatt GM, Denson JS: Needle nerve stimulator locator. Nerve blocks with a new instrument for locating nerves. Anesth Analg 1962;41:599–602.
5. Montgomery SJ, Raj PP, Nettles D, Jenkins MT: The use of the nerve stimulator with standard unsheathed needles in nerve blockade. Anesth Analg 1973;52:827–831.
6. Ford DJ, Pither C, Raj PP: Comparison of insulated and uninsulated needles for locating peripheral nerves with a peripheral nerve stimulator. Anesth Analg 1984;63:925–928.
7. Ford DJ, Pither CE, Raj PP: Electrical characteristics of peripheral nerve stimulators: Implications for nerve localization. Reg Anesth 1984;9:73–77.
8. Pither CE, Ford DJ, Raij PP: The use of peripheral nerve stimulators for regional anesthesia, a review of experimental characteristics, technique, and clinical applications. Reg Anesth 1985;10:49–58.
9. Hadzic A, Vloka JD, Claudio RE, Thys DM, Santos AC: Electrical nerve localization: Effects of cutaneous electrode and duration of the stimulus on motor response. Anesthesiology 2004;100:1526–1530.
10. Kaiser H, Neuburger M: How close is close enough—How close is safe enough? Reg Anesth Pain Med 2002;27:227–228.
11. Neuburger M, Rotzinger M, Kaiser H: Electric nerve stimulation in relation to impulse strength. A quantitative study of the distance of the electrode point to the nerve. Acta Anaesthesiol Scand 2007;51:942–948.
12. Bosenberg AT, Raw R, Boezaart AP: Surface mapping of peripheral nerves in children with a nerve stimulator. Paediatr Anaesth 2002;12:398–403.
13. Urmey WF, Grossi P: Percutaneous electrode guidance. A non-invasive technique for prelocation of peripheral nerves to facilitate peripheral plexus or nerve block. Reg Anesth Pain Med 2002;27:261–267.
14. Urmey WF, Grossi P: Percutaneous electrode guidance and subcutaneous stimulating electrode guidance. Modifications of the original technique. Reg Anesth Pain Med 2003;28:253–255.
15. Capdevilla X, Lopez S, Bernard N, et al: Percutaneous electrode guidance using the insulated needle for prelocation of peripheral nerves during axillary plexus blocks. Reg Anesth Pain Med 2004;29:206–211.
16. Tsui BC, Gupta S, Finucane B: Confirmation of epidural catheter placement using nerve stimulation. Can J Anesth 1998;45:640–644.
17. Tsui BC, Guenther C, Emery D, Finucane B: Determining epidural catheter location using nerve stimulation with radiological confirmation. Reg Anesth Pain Med 2000;25:306–309.
18. Tsui BC, Seal R, Koller J, Entwistle L, Haugen R, Kearney R: Thoracic epidural analgesia via the caudal approach in pediatric patients undergoing fundoplication using nerve stimulation guidance. Anesth Analg 2001;93:1152–1155.
19. Boezaart AP, de Beer JF, du Toit C. van Rooyen K: A new technique of continuous interscalene nerve block. Can J Anesth 1999;46:275–281.
20. Kaiser H. Periphere elektrische Nervenstimulation. In Niesel HC, Van Aken H (eds): Regionalanästhesie, Lokalanästhesie, Regionale Schmerztherapie, 2nd edi. Thieme, 2002.
21. Gadsden J, Latmore M, Levine DM, Robinson A: High opening injection pressure is associated with needle-nerve and needle-fascia contact during femoral nerve block. Reg Anesth Pain Med 2016;41:50–55.
22. Gadsden JC, Choi JJ, Lin E, Robinson A: Opening injection pressure consistently detects needle-nerve contact during ultrasound-guided interscalene brachial plexus block. Anesthesiology 2014;120:1246–1253.
23. Tsui BC, Kropelin B: The electrophysiological effect of dextrose 5% in water on single-shot peripheral nerve stimulation. Anesth Analg 2005;100:1837–1839.
24. Tsui BC: Electrical impedance to distinguish intraneural from extraneural needle placement in porcine nerves during direct exposure and ultrasound guidance. Anesthesiology 2008;109:479–483.
25. Tsui BC, Chin JH: Electrical impedance to warn of intravascular needle placement. Abstract ASRA 2007. Reg Anesth Pain Med 2007;32:A-51.
26. Urmey WF, Grossi P: Use of Sequential Electrical Nerve Stimuli (SENS) for location of the sciatic nerve and lumbar plexus. Reg Anesth Pain Med 2006;31:463–469.
27. Jochum D, Iohom G, Diarra DP, Loughnane F, Dupré LJ, Bouaziz H: An objective assessment of nerve stimulators used for peripheral nerve blockade. Anaesthesia 2006;61:557–564.
28. Denny NM, Barber N, Sildown DJ: Evaluation of an insulated Tuohy needle system for the placement of interscalene brachial plexus catheters. Anaesthesia 2003;58:554–557.

APPENDIX: GLOSSARY OF PHYSICAL PARAMETERS

Voltage, Potential, Current, Resistance/Impedance

Voltage U is the difference in electrical potential between two points carrying different amounts of positive and negative charge. It is measured in volts (V) or millivolts (mV). Voltage can be compared to the filled level of a water tank, which determines the pressure at the bottom outlet (Figure 14–10A). In modern nerve stimulators using constant-current sources, voltage is adapted automatically and cannot (or does not need to) be influenced by the user.

Current I is the measure of the flow of a positive or negative charge. It is expressed in amperes (A) or milliamperes (mA). Current can be compared to the flow of water.

A total charge **Q** applied to a nerve equals the product of the intensity I of the applied current and the duration t of the square pulse of the current: $Q = I \times t$.

The minimum current intensity I required to produce an action potential can be expressed by the relationship

$$I_{Threshold} = \frac{I_{Rheobase}}{1 - e^{-t/c}}$$

where t is the pulse duration, c is the time constant of nerve membrane related to chronaxy.

The **electrical resistance R** limits the flow of current at a given voltage (see Ohm's law) and is measured in ohms (Ω) or kilo-Ohms (kΩ).

If there is capacitance in addition to Ohm's resistance involved (which is the case for any tissue), the resistance becomes a so-called complex resistance or **impedance.** The

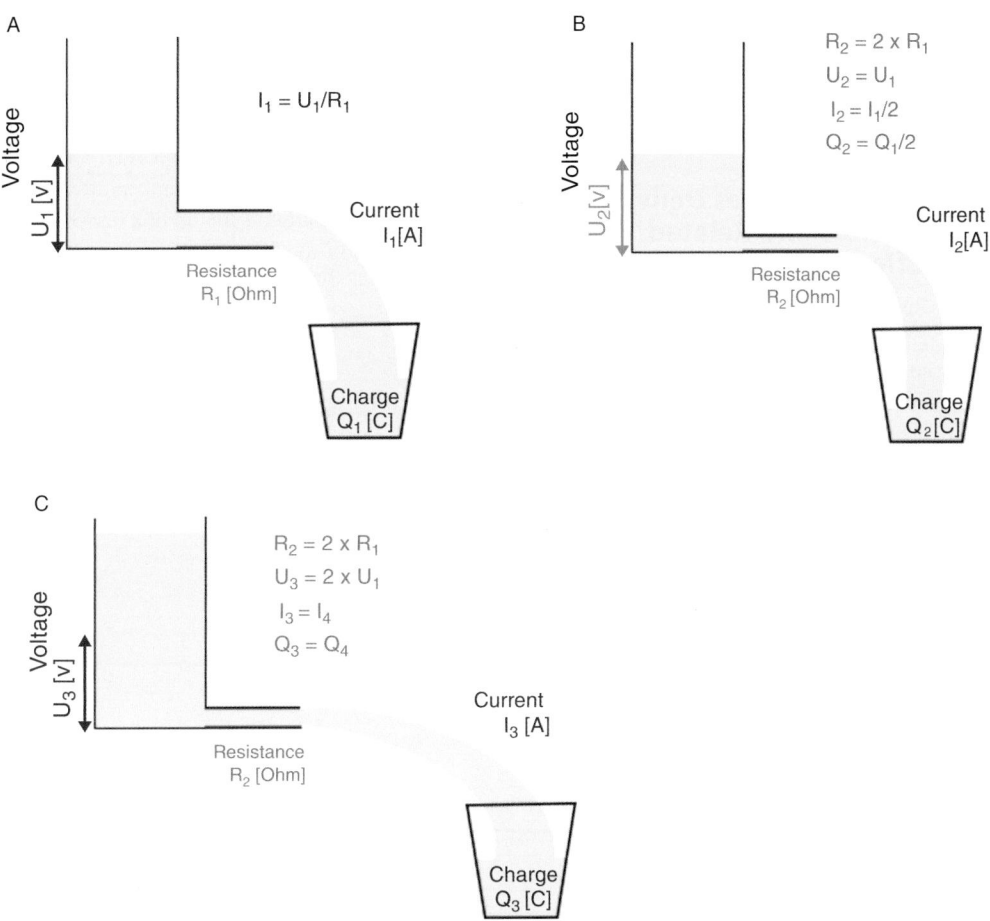

FIGURE 14–10. Ohm's law and principle of a constant-current source. Functional principle of a constant-current source. **A:** Low-resistance R_1 requires voltage U_1 to achieve desired current I_1. **B:** High-resistance $R_2 = 2 \times R_1$ causes current I to decrease to $I_2 = I_1/2$ if voltage U remains constant ($U_2 = U_1$). **C:** Constant-current source automatically increases output voltage to $U_3 = 2 \times U_1$ to compensate for the higher-resistance R_2; therefore, current I increases to the desired level of $I_3 = I_1$.

main difference between the two is that the value of the impedance is dependent on the frequency of the applied voltage/current, which is not the case for an Ohm's resistor. In clinical practice, this means that the impedance of the tissue is higher for low frequencies (ie, a long pulse duration) and lower for higher frequencies (ie, a short pulse duration). Consequently, a constant-current source (which delivers longer-duration impulses, eg, 1 ms vs. 0.1 ms) needs to have a stronger output stage (higher output voltage) to compensate for the higher tissue impedance involved and to deliver the desired current. However, the basic principles of Ohm's law remain the same.

Ohm's Law

Ohm's law describes the relationship between voltage, resistance, and current according to the equation

$$U[V] = R[\Omega] \times I[A]$$

or conversely,

$$I[A] = U[V]/R[\Omega]$$

This means that, at a given voltage, current changes with resistance. If a constant current must be achieved (as needed for

nerve stimulation), the voltage has to adapt to the varying resistance of the entire electrical circuit. For nerve localization in particular, the voltage must adapt to the resistance of the needle tip, the electrode-to-skin interface, and the tissue layers. A constant-current source does this automatically. Ohm's law and the functional principle of a constant-current source are illustrated in Figures 14–10A, 14–10B, and 14–10C.

Coulomb's Law, Electric Field, Current Density, and Charge

According to **Coulomb's law,** the strength of the **electric field,** and therefore the corresponding **current density J**, in relation to the distance from the current source is given by

$$J(r) = k \times I_0/r^2$$

where k is a constant, and I_0 is the initial current. This means that the current (or charge) that reaches the nerve decreases by a factor of 4 if the distance to the nerve is doubled, or conversely, it increases by a factor of 4 if the distance is divided in half (ideal conditions assumed).

The **charge Q** is the product of current multiplied by time and is given in ampere-seconds (As) or coulombs (C). As an example, rechargeable batteries often have an indication of Ah or mAh as the measure of their capacitance of charge (kilo = 1000 or 10^3; milli = 0.001 or 10^{-3}; micro = 0.000001 or 10^{-6}; nano = 0.000000001 or 10^{-9}).

■ Energy of Electrical Impulses Delivered by Nerve Stimulators and Related Temperature Effects

According to a worst-case scenario calculation, the temperature increase caused by a stimulus of 5-mA current and 1-ms duration at a maximum output voltage of 95 V would be less than 0.5 C if all the energy were concentrated within a small volume of only 1 mm³ and no temperature dissipation into the surrounding tissue occurred. This calculation can be applied for the tip of a nerve stimulation needle.

The maximum energy E of the electrical impulse delivered by a common nerve stimulator would be

$$E \leq U \times I \times t = 95 \text{ V} \times 5 \text{ mA} \times 1 \text{ ms} = 0.475 \text{ mWs} = 0.475 \text{ mJ}$$

The caloric equivalent for water is $c_w = 4.19 \text{ J g}^{-1} \text{ K}^{-1}$.

One stimulus creates a temperature difference ΔT within 1 mm³ of tissue around the tip of a nerve stimulation needle. For the calculation that follows, it is assumed that tissue contains a minimum of 50% water, and the mass M of 1 mm³ of tissue is 1 mg.

$$\Delta T \leq 2 \times E/(M \times c_w) = 2 \times 0.475 \times 10^{-3} \text{ J}/(10^{-3} \text{ g} \times 4.19 \text{ g/K})$$
$$= 0.45 \text{ K}$$

That is, the maximum temperature increase in this worst-case scenario calculation is less than 0.5 C. In practice, this means that the temperature effect of normal nerve stimulation on the tissue can be neglected.

| SECTION 4 | Patient Management Considerations |

CHAPTER 15

Developing Regional Anesthesia Pathways

Andrew Neice and Michael J. Barrington

INTRODUCTION

Regional anesthesia is best practiced in the context of a standardized anesthetic and surgical protocols; these plans are generally referred to as anesthetic pathways. For a patient having surgery that uses an anesthetic pathway, many of the decisions about the patient's care are made not at the bedside in the immediate preoperative period, but instead long before the surgery by carefully considering the risks and benefits of various anesthesia and perioperative treatment options.

When well designed, anesthetic pathways can improve patient care by ensuring that patients receive consistent, coordinated, evidenced-based care. They can also reduce costs by eliminating unnecessary interventions and reducing complications. Of course, pathways should not be indiscriminately adhered to as some patients will require modification to atone for specific medical conditions or patient preferences. Regardless, anesthetic pathways allow clinicians to focus on the unique characteristics of a patient instead of the common characteristics of an entire cohort, which were already examined during pathway development.

At their core, anesthetic pathways (or clinical pathways in any field) are a series of medical decisions. As leaders of the perioperative surgical home, anesthesiologists are best suited to lead their design. There are often many subtle issues that arise in the development of a pathway that may not be familiar to anyone other than a clinician who is frequently and personally involved in patient care. In addition, anesthesiologists' working relations with surgeons, administrators, and the entire operating room team are paramount in development and success of patient pathways. Interspecialty coordination is vital to the successful development of anesthetic pathways. Anesthetic decisions will frequently affect patients' ability to rehabilitate in the immediate postoperative period, so anesthetic and surgical pathways must be designed by a team effort.

Because there is evidence that use of regional anesthesia may affect the mortality and morbidity[1-5] of common surgeries, and because pain control in the postoperative period is often challenging, regional anesthesia (either neuraxial or peripheral block) is often a key feature of anesthetic pathways. Therefore, development of pathways is of particular interest to practitioners whose clinical practice includes regional anesthesia.

Designing and implementing clinical pathways require skills often not taught during residency training. Physicians tailor their treatments with the unique characteristics of each patient in mind. This is related to physician training designed to elicit and synthesize data for a specific patient. Clinical pathways, in contrast, must be designed to optimize the average experience of a cohort of patients, often making trade-offs and compromises in the process. Knowledge of epidemiology and statistics are vital to effective clinical pathway design. Numerically estimating probable outcomes, and choosing those that rate most favorably, is central to the development of the pathway.

Benefits of an anesthesia pathway will of course depend on the peculiarities of the pathway itself, the institution, the surgical and anesthetic techniques, and the other health-care providers using the pathway (such as nursing care, physical therapy, etc.). A pathway designed for one institution may not be appropriate for another institution, which is why in this chapter we have chosen to emphasize the process of pathway development instead of presenting specific pathways. Furthermore, the goals of an anesthetic pathway may vary—some pathways may be designed to reduce morbidity or mortality, while others may be focused on reducing cost while maintaining a high level of patient care. Common goals of an anesthetic pathway include reducing in-hospital morbidity and mortality, reducing length of hospital stay, reducing costs, improving patient satisfaction, reducing readmissions, and improving long-term functional outcomes.

Despite this heterogeneity, there is evidence that, generally speaking, clinical pathways improve patient care. A recent meta-analysis of clinical pathways found that they were associated with lower rates of patient complications (eg, wound infections, bleeding, and pneumonia), as well as improved documentation.[6] Most of the studies included in the meta-analysis also showed a reduction in the length-of-stay and hospital costs without increased risk of readmission rates and mortality. However, it is possible that some clinical pathways actually could improve these outcomes as well. The considerable heterogeneity of successful clinical pathways has not allowed investigators to identify features common to successful (or unsuccessful) clinical pathways.[6] Nevertheless, basic principles of risk management may be deployed to aid in the design of clinical pathways, and developing a reusable, common framework for approaching clinical pathways seems likely to increase the probability of success.

In this chapter, we present a framework for developing clinical pathways and review some of the prerequisite knowledge required for this process. We also present case scenarios that illustrate the subtleties in applying existing medical literature to clinical pathways. Finally, we present components of a surgical pathway for total knee arthroplasty.

FRAMEWORK FOR ANESTHETIC PATHWAYS

An example of a single component of a clinical pathway is shown in Table 15–1. This is a component of a larger pathway for total joint arthroplasty, which is further discussed in the final section of this chapter. This component describes the standard oral premedications for the surgery and contains

TABLE 15–1. Example of a pathway item: oral premedication for total knee arthroplasty.

Recommended Oral Premedications Prior to Surgery (Example Only)	
Acetaminophen 1 g by mouth	Avoid in those with cirrhosis, elevated liver function tests
Celecoxib 400 mg by mouth	Avoid in those with sulfa allergy, renal dysfunction
Gabapentin 600 mg by mouth	Avoid in patients with renal dysfunction, outpatients, patients with advanced age or dementia

Note: This is an example of a pathway element only, not a formal recommendation.

TABLE 15–2. Examples of pathway elements.

Enumeration of the goals of the pathway
Criteria for patient selection, preparation for surgery, and education prior to surgery
Preoperative optimization (eg, blood pressure goals, hematocrit goals, associated pharmacologic interventions)
Recommended surgical anesthesia
Recommended systemic multimodal anesthetic technique
Recommended regional anesthesia/analgesia for the treatment of postoperative pain
Recommended prophylactic therapy for postoperative nausea and vomiting
Recommended intraoperative fluid or hematocrit goals or transfusion criteria
Recommended intraoperative management of hemodynamics (eg, preferred blood pressures, preferred pressors, etc.)
Recommended adjuvant drugs (eg, preferred antibiotics, anticoagulation, antifibrinolytics)
Recommended adjuvant monitoring (eg, evoked potentials, bispectral index, cerebral oxygenation)

specific information about dose, common contraindications, and common additions to the pathway that may be needed for some patients. Although developing a clinical pathway often involves lengthy analyses with uncertainties, final pathway elements should be brief and specific. Besides recommended premedications, pathways may have many different elements; for example, see those shown in Table 15–2.

It should be noted that although the pathways developed by anesthesiologists are primarily concerned with the anesthetic management of the patient, they are designed to dovetail with the corresponding surgical pathway. For example, the choice of regional anesthesia may allow the patient to complete physical therapy on postoperative day 1.

A process for developing clinical pathways is shown in Figure 15–1. This process consists of the following:

1. Identifying the goals of the pathway and different treatment options to help achieve those goals. This should include all stages of anesthesia and surgery, including postoperative recovery.
2. Identifying ways in which each treatment interacts with the others (eg, the type of regional anesthesia may affect the patient's ability to perform physical therapy postoperatively, premedications may delay discharge due to sedation).
3. Identifying possible risks, costs, and benefits of each treatment, including mortality, morbidity, patient satisfaction, institutional capabilities, financial cost, and other factors.
4. Making numerical estimates of the risks, costs, and benefits identified in step 3. Some of this information (eg, information on cost) can be gathered and tabulated. However, most of the information cannot be known with

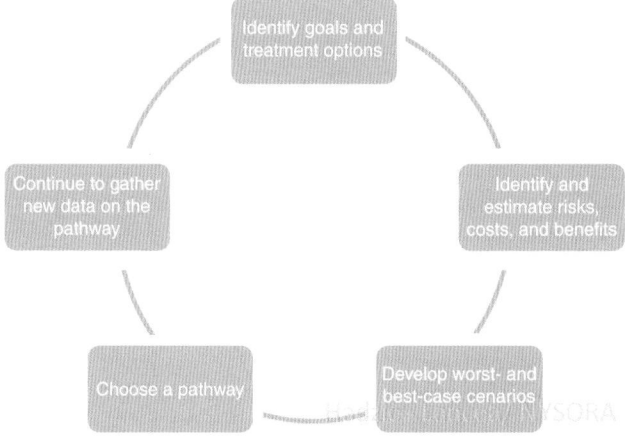

FIGURE 15–1. Summary of steps involved in developing a clinical pathway.

any certainty. In many cases, the medical literature can provide estimates of the probabilities involved, as long as the physician understands the limitations of a particular study.

5. Use the estimates developed in step 4 to develop probable outcomes and worst-case and best-case scenarios for each pathway.

6. Choose the pathway most likely to benefit the patient based on step 5.

7. Continually refine the estimates of the risks, costs, and benefits as new information becomes available and refine the clinical pathways.

If we could quantify the risks and benefits of each intervention as easily as we could quantify the financial costs of procedures and equipment, steps 4, 5, and 6 would be trivial. However, this is rarely the case. In many cases, there may be not adequate published data to guide the process. Sometimes, there may be some incongruity between available studies and the desired information—the only studies available may have been done on similar, but different, patient populations; have analyzed similar, but different, surgical procedures; or may describe interventions that you cannot exactly replicate at your institution. Nevertheless, the closest match to one's institutional conditions can be used to estimate probabilities used in step 5.

Another risk to consider includes those complications that may not manifest until well after the treatment period. For instance, recently introduced drugs, procedures, or therapies by definition will have unknown long-term risks. Recognizing the limitations of the existing evidence for each intervention in the literature is crucial in protocol development. Although inferential statistics enhances a physician's judgment beyond what can be achieved simply by relying on their historical personal observations, unfortunately any given study may have unforeseen biases that may make the study less than an ideal guidance for the protocol being developed. As such, when developing "worst-case" and "best-case" scenarios, one needs to take into account the possibility that a study has made a type I or (more commonly) a type II error.

REVIEW OF STATISTICAL CONCEPTS RELEVANT TO THE DEVELOPMENT OF ANESTHETIC PATHWAYS

A good analogy for the role of statistics in enhancing clinician judgment is comparing it to the role that a magnifying lens plays in enhancing vision. Drugs or interventions that have large, consistent effects (eg, the effect of insulin on glucose or epinephrine on heart rate) can be easily appreciated by the clinician without any sort of corroborating study, just as a magnifying lens is generally not necessary to see frank pus in a wound. Likewise, a study that is underpowered may be unable to detect subtle effects, just as a simple hand lens is not powerful enough to image individual bacteria. While few clinicians would attempt to diagnose a bacterial infection with only a magnifying glass, clinicians frequently make the error of assuming that a reported negative result is synonymous with no effect, without considering the limit of detection of the study. Rare but catastrophic complications are of particular concern as extremely large numbers of patients may be required to properly power a study.

A statistical test may report either that observed data are consistent with random chance (the null hypothesis, a "negative" result) or reject the null hypothesis and assert that there is an association between a treatment and an outcome (a "positive" result). In reality, there may or may not be an association between a treatment and an outcome. There are therefore four possibilities for any statistical test, two of which involve drawing the correct conclusion, and two of which are errors. These are traditionally shown using a 2 × 2 table as shown in Table 15–3.

The two types of possible errors are a type I error (alpha), which involves incorrectly concluding that an association exists when one does not, and a type II error (beta), which involves incorrectly concluding that no association exists when in fact one does. Obviously, the probabilities of making the two types of errors are related. Imagine a statistical test that always asserts there is an association between the treatment and outcome, regardless of the data. This technique will frequently make type I errors but will never make a type II error (because it never asserts a negative result).

By convention, statistical tests compute the probability that a set of data is due to random chance (the p value) and if this is below some fixed threshold (alpha), the notion that the data are due to random chance is rejected. Generally, a confidence interval is reported as well. When alpha is fixed, most commonly at 0.05, beta will be a function of the other features of the statistical test. One of the simpler formulas relating alpha, beta, change in mean, standard deviation of the data, and sample size

TABLE 15–3. Possible outcomes of a statistical test.

	Hypothesis Is True	Hypothesis Is False
Hypothesis is accepted	Correct decision	Type I error (alpha)
Hypothesis is rejected	Type II error (beta)	Correct decision

is shown in Equation 15–1. Equation 15–1 describes power relationships for a test of a large sample of a continuous outcome variable in a single population with known mean and standard deviation:

$$ES = \frac{Z_{1-\alpha/2} + Z_{1-\beta}}{\sqrt{n}} = \frac{|\mu - \mu_0|}{\sigma} \qquad (15-1)$$

where n is sample size, σ is sample standard deviation, μ is the sample mean, μ_0 is the population mean, ES is effect size, and Z is the Z-score corresponding to the value in subscript. Different statistical tests (eg, t tests for continuous variables, t tests for proportions, χ^2 tests, analysis-of-variance [ANOVA] tests, etc.) will have somewhat different formulas for beta, but in general beta (and hence the probability of a type II error) will decrease with larger sample sizes, less-restrictive choices of alpha, smaller standard deviations in the data, and larger effect sizes.

Statistical power is simply $1-\beta$ and is more frequently referenced than β. While alpha is most commonly fixed at 0.05, a statistical power of 0.8 is generally considered adequate for detection of associations, although in some cases[4] this is increased to 0.9. Unfortunately, while the choice of alpha is almost always explicitly stated in a publication, it is often left to the clinician to infer the power of the study, particularly for secondary outcomes. Fortunately, formulas such as Equation 15–1 can be readily found in common textbooks or in statistical software packages. In addition, many academic statistics departments have made online tools available to calculate statistical power (eg, References 7 and 8). Formulas such as Equation 15–1 can be used to calculate the smallest effect size that a particular study is likely to detect. It then falls to the clinician to decide whether this effect size is small enough that smaller effect sizes are clinically irrelevant. If smaller effect sizes are still clinically relevant, then the clinician developing a pathway needs to take into account the possibility that there is a small but real effect size, a type II error was made, and adjust the best- or worst- case scenarios accordingly.

EXAMPLES OF PATHWAY DEVELOPMENT

We now provide a few illustrative examples of the analysis discussed previously. First, we present a case scenario that illustrates the type of analysis described. Then, we review some examples of drugs that were introduced to routine surgical protocols that caused patient harm; this illustrates pitfalls in pathway development. Last, we present components of a pathway for total knee replacement.

Illustrative Case: Adjuvants to Spinal Anesthesia

Suppose a novel drug (drug X) has been developed that increases the duration of spinal anesthesia when added to bupivacaine. Your group performs total hip and knee arthroplasty under spinal anesthesia but occasionally has to convert to general anesthesia due to unexpectedly long surgical times. The total joint pathway currently uses bupivacaine-only spinals but

is considering adding drug X to the total joint pathway to prolong the length of spinal anesthetic and reduce unexpected conversions to general anesthesia.

An initial study compared spinal anesthesia with bupivacaine versus drug X plus bupivacaine, with 500 patients in the treatment group and 500 in the control group. The study found that spinal anesthesia with bupivacaine provided adequate surgical anesthesia only for 180 minutes, while bupivacaine with drug X provided adequate surgical anesthesia for 200 minutes (95% CI 195–205 minutes, $p < .05$). Secondary outcomes included incidence of vomiting on postoperative days 1–3 and urinary retention requiring Foley catheterization. In the control arm, 3% and in the treatment arm 4% of patients vomited postoperatively, but this result was not statistically significant. In the control arm, 2% and in the treatment arm 3% of patients had urinary retention; however, this was also not statistically significant. The drug costs $50 per dose.

Analysis of Costs and Benefits

Even for a relatively simple (and contrived) question such as this, a complete analysis can become complex. We therefore present an abbreviated version of the procedure:

1. **Identify goals and treatment options**. We limit ourselves to the goal of lengthening spinal anesthesia to reduce conversions to general anesthesia. Alternatives to the inclusion of drug X should be explored. Drug X must be evaluated not in a vacuum but instead in competition with other techniques. For example, other drugs may be available that lengthen spinal anesthesia for a comparable time, or simply increasing spinal dosage may be feasible to lengthen surgical anesthesia. Alternatively, the subpopulation likely to have longer operative time may be identified, and these patients could automatically receive general anesthesia or drug X could be reserved for them only. The risks and benefits of each of these options must be individually considered and compared with the routine use of drug X.

2. **Identify ways each treatment interacts with the rest of the pathway**. Although no restrictions were mentioned, we would need to confirm that the use of drug X does not require special postoperative monitoring (such as continuous pulse oximetry), an alteration in nursing care (such as changing fall precautions), or change in physical therapy (such as delaying mobilization) or require alterations to other parts of the anesthetic and surgical pathway. If any restrictions or interactions are identified, they must be accounted for in step 3.

3. **Identify risks, costs, and benefits**. For this illustration, we restrict the analyses to the risks, benefits, and costs alluded to in the study. The primary benefit would be increased duration of surgical anesthesia and a reduced need to convert to general anesthesia, which of course carries a number of attendant risks and costs. The risks include increased risk of urinary retention and postoperative

vomiting. Although the initial study did not link either of these outcomes to drug X, we shall see in step 4 that the worst-case scenario must include the risk that this study made a type II error. The costs are easiest to quantify: This will add $50 in drug costs to each surgery.

4. **Make numerical estimates of the risks, costs, and benefits identified in step 3.** The benefits of this drug will depend on the specifics of your institution. For example, suppose in reviewing your records, you find that you performed 500 total joint arthroplasties in the past year, and 5 of them required unexpected conversion to general anesthesia. The total surgical times for the five cases were 195, 250, 200, 190, and 220 minutes. Using the published confidence interval, use of drug X may have eliminated need to convert to general anesthesia in 2 of the cases (if it lengthens time to 195 minutes) to 3 of the cases (if it lengthens time to 205 minutes).

The costs of this drug, if used on all patients, would be an extra $25,000 annually. If a high-risk subpopulation could be identified for use of the drug, this could potentially be reduced.

The study found no link between urinary retention or postoperative vomiting with drug X, so in the best-case scenario, adding drug X does not introduce any new risks of complications. However, let us consider the power of this study. Presumably, the data on urinary retention and postoperative vomiting were analyzed using a *t* test for proportions.

Using online power calculators or statistics packages,[6] we can estimate the effect size that would be detected. Assuming a baseline rate of urinary retention of 2% (based on the control arm of the study), the drug would need to increase the rate to 5%–6% to achieve a power of approximately 0.8. Effect sizes lower than this will not be reliably detected. For postoperative vomiting, a power of 0.8 corresponds to the drug increasing the rate of vomiting to 7%.

If rates of postoperative vomiting and urinary retention more than doubled, most clinicians would consider that a clinically relevant increase, but it would not be reliably detected by the study discussed. Therefore, we must consider the possibility that the study made a type II error and adjust our worst-case scenario appropriately.

If the study did make a type II error, what should we use for our estimates of effect size? The most reasonable estimate can be obtained by examining the study itself; as subjects are added, the rates converge toward their true values and eventually may cross a threshold of statistical significance. In the study discussed, postoperative vomiting was 3% in the control arm and 4% in the treatment arm, and urinary retention was 2% in the control arm and 3% in the treatment arm. We can use these increases to inform our estimates.

Assuming that our institution has similar rates of vomiting on postoperative days 1–3 (3%) and similar rates of urinary retention (2%), we would estimate that they would increase to 4% and 3%. With a surgical volume of 500 patients per year, this corresponds to 5 extra cases of urinary retention and 5 extra cases of postoperative vomiting per year.

5. **Use the estimates to construct best- and worst-case scenarios.** Best case: Eliminate three conversions to general anesthesia per year. Add $25,000 to health-care costs. Worst case: Eliminate two conversions to general anesthesia per year. Add $25,000 to health-care costs. Create five extra cases of urinary retention and five extra cases of postoperative vomiting.

In this particular case, we note that the benefits of the drug may be improved if we can accurately identify a subpopulation likely to benefit. For example, if the drug is only given to the 10% of patients with the highest risk of long surgical times, both the cost and the morbidity associated with postoperative vomiting and urinary retention would decrease by a factor of 10. If the subpopulation is accurately identified, the number of general anesthesia conversions may be unaffected or minimally affected.

6. **Choose the pathway most likely to benefit the patient.** Depending on the risks involved in conversions to general anesthesia, this drug may or may not be worth adding to the anesthetic pathway. Ultimately, clinical judgment is required to make a decision. However, by using the framework discussed, the clinician is significantly better informed than if the clinician simply made a decision based on intuition alone.

7. **Continually refine the estimates of risks, costs, and benefits.** In this scenario, the institution's annual surgical volume (500) is equal to the number of patients involved in each arm of the study. Given this, if the institution tracks its own complication rates before and after the change, it should be able to quickly ascertain the true risks, benefits, and costs of the intervention and make a more informed decision than the initial analysis.

Surprisingly, it is often the case that the number of patients enrolled in studies in the published literature is much smaller than the number of surgeries performed at even small institutions. For example, a recent meta-analysis on the effects of spinal opioids only included approximately 100–150 subjects and controls for an analysis of postoperative vomiting and urinary retention for intrathecal fentanyl, despite the long and widespread use of fentanyl in spinal anesthesia.[9] Because of this, analysis of internal data is often helpful in evaluating pathway success or failure. Use of internal data also sidesteps the problem of published studies using slightly different patient populations, drugs, or techniques than used at the home institution.

EXAMPLES OF PATHWAYS THAT CAUSED PATIENT HARM

The previous section was a hypothetical illustration of the development of one part of a pathway. In this section, we take a moment to discuss historical instances in which patient harm resulted from the introduction of a new drug as part of routine perioperative care. Although these drugs were introduced before the notion of surgical and anesthetic pathways became common, the experience with these drugs provides insight into some of the hazards of applying new treatments to large patient cohorts.

Enoxaparin and Venous Thromboembolism Prophylaxis

Enoxaparin was the first low molecular weight heparin approved by the United States Food and Drug Administration for general use. Shortly after the drug's approval in May 1993, it entered widespread, routine use as prophylaxis for venous thromboembolism. Because many orthopedic surgeries, including total joint arthroplasty, pose a high risk for venous thromboembolism, and epidural or spinal anesthesia was frequently the preferred anesthetic for these cases, enoxaparin was often used in conjunction with neuraxial anesthesia.

Prior to the development of enoxaparin, unfractionated subcutaneous heparin had been widely used for venous thromboembolism prophylaxis. While the risk of epidural hematoma associated with enoxaparin administration was felt to be comparable to that of subcutaneous heparin administration initially, the pharmacological differences between low molecular weight and unfractionated heparin had been underestimated.[10]

Shortly after introduction, the US Food and Drug Administration began to receive reports of epidural hematoma associated with enoxaparin administration. In December 1997, the administration issued a public health advisory stating that it had received over 30 reports of postneuraxial epidural hematoma associated with enoxaparin and required that enoxaparin carry a black box warning indicating significant risk of patient harm.[11] By April 1998, the number of reports had increased to more than 40.[10,12] The United States Food and Drug Administration approached the American Society of Regional Anesthesia and Pain Medicine to develop new guidelines for use of enoxaparin with neuraxial anesthesia. These guidelines were published in November 1998 and recommended much more conservative use of enoxaparin.[8]

Aprotinin and Reduction of Perioperative Transfusions

Aprotinin is a small peptide molecule that acts as an antifibrinolytic by inhibiting trypsin and related proteolytic enzymes. It was used most commonly in cardiac surgery[13,14], where it was shown to significantly reduce transfusion requirements, and its use was investigated in other types of surgeries, such as orthopedic procedures.[15,16] Although one meta-analysis showed no increased risk of mortality, myocardial infarction, or renal failure,[17] large observational studies[18,19] contradicted these findings and demonstrated an increased risk of postoperative renal failure. Further observational studies[20] focused on long-term follow-up and confirmed increased morbidity and mortality associated with aprotinin, particularly with regard not only renal failure, but also stroke, death, and nonfatal myocardial infarction. Sales of aprotinin were halted in 2008; aprotinin has been largely superseded by tranexamic acid and aminocaproic acid. There remains some controversy regarding whether the observed increases in renal failure were due to the effect of aprotinin or some other confounder.[21]

Discussion

In both of these examples, significant patient harm resulted from the introduction of a new drug into an anesthetic and surgical pathway because there were insufficient data to indicate potential for patient harm. Risks became apparent only after a larger number of patients were treated and significant patient complications had occurred.

In the first case, low molecular weight heparins and neuraxial anesthesia, the difficulty in predicting patient harm was due in large part to the extremely low frequency of the adverse event. If it is assumed that the baseline risk of spinal hematoma is 1:150,000, even a relatively large increase in the risk of hematoma requires large sample sizes to detect an increased risk.[22] Sample sizes this large often cannot be realistically obtained prior to a drug's introduction, and only postapproval surveillance or the development of high-quality clinical registries will detect such uncommon rare, but potentially catastrophic, adverse events.

In the second case, aprotinin and renal failure, a number of factors can be identified. Initial investigations were not focused on increased risk of renal failure and either they did not investigate this risk or the study was underpowered. In addition, some believed that the complications associated with aprotinin were transient in nature,[17] and that there were no long-term risks associated with aprotinin. Obviously, this could not be investigated until years after aprotinin came into use.

These cases highlight the risks associated with new therapeutic agents or old therapeutic agents used in new situations. Preliminary studies may investigate the wrong risks or may be underpowered, or risks may be long term and may not become evident until well after the study period. Given this, when considering the risks and benefits to the patient, the clinician must also consider unknown or unquantified risk and include the agent only if the ratio of known, quantifiable risks and benefits is overwhelmingly positive. For drugs with a long history of use and well-defined risks, less caution is warranted.

COMPONENTS OF A FULL PATHWAY: TOTAL KNEE ARTHROPLASTY

In this section, we present components of a surgical pathway for total knee arthroplasty. This is shown in Table 15-4. However, instead of presenting final recommendations (as would be done in a completed pathway), we highlight the common issues that are faced when developing different aspects of the pathway, as well as drugs and techniques that are frequently employed. This is done to avoid implying that there is a final consensus around the "correct" pathway for total joint arthroplasty—even if such a consensus existed, it would rapidly become out of date as new studies, drugs, and techniques become available. Providers with different patient populations and different subspecialties may develop different pathways appropriate to their institution.

TABLE 15–4. Components of a total knee arthroplasty pathway, highlighting some common decisions that must be made during pathway development. *(Continued)*

Anesthetic Pathway for Total Joint Arthroplasty

Goals of the pathway

The goals of the pathway should be clearly stated and commonly include reduction in mortality, morbidity, and costs; increases in patient satisfaction; and improved pain control. Goals should involve real clinical endpoints when possible and be agnostic to means, for example, *reduce postoperative pain scores* is a more appropriate goal than *reduce postoperative opioid consumption.*

Patient selection

Modifiable risk factors, such as smoking, poorly controlled diabetes, obesity, and recreational drug use, may address when surgery should be delayed to address these factors. In addition, nonmodifiable comorbidities may create an unacceptable surgical risk; criteria for patient selection may be included in a pathway. Obviously, this must be coordinated with orthopedics.

Preoperative education and preadmission planning

Frequently, patients are seen routinely in an anesthesia preoperative clinic. This part of the pathway provides an opportunity to identify patient characteristics that conflict with the default elements in the anesthetic pathway and address them preoperatively. For example, a patient with a penicillin allergy may receive skin-prick testing to determine whether the patient may be administered cephalosporins. In addition, if the pathway includes continuous peripheral nerve catheters, this may provide an opportunity for patient education.

Preprocedure checklist

This element of the pathway frequently includes patient identification, site marking, confirmation of allergies and comorbidities, confirmation of availability of blood products, confirmation of anticoagulation status, and final checks of laboratory values.

Oral premedication/multimodal analgesia

Optimization of pain control must be balanced with undesirable side effects such as excessive sedation. The following lists common agents used, along with their benefits and drawbacks.

Agent	Benefits	Drawbacks
Acetaminophen	Reduce postoperative pain scores, opioid sparing[24]	Hepatotoxicity
Gabapentin/pregabalin	Reduce postoperative pain scores, opioid sparing,[25] may reduce incidence of chronic postsurgical pain[26] and have benefit in patients with existing chronic pain[27]	Increased sedation, particularly in elderly; increased respiratory depression with doses > 300 mg[28]
Cyclooxygenase 2 inhibitors	Reduce postoperative pain scores, opioid sparing[29]	Renal impairment; evidence base weakened by retracted publications
Oral opioids (eg, oxycodone SR)	Reduce postoperative pain scores[30]	Increased risk of respiratory depression with oxycodone dose > 10 mg[28]

(continued)

TABLE 15–4. Components of a total knee arthroplasty pathway, highlighting some common decisions that must be made during pathway development. (*Continued*)

Anesthetic Pathway for Total Joint Arthroplasty

Use of regional anesthesia for postoperative pain control

A wide spectrum of regional anesthetic techniques associated with total knee arthroplasty exists, along with significant variation in cost and efficacy. The choice of technique will affect other elements of the anesthetic and surgical pathway. Furthermore, approaches are rapidly evolving as new techniques, equipment, and agents become available. The following lists common sites used for regional anesthesia, along with benefits and drawbacks.

Technique	Benefits	Drawbacks
Epidural block	Considered the gold standard for postoperative analgesia for a range of surgeries	The side-effect profile may interfere with modern care pathway and small risk of catastrophic outcome (eg, epidural hematoma).[31,32]
Femoral nerve block	Relieves majority of postoperative pain, without drawbacks of epidural[33]; associated with improved outcomes at 6 weeks in one trial[34]	Muscle weakness may interfere with rehabilitation. Small risk (2–4 per 10,000) of long-term nerve injury,[35] but overall choice of anesthetic does change risk of nerve injury.[36]
Sciatic nerve block	Reduced posterior knee pain[37]	Risk of neuropathy similar to femoral nerve block. Results of studies vary, ranging from improving analgesia and early mobilization[38] to adding little or no analgesia to existing femoral block.[39] Sciatic block use is controversial[40] and unlikely to improve long-term outcomes.[41]
Selective tibial nerve block	Reduced likelihood of foot drop[42]	Injection closer to popliteal crease; risk of peroneal nerve injury with lateral-to-medial approach or vascular injury.
Adductor canal	Similar pain relief to femoral nerve block with reduced muscle weakness[43]; effective in treating existing severe pain[44]	Closer to surgical site; evolving technique.
Local infiltration analgesia	Easy and quick to perform, no muscle weakness	Evolving evidence for efficacy in this context.[29] However, experts point to poor quality of some of the existing studies.[45] Success of technique likely operator-dependent. Associated with transient peroneal nerve palsy.[46]

Once a site or sites is chosen for regional anesthesia, the provider may utilize different techniques to obtain postoperative analgesia, summarized next.

Technique	Benefits	Drawbacks
Single shot	Quick to perform; low cost; effective.[33]	Shortest duration (may be benefit if rapid recovery of muscle strength is required for physical therapy).
Nerve catheter	Improved analgesia compared to single-injection technique.[47] Longest duration of analgesia; titratable; control over degree of motor block by changing flow rate.	More difficult and time consuming to perform; more expensive; requires postoperative surveillance.
Extended-release formulations of local anesthetic (eg, liposomal bupivacaine)	As quick to perform as single-shot block, with longer block duration.	Compared with bupivacaine, currently little evidence of efficacy.[48] Costly. Limits ability to redo block. Safety and side-effect profile currently emerging.[49]

Surgical anesthesia

Options for surgical anesthesia are summarized next.

Anesthesia	Benefits	Drawbacks
Spinal	Associated with improved outcomes,[2] decreased requirements for critical care services.[50]	Can be technically difficult on certain patients. Occasional catastrophic outcomes (eg, epidural hematoma).[31,32] Duration of spinal anesthesia may be inadequate for surgery. Patients may be reluctant to be "awake" for surgery.
Epidural	Similar benefits as spinal, but can be used for postoperative analgesia and longer-duration surgeries.	Can be technically difficult on certain patients. Occasional catastrophic outcomes (eg epidural hematoma).[31,32] Patients may be reluctant to be "awake" for surgery.
General	Complete amnesia.	Associated with poor outcomes compared to spinal. Occasional catastrophic outcome (eg, difficult airway); increased risk of respiratory depression.[28]

Neuraxial anesthesia has been associated with improved outcomes[1,2]; however, this modality is not always the preferred modality.[51] If neuraxial anesthesia is employed, decisions regarding the inclusion or exclusion of long- or short-acting opioids must be made; this decision can be complex as it affects many subsequent pathway elements (postoperative monitoring, rehabilitation, etc.). Even patients who receive neuraxial anesthesia usually require sedation, and some pathways may specify the desired agents or levels of sedation, in part to avoid excessively sedating the patients. In addition, some patients are likely unsuited for neuraxial anesthesia, for example, due to expected surgical time for joint revisions; this and other criteria (such as difficult spinal) for proceeding to general anesthesia can be described in this section.

Intraoperative drugs

Intraoperative drugs may include first- and second-line antibiotics, preferred antiemetics for spinal or epidural anesthesia versus general anesthesia, and preferred sedatives if spinal or epidural anesthesia is chosen. Anticoagulation is usually started in the postoperative period by the surgery team but may be commented on here. Of note, intraoperative dexamethasone appears to improve postoperative pain scores as well as providing an effective antiemetic, without increasing risk of infection or other perioperative complications.[52]

(continued)

TABLE 15–4. Components of a total knee arthroplasty pathway, highlighting some common decisions that must be made during pathway development. *(Continued)*

Anesthetic Pathway for Total Joint Arthroplasty

Intraoperative transfusion goals and blood conservation options

Blood transfusion has a number of risks,[53] and one of the goals of the pathway may be to minimize blood loss and hence transfusion requirements. A wide variety of techniques can minimize blood loss, some of which are summarized next.

Technique	Benefits	Drawbacks
Intraoperative hypotension	Reduced blood loss.	Increased vigilance and monitoring required. Risk of end-organ ischemia. Underresuscitation may contribute to postoperative orthostatic intolerance, impairing early mobilization.
Tourniquet use	Reduced blood loss and protocols exist for appropriate use.[54]	Risk of ischemic injury or axonal neuropathy[55-57] or effect on quadriceps function.[58]
Appropriate thermoregulation	Reduced blood loss via maintenance of coagulation cascade, improved recovery.	
Cell scavenging	Reduced allogenic blood product requirements.	Added cost and complexity.
Reinfusion drains	Reduced allogenic blood product requirements.	Added cost and complexity.
Tranexamic acid	Reduced blood loss due to antifibrinolysis.[59]	Association with seizures.[60] No known increased risk of thrombotic events but has only recently come into use in this surgical population.

Postoperative pain control

Pathways often address pain control for patients with chronic pain or opioid use, as well as those without. Generally, this section will comment on both the expected infusion rates for any peripheral nerve catheters, as well as adjuvants such as patient-controlled opioid administration, ketamine, or other agents.

Considerations regarding orthopedic surgical pathway

Pathways sometimes comment on ways in which they interact with the surgeon's pathway to make it clear why particular recommendations are made.

The individual elements of the pathway include such diverse topics as preoperative planning, patient education, intraoperative anesthetic management, postoperative pain management, and fluid and hemodynamic goals. A completed pathway, in addition to containing firm, detailed recommendations on management, would contain an addendum that outlines the evidence that was used to make pathway decisions. As we have seen, however, even after identifying the appropriate literature, there is often a significant amount of analysis and judgment that must be used in applying the literature to the pathway.

A final pathway is only useful if it is distributed widely to all relevant providers. In addition to electronic distribution, pathways can be displayed in the form of a poster. This allows the anesthesia provider to have the steps in the pathway easily available at different phases of the patient's care. Common places to display pathway information include preoperative areas, regional anesthesia bays, operating rooms, and anesthesia workrooms. In addition, with the advent of electronic health record systems, many institutions have the capability to create order sets, which automatically create orders associated with the pathway.

CONCLUSION

Perioperative anesthesia and analgesia pathways provide a unique way of improving patient care and lowering cost by deploying existing resources and technology in an evidence-based way. Pathway development should therefore be considered a vital component of the anesthesiologist's practice.

REFERENCES

1. Pugely AJ, Martin CT, Gao Y, Mendoza-Lattes S, Callaghan JJ: Differences in short-term complications between spinal and general anesthesia for primary total knee arthroplasty. J Bone Joint Surg Am 2013;95(3):193–199.
2. Memtsoudis SG, Sun X, Chiu YL, et al. Perioperative comparative effectiveness of anesthetic technique in orthopedic patients. Anesthesiology 2013;118(5):1046–1058.
3. Stundner O, Chiu YL, Sun X, et al: Comparative perioperative outcomes associated with neuraxial versus general anesthesia for simultaneous bilateral total knee arthroplasty. Reg Anesth Pain Med 2012;37(6):638–644.
4. Memtsoudis SG, Stundner O, Rasul R, et al: Sleep apnea and total joint arthroplasty under various types of anesthesia: A population-based study of perioperative outcomes. Reg Anesth Pain Med 2013;38(4):274–281.
5. Liu J, Ma C, Elkassabany N, Fleisher LA, Neuman MD: Neuraxial anesthesia decreases postoperative systemic infection risk compared with general anesthesia in knee arthroplasty. Anesth Analg 2013;117(4):1010–1016.
6. Rotter T, Kinsman L, James E, et al: Clinical pathways: Effects on professional practice, patient outcomes, length of stay and hospital costs. Cochrane Database Syst Rev 2010(3):CD006632.
7. Shiboski S. Epidemiology and biostatistics. 2015. http://www.epibiostat.ucsf.edu/biostat/samplesize.html. Accessed June 30, 2015.
8. Brant R. Sample size calculations. 2015. http://www.stat.ubc.ca/~rollin/stats/ssize/. Accessed June 30, 2015.
9. Popping DM, Elia N, Marret E, Wenk M, Tramer MR: Opioids added to local anesthetics for single-shot intrathecal anesthesia in patients undergoing minor surgery: A meta-analysis of randomized trials. Pain 2012;153(4):784–793.
10. Horlocker TT, Wedel DJ: Neuraxial block and low-molecular-weight heparin: Balancing perioperative analgesia and thromboprophylaxis. Reg Anesth Pain Med 1998;23(6 Suppl 2):164–177.
11. Nightingale SL. From the Food and Drug Administration. JAMA 1999;282(1):19.
12. Wysowski DK, Talarico L, Bacsanyi J, Botstein P: Spinal and epidural hematoma and low-molecular-weight heparin. N Engl J Med 1998;338(24):1774–1775.
13. Bidstrup BP, Royston D, Sapsford RN, Taylor KM: Reduction in blood loss and blood use after cardiopulmonary bypass with high dose aprotinin (Trasylol). J Thorac Cardiovasc Surg 1989;97(3):364–372.
14. Royston D, Bidstrup BP, Taylor KM, Sapsford RN: Effect of aprotinin on need for blood transfusion after repeat open-heart surgery. Lancet 1987;2(8571):1289–1291.
15. Mahdy AM, Webster NR: Perioperative systemic haemostatic agents. Br J Anaesth 2004;93(6):842–858.
16. Shiga T, Wajima Z, Inoue T, Sakamoto A: Aprotinin in major orthopedic surgery: A systematic review of randomized controlled trials. Anesth Analg 2005;101(6):1602–1607.
17. Sedrakyan A, Treasure T, Elefteriades JA: Effect of aprotinin on clinical outcomes in coronary artery bypass graft surgery: A systematic review and meta-analysis of randomized clinical trials. J Thorac Cardiovasc Surg 2004;128(3):442–448.
18. Mangano DT, Tudor IC, Dietzel C, Multicenter Study of Perioperative Ischemia Research G, Ischemia R, Education F: The risk associated with aprotinin in cardiac surgery. N Engl J Med 2006;354(4):353–365.
19. Shaw AD, Stafford-Smith M, White WD, et al: The effect of aprotinin on outcome after coronary-artery bypass grafting. N Engl J Med 2008;358(8):784–793.
20. Mangano DT, Miao Y, Vuylsteke A, et al: Mortality associated with aprotinin during 5 years following coronary artery bypass graft surgery. JAMA 2007;297(5):471–479.
21. Furnary AP, Wu Y, Hiratzka LF, Grunkemeier GL, Page US 3rd: Aprotinin does not increase the risk of renal failure in cardiac surgery patients. Circulation 2007;116(11 Suppl):I127–I133.
22. Schroeder DR: Statistics: Detecting a rare adverse drug reaction using spontaneous reports. Reg Anesth Pain Med 1998;23(6 Suppl 2):183–189.
23. Peersman G, Laskin R, Davis J, Peterson M: Infection in total knee replacement: A retrospective review of 6489 total knee replacements. Clin Orthop Relat Res 2001(392):15–23.
24. Zhou TJ, Tang J, White PF: Propacetamol versus ketorolac for treatment of acute postoperative pain after total hip or knee replacement. Anesth Analg 2001;92(6):1569–1575.
25. Mishriky BM, Waldron NH, Habib AS: Impact of pregabalin on acute and persistent postoperative pain: A systematic review and meta-analysis. Br J Anaesth. 2015;114(1):10–31.
26. Clarke H, Bonin RP, Orser BA, Englesakis M, Wijeysundera DN, Katz J: The prevention of chronic postsurgical pain using gabapentin and pregabalin: A combined systematic review and meta-analysis. Anesth Analg 2012;115(2):428–442.
27. Sawan H, Chen AF, Viscusi ER, Parvizi J, Hozack WJ: Pregabalin reduces opioid consumption and improves outcome in chronic pain patients undergoing total knee arthroplasty. Phys Sportsmed 2014;42(2):10–18.
28. Weingarten TN, Jacob AK, Njathi CW, Wilson GA, Sprung J: Multimodal analgesic protocol and postanesthesia respiratory depression during phase I recovery after total joint arthroplasty. Reg Anesth Pain Med 2015;40(4):330–336.
29. Lin J, Zhang L, Yang H: Perioperative administration of selective cyclooxygenase-2 inhibitors for postoperative pain management in patients after total knee arthroplasty. J Arthroplasty. 2013;28(2):207–213 e2.
30. Rothwell MP, Pearson D, Hunter JD, et al: Oral oxycodone offers equivalent analgesia to intravenous patient-controlled analgesia after total hip replacement: A randomized, single-centre, non-blinded, non-inferiority study. Br J Anaesth 2011;106(6):865–872.
31. Pumberger M, Memtsoudis SG, Stundner O, et al: An analysis of the safety of epidural and spinal neuraxial anesthesia in more than 100,000 consecutive major lower extremity joint replacements. Reg Anesth Pain Med 2013;38(6):515–519.
32. Bateman BT, Mhyre JM, Ehrenfeld J, et al: The risk and outcomes of epidural hematomas after perioperative and obstetric epidural catheterization: A report from the Multicenter Perioperative Outcomes Group Research Consortium. Anesth Analg 2013;116(6):1380–1385.
33. Paul JE, Arya A, Hurlburt L, et al: Femoral nerve block improves analgesia outcomes after total knee arthroplasty: A meta-analysis of randomized controlled trials. Anesthesiology 2010;113(5):1144–1162.
34. Carli F, Clemente A, Asenjo JF, et al: Analgesia and functional outcome after total knee arthroplasty: Periarticular infiltration vs continuous femoral nerve block. Br J Anaesth 2010;105(2):185–195.

35. Neal JM, Barrington MJ, Brull R, et al: The second ASRA practice advisory on neurologic complications associated with regional anesthesia and pain medicine executive summary 2015. Reg Anesth Pain Med 2015;40(5):401–430.

36. Jacob AK, Mantilla CB, Sviggum HP, Schroeder DR, Pagnano MW, Hebl JR: Perioperative nerve injury after total knee arthroplasty: Regional anesthesia risk during a 20-year cohort study. Anesthesiology 2011;114(2):311–317.

37. Sato K, Adachi T, Shirai N, Naoi N: Continuous versus single-injection sciatic nerve block added to continuous femoral nerve block for analgesia after total knee arthroplasty: A prospective, randomized, double-blind study. Reg Anesth Pain Med 2014;39(3):225–229.

38. Cappelleri G, Ghisi D, Fanelli A, Albertin A, Somalvico F, Aldegheri G: Does continuous sciatic nerve block improve postoperative analgesia and early rehabilitation after total knee arthroplasty? A prospective, randomized, double-blinded study. Reg Anesth Pain Med 2011;36(5):489–492.

39. Abdallah FW, Chan VW, Gandhi R, Koshkin A, Abbas S, Brull R: The analgesic effects of proximal, distal, or no sciatic nerve block on posterior knee pain after total knee arthroplasty: A double-blind placebo-controlled randomized trial. Anesthesiology 2014;121(6):1302–1310.

40. Safa B, Gollish J, Haslam L, McCartney CJ: Comparing the effects of single shot sciatic nerve block versus posterior capsule local anesthetic infiltration on analgesia and functional outcome after total knee arthroplasty: a prospective, randomized, double-blinded, controlled trial. J Arthroplasty 2014;29(6):1149–1153.

41. Wegener JT, van Ooij B, van Dijk CN, et al: Long-term pain and functional disability after total knee arthroplasty with and without single-injection or continuous sciatic nerve block in addition to continuous femoral nerve block: A prospective, 1-year follow-up of a randomized controlled trial. Reg Anesth Pain Med 2013;38(1):58–63.

42. Sinha SK, Abrams JH, Arumugam S, et al: Femoral nerve block with selective tibial nerve block provides effective analgesia without foot drop after total knee arthroplasty: A prospective, randomized, observer-blinded study. Anesth Analg 2012;115(1):202–206.

43. Jaeger P, Zaric D, Fomsgaard JS, et al: Adductor canal block versus femoral nerve block for analgesia after total knee arthroplasty: A randomized, double-blind study. Reg Anesth Pain Med 2013;38(6):526–532.

44. Jaeger P, Grevstad U, Henningsen MH, Gottschau B, Mathiesen O, Dahl JB: Effect of adductor-canal-blockade on established, severe post-operative pain after total knee arthroplasty: A randomised study. Acta Anaesth Scand 2012;56(8):1013–1019.

45. Andersen LO, Kehlet H: Analgesic efficacy of local infiltration analgesia in hip and knee arthroplasty: A systematic review. Br J Anaesth 2014;113(3):360–374.

46. Tsukada S, Wakui M, Hoshino A: Postoperative epidural analgesia compared with intraoperative periarticular injection for pain control following total knee arthroplasty under spinal anesthesia: A randomized controlled trial. J Bone Joint Surg Am 2014;96(17):1433–1438.

47. Bingham AE, Fu R, Horn JL, Abrahams MS: Continuous peripheral nerve block compared with single-injection peripheral nerve block: A systematic review and meta-analysis of randomized controlled trials. Reg Anesth Pain Med 2012;37(6):583–594.

48. Schroer WC, Diesfeld PG, LeMarr AR, Morton DJ, Reedy ME: Does extended-release liposomal bupivacaine better control pain than bupivacaine after TKA? A prospective, randomized clinical trial. J Arthroplasty 2015;30(9 Suppl):64–67.

49. Ilfeld BM, Viscusi ER, Hadzic A, et al: Safety and side effect profile of liposome bupivacaine (Exparel) in peripheral nerve blocks. Reg Anesth Pain Med 2015;40(5):572–582.

50. Memtsoudis SG, Sun X, Chiu YL, et al: Utilization of critical care services among patients undergoing total hip and knee arthroplasty: Epidemiology and risk factors. Anesthesiology 2012;117(1):107–116.

51. Fleischut PM, Eskreis-Winkler JM, Gaber-Baylis LK, et al: Variability in anesthetic care for total knee arthroplasty: An analysis from the anesthesia quality institute. Am J Med Qual 2015;30(2):172–179.

52. Backes JR, Bentley JC, Politi JR, Chambers BT: Dexamethasone reduces length of hospitalization and improves postoperative pain and nausea after total joint arthroplasty: A prospective, randomized controlled trial. J Arthroplasty 2013;28(8 Suppl):11–17.

53. Goodnough LT: Risks of blood transfusion. Crit Care Med 2003;31(12 Suppl):S678–S686.

54. Fitzgibbons PG, Digiovanni C, Hares S, Akelman E: Safe tourniquet use: A review of the evidence. J Am Acad Orthop Surg 2012;20(5):310–319.

55. Nitz AJ, Dobner JJ, Matulionis DH: Pneumatic tourniquet application and nerve integrity: Motor function and electrophysiology. Exp Neurol 1986;94(2):264–279.

56. Kornbluth ID, Freedman MK, Sher L, Frederick RW: Femoral, saphenous nerve palsy after tourniquet use: A case report. Arch Phys Med Rehab 2003;84(6):909–911.

57. Weingarden SI, Louis DL, Waylonis GW: Electromyographic changes in postmeniscectomy patients. Role of the pneumatic tourniquet. JAMA 1979;241(12):1248–1250.

58. Saunders KC, Louis DL, Weingarden SI, Waylonis GW: Effect of tourniquet time on postoperative quadriceps function. Clin Orthop Relat Res 1979(143):194–199.

59. Kagoma YK, Crowther MA, Douketis J, Bhandari M, Eikelboom J, Lim W: Use of antifibrinolytic therapy to reduce transfusion in patients undergoing orthopedic surgery: A systematic review of randomized trials. Thrombosis Res 2009;123(5):687–696.

60. Murkin JM, Falter F, Granton J, Young B, Burt C, Chu M: High-dose tranexamic acid is associated with nonischemic clinical seizures in cardiac surgical patients. Anesth Analg 2010;110(2):350–353.

CHAPTER 16

Infection Control in Regional Anesthesia

Sebastian Schulz-Stübner, Jean M. Pottinger, Stacy A. Coffin, and Loreen A. Herwaldt

INTRODUCTION

Infectious complications related to regional anesthesia are rare. Because most of the information is available in case reports and retrospective surveys, it is likely that these complications are underreported. It is hoped that recent surveillance[1] and prospective registry projects[2] using standardized surveillance definitions and the integration of such in national quality assurance projects (American Society of Regional Anesthesia [ASRA] Acute-POP/AQI)[3] will generate more comprehensive data for risk assessment and evaluation of infection control recommendations in the future. Integration of a structured surveillance tool into the electronic medical record and a hospital's quality management system[4] will ease the workload for clinicians and facilitate surveillance compliance (Table 16–1).

While we have to work on reducing infectious complications associated with regional anesthesia because of the potential severe individual consequences, some studies demonstrate a reduction of surgical site infections with the use of local anesthesia—opening the research arena regarding whether the avoidance of general anesthesia, intrinsic properties of local anesthetics, or a combination of both is responsible for this observation.[5]

The objective of this chapter is to summarize information from the literature on infections complications associated with regional anesthesia, as well as to discuss the mechanism and suggest strategies to prevent these complications.

PATHOGENESIS OF INFECTIONS ASSOCIATED WITH CENTRAL NEURAXIAL BLOCKADE

Microorganisms from exogenous or endogenous sources may gain access to the subarachnoid, epidural, or tissue space surrounding peripheral nerves in several ways. Microorganisms from the patient's or anesthesia practitioner's flora can be inoculated directly when a catheter or needle is inserted into those spaces.[6] Several reports in the literature suggested that infections are on occasion caused by the anesthesia practitioner's flora.[7–9] For example, Trautmann and colleagues reported a case of meningitis caused by a *Staphylococcus aureus* strain that was identical by pulsed-field gel electrophoresis to the *S. aureus* isolated from the anesthesiologist's nose.[8] Rubin et al could trace to a single anesthesiologist *Streptococcus salivarius* as the responsible agent for six cases of meningitis following spinal anesthesia,[10] and the Centers for Disease Control and Prevention (CDC) reported five cases in Ohio and one case in New York between 2008 and 2009 with the same organisms.[11]

Microorganisms can also enter the epidural space by hematogenous spread from other body sites, such as infected skin,[8,12] or by migrating along the catheter tract.[13,14] Several case reports suggested that infection was caused by spread of bacteria from infected sites through the bloodstream to the epidural space.[15–17] Others maintained that infections at distal sites are *not* contraindications to epidural anesthesia. For example, Newman concluded that distal infections did not increase the risk of epidural infection because traumatic injuries are often infected, and no epidural catheter-related infections were identified among over 3000 patients who had epidural neural blockades for postoperative or posttraumatic analgesia.[18] Gritsenko and coworkers analyzed the charts of 474 patients who underwent removal of an infected hip or knee prosthesis under neuraxial anesthesia and found in 0.6% of the cases clinical signs of central neuraxial infections (meningitis or epidural abscess) and three other anesthesia-related complications, including a psoas abscess beside an epidural hematoma and back pain.[19]

TABLE 16–1. Regional anesthesia surveillance system complication definitions.

	A: Essential Criteria	B: Contributory Criteria
Epidural infection		
EI1: Superficial soft tissue infection 2 A and B criteria needed	Swelling Local tenderness	Fever (>38.0°C) Drainage Positive culture from the area Leukocytosis (>12/nL or CRP > 20 mg/L) Local erythema
EI2: Epidural abscess 1 A and 3 B criteria needed	Radiological evidence of a mass in the epidural space consistent with an epidural abscess within 30 days after epidural/spinal needle/catheter placement/catheter removal or attempted epidural/spinal placement	Fever (>38.0°C) Drainage Positive culture from surgical exploration or puncture Leukocytosis (12/nL or CRP > 20 mg/L) Local erythema Local tenderness Focal back pain Neurologic deficit[a]
EI2N[a]	Same as above: Classified as EI 2 N if neurologic deficit is present as a contributory criterion	
EI3: Epidural infection with sepsis 1 A and 4 B criteria needed	Diagnostic criteria of EI1 or EI2 or EI2N[a] puncture site or abscess	Positive blood culture with the same organism isolated from Fever > 38.0°C or hypothermia < 36°C Leukocytosis > 12 nL or leukopenia < 4 nL BP systolic < 90 mm Hg Tachycardia > 90 bpm Respiratory failure (AF > 20, $paCO_2$ < 32 mm Hg, PaO_2 < 70 mm Hg breathing spontaneously or PaO_2/FiO_2 < 175 on mechanical ventilation)
EI3N	Same as above: Classified as EI3N if EI2N[a] criteria are present	
Peripheral nerve block–associated other infection		
OI1: Superficial soft tissue infection	Swelling along the catheter or needle placement track Local tenderness along the catheter or needle placement track	Fever (>38.0°C) Drainage Positive culture from the area Leukocytosis (>12/nL or CRP > 20 mg/L) Local erythema
OI2: Abscess or deep tissue infection	Evidence of an abscess or fluid collection consistent with an infectious process by imaging or surgical exploration within 30 days after peripheral nerve block needle placement/catheter removal or attempted placement	Fever (>38.0°C) Drainage Positive culture from surgical exploration or puncture Leukocytosis (>12/nL or CRP > 20 mg/L) Local erythema Local tenderness Focal back pain Neurologic deficit[a]

(continued)

TABLE 16–1. Regional anesthesia surveillance system complication definitions. (*Continued*)

	A: Essential Criteria	B: Contributory Criteria
OI2N[a]	Same as above: Classified as OI2N if neurologic deficit is present as contributory criterion	Positive blood culture with the same organism isolated from puncture site or abscess Fever > 38.0°C or hypothermia < 36°C Leukocytosis > 12 nL or leukopenia < 4 nL BP systolic < 90 mm Hg Tachycardia > 90 bpm Respiratory failure (AF > 20, $PaCO_2$ < 32 mm Hg, PaO_2 < 70 mm Hg breathing spontaneously or PaO_2/FiO_2 < 175 on mechanical ventilation)
OI3: Infection with sepsis 1 A and 4 B criteria needed	Diagnostic criteria of OI1 or OI2 or OI2N[a]	Positive blood culture with the same organism isolated from puncture site or abscess Fever > 38.0°C or hypothermia < 36°C Leukocytosis > 12 nL or leukopenia < 4 nL BP systolic < 90 mm Hg Tachycardia > 90 bpm Respiratory failure (AF > 20, $PaCO_2$ < 32 mm Hg, PaO_2 < 70 mm Hg breathing spontaneously or PaO_2/FiO_2 < 175 on mechanical ventilation)
OI3N	Same as above: Classified as OI3N if OI2N[a] criteria are present	New onset of central neurologic symptoms Headache Stiff neck Fever > 38.0°C Positive CSF culture Meningitis-specific antibiotic therapy started Spinal or epidural block (catheter insertion/removal) in the past 72 h
Neurologic deficit ND1: Neurologic deficit	Residual sensory and/or motor and/or autonomic block 72 h after last injection of local anesthetic without other identifiable etiology New onset of sensory and/or motor and/or autonomic deficit 24 h after resolution of the original block without other identifiable etiology If regional anesthetic-/analgesia-related infection is present classify, as EIXN/OIXN[a]	Electrophysiological evidence of new nerve damage (MEP, SEP, nerve conduction study, electromyography)
2 A and 1 B criteria needed		New loss of deep tendon reflexes New loss of vibration sensation New onset of neuropathic pain in affected nerve distribution area Paresthesia in affected nerve distribution area Sensory and/or motor and/or autonomic deficit consistent with dermatomes or nerve distribution area

[a]CRP: C-reactive protein; BP: Blood pressure; AF: Air flow (Respiratoty rate); CSF: cerebrospinal fluid; MEP: Motor evoked potentials; SEP: Sensory evoked potentials. If regional anesthetic-/analgesia-related infection is present, classify as EI XN/OI XN.

Source: Adapted with permission from Schulz-Stübner S, Kelley J: Regional Anesthesia Surveillance System: first experiences with a quality assessment tool for regional anesthesia and analgesia. *Acta Anaesthesiol Scand.* 2007 Mar;51(3):305-315.

Clinical Pearls

- Streptococcal species, *S. aureus,* and *Pseudomonas aeruginosa* are the most common causative agents but multiresistant species also emerge as causative pathogens as their endemic impact grows within health-care systems.
- Microorganisms from the patient's or anesthesia practitioner's flora can be inoculated directly when a catheter or needle is inserted into the epidural or subarachnoid space.
- Because it is easy to contaminate the needle or the catheters, aseptic measures.

The anesthetic agents injected into the subarachnoid or epidural space are another possible source of infection. Infections from contaminated multidose vials are likely rare because most anesthetic drugs are weak bases dissolved in acidic solutions that inhibit growth of bacteria and fungi.[20–22] Besides most multidose local anesthetic solutions contain a bacteriostatic agent. Nevertheless, the case report by North and Brophy suggested that contaminated multidose vials still can be a source of infection. These authors reported an infection in which *S. aureus* with matching phage types were isolated from an abscess and a multidose lidocaine vial.[7]

A report by Wong et al[23] described, besides other infection control violations, the use of single-dose medications for multiple patients as the culprit in an outbreak of *Klebsiella pneumoniae* and *Enterobacter aerogenes* bacteremia in a pain clinic. Breaches in aseptic technique for medication preparation can be detrimental, especially if a compound pharmacy is involved: In 2012, more than 200 patients suffered fungal infections with *Exserohilum rostratum* after use of contaminated methypednisolone injections for interventional pain procedures in multiple institutions in the United States.[24]

To assess whether contamination of the anesthetic agent or the equipment (needles, syringes, tubing) is related to subsequent infections, investigators have cultured these items after they have been used with patients or during simulations. In four studies, 0%–29% of used catheters were contaminated,[25–28] and James and coworkers found that 5 of 101 syringes used to inject anesthetic agents were contaminated.[25] Ross and coworkers drew up 0.25% bupivacaine into control syringes and into syringes used to induce continuous lumbar epidural neural blockade (test syringe) in 18 obstetric patients.[29] After each dose from the test syringe, the investigators cultured the contents of both the test and the control syringes. Six of 18 test syringes were contaminated with bacteria, compared with only 1 of 18 control syringes. Raedler and associates cultured 114 spinal and 20 epidural needles after use for single lumbar injections.[30] Twenty-four cultures (17.9%) grew microorganisms: 15.7% coagulase-negative staphylococci; 1.5% yeasts; and 0.8% each enterococci, pneumococci, and micrococci. The authors concluded that it is easy to contaminate the needle, and that anesthesiologists need to improve their hygienic measures. Despite finding contaminated equipment or anesthetic solutions, no infected patient was identified[25–29]; thus, none of the

authors was able to correlate contamination with infection. However, Loftus and coworkers examined the contamination of intravenous stopcocks during general anesthesia and showed, for the first time, postoperative infections with the same organism.[6] It is therefore conceivable that contamination during the placement of a regional block, and, even more likely, during handling of continuous catheter systems, can cause infections. Although the risk for such infections would be less likely than that of manipulating intravenous lines.

INFECTIONS ASSOCIATED WITH EPIDURAL BLOCKADE

The numerous case reports in the literature of infections occurring after epidural neuraxial blockade, attest to the fact that such complications do occur and can be severe (Table 16–2).[7,15,17,30–69] Of 57 patients in these case reports, 41 acquired epidural or intraspinal abscesses, 1 developed a subcutaneous abscess, 2 had meningitis without epidural abscess formation, and 1 developed sepsis. Four patients had injections only, 1 patient had injections and several catheters, and the remaining patients had catheters. Among the 38 patients who had catheters and for whom the duration of catheterization was specified, the median duration of catheterization was 3 days (range 50 minutes to 6 weeks). The median time to onset of the first signs or symptoms of infection was 4 days (range 1 day to 4.8 months) after catheter placement. *Staphylococcus aureus* caused 27 of 43 infections from which bacterial pathogens were isolated. *Pseudomonas aeruginosa* caused five infections and *Streptococcus* spp. caused five. Methicillin-resistant *S. aureus* (MRSA) was isolated in one case; three patients died.

Clinical Pearls

- Epidural catheters inserted for long-term pain control become infected more frequently than those used for short periods of time.
- Malignancy and reduced immunocompetence might be additional risk factors for catheter infection.
- Case reports of infections occurring after epidural neuraxial blockade point out that complications from infection can be severe and often lead to epidural or intraspinal abscesses.

It should be kept in mind that the number of reported cases does not allow us to assess the true frequency of infections after epidural neural blockade. However, several investigators have performed studies to assess this risk. When reviewing 350 reports in the literature, Dawkins in 1969 found no reports of infection after thoracic or lumbar epidural block but identified 8 (0.2%) reports of infection after 3767 sacral epidural blocks used for operative procedures and for obstetrics.[74] More recently, Dawson reviewed the literature and found rates of deep

TABLE 16–2. Infections associated with epidural neural blockade.

Author (Reference)	Year	Indication	Epidural Site	Filter Used	Catheter Duration	Type of Infection	Time From Insertion to Symptoms	Signs and Symptoms	Microorganism	Outcome
Edwards and Hingson[31]	1943	Vaginal delivery	Caudal	NS	NS	Epidural abscess, bacteremia	NS	NS	Staphylococcus aureus	Died 31 days after delivery
Ferguson and Kirsch[32a]	1974	Postoperative analgesia	Thoracic	NS	2 days	Epidural empyema	4 days 10 days 14 days	Fever, headache, meningism Urinary retention Paraparesis	Staphylococcus epidermidis	Sensory impairment, spastic weakness, walks with crutches
Saady[33a]	1976	Postoperative analgesia	Thoracic	Yes	1.7 days	Epidural abscess	4 days 8 days 9 days 10 days 14 days	Fever Chills, abdominal pain right upper quadrant Headache, stiff neck Urinary retention Lower extremity paraparesis, no anal tone	S. aureus	Sensory impairment, walks with minimal assistance
North and Brophy[7]	1979	1. Priapism 2. Fractured ribs, chest injury	Lumbar Thoracic	No Yes	3 days 4 days	Epidural abscess Epidural abscess	1 day 10 days 2 days 4 days	Fever Stiff neck, dysphagia, back pain, absent ankle jerks Fever Stiff neck, sensory loss T2 to T6	S. aureus S. aureus	Full recovery Sensory impairment
Wenningsted-Torgard et al[45b]	1982	Lower back pain	Lumbar	NS	6 days	Skin abscess, spondylitis, bacteremia	10 days	Fever	S. aureus	Wedge formation of two vertebral bodies
McDonogh and Cranney[35]	1984	Fractured ribs	Thoracic	Yes	3.3 days	Epidural abscess	2.5 days 19 days	Fever Paralysis left leg, weakness, right leg, urinary retention, sensory deficit T7 to 8	S. aureus	Residual left-side weakness, uses walking frame, urinary retention

(continued)

TABLE 16–2. Infections associated with epidural neural blockade. (*Continued*)

Author (Reference)	Year	Indication	Epidural Site	Filter Used	Catheter Duration	Type of Infection	Time From Insertion to Symptoms	Signs and Symptoms	Microorganism	Outcome
Konig et al[36]	1985	Knee surgery	Lumbar	NS	4 days	Paravertebral and epidural abscesses, osteomyelitis, phlegmonous duritis, myelitis	2 weeks	Pain, lower extremity paraparesis	*S. epidermidis*	Nearly complete recovery
Sollmann et al[37]	1987	Phantom limb pain	NS	NS	6 weeks	Large encapsulated "spinal" abscess compressing dura at L4–L5	6 weeks, 5 months	Severe back pain Severe sciatica	*Pseudomonas aeruginosa*	Persistent pain
Fine et al[38]	1988	Neuralgic pain syndrome	Thoracic	Yes	3 days	Site infection, epidural abscess	9 days	Fever, chills, urinary retention	No culture obtained	Sensory impairment
Ready and Helfer[39]	1989	1. Vaginal delivery	Lumbar	NS	50 min	Meningitis	1 day	Headache, stiff neck, fever, back pain, nuchal rigidity	*Streptococcus uberis*	Full recovery
		2. Cesarean section	NS	NS	3 days	Cellulitis meningitis	3.5 days 5.5 days	Fever Headache, nuchal rigidity, photophobia, hyperacusis	*Enterococcus faecalis*	Full recovery
Berga and Trierweiler[40]	1989	Vaginal delivery	Lumbar	NS	NS	Meningitis	1 day	Headache	*Streptococcus sanguis*	Full recovery
Goucke and Graziotti[41]	1990	Back pain	Lumbar	NS	3 epidural injections	Bacteremia, epidural abscess	3.3 weeks after last injection	Back pain, fever, urinary retention	*S. aureus*	Died 7 weeks after laminectomy
Lynch and Zech[42]	1990	Intra- and postoperative analgesia	Lumbar	Yes	3 days	Spondylitis	3 days	Fever, chills, headache, back pain	*P. aeruginosa*	9-month recovery, wears lumbar brace, some lumbar pain

Reference	Year	Indication	Level			Diagnosis		Symptoms	Organism	Outcome
Strong[43]	1991	1. Herpes zoster[b]	Thoracic	Yes	2.5 days 3 days[c]	Epidural abscess	4.4 weeks	Pain, headache, stiff neck, fever, right flank pain	S. aureus	Full recovery Full recovery
		2. Reflex sympathetic dystrophy	Cervical	Yes	5 days 5 days[c]	Cellulitis Epidural abscess	16 days 7 weeks	Cellulitis Neck pain radiating to left arm	Culture negative	
Klygis and Reisberg[44]	1991	Vaginal delivery	NS	NS		Epidural abscess	1.5 days	Back pain, paresthesias medial thigh and plantar surface of feet, fever	Group G streptococci	Full recovery
Dawson et al[45]	1991	Postoperative analgesia	Thoracic	Yes	4 days	Epidural abscess	12 days 18 days	Numbness and weakness in leg, urinary incontinence Paraplegia	S. aureus	Loss of motor function, requires indwelling urinary catheter, able to take few steps with help
Waldmann[142]	1991	Cervical radiculopathy	C6	NS	NS	Epidural abscess	72 h	Stiff neck and chills	S. aureus	Quadraparetic with partial function of upper extremities and able to walk
Ferguson[46]	1992	Intra- and postoperative analgesia	Lumbar	Yes	4 days	Cellulitis, epidural infection	7 days	Fever, back pain	S. aureus	Not specified
NganKee and Jones[47]	1992	Cesarean section	Lumbar	Yes	50 h	Epidural abscess	5 days	Fever, back pain, rigors, bacteremia, paresthesias, weakness of both legs	S. aureus	Full recovery after 8 weeks

(continued)

TABLE 16–2. Infections associated with epidural neural blockade. *(Continued)*

Author (Reference)	Year	Indication	Epidural Site	Filter Used	Catheter Duration	Type of Infection	Time From Insertion to Symptoms	Signs and Symptoms	Microorganism	Outcome
Sowter et al[48]	1992	Intra- and postoperative analgesia	Thoracic	Yes	5 days	Epidural abscess	3.6 weeks	Back pain, urinary retention, paresthesias and weakness both legs	S. aureus	Paraplegic with indwelling urethral catheter
Shintani et al[49]	1992	Herpes zoster	Lumbar	NS	3 days	Meningitis, epidural abscess	3 days	Headache, nausea, vomiting, fever, somnolence, back pain	Methicillin-resistant S. aureus	Full recovery
Nordstrom and Sandin[50]	1993	Fractured ribs	Thoracic	Yes	6 days	Epidural abscess	19 days	Back pain, numbness both legs, fever, paresis urethral sphincter	S. aureus	Incomplete recovery of motor function 4 months after laminectomy
Mamourian et al[70]	1993	PVD	L3–L4	NS	48 h	Epidural abscess	72 h	Lower extremity radicular pain and weakness, urinary retention	S. aureus	Full recovery
		Low back pain	NS	NS	Single shot	Epidural abscess	2 weeks	Worsening pain, leg weakness, urinary retention	S. aureus	Died from ventricular tachycardia
		PVD	NS	NS	Single shot	Epidural abscess	24 h, 4 days	Fever, leg spasm	S. aureus	No neurologic deficit
Davis et al[51]	1993	Vaginal delivery	Lumbar	NS	Less than 1 day	Meningitis	1.7 days	Headache, vomiting, confusion, delirium, fever	Group β-hemolytic streptococci	Full recovery
Ania[52b]	1994	Lumbar pain	NS	NS	8 days	Meningitis	1 day; 3 days	Headache, chills, vomiting	S. aureus	Full recovery
Tabo et al[71]	1994	Herpes zoster	L3–L4	NS	3 days	Epidural abscess	4 days	Fever, fatigue, pain	S. aureus	Full recovery
Borum et al[53]	1995	Vaginal delivery	Lumbar	Yes	1 day	Epidural abscess	4 days	Low back pain, tingling both lower extremities	S. aureus	Full recovery
							6 days	Weakness both lower extremities		

Liu and Pope[54]	1996	Extracorporeal shockwave lithotripsy	NS	NS	NS	Meningitis	Headache, photophobia	*Streptococcus pneumoniae*	Full recovery
Dunn et al[55]	1996	Intra- and postoperative analgesia	NS	NS	1 day	Epidural abscess, osteomyelitis	Neck and back pain	*S. aureus*	Mild hip and loin pain 5 months after the operation
					14 days		Back pain, nausea, vomiting, fever		
Cooper and Sharpe[56b]	1996	Chronic back pain	Not specified	NS	Injection	Meningitis, cauda equina syndrome	Increased back pain, chills, profuse sweating	*S. aureus*	Incontinent of stool
					13 days		Leg weakness, incontinent of stool		
Barontini et al[57]	1996	Transurethral resection of prostate	Lumbar	NS	NS	Epidural abscess	Fever, leg weakness Chills, pain, flaccid paraparesis of leg	No culture obtained	Paraplegia
					2 days 4 days				
Pinczower and Gyorke[15]	1996	Postoperative analgesia	Lumbar	NS	4 days	L1 vertebral osteomyelitis	Low back pain	*P. aeruginosa*	Full recovery
					3 weeks				
Wang et al[72]	1996	RSD	L2–L3 and L3–L4 (total of 4 catheters during 4 weeks)	NS	4 weeks	Small epidural abscess with meningeal irritation	Nuchal rigidity, back pain, nausea, photophobia, severe headache	Not identified	Full recovery
					?				
Bengtsson et al[17]	1997	1. Analgesia after a traumatic amputation	L3–L4, T12–L1	Yes	1 day,c 4 days	Meningitis	Fever, pain and erythema at 2nd insertion site, stiff neck	*P. aeruginosa*	Full recovery
					4 days				
		2. Analgesia for phantom pains after an amputation	Lumbar	Yes	3 days	Soft tissue and interspinal abscess	Fever, severe headache, erythema, *S. aureus* and swelling at insertion site, back pain radiating to right thigh	No culture obtained	Radicular pain in lower back
					3 days				

(continued)

TABLE 16–2. Infections associated with epidural neural blockade. (*Continued*)

Author (Reference)	Year	Indication	Epidural Site	Filter Used	Catheter Duration	Type of Infection	Time From Insertion to Symptoms	Signs and Symptoms	Microorganism	Outcome
		3. Analgesia for painful foot ulcers	Lumbar tunneled catheter	Yes	16 days	Psoas abscess at L2 to L5 tracking to L3–L4 intraspinal level	11 days, 14 days	Fever, pain radiating from back	S. aureus	Full recovery
Sarrubbi and Vasquez[58]	1997	1. Analgesia for reflex sympathetic dystrophy	L1–L2	NS	3 days	Epidural abscess	3 days	High fever, cloudy drainage at catheter exit site	S. aureus	Recovered to her baseline
		2. Surgical anesthesia and postoperative analgesia	NS	NS	2 days	Epidural abscess and meningitis	2 days	Bilateral leg weakness and double vision	S. aureus	Ambulated with a walker at 3 months
							5 days	Flaccid paralysis, double vision from 3rd-nerve palsy, meningism, sensory level L1		
Iseki et al[59]	1998	Analgesia for herpes zoster	11 epidural injections then catheters at T6–T7, T8–T9, T7–T8	NS	4 days,c 1 day, 6 days	Epidural abscess at T6–T7 and inflammation of the perivertebral muscles at T5 to T7	6 days after the final catheterization	Fever, elevated white blood count and C-reactive protein	Methicillin-resistant S. aureus	Full recovery
O'Brien and Rawluk[60]	1999	Analgesia for low back pain	1 epidural injection	NS	Not applicable	Epidural abscess	3 months	Back pain, bilateral lower extremity pain	Mycobacterium fortuitum	Full recovery
Halkic et al[61]	2001	Postoperative analgesia	T11–T12	NS	4 days	Spondylodiscitis at L5–S1	4 days	Lumbar pain radiating to the groin	Propionibacterium acnes	Full recovery
Phillips et al[62]	2002	1. Postoperative analgesia	Thoracic	NS	3 days	Epidural abscess	4 days	Fever	S. aureus	Full recovery

(continued)

		2. Postoperative analgesia	Thoracic	NS	3 days		5 days	Low backache, headache, tenderness at insertion site	Methicillin-resistant *S. aureus*	Died of a pulmonary embolus and cardiac arrest
							3 weeks	Pain at insertion site, weakness in lower extremities, urinary retention		
Royakkers et al[63]	2002	1. Postoperative analgesia	L2–L3	Yes	4 days	Epidural abscess	3 days	Fever	*S. aureus*	Full recovery
							4 days	Elevated ESR, WBC, C-reactive protein		
							5 days	Erythema at exit site		
							7 days	Pus at insertion site		
		2. Postoperative analgesia	T7–T8	NS	5 days	Epidural abscess	6 days	Erythema and pus at insertion site	*S. aureus*	Full recovery
		3. Postoperative analgesia	T10–T11	NS	3 days	Epidural abscess	7 days	Signs of local infection, back pain, fever to 39°C	*S. aureus*	Full recovery
Hagiwara et al[64]	2003	Postoperative analgesia	Low thoracic	NS	NS	Epidural abscess	4.8 months	Fever, back pain, neck stiffness, coma, and quadriplegia	Methicillin-resistant *S. aureus*	Nearly full recovery
Evans and Misra[65]	2003	Labor analgesia	Lumbar	Yes	NS	Epidural abscess	7 days	Back and leg pain	NS	Incomplete recovery
							9 days	Hot and cold flushes, flu-like illness, pain from back down both legs		
							11 days	Fever, dehydration, tachycardia		
							12 days	Unable to bear weight or pass urine, sensation decreased below knees		

TABLE 16–2. Infections associated with epidural neural blockade. *(Continued)*

Author (Reference)	Year	Indication	Epidural Site	Filter Used	Catheter Duration	Type of Infection	Time From Insertion to Symptoms	Signs and Symptoms	Microorganism	Outcome
Yue and Tan[66]	2003	Low back pain	Caudal	NS in abstract	NS in abstract	Diskitis	4 weeks	Low back pain, elevated serum acute-phase reactants, radiographic evidence of L4–L5 diskitis	*P. aeruginosa*	Full recovery
Hagiwara et al[69]	2003	Colectomy	Lumbar	NS	NS	Epidural abscess	144 days	Fever, severe back pain	Methicillin-resistant *S. aureus*	Slight gait disturbance
Volk et al[179]	2005	Hip replacement	Lumbar	Yes	3 days	Subdural empyema and paraspinal abscess	16 days	Fever, back pain, mild headache	NS	Full recovery
Aiba et al[67]	2009	NS	NS	NS	NS	Wide epidural abscess	NS	NS	NS	NS
Radif and Dalsgaard[68]	2009	NS	NS	NS	2 days	Subcutaneous abscess and meningitis	2 days	Pain, later fever and neck rigidity	NS	Full recovery
Pitkänen et al[113]	2013	Abdominal surgery	Thoracic	NS	9 days	Epidural abscess	NS	NS	NS	Full recovery
		Herniated disk	NS	NS	Several injections	Epidural abscess	NS	NS	NS	Full recovery
		Multiple trauma	Thoracic	NS	14 days	Epidural abscess	NS	NS	NS	Full recovery
		Chronic pain	NS	NS	NS	Meningitis	NS	NS	NS	Full recovery
		Chronic pain	NS	NS	14 days	Sepsis	NS	NS	NS	Full recovery

ESR = erythrocyte sedimentation rate; NS = not specified; PVD = peripheral vascular disease; WBC = white blood cell count.

[a]Although discrepancies exist in the two reports, these articles may report the same patient.

[b]Patient was given epidural anesthetic agents and epidural steroids.

[c]Patient had more than one epidural catheter.

Source: Adapted with permission from Mayhall CG: *Hospital Epidemiology and Infection Control*, 3rd ed. Philadelphia: Lippincott, Williams and Wilkins; 2004.

infection ranging from 0% to 0.7% and rates of superficial infection ranging from 1.8% to 12%.[75]

Scott and Hibbard surveyed all obstetric units in the United Kingdom and identified one epidural abscess in approximately 506,000 epidural neural blocks.[76] In contrast, Palot and colleagues identified three cases of meningitis in 300,000 patients who had undergone epidural blocks.[77] Three smaller series of obstetric epidural neural blockades (some 12,000 patients) did not identify any infections.[78–80] Similarly, in a recent study by the French SOS group on complications of regional anesthesia, Auroy and coworkers did not identify any infections in 29,732 epidural neural blocks given for obstetrical procedures.[81] Together, the results of these five studies suggest that four or five serious infectious complications (ie, epidural abscesses or meningitis) occur per 1 million obstetric epidural neural blocks.

A number of studies have assessed infections associated with epidural neural blockades performed for operative procedures or for short-term pain relief. However, these studies reported fewer patients than the studies of epidural neural blockade for obstetric procedures. Findings from 10 studies are summarized in Table 16–3.[58,62,81–87] Brooks and collaborators found four infections among 4832 (0.08%) patients undergoing epidural neuraxial blockade for surgical procedures or for labor and delivery.[88] All four infections occurred in healthy young women who underwent cesarean sections; two infections were superficial (0.04%), and two involved the epidural space (0.04%). In contrast, Holt and colleagues reported 53 (1.8%) local infections and 11 (0.4%) central nervous system infections related to approximately 3000 epidural catheters.[89,90] The median duration of catheterization was 8 days for patients with local infections and 15 days for those with generalized symptoms

($p = .01$). Catheters removed from patients with clinical symptoms were more heavily colonized than those removed from asymptomatic patients. However, 59 of 78 catheters with positive cultures were removed because patients were symptomatic, suggesting that this observation may have been affected by ascertainment bias.

Given that the incidence of infections identified in all studies has been low, the results reported by investigators who calculated the upper boundaries of the infection risk associated with epidural neural blockade are particularly important because they provide a better estimate of the true risk than do studies that reported only the number of infections and the number of procedures. For example, Strafford and coworkers did not identify skin infections or epidural abscesses among 1458 pediatric patients who had epidural analgesia to control perioperative pain.[91] These investigators calculated the incidence of clinical infection to be 0 with a 95% confidence interval from 0% to 0.03%, or three infections per 10,000 procedures. Auroy and colleagues, as noted previously, did not identify any infections among 29,732 procedures done for deliveries.[81] They calculated 95% confidence intervals of 0/10,000 to 1/10,000 procedures. Darchy and associates evaluated 75 patients, 9 (12%; incidence density rate of 2.7/100 catheter-days) of whom acquired local infections. None of the patients acquired deep infections.[83] Based on these data, Darchy and associates estimated the upper risk of spinal space infections to be 4.8% for catheters that remained in place for 4 days. Of note, these estimates are considerably higher than those of Strafford and coworkers[91] and higher even than the rates found by Du Pen and collaborators among patients with epidural catheters for long-term pain control.[92]

TABLE 16–3. Infections after epidural neural blockades done for surgical procedures or short-term pain relief.

Author (Reference)	Year Published	Number of Patients	Number of Infections
Hunt et al[28]	1977	102	1 cellulitis
Sethna et al[82]	1992	1200 children	0
Darchy et al[83]	1996	75	9 local infections, 4 of which were associated with catheter infections
McNeeley et al[84]	1997	91	0
Abel et al[85]	1998	4392	0
Grass et al[86]	1998	5193	1 exit site infection
Kost-Byerly et al[87]	1998	210 children	21/170 (12.3%) of caudal catheters, 1/40 (2.5%) lumbar catheters were associated with cellulitis
Phillips et al[62]	2002	2401	3 epidural infections
Auroy et al[81]	2002	5561	1 meningitis
Volk et al[140]	2009	5057	136 exit site infections

Source: Data from Mayhall CG: *Hospital Epidemiology and Infection Control*, 3rd ed. Philadelphia: Lippincott, Williams and Wilkins; 2004.

In general, epidural catheters inserted for long-term pain control become infected more frequently than those used for short periods of time. Du Pen and associates identified 30 superficial (9.3/10,000 catheter-days), 8 deep catheter track (2.5/10,000 catheter-days), and 15 epidural space (4.6/10,000 catheter-days) infections among 350 patients who had long-term epidural catheters.[92] Similarly, Zenz and colleagues identified two cases of meningitis among 139 patients (1.4%, or 2.1/10,000 catheter-days) treated for pain due to malignancy.[93] Coombs reported that 10 of 92 (10.9%) cancer patients acquired local infections, and 2 (2.2%) acquired meningitis.[94] Malignancy and reduced immunocompetence might be additional risk factors in the population with long-term catheters.

Whether newly developed transparent dressings with integrated chlorhexidine patches might be beneficial for this vulnerable population remains to be seen.

INFECTIONS ASSOCIATED WITH SUBARACHNOID BLOCKADE

Case reports in the literature indicated that serious infections can occur as complications of subarachnoid neural blockade (Table 16–4).[8–11,13,14,95–112] Of the 471 infections reported in these case reports, 272 were meningitis, 4 were epidural abscesses, 2 were soft tissue abscesses, 2 were infections of a disk or of a disk space, 1 developed cerebral and spinal abscesses, and 1 was a case of severe necrotizing fasciitis. In the last case mentioned, the authors speculated about a contaminated reused multiuse vial of local anesthetic as the cause.[112] The median time to onset of signs or symptoms of infection was 1 day (range 1 hour to 2 months) for all infections and 18 hours (range 1 hour to 10 days for meningitis). Streptococcal species caused 24 of the 37 infections from which bacterial pathogens were identified; S. aureus caused 2 infections; Pseudomonas spp. caused 4; and an extended spectrum betalactamase Serratia marcescens caused 1. Compared with infections after epidural neural blockade, infections associated with subarachnoid neural blockade were more likely to be caused by streptococci, and patients were more likely to recover fully. Table 16–5 reviews data from 10 studies or reviews that, if taken together, suggest that the rate of infection was approximately 3.5 per 100,000 subarachnoid neural blockades.[81,109,115–123]

INFECTIONS ASSOCIATED WITH COMBINED EPIDURAL AND SUBARACHNOID BLOCKADE

At present, there are few reports in the literature about infectious complications as a result of using combined epidural-subarachnoid (CSE) neural blockade. In 11 case reports of infections with a total number of 12 patients after combined procedures[62,124–130] (Table 16–6), the median time to onset of signs or symptoms of infection was 21 hours (range 8 hours to 9 days) for all infections and 18 hours (range 8 hours to 3 days) for meningitis. Signs or symptoms of epidural abscesses were first noted 1–9 days after the procedures. Streptococcal species caused three of six cases of meningitis, and S. aureus caused all

three epidural abscesses. Ten of twelve patients recovered fully. Cascio and Heath assessed rates of infection associated with combined procedures and identified one case of meningitis after about 700 (≈0.1%) CSE neural blockades.[124]

INFECTIONS ASSOCIATED WITH PERIPHERAL NERVE BLOCKS

Continuous regional anesthetic techniques utilizing peripheral nerve blocks have become more popular in recent years for postoperative pain management, especially for orthopedic procedures.[132,133] Only a few studies have addressed infectious complications related to these procedures. The study by Auroy and coworkers of French anesthesiologists did not identify any infections after 43,946 peripheral blocks.[52] Bergman and colleagues identified 1 patient among 368 patients (405 axillary catheters) who had a local S. aureus skin infection in the axilla after 48 hours of axillary analgesia.[134] The patient recovered fully with antibiotic treatment. Meier and colleagues reported eight superficial skin infections among 91 patients who had continuous interscalene catheters for an average of 5 days.[135] Nseir described a case of fatal streptococcal necrotizing fasciitis following axillary brachial plexus block.[136] Adam reported a psoas abscess complicating a femoral nerve block catheter.[137]

Cuvillion and coworkers obtained cultures of 208 femoral catheters when they were removed after 48 hours.[138] Of the catheters, 54% were colonized with potentially pathogenic bacteria (71% Staphylococcus epidermidis, 10% Enterococcus spp., and 4% Klebsiella spp.). These investigators also reported three episodes of transient bacteremia, but they did not identify any abscesses or episodes of clinical sepsis.[136] None of the groups provided information about the aseptic techniques used for catheter insertion.

Compère reported a single infection in 400 continuous popliteal sciatic nerve blocks (0.25%),[139] while Volk and coworkers from the German regional anesthesia network reported in 2009 a 1.3% incidence of infectious complications for peripheral blocks in 3724 procedures compared to a higher rate for neuraxial techniques (2.7% in 5057 procedures).[140]

Between 2002 and 2009, Reisig[141] and coworkers collected data on 10,549 peripheral catheter procedures in an observations study that included the implementation of a comprehensive infection control bundle. While the definitions of inflammation and infection used in this study remain somewhat vague, they could show a rate of 4.2% for inflammation and 3.2% for infections in 3491 procedures before the intervention and a reduction to 2.6% for inflammation and 0.9% for infections in 7053 procedures after the interventions.

Other reports included cases of osteomyelitis following digital blocks[141] and hematoma block for fracture repair,[142] as well as orbital cellulites from sub-Tenon anesthesia,[143,144] mediastinitis following continuous interscalene block,[145] Aspergillus caldioustus infection after unspecified lower back nerve block,[146] and two cases with sepsis after femoral nerve catheters.[147]

All these reports emphasize the importance of maintaining strict asepsis when performing continuing peripheral nerve blocks.

TABLE 16–4. Infections associated with subarachnoid neural blockade.

Author (Reference)	Year Indication	Indication	Type of Infection	Incubation Period	Signs and Symptoms	Microorganism	Outcome	Comments
Corbett and Rosenstein[96]	1971	1. Vaginal delivery	Meningitis	36 h	Fever, headache, stiff neck	*Pseudomonas aeruginosa*	Full recovery	Three patients infected when a physician rinsed the spinal needle stylet in saline used for consecutive deliveries
		2. Vaginal delivery	Meningitis	3 days	Fever, headache, stiff neck, neck pain, nuchal rigidity	*P. aeruginosa*	Full recovery	
		3. Vaginal delivery	Meningitis	4 days	Fever, headache, nausea	*P. aeruginosa*	Full recovery	
Siegel et al[97]	1974	Vaginal delivery	Left subgluteal abscess	4 h	Buttock pain radiating to thigh	Mimeae	Full recovery	
				14 days	Severe pain sacroiliac joint			
Loarie and Fairley[13]	1978	Debride necrotic heel ulcers	Epidural abscess	2 days	Fever, back pain, urinary retention	*Staphylococcus epidermidis, Bacteroides*	Full recovery	Insulin-dependent diabetic
				15 days	Bilateral lower extremity weakness, absent anal sphincter tone			
Berman and Eisele[14]	1978	Transurethral evacuation of clot from bladder	Meningitis	1 h	Shaking chill, fever, back pain, headache, confusion	*Enterococcus*	Not specified	

(continued)

TABLE 16–4. Infections associated with subarachnoid neural blockade. (*Continued*)

Author (Reference)	Year Indication	Indication	Type of Infection	Incubation Period	Signs and Symptoms	Microorganism	Outcome	Comments
Beaudoin and Klein[98]	1984	Debride and drain infected foot	Epidural abscess	4 days after last subarachnoid neural blockade	Back pain, pain radiating to upper thighs	*Pseudomonas* spp.	Full recovery	35-year-old insulin-dependent diabetic, received 5 subarachnoid neural blockades in 10 days
Abdel-Magid and Kotb[99]	1990	Hemorrhoidectomy	Epidural abscess	15 days	Back pain, leg weakness, urinary retention, fever, bilateral absent ankle reflexes	*Proteus* spp.	Full recovery	
Roberts and Petts[100]	1990	Remove retained placenta	Meningitis	18 h	Headache, photophobia, fever, chills, positive Kernig sign, quadriceps weakness	Culture negative	Full recovery	Antibiotics started before the lumbar puncture
Lee and Parry[101]	1991	Cesarean section	Meningitis	16 h	Severe headache	Culture negative	Full recovery	
				22 h	Nausea, photophobia, decreasing mental status, fever, nuchal rigidity, positive Kernig sign			
Blackmore et al[102]	1993	Herniorrhaphy	Meningitis and bacteremia	16 h	Fever, vomiting, obtundation	*Streptococcus mitis*	Full recovery	
Ezri et al[103]	1994	Hemorrhoidectomy	Meningitis	10 days	Fever	*Escherichia coli*	Full recovery	
				25 days	Malaise, headache, photophobia, dizziness, fever			

(continued)

Study	Year	Procedure	Complication	Onset	Signs/symptoms	Organism	Outcome	Comments
Mahendru et al[104]	1994	Foot amputation	Epidural abscess	3 weeks	Back pain, bilateral lower extremity paresis and weakness	No culture obtained	Died from esophageal carcinoma	Insulin-dependent diabetic
Gebhard and Brugman[105]	1994	Knee arthroscopy	Diskitis	2 months	Back and thigh pain, elevated sedimentation rate	Propionibacterium acnes	Full recovery	
Newton et al[106]	1994	Vaginal delivery	Meningitis	12 h	Headache, photophobia, declining mental status, fever	Streptococcus salivarius	Full recovery	
Schneeberger et al[19]	1996	1. Knee arthroscopy	Meningitis	12 h	Fever, meningeal signs	Streptococcus sanguis	Full recovery	
		2. Knee arthroscopy	Meningitis	12 h / 2 days	Headache / Fever, meningeal signs	S. mitis	Full recovery	
		3. Varicose vein stripping	Meningitis	24 h	Headache, fever, impaired consciousness, meningeal signs	S. salivarius	Full recovery	
		4. Varicose vein stripping	Meningitis	12 h	Headache, fever	Streptococcus cremoris	Communicating hydrocephalus	
Horlocker et al[109]	1997	1. Urologic procedure	Disk space infection	1 day / 4 months	Low back pain / Incapacitating low back pain	Staphylococcus aureus	Full recovery	
		2. Examination under anesthesia	Paraspinal abscess	1 day / 11 days	Low back pain / Fever	S. aureus	Full recovery	Hydrocephalus may have been preexisting

TABLE 16–4. Infections associated with subarachnoid neural blockade. (*Continued*)

Author (Reference)	Year Indication	Indication	Type of Infection	Incubation Period	Signs and Symptoms	Microorganism	Outcome	Comments
Kaiser et al[107]	1997	Hysterectomy	Meningitis	12 h	High fever, severe headache, lumbar pain, lethargy, Glasgow score of 12, nuchal rigidity, positive Kernig and Brudzinski signs	*S. salivarius*	Full recovery	
Laurila et al[73]	1998	Arthroscopy	Meningitis	16 h	Headache, nausea, vomiting	*S. salivarius*	Full recovery	Anesthesiologist wore mask and gloves and used chlorhexidine-alcohol solution for skin preparation
Fernandez et al[108]	1999	Arthroscopic meniscectomy	Meningitis	18 h	Severe headache, nausea, vomiting, high fever, nuchal rigidity	*S. mitis*	Full recovery	
Yaniv and Potasman[95]	2000	Extracorporeal shock wave lithotripsy for ureterolithiasis	Meningitis	12 h	Fever, severe headache, meningeal signs, elevated white blood cell count	*S. salivarius*	Minor sequelae, mild paresthesia of right thigh	Anesthesiologist wore gown, sterile gloves, face mask
Trautmann et al[8]	2002	Arthroscopic knee repair	Meningitis	1 day	Fever, nausea, stiff neck	*S. salivarius*	Full recovery	Both patients underwent their operations the same day
		Arthroscopic knee repair	Meningitis	1 day	Headache, nausea, stiff neck	*S. salivarius*	Full recovery	

Rubin et al[10]	2007	6 surgical cases	Meningitis	NS	Fever, stiff neck	S. salivarius	Full recovery	Single anesthesiologist with possible violation of aseptic technique
Cervero[111]	2009	Surgery	Meningitis	NS	NS	S. salivarius	NS	
CDC[11]	2010	Intrapartum (6 cases)	Meningitis	NS	NS	S. salivarius	Full recovery	Not wearing a mask in 5 cases
Hadzic et al[110]	2012	Orthopedic surgery	Meningitis	1 day	Headache, fever	ESBL Serratia marcescens	Full recovery	Multiresistant organisms need to be considered for empiric treatment depending on local endemic situation
Kundra et al[112]	2012	Cesarean delivery	Necrotizing fasciitis	5 days	Skin necrosis from puncture site to the gluteal region	NS	Full recovery	Reused contaminated multidose vial as likely cause
Pitkänen et al[113]	2013	Knee arthroscopy	Cerebral and spinal abscesses	2 months	Headache, stiff neck	NS	Death	
		Knee surgery	Meningitis	NS	NS	NS	Full recovery	
		Phimosis	Meningitis	NS	NS	NS	Full recovery	
		Knee arthroscopy	Meningitis	NS	NS	NS	Full recovery	
		Prostate hyperplasia	Meningitis	NS	NS	NS	Full recovery	
		Knee arthroscopy	Meningitis	NS	NS	NS	Full recovery	

Source: Adapted with permission from Mayhall CG: *Hospital Epidemiology and Infection Control*, 3rd ed. Philadelphia: Lippincott, Williams and Wilkins; 2004.

TABLE 16–5. Frequency of meningitis after subarachnoid neural blockade.

Author (Reference)	Year	Number of Patients	Number of Infections	Rate of Meningitis
Evans[116]	1945	2500	0	0
Scarborough[117]	1958	5000	0	0
Dripps and Vandam[118]	1954	8460	0	0
Moore and Bridenbaugh[119]	1966	11,574	0	0
Lund and Cwik[120]	1968	>21,000	0	0
Sadove et al[121]	1961	>20,000	3	≈15/100,000
Arner[122]	1952	21,230	1	4.7/100,000
Horlocker et al[109]	1997	4217	0	0
Auroy et al[81]	2002	5640 obstetrical	0	0
Auroy et al[81]	2002	35,439 nonobstetrical	1	2.8/100,000
Pugely et al[123]	2013	6030 Total knee replacements	?	0
Total		>141,090	5	≈3.5/100,000

Source: Adapted with permission from Mayhall CG: *Hospital Epidemiology and Infection Control*, 3rd ed. Philadelphia: Lippincott, Williams and Wilkins; 2004.

PREVENTION OF INFECTIONS ASSOCIATED WITH REGIONAL ANESTHESIA

Anesthesiologists disagree about the necessity of certain infection control precautions.[148–154] For example, several surveys indicated that only 50%–66% of anesthesia staff wore masks when performing epidural and subarachnoid neural blockades.[155–157]

Clinical Pearls

- Wearing a mask during insertion of indwelling neuraxial or peripheral nerve catheters is suggested.
- Sterile gown should be warn during insertion of epidural or nerve block catheters.
- Sterile ultrasound transducer cover should be routinely used with ultrasound-guided procedures.
- Surveillance for catheter site infections is one of the most effective methods for reducing the incidence and consequence of indwelling catheter–related infections.

The review of studies on infections associated with epidural anesthesia indicated that there is no consensus regarding patient risk factors for infectious complications of epidural neural blockade.[133] Few studies assess risk factors for infection associated with epidural or subarachnoid neural blockades, possibly in part because these infections are uncommon. In fact, only one case-control study was performed to evaluate risk factors for infections associated with epidural neural blockade.[158] Dawson and colleagues evaluated epidural neural blockades performed for postoperative pain relief and found that

procedures done between April and August had a sixfold higher risk than those done during other months (95% CI 1.28–28.12, p = .009). The risk of infection was lower if a bag rather than a syringe was used to administer the anesthetic agent (odds ratio 0.17, 95% CI 0.02–1.34, p = .05). Of the two risk factors identified by this study, only the latter, use of syringes, could be addressed by practice changes.

Assuming that the respiratory tract of anesthesia personnel could be a source of infection, Philips and associates conducted a simulation to assess the efficacy of masks.[159] They seated anesthesia staff with and without masks in a room with controlled environment and asked them to speak in front of blood agar plates placed 30 cm away. The number of bacteria on the plates was significantly lower when masks were worn. However, the clinical significance of this finding is unknown.

Chlorhexidine has been shown to reduce the risk of catheter-associated bloodstream infections significantly compared with povidone-iodine.[160] Several investigators have tried to determine whether a particular disinfectant provides more effective skin antisepsis before epidural neural blocks than do other agents.[161–164] However, none of the studies was large enough to assess rates of infection; instead, the outcomes evaluated were catheter or skin colonization.

Kasuda and colleagues randomly assigned 70 patients to have their skin prepared with either a 0.5% alcoholic solution of chlorhexidine or 10% povidone-iodine.[162] After a median of 49 ± 7 hours, the investigators removed the catheters and obtained cultures of the insertion sites and catheter tips. There was no difference in rates of positive cultures.

Kinirons and associates (the only investigators who reported a power calculation) obtained cultures from catheters removed from 96 children who had epidural catheters longer

TABLE 16–6. Infections associated with combined subarachnoid and epidural neural blockade.

Author (Reference)	Year	Indication	Type of Infection	Time of Symptom Onset	Signs and Symptoms	Microorganism	Outcome	Comments
Cascio and Heath[124]	1995	Vaginal delivery	Meningitis	16 h after delivery, ≈ 20 h after insertion	Fever, headache, chills, photophobia, mild nuchal rigidity	*Streptococcus salivarius*	Full recovery	Anesthesiologist wore mask, cap, and sterile gloves and used povidone-iodine spray for skin antisepsis
Harding et al[125]	1994	1. Vaginal delivery	Aseptic meningitis	21 h after the injection	Severe headache, faint feeling, shortness of breath, urinary retention, aphasia, tingling right side of face, neck stiffness, positive Kernig sign, low-grade temperature	No growth	Full recovery	Anesthesiologist scrubbed, wore sterile gown and gloves, and used alcoholic chlorhexidine for skin antisepsis
		2. Vaginal delivery converted to emergency cesarean section	Meningitis	3 days after the operation	Headache, fever, vomiting, severe stiff neck, elevated white blood cell count, hypotension, bradycardia	*Staphylococcus epidermidis*	Full recovery	Alcoholic chlorhexidine used for skin antisepsis
Stallard and Barry[126]	1994	Analgesia during labor, subsequent cesarean section	Meningitis	18 h after the operation	Acute confusion, fever, aphasia, ignored left side, elevated white blood cell count	No growth	Full recovery	Did three procedures to achieve adequate analgesia; anesthesiologist used alcoholic chlorhexidine for skin antisepsis and wore mask, gown, and gloves

(continued)

CHAPTER 16

TABLE 16–6. Infections associated with combined subarachnoid and epidural neural blockade. (Continued)

Author (Reference)	Year	Indication	Type of Infection	Time of Symptom Onset	Signs and Symptoms	Microorganism	Outcome	Comments
Aldebert and Sleth[127]	1996	Vaginal delivery	Meningitis	8 h after puncture	Headache, nausea, fever, agitation, nuchal rigidity, positive Babinski sign	Nonhemolytic streptococcus	Full recovery	Anesthesiologist wore mask, gown, cap, and sterile gloves
Dysart and Balakrishnan[128]	1997	Cesarean section	Epidural abscess	9 days after the operation	Backache, fever, foot drop, weakness of ankle eversion and inversion, absent ankle jerk reflex, decreased pinprick sensation from L5 to perianal region, elevated erythrocyte sedimentation rate	Staphylococcus aureus	Nearly full recovery; patient had residual numbness in L5 distribution	Anesthesiologist wore a mask, gown, and gloves and used chlorhexidine for skin antisepsis
Schroter et al[129]	1997	Anesthesia for vascular surgery	Epidural abscess	1 day after procedure	Back pain, fever, slight nuchal rigidity, erythema and induration at puncture site and purulent drainage from puncture site, elevated white blood cell count	S. aureus	Full recovery	Anesthesiologist wore a mask, surgical hood, sterile gloves, and gown and used povidone-iodine for skin antisepsis
Bouhemad et al[130]	1998	Cesarean section	Meningitis	14 h after delivery	Fever, severe headache, photophobia, drowsiness, stiff neck, positive Kernig sign	S. salivarius	Full recovery	Anesthesiologist wore gown, gloves, face mask, and cap and used tincture of iodine for skin antisepsis
Rathmell et al[114]	2000	Labor analgesia in patient with multiple trauma	Epidural abscess	7 days after catheter placement	Back pain, purulent discharge from insertion site	S. aureus	Full recovery	

Phillips et al[62]	2002	Surgical anesthesia and postoperative analgesia	Epidural abscess Ll–L2	Day 6	Discomfort at the epidural site and severe radicular pain in L2 dermatome, erythema and swelling at site, decreased strength, light touch, and pinprick, and loss of ankle jerk reflex	S. aureus	Discharged from hospital 3 months after first operation	Anesthesiologist wore a cap, gown, and sterile gloves and used 10% povidone-iodine for skin antisepsis
Sandkovsky et al[131]	2009	Delivery	Meningitis	NS	NS	Streptococcus spp.	NS	
Pitkänen et al[113]	2013	Total hip arthroplasty	Epidural abscess	NS	NS	NS	Full recovery	

Source: Adapted with permission from Mayhall CG: *Hospital Epidemiology and Infection Control*, 3rd ed. Philadelphia: Lippincott, Williams and Wilkins; 2004

than 24 hours.[163] The colonization rate was lower for catheters removed from children whose skin was prepared with a 0.5% alcoholic solution of chlorhexidine (1/52 catheters, 0.9/100 catheter-days) than for those removed from children whose skin was prepared with povidone-iodine (5/44 catheters, 5.6/100 catheter-days) (relative risk 0.2, 95% CI 0.1–1.0).

Sato and coworkers enrolled 60 patients who were undergoing back operations under general anesthesia.[164] After preparing the site with either 0.5% alcoholic chlorhexidine or 10% povidone-iodine, the investigators obtained skin biopsies. Cultures from skin prepared with the alcoholic chlorhexidine were less likely to be positive (5.7%) than were cultures from skin prepared with povidone-–iodine (32.4%; $p < .01$). However, microscopy was as likely to identify bacteria in the hair follicles of skin prepared with the alcoholic solution of chlorhexidine (14.3%) as skin prepared with povidone-iodine (11.8%).

This has led to the recommendation to use alcoholic chlorhexidine for skin preparation despite some concerns about potential neurotoxicity. The latter might be the reason American Society of Anesthesiologists (ASA) members were equivocal on the issue during the consensus process, while external experts were in favor of the recommendation.

Sviggum et al published the experiences from the Mayo Clinic analyzing almost 12,000 spinal anesthetics between 2006 and 2010 that used alcoholic chlorhexidine.[165] They did not observe any change in neurological complications, considering the practice to be safe. Unfortunately, no data about infectious complications were reported.

The safety of alcoholic chlorhexidine was underlined in an experimental study by Doan and coworkers. They found damage to neuronal cell cultures with chlorhexidine as well as with 10% iodine they could also show that a relevant toxic concentration of skin disinfectants cannot be reached if the puncture is performed through dry skin.[166] Therefore, allowing the skin to completely dry once disinfected before performing the block is more important than the choice of the solution in order to prevent any neurotoxic effect.

Malhotra et al[167] demonstrated in a study of 309 healthy volunteers that single application of 0.5% chlorhexidine gluconate in 70% ethanol was as effective as two applications.

The fact that infections rarely complicate neuraxial blockades suggests that the infection control practices used for these procedures are usually adequate. Given the very low rates of infection associated with epidural and subarachnoid neural blockade, it will be difficult to prove that additional infection control practices such as wearing masks and using full barrier precautions (ie, the anesthesiologist wears a cap, mask, sterile gloves, and sterile gown and uses a large drape to cover the patient) reduce the risk of infection. However, bacteria that colonize the skin, respiratory tract, or water caused most reported infections after epidural and subarachnoid neural blockades. Masks have been shown to decrease spread of organisms when anesthesiologists are talking.[159] Thus, a mask would allow the anesthesiologist to talk to the patient while doing the procedure and could decrease the risk of contaminating the insertion site with oral or respiratory flora. This has also been incorporated in the ASA "Practice Advisory for the Prevention, Diagnosis, and Management of Infectious Complications Associated With Neuraxial Techniques."[168]

Furthermore, epidural and subarachnoid neural blockades are at least as invasive as placing central venous catheters, and the consequences of subsequent infections are at least as bad as those for catheter-associated bloodstream infections. Because the use of full barrier precautions reduces the incidence of catheter-related bloodstream infections,[169] aseptic measures similar to those used for placing central venous catheters should be used during the placement of catheters that will remain in place for several days or longer.[75] While the ASA practice advisory still uses the term *hand washing* before putting on sterile gown and gloves, hand disinfection with an alcoholic hand rub (with 70% alcohol) is the internationally preferred standard.[4,170]

Anesthesia personnel should observe their patients closely for signs and symptoms of infection so that infections can be diagnosed and treated immediately. Pegues and coworkers reviewed medical records from 1980 to 1992 of patients who had short-term epidural catheters to identify those who acquired infections. They followed patients prospectively from January 1993 until June 1993.[170] In 1990, they introduced a standardized procedure for inspecting temporary epidural catheters. During the entire 12.5-year period, the investigators identified seven infections, all of which occurred after catheters were inspected routinely. The increased incidence of infection could have resulted from ascertainment or misclassification bias associated with the retrospective review or from increased use of epidural catheters for pain management during the later time period. On the other hand, it could indicate that infections were not diagnosed when catheters were not inspected routinely for signs of infection.

Because it may be difficult to draw up opioids in a sterile manner from ampoules, some have suggested that these drugs be drawn through a filter into a syringe, which is then double wrapped and sterilized in ethylene oxide.[171] However, the benefit of such extreme precautions is highly hypothetical.

Brooks and coworkers were among the first to implement and report on structured infection control measures for continuous neuraxial blocks in their hospital.[88] In 2008, we reviewed the literature and compared the infection control recommendations of the ASRA and the German Society of Anesthesiology and Intensive Care (DGAI)[172] and noticed some discrepancies, especially regarding the use of masks and gowns or filters. In 2010, new guidelines by the ASA were developed in a consensus process among ASA members and external experts to clarify some of the issues. However, the evidence supporting many of the recommendations remains sparse, and extrapolation from other areas of practical implementation of infection control is needed.

The ASA "Practice Advisory for the Prevention, Diagnosis, and Management of Infectious Complications Associated With Neuraxial Techniques"[168] has published the following guidelines for the placement of neuraxial blocks:

- Before performing neuraxial techniques, a history and physical examination relevant to the procedure and review of relevant laboratory studies should be conducted to identify patients who may be at risk of infectious complications. Consider alternatives to neuraxial techniques for patients at high risk.
- When neuraxial techniques are indicated in a known or suspected bacteremic patient, consider administering preprocedure antibiotic therapy.

- Selection of neuraxial technique should be determined on a case-by-case basis, including consideration of the evolving medical status of the patient.
- Lumbar puncture should be avoided in the patient with a known epidural abscess.
- Aseptic techniques should always be used during the preparation of equipment (eg, ultrasound) and the placement of neuraxial needles and catheters, including the following:
  - Removal of jewelry (eg, rings and watches); hand washing; and wearing of caps, masks (covering both mouth and nose and consider changing before each new case), and sterile gloves
  - Use of individual packets of antiseptics for skin preparation
  - Use of chlorhexidine (preferably with alcohol) for skin preparation, allowing for adequate drying time
- Sterile draping of the patient.
- Use of sterile occlusive dressings at the catheter insertion site.
- Bacterial filters may be considered during extended continuous epidural infusion.

- Limit the disconnection and reconnection of neuraxial delivery systems to minimize the risk of infectious complications.
- Consider removing unwitnessed accidentally disconnected catheters.

Catheters should not remain in situ longer than clinically necessary.

The following recommendations are given for the diagnosis and management of infectious complications after neuraxial block:

- Daily evaluation of patients with indwelling catheters for early signs and symptoms (eg, fever, backache, headache, erythema, and tenderness at the insertion site) of infectious complications should be performed throughout the patients' stay in the facility.
- To minimize the impact of an infectious complication, promptly attend to signs or symptoms.
- If an infection is suspected:
  - Remove an in situ catheter and consider culturing the catheter tip.

TABLE 16–7. Summary of recommendations for infection control practice.

	Single-Shot PNB	Continuous Catheter PNB	Single-Shot Neuraxial Block	Continuous Neuraxial Catheter	Long-Term Implanted Device/ Catheter (eg, Intrathecal Pump)
2% chlorhexidine in 70% alcohol skin prep[a]	+	+	+	+	+
Small sterile drape	(+)		+		
Large sterile drape		+		+	+
Sterile gloves	+	+	+	+	+
Sterile gown		+ (especially for stimulating catheters)		(+)	+
Mask		+	+	+	+
Hair cover		+	+	+	+
Prophylactic antibiotics	−	−	−	−	+ single perioperative dose
Filter on injection/infusion system	−	(+)	−	(+)	NA
OR or special procedure room					+
Tunneling of catheter		+ (to prevent dislocation)		+ if used for more than 3 days	
Preparation of injection/ infusion solution under sterile conditions (pharmacy)		(+) for continuous infusion		(+) for continuous infusion	

+ strongly recommended; (+) consider; − not recommended; NA = not applicable; PNB = peripheral nerve block.
[a]Alternatively, 10% povidone-iodine or 80% alcohol or a mixture of 70%–80% alcohol with povidone-iodine for at least 3 minutes. Choice of agent also depends on type of block (eg, eye blocks, etc.).

- Order appropriate blood tests.
- Obtain appropriate cultures.
- If an abscess is suspected or neurologic dysfunction is present, imaging studies should be performed, and consultation with other appropriate specialties should be promptly obtained.
- Appropriate antibiotic therapy should always be administered at the earliest sign or symptom of a serious neuraxial infection.
- Consultation with a physician with expertise in the diagnosis and treatment of infectious diseases should be considered.

However, guidelines and standard operating procedures alone are not enough to ensure proper aseptic technique. Friedman and coworkers showed in a videotape analysis of 35 epidural placements by second-year residents a significant increase in manual skills with growing experience, but there was no increase in aseptic technique.[173] This highlights the need for a special focus on aseptic technique in residency and during infection control audits of anesthesia providers.

PERIPHERAL BLOCKS AND PERIPHERAL CONTINUOUS CATHETERS

Recent studies indicated that infection control protocols similar to the recommendations for neuraxial block can reduce the incidence of infectious complications associated with placement of continuous peripheral nerve catheters.[174] Unfortunately, the effectiveness of each step is hard to assess, a problem familiar from all the other recommended approaches in infection control, such as the ones for prevention of central line–associated bloodstream infections[175] or ventilator-associated pneumonia.[176]

With the increasing use of real-time ultrasound, the correct handling of the ultrasound probe becomes an additional concern. To maintain the aseptic field, the cable and the probe should be covered with a sterile sheath to avoid contamination in the case of needle contact. Sterile contact gel or sterile saline should be used within the sheath. Puncture aids fixating the needle to the probe must be sterile.[4] After the procedure, ultrasound probes need to be cleaned removing any residual gel and disinfected with an appropriate disinfectant that cannot damage the probe. Alternative techniques using ultraviolet light to disinfect ultrasound probes are under investigation.[177,178]

SUMMARY

Although rare, infectious complications from regional anesthesia and analgesia do occur and can be serious. Recent guidelines offer practice recommendations especially for neuraxial blocks. Table 16–7 summarizes the key recommendations for decreasing the risk of infections related to regional anesthesia procedures. Surveillance systems should be implemented as part of national quality assurance programs to allow benchmarking and process optimization as well as providing data from large population databases, which would be beneficial in addressing some of the unanswered questions about infections after regional anesthesia procedures.

REFERENCES

1. Schulz-Stübner S, Kelley J: Regional Anesthesia Surveillance System: first experiences with a quality assessment tool for regional anesthesia and analgesia. Acta Anesthesiol Scand 2007;51:305–315.
2. Barrington MJ, Watts SA, Gledhill SR, et al: Preliminary results of the Australasian Regional Anesthesia Collaboration: a prospective audit of more than 7000 peripheral nerve blocks for neurologic and other complications. Reg Anesth Pain Med 2009;34:534–541.
3. Liu SS, Wu CL, Ballantyne JC, et al: Where in the world is ASRA Acute POP? Reg Anesth Pain Med 2009;34:269–274.
4. Schulz-Stübner S, Czaplik M. Quality management in regional anesthesia using the example of the Regional Anesthesia Surveillance System (RASS). Schmerz 2013;27:56–66.
5. Lee JS, Hayanga AJ, Kubus JJ, et al: Local anesthesia: A strategy for reducing surgical site infections. World J Surg 2011;35:2596–2602.
6. Loftus R, Brown JR, Koff M, et al: Multiple reservoirs contribute to intraoperative bacterial transmission. Anesth Analg 2012;114. 1236–1248.
7. North JB, Brophy BP: Epidural abscess: A hazard of spinal epidural anaesthesia. Aust N Z J Surg 1979;49:484–485.
8. Trautmann M, Lepper PM, Schmitz FJ: Three cases of bacterial meningitis after spinal and epidural anesthesia. Eur J Clin Microbiol Infect Dis 2002;21:43–45.
9. Schneeberger PM, Janssen M, Voss A: Alpha-hemolytic streptococci: A major pathogen of iatrogenic meningitis following lumbar puncture. Case reports and a review of the literature. Infection 1996;24: 29–33.
10. Rubin L, Sprecher H, Kabaha A, et al: Meningitis following spinal anesthesia: 6 cases in 5 years. Infect Control Hosp Epidemiol 2007; 28:1187–1190.
11. Centers for Disease Control and Prevention (CDC): Bacterial meningitis after intrapartum anesthesia—New York and Ohio, 2008–2009. MMWR Morb Mortal Wkly Rep 2010;29:65–69.
12. Baker AS, Ojemann RG, Swartz MN, et al: Spinal epidural abscess. N Engl J Med 1975;293:463–468.
13. Loarie DJ, Fairley HB: Epidural abscess following spinal anesthesia. Anesth Analg 1978;57:351–353.
14. Berman RS, Eisele JH: Bacteremia, spinal anesthesia, and development of meningitis. Anesthesiology 1978;48:376–377.
15. Pinczower GR, Gyorke A: Vertebral osteomyelitis as a cause of back pain after epidural anesthesia. Anesthesiology 1996;84:215–217.
16. Wulf H, Striepling E: Postmortem findings after epidural anaesthesia. Anaesthesia 1990;45:357–361.
17. Bengtsson M, Nettelblad H, Sjoberg F: Extradural catheter-related infections in patients with infected cutaneous wounds. Br J Anaesth 1997;79:668–670.
18. Newman B: Extradural catheter-related infections in patients with infected cutaneous wounds. Br J Anaesth 1998;80:566.
19. Gritsenko K, Marcello D, Liguori GA, et al: Meningitis or epidural abscess after neuraxial block for removal of infected hip or knee prosthesis. Br J Anesth 2012;108:485–490.
20. Schmidt RM, Rosenkranz HS: Antimicrobial activity of local anesthetics: Lidocaine and procaine. J Infect Dis 1970;121:597–607.
21. Berry CB, Gillespie T, Hood J, et al: Growth of microorganisms in solutions of intravenous anaesthetic agents. Anaesthesia 1993;48: 30–32.
22. Sosis M, Braverman B: Growth of *Staphylococcus aureus* in four intravenous anesthetics. Anesth Analg 1993;77:766–768.
23. Wong MR, Del Rosso P, Heine L, et al: An outbreak of *Klebsiella pneumoniae* and *Enterobacter aerogenes* bacteremia after interventionsal pain management procedures. New York City 2008. Reg Anesth Pain Med 2010;35:496–499.
24. Kauffmann CA, Pappas PG, Patterson TF: Fungal infections associated with contaminated methylprednisolone infections—preliminary report. NEJM 2012. doi:10.1056/NEJMra1212617.
25. James FM, George RH, Naiem H, et al: Bacteriologic aspects of epidural analgesia. Anesth Analg 1976;55:187–190.
26. Shapiro JM, Bond EL, Garman JK: Use of a chlorhexidine dressing to reduce microbial colonization of epidural catheters. Anesthesiology 1990;73:625–631.
27. Barreto RS: Bacteriological culture of indwelling epidural catheters. Anesthesiology 1962;23:643–646.
28. Hunt JR, Rigor BM, Collins JR: The potential for contamination of continuous epidural catheters. Anesth Analg 1977;56:222–225.

Infection Control in Regional Anesthesia **249**

CHAPTER 16

29. Ross RM, Burday M, Baker T: Contamination of single dose of bupivacaine vials used repeatedly in the same patient [Abstract]. Anesth Analg 1992;74:S257.
30. Raedler C, Lass-Florl C, Puhringer F, et al: Bacterial contamination of needles used for spinal and epidural anaesthesia. Br J Anaesth 1999;83: 657–658.
31. Edwards WB, Hingson RA: The present status of continuous caudai analgesia in obstetrics. N Y Acad Med Bull 1943;19:507–518.
32. Ferguson JF, Kirsch WM: Epidural empyema following thoracic extradural block. Case report. J Neurosurg 1974;41:762–764.
33. Saady A: Epidural abscess complicating thoracic epidural analgesia. Anesthesiology 1976;44:244–246.
34. Wenningsted-Torgard K, Heyn J, Willumsen L: Spondylitis following epidural morphine. Acta Anaesth Scand 1982;26:649–651.
35. McDonogh AJ, Cranney BS: Delayed presentation of an epidural abscess. Anaesth Intensive Care 1984;12:364–365.
36. Konig HJ, Schleep J, Krahling KH: Ein Fall von Querschnittsyndrom nach Kontamination eines Periduralkatheters. Reg Anaesth 1985;8: 60–62.
37. Sollman W-P, Gaab MR, Panning B: Lumbales epidurales Hämatom und spinaler Abszess nach Periduralanästhesie. Reg Anaesth 1987;10: 121–124.
38. Fine PG, Hare BD, Zahniser JC: Epidural abscess following epidural catheterization in a chronic pain patient: A diagnostic dilemma. Anesthesiology 1988;69:422–424.
39. Ready LB, Helfer D: Bacterial meningitis in parturients after epidural anesthesia. Anesthesiology 1989;71:988–990.
40. Berga S, Trierweiler MW: Bacterial meningitis following epidural anesthesia for vaginal delivery: A case report. Obstet Gynecol 1989; 74:437–439.
41. Goucke CR, Graziotti P: Extradural abscess following local anaesthetic and steroid injection for chronic low back pain. Br J Anaesth 1990;65: 427–429.
42. Lynch J, Zech D: Spondylitis without epidural abscess formation following short-term use of an epidural catheter. Acta Anaesthesiol Scand 1990;34:167–170.
43. Strong WE: Epidural abscess associated with epidural catheterization: A rare event? Report of two cases with markedly delayed presentation. Anesthesiology 1991;74:943–946.
44. Klygis LM, Reisberg BE: Spinal epidural abscess caused by group G streptococci. Am J Med 1991;91:89–90.
45. Dawson P, Rosenfeld JV, Murphy MA, et al: Epidural abscess associated with postoperative epidural analgesia. Anesth Intens Care 1991;19: 569–591.
46. Ferguson CC: Infection and the epidural space: A case report. AANA J 1992;60:393–396.
47. NganKee WD, Jones MR, Thomas P, et al: Epidural abscess complicating extradural anaesthesia for caesarean section. Br J Anaesth 1992;69: 647–652.
48. Sowter MC, Burgess NA, Woodsford PV, et al: Delayed presentation of an extradural abscess complicating thoracic extradural analgesia. Br J Anaesth 1992;68:103–105.
49. Shintani S, Tanaka H, Irifune A, et al: Iatrogenic acute spinal epidural abscess with septic meningitis: MR findings. Clin Neurol Neurosurg 1992;94:253–255.
50. Nordstrom O, Sandin R: Delayed presentation of an extradural abscess in a patient with alcohol abuse. Br J Anaesth 1993;70:368–369.
51. Davis L, Hargreaves C, Robinson PN: Postpartum meningitis. Anaesthesia 1993;48:788–789.
52. Ania BJ: *Staphylococus aureus* meningitis after short-term epidural analgesia. Clin Infect Dis 1994;18:844–845.
53. Borum SE, McLeskey CH, Williamson JB, et al: Epidural abscess after obstetric epidural analgesia. Anesthesiology 1995;82:1523–1526.
54. Liu SS, Pope A: Spinal meningitis masquerading as postdural puncture headache [Letter]. Anesthesiology 1996;85:1493–1494.
55. Dunn LT, Javed A, Findlay G, et al: Iatrogenic spinal infection following epidural anaesthesia: case report. Eur Spine J 1996;5:418–420.
56. Cooper AB, Sharpe MD: Bacterial meningitis and cauda equina syndrome after epidural steroid injections. Can J Anaesth 1996;43: 471–475.
57. Barontini F, Conti P, Marello G, et al: Major neurological sequelae of lumbar epidural anesthesia. Report of three cases. Ital J Neurol Sci 1996; 17:333–339.
58. Sarrubi FA, Vasquez JE: Spinal epidural abscess associated with the use of temporary epidural catheters: Report of two cases and review. Clin Infect Dis 1997;25:1155–1158.

59. Iseki M, Okuno S, Tanabe Y, et al: Methicillin-resistant *Staphylococcus aureus* sepsis resulting from infection in paravertebral muscle after continuous epidural infusion for pain control in a patient with herpes zoster. Anesth Analg 1998;87:116–118.
60. O'Brien DPK, Rawluk DJR: Iatrogenic *Mycobacterium* infection after an epidural injection. Spine 1999;24:1257–1259.
61. Halkic N, Blanc C, Corthesy ME, et al: Lumbar spondylodiscitis after epidural anaesthesia at a distant site [Letter]. Anaesthesia 2001;56: 602–603.
62. Phillips JMG, Stedeford JC, Hartsilver E, et al: Epidural abscess complicating insertion of epidural catheters. Br J Anaesth 2002;89:778–782.
63. Royakkers AA, Willigers H, van der Ven AJ, et al: Catheter-related epidural abscesses—Don't wait for neurological deficits. Acta Anaesthesiol Scand 2002;46:611–61553.
64. Hagiwara N, Hata J, Takaba H, et al: Late onset of spinal epidural abscess after spinal epidural cathterization. No To Shinkei 2003;55: 633–636.
65. Evans PR, Misra U: Poor outcome following epidural abscess complicating epidural analgesia for labour. Eur J Obstet Gynecol Reprod Biol 2003;109:102–105.
66. Yue WM, Tan SB: Distant skip level discitis and vertebral osteomyelitis after caudal epidural injection: A case report of a rare complication of epidural injections. Spine 2003;11:E209–E211.
67. Aiba S, Odaka M, Hirata K: Case of spinal epidural abscess with wide lesion after epidural anesthesia. Brain Nerve 2009;61:614–615.
68. Radif A, Dalsgaard LB: Subcutaneous abscess following epidural catheterization. Ugeskr Laeger 2009;171:1938–1939.
69. Hagiwara N, Hata J, Takaba, et al: Late onset of spinal epidural abscess after spinal epidural catheterization.No To Shinkei 2003;55:633–636.
70. Mamourian AC, Dickman CA, Drayer BP, et al: Spinal epidural abscess: Three cases following spinal epidural injection demonstrated with magnetic resonance imaging. Anesthesiology 1993;78:204–207.
71. Tabo E, Ohkuma Y, Kimura S, et al: Successful percutaneous drainage of epidural abscess with epidural needle and catheter. Anesthesiology 1994; 80:1393–1395.
72. Wang JS, Fellows DG, Vakharia S, et al: Epidural abscess—Early magnetic resonance imaging detection and conservative therapy. Anesth Analg 1996;82:1069–1071.
73. Laurila JJ, Kostamovaara PA, Alahuhta S: *Streptococcus salivarius* meningitis after spinal anesthesia. Anesthesiology 1998;89:1579–1580.
74. Dawkins CJM: An analysis of the complications of extradural and caudal block. Anaesthesia 1969;24:554–563.
75. Dawson SJ: Epidural catheter infections. J Hosp Infect 2001;47:3–8.
76. Scott DB, Hibbard BM: Serious non-fatal complications associated with extradural block in obstetric practice. Br J Anaesth 1990;64:537–541.
77. Palot M, Visseaux H, Botmans C, et al: Epidemiologie des complications de l'analgesie peridurale obstetricale. Cah Anesthesiol 1994;42: 229–233.
78. Eisen SM, Rosen N, Winesanker H, et al: The routine use of lumbar epidural anaesthesia in obstetrics: A clinical review of 9,532 cases. Can Anaesth Soc J 1960;7:280–289.
79. Holdcroft A, Morgan M: Maternal complications of obstetric epidural analgesia. Anaesth Intens Care 1976;4:108–112.
80. Abouleish E, Amortegui AJ, Taylor FH: Are bacterial filters needed in continuous epidural analgesia for obstetrics? Anesthesiology 1977;46: 351–354.
81. Auroy Y, Benhamou D, Bargues L, et al: Major complications of regional anesthesia in France: The SOS Regional Anesthesia Hotline Service. Anesthesiology 2002;97:1274–1280.
82. Sethna NF, Berde CB, Wilder RT, et al: The risk of infection from pediatric epidural analgesia is low [Abstract]. Anesthesiology 1992;77(3A): A1158.
83. Darchy B, Forceville X, Bavoux E, et al: Clinical and bacteriologic survey of epidural analgesia in patients in the intensive care unit. Anesthesiology 1996;85:988–998.
84. McNeely JK, Trentadue NC, Rusy LM, et al: Culture of bacteria from lumbar and caudal epidural catheters used for postoperative analgesia in children. Reg Anesth 1997;22:428–431.
85. Abel MD, Horlocker TT, Messick JM, et al: Neurologic complications following placement of 4392 consecutive epidural catheters in anesthetized patients [Abstract]. Reg Anesth Pain Med 1998;23(Suppl 3):3.
86. Grass JA, Haider N, Group M, et al: Incidence of complications related to epidural catheterization and maintenance for postoperative analgesia [Abstract]. Reg Anesth Pain Med 1998;23:108.
87. Kost-Byerly S, Tobin JR, Greenberg RS, et al: Bacterial colonization and infection rate of continuous epidural catheters in children. Anesth Analg 1998;86:712–716.

88. Brooks K, Pasero C, Hubbard L, et al: The risk of infection associated with epidural analgesia. Infect Control Hosp Epidemiol 1995;16: 725–726.

89. Holt HM, Andersen SS, Andersen O, et al: Infections following epidural catheterization. J Hosp Infect 1995;30:253–260.

90. Holt HM, Gahrn-Hansen B, Andersen SS, et al: Infections following epidural catheters [Letter]. J Hosp Infect 1997;35:245.

91. Stafford MA, Wilder RT, Berde CB: The risk of infection from epidural analgesia in children: A review of 1620 cases. Anesth Analg 1995;80: 234–238.

92. Du Pen SL, Peterson DG, Williams A, et al: Infection during chronic epidural catheterization: Diagnosis and treatment. Anesthesiology 1990;73:905–909.

93. Zenz M, Piepenbrock S, Tryba M: Epidural opiates: Long-term experiences in cancer pain. Klin Wochenschr 1985;63:225–229.

94. Coombs DW: Management of chronic pain by epidural and intrathecal opioids: Newer drugs and delivery systems. Int Anesth Clin 1986;24: 59–74.

95. Yaniv LG, Potasman I: Iatrogenic meningitis: An increasing role for resistant viridans streptococci? Case report and review of the last 20 years. Scand J Infect Dis 2000;32:693–696.

96. Corbett JJ, Rosenstein BJ: *Pseudomonas* meningitis related to spinal anesthesia. Report of three cases with a common source. Neurology 1971;21:946–950.

97. Siegel RS, Alicandri FP, Jacoby AW: Subgluteal infection following regional anesthesia [Letter]. JAMA 1974;229:268.

98. Beaudoin MG, Klein L: Epidural abscess following multiple spinal anaesthetics. Anaesth Intens Care 1984;12:163–164.

99. Abdel-Magid RA, Kotb HI: Epidural abscess after spinal anesthesia: A favorable outcome. Neurosurgery 1990;27:310–311.

100. Roberts SP, Petts HV: Meningitis after obstetric spinal anaesthesia. Anaesthesia 1990;45:376–377.

101. Lee JJ, Parry H: Bacterial meningitis following spinal anaesthesia for caesarean section. Br J Anaesth 1991;66:383–386.

102. Blackmore TK, Morley HR, Gordon DL: *Streptococcus mitis*–induced bacteremia and meningitis after spinal anesthesia. Anesthesiology 1993;78:592–594.

103. Ezri T, Szmuk P, Guy M: Delayed-onset meningitis after spinal anesthesia [Letter]. Anesth Analg 1994;79:606–607.

104. Mahendru V, Bacon DR, Lema MJ: Multiple epidural abscesses and spinal anesthesia in a diabetic patient. Case report. Reg Anesth 1994;19: 66–68.

105. Gebhard JS, Brugman JL: Percutaneous disectomy for the treatment of bacterial discitis. Spine 1994;19:855–857.

106. Newton JA Jr, Lesnik IK, Kennedy CA: *Streptococcus salivarius* meningitis following spinal anesthesia [Letter]. Clin Infect Dis 1994;18:840–841.

107. Kaiser E, Suppini A, de Jaureguiberry JP, et al: Meningite aigue a *Streptococcus salivarius* après rachianesthesie. Ann Fr Anesth Reanim 1997;16:47–49.

108. Fernandez R, Paz I, Pazos C, et al: Meningitis producida por *Streptococcus mitis* tras anestesia intradural [Letter]. Enferm Infecc Microbiol Clin 1999;17:150.

109. Horlocker TT, McGregor DG, Matsushige DK, et al: A retrospective review of 4767 consecutive spinal anesthetics: Central nervous system complications. Perioperative Outcomes Group. Anesth Analg. 1997;84: 578–584.

110. Hadzic A, Koluder-Cimic N, Hadzovic-Cengic M, et al: *Serratia marcescens* meningitis following spinal anaesthesia and arthroscopy. Med Arh 2012;66(S1):54–55.

111. Cervero M: *Streptococcus salivarus* meningitis following subarachnoid anesthesia. Enferm Infecc Microbiol Clin 2009;27:371–372.

112. Kundra S, Singh RM, Grewal A, et al: Necrotizing fasciitis after spinal anesthesia. Acta Anesthesiol Scand 2013;257–261.

113. Pitkänen MT, Aromaa U, Cozanitis DA, et al: Serious complications associated with spinal and epidural anaesthesia in Finland from 2000–2009. Acta Anesthesiol Scand 2013;57:553–564. doi:10.1111/aas.12064.

114. Rathmell JP, Garahan MB, Alsofrom GF: Epidural abscess following epidural analgesia. Reg Anesth Pain Med 2000;25:79–82.

115. Herwaldt LA, Pottinger JM, Coffin SA, Schulz-Stübner S: Nosocomial infections associated with anesthesia. In Mayhall CG (ed): *Hospital Epidemiology and Infection Control*, 3rd ed. Lippincott, Williams and Wilkins, 2004, pp 1073–1117.

116. Evans FT: Sepsis and asepsis in spinal analgesia. Proc R Soc Med 1945;39:181–185.

117. Scarborough RA: Spinal anesthesia from the surgeon's standpoint. JAMA 1958;168:1324–1326.

118. Dripps RD, Vandam LD: Long-term follow-up of patients who received 10,098 spinal anesthetics. JAMA 1954;156:1486–1491.

119. Moore DC, Bridenbaugh LD: Spinal (subarachnoid) block. JAMA 1966;195:907–912.

120. Lund PC, Cwik JC: Modern trends in spinal anaesthesia. Can Anaesth Soc J 1968;15:118–134.

121. Sadove MS, Levin MJ, Rant-Sejdinaj I: Neurological complications of spinal anaesthesia. Can Anaesth Soc J 1961;8:405–416.

122. Arner O: Complications following spinal anesthesia. Their significance and a technique to reduce their incidence. Acta Chir Scand 1952;104:336–338.

123. Pugely AJ, Martin CT, Gao Y, et al: Differences in short-term complications between spinal and general anesthesia for primary total knee arthroplasty. J Bone Joint Surg Am 2013;95:193–199.

124. Cascio M, Heath G: Meningitis following a combined spinal-epidural technique in a labouring term parturient. Can J Anaesth 1996;43: 399–402.

125. Harding SA, Collis RE, Morgan BM: Meningitis after combined spinal-extradural anaesthesia in obstetrics. Br J Anaesth 1994;73: 545–547.

126. Stallard N, Barry P: Another complication of the combined extradural-subarachnoid technique [Letter]. Br J Anaesth 1995;75:370–371.

127. Aldebert S, Sleth JC: Meningite bacterienne après anesthesia rachidienne et peridurale combinee en obstetrie. Ann Fr Anesth Reanim 1996;15: 687–688.

128. Dysart RH, Balakrishnan V: Conservative management of extradural abscess complicating spinal-extradural anaesthesia for caesarean section. Br J Anaesth 1997;78:591–593.

129. Schroter J, Wa Djamba D, Hoffmann V, et al: Epidural abscess after combined spinal-epidural block. Can J Anaesth 1997;44:300–304.

130. Bouhemad B, Dounas M, Mercier FJ, et al: Bacterial meningitis following combined spinal-epidural analgesia for labour. Anaesthesia 1998;53:290–295.

131. Sandkovsky U, Mihu MR, Adeyeye A, et al: Iatrogenic meningitis in an obstetric patient after combined spinal-epidural analgesia: Case report and review of the literature. South Med J 2009;102:287–290.

132. Peng PW, Chan VW: Local and regional block in postoperative pain control. Surg Clin North Am 1999;79:345–370.

133. Graf BM, Martin E: Peripheral nerve block. An overview of new developments in an old technique [in German]. Anaesthesist 2001;50: 312–322.

134. Bergman BD, Hebl JR, Kent J, et al: Neurologic complications of 405 consecutive continuous axillary catheters. Anesth Analg 2003;96: 247–252.

135. Meier G, Bauereis C, Heinrich C: Interscalene brachial plexus catheter for anesthesia and postoperative pain therapy. Experience with a modified technique [in German]. Anaesthesist 1997;46:715–719.

136. Nseir S, Pronnier P, Soubrier S, et al: Fatal streptococcal necrotizing fasciitis as a complication of axillary brachial plexus block. Br J Anaesth 2004;92:427–429.

137. Adam F, Jaziri S, Chauvin M: Psoas abscess complicating femoral nerve block catheter. Anesthesiology 2003;99:230–231.

138. Cuvillon P, Ripart J, Lalourcey L, et al: The continuous femoral nerve block catheter for postoperative analgesia: Bacterial colonization, infectious rate and adverse effects. Anesth Analg 2001;93:1045–1049.

139. Compère V, Rey N, Baert O, et al: Major complications after 400 continuous popliteal sciatic nerve blocks for post-operative analgesia. Acta Anesth Scand 2009;53:339–345.

140. Volk T, Engelhardt L, Spies C, et al: Incidence of infection from catheter procedures ro regional anesthesia: First results from the network of DGAI and BDA. Anaesthesist 2009;58:1107–1112.

141. Reisig F, Neuburger M, Zausig YA et al: Successful infection control in regional anesthesia procedures: Observational survey after introduction of the DGAI hygiene recommendations. Anaesthesist 2013;62: 105–112.

142. Davlin LB, Aulicino PL: Osteomyelitis of the metacarpal head following digital block anesthesia. Orthopedics 1999;22:1187–1188.

143. Basu A, Bhalaik V, Stanislas M, et al: Osteomyelitis following a haematoma block. Injury 2003;34:79–82.

144. Dahlmann AH, Appaswamy S, Headon MP: Orbital cellulitis following sub-Tenon's anaesthesia. Eye 2002;16:200–201.

145. Redmill B, Sandy C, Rose GE: Orbital cellulitis following corneal gluing under sub-Tenon's local anaesthesia. Eye 2001;15:554–556.

146. Capdevilla X, Jaber S, Pesonen P, et al: Acute neck cellulits and mediastinitis complicating a continuous interscalene block. Anesth Analg 2008;107:1419–1421.

147. Sato Y, Suzino K, Suzuku A, et al: Case of primary cutaneous aspergillus cadioustus infection caused by nerve block therapy. Med Mycol J 2011;52:239–244.

148. Delfosse F, Pronnier P, Levent T: Infections complicating femoral nerve catheter for postoperative analgesia: About two cases. Ann Fr Anesth Reanim 2011;30:516–520.

149. Wildsmith JA: Regional anaesthesia requires attention to detail [Letter]. Br J Anaesth 1991;67:224–225.

150. Yentis SM: Wearing of face masks for spinal anaesthesia [Letter]. Br J Anaesth 1992;68:224.

151. Wildsmith JA: Wearing of face masks for spinal anaesthesia [Letter]. Br J Anaesth 1992;68:224.

152. O'Kelly SW, Marsh D: Face masks and spinal anaesthesia [Letter]. Br J Anaesth 1993;70:239.

153. Wildsmith JA: Face masks and spinal anaesthesia [Letter]. Br J Anaesth 1993;70:239.

154. Bromage PR: Postpartum meningitis [Letter]. Anaesthesia 1994;49:260.

155. Smedstad KG: Infection after central neuraxial block [Editorial]. Can J Anaesth 1997;44:235–238.

156. Panikkar KK, Yentis SM: Wearing of masks for obstetric regional anaesthesia. A postal survey. Anaesthesia 1996;51:398–400.

157. O'Higgins F, Tuckey JP: Thoracic epidural anaesthesia and analgesia: United Kingdom practice. Acta Anaesthesiol Scand 2000;44: 1087–1092.

158. Sleth JC: Evaluation des mesures d'asepsie lors de la realisation d'un catheterisme epidural et perception de son risqué infectieux. Resultats d'une enquete en Languedoc-Roussillon. Ann Fr Anesth Reanim 1998;17:408–414.

159. Dawson SJ, Small H, Logan MN, et al: Case control study of epidural catheter infections in a district general hospital. Commun Dis Public Health 2000;3:300–302.

160. Philips BJ, Fergusson S, Armstrong P, et al: Surgical face masks are effective in reducing bacterial contamination caused by dispersal from the upper airway. Br J Anaesth 1992;69:407–408.

161. Chaiyakunapruk N, Veenstra DL, Lipsky BA, et al: Vascular catheter site care: The clinical and economic benefits of chlorhexidine gluconate compared with povidone iodine. Clin Infect Dis 2003;37(6):764–771.

162. Adam MN, Dinulescu T, Mathieu P, et al: Comparaison de l'efficacite de deux antiseptiques dans la prevention de l'infection liee aux catheters periduraux. Can Anesthesiol 1996;44:465–467.

163. Kasuda H, Fukuda H, Togashi H, et al: Skin disinfection before epidural catheterization: Comparative study of povidone-iodine versus chlorhexidine ethanol. Dermatology 2002;204(Suppl 1):42–46.

164. Kinirons B, Mimoz O, Lafendi L, et al: Chlorhexidine versus povi-done iodine in preventing colonization of continuous epidural catheters in children. Anesthesiology 2001;94:239–244.

165. Sato S, Sakuragi T, Dan K: Human skin flora as a potential source of epidural abscess. Anesthesiology 1996;85:1276–1282.

166. Sviggum HP, Jacob AK, Arendt KW, et al: Neurologic complications after chlorhexidine antisepsis for spinal anesthesia. Reg Anesth Pain Med 2012;37:139–144.

167. Doan L, Piskoun B, Rosenberg AD, et al: In vitro antiseptic effects on viability of neuronal and Schwann cells. Reg Anesth Pain Med 2012;37:131–138.

168. Malhotra S, Dharmadasa A, Yentis SM: One vs. two applications of chlorhexidine/ethanol for disinfecting the skin: Implications for regional anesthesia. Anaesthesia 2011;574–578.

169. ASA Practice Advisory for the Prevention, Diagnosis, and Management of Infectious Complications Associated With Neuraxial Techniques: A report by the American Society of Anesthesiologists Task Force on Infectious Complications Associated With Neuraxial Techniques. Anesthesiology 2010;112:530–545.

170. Raad II, Hohn DC, Gilbreath BJ, et al: Prevention of central venous catheter-related infections by using maximal sterile barrier precautions during insertion. Infect Control Hosp Epidemiol 1994;15:231–238.

171. Kerwat K, Schulz-Stübner S, Steinfeldt T, Kessler P, Volk T, Gastmeier P, Geffers C, Ermert T, Boschin MG, Wiesmann T, Wulf H. Hygieneempfehlungen für die Regionalanästhesie. Anästh Intensivmed 2015;56:34–40.

172. Pegues DA, Carr DB, Hopkins CC: Infectious complications associated with temporary epidural catheters. Clin Infect Dis 1994;19:970–972.

173. Green BGJ, Pathy GV: Ensuring sterility of opioids for spinal administration [Letter]. Anaesthesia 1999;54:511.

174. Schulz-Stübner S, Pottinger J, Coffin S, Herwaldt L: Nosocomial infections and infection control in regional anesthesia. Acta Anesth Scand 2008;52:1144–1157.

175. Friedman Z, Siddiqui N, Katznelson R, et al: Experience is not enough: repeated breaches in epidural anesthesia aseptic technique by novice operators despite improved skill. Anesthesiology 2008;108:914–920.

176. Reisig F, Neuburger M, Zausig YA, et al: Successful infection control in regional anesthesia procedures: Observational survey after introduction of the DGAI hygiene recommendations [in German]. Anaesthesist 2013;62:105–112. Epub ahead of print.

177. O'Grady NP, Alexander M, Burns LA, et al, and the Healthcare Infection Control Practices Advisory Committee (HICPAC): *Guidelines for the Prevention of Intravascular Catheter-Related Infections.* CDC, 2011.

178. Rosenthal VD, Rodrigues C, Alvarez-Moreno C, et al: Effectiveness of a multidimensional approach for prevention of ventilator-associated pneumonia in adult intensive care units from 14 developing countries of four continents. Findings of the International Nosocomial Infection Control Consortium. Crit Care Med 2012;40:3121–3128.

179. Bloc S, Mercadal L, Garnier T, et al: Evaluation of a new disinfection method for ultrasound probes used for regional anesthesia: Ultraviolet C light. J Ultrasound Med 2011;30:785–788.

180. Kac G, Pdglajen I, Si-Mohamed A, et al: Evaluation of ultraviolet C for disinfection of endocavitary ultrasound transducers persistently contaminated despite probe covers. Infect Control Hosp Epidemiol 2010;31:165–170.

181. Volk T, Hbecker R, Rücker G, et al: Subdural empyema combined with paraspinal abscess after epidural catheter insertion. Anesth Analg 2005;100:122–123.

Local Anesthetics, Regional Anesthesia, and Cancer Recurrence

Alain Borgeat, José Aguirre, and E. Gina Votta-Velis

INTRODUCTION

Surgical excision is the cornerstone of treatment for solid tumors. Metastatic disease is the most important cause of cancer-related death patients affected with cancer. The likelihood of tumor metastases depends on the balance between the metastatic potential of the primary tumor and the antimetastatic host defenses. Among them, cell-mediated immunity and natural killer (NK) cell function are critical components.

A wealth of basic science data supports the hypothesis that the surgical stress response increases the likelihood of cancer dissemination during and after cancer surgery. Therefore, anesthetic management can potentially influence mid- and long-term outcome. Au contraire, surgery can inhibit major host defenses and promote the occurrence of metastases. Anesthetic techniques and drug choice also can affect the immune system. Together, these two interventions can have profound interactions with a patient's immune defenses. The aims of this chapter are to review how the immune system can be influenced by surgery and anesthesia and discuss the possible mechanisms behind a potential benefit of one intervention over the other in this setting.

THE IMMUNE SYSTEM: THE IMPORTANCE OF TH1/TH2 RATIO

Intact immune responses to cancer cells are crucial in preventing and inhibiting tumor occurrence. The modern concept of immunoediting includes these processes: elimination, equilibrium, and escape.[1,2] This implies that impairment in immune surveillance during the elimination process allows the escape of cancer cells from the protective immune attack. The appearance of clinically apparent tumors through the equilibrium

process may occur, rendering the tumor cells more resistant to the immune system.

The NhK, CD4+ Th1 (T helper 1), and CD8+ CTL (cytotoxic lymphocyte) cells are the major antitumor immune effector cells, whereas Th2 (T helper 2), tumor-associated macrophages (TAM), and regulatory T (Treg) cells are the among the most important cells in the promotion of tumor settlement, growth, and progress by inhibiting the immune responses against cancer.[3,4] Other mediators like proinflammatory cytokines,[5] catecholamines,[6] prostaglandins,[6] and high levels of signal transducer and activator of transcription 3 (STAT3) factor activity[7] are also involved in the process of postoperative metastases. NK cells have a crucial role particularly in eliminating metastases without prior sensitization and major histocompatibility complex (MHC) restriction.[8] Therefore, preservation or activation of the function of NK cells is important. In this context, Th1 cells, characterized by interleukin (IL) 2, IL-12, and interferon gamma (IFN-γ) secretions are mandatory to induce antitumor CTL[9] and to activate NK cells.[8] On the other hand, Th2 cells differentiated by IL-4 and IL-10 can induce Th17 cells, Treg cells, TAMs, and myeloid derived suppressor cells (MDSCs),[10] which have a major role in promoting tumor growth and metastasis by inhibiting antitumor immune responses like Th1 induction, CTL function, and NK activity.[11]

The role of proinflammatory cytokines (IL-6, tumor necrosis factor alpha [TNF-α], IL-13) should be outlined because release from infiltrating leukocytes close to the primary tumor site can activate nuclear factor κB (NF-κB) and STAT3 in cancer cells and can contribute to cancer proliferation and survival.[12] NK cell function can also be downregulated by prostaglandins, especially prostaglandin E_2 (PGE_2) by shifting cytokine balance toward Th2 dominance[13] and promoting tumor angiogenesis.[10]

Th1-type responses are necessary for antitumor immunity. It has been shown that, in general, cancer patients have a Th2-dominant status.[14] Surgery per se induces the Th1/Th2 balance toward Th2 immune response.[15] This is explained by the surgical activation of the sympathetic nervous system and the hypothalamic-pituitary-adrenal axis.[16]

ANESTHETIC INTERVENTIONS AND POTENTIAL EFFECTS ON IMMUNOMODULATION

Anesthetic techniques or drugs may have a direct impact on the immune balance of cancer patients. This section reviews the established and hypothetical effects of various anesthetic interventions, pharmacological agents and perioperative occurrences that may affect immunomodulation.

Hypotension, Hypovolemia, and Hypoxia

The occurrence of hypotension/hypovolemia during surgery is are some of the factors responsible for the activation of the sympathetic system. The resulting tissue hypoxia may increase the expression of the intercellular adhesion molecule 1 (ICAM-1) and vascular cell adhesion molecule 1 (VCAM-1) as well as P-selectin and E-selectin in vascular endothelium.[17] This initiates the systemic inflammatory response syndrome (SIRS), responsible for a depressed Th1 response[18] and therefore a shift toward the Th2 response phenotype.

Hypothermia

Hypothermia is a common occurrence during surgery. In vitro human investigation has demonstrated that monocytes incubated at temperature lower than 36°C reduced human leukocyte antigen (HLA)-DR expression, delayed TNF-α clearance, and increased IL-10 release.[19] In vivo animal studies have shown a suppression of NK cell activity.[19]

Hyperglycemia

Hyperglycemia during surgery is the result of the activation of the stress response. Acute hyperglycemia inhibits glucose-6-phosphatase dehydrogenase, the enzyme necessary for the formation of nicotinamide adenine dinucleotide phosphate,[20] which will block the functions of monocytes and neutrophils. The risk of infection is increased, and the occurrence of microvascular inflammation engenders an increased release of proinflammatory cytokines (IL-6, TNF-α) from immune cells.[20]

However, no data showing that perioperative hyperglycemia is associated with tumor spread or metastasis are available.

Blood Transfusion

Allogenic blood transfusion is recognized to have diverse negative immunomodulatory effects. However, blood transfusion is also a marker for sicker patients. In this context, it has been shown that anemia per se also has negative immune effects. Therefore, it is important to find the right balance, and avoiding unnecessary transfusions.

Volatile Anesthetics

Volatile anesthetics have been shown to have suppressive effects on immune cells. Halothane,[21] isoflurane,[22] and sevoflurane[23] suppress NK cell activity. The precise mechanism by which these agents interact with the immune system is not clear. However, a recent study showed that pretreatment with isoflurane can enhance resistance to apoptosis of colon cancer cells after exposure to anticancer drugs in vitro via a caveolin-dependent mechanism.[24]

Propofol

Propofol at a clinical concentration does not appear to have significant effects on NK cells and lymphocytes. Propofol, but not thiopental or ketamine, does not suppress NK cell activity in whole blood and does not increase susceptibility to tumor metastases.[21] A comparison between propofol and isoflurane[25] showed that propofol, but not isoflurane, increased the Th1/Th2 ratio, which is beneficial for patients with cancer. On the other hand, sevoflurane anesthesia[26] increased proinflammatory cytokine IL-17 and decreased the Th1/Th2 ratio. Propofol also has inhibiting activity against cyclooxygenase (COX) 2.[27] This is beneficial because in most human cancer cells COX-2 is overexpressed. COX-2 expression is critical for the production of PGE_2, which promotes tumor progression, VEGF (vascular endothelial growth factor) production in cancer cells, NK cell inhibition, and Th2 polarization.[27]

Midazolam and Ketamine

Midazolam[28] and ketamine[29] impair dendritic cell induction of Th1-type immune response in vitro and in vivo. Dendritic cells and Th1-type cells are important players in host defense against tumor. Ketamine also upregulates PGE_2[30] and increases lung metastases through NK cell inhibition in rat models.

Opioids

Morphine-induced immunosuppression is mediated by its binding to a member of the seven-transmembrane G-protein-coupled μ-opioid receptors (MORs) on immune cells.[31] The μ-receptor, which is morphine sensitive, is responsible for its immunomodulation.[32] Interestingly, fentanyl, despite sharing analgesic properties with morphine, does not bind to μ_3-receptor.[33] However, morphine administration reduces CTL and NK cell functions[31,34] and IL-2 and IFN-γ expression in T cells.[35,36] It also enhances IL-4 expression in T cells[37] favoring Th2 differentiation. Fentanyl was shown to have a suppressive effect on NK activity in nonsurgical individuals but to have a positive effect in operative subjects.[38] In contrast, remifentanil did not impair NK activity.[39]

Epidemiologic studies suggested that patients who receive general anesthesia with opioids rather than local anesthetics (LAs) or regional anesthetics may have a greater rate of cancer recurrence.[40] Beilin et al[41] investigated NK cell cytotoxic activity in 40 patients undergoing major surgery, who were randomized to receive either a high-dose fentanyl anesthesia regimen, including midazolam as a single dose and isoflurane if necessary, or low-dose fentanyl, with isoflurane and nitrous oxide used for anesthetic maintenance. In vitro NKA was suppressed in all patients, but high-dose fentanyl resulted in a slower rate of recovery of NK cell activity compared to low-dose fentanyl.

Sacerdote et al[42] studied the effects of morphine and tramadol in patients undergoing abdominal surgery for uterine carcinoma. Phytohemaglutinin-induced T-lymphocyte proliferation and NKA were evaluated. In the morphine group, lymphoproliferative values were attenuated by surgical stress and stayed depressed after the administration of morphine, whereas in the tramadol group these values came back to baseline after the administration of tramadol. NKA was increased by tramadol.

Gupta et al[43] demonstrated that morphine stimulates angiogenesis by activating proangiogenic signaling via Gi/Go-coupled G-protein receptors and nitric oxide. In clinically relevant plasma concentrations, morphine stimulated human microvascular endothelial cell proliferation and promoted tumor neovascularization in a human breast tumor xenograft model in mice, which led to the progression of the tumor.

Singleton et al[44] showed that μ-opioid agonists in clinical concentrations transactivate the VEGF receptors, and that the opioid-induced angiogenesis was blocked by both naloxone and the peripheral MOR antagonist methylnaltrexone. This group suggested that because μ-opioid agonists can alter the endothelial barrier integrity and affect vascular permeability, during tumor surgery, they could potentially facilitate transmigration of cells through the endothelium. This process was shown to be attenuated by methylnaltrexone.[45]

Mathew et al[46] reported that the expression of MORs was increased in lung cancer cells (Lewis lung carcinoma) and that the silencing of MOR in those cells reduced tumor growth and metastasis in mouse models.

Subsequently, Lennon et al[47] published the results of their more recent study where the effect of overexpression of the MOR on lung cancer progression was examined. The authors tested their hypothesis in vitro (H358 human non-small cell lung cancer [NSCLC] cells) and in vivo (human lung cancer xenograft models/nude mouse model). They demonstrated that MOR1 overexpression in H358 human NSCLC cells increased proliferation, migration, invasion, transendothelial migration, and activation of two serine/threonine kinases implicated in cancer progression (Akt [protein kinase B] and mammalian target of rapamycin [mTOR]). In addition, the same effect of increased tumor growth and lung metastasis was observed in human NSCLC xenografts. The authors suggested that these results may provide a plausible explanation for the differences in recurrence rates observed in different contexts.[40,48–50]

In conclusion, there are currently epidemiologic, animal, and cellular studies that suggest a possible role of MOR on tumor growth and metastasis that warrants further investigation.

REGIONAL ANESTHESIA AND CANCER METASTASES

Local Anesthetics and Cancer In Vitro

In vitro studies have demonstrated the antiproliferative or cytotoxic effect of LAs on cancer cells. Martinsson et al[51] evaluated the effect of ropivacaine on the proliferation of human colon adenocarcinoma cells in vitro. Ropivacaine inhibited the growth of these cells in a dose-dependent manner. The effective concentrations were within the therapeutic range, similar to the ones found in the colon of the patients treated rectally with ropivacaine. In the same study, lidocaine was found to be less potent than ropivacaine in inhibiting cell proliferation.

Sakaguchi et al[52] investigated the effects of lidocaine on proliferation of a human tongue cancer cell line that has a high level of epidermal growth factor receptor (EGFR) expression. Lidocaine in clinical concentrations suppressed EGF-induced proliferation of the malignant cells and inhibited EGF-stimulated tyrosine kinase activity of EGFR without cytotoxicity.

Lucchinetti et al[53] reported the results of the antiproliferative effects of LAs on mesenchymal stem cells (MSCs) and the potential implications for tumor spreading and wound healing. MSCs play a key role in tumor growth and metastasis by releasing growth factors, enhancing angiogenesis, immunomodulation, and epithelial-to-mesenchymal transformation. MSCs also contribute to tissue repair. The authors tested the effect of increasing concentrations of the amide LAs lidocaine, ropivacaine, and bupivacaine on proliferation, colony formation, in vitro wound healing, and bone differentiation assays of culture-expanded bone-marrow–derived murine MSCs. They demonstrated that MSCs are sensitive to the antiproliferative effects of LAs at concentrations of 10–100 μM. Their results suggested that mechanisms involved in this antiproliferative action may include the inhibition of NF-κB-ICAM-1 signaling pathway as well as the inhibition of mitochondrial respiration with adenosine triphosphate (ATP) depletion.

Effects of Anesthetic Techniques on Cellular Immunity

In the absence of surgery, general or epidural anesthesia has only minor effects on immune cell functions.[54] However, several preliminary studies in humans have indicated the beneficial effects of epidural anesthesia on immune cell functions in the setting of surgery-induced tissue trauma/stress.

Koltum et al[55] compared, in 20 patients who underwent colectomy under laparotomy for various diagnosis, the effect of awake epidural anesthesia (AEA) versus general endotracheal anesthesia (GETA) on natural killer cell cytotoxicity (NKCC). They found that AEA significantly preserved perioperative NKCC compared to GETA.

Hole et al[56] evaluated the phagocytic capabilities as well as the ability of monocytes to induce lysis of malignant cells in 18 patients undergoing total hip arthroplasty performed under either general or epidural anesthesia. While the phagocytic function of the monocytes derived from patients in the epidural group was found to be increased, the ability to induce lysis in malignant cells of the monocytes derived from patients who underwent general anesthesia was significantly reduced.

Wada et al[23] demonstrated in a rat model that sevoflurane anesthesia and laparotomy diminished tumoricidal activity in liver mononuclear cells (Th cells). On the contrary, a spinal block attenuated this effect. Bar-Yosef et al[57] showed the beneficial effects of spinal anesthesia on lung tumor retention in rats. The group with laparotomy plus general anesthesia had a

17-fold increase in lung metastasis. Spinal block reduced this effect by 70%. The authors concluded that surgical stress in rats promoted the development of metastasis, which was significantly attenuated by regional anesthesia.

Data from Retrospective Studies

In recent years, a number of retrospective studies suggested that regional anesthesia may have a beneficial effect on reducing cancer recurrence and metastasis.

Such studies are often limited by the accuracy of the available medical records, the lack of control in selection and measurement bias, and multiple uncontrolled confounding factors that could have an impact on cancer recurrence.

In one of the first published retrospective studies indicating the beneficial effects of regional anesthesia, Schlagenhauff et al[58] evaluated the prognostic impact of general and regional anesthesia for the excision of primary cutaneous melanoma. The authors examined follow-up data of 4329 patients. The study concluded that there was a significantly increased risk of death for patients treated with general anesthesia for the primary excision of melanoma, thus favoring regional anesthesia for this procedure.

Exadaktylos et al[59] conducted a small retrospective study based on the review of the medical records from patients that underwent mastectomy and axillary dissection for breast cancer. The patients had received either general anesthesia combined with paravertebral anesthesia/analgesia or general anesthesia combined with patient-controlled morphine analgesia. The authors examined the records of 129 patients who had a follow-up time of 32 ± 5 months. Their results suggested that the use of paravertebral anesthesia and analgesia for breast cancer surgery versus opioid use was associated with a metastasis/recurrence-free survival benefit of 94% versus 77% at 37 months.

Christopherson et al,[48] in a retrospective study, evaluated the long-term survival after resection of colon cancer under general anesthesia with or without epidural anesthesia in 177 patients. Analysis was performed separately for patients with and without metastasis because the presence of distant metastasis had the greatest effect on survival. Their results suggested that the patients with epidural analgesia had an improved survival (p = .012), up to 1.5 years; thereafter, the type of anesthesia did not appear to affect survival (p = .27).

Biki et al[49] evaluated retrospective date for prostate cancer recurrence in patients who received either general anesthesia with epidural anesthesia/analgesia (n = 102) or general anesthesia with postoperative opioid analgesia (n = 123). The primary outcome measure was the incidence of "biochemical recurrence," that is, an increase in prostate-specific antigen (PSA) after radical prostatectomy compared with its immediate postoperative peak value, which was the cause for initiation of adjuvant treatment. Adjustment for confounding factors was performed, and the results showed that patients who received general anesthesia combined with epidural analgesia had a 57% (95% CI, 17%–78%) lower risk of cancer recurrence than patients who had general anesthesia and postoperative opioids.

Tsui et al[50] evaluated the effect of adjunctive epidural LA and opioid infusion on disease recurrence following radical prostatectomy for adenocarcinoma under general anesthesia. This study was a retrospective analysis of a small randomized trial conducted for other purposes, such as pain control, blood loss, and the need for perioperative blood transfusion. The authors conducted a prolonged follow-up chart review to determine clinically evident or biochemical recurrence of prostate cancer. The median follow-up time was 4.5 years, and no difference in disease-free survival between the epidural and the control group was observed. Because the study had a different endpoint, it was significantly underpowered for evaluating cancer recurrence.

Ismail et al[60] examined retrospective data to determine the effect of neuraxial anesthesia in the progression of cervical cancer in 132 patients who were treated with brachytherapy. The use of neuraxial anesthesia during the first brachytherapy (most invasive one) was not associated with a reduced risk of local or systemic recurrence, long-term mortality from tumor recurrence, or all-cause mortality after adjusting for other prognostic factors. The study have failed to demonstrate a difference between the general and the regional anesthesia groups due to the underpowered sample size. Other factors that might have contributed to this result are the minimally invasive nature of the therapeutic procedure used for this treatment and the short duration of the neuraxial anesthesia.

Gottschalk et al[61] reviewed the records of 669 patients undergoing colorectal surgery to determine the association between perioperative epidural analgesia and cancer recurrence. The primary outcome of the study was time to cancer recurrence. In this study, the epidural and nonepidural groups were compared in all available potential confounders, and their relationship with cancer recurrence was analyzed by using a multivariable Cox proportional hazards regression model. Overall, no association between epidural use and recurrence was found (p = .43), with an adjusted estimated hazard ratio (HR) of 0.82 (95% CI 0.49–1.35). However, the authors found that the epidural-by-age interaction was statistically significant (p = .03). Epidural analgesia was associated with reduced cancer occurrence in patients older than 64 years, suggesting that age and tumor type may play an important role.

Wuethrich et al[62] evaluated the effect of anesthetic technique on disease progression and long-term survival in patients receiving general anesthesia plus intraoperative and postoperative thoracic epidural analgesia (n = 103) in comparison to patients receiving general anesthesia alone (n = 158). The patients underwent open retropubic radical prostatectomy with extended lymph node dissection. The authors' assessment was more detailed in that they evaluated biochemical recurrence-free survival, clinical progression-free survival, cancer-specific survival, and overall survival. It was demonstrated that general anesthesia combined with epidural analgesia resulted in improved clinical progression-free survival (HR 0.45, 95% CI 0.27–0.75, p = .002). No significant difference was found between general anesthesia plus postoperative ketorolac-morphine analgesia and general anesthesia plus intraoperative and postoperative thoracic epidural analgesia in biochemical recurrence-free survival, cancer-specific survival, or overall survival. The authors used a historical control group, which represented a limitation.

Myles et al[63] conducted a large (*n* = 503) retrospective study as a follow-up to the Multicenter Australian Study of Epidural Anaesthesia and Analgesia in Major Surgery (MASTER). This multicenter randomized clinical trial tested the hypothesis that combined epidural and general anesthesia reduced the frequency of major postoperative complications compared with general anesthesia and opioid analgesia. The goal was to compare long-term recurrence of cancer and survival in patients who underwent major abdominal surgery under general anesthesia with the supplement consisting of intraoperative and postoperative epidural analgesia (epidural group *n* = 263) or under general anesthesia and postoperative opioids for analgesia (control group *n* = 240). The median time to recurrence of cancer or death was 2.8 (95% CI 0.7 to 8.7) years in the control group and 2.6 (0.7 to 8.7) years in the epidural group (*p* = .61). Recurrence-free survival was similar in both epidural and control groups. However, the fact that 50% of the epidurals did not work is a major weakness of this study and raised serious doubts concerning the validity of the results.

De Oliveira et al,[64] in a recent retrospective study, studied any association between intraoperative neuraxial regional anesthesia and decreased ovarian cancer recurrence. The study reviewed data from 182 patients who underwent primary cytoreductive surgery for ovarian cancer. All the patients received general anesthesia. Of those, 127 received intravenous opioids for postoperative pain control, and 55 received epidural catheters. Of these patients, 26 received epidural anesthesia intra- as well as postoperatively for analgesia. The rest of the patients had the epidural only for postoperative pain control. The authors found that in the intraoperative/postoperative epidural group the mean time to cancer recurrence was 73 (56–91) months, which was longer than for either the epidural postoperative group at 33 (21–45) months (*p* = .002) or the nonepidural group at 38 (30–47) months (*p* = .001).

In a recently published retrospective study, Cummings et al[65] compared the effects of epidural analgesia and traditional pain management on survival and cancer recurrence after colectomy. A cohort of 42,151 patients over 66 years old who underwent colectomy was identified from the Medicare-Surveillance, Epidemiology and End Results database. Of these patients, 22.9% (*n* = 9670) had an epidural at the time of resection. The results of this study demonstrated that the epidural use was associated with improved survival in patients with nonmetastatic colon cancer. Five-year survival was 61% in the epidural group and 55% in the nonepidural one.

Day et al[66] undertook a retrospective analysis of the effect of postoperative analgesia on survival in patients after laparoscopic resection of colorectal cancer. The data of 424 patients were analyzed. The three groups (epidural = 107, spinal block = 144, and patient-controlled analgesia = 173) were similar regarding patient and surgical characteristics. In the epidural group, patients received a mixture of bupivacaine and fentanyl for 48 hours. The authors did not find any difference between the groups in overall survival.

Some of the discussed retrospective studies provided results suggesting that regional anesthesia might have a beneficial affect in reducing cancer recurrence and some did not. The interpretation of the results of these investigations is complex because neither the LAs nor the concentration and the time and duration of application are known. Moreover, some analgesic regimens were a mixture of LA and opioid. Consequently, no clear-cut conclusions or recommendations for clinical care can be made (Table 17–1).

Clinical recommendations are also precluded because the clinical assessment of these results is even more difficult as no information regarding surgical technique is available. Although the possibility that regional anesthesia may reduce the incidence of metastasis is exciting, currently it is a hypothesis as adequately powered prospective randomized clinical trials are needed to validate the current observational results. What is known however, is that LAs have anti-inflammatory properties and do affect the mediators of inflammation at the molecular level. There is also evidence that inflammatory mechanisms may play a role in cancer metastasis.

INFLAMMATION AND CANCER

Epidemiological studies and molecular investigations of genetically modified mice and led to the conclusion that the mechanisms leading to inflammation and cancer may be linked.[67–70] The presence of inflammatory cells and inflammatory mediators in tumors, tissue remodeling, and angiogenesis is similar to that seen in chronic inflammatory responses that precede and constitute the hallmark of cancer-related inflammation.

Cancer and inflammation are connected by two pathways: an intrinsic one and an extrinsic one.[71] The intrinsic pathway is activated by genetic events such as mutations, chromosomal rearrangements, and so on that affect oncogenes. Cells that are transformed by these events produce inflammatory mediators, thereby generating an inflammatory microenviroment in the tumor area. By contrast, in the extrinsic pathway it is the inflammatory or infectious condition that is responsible for the risk of developing cancer at certain sites, such as colon, prostate, and pancreas. The two pathways lead to a common one and follow the activation of the nuclear transcription factor NF-κB and other transcription factors.

These factors regulate the production of inflammatory mediators such as cytokines and chemokines, which in turn recruit and activate various leukocytes. The cytokines activate the same key transcription factors in inflammatory cells, stromal cells, and tumor cells. This results in the subsequent release of more inflammatory mediators and the formation of a cancer-related inflammatory milieu (Figure 17–1).[71]

Role of the ICAM-1 and Src Protein Tyrosine Kinase on Inflammation and Metastasis

The role of cell adhesion molecules (CAMs) such as ICAM-1, VCAM-1, E-selectin, and P-selectin has been studied extensively in the process of inflammation.[72] Similarly, CAMs have been implicated in tumor progression.[73] Some circulating cancer cells have been shown to extravasate to a secondary site using a process similar to inflammatory cells.[74] This process shared by inflammatory and cancer cells may partially explain the link between inflammation and the occurrence of

TABLE 17-1. Retrospective studies.

Study	Which LA	Dosage	Duration	Time of First Application	Results	Remarks
Exadaktylos et al 2006: breast[59]	Levobupi 0.25%	0.2-mL/kg bolus of 0.25% infusion of 0.25% (rate?)	48 h postop	Before surgical cut	++	Retrospective paravertebral block T2–T3
Biki et al 2008: prostate[49]	—	—	48–72 h postop	Before surgical cut	++	Retrospective Epidural T11–T12
Christopherson et al 2008: colon[48]	Bupi 0.5%	Bolus of 5–10 mL as needed	—	Before surgical cut	+ Without metastasis — with metastasis	Retrospective Lumbar or thoracic epidural
Gottschalk et al 2010: colon[61]	—	—	—	—	+ older than 64 — younger than 64	Retrospective Epidural
Tsui et al 2010: prostate[50]	Ropi 0.5%	(Loading dose?) then ropi 0.2% + fentanyl	—	Before surgical cut	—	Retrospective analysis of RCT thoracic or lumbar epidural
Wuethrich et al 2010: prostate[62]	Bupi 0.25%	8–10 mL/h 0.25% perioperative then 0.1% bupi + epi + fentanyl 8–15 mL/h	Perioperative	—	—	Retrospective Thoracic epidural T10–T12 Historical control group
Schlagenhauff et al 2000: melanoma[58]	Local anesthesia	—	—	Before surgical cut	++	Retrospective local anesthesia vs general anesthesia Ø Epidural or spinal
Ismail et al 2010: cervical cancer[60]	—	—	—	Before treatment	—	Retrospective NB: brachytherapy
De Oliveira et al 2011: ovarian cancer[64]	Bupi (?)	Bolus (10 mg) + infusion 12.5 mg/h	48–72 h	Before surgical cut or after the end of surgery	+ If epidural before surgical cut — if after surgical cut	Retrospective Epidural T10–T12
Cummings et al 2012: colon[65]	—	—	—	—	++	Retrospective Epidural (thoracic or lumbar)
Day et al 2012: colorectal[66]	Ep bupi SPA bupi	Ep bupi 0.2% 10 mL + fentanyl then bupi 0.15% + FNT at 4–8 mL/h	48 h	Before surgical cut	—	Retrospective Epidural T9–T12 SPA L2–L4

bupi = bupivacaine; levobupi = levobupivacaine; ropi = ropivacaine.

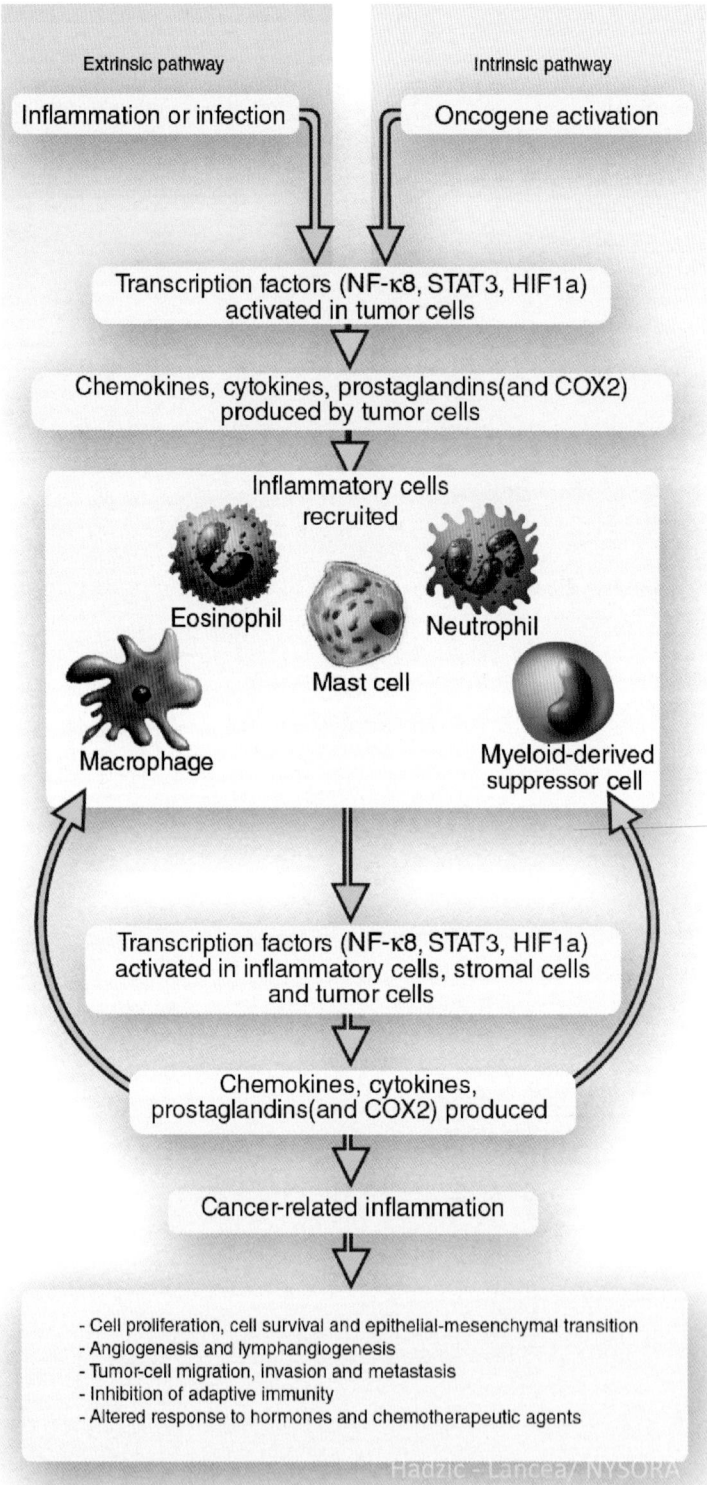

FIGURE 17–1. Pathways that connect inflammation and cancer. Cancer and inflammation are connected by two pathways: the intrinsic pathway and the extrinsic pathway. The intrinsic pathway is activated by genetic events that cause neoplasia. These events include the activation of various types of oncogene by mutation, chromosomal rearrangement or amplification, and the inactivation of tumor suppressor genes. Cells that are transformed in this manner produce inflammatory mediators, thereby generating an inflammatory microenvironment in tumors for which there is no underlying inflammatory condition. By contrast, in the extrinsic pathway, inflammatory or infectious conditions augment the risk of developing cancer at certain anatomical sites. The two pathways converge, resulting in the activation of transcription factors, mainly nuclear factor kappa B (NF-κB), signal transducer and activator of transcription 3 (STAT3), and hypoxia-inducible factor 1α (HIFlα), in tumor cells. (Reproduced with permission from Mantovani A, Allavena P, Sica A, et al: Cancer-related inflammation. *Nature.* 2008 Jul 24;454(7203):436-444.)

metastasis. Furthermore, it may help to understand the therapeutic benefit of anti-inflammatory drugs in cancer treatment.

Scientific evidence has implicated a role of ICAM-1 in tumor invasion in vitro and in metastasis in vivo and hence in the malignant potential of various types of cancer. Kageshita et al[75] have demonstrated that ICAM-1 expression in primary lesions and the serum of patients with malignant melanoma was associated with a reduction in the disease-free interval and survival. Also, a significantly higher level of serum ICAM-1 (sICAM-1) was detected in the patients with liver metastasis, and its levels were increased in serial blood samples obtained from patients with progressing disease. Similar results were reported in a study that examined the role of ICAM-1 in the invasion of human breast cancer cells.[74]

Maurer et al[76] determined that overexpression of ICAM-1, V-CAM-1, and endothelial leukocyte adhesion molecule 1 (ELAM-1) influenced the tumor progression in colorectal cancer. High expression of ICAM-1 in tumors was an indicator of metastatic potential and poor prognosis.[77] Because ICAM-1 is associated with a variety of cancer types and has a role in cancer metastasis, it can be also used as a biomarker for tumor prognosis as well as a target for therapeutic interventions.[78–80]

Current evidence has shown that the binding of apical cell surface associated mucin (MUC-1) on circulating tumor cells to the ICAM-1 on the endothelial cells could represent one of the first crucial steps in metastasis. This molecule is a mucin-glycosylated phosphoprotein that lines the apical surface of epithelial cells in the lung and several other organs. Roland et al[81] proposed that this binding results in a release of cytokines and chemokines that attract macrophages and upregulate tumor production of ICAM-1. Macrophages produce more cytokines that attract neutrophils (polymorphonuclear neutrophils, PMNs), which adhere to the ICAM-1 of the tumor cell surface. This interaction causes degranulation of the PMNs, releasing proteases, with subsequent deterioration of the endothelial barrier promoting extravasation of the tumor cells and formation of metastatic sites.[82–85]

Another potent regulator of endothelial permeability and the inflammatory responses in tissue cells is Src kinase.[86] Src protein tyrosine kinase (PTK) family members have been identified as essential for the recruitment and activation of monocytes, macrophages, neutrophils, and other immune cells.[87] The Src family of nonreceptor protein tyrosine kinases plays a critical role in a variety of cellular signal transduction pathways, regulating such diverse processes as cell division, motility adhesion, angiogenesis, and survival. Activation of Src family kinases is common in a variety of human cancers, may occur through different mechanisms, and is frequently a critical event in tumor progression. Src kinases appear to be important in the proliferation of the tumor, disruption of cell/cell contacts, migration, invasiveness, and resistance to apoptosis. Src family kinases are thus attractive targets for use as anticancer theurapeutics.[88]

It has been demonstrated that once tumor cells leave their primary site, they enter the blood vessels and again they extravasate to form satellite lesions. It was shown in mice that endothelial barrier disruption by VEGF-mediated Src activation potentiated tumor cell extravasation and metastasis. Some of the metastatic tumor cells secrete VEGF, which subsequently activates Src and compromises the endothelial barrier by disrupting a VE-/-β-catenin complex in lung endothelial cell-cell junctions. This is supported by the findings that mice genetically deficient in the c-Src are resistant to tumor cell metastasis.[89] Src is also an upstream regulator of Rho family GTPases (guanosine triphosphatases) such as Rac and Rho, which together regulate dynamic changes in the cytoskeleton and control the disassembly of actin-based cytoskeletal structures and cell-matrix adhesions.[90]

Finally, another protein that plays a role in inflammation by attracting monocytes and macrophages to the site is the monocyte chemoattractant protein 1 (MCP-1). This is a chemokine that exerts strong chemoattractant activities on monocytes, T cells, and NK cells.[91] In addition to promoting the transmigration of circulating monocytes into tissues, MCP-1 exerts various other effects on these cells, including superoxide anion induction chemotaxis and calcium flux.[92] Its production is also associated with angiogenesis and tumor invasion. Goede et al[93] analyzed the angiogenesis-inducing capability of MCP-1 and found it was a potent angiogenic factor when implanted into the rabbit cornea, with an effect similar to the specific angiogenic VEGF. Moreover, serum levels of MCP-1 have been found to be elevated in lung cancer patients with bone metastases.[94]

Evidence of Antimetastatic Effect of Local Anesthetics

Anti-inflammatory properties of ropivacaine have been demonstrated in different experimental models of lung injury.[95] Lidocaine also has well-documented anti-inflammatory properties and a safer profile for systemic toxicity. As mentioned, inflammatory processes involving Src tyrosine protein kinase and ICAM-1 play a role in cancer metastasis. It could be hypothesized that the amide LAs might attenuate the metastatic process of cancer cells in a similar manner to the inflammatory one.

In a recent study, we showed that lidocaine and ropivacaine may inhibit inflammatory cytokine signaling, proliferation, and migration of lung adenocarcinoma cells.[96] The following in vitro study was performed: NCI-H838 lung cancer cells were incubated with TNF-α in the absence/presence of ropivacaine or lidocaine (1 nM, 1 μM, 10 μM, 100 μM). Cell lysates were analyzed for Src activation (phosphor-Y419 Src) and ICAM-1 phosphorylation (phosphor-Y512 ICAM-1) via Western blot. MCP-1 production, cell proliferation, and migration were also evaluated. The results of this work showed that both lidocaine and ropivacaine inhibited Src activation induced by inflammatory mediators TNF-α (Figures 17–2 and 17–3). We also showed that both lidocaine and ropivacaine attenuated TNF-α-induced MCP-1 production in H838 cancer cells, and that they inhibited their proliferation and migration as well (Figure 17–4). Interestingly, the ester LA chloroprocaine did not demonstrate these properties, suggesting these effects were specific to the amide type of LAs.

To support the direct inhibition of Src tyrosine protein kinase by the amide LAs, the cells were treated with veratridine, a sodium channel activator and tetrodotoxin (TTX), a non-LA

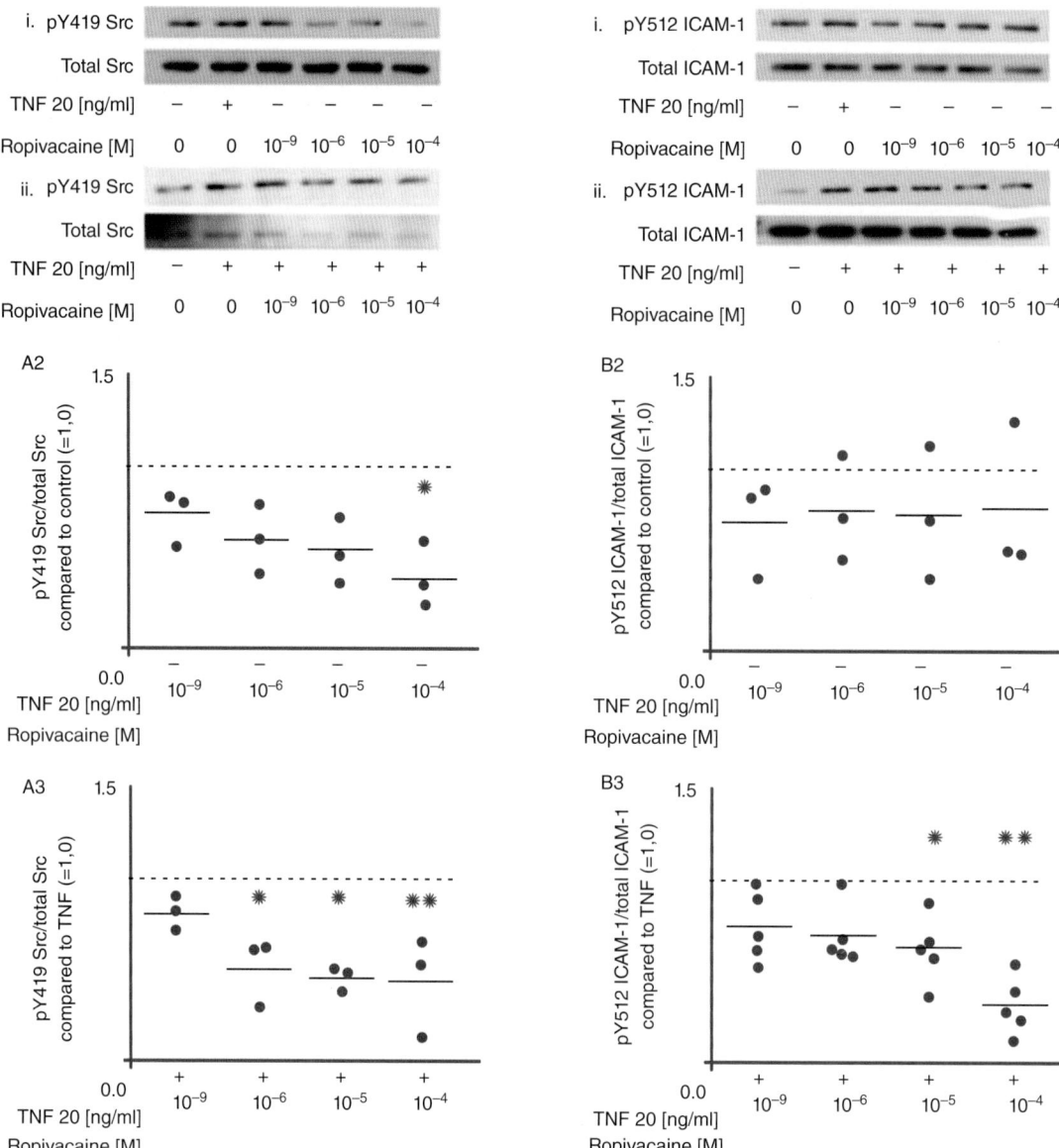

FIGURE 17–2. A: Effect of ropivacaine on the phosphorylation status of Src in NCI-H838 lung cancer cells. A. (i) Representative Western blot of NCI-H838 cell Src, phosphorylated at tyrosine 419 (pY419 Src, row 1) and total Src (row 2) after treatment with either tumor necrosis factor alpha (TNF-α) (20 ng/mL) or with different concentrations of ropivacaine (1 nM, 1 μM, 10 μM, 100 μM) for 20 minutes. (ii) Representative blot of NCI-H838 lung cancer cell pY419 Src (row 1) and total Src (row 2) after treatment with TNF-α (20 ng/mL) with or without different concentrations of ropivacaine (1 nM, 1 μM, 10 μM, 100 μM) for 20 minutes. B. Relative density of the Western blot bands of pY419 Src normalized to the densitometry values of total Src compared with control (= 1.0, dashed line) in the absence of TNF-α expressed. Data from three independent experiments shown as scatter plot ($n = 3$). Horizontal line indicates mean for each group; $*p < .05$ versus control. C. Relative density of the Western blot bands of pH419 Src normalized to the densitometry values of total Src after coincubation of ropivacaine with TNF-α (20 ng/mL) compared with TNF-α alone (= 1.0, dashed line). Data from three independent experiments shown as scatter plot ($n = 3$). Horizontal line indicates mean for each group; $*p > .05$ versus TNF-α. $**p > .01$ versus TNF-α. (Reprinted by permission from Wolters Kluwer Health: Anesthesiology, Piegeler T, Votta-Velis EG, Liu G, et al: Antimetastatic potential of amide-linked local anesthetics: Inhibition of lung adenocarcinoma cell migration and inflammatory Src signaling independent of sodium channel blockade. Anesthesiology 2012;117:548–559, copyright 2012.) **B:** Effect of ropivacaine on the phosphorylation status of intercellular adhesion molecule 1 (ICAM-1) in NCI-H838 lung cancer cells. A. (i) Representative Western blot of NCI-H838 lung cancer cell ICAM-1, phosphorylated at tyrosine 512 (pY512 ICAM-1, row 1) and total ICAM-1 (row 2) after treatment with either TNF-α (20 ng/mL) or different concentrations of ropivacaine (1 nM, 1 μM, 10 μM, 100 μM) for 20 minutes. (ii) Representative blot of NCI-H838 cell pY512 ICAM-1 (row 1) and total ICAM-1 (row 2) after treatment with TNF-α (20 ng/mL) in the presence or absence of different concentrations of ropivacaine (1 nM, 1 μM, 10 μM, 100 μM) for 20 minutes. B. Relative density of the Western blot bands of pY512 ICAM-1 normalized to the densitometry values of total ICAM-1 compared with control (= 1.0, dashed line) in the absence of TNF-α. Data from three independent experiments shown as scatter plot ($n = 3$). Horizontal line indicates mean for each group. C. Relative density of the Western blot bands of pY512 ICAM-1 normalized to the densitometry values of total ICAM-1 after coincubation of ropivacaine with TNF-α (20 ng/mL) compared with TNF-α alone (= 1.0 dashed line). Data from five independent experiments shown as scatter plot ($n = 5$). Horizontal line indicates mean for each group; $*p < .05$ versus TNF-α. $**p < .01$ versus TNF-α. (Reproduced with permission from Piegeler T, Votta-Velis EG, Liu G, et al: Antimetastatic potential of amide-linked local anesthetics: inhibition of lung adenocarcinoma cell migration and inflammatory Src signaling independent of sodium channel blockade. *Anesthesiology.* 2012 Sep;117(3):548-559.)

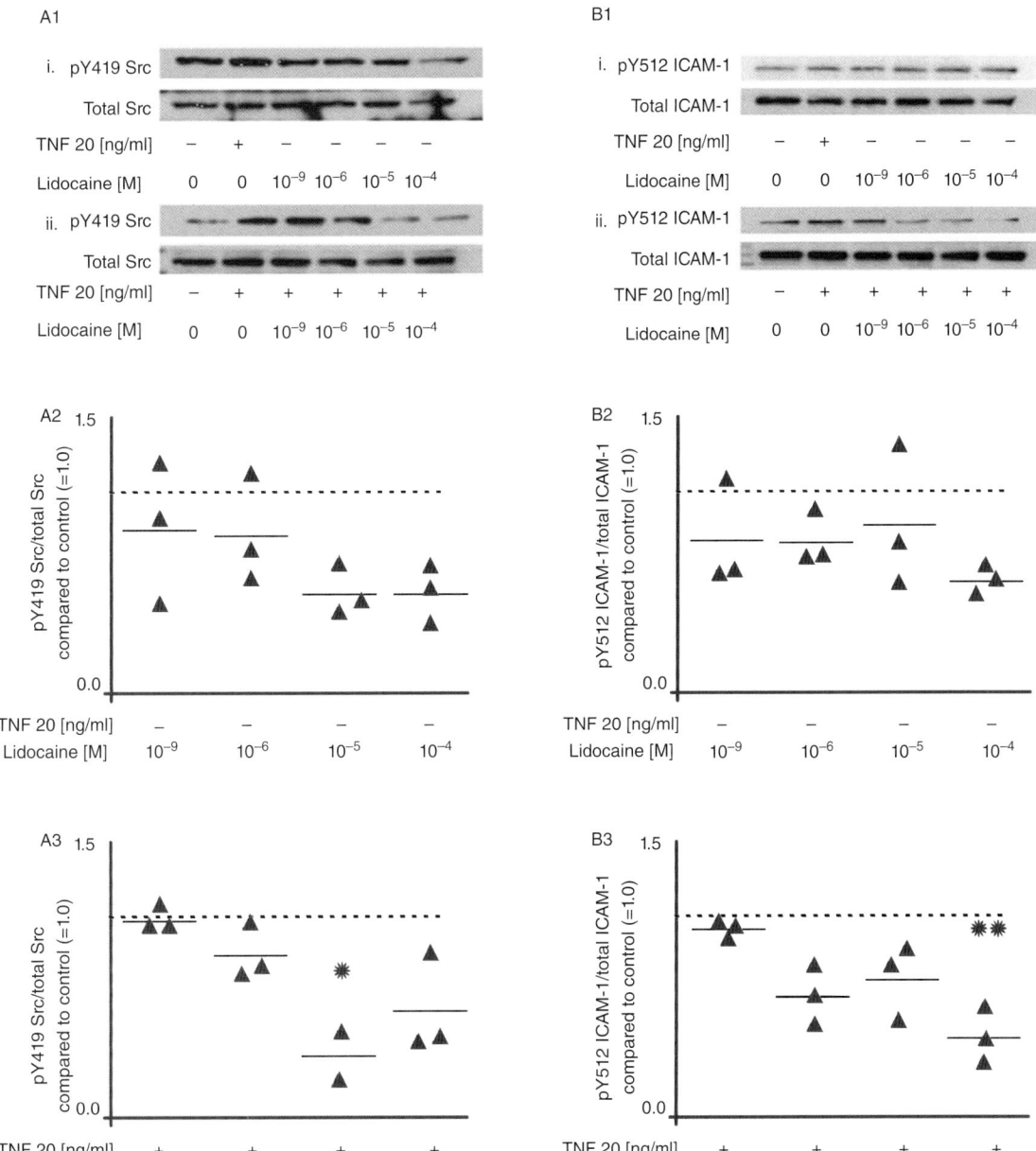

FIGURE 17–3. A: Effect of lidocaine on the phosphorylation status of Src in NCI-H838 lung cancer cells. A. (i) Representative Western blot of NCI-H838 cell Src, phosphorylated at tyrosine 419 (pY419 Src, row 1) and total Src (row 2) after treatment with either tumor necrosis factor alpha (TNF-α) (20 ng/mL) or with different concentrations of lidocaine (1 nM, 1 μM, 10 μM, 100 μM) for 20 minutes. (ii) Representative blot of NCI-H838 lung cancer cell pY419 Src (row 1) and total Src (row 2) after treatment with TNF-α (20 ng/mL) with or without different concentrations of lidocaine (1 nM, 1 μM, 10 μM, 100 μM) for 20 minutes. B. Relative density of the Western blot bands of pY419 Src normalized to the densitometry values of total Src compared with control (= 1.0, dashed line) in the absence of TNF-α. Data from three independent experiments shown as scatter plot ($n = 3$). Horizontal line indicates mean for each group. C. Relative density of the Western blot bands of pY419 Src normalized to the densitometry values of total Src after coincubation of lidocaine with TNF-α (20 ng/mL) compared with TNF-α alone (= 1.0 dashed line). Data from three independent experiments shown as scatter plot ($n = 3$). Horizontal line indicates mean for each group; *$p < .05$ versus TNF-α. (Reprinted by permission from Wolters Kluwer Health: Anesthesiology, Piegeler T, Votta-Velis EG, Liu G, et al: Antimetastatic potential of amide-linked local anesthetics: Inhibition of lung adenocarcinoma cell migration and inflammatory Src signaling independent of sodium channel blockade. Anesthesiology 2012;117:548–559, copyright 2012.) **B:** Effect of lidocaine on the phosphorylation status of intercellular adhesion molecule 1 (ICAM-1) in NCI-H838 lung cancer cells. A. (i) Representative Western blot of NCI-H838 lung cancer cell ICAM-1, phosphorylated at tyrosine 512 (pY512 ICAM-1, row 1) and total ICAM-1 (row 2) after treatment with either TNF-α (20 ng/mL) or different concentrations of lidocaine (1 nM, 1 μM, 10 μM, 100 μM) for 20 minutes. (ii) Representative blot of NCI-H838 cell pY512 ICAM-1 (row 1) and total ICAM-1 (row 2) after treatment with TNF-α (20 ng/mL) in the presence or absence of different concentrations of lidocaine (1 nM, 1 μM, 10 μM, 100 μM) for 20 minutes. B. Relative density of the Western blot bands of pY512 ICAM-1 normalized to the densitometry values of total ICAM-1 compared with control (= 1.0, dashed line) in the absence of TNF-α. Data from three independent experiments shown as scatter plot ($n = 3$). Horizontal line indicates mean for each group. C. Relative density of the Western blot bands of pY512 ICAM-1 normalized to the densitometry values of total ICAM-1 after coincubation of lidocaine with TNF-α (20 ng/mL) compared with TNF-α alone (= 1.0, dashed line). Data from three independent experiments shown as scatter plot ($n = 3$). Horizontal line indicates mean for each group. **$p < .01$ versus TNF-α. (Reproduced with permission from Piegeler T, Votta-Velis EG, Liu G, et al: Antimetastatic potential of amide-linked local anesthetics: inhibition of lung adenocarcinoma cell migration and inflammatory Src signaling independent of sodium channel blockade. *Anesthesiology.* 2012 Sep;117(3):548-559.)

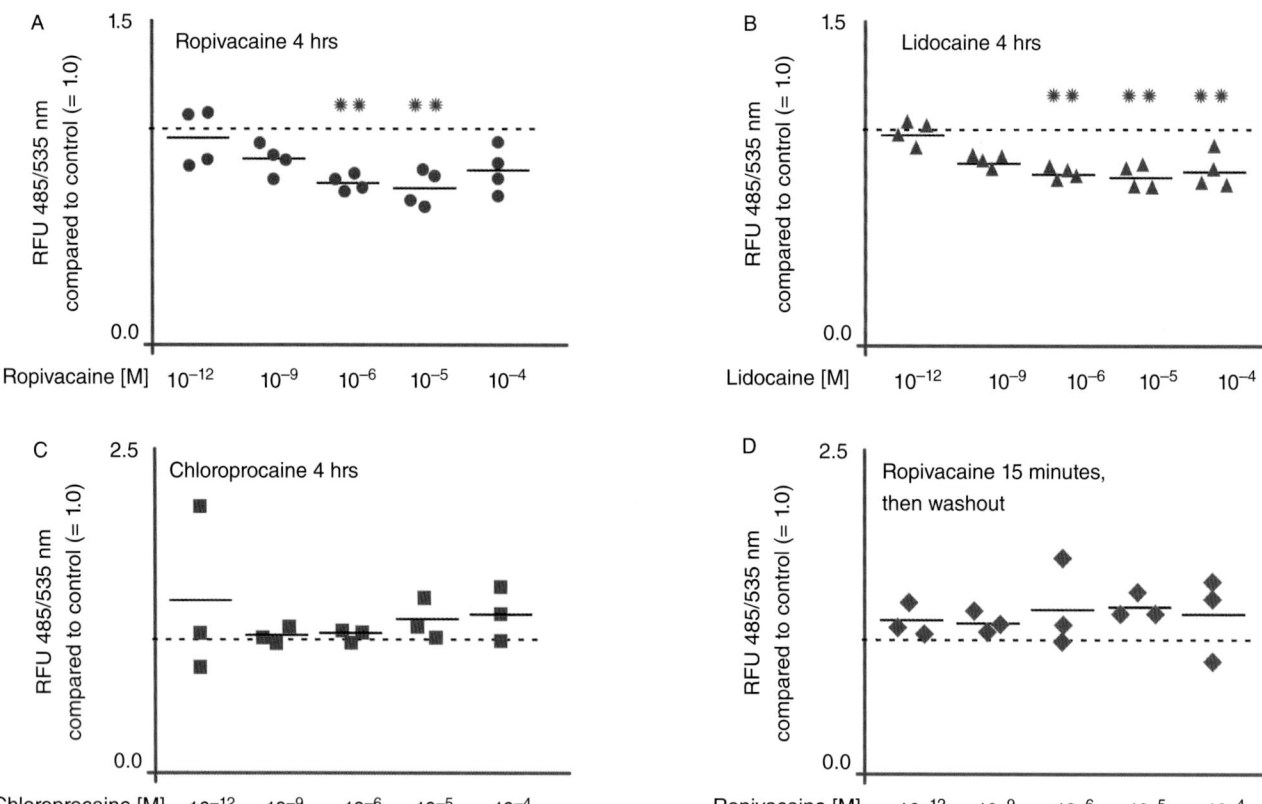

FIGURE 17–4. Migratory ability of NCI-H838 lung cancer cells in the presence of ropivacaine, lidocaine, and chloroprocaine. Determination of in vitro transmigration of NCI-H838 cells through a polycarbonate membrane after 4 hours in the absence or presence of different concentrations (1 pm, 1 nM, 1 μM, 10 μM, 100 μM) of **A**, ropivacaine; **B**, lidocaine; and **C**, chloroprocaine. **D**. Determination of in vitro transmigration of NCI-H838 cells through a polycarbonate membrane after 4 hours in the absence or presence of different concentrations (1 pm, 1 nM, 1 μM, 10 μM, 100 μM) of ropivacaine for only 15 minutes followed by a wash of the cells with fresh medium right before the start of the assay. Cells were stained with a fluorescent dye before the start of the assay and lysed after migration through the membrane. Fluorescence was measured at 435/535 nM (excitation/emission). Values for untreated cells were set as 1.0 (dashed line). Data from four (A and B) or three (C and D) independent experiments shown as scatter plot. Horizontal line indicates mean for each group. **$p < .01$ versus control. RFU = relative fluorescence units. (Reproduced with permission from Piegeler T, Votta-Velis EG, Liu G, et al: Antimetastatic potential of amide-linked local anesthetics: inhibition of lung adenocarcinoma cell migration and inflammatory Src signaling independent of sodium channel blockade. *Anesthesiology.* 2012 Sep;117(3):548-559.)

sodium channel inhibitor. We did not observe any alteration in the phosphorylation status of Src and ICAM-1 after treatment with veratridine compared to untreated cells, indicating that the phosphorylation of these two proteins was independent from sodium channel activation. The application of TTX had no effect on the phosphorylation status of these proteins, neither after treatment with TTX alone compared to untreated cells nor after coincubation with TNF-α compared to TNF-α alone. Taken together with the results obtained in the experiments with veratridine, we postulated that the observed effects of the inhibition of Src and ICAM-1 phosphorylation were independent of sodium channel inhibition.

Metastatic disease after cancer surgery remains a crucial issue. Cancer dissemination is a multistep process in which many cellular and molecular regulatory mechanisms may be involved and are targets for therapeutic interventions.

Traditional systemic therapy is delayed for weeks after major surgery to allow wound healing and thus avoiding the risks of immunosuppression and postoperative infections. However,

recent studies demonstrated that cellular and molecular events that are critical to the metastatic process may be significantly influenced during and immediately after surgery.[97] The perioperative period may be a window of therapeutic opportunity because metastasis may be initiated during this period. Preliminary studies using LAs have shown encouraging results for cancer outcomes. So far, the potential beneficial effect of regional anesthesia to improve long-term outcome after cancer surgery has contributed mainly to the inhibition of the neuroendocrine stress response to surgery and to the reduction in the requirements of the volatile anesthetics and opioids.

CONCLUSION

The amide LAs block TNF-α-induced Src activation and ICAM-1 phosphorylation in vitro. Both of these processes may favor the extravasation of tumor cancer cells and metastasis. Cytokines such as TNF-α increase the expression of

ICAM-1 in the H838 NSCLC. Src protein tyrosine kinase, which lies both upstream and downstream of activated ICAM-1, functions as a regulator of endothelial permeability and is also involved in signaling epithelial-to-mesenchymal transformation and extravasation of cancer cells, a process necessary for tumor metastasis. The activity of these two systems is significantly inhibited in vitro by the application of amide-type LAs. The immediate postoperative period is a crucial time in surgical oncology because no treatment will be started for a few weeks. The application of amide-type LAs in the perioperative period may be beneficial in preventing metastasis. However, the current preliminary data require further studies before any clinical recommendations can be made.

REFERENCES

1. Dunn GP, Old LJ, Schreiber RD: The immunobiology of cancer immunosurveillance and immunoediting. Immunity 2004;21:137–148.
2. Schreiber RD, Old LJ, Smyth MJ: Cancer immunoediting: integrating immunity's roles in cancer suppression and promotion. Science 2011;331: 1565–1570.
3. Knutson KL, Disis ML: Tumor antigen-specific T helper cells in cancer immunity and immunotherapy. Cancer Immunol Immunother 2005;54: 721–728.
4. Zamarron BF, Chen W: Dual roles of immune cells and their factors in cancer development and progression. Int J Biol Sci 2011;7:651–658.
5. Mantovani A, Marchesi F, Porta C, Sica A, Allavena P: Inflammation and cancer: Breast cancer as a prototype. Breast 2007;16(Suppl 2): S27–S33.
6. Goldfarb Y, Sorski L, Benish M, Levi B, Melamed R, Ben-Eliyahu S: Improving postoperative immune status and resistance to cancer metastasis: a combined perioperative approach of immunostimulation and prevention of excessive surgical stress responses. Ann Surg 2011;253: 798–810.
7. Yaguchi T, Sumimoto H, Kudo-Saito C, et al: The mechanisms of cancer immunoescape and development of overcoming strategies. Int J Hematol 2011;93:294–300.
8. Stojanovic A, Cerwenka A: Natural killer cells and solid tumors. J Innate Immun 2011;3:355–364.
9. Kennedy R, Celis E: Multiple roles for CD4+ T cells in anti-tumor immune responses. Immunol Rev 2008;222:129–144.
10. Mantovani A, Sica A: Macrophages, innate immunity and cancer: Balance, tolerance, and diversity. Curr Opin Immunol 2010;22: 231–237.
11. Ostrand-Rosenberg S, Sinha P: Myeloid-derived suppressor cells: Linking inflammation and cancer. J Immunol 2009;182:4499–4506.
12. Grivennikov SI, Greten FR, Karin M: Immunity, inflammation, and cancer. Cell 2010;140:883–899.
13. Kuroda E, Yamashita U: Mechanisms of enhanced macrophage-mediated prostaglandin E2 production and its suppressive role in Th1 activation in Th2-dominant BALB/c mice. J Immunol 2003;170:757–764.
14. Becker Y: Molecular immunological approaches to biotherapy of human cancers—a review, hypothesis and implications. Anticancer Res 2006;26:1113–1134.
15. Ishikawa M, Nishioka M, Hanaki N, et al: Perioperative immune responses in cancer patients undergoing digestive surgeries. World J Surg Oncol 2009;7:7.
16. Gottschalk A, Sharma S, Ford J, Durieux ME, Tiouririne M: Review article: The role of the perioperative period in recurrence after cancer surgery. Anesth Analg 2010;110:1636–1643.
17. van Meurs M, Wulfert FM, Jongman RM, et al: Hemorrhagic shock-induced endothelial cell activation in a spontaneous breathing and a mechanical ventilation hemorrhagic shock model is induced by a proinflammatory response and not by hypoxia. Anesthesiology 2011;115: 474–482.
18. Eltzschig HK, Carmeliet P: Hypoxia and inflammation. N Engl J Med 2011;364:656–665.
19. Qadan M, Gardner SA, Vitale DS, Lominadze D, Joshua IG, Polk HC Jr: Hypothermia and surgery: Immunologic mechanisms for current practice. Ann Surg 2009;250:134–140.
20. Turina M, Fry DE, Polk HC Jr: Acute hyperglycemia and the innate immune system: Clinical, cellular, and molecular aspects. Crit Care Med 2005;33:1624–1633.
21. Melamed R, Bar-Yosef S, Shakhar G, Shakhar K, Ben-Eliyahu S: Suppression of natural killer cell activity and promotion of tumor metastasis by ketamine, thiopental, and halothane, but not by propofol: Mediating mechanisms and prophylactic measures. Anesth Analg 2003; 97:1331–1339.
22. Markovic SN, Knight PR, Murasko DM: Inhibition of interferon stimulation of natural killer cell activity in mice anesthetized with halothane or isoflurane. Anesthesiology 1993;78:700–706.
23. Wada H, Seki S, Takahashi T, et al: Combined spinal and general anesthesia attenuates liver metastasis by preserving TH1/TH2 cytokine balance. Anesthesiology 2007;106:499–506.
24. Kawaraguchi Y, Horikawa YT, Murphy AN, et al: Volatile anesthetics protect cancer cells against tumor necrosis factor-related apoptosis-inducing ligand-induced apoptosis via caveolins. Anesthesiology 2011; 115:499–508.
25. Ren XF, Li WZ, Meng FY, Lin CF: Differential effects of propofol and isoflurane on the activation of T-helper cells in lung cancer patients. Anaesthesia 2010;65:478–482.
26. Tylman M, Sarbinowski R, Bengtson JP, Kvarnstrom A, Bengtsson A: Inflammatory response in patients undergoing colorectal cancer surgery: The effect of two different anesthetic techniques. Minerva Anestesiol 2011;77:275–282.
27. Inada T, Kubo K, Shingu K: Possible link between cyclooxygenase-inhibiting and antitumor properties of propofol. J Anesth 2011;25: 569–575.
28. Ohta N, Ohashi Y, Takayama C, Mashimo T, Fujino Y: Midazolam suppresses maturation of murine dendritic cells and priming of lipopolysaccharide-induced t helper 1-type immune response. Anesthesiology 2011;114:355–362.
29. Ohta N, Ohashi Y, Fujino Y: Ketamine inhibits maturation of bone marrow-derived dendritic cells and priming of the Th1-type immune response. Anesth Analg 2009;109:793–800.
30. Son KA, Kang JH, Yang MP: Ketamine inhibits the phagocytic responses of canine peripheral blood polymorphonuclear cells through the upregulation of prostaglandin E2 in peripheral blood mononuclear cells in vitro. Res Vet Sci 2009;87:41–46.
31. Al-Hasani R, Bruchas MR: Molecular mechanisms of opioid receptor-dependent signaling and behavior. Anesthesiology 2011;115:1363–1381.
32. Welters ID, Menzebach A, Goumon Y, et al: Morphine suppresses complement receptor expression, phagocytosis, and respiratory burst in neutrophils by a nitric oxide and mu(3) opiate receptor-dependent mechanism. J Neuroimmunol 2000;111:139–145.
33. Bilfinger TV, Fimiani C, Stefano GB: Morphine's immunoregulatory actions are not shared by fentanyl. Int J Cardiol 1998;64(Suppl 1):S61–S66.
34. Mojadadi S, Jamali A, Khansarinejad B, Soleimanjahi H, Bamdad T: Acute morphine administration reduces cell-mediated immunity and induces reactivation of latent herpes simplex virus type 1 in BALB/c mice. Cell Mol Immunol 2009;6:111–116.
35. Borner C, Warnick B, Smida M, et al: Mechanisms of opioid-mediated inhibition of human T cell receptor signaling. J Immunol 2009;183: 882–889.
36. Wang J, Barke RA, Charboneau R, Loh HH, Roy S: Morphine negatively regulates interferon-gamma promoter activity in activated murine T cells through two distinct cyclic AMP-dependent pathways. J Biol Chem 2003;278:37622–37631.
37. Roy S, Wang J, Charboneau R, Loh HH, Barke RA: Morphine induces CD4+ T cell IL-4 expression through an adenylyl cyclase mechanism independent of the protein kinase A pathway. J Immunol 2005;175: 6361–6367.
38. Page GG, Blakely WP, Ben-Eliyahu S: Evidence that postoperative pain is a mediator of the tumor-promoting effects of surgery in rats. Pain 2001;90:191–199.
39. Cronin AJ, Aucutt-Walter NM, Budinetz T, et al: Low-dose remifentanil infusion does not impair natural killer cell function in healthy volunteers. Br J Anaesth 2003;91:805–809.
40. Bovill JG: Surgery for cancer: does anesthesia matter? Anesth Analg 2010;110:1524–1526.
41. Beilin B, Shavit Y, Hart J, et al: Effects of anesthesia based on large versus small doses of fentanyl on natural killer cell cytotoxicity in the perioperative period. Anesth Analg 1996;82:492–497.
42. Sacerdote P, Bianchi M, Gaspani L, et al: The effects of tramadol and morphine on immune responses and pain after surgery in cancer patients. Anesth Analg 2000;90:1411–1414.

43. Gupta K, Kshirsagar S, Chang L, et al: Morphine stimulates angiogenesis by activating proangiogenic and survival-promoting signaling and promotes breast tumor growth. Cancer Res 2002;62: 4491–4498.

44. Singleton PA, Lingen MW, Fekete MJ, Garcia JG, Moss J: Methylnaltrexone inhibits opiate and VEGF-induced angiogenesis: role of receptor transactivation. Microvasc Res 2006;72:3–11.

45. Singleton PA, Moreno-Vinasco L, Sammani S, Wanderling SL, Moss J, Garcia JG: Attenuation of vascular permeability by methylnaltrexone: role of mOP-R and S1P3 transactivation. Am J Respir Cell Mol Biol 2007; 37:222:231.

46. Mathew B, Lennon FE, Siegler J, et al: The novel role of the mu opioid receptor in lung cancer progression: a laboratory investigation. Anesth Analg 2011;112:558–567.

47. Lennon FE, Mirzapoiazova T, Mambetsariev B, Salgia R, Moss J, Singleton PA: Overexpression of the mu-opioid receptor in human non-small cell lung cancer promotes Akt and mTOR activation, tumor growth, and metastasis. Anesthesiology 2012;116:857–867.

48. Christopherson R, James KE, Tableman M, Marshall P, Johnson FE: Long-term survival after colon cancer surgery: A variation associated with choice of anesthesia. Anesth Analg 2008;107:325–332.

49. Biki B, Mascha E, Moriarty DC, Fitzpatrick JM, Sessler DI, Buggy DJ: Anesthetic technique for radical prostatectomy surgery affects cancer recurrence: A retrospective analysis. Anesthesiology 2008;109: 180–187.

50. Tsui BC, Rashiq S, Schopflocher D, et al: Epidural anesthesia and cancer recurrence rates after radical prostatectomy. Can J Anaesth 2010; 57: 107–112.

51. Martinsson T: Ropivacaine inhibits serum-induced proliferation of colon adenocarcinoma cells in vitro. J Pharmacol Exp Ther 1999;288: 660–664.

52. Sakaguchi M, Kuroda Y, Hirose M: The antiproliferative effect of lidocaine on human tongue cancer cells with inhibition of the activity of epidermal growth factor receptor. Anesth Analg 2006;102: 1103–1107.

53. Lucchinetti E, Awad AE, Rahman M, et al: Antiproliferative effects of local anesthetics on mesenchymal stem cells: Potential implications for tumor spreading and wound healing. Anesthesiology 2012;116:841–856.

54. Procopio MA, Rassias AJ, DeLeo JA, Pahl J, Hildebrandt L, Yeager MP: The in vivo effects of general and epidural anesthesia on human immune function. Anesth Analg 2001;93:460–465.

55. Koltun WA, Bloomer MM, Tilberg AF, et al: Awake epidural anesthesia is associated with improved natural killer cell cytotoxicity and a reduced stress response. Am J Surg 1996;171:68–72.

56. Hole A, Unsgaard G, Breivik H: Monocyte functions are depressed during and after surgery under general anaesthesia but not under epidural anaesthesia. Acta Anaesthesiol Scand 1982;26:301–307.

57. Bar-Yosef S, Melamed R, Page GG, Shakhar G, Shakhar K, Ben-Eliyahu S: Attenuation of the tumor-promoting effect of surgery by spinal blockade in rats. Anesthesiology 2001;94:1066–1073.

58. Schlagenhauff B, Ellwanger U, Breuninger H, Stroebel W, Rassner G, Garbe C: Prognostic impact of the type of anaesthesia used during the excision of primary cutaneous melanoma. Melanoma Res 2000;10: 165–169.

59. Exadaktylos AK, Buggy DJ, Moriarty DC, Mascha E, Sessler DI: Can anesthetic technique for primary breast cancer surgery affect recurrence or metastasis? Anesthesiology 2006;105:660–664.

60. Ismail H, Ho KM, Narayan K, Kondalsamy-Chennakesavan S: Effect of neuraxial anaesthesia on tumour progression in cervical cancer patients treated with brachytherapy: A retrospective cohort study. Br J Anaesth 2010;105:145–149.

61. Gottschalk A, Ford JG, Regelin CC, et al: Association between epidural analgesia and cancer recurrence after colorectal cancer surgery. Anesthesiology 2010;113:27–34.

62. Wuethrich PY, Hsu Schmitz SF, Kessler TM, et al: Potential influence of the anesthetic technique used during open radical prostatectomy on prostate cancer-related outcome: A retrospective study. Anesthesiology 2010;113:570–576.

63. Myles PS, Peyton P, Silbert B, Hunt J, Rigg JR, Sessler DI: Perioperative epidural analgesia for major abdominal surgery for cancer and recurrence-free survival: Randomised trial. BMJ 2011;342:d1491.

64. de Oliveira GS Jr, Ahmad S, Schink JC, Singh DK, Fitzgerald PC, McCarthy RJ: Intraoperative neuraxial anesthesia but not postoperative neuraxial analgesia is associated with increased relapse-free survival in ovarian cancer patients after primary cytoreductive surgery. Reg Anesth Pain Med 2011;36:271–277.

65. Cummings KC 3rd, Xu F, Cummings LC, Cooper GS: A comparison of epidural analgesia and traditional pain management effects on survival and cancer recurrence after colectomy: A population-based study. Anesthesiology 2012;116:797–806.

66. Day A, Smith R, Jourdan I, Fawcett W, Scott M, Rockall T: Retrospective analysis of the effect of postoperative analgesia on survival in patients after laparoscopic resection of colorectal cancer. Br J Anaesth 2012;109: 185–190.

67. Balkwill F, Mantovani A: Inflammation and cancer: back to Virchow? Lancet 2001;357:539–545.

68. Balkwill F, Charles KA, Mantovani A: Smoldering and polarized inflammation in the initiation and promotion of malignant disease. Cancer Cell 2005;7:211–217.

69. Coussens LM, Werb Z: Inflammation and cancer. Nature 2002;420: 860–867.

70. Karin M: Nuclear factor-kappaB in cancer development and progression. Nature 2006;441:431–436.

71. Mantovani A, Allavena P, Sica A, Balkwill F: Cancer-related inflammation. Nature 2008;454:436–444.

72. Kim I, Moon SO, Kim SH, Kim HJ, Koh YS, Koh GY: Vascular endothelial growth factor expression of intercellular adhesion molecule 1 (ICAM-1), vascular cell adhesion molecule 1 (VCAM-1), and E-selectin through nuclear factor-kappa B activation in endothelial cells. J Biol Chem 2001;276:7614–7620.

73. Johnson JP. Cell adhesion molecules in the development and progression of malignant melanoma. Cancer Metastasis Rev 1999;18:345–357.

74. Rosette C, Roth RB, Oeth P, et al: Role of ICAM1 in invasion of human breast cancer cells. Carcinogenesis 2005;26:943–950.

75. Kageshita T, Yoshii A, Kimura T, et al: Clinical relevance of ICAM-1 expression in primary lesions and serum of patients with malignant melanoma. Cancer Res 1993;53:4927–4932.

76. Maurer CA, Friess H, Kretschmann B, et al: Over-expression of ICAM-1, VCAM-1 and ELAM-1 might influence tumor progression in colorectal cancer. Int J Cancer 1998;79:76–81.

77. Natali PG, Hamby CV, Felding-Habermann B, et al: Clinical significance of alpha(v)beta3 integrin and intercellular adhesion molecule-1 expression in cutaneous malignant melanoma lesions. Cancer Res 1997;57: 1554–1560.

78. Hayes SH, Seigel GM: Immunoreactivity of ICAM-1 in human tumors, metastases and normal tissues. Int J Clin Exp Pathol 2009;2:553–560.

79. Maruo Y, Gochi A, Kaihara A, et al: ICAM-1 expression and the soluble ICAM-1 level for evaluating the metastatic potential of gastric cancer. Int J Cancer 2002;100:486–490.

80. Huang WC, Chan ST, Yang TL, Tzeng CC, Chen CC: Inhibition of ICAM-1 gene expression, monocyte adhesion and cancer cell invasion by targeting IKK complex: Molecular and functional study of novel alpha-methylene-gamma-butyrolactone derivatives. Carcinogenesis 2004;25: 1925–1934.

81. Roland CL, Harken AH, Sarr MG, Barnett CC Jr: ICAM-1 expression determines malignant potential of cancer. Surgery 2007;141: 705–707.

82. Rahn JJ, Shen Q, Mah BK, Hugh JC: MUC1 initiates a calcium signal after ligation by intercellular adhesion molecule-1. J Biol Chem 2004;279: 29386–29390.

83. Pollard JW: Tumour-educated macrophages promote tumour progression and metastasis. Nat Rev Cancer 2004;4:71–78.

84. Barnett CC Jr, Moore EE, Mierau GW, et al: ICAM-1-CD18 interaction mediates neutrophil cytotoxicity through protease release. Am J Physiol 1998;274: C1634–C1644.

85. Wu QD, Wang JH, Condron C, Bouchier-Hayes D, Redmond HP: Human neutrophils facilitate tumor cell transendothelial migration. Am J Physiol Cell Physiol 2001;280:C814–C822.

86. Hu G, Minshall RD: Regulation of transendothelial permeability by Src kinase. Microvasc Res 2009;77:21–25.

87. Okutani D: [Src protein tyrosine kinase family and acute lung injury]. Nihon Rinsho Meneki Gakkai Kaishi 2006;29:334–341.

88. Summy JM, Gallick GE: Src family kinases in tumor progression and metastasis. Cancer Metastasis Rev 2003;22:337–358.

89. Weis S, Cui J, Barnes L, Cheresh D: Endothelial barrier disruption by VEGF-mediated Src activity potentiates tumor cell extravasation and metastasis. J Cell Biol 2004;167:223–229.

90. Guarino M: Src signaling in cancer invasion. J Cell Physiol 2010; 223: 14–26.

91. Rollins BJ: Monocyte chemoattractant protein 1: A potential regulator of monocyte recruitment in inflammatory disease. Mol Med Today 1996;2: 198–204.

92. Rollins BJ, Walz A, Baggiolini M: Recombinant human MCP-1/JE induces chemotaxis, calcium flux, and the respiratory burst in human monocytes. Blood 1991;78:1112–1116.

93. Goede V, Brogelli L, Ziche M, Augustin HG: Induction of inflammatory angiogenesis by monocyte chemoattractant protein-1. Int J Cancer 1999;82:765–770.

94. Cai Z, Chen Q, Chen J, et al: Monocyte chemotactic protein 1 promotes lung cancer-induced bone resorptive lesions in vivo. Neoplasia 2009;11:228–236.

95. Blumenthal S, Borgeat A, Pasch T, et al: Ropivacaine decreases inflammation in experimental endotoxin-induced lung injury. Anesthesiology 2006;104:961–969.

96. Piegeler T, Votta-Velis EG, Liu G, et al: Antimetastatic potential of amide-linked local anesthetics: Inhibition of lung adenocarcinoma cell migration and inflammatory Src signaling independent of sodium channel blockade. Anesthesiology 2012;117:548–559.

97. Peach G, Kim C, Zacharakis E, Purkayastha S, Ziprin P: Prognostic significance of circulating tumour cells following surgical resection of colorectal cancers: A systematic review. Br J Cancer 2010;102:1327–1334.

Perioperative Regional Anesthesia and Analgesia: Effects on Cancer Recurrence and Survival After Oncological Surgery

Zoe S. Gan, Yanxia Sun, and Tong J. Gan

INTRODUCTION

The effects of perioperative regional anesthesia (RA) on cancer recurrence and overall survival after surgery have been a subject of much interest and controversy. This chapter discusses the available evidence and possible mechanisms by which RA could have beneficial effects in these patients.

Surgical treatment of cancer is well established. An important consideration with oncological surgery is that the procedure may disseminate tumor cells in patients with micrometastases.[1,2] Metastatic recurrence, rather than the primary cancer, accounts for approximately 90% of cancer-related deaths.[3] Cancer cell development in local and metastatic recurrence is dependent on the interplay between the host defenses and the tumor's ability to seed, proliferate, and attract new blood vessels.[4,5] However, these in turn may be influenced by surgery, general anesthesia, and opioid administration, which are three of several perioperative factors that may contribute to metastatic spread.

There are several mechanisms through which these perioperative factors potentially affect cancer cell evolution. Surgery itself is a major physiological stress that may depress cell-mediated immunity, particularly the activity of natural killer (NK) cells and macrophages that would otherwise destroy various tumor cells.[6] This immunosuppression may be induced by factors such as neuroendocrine stress responses,[7] blood transfusion,[8] and hypothermia.[9] Surgery may also reduce antiangiogenic factors while increasing proangiogenic[10] and growth factors that cause malignant cells to proliferate.[11,12] In addition, general anesthesia with halogenated volatile agents or intravenous drugs such as thiopental may contribute to postoperative immune suppression by inhibiting the function of NK cells, neutrophils,

dendritic cells, and macrophages.[12,13] Intraoperative and postoperative opioid use has been shown to interfere with immune function, specifically by altering the levels of NK cells, B cells, and T lymphocytes, as well as stimulate angiogenesis via alterations in cytokine levels.[13] Thus, these perioperative factors may complicate surgical treatment of cancer by increasing growth factors and modulating host immunity (Figure 18–1).

Regional anesthesia and analgesia are commonly used for perioperative pain management and may have implications in both short- and long-term outcomes following oncological surgery. Regional anesthesia could potentially attenuate the stress response related to surgery, preserve immune function, and slow the surgical promotion of metastases.[6,14] Furthermore, it decreases the intraoperative use of volatile anesthetics and perioperative opioids.[15] In combination, these effects may lead to better preservation of perioperative immune function and a reduced incidence of cancer recurrence.

A recently published systematic review and meta-analysis evaluated these effects.[16] The meta-analysis included studies that compared the effects of RA on cancer recurrence and mortality with those of general anesthesia.

A total of 20 studies published between 2006 and 2014 met inclusion criteria and yielded 54,541 patients; 16,618 of these individuals received perioperative RA, with study sample sizes ranging from 94 to 42,151 (Table 18–1). Studies were most frequently excluded for the following reasons: not investigating RA for recurrence-free survival or overall survival; lacking original data; lacking cancer-related outcomes (time to cancer recurrence, all-cause mortality, disease-free survival, or cancer recurrence-free survival); or performing repeated analysis in a single population.

Perioperative Regional Anesthesia and Analgesia: Effects on Cancer Recurrence and Survival After Oncological Surgery **267**

CHAPTER 18

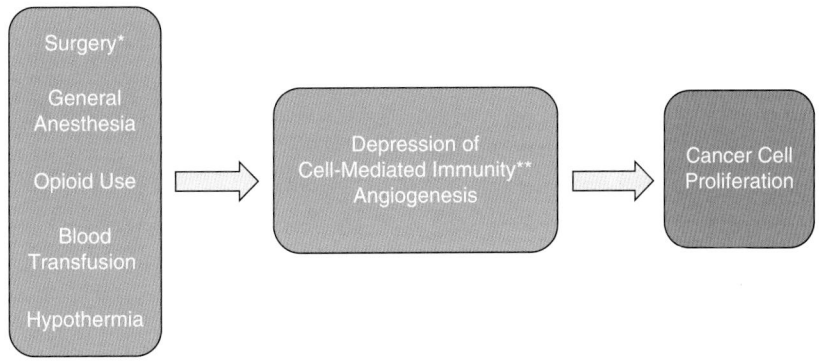

FIGURE 18–1. Perioperative factors affecting cancer cell evolution.

OVERALL PATIENT SURVIVAL

Overall survival was assessed in 13 studies.[17–27] There was a significantly positive association between RA and overall survival (hazard ratio [HR] = 0.84, 95% CI 0.75 to 0.94, I^2 = 41%) (Figure 18–2). This association held true when different cancer types were analyzed, including colorectal cancer (HR = 0.80, 95% CI 0.66 to 0.97); prostate cancer (HR = 0.77, 95% CI 0.61 to 0.97); and ovarian cancer (HR = 0.83, 95% CI 0.71 to 0.97).

CANCER RECURRENCE

The effect of RA on cancer recurrence-free survival was analyzed among 15 studies.[17,19,21,22,24–34] There was no overall effect on cancer recurrence-free survival among the RA and control groups (HR = 0.93, 95% CI 0.79 to 1.10, I^2 = 70%) (Figure 18–3). Subgroup analyses showed that different types of cancer had slightly different pooled HRs, but the differences were not statistically significant. Cancer types analyzed included colorectal cancer (0.86, 95% CI 0.67 to 1.12); ovarian cancer (0.73, 95% CI 0.39 to 1.37); and prostate cancer (0.82, 95% CI 0.58 to 1.14). Based on influence analyses, no individual study substantially influenced the pooled HR.

Perioperative RA may improve overall survival following oncologic surgery (HR = 0.84, 95% CI 0.75 to 0.94, I^2 = 41%). However, there was no positive association found between RA and reduced cancer recurrence (HR = 0.91, 95% CI 0.70 to 1.18, I^2 = 83%).

There are several potential explanations for the discrepancy between overall survival and cancer recurrence. First, some experimental studies have suggested that RA may not significantly influence recurrence, but rather slows cancer progression by reducing surgery-induced immunosuppression and postoperative pain, resulting in prolonged survival.[35,36] Second, RA may increase survival through means that are independent of the underlying disease, such as better rehabilitation, anti-inflammatory properties, and less chronic pain.[37] Finally, lack of statistical power could limit the demonstration of a true association between RA and cancer recurrence. This issue may be addressed in the future with additional prospective trials.

There is considerable variation in tumor biology from organ to organ, and it is likely that any potential effects of RA may vary from site to site. Although the effects of RA on cancer recurrence may be specific to certain tumors, subgroup analyses indicated that the absence of an effect was consistent for different types of cancer (colorectal, prostate, and ovarian cancer). It appears that RA does not differentially affect recurrence or overall survival for various cancer types.

Of several recently published trials on this topic, the meta-analysis by Sun et al[16] provides the most up-to-date analysis of the effects of RA on cancer recurrence and survival. It includes seven recently published studies[17,26,27,32,33,38,39] with higher-quality scores that were not identified in the previous meta-analysis, as well as five new studies[17,26,27,32,33] and three studies[21,22,25] excluded by previous meta-analysis. Importantly, the findings discussed in this chapter are consistent with those of prior meta-analyses.

While meta-analysis allows for a more comprehensive assessment of RA's potential effects on cancer recurrence and survival, several limitations should be kept in mind. First, because the included studies were retrospective, meta-analysis of these studies may have been susceptible to biases and confounding factors present in the original studies.[40] When available, adjusted estimates were used to control for possible sources of confounding factors. Unfortunately, the estimates could not be consistent in all studies. Sensitivity analyses were conducted for previous randomized controlled trials (RCTs) with limited bias. However, initial randomization in those RCTs was not stratified for tumor characteristics, and there may have been residual confounding factors or bias.

Finally, heterogeneity across studies may have affected the pooled estimates. Factors contributing to heterogeneity include type of surgical procedure, type of cancer, differences in study populations, assessment of covariates, and the definition and validation of survival endpoints. Several of the studies may have had follow-up periods of varying duration. Outcomes may have also been affected by the use of different RA strategies across studies. For example, one included study[34] found that intraoperative, rather than postoperative, use of epidural anesthesia led to delayed cancer recurrence following surgery in ovarian

TABLE 18–1. Characteristics of included studies.

Trials	Date of Surgery/ Follow-up Period	NOS Score	Type of Tumor	Technique RA (n)	Technique GA (n)	Study Design	Type of Procedure	Main Outcomes (RA/GA) Adjusted Risk Estimate (95% CI)
Scavonetto et al 2014[27]	1991.1– 2005.12 8.6 yr	7	Prostate cancer	GA + SPA/EDA (1642): SPA single injection before surgery; EDA: initiated before surgery and lasted 48/72 h after surgery	GA + opioid analgesia (1642)	Retrospective cohort study	Radical retropubic prostatectomy	RFS: 1.00 (0.83–1.21) OS: 0.76 (0.56–1.00)
Roiss et al 2014[26]	2002–2007 NA	7	Prostate cancer	GA + SPA (3047): single injection before surgery	GA (1725)	Retrospective cohort study	Radical retropubic prostatectomy	RFS: 1.09 (0.85–1.41) OS: 0.90 (0.51–1.6)
Merquiol et al 2013[33]	1984.1– 2008.12 54 months	7	Laryngeal and hypopharyngeal cancer	GA + EDA (111): initiated before surgery and lasted 48 h after surgery	GA + opioid analgesia (160)	Retrospective cohort study	Total pharyngo-laryngectomy; reconstructive laryngectomy	RFS: 0.49 (0.25–0.96) OS: 0.61 (0.39–0.96)
Binczak et al 2013[32]	1990.2– 1991.4 17.3 yr (median)	7	Various abdominal malignancies	GA + EDA (69): initiated before surgery and lasted until the fifth postoperative day	GA + opioid analgesia (63)	Previous RCT[a]	Major abdominal surgery for cancer	RFS: 0.81 (0.52–1.26) OS: 0.71 (0.47–1.07)
Lin et al 2011[23]	1994.1– 2006.10 2.0–14.5 yr	6	Ovarian serous adenocarcinoma	EDA (106): initiated before surgery and lasted 48 h after surgery	GA + opioid analgesia (37)	Retrospective cohort study	Laparotomy for ovarian carcinoma	OS: 0.82 (0.70–0.96)
Biki et al 2008[28]	1994.1– 2003.12 2.8–12.8 yr	6	Prostate cancer	GA + EDA (102): initiated before surgery and continued an infusion for 48–72 h after surgery	GA + opioid analgesia (123)	Retrospective cohort study	Radical prostatectomy	RFS: 0.43 (95% CI 0.22–0.83)
Gottschalk et al 2010[30]	2000.1–2007.3 1.8 yr (median)	7	Colorectal cancer	GA + EDA (256): perioperatively	GA (253)	Retrospective cohort study	Open colectomy	RFS: 0.82 (0.49–1.35)

Study		Dates / Follow-up	Cancer type	Regional group	Comparison group	Study type	Surgery	Results
Gottschalk et al 2012[38]	6	1998.2–2005.4; 52.5 months (mean)	Malignant melanoma	Spinal anesthesia (52): intraoperatively	GA-sevoflurane/sufentanil (118); TIVA (103)	Retrospective cohort study	Lymph node dissection for malignant melanoma	OS: A trend longer survival in spinal group (p = .087)
Tsui et al 2010[31]	6	2000–2001; At least 5 yr	Prostate cancer	EA + GA (49): intraoperatively	GA (50)	Previous RCT[a]	Radical prostatectomy	RFS: 1.33 (0.64–2.77)
Christopherson et al 2008[18]	7	1992.3–1994.8; 8.3–10.8 yr[b]	Colon cancer	GA + EDA (85): initiated before surgery and lasted as long as judged clinically appropriate after surgery	GA + opioids (92)	Previous RCT[a]	Open colectomy	OS (nonmetastasis subgroup): in the first 1.46 yr: 0.22 (0.07–0.69); Patient survival > 1.46 yr: 1.43 (0.75–2.70); OS (metastasis subgroup): 0.70 (0.40–1.24)
Myles et al 2011[24]	7	1995.7–2001.5; 9.0–14.8 yr[b]	Various abdominal malignancies	GA + EDA (230): initiated before surgery and lasted 74 h after surgery	GA + PCA (216)	Previous RCT[a]	Major abdominal surgery	RFS: 0.95 (0.76–1.17); OS: 0.95 (0.77–1.18)
Day et al 2012[39]	6	2003.10–2010.12; EDA (median): 37 months; PCA (median): 28 months	Bowel cancer	GA + EDA (107)/GA + SPA (144): EDA: initiated before surgery and lasted 48 h after surgery	GA + PCA (173)	Retrospective cohort study	Laparoscopic colorectal resection	No significant difference in overall survival (p = .622) or disease-free survival (p = 0.490) at 5 yr between the three groups
Gupta et al 2011[20]	6	2004.1–2008.1; 1–5yr	Colorectal cancer	GA + EDA (562): initiated before surgery and lasted 2–5 days after surgery	GA + PCA (93)	Retrospective cohort study	Open colectomy	OS (rectal cancer): 0.45 (0.22–0.90); OS (colon cancer): 0.82 (0.30–2.19)
Wuethrich et al 2010[25]	7	1994.1–2000.12; GA (median): 8.5 yr; EDA (median): 11.9 yr	Prostate	GA + EDA (103): initiated before surgery and lasted at least 48 h after surgery	GA + morphine (158)	Retrospective cohort study	Radical prostatectomy	RFS: 1.14 (0.84–1.54); OS: 0.61 (0.29–1.28)

(continued)

CHAPTER 18

TABLE 18–1. Characteristics of included studies. (*Continued*)

Trials`	Date of Surgery/ Follow-up Period	NOS Score	Type of Tumor	Technique RA (n)	Technique GA (n)	Study Design	Type of Procedure	Main Outcomes (RA/GA) Adjusted Risk Estimate (95% CI)
Exadaktylos et al 2006[29]	2001.9-2002.12 2.5–4.0 yr	6	Breast cancer	GA + paravertebral block (50): initiated before surgery and an infusion lasted for 48 h after surgery	GA + opioid (79)	Retrospective cohort study	Mastectomy	RFS: 0.21 (0.06–0.71)
Ismail et al 2010[21]	1996–2003 NA	6	Cervical cancer	Neuraxial anesthesia (69): intraoperatively	GA (63)	Retrospective cohort study	Brachytherapy	RFS: 0.95 (0.54–1.67) OS: 1.46 (0.81–2.61)
Cummings et al 2012[19]	1996–2005 5.3 yr (median) in EDA; 4.8 yr in the control group	8	Colorectal cancer	GA + EDA (9670): perioperatively	GA + opioid pain management (32,481)	Retrospective cohort study	Open colectomy	RFS: 1.05 (0.95–1.15) OS: 0.91 (0.87–0.94)
Lai et al 2012[22]	1999.8-2008.12 2.1–11.4 yr[b]	7	Hepatocellular carcinoma	EDA (62): intraoperatively	GA (117)	Retrospective cohort study	Radio-frequency ablation of hepatocelluar carcinoma	RFS 4.31 (2.24–8.29) OS: 1.26 (0.81–1.97)
de Oliveira et al 2011[34]	2000.1-2006.10 42 months (median)	7	Ovarian cancer	GA + postop EDA (29)/GA + EDA (26)	GA + PCA (127)	Retrospective cohort study	Debulking surgery for ovarian cancer	RFS (postop EDA): 0.86 (0.52–1.14); RFS (intraop EDA): 0.37 (0.19–0.73)
Capmas et al 2012[17]	2007.1-2009.12 NA	6	Ovarian cancer	GA + postop EDA (47)	GA (47)	Retrospective cohort study	Complete cytoreduction	RFS: 1.18 (0.61–2.31) OS: 1.25 (0.39–4.04)

EDA = epidural anesthesia and analgesia; GA = general anesthesia; HR = hazard ratio; NA = not available; NOS = Newcastle-Ottawa Scale; OS = overall survival; PCA = patient-controlled analgesia; RCT = randomized control trial; RFS = recurrence-free survival; SPA = spinal anesthesia.

aCurrent study based on previous RCT study that was designed initially to investigate the association between RA and other outcomes.

bCalculated from evaluation date minus date of surgery.

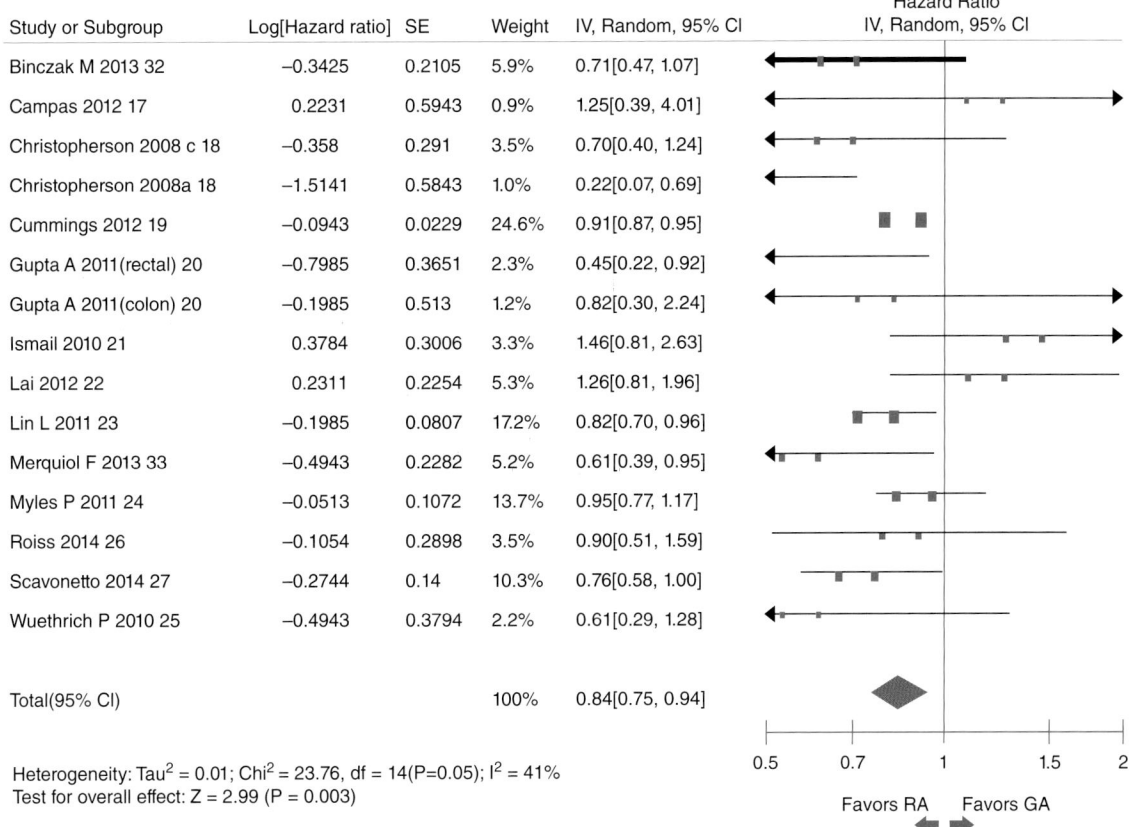

FIGURE 18–2. Meta-analysis and pooled hazard ratio (HR) of the effect of perioperative regional anesthesia and analgesia on overall survival after cancer surgery. a = patients without distant metastasis before surgery. c = patients with distant metastases before surgery; RA = regional anesthesia and analgesia; GA = general anesthesia; IV = inverse variance.

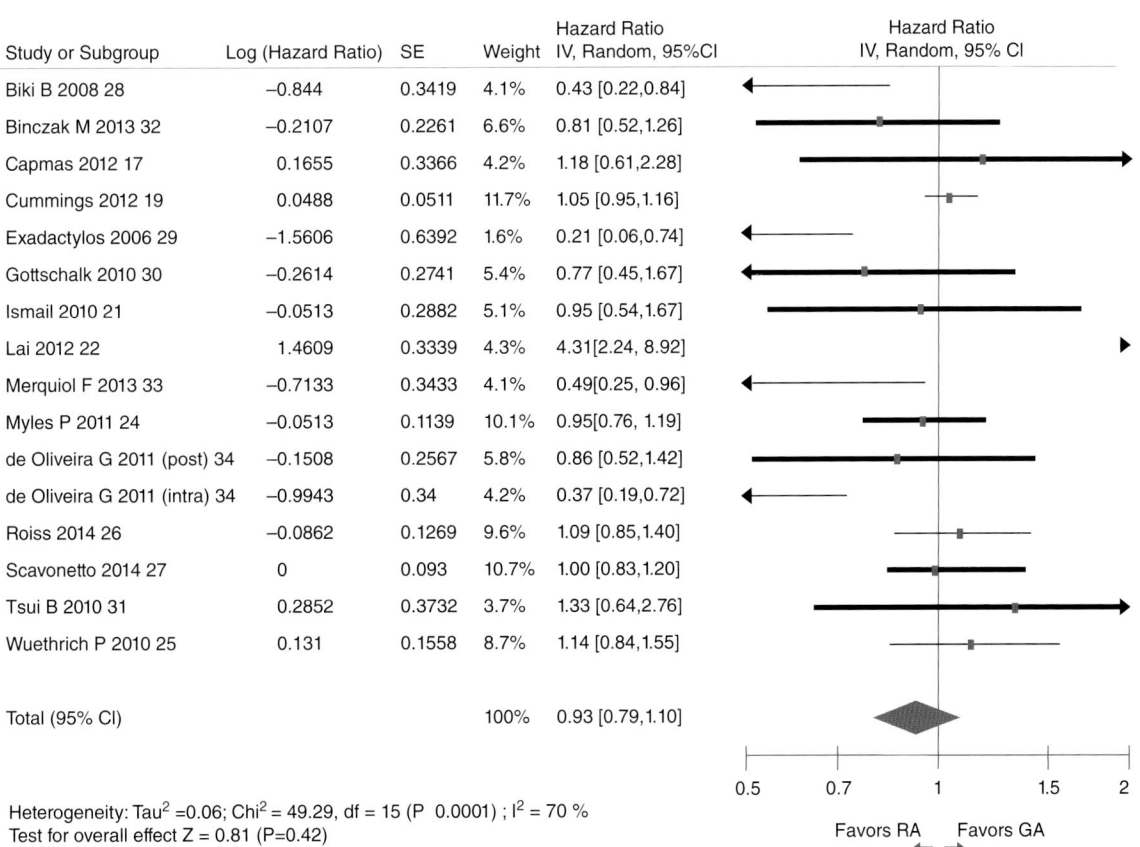

FIGURE 18–3. Meta-analysis and pooled hazard ratio (HR) of the effect of perioperative regional anesthesia and analgesia on cancer recurrence-free survival after cancer surgery. GA = general anesthesia; intra = epidural anesthesia initiated during surgery; post = epidural anesthesia initiated after surgery; RA = regional anesthesia and analgesia.

cancer patients. However, neither subgroup analyses nor meta-regression based on RA strategy were conducted due to the limited number of studies included.

Publication bias also remains a limitation of any meta-analysis. The Begg's test and Egger's test conducted in this analysis did not exhibit significant asymmetry, thus indicating that there was no significant evidence of publication bias for either overall survival or cancer recurrence-free survival. However, this cannot completely rule out publication bias.[41] Finally, because the findings do not necessarily suggest causation, one cannot simply deduce that the use of perioperative RA would improve prognoses for cancer patients.

CONCLUSIONS

Based on the available data, it is possible that the use of RA perioperatively may improve overall survival after oncologic surgery. However, the current data do not suggest a positive association between RA and cancer recurrence-free survival. Based on the biological and clinical effects of local anesthetics and RA, RA may be beneficial in some patients undergoing cancer surgery, most likely through preservation of the immune system and attenuation of the stress response to surgery. Understanding the true clinical implications of RA, however, awaits additional well-designed, higher-powered prospective clinical trials.

REFERENCES

1. Camara O, Kavallaris A, Noschel H, Rengsberger M, Jorke C, Pachmann K: Seeding of epithelial cells into circulation during surgery for breast cancer: The fate of malignant and benign mobilized cells. World J Surg Oncol 2006;4:67.
2. Denis MG, Lipart C, Leborgne J, et al: Detection of disseminated tumor cells in peripheral blood of colorectal cancer patients. Int J Cancer 1997;74:540–544.
3. Gupta GP, Massague J: Cancer metastasis: Building a framework. Cell 2006;127:679–695.
4. Colacchio TA, Yeager MP, Hildebrandt LW: Perioperative immunomodulation in cancer surgery. Am J Surg 1994;167:174–179.
5. Shakhar G, Ben-Eliyahu S: Potential prophylactic measures against postoperative immunosuppression: Could they reduce recurrence rates in oncological patients? Ann Surg Oncol 2003;10:972–992.
6. Bar-Yosef S, Melamed R, Page GG, Shakhar G, Shakhar K, Ben-Eliyahu S: Attenuation of the tumor-promoting effect of surgery by spinal blockade in rats. Anesthesiology 2001;94:1066–1073.
7. Ben-Eliyahu S: The promotion of tumor metastasis by surgery and stress: Immunological basis and implications for psychoneuroimmunology. Brain Behav Immun 2003;17(Suppl 1):S27–S36.
8. Klein HG: Immunomodulatory aspects of transfusion: a once and future risk? Anesthesiology 1999;91:861–865.
9. Ben-Eliyahu S, Shakhar G, Rosenne E, Levinson Y, Beilin B: Hypothermia in barbiturate-anesthetized rats suppresses natural killer cell activity and compromises resistance to tumor metastasis: A role for adrenergic mechanisms. Anesthesiology 1999;91:732–740.
10. Zetter BR. Angiogenesis and tumor metastasis. Annu Rev Med 1998;49:407–424.
11. O'Reilly MS, Boehm T, Shing Y, et al: Endostatin: An endogenous inhibitor of angiogenesis and tumor growth. Cell 1997;88:277–285.
12. Melamed R, Bar-Yosef S, Shakhar G, Shakhar K, Ben-Eliyahu S: Suppression of natural killer cell activity and promotion of tumor metastasis by ketamine, thiopental, and halothane, but not by propofol: Mediating mechanisms and prophylactic measures. Anesth Analg 2003;97:1331–1339.
13. Brand JM, Kirchner H, Poppe C, Schmucker P: The effects of general anesthesia on human peripheral immune cell distribution and cytokine production. Clin Immunol Immunopathol 1997;83:190–194.
14. O'Riain SC, Buggy DJ, Kerin MJ, Watson RW, Moriarty DC: Inhibition of the stress response to breast cancer surgery by regional anesthesia and analgesia does not affect vascular endothelial growth factor and prostaglandin E2. Anesth Analg 2005;100:244–249.
15. Hansdottir V, Philip J, Olsen MF, Eduard C, Houltz E, Ricksten SE: Thoracic epidural versus intravenous patient-controlled analgesia after cardiac surgery: A randomized controlled trial on length of hospital stay and patient-perceived quality of recovery. Anesthesiology 2006;104:142–151.
16. Sun Y, Li T, Gan TJ: The effects of perioperative regional anesthesia and analgesia on cancer recurrence and survival after oncology surgery: A systematic review and meta-analysis. Reg Anesth Pain Med 2015;40:589–598.
17. Capmas P, Billard V, Gouy S, et al: Impact of epidural analgesia on survival in patients undergoing complete cytoreductive surgery for ovarian cancer. Anticancer Res 2012;32:1537–1542.
18. Christopherson R, James KE, Tableman M, Marshall P, Johnson FE: Long-term survival after colon cancer surgery: A variation associated with choice of anesthesia. Anesth Analg 2008;107:325–332.
19. Cummings KC 3rd, Xu F, Cummings LC, Cooper GS: A comparison of epidural analgesia and traditional pain management effects on survival and cancer recurrence after colectomy: A population-based study. Anesthesiology 2012;116:797–806.
20. Gupta A, Bjornsson A, Fredriksson M, Hallbook O, Eintrei C: Reduction in mortality after epidural anaesthesia and analgesia in patients undergoing rectal but not colonic cancer surgery: A retrospective analysis of data from 655 patients in central Sweden. Br J Anaesth 2011;107:164–170.
21. Ismail H, Ho KM, Narayan K, Kondalsamy-Chennakesavan S: Effect of neuraxial anaesthesia on tumour progression in cervical cancer patients treated with brachytherapy: A retrospective cohort study. Br J Anaesth 2010;105:145–149.
22. Lai R, Peng Z, Chen D, et al: The effects of anesthetic technique on cancer recurrence in percutaneous radiofrequency ablation of small hepatocellular carcinoma. Anesth Analg 2012;114:290–296.
23. Lin L, Liu C, Tan H, Ouyang H, Zhang Y, Zeng W: Anaesthetic technique may affect prognosis for ovarian serous adenocarcinoma: a retrospective analysis. Br J Anaesth 2011;106:814–822.
24. Myles PS, Peyton P, Silbert B, Hunt J, Rigg JR, Sessler DI: Perioperative epidural analgesia for major abdominal surgery for cancer and recurrence-free survival: Randomised trial. BMJ 2011;342:d1491.
25. Wuethrich PY, Hsu Schmitz SF, Kessler TM, et al: Potential influence of the anesthetic technique used during open radical prostatectomy on prostate cancer-related outcome: A retrospective study. Anesthesiology 2010;113:570–576.
26. Roiss M, Schiffmann J, Tennstedt P, et al: Oncological long-term outcome of 4772 patients with prostate cancer undergoing radical prostatectomy: Does the anaesthetic technique matter? Eur J Surg Oncol 2014;40(12):1686–1692.
27. Scavonetto F, Yeoh TY, Umbreit EC, et al: Association between neuraxial analgesia, cancer progression, and mortality after radical prostatectomy: A large, retrospective matched cohort study. Br J Anaesth 2014;113(Suppl 1):i95–i102.
28. Biki B, Mascha E, Moriarty DC, Fitzpatrick JM, Sessler DI, Buggy DJ: Anesthetic technique for radical prostatectomy surgery affects cancer recurrence: A retrospective analysis. Anesthesiology 2008;109:180–187.
29. Exadaktylos AK, Buggy DJ, Moriarty DC, Mascha E, Sessler DI: Can anesthetic technique for primary breast cancer surgery affect recurrence or metastasis? Anesthesiology 2006;105:660–664.
30. Gottschalk A, Ford JG, Regelin CC, et al: Association between epidural analgesia and cancer recurrence after colorectal cancer surgery. Anesthesiology 2010;113:27–34.
31. Tsui BC, Rashiq S, Schopflocher D, Murtha A, Broemling S, Pillay J, Finucane BT: Epidural anesthesia and cancer recurrence rates after radical prostatectomy. Can J Anaesth 2010;57:107–112.
32. Binczak M, Tournay E, Billard V, Rey A, Jayr C: Major abdominal surgery for cancer: Does epidural analgesia have a long-term effect on recurrence-free and overall survival? Ann Fr Anesth Reanim 2013;32:e81–e88.
33. Merquiol F, Montelimard AS, Nourissat A, Molliex S, Zufferey PJ: Cervical epidural anesthesia is associated with increased cancer-free survival in laryngeal and hypopharyngeal cancer surgery: A retrospective propensity-matched analysis. Reg Anesth Pain Med 2013;38:398–402.
34. de Oliveira GS Jr, Ahmad S, Schink JC, Singh DK, Fitzgerald PC, McCarthy RJ: Intraoperative neuraxial anesthesia but not postoperative neuraxial analgesia is associated with increased relapse-free survival in ovarian cancer patients after primary cytoreductive surgery. Reg Anesth Pain Med 2011;36:271–277.

35. Page GG, Blakely WP, Ben-Eliyahu S: Evidence that postoperative pain is a mediator of the tumor-promoting effects of surgery in rats. Pain 2001;90:191–199.
36. Santamaria LB, Schifilliti D, La Torre D, Fodale V: Drugs of anaesthesia and cancer. Surg Oncol 2010;19:63–81.
37. Beloeil H, Asehnoune K, Moine P, Benhamou D, Mazoit JX: Bupivacaine's action on the carrageenan-induced inflammatory response in mice: Cytokine production by leukocytes after ex-vivo stimulation. Anesth Analg 2005;100:1081–1086.
38. Gottschalk A, Brodner G, Van Aken HK, Ellger B, Althaus S, Schulze HJ: Can regional anaesthesia for lymph-node dissection improve the prognosis in malignant melanoma? Br J Anaesth 2012;109:253–259.
39. Day A, Smith R, Jourdan I, Fawcett W, Scott M, Rockall T: Retrospective analysis of the effect of postoperative analgesia on survival in patients after laparoscopic resection of colorectal cancer. Br J Anaesth 2012;109:185–190.
40. Egger M, Schneider M, Davey Smith G: Spurious precision? Meta-analysis of observational studies. BMJ 1998;316:140–144.
41. Ioannidis JP, Trikalinos TA: The appropriateness of asymmetry tests for publication bias in meta-analyses: A large survey. CMAJ 2007;176:1091–1096.

CHAPTER 18

CLINICAL PRACTICE OF REGIONAL ANESTHESIA

LOCAL AND INFILTRATIONAL ANESTHESIA

Intra-articular and Periarticular Infiltration of Local Anesthetics

Johan Raeder and Ulrich J. Spreng

INTRODUCTION

Infiltration or instillation of local anesthetics around and into the joint as an analgesic adjunct for postoperative joint surgery pain has been used for decades. However, there has been a renewed interest in local infiltration analgesia (LIA), partly due to the work in 2008 of Kerr and Kohan,[1] who demonstrated superior analgesia after total knee or hip arthroplasty with extended, diluted infiltration of local anesthesia with epinephrine and ketorolac added and repeated injections through intra-articular catheters. The interest in using LIA in knee and hip surgery may be also due to the lack of the simpler regional anesthesia alternatives that exist for other joints. For instance, analgesia after shoulder and upper extremity surgery can be accomplished with a simple, single injection block of the brachial plexus, whereas analgesia for hip and knee joints requires multiple and more technically challenging nerve blocks. Also, while motor weakness is common with nerve blocks, infiltration analgesia typically spares the motor function.

THE CONCEPT OF LOCAL INFILTRATION ANALGESIA

There are three basic components of the LIA concept: high volume of diluted, long-acting local anesthetic; nonlocal anesthetic adjuvants; and catheter bolus injections (top-ups) for 1–3 days.

High Volume of Diluted Long-Acting Anesthetic Drug

A problem with local anesthetic infiltration for major surgery is that many different structures and layers must be infiltrated. In doing so, a certain minimum volume of local anesthetic is required for an effective local infiltration to cover all relevant structures. With conventional concentrations of local anesthetic solutions, such high volumes carry an unacceptable risk of systemic toxicity (see Chapter 65, Local Anesthetic Systemic Toxicity). However, anesthesia of the small nerve endings in and around joints does not require high-concentration local anesthetic. Thus, the concentration of local anesthetic may be lowered and the volume increased, keeping the total dose within safe limits. Further, as the major joints are devoid of major blood vessels, the risk of inadvertent injection of a large bolus directly into circulation is small.

Nonlocal Anesthetic Adjuvants

As careful injections of local anesthetic are made close to the site of surgical injury, there is a potential for targeting the source of pain caused by local inflammation and pain to supply effective treatment close to the origin of pain. This is an alternative to the systemic approach to analgesia by which a potentially higher total dose of drug is needed and carries a higher potential of general side effects. Nonlocal anesthetic adjuvants such as anti-inflammatory agents, nonsteroidal anti-inflammatory drugs (NSAIDs—traditional or cyclooxygenase [COX] 2 inhibitors) and steroids, as well as opioids and ketamine have all been used.

The role of epinephrine or clonidine in the LIA mixture, however, has not been well studied. While both drugs have an analgesic effect on the spinal α_2 receptors when given epidurally or spinally, there is no documentation on any specific analgesic effect or target mechanism of these drugs when used peripherally.[2] Epinephrine is often empirically included "just in case" due to the potential to prolong effect of other locally active drugs as their clearance from the local site is delayed due to the epinephrine-induced vasoconstriction.[3]

Catheter Top-ups for 1 to 3 Days

Long-acting local anesthetics used for infiltration, perioperative injections, and infiltration all have a limited duration and wear off within a few hours after injection. Because repeated injection of the local anesthetic is painful or inconvenient, one approach is to leave one or more catheters in the wound or joint to provide the vehicle for boluses or continuous infusion of local anesthetics. The use of catheters in a setting of major joint replacement, however, is controversial because of the potential for infection.[4] The routine use of catheter is also challenged in the United States by the recent development and FDA approval of long-acting depot bupivacaine, (liposomal bupivacaine) although the role and potential of this drug in the LIA concept requires more scrutiny.[5]

EVIDENCE-BASED INFORMATION ON EFFICACY AND SAFETY OF LOCAL INFILTRATION ANALGESIA

As often is the case with new methods and techniques, the initial enthusiasm for LIA expressed in clinical practices, professional gatherings, and case reports,[1] awaits evidence-based scrutiny before recommendations for everyday clinical use can be made.[6,7] The following are important questions that need scrutiny:

1. Is the method sufficiently efficacious?
2. What components of the new method are efficient?
3. How does LIA compare to other common methods in terms of safety, quality, and cost?

If a new method is tested as a component of a multimodal regimen and shows superiority versus controls, we may have the answer to the first question, but questions 2 and 3 remain unanswered. The logical next steps are to put to test each component individually (keeping all the rest unchanged and standardized) in controlled and standardized conditions to elucidate which components of the multimodal protocol are actually beneficial. The LIA should be compared with the best potential alternatives used under optimal conditions: intrathecal opioid, epidural analgesia, femoral nerve block, other nerve blocks, or just optimal multimodal analgesia, including local anesthesia wound infiltration.

We do know that infiltration of local anesthetics confers analgesia after knee replacement surgery, assuming that local anesthetic is skillfully infiltrated in all relevant tissues.[8] In a study of hernia repair with bupivacaine infiltration analgesia, Aasboe et al showed improved pain relief for as much as 1 week after the procedure.[9] Still, such results are to some extent procedure specific and not reproduced with LIA by others. In the study of Andersen et al on knee arthroplasty, the preoperative ropivacaine infiltration was superior to placebo at 6 hours but not at 24 hours.[4] The success of LIA may be dependent on how extensive the local infiltration technique is performed in terms of including all relevant structures, not only the superficial wound layers.[5]

With all new concepts, one must find a balance between rapidly incorporating the benefits into everyday practice while waiting for objective documentation from quality studies. The studies done so far on the efficacy of LIA do not have the power, standardization, or quality to provide a clear answer or even provide quality pooled data for meta-analyses.[6] One reason for the paucity of the evidence is that randomized, blinded studies incorporating LIA are somewhat difficult to design because all injections, catheters, and refilling, need to be done in the placebo group as well.[10] Even then,[8] such a placebo group would not be relevant because in clinical practice saline injections in wound structures and catheters would not occur, and yet, saline injections alone may have analgesic benefits.[11] This is because infiltration of saline into the knee joint has analgesic effect,[10,11] possibly by cooling and dilution of inflammatory local proteins, or placebo.

As there are many confounders, ideal studies on the efficacy of LIA should address only one or a few specific items at a time, controlling or standardizing the others. Such specific items include one specific type of surgery, systemic controls for all active drugs in the LIA mixture, and sham or placebo infusions or top-ups when testing postoperative LIA.

Analgesic effects of ketorolac[12] and ropivacaine when given systemically are well known. Likewise, intra-articular administration will also result in systemic absorption and systemic effects. It should be remembered that LIA may never be well standardized as a defined dose of a single intravenous drug or a specific nerve block for a few reasons. First, different types of surgery and joints vary in anatomical composition, acceptability for and spread of LIA, and degree of postoperative pain.[13] Second, differences in infiltration techniques may influence the analgesic benefits.

Clinical impression suggests that the morning injection the day after surgery seems to have an analgesic effect on patients in pain, although this was not demonstrated convincingly in controlled studies.[7,8,10] This may be because control patients in studies usually receive a placebo injection and often have low-to-moderate pain and thus not much potential or statistical power for showing improvements for the whole group.

Two further aspects of clinical interpretation of studies are important: If the control group receives an effective multimodal analgesic regimen resulting in low pain scores, it makes it difficult to demonstrate additional benefits of a new method. However, if a new method is equally effective but not better, it does not mean that the new method is of no value. In contrast, this simply provides a choice of two different methods with differences in side-effect profile, risks, and practical and economic aspects.

The benefits of LIA may be in various aspects of nursing care, less need for patient compliance, lower total dose of NSAID, lower need for opioids, lower need for gabapentinoids and their potential side effects, and so on. Still, the number of patients in many studies is too low to address the questions of safety and less-frequent side effects. Studies must carefully examine serious, but rare, side effects, as well as how to use LIA as a tool to improve rehabilitation, shorten hospital stay, and achieve a better functional outcome.

What are the alternatives to LIA for knee or hip arthroplasty? In terms of "most effective" pain relief, it is hard to better epidural analgesia.[14] However, epidural analgesia does not provide any analgesic benefits beyond the period of active use. In addition, during the analgesic treatment, the technique is resource demanding and impairs mobilization and physiotherapy.[14] There are also risks of urinary retention, hypotension, and epidural hematoma.

The femoral nerve block for knee arthroplasty provides more specific treatment but does not cover all nerves involved in knee innervation and results in quadriceps muscle weakness. As with epidural block, this technique may be associated with very rare but serious nerve damage. In a recent study comparing LIA and femoral block for knee arthroplasty, Affas et al showed less pain with activity with LIA at 24 hours and an advantage in terms of ease of performance and lower costs.[15] Other nerve blocks may provide more focused single-knee pain relief without motor block, such as an adductor canal block of the saphenous and obturator nerves.[16]

Intrathecal opioid, as used in the study of Essving et al[17] may be beneficial as well. Morphine appears to be the best drug in terms of prolonged effect after a single shot. However, a dose higher than 0.1 mg may in some cases prolong the effect, but with a higher risk of side effects.[18]

The expert, evidence-based, procedure-specific recommendation for knee arthroplasty (see http://www.postoppain.org/image.aspx?imgid=654) is the combination of either spinal anesthesia without opioid or general anesthesia with femoral block as the first choice for anesthesia. Either should be supplemented with acetaminophen plus NSAID plus an opioid for breakthrough pain. The recommendation for avoiding intrathecal morphine was based on nausea in a study with a morphine dose of 0.25 mg[18] and may not be relevant with the 0.1-mg dose used by Essving et al.[17] Although used by some, there are no convincing data that steroids[19] or gabapentinoid[20] confer additional analgesic benefits.

POTENTIAL AND DOCUMENTED PROS AND CONS OF LOCAL INFILTRATION ANALGESIA AND ALTERNATIVES

Pros

A major benefit of LIA is the lack of motor impairment often seen with alternative techniques of nerve blocks, such as femoral or sciatic nerve blocks, or epidural analgesia. With LIA, there is also a minor risk of hematoma formation, which is a feared complication of deep blocks, such as lumbar block or epidural analgesia. Also, LIA is not contraindicated in cases of increased bleeding risk from other causes, such as therapeutic anticoagulation, platelet inhibition, or even use of traditional NSAIDs or low-dose acetylsalicylic acid.

Another argument for LIA is its simplicity; the infiltration is can be done by the surgeon intraoperatively or anesthesia providers using ultrasound. Postoperative top-ups of one or more catheters may be done easily by a nurse on the ward.

Cons

Some of the specific cons of LIA have to do with the potential dangers of supplying a potent drug close to delicate joint structures. The local anesthetic may be neurotoxic to small nerves when supplied repeatedly, although diluted ropivacaine has proven to be safe for 2–3 days of continuous infusion.[21] A more serious concern may be the chondrotoxic effect, especially with bupivacaine.[22] Because in most hip and knee replacement surgeries the cartilage is removed as a part of the procedure, this consideration may not be of practical concern.

Adding NSAIDs, COX-2 inhibitors, or glucocorticoids may slow or impair tissue healing or growth, although practical impact has not yet been shown in human clinical studies in patients having hip or knee replacement. A concern has been voiced regarding a potential for increased risk of infection with LIA. This concern arises mainly from the postoperative use of a catheter with the risk of contamination from multiple injections as well as bacteria migration along the indwelling catheter, rather than from the sterile infiltration done during surgery. It is also theorized that epinephrine may impede circulation, oxygenation, and macrophage function. To minimize the risk of infection, it is important to use strict aseptic procedures for all top-ups and refills of infusions.

LOCAL INFILTRATION ANALGESIA FOR HIP ARTHROPLASTY

Kehlet et al[6] reviewed six available studies in 2011, whereas McCarthy and Iohom[23] extended the review by including additional additional studies. Since then, the two studies of Rikalainen-Salimi[26] and Murphy et al[25] have also been published.

The early studies of Kerr and Kohan et al[1] and Otte et al[26] reported favorable analgesia and rapid mobilization with LIA; however, there were no control groups. In the Parvataneni et al[27] and Busch et al[28] studies, LIA was compared to intravenous opioid analgesia. Both studies reported lower pain scores with LIA; the Parvataneni et al study reduced hospital stay by 1 day with LIA.

Four studies have compared LIA versus placebo. The first placebo-controlled trial of Bianconi et al[29] from 2003 used only 40 mL of ropivacaine 5 mg/mL were used for infiltration, but infusion of 10 mg/h continued for 35 hours. The LIA group had lower pain scores at rest and during mobilization up to 72 hours postoperatively and a lower need for opioids. The study of Andersson et al[30] used infiltration, followed by bolus the next day, and demonstrated less pain and opioid consumption from 4 hours postoperatively up to 2 weeks, whereas joint function was improved at 1 week. Murphy et al[25] compared infiltration with 60 mL levobupivacaine 2.5 mg/mL versus placebo. The morphine consumption was reduced by 4% in the LIA group during the first 12 hours, but quality of analgesia and side effects were similar. In the placebo-controlled study of Lunn et al,[31] the placebo group received an optimal multimodal analgesic regimen of acetaminophen, celecoxib, and gabapentin with equal results as in the LIA group.

Andersen et al[32] compared LIA with top-up injections to epidural analgesia and found less opioid consumption, better mobilization, and shorter hospital stay with LIA. Specht et al[33] found that a top-up bolus at 10 and 22 hours was no better than placebo in patients who received perioperative LIA.

Rikalainen-Salmi et al[24] compared LIA with a top-up morning after surgery to morphine 0.1 mg given as a part of the spinal anesthetic. The LIA technique resulted in less opioid consumption on the day of surgery and better early mobilization, without any difference in pain scores and patient satisfaction; the LIA top-up, however, did not confer any benefit. Taken together, LIA appears to be better than placebo for hip replacement surgery, whereas in comparison with other optimized methods, the results are mixed.

Whether the adjuncts in the LIA solutions have a specific local effect compared with systemic administration has not been studied properly in hip surgery.

LOCAL INFILTRATION ANALGESIA FOR KNEE ARTHROPLASTY

A wide range of LIA techniques for total knee arthroplasty have been described in recent literature. In earlier studies, the volume of the mixture of local anesthetics and adjuvants used was lower than 50 mL.[29,34-36]

In the study of Kerr and Kohan, a mixture of ropivacaine (2 mg/mL, maximum 300 mg), ketorolac (30 mg), and epinephrine (10 μg/mL) was diluted with saline to a volume of 150–170 mL. The mixture was injected into the different knee structures during the knee arthroplasty in three stages: after preparation of bone surfaces (30–50 mL), after insertion of the prosthesis components (35–50 mL), and into subcutaneous tissue (25–50 mL). At the end of surgery, an 18-gauge epidural catheter was inserted with the catheter tip placed anterior to the posterior capsule, and 10–15 mL of the mixture were injected. This catheter was used for a further injection 15–20 hours postoperatively, when another 50 mL of the mixture were injected through the catheter.

To our knowledge, the first randomized studies regarding high-volume intra- or periarticular multimodal drug injection in total knee arthroplasty were published by Busch et al[37] and Vendittoli el al.[38] Several reviews regarding LIA following total knee arthroplasty have been published recently.[6,39,40] The most recent review by Gibbs et al[41] included a total of 29 randomized studies. However, this number in Gibbs and colleagues' review also included some local infiltration studies in which low volumes of LIA (<100 mL) were used.[34,36] Most of the individual studies lacked adequate blinding. However, when comparing different treatment modalities (eg, LIA vs. epidural analgesia), a proper trial would require invasive procedures in the placebo group, which may be unethical and therefore difficult to execute. Andersen and colleagues conducted a double-blind, placebo-controlled study in patients undergoing bilateral total knee arthroplasty and demonstrated the effectiveness of the LIA technique.[42]

However, based on the current information, effectiveness of a postoperative top-up dose is questionable and may carry a risk of infection.[7] Regardless, several authors reported that postoperative top-up injections are associated with less opioid consumption and lower pain scores.[8,14,43,44] To date, no study reported an increased incidence of postoperative infections with LIA catheters.

Clinical Pearls

Is LIA of sufficient clinical benefit to warrant routine clinical use?
A. Hip replacement surgery
   LIA is not better than preoperative spinal anesthesia followed by multimodal analgesia with acetaminophen + NSAID/COX-2 inhibitor + either glucocorticoid or gabapentinoid.
   In patients in whom multimodal therapy is contraindicated LIA may be a valuable analgesic method, reducing the need for rescue opioids.
B. Knee replacement surgery
   Yes, even with an optimal preoperative spinal (or other nerve blocks) and three-component systemic multimodal analgesia, preoperative LIA still provides additional analgesia for 24–48 hours.

Compared to no injections or saline injections, all studies showed LIA had a beneficial analgesic effect.[8,37,38,43,45] The two studies comparing LIA to femoral nerve block, however, showed conflicting results. While Toftdahl and colleagues[44] concluded that LIA was superior to a continuous femoral nerve block regarding opioid consumption and pain scores during the first postoperative day, Carli et al[46] suggested that the femoral nerve is better. Of note, patients in the Carli et al study received an infiltration with ropivacaine, ketorolac, and epinephrine into the posterior capsule of the knee joint during surgery (in addition to LIA or femoral nerve block).

Both studies comparing LIA with epidural analgesia (Table 19–1) demonstrated that LIA can reduce both postoperative opioid consumption and postoperative pain scores.[14,47] Moreover, LIA was associated with faster mobilization and earlier readiness for hospital discharge.[14]

The LIA recipe (ie, volume, content, as well as the use of adjuvants) is not well defined. Two recently published studies have shown that ketorolac is an important factor in the LIA mixture.[14,48] Moreover, Spreng and colleagues showed that local administration of ketorolac and morphine may also have a local effect.[14]

Application of a compression bandage for 24 hours postoperatively[49] and infiltration of superficial layers in the knee joint with local anesthetics are also important for the effectiveness of the LIA.[42]

Several recent studies have been published regarding continuous infusion of local anesthetics with or without adjuvants.[50,51] Gomez-Cardero and Rodriguez-Merchán[50] compared continuous LIA for 60 hours (ropivacaine) with placebo and found reduced opioid consumption and pain scores for the first 3 days after surgery. Ong and colleagues[51] examined the use of continuous intra-articular infusion or bolus dose and demonstrated reduced opioid consumption and lower pain scores compared to intravenous pain treatment only.

TABLE 19–1. Comparison of local infiltration analgesia with other techniques.

Author (Reference Number)	Patients (n)	Groups Intraoperative	Treatment Intraoperative	Groups Postoperative	Treatment Postoperative	Findings of LIA
1. Studies Comparing LIA With No Injections or Saline Injections						
Busch et al (2006)[37]	64	LIA (100 mL) / No injection	400 mg ropivacaine / 30 mg ketorolac / 5 mg epimorphine / 0.6 mg epinephrine	All patients	No injections into the knee / Morphine PCA	Opioid consumption ↓ (0–24 h) / Pain ↓ (0–4 h)
Vendittoli et al (2006)[38]	42	LIA (160 mL) / No injection	275 mg ropivacaine / 30 mg ketorolac / 0.5 mg epinephrine	LIA (15 mL) / No injection	150 mg ropivacaine after 16–24 h	Opioid consumption ↓ (0–48 h) / Pain ↓ (0–48 h)
Andersen et al (2008)[8]	12 (24 knees)	LIA (170 mL) / Control	340 mg ropivacaine / 1.7 mg epinephrine / Saline (170 mL)	LIA / Control	8 h: 40 mg ropivacaine + 0.2 mg epinephrine (20 mL) / 24 h: 100 mg ropivacaine + 0.5 mg epinephrine (50 mL) / 8 h + 24 h: saline (20 + 50 mL)	Pain ↓ (0–24 h)
Kazak et al (2010)[45]	60	LIA (150 mL) / LIA (150 mL) / Control	200 mg bupivacaine 0.5 mg epinephrine / 200 mg levobupivacaine 0.5 mg epinephrine / Saline (150 mL)	LIA (25 mL) / LIA (25 mL) / Control	10 h + 22 h: 120 mg bupivacaine / 10 h + 22 h: 120 mg levobupivacaine + 0.5 mg epinephrine / 10 h + 22 h: saline (25 mL + 25 mL)	Opioid consumption ↓ (0–48 h) / Pain ↓ (0–48 h)
Essving et al (2010)[43]	48	LIA (166 mL) / No injection	400 mg ropivacaine / 30 mg ketorolac / 0.5 mg epinephrine	LIA (22 mL) / Control	21 h: 200 mg ropivacaine + 30 mg ketorolac + 0.1 mg epinephrine / 21 h: saline (22 mL)	Opioid consumption ↓ (0–48 h) / Pain ↓ (0–27 h)
2. Studies Comparing LIA With Femoral Nerve Block						
Carli et al (2010)[46]	40	LIA (102 mL) → peri- and intra-articularly FNB (8mL) / *All patients:* → Infiltration postoperative capsule (51 mL)	200 mg ropivacaine / 30 mg ketorolac / 0.5 mg epinephrine + 8 mL saline in femoral catheter / 16 mg ropivacaine + 100 mL saline into periarticular catheter / 100 mg ropivacaine / 15 mg ketorolac / 0.25 mg epinephrine	LIA (50) mL / FNB	24 h: 250 mg ropivacaine + 30 mg ketorolac + 0.25 mg epinephrine + 8 mL/h saline through femoral catheter for 48 h / Ropivacaine 2 mg/mL 8mL/h for 48 h + 50 mL saline into periarticular catheter 24 h after surgery	Opioid consumption ↑ (0–48 h) for LIA group (peri- and intra-articular infiltrations)

Study	N	Group (volume)	Initial dose	Subsequent/infusion dose	Outcome
Toftdahl et al (2007)[44]	77	LIA (152 mL)	300 mg ropivacaine, 30 mg ketorolac, 0.5 mg epinephrine, 200 mg ropivacaine, 4 mg morphine + 50 mg bupivacaine through drain (intra-articular)	12 h + 24 h: 200 mg ropivacaine + 30 mg ketorolac + 0.5 mg epinephrine	Opioid consumption ↓ (0–24 h), Pain ↓ (0–24 h)
		FNB (20 mL)		Ropivacaine 2 mg/mL at 10 mL/h for 48 h	

3. Studies Comparing LIA With Epidural Analgesia

Study	N	Group (volume)	Initial dose	Subsequent/infusion dose	Outcome
Andersen et al (2010)[47]	40	LIA (152 mL)	300 mg ropivacaine, 30 mg ketorolac, 0.5 mg epinephrine	Continuous infusion at 4 mL/h for 48 h (380 mg ropivacaine, 60 mg ketorolac)	Opioid consumption ↓ (0–48 h), Pain ↓ (0–72 h)
		EDA	Test dose 3 mL: lidocaine + epinephrine	Continuous infusion at 4 mL/h for 48 h (ropivacaine 2 mg/mL), Ketorolac 15 mg IV × 6	
Spreng et al (2010)[14]	99	LIA (150 mL)	150 mg ropivacaine, 30 mg ketorolac, 5 mg morphine, 0.5 mg epinephrine, 6 mL saline IV	22–24 h: 142.5 mg ropivacaine + 30 mg ketorolac, 1 mL saline IV	Opioid consumption ↓ (0–72 h), Pain ↓ (24–72 h)
		LIA IV (150mL)	150 mg ropivacaine, 0.5 mg epinephrine, 6 mL saline (LIA), 30 mg ketorolac IV, 5 mg morphine IV	22–24 h: 142.5 mg ropivacaine + 1 mL saline (LIA), 1 mL ketorolac IV	
		EDA	Test dose 3 mL: lidocaine + epinephrine	6–10 mL/h for 48h: fentanyl 2 µg/mL + bupivacaine 1 mg/mL + epinephrine 1 µg/mL	

4. Studies Comparing Different LIA Techniques

Study	N	Group (volume)	Initial dose	Subsequent/infusion dose	Outcome
Andersen et al (2008)[49]	48	LIA ± compression bandage	340 mg ropivacaine, 1 mg epinephrine (170 mL)	6 h + 12 h: 40 mg ropivacaine + 0.2 mg epinephrine (20 mL), 24 h: 100 mg epinephrine (50 mL)	Pain ↓ (0–8h) with compression bandage
Andersen et al (2010;p984)	43	All patients: LIA (150 mL)	300 mg ropivacaine, 1 mg epinephrine	6 h + 24 h: ropivacaine 5 mg/mL	No differences between the groups
		LIA (10 mL)		6 h + 24 h: ropivacaine 10 mg/mL	
Andersen et al (2010;p543)[42]	16 (32 knees)	LIA (150 mL)	200 mg ropivacaine, 1 mg epinephrine, 100 mg ropivacaine to superficial layers	24 h: 100 mg ropivacaine subcutaneously	Pain ↓ (0–6 h) with infiltration of superficial layers, but no difference after 24 h
		Control (100 mL)	200 mg ropivacaine, 1 mg epinephrine, 50 mL saline to superficial layers	24 h: saline subcutaneously	

(continued)

TABLE 19–1. Comparison of local infiltration analgesia with other techniques. *(Continued)*

Author (Reference Number)	Patients (n)	Groups Intraoperative	Treatment Intraoperative	Groups Postoperative	Treatment Postoperative	Findings of LIA
Andersen et al (2010;p904)	60	*All patients:* LIA (150 mL)	300 mg ropivacaine 1 mg epinephrine	LIA (20 mL) intracapsular; LIA (20 mL) intra-articular	6 h + 24 h: 100 mg ropivacaine	No differences between the groups
Andersen et al (2008;p800)[49]	32	*All patients:* LIA (170 mL)	340 mg ropivacaine 1.2 mg epinephrine	LIA; LIA	6 h + 12 h + 24 h: 40 mg ropivacaine + 0.2 mg epinephrine (20 mL). Additional 60 mg ropivacaine + 0.3 mg epinephrine (30 mL) during catheter retraction; 6 h + 12 h + 24 h: 40 mg ropivacaine + 0.2 mg epinephrine (20 mL). Additional 30 mL saline during catheter retraction	No differences between the groups
Spreng et al (2010)[14]	99	LIA (150 mL); LIA IV (150 mL); EDA	150 mg ropivacaine 30 mg ketorolac 5 mg morphine 0.5 mg epinephrine 6 mL saline IV; 150 mg ropivacaine 0.5 mg epinephrine 6 mL saline (LIA) 30 mg ketorolac IV 5 mg morphine IV; Test dose 3 mL: lidocaine + epinephrine	LIA (20 mL); LIA IV (20 mL); EDA	22–24 h: 142.5 mg ropivacaine + 30 mg ketorolac 1 mL saline IV; 22–24 h: 142.5 mg ropivacaine + 1 mL saline (LIA) 1 mL ketorolac IV; 6–10 mL/h for 48 h (fentanyl 2 µg/mL + bupivacaine 1 mg/mL + epinephrine 1 µg/mL)	Opioid consumption ↓ (0–72 h) when ketorolac and morphine were infiltrated into the knee; Pain ↓ (0–72 h) when ketorolac and morphine were infiltrated into the knee
Andersen et al (2013)[48]	60	LIA (151 mL); LIA (151 mL)	300 mg ropivacaine 30 mg ketorolac; 300 mg ropivacaine 1 mL saline	LIA (10 mL); LIA (10 mL)	Every 6 h for 48 h: 100 mg ropivacaine + 15 mg ketorolac; Every 6 h for 48 h: 100 mg ropivacaine + 1 mL	Opioid consumption ↓ (0–48 h) in the ketorolac group; Pain ↓ (0–48 h) in the ketorolac group

EDA = epidural analgesia; IV = intravenous; LIA = local infiltration analgesia; FNB = femoral nerve block; PCA = patient-controlled analgesia.

LOCAL INFILTRATION ANALGESIA RECIPES

LIA in Total Knee Arthroplasty

The LIA Recipe

The solution, which is infiltrated into the knee, should be prepared under aseptic conditions (Figure 19–1). The total volume of the solution is 150 mL and contains the following:

- 200 mg ropivacaine (2 mg/mL) (amount of infiltrated ropivacaine in published studies varied: 150 mg,[14] 200 mg,[52] 300 mg,[1] 400 mg[37])
- 30 mg ketorolac (30 mg/mL)
- 0.5 mg epinephrine (1 mg/mL)
- Isotonic saline (dilution to 150 mL total)

Clinical Pearls

Although there are numerous recipes, the following formula is efficacious for both knee and hip replacement surgery:

- Total volume 150 mL (add normal saline according to the number of milliliters used by the other drugs)
- 200 mg ropivacaine (use any practical preparation: 2, 5, 7.7 mg/mL, dilute)
- 30 mg ketorolac

The addition of epinephrine (eg, 0.5 mg in 150 mL) may have a beneficial effect on hemostasis.

The solution, which is infiltrated into the knee catheter postoperatively (top-up dose), should also be prepared under aseptic conditions. The total volume of the solution should be 15–20 mL for each injection and contains the following:

- 150 mg ropivacaine (5–7.5 mg/mL)
- 30 mg ketorolac (30 mg/mL)
- Isotonic saline (dilution to 15–20 mL total)

Injection Technique

- After surgical preparation of the knee joint, 40 mL of the LIA solution are infiltrated into posterior capsule structures by the orthopedic surgeon. A "moving needle technique" is preferable (Figure 19–2, area marked I).
- After the joint replacement, 50–60 mL of the solution are infiltrated circularly around the prosthesis (Figure 19–2, area marked IIa and IIb).
- An 18-gauge epidural catheter with a bacterial filter can be placed from the lateral side into the knee joint (optional) (Figure 19–2, sinusoidal line, marked III; Figure 19–3).
- After closure of the capsule, another 50 mL of the solution are infiltrated into the fascia and subcutis (Figure 19–4).
- If a catheter is used, 10 mL of the solution are injected through the knee catheter at the end of surgery to verify fluid flow (Figure 19–5).

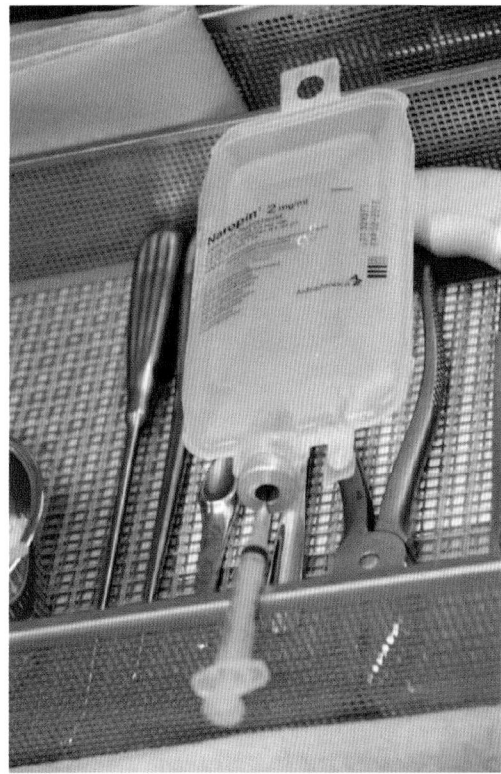

FIGURE 19–1. In the operating room, a sterile bag with ropivacaine from the pharmacy receives the addition of 30 mg (1 mL) ketorolac and 0.5 mg (0.5 mL) epinephrine.

- Aseptic top-up injections into the knee catheter (15–20 mL, according to the actual knee size) after 8, 16, and 24 hours (Figure 19–6).
- The knee catheter is removed during the last injection with subsequent spread into the fascia and subcutis.

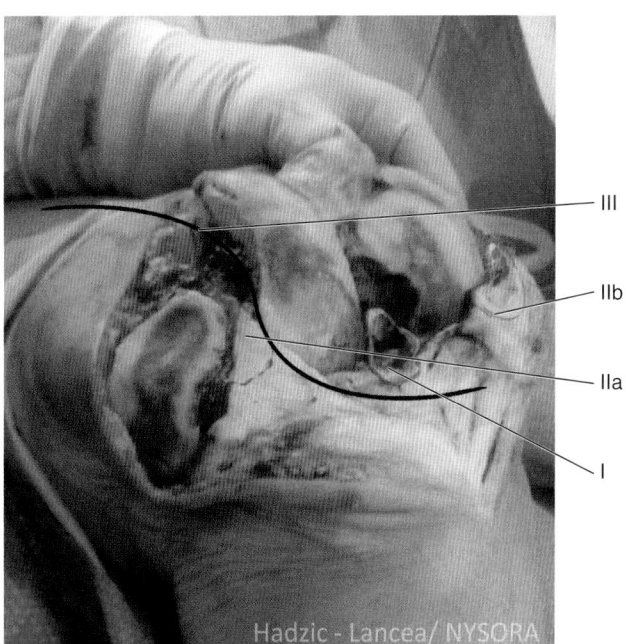

FIGURE 19–2. Four steps LIA injection technique in patients having knee replacement.

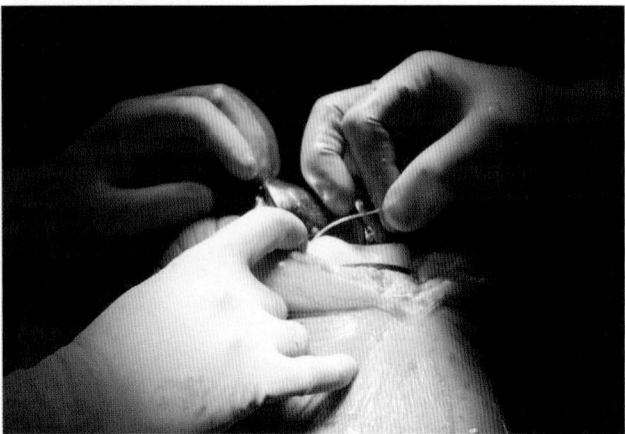

FIGURE 19–3. The catheter is placed into the knee laterally.

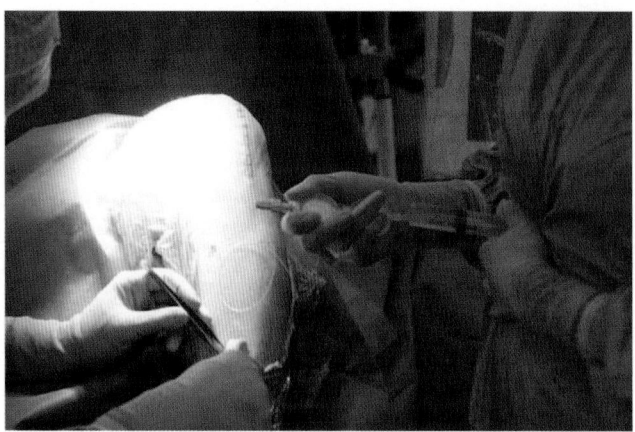

FIGURE 19–5. The last injection through the catheter: 10 mL for analgesia and for testing the catheter.

LIA in Total Hip Arthroplasty
The LIA Cocktail

The LIA cocktail solution, which is infiltrated into the hip, should be prepared under aseptic conditions (Figure 19–1). The total volume of the solution is 100 mL and contains the following:

- 200 mg ropivacaine (2 mg/mL)
- 30 mg ketorolac (30 mg/mL)
- 0.5 mg epinephrine (1 mg/mL)
- Isotonic saline (dilution to 100 mL total)

Injection Technique

Depending on the size of the surgical incision and choice of surgical approach, 100 mL of the LIA solution are injected in two stages:

- After surgical preperation of the acetabulum, 50 mL of the solution are infiltrated into capsule structures (if remaining), into adductor muscles and into the gluteus medius muscle.

Clinical Pearls

Should we include catheters for peri- or intra-articular infusion/top-ups when using LIA?

- No, there is strong evidence for no benefit of catheter after hip prosthesis.
- After knee prosthesis, the evidence is more conflicting, mostly indicating no extra effect when compared with optimal multimodal systemic analgesia, but some effect if not all components of the multimodal regimes are used.
- A recent report of an increased rate of infections[55] with catheters, added to anecdotal reports of similar results, added to the evidence in disfavor of catheter use.

- After insertion of the femoral component, another 50 mL are infiltrated into the external rotators (quadratus femoris muscle, obturator muscle, and the tendon of the gluteus maximus muscle) (Figure 19–6).

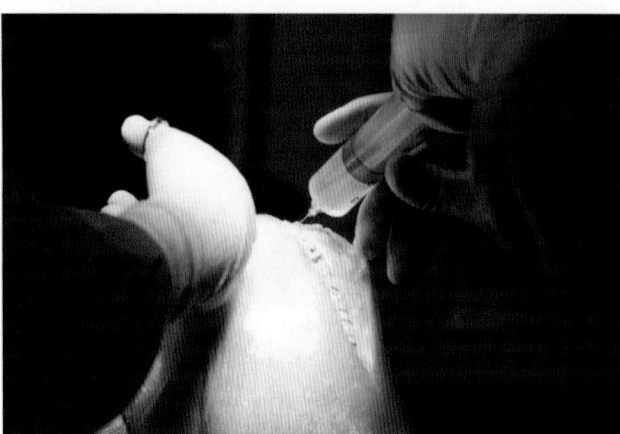

FIGURE 19–4. The fascia and subcutaneous tissue are infiltrated with 50 ml. of LIA solution.

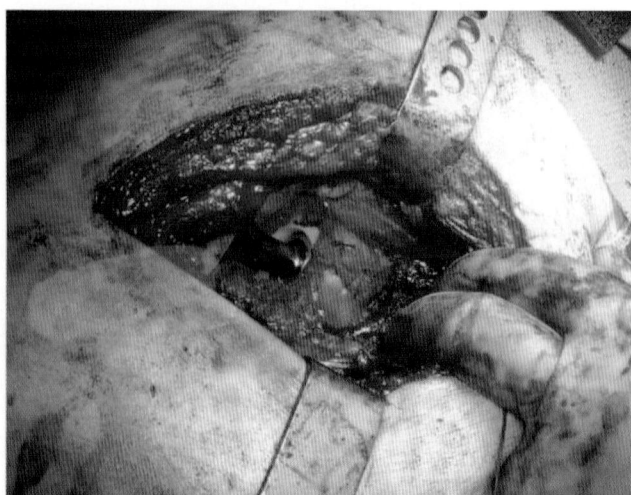

FIGURE 19–6. Sites for infiltration of LIA in hip arthroplasty: transparent blue area for first injection (see text) and transparent green area for the second injection.

REFERENCES

1. Kerr DR, Kohan L: Local infiltration analgesia: A technique for the control of acute postoperative pain following knee and hip surgery: A case study of 325 patients. Acta Orthop 2008;79:174–183.

2. Goodwin RC, Amjadi F, Parker RD: Short-term analgesic effects of intra-articular injections after knee arthroscopy. Arthroscopy 2005;21: 307–312.

3. Brummett CM, Williams BA: Additives to local anesthetics for peripheral nerve blockade. Int Anesthesiol Clin 2011;49:104–116.

4. Ilfeld BM: Continuous peripheral nerve blocks: A review of the published evidence. Anesth Analg 2011;113:904–925.

5. Smoot JD, Bergese SD, Onel E, et al: The efficacy and safety of DepoFoam bupivacaine in patients undergoing bilateral, cosmetic, submuscular augmentation mammaplasty: A randomized, double-blind, active-control study. Aesthet Surg J 2012;32:69–76.

6. Kehlet H, Andersen LO: Local infiltration analgesia in joint replacement: The evidence and recommendations for clinical practice. Acta Anaesthesiol Scand 2011;55:778–784.

7. Raeder J, Spreng UJ: Local-infiltration anaesthesia (LIA): Post-operative pain management revisited and appraised by the surgeons? Acta Anaesthesiol Scand 2011;55:772–774.

8. Andersen LO, Husted H, Otte KS, et al: High-volume infiltration analgesia in total knee arthroplasty: A randomized, double-blind, placebo-controlled trial. Acta Anaesthesiol Scand 2008;52:1331–1335.

9. Aasbo V, Thuen A, Raeder J: Improved long-lasting postoperative analgesia, recovery function and patient satisfaction after inguinal hernia repair with inguinal field block compared with general anesthesia. Acta Anaesthesiol Scand 2002;46:674–678.

10. Parker RD, Streem K, Schmitz L, Martineau PA: Efficacy of continuous intra-articular bupivacaine infusion for postoperative analgesia after anterior cruciate ligament reconstruction: A double-blinded, placebo-controlled, prospective, and randomized study. Am J Sports Med 2007; 35:531–536.

11. Rosseland LA, Helgesen KG, Breivik H, Stubhaug A: Moderate-to-severe pain after knee arthroscopy is relieved by intraarticular saline: a randomized controlled trial. Anesth Analg 2004;98:1546–1551, table.

12. Lenz H, Raeder, Heyerdahl F, et al: Modulation of remifentanil-induced postinfusion hyperalgesia by parecoxib or ketorolac in humans. Pain 2011;100–110.

13. Dye SF: The pathophysiology of patellofemoral pain: A tissue homeostasis perspective. Clin Orthop Relat Res 2005;100–110.

14. Spreng UJ, Dahl V, Hjall A, et al: High-volume local infiltration analgesia combined with intravenous or local ketorolac + morphine compared with epidural analgesia after total knee arthroplasty. Br J Anaesth 2010;105: 675–682.

15. Affas F, Nygards EB, Stiller CO, et al: Pain control after total knee arthroplasty: A randomized trial comparing local infiltration anesthesia and continuous femoral block. Acta Orthop 2011;82(4):441–447.

16. Lund J, Jenstrup MT, Jaeger P, et al: Continuous adductor-canal-blockade for adjuvant post-operative analgesia after major knee surgery: Preliminary results. Acta Anaesthesiol Scand 2011;55:14–19.

17. Essving P, Axelsson K, Åberg E, et al: Local infiltration analgesia (LIA) vs. intrathecal morphine for postoperative pain management following total knee arthroplasty. A randomized, controlled trial. Anesth Analg 2011;113: 926–933.

18. Sites BD, Beach M, Gallagher JD, et al: A single injection ultrasound-assisted femoral nerve block provides side effect-sparing analgesia when compared with intrathecal morphine in patients undergoing total knee arthroplasty. Anesth Analg 2004;99:1539–1543.

19. Hval K, Thagaard KS, Schlichting E, Raeder J: The prolonged postoperative analgesic effect when dexamethasone is added to a nonsteroidal antiinflammatory drug (rofecoxib) before breast surgery. Anesth Analg 2007;105:481–486.

20. Zhang J, Ho KY, Wang Y: Efficacy of pregabalin in acute postoperative pain: A meta-analysis. Br J Anaesth 2011;106:454–462.

21. Banks A: Innovations in postoperative pain management: Continuous infusion of local anesthetics. AORN J 2007;85:904–914.

22. Piper SL, Kramer JD, Kim HT, Feeley BT: Effects of local anesthetics on articular cartilage. Am J Sports Med 2011;39:2245–2253.

23. McCarthy D, Iohom G: Local infiltration analgesia for postoperative pain control following total hip arthroplasty: A systematic review. Anesthesiol Res Pract 2012;2012:709531.

24. Rikalainen-Salmi R, Forster JG, Makela K, et al: Local infiltration analgesia with levobupivacaine compared with intrathecal morphine in total hip arthroplasty patients. Acta Anaesthesiol Scand 2012;56: 695–705.

25. Murphy TP, Byrne DP, Curtin P, et al: Can a periarticular levobupivacaine injection reduce postoperative opiate consumption during primary hip arthroplasty? Clin Orthop Relat Res 2012;470:1151–1157.

26. Otte K, Husted H, Andersen L, et al: Local infiltration analgesia in total knee arthroplasty and hip resurfacing: A methodological study. Acute Pain 2008;10:111–116.

27. Parvataneni HK, Shah VP, Howard H, et al: Controlling pain after total hip and knee arthroplasty using a multimodal protocol with local periarticular injections: A prospective randomized study. J Arthroplasty 2007;22:33–38.

28. Busch CA, Whitehouse MR, Shore BJ, et al: The efficacy of periarticular multimodal drug infiltration in total hip arthroplasty. Clin Orthop Relat Res 2010;468:2152–2159.

29. Bianconi M, Ferraro L, Traina GC, et al: Pharmacokinetics and efficacy of ropivacaine continuous wound instillation after joint replacement surgery. Br J Anaesth 2003;91:830–835.

30. Andersen LJ, Poulsen T, Krogh B, Nielsen T: Postoperative analgesia in total hip arthroplasty: A randomized double-blinded, placebo-controlled study on peroperative and postoperative ropivacaine, ketorolac, and adrenaline wound infiltration. Acta Orthop 2007;78:187–192.

31. Lunn TH, Husted H, Solgaard S, et al: Intraoperative local infiltration analgesia for early analgesia after total hip arthroplasty: A randomized, double-blind, placebo-controlled trial. Reg Anesth Pain Med 2011;36: 424–429.

32. Andersen KV, Pfeiffer-Jensen M, Haraldsted V, Soballe K: Reduced hospital stay and narcotic consumption, and improved mobilization with local and intraarticular infiltration after hip arthroplasty: A randomized clinical trial of an intraarticular technique versus epidural infusion in 80 patients. Acta Orthop 2007;78:180–186.

33. Specht K, Leonhardt JS, Revald P, et al: No evidence of a clinically important effect of adding local infusion analgesia administrated through a catheter in pain treatment after total hip arthroplasty. Acta Orthop 2011;82:315–320.

34. Badner NH, Bourne RB, Rorabeck CH, et al: Intra-articular injection of bupivacaine in knee-replacement operations. Results of use for analgesia and for preemptive blockade. J Bone Joint Surg Am 1996;78:734–738.

35. Mauerhan DR, Campbell M, Miller JS, et al: Intra-articular morphine and/or bupivacaine in the management of pain after total knee arthroplasty. J Arthroplasty 1997;12:546–552.

36. Ritter MA, Koehler M, Keating EM, et al: Intra-articular morphine and/or bupivacaine after total knee replacement. J Bone Joint Surg Br 1999; 81:301–303.

37. Busch CA, Shore BJ, Bhandari R, et al: Efficacy of periarticular multimodal drug injection in total knee arthroplasty. A randomized trial. J Bone Joint Surg Am 2006;88:959–963.

38. Vendittoli PA, Makinen P, Drolet P, et al: A multimodal analgesia protocol for total knee arthroplasty. A randomized, controlled study. J Bone Joint Surg Am 2006;88:282–289.

39. Morin AM, Wulf H: High volume local infiltration analgesia (LIA) for total hip and knee arthroplasty: A brief review of the current status [in German]. Anasthesiol Intensivmed Notfallmed Schmerzther 2011;46: 84–86.

40. Ganapathy S, Brookes J, Bourne R: Local infiltration analgesia. Anesthesiol Clin 2011;29:329–342.

41. Gibbs DM, Green TP, Esler CN: The local infiltration of analgesia following total knee replacement: A review of current literature. J Bone Joint Surg Br 2012;94:1154–1159.

42. Andersen LO, Husted H, Kristensen BB, et al: Analgesic efficacy of subcutaneous local anaesthetic wound infiltration in bilateral knee arthroplasty: A randomised, placebo-controlled, double-blind trial. Acta Anaesthesiol Scand 2010;54:543–548.

43. Essving P, Axelsson K, Kjellberg J, et al: Reduced morphine consumption and pain intensity with local infiltration analgesia (LIA) following total knee arthroplasty. Acta Orthop 2010;81:354–360.

44. Toftdahl K, Nikolajsen L, Haraldsted V, et al: Comparison of peri- and intraarticular analgesia with femoral nerve block after total knee arthroplasty: A randomized clinical trial. Acta Orthop 2007;78: 172–179.

45. Kazak BZ, Aysu SE, Darcin K, et al: Intraarticular levobupivacaine or bupivacaine administration decreases pain scores and provides a better recovery after total knee arthroplasty. J Anesth 2010;24:694–699.

46. Carli F, Clemente A, Asenjo JF, et al: Analgesia and functional outcome after total knee arthroplasty: Periarticular infiltration vs continuous femoral nerve block. Br J Anaesth 2010;105:185–195.

47. Andersen KV, Bak M, Christensen BV, et al: A randomized, controlled trial comparing local infiltration analgesia with epidural infusion for total knee arthroplasty. Acta Orthop 2010;81:606–610.

48. Andersen KV, Nikolajsen L, Haraldsted V, et al: Local infiltration analgesia for total knee arthroplasty: Should ketorolac be added? Br J Anaesth 2013;111:242–248.

49. Andersen LO, Husted H, Otte KS, et al: A compression bandage improves local infiltration analgesia in total knee arthroplasty. Acta Orthop 2008;79:806–811.

50. Gomez-Cardero P, Rodriguez-Merchan EC: Postoperative analgesia in TKA: Ropivacaine continuous intraarticular infusion. Clin Orthop Relat Res 2010;468:1242–1247.

51. Ong JC, Chin PL, Fook-Chong SM, et al: Continuous infiltration of local anaesthetic following total knee arthroplasty. J Orthop Surg (Hong Kong) 2010;18:203207.

52. Essving P, Axelsson K, Kjellberg J, et al: Reduced hospital stay, morphine consumption, and pain intensity with local infiltration analgesia after unicompartmental knee arthroplasty. Acta Orthop 2009;80:213–219.

53. Ali A, Sundberg M, Hansson U, Malmvik J, Flivik G: Doubtful effect of continuous intraarticular analgesia after total knee arthroplasty. Acta Orthop 2015;86:373–377.

Regional and Topical Anesthesia for Awake Endotracheal Intubation

Imran Ahmad

INTRODUCTION

Awake endotracheal intubation can be achieved using a variety of equipment, such as video laryngoscopes, optical stylets, and fiber-optic scopes. Appropriate anesthesia of the airway and sedation can enable any of these techniques to be used successfully.

The commonest method used to perform an awake endotracheal intubation is with a flexible fiberscope, and an awake fiber-optic intubation is regarded as the gold standard for the endotracheal intubation of patients with an anticipated difficult airway. This procedure requires skills and knowledge that should be familiar to all anesthesiologists.

Recently, there have been many advances in regional anesthesia, allowing for more complicated and innovative procedures to be done under regional block techniques; however, not all of these cases can be done solely under regional anesthesia. Often, a combination of regional and general anesthesia is required; therefore, all anesthesiologists must be familiar with awake intubation techniques, especially if the patient has an anticipated difficult airway. Anesthetizing patients with an anticipated difficult airway is often a source of anxiety and trepidation, but appropriate airway topicalization and sedation techniques can create the appropriate conditions for a safe and stress-free procedure for both the patient and the anesthesiologist.

It is difficult to give precise figures on the incidence of difficult airways due to a variety of reasons, including population differences, operator skill variation, operator reporting, and an inconsistency in the definition of a difficult airway. In the general population, the approximate figures for the incidence of Cormack and Lehane laryngoscopy grades 3 and 4 is 10%, difficult intubation is 1%, and difficult bag mask ventilation is 0.08%–5%.[1–4]

Endotracheal intubation is usually performed under general anesthesia, but if a difficult airway is anticipated, then this should ideally be done under regional anesthesia (with or without sedation) as this allows the patient to breathe spontaneously, maintain airway patency, and cooperate with the operator. If any untoward difficulties are experienced, then the procedure can be abandoned with minimum risk to the patient. There are obvious exceptions to performing an awake intubation, such as patient refusal, young children, and uncooperative patients (due to confusion or learning disabilities).

To successfully perform an awake endotracheal intubation, one should be familiar with the following:

- Sensory innervation of the upper airway
- Agents available for topicalization
- Application techniques available to topicalize the airway
- Regional anesthesia techniques, landmark or ultrasound guided
- Safe sedation techniques

SENSORY INNERVATION OF THE AIRWAY

The upper airway is divided into the nasal and oral cavities, the pharynx, and the larynx. The sensory innervation to the upper airway is supplied by the trigeminal, glossopharyngeal, and vagus nerves (Figure 20–1).

Nose

The nose is entirely innervated by branches of the trigeminal nerve. Septum and anterior parts of the nasal cavity are affected by the anterior ethmoidal nerve (a branch of the ophthalmic nerve). The rest of the nasal cavity is innervated by the greater and lesser palatine nerves (branches of the maxillary nerve).

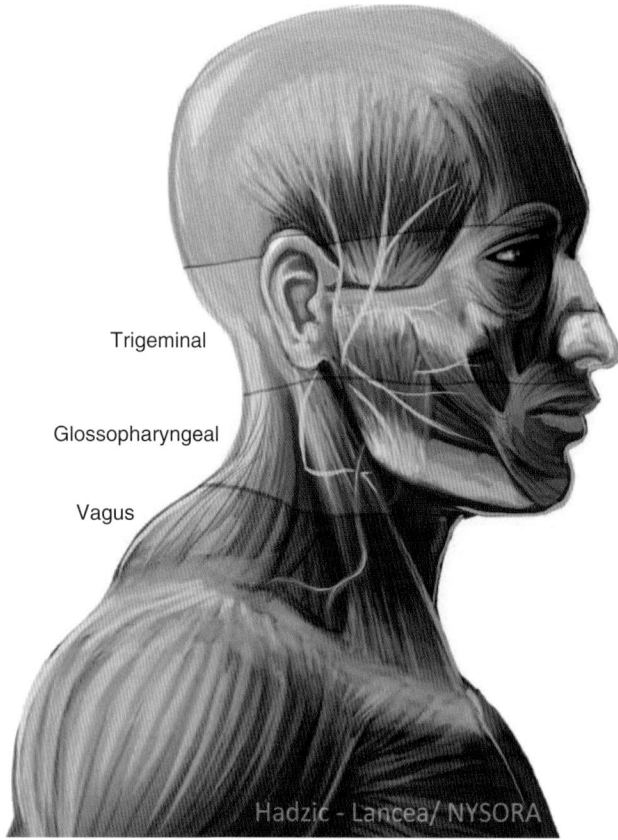

Hadzic - Lancea/ NYSORA

FIGURE 20–1. Innervation of the upper airway.

The palatine nerves are relayed through the pterygopalatine ganglion, found in the pterygopalatine fossa, which is situated close to the sphenopalatine fossa, located just posterior to the middle turbinate.

Pharynx

The pharynx is largely innervated by the glossopharyngeal nerve. Innervation of the whole pharynx, posterior third of tongue, the fauces, tonsils, and epiglottis is from the glossopharyngeal nerve.

Oropharynx

The oropharynx is innervated by branches of the vagus, trigeminal, and glossopharyngeal nerves. The posterior third of the tongue, vallecula, and anterior surface of the epiglottis are innervated by the tonsillar nerve (a branch of the glossopharyngeal nerve). The posterior and lateral wall of the pharynx are innervated by the pharyngeal nerve (a branch of the vagus nerve). The tonsillar nerve affects the tonsils. The anterior two-thirds of the tongue are innervated by the lingual nerve (branch of the mandibular division of the trigeminal nerve).

Larynx

The larynx is innervated by the vagus nerve (Figure 20–2). Above the vocal cords (base of tongue, posterior epiglottis, aryepiglottic folds, and arytenoids), the internal branch of the superior laryngeal nerve (a branch of the vagus nerve) supplies innervation. For the vocal cords and below the vocal cords, the recurrent laryngeal nerve (a branch of the vagus nerve) is the supplier.

Clinical Pearls

- The greater and lesser palatine nerves provide sensation to the nasal turbinates and posterior two-thirds of the nasal septum.
- The anterior ethmoid nerve innervates the remainder of the nasal passage.
- The glossopharyngeal nerve provides sensory innervation to the posterior third of the tongue, the vallecula, the anterior surface of the epiglottis (lingual branch), the walls of the pharynx (pharyngeal branch), and the tonsils (tonsillar branch).
- The superior laryngeal nerve innervates the base of the tongue, posterior surface of the epiglottis, aryepiglottic fold, and the arytenoids.
- The recurrent laryngeal nerve provides sensory innervation to the trachea and vocal folds.

TOPICAL ANESTHESIA

Cocaine

Cocaine is the only local anesthetic with vasoconstrictor properties; therefore, it is particularly useful for topical anesthesia of the nasopharynx, which is highly vascular. Cocaine is available as a 5% or 10% solution and in paste form; the maximum recommended dose is 1.5 mg/kg. It should be used with caution in patients with coronary artery disease, hypertension, and pseudocholinesterase deficiency.

The mixture of 2 mL of 10% cocaine, 1 mL 1:1000 adrenaline, 2 mL sodium bicarbonate, and 5 mL sodium chloride makes 10 mL of Moffett's solution.[5] This is commonly used in rhinological procedures to provide local anesthesia, vasoconstriction, and decongestion. It is also used to topicalize the nasal mucosa to provide the optimal conditions for nasal intubations.

Lidocaine

Lidocaine is the most commonly used local anesthetic for airway topicalization. The 4% solution and 10% spray are most often used (Figure 20–3). Systemic absorption from topical application to the upper airways is lower than expected, so in practice higher doses can be used than the recommended 2 mg/kg.[3,6]

Vasoconstrictors

Vasoconstrictors should be used when the nasal mucosa is being anesthetized; this is because the mucosa is highly vascular, and bleeding can readily occur on instrumentation, which can obscure the view seen on the fiberscope.

As mentioned, cocaine has inherent vasoconstrictor properties, so it is a suitable agent to use for the nasal mucosa. Vasoconstrictor agents such as xylometazoline and phenylephrine are prepared with lidocaine to produce local anesthesia and vasoconstriction. These mixtures are also suitable agents for preparation of the nasal mucosa.[6]

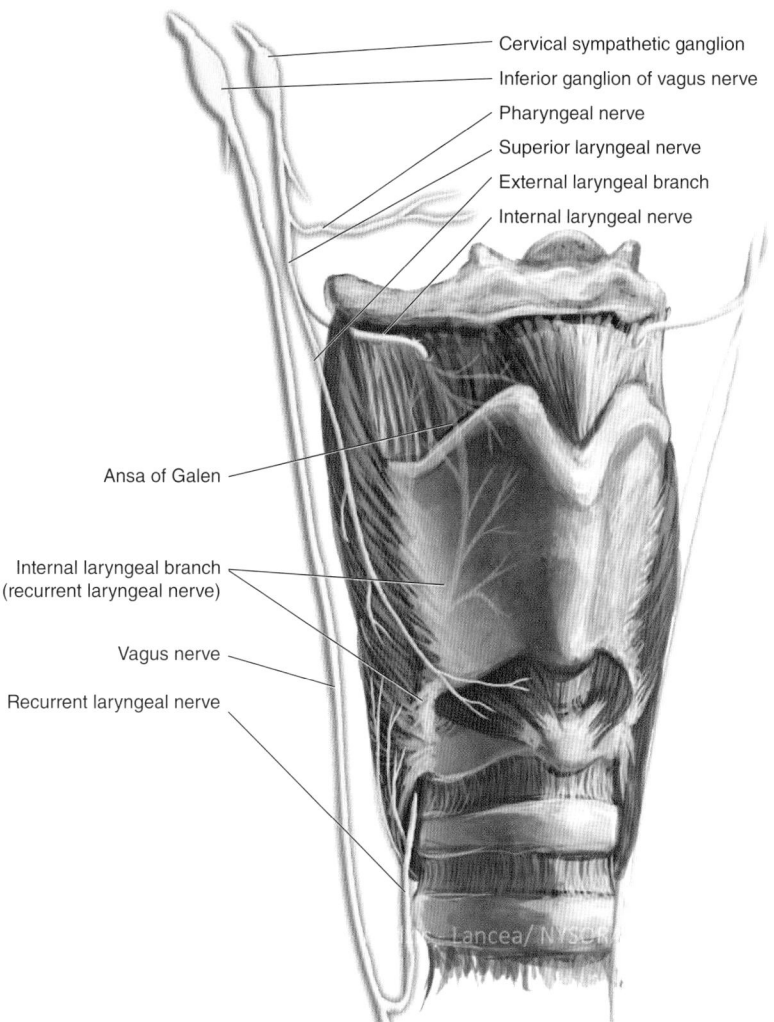

FIGURE 20–2. Innervation of the larynx.

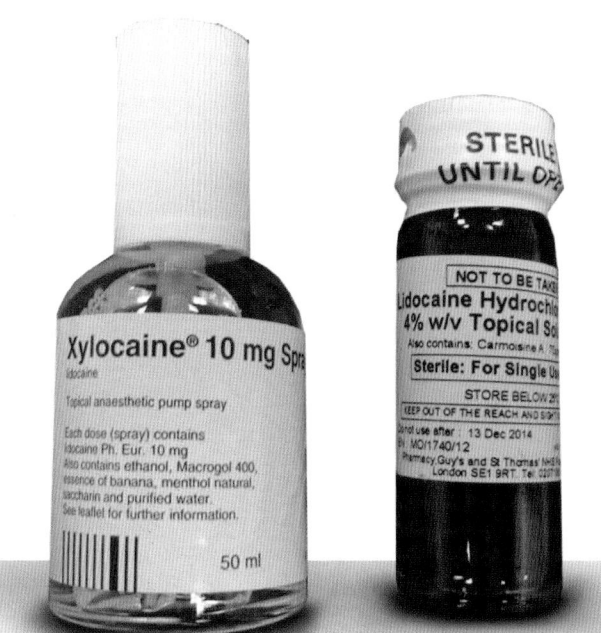

FIGURE 20–3. Lidocaine, 10% and 4%.

Clinical Pearls

• The use of vasoconstrictors reduces the bleeding "shrinks" the nasal mucosa resulting in better surgical exposure.
• Shrinking of the nasal mucosa increases the size of the nasal airway passages, creating more space for the fiberscope and endotracheal tube.
• Appropriate time should be allowed for the vasoconstrictor to take effect before commencing fiberoscopy

APPLICATION TECHNIQUES

There are various techniques available to topicalize the upper airway in preparation for awake intubation.[7,8] The nasopharynx and oropharynx can be sprayed directly from the container of local anesthetic preparations, sprayed using the McKenzie technique, or sprayed via a mucosal atomization device (MAD).

The McKenzie technique uses a 20-gauge cannula attached to oxygen bubble tubing via a three-way tap. The other end of

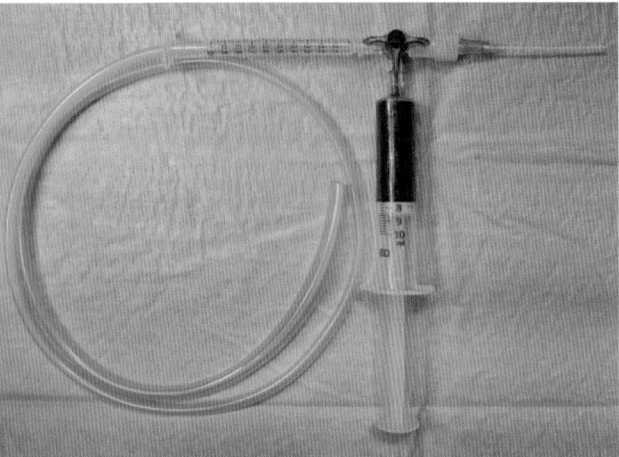

FIGURE 20–4. Setup for McKenzie technique.

bubble tubing is then attached to an oxygen source, which is turned on to deliver a flow of 2–4 L/min. As the local anesthetic is slowly administered via a 5-mL syringe attached to the top port of the cannula, a jetlike spray effect is seen, which greatly increases the surface area of the local anesthetic and allows directed topicalization of the nasal and oral mucosa (Figure 20–4).

Clinical Pearls

- Maintain a tight seal between the tubing and the cannula to prevent leakage of local anesthetic from these areas.
- Slow, continuous pressure on the 5-mL syringe containing local anesthesia will result in a "hissing" sound as a fine mist is sprayed out of the cannula.

Commercially available mucosal atomizers allow a similar mistlike effect as seen with the McKenzie technique by just attaching them to the end of a syringe (Figure 20–5). These devices are available for nasal and oral applications.[6]

Adding approximately 5 mL of 4% lidocaine to a nebulizer, then delivering it with oxygen for up to 30 minutes is a safe and noninvasive way to topicalize the airway all the way down to the trachea (Figure 20–6). It is well tolerated and is a useful technique to topicalize the whole airway. It also allows the topicalization of patients with limited mouth opening, where atomizers cannot be passed into the mouth to topicalize the oropharynx.[6]

The vocal cords can also be sprayed directly with local anesthetic using the spray-as-you-go (SAYGO) technique.[9] Here, the distal end of a 16-gauge epidural catheter is cut 3 cm from the end and then fed through the working channel of a fiberscope. The Luer lock connector is connected to the proximal end of the catheter and then attached to a 5-mL syringe prepared with 4% lidocaine. The distal end should protrude out of the fiberscope, so that the tip is just visible. The local anesthetic is then dripped onto the vocal cords prior to the fiberscope being introduced into the trachea. This reduces patient discomfort and coughing when the fiberscope and endotracheal tube are introduced into the trachea.

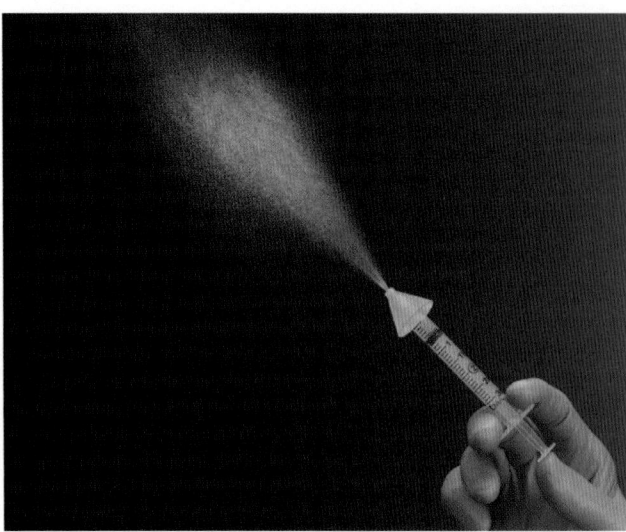

FIGURE 20–5. Mucosal atomization device (MAD).

Usually, a combination of techniques (Table 20–1) is used to deliver local anesthetic to the airway mucosa in preparation for awake intubation. For example, to prepare the nasopharynx, preprepared local anesthetic solution can be sprayed into the nasal mucosa using the nozzle from the container. The oropharynx could be prepared using local anesthetic sprayed using the McKenzie technique, and the vocal cords could be sprayed using the SAYGO method. Alternatively, the MADs can be used to spray the nasal and oral mucosa. Whichever technique or combination of techniques is used, the aim should be to have an airway adequately anesthetized in preparation for instrumentation.

Clinical Pearls

- Sitting the patient in an upright position will help with oxygenation and topicalization.
- Always administer supplementary oxygen.
- Start and establish the sedation before commencing the topicalization process, which can be uncomfortable.
- Asking the patient to "sniff" while spraying the nasopharynx can aid in the distribution of local anesthetic.

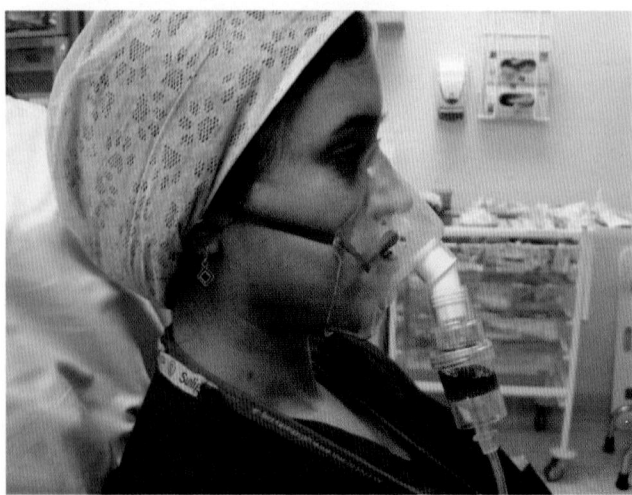

FIGURE 20–6. Administration of nebulized lidocaine.

TABLE 20–1. Application techniques.

Spray from container
Local anesthetic soaked in ribbon gauze
Cotton applicators
McKenzie technique
Mucosal atomization device
Inhalation of nebulized lidocaine
"Spray as you go" via epidural catheter

REGIONAL ANESTHESIA TECHNIQUES

Nerve blocks can provide anesthesia for awake intubation but can be technically more challenging to perform than topical anesthesia of the airway. They do carry a higher risk of complications, such as intravascular injection and nerve damage, and more than one nerve needs to be blocked. These are the glossopharyngeal, superior laryngeal, and recurrent laryngeal nerves, as they supply the innervation to the oropharynx and larynx. Therefore, the nerve blocks required to anesthetize the airway are the glossopharyngeal, superior laryngeal, and translaryngeal blocks.

The nasal passages are supplied by the palatine nerves and anterior ethmoidal nerve. These nerves need to be blocked to allow for awake nasal fiber-optic intubation. These nerves are usually blocked by the topical application of local anesthetic to the nasal passages, usually by inhalation, spray topicalization, or the application of cotton applicators soaked in anesthetic.

Landmark Technique
Glossopharyngeal Nerve Block

The glossopharyngeal nerve provides sensation to the posterior third of the tongue and the vallecula and provides the sensory limb for the gag reflex; therefore, this block is particularly useful in abolishing this reflex. There are two approaches described for this block: intraoral and peristyloid.

For the intraoral approach, the patient requires sufficient mouth opening to allow adequate visualization and access to the base of the posterior tonsillar pillars (palatopharyngeal arch) (Figure 20–7). After adequate topical anesthesia (lidocaine spray) has been applied, the tongue is retracted medially with a laryngoscope blade or a tongue depressor, allowing access to the posterior tonsillar pillar. Then, using a 22- or 25-gauge needle, 2–5 mL of 2% lidocaine are injected submucosally, after negative aspiration. The point of injection is at the caudal aspect of the posterior tonsillar pillar (approximately 0.5 cm lateral to the lateral edge of the tongue where it joins the floor of the mouth; Figure 20–8). This is then repeated on the other side.

Alternatively, a gauze soaked in local anesthetic can be firmly applied to this region for a few minutes. This method avoids the risk of intravascular injection but is not as successful as when the local anesthetic is injected.

The peristyloid approach aims to infiltrate local anesthetic just posterior to the styloid process where the glossopharyngeal nerve lies. In close proximity to this is the internal carotid artery, so care must be taken when using this approach.

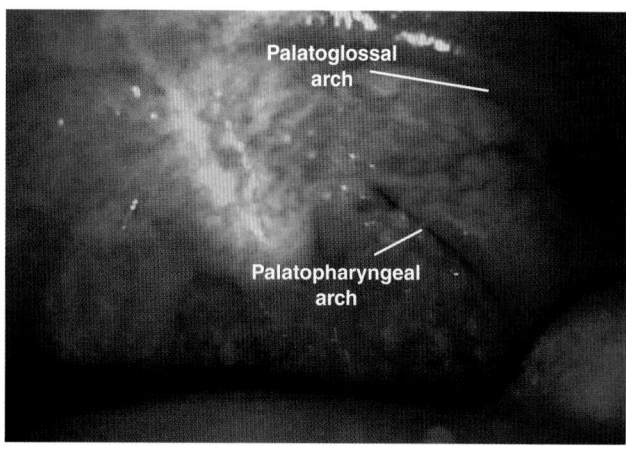

FIGURE 20–7. Palatopharyngeal arch.

The patient should be placed in a supine position with the head placed neutrally. The styloid process is located at the midpoint of a line drawn from the angle of the jaw to the tip of the mastoid process. It can be palpated using deep pressure, but this may be uncomfortable for the patient; a needle is inserted perpendicular to the skin, aiming to hit the styloid process. Once contact has been made (usually 1–2 cm deep), the needle should be reangled posteriorly and walked off the styloid process until contact is lost, then 5–7 mL of 2% lidocaine can be injected after negative aspiration. This is then repeated on the other side.

Clinical Pearls

- The glossopharyngeal nerve is most easily blocked where it crosses the palatoglossal arch.
- It can be blocked by spraying local anesthetic, by applying gauze or pledgets soaked in local anesthetic directly over the nerve, or by direct injection of local anesthetic around the nerve.
- This helps to abolish the gag reflex, but this block on its own will not provide adequate conditions for an awake fiber-optic intubation.

Superior Laryngeal Nerve Block

The superior laryngeal nerve provides sensation to the laryngeal structures above the vocal cords and lies inferior to the greater cornu of the hyoid bone; here, it splits into the internal and external branches. The internal branch then penetrates the thyrohyoid membrane about 2–4 mm inferior to the greater cornu, continuing submucosally in the piriform recess (Figure 20–9 and Figure 20–10). The external branch does not penetrate the thyrohyoid membrane; it descends on the larynx deep to the sternothyroid muscle. The superior laryngeal nerve can be blocked using the external or internal approach.

To perform the block using the external approach, the patient is placed in the supine position and will need a degree of neck extension to facilitate identification of the hyoid bone. Once identified, the hyoid bone is gently displaced to the side where the block is to be performed and a 25-gauge needle is

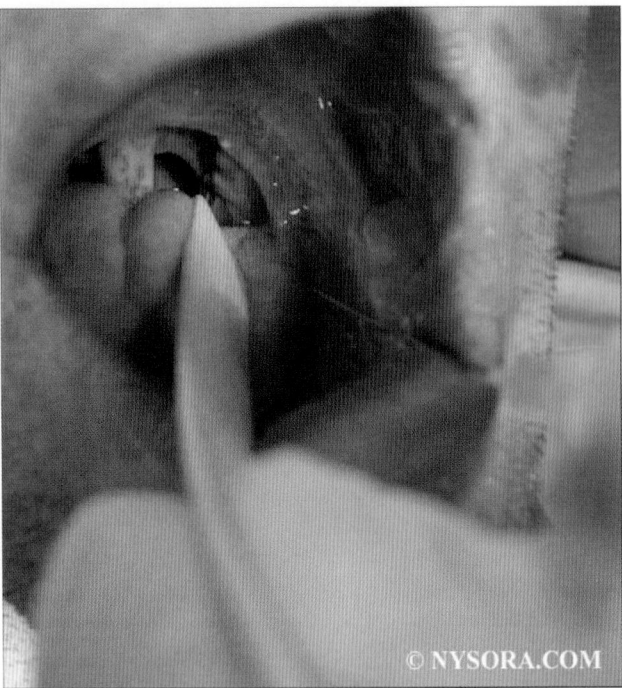

FIGURE 20–8. Glossopharyngeal nerve block.

inserted from the lateral side of the neck, aiming toward the greater cornu.[10] Once contact has been made, the needle is walked off the bone inferiorly, and injecting 2 mL of 2% lidocaine here will block both the internal and the external branches of the superior laryngeal nerve (Figure 20–11). If the

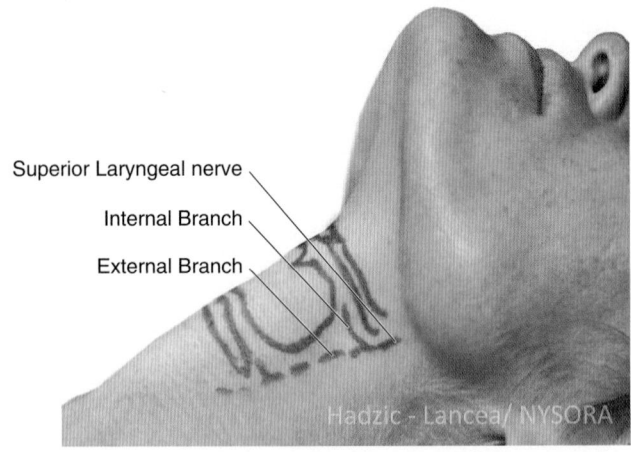

FIGURE 20–10. Surface anatomy of superior laryngeal nerve and branches.

needle is advanced a few millimeters, it will pierce the thyrohyoid membrane, and a "give" is felt. Injecting local anesthetic here will result in only the internal branch of the superior laryngeal nerve being blocked. As with all blocks, careful aspiration must be performed prior to injection, especially as the carotid artery is in close proximity.

If it is difficult to identify the hyoid bone, the superior cornu of the thyroid cartilage can be identified instead. This is located by identifying the thyroid notch, tracing the upper edge posteriorly until the superior cornu can be palpated as a small round structure. This lies just inferior to the greater cornu of the hyoid bone. The needle can be inserted, aiming for the superior cornu of the thyroid cartilage, then walked cephalad, then local anesthetic is injected once the needle loses contact with the superior cornu. If the thyrohyoid membrane is pierced, then inject 2 mL of local anesthetic here and a further 2 mL as the needle is withdrawn; this will increase the chances of both the internal and external branches of the superior laryngeal nerve being blocked.[11]

The internal approach uses gauze or pledgets soaked in local anesthetic and placed in the piriform fossae using Krause's forceps. These need to be kept in place for 5-10 minutes to allow sufficient time for the local anesthetic to take effect.[12]

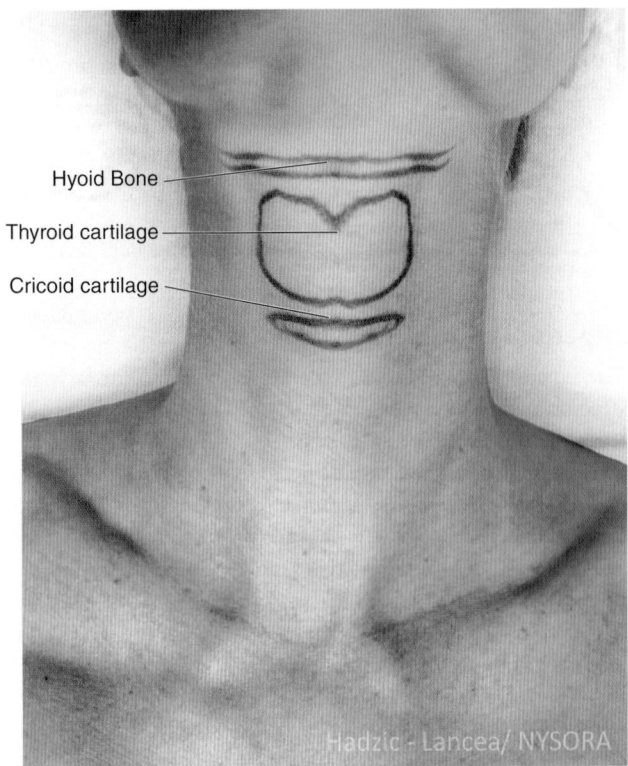

FIGURE 20–9. Surface anatomy of hyoid bone, thyroid, and cricoid cartilages.

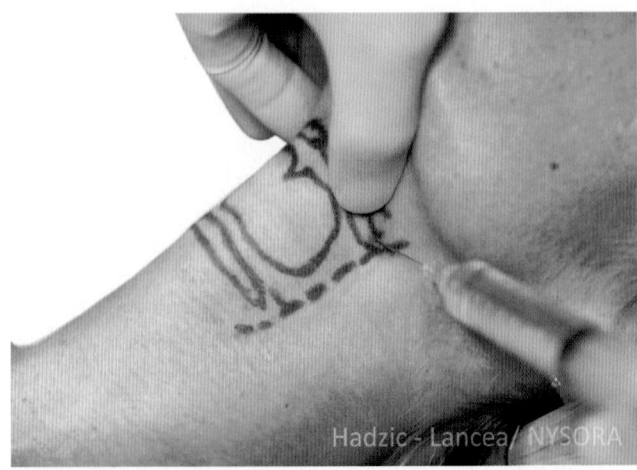

FIGURE 20–11. Superior laryngeal nerve block.

Recurrent Laryngeal Nerve Block

The sensory innervation of the vocal cords and trachea is supplied by the recurrent laryngeal nerves. These ascend along the tracheoesophageal groove and also provide the motor supply to all the intrinsic muscles of the larynx except the cricothyroid muscle. Direct recurrent laryngeal nerve blocks are not performed as they can result in bilateral vocal cord paralysis and airway obstruction, as both the motor and the sensory fibers run together. Therefore, this nerve is blocked using the translaryngeal block.[13]

To perform this, the patient should be supine, with the neck extended be identified in the midline, then the palpating finger should be moved in a caudad direction until the cricoid cartilage is palpated. The cricothyroid membrane lies between these two structures, immediately above the cricoid cartilage. The thumb and third digit of one hand should stabilize the trachea at the level of the thyroid cartilage, then a 22 or 20 gauge needle should be inserted perpendicular to the skin with the aim to penetrate the cricothyroid membrane (above the cricoid cartilage) (Figure 20–12). This should be done with continuous aspiration of the syringe, as the appearance of bubbles will indicate that the needle tip is now in the trachea. At this point, immediately stop advancing the needle; otherwise, the posterior laryngeal wall can be punctured. Rapid injection (and then removal of the needle) of 5 mL of 4% lidocaine will result in coughing, which will help to disperse the local anesthetic and blockade of the recurrent laryngeal nerve.

Clinical Pearls

- Appropriate position of the patient will aid in the correct identification of the cricoid and thyroid cartilages and the cricothyroid membrane.
- The neck should be extended, which makes these structures more prominent.
- Placing a liter bag of infusion fluids between the shoulder blades can help achieve this position.

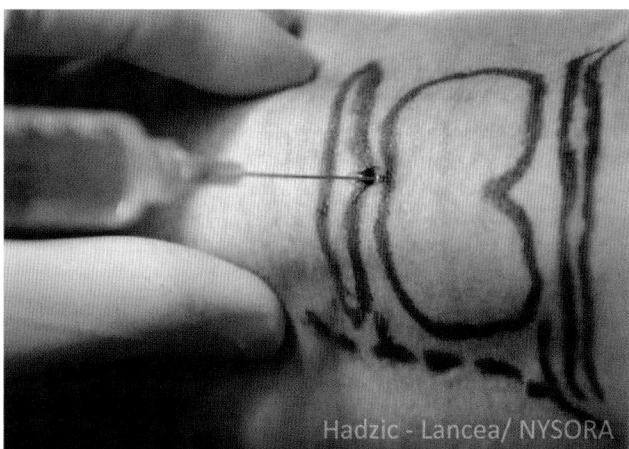

FIGURE 20–12. Translaryngeal block.

TABLE 20–2. Structures that can be identified on ultrasound.
Hyoid bone
Thyroid cartilage
Thyrohyoid membrane
Superior laryngeal artery
Superior laryngeal nerve

Ultrasound-Guided Techniques

Ultrasound can be used to help increase the success rate of performing some of the blocks described (Table 20–2). Ultrasound can increase the accuracy of the deposition of local anesthetic around the greater cornu of the hyoid bone for the superior laryngeal nerve block and can be used to identify the cricothyroid membrane for translaryngeal blocks.[14–16]

Superior Laryngeal Nerve Block

Sometimes, it can be difficult to identify the landmarks (eg, in obese patients) when trying to perform this block. Ultrasound can therefore be used to facilitate the deposition of local anesthetic to the correct place. The hyoid bone can be visualized on ultrasound (Figure 20–13), and an in-plane technique can be used to deposit local anesthetic around the surface of the greater cornu of the hyoid bone to achieve the block.[17]

Place the transducer probe in the sagittal plane to identify the greater cornu of the hyoid bone; the transducer is then rotated transversely to identify the superior lateral aspect of the thyrohyoid membrane. The superior laryngeal nerve can be seen superficial to the thyrohyoid membrane when the medial aspect of the probe is rotated cephalad. The internal branch of the superior laryngeal nerve runs along with the superior laryngeal artery, just below the greater cornu of the hyoid bone.

An alternative approach is to identify the hyoid bone, which appears as a hyperechoic curved bright structure on ultrasound in the midline. If the probe is moved laterally, the greater cornu of the hyoid bone can be seen as a bright structure medial to the superior laryngeal artery. The internal branch of the superior laryngeal nerve runs with the superior laryngeal artery just below the level of the greater cornu of the hyoid bone. Using an in-plane technique, a needle is passed perpendicular to the skin, aiming just below the greater cornu of the hyoid bone. Then, 1–2 mL of local anesthetic can be injected here after negative aspiration[18] (Figure 20–14).

This technique has been shown to have a success rate of over 90%. Failure is thought to be due to variations in the anatomical position of the superior laryngeal nerve in relation to the hyoid bone.

Translaryngeal Block

Sometimes, the correct location of the cricothyroid membrane is difficult to identify by palpation only. Ultrasound can be used to identify the thyroid and cricoid cartilages and the cricothyroid membrane (Table 20–3), ensuring that the local anesthetic is deposited correctly and a successful translaryngeal block is achieved[19] (Figure 20–15).

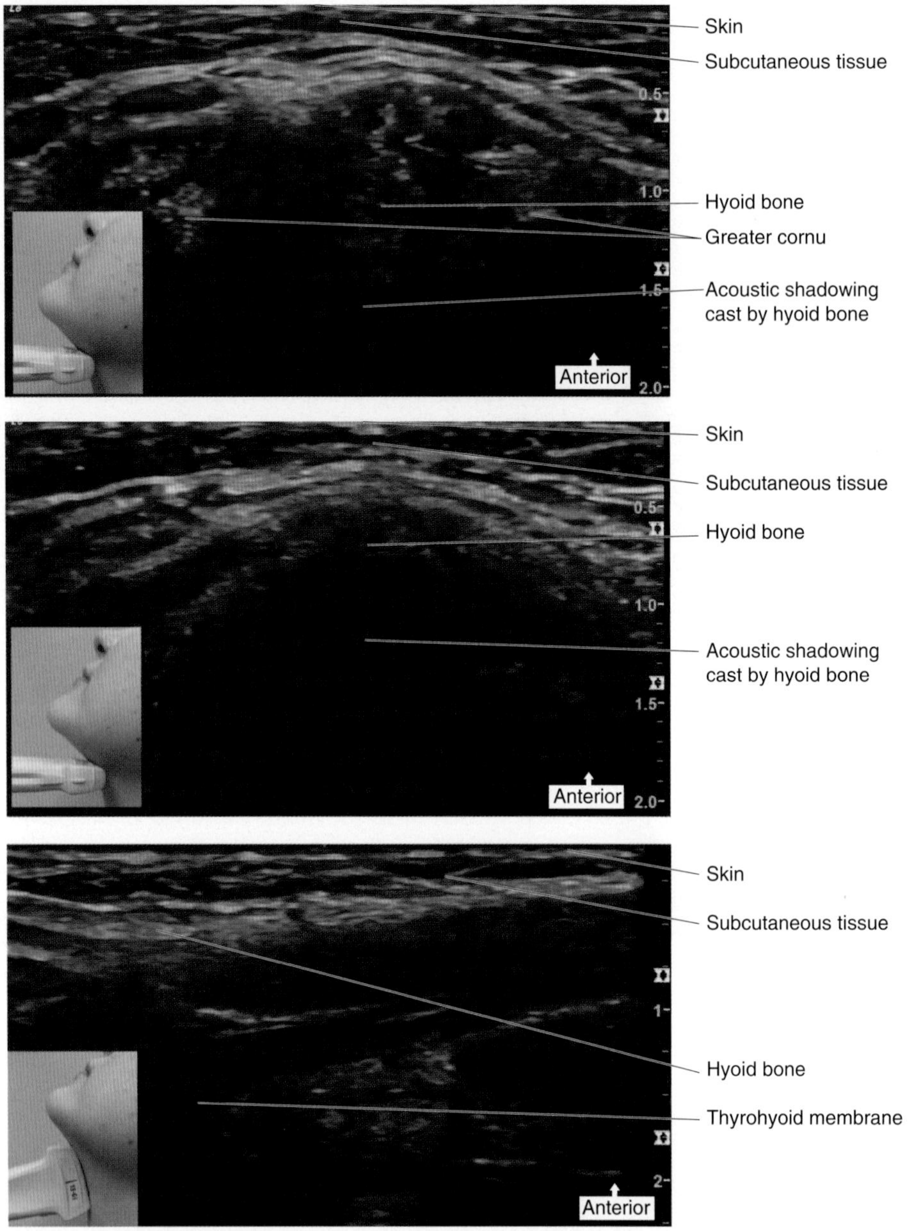

Skin
Subcutaneous tissue
Hyoid bone
Greater cornu
Acoustic shadowing cast by hyoid bone
Anterior
Skin
Subcutaneous tissue
Hyoid bone
Acoustic shadowing cast by hyoid bone
Anterior
Skin
Subcutaneous tissue
Hyoid bone
Thyrohyoid membrane
Anterior

FIGURE 20–13. Ultrasound images of hyoid bone.

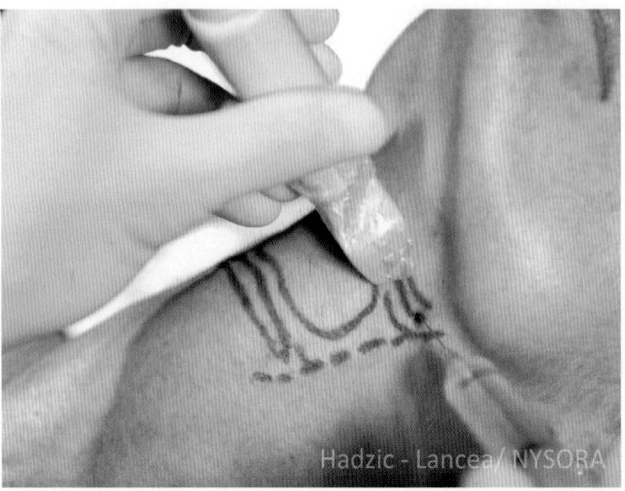

Hadzic - Lancea / NYSORA

FIGURE 20–14. Ultrasound-guided superior laryngeal nerve block.

If the probe is placed longitudinally in the midline of the neck, the tracheal rings can be seen. If the probe is then advanced cranially, the cricoid cartilage can be seen next; this is a slightly elongated structure that is larger and more superficial than the tracheal rings. If the probe is further advanced cranially, the thyroid cartilage can be seen. The cricothyroid membrane lies between the caudal border of the thyroid cartilage and the cephalad border of the cricoid cartilage. Keep the probe in the midline with the cricothyroid membrane in the middle

TABLE 20–3. Readily identifiable structures.
Tracheal rings
Cricoid cartilage
Thyroid cartilage
Cricothyroid membrane

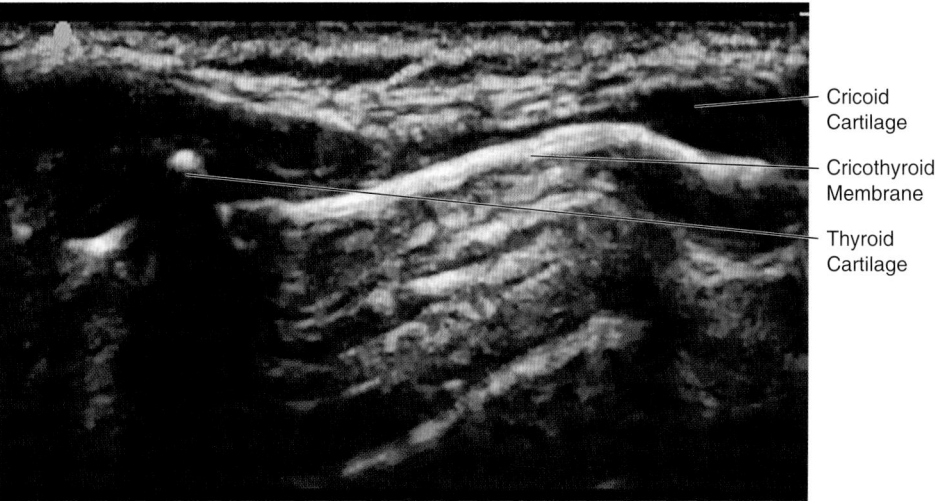

FIGURE 20–15. Ultrasound image of cricoid cartilage, thyroid cartilage, saggital plane, and cricothyroid membrane.

Cricoid Cartilage

Cricothyroid Membrane

Thyroid Cartilage

of the image seen on the monitor; then, the exact location on the patient's neck can be marked using a marker pen. Now that the position of the cricothyroid membrane has been located, the translaryngeal block can be performed.

The block can also be performed under real-time sonography by simply tilting the probe from the midline to a parasagittal position, keeping the cricoid cartilage in view. The needle entry point should be just cranial to the cricoid cartilage and can be seen on the ultrasound monitor (Figure 20–16). Once air is aspirated, this confirms that the needle is through the membrane and in the trachea.

SEDATION TECHNIQUES

Awake endotracheal intubation can be an unpleasant experience for the patient, even if thorough topicalization of the airway has been done. The aim of conscious sedation is not only to allow the patient to tolerate the procedure but also to provide optimal intubating conditions. There are various techniques

available to achieve the desired level of sedation; whichever is used, the priority is to avoid oversedation of the patient. Oversedation could lead to an unresponsive patient with loss of airway, which could result in serious consequences.

The ideal sedation conditions would involve a comfortable patient responsive to commands with a maintained airway, spontaneous breathing, and a degree of amnesia (Table 20–4).[20]

Two drugs are becoming increasingly popular and have growing evidence to support their use for conscious sedation: remifentanil and dexmedetomidine.[20] Remifentanil is an ultrashort-acting opioid, and dexmedetomidine is a highly selective α_2 agonist (Table 20–5).

Remifentanil has been found to provide good intubating conditions, is well tolerated, and has high patient satisfaction scores, although there is a high incidence of recall when used as a solo agent. Best results are seen when a target controlled infusion (TCI) technique is used.[21–23]

The advantage of dexmedetomidine is that a state of cooperative sedation is achieved; it also has antisialagogue effects. There is level 1 evidence to support its use for good intubating conditions, patient tolerance, and patient satisfaction. It is usually administered as a slow bolus over 120 minutes followed by an infusion.[24–26]

Benzodiazepines are usually administered in combination with an opioid as intermittent boluses and have been used as a sedative for awake fiber-optic intubation. The disadvantage of

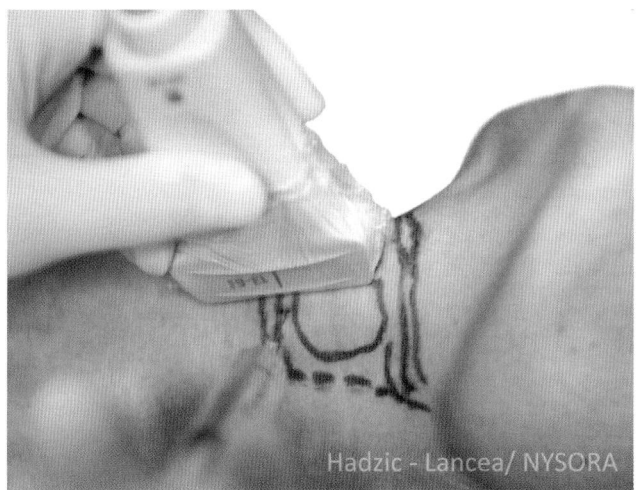

Hadzic - Lancea/ NYSORA

FIGURE 20–16. Ultrasound-guided translaryngeal block.

TABLE 20–4. Ideal sedation conditions.

Anxiolysis
Amnesia
Analgesia
Suppression of gag and cough reflexes
Easily titratable
Minimal respiratory side effects
Rapidly reversible

TABLE 20–5. Examples of sedation techniques.

Boluses of benzodiazepines (eg, diazepam, midazolam)
Boluses of opioids (eg, fentanyl, alfentanyl, morphine)
Boluses of α_2 agonists (eg, clonidine, dexmedetomidine)
Boluses of anesthetic agents (propofol, ketamine)
Combination of agents (eg, benzodiazepines and opioids)
Intravenous infusion (propofol, remifentanil, dexmedetomidine)
Combination of intravenous infusions (propofol and remifentanil)

using boluses of benzodiazepines is that intermittent boluses are associated with overshooting; therefore, there is a risk of oversedation and apnea.[27,28]

Propofol can be administered as intermittent boluses or as an infusion. Both techniques have been shown to be safe and well tolerated by patients. There is now increasing popularity of administering propofol as a TCI, either as a sole agent or in combination with remifentanil. Whichever technique is used, it is important to maintain a balance of an appropriate level of sedation and avoidance of underdosing or overdosing.[29]

The combination of propofol and remifentanil TCI has proven to be a safe technique for fiber-optic intubation with consistent pharmacodynamic effects and allows for a more predictable level of sedation.[29]

Clinical Pearls

- Safe sedation can be achieved by slowly administering the sedative drugs and continually communicating with the patient.
- Bispectral Index (BIS) monitoring can also be used to aid and guide sedation level.

AUTHOR'S PREFERRED TECHNIQUE FOR PERFORMING AN AWAKE FIBER-OPTIC INTUBATION

There are numerous techniques available for performing an awake fiber-optic intubation. Next is described a well-accepted and successful technique I use on a regular basis:

- Sit patient as upright as tolerable.
- Administer supplemental oxygen (via Hudson mask or nasal cannulae).
- Attach full monitoring.
- Start remifentanil (1–3 ng/mL) and propofol (0.5–1 µg/mL) TCI infusion. Do *not* give a bolus dose. Titrate the dose according to the patient's level of sedation.
- Start to topicalize the nasopharynx with Moffett's solution sprayed via MAD.
- Topicalize the oropharynx with 4% lidocaine using a MAD.

- After topicalization, suction any secretions using a soft suction catheter; this also tests the effectiveness of the local anesthetic.
- If patient does not tolerate the suction catheter, spray oropharynx with 2–4 sprays of 10% lidocaine.
- Preload the fiberscope with a nasal endotracheal tube (ETT) (size 6/6.5 outer diameter [OD]).
- Start fiberoscopy via the nasopharynx and visualize the vocal cords.
- Pass the fiberscope into the trachea.
- "Railroad" the lubricated ETT over the scope gently into the trachea, trying not to touch the carina with the fiberscope.
- Confirm correct placement of the ETT by visualizing the carina and ETT.
- Connect the ETT to the anesthetic circuit and capnography.
- Gently inflate the cuff of the ETT.
- Keep hold of the ETT until it has been safely secured.
- Patient is now safe to anesthetize.

SUMMARY

To successfully perform awake intubation in a patient with an anticipated difficult airway, it is important that you have an understanding of and are competent in all of the following:

- Innervation of the upper airway
- Knowledge of appropriate local anesthetic techniques and vasoconstrictor drugs
- Techniques available to topicalize/anesthetize the upper airway
- Prudent sedation techniques
- Oxygenation techniques during the procedure
- Techniques used for the correct placement of the endotracheal tube

This will enable a safe, stress-free, and successful awake intubation with high levels of patient satisfaction.

REFERENCES

1. Cheney FW, Posner KL, Caplan RA: Adverse respiratory events infrequently leading to malpractice suits. A closed claims analysis. Anaesthesiology 1991;75:932–939.
2. Cheney FW, Posner KL, Lee LA, Caplan RA, Domino KB: Trends in anaesthesia-related death and brain damage: A closed claims analysis. Anaesthesiology 2006;105:1081–1086.
3. Popat M (ed). *Difficult Airway Management*. Oxford University Press, 2009.
4. Rose DK, Cohen MM: The airway: Problems and predictions in 18,500 patients. Can J Anaesth 1994;41:372–383.
5. Benjamin E, Wong DK, Choa D: "Moffett's" solution: A review of the evidence and scientific basis for the topical preparation of the nose. Clin Otolaryngol Allied Sci 2004;29(6):582–587.
6. Simmons ST, Schleich AR: Airway regional anaesthesia for awake fiberoptic intubation. Reg Anesth Pain Med 2002;27:180–192.
7. Curran J, Hamilton C, Taylor T: Topical analgesia before tracheal intubation. Anaesthesia 1975;30:765–768.
8. Morris IR: Fibreoptic intubation. Can J Anaesth 1994;41:996–1008.
9. Vloka JD, Hadzic A, Kitain E: A simple adaptation to the Olympus LF1 and LF2 fiberoptic bronchoscopes for instillation of local anesthetic. Anesthesiology 1995;82:792.

10. Furlan JC: Anatomical study applied to anesthetic block technique of the superior laryngeal nerve. Acta Anaesthesiol Scand 2002;46:199–202.

11. Wheatley JR, Brancatisano A, Engel LA: Respiratory-related activity of cricothyroid muscle in awake normal humans. J Appl Physiol 1991;70:2226–2232.

12. Curran J, Hamilton C, Taylor T: Topical analgesia before tracheal intubation. Anaesthesia 1975;30:765–768.

13. Tsui BC, Dillane D: Finucane. Neural blockade for surgery to the neck and head: Clinical applications. In: Cousins MJ, Bridenbaugh PO, Carr D, et al (eds). *Cousin and Bridenbaugh's Neural Blockade in Clinical Anesthesia and Management of Pain*, 4th ed. Lippincott Williams and Wilkins; 2008:479-491.

14. Green JS, Tsui BCH: Applications of ultrasonography in ENT: Airway assessment and nerve blockade. Anaesthesiology Clin 2010;28:541–553.

15. Singh M, Chin KJ, Chan VWS, Wong DT, Prasad GA, Yu E: Use of sonography for airway assessment. An observational study. J Ultrasound Med 2010;29:79–85.

16. Kristensen MS: Ultrasonography in the management of the airway. Acta Anaesthesiol Scand 2011;55:1155–1173.

17. Manikandan S, Neema PK, Rathod RC: Ultrasound-guided bilateral superior laryngeal nerve block to aid awake endotracheal intubation in a patient with cervical spine disease for emergency surgery. Anaesth Intensive Care 2010;38:946–948.

18. Kaur B, Tang R, Sawka A, Krebs C, Vaghadia H: A method for ultrasonographic visualization and injection of the superior laryngeal nerve: Volunteer study and cadaver simulation. Anaesth Analg 2012;115(5):1242–1245.

19. De Oliveira GS Jr, Fitzgerald P, Kendall M: Ultrasound-assisted translaryngeal block for awake fibreoptic intubation. Can J Anesth/J Can Anesth 2011;58:664–665.

20. Johnson KD, Rai MR; Conscious sedation for awake fibreoptic intubation: A review of the literature. Can J Anaesth 2013;60(6):584–599.

21. Rai MR, Parry TM, Dombrovskis A, Warner OJ: Remifentanil target controlled infusion vs propofol target-controlled infusion for conscious sedation for awake fibreoptic intubation: A double blond randomized controlled trial. Br J Anaesth 2008;100:125–130.

22. Puchner W, Egger P, Punringer F, Lockinger A, Obwegeser J, Gombotz H: Evaluation of remifentanil as a single drug for awake fibreoptic intubation. Acta Anaesthesiol Scand 2002;46:350–354.

23. Mingo OH, Ashpole KJ, Irving CJ, Rucklidge MW: Remifentanil sedation for awake fibreoptic intubation with limited application of local anaesthetic in patients for elective head and neck surgery. Anaesthesia 2008;63:1065–1069.

24. Maroof M, Khan RM, Jain D, Ashraf M: Dexmedetomidine is a useful adjunct for awake intubation. Can J Anesth 2005;52:776–777.

25. Unger RJ, Gallagher CJ: Dexmedetomidine sedation for awake fibreoptic intubation. Semin Anesth Perioper Med Pain 2006;25:65–70.

26. Bergese SD, Khabiri B, Roberts WD, Howie MB, McSweeney TD, Gerhardt MA: Dexmedetomidine for conscious sedation in difficult awake fibreoptic intubation cases. J Clin Anesth 2007;19:141–144.

27. Sidhu VS, Whitehead EM, Ainsworth QP, Smith M, Calder I: A technique for awake fibreoptic intubation. Experience in patients with cervical spine disease. Anaesthesia 1993;48:910–913.

28. JooHS, Kapoor S, Rose DK, Naik VN: The intubating laryngeal mask airway after induction of anaesthesia versus awake fibreoptic intubation in patients with difficult airways. Anesth Analg 2001;92:1342–1346.

29. Lallo A, Billard V, Bourgain JL: A comparison of propofol and remifentanil target-controlled infusions to fascilitate fibreoptic nasotracheal intubation. Anesth Analg 2009;108:852–857.

INTRAVENOUS REGIONAL BLOCK FOR UPPER & LOWER EXTREMITY

CHAPTER 21

Intravenous Regional Block for Upper and Lower Extremity Surgery

Kenneth D. Candido, Anthony R. Tharian, and Alon P. Winnie

INTRODUCTION

The technique of intravenous regional anesthesia (IVRA), or "Bier block," was first introduced in 1908 by the German surgeon August Bier.[1] A Bier block essentially consists of injecting local anesthetic solutions into the venous system of an upper or lower extremity that has been exsanguinated by compression or gravity and that has been isolated by means of a tourniquet from the central circulation. In Bier's original technique, the local anesthetic procaine in concentrations of 0.25% to 0.5% was injected through an intravenous cannula, which had been placed between two Esmarch bandages utilized as tourniquets to divide the arm into proximal and distal components.[2-4] After injecting the local anesthetic, Bier noted two distinct types of anesthesia: an almost-immediate onset of "direct" anesthesia between the two tourniquets and then, after a delay of 5 to 7 minutes, an "indirect" anesthesia distal to the distally placed tourniquet. By performing dissections of the venous system of the upper extremity in cadavers after injecting methylene blue, Bier was able to determine that the direct anesthesia was the result of local anesthesia bathing bare nerve endings in the tissues, whereas the indirect anesthesia was most probably due to local anesthesia being transported to the substance of the nerves via the vasa nervorum, where a typical conduction block occurs. Bier's conclusion was that two mechanisms of anesthesia were associated with this technique: peripheral infiltration block and conduction block. The technique, as originally described by Bier, remains essentially unchanged in modern practice for the past 106 years, except for the introduction of the pneumatic-type double-tourniquet preparation used in current clinical practice[5-7] (Figure 21-1).

A Bier block can be used for brief surgical procedures or manipulations of the upper or lower extremity. However, the technique has found its greatest acceptance for use for the upper extremity because tourniquet problems and other safety issues seem to arise more frequently when IVRA is used on the lower extremities. Bier block is also a procedure that has found utility as a treatment adjunct for patients suffering from complex regional pain syndromes (CRPSs) (formerly known as reflex sympathetic dystrophy, with sympathetically maintained pain) as an alternative to repeated sympathetic ganglion blocks. In this regard, IVRA has been shown to decrease neurogenic inflammation, a phenomenon possibly associated with CRPS, with little impairment of sensory function, at least when mepivacaine is the local anesthetic chosen for the block. Sensibility to cold is significantly decreased 10 to 30 minutes after the block, even with a reduction in the skin temperature on the blocked side.[8] Chemical sympathectomy using IVRA with agents such as guanethidine or bretylium may last up to 5 days, as compared with local anesthetic blocks, which typically provide analgesia lasting only several hours. Quantitative sensory testing (QSART, quantitative sudomotor axon reflex testing) before and after such blocks demonstrated that it is possible to predict which patients will have long-lasting pain alleviation using IVRA guanethidine blocks following traumatic injury or surgery.[9]

Although IVRA is a safe and effective method of administering local anesthetics for extremity block both for surgery and for pain control, one large published survey noted that most third-year (CA-3) anesthesia residents had performed fewer than 10 such blocks during the entire course of their training.[10]

ANATOMY

The only relevant anatomy is the location and distribution of the veins of the hand, of the antecubital fossa, and of the foot and ankle region.

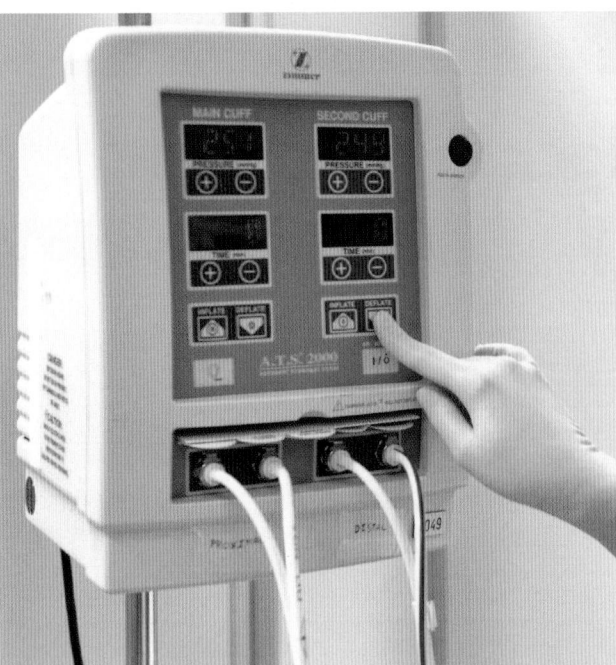

FIGURE 21-1. Double pneumatic tourniquet system for use in intravenous regional anesthesia of the upper or lower extremity.

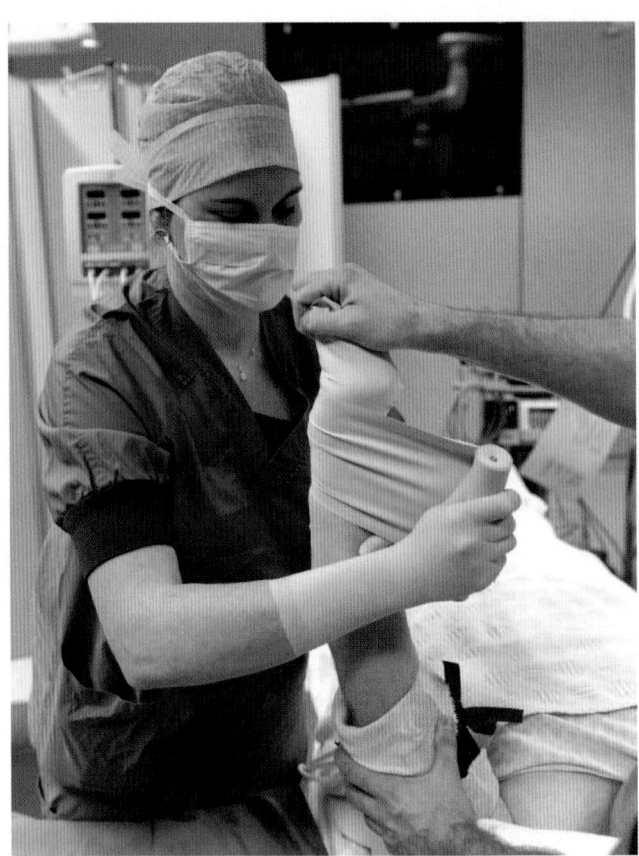

FIGURE 21-2. Beginning of the exsanguination process of the elevated left upper extremity using a tightly wrapped Esmarch bandage from the distal hand to the proximal upper extremity at the base of the distal tourniquet.

INDICATIONS

Upper Extremity

Intravenous regional anesthesia using local anesthetic, most commonly lidocaine 0.5%–1% (prilocaine 1% in Europe), is appropriate for surgery and manipulation of the extremities requiring anesthesia of up to 1 hour's duration. It is most suited for peripheral, soft tissue operations such as ganglionectomy, carpal tunnel release, Dupuytren's contracture surgery, or reduction of fractures. However, the necessity of exsanguinating the extremity using an Esmarch bandage, a potentially painful maneuver, may preclude certain procedures from being undertaken with this technique (Figures 21–2 and 21–3). Likewise, manipulations of the ulnar, median or radial nerves may cause paresthesias, which may require the use of adjuvant parenteral analgesics or sedatives. A novel use of IVRA is for anesthetizing the hand prior to injecting botulinum toxin A (BTX-A) for the treatment of hyperhidrosis. BTX-A significantly reduces sweat production, as measured by Minor's test and as quantified by corneometer analysis, but the injection is painful unless the hand is anesthetized beforehand; IVRA has been found to be suitable for this purpose.[11,12] According to a recent study, there was no difference in the degree and duration of analgesia between IVRA and stellate ganglion block (SGB) using a combination of 70 mg of lidocaine and 30 µg of clonidine in patients with CRPS type 1 affecting the upper extremities. The study concluded that IVRA was preferable to SGB in this setting due to its lower risk of undesirable side effects and easier execution than SGB.[13]

Upper extremity IVRA has been utilized occasionally for prolonged analgesia/anesthesia (ie, surgeries expected to persist for longer than 1 hour), with a mandatory tourniquet deflation period of at least 1 minute prior to reestablishing the anesthetized state.[14]

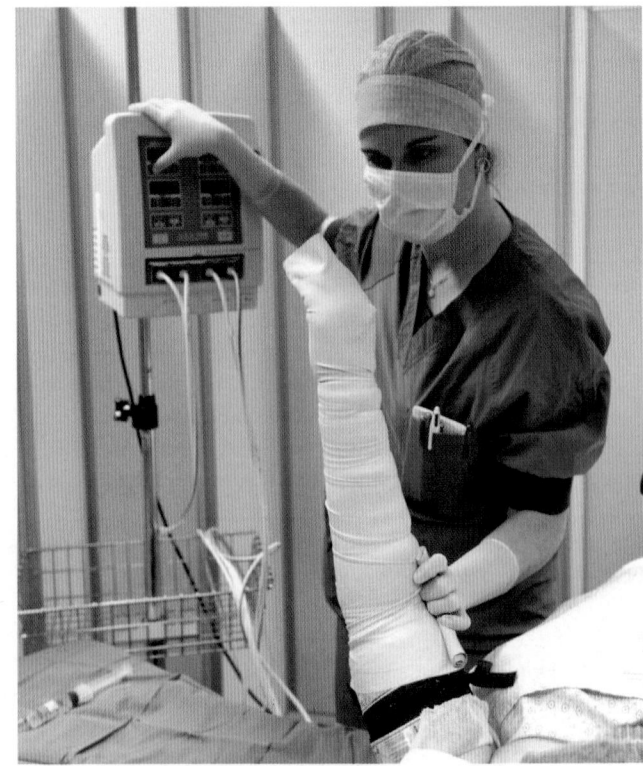

FIGURE 21-3. Keeping the Esmarch bandage tightly wrapped, first distal, then proximal tourniquets are to 50-100 mm Hg above the systolic arterial blood pressure.

Lower Extremity

Intravenous regional anesthesia may be used for brief surgical interventions of the lower extremity in a manner analogous to that described for upper extremity surgery. Surgical procedures that may be completed using this approach include excision of a mass; digital nerve repair; phalangeal fracture/dislocation surgery; and accessory navicular excision. Any foot, ankle, or distal lower extremity orthopedic procedure requiring approximately 45 minutes or less to complete may be amenable to this modality. Although IVRA has been associated with an increased incidence of compartment syndrome when treating tibial shaft fractures and has therefore been deemed contraindicated in such cases, a study in volunteers showed no significant difference in tissue pressures before and after tourniquet inflation regardless of the volume of saline used (≤1.5 mL/kg) or as a function of time following saline injection during tourniquet inflation. The authors concluded that, in the normal atraumatic limb, simulated IVRA using normal saline (NS) does not increase tissue pressure within the anterior compartment of the leg.[15]

Pediatrics

Intravenous regional anesthesia has been an acceptable choice in selected pediatric patients for the reduction of fractures of the upper extremity. A retrospective study comparing IVRA and conscious sedation for the reduction of pediatric forearm fractures found IVRA to be a safe, efficient, and cost-effective method of reducing pediatric forearm fractures.[16] There were 600 patients in the IVRA group and 645 patients in the conscious sedation group. No patient experienced compartment syndrome or a need for readmission secondary to cast application. Some intervention to their cast because of tightness was needed by 28 patients (4.34%) in the procedural sedation group and 13 patients (2.16%) in the IVRA group.[16]

CONTRAINDICATIONS

The only absolute contraindication to IVRA is patient refusal. Relative contraindications include the following:

- Crush injuries of an extremity
- Inability to locate peripheral veins
- Local skin infections
- Cellulitis
- Compound fractures
- Patients with convincing history of allergy to local anesthetics
- Patients with severe vascular injuries to the extremity
- Preexisting vascular arteriovenous shunts and patients in whom a tourniquet is unsuitable (ie, patients with severe peripheral vascular disease)
- Sickle cell disease
- Surgery planed for >1 hour are typically not good indication for IV regional anesthesia due to occurrence of Tourniquet pain.

EQUIPMENT

Figures 21–1 to 21–8 show equipment used in IVRA.

1. Local anesthetic agents: lidocaine HCl, 0.25%–0.1% (alternative is prilocaine, 0.5%)
2. One rubber tourniquet (Penrose drain) 12–18 in. in length (30–45 cm) and 7/8-in. wide (2.3 cm) for use prior to placing the intravenous cannula
3. One 20- or 22-gauge intravenous extracatheter (catheter over needle) (Figure 21–5)
4. One 500-mL or 1-L bag of intravenous solution connected to an infusion set (vs. a hep lock) to be connected to the intravenous cannula to maintain its patency until the anesthetic solution is injected in the isolated extremity (may substitute a saline-flushed intravenous port instead)
5. Standard American Society of Anesthesiologists (ASA) monitors (electrocardiograph, blood pressure, pulse oximeter)
6. Resuscitation equipment (intravenous catheter, crystalloid solution, and infusion set for the contralateral upper extremity) (for upper extremity IVRA)
7. Two pneumatic tourniquets of appropriate size for the selected extremity (Figures 21–6 and 21–9)
8. One Esmarch bandage 60 in. in length (152 cm) *and* 4 in. wide (10 cm) for exsanguinating the arm (Figures 21–2, 21–3, and 21–7)

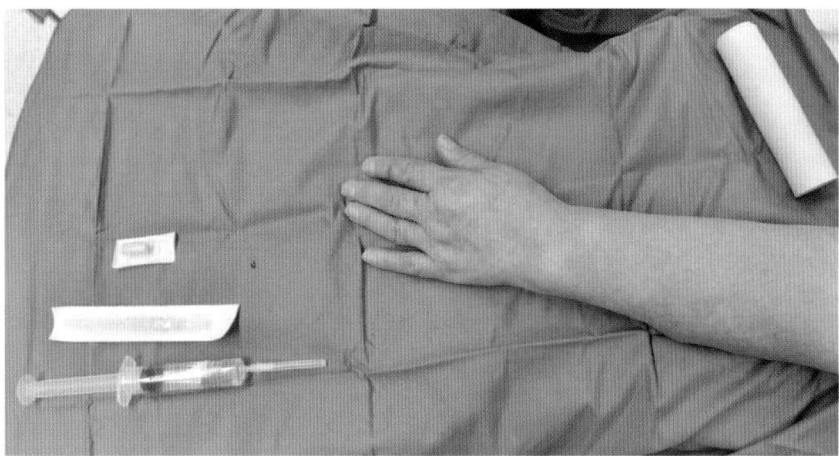

FIGURE 21–4. Equipment for IVRA consists of Esmarch bandage, local anesthetic vials, rubber tourniquet, intravenous (IV) extracatheter (catheter over needle), alcohol swabs, and a syringe to draw up local anesthetic.

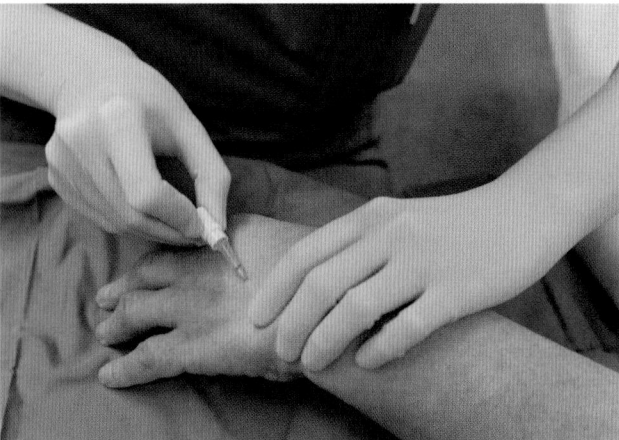

FIGURE 21–5. Intravenous cannula and Hep-Lock placed in a distal vein of the hand in preparation for IVRA.

9. Sterile skin preparatory set
10. A 30- or 50-mL Luer lock syringe
11. One graduated measuring cup for the mixing of solution, preferably with a 100-mL capacity
12. Adhesive tape, various sizes

PATIENT PREPARATION

The patient lies in the dorsal recumbent position as long as the vein selected for placement is readily accessible. The resuscitative equipment is checked, and the pneumatic tourniquets are tested and prepared for use. For surgery on the elbow, the needle will be placed in the forearm or antecubital fossa. For procedures on the hand or forearm, a vein in the dorsum of the hand is best selected (Figure 21–5).

For lower extremity procedures, a vein on the foot, ankle, or lower leg is chosen. After obtaining intravenous access in a nonoperated extremity (alternatively, a central venous access may be secured), a full complement of ASA monitors is

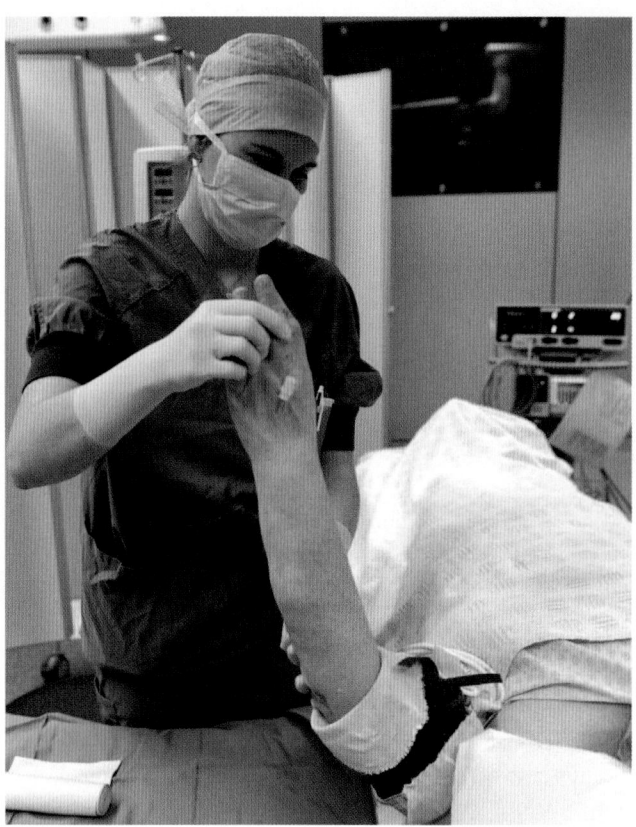

FIGURE 21–7. Elevation of the extremity to allow passive exsanguination.

applied, and baseline vital signs are assessed. If the patient is in severe pain, small aliquots of intravenous analgesics may now be administered (ie, fentanyl 1–2 µg/kg) to facilitate the exsanguination process. Because total patient cooperation is not essential to be successful, small doses of water-soluble benzodiazepine (ie, midazolam 15–25 µg/kg) may alternatively be administered for anxiolysis. An important benefit to choosing a benzodiazepine is the suppression of the convulsant response associated with local anesthetic toxicity, a valid concern in the patient undergoing IVRA due to the large volume of the agent being directly administered into the vascular system.

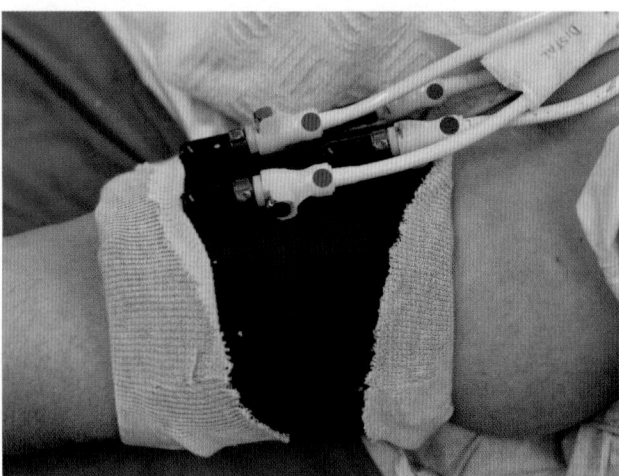

FIGURE 21–6. Clearly labeled proximal (RED) and distal (BLUE) tourniquet of the double tourniquet system. The tourniquet is always inflated in the following order: Distal, Proximal. Once the functionality is checked, the distal tourniquet (BLUE) is deflated.

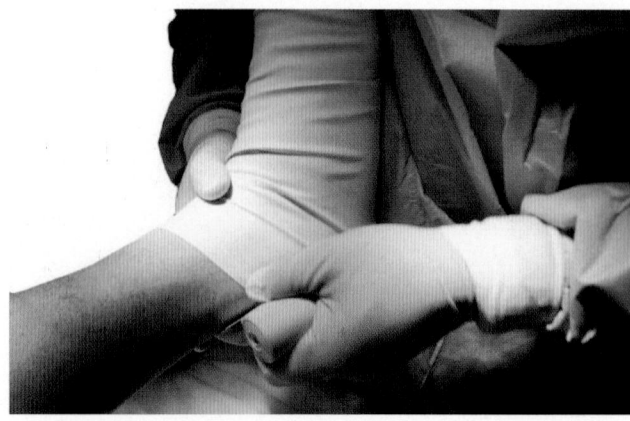

FIGURE 21–8. The elevated right lower extremity is wrapped with a tightly wound Esmarch bandage to the tourniquet.

TECHNIQUE

Upper Extremity IVRA

The following is the technique for IVRA for upper extremity procedures:

1. **An indwelling plastic catheter is inserted** into a peripheral vein as far distally as possible under strict aseptic precautions (Figure 21–5).

2. **A double-pneumatic tourniquet is placed on the proximal cuff high on the upper arm** (Figures 21–6 and 21–7). While by convention the tourniquets are placed on the biceps area, one study found that the dosage of lidocaine could be almost halved when the tourniquet was placed in the forearm instead of the upper arm.[17] Twenty patients undergoing forearm and hand surgeries received IVRA with a combination of lidocaine 1.5 mg/kg and ketorolac 0.15 mg/kg with a tourniquet placed on the forearm. Another 20 patients undergoing similar procedures received IVRA with double the dose of the same medications and with the tourniquet placed on the upper arm. Surgical anesthesia was assessed as excellent in all 20 patients in the upper arm tourniquet group, while it was rated as excellent in 19/20 patients in the forearm tourniquet group. Onset as well as regression of sensory block were similar in both groups.[17] A recent study comparing forearm tourniquet placement (n = 28) with 8 mL of 2% lidocaine and 10 mg ketorolac and upper arm tourniquet placement (n = 28) with 15 mL of 2% lidocaine and 20 mg ketorolac found that patients in the forearm tourniquet group experienced less discomfort, fewer sedation interventions, and a greater likelihood of bypassing the postanesthesia care unit (PACU) when compared with the group with the upper arm tourniquet.[18]

3. **The entire arm is elevated to allow passive exsanguination** (Figure 21–7), and a rubber Esmarch bandage is wound around the arm spirally from the fingertips of the hand to the distal cuff of the double tourniquet to exsanguinate the arm (Figures 21–2 and 21–3).

4. **The axillary artery is digitally occluded**, and while pressure is maintained on it, the proximal pneumatic cuff is inflated to 50–100 mm Hg above the systolic arterial blood pressure, after which the Esmarch bandage is removed.

5. **Following inflation of the proximal cuff and removal of the Esmarch bandage, 30–50 mL of 0.5% lidocaine HCl are injected** via the indwelling plastic catheter, the volume depending on the size of the arm being anesthetized.

6. To the level of the procedure table, the intravenous cannula in the surgical extremity is withdrawn, and pressure is quickly applied over the site using sterile gauze.

7. **About 25–30 minutes after the onset of anesthesia or when a patient complains of tourniquet pain, the distal cuff is inflated and the proximal cuff is deflated** to minimize the development of tourniquet pain.

Lower Extremity IVRA

The only significant difference in IVRA for the upper and lower extremities is that the IVRA technique for the lower extremity requires relatively larger volumes of local anesthetic solutions by virtue of the obvious size disparity between upper and lower extremities. This is necessary to more completely fill the larger vascular compartment of the lower extremity from the distally placed intravenous cannula to the proximal tourniquet (100 mL vs. 50 mL).

PHARMACOLOGIC CONSIDERATIONS

Local Anesthetic Considerations

Lidocaine is the prototypical local anesthetic used for IVRA in the United States. In Europe, however, prilocaine may be more commonly used and in fact has been the subject of most clinical trials. Attempts have been made to maximize the efficacy of lidocaine while minimizing side effects or toxicity of the agent. Alkalinization of 0.5% lidocaine (using 1.4% sodium bicarbonate) for IVRA was studied in 31 patients. The authors found no clinical advantage to the practice of alkalinization of lidocaine with respect to sensory block, motor block, or the appearance of postoperative pain.[19] When lidocaine was compared with alkalinized and nonalkalinized 2-chloroprocaine, both used as 0.5% concentrations and used exclusively for hand surgery, alkalinized chloroprocaine behaved similarly to lidocaine, but plain chloroprocaine offered no benefit and produced more side effects than seen with lidocaine.[20]

Another study comparing IVRA with low-concentration/high-volume lidocaine (0.5% concentration of 30–50 mL lidocaine) and higher-concentration/low-volume lidocaine (2% concentration of 12–15 mL lidocaine) in patients undergoing upper extremity surgery showed a faster onset and delayed regression of sensory block in the higher-concentration/low-volume group. There were no significant differences in hemodynamic data such as systolic and diastolic blood pressure, mean blood pressure, and heart rate between the two groups.[21]

Lidocaine has been compared with ropivacaine for upper extremity IVRA in two separate studies. Two doses of ropivacaine (1.2 and 1.8 mg/kg) were compared with one dose of lidocaine (3.0 mg/kg) in 15 volunteers. Recovery of sensory and motor block after tourniquet release was slowest with the high-dose ropivacaine group. More patients in the lidocaine group (5 of 5) experienced light-headedness following tourniquet release, versus only 1 in the high-dose ropivacaine group.[22] In the second study, 51 patients were randomized to receive either ropivacaine 0.375% or lidocaine 0.5% in a volume of 0.4 mL/kg up to 25 mL. Postoperative analgesia as measured by first request for analgesics was superior in the ropivacaine group.[23]

The progression of sensory blockade in the hand following IVRA with 20 mL of 0.3% ropivacaine and a double tourniquet placed in the forearm was studied in 10 healthy volunteers.[22] The local anesthetic was injected through a 22-gauge intravenous catheter placed in a prominent vein on the dorsum of the hand after exsanguination of the hand using an Esmarch bandage and sequentially inflating the distal tourniquet to

150 mm Hg or 20 mm Hg above the systolic blood pressure (whichever was higher) and the proximal tourniquet to 250 mm Hg. The distal tourniquet was then deflated, and the Esmarch bandage was removed. Baseline values for cold and touch sensation were determined before the block, and updated values were obtained repeatedly and continuously, beginning 5 minutes after the local anesthetic injection and continuing until loss of sensation was obtained in all areas. There was an almost-immediate loss of cold perception followed by a delayed and uneven spread of loss of touch sensation. The initial spread of anesthesia was noted both proximally and distally in the dorsum of the hand and then progressed to the fingertips, with a delayed proximal spread over the palmar surface of the hand to the wrist.[24]

Prilocaine has been compared with lidocaine, as well as with other local anesthetics used for IVRA. While evaluating the onset of sensory and motor block, 40 mL of 0.5% prilocaine (100 mg) was compared with the same volume and same concentration of chloroprocaine in 10 volunteers undergoing IVRA. Motor block onset did not differ between groups, and sensation was recovered almost equally well. However, recovery of motor function was shorter in the prilocaine group, and more chloroprocaine patients demonstrated signs of venous irritation or antecubital urticaria for 30–45 minutes after tourniquet deflation. Heart rate changes were also more notable in the chloroprocaine group.[25] The same group of investigators expanded their study to include 60 patients, 30 in each of the respective groups detailed previously. Now, the investigators found that complete recovery of sensory block was faster in the prilocaine group (7.1 vs. 9.8 minutes). Otherwise, the incidence of side effects remained higher in the chloroprocaine group.[26]

Next, these investigators compared 0.5% prilocaine with the same concentration of articaine (a newer amino amide-type local anesthetic that contains thiophene and is pharmacologically similar to mepivacaine) for upper extremity IVRA. Articaine, a potent local anesthetic with a low degree of toxicity by virtue of its rapid metabolism with esterases, was felt to be a suitable alternative to prilocaine. Ten volunteers participated in this double-blind, crossover comparison of the two agents. They found no significant difference between the two with respect of onset of anesthesia or motor block or in recovery of sensory or motor function. However, 80% of the subjects experienced skin rashes after receiving articaine, versus 20% in the prilocaine group.[27]

When 0.5% prilocaine was compared with the same concentrations of articaine or lidocaine in three groups of 10 patients each for IVRA, it was found that the onset of sensory block was significantly shorter in the articaine group, which also had the lowest peak plasma concentrations of local anesthetic following tourniquet release.[28] Plain prilocaine 1% has been compared with the same local anesthetic combined with four different additives for IVRA: bupivacaine 0.25%, clonidine 150 μg, sufentanil 25 μg, or tenoxicam 20 mg. The sufentanil-added group demonstrated the most rapid onset of sensory block; postoperative pain scores were improved by adding either clonidine or tenoxicam. Otherwise, there were no significant differences among the five groups with respect to

onset and duration of sensory block.[29] Unlike the situation noted for lidocaine with addition of bicarbonate as an adjuvant, the addition of bicarbonate to prilocaine does seem to shorten onset time and prolong the duration of anesthesia during IVRA.[30,31]

The use of mepivacaine for IVRA has been studied. Sixteen patients were evaluated using 1.4 mg/kg in 40 mL total for IVRA versus saline blocks performed in the same individuals on the contralateral arm. Arterial occlusion was maintained for 20 minutes. Reactive hyperemia was attenuated in the mepivacaine-treated arm for the 60-minute evaluation period, indicating that mepivacaine is a potent vasoconstrictor having a long duration of action. This finding has implications for the use of mepivacaine in individuals either with compromised upper extremity blood flow or with CRPS, for whom it probably should not be considered the local anesthetic of choice.[32]

The same study group evaluated the effects of mepivacaine IVRA on intracutaneous capsaicin-induced burning pain and on microvascular skin blood flow as measured by Doppler perfusion imaging. The reactive hyperemia was less in the mepivacaine-treated arm 10 minutes after tourniquet release, and the area of the flare was smaller after capsaicin in the mepivacaine-treated arms. The authors concluded that mepivacaine IVRA had no effects on post-IVRA sensory function of thin afferent fibers, but differentially decreased the spread of capsaicin-induced flare.[33]

Clinical Pearls

- Lidocaine is the prototypical drug used for IVRA in the United States; prilocaine is favored in Europe.
- Alkalinization of lidocaine confers minimal, if any, advantage to commercial lidocaine for IVRA.
- The potent vasoconstrictive properties of mepivacaine detract from its overall attractiveness as a primary agent for IVRA.

Adjuncts to Local Anesthetics for IVRA

A systematic review of the literature was undertaken to evaluate the use of adjuncts to local anesthetics for IVRA. Twenty-nine studies met the criteria of being randomized, double blind, and controlled. Data on 1217 study subjects were reviewed, and the agents studied included opioids (fentanyl, sufentanil, meperidine, and morphine); clonidine; muscle relaxants (atracurium, pancuronium, mivacurium); tramadol; nonsteroidal anti-inflammatory agents (NSAIDs) (ketorolac, tenoxicam, acetylsalicylate); alkalinization using sodium bicarbonate; the addition of potassium; and temperature alterations. The authors found solid evidence supporting the use of NSAIDs in general and ketorolac in particular for improving postoperative analgesia and prolonging tourniquet tolerance during IVRA. Opioids fared poorly when used for IVRA, with only meperidine in doses of 30 mg or greater showing substantial postoperative benefits at the expense of postdeflation nausea, vomiting, and dizziness. Muscle relaxants improved postoperative motor block and were beneficial in fracture reduction in which muscular relaxation is imperative for good results.[34]

Alpha₂ Agonists (Clonidine and Dexmedetomidine)

Clonidine has been added to both prilocaine and lidocaine as an adjunct to IVRA for extremity surgery. When 2 μg/kg were added to prilocaine 0.5% in a randomized, double-blind fashion in 56 patients undergoing upper extremity surgery, there was no difference between groups regarding sensory or motor block onset or duration. The patients who had clonidine had a significant reduction in arterial blood pressure after tourniquet release (24%–48%), while heart rates remained unchanged. The authors concluded that clonidine was of limited benefit as an adjunct to local anesthetics.[35] The addition of clonidine to prilocaine dramatically suppressed tourniquet pain, but it did not alter postoperative pain following tourniquet deflation.[36] Clonidine was found to provide no measurable benefits when added to lidocaine for IVRA in patients undergoing carpal tunnel release.[37]

Dexmedetomidine is appropriately eight times more selective toward the α-adrenoreceptors than clonidine. As such, it has been used in IVRA to determine if it might advance some of the beneficial findings noted with the latter agent. Thirty patients undergoing hand surgery under IVRA received 0.5% lidocaine alone or lidocaine plus dexmedetomidine 0.5 μg/kg. The dexmedetomidine group showed a more rapid onset of sensory and motor block; prolonged sensory and motor block recovery; prolonged tolerance for the tourniquet; and improved quality of analgesia compared with the group that received local anesthetic only.[38]

A shortened sensory block onset time; prolonged sensory and motor block recovery times; prolonged duration of analgesia for tourniquet; and prolonged postoperative analgesia were noted in patients undergoing IVRA with dexmedetomidine in another randomized, double-blind study comparing the effects of lornoxicam or dexmedetomidine in IVRA with prilocaine in patients undergoing hand or forearm surgery. In this study, IVRA was achieved with 2% prilocaine at 3 mg/kg in the control group (n = 25), 2% prilocaine at 3 mg/kg plus dexmedetomidine 0.5 μg/kg in the dexmedetomidine group (n = 25), and 2% prilocaine at 3 mg/kg plus lornoxicam 8 mg in the lornoxicam group (n = 25). In each group, the drugs were diluted with 0.9% normal saline to a total volume of 40 mL.[39]

A more recent study comparing the effects of dexmedetomidine when added to lidocaine for IVRA and when administered parenterally as premedication before IVRA found that both these groups had similarly improved quality of anesthesia and perioperative analgesia. This study was done on patients undergoing carpal tunnel release randomized into three groups. IVRA was done using 40 mL of 0.5% lidocaine. A single dose of dexmedetomidine 0.5 μg/kg and placebo (saline) solution in a total volume of 20 mL was administered to group P (n = 15) and group S (n = 15), respectively, before IVRA. Dexmedetomidine at 0.5 μg/kg of was added to lidocaine in group A (n = 15) during IVRA. The onset and recovery time of sensory and motor block, intraoperative-postoperative visual analog scale

(VAS), Ramsay sedation score (RSS), analgesic requirements, hemodynamic variables, and side effects were noted. Significantly shortened sensory block onset and recovery time in groups P and A, shortened motor block onset time in group P, and decreased intraoperative VAS scores and analgesic requirement in groups P and A were found. Intraoperative RSS in group P and postoperative RSS in groups P and A were higher than in group S. Intraoperative and postoperative heart rate and postoperative mean arterial blood pressure (MAP) of group P were significantly lower than in groups A and S, respectively.[40]

Opioids

Because opiate receptors were discovered to exist in the peripheral nervous system[41,42] and with the demonstration that opioids may produce effective, long-lasting analgesia when injected in conjunction with local anesthetics for brachial plexus block,[43-47] several investigators have attempted to decrease the potential for toxicity from local anesthetic–only IVRA by adding opioids to reduce the concentration of lidocaine. Although it has not been proven that the addition of fentanyl to lidocaine for IVRA results in improved analgesia while reducing the risks,[48,49] the addition of fentanyl in 200-μg doses to prilocaine 0.5% did result in more complete analgesia than in patients who had 100 μg added, or when plain prilocaine was used for IVRA. Postoperative nausea and central nervous system side effects were higher in the fentanyl-added groups versus those who received local anesthetic alone.[50] Two other studies, however, found that the addition of opioids to prilocaine did not improve success with the technique.[51,52] More research on the effects of the addition of opioids to prilocaine for IVRA may ultimately resolve this discrepancy.

Some investigators have found that adding opioids and muscle relaxants to 0.25% lidocaine provides the same analgesia and muscular relaxation as that provided by 0.5% lidocaine alone, while reducing the likelihood of systemic toxicity. Adjuvants added to lidocaine have included fentanyl 50 μg plus pancuronium 0.5 mg,[53,54] fentanyl plus rocuronium,[55] fentanyl plus D-tubocurarine,[56] and fentanyl plus vecuronium.[57] In each case, the authors reported outstanding operating conditions, and because the lidocaine concentration was able to be reduced to 0.20% (ie, more than one-half the normal used), the potential for systemic toxicity was at least halved.

When meperidine 0.25%, 40 mL (100 mg), was used as a solitary agent for IVRA, complete motor block was produced, just as effective as that produced by lidocaine. Motor block onset was as rapid as or more rapid than sensory block onset in each of the 15 patients in this study group. However, when compared with plain lidocaine in this study, there was a higher incidence of dizziness, nausea, and pain at the injection site.[58]

Tramadol

Tramadol has been evaluated for use in IVRA of the upper extremity. Sixty volunteers divided into four groups of 15 patients each received IVRA with 40 mL of tramadol 0.25% (100 mg), 0.9% normal saline, lidocaine 0.5%, or lidocaine plus tramadol 0.25%. The onset and recovery of sensory and motor block were similar between the tramadol and normal saline–only groups. However, the addition of tramadol to lidocaine resulted in faster onset of sensory block at the expense of an increase in skin rash and painful burning sensations at the injection site. The conclusion of the authors was that tramadol alone does not possess local anesthetic effects but might modify the effects if added to a local anesthetic such as lidocaine.[59]

In another study comparing 0.5% lidocaine with and without 50 mg of tramadol for upper extremity IVRA, the tramadol-added group experienced less tourniquet pain than the local-only group, but as in the study mentioned previously, there were several cases of skin urticaria in the tramadol group but not in the lidocaine-only group.[60] Tramadol (100 mg) added to lidocaine for IVRA for upper extremity anesthesia acted similarly to sufentanil (25 µg) or clonidine (1 µg/kg) added to the local anesthesia with respect to intraoperative hemodynamic data, time to recovery of sensory block, onset and recovery of motor block, sedation scores, and postoperative pain.[61] In summary, tramadol is ineffective as a solo agent for IVRA but may confer some advantage when added to lidocaine. This advantage, however, may be offset by the significant incidence of dermatologic side effects of tramadol given intravenously in an exsanguinated extremity.

Muscle Relaxants

A small dose of nondepolarizing muscle relaxant may be chosen as an adjunct to the local anesthetic administered for IVRA; however, because D-tubocurarine releases histamine even in judicious doses, it is probably best to avoid this agent altogether. Atracurium has been added to lidocaine in an effort to improve muscular relaxation during IVRA, particularly during the reduction of upper extremity fractures and dislocations. Adding 3 mg of atracurium to lidocaine for IVRA resulted in a decrease in the onset time of analgesia in the hand, but not at the tourniquet site. There was no added benefit to adding this agent or adding alfentanil to lidocaine in the same study.[62] A study using 2 mg of atracurium added to 40 mL of 0.5% lidocaine for IVRA for hand surgery in 40 patients randomized to one of two groups found that the addition of the atracurium provided a greater degree of muscle relaxation, easier reduction of fractures, and better operating conditions, as well as less pain after surgery.[63]

Neostigmine

Neostigmine has been suggested as a coanalgesic when used for epidural and intrathecal analgesia and anesthesia, but evidence of its benefit in the peripheral nervous system is lacking. In two studies, one using neostigmine added to lidocaine and the other using the adjuvant added to prilocaine, there have been conflicting findings. When neostigmine (1 mg) was added to 0.5% lidocaine for IVRA in a study of 54 volunteers randomized into one of three study groups, it was found that the addition of the adjuvant provided no benefit in terms of analgesia or anesthesia compared with controls.[64] When one-half of the dose of neostigmine (0.5 mg) was added to prilocaine (3 mg/kg) for IVRA in 30 patients randomized to one of two treatment groups, it was found that the adjuvant group demonstrated shortened sensory and motor block onset times, prolonged sensory and

motor block recovery times, improved quality of anesthesia, and prolonged time to first analgesic requirement versus the plain prilocaine group.[65]

A more recent study looking at the effect of adding 0.5 mg neostigmine to 40 mL of 0.5% lidocaine for IVRA in patients undergoing elective or emergency forearm and hand surgeries randomized into two groups, with 1 mL of isotonic saline added to 40 mL of 0.5% lidocaine in the control group, noted significantly shorter sensory and motor block onset times and longer recovery times in the neostigmine group when compared to the control group. The quality of intraoperative anesthesia and frequency of tourniquet pain were similar in both groups.[66] It appears that the conflicting findings with two different doses of neostigmine added to lidocaine for IVRA will need to be confirmed by additional work incorporating larger patient sample sizes to resolve the discrepancy in the two small studies mentioned previously.

Nonsteroidal Anti-inflammatory Agents

Other attempts to improve IVRA with lidocaine have included using NSAIDs to suppress tourniquet pain while enhancing postoperative analgesia. Although ketorolac has shown some efficacy, other NSAIDs have not fared as favorably. Ketorolac was studied as an adjuvant to lidocaine using either a forearm or an upper arm tourniquet in patients undergoing hand or forearm surgery.[67] In this study, the patients were randomized into two groups: group UA, consisting of 20 patients undergoing IVRA with an upper arm tourniquet; and group FA, consisting of 20 patients undergoing IVRA with a forearm tourniquet. Patients in the upper arm tourniquet group received IVRA with 0.5% lidocaine at the dose of 3 mg/kg plus ketorolac 0.3 mg/kg. IVRA in the forearm tourniquet group was established with 0.5% lidocaine at 0.15 mg/kg plus ketorolac 0.15 mg/kg. There was no statistically significant difference in the onset and duration of sensory block and the need for analgesic supplementation between the two groups. Postoperative pain scores were also similar between the two groups. The authors concluded that forearm tourniquet IVRA with 0.5% lidocaine at a dose of 1.5 mg/kg plus ketorolac 0.15 mg/kg is a safe and clinically viable option that provides similar perioperative anesthesia and analgesia as that provided by upper arm tourniquet IVRA with 0.5% lidocaine at a dose of 3 mg/kg plus ketorolac 0.3 mg/kg, while reducing the dose of lidocaine and ketorolac by half.[67]

Another NSAID, tenoxicam, was added to prilocaine in one study of 45 total patients. A 20-mg dose of the NSAID was used in patients undergoing IVRA for reduction of Colles fractures, with patients divided into three groups. One group received local anesthetic only; one received local plus tenoxicam; and one group had IVRA with local anesthetic only plus an intravenous NSAID. In this last group, the tenoxicam (20 mg) was injected in the contralateral arm, opposite the IVRA procedure arm. The group receiving the NSAID added to the local anesthetic had superior analgesia and lower pain scores than either of the other two groups of patients.[68]

A more recent study comparing the intraoperative and postoperative analgesic effects of lornoxicam and fentanyl when added to lidocaine for IVRA in patients undergoing hand surgery showed increased sensory block recovery time and first analgesic requirement time in the lornoxicam group, with no increased incidence of side effects, when compared to the lidocaine-only group and the lidocaine with fentanyl group. In this study, a total of 45 patients were randomized into three groups. Patients in group 1 received 3 mg/kg of 2% lidocaine (40 mL); group 2 received 3 mg/kg lidocaine, 38 mL plus lornoxicam 2 mL (4 mg/mL); and group 3 received 3 mg/kg lidocaine, 38 mL plus 2 mL fentanyl (0.05 mg/mL). This study also concluded that addition of fentanyl to lidocaine IVRA (group 3) seemed to be superior to lidocaine IVRA (group 1) and lornoxicam added to lidocaine IVRA (group 2) in decreasing tourniquet pain; however, this was at the expense of increasing side effects like itching.[69]

Dexketoprofen is another NSAID that has been studied as an adjunct to lidocaine for IVRA. In this prospective, randomized, placebo-controlled study, patients scheduled for elective hand or forearm soft tissue surgery were randomly divided into three groups. All 45 patients received 0.5% lidocaine as IVRA. Dexketoprofen 50 mg was given either intravenously or added into the IVRA solution, and the control group received an equal volume of saline both intravenously and as part of the IVRA. The times of sensory and motor block onset, recovery time, and postoperative analgesic consumption were recorded. Compared with controls, the addition of dexketoprofen to the IVRA solution resulted in more rapid onset of sensory and motor block, longer recovery time, decreased intra- and postoperative pain scores, and decreased postoperative analgesic requirements. The pharmacological formulation of dexketoprofen used in this study contained ethanol as an excipient. The authors stated that the neurolytic effect of ethanol may have contributed to the faster development of sensory and motor blockade and longer recovery times in the IVRA group in this study.[70]

Other Specific Agents: Corticosteroids

The anti-inflammatory properties of glucocorticoid-type steroids have been evaluated when these agents have been added to local anesthetics for IVRA in patients with rheumatoid arthritis (RA). In a randomized, double-blind, crossover, placebo-controlled study, 20 patients with RA received either 50 mg methylprednisolone in mepivacaine 0.25% or mepivacaine plain for upper extremity IVRA. The other extremity received the opposite treatment. One week later, the same medications were injected into the contralateral extremities, respectively. Fifty percent of patients reported subjective improvement at 1 and 6 weeks; objective parameters like grip strength did not change until the 6-week evaluation, at which time a significant increase was noted, as was the reduction in grip diastasis and movement-invoked pain. This report suggested that corticosteroids administered by IVRA may provide sustained analgesia in certain RA sufferers.[71]

Steroid IVRA has also been used as adjunctive treatment of CRPS type 1. Methylprednisolone (40 mg) was added to lidocaine for IVRA in a randomized, double-blind, placebo-controlled fashion in 22 patients. Treatments were applied once per week, for up to three sessions of blocks. The investigators found no benefit in adding the steroid to the local with regard to improvement in pain severity or shortening the course of the disease.[72]

Interestingly, a case series involving 168 patients with CRPS type 1 of the upper extremity treated with IVRA using 25 mL of 0.5% lidocaine and 125 mg of methylprednisolone diluted in 10 mL of normal saline and followed up over a 5-year period reported complete absence of pain in 92% of patients at the end of the follow-up period. IVRA was performed with the tourniquet kept inflated for 20 minutes, during which time the affected extremity was manipulated in an attempt to increase the range of motion. The tourniquet was then gradually deflated to avoid rapid entry of the injected agents to the circulation. The same process was repeated once or twice a week depending on the intensity and persistence of the patient's symptoms, and in between sessions patients were kept under mild physical therapy, which was not prolonged or stressful. An average of 4.8 sessions was needed to relieve the symptoms and to provide a functional extremity. The authors attributed the clinical results to the early stage of CRPS type 1 on initiating treatment and the increased dosing of methylprednisolone when compared to previous studies.[73]

Acetaminophen

Because of its known analgesic effects, acetaminophen (APAP) (paracetamol) has been studied as an adjuvant to local anesthetics in patients undergoing hand surgery under IVRA. Sixty patients undergoing hand surgery were randomized into three groups. All groups received IVRA lidocaine (3 mg/kg) diluted with normal saline to a total volume of 40 mL. Group 1 received IVRA lidocaine plus intravenous saline. Group 2 received IVRA lidocaine and an APAP (300 mg) admixture plus intravenous saline; and group 3 received IVRA lidocaine plus intravenous APAP (300 mg). Sensory and motor block onset time, tourniquet pain, and analgesic use were assessed during surgery. After tourniquet deflation, VAS scores at 1, 2, 4, 6, 12, and 24 hours; the time to first analgesic requirement; total analgesic consumption in first 24 hours; and side effects were noted. There was no significant difference in the onset of sensory blocks between the three groups; however, the duration of sensory block was significantly longer in group 2. Motor block onset time was shorter and duration of motor block was longer in group 2. Tourniquet pain was reduced and the quality of anesthesia scores as reported by the anesthesiologist, who was blinded to the study drug, was also significantly higher in group 2. There was no demonstrable decrease in postoperative pain scores between the three groups. The authors did point out the arbitrary dosing of APAP (300 mg) as a deficiency of the study. Further dose-ranging studies are required to optimize the dosing of paracetamol when used as an adjuvant to lidocaine for IVRA.[74]

Another study evaluating the effect of APAP, when added to lidocaine in IVRA, on sensory and motor block onset time, tourniquet pain, and postoperative analgesia found a shorter sensory block onset time; delayed tourniquet pain onset time; and reduced postoperative pain scores and analgesic consumption. The dosing of acetaminophen was identical to the earlier study (0.5% lidocaine diluted with 300 mg of intravenous APAP to a total volume of 40 mL). The control group received

0.5% lidocaine diluted with 0.9% normal saline to a total volume of 40 mL. Time of onset and duration of motor block were not assessed in this study. In an attempt to explain the faster onset time of the sensory block in the lidocaine-acetaminophen group, the authors investigated the pH of the lidocaine-acetaminophen mixture and found that the pH value of this mixture was 5.88, which was lower than the pH of the lidocaine–normal saline mixture, which was 6.16. This contradicts the fact that the higher the pH of the local anesthetic, the greater the nerve penetration and hence faster onset of neural blockade. In this study, the authors attributed the faster onset of sensory blockade to possible antinociceptive effects of APAP at peripheral sites.[75]

Nitroglycerine

The effect of nitroglycerine (NTG), when added to lidocaine for IVRA, was studied in a prospective, randomized, double-blind study.[76] Thirty patients undergoing hand surgery were randomly assigned to two groups. The control group (group C, n = 15) received a total dose of 40 mL with 3 mg/kg of lidocaine diluted with normal saline, and the NTG group (group NTG, n = 15) received an additional 200 μg NTG. Shortened sensory and motor block onset times; prolonged sensory and motor block recovery times; decreased tourniquet pain; and improved quality of anesthesia were noted in the NTG group. Postoperative analgesic requirements were also significantly decreased in the NTG group. The authors attributed the shorter onset time of sensory and motor blockade to the vasodilatory effects of NTG that promotes the distribution of local anesthetic to the nerves. Some of the other mechanisms that may contribute to the improved analgesia with NTG may include the metabolism of NTG to nitric oxide, which in turn causes an increase in the intracellular concentration of cyclic guanosine monophosphate, which produces pain modulation in the central and peripheral nervous system.[77,78] Nitric oxide generators have also been shown to induce anti-inflammatory effects and analgesia by blocking hyperalgesia and the neurogenic component of inflammatory edema by topical application.[79]

Midazolam

Midazolam has been shown to hasten the onset of sensory and motor blockade and improve postoperative analgesia when added to bupivacaine for brachial plexus block.[80,81] Midazolam was shown to have analgesic effects mediated through GABA (γ-aminobutyric acid) receptors in the spinal cord in animal studies.[82] GABA receptors have also been found in peripheral nerves.[83–85] Midazolam was also shown to reduce A-delta and C-fiber activity.[86]

In a study designed to evaluate the effect of midazolam when added to lidocaine for IVRA, 40 patients undergoing hand surgery were randomly assigned to two groups. The control group received 3 mg/kg lidocaine 2% diluted with saline to a total volume of 40 mL, and the midazolam group received an additional 50 μg/kg of midazolam. There were no statistically significant differences in the sensory and motor block onset and recovery times between the two groups. However, a subjective pain assessment score using the numeric rating scale (NRS) for tourniquet pain was significantly decreased in the midazolam group. Anesthesia quality as evaluated by the patient and the surgeon was also significantly better in the midazolam group. Postoperative NRS pain scores were also significantly lower in the midazolam group for the initial 2 hours postoperatively. However, postoperative sedation scores were also higher in the midazolam group. The authors indicated that the enhanced postoperative analgesia after tourniquet deflation may be explained by the systemic effect of midazolam in addition to the peripheral analgesic effect.[87]

Another study involved 60 patients undergoing hand surgery randomized into two groups, with the control group and the midazolam group receiving IVRA with exactly identical dosing of lidocaine and midazolam as in the previous study. This study showed shortened sensory and motor block onset times and prolonged sensory and motor block recovery times in addition to decreased tourniquet pain scores and postoperative pain scores.[88] The conflicting findings with regard to the sensory and motor block onset times may warrant further studies with greater sample sizes to resolve the discrepancy. At present, all that can be stated is that midazolam appears to hold some promise as an adjunct to local anesthetic when used for upper extremity IVRA.

Ketamine

Ketamine is a potent analgesic agent whose principal mechanism of action is antagonism of N-methyl-D-aspartate (NMDA) glutamate receptors that play a crucial role in the pain-processing mechanism at the level of the spinal cord. Animal studies have indicated the presence of NMDA receptors in peripheral nerves.[89] Ketamine has also been shown to produce transient blockade of peripheral nerve sodium and potassium channels.[90] The possible presence of NMDA receptors in peripheral nerves as well as the ability of ketamine to block sodium channels locally points to a possible peripheral site of action for ketamine, in addition to its well-established central sites of action.

Ketamine was studied as an adjuvant in lidocaine IVRA in patients undergoing hand surgery and its efficacy in controlling intraoperative tourniquet pain, postoperative analgesia, and side effects was compared to the same dosage of ketamine administered systemically. In this randomized, double-blind, systemic control study, 40 patients undergoing outpatient hand surgery were randomized into two groups. In group "IVRA," 0.1 mg/kg ketamine in 1 mL of normal saline was added to the IVRA lidocaine, and 1 mL of normal saline was administered via a peripheral intravenous line. In group "systemic," 1 mL of normal saline was added to the IVRA syringe, and 0.1 mg/kg ketamine in 1 mL of normal saline was administered via a peripheral intravenous line. Both groups received 40 mL of 0.5% lidocaine for IVRA. The study found no difference between the groups in the study parameters mentioned, and the authors concluded that IVRA ketamine and systemic intravenous ketamine were indistinguishable in terms of intraoperative tourniquet pain and postoperative analgesic consumption. The speed of onset and the duration of sensory and motor block were not measured in this study.[91]

Another study comparing the efficacy of ketamine and clonidine when they are added separately to 40 mL of 0.5% lidocaine for IVRA in patients undergoing hand or forearm surgery found delayed onset of tourniquet pain and decreased analgesic consumption in both these groups when compared to the control group receiving 40 mL of 0.5% lidocaine with saline added to it. Ketamine had a more potent effect on the study parameters when compared to clonidine. In this study involving 45 patients randomized into three groups, IVRA was performed using 40 mL of 0.5% lidocaine and saline, 1 μg/kg clonidine, or 0.1 mg/kg ketamine.[92]

Specific IVRA Treatments for CRPS

Adrenergic blocking agents or antagonists, particularly those effective at the α receptor, have shown promise in the treatment of CRPS, particularly when these agents are used for IVRA. Other adrenergic adjuvants release and then subsequently prevent the reuptake of norepinephrine at the neurovascular junction. Their use in CRPS is intuitive because the pathophysiology of the disease is suspected to include the α receptor and to be mediated by norepinephrine. However, there is significant controversy regarding this topic, particularly when current research is compared with the findings of studies conducted almost 40 years ago. Guanethidine, reserpine, and bretylium have all been evaluated for IVRA for CRPS. When 15 mg guanethidine were added to 0.5% prilocaine in a group of 57 patients with CRPS of the upper extremity and hand, the guanethidine was not found more effective than normal saline in treating allodynia and burning pain of CRPS following distal radius fractures.[93]

These findings corroborated work done in a double-blind, randomized, multicenter study 7 years earlier. Sixty patients with Reflex sympathetic dystrophy (RSD)/causalgia received four IVRA blocks at 4-day intervals with either guanethidine or placebo in 0.5% lidocaine. Long term, there was no difference noted between the placebo group and the guanethidine group, and only 35% of patients overall in all groups had a resolution of their problem.[94]

Bretylium has been used as well in CRPS. In a randomized, controlled trial, 0.5% lidocaine was compared with the same local anesthetic to which bretylium 1.5 mg/kg were added. A decrease in pain of 30% or more was considered significant. The bretylium-local group had pain relief for 20 ± 17.5 days, as opposed to the lidocaine-only group, wherein analgesia persisted for only 2.7 ± 3.7 days. The bretylium was far superior to the local anesthetic alone in treating CRPS in this study.[95]

Intravenous regional anesthesia with bretylium was utilized to demonstrate that a reduction in sympathetic tone of exercising forearm muscles would increase blood flow, reduce muscle acidosis, and attenuate reflex responses. IVRA with bretylium increased blood flow as well as oxygen consumption in the exercising forearm, although both venous potassium and hydrogen ion content were elevated during the exercise phase, implying that reflex effects were unaffected by bretylium block.[96]

COMPLICATIONS

Complications due to IVRA may be classified either as drug or equipment (ie, tourniquet) related. Drug-related complications depend on the agents, including local anesthetics and adjuvants, being administered directly into the vascular system. Equipment-related complications include all devices and techniques used to

isolate the vascular space from the systemic circulation. Inadvertent or unintentional deflation of the cuff, cuff failure, a sudden increase in venous pressure within the occluded tissue to a level higher than cuff pressure, and an intact interosseous circulation may all contribute to complications of IVRA.

Lidocaine is the most commonly utilized local anesthetic for IVRA and is therefore the agent about which most complications have been reported. Fortunately, lidocaine does not accumulate to any great extent at sodium channels at therapeutic plasma concentrations, and because it both rapidly binds to and dissociates from the channel, toxic accumulations of the drug at the channel are atypical.[97,98] Excessive plasma concentrations of lidocaine, as are associated with intravenous boluses of large doses with a faulty tourniquet system, result in peripheral vasodilation and diminished cardiac contractility, usually seen clinically as hypotension. The usual onset of IVRA using lidocaine in 0.5% concentrations is rapid (about 4.5 ± 0.3 minutes), and the termination of anesthesia once the tourniquet has been deflated is also rapid (5.8 ± 0.5 minutes).[99] Usually, there are no signs or symptoms of cardiovascular or central nervous system toxicity if the tourniquet is deflated at least 30 minutes after the drug is injected into the venous system, although tinnitus has been noted at the 20- and 27-second postdeflation periods following standard inflation times.[100]

However, a literature search in the American National Library of Medicine's PubMed*, in Embase*, and in MEDLINE*, spanning the period from 1950 to 2007 revealed 24 cases of seizures, with seizures reportedly occurring in 12 cases while the cuff was still inflated and in 9 cases after the cuff was deflated. Information was not available in three cases. Seizures occurring during tourniquet inflation were reported with tourniquet pressure exceeding the initial systolic arterial blood pressure by 150 mm Hg. Seizures occurring after tourniquet deflation were reported with tourniquet times as long as 60 minutes and with a delay of up to 10 minutes after tourniquet deflation. The lowest dose of local anesthetic associated with a seizure was 1.4 mg/kg for lidocaine, 4 mg/kg for prilocaine, and 1.3 mg/kg for bupivacaine.[101]

Although about 70% of the administered lidocaine dose remains within the tissues of the isolated limb after tourniquet deflation, the remaining 30% enters the systemic circulation during the ensuing 45 minutes.[98] Much more drug is released from the tissues of the isolated limb into the circulation after tourniquet deflation if the limb is inadvertently exercised, emphasizing the importance of maintaining the previously anesthetized extremity quiescent for some time immediately following tourniquet deflation.

The other commonly utilized local anesthetic used for IVRA, prilocaine, is associated with the formation of methemoglobin (MetHb), which occurs about 4 to 8 hours after its administration.[97] Fortunately, significant methemoglobinemia has not been reported when prilocaine has been used for IVRA. Prilocaine (0.5%) administered for IVRA has an onset of analgesia of about 11 minutes (±6.8 minutes), and termination of analgesia following tourniquet deflation averages 7.2 minutes (±4.6 minutes).[25] The use of this agent for IVRA appears to be extraordinarily safe. Indeed, in one survey of 45,000 prilocaine IVRA blocks, there were no serious side effects and no deaths from using this drug via this technique.[102] In terms of effectiveness, prilocaine seems to be equivalent to lidocaine when used for IVRA.

When opioids are administered in combination with local anesthetics for IVRA in an attempt to prolong analgesia following cuff deflation, occasional side effects typically attributed to opioids administered systemically may be noted following cuff deflation. These include nausea, vomiting, and mild sedation.[48,51] When neurovascular blocking drugs are administered in conjunction with local anesthetics to improve surgical conditions in patients undergoing fracture reduction, there have been no reports of complications from these adjuvants.

Clinical Pearls

- An intact tourniquet system is essential for the successful and safe performance of IVRA.
- Unintentional deflation of the tourniquet or the presence of a vascular communication even with an intact, functioning tourniquet may result in severe systemic toxicity.
- When the surgical procedures is shorter than 30 minutes, intermittent cuff deflation and inflation may effectively prolong the time to achieve peak arterial concentrations of the local anesthetic but may not be entirely reliable in minimizing toxicity due to release of local anesthetic into the circulation.[103]
- The tourniquet should not be deflated until at least 30 minutes has elapsed from the time local anesthetic (and adjuvants, if used) is injected into the isolated venous system.

In addition, the tourniquet itself may be a source of complications because it may cause ischemic pain and discomfort. Systemic hypertension may result from tourniquet inflation that is sustained or prolonged. Equipment misuse or malfunction is an important, and avoidable, source of complications due to this technique. Even an intact, fully functional tourniquet may be associated with leakage of administered drugs from a supposedly isolated extremity into the systemic circulation.[104,105]

Lower limb IVRA has an almost 100% incidence of local anesthetic leakage from beneath the tourniquet, versus about a 25% incidence for upper extremity block.[106] As a corollary to this leakage phenomenon, the use of IVRA for lower extremity analgesia has an associated high incidence of poor-quality block (almost 40% in one prospective study).[107] Drug may leak past an apparently fully functioning cuff and gain access to the systemic circulation via the interosseous circulation, which is not affected by the occlusion of muscles, soft tissues, and the accompanying vascular channels included therein. This factor has been recognized for almost 50 years, yet it does not appear to be significant in the production of complications due to IVRA.[108]

Tourniquet deflation after IVRA is associated with signs and symptoms of systemic local anesthetic toxicity, ranging from mild events related to the central nervous system, such as tinnitus and perioral numbness, to seizures, and finally to devastating cardiovascular collapse. These correlate with local anesthetic concentrations in arterial blood and not to venous concentrations.[103,109]

Another complication due to IVRA is tourniquet pain, which not uncommonly occurs if a double pneumatic device is not utilized[105] (Figures 21–1 and 21–9). We recommend the use of such a tourniquet for any procedure performed using IVRA that is expected to last longer than 30 minutes. Even when such guidelines are followed, however, untoward events occur following tourniquet deflation after a "safe" time interval.[101]

Very rare, isolated reports of neurologic complications, including damage to the median, ulnar, and musculocutaneous nerves, are associated with IVRA.[110] The cause of such complications appears to be direct pressure of the tourniquet applied to these nerves, which subsequently exhibit histologic changes resembling crush injuries. It is recommended that tourniquet time not exceed 2 hours to reduce the likelihood of capillary and muscle damage secondary to tissue acidosis.[110,111]

Compartment syndrome may occur rarely following IVRA, especially when IVRA is used for reduction of long-bone lower extremity fractures, and may be due both to the large volume of local anesthetic injected to effect analgesia and to inadequate or incomplete exsanguination of the limb prior to performing the block.[112,113] There is a case report of this complication following inadvertent injection of hypertonic saline solution when local anesthetic was intended to be injected.[114]

A 33-year-old pregnant patient undergoing IVRA for endoscopic carpal tunnel release experienced a severe episode of phantom limb sensation after the injection of the local anesthetic. The symptoms resolved on dissipation of the IVRA.[115] There is one report of the devastating necessity for amputation of the arm in a 28-year-old patient whose radial and ulnar arteries thrombosed following IVRA after a brief tourniquet occlusion time.[116] Whether this resulted from unsuspected intraarterial injection of drug, a drug administration error, or perhaps an idiosyncratic drug reaction is purely speculative. Three cases including either death or permanent brain damage associated with IVRA were reported in the ASA Closed Claims Project for the years 1980 to 1999. Specifics of these cases are not known.[117]

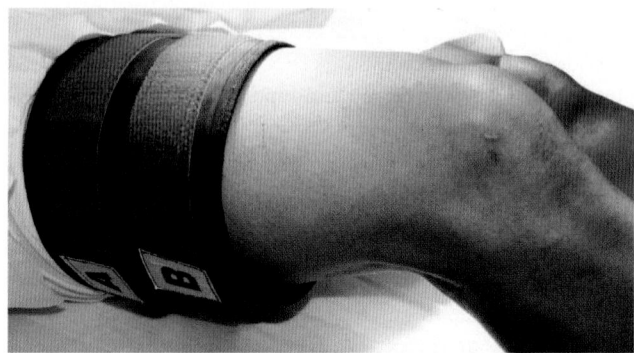

FIGURE 21–9. The double tourniquet system is placed on the proximal right thigh, in preparation for IVRA of the right lower extremity.

Local Anesthetic Toxicity

Although lidocaine is the most commonly utilized local anesthetic agent for IVRA in the United States, in Europe prilocaine 0.5% is more routinely chosen. Prilocaine, however, is metabolized to orthotoluidine, an oxidizing compound capable of converting hemoglobin to MetHb. This is usually only of concern when the dose of prilocaine exceeds 600 mg, which, even for lower extremity IVRA in which volumes as large as 100 mL are utilized, should not be attained (ie, 100 mL × 0.5% prilocaine = 500 mg).

Clinical Pearls

- Severe methemoglobinemia is a medical emergency requiring prompt recognition and appropriate treatment.
- A good history and high level of suspicion are required to make the diagnosis.
- For methemoglobinemia due to drug exposure, traditional first-line therapy consists of the infusion of methylene blue (MB).
- Dextrose should be given because the major source of NADH (reduced [hydrogenated] nicotinamide adenine dinucleotide) in the red blood cells is the catabolism of sugar through glycolysis. Dextrose is also necessary to form NADPH (reduced [hydrogenated] NAD phosphate) through the hexose monophosphate shunt, which is necessary for MB to be effective.
- The dose of MB is 1 to 2 mg/kg IV over 5 minutes (total dose should not exceed 7–8 mg/kg).
- MB can cause dyspnea, chest pain, or hemolysis.
- MB provides an artificial electron transporter for the reduction of MetHb via the NADPH-dependent pathway. The response is rapid; the dose may be repeated in 1 hour if the level of MetHb is still high 1 hour after the initial infusion.
- Rebound methemoglobinemia may occur up to 18 hours after MB administration due to prolonged absorption of lipophilic agents (benzocaine) from adipose tissue. It is reasonable to perform serial measurements of MetHb levels following treatment with MB. MB should not be administered to patients with glucose-6-phosphate dehydrogenase (G6PD) deficiency because the reduction of MetHb by MB is dependent on NADPH generated by G6PD (hemolysis). An alternative treatment for these patients is ascorbic acid (2 mg/kg).
- Blood transfusion or exchange transfusion may be helpful in patients who are in shock. Hyperbaric oxygen has been used with anecdotal success in severe cases.

Deflation of the tourniquet after surgery is a critical step in minimizing the possibility of toxicity associated with IVRA. First, it is absolutely mandatory that the tourniquet not be deflated unless at least 30 minutes have elapsed since the injection of the local anesthetic,[33] even if the duration of surgery or of the manipulation has been brief. If the surgery is brief, and the patient needs to recover in the PACU, it is acceptable to clamp off the distal tourniquet while it is inflated, remove the patient from the operating area (with the tourniquet inflated), and transfer the patient to a monitored care setting. At no time should anyone remove the clamped tourniquet, however, until the 30-minute period commencing with the injection of local anesthetic solution has elapsed. At such time, the patient should be continually monitored for at least 15 minutes following tourniquet unclamping in the PACU. At least one case of cardiac arrest has been reported when the tourniquet was released soon after the injection of local anesthetic, where the duration of surgery was extremely short.[118]

Second, it is absolutely essential that the tourniquet deflation be accomplished in a "cyclical" fashion as follows: The cuff is deflated (after a minimum of 30 minutes) and is immediately reinflated. The patient is observed or questioned carefully for the occurrence of symptoms associated with local anesthetic toxicity, such as tinnitus, light-headedness, metallic taste in the mouth, and so on. Obviously, signs of stimulation of the central nervous system may also represent local anesthetic toxicity and must also be sought. If there are no such signs or symptoms after about 1 minute, the cuff is once again deflated and again immediately reinflated for a period of about 1 to 2 minutes, with the patient being observed and queried for systemic local anesthetic toxicity. If none appears by this time, the tourniquet may be safely deflated and removed from the extremity. The safety of such cycled deflating/reinflating is that, with each deflation, only a small fraction of the administered (and unbound) local anesthetic is allowed to enter the systemic circulation, minimizing the possibility of a sudden, sustained increase in the blood level of the local aneshtetic.[103]

SUMMARY

Intravenous regional anesthesia is a valuable adjunct to the armamentarium of clinicians in any specialty dealing with the acutely injured patient. The simplicity of the technique and the relative safety (if strict adherence to the previously listed protocol is maintained) make it an attractive alternative to brachial plexus block (for upper extremity surgery or manipulation) and spinal or epidural block (for lower extremity surgery or manipulation). Simply being able to identify and access a peripheral vein and apply a pneumatic tourniquet make this one of the most "user-friendly" regional block modalities in clinical practice. There is no requirement for being facile with a peripheral nerve stimulator or interpreting images obtained from an ultrasound machine. One of the only potential disadvantages associated with IVRA is the finite duration of anesthesia/analgesia associated with its use. A relative inability to prolong analgesia long into the postprocedure period detracts from its utility. For those occasions, continuous catheter insertion and maintenance by way of plexus anesthesia ensures offering an attractive alternative.

REFERENCES

1. Bier A: Uber einen neun weg local anaesthesia an den gliedmassen zuerzeugen. Arch Klin Chir 1908;86:1007–1016.
2. Bier A: On a new method of local anesthesia. Muench Med Wschir 1909; 56:589.

3. Bier A: Concerning venous anesthesia. Berl Klin Wschr 1909;46: 477–489.

4. Bier A: On local anesthesia with special reference to vein anesthesia. Edinburgh Med J 19105:103–123.

5. Morrison J: Intravenous local anesthesia. Br J Surg 1930–1931;18:641–647.

6. Herreros L: Regional anesthesia by the intravenous route. Anesthesiology 1946;7:558–560.

7. Holmes CMcK: Intravenous regional analgesia. Lancet 1963;1:245–247.

8. Kalman S, Svenson H, Lisander B, et al: Quantitative sensory changes in humans after intravenous regional block with mepivacaine. Reg Anesth Pain Med 1999;24:236–241.

9. Wahren L, Torebjork E, Nystorm B: Quantitative sensory testing before and after regional guanethidine block in patients with neuralgia in the hand. Pain 1991;46:23–30.

10. Smith M, Sprung J, Zura A, et al: A survey of exposure to regional anesthesia techniques in American anesthesia residency training programs. Reg Anesth Pain Med 1999;24:11–16.

11. Blaheta H, Vollert B, Zuder D, et al: Intravenous regional anesthesia (Bier's block) for botulinum toxin therapy of palmar hyperhidrosis is safe and effective. Dermatol Surg 2002;28:666–671.

12. Bosdotter Enroth S, Rystedt A, Covaciu L, et al: Bilateral forearm intravenous regional anesthesia with prilocaine for botulinum toxin treatment of palmar hyperhidrosis.. J Am Acad Dermatol 2010;63(3): 466–474.

13. Nascimento MSA, Klamt JG, and Prado WA: Intravenous regional block is similar to sympathetic ganglion block for pain management in patients with complex regional pain syndrome type 1. Braz J Med Biol Res 2010; 43(12):1239–1244.

14. Glickman L, Mackinnon S, Rao T, et al: Continuous intravenous regional anesthesia. J Hand Surg 1992;17:82–86.

15. Mabee J, Shean C, Orlinsky M, et al: The effects of simulated Bier block IVRA on intracompartmental tissue pressure. Acta Anaesthesiol Scand 1997;41:208–213.

16. Aarons CE, Fernandez MD, Willsey M, Peterson B, Key C, Fabregas J: Bier block regional anesthesia and casting for forearm fractures: Safety in the pediatric emergency department setting. J Pediatr Orthop 2014;34:45–49.

17. Singh R, Bhagawat A, Bhadoria P, Kohli A: Forearm IVRA, using 0.5% lidocaine in a dose of 1.5 mg/kg with ketorolac 0.15 mg/kg for hand and wrist surgeries. Minerva Anestesiol 2010;76:109–114.

18. Chiao FB, Chen J, Lesser JB, Resta-Flarer F, Bennett H: Single-cuff forearm tourniquet in intravenous regional anesthesia results in less pain and fewer sedation requirements than upper arm tourniquet. Br J Anaesth 2013;111(2):271–275.

19. Benlabed M, Jullien P, Guelmi K, et al: Alkanization of 0.5% lidocaine for intravenous regional anesthesia. Reg Anesth 1990;15:59–60.

20. Lavin P, Henderson C, Vaghadia H: Non-alkalinized and alkalinized 2-chloroprocaine versus lidocaine for intravenous regional anesthesia during outpatient hand surgery. Can J Anaesth 1999;46:939–945.

21. Ulus A, Gurses E, Oztrurk I, Serin S: Comparative evaluation of two different volumes of lidocaine in intravenous regional anesthesia. Med Sci Monit 2013;19:978–983.

22. Chan V, Weisbrod M, Kaszas Z, et al: Comparison of ropivacaine and lidocaine for intravenous regional anesthesia in volunteers: A preliminary study on anesthetic efficacy and blood level. Anesthesiology 1999;90: 1602–1608.

23. Peng P, Coleman M, McCartney C, et al: Comparison of anesthetic effect between 0.375% ropivacaine versus 0.5% lidocaine in forearm intravenous regional anesthesia. Reg Anesth Pain Med 2002;27;595–599.

24. Horn JL, Cordo P, Kunster D, et al: Progression of forearm intravenous regional anesthesia with ropivacaine. Reg Anesth Pain Med 2011;36(2): 177–180.

25. Pitkanen M, Suzuki N, Rosenberg P: Intravenous regional anesthesia with 0.5% prilocaine or 0.5% chloroprocaine. A double blind comparison in volunteers. Anaesthesia 1992;47:618–619.

26. Pitkanen M, Kytta J, Rosenberg P: Comparison of 2-chloroprocaine and prilocaine for intravenous regional anesthesia of the arm: A clinical study. Anaesthesia 1993;48:1091–1093.

27. Pitkanen M, Xu M, Haasio J, et al: Comparison of 0.5% articaine with 0.5% prilocaine in intravenous regional anesthesia of the arm: A cross over study in volunteers. Reg Anesth Pain Med 1999;24:131–135.

28. Simon M, Gielen M, Albernik N, et al: Intravenous regional anesthesia with 0.5% articaine, 0.5% lidocaine, or 0.5% prilocaine. A double-blind randomized clinical study. Reg Anesth 1997;22:29–34.

29. Hoffman V, Vercauteren M, Van Steenberge A, et al: Intravenous regional anesthesia. Evaluation of four different additives to prilocaine. Acta Anaesthesiol Belg 1997;48:71–76.

30. Armstrong P, Brockway M, Wildsmith J: Alkalinization of prilocaine for intravenous regional anesthesia. Anaesthesia 1990;45:11–13.

31. Solak M, Akturk G, Erciyes N, et al: The addition of sodium bicarbonate to prilocaine solution during IV regional anesthesia. Acta Anaesthesiol Scand 1991;35:572–574.

32. Kalman S, Bjorn K, Tholen E, et al: Mepivacaine as an intravenous regional block interferes with reactive hyperemia and decreases steady state blood flow. Reg Anesth 1997;22:552–556.

33. Kalman S, Liderfalk C, Wardell K, et al: Differential effect on vasodilation and pain after intradermal capsaicin in humans during decay of intravenous regional anesthesia with mepivacaine. Reg Anesth Pain Med 1998;23:402–408.

34. Choyce A, Peng P: A systematic review of adjuncts for intravenous regional anesthesia for surgical procedures. Can J Anaesth 2002;49: 32–45.

35. Kleinschmidt S, Stockl W, Wilhelm W, et al: The addition of clonidine to prilocaine for intravenous regional anesthesia. Eur J Anaesthesiol 1997;14:40–46.

36. Cucchia G, Chasot-Di Dio V, et al: Effect of addition of clonidine to local anesthetic during the Bier block on the pre- and postoperative analgesia. Br J Anaesth 1997;78(Suppl 1):78–79.

37. Ivie CS, Viscomi CM, Adams DC, Friend AF, Murphy TR, Parker CJ: Clonidine as an adjunct to intravenous regional anesthesia: A randomized, double-blind, placebo controlled dose ranging study. Anaesthesiol Clin Pharmacol 2011;27(3):323–327.

38. Memis D, Turan A, Karamanlioglu B, et al: Adding dexmedetomidine to lidocaine for intravenous regional anesthesia. Anesth Analg 2004;98: 835–840.

39. Kol IO, Ozturk H, Kaygusuz K, Gursoy S, Comert B, Mimaroglu C: Addition of dexmedetomidine or lornoxicam to prilocaine in intravenous regional anesthesia for hand or forearm surgery: A randomized controlled study. Clin Drug Investig 2009;29(2):121–129.

40. Mirzak A, Gul R, Erkutlu I, Alptekin M, Oner U: Premedication with dexmedetomidine alone or together with 0.5% lidocaine for IVRA. J Surg Res 2010;164(2):242–247.

41. Fields H, Emson P, Leigh B, et al: Multiple opiate receptor sites on primary afferent fibers. Nature 1980;284:351–353.

42. Young W, Wamsley J, Zarbin M, et al: Opioid receptors undergo axonal flow. Science 1980;210:76–78.

43. Boogaerts J, Balatoni E, Lafont N, et al: Utilisation des morphiniques dans les blocs nerveux peripheriques. Congres Ser Ars Medicina 1985; 3:143–150.

44. Gobeaux D, Landais A: Utilisation de deux morphiniques dans les blocs du plexus brachial. J Can Anesth 1988;36:437–440.

45. Gobeaux D, Landais A, Bexon G, et al: Adjonction de fentanyl la lidocaine adrenaline pour le blocage du plexus brachial. J Can Anesth 1987;35:195–199.

46. Viel E, Eledjam J, de la Coussaye J, et al: Brachial plexus block with opioids for postoperative pain relief: Comparison between buprenorphine and morphine. Reg Anesth 1989;14:274–278.

47. Candido K, Khan M, Raja D, et al: Brachial plexus block for postoperative pain relief. Reg Anesth 2000;25:23.

48. Arhtur J, Mian T, Heavner J, et al: Fentanyl and lidocaine versus lidocaine for Bier block. Reg Anesth 1992;17:223–227.

49. Bobart V, Hartmannsgruber M, Atanassoff P, et al: Analgesia/anesthesia after fentanyl plus lidocaine vs. plain lidocaine for intravenous regional anesthesia. Anesth Analg 1998:86:S-3.

50. Pitkanen M, Rosenberg P, Pere P, et al: Fentanyl- prilocaine mixture for intravenous regional anesthesia in patients undergoing surgery. Anaesthesia 1992;47:395–398.

51. Armstrong P, Power I, Wildsmith J: Addition of fentanyl to prilocaine for intravenous regional anesthesia. Anaesthesia 1991;46:278–280.

52. Gupta A, Begntsson M, Bjornsson A, et al: Lack of peripheral analgesic effect of low-dose morphine during intravenous regional anesthesia. Reg Anesth 1993;18:250–253.

53. Abdulla W, Fadhil N: A new approach to intravenous regional anesthesia. Anesth Analg 1992;75:597–601.

54. Sztark F, Thicoipe M, Favarel-Garriques J, et al: The use of 0.25% lidocaine with fentanyl and pancuronium for intravenous regional anesthesia. Anesth Analg 1997;84:777–779.

55. Subxedar D, Gevirtz C, Malik V, et al: Intravenous regional anesthesia: Prospective evaluation of 0.25% lidocaine with fentanyl and rocuronium. Reg Anesth 1997;22:41.

56. Thapar P, Skerman J: Evaluation of 0.2% lidocaine with fentanyl and D-tubocurarine for intravenous regional anesthesia. Reg Anesth 1997; 84: S342.

57. Santhosh MC, Rohini BP, Roopa S, Raghavendra PR: Study of 0.5% lidocaine alone and combination of 0.25% lidocaine with fentanyl and vecuronium in intravenous regional anesthesia for upper limb surgeries. Rev Bras Anestesiol 2013;63(3):254–257.

58. Acalovschi I, Cristea T: Intravenous regional anesthesia with meperidine. Anesth Analg 1995;81:539–543.

59. Acalovschi I, Cristea T, Margarit S, et al: Tramadol added to lidocaine for intravenous regional anesthesia. Anesth Analg 2001;92:209–214.

60. Tan S, Pay L, Chan S: Intravenous regional anesthesia using lignocaine and tramadol. Ann Acad Med Singapore 2001;30:516–519.

61. Alayurt S, Memis D, Pamucku Z: The addition of sufentanil, tramadol or clonidine to lignocaine for intravenous regional anaesthesia. Anaesth Intensive Care 2004;32:22–27.

62. Kurt N, Kurt I, Aygunes B, et al: Effects of adding alfentanil or atracurium to lidocaine solution for intravenous regional anesthesia. Eur J Anaesthesiol 2002;19:522–525.

63. Elhakim M, Sadek R: Addition of atracurium to lidocaine for intravenous regional anesthesia. Acta Anaesthesiol Scand 1994;38:542–544.

64. McCartney C, Brill S, Rawson R, et al: No anesthetic or analgesic benefit of neostigmine 1 mg added to intravenous regional anesthesia with lidocaine 0.5% for hand surgery. Reg Anesth Pain Med 2003;28:414–417.

65. Turan A, Karamanlyoglu B, Memis D, et al: Intravenous regional anesthesia using prilocaine and neostigmine. Anesth Analg 2002;95:1419–1422.

66. Sethi D, Wason R: Intravenous regional anesthesia using lidocaine and neostigmine for upper limb surgery. J Clin Anesth 2010;22(5):324–328.

67. Singh R, Bhagwat A, Bhadoria P, Kohli A: Forearm IVRA, using 0.5% lidocaine in a dose of 1.5 mg/kg with ketorolac 0.15 mg/kg for hand and wrist surgeries. Minerva Anestesiol 2010;76(2):109–114.

68. Jones N, Pugh S: The addition of tenoxicam to prilocaine for intravenous regional anaesthesia. Anaesthesia 1996;51:446–448.

69. Sertoz N, Kocaoglu N, Ayanoglu HO: Comparison of lornoxicam and fentanyl when added to lidocaine in intravenous regional anesthesia. Rev Bras Anestesiol 2013;63(4):311–316.

70. Yurtlu S, Hanci V, Kargi E, Erdogan G, et al: The analgesic effect of dexketoprofen when added to lidocaine for intravenous regional anesthesia: A prospective, randomized, placebo-controlled study. J Int Med Res 2011;39(5):1923–1931.

71. Bengtsson A, Bengtsson M, Nilsson I, et al: Effects of intravenous regional administration of methylprednisolone plus mepivacaine in rheumatoid arthritis. Scand J Rheumatol 1998;27:277–280.

72. Taskaynatan M, Ozgul A, Tan A, et al: Bier block with methylprednisolone and lidocaine in CRPS Type 1: A randomized, double-blinded placebo controlled study. Reg Anesth Pain Med 2004;29:408–412.

73. Varitimidis SE, Papatheodorou LK, Dailiana ZH, Poultsides L, Malizos KN: Complex regional pain syndrome type I as a consequence of trauma or surgery to upper extremity: Management with intravenous regional anesthesia, using lidocaine and methylprednisolone. J Hand Surg Eur 2011;36(9):771–777.

74. Sen H, Kulachi Y, Bicerer E, Ozkan S, Dagli G, Turan A: The analgesic effect of paracetamol when added to lidocaine for intravenous regional anesthesia. Anesth Analg 2009;109(4):1327–1330.

75. Ko MJ, Lee JH, Cheong SH, et al: Comparison of the effects of acetaminophen to ketorolac when added to lidocaine for intravenous regional anesthesia. Korean J Anesthesiol 2010;58(4):357–361.

76. Sen S, Ugur B, Aydin ON, et al: The analgesic effect of nitroglycerin added to lidocaine on intravenous regional anesthesia. Anesth Analg 2006;102(3):916–920.

77. Lauretti GR, Perez MV, Reis MP, Pereira NL: Double-blind evaluation of transdermal nitroglycerine as an adjuvant to oral morphine for cancer pain management. J Clin Anesth 2002:14:83–86).

78. Lauretti GR, de Olivera R, Reis MP, et al: Transdermal nitroglycerine enhances spinal sufentanil postoperative analgesia following orthopedic surgery. Anesthesiology 1999;90:734–739.

79. Ferreira SH, Lorenzette BB, Faccioli LH: Blockade of hyperalgesia and neurogenic edema by topical application of NTG. Eur J Pharmacol 1992;217:207–209.

80. Jaro K, Batra YK, Panda NB: Brachial plexus block with midazolam and bupivacaine improves analgesia. Can J Anaesth 2005;52:822–826.

81. Laig N, Khan MN, Arif M, Khan S: Midazolam with bupivacaine for improving analgesia quality in brachial plexus block for upper limb surgeries. J Coll Physicians Surg Pak 2008;18:674–678.

82. Nishiyama T, Tamai H, Hanaoka K: Serum and cerebrospinal fluid concentrations of midazolam after epidural administration in dogs. Anesth Analg 2003;96:159–162.

83. Bhisitkul RB, Villa JE, Kocsis JD: Axonal GABA receptors are selectively present in normal and regenerated sensory fibers in rat peripheral nerves. Exp Brain Res 1987:66:659–663.

84. Brown DA, Marsh S: Axonal GABA receptors in mammalian peripheral nerve trunks. Brain Res 1978;156:187–191.

85. Cairns BE, Sessle BJ, Hu JW: Activation of peripheral GABA-A receptors inhibits temporomandibular joint-evoked jaw muscle activity. J Neurophysiol 1999;81:1966–1969.

86. Kontinen VK, Dickenson AH: Effects of midazolam in the spinal nerve ligation model of neuropathic pain in rats. Pain 2000;85:425–431.

87. Farouk S, Aly AJ: Quality of lidocaine analgesia with and without midazolam for intravenous regional anesthesia. J Anesth 2010;24(6):864–868.

88. Kashefi P, Montazeri K, Honarmand A, Safavi M, Hosseini HM: The analgesic effect of midazolam when added to lidocaine for intravenous regional anesthesia. J Res Med Sci 2011;16(9):1139–1148.

89. Carlton SM, Hargett GL, Coggeshall RE: Localization and activation of glutamate receptors in ummyelinated axons of rat glabrous skin. Neurosci Lett 1995;197:25–28.

90. Brau ME, Sander F, Vogel W, Hempelmann G: Blocking mechanisms of ketamine and its enantiomers in enzymatically demyelinated peripheral nerve as revealed by single-channel experiments. Anesthesiology 1997;86:394–404.

91. Viscomi CM, Friend C, Parker C, Murphy T, Yarnell M: Ketamine as an adjuvant in lidocaine intravenous regional anesthesia: A randomized, double-blind, systemic control trial. Reg Anesth Pain Med 2009;34(2):130–133.

92. Georgias NK, Maidatsi PG, Kyriakidis AM, et al: Clonidine versus ketamine to prevent tourniquet pain during intravenous regional anesthesia with lidocaine. Reg Anesth Pain Med 2001;26(6):512–517.

93. Livingstone J, Atkins R: Intravenous regional guanethidine blockade in the treatment of posttraumatic complex regional pain syndrome 1(algodystrophy) of the hand. J Bone Joint Surg Br 2002;84:380–386.

94. Ramamurthy S, Hoffman J: Intravenous regional guanethidine in the treatment of reflex sympathetic dystrophy/causalgia. A randomized, double-blind study. Guanethidine Study Group. Anesth Analg 1995;81:718–723.

95. Hord A, Rooks M, Stephens B, et al: Intravenous regional bretylium and lidocaine for treatment of reflex sympathetic dystrophy: A randomized, double-blind study. Anesth Analg 1992;74:818–821.

96. Lee F, Shoemaker J, McQuillan P, et al: Effects of forearm Bier block with bretylium on the hemodynamic and metabolic responses to handgrip. Am J Physiol Heart Circ 2000;279:H586–H593.

97. Bader A, Concepcion M, Hurley R, et al: Comparison of lidocaine and prilocaine for intravenous regional anesthesia. Anesthesiology 1988;69:409–412.

98. Tucker G, Boas R: Pharmacokinetic aspects of intravenous anesthesia. Anesthesiology 1971;34:538–549.

99. Ware R: Intravenous regional anesthesia using bupivacaine. A double blind comparison with lignocaine. Anaesthesia 1979;34:231–235.

100. Smith C, Steinhaus J, Haynes C: The safety and effectiveness of intravenous regional anesthesia. South Med J 1968;61:1057–1060.

101. Guay J: Adverse events associated with intravenous regional anesthesia (Bier Block): A systematic review of complications. J Clin Anesth 2009;21:585–594.

102. Bartholomew K, Sloan J: Prilocaine for Bier's block: How safe is safe? Arch Emerg Med 1990;7:189–195.

103. Sukhani R, Garcia C, Munhall R, et al: Lidocaine disposition following intravenous regional anesthesia with different deflation techniques Anesth Analg 1989;68:633–637.

104. Mazze R, Dunbar R: Plasma lidocaine concentrations after caudal, lumbar epidural, axillary block and intravenous regional anesthesia. Anesthesiology 1966;27:574–579.

105. Dunbar R, Mazze R: Intravenous regional anesthesia: Experience with 779 cases. Anesth Analg 1967;46:806–813.

106. Davies J, Walford A: Intravenous regional anesthesia for foot surgery. Acta Anaesthesiol Scand 1986;30:145–147.

107. Kim D, Shuman C, Sadr B: Intravenous regional anesthesia for outpatient foot and ankle surgery. A prospective study. Orthopedics 1993:16; 1109–1113.

108. Cotev S, Robin G: Experimental studies on intravenous regional anesthesia using radioactive lignocaine. Br J Anaesth 1966;38:936–940.

109. Hargrove R, Hoyle J, Parker J: Blood lidocaine levels following intravenous regional analgesia. Anaesthesia 1996;21:37–41.

110. Larsen U, Hommelgaard P: Pneumatic tourniquet paralysis following intravenous regional anesthesia. Anaesthesia 1987;42:526–528.

111. Shaw-Wilgis E: Observations on the effects of tourniquet ischemia. J Bone Joint Surg 1971;1104:190.
112. Mabee J, Bostwick T, Burke M: Iatrogenic compartment syndrome from hypertonic saline injection in Bier block. J Emerg Med 1994;12: 473–476.
113. Quigley J, Popich G, Lanz U: Compartment syndrome of the forearm and hand: A case report. Clin Orthop 1981;161:247–251.
114. Hastings H 2nd, Misamore G: Compartment syndrome resulting from intravenous regional anesthesia. J Hand Surg 1987;12:559–562.
115. Dominguez E: Distressing upper extremity phantom limb sensation during intravenous regional ansthesia. Reg Anesth Pain Med 2001;26:72–74.
116. Luce E, Mangubat E: Loss of hand and forearm following Bier block: A case report. J Hand Surg 1983;8:280–283.
117. Lee LA, Posner K, Domino KB, et al: Injuries associated with regional anesthesia in the 1980's and 1990's. A closed claims analysis. Anesthesiology 2004;101:143–152.
118. Kennedy B, Duthie A, Parbrook G, Carr T: Intravenous regional anesthesia: An appraisal. Br Med J 1965;5440:954–957.

NEURAXIAL ANESTHESIA

CHAPTER 22

Neuraxial Anatomy (Anatomy Relevant to Neuraxial Anesthesia)

Steven L. Orebaugh and Hillenn Cruz Eng

INTRODUCTION

The vertebral column forms part of the axis of the human body, extending in the midline from the base of the skull to the pelvis. Its four primary functions are protection of the spinal cord, support of the head, provision of an attachment point for the upper extremities, and transmission of weight from the trunk to the lower extremities. Pertinent to regional anesthesia, the vertebral column serves as the landmark for a wide variety of regional anesthesia techniques. It is important, therefore, that the anesthesiologist be able to develop a three-dimensional mental image of the structures comprising the vertebral column.

ANATOMIC CONSIDERATIONS

The vertebral column consists of 33 vertebrae (7 cervical, 12 thoracic, 5 lumbar, 5 sacral, and 4 coccygeal segments) (Figure 22–1). In the embryonic period, the spine curves into a C shape, forming two primary curvatures with their convex aspect directed posteriorly. These curvatures persist through adulthood as the thoracic and sacral curves. The cervical and lumbar lordoses are secondary curvatures that develop after birth as a result of extension of the head and lower limbs when standing erect. The secondary curvatures are convex anteriorly and augment the flexibility of the spine.

Vertebrae

A typical vertebra consists of a vertebral **arch** posteriorly and a **body** anteriorly. This holds true for all vertebrae except C1. Two **pedicles** arise on the posterolateral aspects of each vertebra and fuse with the two **laminae** to encircle the **vertebral foramen**[1] (Figures 22–2A, 22–2B). These structures form the vertebral canal, which contains the spinal cord, spinal nerves, and epidural space. Fibrocartilaginous disks containing the **nucleus pulposus**, an avascular gelatinous body surrounded by the collagenous lamellae of the annular ligament, join the vertebral bodies. The **transverse processes** arise from the laminae and project laterally, whereas the **spinous process** projects posteriorly from the midline union of the laminae (Figures 22–2A, 22–2B). The spinous process is frequently bifid at the cervical level and serves as an attachment for muscles and ligaments.

C1 (**atlas**), C2 (**axis**), and C7 (**vertebra prominens**) are described as *atypical* cervical vertebrae due to their unique features. C1 is a ringlike bone that has no body or spinous process. It is formed by two lateral masses with facets that connect anteriorly to a short arch and posteriorly to a longer, curved arch. The anterior arch articulates with the dens, and the posterior arch has a groove where the vertebral artery passes (Figure 22–3A). The odontoid process (dens) of C2 protrudes superiorly, hence the name axis (Figure 22–3B). Together, the atlas and axis form the axis of rotation for the atlantoaxial joint. The C7 (vertebra prominens) has a long, nonbifid spinous process that serves as a useful landmark for a variety of regional

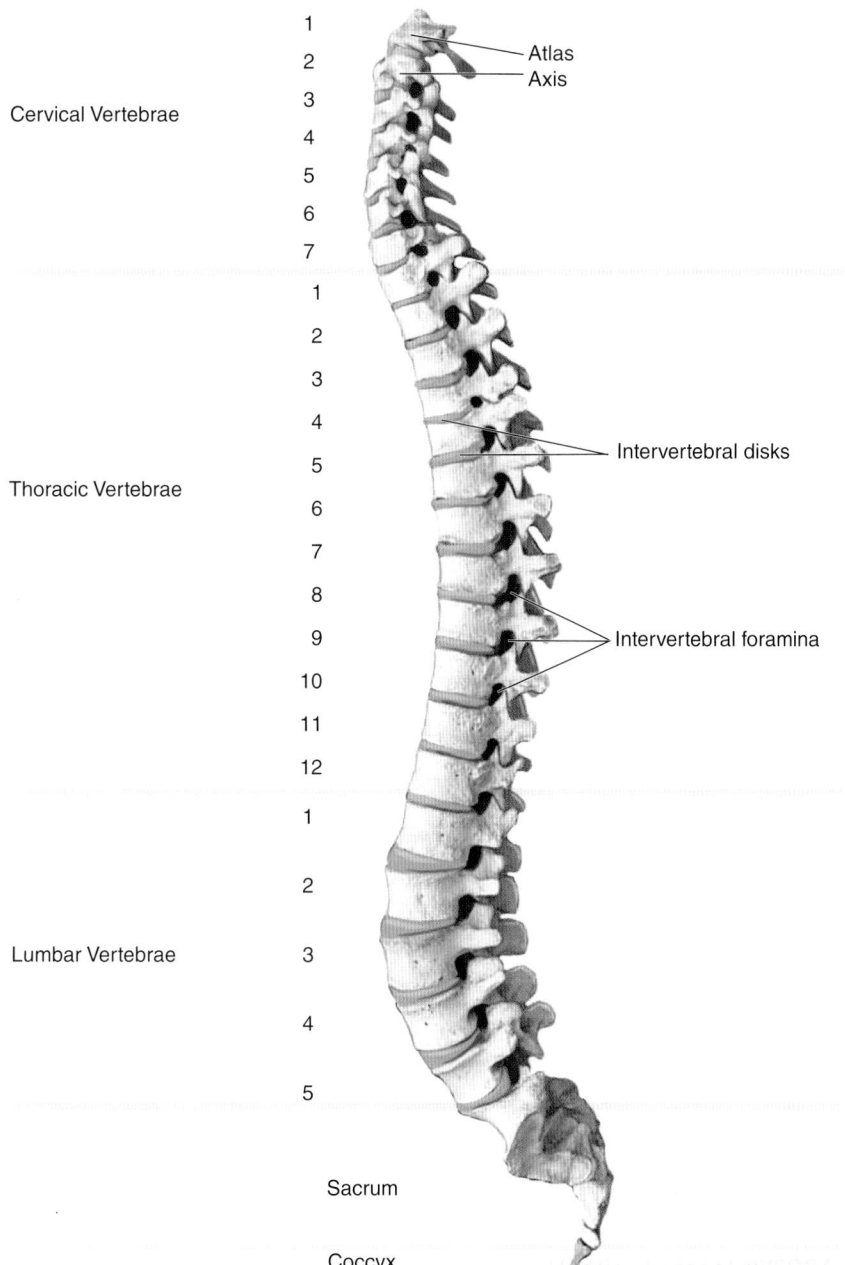

Cervical Vertebrae

1
2   Atlas
3   Axis
4
5
6
7

Thoracic Vertebrae

1
2
3
4
5   Intervertebral disks
6
7
8
9   Intervertebral foramina
10
11
12

Lumbar Vertebrae

1
2
3
4
5

Sacrum

Coccyx

FIGURE 22–1. The vertebral column and the curvatures of the adult spine, lateral view.

anesthesia procedures (Figure 22–3C). The C7 transverse process is large and has only one posterior tubercle.

The interlaminar spaces in the thoracic spine are narrow and more challenging to access with a needle due to overlapping laminae. In contrast, the laminae of the five lumbar vertebrae do not overlap. The interlaminar space between adjacent lumbar vertebrae is rather large.[2]

Vertebral **facet** (**zygapophyseal**) **joints** articulate posterior elements of adjacent vertebrae. The junction of the lamina and pedicles gives rise to **inferior** and **superior articular processes** (Figures 22–2A, 22–2B). The inferior articular process protrudes caudally and overlaps the inferiorly adjacent vertebra's superior articular process. This alignment is important to

understand when performing interventional pain procedures such as facet joint injections, intra-articular steroid injections or radio-frequency denervation. Joint surfaces in the cervical spine are oriented halfway between the axial and coronal planes. This alignment allows an ample degree of rotation, flexion, and extension but little resistance to backward and forward shearing forces. Facet joints in the thoracic region are oriented in a more coronal plane, which provides greater protection against shearing forces but reduced rotation, flexion, and extension.

In the lumbar spine, joint surfaces are curved, with a coronal orientation of the anterior portion and a sagittally oriented posterior portion.[3] Thoracic facets are located anterior to the

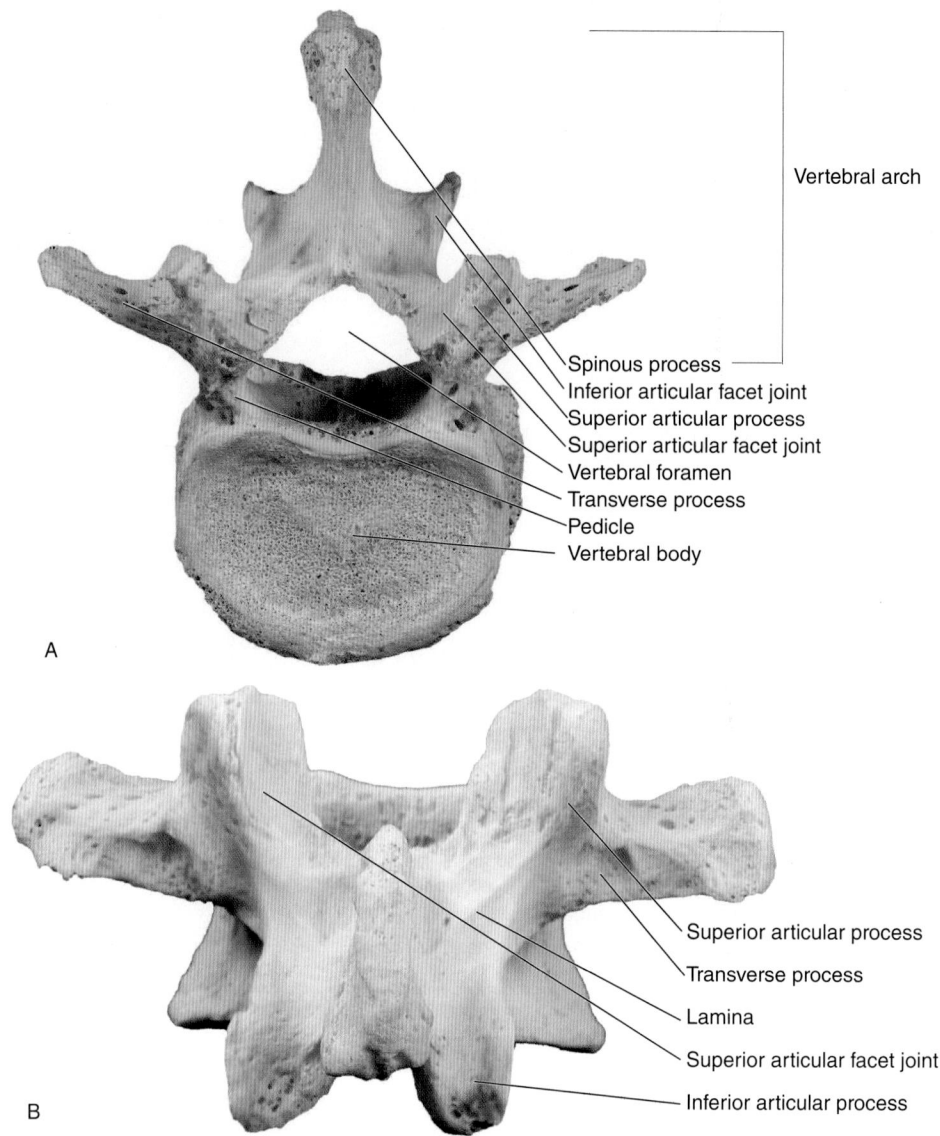

Vertebral arch

Spinous process
Inferior articular facet joint
Superior articular process
Superior articular facet joint
Vertebral foramen
Transverse process
Pedicle
Vertebral body

A

Superior articular process

Transverse process

Lamina

Superior articular facet joint

Inferior articular process

B

FIGURE 22–2. A typical vertebra. **A:** Superior view of the L5 vertebra. **B:** Posterior view of the L5 vertebra.

transverse processes, whereas cervical and lumbar facets are located posterior to their transverse processes. Five sacral vertebrae fuse to form the wedge-shaped **sacrum**, which connects the spine with the iliac wings of the pelvis[4] (Figures 22–4A, 22–4B). In childhood, the sacral vertebrae are connected by cartilage, which progresses to osseous fusion after puberty, with only a narrow remnant of sacral disk remaining in adulthood. Fusion is generally complete through the S5 level, although there can be complete lack of any posterior bony roof over the sacral vertebral canal. The **sacral hiatus** is an opening formed by the incomplete posterior fusion of the fifth sacral vertebra. It lies at the apex of the coccyx, which is formed by the union of the last four vertebrae (Figure 22–4C). This hiatus provides a convenient access to the caudal ending of the epidural space, especially in children. The **sacral cornu** are bony prominences on each side of the hiatus that are easily palpated in small children and serve as landmarks for a caudal epidural block.

Intervertebral Ligaments

The vertebral column is stabilized by a series of ligaments. The **anterior** and **posterior longitudinal ligaments** run along the anterior and posterior surfaces of the vertebral bodies, respectively, reinforcing the vertebral column. The **supraspinous ligament**, a heavy band that runs along the tips of the spinous processes, becomes thinner in the lumbar region (Figure 22–5). This ligament continues as the **ligamentum nuchae** above T7 and attaches to the occipital external protuberance at the base of the skull.[5] The **interspinous ligament** is a narrow web of tissue that attaches between spinous processes; anteriorly it fuses with the ligamentum flavum and posteriorly with the supraspinous ligament (Figure 22–5).

The **ligamentum flavum** is a dense, homogenous structure, composed mostly of elastin which connects the lamina of adjacent vertebrae[5,6] (Figure 22–5). The lateral edges of the ligamentum flavum surround facet joints anteriorly, reinforcing their

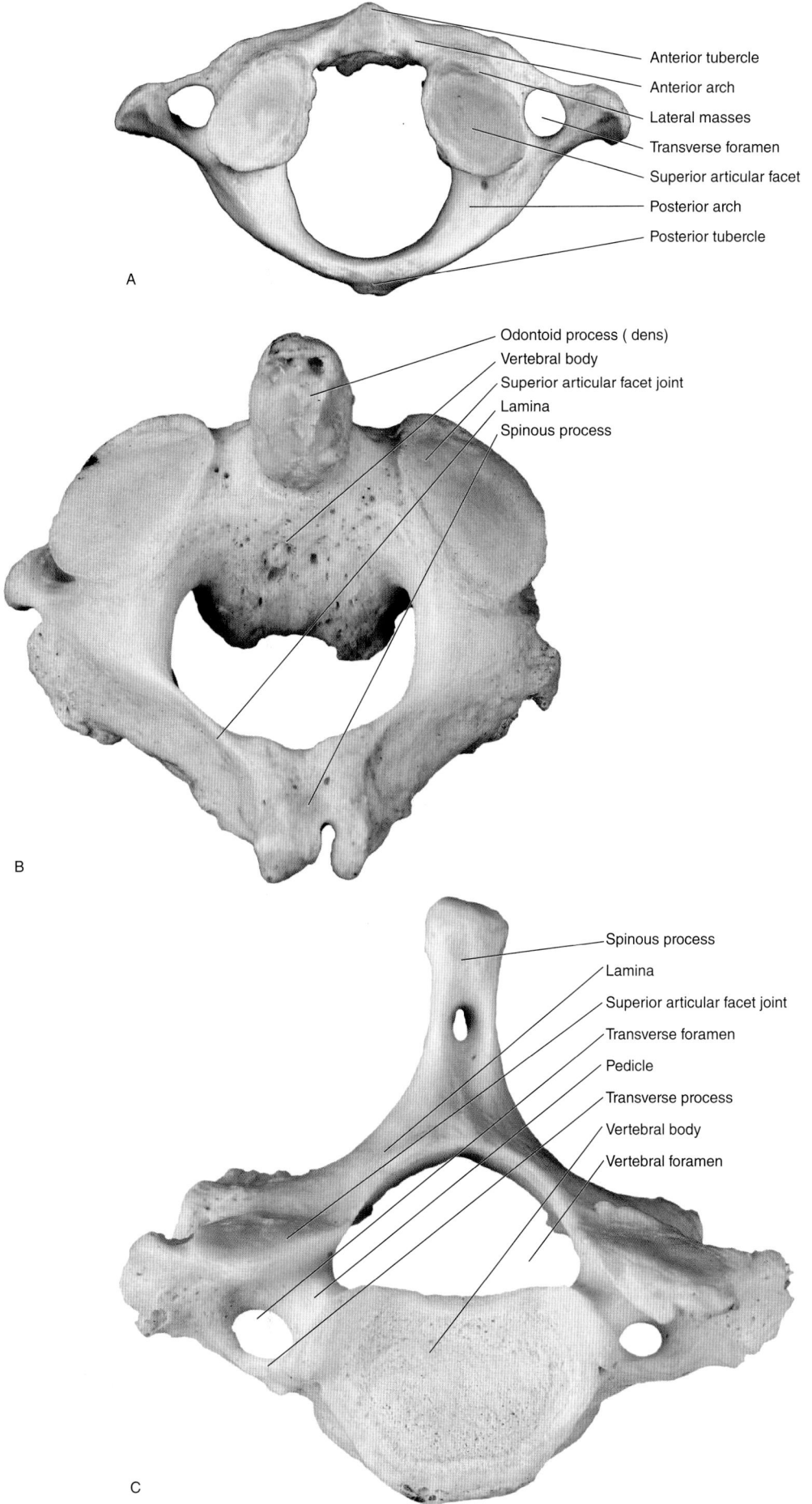

Anterior tubercle
Anterior arch
Lateral masses
Transverse foramen
Superior articular facet
Posterior arch
Posterior tubercle

A

Odontoid process (dens)
Vertebral body
Superior articular facet joint
Lamina
Spinous process

B

Spinous process
Lamina
Superior articular facet joint
Transverse foramen
Pedicle
Transverse process
Vertebral body
Vertebral foramen

C

FIGURE 22–3. The atypical vertebrae. **A:** Superior view of the C1 vertebra (atlas). **B:** Superior view of the C2 vertebra (axis) with a bifid spinous process. **C:** Superior view of the C7 vertebra; the spinous process is nonbifid.

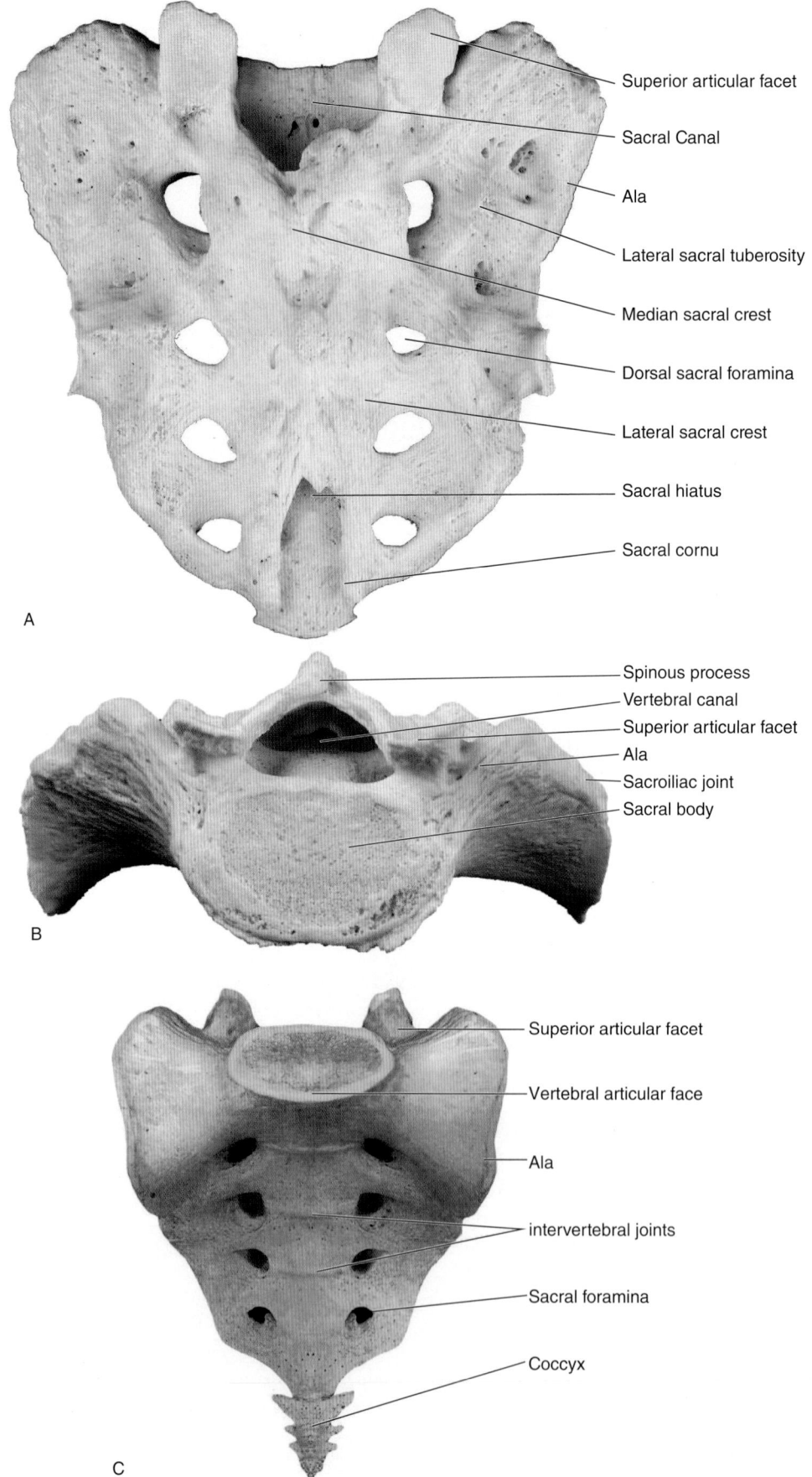

FIGURE 22–4. The sacrum and coccyx. **A:** Posterior view of the sacrum; the sacrum curves anteriorly proximal to its narrowing tip where it articulates with the coccyx. **B:** The base of the sacrum is directed upward and forward. **C:** Anterior view of the coccyx.

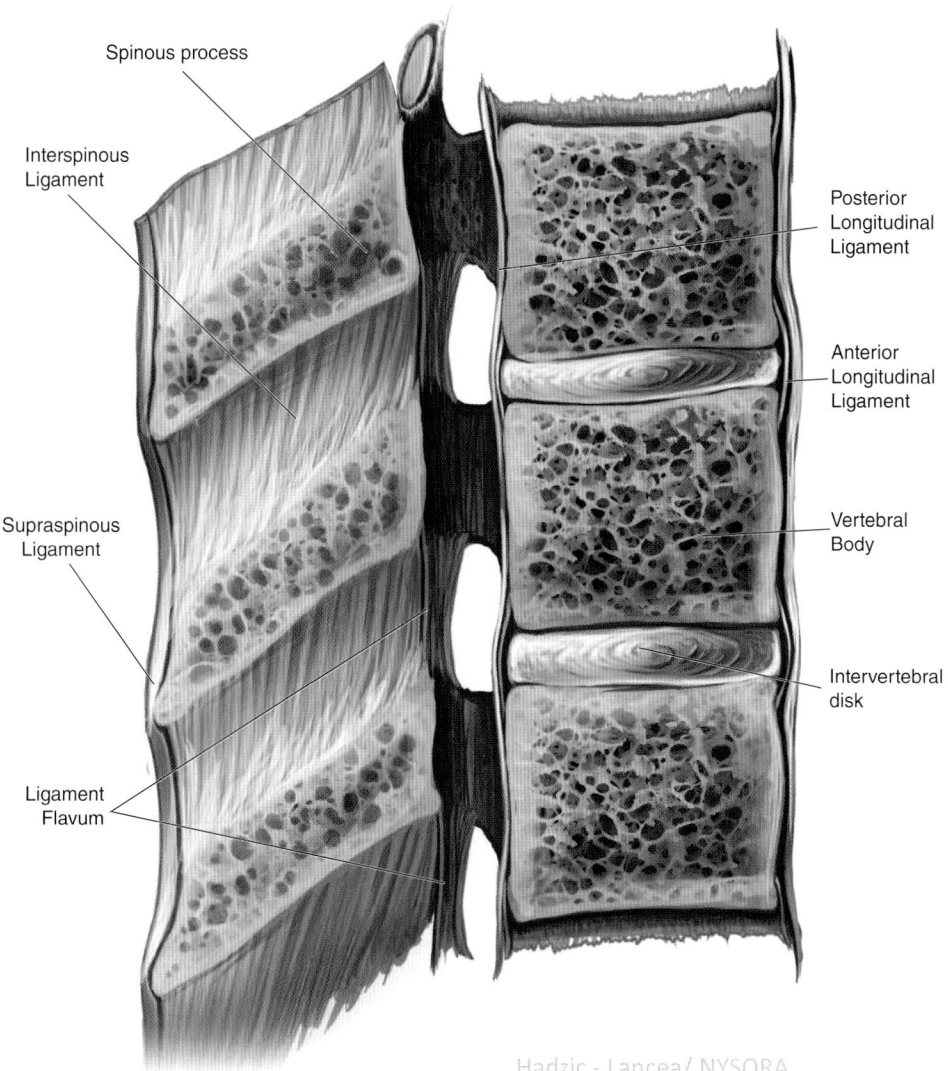

FIGURE 22–5. A cross-sectional view of the vertebral canal with the intervertebral ligaments, vertebral body, and spinous process.

joint capsule. When a needle is advanced toward the epidural space, there is an easily perceptible *increase in resistance* when the ligamentum flavum is encountered. More importantly for the practice of neuraxial anesthesia, a perceptible, sudden *loss of resistance* is encountered when the tip of the needle passes through the ligamentum and enters the epidural space.

The ligamentum flavum consists of right and left halves that join at an angle of less than 90°. Importantly, this midline fusion may be absent to a variable degree depending on the vertebral level.[2] These fusion gaps allow for veins to connect to vertebral venous plexuses.[7] Of note, the fusion gaps are more prevalent at cervical and thoracic levels. Yoon et al reported that midline gaps between C3 and T2 occur in 87%–100% of individuals. The incidence of the midline gap decreases at lower vertebral levels, with T4–T5 the lowest (8%).[7] In theory, a midline gap poses a risk of failure to recognize a loss of resistance at the cervical and high thoracic levels when using the midline approach, resulting in an inadvertent dural puncture.

The ligamentum flavum is thinnest in the cervical and upper thoracic regions and thickest in the lower thoracic and lumbar regions.[8,9] As a result, resistance to needle advancement is easier to appreciate when a needle is introduced at a lower level (eg, lumbar).[7,8] At the L2–L3 interspace, the ligamentum flavum is 3- to 5-mm thick. At this level, the distance from the ligamentum to the spinal meninges is 4–6 mm.[6] Consequently, a midline insertion of an epidural needle at this level is least likely to result in an inadvertent meningeal puncture with epidural anesthesia-analgesia.

The lateral wall of the vertebral canal has gaps between consecutive pedicles known as **intervertebral foramina** (Figure 22–1A). Because the pedicles attach more cephalad of the middle of the vertebral body, the intervertebral foramina are centered opposite the lower half of the vertebral body, with the vertebral disk at the caudal end of the foramen. As a consequence, the borders of the intervertebral foramina are the pedicle at the cephalad and caudal ends, the vertebral body (cephalad) and the disk (caudally) on the anterior aspect, a portion of the next vertebral body most inferiorly, and posteriorly the lamina, facet joint, and ligamentum flavum.

Spinal Meninges

The spinal cord is an extension of the medulla oblongata. It has three covering membranes: the dura, arachnoid, and pia maters (Figure 22–6A). These membranes concentrically divide the vertebral canal into three distinct compartments: the epidural, subdural, and subarachnoid spaces. The epidural space contains fat, epidural veins, spinal nerve roots, and connective tissue (Figure 22–6B) The subdural space is a "potential" space between the dura and the arachnoid and contains a serous fluid. The subdural compartment is formed by flat neuroepithelial cells that have long interlacing branches. These cells are in close contact with the inner dural layers. This space can be expanded

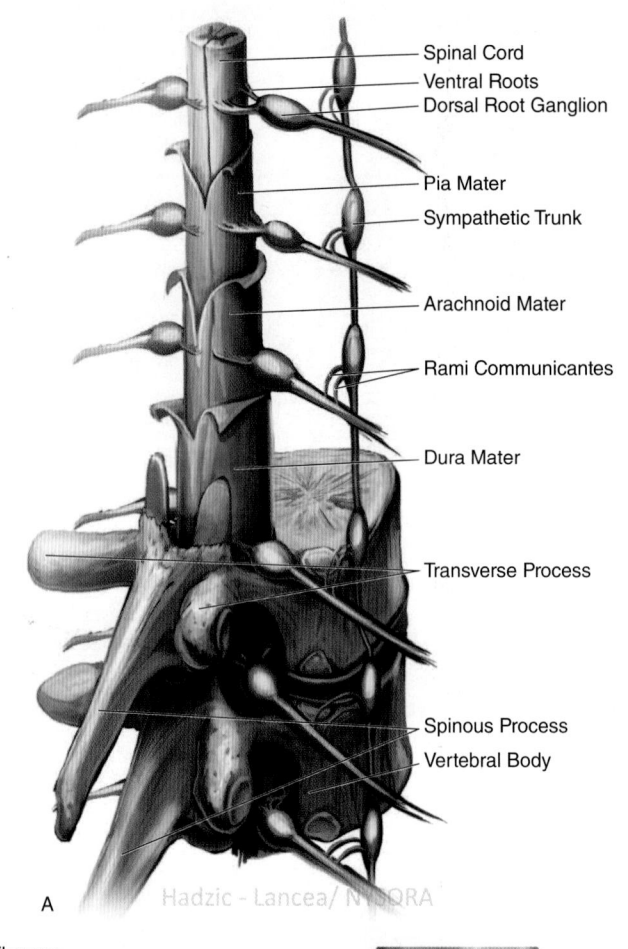

Spinal Cord
Ventral Roots
Dorsal Root Ganglion

Pia Mater

Sympathetic Trunk

Arachnoid Mater

Rami Communicantes

Dura Mater

Transverse Process

Spinous Process
Vertebral Body

A

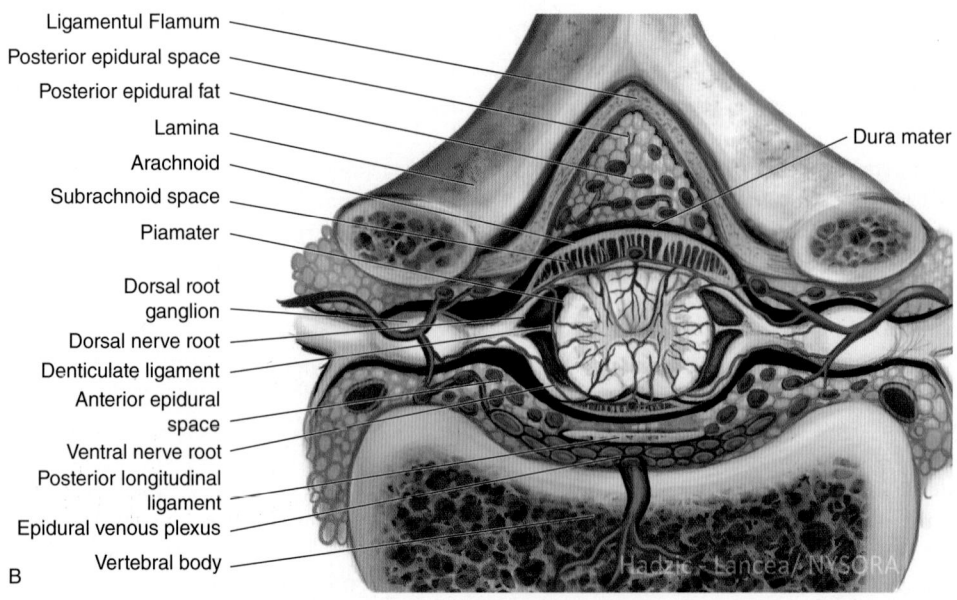

Ligamentul Flamum
Posterior epidural space
Posterior epidural fat
Lamina
Arachnoid
Subrachnoid space
Piamater

Dorsal root ganglion
Dorsal nerve root
Denticulate ligament
Anterior epidural space
Ventral nerve root
Posterior longitudinal ligament
Epidural venous plexus
Vertebral body

Dura mater

B

FIGURE 22–6. A. Sagittal view of the spinal cord with meningeal layers, dorsal root ganglia, spinal nerves, and sympathetic trunk. **B.** Cross-sectional view of the spinal cord depicting the ligamentum flavum in respect to the posterior epidural space. Notice the close proximity of the posterior epidural space to the subarachnoid space.

by shearing the neuroepithelial cell layer connections with the collagen fibers of the dura mater. This expansion of the subdural space can be caused mechanically by injecting air or a liquid such as contrast media or local anesthetics, which, by applying pressure in the space, separates the cell layers.[10] The subarachnoid space is traversed by threads of connective tissue extending from the arachnoid mater to the pia mater. It contains the spinal cord, dorsal and ventral nerve roots, and cerebrospinal fluid (CSF). The subarachnoid space ends at the S2 vertebral level.

Spinal Cord

There are eight cervical neural segments. The eighth segmental nerve emerges between the seventh cervical and first thoracic vertebrae, whereas the remaining cervical nerves emerge above their same-numbered vertebrae. Thoracic, lumbar, and sacral nerves emerge from the vertebral column below the same-numbered bony segment[1] (Figure 22–6A). Anterior and posterior spinal nerve roots arise from rootlets along the spinal cord. The roots of the upper and lower extremity plexuses (brachial and lumbosacral) are significantly larger compared to other levels.[11]

The dural sac is continuous from the foramen magnum to the sacral region, where it spreads distally to cover the filum terminale.

In children, the dural sac terminates lower, and in some adults, the sac termination can be as high as L5. The vertebral canal contains the dural sac, which adheres superiorly to the foramen magnum, to the posterior longitudinal ligament anteriorly, the ligamentum flavum and laminae posteriorly, and the pedicles laterally.

The spinal cord tapers and ends as the **conus medullaris** at the level of the L1–L2 intervertebral disk (Figure 22–7A). The **filum terminale**, a fibrous extension of the spinal cord, extends caudally to the coccyx. The **cauda equina** is a bundle of nerve roots in the subarachnoid space distal to the conus medullaris[12] (Figure 22–7A).

The spinal cord receives blood primarily from one **anterior** and two **posterior spinal arteries** that derive from the **vertebral arteries** (Figure 22–7B). Other major arteries that supplement blood supply to the spinal cord include the **vertebral, ascending cervical, posterior intercostal, lumbar**, and **lateral sacral arteries**. The single anterior spinal artery and two posterior spinal arteries run longitudinally along the length of the cord and combine with segmental arteries in each region. The **major segmental artery (Adamkiewicz)** is the largest segmental artery and is found between the T8 and L1 vertebral segments. The Adamkiewicz artery is the major blood supplier to two-thirds of the spinal cord. Injury of this artery may result

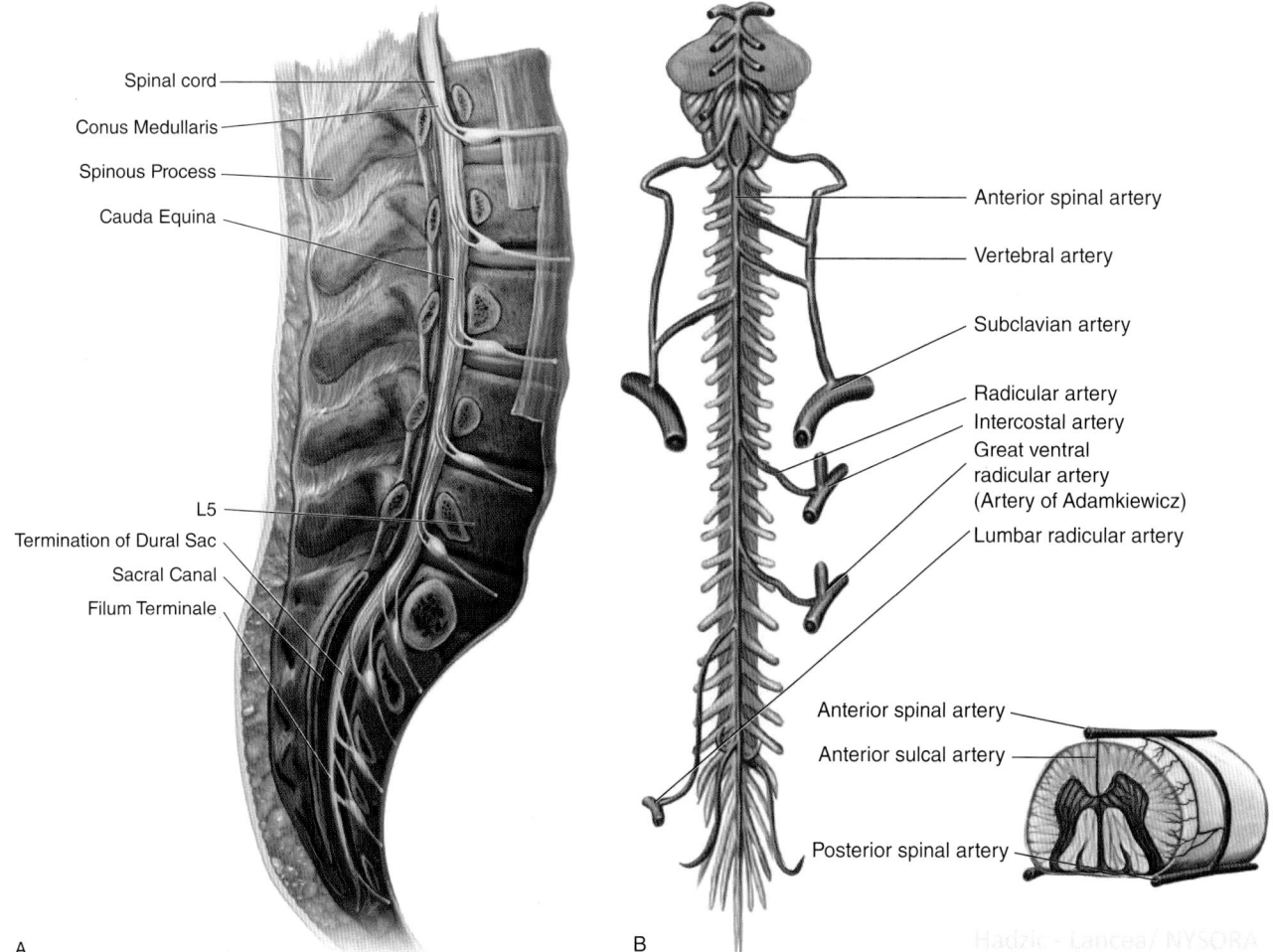

FIGURE 22–7. A. Sagittal view of the lumbar vertebrae. The spinal cord terminates at the L1-L2 interspace. **B.** Arterial supply to the anterior spinal cord. The Artery of Adamkiewicz emerges from T8-L1 vertebral segments. The small insert demonstrates the blood supply to the spinal cord (one anterior and two posterior arteries).

in *anterior spinal artery syndrome,* characterized by loss of urinary and fecal continence as well as impaired motor function of the legs.[1] The **radicular arteries** are branches of the spinal arteries and run within the vertebral canal and supply the vertebral column. **Radicular veins** drain blood from the vertebral venous plexus and eventually drain into the major venous system: the **superior** and **inferior vena cava** and the **azygos venous system of the thorax**.[1]

MOVEMENTS OF THE SPINE

The fundamental movements through the vertebral column are flexion, extension, rotation, and lateral flexion in the cervical and lumbar spine. Movement between individual vertebrae is relatively limited, although the effect is compounded along the entire spine. Thoracic vertebrae, in particular, have limited mobility due to the rib cage. Flexion is greatest in the cervical spine, whereas extension is greatest in the lumbar region. The thoracic and sacral regions are the most stable.

SPECIAL CONSIDERATIONS

In the United States and most developed countries, there is an increase in aging population. This trend carries with it an increased prevalence of spinal deformities, such as spinal stenosis, scoliosis, hyperkyphosis, and hyperlordosis. Elderly patients present anesthetic challenges when neuraxial techniques are required. With advancing age, a diminishing thickness of intervertebral disks results in decreased height of the vertebral column. Thickened ligaments and osteophytes also contribute to difficulty in accessing both the subarachnoid and epidural spaces. The frequency of spinal deformities in older adults can be as high as 70%.[13]

Adult scoliosis, in particular, is frequently encountered in older adults. In fact, Schwab et al demonstrated that scoliosis was present in 68% of an asymptomatic volunteer population older than 60 years of age. A thorough understanding of the scoliotic spine will aid in successfully performing central neuraxial blockade in this patient population. In the scoliotic spine, vertebral bodies are rotated toward the convexity of the curve, and their spinous processes face *into* the concavity of the curve[14] (Figure 22–8).

The diagnosis of scoliosis is made when there is a Cobb angle of greater than 10° in the coronal plane of the spine in a skeletally mature patient.[15] The Cobb angle, which is used to measure the magnitude of scoliosis, is formed between a line drawn parallel to the superior endplate of one vertebra above the curve deformity and a line drawn parallel to the inferior endplate of the vertebra one level below the curve deformity[16] (Figure 22–8). In untreated patients, there is a strong linear relationship between the Cobb angle and the degree of vertebral rotation in both thoracic and lumbar curves, with maximum rotation occurring at the apex of the scoliotic curve.[17,18] A compensatory curvature of the spine always occurs in the opposite direction of the scoliotic curve.

Scoliosis usually presents in childhood or adolescence and is diagnosed during routine physical examination. Untreated, it may become progressive and result in respiratory impairment and gait disturbances. Scoliosis may also go undiagnosed and present later in life as back pain.[15,19]

Treatment depends on the severity of the scoliosis. Mild scoliosis (11°–25°) is usually observed. Moderate scoliosis (25°–50°) in the skeletally immature patient frequently progresses and therefore is most often braced. Patients with severe scoliosis (>50°) are usually treated surgically.[20]

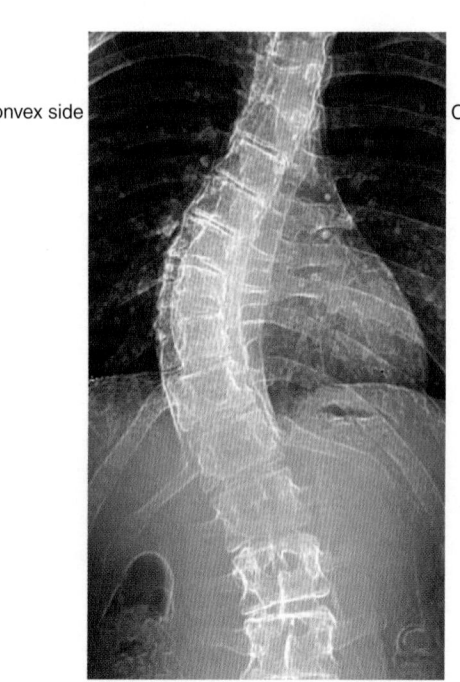
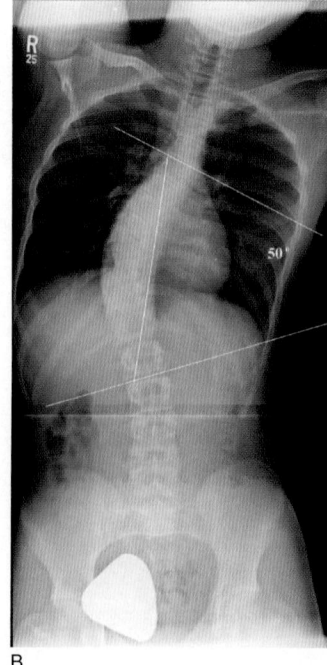

FIGURE 22–8. Adolescent scoliotic spine. **A:** S-shaped scoliosis of the thoracolumbar spine. **B:** Cobb angle of 50°.

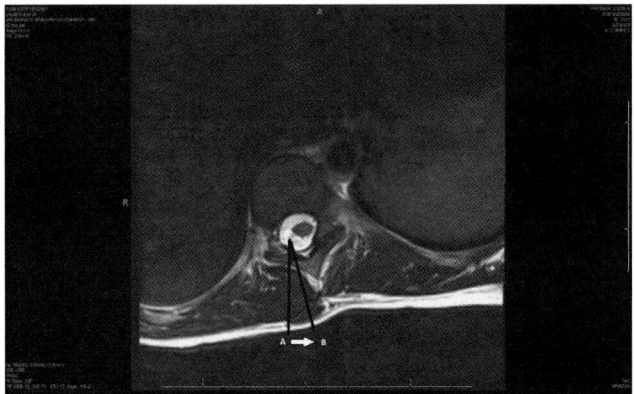

FIGURE 22–9. Paramedian approach in a scoliotic spine; arrow B represents the needle realignment towards the convex side of the scoliotic spine compared to arrow A, which depicts the usual paramedian approach in a normal spine.

The degree of vertebral body rotation along the long axis of the spine influences the orientation of a needle during insertion for neuraxial anesthesia. In the patients with scoliosis, the vertebral body rotates toward the convex side of the curve. As a result of this rotation, the spinous processes point toward the midline (the concave side). This results in a larger interlaminar space on the convex side of the spine.[21,22] A direct path to the neuraxial space is created by this vertebral body rotation, allowing the use of a paramedian approach from the convex side of the curve (Figure 22–9). Surface landmarks, particularly the spinous process, may be difficult to identify in the severe scoliotic spine. X-rays, and most recently preprocedural ultrasound scanning, may be useful to determine the longitudinal angulation of the spine, the location and orientation of the spinous process, as well as the depth of the lamina.[23–25]

Clinical Pearls

- The spinal cord ends at the L1-to-L2 level; performing spinal anesthesia at or above this level is not recommended.
- Failure of the ligamentum flavum to fuse in the cervical and upper thoracic levels may reduce the sense of *loss of resistance* with a midline approach to epidural anesthesia. A paramedian approach may be more suitable at these levels because the needle is advanced to a point where the presence of a ligamentum flavum is most reliable, enabling successful access to the epidural space.
- In patients with scoliosis, a paramedian approach from the convex side may be more successful.

REFERENCES

1. Standring S (ed): *Gray's Anatomy: The Anatomical Basis of Clinical Practice*, 40th ed. Churchill Livingston, Elsevier Health, 2008.
2. Hogan QH: Lumbar epidural anatomy. A new look by cryomicrotome section. Anesthesiology 1991;75:767-775.
3. Scapinelli R: Morphological and functional changes of the lumbar spinous processes in the elderly. Surg Radiol Anat 1989;11:129.
4. Aggarwal A, Kaur H, Batra YK, et al: Anatomic consideration of caudal epidural space: A cadaver study. Clin Anat 2009;22:730.
5. Hogan QH: Epidural anatomy: New observations. Can J Anaesth 1998; 45:40.
6. Zarzur E: Anatomic studies of the human lumbar ligamentum flavum. Anesth Analg 1984;63:499.
7. Yoon SP, Kim HJ, Choi YS: Anatomic variations of cervical and high thoracic ligamentum flavum. Korean J Pain 2014;27:321.
8. Lirk P, Colvin J, Steger B, et al: Incidence of lower thoracic ligamentum flavum midline gaps. Br J Anaesth 2005;94:852.
9. Lirk P, Kolbitsch C, Putz G, et al. Cervical and high thoracic ligamentum flavum frequently fails to fuse in the midline. Anesthesiology 2003; 99:1387.
10. Reina MA, Lopez Garcia A, de Andres JA, Villanueva MC, Cortes L: Does the subdural space exist? Rev Esp Anestesiol Reanim 1998;45:367.
11. Kostelic JK, Haughton VM, Sether LA: Lumbar spinal nerves in the neural foramen: MR appearance. Radiology 1991;178:837.
12. MacDonald A, Chatrath P, Spector T, et al: Level of termination of the spinal cord and the dural sac: A magnetic resonance study. Clin Anat 1999;12:149.
13. Schwab F, Dubey A, Gamez L, et al: Adult scoliosis: prevalence, SF-36, and nutritional parameters in an elderly volunteer population. Spine 2005;30:1082.
14. McLeod A, Roche A, Fennelly M: Case series: Ultrasonography may assist epidural insertion in scoliosis patients. Can J Anaesth 2005;52:717.
15. Aebi M: The adult scoliosis. Eur Spine J 2005;14:925.
16. Smith JS, Shaffrey CI, Fu KM, et al: Clinical and radiographic evaluation of the adult spinal deformity patient. Neurosurg Clin N Am 2013;24:143.
17. White AA, Panjab MM: *Clinical Biomechanics of the Spine*, 2nd ed. Lippincott, 1990.
18. Suzuki S, Yamamuro T, Shikata J, et al: Ultrasound measurement of vertebral rotation in idiopathic scoliosis. J Bone Joint Surg Br 1989;71:252.
19. Glassman SD, Berven S, Bridwell K, et al: Correlation of radiographic parameters and clinical symptoms in adult scoliosis. Spine 2005;30:682.
20. Bowens C, Dobie KH, Devin CJ, et al: An approach to neuraxial anaesthesia for the severely scoliotic spine. Br J Anaesth 2013;111:807.
21. Huang J: Paramedian approach for neuraxial anesthesia in parturients with scoliosis. Anesth Anal 2010;111:821.
22. Ko JY, Leffert LR: Clinical implications of neuraxial anesthesia in the parturient with scoliosis. Anesth Analg 2009;09:1930.
23. Chin KJ, Perlas A, Chan V, et al: Ultrasound Imaging facilitates spinal anesthesia in adults with difficult surface anatomic landmarks. Anesthesiology 2001;115:94.
24. Chin KJ, Karmakar MK, Peng P: Ultrasonography of the adult thoracic and lumbar spine for cetral neuraxial blockade. Anesthesiology 2011; 114:1459.
25. Chin KJ, MacFarlane AJR, Chan V, Brull R: The use of ultrasound to facilitate spinal anesthesia in a patient with previous lumbar laminectomy and fusion: A case report. J Clin Ultrasound 2009;37:482.

CHAPTER 23

Spinal Anesthesia

Adrian Chin and André van Zundert

THE HISTORY OF SPINAL ANESTHESIA

Carl Koller, an ophthalmologist from Vienna, in 1884 first described the use of topical cocaine for analgesia of the eye.[1] William Halsted and Richard Hall, surgeons at Roosevelt Hospital in New York City, took the idea of local anesthesia a step further by injecting cocaine into human tissues and nerves to produce anesthesia for surgery.[2] James Leonard Corning, a neurologist in New York City, in 1885 described the use of cocaine for spinal anesthesia.[3] Because Corning was a frequent observer at Roosevelt Hospital, the idea of using cocaine in the subarachnoid space may have come from observing Halsted and Hall performing cocaine injections. Corning first injected cocaine intrathecally into a dog and within a few minutes the dog had marked weakness in the hindquarters.[4] Next, Corning injected cocaine into a man at the T11–T12 interspace into what he thought was the subarachnoid space. Because Corning did not notice any effect after 8 minutes, he repeated the injection. Ten minutes after the second injection, the patient complained of sleepiness in his legs but was able to stand and walk. Because Corning made no mention of cerebrospinal fluid (CSF) efflux, most likely he inadvertently gave an epidural rather than a spinal injection to the patient.

The presence of a neuraxial fluid was first noted by Galen in AD 200, and CSF was later studied in the 1500s by Antonio Valsalva.[5] Dural puncture was described in 1891 by Essex Wynter[6] followed shortly by Heinrich Quincke 6 months later.[7] Augustus Karl Gustav Bier, a German surgeon, used cocaine intrathecally in 1898 on six patients for lower extremity surgery.[8,9] In true scientific fashion, Bier decided to experiment on himself and developed a postdural puncture headache (PDPH) for his efforts. His assistant, Dr. Otto Hildebrandt, volunteered to have the procedure performed after Bier was unable to continue due to the PDPH. After injection of spinal cocaine into Hildebrandt, Bier conducted experiments on the lower half of Hildebrandt's body. Bier described needle pricks and cigar

burns to the legs, incisions on the thighs, avulsion of pubic hairs, strong blows with an iron hammer to the shins, and torsion of the testicles. Hildebrandt reported minimal to no pain during the experiments; however, afterward he suffered nausea, vomiting, PDPH, and bruising and pain in his legs. Bier attributed the PDPH to loss of CSF and felt the use of small-gauge needles would help prevent the headache.[10]

Dudley Tait and Guido Caglieri performed the first spinal anesthetic in the United States in San Francisco in 1899. Their studies included cadavers, animals, and live patients to determine the benefits of lumbar puncture, especially in the treatment of syphilis. Tait and Caglieri injected mercuric salts and iodides into the CSF, but worsened the condition of one patient with tertiary syphilis.[11] Rudolph Matas, a vascular surgeon in New Orleans, described the use of spinal cocaine on patients and possibly was the first to use morphine in the subarachnoid space.[12,13] Matas also described the complication of death after lumbar puncture. Theodore Tuffier, a French surgeon in Paris, studied spinal anesthesia and reported on it in 1900. Tuffier felt that cocaine should not be injected until CSF was recognized.[14] Tuffier taught at the University of Paris at the same time that Tait was a medical student there and most likely was one of Tait's mentors. Tuffier's demonstrations in Paris helped popularize spinal anesthesia in Europe.

Arthur Barker, a professor of surgery at the University of London, reported on the advancement of spinal techniques in 1907, including the use of a hyperbaric spinal local anesthetic, emphasis on sterility, and ease of midline over paramedian dural puncture.[15] Advancement of sterility and the investigation of decreases in blood pressure after injection helped make spinal anesthesia safer and more popular. Gaston Labat was a strong proponent of spinal anesthesia in the United States and performed early studies on the effects of Trendelenburg position on blood pressure after spinal anesthesia.[16] George Pitkin attempted to use a hypobaric local anesthetic to control the level of spinal block by mixing procaine with alcohol.[17] Lincoln

Sise, an anesthesiologist at the Lahey Clinic in Boston, used Barker's technique of hyperbaric spinal anesthesia with both procaine and tetracaine.[18–20]

Spinal anesthesia became more popular as new developments occurred, including the introduction in 1946 of saddle block anesthesia by Adriani and Roman-Vega.[21] However, in 1947 the well-publicized case of Woolley and Roe (United Kingdom) resulted in two patients becoming paraplegic in one day.[22] Across the Atlantic, reports of paraplegia in the United States similarly caused anesthesiologists to discontinue the use of spinal anesthesia.[23] The development of novel intravenous anesthetic agents and neuromuscular blockers coincided with the decreased use of spinal anesthesia. In 1954, Dripps and Vandam described the safety of spinal anesthetics in more than 10,000 patients,[24] and spinal anesthesia was revived.

In the field of obstetrics, over 500,000 spinals had been performed on American women by the mid-1950s.[25] Despite spinal anesthesia being the most frequently used technique for vaginal delivery and cesarean section in the 1950s, subsequent improvements in epidural technology resulted in a decline in obstetric spinal anesthesia in the late 1960s. The Third National Audit Project (NAP3) estimated 133,525 obstetric spinals were performed in 2006 in the United Kingdom.[26]

The early development of spinal needles paralleled the early development of spinal anesthesia. Corning chose a gold needle that had a short bevel point, flexible cannula, and set screw that fixed the needle to the depth of dural penetration. Corning also used an introducer for the needle, which was right angled. Quincke used a beveled needle that was sharp and hollow. Bier developed his own sharp needle that did not require an introducer. The needle was larger bore (15 or 17 gauge) with a long, cutting bevel. The main problems with Bier's needle were pain on insertion and the loss of local anesthetic due to the large hole in the dura after dural puncture. Barker's needle did not have an inner cannula, was made of nickel, and had a sharp, medium-length bevel with a matching stylet. Labat developed an unbreakable nickel needle that had a sharp, short-length bevel with a matching stylet. Labat believed that the short bevel minimized damage to the tissues when inserted into the back.

Herbert Greene realized that loss of CSF was a major problem in spinal anesthesia and developed a smooth-tip, smaller-gauge needle that resulted in a lower incidence of PDPH.[27] Barnett Greene described the use of a 26-gauge spinal needle in obstetrics with a decreased incidence of PDPH.[28] The Greene needle was popular until the introduction of the Whitacre needle. Hart and Whitacre[29] used a pencil-point needle to decrease PDPH from 5%–10% to 2%. Sprotte modified the Whitacre needle and in 1987 published his trial of over 34,000 spinal anesthetics.[30] Modifications of the Sprotte needle occurred the 1990s to produce the needle that is in use today.[31]

Spinal anesthesia has progressed greatly since 1885. Every aspect, from improved equipment and pharmacological agents, to greater understanding of physiology and anatomy, have made spinal anesthesia increasingly safer. Changing clinical knowledge has seen shifts in what is considered a contraindication to spinal anesthesia, and the evolution of novel techniques,

such as the use of ultrasound, have allowed spinal anesthesia in what would once have been thought impossible situations. Nonetheless, no technique is risk free, and every effort must be made to prevent complications. Learning how to perform spinal anesthesia is an invaluable skill that all anesthesiologists should have in their armamentarium.

THE RISKS AND BENEFITS OF SPINAL ANESTHESIA

Before offering a patient spinal anesthesia, an anesthesiologist not only must be aware of the indications and contraindications of spinal anesthesia but also must be able to weigh the risks and benefits of performing the procedure. This requires a thorough understanding of the available evidence, in particular how the risk-benefit ratio compares to that of any alternative, and an ability to apply the evidence to a given clinical scenario. Thus, an informed anesthesiologist can facilitate the patient in making an informed decision.

Contraindications and Risks of Spinal Anesthesia

Contraindications to Spinal Anesthesia

There are absolute and relative contraindications to spinal anesthesia (see Table 23–1). Absolute contraindications include patient refusal; infection at the site of injection; severe, uncorrected hypovolemia; true allergy to any of the drugs; and increased intracranial pressure, except in cases of pseudo–tumor cerebri (idiopathic intracranial hypertension). High intracranial pressure increases the risk of uncal herniation when CSF is lost through the needle. Spinal anesthesia is also contraindicated when the operation is expected to take longer than the duration of the block or result in blood loss such that the development of severe hypovolemia is likely.

Coagulopathy, previously considered an absolute contraindication, may be considered depending on the level of derangement. Another relative contraindication of spinal anesthesia is sepsis distinct from the anatomic site of puncture (eg, chorioamnionitis or lower extremity infection). If the patient is on antibiotics and the vital signs are stable, spinal anesthesia may be considered. Spinal anesthesia is relatively contraindicated in cardiac diseases with fixed cardiac output (CO) states. Aortic stenosis, once considered to be an absolute contraindication for

TABLE 23–1. Contraindications to spinal anesthesia.

Absolute Contraindications	Relative Contraindications
• Patient refusal	• Coagulopathy
• Infection at the site of injection	• Sepsis
• Uncorrected hypovolemia	• Fixed cardiac output states
• Allergy	• Indeterminate neurological disease
• Increased intracranial pressure	

spinal anesthesia, does not always preclude a carefully conducted spinal anesthetic.[32–34]

Indeterminate neurological disease is a relative contraindication. Multiple sclerosis and other demyelinating diseases are challenging. In vitro experiments suggest that demyelinated nerves are more susceptible to local anesthetic toxicity. However, no clinical study has convincingly demonstrated that spinal anesthesia worsens such neurologic diseases. Indeed, with the knowledge that pain, stress, fever, and fatigue exacerbate these diseases, a stress-free central neuraxial block (CNB) may be preferred for surgery.[35–39]

Spinal anesthesia in the immunocompromised patient also presents a challenge for the anesthesiologist and is the subject of a consensus statement.[40] Although this consensus statement does not provide prescriptive advice for every situation, it does summarize the available evidence. Previous spinal surgery was once thought to be a contraindication. Dural puncture may be difficult, and spread of local anesthetic may be restricted by scar tissue. However, there are case reports of successful spinal anesthesia in this setting, particularly with the assistance of ultrasound.[41–43] There are theoretical risks in inserting a hollow-body needle through tattoo ink.[44] However, there are no reported complications from inserting a spinal or epidural needle through a tattoo.[45] Stylets may decrease the likelihood of transmitting a core of tissue to the subarachnoid space, and if concerned, a small skin incision may be made prior to needle insertion. Introducers serve to prevent contamination of the CSF with small pieces of epidermis, which could lead to the formation of dermoid spinal cord tumors.

Risks of Spinal Anesthesia: Complications

Complications of spinal blockade are often divided into major and minor complications. Reassuringly, most major complications are rare. Minor complications, however, are common and therefore should not be dismissed. Minor complications include nausea, vomiting, mild hypotension, shivering, itch, hearing impairment, and urinary retention. PDPH and failed spinal blockade are significant, and not uncommon, complications of spinal anesthesia. We therefore consider them as moderate complications (see Table 23–2). Failure of spinal anesthesia has been mentioned as between 1% and 17% and is discussed further in this chapter.

Minor Complications of Spinal Anesthesia

Nausea and Vomiting Nausea and vomiting presenting after spinal anesthesia are distressing for the patient and may impede the surgeon. Incidence of intraoperative nausea and vomiting (IONV) in nonobstetric surgery can be up to 42% and may be as high as 80% in parturients.[46]

Causes are complex and multifactorial. Causes unrelated to the spinal may include patient factors (eg, anxiety, reduced lower esophageal sphincter tone, increased gastric pressure, vagal hyperactivity, hormonal changes); surgical factors (exteriorization of the uterus, peritoneal traction); and other factors (eg, systemic opioids, uterotonic drugs, antibiotics, movement).[46,47] Spinal anesthesia itself may cause IONV or postoperative nausea and vomiting (PONV) via a variety of mechanisms, including hypotension, intrathecal additives, inadequate block, or high block. Risks factors for IONV under spinal include peak block height greater than T6, baseline heart rate (HR) 60 beats/minute or more, a history of motion sickness, and previous hypotension after spinal block.[48]

Hypotension must be the *first* consideration when a patient complains of nausea, especially immediately after onset of spinal anesthesia. This has been long known. Evans, in his 1929 textbook on spinal anesthesia, noted that "the sudden fall in blood pressure is followed by nausea."[49] Mechanisms and management of hypotension are covered in greater detail elsewhere (see section on cardiovascular effects of spinal anesthesia).

A variety of intrathecal additives have been shown to increase IONV or PONV. Intrathecal morphine, diamorphine, clonidine, and neostigmine all increase nausea and vomiting. Intrathecal fentanyl, however, reduces IONV, perhaps by improving block quality, decreasing supplemental opioids, or decreasing hypotension.[46]

While low spinal block can cause nausea from surgical stimulation, high sympathetic spinal block (with relative parasympathetic overactivity) can also result in nausea. Glycopyrrolate was shown to be better than placebo in reducing nausea during cesarean section, although the rate of nausea was still high (42%).[50] However, prophylactic glycopyrrolate can increase hypotension after spinal anesthesia.[46]

A recent meta-analysis suggested metoclopramide (10 mg) was effective and safe for prevention of IONV and PONV in the setting of cesarean delivery under neuraxial block.[47]

TABLE 23–2. Complications of spinal anesthesia.

Minor	Moderate	Major
• Nausea and vomiting	• Failed spinal	• Direct needle trauma
• Mild hypotension	• Postdural puncture headache	• Infection (abscess, meningitis)
• Shivering		• Vertebral canal hematoma
• Itch		• Spinal cord ischemia
• Transient mild hearing impairment		• Cauda equina syndrome
• Urinary retention		• Arachnoiditis
		• Peripheral nerve injury
		• Total spinal anesthesia
		• Cardiovascular collapse
		• Death

Another meta-analysis showed the serotonin 5-HT$_3$ receptor antagonists reduced the incidence of nausea and vomiting and the need for postoperative rescue antiemetic when intrathecal morphine was used for cesarean section.[51]

Despite some studies showing a benefit of P6 (pericardium 6 nei guan point) stimulation, based on Chinese acupuncture, a 2008 systematic review found inconsistent results in preventing IONV and PONV.[52]

Hypotension Mechanisms and management of hypotension are covered elsewhere (see section on cardiovascular effects of spinal anesthesia).

Shivering Crowley et al reviewed shivering and neuraxial anesthesia.[53] Spinal and epidural anesthesia, and indeed general anesthesia, may induce shivering. The incidence of shivering secondary to neuraxial block is difficult to assess given the heterogeneity of studies but is about 55%. In the first 30 minutes after block, spinal anesthesia decreases core body temperature faster than epidural anesthesia. After 30 minutes, both techniques cause temperature to fall at the same rate. Despite this, shivering after spinal anesthesia is no greater than after epidural anesthesia.[54] Indeed, the intensity of shivering seems to be higher with epidurals. Postulated mechanisms for this include an inability to shiver due to more pronounced motor blockade with spinal anesthesia and a decreased shivering threshold with more dermatomes (and thus thermoregulatory afferents) blocked during spinal anesthesia. Several strategies have been suggested to reduce neuraxial shivering (see Table 23–3).

Itch Pruritis is a well-known side effect of opiates and is more common with administration via the spinal route (46%) compared with epidural (8.5%) and systemic routes.[55] The severity of pruritis is proportional to intrathecal morphine dose but not epidural morphine dose.[56] Pruritis associated with neuraxial opioids is often distributed around the nose and face. Although symptoms may not be mediated via opioid receptors, pruritis can be treated with the opioid receptor antagonist naloxone.[55]

TABLE 23–3. Suggested strategies to prevent and treat neuraxial anesthesia shivering.

Prevention	Treatment
• Prewarm with forced air warmer for 15 minutes	• Intravenous meperidine 50 mg
• Avoid cold epidural or intravenous fluids	• Intravenous tramadol 0.25 mg/kg or 0.5 mg/kg or 1 mg/kg
• Intrathecal fentanyl 20 μg	• Intravenous clonidine 30, 60, 90, or 150 μg
• Intrathecal meperidine 0.2 mg/kg or 10 mg	
• Intravenous ondansetron 8 mg	
• Epidural fentanyl	
• Epidural meperidine	

Source: Adapted with permission from Crowley LJ, Buggy DJ: Shivering and neuraxial anesthesia. *Reg Anesth Pain Med.* 2008;May/June;33(3):241–252.

There are reports of ondansetron being used for opioid-induced pruritis, suggesting a role of serotonin receptors in morphine-induced pruritis.[57] A 2009 meta-analysis of obstetric patients who had received intrathecal morphine showed that 5-HT$_3$ receptor antagonists did not reduce the incidence of pruritis but did reduce the severity of itching and the need to treat pruritis. The 5-HT$_3$ receptor antagonists were useful in treating established pruritis (number needed to treat [NNT] = 3).[51]

Hearing Impairment Hearing loss, particularly in the low-frequency range, has been reported after spinal anesthesia. Quoted incidences vary widely (3%–92%).[58] Otoacoustic emissions, an objective measurement of hearing that reflects outer hair cell function, demonstrated hearing loss to be more common than suspected, but transient, with full recovery occurring in 15 days.[59] Other authors have similarly concluded that hearing loss commonly disappears spontaneously.[58] A comparison of hearing loss after general and spinal anesthesia concluded that hearing loss occurs irrespective of technique.[58] Hearing loss may or may not be associated with PDPH and may improve with an epidural blood patch.[60] Hearing loss after spinal block may be related to needle gauge[61] and may be less common in the obstetric population.[62] Finegold showed that hearing loss did not occur in women having elective cesarean sections when 24-gauge Sprotte needles or 25-gauge Quincke needles were used.[62] It has been suggested that consent for spinal anesthesia should include a discussion for medicolegal reasons of possible hearing loss.[59,63]

Postoperative Urinary Retention Micturition is the product of a complex interplay of physiology. Postoperative urinary retention (POUR), therefore, is often multifactorial in origin. Patient risk factors for POUR include male sex and previous urologic dysfunction. Surgical risk factors include pelvic or prolonged surgery. Anesthetic factors include anticholinergic drugs, opioids, and fluid administration (>1000 mL).[64] POUR can occur with both neuraxial and general anesthesia.

Occurrence of POUR after neuraxial block is due to neural interruption of the micturition reflex as well as bladder overdistention. Neuraxial opioids exert an effect at the spinal cord and the pontine micturition center. The parasympathetic blockade induced by spinal anesthesia must end before voiding occurs. This usually corresponds with return of the S2–S4 segments.[64] The type and dose of local anesthetic, as well as the use of neuraxial opioid, influence the return of spontaneous micturition. Time to micturition is quickest with 2-chloroprocaine and slowest with bupivacaine.[65]

A recent systematic review found six studies that compared the effect of neuraxial anesthesia with other techniques.[65] Four studies compared local infiltration with intrathecal anesthesia; three of these found lower incidences of urinary retention with local infiltration. The other two studies found no difference in time to micturition when intrathecal anesthesia was compared with general anesthesia in the first instance and general anesthesia and peripheral nerve block in the second instance.

Postdural Puncture Headache Postdural puncture headache, often classified as a minor[66] (or at least not a major[26]) complication, can be severe and debilitating and has been considered *the* neurological complication of spinal anesthesia.[67] It is a common cause for medicolegal claims. The incidence of PDPH is influenced by patient demographics and is less common in elderly patients.[68] In a high-risk group, such as obstetric patients, the risk after lumbar puncture with a Whitacre 27-gauge needle is about 1.7%.[69] Needle size and type influence PDPH rate. Other risk factors include lesser body mass index (BMI), female gender, history of recurrent headaches, and previous PDPH.[5]

Postdural puncture headache should be thought of as neither a common "minor" complication nor a rare "major" complication, but as a not uncommon "moderate" complication. The reader is referred to Chapter 27 for further detailed information.

Major Complications of Spinal Anesthesia
Major complications of spinal anesthesia include direct needle trauma, infection (meningitis or abscess formation), vertebral canal hematoma, spinal cord ischemia, cauda equina syndrome (CES), arachnoiditis, and peripheral nerve injury. The end result of these complications may be permanent neurologic disability. Other major complications include total spinal anesthesia (TSA), cardiovascular collapse, and death.

Direct Needle Trauma
Neurologic injury can occur after needle introduction into the spinal cord or nerves. Although the elicitation of paresthesias during spinal anesthesia has been implicated as a risk factor for persistent neurologic injury, it is not known whether an intervention after paresthesia can prevent development of neurologic complications.[70] A retrospective analysis found 298 of 4767 (6.3%) patients experienced paresthesia during spinal needle insertion. Of the 298, four patients had persistent paresthesia postoperatively. A further two patients with postoperative paresthesia did not have paresthesia during needle insertion. All six patients had resolution of symptoms by 24 months.[71] When paresthesia occurs, the spinal needle may be adjacent to or penetrating neural tissue; if the latter is the case, injection of local anesthetic into the spinal nerve may result in permanent neurologic damage. Analogous controversies exist with peripheral nerve blockade; the implications of paresthesia techniques and extraneural and intraneural injection are the subject of much debate.[72]

Meningitis
Meningitis, either bacterial or aseptic, can occur after spinal anesthesia is performed.[73] Sources of infection include contaminated spinal trays and medication, oral flora of the anesthesiologist, and patient infection. Most cases of meningitis after spinal anesthesia in the first half of the 20th century were aseptic and could be traced to chemical contamination and detergents.[74,75] Marinac showed that causes of drug- and chemical-induced meningitis include nonsteroidal anti-inflammatory drugs, certain antibiotics, radiographic agents, and muromonab-CD3. There also appears to be an association between the occurrence of the hypersensitivity-type reactions and underlying collagen, vascular, or rheumatologic disease.[76] Carp and Bailey performed lumbar puncture in bacteremic rats, and only those with a circulating

Escherichia coli count greater than 50 CFU/mL at the time of lumbar puncture developed meningitis.[77] Although meningitis after lumbar puncture has also been described in bacteremic children,[78] the incidence of meningitis after diagnostic lumbar puncture is not significantly different in bacteremic patients compared with spontaneous incidence of meningitis.[79] Oral flora can contaminate the CSF when a spinal anesthetic is being performed, underlying the importance of wearing a mask. *Streptococcus salivarius*, *Streptococcus viridans*, *Staphylococcus aureus*, *Pseudomonas aeruginosa*, *Acinetobacter*, and *Mycobacterium tuberculosis* have all been isolated in cases of bacterial meningitis after spinal anesthesia or lumbar puncture.[80–83]

Vertebral Canal Hematoma
Vertebral canal hematoma formation is a rare but devastating complication after spinal anesthesia. Although most spinal hematomata occur in the epidural space due to the prominent epidural venous plexus, a few reports have mentioned subarachnoid bleeding as the cause of neurologic deficits. The source of the bleeding can be from either an injured artery or an injured vein. Spinal hematoma and spinal cord ischemia have a poorer prognosis than infective complications.[26] If new or progressive neurologic symptoms develop, an immediate neurosurgery consultation should be obtained, and magnetic resonance imaging (MRI) of the spine should be performed as soon as possible.

Spinal Cord Ischemia
The superficial arterial system of the spinal cord consists of three longitudinal arteries (the anterior spinal artery and two posterior spinal arteries) and a pial plexus.[84] The posterior cord is relatively protected from ischemia by abundant anastomoses. The central area of the anterior spinal cord is reliant on the anterior spinal artery and therefore more prone to ischemia. Proposed mechanisms for spinal cord ischemia secondary to spinal blockade include prolonged hypotension, the addition of vasoconstrictors to local anesthetics, and compression of arterial supply by vertebral canal hematoma.[70]

Cauda Equina Syndrome
Cauda equina syndrome (CES) has been reported with the use of continuous spinal microcatheters.[85–88] The use of hyperbaric 5% lidocaine for spinal anesthesia is associated with an increased incidence of CES,[89–91] although other local anesthetics have been implicated.[92–95] Other risk factors for CES include lithotomy position, repeated dosing of local anesthetic solution through continuous spinal catheters, and possibly multiple single-injection spinal anesthetics. Suggestions for prevention of CES from spinal anesthesia include aspiration of CSF before and after local anesthetic injection. Some suggest that when CSF cannot be aspirated after half the dose is injected, a full dose not be administered. Limiting the amount of local anesthetic given in the subarachnoid space may help prevent CES.

Arachnoiditis
Arachnoiditis can occur after spinal injection of local anesthetic solution but is also known to occur after intrathecal steroid injection.[96–99] Causes of arachnoiditis include infection; myelograms from oil-based dyes; blood in the intrathecal space; neuroirritant, neurotoxic, or neurolytic substances; surgical interventions in the spine; intrathecal corticosteroids;

and trauma. Arachnoiditis has been reported after traumatic dural puncture and after unintentional intrathecal injection of local anesthetics, detergents, antiseptics, or other substances.[100]

Peripheral Nerve Injury Spinal anesthesia may indirectly result in peripheral nerve injury. The sensory block induced by spinal anesthesia temporarily abolishes normal protective reflexes. Therefore, care must be taken with appropriate positioning, avoidance of tight plaster casts, and observation of distal circulation. Hence, it is imperative that there is good nursing care of limbs rendered insensate by spinal anesthesia.

Total Spinal Anesthesia Total spinal anesthesia (TSA) results in respiratory depression, cardiovascular compromise, and loss of consciousness. This may or may not be preceded by numbness, paresthesia, or weakness of the upper limb; shortness of breath; nausea; or anxiety. The mechanism of TSA is unclear.

The importance of providing cardiorespiratory support and anxiolysis is illustrated by the management of *intentional* TSA. Total spinal anesthesia has been used therapeutically for intractable pain.[101] After injection of 20 mL of 1.5% lidocaine at the L3–L4 level, patients were tilted head down. Thiopental was given to prevent unpleasant sensations. After loss of consciousness, paralysis (without muscle relaxant), and pupil dilation, a laryngeal mask airway (LMA) was inserted and positive pressure ventilation applied. Ephedrine and atropine were used for cardiovascular support if required. Mechanical ventilation was required for about an hour, after which the LMA was removed.

Cardiovascular Collapse Cardiovascular collapse can occur after spinal anesthesia, although it is a rare event. Auroy and coworkers reported 9 cardiac arrests in 35,439 spinal anesthetics performed.[102] Refer to the section on Cardiovascular Effects of Spinal Anesthesia.

Estimating the Risks of the Major Complications of Spinal Anesthesia

While minor risks are often thought of as side effects, major complications are of more concern to clinicians and patients. Perception of risk can be influenced by sensational case reports, such as given by Woolley and Roe.[22] Early efforts to assess risk were hampered by lack of good numerator (number of complications) and denominator (number of spinal blocks) data. Vandam and Dripps, in an attempt to redress "unsubstantiated clinical impressions" of mid-20th century anesthesiologists, examined the records of over 10,000 spinal anesthetics.[103] They concluded that objections to spinal anesthesia were undeserved. Retrospective evidence from Finland for the period 1987–1993 estimated the risk of major complication following spinal anesthesia at 1 in 22,000.[104] A no-fault compensation scheme was thought to increase data veracity. Swedish data (Moen)[92] from the period 1990–1999 found a similar risk of 1 in 20,000–30,000. Although good evidence at the time, the Scandinavian evidence was criticized because of retrospective design, which risks underreporting. Moreover, numerator data sourced from administrative databases may not indicate either causation or final outcome.

Auroy attempted to address weaknesses of an earlier study[105] by setting up a telephone hotline, allowing contemporaneous assessment of causality.[102] This prospective study from 1998 to 1999 investigated complications from any type of regional anesthesia. Auroy's results relied on voluntary contribution by French anesthesiologists (<6% participation rate) and may have been skewed by differing complication rates in those willing to participate. A 2007 review found a much higher incidence of neurological complications after spinal anesthesia in Auroy's work (3.7–11.8 per 10,000) compared with Moen's work (0.4 per 10,000).[106] Auroy, unlike Moen, included peripheral neuropathy and radiculopathy in the numerator data.

Designing a prospective study to accurately quantify the risk of spinal anesthesia has been difficult due to the low incidence of major complications. The NAP3 of the Royal College of Anaesthetists is the best evidence to date on major complications after CNB.[26] NAP3 is notable for a variety of reasons: It is the largest prospective audit of CNB to date; it achieved a 100% return rate; and it gathered numerator and denominator data from a variety of sources. It also investigated causality and outcome.

Numerator data in NAP3 pertained to major complications over a 12-month period (2006–2007). Reports came from local hospital reporters and clinicians. Litigation authorities, medical defense organizations, journals, and even Google searches of media reports were reviewed to identify missed complications. Complications were classified as infections, hematomata, nerve injuries, cardiovascular collapses, and wrong-route errors. Notably, PDPH was not included as a major complication. Complications were examined by a panel, and the likelihood of CNB as the cause was established. Denominator data were sourced from a 2-week census and validated by contacting a number of organizations and databases.

The findings of permanent harm were presented optimistically or pessimistically (see Table 23–4). Optimistic figures

---

TABLE 23–4. Useful numbers for quoting risk to patients.

Central Neuraxial Blockade	Risk (Pessimistic)	Risk (Optimistic)
Permanent harm from major complication	1 in 25,000	1 in 50,000
Death and paraplegia	1 in 50,000	1 in 150,000

The following summarize the risks of central neuraxial blockade:

Figures have been simplified to aid memory. See text for actual risks.

Risk quoted as "pessimistic" or "optimistic" based on interpretation of NAP3 data.

Major complications include spinal infection or bleeding, major nerve damage, wrong-route injection error, and death.

Figures relate to all neuraxial blocks and therefore are not limited to spinal anesthesia. The incidence of complications from epidural and combined spinal-epidural blocks were at least twice those of spinal or caudal blocks.

excluded complications where recovery was likely or causality tenuous. Permanent harm after *any type of* CNB was pessimistically 1:23,500 and optimistically 1:50,500. The risk of death or paraplegia after *any type of* CNB was pessimistically 1:54,500 and optimistically 1:141,500. The incidences of complications of spinals and caudals were at least half that of epidurals and combined spinal-epidural (CSE) blocks. Of approximately 700,000 CNBs, 46% were spinals. Although the authors cautioned against subgroup analysis, the obstetric setting was found to have a low incidence of complications, while the adult perioperative setting had the highest complications. Complete or near-complete neurological recovery occurred in 61% of cases.

Importantly, NAP3 did not examine minor complications or major complications without permanent harm. For example, patients may have had cardiovascular collapse requiring intensive care or have had meningitis, but as they made a full recovery were excluded from even the pessimistic calculation. These are complications a patient would consider severe. The authors did acknowledge their figures represent a minimum possible incidence of complications; however, others have speculated that they may have overestimated risk.[107] As there was no control group, NAP3 cannot answer if CNB is safer than other techniques such as general anesthesia.

The NAP3 study reassured us that permanent harm as a result of spinal anesthesia is rare. The large scope and excellent methodology of NAP3 mean a similar audit is unlikely to be repeated soon. Efforts should be made in ameliorating "minor" and "moderate" complications that are more likely to trouble our patients. In particular, PDPH deserves special attention.

Major complications, nonetheless, do happen, and every effort must be made to prevent them. Awareness of the low risk of serious complications should not give rise to complacency. Indeed, a given complication may become so rare that a single anesthesiologist is unlikely to encounter it in a lifetime of practice. However, given the catastrophic nature of such complications, ongoing vigilance is of paramount importance.

Indications and Benefits of Spinal Anesthesia

Indications

Spinal anesthesia provides excellent operating conditions for surgery below the umbilicus. Thus, it has been used in the fields of urological, gynecological, obstetric, and lower abdominal and perineal general surgery. Likewise, it has been used in lower limb vascular and orthopedic surgery. More recently, spinal anesthesia has been used in surgery above the umbilicus (see section on laparoscopic surgery).[108–113]

Benefits of Spinal Anesthesia

Although spinal anesthesia is a commonly used technique, with an estimated 324,950 spinal anesthetics each year in the United Kingdom alone,[26] mortality and morbidity benefits are difficult to prove or disprove. It was hypothesized that due to beneficial modulation of the stress response, regional anesthesia would be safer than general anesthesia. However, clinical trials have been contradictory, and debates continue over the superiority of one technique over the other. Evaluations of the benefits of spinal

blockade are troubled by the heterogeneity of studies and arguments about whether analysis should include intention to treat.[114] In addition, much of the evidence for the benefits of neuraxial blockade pertains to epidurals, and some reviews do not differentiate between spinal and epidural anesthesia. For example, CNB has been shown to reduce blood loss[115] and thromboembolic events.[116] However, the authors of these studies were wise not to analyze spinal and epidural anesthesia individually, as the subgroup sample size would have been inadequate. Further studies are required to elucidate the relative benefits of each technique.

An obvious benefit of spinal anesthesia is the avoidance of the many risks of general anesthesia. However, it must be remembered that there is always the possibility of conversion to general anesthesia, and an emergent general anesthesia may be riskier than a planned general anesthesia.

Spinal anesthesia is advantageous in certain clinical settings. It is now commonplace for women having cesarean delivery to have a neuraxial block. Spinal anesthesia avoids the problems associated with general anesthesia in the pregnant patient, notably risks of difficult airway, awareness, and aspiration. Maternal blood loss has been found to be lower with spinal compared with general anesthesia.[117] Falling maternal mortality rates have been attributed to the increase in the practice of regional anesthesia. Moreover, regional anesthesia allows a mother to be awake for childbirth and a partner to be present if desired. However, a Cochrane review found no evidence of the superiority of regional anesthesia over general anesthesia with regard to major maternal or neonatal outcomes.[117] Likewise, a 2005 meta-analysis showed cord pH, an indicator of fetal well-being, to be lower with spinal compared with epidural and general anesthesia, although this may have been due to the use of ephedrine in the studies analyzed.[118] Nonetheless, spinal anesthesia remains the technique of choice for many obstetric anesthesiologists because of safety, reliability, and patient expectation.

A 2005 review of "best practice" for hip fractures found spinal anesthesia to have consistent benefits, and recommended the use of regional anesthesia "whenever possible."[119] Benefits cited included reduced mortality, deep vein thrombosis (DVT), transfusion requirements, and pulmonary complications. However, these recommendations, based on two reviews, illustrate the shortcomings of the available evidence. The first review had a heterogeneous population and limited power for subgroup analysis; extrapolating the findings to spinal anesthesia for hip fracture surgery is therefore questionable.[120] The second review found only a borderline difference in mortality at 1 month and no difference at 3 months. Moreover, all included studies had methodological flaws.[121]

The stress response to cardiac surgery is reduced by intrathecal bupivacaine in combination with general anesthesia[122] and partially attenuated by intrathecal morphine.[123] Low-dose intrathecal morphine (259 ± 53 μg) has been shown to facilitate early extubation after cardiac surgery.[124] A meta analysis of intrathecal morphine in cardiac surgery showed a modest decrease in morphine use and pain scores, although earlier extubation was only seen in a subset of patients receiving less than 500 μg of intrathecal morphine.[125]

As modern anesthesia and perioperative care become safer, it will become increasingly more difficult to prove an advantage of one technique over another. The ideal technique may in fact be a permutation of general anesthesia, neuraxial block, peripheral nerve blockade, or local infiltration analgesia.

Spinal Anesthesia: The Final Risk-Benefit Analysis

Once armed with the evidence regarding the risks and benefits of spinal anesthesia, the anesthesiologist must decide whether the evidence applies to the individual patient and clinical situation. Although complications can be devastating, NAP3 reassured us that major complications from spinal anesthesia are rare. Compelling benefits are harder to prove, yet there are advantages in certain clinical situations. Furthermore, the risk-benefit ratio must be compared with the risk-benefit ratio of available alternatives. The historical rise in safety of spinal anesthesia has been paralleled by a rise in safety of alternative techniques, including epidural anesthesia, peripheral nerve blockade, local infiltration analgesia, and of course general anesthesia. This competition between alternate techniques is likely to continue. Moreover, different modalities can be used in conjunction, complicating the final decision. The modern anesthesiologist must consider this matrix of risk-benefit ratios, which is beyond the scope of this chapter.

FUNCTIONAL ANATOMY OF SPINAL BLOCKADE

In reviewing the functional anatomy of spinal blockade, an intimate knowledge of the spinal column, spinal cord, and spinal nerves must be present. This chapter briefly reviews the anatomy, surface anatomy, and sonoanatomy of the spinal cord.

The vertebral column consists of 33 vertebrae: 7 cervical, 12 thoracic, 5 lumbar, 5 sacral, and 4 coccygeal segments. The vertebral column usually contains three curves. The cervical and lumbar curves are convex anteriorly, and the thoracic curve is convex posteriorly. The vertebral column curves, along with gravity, baricity of local anesthetic, and patient position, influence the spread of local anesthetics in the subarachnoid space. Figure 23–1 depicts the spinal column, vertebrae, and intervertebral disks and foramina.

Five ligaments hold the spinal column together (Figure 23–2). The supraspinous ligaments connect the apices of the spinous processes from the seventh cervical vertebra (C7) to the sacrum. The supraspinous ligament is known as the ligamentum nuchae in the area above C7. The interspinous ligaments connect the spinous processes together. The ligamentum flavum, or yellow ligament, connects the laminae above and below together. Finally, the posterior and anterior longitudinal ligaments bind the vertebral bodies together.

The three membranes that protect the spinal cord are the dura mater, arachnoid mater, and pia mater. The dura mater, or tough mother, is the outermost layer. The dural sac extends to the second sacral vertebra (S2). The arachnoid mater is the middle layer, and the subdural space lies between the dural

mater and arachnoid mater. The arachnoid mater, or cobweb mother, also ends at S2, like the dural sac. The pia mater, or soft mother, clings to the surface of the spinal cord and ends in the filum terminale, which helps to hold the spinal cord to the sacrum. The space between the arachnoid and pia mater is known as the subarachnoid space, and spinal nerves run in this space, as does CSF. Figure 23–3 depicts the spinal cord, dorsal root ganglia and ventral rootlets, spinal nerves, sympathetic trunk, rami communicantes, and pia, arachnoid, and dura maters.

When performing a spinal anesthetic using the midline approach, the layers of anatomy that are traversed (from posterior to anterior) are skin, subcutaneous fat, supraspinous ligament, interspinous ligament, ligamentum flavum, dura mater, subdural space, arachnoid mater, and finally the subarachnoid space. When the paramedian technique is applied, the spinal needle should traverse the skin, subcutaneous fat, paraspinous muscle, ligamentum flavum, dura mater, subdural space, and arachnoid mater and then pass into the subarachnoid space.

Clinical Pearls

When performing a spinal anesthetic using the midline approach, the layers of anatomy that are traversed (from posterior to anterior) are

- Skin
- Subcutaneous fat
- Supraspinous ligament
- Interspinous ligament
- Ligamentum flavum
- Dura mater
- Subdural space
- Arachnoid mater
- Subarachnoid space

When performing a spinal anesthetic using the paramedian approach, the spinal needle should traverse

- Skin
- Subcutaneous fat
- Paraspinous muscle
- Ligamentum flavum
- Dura mater
- Subdural space
- Arachnoid mater
- Subarachnoid space

The anatomy of the subdural space requires special attention. The subdural space is a meningeal plane that lies between the dura and the arachnoid mater, extending from the cranial cavity to the second sacral vertebrae.[126] Ultrastructural examination has shown this is an acquired space that only becomes real after tearing of neurothelial cells within the space.[127] The subdural space extends laterally around the dorsal nerve root and ganglion. There is less potential capacity of the subdural space adjacent to the ventral nerve roots. This may explain the sparing of anterior motor and sympathetic fibers during subdural block (SDB) (Figure 23–4).[126]

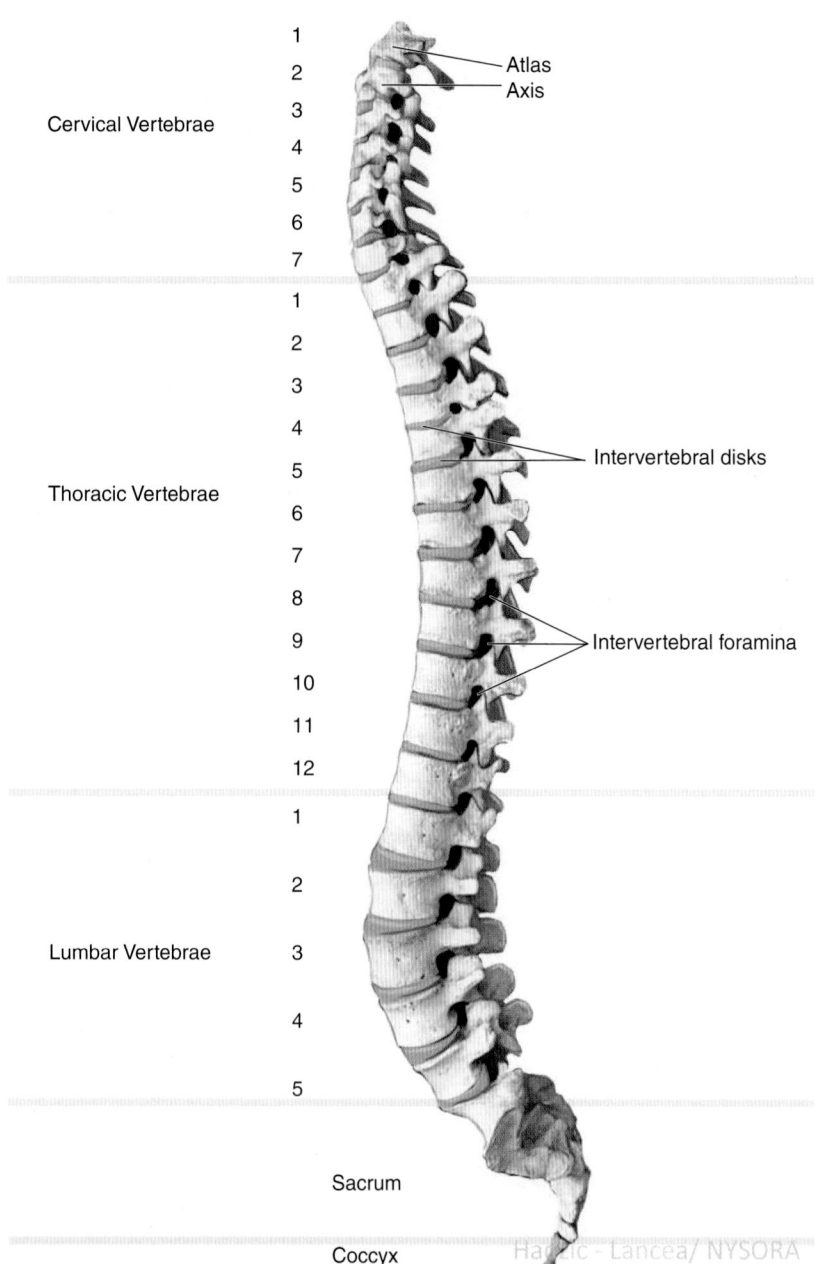

Cervical Vertebrae
1
2 — Atlas
3 — Axis
4
5
6
7

Thoracic Vertebrae
1
2
3
4 — Intervertebral disks
5
6
7
8
9 — Intervertebral foramina
10
11
12

Lumbar Vertebrae
1
2
3
4
5

Sacrum

Coccyx

FIGURE 23–1. Spinal column, vertebrae, and intervertebral disks and foramina.

The length of the spinal cord varies according to age. In the first trimester, the spinal cord extends to the end of the spinal column, but as the fetus ages, the vertebral column lengthens more than the spinal cord. At birth, the spinal cord ends at approximately L3. In the adult, the terminal end of the cord, known as the conus medullaris, lies at approximately L1. However, MRI and cadaveric studies have reported a conus medullaris below L1 in 19%–58% and below L2 in 0%–5%.[128] The conus medullaris may lie anywhere between T12 and L3.[129] Figure 23–5 shows a cross section of the lumbar vertebrae and spinal cord. The typical position of the conus medullaris, cauda equina, termination of the dural sac, and filum terminale are shown. A sacral spinal cord in an adult has been reported, although this is extremely rare.[130] The length of the spinal cord

must always be kept in mind when a neuraxial anesthetic is performed, as injection into the cord can cause great damage and result in paralysis.[131]

There are eight cervical spinal nerves and seven cervical vertebrae. Cervical spinal nerves 1 to 7 are numbered according to the vertebral body *below*. The eighth cervical nerve exits from below the seventh cervical vertebral body. Below this, spinal nerves are numbered according to the vertebral body *above*. The spinal nerve roots and spinal cord serve as the target sites for spinal anesthesia.

Surface Anatomy

When preparing for spinal anesthetic blockade, it is important to accurately identify landmarks on the patient.

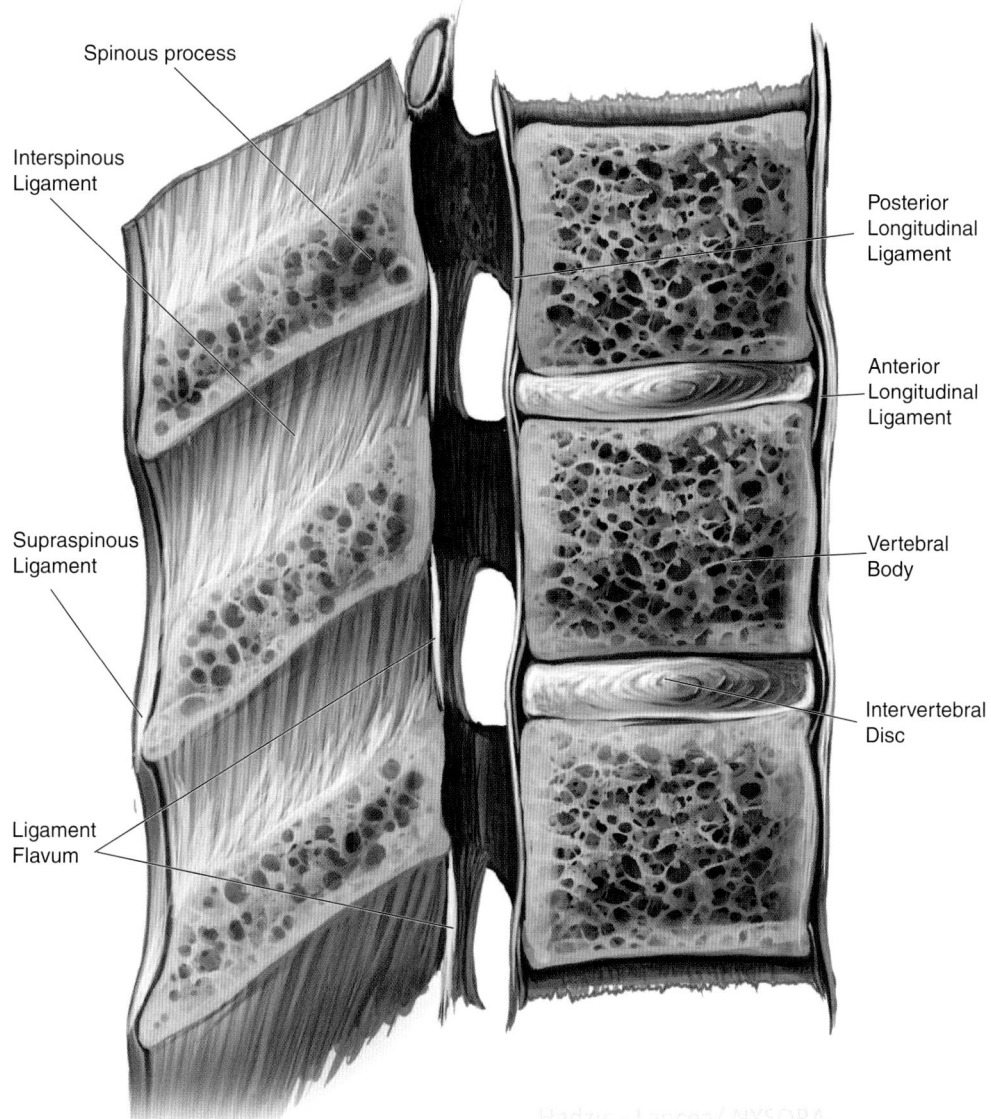

Spinous process

Interspinous
Ligament

Supraspinous
Ligament

Ligament
Flavum

Posterior
Longitudinal
Ligament

Anterior
Longitudinal
Ligament

Vertebral
Body

Intervertebral
Disc

Hadzic - Lancea/ NYSORA

FIGURE 23–2. Cross section of the spinal canal and adjacent ligaments. (Reproduced with permission from Leffert LR, Schwamm LH: Neuraxial anesthesia in parturients with intracranial pathology: a comprehensive review and reassessment of risk. *Anesthesiology*. 2013 Sep;119(3):703-718.)

The midline is identified by palpating the spinous processes. The iliac crests usually are at the same vertical height as the fourth lumbar spinous process or the interspace between the fourth and fifth lumbar vertebrae. An intercristal line can be drawn between the iliac crests to help locate this interspace. Care must be taken to feel for the soft area between the spinous processes to locate the interspace. Depending on the level of anesthesia necessary for the surgery and the ability to feel for the interspace, the L3–L4 interspace or the L4–L5 interspace can be used to introduce the spinal needle. Because the spinal cord commonly ends at the L1-to-L2 level, it is conventional not to attempt spinal anesthesia at or above this level. More recently, segmental thoracic spinal anesthesia has been described.[108,109]

It would be incomplete to discuss surface anatomy without mentioning the dermatomes that are important for spinal anesthesia. A dermatome is an area of skin innervated by

sensory fibers from a single spinal nerve. The tenth thoracic (T10) dermatome corresponds to the umbilicus, the sixth thoracic (T6) dermatome the xiphoid, and the fourth thoracic (T4) dermatome the nipples. Figure 23–6 illustrates the dermatomes of the human body. To achieve surgical anesthesia for a given procedure, the extent of spinal anesthesia must reach a certain dermatomal level. Dermatomal levels of spinal anesthesia for common surgical procedures are listed in Table 23–5.

Clinical Pearls

- T10 dermatome corresponds to the umbilicus.
- T6 dermatome corresponds to the xiphoid.
- T4 dermatome corresponds to the nipples.

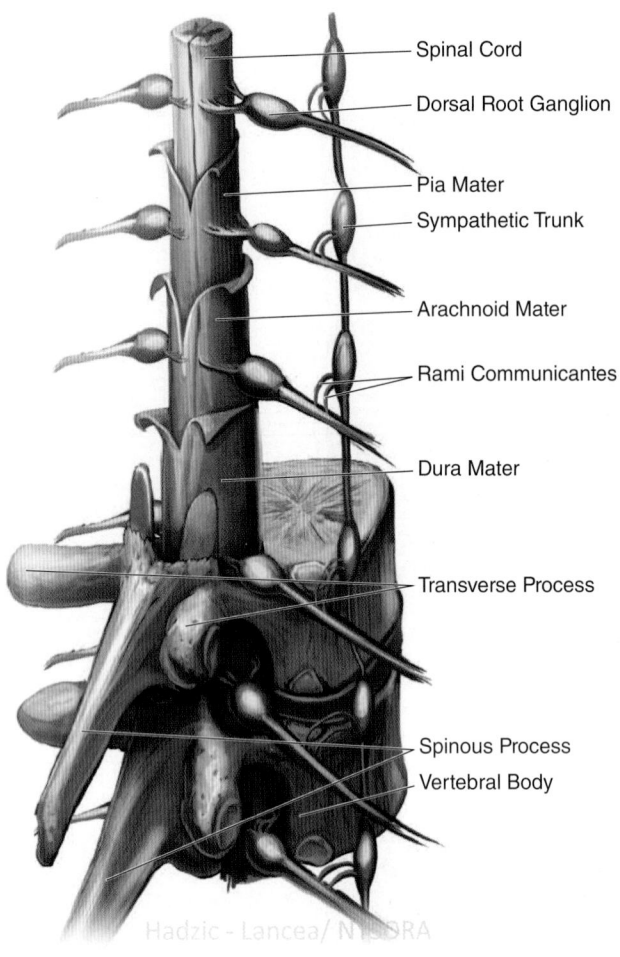

FIGURE 23–3. Spinal cord with meningeal layers, dorsal root ganglia, and the sympathetic nerve trunk.

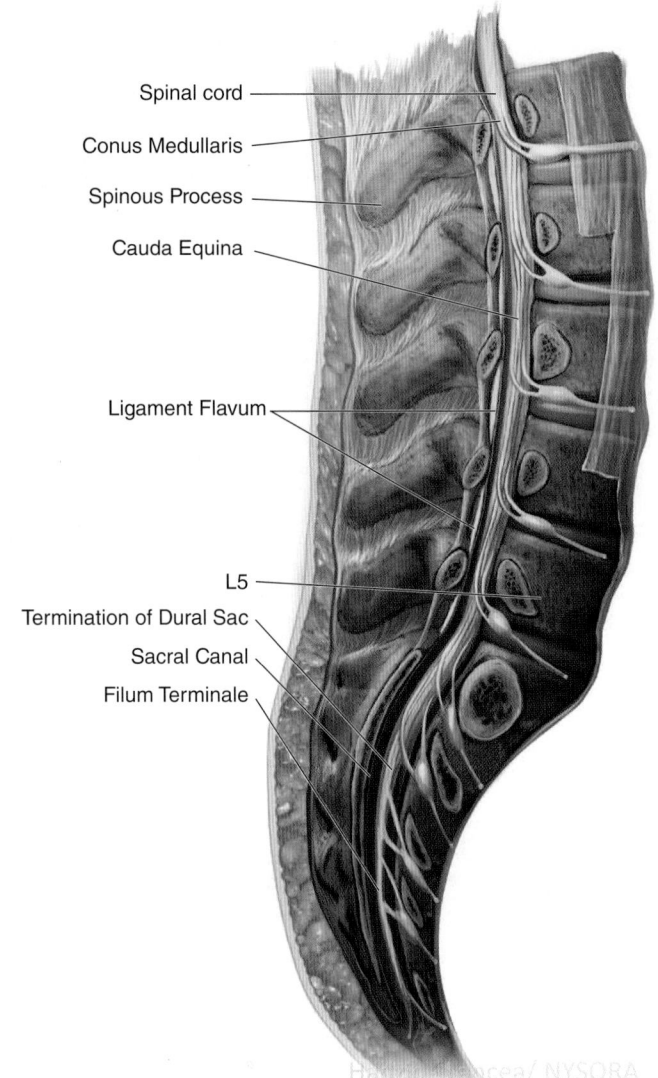

FIGURE 23–5. Cross section of the lumbar vertebrae.

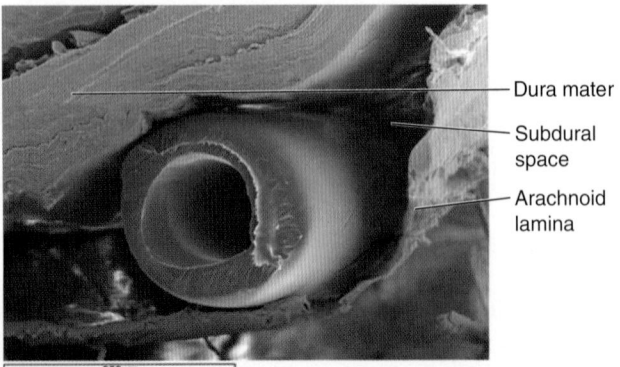

FIGURE 23–4. Epidural catheter in subdural space. Enhanced view of an epidural catheter inside a subdural space obtained from a cadaver under scanning electron microscopy. Magnification ×20. (Reproduced with permission from Reina MA, Collier CB, Prats-Galino A, et al: Unintentional subdural placement of epidural catheters during attempted epidural anesthesia: an anatomic study of spinal subdural compartment. *Reg Anesth Pain Med.* 2011 Nov-Dec;36(6):537-541.)

▮ Sonoanatomy

"Surface" anatomy refers to structures close enough to the integument that they are palpable. However, due to body habitus, this may not be possible.[128,132] Neuraxial ultrasound allows sonoanatomical visualization of these structures and deeper structures. However, as the ultrasound beam cannot penetrate the bony vertebrae, specialized ultrasonic windows are required to visualize the neuraxis. The technique of neuraxial ultrasound is discussed elsewhere (see section on recent developments in spinal anesthesia).

PHARMACOLOGY

The choice of local anesthetic is based on potency of the agent, onset and duration of anesthesia, and side effects of the drug. Two distinct groups of local anesthetics are used in spinal anesthesia, esters and amides, which are characterized by the bond that connects the aromatic portion and the

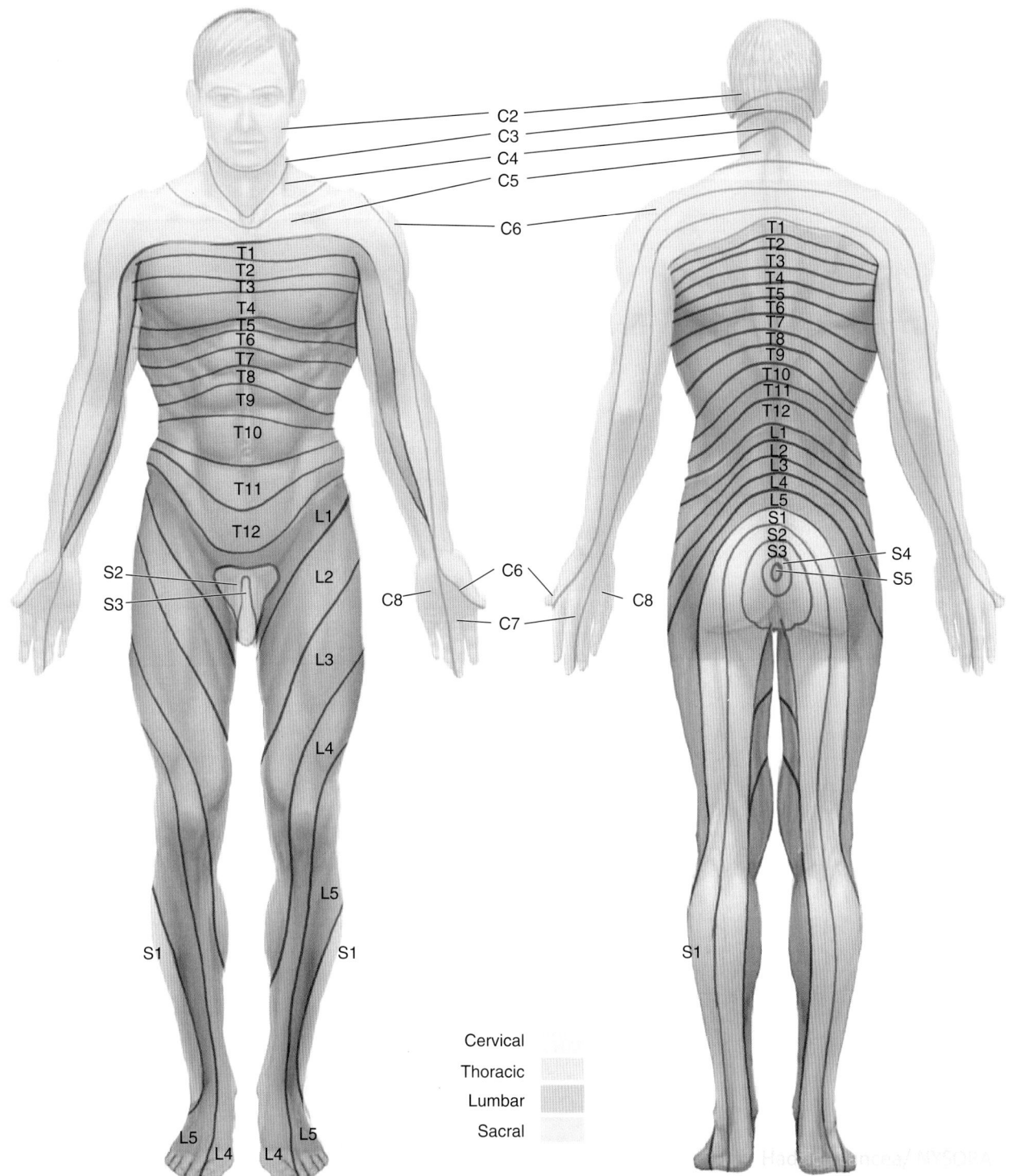

FIGURE 23–6. Dermatomes of the human body.

intermediate chain. Esters contain an ester link between the aromatic portion and the intermediate chain, and examples include procaine, chloroprocaine, and tetracaine. Amides contain an amide link between the aromatic portion and the intermediate chain, and examples include bupivacaine, ropivacaine, etidocaine, lidocaine, mepivacaine, and prilocaine. Although metabolism is important for determining activity of local anesthetics, lipid solubility, protein binding, and pK_a also influence activity.[133]

Clinical Pearls

- Potency of local anesthetics is related to lipid solubility.
- The duration of action of a local anesthetic is affected by the protein binding.
- The onset of action is related to the amount of local anesthetic available in the base form.

TABLE 23–5. Dermatomal levels of spinal anesthesia for common surgical procedures.

Procedure	Dermatomal Level
Upper abdominal surgery	T4
Intestinal, gynecologic, and urologic surgery	T6
Transurethral resection of the prostate	T10
Vaginal delivery of a fetus and hip surgery	T10
Thigh surgery and lower leg amputations	L1
Foot and ankle surgery	L2
Perineal and anal surgery	S2 to S5 (saddle block)

Lipid solubility relates to the potency of local anesthetics. Low lipid solubility indicates that higher concentrations of local anesthesia must be given to obtain nerve blockade. Conversely, high lipid solubility produces anesthesia at low concentrations. Protein binding affects the duration of action of a local anesthetic. Higher protein binding results in longer duration of action. The pK_a of a local anesthetic is the pH at which ionized and nonionized forms are present equally in solution, which is important because the nonionized form allows the local anesthetic to diffuse across the lipophilic nerve sheath and reach the sodium channels in the nerve membrane. The onset of action relates to the amount of local anesthetic available in the base form. Most local anesthetics follow the rule that the lower the pK_a, the faster the onset of action and vice versa. Please refer to Chapter 7 (Clinical Pharmacology of Local Anesthetics).

Pharmacokinetics of Local Anesthetics in the Subarachnoid Space

Pharmacokinetics of local anesthetics includes uptake and elimination of the drug. Four factors play a role in the uptake of local anesthetics from the subarachnoid space into neuronal tissue: (1) concentration of local anesthetic in CSF, (2) surface area of nerve tissue exposed to CSF, (3) lipid content of nerve tissue, and (4) blood flow to nerve tissue.[134,135]

The uptake of local anesthetic is greatest at the site of highest concentration in the CSF and is decreased above and below this site. As discussed previously, uptake and spread of local anesthetics after spinal injection are determined by multiple factors, including dose, volume, and baricity of local anesthetic and patient positioning.

Both the nerve roots and the spinal cord take up local anesthetics after injection into the subarachnoid space. The more surface area of the nerve root exposed, the greater the uptake of local anesthetic.[136–139] The spinal cord has two mechanisms for uptake of local anesthetics. The first mechanism is by diffusion from the CSF to the pia mater and into the spinal cord, which is a slow process. Only the most superficial portion of the spinal cord is affected by diffusion of local anesthetics. The second method of local anesthetic uptake is by extension into the spaces of Virchow-Robin, which are the areas of pia mater that surround the blood vessels that penetrate the central nervous system. The spaces of Virchow-Robin connect with the perineuronal clefts that surround nerve cell bodies in the spinal

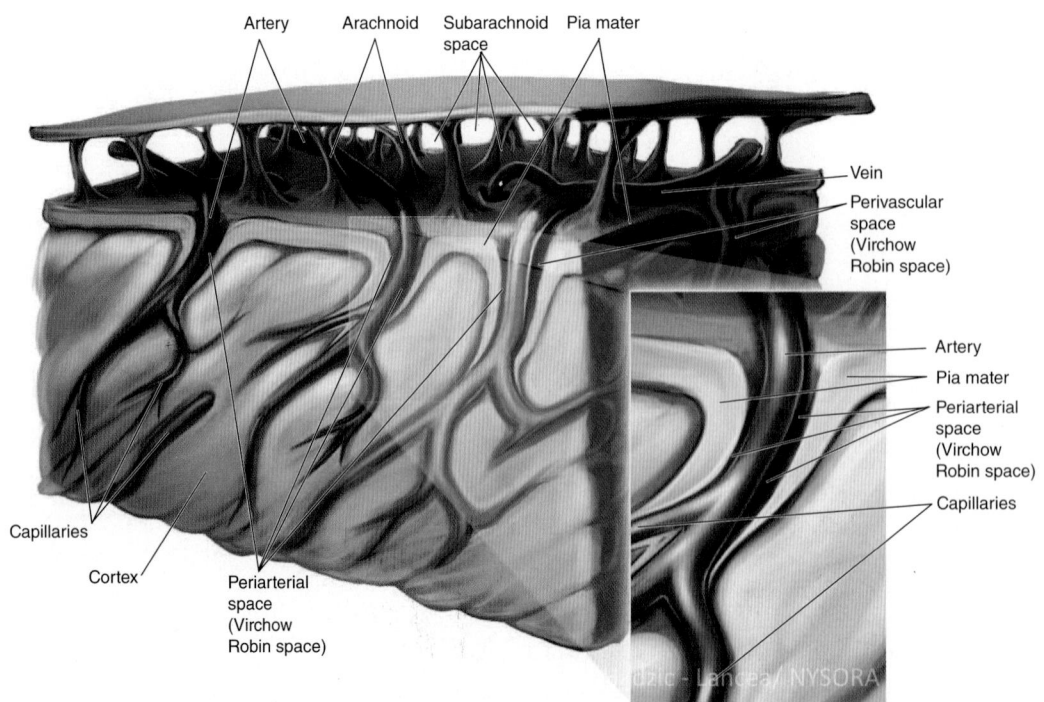

FIGURE 23–7. Virchow-Robin space.

cord and penetrate through to the deeper areas of the spinal cord. Figure 23–7 is a representation of the periarterial Virchow-Robin spaces around the spinal cord.

Clinical Pearls

The three most important modifiable factors in determining distribution of local anesthetics are

- Baricity of the local anesthetic solution
- Position of the patient during and just after injection
- Dose of the anesthetic injected

Lipid content determines uptake of local anesthetics. Heavily myelinated tissues in the subarachnoid space contain higher concentrations of local anesthetics after injection. The higher the degree of myelination, the higher the concentration of local anesthetic, as there is a high lipid content in myelin. If an area of nerve root does not contain myelin, an increased risk of nerve damage occurs in that area.[140]

Blood flow determines the rate of removal of local anesthetics from spinal cord tissue. The faster the blood flows in the spinal cord, the more rapid the anesthetic is washed away. This may partly explain why the concentration of local anesthetics is greater in the posterior spinal cord than in the anterior spinal cord, even though the anterior cord is more readily accessed by the Virchow-Robin spaces. After a spinal anesthetic is administered, blood flow may be increased or decreased to the spinal cord, depending on the particular local anesthetic administered; for example, tetracaine increases cord flow, but lidocaine and bupivacaine decrease it, which affects elimination of the local anesthetic.[141–143]

Elimination of local anesthetic from the subarachnoid space is by vascular absorption in the epidural space and the subarachnoid space. Local anesthetics travel across the dura in both directions. In the epidural space, vascular absorption can occur, just as in the subarachnoid space. Vascular supply to the spinal cord consists of vessels located on the spinal cord and in the pia mater. Because vascular perfusion to the spinal cord varies, the rate of elimination of local anesthetics varies.[134]

Distribution

The distribution and decrease in concentration of local anesthetics is based on the area of highest concentration, which can be independent of the injection site. Many factors affect the distribution of local anesthetics in the subarachnoid space. Table 23–6 lists some of these factors.[144]

Baricity plays an important role in determining the spread of local anesthetic in the spinal space and is equal to the density of the local anesthetic divided by the density of the CSF at 37°C.[145–152] Local anesthetics can be hyperbaric, hypobaric, or isobaric when compared to CSF, and baricity is the main determinant of how the local anesthetic is distributed when injected into the CSF. Table 23–7 compares the density,

TABLE 23–6. Determinants of local anesthetic spread in the subarachnoid space.

Properties of local anesthetic solution
- Baricity
- Dose
- Volume
- Specific gravity

Patient characteristics
- Position during and after injection
- Height (extremely short or tall)
- Spinal column anatomy
- Decreased cerebrospinal fluid volume (increased intra-abdominal pressure due to increased weight, pregnancy, etc.)

Technique
- Site of injection
- Needle bevel direction

specific gravity, and baricity of different substances and local anesthetics.[144,145,147,153,154]

Hypobaric solutions are less dense than CSF and tend to rise against gravity. Isobaric solutions are as dense as CSF and tend to remain at the level at which they are injected. Hyperbaric solutions are more dense than CSF and tend to follow gravity after injection.

Hypobaric solutions have a baricity of less than 1.0 relative to CSF and are usually made by adding distilled sterile water to the local anesthetic. Tetracaine, dibucaine, and bupivacaine have all been used as hypobaric solutions in spinal anesthesia. Patient positioning is important after injection of a hypobaric spinal anesthetic because it is the first few minutes that determine the spread of anesthesia. If the patient is in Trendelenburg position after injection, the anesthetic will spread in the caudal direction and if the patient is in reverse Trendelenburg position, the anesthetic will spread cephalad after injection.

The baricity of isobaric solutions is equal to 1.0. Tetracaine and bupivacaine have both been used with success for isobaric spinal anesthesia. Gravity does not play a role in the spread of isobaric solutions, unlike with hypo- or hyperbaric local anesthetics. Therefore, patient positioning does not affect spread of isobaric solutions. Injection can be made in any position, and then the patient can be placed into the position necessary for surgery.

Hyperbaric solutions have baricity greater than 1.0. A local anesthetic solution can be made hyperbaric by adding dextrose or glucose. Bupivacaine, lidocaine, and tetracaine have all been used as hyperbaric solutions in spinal anesthesia. Patient positioning affects the spread of the anesthetic. A patient in Trendelenburg position would have the anesthetic travel in a cephalad direction and vice versa.

Dose and volume both play a role in distribution of local anesthetics after spinal injection. For further information, please refer to the section Volume, Concentration, and Dose of Local Anesthetic.

TABLE 23–7. Density, specific gravity, and baricity of different substances and local anesthetics.

		Density	Specific Gravity	Baricity
Water		0.9933	1.0000	0.9930
Cerebrospinal fluid		1.0003	1.0069	1.0000
Hypobaric				
• Tetracaine	0.33% in water	0.9980	1.0046	0.9977
• Lidocaine	0.5% in water	N/A	1.0038	0.9985
Isobaric				
• Tetracaine	0.5% in 50% CSF	0.9998	1.0064	0.9995
• Lidocaine	2% in water	1.0003	1.0066	1.0003
• Bupivacaine	0.5% in water	0.9993	1.0059	0.9990
Hyperbaric				
• Tetracaine	0.5% in 5% dextrose	1.0136	1.0203	1.0133
• Lidocaine	5% in 7.5% dextrose	1.0265	1.0333	1.0265
• Bupivacaine	0.5% in 8% dextrose	1.0210	1.0278	1.0207
• Bupivacaine	0.75% in 8% dextrose	1.0247	1.0300	1.0227

Effects of the Volume of the Lumbar Cistern on Block Height

Cerebrospinal fluid is produced in the brain at 0.35 mL/min and fills the subarachnoid space. This clear, colorless fluid has an approximate adult volume of 150 mL, half of which is in the cranium and half in the spinal canal. However, CSF volume varies considerably, and decreased CSF volume can result from obesity, pregnancy, or any other cause of increased abdominal pressure.[155] This is partly due to compression of the intervertebral foramen, which displaces the CSF.

Clinical Pearl

- Due to the wide variability in CSF volume, the ability to predict the level of the spinal blockade after local anesthetic injection is very poor, even if BMI is calculated and used.

Multiple factors affect the distribution of local anesthesia after spinal blockade,[144] one being CSF volume. Carpenter showed that lumbosacral CSF volume correlated with peak sensory block height and duration of surgical anesthesia.[156] The density of CSF is related to peak sensory block level, and lumbosacral CSF volume correlates to peak sensory block level and onset and duration of motor block.[157] However, due to the wide variability in CSF volume, the ability to predict the level of the spinal blockade after local anesthetic injection is poor, even if BMI is calculated and used.

Local Anesthetics

Cocaine was the first spinal anesthetic used, and procaine and tetracaine soon followed. Lidocaine, 2-chloroprocaine, bupivacaine, mepivacaine, and ropivacaine have also been used intrathecally. In addition, there is a growing interest in medications that produce anesthesia and analgesia while limiting side effects. A variety of medications, including vasoconstrictors, opioids, α_2-adrenergic agonists, and acetylcholinesterase inhibitors, have been added to spinal medications to enhance analgesia while reducing the motor blockade produced by local anesthetics.

Lidocaine was first used as a spinal anesthetic in 1945, and it has been one of the most widely used spinal anesthetics since. Onset of anesthesia occurs in 3 to 5 minutes with a duration of anesthesia that lasts for 1 to 1.5 hour. Lidocaine spinal anesthesia has been used for short-to-intermediate length operating room cases. The major drawback of lidocaine is the association with transient neurologic symptoms (TNSs), which present as low back pain and lower extremity dysesthesias with radiation to the buttocks, thighs, and lower limbs after recovery from spinal anesthesia. TNSs occur in about 14% of patients receiving lidocaine spinal anesthesia.[158,159] Lithotomy position is associated with a higher incidence of TNSs. Because of the risk of TNSs, lidocaine has mostly been replaced by other local anesthetics.

Intrathecal use of 2-chloroprocaine was described in 1952. In the 1980s, concerns were raised regarding neurotoxicity with the use of 2-chloroprocaine. Studies have suggested that sodium bisulfite, an antioxidant used in combination with 2-chloroprocaine, is responsible. Chronic neurologic deficits have been reported in rabbits when sodium bisulfite was injected into the lumbar subarachnoid space, but when preservative-free 2-chloroprocaine was injected, no permanent neurologic sequelae were noted.[160] Results from clinical trials have shown preservative-free 2-chloroprocaine to be safe, short acting, and acceptable for outpatient surgery.[161,162] However, addition of epinephrine is not recommended due to an association with flu-like symptoms and back pain.[161] Intrathecal 2-chloroprocaine is not currently approved by the Food and

Drug Administration (FDA), although package labeling states it may be used for epidural anesthesia.[163] Onset time is fast, and the duration is around 100 to 120 minutes. The dose ranges from 20 to 60 mg, with 40 mg as a usual dose.

Procaine is a short-acting ester local anesthetic. Procaine has an onset time of 3 to 5 minutes and a duration of 50 to 60 minutes. A dose of 50 to 100 mg has been suggested for perineal and lower extremity surgery. However, there is a 14% incidence of block failure associated with procaine 10%.[164] Concerns about the neurotoxicity of procaine have limited its use.[165] For all these reasons, procaine is currently rarely used for spinal anesthesia.

Bupivacaine is one of the most widely used local anesthetics for spinal anesthesia and provides adequate anesthesia and analgesia for intermediate-to-long-duration operating room cases. Bupivacaine has a low incidence of TNSs.[166–168] Onset of anesthesia occurs in 5 to 8 minutes, with a duration of anesthesia that lasts from 90 to 150 minutes. For outpatient spinal anesthesia, small doses of bupivacaine are recommended to avoid prolonged discharge time due to duration of block. Bupivacaine is often packaged as 0.75% in 8.25% dextrose. Other forms of spinal bupivacaine include 0.5% with or without dextrose and 0.75% without dextrose.

Clinical Pearls

- Use of intrathecal lidocaine is limited by TNSs.
- Bupivacaine has a very low incidence of TNSs.
- Onset of anesthesia occurs in 5 to 8 minutes with bupivacaine and a duration of anesthesia that lasts from 210 to 240 minutes; thus, it is appropriate for intermediate-to-long operating room cases.

Tetracaine has an onset of anesthesia within 3 to 5 minutes and a duration of 70 to 180 minutes and, like bupivacaine, is used for cases that are intermediate to longer duration. The 1% solution can be mixed with 10% glucose in equal parts to form a hyperbaric spinal anesthetic that is used for perineal and abdominal surgery. With tetracaine, TNSs occur at a lower rate than with lidocaine spinal anesthesia. The addition of phenylephrine may play a role in the development of TNSs.[169–171]

Mepivacaine is similar to lidocaine and has been used since the 1960s for spinal anesthesia. The incidence of TNSs reported after mepivacaine spinal anesthesia varies widely, with rates from 0% to 30%.[172–174]

Ropivacaine was introduced in the 1990s. For applications in spinal anesthesia, ropivacaine has been found to be less potent than bupivacaine.[175] Dose range-finding studies have demonstrated the ED95 of spinal ropivacaine in lower limb surgery (11.4 mg),[176] pregnant patients (26.8 mg),[177] and neonates (1.08 mg/kg).[178] Intrathecal use of ropivacaine is not widespread, and large-scale safety data are awaited. An early study identified back pain in 5 of 18 volunteers injected with intrathecal hyperbaric ropivacaine.[179] TNSs have been reported with spinal ropivacaine,[175] although the incidence is not as common as seen with lidocaine.[159] Other small studies have not demonstrated any major side effects.[180–182]

Table 23–8 shows some of the local anesthetics used for spinal anesthesia and dosage duration and concentration for different levels of spinal blockade.[161,183–191]

Additives to Local Anesthesia

Vasoconstrictors have been added to local anesthetics, and both epinephrine and phenylephrine have been studied. Anesthesia is intensified and prolonged with smaller doses of local anesthetics when epinephrine or phenylephrine is added. Tissue vasoconstriction is produced, thus limiting the systemic reabsorption of the local anesthetic and prolonging the duration of action by keeping the local anesthetic in contact with the nerve fibers. However, ischemic complications can occur after the use of vasoconstrictors in spinal anesthesia. In some studies, epinephrine was implicated as the cause of CES because of anterior spinal artery ischemia. Regardless, many studies do not demonstrate an association between the use of vasoconstrictors for spinal anesthesia and the incidence of CES.[192,193] Phenylephrine has been shown to increase the risk of TNSs and may decrease block height.[171,194]

Epinephrine is thought to work by decreasing local anesthetic uptake and thus prolonging the spinal blockade of some local anesthetics. However, vasoconstrictors can cause ischemia, and there is a theoretical concern of spinal cord ischemia when epinephrine is added to spinal anesthetics. Animal models have

TABLE 23–8. Dose, duration, and onset of local anesthetics used in spinal anesthesia.

	Dose (mg)		Duration (minutes)		Onset (minutes)
	To T10	to T4	Plain	With Epinephrine	
Commonly used Bupivacaine 0.75%	8–12	14–20	90–110	100–150	5–8
Less commonly used					
• Lidocaine 5%	50–75	75–100	60–70	75–100	3–5
• Tetracaine 0.5%	6–10	12–16	70–90	120–180	3–5
• Mepivacaine 2%	N/A	60–80	140–160	N/A	2–4
• Ropivacaine 0.75%	15–17	18–20	140–200	N/A	3–5
• Levobupivacaine 0.5%	10–15	N/A	135–170	N/A	4–8
• Chloroprocaine 3%	30	45	80–120	N/A	2–4

not shown any decrease in spinal cord blood flow or increase in spinal cord ischemia when epinephrine is given for spinal blockade, even though some neurologic complications associated with the addition of epinephrine exist.[141,143,195,196]

Clinical Pearls

- Adding 0.1 mL of 1:1000 epinephrine to 10 mL of local anesthetic yields a 1:100,000 concentration of epinephrine.
- Adding 0.1 mL of 1:1000 epinephrine to 20 mL of local anesthetic yields a 1:200,000 concentration and so on (0.1 mL in 30 mL = 1:300,000).

Dilution of epinephrine with local anesthetic is a potential source of drug error, with mistakes potentially incorrect by a factor of 10 or 100. If using epinephrine packaged as 1 mg in 1 mL, which is a 1:1000 solution, a simple rule can be followed. Adding 0.1 mL of epinephrine to 10 mL of local anesthetic yields a 1:100,000 concentration of epinephrine. Adding 0.1 mL of epinephrine to 20 mL of local anesthetic yields a 1:200,000 concentration, and so on (0.1 mL in 30 mL = 1:300,000).

Epinephrine prolongs the duration of spinal anesthesia.[197–199] In the past, it was thought that epinephrine had no effect on hyperbaric spinal bupivacaine using two-segment regression to test neural blockade.[200] However, another study showed that epinephrine prolongs the duration of hyperbaric spinal bupivacaine when pinprick, transcutaneous electrical nerve stimulation (TENS) equivalent to surgical stimulation, and tolerance of a pneumatic thigh tourniquet were used to determine neural blockade.[201] There is controversy regarding prolongation of spinal bupivacaine neural blockade when epinephrine is added.[202–205] The same controversy exists about the prolongation of spinal lidocaine with epinephrine.[206–210]

All four types of opioid receptors are found in the dorsal horn of the spinal cord and serve as the target for intrathecal opioid injection. Receptors are located on spinal cord neurons and terminals of afferents originating in the dorsal root ganglion. Fentanyl, sufentanil, meperidine, and morphine have all been used intrathecally. Side effects that may be seen include pruritus, nausea and vomiting, and respiratory depression.[211–215]

The α_2-adrenergic agonists can be added to spinal injections of local anesthetics to enhance pain relief and prolong sensory and motor block. Enhanced postoperative analgesia has been demonstrated in cesarean deliveries, fixation of femoral fractures, and knee arthroscopies when clonidine was added to the local anesthetic solution. Clonidine prolongs the sensory and motor blockade of a local anesthetic after spinal injection.[216–218] Sensory blockade is thought to be mediated by both presynaptic and postsynaptic mechanisms. Clonidine induces hyperpolarization at the ventral horn of the spinal cord and facilitates the action of the local anesthetic, thus prolonging motor blockade when used as an additive. However, when used alone in intrathecal injections, clonidine does not cause motor block or

weakness.[219] Side effects can occur with the use of spinal clonidine and include hypotension, bradycardia, and sedation. Neuraxial clonidine has been used for the treatment for intractable pain.[220,221]

Acetylcholinesterase inhibitors prevent the breakdown of acetylcholine and produce analgesia when injected intrathecally. The antinociceptive effects are due to increased acetylcholine and generation of nitric oxide. It has been shown in a rat model that diabetic neuropathy can be alleviated after intrathecal neostigmine injection.[222] Side effects of intrathecal neostigmine include nausea and vomiting, bradycardia requiring atropine, anxiety, agitation, restlessness, and lower extremity weakness.[223–225] Although spinal neostigmine provides extended pain control, the side effects that occur do not allow its widespread use.

PHARMACODYNAMICS OF SPINAL ANESTHESIA

The pharmacodynamics of spinal injection of local anesthesia are wide ranging. The cardiovascular, respiratory, gastrointestinal, hepatic, and renal effect consequences of spinal anesthesia are discussed next.

Cardiovascular Effects of Spinal Anesthesia

It is well recognized that spinal anesthesia results in hypotension. In fact, a degree of hypotension often reassures the anesthesiologist that the block is indeed spinal. However, hypotension may cause nausea and vomiting, ischemia of critical organs, cardiovascular collapse, and in the case of the pregnant mother may endanger the fetus. Historically, there have been shifts in the definitions, suggested mechanisms, and management of hypotension.

Defining hypotension is troublesome. One study found 15 different definitions of hypotension in 63 publications.[226] Some definitions used a single criterion (decrease of 80% from baseline), while others used combinations (a fall of 80% from baseline *or* a systolic blood pressure less than 100 mm Hg). The incidence of hypotension in a single cohort of patients varied from 7.4% to 74.1% depending on the definition used.

There have been many suggested mechanisms for spinal anesthesia–induced hypotension, including direct circulatory effects of local anesthetics, relative adrenal insufficiency, skeletal muscle paralysis, ascending medullary vasomotor block, and concurrent respiratory insufficiency. The primary insult, however, is the preganglionic sympathetic block produced by spinal anesthesia.[227,228] It therefore follows that because the block height determines the extent of sympathetic blockade, this in turn determines the amount of change in cardiovascular parameters. However, this relationship cannot be predicted. Sympathetic block may be variably between two and six dermatomes above the sensory level and incomplete below this level.[227] The sudden sympathetic block with spinal anesthesia gives little time for cardiovascular compensation, which may account for a similar sympathetic block with epidural anesthesia, but less hypotension.[229]

Clinical Pearls

- Spinal anesthesia block the sympathetic chain, which is the main mechanism of cardiovascular changes.
- The block height determines the level of sympathetic blockade, which determines the degree of change in cardiovascular parameters.

Sympathetic block causes hypotension via its effects on preload, afterload, contractility, and HR—in other words, the determinants of cardiac output (CO)—and by decreasing systemic vascular resistance (SVR). Preload is decreased by sympathetic block-mediated venodilation, resulting in pooling of blood in the peripheries and decreased venous return.[229] During sympathetic block, the venous system is maximally vasodilated and therefore reliant on gravity to return blood to the heart. Thus, patient positioning, and aortocaval compression in the case of a gravid uterus, markedly influences venous return during spinal anesthesia.[227,230]

Arterial vasomotor tone can also be decreased by sympathetic block, decreasing SVR, and afterload. Arterial vasodilation, unlike venodilation, is not maximal after spinal blockade, and vascular smooth muscle continues to retain some autonomic tone after sympathetic denervation. This residual vascular tone can be lost in the presence of hypoxia and acidosis, which may account for cardiovascular collapse after high spinal anesthesia without cardiorespiratory support.[227] Although there is vasodilation below the level of spinal blockade, there is compensatory vasoconstriction above, mediated by carotid and aortic arch baroreceptors. This is important for two reasons. First, blockade at higher dermatomal levels may result in less compensation. Second, use of vasodilatory drugs such as glyceryl trinitrate (GTN), sodium nitroprusside, or volatile anesthetics may abolish this compensatory mechanism and worsen hypotension or even result in cardiac arrest.[231]

There may be an initial increase in CO associated with a decreased afterload.[229] Alternatively, CO may fall due to decreased preload.[232] Some studies have shown that CO is unchanged or slightly reduced during onset of spinal anesthesia. Others, in elderly patients, have shown a biphasic change in CO with an initial increase in the first 7 minutes, followed by a fall (Figure 23–8).[233] This may be attributed to a fall in afterload preceding a fall in preload.

Contractility may be affected by blockade of the upper thoracic sympathetic nerves.[227] Interestingly, a study investigating the common phenomenon of ST segment depression in healthy women undergoing cesarean section (25-60%) found ST depression to be associated with a hyperkinetic contractile state.[234]

The effect of spinal anesthesia on HR is complex. HR may increase (secondary to hypotension via the baroreceptor reflex) or decrease (either from sympathetic block of cardiac accelerator fibers originating from T1–T4 spinal segments, or via the *reverse* Bainbridge reflex).[228] The reverse Bainbridge reflex is a decrease in HR due to decreased venous return, detected by stretch receptors in the right atrium, and is weaker than the baroreceptor reflex. The Bezold-Jarisch reflex (BJR) is another reflex that decreases HR. The BJR has been implicated as a cause

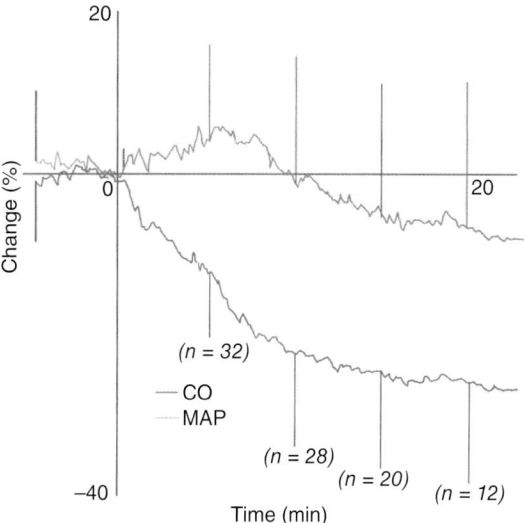

FIGURE 23–8. Figure from the work of Meyhoff et al showing a fall in mean arterial pressure (MAP) and biphasic cardiac output (CO) after spinal anesthesia. Average CO and MAP changes plus or minus standard deviation during onset of spinal anesthesia in elderly patients. Subarachnoid injection is given at time = 0 minutes. After termination of data collection, the last CO and MAP recording are still represented in the average throughout the rest of the graph. Each line is thus hypothetical as it consists of averages of 32 patients even after data termination; this is done for illustration purposes only. (Reproduced with permission from Meyhoff CS, Hesselbjerg L, Koscielniak-Nielsen Z, et al: Biphasic cardiac output changes during onset of spinal anaesthesia in elderly patients. *Eur J Anaesthesiol.* 2007 Sep;24(9):770-775.)

of bradycardia, hypotension, and cardiovascular collapse after central neuraxial anesthesia, in particular spinal anesthesia.[235,236] The BJR is a cardioinhibitory reflex and is usually not a dominant reflex. The association with spinal anesthesia is probably weak.[237,238] The BJR has been blamed for bradycardia after spinal anesthesia, especially after hemorrhage.[239] Vigorous contractions of an underfilled heart may initiate the BJR. This is more likely with the use of ephedrine rather than phenylephrine.[228]

Young, healthy (American Society of Anesthesiologists class 1) patients have a higher risk of bradycardia. Beta-blocker use also increases the risk of bradycardia. The incidence of bradycardia in the nonpregnant population is about 13%.[48] Even though bradycardia is usually well tolerated, asystole and second- and third-degree heart block can occur, so it is wise to be vigilant when monitoring a patient after spinal anesthesia and treat promptly.[240]

Risk factors associated with hypotension include hypovolemia, preoperative hypertension, high sensory block height, age older than 40 years, obesity, combined general and spinal anesthesia, chronic alcohol consumption, elevated BMI, and urgency of nonobstetric surgery.[48,241–243] Hypotension is less likely in women who are in labor compared with those undergoing elective cesarean section.[244]

Management of Hypotension After Spinal Anesthesia

Changing Beliefs Shifting beliefs in the theoretical basis of spinal-induced hypotension have been echoed by changes in management. For example, if decreased preload is believed to be of primary importance, then positioning and fluid therapy are the treatments of choice,[245] and similarly if vasodilation is the culprit, then a vasoconstrictor should be first line.[228] This has led to vigorous debate.[246] In the 1970s, it was suggested not to give vasopressors until "all other methods of combating hypotension" were utilized,[245] underlining the importance of preload. Evidence to support this was extrapolated from flawed studies on pregnant ewes undergoing general anesthesia, which suggested vasopressors adversely effected the uteroplacental circulation. The title *vasopressor of choice* has similarly generated much controversy. Ephedrine was traditionally nominated as it preserved uterine blood flow (in the aforementioned animal studies). Work by Ngan Kee, among others, has suggested phenylephrine may be the vasopressor of choice,[228] at least in the elective obstetric setting.

Management Management of hypotension following spinal anesthesia should include frequent (every minute initially) monitoring of blood pressure, in addition to electrocardiogram (ECG), oxygen saturation, and fetal monitoring in the case of a pregnant patient. Consideration should be given to invasive blood pressure monitoring if the patient has significant cardiac comorbidities. Fluid therapy should be used in a dehydrated patient to restore volume prior to commencing spinal anesthesia.

Nonpharmacological methods to treat hypotension include positioning, leg compression, and uterine displacement. Trendelenburg positioning can increase venous return to the heart. This position should not exceed 20° because extreme Trendelenburg can lead to a decrease in cerebral perfusion and blood flow due to increases in jugular venous pressure. If the level of spinal anesthesia is not fixed, the Trendelenburg position can alter the level of spinal anesthesia and cause a high level of spinal anesthesia in patients receiving hyperbaric local anesthetic solutions.[247] This can be minimized by raising the upper part of the body with a pillow under the shoulders while keeping the lower part of the body elevated above heart level. A Cochrane review in pregnant women found lower limb compression to have some benefit, although different methods had varying efficacies.[248] Aortocaval compression from a gravid uterus should be avoided. Full lateral positioning results in less hypotension than left lateral tilt, although this may not be practical. A wedge under the right hip, or a tilting table, can be used to achieve left lateral tilt. However, the optimal degree of tilt is unknown, and there may be considerable variability among different patients.[229]

There have been conflicting opinions on appropriate fluid management during spinal anesthesia. Early studies suggested crystalloid "preloading" prior to spinal blockade was effective. More recent work showed minimal effect of preloading.[249,250] Colloid preloading does seem to be effective,[251] although this must be balanced against the risk of allergic reactions and increased costs. "Coloading" (rapid administration of fluid immediately after spinal anesthesia) with crystalloid is better than preloading at preventing hypotension.[252]

Hypotension can be limited by lowering the dose of spinal local anesthetic. One review found 5–7 mg of bupivacaine to

be sufficient for cesarean section. However, complete motor block was rare, duration was limited, and an epidural catheter for early top-up doses was essential.[253] A meta-analysis in 2011 found lower doses of bupivacaine to be associated with lower anesthetic efficacy but less hypotension and nausea.[254]

Conflicting opinions exist regarding the vasopressor of choice for spinal-induced hypotension. Ephedrine and phenylephrine have been the two main contenders; however, others have been used. Ephedrine is a direct and indirect α- and β-receptor agonist. It was felt to be safer than phenylephrine because it limited vasoconstriction of the uteroplacental circulation in early animal studies. However, ephedrine has a slow onset of action, is subject to tachyphylaxis, and has limited efficacy in treating hypotension.[229] Of more concern is the increased risk of fetal acidosis.[255] Whether this translates to poorer clinical outcomes is uncertain.

Phenylephrine is an direct α_1-receptor agonist. It was used successfully in the 1960s for spinal anesthesia in New York,[256] but fell out of favor due to concerns about poor tissue perfusion. In particular, uteroplacental vasoconstriction was noted in (somewhat-flawed) pregnant animal models. Recent work has shown that fetal acidosis does not occur when usual doses are used.[257] In addition, phenylephrine seems superior to ephedrine in reducing hypotension and nausea.[228] Phenylephrine has been used as a bolus or as an infusion and has been used to treat hypotension prophylactically as well as reactively (Table 23–9). Optimal dosing regimens are yet to be established. Ngan Kee effectively prevented hypotension in elective obstetric patients by using a combination of crystalloid coload with a prophylactic infusion of phenylephrine.[258]

Phenylephrine is the current vasopressor of choice for spinal hypotension, at least in the elective obstetric setting. There are, however, drawbacks. First, phenylephrine results in decreased CO, although the significance of this is uncertain.[228,259] Second, intravenous phenylephrine has been shown to decrease spinal block height in pregnant[228] and nonpregnant patients.[260] Third, Cooper referred to two case reports of hypertensive crisis involving phenylephrine and atropine, resulting in significant morbidity.[228] It is suggested that hypertension induced by vasopressors is limited by a reflex decrease in HR. Atropine, *in this setting*, can therefore result in hypertensive crisis. Finally, the usual presentation of phenylephrine is highly concentrated (10 mg/mL) and needs to be diluted in a 100-mL bag of saline (100 μg/mL). Anesthesiologists more familiar with ephedrine may find this tiresome or, worse still, may commit a drug concentration error. Moreover, as a usual case requires much less than a 100-mL bag of phenylephrine, there is a risk of cross contamination if bags are reused.

Cardiovascular collapse can occur after spinal anesthesia, although it is a rare event. Auroy and coworkers reported 9 cardiac arrests in 35,439 spinal anesthetics performed.[102] Bradycardia usually precedes cardiac arrest,[236,261-263] and early, aggressive treatment of bradycardia is warranted. Treatment of bradycardia includes intravenous atropine, ephedrine, and epinephrine. In cases of cardiac arrest after spinal anesthesia, epinephrine should be used early, and the Advanced Cardiac Life Support (ACLS) protocol should be initiated.[264]

Further work on spinal-induced hypotension is required. Although treatment is usually aimed at systolic blood pressure,

TABLE 23–9. Phenylephrine Infusion Regimen.

1. Cycle blood pressure measurement at 1-minute intervals until delivery of baby.
2. Prepare phenylephrine solution 0.1 mg/mL: Add 1 ampoule of phenylephrine 10 mg to 100 mL normal saline.
3. Draw this solution into 20- or 50-mL syringe to be delivered via infusion pump.
4. At completion of injection of spinal drug, start phenylephrine infusion at 60 mL per hour.
5. Commence rapid intravenous infusion of 1 L of crystalloid.
6. Subsequent phenylephrine infusion can be given by a variety of regimens:

A. On/off infusion regimen:
For first 2 minutes:
   ON: unless systolic blood pressure was greater than 120% of baseline
Second minute until the time of uterine incision:
   ON: If systolic blood pressure equal to or less than baseline
   OFF: If systolic blood pressure greater than baseline.

B. Sliding scale infusion regimen:

Systolic Blood Pressure (mm Hg)	Infusion rate (mL/h)
≥140	0
≥120	15
≥100	30
≥80	45
≥60	60

Bolus Regimen

Prepare phenylephrine solution 0.1 mg/mL:
Add 1 ampoule of phenylephrine 10 mg to 100 mL normal saline.
Draw this solution into a 10-mL syringe:
   If systolic blood pressure is less than 80%, baseline, give 1 mL together with bolus intravenous field.

Source: Reproduced with permission from Khaw KS, Ngan Kee WD, Lee SW: Hypotension during spinal anaesthesia for Caesarean section: Implications, detection, prevention and treatment. *Fetal Matern Med Rev.* 2006;17(2):157-183.

mean blood pressure may be a better target.[265] Different receptors may also be targeted. For example, prophylactic intravenous ondansetron has been shown to reduce hypotension, perhaps by modulating the BJR.[266] Different patient subpopulations may require different therapies. Most evidence pertains to the elective, healthy obstetric setting, and the extent to which this can be extrapolated to other groups remains to be seen. Last, despite published evidence of the benefits of phenylephrine over ephedrine for elective cesarean section, there is reluctance to change practice.[267] Psychological and institutional barriers to change need to be addressed.

Respiratory Effects of Spinal Anesthesia

In patients with normal lung physiology, spinal anesthesia has little effect on pulmonary function.[268] Lung volumes, resting minute ventilation, dead space, arterial blood gas tensions, and shunt fraction show minimal change after spinal anesthesia. The main respiratory effect of spinal anesthesia occurs during high spinal blockade when active exhalation is affected due to paralysis of abdominal and intercostal muscles. During high spinal blockade, expiratory reserve volume, peak expiratory flow, and maximum minute ventilation are reduced. Patients with obstructive pulmonary disease who rely on accessory muscle use for adequate ventilation should be monitored carefully after spinal blockade. Patients with normal pulmonary function and a high spinal block may complain of dyspnea, but if they are able to speak clearly in a normal voice, ventilation is usually adequate. The dyspnea is usually due to the inability to feel the chest wall move during respiration, and simple assurance is usually effective in allaying the patient's distress.

Clinical Pearls

- Arterial blood gas measurements do not change during high spinal anesthesia in patients who are spontaneously breathing room air.
- Because a high spinal usually does not affect the cervical area, sparing of the phrenic nerve and normal diaphragmatic function occurs, and inspiration is minimally affected.

Arterial blood gas measurements do not change during high spinal anesthesia in patients who are spontaneously breathing room air. The main effect of high spinal anesthesia is on expiration, as the muscles of exhalation are impaired. Because a high spinal usually does not affect the cervical area, sparing of the phrenic nerve and normal diaphragmatic function occurs, and inspiration is minimally affected. Although Steinbrook and colleagues found that spinal anesthesia was not associated with significant changes in vital capacity, maximal inspiratory pressure, or resting end-tidal PCO_2, an increased ventilatory responsiveness to CO_2 with bupivacaine spinal anesthesia was seen.[269]

Gastrointestinal Effects of Spinal Anesthesia

The sympathetic innervation to the abdominal organs arises from T6 to L2. Due to sympathetic blockade and unopposed parasympathetic activity after spinal blockade, secretions increase, sphincters relax, and the bowel becomes constricted.

Increased vagal activity after sympathetic block causes increased peristalsis of the gastrointestinal tract, which can lead to nausea. Nausea may also result from hypotension-induced gut ischemia, which produces serotonin and other emetogenic substances.[46] The incidence of IONV in nonobstetric surgery can be up to 42% and may be as high as 80% in parturients.[46]

Hepatic and Renal Effects of Spinal Anesthesia

Hepatic blood flow correlates to arterial blood flow. There is no autoregulation of hepatic blood flow; thus, as arterial blood flow decreases after spinal anesthesia, so does hepatic blood flow.[270] If the mean arterial pressure (MAP) after placing a spinal anesthetic is maintained, hepatic blood flow will also be maintained. Patients with hepatic disease must be carefully monitored, and their blood pressure must be controlled during anesthesia to maintain hepatic perfusion. No studies have conclusively shown the superiority of regional or general anesthesia in patients with liver disease.[271–275] In patients with liver disease, either regional or general anesthesia can be given, as long as the MAP is kept close to baseline.

Clinical Pearls

- If mean blood pressure is maintained after placing a spinal anesthetic, neither hepatic nor renal blood flow will decrease.
- Spinal anesthesia does not alter autoregulation of renal blood flow.

Renal blood flow is autoregulated. The kidneys remain perfused when the MAP remains above 50 mm Hg. Transient decreases in renal blood flow may occur when MAP is less than 50 mm Hg, but even after long decreases in MAP, renal function returns to normal when blood pressure returns to normal. Again, attention to blood pressure is important after placing a spinal anesthetic, and the MAP should be as close to baseline as possible. Spinal anesthesia does not affect autoregulation of renal blood flow. It has been shown in sheep that renal perfusion changed little after spinal anesthesia.[276–279]

FACTORS AFFECTING LEVEL OF SPINAL BLOCKADE

Many factors have been suggested as possible determinants of spinal blockade level.[144] The four main categories of factors are (1) characteristics of the local anesthetic solution, (2) patient characteristics, (3) technique of spinal blockade, and (4) diffusion. Characteristics of local anesthetic solution include baricity, dose, concentration, and volume injected. Patient characteristics include age, weight, height, gender, intra-abdominal pressure, anatomy of the spinal column, spinal fluid characteristics, and patient position.[280] Techniques of spinal blockade include site of injection, speed of injection, direction of needle bevel, force of injection, and addition of vasoconstrictors. Although all these factors have been postulated as affecting spinal spread of anesthetic, not many have been shown to change the distribution of blockade when all other factors that affect blockade are kept constant.

Site of Injection

The site of injection of local anesthetics for spinal anesthesia can determine the level of blockade. In some studies, isobaric spinal 0.5% bupivacaine produces sensory blockade that is reduced by two dermatomes per interspace when injection at L2–L3, L3–L4, and L4–L5 interspaces are compared.[281,282] However, no difference in block height exists when hyperbaric bupivacaine or dibucaine is injected as a spinal anesthetic in different interspaces.[283–285]

Age

Some studies have reported changes in block height after spinal anesthesia in the elderly patient as compared with the young patient, but other studies have reported no difference in block height.[286–289] These studies were performed with both isobaric and hyperbaric 0.5% bupivacaine.

Clinical Pearl

- Baricity plays a major role in determining block height after spinal anesthesia in older populations.

Isobaric bupivacaine appears to increase block height, and hyperbaric bupivacaine does not appear to change block height with increasing age. If there is a correlation between increasing age and spinal anesthesia height, it is not strong enough by itself to be a reliable predictor in the clinical setting.[290,291] Just as with site of injection, it appears that baricity plays a major role in determining block height after spinal anesthesia in older populations, and age is not an independent factor.

Position

Positioning of the patient is important for determining level of blockade after hyperbaric and hypobaric spinal anesthesia, but not for isobaric solutions. Sitting, Trendelenburg, and prone jackknife positions can greatly change the spread of the local anesthetic due to effect of gravity.[292–294]

Clinical Pearl

- Positioning of the patient is important for determining level of blockade after hyperbaric and hypobaric spinal anesthesia, but not for isobaric solutions.

The combination of baricity of the local anesthetic solution and patient positioning determines spinal block height.[295] The sitting position in combination with a hyperbaric solution can produce analgesia in the perineum. Trendelenburg positioning will also affect spread of hyperbaric and hypobaric local anesthetics due to the effect of gravity.[247,296] Prone jackknife positioning is used for rectal, perineal, and lumbar procedures with a hypobaric local anesthetic.[153,297] This prevents rostral spread of the spinal blockade after injection.

Flexion of the supine patient's hips and knees flattens lumbar lordosis and decreases sacral pooling of local anesthetic. Combined with Trendelenburg positioning, this may help cephalad spread.[298] This position may inadvertently be attained when a urinary catheter is placed after spinal insertion.

Speed of Injection

Speed of injection has been reported to affect spinal block height, but the data available in the literature are conflicting.[299] In studies using isobaric bupivacaine, there is no difference in spinal block height with different speeds of injection.[300–302] Even though spinal block height does not change with speed of injection, a smooth, slow injection should be used when giving a spinal anesthetic. If a forceful injection is given and the syringe is not connected tightly to the spinal needle, the needle might disconnect from the syringe with loss of local anesthetic.

Volume, Concentration, and Dose of Local Anesthetic

It is difficult to maintain volume, concentration, or dose of local anesthetic constant without changing any of the other variables; thus, it is difficult to produce high-quality studies that investigate these variables singly. Axelsson and associates showed that volume of local anesthetic can affect spinal block height and duration when equivalent doses are used.[303]

Peng and coworkers showed that concentration of local anesthetic is directly related to dose when determining effective anesthesia.[304] However, dose of local anesthetic plays the greatest role in determining spinal block duration, as neither volume nor concentration of isobaric bupivacaine or tetracaine alter spinal block duration when the dose is held constant.[305,306] Studies have repeatedly shown that spinal block duration is longer when higher doses of local anesthetic are given.[148,303,307–309] When performing a spinal anesthetic, be cognizant of not only the dose of local anesthetic but also the volume and concentration so the patient is not overdosed or underdosed.

The use of hyperbaric solutions minimizes the importance of dose and volume except when doses of hyperbaric bupivacaine equal to or less than 10 mg are used. In those cases, there is less cephalad spread and a shorter duration of action.[293] A dose of hyperbaric bupivacaine between 10 and 20 mg results in similar block height.[283] When using hyperbaric solutions, it is important to note that patient positioning and baricity are the most influential factors on block height, except when low doses of hyperbaric bupivacaine are used.

EQUIPMENT FOR SPINAL ANESTHESIA

Maintaining Asepsis

No single intervention guarantees asepsis. Therefore, a multiprong approach is advisable.

In the past, most institutions had reusable trays for spinal anesthesia. These trays required preparation by anesthesiologists or anesthesia personnel to ensure that bacterial and chemical contamination would not occur. Currently, commercially prepared, disposable spinal trays are available and are in use by most institutions. These trays are portable, sterile, and easy to use. Figure 23–9 shows the contents of a standard, commercially prepared spinal anesthetic tray.

The ideal skin preparation solution should be bactericidal and have a quick onset and long duration. Chlorhexidine is superior to povidone iodine in all these respects.[114] In addition, the ideal agent should not be neurotoxic. Unfortunately, bactericidal agents are neurotoxic. It is therefore prudent to use the lowest effective concentration and allow the preparation to dry. Although subject to debate, 0.5% chlorhexidine in alcohol 70% is currently recommended by some groups.[310] Contamination of equipment with skin preparation can theoretically lead to the introduction of neurotoxic substances into neural tissue. Of more concern is accidental neuraxial injection of antiseptic solution, possibly from antiseptic solution and local anesthetic being placed in adjacent pots. Therefore, after skin preparation, unused antiseptic should be discarded before commencement of the procedure (and intrathecal drugs should be drawn directly from sterile ampules). Tinted antiseptic solutions may decrease the likelihood of drug error and allow easy identification of missed skin during application.

Proving a benefit of individual infection control measures is difficult due to the rarity of infectious complications. Past evidence has been contradictory. For example, it has been suggested that shedding of skin scales from mask "wiggling" may occur,[311] increasing bacterial contamination. Yet, in 1995 there were calls for

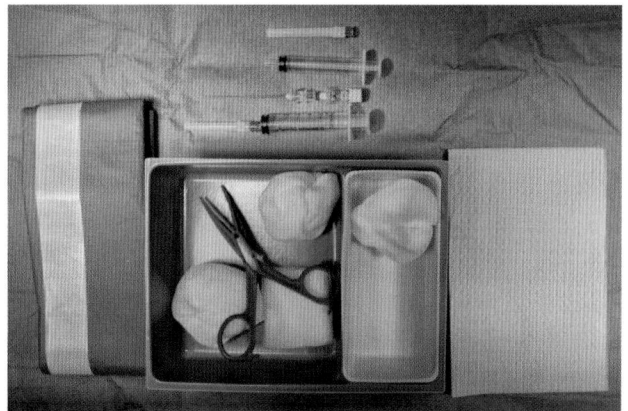

FIGURE 23–9. Contents of a standard, commercially prepared spinal anesthetic tray.

routine face mask use after it was unambiguously proven, using polymerase chain reaction (PCR) fingerprinting, that a case of *Streptococcus salivarius* meningitis originated in the throat of the doctor who had performed a lumbar puncture.[312] It is our strong belief that face mask wearing should be mandatory when performing spinal anesthesia. A 2006 American Society of Regional Anesthesia and Pain Medicine (ASRA) practice advisory recommended mask wearing in addition to removing jewelry, thorough hand washing, and sterile surgical gloves for all regional anesthesia techniques. Major components of an aseptic technique also included a surgical hat and sterile draping.[313] Other international professional bodies have similar guidelines.[314]

Prophylactic antibiotics are unnecessary for spinal anesthesia. If, as it happens, antibiotic prophylaxis is required for the prevention of surgical site infection, it may be prudent to administer antibiotics before insertion of a spinal needle.

The reader is referred to Chapter 16 (Infection Control in Regional Anesthesia) for more information.

Resuscitation and Monitoring

Resuscitation equipment must be available whenever a spinal anesthetic is performed. This includes equipment and medication required to secure an airway, provide ventilation, and support cardiac function. All patients receiving spinal anesthesia should have an intravenous line.

The patient must be monitored during the placement of the spinal anesthetic with a pulse oximeter, blood pressure cuff, and ECG. Fetal monitoring should be used in the case of a pregnant patient. Noninvasive blood pressure should be measured at 1-minute intervals initially, as hypotension may be sudden. Shivering and body habitus may make noninvasive blood pressure measurement difficult. Consideration should be given to invasive blood pressure monitoring if the patient has significant cardiovascular disease.

Needles

Needles of different diameters and shapes have been developed for spinal anesthesia. The ones currently used have a close-fitting, removable stylet, which prevents skin and adipose tissue from plugging the needle and possibly entering the subarachnoid space. Figure 23–10 shows the different types of needles used along with the type of point at the end of the needle.

The pencil-point needles (Sprotte and Whitacre) have a rounded, noncutting bevel with a solid tip. The opening is located on the side of the needle 2–4 mm proximal to the tip of the needle. The needles with cutting bevels include the Quincke and Pitkin needles. The Quincke needle has a sharp point with a medium-length cutting needle, and the Pitkin has a sharp point and short bevel with cutting edges. Finally, the Greene spinal needle has a rounded point and rounded noncutting bevel. If a continuous spinal catheter is to be placed, a Tuohy needle can be used to find the subarachnoid space before placement of the catheter.

Pencil-point needles provide a better tactile sensation of the layers of ligament encountered but require more force to insert than bevel-tip needles. The bevel of the needle should be

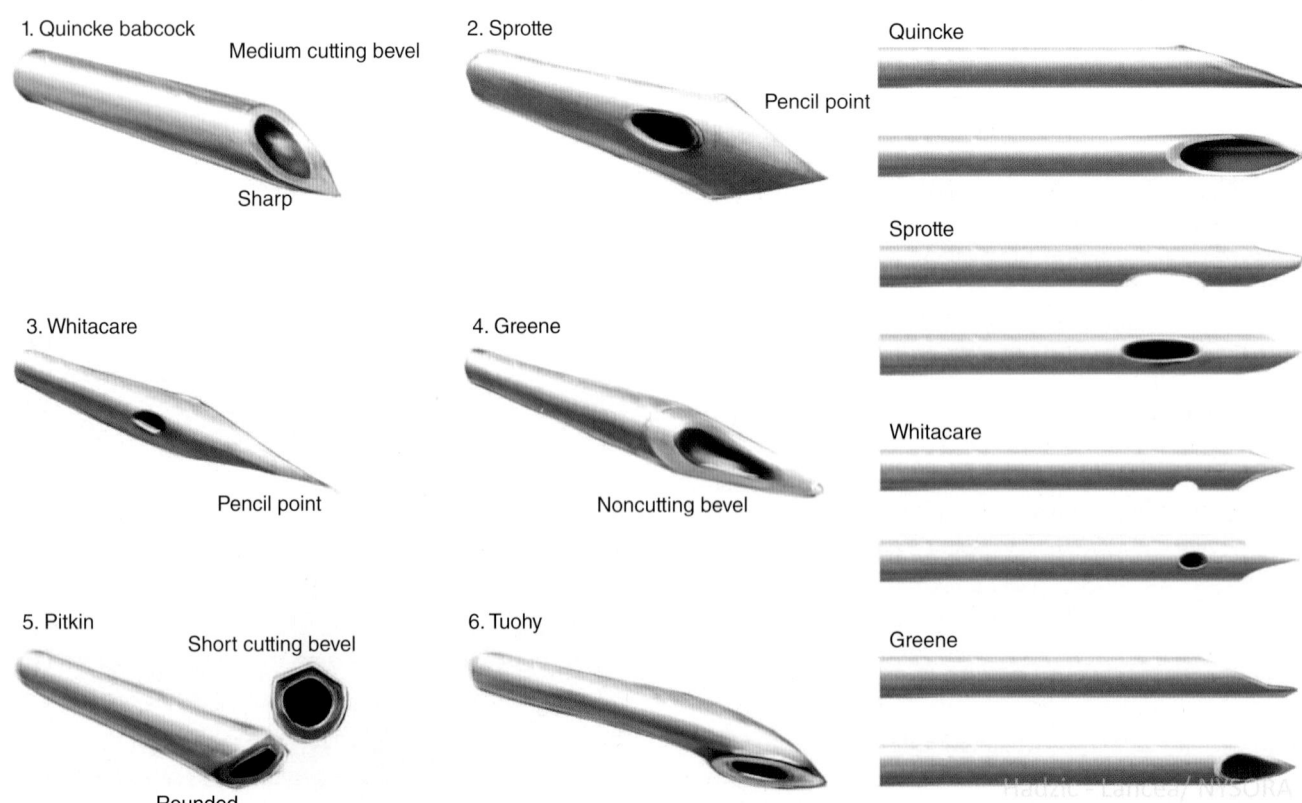

FIGURE 23–10. Different types of needles.

directed longitudinally to decrease the incidence of PDPH.[315] Small-gauge needles and needles with rounded, noncutting bevels also decrease the incidence of PDPH but are more easily deflected than larger-gauge needles. The reader is referred to Chapter 6 (Ultrastructural Anatomy of the Spinal Meninges and Related Structures) and Chapter 23 (Postdural Puncture Headache).

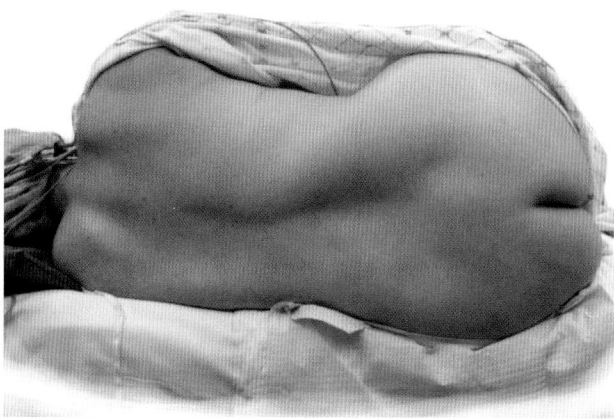

FIGURE 23–11. Patient in lateral decubitus position.

Clinical Pearls

- Pencil-point needles provide a better tactile sensation of the layers of ligament encountered but require more force to insert than bevel-tip needles.
- The use of introducers help preventing the passage of epidermic contaminants to the CSF.

Introducers have been designed to assist with the placement of spinal needles into the subarachnoid space due to the difficulty in directing needles of small bore through the tissues. Introducers also serve to prevent contamination of the CSF with small pieces of epidermis, which could lead to the formation of dermoid spinal cord tumors. The introducer is placed into the interspinous ligament in the intended direction of the spinal needle, and the spinal needle is then placed through the introducer.

POSITION OF THE PATIENT

Proper positioning of the patient for spinal anesthesia is essential for a fast, successful block. It has been shown to be an independent predictor for successful first attempt at neuraxial block.[316] Many factors come into play for positioning of the patient. Before beginning the procedure, both the patient and the anesthesiologist should be comfortable. This includes positioning the height of the operating room table, providing adequate blankets or covers for the patient, ensuring a comfortable room temperature, and providing sedation for the patient if required. Personnel trained in positioning patients are invaluable, and commercial positioning devices may be useful.

When providing sedation, it is important to avoid oversedation. The patient should be able to cooperate before, during, and after administration of the spinal anesthetic. There are three main positions for administering a spinal anesthetic: the lateral decubitus, sitting, and prone positions.

Lateral Decubitus Position

A commonly used position for placing a spinal anesthetic is the lateral decubitus position. Ideal positioning consists of having the back of the patient parallel to the edge of the bed closest to the anesthesiologist, with the patient's knees flexed to the abdomen and neck flexed. Figure 23–11 shows a patient in the lateral decubitus position.

It is beneficial to have an assistant to help hold and encourage the patient to stay in this position. Depending on the operative site and operative position, a hypo-, iso-, or hyperbaric solution of local anesthetic can be injected.

Clinical Pearls

- A commonly used position for placing a spinal anesthetic is the lateral decubitus position.
- Ideal positioning consists of having the back of the patient parallel to the edge of the bed closest to the anesthesiologist, knees flexed to the abdomen, and neck flexed.

Sitting Position and "Saddle Block"

Strictly speaking, the sitting position is best utilized for low lumbar or sacral anesthesia and in instances when the patient is obese and there is difficulty in finding the midline. In practice, however, many anesthesiologists prefer the sitting position in all patients who can be positioned this way. The sitting position avoids the potential rotation of the spine that can occur with the lateral decubitus position. Using a stool for a footrest and a pillow for the patient to hold can be valuable in this position. The patient should flex the neck and push out the lower back to open up the lumbar intervertebral spaces. Figure 23–12 depicts a patient in the sitting position, and the L4–L5 interspace is marked.

When performing a "saddle block," the patient should remain in the sitting position for at least 5 minutes after a hyperbaric spinal anesthetic is placed to allow the spinal anesthetic to settle into that region. If a higher level of blockade is necessary, the patient should be placed supine immediately after spinal placement and the table adjusted accordingly.

Clinical Pearls

- The sitting position is utilized for low lumbar or sacral anesthesia and in instances when the patient is obese and there is difficulty in finding the midline in the lateral position.
- When performing a saddle block, the patient should remain in the sitting position for at least 5 min after a hyperbaric spinal anesthetic is placed to allow the spinal to settle into that region.

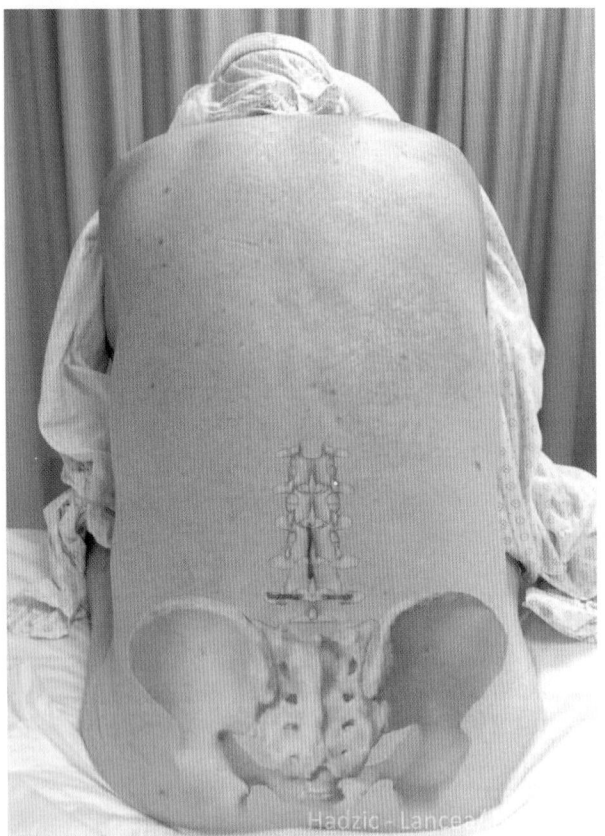

FIGURE 23–12. Patient in sitting position with the L4–L5 interspace marked.

Prone Position

The prone position can be utilized for induction of spinal anesthesia if the patient needs to be in this position for the surgery, such as for rectal, perineal, or lumbar procedures. A hypobaric or isobaric solution of local anesthetic is preferred in the prone jackknife position for these procedures. This avoids rostral spread of the local anesthetic and decreases the risk of high spinal anesthesia.

Clinical Pearl

- The prone position is utilized for spinal anesthesia if the patient needs to be in this position for the surgery, such as for rectal, perineal, or lumbar procedures.

Another, less-elegant solution is to inject a hyperbaric solution of local anesthetic with the patient in the *sitting* position and wait until the spinal anesthesia "sets in," which is typically 15–20 minutes after injection. The patient is then positioned in the prone position with vigilant monitoring, including frequent verbal communication with the patient.

TECHNIQUE OF LUMBAR PUNCTURE

When performing a spinal anesthetic, appropriate monitors should be placed, and airway and resuscitation equipment should be readily available. All equipment for the spinal blockade should be ready for use, and all necessary medications should be drawn up prior to positioning the patient for spinal anesthesia. Adequate preparation for the spinal reduces the amount of time needed to perform the block and assists with making the patient comfortable.

Proper positioning is the key to making the spinal anesthetic quick and successful. Once the patient is correctly positioned, the midline should be palpated. The iliac crests are palpated, and a line is drawn between them to find the body of L4 or the L4–L5 interspace. Other interspaces can be identified, depending on where the needle is to be inserted.

The skin should be cleaned with skin preparation solution such as 0.5% chlorhexidine, and the area should be draped in a sterile fashion. The skin preparation solution should be allowed to dry, and unused skin preparation solution must be removed from the anesthesiologist's workspace. A small wheal of local anesthetic is injected into the skin at the planned site of insertion. More local anesthetic is then administered along the intended path of the spinal needle insertion to the estimated depth of the supraspinous ligament. This serves a dual purpose: additional anesthesia for the spinal needle insertion and identification of the correct path for spinal needle placement. Care must be taken in thin patients to avoid dural puncture, and inadvertent spinal anesthesia, at this stage.

Clinical Pearls

- When performing a spinal anesthetic, appropriate monitors should be placed, and airway and resuscitation equipment should be readily available.
- All equipment for the spinal blockade should be ready for use, and all necessary medications should be drawn up prior to positioning the patient for spinal anesthesia.

Midline Approach

If the midline approach is used, palpate the desired interspace and inject local anesthetic into the skin and subcutaneous tissue. The introducer needle is placed with a slight cephalad angle of 10° to 15°. Next, the spinal needle is passed through the introducer. The needle passes through the subcutaneous tissue, supraspinous ligament, interspinous ligament, ligamentum flavum, epidural space, dura mater, and subarachnoid mater to reach the subarachnoid space.

Resistance changes as the spinal needle passes through each level on the way to the subarachnoid space. Subcutaneous tissue offers less resistance to the spinal needle than ligaments. When the spinal needle goes though the dura mater, a "pop" is often appreciated. Once this pop is felt, the stylet should be removed from the needle to check for flow of CSF. For spinal needles of higher gauge (26–29 gauge), this usually takes 5–10 seconds, but in some patients, it can take a minute or longer. If there is no flow, some suggest rotating the needle 90° as the needle orifice might be obstructed. Debris can obstruct the orifice of the spinal needle. If necessary, withdraw the needle and clear the orifice before attempting the spinal anesthetic again. A common cause of failure to obtain CSF flow is the spinal needle being off the midline. The midline should be reassessed and the needle repositioned.

If the spinal needle contacts bone, the depth of the needle should be noted and the needle placed more cephalad. If bone is contacted again, the needle depth should be compared with that of the last bone contact to determine what structure is being contacted. For instance, if bone contact is deeper than the first insertion, the needle should be redirected more cephalad to avoid the inferior spinous process. If bone contact is at roughly the same depth as the original insertion, it may be lamina being contacted, and the midline should be reassessed. If bone contact is shallower than the original insertion, the needle should be redirected caudally to avoid the superior spinous process.

Clinical Pearls

- When the spinal needle goes though the dura mater, a "pop" is often appreciated.
- Once this pop is felt, the stylet should be removed from the introducer to check for flow of CSF.
- For spinal needles of a higher gauge (26–29 gauge), this usually takes 5–10 seconds, but in some patients, it can take longer.
- If there is no flow, the needle might be obstructed by a nerve root and rotating it 90° may be helpful.

When the spinal needle needs to be reinserted, it is important to withdraw the needle back to the skin level before redirection. Only make small changes in the angle of direction when reinserting the spinal needle as small changes at the surface lead to large changes in direction when the needle reaches greater depths. Bowing and curving of the spinal needle when inserting through the skin or introducer can also steer the needle off course when attempting to contact the subarachnoid space.

Paresthesias may be elicited when passing a spinal needle. The stylet should be removed from the spinal needle, and if CSF is seen and the paresthesia is no longer present, it is safe to inject the local anesthetic. A cauda equina nerve root may have been encountered. If there is no CSF flow, it is possible that the spinal needle has contacted a spinal nerve root traversing the epidural space. The needle should be removed and redirected toward the side opposite the paresthesia.

After free flow of CSF is established, inject the local anesthetic slowly at a speed of less than 0.5 mL/s. Additional aspiration of CSF at the midpoint and end of injection can be attempted to confirm continued subarachnoid administration but may not always be possible when small needles are used. Once local anesthetic injection is complete, the introducer and spinal needle are removed as one unit from the back of the patient. The patient should then be positioned according to the surgical procedure and baricity of local anesthetic given. The table can be tilted in either the Trendelenburg or the reverse Trendelenburg position as needed to adjust the height of the block after testing the sensory level. The anesthesiologist should carefully monitor and support vital signs.

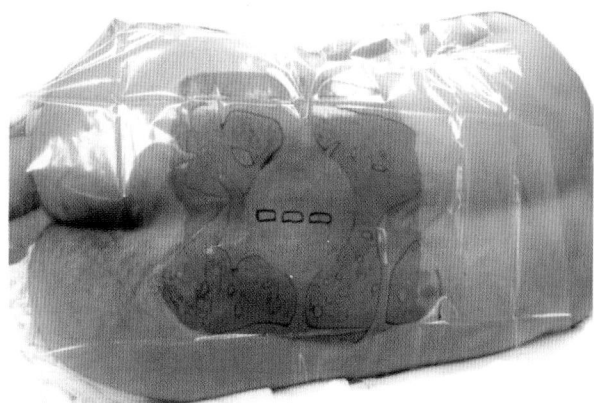

FIGURE 23–13. Landmarks used in a paramedian approach to spinal anesthesia.

Paramedian (Lateral) Approach

If the patient has a calcified interspinous ligament or difficulty in flexing the spine, a paramedian approach to achieve spinal anesthesia can be utilized. The patient can be in any position for this approach: sitting, lateral, or even prone jackknife. After palpating the superior and inferior lumbar spinous processes of the desired interspace, local anesthetic is infiltrated 1 cm lateral to the superior aspect of the inferior spinous process. The needle should be directed slightly medially. A 10° and 15° medial angulation of the needle will reach the midline at a depth of about 5.7 cm (tan 80°) and 3.7 cm (tan 75°), respectively. This demonstrates that small changes in angulation can have pronounced effects on needle-tip placement. Although slight cephalad angulation is also required, a common error is too steep an initial approach. If lamina is contacted, the needle should then be angled cephalad and "walked off" the lamina into the subarachnoid space.

Other methods have been described. All techniques involve a similar vertical axis for the puncture site (1–1.5 cm from the midline). They differ in the horizontal axis (eg, 1 cm lateral to the spinous process, 1 cm lateral to the interspace, 1 cm lateral and 1 cm inferior to the interspace, 1 cm lateral and 1 cm inferior to the inferior aspect of the superior spinous process) and the degree of cephalad angulation required.

Figure 23–13 shows the landmarks used for a paramedian approach to spinal anesthesia. Figure 23–14 depicts successful performance of a paramedian spinal anesthetic.

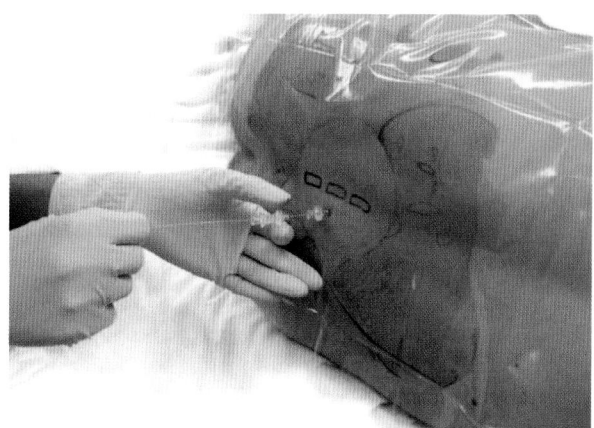

FIGURE 23–14. Paramedian approach: needle placement.

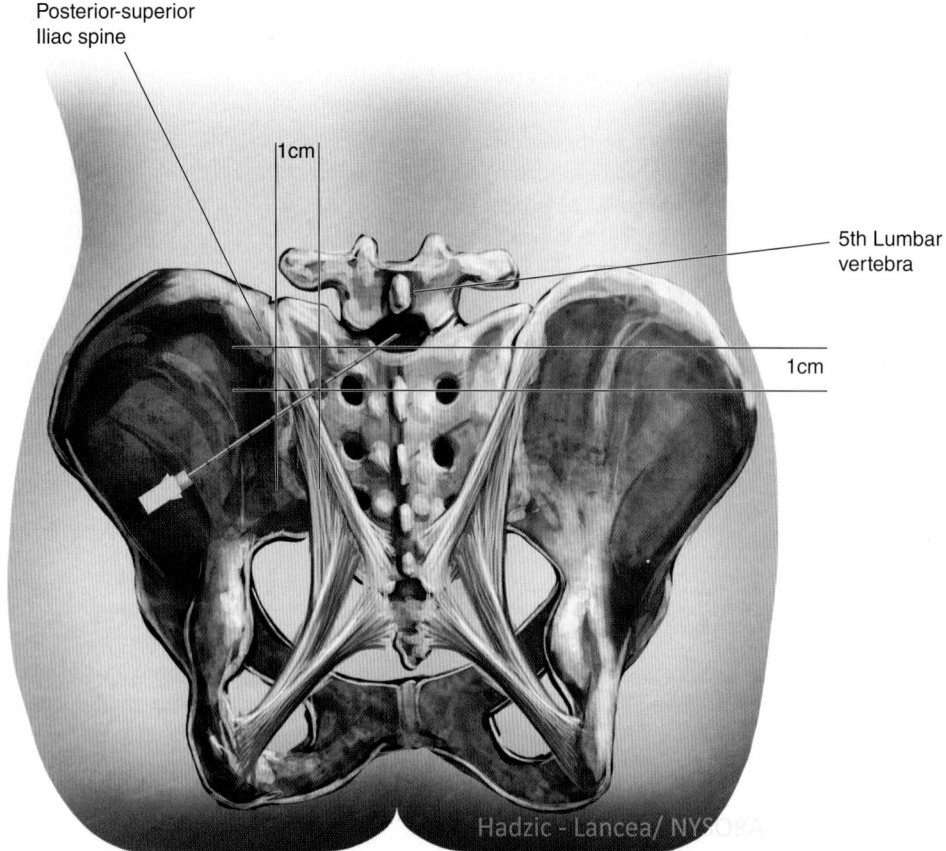

Posterior-superior
Iliac spine

1cm

5th Lumbar
vertebra

1cm

Hadzic - Lancea/ NYSORA

FIGURE 23–15. Taylor approach to spinal anesthesia.

Clinical Pearls

For the paramedian approach:

- After palpating the superior and inferior lumbar spinous processes of the desired interspace, local anesthetic is infiltrated 1 cm lateral to the superior aspect of the inferior spinous process.
- The needle should be angled in a slight medial and cephalad direction.
- If lamina is contacted, the needle should then be angled cephalad and "walked off" the lamina into the subarachnoid space.
- The ligamentum flavum is usually the first resistance identified.

Taylor Approach

The Taylor, or lumbosacral, approach to spinal anesthesia is a paramedian approach directed toward the L5–S1 interspace. Because this is the largest interspace, the Taylor approach can be used when other approaches are not successful or cannot be performed. As with the paramedian approach, the patient can be in any position for this approach: sitting, lateral, or prone.

The needle should be inserted at a point 1 cm medial and inferior to the posterior superior iliac spine, then angled cephalad 45°–55° and medially. This angle should be medial enough to

reach the midline at the L5–S1 interspace. After needle insertion, the first significant resistance felt is the ligamentum flavum, and then the dura mater is punctured to allow free flow of CSF as the subarachnoid space is entered. Figure 23–15 shows the Taylor approach to spinal anesthesia. Real-time ultrasound-guided prone spinal anesthesia via the Taylor approach has been described[317] and may improve patient comfort and compliance during the procedure.

Clinical Pearls

For the Taylor approach:

- The needle should be inserted at a point 1 cm medial and inferior to the posterior superior iliac spine, then angled cephalad 45°–55° and medially.
- This angle should be medial enough to reach the midline at the L5–S1 interspace.
- After needle insertion, the first significant resistance felt is the ligamentum flavum.

CONTINUOUS CATHETER TECHNIQUES

An indwelling catheter can be placed for continuous spinal anesthesia. Local anesthetics can be dosed repeatedly through the catheter and the level and duration of anesthesia adjusted as necessary for the surgical procedure. Placement of a continuous spinal catheter occurs in a similar fashion as a regular spinal anesthetic except that a larger-gauge needle, such as a Tuohy, is used to enable the passage of the catheter. After insertion of the Tuohy needle, the subarachnoid space is found, and the spinal catheter is passed 2–3 cm into the subarachnoid space. If there is difficulty in passing the catheter, attempt to rotate the Tuohy needle 180°. Never withdraw the catheter back into the needle shaft because there is a risk of shearing the catheter and leaving a piece of it in the subarachnoid space. If the catheter needs to be withdrawn, withdraw the catheter and needle together and attempt the continuous spinal at another interspace. Communication is critical to avoid a spinal catheter being mistaken for the more common epidural catheter. This involves labeling, documentation, handover, and vigilance.

Clinical Pearls

- After insertion of the Tuohy needle, the subarachnoid space is entered and the spinal catheter is passed 2–3 cm into the subarachnoid space.
- If there is difficulty in passing the catheter, attempt to rotate the Tuohy needle 180°.
- Communication is critical to avoid a spinal catheter being mistaken for the more common epidural catheter.

Because the needle used to pass the spinal catheter is a large-bore needle, there is a much higher risk of PDPH, especially in young female patients. Cauda equina syndrome can occur with small spinal catheters, so the FDA has advised against using catheters smaller than 24 gauge for continuous spinal anesthetics.[85–88,318]

In 2008, a randomized clinical trial (FDA Investigational Device Exemption) reported on the safety of continuous spinal "microcatheters" in obstetric patients. A 28-gauge catheter was placed in 329 patients; there were no reported permanent neurological outcomes. The trial compared continuous spinal analgesia with epidural analgesia and found lower initial pain scores, higher patient satisfaction, and less motor block in the spinal group, with no difference in neonatal or obstetric outcomes.[319] However, the spinal group had higher pruritis scores and a trend toward more PDPH (9% compared with 4% in the epidural group). Intrathecal catheters were more difficult to remove than epidural catheters. One patient had an intrathecal catheter broken on removal, albeit by an untrained individual, leaving a fragment in the patient's back.

CLINICAL SITUATIONS ENCOUNTERED IN THE PRACTICE OF SPINAL ANESTHESIA

The Difficult and Failed Spinal

Spinal anesthesia has long been considered a reliable block, with failure rates less than 1%. Conversion to general anesthesia was as low as 0.5% in a prospective cohort study of obstetric patients.[320] However, failure rates as high as 17%

have been reported.[321] Failed spinal anesthesia may present as complete absence of block, partial block, or inadequate duration of block.

Although expertise may reduce the chance of a failed spinal, even experienced clinicians will be confronted with failed spinal blocks. After being reassured by the appearance of CSF, a subsequent failed or patchy block can leave an anesthesiologist frustrated and bewildered. A methodical approach is required when managing failed spinal blockade.

In an excellent review article, Fettes et al classified failure of spinal anesthesia into five groups: failure of lumbar puncture, failure of solution injection, solution spread in the CSF, drug action on the nerve roots and cord, and patient management.[298] Their review is summarized next.

Failed Lumbar Puncture

Whenever there are problems with placing a spinal anesthetic, the anesthesiologist should reassess the position of the patient. A member of the operating room personnel who is trained to assist with patient positioning should be used. Alternatively, positioning of the patient can be enhanced with commercially available positioning devices. These devices can help maintain spinal flexion and create a stable support for the patient, which can be useful if no trained operating room personnel are available to assist with positioning.

If the proposed interspace cannot be found, the interspace above or below the original site of spinal injection can be attempted. When the sitting position cannot be used or is unsuccessful, the lateral decubitus position can be used. Either the midline or the lateral paramedian technique can be attempted. The largest interlaminar space is at L5, and this can be sought via Taylor's approach, described previously in this chapter.

Three independent predictors of success when performing neuraxial block have been identified: adequate positioning, the anesthesiologist's experience, and the ability to palpate anatomical landmarks.[316] Improper positioning may be due to patients' inability to flex the spine rather than anesthesiologists' failure to encourage flexion. A predictably difficult back should not be used to teach inexperienced trainees. If anatomical landmarks are imperceptible spinal ultrasonography can be used to assist lumbar puncture (see section on neuraxial ultrasound).

Failure of Solution Injection

Because of the small volumes of injectate used in spinal anesthesia, apparently trivial reductions in the volume of solution may result in a less-than-adequate block. Reductions in solution injected may be the result of loss of injectate when the spinal syringe is attached to the needle hub or loss into tissues adjacent to the subarachnoid space due to needle orifice migration or the orifice straddling a number of potential spaces (eg, the subarachnoid and subdural or epidural spaces). Intentional reductions in dose, usually to decrease side effects, may also result in decreased efficacy.[254]

Failure of Solution Spread Within the CSF

Failure of solution spread within the CSF may be due to spinal deformities such as kyphosis or scoliosis, previous surgery, transverse or longitudinal spinal septae, spinal stenosis, or extradural cysts. Tarlov cysts are a type of extradural cyst seen incidentally on MRI scans and have an incidence as high as 9%. Although usually asymptomatic, they contain CSF and may account for positive aspiration of CSF yet failure of complete block.[322] Lumbar CSF volume is an important determinant of spread.[156]

Failure of Drug Action

Failure of drug action may result from the incorrect drug being administered. The correct drug may be inactive as the result of physicochemical instability (less likely with modern agents) or may be impaired due to chemical incompatibilities when two or more agents are used. The phenomenon of local anesthetic resistance has been questioned in the literature.

Failure of Patient Management

Descartes's classic 17th-century picture of pain showing a connection between a boy's burning foot and his brain via the middle of his back—"just as when you pull one end of a string, you cause a bell hanging at the other end to ring"—could lead one to believe spinal anesthesia can cure all pain. However, pain perception is far more complex, and despite perfect spinal blockade, a patient may experience discomfort or pain. Patients should be counseled preoperatively about expected "normal" sensations such as pulling, pushing, and stretching. Preoperative testing of spinal blockade to reassure both the patient and the anesthesiologist may paradoxically distress the patient if performed too early. Intraoperatively, a patient may require supplemental anxiolysis and analgesia or general anesthesia.

Management of a failed spinal block will depend on whether it occurs preoperatively or intraoperatively and the nature of the failure. Options to optimize spinal anesthesia include changing the patient's position to improve spread and repeating the spinal block. Two important principles must be remembered when repeating a spinal block. First, the second attempt must not be identical to the first. This is not only to avoid a repeat failure but also perhaps to prevent a second dose of local anesthetic accumulating in a restricted space, which can lead to neurological injury. Second, a repeat dose may result in excessive spread of local anesthetic. Alternatives such as epidural anesthesia, peripheral nerve blockade, local infiltration, systemic analgesia, and general anesthesia should be considered based on the merits of the case and are beyond the scope of this chapter.

Inadvertent Subdural Block

Failed subarachnoid block may be the result of inadvertent subdural injection and deserves special attention. The subdural space is a potential space that only becomes real after tearing of neurothelial cells within the space[127] as a result of iatrogenic needle insertion and fluid injection (see Figure 23–4). Characteristic features of a SDB are a high sensory level with motor and sympathetic sparing. This may be the result of the limited ventral capacity of the space, which results in sparing of the anterior motor and sympathetic fibers. However, a SDB may also present in a number of different ways: failed block, unilateral block, Horner syndrome, trigeminal nerve palsy, respiratory insufficiency, or unconsciousness due to brainstem involvement.[126] Onset of nerve blockade is slower than subarachnoid block but faster than epidural block and usually resolves after 2 hours.

The incidence of subdural injection after contrast myelography ranges between 1% and 13%. The incidence of SDB after attempted spinal anesthesia is unknown.[126] Because the dura is intentionally breached during attempted spinal anesthesia, the incidence of SDB may be higher compared with epidural block (variously quoted as between 0.024% and 0.82%). The size of the acquired subdural space is probably proportional to the volume of fluid injected. Therefore, typical volumes used with spinal anesthesia may not be as significant as volumes used with epidural anesthesia.[323]

Outpatient Spinal Anesthesia

Each year, the number of surgeries increase, and more are performed on an outpatient basis. As anesthesiologists, we are always looking for new ways to provide efficient anesthetic care that is safe, controls pain, allows the patient to be discharged home in a timely fashion as per postanesthesia care unit protocol, and is easily performed and reproducible. It has previously been suggested that spinal anaesthesia may be incorporated into the outpatient surgery model.[324]

Unilateral Spinal Block

Use of a unilateral spinal block for elderly patients and outpatient surgery has undergone a resurgence. Unilateral spinal anesthesia was described in 1950 by Ruben and Kamsler. Their report concerned 116 patients for surgical reduction of hip fracture performed under unilateral spinal blockade.[325] No deaths were reported, and no increase in the hazard of operation was found. Recently, attention has returned to the use of unilateral spinal anesthesia in elderly patients[326] and for outpatient surgery.[327]

Use of unilateral spinal anesthesia results in decreased changes in systolic, mean and diastolic pressures, or oxygen saturation in elderly trauma patients (eg, hip fracture). Keeping the operative side up and using a hypobaric spinal solution in a low dose for these cases results in excellent anesthesia and remarkable hemostability when the patient is kept in the lateral position for 5–10 minutes before repositioning supine. When using hyperbaric solutions, the operative side should be dependent.

Outpatient surgery using hyperbaric 0.5% bupivacaine takes about 16 minutes for development of surgical anesthesia from time of injection with unilateral spinal anesthesia and 13 minutes with traditional bilateral spinal anesthesia. Less hemodynamic changes are found in the unilateral spinal anesthesia group, with quicker regression of the block and equal time to discharge home.[328]

Compared with other outpatient surgery, less motor block is required for knee arthroscopy. Doses of hyperbaric bupivacaine as low as 4–5 mg are effective when combined with unilateral positioning. Higher doses delay recovery. Addition of intrathecal opioids improves analgesia but increases opioid-related side effects. Ropivacaine does not improve recovery time.[329]

In performing unilateral spinal anesthesia, use of a pencil-point 25-gauge or 27-gauge needle with the orifice directed at the operative side is suggested. Low-dose bupivacaine should be used, with hyperbaric bupivacaine (operative side down) in outpatient surgery and hypobaric bupivacaine (operative side up) in the elderly trauma patient.[330] A slow injection rate should be used to produce laminar flow that will assist in producing a unilateral blockade. There is little evidence that keeping a patient in the lateral position for more than 15 minutes is helpful.

The Obstetric Patient

In 1901, Kreis described the first spinal anesthetic for vaginal delivery.[331] The following year, Hopkins performed the first successful spinal anesthetic for cesarean section in a woman with placenta previa.[229] Spinal anesthesia for labor and delivery has progressed greatly since that time. Although many arguments are made against general anesthesia in the pregnant woman due to increased risk of aspiration and difficult intubation, the anesthesiologist must be prepared to induce general anesthesia in the face of a failed or total spinal anesthetic.

Obstetric regional anesthesia is a topic in itself, and as such is covered in Chapter 41 (Obstetric Regional Anesthesia). Examples of how spinal anesthesia differs in the obstetric population are listed in Table 23–10.

The Anticoagulated Patient

As the population ages, more patients are presenting for surgery with pre-, intra-, or postoperative requirements for antiplatelet, anticoagulant, or thrombolytic therapy. Novel agents continue to be developed, giving rise to concerns in patients undergoing spinal anesthesia. These concerns led to the evolution of the ASRA evidence-based guidelines on regional anesthesia in the patient receiving antithrombotic or thrombolytic therapy, now up to its third edition.[332]

The reader is referred to Chapter 52 (Neuraxial Anesthesia and Peripheral Nerve Blocks in Patients on Anticoagulants) for an in-depth discussion on the use of neuraxial anesthesia in the anticoagulated patient.

Other Clinical Situations

Spinal anesthesia in the pediatric patient and the patient with preexisting neurology are covered in Chapters 43 and 49, respectively.

RECENT DEVELOPMENTS IN SPINAL ANESTHESIA

Neuraxial Ultrasound

Conventional palpation of surface anatomy has been shown to be unreliable.[128,132] Neuraxial ultrasound aims to overcome the inaccuracies of surface anatomy with sonoanatomy. The first

description of ultrasound-assisted lumbar puncture[333] was in 1971. More recently, neuraxial ultrasound has been used as a preprocedure scan and for real-time needle placement. Much of the evidence regarding neuraxial ultrasound pertains to preprocedural scanning prior to epidural insertion, especially in the setting of obstetric anesthesia, and has been produced by a limited number of specialized centers. This evidence shows that scanning decreases needle attempts, accurately predicts depth to the epidural space, and may improve the success rate of junior trainees.[334–336]

Spinal ultrasonography in the setting of single-shot spinal anesthesia is less well studied. Ultrasonography allows increased accuracy at identifying lumbar interspaces.[334] This is important as palpation of the lumbar spine is likely to generate a higher interspace than expected,[128] and the conus medullaris has been shown to be at times lower than the conventionally taught L1 level. These two facts not only pose a theoretical risk but also have resulted in persistent neurological injury.[132] An observational study in orthopedic patients demonstrated accurate ultrasonographic prediction of the depth to the dura prior to spinal insertion.[337] Preprocedural ultrasonography has been used to achieve spinal anesthesia in clinically difficult situations such as obesity, kyphoscoliosis, and previous spinal surgery, including Harrington rods.[41–43,338] Real-time ultrasound-guided spinal anesthesia has been described in technically difficult patients[339] and in the prone position via Taylor's approach.[317] A randomized trial comparing preprocedural scanning with standard palpation for spinal anesthesia in patients with difficult surface anatomical landmarks showed a twofold difference in first attempt success (62% ultrasound vs. 32% control).[340]

Ultrasound scanning of the neuraxis is best learned in tailored workshops and simulations. Real-time ultrasound advancement of a spinal needle into the subarachnoid space is an expert skill, and practitioners should possess considerable probe and needle skills. Preprocedure scanning and marking of a patient's back require less hand-eye coordination but may also be difficult to learn.[341] Competence at identifying designated spinous processes has been achieved after scanning 22–36 patients.[342] Here, we outline six sonoanatomical views of the lumbar spine and a simplified method for performing a neuraxial preprocedure scan and outline common beginner pitfalls.

Sonoanatomy

Different researchers have described varying numbers of necessary sonographic views, often associated with fanciful monikers. Karmakar refers to "horse heads," "camel humps," and "trident" signs (longitudinal paramedian views), whereas Carvalho refers to a "saw" (longitudinal view) and a "flying bat" (transverse view).[343] The novice should not become bewildered by the varying nomenclature, as they are simply tools of pattern recognition.

Specialized ultrasonic windows are required to visualize the neuraxis due to the bony structures that encase it. Six basic views are shown in Table 23–11.

The anterior and posterior complexes are useful terms for identifying structures. The anterior complex represents the *anterior* dura, posterior longitudinal ligament, and posterior vertebral body. The posterior complex represents the

TABLE 23–10. Spinal anesthesia in the obstetric patient.

Consent	• May be difficult to obtain truly informed consent in a laboring patient.
Risks	• Lower risk of major permanent complications compared with neuraxial blockade for nonobstetric surgery.[26] • Higher risk of postdural puncture headache. • A 2005 meta-analysis showed cord pH, an indicator of fetal well-being, to be lower with spinal compared with epidural and general anesthesia, although this may be attributed to the use of ephedrine in the studies analyzed.[118]
Benefits	• Avoidance of maternal risks of general anesthesia, in particular the three As: aspiration, awareness, and difficult airway. • Avoidance of fetal exposure to general anesthesia drugs. • Early maternal bonding with the newborn. • Partner or support person may be present.
Indications	• Spinal anesthesia may be used for labor analgesia, forceps delivery, cesarean delivery, manual removal of placenta, perineal repair, or nonobstetric surgery in the obstetric patient.
Anatomy	• Exaggerated lumbar lordosis during pregnancy can increase the height of the intercristal line such that 6% of term women have an intercristal line at or above L3.[352] • The pronounced lumbar flexion required to perform spinal anesthesia may be difficult due to the gravid uterus.
Physiology	• Aortocaval compression from a gravid uterus may worsen spinal-induced hypotension, posing risks for both mother and fetus.
Pharmacology	• Pregnant women require less local anesthetic to achieve the same level of anesthesia as nonpregnant women. This observation is likely due to both hormonal and mechanical factors.
Technique	• Be prepared to convert to general anesthesia. Prior to placement of a spinal anesthetic, the pregnant patient should receive 30 mL of 0.3 M sodium citrate orally to decrease stomach acidity. Equipment and drugs necessary to administer general anesthesia should be readily available. • After the spinal anesthetic is given, the patient should be in the supine position with left uterine displacement. Fetal heart rate should be monitored by Doppler or fetal scalp electrocardiogram (ECG). • A T4-level block is usually required for a cesarean section due to traction on the peritoneum and uterine exteriorization. • Some patients complain of dyspnea due to abdominal and intercostal motor blockade, but if the patient is able to speak clearly, reassurance and monitoring is usually all that is required. Sensory loss in the upper limb or inability to extend the forearm (C7/C8) should warn the clinician regarding impending diaphragmatic paralysis (C3/C4/C5). • If the mother wants to nurse the newborn, an assessment of upper limb strength should be made. Adequate staffing should allow someone other than the anesthesiologist to be responsible for the well-being of the newborn. • Hypotension and nausea are common, especially in the elective setting (see section on management of hypotension after spinal anesthesia). Prophylactic phenylephrine and "coloading" with fluid effectively prevents hypotension and nausea. Table 23–9 provides a suggested regimen for managing hypotension during elective cesarean section.

ligamentum flavum, epidural space, and posterior dura. While the "target" of spinal anesthesia is the posterior complex, the visualization of the anterior complex denotes a clear ultrasonographic window through the interlaminar space.[335]

Neuraxial Ultrasound Preprocedure Scan

1. After positioning the patient in a conventional manner, **apply a low-frequency (2- to 5-MHz) curved array probe** to the middle of the patient's lower back in a transverse orientation.

2. **Optimize the image** for depth, frequency, and time-gain compensation.

3. **Mark the midline.** This is done by simply aligning the transversely oriented probe such that there is symmetry of the ultrasound appearance (left side of screen being a mirror of the right side). This will correspond to either the transverse spinous process or transverse interlaminar view. Sliding the transversely applied probe in a cephalad direction, a marking pen is used at intervals to mark the skin adjacent to the middle of the long edge of the probe.

TABLE 23–11. Sonoanatomical views of the lumbar spine.

View	Probe Footprint	Ultrasound View	Pattern Recognition Image	Notes
Transverse spinous process view				A distinct midline shadow is cast by the spinous process. Note the laminae (L) are visible, but the anterior and posterior complexes are obscured.
Transverse interlaminar (interspinous) view				"Flying Bat" The articular processes/ facet joints (APFJ) and transverse processes (TP) are visible. Tilting the probe will highlight the posterior (PC) and anterior (AC) complexes.
Paramedian sagittal transverse process view				The "trident" sign represents finger-like shadowing behind the transverse processes.

(continued)

TABLE 23–11. Sonoanatomical views of the lumbar spine. (*Continued*)

View	Probe Footprint	Ultrasound View	Pattern Recognition Image	Notes
Paramedian sagittal articular process view				"Camel humps" represent continuous hyperechoic bone due to vertebrae being "connected" by articular processes. The anterior and posterior complexes are not seen.
Paramedian sagittal laminar view				"Horse heads" "Sawtooth" The hyperechoic bone is not continuous due to the interlaminar space. This space allows visualization of the posterior and anterior complexes.
Paramedian sagittal oblique view			Dura / AC	Slight medial tilt optimizes the view of the posterior and anterior complexes (AC). The dura is seen as a thin hyperechoic line. This view can be used for real-time ultrasound-guided needle advancement.

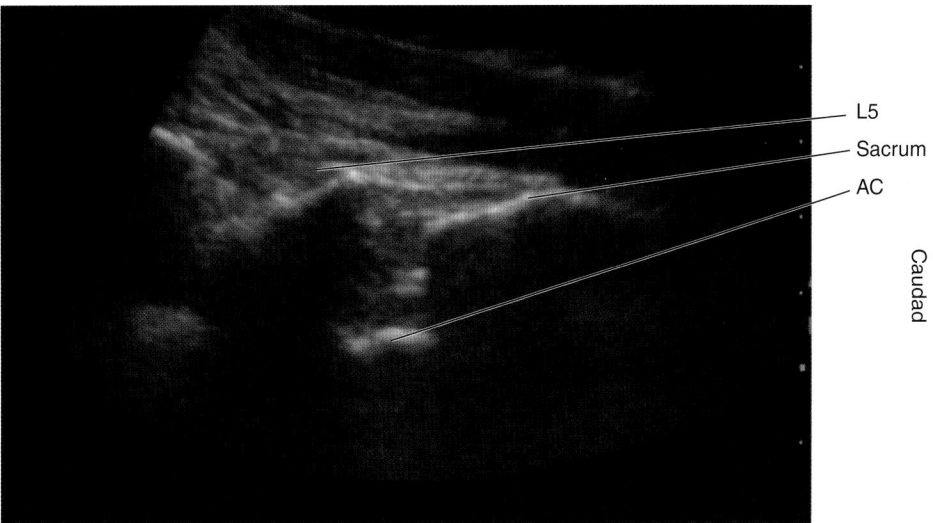

FIGURE 23-16. Ultrasound image of the lumbosacral junction. A continuous hyperechoic line (sacrum) is seen. An anterior complex (AC) should be seen between the sacrum and fifth lumbar lamina.

Practically, it helps to start low and mark above the probe on skin free of ultrasound gel. This technique assumes there is actual symmetry in the patient's anatomy (no scoliosis, rotation, or metalwork).

4. **Identify the lumbosacral junction.** The probe is oriented to obtain a paramedian sagittal laminar view. After identifying the lamina, the probe is slid caudally until a continuous hyperechoic line (sacrum) is seen. An anterior complex should be seen between the sacrum and fifth lumbar lamina (see Figure 23–16).

5. **Mark the lamina** of L1–L5. The probe, maintaining a paramedian orientation, can then be moved cephalad as a marking pen, again at the midpoint of the long edge of the probe, and is used to mark the lamina or interlaminar spaces.

6. **Obtain a transverse interlaminar view at the desired level.** The probe is rotated transversely at the desired level (eg, L3–L4). Slight cephalad-caudal tilting and sliding are necessary to optimize the appearance of the posterior and anterior complex.

7. **Identify the dura** (posterior complex) and mark the depth with calipers.

8. **Note the tilt of the probe** (usually slightly cephalad). This indicates the required angulation of the needle once inserted at the optimal insertion point.

9. **Mark the optimal needle insertion point.** A pen is used to mark the four midpoints of the long and short edges of the probe. The probe is put down, and a horizontal and vertical line is constructed. Where they intersect is the optimal needle insertion point. The vertical line should correspond with the previously marked midline.

10. **Check the optimal insertion point by reapplying probe** and ensuring a good view of the anterior complex.

Additional views of the spine can be obtained by placing the probe in a paramedian sagittal orientation and sliding laterally through the paramedian laminar, articular process, and transverse process views. The paramedian oblique view is obtained by tilting the probe medially, aiming to highlight the posterior and anterior complexes through the interlaminar space. This view can be used for real-time ultrasound-guided spinal anesthesia.

Pitfalls

The most significant pitfall is, after initial training, waiting for the difficult patient before attempting neuraxial ultrasound. Ultrasound scanning requires pattern recognition, and skills need to be attained by scanning "easy" backs. Imprecise skin marking has been postulated as a reason for failure.[341] Care should be taken to ensure the curved array probe is perpendicular to the skin when using a marking pen. Confusing the anterior complex for the posterior complex risks gross overestimation of the depth to the (posterior) dura. When measuring dural depth, the probe may indent the skin, thereby underestimating depth. Misidentification of the lumbosacral junction or failing to recognize anomalies of the junction, present in 12% of the population,[344] will result in incorrect labeling of the interlaminar spaces. Last, ultrasound gel should be cleaned from the skin prior to performing neuraxial block.

Laparoscopic Surgery With Lumbar Spinal Anesthesia

Lumbar spinal anesthesia has been used in the settings of laparoscopic extraperitoneal[345] and intraperitoneal[346] inguinal hernia repair, outpatient gynecological laparoscopy,[347] laparoscopic cholecystectomy,[110,111] and laparoscopic ventral hernia repair.[348] Laparoscopic surgery with an awake patient requires some special considerations. First, patient selection and education are paramount. Caution should be used when interpreting general anesthesia conversion rates in clinical trials as patients who consent to the trial may be more likely to tolerate an awake procedure. Anxiolysis should be offered, and patients should be counseled about expected sensations. Pneumoperitoneum can be perceived as a weight on the abdomen.[347] The possibility of conversion to general anesthesia, which is often due to shoulder tip pain, should be discussed.

Surgical technique and trocar sites may need to be modified.[110] Pneumoperitoneum with nitrous oxide insufflation has been used to avoid peritoneal irritation and pain thought to be associated with conventional carbon dioxide insufflation.[110] However, carbon dioxide insufflation has subsequently been used.[111,113] Avoidance of head-up left lateral tilt that is associated with diaphragmatic irritation has been suggested.[112] Some studies have limited insufflation to less than 11 mm Hg and used a nasogastric tube to decompress the stomach and reduce aspiration risk.[110,111] Others did not modify surgical technique except for low-flow insufflation (nasogastric tubes were avoided and maintained carbon dioxide insufflation at 15 mm Hg).[113] Addition of intrathecal fentanyl[349] or clonidine[350] may decrease shoulder tip pain.

The main two drawbacks of spinal anesthesia for laparoscopic cholecystectomy seemed to be shoulder tip pain resulting in patient dissatisfaction or conversion to general anesthesia and a high rate of PDPH (up to 10%).[349] Due to the small numbers and heterogeneous techniques in previous studies, it has been difficult to establish the ideal technique.

Tzovaras and colleagues in 2008 published an interim analysis of a randomized trial.[112] One hundred patients were randomized to either general or spinal anesthesia for laparoscopic cholecystectomy. Both arms of the study had nasogastric tubes and carbon dioxide insufflation to a maximum of 10 mm Hg. The spinal group had 3 mL of 0.5% hyperbaric bupivacaine, 250 µg morphine, and 20 µg fentanyl injected at the L2–L3 level via a 25-gauge pencil-point needle in the right lateral decubitus position. The patient was then placed in the Trendelenburg position for 3 minutes. Despite intraoperative shoulder tip discomfort or pain in 43% patients of the spinal group, only half of these patients required fentanyl, and no patient required conversion to general anesthesia. Of those in the spinal and general anesthesia groups, 96% and 94%, respectively, were highly or fairly satisfied with their procedure. Moreover, postoperative pain was less in the spinal group compared with the general anesthesia group. The trial was discontinued as the primary endpoint (pain) was reached with the first 100 patients. No patient in the spinal group had a classic PDPH (G. Tzovaras, personal communication, 2012).

Thoracic Spinal Anesthesia

Thoracic spinal anesthesia was described in the early 1900s by Professor Thomas Jonnesco, although he was criticized by his contemporaries, including Professor Bier.[351] He called his technique "general spinal analgesia" and described two puncture sites, the T1–T2 and T12–L1 interspaces, depending on the surgery required. In his article, he made astounding claims of being able to perform head and neck surgery, including total laryngotomy, under high-thoracic analgesia and incorrectly predicted in 1909 that his technique would "in a short time be universally accepted."

In 2006, thoracic spinal anesthetic for a patient requiring laparoscopic cholecystectomy was reported.[109] Segmental thoracic

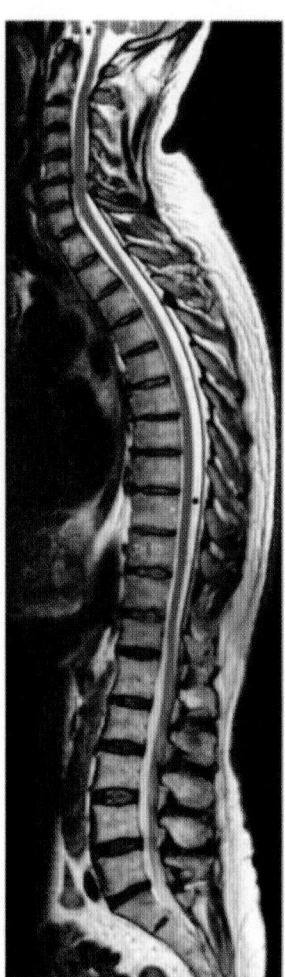

FIGURE 23–17. Midline MRI of the spinal column. In the thoracic segments, the spinal cord is positioned anteriorly leaving a significant space (*) between the posterior dura and the spinal cord. At the lumbar level, the space disappears almost completely. (Reproduced with permission from van Zundert AA, Stultiens G, Jakimowicz JJ, et al: Segmental spinal anaesthesia for cholecystectomy in a patient with severe lung disease. *Br J Anaesth.* 2006 Apr;96(4):464-466.)

spinal anesthesia for laparoscopic cholecystectomy was shown to be effective in a small number of healthy patients, although the authors cautioned that the technique, still in its infancy, should not be used in routine practice.[108]

Spinal anesthesia is traditionally performed in the lumbar region below the level of the conus medullaris to avoid injury to the spinal cord. However, MRI images, albeit in a supine position, have shown that the mid- to lower thoracic segment of the cord lies anteriorly, such that there is a CSF-filled space between the dura and the cord (see Figure 23–17).

SUMMARY

Spinal anesthesia is a reliable, safe, and effective form of anesthesia. Much has changed since its beginnings in the late 19th century. Mastery of spinal anesthesia comes with practice, diligence, and knowledge of physiology, pharmacology, and anatomy.

Patient safety must always be at the forefront when considering performing a spinal anesthetic. Spinal anesthesia is an indispensable technique in the practice of modern anesthesia.

REFERENCES

1. Koller C: Vorlaufige Mittheilung über locale Anasthesirung am Auge. Klin Mbl Augenheilk 1884;22:60–63.
2. Halsted WS: Practical comments on the use and abuse of cocaine; suggested by its invariably successful employment in more than a thousand minor surgical operations. NY Med J 1885;42:294.
3. Corning JL: Spinal anaesthesia and local medication of the cord. NY Med J 1885;42:483–485.
4. Gorelick PB, Zych D: James Leonard Corning and the early history of spinal puncture. Neurology 1987;37(4):672–674.
5. Arendt K, Demaerschalk BM, Wingerchuk DM, Camann W: Atraumatic lumbar puncture needles: After all these years, are we still missing the point? Neurologist 2009;15(1):17–20.
6. Wynter E: Four cases of tubercular meningitis in which paracentesis of the theca vertebralis was performed for relief of fluid pressure. Lancet 1891;981–982.
7. Ball C, Westhorpe R: Local anaesthesia—early spinal anaesthesia. Anaesth Intensive Care 2003;31(5):493.
8. Bier A: Experiments regarding the cocainization of the spinal cord. Dtsch Z Chir 1899;51:361–369.
9. Marx GF: The first spinal anesthesia. Who deserves the laurels? Reg Anesth 1994;19(6):429–430.
10. Wulf HF: The centennial of spinal anesthesia. Anesthesiology 1998;89(2):500–506.
11. Larson MD: Tait and Caglieri. The first spinal anesthetic in America. Anesthesiology 1996;85(4):913–919.
12. Matas R: Local and regional anesthesia with cocaine and other analgesic drugs, including the subarachnoid method, as applied in the general surgical practice. Phil Med J 1900;6:820–843.
13. Vandam LD: On the origins of intrathecal anesthesia. Reg Anesth Pain Med 1998;23(4):335–339; discussion 84–87.
14. Tuffier T: Anesthesie medullaire chirurgicale par injection sous-arachnoidienne lombaire de cocaine; technique et resultats. Semin Med 1900;20:167.
15. Barker AE: A report on clinical experiences with spinal analgesia in 100 cases and some reflections on the procedure. BMJ 1907;1:665–674.
16. Labat G: Circulatory disturbances associated with subarachnoid nerve block. Long Island Med J 1927;21:573.
17. Pitkin G: Controllable spinal anesthesia. Am J Surg 1928;5:537.
18. Sise LF: Spinal anesthesia for upper and lower abdominal operations. N Engl J Med 1928;199:61.
19. Sise LF: Pontocaineglucose for spinal anesthesia. Surg Clin North Am 1935;15:1501.
20. Brown DL, Fink BR: The history of neural blockade and pain management. In Cousins MJ, Bridenbaugh PO (eds): *Neural Blockade*, 3rd ed. Lippincott-Raven, 1998, pp 3–27.
21. Adriani J, Roman-Vega D: Saddle block anesthesia. Am J Surg 1946;71:12.
22. Maltby JR, Hutter CD, Clayton KC: The Woolley and Roe case. Br J Anaesth 2000;84(1):121–126.
23. Kennedy F, Effron AS, Perry G: The grave spinal cord paralyses caused by spinal anesthesia. Surg Gynecol Obstet 1950;91(4):385–398.
24. Dripps RD, Vandam LD: Long-term follow-up of patients who received 10,098 spinal anesthetics: Failure to discover major neurological sequelae. JAMA 1954;156(16):1486–1491.
25. Morgan P: Spinal anaesthesia in obstetrics. Can J Anaesth 1995;42(12):1145–1163.
26. Cook TM, Counsell D, Wildsmith JA: Major complications of central neuraxial block: Report on the Third National Audit Project of the Royal College of Anaesthetists. Br J Anaesth 2009;102(2):179–190.
27. Greene HM: Lumbar puncture and the prevention of postdural puncture headache. JAMA 1926;86:391–392.
28. Greene BA: A 26 gauge lumbar puncture needle: Its value in the prophylaxis of headache following spinal analgesia for vaginal delivery. Anesthesiology 1950;11:464–469.
29. Hart JR, Whitacre RJ: Pencil-point needle in prevention of postspinal headache. JAMA 1951;147(7):657–658.
30. Sprotte G, Schedel R, Pajunk H: [An "atraumatic" universal needle for single-shot regional anesthesia: clinical results and a 6 year trial in over 30,000 regional anesthesias]. Reg Anaesth 1987;10(3):104–108.
31. Calthorpe N: The history of spinal needles: Getting to the point. Anaesthesia 2004;59(12):1231–1241.
32. McDonald SB: Is neuraxial blockade contraindicated in the patient with aortic stenosis? Reg Anesth Pain Med 2004;29(5):496–502.
33. O'Keefe JH Jr, Shub C, Rettke SR: Risk of noncardiac surgical procedures in patients with aortic stenosis. Mayo Clin Proc 1989;64(4):400–405.
34. Collard CD, Eappen S, Lynch EP, Concepcion M: Continuous spinal anesthesia with invasive hemodynamic monitoring for surgical repair of the hip in two patients with severe aortic stenosis. Anesth Analg 1995;81(1):195–198.
35. Bamford C, Sibley W, Laguna J: Anesthesia in multiple sclerosis. Can J Neurol Sci 1978;5(1):41–44.
36. Kytta J, Rosenberg PH: Anaesthesia for patients with multiple sclerosis. Ann Chir Gynaecol 1984;73(5):299–303.
37. Bouchard P, Caillet JB, Monnet F, Banssillon V: [Spinal anesthesia and multiple sclerosis]. Ann Fr Anesth Reanim 1984;3(3):194–198.
38. Levesque P, Marsepoil T, Ho P, Venutolo F, Lesouef JM: [Multiple sclerosis disclosed by spinal anesthesia]. Ann Fr Anesth Reanim 1988;7(1):68–70.
39. Vadalouca A, Moka E, Sykiotis C: Combined spinal-epidural technique for total hysterectomy in a patient with advanced, progressive multiple sclerosis. Reg Anesth Pain Med 2002;27(5):540–541.
40. Horlocker TT, Wedel DJ: Regional anesthesia in the immunocompromised patient. Reg Anesth Pain Med 2006;31(4):334–345.
41. Chin KJ, Macfarlane AJ, Chan V, Brull R: The use of ultrasound to facilitate spinal anesthesia in a patient with previous lumbar laminectomy and fusion: A case report. J Clin Ultrasound 2009;37(8):482–485.
42. Prasad GA, Tumber PS, Lupu CM: Ultrasound guided spinal anesthesia. Can J Anaesth 2008;55(10):716–717.
43. Costello JF, Balki M: Cesarean delivery under ultrasound-guided spinal anesthesia [corrected] in a parturient with poliomyelitis and Harrington instrumentation. Can J Anaesth 2008;55(9):606–611.
44. Douglas MJ, Swenerton JE: Epidural anesthesia in three parturients with lumbar tattoos: A review of possible implications. Can J Anaesth 2002;49(10):1057–1060.
45. Mavropoulos A, Camann W: Use of a lumbar tattoo to aid spinal anesthesia for cesarean delivery. Int J Obstet Anesth 2009;18(1):98–99.
46. Balki M, Carvalho JC: Intraoperative nausea and vomiting during cesarean section under regional anesthesia. Int J Obstet Anesth 2005;14(3):230–241.
47. Mishriky BM, Habib AS: Metoclopramide for nausea and vomiting prophylaxis during and after caesarean delivery: A systematic review and meta-analysis. Br J Anaesth 2012;108(3):374–383.
48. Carpenter RL, Caplan RA, Brown DL, Stephenson C, Wu R: Incidence and risk factors for side effects of spinal anesthesia. Anesthesiology 1992;76(6):906–916.
49. Evans CH: *Spinal Anesthesia <Subarachnoid Radicular Conduction Block> Principles and Technique.* Hoeber, 1929.
50. Ure D, James KS, McNeill M, Booth JV: Glycopyrrolate reduces nausea during spinal anaesthesia for caesarean section without affecting neonatal outcome. Br J Anaesth 1999;82(2):277–279.
51. George RB, Allen TK, Habib AS: Serotonin receptor antagonists for the prevention and treatment of pruritus, nausea, and vomiting in women undergoing cesarean delivery with intrathecal morphine: A systematic review and meta-analysis. Anesth Analg 2009;109(1):174–182.
52. Allen TK, Habib AS: P6 stimulation for the prevention of nausea and vomiting associated with cesarean delivery under neuraxial anesthesia: A systematic review of randomized controlled trials. Anesth Analg 2008;107(4):1308–1312.
53. Crowley LJ, Buggy DJ: Shivering and neuraxial anesthesia. Reg Anesth Pain Med 2008;33(3):241–252.
54. Saito T, Sessler DI, Fujita K, Ooi Y, Jeffrey R: Thermoregulatory effects of spinal and epidural anesthesia during cesarean delivery. Reg Anesth Pain Med 1998;23(4):418–423.
55. Ballantyne JC, Loach AB, Carr DB: Itching after epidural and spinal opiates. Pain 1988;33(2):149–160.
56. Bauchat JR: Focused review: Neuraxial morphine and oral herpes reactivation in the obstetric population. Anesth Analg 2010;111(5): 1238–1241.
57. Crighton IM, Hobbs GJ, Reid MF: Ondansetron for the treatment of pruritus after spinal opioids. Anaesthesia 1996;51(2):199–200.
58. Schaffartzik W, Hirsch J, Frickmann F, Kuhly P, Ernst A: Hearing loss after spinal and general anesthesia: A comparative study. Anesth Analg 2000;91(6):1466–1472.
59. Karatas E, Goksu S, Durucu C, Isik Y, Kanlikama M: Evaluation of hearing loss after spinal anesthesia with otoacoustic emissions. Eur Arch Otorhinolaryngol 2006;263(8):705–710.

60. Lee CM, Peachman FA: Unilateral hearing loss after spinal anesthesia treated with epidural blood patch. Anesth Analg 1986;65(3):312.
61. Fog J, Wang LP, Sundberg A, Mucchiano C: Hearing loss after spinal anesthesia is related to needle size. Anesth Analg 1990;70(5):517–522.
62. Finegold H, Mandell G, Vallejo M, Ramanathan S: Does spinal anesthesia cause hearing loss in the obstetric population? Anesth Analg 2002;95(1):198–203; table of contents.
63. Michel O, Brusis T: Hearing loss as a sequel of lumbar puncture. Ann Otol Rhinol Laryngol 1992;101(5):390–394.
64. Mulroy MF, Alley EA: Management of bladder volumes when using neuraxial anesthesia. Int Anesthesiol Clin 2012;50(1):101–110.
65. Choi S, Mahon P, Awad IT: Neuraxial anesthesia and bladder dysfunction in the perioperative period: A systematic review. Can J Anaesth 2012;59(7):681–703.
66. Lambert DH: Complications of spinal anesthesia. Int Anesthesiol Clin 1989;27(1):51–55.
67. Harrington BE: Postdural puncture headache and the development of the epidural blood patch. Reg Anesth Pain Med 2004;29(2):136–163; discussion 35.
68. Vandam LD, Dripps RD: Long-term follow-up of patients who received 10,098 spinal anesthetics; syndrome of decreased intracranial pressure (headache and ocular and auditory difficulties). JAMA 1956;161(7):586–591.
69. Choi PT, Galinski SE, Takeuchi L, Lucas S, Tamayo C, Jadad AR: PDPH is a common complication of neuraxial blockade in parturients: A meta-analysis of obstetrical studies. Can J Anaesth 2003;50(5):460–469.
70. Horlocker TT: Complications of spinal and epidural anesthesia. Anesthesiol Clin North Am 2000;18(2):461–485.
71. Horlocker TT, McGregor DG, Matsushige DK, Schroeder DR, Besse JA: A retrospective review of 4767 consecutive spinal anesthetics: central nervous system complications. Perioperative Outcomes Group. Anesth Analg 1997;84(3):578–584.
72. Reiss W, Shariat AN, Kurapati S, Hadzic A: Intraneural injections. Reg Anesth Pain Med 2011;36(1):97–98.
73. Burke D, Wildsmith JA: Meningitis after spinal anaesthesia. Br J Anaesth 1997;78(6):635–636.
74. Goldman WW Jr, Sanford JP: An "epidemic" of chemical meningitis. Am J Med 1960;29:94–101.
75. Hurst EW: Adhesive arachnoiditis and vascular blockage caused by detergents and other chemical irritants: An experimental study. J Pathol Bacteriol 1955;70(1):167–178.
76. Marinac JS: Drug- and chemical-induced aseptic meningitis: A review of the literature. Ann Pharmacother 1992;26(6):813–822.
77. Carp H, Bailey S: The association between meningitis and dural puncture in bacteremic rats. Anesthesiology 1992;76(5):739–742.
78. Teele DW, Dashefsky B, Rakusan T, Klein JO: Meningitis after lumbar puncture in children with bacteremia. N Engl J Med 1981;305(18):1079–1081.
79. Eng RH, Seligman SJ: Lumbar puncture-induced meningitis. JAMA 1981;245(14):1456–1459.
80. Conangla G, Rodriguez L, Alonso-Tarres C, Avila A, de la Campa AG: [*Streptococcus salivarius* meningitis after spinal anesthesia]. Neurologia 2004;19(6):331–333.
81. Pandian JD, Sarada C, Radhakrishnan VV, Kishore A: Iatrogenic meningitis after lumbar puncture—A preventable health hazard. J Hosp Infect 2004;56(2):119–124.
82. Kocamanoglu IS, Sener EB, Tur A, Ustun E, Sahinoglu H: Streptococcal meningitis after spinal anesthesia: Report of a case. Can J Anaesth 2003;50(3):314–315.
83. Yaniv LG, Potasman I: Iatrogenic meningitis: An increasing role for resistant viridans streptococci? Case report and review of the last 20 years. Scand J Infect Dis 2000;32(6):693–696.
84. Santillan A, Nacarino V, Greenberg E, Riina HA, Gobin YP, Patsalides A: Vascular anatomy of the spinal cord. J Neurointerv Surg 2012;4(1):67–74.
85. Ilias WK, Klimscha W, Skrbensky G, Weinstabl R, Widhalm A: Continuous microspinal anaesthesia: Another perspective on mechanisms inducing cauda equina syndrome. Anaesthesia 1998;53(7):618–623.
86. Rigler ML, Drasner K, Krejcie TC, et al: Cauda equina syndrome after continuous spinal anesthesia. Anesth Analg 1991;72(3):275–281.
87. Benson JS: US Food and Drug Administration safety alert: Cauda equina syndrome associated with use of small-bore catheters in continuous spinal anesthesia. AANA J 1992;60(3):223.
88. Mollmann M, Holst D, Lubbesmeyer H, Lawin P: Continuous spinal anesthesia: Mechanical and technical problems of catheter placement. Reg Anesth 1993;18(6 Suppl):469–472.
89. Loo CC, Irestedt L: Cauda equina syndrome after spinal anaesthesia with hyperbaric 5% lignocaine: A review of six cases of cauda equina syndrome reported to the Swedish Pharmaceutical Insurance 1993–1997. Acta Anaesthesiol Scand 1999;43(4):371–379.
90. Panadero A, Monedero P, Fernandez-Liesa JI, Percaz J, Olavide I, Iribarren MJ: Repeated transient neurological symptoms after spinal anaesthesia with hyperbaric 5% lidocaine. Br J Anaesth 1998;81(3):471–472.
91. Pavon A, Anadon Senac P: [Neurotoxicity of intrathecal lidocaine]. Rev Esp Anestesiol Reanim 2001;48(7):326–336.
92. Moen V, Dahlgren N, Irestedt L: Severe neurological complications after central neuraxial blockades in Sweden 1990–1999. Anesthesiology 2004;101(4):950–959.
93. Akioka K, Torigoe K, Maruta H, et al: A case of cauda equina syndrome following spinal anesthesia with hyperbaric dibucaine. J Anesth 2001;15(2):106–107.
94. Lopez-Soriano F, Lajarin B, Verdu JM, Rivas F, Lopez-Robles J: [Cauda equina hemisyndrome after intradural anesthesia with bupivacaine for hip surgery]. Rev Esp Anestesiol Reanim 2002;49(9):494–496.
95. Vianna PT, Resende LA, Ganem EM, Gabarra RC, Yamashita S, Barreira AA: Cauda equina syndrome after spinal tetracaine: Electromyographic evaluation—20 years follow-up. Anesthesiology 2001;95(5):1290–1291.
96. Woods WW, Franklin RG: Progressive adhesive arachnoiditis following spinal anesthesia. Calif Med 1951;75(3):196–198.
97. Joseph SI, Denson JS: Spinal anesthesia, arachnoiditis, and paraplegia. JAMA 1958;168(10):1330–1333.
98. Parnass SM, Schmidt KJ: Adverse effects of spinal and epidural anaesthesia. Drug Saf 1990;5(3):179–194.
99. Roche J: Steroid-induced arachnoiditis. Med J Aust 1984;140(5):281–284.
100. Aldrete JA: Neurologic deficits and arachnoiditis following neuroaxial anesthesia. Acta Anaesthesiol Scand 2003;47(1):3–12.
101. Yokoyama M, Itano Y, Kusume Y, Oe K, Mizobuchi S, Morita K: Total spinal anesthesia provides transient relief of intractable pain. Can J Anaesth 2002;49(8):810–813.
102. Auroy Y, Benhamou D, Bargues L, et al: Major complications of regional anesthesia in France: The SOS Regional Anesthesia Hotline Service. Anesthesiology 2002;97(5):1274–1280.
103. Vandam LD, Dripps RD: Long-term follow-up of patients who received 10,098 spinal anesthetics. IV. Neurological disease incident to traumatic lumbar puncture during spinal anesthesia. JAMA 1960;172:1483–1487.
104. Aromaa U, Lahdensuu M, Cozanitis DA: Severe complications associated with epidural and spinal anaesthesias in Finland 1987–1993. A study based on patient insurance claims [see comment]. Acta Anaesthesiol Scand 1997;41(4):445–452.
105. Auroy Y, Narchi P, Messiah A, Litt L, Rouvier B, Samii K: Serious complications related to regional anesthesia: Results of a prospective survey in France. Anesthesiology 1997;87(3):479–486.
106. Brull R, McCartney CJ, Chan VW, El-Beheiry H: Neurological complications after regional anesthesia: Contemporary estimates of risk. Anesth Analg 2007;104(4):965–974.
107. Buggy DJ: Central neuraxial block: Defining risk more clearly. Br J Anaesth 2009;102(2):151–153.
108. van Zundert AA, Stultiens G, Jakimowicz JJ, et al: Laparoscopic cholecystectomy under segmental thoracic spinal anaesthesia: A feasibility study. Br J Anaesth 2007;98(5):682–686.
109. van Zundert AA, Stultiens G, Jakimowicz JJ, van den Borne BE, van der Ham WG, Wildsmith JA: Segmental spinal anaesthesia for cholecystectomy in a patient with severe lung disease. Br J Anaesth 2006;96(4):464–466.
110. Hamad MA, El-Khattary OA: Laparoscopic cholecystectomy under spinal anesthesia with nitrous oxide pneumoperitoneum: A feasibility study. Surg Endosc 2003;17(9):1426–1428.
111. Tzovaras G, Fafoulakis F, Pratsas K, Georgopoulou S, Stamatiou G, Hatzitheofilou C: Laparoscopic cholecystectomy under spinal anesthesia: A pilot study. Surg Endosc 2006;20(4):580–582.
112. Tzovaras G, Fafoulakis F, Pratsas K, Georgopoulou S, Stamatiou G, Hatzitheofilou C: Spinal versus general anesthesia for laparoscopic cholecystectomy: Interim analysis of a controlled randomized trial. Arch Surg 2008;143(5):497–501.
113. Yuksek YN, Akat AZ, Gozalan U, et al: Laparoscopic cholecystectomy under spinal anesthesia. Am J Surg 2008;195(4):533–536.
114. Cook TM: Report and findings of the 3rd National Audit Project of the Royal College of Anaesthetists. 2009:17–26.
115. Guay J: The effect of neuraxial blocks on surgical blood loss and blood transfusion requirements: A meta-analysis. J Clin Anesth 2006;18(2):124–128.

116. Mauermann WJ, Shilling AM, Zuo Z: A comparison of neuraxial block versus general anesthesia for elective total hip replacement: A meta-analysis. Anesth Analg 2006;103(4):1018–1025.

117. Afolabi BB, Lesi FE, Merah NA: Regional versus general anaesthesia for caesarean section. Cochrane Database Syst Rev 2006(4):CD004350.

118. Reynolds F, Seed PT: Anaesthesia for Caesarean section and neonatal acid-base status: A meta-analysis. Anaesthesia 2005;60(7):636–653.

119. Beaupre LA, Jones CA, Saunders LD, Johnston DW, Buckingham J, Majumdar SR: Best practices for elderly hip fracture patients. A systematic overview of the evidence. J Gen Intern Med 2005;20(11):1019–1025.

120. Rodgers A, Walker N, Schug S, et al: Reduction of postoperative mortality and morbidity with epidural or spinal anaesthesia: Results from overview of randomised trials. BMJ 2000;321(7275):1493.

121. Parker MJ, Handoll HH, Griffiths R: Anaesthesia for hip fracture surgery in adults. Cochrane Database Syst Rev 2004(4):CD000521.

122. Lee TW, Grocott HP, Schwinn D, Jacobsohn E: High spinal anesthesia for cardiac surgery: Effects on beta-adrenergic receptor function, stress response, and hemodynamics. Anesthesiology 2003;98(2):499–510.

123. Hall R, Adderley N, MacLaren C, et al: Does intrathecal morphine alter the stress response following coronary artery bypass grafting surgery? Can J Anaesth 2000;47(5):463–466.

124. Parlow JL, Steele RG, O'Reilly D: Low dose intrathecal morphine facilitates early extubation after cardiac surgery: results of a retrospective continuous quality improvement audit. Can J Anaesth 2005;52(1):94–99.

125. Liu SS, Block BM, Wu CL: Effects of perioperative central neuraxial analgesia on outcome after coronary artery bypass surgery: A meta-analysis. Anesthesiology 2004;101(1):153–161.

126. Agarwal D, Mohta M, Tyagi A, Sethi AK: Subdural block and the anaesthetist. Anaesth Intensive Care 2010;38(1):20–26.

127. Reina MA, De Leon Casasola O, Lopez A, De Andres JA, Mora M, Fernandez A: The origin of the spinal subdural space: Ultrastructure findings. Anesth Analg 2002;94(4):991–995; table of contents.

128. Broadbent CR, Maxwell WB, Ferrie R, Wilson DJ, Gawne-Cain M, Russell R: Ability of anaesthetists to identify a marked lumbar interspace. Anaesthesia 2000;55(11):1122–1126.

129. Saifuddin A, Burnett SJ, White J: The variation of position of the conus medullaris in an adult population. A magnetic resonance imaging study. Spine (Phila Pa 1976) 1998;23(13):1452–1456.

130. Reiman A, Anson B: Vertebral termination of the spinal cord with report of a case of sacral cord. Anat Rec 1944;88:127.

131. Bromage PR: Neurological complications of subarachnoid and epidural anaesthesia. Acta Anaesthesiol Scand 1997;41(4):439–444.

132. Reynolds F: Damage to the conus medullaris following spinal anaesthesia. Anaesthesia 2001;56(3):238–247.

133. Covino BG: Pharmacology of local anaesthetic agents. Br J Anaesth 1986;58(7):701–716.

134. Greene NM: Uptake and elimination of local anesthetics during spinal anesthesia. Anesth Analg 1983;62(11):1013–1024.

135. Stienstra R, Greene NM: Factors affecting the subarachnoid spread of local anesthetic solutions. Reg Anesth 1991;16(1):1–6.

136. Cohen EN: Distribution of local anesthetic agents in the neuraxis of the dog. Anesthesiology 1968;29(5):1002–1005.

137. Schell RM, Brauer FS, Cole DJ, Applegate RL 2nd: Persistent sacral nerve root deficits after continuous spinal anaesthesia. Can J Anaesth 1991;38(7):908–911.

138. Hogan Q: Size of human lower thoracic and lumbosacral nerve roots. Anesthesiology 1996;85(1):37–42.

139. Kaneko S, Matsumoto M, Tsuruta S, Hirata T, Gondo T, Sakabe T: The nerve root entry zone is highly vulnerable to intrathecal tetracaine in rabbits. Anesth Analg 2005;101(1):107–114; table of contents.

140. Takenami T, Yagishita S, Asato F, Hoka S: Neurotoxicity of intrathecally administered tetracaine commences at the posterior roots near entry into the spinal cord. Reg Anesth Pain Med 2000;25(4):372–379.

141. Kristensen JD, Karlsten R, Gordh T: Spinal cord blood flow after intrathecal injection of ropivacaine and bupivacaine with or without epinephrine in rats. Acta Anaesthesiol Scand 1998;42(6):685–690.

142. Dohi S, Matsumiya N, Takeshima R, Naito H: The effects of subarachnoid lidocaine and phenylephrine on spinal cord and cerebral blood flow in dogs. Anesthesiology 1984;61(3):238–244.

143. Kozody R, Palahniuk RJ, Cumming MO: Spinal cord blood flow following subarachnoid tetracaine. Can Anaesth Soc J 1985;32(1):23–29.

144. Greene NM: Distribution of local anesthetic solutions within the subarachnoid space. Anesth Analg 1985;64(7):715–730.

145. Horlocker TT, Wedel DJ: Density, specific gravity, and baricity of spinal anesthetic solutions at body temperature. Anesth Analg 1993;76(5):1015–1018.

146. Hallworth SP, Fernando R, Columb MO, Stocks GM: The effect of posture and baricity on the spread of intrathecal bupivacaine for elective cesarean delivery. Anesth Analg 2005;100(4):1159–1165.

147. McLeod GA: Density of spinal anaesthetic solutions of bupivacaine, levobupivacaine, and ropivacaine with and without dextrose. Br J Anaesth 2004;92(4):547–551.

148. Brown DT, Wildsmith JA, Covino BG, Scott DB: Effect of baricity on spinal anaesthesia with amethocaine. Br J Anaesth 1980;52(6):589–596.

149. Siker ES, Wolfson B, Stewart WD, Pavilack P, Pappas MT: Mepivacaine for spinal anesthesia: Effects of changes in concentration and baricity. Anesth Analg 1966;45(2):191–196.

150. Chambers WA, Edstrom HH, Scott DB: Effect of baricity on spinal anaesthesia with bupivacaine. Br J Anaesth 1981;53(3):279–282.

151. Denson DD, Bridenbaugh PO, Turner PA, Phero JC: Comparison of neural blockade and pharmacokinetics after subarachnoid lidocaine in the rhesus monkey. II: Effects of volume, osmolality, and baricity. Anesth Analg 1983;62(11):995–1001.

152. Hare GM, Ngan JC: Density determination of local anaesthetic opioid mixtures for spinal anaesthesia. Can J Anaesth 1998;45(4):341–346.

153. Bodily MN, Carpenter RL, Owens BD: Lidocaine 0.5% spinal anaesthesia: a hypobaric solution for short-stay perirectal surgery. Can J Anaesth 1992;39(8):770–773.

154. Lui AC, Polis TZ, Cicutti NJ: Densities of cerebrospinal fluid and spinal anaesthetic solutions in surgical patients at body temperature. Can J Anaesth 1998;45(4):297–303.

155. Hogan QH, Prost R, Kulier A, Taylor ML, Liu S, Mark L: Magnetic resonance imaging of cerebrospinal fluid volume and the influence of body habitus and abdominal pressure. Anesthesiology 1996;84(6):1341–1349.

156. Carpenter RL, Hogan QH, Liu SS, Crane B, Moore J: Lumbosacral cerebrospinal fluid volume is the primary determinant of sensory block extent and duration during spinal anesthesia. Anesthesiology 1998;89(1):24–29.

157. Higuchi H, Hirata J, Adachi Y, Kazama T: Influence of lumbosacral cerebrospinal fluid density, velocity, and volume on extent and duration of plain bupivacaine spinal anesthesia. Anesthesiology 2004;100(1):106–114.

158. Schneider M, Ettlin T, Kaufmann M, et al: Transient neurologic toxicity after hyperbaric subarachnoid anesthesia with 5% lidocaine. Anesth Analg 1993;76(5):1154–1157.

159. Zaric D, Christiansen C, Pace NL, Punjasawadwong Y: Transient neurologic symptoms after spinal anesthesia with lidocaine versus other local anesthetics: A systematic review of randomized, controlled trials. Anesth Analg 2005;100(6):1811–1816.

160. Wang BC, Hillman DE, Spielholz NI, Turndorf H: Chronic neurological deficits and Nesacaine-CE—an effect of the anesthetic, 2-chloroprocaine, or the antioxidant, sodium bisulfite? Anesth Analg 1984;63(4):445–447.

161. Smith KN, Kopacz DJ, McDonald SB: Spinal 2-chloroprocaine: a dose-ranging study and the effect of added epinephrine. Anesth Analg 2004;98(1):81–88; table of contents.

162. Hejtmanek MR, Pollock JE: Chloroprocaine for spinal anesthesia: A retrospective analysis. Acta Anaesthesiol Scand 2011;55(3):267–272.

163. Pollock JE: Intrathecal chloroprocaine—not yet "safe" by US FDA parameters. Int Anesthesiol Clin 2012;50(1):93–100.

164. Le Truong HH, Girard M, Drolet P, Grenier Y, Boucher C, Bergeron L: Spinal anesthesia: A comparison of procaine and lidocaine. Can J Anaesth 2001;48(5):470–473.

165. Johnson ME: Neurotoxicity of spinal procaine—a caution. Reg Anesth Pain Med 2001;26(3):288.

166. Hampl KF, Schneider MC, Ummenhofer W, Drewe J: Transient neurologic symptoms after spinal anesthesia. Anesth Analg 1995;81(6):1148–1153.

167. Hampl KF, Heinzmann-Wiedmer S, Luginbuehl I, et al: Transient neurologic symptoms after spinal anesthesia: a lower incidence with prilocaine and bupivacaine than with lidocaine. Anesthesiology 1998;88(3):629–633.

168. Keld DB, Hein L, Dalgaard M, Krogh L, Rodt SA: The incidence of transient neurologic symptoms (TNS) after spinal anaesthesia in patients undergoing surgery in the supine position. Hyperbaric lidocaine 5% versus hyperbaric bupivacaine 0.5%. Acta Anaesthesiol Scand 2000;44(3):285–290.

169. Freedman JM, Li DK, Drasner K, Jaskela MC, Larsen B, Wi S: Transient neurologic symptoms after spinal anesthesia: An epidemiologic study of 1863 patients. Anesthesiology 1998;89(3):633–641.

170. Sumi M, Sakura S, Kosaka Y: Intrathecal hyperbaric 0.5% tetracaine as a possible cause of transient neurologic toxicity. Anesth Analg 1996;82(5):1076–1077.

171. Sakura S, Sumi M, Sakaguchi Y, Saito Y, Kosaka Y, Drasner K: The addition of phenylephrine contributes to the development of transient neurologic symptoms after spinal anesthesia with 0.5% tetracaine. Anesthesiology 1997;87(4):771–778.

172. Liguori GA, Zayas VM, Chisholm MF: Transient neurologic symptoms after spinal anesthesia with mepivacaine and lidocaine. Anesthesiology 1998;88(3):619–623.

173. Salazar F, Bogdanovich A, Adalia R, Chabas E, Gomar C: Transient neurologic symptoms after spinal anaesthesia using isobaric 2% mepivacaine and isobaric 2% lidocaine. Acta Anaesthesiol Scand 2001;45(2):240–245.

174. Eberhart LH, Morin AM, Kranke P, Geldner G, Wulf H: [Transient neurologic symptoms after spinal anesthesia. A quantitative systematic overview (meta-analysis) of randomized controlled studies]. Anaesthesist 2002;51(7):539–546.

175. Ganapathy S, Sandhu HB, Stockall CA, Hurley D: Transient neurologic symptom (TNS) following intrathecal ropivacaine. Anesthesiology 2000;93(6):1537–1539.

176. Lee YY, Ngan Kee WD, Chang HK, So CL, Gin T: Spinal ropivacaine for lower limb surgery: A dose response study. Anesth Analg 2007;105(2):520–523.

177. Khaw KS, Ngan Kee WD, Wong EL, Liu JY, Chung R: Spinal ropivacaine for cesarean section: a dose-finding study. Anesthesiology 2001;95(6):1346–1350.

178. Frawley G, Skinner A, Thomas J, Smith S: Ropivacaine spinal anesthesia in neonates: A dose range finding study. Paediatr Anaesth 2007;17(2):126–132.

179. McDonald SB, Liu SS, Kopacz DJ, Stephenson CA: Hyperbaric spinal ropivacaine: A comparison to bupivacaine in volunteers. Anesthesiology 1999;90(4):971–977.

180. Wahedi W, Nolte H, Klein P: [Ropivacaine for spinal anesthesia. A dose-finding study]. Anaesthesist 1996;45(8):737–744.

181. van Kleef JW, Veering BT, Burm AG: Spinal anesthesia with ropivacaine: A double-blind study on the efficacy and safety of 0.5% and 0.75% solutions in patients undergoing minor lower limb surgery. Anesth Analg 1994;78(6):1125–1130.

182. Hughes D, Hill D, Fee JP: Intrathecal ropivacaine or bupivacaine with fentanyl for labour. Br J Anaesth 2001;87(5):733–737.

183. Breebaart MB, Vercauteren MP, Hoffmann VL, Adriaensen HA: Urinary bladder scanning after day-case arthroscopy under spinal anaesthesia: Comparison between lidocaine, ropivacaine, and levobupivacaine. Br J Anaesth 2003;90(3):309–313.

184. Brown DL: Spinal, epidural, and caudal anesthesia. In Miller RD (ed). *Anesthesia*, 4th ed. Churchill Livingston, 1994, pp 1505–1533.

185. Pawlowski J, Sukhani R, Pappas AL, et al: The anesthetic and recovery profile of two doses (60 and 80 mg) of plain mepivacaine for ambulatory spinal anesthesia. Anesth Analg 2000;91(3):580–584.

186. Kallio H, Snall EV, Kero MP, Rosenberg PH: A comparison of intrathecal plain solutions containing ropivacaine 20 or 15 mg versus bupivacaine 10 mg. Anesth Analg 2004;99(3):713–717; table of contents.

187. McNamee DA, Parks L, McClelland AM, et al: Intrathecal ropivacaine for total hip arthroplasty: Double-blind comparative study with isobaric 7.5 mg ml(-1) and 10 mg ml(-1) solutions. Br J Anaesth 2001;87(5):743–747.

188. Burke D, Kennedy S, Bannister J: Spinal anesthesia with 0.5% S(-)-bupivacaine for elective lower limb surgery. Reg Anesth Pain Med 1999;24(6):519–523.

189. Glaser C, Marhofer P, Zimpfer G, et al: Levobupivacaine versus racemic bupivacaine for spinal anesthesia. Anesth Analg 2002;94(1):194–198; table of contents.

190. Alley EA, Kopacz DJ, McDonald SB, Liu SS: Hyperbaric spinal levobupivacaine: A comparison to racemic bupivacaine in volunteers. Anesth Analg 2002;94(1):188–193; table of contents.

191. Bridenbaugh PO, Greene NM, Brull SJ: Spinal (subarachoid) neural blockade. In Cousins MJ, Bridenbaugh PO (eds). *Neural Blockade*, 3rd ed. Lippincott-Raven, 1998.

192. Tetzlaff JE, Dilger J, Yap E, Smith MP, Schoenwald PK: Cauda equina syndrome after spinal anaesthesia in a patient with severe vascular disease. Can J Anaesth 1998;45(7):667–669.

193. Lee DS, Bui T, Ferrarese J, Richardson PK: Cauda equina syndrome after incidental total spinal anesthesia with 2% lidocaine. J Clin Anesth 1998;10(1):66–69.

194. Maehara Y, Kusunoki S, Kawamoto M, et al: A prospective multicenter trial to determine the incidence of transient neurologic symptoms after spinal anesthesia with phenylephrine added to 0.5% tetracaine. Hiroshima J Med Sci 2001;50(2):47–51.

195. Kozody R, Palahniuk RJ, Wade JG, Cumming MO, Pucci WR: The effect of subarachnoid epinephrine and phenylephrine on spinal cord blood flow. Can Anaesth Soc J 1984;31(5):503–508.

196. Porter SS, Albin MS, Watson WA, Bunegin L, Pantoja G: Spinal cord and cerebral blood flow responses to subarachnoid injection of local anesthetics with and without epinephrine. Acta Anaesthesiol Scand 1985;29(3):330–338.

197. Concepcion M, Maddi R, Francis D, Rocco AG, Murray E, Covino BG: Vasoconstrictors in spinal anesthesia with tetracaine—A comparison of epinephrine and phenylephrine. Anesth Analg 1984;63(2):134–138.

198. Armstrong IR, Littlewood DG, Chambers WA: Spinal anesthesia with tetracaine—effect of added vasoconstrictors. Anesth Analg 1983;62(9):793–795.

199. Rice LJ, DeMars PD, Whalen TV, Crooms JC, Parkinson SK: Duration of spinal anesthesia in infants less than one year of age. Comparison of three hyperbaric techniques. Reg Anesth 1994;19(5):325–329.

200. Chambers WA, Littlewood DG, Scott DB: Spinal anesthesia with hyperbaric bupivacaine: effect of added vasoconstrictors. Anesth Analg 1982;61(1):49–52.

201. Moore JM, Liu SS, Pollock JE, Neal JM, Knab JH: The effect of epinephrine on small-dose hyperbaric bupivacaine spinal anesthesia: clinical implications for ambulatory surgery. Anesth Analg 1998;86(5):973–977.

202. Racle JP, Poy JY, Benkhadra A, Jourdren L, Fockenier F: [Prolongation of spinal anesthesia with hyperbaric bupivacaine by adrenaline and clonidine in the elderly]. Ann Fr Anesth Reanim 1988;7(2):139–144.

203. Vercauteren MP, Jacobs S, Jacquemyn Y, Adriaensen HA: Intrathecal labor analgesia with bupivacaine and sufentanil: The effect of adding 2.25 microg epinephrine. Reg Anesth Pain Med 2001;26(5):473–477.

204. Goodman SR, Kim-Lo SH, Ciliberto CF, Ridley DM, Smiley RM: Epinephrine is not a useful addition to intrathecal fentanyl or fentanyl-bupivacaine for labor analgesia. Reg Anesth Pain Med 2002;27(4):374–379.

205. Gautier PE, Debry F, Fanard L, Van Steenberge A, Hody JL: Ambulatory combined spinal-epidural analgesia for labor. Influence of epinephrine on bupivacaine-sufentanil combination. Reg Anesth 1997;22(2):143–149.

206. Chambers WA, Littlewood DG, Logan MR, Scott DB: Effect of added epinephrine on spinal anesthesia with lidocaine. Anesth Analg 1981;60(6):417–420.

207. Chiu AA, Liu S, Carpenter RL, Kasman GS, Pollock JE, Neal JM: The effects of epinephrine on lidocaine spinal anesthesia: A cross-over study. Anesth Analg 1995;80(4):735–739.

208. Racle JP, Benkhadra A, Poy JY: Subarachnoid anaesthesia produced by hyperbaric lignocaine in elderly patients. Prolongation of effect with adrenaline. Br J Anaesth 1988;60(7):831–835.

209. Spivey DL: Epinephrine does not prolong lidocaine spinal anesthesia in term parturients. Anesth Analg 1985;64(5):468–470.

210. Moore DC, Chadwick HS, Ready LB: Epinephrine prolongs lidocaine spinal: Pain in the operative site the most accurate method of determining local anesthetic duration. Anesthesiology 1987;67(3):416–418.

211. Glynn CJ, Mather LE, Cousins MJ, Wilson PR, Graham JR: Spinal narcotics and respiratory depression. Lancet 1979;2(8138):356–357.

212. Cunningham AJ, McKenna JA, Skene DS: Single injection spinal anaesthesia with amethocaine and morphine for transurethral prostatectomy. Br J Anaesth 1983;55(5):423–427.

213. Nordberg G, Hedner T, Mellstrand T, Dahlstrom B: Pharmacokinetic aspects of intrathecal morphine analgesia. Anesthesiology 1984;60(5):448–454.

214. Abouleish E, Rawal N, Rashad MN: The addition of 0.2 mg subarachnoid morphine to hyperbaric bupivacaine for cesarean delivery: A prospective study of 856 cases. Reg Anesth 1991;16(3):137–140.

215. Borgeat A, Singer T: Nausea and vomiting after spinal anaesthesia with morphine. Acta Anaesthesiol Scand 1998;42(10):1231.

216. Bonnet F, Buisson VB, Francois Y, Catoire P, Saada M: Effects of oral and subarachnoid clonidine on spinal anesthesia with bupivacaine. Reg Anesth 1990;15(4):211–214.

217. Dobrydnjov I, Axelsson K, Thorn SE, et al: Clonidine combined with small-dose bupivacaine during spinal anesthesia for inguinal herniorrhaphy: A randomized double-blinded study. Anesth Analg 2003;96(5):1496–1503; table of contents.

218. Strebel S, Gurzeler JA, Schneider MC, Aeschbach A, Kindler CH: Small-dose intrathecal clonidine and isobaric bupivacaine for orthopedic surgery: a dose-response study. Anesth Analg 2004;99(4):1231–1238; table of contents.

219. Filos KS, Goudas LC, Patroni O, Polyzou V: Hemodynamic and analgesic profile after intrathecal clonidine in humans. A dose-response study. Anesthesiology 1994;81(3):591–601; discussion 27A–28A.

220. Hassenbusch SJ, Gunes S, Wachsman S, Willis KD: Intrathecal clonidine in the treatment of intractable pain: A phase I/II study. Pain Med 2002;3(2):85–91.

221. Ackerman LL, Follett KA, Rosenquist RW: Long-term outcomes during treatment of chronic pain with intrathecal clonidine or clonidine/opioid combinations. J Pain Symptom Manage 2003;26(1):668–677.

222. Chen SR, Khan GM, Pan HL: Antiallodynic effect of intrathecal neostigmine is mediated by spinal nitric oxide in a rat model of diabetic neuropathic pain. Anesthesiology 2001;95(4):1007–1012.

223. Ho KM, Ismail H, Lee KC, Branch R: Use of intrathecal neostigmine as an adjunct to other spinal medications in perioperative and peripartum analgesia: A meta-analysis. Anaesth Intensive Care 2005;33(1):41–53.

224. Yegin A, Yilmaz M, Karsli B, Erman M: Analgesic effects of intrathecal neostigmine in perianal surgery. Eur J Anaesthesiol 2003;20(5):404–408.

225. Tan PH, Kuo JH, Liu K, Hung CC, Tsai TC, Deng TY: Efficacy of intrathecal neostigmine for the relief of postinguinal hemiorrhaphy pain. Acta Anaesthesiol Scand 2000;44(9):1056–1060.

226. Klohr S, Roth R, Hofmann T, Rossaint R, Heesen M: Definitions of hypotension after spinal anaesthesia for caesarean section: Literature search and application to parturients. Acta Anaesthesiol Scand 2010;54(8):909–921.

227. Mark JB, Steele SM: Cardiovascular effects of spinal anesthesia. Int Anesthesiol Clin 1989;27(1):31–39.

228. Cooper DW: Caesarean delivery vasopressor management. Curr Opin Anaesthesiol 2012;25(3):300–308.

229. Khaw KS, Ngan Kee WD, Lee SW: Hypotension during spinal anaesthesia for Caesarean section: Implications, detection, prevention and treatment. Fetal Matern Med Rev 2006;17(2):157–183.

230. Shimosato S, Etsten BE: The role of the venous system in cardiocirculatory dynamics during spinal and epidural anesthesia in man. Anesthesiology 1969;30(6):619–628.

231. Cooper J: Cardiac arrest during spinal anesthesia. Anesth Analg 2001;93(1):245.

232. Salinas FV, Sueda LA, Liu SS: Physiology of spinal anaesthesia and practical suggestions for successful spinal anaesthesia. Best Pract Res Clin Anaesthesiol 2003;17(3):289–303.

233. Meyhoff CS, Hesselbjerg L, Koscielniak-Nielsen Z, Rasmussen LS: Biphasic cardiac output changes during onset of spinal anaesthesia in elderly patients. Eur J Anaesthesiol 2007;24(9):770–775.

234. Roy L, Ramanathan S: ST-segment depression and myocardial contractility during cesarean section under spinal anesthesia. Can J Anaesth 1999;46(1):52–55.

235. Ou CH, Tsou MY, Ting CK, Chiou CS, Chan KH, Tsai SK: Occurrence of the Bezold-Jarisch reflex during Cesarean section under spinal anesthesia—A case report. Acta Anaesthesiol Taiwan 2004;42(3):175–178.

236. Mackey DC, Carpenter RL, Thompson GE, Brown DL, Bodily MN: Bradycardia and asystole during spinal anesthesia: A report of three cases without morbidity. Anesthesiology 1989;70(5):866–868.

237. Campagna JA, Carter C: Clinical relevance of the Bezold-Jarisch reflex. Anesthesiology 2003;98(5):1250–1260.

238. Lesser JB, Sanborn KV, Valskys R, Kuroda M: Severe bradycardia during spinal and epidural anesthesia recorded by an anesthesia information management system. Anesthesiology 2003;99(4):859–866.

239. Kinsella SM, Tuckey JP: Perioperative bradycardia and asystole: Relationship to vasovagal syncope and the Bezold-Jarisch reflex. Br J Anaesth 2001;86(6):859–868.

240. Bernards CM, Hymas NJ: Progression of first degree heart block to high-grade second degree block during spinal anesthesia. Can J Anaesth 1992;39(2):173–175.

241. Tarkkila P, Isola J: A regression model for identifying patients at high risk of hypotension, bradycardia and nausea during spinal anesthesia. Acta Anaesthesiol Scand 1992;36(6):554–558.

242. Klasen J, Junger A, Hartmann B, et al: Differing incidences of relevant hypotension with combined spinal-epidural anesthesia and spinal anesthesia. Anesth Analg 2003;96(5):1491–1495; table of contents.

243. Hartmann B, Junger A, Klasen J, et al: The incidence and risk factors for hypotension after spinal anesthesia induction: an analysis with automated data collection. Anesth Analg 2002;94(6):1521–1529; table of contents.

244. Ngan Kee WD, Khaw KS, Lau TK, Ng FF, Chui K, Ng KL: Randomised double-blinded comparison of phenylephrine versus ephedrine for maintaining blood pressure during spinal anaesthesia for non-elective Caesarean section. Anaesthesia 2008;63(12):1319–1326.

245. James FM 3rd, Greiss FC Jr, Kemp RA: An evaluation of vasopressor therapy for maternal hypotension during spinal anesthesia. Anesthesiology 1970;33(1):25–34.

246. Wildsmith JA: Management of hypotension during spinal anesthesia. Reg Anesth Pain Med 2000;25(3):322.

247. Sinclair CJ, Scott DB, Edstrom HH: Effect of the trendelenberg position on spinal anaesthesia with hyperbaric bupivacaine. Br J Anaesth 1982;54(5):497–500.

248. Cyna AM, Andrew M, Emmett RS, Middleton P, Simmons SW: Techniques for preventing hypotension during spinal anaesthesia for caesarean section. Cochrane Database Syst Rev 2006(4):CD002251.

249. Husaini SW, Russell IF: Volume preload: Lack of effect in the prevention of spinal-induced hypotension at caesarean section. Int J Obstet Anesth 1998;7(2):76–81.

250. Jackson R, Reid JA, Thorburn J: Volume preloading is not essential to prevent spinal-induced hypotension at caesarean section. Br J Anaesth 1995;75(3):262–265.

251. Dahlgren G, Granath F, Pregner K, Rosblad PG, Wessel H, Irestedt L: Colloid vs. crystalloid preloading to prevent maternal hypotension during spinal anesthesia for elective cesarean section. Acta Anaesthesiol Scand 2005;49(8):1200–1206.

252. Dyer RA, Farina Z, Joubert IA, et al: Crystalloid preload versus rapid crystalloid administration after induction of spinal anaesthesia (coload) for elective caesarean section. Anaesth Intensive Care 2004;32(3):351–357.

253. Roofthooft E, Van de Velde M: Low-dose spinal anaesthesia for Caesarean section to prevent spinal-induced hypotension. Curr Opin Anaesthesiol 2008;21(3):259–262.

254. Arzola C, Wieczorek PM: Efficacy of low-dose bupivacaine in spinal anaesthesia for Caesarean delivery: Systematic review and meta-analysis. Br J Anaesth 2011;107(3):308–318.

255. Ngan Kee WD, Lee A: Multivariate analysis of factors associated with umbilical arterial pH and standard base excess after Caesarean section under spinal anaesthesia. Anaesthesia 2003;58(2):125–130.

256. Labartino L, Mojdehi E, Mauro AL: Management of hypotension following spinal anesthesia for cesarean section. Anesth Analg 1966;45(2):179–182.

257. Ngan Kee WD, Khaw KS, Ng FF: Comparison of phenylephrine infusion regimens for maintaining maternal blood pressure during spinal anaesthesia for caesarean section. Br J Anaesth 2004;92(4):469–474.

258. Ngan Kee WD, Khaw KS, Ng FF: Prevention of hypotension during spinal anesthesia for cesarean delivery: An effective technique using combination phenylephrine infusion and crystalloid cohydration. Anesthesiology 2005;103(4):744–750.

259. Habib AS: A review of the impact of phenylephrine administration on maternal hemodynamics and maternal and neonatal outcomes in women undergoing cesarean delivery under spinal anesthesia. Anesth Analg 2012;114(2):377–390.

260. Park YH, Ryu T, Hong SW, Kwak KH, Kim SO: The effect of the intravenous phenylephrine on the level of spinal anesthesia. Korean J Anesthesiol 2011;61(5):372–376.

261. Caplan RA, Ward RJ, Posner K, Cheney FW: Unexpected cardiac arrest during spinal anesthesia: A closed claims analysis of predisposing factors. Anesthesiology 1988;68(1):5–11.

262. Lovstad RZ, Granhus G, Hetland S: Bradycardia and asystolic cardiac arrest during spinal anaesthesia: A report of five cases. Acta Anaesthesiol Scand 2000;44(1):48–52.

263. Pan PH, Moore CH, Ross VH: Severe maternal bradycardia and asystole after combined spinal-epidural labor analgesia in a morbidly obese parturient. J Clin Anesth 2004;16(6):461–464.

264. Pollard JB: Cardiac arrest during spinal anesthesia: common mechanisms and strategies for prevention. Anesth Analg 2001;92(1):252–256.

265. Cooper DW: Effect of vasopressors on systolic, mean and diastolic arterial pressure during spinal anaesthesia in pregnancy. Int J Obstet Anesth 2008;17(1):90–92.

266. Sahoo T, SenDasgupta C, Goswami A, Hazra A: Reduction in spinal-induced hypotension with ondansetron in parturients undergoing caesarean section: A double-blind randomised, placebo-controlled study. Int J Obstet Anesth 2012;21(1):24–28.

267. Smiley RM: Burden of proof. Anesthesiology 2009;111(3):470–472.

268. Greene NM, Brull SJ: *Physiology of Spinal Anesthesia*, 4th ed. Williams & Wilkins, 1981.

269. Steinbrook RA, Concepcion M, Topulos GP: Ventilatory responses to hypercapnia during bupivacaine spinal anesthesia. Anesth Analg 1988;67(3):247–252.

270. Nakayama M, Kanaya N, Fujita S, Namiki A: Effects of ephedrine on indocyanine green clearance during spinal anesthesia: Evaluation by the finger piece method. Anesth Analg 1993;77(5):947–949.

271. Zinn SE, Fairley HB, Glenn JD: Liver function in patients with mild alcoholic hepatitis, after enflurane, nitrous oxide-narcotic, and spinal anesthesia. Anesth Analg 1985;64(5):487–490.

272. Igarashi M, Kawana S, Iwasaki H, Namiki A: [Anesthetic management for a patient with citrullinemia and liver cirrhosis]. Masui 1995;44(1):96–99.

273. Fukuda T, Okutani R, Kono K, Yoshimura Y, Ochiai N: [Anesthetic management for cesarean section of a patient with transient diabetes insipidus and acute severe liver dysfunction]. Masui 1993;42(10):1511–1516.

274. McNeill MJ, Bennet A: Use of regional anaesthesia in a patient with acute porphyria. Br J Anaesth 1990;64(3):371–373.

275. Consolo D, Ouardirhi Y, Wessels C, Girard C: [Obstetrical anaesthesia and porphyrias]. Ann Fr Anesth Reanim 2005;24(4):428–431.

276. Runciman WB, Mather LE, Ilsley AH, Carapetis RJ, Upton RN: A sheep preparation for studying interactions between blood flow and drug disposition. III: Effects of general and spinal anaesthesia on regional blood flow and oxygen tensions. Br J Anaesth 1984;56(11):1247–1258.

277. Runciman WB, Mather LE, Ilsley AH, Carapetis RJ, Upton RN: A sheep preparation for studying interactions between blood flow and drug disposition. IV: The effects of general and spinal anaesthesia on blood flow and cefoxitin disposition. Br J Anaesth 1985;57(12):1239–1247.

278. Runciman WB, Mather LE, Ilsley AH, Carapetis RJ, Upton RN: A sheep preparation for studying interactions between blood flow and drug disposition. VI: Effects of general or subarachnoid anaesthesia on blood flow and chlormethiazole disposition. Br J Anaesth 1986;58(11):1308–1316.

279. Mather LE, Runciman WB, Ilsley AH, Carapetis RJ, Upton RN: A sheep preparation for studying interactions between blood flow and drug disposition. V: The effects of general and subarachnoid anaesthesia on blood flow and pethidine disposition. Br J Anaesth 1986;58(8): 888–896.

280. Taivainen T, Tuominen M, Rosenberg PH: Influence of obesity on the spread of spinal analgesia after injection of plain 0.5% bupivacaine at the L3–4 or L4–5 interspace. Br J Anaesth 1990;64(5):542–546.

281. Tuominen M, Taivainen T, Rosenberg PH: Spread of spinal anaesthesia with plain 0.5% bupivacaine: Influence of the vertebral interspace used for injection. Br J Anaesth 1989;62(4):358–361.

282. Tuominen M, Kuulasmaa K, Taivainen T, Rosenberg PH: Individual predictability of repeated spinal anaesthesia with isobaric bupivacaine. Acta Anaesthesiol Scand 1989;33(1):13–14.

283. Sundnes KO, Vaagenes P, Skretting P, Lind B, Edstrom HH: Spinal analgesia with hyperbaric bupivacaine: Effects of volume of solution. Br J Anaesth 1982;54(1):69–74.

284. Konishi R, Mitsuhata H, Saitoh J, Hirabayashi Y, Shimizu R: [The spread of subarachnoid hyperbaric dibucaine in the term parturient]. Masui 1997;46(2):184–187.

285. Veering BT, Ter Riet PM, Burm AG, Stienstra R, Van Kleef JW: Spinal anaesthesia with 0.5% hyperbaric bupivacaine in elderly patients: Effect of site of injection on spread of analgesia. Br J Anaesth 1996;77(3):343–346.

286. Cameron AE, Arnold RW, Ghorisa MW, Jamieson V: Spinal analgesia using bupivacaine 0.5% plain. Variation in the extent of the block with patient age. Anaesthesia 1981;36(3):318–322.

287. Pitkanen M, Haapaniemi L, Tuominen M, Rosenberg PH: Influence of age on spinal anaesthesia with isobaric 0.5% bupivacaine. Br J Anaesth 1984;56(3):279–284.

288. Veering BT, Burm AG, Vletter AA, van den Hoeven RA, Spierdijk J: The effect of age on systemic absorption and systemic disposition of bupivacaine after subarachnoid administration. Anesthesiology 1991;74(2):250–257.

289. Racle JP, Benkhadra A, Poy JY, Gleizal B: Spinal analgesia with hyperbaric bupivacaine: Influence of age. Br J Anaesth 1988;60(5):508–514.

290. Schiffer E, Van Gessel E, Gamulin Z: Influence of sex on cerebrospinal fluid density in adults. Br J Anaesth 1999;83(6):943–944.

291. Pargger H, Hampl KF, Aeschbach A, Paganoni R, Schneider MC: Combined effect of patient variables on sensory level after spinal 0.5% plain bupivacaine. Acta Anaesthesiol Scand 1998;42(4):430–434.

292. Povey HM, Jacobsen J, Westergaard-Nielsen J: Subarachnoid analgesia with hyperbaric 0.5% bupivacaine: Effect of a 60-min period of sitting. Acta Anaesthesiol Scand 1989;33(4):295–297.

293. Alston RP, Littlewood DG, Meek R, Edstrom HH: Spinal anaesthesia with hyperbaric bupivacaine: Effects of concentration and volume when administered in the sitting position. Br J Anaesth 1988;61(2):144–148.

294. Alston RP: Spinal anaesthesia with 0.5% bupivacaine 3 mL: Comparison of plain and hyperbaric solutions administered to seated patients. Br J Anaesth 1988;61(4):385–389.

295. Mitchell RW, Bowler GM, Scott DB, Edstrom HH: Effects of posture and baricity on spinal anaesthesia with 0.5% bupivacaine 5 ml. A double-blind study. Br J Anaesth 1988;61(2):139–143.

296. Povey HM, Olsen PA, Pihl H: Spinal analgesia with hyperbaric 0.5% bupivacaine: Effects of different patient positions. Acta Anaesthesiol Scand 1987;31(7):616–619.

297. Maroof M, Khan RM, Siddique M, Tariq M: Hypobaric spinal anaesthesia with bupivacaine (0.1%) gives selective sensory block for ano-rectal surgery. Can J Anaesth 1995;42(8):691–694.

298. Fettes PD, Jansson JR, Wildsmith JA: Failed spinal anaesthesia: mechanisms, management, and prevention. Br J Anaesth 2009;102(6):739–748.

299. Tuominen M, Pitkanen M, Rosenberg PH: Effect of speed of injection of 0.5% plain bupivacaine on the spread of spinal anaesthesia. Br J Anaesth 1992;69(2):148–149.

300. Van Gessel EF, Praplan J, Fuchs T, Forster A, Gamulin Z: Influence of injection speed on the subarachnoid distribution of isobaric bupivacaine 0.5%. Anesth Analg 1993;77(3):483–487.

301. Stienstra R, Van Poorten F: Speed of injection does not affect subarachnoid distribution of plain bupivacaine 0.5%. Reg Anesth 1990;15(4):208–210.

302. Bucx MJ, Kroon JW, Stienstra R: Effect of speed of injection on the maximum sensory level for spinal anesthesia using plain bupivacaine 0.5% at room temperature. Reg Anesth 1993;18(2):103–105.

303. Axelsson KH, Edstrom HH, Sundberg AE, Widman GB: Spinal anaesthesia with hyperbaric 0.5% bupivacaine: Effects of volume. Acta Anaesthesiol Scand 1982;26(5):439–445.

304. Peng PW, Chan VW, Perlas A: Minimum effective anaesthetic concentration of hyperbaric lidocaine for spinal anaesthesia. Can J Anaesth 1998;45(2):122–129.

305. Alfonsi P, Brusset A, Levy R, Gauneau P, Chauvin M: [Spinal anesthesia with bupivacaine without glucose in the elderly: Effect of concentration and volume on the hemodynamic profile]. Ann Fr Anesth Reanim 1991;10(6):543–547.

306. Pflug EA, Aasheim GM, Beck HA: Spinal anesthesia: bupivacaine versus tetracaine. Anesth Analg 1976;55(4):489–492.

307. Sheskey MC, Rocco AG, Bizzarri-Schmid M, Francis DM, Edstrom H, Covino BG: A dose-response study of bupivacaine for spinal anesthesia. Anesth Analg 1983;62(10):931–935.

308. Kopacz DJ: Spinal 2-chloroprocaine: Minimum effective dose. Reg Anesth Pain Med 2005;30(1):36–42.

309. Van Zundert AA, Grouls RJ, Korsten HH, Lambert DH: Spinal anesthesia. Volume or concentration—What matters? Reg Anesth 1996;21(2):112–118.

310. Cook TM, Fischer B, Bogod D, et al: Antiseptic solutions for central neuraxial blockade: Which concentration of chlorhexidine in alcohol should we use? Br J Anaesth 2009;103:456–457.

311. Schweizer RT: Mask wiggling as a potential cause of wound contamination. Lancet 1976;2(7995):1129–1130.

312. Veringa E, van Belkum A, Schellekens H: Iatrogenic meningitis by *Streptococcus salivarius* following lumbar puncture. J Hosp Infect 1995;29(4):316–318.

313. Hebl JR: The importance and implications of aseptic techniques during regional anesthesia. Reg Anesth Pain Med 2006;31(4):311–323.

314. Association of Anaesthetists of Great Britain and Ireland. Infection control in anaesthesia. Anaesthesia 2008;63(9):1027–1036.

315. Ross BK, Chadwick HS, Mancuso JJ, Benedetti C: Sprotte needle for obstetric anesthesia: Decreased incidence of post dural puncture headache. Reg Anesth 1992;17(1):29–33.

316. de Filho GR, Gomes HP, da Fonseca MH, Hoffman JC, Pederneiras SG, Garcia JH: Predictors of successful neuraxial block: A prospective study. Eur J Anaesthesiol 2002;19(6):447–451.

317. Lee PJ, Tang R, Sawka A, Krebs C, Vaghadia H: Brief report: Real-time ultrasound-guided spinal anesthesia using Taylor's approach. Anesth Analg 2011;112(5):1236–1238.

318. Palmer CM: Continuous spinal anesthesia and analgesia in obstetrics. Anesth Analg 2010;111(6):1476–1479.

319. Arkoosh VA, Palmer CM, Yun EM, et al: A randomized, double-masked, multicenter comparison of the safety of continuous intrathecal labor analgesia using a 28-gauge catheter versus continuous epidural labor analgesia. Anesthesiology 2008;108(2):286–298.

320. Sng BL, Lim Y, Sia AT: An observational prospective cohort study of incidence and characteristics of failed spinal anaesthesia for caesarean section. Int J Obstet Anesth 2009;18(3):237–241.

321. Levy JH, Islas JA, Ghia JN, Turnbull C: A retrospective study of the incidence and causes of failed spinal anesthetics in a university hospital. Anesth Analg 1985;64(7):705–710.

322. Hoppe J, Popham P: Complete failure of spinal anaesthesia in obstetrics. Int J Obstet Anesth 2007;16(3):250–255.

323. Reina MA, Collier CB, Prats-Galino A, Puigdellivol-Sanchez A, Maches F, De Andres JA: Unintentional subdural placement of epidural catheters during attempted epidural anesthesia: An anatomic study of spinal subdural compartment. Reg Anesth Pain Med 2011;36(6):537–541.

324. Capdevila X, Dadure C: Perioperative management for one day hospital admission: Regional anesthesia is better than general anesthesia. Acta Anaesthesiol Belg 2004;55(Suppl):33–36.

325. Ruben JE, Kamsler PM: Unilateral spinal anesthesia for surgical reduction of hip fractures. Am J Surg 1950;79(2):312–317.

326. Khatouf M, Loughnane F, Boini S, et al: [Unilateral spinal anaesthesia in elderly patient for hip trauma: A pilot study]. Ann Fr Anesth Reanim 2005;24(3):249–254.

327. Cappelleri G, Aldegheri G, Danelli G, et al: Spinal anesthesia with hyperbaric levobupivacaine and ropivacaine for outpatient knee arthroscopy: A prospective, randomized, double-blind study. Anesth Analg 2005;101(1):77–82; table of contents.

328. Fanelli G, Borghi B, Casati A, Bertini L, Montebugnoli M, Torri G: Unilateral bupivacaine spinal anesthesia for outpatient knee arthroscopy. Italian Study Group on Unilateral Spinal Anesthesia. Can J Anaesth 2000;47(8):746–751.

329. Nair GS, Abrishami A, Lermitte J, Chung F: Systematic review of spinal anaesthesia using bupivacaine for ambulatory knee arthroscopy. Br J Anaesth 2009;102(3):307–315.

330. Casati A, Fanelli G: Unilateral spinal anesthesia. State of the art. Minerva Anestesiol 2001;67(12):855–862.

331. Schneider MC, Holzgreve W: [100 years ago: Oskar Kreis, a pioneer in spinal obstetric analgesia at the University Women's Clinic of Basel]. Anaesthesist 2001;50(7):525–528.

332. Horlocker TT, Wedel DJ, Rowlingson JC, et al: Regional anesthesia in the patient receiving antithrombotic or thrombolytic therapy: American Society of Regional Anesthesia and Pain Medicine evidence-based guidelines (third edition). Reg Anesth Pain Med 2010;35(1):64–101.

333. Bogin IN, Stulin ID: [Application of the method of 2-dimensional echospondylography for determining landmarks in lumbar punctures]. Zh Nevropatol Psikhiatr Im S S Korsakova 1971;71(12):1810–1811.

334. Perlas A: Evidence for the use of ultrasound in neuraxial blocks. Reg Anesth Pain Med 2010;35(2 Suppl):S43–S46.

335. Chin KJ, Karmakar MK, Peng P: Ultrasonography of the adult thoracic and lumbar spine for central neuraxial blockade. Anesthesiology 2011;114(6):1459–1485.

336. Chin KJ, Perlas A: Ultrasonography of the lumbar spine for neuraxial and lumbar plexus blocks. Curr Opin Anaesthesiol 2011;24(5):567–572.

337. Chin KJ, Perlas A, Singh M, et al: An ultrasound-assisted approach facilitates spinal anesthesia for total joint arthroplasty. Can J Anaesth 2009;56(9):643–650.

338. O'Donnell D, Prasad A, Perlas A: Ultrasound-assisted spinal anesthesia in obese patients. Can J Anaesth 2009;56(12):982–983.

339. Chin KJ, Chan VW, Ramlogan R, Perlas A: Real-time ultrasound-guided spinal anesthesia in patients with a challenging spinal anatomy: Two case reports. Acta Anaesthesiol Scand 2010;54(2):252–255.

340. Chin KJ, Perlas A, Chan V, Brown-Shreves D, Koshkin A, Vaishnav V: Ultrasound imaging facilitates spinal anesthesia in adults with difficult surface anatomic landmarks. Anesthesiology 2011;115(1):94–101.

341. Margarido CB, Arzola C, Balki M, Carvalho JC: Anesthesiologists' learning curves for ultrasound assessment of the lumbar spine. Can J Anaesth 2010;57(2):120–126.

342. Halpern SH, Banerjee A, Stocche R, Glanc P: The use of ultrasound for lumbar spinous process identification: A pilot study. Can J Anaesth 2010;57(9):817–822.

343. Carvalho JC: Ultrasound-facilitated epidurals and spinals in obstetrics. Anesthesiol Clin 2008;26(1):145–158, vii–viii.

344. Bron JL, van Royen BJ, Wuisman PI: The clinical significance of lumbosacral transitional anomalies. Acta Orthop Belg 2007;73(6):687–695.

345. Spivak H, Nudelman I, Fuco V, et al: Laparoscopic extraperitoneal inguinal hernia repair with spinal anesthesia and nitrous oxide insufflation. Surg Endosc 1999;13(10):1026–1029.

346. Schmidt J, Carbajo MA, Lampert R, Zirngibl H: Laparoscopic intraperitoneal onlay polytetrafluoroethylene mesh repair (IPOM) for inguinal hernia during spinal anesthesia in patients with severe medical conditions. Surg Laparosc Endosc Percutan Tech 2001;11(1):34–37.

347. Vaghadia H, Viskari D, Mitchell GW, Berrill A: Selective spinal anesthesia for outpatient laparoscopy. I: Characteristics of three hypobaric solutions. Can J Anaesth 2001;48(3):256–260.

348. Tzovaras G, Zacharoulis D, Georgopoulou S, Pratsas K, Stamatiou G, Hatzitheofilou C: Laparoscopic ventral hernia repair under spinal anesthesia: A feasibility study. Am J Surg 2008;196(2):191–194.

349. Chilvers CR, Vaghadia H, Mitchell GW, Merrick PM: Small-dose hypobaric lidocaine-fentanyl spinal anesthesia for short duration outpatient laparoscopy. II. Optimal fentanyl dose. Anesth Analg 1997;84(1):65–70.

350. Ghodki PS, Sardesai SP, Thombre SK: Evaluation of the effect of intrathecal clonidine to decrease shoulder tip pain in laparoscopy under spinal anaesthesia. Indian J Anaesth 2010;54(3):231–234.

351. Jonnesco T. Remarks ON GENERAL SPINAL ANALGESIA. Br Med J 1909;2(2550):1396–1401.

352. Lee AJ, Ranasinghe JS, Chehade JM, Arheart K, Saltzman BS, Penning DH, et al: Ultrasound assessment of the vertebral level of the intercristal line in pregnancy. Anesth Analg 2011;113(3):559–564.

Mechanisms and Management of Failed Spinal Anesthesia

John D. Rae and Paul D. W. Fettes

INTRODUCTION

In busy clinical practice it is not uncommon that an intrathecal injection of local anesthetic in attempt to accomplish spinal anesthesia, perfectly performed, fails. Indeed, despite the reliability of the technique, the possibility of failure can never be completely eliminated. Managing a patient with an ineffective or inadequate spinal anesthetic can be challenging, and prevention is better than cure.

In this chapter, we discuss systematically the potential mechanisms by which spinal anesthesia may fail: detail strategies to decrease the failure rate and protocols for managing an incomplete spinal anesthetic.

Clinical Pearl

- Inability to reach the subarachnoid space, errors in drug preparation or injection, unsatisfactory spread of the injectate within the cerebrospinal fluid (CSF), ineffective drug action on neural tissue, and difficulties relating to patient expectations and psychology rather than genuine block failure.

The dense neuraxial blockade obtained by the administration of a spinal (intrathecal) injection of local anesthetic is widely held to be among the most reliable regional techniques. The anatomy is usually straightforward to palpate and identify, the technique for needle insertion simple and easy to teach, and the presence of CSF acts as both a definite endpoint for needling and a medium for carriage of local anesthetic within the subarachnoid space. The simplicity of the procedure was succinctly described by Labat, one of the pioneers of regional anesthesia, almost 100 years ago.[1]

> Two conditions are, therefore, absolutely necessary to produce spinalanaesthesia: Puncture of the dura mater and subarachnoid injection of an anesthetic agent.
>
> Gaston Labat, 1922

Yet, despite this simplicity, failure is not uncommon. What constitutes failure? At the most basic level, a spinal anesthetic has been attempted but the satisfactory conditions for proceeding with surgery are not obtained. Failure encompasses a spectrum that includes the total absence of any neuraxial block or the development of a partial block that is of insufficient height, duration, or quality.

In experienced hands, most anesthesiologists would expect the failure rate of spinal anesthesia to be low, probably less than 1%. A retrospective analysis of almost 5000 spinal anesthetics by Horlocker and colleagues[2] reported inadequate anesthesia in less than 2% of cases, and failure rates of under 1% have been described.[3] Yet, the "failed spinal" demonstrates remarkable interinstitutional variation, and in some published reports, it may be much higher. One American teaching hospital quoted a surprising failure rate of 17%, with the majority of failures deemed "avoidable."[4] A second institution reported a 4% failure rate—more in keeping with expectations, but nonetheless significant.[5] Analyzing their failures, "errors of judgement" were felt to be the main causative factor. The suggestion from these reports is that with meticulous attention to detail and appropriate management, most failures of spinal anesthesia could be prevented.

Patients undergoing an operation under spinal block expect reliable surgical anesthesia, and an inadequate block will generate anxiety for both patient and clinician. In addition, by conducting this invasive procedure, such as spinal anesthesia, we subject patients to small but well-established risks. For these reasons and to improve our own clinical practice, we must strive to minimize the incidence of failure, and to do this we must understand why failure occurs. Broadly, there are three areas where shortfalls may occur: faulty technique, lack of sufficient experience to troubleshoot "on the go" and the lack of attention to detail.[6] It is helpful to distill the procedure into five distinct phases and analyze the keys to success at each stage. In sequence, these phases are lumbar puncture, injection of local anesthetic solution, spread of solution through the CSF, drug action on neural tissue, and patient management.

MECHANISMS OF FAILURE

Unsuccessful Lumbar Puncture

The most evident cause of failure is an inability to successfully access the subarachnoid space. This may occur due to incorrect needling technique, poor patient positioning, anatomical abnormality, or equipment-related factors. The first two factors are operator and experience dependent and therefore can be considered modifiable. Anatomical difficulties such as scoliosis, kyphosis, vertebral collapse, calcified ligaments, or obesity may increase the difficulty of lumbar puncture, particularly in the geriatric population, but can be overcome at least to some degree by good positioning and clinical experience. Issues with equipment may result in a lack of CSF flow despite correct placement of the needle within the subarachnoid space. Manufacturing problems resulting in a needle with a blocked lumen are a theoretical possibility, but obstruction of the lumen by clot or tissue is more likely. For these reasons, the needle and stylet should be visually checked before starting the procedure, and to prevent blockage, the stylet should always be in place when the needle is advanced.

Clinical Pearls

- The needle and stylet should be visually checked before starting the procedure.
- Failure to obtain CSF flow despite an apparently successful needle placement(s) should raise the suspicion of needle blockage and prompt needle withdrawal and "flush test" to assure patency.

Positioning

Optimal positioning is vital to facilitate needle placement, particularly in more challenging cases. The choice of sitting or lateral position is of personal preference. Sitting may allow easier identification of the midline, particularly in the obese, and is often seen as the position of choice for "difficult" spinals; however, the reverse may also be true. In any event, the patient should be on a firm, level gurney or bed that can be adjusted in height for ergonomic ease. The patient should be asked to curl up, flexing the entire spine to maximize the space for needle

insertion between spinous processes. Flexing of the hips, knees, and neck increases the effectiveness of this procedure. The presence of a skilled assistant to "coach" the patient and discourage any lateral or rotational movement is invaluable.[7]

Clinical Pearls

- A useful position tip is to ask the patient to "try to touch their knees with their chin".
- This typically leads to a satisfactory flexing of the spine and facilitates needle passage into epidural or subarachnoidal space.

Needle Insertion

The classically described site for lumbar puncture is in the midline between the spinous processes of the third and fourth lumbar vertebrae. This level can be estimated by drawing a line between the anterior superior iliac spines: Tuffier's line. Evidence has shown that this landmark may be very accurate at estimating their level of needle insertion,[8] and more detailed palpation and making sure that the presumptive L3/4 level makes sense ("reality check"). It must be emphasized that great care must be taken to insert needle below the conus medullaris, which in some individuals may be as low as the second lumbar interspace. The needle should be perpendicular to the skin in both planes and advanced with caution. Fine adjustments to the needle angle may be required if an obstruction is encountered, with a slight cephalad angulation most commonly required. Lateral alterations in needle angle may be required, especially in patients with significant scoliosis and when needle-bone contact occurs at a greater depth (beyond spinal process), suggesting needle-contact with the laminae and the need to re-adjust the needle path lateral-medial. A clear knowledge of vertebral 3D-spacial anatomy and a mental image of where the needle tip is thought to lie will assist the operator in interpreting tactile feedback from the needle and guide alterations in needle angle.

In addition to the midline technique, lateral or paramedian approaches can be used. These have the advantage of avoiding ossified midline ligaments, particularly a problem in the elderly, but are more technically challenging procedures. If difficulty should be encountered, the same basic principles apply: Ensuring the patient is optimally positioned and a thorough understanding of the path of the needle and the likely obstacle may yield results.

Adjuncts

The ideal means of achieving the optimal spinal position is with a patient who is comfortable and calm, understands what is being asked of him or her, and has full trust in the anesthesia provider. Preprocedure counseling, establishment of rapport, and a reassuring, professional manner can facilitate this during the spinal procedure. A small dose of anxiolytic medication may assist proceedings, but sedation should be titrated carefully on the basis that it is easier to give more drug than to mitigate the effects of overdosing. Care must be taken to infiltrate local anesthetic to provide effective analgesia without distorting the spinal anatomy; an initial intradermal injection will help to facilitate this. The purpose of these adjuncts is to attain the ideal position, allay patient concern, and minimize movement, thus providing the best possible conditions for lumbar puncture.

Ultrasound

The ubiquitous use of ultrasound in regional anesthesia has not been adopted as a routine neuraxial procedure but has several advantages to offer over a landmark technique. A preprocedure scan can be useful in patients with abnormal or impalpable anatomy to identify the midline and level of injection and to assess the depth of dura from the skin. Its use in epidural techniques has been shown to increase success rates, reduce the need for multiple punctures, and improve patient comfort; it seems logical that this would translate to increased success with spinal anesthesia.[9] Real-time scanning of needle placement for epidural insertion has been described but is not a technique in widespread use. The main obstacles to uptake of ultrasound in neuraxial block are lack of awareness of the technique and limited training in this area, with the technique requiring knowledge of the sonoanatomy of the spine and a high degree of dexterity.

Pseudosuccessful Lumbar Puncture

Rarely, the flow of a clear fluid of noncerebrospinal origin through the spinal needle may mimic successful lumbar puncture without this having occurred. There are two scenarios in which this may occur. "Topping up" a lumbar epidural in obstetric practice for cesarean section may result in a reservoir of local anesthetic in the epidural space. Epidural spread of injectate has also been reported following lumbar plexus block.[10] This may be mistaken for CSF at subsequent spinal injection.

Traditionally, bedside testing for glucose has been advocated to distinguish this fluid from CSF; however, a positive glucose test does not definitely confirm the presence of CSF as the fluid in the epidural space will rapidly equilibrate with extracellular fluid. Another, potential source of fluid mimicking CSF is the presence of a congenital arachnoid cyst.[11] Tarlov cysts are meningeal dilatations of the posterior spinal nerve root, reportedly present in 4.5%–9% of the population.[12] Such a cyst could result in CSF flow through the needle, but anesthetic injected may fail to result in anesthesia. The actual clinical relevance and occurrence of failed spinal anesthesia due to the "false CSF" flow from arachnoidal cysts is unknown.

Solution Injection Errors

Successful lumbar puncture is an absolute requirement for spinal anesthesia but does not preclude failure by a number of other mechanisms. To ensure a block suitable for surgery, a proper dose of local anesthetic must be calculated, prepared, and delivered to the site of action.

Dose Selection

Research into intrathecal drug spread has demonstrated that, providing a dose within the therapeutic range is selected, alterations in drug dose have a relatively minor part to play in the height of spinal block achieved but are significant in governing the duration and quality of the result.[13,14] The dose selected is dictated by a number of factors, including choice of local anesthetic, baricity of the solution, patient positioning, the nature of block desired, and the extent and length of planned surgery. To choose a suitable dose, the clinician must have knowledge of the clinical characteristics and pharmakokinetics of the intrathecally injected local anesthetics.

Trials of drug dosing during continuous intrathecal anesthesia have demonstrated that a satisfactory block can be achieved with relatively low anesthetic doses.[15] Given that failure of a "single-shot" spinal is distressing for the patient and can be associated with increased morbidity (eg, the requirement for general anesthesia and airway management during cesarean section), doses used in practice are often deliberately in excess of the bare minimum required. The clinician must weigh the difficulties of managing hypotension or prolonged anesthesia versus the risk of block failure.

Studies have shown that in many circumstances, lower than commonly-used doses (ie, 5–10 mg rather than 15 mg of hyperbaric bupivacaine) can be used sufficient to achieve effective blockade.[16] This has the advantage of potentially lessening hypotension and, by increasing the speed of block regression, aiding postoperative mobility or decreasing the need for bladder catheterization. While these techniques can be successfully used in experienced hands and appropriately selected cases, the margin for error is significantly decreased. It becomes imperative that the entire volume of the syringe is successfully delivered into the subarachnoid space. Loss of even a small amount of injectate either via spillage (see the next section) or simply in the dead space of the needle and hub may result in an ineffective anesthetic.

Loss of Injectate

Leakage may occur at the Luer connection between needle and syringe or from a deficiency at the joint between needle hub and shaft.[17] Considering the small volumes involved, even the smallest leak of solution may result in a significant decrease in the dose of drug delivered. This pitfall can be avoided by ensuring a good connection between the syringe and needle hub and visually verifying that no leak is occurring.

Misplaced Injection

It is crucial that during the process of ensuring a leak-tight connection between needle and syringe, meticulous attention is paid to avoid accidental movement of the needle. Once the syringe is securely connected, aspiration of CSF can be used to confirm that the tip is still within the subarachnoid space. This maneuver in itself carries potential for needle displacement, as does the injection of anesthetic solution. For this reason, it is imperative that the operator secure the needle position prior to any further manipulation. This can be achieved by stabilizing the dorsum of one hand against the patient's back and anchoring the hub of the needle between thumb and forefinger while the other hand has control of the syringe.[18] Many anesthesiologists would advocate aspirating CSF postinjection to ensure the needle position has not moved during the process. Although there is no evidence to suggest this reduces the failure rate, it may at least alert the anesthetist to the possibility that not all of the drug has reached its intended destination.

Clinical Pearl

The following steps can be undertaken to assure that the needle has been in the subarachnoidal space throughout the cycle of injection:

- Gentle aspiration of 0.5-1 ml before injection to assure CSF retrieval from the subarachnoidal space.
- Gentle aspiration of 0.5-1ml at the end of the spinal injection can be done to assure that the needle tip stayed in the subarachnoidal space throughout the injection process.
- The aspirated 0.5ml-1ml is then re-injected and the needle is withdrawn.

Stabilization of the needle during injection is important with all types of spinal needle but particularly so with "pencil-point" needles commonly in use. In these needles, the opening through which injectate emerges is some distance proximal to the tip; therefore, minimal posterior displacement of the needle can result in this opening being outside the subarachnoid space and subsequent block failure.[19] As the length of the opening of pencil-point needles is significantly longer than the bevel of a Quincke needle, it is also possible for the dura to bridge this opening[20] (Figure 23A–1). This problem may be compounded by the dura mater working as a flap valve. The opening CSF pressure results in an initial successful flow of CSF through the

needle (Figure 23A–2a), but on injection, the dura moves forward and a portion of the solution flows into the epidural space (Figure 23A–2b). As with leakage between the needle and syringe, given the small volumes involved, loss of even a small amount of injectate may substantially influence the quality of the block.

If the needle tip is misplaced such that the arachnoid mater acts as the flap valve, local anesthetic will spread into the subdural space (Figure 23A–2c). Subdural block is well recognized as a potential side effect of epidural anesthesia[21] (where it may result in a more extensive, prolonged, or unpredictable effect because of the larger volume of local anesthetic used for epidural anesthesia), but it has also been recorded as a consequence of attempted spinal anesthesia.[22,23] Subdural injection is seen relatively frequently during myelography and its occurrence in daily clinical practice of anesthesiology is likely underestimated.[24]

Due to the initial flow of CSF and minute distances between the layers of the dura, these subtle misplacements are difficult to identify or eliminate. One suggested solution, once CSF has been successfully located, is to rotate the needle a full 360° before aspirating. Theoretically, this may lessen the chance of the dura layers catching on the opening of the needle.

Inadequate Intrathecal Spread

Even when the entire volume of injectate is successfully delivered to the intrathecal space, the spread of solution within the CSF can be somewhat unpredictable.[25] The practitioner must have an understanding of the common factors affecting intrathecal spread and the degree to which they may be manipulated.

Anatomical Abnormality

Dispersion of injectate within the CSF is dictated by the complex interaction between the anatomy of the spinal canal, the physical properties of the solution, and gravity.

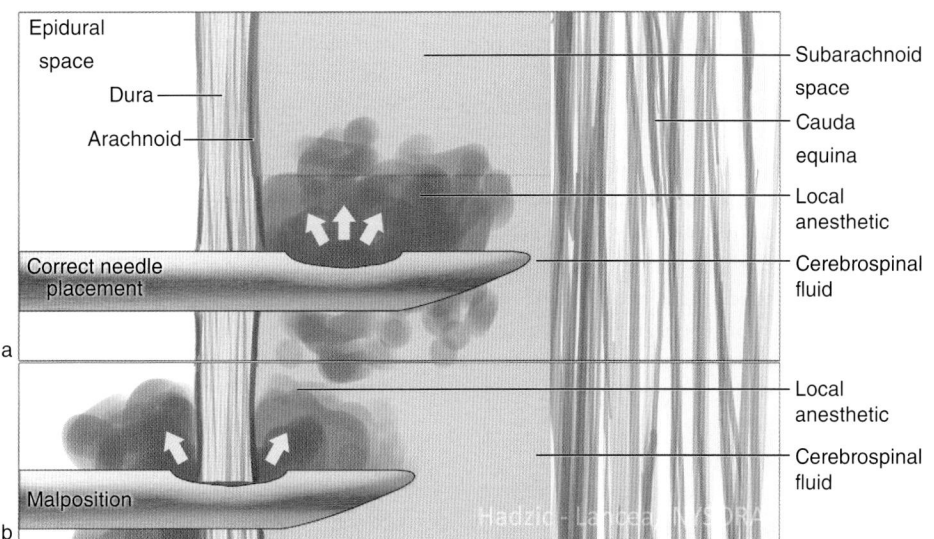

FIGURE 23A–1. Correct needle placement with (**A**) all drug delivered to CSF and (**B**) malposition where some of the drug is lost into the epidural space.

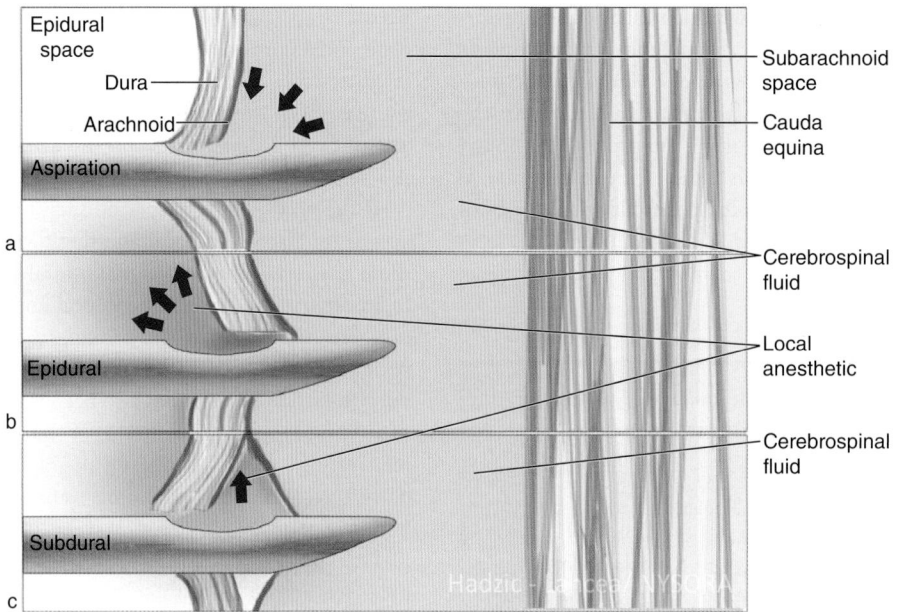

FIGURE 23A–2. The flap valve effect: (**A**) CSF is aspirated but on injection the meningeal layers move, resulting in (**B**) epidural or (**C**) subdural injection of drug.

The normal kyphotic and lordotic curvatures of the vertebral column are important anatomical factors affecting the spread of solution, and the presence of anatomical abnormality, including scoliosis, will alter this. Preoperative examination of the patient may allow identification of such anatomical abnormalities. The actual effect of anatomical deviations on the block quality is unpredictable; variability in the block height is probably more common than block failure.

To achieve a uniform symmetrical block, the local anesthetic should diffuse freely within CSF, without anatomical barriers. For instance, it is also possible for the ligaments that support the spinal cord to form a barrier to the spread of anesthetic within the subarachnoid space. By acting as septae, these anomalies, although uncommon, may cause a unilateral block,[26] or limited cephalad spread. Other examples of spinal pathologies that may impede the spread or effect of injectate include spinal stenosis and adhesions from spinal surgery or from previous administration of intrathecal chemotherapy.[27,28]

In one case report, two occurrences of failed spinal anesthesia in the same patient were investigated with magnetic resonance imaging (MRI) and revealed larger-than-normal CSF volume in the dural sac below the termination of the cord.[29] The volume of CSF within the subarachnoid space has since been shown to be an important cause of the interindividual variation in the degree of cephalad spread of anesthetic.[30] MRI studies found negative correlation between lumbosacral CSF volume and peak sensory block height. A similar picture may be encountered in patients with connective tissue diseases, including Marfan syndrome, who may develop dural ectasia, a pathological enlargement of the dura.[31]

Density of the Local Anesthetic Solution

Density of the injected solution relative to the CSF is another important determinant of intrathecal spread. "Plain" bupivacaine is commonly regarded as isobaric, although it is in fact slightly hypobaric compared to CSF at 37°C. Its spread through CSF is by local turbulent currents and diffusion, which results in a block of somewhat unpredictable spread (in some cases no higher than the second lumbar dermatome[32]) with a relatively slow onset to maximal block height. However, it tends to give reliable anesthesia to the lower extremities with limited spread to the thoracic level. The combination of the slow onset and lower block height results in less risk of cardiovascular instability.[33]

The use of hyperbaric solutions to influence the spread within CSF was described more than 100 years ago by Barker, an early proponent of neuraxial blockade in the United Kingdom.[34] This is typically achieved by addition of dextrose to accomplish a density higher than that of the CSF. Commercial preparations of hyperbaric local anesthetic contain up to 8% glucose, although even preparations containing 1% glucose will result in a predictable block. Following the injection of a hyperbaric solution at the level of L3/L4 in a supine subject, this solution travels predominantly by bulk flow under the influence of gravity "downward" along the curvature of the spine. It naturally moves to the concavity of the thoracic curve (Figure 23A–3), exposing the neuraxial tissue to local anesthetic. If, however, the level of injection is more caudal, the hyperbaric solution may be descend below the lumbar lordosis and fail to spread more cephalad (Figure 23A–4), particularly if the injection is performed while sitting and the patient is not quickly placed supine.

This manifests clinically as a block of only the sacral nerve roots, as reported with a caudally placed spinal catheters.[35] In some circumstances, a "saddle" block is intentionally sought.

Drug Failure

Assuming successful lumbar puncture, adequate drug delivery, and normal anatomy, the final possible cause of an ineffective

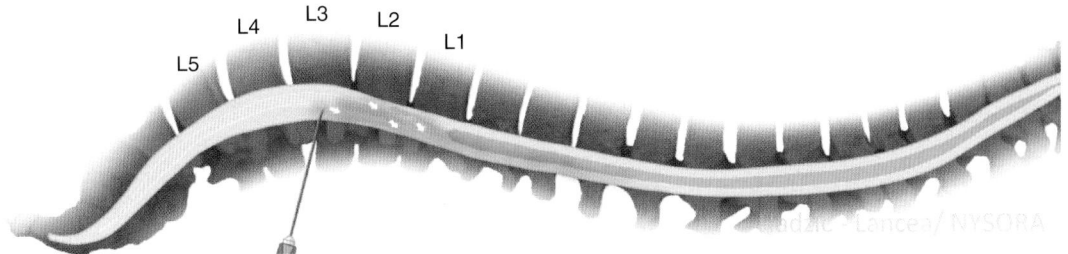

FIGURE 23A–3. Injection at the second or third lumbar interspace will normally result in a significant fraction of the drug spreading cranially from the point of injection (but too high an injection risks inadvertent damage to the spinal cord).

spinal anesthetic is a failure of drug to exhibit blockade on the neural tissue.

Injection of Incorrect Drug

Anesthetics for intrathecal use are commonly supplied in ampoules of aqueous solution, ready for use. Preparations of local anesthetics specifically made for use in spinal anesthesia minimize the opportunity for errors during drug preparation. Nevertheless, the presence of other clear solutions on the spinal tray gives the potential for confusion and inadvertent injection of the wrong drug, with consequent block failure or neurotoxicity. Local anesthetic used for skin preparation is the common culprit; chlorhexidine solution may also be present, although recent guidelines advise separating this from the procedural area due to the risk of contamination and possible adhesive arachnoiditis. The relatively high incidence of so-called syringe swaps in general anesthetic practice has led to almost-universal use of syringe labels. The potential for syringe swaps can be further decreased by meticulous preparation, reducing the number of unnecessary drug ampoules on the tray, and adopting a consistent system for drawing up solutions—for example, always using a certain size of syringe for each particular drug.

Physicochemical Incompatibility

The common practice of utilizing adjuvants to local anesthetic in spinal injections necessitates the mixing of solutions, introducing the possibility of a chemical reaction, potentially reducing efficacy. Clinical experience has shown that the commonly used opioids appear compatible with local anesthetics, but there are few hard data to support this and even fewer for mixing with other adjuncts, such as midazolam, clonidine, or ketamine.

The mixing of three substances for intrathecal injection, not uncommon in today's practice, must further raise the opportunity for chemical interaction. This reaction could result in formation of a precipitate, which would be obvious within the syringe, but less evident would be a reduction in pH of the solution. This could decrease the fraction of un-ionized drug within the injectate, thereby reducing the mass of local anesthetic capable of diffusing into neural tissue and available for neural blockade. One example of this effect may be illustrated by a case report of a higher failure rate following addition of vasoconstrictor to the local anesthetic solution.[36]

Inactive Local Anesthetic Solution

Amide local anesthetics such as bupivacaine, ropivacaine, and lidocaine are stable compounds, which are heat sterilized in solution and may be stored for years without significant impact on their efficacy. Regardless, several cases of spinal anesthetic failure thought to be related to local anesthetic inactivity have been published.[37–40] Local anesthetic inactivity may be more common with ester-type anesthetic agents, which are less chemically stable and over time may undergo hydrolysis, degrading their effectiveness.

Local Anesthetic Resistance

Several cases of failed spinal anesthesia have been attributed to local anesthetic resistance.[41,42] These authors postulated that the causes were altered activity of local anesthetic at the sodium channel as a result of mutation of the sodium channel. This altered activity, however, has not been demonstrated at cellular level, nor mutations found in the patients described. Mutations of sodium channels (channelopathies) do occur but they are rare, and are associated with significant neurological disease.

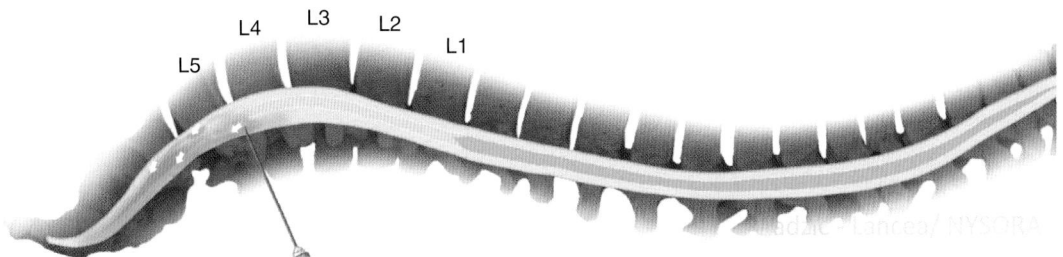

FIGURE 23A–4. Injection at the fourth interspace or lower reduces the risk of cord damage, but it may result in predominantly caudal spread of the drug and an inadequate block for surgery.

Specifically Na$_v$1.1 mutations are associated with intractable epilepsy[43] and Na$_v$1.7 mutations are associated with chronic pain.[43, 44] To our knowledge mutations of the sodium channel, however, do not exist in asymptomatic individuals.

Failure of Subsequent Management

A well executed spinal anesthetic typically results in reliable anesthesia. However, perioperative management of a patient under spinal anesthesia is just as important for success. For instance, the patient may perceive unblocked sensations of movement, pressure, or traction experienced intraoperatively to be painful or uncomfortable experiences. This likelihood is heightened by awareness of the clinical environment and the patient's underlying views, fears, and expectations of the hospital setting, potentiated by the stress of undergoing a surgical procedure. Failure to address these psychological aspects of spinal anesthesia can lead to anxiety, distress, and the need to convert an adequate spinal anesthetic to general anesthesia.

Even for the most composed patients, lying supine in operating theater completely awake while undergoing an operative procedure may be unnatural and anxiety-provoking experience. The surgery being performed may require the patient to lie in an awkward position for a considerable time (eg, during hip arthroplasty). Operating tables are primarily designed to provide good surgical conditions and are often narrow and uncomfortable. Manipulation of the intra-abdominal viscera may result in activation of unblocked parasympathetic nerves and the experience of unpleasant sensations. Patient selection and expectation management are also important to success. Adequate preprocedure patient counseling, positive suggestion, and a supportive, reassuring manner intraoperatively are all essential ingredients to success. A judicious use of sedative adjunctive medications such as benzodiazepines and intraoperative infusions of propofol and remifentanil can further contribute to the patient acceptance of the spinal anesthesia, satisfaction and improve overall perioperative experience. With appropriate monitoring and cautious dosing, there are few situations outside obstetric anesthesia for which sedation would be contraindicated. Some patients can also benefit from or prefer alternative distraction techniques, such as listening to music.

Testing the Block

There are wide variations in practice regarding the assessment of adequacy of a spinal anesthetic, but some form of test is commonly carried out, particularly in obstetric anesthesia. Common techniques include testing for motor effect by asking the patient to move his or her legs and then testing the different sensory modalities, such as light touch, cold, or pinprick sensation. Carried out well, this can be a confidence-building procedure; however, it also may instill doubt in the patient about the quality of the block or the anesthetist. If testing is commenced prematurely, without allowing adequate time for the spinal anesthesia to "set in", the patient may assume that the anesthetic failed and become anxious. For similar reasons, it is recommended that testing should start in the lower dermatomes, where the onset of the block will be the most rapid. By moving

cephalad from this point, the development of anesthesia can be demonstrated and anxiety prevented.

It should be noted that achievement of a block *height* adequate for surgery does not guarantee that the *quality* of the block is sufficient for surgery, particularly when pinprick or perception to cold are used as testing modalities. Provided the patient is not deeply sedated, block quality can be assessed by asking the operator to covertly apply a painful stimulus prior to incision without warning the patient. This can be achieved by pinching the skin with surgical forceps out of the patient's line of sight.

Combined Spinal-epidural and Catheter Techniques

Most commonly, intrathecal anesthetic techniques utilize a one-off injection that, as discussed, may not always provide satisfactory surgical anesthesia. The placement of an intrathecal catheter or a combined spinal-epidural (CSE) technique can be useful to extend the height of the block or prolong its duration, which adds an versatility. The presence of an accurately placed catheter will allow an inadequate block to be supplemented or infusion of local anesthetic can be used to provide continuous analgesia. Placement and maintenance of these catheters however, requires a higher level of knowledge and technical expertise on the part of the operator. The subarachnoidal injection during CSE requires small volume of local anesthetic thus, the discussed issues whereby a proportion of the injectate is lost via leakage or dead-space remain pertinent. Use of intrathecal catheters has declined as of late because of the increased potential for infection with the introduction of a catheter into the CSF and because of case reports of arachnoiditis resulting from the concentrated effect of local anesthetic on nerve roots.[45] Insertion can be technically challenging, and leaving an excessive length of catheter in situ may result in local anesthetic pooling in the caudal portion of the dural sac. Finally, the relatively uncommon use of the spinal catheters may be related to the potential risk of error whereby intrathecal catheter could be confused with an epidural catheter, which is much more commonly used in clinical practice. This may lead to an error in "toping up" and overdose with consequent development of high spinal anesthesia.

FAILED SPINAL ANESTHESIA

Despite meticulous technique and local anesthetic and dose selection, subarachnoidal injection caries a small risk of failed spinal anesthesia. Moreover, even when the level of spinal blockade appears to be adequate during testing, spinal anesthesia can fail to provide adequate operating conditions intraoperatively. To the patient, this may be a source of pain, anxiety, and psychological trauma and to the anesthesia provider one of stress, complaints, and potential medicolegal sequelae. For that reason, the possibility of block failure should be discussed with all patients as part of the consent process to ensure that both parties are cognizant of the possibility of this occurring and the steps to be taken if it does. If the duration or extent of the planned procedure is unclear, an alternative technique should be considered. In patients with severe comorbidities, respiratory compromise or a difficult airway, the traditional conversion to general anesthesia may be hazardous. For these reasons, prevention is better than cure, and meticulous attention to detail is crucial.

Management of the Failed Spinal Anesthesia

The strategy for managing an inadequate spinal anesthetic is dictated by two factors: the time at which failure is detected and the nature of the failure. After the subarachnoidal injection, the anesthesia provider should closely monitor the patient for the expected signs of neuraxial blockade. The consequences of autonomic nervous system blockade, such as decrease of blood pressure with or without the presence of compensatory tachycardia provide early clue of onset of spinal anesthesia even without any formal testing. Lack of autonomic response or slower-than-expected development of motor or sensory block should alert the clinician to potential of inadequate or failed spinal anesthesia. Although usually swift, the development of anesthesia can be more gradual in some patients,[6] and additional observation time should be contemplated before starting surgery or assuming failure. If 15 minutes have lapsed since intrathecal injection and the spinal block does not follow a typical onset pattern, anticipated, it is highly likely that the spinal anesthetic will be inadequate for surgery and additional anesthetic interventions will be required. The possible flaws in the block, their likely origins, and suggested solutions are outlined (Table 23A–1):

1. *No block*: An incorrect solution was injected, the solution was injected into an incorrect anatomical location, or the local anesthetic is defective. The options are to repeat the process or administer a general anesthetic. If repeating the spinal injection, sufficient time (20 minutes) must be allowed to pass to ensure that there is truly no block developing. If a second injection is performed after a successful but slowly developing first procedure, a "total spinal" may result.

2. *Spinal block of insufficient height*: Potential causes are that the local anesthetic has been lost during injection (eg, leakage at needle-syringe connection), lumbar puncture was in too low a lumbar interspace, or an anatomical barrier is preventing diffusion of anesthetic. Manipulating posture and utilizing gravity may overcome these difficulties. If hyperbaric formulation was used, the patient should be placed in Trendelenburg position with the hips and knees flexed. This will flatten the lumbar lordosis, allowing injectate to travel cephalad. Change in position after injection of isobaric bupivacaine is unlikely to be successful.

3. *Unilateral block*: The most common problem is patient position, although an anatomical barrier to spread formed by the longitudinal ligaments could lead to unilateral spinal anesthesia. Bilateral spread of the block can be encouraged by moving the patient so that the unblocked side is downward (although again positional change is less likely to be helpful when plain solutions have been used). A unilateral block should be sufficient for ipsilateral lower limb surgery, but the surgeon must be warned that the other limb is not anesthetized.

4. *Patchy block*: This describes a block that appears to have spread adequately but is of inconsistent quality with variable sensory and motor blockade. There are multiple possible explanations but most common is administration of an insufficient dose of anesthetic drug, either due to underdosing or solution not reaching the target. Additional sedation and opiate analgesia, may prove successful particularly if anxiety is a prominent factor. Alternatively, conversion to general anesthesia may be required.

TABLE 23A–1. Mechanisms of failure and suggested management.

Clinical Presentation	Possible Cause	Suggested Management
No block	Injection not into CSF Syringe swap Faulty local anesthetic	Repeat injection (with caution) General anesthesia
Insufficient block height or density	Insufficient drug delivered Injection site too low Anatomical abnormality	Postural maneuvers Intravenous analgesia/sedation
Unilateral block	Patient positioning Anatomical abnormality	Postural maneuvers Proceed with care (if correct side blocked)
Patchy block	Insufficient drug delivered Anatomical abnormality	Repeat injection (with caution) Intravenous analgesia/sedation General anesthesia
Inadequate duration	Insufficient drug delivered Syringe swap Lengthy procedure	Intravenous analgesia/sedation General anesthesia

5. *Inadequate duration*: The most likely culprit is the delivery of an insufficient dose of local anesthetic. Another possibility is a "syringe swap" by which a short-acting agent such as lidocaine is injected instead of the intended bupivacaine. Last, the procedure may have lasted longer than anticipated. As previously stated, the only realistic solutions are additional intravenous analgesia, sedation, or general anesthesia.

In all these scenarios, judicious use of analgesia and sedation will prove invaluable in the management of unsatisfactory block. Intravenous infusions of propofol and remifentanil, can be used at low concentrations to good effect. Postoperative documentation of events and patient follow-up are important.

Repeating the Block

If no appreciable block is seen at 15–20 minutes, then the most logical step is to repeat the injection, taking steps to eliminate the proposed cause of previous failure. Unless the previous injection is complete failure, repeating subarachnoidal injection should not be done routinely. This is because high concentrations of local anesthetic intrathecally can be neurotoxic, and repeating the procedure may lead to such a concentration,[46] particularly if there is an anatomical barrier preventing spread. Lesions of the cauda equina have been reported following multiple injections via an indwelling an intrathecal catheter.[47] Repeating the procedure, particularly in the context of a patchy or low block, can lead to unpredictable extensive cephalad spread[48] with the potential for cardiovascular instability, respiratory embarrassment, or total spinal anesthesia.

Moreover, if block failure is secondary to anatomical factors, then repeat injection is unlikely to produce a more favorable result. A unilateral block thought secondary to a longitudinal anatomical barrier may tempt the anesthetist into performing a second injection on the opposite side, but there is no guarantee that this will not follow the path of the first attempt. An obstruction to intrathecal spread may also distort the epidural space, so epidural anesthesia may prove no more successful.

Postoperative Management
Documentation and Follow-up

At the postoperative visit, the patient should be given a full explanation of events. A detailed account of proceedings should be documented in the medical record to inform future anesthetic procedures. Rarely, unusual patterns of failure may signal the presence of serious neurological pathology, and if there are other signs or symptoms, then neurology consultation is advised. If a patient has experienced failure of spinal anesthesia on more than one occasion, MRI of the spine may be used to exclude or delineate abnormal anatomy.

Investigating "Faulty" Local Anesthetic

Although spinal anesthetic failure is an uncommon occurrence, certain circumstances may lead the anesthetist to closely scrutinize the local anesthetic agent. Lack of effect following a technically undemanding procedure or multiple failures within the same theater or department raises the possibility of a faulty batch of local anesthetic. Hyperbaric bupivacaine is the most commonly reported culprit, most likely due to its prevalence in current practice.[37–40] Amide local anesthetics are chemically stable compounds that undergo heat sterilization as part of normal preparation. In addition to this, modern quality control procedures mean that drug failure is a rare occurrence, but if all other factors are eliminated, it must be considered. If the anesthetic used in the procedure has been retained, some authorities advocate infiltrating the skin to test its efficacy. Corroboration with reports from colleagues, pharmacy, and other hospitals will help to establish if others have had similar problems, although concerns of anesthetic failure have rarely been borne out by case reports.

SUMMARY

With proper technique, training, and meticulous attention to detail, failure rate of spinal anesthesia should be less than 1%. Good communication and appropriate management can mitigate against many of the common difficulties. Even best practice cannot completely eliminate the possibility of failure; thus, the careful assessment of the adequacy of the spinal blockade and management strategy should the failure occur intraoperatively should always be contemplated.

REFERENCES

1. Labat G: *Regional Anesthesia: Its Technic and Clinical Application.* Saunders, 1922.
2. Horlocker TT, McGregor DG, Matsushige DK, Schroeder DR, Besse JA: A retrospective review of 4767 consecutive spinal anesthetics: Central nervous system complications. Anesth Analg 1997;84:578–584.
3. Harten JM, Boyne I, Hannah P, Varveris D, Brown A: Effects of height and weight adjusted dose of local anaesthetic for spinal anaesthesia for elective caesarean section. Anaesthesia 2005;60:348–353.
4. Levy JH, Islas JA, Ghia JN, Turnbull C: A retrospective study of the incidence and causes of failed spinal anesthetics in a university hospital. Anesth Analg 1985;64:705–710.
5. Munhall RJ, Sukhani R, Winnie AP: Incidence and etiology of failed spinal anesthetics in a university hospital. Anesth Analg 1988;67:843–848.
6. Charlton JE. Managing the block. In Wildsmith JAW, Armitage EN, McClure JH (eds): *Principles and Practice of Regional* Anaesthesia, 3rd ed. Churchill Livingstone, 2003; 91–109.
7. Rubin AP. Spinal anaesthesia. In Wildsmith JAW, Armitage EN, McClure JH, eds: *Principles and Practice of Regional Anaesthesia*, 3rd ed: Churchill Livingstone, 2003: 125–138.
8. Broadbent CR, Maxwell WB, Ferrie R, Wilson DJ, Gawne-Cain M, Russell R: Ability of anaesthetists to identify a marked lumbar interspace. Anaesthesia 2000;55:1106–1126.
9. Kwok WH, Karmakar M: Spinal and Epidural Block. New York School of Regional Anesthesia. September 20, 2013. http://www.nysora.com/techniques/neuraxial-and-perineuraxial-techniques/ultrasound-guided/3276-spinal-and-epidural-block.html.
10. Lang SA, Prusinkiewicz C, Tsui BCH: Failed spinal anesthesia after a psoas compartment block. Can J Anesth 2005;52:74–78.
11. Stace JD, Gaylard DG: Failed spinal anaesthesia. Anaesthesia 1996;51:892–893.
12. Acosta L, Quinones-Hinojosa A, Schmidt MH, Weinstein PR: Diagnosis and management of sacral Tarlov cysts. Case report and review of the literature. Neurosurg Focus 2003;15:E15.
13. Lee JA, Atkinson RS: *Sir Robert Macintosh's Lumbar Puncture and Spinal Analgesia.* Churchill Livingstone, 1978.
14. Hocking G, Wildsmith JAW: Intrathecal drug spread. Br J Anaesth 2004; 93:568–578.

15. Hurley RJ, Lambert DH: Continuous spinal anesthesia with a microcatheter technique: Preliminary experience. Anesth Analg 1990;70: 97–102.

16. Atallah MM, Shorrab AA, Abdel Mageed YM, Demian AD: Low-dose bupivacaine spinal anaesthesia for percutaneous nephrolithotomy: The suitability and impact of adding intrathecal fentanyl. Acta Anaesthesiol Scand 2006;50:798–803.

17. Ben-David B, Levin H, Tarhi D: An unusual explanation for a failed spinal. Can J Anaesth 1995;45:448–449.

18. Tarkkila PJ: Incidence and causes of failed spinal anesthetics in a university hospital: A prospective study. Reg Anesth 1991;16:48–51.

19. Crone W: Failed spinal anesthesia with the Sprotte needle. Anesthesiology 1991;75:717–718.

20. Thomson GE, McMahon D: Spinal needle manufacture, design and use. Bailliere's Clin Anaesthesiol 1993;7:817–830.

21. Collier CB: Accidental subdural injection during attempted lumbar epidural block may present as a failed or inadequate block: Radiological evidence. Reg Anesth Pain Med 2004;29:45–51.

22. Singh B, Sharma P: Subdural block complicating spinal anesthesia. Anesth Analg 2002;94:1007–1009.

23. Gershon RY: Local anesthesia for caesarean section with a subdural catheter. Can J Anaesth 1996;43:1068–1071.

24. Jones MD, Newton TH: Inadvertent extra-arachnoid injection in myelography. Radiology 1963;80:818–822.

25. Bier A: Versuche ueber Cocainiserung des Rueckenmarkes. Dtsche Z Chir 1899;51:361–369.

26. Armstrong PJ: Unilateral subarachnoid anaesthesia. Anaesthesia 1989;44: 918–919.

27. Adler R, Lenz G: Neurological complaints after unsuccessful spinal anaesthesia as a manifestation of incipient syringomyelia. Eur J Anaesthesiol 1998;15:105–105.

28. Westphal M, Gotz T, Booke M: Failed spinal anaesthesia after intrathecal chemotherapy. Eur J Anaesthesiol 2005;22:235–236.

29. Hirabayashi Y, Fukuda H, Saitoh K, Inoue S, Mitsuhata H, Shimizu R: Failed spinal anaesthesia: Cause identified by MRI. Can J Anaesth 1996;43:1072–1075.

30. Carpenter RL, Hogan QH, Liu SS, Crane B, Moore J: Lumbosacral cerebrospinal fluid volume is the primary determinant of sensory block extent and duration during spinal anesthesia. Anesthesiology 1998;89: 24–29.

31. Lacassie HJ, Millar S, Leithe LG, et al: Dural ectasia: A likely cause of inadequate spinal anaesthesia in two parturients with Marfan's syndrome. Br J Anaesth 2005;94:500–504.

32. Logan ML, McClure JH, Wildsmith JAW: Plain bupivacaine—An unpredictable spinal anaesthetic agent. Br J Anaesth 1986;58:292–296.

33. Wildsmith JAW, McClure JH, Brown DT, Scott DB: Effects of posture on the spread of isobaric and hyperbaric amethocaine. Br J Anaesth 1981;53: 273–278.

34. Barker AE: A report on clinical experiences with spinal analgesia in 100 cases. BMJ 1907;i:665–674.

35. Morrison LMM, McClure JH, Wildsmith JAW: Clinical evaluation of a spinal catheter technique in femoro-popliteal graft surgery. Anaesthesia 1991;46:576–578.

36. Manchikanti L, Hadley C, Markwell SJ, Colliver JA: A retrospective analysis of failed spinal anesthetic attempts in a community hospital. Anesth Analg 1987;66:363–366.

37. Wood M, Ismail F: Inadequate spinal anaesthesia with 0.5% Marcaine Heavy (batch 1961). Int J Obs Anaesth 2003;12:310–311.

38. Harris RW, McDonald P: Inadequate spinal anaesthesia with 0.5% Marcaine Heavy (batch DK-1961). Int J Obs Anaesth 2004;13: 130–131.

39. Calthorpe N: Inadequate spinal anaesthesia with 0.5% Marcaine Heavy (batch DK 2016). Int J Obs Anaesth 2004;13:131.

40. Smiley RM, Redai I: More failed spinal anesthetics with hyperbaric bupivacaine. Int J Obs Anaesth 2004;13:131–134.

41. Kavlock R, Ting PH. Local anesthetic resistance in a pregnant patient with lumbosacral plexopathy. BMC anesthesiology. 2004 Jan 16;4(1):1.

42. Batas D, Nejad MRG, Prabhu P: Resistance to local anaesthetics: A case report. Br J Anaesth. 2007. http://bja.oxfordjournals.org/cgi/qa-display/short/brjana_el;1576.

43. Catterall WA, Sulayman D-H, Meisler MH, Pietrobon D: Inherited Neuronal Ion Channelopathies: New Windows on Complex Neurological Diseases. J Neurosci 2008;28:11768–11777.

44. Sheets PL, Jackson JO, Waxman SG et al: A Na$_v$1.7 mutation associated with hereditary erythromyalgia contributes to neuronal hyperexcitability and displays reduced lidocaine sensitivity. J Physiol 2007;581:1019–1031.

45. Schell RM, Brauer FS, Cole DJ, Applegate RL. Persistent sacral nerve root deficits after continuous spinal anaesthesia. Can J Anaesth 1991;38: 90–111.

46. Hirabayashi Y, Konishi R, Shimizu R: Neurologic symptom associated with a repeated injection after failed spinal anesthesia. Anesthesiology 1998;89:1294–1295.

47. Rigler ML, Drasner K, Krejce TC, Yelich SJ, Scholnick FT, DeFontes JA: Cauda equine syndrome after continuous spinal anesthesia. Anesth Analg 1991;72:275–281.

48. Deshpande S, Idriz R: Repeat dose after an inadequate spinal block. Anaesthesia 1996;51:892.

CHAPTER 24

Epidural Anesthesia and Analgesia

*Roulhac D. Toledano and Marc Van de Velde**

INTRODUCTION

Clinical indications for epidural anesthesia and analgesia have expanded significantly over the past several decades. Epidural analgesia is often used to supplement general anesthesia (GA) for surgical procedures in patients of all ages with moderate-to-severe comorbid disease; provide analgesia in the intraoperative, postoperative, peripartum, and end-of-life settings; and can be used as the primary anesthetic for surgeries from the mediastinum to the lower extremities. In addition, epidural techniques are used increasingly for diagnostic procedures, acute pain therapy, and management of chronic pain. Epidural blockade may also reduce the surgical stress response, the risk of cancer recurrence, the incidence of perioperative thromboembolic events, and, possibly, the morbidity and mortality associated with major surgery.

This chapter covers the essentials of epidural anesthesia and analgesia. After a brief history of the transformation from single-shot to continuous epidural catheter techniques, it reviews (1) indications for and contraindications to epidural blockade; (2) basic anatomic considerations for epidural placement; (3) physiologic effects of epidural blockade; (4) pharmacology of drugs used for epidural anesthesia and analgesia; (5) techniques for successful epidural placement; and (6) major and minor complications associated with epidural blockade. This chapter also addresses several areas of controversy concerning epidural techniques. These include controversies about epidural space

anatomy, the traditional epinephrine test dose, methods used to identify the epidural space, and whether particular clinical outcomes may be improved with epidural techniques when compared to GA. More detailed information about local anesthetics (LAs), the mechanism of neuraxial blockade, the combined spinal-epidural (CSE) technique, obstetric anesthesia, and complications of central neuraxial blockade is provided elsewhere in this textbook.

BRIEF HISTORY

The neurologist J. Leonard Corning proposed injecting an anesthetic solution into the epidural space in the 1880s, but devoted his research primarily to subarachnoid blocks. Despite coining the term *spinal anesthesia*, he may unknowingly have been investigating the epidural space. The French physicians Jean Sicard and Fernand Cathelin are credited with the first intentional administration of epidural anesthesia. At the turn of the 20th century, they independently introduced single-shot caudal blocks with cocaine for neurologic and genitourinary procedures, respectively.[1] Nineteen years later, the Spanish surgeon Fidel Pagés Miravé described a single-shot thoracolumbar approach to "peridural" anesthesia, identifying the epidural space through subtle tactile distinctions in the ligaments.[2] Within a decade and seemingly without the knowledge of Pagés's work, the Italian surgeon Achille Dogliotti popularized a reproducible loss-of-resistance (LOR) technique to identify the epidural space.[3] Contemporaneously, the Argentine surgeon Alberto Gutiérrez described the "sign of the drop" for identification of the epidural space.

---

*The authors would like to thank Michael A. Maloney, MB, BAO, ChB, for his help with the tables and figures.

A number of innovations by Eugene Aburel, Robert Hingson, Waldo Edwards, and James Southworth, among others, attempted to prolong the single-shot epidural technique. However, Cuban anesthesiologist Manual Martinez Curbelo is credited with adapting Edward Tuohy's continuous subarachnoid technique for the epidural space in 1947. His efforts were facilitated by an extensive knowledge of anatomy, a first-hand experience observing Tuohy at the Mayo Clinic, and the availability of 16-gauge Tuohy needles and small, gradated 3.5-French ureteral catheters, which curved as they exited the tip of the needle.[4] Several modifications of the Tuohy needle, itself a modification of the Huber needle, have since emerged.

The epidural catheter has also evolved from its origins as a modified ureteral catheter. Several manufacturers currently use nylon blends to produce thin, kink-resistant catheters of appropriate tensile strength and stiffness. The wire-reinforced catheter represents the most recent technological advance in epidural catheter design. The addition of a circumferential stainless steel coil within a nylon or polyurethane catheter confers greater flexibility compared to standard nylon catheters and may decrease the incidence of venous cannulation, intrathecal placement, catheter migration, and paresthesias.

INDICATIONS

This section presents common and controversial indications for the use of lumbar and thoracic epidural blockade in lower extremity, genitourinary, vascular, gynecologic, colorectal, and cardiothoracic surgery. It also reviews less common and novel indications for epidural anesthesia and analgesia, including for the treatment of patients with sepsis and uncommon medical disorders (Table 24–1). The use of neuraxial blockade for obstetric patients, pediatric surgery, and chronic pain and in the ambulatory setting is covered in greater detail elsewhere in this textbook.

Lumbar Epidural Blockade

Epidural anesthesia has been administered most commonly for procedures involving the lower limbs, pelvis, perineum, and lower abdomen but is increasingly being used as the sole anesthetic or as a complement to GA for a greater diversity of procedures. This section examines several common indications for lumbar epidural blockade, including lower extremity orthopedic surgery, infrainguinal vascular procedures, and genitourinary and vaginal gynecologic surgeries. When applicable, it reviews the benefits and drawbacks of the use of neuraxial techniques versus GA for specific procedures.

Lower Extremity Major Orthopedic Surgery

Both perioperative anticoagulant thromboprophylaxis and the increasing reliance on peripheral nerve blocks have influenced the current use of continuous lumbar epidural blockade for lower extremity surgery. Nonetheless, neuraxial blockade as a sole anesthetic or as a supplement to either GA or peripheral techniques is still widely used for major orthopedic surgeries of the lower extremities. The effective postoperative pain control

TABLE 24–1. Examples of applications for epidural blockade.

Specialty	Surgical Procedure
Orthopedic surgery	Major hip and knee surgery, pelvic fractures
Obstetric surgery	Cesarean delivery, labor analgesia
Gynecologic surgery	Hysterectomy, pelvic floor procedures
General surgery	Breast, hepatic, gastric, colonic surgery
Pediatric surgery	Inguinal hernia repair, orthopedic surgery
Ambulatory surgery	Foot, knee, hip, anorectal surgery
Cardiothoracic surgery	Thoracotomy, esophagectomy, thymectomy, coronary artery bypass grafting (on and off pump)
Urologic surgery	Prostatectomy, cystectomy, lithotripsy, nephrectomy
Vascular surgery	Amputation of lower extremity, revascularization procedures
Medical conditions	Autonomic hyperreflexia, myasthenia gravis, pheochromocytoma, known or suspected malignant hyperthermia

provided by either peripheral or neuraxial blocks, or a combination of the two techniques, improves patient satisfaction, permits early ambulation, accelerates functional recuperation, and may shorten hospital stay, particularly after major knee surgery. Other potential benefits of the use of neuraxial blockade in lieu of GA include the reduced incidence of deep vein thrombosis (DVT) in patients undergoing total hip[5] and knee[6] replacement surgery, improved postoperative cognitive function, and decreased intraoperative blood loss and transfusion requirements.[7] A recent meta-analysis also demonstrated a statistically significant reduction in operative time when neuraxial blockade was used in patients undergoing elective total hip replacement, although the authors did not distinguish between spinal and epidural techniques.[8]

Major orthopedic procedures that can be performed under epidural, CSE, or integrated epidural and GA include primary hip or knee arthroplasty, surgery for hip fracture, revision arthroplasty, bilateral total knee arthroplasty, acetabular bone grafting, and insertion of long-stem femoral prostheses (Table 24–2). Spinal anesthesia may be the preferred technique in some of these cases, particularly if anticipated postoperative pain is slight or negligible (eg, total hip arthroplasty) or if a

TABLE 24–2. Orthopedic surgeries suitable for epidural, combined spinal-epidural, or integrated epidural–general anesthesia.

Procedure	Sensory Level Required
Closed reduction and external fixation of pelvis	Neuraxial technique seldom adequate for surgery; epidural useful for postoperative analgesia
Hip arthroplasty, arthrodesis, synovectomy	T10
Open reduction internal fixation of acetabular fracture	T10
Open reduction internal fixation of femur, tibia, ankle, or foot	T12
Closed reduction and external fixation of femur and tibia	T12
Above- and below-knee amputation	T12 (T8 with tourniquet)
Knee arthrotomy	T12 (T8 with tourniquet)
Arthroscopy of knee	T12
Repair/reconstruction of knee ligaments	T12
Total knee replacement	T12 (T8 with tourniquet)
Distal tibia, ankle, and foot procedures	T12
Ankle arthroscopy, arthrotomy, arthrodesis	T12
Transmetatarsal amputation	T12

supplemental peripheral nerve block is planned. Anesthesia to T10 with needle placement at L3 to L4 is adequate for most of these procedures.

The use of neuraxial anesthesia for major orthopedic surgery is not without risks and challenges. Elderly patients, trauma victims, and individuals with hemophilia who develop complications from recurrent bleeding into their joints may not be appropriate candidates for regional blockade. In general, epidural procedures are well tolerated in patients with age-related comorbidities, such as restrictive pulmonary disease, prolonged hepatic clearance of drugs, hypertension (HTN), coronary artery disease (CAD), and renal insufficiency. Elderly patients may benefit from the decreased postoperative confusion and delirium associated with regional anesthesia, provided intraoperative hypotension is kept to a minimum.[9] However,

prevention of excessive sympathectomy-induced hemodynamic changes can be challenging, as these patients are both less capable of responding to hypotension and more prone to cardiac decompensation and pulmonary edema in response to rapid fluid administration. An epidural technique with a sensory level below T10, as appropriate for many orthopedic surgeries, and judicious administration of fluids and vasopressors may minimize these risks.

Elderly patients commonly present for surgery on anticoagulant or antiplatelet medications and may pose a risk for neurologic injury related to central neuraxial blockade. If an epidural technique is selected for these or other high-risk patients, appropriate timing of both blockade initiation and catheter removal relative to the timing of anticoagulant drug administration must be taken into account. For trauma patients, attaining proper positioning for administration of epidural anesthesia may present a challenge. Initiation of neuraxial blockade in the lateral position may improve chances of success.

Intraoperatively, tourniquet pain can be anticipated with either spinal or epidural blockade, but occurs more frequently with the latter. While the mechanism remains poorly understood, it commonly presents within an hour of tourniquet inflation, increases in intensity over time, and is accompanied by tachycardia and elevated blood pressure. The administration of intrathecal or epidural preservative-free morphine may delay the onset of tourniquet pain.[10]

Lower Limb Vascular Surgery

There are several potential benefits of the use of neuraxial anesthesia and analgesia for lower extremity vascular procedures. Patients undergoing vascular surgery commonly have multiple major systemic diseases, such as CAD, cerebrovascular disease (CVD), diabetes mellitus (DM), chronic renal insufficiency, chronic HTN, and chronic obstructive pulmonary disease (COPD). Patients who present for arterial embolectomy may also have conditions that predispose them to intracardiac thrombus formation, such as mitral stenosis or atrial fibrillation. Avoiding GA in this high-risk patient population possibly enhances graft patency, reducing the need for reexploration and reducing the risk of thromboembolic complications; these are some of the advantages of using regional anesthesia. However, management of these individuals is often complicated by the high probability that they are taking presurgical antiplatelet or anticoagulant medications and will require additional systemic anticoagulation intraoperatively and postoperatively. Thus, these patients are considered at an increased risk for epidural hematoma; a careful risk-benefit analysis is necessary prior to initiating epidural blockade. Consideration must also be given to the type of vascular procedure to be performed, the anticipated length of the procedure, the possible need for invasive monitoring, and the timely removal of the epidural catheter before transitioning to oral anticoagulation therapy. Maintaining normothermia, ensuring that motor strength can be promptly assessed postoperatively, and providing appropriate sedation during lengthy procedures are additional challenges.

Infrainguinal vascular procedures that are suitable for epidural blockade include arterial bypass surgeries, arterial embolectomy, and venous thrombectomy or vein excision

TABLE 24–3. Examples of vascular procedures performed with epidural blockade.

Abdominal aortic aneurysm repair (neuraxial technique seldom adequate as sole anesthetic)

Aortofemoral bypass

Renal artery bypass

Mesenteric artery bypass

Infrainguinal arterial bypass with saphenous vein or synthetic graft

Embolectomy

Thrombectomy

Endovascular procedures (intraluminal balloon dilation with stent placement; aneurysm repair)

TABLE 24–4. Benefits of central neuraxial blockade versus general anesthesia for transurethral resection of the prostate.

Early detection of mental status changes

Early detection of breakthrough pain (indicative of capsular/bladder perforation)

Reduced blood loss

Decreased incidence of deep vein thrombosis

Decreased incidence of circulatory overload

Improved postoperative pain control

(Table 24–3). Slow titration of LAs to attain a T8–T10 level, while maintaining hemodynamic stability, is optimal. The addition of epinephrine to LAs is controversial due to concerns that its vasoconstrictive effect may jeopardize an already-tenuous blood supply to the spinal cord. Studies to date have failed to demonstrate a difference in cardiovascular and pulmonary morbidity and mortality with the use of epidural anesthesia as compared with GA for these procedures,[11] although epidural techniques may be superior for promoting graft survival.

Lower Genitourinary Procedures

Lumbar epidural blockade as either a primary anesthetic or as an adjunct to GA is an appropriate option for a variety of genitourinary procedures. Epidural anesthesia with a T9–T10 sensory level can be used for transurethral resection of the prostate (TURP), although spinal anesthesia may be preferred due to its improved sacral coverage, denser sensory blockade, and shorter duration. Both techniques are considered superior to GA for several reasons, including earlier detection of mental status changes associated with TURP syndrome; the ability of the patient to communicate breakthrough pain if an untoward complication such as perforation of the prostatic capsule or bladder occurs; the potential for decreased bleeding; and the decreased risks of perioperative thromboembolic events and fluid overload (Table 24–4).[12] In addition, patients presenting for this and other prostate surgeries are generally elderly, with multiple comorbidities, and have a low risk for certain complications of neuraxial blockade, such as postdural puncture headache (PDPH).

Other transurethral procedures, such as cystoscopy and ureteral stone extraction, can be performed under GA, topical anesthesia, or neuraxial blockade, depending on the extent and complexity of the procedure, patient comorbidities, and patient, anesthesiologist, and surgeon preference. Of note, paraplegic and quadriplegic patients comprise a subset of patients who present for repeated cystoscopies and stone extraction procedures; neuraxial anesthesia is often preferred in these patients

because of the risk of autonomic hyperreflexia (AH) (see separate section on this topic). Because these procedures are done on an outpatient basis, lengthy residual epidural blockade should be avoided. Although there is some interindividual variability, a sensory level as high as T8 is required for procedures involving the ureters, while a T9–T10 sensory level is appropriate for procedures involving the bladder (Table 24–5).

Vaginal Gynecologic Surgeries

Several vaginal gynecologic surgeries can be performed with epidural blockade, although single-shot spinal or GA and, in some cases, paracervical block or topical anesthesia may be more appropriate (Table 24–6). A dilation and curettage (D&C) can be performed under paracervical block, GA, or

TABLE 24–5. Sensory level required for genitourinary procedures.

Procedure	Sensory Level Required
Nephrectomy	Consider combined general-epidural anesthesia
Cystectomy	T4
Extracorporeal shock wave lithotripsy	T6
Open prostatectomy	T8
Ureteral stone extraction	T8
Cystoscopy	T9
Transurethral resection of prostate	T9
Surgery involving testes	T10
Surgery involving penis	L1
Urethral procedures	Sacral block

TABLE 24–6. Vaginal gynecologic procedures suitable for epidural blockade.

Dilation and curettage

Hysteroscopy (with or without distention media)

Urinary incontinence procedures

Hysterectomy

neuraxial blockade. If neuraxial anesthesia is selected, a T10 sensory level is appropriate. While outpatient diagnostic hysteroscopy can be performed under LA,[13] hysteroscopy with distention media typically requires general or neuraxial anesthesia. Epidural anesthesia may have the disadvantage of increased glycine absorption compared to GA.[14] However, mental status changes related to absorption of the hypotonic irrigation solution are more easily detected in awake patients. For urinary incontinence procedures, epidural anesthesia offers the advantage of permitting the patient to participate in the intraoperative cough test, which theoretically decreases the risk of postoperative voiding dysfunction, although the incidence of this untoward outcome does not appear to be increased under GA.[15] A T10 sensory level provides sufficient anesthesia for bladder procedures, but the level should be extended to T4 if the peritoneum is opened. Vaginal hysterectomy can be performed under general or neuraxial (most commonly spinal) anesthesia. A T4–T6 sensory level is appropriate for uterine procedures.

Thoracic Epidural Anesthesia and Analgesia

The benefits of and indications for thoracic epidural anesthesia (TEA) are expanding (Table 24–7). TEA offers superior perioperative analgesia compared with systemic opioids,[16] decreases postoperative pulmonary complications,[17] decreases the duration of postoperative ileus,[18] and decreases mortality in patients with multiple rib fractures, among other things.[19] This section explores the role of TEA as either a primary anesthetic or as an adjuvant to GA for cardiac, thoracic, abdominal, colorectal, genitourinary, and gynecologic surgery (Figure 24–1). It also reviews the expanding role of TEA for video-assisted thoracic surgery (VATS) and laparoscopic surgery.

TABLE 24–7. Benefits of thoracic epidural anesthesia and analgesia.

Improved perioperative analgesia compared with other modalities

Decreased postoperative pulmonary complications

Decreased duration of postoperative ileus

Decreased duration of mechanical ventilation

Decreased mortality in patients with rib fractures

Cardiac Surgery

High TEA (blockade of the upper five thoracic segments) as an adjuvant to GA in cardiac surgery with cardiopulmonary bypass (CPB) has gained interest over the past several decades. Purported benefits include improved distribution of coronary blood flow,[20] reduced oxygen demand, improved regional left ventricular function, a reduction in the incidence of supraventricular arrhythmias,[21] attenuation of the surgical stress response,[22] improved intraoperative hemodynamic stability, faster recovery of awareness, improved postoperative analgesia, and a reduction of postoperative renal and pulmonary complications. Several of these potential benefits can be attributed to selective blockade of cardiac sympathetic innervation (the T1–T4 spinal segments). However, the insertion of an epidural catheter in patients requiring full heparinization for CPB carries the risk of epidural hematoma.

The evidence in support of high TEA for cardiac surgery is not conclusive. A study by Liu and colleagues comparing TEA with traditional opioid-based GA for coronary artery bypass grafting (CABG) with CPB found no difference in the rates of mortality or myocardial infarction, but demonstrated a statistically significant reduction in the risk of postoperative cardiac arrhythmias and pulmonary complications, improved pain scores, and earlier tracheal extubation in the TEA group.[23] In contrast, a recent randomized control trial comparing the clinical effects of fast-track GA with TEA versus fast-track GA alone in over 600 patients undergoing elective cardiac surgery (both on pump and off pump) found no statistically significant difference in 30-day survival free from myocardial infarction, pulmonary complications, renal failure, or stroke.[24] The duration of mechanical ventilation, length of intensive care unit (ICU) stay, length of hospital stay, and quality of life at 30-day follow-up were also similar for the two groups. Overall, the role of TEA as an adjuvant to GA for cardiac surgery with CPB remains controversial.

The role of high TEA in off-pump coronary artery bypass (OPCAB) surgery is also debated in the literature. TEA offers the advantages of avoiding intubation of the trachea in selected CABG cases, earlier extubation in patients receiving GA, and reduced postoperative pain and morbidity. But, concerns remain about compromised ventilation with a high sensory blockade, hypotension due to sympathicolysis, and epidural hematoma, despite the vastly reduced heparin dose compared with CPB cases. A recent prospective, randomized controlled trial of more than 200 patients undergoing OPCAB surgery found that the addition of high TEA to GA significantly reduced the incidence of postoperative arrhythmias, improved pain control, and improved the quality of recovery.[25] Until more definitive outcome data are available, the role of neuraxial techniques in OPCAB surgery remains uncertain.

Thoracic and Upper Abdominal Surgical Procedures

Epidural anesthesia and analgesia are commonly used for upper abdominal and thoracic surgery, including gastrectomy, esophagectomy, lobectomy, and descending thoracic aorta procedures

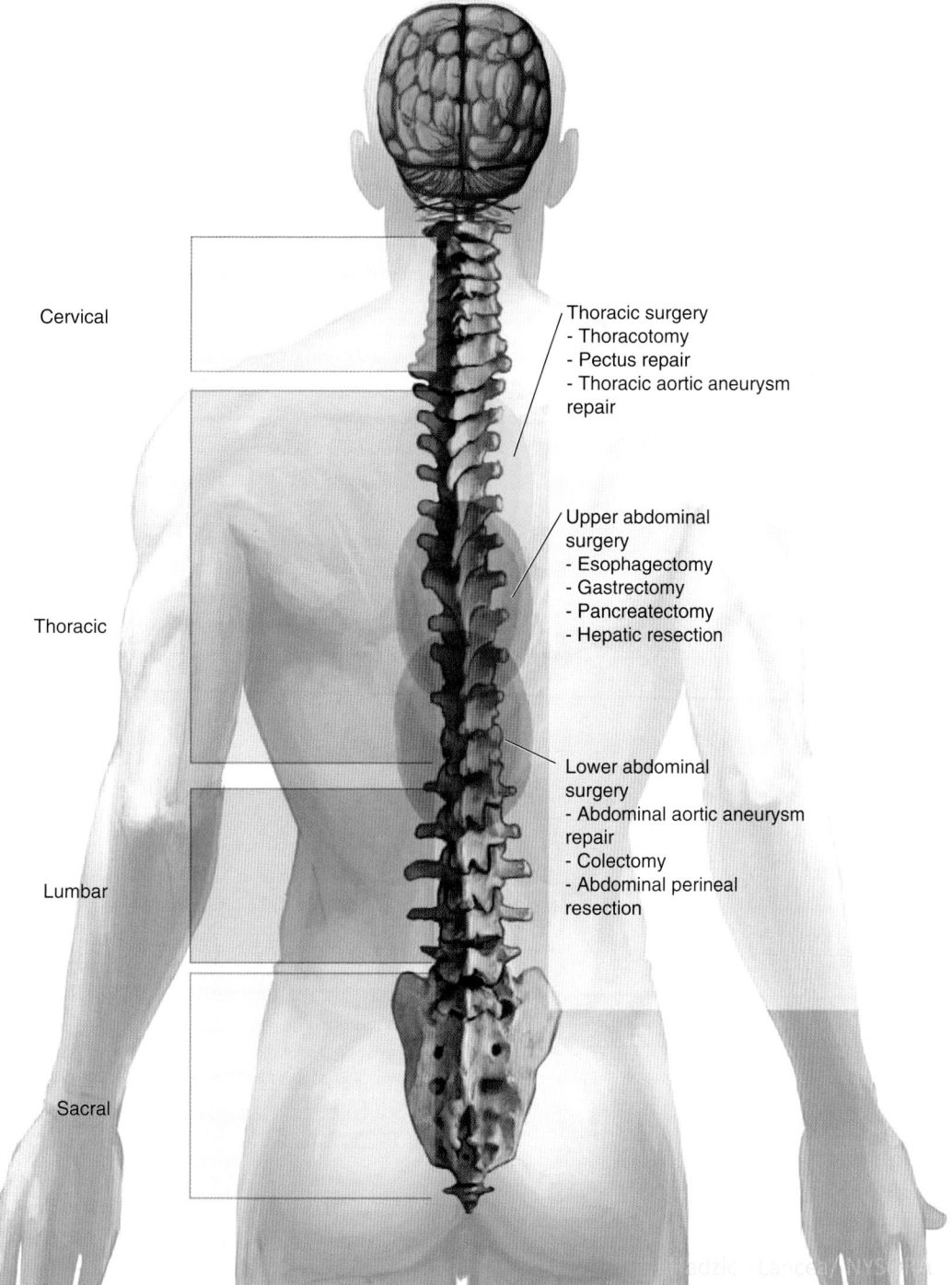

Cervical

Thoracic surgery
- Thoracotomy
- Pectus repair
- Thoracic aortic aneurysm repair

Upper abdominal surgery
- Esophagectomy
- Gastrectomy
- Pancreatectomy
- Hepatic resection

Thoracic

Lower abdominal surgery
- Abdominal aortic aneurysm repair
- Colectomy
- Abdominal perineal resection

Lumbar

Sacral

FIGURE 24–1. Level of placement in surgeries performed with thoracic epidural anesthesia and analgesia.

(Table 24–8). It is less commonly used for VATS, unless conversion to an open procedure is highly anticipated or if the patient is at high risk for complications from GA. Epidural blockade for many of these procedures commonly serves as an adjuvant to GA and as an essential component of postoperative pain management. Concurrent administration of high TEA with GA, however, carries risks of intraoperative bradycardia, hypotension, and changes in airway resistance. There is some debate regarding whether intraoperative activation of epidural blockade is required to appreciate the analgesic benefits of TEA

or if postoperative activation produces equivalent benefits. A systematic review by Møiniche and colleagues found that the timing of several types of analgesia, including epidurals, intravenous opioids, and peripheral LAs, did not influence the quality of postoperative pain control.[26]

Thoracic epidural anesthesia initiated at the mid- to upper thoracic region can also be used for breast procedures. Benefits may include superior postoperative analgesia, decreased incidence of postoperative nausea and vomiting (PONV), improved patient satisfaction, and avoiding tracheal intubation in patients

TABLE 24–8. Indications for thoracic epidural anesthesia and analgesia.

Anatomic Region	Procedure
Thorax	Thoracotomy
	Pectus repair
	Thoracic aneurysm repair
	Thymectomy
	Video-assisted thoracic surgery
Upper abdomen	Esophagectomy
	Gastrectomy
	Pancreatectomy
	Cholecystecomy
	Hepatic resection
Lower abdomen	Abdominal aortic aneurysm repair
	Colectomy
	Bowel resection
	Abdominal perineal resection
Urogenital/ gynecologic	Cystectomy
	Nephrectomy
	Ureteral repair
	Radical abdominal prostatectomy
	Ovarian tumor debulking
	Pelvic exenteration
	Total abdominal hysterectomy

with moderate-to-severe comorbidities.[27] The sensory level required depends on the procedure: A level extending from T1–T7 is adequate for breast augmentation; C5–T7 is required for modified radical mastectomy; and C5–L1 is required for mastectomy with transverse rectus abdominis myocutaneous (TRAM) flap reconstruction (Table 24–9).[28] The epidural catheter can be introduced at T2–T4 to achieve segmental

TABLE 24–9. Sensory level required for breast procedures.

Surgery	Segmental Blockade
Modified radical mastectomy	C5–T7
Mastectomy with transverse rectus abdominus flap	C5–L1
Partial mastectomy; breast augmentation	T1–T7

blockade of the thoracic dermatomes for most breast procedures; placement at T8–T10 is appropriate for TRAM flap reconstruction.

Epidural blockade provides a useful adjuvant to GA for procedures within the thoracic cavity, such as lung and esophageal surgery. The benefits of TEA for these procedures include enhanced postoperative analgesia; reduced pulmonary morbidity (eg, atelectasis, pneumonia, and hypoxemia); swift resolution of postoperative ileus; and decreased postoperative catabolism, which may spare muscle mass. Segmental epidural blockade of T1–T10 provides sensory blockade of the thoracotomy incision and the chest tube insertion site.

Upper abdominal surgeries that can be performed with epidural anesthesia and analgesia include esophagectomy, gastrectomy, pancreatectomy, hepatic resection,[29] and cholecystectomy. Laparoscopic cholecystectomy with epidural blockade[30] and distal gastrectomy with a combined general-epidural anesthetic have also been reported.[31] Midthoracic epidural catheter placement with segmental blockade extending from T5 (T4 for laparoscopic surgery) to T8 is appropriate for most upper abdominal procedures and, due to lumbar and sacral nerve root sparing, has minimal risk of lower extremity motor deficits, urinary retention, hypotension, and other sequelae of lumbar epidural anesthesia.

Suprainguinal Vascular Procedures

An upper midthoracic epidural can be used as an adjuvant to GA for surgeries of the abdominal aorta and its major branches. Epidural blockade for aortofemoral bypass, renal artery bypass, and repair of abdominal aortic aneurysms may provide superior postoperative pain control, facilitate early extubation of the trachea, permit early ambulation, and decrease the risk of thromboembolic events in patients who are at particularly high risk for this untoward complication. However, intraoperative epidural blockade may complicate management of hemodynamic changes associated with aortic cross-clamping and unclamping, as well as compromise early assessment of motor function in the immediate postoperative period. A sensory level from T6 to T12 is necessary for an extensive abdominal incision; a level extending from T4–T12 is required to attain denervation of the viscera.

Extracorporeal Shock Wave Lithotripsy, Prostatectomy, Cystectomy, Nephrectomy

Extracorporeal shock wave lithotripsy (ESWL) with or without water immersion can be performed under general or neuraxial anesthesia. A T6–T12 sensory level is necessary when neuraxial techniques are selected. Epidural blockade is associated with less intraoperative hypotension than a single-shot spinal, although both techniques serve to avoid GA in potentially high-risk patients.

Open prostate surgery, radical cystectomy and urinary diversion, and simple, partial, and radical nephrectomy can be performed under neuraxial blockade, either alone or in combination with GA, depending on the procedure. Some potential advantages of neuraxial compared with GA for radical retropubic prostatectomy include decreased intraoperative blood loss and transfusions,[32] a decreased incidence of postoperative thromboembolic events, improved analgesia and level of activity up to

9 weeks postoperatively,[33] faster return of bowel function,[34] and several other still-disputed advantages of neuraxial anesthesia, such as faster time to hospital discharge and reduced hospital costs. For the open procedure, patients may require generous sedation in the absence of a combined general-neuraxial technique. A T6 sensory level is required, with catheter placement in the midthoracic region. Radical cystectomy is performed on patients with invasive bladder cancer and may have improved outcomes with a combined general-epidural anesthetic compared to GA alone. Epidural blockade can provide controlled hypotension intraoperatively, contributing to decreased blood loss, and optimize postoperative pain relief.[35] A midthoracic epidural with a T6 sensory level is appropriate. Although GA is often required for radical nephrectomy due to concerns for patient positioning, intraoperative hypotension, and the potential for significant intraoperative blood loss, epidural analgesia provides more effective postoperative pain relief than systemic opioids while avoiding the adverse effects of the latter.

Several other urologic-related surgeries can be performed with neuraxial blockade as the sole anesthetic or as an adjuvant to GA. The use of a combined GA-epidural technique in patients with functional adrenal tumors undergoing laparoscopic adrenalectomy is safe and effective and may have the added benefit of minimizing fluctuations in hormone levels. Of note, however, epidural blockade may not diminish the pressor effects of direct tumor stimulation. The use of epidural anesthesia for retroperitoneal laparoscopic biopsy for patients who are not candidates for percutaneous biopsy has also been reported.[36]

Lower Abdominal and Gynecologic Surgeries

Total abdominal hysterectomy is often performed under GA, a combined general-epidural anesthetic, or neuraxial anesthesia with or without sedation. Although still not routine, gynecologic laparoscopy is increasingly being performed under neuraxial anesthesia, commonly with decreased Trendelenburg tilt, reduced CO_2 insufflation pressures (below 15 mm Hg), and supplemental opioids or nonsteroidal anti-inflammatory drugs (NSAIDs) to minimize referred shoulder pain. Epidural blockade for open procedures has the advantages of providing prolonged postoperative analgesia, decreasing the incidence of PONV and perioperative thromboembolic events, and potentially influencing perioperative immune function and, relatedly, the recurrence of cancer in patients undergoing hysterectomy for ovarian or related cancer. The proposed preemptive analgesia effect provided by neuraxial blockade during abdominal hysterectomy requires further investigation.[37] A sensory level extending to T4 or T6 provides sufficient anesthesia for procedures involving the uterus. Either epidural catheter insertion in the lumbar region with high volumes of LAs to raise the sensory level or low- to midthoracic placement is appropriate. The visceral pain associated with bowel and peritoneal manipulation decreases as the level of the blockade is increased; a T3–T4 level may be optimal.[38]

Open and laparoscopic colectomy, sigmoidectomy, and appendectomy are among other lower abdominal surgeries that can be performed under neuraxial anesthesia, with or without GA. Of particular interest in patients undergoing bowel surgery,

thoracic epidural blockade decreases the duration of postoperative ileus, possibly without affecting anastomotic healing and leakage.[39] The superior postoperative analgesia associated with continuous epidural infusions, with or without opioids, most likely improves postoperative lung function in patients undergoing gastrointestinal (GI) surgery, although specific randomized controlled trials have not been conducted. In combination with early feeding and ambulation, TEA plays a role in early hospital discharge after certain GI surgeries.[40] A similar outcome has been demonstrated after laparoscopic colonic resection, followed by epidural analgesia for 2 days and early oral nutrition and mobilization (ie, multimodal rehabilitation).[41] Epidural catheter placement between T9 and T11 is usually appropriate for lower abdominal procedures; a sensory blockade extending to T7 or T9 is required for most colonic surgeries (sigmoid resection, ileotransversostomy, hemicolectomy).

Uncommon Medical Disorders and Clinical Scenarios

Epidural anesthesia and analgesia may also be indicated in the perioperative management of patients with specific medical conditions or coexisting disease, such as myasthenia gravis (MG), AH, malignant hyperthermia (MH), COPD, pheochromocytoma (see previous discussion), and sepsis. Several other subsets of patients may benefit from continuous epidural catheter techniques, including palliative care patients, parturients with comorbidities, and patients at risk for recurrent malignancy.

Myasthenia Gravis

Patients with MG pose particular challenges to anesthesiologists, including abnormal responses to depolarizing and nondepolarizing neuromuscular blocking agents; potential difficulty reversing residual neuromuscular blockade in patients taking cholinesterase inhibitors; prolonged postoperative mechanical ventilation requirements; risk of postsurgical respiratory failure; and postoperative pain management concerns.[42] Epidural blockade eliminates the need for intraoperative muscle relaxants in myasthenic patients and provides superior postoperative pain relief compared with opioids, while minimizing the risk of opioid-induced respiratory depression and pulmonary dysfunction.[43] Due to the possibility that ester LA metabolism may be prolonged in patients taking cholinesterase inhibitors, amide LAs may be preferred for the management of myasthenic patients. Reduced doses of LAs may also be appropriate. Concerns for compromising a myasthenic patient's respiratory function with a high epidural appear to be unfounded.[44]

Autonomic Hyperreflexia

Epidural techniques are appropriate for the perioperative management of patients with AH. AH occurs in up to 85% of patients with spinal cord injuries at or above T4–T7 as a result of uninhibited sympathetic activity. In response to visceral or cutaneous stimulation below the level of the lesion and in the absence of descending central inhibition, patients may develop acute, extreme sympathetic hyperactivity. Generally, intense vasoconstriction occurs below the level of the spinal cord lesion, with vasodilation above. Patients may experience sweating, nausea, flushing, pallor, shivering, nasal obstruction, blurred vision, headache, difficulty breathing, seizures, and cardiac arrhythmias. Reflex bradycardia is seen in the majority of cases. Severe life-threatening HTN can result in intracranial hemorrhage, myocardial ischemia, pulmonary edema, and death. Epidural blockade as the sole anesthetic, as a supplement to GA, or for labor analgesia attenuates the physiologic perturbations associated with AH, although incomplete block of sacral segments or missed segments may contribute to a high failure rate.[45] Spinal anesthesia, which blocks the afferent limb of this potentially lethal reflex, and deep GA more reliably prevent AH.[46]

Malignant Hyperthermia

The anesthetic management of MH presents a challenge to the anesthesiologist. MH is a clinical syndrome of markedly accelerated metabolism triggered primarily by volatile agents and the depolarizing agent succinylcholine. Susceptible patients may develop fever, tachycardia, hypercarbia, tachypnea, arrhythmias, hypoxemia, profuse sweating, HTN, myoglobinuria, mixed acidosis, and muscle rigidity in response to exposure to volatile agents or succinylcholine, although cases have been reported in which there is no evident triggering agent. Late complications may include consumptive coagulopathy, acute renal failure, muscle necrosis, pulmonary edema, and neurologic sequelae. Avoiding exposure to triggering agents is a cornerstone in the management of MH-susceptible patients. Whenever suitable, local, peripheral, or central neuraxial blocks are recommended, as these techniques are reported to be safer than the use of GA.[47] Both ester and amide LAs are considered safe in MH-susceptible patients, as is epinephrine, although controversy remains in the literature.

Chronic Obstructive Pulmonary Disease

Epidural blockade is a reasonable anesthetic option for patients with COPD undergoing major surgery due to concerns for prolonged mechanical ventilation. However, whether epidural techniques reduce pulmonary complications in patients with COPD is not known. In a recent propensity-controlled analysis of more than 500 patients with COPD undergoing abdominal surgery, epidural analgesia as an adjunct to GA was associated with a statistically significant reduction in the risk of postoperative pneumonia.[48] Patients with the most severe type of COPD benefited disproportionately. The study also found a nonsignificant beneficial effect of epidural analgesia on 30-day mortality, a trend that has been demonstrated in other studies.[7]

Pediatric Surgery

There is a considerable body of literature dedicated to the use of regional anesthesia for pediatric surgery in both the inpatient and the ambulatory settings. Advantages of neuraxial blockade for the pediatric population include optimal postoperative analgesia, which is particularly important in extensive scoliosis repair, repair of pectus excavatum, and major abdominal and thoracic procedures; decreased GA requirements; earlier awakening; and earlier discharge in the ambulatory setting. Certain

subsets of pediatric patients, such as those with cystic fibrosis, a family history of MH, or a history of prematurity, also benefit from the use of neuraxial anesthesia in lieu of GA. However, parental refusal, concerns about performing regional blocks in anesthetized patients, and airway concerns in patients with limited oxygen reserves pose challenges to the routine use of neuraxial blockade in this patient population.

The single-shot caudal approach to the epidural space, with or without sedation, is commonly used in pediatric patients for a variety of surgeries, including circumcision, hypospadias repair, inguinal herniorrhaphy, and orchidopexy. Continuous caudal catheters may be advanced cephalad to higher vertebral levels and used as the sole anesthetic or as an adjuvant to GA. Lumbar anesthesia and TEA provide a more reliable sensory blockade at higher segmental levels in older children. See Chapter 42 on pediatric regional anesthesia for a more detailed discussion of caudal blocks.

Ambulatory Surgery

Spinal anesthesia or peripheral nerve blocks are preferred over epidural techniques for most clinical scenarios in the ambulatory setting due to concerns for the relatively slow onset of epidural blockade, urinary retention, prolonged immobility, PDPH, and delayed discharge. The use of short-acting LAs, when appropriate, may obviate these concerns. Epidural techniques have the advantages of permitting slow titration of LAs, the ability to tailor block height and duration to the surgical procedure, and a decreased risk of transient neurologic symptoms (TNS) when compared with spinal anesthesia. Total hip arthroplasty, knee arthroscopy, foot surgery, inguinal herniorrhaphy, pelvic laparoscopy, and anorectal procedures are among the many outpatient surgeries that can be performed with neuraxial blockade as the primary anesthetic.[49] Regional blockade in the ambulatory setting is discussed in greater detail elsewhere in this volume.

Labor Analgesia and Anesthesia

Parturients comprise the single largest group to receive epidural analgesia. For adequate pain relief during the first stage of labor, coverage of the dermatomes from T10 to L1 is necessary; analgesia should extend caudally to S2–S4 (to include the pudendal nerve) during the second stage of labor. Epidural placement at the L3–L4 interspace is most common in laboring patients. However, surface anatomic landmarks may be difficult to appreciate in obstetric patients and may not reliably identify the intended interspace in this subset of patients due to both the anterior rotation of the pelvis and exaggerated lumbar lordosis. Several other factors may affect the ease of epidural placement and spread of epidurally administered LAs in parturients, including engorgement of epidural veins, elevated hormonal levels, and excessive weight gain. Refer to Chapter 41 for additional information on epidural techniques in laboring patients.

Miscellaneous

Several nonanesthetic applications for epidural procedures have emerged. Epidural catheter infusion techniques are being used increasingly for pain control at the end of life in both children and adults, including those with cancer-related pain.[50] There is also an evolving interest in whether epidural anesthesia and analgesia may have a protective role in sepsis. Of particular interest is whether critically ill patients may benefit from the increased splanchnic organ perfusion and oxygenation, as well as immunomodulation, seen in healthy patients who have received epidural anesthesia. However, additional studies are needed to evaluate the risk and benefits of epidural techniques in sepsis.[51] Another novel application for epidural LAs proposes that continuous infusions may improve placental blood flow in parturients with chronically compromised uterine perfusion and intrauterine growth restriction.[52]

There is a growing body of literature devoted to the potential beneficial effects of epidural analgesia in patients with cancer, although the data are preliminary and at times contradictory. Surgical stress and certain anesthetic agents suppress the host's immune function, including its ability to eliminate circulating tumor cells, and can predispose patients with cancer to postoperative infection, tumor growth, and metastasis. Recent studies have demonstrated improved perioperative immune function with the use of TEA in patients undergoing elective laparoscopic radical hysterectomy for cervical cancer.[53] Regional adjuncts to anesthesia have also been shown to have beneficial effects against recurrence of breast[54] and prostate[55] cancer. These protective effects may reflect both the decreased opioid requirements and the reduced neurohumoral stress response associated with epidural blockade.[56]

CONTRAINDICATIONS

Serious complications of epidural techniques are rare. However, epidural hematomas, epidural abscesses, permanent nerve injury, infection, and cardiovascular collapse, among other adverse events, have been attributed to neuraxial blockade. As a result, an understanding of the conditions that may predispose certain patient populations to these and other complications is essential. This section reviews the absolute, relative, and controversial contraindications to epidural placement (Table 24–10). Ultimately, a risk-benefit analysis with particular emphasis on patient comorbidities, airway anatomy, patient preferences, and type and duration of surgery is recommended prior to initiation of epidural blockade.

Absolute Contraindications

Although the contraindications to epidural blockade have been classified historically as absolute, relative, and controversial, opinions regarding absolute contraindications have evolved with advances in equipment, techniques, and practitioner experience. Currently, patient refusal may be considered the only absolute contraindication to epidural blockade. Although coagulopathy is considered a relative contraindication, initiating neuraxial blockade in the presence of severe coagulation abnormalities, such as frank disseminated intravascular coagulation (DIC), is contraindicated. Most other pathologic conditions comprise relative or controversial contraindications and require careful risk-benefit analysis prior to initiation of epidural blockade.

TABLE 24–10. Contraindications to epidural blockade.

Absolute	Patient refusal
	Severe coagulation abnormalities (eg, frank disseminated intravascular coagulation)
Relative and controversial	Sepsis
	Elevated intracranial pressure
	Anticoagulants
	Thrombocytopenia
	Other bleeding diatheses
	Preexisting central nervous system disorders (eg, multiple sclerosis)
	Fever/infection (eg, varicella zoster virus)
	Preload dependent states (eg, aortic stenosis)
	Previous back surgery, preexisting neurologic injury, back pain
	Placement in anesthetized adults
	Needle placement through tattoo

Relative and Controversial Contraindications

Sepsis

There is growing interest in using epidural anesthesia and analgesia to modulate inflammatory responses and to prevent or treat myocardial ischemia, respiratory dysfunction, and splanchnic ischemia in septic patients. However, there is insufficient evidence to determine whether epidural blockade is harmful or protective in sepsis.[57] Despite the potential benefits of regional techniques in this setting, many anesthesiologists may be reluctant to initiate epidural blockade in septic patients due to concerns for relative hypovolemia, refractory hypotension, coagulopathy, and the introduction of blood-borne pathogens into the epidural or subarachnoid space. If regional anesthesia is selected, a slow-onset dosing technique after or with concurrent antibiotic, intravenous fluid, and vasopressor administration may be feasible.

Increased Intracranial Pressure

Accidental dural puncture (ADP) in the setting of elevated intracranial pressure (ICP) with radiologic evidence of obstructed cerebrospinal fluid (CSF) flow or mass effect with or without midline shift can place patients at risk of cerebral herniation and other neurological deterioration.[58] Patients with increased ICP

TABLE 24–11. Signs and symptoms of elevated intracranial pressure.

Headache

Drowsiness

Nausea and vomiting

New-onset seizures

Decreased level of consciousness

Papilledema

Pupillary changes

Focal neurologic signs

at baseline may also experience an additional increase in pressure on epidural drug injection.[59] Consultation with a neurologic expert is strongly recommended, and localizing neurologic signs and symptoms should be ruled out by history and physical examination prior to initiation of neuraxial blockade in patients with new neurologic symptoms or known intracranial lesions[60] (Table 24–11). A decision tree may aid in assessing whether it is safe to proceed with neuraxial techniques in the presence of intracranial space-occupying lesions (Figure 24–2).

Coagulopathy

Coagulopathy is a relative contraindication to epidural placement, although thorough consideration of the etiology and severity of the coagulopathy is warranted on a case-by-case basis. Anticoagulants increase the risk of epidural hematoma and should be withheld in a timely fashion before initiation of epidural blockade. Precautions should also be taken before epidural catheter removal, as catheter removal may be as traumatic as catheter placement.[61]

Clinical Pearl

- Epidural needle and catheter placement both carry a risk of epidural hematoma in patients on anticoagulants. Similar precautions should be observed during placement and removal of epidural catheters.

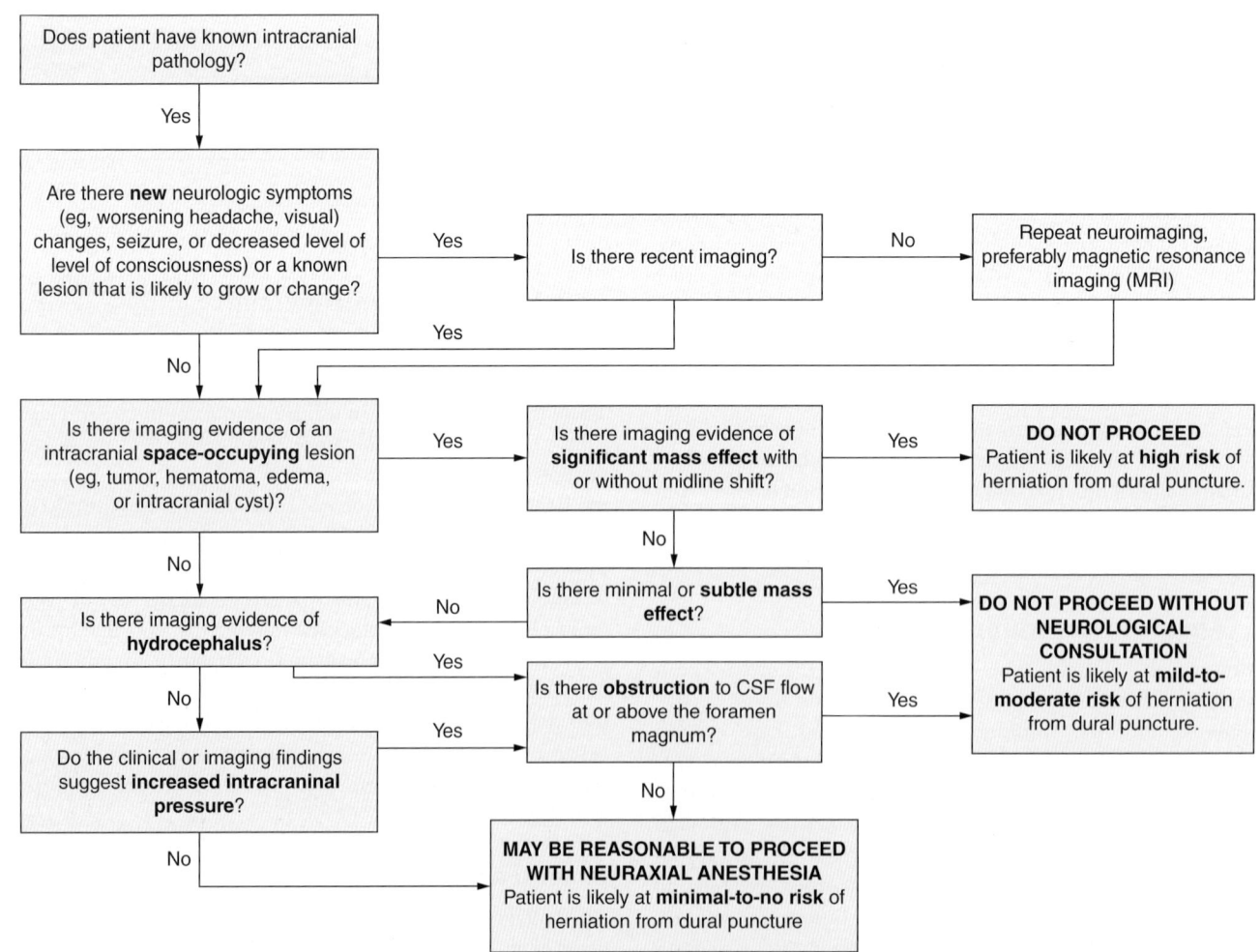

FIGURE 24–2. Safety algorithm for neuroaxial blockade in patients with intracranial space-occupying lesions. CSF = cerebrospinal fluid. (Reproduced with permission from Leffert LR, Schwamm LH: Neuraxial anesthesia in parturients with intracranial pathology: a comprehensive review and reassessment of risk. *Anesthesiology.* 2013 Sep;119(3):703-718.)

TABLE 24–12. Epidural blockade in patients receiving antithrombotic therapy.

NSAIDs (aspirin)	No contraindication
Clopidogrel	Wait 7 days before epidural placement
5000 U subcutaneous UFH every 12 hours	No contraindication
>10,000 U subcutaneous UFH daily	Safety not established
Intravenous heparin	Wait at least 60 minutes after instrumentation before administration of heparin; consider aPTT and wait 2–4 hours prior to catheter removal
LMWH thromboprophylactic dose	Wait 12 hours before epidural placement
LMWH therapeutic dose	Wait 24 hours before epidural placement
Warfarin	Wait for INR to normalize before neuraxial block; remove neuraxial catheter when INR < 1.5

INR = international normalized ratio; LMWH = low molecular weight heparin; NSAIDs = nonsteroidal anti-inflammatory drugs; UFH = unfractionated heparin.

The American Society of Regional Anesthesia and Pain Medicine periodically updates its guidelines for the initiation of regional anesthesia in patients receiving antithrombotic or thrombolytic therapy.[62] Briefly, neuraxial techniques in patients receiving subcutaneous unfractionated heparin (UFH) with dosing regimens of 5000 U every 12 hours are considered safe (Table 24–12). The risks and benefits of thrice-daily UFH or more than 10,000 U daily should be assessed on an individual basis; vigilance should be maintained to detect new or worsening neurodeficits in this setting. For patients receiving heparin for more than 4 days, a platelet count should be assessed before neuraxial block or catheter removal due to concerns for heparin-induced thrombocytopenia (HIT). In patients who receive systemic heparinization, it is recommended to assess the activated plasma thromboplastin time (aPTT) and discontinue heparin for 2 to 4 hours prior to catheter manipulation or removal. Administration of intravenous heparin intraoperatively should be delayed for at least 1 hour after epidural placement; a delay before administration of subcutaneous heparin is not required. In cases of full heparinization for CPB, additional precautions include delaying surgery for 24 hours in the event of a traumatic tap, tightly controlling the heparin effect and reversal, and removing catheters when normal coagulation is restored.

Epidural blockade in patients taking aspirin and nonaspirin NSAIDs is considered safe, as the risk of epidural hematoma is low. Needle placement should be delayed for 12 hours in patients receiving low molecular weight heparin (LMWH) thromboprophylaxis and for 24 hours in those receiving therapeutic doses. It is recommended that warfarin be discontinued for several days prior to surgery and that the international normalized ratio (INR) return to baseline prior to initiation of epidural techniques. An INR below 1.5 is considered sufficient for catheter removal, although many clinicians may be comfortable manipulating catheters with higher INR values. Refer to Chapter 52 for more detailed information on these and newer agents.

Neuraxial techniques are contraindicated in the setting of DIC, which may complicate sepsis, trauma, liver failure, placental abruption, amniotic fluid embolism, and massive transfusion, among other disease processes (Table 24–13). If DIC develops after epidural placement, the catheter should be removed once normal clotting parameters have been restored.

Thrombocytopenia and Other Common Bleeding Disorders

Thrombocytopenia, which may be caused by several pathologic conditions, is a relative contraindication to neuraxial anesthesia.

TABLE 24–13. Conditions associated with disseminated intravascular coagulation.

Sepsis
Trauma (head injury, extensive soft tissue injury, fat embolism, massive hemorrhage)
Massive transfusion
Malignancy (pancreatic carcinoma, myeloproliferative disease)
Peripartum (amniotic fluid embolism, placental abruption, HELLP [hemolysis, elevated liver enzymes, and low platelet count] syndrome, abnormal placentation)
Vascular disorders (aortic aneurysm, giant hemangioma)
Immunologic disorders (hemolytic transfusion reaction, transplant rejection, severe allergic reaction)
Liver failure

While there is currently no universally accepted platelet count below which epidural placement should be avoided, many clinicians are comfortable with a platelet count above 70,000 mm^3 in the absence of clinical bleeding.[63] The cutoff may be higher or lower, however, depending on the etiology of the thrombocytopenia, the bleeding history, the trend in platelet number, individual patient characteristics (eg, a known or suspected difficult airway), and provider expertise and comfort level. In general, platelet function is normal in conditions such as gestational thrombocytopenia and immune thrombocytopenic purpura (ITP).

Clinical Pearl

- The etiology of thrombocytopenia, the patient's bleeding history, and the trend in platelet count must be taken into account when determining the safety of initiation of epidural blockade in thrombocytopenic patients. Certain conditions, such as ITP and gestational thrombocytopenia, are associated with functioning platelets despite a low platelet count.

A platelet count below 50,000 mm^3 in the setting of ITP may respond to corticosteroids or intravenous immunoglobulin (IVIG), when necessary. Functional platelet defects may be present in several less-common conditions, such as HELLP syndrome (hemolysis, elevated liver enzymes, and low platelet count); thrombotic thrombocytopenic purpura (TTP); and hemolytic uremic syndrome (HUS). Other conditions such as systemic lupus erythematous (SLE), antiphospholipid syndrome, type 2B von Willebrand disease (vWD), HIT, and DIC are associated with thrombocytopenia of varying degrees (Table 24–14).

A standard platelet count has not been established for catheter removal. While some sources suggest 60,000 mm^3 is appropriate, catheter removal without adverse sequelae has been reported at counts below that cutoff.[64] If platelet number or function is impaired after an epidural catheter has been placed, such as in the case of intraoperative DIC, the catheter should remain in situ until the coagulopathy has resolved.

Other common bleeding diatheses that comprise relative contraindications to the initiation of epidural blockade include hemophilia, vWD, and disorders related to lupus anticoagulants and anticardiolipin antibodies. Hemophilia A and B are X-linked diseases characterized by deficiencies in factors VIII and IX, respectively. Although specific guidelines are lacking, neuraxial procedures are considered safe in carriers of the disease with normal factor levels and no bleeding complications. Neuraxial techniques have been performed without adverse sequelae in homozygous patients after factor replacement therapy once factor levels and the aPTT have normalized. Patients with lupus anticoagulants and anticardiolipin antibodies are predisposed to platelet aggregation, thrombocytopenia, and, because of interactions between antibodies and platelet membranes, thrombosis. As a result, many of these patients are anticoagulated with heparin in the peripartum or perioperative

TABLE 24–14. Causes of thrombocytopenia.

Autoimmune	Idiopathic thrombocytopenic purpura
	Thrombotic thrombocytopenic purpura
	Antiphospholipid syndrome
	Systemic lupus erythematosus
Peripartum	Gestational thrombocytopenia
	Preeclampsia (HELLP [hemolysis, elevated liver enzymes, and low platelet count] syndrome)
von Willebrand disease	Type 2B
Drug related	Heparin-induced thrombocytopenia
	Methyldopa
	Sulfamethoxazole
Lymphoproliferative disorders	
Hemolytic uremic syndrome	

period. Heparin levels should be monitored with a blood heparin assay, thrombin time, or activated clotting test prior to performing neuraxial blockade. Of note, the aPTT is elevated at baseline in these patients and is likely to remain elevated after discontinuation of heparin due to interactions between the circulating antibodies and the coagulation tests.

Von Willebrand disease is the most common inherited bleeding disorder. It is characterized by either a quantitative (type 1 and type 3) or qualitative (type 2) deficiency in von Willebrand factor (vWF), a plasma glycoprotein that binds to and stabilizes factor VIII and mediates platelet adhesion at sites of vascular injury. The clinical presentation of vWD varies: Patients with type 1, the most common type, experience mucocutaneous bleeding, easy bruising, and menorrhagia; patients with type 2 vWD may experience moderate-to-severe bleeding and, in the case of type 2B, thrombocytopenia; type 3, which is rare, presents with severe bleeding, including hemarthroses (Table 24–15). Both treatment options and the decision to proceed with neuraxial blockade also vary with the different disease presentations. Type I responds to desmopressin (DDAVP), which promotes secretion of stored vWF from endothelial cells and results in a rapid rise in both plasma vWF and factor VIII. Factor VIII concentrates and cryoprecipitate are treatment options for type 2 and type 3 vWD. Specialized laboratory tests may help confirm the diagnosis and type of vWD but are not widely available; standard coagulation tests may serve to rule out other bleeding disorders. In addition to a thorough history and physical examination, collaboration with a hematologist and other team

TABLE 24–15. Classification of von Willebrand disease.

Type	Underlying disorder	Clinical Presentation/Characteristics
1	Deficient quantity of vWF	Mucocutaneous bleeding, epistaxis, easy bruising, menorrhagia
2A	Defect in quality of vWF	Moderate bleeding
2B	Abnormal vWF	Moderate bleeding; thrombocytopenia; risk of thrombosis
2M	Abnormal vWF binding	Rare; significant bleeding
2N	Inactive vWF binding sites	May see low factor VIII and normal vWF levels
3	Severe deficiency of vWF	Severe bleeding, hemarthroses, muscle hematomas

vWF = von Willebrand factor.

members, and a review of any pertinent laboratory results, a risk-benefit analysis should be performed prior to initiation of epidural procedures in patients with vWD.

Preexisting Central Nervous System Disorders

Historically, the administration of neuraxial blockade has been contraindicated in patients with preexisting central nervous system (CNS) disease, including multiple sclerosis (MS), postpolio syndrome (PPS), and Guillain-Barré syndrome (GBS). In the case of MS, demyelinated nerves were thought to be more vulnerable to LA-induced neurotoxicity. An early study by Bader and colleagues suggested an association between MS relapse and higher concentrations of epidural LA among parturients,[65] although a subsequent study in the same patient population failed to demonstrate an adverse effect of epidural anesthesia on either the rate of relapse or the progression of disease.[66] A more recent retrospective study by Hebl and colleagues found no evidence of MS relapse after spinal or epidural anesthesia in 35 patients, 18 of whom received epidural blockade.[67] While it is unlikely that epidural anesthesia and analgesia cause MS exacerbations, definitive studies on pharmacological properties of LAs in MS, optimal dosing regimens, and whether LAs interact directly with MS lesions are lacking.[68] Until further data are available, it is reasonable to use low-concentration LAs and perform a thorough assessment and documentation of disease severity and neurologic status prior to initiation of central neuraxial blockade in patients with MS. These patients should also be informed of possible aggravation of symptoms, irrespective of anesthetic technique.

The decision to perform epidural anesthesia in patients with PPS, the most prevalent motor neuron disease in North America, requires careful analysis of the potential risks and benefits on a case-by-case basis. PPS is a late-onset manifestation of acute poliomyelitis infection that presents with fatigue, joint pain, and muscle atrophy in previously affected muscle groups. Epidural techniques in this patient population can be complicated by difficult puncture related to abnormal spinal anatomy, potential worsening of symptoms, and transient respiratory weakness. Alternatively, GA presents challenges related to sensitivity to muscle relaxants and sedatives and risks of respiratory compromise and aspiration. Although data are limited, there is no evidence that epidural techniques contribute to worsening of neurologic symptoms in patients with PPS.

Evidence linking epidural techniques to either activation or recurrence of GBS is also lacking. GBS presents with progressive motor weakness, ascending paralysis, and areflexia, most likely attributable to a postinfection inflammatory response. Older age at onset and severe initial disease are among the risk factors for prolonged neurologic dysfunction. Epidural anesthesia has been used successfully in patients with GBS, most commonly in obstetric patients, although exaggerated hemodynamic responses (hypotension and bradycardia), higher-than-normal spread of LAs, and worsening of neurologic symptoms have been reported.[69] As always, a risk-benefit analysis is warranted prior to performance of epidural blockade in patients with GBS, as are assessment and documentation of neurologic examination of the patient and a thorough discussion of the risks of anesthesia. It is reasonable to avoid regional techniques during periods of acute neuronal inflammation.

Patients with spina bifida may also present a unique challenge to anesthesiologists. Spina bifida occulta occurs when the neural arch fails to close without herniation of the meninges or neural tissues. It is most commonly limited to one vertebra, although a small percentage of affected individuals have involvement of two or more vertebrae with associated neurologic abnormalities, underlying cord abnormalities, and scoliosis. In general, the use of epidural techniques is not contraindicated in patients with spina bifida occulta, although placement at the level of the occulta lesion, most commonly at L5 to S1, may have an increased risk of dural puncture and patchy or higher-than-normal response to LAs. In contrast, epidural placement in patients with spina bifida cystica has several potential risks, including risk of direct injury to the cord due to a low-lying conus medullaris, unpredictable or higher-than-expected spread of LAs, and increased risk of dural puncture.

Fever or Infection

Controversy exists regarding the administration of neuraxial anesthesia in febrile patients and in individuals infected with human immunodeficiency virus (HIV), herpes simplex virus type 2 (HSV-2), and varicella zoster virus (VZV). The use of regional anesthesia in the presence of a low-grade fever of infectious origin is controversial due to concerns of spreading the infectious agent to the epidural or subarachnoid space, with subsequent meningitis or epidural abscess formation. Fortunately, infectious complications of regional anesthesia are rare, and studies to date have failed to demonstrate a causal relationship between neuraxial procedures, with or without dural puncture, and subsequent neurologic complications. While no universal guidelines exist, available data suggest that fever does not preclude the safe administration of epidural anesthesia and analgesia. The anesthetic management of febrile patients should be based on an individual risk-benefit analysis. Whether general or regional anesthesia is chosen, antibiotic therapy should be either completed prior to or underway during initiation of the anesthetic. Adherence to strict aseptic techniques and postprocedure monitoring to detect and treat any complications are essential.

Historically, there have been concerns about the safety of neuraxial procedures in individuals infected with HIV due to both the theoretical risk of inoculation of the virus into the CNS and the possibility that neurologic manifestations of HIV may be attributed to the anesthetic technique.[70] However, the CNS is infected early in the course of HIV infection, and there is no evidence that neuraxial instrumentation, including an epidural blood patch (EBP) for the treatment of PDPH, confers additional risk of viral spread to the CNS. There also is no evidence that the introduction of HIV-infected blood into the CSF might exacerbate a preexisting CNS infection, such as meningitis. Concerns that neurologic sequelae of HIV might be attributed to the neuraxial technique also appear to be unsubstantiated, as a temporal relationship between the epidural placement and the onset of neurologic deficits is unlikely. Nonetheless, thorough documentation of any preexisting neurologic deficit is recommended, given that neurologic complications of HIV are not uncommon and that HIV-positive individuals are at high risk for other sexually transmitted diseases that affect the CNS. Potential risks should be discussed in advance, and, as always, strict aseptic technique to protect both the patient and the anesthesiology provider must be maintained.

Areas of concern regarding the use of regional anesthesia in patients with HSV-2 include the risk of introducing the virus into the CNS during administration of neuraxial anesthesia; the possibility that a disseminated infection that develops after a regional anesthetic might be ascribed to the anesthetic itself, despite the lack of a causal relationship; and the safety of neuraxial techniques in primary HSV-2 outbreaks, which may be silent and difficult to distinguish from secondary outbreaks, but more commonly present with viremia, constitutional symptoms, genital lesions, and, in a small percentage of patients, aseptic meningitis. There are no documented cases of septic or neurologic complications following neuraxial procedures in patients with secondary (ie, recurrent) HSV infection; however, the safety of regional anesthesia in patients with primary infection has not been established. Crosby and colleagues conducted a 6-year retrospective analysis of 89 patients with secondary HSV infection who received epidural anesthesia for cesarean delivery and reported that no patients suffered septic or neurologic complications.[71] Similarly, in their retrospective survey of 164 parturients

with secondary HSV infection who received spinal, epidural, or GA for cesarean delivery, Bader et al reported no adverse outcomes related to the anesthetic.[72] Based on the findings in these and other reported series, it appears safe to use spinal or epidural anesthesia in patients with secondary HSV infection. Pending more conclusive data, however, it seems prudent to avoid neuraxial blockade in patients with HSV-2 viremia.

Concerns also exist regarding the use of regional anesthesia in adults with either primary or recurrent VZV infections, such as herpes zoster (ie, shingles) and postherpetic neuralgia (PHN). However, neuraxial procedures, including epidural steroid injections, are not uncommonly used to treat acute herpes zoster, prevent PHN, and treat the pain associated with PHN, often in conjunction with antiviral therapy. The presence of active lesions at the site of injection is considered a contraindication to these and other neuraxial techniques. For the small subset of patients who are infected with primary VZV as adults, severe complications such as aseptic meningitis, encephalitis, and varicella pneumonia may result. The performance of regional anesthesia in this setting is more controversial but may be preferable to GA in some cases, primarily due to concerns for pneumonia.[73] Ultimately, a careful risk-benefit analysis, in addition to assessment and documentation of any preexisting neurologic deficits, is recommended prior to initiation of neuraxial blockade in these patients.

Localized skin infection at the site of intended needle puncture is another relative contraindication to neuraxial blockade, primarily due to concerns that spinal epidural abscess (SEA) or meningitis may result. Hematogenous spread of a localized infection has been implicated in SEA, although a causal relationship is not clearly established in the reported cases. Maintenance of strict sterile precautions and a low index of suspicion in the presence of neurologic signs may minimize the risk. Needle insertion should be attempted after appropriate antibiotic administration, and a site remote from the localized infection is recommended.

Previous Back Surgery, Preexisting Neurologic Injury, and Back Pain

Traditionally, a history of previous back surgery was considered a relative contraindication to neuraxial blockade due to concerns for infection, exacerbation of preexisting neurologic deficits, and an increased likelihood of difficult or unsuccessful block. Technical difficulties may be related to degenerative changes above or below the level of fusion, adhesions in the epidural space, epidural space obliteration, dense scar tissue at the point of intended needle entry on the skin surface, the presence of graft material, and the presence of extensive rods that preclude identification of or access to midline. Despite these concerns, one large retrospective study of patients with a history of spinal stenosis, peripheral neuropathy, or lumbar radiculopathy found that previous spinal surgery did not affect the success rate or frequency of technical complications.[74] In patients with metal rods (eg, Harrington rods), anteroposterior and lateral radiographs or a copy of the operative report may help to identify the extent of instrumentation, as well as the presence of additional anatomic abnormalities. Ultrasound may aid in the identification of midline in challenging epidural cases. Potential complications, such as irregular, limited, or excessive cranial spread of LAs and an increased risk of PDPH if multiple attempts at placement are required, should be discussed with the patient during the informed consent process. Of note, similar technical difficulties encountered during the original technique can be expected during an EBP procedure. Because of these and other concerns, spinal anesthesia may be preferred, when appropriate, over epidural blockade.

Back pain is a ubiquitous problem that should not be considered a contraindication to neuraxial blockade and, rather, is a relatively common indication for epidural steroid and LA injections. One recent study found a higher than previously reported rate of new neurologic deficits and worsening of preexisting symptoms in patients with compressive radiculopathy or multiple neurologic disorders (spinal stenosis or lumbar disk disease) who received neuraxial anesthesia.[74] However, a causal relationship was not clearly established. Many of the concerns regarding neuraxial procedures in patients with back pain can be addressed prior to initiation of neuraxial anesthesia with a thorough history and physical examination; not uncommonly, the cause of back pain is not neurologic in origin. In these cases, regional techniques are not associated with new-onset back pain and are unlikely to exacerbate the preexisting condition. Because patients with preexisting neurologic conditions may be at increased risk of postoperative neurologic complications after neuraxial techniques, a careful risk-benefit analysis is warranted on a case-by-case basis. Preexisting neurologic deficits or symptoms and their severity should be documented.

Preload-Dependent States

Traditionally, neuraxial blockade has been considered contraindicated in patients with severe aortic stenosis (AS) and other preload-dependent conditions, such as hypertrophic obstructive cardiomyopathy (asymmetric septal hypertrophy, ASH), due to the risk of acute decompensation in response to decreased systemic vascular resistance (SVR). The later stages of AS are associated with decreased diastolic compliance, impaired relaxation, increased myocardial oxygen demand, and decreased perfusion of the endocardium.[75] Decreased SVR in the setting of either GA or neuraxial blockade leads to decreased coronary perfusion and contractility, with a further reduction in cardiac output (CO) and worsening hypotension. Bradycardia, tachycardia, and other dysrhythmias are also poorly tolerated. The current evidence regarding regional anesthesia in patients with AS is based on case reports and lacks the scientific validity provided by randomized controlled trials. However, it appears that carefully titrated CSE and continuous epidural and spinal techniques, most commonly with invasive monitoring, may be acceptable options for patients with AS. Single-shot spinal anesthetics are generally contraindicated, as gradual onset of sympathetic blockade is essential.

Anesthetic goals for patients with ASH are similar, with emphasis on maintaining preload, afterload, euvolemia, and vascular resistance, while avoiding tachycardia and enhanced contractility. Invasive monitoring and, if necessary, intermittent

transthoracic echocardiography may help guide fluid and vasopressor requirements, as well as guide management in the event of acute decompensation.[76]

Epidural Placement in Anesthetized Patients

Initiation of epidural blockade in adults under GA is controversial due to concerns that these patients cannot respond to pain and may therefore be at increased risk for neurologic complications. Indeed, paresthesias during block performance and pain on LA injection have been identified as risk factors for serious neurologic deficits after regional techniques. Consequently, some experts consider close communication with the patient an essential component of safe epidural performance.[77] Current data support the practice of epidural insertion in awake or minimally sedated patients, but needle and catheter placement in anesthetized adults may be an acceptable alternative in selected cases. Studies of lumbar epidural insertion while patients are undergoing GA have demonstrated that the risk of neurologic complications is small.[78] Overall, the relative risk of administration of epidural blockade in anesthetized patients, compared with epidural placement in awake patients, is unknown due to the low overall incidence of serious neurologic complications associated with regional anesthesia.

Needle Insertion Through a Tattoo

Concerns that puncturing a tattoo during epidural placement may have adverse sequelae appear unsubstantiated in the literature. Theoretical risks are related primarily to the introduction of a potentially toxic or carcinogenic pigment into the epidural, subdural, or subarachnoid space. However, to date no significant complications related to inserting a needle through a tattoo have been reported in the literature, although potential long-term consequences cannot be dismissed.

ANATOMY

An understanding of the anatomy of the vertebral column, spinal canal, epidural space and its contents, and commonly encountered anatomic variations among individuals is essential for the safe and effective initiation of epidural blockade. A three-dimensional mental image of vertebral column anatomy also aids in troubleshooting when identification of the epidural space is equivocal or when complications of epidural catheterization, such as unilateral blockade, intravascular cannulation, or catheter migration, occur. This section presents the basic anatomic considerations for successful epidural anesthesia and analgesia and reviews several controversies in the field of applied anatomy, including the accuracy of anatomic landmarks to estimate the spinous process level, the existence (or lack thereof) of a subdural compartment, and the contents of the epidural space.

Vertebral Column
General Appearance

Seven cervical, 12 thoracic, 5 lumbar, 5 fused sacral, and 3 to 5 (most commonly 4) fused coccygeal vertebrae comprise the

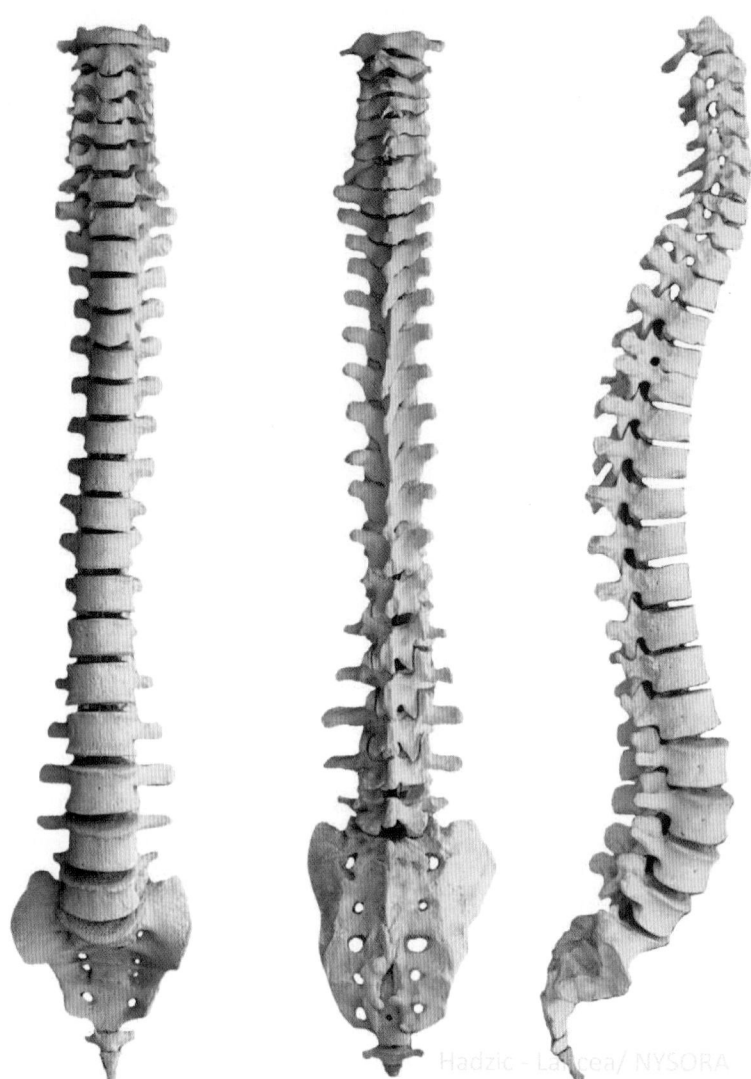

FIGURE 24–3. Physiologic spinal curves: anterior, posterior, and lateral views (left to right).

vertebral column. The vertebral column is straight when viewed dorsally or ventrally. When viewed from the side, the cervical and lumbar regions are concave posteriorly (lordosis), and the thoracic and sacral regions are concave anteriorly (kyphosis) (Figure 24–3). The four physiologic spinal curves are fully developed by 10 years of age and become more pronounced during pregnancy and with aging. In the supine position, C5 and L3 are positioned at the highest points of the lordosis; the peaks of kyphosis occur at T5 to T7 and at S2.

Clinical Pearl

- C5 and L3 comprise the highest points of lordosis in the supine position; the highest points of kyphosis are T5 to T7 and S2.

Structure of Vertebrae

With the exceptions of C1 and C2 and the fused sacral and coccygeal regions, the general structure of each vertebra consists of an anterior vertebral body (corpus, centrum) and a posterior bony arch. The arch is formed by the laminae; the pedicles, which extend from the posterolateral margins of the vertebral body; and the posterior surface of the vertebral body itself. In addition to the spinous processes, which are formed by the fusion of the laminae at midline, the vertebral arch supports three pairs of processes that emerge from the point where the laminae and pedicles join: two transverse processes, two superior articular processes, and two inferior articular processes. Adjacent vertebral arches enclose the vertebral canal and surround portions of the longitudinal spinal cord. The spinal canal communicates with the paravertebral space by way of gaps between the pedicles of successive vertebrae. These intervertebral foramina serve as passageways for the segmental nerves, arteries, and veins.

There is substantial variation in the size and shape of the vertebral bodies, the spinous processes, and the spinal canal at different levels of the vertebral column (Figure 24–4). C3 through C7 have the smallest vertebral bodies, while the spinal canal at this level is wide, measuring 25 mm. These cervical vertebrae, with the exception of C7, have short, bifurcated spinous processes. C7, the vertebra prominens, has a long, slender,

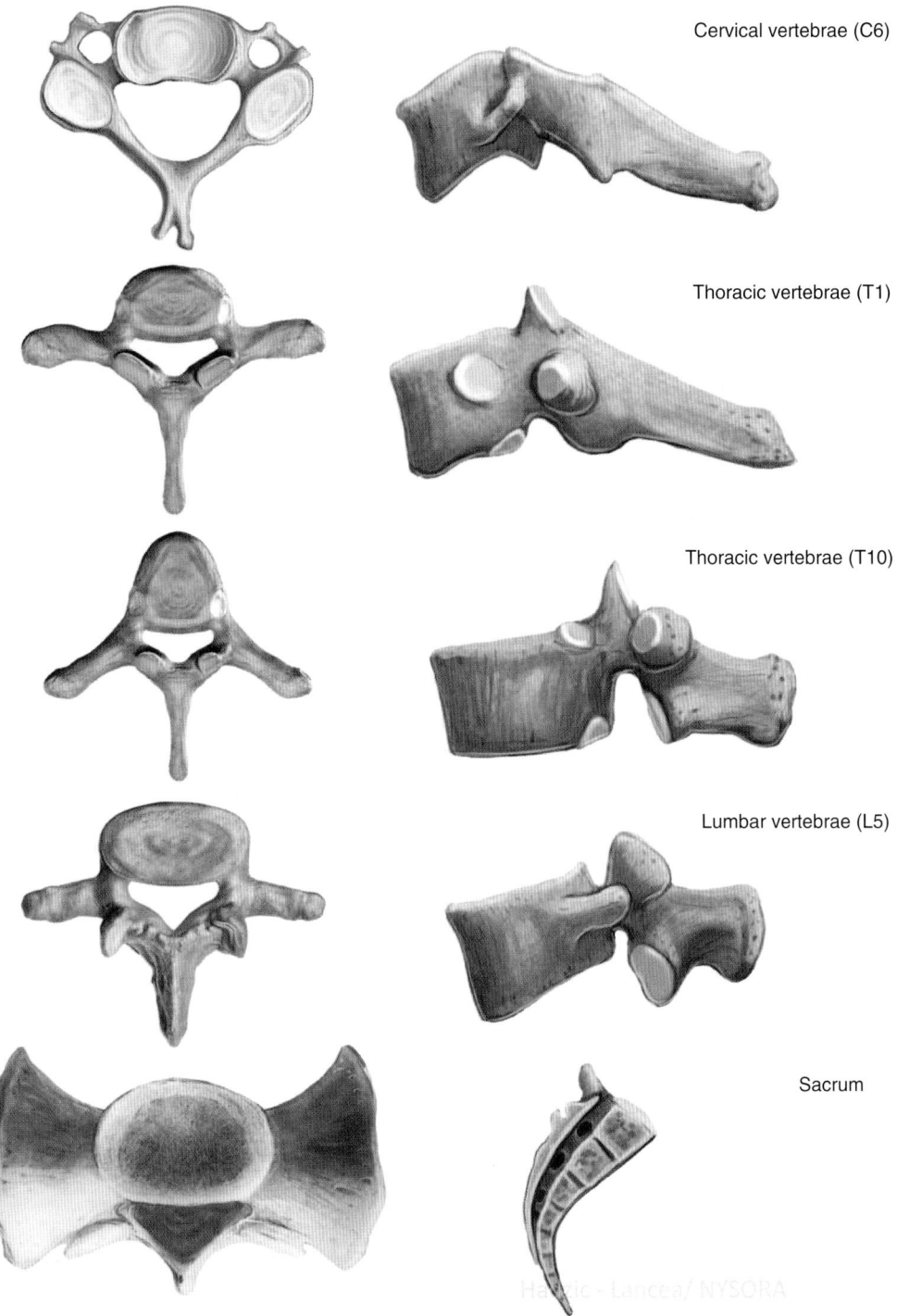

Cervical vertebrae (C6)

Thoracic vertebrae (T1)

Thoracic vertebrae (T10)

Lumbar vertebrae (L5)

Sacrum

FIGURE 24–4. Size and shape of the vertebral bodies at different spinal levels.

and easily palpable horizontal spinous process protruding at the base of the neck that often serves as a surface landmark during epidural procedures. However, the first thoracic spinous process may be equally or more prominent than C7 in up to one-third of male individuals, as well as in thin patients and in patients with scoliosis and degenerative diseases.[79] The vertebra prominens may also be difficult to distinguish from C6 in up to half of individuals, most commonly females.[80]

The thoracic vertebral bodies are larger than the cervical vertebral bodies and are wider in the posterior than anterior

dimension, contributing to the characteristic thoracic curvature. The long and slender thoracic spinous processes, with tips that point caudally, are most sharply angled between T4 and T9, making insertion of the epidural needle in the midline more difficult in the midthoracic region. Beyond T10, they increasingly resemble those in the lumbar region. Each thoracic vertebra articulates with ribs along the dorsolateral border of its body, a feature that may help distinguish the lower thoracic and upper lumbar regions. The inferior angle of the scapula and the 12th rib are widely used in clinical practice to estimate the level of the

TABLE 24–16. Anatomic landmarks to identify vertebral levels.

Vertebra prominens	C7
Root of spine of scapula	T3
Inferior angle of scapula	T7
Rib margin	L1
Superior aspect of iliac crest	L3, L4
Posterior superior iliac spine	S2

spinous processes of T7 and T12, respectively. The imaginary line connecting the caudal-most margin of the 12th ribs is often presumed to cross the L1 spinous process (Table 24–16).

The lumbar vertebrae are the largest movable segments, with thicker anterior than posterior dimensions that contribute to the characteristic lumbar curvature. The spinous processes in this region are blunt and large, with tips that point posteriorly. Anatomic variations in the lumbosacral region that may have clinical implications are not uncommon. Sacralization of the last lumbar vertebra, marked by fusion of L5 to the sacral bone, and lumbarization of S1 and S2, in which fusion is incomplete, may make numbering and identification of the correct lumbar level difficult.[81] Although probably not of clinical significance, patients with sacralization have also been found to have a higher position of the conus medullaris, which demarcates the cone-shaped terminus of the spinal cord, than those with lumbarization or without lumbosacral transitional vertebrae.[82] In the absence of these transitional vertebrae, the largest and most easily palpable interspace corresponds to L5 to S1.

Surface Anatomic Landmarks to Identify the Spinal Level

Surface landmarks are often used to identify the intended spinal level during initiation of epidural anesthesia (Figure 24–5). However, palpation and inspection of surface anatomical landmarks may fail to help localize the correct intervertebral space, particularly when considering individual variations in the vertebral level of these landmarks, the varying termination of the conus medullaris between the middle third of T12 and the upper third of L3,[83] and anesthesiologists' poor record of identifying the correct interspace.

Common pitfalls to using skeletal landmarks to identify the level of puncture include the following: The vertebra prominens is commonly confused with C6 and T1; the scapula may be difficult to identify during TEA placement in obese patients; tracing the vertebra attached to the 12th rib can be misleading, particularly in obese patients; and the line connecting the posterior superior iliac spines, often used to identify S2, commonly crosses the midline at variable levels between L5 and S1.[84] Several studies have demonstrated that Tuffier's line (also known as Jacoby's line or the intercristal line), which joins the superior aspect of the iliac crests, may cross midline at least one, and

perhaps two, levels higher than the predicted L4–L5 interspace,[85] particularly in pregnant,[86] elderly, and obese patients.

Anesthesiologists have a poor record of estimating the correct interspace based on external landmarks. Van Gessel and colleagues found that the level of lumbar puncture is misidentified up to 59% of the time.[87] In a more recent study, Broadbent and coworkers found that practitioners identify the correct lumbar level in only 29% of cases; the space is misidentified by two spinal levels, with the actual level higher than that predicted, in 14% of cases.[88] Lirk et al confirmed the tendency of trained anesthetists to place the epidural needle more cranially than intended, most often within one interspace of the predicted level, also in the cervical and thoracic spinal column.[89] Overall, given the importance of selecting the correct site of puncture, caution is advised when using surface anatomic landmarks to identify intervertebral spaces. The increasing reliance on ultrasound determination of the spinal level may decrease the incidence of complications related to misidentification of the intended interspace.

Joints and Ligaments of the Vertebral Column
General

Adjacent vertebrae of the cervical, thoracic, and lumbar regions, excluding C1 and C2, are separated and cushioned by fibrocartilaginous intervertebral disks. The soft, elastic core of each disk, the nucleus pulposus, is composed primarily of water, as well as scattered elastic and reticular fibers. The fibrocartilaginous annulus fibrosis surrounds the nucleus pulposus and attaches the disks to the bodies of adjacent vertebrae. The disks, which account for up to one-quarter of the length of an adult vertebral column, lose their water content as we age, contributing to the shortening of the vertebral column, reducing their effectiveness as cushions, and rendering them more prone to injury, particularly in the lumbar region.

The articular processes arise at the junction between the pedicles and laminae. Superior and inferior articular processes project cranially and caudally, respectively, on both sides of each vertebra. The vertebral arches are connected by facet joints, which link the inferior articular processes of one vertebra with the superior articular processes of the more caudal vertebra. The facet joints are heavily innervated by the medial branch of the dorsal ramus of the spinal nerves. This innervation serves to direct contraction of muscle that moves the vertebral column.

The Longitudinal Ligaments

The anterior and posterior longitudinal ligaments support the vertebral column, binding the vertebral bodies and intervertebral disks together (Figure 24–6). The posterior longitudinal ligament, which forms the anterior wall of the vertebral canal, is less broad than its anterior counterpart and weakens with age and other degenerative processes. Clinically, disk herniation occurs primarily in the paramedian portion of the posterior disk, at weak points in the posterior longitudinal ligament. This area comprises the anterior epidural space, as opposed to the more clinically relevant posterior epidural space, and should not interfere with epidural needle placement.

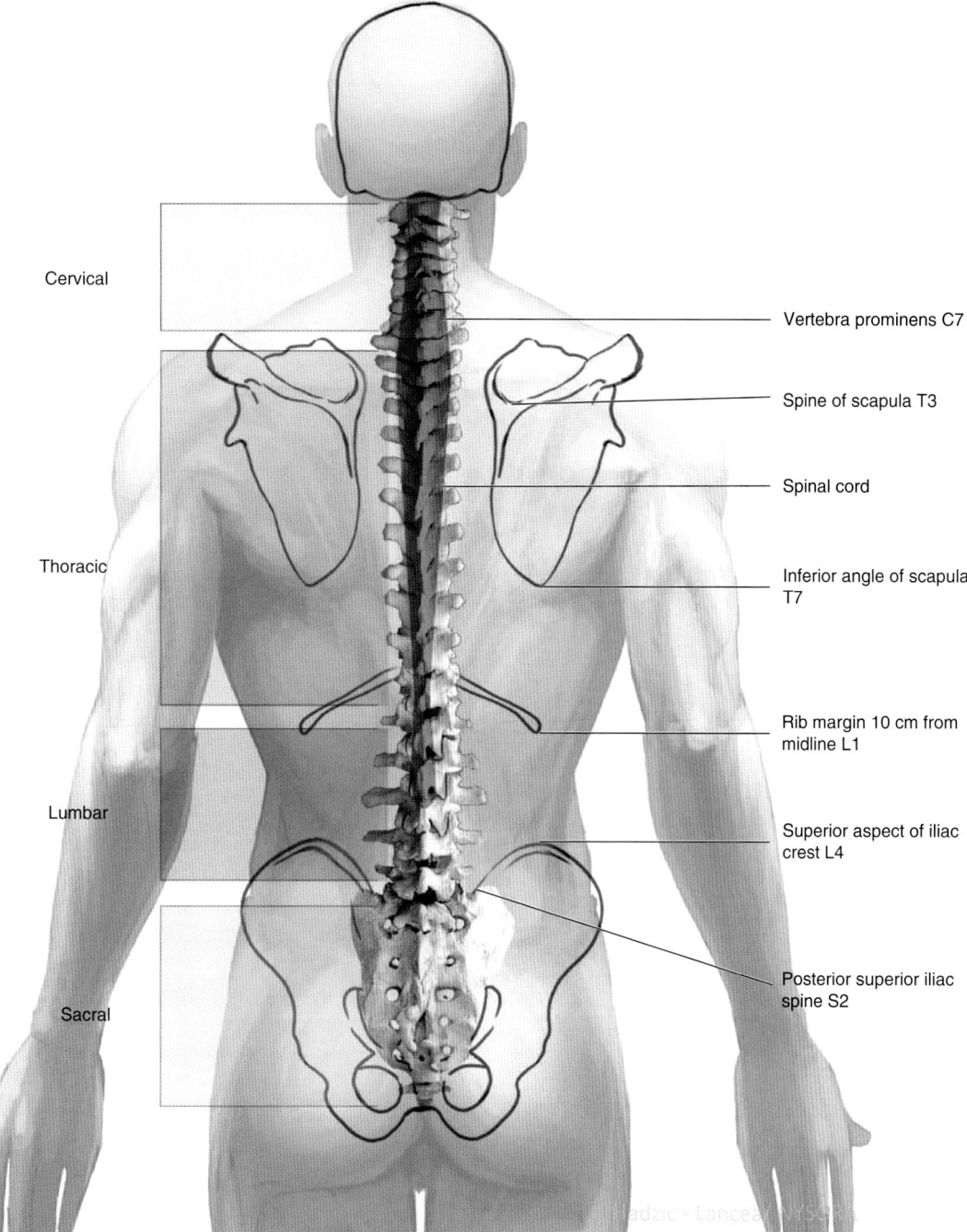

FIGURE 24–5. Skeletal landmarks used to determine the level of epidural placement.

Clinical Pearl

• Disk herniation occurs primarily at weak points in the posterior longitudinal ligament in an area that comprises the anterior epidural space, as opposed to the more clinically relevant posterior epidural space.

Nonetheless, thorough documentation of preexisting pain and neurologic deficits in patients with known disk herniation is recommended prior to initiation of epidural anesthesia. Also of clinical relevance, a membranous lateral extension of

the posterior longitudinal ligament may serve as a barrier to the spread of epidural solutions and appears to cordon the veins anterior to the dura away from the rest of the epidural space.[90]

Clinical Pearl

• A membranous lateral extension of the posterior longitudinal ligament appears to cordon off the veins in the anterolateral epidural space, where epidural vein puncture and catheter cannulation are more likely to occur.

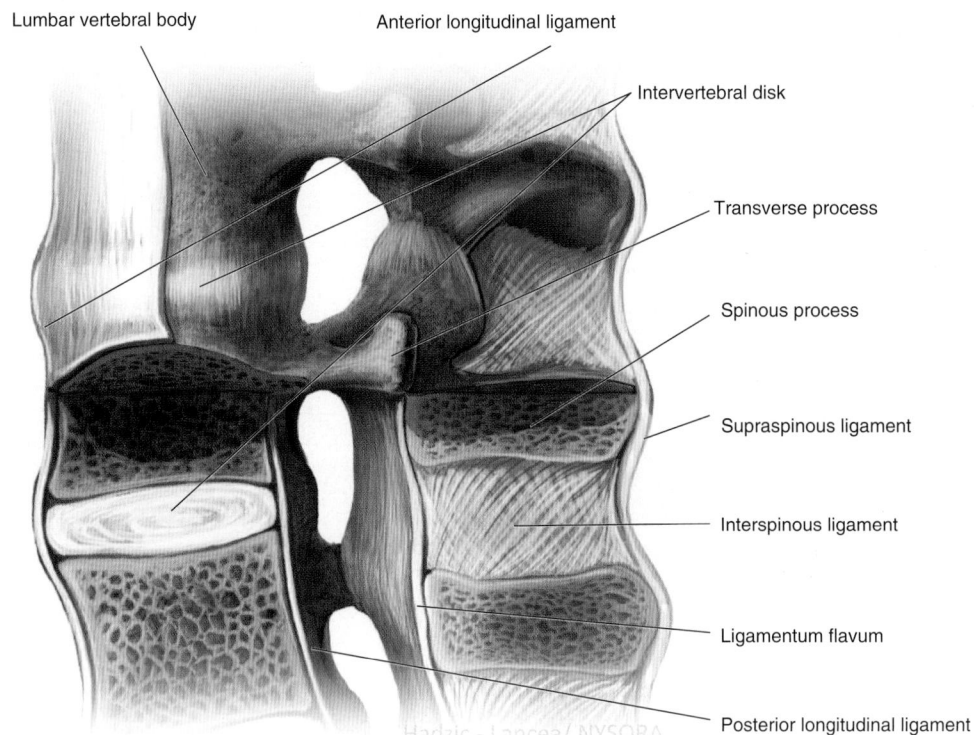

FIGURE 24–6. Ligaments of the vertebral canal.

The Supraspinous and Interspinous Ligaments

Several other ligaments that support the vertebral column serve as key anatomic landmarks during epidural needle placement. The supraspinous ligament connects the tips of the spinous processes from C7 to L5; above C7 and extending to the base of the skull, it is called the ligamentum nuchae. This relatively superficial, inextensible ligament is most prominent in the upper thoracic region and becomes thinner and less conspicuous toward the lower lumbar region.[91] The interspinous ligament, directly anterior to the supraspinous ligament, traverses the space between adjacent spinous processes in a posterocranial direction. It is less developed in the cervical region, which may contribute to a false LOR during cervical epidural procedures.[92] On histological examination, the interspinous ligament appears to have intermittent midline cavities filled with fat.

Both the supra- and interspinous ligaments are composed of collagenous fibers that make a characteristic "crunching" sound or distinct tactile sensation as the epidural needle advances. During initiation of epidural placement via the midline approach, these ligaments serve as appropriate sites to engage the needle, although some practitioners may engage the needle closer to the epidural space, in the ligamentum flavum. A "floppy" epidural needle that angles laterally prior to attachment of the LOR syringe may indicate an off-midline approach, away from the supra- or interspinous ligaments.

The Ligamentum Flavum

The ligamentum flavum connects the lamina of adjacent vertebrae from the inferior border of C2 to the superior border of S1. Laterally, it extends into the intervertebral foramina, where it joins the capsule of the articular process. Anteriorly, it limits the vertebral canal and forms the posterior border of the epidural space. At each spinal level, the right and left ligamentum flava join discontinuously in an acute angle with the opening oriented in the ventral direction, occasionally forming midline gaps filled with epidural fat.[93] In contrast to the collagenous inter- and supraspinous ligaments, the ligamentum flavum comprises primarily thick, elastic fibers arranged longitudinally in a tight network. Areas of ossification of the ligamentum flavum occur at different levels of the vertebral canal and appear to be a normal variant. These bony spurs, which may contribute to preexisting neurological symptoms and could potentially impede epidural needle advancement, are most commonly encountered in the lower thoracic region, between T9 and T11, and diminish in both frequency and size in the caudal and cranial directions.[94]

The ligamentum flavum has variable characteristics, many of which are disputed in the literature, at different vertebral levels. First, its thickness varies at different levels and, possibly, in different physiologic states, with a range of 1.5–3.0 mm in the cervical segment, 3.0–5.0 mm in the thoracic segment, 5.0–6.0 mm in the lumbar segment, and 2.0–6.0 mm in the caudal region (Table 24–17).[95] In isolated pregnant patients, the ligamentum flavum has been reported to be as thick as 10 mm, presumably due to edema.[96] Also of note, the flavum's thickness varies within the interspace itself, with the caudal region being significantly thicker than the rostral.

TABLE 24–17. Thickness of the ligamentum flavum at different vertebral levels.

Vertebral Level	Thickness (mm)
Cervical	1.5–3.0
Thoracic	3.0–5.0
Lumbar	5.0–6.0
Caudal	2.0–6.0

Clinical Pearl

- The ligamentum flavum varies in thickness at different spinal levels and is thickest in the lumbar region. Its thickness also varies within each interspace.

Clinically, these varying degrees of thickness may influence the risk of inadvertent dural puncture or determine whether injection of an anesthetic solution into the epidural space is possible with the skin infiltration needle.

Another controversy concerns the incidence and location of gaps formed by the incomplete fusion of the right and left ligamentum flava. In their study of 52 human cadavers, Lirk and colleagues found that up to 74% of the flava in the cervical region are discontinuous at midline.[97] These gaps vary in location, with some occupying the entire height of the ligamentum flavum between successive vertebral arches and others occupying the caudal third portion only (Figure 24–7). Veins connecting the posterior external and internal vertebral venous plexuses not uncommonly traverse the caudal portion of the gaps. In another cadaveric study, Lirk et al determined that thoracic midline gaps were less frequent than cervical gaps but more frequent than those in the lumbar region, with an incidence as high as 35.2% at T10 to T11.[98] In cadaveric studies of the lumbar ligamentum flavum, gaps were found most commonly at L1 and L2 (22.2%) and decreased caudally (11.4% at L2 to L4; 9.3% at L4 to L5; 0% at L5 to S1).[99] Clinically, these gaps may contribute to failure to identify the epidural space using the LOR technique at midline. The characteristic "pop" sound and tactile sensation conferred by penetration of the elastic fibers of the ligamentum flavum may be absent in the setting of a discontinuous ligamentous arch. The depth to the epidural space at midline may also be affected.

Clinical Pearl

- Ligamentum flavum midline gaps represent incomplete fusion of the right and left ligamentum flava. They are common in the cervical spine and decrease in frequency in the thoracic and lumbar regions. The variable thickness of the ligamentum flavum and the presence of midline gaps may contribute to failure to identify the epidural space.

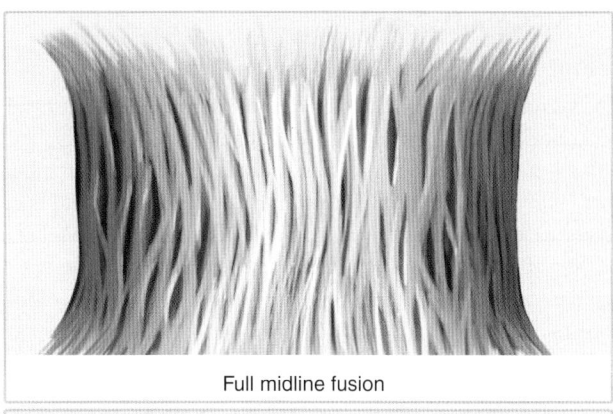

Full midline fusion

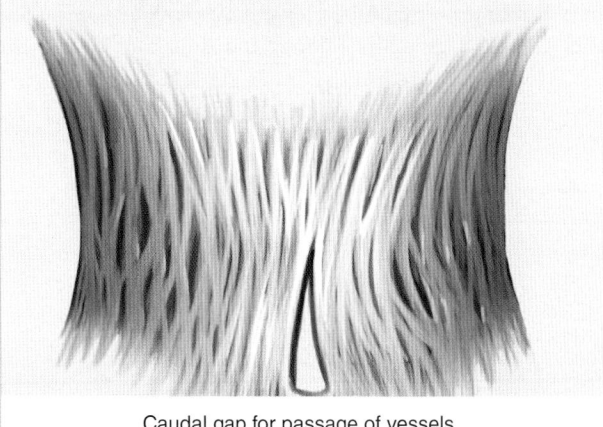

Caudal gap for passage of vessels

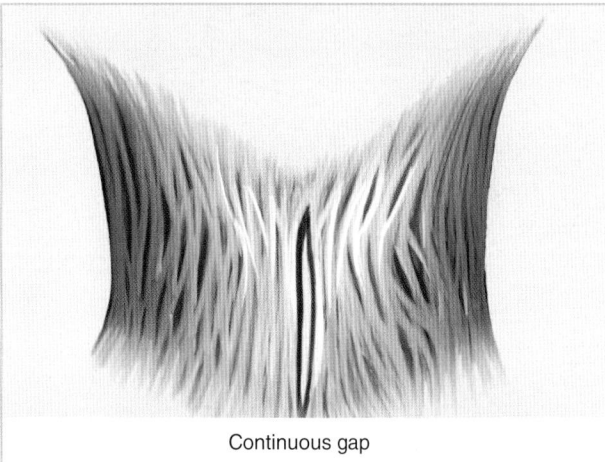

Continuous gap

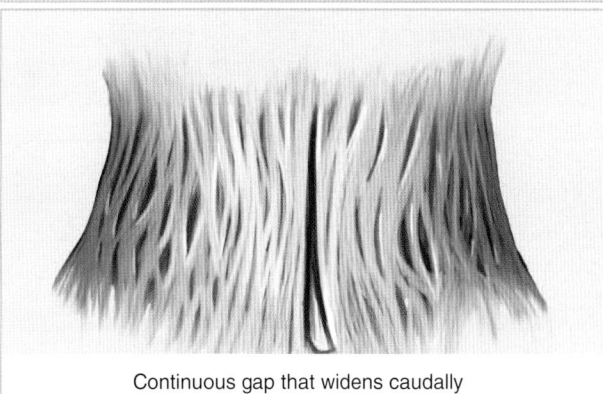

Continuous gap that widens caudally

FIGURE 24–7. Ligamentum flavum with different types of midline gaps.

The Spinal Canal
General

The vertebrae serve primarily to support the weight of the head, neck, and trunk; transfer that weight to the lower limbs; and protect the contents of the spinal canal, including the spinal cord. An extension of the medulla oblongata, the spinal cord serves as the conduit between the CNS and the peripheral nerves via 31 pairs of spinal nerves (8 cervical, 12 thoracic, 5 lumbar, 5 sacral, and 1 coccygeal) (Figure 24–8). The adult cord measures approximately 45 cm or 18 inches and has two regions of enlarged diameter at C2–T2 and at T9–L2, areas that correspond with the origin of the nerve supplies to the upper and lower extremities. However, its level of termination varies with age, as well as among individuals of similar age

groups. As a result of a discrepancy in the pace of growth of the spinal cord and vertebral column during development, the spinal cord at birth ends at approximately L3. By 6–12 months of age, the level of termination parallels that of adults, most commonly at L1. Below the conus medullaris, the long dorsal and ventral roots of all the spinal nerves below L1 form a bundle known as the cauda equina, or horse's tail. A collection of strands of neuron-free fibrous tissue enveloped in pia mater comprises the filum terminale and extends from the inferior tip of the conus medullaris to the second or third sacral vertebra.

Spinal Nerves

Spinal nerves are classified as mixed nerves because they contain both a sensory and a motor component and, in many cases, autonomic fibers. Each nerve forms from the fusion of dorsal (sensory) and ventral (somatic and visceral motor) nerve roots as they exit the vertebral canal distal to the dorsal root ganglia, which contain the cell bodies of sensory neurons on either side of the spinal cord and lie between the pedicles of adjacent vertebrae. In general, dorsal roots are larger and more easily blocked than ventral roots, a phenomenon that may be explained in part by the larger surface area for exposure to LAs provided by the bundled dorsal roots.

At the cervical level, the first pair of spinal nerves exits between the skull and C1. Subsequent cervical nerves continue to exit above the corresponding vertebra, assuming the name of the vertebra immediately following them. However, a transition occurs between the seventh cervical and first thoracic vertebrae, where an eighth pair of cervical nerves exits; thereafter, the spinal nerves exit below the corresponding vertebra and take the name of the vertebra immediately above. The spinal nerves divide into the anterior and posterior primary rami soon after they exit the intervertebral foramina. The anterior (ventral) rami supply the ventrolateral side of the trunk, structures of the body wall, and the limbs. The posterior (dorsal) primary rami innervate specific regions of the skin that resemble horizontal bands extending from the origin of each pair of spinal nerves, called dermatomes, and the muscles of the back. Clinically, knowledge of dermatomes is essential when planning anesthetics to specific cutaneous regions (Figure 24–9), although anesthesia may not be conferred reliably to the underlying viscera due to a separate innervation, and there is significant overlap in spinal nerve innervation of adjacent dermatomes (Table 24–18).

An intricate relationship exists between the spinal nerves and the autonomic nervous system (Figure 24–10). Preganglionic sympathetic nerve fibers originate in the spinal cord from T1 to L2 and are blocked to varying degrees during epidural anesthesia. They exit the spinal cord with spinal nerves and form the sympathetic chain, which extends the entire length of the spinal column on the anterolateral aspects of the vertebral bodies. The chain gives rise to the stellate ganglion, splanchnic nerves, and the celiac plexus, among other things. There are potential benefits and marked drawbacks to epidural blockade of the sympathetic nervous system. TEA appears to increase GI mobility by blocking the sympathetic supply to the inferior mesenteric ganglia, thereby reducing the incidence of postoperative ileus. Epidural anesthesia may also block the systemic stress response

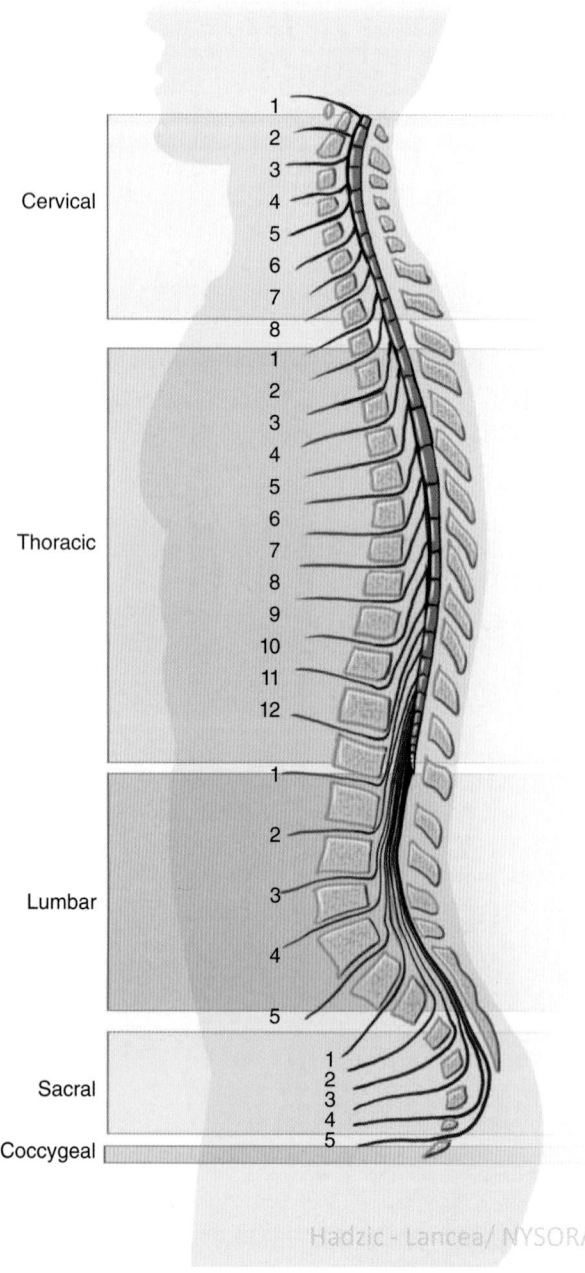

FIGURE 24–8. Vertebral column with spinal nerves.

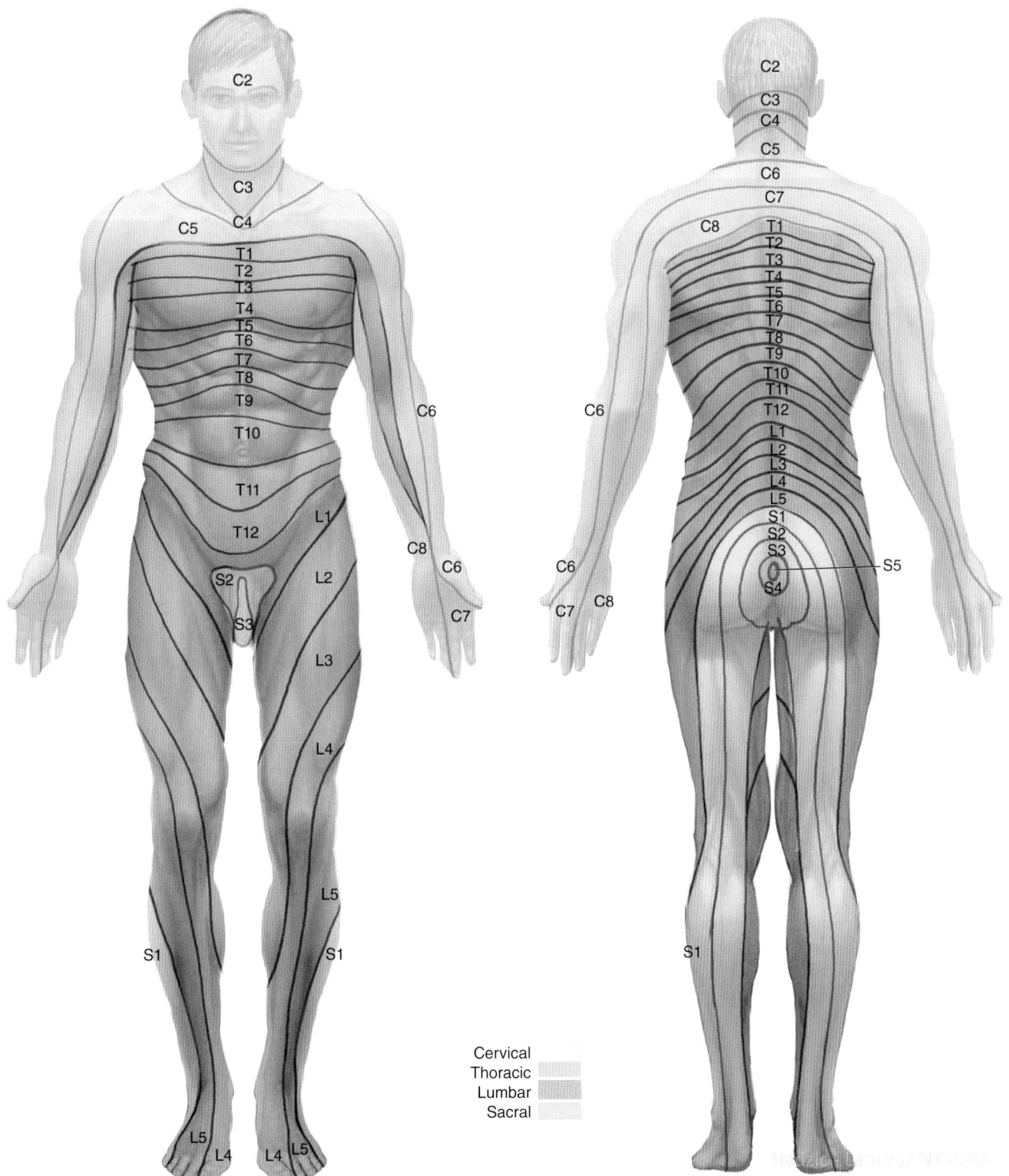

FIGURE 24–9. Distribution of dermatomes.

to surgery, in part by blockade of the sympathetic nervous system. However, mid- to low-thoracic sympathetic blockade may be associated with dilation of the splanchnic vascular beds, a marked increase in venous capacitance, a decrease in preload to the right heart, and many of the other undesirable effects (see Physiologic Effects of Epidural Blockade).

Cranial and sacral components comprise the parasympathetic nervous system. The vagus nerve, in particular, provides parasympathetic innervation to a broad area, including the head, neck, the thoracic organs and parts of the digestive tract. Parasympathetic innervation of the bladder, the descending large intestine, and the rectum originate at spinal cord levels S2 to S4.

TABLE 24–18. Surface landmark correlation to dermatomal level.

Level of Blockade	Anatomic Landmark
C6	Thumb
C8	Fifth finger
T1	Inner aspect of arm
T4	Nipple
T6	Xiphoid process
T10	Umbilicus
T12	Inguinal ligament
S1	Lateral aspect of foot
S2–S4	Perineum

Spinal Meninges

Spinal meninges cover the cord and nerve roots and are continuous with the cranial meninges that surround and protect the brain (Figure 24–11). The tough, predominantly collagenous outermost layer, the dura mater, encloses the CNS and provides localized points of attachment to the skull, sacrum, and vertebrae to anchor the spinal cord within the vertebral canal. Cranially, the spinal dura mater fuses with periosteum at the level of the foramen magnum; caudally, it fuses with elements of the filum terminale and contributes to formation of the coccygeal ligament; laterally, the dura mater surrounds nerve roots as they exit the intervertebral foramina. The dura mater touches the spinal canal in areas, but does not adhere to it except in pathologic conditions. It also confers both permeability and mechanical resistance to the dural sac, which terminates at S1 to S2 in adults and S3 to S4 in babies. The spinal nerve root cuffs, which have been postulated to play a role in the uptake of epidurally administered LAs, are lateral projections of both the dura mater and the underlying arachnoid lamina.[100]

The flexible arachnoid mater, the middle meningeal layer, is loosely attached to the inner aspect of the dura and encloses the spinal cord and surrounding CSF within the subarachnoid space. It is composed of layers of epithelial-like cells connected by tight and occluding junctions, which impart its low permeability. The cell layers of the arachnoid mater are oriented parallel to the long axis of the spinal cord (cephalocaudad), a finding that has led some investigators to claim that the architecture of the arachnoid mater, rather than the dura mater, accounts for the difference in headache rates between perpendicular and parallel insertions of beveled spinal needles.[101] By virtue of its flexibility, the arachnoid mater may "tent" and resist puncture by an advancing needle during initiation of spinal or CSE anesthesia. A discontinuous subarachnoid septum (septum posticum) that stretches from the posterior spinal cord to the arachnoid may contribute to irregular spread of LAs in the subarachnoid space.

The innermost meningeal layer, the pia mater, closely invests the underlying spinal cord and its blood vessels, as well as nerve roots and blood vessels in the subarachnoid space, and appears to have fenestrated areas that may influence the transfer of LAs during subarachnoid blocks.[102] Caudally, the pia mater continues from the inferior tip of the conus medullaris as the filum terminale and fuses into the sacrococcygeal ligament.

It is possible that a cavity can be created at the arachnoid-dura interface that may explain patchy or failed epidural blocks with higher-than-expected cephalad spread (so-called subdural blocks). Early research suggested that the subdural extra-arachnoid space comprised a true potential space, with serous fluid that permitted movement of the dura and arachnoid layers alongside each other. Blomberg used spinaloscopy in cadaver studies to demonstrate its existence in up to 66% of humans.[103] However, recent evidence suggests that, unlike a potential space, this arachnoid-dura interface is an area prone to mechanical stress that shears open only after direct trauma, such as air or fluid injection.[104] It is also possible that these clefts may actually occur between layers of arachnoid instead of between dural border cells at the arachnoid-dura interface. More information on spinal meninges and related structures are detailed in Chapter 6.

Clinical Pearl

- Clefts may form at the arachnoid-dura interface as a result of mechanical stress and direct trauma. Injection of a large volume of LA intended for the epidural space in this area may result in a subdural block.

Blood Supply

Vertebral and segmental arteries supply the spinal cord. A single anterior spinal artery and two posterior spinal arteries, and their offshoots, arise from the vertebral arteries and supply the anterior two-thirds of the spinal cord and the remainder of the cord, respectively (Figure 24–12). The anterior artery is thin at the midthoracic level of the spinal cord, an area that also has limited collateral blood supply. Segmental arteries, which emerge from branches of the cervical and iliac arteries, among others, spread along the entire length of the spinal cord and anastomose with the anterior and posterior arteries. The artery of Adamkiewicz is among the largest segmental arteries and is most commonly unilateral, arising from the left side of the aorta between T8 and L1. With regard to the venous system, anterior and posterior spinal veins, which anastomose with the internal vertebral plexus in the epidural space, drain into the azygos, the hemiazygos, and internal iliac veins, among other segmental veins, via intervertebral veins. The internal vertebral venous plexus consists of two anterior and two posterior longitudinal vessels with a variable distribution and is postulated to be involved in bloody or traumatic epidural needle and catheter placements.[105]

Epidural Space

The epidural space surrounds the dura mater circumferentially and extends from the foramen magnum to the sacrococcygeal ligament. The space is bound posteriorly by the ligamentum flavum, laterally by the pedicles and the intervertebral foramina, and anteriorly by the posterior longitudinal ligament. Of the

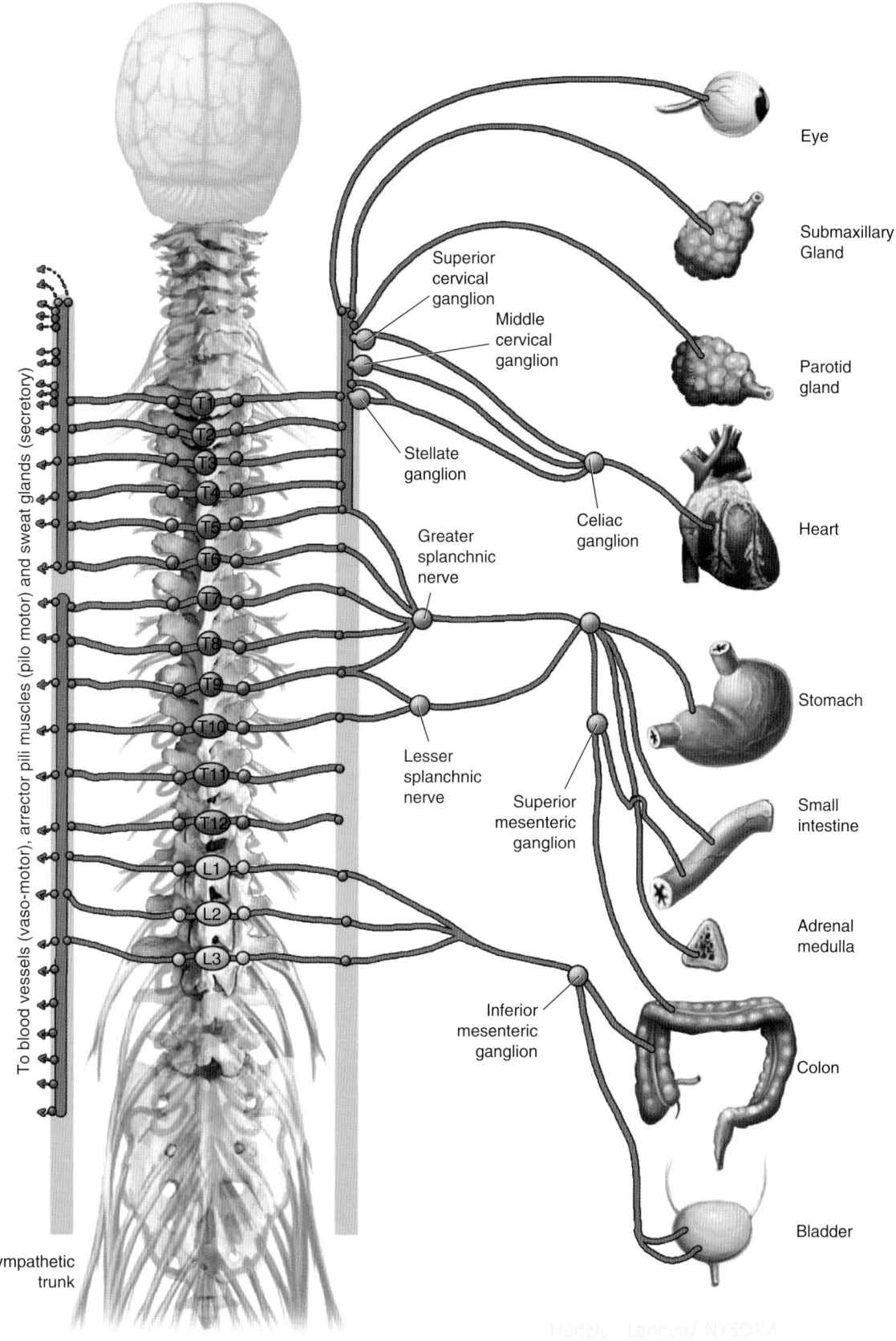

FIGURE 24-10. Sympathetic nervous system.

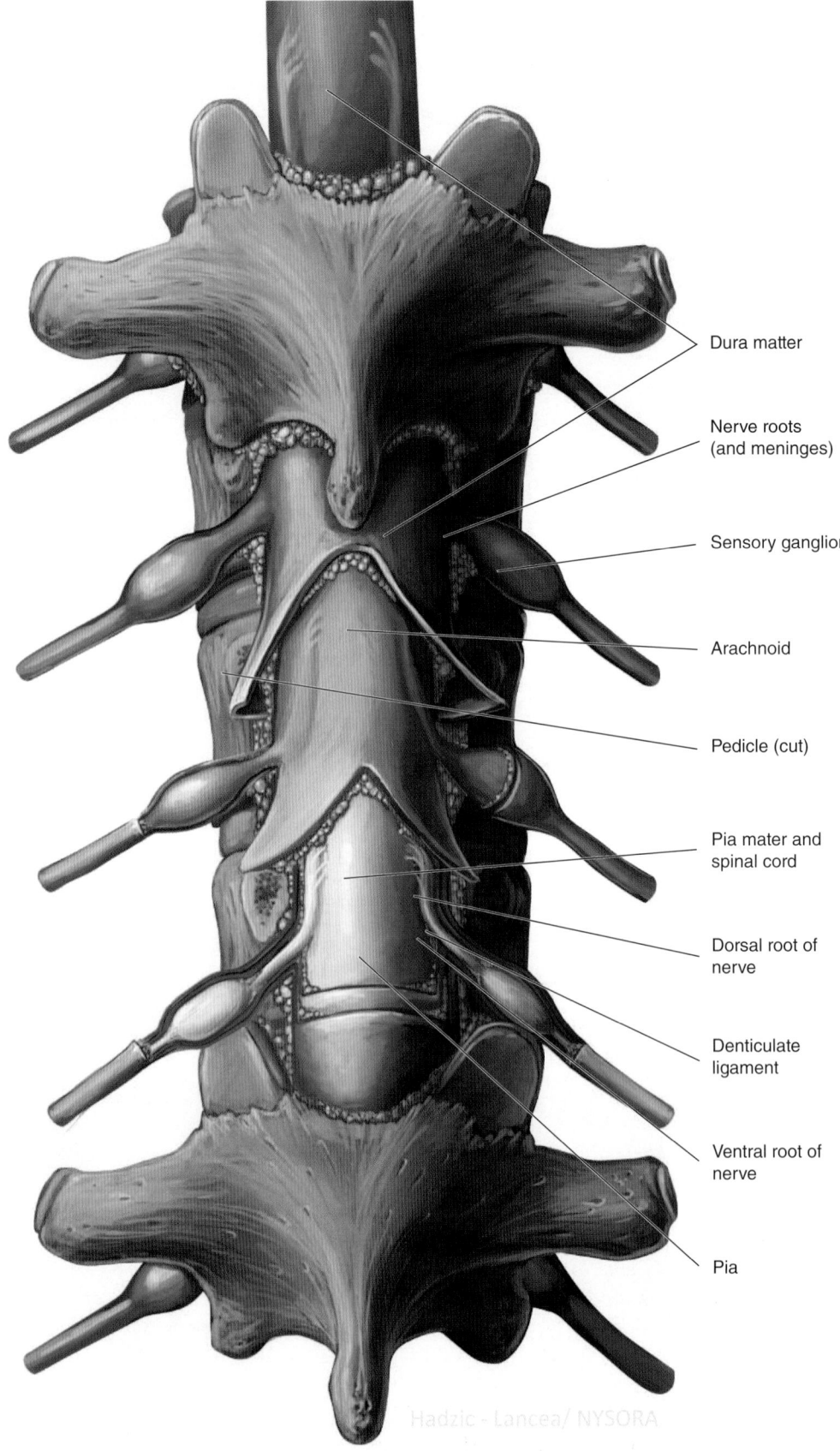

Dura matter

Nerve roots
(and meninges)

Sensory ganglion

Arachnoid

Pedicle (cut)

Pia mater and
spinal cord

Dorsal root of
nerve

Denticulate
ligament

Ventral root of
nerve

Pia

FIGURE 24–11. Spinal meninges.

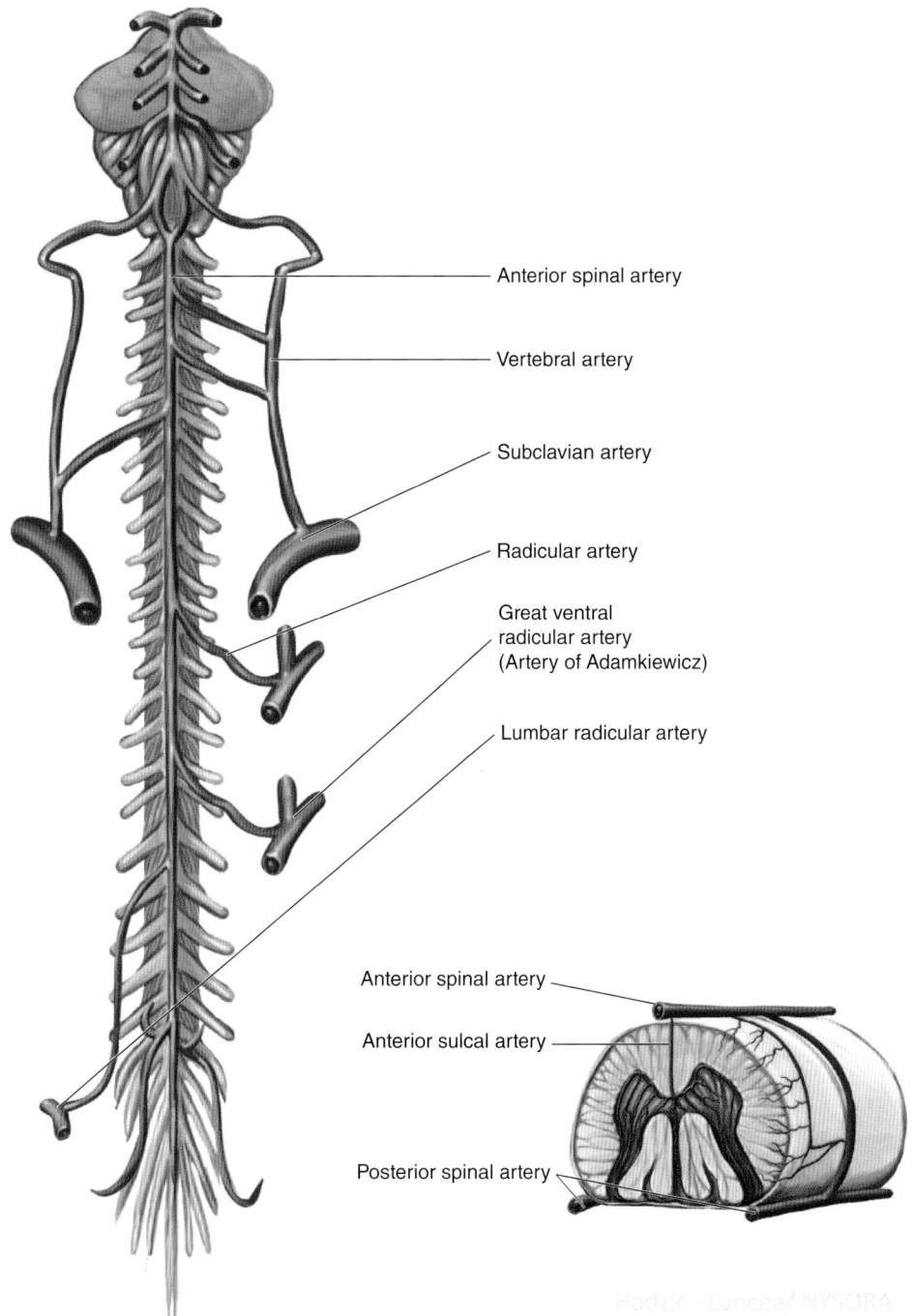

Anterior spinal artery

Vertebral artery

Subclavian artery

Radicular artery

Great ventral
radicular artery
(Artery of Adamkiewicz)

Lumbar radicular artery

Anterior spinal artery

Anterior sulcal artery

Posterior spinal artery

FIGURE 24–12. Blood supply of the spinal cord.

three epidural space compartments (posterior, lateral, and ante-rior), the posterior epidural space is most relevant clinically. The epidural space in general contains adipose tissue, blood vessels, nerve roots, and loose connective tissue in a nonuniform distri-bution. The veins in the space are continuous with the iliac vessels in the pelvis and the azygos system in the abdominal and thoracic body walls. Because the plexus is valveless, blood from any of the connected systems can flow into the epidural vessels. In contrast to traditional dogma, these vessels are located pri-marily in the anterior epidural space, where they are largely confined by the membranous extension of the posterior longi-tudinal ligament[106] (Figure 24–13). This area is probably a

common site of epidural catheter blood vessel puncture. Also of clinical significance, the subatmospheric pressure of the epidural space diminishes significantly in the lumbar region, potentially affecting both the hanging-drop and the epidural pressure wave-form techniques of identification of the epidural space.

The contents of the epidural space and their clinical impli-cations have been debated extensively in the literature. The amount of adipose tissue in the epidural space appears to affect the spread of LA, but it remains unclear whether epidural fat prolongs block duration by serving as a reservoir or decreases the amount of available drug, thereby slowing onset, or both.[107] The reduction of adipose tissue with age is speculated to

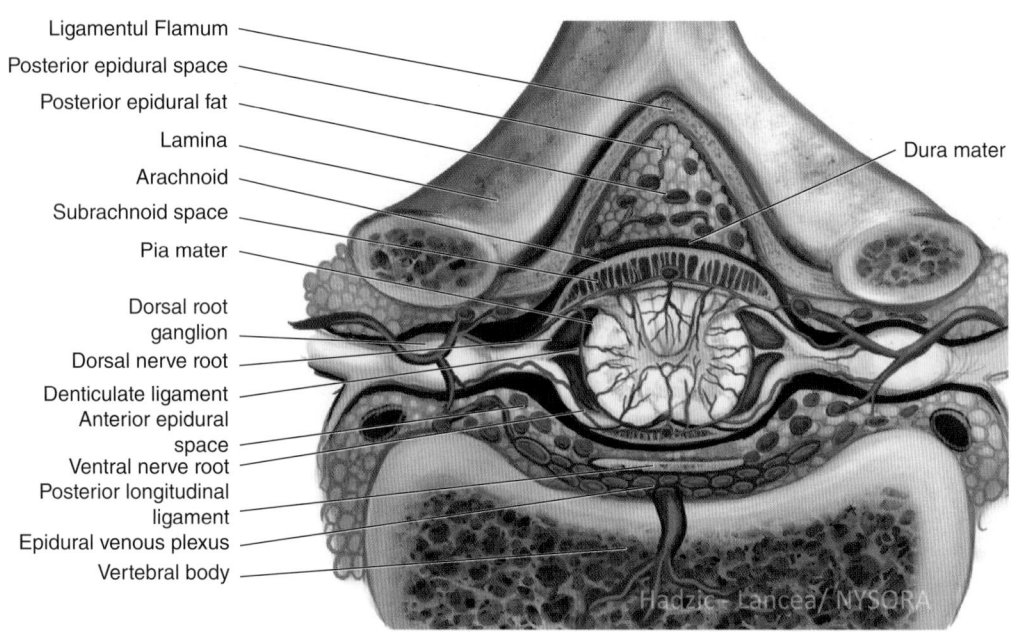

Ligamentul Flamum
Posterior epidural space
Posterior epidural fat
Lamina
Arachnoid
Subrachnoid space
Pia mater
Dorsal root ganglion
Dorsal nerve root
Denticulate ligament
Anterior epidural space
Ventral nerve root
Posterior longitudinal ligament
Epidural venous plexus
Vertebral body
Dura mater

FIGURE 24–13. Epidural vein distribution in the lumbar region.

account in part for the higher levels and faster onset of epidural anesthesia in the elderly.[108] Similarly, the increase in adipose tissue in the lower lumbar area where the dural sac tapers may contribute to the variable effects of LA injections below L4–L5. Finally, adipose tissue in the midline gap, where the ligamentum flava fuse, may alter the tactile sensation that is normally appreciated during the LOR technique.

Another anatomic controversy of the epidural space concerns whether septae, alternately described as sparse strands and as a continuous membrane that attaches the dura to the ligamentum flavum,[109] obstruct catheter advancement, affect the spread and onset of LAs, and contribute to unilateral blocks and unintentional dural punctures. However, these septae have more recently been identified as an artifact of the midline posterior epidural fat pad.[110] These fatty midline attachments do not appear to have a clinically significant effect on the spread of LAs.[106] Rather, Hogan has postulated that the distribution of solution is non-uniform and directed among paths between structures in the epidural space according to differential pressures.[111]

Distance From Skin to Epidural Space

The distance from the skin to the epidural space varies at different levels of the vertebral column. In the cervical region, Han and colleagues found that the average skin-to-epidural space depth (via the midline approach) was shallowest at C5 and C6 and increased in the caudal direction.[92] Fujinaka et al noted that it is difficult to predict the actual depth of the cervical epidural space based on clinical characteristics.[112] In contrast, Aldrete and coworkers, using magnetic resonance imaging (MRI) to measure the depth from the skin to the inner ligamentum flavum, noted the greatest depth at the C6-to-T1 levels, with a mean of 5.7 cm, possibly due to the presence of fatty tissue (the so-called hump pad) in the area.[113] The depth to space in the midthoracic region from midline is influenced primarily by the sharp caudal angle of the spinous processes. As a result of the steep angle and bony

impediments in this region, the paramedian approach is often preferred for midthoracic epidural placement.

Several studies have sought to measure the depth to the epidural space at the lumbar level. Studies of parturients show a range of depth from skin to space of 2 to 9 cm, with 89% in the range of 3.5–7.5 cm.[114] In their search for a multivariate model to predict the distance in an obstetric population, Segal and colleagues confirmed previously reported associations between increased weight and increased depth, as well as between oriental race and shallower spaces, with no independent association between race and depth after controlling for weight.[114] In an earlier study, Sutton and Linter recorded that the skin to extradural space in 3011 parturients was 4 to 6 cm in 76% of the study participants.[115] Patients with a shallow depth of 2 to 4 cm, comprising 16% of the study population, were found to be at a threefold higher risk of unintentional dural puncture. Of note, the shallow depth falls within the range of length of the LA infiltration needle. Overall, estimates of the depth to epidural space cannot be applied to the population at large, as independent variables, such as degree of flexion, patient positioning, dimpling and edema at the skin and subcutaneous tissue, and the angle of needle insertion, among other things, are difficult to quantitate and control. In the near future, routine ultrasound determination of depth to space on an individual basis prior to or during epidural needle placement might provide the most reliable means of diminishing the risk of inadvertent dural puncture and other complications of epidural anesthesia. Fluoroscopy is most appropriate in the cervical region, where spinal cord injury, total spinal anesthesia, and intra-arterial injection are among the possible complications.

The variable depth of the posterior epidural space is another clinically relevant measure that may influence the incidence of inadvertent dural puncture. The posterior epidural space viewed in the midline sagittal plane has been described as sawtoothed, characterizing its segmented shape.[116] While studies are conflicting, at each segmental level, the depth of the posterior epidural space appears shallower at the caudal end. These variations notwithstanding, the distance between the ligamentum flavum and the dura is typically estimated as 7 mm, with a broad range from 2 mm to 2.5 cm.[106] This anterior-posterior distance is largest in the lumbar region, at L3–L4, decreases in the thoracic region, and is absent in the cervical region.[117]

PHYSIOLOGIC EFFECTS OF EPIDURAL BLOCKADE

Epidural blockade provides surgical anesthesia, intraoperative muscle relaxation, and intrapartum and postoperative pain relief with widespread direct and indirect effects on several physiologic systems. The extent of these physiologic effects depends on the level of placement and the number of spinal segments blocked. In general, high thoracic epidural blocks (ie, above T5) and extensive epidural blocks are associated with more profound physiologic changes than blocks with low sensory levels (ie, below T10). This section reviews the physiologic alterations related to epidural anesthesia and analgesia.

Differential Blockade

Differential blockade occurs when sensory, motor, and sympathetic nerve functions are obtunded at different rates and to different degrees. It may be observed at both onset and regression of the block. In general, sympathetic blockade, which is not uncommonly incomplete, extends two to six dermatomes higher than sensory blockade, which in turn is higher than the motor blockade. Sensory blockade also occurs with a lower concentration or total dose of LA and develops faster than motor blockade. Among sensory functions, temperature is blocked first, followed by pinprick and, finally, touch.

Although the mechanism of differential blockade has not been fully elucidated, it may be attributed to anatomic features of blocked nerves (eg, diameter and presence or absence of myelin), the length of blocked nervous tissue (a minimal length of blocked nerve is required for effective neuronal blockade), differences in nerve lipid membrane and ion channel composition, concurrent axonal activity during block onset, and LA type and concentration. These and several other mechanisms may collectively contribute to differential blockade.

Central Nervous System Effects

Cerebral blood flow (CBF) is autoregulated and is not affected by epidural blockade unless the patient experiences pronounced hypotension. However, neuraxial anesthesia does appear to have a sedative effect and to reduce anesthetic requirements for several agents, including midazolam, propofol, thiopental, fentanyl, and volatile agents. The degree of sedation and minimum alveolar concentration (MAC) sparing effect appear to correlate with the height and level of the sensory block; blockade of the middle thoracic dermatomes is associated with greater sedative effects than blockade of the lower lumbar segments.[118] Although data are conflicting, higher-concentration LAs may contribute to a greater MAC-sparing effect.[119] The addition of opioid adjuvants, such as morphine, to the epidural LA solution does not

appear to reduce volatile agent requirements any further, although it does contribute to better postoperative pain scores.[120] Overall, decreased anesthetic requirements have most commonly been attributed to decreased afferent input induced by the neuraxial block rather than to systemic effects of LAs, altered pharmacokinetics, or direct action of LAs on the brain.[121]

Several studies have demonstrated reduced hypnotic and anesthetic requirements after central neuraxial blockade. In an early study of 53 American Society of Anesthesiologists (ASA) physical status I and II adult males, Tverskoy and colleagues determined that subarachnoid bupivacaine blockade decreased hypnotic requirements for both midazolam and thiopental.[122] A study that followed, also in ASA physical status I and II patients, determined that epidural bupivacaine profoundly decreased midazolam hypnotic requirements.[123] Similarly, in a small prospective, randomized, double-blind, placebo-controlled trial, Hodgson and colleagues found that lidocaine epidural anesthesia reduced the MAC of sevoflurane by up to 50%.[124] More recently, epidural bupivacaine administered via the caudal route has been shown to have a sparing effect on both intravenous fentanyl and sevoflurane requirements during orthopedic surgery in children.[125]

Cardiovascular and Hemodynamic Effects

Cardiovascular changes associated with epidural anesthesia and analgesia result primarily from blockade of sympathetic nerve fiber conduction. These changes include venous and arterial vasodilation, reduced SVR, changes in chronotropy and inotropy, and associated alterations in blood pressure and CO. The type and intensity of these changes are related to the level of block, the total number of dermatomes blocked, and, relatedly, the type and dose of LA administered. In general, lumbar epidural or low thoracic blocks are not associated with significant hemodynamic changes, while higher thoracic blocks (particularly those involving the T1–T4 sympathetic fibers) can cause more marked changes, not all of which are detrimental. However, factors such as pregnancy, age, comorbidities, patient positioning, and hypovolemia can complicate the clinical scenario and the anticipated cardiovascular effects.

Hypotension

Hypotension associated with neuraxial blockade results primarily from vasodilation and increased vascular bed capacitance.[126] Both direct inhibition of the sympathetic outflow to the nerves innervating the blood vessels and a decrease in endogenous catecholamine release from the adrenal glands contribute to arterial and venous vasodilation. In general, arteriolar smooth muscle maintains autonomous tone, even in the setting of complete sympathectomy, while veins and venules dilate maximally. However, a degree of arteriolar vasodilation does occur. The venodilatory effect also predominates because of the large amount of blood in the venous system compared to the arterial system.

The degree of hypotension associated with epidural blockade correlates with the sensory level. For example, a more marked increase in venous capacitance occurs with blockade of the sympathetic outflow to the splanchnic veins (T6 to L1) due to dilation of the extensive splanchnic bed. With low epidural blocks, vasoconstriction of unblocked areas and release of catecholamines from the adrenal medullary system partially compensate for venous and arteriolar pooling and reductions in mean arterial pressure.[127] Overall, healthy, normovolemic patients experience a nominal decrease in peripheral resistance and blood pressure during initiation and maintenance of epidural blockade.

Risk factors for appreciable hypotension during neuraxial anesthesia include sensory level above T5, low baseline pressure, increasing age, and combined general-neuraxial anesthesia. Severely hypovolemic patients and cardiac-compromised patients are also more likely to experience significant hypotension requiring vasopressor and inotropic support. Hypotension occurs more commonly with spinals than with epidurals, despite equivalent degrees of sympathetic blockade.

Heart Rate and Cardiac Function

In general, changes in heart rate and ventricular function vary with level of blockade, with more pronounced changes as the level increases. When the cardiac sympathetic fibers from T1 to T4 are blocked, decreased cardiac contractility and bradycardia ensue, resulting in decreased CO. Bradycardia also results from the decreased atrial stretch receptor activity attributed to decreased right atrial pressure. Venous pooling also contributes to the reduction in CO, particularly with higher blocks. Missant et al studied the effects of epidural anesthesia on left and right ventricular function in a pig model and found that lumbar epidural anesthesia reduced SVR without affecting left or right ventricular function.[128] However, TEA reduced left ventricular contractility and minimally reduced SVR, while preserving right ventricular function.

Neuraxial blockade appears to have certain beneficial effects on the cardiovascular system, such as improved myocardial blood flow and myocardial oxygen balance. Tissue oxygenation has been observed to improve with high TEA under certain circumstances, particularly with intravenous fluid administration.[129,130] TEA also appears to have antianginal effects,[131,132] improve coronary perfusion,[20] and improve recovery from reversible myocardial ischemia.[133,134] Whether this results in improved perioperative cardiac outcome following major cardiac or thoracic surgery, however, is the subject of ongoing debate.[135] Several authors have hypothesized that TEA may also protect against postoperative arrhythmias and atrial fibrillation after major cardiac and thoracic surgeries. However, data are conflicting. Svircevic et al performed a meta-analysis comparing GA and TEA for cardiac surgery and noted fewer postoperative supraventricular arrhythmias.[136] However, Gu et al, in another recent meta-analysis, could not support such an effect.[137]

Pulmonary Effects

The motor and sympathetic changes associated with epidural anesthesia may affect lung function, depending on the level of blockade. In general, tidal volume remains unchanged even during high neuraxial blocks, while vital capacity may be reduced due to the decrease in expiratory reserve volume that occurs as accessory muscles involved in expiration are blocked. The ability to cough and clear respiratory secretions may also be impaired, particularly in patients with severely compromised respiratory function at baseline. However, inspiratory muscle function is unaffected and should remain sufficient to provide adequate ventilatory function.

Higher sensory levels may result in more marked changes in lung function. In a sentinel study, Freund et al inserted a lumbar epidural catheter and administered a mean volume of 20 mL of 2% lidocaine.[138] An extensive block to T4 was achieved, but the decrease in vital capacity was minimal. However, catheter insertion at higher levels, with concomitant higher spread of LA, results in more pronounced pulmonary derangement.[139] In contrast, when TEA is used postoperatively, a net positive effect on lung function can be observed, most likely because the enhanced pain relief prevents splinting. In a recent review article, Lirk and Hollmann determined the role of TEA and confirmed the benefits in major abdominal and thoracic surgery.[140]

The rare occurrence of respiratory arrest after high epidural or spinal blockade can be attributed to hypoperfusion of the respiratory center in the brainstem rather than to direct LA effects on either the phrenic nerve or the CNS.

Gastrointestinal Effects

The sympathetic outflow to the GI tract arises from T5 to T12, while parasympathetic innervation is supplied by the vagus nerve. Sympathectomy associated with epidural blockade in the mid- to low-thoracic levels results in unopposed vagal tone, which manifests clinically with increased peristalsis, relaxed sphincters, an increase in GI secretions, and, likely, more rapid restoration of GI motility in the postoperative phase. Nausea and vomiting commonly accompany hyperperistalsis and can be treated effectively with intravenous atropine. Theoretically, increased intestinal motility could contribute to breakdown of surgical anastomoses, but this has not been demonstrated in the literature. Rather, TEA may decrease the risk of anastomotic leakage and improve perioperative intestinal perfusion, although the data are somewhat conflicting. Numerous experimental and clinical studies have demonstrated that TEA protects against splanchnic hypoperfusion and reduces postoperative ileus.[141] However, similar benefits are not seen with lumbar epidural anesthesia.[141]

Renal/Genitourinary Effects

Because renal blood flow (RBF) is maintained through autoregulation, epidural anesthesia has little effect on renal function in healthy individuals. Compensatory and feedback mechanisms (afferent arteriolar dilation and efferent arteriolar vasoconstriction) ensure constant RBF over a broad range of pressures (50–150 mm Hg). During transient periods of hypotension below 50 mm Hg, oxygen delivery to the kidneys is adequately maintained.

Neuraxial blockade at the lumbar level has been postulated to impair control of bladder function secondary to blockade of the S2–S4 nerve roots, which carry the sympathetic and parasympathetic nerves that innervate the bladder. Urinary retention may occur until the block wears off. The clinician should avoid administering an excessive volume of intravenous fluids if a urinary catheter is not in place.

Neuroendocrine Effects

Surgical stress produces a variety of changes in the host's humoral and immune response. Increased protein catabolism and oxygen consumption are common. Increased plasma concentrations of catecholamines, vasopressin, growth hormone, renin, angiotensin, cortisol, glucose, antidiuretic hormone, and thyroid-stimulating hormone have been documented after sympathetic stimulation associated with both minimally invasive and major open surgery. Perioperative manifestations of the surgical stress response may include HTN, tachycardia, hyperglycemia, suppressed immune function, and altered renal function. Increased catecholamine levels can also cause increased left ventricular afterload and, in combination with other pathologic responses to stress (eg, proinflammatory responses that may lead to plaque instability via activation of matrix metalloproteinase; raised corticotropin-releasing hormone levels that reduce cardiac nitric oxide release, increase endothelin production, and aggravate coronary endothelial dysfunction), trigger acute coronary syndromes and myocardial infarctions in patients with coexisting cardiac disease. Afferent sensory information from the surgical site is thought to play a pivotal role in this response.

The surgical stress response can be influenced by sympathetic blockade during epidural anesthesia and analgesia. The mechanisms involved are unresolved but most likely include both direct blockade of afferent and efferent signals during surgical stress and direct effects of LA agents. Brodner et al demonstrated that TEA combined with GA resulted in a reduced surgical stress response when compared to GA alone.[142]

The most critical effect of neuroendocrine activation in the perioperative period is the increase in plasma norepinephrine, which peaks roughly 18 hours after the surgical stimulus is initiated. The increase in plasma norepinephrine is associated with activation of nitric oxide in the endothelium of patients with atherosclerotic disease, producing paradoxical vasospasm. Thus, in patients with significant atherosclerotic disease, the combination of vasospasm and a hypercoagulable state may be the factors modulated by the cardioprotective effects of TEA. Indeed, studies indicated that coronary artery blood flow is improved with TEA.[20]

Thermoregulation

Hypothermia has significant side effects, such as increased cardiac morbidity, impaired coagulation, increased blood loss, and increased risk for infection. The rate and severity of hypothermia associated with epidural anesthesia is similar to that observed during cases under GA.[143] Hypothermia associated with neuraxial anesthesia is primarily due to peripheral vasodilation resulting in heat redistribution from the core to the periphery.[144] In addition, reduced heat production (due to reduced metabolic activity) results in a negative heat balance due to unchanged heat loss. Finally, thermoregulatory control is impaired. Of note, rewarming with forced air warming devices occurs more rapidly with neuraxial anesthesia as compared to GA due to peripheral vasodilation.[145]

Coagulation System

The postoperative period is a marked hypercoagulable state. Neuraxial blockade is associated with a decreased risk of DVT and pulmonary embolism, as well as a decreased risk of arterial and venous thrombosis.

PHARMACOLOGY OF EPIDURAL BLOCKADE

An understanding of the physiology of nerve conduction and the pharmacology of LAs is essential for successful epidural blockade. Potency and duration of LAs, preferential blockade of sensory and motor fibers, and the anticipated duration of surgery or need for postoperative analgesia are factors that should be considered before initiating epidural blockade. This section covers several practical aspects of attaining effective epidural anesthesia and analgesia.

Epidural solutions may contain an LA with or without an adjuvant drug. Dose, volume, and concentration, as well as site of injection, of the LA solution vary, resulting in different pharmacodynamic effects. A, B, and C nerve fibers vary in size and in the presence of a myelin sheath. A-delta and C fibers are responsible for temperature and pain transmission. B fibers are autonomic fibers. The larger A fibers (especially A-alpha fibers) are motor fibers. C fibers are unmyelinated and smallest in size. Because they lack a protective myelin sheath and diffusion barrier, they are blocked rapidly. A and B fibers are myelinated and larger in size than C fibers. B fibers are responsible for autonomic nervous system transmission. They are smaller in size than A-delta fibers, but larger than C fibers. It is widely accepted that autonomic fibers are more susceptible to LA block than sensory fibers. Epidurally administered LA preferentially blocks sympathetic neural function; this explains the more extensive sympathetic dermatomal blockade when compared with sensory and motor blocks.[146–149] However, Ginosar et al recently suggested that sensory function was more susceptible to blockade than sympathetic function.[150] Several other studies concurred.[151,152] The dose and concentration of LA used may account for the different findings in these studies. Because of their thick myelin sheath, motor fibers require much more LA and much more time before an adequate block is achieved.

Local anesthetics produce reversible nerve blockade by blocking sodium passage through the nerve membrane. When LA is injected into the epidural space, several things occur. Most of the injected LA is absorbed into the venous blood, and a large part is retained in epidural fatty tissue. The primary sites of action of an epidurally administered LA are the ventral and dorsal nerve roots that pass through the epidural space. However, based on studies using labeled LAs, LAs can cross the dura and penetrate the spinal cord, but to a lesser extent than their penetration into the spinal nerve roots.[153] The segmental nerve roots are mixed sensory, motor, and sympathetic nerve fibers. Hence, all three types of fibers will be affected (to varying degrees).

Choice of Local Anesthetics

Drugs used for epidural blockade can be categorized into short-, intermediate-, and long-acting LAs. Onset of epidural blockade in the dermatomes immediately surrounding the site of injection can usually be detected within 5 or 10 minutes, if not sooner. The time to peak effect varies with the type of LA and the dose/volume administered (Table 24–19).

TABLE 24–19. Commonly used local anesthetics for epidural anesthesia and analgesia.

Drug	Concentration (%)	Onset Time (min)	Duration (min)
2-Chloroprocaine	3	5–15	30–90
Lidocaine	2	10–20	60–120
Bupivacaine	0.0625–0.5	15–20	160–220
Ropivacaine	0.1–0.75	15–20	140–220
Levobupivacaine	0.0625–0.5	15–20	150–225

Duration of blockade can be prolonged by addition of epinephrine, typically 1:200:000 to 1:400:000.

The shortest-acting LA for neuraxial blockade is chloroprocaine, an ester. In the past, chloroprocaine was associated with adhesive arachnoiditis when large volumes were accidentally administered into the subarachnoid space.[154] In addition, severe back pain was not uncommonly reported when large volumes were administered in the epidural space, most likely due to the ethylenediaminetetraacetic acid (EDTA) and bisulfite preservatives in the solution. Since 1996, preservative-free chloroprocaine has been available and has not been associated with either neurotoxic effects or back pain. In ambulatory settings and for emergency cesarean deliveries with in situ epidurals, chloroprocaine can provide excellent surgical anesthesia quickly, without delaying recovery room discharge.

Delivered via the epidural route, 2% lidocaine is an intermediate-acting LA commonly used for surgical anesthesia. When epinephrine is added to the solution (1:200,000), it prolongs the duration of action by up to 60%.

Long-acting LAs used for epidural blockade are bupivacaine, levobupivacaine (no longer available in the United States), and ropivacaine. Dilute concentrations (eg, 0.1% to 0.25%) can be used for analgesia, while higher concentrations (eg, 0.5%) may be more appropriate for surgical anesthesia. The addition of epinephrine to these solutions can prolong the duration of action, although this effect is less reliable with long- versus intermediate-acting agents. Severe cardiotoxic reactions (hypotension, atrioventricular block, ventricular fibrillation, and torsades de pointes) refractory to usual resuscitation methods can result from accidental intravascular injection of bupivacaine. The rationale for the resistance to resuscitative measures lies in its high degree of protein binding and more pronounced effect on cardiac sodium channel blockade.[155,156] Levobupivacaine, the S-enantiomer of bupivacaine, has a similar profile to bupivacaine but with less-pronounced cardiotoxic effects. Ropivacaine, a mepivacaine analogue, has a similar profile of action to bupivacaine. In most studies, ropivacaine has demonstrated a slightly shorter duration of action than bupivacaine, potentially with a less-dense motor block at equipotent doses. A deterrent to the broader use of ropivacaine in clinical practice is its higher cost.[157,158]

Onset and Duration of Local Anesthetics

Alkalinization of the LAs, which are marketed in a water-soluble, ionized state, hastens onset. By increasing the concentration of the nonionized form, more lipid-soluble LA is available to penetrate the neural sheath and nerve membrane. Adding sodium bicarbonate immediately before injection of lidocaine, mepivacaine, or chloroprocaine produces a clinically significant faster onset of anesthesia and may also contribute to a denser block.[159] However, ropivacaine and bupivacaine will precipitate with the addition of bicarbonate unless a very low concentration is used. Combining short- and long-acting drugs for rapid onset and a prolonged sensory block has not been proven to be effective. For example, mixing 2-chloroprocaine with bupivacaine for the rapid onset of the former and long duration of the latter results in shortening the duration and effectiveness of the bupivacaine.[160] Continuous drug administration and the use of additives obviate the need for mixing LAs.

Clinical Pearl

- Combining short- and intermediate- or long-acting LAs for rapid onset with prolonged duration of action has not been proven to be effective. Continuous drug administration and the use of additives obviate the need for mixing LAs.

Adding epinephrine to certain LAs can increase the duration of action, most likely by decreasing vascular absorption. The effect is greatest with 2-chloroprocaine, lidocaine, and mepivacaine and is less effective with the longer-acting agents. Other vasoconstrictors, such as phenylephrine, have not been proven to be as effective in reducing the peak blood levels of LAs as epinephrine.[161]

Adjuvants to Local Anesthetics in the Epidural Space

A variety of other classes of drugs have been studied more recently to try to improve the quality of neuraxial blockade. In addition to several opioids (eg, fentanyl, sufentanil, and preparations of morphine); α-adrenergic agonists; cholinesterase inhibitors; semisynthetic opioid agonist-antagonists; ketamine; and midazolam have been studied, with mixed results.

The administration of clonidine in the epidural space has been studied extensively. An α_2-adrenergic agonist, clonidine appears to prolong the duration of action of LAs, although the mechanism remains unclear. Animal studies have shown that clonidine reduces regional spinal cord blood flow, therefore slowing the rate of drug elimination.[162] Kroin and colleagues demonstrated that the mechanism by which clonidine prolongs the duration of a block when mixed with LAs is not mediated by α-adrenoreceptors; rather, it is more likely related to the hyperpolarization-activated cation current I_h.[163]

Some of the potential benefits of the administration of clonidine in the epidural space may include the following:

1. Prolongation and enhancement of the effects of epidural LAs without an additional risk of hypotension
2. Reduction in LA dose requirements for labor epidural analgesia[164,165]
3. Effective analgesia without motor impairment[162]
4. Synergistic effect with opioids and opioid agonist-antagonists
5. Modulation of the stress response to thoracic surgery[166]
6. Preservation of lung function after thoracotomy[167]
7. Possible reduction in cytokine response, further reducing pain sensitivity[168]

Side effects that are commonly associated with epidural clonidine include dose-independent hypotension, bradycardia, sedation, and dry mouth. Combining clonidine with other agents, such as opioids, anticholinergics, opioid agonist-antagonists, and ketamine, may enhance the beneficial effects of these drugs while minimizing adverse side effects.[169,170]

Neostigmine, a cholinesterase inhibitor, is a more recent addition to the list of epidural additives for selective analgesia. The mechanism of action for its analgesic effect appears to be the inhibition of the breakdown of acetylcholine and the indirect stimulation of muscarinic and nicotinic receptors in the spinal cord. Although experience with epidural neostigmine is limited, it has been reported to provide postoperative pain relief without inducing respiratory depression, motor impairment, or hypotension.[169] When combined with other opioids, clonidine, and LAs, it may provide benefits similar to clonidine without the side-effect profile of any of these drugs given alone.[171–173] Observations in patients with cancer pain showed promise that its use might be associated with less nausea and vomiting than the intrathecal application.[174] In an investigation randomizing 48 patients to receive 0, 1, 2, or 4 μg/kg of epidural neostigmine in addition to a bupivacaine spinal anesthetic for minor knee surgery, no case of intraoperative nausea or vomiting was observed, and postoperative nausea scores did not differ between groups.[175] These results need to be corroborated by further studies before epidural neostigmine can be recommended for daily practice.

Other agents, such as ketamine, tramadol, droperidol, and midazolam, have been considered for epidural administration, with mixed results. Considerable controversy surrounds the use of midazolam intrathecally. Despite multiple publications recommending its use,[176–178] recent studies have demonstrated that even a single dose of intrathecal midazolam may have neurotoxic effects.[179] Until its safety profile can be ensured in human subjects, it is not recommended for neuraxial use at this time.[180]

One agent that shows promise is the extended-release formulation of one of the oldest opioids, morphine. DepoDur®, the brand name for extended-release epidural morphine, uses a drug-release delivery system called DepoFoam®. DepoFoam is composed of microscopic lipid-based particles with internal vesicles that contain the active drug and slowly release it. Recent studies have demonstrated effective pain relief with relatively minor side effects for up to 48 hours when appropriately dosed.[181–183] However, concerns about delayed respiratory depression have limited its clinical use in this early stage of its clinical use.

Other Factors Affecting Epidural Blockade

Injection Site

The epidural blockade is most effective when the block or the catheter is inserted in a location that corresponds to the dermatomes covered by the surgical incision. The most rapid onset and the densest block occur at the site of injection. By inserting the catheter closer to the dermatomal distribution of the surgical site, a lower dose of drug can be given, thereby reducing side effects.[184,185] This concept is especially important when thoracic epidural analgesia is used for postoperative analgesia.

After lumbar epidural injection, the analgesic and anesthetic effects spread to a greater degree cranially then caudally. Of note, there is a delay in onset of anesthesia at the L5–S1 segments secondary to the larger size of these nerve roots.[186] With thoracic injection, the LA spreads evenly from the site of injection, but meets resistance to blockade in the lumbar region because of the larger nerve roots. By controlling the dose in the thoracic region, a true segmental blockade affecting only the thoracic region can be established. Lumbar and sacral regions will be spared, thereby avoiding more extensive sympathetic blockade and subsequent associated hypotension and bladder dysfunction, as well as lower limb motor blockade.

Dose, Volume, and Concentration

The dose of LAs necessary for epidural anesthesia or analgesia is a function of the concentration of the solution and the volume injected. Concentration of the drug affects the density of the block; the higher the concentration, the more profound the motor and sensory block. Lower concentrations can selectively produce a sensory block.[187]

Volume and total LA dose are the variables that affect the degree of spread of the block. A larger volume of the same concentration of LA will block a greater number of segments. However, if the total dose of LA is unchanged but the concentration is doubled, the volume can be halved to achieve similar spread of LA.[188] A generally accepted guideline for dosing epidural anesthesia in adults is 1–2 mL per segment to be blocked. This guideline should be adjusted for shorter patients and for very tall patients. For example, to achieve a T10 sensory level from an L3–L4 injection, approximately 8 mL of LA should be administered. Below concentrations of the equivalent of 1% lidocaine, motor block is minimal, regardless of the volume of the LA injected, unless doses are given at repeating intervals.

Time to repeat a dose of LAs depends on the duration of the drug. Doses should be administered before the block regresses to the point the patient experiences pain, commonly referred to as "time to two-segment regression." This is defined as the time it takes for the sensory block to regress by two dermatome levels. When two-segment regression has occurred, one-third to one-half of the initial loading dose can safely be administered

TABLE 24–20. Redosing local anesthetics.

Drug	Concentration (%)	Time to Two-Segment Regression (min)	Recommended Time for "Top-Up" Dose From Initial Dose (min)
2-Chloroprocaine	3	45–75	45
Lidocaine	2	60–140	60
Bupivacaine	0.10	180–260	120
Ropivacaine	0.10	180–260	120

to maintain the block. For example, the time to two-segment regression of lidocaine is 60–140 minutes (Table 24–20).

Patient Positioning

Patient positioning during initiation of epidural blockade does not appear to affect the resultant spread of analgesia or anesthesia. The patient may be placed in either the lateral or sitting position. The midline of the spine is easier to palpate when the patient is sitting, especially in the obese patient, therefore making the block technically easier. Whether the patient is in the sitting or the lateral position, there is no significant difference in block height.[189] It has been suggested in a study by Seow and associates that there is slightly faster onset time, duration, and density of motor block on the dependent side when the epidural is placed with the patient in the lateral position.[190]

Patient Characteristics: Age, Weight, Height, and Pregnancy

With advancing age, the LA dose required to attain a specific block is reduced. Some studies have observed a nonclinically significant difference in block height (between one and four segments higher) with a fixed volume and concentration of LA in patients older than age 50.[191–193] Greater spread in the elderly may be related to the reduced size of the intervertebral foramina, which theoretically limits the egress of LAs from the epidural space. Decreased epidural fat, which allows more of the drug to bathe the nerves, and changes in the compliance of the epidural space, which may lead to enhanced cephalad spread, have also been proposed.[194]

There is little correlation between the spread of analgesia and the weight of the patient. However, in morbidly obese patients, there may be compression of the epidural space related to increased intra-abdominal pressure; a higher block may be attained with a given dose of LA.

Height appears to play little role in LA requirements. For short patients (≤5 ft 2 in.), the common practice has been to reduce the dose to 1 mL per segment to be blocked (instead of 2 mL per segment). Bromage suggested a more precise dosing regimen of increasing the dose of LA by 0.1 mL per segment for every 2 in. above 5 ft of height.[195] The safest practice is to use incremental dosing and monitor the effect to avoid excessively high anesthetic levels.

Pregnancy causes an increased sensitivity to both LAs and general anesthetics, although the studies regarding the causes are conflicting. Elevated levels of progesterone and endogenous

endorphins may contribute. Conflicting evidence regarding the spread of LA in pregnant versus nonpregnant individuals has been published.[196,197]

Intermittent Versus Continuous Epidural Block

The decision whether to use intermittent dosing after the initial loading dose, a continuous infusion, or patient-controlled or programmed intermittent bolus dosing may be influenced by the nature of the surgery or procedure, staffing, and equipment. All of these options can provide safe and effective epidural analgesia or anesthesia. Advantages of continuous infusion include greater cardiovascular stability, fewer labor requirements, decreased incidence of tachyphylaxis, decreased frequency and severity of side effects related to bolus injections, less rostral spread, decreased risk of the potential for contamination, and the ability to achieve a steady state of anesthesia. Intermittent manual bolus dosing, on the other hand, is simple and does not require additional equipment (eg, infusion devices).

EPIDURAL TECHNIQUE

Several factors influence the success of epidural blockade, including the clinician's experience and knowledge of anatomy, patient preparation and positioning, the level of epidural catheter insertion, and the technique used to initiate the procedure. This section reviews factors that contribute to successful epidural placement, starting with patient selection and preparation, equipment requirements, and current recommendations for the prevention of infectious complications associated with neuraxial techniques. It then presents technical aspects of cervical, thoracic, and lumbar epidural placement and addresses various controversies related to the technique of neuraxial blockade, such as the optimal method to identify the epidural space and the efficacy of the epidural test dose.

Patient Evaluation

As in the case with any anesthetic, the risks and benefits of epidural placement should be discussed with the patient in a manner consistent with informed consent. Any concerns and questions should be addressed prior to the administration of premedication. When a language barrier exists, trained interpreters or telephone translation services should be utilized.

The patient's medical history and active medication list should be reviewed prior to the initiation of epidural blockade, with particular emphasis on the presence of conditions that may predispose the patient to serious complications. Drug therapy that influences the patient's clotting function or physiologic response to blockade of the sympathetic preganglionic fibers should be taken into consideration, including when the last dose was administered. The patient's last oral intake should also be documented. For those patients receiving epidural blockade as the sole anesthetic or as an adjuvant to GA for elective surgical procedures, the ASA guidelines for nothing by mouth should be enforced. Patients with medical conditions that worsen with reduced afterload or preload (eg, severe AS, mitral stenosis, hypertrophic cardiomyopathy) and patients who may experience worsening shortness of breath, such as those with restrictive lung disease or severe COPD, may require additional testing. Clinical conditions that predispose patients to neuraxial infections, such as immunosuppression, DM, pancreatitis, and alcohol or drug abuse, may require further evaluation or laboratory studies. Preexisting neurologic deficits or CNS disorders should be assessed and documented. History of sensitivity or adverse reaction to opioids or LAs and complications related to prior epidural procedures require further investigation.

Physical examination should include an evaluation of the spine for evidence of scoliosis or prior back surgery, focal infection, severely limited range of motion, or other findings that may make epidural placement more challenging or impossible. Obesity, especially central obesity, may obscure surface landmarks.

Routine laboratory studies are not required for epidural placement in healthy patients for routine procedures. Many clinicians may choose to obtain a complete blood cell count (CBC), particularly when appreciable blood loss is expected or when the patient is known to be anemic. Baseline assessment of the patient's coagulation status or platelet count should be obtained in patients with known or suspected coagulation disorders, bleeding diatheses, and thrombocytopenia, as well as in patients receiving antithrombotic or thrombolytic therapy or any medications known to affect platelet quality or function (besides routine NSAIDs).

Clinical Pearls

- Routine laboratory studies are not required for initiation of epidural blockade in healthy patients for routine procedures.
- Patients with known or suspected bleeding disorders and those receiving antithrombotic or thrombolytic therapy require assessment of baseline coagulation status or platelet count (and possibly platelet function).
- Patients undergoing surgeries with anticipated blood loss or hemodynamic changes may require additional workup, including a CBC.

Preparation

A large-bore intravenous catheter for fluid or emergency drug administration must be secured prior to initiation of epidural blockade. Fluid preloading is not required and may be harmful in certain subsets of patients with decreased serum colloid

TABLE 24-21. Emergency equipment and drugs for initiation of neuraxial blockade.

Airway equipment	Ambu bag with mask
	Oxygen source
	Oral and nasal airways
	Laryngoscope handles and blades
	Endotracheal tubes
	Eschmann stylet/bougie
	Syringes and needles
Emergency drugs	Ephedrine
	Phenylephrine
	Epinephrine
	Atropine
	Sedative/hypnotic
	20% lipid emulsion
	Succinylcholine

oncotic pressure (eg, those with burns, preeclamptic patients).[198] However, reversible conditions, such as severe hypovolemia, should be managed prior to block placement and dosing.

Appropriate monitoring during performance of epidural blockade depends on the purpose of the epidural block and when and where the epidural is to be dosed. Epidural blocks for analgesia, such as for labor analgesia, require intermittent blood pressure monitoring during placement and for the duration of the epidural infusion, as well as continuous pulse oximetry with heart rate monitoring during placement and block initiation. Electrocardiogram (ECG) monitoring should be available. In laboring patients, fetal heart rate monitoring before and after placement is recommended if continuous monitoring is not feasible.

Sedatives or analgesics are not uncommonly administered to alleviate patient stress and discomfort during epidural placement and may require additional monitors and equipment, such as a nasal cannula. If premedications are administered, medical personnel who can provide continuous monitoring should be present. Of note, excessive sedation should be avoided to ensure patient cooperation during positioning, to detect the presence of paresthesias during placement, and to evaluate the level of sensory blockade and the effect of the test dose (if administered). Standard ASA monitors are required for initiation and intraoperative management of epidural anesthesia. Emergency drugs and equipment must be readily available during initiation of all central neuraxial procedures (Table 24-21).

Communication With Surgical Staff

A discussion with the surgical staff regarding the operative approach, the desired positioning of the patient, the estimated length of the surgical procedure, the anesthetic or analgesic goals of the blockade, and postoperative analgesic requirements can help to determine whether a continuous epidural, a single-shot epidural, or a CSE is preferable. The surgical staff can also share information about the patient that is not readily available in the chart or immediately apparent during the preoperative interview.

When feasible, to minimize unnecessary delays the block can be initiated in the preoperative area or in the operating room while the nursing staff is setting up the surgical equipment. Wherever the block is performed, sufficient space for the anesthesiologist and, optimally, an assistant, as well as adequate lighting, monitoring, and resuscitation equipment are essential.

Equipment

Commercially prepared, sterile, disposable epidural trays are available from several manufacturers. A standard kit typically includes the following: a sterile drape; prep swabs; 4 × 4 gauze sponges; a paper towel; povidone-iodine solution; an ampoule of 0.9% preservative-free sodium chloride; a 5-mL ampoule of 1.5% lidocaine with epinephrine 1:200,000; a 5-mL ampoule of 1% lidocaine for skin infiltration; a filtering device (needle or straw); a bacterial filter; needles and syringes of various sizes; a styletted epidural needle with cm markings; a 5- or 10-mL glass or plastic LOR syringe (either Luer lock or Luer slip); a catheter connector securing device; an epidural catheter with

centimeter gradations and a connector/adapter; a thread assist device (TAD); a needle guard for sharps disposal; and labels.

In an adult epidural kit, the epidural needle is typically 17 or 18 gauge and 9 cm (roughly 3.5 in.) in length, with surface markings at 1-cm intervals. Longer needles up to 15 cm (6 in.) in length are available for obese patients. The Tuohy needle, which is commonly supplied in noncustom kits, has a curved tip with a blunt bevel designed to permit easier identification of tissue as the needle advances and facilitate passage of the epidural catheter. Wings at the junction of the needle shaft and hub may allow for better control as the needle is passed through tissue, particularly when using the "hanging drop" technique for epidural space identification, although some practitioners may prefer epidural needles without wings or with attachable wings (Figure 24–14). Epidural needles with a back-eye opening for exit of a spinal needle (for CSEs) and double-lumen needles with separate openings for the spinal needle and catheter are also available.

Epidural catheters vary in diameter, materials, and tip design. In commercially prepared kits, 19-gauge catheters are usually paired with 17-gauge epidural needles; 20-gauge catheters are paired with 18-gauge needles. Many currently available epidural catheters are nylon blends with varying degrees of stiffness to facilitate threading. Some stiff nylon catheters have specially designed flexible tips intended to veer away from veins, nerves, and other obstacles encountered in the epidural space. Wire-reinforced catheters embedded in either a

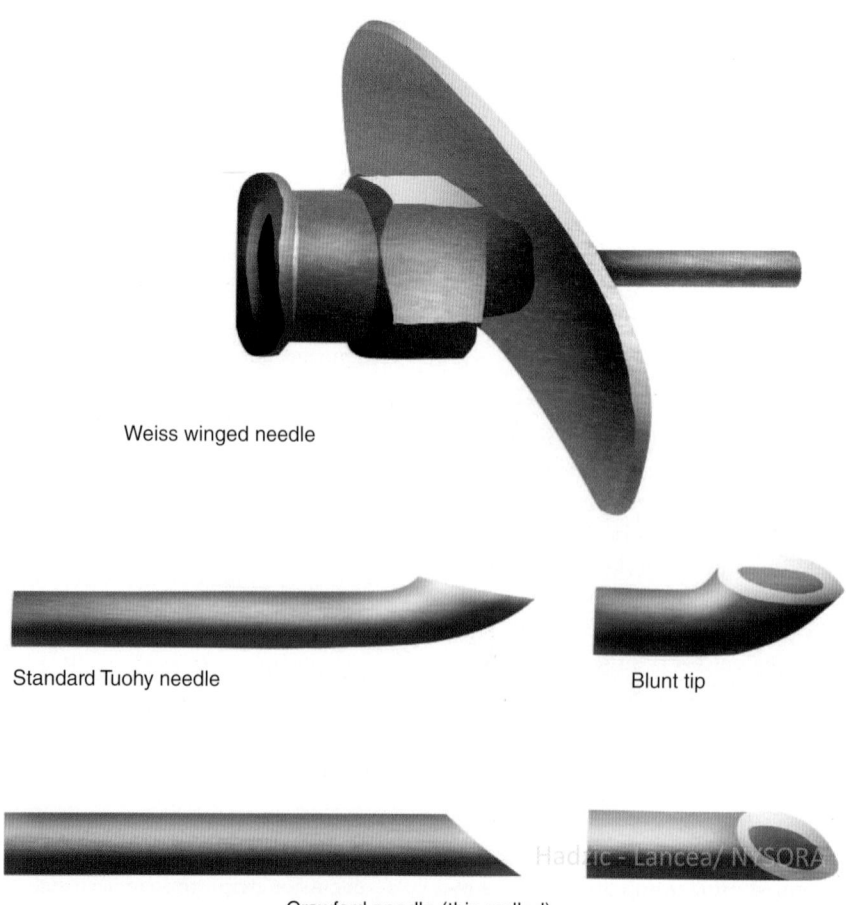

Weiss winged needle

Standard Tuohy needle

Blunt tip

Crawford needle (thin walled)

FIGURE 24–14. Epidural needles: bevel and wing configuration.

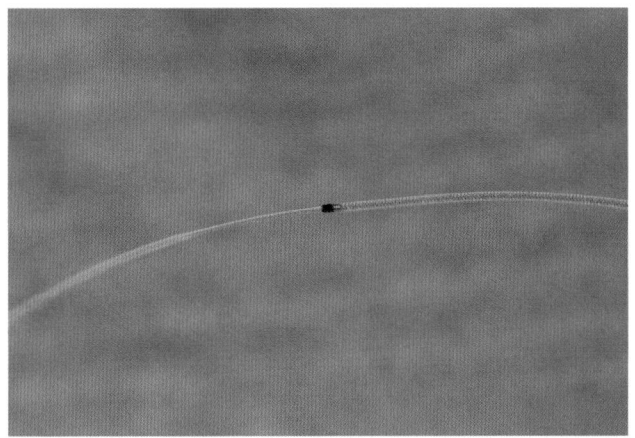

FIGURE 24–15. Single end-hole wire-reinforced catheter. (Used with permission from Epimed International.)

polyurethane or nylon-blend catheter represent a more recent technological advance and are becoming increasingly popular (Figure 24–15). Adult versions are 19 gauge in diameter and designed for use with a 17-gauge epidural needle; pediatric versions are available from some manufacturers.

Many commercially available nylon and wire-reinforced catheters are manufactured in both single end-hole and multiorifice versions (Figure 24–16). A lack of robust data precludes a full assessment of whether clinical outcomes, such as the incidence of paresthesias, epidural vein cannulation, intrathecal migration, and adequate analgesia, are improved with the uniport or multiport design. However, a 2009 prospective, single-blind, randomized controlled trial by Spiegel et al investigated the success of labor analgesia, the number of episodes of breakthrough pain requiring supplemental medicine, and the occurrence of complications, such as paresthesias and intravascular and intrathecal catheter placement, in 493 parturients who received either a single end-hole, wire-reinforced polyurethane catheter or a multiorifice, wire-reinforced nylon catheter.[199] The authors found no statistically significant difference in outcomes between the two groups and postulated that the flexibility afforded by the wire coil may eliminate any of the potential advantages of the multiport design.

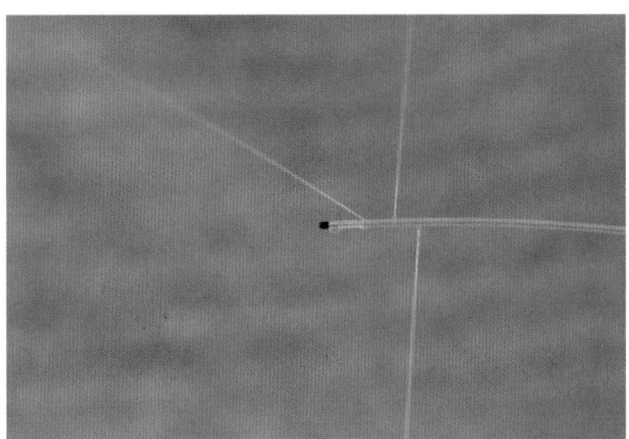

FIGURE 24–16. Multiorifice wire-reinforced catheter. (Used with permission from Epimed International.)

Clinical Pearls

- The use of wire-reinforced epidural catheters appears to reduce the incidence of complications associated with epidural techniques, including epidural vein cannulation, paresthesias, and inadequate analgesia.
- Current data suggest that clinical outcomes are similar with the use of uniport and multiport spring-wound catheters; the flexibility afforded by the stainless steel coil appears to negate any potential benefits of a multiport design.

Additional equipment that may be needed for initiation of epidural procedures includes 0.5% chlorhexidine with ethanol (Hydrex®) or 2% chlorhexidine with 70% isopropyl alcohol (ChloraPrep®), which is not supplied in epidural trays; a transparent sterile, occlusive dressing for the puncture site; and tape to secure the catheter. To minimize the remote risk of chemical arachnoiditis, the skin disinfection solution should not make contact with the epidural drugs or equipment and should be given adequate time to dry. Usually a large clear dressing (eg, Tegaderm") and adhesive tape are sufficient to prevent catheter dislodgement and to keep the epidural insertion site visible and clean. A sterile pen to label medications and a 25- or 27-gauge spinal needle (for CSEs) can be dropped onto the sterile field.

Clinical Pearls

- A clear sterile occlusive dressing is recommended to prevent catheter dislodgement.
- The catheter and its centimeter markings should be visible to the anesthesia provider to ensure that the catheter remains at the original insertion site and that CSF and heme return are absent prior to dosing.

Analgesia and Sedation During Block Initiation

Analgesia or sedation can be provided to improve patient comfort during neuraxial blockade. However, there is emerging evidence that intravenous sedatives may increase pain perception in an agent-type- and pain-type-specific manner.[200] Light sedation with a benzodiazepine (most commonly midazolam) or a short-acting opioid prior to epidural placement is usually sufficient. This may also be appropriate for obstetric patients. In a small, double-blind randomized study, Frölich and colleagues found that maternal analgesia and sedation with fentanyl and midazolam prior to spinal placement was not associated with adverse neonatal effects.[201] Importantly, mothers in both the group that received premedication and the control group showed no difference in their ability to recall the births of their babies.

For those who prefer to be "asleep" during epidural placement, a propofol infusion can be titrated to maintain sedation without respiratory impairment in selected clinical settings.

However, it is preferable to have adult patients awake and cooperative enough to alert the anesthesia provider to the presence of paresthesias during initiation of neuraxial blockade and to participate in assessment of the sensory level. In clinical scenarios in which the administration of premedication prior to epidural placement may not be appropriate, there appears to be a placebo effect from the use of gentler, more reassuring words during lidocaine skin wheal administration, which is often considered the most painful part of the procedure.[202] Studies suggest that the following tips may also serve to reduce pain on injection of LA: Chloroprocaine (with or without sodium bicarbonate) may be less painful than lidocaine for skin infiltration[203]; adjusting the pH of lidocaine to approximate physiologic pH reduces pain on injection[204]; and cryoanalgesia (skin cooling) may be as effective as buffering the LA solution with sodium bicarbonate.[205]

Clinical Pearls

The following tips may serve to reduce pain on injection of LA for skin infiltration:

- Communication with the patient during the procedure and verbal reassurance
- Adjusting the pH of lidocaine with the addition of sodium bicarbonate to more closely approximate physiologic pH
- Skin cooling (cryoanalgesia) or topical anesthetic before skin puncture

Patient Positioning

Optimal patient positioning is essential for successful epidural placement. Depending on the patient's medical status (eg, body habitus and ability to cooperate), the planned procedure, the anesthesia provider's experience, the baricity of the intrathecal solution (for CSE placement), and several other factors, the sitting, lateral decubitus, jackknife, or prone position can be used. Each position has advantages and disadvantages. Regardless of which position is selected for the initiation of neuraxial procedures, it is useful to have an assistant to help maintain the position until the procedure is complete. Overall, while epidural block can be initiated with the patient in any position that permits access to the back, improper positioning can turn an otherwise-easy epidural placement into a needlessly challenging one. Several positioning devices are available commercially to facilitate patient positioning without the aid of nursing personnel.

Sitting Position

In general, it is technically easier to identify the midline in the sitting position, particularly in obese and scoliotic patients. Anesthesia providers may also be more experienced and more comfortable performing neuraxial procedures in the sitting position. The sitting position has also been observed to provide the most direct route to the epidural space, with shorter distance from skin to space[206] and, in the case of CSEs with dextrose-free LA and hypobaric intrathecal opioids, greater cephalad spread of the sensory block.[207] However, elderly patients, parturients in

TABLE 24–22. Advantages of sitting position for initiation of neuraxial blockade.

Easier to identify midline, particularly in obese and scoliotic patients

Practitioners more experienced in sitting position

Shorter procedure time

Shorter distance from skin to epidural space

Greater cephalad spread of hypobaric solutions

advanced stages of labor, patients with hip fractures, heavily sedated patients, and uncooperative patients may not be able to assume or maintain the sitting position (Table 24–22).

If the sitting position is chosen, the patient should be assisted to sit on the operating room table or bed with the backs of the knees touching the edge of the bed and the feet resting on a stool or hanging over the bed. The patient should relax the shoulders and curve the back out toward the clinician, assuming a "slouched" or "mad-cat" position. It is useful to have an assistant stand in front of the patient and help the patient attain maximal spinal flexion (Figure 24–17). Flexing the neck should help to flex the lower spine and open the vertebral spaces (Figure 24–18). Asking the patient to hug a pillow may also help with positioning.

Lateral Decubitus Position

The lateral decubitus position may be more appropriate for patients who cannot comfortably assume the sitting position. Additional benefits include the following: Sedation can be used more liberally; vagal reflexes can be minimized; hemodynamic changes may be better tolerated; there may be less need for a well-trained assistant to help maintain positioning; and there appears to be a reduced incidence of unintentional epidural vein cannulation and dural puncture (Table 24–23).[208] Finally, in the case of CSEs with hyperbaric LAs, unilateral blocks for certain orthopedic procedures may be more easily attained in the lateral position.

In the lateral decubitus position, the patient's back should be fully aligned with the edge of the table or bed (Figure 24–19). The left lateral recumbent position may be preferable for right-handed physicians and may provide improved hemodynamic stability for parturients. The coronal plane of the patient should be perpendicular to the floor, with the tips of the spinous processes pointing toward the wall. The thighs should be flexed toward the abdomen and the knees drawn to the chest; the neck should be in a neutral position or flexed so that the chin rests on the chest. Asking the patient to "assume the fetal position" may help maximally flex the spine. The hips should be aligned one above the other, and the nondependent arm should extend toward and rest on the nondependent hip. The patient's head may need to be elevated with a pillow to avoid rotation of the spine. Obese patients or those with larger hips may require additional pillows to maintain proper alignment. Directing the needle toward an imaginary line that extends cephalad and

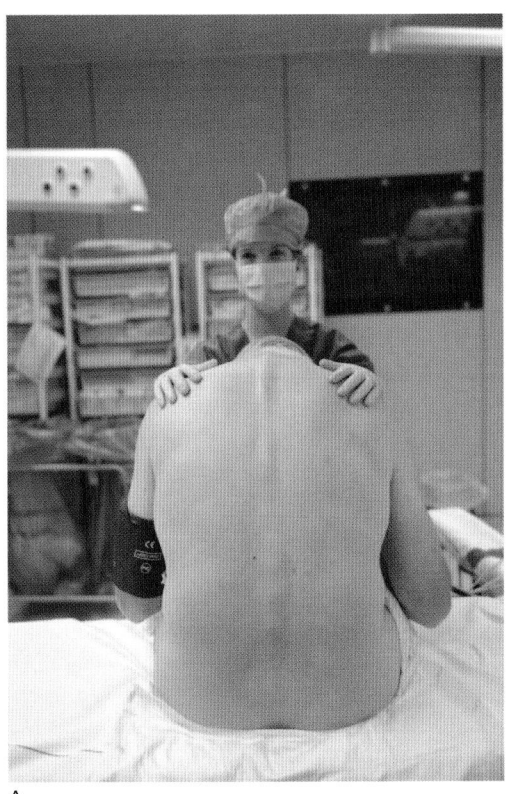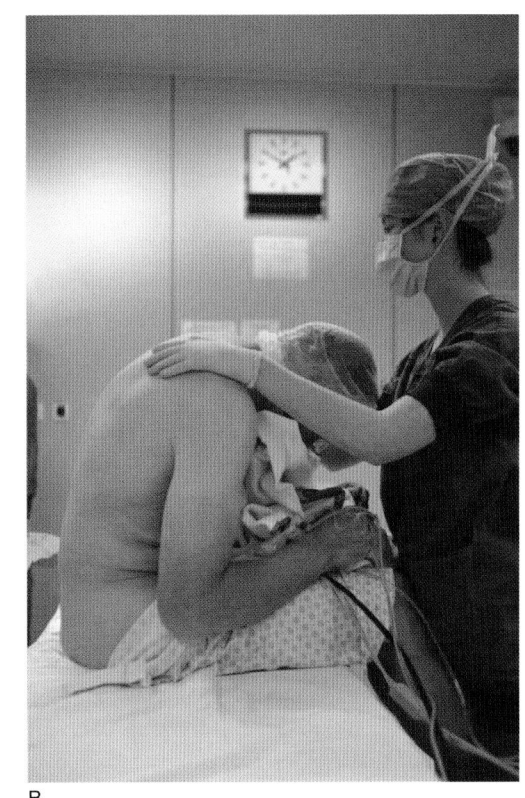

A   B

FIGURE 24–17. A, B: Epidural placement in the sitting position with assistant helping to position the patient.

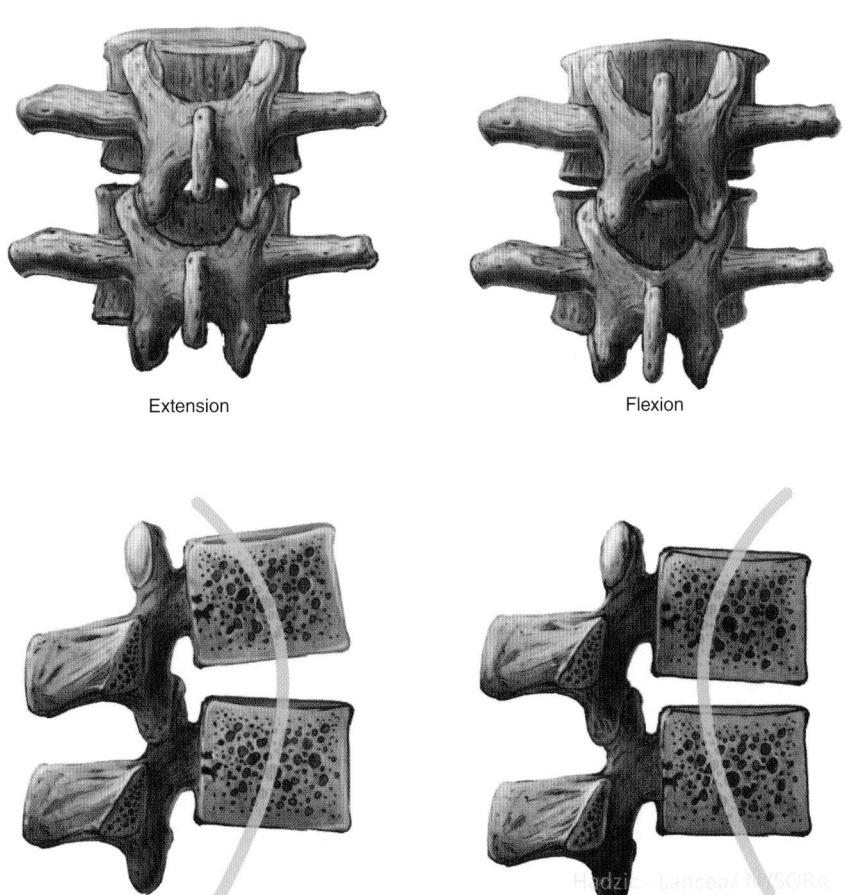

Extension   Flexion

Extension   Flexion

FIGURE 24–18. Flexion versus extension during epidural placement.

TABLE 24–23. Advantages of lateral position for initiation of neuraxial blockade.

Sedation can be used more liberally
Reduced patient movement
Increased patient comfort
Improved patient cooperation
Improved patient satisfaction
Reduced catheter displacement
Decreased incidence of epidural vein cannulation
Attenuation of vagal reflexes
Hemodynamic changes better tolerated
Bedside assistance may not be required
Intentional unilateral block for surgical procedures feasible

caudad from the umbilicus may optimize chances of midline insertion, which is particularly important during initiation of CSEs (Table 24–24). The bevel of the epidural needle is directed toward the patient's head.

Infection Control

Adherence to strict aseptic techniques is essential during initiation and maintenance of neuraxial blockade. The ASA Task Force on Infectious Complications Associated With Neuraxial Techniques advises the following measures: remove jewelry on fingers and wrists; use careful hand washing before gloving; use caps, masks (changed with each new patient encounter), and sterile gloves; use chlorhexidine with alcohol for skin preparation; drape the patient under sterile conditions; and cover the catheter insertion site with a sterile occlusive dressing.[209] A single application of chlorhexidine with alcohol appears as efficacious as two applications for skin disinfection.[210] When chlorhexidine, which is not supplied in epidural kits, is not available, the use of povidone-iodine with alcohol is preferable to povidone-iodine alone. All antiseptic solutions are considered neurotoxic if they come into direct contact with the meninges[211]; care should be taken to keep needles and drugs in the epidural tray separate

from the skin disinfectants. Bacterial filters may be helpful for patients with chronic or extended continuous epidural infusions, but there are no data to support that they decrease the incidence of catheter-related infections. The catheter should remain in place no longer than necessary, and catheter disconnects and filter changes should be kept to a minimum. The data are insufficient to support wearing a surgical gown during initiation of epidural procedures (Table 24–25).

Techniques to Identify the Epidural Space

Three techniques can be used to identify the epidural space: LOR, hanging drop, and ultrasonography. Despite increasing interest in ultrasound-assisted neuraxial procedures, the LOR technique, which relies on the different tissue densities as the needle passes through ligaments into the epidural space, is the most commonly used technique. Both LOR to fluid, with or without an air bubble, and air are recognized as acceptable means of identifying the epidural space. Randomized trials comparing saline to air for LOR have suggested that saline is superior. However, these trials may overstate the difference between the two media by forcing the anesthesia provider to use a less-preferred technique.[212] Regardless of which technique is used during routine epidural placement, it is important to bear in mind that LOR to air is not recommended for EBP procedures.

Evidence in the literature is lacking concerning the best method to identify the epidural space in children, who are commonly anesthetized during placement. Recently, the use of ultrasound has been advocated. However, the technique can be cumbersome and requires experience with ultrasound imaging. With refinements in technology and expanding practitioner experience, ultrasound guidance may facilitate placement of epidural catheters in this patient population.

Loss of Resistance to Air

The LOR to air technique is associated with several complications (Table 24–26). Air is compressible and may result in a false LOR and, relatedly, an increased incidence of ADP. ADP in the setting of LOR to air may result in pneumocephalus, a severe headache that develops immediately after injection of air into the subarachnoid space.[213] Pneumocephalus, in turn, can result in serious neurologic injury, such as hemiparesis and generalized convulsions, as well as nausea and vomiting and delayed recovery

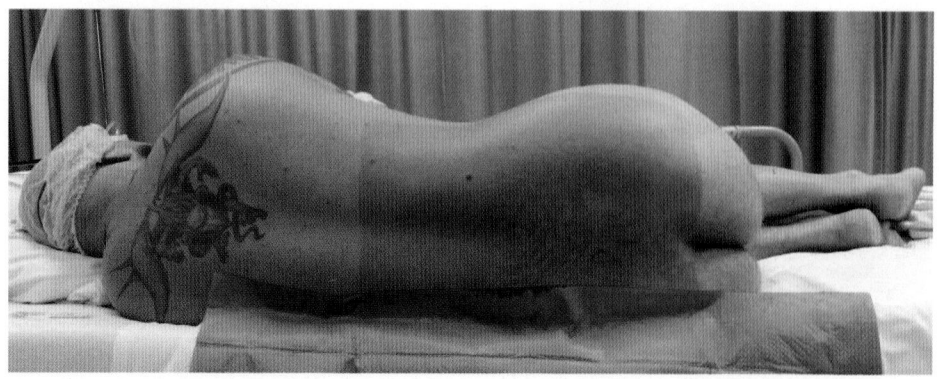

FIGURE 24–19. Epidural placement in the lateral position.

TABLE 24–24. Tips for attaining optimal lateral position.

Align patient's back with edge of table or bed

Align coronal plane perpendicular to floor

Flex thighs toward abdomen

Neck should be neutral or flexed

Align hips one above the other

Rest nondependent arm on nondependent hip

Elevate head with pillow to avoid rotation of the spine

TABLE 24–26. Complications associated with loss of resistance to air.

Pneumocephalus

Increased risk of accidental dural puncture

Faster onset of signs and symptoms of PDPH

Higher incidence of PDPH

Incomplete/patchy block

Spinal cord or nerve root compression by air

Venous air embolism

Subcutaneous emphysema

Increased incidence of epidural vein cannulation

Difficult catheter insertion

PDPH = postdural puncture headache.

from GA.[214] The incidence of PDPH and the onset of symptoms may also be higher when the LOR to air technique is used to identify the epidural space. In addition, the LOR to air technique has been associated with a higher incidence of unblocked segments or patchy pain relief and neurologic deficits related to compression of nerve roots or the spinal cord by air bubbles.[215] Venous air embolism (VAE) in the presence of tears in the epidural venous plexus or if the pressure from the air source is higher than the venous pressure has been reported.[216] Finally, both an increased incidence of epidural venous cannulation and difficult catheter insertion have been associated with LOR to air, particularly in the absence of fluid predistension of the epidural space, although the data are conflicting.[217]

Advocates of LOR to air feel that it is easier to detect ADP if air alone is used, as any fluid return is undeniably CSF in the absence of saline injection. In the event of an equivocal ADP, CSF can be distinguished from saline with the use of a urine reagent strip to check for glucose and protein; if positive, the diagnosis of CSF can be made. CSF can also be distinguished from saline or LA by the temperature differential; CSF is expected to be body temperature. Advocates of the LOR to air approach also point to the inadequate sensory block and delay in block onset that may occur if large volumes of saline are injected into the epidural space, presumably due to a dilutional effect. This, however, can be avoided by limiting the amount of saline injected. For practitioners who routinely perform CSEs, an argument could also be

made that injecting saline complicates the identification of CSF prior to the administration of intrathecal medications.

To identify the epidural space with the LOR to air technique, advance the needle slowly, exerting either continuous or intermittent pressure on the LOR syringe. As the needle enters the ligamentum flavum, there is usually a distinct sensation of increased resistance followed by a subtle "give" when light pressure is exerted on the plunger. Avoid injecting air on identifying the epidural space due to concerns for pneumocephalus (in the event of ADP) and patchy, inadequate analgesia.

Loss of Resistance to Saline With or Without an Air Bubble

The syringe is filled with 2–3 mL of saline or saline with a clearly visible air bubble. The bubble provides a gauge of the appropriate pressure to be applied on the LOR syringe; it will compress and provide some resistance if the epidural needle tip is engaged in ligament but will dissipate effortlessly with only light pressure once the needle enters the epidural space. The saline can be injected directly for fluid predistension. The small air bubble should not result in complications associated with LOR to air if it also is injected. Omit the air bubble when performing an EBP due to the remote possibility that the air could be introduced into the subarachnoid space via the meningeal breach.

With LOR to saline with or without air, the needle is advanced in the same fashion as with air. Continuous or intermittent pressure can be exerted on the plunger of the needle.

The Hanging Drop Technique

The hanging drop technique relies on the subatmospheric pressure of the epidural space, which is more pronounced and reliable in the cervical and thoracic regions than in the lumbar segments. Dural tenting from the advancing epidural needle also contributes to the pressure that appears to "suck in" the drop of fluid. To identify the epidural space with this approach, an epidural needle with wings is required. A drop of saline is placed at the hub of the needle once the needle is engaged in

TABLE 24–25. Aseptic technique during epidural blockade initiation and maintenance.

Remove jewelry on fingers and wrists

Perform careful hand washing before gloving

Use cap, mask, and sterile gloves

Use chlorhexidine with alcohol for skin preparation

Drape the patient under sterile conditions

Cover catheter insertion site with sterile, occlusive dressing

Keep catheter in place no longer than necessary

Keep catheter disconnection and filter changes to a minimum

ligament. The needle is advanced continuously with the thumb and index fingers firmly grasping the wings and the third through fifth fingers of both hands positioned against the patient's back. Entry into the epidural space is signaled by entry of the drop into the hub of the needle.

The hanging drop technique is most effective in the thoracic region, where the subatmospheric pressure is more notable. However, this technique carries a higher risk of meningeal tear, in part because of the epidural needle's proximity to the dura. Also, patients with severe obstructive lung disease may have attenuated subatmospheric pressure, even in the thoracic region; the hanging drop technique may not be appropriate in this setting.

Ultrasonography

Ultrasound technology is being used increasingly to aid in the identification of the epidural space. Studies suggest that the use of ultrasonography to identify the anticipated depth to space, particularly in obese parturients,[218] and to identify the midline prior to placement reduces the number of attempts, minimizes the risk of complications, and facilitates the procedure without significantly prolonging the procedure. Ultrasound guidance also serves to help identify the correct interspace, which may be difficult based on anatomic landmarks alone. See Chapter 40 for more detailed information about ultrasound-guided neuraxial techniques.

■ Technique of Epidural Blockade

There are four common approaches to the epidural space: midline, paramedian, Taylor (modified paramedian), and caudal. Clinical expertise in each of these techniques gives the anesthesiologist more flexibility when performing epidural blockade. For all approaches, monitors should be in place and the skin should be prepped and draped in a sterile fashion before initiation of the procedure. Emergency equipment and medication must be immediately available. Sedation may be used, as appropriate. In general, the epidural needle bevel should be facing cephalad regardless of the approach used to access the epidural space unless an intentional unilateral block is desired (eg, for lower extremity orthopedic procedures performed under CSE).

Midline Approach

This approach is most commonly used for epidural placement in the sitting position and for epidural procedures in the lumbar, low thoracic, and cervical spine region.

1. An epidural tray can be placed to the anesthesiologist's right for right-handed and left for left-handed clinicians.
2. Identify the desired interspace by surface anatomic landmarks and palpation or with ultrasonography. The needle used to anesthetize the skin can also be used as a "finder needle" to help identify bony landmarks, particularly in obese patients.
3. Infiltrate the skin and subcutaneous tissue with LA (most commonly 1% lidocaine) along the intended path of the epidural needle between adjacent spinous processes. A large

skin wheal with a smaller volume of LA in the subcutaneous tissue will serve to anesthetize the skin adequately without obscuring landmarks.

4. Insert the styletted epidural needle along the same track with the bevel oriented cephalad. During needle insertion, the dorsum of the anesthesiologist's noninjecting hand can rest on the patient's back with the thumb and index finger holding the hub of the epidural needle. A modified approach is to advance with the dominant hand firmly wrapped around the hub of the epidural needle while the index finger and thumb of the nondominant hand grasp and guide the needle shaft. Placing the tips of the middle fingers on the patient's back and grasping the needle wings with both thumbs and forefingers is an alternative method to engage the needle.

To engage the epidural needle properly, advance through the skin, subcutaneous tissue, fatty tissue, supraspinous ligament, interspinous ligament, and, possibly, into the ligamentum flavum; at that point, the needle should sit firmly in the midline (Figure 24–20). If the needle shaft wobbles or deviates sideways, it is not properly anchored in ligament. The epidural needle can be engaged in the interspinous ligament or the ligamentum flavum.

Clinical Pearls

- The epidural needle advances through skin, subcutaneous tissue, supraspinous ligament, interspinous ligament, and ligamentum flavum before reaching the epidural space.
- The needle can be engaged in either the interspinous ligament or the ligamentum flavum during initiation of epidural blockade.
- Lateral deviation or a "wobbly" needle indicates that the needle is not properly engaged in ligament, necessitating withdrawal and re-direction toward midline.

Determining which ligaments are traversed is an acquired skill. The interspinous ligament may feel "gritty" against the advancing needle, while the ligamentum flavum offers more resistance. However, midline gaps in the ligamentum flavum are not uncommon, and obstetric patients may have softer ligaments. The depth from the skin to the ligamentum flavum generally ranges from 4 to 6 cm in normal-size adults, although there is a great deal of variability.

After the ligaments are penetrated, it is no longer advisable to change the direction of the needle tip without withdrawing the needle several centimeters or to the skin level. The stylet should be placed in the epidural needle while redirecting to avoid the accumulation of bony debris or soft tissue plugs that may hinder the flow of CSF in the event of an ADP.

5. Remove the stylet from the epidural needle and attach the LOR syringe with air or saline (with or without an air bubble) firmly to the hub of the needle. Glass or low-resistance plastic LOR syringes are appropriate. Care should be taken to ensure that glass syringes are not "sticky."

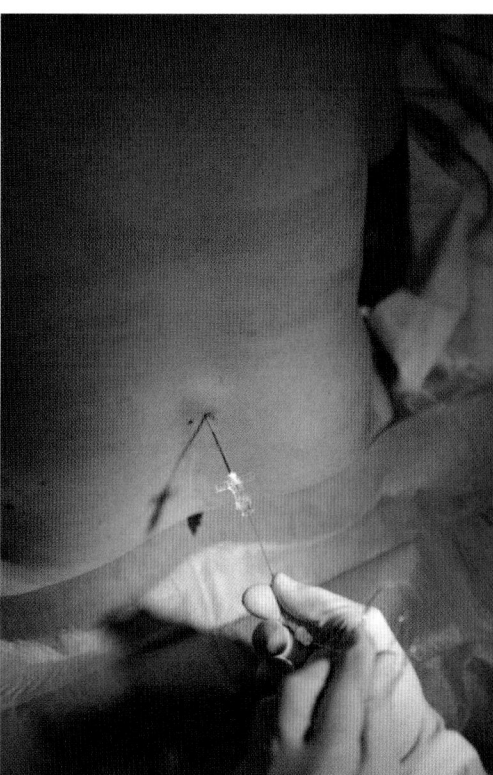

FIGURE 24–20. Epidural needle engaged in midline ligament.

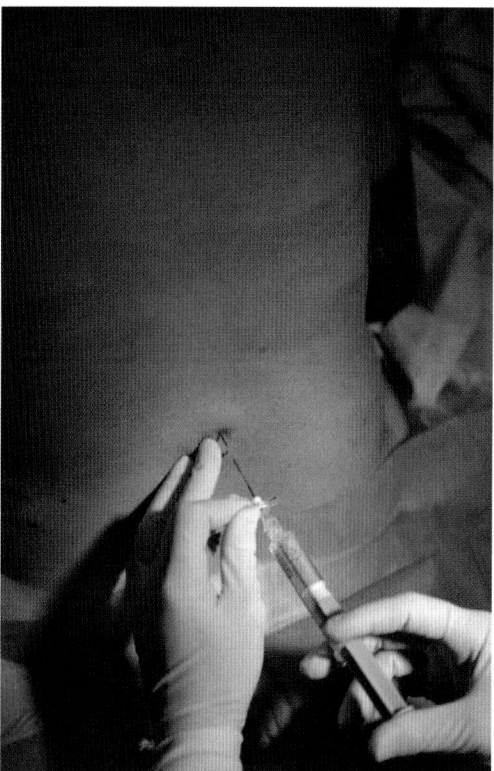

FIGURE 24–21. Advancing epidural needle: nondominant hand on patient's back with thumb and forefinger on needle hub.

Multiple hand positions are appropriate to advance the epidural needle into the epidural space: The back of the nondominant hand can rest firmly on the patient's back, with the thumb and forefinger grasping the needle shaft, while pressure is exerted on the LOR plunger either continuously or intermittently by the thumb of the dominant hand. The nondominant hand can rest on the patient's back with the thumb and forefinger extending to and stabilizing the needle hub, while the thumb of the dominant hand applies pressure (Figure 24–21). Or, the middle through fourth or fifth fingers of the nondominant hands can rest on the back, with both thumbs and forefingers grasping the wings of the epidural needle and the dominant hand intermittently releasing its position and exerting pressure on the LOR syringe plunger (Figure 24–22).

As the needle enters the epidural space, the plunger of the LOR syringe suddenly "gives." Avoid injecting the full contents of the syringe, particularly with LOR to air, if possible. For continuous epidurals, a small volume of saline can be injected into the epidural space to dilate the space, thereby reducing the risk of epidural vein cannulation and facilitating catheter insertion. Note the depth of the needle at the skin. The marking on the needle at the skin represents the depth from the skin to the epidural space. Because the centimeter markings are not numbered, it may help to count the number of centimeter markings between the skin and the epidural needle hub and subtract that number from the length of the needle. For example, if 4 markings remain visible between the skin and the needle hub, subtract 4 from 9

(the common length of an epidural needle) to determine that the depth to epidural space is 5 cm.

6. Insert the catheter with the assistance of the insertion device that fits into the epidural needle hub until the 15-cm mark is visualized entering the needle hub; then, remove the needle without dislodging the catheter (Figure 24–23). The catheter should be threaded no more than 5–6 cm into the epidural space; 2–3 cm is appropriate for short surgical procedures. To determine where the catheter should be secured at the skin, add 2–6 cm, depending on the distance the catheter is to be threaded, to the previously calculated depth to epidural space. For example, if the needle entered the epidural space at 7 cm, the catheter should be secured at the 12-cm mark at the skin to ensure that 5 cm of the catheter rests in the epidural space.

Clinical Pearl

- An easy way to measure depth to epidural space when using the LOR technique is to count the number of centimeter markings that are visible between the skin and the needle hub. Subtract that number from the length of the needle. For example, most epidural needles are 9 cm in length. If 4 centimeter markings are visible after epidural space identification, subtract 4 from 9 to conclude that the depth to space is 5 cm. The epidural catheter should be inserted no more than 5 or 6 cm beyond that distance (ie, taped at 10–11 cm at the skin).

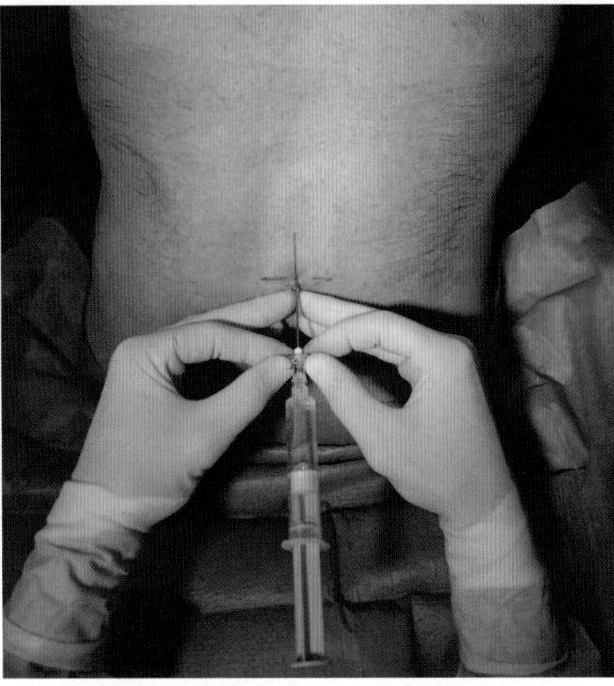

FIGURE 24–22. Advancing epidural needle: thumbs and index fingers grasping wings.

For the less-common single-shot epidural technique, the LA may be administered directly through the needle in divided doses over several minutes. This technique, however, requires that the patient remain immobile during dosing and may result in painful pressure with large

volumes. For the continuous catheter technique, administering LA through the needle is not recommended, as correct catheter placement cannot be verified.

7. A clear occlusive dressing should be applied over the insertion site to allow inspection of the catheter. The catheter should be secured to the patient's back with the connector at the patient's shoulder. Using clear tape has the advantage of permitting the practitioner to visualize the proximal and distal "flashback" windows of the catheter prior to administering boluses of LA.

Paramedian Approach

The paramedian approach offers a larger opening into the epidural space than the midline approach and is particularly useful for patients who cannot be positioned easily or who cannot flex the spine during epidural placement; for patients with calcified ligaments or spinal deformities (eg, kyphoscoliosis, prior lumbar surgery); and for epidural techniques in the low- to midthoracic area. The spinous processes from T4–T9 are sharply angled and have tips that point caudally, making midline insertion of the epidural needle more difficult.

The "feel" of the paramedian approach is different from that of the midline approach because different tissues are penetrated. The supraspinous and interspinous ligaments are midline structures that are not traversed in the paramedian approach. Instead, the epidural needle penetrates paraspinous tissue with little resistance before entering the ligamentum flavum. Several approaches to the paramedian technique have been described. Essentially, needle entry is directed caudal and lateral to the inferior aspect of the superior spinous process of the desired interspace and walked off the lamina in a cephalad direction (Figure 24–24).

1. Identify the intended interspace with surface landmarks, palpation, or ultrasound guidance. Raise a skin wheal roughly 1 cm lateral and 1 cm caudad to the inferior aspect of the superior spinous process of the desired spinal level.
2. The epidural needle is inserted 15° off the sagittal plane, angled toward midline with a cephalad tilt.

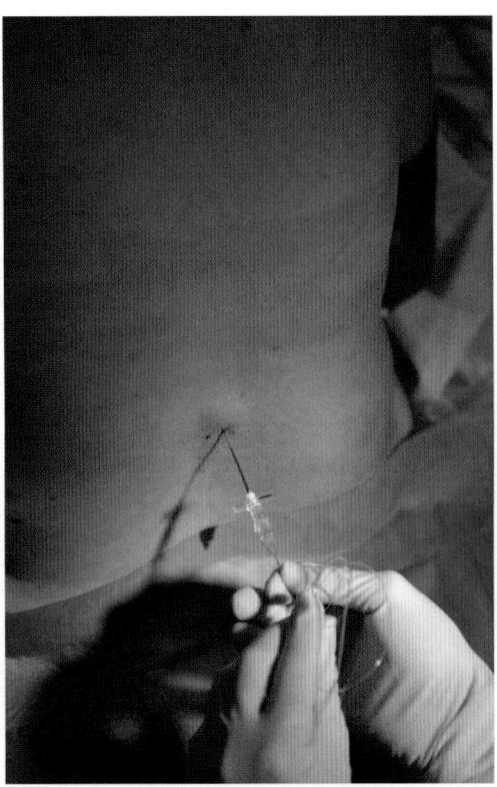

FIGURE 24–23. Inserting the epidural catheter.

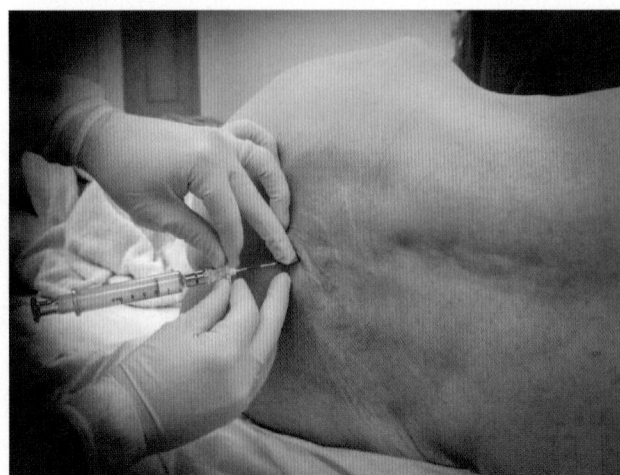

FIGURE 24–24. Paramedian epidural technique.

3. If bone (most likely lamina, if depth and angle of approach are appropriate) is encountered, the needle is redirected in a cephalad and medial direction (See Part VI, Pediatric Anesthesia). If the lateral aspect of the spinous process is encountered, the needle should be redirected laterally and cephalad.

Taylor Approach

The Taylor approach is a modified paramedian approach utilizing the large L5–S1 interspace. It is an excellent approach for hip surgery or for any lower extremity surgery in trauma patients who cannot tolerate the sitting position. This approach may provide the only available access to the epidural space in patients with ossified ligaments.

1. With the patient in the sitting or lateral position, a skin wheal is placed 1 cm medial and 1 cm caudad to the posterior superior iliac spine.
2. The epidural needle is inserted into this site in a medial and cephalad direction at a 45° to 55° angle.
3. As in the classic paramedian approach, the first resistance felt before entry to the epidural space is on entry into the ligamentum flavum.
4. If the needle contacts bone (usually the sacrum), the needle should be walked off the bone into the ligament and then into the epidural space in progressively more medial and cephalad directions.

Caudal Approach

The caudal approach is commonly used in pediatrics for single-shot or continuous epidural catheter placement for intraoperative and postoperative analgesia (see Chapter 25). In adults, it is usually reserved for procedures requiring blockade of the sacral and lumbar nerves (eg, anal and vaginal surgeries, inguinal herniorrhaphy, cystoscopy); epidurography; and lysis of adhesions in patients with low-back pain with radiculopathy after spinal surgery.

The sacrum is a triangular-shaped bone formed by the fusion of the sacral vertebrae. Nonfusion of the fifth sacral vertebral arch creates the structure known as the sacral hiatus, which is covered by the sacrococcygeal ligament (an extension of the ligamentum flavum) and bordered by bony prominences known as the sacral cornua. The sacral hiatus is the point of access into the sacral epidural space. It is usually identified as a groove above the coccyx (Figure 24–25). If fluoroscopy is not used, there are two methods to identify the hiatus:(1) The sacral hiatus lies at the apex of an equilateral triangle connecting the posterior superior iliac spines and pointing caudad. (2) The bony protuberances (the sacral cornua) that surround the sacral hiatus can be palpated by applying firm pressure with the index finger as it moves cephalad from the coccyx.

1. Place the patient in a lateral or prone position (with pillow under pelvis and hips internally rotated, if prone). In the lateral position, the dependent leg is flexed slightly, while the nondependent leg is flexed to a greater degree (until the knee contacts the bed).
2. Advance the needle at a 45° tilt (relative to the skin surface).
3. A distinct "pop" or "snap" is felt when the needle pierces the sacrococcygeal membrane.
4. If the dorsal aspect of the ventral plate of the sacrum is encountered, withdraw the needle slightly, decrease the

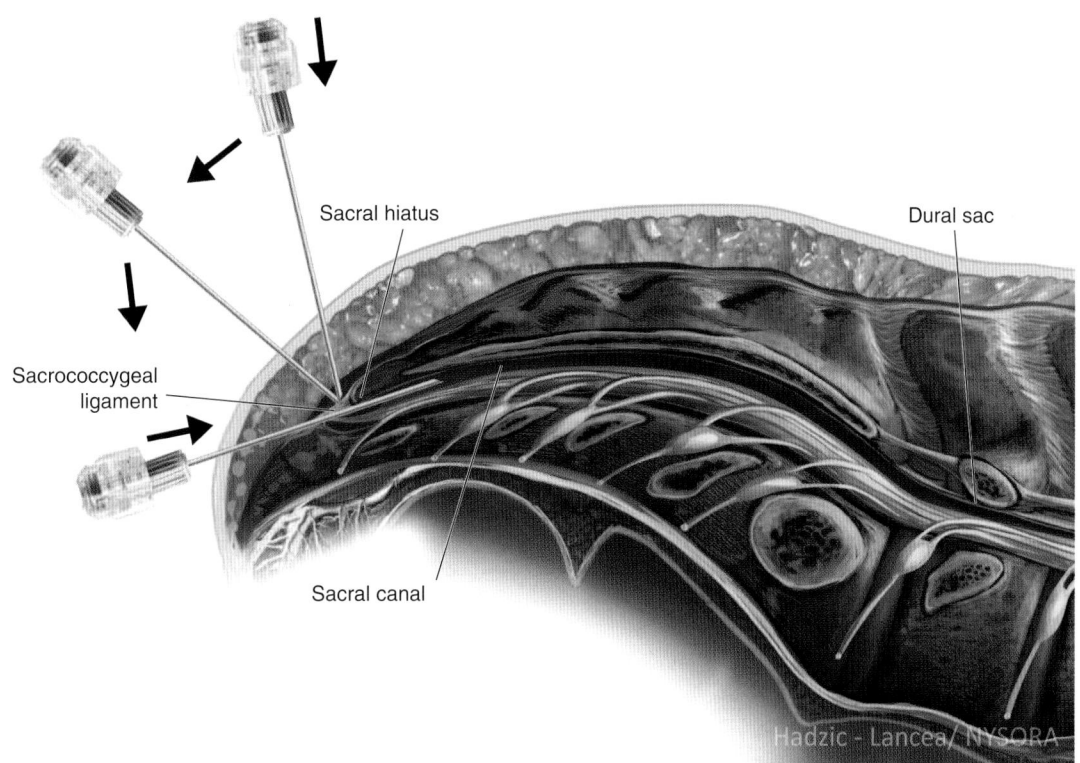

FIGURE 24–25. Caudal approach for epidural catheter placement.

angle of insertion, and advance again. The needle angle is lowered until it is almost flat against the skin (ie, parallel to the coronal plane) for male patients. Female patients may require a 15° tilt.

5. After LOR is encountered, advance the needle slightly into the caudal canal. Advancing too far may lead to ADP or unintended intravascular injection or epidural vein cannulation during catheter placement. If LOR is equivocal, several milliliters of saline can be injected through the caudal needle while palpating the skin overlying the sacrum. The needle is likely positioned correctly if a skin bulge does not develop.

6. Aspirate for blood or CSF before injecting LA.

7. An epidural catheter can be inserted through the needle and advanced to the desired level.

Cervical Epidural Blockade

Single-shot or continuous cervical epidural techniques are used for a variety of surgical and pain procedures, including carotid endarterectomy, thyroidectomy, and chronic neck pain conditions. Both the midline and paramedian approaches are used to perform cervical procedures, although fluoroscopic guidance is becoming increasingly common. Cervical epidural blockade can be initiated in the prone, lateral, or sitting position. The prone position is used most commonly for fluoroscopic-assisted procedures, although the sitting position can be used. Whichever position is used, flexion of the neck serves to increase the distance from the ligamentum flavum to the dura mater, increasing the margin of safety for these procedures, and to expand the interlaminar space.

As in the case of lumbar and thoracic epidural procedures, both the LOR and the hanging drop techniques are suitable methods to identify the epidural space. Either air (preferably a small volume) or saline (with or without an air bubble) can be used for LOR. However, the ligamentum flavum is discontinuous at midline in the cervical region in a large percentage of patients, contributing to a false LOR. Also, it is important to bear in mind that the ligamentum flavum is thinner at this level (1.5–3 mm) than at the lumbar and thoracic levels.

In the cervical region, the C7–T1 interspace is widest and easiest to access. In addition, the depth from the skin to the epidural space is larger at this interspace, and the distance from the epidural space to the dural sac is greater than at other cervical levels. However, using palpation and surface landmarks to identify the C7–T1 level is not always reliable; the vertebra prominens (presumed to be C7) is not uncommonly confused with C6 and T1 in certain patient populations. Single-shot injections at this level should be administered slowly. For continuous catheter techniques, the catheter is usually threaded no more than 2–3 cm.

Initiation and Management of Epidural Blockade

Test Dose

Before administering medications through the epidural catheter, subarachnoid, intravascular, and subdural placement should be ruled out. Although rare, catheter migration may occur after initial confirmation that the catheter is in the epidural space; each bolus should be preceded by confirmation of proper catheter location.

Although the efficacy of LA with epinephrine in detecting misplaced catheters has been questioned, many clinicians still routinely rely on the pharmacologic test dose. The classical dose combines 3 mL of 1.5% lidocaine with 15 μg of epinephrine. The intrathecal injection of 45 mg of lidocaine should produce a significant motor block if the catheter is in the subarachnoid space, although recent evidence suggests that this is not always reliable.[219] A change in heart rate of 20% or greater (or, alternatively, an increase in heart rate of 10 to 25 beats per minute) within 1 minute suggests that the catheter has been placed in (or has migrated into) a vessel and should be replaced. If the heart rate does not increase by 20% or greater or if a significant motor block does not develop within 5 minutes, the test dose is considered negative. Exceptions to this rule have been observed in laboring patients, anesthetized patients, and patients receiving β-adrenergic blocking agents. Relying on ECG changes after the test dose and the use of nerve stimulators[220] have been advocated as alternative methods to confirm epidural placement, although these methods also have shortcomings.

The safety and efficacy of the traditional test dose is debated in the literature. In laboring patients, a change in heart rate attributed to the epinephrine may in fact be due to a painful contraction, contributing to a false-positive interpretation. Alternatively, a true-positive test result in this patient population can result in an epinephrine-induced decrease in uterine blood flow. Patients with HTN, including women with preeclampsia, can experience a severe increase in blood pressure that may not be well tolerated after an intravenous dose of 15 μg of epinephrine. Volatile general anesthetics may interfere with the response to epinephrine and contribute to a high percentage of false-negative results in children, who are most commonly anesthetized during epidural placement. In patients on β-adrenergic blocking agents, heart rate changes may not be reliable. An increase in systolic blood pressure greater than 20 mm Hg has been used as an indicator of intravascular injection in this patient population.

Additional studies are needed to determine the optimal strategy to detect intrathecal and intravascular catheter placement. Fortunately, with the widespread use of low-concentration LA infusions for epidural analgesia, the risk of systemic LA toxicity is vastly reduced; the utility of a traditional test dose to evaluate for intravascular cannulation in this setting is limited. In addition, epidural catheter design innovations over the past several decades, particularly the introduction of flexible catheters, have contributed to a marked decrease in the incidence of both intrathecal catheter migration and epidural venous cannulation or migration. Nonetheless, incremental dosing of LA (ie, 3- to 5-mL aliquots), with simultaneous aspiration for blood and CSF and careful observation, is required when dosing an epidural. In the future, new methods of detecting misplaced catheters, such as acoustic signal guidance, nerve stimulation, and ultrasound-guided insertion, may replace the classical test dose.

Dosing Regimen

After the epidural catheter has been aspirated to check for blood or CSF or after a negative test dose, the catheter can be dosed to provide analgesia or anesthesia. As mentioned, LA concentration determines the density of block, while the volume and total dose of LA determine the spread. As a general guideline, the initial loading dose can be determined as follows: 1–2 mL of LA per segment to be blocked in a lumbar epidural, 0.7 mL per segment for a thoracic epidural, and 3 mL per segment for a caudal epidural. The loading dose should be administered through the catheter in 3- to 5-mL aliquots at 3- to 5-minute intervals, permitting time to assess the patient's response to dosing and to avoid systemic toxicity. Appropriate loading doses for postoperative analgesia include 10 mL of 0.2%–0.25% bupivacaine, levobupivacaine, or ropivacaine with or without adjuvants; however, patients may experience varying degrees of motor block. Recent evidence suggests that higher volumes of lower-concentration LAs may provide better spread and improved analgesia.[221] Up to 20 mL of 0.0625%–0.125% bupivacaine or the equipotent dose of ropivacaine may be administered incrementally as a loading dose. Higher-concentration LAs are required for surgical anesthesia. Up to 20 mL of 2% lidocaine, with or without epinephrine 1:200,000 and sodium bicarbonate, or 15 mL of 0.5% bupivacaine or ropivacaine may be used to initiate epidural anesthesia in the lumbar region.

Maintenance of the desired level of anesthesia can be accomplished through intermittent or continuous dosing after the initial loading dose. With manual boluses, one-quarter to one-third of the initial amount can be administered at timed intervals, depending on duration of action of the initial LA (ie, short, intermediate, or long acting), although several maintenance regimens are appropriate. Manual boluses are usually given during prolonged surgery; a continuous infusion, however, can be started after the initial bolus to maintain surgical anesthesia. Continuous infusions require the same diligent attention to the patient as any other anesthetic. The usual infusion rate is between 4 and 15 mL/h. The wide range is usually dependent on the age, weight, extent of sensory or motor blockade desired in a particular patient; site of catheter insertion; and the type and dose of LA. Thus, individualization is necessary, and a fixed rule cannot be applied for this purpose.

Patient-controlled epidural analgesia (PCEA), most commonly with infusions of low-concentration LAs and opioid adjuncts, are increasingly used for postoperative analgesia and for laboring patients. A demand bolus at timed intervals, with or without a loading dose and a background infusion, can be programmed to optimize patient comfort with less LA consumption.[222] Pumps that deliver automated mandatory boluses at timed intervals, with or without a basal infusion, have been developed, although they are not yet widely available.

For thoracic epidural blockade, several dosing regimens can be used to minimize hemodynamic changes and respiratory impairment (in awake patients). An initial dose of 3 to 6 mL of dilute bupivacaine 0.125%–0.25% or 0.1%–0.2% ropivacaine with or without fentanyl, hydromorphone, or preservative-free morphine can be followed by 3 mL of 0.25%–0.5% bupivacaine every 30 min. An alternative regimen is as follows: Administer a loading dose with 3–6 mL of 0.125% bupivacaine or 0.1%–0.2% ropivacaine with an opioid (fentanyl 2 µg/mL or hydromorphone 20 µg/mL) at least 30 minutes before the end of the case, as tolerated. Start an infusion of bupivacaine 0.0625% or 0.1% ropivacaine with fentanyl or hydromorphone at 3–5 mL/h before the patient leaves the operating room.

The level and duration of epidural anesthesia depends primarily on the injection site and the volume and concentration of the drug. Other factors such as age, pregnancy, and sex are less important factors but need to be considered. The addition of fresh epinephrine and 8.4% sodium bicarbonate to lidocaine, mepivacaine, and chloroprocaine will decrease the latency, improve the quality, and prolong the duration of the block. Epinephrine is less effective with the long-acting LAs. Adding bicarbonate to ropivacaine and bupivacaine can cause precipitation. The addition of opioids (eg, fentanyl) has been shown to improve the quality of the block without any effect on duration.

Top-Up Dosing

Repeat doses, commonly referred to as "top-ups," should be administered before the level of the block has receded more than two dermatomes. One-quarter to one-third or more of the original loading dose of LA can be administered for each repeat dose, although different top-up doses may be required for different clinical scenarios. For example, if the patient is comfortable but the sensory level is not adequate, a high-volume, low-concentration LA top-up may be appropriate. This may also be the case if the blockade is unilateral or patchy but the patient desires to maintain motor strength. However, if the patient requires a denser block for surgical anesthesia or for the second stage of labor, for example, less volume of a higher-concentration LA may be a better choice. Overall, the anesthesiologist must have a working knowledge of the characteristics of the LA used to properly implement a redosing protocol.

Problem Solving

Epidural placement presents unique challenges that are directly related to practitioner experience, the clinical scenario, and patient characteristics, among other things. Most of these problems can be overcome if the clinician recognizes the problem, is familiar with vertebral column anatomy, and knows how to make adjustments in technique (Table 24–27).

Difficulty Identifying the Epidural Space

Several troubleshooting measures may help if equivocal LOR occurs while trying to identify the epidural space. First, ensure that the LOR syringe is tightly connected to the epidural needle. If using the LOR to air technique, next put 2–3 mL of saline into the LOR syringe and push gently (ie, with the little finger). If using LOR to saline, omit the bubble for this step. The saline will flow easily if the tip of the epidural needle is in

TABLE 24–27. Problem solving during initiation of epidural blockade.

Problem	Possible Explanation	Action
Needle floppy; needle angles laterally	Entry off midline; missed supraspinous ligament	Reassess midline; redirect needle
Bone contact at < 2 cm	Contacted spinous process; spinal flexion inadequate	Reidentify interspace; place needle in caudal region of interspace
Bone contact at ≥ 4 cm	Needle entry too lateral; contacted lamina	Redirect needle toward midline
Bony resistance throughout	Ossified ligaments; arthritic spine	Consider paramedian approach
Inability to advance catheter	False loss of resistance; narrow epidural space; needle too close to dura mater; obstructed needle orifice	Fluid predistention; rotate needle bevel; use stiffer catheter; advance epidural needle slightly; attempt new placement at different interspace; withdraw needle to ligamentum flavum and readvance
Heme in catheter	Epidural vein cannulation; needle entry too lateral; engorged epidural veins	Withdraw catheter 1–2 cm and flush with saline; perform new placement if heme persists; consider initiating epidural procedure in lateral position
Warm, clear fluid return in needle or catheter	Accidental dural puncture; intrathecal placement	Distinguish cerebrospinal fluid from saline or local anesthetic; if cerebrospinal fluid, consider continuous spinal or new placement at different interspace
Pain/paresthesia on catheter insertion	Catheter advanced > 6 cm into epidural space; catheter near nerve root	Withdraw catheter to < 6 cm in epidural space (2–3 cm for short surgical procedures); perform new placement if pain persists
Inability to palpate spinous processes	Obesity; severe arthritis; patient with previous back surgery	Optimize patient position; consider midline approach for obese patients; use long finder needle to help identify bony landmarks; consider placement in lateral position if patient unable to flex spine; use ultrasonography
Inability to flex spine	Elderly; arthritis; patient with previous spinal instrumentation	Consider paramedian approach; consider placement in lateral position
Curvature of spine	Scoliosis	Use ultrasonography; if possible, perform procedure below level of curvature (otherwise direct needle into curve)

the epidural space but will encounter resistance if the needle tip is in soft tissue. If resistance is met, continue injecting the saline into the soft tissue and then resume the original LOR technique. Often, the familiar feedback from the LOR syringe returns after saline has dissipated throughout the soft tissue planes.

Another method to distinguish between soft tissue and the epidural space during the LOR to saline technique is to place a small bubble in the LOR syringe. The bubble should compress to varying degrees when the epidural needle is in soft tissue or ligament but will inject effortlessly if the needle is in the epidural space.

If LOR is still equivocal, insert a 25- or 27-gauge spinal needle through the epidural needle to puncture the dura. If

CSF is visible in the spinal needle, the epidural needle is properly placed. The absence of CSF indicates that the epidural space has not yet been encountered or that the epidural needle is off midline, in the lateral epidural space.

If LOR remains equivocal, attempt to thread the catheter. Many catheters, particularly flexible or wire-reinforced versions, will not advance if the epidural needle is not fully in the epidural space.

Paresthesias During Epidural Needle or Catheter Placement

Patients not uncommonly report paresthesias during epidural procedures, particularly on direct questioning by the clinician. Because a paresthesia indicates that the needle or catheter is near a nerve, the needle should be withdrawn and redirected if the sensation persists. Alternatively, the epidural procedure can be initiated at another interspace. Most often, however, the needle can simply be redirected away from the side where the paresthesia was detected. During catheter placement, fluid predistention may help to reduce the incidence of paresthesias, although the data are conflicting. Threading the catheter no more than 5–6 cm appears to reduce the risk of paresthesias. The use of flexible catheters and, in particular, wire-reinforced catheters also appears to reduce the incidence of paresthesias. If a paresthesia is transient, it is acceptable to continue advancing the needle or threading the catheter.

Accidental Dural Puncture

Accidental dural puncture complicates an estimated 1% of epidural procedures, although the reported incidence varies substantially in the literature. Management options include placing a continuous spinal catheter or withdrawing the epidural needle and repeating the epidural procedure at a different interspace. Whether a spinal catheter is placed or a new epidural placement is performed, the choice should be made quickly to avoid excessive egress of CSF through the large-bore epidural needle. A continuous spinal technique may have the slight advantage of reducing the incidence of PDPH and the need for an EBP (see discussion that follows), although the data are limited and conflicting.[223,224] In cases in which identification of the epidural space was difficult or with high-risk patients (eg, obese parturients with a high likelihood of conversion to cesarean delivery and surgical patients with anticipated difficult airways), placing a continuous spinal catheter may also be advantageous. This option avoids the risk of a second dural puncture and has been reported to provide reliable analgesia and anesthesia, although the data are conflicting. Disadvantages of threading a continuous spinal catheter include the risk of an accidental injection of large doses of LA intended for the epidural space and, possibly, an increased risk of infection. Protocols should be in place to alert all providers when a spinal catheter has been placed.

If the practitioner elects to place the epidural at another interspace, he or she incurs the risk of a second ADP. Also, there is a concern for LA passage from the epidural to the subarachnoid space via the dural breach, resulting in a higher-than-anticipated block. Although it may not be necessary, it is reasonable to reduce the basal rate for continuous or PCEA pumps; as always, use caution when injecting boluses of LA or epidural morphine. The evidence does not support the use of the epidural catheter for a prophylactic EBP,[225] although more recent studies may demonstrate some benefit. More elaborate considerations of the anatomy, pathophysiology, and treatment of PDPH are discussed in Chapter 27.

Difficulty Threading the Catheter

Difficulty threading the catheter is not uncommon, even if the needle is properly engaged in the epidural space. This problem is more common with flexible, soft-tipped catheters. Troubleshooting measures include confirming that the epidural needle is properly positioned in the epidural space (see previous discussion); injecting several milliliters of saline to "open" the epidural space; advancing the epidural needle slightly so that the entire bevel is engaged in the epidural space (the LOR syringe with saline without an air bubble should be attached during this step); rotating the bevel of the epidural needle; inserting a different, less-flexible catheter; retracting the needle to the ligament and identifying the epidural space again; and repeating the epidural procedure at a different spinal level. Occasionally, the epidural needle is plugged with tissue debris that blocks the passage of the catheter. Replacing and then removing the stylet may serve to remove the obstructing debris. The subatmospheric pressure is variable in the lumbar region; asking the patient to take a deep breath is unlikely to facilitate catheter threading, particularly when with flexible, wire-reinforced catheters. Overall, performing a new placement at another interspace appears to confer less risk of ADP than rotating the needle or cautiously advancing the epidural needle. If electing to start over at another interspace, withdraw the needle and the catheter simultaneously to avoid shearing of the catheter.

Unilateral Block

After an epidural has been dosed adequately, the patient may complain that one side is densely blocked, while the opposite side has intact pain and motor function. The most common explanation for a unilateral block is that the catheter has advanced too far into the epidural space, permitting the tip of the catheter to enter the intervertebral foramen or be in close proximity to a nerve. Current data suggest that there is no indication to advance a catheter (either single end hole or multiorifice) more than 6 cm into the epidural space. If a unilateral block persists despite appropriate depth of insertion, consider pulling the catheter back 1–2 cm, leaving 3–4 cm (2–3 cm for short procedures) in the epidural space. If the patient remains uncomfortable despite catheter manipulation, place the patient in the lateral position with the unblocked side down and administer several milliliters of dilute LA. If these maneuvers have no effect, replace the catheter.

Blood in the Epidural Needle or Catheter

Epidural vein cannulation is not uncommon, although the incidence has declined substantially with the widespread use of flexible catheters. The epidural veins lie primarily in the anterior epidural space, cordoned off by the posterior longitudinal ligament and its fascia. A bloody tap may be an indication that needle or catheter insertion is too lateral and should be redirected toward midline. Other measures to minimize the risk of epidural vein cannulation during catheter insertion include the use of wire-reinforced catheters, the administration of fluid to open the epidural space prior to threading the catheter, and avoiding catheter insertion beyond 5–6 cm, among others (see Local Anesthetic Systemic Toxicity). If blood returns through the catheter despite these measures, the catheter can be withdrawn slightly and flushed with saline. This can be repeated until either the blood ceases to return or there is insufficient length of catheter in the epidural space, at which point the catheter must be replaced.

Pain Despite Adequate Block Height and Density

Persistent pain despite adequate block height and density may be a result of incomplete blockade ("window" of pain), "patchy" blockade, or poor sacral spread. A window of pain in which a distinct, small area remains unblocked despite an otherwise dense block may be difficult to troubleshoot. It is reasonable to administer top-ups and turn the patient with the window side of the catheter down. Injecting opioids into the epidural space may also help. However, performing a CSE technique that provides density from the spinal portion or replacing the epidural at another interspace may be required. Extreme caution should be exercised when deciding to perform CSE anesthetic in case of failed epidural anesthesia as there may be a higher risk of high spinal anesthesia. Wherever possible, a continuous spinal catheter with gradual dosing of the spinal anesthetic should be considered.

A "spotty" or "patchy" block may result from the injection of air when using the LOR to air technique, from individual anatomic variations that contribute to "missed" dermatomes, or from catheter migration. Administering additional LA, with or without an opioid, after a sufficient amount of time has elapsed since the initial dose is appropriate. It may also help to withdraw the catheter 1–2 cm and place the patient with the less-blocked side in the dependent position. However, it is also reasonable to replace the catheter, particularly if multiple top-ups have been administered and if there is a high likelihood of conversion to surgical anesthesia.

In the case of poor sacral spread, the following measures may help: Raise the head of the bed and redose the catheter with a more highly concentrated LA; administer 100 µg of epidural fentanyl to improve the quality of the block; or inject preservative-free neostigmine 500–750 µg or clonidine 75 µg epidurally. Replacing a stand-alone epidural with a CSE also improves sacral analgesia, as the sacral nerve is large and occasionally difficult to block with LAs administered in the epidural space.

Inadequate Analgesia Despite Fully Dosed Epidural Catheter

Most often, the best strategy is to replace the epidural catheter. To assess whether an epidural is functioning properly, feel whether both legs are warm to touch (LA-induced vasodilation should make the lower extremities warm if the epidural is properly placed and fully functioning). Assess also whether the patient has decreased temperature perception and decreased response to pinprick in the dermatomes that correspond to the expected sensory blockade. Consider administering a definitive dose of LA (eg, 5–10 mL of 2% lidocaine with or without epinephrine in incremental doses) to determine whether the catheter is functioning, provided that the resulting motor blockade is not contraindicated. Evaluate the patient's motor strength and temperature and pain perception after each dose. Monitor vital signs for any indication of sympathectomy-induced hypotension. It is advisable not to administer more than 10 mL of LA if the catheter remains equivocal; removing the catheter and performing a spinal anesthetic incurs the risk of a high or total spinal if an excessive amount of LA has already been administered epidurally. Recent evidence suggests that the number of

top-ups is a reliable indicator of whether an epidural used for analgesia can be successfully used for surgical anesthesia.[226] If several top-ups have been administered and the degree of analgesia remains equivocal, the catheter should be removed and replaced.

Dissipating Block Requiring Larger Doses

This problem occurs for several possible reasons. Patients who received CSEs with either spinal fentanyl or a combination of opioid and LA may experience an abrupt transition from relief to an inadequate epidural block, particularly if the spinal anesthetic has resolved before a sufficient volume of the epidural infusion has accumulated. Increasingly larger doses of LA per epidural may be required to compensate for the inadequate epidural loading dose and to meet high patient expectations after experiencing the comfort of the spinal portion. Alternatively, if the epidural catheter has been used for analgesia and has been dosed frequently, tachyphylaxis to the LA can occur. Another possibility is that the catheter has migrated into a vessel (see previous discussion) or become completely dislodged from the epidural space. If the catheter remains in its initial insertion site, administer a bolus of higher-concentration LA and increase the infusion rate (if continuous). Consider adding an opioid or clonidine to enhance the quality of the block.

Failed Epidural Analgesia

The problem of failed epidural analgesia is often seen in obstetrics. An epidural catheter is placed and dosed, but the patient remains uncomfortable. More LA is administered, with subjective improvement. Subsequently, the patient is taken to the operating room for cesarean delivery, which requires a dense T4 sensory level, and the block is inadequate.

Several options exist if an epidural fails despite troubleshooting measures. In elective situations, the epidural catheter can be replaced, preferably at a different interspace, and cautiously redosed to decrease the risk of high epidural blockade. For more urgent procedures, a CSE can be performed. A reduced dose of spinal medication is necessary if a large volume of epidural LA was administered while troubleshooting or if the patient has a partial block. With a CSE, the sensory level can be raised as necessary with supplemental epidural dosing. A reduced dose single-shot spinal may also be appropriate if speed of onset is a concern. However, replacing a failed epidural with a spinal technique incurs the risk of high or total spinal anesthesia. Infiltrating the skin and subcutaneous tissue with LA or performing a peripheral nerve block, depending on the time remaining in the surgery and the type of surgery, may provide alternatives. Conversion to GA is appropriate if there is insufficient time to repeat the neuraxial technique or to place a peripheral block or if performing another neuraxial procedure presents undue risk.

Optimally, a nonfunctioning epidural will be recognized and replaced before large doses of LA have been administered and before alternative anesthetic techniques are required. The number of boluses required to maintain adequate analgesia is a reliable indicator that an epidural used for analgesia may fail on conversion to surgical anesthesia. As a general rule, if catheter function remains equivocal during dosing, stop injecting after a predetermined volume (eg, 10 mL) to ensure that performing another regional technique does not lead to high or total spinal anesthesia or to LA systemic toxicity (LAST).

Difficulty Removing the Epidural Catheter

Occasionally, resistance is met on attempted removal of the epidural catheter. Using excessive force may lead to catheter breakage and retained catheter fragments. In the event of catheter entrapment, placing the patient in the lateral decubitus position or in the original insertion position and applying continuous, gentle traction may facilitate removal. Sometimes, positioning the patient in the identical position in which the catheter was inserted may be necessary. Taping the catheter to the skin under traction and reattempting removal later, threading a stylet, and injecting saline into a wire-reinforced catheter have also been observed to assist in removal. Reports of neurologic sequelae from retained fragments are rare, suggesting that surgical removal is unwarranted in the asymptomatic patient.

COMPLICATIONS AND COMMON SIDE EFFECTS

Complications of epidural blockade can be classified broadly as either drug or procedure related. Potential drug-related complications include LAST, allergy to LAs, direct LA-induced nervous tissue injury, and drug or mode of delivery errors. Procedure-related complications may be mild to moderate or transient, such as back pain, pneumocephalus, and PDPH. Potentially life-threatening complications include subdural injection of LAs, total or high spinal, infectious or aseptic meningitis, cardiac arrest, SEA, epidural hematoma formation, and permanent neurologic injuries. In contrast to complications, several known or expected side effects accompany initiation and maintenance of epidural blockade without adversely affecting long-term patient outcomes. This section reviews both the complications and the common side effects associated with epidural blockade, with emphasis on risk factors, preventive measures, and treatment. Several of the complications are covered in greater detail elsewhere in this textbook.

Local Anesthetic Systemic Toxicity

Local anesthetic systemic toxicity results from excessive plasma concentration in the blood due to unintentional intravascular injection or, less commonly, systemic absorption from the injection site.[227] Direct intravascular injection can occur with unintentional epidural vein cannulation during catheter placement or subsequent catheter migration into a vessel. Risk factors for intravascular cannulation include trauma to the epidural vessels during block initiation, the use of stiff catheters, pregnancy, and patient positioning during epidural placement, among others (Table 24–28). The risk of epidural vein cannulation in obstetric patients may be reduced with initiation of epidural blockade in the lateral position, the use of wire-reinforced catheters, the use of a single end-hole (versus multiorifice) catheters, fluid predistention with normal saline prior to threading the catheter, and limiting the depth of catheter

TABLE 24–28. Risk factors for epidural vein cannulation.

Trauma to epidural vessels during block initiation
Multiple attempts at placement
Stiff, nonflexible catheter
Engorged epidural veins (eg, pregnancy)
Sitting position

insertion to 6 cm or less (Table 24–29).[228] Limiting the number of attempts at epidural placement; avoiding the lateral epidural space, where vessel puncture is more likely; and avoiding direct administration of LAs through the epidural needle may also reduce the risk of direct intravascular injection.

Although the data are inconclusive regarding the role of catheter material and tip configuration, the use of flexible catheters may reduce the risk of subsequent catheter migration into a vessel. Because of preferential efflux from the proximal port of multiport catheters during continuous infusion techniques, there remains a remote possibility that a distal port may migrate into a vessel unnoticed until a manual bolus is administered. This can be avoided with the use of a single-orifice catheter.

Dosing the epidural catheter in 3- to 5-mL increments with frequent negative aspiration for blood and CSF is recommended to detect misplaced catheters. Most commercially available epidural catheters have distal and proximal "flashback" windows to facilitate visualization of blood or CSF on aspiration. The use of a transparent dressing and tape improves visualization of these windows. Although the use of the traditional epinephrine test dose is controversial, a test dose may be used to assess whether the catheter tip is in a blood vessel.

The degree of systemic absorption is determined in part by the site of injection, the dose and concentration of LA injected, properties of the LA administered, the vascularity of the injection site, and the presence or absence of epinephrine in the solution. Certain conditions and comorbidities, such as advanced age, liver failure, low plasma protein concentration, severe cardiac dysfunction, ischemic heart disease, cardiac conduction abnormalities, and metabolic and respiratory acidosis, may also predispose patients to systemic toxicity.[229] In general, systemic absorption from the epidural space is less likely to

TABLE 24–29. Strategies to avoid epidural vein cannulation.

Placement in lateral position
Use of flexible, wire-reinforced catheter
Use of single- versus multiorifice catheter
Fluid predistention prior to threading the catheter
Limit depth of catheter insertion to < 6 cm

TABLE 24–30. Relative order of peak plasma concentration of local anesthetic associated with regional anesthesia (descending order).

Intercostal

Caudal

Paracervical

Epidural

Brachial plexus

Sciatic/femoral

TABLE 24–31. Signs and symptoms of local anesthatic systemic toxicity.

Central Nervous System Toxicity	Cardiovascular Toxicity
Perioral tingling and numbness	Hypotension
Lightheadedness/dizziness	Peripheral vasodilation
Tinnitus	Bradycardia, conduction delays
Visual disturbances	Ventricular dysrhythmias
Restlessness, agitation	Cardiac arrest
Slurred speech	
Shivering	
Generalized seizures	
Respiratory depression/arrest	

occur than from areas of higher vascularity. The areas of highest plasma concentration from absorption in descending order are as follows: intercostal, caudal, paracervical, epidural, brachial plexus, and sciatic/femoral (Table 24–30). However, trauma to the vessels during initiation of the epidural procedure may lead to more rapid intravascular absorption from the epidural space than anticipated. The addition of epinephrine to the LA solution diminishes systemic absorption but may not be appropriate in highly vascular areas, where systemic absorption is likely, or for all patient populations. Epinephrine may also unnecessarily prolong the duration of action of LAs. Toxicity associated with systemic absorption of LAs can be reduced by careful patient selection, remaining vigilant for signs and symptoms of toxicity, limiting the total dose of LA administered, use of appropriate LA concentrations, and, possibly, by using the newer amide LAs, such as ropivacaine and levobupivacaine. Racemic bupivacaine has been associated with greater cardiotoxicity due to enhanced binding to and slower dissociation from ion channels in the myocardium.

Early CNS signs and symptoms of LA toxicity include lightheadedness, dizziness, tinnitus, perioral numbness and tingling, slurred speech, diplopia or blurred vision, restlessness, and confusion. Muscle twitching, tremors of the facial muscles and extremities, shivering, and generalized seizures occur at higher plasma concentrations, followed by global CNS depression, as manifested by drowsiness, unconsciousness, and respiratory arrest. Acidosis, hypercarbia, and hypoxia both predispose to and exacerbate CNS toxicity. Cardiovascular manifestations at high plasma concentrations include hypotension, bradycardia and other arrhythmias, and cardiac arrest (Table 24–31).

When LAST is recognized or suspected, refrain from administering additional LA and call for assistance. Treatment requires immediate attention to airway support, suppression of seizure activity, and preparedness for cardiopulmonary resuscitation and, possibly, CPB. Current guidelines recommend limiting individual epinephrine doses to less than 1 μg/kg during resuscitative efforts. Lipid emulsion (20%) therapy should be commenced with an initial loading dose of 1.5 mL/kg, followed by a continuous infusion of 0.25 mL/kg/min for a minimum of 10 minutes after circulatory stability has been restored.[229] Refer to Chapter 65 for a more detailed discussion of LAST.

Allergy to Local Anesthetics

True allergic reactions to LAs can occur, but fortunately are rare. Most documented reactions are not mediated by immunoglobulin E (IgE) and can be attributed to reactions to other agents administered concomitantly (eg, additives, epinephrine, preservatives, antibiotics) or to a delayed type IV hypersensitivity reaction (ie, mild contact dermatitis). Alternatively, reported reactions may be due to anxiety, a vasovagal episode, endogenous sympathetic stimulation, or an adverse patient response to the surgical, dental, ophthalmic, or obstetric procedure itself. Based on an extensive review of the literature, Bhole and colleagues estimated the prevalence of true IgE-mediated allergy to be less than 1%.[230] An immune complex–mediated reaction associated with reduced or depleted serum complement levels is even rarer.

When a patient reports a history of allergy to LAs, it is important to elicit a detailed history, including which LA was implicated, the dose and route of administration, the reaction that occurred, and the clinical setting. True allergic reactions may present with a range of dermatologic, cardiac, or respiratory signs and symptoms, such as hives, pruritus, angioedema, hypotension, shock, and bronchospasm. Although the current literature suggests that allergic reactions to amide LAs are more common than reactions to ester-linkage-type LAs, this may reflect the current preferential use of the former. Historically, adverse reactions, especially contact dermatitis, have been reported more often with ester agents, such as procaine, benzocaine, tetracaine, and chloroprocaine. This may be partly attributable to the fact that ester compounds are derivatives of para-aminobenzoic acid (PABA), an additive found in many household items (eg, lotion, sunscreen, cosmetics); previous exposure to PABA has been hypothesized to sensitize individuals to ester LAs. Alternatively, methylparaben, a preservative in both amide and ester LAs that is metabolized to

PABA, may account for many of the reported allergic reactions. Cross-reactivity between the amide and ester groups has been reported, but is exceedingly rare and likely attributable to a common preservative. Cross-reactivity can occur between ester LAs and, less commonly, between amide LAs.

Reliable tests to identify sensitivity to LAs are currently lacking. The presence of serum mast cell tryptase can confirm an anaphylactic reaction in the immediate aftermath, while skin prick testing, intradermal testing, and subcutaneous challenge tests may help identify the causative agent. Management of an allergic reaction to LAs includes removing the offending agent; early administration of intravenous epinephrine to treat hypotension and cardiovascular collapse; airway support, if necessary; and, possibly, intravenous administration of histamine-1 and -2 receptor blockers, bronchodilators, and corticosteroids.

Arachnoiditis

Arachnoiditis is a rare disorder marked by inflammatory changes in the arachnoid mater. Although the precise mechanism remains unclear, fibrosis develops and adhesions form between the nerve roots and the membranes that surround the brain, spinal cord, and cauda equina. In chronic, adhesive cases, collagen deposits ultimately encapsulate the nerve roots, creating nerve root atrophy as a result of an interruption to the blood supply.[231] Trauma, surgery, infections, contaminants, disinfectants, contrast media, tumors, subarachnoid hemorrhage, and the subarachnoid administration of irritants (eg, steroids) can precipitate these inflammatory changes. Accidental intrathecal administration of large volumes of chloroprocaine containing the preservative sodium bisulfite has also been linked to arachnoiditis, although the role of the preservative has been called into question in recent studies.[232]

A link between epidural block or catheter placement and arachnoiditis has not been clearly established in the literature. No data exist on the risk of arachnoiditis with the use of the antiseptic solution chlorhexidine in humans[233]; nonetheless, it is prudent to keep the solution away from all drugs and equipment in the spinal and epidural kits and to permit it to dry before initiating neuraxial procedures. Chlorhexidine in alcohol remains the solution of choice for skin disinfection prior to initiation of central neuraxial blockade.

The clinical presentation of arachnoiditis is complex, with varied symptomatology, and may be delayed for several months. The most common clinical features are back pain that radiates to the lower extremities and increases on exertion; buttocks pain; muscle spasms; decreased range of motion of the trunk; sensory abnormalities; motor weakness or paralysis below the level of injury that does not typically progress; and urinary sphincter dysfunction (Table 24–32).[234]

Unfortunately, the mixed clinical presentation can lead to misdiagnosis, and arachnoiditis may be attributed incorrectly to spinal stenosis, lumbar disk disease, spinal tumors, or other compressive lesions of the spine. Diagnosis can be confirmed by myelography, computed tomography (CT), or MRI. Characteristic MRI findings show conglomerations of roots residing centrally in the dural sac, adhesions tethering the nerve roots peripherally, and soft tissue replacing the subarachnoid space.[235]

TABLE 24–32. Clinical presentation of arachnoiditis.

Back pain radiating to lower extremities, worsens with activity

Buttocks pain

Muscle spasms

Motor weakness/paralysis

Decreased range of motion of trunk

Urinary sphincter dysfunction

Unfortunately, significant neurologic improvement is unlikely with current therapies, including intravenous corticosteroids, NSAIDs, and antibiotic therapy. Deficits may progress to severe and permanent disability.

Backache

Back pain is a common postoperative complaint, with an incidence that ranges from 3% to 31% after nonobstetric surgery, regardless of the anesthetic technique.[236] Although the etiology is multifactorial, both postoperative and peripartum back pain are often attributed to neuraxial techniques when a temporal association exists.

Backache after epidural blockade is more common, more severe, and longer lasting than after spinal procedures. Local trauma, inflammation of the ligaments, needle puncture of an intervertebral disk, stretching of the joint capsules and ligaments beyond their physiologic range, and muscle spasm may account for some of the reported postepidural back pain. The use of larger needles, the insertion of catheters, and the increased volume of LAs, when compared with spinal techniques, may also play a role. Large epidural doses of 2-chloroprocaine containing the preservative EDTA have also been associated with back pain[237]; similar complications have not been observed with preservative-free 2-chloroprocaine. In a recent study, Hakim and colleagues identified the following independent risk factors for persistent (ie, ≥3 months) low-back pain after nonobstetric surgery with epidural anesthesia: multiple attempts at epidural placement, higher body mass index (BMI), surgery in the lithotomy position, and surgical time exceeding 2.5 hours.[238]

Back pain after epidural blockade is usually self-limiting and should resolve within 7–10 days. Patients should be encouraged to refrain from bed rest. NSAIDs, acetaminophen, or heat may provide symptomatic relief. If pain persists, progresses, or is out of proportion to what might be expected, other etiologies, such as TNS, herniated disk, spinal stenosis, arachnoiditis, sacroiliitis, musculoskeletal injury, nerve injury, epidural abscess, and epidural hematoma, should be considered. Prophylactic interventions that may help prevent back pain associated with epidural procedures include performing a field block to anesthetize the recurrent spinal nerves that innervate the interspinous ligaments and muscles prior to initiating epidural blockade[239]; adding NSAIDs to the LA used for skin infiltration[236]; and administering epidural dexamethasone.[240]

Despite the widespread association between musculoskeletal back pain and neuraxial procedures, studies of pregnant women who have received epidural analgesia for labor pain provide compelling evidence that back pain is unrelated to neuraxial techniques. Several randomized controlled trials and prospective cohort studies have shown that new, long-term postpartum back pain is not caused by intrapartum epidural analgesia.[241]

Postdural Puncture Headache

Postdural puncture headache is a common complication of spinal anesthesia, lumbar punctures ("spinal taps"), and epidural procedures complicated by ADP or unrecognized dural tear. The incidence of ADP is generally accepted to be at or below 1%; up to 80% of patients may experience PDPH following ADP. Although the precise mechanism remains poorly understood, signs and symptoms of PDPH appear to result from CSF leakage through the dural hole. In the upright position, the brain tissue sags in the cranial vault, creating painful traction on the dura, falx cerebri, cerebral blood vessels, tentorium, cranial nerves, and nerve roots.[242] This traction also contributes to the cranial nerve palsies that are not uncommonly seen in patients with PDPH.[243] Compensatory cerebral vasodilation in response to the decrease in CSF also appears to play a role in the genesis and severity of PDPH.

A universally accepted definition of PDPH is lacking in the literature. According to the International Headache Society, a PDPH develops within 5 days of a lumbar puncture, is usually accompanied by neck stiffness or subjective hearing symptoms, and resolves spontaneously within 2 weeks or after effective treatment with an EBP.[244] Clinically, patients commonly complain of a fronto-occipital headache that is mild or absent in the supine position and intensifies when the head is elevated. The pain may extend into the neck, shoulders, and upper extremities and may be accompanied by nausea and vomiting, dizziness, diplopia, tinnitus, blurred vision, nystagmus, and hearing loss. Cranial nerve involvement should prompt expeditious evaluation and treatment. The headache develops within 48 hours in the vast majority of cases (most commonly in the first 24 hours) (Table 24–33). Headaches that occur during or immediately after epidural procedures are more likely due to

accidental injection of air during identification of the epidural space with the LOR to air technique (pneumocephalus). PDPH typically resolves spontaneously within 1 to 2 weeks but may last months or even years; a substantial percentage of patients may develop chronic headaches after ADP with a large-bore Tuohy needle.[245]

Risk factors for PDPH include younger age, female gender, lower BMI, pregnancy, pushing during the second stage of labor, the use of cutting versus atraumatic spinal needles, and the use of larger-gauge needles (Table 24–34). There is less-compelling evidence regarding the role of needle bevel orientation, the number of dural punctures, the approach used to enter the epidural space (paramedian vs. midline), patient positioning during initiation of the epidural procedure, and the technique used to identify the epidural space (LOR to air versus saline with or without an air bubble).

Several interventions for the prevention or treatment of PDPH have been proposed. There appears to be little benefit from conservative measures, such as bed rest and aggressive fluid administration. However, symptomatic relief may be obtained with analgesics, pharmacologic agents with vasoconstricting properties (caffeine, theophylline, sumatriptan), and, possibly, corticotropin (ACTH). In a quantitative systematic review of available evidence for measures to prevent PDPH, Apfel et al found that the administration of epidural morphine prior to removal of the catheter may confer some advantage, but this conclusion was based on one small randomized controlled trial.[246] In a recent meta-analysis, Heesen et al. suggested that insertion of an intrathecal catheter following ADP may protect against PDPH and may reduce the need for an EBP, but additional studies are warranted.[223] The evidence to date regarding the routine use of prophylactic EBP is not conclusive.[225] There are limited data to support epidural patching with normal saline, dextran 40, and gelatin and fibrin glue.

Epidural blood patch, preferably early in the course of the headache, remains the gold standard for treatment. Observational studies reported rapid recovery in over 90% of patients after EBP, although relief may be transient in a small percentage of these patients.[247] A well-designed, randomized controlled trial in neurology patients demonstrated that EBP offers complete resolution of symptoms in a large percentage of patients and reduces the severity of symptoms in those who do not experience complete resolution.[248] In addition, early treatment with an EBP

TABLE 24–33. Signs and symptoms of postdural puncture headache.

Fronto-occipital headache; intensifies when head is elevated
Neck stiffness
Neck, shoulder, and/or arm pain
Tinnitus, hearing loss
Nausea, vomiting, dizziness
Diplopia, blurred vision, nystagmus

TABLE 24–34. Risk factors for postdural puncture headache.

Younger age
Female gender
Low body mass index
Loss of resistance to air
Pushing during second stage of labor
Use of cutting needle
Use of larger-gauge needle

decreases the length of hospital stay and emergency room visits and permits patients to resume their activities of daily living sooner than otherwise feasible with expectant management.[249]

Prior to performing an EBP, other causes of headache, such as preeclampsia/eclampsia and meningitis, should be ruled out. In certain clinical scenarios, it may also be necessary to rule out elevated ICP. Using sterile techniques, the epidural space at or below the level of prior ADP is identified using LOR to normal saline. The air bubble is omitted due to the concern that air may enter the dural breach, leading to pneumocephalus. Up to 20 mL of the patient's blood (drawn aseptically) is slowly injected into the space; the clinician should stop injecting blood if the patient experiences moderate-to-severe pain or pressure in the lower back or neck region. Although the optimal volume of blood remains to be determined, injection of more than 20 mL appears to confer no additional benefit.[250] The patient typically remains supine for at least 1 hour after the EBP. Back pain and, less frequently, neck pain are commonly experienced during the procedure and, when severe, may alert the clinician to stop injecting blood. To minimize the risk of infections and related sequelae, both the acquisition of autologous blood and identification of the epidural space should be performed using strict aseptic techniques. For a more in-depth discussion of PDPH, refer to Chapter 27.

Subdural Injection

The subdural space has been described historically as a potential space between the normally closely adherent arachnoid mater and the overlying dura mater, although it may represent a cleft along the dural border cell layer that results only from direct tissue damage.[251] Injection of a small dose of LA into the area can have profound hemodynamic and sympatholytic effects.

Subdural injection is a relatively rare occurrence, with an estimated incidence of 0.1%–0.82% of epidural injections.[252] Clinical features that may help to distinguish subdural from epidural or spinal anesthesia include a higher-than-expected sensory blockade with poor caudal spread and sacral sparing; a higher-than-anticipated level of motor blockade of variable density; and a speed of onset that more closely resembles epidural anesthesia (10–20 minutes). Subdural injections commonly result in bilateral blockade, although unilateral or patchy blocks can occur, with more notable sensory and motor changes in the upper extremities and inadequate analgesia and anesthesia in the lower extremities. Patients may develop Horner syndrome (ptosis, miosis, and anhidrosis), facial and corneal anesthesia, and dyspnea. In addition, mild-to-moderate hypotension may develop (Table 24–35). Treatment may require cardiovascular and respiratory support, including the administration of intravenous fluid and vasopressors and, possibly, endotracheal intubation with mechanical ventilation. However, case reports have described the use of subdural catheters to attain surgical anesthesia.

Total Spinal Anesthesia

Total spinal blockade, which complicates an estimated 1 in 1400 attempted epidural procedures[253] may result from

TABLE 24–35. Clinical presentation of a subdural block.

Higher-than-expected sensory blockade

Poor caudal spread, sacral sparing

Higher-than-expected motor blockade of variable density

Blockade usually bilateral, but may be unilateral or asymmetric

Horner syndrome (ptosis, miosis, anhidrosis)

Facial and corneal anesthesia

Dyspnea

Hypotension

unrecognized ADP with unintentional injection of an epidural dose of LA, the administration of a large dose of LA into the subdural compartment, and undetected migration of the epidural catheter tip into the subarachnoid space. It has also been observed when one hole of a multiorifice catheter is lodged in the subarachnoid space; with translocation of LA through an accidental or intentional dural breach; after CSE techniques; and after a failed epidural blockade is replaced with a spinal technique.[254]

Total spinal anesthesia usually develops within minutes of LA administration, although it may occur unexpectedly later with changes in patient positioning or after a previously functioning epidural catheter has migrated into the subarachnoid space. During total spinal blockade, the LA spreads high enough to block the entire spinal cord and, occasionally, the brainstem. Ascending sensory and motor changes develop rapidly, followed by profound hypotension, bradycardia, dyspnea, and difficulty phonating and swallowing. Unconsciousness and apnea may result from direct LA action on the brainstem, respiratory muscle paralysis, and cerebral hypoperfusion. Treatment includes airway support and, if necessary, endotracheal intubation; the administration of 100% oxygen; and hemodynamic support with intravenous fluids and vasopressors. Epinephrine should be used early and in escalating doses to stabilize the heart rate and blood pressure in unstable patients. As the block recedes, the patient will regain consciousness and control of breathing followed by recovery of motor and sensory function. The administration of sedation until the block regresses may be appropriate once the patient is stable.

Total spinal anesthesia can usually be avoided during continuous epidural catheter techniques by careful administration of LA in small, divided doses, with frequent aspiration and, possibly, the use of an epidural test dose. Patients should be monitored during top-ups, during incremental dosing to attain surgical anesthesia, and while on PCEAs. Unusual patient complaints and unexpected hemodynamic changes may warrant immediate removal and replacement of the catheter. If unintentional dural puncture is recognized during needle placement, the needle can be removed and placed at another interspace or a spinal catheter can be inserted. If ADP is recognized after catheter insertion, either proceeding with a continuous spinal technique or repeating the epidural procedure at another interspace is appropriate. A reduced dose of LA may be required if a catheter is successfully placed at a different spinal level after a prior dural puncture. If a spinal catheter is placed, the catheter should be clearly labeled, the infusion pump should be labeled and configured at a reduced dose, and all practitioners involved should be informed. Optimally, procedures and policies should be in place regarding management of spinal catheters.

Spinal Epidural Abscess

Spinal epidural abscess is a rare disorder that affects elderly and immunocompromised patients disproportionately.[255] Individuals with prolonged intensive care unit stays, intravenous drug users, and patients with bacteremia, DM, alcohol dependence, cancer, HIV, and end-stage renal disease are at increased risk compared with the general population (Table 24–36). In recent decades, the incidence of SEA has increased, in part due to the increase in spinal instrumentation, the rise of illicit drug use, and the aging population.[256,257]

An estimated 5% of SEAs are associated with epidural procedures.[258] Risk factors for this rare complication include extended epidural catheter infusions and localized or systemic infection at the time of initiation of the block. The site of epidural placement also appears to place some patients at higher risk for SEA formation, with thoracic and lumbar catheters implicated more often than cervical catheters.[256] Poor adherence to sterile technique and, possibly, multiple attempts at epidural placement may place patients at additional risk.

Bacteria gain access to the epidural space through either hematogenous spread (most commonly) or contiguous spread; the source of access is not identified in the remainder of the cases. *Staphylococcus aureus* and, increasingly, methicillin-resistant *S. aureus* (MRSA) account for the vast majority of the SEA cases. Pathogens that are less commonly involved include *Escherichia coli*, *Pseudomonas aeruginosa*, and *Staphylococcus*

epidermidis, with the last more commonly associated with neuraxial procedures, including epidural blockade and epidural steroid injections. The infection appears to injure the spinal cord via direct mechanical compression or thrombosis (vascular occlusion from septic thrombophlebitis) or a combination of the two, although the precise mechanism has not been elucidated.

Early diagnosis, prompt treatment, and consistent follow-up are essential to avoid irreversible neurologic damage from SEA. The most common clinical symptoms are back pain, fever, and neurologic changes, such as leg weakness or sensory deficits, but a majority of patients do not present with this triad. Instead, patients may present with bladder dysfunction, sepsis, meningitis, paraplegia or quadriplegia, urinary tract infection (UTI), mental status changes, inflammation at the catheter site, headache, neck stiffness, or nausea and vomiting. Symptoms most commonly present within 7 days but may be delayed for 60 days or more.[259] Elevated white blood cell (WBC) count and elevated erythrocyte sedimentation rate (ESR) or C-reactive protein may also be present, but these laboratory findings are nonspecific. If SEA is suspected, gadolinium-enhanced MRI is the diagnostic tool of choice. Some investigators have proposed that MRI scanning be considered in patients who have received epidural catheters if systemic and local signs of infection (eg, pus or erythema at the epidural insertion site) develop, even in the absence of neurologic deficits.

Broad-spectrum intravenous antibiotic administration, ultimately tailored to blood or tissue cultures, without surgical drainage may be appropriate treatment for SEA in the absence of neurologic symptoms. However, prompt surgical intervention (decompressive laminectomy, debridement of infected tissue, and abscess drainage) may be required, depending on the clinical presentation. Most likely owing to a delay in diagnosis or an initial misdiagnosis, morbidity associated with SEA remains high at 33%–47%, while mortality is estimated to be 5%.[257] Neurologic status prior to intervention is the strongest predictor of final outcome.[260] There is also a strong association between poor outcome and age greater than 70 years, MRSA strain infection, and the presence of DM or adrenal insufficiency.[261]

The risk and long-term sequelae of SEA can be reduced with careful patient selection, maintenance of strict sterile techniques during initiation of epidural procedures, the administration of antibiotics prior to initiation of neuraxial blockade in patients with fever or localized infection, removal of indwelling catheters at the earliest sign of infection at the puncture site, and maintenance of a high index of suspicion in patients with risk factors who present with nonspecific neurologic complaints or local and systemic signs of infection, possibly several weeks after an epidural procedure.

TABLE 24–36. Predisposing conditions for spinal epidural abscess.	
Elderly	Steroid injection
Diabetes mellitus	Alcoholism
HIV/AIDS	Liver disease
Chronic steroid use	Renal failure
Adrenal insufficiency	Rheumatoid arthritis
Chronic epidural catheter	Cellulitis
Prolonged urinary catheterization	Psoas abscess
Indwelling vascular device	Intravenous drug use
Recent spinal instrumentation	Osteomyelitis

Meningitis

Bacterial meningitis following epidural anesthesia is a rare event. Microorganisms can be transmitted via syringes, catheters, needles, infusion tubing, and medications injected into the epidural space, as well as from the clinician or patient. Similar infectious complications can occur with nonanesthetic procedures, such as EBP, myelography, epidural steroid injection, and diagnostic lumbar puncture. Most cases appear to be caused by contamination of the puncture site by organisms from the naso- or oropharynx of the health care provider. Less commonly, contaminants from incompletely sterilized skin and direct or hematogenous spread from an endogenous infectious site are implicated.[262] A dural puncture, such as in the setting of a CSE, spinal, or an ADP, is believed to place patients at higher risk by allowing transfer of blood-borne pathogens across the blood-brain barrier.[263] However, the incidence of bacterial meningitis remains low despite the increasing use of CSE and spinal techniques. Also, diagnostic lumbar puncture in the setting of bacteremia is rarely associated with meningitis. Additional risk factors include breaches in aseptic technique, reinsertion of the stylet that has been exposed to ambient air, difficulty performing the neuraxial procedure, and, relatedly, multiple attempts at spinal or epidural placement.

Signs and symptoms of meningitis include fever, headache, lethargy, confusion, nuchal rigidity, nausea/vomiting, photophobia, and Kernig sign (Table 24–37). Symptoms usually present within 6 to 36 hours after the anesthetic procedure. Because the initial clinical presentation is similar to that of a PDPH, the diagnosis of meningitis can be delayed. Meningitis can be distinguished from PDPH by the presence of a fever, mental status changes (ie, lethargy and confusion), and a headache that is not positional in nature. The diagnosis is confirmed with CSF analysis and culture with or without prior head CT. The CSF is often cloudy, with leukocytosis (predominantly neutrophils), elevated protein content, and low glucose concentration. Early diagnosis is essential. Common pathogens include *Streptococcus salivarius* and other strains of viridans streptococci, *S. aureus*, *P. aeruginosa*, *Neisseria meningitidis*, and *Enterococcus faecalis*. In many cases, no organism is isolated. Treatment of bacterial meningitis includes immediate empiric broad-spectrum antibiotic therapy, such as vancomycin with a third-generation cephalosporin, ultimately tailored to blood or CSF culture results. Neurologic sequelae may include cranial nerve palsies, hemiparesis, quadriparesis, and

TABLE 24–37. Signs and symptoms of bacterial meningitis.

Fever

Mental status changes (lethargy, confusion)

Headache

Nuchal rigidity

Nausea, vomiting

Backache

Photophobia

Seizures

Focal neurologic deficits

Kernig sign

Brudzinski sign

aphasia. If diagnosis and treatment are delayed, death may result. Adherence to full aseptic precautions, including removal of jewelry, hand washing, appropriate skin preparation with individual packets of antiseptic solution (preferably chlorhexidine with alcohol), the use of a sterile drape and dressing, and, at a minimum, the use of caps, sterile gloves, and face masks (changed between each patient encounter), is critical to minimize the risk of bacterial meningitis associated with neuraxial instrumentation. Alternatives to neuraxial techniques should be offered to patients at high risk for infectious complications, and patients with known or suspected bacteremia should be started on antibiotic therapy prior to neuraxial instrumentation.

Spinal Cord and Nerve Root Injury

Neurologic deficits can be caused by direct trauma to the spinal cord or spinal nerves, from spinal cord ischemia, from accidental injection of neurotoxic drugs or chemicals, or from hematomas or abscesses.[264] Fortunately, serious neurologic injury is an extremely rare complication of neuraxial anesthesia, with an estimated incidence of 0.03%–0.1%. Horlocker and colleagues evaluated the records of over 4000 patients who had received lumbar epidurals for thoracic surgery while under GA and found no cases of neurologic complications. In another extensive review of 45,000 patients undergoing epidural placement, 40 cases of neurologic injuries were reported. Of note, 22 of these patients experienced paresthesias during the epidural procedure.[265] There have been a few case reports of myelopathy and paraplegia occurring with thoracic epidurals placed in anesthetized patients, but these complications are exceedingly rare.[266] Most peripheral neuropathies associated with neuraxial techniques resolve spontaneously. Those that become permanent are usually limited to persistent paresthesias and limited motor weakness.

Cauda Equina Syndrome

Cauda equina syndrome (CES), a rare state of neurologic compromise due to lumbosacral root compression, is characterized by bowel and bladder dysfunction, low-back pain, perineal sensory loss and other patchy sensory deficits, unilateral or bilateral sciatica, and lower extremity motor weakness. It has been associated with trauma, infection, lithotomy position, and ischemic compression by a hematoma, abscess, tumor, prolapsed intervertebral disk, or spondylolisthesis.[267] CES has also been linked to direct neurotoxicity from large volumes or high concentrations of hyperbaric LAs in the sacral CSF. The nerve roots of the cauda equina have a poorly developed epineurium and limited blood flow and appear to be particularly susceptible to the pooling of LAs that may accompany continuous spinal infusions with microbore catheters, accidental intrathecal injection of large doses of LA intended for epidural anesthesia, and repeat intrathecal injections after failed spinal block.[268] Cases of CES have also been reported after single-shot spinals.[269]

Whether intrinsic neurotoxicity of LAs, microenvironmental factors, excessively large doses of LAs, the microbore catheter used for continuous spinal anesthesia, patient positioning, the surgical procedure, or a combination of these factors is primarily responsible for CES has not been fully elucidated in the literature. The US Food and Drug Administration (FDA) removed small-bore continuous spinal catheters from the market in the early 1990s after a series of reports of CES in association with their use.[270] However, continuous spinal anesthesia remains a useful technique. The use of lower concentrations of LAs, limiting the total dose of LA, limiting the depth of insertion of the spinal catheter, and using maneuvers to increase the spread of LA if maldistribution is suspected may minimize the risk of CES.[271] Some investigators have also advocated using alternatives to hyperbaric 5% lidocaine given that safe alternatives exist.[272] Unfortunately, CES is a permanent disability. Symptoms consistent with this syndrome should prompt an early neurology consult and imaging studies. High-dose corticosteroids; surgical decompression (eg, in the case of a lumbar synovial cyst, hemangioma, or metastatic tumors); and treatment of the underlying disorder with chemotherapeutic agents or antibiotics (eg, in the case of malignancy or abscess formation) have been used, but limited data are available on optimal therapies and the course of recovery.

Epidural Hematoma

Epidural hematoma is a rare occurrence that can lead to cord compression, cord ischemia, or myelopathy similar to that caused by a space-occupying tumor. The incidence of hematoma associated with epidural blockade is estimated at 1:150,000, somewhat higher than that of spinal anesthetics (1:220,000). However, the incidence varies dramatically with the patient population and may be significantly higher in a subset of patients with a less-compliant epidural space and a greater likelihood of coagulation disorders. Indeed, hemostatic abnormalities during either initiation of epidural blockade or removal of the epidural catheter are present in the majority of reported cases, although a large proportion of the documented cases also occur spontaneously, with no predisposing factors. Complicated epidural needle or catheter placement also appears to place the patient at risk for epidural hematoma formation.

Coagulation disturbances that predispose patients to the development of epidural hematoma may be iatrogenic or secondary to underlying disease. Iatrogenic disturbances that may predispose patients to epidural hematoma formation are often associated with antithrombotic or thrombolytic therapy. The most recent American Society of Regional Anesthesia and Pain Medicine guidelines can be used to assist the anesthesiologist in determining the most appropriate and safest period for initiating epidural blockade in anticoagulated patients (see Chapter 52). Thrombocytopenia is a relatively common cause of coagulopathy and may be related to pregnancy (gestational thrombocytopenia, HELLP syndrome, or preeclampsia/eclampsia), immune disorders (eg, ITP), or hepatic dysfunction, among other things. Unfortunately, there is no universally accepted platelet count that can be considered safe for performance of neuraxial blockade, and there is no widely available bedside test to assess platelet function. The nature of the underlying disorder must be taken into account (eg, Is the process dynamic, with rapidly dropping platelets? Is platelet function intact despite a low

number? Is the patient on concomitant antiplatelet therapy? Does he or she have another disorder affecting coagulation? and so on), and patients with thrombocytopenia should be approached with caution prior to initiation of neuraxial blockade.

Signs and symptoms of epidural hematoma may progress rapidly from mild sensory or motor deficits to devastating paraplegia and incontinence. Early signs include back pain and pressure, with motor and sensory deficits. The back pain associated with epidural hematoma may be severe and persistent. Bowel and bladder incontinence, radicular pain, and worsening lower extremity neurologic deficits ensue. The onset of symptoms is usually within 12 hours to 2 days of initiation of neuraxial blockade or removal of an epidural catheter. Unfortunately, motor and sensory deficits within this timeframe may be mistaken for residual epidural blockade. Recurrence of motor and sensory blockade after partial or total resolution or, alternatively, prolonged block should raise concerns for an epidural hematoma and prompt immediate consultation with a neurologist or neurosurgeon, as well as prompt MRI scanning. A negative MRI cannot rule out a developing hematoma, which may not be recognized by an inexperienced radiologist.[273] Surgical decompression within 8 hours is advocated to minimize the risk of permanent neurologic injury.

Anterior Spinal Artery Syndrome

Anterior spinal artery syndrome (ASAS) occurs most commonly in patients with vascular disease and concomitant decreased spinal blood flow due to obstruction, compression, or hypotension. However, it has also been described in the setting of acute thoracic disk herniation, spondylosis, arteriovenous malformation, and similar pathologic conditions that can disrupt the tenuous blood flow in the anterior spinal artery distribution. ASAS is the most common neurologic complication after abdominal aortic surgery but has also been reported after surgery on the thoracic spine. Massive blood loss and persistent hypotension induced by neuraxial anesthesia have been implicated in the intraoperative development of this potentially life-threatening syndrome. ASAS presents with immediate, painless paraplegia and loss of lower extremity sensory function. Proprioception and vibration sense are spared. Prognosis is poor, with permanent and disabling neurologic deficits. Correction of intraoperative hypotension is essential in patients at high risk for ASAS.

Cardiac Arrest

Cardiac arrest resulting in death or brain damage is a rare complication of epidural blockade.[274] Causes include unintentional total spinal anesthesia, LAST, myocardial ischemia, respiratory compromise, or any of several circulatory events that do not fall within these categories, such as complete blockade of the preganglionic cardiac accelerator fibers or vagal predominance in the setting of sympathetic blockade.[275] Although the mechanism of increased vagal tone has not been fully elucidated, blockade of the sympathetic efferents results in vasodilation and a decrease in venous return. Decreased preload, in turn, may enhance cardiac vagal tone. Bradycardia, reduced CO, and cardiac arrest may result and can be attributed in part to reflex activity. The paradoxical Bezold-Jarisch reflex, for example, triggers slowing of the heart rate in response to decreased ventricular volume to permit more time for complete filling of the heart.

To minimize the risk of cardiac arrest associated with vagal predominance after neuraxial procedures, Pollard and colleagues proposed maintenance of adequate preload, the use of vagolytic drugs and pressor agents, if necessary, appropriate patient selection, and caution when changing patient positioning.[276] Early epinephrine administration is recommended if bradycardia is marked. Vasopressin may be more effective than epinephrine for cardiopulmonary resuscitation during epidural anesthesia due to its longer-lasting effect and the improved acid-base profile after multiple doses,[277] although adherence to the most current advanced cardiovascular life support (ACLS) protocol is recommended. Patient-related risk factors for cardiac arrest after neuraxial anesthesia include male gender, ASA I physical status, a low baseline heart rate (below 60), a sensory level above T6, age below 50, the use of β-adrenergic blocking agents, and prolonged PR interval. Rapid onset of action of LAs, the use of LAs that cause a more profound sympathetic block, and a broader spread of block have also been associated with hypotension and bradycardia after epidural blockade.[278] Ligouri and colleagues have identified the following secondary factors that may precipitate or contribute to the severity of the increased vagal tone associated with bradycardia and asystole during epidural anesthesia: opioid administration, hypoxemia, sedation, hypercarbia, chronic medication use, and coexisting medical disease.[279]

Side Effects

Several common side effects accompany epidural procedures, including transient fever in obstetric patients, nausea and vomiting, pruritus associated with neuraxial opioids, shivering, and urinary retention. Numerous studies have found an association between epidural labor analgesia and new-onset maternal intrapartum fever, although the relationship may not be causal. The increase in maternal temperature is often subclinical and self-limited and does not appear to have an adverse effect on the fetus.[281]

Nausea and vomiting are common after both GA and neuraxial blockade. In the setting of epidural anesthesia and analgesia, nausea and vomiting may be attributed to hypotension or to the epidural adjuvants, such as opioids. Lipophilic opioids, such as fentanyl and sufentanil, administered epidurally appear to confer some decreased risk of nausea and vomiting when compared to epidural morphine.[281] The administration of intravenous ondansetron (possibly in combination with other antiemetic agents), supplemental oxygen, and anxiolytics, as well as prompt correction of hypotension and hypovolemia, is recommended in the multimodal approach to therapy. Intravenous dexamethasone also appears to be effective in reducing nausea and vomiting associated with epidural morphine.[282] Ephedrine, which is thought to have antiemetic effects unrelated to its hemodynamic effects, antihistamines, and anticholinergics also show promise.

Pruritus, a common side effect of neuraxial opioids, is observed more often during spinals than epidurals. It is usually transient and most commonly affects the nose and other areas of the face. The pure opioid antagonist naloxone effectively reverses opioid-induced pruritus, but at the cost of reversing the analgesia. The partial agonist-antagonist nalbuphine appears to be the most effective treatment of opioid-induced pruritus. A single 5-mg dose is often sufficient; a second 5-mg dose is occasionally necessary. Antihistamines are ineffective; opioid-induced pruritus is not a histamine-mediated reaction.

Shivering is another common side effect of neuraxial analgesia and anesthesia, occurring more quickly and more intensely in spinal versus epidural anesthesia. The mechanism remains unclear but may be related in part to impairment of central thermoregulatory control and redistribution of body heat.

Hypotension, as defined by a greater than 20% reduction in systolic, diastolic, or mean blood pressure, is common following epidural blockade. High thoracic blocks, obesity, concurrent general and neuraxial anesthesia, hypovolemia, and excessive intraoperative blood loss are among the risk factors. Patients may present with nausea, vomiting, light-headedness, mental status changes, shortness of breath, difficulty breathing, and cardiac arrhythmias. Cardiovascular collapse may accompany severe cases. Optimally, the blood pressure should be maintained within 20% of the patient's resting baseline. Proposed methods to reduce the incidence of hypotension after neuraxial blockade include the judicious administration of vasopressors (most commonly, ephedrine or phenylephrine); volume expansion with a crystalloid or colloid solution at the time of initiation of the block (ie, a coload); maintenance of left uterine displacement after 18 to 20 weeks' gestation in obstetric patients; changing patient positioning (eg, from supine to sitting) gradually; placing the block at a lower spinal segment, when feasible; slow titration of epidural LAs; and reducing the dose of intrathecal or epidural LA. In cases of severe hypotension, elevating the lower extremities or placing military antishock trousers will reduce venous pooling. Alternative α- and β-adrenergic pressor agents, such as norepinephrine and epinephrine, should also be considered. Positioning the patient in reverse Trendelenburg in an attempt to limit the spread of the LA should be avoided; Trendelenburg will serve to alleviate venous pooling in the lower extremities and improve blood flow to the heart and brain (Table 24–38). Many of these measures to reduce the incidence and severity of hypotension following neuraxial blockade remain under debate in the literature and are beyond the purview of this chapter.

SUMMARY

Both the indications for neuraxial techniques and the patient population that is considered appropriate for these procedures have expanded over the past several decades. Epidural blockade is currently being advocated as an adjuvant to GA for cardiothoracic, major vascular, and other high-risk surgeries; as the sole anesthetic in surgeries that were previously performed exclusively under GA; and for acute and chronic pain management. Neuraxial techniques are also increasingly being used in the ambulatory setting, where the decrease in PONV and

TABLE 24–38. Treatment of hypotension following neuraxial blockade.

Discontinue epidural infusion, if applicable

Volume expansion with intravenous fluid administration

Intravenous vasopressor administration (phenylephrine and/or ephedrine)

Place patient in Trendelenburg position

Ensure uterine displacement after 18–20 weeks' gestation

Elevate lower extremities

Administer atropine 0.4–0.5 mg IV with concurrent bradycardia

Wrap legs with thromboembolic deterrent stockings/pneumatic compression hose; place military antishock trousers

Norepinephrine or epinephrine administration as needed

improved pain relief permit earlier discharge; for a variety of diagnostic procedures; and to alleviate pain in adults and children in the end-of-life setting.

The benefits of epidural blockade are well established. Epidural techniques provide optimal pain relief following major surgeries and have been associated with fewer cardiovascular, respiratory, GI, and hematologic complications when compared with GA.[283] The incidence of perioperative thromboembolic events, the time to return of GI function, and length of intensive care stay, among other things, appear to be reduced with epidural blockade. In addition, epidural anesthesia has been associated with prolonged survival and decreased cancer recurrence rates in patients with breast, localized colon, prostate, and ovarian cancers.[284] However, the potential role of epidural blockade in reducing mortality after major surgery is still debated in the literature.

Despite the many potential advantages of epidural blockade, neuraxial techniques are not without risks, although major complications are rare. A risk-benefit analysis on a case-by-case basis and informed patient consent are warranted prior to initiation of epidural blockade.

REFERENCES

1. Frölich MA, Caton D: Pioneers in epidural needle design. Anesth Analg 2001;93:215–220.
2. Cortés RC: Lumbar epidural anesthesia, 1931–1936: A second debut. Rev Esp Anestesiol Reanim 2005;52:159–168.
3. Dogliotti AM: Segmental peridural spinal anesthesia: A new method of block. Am J Surg 1933;20:107–118.
4. Curbelo MM: Continuous peridural segmental anesthesia by means of a ureteral catheter. Curr Res Anesth Analg 1949;28:13–23.
5. Modig J, Borg T, Karlström G, et al: Thromboembolism after total hip replacement: Role of epidural and general anesthesia. Anesth Analg 1983;62:174–180.
6. Jørgensen LN, Rasmussen LS, Nielsen P, et al: Antithrombotic efficacy of continuous extradural analgesia after knee replacement. Br J Anaesth 1991;66:8–12.
7. Rodgers A, Walker N, Schug S, et al: Reduction of postoperative mortality and morbidity with epidural or spinal anaesthesia: Results from overview of randomised trials. BMJ 2000;321:1–12.
8. Mauermann WJ, Shilling AM, Zuo Z: A comparison of neuraxial block versus general anesthesia for elective total hip replacement: A meta-analysis. Anesth Analg 2006;103:1018–1025.
9. Schindler I: Regional anesthesia in the elderly: Indications and contraindications. Acta Anaesthesiol Scand Suppl 1997;111:209–211.
10. Cherng CH, Wong CS, Chang FL, et al: Epidural morphine delays the onset of tourniquet pain during epidural lidocaine anesthesia. Anesth Analg 2002;94:1614–1616.
11. Christopherson R, Beattie C, Frank SM, et al: Perioperative morbidity in patients randomized to epidural or general anesthesia for lower extremity vascular surgery. Anesthesiology 1993;79:422–434.
12. Sproviero M: Neuraxial anesthesia for adult genitourinary procedures. In Wong CA (ed): *Spinal and Epidural Anesthesia*. McGraw-Hill, 2007, pp 229–236.
13. Soriano D, Ajaj S, Chuong T, et al: Lidocaine spray and outpatient hysteroscopy: Randomized placebo-controlled trial. Obstet Gynecol 2000;96:661–664.
14. Goldenberg M, Cohen SB, Etchin A, et al: A randomized prospective comparative study of general versus epidural anesthesia for transcervical hysteroscopic endometrial resection. Am J Obstet Gynecol 2001;184:273–276.
15. Murphy M, Heit MH, Fouts L, et al. Effect of anesthesia on voiding function after tension-free vaginal tape procedure. Obstet Gynecol 2003;101:666–670.
16. Block BM, Liu SS, Rowlingson AJ, et al: Efficacy of postoperative epidural analgesia: A meta-analysis. JAMA 2003;290:2455–2463.
17. Ballantyne JC, Carr DB, deFerranti S, et al: The comparative effects of postoperative analgesic therapies on pulmonary outcome: Cumulative meta-analyses of randomized, controlled trials. Anesth Analg 1998;86:598–612.
18. Liu SS, Wu CL: Effect of postoperative analgesia on major postoperative complications: A systemic update of the evidence. Anesth Analg 2007;104:689–702.
19. Manion SC, Brennan TJ: Thoracic epidural analgesia and acute pain management. Anesthesiology 2011;115:181–188.
20. Nygård E, Kofoed KF, Freiburg J, et al: Effects of high thoracic epidural analgesia on myocardial blood flow in patients with ischemic heart disease. Circulation 2005;111:2165–2170.
21. Scott NB, Turfrey DJ, Ray DA, et al: A prospective randomized study of the potential benefits of thoracic epidural anesthesia and analgesia in patients undergoing coronary artery bypass grafting. Anesth Analg 2001;93:528–535.
22. Loick HM, Schmidt C, Van Aken H, et al: High thoracic epidural anesthesia, but not clonidine, attenuates the perioperative stress response via sympatholysis and reduces the release of troponin T in patients undergoing coronary artery bypass grafting. Anesth Analg 1999;88:701–709.
23. Liu SS, Block BM, Wu CL: Effects of perioperative central neuraxial analgesia on outcome after coronary artery bypass surgery: A meta-analysis. Anesthesiology 2004;101:153–161.
24. Svircevic V, Nierich AP, Moons KG, et al: Thoracic epidural anesthesia for cardiac surgery: A randomized trial. Anesthesiology 2011;114:262–270.
25. Caputo M, Alwair H, Rogers CA, et al: Thoracic epidural anesthesia improves early outcomes in patients undergoing off-pump coronary artery bypass surgery: A prospective, randomized, controlled trial. Anesthesiology 2011;114:380–390.
26. Møiniche S, Kehlet H, Dahl JB: A qualitative and quantitative systematic review of preemptive analgesia for postoperative pain relief: The role of timing of analgesia. Anesthesiology 2002;96:725–741.
27. Groeben H, Schäfer B, Pavlakovic G, et al: Lung function under high thoracic segmental epidural anesthesia with ropivacaine or bupivacaine in patients with severe obstructive pulmonary disease undergoing breast surgery. Anesthesiology 2002;96:536–541.
28. Diaz N, Wong CA: Neuraxial anesthesia for general surgery. In Wong CA (ed): *Spinal and Epidural Anesthesia*. McGraw-Hill, 2007, pp 221–227.
29. Matot I, Scheinin O, Eid A, et al: Epidural anesthesia and analgesia in liver resection. Anesth Analg 2002;95:1179–1181.
30. Zhang HW, Chen YJ, Cao MH, et al: Laparoscopic cholecystectomy under epidural anesthesia: A retrospective comparison of 100 patients. Am Surg 2012;78:107–110.
31. Asakura K, Nakazawa K, Tanaka N, et al. Case of cardiac arrest due to coronary spasm during laparoscopic distal gastrectomy. Masui 2011;60:75–79.

32. Shir Y, Raja SN, Frank SM, et al: Intraoperative blood loss during radical retropubic prostatectomy. Epidural versus general anesthesia. Urology 1995;45:993–999.

33. Gottschalk A, Smith DS, Jobes DR, et al: Preemptive epidural analgesia and recovery from radical prostatectomy: A randomized controlled trial. JAMA 1998;279:1076–1082.

34. Stevens RA, Mikat-Stevens M, Flanigan R, et al: Does the choice of anesthetic technique affect the recovery of bowel function after radical prostatectomy? Urology 1998;52:213–218.

35. Ozyuvaci E, Altan A, Karadeniz T, et al: General anesthesia versus epidural and general anesthesia in radical cystectomy. Urol Int 2005;74:62–67.

36. Micali S, Jarrett TW, Pappa P, et al: Efficacy of epidural anesthesia for retroperitoneoscopic renal biopsy. Urology 2000;55:590.

37. Richards JT, Read JR, Chambers WA. Epidural anaesthesia as a method of pre-emptive analgesia for abdominal hysterectomy. Anaesthesia 1998;53:296–298.

38. Mihic DN, Abram SE: Optimal regional anaesthesia for abdominal hysterectomy: Combined subarachnoid and epidural block compared with other regional techniques. Eur J Anaesthesiol 1993;10:297–301.

39. Holte K, Kehlet H: Epidural analgesia and risk of anastomotic leakage. Reg Anesth Pain Med 2001;26:111.

40. Kehlet H, Mogensen T: Hospital stay of 2 days after open sigmoidectomy with a multimodal rehabilitation programme. Br J Surg 1999;86:227–230.

41. Bardram L, Funch-Jensen P, Kehlet H: Rapid rehabilitation in elderly patients after laparoscopic colonic resection. Br J Surg 2000;87: 1540–1545.

42. Blichfeldt-Lauridsen L, Hansen BD: Anesthesia and myasthenia gravis. Acta Anaesthesiol Scand 2012;56:17–22.

43. Kirsh JR, Diringer MN, Borel CO, et al: Preoperative lumbar epidural morphine improves postoperative analgesia and ventilatory function after transsternal thymectomy in patients with myasthenia gravis. Crit Care Med 1991;19:1474–1479.

44. Bagshaw O: A combination of total intravenous anesthesia and thoracic epidural for thymectomy in juvenile myasthenia gravis. Paediatr Anaesth 2007;17:370–374.

45. Hambly PR, Martin B: Anaesthesia for chronic spinal cord lesions. Anaesthesia 1998;53:273–289.

46. Lambert DH, Deane RS, Mazuzan JE: Anesthesia and the control of blood pressure in patients with spinal cord injury. Anesth Analg 1982;61:344–348.

47. Ording H: Incidence of malignant hyperthermia in Denmark. Anesth Analg 1985;64:700–704.

48. van Lier F, van der Geest PJ, Hoeks SE, et al: Epidural analgesia is associated with improved health outcomes of surgical patients with chronic obstructive pulmonary disease. Anesthesiology 2011;115:315–321.

49. Mulroy MF, Salinas FV: Neuraxial techniques for ambulatory anesthesia. Int Anesthesiol Clin 2005;43:129–141.

50. Anghelescu DL, Faughnan LG, Baker JN, et al: Use of epidural and peripheral nerve blocks at the end of life in children and young adults with cancer: The collaboration between a pain service and a palliative care service. Paediatr Anaesth 2010;20:1070–1077.

51. Sielenkämper AW, Van Aken H: Epidural analgesia in sepsis: Too early to judge a new concept. Intensive Care Med 2004;30:1987–1989.

52. Strümper D, Louwen F, Durieux ME, et al: Epidural local anesthetics: A novel treatment for fetal growth retardation? Fetal Diagn Ther 2005; 20:208–213.

53. Hong JY, Lim KT: Effect of preemptive epidural analgesia on cytokine response and postoperative pain in laparoscopic radical hysterectomy for cervical cancer. Reg Anesth Pain Med 2008;33:44–51.

54. Exadaktylos AK, Buggy DJ, Moriarty DC, et al: Can anesthetic technique for primary breast cancer surgery affect recurrence or metastasis? Anesthesiology 2006;105:660–664.

55. Biki B, Mascha E, Moriarty DC, et al. Anesthetic technique for radical prostatectomy surgery affects cancer recurrence: A retrospective analysis. Anesthesiology 2008;109:180–187.

56. Freise H, Van Aken H: Risks and benefits of thoracic epidural anaesthesia. Br J Anaesth 2011;107:859–868.

57. Mutz C, Vagts DA: Thoracic epidural anesthesia in sepsis—is it harmful or protective? Crit Care 2009;13:182.

58. Su TM, Lan CM, Yang LC, et al: Brain tumor presenting with fatal herniation following delivery under epidural anesthesia. Anesthesiology 2002;96:508–509.

59. Grocott HP, Mutch WA: Epidural anesthesia and acutely increased intracranial pressure: Lumbar epidural space hydrodynamics in a porcine model. Anesthesiology 1996;85:1086–1091.

60. Leffert LR, Schwamm LH: Neuraxial anesthesia in parturients with intracranial pathology: A comprehensive review and reassessment of risk. Anesthesiology 2013;119:703–718.

61. Vandermeulen EP, Van Aken H, Vermylen J: Anticoagulants and spinal-epidural anesthesia. Anesth Analg 1994;79:1165–1177.

62. Horlocker TT, Wedel DJ, Rowlingson JC, et al: Regional anesthesia in the patient receiving antithrombotic or thrombolytic therapy: American Society of Regional Anesthesia and Pain Medicine evidence-based guidelines (third edition). Reg Anesth Pain Med 2010;35:64–101.

63. O'Rourke, N, Khan K, Hepner DL: Contraindications to neuraxial anesthesia. In Wong CA (ed): *Spinal and Epidural Anesthesia*. McGraw-Hill, 2007, pp 127–149.

64. Choi S, Brull R: Neuraxial techniques in obstetric and non-obstetric patients with common bleeding diatheses. Anesth Analg 2009;109: 648–660.

65. Bader AM, Hunt CO, Datta S, et al: Anesthesia for the obstetric patient with multiple sclerosis. J Clin Anesth 1988;1:21–24.

66. Confavreux C, Hutchinson M, Hours MM, et al: Rate of pregnancy-related relapse in multiple sclerosis. Pregnancy in Multiple Sclerosis Group. N Engl J Med 1998;339:285–291.

67. Hebl JR, Horlocker TT, Schroeder DR: Neuraxial anesthesia and analgesia in patients with preexisting central nervous system disorders. Anesth Analg 2006;103:223–228.

68. Lirk P, Birmingham B, Hogan Q: Regional anesthesia in patients with preexisting neuropathy. Int Anesthesiol Clin 2011;49:144–165.

69. Wiertlewski S, Magot A, Drapier S, et al: Worsening of neurologic symptoms after epidural anesthesia for labor in a Guillain-Barré patient. Anesth Analg 2004;98:825–827.

70. Toledano RD, Pian-Smith MC: Human immunodeficiency virus: Maternal and fetal considerations and management. In Suresh MS, Segal BS, Preston RL, et al (eds): *Shnider and Levinson's Anesthesia for Obstetrics*, 5th ed. Lippincott Williams & Wilkins, 2013, pp 595–605.

71. Crosby ET, Halpern SH, Rolbin SH: Epidural anaesthesia for caesarean section in patients with active recurrent genital herpes simplex infections: A retrospective review. Can J Anaesth 1989;36:701–704.

72. Bader AM, Camann WR, Datta S: Anesthesia for cesarean delivery in patients with herpes simplex virus type-2 infections. Reg Anesth 1990; 15:261–263.

73. Brown NW, Parsons APR, Kam PCA: Anaesthetic considerations in a parturient with varicella presenting for caesarean section. Anaesthesia 2003;58:1092–1095.

74. Hebl JR, Horlocker TT, Kopp SL, et al: Neuraxial blockade in patients with preexisting spinal stenosis, lumbar disk disease, or prior spine surgery: Efficacy and neurologic complications. Anesth Analg 2010;111: 1511–1519.

75. McDonald SB: Is neuraxial blockade contraindicated in the patient with aortic stenosis? Reg Anesth Pain Med 2004;29:496–502.

76. Ferguson EA, Paech MJ, Veltman MG: Hypertrophic cardiomyopathy and caesarean section: Intraoperative use of transthoracic echocardiography. Int J Obstet Anesth 2006;15:311–316.

77. Rosenquist RW, Birnbach DJ: Epidural insertion in anesthetized adults: Will your patients thank you? Anesth Analg 2003;96:1545–1546.

78. Horlocker TT, Abel MD, Messick JM, et al: Small risk of serious neurologic complications related to lumbar epidural catheter placement in anesthetized patients. Anesth Analg 2003;96:1547–1552.

79. Han KR, Kim C, Park SK, et al: Distance to the adult cervical epidural space. Reg Anesth Pain Med 2003;28:95–97.

80. Stonelake PS, Burwell RG, Webb JK: Variation in vertebral levels of the vertebra prominens and sacral dimples in subjects with scoliosis. J Anat 1988;159:165–172.

81. Hughes RJ, Saifuddin A: Imaging of lumbosacral transitional vertebrae. Clin Radiol 2004;59:984–991.

82. Kim JT, Bahk JH, Sung J: Influence of age and sex on the position of the conus medullaris and Tuffier's line in adults. Anesthesiology 2003;99: 1359–1363.

83. Saifuddin A, Burnett SJ, White J: The variation of position of the conus medullaris in an adult population. A magnetic resonance imaging study. Spine 1998;23:1452–1456.

84. Vandermeersch E, Kick O, Mollmann M, et al: CSE—The combination of spinal and epidural anesthesia. Reg Anaesth 1991;14:108–112.

85. Lirk P, Hogan Q: Spinal and epidural anatomy. In Wong CA (ed): *Spinal and Epidural Anesthesia*. McGraw-Hill, 2007, 1–25.

86. Lee AJ, Ranasinghe JS, Chehade JM, et al: Ultrasound assessment of the vertebral level of the intercristal line in pregnancy. Anesth Analg 2011;113:559–564.

87. Van Gessel EF, Forster A, Gamulin Z: Continuous spinal anesthesia: Where do spinal catheters go? Anesth Analg 1993;76:1004–1007.

88. Broadbent CR, Maxwell WB, Ferrie R, et al: Ability of anaesthetists to identify a marked lumbar interspace. Anaesthesia 2000;55: 1122–1126.
89. Lirk P, Messner H, Deibl M, et al: Accuracy in estimating the correct intervertebral space level during lumbar, thoracic and cervical anaesthesia. Acta Anaesthesiol Scand 2004;48:347–349.
90. Hogan QH: Lumbar epidural anatomy. A new look by cryomicrotome section. Anesthesiology 1991;75:767–775.
91. Heylings DJ: Supraspinous and interspinous ligaments of the human lumbar spine. J Anat 1978;125:127–131.
92. Han KR, Kim C, Park SK, et al: Distance to the adult cervical epidural space. Reg Anesth Pain Med 2003;28:95–97.
93. Zarzur E: Anatomic studies of the human ligamentum flavum. Anesth Analg 1984;63:499–502.
94. Williams DM, Gabrielsen TO, Latack JT, et al: Ossification in the cephalic attachment of the ligamentum flavum. An anatomical and CT study. Radiology 1984;150:423–426.
95. Brown DL: Spinal, epidural, and caudal anesthesia. In Miller RD, Fleisher LE, Johns RA, et al (eds): *Miller's Anesthesia*, 6th ed. Elsevier, 2005, pp 1653–1683.
96. Westbrook JL, Renowden SA, Carrie LE: Study of the anatomy of the extradural region using magnetic resonance imaging. Br J Anaesth 1993; 71:495–498.
97. Lirk P, Kolbitsch C, Putz G, et al: Cervical and high thoracic ligamentum flavum frequently fails to fuse in the midline. Anesthesiology 2003;99: 1387–1390.
98. Lirk P, Colvin J, Steger B, et al: Incidence of lower thoracic ligamentum flavum midline gaps. Br J Anaesth 2005;94:852–855.
99. Lirk P, Moriggl B, Colvin J, et al: The incidence of lumbar ligamentum flavum midline gaps. Anesth Analg 2004;98:1178–1180.
100. Reina MA, Villanueva MC, Machés F, et al: The ultrastructure of the human spinal nerve root cuff in the lumbar spine. Anesth Analg 2008; 106:339–344.
101. Bernards CM: Sophistry in medicine: Lessons from the epidural space. Reg Anesth Pain Med 2005;30:56–66.
102. Reina MA, De León Casasola O, Villanueva MC, et al: Ultrastructural findings in human spinal pia mater in relation to subarachnoid anesthesia. Anesth Analg 2004;98:1479–1485.
103. Blomberg RG: The lumbar subdural extraarchnoid space of humans: An anatomical study using spinaloscopy in autopsy cases. Anesth Analg 1987;66:177–180.
104. Haines DE: On the question of a subdural space. Anat Rec 1991;230: 3–21.
105. Boon JM, Abrahams PH, Meiring JH, et al: Lumbar puncture: Anatomical review of a clinical skill. Clin Anat 2004;17:544–553.
106. Hogan QH: Epidural anatomy: New observations. Can J Anaesth 1998;45:R40–48.
107. Bernards CM: Epidural anesthesia. In Mulroy MF, Bernards CM, McDonald SB, et al (eds): *A Practical Approach to Regional Anesthesia*, 4th ed. Lippincott Williams & Wilkins, 2009, p 104.
108. Igarashi T, Hirabayashi Y, Shimizu R, et al: The lumbar extradural structure changes with increasing age. Br J Anaesth 1997;78:149–152.
109. Blomberg R: The dorsomedian connective tissue band in the lumbar epidural space of humans: An anatomical study using epiduroscopy in autopsy cases. Anesth Analg 1986;65:747–752.
110. Hogan QH, Toth J: Anatomy of soft tissues of the spinal canal. Reg Anesth Pain Med 1999;24:303–310.
111. Hogan QH: Distribution of solution in the epidural space: Examination by cryomicrotome section. Reg Anesth Pain Med 2002;27:150–156.
112. Fujinaka MK, Lawson EF, Schukteis G, Wallace MS: Cervical epidural depth: correlation between needle angle, cervical anatomy, and body surface area. Pain Med 2012;13:665–669.
113. Aldrete JA, Mushin AU, Zapata JC, et al: Skin to cervical epidural space distances as read from magnetic resonance imaging films: Consideration of the "hump pad." J Clin Anesth 1998;10:309–313.
114. Segal S, Beach M, Eappen S: A multivariate model to predict the distance from the skin to the epidural space in an obstetric population. Reg Anesth 1996;21:451–455.
115. Sutton DN, Linter SP: Depth of extradural space and dural puncture. Anaesthesia 1991;46:97–98.
116. Reynolds AF, Roberts PA, Pollay M, et al: Quantitative anatomy of the thoracolumbar epidural space. Neurosurgery 1986;17:905–907.
117. Hogan QH: Epidural anatomy examined by cryomicrotome section. Influence of age, vertebral level, and disease. Reg Anesth 1996;21: 395–406.
118. Toprak HI, Ozpolat Z, Ozturk E, et al: Hyperbaric bupivacaine affects the doses of midazolam required for sedation after spinal anaesthesia. Eur J Anaesthesiol 2005;22:904–906.
119. Shono A, Sakura S, Saito Y, et al: Comparison of 1% and 2% lidocaine epidural anaesthesia combined with sevoflurane general anaesthesia utilizing a constant bispectral index. Br J Anaesth 2003;91:825–829.
120. Koo M, Sabaté A, Dalmau A, et al: Sevoflurane requirements during coloproctologic surgery: Difference between two different epidural regimens. J Clin Anesth 2003;15:97–102.
121. Eappen S, Kissin I: Effect of subarachnoid bupivacaine block on anesthetic requirements for thiopental in rats. Anesthesiology 1998;88: 1036–1042.
122. Tverskoy M, Shagal M, Finger J, et al: Subarachnoid bupivacaine blockade decreases midazolam and thiopental hypnotic requirements. J Clin Anesth 1994;6:487–490.
123. Tverskoy M, Shifrin V, Finger J, et al: Effect of epidural bupivacaine block on midazolam hypnotic requirements. Reg Anesth 1996;21: 209–213.
124. Hodgson PS, Liu SS, Gras TW: Does epidural anesthesia have general anesthetic effects? A prospective, randomized, double-blind, placebo-controlled trial. Anesthesiology 1999;91:1687–1692.
125. Reinoso-Barbero F, Martínez-García E, Hernández-Gancedo MC, et al: The effect of epidural bupivacaine on maintenance requirements of sevoflurane evaluated by bispectral index in children. Eur J Anaesthesiol 2006;23:460–464.
126. Holte K, Foss NB, Svensén C, et al: Epidural anesthesia, hypotension, and changes in intravascular volume. Anesthesiology 2004;100:281–286.
127. Meisner A, Rolf A, Van Aken H: Thoracic epidural anesthesia and the patient with heart disease: Benefits, risks, and controversies. Anesth Analg 1997;85, 517–528.
128. Missant C, Claus P, Rex S, Wouters PF: Differential effects of lumbar and thoracic epidural anaesthesia on the haemodynamic response to acute right ventricular pressure overload. Br J Anaesth 2010;104:143–149.
129. Buggy DJ, Doherty WL, Hart EM, Pallet EJ: Postoperative wound oxygen tension with epidural or intravenous analgesia: A prospective, randomized, single-blind clinical trial. Anesthesiology 2002;97:952–958.
130. Kabon B, Fleischmann E, Treschan T, et al: Thoracic epidural anesthesia increases tissue oxygenation during major abdominal surgery. Anesth Analg 2003;97:1812–1817.
131. Olausson K, Magnusdottir H, Lurje L, et al: Anti-ischemic and anti-anginal effects of thoracic epidural anesthesia versus those of conventional medical therapy in the treatment of severe refractory unstable angina pectoris. Circulation 1997;96:2178–2182.
132. Richter A, Cederholm I, Fredrikson M, et al: Effect of long-term thoracic epidural analgesia on refractory angina pectoris: A 10 year experience. J Cardiothorac Vasc Anesth 2012;26:822–828.
133. Rolf N, Van de Velde M, Wouters PF, et al: Thoracic epidural anesthesia improves functional recovery from myocardial stunning in conscious dogs. Anesth Analg 1996;83:935–940.
134. Rolf N, Meissner A, Van Aken H, et al: The effects of thoracic epidural anesthesia on functional recovery from myocardial stunning in propofol anesthetized dogs. Anesth Analg 1997;84:723–729.
135. Freise H, Van Aken HK: Risks and benefits of thoracic epidural anaesthesia. Br J Anaesth 2011;107:859–868.
136. Svircevic V, van Dijk D, Nierich AP, et al: Meta-analysis of thoracic epidural anesthesia versus general anesthesia for cardiac surgery. Anesthesiology 2011;114:271–282.
137. Gu WJ, Wei CY, Huang DQ, et al: Meta-analysis of randomized controlled trials on the efficacy of thoracic epidural anesthesia in preventing atrial fibrillation after coronary artery bypass grafting. BMC Cardiovasc Disord 2012;12:1–7.
138. Freund FG, Bonica JJ, Ward RJ, et al: Ventilatory reserve and level of motor block during high spinal and epidural anesthesia. Anesthesiology 1967;28:834–837.
139. Groeben H: Epidural anesthesia and pulmonary function. J Anesth 2006;20:290–299.
140. Lirk P, Hollmann MW: Outcome after regional anesthesia: Weighing risks and benefits. Minerva Anestesiol 2014;80:610–618.
141. Sielenkämper AW, Van Aken H: Thoracic epidural anesthesia: More than just anesthesia/analgesia. Anesthesiology 2003;99:523–525.
142. Brodner G, Van Aken H, Hertle L, et al: Multimodal perioperative management—combining thoracic epidural analgesia, forced mobilization, and oral nutrition—reduces hormonal and metabolic stress and improves convalescence after major urologic surgery. Anesth Analg 2001;92:1594–1600.
143. Frank SM, Beattie C, Christopherson R, et al: Epidural versus general anesthesia, ambient operating room temperature, and patient age as predictors of inadvertent hypothermia. Anesthesiology 1992;77: 252–257.
144. Matsukawa T, Sessler DI, Christensen R, et al: Heat flow and distribution during epidural anesthesia. Anesthesiology 1995;83: 961–967.

145. Szmuk P, Ezri T, Sessler D, et al: Spinal anesthesia speeds active postoperative rewarming. Anesthesiology 1997;87:1050–1054.

146. Backman SB: Regional anesthesia: sympathectomy-mediated vasodilation. Can J Anaesth 2009;56:702–703.

147. Greene NM: Area of differential block in spinal anesthesia with hyperbaric tetracaine. Anesthesiology 1958;19:45–50.

148. Brull SJ, Greene NM: Zones of differential sensory block during extradural anaesthesia. Br J Anaesth 1991;66:651–655.

149. Valley MA, Bourke DL, Hamil MP, et al: Time course of sympathetic blockade during epidural anesthesia: Laser Doppler flowmetry studies or regional skin perfusion. Anesth Analg 1993;76:289–294.

150. Ginosar Y, Weiniger CF, Kurz V, et al: Sympathectomy mediated vasodilation: A randomized concentration ranging study of epidural bupivacaine. Can J Anaesth 2009;56:213–221.

151. Bengsston M: Changes in skin blood flow and temperature during spinal analgesia evaluated by laser Doppler flowmetry and infrared thermography. Acta Anaesthesiol Scand 1984;28:625–630.

152. Kimura T, Goda Y, Kemmotsu O, et al: Regional differences in skin blood flow and temperature during total spinal anaesthesia. Can J Anaesth 1992;39:123–127.

153. Bromage PR, Joyal AC, Binney JC: Local anesthetic drugs: penetration from the spinal extradural space into the neuraxis. Science 1963; 140: 392–394.

154. Moore D, Spierdijk J, VanKleef J, et al: Chloroprocaine neurotoxicity: Four additional cases. Anesth Analg 1982;61:155–159.

155. Lynch C 3rd: Depression of myocardial contractility in vitro by bupivacaine, etidocainem, and lidocaine. Anesth Analg 1986;65: 551–559.

156. Graf B, Martin E, Bosnjak Z: Stereospecific effect of bupivacaine isomers on atrioventricular conduction in the isolated perfused guinea pig heart. Anesthesiology 1997;86:410–419.

157. McClure JH: Ropivacaine. Br J Anaesth 1996;76:300–307.

158. Bader AM, Datta A, Flanagan H, et al: Comparison of bupivacaine- and ropivacaine-induced conduction blockade in isolated rabbit vagus nerve. Anesth Analg 1989;68:724–727.

159. Curatolo M, Petersen-Felix S, Arendt-Nielsen L, et al: Adding sodium bicarbonate to lidocaine enhances the depth of epidural blockade. Anesth Analg 1998;86:341–347.

160. Corke BC, Carlson CG, Dettbarn WD: The influence of 2-chloroprocaine on the subsequent analgesic potency of bupivacaine. Anesthesiology 1984;60:25–27.

161. Stanton-Hicks M, Berges PU, Bonica JJ: Circulatory effects of peridural block. IV. Comparison of the effects of epinephrine and phenylephrine. Anesthesiology 1973;39:308–314.

162. Bouguet D: Caudal clonidine added to local anesthetics enhances postoperative analgesia after anal surgery in adults. Anesthesiology 1994; 81:A942.

163. Kroin JS, Buvanendran A, Beck DR, et al: Clonidine prolongation of lidocaine analgesia after sciatic nerve block in rats is mediated via the hyperpolarization-activated cation current, not by alpha-adrenoreceptors. Anesthesiology 2004;101:488–494.

164. Landau R, Schiffer E, Morales M, et al: The dose-sparing effect of clonidine added to ropivacaine for labor epidural analgesia. Anesth Analg 2002;95:728–734.

165. Kayacan N, Arici G, Karsli B, et al: Patient-controlled epidural analgesia in labour: The addition of fentanyl or clonidine to bupivacaine. Agri 2004;16:59–66.

166. Novak-Jankovic V, Paver-Eržen V, Bovill JG, et al: Effect of epidural and intravenous clonidine on the neuro-endocrine and immune stress response in patients undergoing lung surgery. Eur J Anaesthiol 2000; 17:50–56.

167. Matot I, Drenger B, Weissman C, et al: Epidural clonidine, bupivacaine and methadone as the sole analgesic agent after thoracotomy for lung resection. Anaesthesia 2004;59:861–866.

168. Wu CT, Jao SW, Borel CO: The effect of epidural clonidine on perioperative cytokine response, postoperative pain, and bowel function in patients undergoing colorectal surgery. Anesth Analg 2004;99: 502–509.

169. Roelants F, Lavand'homme PM, Mercier-Fuzier V: Epidural administration of neostigmine and clonidine to induce labor analgesia: Evaluation of efficacy and local anesthetic-sparing effect. Anesthesiology 2005;102:1205–1210.

170. Boogmans T, Vertommen J, Valkenborgh T, et al: Epidural neostigmine and clonidine improves the quality of combined spinal epidural analgesia in labour: A randomised, double-blind controlled trial. Eur J Anaesthesiol 2014;31:190–196.

171. Roelants F, Lavand'homme PM: Epidural neostigmine combined with sufentanil provides balanced and selective analgesia in early labor. Anesthesiology 2004;101:439–444.

172. Omais M, Lauretti G, Paccola CA: Epidural morphine and neostigmine for postoperative analgesia after orthopedic surgery. Anesth Analg 2002;95:1698–1701.

173. Habib AS, Gan TJ. Use of neostigmine in the management of acute postoperative pain and labour pain: A review. CNS Drugs 2006;20: 821–839.

174. Lauretti GR, Gomes JM, Reis MP, Pereira NL:. Low doses of epidural ketamine or neostigmine, but not midazolam, improve morphine analgesia in epidural terminal cancer pain therapy. J Clin Anesth 1999; 11(8):663–668.

175. Lauretti GR, de Oliveira R, Perez MV, et al: Postoperative analgesia by intraarticular and epidural neostigmine following knee surgery. J Clin Anesth 2000;12:444–448.

176. Johansen MJ, Gradert TL, Sattefield WC, et al: Safety of continuous intrathecal midazolam infusion in the sheep model. Anesth Analg 2004;98:1528–1535.

177. Bharti N, Madan R, Mohanty PR, et al: Intrathecal midazolam added to bupivacaine improves the duration and quality of spinal anaesthesia. Acta Anaesthesiol Scand 2003;47:1101–1105.

178. Tucker AP, Mezzatesta J, Nadeson R, et al: Intrathecal midazolam II: Combination with intrathecal fentanyl for labor pain. Anesth Analg 2004;98:1521–1527.

179. Ugur B, Basaloglu K, Yurtseven T, et al: Neurotoxicity with single dose intrathecal midazolam administration. Eur J Anaesthiol 2005;22: 907–912.

180. Yaksh TL, Allen JW: Preclinical insights into the implementation of intrathecal midazolam: a cautionary tale. Anesth Analg 2004;98: 1509–1511.

181. Gambling D, Hughes T, Martin G, et al: A comparison of Depodur, a novel, single-dose extended-release epidural morphine, with standard epidural morphine for pain relief after lower abdominal surgery. Anesth Analg 2005;100:1065–1074.

182. Viscusi ER, Martin G, Hartrick CT, et al: Forty-eight hours of postoperative pain relief after total hip arthroplasty with a novel, extended-release epidural morphine formulation. Anesthesiology 2005;102:1014–1022.

183. Carvalho B, Riley E, Cohen SE, et al: Single-dose, sustained release epidural morphine in the management of postoperative pain after elective cesarean delivery: Results of a multicenter randomized controlled study. Anesth Analg 2005;100:1150–1158.

184. Magnusdottir H, Kimo K, Ricksten S: High thoracic epidural analgesia does not inhibit sympathetic nerve activity in the lower extremities. Anesthesiology 1999;91:1299–1304.

185. Basse L, Werner M, Kehlet H: Is urinary drainage necessary during continuous epidural anesthesia after colonic resection. Reg Anesth Pain Med 2000;25:498–501.

186. Galindo A, Hernandez J, Benavides O, et al: Quality of spinal extradural anesthesia: The influence of spinal nerve root diameter. Br J Anaesth 1975;47:41–47.

187. Duggan J, Bowler GM, McClure JH, et al: Extradural block with bupivacaine: Influence of dose, volume, concentration and patient characteristics. Br J Anaesth 1998;61:324–331.

188. Sakura S, Sumi M, Kushizaki H, et al: Concentration of lidocaine affects intensity of sensory block during lumbar epidural anesthesia. Anesth Analg 1999;88:123–127.

189. Hodgkinson R, Husain FJ: Obesity, gravity, and spread of epidural anesthesia. Anesth Analg 1981;60:421–424.

190. Seow LT, Lips FJ, Cousins MJ: Effect of lateral position on epidural blockade for surgery. Anaesth Intensive Care 1983;11:97–102.

191. Park WY, Hagins FM, Rivat EL, et al: Age and epidural dose response in adult men. Anesthesiology 1982;56:318–320.

192. Park WY, Massengale M, Kim SI, et al: Age and spread of local anesthetic solutions in the epidural space. Anesth Analg 1980;59:768–771.

193. Veering BT, Burm AG, van Kleef JW, et al: Epidural anesthesia with bupivacaine: Effects of age on neural blockade and pharmacokinetics. Anesth Analg 1987;66:589–593.

194. Hirabayashi Y, Shimizu R, Matsuda I, et al: Effect of extradural compliance and resistance on spread of extradural analgesia. Br J Anaesth 1990;65:508–513.

195. Bromage PR, Bufoot MF, Crowell DE, et al: Quality of epidural blockade. I. Influence of physical factors. Br J Anaesth 1964;36: 342–352.

196. Grundy EM, Zamora AM, Winnie AP: Comparison of spread of epidural anesthesia in pregnant and nonpregnant women. Anesth Analg 1978;57:544–546.

197. Arakawa M: Does pregnancy increase the efficacy of lumbar epidural anesthesia? Int J Obstet Anesth 2004;13:86–90.

198. Henke VG, Bateman BT, Leffert LR: Spinal anesthesia in severe preeclampsia. Anaesth Analg 2013;117:686–693.

199. Spiegel JE, Vasudevan A, Li Y, et al: A randomized prospective study comparing two flexible epidural catheters for labour analgesia. Br J Anaesth 2009;103:400–405.

200. Frölich MA, Zhang K, Ness TJ: Effect of sedation on pain perception. Anesthesiology 2013;118:611–621.

201. Frölich MA, Burchfield DJ, Euliano TY, et al: A single dose of fentanyl and midazolam prior to Cesarean section have no adverse neonatal effects. Can J Anaesth 2006;53:79–85.

202. Varelmann D, Pancaro C, Cappiello EC, et al: Nocebo-induced hyperalgesia during local anesthetic injection. Anesth Analg 2010;110:868–870.

203. Marica LS, O'Day T, Janosky J, et al: Chloroprocaine is less painful than lidocaine for skin infiltration anesthesia. Anesth Analg 2002;94:351–354.

204. Cepeda MS, Tzortzopoulou A, Thackrey M, et al: Adjusting the pH of lidocaine for reducing pain on injection. Cochrane Database Syst Rev 2010;12:CD006581.

205. Al Shahwan MA: Prospective comparison between buffered 1% lidocaine-epinephrine and skin cooling in reducing the pain of local anesthetic infiltration. Dermatol Surg 2012;38:1654–1659.

206. Hamilton CL, Riley ET, Cohen SE: Changes in the position of epidural catheters associated with patient movement. Anesthesiology 1997;86:778–784.

207. Richardson MG, Thakur R, Abramowicz JS, et al: Maternal posture influences the extent of sensory block produced by intrathecal dextrose-free bupivacaine with fentanyl for labor analgesia. Anesth Analg 1996;83:1229–1233.

208. Tsen LC: Neuraxial techniques for labor analgesia should be placed in the lateral position. Int J Obstet Anesth 2008;17:146–149.

209. American Society of Anesthesiologists Task Force on Infectious Complications Associated With Neuraxial Techniques: Practice advisory for the prevention, diagnosis, and management of infectious complications associated with neuraxial techniques. Anesthesiology 2010;112:530–545.

210. Malhotra S, Dharmadasa A, Yentis SM: One vs two applications of chlorhexidine/ethanol for disinfecting the skin: Implications for regional anaesthesia. Anaesthesia 2011;66:574–578.

211. Bogod DS: The sting in the tail: Antisepsis and the neuraxis revisited. Anaesthesia 2012;67:1305–1309.

212. Segal S, Arendt KW: A retrospective effectiveness study of loss of resistance to air or saline for identification of the epidural space. Anesth Analg 2010;110:558–563.

213. Laviola S, Kirvelä M, Spoto M: Pneumocephalus with intense headache and unilateral pupillary dilatation after accidental dural puncture during epidural anesthesia for cesarean section. Anesth Analg 1999;88:582–583.

214. Van de Velde M: Identification of the epidural space: Stop using the loss of resistance to air technique! Acta Anaesthiol Belg 2006;57:51–54.

215. Dalens B, Bazin JE, Haberer JP: Epidural bubbles as a cause of incomplete analgesia during epidural anesthesia. Anesth Analg 1987;66:679–683.

216. Naulty JS, Ostheimer GW, Datta S, et al: Incidence of venous air embolism during epidural catheter insertion. Anesthesiology 1982;57:410–412.

217. Evron S, Sessler D, Sadan O, et al: Identification of the epidural space: Loss of resistance with air, lidocaine, or the combination of air and lidocaine. Anesth Analg 2004;99:245–250.

218. Balki M, Lee Y, Halpern S, et al: Ultrasound imaging of the lumbar spine in the transverse plane: The correlation between estimated and actual depth to the epidural space in obese parturients. Anesth Analg 2009;108:1876–1881.

219. Mhyre JM: Why do pharmacologic test doses fail to identify the unintended intrathecal catheter in obstetrics? Anesth Analg 2013;116:4–7.

220. Tsui B, Gupta S, Finucane B: Confirmation of epidural catheter placement using nerve stimulation. Can J Anaesth 1998;45: 640–644,1998.

221. Lyons GR, Kocarev MG, Wilson RC, et al: A comparison of minimum local anesthetic volumes and doses of epidural bupivacaine (0.125% w/v and 0.25% w/v) for analgesia in labor. Anesth Analg 2007;104:412–415.

222. Wong CA, Ratliff JT, Sullivan JT, et al: A randomized comparison of programmed intermittent epidural bolus with continuous epidural infusion for labor analgesia. Anesth Analg 2006;102:904–909.

223. Heesen M, Klohr S, Rossaint R, et al: Can the incidence of accidental dural puncture in laboring women be reduced? A systematic review and meta-analysis. Minerva Anestesiol 2013;79:1187–1197.

224. Van de Velde M, Schepers R, Berends N, et al: Ten years of experience with accidental dural puncture and post-dural puncture headache in a tertiary obstetric anaesthesia department. Int J Obstet Anesth 2008;17:329–335.

225. Agerson AN, Scavone BM: Prophylactic epidural blood patch after unintentional dural puncture for the prevention of postdural puncture headache in parturients. Anesth Analg 2012;115:133–136.

226. Bauer ME, Kountanis JA, Tsen LC, et al: Risk factors for failed conversion of labor epidural analgesia to cesarean delivery anesthesia: A systematic review and meta-analysis of observational trials. Int J Obstet Anesth 2012;21:294–309.

227. Toledano RD, Kodali BS, Camann WR: Anesthesia drugs in the obstetric and gynecologic practice. Rev Obstet Gynecol 2009;2:93–100.

228. Mhyre JM, Greenfield ML, Tsen LC, et al: A systematic review of randomized controlled trials that evaluate strategies to avoid epidural vein cannulation during obstetric epidural catheter placement. Anesth Analg 2009;108:1232–1242.

229. Neal JM, Mulroy MF, Weinberg GL: American Society of Regional Anesthesia and Pain Medicine checklist for managing local anesthetic systemic toxicity: 2012 version. Reg Anesth Pain Med 2012;37:16–18.

230. Bhole MV, Manson AL, Seneviratne SL, et al: IgE-mediated allergy to local anaesthetics: Separating fact from perception: A UK perspective. Br J Anaesth 2012;108:903–911.

231. Rice I, Wee MY, Thomson K: Obstetric epidurals and chronic adhesive arachnoiditis. Br J Anaesth 2004;92:109–120.

232. Taniguchi M, Bollen AW, Drasner K: Sodium bisulfite: Scapegoat for chloroprocaine neurotoxicity? Anesthesiology 2004;100:85–91.

233. Checketts MR: Wash & go—but with what? Skin antiseptic solutions for central neuraxial block. Anaesthesia 2012;67:819–822.

234. Na EH, Han SJ, Kim MH: Delayed occurrence of spinal arachnoiditis following a caudal block. J Spinal Cord Med 2011;34:616–619.

235. Ross JS, Masaryk T, Modic M, et al: MR imaging of lumbar arachnoiditis. Am J Roentgenol 1987;149:1025–1032.

236. Wang YL, Hsieh JR, Chung HS, et al: The local addition of tenoxicam reduces the incidence of low back pain after lumbar epidural anesthesia. Anesthesiology 1998;89:1414–1417.

237. Stevens RA, Urmey WF, Urquhart, et al: Back pain after epidural anesthesia with chloroprocaine. Anesthesiology 1993;78:492–497.

238. Hakim SH, Narouze S, Shaker NN, et al: Risk factors for new-onset persistent low-back pain following nonobstetric surgery performed with epidural anesthesia. Reg Anesth Pain Med 2012;37:175–182.

239. Wilkinson HA: Field block anesthesia for lumbar puncture. JAMA 1983;249:2177.

240. Wang YL, Tan PP, Yang CH, et al: Epidural dexamethasone reduces the incidence of backache after lumbar epidural anesthesia. Anesth Analg 1997;84:376–378.

241. Breen TW: Epidural analgesia and back pain. In Halpern Sh, Douglas MJ (eds): Evidence-Based Obstetric Anesthesia. BMJ Books, 2005, pp 208–216.

242. Arendt K, Demaerschalk BM, Wingerchuck DM, et al: Atraumatic lumbar puncture needles: After all these years, are we still missing the point? Neurologist 2009;15:17–20.

243. Brownridge P: The management of headache following accidental dural puncture in obstetric patients. Anaesth Intensive Care 1983;11:4–15.

244. Headache Classification Committee of the International Headache Society: The international classification of headache disorders, third edition. Cephalalgia 2013;33:629–808.

245. Webb CA, Weyker PD, Zhang L, et al: Unintentional dural puncture with a Tuohy needle increases risk of chronic headache. Anesth Analg 2012;115:124–132.

246. Apfel CC, Saxena A, Cakmakkaya OS, et al: Prevention of postdural puncture headache after accidental dural puncture: A quantitative systematic review. Br J Anaesth 2010;105:255–263.

247. Oedit R, van Kooten F, Bakker SL, et al: Efficacy of the epidural blood patch for the treatment of post lumbar puncture headache BLOPP: A randomised, observer-blind, controlled clinical trial. BMC Neurol 2005;5:12.

248. van Kooten F, Oedit R, Bakker SL, et al: Epidural blood patch in post dural puncture heachache: A randomized, observed-blind, controlled clinical trial. J Neurol Neurosurg Psychiatry 2008;79:553–559.

249. Angle P, Tang SL, Thompson D, et al: Expectant management of postdural puncture headache increases hospital length of stay and emergency room visits. Can J Anaesth 2005;52:397–402.

250. Paech MJ, Doherty DA, Christmas T, et al: The volume of blood for epidural blood patch in obstetrics: A randomized, blinded clinical trial. Anesth Analg 2011;113:126–133.

251. Haines DE: On the question of a subdural space. Anat Rec 1991; 230:3–21.

252. Lubenow T, Keh-Wong E, Kristof K, et al: Inadvertent subdural injection: A complication of epidural block. Anesth Analg 1988;67: 175–179.

253. Paech MJ, Godkin R, Webster S: Complications of obstetric epidural analgesia and anaesthesia: A prospective analysis of 10,995 cases. Int J Obstet Anesth 1998;7:5–11.

254. Cappiello E, Tsen LC: Complications and side effects of central neuraxial techniques. In Wong CA (ed): *Spinal and Epidural Anesthesia*. McGraw-Hill, 2007, pp 152–182.

255. Grewal S, Hocking G, Wildsmith JA: Epidural abscesses. Br J Anaesth 2006;96:292–302.

256. Darouiche R, Spinal epidural abscess: N Engl J Med 2006;355: 2012–2020.

257. Connor DE, Chittiboina P, Caldito G, et al: Comparison of operative and nonoperative management of spinal epidural abscess: A retrospective review of clinical and laboratory predictors of neurologic outcome. J Neurosurg Spine 2013;19:119–127.

258. Curry WT, Hoh BL, Amin-Hanjani S, et al: Spinal epidural abscess: Clinical presentation, management, and outcome. Surg Neurol 2005;63:364–371.

259. Okano K, Kondo H, Tsuchiya R, et al: Spinal epidural abscess associated with epidural catheterization: Report of a case and a review of the literature. Jpn J Clin Oncol 1999;29:49–52.

260. Danner RL, Hartman BJ: Update on spinal epidural abscess: 35 cases and review of the literature. Rev Infect Dis 1987;9:265–274.

261. Huang PY, Chen SF, Chang WN, et al: Spinal epidural abscess in adults caused by *Staphylococcus aureus*: Clinical characteristics and prognostic factors. Clin Neurol Neurosurg 2012;114:572–576.

262. Baer ET: Post-dural puncture bacterial meningitis. Anesthesiology 2006; 105:381–393.

263. Reynolds F: Neurological infections after neuraxial anaesthesia. Anesthesiol Clin 2008;26:23–52.

264. Usubiaga JE: Neurological complications following epidural anesthesia. Int Anaesthesiol 1975;13:1–153.

265. Kane RE: Neurologic deficits following epidural or spinal anesthesia. Anesth Analg 1981;60:150–161.

266. Kao M, Tsai S, Tsou M, et al: Paraplegia after delayed detection of inadvertent spinal cord injury during thoracic epidural catheterization in an anesthetized elderly patient. Anesth Analg 2004;99:580–583.

267. Loo CC, Irestedt L: Cauda equina syndrome after spinal anaesthesia with hyperbaric 5% lignocaine: A review of six cases of cauda equina syndrome reported to the Swedish Pharmaceutical Insurance 1993–1997. Acta Anaesthesiol Scand 1999;43:371–379.

268. Lambert DH, Hurley RJ: Cauda equina syndrome and continuous spinal anesthesia. Anesth Analg 1991;72:817–819.

269. Gerancher JC: Cauda equina syndrome following a single spinal administration of 5% hyperbaric lidocaine through a 25-gauge Whitacre needle. Anesthesiology 1997;87:687–689.

270. Benson JS: US Food and Drug Administration safety alert: Cauda equine syndrome associated with the use of small-bore catheters in continuous spinal anesthesia. AANA J 1992;60:223.

271. Rigler ML, Drasner K, Krejcie, TC, et al: Cauda equina syndrome after continuous spinal anesthesia. Anesth Analg 1991;72:275–281.

272. Gaiser RR: Should intrathecal lidocaine be used in the 21st century? J Clin Anesth 2000;12:476–481.

273. Walters MA, Van de Velde M, Wilms G: Acute intrathecal haematoma following neuraxial anaesthesia: Diagnostic delay after apparently normal radiological imaging. Int J Obstet Anesth 2012;21:181–185.

274. Auroy Y, Narchi P, Messiah A, et al: Serious complications related to regional anesthesia: Results of a prospective survey in France. Anesthesiology 1997;87:479–486.

275. Pollard JB: Common mechanisms and strategies for prevention and treatment of cardiac arrest during epidural anesthesia. J Clin Anesth 2002;14:52–56.

276. Pollard JB: Cardiac arrest during spinal anesthesia: Common mechanisms and strategies for prevention. Anesth Analg 2001;92:252–256.

277. Krismer AC, Hogan QH, Wenzel V, et al: The efficacy of epinephrine or vasopressin for resuscitation during epidural anesthesia. Anesth Analg 2001;93:734–742.

278. Curatolo M, Scaramozzino P, Venuti FS, et al: Factors associated with hypotension and bradycardia after epidural blockade. Anesth Analg 1996;83:1033–1040.

279. Liguori GA, Sharrock NE: Asystole and severe bradycardia during epidural anesthesia in orthopedic patients. Anesthesiology 1997;86: 250–257.

280. Camann WR, Hortvet LA, Hughes N, et al: Maternal temperature regulation during extradural analgesia for labour. Br J Anaesth 1991;67: 565–568.

281. Borgeat A, Ekatodramis G, Schenker CA: Postoperative nausea and vomiting in regional anesthesia: A review. Anesthesiology 2003;98: 530–547.

282. Allen TK, Jones CA, Habib AS: Dexamethasone for the prophylaxis of postoperative nausea and vomiting associated with neuraxial morphine administration: A systematic review and meta-analysis. Anesth Analg 2012;114:813–822.

283. Turnbull J, Mooneshinghe R: Perioperative epidurals: The controversy goes on. Br J Hosp Med 2011;72:538.

284. Dong H, Zhang Y, Xi H: The effects of epidural anaesthesia and analgesia on natural killer cell cytotoxicity and cytokine response in patients with epithelial ovarian cancer undergoing radical resection, J Int Med Research 2012;40:1822–1829.

Caudal Anesthesia

Kenneth D. Candido, Anthony R. Tharian, and Alon P. Winnie

INTRODUCTION

Caudal anesthesia was described at the turn of last century by two French physicians, Fernand Cathelin and Jean-Anthanase Sicard. The technique pre-dated the lumbar approach to epidural block by several years.[1] Caudal anesthesia, however, did not gain in popularity immediately following its inception. One of the major reasons caudal anesthesia was not embraced is the wide anatomical variations of sacral bones and the consequent failure rate associated with attempts to locate the sacral hiatus. The failure rate of 5% to 10% made caudal epidural anesthesia unpopular until a resurgence of interest in the 1940s, led by Hingson and colleagues, who used it in obstetrical anesthesia. Caudal epidural anesthesia has many applications, including surgical anesthesia in children and adults, as well as the management of acute and chronic pain conditions. Success rates of 98%–100% can be achieved in infants and young children before the age of puberty, as well as in lean adults.[1] The technique of caudal epidural block in pain management has been greatly enhanced by the use of fluoroscopic guidance and epidurography, in which high success rates can be attained.

Unfortunately, clinical indications, and especially therapeutic interventions for the relief of chronic pain in individuals with failed back surgery syndrome, are often most prevalent in patients with difficult caudal landmarks. It has been suggested that traditional lumbar peridural block should not be attempted employing an approach requiring needle placement through a spinal surgery scar due to the likelihood of tearing the dura and the possibility of inducing hematoma formation over the cauda equina when blood from the procedure becomes trapped

between the layers of scar and connective tissues.[2] Under these circumstances, it is recommended that fluoroscopically guided caudal epidural block be performed in lieu of the traditional palpation approach. Alternatively, the use of ultrasound may be appropriate to identify the sacral hiatus, and this technique has recently been described. The second resurgence in popularity of caudal anesthesia has paralleled the increasing need to find safe alternatives to conventional lumbar epidural block in selected patient populations, such as individuals with failed back surgery syndrome.

ANATOMIC CONSIDERATIONS

The sacrum is a large triangularly shaped bone formed by the fusion of the five sacral vertebrae. It has a blunted, caudal apex that articulates with the coccyx. Its superior, wide base articulates with the fifth lumbar vertebra at the lumbosacral angle (see Figure 25–1A). Its dorsal surface is convex and has a raised interrupted median crest with four (sometimes three) spinous tubercles representing fused sacral spines. Flanking the median crest, the posterior surface is formed by fused laminae. Lateral to the median crest, four pairs of dorsal foramina lead into the sacral canal through intervertebral foramina, each of which transmits the dorsal ramus of a sacral spinal nerve (see Figure 25–1A). Below the fourth (or third) spinous tubercle, an arched sacral hiatus is identified in the posterior wall of the sacral canal due to the failure of the fifth pair of laminae to meet, exposing the dorsal surface of the fifth sacral vertebral body. The caudal opening of the canal is the sacral hiatus (see Figures 25–1B and 25–1C) roofed by the firm elastic membrane, the sacrococcygeal ligament, which is

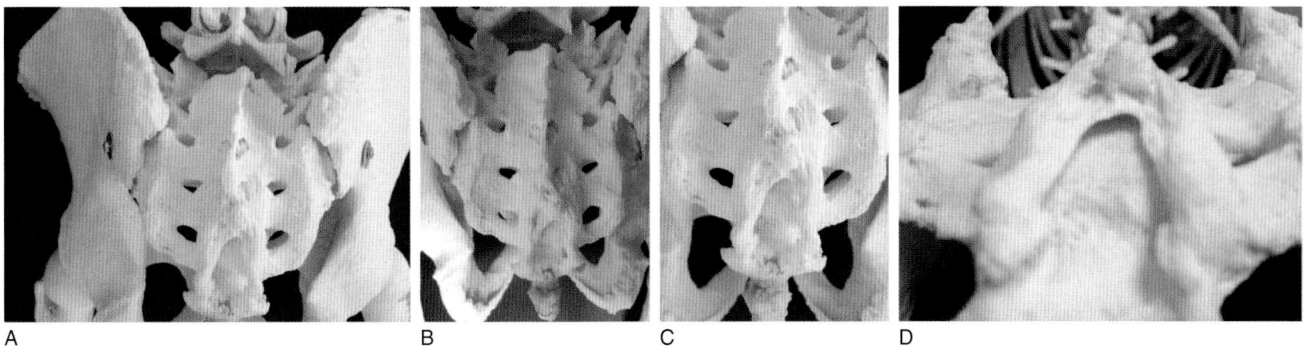

FIGURE 25–1. A: Skeletal specimen of the sacrum viewed from craniad to caudad demonstrating the four pairs of dorsal foramina, situated bilaterally. **B:** Skeletal model demonstrating the sacral hiatus and its relationship to the coccyx and the sacrum. The fifth inferior articular processes project caudally and flank the sacral hiatus as sacral cornua. **C:** Skeletal model showing the sacral hiatus with the exposed dorsal surface of the fifth sacral vertebral body. **D:** Skeletal specimen viewed from inferior to the sacral hiatus.

an extension of the ligamentum flavum. The fifth inferior articular processes project caudally and flank the sacral hiatus as sacral cornua, connected to the coccygeal cornua by intercornual ligaments.

The sacral canal is triangular in shape. It is a continuation of the lumbar spinal canal. Each lateral wall presents four intervertebral foramina, through which the canal is in contiguous with the pelvic and dorsal sacral foramina. The posterior sacral foramina are smaller than their anterior counterparts. The sacral canal contains the cauda equina (including the filum terminale) and the spinal meninges. Near its midlevel (typically the middle one-third of S2, but varying from the midpoint of S1 to the midpoint of S3), the subarachnoid and subdural spaces cease to exist, and the lower sacral spinal roots and filum terminale pierce the arachnoid and dura maters.[3,4] However, variations in the termination of the dural sac as well as pathologic conditions like sacral meningocele or sacral perineural cysts can increase the chances of inadvertent dural puncture when performing caudal block in such patients with abnormal anatomy.[5]

The lowest margin of the filum terminale emerges at the sacral hiatus and traverses the dorsal surface of the fifth sacral vertebra and sacrococcygeal joint to reach the coccyx. The fifth sacral nerve roots also emerge through the hiatus medial to each of the sacral cornua. The sacral canal contains the epidural venous plexus, which generally terminates at S4 but which may continue more caudally. Most of these vessels are concentrated in the anterolateral portion of the canal. The remainder of the sacral canal is filled with adipose tissue, which is subject to an age-related decrease in its density. This change may be responsible for the transition from the predictable spread of local anesthetics administered for caudal anesthesia in children to the limited and unpredictable segmental spread seen in adults.[6]

Considerable variability occurs in sacral hiatus anatomy among individuals of seemingly similar backgrounds, race, and stature.[1] As individuals age, the overlying ligaments and the cornua thicken significantly. The hiatal margins often defy recognition by even skilled fingertips. The practical problems related to caudal anesthesia are mainly attributable to wide anatomical variations in size, shape, and orientation of the

sacrum. Trotter[3] summarized the major anatomical variations of the sacrum. The sacral hiatus may be almost closed, asymmetrically open, or widely open secondary to anomalies in the pattern of fusion of the laminae of the sacral arches. Sacral spina bifida was noted in about 2% of males and in 0.3% of females. The anteroposterior depth of the sacral canal may vary from less than 2 mm to greater than 1 cm. Individuals with sacral canals having anterior-posterior (A-P) diameters less than about 3 mm may not be able to accommodate anything larger than a 21-gauge needle (5% of the population).[1]

In addition, the lateral width of the sacral canal varies significantly. Because the depth and width may vary, the volume of the canal itself may also vary. Trotter found that sacral volumes varied between 12 and 65 mL, with a mean volume of 33 mL.[3] A magnetic resonance imaging (MRI) study in 37 adult patients found the volume (excluding the foramina and dural sac) was 14.4 mL, with a range of 9.5 to 26.6 mL.[7] Patients with smaller capacities may not be able to accommodate the typical volumes of local anesthetics administered for epidural anesthesia via the caudal route.

In a cadaver study of 53 specimens, the mean distance between the tip of the dural sac and the upper edge of the sacral hiatus as denoted by the sacrococcygeal membrane was 45 mm, with a range of 16–75 mm[3]. In the MRI study mentioned, the mean distance was found to be 60.5 mm, with a range of 34–80 mm.[7]

The sacrococcygeal membrane could not be identified in 10.8% of subjects using MRI.[7] An anatomical evaluation of 92 isolated sacra found that 42% of cases had both a hiatus and cornua; 4% of the cases showed an absent hiatus. The apex of the sacral hiatus, in that study, was noted in 64% of cases to exist at the S4 level. The hiatus was closed in 3% of cases.[8]

The sacral foramina afford anatomical passages that permit the spread of injected solutions, such as local anesthetics and adjuvants (see Figure 25–1A). The posterior sacral foramina are essentially sealed by the multifidus and sacrospinalis muscles, but the anterior foramina are unobstructed by muscles and ligaments, permitting ready egress of solutions through them.[9] The sacral curvature varies substantially.[10] In a cadaver study, looking at the anatomy of caudal epidural space, the sacral cornua were not palpable bilaterally in 14.3% and palpable unilaterally in 24.5% of specimens. The level of maximum curvature of the sacrum was at S3 in 69.4% of cases.[11] This variability tends to be more severe in males than in females.

The clinical significance of this finding is that a noncurving epidural needle will more likely pass easily into the canal of females than males. The angle between the axis of the lumbar canal and the sacral canal varies between 7° and 70° in subjects with marked lordosis. The clinical implication of this finding is that the cephalad flow of caudally injected solutions may be more limited in lordotic patients with exaggerated lumbosacral angles than in those with flatter lumbosacral angles, in whom the axes of the lumbar and sacral canals are more closely aligned.

Clinical Pearls

- Considerable variability occurs in sacral hiatus anatomy.
- With advancing age, the overlying ligaments and the cornua thicken; consequently, identification of the sacral hiatal margins becomes more challenging.
- The success rate of caudal anesthesia is largely dependent on anatomic variations in size, shape, and orientation of the sacrum.

INDICATIONS FOR CAUDAL EPIDURAL BLOCK

The indications for caudal epidural block are essentially the same as for lumbar epidural block, but its use may be preferred when sacral nerve spread of anesthetics and adjuvants is preferred over lumbar nerve spread. The unpredictability cephalad spread of anesthetics administered into the caudal canal limits the use of this technique in situations where it is essential to provide lower thoracic and upper abdominal neuraxial blockade. Although this modality is described for perioperative use (diminishing role) and for managing chronic pain scenarios in adults (increasing role), caudal block has a wide range of indications[12–15] (Table 25–1). Successful treatment of postdural puncture headache by performing an epidural blood patch through a caudally placed needle has been reported.[16]

Clinical Pearls

- The indications for caudal epidural block are essentially the same as those for lumbar epidural block.
- Caudal block may be preferred over lumbar epidural block when sacral nerve spread of anesthetics and adjuvants is preferred over lumbar nerve spread.
- The unpredictability of ascertaining consistent cephalad spread of anesthetics administered through the caudal canal limits the usefulness of this technique when it is essential to provide lower thoracic and upper abdominal neuraxial blockade.

TABLE 25–1. Indications for caudal epidural block.

Surgical, Obstetric, Diagnostic, and Prognostic
1. Surgical anesthesia
2. Obstetric anesthesia
3. Differential neural blockade to evaluate pelvic, bladder, perineal, genital, rectal, anal, and lower extremity pain
4. Prognostic indicator before destruction of sacral nerves

Acute Pain
1. Acute low back pain
2. Acute lumbar radiculopathy
3. Palliation in acute pain emergencies
4. Postoperative pain
5. Pelvic and lower extremity pain secondary to trauma
6. Pain of acute herpes zoster
7. Acute vascular insufficiency of the lower extremities
8. Hidradenitis suppurativa

Chronic Benign Pain
1. Lumbar radiculopathy
2. Spinal stenosis
3. Low back syndrome
4. Vertebral compression fractures
5. Diabetic polyneuropathy
6. Postherpetic neuralgia
7. Reflex sympathetic dystrophy
8. Orchialgia
9. Proctalgia
10. Pelvic pain syndromes

Cancer Pain
1. Pain secondary to pelvic, perineal, genital, or rectal malignancy
2. Bony metastases to pelvis
3. Chemotherapy-related peripheral neuropathy

Special Situations
Patients with previous lumbar spine surgery
Patients who are "anticoagulated" or have coagulopathy

Source: Modified with permission from Waldman S: *Pain Management*, 2nd ed. Philadelphia: Elsevier Saunders; 2011.

Other, newer indications in adults deserve mention and are described further in this chapter, including the performance of percutaneous epidural neuroplasty[17,18]; the use of caudal analgesia following lumbar spinal surgery[19]; caudal analgesia after orthopedic lower extremity surgery[20]; local anesthetic adjuvants for postoperative analgesia[21]; and caudal block for performing neurolysis for treatment intractable cancer pain.[22]

THE TECHNIQUE OF CAUDAL EPIDURAL BLOCK

The classical technique of caudal epidural block involves palpation, identification, and puncture.[1] Patients are evaluated as for any epidural block, and the indications and relative and absolute contraindications to its performance are identical. A full complement of noninvasive monitors is applied, and baseline vital signs are assessed. One must decide whether a continuous or single-shot technique will be employed. For continuous techniques, a Tuohy-type needle with a lateral-facing orifice is preferred.

Patient Positioning

Several positions can be used in adults, compared with the lateral decubitus position in neonates and children. The lateral position is often preferred in pediatrics because it permits easy access to the airway when general anesthesia or heavy sedation has been administered prior to performing the block. In pediatric patients, blocks may be performed with the patient fully anesthetized; this is not recommended for older children and adults. In adults, the prone position is the most frequently utilized, but the lateral decubitus position or the knee-chest (also known as "knee-elbow") position may be employed. In the prone position, the procedure table or operating room table should be flexed, or a pillow may be placed beneath the symphysis pubis and iliac crests to produce slight flexion of the hips. This maneuver makes palpation of the caudal canal easier. The legs are separated with the heels rotated outward to smooth out the upper part of the anal cleft, while simultaneously relaxing the gluteal muscles. For placement of caudal epidural block in the parturient, the lateral (Sim's position) and the knee-elbow position are most commonly used.

Anatomical Landmarks

A dry gauze swab is placed in the intergluteal cleft to protect the anal area and genitalia from povidone iodine or other disinfectants (especially alcohol) used to desinfect the skin. Anatomical landmarks are next assessed. The skinfolds of the buttocks are useful guides in locating the underlying sacral hiatus. Alternatively, a triangle may be marked on the skin over the sacrum, using the posterior superior iliac spines (PSISs) as the base, with the apex pointing inferiorly (caudally). Normally, this apex sits over or immediately adjacent to the sacral hiatus. However, a recent study indicated that identification of the sacral hiatus using this method may be inaccurate because the actual triangle formed by the sacral hiatus and PSISs is not equiangular.[23] Once the hiatus is marked, the tip of the index finger is placed on the tip of the coccyx in the intergluteal cleft while the thumb of the same hand palpates the two sacral cornua located 3–4 cm more rostrally at the upper end of the intergluteal cleft. The sacral cornua may be identified by gently moving the palpating index finger from side to side (Figure 25–2). The palpating thumb should sink into the hollow between the two cornua, as if between two knuckles of a fist.[1] Sterile skin preparation and draping of the entire region are performed in the usual fashion.

Technique Using Fluoroscopy

A small-gauge 1.5-inch needle is then utilized to infiltrate the skin over the sacral hiatus using 3–5 mL of 1%–1.5% plain

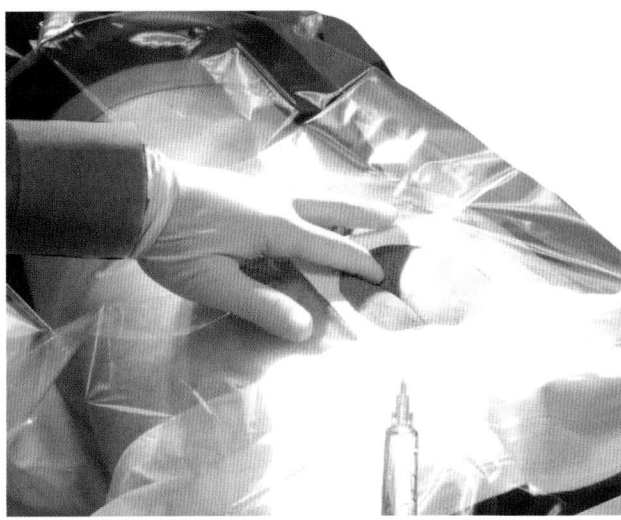

FIGURE 25–2. Technique of palpating the midline over the sacral hiatus. The palpating index and middle fingers are spread over the fifth sacral vertebral body. The sacrococcygeal ligament lies directly beneath the palpating finger.

lidocaine HCl (Figure 25–3). If fluoroscopy is utilized, a lateral view is obtained to demonstrate the anatomic boundaries of the sacral canal. We routinely leave the local anesthetic infiltration needle in situ for this view because it demonstrates whether the approach is at the appropriate level for subsequent advancement of the epidural needle. With fluoroscopy, the caudal canal appears as a translucent layer posterior to the sacral segments. The median sacral crest is visualized as an opaque line posterior to the caudal canal. The sacral hiatus is usually visualized as a translucent opening at the base of the caudal canal. The coccyx may be seen articulating with the inferior surface of the sacrum (Figure 25–4).

Once the tissues overlying the hiatus have been anesthetized, a 17- or 18-gauge Tuohy-type needle is inserted either in the midline or, using a lateral approach, into the caudal canal (Figure 25–5, Figure 25–6). A feeling of a slight "snap" may be

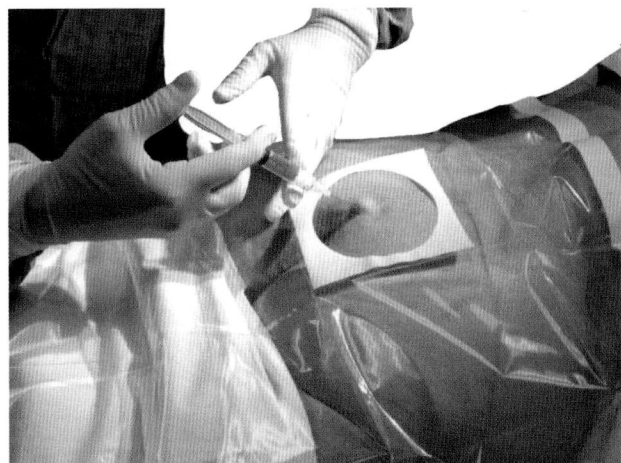

FIGURE 25–3. Technique of skin infiltration with local anesthetic. The needle is inserted first above and then into the substance of the sacrococcygeal ligament.

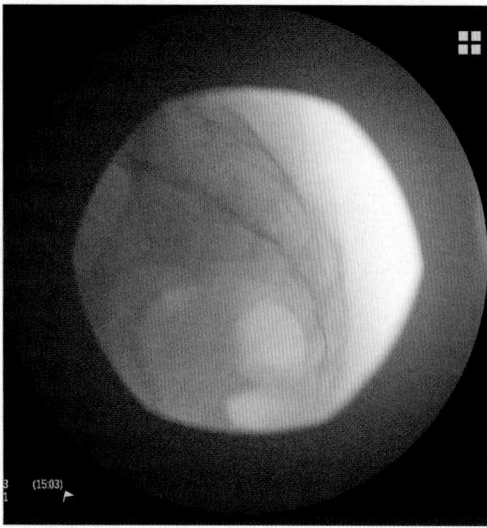

FIGURE 25–4. Lateral fluoroscopic image demonstrating the boundaries of the caudal canal.

appreciated when the advancing needle pierces the sacrococcygeal ligament. Once the needle reaches the ventral wall of the sacral canal, it is slowly withdrawn and reoriented, directing it more cranially (by depressing hub and advancing) for further insertion into the canal. We utilize the anteroposterior view once the epidural needle is safely situated within the canal, and the epidural catheter is advanced cephalad (Figure 25–7, Figure 25–8). In this projection, the intermediate sacral crests appear as opaque vertical lines on either side of the midline. The sacral foramina are visualized as translucent and nearly circular areas lateral to the intermediate sacral crests. The presence of intestinal gas may obscure the recognition of these structures. A syringe loaded with either air or saline containing a small air bubble is then attached to the needle, and the loss-of-resistance technique is used to establish entry into the epidural space.

Clinical Pearls

- The needle tip should stay below the S2 level to avoid tearing the dura.
- The needle should never be advanced in the space too deep.
- The skin corresponding to about 1 cm inferior to the PSISs indicates the S2 level (caudal-most extension of the dura mater).
- The dural sac extends lower in children than in adults, and epidural needles should be carefully advanced no deeper than the S3 or S4 level.

An acoustic test, also called the "whoosh" test has been described for identifying correct needle placement in the caudal canal. This characteristic sound has been noted during auscultation of the thoracolumbar region during the injection of 2–3 mL of air into the caudal epidural space.[24] The "swoosh test," described by Orme and Berg, substitutes saline or local anesthestic instead of air as the injectate. Of the 108 patients with a successful block in one study, 98 had a positive test, with no false-positive results.[25] Once the correct placement of the needle is confirmed, a catheter is inserted into the desired location (depth) and its position confirmed fluoroscopically when desired (Figure 25–9). Color Doppler ultrasonography has also been described for guiding the needle insertion into the epidural space and to confirm any intravascular injection.[26]

ULTRASOUND-GUIDED CAUDAL BLOCK

Ultrasound has played an increasing role in regional anesthesia and pain management, ultrasound guidance can be utilized to identify the sacral hiatus, thereby facilitating needle entry into the hiatus, as well as to visualize the advancing needle in the caudal canal. Because caudal blocks are relatively easy to perform in the pediatric population, ultrasound may not be

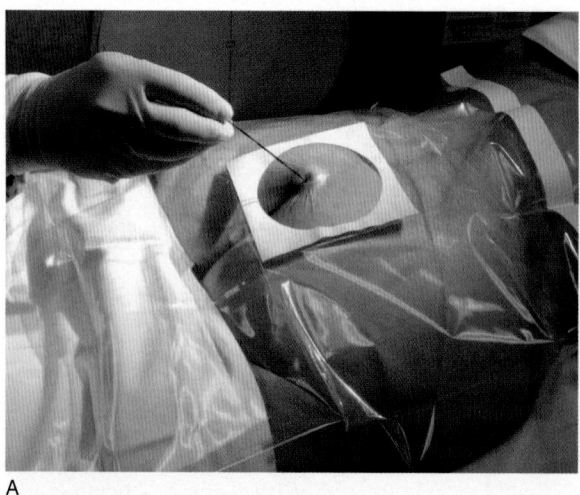

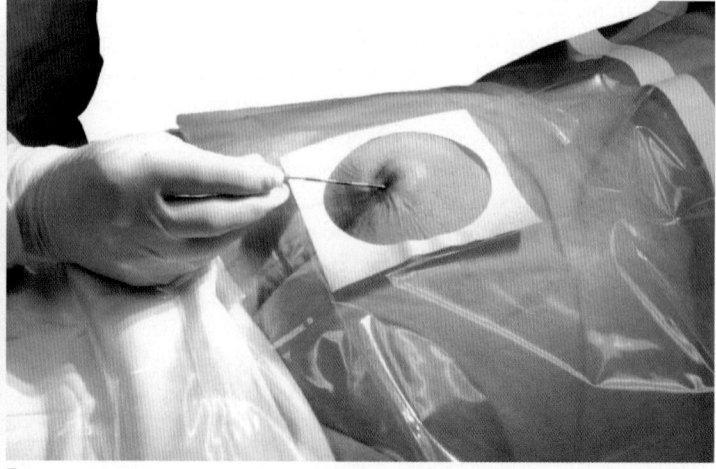

A   B

FIGURE 25–5. An 18-gauge, Tuohy-type needle is advanced from the skin into the sacral hiatus through the sacrococcygeal ligament. Usually, when fluoroscopy is not available to verify correct needle placement, a syringe loaded with air or saline is attached to the needle, and the loss-of-resistance technique is employed to identify the epidural space.

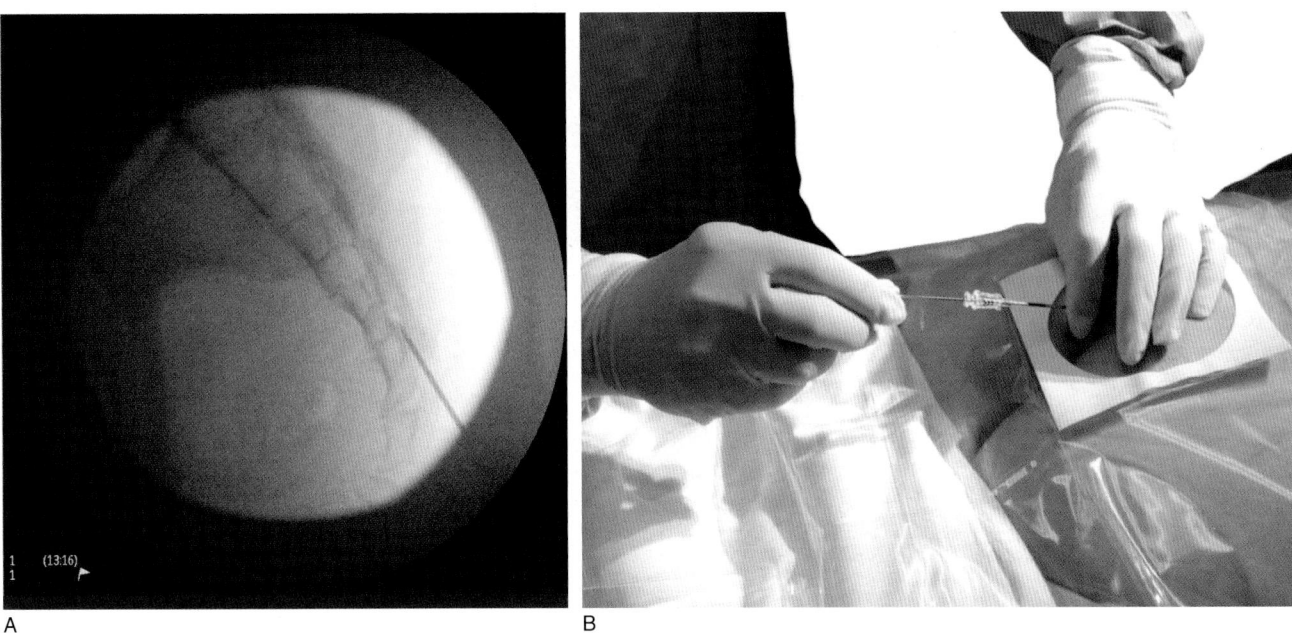

A   B

FIGURE 25–6. Lateral fluoroscopic image depicting the 18-gauge Tuohy needle correctly seated in the caudal epidural space.

significantly advantageous over landmark-based techniques. However, in adult patients, for whom the anatomy of the sacral hiatus, caudal canal, and dural sac are variable, ultrasound guidance may prove to be helpful in reducing the risk of complications such as tissue trauma, dural puncture, local anesthetic toxicity, and vascular compromise.

Technique

With the patient in the prone position, the sacral cornua are identified by palpation using the technique described in the section on anatomic landmarks. Sterile skin preparation and draping of the entire region are performed. A low-frequency curvilinear probe, is placed in the transverse plane across the two sacral cornua (Figure 25–10). The sacral cornua can be visualized as two symmetric hyperechoic arches, with a hypoechoic shade underneath both lines, bridging these two structures. Traversing this hypoechoic area are two hyperechoic lines, the superficial one being the sacrococcygeal ligament and the

deeper one line being the dorsal bony surface of the sacrum (Figure 25–11). A 22-gauge needle is inserted into the space between the two cornua. A distinct "pop" is felt as the needle tip penetrates the sacrococcygeal ligament.

At this point, the orientation of the probe is changed into the sagittal plane (Figure 25–12), and the caudal canal is identified as a hypoechoic canal tapering off caudally and bordered by dorsal and ventral hyperechoic bands. The dorsal band is formed by the dorsal bony aspect of the caudal canal cranially and the sacrococcygeal ligament caudally. The ventral band is formed by the ventral bony surface of the caudal canal (Figure 25–13).

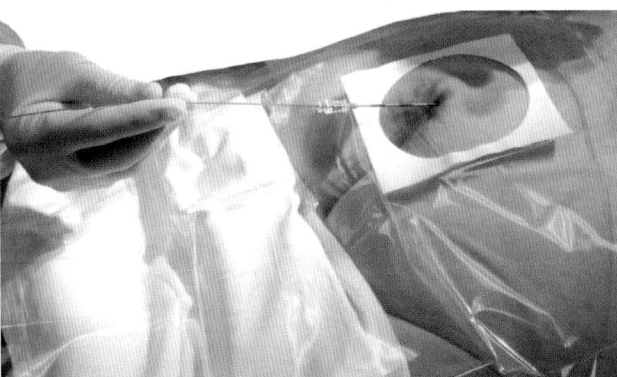

FIGURE 25–7. A continuous catheter with a stylet in place is being advanced through the 18-gauge Tuohy needle placed in the canal.

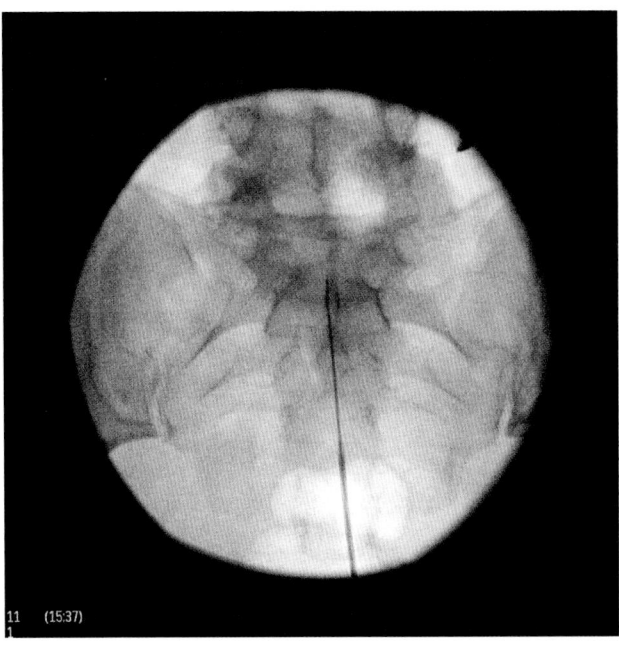

FIGURE 25–8. Anteroposterior fluoroscopic imaging depicting proper placement of the needle.

PART 3

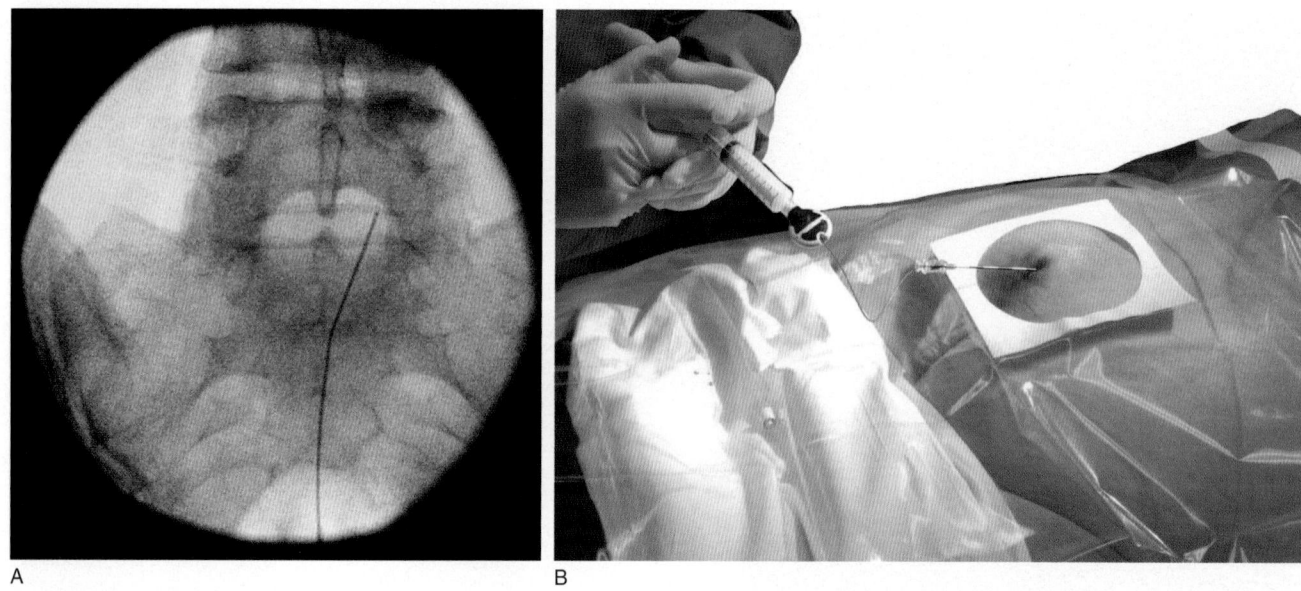

A   B

FIGURE 25–9. Anteroposterior fluoroscopic image depicting the catheter advanced to the L5–S1 interspace.

Once the needle is within the caudal canal, aspiration is undertaken to ensure there is no CSF or blood. Once negative aspiration is confirmed, injection is carried out under real-time ultrasonography. The spread of the injectate can be visualized as turbulence within the caudal canal.[27]

The major limitation of the ultrasound-guided caudal block is the difficulty in identifying intrathecal or intravascular injection. Although color Doppler has been described[26] to detect intrathecal or intravascular injection, the turbulence created by the injectate in the caudal canal produces variable color patterns, which makes interpretation unreliable. Contrast fluoroscopy is still the best technique to rule out inadvertent intrathecal or intravascular injection.

Clinical Pearls

- In pediatric patients, electrical stimulation has been used to ascertain correct needle placement in the caudal canal. Anal sphincter contraction (corresponding to stimulation of S2–S4) is sought with 1- to 10-mA currents.[28]
- If the needle has been inserted correctly, moving the hub from side to side, while the shaft is held at the sacrococcygeal membrane will allow the tip swinging freely in the sacral canal like a fulcrum.

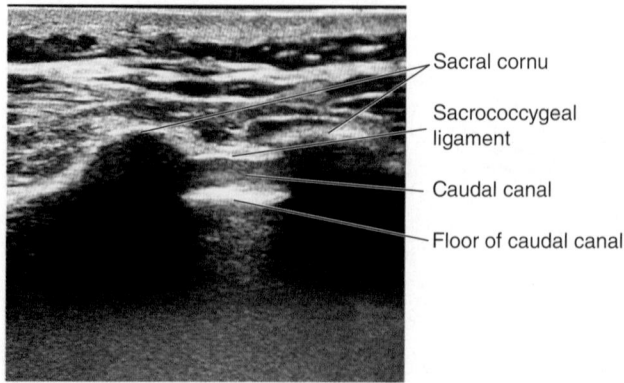

Sacral cornu

Sacrococcygeal ligament

Caudal canal

Floor of caudal canal

FIGURE 25–10. A low-frequency curvilinear ultrasound probe ensheathed in a sterile probe cover containing gel being placed in the transverse plane across the two sacral cornua.

FIGURE 25–11. Ultrasound image along the short axis of the caudal canal, depicting the sacral cornua, sacrococcygeal ligament, and the caudal canal.

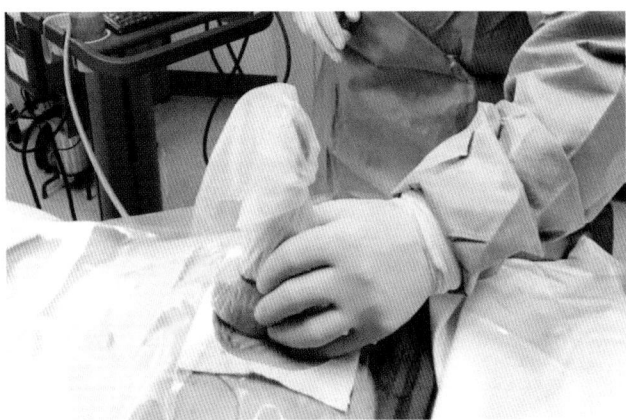

FIGURE 25–12. The low-frequency curvilinear probe placed in the sagittal plane along the long axis of the caudal canal.

- If cerebrospinal fluid (CSF) is obtained after aspiration, the needle should be withdrawn and injection should not be undertaken.
- If blood is aspirated, the needle should be withdrawn and reinserted until no blood is apparent at the hub.
- When injection of air (or saline) for the loss-of-resistance technique results in bulging over the sacrum, the needle tip most probably lies dorsal to the sacrum in the subcutaneous tissues.
- If the needle tip is subperiosteal, the injection will meet with significant resistance, resulting is significant patient discomfort. The cortical layer of the sacral bone is often thin, particularly in infants and older subjects, and its penetration can easily occur especially if force is exerted while advancing the needle. The sensation of entering cancellous bone is not unlike penetrating the sacrococcygeal membrane; there is a feeling of resistance that is suddenly overcome, and the needle advances more freely and subsequent injection is unhampered.

Several complications related to the technique procedure have been described. Injected solutions may be absorbed rapidly from bone marrow, and toxic drug reactions result. In this situation, pain is typically noted over the caudal part of the sacrum during the injection. If this occurs, the needle should be withdrawn slightly and rotated on its axis until it can be reinserted in a slightly different direction.[29–31]

If injection is made anterior to the sacrum, it is possible to perforate the rectum, or, in parturients, the baby's head may be injured. This limits the use of caudal block in laboring women once the presenting part has descended into the perineum. Inadvertent venous puncture may also occur, and the incidence of this has been reported to be about 0.6%.[32]

Caudal block may be used with a single-shot or continuous catheter technique. For continuous block, the catheter may be advanced anterograde (conventionally) or retrograde. Continuous caudal block may be performed in retrograde fashion using needle insertion into the lumbar epidural space, but directed inferiorly instead of superiorly. In one study of 10 patients, epidural catheters were advanced through 18-gauge Tuohy-type epidural needles in retrograde fashion from the L4–L5 interspace. This technique was associated with a 20% failure rate, with the catheter going into the paravertebral or retrorectal spaces, despite easy epidural space entry.[33] Using the conventional approach, a Huber-tipped Tuohy needle is used as a conduit to pass the epidural catheter into the canal. This needle has a curved bevel tip that limits it being caught or snagged on the sacral periosteum. The needle is inserted with its shoulder facing anteriorly and its orifice dorsally. Alternatively, a standard 16- or 17-gauge catheter-over-needle assemblage (angiocatheter) may serve as the introducing needle for subsequent catheter placement. The catheter is advanced under fluoroscopic guidance, especially when it is performed for chronic pain management in failed back surgery syndrome. The catheters should be advanced gently because there have been reports of dural puncture with rapid or aggressive advancement. A lateral and anteroposterior fluoroscopic views should be obtained

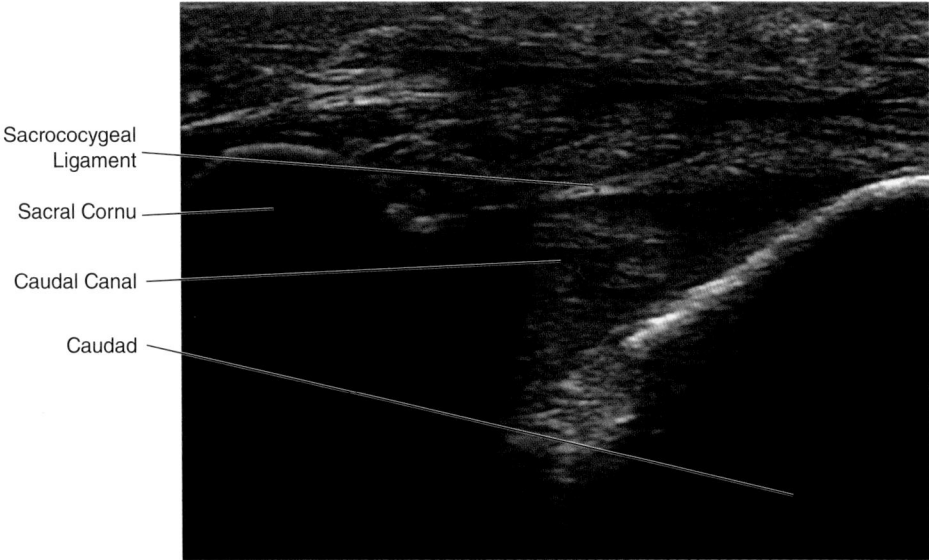

Sacrococcygeal Ligament

Sacral Cornu

Caudal Canal

Caudad

FIGURE 25–13. Ultrasonographic image along the long axis of the caudal canal depicting the long-axis view of the caudal canal.

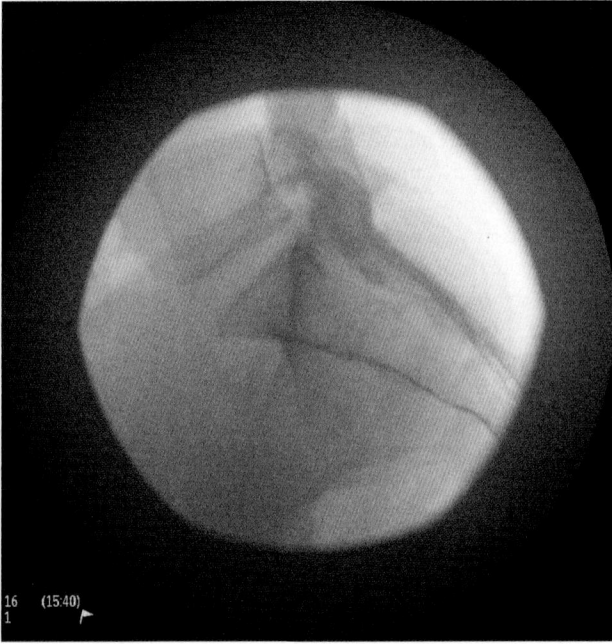

FIGURE 25–14. Lateral fluoroscopic image depicting radiopaque contrast medium in the caudal and lower lumbar epidural spaces. The image shows considerable spread, both anteriorly and posteriorly, following the injection of 2 mL of dye.

to demonstrate placement of the catheter in the epidural space (Figures 25–14 and 25-9) and to follow its path in a cephalad or cephalolateral direction. When the desired level is attained, iodinated nonionic contrast media may be injected, followed by the injection of local anesthetics, corticosteroids, or adjuncts (Figure 25–15). Usually, the catheter is not advanced higher than the level of L4 vertebral body, although it could be advanced to the L1 or L2 levels for specific indications. Some

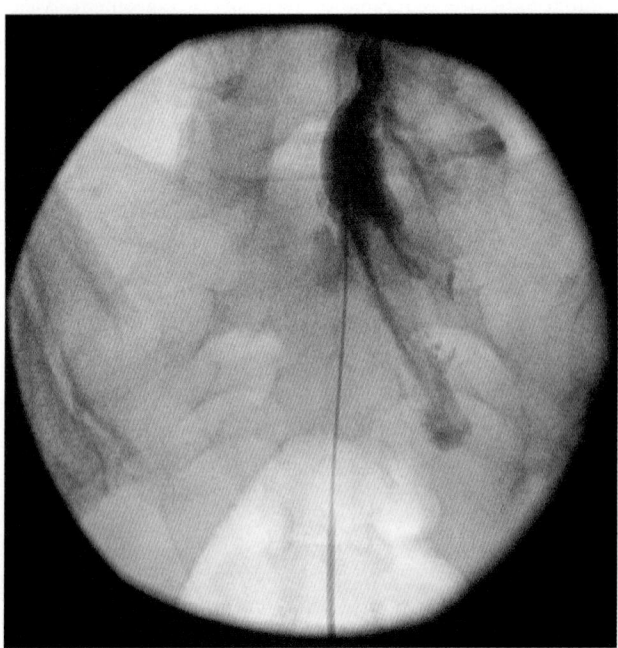

FIGURE 25–15. Anteroposterior fluoroscopic image depicting radiopaque contrast medium in the epidural space.

authors recommend not to advance the catheter more than 8–12 cm cephalad.

Clinical Pearls

- Spread of the local anesthetic solutions injected into the caudal epidural space in adults is influenced by injected volume, speed of injection, and patient positioning.
- There is no correlation between the speed of injection and spread of the local anesthetic in children undergoing caudal anesthesia.[34]

CHARACTERISTICS OF CAUDAL EPIDURAL BLOCK IN ADULTS

Caudal epidural block results in sensory and motor block of the sacral roots and limited autonomic block. The sacral contribution of the parasympathetic nervous system is blocked causing loss of visceromotor function of the bladder and intestines distal to the colonic splenic flexure. Sympathetic block, although limited compared to the lumbar or thoracic epidural block, does occur. However, the sympathetic outflow from the preganglionic sympathetic fibers of the spinal cord ends at the L2 level; therefore, caudal block should not routinely result in peripheral vasodilatation of the lower extremities to the degree witnessed with lumbar epidural blockade. Caudal epidural local anesthetic block in adults may be chosen for surgeries of the lower abdomen, perineum, or lower extremities. The local anesthetic mixtures and doses are similar to those for lumbar epidural block (Table 25–2). One recent study looking at the effect of gender on the minimal local anesthetic concentrations (MLACs) of ropivacaine for caudal anesthesia in patients undergoing anorectal surgery found that the MLAC for caudal anesthesia in female patients is 31% higher than in male patients.[35]

Spread of Local Anesthetic Solutions

The large capacity of the sacral canal accommodates correspondingly large volumes of solution; significant volumes may be lost through the wide anterior sacral foramina. Therefore, the caudal dose requirements of local anesthetics to achieve the same segmental spread are significantly larger than are the corresponding lumbar doses. Roughly twice the lumbar epidural local anesthetic dose is needed for caudal blockade to attain similar levels of analgesia and anesthesia, and solutions injected in the caudal space take longer to spread (Table 25–2). Bromage noted that age is not correlated with caudal segmental spread in adults, and the upper level of analgesia resulting from 20-mL doses of local anesthetic solution varies widely between S2 and T8.[1] This unpredictability limits the usefulness of applying caudal anesthesia for surgical procedures that require cephalad analgesia levels above the pelvic level or the umbilicus. A more recent study confirmed Bromage's findings. In 172 women undergoing minor gynecologic surgery using caudal anesthesia with 20 mL of 1.5% lidocaine,[36] the highest sensory dermatome level reached was below T10.

TABLE 25–2. Local anesthetics commonly used for caudal anesthesia in adults

Agent	Concentration	Dose (mg)	Sensory Onset (4-Segment Spread)	Duration (2-Segment Regression)
Lidocaine	1.5%–2%	300–600	10–20 min	90–150 min
Chloroprocaine	2%–3%	400–900	8–15 min	45–80 min
Mepivacaine	2%%	400–600	10–20 min	90–240 min
Ropivacaine	0.75%–1%	150–300	15–25 min	120–210 min
Bupivacaine/ levobupivacaine	0.5%–0.75%	100–225	10–25 min	180–270 min

All solutions with epinephrine 1:200,000, except ropivacaine.

Clinical Pearls

- The sacral canal contains the cauda equina (including the filum terminale), the spinal meninges, adipose tissue, and sacral venous plexus.
- The volume of the sacral canal averages 14.4 mL.
- The indications for caudal epidural block are the same as for a lumbar epidural block.
- Percutaneous epidural neuroplasty is a technique of administering local anesthetics, corticosteroids, hyaluronidase, and hypertonic saline through a caudal catheter for the purpose of lysing epidural adhesions.
- Adult patients are typically placed prone for the block, whereas the lateral decubitus position is preferred for pediatrics.
- Caudal blockade in pediatrics is used primarily for perioperative pain control, whereas in adults it is primarily for chronic pain management.
- In adults, roughly twice the local anesthetic dose is required to attain the same segmental spread with caudal block compared with the dose used for lumbar epidural block.

Indications for Caudal Epidural Analgesia in Adults

A caudal epidural block is indicated whenever the area of surgery involves the sacral and lower lumbar nerve roots. The technique is suitable for anal surgery (hemorrhoidectomy and anal dilation), gynecologic procedures, surgery on the penis or scrotum, and lower limb surgeries. Using a catheter technique, it is possible to use the caudal epidural block for cesarean section, vaginal hysterectomy, and inguinal herniorrhaphy.

A caudal epidural block is used less frequently than the lumbar or thoracic epidural block for perioperative analgesia in adults. The pelvis enlarges markedly in puberty, while the epidural fat in the lumbosacral region undergoes compaction and increased fibrous content. This hinders cephalad spread of solutions, particularly when compared with the spread in children.

As an alternative to the caudal epidural block in adults, one might consider a median approach to transsacral epidural block. In the original description of that technique, 87% of blocks were successful for transurethral resection of bladder tumors versus 100% success for sacral procedures. Anesthesia level, side effects, and hemodynamics were similar between the two groups studied in the initial report.[37]

CAUDAL BLOCK FOR LABOR ANALGESIA

The sacral canal shares in the general engorgement of extradural veins that occurs in late pregnancy or in any clinical condition in which the inferior vena cava (IVC) is partially obstructed. Because the effective volume of the caudal canal is markedly diminished during the latter part pregnancy, the caudal dosage should be reduced proportionately in women at term. The segmental spread of local anesthetics may increase substantially in pregnant women at term, necessitating a 28% to 33% decrease of dose requirement in this patient population.[1] The choice of a continuous catheter or a single-shot technique during active labor is limited by the relative lack of sterility at the sacral hiatus, which may be contaminated by feces and meconium.

Rare cases of Horner syndrome have been reported when large doses of local anesthetics are injected caudally during labor analgesia administration.[1] This is most likely to occur if injection is made with the patient on her back (engorgement of epidural venous plexus and IVC compression are maximal).

The so-called dual technique (lumbar and caudal) of epidural block for labor is no longer widely used. Because the pain of uterine contractions is mediated by sympathetic nervous system fibers originating from the T10 to L2 spinal segments, a lumbar epidural catheter suffices for both stage I and stage II of parturition, with dosage adjustments made depending on the exact circumstances and requirements (see Chapter 41, Obstetric Regional Anesthesia).

INDICATIONS FOR CAUDAL EPIDURAL ANALGESIA IN CHILDREN

Characteristics of the Blockade

The sacral hiatus is usually easy to palpate in infants and children, which makes this technique much easier and predictable. Consequently, in many institutions with large numbers of pediatric patients, caudal epidural block is an integral part of the intra- and postoperative pain management for children undergoing a wide range of surgical procedures both below and above the diaphragm. The technique is easily learned; one study demonstrated an 80% success rate in resident trainees after completing 32 procedures performed without fluoroscopic guidance.[38] In infants and small children, a 21-gauge, short-bevel, 1-inch needle may be used for single-injection techniques. For continuous blocks, a standard epidural catheter may be advanced through an 18-gauge angiocatheter or through a thin-wall 18-gauge epidural needle. It has been noted that by 4 or 5 years of age the sacral canal is usually large enough to accept such a needle for passage of a catheter.[1] The electrocardiogram has been used to verify appropriate thoracic catheter tip placement (epidural electrocardiography).[39]

Spread of Local Anesthetic Solutions

The segmental spread of analgesia following caudal administration is more predictable in children up to about 12 years of age.[40] Some studies suggested that the cephalad spread of caudal solutions in children is not hampered by the same anatomical constraints that develop from puberty onward. Before puberty, anatomical barriers at the lumbosacral junction have not yet developed to a marked degree, and caudal solutions can flow freely upward into the higher recesses of the spinal canal. As a consequence, the rostral spread of caudal anesthesia is more extensive and more predictable in children than in adults.

Indications in Children

In children, caudal block is usually combined with light general anesthesia with spontaneous ventilation. During lower abdominal and genitourinary surgery in children, caudal block with 0.25% bupivacaine (2 mg/kg) was shown to lower the metabolic and endocrine responses to stress, as measured by glucose concentrations; mean prolactin levels; insulin; and cortisol concentrations, as compared with general anesthesia alone.[41] Thoracic placement of catheters is possible in neonates and small children. However, one radiographic study of 115 infants found 10 caudally placed catheters to be in the high thoracic or low cervical region, when their intended site was in the lower thoracic segments.[42]

The three groups of indications for caudal epidural block in children are the following:

1. Patients requiring sacral block (circumcision, anal surgery)
2. Patients requiring lower thoracic block (inguinal herniorrhaphy)
3. Patients requiring analgesia of the upper thoracic dermatomes (thoracic surgery)

Pharmacologic Considerations for Caudal Epidural Anesthesia in Children

Caudal block with bupivacaine (4 mg/kg) and morphine (150 µg/kg) was found to lower fentanyl requirements during cardiac surgery and shorten extubation times in a group of 30 pediatric patients randomized to receive general anesthesia alone or a combination of general or caudal block.[43]

Anesthetic dose requirements are about 0.1 mL/segment per year for 1% lidocaine or 0.25% bupivacaine.[1] The dose may also be calculated based on body weight. The relationship between age and dose requirements is strictly linear, with a high degree of correlation up to 12 years old.[1] A recent study using fluoroscopy with 0.2% ropivacaine containing radiopaque dye at a ratio of 1:4 showed that the weight-based doses for caudally administered 0.2% bupivacaine were applicable to 0.2% ropivacaine as well.[44] Plasma bupivacaine concentrations in children receiving caudal block with 0.2% of the local anesthetic (2 mg/kg) were less than equivalent doses administered via ilioinguinal-iliohypogastric block for pain control following herniotomy or orchidopexy. In addition, the times to peak plasma concentrations were faster in the peripheral nerve block group, indicating that caudal block is a safe alternative to local infiltration techniques in inguinal surgery.[45]

In a study of children 1 to 6 years of age who underwent orchidopexy, a caudal block using larger volumes of dilute bupivacaine (0.2%) was shown to be more effective than a smaller volume of the standard (0.25%) concentration for blocking the peritoneal response to spermatic cord traction, with no change in the quality of postoperative analgesia. In that study, the total bupivacaine dose was identical in both groups (20 mg).[46] Ropivacaine 0.5% was shown to provide a significantly longer duration of analgesia following inguinal herniorrhaphy in children aged 1.5–7 years when compared to 0.25% ropivacaine or 0.25% bupivacaine.[47] All children received 0.75 mL/kg of the local anesthetic. However, the times to first voiding and to standing were significantly delayed in the group receiving 0.5% ropivacaine, and there was one case of motor block of the lower extremities.

Another study compared high-volume/low-concentration (1.5 mL/kg of 0.15% solution) and low-volume/high-concentration ropivacaine (1.0 mL/kg 0.225% solution) for caudal analgesia in children aged 1–5 years of age undergoing orchiopexy. This study showed that a larger volume of diluted ropivacaine provided better quality and longer duration of analgesia after discharge than a smaller volume of more concentrated ropivacaine.[48]

Ropivacaine has also been used for caudal block for hypospadias repair in a double-blind, randomized study in 26 children. The minimal effective local anesthetic concentration of ropivacaine was found to be 0.11%, to provide effective caudal analgesia in children under general anesthesia with 0.5 minimum alveolar concentration of enflurane.[49]

Plasma concentrations of ropivacaine after caudal block in 20 children 1 to 8 years of age, using 2 mg/mL, 1 mL/kg, demonstrated free fractions of 5%, clearance of 7.4 mL/kg/min, and terminal half-life of 3.2 hours, well below those associated with toxic symptoms in adults.[50] Another study looking at the minimum local analgesic concentration of ropivacaine for intraoperative caudal analgesia in preschool and school-age children undergoing hypospadias repair found that a higher concentration of ropivacaine was needed for school-age children than preschool age children to provide intraoperative caudal analgesia when combined with general anesthesia.[51] Of the three commonly used local anesthetics for single-shot caudal anesthesia (bupivacaine, ropivacaine, and levobupivacaine), no superiority in terms of clinical efficacy was found for any of these drugs in a meta-analysis of 17 randomized controlled trials that concerned single-shot pediatric caudal anesthesia with at least two of the three drugs in question. Bupivacaine and ropivacaine showed the highest and lowest incidence of motor block, respectively.[52]

A quantitative systematic review of randomized controlled trials looking at the safety and efficacy of clonidine as an additive for caudal regional anesthesia suggested that clonidine may provide extended duration of analgesia with a decreased incidence for analgesic rescue requirements and few adverse effects compared to caudal local anesthetics alone. Data from 20 randomized controlled trials were used in this meta-analysis to assess the safety and efficacy of caudal clonidine added to local anesthetics versus local anesthetics alone in children undergoing urological, lower abdominal, or lower limb surgery.[53] Dexmedetomidine (1 μg/kg) was shown to provide extended duration of pain relief when added to bupivacaine 2.5 mg/mL, 1 mL/kg, when compared to an identical dose of bupivacaine alone in children aged 1–6 years undergoing unilateral inguinal hernia repair/orchidopexy.[54] Another study compared the analgesic effects and side effects of dexmedetomidine and clonidine added to bupivacaine in pediatric patients undergoing lower abdominal surgeries. Sixty patients aged 6 months to 6 years were evenly and randomly assigned into three groups in a double-blinded manner. Each patient received a single caudal dose of bupivacaine 0.25% (1 mL/kg) combined with dexmedetomidine 2 μg/kg in normal saline 1 mL, clonidine 2 μg/kg in normal saline 1 mL, or a corresponding volume of normal saline.[55] The results demonstrated that while both additives increased the period of analgesia, there was no significant advantage of selecting dexmedetomidine over clonidine.

The local anesthetics typically administered for single-shot caudal blocks in pediatric patients are listed in Table 25–3.

Clinical Pearls

- Relaxation of the anal sphincter following local anesthetic injection may predict the success for a caudal block.
- This is particularly useful in children because most caudal blocks are performed while the child is anesthetized, and it is not possible to assess the effectiveness of the block by testing for sensory analgesia levels.
- One study demonstrated that the presence of a lax anal sphincter at the termination of surgery correlated with the reduced need to administer opioids perioperatively.[56]

Other Considerations for Use of Caudal Epidural Anesthesia in Children

Although the caudal block is a mainstay of perioperative pain management in pediatric surgery and represents probably 60% of all regional anesthetic techniques performed in this patient population, not all studies have demonstrated a marked benefit of caudal block for postoperative analgesia when compared with other modalities. Following unilateral inguinal herniorrhaphy, the caudal block was shown to provide effective, but not superior, pain management when compared with local wound infiltration in 54 children. The side effects and rescue analgesia requirements did not differ between the two groups.[57]

Caudal epidural block in children may induce significant changes in descending aortic blood flow while maintaining heart rate and mean arterial blood pressure. In a study of 10 children aged 2 months to 5 years, a transesophageal Doppler probe was used to calculate hemodynamic variables after the injection of 1 mL/kg of 0.25% bupivacaine with epinephrine 5 μg/mL. The aortic ejection volume increased, and aortic vascular resistance decreased by about 40%.[58] Another study that looked at peripheral hemodynamics using Doppler ultrasonography in sevoflurane-anesthetized children before and after a caudal block showed significantly altered flow patterns after the block. The peak velocity increased by 24%; volume flow increased by 76%; and the diameter of the dorsalis pedis

TABLE 25–3. Typical local anesthetics for caudal block in pediatrics (single shot).

Agent	Concentration (%)	Dose	Onset (minutes)	Duration of Action (minutes)
Ropivacaine[74]	0.2	2 mg/kg	9	520
Bupivacaine[74]	0.25	2 mg/kg	12	253
Ropivacaine[75]	0.2	0.7 mg/kg	11.7	491
Bupivacaine[75]	0.25	0.7 mg/kg	13.1	457
Ropivacaine[76]	0.2	1 mL/kg	8.4	Not available
Levobupivacaine[76]	0.25	1 mL/kg	8.8	Not available
Bupivacaine[76]	0.25	1 mL/kg	8.8	Not available

artery increased by 20%. However, blood pressures and heart rates were not significantly affected by caudal block.[59] These data suggest that caudal block results in vasodilatation secondary to sympathetic nervous system blockade.

APPLICATIONS OF CAUDAL EPIDURAL BLOCK IN ACUTE AND CHRONIC PAIN MANAGEMENT

Radiculopathy Refractory to Conventional Therapy

In cases of radiculopathy refractory to conventional analgesic therapies, caudal epidural analgesic techniques can significantly and reliably reduce pain. One such technique is percutaneous epidural neuroplasty: A caudal catheter is left in place for up to 3 days for the purpose of injecting hypertonic solutions into the epidural space to treat radiculopathy with low back pain and associated epidural scarring, typically from previous lumbar spinal surgery. In addition to local anesthetics and corticosteroids, hypertonic saline and hyaluronidase are added to the injectate. The technique requires use of fluoroscopic guidance and caudal epidurography because of its efficacy in correlating a filling defect of injected iodinated nonionic contrast medium with a patient's reported level of pain.[18]

Injection of solutions into the epidural space of a patient with meningeal adhesions is usually painful because of stretching of affected nerve roots.[14] Dexamethasone or betamethasone have been recommended instead of methylprednisolone or triamcinolone because particulate steroids may occlude an epidural catheter or possibly cause spinal ischemia following unintentional intravascular injection.

Hypertonic saline is used to prolong pain relief due to its local anesthetic effects and its ability to reduce edema in previously scarred or inflamed nerve roots.[17] A lateral needle approach is recommended into the caudal canal, directing the needle and catheter toward the affected side. Lateral placement tends to minimize the likelihood of penetrating the dural sac or injecting subdural. When 5–10 mL of contrast media are injected into the caudal canal through an epidural catheter, a "Christmas tree" appearance develops as dye spreads into the perineural structures inside the bony canal and along the nerves as they exit the vertebral column.[17] Epidural adhesions prevent the spread of the dye, so the involved nerves are not outlined by the contrast. Once correct catheter placement in the epidural space is ensured, 1500 units of hyaluronidase in 10 mL of preservative-free saline is injected rapidly. This is followed by an injection of 10 mL of 0.2% ropivacaine and 40 mg of triamcinolone. After these two injections, an additional volume of 9 mL of 10% hypertonic saline is infused over 20–30 minutes. On the second and third days, the local anesthetic (ropivacaine) injection is followed by the hypertonic saline solution.

A study compared the effectiveness of percutaneous epidural adhesiolysis utilizing an injection of 5 mL of preservative-free 2% lidocaine, followed by 6 mL of 10% sodium chloride solution and 6 mg of nonparticulate betamethasone via a fluoroscopically guided, targeted placement of a caudal catheter (group 1) versus an injection of the same solution with 6 mL of 0.9% sodium chloride solution instead of the hypertonic saline via a catheter placed in the caudal canal with its tip at the S3 level (group 2). The study found significant pain relief (76%) in the hypertonic saline group at 1-year follow-up, compared to 4% of patients in the normal saline group.[60]

A prospective, double-blind, randomized study looking at the role of adding hyaluronidase to fluoroscopically guided caudal epidural steroid and hypertonic saline injections in patients with failed back surgery syndrome showed a significant improvement in long-term pain relief in patients who received hyaluronidase. A total of 38 patients were enrolled in the study. Twenty patients received fluoroscopically guided caudal injections of 10 mL of 0.25% bupivacaine solution containing 80 mg of methylprednisolone and 30 mL of 3% hypertonic saline (group 1). Eighteen patients received the same amount of local anesthetic and steroids, followed by 1500 IU of hyaluronidase (which was replaced by an equivalent volume of normal saline in group 1 patients) and 30 mL of 3% hypertonic saline (group 2).[61]

Another randomized, controlled, double-blind trial of fluoroscopically guided caudal epidural injections compared 10 mL of lidocaine 0.5% and 9 mL of lidocaine 0.5% mixed with either 6 mg of betamethasone or 40 mg of methylprednisolone (total volume 10 mL). This study showed a potential superiority of steroids when compared with local anesthetic alone at 1-year follow-up.[62]

Postoperative Analgesia in Patients Undergoing Lumbar Spine Surgery

Another unique application of caudal block is the provision of postoperative analgesia in patients undergoing lumbar spine surgeries. In one case series, patients received 20 mL of 0.25% bupivacaine with 0.1 mg buprenorphine via the caudal epidural approach, performed prior to surgical incision. The patients underwent posterior interbody fusion and laminotomy for spinal stenosis, and postoperative pain control was compared in the caudal group with a group treated with conventional parenteral opioids. The caudal group required fewer rescue analgesic medication doses for the first 12 hours following surgery.[19] A reduction in blood pressure in the caudal group patients undergoing laminotomy, but not fusion, was noted in the patients with prolonged duration (24 hours) of postoperative analgesia.

Other Applications

Caudal epidural block has also been compared with intramuscular opioids in the treatment of pain after emergency lower extremity orthopedic surgery. The caudal group who received 20 mL of 0.5% bupivacaine had 8 hours of superior analgesia and also had a significant reduction in the need for rescue opioid medications.[20]

Caudal injection of clonidine (75 µg with 7 mL bupivacaine 0.5% and 7 mL lidocaine 2% with epinephrine 5 µg/mL) has been used for postoperative analgesia after elective hemorrhoidectomy. Thirty-two adults received the clonidine-local combination, while a control group received local anesthetic alone.

Analgesia averaged 12 hours in the clonidine group, compared to less than 5 hours in the group receiving only local anesthetic. Bradycardia occurred in about 22% of patients in the clonidine group.[18] This contrasts with the results of an evaluation of clonidine used as an adjunct for pediatric caudal anesthesia as noted previously.[63]

Caudal injections of alcohol or phenol have been used to treat intractable pain due to cancer. In a study of 67 blocks, it was found that the lower sacral roots were easily reached with the caudal injection, and that the S1 and S2 roots (contribution from the lumbosacral plexus) were spared.[22]

COMPLICATIONS ASSOCIATED WITH CAUDAL EPIDURAL BLOCK

The complications of caudal block are the same as those occurring following lumbar epidural block and may include those related to the technique itself and those related to the injectate (local anesthetic or other injected substance). Fortunately, serious complications occur infrequently. The list of potential complications includes epidural abscess, meningitis, epidural hematoma, dural puncture and postdural puncture headache, subdural injection, pneumocephalus and air embolism, back pain,[64] and broken or knotted epidural catheters. Other rare complications that have been reported with caudal anesthesia include unilateral parotid swelling,[65] persistent hiccups following continuous caudal infusion of 0.1% ropivacaine,[66] and intracranial hypotension headache after uncomplicated caudal epidural injection.[67]

Systemic Toxicity of Local Anesthetics

The incidence of local anesthetic–induced seizures following caudal block seems to be higher that of lumbar or thoracic approaches. In a retrospective study of 25,697 patients who received brachial plexus blocks, caudal epidural blocks, or lumbar epidural blocks from 1985 to 1992, Brown noted 26 seizure episodes.[68] The frequency of seizures in adults by decreasing order was caudal, brachial plexus block, lumbar, or thoracic epidural block. Nine cases were attributed to caudal blocks, eight occurring with chloroprocaine and one with lidocaine. There was a 70-fold increased incidence of local anesthetic toxic reactions with caudal epidural anesthesia (0.69%) than with lumbar or thoracic epidural anesthesia in adults.

Clinical Pearls

- The incidence of local anesthetic–induced seizures following caudal epidural block is higher than following lumbar or thoracic approaches.
- The relative risk of local anesthetic toxicity follows this order: caudal > brachial plexus block > lumbar or thoracic epidural block.
- Elevation of heart rate by more than 10 beats per minute or an increase in systolic blood pressure of more than 15 mm Hg after injection of epinephrine-containing local anesthetic is suggestive of intravascular injection.

In children, however, one retrospective review identified only two toxic reactions (ie, local anesthetic–induced seizures) in 15,000 caudal blocks.[69] Dalens's group found that unintentional intravascular injection occurs in up to 0.4% of pediatric caudal blocks,[70] demonstrating the importance of performing epinephrine-containing test dosing in this age group. It has been suggested that an elevation of heart rate by more than 10 beats per minute or an increase in systolic blood pressure of more than 15 mm Hg should be taken as indicative of systemic injection. T-wave changes on the ECG occur earliest following intravascular injection, followed by heart rate changes and finally by blood pressure changes. These changes may be delayed for up to 90 seconds following the injection.[70]

Occurrence of Total Spinal Anesthesia

Total spinal anesthesia can occur when an injected dose of local anesthetic intended for the epidural space gains access to the subarachnoid space. In the case report of an 18-month-old child weighing 10 kg who received a caudal block postoperatively after undergoing emergency repair of a recurrent diaphragmatic hernia, 4 mL of 0.5% bupivacaine and 2.5 µg/kg of buprenorphine were injected in a total volume of 10 mL. Eye opening and hand movement were delayed for 3 hours following this complication.[71] In another infant undergoing revision of a Nissen fundoplication, a caudally placed catheter was unintentionally advanced to the cervical spinal region. Electrical stimulation of the catheter (Tsui test) resulted in phrenic nerve stimulation. The catheter was successfully repositioned and further care was uncomplicated. This case report illustrates the relative ease of passing the catheter to high vertebral levels in infants as opposed to adults.[72]

Infection

One case report documented the rare occurrence of distant diskitis and vertebral osteomyelitis involving skip levels and without the development of epidural abscess formation in an elderly woman who received caudal epidural steroid and local anesthetic for degenerative spondylolisthesis. One month later, she developed an L2–L3 and L4–L5 infective diskitis, together with adjacent vertebral osteomyelitis. Cultures demonstrated *Pseudomonas aeruginosa* growth, which was treated with antibiotics.[73]

SUMMARY

Caudal epidural block is a technique of providing analgesia and anesthesia of the lumbosacral nerve roots that pre-dates conventional lumbar approaches. The block has undergone several periods of acceptability, and although it is infrequently applied to routine surgical cases in adults, it is the most commonly performed regional anesthetic technique in infants and children. Caudal block in adult patients has enjoyed a resurgence lately, mainly because it provides an alternative route to the lumbar epidural space when direct access is limited by previous surgeries and for performing epiduroscopy. Clinicians who routinely utilize fluoroscopy and ultrasound imaging will find that it has many applications, for both routine and complicated cases.

REFERENCES

1. Bromage PR: *Epidural Analgesia*. Saunders, 1978, pp 258–282.
2. Racz G: Personal communication, October 12, 2003, American Society of Anesthesiologists Annual Meeting, San Francisco.
3. Trotter M: Variations of the sacral canal: Their significance in the administration of caudal analgesia. Anesth Analg 1947;26:192–202.
4. MacDonald A, Chatrath P, Spector T, et al: Level of termination of the spinal cord and the dural sac: A magnetic resonance study. Clin Anat; 1999;12:149–152.
5. Joo J, Kim J, Lee J: The prevalence of anatomical variations that can cause inadvertent dural puncture when performing caudal block in Koreans: A study using magnetic resonance imaging. Anesthesia 2010;65 (1):23–26.
6. Igarashi T, Hirabayashi Y, Shimizu R, et al: The lumbar extradural structure changes with increasing age. Br J Anaest 1997;78:149–152.
7. Crighton I, Barry B, Hobbs G: A study of the anatomy of the caudal space using magnetic resonance imaging. Br J Anaesth 1997;78:391–395.
8. Sekiguchi M, Yabuki S, Satoh K, et al: An anatomic study of the sacral hiatus. A basis for successful epidural block. Clin J Pain 2004;20:51–54.
9. Bryce-Smith R: The spread of solutions in the extradural space. Anaesthesia 1954;9:201–205.
10. Brenner E: Sacral anesthesia. Ann Surg 1924;79:118–123.
11. Aggarwal A, Kaur H, Batra YK, et al: Anatomic consideration of caudal epidural space: A cadaver study. Clin Anat 2009;22(6):730–737.
12. Waldman S: Caudal epidural nerve block. In Waldman S (ed): *Interventional Pain Management*, 2nd ed. Saunders, 2001, p 520.
13. Winnie A, Candido KD: Differential neural blockade for the diagnosis of pain. In Waldman S (ed): *Interventional Pain Management*, 2nd ed. Saunders, 2001, pp 162–173.
14. Candido KD, Stevens RA: Intrathecal neurolytic blocks for the relief of cancer pain. Best Pract Res Clin Anaesthesiol 2003;17:407–428.
15. Lou L, Racz G, Heavner J: Percutaneous epidural neuroplasty. In Waldman S (ed): *Interventional Pain Management*, 2nd ed. Saunders, 2001, pp 434–445.
16. Cook RA, Driver RP Jr: Epidural blood patch. W V Med J 2009;105(5): 28–29.
17. Heavner J, Racz G, Raj P: Percutaneous epidural neuroplasty: Prospective evaluation of 0.9% NaCl versus 10% NaCl with or without hyaluronidase. Reg Anesth Pain Med 1999;24:202–207.
18. Manchikanti L, Bakhit C, Pampati V: Role of epidurography in caudal neuroplasty. Pain Digest 1998;8:277–281.
19. Kakiuchi M, Abe K: Pre-incisional caudal epidural blockade and the relief of pain after lumbar spine operations. Int Orthop 1997;21:62–66.
20. McCrirrick A, Ramage D: Caudal blockade for postoperative analgesia: A useful adjunct to intramuscular opiates following emergency lower leg orthopaedic surgery. Anaesth Intensive Care 1991;19:551–554.
21. Van Elstraete A, Pastureau F, Lebrun T, et al: Caudal clonidine for postoperative analgesia in adults. Br J Anaesth 2000;84:401–402.
22. Porges P, Zdrahal F: [Intrathecal alcohol neurolysis of the lower sacral roots in inoperable rectal cancer]. Anaesthetist 1985;34:627–629.
23. Ivani G, DeNegri P, Conio A, et al: Comparison of racemic bupivacaine, ropivacaine and levobupivacaine for pediatric caudal anesthesia. Effects on postoperative analgesia and motor blockade. Reg Anesth Pain Med 2002;27:157–161.
24. Chan S, Tay H, Thomas E: "Whoosh" test as a teaching aid in caudal block. Anaesth Intensive Care 1993;21:414–415.
25. Orme R, Berg S: The "swoosh" test—an evaluation of a modified "whoosh" test in children. Br J Aneaesth 2003;90:62–65.
26. Kim MS, Han KH, Kim EM, et al: The myth of the equilateral triangle for identification of sacral hiatus in children disproved by ultrasonography. Reg Anesth Pain Med 2013;38(3):243–247.
27. Yoon JS, Sim KH, Kim SJ, Kim WS, Koh SB, Kim BJ: The feasibility of color Doppler ultrasonography for caudal epidural steroid injection. Pain 2005;118:210–214.
28. Tsui B, Tarkkila P, Gupta S, Kearney R: Confirmation of caudal needle placement using nerve stimulation. Anesthesiology 1999;91:374–378.
29. Digiovanni A: Inadvertent interosseous injection—a hazard of caudal anesthesia. Anesthesiology 1971;34:92–94.
30. Lofstrom B: Caudal anaesthesia. In Ejnar Eriksson (ed): *Illustrated Handbook in Local Anaesthesia*. Astra, 1969, pp 129–134.
31. Caudal block. In Covino BG, Scott DB (eds): *Handbook of Epidural Anaesthesia and Analgesia*. Grune & Stratton, 1985, pp 104–108.
32. Dawkins C: An analysis of the complications of extradural and caudal block. Anaesthesia 1969;24:554–563.
33. Chung Y, Lin C, Pang W, et al: An alternative continuous caudal block with caudad catheterization via lower lumbar interspace in adult patients. Acta Anaesthesiol Scand 1998;36:221–227.
34. Triffterer L, Machata AM, Latzke D, et al: Ultrasound assessment of cranial spread during caudal blockade in children: effect of the speed of injection of local anesthetics. Br J Anaesth 2012;108(4):670–674.
35. Li Y, Zhou Y, Chen H, Feng Z: The effect of sex on the minimum local analgesic concentration of ropivacaine for caudal anesthesia in anorectal surgery. Anesth Analg 2010;110:1490–1493.
36. Wong S, Li J, Chen C, et al: Caudal epidural block for minor gynecologic procedures in outpatient surgery. Chang Gung Med J 2004;27:116–121.
37. Nishiyama T, Hanaoka K, Ochiai Y: The median approach to transsacral epidural block. Anesth Analg 2002;95:1067–1070.
38. Schuepfer G, Konrad C, Schmeck J, et al: Generating a learning curve for pediatric caudal epidural blocks: An empirical evaluation of technical skills in novice and experienced anesthesiologists. Reg Anesth Pain Med 2000;25:385–388.
39. Tsui B, Seal R, Koller J: Thoracic epidural catheter placement via the caudal approach in infants by using electrocardiographic guidance. Anesth Analg 2002;95:326–330.
40. Lundblad M, Lonnqvist PA, Eksborg S, Marhofer P: Segmental distribution of high-volume caudal anesthesia in neonates, infants and toddlers as assessed by ultrasonography. Paediatr Anaesth 2011;21(2): 121–127.
41. Tuncer S, Yosunkaya A, Reisli R, et al: Effect of caudal block on stress response in children. Pediatr Int 2004;46:53–57.
42. Valairucha S, Seefelder C, Houck C: Thoracic epidural catheters placed by the caudal route in infants: The importance of radiographic conformation. Paediatr Anaest 2002;12:424–428.
43. Rojas-Perez E, Castillo-Zamora C, Nava-Ocampo A: A randomized trial of caudal block with bupivacaine 4 mg x kg⁻¹(1.8ml x kg⁻¹) vs general anesthesia with fentanyl for cardiac surgery. Paediatr Anaesth 2003; 13:311–317.
44. Koo BN, Hong JY, Kil HK: Spread of ropivacaine by a weight-based formula in a pediatric caudal block: A fluoroscopic examination. Acta Anaesthesiol Scand 2010;54(5):562–565.
45. Stow P, Scott A, Phillips A, et al: Plasma bupivacaine concentrations during caudal analgesia and ilioinguinal-iliohypogastric nerve block in children. Anaesthesia 1998;43:650–653.
46. Verghese S, Hannallah R, Rice LJ, et al: Caudal anesthesia in children: Effect of volume versus concentration of bupivacaine on blocking spermatic cord traction response during orchidopexy. Anesth Analg 2002;95: 1219–1223.
47. Koinig H, Krenn C, Glaser C, et al: The dose-response of caudal ropivacaine in children. Anesthesiology 1999;90:1339–1344.
48. Jeong-Yeon Hong MD, Sang W, Han MD, et al: A comparison of high volume/low concentration and low volume/high concentration ropivacaine in caudal analgesia for pediatric orchiopexy. Anesth Analg 2009;109: 1073–1078.
49. Deng S, Xiao, W, Tang G, et al: The minimum local anesthetic concentration of ropivacaine for caudal analgesia in children. Anesth Analg 2002;94:1465–1468.
50. Lonnqvist P, Westrin P, Larsson B, et al: Ropivacaine pharmacokinetics after caudal block in 1-8 year old children. Br J Anaesth 2000;85: 506–511.
51. Deng XM, Xiao WJ, Tang GZ, Luo MP, Xu KL: Minimum local analgesic concentration of ropivacaine for intra-operative caudal analgesia in pre-school and school age children. Anesthesia 2010;65(10):991–995.
52. Dobereiner EF, Cox RG, Ewen A, Lardner DR: Evidence-based clinical update: Which local anesthetic drug for pediatric caudal block provides optimal efficacy with the fewest side effects? Can J Anaesth 2010;57(12):1102–1110.
53. Schnabel A, Poepping DM, Pogatzki-Zahn EM, Zahn PK: Efficacy and safety of clonidine as additive for caudal regional anesthesia: A quantitative systematic review of randomized controlled trials. Pediatr Anesth 2011;21:1219–1230.
54. Saadawy I, Bolker A, Elshahawy MA, et al: Effect of dexmedetomidine on the characteristics of bupivacaine in a caudal block in pediatrics. Acta Anaesthesiol Scand 2009;53:251–256.
55. El-Hennawy M, Abd-Elwahab AM, Abd-Elmaksoud AM, et al: Addition of clonidine or dexmedetomidine to bupivacaine prolongs caudal analgesia in children. Br J Anaesth 2009;103(2):268–274.
56. Verghese S, Mostello L, Patel R: Testing anal sphincter tone predicts the effectiveness of caudal analgesia in children. Anesth Analg 2002;94: 1161–1164.
57. Schindler M, Swann M, Crawford M: A comparison of postoperative analgesia provided by wound infiltration or caudal analgesia. Anesth Intensive Care 1991;19:46–49.

58. Larousse E, Asehnoune K, Dartayet B, et al: The hemodynamic effects of pediatric caudal anesthesia assessed by esophageal Doppler. Anesth Analg 2002;94:1165–1168.

59. Hong JY, Ahn S, Kil HK: Changes of dorsalis pedis artery flow pattern after caudal block in children: observational study using a duplex sonography. Pediatr Anesth 2011;21:116–120.

60. Manchikanti L, Cash KA, McManus CD, et al. The preliminary results of a comparative effectiveness evaluation of adhesiolysis and caudal epidural injections in managing chronic low back pain secondary to spinal stenosis: A randomized, equivalence controlled trial. Pain Physician 2009; 12:E341–E354.

61. Yousef AA, El-Deen AS, Al-Deeb AE: The role of adding hyaluronidase to fluroscopically guided caudal steroid and hypertonic saline injection in patients with failed back surgery syndrome: A prospective, double-blinded, randomized study. Pain Pract 2010;10(6):548–553.

62. Manchikanti L, Singh V, Cash KA, Pampati V: A randomized, controlled, double-blind trial of fluoroscopic caudal epidural injections in the treatment of lumbar disc herniation and radiculitis. Spine 2011;36(23): 1897–1905.

63. Joshi W, Connelly R, Freeman K, et al: Analgesic effect of clonidine added to bupivacaine 0.125% in pediatric caudal blockade. Paediatr Anaesth 2004;14:483–486.

64. Valois T, Otis A, Ranger M, Muir JG: Incidence of self-limiting back pain in children following caudal blockade: an exploratory study. Pediatr Anesth 2010;20:844–850.

65. Lin J, Zuo YX: Unilateral parotid swelling, following caudal block without airway device placement. Pediatr Anesth 2011;21:169–178.

66. Bagdure DN, Reiter PD, Bhoite GR, et al: Persistent hiccups associated with epidural ropivacaine in a newborn. Ann Pharmacother 2011; 45(6):e35.

67. Thomas R, Thanthulage S: Intracranial hypotension headache after uncomplicated caudal epidural injection. Anaesthesia 2012;67: 416–419.

68. Brown D, Ransom D, Hall J, et al: Regional anesthesia and local anesthetic-induced systemic toxicity: Seizure frequency and accompanying cardiovascular changes. Anesth Analg 1995;81:321–328.

69. Giaufre E, Dalens B, Gombert A: Epidemiology and morbidity of regional anesthesia in children: A one year prospective survey of the French–language Society of Pediatric Anesthesiologists. Anesth Analg 1996:83: 904–912.

70. Dalens B, Hansanoui A: Caudal anesthesia in pediatric surgery: Success rate and adverse effects in 750 consecutive patients. Anesth Analg 1989;8:83–89.

71. Afshan G, Khan F: Total spinal anaesthesia following caudal block with bupivacaine and buprenorphine. Paediatr Anaesth 1996;6:239–242.

72. Tsui B, Malherbe S: Inadvertent cervical epidural catheter placement via the caudal route using electrical stimulation. Anesth Analg 2004;99: 259–261.

73. Yue W, Tan S: Distant skip level discitis and vertebral osteomyelitis after caudal epidural injection: A case report of a rare complication of epidural injections. Spine 2003;1:209–211.

74. Ivani G, Mereto N, Lampugnani E, et al: Ropivacaine in paediatric surgery: Preliminary results [Abstract]. Paediatr Anaesth 1998;8: 127–129.

75. Ivani G, Lampugnani E, De Negri P, et al: Ropivacaine vs. bupivacaine in major surgery in infants [abstract]. Can J Anaesth 1999;46: 467–469.

76. Ivani G, De Negri P, Conio A, et al: Comparison of racemic bupivacaine, ropivacaine and levobupivacaine for pediatric cauda anesthesia. Effects on postoperative analgesia and motor blockade. Reg Anesth Pain Med 2002;27:157–161.

CHAPTER 26

Combined Spinal-Epidural Anesthesia

J. Sudharma Ranasinghe, Elyad Davidson, and David J. Birnbach

INTRODUCTION

In recent years, regional anesthesia techniques for surgery, obstetrics, and postoperative pain management have been used with increasing frequency.[1–3] The combined spinal-epidural (CSE) technique, a comparatively new anesthetic choice, includes an initial subarachnoid injection followed by epidural catheter placement and subsequent administration of epidural medications. This allows for rapid relief of pain or induction of regional anesthesia by the rapid onset of the spinal drugs and subsequent administration of medications for prolonged anesthesia. In addition, postoperative analgesia via the epidural catheter can be delivered for extended periods.

Clinical studies have demonstrated that the CSE technique provides excellent surgical conditions as quickly as the single-shot subarachnoid block and with advantages in comparison to the conventional epidural block.[4–6] The advantage lies in the fact that CSE anesthesia offers benefits of both spinal and epidural anesthesia.

Although the CSE technique has become increasingly popular over the past two decades, it is a more complex technique that requires comprehensive understanding of epidural and spinal physiology and pharmacology.

This chapter discusses the technical aspects, advantages, potential complications, and limitations of the CSE technique for surgery, postoperative pain management, and labor analgesia.

CLINICAL APPLICATIONS OF CSE

The results of a survey conducted by Blanshard and Cook demonstrated wide variation in CSE anesthesia use and practice among experienced anesthesiologists,[7] reflecting concern over the frequency of CSE-related complications,[8,9] controversy over the technique,[10,11] and the potential for higher failure rates with the CSE technique compared with individual spinal or other anesthetic techniques.[12]

General Surgery

The CSE technique has been described in the medical literature for use in general surgery, orthopedics, trauma surgery of a lower limb, and urological and gynecological surgery. Clinical studies have demonstrated that the CSE technique provides excellent surgical conditions as quickly as with single-shot subarachnoid block—conditions that are better than with epidural block alone.[4,13] With the CSE technique, surgical anesthesia is established rapidly, saving 15–20 minutes compared with epidural anesthesia. Furthermore, epidural catheterization provides the possibility of supplementing the subarachnoid anesthesia, which may be insufficient when used alone.

This was recently illustrated by Mane et al,[14] who presented a case series of laparoscopic appendectomy successfully performed under CSE anesthesia. CSE anesthesia in their series was performed using separate needles at two different interspaces. Spinal anesthesia was performed at the L2–L3 interspace using 2 mL 0.5% (10 mg) hyperbaric bupivacaine mixed with 25 µg fentanyl. The epidural catheter was inserted at the T10–T11 interspace to supplement spinal anesthesia and for postoperative pain relief. In an obstetrics-related article, it was also observed that various needles can be used in different combinations when performing the CSE technique and may have different advantages and disadvantages for different patients and situations.[15] This is discussed further in the chapter.

Labor Analgesia

The CSE technique is widely used in obstetric practice to provide optimal analgesia for parturients. It offers effective, rapid-onset analgesia with minimal risk of toxicity or motor block.[16] In addition, this technique provides the ability to prolong the duration of analgesia, as often is required in labor, through the use of an epidural catheter. Furthermore, should an operative delivery become necessary, that same epidural catheter can be used to provide operative anesthesia. The onset of spinal analgesia is almost immediate, and the duration is between 2 and 3 hours, depending on which agent or agents are chosen.

The duration of spinal analgesia, however, has been found to be decreased when administered to a woman in advanced labor versus one in early labor.[17] Laboring patients may have greater satisfaction with CSE anesthesia than with standard epidurals, perhaps because of a greater feeling of self-control.[18] The original descriptions of spinal labor analgesia utilized sufentanil or fentanyl,[19] but the addition of isobaric bupivacaine to the opioid produces a greater density of sensory blockade while still minimizing motor blockade.[20] Originally, 25 µg of fentanyl or 10 µg of sufentanil were advocated, but subsequent studies suggested the use of smaller doses of opioid combined with a local anesthetic.[21] For example, many clinicians are now routinely using 10–15 µg of intrathecal fentanyl. Several studies have suggested that ropivacaine and levobupivacaine can be substituted for intrathecal bupivacaine, especially when added to an opioid, to provide labor analgesia.[22–24] The CSE technique has also made ambulation possible for many women receiving neuraxial analgesia, although ambulation may also be possible with other techniques. Wilson et al[25] showed that significantly more women maintained superior leg power for a longer period with CSE anesthesia than with low-dose infusion of standard epidural. In addition to the advantage of rapid onset of pain relief, the CSE technique may reduce the incidence of several potential problems associated with the conventional epidural technique, including incomplete (patchy) blockade, motor block, and poor sacral spread.

Another potential advantage of the CSE technique is that it may be associated with a significant reduction in the duration of the first stage of labor in primiparous parturients.[26,27] However, according to a more recent study by Pascual-Ramirez et al,[28] when compared with conventional epidural analgesia, the CSE technique did not shorten total labor duration but did reduce local anesthetic requirement and motor weakness. Reduction of motor blockade is advantageous for parturients, even those who will not ambulate.

Combined Spinal-Epidural Technique for Cesarean Delivery

The CSE technique, first reported as an option for cesarean delivery in 1984,[29] has recently increased dramatically in popularity. The advantage of this technique is that it provides rapid onset of dense surgical anesthesia while allowing the ability to prolong the block with an epidural catheter. In addition, because the block can be supplemented at any time, the CSE technique allows the initial use of smaller doses of spinal local anesthetics, which may in turn reduce the incidence of high

spinal block or prolonged hypotension.[30] It may also reduce the duration of postanesthesia care unit (PACU) stay. Potential problems of the CSE technique for cesarean delivery include an inability to test the catheter, the possibility of a failed epidural catheter after spinal injection, and the risk of enhanced spread of previously injected spinal drug after use of the epidural catheter.[31]

Combined Spinal-Epidural Technique for External Cephalic Version of Breech Presentation

Neuraxial analgesia has been used to reduce the maternal pain during external cephalic version (ECV) for breech presentation. A potential benefit of the CSE technique is the ability to provide fast and effective pain relief for ECV and convert to neuraxial anesthesia for emergency delivery, if required. Kawase et al[32] reported a successful case of ECV under CSE technique followed by vaginal delivery. Sullivan and colleagues[33] studied the effect of the CSE technique on the success of ECV when compared with systemic opioid analgesia and found no difference; however, the pain scores were lower and satisfaction was higher with CSE analgesia.

ADVANTAGES OF THE COMBINED SPINAL-EPIDURAL TECHNIQUE

Onset of the Block

When CSE block was compared with either epidural or subarachnoid block for hip or knee arthroplasty, CSE anesthesia was found to be superior to epidural anesthesia. With the CSE technique, surgical anesthesia was rapidly established, saving 15–20 minutes compared with epidural anesthesia. Furthermore, the epidural catheter provided the possibility of supplementing insufficient subarachnoid anesthesia. Patients who received the CSE technique had more intense motor blockade than those who received epidural anesthesia alone.[4]

Failure Rate

It has been reported that the CSE technique decreases the failure rate and incidence of several other adverse events associated with neuraxial analgesia.[34] In a retrospective analysis of almost 20,000 deliveries (75% neuraxial labor analgesia rate), the overall failure rate with this technique was 12%. The patients had adequate analgesia from initial placement, but 6.8% of patients had subsequent inadequate analgesia during labor and required epidural catheter replacement. Ultimately, 98.8% of all patients in Pan's report received adequate analgesia, even though 1.5% of patients had one or more epidural catheter replacements.[34] However, when compared with epidural analgesia alone for labor, the incidents of overall failure, accidental intravascular epidural catheters, accidental dural punctures, inadequate epidural analgesia, and catheter replacements were repeatedly shown to be significantly lower in patients receiving CSE analgesia.[16,34,35] In addition, Eappen et al reported that CSE had a higher success rate compared to the conventional epidural technique.[35] This difference may be due to the ability to confirm questionable epidural location by successful spinal placement and observation of cerebrospinal fluid (CSF).

Local Anesthetic Requirement

During Surgery CSE enables low-dose spinal anesthesia for cesarean delivery.[36–40] When using single-shot spinal (SSS) anesthesia for ambulatory surgery, many anesthesiologists tend to administer more medication than is needed because there is only one chance to ensure an effective spinal block. The presence of an epidural catheter as a "safety net" allows the anesthesiologist to use the lowest effective dose of local anesthetic. Urmey et al used the CSE technique to investigate the appropriate dose of intrathecal isobaric lidocaine 2% for day case arthroscopy.[41] The CSE technique provided excellent anesthesia for all 90 patients in his study. Patients receiving the smallest dose (40 mg) had a significantly shorter duration of anesthesia, which allowed quicker discharge than for the patients receiving 60 or 80 mg of intrathecal lidocaine.

Norris et al suggested the use of a CSE technique with intrathecal sufentanil alone for outpatient shock-wave lithotripsy, reserving the use of epidural catheter for patients who did not achieve adequate analgesia.[42]

During Labor Analgesia Patel et al[43] studied the impact of spinal medication administered as part of a CSE technique on the subsequent epidural bupivacaine requirement. In a prospective, randomized, double-blind study, the MLAC (minimum local analgesic concentration) of epidural bupivacaine for labor analgesia was assessed following initial intrathecal (CSE) or epidural medication (standard epidural). They reported that the MLAC of epidural bupivacaine was not reduced by the use of intrathecal medication, but actually increased by a factor of 1.45. (MLAC in the standard epidural group was 0.032% wt/vol and for the CSE group was 0.047% wt/vol.) This suggests that CSE analgesia may not offer a quantitative analgesia advantage over standard epidural analgesia beyond the initial dose.

Epidural Volume Extension: A Modification of the CSE

During CSE anesthesia, it has been shown that supplementation of the epidural space with epidural saline ("epidural volume extension," EVE) may influence the anesthetic level and quality of spinal anesthesia. The proposed mechanism for this augmentation is a compressive effect on the subarachnoid space that promotes the cephalad spread of local anesthetic.

Takiguschi et al,[44] in a study using myelography on human volunteers, demonstrated that the contrast medium in the subarachnoid space was displaced cranially after lumbar epidural saline injection and the diameter of the subarachnoid space was narrowed due to the volume effect. This is a time-dependent phenomenon with maximum benefit if performed early.

Similarly, Blumgart et al showed that EVE with 10 mL of normal saline resulted in an increase in sensory block height of four segments following the administration of 8–9 mg of subarachnoid hyperbaric bupivacaine in women undergoing cesarean delivery.[45] However, a more recent study by Loubert et al

failed to show a difference in sensory block height after EVE with 5 mL of normal saline.[46] It is possible that the 5-mL volume was insufficient in this patient population, although the volume of normal saline that has been previously shown to be effective for EVE is approximately 5–10 mL.[47]

The results may also be due to a positional effect; in both studies, the CSE technique was performed in the sitting position. However, Blumgart injected 10 mL of saline epidurally through the catheter within 5 minutes of hyperbaric spinal medication only after the patient was turned supine with a 15° left lateral tilt. In Loubert's study, 5 mL of normal saline were injected through the Tuohy needle immediately after the spinal hyperbaric medication while the patients were still in the sitting position. Finally, the epidural catheter was threaded and the patients were helped into the supine 15° left lateral tilt.

Is the baricity of the local anesthetic a factor? A study by Tyagi et al demonstrated (in nonobstetric patients) that EVE was more effective with plain bupivacaine compared to hyperbaric bupivacaine, requiring a smaller dose while producing a higher sensory block with an earlier onset.[48] They attributed this difference to the restricted spread of hyperbaric local anesthetics in the subarachnoid space compared to the plain solution. Another study by Tyagi et al found that the intrathecal block level was similar in duration and extent with hyperbaric bupivacaine whether given as a SSS or a CSE administration with or without EVE on parturients undergoing elective cesarean delivery.[49]

Many factors seem to affect EVE. These include timing, volume of saline, features of the local anesthetic (hyperbaric vs. hypobaric), position during or after spinal anesthesia, and obstetric versus nonobstetric patients. Although it has been proposed that EVE may allow a reduced subarachnoid dose of local anesthetic for surgery and consequently reduce the incidence of hemodynamic effects associated with spinal block, there is a lack of uniformity between protocols and study results. Therefore, the influence of epidural saline injection on the quality of spinal anesthesia remains unclear.

Sequential CSE

In a study by Fan et al, four different intrathecal doses of hyperbaric bupivacaine (2.5, 5, 7.5, and 10 mg) were compared in patients undergoing cesarean delivery under sequential CSE block, a technique that involves administration of a relatively small subarachnoid block that may be supplemented as needed by epidural local anesthetics. The authors demonstrated that 5 mg intrathecal bupivacaine combined with an appropriate dose of epidural lidocaine provided adequate surgical analgesia while maintaining optimal hemodynamic stability. Higher doses of intrathecal bupivacaine were associated with typical adverse effects of high subarachnoid block, such as nausea, vomiting, and dyspnea.[50]

Macfarlane et al demonstrated that CSE anesthesia appears to offer no hemodynamic benefits compared with SSS anesthesia during cesarean delivery when the same dose of local anesthetic is administered. Hemodynamic stability was studied directly by measuring noninvasive blood pressure and indirectly by the ephedrine requirement, systemic vascular resistance index, and cardiac index using thoracic impedance cardiography.[51]

Combined Spinal-Epidural for High-Risk Patients

The sequential CSE technique may be particularly advantageous in high-risk patients, such as those with cardiac disease, when slower onset of sympathetic blockade is desirable.[52,53] Most spinal anesthetics are administered as a single-injection procedure, and rapid onset of sympathetic blockade may result in abrupt, severe hypotension. Traditionally, high-risk patients are managed with the slow onset of controlled epidural anesthesia, which requires much higher total dosages of local anesthetic than is the case with sequential CSE. With careful positioning of the patient prior to induction of the subarachnoid block, and by allowing titration with small incremental epidural doses to the precise level of anesthesia desired, the sequential CSE technique may enhance the safety of the neuraxial block.

Agarwal et al reported successful management of hysterectomy in a patient with ventricular septal defect and pulmonary atresia (VSD-PA) using CSE with the EVE technique.[54] Along similar high-risk lines, Month et al presented two parturients with idiopathic intracranial hypertension who achieved both labor analgesia and symptomatic relief using the CSE technique with small-volume CSF withdrawal.[55]

In summary, CSE can reduce or eliminate many of the disadvantages of subarachnoid or epidural anesthesia alone while preserving their respective advantages. The CSE block offers the speed of onset, efficacy, and minimal toxicity of a subarachnoid block combined with the potential of improving an inadequate block or prolonging the duration of anesthesia with epidural supplements; with the epidural, one may extend the analgesia well into the postoperative period. Although the sequential CSE technique will take somewhat longer than the standard CSE technique, the use of minimal doses of local anesthetics has been shown to reduce the frequency and severity of hypotension when compared with epidural or spinal techniques.[56]

Despite numerous studies advocating CSE, a 2007 Cochrane review of 19 randomized trials involving 2658 laboring women concluded that CSE offers little benefit when compared to conventional epidural analgesia, and there was no difference in the overall satisfaction of the women between the two techniques.[57] However, the authors did acknowledge that CSE produced slightly faster onset of effective pain relief and less need for rescue analgesia and was associated with less urinary retention. Later, Van de Velde[58] criticized this Cochrane review, stating that a number of well-performed studies were excluded from analysis. He wrote, "With conventional epidural analgesia, a wider interpatient variability exists with respect to onset time of analgesia. With CSE, onset time is short in all patients irrespective of the other factors."

FUNCTIONAL ANATOMY RELATED TO CSE

When performing an epidural block, skin-to-epidural space distance (SED) and the posterior epidural space distance (PED) are measures that can help reduce the inadvertent penetration of the dura and injury to neural structures.[59,60] The knowledge of these distances is also important in the success rate of epidural blocks. The PED, a measure of the epidural space depth, is particularly important with the CSE needle-through-needle (NTN) technique. Underestimation of this distance (short protrusion of the spinal needle through the epidural needle) will result in a higher incidence of spinal block failure. Any nonmidline approach also would increase the risk of not reaching the subarachnoid space because the dural sac has a triangular shape with the top pointing dorsally. Overestimation of PED will cause over protrusion of the spinal needle, which may increase the risk of neural damage.[61] These distances have been measured using various methods,[62] including magnetic resonance imaging (MRI), computed tomography (CT), ultrasound, and measurement of CSE tip-to-tip distance or the amount of protrusion of the spinal needle beyond the Tuohy needle.

The distance from the SED is most commonly 4 cm (50%) and is 4–6 cm in 80% of the population according to detailed records of 3200 cases.[62] The width of the PED varies with vertebral level, being the widest in the midlumbar region (5–6 mm) and decreasing toward the cervical vertebral column. In the midthoracic region, it is 3–5 mm in the midline and narrows laterally. In the lower cervical region, it is only 1.5–2 mm in the midline.[63] These spaces also correlate with the weight/height ratio and body mass index (BMI).[64] Based on these measures, the present design of spinal needle protrusion varies between 10 and 15 mm beyond the epidural needle.

Epidural Space and Ligament Flavum

The thickness of the ligamentum flavum, distance to dura, and skin-to-dura distance vary with the area of vertebral canal (see Table 26–1).

The two ligamenta flava are variably joined (fused) in the midline, and this fusion or lack of fusion of the ligamenta flavum occurs at different vertebral levels in individual patients. Lirk et al investigated the incidence of lumbar ligamentum flavum midline gaps in embalmed cadavers.[65] Vertebral column specimens were obtained from 45 human cadavers. The gaps in the lumbar ligamentum flavum are most frequent between L1 and L2 (22.2%) but are rare below this level (L2–L3 = 11.4%, L3–L4 = 11.1%, L4–L5 = 9.3%, L5–S1 = 0). Therefore, when using a midline approach, one

TABLE 26–1. Characteristics of ligamentum flavum at different vertebral levels.

Site	Skin to Ligament (cm)	Thickness of Ligament (mm)
Cervical	—	1.5–3.0
Thoracic	—	3.0–5.0
Lumbar	3.0–8.0	5.0–6.0
Caudal	Variable	2.0–6.0

Source: Data from Miller RD: *Anesthesia*, 6th ed. Philadelphia: Churchill Livingstone; 2005.

cannot rely on the ligamentum flavum to impede entering the epidural space in all patients.

TECHNIQUE

A number of reviews have discussed the technical factors related to the performance and success of CSE.[66–68] Although CSE is considered a relatively new technique, in 1937 Soresi actually described the intentional injection of anesthetic agents outside and within the subarachnoid space.[69] Somewhat different from current practice, Soresi intentionally used a single needle. He first injected some local anesthetic into the epidural space and then advanced the needle and injected the rest of the medication to cause a subarachnoid block. Although this technique included both spinal and epidural anesthesia, no catheter was used.

In 1979, Curelaru[70] reported the first CSE with an introduction of an epidural catheter through a Tuohy needle. Catheter insertion was followed by a test dose and then a traditional dural puncture, which was performed at a different interspace using a 26-gauge spinal needle. That same year, Brownridge suggested the use of CSE for obstetrics. He described successful use of CSE for elective cesarean section in 1981.[71,72]

In 1982, the NTN CSE technique was first described independently by Coates and Mumtaz, and its active use in obstetric practice was first published in 1984 by Carrie.[73–75] Popularity of the technique began in the late 1990s. Several approaches for initiation of CSE have been described in the recent literature.

Needle-Through-Needle Technique

In contrast to Soresi's initial description of CSE, in which a single needle was introduced into the epidural space and then advanced into the subarachnoid space, the currently preferred NTN technique includes use of separate epidural and spinal needles. Typically, the epidural space is located with a conventional epidural needle and technique, and then a long spinal needle is passed through the epidural needle until CSF appears in the hub of the spinal needle. Drug is administered via the spinal needle into the subarachnoid space, the spinal needle is removed, and finally an epidural catheter is inserted into the epidural space. Although several different CSE techniques are used in clinical practice (including the two-needle, two-interspace technique), NTN is the most widely used CSE technique in the United States.

Separate Needle Technique

The CSE technique may be performed using two separate needles with the separate needle technique (SNT), with spinal block and epidural catheter placement at either a single[76,77] or two different interspaces.[78–80] If the epidural catheter is placed first, proper placement can be tested before administration of spinal medications, potentially decreasing the risk of accidental intravascular or intrathecal catheter migration. Placing the epidural catheter first may also reduce the risk of neural damage, which may occur when the catheter is inserted after subarachnoid block, because paresthesia and other warning signs of

improper needle placement may be absent after administration of spinal medications. However, there is also the risk of striking the epidural catheter with the spinal needle.[81–83] Some authors consider this to be a purely hypothetical risk and have demonstrated that it is not possible to perforate an epidural catheter with commonly used spinal needles.[84,85]

Cook et al[86] reported a series of 201 consecutive CSEs performed with a novel SNT. The study was designed to avoid potential and actual problems associated with the CSE technique. Cook et al placed the spinal needle in the subarachnoid space and then replaced the spinal needle stylet to stop the CSF leak. Next, the epidural catheter was placed through a different interspace and then returned to the spinal needle to inject the subarachnoid drug, thus avoiding epidural catheter insertion in an anesthetized patient. This method of CSE anesthesia, although much more work, may be associated with high success and low complication rates.

Regardless of which component is performed first, the major disadvantage of the two-needle, two-interspace technique is that it takes longer to perform and requires two separate injections.

Comparison of Techniques

The SNT technique has a few theoretical advantages compared to the NTN technique. It enables placement of the epidural catheter prior to initiation of the spinal block. The SNT may thus theoretically reduce the risk for neurological injury because paresthesia and other symptoms are not masked. Because the epidural catheter is placed early, problems that may occur due to delayed catheter placement (technical problems) after the injection of a hyperbaric spinal solution (such as unilateral, sacral, or low lumbar regional neuraxial block) are avoided.[87–89]

Several studies have compared NTN and SNT techniques.[90–93] Some have reported better success and lower failure rates with the SNT. However, these studies also reported greater patient acceptance and less discomfort with the NTN technique. Backe et al, in a prospective randomized study,[94] compared the outcomes and techniques of NTN and SNT (double space) CSE in 200 elective cesarean delivery patients. Successful blocks to T5 with the double-space and the NTN techniques were 80 versus 54, respectively, odds ratio 0.29. SNT had a greater success rate than the NTN technique; the T5 dermatome was reached with fewer corrective manipulations (epidural augmentation or repeated blocks). Failure to enter the intrathecal space once the epidural space had been located occurred in 29 patients in the NTN group. Time to readiness for surgery, however, was slightly increased with SNT (15 minutes with SNT vs. 12.9 minutes with NTN).

Sadashivaiah et al[95] retrospectively analyzed data from 3519 elective cesarean deliveries performed under the SNT technique. They reported a lower rate of conversion to general anesthetic due to failed neuraxial block (0.23%) than previously reported (0.8%–1.3%).

One of the problems with the NTN technique is that many patients complain of paresthesia/dysesthesia or respond (movement, grimacing, vocalization) to dural puncture during insertion of a pencil-point needle. Van den Berg et al[96] compared the effects of saline versus air for loss of resistance (LOR) on the occurrence of this discomfort and reported that use of saline is associated with fewer patient (18% vs. 44%) responses at the moment of thecal penetration. Although the mechanism of this reduced response with saline for LOR is not clear, the authors postulated that perhaps the placement of saline in the epidural space modulated dural sensitivity.

Techniques to Improve the Success and Safety of Combined Spinal-Epidural

The success of a CSE block is heavily dependent on accurate cannulation of the epidural space. The identification of the epidural space is traditionally achieved by a blind LOR technique. With this handling of the needles, where the feedback to the operator is merely tactile, deviation of the axis of the needle trajectory may occur. Because of the triangular form of the dural sac, deviation of the spinal needle from the midline will cause the dural sac to be missed, leading to spinal component failure or unsuccessful dural puncture.

Grau et al performed real-time ultrasound scanning of the lumbar spine to provide accurate reading of the location of the needle tip and to facilitate the performance of CSE anesthesia.[97] Their aim was to establish a less-invasive method to monitor the advancement of the needle in real time. Thirty parturients scheduled for cesarean delivery were randomized to three equal groups. Ten control patients received CSE anesthesia performed in a conventional manner. Ten received ultrasound scans by an off-line technique. The remaining 10 received online imaging of the lumbar region during puncture. The Tuohy needle was inserted using the midline approach in all three groups. In the control group, CSE was performed using A single-space NTN technique with the standard LOR to saline method.

In the off-line group, ultrasound images were taken just before the puncture to improve needle trajectory. In the online group, ultrasonic images were taken to monitor and identify needle trajectory in real time.

The authors reported that in both ultrasound groups, a significant reduction in the number of necessary puncture attempts was found ($p < .036$); the number of interspaces necessary for puncture was reduced ($p < .036$); and the number of spinal needle manipulations was significantly reduced ($p < .036$). Dural tenting was observed in 9 of 10 of the online group (tenting length 2.4 mm). Asymmetric block was observed in 10% of those in the control group, but not in any of those in the ultrasound groups. The authors concluded that the use of ultrasound imaging was obviously helpful in finding the ideal needle trajectory and to improve puncture conditions by demonstration of the relevant anatomy.

In the CSE NTN technique, there is no practical test to confirm correct epidural catheter placement. Tsui and colleagues proposed the use of nerve stimulators to confirm the proper placement of epidural catheter.[98] They studied 39 obstetric patients in labor, receiving epidural catheters (not CSE) for analgesia. A low-current (1- to 10-mA) electrical stimulation was used to confirm the correct placement of the epidural catheter (19-gauge Arrow Flextip plus). A positive motor response (truncal or limb) indicated that the catheter was in the epidural space. They reported that the sensitivity and specificity of this test were 100% and 100%, respectively, with 38 true positive tests and 1 true negative test. A case of intravascular epidural catheter migration was detected using this new test and was subsequently confirmed by a positive epinephrine test. If the motor response only occurs with larger currents (>10 mA) or does not respond at all (before receiving any local anesthetics), the catheter is most likely outside the epidural space. If a positive response occurs at an unusually low milliamperage (<1 mA), intrathecal placement is likely.

The electrical stimulation test may not be applicable when the CSE technique is used for surgery, where anesthetic doses of local anesthetics are administered intrathecally prior to the placement of the epidural catheter. When using the CSE technique for labor analgesia, this test may be utilized as a simple and practical method to determine the epidural catheter placement. The standard test dose utilized in the United States (3 mL of 1.5% lidocaine with 1:200,000 epinephrine) may help to identify intravascular and intrathecal placement, but it does not verify appropriate epidural placement or function.

DRUGS FOR COMBINED SPINAL-EPIDURAL

Sufentanil and fentanyl, with or without local anesthetics, are most often administered intrathecally to provide analgesia for the laboring woman receiving CSE. The usual doses of sufentanil are 2.5–10 µg; however, most practitioners are now using 2.5 or 5 µg. The ED_{50} and ED_{95} for laboring patients were found to be 2.6 and 8.9 µg respectively.[99] The doses of fentanyl used are typically 10–25 µg. The median effective dose (ED_{50}) and effective dose in 95% of the population (ED_{95}) for laboring patients have been reported to be 5.5 and 17.4 µg, respectively.[100] Although the original studies used much higher doses of intrathecal opioids (10 µg sufentanil and 25–50 µg of fentanyl), subsequent studies have suggested the use of smaller doses, with reduced side effects and similar analgesic effect.[101]

Morphine, a highly ionized, water-soluble opioid, produces analgesia of long duration but slow onset (approximately 60 minutes between neuraxial injection and onset). In addition, it may be associated with an unacceptably high incidence of side effects, such as nausea, vomiting, pruritus, as well as the potential for delayed respiratory depression. These side effects, coupled with the slow onset of pain relief, limit the usefulness of intrathecal morphine for labor analgesia. Intrathecal meperidine (10 mg) may provide reliable analgesia in advanced labor[102] but has been associated with a high incidence of nausea, vomiting, hypotension, and need for low blood pressure management. In addition, it is the only opioid that has intrinsic local anesthetic properties at clinically appropriate doses[102] by blocking nerve conduction at the proximal end of the dorsal root[103] via a mechanism other than sodium channel blockade.[104] This nerve conduction blockade is not reversible with naloxone.[103]

In many patients, a single intrathecal injection of a lipid-soluble opioid is insufficient to produce analgesia for the entire duration of labor. If the second stage of labor is imminent, to achieve a greater depth of pain relief, the subarachnoid administration of local anesthetic plus opioid should be considered.

The combination of 2.5–5 µg sufentanil plus 2.5 mg bupivacaine provides rapid analgesia without motor block, alleviates the pain of the second stage of labor, and lasts longer than sufentanil alone.[105] Although the original reports[106] recommended the use of 10 µg of sufentanil, Sia and colleagues showed that adequate labor pain relief could be safely provided by administering half that dose of intrathecal sufentanil plus bupivacaine.[107]

Previous studies[108] have attempted to determine the ED_{50} of intrathecal bupivacaine, defined as minimum local anesthetic dose (MLAD) or ED_{50} and then use this to assess the effect of different doses of fentanyl. The MLAD of intrathecal bupivacaine has been found to be 1.99 mg, and the addition of 5 µg intrathecal fentanyl offered a similar significant sparing effect to 15 or 25 µg of fentanyl, resulting in less pruritus but with a shortened duration of action. ED_{95} was estimated from those studies.

Whitty et al[109] performed an up-down dose-finding study to determine the ED_{95} for intrathecal bupivacaine (more clinically relevant than that calculated from ED_{50}) when combined with a fixed amount of fentanyl. They recommended 1.75 mg of bupivacaine with 15 µg of fentanyl to reliably and rapidly relieve pain of parturients in the active phase of labor. At Jackson Memorial Hospital (Miami, FL), we currently use 1.25 mg bupivacaine plus 15 µg fentanyl as our spinal drug.

Levin et al compared a standard dose of intrathecal bupivacaine with sufentanil for CSE analgesia using two doses of ropivacaine (2 and 4 mg) with sufentanil. They concluded that both local anesthetics provided similar labor analgesia duration with equivalent side effects.[110]

COMPLICATIONS AND CONCERNS OF THE CSE TECHNIQUE

Failure of the Spinal Component

The most common method of performing a CSE is the single-interspace NTN technique. Failure to achieve a spinal block with this technique has been reported in 10%–15% of cases in the past,[111,112] although in experienced hands this risk may be as low as 2%–5%.[113]

Possible causes for failure of CSE include the following:

1. *Spinal needle too short.* The needle does not extend far enough beyond the epidural tip or tents the dura.[111] Holloway and Telford observed the distance from identification of the epidural space to penetration of the dura in 31 patients during the use of a Tuohy needle to perform deliberate dural puncture for the insertion of lumbar drains.[114] Although many reference textbooks indicate lesser distances[115] from location of the epidural spaces to dural puncture, these authors found an unexpectedly large distance of up to 2.25 cm[114] and postulated that tenting of the dura by the blunt atraumatic spinal needle might be the cause of this finding.

2. *Failure to enter the dura.* This may occur with very small caliber needles that lack the rigidity to puncture the dura.[116] As postulated by Holloway and Telford,[114] the absence of negative epidural space pressure limits the transdural pressure gradient and minimizes the reactive forces across the

dura. Therefore, penetration of the dura (a relatively tough membrane) requires a substantial reactive force.[117]

3. *Divergence from the midline.* This may cause the spinal needle to pass by the dura,[92,97] despite the fact the epidural space has been identified.

4. *Use of a long small-gauge spinal needle.* A long small-gauge spinal needle may penetrate the dura and then be advanced too far (to the anterior epidural space) due to the delay in the reflux of CSF.[118–120]

5. *Use of a long pencil-point spinal needle.* Another potential problem may occur with the long pencil-point spinal needles currently being used. The spinal needle may be poorly anchored because it is located in the epidural needle and not held firmly in tissue. Therefore, with the spinal needle likely to move during injection, the medication may be only partially administered to the subarachnoid space.[121–123] The ability to hold the spinal needle steadily takes practice but is easily learned.

6. *Delay while placing the epidural catheter.* After subarachnoid drug has been administered, there can be a delay while placing the epidural catheter. This is usually brief and without consequences, but according to some authors,[124,125] it may alter the final characteristics of the block. This complication is of greater clinical significance when performing CSE for cesarean delivery. However, should a delay occur and the block not reach optimum height, the epidural catheter can be used to supplement the block.

Most current needle designs allow extension of the spinal needle 12–15 mm beyond the tip of the Tuohy needle. Excessively long needles, however, pose problems of handling and depth of placement. Deviation from midline will lengthen the epidural-dural distance and may also cause the spinal needle to miss the spinal space laterally (Figures 26–1 and 26–2). In addition, preservative-free normal saline used to identify the epidural space may be misinterpreted as CSF.

Complications Associated With Spinal Migration of the Epidural Catheter or Intrathecal Administration of Epidural Drugs

Subarachnoid Placement of Intended Epidural Catheter

One of the concerns with the CSE technique is that the epidural catheter may unintentionally pass through the dural puncture hole into the subarachnoid space during the CSE technique. This seems more likely with the NTN CSE technique than the SNT or with epidural needles with back holes (Figure 26–3). Although this may seem a rare theoretical problem, several publications have reported its occurrence.[126–129]

Angle et al[130] studied factors contributing to unintentional subarachnoid catheter passage after epidural placement with an in vitro model using human dural tissue. In that study, the dura was punctured with 25-gauge Whitacre® spinal needles. The likelihood of the catheter to enter into the subarachnoidal space was compared between the intact dura, versus the dura with obvious epidural needle punctures, and single 25-gauge

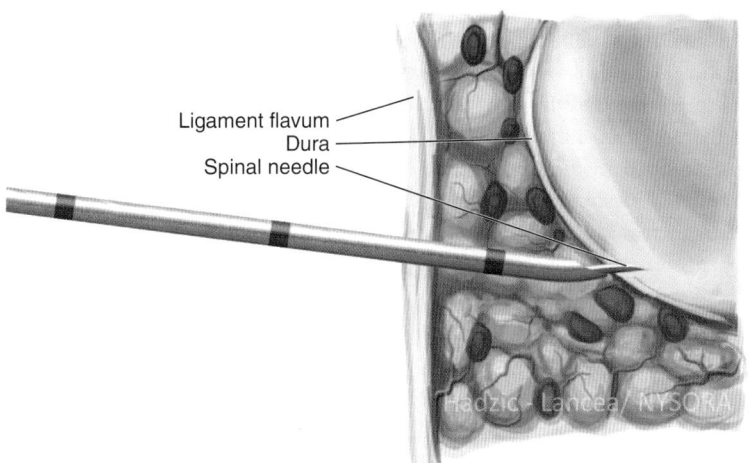

FIGURE 26–1. Deviation of the epidural needle laterally.

Whitacre spinal needle punctures after a CSE technique. Their conclusion was that the catheter passage is unlikely to occur in the presence of an intact dura or after an uncomplicated CSE technique. Therefore, unintentional subarachnoid passage of the epidural catheter suggests dural damage with the epidural needle.

Holtz et al investigated the possible passage of the epidural catheter into the subarachnoid space in an anatomical preparation.[131] In 10 series of experiments, the epidural compartment was entered with an 18-gauge Tuohy needle. The spinal puncture (27- or 29- gauge Quincke needle) was performed with the NTN technique. Subsequently, the internal side of the intrathecal compartment was examined endoscopically for penetration of the epidural catheter. In a similar way, the endoscope was inserted epidurally to visualize the movements of the epidural catheter in the epidural compartment. In this model of simulated physiologic intrathecal conditions, using one space NTN technique, they could not detect intrathecal passage of the epidural catheter.

Holmstrom and colleagues, in a percutaneous epiduroscopy study using fresh cadavers, also reported that it was impossible to force an epidural catheter into the subarachnoid space after a single perforation of the dura with a small-gauge spinal needle. However, they found that the risk of intrathecal catheter migration increased to approximately 5% after multiple dural punctures with the spinal needle. Dural penetration of the epidural catheter after a dural puncture with a Tuohy needle was clearly demonstrated in the same study.[132]

Whether the incidence of an unintentional passage of the epidural catheter into the subarachnoid space is increased with CSE as compared to standard epidural technique alone is controversial. Therefore, regardless of technique used, all epidural medications should be given in incremental doses.

Subarachnoid Spread of Epidurally Administered Drugs

Leighton and colleagues reported that, following a CSE, a dose of epidural local anesthetic will produce a higher dermatomal level than expected, presumably due to subarachnoid flux of the drug.[133] However, when used for labor analgesia, unless the dura is breached with the epidural needle or large bolus volumes are administered,[134] flux should not be clinically significant. Suzuki et al found, in nonpregnant patients, that dural puncture using a 26-gauge Whitacre spinal needle before the epidural injection increased caudal spread of analgesia induced by epidural local anesthetics with no change in the cephalad spread.[135]

Holtz et al endoscopically investigated the possible passage of epidural anesthetic through the dural puncture hole into the CSF compartment in an anatomical preparation.[131] Even 1 hour after epidural administration of 20 mL of methylene blue–dyed local anesthetic (bupivacaine 0.5%, isobaric), no passage of local anesthetic into the intrathecal compartment could be detected under continuous endoscopic monitoring.

A study by Kamiya et al[136] measured the lidocaine concentration in CSF after epidural administration at different interspaces with or without preceding spinal anesthesia. They concluded that there was no difference in the lidocaine concentrations in CSF with or without a meningeal hole. The authors explained the possible reason for the lack of difference in lidocaine concentration as follows: Lidocaine readily penetrates through meningeal tissue, and this transfer efficiency was most likely not affected by the presence of a small meningeal hole. The equilibrium of the lidocaine concentration in CSF, close to the administration site, would be attained within a few minutes

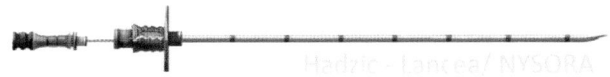

FIGURE 26–2. Spinal needle threaded into epidural needle.

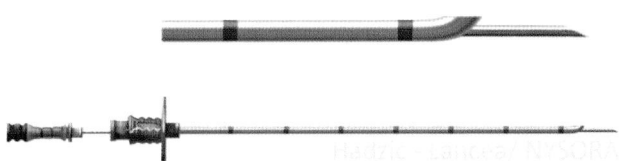

FIGURE 26–3. Epidural needle with back hole.

due to this rapid penetration. Stated differently, the amount of local anesthetic that crosses through the small hole in the dura is trivial when compared with the amount that crosses through the meninges. This study confirmed that CSE is safe, and that the dural holes have no clinically significant influence on duration or extent of the spinal blocks in patients undergoing cesarean delivery. The data from several clinical studies of the CSE technique have not indicated an increase in spread of sensory block due to subarachnoid leakage of epidurally administered medications.[131,137–139]

However, the magnitude of flux is a function of the diameter of the spinal needle, and the risk may be increased by using a larger spinal needle or in the presence of a hole made with a Tuohy needle. The possibility of this hazard is supported by reports of high or total spinal block during epidural anesthesia administered following unintentional dural perforation with the epidural needle.[140,141]

The administration of a test dose for spinal placement of an epidural catheter may be problematic and aspiration may fail, but test doses have been found to detect more intrathecal catheters than aspiration alone during labor analgesia.[142] Despite studies that have reported that intrathecal migration is very rare and that the flux should not produce clinically relevant complications, the reader is cautioned that epidural drugs or catheters may migrate into the spinal space following CSE. Therefore, all epidural doses should be incremental, and patients receiving continuous epidural infusions for analgesia should be checked approximately every hour to rule out excessive motor or sensory block that may be indicative of unintentional intrathecal administration of drugs.

Hypotension

Does subarachnoid block induced by CSE (using LOR to air) render a higher level of sensory anesthesia than SSS when an identical mass of intrathecal anesthetic was injected? Goy et al performed a prospective randomized study comparing CSE (using LOR to air) versus SSS on 60 patients who were undergoing minor gynecological procedures and concluded that subarachnoid block induced by CSE produces greater sensorimotor anesthesia ($p < .01$) and prolonged recovery ($p < .05$) than SSS.[143] They also found a more frequent incidence of hypotension and vasopressor use in the CSE group ($p < .05$), despite using identical doses of intrathecal medications.[143]

Another study reported similar findings when only 4 mL of air were used as part of the LOR technique.[144] The objective of that study was to determine the ED_{50} of intrathecal hyperbaric bupivacaine for CSE and SSS by using the up-down sequential allocation technique. Sixty participants were allocated into two groups in a double-blind, randomized, prospective study design. They concluded that, under similar clinical conditions, the ED_{50} of intrathecal hyperbaric bupivacaine in CSE was 20% less than that in SSS. Although the mechanism that accounts for this finding has not been determined, one possible explanation is that the LOR to air technique in CSE could introduce air pockets within the epidural space. MRI has demonstrated residual air pockets to extend up to three lumbar vertebral segments and compress the lumbar thecal sac dorsally

and laterally.[145] This could potentially result in a reduction of the lumbosacral CSF volume and enhance the extent of sensory anesthesia.[146]

Epidural administration of drugs seems to affect the thecal contents and therefore influence the spread of earlier induced subarachnoid block.[147,148] The magnitude of this effect depends on the time interval between the injections and the volume of the epidural injectate. Initially, the proposed mechanism for this effect was the subarachnoid leak of epidurally administered medications.

Hypotension can occur following the administration of intrathecal fentanyl or sufentanil, even if sympathetic blockade does not occur. However, the hemodynamic effects of intrathecal fentanyl are usually benign in nature and may actually be due to a decrease in catecholamines secondary to pain relief. Vasodilation due to sympathectomy, however, causes a decrease in preload, end diastolic index, and stroke index and an increase in heart rate. Because the end diastolic index and stroke index remained relatively stable and the heart rate decreased in a study by Mandell and colleagues, these authors concluded that the observed hypotension was not due to vasodilation.[149] The hypotensive episodes following administration of neuraxial opioids for labor are transient, easily treated, and not necessarily associated with adverse fetal heart rate changes.

Neurological injury

Neurological complications directly related to spinal anesthesia may be caused by trauma, cord ischemia, infection, and neurotoxicity.

Needle Trauma

Needle- or catheter-induced trauma rarely results in permanent neurological injury. However, Horlocker et al, in a retrospective review of 4767 consecutive spinal anesthetics for central nervous system complications, concluded that the presence of a paresthesia during needle placement significantly increased the risk of persistent paresthesia ($p < .001$). In that review, paresthesia was elicited during needle placement in 298 (6.3%) cases. Six patients reported pain (persistent paresthesia) on resolution of the spinal anesthetic; four of these individuals had pain that resolved within 1 week, and the pain of the remaining two resolved in 18–24 months.[150] According to a more recent study by Bigeleisen on peripheral nerve blockade, nerve puncture and intraneural injection did not invariably lead to neurological injury.[151]

There are a few reasons for a possible increase in the risk of neurological sequelae following the CSE technique. In the single-space, NTN technique of CSE, the insertion of the epidural needle and catheter after administration of spinal local anesthetics may prevent identification of paresthesias that may warn the anesthesiologist about needle misplacement. Higher incidence of paresthesia during CSE is a recognized factor. In fact, it has been reported that paresthesias occur in up to 11% of patients undergoing CSE.[152] Browne et al reported a 14% incidence of paresthesias with the Espocan needle (18-gauge Tuohy epidural needle with an extra lumen in the needle bevel) and a 42% incidence with a conventional Tuohy epidural needle.[15]

In a randomized prospective study, McAndrew et al similarly reported that 37% (17 of 46) of women in the NTN CSE group and only 9% (4 of 43) in the SSS group had paresthesia on spinal needle insertion ($p < 0.05$). The equipment used was a 16-gauge/26-gauge CSE kit and a 26-gauge pencil-point spinal needle with introducer (both Sims Portex, Australia). They postulated that the higher incidence of paresthesias may be related to deeper penetration of the subarachnoid space with the CSE technique. Interestingly, in that study, none of the patients had persistent neurological symptoms on examination at postoperative day 1.[153]

Holloway et al conducted a pilot survey of anesthetists' experiences of neurological sequelae following spinal and CSE anesthesia in the obstetric units in the United Kingdom.[154] Because of the retrospective nature of the survey, many neurological problems that were reported lacked detail. However, there were no obvious differences in incidence of problems associated with CSE versus the SSS techniques.

Turner and Shaw suggested the possibility that painful insertion and subsequent root damage might be increased by the use of atraumatic pencil-point spinal needles.[155] In that survey, problems were reported with both Whitacre and Sprotte needles, but none with Quincke needles. However, the numbers using Quincke needles were too small to allow statistical analysis.

More dangerous than root damage is damage to the spinal cord itself, and in that survey,[155] there were two cases of conus damage, one with CSE and one with SSS. This complication is not a fault of atraumatic needles, but rather of the technique. It is important to remember that in 19% of patients, the spinal cord terminates below L1. Even more worrisome, in more than 50% of cases, the chosen space is incorrectly identified.[156] Therefore, a space L3/L4 or below should be selected for CSE or SSS.

Risk of Metal Toxicity in CSE

It has been alleged that during the NTN CSE technique, tiny metal particles abraded by the spinal needle from the inner edge of the Tuohy needle may be introduced into the epidural or spinal compartment.[157] To examine this concern, Holst and colleagues simulated the NTN technique in an in vitro model.[131] They used atomic absorption spectrography (AAS) to identify abraded metal particles. The needles were then examined under an electron microscope. They reported no increased alloy components detected in the rinse solution after either twofold or fivefold puncture compared with the control measurements. After five punctures and handling the needle as in normal practice, no traces of use could be detected by electron microscopy on the inner ground edge of the Tuohy needle.[131]

Tissue Coring

Tissue coring is a phenomenon that may occur during lumbar puncture, in which pieces of tissue are removed by the needle as it passes through the tissue and deposits the pieces in the subarachnoid space. Although rare, adverse outcomes such as intraspinal iatrogenic epidermoid tumors may be associated with this phenomenon. Sharma et al[158] postulated that the CSE technique introduces fewer epithelial cells in the subarachnoid space when compared with the SSS without the use of an introducer. However, this study did not support the hypothesis. Significant tissue coring occurred with both techniques (CSE 88% and SSS 96%).

Infectious Neurological Complications

Although overall incidence of infections and their sequelae following placement of CSE is perceived to be extremely low, the relative risk compared to either a spinal or epidural techniques alone is not known. In a classic study, Dripps and Vandam prospectively reported no cases of meningitis after 10,098 spinal anesthetics.[159] Phillips et al also reported no cases after a prospective review of 10,440 such cases.[160] These studies included patients undergoing obstetric and urological operations, which are known to be associated with perioperative bacteremia. However, case reports of meningitis following CSEs appeared in the journals beginning mid1990s.[161,162]

Theoretically, CSE is thought to be associated with an increased risk of meningitis compared to epidural alone because the dura (protective barrier for the central nervous system) is punctured deliberately during CSE, and then a foreign body, an epidural catheter, is placed nearby. The epidural catheter can lie close to the dural hole and is a potential focus of infection, especially following bacteremia.[163] Contamination of the subarachnoid space may occur from bleeding due to needle trauma in a bacteremic patient or from failure of aseptic technique.

Several studies have shown that face masks prevent forward dispersal of organisms from the upper airway and downward dispersal during talking and head turning.[164,165] Despite this, in 1996 a postal survey of members of the Obstetric Anaesthetists Association in the United Kingdom found that over half those surveyed did not routinely wear face masks when performing neuraxial anesthesia.[166]

In 2007, for the first time, the Healthcare Infection Control Practices Advisory Committee (HICPAC) recommended that surgical masks be worn during spinal procedures to prevent infections.[167] This recommendation was made in response to several reports of meningitis following myelography procedures. In 2008, three bacterial meningitis cases in postpartum women were reported to the New York State Department of Health. All three women received CSE for labor. *Streptococcus salivarius* (a normal commensal of oral flora) was cultured from the CSF of two patients. The anesthesiologist responsible for all three cases reported routine use of masks during neuraxial procedures. However, the staff reported that it was common to have unmasked visitors present in the room during these procedures. The hospital instituted new policies to minimize visitors and to require masks for all persons in the room during neuraxial labor analgesia procedures. In 2009, two similar cases were reported to the Ohio Department of Health. The anesthesiologist responsible for these two cases did not wear a mask. CSF cultures from both patients revealed *S. salivarius*, and one of them died from suppurative meningoencephalitis.[168] In 2009, Sankovsky et al[169] also reported a case of *S. salivarius* meningitis subsequent to CSE for labor in a healthy primigravid patient. The anesthesiologist was wearing sterile gloves and a mask, but the mask had been worn during prior procedures.

These cases highlight the importance of adhering to established infection control recommendations during neuraxial procedures, which include the use of masks, washing hands, and adherence to aseptic technique. It is important that the face mask be tightly attached to cover the mouth and nose and not be reused.

Headache and neck pain or neck stiffness in a patient who recently received spinal anesthesia is often attributed to post-dural puncture headache (PDPH). One case report highlighted the dangers associated with missed diagnosis of meningitis. The patient was misdiagnosed as having endometritis when presenting with headache, vomiting, and fever for 2 days after uncomplicated epidural analgesia for labor. Her condition rapidly deteriorated, and meningitis was not considered as a diagnosis until it was too late. She subsequently died in intensive care.[170]

Cauda Equina Syndrome

Hyperbaric bupivacaine is frequently administered intrathecally during CSE anesthesia. Although neurological problems are mostly reported following administration of lidocaine or mepivacaine, a few cases of cauda equina syndrome following ordinary doses of intrathecal bupivacaine in a CSE technique have been reported.

Tariq[171] reported a case of an 83-year-old man who developed cauda equina syndrome after uneventful CSE anesthesia for elective knee arthroplasty. Takasu et al[172] reported a 29-year-old parturient who developed cauda equina syndrome following uneventful CSE with hyperbaric bupivacaine for cesarean delivery. Kubina et al[173] also described two cases of cauda equina following uneventful CSE with hyperbaric bupivacaine. One of the patients, however, suffered from spinal stenosis, which could explain this complication. Kato et al described a case of cauda equina syndrome following CSE with an ordinary dose of hyperbaric bupivacaine in an older patient without spinal stenosis.[174] It is thought that the lack of a protective sheath in the cauda equina as the spinal nerves and roots pass through the dura makes them particularly prone to injury from high concentration of local anesthetics.

Postdural Puncture Headache

The incidence of PDPH after CSE technique is controversial; some authors have reported decreased incidence when compared with epidural technique alone,[175] while others report an increased incidence.[176] Balestrieri reported that the patients who received conventional epidural analgesia were more likely to suffer an accidental dural puncture (twofold increase; epidural vs. CSE = 4.2% vs. 1.7%). They offered two possible explanations for this result. The first reason was that they usually chose CSE for women who were most often in early labor and reserved epidural analgesia for patients in the more painful active phase of labor. Therefore, the patients in the epidural group were more likely to move during the procedure and thus cause a "wet tap." Second, during CSE if uncertain of the location of the epidural needle, the spinal needle could be inserted to look for CSF[177] and the epidural needle advanced no further after seeing CSF in the spinal needle.

There are other factors that may also decrease the incidence of PDPH following the CSE technique. Administration of intrathecal opioids has been shown to decrease the incidence of PDPH.[178] Subsequent infusion of epidural local anesthetic increases the subarachnoid pressure and may help to decrease the incidence of PDPH following CSE. Dunn et al. argued that the intentional dural puncture involved in the CSE technique would increase the risk of PDPH in obstetric patients compared to epidural analgesia alone.[176] The use of small-gauge atraumatic pencil-point spinal needles (such as Whitacre, Pencan, Sprotte, and Gertie Marx) will greatly reduce the incidence of PDPH in patients receiving CSE.[175,179]

Chan and Paech reported three cases of persistent CSF leak following uneventful CSE analgesia for labor.[180] It was confirmed that the leaking fluid was CSF in two cases by β_2-trasferrin immunofixation assay.[181] None of the patients developed PDPH or any other complications. Howes and Lenz also reported a CSF cutaneous fistula in two patients following epidural anesthesia (not CSE) for postoperative pain relief. Both patients developed PDPH only after removal of the catheters and were treated successfully with autologous blood patch.[182]

Complications Related to Labor Analgesia
Fetal Bradycardia

Reports in the literature suggested an increased frequency of nonreassuring fetal heart rate (FHR) tracings and fetal bradycardia associated with CSE.[183–185] The etiology of fetal bradycardia after CSE remains elusive but may be related to an acute reduction in circulating maternal catecholamine levels after the almost-immediate onset of analgesia. In addition, it has been postulated that an imbalance between epinephrine and norepinephrine levels (decreased epinephrine levels in the continuing presence of high norepinephrine levels) causes unopposed α-adrenoceptor effects on uterine tone with increased uterine vascular resistance leading to decreased uterine blood flow.

A meta-analysis by Mardirosoff and colleagues found a relative risk of 1.81 of having FHR abnormalities when intrathecal opioids were used. However, the risk of subsequent cesarean delivery was not increased.[186] There is evidence of a dose relationship and greater occurrence of worrisome FHR abnormalities with higher doses of opioids.[187] Nicolet et al performed a prospective study to identify maternal factors implicated in fetal bradycardia after CSE for labor pain. They found that the level of maternal pain scores at the time of labor analgesia request and maternal age were independent predictors of fetal bradycardia after neuraxial analgesia for labor.[188]

The resulting fetal bradycardia was usually short lived and typically resolved within 5–8 minutes.[189] A retrospective study of 1240 patients who received regional labor analgesia (mostly CSE) and 1140 patients who received systemic medication or no analgesia demonstrated no significant difference in the rate of cesarean delivery, with rates of 1.3% and 1.4%, respectively. That study also reported that no emergency cesarean deliveries for acute fetal "distress" were necessary in the absence of obstetric indications up to 90 minutes after intrathecal sufentanil administration.[190] A prospective randomized study by Skupski et al[191] also found no difference in the rate of prolonged deceleration between labor epidural versus CSE for labor (3.2% vs. 6.2%, respectively; $p = 0.43$).

EQUIPMENT

The CSE technique has gained popularity and acceptance, especially in obstetrics. Special kits have been produced for CSE (eg, B Braun Medical Ltd. comprising the standard 16-gauge, 8-cm Tuohy needle with a 26-gauge Quincke spinal needle). Various concerns of the CSE technique have led to some modification of the needles used.

To direct the epidural catheter away from the dural puncture site, Rawal et al recommended rotation of the epidural needle 180° following dural puncture. This maneuver directs the epidural catheter 2–2.5 mm away from the dural puncture site.[192] However, Meikljohn, using postmortem dura mater, demonstrated that rotation of the epidural needle significantly decreased the force required to puncture the dura[117] and thus might result in a wet tap.

Recently, CSE kits designed with an orifice in the back curve (back hole) of the epidural needle for separate spinal needle passage have been made available[15] (Figure 26–4). This needle and others like it may reduce the likelihood of dural passage of the epidural catheter by directing the catheter away from the dural puncture site. However, the spinal needle may not always go through the spinal needle orifice and may exit through the Huber tip, thus losing the advantage of the back hole[15] (Figure 26–5).

Joshi and McCarroll suggested a technique to enhance the spinal needle exit through the spinal needle orifice.[111,193] The modified technique consisted of first aligning the bevel orifice of the spinal needle to the same direction as the Tuohy bevel and then bending the spinal needle 10° toward the Tuohy bevel while advancing through the Tuohy needle. This technique guides the spinal needle tip to exit through the back hole. Pan, in a prospective randomized study, evaluated the success rate of

the spinal needle exiting through the spinal needle orifice in two commonly available single-lumen, dual-orifice, CSE needle kits.[194] The CSE kits studies were first the Espocan CSE kit (Braun Medical Ltd.) that consists of a standard 18-gauge Tuohy needle with a 26-gauge sleeved Quincke spinal needle that extends 12 mm beyond the tip of the Tuohy needle through the back hole. The sleeve on the spinal needle was designed to guide the spinal needle to exit through the back hole. Second was the Espocan CSE kit (Braun Medical Ltd.), which consists of the same epidural needle with a 27-gauge nonsleeved Sprotte spinal needle that extends 13 mm beyond the tip of the Tuohy needle through the back hole. They performed 1600 attempts, which included the modified technique described by Joshi and McCarroll. The modified technique improved the success rate of spinal needle exiting through the back hole from 67% to 94% for the first kit and 50% to 81% for the second kit; cephalad orientation of the Tuohy needle bevel further improved the success rate to 96% and 91%, respectively. Overall, the sleeved spinal needle had a better success rate than the unsleeved spinal needle.

The failure of the spinal needle to exit through the back hole may also result in bending of the spinal needle and less protrusion beyond the tip of the Tuohy needle. This may contribute to the increased failure rate of dural puncture. The ideal length of spinal needle protrusion is reported to be at least 12–13 mm. In a prospective randomized study of 40 patients, Joshi and McCarroll reported a 15% failure rate of CSF return when the spinal needle protruded only 10 mm beyond the tip of the Tuohy needle and 0% with a 13-mm protrusion.[111] Riley et al reported[195] similar results comparing 24-gauge Sprotte (9-mm protrusion past the tip of the Tuhoy and 17% failure to obtain CSF) and Gertie Marx (protrusion 17 mm and 0% failure rate). The number of patients developing PDPH and requiring blood

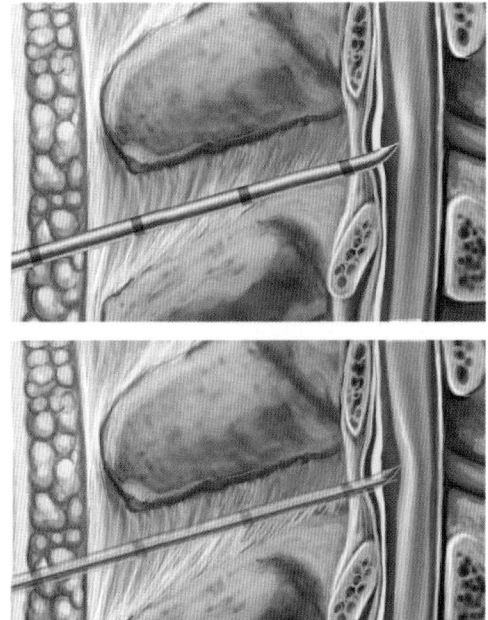
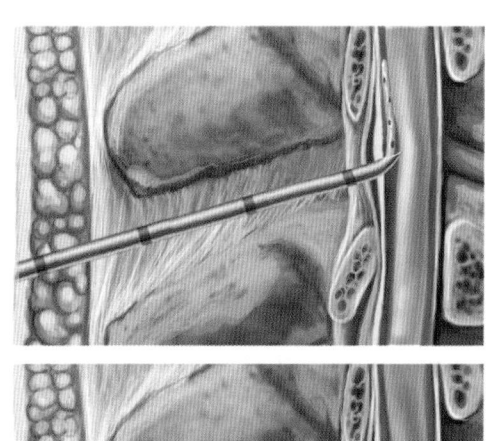
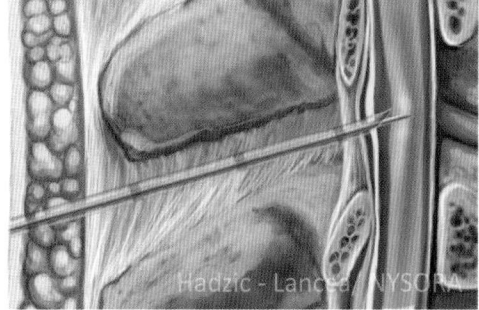

FIGURE 26–4. Combined spinal-epidural kit with an orifice in the back curve for separate spinal needle passage.

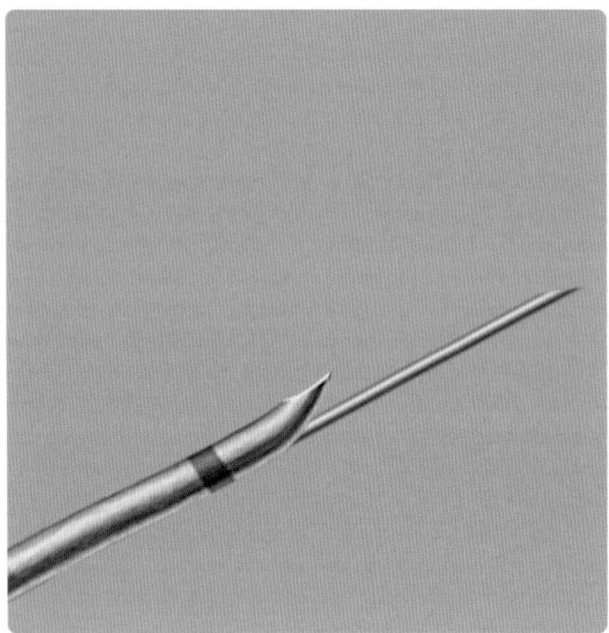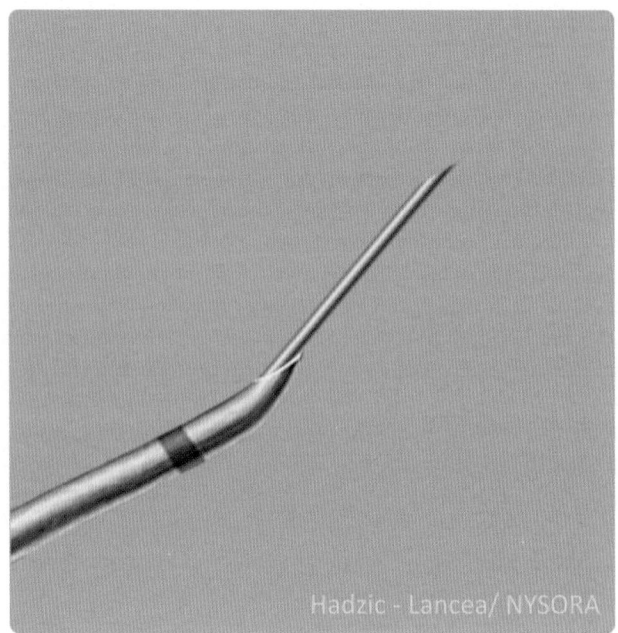

FIGURE 26–5. Combined spinal-epidural kit with spinal needle exiting the back hole and the Huber tip.

patch was greater with Gertie Marx than the Sprotte needle. However, this difference was not statistically significant. It is possible that the longer spinal needle also punctured the anterior aspect of the dura and thus might have caused a greater CSF leak. Greater rates of paresthesia were also noted (anecdotal) with the 127-mm needle, and the 124-mm Gertie Marx needle was suggested as an excellent compromise.

Herbstman et al compared four pencil-point spinal needles commonly used in the CSE technique and reported that longer spinal needles were associated with significantly more transient paresthesias (Gertie Marx 15-mm protrusion with 29% incidence; Whitacre 10-mm protrusion with 17% incidence). Success in obtaining CSF and the incidence of PDPH did not differ among the four needles.[196]

The conventional spinal needle in the CSE kit, which does not lock within the epidural needle, may be difficult to handle and stabilize during injection of spinal medication. The displacement of the spinal needle during aspiration of the CSF and injection may result in failed anesthesia or may push the spinal needle deeper, leading to nerve damage or anterior dural perforation. To overcome this problem, Simsa suggested an external fixation device.[197] This device, however, is somewhat complicated to handle.

Recently, spinal needles with an adjustable locking device have been introduced (CSEcure and Adjustable Durasafe CSE needle). Studies of the lockable extensions reported them to provide safe and stable conditions during placement of the syringe and injection.[62,198] However, both studies reported frequent inability to feel dural perforation with the locking needles (15.3% with CSFcure and 25% with Adjustable Durasafe). There was no clear explanation for this.

In a CSE technique, sometimes the epidural catheter cannot be threaded or threaded intravascularly after the intrathecal drugs have been injected. To overcome this problem, a dual-lumen, dual-orifice CSE kit was developed in which an epidural catheter can be inserted in place prior to inserting the spinal needle and medication.[199,200] This is possible because there are two separate lumens for the catheter and the spinal needle (Figure 26–6).

Recently, a dual-lumen CSE needle was commercialized in Europe (Epistar; Medimex, Germany).

CONTROVERSIAL TOPICS IN CSE TECHNIQUE

Test Dose

The issue of whether a test dose is needed when administering labor epidural analgesia is controversial.[201,202] Because very dilute solutions of LAs are commonly used and aspiration is often diagnostic, some authors believe that a conventional test dose is unnecessary.[203] However, because catheter aspiration is not always predictive (especially when using a single-orifice epidural catheter), others maintain the importance of a test dose to improve detection of intrathecal or intravascular placement of an epidural catheter.[204]

Part of the controversy surrounding the testing of epidural catheters involves the use of epinephrine. Epinephrine has been shown to produce a reliable increase in heart rate in volunteers and surgical patients when the epidural has been sited in a blood vessel.[204] However, in laboring women, maternal heart rate variability from the pain of uterine contractions may confuse interpretation of the heart rate response, and intravenous epinephrine may have deleterious effects on uterine blood flow.[205]

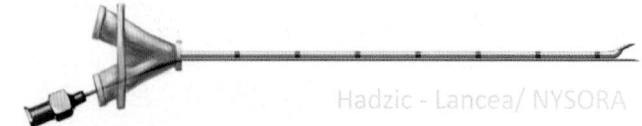

FIGURE 26–6. Dual-lumen, dual-orifice CSE kit.

Means to improve the reliability of an epinephrine test dose include injecting the dose between uterine contractions and repeating the test dose when the response is equivocal. However, the lack of sensitivity and specificity of the test dose calls into question its usefulness as a diagnostic tool.

Leighton and colleagues have described an alternative means of testing an epidural catheter for intravascular placement. They advocated the injection of 1–2 mL of air into the epidural catheter while listening over the precordium with the maternal external Doppler monitor for evidence of air.[206]

With reports of subarachnoid administration of chloroprocaine,[207] it is possible that in the future this agent will be utilized for testing epidural catheters. Caution, however, is necessary because preservative-containing chloroprocaine is also commercially available. If continuous infusion of dilute local anesthetic is administered and the patient remains comfortable without a motor block, proper epidural catheter placement is highly likely. That is, if the epidural catheter were intravascular, the patient should have inadequate pain relief, and if the catheter were subarachnoid, a solid motor block would develop. Although infusions of ultradilute local anesthetics do not pose a serious threat, such is not true of concentrated local anesthetics used for operative delivery. Some authors have suggested that a test dose is essential for any parturient receiving epidural anesthesia.[204] Regardless of the technique used, the safe practice of administering labor epidural analgesia dictates initial catheter aspiration, incremental injections, and continuous monitoring for evidence of local anesthetic toxicity.

Positioning for CSE

Neuraxial blocks are often performed with the patients in the sitting position, especially obese individuals, because the midline is easily recognized. The sitting position has been shown to allow better spinal flexion in the parturients.[208] In addition, the distance from the skin to the epidural space was shown to be significantly greater when epidural puncture was performed in the lateral position as compared with the sitting position. This change in distance may cause catheter dislodgment when the patient is turned from the sitting position to lateral, with consequent inadequate analgesia.

Yun et al compared the effects of induction of CSE anesthesia in the sitting versus lateral position in healthy women undergoing elective cesarean delivery.[209] The severity of hypotension, measured by the maximal percentage decrease in systolic blood pressure from control, as well as its duration were significantly greater in the sitting group ($p < 0.05$). Patients in the sitting group required twice as much ephedrine to treat hypotension than those in the lateral recumbent group. The reason for the difference in the severity of hypotension was not clear. They postulated it to be related to a slower recovery from venous pooling in the lower extremities when assuming a supine position from the initial sitting position. These authors concluded that the position used for induction of CSE should be considered in cases associated with greater maternal or fetal risk from hypotension.

Traditional teaching is that the spread of hyperbaric intrathecal solutions follows gravity. Lewis et al compared the development of spinal blocks in the left lateral position versus a supine wedge position after performing the CSE in the sitting position.[210] The intrathecal medications consisted of 2 mL of 0.5% hyperbaric bupivacaine with 15 μg fentanyl. The left lateral position did not produce unilateral blockade. The left lateral position was associated with slower block onset ($p = .004$) but eventually produced a spinal block similar in characteristics to that obtained in the supine wedge position. The left lateral position is known to improve maternal cardiac output, and slower onset may be outweighed by the possible benefit to the fetus.

SUMMARY

The CSE technique is well established method[10,58] for various types of surgery, particularly in obstetrics. In our institution, the CSE technique is the most commonly performed regional technique for labor analgesia (97%) as well as cesarean delivery (54%). CSE offers many advantages; it provides a method to administer neuraxial anesthesia and analgesia in numerous clinical situations.

The CSE technique offers the advantages of both spinal and epidural techniques and therefore has a high success rate in providing regional anesthesia. CSE provides rapid onset and the ability to titrate to a desired sensory level, control the duration of the block, and deliver postoperative analgesia. Another advantage of CSE is the facilitation of the spinal needle entrance into the subarachnoid space. The Tuohy needle serves as a guide for the spinal needle almost to the subarachnoid space. This allows for use of the smaller-gauge atraumatic spinal needles, with which the PDPH is absent or rare.[179]

The disadvantages of the CSE are that, the combined technique introduces potential side effects such as PDPH, the increased risk of catheter migration into the subarachnoid space, and transient paresthesias from the spinal needle. Although the risk is low, a number of equipment modifications have been suggested and developed to avoid penetration of the epidural catheter through the dural hole made by the spinal needle.

The ideal length of spinal needle protrusion beyond the tip of the epidural needle is reported to be at least 12–13 mm. Longer spinal needles were shown to be associated with significantly higher incidence of transient paresthesias. Inability to obtain CSF through the spinal needle may occur with shorter needles (<10 mm of protrusion) and result in failure of the spinal component of the technique. CSE failure is also related to a faulty puncture site or axis deviation during needle advancement. The risk of infection, hematoma, and neurological damage increases with multiple attempts and multiple manipulations of the needles, but it is not clear if the CSE technique increases these risks.

REFERENCES

1. Rodgers A, Walker N, Schug S, et al. Reduction of postoperative mortality and morbidity with epidural or spinal anaesthesia: Results from overview of randomised trials. BMJ 2000;321:1493–1504.
2. Buhre W, Rossaint R: Perioperative management and monitoring in anaesthesia. Lancet 2003;362:1839–1846.
3. Kehlet H, Wilmore DW: Multimodal strategies to improve surgical outcome. Am J Surg 2002;183:630–641.

4. Holmström B, Laugaland K, Rawal N, et al: Combined spinal epidural block versus spinal and epidural block for orthopaedic surgery. Can J Anesth 1993;40:601–606.

5. Stienstra R, Dahan A, Alhadi ZRB, et al: Mechanism of action of an epidural top-up in combined spinal epidural anaesthesia. Anesth Analg 1996;83:382–386.

6. Stienstra R, Dilrosun-Alhadi BZR, Dahan A, et al: The epidural top-up in combined spinal-epidural anaesthesia: The effect of volume versus dose. Anesth Analg 1999;88:810–814.

7. Blanshard HJ, Cook TM: Use of combined spinal-epidural by obstetric anaesthetists. Anaesthesia 2004;59(9):922–923.

8. Norris MC. Are combined spinal epidural catheters reliable. Int J Obsted Anaesth 2000;9:3–6.

9. Reynolds F: Damage to the conus medullaris following spinal anaesthesia. Anaesthesia 2001;56:238–247.

10. Cook TM: Combined spinal-epidural techniques. Anaesthesia 2000; 55:42–64.

11. Hughes D, Simmons SW, Brown J, Cyna AM: Combined spinal-epidural versus epidural analgesia in labour. Cochrane Database Syst Rev 2003;(4):CD003401.

12. Poulakka R, Pitkanen MT, Rosenberg PH: Comparison of technical and block characteristics of different combined spinal and epidural anesthesia techniques. Reg Anesth Pain Med 2001;26:17–23.

13. Cherng YG, Wang YP, Liu CC, Shi JJ, Huang CC: Combined spinal and epidural anesthesia for abdominal hysterectomy in a patient with myotonic dystrophy. Case report. Reg Anesth 1994;19(1):69–72.

14. Mane RS, Patil MC, Kedareshvara KS, Sanikop CS: Combined spinal epidural anesthesia for laparoscopic appendectomy in adults: A case series. Saudi J Anaesth 2012;6:27–30.

15. Browne IM, Birnbach DJ, Stein DJ, O'Gorman DA: A comparison of Espocan and Tuohy needles for the combined spinal-epidural technique for labor analgesia. Anesth Analg 2005;101:535–540.

16. Hermanides J, Hollmann MW, Stevens MF, Lirk P: Failed epidural: Causes and management. Br J Anaesth 2012;109:144–154.

17. Viscomi CM, Rathmell JP, Pace NL: Duration of intrathecal labor analgesia. Early versus advanced labor. Anesth Analg 1997;84:1108–1112.

18. Collis RE, Davies DW, Aveling W: Randomised comparison of combined spinal epidural and standard epidural analgesia in labour. Lancet 1995;345:1413–1416.

19. Palmer CM, Randall CC, Hays R, et al: The dose-response relation of intrathecal fentanyl for labor analgesia. Anesthesiology 1998;88:355–361.

20. Campbell DC, Camann WR, Datta S, et al: The addition of bupivacaine to intrathecal sufentanil for labor analgesia. Anesth Analg 1995;81: 305–309.

21. Sia AT, Chong JL, Chiu JW: Combination of intrathecal sufentanil 10 mcg plus bupivacaine 2.5 mg for labor analgesia. Is half the dose enough? Anesth Analg 1999;88:362–366.

22. Hughes D, Hill D, Fee JP: Intrathecal ropivacaine or bupivacaine with fentanyl for labour. Br J Anaesth 2001;87:733–737.

23. Vercauteren MP, Haus G, De Decker K, et al: Levobupivacaine combined with sufentanil for intrathecal labor analgesia: A comparison with racemic bupivacaine. Anesth Analg 2001;93:996–1000.

24. Van de Velde M, Dreelinck R, Dubois J, et al. Determination of the full dose-response relation of intrathecal bupivacaine, levobupivacaine, and ropivacaine, combined with sufentanil, for labor analgesia. Anesthesiology 2007;106:149–156.

25. Wilson MJ, MacArthur C, Cooper GM, Shennan A; COMET Study Group UK: Ambulation in labour and delivery mode: A randomised controlled trial of high-dose vs mobile epidural analgesia. Anaesthesia 2009;64:266–272.

26. Tsen L, Thue B, Datta S, et al: Is combined spinal-epidural analgesia associated with more rapid cervical dilation in nulliparous patients when compared with conventional epidural analgesia? Anesthesiology 1999;91: 920–925.

27. Wong CA, Scavon BM, Peaceman AM, et al: The risk of cesarean delivery with neuraxial analgesia given early versus late in labor. N Engl J Med 2005;352(7):655–665.

28. Pascual-Ramirez J, Haya J, Pérez-López FR, et al: Effect of combined spinal epidural analgesia versus epidural analgesia on labor and delivery duration. Int J Gynaecol Obstet 2011;114:246–250.

29. Carrie LES, O'Sullivan GM: Subarachnoid bupivacaine 0.5% for cesarean section. Eur J Anaesthesiol 1984;1:275–283.

30. Crowhurst J, Birnbach DJ: Low dose neuraxial block. Heading towards the new millennium. Anesth Analg 2000;90:241–242.

31. Blumgart CH, Ryall D, Dennison B, et al: Mechanism of extension of spinal anaesthesia by extradural injection of local anesthetic. Br J Anaesth 1992;169:457.

32. Kawasw H, Sumikura H, Kamada T, et al: Case of external cephalic version under combined spinal-epidural anesthesia followed by vaginal delivery. Masui 2009;58:637–640.

33. Sullivan JT, Grobman WA, Bauchat JR, et al: A randomized controlled trial of the effect of combined spinal-epidural analgesia on the success of external cephalic version for breech presentation. Int J Obstet Anesth 2009;18:328–334.

34. Pan PH, Bogard TD, Owen MD: Incidence and characteristics of failures in obstetric neuraxial analgesia and anesthesia: A retrospective analysis of 19,259 deliveries. Int J Obstet Anesth 2004;13(4):227–233.

35. Eappen S, Blinn A, Segal S: Incidence of epidural catheter replacement in parturients: A retrospective chart review. Int J Obstet Anesth 1998;7: 220–225.

36. Choi DH, Park YD: Comparison of combined spinal–epidural anaesthesia and spinal anaesthesia for caesarean section. IMRAPT 2002;14:A129.

37. Reyes M, Pan PH:. Very low-dose spinal anesthesia for cesarean section in a morbidly obese preeclamptic patient and its potential implications. Int J Obstet Anesth 2004;13:99–102.

38. Ranasinghe JS, Steadman J, Toyama T, Lai M: Combined spinal epidural anaesthesia is better than spinal or epidural alone for caesarean delivery. Br J Anaesth 2003;91:299–300.

39. Lim Y, Loo CC, Goh E: Ultra low dose combined spinal and epidural anesthesia for cesarean section. Int J Obstet Anesth 2004;13:198–200.

40. Peng PW, Chan VW, Perks A: Minimum effective anaesthetic concentration of hyperbaric lidocaine for spinal anaesthesia. Can J Anesth 1998;45:122–129.

41. Urmey WF, Stanton J, Peterson M, et al: Combined spinal–epidural anaesthesia for outpatient surgery. Dose-response characteristics of intrathecal isobaric lidocaine using a 27-gauge Whitacre needle. Anesthesiology 1995;83:528–534.

42. Norris MC, Combined spinal–epidural anaesthesia for urological and lower extremity vascular procedures. Tech Reg Anaesth Pain Manag 1997;1:131–136.

43. Patel NP, Armstrong SL, Fernando R, et al: Combined spinal epidural vs epidural labour analgesia: Does initial intrathecal analgesia reduce the subsequent minimum local analgesic concentration of epidural bupivacaine? Anaesthesia 2012;67:584–593.

44. Takiguchi T, Okano T, Egawa H, et al: The effect of epidural saline injection on analgesic level during combined spinal and epidural anesthesia assessed clinically and myelographically. Anesth Analg 1997; 85:1097–1100.

45. Blumgart CH, Ryall D, Dennison B, et al: Mechanism of extension of spinal anaesthesia by extradural injection of local anaesthetic. Br J Anaesth 1992;69:457–460.

46. Loubert C, Hallworth S, Fernando R, et al: Epidural volume extension in combined spinal epidural anaesthesia for elective caesarean section: a randomised controlled trial. Anesth Analg 2011;113:811–817.

47. Doganci N, Apan A, Tekin O, Kaymak C: Epidural volume expansion: Is there a ceiling effect? Minerva Anestesiol 2010;76:334–339.

48. Tyagi A, Kumar A, Sethi AK, Mohta M: Epidural volume extension and intrathecal dose requirement: Plain versus hyperbaric bupivacaine. Anesth Analg 2008;107:333–338.

49. Tyagi A, Girotra G, Kumar A, et al: Single-shot spinal anaesthesia, combined spinal-epidural and epidural volume extension for elective caesarean section: A randomized comparison. Int J Obstet Anesth 2009; 18:231–236.

50. Fan SZ, Suseti L, Wang YP, et al: Low dose of intrathecal hyperbaric bupivacaine combined with epidural lidocaine for caesarean section—a balance block technique. Anesth Analg 1994;78:474–477.

51. Macfarlane A, Pryn A, Litchfield K, et al: Randomised controlled trial of combined spinal epidural vs. spinal anaesthesia for elective caesarean section: Vasopressor requirements and cardiovascular changes. Eur J Anaesth 2009;26:47–51.

52. Landau R, Giraud R, Morales M, Kern C, Trindade P: Sequential combined spinal-epidural anesthesia for cesarean section in a woman with a double-outlet right ventricle. Acta Anaesthesiol Scand 2004; 48: 922–926.

53. Parneix M, Fanou L, Morau E, Colson P: Low dose vombined spinal-epidural anesthesia for cesarean section in a patient with Eisenmenger's syndrome. Int J. Obstet Anesth 2009;18:81–84.

54. Agarwal A, Garg R, Joshi A, Verma S: Combined spinal epidural anesthesia with epidural volume extension technique for hysterectomy in patient with unpalliated cyanotic heart disease—A case-report. Acta Anaesthesiol Belg 2010;61:159–161.

55. Month RC, Vaida SJ: A combined spinal-epidural technique for labor analgesia and symptomatic relief in two parturients with idiopathic intracranial hypertension. Int J Obstet Anesth 2012;21:192–194.

56. Thorén T, Holmström B, Rawal N, et al: Sequential combined spinal epidural block versus spinal block for Caesarean section: Effects on maternal hypotension and neurobehavioral function of the newborn. Anesth Analg 1994;78:1087–1092.

57. Simmons SW, Cyna AM, Dennis AT, Hughes D: Combined spinal-epidural versus epidural analgesia in labour. Cochrane Database Syst Rev 2007;(3):CD003401.

58. Van De Velde M: Combined spinal epidural analgesia for labor and delivery: A balanced view based on experience and literature. Acta Anaesth Belg 2009;60:109–122.

59. Hoffmann VL, Vercauteren MP, Vreugde JP, Hans GH, Coppejans HC, Adriaensen HA: Posterior epidural space depth: Safety of the loss of resistance and hanging drop techniques. Br J Anaesth 1999;83: 807–809.

60. Han KR, Kim C, Park SK, Kim JS: Distance to the adult cervical epidural space. Reg Anesth Pain Med 2003;28:95–97.

61. McAndrew CR, Harms P: Paraesthesiae during needle-through-needle combined spinal epidural versus single-shot spinal for elective caesarean section. Anaesth Intensive Care 2003;31:514–517

62. Hoffmann VL, Vercauteren MP, Buczkowski PW, Vanspringel GL: A new combined spinal-epidural apparatus: Measurement of the distance to the epidural and subarachnoid spaces. Anaesthesia 1997;52:350–355.

63. Cousins MJ, Bridenbaugh PO: *Neural Blockade in Clinical Anesthesia and Management of Pain*, 3rd ed. Lippincott-Raven, 1998, pp 252–255.

64. Watts RW: The influence of obesity on the relationship between body mass index and the distance to the epidural space from the skin. Anesth Intensive Care 1993;21;309–310.

65. Lirk P, Moriggl B, Colvin J, et al: The incidence of lumbar Ligamentum flavum midline gaps. Anesth Analg 2004;98:1178–1180.

66. Cook TM: Combined spinal-epidural techniques. Anaesthesia 2000;55: 42–64.

67. Landau R: Combined spinal-epidural analgesia for labor: Breakthrough or unjustified invasion? Semin Perinatol 2002;26:109–121.

68. Rawal N, Holmstrom B: The combined spinal-epidural technique. Best Pract Res Clin Anaesthesiol 2003;17:347–364.

69. Soresi AL: Episubdural anesthesia. Anesth Analg 1937;16:306–310.

70. Curelaru I: Long duration subarachnoid anesthesia with continuous epidural block. Prak Anaesth 1979;14:71–78.

71. Brownridge P: Central neural blockade and cesarean section, part 1. Review and case series. Anaesth Intensive Care 1979;7:33–41.

72. Brownridge P: Epidural and subarachnoid analgesia for elective cesarean section. Anaesthesia 1981;36:70.

73. Coates MB: Combined subarachnoid and epidural techniques. Anaesthesia. 982;37:89–90.

74. Mumtaz MH, Daz M, Kuz M: Another single space technique for orthopaedic surgery. Anaesthesia 1982;37:90.

75. Carrie LES, O'Sullivan GM: Subarachnoid bupivacaine 0.5% for cesarean section. Eur J Anaesth 1984;1:275–283.

76. Turner MA, Reifenberg NA. Combined spinal epidural analgesia. The single space double-barrel technique. Int J Obstet Anesth 1995;55: 158–160.

77. Cook TM: A new combined spinal-epidural technique. Int J Obstet Anesth 1999;55:3–6.

78. Brownridge P: Epidural and subarachnoid analgesia for elective caesarean section. Anaesthesia 1981;55:70.

79. Carrie LES: Epidural versus combined spinal epidural block for caesarean section. Acta Anaesth Scand 1988;55:5956.

80. Morris GN, Kinsella M, Thomas TA: Pencil-point needles and combined spinal epidural block. Why needle through needle? Anaesthesia 1998;55: 1132.

81. Kestin IG: Spinal anaesthesia in obstetrics. Br J Anaesth 1991;55:663.

82. Eldor J: Combined spinal–epidural anaesthesia through the Portex set. Anaesthesia 1993;55:836.

83. Soni AK, Sarna MC. Combined spinal epidural analgesia. The single space double-barrel technique. Int J Obstet Anesth 1996;55:206–207.

84. Sakuma N, Hori M, Suzuki H, et al: A sheared off and sequestered epidural catheter: A case report. Masui 2004;53(2):198–200.

85. Roberts E, Brighouse D: Combined spinal-epidural anesthesia for caesarean section. Anaesthesia 1992;55:1006.

86. Cook TM: 201 combined spinal-epidurals for anaesthesia using a separate needle technique. Eur J Anaesthiol 2004;21:679–683.

87. Levin A, Segal S, Datta S: Does combined spinalepidural analgesia alter the incidence of paraesthesia during epidural catheter insertion? Anesth Analg 1998;55:44551.

88. Familton MJG, Morgan BM: "Needle-through-needle" technique for combined spinal–extradural anaesthesia in obstetrics. Br J Anaesth 1992; 55:327.

89. Patel M, Samsoon G, Swami A, Morgan B: Posture and the spread of hyperbaric bupivacaine in parturients using the combined spinal epidural technique. Can J Anaesth 1993;55:943–946.

90. McAndrew CR, Harms P: Paraesthesiae during needle-through-needle combined spinal epidural versus single-shot spinal for elective caesarean section. Anaesth Intensive Care 2003;31:514–517.

91. Lyons G, Macdonald R, Mikl B: Combined epiduralspinal anaesthesia for Caesarean section. Through the needle or in separate spaces? Anaesthesia 1992;55:199–201.

92. Casati A, D'ambrosio A, De Negri P, Fanelli G, Tageriello V, Tarantino F: A clinical comparison between needle-through-needle and double segment techniques for combined spinal and epidural anesthesia. Reg Anesth Pain Med 1998;55:3904.

93. Rawal N, Van Zundert A, Holmström B, Crowhurst JA: Combined spinalepidural technique. Reg Anesth 1997;55:40623.

94. Backe SK, Sheikh Z, Wilson R, Lyons GR: Combined epidural/spinal anaesthesia: Needle-through-needle or separate spaces? Eur J Anaesthesiol 2004;21:854–857.

95. Sadashivaiah J, Wilson R, McLure H, Lyons G: Double-space combined spinal-epidural technique for elective caesarean section: A review of 10 years' experience in a UK teaching maternity unit. Int J Obstet Anesth 2010;19:183–187.

96. Van den Berg AA, Ghatge S, Wang S: Loss of resistance to saline reduces responses accompanying spinal needle insertion during institution of "needle-through-needle" combined spinal-epidural analgesia. Anaesth Intensive Care 2010;38:1013–1017.

97. Grau T, Leipold RW, Fatehi s, Martin E, Motsch J: Real-time ultrasonic observation of combined spinal-epidural anaesthesia. Eur J Anaesthesiol 2004;21:25–31.

98. Tsui BC, Gupta S, Finucane B: Determination of epidural catheter placement using nerve stimulation in obstetric patients. Reg Anesth 1999;24:17–23.

99. Herman NL, Calicott R, Van Decar TK, et al: Determination of the dose-response relationship for intrathecal sufentanil in laboring patients. Anesth Analg 1997;84:1256–1261.

100. Herman NL, Choi KC, Affleck PJ, et al: Analgesia, pruritus, and ventilation exhibit in parturients receiving intrathecal fentanyl during labor. Anesth Analg 1999;89:378–383.

101. Palmer CM, Randall CC, Hays R, et al: The dose-response relation of intrathecal fentanyl for labor analgesia. Anesthesiology 1998;88:355–361.

102. Honet JE, Arkoosh VA, Norris MC, et al: Comparison among intrathecal fentanyl, meperidine, and sufentanil for labor analgesia. Anesth Analg 1992;75:734–739.

103. Jaffe RA, Rowe MA: Comparison of the local anesthetic effects of meperidine, fentanyl, and sufentanil on dorsal root axons. Anesth Analg 1996;83:776–781.

104. Flanagan MT, Walker FO, Butterworth J: Failure of meperidine to anesthetize human median nerve. A blinded comparison with lidocaine and saline. Reg Anesth 1997;22:73–79.

105. Abouleish A, Abouleish E, Camann W: Combined spinal-epidural analgesia in advanced labor. Can J Anaesth 1994;41:575–578.

106. Campbell DC, Camann WR, Datta S: The addition of bupivacaine to intrathecal sufentanil for labor analgesia. Anesth Analg 1995;81: 305–309.

107. Sia ATH, Chong JL, Chiu JW: Combination of intrathecal sufentanil 10 μg plus bupivacaine 2.5mg for labor analgesia: Is half the dose enough? Anesth Analg 1999;88:362–366.

108. Stocks GM, Hallworth SP, Fernando R, et al: Minimum local analgesic dose of intrathecal bupivacaine in labor and the effect of intrathecal fentanyl. Anesthesiology 2001, 94:593–598.

109. Whitty R, Goldszmidt E, Parkes RK, Carvalho JC: Determination of the ED95 for intrathecal plain bupivacaine combined with fentanyl in active labor. Int J Obstet Anesth 2007;16:341–345.

110. Levin A, Datta S, Camann W: Intrathecal ropivacaine for labor analgesia: A comparison with bupivacaine. Anesth Analg 1998;87:624–627.

111. Joshi GP, McCarroll SM: Evaluation of combined spinal-epidural anaesthesia using two different techniques. Reg Anaesth 1994;55:16974.

112. Collis RE, Baxandall ML, Srikantharajah ID, Edge G, Kadim MY, Morgan BM: Combined spinal epidural analgesia with ability to walk throughout labour. Lancet 1993;55:7678.

113. Hoffmann VLH, Vercauteran MP, Buczkowski PW, Vanspringel GLJ: A new combined spinal epidural apparatus: Measurement of the distance to the epidural and subarachnoid spaces. Anaesthesia 1997;55:350–355.

114. Holloway TE, Telford RJ: Observations on deliberate dural puncture with a Touhy needle: Depth measurement. Anesthesia 1991;46:722–724.

115. Cousins MJ, Bridenhagh PO: *Neural Blockade in Clinical Anesthesia and Management of Pain*, 3rd ed. Lippincott-Raven, 1998, pp 255.

116. Brighouse D, Wilkins A: Failure of pencil-point spinal needles to enter the subarachnoid space. Anaesthesia 1994;55:176.

117. Meiklejohn BH: The effect of rotation of an epidural needle: An in vitro study. Anaesthesia 1987;42:1180–1182.

118. Husemeyer RP, White DC: Topography of the lumbar epidural space. Anaesthesia 1980;55:7–11.

119. Waldman SA, Liguori GA: Comparison of the flow rates of 27-Gauge Whitacre and Sprotte needles for combined spinal and epidural anesthesia. Reg Anesth 1996;55:378–379.

120. Vandermeersch E: Combined spinal-epidural anaesthesia. Balliere's Clin Anaesth 1993;7:691–708.

121. Fukishige T, Sano T, Kano T: Lumbar dural sac deformation after epidural injection. Anesthesiology 1998;55:A870.

122. Norris MC, Grieco WM, Borkowski M, et al: Complications of labor analgesia: Epidural versus combined spinal epidural techniques. Anesth Analg 1994;55:529–537.

123. Lesser P, Bembridge M, Lyons G, Macdonald R: An evaluation of a 30-gauge needle for spinal anaesthesia for Caesarean section. Anaesthesia 1990;55:76–78.

124. Dennison B: Combined subarachnoid and epidural block for caesarean section. Can J Anaesth 1987;55:105.

125. Patel M, Swami M: Combined spinal-extradural anaesthesia for Caesarean section. Anaesthesia 1992;55:1005–1006.

126. Robbins PM, Fernando R, Lim GH: Accidental intrathecal insertion of an extradural catheter during combined spinal-extradural anaesthesia for Caesarean section. Br J Anaesth 1995;75:355–357.

127. Vucevic M, Russell IF: Spinal anaesthesia for caesarean section: 0.125% plain bupivacaine 12mL compared with 0.5% plain bupivacaine 3 ml. Br J Anaesth 1992;55:590–595.

128. Ferguson DJM: Dural puncture and epidural catheters. Anaesthesia 1992;55:272.

129. Muranaka K, Tsutsui T: Comparison of clinical usefulness of the two types of combined spinal epidural needles. Masui 1994;55:1714–1717.

130. Angle P, Kronberg JE, Thompson DE, Duffin J, et al: Epidural catheter penetration of human dura tissue: In vitro investigation. Anesthesiology 2004;100(6);141–146.

131. Holtz D, Mollman M, Schymroszcyk B, Ebel C, Wendt M: No risk of metal toxicity in combined spinal-epidural anesthesia. Anesth Analg 1999;88(2):393–397.

132. Holmstrom B, Rawal N, Axelsson K, et al: Risk of catheter migration during combined spinal epidural block-percutaneous epiduroscopy study. Anesth Analg 1995;80:747–753.

133. Leighton BL, Arkoosh VA, Huffnagle S, et al: The dermatomal spread of epidural bupivacaine with and without prior intrathecal sufentanil. Anesth Analg 1996;83:526–529.

134. Stienstra R, Dilrosun-Alhadi BZ, Dahan A, van Kleef JW, Veering BT, Burm AG: The epidural "top-up" in combined spinal-epidural anaesthesia: The effect of volume versus dose. Anesth Analg 1999;88:810–814.

135. Suzuki N, Koganemaru M, Onizuka S, Takasaki M: Dural puncture with a 26G spinal needle affects spread of epidural anesthesia. Anesth Analg 1996;82:1040–1042.

136. Kamiya Y, Kikuchi T, Inagawa G, et al: Lidocaine concentration in cerebrospinal fluid after epidural administration: A comparison between epidural and combined spinal-epidural anesthesia. Anesthesiology 2009;110:1127–1132.

137. Leach A, Smith GB: Subarachnoid spread of epidural local anaesthetic following dural puncture. Anaesthesia 1988;43:671–674.

138. Gaiser RR, Lewin SB, Cheek TG, Gutsche BB: Effects of immediately initiating an epidural infusion in the combined spinal and epidural technique in nulliparous parturients. Reg Anesth Pain Med 2000;25:223–227.

139. Beaubien G, Drolet P, Girard M, Grenier Y: Patient-controlled epidural analgesia with fentanyl-bupivacaine: Influence of prior dural puncture. Reg Anesth Pain Med 2000;25:254–258.

140. Hodgkinson R: Total spinal block after epidural injection into an interspace adjacent to an inadvertent dural perforation. Anesthesiology 1981;55:593–595.

141. Eldor J, Guedj P, Levine S. Delayed respiratory arrest in combined spinal-epidural anesthesia. Case report. Reg Anesth 1994;19;418–422.

142. Kuczkowski KM, Birnbach DJ, O'Gorman DA, Stein DJ, Santos AC: Does a test dose increase the likelihood of identifying intrathecal placement of epidural catheters during labor analgesia? Abstract of Scientific Papers SOAP. Anesthesiology 2000;A26.

143. Goy RW, Sia AT. Sensorimotor anesthesia and hypotension after subarachnoid block: Combined spinal-epidural versus single-shot spinal technique. Anesth Analg 2004;98(2):491–496.

144. Goy RWL, Chee-Seng Y: The median effective dose of intrathecal hyperbaric bupivacaine is larger in the single-shot spinal as compared with the combined spinal-epidural technique. Anesth Analg 2005; 100:1499–1502.

145. Gaur V, Gupta RK, Agarwal A, et al: Air or nitrous oxide for loss-of-resistance epidural technique? Can J Anaesth 2000;47:503–505.

146. Carpenter RL, Hogan QH, Liu SS, et al: Lumbosacral cerebrospinal fluid volume is the primary determinant of sensory block extent and duration during spinal anesthesia. Anesthesiology 1998;89:24–29.

147. Rawal N, Schollin J, Wesström G: Epidural versus combined spinal epidural block for caesarean section. Acta Anaesth Scand 1988;32:61–66.

148. Kumar C: Combined subarachnoid and epidural block for caesarean section. Can J Anesth 1987;34:329–330.

149. Mandell GL, Jamnback L, Ramanathan S: Hemodynamic effects of subarachnoid fentanyl in laboring parturients. Reg Anesth 1995;21(2):103–111.

150. Horlocker TT, McGregor DG, Matsushige DK, Schroeder DR, Besse JA: A retrospective review of 4767 consecutive spinal anesthetics: Central nervous system complications. Anesth Analg 1997;55:578–584.

151. Bigeleisen PE: Nerve puncture and apparent intraneural injection during ultrasound-guided axillary block does not invariably result in neurologic injury. Anesthesiology 2006;105:779–783.

152. Simsa J: Use of 29-G spinal needle s and a fixation device with combined spinal epidural technique. Acta Anaesth Scand 1994;38:439–441.

153. McAndrew CR, Harms P: Paraesthesiae during needle-through-needle combined spinal epidural versus single-shot spinal for elective caesarean section. Anaesth Intensive Care 2003;31(5):514–517.

154. Holloway J, Seed PT, O'Sullivan G, Reynolds F: Paraesthesiae and nerve damage following combined spinal epidural and spinal anaesthesia: A pilot survey. Int J Obstet Anesth 2000;9(3):151–155.

155. Turner MA, Shaw M: Atraumatic spinal needlea [letter]. Anaesthesia 1993;48:452.

156. Broadbent CR, Maxwell WB, Ferrie R, et al: Ability of anaesthetists to identify a marked lumbar interspace. Anaesthesia 2000;55:1106–1126.

157. Eldor J: Metallic fragments and the combined spinal-extradural technique. Br J Anaesth 1992;69:663.

158. Sharma B, Gupta S, Jain N, Handoo A, Sood J: Cerebrospinal fluid cytology in patients undergoing combined spinal epidural versus spinal anaesthesia without an introducer. Anaesth Intensive Care 2011; 39:914–918.

159. Dripps Rd, Vandem LD: Long-term follow-up of patients who received 10,098 spinal anaesthetics. JAMA 1954;156:1486–1491.

160. Phillips OC, Ebner H, Melson AT, Black MH: Neurological complications following spinal anesthesia with lidocaine: A prospective review of 10,440 cases. Anesthesiology 1969;30:284–289.

161. Harding SA, Collis RE, Morgan BM: Meningitis after combined spinal extradural anaesthesia in obstetrics. Br J Anaesth 1994;73:545–547.

162. Cascio M: Meningitis following a combined spinal-epidural technique in a labouring term parturient. Can J Anaesth 1996;43:399–402.

163. Pinder AJ, Dresner M: Meningococcal meningitis after combined spinal-epidural analgesia. Int J Obstet Anesth 2003;12:183–187.

164. McLure HA, Talboys CA, Yentis SM, Azadian BS: Surgical facemesks and downward dispersal of bacteria. Anaesthesia 1998;53:624–626.

165. Phillips BJ, Fergusson S, Armstrong P, Anderson FM, Wildsmith JAW: Surgical facemasks are effective in reducing bacterial contamination caused by dispersal from the upper airway. Br J Anaesth 1992;69:407–408.

166. Burnstein R, Buckland R, Pickett JA: A survey of epidural analgesia for labour in the United Kingdom. Anesthesia 1999;54:634–650.

167. Siegel J, Rhinehart E, Jackson M, Chiarello L; and the Healthcare Infection Control Practices Advisory Committee. Guideline for isolation precautions: Preventing transmission of infectious agents in healthcare settings, June 2007. http://www.premierinc.com/safety/topics/guidelines/downloads/cdc-isolation-2007.pdf.

168. Centers for Disease Control and Prevention. Bacterial meningitis after spinal anesthesia during labor—Ohio and New York, 2008–2009. MMWR Morb Mortal Wkly Rep 2010;59:65–69.

169. Sandkovsky U, Mihu MR, Adeyeye A, et al: Iatrogenic meningitis in an obstetric patient after combined spinal-epidural analgesia: Case report and review of the literature. South Med J 2009;102:287–290.

170. Choy JC: Mortality from peripartum meningitis. Anaesth Intensive Care 2000;28:328–330.

171. Tariq A: Neurological deficit following combined spinal-epidural anesthesia for knee arthroplasty. Middle East J Anesthesiol 2010;20:759–762.

172. Takasu, M, Okita M, Araki m, et al: Gadolinium enhancement of cauda equina after combined spinal-epidural anaesthesia. Br J Radiol 2010;83:192–194.

173. Kubina P, Gupta A Oscarsson A, et al: Two cases of cauda equina syndrome following spinal-epidural anesthesia. Reg Anesth 1997;22: 447–450.

174. Kato J, Konishi J, Yoshida H, et al: Cauda equina syndrome following combined spinal and epidural anesthesia: A case report. Can J Anaesth 2011;58:638–641.

175. Rawal N, Holmstrom B, Croehurst JA, Van Zundert A: The combined spinal-epidural technique. Anaesthsiol Clin North America 2000;18: 267–295.

176. Dunn SM, Connelly NR, Parker RK: Postdural puncture headache (PDPH) and combined spinal anesthesia (CSE). Anesth Analg 2000;90: 1249–1250.

177. Balestrieri PJ: The incidence of postdural puncture headache and combined spinal-epidural: Some thoughts. Int J Obstet Anesth 2003; 12(4):305–306.

178. Brownridge P. Spinal anaesthesia in obstetrics. Br J Anaesth 1991;67: 663–667.

179. Geurts JW, Haanschoten MC, Van Wijk RM, Kraak H, Besse TC: Postdural puncture headache in young patients. A comparative study between the use of 0.52 mm (25-gauge) and 0.33 mm (29-gauge) spinal needles. Acta Anaesthesiol Scand 1990;34:350–353.

180. Chan BO, Paech MJ: Persistent cerebrospinal fluid leak: A complication of the combined spinal-epidural technique. Anesth Analg 2004;98(3): 828–830.

181. Reisinger PWM, Hochstrasser K: The diagnosis of CSF fistulae on the basis of detection of beta2-transferrin by polyacrylamide gel electrophoresis and immunoblotting. J Clin Chem Clin Biochem 1989; 27:169–172.

182. Howes J, Lenz R: Cerebrospinal fluid cutaneous fistula—An unusual complication of epidural anaesthesia. Anaesthesia 1994;49:221–222.

183. Pan PH, Moore CH, Ross VH: Severe maternal bradycardia and asystole after combined spinal-epidural labor analgesia in a morbidly obese parturient. J Clin Anesth 2004;16(6):461–464.

184. Kuczkowski KM: Severe persistent fetal bradycardia following subarachnoid administration of fentanyl and bupivacaine for induction of a combined spinal-epidural analgesia for labor pain. J Clin Anesth 2004;16(1):78–79.

185. D'Angelo R, Eisenach JC: Severe maternal hypotension and fetal bradycardia after a CSE. Anesthesiology 1997;81:116–118.

186. Mardirosoff C, Dumont L, Boulvain M, Tramèr MR: Fetal bradycardia due to intrathecal opioids for labour analgesia: A systematic review. BJOG 2002;109:274–281.

187. Van de Velde M: Neuraxial analgesia and fetal bradycardia. Curr Opin Anaesthesiol 2005;18:253–256.

188. Nocolet J, Miller A, Kaufman I, et al: Maternal factors implicated in fetal bradycardia after combined spinal epidural for labour pain. Eur J Anaesth 2008;25:721–725.

189. Clarke VT, Smiley RM, Finster M: Uterine hyperactivity after intrathecal injection of fentanyl for analgesia durign labor: A cause of fetal brady cardia? Anesthesiology 1994;81:1083.

190. Albright GA, Forster RM: Does combined spinal-epidural analgesia with subarachnoid sufentanil increase the incidence of emergency cesarean delivery? Reg Anesth Pain Med 1997;22:400–405.

191. Skupski DW, Abramovitz S, Samuels J, et al: Adverse effects of combined spinal-epidural versus traditional epidural analgesia during labor. Int J. Gynecol Obstet 2009;106:242–245.

192. Rawal N, Schollin J, Wesstrom G: Epidural versus combined spinal epidural block for cesarean section. Acta Anaesthesiol Scand 1988;32: 61–66.

193. Joshi GP, MaCarroll SM: Combined spinal–epidural anesthesia using needle-through-needle technique [Letter]. Anesthesiology 1993;78: 406–407.

194. Pan PH: Laboratory evaluation of single-lumen, dual-orifice combined spinal-epidural needles: Effects of bevel orientation and modified technique. J Clin Anesth 1998;10(4):286–290.

195. Riley ET, Hamilton CL, Ratner EF, Cohen S: A comparison of the 24-gauge Sprotte and Gertie Marx spinal needles for combined spinal-epidural analgesia during labor. Anesthesiology 2002;97:574–577.

196. Herbstman CH, Jaffe JB, Tuman KJ, et al: An in vivo evaluation of four spinal needles used for the combined spinal-epidural technique. Anesth Analg 1998;86(3):520–522.

197. Simsa J: Needle fixation with combined spinalepidural anaesthesia. Acta Anaesth Scand 1995;55:275.

198. Stocks GM, Hallworth SP, Fernando R: Evaluation of a spinal needle locking device for use with the combined spinal epidural technique. Anaesthesia 2000;55(12):1185–1188.

199. Eldor J, Chaimsky G: The Eldor combined-spinal epidural needle. Anesthesia 1993;48:173.

200. Torrieri A, Aldrete JA: Combined spinal-epidural needle. Acts Anaesth Belg 1998;39:65–66.

201. Birnbach DJ, Chestnut DH: The epidural test dose in obstetric practice: Has it outlived its usefulness? Anesth Analg 1999;88:971.

202. Steffek M, Owczuk R, Szlyk-Augustyn M, Lasinska-Kowara M, Wujtewicz M: Total spinal anaesthesia as a complication of local anaesthetic test-dose administration through an epidural catheter. Acta Anaesthesiol Scand 2004;48(9):1211–1213.

203. Norris MC, Ferrenbach D, Dalman H, et al: Does epinephrine improve the diagnostic accuracy of aspiration during labor epidural analgesia? Anesth Analg 1999;88;1073.

204. Moore DC, Batra MS: The components of an effective test dose prior to epidural block. Anesthesiology 1981;55:693.

205. Hood DD, Dewan DM, James FM III: Maternal and fetal effect of epinephrine in gravid ewes. Anesthesiology 1986;64:610.

206. Leighton BL, Norris MC, DeSimone CA, et al: The air test as a clinically useful indicator of intravenously placed epidural catheters. Anesthesiology 1990;73:610.

207. Kopacz DJ: Spinal 2-chloroprocaine: Minimum effective dose. Reg Anesth Pain Med 2005;30(1):36–42.

208. Hamza J, Smida M, Benhamou D, Cohen SE: Parturient's poture during epidural puncture affects the distance from skin to epidural space. J Clin Anesth 1995;7:1–4.

209. Yun EM, Marx GF, Santos AC: The effects of maternal position during induction of combined spinal-epidural anesthesia for caesarean delivery. Anesth Analg 1998;87:614–618.

210. Lewis NL, Ritchie EL, Downer JP, Nel MR: Left lateral vs. supine, wedged position for development of block after combined spinal-epidural anaesthesia for caesarean section. Anaesthesia 2004;59: 894–898.

CHAPTER 27

Postdural Puncture Headache

Brian E. Harrington and Miguel Angel Reina

INTRODUCTION

Postural headaches following interventions that disrupt meningeal integrity are most commonly labeled *postdural puncture headaches* (PDPHs). This terminology has been officially adopted in the International Classification of Headache Disorders[1] and is used in this chapter. However, use of the word *postdural* has been criticized as confusing[2] and probably inaccurate,[3] resulting in the proposal of an alternate term, *meningeal puncture headache* (MPH), which readers may increasingly encounter.[4,5] It is also important to acknowledge that references to "dural puncture" throughout the medical literature (including this chapter) actually describe puncture of the dura-arachnoid and are more correctly termed and thought of as "meningeal puncture."

Regardless of terminology, the PDPH is well known to the many clinicians whose practice includes procedures that access the subarachnoid space. Yet, our understanding of this serious complication remains surprisingly incomplete. This chapter summarizes the current state of knowledge regarding this familiar iatrogenic problem as well as the closely related topics of accidental, or unintentional, dural puncture (ADP or UDP, respectively), and the epidural blood patch (EBP).

HISTORY AND CURRENT RELEVANCE

As one of the earliest recognized complications of regional anesthesia, PDPH has a long and colorful history.[6] Dr. August Bier noted this adverse effect in the first patient to undergo successful spinal anesthesia on August 16, 1898 (Figure 27–1).

Bier observed: "Two hours after the operation his back and left leg became painful and the patient vomited and complained of severe headache. The pain and vomiting soon ceased, but *headache was still present the next day*" (italics added).[7] The following week, Bier and his assistant, Dr. August Hildebrandt, performed experiments with cocainization of the spinal cord on themselves. In a description of PDPH scarcely improved on in an intervening century, Bier later reported firsthand his experience in the days to follow: "I had a feeling of very strong pressure on my skull and became rather dizzy when I stood up rapidly from my chair. All these symptoms vanished at once when I lay down flat, but returned when I stood up. ... I was forced to take to bed and remained there for nine days, because all the manifestations recurred as soon as I got up. ... The symptoms finally resolved nine days after the lumbar puncture."[7] In medical history, few complications have come to be associated as closely to a specific technique as PDPH with spinal anesthesia.

Employing the methods of the early 20th century, spinal anesthesia was frequently followed by severe and prolonged headache, casting a long shadow over the development and acceptance of this modality. Investigations into the cause of these troubling symptoms eventually led to the conclusion that they were due to persistent cerebrospinal fluid (CSF) loss through the rent created in the meninges. The most notable successful efforts to minimize the loss of CSF were through the use of smaller-gauge and "noncutting" needles (as convincingly demonstrated in the 1950s by Vandam and Dripps[8] and Hart and Whitacre,[9] respectively). Despite these significant advances in prevention, PDPH remained a frustratingly common occurrence.

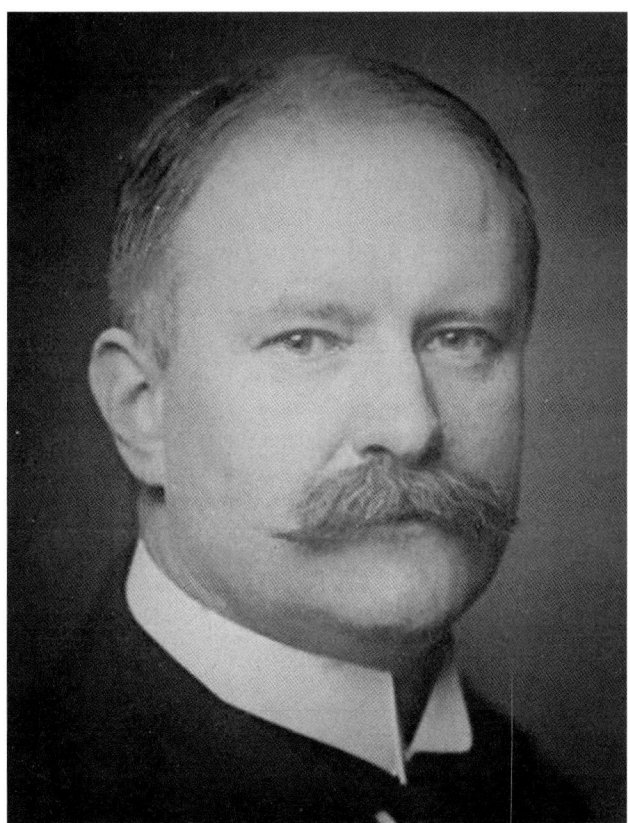

FIGURE 27–1. Dr. August Bier.

The extensive search for effective treatments for PDPH dates to Bier's time. Yet, efforts through the first half of the 20th century, while often intensive and creative, were questionably worthwhile. In a monograph intended to be a comprehensive review of PDPH from the 1890s through 1960, Dr. Wallace Tourette and colleagues cited dozens of separate and far-ranging treatment recommendations, including such interventions as intravenous ethanol, x-rays to the skull, sympathetic blocks, and manipulation of the spine.[10] Unfortunately, prior to the introduction of the EBP there were no treatment measures that could be described as significant improvements over the simple passage of time. In his 1955 textbook, *Complications of Regional Anesthesia*, Dr. Daniel C. Moore described in detail a full 3-day treatment protocol for PDPH. He concluded by noting that 3 days was the usual duration of untreated mild-to-moderate headaches, but that, "Nevertheless, the patient feels an attempt to help his problem is being made."[11]

The EBP, a startlingly unique medical procedure, proved to be the major breakthrough in the treatment of PDPH. The concept of using autologous blood to "patch" a hole in the meninges was introduced in late 1960 by Dr. James Gormley, a general surgeon.[12] Yet, Gormley's brief report went largely unnoticed for nearly a decade because, to the practitioners of the day, an iatrogenic epidural hematoma raised serious concerns of scarring, infection, and nerve damage. The procedure was only later popularized in anesthesiology circles, and performed as a true epidural injection, largely through the work of Drs. Anthony DiGiovanni and Burdett Dunbar.[13] The EBP procedure was further refined through the 1970s as the volume

of blood commonly utilized increased to 20 mL.[14] Today, the EBP is nearly universally employed as the cornerstone for treatment for severe PDPH.[15]

Postdural puncture headache remains a prominent clinical concern to the present day. Largely due to modifications in practice that followed the identification of risk factors, rates of PDPH following spinal anesthesia have steadily declined, from an incidence exceeding 50% in Bier's time, to around 10% in the 1950s,[8] until currently a rate of 1% or less can be reasonably expected. However, as perhaps the highest-risk group, an unfortunate 1.7% of obstetric patients continue to experience PDPH after spinal anesthesia using 27-gauge Whitacre needles.[16] Intending to avoid meningeal puncture, epidural techniques are an attractive alternative to spinal anesthesia. Yet, occasional ADP, with either the needle or the catheter, is unavoidable (and may be unrecognized at the time in over 25% of patients who eventually develop PDPH[17]). In nonobstetric situations (eg, interlaminar epidural steroid injections), the rate of ADP should be less than 0.5%. However, ADP is of greatest concern in the obstetric anesthesia setting, where the incidence of this adverse event is around 1.5%.[16] Over half of all patients who experience ADP with epidural needles will eventually develop headache symptoms, with many studies in obstetric populations reporting PDPH rates of 75% or greater. Of further concern, ADP in parturients has also been noted to be associated with chronic headache and back pain that is reduced, but not entirely eliminated, by EBP.[18] In addition to anesthesia interventions, PDPH remains a too-common iatrogenic complication following myelography and diagnostic/therapeutic lumbar puncture (LP). In these situations, rates of MPH of around 10% are still commonly cited as practitioners often continue to use large-gauge Quincke needles—considered necessary due to the viscosity of contrast material and to facilitate the timely collection of CSF.[19] Consequently, there is evidence to suggest that the majority of instances of PDPH now have a non-anesthesia-related origin.[20]

Clinical Pearls

- PDPH may carry a risk of medicolegal liability.
- ADP may result in chronic headache and back pain.
- Anesthetic procedures with risk of PDPH require proper informed consent.

The practical significance of PDPH is illustrated by notation in the American Society of Anesthesiologists Closed Claims Project database as one of the most frequent claims for malpractice involving obstetric anesthesia,[21] regional anesthesia,[22] and chronic pain management.[23] Justifiably, headache is the most commonly disclosed risk when obtaining consent for spinal and epidural anesthesia.[24] The potentially serious nature of this complication necessitates inclusion in informed consent involving any procedure that may result in PDPH. As part of this discussion, patients should also be apprised of the normal delayed onset of symptoms and be given clear instructions for the timely provision of advice or management should they experience adverse effects.

PATHOPHYSIOLOGY

It has long been accepted that PDPH results from a disruption of normal CSF homeostasis. However, despite a great deal of research and observational data, the pathophysiology of PDPH remains incompletely understood.[25] Cerebrospinal fluid is produced primarily in the choroid plexus at a rate of approximately 0.35 mL/min and reabsorbed through the arachnoid villa. The total CSF volume in adults is maintained around 150 mL, of which approximately half is extracranial, and gives rise to normal lumbar opening pressures of 5–15 cm H_2O in the horizontal position (40–50 cm H_2O in the upright position). It has been shown experimentally that the loss of approximately 10% of total CSF volume predictably results in the development of typical PDPH symptoms, which resolve promptly with reconstitution of this deficit.[26] It is generally agreed that PDPH is due to the loss of CSF through a persistent leak in the meninges. In this regard, it has been postulated that the cellular arachnoid mater (containing frequent tight junctions and occluding junctions) is perhaps more important than the more permeable and acellular dura mater in the generation of symptoms.[3] In fresh cadavers, Reina et al studied lesions of the human dural sac produced by different spinal needles and different bevel orientations. The dura mater has a thickness around 400 μm, and it is formed by randomly distributed fibers, arranged around 80 concentric layers, known as dural laminas, while the arachnoid layer has a thickness around 40 μm[1-9] (Figure 27–2).

Recently, these authors reported on the possible importance of the arachnoid layer in the closure of dural and arachnoid

A. Dura mater

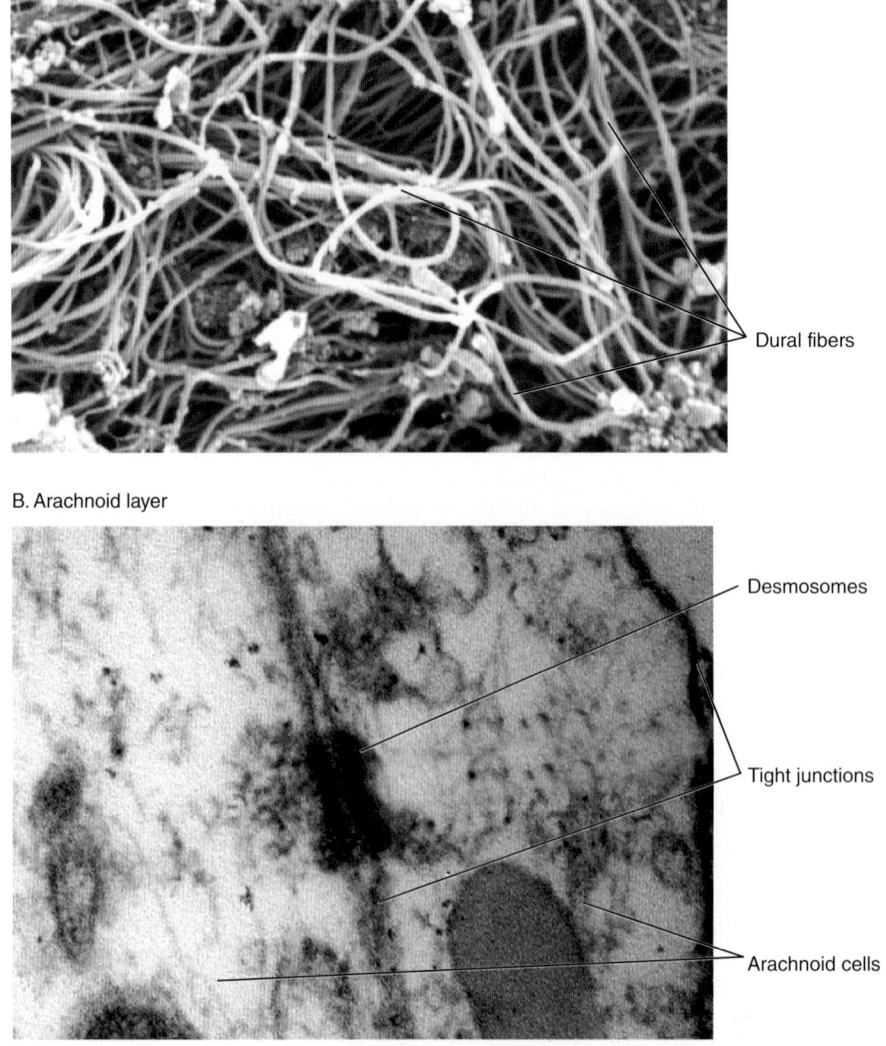

B. Arachnoid layer

FIGURE 27-2. A: Human spinal dura mater. Collagen fibers in random direction. Scanning electron microscopy. Magnification x6500. Reproduced with permission from Dittmann M, Reina MA, López García A: New results in the visualization of the spinal dura mater with scanning electron microscopy. *Anaesthesist.* 1998 May;47(5):409-413. **B:** Human spinal arachnoid layer. Arachnoid cells. Transmission electron microscopy. Magnification x150000. Reproduced with permission from Reina MA1, Prats-Galino A, Sola RG, et al: Structure of the arachnoid layer of the human spinal meninges: a barrier that regulates dural sac permeability. *Rev Esp Anestesiol Reanim.* 2010 Oct;57(8):486–492.

lesions.[1,2] The arachnoid membrane may exhibit tissue closure in relation to the dura because its main function is to act as a barrier; therefore, it may lack the elastic properties of the dural layer. The arachnoid layer limits the escape of fluid, so the amount of CSF lost through the punctured orifice is likely related to the speed of closure of the arachnoid lesion (Figures 27–3 to 27–6).

Thus, the anatomically supported term *meningeal puncture headache* (MPH) has been proposed as an alternative to the rather ambiguous *postdural puncture headache* (PDPH). The apparent role of the arachnoid mater in this disorder further calls into question the significance of many published studies that involve isolated dura mater in vitro.

The actual means by which CSF hypotension generates headache is somewhat controversial and currently ascribed to a bimodal mechanism involving both loss of intracranial support and cerebral vasodilation (predominantly venous). Diminished buoyant support is thought to allow the brain to sag in the upright position, resulting in traction and pressure on pain-sensitive structures within the cranium (dura, cranial nerves,

bridging veins, and venous sinuses). Adenosine-mediated vasodilation may occur secondary to diminished intracranial CSF (in accordance with the Monro-Kellie hypothesis, which states that intracranial volume must remain constant) and reflexively secondary to traction on intracranial vessels.

Multiple neural pathways are involved in generating the symptoms of PDPH. These include the ophthalmic branch of the trigeminal nerve (cranial nerve [CN] V_1) in frontal head pain, cranial nerves IX and X in occipital pain, and cervical nerves C1–C3 in neck and shoulder pain.[27] Nausea is attributed to vagal stimulation (CN X). Auditory and vestibular symptoms are secondary to the direct communication between the CSF and the perilymph via the cochlear aqueduct, which results in decreased perilymphatic pressures in the inner ear and an imbalance between the endolymph and perilymph.[28,29] Significant visual disturbances are thought to represent a transient palsy of the nerves supplying the extraocular muscles of the eye (CN III, IV, and VI). Here, the lateral rectus muscle is most often involved, which is attributed to the long, vulnerable intracranial course of the abducens nerve (CN VI).[30,31] Other, much

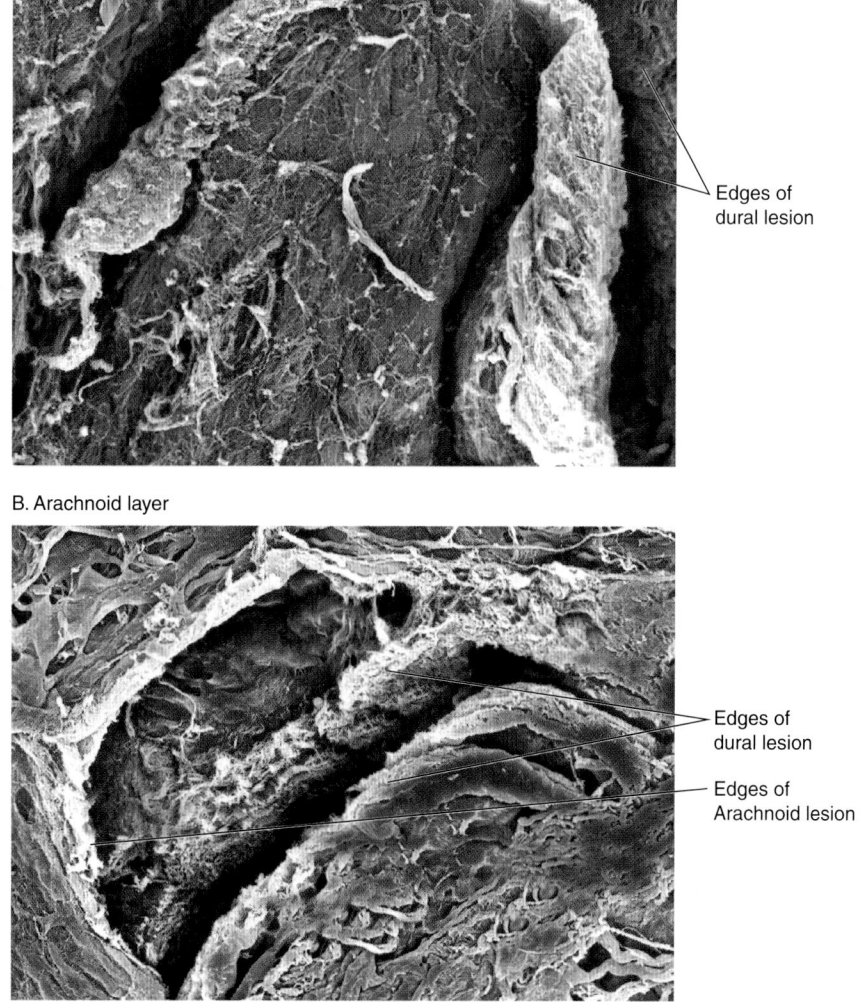

FIGURE 27–3. Human dura mater. Dura-arachnoid lesion produced by 25-gauge Quincke needle. Scanning electron microscopy. Magnification ×200. **A:** Dural surface. **B:** Arachnoid surface.

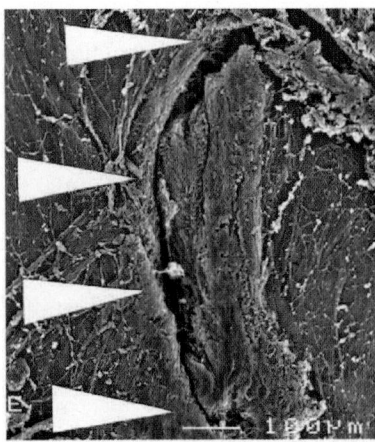
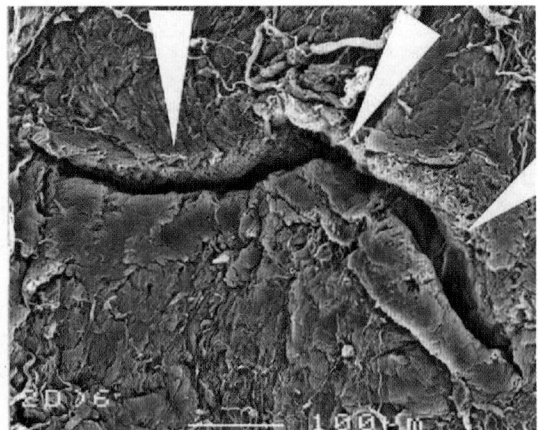

A. Dura mater

B. Dura mater

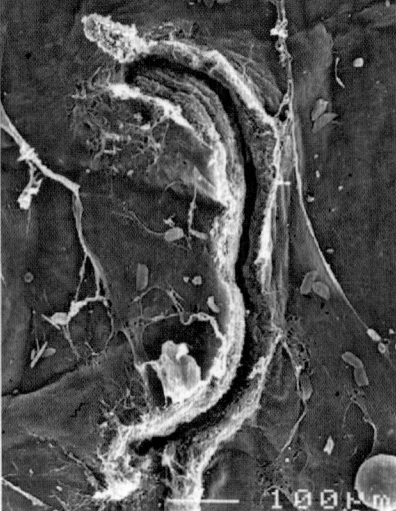
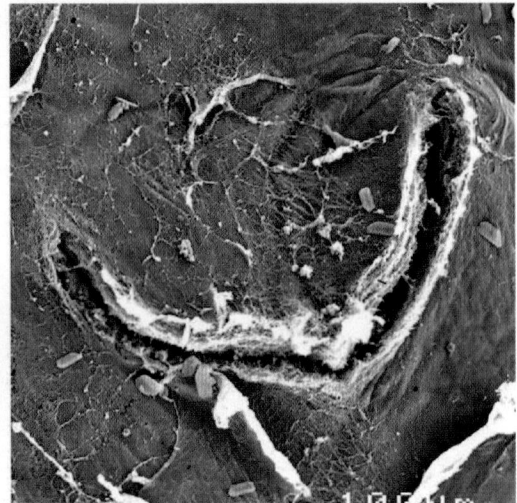

C. Arachnoid layer

D. Arachnoid layer

FIGURE 27–4. Human dura-arachnoid lesion produced by 22-gauge Quincke needle. Scanning electron microscopy. Magnification ×100. **A and B:** Dural surface. **C and D:** Arachnoid surface. (Reproduced with permission from Reina MA, López A, Badorrey V, et al: Dura-arachnoid lesions produced by 22 gauge Quincke spinal needles during a lumbar puncture. *J Neurol Neurosurg Psychiatry.* 2004 Jun;75(6):893–897.)

less-frequent cranial nerve palsies of the trigeminal (CN V), facial (CN VII), and auditory (CN VIII) nerves have also been reported.[32]

CLINICAL PRESENTATION AND CHARACTERISTICS

Although many clinical variations have been described, most cases of PDPH are characterized by their typical onset, presentation, and associated symptoms.

> ### Clinical Pearls
>
> Most cases of PDPH will be typical (see text for details) in
>
> - Onset—often delayed, but within 48 hours
> - Presentation—symmetric, bilateral headache
> - Associated symptoms—more likely with severe headache

Onset

Onset of symptoms is generally delayed, with headache usually beginning 12–48 hours and rarely more than 5 days following meningeal puncture. In their landmark observational study, Vandam and Dripps reported onset of headache symptoms within 3 days of spinal anesthesia in 84.8% of patients for whom such data were available.[8] More recently, Lybecker and colleagues performed a detailed analysis of 75 consecutive patients with PDPH following spinal anesthesia (primarily using 25-gauge cutting-point needles). While none of their patients noted the onset of symptoms during the first hour following meningeal puncture, 65% experienced symptoms within 24 hours and 92% within 48 hours.[33] An onset of symptoms within 1 hour of neuraxial procedures is suspicious for pneumocephalus, especially in the setting of an epidural loss-of-resistance technique using air.[34] Occasional reports of unusually delayed onset of PDPH highlight the importance of seeking a history of central neuraxial instrumentation whenever positional headaches are evaluated.[35]

A. Dura mater

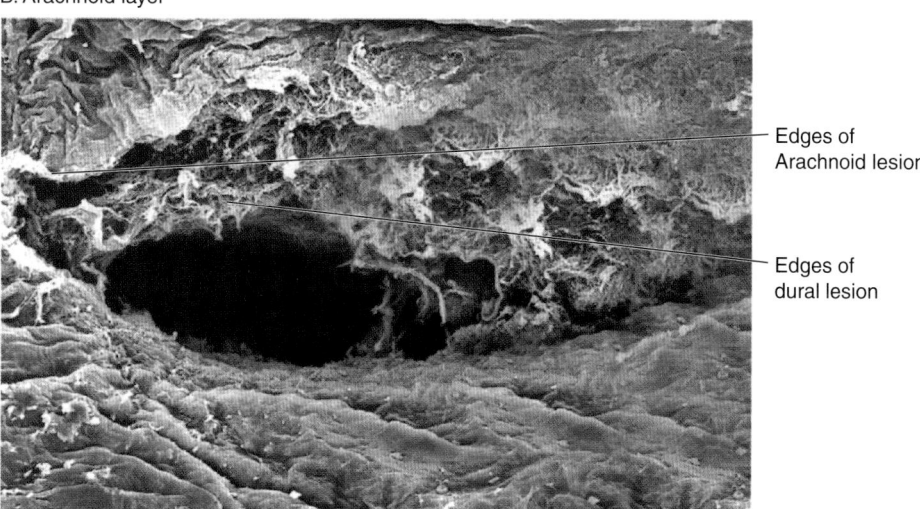

Edges of
dural lesion

B. Arachnoid layer

Edges of
Arachnoid lesion

Edges of
dural lesion

FIGURE 27–5. Human dura-arachnoid lesion produced by 25-gauge Whitacre needle. Scanning electron microscopy. Magnification ×200.
A: Dural surface. **B:** Arachnoid surface. (Reproduced with permission from Reina MA, López-García A, de Andrés-Ibáñez JA, et al: Electron microscopy of the lesions produced in the human dura mater by Quincke beveled and Whitacre needles. *Rev Esp Anestesiol Reanim.* 1997 Feb; 44(2):56–61)

Presentation

The cardinal feature of PDPH is its postural nature, with headache symptoms worsening in the upright position and relieved, or at least improved, with recumbency. The International Headache Society (IHS) diagnostic criteria further describe this positional quality as worsening within 15 minutes of sitting or standing and improving within 15 minutes after lying.[1] Headache is always bilateral, with a distribution that is frontal (25%), occipital (27%), or both (45%).[33] Headaches are typically described as "dull/aching," "throbbing," or "pressure type."

The severity of headache symptoms, a feature with important ramifications for treatment, varies considerably among patients. Although there is no universally accepted severity scale, one practical approach is to have patients simply rate their headache intensity using a 10-point analog scale, with 1–3 classified as "mild," 4–6 "moderate," and 7–10 "severe."

Lybecker et al further categorized patients according to restriction in physical activity, degree of confinement to bed, and presence of associated symptoms.[33] Using this classification system, they prospectively determined that 11% of their PDPH cases after spinal anesthesia were mild, 23% moderate, and 67% severe.

Associated Symptoms

The IHS criteria for PDPH require that headache be accompanied by at least one of the following symptoms: neck stiffness, tinnitus, hypoacusia, photophobia, and nausea. However, these criteria may need to be revisited as many patients (29% in one recent study)[36] have been noted to suffer from PDPH in the absence of any symptoms apart from the headache itself. It can be said that the more severe the headache, the more likely it is to be accompanied by associated symptoms.

A. Dura mater

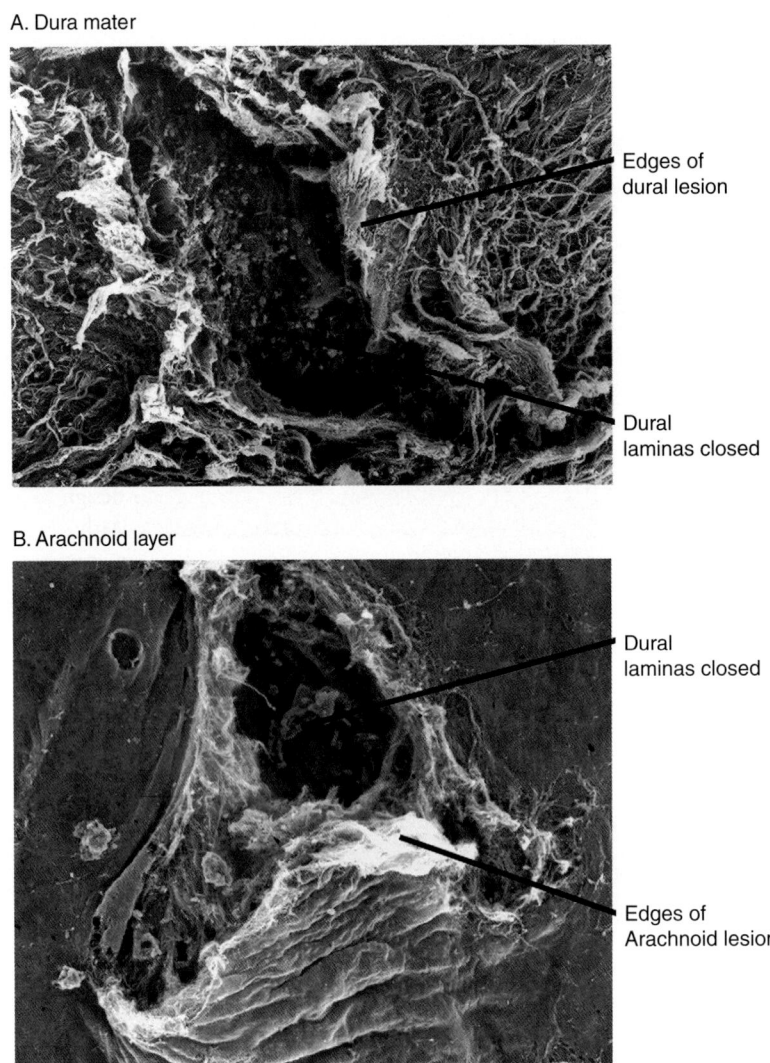

Edges of
dural lesion

Dural
laminas closed

B. Arachnoid layer

Dural
laminas closed

Edges of
Arachnoid lesion

FIGURE 27–6. Human spinal dura mater. Dura-arachnoid lesion produced by 25-gauge Whitacre needle. Scanning electron microscopy. Magnification ×200. **A:** Dural surface. **B:** Arachnoid surface. (Reproduced with permission from Reina MA, de Leon-Casasola OA, Lopez A, et al: An in vitro study of dural lesions produced by 25-gauge Quincke and Whitacre needles evaluated by scanning electron microscopy. *Reg Anesth Pain Med.* 2000 Jul-Aug;25(4):393–402.)

Clinical Pearl

The IHS criteria for PDPH are as follows:
- Headache accompanied by at least one of these symptoms:
  - neck stiffness
  - tinnitus
  - hypoacusia
  - photophobia
  - nausea

The most common associated symptom is nausea, which may be reported by a majority of patients (especially if questioned specifically) and can lead to vomiting.[33] Pain and stiffness in the neck and shoulders are also common and are seen in nearly half of all patients experiencing PDPH.[37] Uncommonly, patients may experience auditory or visual symptoms, and the risk for either appears to be directly related to needle size.[30,38]

In Vandam and Dripps's large observational study of PDPH, auditory and visual symptoms were each seen in 0.4% of patients.[8] Auditory symptoms include hearing loss, tinnitus, and even hyperacusis, and can be unilateral. It is interesting to note that subclinical hearing loss, especially in the lower frequencies, has been found to be common following spinal anesthesia, even in the absence of PDPH.[38] Closely associated with auditory function, vestibular disturbances (dizziness or vertigo) may also occur. Visual problems include blurred vision, difficulties with accommodation, mild photophobia, and diplopia.[30] In contrast to headache complaints, which are consistently bilateral, nearly 80% of episodes of diplopia secondary to meningeal puncture involve unilateral cranial nerve palsies.

RISK FACTORS

Risk factors for PDPH can be broadly categorized into patient characteristics and procedural details.

Patient Characteristics

The patient characteristic having the greatest impact on risk of PDPH is age. Uncommonly reported in children less than 10 years of age, PDPH has a peak incidence in the teens and early 20s.[39] The incidence then declines over time, becoming much less frequent in patients over 50 years of age.

Gender is also a significant risk factor, with nonpregnant females having approximately twice the risk for PDPH when compared with age-matched male subjects.[40] While the etiology behind this gender difference has not been convincingly elucidated, a number of physiological, anatomical, social, perceptual, and behavioral explanations have been proposed.[36]

Clinical Pearl

Major patient related risk factors for PDPH include:
- Age: It is uncommon in patients less than 10 years of age; peak incidence is in the teens and early 20s.
- Gender: Nonpregnant females have twice the risk compared to age-matched men.

Pregnancy has traditionally been regarded as a risk factor for PDPH,[8] but this consideration largely reflects a young female cohort as well as the high incidence of ADP in the gravid population. Although controversial, pushing during the second stage of labor, thought to promote the loss of CSF through a hole in the meninges, has been reported to influence the risk of PDPH following ADP. Angle and colleagues noted that the cumulative duration of bearing down correlated with the risk of developing PDPH in patients who had experienced ADP.[41] They also found that patients who avoided pushing altogether (proceeded to cesarean delivery prior to reaching second-stage labor) had a much lower incidence of PDPH (10%) than those who pushed (74%). Furthermore, they noted a marked difference in the requirement for EBP to treat PDPH between those who pushed and those who did not (81% vs. 0%).

Body mass index (BMI) appears to be a mixed-risk factor. Morbid obesity presents obvious technical difficulties for central neuraxial procedures, increasing the likelihood of multiple needle passes and ADP.[42] Yet, low BMI has been reported to be an independent risk factor for PDPH,[43] and high BMI (ie, obesity) may actually decrease risk, possibly secondary to a beneficial effect of increased intra-abdominal pressure.[44]

Recently, a retrospective analysis reported cigarette smoking to be associated with a lower risk of PDPH.[45] It can be hoped that this observation will promote further insights into the mechanism of PDPH symptoms and pharmacologic treatment options.

Postdural puncture headaches appear to have an interesting association with other headaches. Patients who report having had a headache within the week prior to LP have been observed to have a higher incidence of PDPH.[43] On further analysis, only those with chronic bilateral tension-type headaches were found to be at increased risk.[46] A history of unilateral headache[46] or migraine[47] has not been linked to an increased risk of PDPH. Menstrual cycle, a factor in migraine headaches,

did not influence the rate of PDPH in one small pilot study.[48] Patients with a history of previous PDPH, particularly women, appear to have an increased risk for new PDPH after spinal anesthesia.[36] With epidural procedures, patients with a history of ADP have been shown to be at slightly increased risk for another ADP (and subsequent PDPH).[49]

Procedural Details

Needle size and tip design are the most important procedural factors related to PDPH.[50] Needle size is directly related to the risk of PDPH. Meningeal puncture with larger needles is associated with a higher incidence of PDPH,[8] more severe headaches, more associated symptoms,[50] a longer duration of symptoms,[51] and a greater need for definitive treatment measures.[52] Needle tip design is also a major influence, with "noncutting" needles clearly associated with a reduced incidence of PDPH when compared with "cutting" (usually Quincke) needles of the same gauge (Figure 27–7). In general, noncutting needles have an opening set back from a tapered ("pencil-point") tip and include the Whitacre, Sprotte, European, Pencan, and Gertie Marx needles. Adding to this somewhat-confusing terminology, noncutting needles are sometimes still incorrectly referred to as "atraumatic" needles, this despite being shown with electron microscopy to produce a more traumatic rent in the dura than cutting needles (perhaps resulting in a better inflammatory healing response).[53] The influence of needle size on risk of PDPH appears to be greatest for cutting needles (in other words, the reduction seen in the incidence of PDPH between 22- and 26-gauge sizes is greater for cutting than noncutting needles). Insertion of cutting needles with the bevel parallel to the long axis of the spine significantly reduces the incidence of PDPH.[54] This observation was for many years attributed to spreading rather than cutting of longitudinally oriented dural fibers. However, scanning electron microscopy revealed the dura to be made of many layers of concentrically

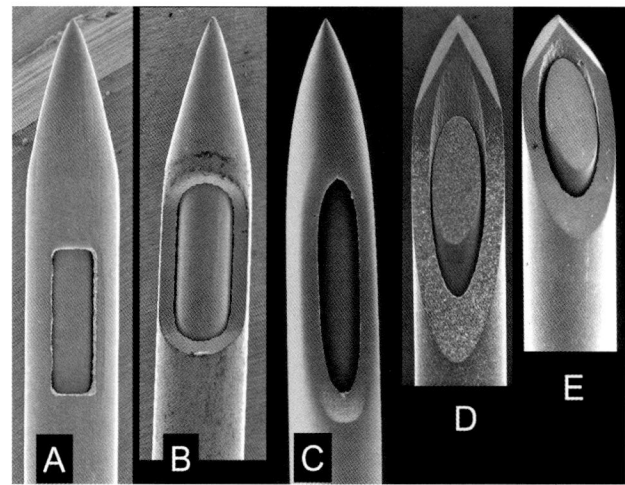

FIGURE 27–7. Spinal needles of different manufacturers with same external diameter. **A:** Whitacre type. **B:** Spinal type. **C:** Sprotte type. **D, E:** Quincke type. Scanning electron microscopy. Magnification ×40. (Reproduced with permission from Reina MA: *Atlas of Functional Anatomy for Regional Anesthesia and Pain Medicine.* Heidelberg: Springer; 2015.)

directed fibers,[55] and the importance of needle bevel insertion is now thought to be due to longitudinal tension on the meninges, particularly in the upright position, and its influence on CSF leakage through holes having differing orientations.

Clinical Pearl

- The most important equipment-related details for risk of PDPH are needle gauge (larger > smaller) and needle tip design (cutting > noncutting).

Not surprisingly, the experience/comfort/skill of the operator appear to be significant factors in the development of PDPH. A larger number of meningeal punctures, frequently associated with inexperience, have been shown to increase the rate of PDPH.[56] De Almeida et al noted higher rates of PDPH when LP was performed by inexperienced providers.[57] Higher rates of ADP have been consistently reported when epidural procedures are performed by residents.[58,59] The risk of ADP also appears to be higher for procedures done at night, strongly suggesting a significant contribution of operator fatigue.[60]

A number of procedural details do not appear to influence the rate of development of PDPH, including patient position at the time of meningeal puncture, "bloody tap" during spinal anesthesia, addition of opiates to the spinal block, and volume of CSF removed (for diagnostic purposes).[6]

PREVENTION

Although prophylaxis is most simply thought of as preventing any symptoms of PDPH, in the clinical context this issue is deceptively complex. It is important to appreciate that significant "prevention" may encompass a number of other endpoints, such as a reduced incidence of severe PDPH, a shorter duration of symptoms, or decreased need for EBP. Unfortunately, despite the clear relevance of this issue, the overall quality of evidence for preventive measures is generally weak.[61–63]

General Measures

As with all regional techniques, appropriate patient selection is crucial in minimizing complications. As age is a major risk factor, indications for spinal anesthesia should be weighed against the risks of PDPH in patients under 40 years of age unless the benefits are sufficiently compelling (such as in the obstetric population). Practitioners (and patients alike) may also wish to carefully consider central neuraxial techniques in those with a previous history of ADP or PDPH (particularly females). Other patient-related factors (eg, obesity) should be considered on a case-by-case basis, weighing the risks of PDPH with the benefits of regional anesthesia.

While only recently utilized for neuraxial techniques, the use of ultrasound for regional anesthesia holds some promise in reducing the risk of PDPH. Ultrasound can decrease the number of needle passes required for regional procedures and has been shown to accurately predict the depth of the epidural

space.[64] Further study is ongoing to define this potential for ultrasound to reduce the incidence of ADP and PDPH.

While multiple pharmacologic agents have been tried and investigated for prevention of PDPH, the efficacy of various strategies remains unclear. As an example, intravenous dexamethasone has recently been shown in randomized controlled trials (RCTs) to decrease,[65] but not influence,[66] and even increase the risk of PDPH.[67]

A recent review of drug therapy for preventing PDPH identified only 10 RCTs for review.[68] The primary outcome, a reduction in the number of patients affected by PDPH of any severity, was affected by administration of intrathecal morphine sulfate or fentanyl, oral caffeine, rectal indomethacin, or intravenous dexamethasone. Although a reduction in the incidence of PDPH was seen with epidurally administered morphine (relative risk [RR] 0.25),[69] intravenous cosyntropin (RR 0.49),[70] and intravenous aminophylline (RR 0.21 at 48 hours),[71] the benefit of each was only demonstrated in a single study.

Regardless, despite the paucity of evidence, pharmacologic measures—particularly caffeine—continue to be widely used in hopes of decreasing the incidence or severity of PDPH following meningeal puncture.[15] However, no pharmacologic prophylaxis for PDPH has been independently confirmed, and various regimens used have been associated with adverse events.

A recent survey of US anesthesiologists reported that bed rest and aggressive oral and intravenous hydration continue to be suggested by a sizable majority as prophylactic measures against PDPH.[15] However, a systematic review of the literature regarding bed rest versus early mobilization after dural puncture failed to show any evidence of benefit from bed rest and suggested that the risk of PDPH may actually be decreased by early mobilization.[72] It is notable that the practice of US anesthesiologists regarding bed rest is in contrast to that in UK maternity units, where a survey indicated that 75% of UK consultants encourage mobilization as early as possible following ADP as prophylaxis against PDPH.[73] Likewise, in a randomized prospective trial, increased oral hydration following LP failed to decrease the incidence or duration of PDPH.[74] In summary, at this time there is no evidence to support the common practice of recommending bed rest and aggressive hydration in the prevention of PDPH.

Clinical Pearl

- There is no evidence to support the common practice of recommending bed rest and aggressive hydration in the prevention of PDPH.

Spinal Technique

Needle selection is critical for reducing the incidence of PDPH. Given the strong association between needle gauge and PDPH, spinal procedures should be performed with needles having the smallest gauge reasonably possible. However, it should be acknowledged that needles of extremely small gauge can be more difficult to place, have a slow return of CSF, may be associated with multiple unrecognized punctures of the dura, and can result in a higher rate of failed block. Attention to needle tip design is another important technical means of reducing the risk of PDPH with spinal anesthesia. If available, noncutting needles should routinely be employed as they appear to be associated with fewer adverse events at a lower overall cost.[75] These factors generally make a 24- to 27-gauge noncutting needle the ideal choice for spinal anesthesia. If cutting-tip needles are used, the bevel should be directed parallel to the long axis of the spine (Figure 27–7).

Replacing the stylet after CSF collection but prior to needle withdrawal has been shown to be an effective means of lowering the incidence of PDPH after LP. In a prospective, randomized study of 600 patients with procedures using 21-gauge Sprotte needles, replacing the stylet reduced the incidence of PDPH from 16.3% to 5.0% ($p < .005$).[76] This safe-and-simple maneuver is theorized to decrease the possibility of a wicking strand of arachnoid mater from extending across the dura. However, in a more recent study of 630 patients having spinal anesthesia using 25-gauge Quincke needles, replacing the stylet did not affect the incidence of PDPH.[77] The disparity in these results may be related to the needle gauges used as well as fundamental differences between the techniques of lumbar puncture (drainage of CSF) and spinal anesthesia (injection of anesthetic agent).

Continuous spinal anesthesia (CSA) has been reported by some to be associated with surprisingly low incidences of PDPH compared with single-dose spinal techniques using similar-gauge needles.[78] This observation has been attributed to reaction to the catheter, which may promote better sealing of a breach in the meninges. CSA with small-gauge needles and catheters ("microcatheters") is an appealing option when titration of spinal drug is desirable and duration of surgery is uncertain, but microcatheters are currently unavailable in the United States, where the risk of PDPH with CSA remains concerning when using about 20-gauge "macrocatheters." For this reason, although the technique may have clinical advantages, deliberate CSA has been investigated almost exclusively in low-risk populations.

As mentioned, aminophylline has been demonstrated in one RCT to reduce the incidence of PDPH.[71] Patients undergoing cesarean delivery under spinal anesthesia were randomized to receive intravenous aminophylline (1 mg/kg) or placebo after cord clamping. At 48 hours after surgery, 3 of 60 patients (5%) receiving aminophylline versus 14 of 60 patients (23.3%) in the control group experienced PDPH. No patients in either group required EBP.

Epidural Technique

Although epidural options are limited, especially with catheter techniques, the risk of PDPH following ADP can be reduced by using the smallest feasible epidural needles. Simply decreasing the size of epidural needles from 16 to 18 gauge has been reported to reduce the incidence of PDPH from 88% to 64%.[79]

The issue of air versus liquid for identification of the epidural space with the loss-of-resistance technique has long been a source of controversy. Each method has acknowledged advantages and disadvantages, but neither has been shown convincingly to result in a lower risk of ADP.[80] In this case, operator preference and experience would be expected to strongly influence performance, and the overriding significance of this factor is illustrated in fewer instances of ADP noted when the medium is chosen at the anesthesiologist's discretion.[81]

Bevel orientation for epidural needle insertion remains a matter of debate. Norris et al found the incidence of moderate-to-severe PDPH after ADP was only 24% when the needle bevel was oriented parallel to the long axis of the spine (compared to 70% with perpendicular insertion).[82] This resulted in fewer therapeutic EBPs administered to patients in the parallel group ($p < .05$). However, this technique necessitates a controversial 90° rotation of the needle for catheter placement.[83] It appears that a number of concerns regarding parallel needle insertion (lateral needle deviation, difficulties with catheter insertion, and dural trauma with needle rotation) are of greater concern to practitioners. Most respondents (71.3%) to a survey of US anesthesiologists preferred to insert epidural needles with the bevel perpendicular to the long axis of the spine (consistent with the intended direction of catheter travel).[15]

Combined spinal-epidural (CSE) techniques have been reported to be associated with a low incidence of PDPH. While providing the advantages of a spinal anesthetic, CSE appears to have no increased incidence of PDPH or need for EBP when compared to conventional epidural analgesia.[84] This observation may be due to several factors, including the ability to successfully use extremely small (eg, 27-gauge) noncutting spinal needles and tamponade provided by epidural infusions.

Measures to Reduce the Risk of PDPH After ADP

The risk-to-benefit ratio of prophylaxis should be most favorable in situations having the greatest likelihood of developing severe PDPH. Therefore, most efforts to reduce the risk of PDPH after ADP have been in the obstetric patient population. Several prophylactic measures, discussed in the material that follows, are worthy of consideration and have been utilized alone or in combination.[85] However, because not all patients who experience ADP will develop PDPH, and only a portion of those who do will require definitive treatment with an EBP, a cautious approach in this regard is still generally warranted. It should be acknowledged that the efficacy of all the measures discussed next is debatable. Therefore, it is critical that in the event of recognized ADP, these patients at the very least be clearly informed of the high risk of PDPH development and be followed daily until discharge (or called at home if discharged within 48 hours).

Stylet Replacement

Although there have not been any studies to support the use of the stylet replacement technique in the setting of ADP, replacing the stylet is a simple and effective means of lowering the incidence of PDPH after LP.[76] Given the innocuous nature of this maneuver, if no other prophylactic measures are taken, there appears to be little reason not to replace the stylet prior to epidural needle removal in the event of ADP.

Subarachnoid Saline

Limited evidence indicates that the subarachnoid injection of sterile preservative-free saline following ADP may be associated with a significant reduction in the incidence of PDPH and need for EBP. In one small study (*n* = 43), immediate injection of 10 mL saline through the epidural needle substantially reduced the incidence of PDPH (32%, compared with 62% in a matched control group) and resulted in a significant reduction in the need for EBP (*p* = 0.004).[86] The injection of saline and the reinjection of CSF have been speculated as important in the prevention of PDPH by maintaining CSF volume.[85] However, given the relatively rapid rate of CSF regeneration, it may be that the benefit of fluid injection following ADP is actually in preventing a wicking strand of arachnoid (as proposed for stylet replacement after LP). Further investigation into this issue is needed.

Intravenous Cosyntropin

As mentioned, there is no convincing evidence that systemic pharmacologic measures are beneficial in the prevention of PDPH. However, based on a number of theoretical mechanisms, corticotropin (adrenocorticotrophic hormone, ACTH) and its analogues have long been used in the treatment of PDPH.[87] Hakim recently reported randomizing 90 parturients experiencing ADP to receive either 1 mg cosyntropin or saline intravenously 30 minutes after delivery.[70] The incidence of PDPH and EBP was 33% and 11% in the cosyntropin group versus 69% and 30% in the saline group. No serious reactions were associated with cosyntropin use. These limited data are encouraging but will need to be supported through further study.

Limiting/Avoiding Pushing

In the event of ADP, limiting the duration of the second stage of labor (usually to 30–60 minutes) and avoiding pushing at that time may reduce the risk of PDPH. While these measures are not uncommonly recommended in UK maternity units,[73] such management is rare in US practice.[15]

Intrathecal Catheters

Following ADP in an obstetric setting, Russell noted a 41% incidence of at least two additional attempts at epidural placement and a 9% risk of a second dural puncture.[88] Immediately placing an intrathecal catheter (ITC) after ADP has the advantages of being able to rapidly provide spinal analgesia as well as eliminate the possibility of another ADP under challenging clinical circumstances. However, the potential benefits of ITC use must be weighed against the readily appreciated risks involved (accidental use, misuse, and infection).

Although evidence is extremely limited, ITC use has also been proposed to reduce the risk of PDPH after ADP.[62] The mechanism of benefit from ITCs is unclear but may be due to reaction to the catheter, with inflammation or edema preventing further CSF loss after removal. Ayad and colleagues placed and maintained an ITC for 24 hours following ADP.[89] In their obstetric population, catheter placement resulted in a PDPH rate of only 6.2%, with an expected incidence of greater than 50% in this setting. However, this impressive reduction in the incidence of PDPH has generally not been duplicated. A recent meta-analysis of nine studies concluded that ITC insertion following ADP failed to statistically decrease the incidence of

PDPH (RR = 0.82, 95% CI 0.67–1.01, *p* = .06) but did, however, significantly reduce the need for EBP (RR = 0.64, 95% CI 0.49-0.84, *p* = 0.001).[90] It should be noted that benefits have often not been reported in studies where catheters have been left in situ for less than 24 hours. There are also preliminary data to suggest that the incidence of PDPH may be further reduced by the injection of preservative-free saline through an ITC immediately prior to removal.[86] With some accepted and other possible benefits, rates of ITC use following ADP have clearly increased during the past decade. Recent surveys of US, UK, and Australian practice have noted rates of routine intrathecal catheterization following ADP in obstetric patients of 18%, 28%, and 35%, respectively.[15,73,91]

Although ITC use has become more common, reattempting an epidural at an adjacent interspace remains the preferred action following ADP.[15] Provided an epidural catheter can be successfully placed, several epidural approaches have been used in hope of reducing the incidence and severity of PDPH.

Epidural Saline

Efforts regarding epidural saline have included both bolus (usually around 50 mL as a single or repeated injection) and continuous infusion techniques (commonly 600–1000 mL over 24 hours). As these measures are resource intensive and may only serve to delay the inevitable onset of symptoms, they have generally not been continued beyond 36 hours. In one large analysis (*n* = 241), Stride and Cooper reported a reduction in the incidence of PDPH from 86% in a conservatively treated control group to 70% with epidural saline infusion.[92] Trivedi and colleagues noted a similar reduction in PDPH (from 87% to 67%) in 30 patients who received a single prophylactic "saline patch" (40–60 mL) following completion of an obstetric procedure.[93] Other studies of epidural saline have noted this modest decrease in the incidence of PDPH. Stride and Cooper also reported a lower incidence of severe headache (from 64% to 47%), but this effect has been inconsistently seen by other investigators, and there is no convincing evidence that epidural saline reduces the eventual need for EBP.

Epidural Opiates

Epidural opiates (especially morphine), while long utilized for the treatment of PDPH, have been thought unlikely to influence the natural history of the disorder. However, recently revisiting the issue of opiates as prophylaxis after ADP, Al-metwalli found two epidural injections of morphine (3 mg in 10 mL), compared with epidural injections of an equal volume of saline, resulted in fewer episodes of PDPH (*p* = 0.014) and decreased the need for EBP (*p* = 0.022).[69] Due to the small number of patients involved (*n* = 25), further prospective investigation is warranted.

Prophylactic Epidural Blood Patch

The impressive efficacy of the EBP when used as treatment for PDPH has fueled interest in the technique for prophylaxis. Research into the efficacy of the EBP for prophylaxis has yielded mixed results, and closer scrutiny indicates that optimism should be guarded. The strongest investigation to date has been by Scavone and colleagues, who performed a prospective, randomized, double-blind study in 64 parturients comparing the prophylactic EBP (PEBP) to a sham EBP.[94] In this study, an identical 56% of patients in each group went on to develop PDPH. Although there was a trend toward fewer therapeutic EBPs recommended and performed in the prophylactic group, the difference was not statistically significant ($p = 0.08$). The primary benefit of the PEBP was a shorter total duration of symptoms (from a median of approximately 5 days to 2 days) and, consequently, a reduction in the overall pain burden.

While there are studies that have shown greater benefit from PEBP, systematic reviews of the evidence have repeatedly noted the inferior methodology of these other studies when compared with that of Scavone et al.[63,95,96] With such inconclusive support, the PEBP is not currently recommended as a routine measure based on available evidence.[62,97] Due to concerns of exposing patients to a potentially unnecessary and marginally beneficial procedure, prophylactic application of the EBP has declined substantially in recent years.[15,73,98] If used for prophylaxis, the EBP should be performed only after any spinal or epidural local anesthetic has worn off, as premature administration has been associated with excessive cephalad displacement of local anesthetic.[99] Residual epidural local anesthetic may also inhibit coagulation of blood, further decreasing the efficacy of the EBP.[100]

DIAGNOSTIC EVALUATION

Postdural puncture headache remains a diagnosis of exclusion. Although headache following meningeal puncture will naturally be suspected to be PDPH, it remains critical to rule out other etiologies (Table 27–1). Fortunately, a careful history with a brief consideration of other possible diagnoses is usually all that is necessary to differentiate PDPH from other causes of headache. While numerous clinical variations have been reported, most cases of PDPH will have (a) a history of known

TABLE 27–1. Differential diagnosis of non-PDPH following meningeal puncture.

Benign etiologies
  Nonspecific headache
  Exacerbation of chronic headache
    (eg, tension-type headache)
  Hypertensive headache
  Pneumocephalus
  Sinusitis
  Drug-related side effect
  Spontaneous intracranial hypotension
  Other
Serious etiologies
  Meningitis
  Subdural hematoma (SDH)
  Subarachnoid hemorrhage
  Preeclampsia/eclampsia
  Intracranial venous thrombosis (ICVT)
  Other

or possible meningeal puncture, (b) delayed onset of symptoms (but within 48 hours), and (c) bilateral postural headache (possibly accompanied by associated symptoms if moderate or severe). Importantly, most non-MPHs will not have a strong positional nature. Laboratory studies are usually not necessary for the diagnosis of PDPH and, if obtained, are generally unremarkable (most commonly, MRI may show meningeal enhancement and LP may reveal low opening pressures and increased CSF protein).

Physical examination plays a limited role in the diagnosis of PDPH. Vital signs (normal blood pressure and absence of fever) and a basic neurologic exam (gross motor and sensory function plus ocular and facial movements) should be documented. Firm bilateral jugular venous pressure, applied briefly (10–15 seconds), tends to worsen headaches secondary to intracranial hypotension.[26] Conversely, the "sitting epigastric pressure test" may result in transient relief of PDPH symptoms.[101] For this test, the patient is placed in a sitting position until headache symptoms become manifest. Firm, continuous abdominal pressure is applied with one hand, while the other hand is secure against the patient's back. In cases of PDPH, some improvement is usually noted within 15–30 seconds with prompt return of symptoms on release of abdominal pressure.

It must be appreciated that benign headaches are frequently encountered in the perioperative setting, even in the absence of meningeal puncture, but have generally been noted to be less severe than PDPH (common etiologies include dehydration, hypoglycemia, anxiety, and caffeine withdrawal). With spinal anesthesia, the specific local anesthetic used and the addition of dextrose or epinephrine may influence the occurrence of nonspecific headache but do not affect the rate of true PDPH.[102] The majority of headaches following meningeal puncture will be benign, nonspecific headaches. In a careful analysis of headache following spinal anesthesia for ambulatory surgery in the general population using strict criteria for PDPH, Santanen and colleagues found an incidence of non-MPH of 18.5%, with an incidence of true PDPH of only 1.5%.[103] Headaches and neck/shoulder pain are also common in the postpartum period.[37] In one study, 39% of postpartum patients were noted to be symptomatic, but over 75% of these issues were determined to be primary headaches (migraine, tension type, cervicogenic, and cluster).[59] In this analysis, while 89% of patients received neuraxial anesthesia, only 4.7% of postpartum headaches were PDPH.

Benign headaches can often be differentiated from PDPH by their characteristic features. Exacerbation of chronic headache (eg, tension type, cluster, or migraine) is usually notable for a history of similar headaches. In the study cited immediately in the preceding paragraph, a previous headache history was a significant risk factor for postpartum headache (adjusted odds ratio = 2.25, if > 12 episodes per year).[59] Significant hypertension may cause headaches and should be detected through routine vital sign assessment.

Stella et al studied severe and unrelenting postpartum headaches with onset more than 24 hours from the time of delivery and found that 39% were tension-type headaches, 24% were due to preeclampsia/eclampsia, and only 16% were PDPHs (despite neuraxial anesthesia in 88% of patients).[104] Based on this observation, they recommended treatment of tension/migraine headache prior to consideration of PDPH.

Pneumocephalus can produce a positional headache that can be difficult to distinguish from PDPH and does not respond to EBP but is readily diagnosed with computerized tomography (CT).[105] Sinusitis may be associated with purulent nasal discharge and tenderness over the affected sinus and is often improved with assuming an upright position. It should be kept in mind that headache is also a side effect of some commonly utilized pharmacologic agents, such as ondansetron.[106] Although certainly unusual, classic PDPH symptoms may even conceivably represent a coincidental case of spontaneous intracranial hypotension (SIH).[107] A number of other benign etiologies are possible.

Serious causes of headache will be rare but must be excluded. It is important to remember that lateralizing neurologic signs (with the exception of cranial nerve palsies), fever/chills, seizures, or changes in mental status are not consistent with a diagnosis of PDPH. Meningitis tends to be associated with fever, leukocytosis, changes in mental status, and meningeal signs (such as nuchal rigidity).[108]

Subdural hematoma (SDH) is a recognized complication of dural puncture and is believed under these circumstances to be due to intracranial hypotension resulting in excessive traction on cerebral vessels, leading to their disruption. Practitioners must maintain a high index of suspicion for SDH, which is often preceded by typical PDPH symptoms but progresses to lose its postural component and may evolve to include disturbances in mentation and focal neurologic signs. It has been proposed that early definitive treatment of severe PDPH may serve to prevent SDH.[109]

Subarachnoid hemorrhage, most commonly due to rupture of a cerebral aneurysm or arteriovenous malformation, is usually associated with the sudden onset of excruciating headache followed by a decreased level of consciousness or coma.[110] Preeclampsia/eclampsia often presents with headache and may only become evident in the postpartum period.[111] Intracranial venous thrombosis (ICVT) is most often seen in the postpartum obstetric population, where headache symptoms are easily confused with PDPH but may progress to seizures, focal neurologic signs, and coma.[112,113] Predisposing factors for ICVT include hypercoagulability, dehydration, and inflammatory and infectious diseases. Reports of other intracranial pathology (intracranial tumor, intracerebral hemorrhage, etc.) misdiagnosed as PDPH are extremely uncommon and will be detected with a thorough neurological evaluation.[114]

Diagnosis of PDPH can be particularly challenging in patients who have undergone LP as part of a diagnostic workup for headache. In these situations, a change in the quality of headache, most commonly a new postural nature, points toward PDPH. Occasionally, if the benign diagnostic possibilities cannot be narrowed down with certainty, a favorable response to EBP can provide definitive evidence for a diagnosis of PDPH.

TREATMENT

Once a diagnosis of PDPH has been made, patients should be provided a straightforward explanation of the presumed etiology, anticipated natural course (factoring in the time from

meningeal puncture), and a realistic assessment of treatment options (with consideration of needle gauge). Treatment considerations are presented individually next. Although surveys indicate that formal protocols for management of PDPH are common practice in the United Kingdom, such plans remain the exception in North American practice.[98] A treatment algorithm, based primarily on the severity of symptoms, can serve as a useful guide for management (Figure 27–8).

Time

Because PDPH is a complication that tends to resolve spontaneously, the simple passage of time plays an important role in the appropriate management of this disorder. Prior to the introduction of the EBP as definitive therapy, the natural history of PDPH was documented by Vandam and Dripps as they followed 1011 episodes of PDPH after spinal anesthesia using cutting needles of various sizes.[8] While their analysis was flawed by a lack of information regarding duration in 9% of patients, if one considers their observed data, spontaneous resolution of PDPH was seen in 59% of cases within 4 days and 80% within 1 week.

More recently, Lybecker et al closely followed 75 episodes of PDPH after spinal anesthesia and, while providing an EBP to 40% of their patients (generally to those having the most severe symptoms), observed in the untreated patients a median duration of symptoms of 5 days with a range of 1–12 days.[33] van Kooten et al, in a small but prospective, randomized, blinded study of patients with moderate or severe PDPH following LP primarily using 20 gauge needles, noted 18 of 21 patients (86%) in the control treatment group (24-hour bed rest, at least 2 L of fluids by mouth daily, and analgesics as needed) still having headache symptoms at 7 days, with over half of these still rating symptoms as moderate or severe[115] (Figure 27–9).

These data serve to illustrate the unpredictable and occasionally prolonged duration of untreated PDPH. Indeed, Vandam and Dripps reported 4% of patients still experiencing symptoms 7–12 months after spinal anesthesia.[8] Given this reality, it is not surprising that there are a number of case reports of successful treatment of PDPH months and even years after known or occult meningeal puncture.

Largely due to the self-limited nature of PDPH, the optimal time course of treatment has not been well defined. Clinically, the practical issue is how long definitive therapy (ie, the EBP) can appropriately be delayed. Many practitioners currently advocate a trial, most commonly 24–48 hours, of conservative management.[15] However, the rationale behind this approach is questionable given the often severely disabling nature of symptoms, particularly in the postpartum period when newborn care may be significantly impaired.

Supportive Measures

Reassurance and measures directed toward minimizing symptoms, while not expected to alter the natural course of the disorder, are advised for all patients. By definition, the majority of patients with moderate-to-severe PDPH will naturally seek a recumbent position for symptomatic relief. Despite a lack of

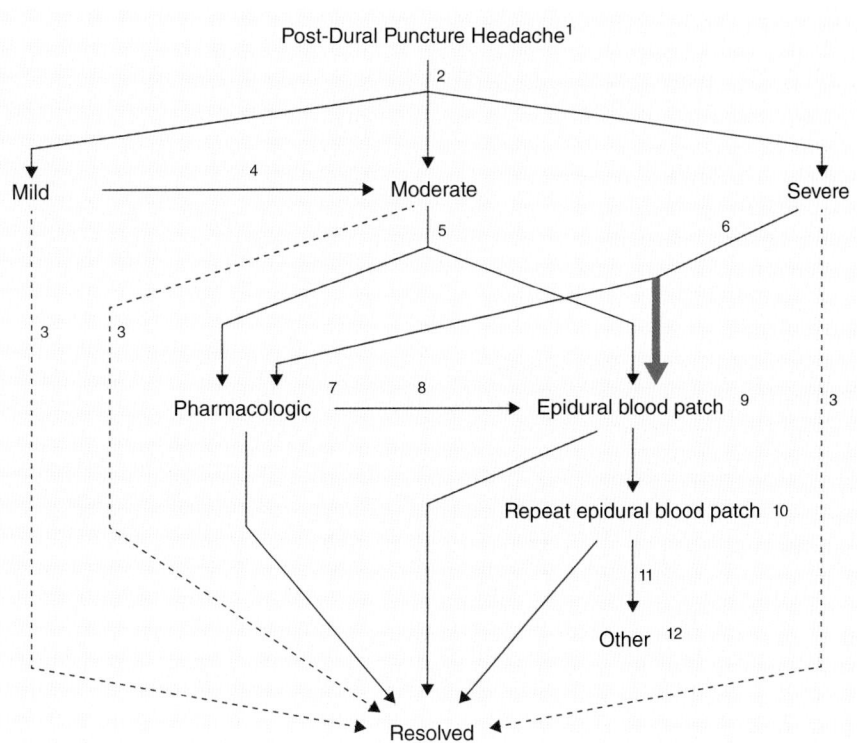

FIGURE 27–8. Treatment algorithm for established PDPH (see text for further details). (1) Patient education, reassurance, and supportive measures. (2) Triage by severity of symptoms. (3) Resolution over time without further treatment. (4) Worsening symptoms or failure to improve substantially within 5 days. (5) Choice of EBP or pharmacologic measures based on patient preference. (6) Definitive treatment (EBP) is recommended (bold arrow). (7) Caffeine or other agents. (8) Failure, worsening of symptoms, or recurrence. (9) Patch materials other than blood remain preliminary. (10) Generally performed no sooner than 24 hours after a first EBP. (11) Serious reconsideration of diagnosis. (12) Radiologic guidance is recommended if another epidural blood patch (EBP). (Reproduced with permission from Neal JM, Rathmell JP: *Complications in Regional Anesthesia and Pain Medicine*, 2nd ed. Philadelphia: Lippincott Williams & Wilkins; 2013.)

supportive evidence, aggressive hydration continues to be the most frequently recommended practice utilized in treatment of PDPH.[15] Although aggressive hydration does not appear to influence the duration of symptoms,[74] patients should and often must be encouraged to avoid dehydration.

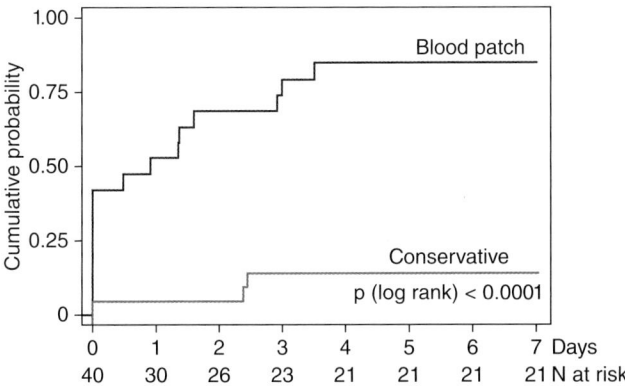

FIGURE 27–9. Cumulative probability of recovery from PDPH. Recovery from moderate-to-severe PDPH after diagnostic LP in 40 patients. At 7 days, only 3 of 21 conservatively treated patients had fully recovered (no headache symptoms) versus 16 of 19 patients treated with EBP ($p < .0001$). (Reproduced with permission from van Kooten F, Oedit R, Bakker SL, et al: Epidural blood patch in post dural puncture headache: a randomised, observer-blind, controlled clinical trial. *Neurol Neurosurg Psychiatry*. 2008 May;79(5):553–558.)

Analgesics (acetaminophen, nonsteroidal anti-inflammatory drugs [NSAIDs], opiates, etc.) may be administered by a number of different routes and are commonly used, yet the relief obtained is often unimpressive, especially with severe headaches. Antiemetics and stool softeners should be prescribed when indicated. Abdominal binders have been advocated but are uncomfortable and seldom used in modern practice. Alternative measures that have been suggested in the management of PDPH include acupuncture[116] and bilateral greater occipital nerve block.[117,118]

Pharmacologic Therapies

Many pharmacologic agents have been advocated as treatments for PDPH. Reports of successful use of pharmacologic agents for treatment of PDPH are intriguing, but their proper place in the management of PDPH awaits further study of efficacy and safety. While appealing, these options have generally been poorly studied and are of questionable value due to the small number of patients treated, methodological flaws in published reports, publication bias, and the self-limited nature of the disorder.

A recent review of RCTs assessing the effectiveness of any pharmacological drug used for treating PDPH only included[118] seven studies with a total of 200 participants (primarily parturients).[119] Given the initial optimistic but eventually disproven role for so many treatments through the years, practitioners are advised to have guarded expectations in this regard, especially when dealing with severe PDPH. A detailed review of pharmacologic therapies for PDPH is beyond the scope of this chapter, but some popular or recently investigated options include the following:

1. *Methylxanthines.* Due to known cerebral vasoconstrictive effects, this class of drugs has become the most commonly used pharmacologic approach to PDPH. These agents include aminophylline, theophylline, and—the most familiar—caffeine. Experimentally, caffeine has been used intravenously (usually 500 mg caffeine sodium benzoate, which contains 250 mg caffeine) and orally (eg, 300 mg). Published studies of caffeine for PDPH consistently demonstrated improvement at 1–4 hours in over 70% of patients treated.[120] However, a single oral dose of 300 mg caffeine for treatment of PDPH is statistically no better than placebo at 24 hours.[121] With a terminal half-life usually less than 6 hours, repeated doses of caffeine would seem necessary for treatment of PDPH, yet few studies have evaluated more than 2 doses for efficacy or safety (of particular concern in the nursing parturient). Furthermore, there is no convincing evidence that caffeine, or any pharmacologic agents, reduce the eventual need for EBP. Overall, the use of caffeine for PDPH does not appear to be supported by the available literature.[122] Nevertheless, surveys indicated that it continues to be widely used in the treatment of PDPH.[15,73,98] Clinically, encouraging unmonitored caffeine intake is of extremely uncertain value, especially considering the widespread lack of awareness of caffeine content in readily available beverages and medications. The temporary benefit often observed with caffeine would indicate that, if used, it is perhaps most appropriate for the treatment of PDPH of moderate (and possibly mild or severe) intensity while awaiting spontaneous resolution of the condition. While the familiarity of caffeine for nonmedical purposes would argue for its general safety, practitioners should note that its use is contraindicated in patients with seizure disorders, pregnancy-induced hypertension, or a history of supraventricular tachyarrhythmias.

2. *Serotonin type 1d receptor agonists.* These agents cause cerebral vasoconstriction and are commonly used for migraine headache. Despite anecdotal reports of success, sumatriptan was ineffective for treatment of severe PDPH in a small randomized, prospective study.[123]

3. *Ergot alkaloids.* These cerebral vasoconstrictive agents are also commonly used for migraine headache. A small, uncontrolled pilot study suggested that methylergonovine (0.25 mg orally three times daily for 24–48 hours) may hasten resolution of PDPH.[124]

4. *Corticosteroidogenics (corticotropin [ACTH] and its synthetic analogues [ie, cosyntropin/tetracosactin]).* Although the mechanism of action remains speculative, ACTH is known to have multiple physiologic effects that could theoretically improve symptoms of PDPH.[87] However, a synthetic ACTH analogue was ineffective for treatment of severe PDPH in a small randomized, prospective study.[125]

5. *Corticosteroids.* Similar to corticosteroidogenics, corticosteroids have multiple physiologic effects that could theoretically improve symptoms of PDPH. In a randomized, prospective study of 60 patients with severe PDPH after spinal anesthesia using 25-gauge Quincke needles for cesarean delivery, addition of hydrocortisone (200 mg IV initially, followed by 100 mg every 8 hours for 6 doses) resulted in significantly lower headache intensity.[126] Only one patient in this study (in the conventionally treated group) required EBP. A similar randomized study in 60 nonobstetric surgery patients experiencing PDPH after spinal anesthesia showed significant reductions in headache intensity in the hydrocortisone group.[127]

6. *Anticonvulsants.* Several membrane-stabilizing agents are widely used for various pain syndromes. Some reports have suggested that gabapentin may be useful in the setting of PDPH. In an uncontrolled case series of 17 postpartum patients with severe PDPH, 9 (53%) experienced "excellent" (visual analog scale [VAS] < 2 of 10 plus resumption of normal activity) relief with gabapentin (200 mg initially, followed by 100–300 mg three times daily, with dose adjusted to tolerance and efficacy).[128] In a randomized, placebo-controlled study, pregabalin (75 mg twice a day for 2 days, then 150 mg twice a day for 2 days) was demonstrated to result in lower pain scores and analgesic consumption in patients with PDPH following spinal anesthesia or LP.[129] It is interesting to note that, despite starting with mean VAS scores of greater than 8 of 10, none of the 40 patients in this study required EBP.

Epidural Therapies

While not a contraindication to epidural treatments, a history of significant technical difficulties with attempted neuraxial techniques should naturally encourage a trial of less-invasive measures. However, the appeal of epidural approaches is evident if access to the epidural space is deemed reasonable or if the patient already has a correctly placed catheter in situ.

Epidural Saline

Epidural saline, as bolus and infusion, has a long history of use for treatment of PDPH. Bolus injections of epidural saline (usually 20–30 ml, repeated as necessary if a catheter is present) have been reported to produce prompt and virtually universal relief of PDPH, yet the practice is plagued by an extremely high rate of headache recurrence. This transient effect is not surprising as increases in epidural pressure following bolus administration of saline have been demonstrated to return to baseline within 10 minutes.[130] Favorable results achieved with this approach have been speculated to represent the mechanical reapproximation of a dural flap (the "tin-lid" phenomenon).[6] However, bolus administration of saline for treatment of PDPH has been convincingly shown to be inferior to the EBP, especially when headaches are secondary to large-bore needle punctures.[131] Overall, epidural saline appears to be of limited value for established PDPH.[62] Nevertheless, the successful use of epidural saline, administered as bolus or infusion, continues to be reported occasionally under exceptional circumstances.[132,133]

Epidural Blood Patch

During the past several decades, the EBP has emerged as the "gold standard" for treatment of PDPH (Figure 27–10).[6] A Cochrane review (a systematic assessment of the evidence) regarding the EBP concluded that the procedure now has proven benefit over more conservative treatment.[97] The mechanism of action of the EBP, while not entirely elucidated, appears to be related to the ability to stop further CSF loss by the formation of clot over the defect in the meninges as well as a tamponade effect with cephalad displacement of CSF (the "epidural pressure patch").[134]

The appropriate role of the EBP in individual situations will depend on multiple factors, including the duration and severity of headache and associated symptoms, type and gauge of original needle used, and patient wishes. The EBP should be encouraged in patients experiencing ADP with an epidural needle and those whose symptoms are categorized as severe (ie, pain score > 6 on a 1–10 scale). Informed consent for the EBP should include a discussion with the patient regarding the common as well as serious risks involved, true success rate, and anticipated side effects. Finally, patients should be provided clear instructions for the provision of timely medical attention should they experience a recurrence of symptoms.

A number of controversies surround the EBP, reflecting the scarcity of adequately powered, randomized trials. The procedure itself has been well described and consists of the sterile injection of fresh autologous blood near the previous dural puncture (Table 27–2). An MRI study of the EBP in 5 young patients (ages 31–44) using 20 mL blood noted a spread of 4.6 ± 0.9 intervertebral spaces (mean ± SD), averaging 3.5 levels above and 1 level below the site of injection.[134] This and other observations of a preferential cephalad spread of blood in the lumbar epidural space has led to the common recommendation to perform the EBP "at or below" the meningeal puncture level. However, the influence of the level of placement and use of an

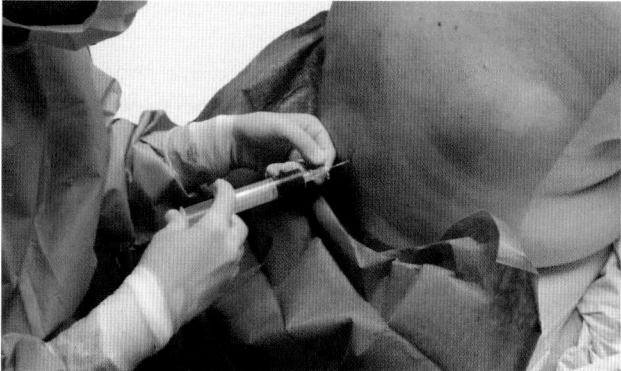

FIGURE 27–10. Blood patch. Administration of an epidural blood patch using 20 mL of freshly drawn blood. The blood is injected until 20 mL are reached or the patient perceives significant pain or pressure in the back, whichever comes first.

TABLE 27–2. Epidural blood patch procedure.

Obtain written informed consent.

Establish intravenous access. An 18-gauge or larger saline lock is sufficient.

Position the patient for epidural needle placement (mindful that a lateral decubitus position may be more comfortable than sitting for the patient).

Using standard sterile technique, place an epidural needle into the epidural space at or below the level of previous meningeal puncture.

Collect 20 mL fresh autologous venous blood using strict sterile technique (this is usually readily accomplished using the previously placed saline lock).

Without delay, steadily inject blood through the epidural needle until the patient reports fullness or discomfort in the back, buttocks, or neck.

Maintain the patient in a recumbent position for a period of time (1–2 hours may result in more complete resolution of symptoms). Intravenous infusion of 1 L crystalloid during this interval is often helpful.

Instructions for discharge:

Encourage over-the-counter analgesics (eg, acetaminophen, ibuprofen) as needed for any mild residual discomfort.

Prescribe stool softeners or cough suppressants if indicated.

Avoid lifting, straining, or air travel for 24 hours.

Provide clear instructions on how to contact anesthesia personnel for inadequate relief or recurrence of symptoms.

epidural catheter (often situated considerably cephalad to a meningeal puncture) on efficacy for EBP has never been clinically evaluated.

The optimal timing of the EBP is a matter of debate. After diagnosis, most practitioners prefer to delay performing the EBP, possibly to further confirm the diagnosis as well as to allow an opportunity for spontaneous resolution. A 1996 survey of UK neurological departments found that only 8% would consider the EBP before 72 hours had passed following LP.[135] A recent survey of UK maternity units reported that 71% would perform the EBP only "after the failure of conservative measures."[73] Likewise, the majority of respondents to recent surveys of practice in the United States and Nordic countries usually waited at least 24 hours from the onset of symptoms before performing the EBP.[15,136]

Several studies have suggested that the EBP procedure may become more effective with the passage of time.[137,138] Safa-Tisseront et al. found a delay of less than 4 days from meningeal puncture before performing an EBP to be an independent risk factor for failure of the procedure.[138] Yet, these authors were careful to state that failure of the EBP may be primarily related to the severity of the CSF leak (with larger, harder-to-treat situations demanding earlier attention), and that their study should not be grounds for delaying the EBP.

Sandesc and colleagues performed a prospective, randomized, double-blind study of the EBP versus conservative management (intravenous or oral fluids up to 3 L/d, NSAIDS, and caffeine sodium benzoate 500 mg IV every 6 hours) in 32 patients with severe PDPH symptoms (mean pain intensity = 8.1).[139] At the time treatment was initiated, none of these patients had experienced symptoms for longer than 24 hours. While all patients in the EBP group had satisfactory resolution of symptoms at 24-hour follow-up, the control group was essentially unchanged (mean pain intensity = 7.8). Notably, 14 of 16 patients in the conservatively treated group then elected for EBP treatment. These investigators concluded that there was no reason to delay the EBP for more than 24 hours after making a diagnosis of severe PDPH. This recommendation was further supported by a prospective analysis of 79 patients with PDPH that determined early EBP in those with moderate-to-severe symptoms minimized overall patient suffering.[140]

The ideal volume of blood for EBP has been an evolving issue that is becoming more clearly understood. Conceptually, the volume of blood used should be sufficient to form an organized clot over the meningeal defect as well as produce some degree of epidural tamponade.[134] When performing the EBP, anesthesiologists commonly inject as much blood as was drawn (usually around 20 mL), stopping when the patient complains of discomfort or fullness in the back, buttocks, or neck.

There appear to be geographic preferences regarding blood volume. The largest analysis of the EBP to date (n = 504) utilized a blood volume of 23 ± 5 ml (mean ± SD).[137] Importantly, this French study found no significant difference in blood volumes between successful and failed EBP. Notably, they reported "discomfort" in 78% of injections with 19 ± 5 mL and "pain" in 54% with 21 ± 5 mL, with the only independent risk factor for pain during EBP being age less than 35 years. A recent survey of US anesthesiologists reported general unanimity for a smaller blood volume, with two-thirds (66.8%) most commonly using between 16 and 20 mL.[15]

As previously mentioned, there may be some experimental support for using a blood volume of 15–20 mL, as early studies of CSF drainage in volunteers reported consistently producing positional headache symptoms with loss of 10% of total CSF volume (approximately 15 mL).[26] Furthermore, the reduction in CSF pressures produced by this degree of fluid loss would be expected to reduce or eliminate transmeningeal driving pressure, resulting at that point in a relative CSF volume homeostasis (in the supine position).

Two RCTs have been performed to determine the optimum volume of blood for EBP in obstetric patients with PDPH following ADP. The first, which compared 7.5 to 15 mL in 33 Taiwanese women, reported similar efficacy with the two volumes and failed to find any advantage with the larger volume.[142] The second was a larger, multicenter study that looked at three volumes of blood for EBP (15, 20, and 30 mL).[143] This trial found that patients receiving 15 mL had less-complete relief of symptoms than those receiving 20 or 30 mL, with no difference in efficacy between 20 and 30 mL. These investigators also found that only 54% of patients randomized to the highest volume were able to tolerate the full 30 mL (compared with 81% in the 20-mL group).

While these two studies failed to definitively determine the ideal volume of blood for EBP, they both indicated that it does not appear necessary to use volumes greater than 20 mL. It is notable that although the utility of the EBP in the treatment of SIH is uncertain,[62] much larger blood volumes (up to 100 mL) are commonly recommended for this indication.[143] However, recent case reports highlighted some potential complications, such as severe radiculopathy, from large-volume EBP,[144,145] and practitioners are therefore generally encouraged to use the smallest effective blood volume.

To allow for clot organization and regeneration of CSF (approximately 0.35 mL/minute), it is common practice to have patients remain recumbent for a period of time following the EBP. While the optimal duration of bed rest immediately following an EBP remains unknown, one small study suggested that maintaining the decubitus position for at least 1 and preferably 2 hours may result in a more complete resolution of symptoms.[146] Patients are also usually advised to avoid lifting, Valsalva maneuvers (eg, straining with bowel movement), and air travel for 24–48 hours after EBP to minimize the risk of patch disruption.

Modifications have been made to the standard EBP technique in special circumstances. To accommodate the religious beliefs of Jehovah's Witness patients, techniques have been described that keep autologous blood within a continuous circuit.[147] The EBP has been repeatedly demonstrated to be safe and effective for treatment of PDPH in the pediatric population.[148,149] A blood volume of 0.2–0.3 mL/kg appears appropriate for young children as well as adolescents. The EBP is also performed with decreased blood volumes at extralumbar sites (eg, cervical spine).[150]

Contraindications to the EBP are similar to those of any epidural needle placement: coagulopathy, systemic sepsis, fever, infection at the site, and patient refusal. Theoretical concerns have been expressed regarding the possibility of neoplastic seeding of the central nervous system in patients with cancer.[151] It has been suggested that special care, in the form of slower injections of smaller blood volumes, may be prudent in patients whose central nervous system may be vulnerable to injury produced by increased epidural pressures generated with EBP, such as those with multiple sclerosis.[152] Although not free from concern and controversy, the EBP has been safely provided to patients with HIV infection[153] and acute varicella.[154]

Minor side effects are common following the EBP. Patients should be warned to expect aching in the back, buttocks, or legs (seen in approximately 25% of patients).[137] While usually short-lived, backache was noted to be persistent in 16% of patients following EBP and lasted 3–100 days (with a mean duration in this subgroup of 27.7 days).[155] Despite these lingering symptoms, patient satisfaction with the EBP is high. Other frequent but benign aftereffects of the EBP include transient neckache,[155] bradycardia,[156] and modest temperature elevation.[155]

Largely through extensive clinical experience, the EBP has been sufficiently proven to be safe. Risks are essentially the same as with other epidural procedures (infection, bleeding, nerve damage, and ADP). Although some patients may develop temporary back and lower extremity radicular pain as mentioned, such complications are uncommon. With proper technique, infectious complications are vanishingly rare. In general, a previous EBP does not appear to significantly influence the success of future epidural interventions,[157] but case reports suggest that the EBP may occasionally result in clinically significant scarring.[158] Serious complications secondary to the EBP do occur but have usually consisted of isolated case reports and have often been associated with significant deviations from standard practice.[6]

Alternative Treatment Options to EBP

A number of alternatives to blood have been promoted as patch materials. The various rationales for using alternative agents include situations for which the use of blood has been ineffective or is contraindicated.[159] The most commonly proposed materials (dextran 40, hydroxyethylstarch, gelatin, and fibrin glue) have been adapted for a perceived ability to provide prolonged epidural tamponade or result in sealing of a meningeal rent. In a rat model, experimental support for a "blood-like" effect was best shown for fibrin glue.[130] Yet, clinical use of these alternatives is limited to case reports and small series, and their use is uncommon in the United States.[15] While not necessarily without merit, these options remain poorly defined and are not without potential for serious risk (eg, allergic reactions to dextran), and reports of their use should still be considered preliminary.

PERSISTENT OR RECURRENT PDPH

Early reports of the EBP frequently cited success rates between 90% and 100% but often did not include a strict definition of "success," had little or no follow-up, and failed to consider the influence of such confounding factors as needle size and tip design, severity of symptoms, or natural history of PDPH. The true efficacy of the EBP procedure is now known to be significantly lower than once thought. Persistent or recurrent headaches following the EBP, while not necessarily requiring consultation, warrant follow-up and thoughtful reevaluation.

The EBP is associated with nearly immediate symptomatic relief in greater than 90% of cases, but appropriate follow-up reveals a number of patients experiencing incomplete relief, failure, or recurrence of symptoms. In an uncontrolled, prospective, observational study of 504 consecutive patients treated with EBP following meningeal puncture with needles of various sizes, Safa-Tisseront et al reported that some relief of symptoms occurs in 93% of patients.[138] On closer analysis, however, complete relief of symptoms was seen in only 75% of patients, with 18% experiencing incomplete relief. They also found that the EBP was more likely to fail if the original meningeal puncture was made with needles larger than 20 gauge. For needles larger than 20 gauge, the unqualified success rate of the EBP was only 62%, with 17% of patients reporting incomplete relief of symptoms and 21% experiencing failure. Not surprisingly, the majority of these large needles were Tuohy epidural needles.

Expectations of success with the EBP must be further tempered in obstetric patients (all young and female) following ADP with epidural needles. Under these circumstances,

Williams et al noted complete relief of symptoms with EBP in only 34% of patients, partial relief in 54%, and no relief in 7% (results unknown in 5%).[160] If performed, a second EBP resulted in complete relief in 50%, partial relief in 36%, and no relief in 14%. In a similar patient population, Banks and colleagues, despite initially observing complete or partial relief with EBP in 95% of patients, reported the return of moderate-to-severe symptoms in 31%, with a mean time to development of recurrent headache of 31.8 hours (range 12–96 hours).[137] The rates of repeat EBP for the Williams and Banks studies were 27% and 19%, respectively. These studies clearly demonstrated the reduced efficacy of the EBP following meningeal punctures made with large needles, which not uncommonly make it necessary to consider repeating the procedure.

Overall, success rates of a second EBP appear to be approximately equal to that of a first. The ideal timing and blood volume for repeat EBP are even more uncertain than for a primary procedure. A majority of US anesthesiologists would wait at least 24 hours after recurrence of PDPH symptoms before performing a second EBP.[15] If more than one EBP is performed within a short period of time, practitioners should remain cognizant of the cumulative amount of blood used as excessive volumes under these circumstances have been implicated in adverse outcomes.[144,145]

Insufficient evidence exists to guide management following a second failed EBP. Given the frequency of PDPH and significant failure rate of the EBP, instances of sequential EBP failure are not unheard of, especially following large-gauge meningeal punctures. In an analysis of outcomes following ADP with 18-gauge Tuohy needles in an obstetric unit, Sadashivaiah reported 3 of 48 patients (6.25%) requiring a third EBP to relieve the headache.[161] Obviously, each failure of the EBP necessitates an even more critical reconsideration of the diagnosis.

While experiences with managing repeated EBP failure have been published,[162] such sporadic case reports are insufficient to guide others. However, one frequently cited and logical recommendation regarding repeat EBP, and particularly a third EBP, is to use some form of radiologic guidance to ensure accurate epidural blood placement (eg, fluoroscopy). Other measures under these difficult circumstances may include any of the aforementioned "treatments," with open surgical repair constituting a last resort.

WHEN TO SEEK FURTHER CONSULTATION

Because PDPH tends to improve even without specific treatment and the EBP has a relatively high rate of success, many practitioners reasonably seek neurological consultation if symptoms have failed to resolve after an arbitrary duration (eg, 7–10 days) or number of EBPs (usually two or three).

Consultation is always indicated if serious non-PDPH is suspected or cannot reasonably be ruled out. As previously mentioned, lateralizing neurologic signs, fever/chills, seizures, or change in mental status are not consistent with a diagnosis of PDPH or benign headache. Consultation is also appropriate for any headaches with atypical features. Proceeding with treatment measures directed toward PDPH under uncertain circumstances may hinder a correct diagnosis, cause critical delays in proper treatment, and can prove harmful. The EBP, for example, has occasionally been reported to produce detrimental increases in intracranial pressure.

Because PDPH can be anticipated to resolve spontaneously, headaches that worsen over time and no longer have a positional nature should be strongly suspected to be secondary to SDH (especially if there are focal neurologic signs or decreases in mental status). Under these circumstances, a neurological consultation should be obtained and diagnostic radiologic studies performed.

Although headache and most associated symptoms, including auditory symptoms,[38] resolve quickly following EBP, cranial nerve palsies generally resolve slowly (within 6 months) and may appropriately prompt a neurology consult for ongoing management and reassurance.[30] Although there are no accepted treatments for cranial nerve palsy associated with PDPH, it seems reasonable to treat these conditions similar to idiopathic facial nerve (CN VII) palsy ("Bell's palsy"). There is some evidence, for example, to suggest that corticosteroids administered early (within 72 hours of onset) may hasten resolution of symptoms from Bell's palsy,[163] and similar treatment has been suggested for cranial nerve palsy following meningeal puncture.[32]

SUMMARY

Over a century after being first described, PDPH remains a significant clinical concern for a number of medical specialties. As with any complication, prevention is preferable to treatment. Identification and consideration of the risk factors for PDPH have resulted in an impressive reduction in the incidence of this persistent iatrogenic problem.

Accidental meningeal puncture with epidural needles continues to be a major concern and challenge. The consequent PDPH symptoms tend to be more severe, of longer duration, and more difficult to treat than those seen with smaller-gauge needles. It should be noted that there is no evidence to support the two most commonly practiced prophylactic measures in this setting: aggressive hydration and encouraging bed rest. Although some prophylactic measures have shown promise, none to this point appears to be a definitive measure.

Many episodes of PDPH, especially those of mild-to-moderate severity, will resolve in a timely manner without specific treatment. Despite being commonly advised, hydration, bed rest, and caffeine are all of questionable value in the treatment of established PDPH. Although alternatives have been proposed, the EBP remains the only proven treatment for PDPH and therefore can be encouraged and performed early (within 24 hours of diagnosis) if symptoms are severe.

Unfortunately, the published literature concerning PDPH has generally been of poor quality.[62,97,164] Many questions remain regarding the optimal means of preventing and treating this troublesome complication. Even much of what is "known" to this point has not been confirmed in follow-up studies. It is anticipated that these issues will be resolved in the future through well-designed clinical investigations.

REFERENCES

1. Van Zundert AAJ, Reina MA, Lee RA. Prevention of post-dural puncture headache (PDPH) in parturients. Contributions from experimental research. Acta Anaesthesiol Scand. 2013;57:947–9.
2. Reina MA, Prats-Galino A, Sola RG, Puigdellívol-Sánchez A, Arriazu Navarro R, De Andrés JA. Structure of the arachnoid layer of the human spinal meninges: a barrier that regulates dural sac permeability. Rev Esp Anestesiol Reanim. 2010;57:486–92. Spanish.
3. Reina MA, López A, Badorrey V, De Andrés JA, Martín S. Dura-arachnoid lesions produced by 22 gauge Quincke spinal needles during a lumbar puncture. J Neurol Neurosurg Psychiatry. 2004;75893–7.
4. Reina MA, de Leon-Casasola OA, Lopez A, De Andres J, Martin S, Mora M. An in vitro study of dural lesions produced by 25-gauge Quincke and Whitacre needles evaluated by scanning electron microscopy. Reg Anesth Pain Med. 2000;25:393–402.
5. Dittmann M, Reina MA, López García A. New results in the visualization of the spinal dura mater with scanning electron microscopy. Anaesthesist. 1998;47:409–13. German.
6. Reina MA, Dittmann M, López Garcia A, van Zundert A. New perspectives in the microscopic structure of human dura mater in the dorsolumbar region. Reg Anesth. 1997;22:161–6.
7. Reina MA, López-García A, de Andrés-Ibáñez JA, Dittmann M, Cascales MR, del Caño MC, Daneri J, Zambrano O. Electron microscopy of the lesions produced in the human dura mater by Quincke beveled and Whitacre needles. Rev Esp Anestesiol Reanim. 1997;44:56–61. Spanish.
8. Reina MA, López A, van Zundert A, De Andrés JA. Ultrastructure of dural lesions produced in lumbar punctures. In: Reina MA. Atlas of functional anatomy of regional anesthesia and pain medicine. New York: Springer; 2015. p.767–794.
9. Reina MA, Castedo J, López A. Postdural puncture headache. Ultrastructure of dural lesions and spinal needles used in lumbar punctures. Rev Arg Anestesiol 2008;66:6–26.
10. Tourtellotte WW, Haerer AF, Heller GL, Somers JE: *Post-Lumbar Puncture Headaches*. Thomas, 1964.
11. Moore DC: Headache. In *Complications of Regional Anesthesia*. Thomas, 1955, pp 177–196.
12. Gormley JB: Treatment of postspinal headache. Anesthesiology 1960; 21:565–566.
13. DiGiovanni AJ, Dunbar BS: Epidural injections of autologous blood for postlumbar-puncture headache. Anesth Analg 1970;49:268–271.
14. Crawford JS: Experiences with epidural blood patch. Anaesthesia 1980;35:513–515.
15. Harrington BE, Schmitt AM: Meningeal (postdural) puncture headache, unintentional dural puncture, and the epidural blood patch. A national survey of United States practice. Reg Anesth Pain Med 2009;34:430–437.
16. Choi PT, Galinski SE, Takeuchi L, et al: PDPH is a common complication of neuraxial blockade in parturients: A meta-analysis of obstetrical studies. Can J Anesth 2003;50:460–469.
17. Paech M, Banks S, Gurrin L: An audit of accidental dural puncture during epidural insertion of a Tuohy needle in obstetric patients. Int J Obstet Anesth 2001;10:162–167.
18. Webb CA, Weyker PD, Zhang L, et al: Unintentional dural puncture with a Tuohy needle increases risk of chronic headache. Anesth Analg 2012;115:124–132.
19. Stendell L, Fomsgaard JS, Olsen KS: There is room for improvement in the prevention and treatment of headache after lumbar puncture. Dan Med J 2012;59:1–5.
20. Vercauteren MP, Hoffmann VH, Mertens E, et al: Seven-year review of requests for epidural blood patches for headache after dural puncture: referral patterns and the effectiveness of blood patches. Eur J Anaesth 1999;16:298–303.
21. Davies JM, Posner KL, Lee LA, et al: Liability associated with obstetric anesthesia. A closed claims analysis. Anesthesiology 2009;110:131–139.
22. Lee LA, Posner KL, Domino KB, et al: Injuries associated with regional anesthesia in the 1980s and 1990s: A closed claims analysis. Anesthesiology 2004;101:143–152.
23. Fitzgibbon DR, Posner KL, Domino KB, et al: Chronic pain management: American Society of Anesthesiologists Closed Claims Project. Anesthesiology 2004;100:98–105.
24. Brull R, McCartney CJL, Chan VWS, et al: Disclosure of risks associated with regional anesthesia: A survey of academic regional anesthesiologists. Reg Anesth Pain Med 2007;32:7–11.
25. Levine DN, Rapalino O: The pathophysiology of lumbar puncture headache. J Neurol Sci 2001;192:1–8.

26. Kunkle EC, Ray BS, Wolff HG: Experimental studies on headache. Analysis of the headache associated with changes in intracranial pressure. Arch Neurol Psychiatry 1943;49:323–358.

27. Larrier D, Lee A: Anatomy of headache and facial pain. Otolaryngol Clin N Am 2003;36:1041–1053.

28. Day CJE, Shutt LE: Auditory, ocular, and facial complications of central neural block. A review of possible mechanisms. Reg Anesth 1996; 21:197–201.

29. Pogodzinski MS, Shallop JK, Sprung J, et al: Hearing loss and cerebrospinal fluid pressure: Case report and review of the literature. Ear Nose Throat J 2009;87:144–147.

30. Nishio I, Williams BA, Williams JP: Diplopia. A complication of dural puncture. Anesthesiology 2004;100:158–164.

31. Yaman ME, Ayberk G, Eylen A, et al: Isolated abducens nerve palsy following lumbar puncture: Case report and review of the mechanism of action. J Neurosurg Sci 2010;54:119–123.

32. Fang JY, Lin JW, Li Q, et al: Trigeminal nerve and facial nerve palsy after combined spinal-epidural anesthesia for cesarean section. J Clin Anesth 2010;22:56–58.

33. Lybecker H, Djernes M, Schmidt JF: Postdural puncture headache (PDPH): Onset, duration, severity, and associated symptoms. An analysis of 75 consecutive patients with PDPH. Acta Anaesthesiol Scand 1995;39:605–612.

34. Aida S, Taga K, Yamakura T, et al: Headache after attempted epidural block: The role of intrathecal air. Anesthesiology 1998;88:76–81.

35. Reamy BV: Post-epidural headache: how late can it occur? J Am Board Fam Med 2009;22:202–205.

36. Amorim JA, Gomes de Barros MV, Valenca MM: Post-dural (post-lumbar) puncture headache: Risk factors and clinical features. Cephalalgia 2012;32:916–923.

37. Chan TM, Ahmed E, Yentis SM, et al: Postpartum headaches: Summary report of the National Obstetric Anaesthetic Database (NOAD) 1999. Int J Obstet Anesth 2003;12:107–112.

38. Sprung J, Bourke BA, Contreras MG, et al: Perioperative hearing impairment. Anesthesiology 2003;98:241–257.

39. Lybecker H, Moller JT, May O, et al: Incidence and prediction of postdural puncture headache: A prospective study of 1021 spinal anesthesias. Anesth Analg 1990;70:389–394.

40. Wu CL, Rowlingson AJ, Cohen SR, et al: Gender and post-dural puncture headache. Anesthesiology 2006;105:613–618.

41. Angle P, Thompson D, Halpern S, et al: Second stage pushing correlates with headache after unintentional dural puncture in parturients. Can J Anesth 1999;46:861–866.

42. Vallejo MC: Anesthetic management of the morbidly obese parturient. Curr Opin Anaesthesiol 2007;20:175–180.

43. Kuntz KM, Kokmen E, Stevens JC, et al: Post-lumbar puncture headaches: Experience in 501 consecutive procedures. Neurology 1992; 42:1884–1887.

44. Faure E, Moreno R, Thisted R: Incidence of postdural puncture headache in morbidly obese parturients. Reg Anesth 1994;19:361–363.

45. Dodge HS, Ekhator NN, Jefferson-Wilson L, et al: Cigarette smokers have reduced risk for post-dural puncture headache. Pain Physician 2013;16:e25–e30.

46. Hannerz J: Postlumbar puncture headache and its relation to chronic tension-type headache. Headache 1997;37:659–662.

47. van Oosterhout WPJ, van der Plas AA, van Zwet EW, et al: Postdural puncture headache in migraineurs and nonheadache subjects. A prospective study. Neurology 2013;80:941–948.

48. Echevarria M, Caba F, Rodriguez R: The influence of the menstrual cycle in postdural puncture headache. Reg Anesth Pain Med 1998;23: 485–490.

49. Blanche R, Eisenach JC, Tuttle R, et al: Previous wet tap does not reduce success rate of labor epidural analgesia. Anesth Analg 1994;79: 291–294.

50. Halpern S, Preston R: Postdural puncture headache and spinal needle design. Metaanalysis. Anesthesiology 1994;81:1376–1383.

51. Kovanen J, Sulkava R: Duration of postural headache after lumbar puncture: Effect of needle size. Headache 1986;26:224–226.

52. Lambert DH, Hurley RJ, Hertwig L, et al: Role of needle gauge and tip configuration in the production of lumbar puncture headache. Reg Anesth 1997;22:66–72.

53. Reina MA, de Leon-Casasola OA, Lopez A, et al: An in vitro study of dural lesions produced by 25-gauge Quincke and Whitacre needles evaluated by scanning electron microscopy. Reg Anesth Pain Med 2000; 25:393–402.

54. Richman J, Joe E, Cohen S, et al: Bevel direction and postdural puncture headache. A meta-analysis. Neurologist 2006;12:224–228.

55. Reina MA, Dittmann M, Garcia AL, et al: New perspectives in the microscopic structure of human dura mater in the dorsolumbar region. Reg Anesth 1997;22:161–166.

56. Seeberger MD, Kaufmann M, Staender S, et al: Repeated dural punctures increase the incidence of postdural puncture headache. Anesth Analg 1996;82:302–305.

57. De Almeida SM, Shumaker SD, LeBlanc SK, et al: Incidence of postdural puncture headache in research volunteers. Headache 2011;51:1503–1510.

58. Singh S, Chaudry SY, Phelps AL, et al: A 5-year audit of accidental dural punctures, postdural puncture headaches, and failed regional anesthetics at a tertiary-care medical center. TheScientificWorldJournal 2009;9: 715–722.

59. Goldszmidt E, Kern R, Chaput A, et al: The incidence and etiology of postpartum headaches: A prospective cohort study. Can J Anesth 2005; 52:971–977.

60. Aya AGM, Manguin R, Robert C, et al: Increased risk of unintentional dural puncture in night-time obstetric epidural anaesthesia. Can J Anesth 1999;46:665–669.

61. Paech MJ, Whybrow T: The prevention and treatment of post dural puncture headache. ASEAN J Anaesthesiol 2007;8:86–95.

62. Warwick WI, Neal JM: Beyond spinal headache: Prophylaxis and treatment of low-pressure headache syndromes. Reg Anesth Pain Med 2007;32:455–461.

63. Apfel CC, Saxena OS, Cakmakkaya OS, et al: Prevention of postdural puncture headache after accidental dural puncture: A quantitative systematic review. Br J Anaesth 2010;105:255–263.

64. Perlas A: Evidence for the use of ultrasound in neuraxial blocks. Reg Anesth Pain Med 2010;35 (Suppl. 1):S43–S46.

65. Hamzei A, Basiri-Moghadam M, Pasban-Noghabi S: Effect of dexamethasone on incidence of headache after spinal anesthesia in cesarean section. A single blind randomized controlled trial. Saudi Med J 2012;33:948–953.

66. Doroudian MR, Norouzi M, Esmailie M, et al: Dexamethasone in preventing post-dural puncture headache: A randomized, double-blind, placebo-controlled trial. Acta Anaesth Belg 2011;62:143–146.

67. Yousefshahi F, Dahmardeh AR, Khajavi M, et al: Effect of dexamethasone on the frequency of postdural puncture headache after spinal anesthesia for cesarean section: A double-blind randomized clinical trial. Acta Neurol Belg 2012;112:345–350.

68. Basurto Ona X, Uriona Tuma SM, Martinez Garcia L, et al: Drug therapy for preventing post-dural puncture headache. Cochrane Database Syst Rev 2013;(2):CD001792.

69. Al-metwalli RR: Epidural morphine injections for prevention of post dural puncture headache. Anaesthesia 2008;63:847–850.

70. Hakim SM: Cosyntropin for prophylaxis against postdural puncture headache after accidental dural puncture. Anesthesiology 2010;113:413–420.

71. Sadeghi SE, Abdollahifard G, Nasabi NA, et al: Effectiveness of single dose aminopylline administration on prevention of post dural puncture headache in patients who received spinal anesthesia for elective cesarean section. World J Med Sci 2012;7:13–16.

72. Jacobus CH: Does bed rest prevent post-lumbar puncture headache? Ann Emerg Med 2012;59:139–140.

73. Baraz R, Collis R: The management of accidental dural puncture during labor epidural analgesia: A survey of UK practice. Anaesthesia 2005;60: 673–679.

74. Sudlow C, Warlow C: Posture and fluids for preventing postdural puncture headache. Cochrane Database Syst Rev 2002;(2):CD001790.

75. Dakka Y, Warra N, Albadareen RJ, et al: Headache rate and cost of care following lumbar puncture at a single tertiary care hospital. Neurology 2011;77:71–74.

76. Strupp M, Brandt T, Muller A: Incidence of post-lumbar puncture syndrome reduced by reinserting the stylet: A randomized prospective study of 600 patients. J Neurol 1998;245:589–592.

77. Sinikoglu NS, Yeter H, Gumus F, et al: Reinsertion of the stylet does not affect incidence of post dural puncture headaches (PDPH) after spinal anesthesia. Rev Bras Anestesiol 2013;63:188–192.

78. Moore JM: Continuous spinal anesthesia. Am J Ther 2009;16: 289–294.

79. Sadashivaiah J, McClure H: 18-g Tuohy needle can reduce the incidence of severe post dural puncture headache. Anaesthesia 2009;64: 1379–1380.

80. Schier R, Guerra D, Aguilar J, et al: Epidural space identification: A meta-analysis of complications after air versus liquid as the medium for loss of resistance. Anesth Analg 2009;109:2012–2021.

81. Segal S, Arendt KW: A retrospective effectiveness study of loss of resistance to air or saline for identification of the epidural space. Anesth Analg 2010;110:558–563.

82. Norris MC, Leighton BL, DeSimone CA: Needle bevel direction and headache after inadvertent dural puncture. Anesthesiology 1989;70:729–731.

83. Duffy B: Don't turn the needle! Anaesth Intensive Care 1993;21:328–330.

84. Simmons SW, Cyna AM, Dennis AT, et al: Combined spinal-epidural versus epidural analgesia in labour. Cochrane Database Syst Rev 2009;(1):CD003401.

85. Kuczkowski KM, Benumof JL: Decrease in the incidence of post-dural puncture headache: Maintaining CSF volume. Acta Anaesthesiol Scand 2003;47:98–100.

86. Charsley MM, Abram SE: The injection of intrathecal normal saline reduces the severity of postdural puncture headache. Reg Anesth Pain Med 2001;26:301–305.

87. Carter BL, Pasupuleti R: Use of intravenous cosyntropin in the treatment of postdural puncture headache. Anesthesiology 2000;92:272–274.

88. Russell IF: A prospective controlled study of continuous spinal anesthesia versus repeat epidural analgesia after accidental dural puncture in labour. Int J Obstet Anesth 2012;21:7–16.

89. Ayad S, Bemian Y, Narouze S, et al: Subarachnoid catheter placement after wet tap for analgesia in labor: Influence on the risk of headache in obstetric patients. Reg Anesth Pain Med 2003;28:512–515.

90. Heesen M, Klohr S, Rossaint R, et al: Insertion of an intrathecal catheter following accidental dural puncture: A meta-analysis. Int J Obstet Anesth 2013;22:26–30.

91. Newman M, Cyna A: Immediate management of inadvertent dural puncture during insertion of a labour epidural: A survey of Australian obstetric anaesthetists. Anaesth Intensive Care 2008;36:96–101.

92. Stride PC, Cooper GM: Dural taps revisited: A 20-year survey from Birmingham Maternity Hospital. Anaesthesia 1993;48:247–255.

93. Trivedi NS, Eddi D, Shevde K: Headache prevention following accidental dural puncture in obstetric patients. J Clin Anesth 1993;5:42–45.

94. Scavone BM, Wong CA, Sullivan JT, et al: Efficacy of a prophylactic epidural blood patch in preventing post dural puncture headache in parturients after inadvertent dural puncture. Anesthesiology 2004;101:1422–1427.

95. Bradbury CL, Singh SI, Badder SR, et al: Prevention of post-dural puncture headache in parturients: A systematic review and meta-analysis. Acta Anaesthesiol Scand 2013;57:417–430.

96. Agerson AN, Scavone BM: Prophylactic epidural blood patch after unintentional dural puncture for the prevention of postdural puncture headache in parturients. Anesth Analg 2012;115:133–136.

97. Boonmak P, Boonmak S: Epidural blood patching for preventing and treating post-dural puncture headache. Cochrane Database Syst Rev 2010;(1):CD001791.

98. Baysinger CL, Pope JE, Lockhart EM, et al: The management of accidental dural puncture and postdural puncture headache: A North American survey. J Clin Anesth 2011;23:349–360.

99. Leivers D: Total spinal anesthesia following early prophylactic epidural blood patch. Anesthesiology 1990;73:1287–1289.

100. Tobias MD, Pilla MA, Rogers C, et al: Lidocaine inhibits blood coagulation: implications for epidural blood patch. Anesth Analg 1996;82:766–769.

101. Gutsche BB: Lumbar epidural analgesia in obstetrics: Taps and patches. In: Reynolds F (ed): *Epidural and Spinal Blockade in Obstetrics*. Balliere Tindall, 1990, pp 75–106.

102. Naulty JS, Hertwig L, Hunt CO, et al: Influence of local anesthetic solution on postdural puncture headache. Anesthesiology 1990;72:450–454.

103. Santanen U, Rautoma P, Luurila H, et al: Comparison of 27-gauge (0.41-mm) Whitacre and Quincke spinal needles with respect to post-dural puncture headache and non-dural puncture headache. Acta Anaesthesiol Scand 2004;48:474–479.

104. Stella CL, Jodicke CD, How HY, et al: Postpartum headache: is your work-up complete? Am J Obstet Gynecol 2007;196:318.e1–318.e7.

105. Somri M, Teszler CB, Vaida SJ, et al: Postdural puncture headache: An imaging-guided management protocol. Anesth Analg 2003;96:1809–1812.

106. Sharma R, Panda A: Ondansetron-induced headache in a parturient mimicking postdural puncture headache. Can J Anesth 2010;57:187–188.

107. Hurlburt L, Lay C, Fehlings MG, et al: Postpartum workup of postdural puncture headache leads to diagnosis and surgical treatment of thoracic pseudomeningocele: A case report. Can J Anesth 2013;60:294–298.

108. National Institute of Neurological Disorders and Stroke. Meningitis and encephalitis fact sheet. http://www.ninds.nih.gov/disorders/encephalitis_meningitis/detail_encephalitis_meningitis.htm. Accessed June 28, 2013.

109. Machurot PY, Vergnion M, Fraipont V, et al: Intracranial subdural hematoma following spinal anesthesia: Case report and review of the literature. Acta Anaesth Belg 2010;61:63–66.

110. Bleeker CP, Hendriks IM, Booij LHDJ: Postpartum post-dural puncture headache: Is your differential diagnosis complete? Br J Anaesth 2004;93:461–464.

111. Matthys LA, Coppage KH, Lambers DS, et al: Delayed postpartum preeclampsia: An experience of 151 cases. Am J Obstet Gynecol 2004;190:1464–1466.

112. Lockhart EM, Baysinger CL: Intracranial venous thrombosis in the parturient. Anesthesiology 2007;107:652–658.

113. Wittmann M, Dewald D, Urbach H, et al: Sinus venous thrombosis: A differential diagnosis of postpartum headache. Arch Gynecol Obstet 2012;285:93–97.

114. Vanden Eede H, Hoffmann VLH, Vercauteren MP: Post-delivery postural headache: Not always a classical post-dural puncture headache. Acta Anaesthesiol Scand 2007;51:763–765.

115. van Kooten F, Oedit R, Bakker SLM, et al: Epidural blood patch in post dural puncture headache: A randomized, observer-blind, controlled clinical trial. J Neurol Neurosurg Psychiatry 2008;79:553–558.

116. Sharma A, Cheam E: Acupuncture in the management of post-partum headache following neuraxial analgesia. Int J Obstet Anesth 2009;18:417–419.

117. Takmaz SA, Kantekin CU, Kaymak C, et al: Treatment of post-dural puncture headache with bilateral greater occipital nerve block. Headache 2010;50:869–872.

118. Cohen S, Ramos D, Grubb W, et al. Reg Anesth Pain Med 2014;39:563.

119. Basurto Ona X, Martinez Garcia L, Sola I, et al: Drug therapy for treating post-dural puncture headache. Cochrane Database Syst Rev 2011;(8):CD007887.

120. Choi A, Laurito CE, Cummingham FE: Pharmacologic management of postdural puncture headache. Ann Pharmacother 1996;30:831–839.

121. Camann WR, Murray RS, Mushlin PS, et al: Effects of oral caffeine on postdural puncture headache. A double-blind, placebo-controlled trial. Anesth Analg 1990;70:181–184.

122. Halker RB, Demaerschalk BM, Wellik KE, et al: Caffeine for the prevention and treatment of postdural puncture headache: debunking the myth. Neurologist 2007;13:323–327.

123. Connelly NR, Parker RK, Rahimi A, et al: Sumatriptan in patients with postdural puncture headache. Headache 2000;40:316–319.

124. Hakim S, Khan RM, Maroof M, et al: Methylergonovine maleate (methergine) relieves postdural puncture headache in obstetric patients. Acta Obstet Gynecol Scand 2005;84:100.

125. Rucklidge MWM, Yentis SM, Paech MJ, et al: Synacthen Depot for the treatment of postdural puncture headache. Anaesthesia 2004;59:138–141.

126. Noyan Ashraf MA, Sadeghi A, Azarbakht Z, et al: Hydrocortisone in post-dural puncture headache. Middle East J Anesthesiol 2007;19:415–422.

127. Rabiul A, Aminur R, Reza E: Role of very short-term intravenous hydrocortisone in reducing postdural puncture headache. J Anaesthesiol Clin Pharmacol 2012;28:190–193.

128. Wagner Y, Storr F, Cope S: Gabapentin in the treatment of post-dural puncture headache: A case series. Anaesth Intensive Care 2012;40:714–718.

129. Huseyinoglu U, Huseyinoglu N, Hamurtekin E, et al: Efect of pregabalin on post-dural-puncture headache following spinal anesthesia and lumbar puncture. J Clin Neurosci 2011;18:1365–1368.

130. Kroin JS, Nagalla SKS, Buvanendran, et al: The mechanisms of intracranial pressure modulation by epidural blood and other injectates in a postdural puncture rat model. Anesth Analg 2002;95:423–429.

131. Bart AJ, Wheeler AS: Comparison of epidural saline placement and epidural blood placement in the treatment of post-lumbar-puncture headache. Anesthesiology 1978;48:221–223.

132. Liu SK, Chen KB, Wu RSC, et al: Management of postdural puncture headache by epidural saline delivered with a patient-controlled pump—A case report. Acta Anaesthesiol Taiwan 2006;44:227–230.

133. Kara I, Ciftci I, Apiliogullari S, et al: Management of postdural puncture headache with epidural saline patch in a 10-year-old child after inguinal hernia repair: A case report. J Pediatr Surg 2012;47:E55–E57.

134. Vakharia SB, Thomas PS, Rosenbaum AE, et al: Magnetic resonance imaging of cerebrospinal fluid leak and tamponade effect of blood patch in postdural puncture headache. Anesth Analg 1997;84:585–590.

135. Serpell MG, Haldane GJ, Jamieson DR, et al: Prevention of headache after lumbar puncture: Questionnaire survey of neurologists and neurosurgeons in United Kingdom. Br Med J 1998;316:1709–1710.

136. Darvish B, Gupta A, Alahuhta S, et al: Management of accidental dural puncture and post-dural puncture headache after labour: A Nordic survey. Acta Anaesthesiol Scand 2011;55:46–53.

137. Banks S, Paech M, Gurrin L: An audit of epidural blood patch after accidental dural puncture with a Tuohy needle in obstetric patients. Int J Obstet Anesth 2001;10:172–176.

138. Safa-Tisseront V, Thormann F, Malassine P, et al: Effectiveness of epidural blood patch in the management of post-dural puncture headache. Anesthesiology 2001;95:334–339.

139. Sandesc D, Lupei MI, Sirbu C, et al: Conventional treatment or epidural blood patch for the treatment of different etiologies of post dural puncture headache. Acta Anaesth Belg 2005;56:265–269.

140. Vilming ST, Kloster R, Sandvik L: When should an epidural blood patch be performed in postlumbar puncture headache? A theoretical approach based on a cohort of 79 patients. Cephalalgia 2005;25:523–527.

141. Chen LK, Huang CH, Jean WH, et al: Effective epidural blood patch volumes for postdural puncture headache in Taiwanese women. J Formos Med Assoc 2007;106:134–140.

142. Paech MJ, Doherty DA, Christmas T, et al: The volume of blood for epidural blood patch in obstetrics: A randomized, blinded clinical trial. Anesth Analg 2011;113:126–133.

143. Schievink WI: Spontaneous spinal cerebrospinal fluid leaks and intracranial hypotension. JAMA 2006;295:2286–2296.

144. Riley CA, Spiegel JE: Complications following large-volume epidural blood patches for postdural puncture headaches. Lumbar subdural hematoma and arachnoiditis: Initial cause or final effect? J Clin Anesth 2009;21:355–359.

145. Desai MJ, Dave AP, Martin MB: Delayed radicular pain following two large volume epidural blood patches for post-lumbar puncture headache: A case report. Pain Physician 2010;13:257–262.

146. Martin R, Jourdain S, Clairoux M, et al: Duration of decubitus position after epidural blood patch. Can J Anaesth 1994;41:23–25.

147. Jagannathan N, Tetzlaff JE: Epidural blood patch in a Jehovah's Witness patient with post-dural puncture cephalgia. Can J Anaesth 2005;52:113.

148. Janssens E, Aerssens P, Alliet P, et al: Post-dural puncture headaches in children: A literature review. Eur J Pediatr 2003;162:117–121.

149. Kokki M, Sjovall S, Kokki H: Epidural blood patches are effective for postdural puncture headache in pediatrics—A 10-year experience. Pediatr Anesth 2012;22:1205–1210.

150. Waldman SD, Feldstein GS, Allen ML: Cervical epidural blood patch: A safe effective treatment for cervical post-dural puncture headache. Anesth Rev 1987;14:23–24.

151. Bucklin BA, Tinker JH, Smith CV: Clinical dilemma: A patient with postdural puncture headache and acute leukemia. Anesth Analg 1999;88:166–167.

152. Koeva V, Bar-Or A, Gendron D, et al: Epidural blood patch in a patient with multiple sclerosis: Is it safe? Can J Anaesth 2013;60:479–483.

153. Tom DJ, Gulevich SJ, Shapiro HM, et al: Epidural blood patch in the HIV-positive patient. Anesthesiology 1992;76:943–947.

154. Martin DP, Bergman BD, Berger IH: Epidural blood patch and acute varicella. Anesth Analg 2004;99:1760–1762.

155. Abouleish E, de la Vega S, Blendinger I, et al: Long-term follow-up of epidural blood patch. Anesth Analg 1975;54:459–463.

156. Andrews PJD, Ackerman WE, Juneja M, et al: Transient bradycardia associated with extradural blood patch after inadvertent dural puncture in parturients. Br J Anaesth 1992;69:401–403.

157. Hebl JR, Horlocker TT, Chantigian RC, et al: Epidural anesthesia and analgesia are not impaired after dural puncture with or without epidural blood patch. Anesth Analg 1999;89:390–394.

158. Collier CB: Blood patches may cause scarring in the epidural space: Two case reports. Int J Obstet Anesth 2011;20:347–351.

159. Vassal O, Baud MC, Bolandard F, et al: Epidural injection of hydroxyethyl starch in the management of postdural puncture headache. Int J Obstet Anesth 2013;22:153–155.

160. Williams EJ, Beaulieu P, Fawcett WJ, et al: Efficacy of epidural blood patch in the obstetric population. Int J Obstet Anesth 1999;8: 105–109.

161. Sadashivaiah J: 18-G Tuohy needle can reduce the incidence of severe post dural puncture headache. Anaesthesia 2009;64:1379–1380.

162. Ho KY, Gan TJ: Management of persistent post-dural puncture headache after repeated epidural blood patch. Acta Anaesthesiol Scand 2007;51:633–636.

163. Sullivan FM, Swan IRC, Donnan PT, et al: Early treatment with prednisone or acyclovir in Bell's palsy. N Engl J Med 2007;357: 1598–1607.

164. Choi PTL, Galinski SE, Lucas S, et al: Examining the evidence in anesthesia literature: A survey and evaluation of obstetrical post-dural puncture headache reports. Can J Anaesth 2002;49:49–56.

CHAPTER 27

ULTRASOUND-GUIDED NERVE BLOCKS

CHAPTER 28

Physics of Ultrasound

Daquan Xu

INTRODUCTION

Ultrasound application allows for noninvasive visualization of tissue structures. Real-time ultrasound images are integrated images resulting from reflection of organ surfaces and scattering within heterogeneous tissues. Ultrasound scanning is an interactive procedure involving the operator, patient, and ultrasound instruments. Although the physics behind ultrasound generation, propagation, detection, and transformation into practical information is rather complex, its clinical application is much simpler. Because ultrasound imaging has improved tremendously over last decade, it can provide anesthesiologists opportunity to directly visualize target nerve and relevant anatomical structures. Ultrasound-guided nerve block is a critical growth area for new applications of ultrasound technology and become an essential part of regional anesthesia. Understanding the basic ultrasound physics presented in this chapter will be helpful for anesthesiologists to appropriately select the transducer, to set the ultrasound system, and then to obtain a pleasing imaging.

HISTORY OF ULTRASOUND

In 1880, French physicists Pierre Curie and his elder brother, Paul-Jacques Curie, discovered the piezoelectric effect in certain crystals.[1] Paul Langevin, a student of Pierre Curie, developed piezoelectric materials, which can generate and receive mechanical vibrations with high frequency (therefore *ultra*sound).[2] During World War I, ultrasound was introduced in the navy as a means to detect enemy submarines.[3] In the medical field,

however, ultrasound was initially used for therapeutic rather than diagnostic purposes. In the late 1920s, Paul Langevin discovered that high-power ultrasound could generate heat in bone and disrupt animal tissues.[4] As a result, throughout the early 1950s ultrasound was used to treat patients with Ménière disease, Parkinson disease, and rheumatic arthritis.[5]

Diagnostic applications of ultrasound began through the collaboration of physicians and sonar (sound navigation ranging) engineers. In 1942, Karl Dussik, a neuropsychiatrist, and his brother, Friederich Dussik, a physicist, described ultrasound as a medical diagnostic tool to visualize neoplastic tissues in the brain and the cerebral ventricles.[6,7] However, limitations of ultrasound instrumentation at the time prevented further development of clinical applications until the mid-1960s. The real-time B-scanner was developed in 1965 and was first introduced in obstetrics.[8,9] In 1976, the first ultrasound machines coupled with Doppler measurements were commercially available.[10]

With regard to regional anesthesia, as early as 1978, La Grange and his colleagues were the first anesthesiologists to publish a case series report of ultrasound application for peripheral nerve blockade.[11] They simply used a Doppler transducer to locate the subclavian artery and performed supraclavicular brachial plexus block in 61 patients (Figures 28–1A and 28–1B). Reportedly, Doppler guidance led to a high block success rate (98%) and absence of complications such as pneumothorax, phrenic nerve palsy, hematoma, convulsion, recurrent laryngeal nerve block, and spinal anesthesia. In 1989, Ting and Sivagnanaratnam reported the use of B-mode ultrasonography to demonstrate the anatomy of the axilla and to observe the spread of local anesthetics during axillary brachial plexus block.[12]

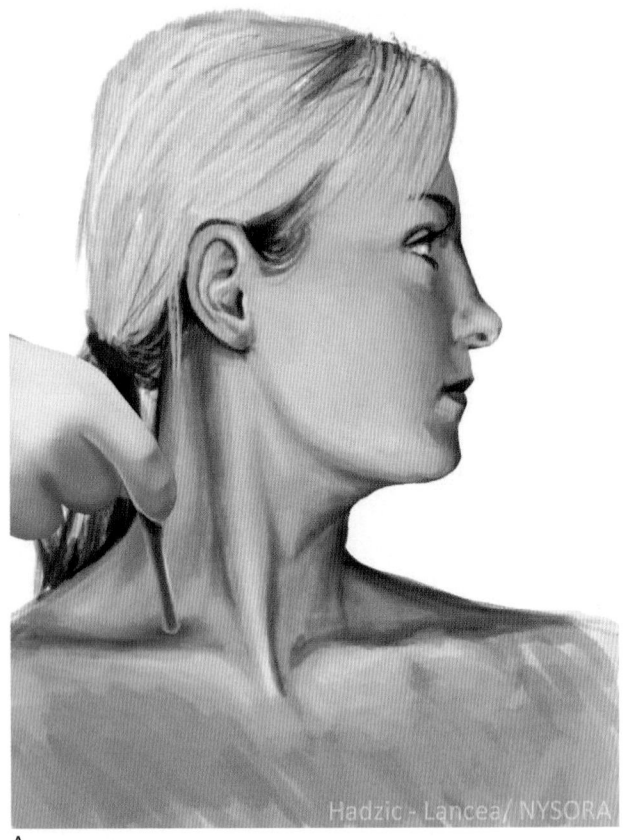
A

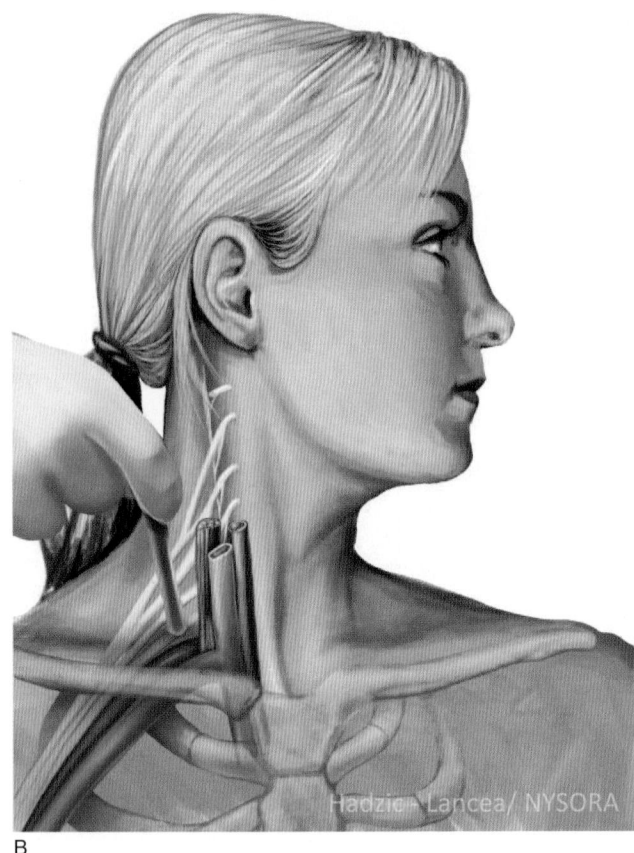
B

FIGURE 28–1. A: Early application of Doppler ultrasound by LaGrange to perform supraclavicular brachial block. **B:** Relationship of the brachial plexus of nerves and the subclavian artery.

In 1994, Stephan Kapral and colleagues systematically explored brachial plexus with B-mode ultrasound. Since that time, multiple teams worldwide have worked tirelessly to define and improve the application of ultrasound imaging in regional anesthesia.[13] Ultrasound-guided nerve blockade is currently used routinely in the practice of regional anesthesia in many centers worldwide.

Here is a summary of ultrasound quick facts:

- 1880: Pierre and Jacques Curie discovered the piezoelectric effect in crystals.
- 1915: Ultrasound was used by the navy for detecting submarines.
- 1920s: Paul Langevin discovered that high-power ultrasound can generate heat in osseous tissues and disrupt animal tissues.
- 1942: The Dussik brothers described ultrasound use as a diagnostic tool.
- 1950s: Ultrasound was used to treat patients with Ménière disease, Parkinson disease, and rheumatic arthritis.
- 1965: The real-time B-scan was developed and was introduced in obstetrics.
- 1978: La Grange published the first case series of ultrasound application for placement of needles for nerve blocks.
- 1989: Ting and Sivagnanaratnam used ultrasonography to demonstrate the anatomy of the axilla and to observe the spread of local anesthetics during axillary block.
- 1994: Steven Kapral and colleagues explored brachial plexus blockade using B-mode ultrasound.

Definition of Ultrasound

Sound travels as a mechanical longitudinal wave in which back-and-forth particle motion is parallel to the direction of wave travel. Ultrasound is high-frequency sound and refers to mechanical vibrations above 20 kHz. Human ears can hear sounds with frequencies between 20 Hz and 20 kHz. Elephants can generate and detect sound with frequencies less than 20 Hz for long-distance communication; bats and dolphins produce sounds in the range of 20 to 100 kHz for precise navigation (Figures 28–2A and 28–2B). Ultrasound frequencies commonly used for medical diagnosis are between 2 and 15 MHz. However, sounds with frequencies above 100 kHz do not occur naturally; only human-developed devices can both generate and detect these frequencies, or ultrasounds.

Piezoelectric Effect

Ultrasound waves can be generated by material with a piezoelectric effect. The piezoelectric effect is a phenomenon exhibited by the generation of an electric charge in response to a mechanical force (squeeze or stretch) applied on certain materials. Conversely, mechanical deformation can be produced when an electric field is applied to such material, also known as the piezoelectric effect (Figure 28–3). Both natural and human-made materials, including quartz crystals and ceramic materials, can demonstrate piezoelectric properties. Recently, lead zirconate titanate has been used as piezoelectric material for

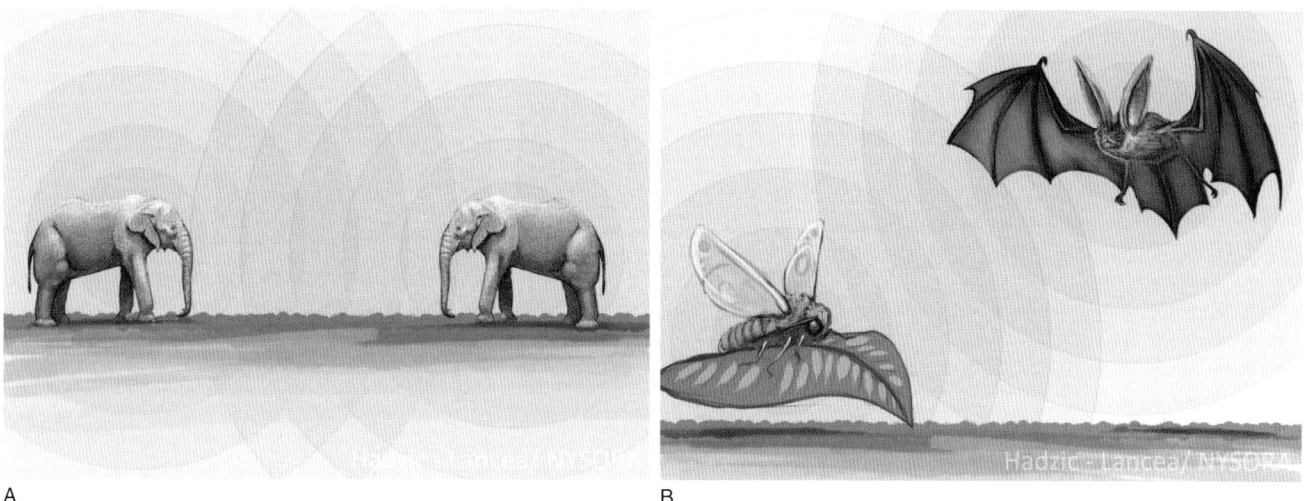

A B

FIGURE 28–2. A: Elephants can generate and detect the sound of frequencies less than 20 Hz for long-distance communication. **B:** Bats and dolphins produce sounds in the range of 20–100 kHz for navigation and spatial orientation.

medical imaging. Lead-free piezoelectric materials are also under development. Individual piezoelectric materials produce a small amount of energy. However, by stacking piezoelectric elements into layers in a transducer, the transducer can convert electric energy into mechanical oscillations more efficiently. These mechanical oscillations are then converted into electric energy.

Ultrasound Terminology

Period is the time for a sound wave to complete one cycle; the period unit of measure is the microsecond (μs).

Wavelength is the length of space over which one cycle occurs; it is equal to the travel distance from the beginning to the end of one cycle.

Frequency is the number of cycles repeated per second and measured in hertz (Hz).

Acoustic velocity is the speed at which a sound wave travels through a medium. It is equal to the frequency times the wavelength. Speed c is determined by the density ρ and stiffness κ of the medium ($c = (\kappa/\rho)^{1/2}$). *Density* is the concentration of a medium. *Stiffness* is the resistance of a material to compression. Propagation speed increases if the stiffness is increased or the density is decreased.

The average propagation speed in soft tissues is 1540 m/s (ranges from 1400 to 1640 m/s). However, ultrasound cannot penetrate lung or bone tissues.

Acoustic impedance z is the degree of difficulty demonstrated by a sound wave being transmitted through a medium; it is equal to density ρ multiplied by acoustic velocity c ($z = \rho c$). It increases if the propagation speed or the density of the medium is increased.

Attenuation coefficient is the parameter used to estimate the decrement of ultrasound amplitude in certain media as a function of ultrasound frequency. The attenuation coefficient increases with increasing frequency; therefore, a practical consequence of attenuation is that the penetration decreases as frequency increases (Figure 28–4).

Ultrasound waves have a self-focusing effect, which refers to the natural narrowing of the ultrasound beam at a certain travel distance in the ultrasonic field. It is a transition level between *near field* and *far field*. The beam width at the transition level is equal to half the diameter of the transducer. At the distance of two times the near-field length, the beam width reaches the transducer diameter. The self-focusing effect amplifies ultrasound signals by increasing acoustic pressure.

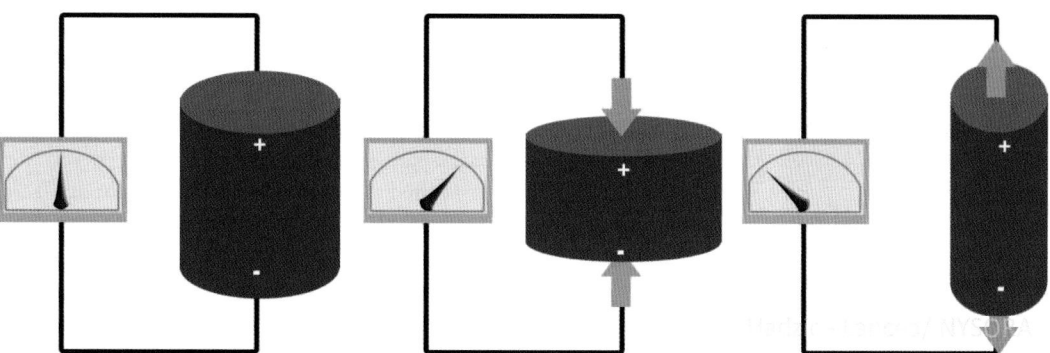

FIGURE 28–3. The piezoelectric effect. Mechanical deformation and consequent oscillation caused by an electrical field applied to certain material can produce a sound of high frequency.

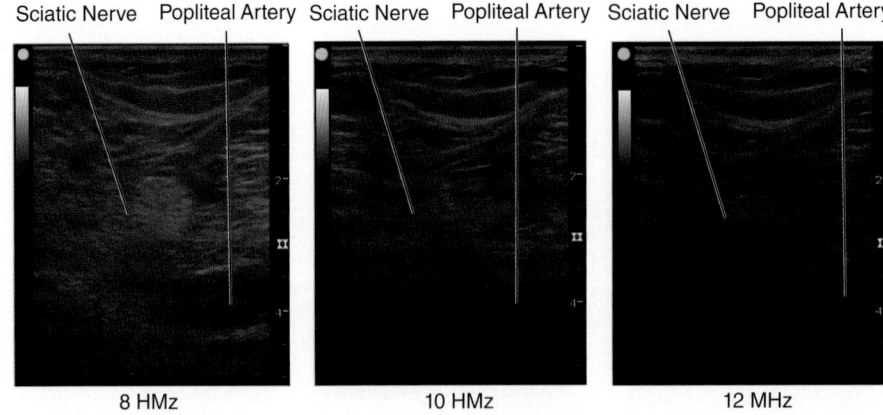

Sciatic Nerve   Popliteal Artery   Sciatic Nerve   Popliteal Artery   Sciatic Nerve   Popliteal Artery

8 HMz   10 HMz   12 MHz

FIGURE 28–4. The ultrasound amplitude decreases in certain media as a function of ultrasound frequency, a phenomenon known as the attenuation coefficient. (Adapted with permission from Hadzic A: *Hadzic's Peripheral Nerve Blocks and Anatomy for Ultrasound-Guided Regional Anesthesia*, 2nd ed. New York: McGraw-Hill, Inc; 2011.)

In ultrasound imaging, there are two aspects of spatial resolution: axial and lateral. *Axial resolution* is the minimum separation of above-below planes along the beam axis. It is determined by spatial pulse length, which is equal to the product of wavelength and the number of cycles within a pulse. It can be presented in the following formula:

$$\text{Axial resolution} = \text{Wavelength } \lambda \times \text{Number of cycles}$$
$$\text{per pulse } n \div 2$$

The number of cycles within a pulse is determined by the damping characteristics of the transducer. The number of cycles within a pulse is usually set between 2 and 4 by the manufacturer of the ultrasound machines. As an example, if a 2-MHz ultrasound transducer is theoretically used to do the scanning, the axial resolution would be between 0.8 and 1.6 mm, making it impossible to visualize a 21-gauge needle. For a constant acoustic velocity, higher-frequency ultrasound can detect smaller objects and provide an image with better resolution. The axial resolution of current ultrasound systems is between 0.05 and 0.5 mm. Figure 28–5 shows images at different resolutions when a 0.5-mm diameter object is visualized with three different frequency settings.

Lateral resolution is another parameter of sharpness to describe the minimum side-by-side distance between two objects. It is determined by both ultrasound frequency and beam width. The higher frequencies have narrower focus and provide better axial and lateral resolution. Lateral resolution can also be improved by adjusting focus to reduce the beam width.

Temporal resolution is also important for observing a moving object such as blood vessels and heart. Like a movie or cartoon video, the human eye requires that the image be updated at a rate of approximately 25 times a second or higher for an ultrasound image to appear continuous. However, imaging resolution will be compromised by increasing the frame rate. Optimizing the ratio of resolution to the frame rate is essential for providing the best possible image.

INTERACTIONS OF ULTRASOUND WITH TISSUES

As the ultrasound wave travels through tissues, it is subject to a number of interactions. The most important features are as follows:

- Reflection
- Scatter
- Absorption

When ultrasound encounters boundaries between different media, part of the ultrasound is reflected and the other part is transmitted. The reflected and transmitted directions are given by the reflection angle θ_r and transmission angle θ_t, respectively (Figure 28–6).

Reflection of sound waves is similar to optical reflection. Some of its energy is sent back into the medium from which it came. In a true reflection, the reflection angle θ_r must equal the incidence angle θ_i. The strength of the reflection from an interface is variable and depends on the difference of impedances

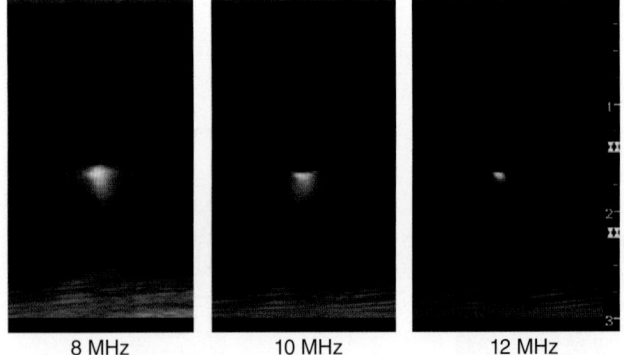

8 MHz   10 MHz   12 MHz

FIGURE 28–5. Ultrasound frequency affects the resolution of the imaged object. Resolution can be improved by increasing frequency and reducing the beam width by focusing. (Reproduced with permission from Hadzic A: *Hadzic's Peripheral Nerve Blocks and Anatomy for Ultrasound-Guided Regional Anesthesia*, 2nd ed. New York: McGraw-Hill, Inc; 2011.)

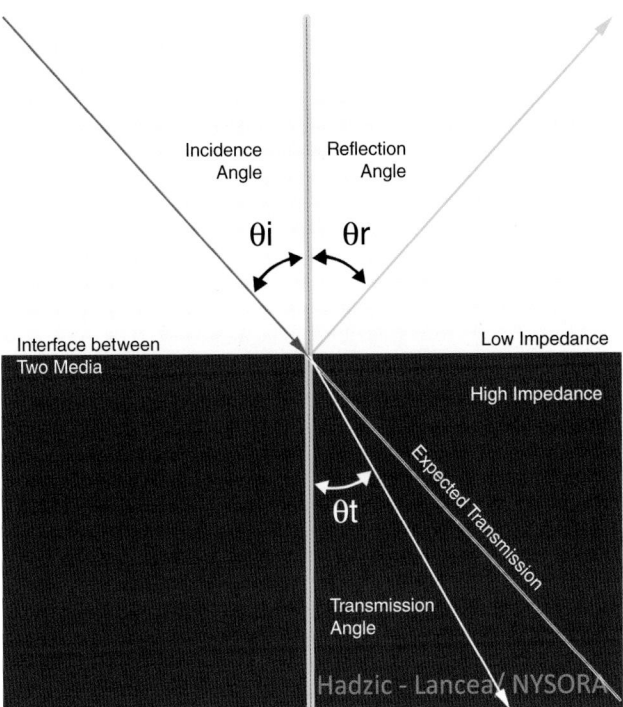

FIGURE 28-6. The interaction of ultrasound waves through the media in which they travel is complex. When ultrasound encounters boundaries between different media, part of the ultrasound is reflected and part is transmitted. The reflected and transmitted directions depend on the respective angles of reflection and transmission. (Adapted with permission from Hadzic A: *Hadzic's Peripheral Nerve Blocks and Anatomy for Ultrasound-Guided Regional Anesthesia*, 2nd ed. New York: McGraw-Hill, Inc; 2011.)

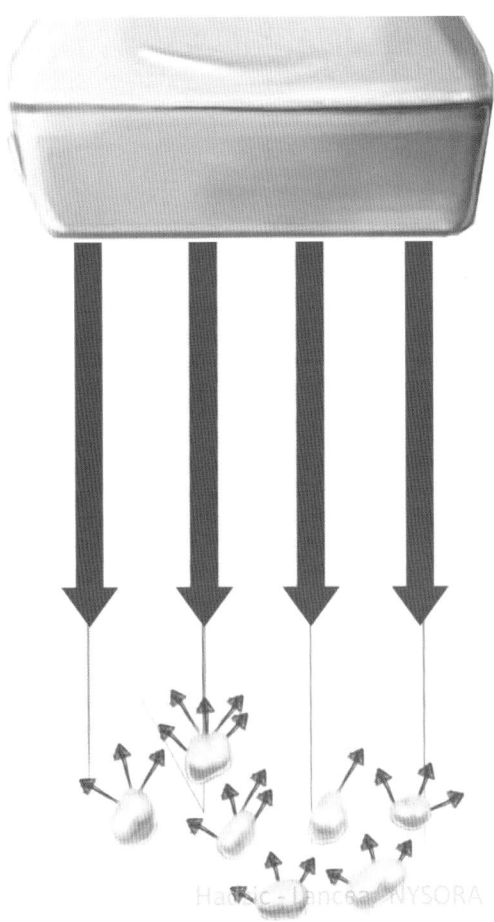

FIGURE 28-7. Scattering is the redirection of ultrasound in any direction caused by rough surfaces or by heterogeneous media. (Adapted with permission from Hadzic A: *Hadzic's Peripheral Nerve Blocks and Anatomy for Ultrasound-Guided Regional Anesthesia*, 2nd ed. New York: McGraw-Hill, Inc; 2011.)

between two affinitive media and the incident angle at the boundary. If the media impedances are equal, there is no reflection (no echo). If there is a significant difference between media impedances, there will be nearly complete reflection. For example, an interface between soft tissues and either lung or bone involves a considerable change in acoustic impedance and creates strong echoes. This reflection intensity is also highly angle dependent. In practical terms, it means that the ultrasound transducer must be placed perpendicular to the target nerve to visualize it clearly. A change in sound direction when crossing the boundary between two media is called *refraction*. If the propagation speed through the second medium is slower than that through the first medium, the refraction angle is smaller than the incident angle. Refraction can cause the artifact that occurs beneath large vessels on the image.

During ultrasound scanning, a coupling medium must be used between the transducer and the skin to displace air from the transducer-skin interface. A variety of gels and oils are applied for this purpose. Moreover, they can act as lubricants, making a smooth scanning performance possible. Most scanned interfaces are somewhat irregular and curved. If the boundary dimensions are significantly less than the wavelength or not smooth, the reflected waves will be diffused.

Scattering is the redirection of sound in any directions by rough surfaces or by heterogeneous media (Figure 28–7).

Normally, scattering intensity is much less than mirror-like reflection intensities and is relatively independent of the direction of the incident sound wave; therefore, the visualization of the target nerve is not significantly influenced by other nearby scattering.

Absorption is defined as the direct conversion of the sound energy into heat. In other words, ultrasound scanning generates heat in the tissue. Higher frequencies are absorbed at a greater rate than lower frequencies. However, a higher scanning frequency gives better axial resolution. If the ultrasound penetration is not sufficient to visualize the structures of interest, a lower frequency is selected to increase the penetration. The use of longer wavelengths (lower frequency) results in lower resolution because the resolution of ultrasound imaging is proportional to the wavelength of the imaging wave. Frequencies between 6 and 12 MHz typically yield adequate resolution for imaging in peripheral nerve blockade, whereas frequencies between 2 and 5 MHz are usually needed for imaging of neuraxial structures. Frequencies of less than 2 MHz or higher than 15 MHz are rarely used because of insufficient resolution or the insufficient penetration depth in most clinical applications.

ULTRASOUND IMAGE MODES

A-Mode

The A-mode is the oldest ultrasound technique and was invented in 1930.[14] The transducer sends a single pulse of ultrasound into the medium. Consequently, a one-dimensional simplest ultrasound image is created on which a series of vertical peaks is generated after ultrasound beams encounter the boundary of the different tissue. The distance between the echoed spikes (Figure 28–8) can be calculated by dividing the speed of ultrasound in the tissue (1540 m/s) by half the elapsed time, but it provides little information on the spatial relationship of imaged structures. Therefore, A-mode ultrasound is not applicable in regional anesthesia.

B-Mode

The B-mode is a two-dimensional (2D) image of the area that is simultaneously scanned by a linear array of 100–300 piezoelectric elements rather than a single one as in A-mode (Figure 28–9). The amplitude of the echo from a series of A-scans is converted into dots of different brightness in B-mode imaging. The horizontal and vertical directions represent real distances in tissue, whereas the intensity of the grayscale indicates echo strength (Figure 28–10). B-mode can provide an image of a cross section through the area of interest, and it is the primary mode currently used in regional anesthesia.

Doppler Mode

The Doppler effect is based on the work of Austrian physicist Johann Christian Doppler.[15] The term describes a change in the frequency or wavelength of a sound wave resulting from relative motion between the sound source and the sound receiver. In other words, at a stationary position, the sound frequency is constant. If the sound source moves toward the sound receiver,

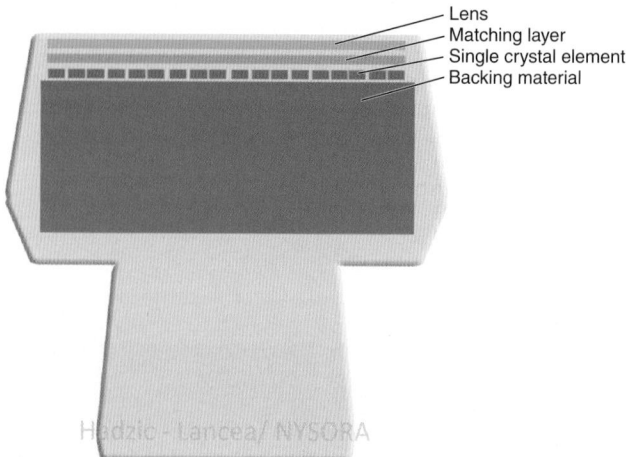

FIGURE 28–9. The B-mode transducer incorporates numeric piezoelectric elements that are electrically connected in parallel.

the sound waves have to be squeezed, and a higher-pitch sound occurs (positive Doppler shift); if the sound source moves away from the receiver, the sound waves have to be stretched, and the received sound has a lower pitch (negative Doppler shift) (Figure 28–11). The magnitude of Doppler shift depends on the incident angle between the directions of emitted ultrasound beam and moving reflectors. With a 90° angle there is no Doppler shift. If the angle is 0° or 180°, the largest Doppler shift can be detected. In medical settings, the Doppler shifts usually fall in the audible range.

Color Doppler produces a color-coded map of Doppler shifts superimposed onto a B-mode ultrasound image. Blood flow direction depends on whether the motion is toward or away from the transducer. Selected by convention, red and blue colors provide information about the direction and velocity of the blood flow. According to the color map (color bar) in the upper left-hand corner of the figure (Figure 28–12), the red color on the top of the bar denotes the flow coming toward the ultrasound probe, and the blue color on the bottom of the bar indicates the flow away from the probe.

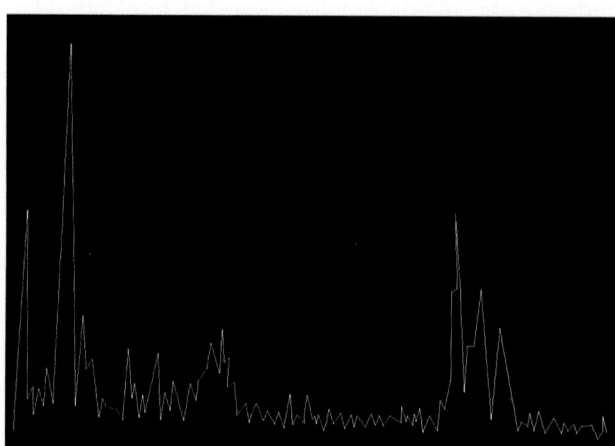

FIGURE 28–8. The A-mode of ultrasound consists of a one-dimensional ultrasound image displayed as a series of vertical peaks corresponding to the depth of structures the ultrasound encounters in different tissues. (Reproduced with permission from Hadzic A: *Hadzic's Peripheral Nerve Blocks and Anatomy for Ultrasound-Guided Regional Anesthesia*, 2nd ed. New York: McGraw-Hill, Inc; 2011.)

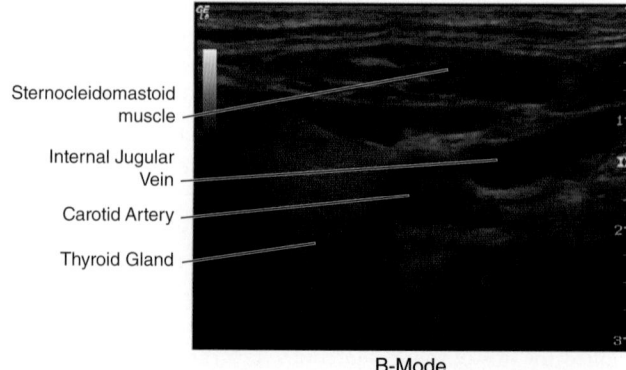

FIGURE 28–10. An example of B-mode imaging. The horizontal and vertical directions represent distances and tissues, whereas the intensity of the grayscale indicates echo strength. (Adapted with permission from Hadzic A: *Hadzic's Peripheral Nerve Blocks and Anatomy for Ultrasound-Guided Regional Anesthesia*, 2nd ed. New York: McGraw-Hill, Inc; 2011.)

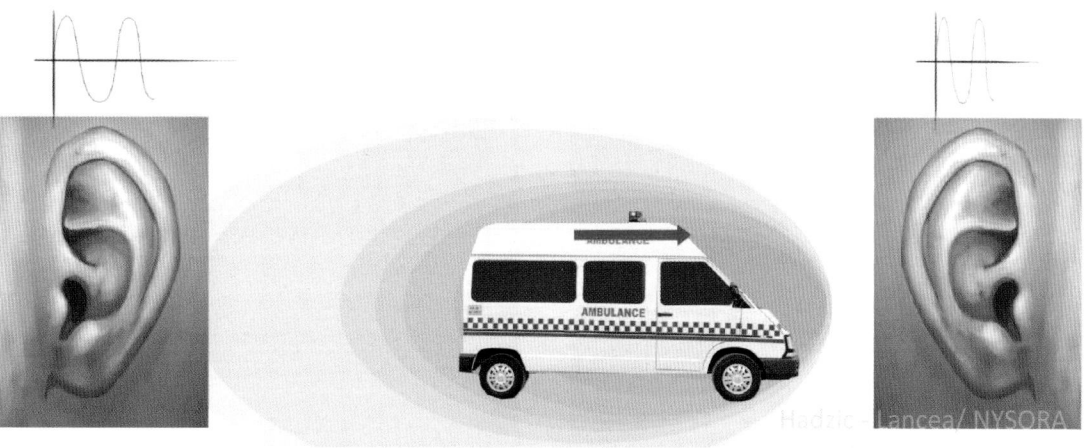

FIGURE 28–11. The Doppler effect. When a sound source moves away from the receiver, the received sound has a lower pitch and vice versa. (Adapted with permission from Hadzic A: *Hadzic's Peripheral Nerve Blocks and Anatomy for Ultrasound-Guided Regional Anesthesia*, 2nd ed. New York: McGraw-Hill, Inc; 2011.)

In ultrasound-guided peripheral nerve blocks, color Doppler mode is used to detect the presence and nature of the blood vessels (artery vs. vein) in the area of interest. When the direction of the ultrasound beam changes, the color of the arterial flow switches from blue to red, or vice versa, depending on the convention used (Figures 28–13, 28–14A, 28–14B, and 28–14C). Power Doppler is up to five times more sensitive in detecting blood flow than color Doppler, and it is less dependent on the scanning angle. Thus, power Doppler can be used to identify the smaller blood vessels more reliably. The drawback is that power Doppler does not provide any information on the direction and speed of blood flow (Figure 28–15).

M-Mode

A single beam in an ultrasound scan can be used to produce a picture with a motion signal, where movement of a structure such as a heart valve can be depicted in a wave-like manner. M-mode is used extensively in cardiac and fetal cardiac imaging; however, its present use in regional anesthesia is negligible (Figure 28–16).

ULTRASOUND INSTRUMENTS

Ultrasound machines convert the echoes received by the transducer into visible dots, which form the anatomic image on an ultrasound screen. The brightness of each dot corresponds to the echo strength, producing what is known as a grayscale image.

Two types of scan transducers are used in regional anesthesia: linear and curved. A linear transducer can produce parallel scan lines and a rectangular display, called a linear scan, whereas a curved transducer yields a curvilinear scan and an arc-shaped image (Figures 28–17A and 28–17B). In clinical scanning, even a very thin layer of air between the transducer and skin

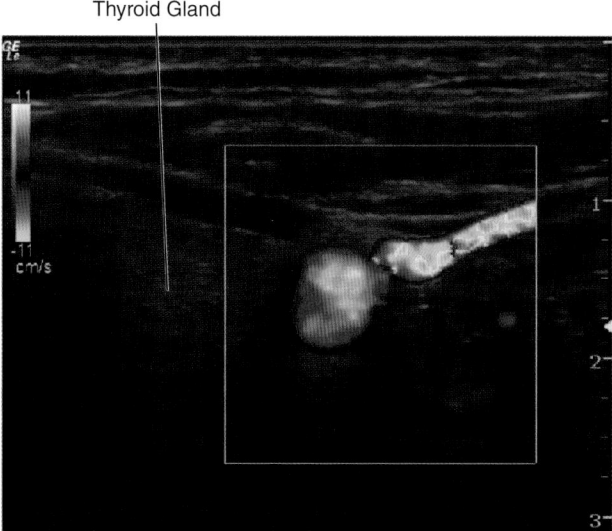

Color Doppler

FIGURE 28–12. Color Doppler produces a color-coded map of Doppler shapes superimposed onto a B-mode ultrasound image. Selected by convention, red and blue colors provide information about the direction and velocity of the blood flow. (Adapted with permission from Hadzic A: *Hadzic's Peripheral Nerve Blocks and Anatomy for Ultrasound-Guided Regional Anesthesia*, 2nd ed. New York: McGraw-Hill, Inc; 2011.)

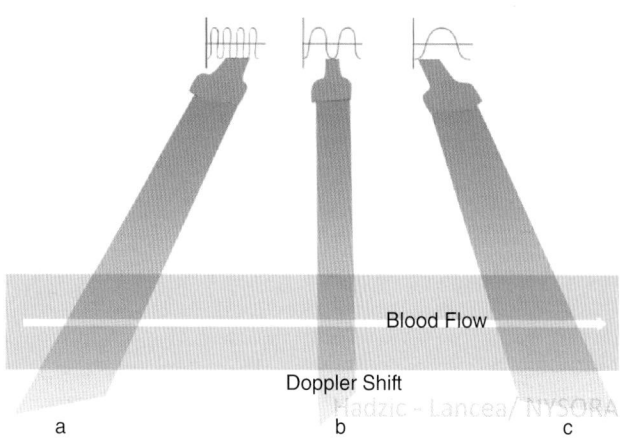

FIGURE 28–13. Color Doppler mode is used to detect the direction of the blood vessel.

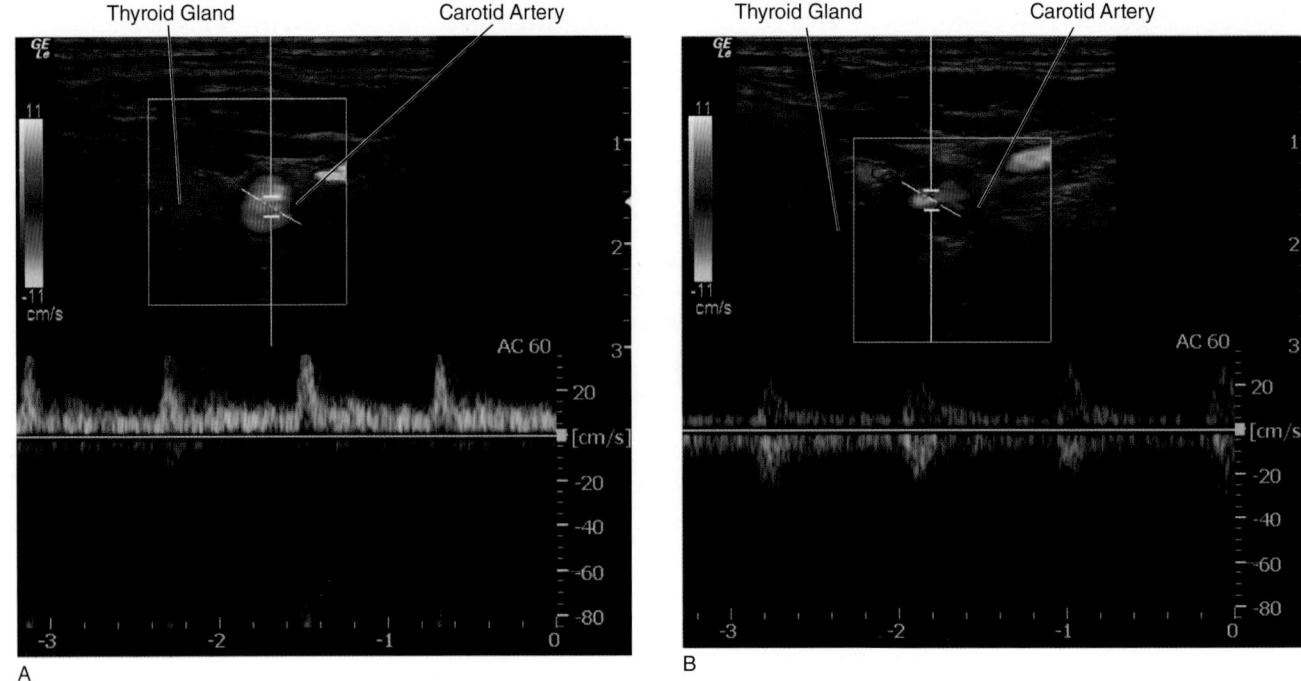

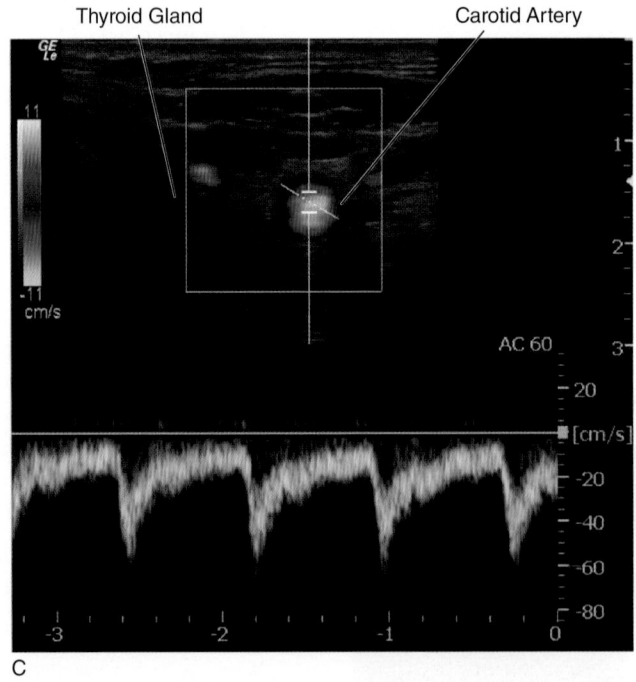

FIGURE 28–14. A: Carotid artery displays red color when the blood flows toward the transducer. **B:** Carotid artery displays ambiguous color at a 90° Doppler angle; the equal waveform can be seen on both sides of the baseline. **C:** Carotid artery displays blue color when the blood flows away from the transducer.

may reflect virtually all the ultrasound, hindering any penetration into the tissue. Therefore, a coupling medium, usually an aqueous gel, is applied between surfaces of the transducer and skin to eliminate the air layer. The ultrasound machines currently used in regional anesthesia provide a 2D image, or "slice." Machines capable of producing three-dimensional (3D) images have recently been developed. Theoretically, 3D imaging should help in understanding the relationship of anatomic structures and spread of local anesthetics. There are three major types of 3D ultrasound imaging: (1) Freehand 3D is based on a set of 2D cross-sectional ultrasound images acquired from a sonographer sweeping the transducer over a region of interest (Figures 28–18A and 28–18B). (2) Volume 3D provides 3D volumetric images using a dedicated 3D transducer. The transducer elements automatically sweep through the region of interest during the scanning; the sonographer is not required to

Power Doppler

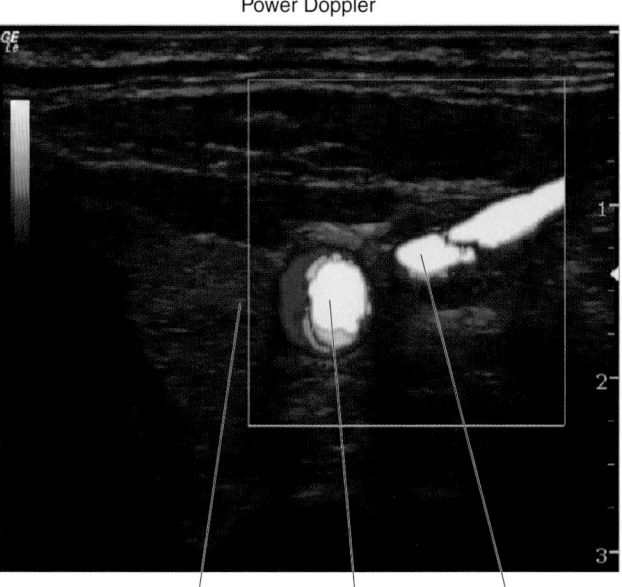

Thyroid Gland   Artery   Vein

FIGURE 28–15. Although the power Doppler may be useful in identifying smaller blood vessels, the drawback is that it does not provide information on the direction and speed of blood flow. (Adapted with permission from Hadzic A: *Hadzic's Peripheral Nerve Blocks and Anatomy for Ultrasound-Guided Regional Anesthesia*, 2nd ed. New York: McGraw-Hill, Inc; 2011.)

A

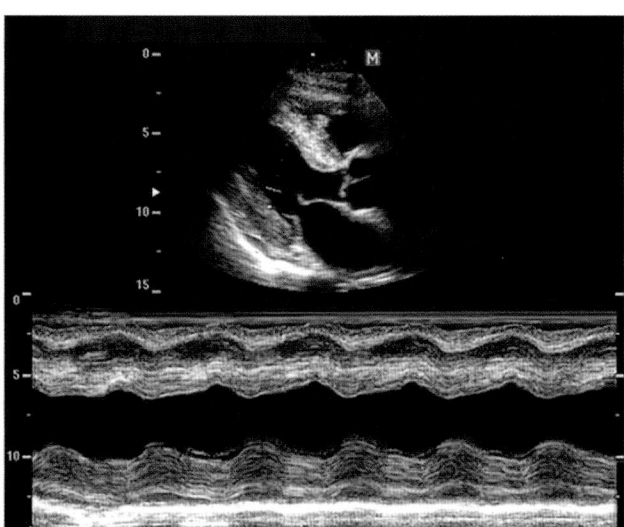

FIGURE 28–16. M-mode consists of a single beam used to produce an image with a motion signal. Movement of a structure can be depicted in a wavelike matter. (Reproduced with permission from Hadzic A: *Hadzic's Peripheral Nerve Blocks and Anatomy for Ultrasound-Guided Regional Anesthesia*, 2nd ed. New York: McGraw-Hill, Inc; 2011.)

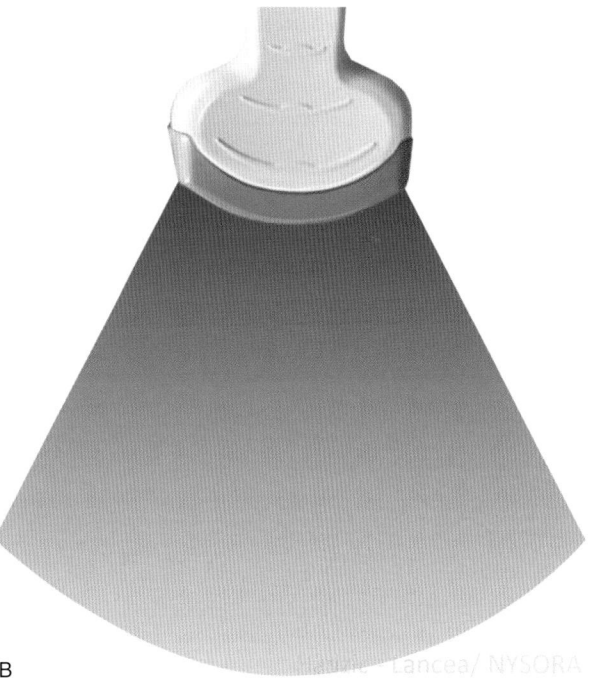

B

FIGURE 28–17. A: Rectangular scan field given by linear transducer. **B:** Arc-shaped scan field given by curved transducer. (Adapted with permission from Hadzic A: *Hadzic's Peripheral Nerve Blocks and Anatomy for Ultrasound-Guided Regional Anesthesia*, 2nd ed. New York: McGraw-Hill, Inc; 2011.)

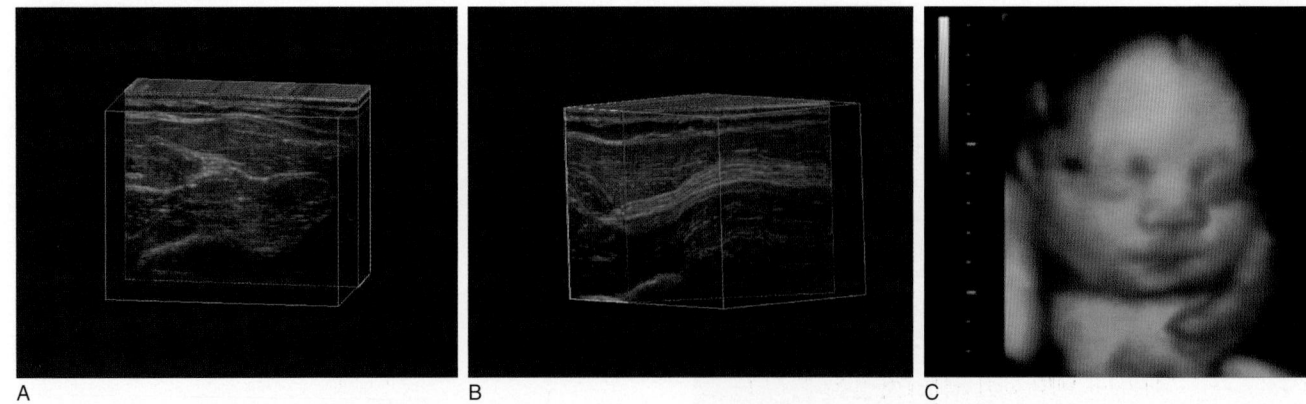

A   B   C

FIGURE 28–18. A: Freehand 3D imaging. A linear transducer produces parallel scan lines and a rectangular display; linear scan. **B:** Freehand 3D imaging. A curved "phase array" transducer results in a curvilinear scan and an arch-shaped image. **C:** Fetal face viewed by volume 3D imaging. (Reproduced with permission from Hadzic A: *Hadzic's Peripheral Nerve Blocks and Anatomy for Ultrasound-Guided Regional Anesthesia*, 2nd ed. New York: McGraw-Hill, Inc; 2011.)

perform hand motions (Figure 28–18C). (3) Real-time 3D takes multiple images at different angles, allowing the sonographer to see the 3D model moving in real time. However, typical spatial resolution of 3D imaging is about 0.34–0.5 mm. At present, 3D imaging systems still lack the resolution and simplicity of 2D images, so their practical use in regional anesthesia is limited.

TIME-GAIN COMPENSATION

The echoes exhibit a steady decline in amplitude with increasing depth. This occurs for two reasons: First, each successive reflection removes a certain amount of energy from the pulse, decreasing the generation of later echoes. Second, tissue absorbs ultrasound, so there is a steady loss of energy as the ultrasound pulse travels through the tissues. This can be corrected by manipulating time-gain compensation (TGC) and compression functions. *Gain* is the ratio of output to input electric power; it controls the brightness of the image. The gain is usually measured in decibels (dB). Increasing the gain amplifies not only the returning signals, but also the background noise within the system in the same manner. TGC is time-dependent amplification. TGC function can be used to increase the amplitude of incoming signals from various tissue depths.

The layout of the TGC controls varies from one machine to another. A popular design is a set of slider knobs. Each knob in the slider set controls the gain for a specific depth, which allows for a well-balanced gain scale on the image (Figures 28–19A, 28–19B, and 28–19C).

Amplification is the conversion of the small voltages received from the transducer into larger ones that are suitable for further processing and storage. There are two amplification processes considered to increase the magnitude of ultrasound echoes: linear and nonlinear amplification. Currently, the ultrasonic imaging system with linear amplifiers is commonly used in medical diagnostic applications. However, strength of echoes attenuates exponentially as the distance between the transducer and the reflector increases. Ultrasonic imaging instruments equipped with logarithmic amplifiers can display echo signals with a wider dynamic range than a linear amplifier and remarkably improve the sensitivity for a small magnitude of echoes on the screen.

Dynamic range is the range of amplitudes from largest to the smallest echo signals that an ultrasound system can detect. The wider/higher dynamic range presents a larger number of grayscale levels, and it creates a softer image; the image with a narrower/lower dynamic range appears with more contrast (Figures 28–20A and 28–20B). Dynamic range less than 50 dB or greater than 100 dB is probably too low or too high in terms of visualization of peripheral nerve. *Compression* is the process of decreasing the differences between the smallest and largest echo-voltage amplitudes; the optimal compression is between 2 and 4 for a maximal scale equal to 6.

FOCUSING

As previously discussed, it is common to use electronic means to narrow the width of the beam at some depth and achieve a focusing effect similar to that obtained using a convex lens (Figure 28–21). There are two types of focusing: annular and linear. These are illustrated in Figures 28–22A and 28–22B, respectively.

Adjusting focus improves the spatial resolution on the plane of interest because the beam width is converged. However, the reduction in beam width at the selected depth is achieved at the expense of degradation in beam width at other depths, resulting in poorer images below the focal zone.

BIOEFFECT AND SAFETY

The mechanisms of action by which an ultrasound application could produce a biologic effect can be conceptually categorized into two aspects: heating and mechanical. In reality, these two

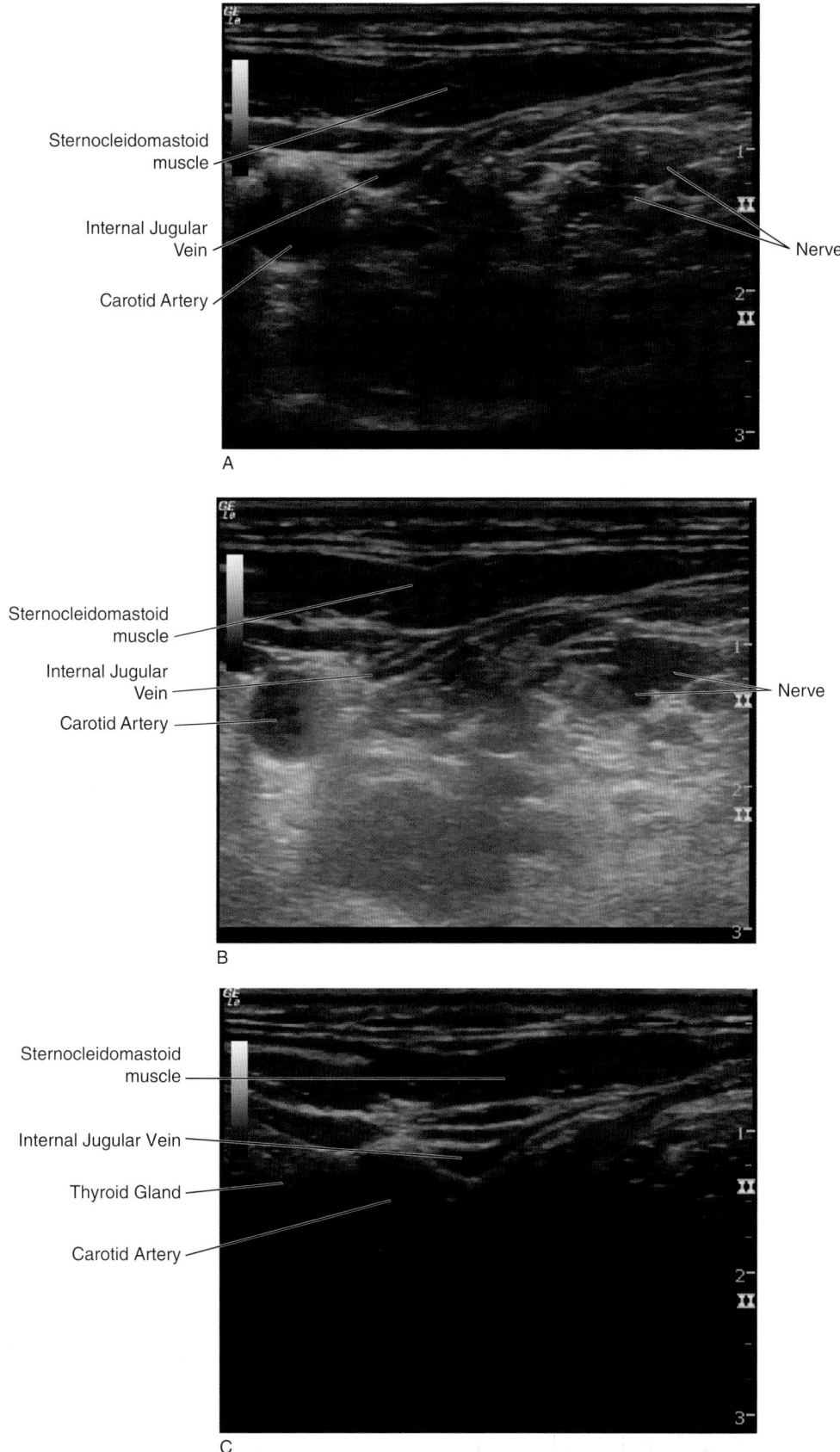

FIGURE 28–19. A, B, and **C:** The effect of the time-gain compensation settings. Time-gain compensation is a function that allows time-(depth) dependent amplification of signals returning from different depths. (Adapted with permission from Hadzic A: *Hadzic's Peripheral Nerve Blocks and Anatomy for Ultrasound-Guided Regional Anesthesia*, 2nd ed. New York: McGraw-Hill, Inc; 2011.)

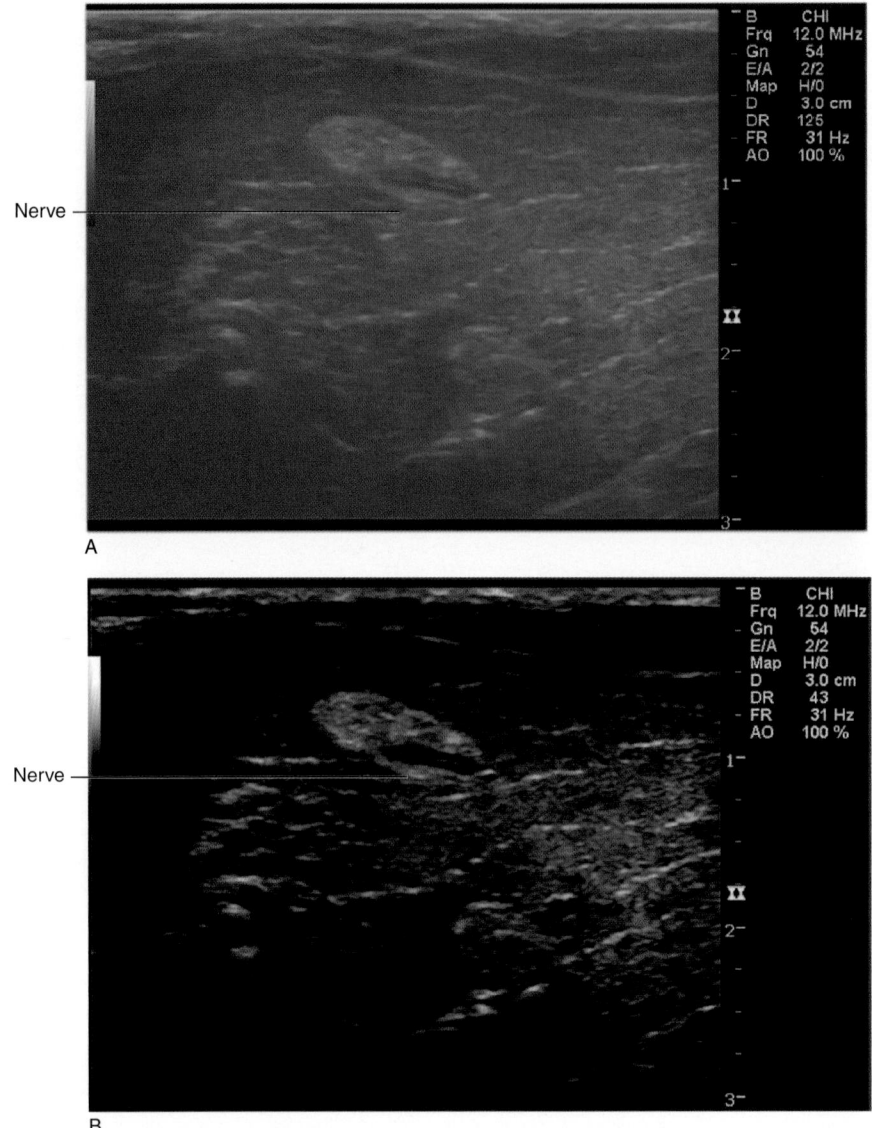

FIGURE 28–20. A: A softer image provided by a higher dynamic range. **B:** An image with more contrast provided by a lower dynamic range.

effects are rarely separable except for extracorporeal lithotripsy, the therapeutic application of mechanical bioeffects alone. The generation of heat increases as ultrasound intensity or frequency is increased. For similar exposure conditions, the expected temperature increase in bone is significantly greater than in soft tissues. In in vivo experiments, high-intensity ultrasound (usually > 2 W/cm²) is used to evaluate harmful biological effect; it is 5 to 20 times larger than therapeutic intensities (0.08–0.5 W/cm²) and 8 to 100 times larger than diagnostic intensities (color flow mode 0.25 W/cm², B-mode scan 0.02 W/cm²). Reports in animal models (mice and rats) suggest that application of ultrasound may result in a number of undesired effects, such as fetal weight reduction, postpartum mortality, fetal abnormalities, tissue lesions, hind limb paralysis, blood flow stasis, and tumor regression. Other reported undesired effects in mice are abnormalities in B-cell development and ovulatory response and teratogenicity.[16,17]

In general, adult tissues are more tolerant of rising temperature than fetal and neonatal tissues. A modern ultrasound machine displays two standard indices: thermal and mechanical. The thermal index (TI) is defined as the transducer acoustic output power divided by the estimated power required to raise tissue temperature by 1°C. The mechanical index (MI) is equal to the peak rarefactional pressure divided by the square root of the center frequency of the pulse bandwidth. TI and MI indicate the relative likelihood of thermal and mechanical hazard in vivo, respectively. Either TI or MI greater than 1.0 is hazardous.[18,19]

Biologic effect due to ultrasound also depends on tissue exposure time. The researchers usually use pregnant mice to expose to ultrasound with a minimum intensity of 1 W/cm² for 60 to 420 minutes to evaluate the time-dependent adverse events that happen in rodent fetuses.[20] Fortunately, ultrasound-guided nerve block requires the use of only low TI and MI values on the patient for a short period of time. Based on in vitro and in vivo experimental study results to date, there is no evidence that the use of diagnostic ultrasound in routine clinical practice is associated with any biologic risks.

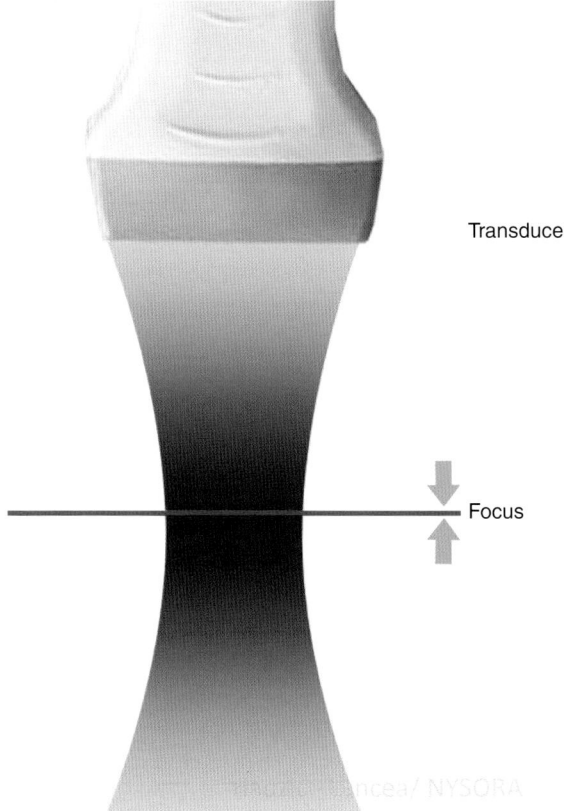

FIGURE 28–21. A demonstration of focusing effect. An electronic means can be used to narrow the width of the beam at a specific depth, resulting in the focusing effect and greater resolution at a chosen depth. (Adapted with permission from Hadzic A: *Hadzic's Peripheral Nerve Blocks and Anatomy for Ultrasound-Guided Regional Anesthesia*, 2nd ed. New York: McGraw-Hill, Inc; 2011.)

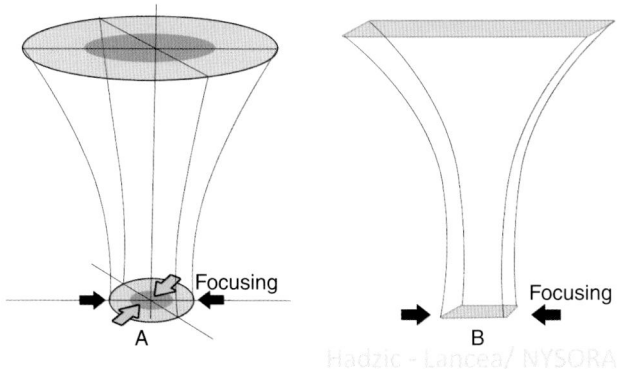

FIGURE 28–22. A: Annular focusing is electronic focusing from all directions in the scan plane given by an annular transducer that contains several ring elements arranged concentrically. **B:** Linear focusing is electronic focusing applied along both lateral sides in the scan plane.

REFERENCES

1. Curie J, Curie P: Développement par pression de l'électricite polaire dans les cristaux hémièdres à faces inclinées. CR Acad Sci (Paris) 1880;91:294.
2. Langevin P: French Patent No. 505,703. Filed September 17, 1917. Issued August 5, 1920.
3. Thompson J: Unrestricted U-boat warfare: The Royal Navy nearly loses the war. In *Imperial War Museum Book of the War at Sea 1914–18*. Pan Books, 2006, Chapter 10.
4. Langévin MP: Lés ondes ultrasonores. Rev Gen Elect 1928;23:626.
5. Ensminger D, Bond LJ: *Ultrasonics: Fundamentals, Technologies, and Applications*, 3rd ed. Francis Group, 2012.
6. Dussik KT: On the possibility of using ultrasound waves as a diagnostic aid. Neurol Psychiat 1942;174:153–168.
7. Dussik KT, Dussik F, Wyt L. Auf dem Wege Zur Hyperphonographie des Gehirnes. Med Wochenschr 1947;97:425–429.
8. Kossoff G, Robinson DE, Garrett WJ: Ultrasonic two-dimensional visualization techniques. IEEE Trans Sonics Ultrason 1965;SU12:31–37.
9. Thompson HE, Holmes JH, Gottesfeld KR, Taylor ES: Fetal development as determined by ultrasound pulse-echo techniques. Am J Obstet Gynecol 1965;92:44–53.
10. US federal trademark registration filed for ECHO-DOPPLER by Advanced Technology Laboratories Inc. Ultrasound apparatus for diagnostic medicine. Trademark serial number 73085203. April 26, 1976.
11. La Grange PDP, Foster PA, Pretorius LK: Application of the Doppler ultrasound blood flow detector in supraclavicular brachial plexus block. Br J Anesth 1978;50:965–967.
12. Ting PL, Sivagnanaratnam V: Ultrasonographic study of the spread of local anaesthetic during axillary brachial plexus block. Br J Anesth 1978; 63:326–329.
13. Kapral S, Krafft P, Eibenberger K, Fitzgerald R, Gosch M, Weinstabl C: Ultrasound-guided supraclavicular approach for regional anesthesia of the brachial plexus. Anesth Analg 1994;78:507–513.
14. Sokolov SY, inventor: Means for indicating flaws in materials. United States patent 2164125. 1937.
15. White DN: Johann Christian Doppler and his effect—A brief history. Ultrasound Med Biol 1982;8(6):583–591.
16. O'Brien WD Jr. Biological effects in laboratory animals. In *Biological Effects of Ultrasound*. Churchill Livingstone, 1985, 77–84.
17. Kerry BG, Robertson VJ, Duck FA: A review of therapeutic ultrasound: Biophysical effects. Phys Ther 2001;81:1351–1358.
18. American Institute of Ultrasound in Medicine, National Electrical Manufacturers Association: *Standard for Real-Time Display of Thermal and Mechanical Acoustic Output Indices on Diagnostic Ultrasound Equipment*, Revision 2. American Institute of Ultrasound in Medicine and National Electrical Manufacturers Association, 2004.
19. British Medical Ultrasound Society: Guidelines for the safe use of diagnostic ultrasound equipment. Ultrasound 2010 May 18:52–59.
20. Ang ES Jr, Gluncic V, Duque A, Schafer ME, Rakic P: Prenatal exposure to ultrasound waves impacts neuronal migration in mice. Proc Natl Acad Sci U S A 2006;103(34):12903–12910.

CHAPTER 29

Optimizing an Ultrasound Image

Daquan Xu, Shaun De Meirsman, and Ruben Schreurs

INTRODUCTION

Optimizing an ultrasound image is an essential skill during ultrasound-guided nerve blockade. Anatomically, a peripheral nerve is always located in the vicinity of an artery between fascial layers. The echotexture of normal nerve shows a hyperechoic, hypoechoic, or honeycomb pattern (Figure 29–1).[1,2] There are several scanning steps to obtain adequate nerve imaging, including the selection of sonographic modes, adjustment of function keys, needle visualization, and interpretation of image artifacts.

Clinical Pearl

- It is often easier to identify easily recognizable structures in the vicinity of the nerve, then to look for the nerve structures upfront.

Common sonographic imaging modes used for medical diagnostics, such as, conventional imaging, compound imaging, and tissue harmonic imaging (THI) can all be utilized in imaging of peripheral nerves. Conventional imaging is generated from a single-element angle beam at a primary frequency designated by the transducer. Compound imaging is implemented by acquiring several (usually three to nine) overlapping frames from different frequencies or from different angles.[3] THI acquires the information from harmonic frequencies generated by ultrasound beam transmission through tissue. Harmonic frequencies are multiples of the primary frequency. THI improves axial resolution and boundary detection by suppression of scattering signals from tissue interfaces, especially for obese patients.

Currently, THI has been set as the default mode by many, if not most, US manufacturers. Compound imaging with THI can provide images with better resolution, penetration, and interfaces and margin enhancement compared with conventional sonography. In Figure 29–2, both compound imaging and conventional imaging were employed to visualize an interscalene brachial plexus. There is clear margin definition of two hypoechoic oval-shaped nerve structures in compound imaging; the contrast resolution between anterior scalene muscle and surrounding adipose tissue is increased in comparison with conventional imaging.

Five function keys on an ultrasound machine are of crucial importance to achieve an optimal image during the performance of peripheral nerve imaging (Figure 29–3).[4]

1. *Depth*: The depth of the nerve is the first consideration when an ultrasound-guided nerve block is performed. Peripheral nerve branches have a great variation of depth, which depends on patients' habitus; the optimal depth setting can provide good focusing properties for imaging. Table 29–1 recommends the initial depth and frequency settings for common peripheral nerve blockades. The target nerve should be at the center of ultrasound imaging because it not only has the best resolution of the nerve but also reveals the other anatomical structures in the vicinity of the nerve. For example, ultrasound imaging during supraclavicular or infraclavicular brachial plexus blockade must require that the first rib and pleura are observed simultaneously to avoid lung puncture with the needle.

2. *Frequency*: The ultrasound transducer with the optimal frequency range should be selected to best visualize the target nerves. Ultrasound energy is absorbed gradually by the transmitted tissue; the higher the frequency of ultrasound, the more rapid the absorption and the less distance propagation. Therefore, a low-frequency transducer is used to scan structures at a deeper location; unfortunately, this is at the expense of reduced image resolution. In some particular cases, like lumbar plexus block, a lower-frequency transducer with a Doppler setting is useful for identifying the vasculature close to the lumbar plexus in obese patients.

Echotexture of Peripheral Nerve

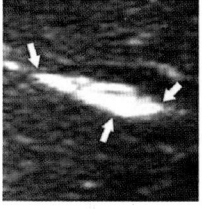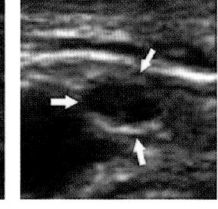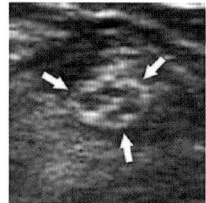

Hyperechoic (Musculocutaneous Nerve)   Hypoechoic (Ulnar Nerve)   Honeycomb (Median Nerve)

FIGURE 29–1. Echotexture of peripheral nerves. (Reproduced with permission from Hadzic A: *Hadzic's Peripheral Nerve Blocks and Anatomy for Ultrasound-Guided Regional Anesthesia*, 2nd ed. New York: McGraw-Hill, Inc.; 2011.)

3. *Focusing*: Lateral resolution can be improved by choosing a higher frequency as well as by focusing the ultrasound beam. In clinical practice, the focus is adjusted at the level of the target nerve; the best image quality for a given nerve is obtained by choosing an appropriate frequency transducer and the focal zone (Figure 29–4A). Furthermore, when possible, selecting no more than two focus zones yields better image because multiple focal zones can slow the frame rate and decrease the temporal resolution.

4. *Gain*: Screen brightness can be adjusted manually by two function buttons—gain and time-gain compensation

(TGC)—on ultrasound machines that have TGC built in. Excessive or inadequate gain can cause blurring of tissue boundaries and loss of information. Optimal gain for scanning peripheral nerves is typically the gain at which the best contrast is obtained between the muscles and the adjacent connective tissue. This is because muscles are well-vascularized tissue invested with connective tissue fibers, whereas the echo texture of connective tissue is similar to that of nerves. In addition, increasing gain below the focus works well with the TGC control to visualize both the target nerve and the structures below it. Figure 29–4B shows the same section with both correct and incorrect gain and TGC settings. TGC sliders aligned in a curve can lead to a desirable image with appropriate gain.

5. *Doppler*: In regional anesthesia, Doppler ultrasound is used to detect vascular structures or the location of the spread of the local anesthetic injection. Doppler velocity scale is best set between 15 and 35 cm/s to reduce aliasing of color Doppler imaging and artifacts of color (Figure 29–5). Of note, power Doppler is more sensitive for detecting blood flow than color Doppler. The gate size is another common setting when color Doppler is used. It should be as small as possible to overlay the area of interest. An appropriate small gate not only can exclude distractive signals from adjacent tissues but also can improve temporal resolution by increasing the frame rate.

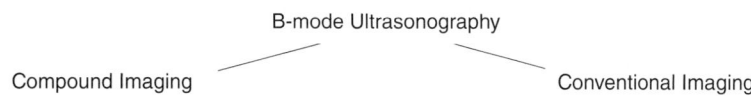

B-mode Ultrasonography

Compound Imaging

Enhances the signals from tissue margins, and reduces speckle. Spatial compounding combines multiple frames from different angles. Frequency compounding combines two images with different frequencies decreasing the speckle.

Conventional Imaging

The imaging is obtained from one single linear array

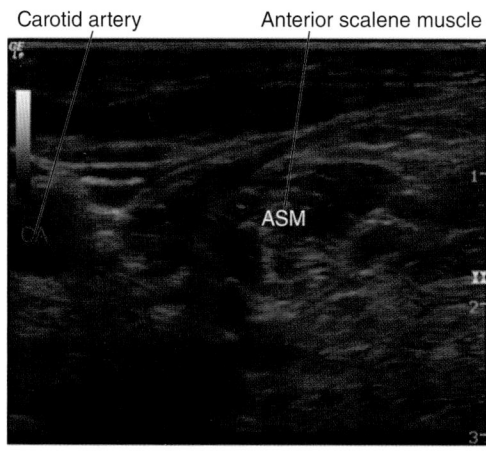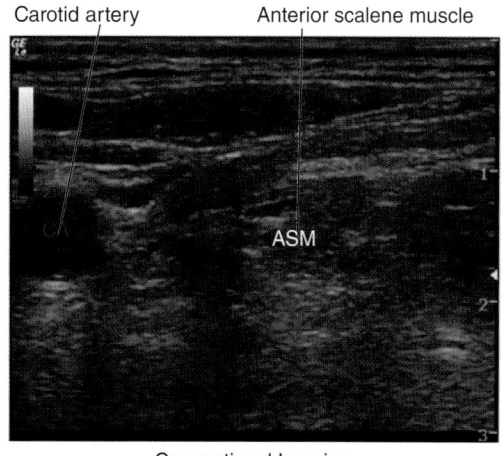

Compound Imaging   Conventional Imaging

FIGURE 29–2. Examples of image quality typically obtained with conventional versus compound imaging. (Reproduced with permission from Hadzic A: *Hadzic's Peripheral Nerve Blocks and Anatomy for Ultrasound-Guided Regional Anesthesia*, 2nd ed. New York: McGraw-Hill, Inc.; 2011.)

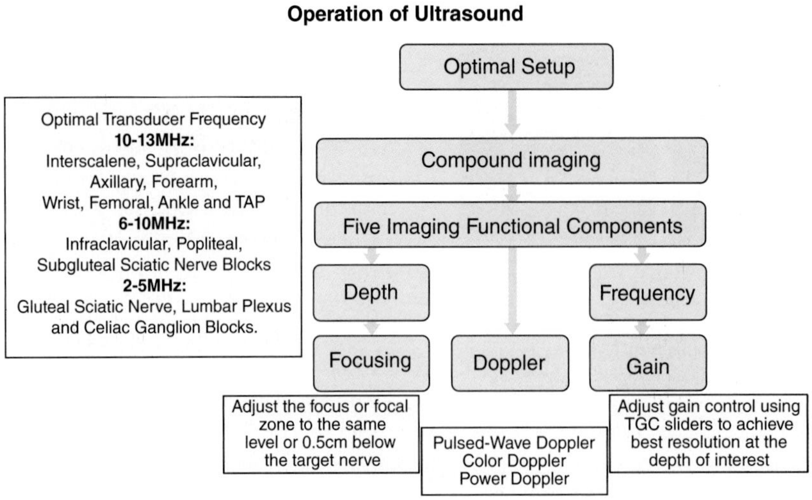

Operation of Ultrasound

```
                              ┌──────────────────────┐
                              │    Optimal Setup     │
                              └──────────────────────┘
                                        │
  ┌─────────────────────────────┐       ▼
  │ Optimal Transducer Frequency│ ┌──────────────────────┐
  │        10-13MHz:            │ │  Compound imaging    │
  │ Interscalene, Supraclavicular,│ └──────────────────────┘
  │   Axillary, Forearm,        │
  │ Wrist, Femoral, Ankle and TAP│ ┌────────────────────────────────┐
  │        6-10MHz:             │ │ Five Imaging Functional Components│
  │ Infraclavicular, Popliteal, │ └────────────────────────────────┘
  │ Subgluteal Sciatic Nerve Blocks│
  │        2-5MHz:             │  ┌──────────┐          ┌──────────┐
  │ Gluteal Sciatic Nerve, Lumbar Plexus│ │  Depth   │          │Frequency │
  │  and Celiac Ganglion Blocks.│  └──────────┘          └──────────┘
  └─────────────────────────────┘
```

Optimal Transducer Frequency
10-13MHz:
Interscalene, Supraclavicular, Axillary, Forearm, Wrist, Femoral, Ankle and TAP
6-10MHz:
Infraclavicular, Popliteal, Subgluteal Sciatic Nerve Blocks
2-5MHz:
Gluteal Sciatic Nerve, Lumbar Plexus and Celiac Ganglion Blocks.

Optimal Setup → Compound imaging → Five Imaging Functional Components → Depth / Frequency

Focusing — Doppler — Gain

Adjust the focus or focal zone to the same level or 0.5cm below the target nerve

Pulsed-Wave Doppler / Color Doppler / Power Doppler

Adjust gain control using TGC sliders to achieve best resolution at the depth of interest

FIGURE 29–3. Optimizing an ultrasound image using five key functional adjustments and specific tips on adjusting the focus and gain. Some ultrasound models are specifically optimized for regional anesthesia application and may not incorporate user-adjustable focus or time-gain compensation (TGC). (Reproduced with permission from Hadzic A: *Hadzic's Peripheral Nerve Blocks and Anatomy for Ultrasound-Guided Regional Anesthesia*, 2nd ed. New York: McGraw-Hill, Inc.; 2011.)

Clinical Pearl

- When excessive pressure is applied on the transducer during imaging, small- and medium-size vessels may collapse and not be detected with Doppler.

Two needle insertion techniques with relevance to the needle-transducer relationship are commonly used in ultrasound-guided nerve block: the in-plane and out-of-plane techniques (Figure 29–6). An in-plane technique means the needle is placed in the plane of the ultrasound beam; as a result, the needle

shaft and the tip can be observed in the longitudinal view in real time as the needle is advanced toward the target nerve. When the needle path is not seen on the image, the needle advancement should be paused; tilting, sliding or rotating the transducer can bring the ultrasound beam into alignment with the needle. In addition, a subtle, fast needle shake and or injection of a small amount of injectate may help depict the needle location.

The out-of-plane technique involves needle insertion perpendicular or any other angle to the transducer to the transducer. The needle shaft is imaged in a cross-sectional plane and often can be identified as a bright dot in the image. Visualization of the tip of the needle, however, requires higher degree of skill. The method used to visualize the tip of the needle is as follows: Once a bright dot (shaft) is seen in the image, the needle can be shaken slightly or the transducer can be tilted toward the direction of needle insertion simultaneously until the dot disappears. Shaking the needle helps differentiate the echo as emanating from the needle or from the surrounding tissue. The last capture of the hyperechoic dot is its tip. A small amount of injectate can be used to confirm the location of the needle tip. Whenever injectate is used to visualize the needle tip, attention must be paid to avoid resistance (pressure) to injection because when the needle-nerve interface is not well seen, there is a risk for the needle to be against the nerve or to inject intrafascicularly.[5]

TABLE 29–1. Suggested optimal imaging depth and frequency for common peripheral nerve blocks.

Field Depth (cm)	Frequency (MHz)	Peripheral Blockades
<2.0	12–15	Wrist, ankle block
2.0–3.0	10–12	Interscalene, supraclavicular, axillary brachial plexus block
3.0–4.0	10–12	Femoral nerve block, TAP block
4.0–7.0	5–10	Infraclavicular, popliteal, subgluteal sciatic nerve blocks
7.0–10.0	5–10	Pudendal, gluteal sciatic nerve, lumbar plexus block
>10.0	3–5	Anterior approach to sciatic nerve, celiac ganglion block

Source: Reproduced with permission from Hadzic A: *Hadzic's Peripheral Nerve Blocks and Anatomy for Ultrasound-Guided Regional Anesthesia*, 2nd ed. New York: McGraw-Hill, Inc.; 2011.

Clinical Pearls

- If the needle trajectory is lost visually, the operator should stop advancing the needle and then tilt the transducer to visualize the needle.
- When the spread of the local anesthetic is not seen during the injection process, the operator should stop the injection, tilt the transducer, and inject a tiny amount of local anesthetic (or air) to locate the needle tip and spread of injectate.

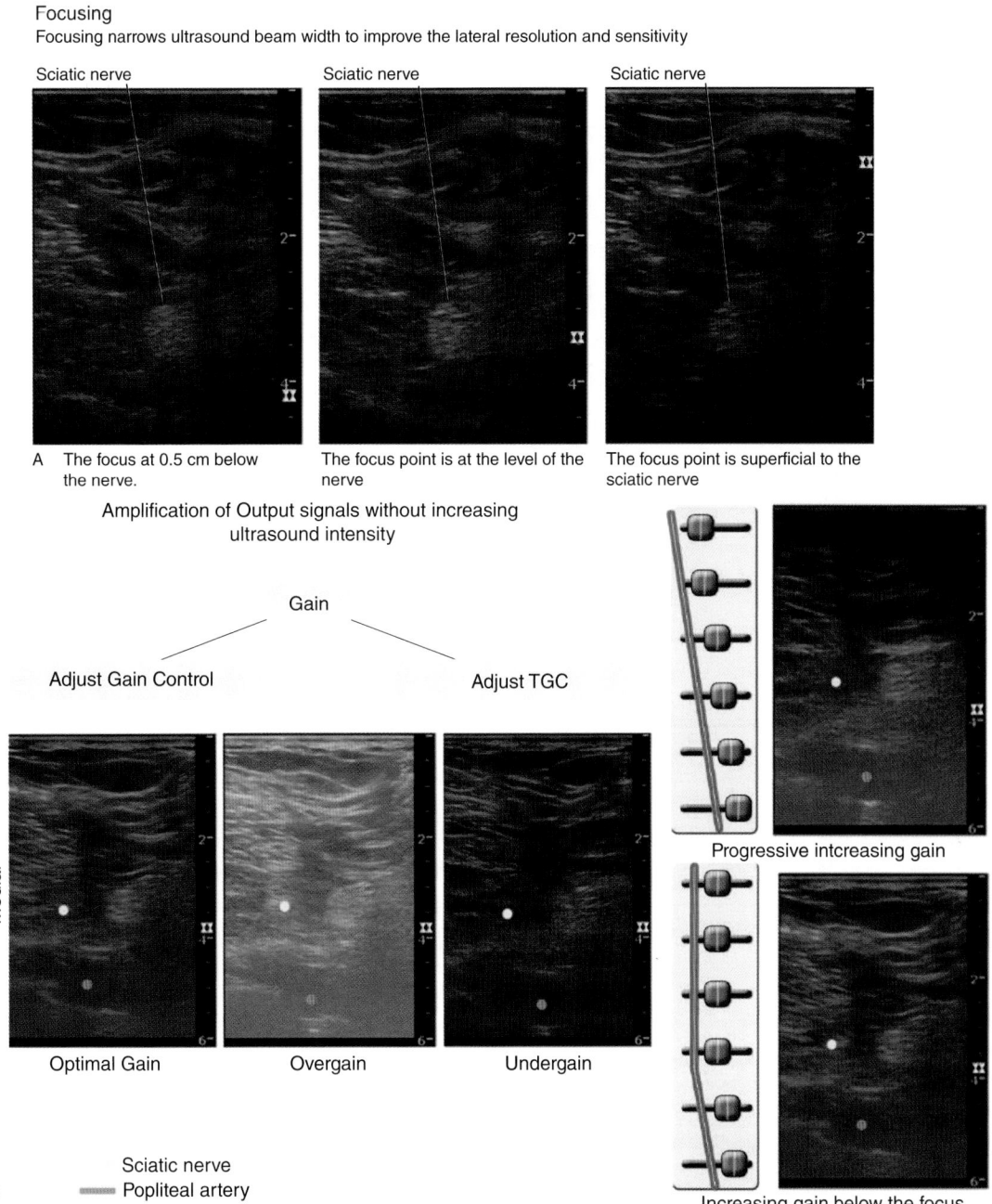

Focusing
Focusing narrows ultrasound beam width to improve the lateral resolution and sensitivity

Sciatic nerve   Sciatic nerve   Sciatic nerve

A   The focus at 0.5 cm below   The focus point is at the level of the   The focus point is superficial to the
      the nerve.   nerve   sciatic nerve

Amplification of Output signals without increasing
ultrasound intensity

Gain

Adjust Gain Control   Adjust TGC

Medial

Optimal Gain   Overgain   Undergain

Progressive intcreasing gain

Sciatic nerve
B   ▭▭ Popliteal artery

Increasing gain below the focus

FIGURE 29–4. A: Focusing narrows ultrasound beam width to improve the lateral resolution and sensitivity. Shown are three examples of focusing when imaging the sciatic nerve: below the nerve, at the level of the nerve, and superficial to the nerve. **B:** Optimal and incorrect gain and TGC settings. (Reproduced with permission from Hadzic A: *Hadzic's Peripheral Nerve Blocks and Anatomy for Ultrasound-Guided Regional Anesthesia*, 2nd ed. New York: McGraw-Hill, Inc.; 2011.)

Continuous peripheral nerve blocks (CPNBs) have become a common practice; however, the visualization of the catheter tip can be challenging. Direct visualization of the catheter tip can be obtained when the catheter is introduced at a short distance from the needle tip (eg, 2 cm past the needle tip) (Figure 29–7). However, when the catheter is inserted 3–5 cm past the needle tip, the needle, nerve, and catheter are never in the same plane of the ultrasound beam, therefore becoming challenging to image. There are two ways to confirm the catheter tip: (1) The operator can tilt or slightly slide the transducer to see a "bright

dot," which is the transverse view of the catheter. The position of the catheter tip can be detected by observing the spread of 1–2 mL injectate through the catheter, and the use of color Doppler may help visualize the spread more significantly (Figures 29–8A and 29–8B). (2) In some cases, the bright dot may not be obviously visualized or ensured; the operator has to slide the transducer within a certain distance away from the needle tip, with the distance based on the length of catheter threaded past the needle tip. Injection of 0.5 mL air can be beneficial to ascertain the position of the catheter tip with a

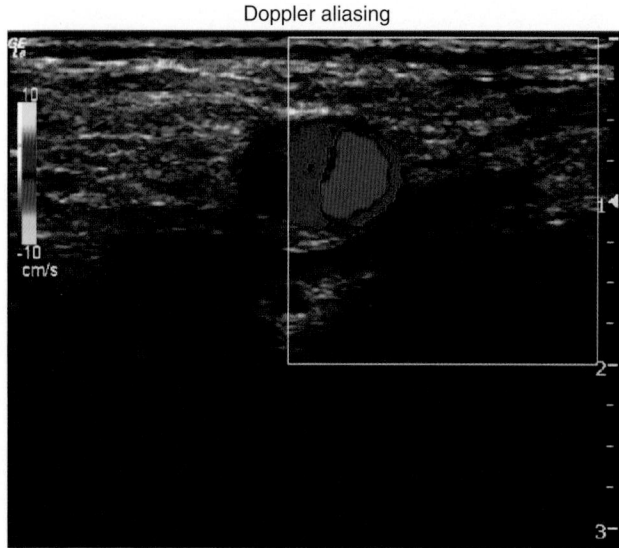

FIGURE 29–5. Color Doppler aliasing occurs when the velocity scale for color Doppler is set too low.

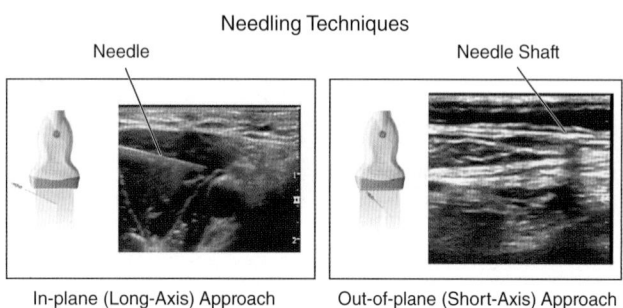

Needling Techniques

Needle / Needle Shaft

In-plane (Long-Axis) Approach   Out-of-plane (Short-Axis) Approach

FIGURE 29–6. In-plane and out-of-plane needle insertion and the appearance in a corresponding ultrasound image.

sharp echoic contrast on the ultrasound image (Figures 29–9A and 29–9B). The obvious drawback is that injection of air may degrade the image for other purposes.

Clinical Pearl

- Catheters often cannot be visualized by ultrasound because they coil within the tissue sheaths. Visualization of the spread of injectate is the most convenient and important method to ascertain the position of the catheter tip in the desired tissue plane.

Ultrasound artifacts occur commonly and, in fact, are an intrinsic part of ultrasound imaging. By definition, an ultrasound artifact is any image aberration that does not represent the correct anatomic structures. Most artifacts are undesirable, and operators must learn how to recognize them during nerve blockade. The five artifacts most commonly seen in regional anesthesia practice (Figure 29–10) are the following[6–8]:

1. *Shadowing* is a significant attenuation of ultrasound signal deep to tissues and structures that absorb or reflect most of the ultrasound waves, as bones, calcifications or air. This is manifested by a weak or absent echo area which appears as a shadow on the imaging behind a bright, hyperechoic interface. Acoustic shadowing has a favorable diagnostic value for detection of calcified lesions, such as gallstones, scar tissue, and the like. However, the shadowing may interfere with nerve visualization in regional anesthesia. Changing the scanning plane to find the best acoustic window is the best strategy to avoid shadowing when necessary.

2. *Enhancement* manifests as overly intense echogenicity behind an object (a fluid-filled structure, such as a vessel or cyst)

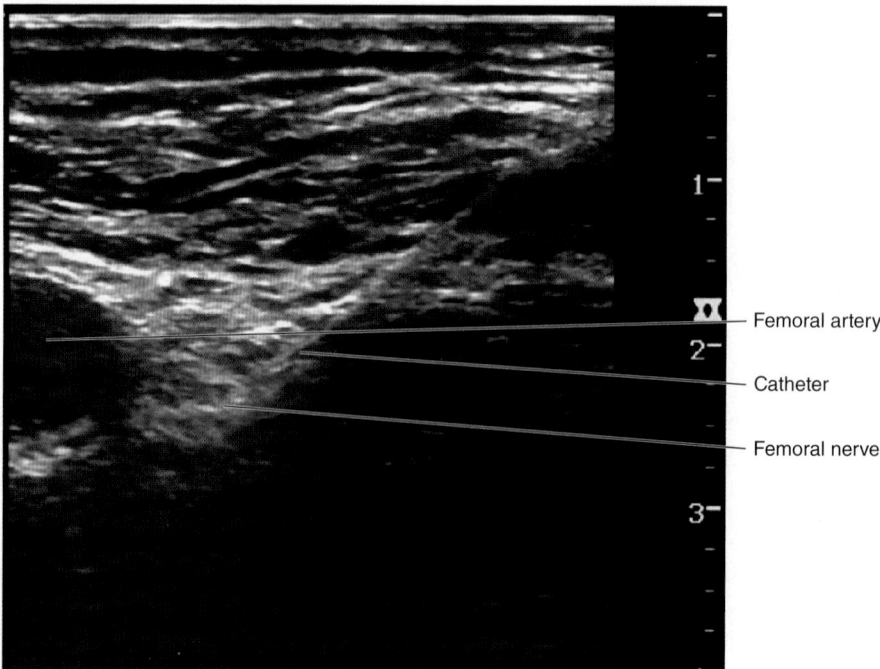

Femoral artery
Catheter
Femoral nerve

FIGURE 29–7. The catheter tip can be directly seen just beneath femoral nerve.

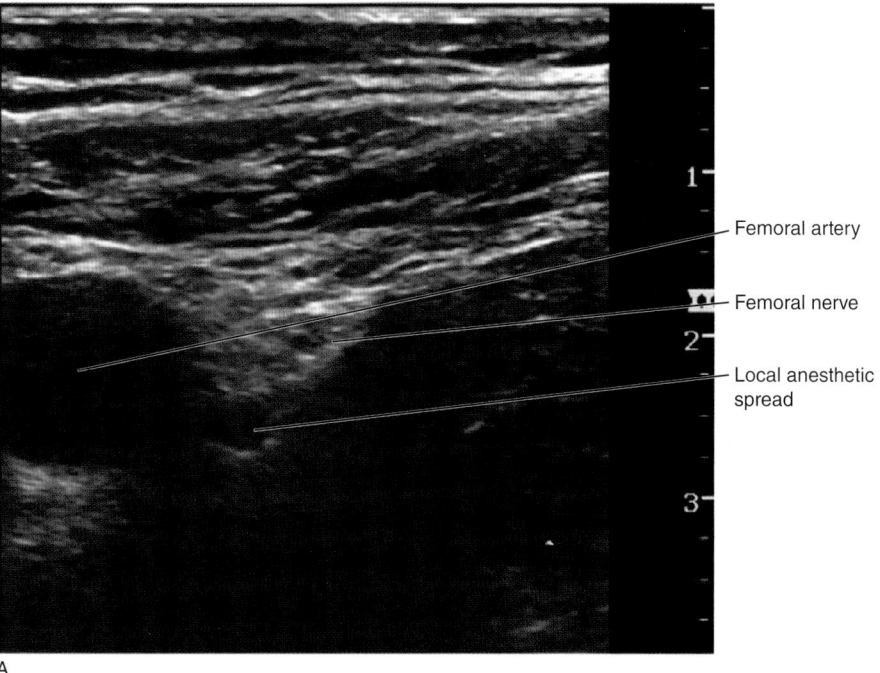

Femoral artery

Femoral nerve

Local anesthetic spread

A

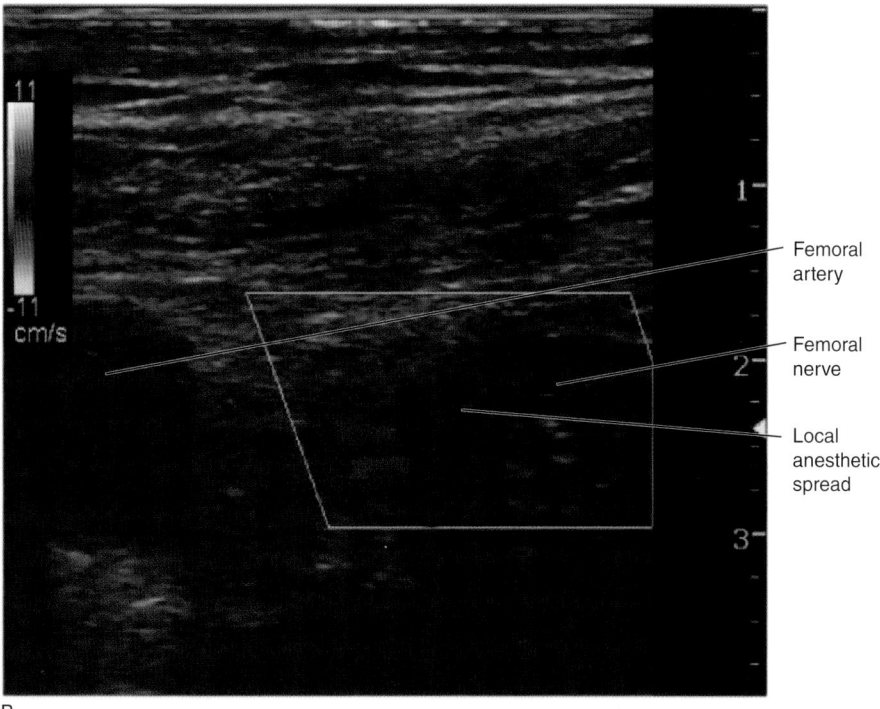

Femoral artery

Femoral nerve

Local anesthetic spread

B

FIGURE 29–8. A: The position of catheter tip can be estimated by observing the spread of injectate. **B:** Doppler can be used to confirm the location of the spread.

that is less attenuating than the surrounding soft tissues. Enhancement occurs when the echo signals are overamplified in brightness disproportional to the echo strength at the same depth. Scanning from different angles or from different planes may help to decrease shadowing/enhancement artifacts and to visualize the target nerve; using automatic TGC may make enhancement artifact less apparent as well.

3. *Reverberation* displays in the form of parallel, equally spaced bright linear echoes behind the reflectors in the near field of the image. The multiple echoes occur when the ultrasound beam bounces repeatedly between the interfaces of the transducer and a strong reflector, especially when these two interfaces are parallel to each other. It may be attenuated or eliminated when the scanning direction is changed slightly or the ultrasound frequency is decreased.

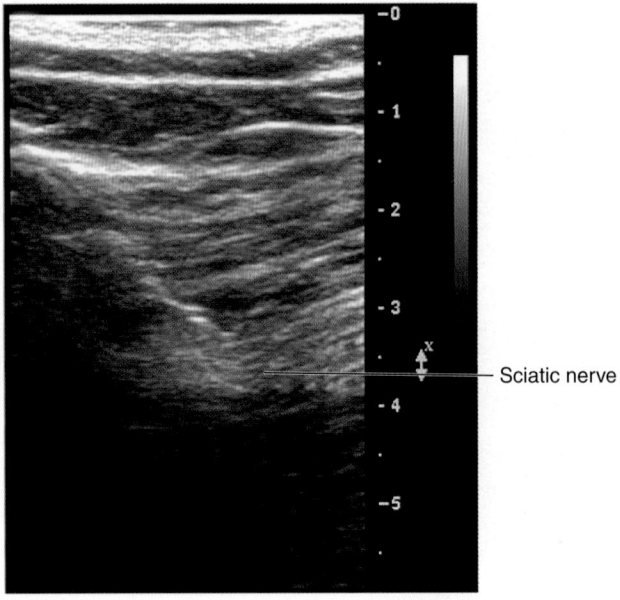

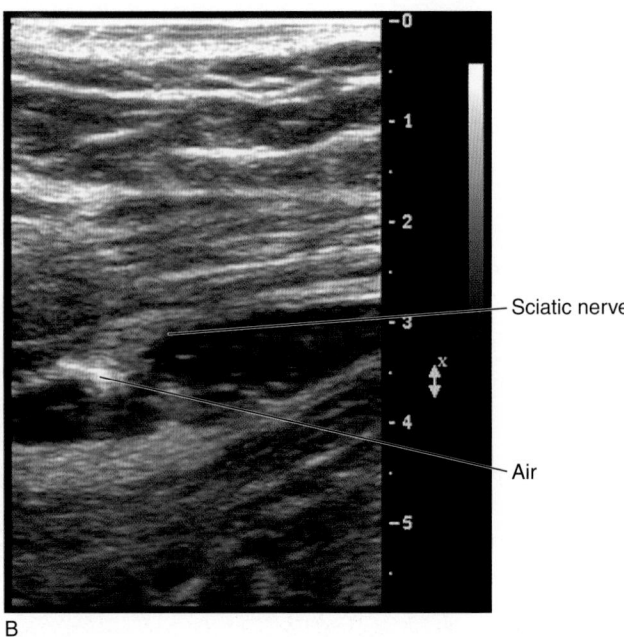

FIGURE 29–9. A: The location of the catheter tip cannot be visualized before a small amount of air is injected. **B:** The discernable brightness indicates the location of the catheter tip when 0.3–0.5 mL air is injected.

4. *Mirror* image artifact results from an object located on one side of a highly reflective linear boundary that acts like an acoustic "mirror," appearing on the other side as well. The transducer receives both direct echoes from the object and indirect echoes from the mirror (Figure 29–11). Both virtual and artifactual images have an equal distance to the mirror from opposite directions. The duplicated artifactual image is always less bright and deeper than the real image because indirect echoes transmit a longer distance and attenuate more wave energy. Changing the scanning direction may decrease the artifact.

Velocity error is the displacement of the interface, which is caused by the difference of actual velocity of ultrasound in human soft tissue, compared with the calibrated speed, which is assumed to be a constant velocity of 1540 m/s set by the ultrasound system. Consequently, a reflector is displaced toward the transducer by a significant error in distance calculations. The inherent artifact in the process of scanning cannot be completely eliminated in all cases by manipulating ultrasound devices or changing the settings. However, recognizing and understanding ultrasound artifacts help the operator avoid misinterpretation of images.

PREPARING TO SCAN

An acronym, SCANNING, can be used by operators to prepare for scanning:

S: Supplies
C: Comfortable positioning
A: Ambiance
N: Name and procedure

N: Nominate transducer
I: Infection control
N: Note lateral/medial/superior/inferior orientation on screen
G: Gain depth

1. Gather supplies: All equipment necessary for ultrasound scanning should be prepared. Equipment may differ slightly depending on the area to be scanned; however, some necessary equipment includes the following:
   a. Ultrasound machine
   b. Transducer covers
   c. Nerve block kit, nerve stimulator
   d. Sterile work trolley
   e. Local anesthetic drawn up and labeled
   f. Whenever possible, connect the ultrasound machine to the power outlet to prevent the machine from powering down during a procedure. Although many point-of-care ultrasound machines are equipped with batteries, these run out of power during the most importunate part of the procedure.
2. Comfortable patient position: The patient should be positioned in such a way that the patient, the anesthesiologist, the ultrasound machine, and the sterile block tray are all arranged ergonomically to allow for time-efficient performance of the procedure.
   a. The ultrasound machine should be set up on the opposite side of the patient from the operator with the screen at the operator's eye level.
   b. The block tray should be positioned close enough to the operator can easily reach for needle, gel, and other supplies without interference with the scanning procedure.

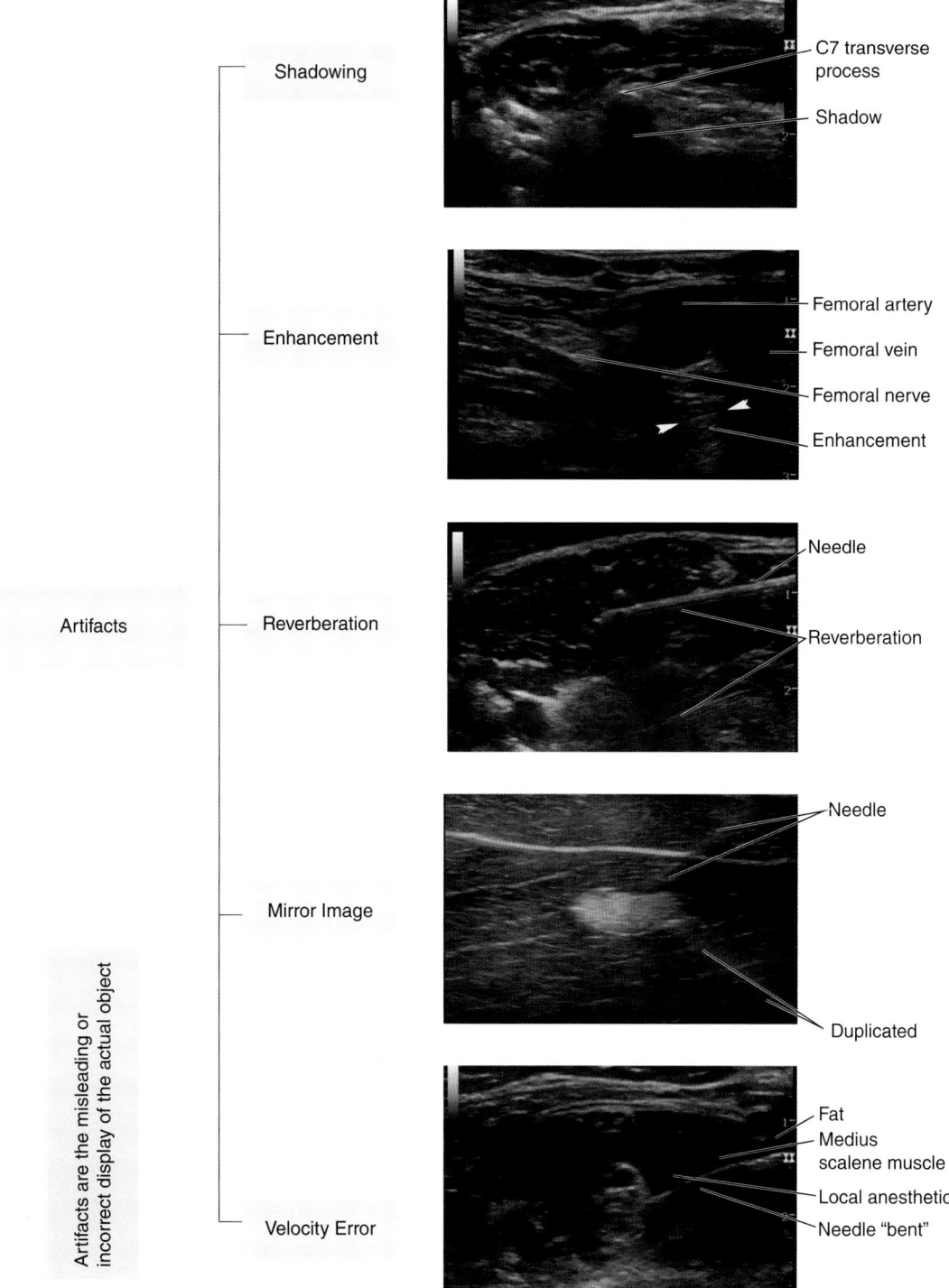

FIGURE 29–10. Five common ultrasound artifacts during ultrasound-guided peripheral nerve block. (Reproduced with permission from Hadzic A: *Hadzic's Peripheral Nerve Blocks and Anatomy for Ultrasound-Guided Regional Anesthesia*, 2nd ed. New York: McGraw-Hill, Inc.; 2011.)

3. Ambiance set room settings: Adjust the lights in the room to view the ultrasound machine and procedural site adequately.
   a. Dim lighting optimizes visualization of the image on the screen; more lighting may be needed for the procedural site.
   b. Adjust the room light settings to allow for proper lighting to both areas, as well as for safe monitoring of the patient.

4. Name of patient, procedure, and site of procedure: Before performing a scan take a "time-out" to ensure patient information is correct, the operation being done is confirmed, and the side in which the procedure is being done is validated. The New York School of Regional Anesthesia (NYSORA) team uses the acronym ECT for the time-out procedure: E for equipment for patient monitoring and needle-nerve monitoring; C for the

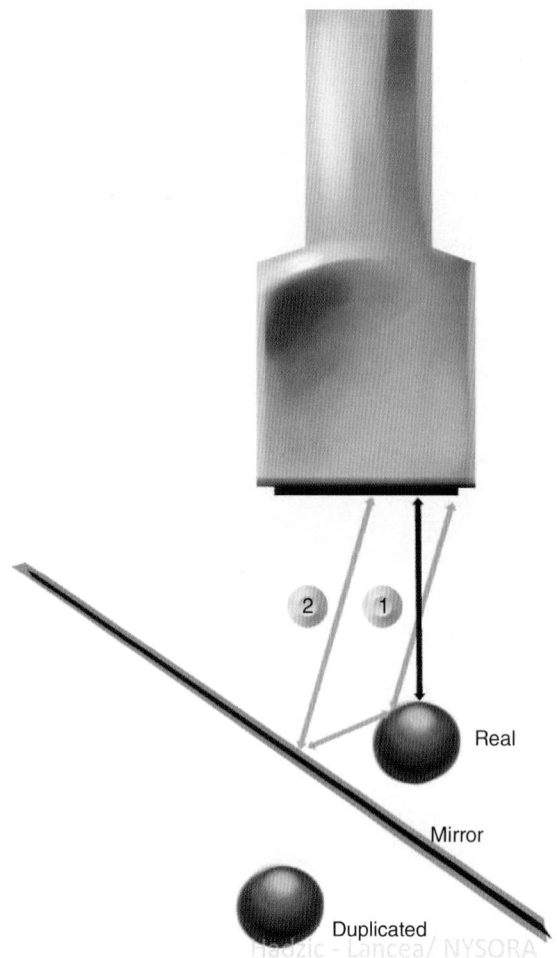

FIGURE 29–11. Mirror image artifact: Transducer receives both direct echoes from the object (1) and indirect echoes from the "mirror" (2).

patient's consent for the procedure; and T for the time for the time-out to identify the patient and ensure correct laterality. Checking that patient information is entered into the ultrasound machine and matches the information on the patient's wristband not only confirms identity but also allows for images to be saved during the scanning process for documentation.

5. Select transducer: Select the transducer that best fits the scheduled procedure. A linear transducer is best for scanning superficial anatomic structures; a curved (phased-array) transducer displays a sector image and is typically better for deeper-positioned structures. A hockey stick ultrasound transducer is an ideal choice for vascular access or a superficial block with limited space, such as an ankle block.

6. Disinfection: Disinfect the patient's skin using a disinfectant solution to reduce the risk of contamination and infection.
7. Orient transducer and apply gel: The operator should orient the transducer to match the medial-lateral orientation of the patient. This is conventionally not done by radiologists/sonographers, but it is useful for intervention-oriented regional anesthesia procedures.
   a. Touch one edge of the transducer to orient the side of the transducer so the medial-lateral orientation on the patient corresponds to that on the screen.
   b. A sufficient amount of gel is applied to either the transducer or the patient's skin to allow for transmission of the ultrasound. A copious amount of disinfectant solution can be used instead of gel in many instances.
   c. Insufficient quality of gel will decrease reflection-absorption rates and may result in unclear/blurry images on the ultrasound image being displayed.
8. Place the transducer on the patient's skin and adjust the ultrasound machine settings:
   a. The gain should be adjusted with the general gain setting or by using TGC.
   b. The depth is adjusted to optimize imaging of the structures of interest.
   c. Where available, focus point level.
   d. Scanning mode can be switched to assist in the recognition of the structures as necessary. Power Doppler can help depict blood vessels; color mode can distinguish between arteries and veins.

REFERENCES

1. Silvestri E, Martinoli C, Derchi LE, Bertolotto M, Chiaramondia M, Rosenberg I: Echotexture of peripheral nerves: Correlation between US and histologic findings and criteria to differentiate tendons. Radiology 1995;197(1):291–296.
2. Stuart RM, Koh E, Breidahl WH: Sonography of peripheral nerve pathology. AJR Am J Roentgenol 2004;182(1):123–129.
3. Jespersen SK, Wilhjelm JE, Sillesen H: Multiangle compound imaging. Ultrason Imaging 1998;20:81–102.
4. Tempkin BB: *Ultrasound Scanning: Principles and Protocols*, 3rd ed. Saunders Elsevier, 2009.
5. Gadsden JC, Choi JJ, Lin E, Robinson A: Opening injection pressure consistently detects needle-nerve contact during ultrasound-guided interscalene brachial plexus block. Anesthesiology 2014;120(5): 1246–1253.
6. Sites BD, Brull R, Chan VW, et al: Artifacts and pitfall errors associated with ultrasound -guided regional anesthesia. Part 1: Understanding the basic principles of ultrasound physics and machine operations. Reg Anesth Pain Med 2007;32(5):412–418.
7. Sites BD, Brull R, Chan VW, et al: Artifacts and pitfall errors associated with ultrasound-guided regional anesthesia. Part II: A pictorial approach to understanding and avoidance. Reg Anesth Pain Med 2007;32(5): 419–433.
8. Bushberg JT, Seibert JA, Leidholdt E Jr, Boone JM. Ultrasound image quality and artifacts. In *The Essential Physics of Medical Imaging*, 3rd ed. Lippincott Williams & Wilkins, 2012, pp 560–567.

CHAPTER 30

Introduction to Ultrasound-Guided Regional Anesthesia

Steven L. Orebaugh and Kyle R. Kirkham

INTRODUCTION

Ultrasonography (US) as a means to guide peripheral nerve blockade (PNB) was first explored by anesthesiologists at the University of Vienna in the mid-1990s.[1] Although radiologists had made use of ultrasound technology to guide needles for biopsy, the application of this imaging modality for PNB was novel at that time.[2] The utility of ultrasound to facilitate a range regional anesthesia techniques including brachial plexus and femoral blocks was demonstrated.[1,3] A decade later, colleagues from the University of Toronto, Canada, began to embrace this technology, further demonstrating its utility and describing in detail the sonoanatomy of the brachial plexus.[4] A number of advances in technology took place in the meantime, including smaller and more mobile ultrasound platforms, improved resolution, and needle recognition software, all cumulatively leading to increased bedside utility of ultrasound by anesthesiologists.[5]

ADVANTAGES OF ULTRASOUND GUIDANCE

The previously used surface anatomy-based techniques, such as nerve stimulation, palpation of landmarks, fascial "clicks," paresthesias, and transarterial approaches, did not allow for the monitoring of the disposition of the local anesthetic injectate. Ultrasound guidance, however, offers a number of important practical advantages for nerve blockade. Ultrasound allows visualization of the anatomy of the region of interest. This allows more informed guidance for the needle pathway to the target while avoiding structures that might be damaged by the needle.[6] Ultrasound also allows visualization of the needle tip as it is passed through the tissues, confirming alignment with the intended path, again reducing the likelihood of inadvertent needle trauma to unintended structures. Perhaps most important, real-time ultrasound imaging permits continual visualization of local anesthetic solution delivery to ensure proper distribution, with the potential for adjustment of the needle tip position as necessary to optimize local anesthetic distribution.[7]

Introduction of ultrasound guidance in regional anesthesia has led to refinement of many nerve block techniques, expanded use of PNB, and greater acceptance by surgical colleagues and patients.

ULTRASOUND AND SONOANATOMY

Ultrasound-guided PNB may be broken down into two fundamental aspects: imaging structures in the plane of section, including the target nerve, and guiding the needle. Understanding and recognition of three-dimensional anatomic structures on a two-dimensional image requires training in the technology and sonoanatomy pattern recognition (Table 30–1). As anatomic recognition remains essential to placing blocks, even with real-time visual guidance, specialty society guidelines for training residents and fellows continue to stress the importance of anatomical dissection and gross anatomy training as an inherent component of learning ultrasound-guided regional anesthesia (UGRA).[8] In a study conducted over a 1-month regional anesthesia rotation, residents demonstrated markedly improved recognition of relevant structures at the sites of several different PNBs, using ultrasound imaging.[9] In an evaluation of ultrasound-guided interscalene block instruction, residents demonstrated increasing efficiency of sonoanatomy recognition as their experience over the course of the rotation increased.[10]

More innovative methods of training have shown promise as well.[11] Integrating an anatomic program into the software of a bedside ultrasound machine has been shown to improve scores on a written test of anatomy.[12] After exposure to a multimedia anatomy presentation, residents and community anesthesiologists demonstrated increased knowledge of ultrasound anatomy on a posttest, although they were not able to improve scores on a practical examination of sonoanatomy on live models.[13] However, the optimal link between anatomic knowledge and recognition of two-dimensional anatomic patterns on ultrasound has not yet been adequately explored.

TABLE 30–1. Optimizing sonoanatomy visualization.

Choose appropriate transducer/frequency
Understand underlying anatomic relationships
Apply varying degree of pressure with transducer
Align transducer with underlying nerve target
Rotate transducer to fine-tune image
Tilt the transducer to optimize image

Certain basic tenets of optimizing an ultrasound image are applicable to all nerve blocks. For instance, sonography requires an understanding of mechanics and ergonomics. Novices are subject to errors such as probe fatigue, reversing probe orientation, and inadequate equipment preparation.[14] To optimize the ultrasound image, the mnemonic PART (pressure, alignment, rotation, tilting) has been recommended.[8] Pressure is necessary to minimize the distance to the target and compress underlying subcutaneous adipose tissues. Alignment refers to placing the transducer in a position over the extremity (or trunk) at which the underlying nerve is expected to be in the field of view. Rotation allows fine-tuning of the view of the target structure. Tilting helps to bring the face of the probe into a perpendicular arrangement with the underlying target to maximize the number of returning echoes and thus provide the best image (Figure 30–1). In-depth discussion on optimizing ultrasound imaging is discussed in Chapter 29.

Clinical Pearl

- To optimize the ultrasound image, the mnemonic PART has been recommended: pressure, alignment, rotation, tilting.

Clinical Pearls

- Recognition and understanding of sonoanatomy requires knowledge of the underlying three-dimensional anatomy.
- Optimum visualization of the target nerve requires appropriate transducer pressure, alignment with nerve, and rotation and tilting of the probe to fine-tune the image.

OPTIMIZING NERVE AND NEEDLE IMAGING WITH ULTRASOUND-CLINICAL SCENARIOS

Nerve imaging may be performed in either short-axis (probe face perpendicular to axis of nerve) or long-axis (probe face parallel to axis of nerve) position (Figure 30–2). It is frequently easier to recognize the round, often-hyperechoic, neural element with short-axis imaging, especially for a beginner. Because most nerve blocks are conducted in the extremities, this orientation results in a transducer position that is transverse, across the long axis of the arm or leg. In general, understanding the course of the nerves, based on knowledge of gross anatomy, allows one to align and rotate the transducer perpendicular to the course of the nerve subsequently adjusting the tilt as described previously to optimize the image.

Once the nerve and surrounding anatomy are identified, a needle path may be chosen so that it is imaged either in plane (needle parallel to long axis of probe) or out of plane (needle perpendicular to long axis of probe) to the ultrasound beam. While neither method has been shown superior for either block success or patient safety, the preferred approach may vary with anatomic or technical considerations. However, with in-plane imaging, it is possible to maintain an image of the entire needle, including the tip, although it can be challenging to keep the needle entirely in the viewing plane of the transducer.[15] This method is especially beneficial during instruction, as the supervisor has continual visualization of the needle tip as it is advanced through the tissues. During out-of-plane imaging, the observer is able to see only the cross section of the needle, which appears as a small hyperechoic dot, at any plane along its entire length, so that distinguishing the tip from the shaft is much more difficult.[15]

Guiding the needle tip to the target while maintaining the entire needle in the plane of imaging, however, can be challenging (Table 30–2). Appropriate adjustment of the bed height and ergonomic placement of the ultrasound so that operator's eyes can easily and rapidly shift from the image to the field (Figure 30–3), where needle alignment with the long axis of the probe can be ensured, is beneficial. It is surprisingly easy for the transducer to wander away from the plane of the needle while one's vision is fixed on the ultrasound screen. This is more likely if the operator has the probe and needle aligned perpendicular to his or her own axis of viewing, as opposed to aligning the needle and probe with the viewing axis.

In a study of novice medical students learning the basics of UGRA, Speer et al found that the subjects required less time to locate the target, and were better able to keep the needle visualized in plane on the ultrasound image, when eyes, needle, probe, and viewing screen were aligned.[16] Needle guides may also permit improved imaging of the needle during approach to the target, although more work has been done in vascular access.[17] One disadvantage of needle guides is that they restrict needle motion to one plane, which may not be always desirable.

Nerves in short axis have an appearance that is to some extent determined by their proximity to the neuraxis. Although in most areas nerves are round, they may appear fusiform, such as the musculocutaneous nerve in the proximal arm,[18] or oval-shaped, such as the sciatic nerve in the infragluteal region.[19] In close association with the spine, nerves and nerve roots are comprised primarily of neural tissue, with minimal connective tissue.[20] Because neural tissue appears hypoechoic on ultrasound imaging, while the connective tissue between fascicles is hyperechoic, nerves near the neuraxis appear as dark nodules.[21] As nerves course peripherally, the number of fascicles increases, although they diminish in size, while the amount of connective tissue also increases.[22] These changes lead to an increasingly complex "honeycomb" appearance on ultrasound in short-axis viewing[21] (Figure 30–4). Unfortunately, because of the technology limitations of the current ultrasound machines, the number

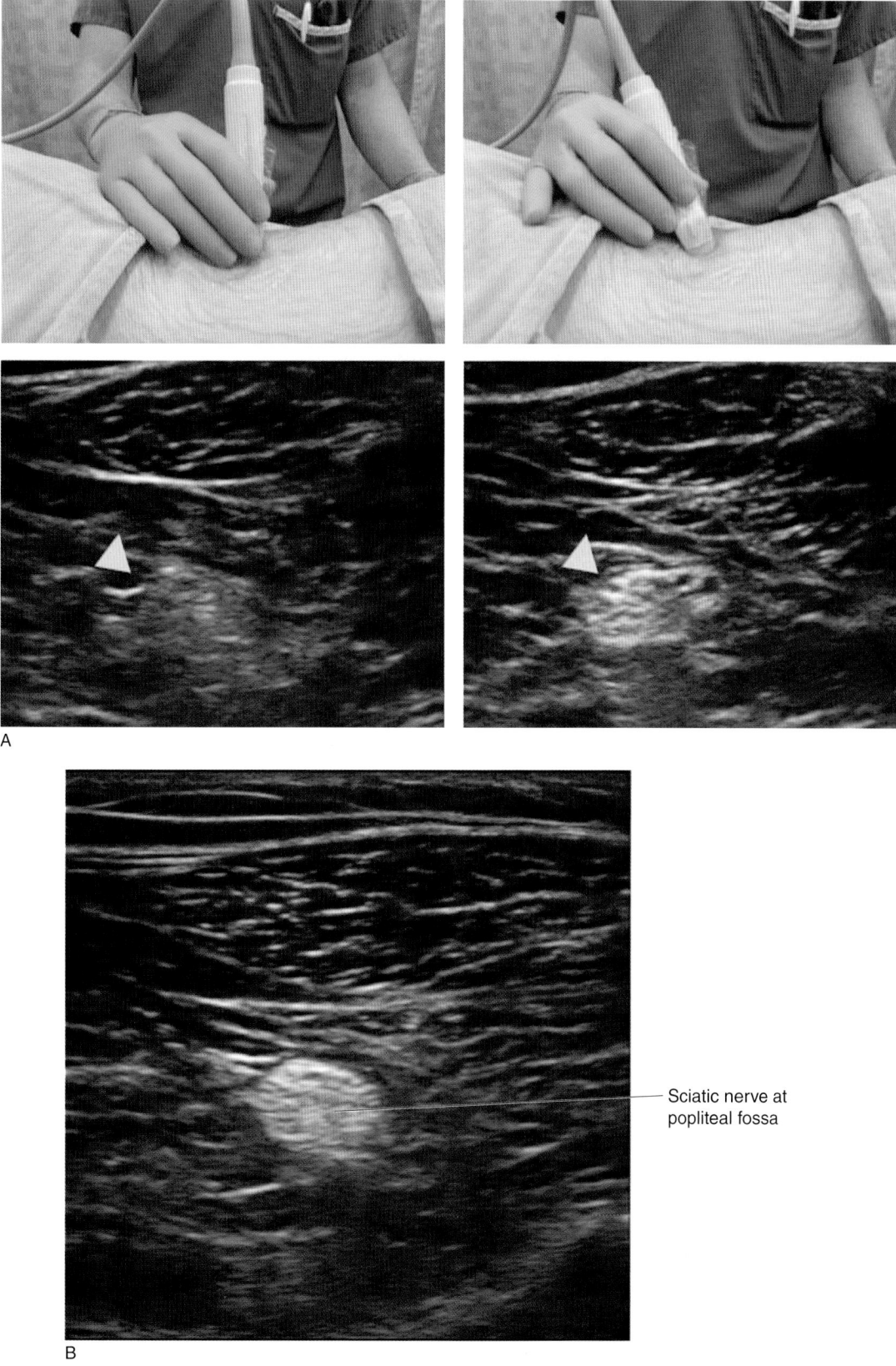

FIGURE 30–1. Fine adjustment of the probe tilt is necessary to optimize echo return from the target structure and enhance image resolution (yellow arrowheads indicate sciatic nerve at the popliteal fossa).

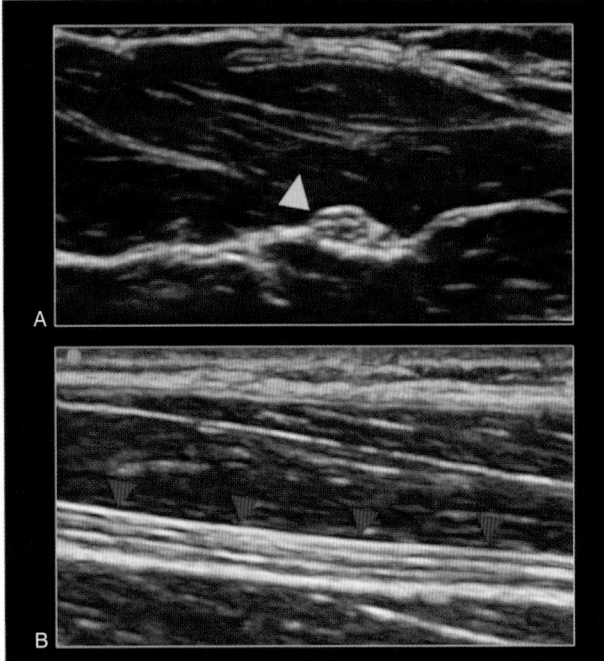

FIGURE 30–2. The median nerve. **A:** Cross-section (target structure out of plane to ultrasound beam; yellow arrowhead). **B:** Longitudinal section (target structure in plane to ultrasound beam; red arrowheads).

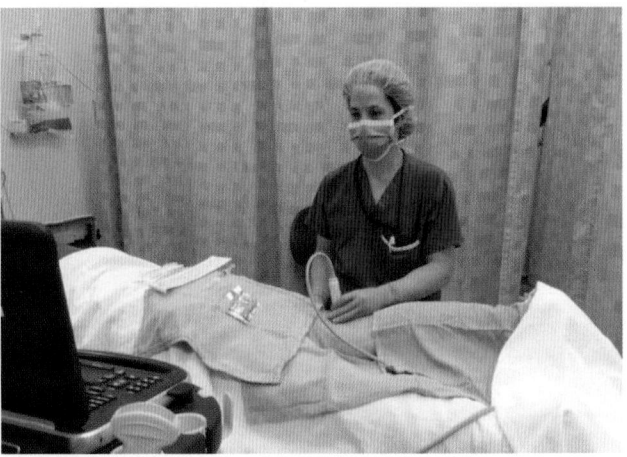

FIGURE 30–3. Ergonomic positioning for bed height and ultrasound position.

and arrangement of fascicles within a peripheral nerve may not be accurately portrayed.[23]

While different tissues have characteristic appearances on ultrasound, nerve may not be easily be distinguished from tendon when both are viewed in short axis. However, using knowledge of anatomy, the operator can follow the course of the structure caudad-cephalad to determine the nature of the structure imaged. The tendons will eventually disappear into the muscle of origin or insert into bones. A good example is the median nerve at the wrist, where it is difficult to discern the neural structure from the many tendons in the carpal tunnel, versus at the midforearm, where the nerve is much more visually distinct, as it is situated between two layers of muscle, with no surrounding tendons[24] (Figure 30–5).

An important aspect of preparing for a block is to obtain the preferred imaging plane while planning the route for needle path. The operator should make certain that no vulnerable

TABLE 30-2. Optimizing needle imaging with ultrasound.

Utilize a shallow angle of approach, if possible
"Heel" the transducer to make the face more parallel to the needle
Rotate the transducer to ensure the entire needle is seen
Tilt the transducer as necessary
Choose an "echogenic" needle
Apply needle recognition software, if available
"Hydrolocation" may help ascertain needle tip location

structures are in the projected course, such as a blood vessel, the pleura, or sensitive structures such as periosteum. This process is referred to as a "preblock scan," which can contribute to patient safety and block success.[6] In addition to two-dimensional imaging, the color Doppler setting should be utilized to identify small vessels, which may readily be confused with nerve structures (particularly roots) when viewed in short axis[25] (Figure 30–6).

To maintain the view of the needle tip and shaft, several techniques can be used. The more parallel the needle is to the face of the probe, the more echoes are transmitted back to the transducer, resulting in a superior image. This can be accomplished by gently indenting the skin at the needle insertion site or by moving the insertion site further away from the probe, resulting in a less-acute angle of insertion (Figure 30–7). The limitation of this approach is that a longer needle may be required, and more tissue is traversed en route to the target.[26]

Another technique, referred to as *heeling*, involves pressing in on the edge of the transducer opposite the side of needle insertion, which results in a more parallel alignment of the probe face with the needle. In addition, the needle itself may be structurally altered to increase its echogenicity; commercially available versions of these "echogenic needles" usually have been etched on the surface of the shaft with crosshatches to create a greater degree of scatter of the ultrasound beam.[27]

As noted, needle guides may be utilized to improve needle imaging, though at the cost of constraint of movement.[28] Laser guidance systems have also been created to improve alignment, with some success.[29] One novel, alternative method of targeted needle placement and local anesthetic delivery utilizes a GPS guidance system, which may be especially useful when imaging is made difficult by steep needle angles.[30] Proprietary software for needle localization at steep angles makes use of spatial compound imaging, which combines images of different angles of insonation. This results in enhanced needle imaging with both standard and echogenic block needles.[31] Finally, localization of the needle tip may be accomplished with "hydrolocation," in which small volumes of either dextrose solution or local anesthetic are injected to visualize spread within tissues, which typically reveals the position of the needle tip.[26]

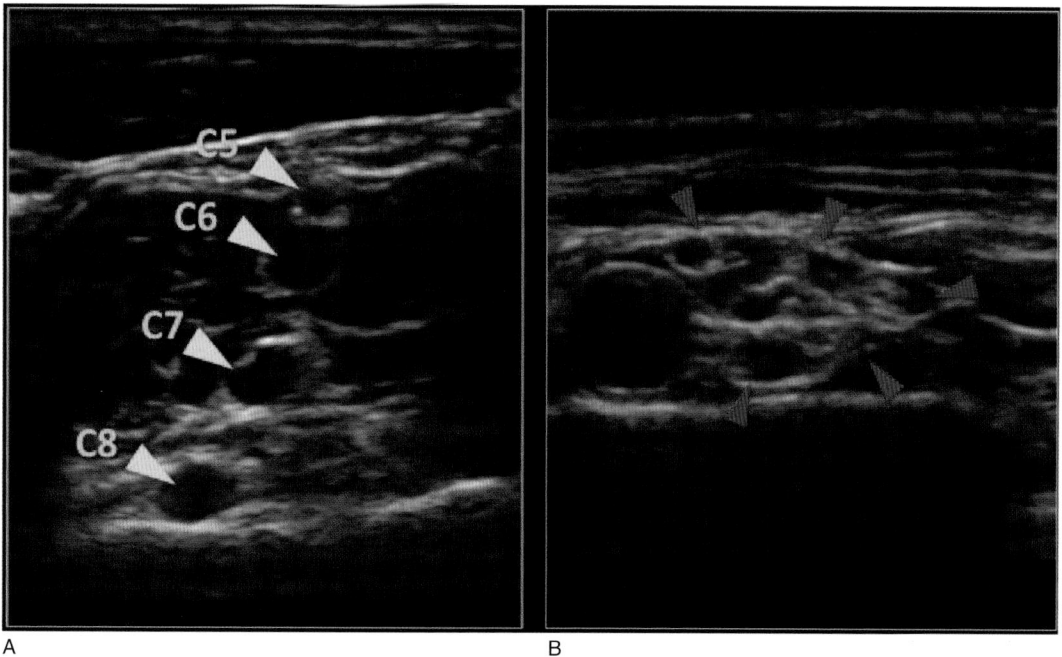

FIGURE 30–4. A: Proximal nerve appearance in the interscalene groove (yellow arrows indicate nerve roots) with little echogenic connective tissue. **B:** More distal in the supraclavicular fossa (red arrows indicate brachial plexus trunks) with "honeycomb" appearance.

Clinical Pearls

- Several different techniques are useful to maintain visualization of the needle with ultrasound imaging, including use of a shallow angle of approach, "heeling" the transducer, commercially available echogenic needles, and physical measures such as rotation and tilting of the transducer.
- In addition, hydrolocation with a small injection of fluid can be utilized to facilitate localization of the needle in difficult situations.

Clinical Pearls

- The needle should be advanced with continuous visualization to avoid injury to anatomic structures.
- A preblock scan, including use of the color Doppler function, helps plan the course of the needle.
- Passage of the needle tip through fascial planes that abut a nerve should be conducted in a tangential fashion to avoid impaling the nerve when the fascia "releases" the needle.

SAFE NEEDLE GUIDANCE WITH ULTRASOUND

In advancing the needle tip toward the targeted nerve with in-plane imaging, one should be cautious and deliberate, attempting to maintain the needle in plane at all times

(Table 30–3). The in-plane needle tip is characterized by a double-echo return generated from the beveled surface. Ultrasound is reflected from both the superficial and the deep walls of the needle, resulting in a step appearance that can be distinguished from the single return of the needle shaft. A subtle sliding motion of the ultrasound probe can aid in confirming the location of the tip as the beam walks up and down the needle shaft.

Commonly, fascial planes will be encountered that resist advance of the needle. These tough layers of connective tissue may be seen to "tent" as the tip pushes against them, suddenly giving way and snapping back to their original position. This abrupt change may have two consequences: First, the needle may advance quickly and inadvertently beyond the intent of the operator (unless this is anticipated); second, the needle may move out of plane. At this point, the forward motion of the needle should be stopped until the in-plane image is once again optimized. It is common for such fascial planes to lie just superficial or adjacent to the nerve target, as at the interscalene groove, the axillary neurovascular bundle, or the femoral nerve.[22,32] This motion may actually result in the needle thrusting forward and encountering the nerve if the sudden give of the fascial plane is not anticipated. For this reason, it is recommended to approach nerves tangentially, projecting the advance of the needle so that its tip will lie adjacent to the nerve, but not aiming for its center.[33]

The resistance encountered by these tough facial planes may also inadvertently redirect a needle when approached at a shallow angle. Temporarily steepening the needle angle may permit an easier and more controlled passage. Unfortunately, ultrasound guidance does not always produce clear images that allow one to distinguish the nerve tissue from surrounding tissue. In such situations, as the needle is advanced,

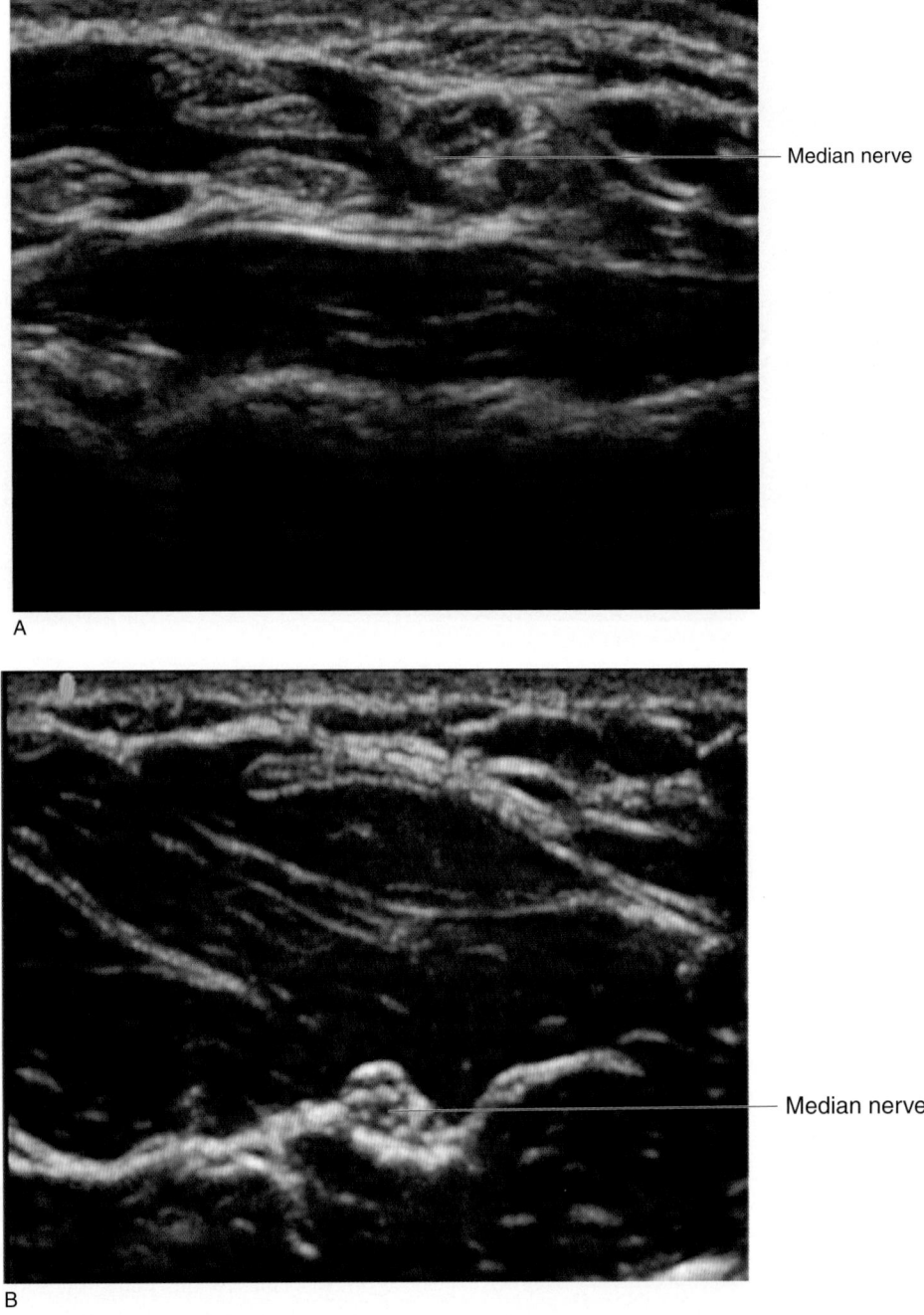

A

B

FIGURE 30–5. A: The median nerve at the wrist among many tendons within the carpal tunnel. **B:** The median nerve more proximal in the forearm surrounded by muscle.

"hydrodissection" (deliberate injection of fluid into tissue planes) can be utilized to separate structures, allowing better clarity in imaging, with either dextrose or local anesthetic solution. In addition, the behavior of tissues can be observed as the needle is advanced to help localize the needle tip in relation to neural tissue.

While it was once held that contacting a nerve with a needle tip would likely result in paresthesia, and, indeed, this was considered an appropriate nerve localization technique, we now know that paresthesia is not consistently elicited with needle-nerve contact. This emphasizes the need to accurately localize the needle tip with ultrasound imaging as well as using additional monitoring during PNBs to detect hazardous

needle-nerve relationships, such as nerve stimulation and injection pressure monitoring.[34,35]

Clinical Pearls

- Deposition of local anesthetic solution should be optimized by taking advantage of fascial planes or sheaths that can contain or channel the drug around the nerve and longitudinally along its course.
- For nerves without such local fascial containment, the solution should be injected in a circumferential manner to hasten onset of the block.

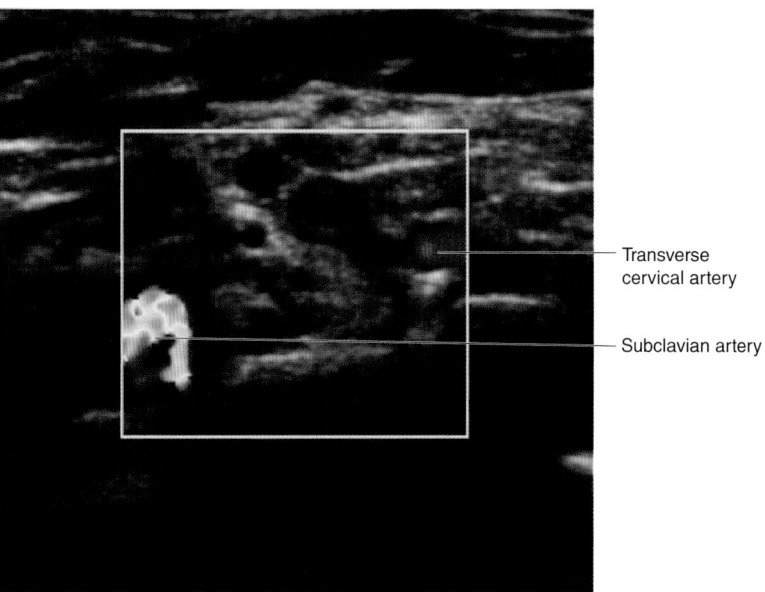

FIGURE 30–6. The supraclavicular brachial plexus with surrounding vasculature. The subclavian artery is indicated by the multicolor area, with the transverse cervical artery indicated by the red area.

Transverse
cervical artery

Subclavian artery

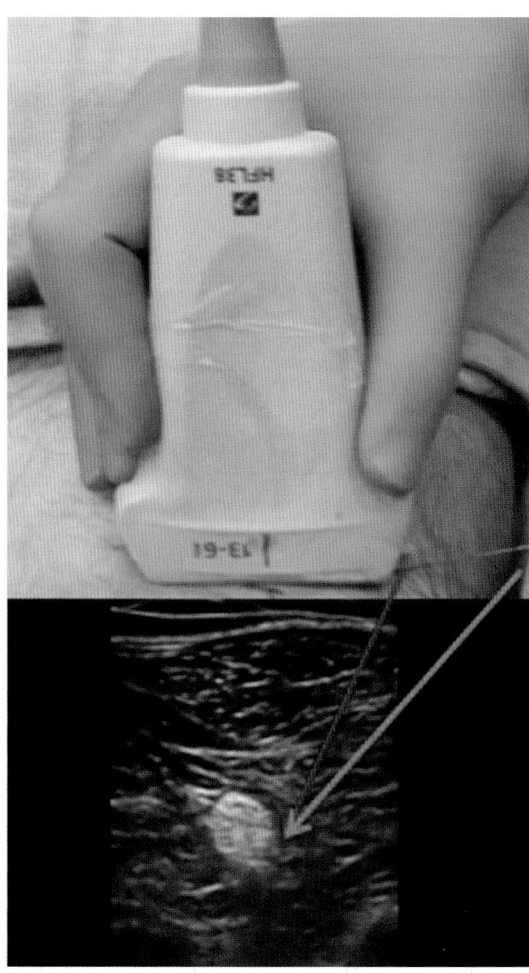

FIGURE 30–7. Needle insertion directly beside the ultrasound probe may result in difficult visualization. Insertion at a distance from the probe permits a shallower approach, allowing for stronger echo return and better visualization of the needle (green arrow) although traversing a longer tissue path.

USE OF PERIPHERAL NERVE STIMULATION WITH ULTRASOUND

The peripheral nerve stimulator (PNS) has been a standard tool in nerve localization during PNBs for several decades, with a high degree of success and low complication rate.[36] However, the widespread adoption of ultrasound imaging has called into question its ongoing role in PNB. Over a decade ago, Perlas et al evaluated the sensitivity of upper extremity peripheral nerves to peripheral nerve stimulation during ultrasound imaging of needle to nerve contact.[37] The authors reported that, despite visualizing the needle tip indenting the surface of the nerve, with the stimulator set to deliver a current of 0.5 mA or less, no motor stimulation occurred over 25% of the time.

Several studies, with a variety of different blocks, have been performed to assess the utility of this localization tool in

TABLE 30–3. Safety tips during ultrasound-guided nerve blocks.

Perform a "preblock scan" to ascertain anatomy
Utilize the color Doppler setting to identify blood vessels
Do not advance needle if tip is not localized
"Hydrodissection" can be utilized to delineate anatomy
When pushing through fascia toward a nerve, approach tangentially
Pass through fascia slowly, awaiting a "pop" or sudden release
Reoptimize image of needle tip after passing through fascia
When in doubt about needle-nerve interface, gently move needle to ascertain that the nerve does not move with it (indicating that tip is embedded within epineurium)

association with UGRA. Whether for supraclavicular block,[38] for axillary block,[39] or for femoral block[40] authors have shown that addition of the nerve stimulator as a nerve localization tool during ultrasound-guided PNB was not contributory to success. Moreover, Robards et al found that absence of a motor response to PNS between 0.2 and 0.5 mA during popliteal block did not always exclude placement of the needle within the nerve, and that stimulation might actually lead to unnecessary manipulation of the needle into the nerve.[41]

However, the stimulator may be useful as an adjunct to UGRA for reasons other than ensuring block efficacy. Because it has been well established that a threshold of nerve stimulation lower than 0.2 mA indicates high likelihood of needle tip placement within the nerve, the stimulator may be employed during UGRA as a safety monitor.[34] The nerve stimulator is particularly necessary during US-guided block of the deep nerves, or when the ultrasound image is less precise than desired. In this setting, an evoked motor response could warn against intrafascicular injection of local anesthetic.

Moreover, in some circumstances, it may be desirable to identify different nerves with more precision, as during axillary block, for which the PNS serves to delineate the nerves by their specific motor response to electrical stimulation. There may be, in some anatomic locations, neural structures that can be challenging to identify by visualization alone, whether they are the target of blockade[42] or one simply wishes to avoid them with the needle[43]; in these cases, a PNS may be invaluable to provide this identification.

Finally, there are nerves that do not lend themselves readily to ultrasound visualization, primarily because of depth or osseous interference with ultrasound transmission. The most common

example of this is the posterior approach to the lumbar plexus, in which ultrasound can be used to identify local osseous structures to guide the block, but for which the PNS remains a valuable tool for guidance of the needle tip into proximity with the nerves of the plexus.[44]

Taken overall, a plethora of data indicate that routine use of a nerve stimulator during ultrasound-guided nerve blocks yields clinically relevant safety information that can influence the clinical decision making and positively affect patient safety. However, the primary purpose of the suggested *routine* use of nerve stimulation with UGRA is for safety monitoring, rather nerve localization (Figure 30–8). In this capacity, the nerve stimulator can be simply set at 0.5 mA (0.1 ms), 2 Hz, without changing the current intensity throughout the procedure. While the motor response is not sought, occurrence of the motor response should necessitate cessation of the needle advancement and slight withdrawal of the needle as a motor response at this current delivery setting almost always indicates needle-nerve contact or intraneural needle placement.[45,46]

OPTIMIZING THE DELIVERY OF LOCAL ANESTHETIC NEAR THE TARGET NERVE

After accurate needle placement near the target nerve, and after ascertaining that aspiration is negative for intravascular needle placement, injection of the local anesthetic is made in the tissue plane that contains the nerve(s) to be anesthetized (Table 30–4). Brull et al evaluated the long-held notion that the local anesthetic solution should be directed in a circumferential manner around the visible nerve, with change of needle position if

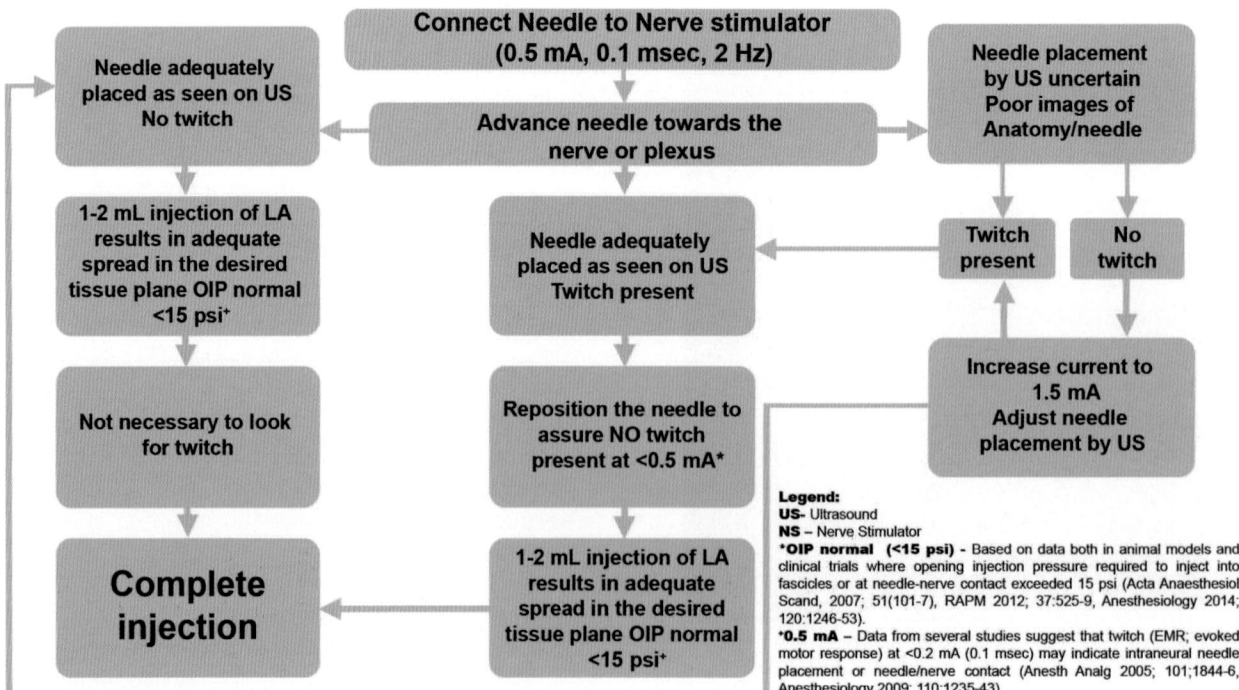

FIGURE 30–8. Algorithm: The primary purpose of the suggested *routine* use of nerve stimulation with UGRA is for the purpose of safety monitoring, rather than nerve localization.

TABLE 30–4. Optimizing local anesthetic deposition.

Inject local anesthetic solution in small aliquots
Observe for pain or high pressure during injection
Make certain that spread of fluid is observed at needle tip during injection
Aspirate between injections
Be aware of intervening fascial planes that may sequester or channel the solution
Avoid deposition of local anesthetic into muscle
For solitary nerves in extremities, seek to create a "donut" or "halo" around nerve
For nerves within a fascial enclosure, seek to "fill" the fascial confines with solution[a]

[a]Specific situations are discussed in chapters covering individual nerve blocks.

necessary, in comparison to simply allowing the solution to accumulate along one aspect of the nerve with one needle position.[47] They found that the resultant block set up 33% more rapidly with the former than with the latter. While the creation of a "donut" or "halo" around the nerve may be suggested as a general recommendation, some nerves, by virtue of their anatomical situation, may not require such deliberate circumferential placement. This is typically dictated by the location and configuration of overlying or surrounding fascial planes, such as in the interscalene groove[48] and at the femoral triangle.[32] Optimal delivery of local anesthetic around each nerve is described in subsequent specific UGRA chapters.

Real-time imaging of local anesthetic injection permits assessment of correct disposition of the fluid. The injection phase should be carried out with small aliquots of local anesthetic (3–5 mL), with a short period allowed to elapse between each, to allow evidence of any symptoms of local anesthetic systemic toxicity (LAST) to be manifest before continuing to administer the drug, as recommended by the American Society of Regional Anesthesia and Pain Medicine (ASRA) guidelines.[49] In addition, delivery of each aliquot should be preceded by aspiration and should progress with attention to opening injection pressures or complaints of pain or paresthesia in the distribution of the target nerve.

While ultrasound has been shown to produce a lower likelihood of intravascular needle placement,[50] intravascular injection with LAST may still occur.[51] It is thus imperative to be aware of the location of vessels, which have a distending pressure so low that ordinary pressure at the body surface with a transducer obliterates their lumen entirely.[4] Therefore, it is helpful to screen for the presence of vessels using color Doppler during the preblock scan. However, small vessels may be missed, and Doppler function deteriorates at greater depths. Thus, it is imperative to observe the ultrasound image throughout the injection for evidence of tissue spread by the local anesthetic solution at the tip of the needle. Failure to visualize such spread suggests that the tip of the needle either is out of plane or is in the lumen of a vessel.

Errant needle placement has been described both into vessels[52] and into nerves.[53,54] Moayeri et al in a cadaver-based study, have

shown that ultrasound imaging is sensitive to injection into peripheral nerve, with as little as 0.5 mL causing visible evidence of nerve distension.[55] Such visualization allows immediate withdrawal of the needle, which may reduce the chance for nerve injury, compared to injection of a large volume of local anesthetic.

CONCLUSION

Ultrasonography has revolutionized the field of regional anesthesia. The effective application of this technology requires understanding of two-dimensional anatomy, optimal imaging of the nerves and anatomical structures, accurate real-time needle guidance, and precise local anesthetic delivery. The combination of these elements ensures that the most benefit can be derived from this powerful imaging modality, ensuring high nerve block success and improved patient safety, particularly with regard to LAST. Individual ultrasound-guided blocks are discussed in detail in Chapters 31 through 35.

REFERENCES

1. Kapral S, Krafft P, Eibenberger K, et al: Ultrasound-guided supraclavicular approach for regional anesthesia of the brachial plexus. Anesth Analg 1994;78:507–513.
2. Marhofer P, Schrogendofer K, Koinig H, et al: Ultasonographic guidance improves sensory block and onset time of three-in-one blocks. Anesth Analg 1997;85:854–857.
3. Marhofer P, Schrogendofer K, Wallner T, et al: Ultasonographic guidance reduces the amount of local anesthetic for 3-in-1 blocks. Reg Anesth Pain Med 1998;23:584–588.
4. Perlas A, Chan VW, Simons M: Brachial plexus examination and localization using ultrasound and electrical stimulation. Anesthesiology 2003;99:429–435.
5. Gray AT: Ultrasound-guided regional anesthesia. Anesthesiology 2006;104:368–373.
6. Manickam BP, Perlas A, Chan VW, et al: The role of a preprocedure systematic survey in ultrasound-guided regional anesthesia. Reg Anesth Pain Med 2008;33:566–570.
7. Sites BD, Brull R: Ultrasound guidance in peripheral regional anesthesia: Philosophy, evidence-based medicine, and techniques. Curr Opin Anesth 2006;19:630–639.
8. Sites BD, Chan VW, Neal JM, et al: The American Society of Regional Anesthesia and Pain Medicine and the European Society of Regional Anaesthesia and Pain Therapy Joint Committee recommendations for education and training in ultrasound-guided regional anesthesia. Reg Anesth Pain Med 2010;35(Suppl 1):S74–80.
9. Orebaugh SL, Bigeleisen PE, Kentor ML: Impact of a regional anesthesia rotation on ultrasonographic identification of anatomic structures by anesthesiology residents. Acta Anaesth Scand 2009;53:364–368.
10. Orebaugh SL, Williams BA, Kentor ML, et al: Interscalene block using ultrasound guidance: Impact of experience on resident performance. Acta Anaesth Scand 2009;53:1268–1274.
11. Adhikary SD, Hadzic A, McQuillan PM: Simulator for teaching hand-eye coordination during ultrasound-guided regional anaesthesia. Br J Anaesth 2013;111(5):844–845.
12. Wegener JT, van Doorn T, Eshuis JH, et al: Value of an electronic tutorial for image interpretation in ultrasound-guided regional anesthesia. Reg Anesth Pain Med 2013;38:44–49.
13. Woodworth GE, Chen EM, Horn JL, et al: Efficacy of computer-based video and simulation in ultrasound-guided regional anesthesia training. J Clin Anesth 2014;26:212–221.
14. Sites BD, Spence BC, Gallagher JD, et al: Characterizing novice behavior associated with learning ultrasound-guided peripheral regional anesthesia. Reg Anesth Pain Med 2007;32:107–115.
15. Sites BD, Spence BC, Gallagher J, et al: Regional anesthesia meets ultrasound: A specialty in transition. ACTA Anaesthes Scand 2008;52:456–466.

16. Speer M, McLennan N, Nixon C: Novice learner in-plane ultrasound imaging. Reg Anesth Pain Med 2013;38:350–352.

17. Ball RD, Scouras NE, Orebaugh S, et al: Randomized, prospective observational simulation study comparing residents' needle-guided vs. free-hand ultrasound techniques for central venous catheter access. Br J Anaesth 2012;108:72–79.

18. Schafhalter-Zoppoth I, Gray AT: The musculocutaneous nerve: Ultrasound appearance for peripheral nerve block. Reg Anesth Pain Med 2005;30:385–390.

19. Moayeri N, van Geffen GJ, Bruhn J, et al: Correlation among ultrasound, cross-sectional anatomy and histology of the sciatic nerve. Reg Anesth Pain Med 2010;35:442–449.

20. Bonnel F: Microscopic anatomy of the adult human brachial plexus: An anatomical and histological basis for microsurgery. Microsurgery 1984; 5:107–118.

21. van Geffen GJ, Moayeri N, Bruhn J, et al: Correlation between ultrasound imaging, cross-sectional anatomy, and histology of the brachial plexus. Reg Anesth Pain Med 2009;34:490–497.

22. Moayeri N, Bigeleisen PE, Groen GJ: Quantitative architecture of the brachial plexus and surrounding compartments, and their possible significance for plexus blocks. Anesthesiology 2008;108:299–304.

23. Sylvestri E, Martinoli C, Derchi LE, et al: Echotexture of peripheral nerves: Correlations between US and histologic findings and criteria to differentiate tendons. Radiology 1995;197:291–296.

24. McCartney CJ, Xu D, Constantinescu C, et al: Ultrasound examination of peripheral nerves in the forearm. Reg Anesth Pain Med 2007;32:434–439.

25. Sites BD, Brull R, Chan VW, et al: Artifacts and pitfall errors associated with ultrasound-guided regional anesthesia. Reg Anesth Pain Med 2007;32:419–433.

26. Chin KJ, Perlas A, Chan VW, et al: Needle visualization in ultrasound-guided regional anesthesia: Challenges and solutions. Reg Anesth Pain Med 2008;33:532–544.

27. Hebard S, Hocking G: Echogenic technology can improve needle visibility during ultrasound-guided regional anesthesia. Reg Anesth Pain Med 2011;36:185–189.

28. Rettig HC, Gielen MJ: Free-handing technique or mechanical needle guide device? [letter] Reg Anesth Pain Med 2009;34:608–609.

29. Tsui, BC: Facilitating needle alignment in-plane to an ultrasound beam using a portable laser unit. Reg Anesth Pain Med 2007;32:84–88.

30. Wong SW, Niazi AU, Chin KJ, et al: Real-time ultrasound guided spinal anesthesia using the SonixGPS needle tracking system. Can J Anaesth 2013;60:50–53.

31. Wiesmann T, Borntrager A, Zoremba M, et al: Compound imaging technology and echogenic needle design. Reg Anesth Pain Med 2013; 38:452–455.

32. Soong J, Schafhalter-Zoppoth I, Gray AT: The importance of transducer angle to ultrasound visibility of the femoral nerve. Reg Anesth Pain Med 2005;30:505.

33. Alakkad H, Chin KJ: The importance of good needling technique in ultrasound-guided axillary block. Reg Anesth 2013;38(2):166.

34. Bigeleisen PE1, Moayeri N, Groen GJ. Extraneural versus intraneural stimulation thresholds during ultrasound-guided supraclavicular block. Anesthesiology. 2009;110:1235–43.

35. Hadzic A, Dilberovic F, Shah S, Kulenovic A, Kapur E, Zaciragic A, Cosovic E, Vuckovic I, Divanovic KA, Mornjakovic Z, Thys DM, Santos AC. Combination of intraneural injection and high injection pressure leads to fascicular injury and neurologic deficits in dogs. Reg Anesth Pain Med 2004;29:417–23.

36. Auroy Y, Benhamou D, Bargues L: Major complications of regional anesthesia in France. Anesthesiology 2002;97:1274–1280.

37. Perlas A, Niazi A, McCartney C, et al: The sensitivity of motor response to nerve stimulation and paresthesia for nerve localization as evaluated by ultrasound. Reg Anesth Pain Med 2006;31:445–450.

38. Beach ML, Sites BD, Gallagher JD: Use of a nerve stimulator does not improve the efficacy of ultrasound-guided supraclavicular block. J Clin Anesth 2006;18:580–584.

39. Chan VW, Perlas A, McCartney CJ, et al: Ultrasound guidance improves the success rate of axillary brachial plexus block. Can J Anaesth 2007; 54:176–182.

40. Sites BD, Beach ML, Chinn CD, et al: A comparison of sensory and motor loss after a femoral nerve block conducted with ultrasound versus ultrasound and nerve stimulation. Reg Anesth Pain Med 2009;34: 508–513.

41. Robards C, Hadzic A, Somasundraram L, et al: Intraneural injectin with low-current stimulation during popliteal sciatic nerve block. Anesth Analg 2009;109:673–677.

42. Sigenthaler A, Moriggl B, Mlekusch S, et al: Ultrasound-guided suprascapular nerve block: Description of a novel supraclavicular approach. Reg Anesth Pain Med 2012;37:325–328.

43. Hanson NA, Auyong DB: Systematic ultrasound identification of the dorsal scapular and long thoracic nerves during interscalene block. Reg Anesth Pain Med 2013;38:54–57.

44. Karmakar MK, Ho AM, Li X, et al: Ultrasound-guided lumbar plexus block through the acoustic window of the lumbar ultrasound trident. Br J Anaesth 2008;100:533–537.

45. Gadsden J, Latmore M, Levine DM, Robinson A: High opening injection pressure is associated with needle-nerve and needle-fascia contact during femoral nerve block. Reg Anesth Pain Med 2016;41(1):50–55.

46. Gadsden JC, Choi JJ, Lin E, Robinson A: Opening injection pressure consistently detects needle-nerve contact during ultrasound-guided interscalene brachial plexus block. Anesthesiology 2014;120(5): 1246–1253.

47. Brull R, MacFarlane AJ, Parrington SJ, et al: Is circumferential injection advantageous for ultrasound-guided popliteal sciatic nerve block? Reg Anesth Pain Med 2011;36:266–270.

48. Spence BC, Beach ML, Gallagher JD, et al: Ultrasound-guided interscalene blocks: Understanding where to inject the local anesthetic. Anaesthesia 2011;66(6):509–514.

49. Neal JM, Bernards CM, Butterworth JF, et al: ASRA practice advisory on local anesthetic systemic toxicity. Reg Anesth Pain Med 2010;35: 350–352.

50. Abrahams MS, Aziz MF, Fu RF, et al: Ultrasound guidance compared with electrical neurostimulation for peripheral nerve block: A systematic review and meta-analysis of randomized controlled trials. Anaesth 2009; 102:408–417.

51. Zetlaoui PJ, Labbe J-P, Benhamou D: Ultrasound guidance for axillary plexus block does not prevent intravascular injection [letter]. Anesthesiology 2008;109:761.

52. VadeBancouer TR, Weinberg GL, Oswald S, et al: Early detection of intravascular injection during ultrasound-guided supraclavicular brachial plexus block. Reg Anesth Pain Med 2008;33:278–279.

53. Liu SS, YaDeau JT, Shaw PM, et al: Incidence of unintentional intraneural injection and postoperative neurological complications with ultrasound-guided interscalene and supraclavicular nerve blocks. Anaesthesia 2011; 66:1365–2044.

54. Hara K, Sakura S, Yokokawa N, et al: Incidence and effects of unintentional intraneural injection during ultrasound-guided subgluteal sciatic nerve block. Reg Anesth Pain Med 2012;37:289–293.

55. Krediet AC, Moayer N, Bleys RL, et al: Intraneural or extraneural: Diagnostic accuracy or ultrasound assessment of localizing low-volume injection. Reg Anesth Pain Med 2014;39:409–413.

Ultrasound-Guided Head and Neck Nerve Blocks

CHAPTER 31

Nerve Blocks of the Face

Chrystelle Sola, Christophe Dadure, Olivier Choquet, and Xavier Capdevila

INTRODUCTION

Regional anesthesia is commonly used for postoperative pain management to decrease postoperative pain and opioid consumption following head and neck surgery. Myriad techniques can be used for both acute and chronic pain management either diagnostic or therapeutic procedures. Because of the vicinity of cranial and cervical nerves to many vital structures in a compact area, the efficacy and safety of cephalic blocks are based on precise and detailed knowledge of the anatomical relationships of the selected nerve, its deep and superficial courses, and the final sensory territories.

Sensory innervation of the face and neck is supplied by the trigeminal nerve (fifth cranial or V) and the C2–C4 cervical nerve roots that constitute the superficial cervical plexus (Figure 31–1A).

This chapter outlines clinically applicable regional blocks of the face that for perioperative and chronic pain management. For each block, practical anatomy, indications, technique, and type of complications are specifically described.

TRIGEMINAL NERVE

The fifth cranial nerve carries both sensory and motor components. The trigeminal ganglion (semilunar or Gasserian ganglion) lies in Meckel's cave, an invagination of the dura mater near the apex of the petrous part of the temporal bone in the posterior cranial fossa. Postganglionic fibers exit the ganglion to form three nerves:

- The ophthalmic nerve (V1), a sensory nerve, divides into three branches (lacrimal, frontal, and nasociliary nerves) before entering the orbit through the superior orbital fissure. It innervates the forehead, eyebrows, upper eyelids, and anterior area of the nose (Figure 31–1B).
- The maxillary nerve (V2), a purely sensory nerve, exits the middle cranial fossa via the foramen rotundum, passes forward and laterally through the pterygopalatine fossa, and reaches the floor of the orbit by the infraorbital foramen. It innervates the lower eyelid, the upper lip, the lateral portion of the nose and nasal septum, cheek, roof of the mouth, bone, teeth and sinus of the maxilla, and the soft and hard palates (Figure 31–1B).
- The mandibular nerve (V3) is a mixed sensory and motor (for the mastication muscles) nerve. After exiting the cranium through the foramen ovale, it delivers sensory branches that supply the front of the ear, the temporal area, the anterior two-thirds of the tongue and the skin, mucosa, and teeth and bone of the mandible (Figure 31–1B).

These sensory nerves can be blocked either at their emergence point from the cranium (V2 and V3) or, more distally and superficially, at their exit from the facial bones (V1, V2, V3) (Figure 31–1).

Clinical Pearls

- Neural blockade of the trigeminal ganglion is reserved for patients with trigeminal neuralgia who do not respond to pharmacologic therapy.
- Block of the trigeminal ganglion and its primary divisions is often used as a diagnostic test to predict response to neural blockade prior to proceeding with neurolysis.

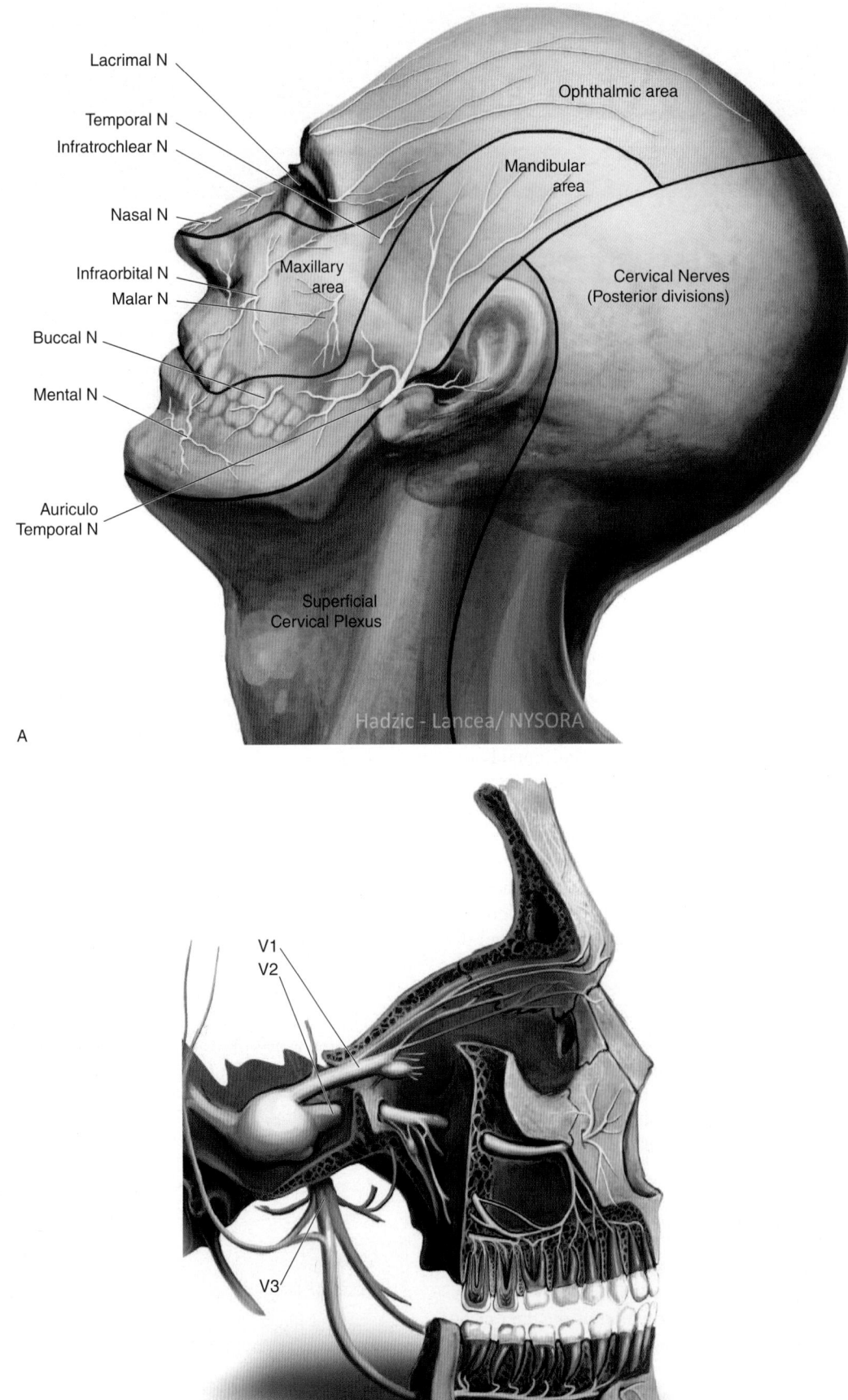

FIGURE 31–1. Innervation of the face. **A:** Dermatomes of the head, neck, and face. **B:** Distribution of the three branches of the trigeminal nerve.

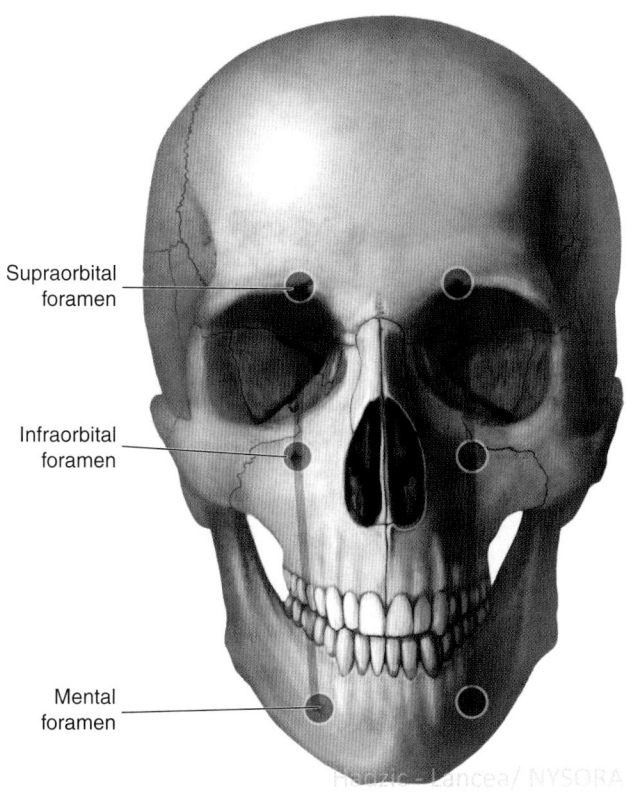

FIGURE 31–2. Terminal sensory branches of the trigeminal nerve exit the facial bone through the supraorbital, infraorbital, and mental foramen, which are at the intersection with the vertical line passing over the ipsilateral centered pupil.

The Superficial Trigeminal Nerve Blocks

For superficial trigeminal nerve blocks, the local anesthetic solution should be injected in close proximity to the three individual terminal superficial branches of the trigeminal nerve divisions: frontal nerve (of the ophthalmic nerve, V1 division); infraorbital nerve (of the maxillary nerve, V2 division); and mental nerve (sensory terminal branch of the mandibular nerve, V3 division). Each nerve is anatomically close to its respective foramen, usually located on a line drawn sagittally through the pupil (Figure 31–2).

Block of the Frontal Nerve (Supraorbital and Supratrochlear Branches)

Anatomy The frontal nerve enters the orbit at the superior orbital fissure and divides into the supraorbital and supratrochlear branches. The supraorbital nerve exits with its vessels through the supraorbital foramen and continues superiorly between the elevator palpebrae superioris and the periosteum. The supratrochlear nerve appears more medial through the supraorbital notch. These two branches supply the sensory innervation to the frontal scalp and forehead, the medial part of the upper eyelid, and the root of the nose (Figures 31–3A and 31–3B).

Indication The block of the frontal nerve is useful for lower forehead and upper eyelid surgery such as repair of a laceration, frontal craniotomies, frontal ventriculoperitoneal shunt placement, Ommaya reservoir placement,[1] and plastic surgical

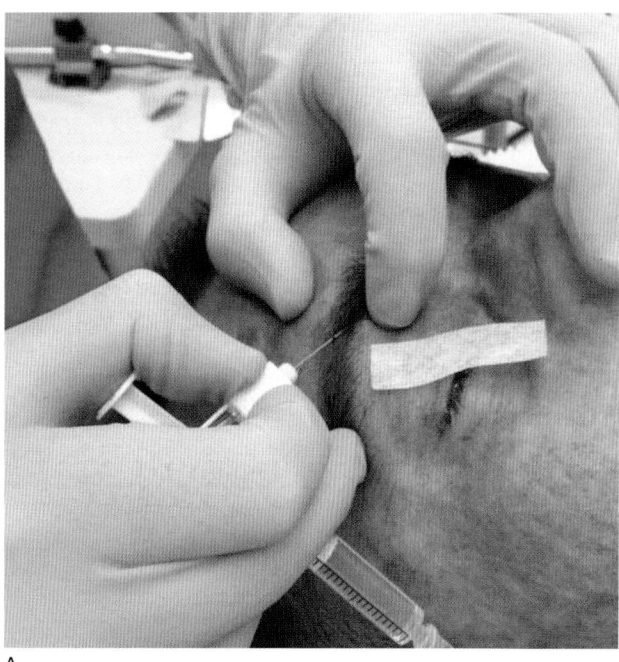

A

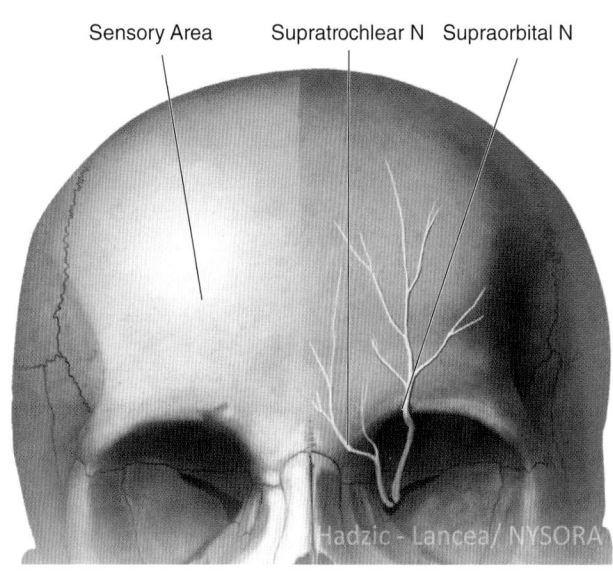

B

FIGURE 31–3. A: Supraorbital and supratrochlear block. **B:** Sensory area of the supraorbital and supratrochlear nerves.

procedures, including excision of anterior scalp pigmented nevus, benign tumor with skin grafting, or dermoid cyst excision.[2] Frequently, surgery on one side of the forehead requires a supplemental block of the contralateral supratrochlear nerve because of overlapping distributions of the nerves.

Block of branches of the ophthalmic nerve has been described for the management of acute migraine headache attacks localized to the ocular and retro-ocular region[3] and in the treatment of pain related to acute zherpesoster.[4]

Classical Landmark Technique The supraorbital foramen can easily be palpated by following the orbit rim 2 cm from the midline in adults (intersection of the medial one-third and the lateral two-thirds). It is located approximately at the same sagittal plane as the pupil in most patients. The needle (25-gauge intradermal needle in adults, 30 gauge in children) is introduced 0.5 cm under the inferior edge of the eyebrow and is directed medially and cephalad. When the needle tip is near the supraorbital notch, after test aspiration, and with caution not to penetrate the foramen, local anesthetic solution (0.5–1 mL) can be injected, creating a subcutaneous wheal. For a supratrochlear block, the landmark is at the top of the angle formed by the eyebrow and the nasal spine where the nerve is in contact with the bone. The supratrochlear nerve can be blocked immediately following supraorbital nerve block, without removing the needle, by directing the needle about 1 cm toward the midline and injecting an additional 0.5 mL of local anesthetic.

After the injection, firm pressure is applied for better anesthetic spread and prevention of ecchymosis.

Complications Complications are rarely reported during the performance of this block, and may include hematoma, intravascular injection, and eye globe damage.

Clinical Pearls

The following are specific complications associated with head and neck blocks:

- Subarachnoid or epidural placement of local anesthetic may lead to high spinal and brainstem anesthesia.
- Generalized seizures may occur with the injection of even small intra-arterial volumes of local anesthetic (0.5 mL or less) as the arterial blood flow continues directly from the arteries in the head and neck to the brain.
- Hematoma formation.
- Respiratory distress may result from block of the phrenic or recurrent laryngeal nerves, pneumothorax, or loss of sensory or motor function of the nerves to the airway.

Block of the Infraorbital Nerve

Anatomy The terminal branch of the maxillary nerve (V2, the second division of the trigeminal nerve) is called the infraorbital nerve when it reaches the infraorbital fossa. It exits the cranium through the infraorbital foramen in a caudad and medial direction and divides into several sensory branches: the inferior palpebral, the lateral nasal, and the superior labial nerves. The infraorbital artery and vein run parallel in close proximity to the nerve. Territories of the infraorbital nerve include the skin and mucous membrane of the upper lip and lower eyelid and the cheek between them and to the lateral side of the nose (Figures 31–4A and 31–4B).

Indications Infraorbital nerve block is commonly used in neonates, infants, and older children undergoing cleft lip repair to provide early postoperative analgesia without the potential risk of respiratory depression that may occur when opioid analgesics are used.[5-7] The other main indications are surgeries of the lower eyelid, the upper lip, the median cheek, endoscopic

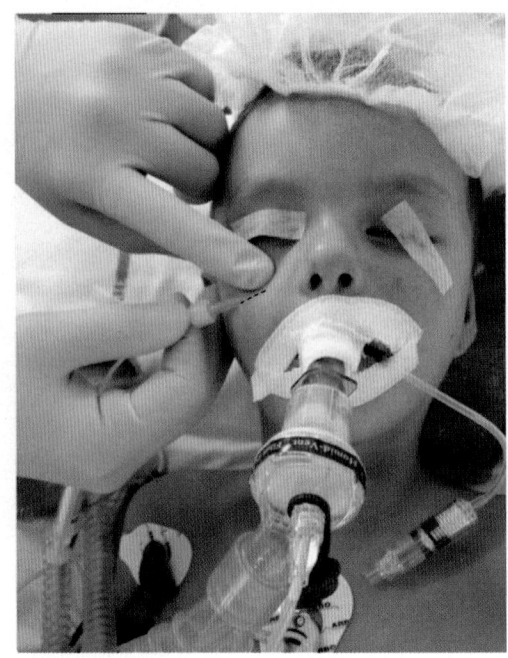

A

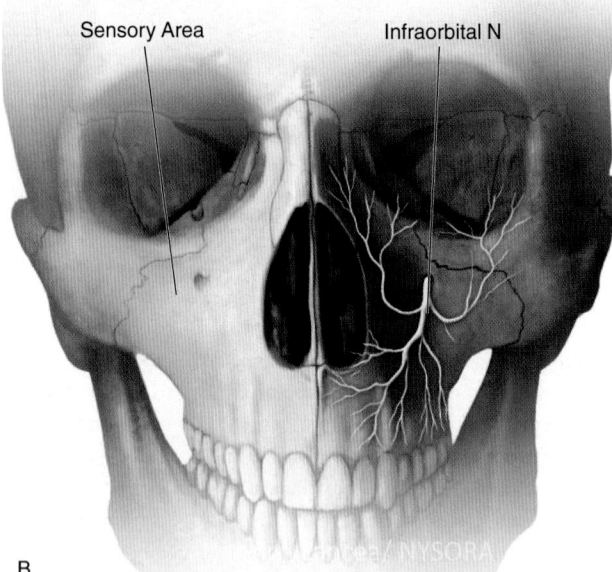

B

FIGURE 31–4. A: Infraorbital nerve block. **B:** Sensory area of the infraorbital nerve.

sinus surgery,[8] rhinoplasty or nasal septal repair, and transsphenoidal hypophysectomy.[9]

Clinical Pearls

- The infraorbital nerve is sensory nerve. As the nerve exits the infraorbital foramen, it supplies the skin of the lower eyelid, nose, cheek, and upper lip.
- It is accompanied by the infraorbital artery and vein.

Classical Landmark Techniques For the classical landmark techniques, two approaches can be used to perform this block: the intraoral and extraoral approaches. Regardless of the chosen technique, it is necessary to prevent the penetration of the foramen to prevent damage to the eyeball. This can be done by keeping a finger on the foramen throughout the procedure.

• For the intraoral approach, the first landmark is the infraorbital foramen, which is localized just below the orbital rim, at the intersection of a vertical line drawn caudally through the center of the pupil and a horizontal line through the nasal alae. The incisor and the first premolar are then palpated. A 25- to 27-gauge needle is inserted into the buccal mucosa in the subsulcal groove at the level of the canine or the first premolar and directed upward and outward into the canine fossa. A finger is kept over the infraorbital foramen to assess the proper location of the needle tip and to avoid damage of the eyeball by accidental cephalad advancement of the needle into the orbit. Then, 1–3 mL of local anesthetic is injected after negative aspiration.

• For the extraoral approach, the infraorbital foramen is palpated (see preceding discussion). A 25- to 27-gauge needle is advanced perpendicularly with a cephalic and medial direction toward the foramen until bony resistance is appreciated. Because the axis of the infraorbital foramen is oriented caudally and medially, a lateral-to-medial approach reduces the risk of penetration of the foramen. A finger is always placed at the level of the infraorbital foramen to avoid further cephalad advancement of the needle, and gentle pressure is recommended to prevent hematoma formation.

Complications Hematoma formation, persistent paresthesia of the upper lip, prolonged numbness of the upper lip, and intravascular placement are possible. A serious (but rare) risk is penetration of the foramen, which may result in nerve damage by compression in the narrow infraorbital canal, or needle penetration of the flimsy orbital floor and damage to the orbital contents. The intraoral approach is not advised in neonates and small infants because of the proximity of the orbit.

Block of the Mental Nerve

Anatomy The mental nerve is the terminal branch of the alveolar nerve (the largest branch of the mandibular nerve, V3). It emerges at the mental foramen and divides into three branches: a descending branch to the skin of the chin and two ascending branches to the skin, labial mucosae of the lower lip, as well as the anterior teeth (Figures 31–5A and 31–5B).

Indications Procedures involving hemangiomata, laceration repair, and other surgery involving the lower lip, skin of the chin, and the incisive and canine teeth.

Classical Landmark Technique For the classical landmark technique, the mental foramen is located in line with the pupil on the mental process of the mandible, in regard to the inferior premolar tooth. Puncture with a 25- to 27-gauge needle is performed 1 cm lateral to the foramen palpated. The needle is directed with a lateral-to-medial direction to avoid foramen penetration.

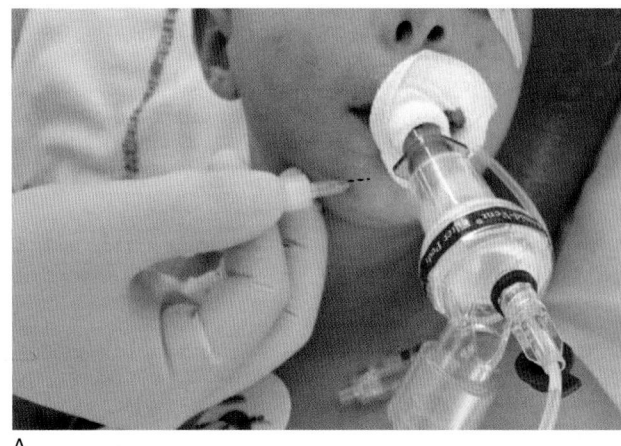

A

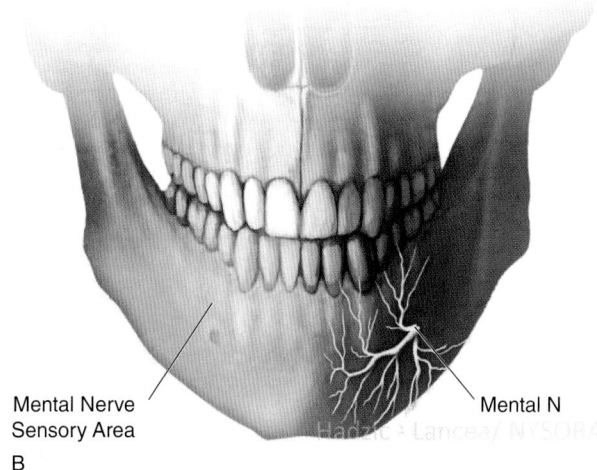

B

FIGURE 31–5. A: Mental nerve block. **B:** Sensory area of the mental nerve.

Similar to the infraorbital nerve block, an intraoral route can be utilized: The lower lip is retracted, and the needle is introduced through the mucosa in front of the first inferior premolar tooth. The needle is directed downward and outward toward the mental foramen palpated with the finger.

Complications Hematoma formation and persistent paresthesia have been reported. Less commonly, penetration of the foramen occurs, which may result in permanent nerve damage or vascular injection.

Ultrasound Guidance Technique for Superficial Trigeminal Nerve Blocks

The ultrasound-guided approach to locate the landmark foramina for superficial trigeminal nerve block is feasible.[10] Using a high-frequency linear transducer, bone appears as a hyperechoic linear edge (white line) with an underlying anechoic (dark) shadow. At the foramina of these three nerves, disruption within the hyperechoic line indicates a discontinuity in the bone ("bone gap"). In addition, ultrasound can visualize satellite vessels close to each nerve using the color Doppler function. The real-time view of the injection spread can help avoid intravascular injection, nerve injury by the needle, or injection into the foramen.

To localize the supraorbital notch (foramen), the probe is located transversely above the orbital rim (Figure 31–6A).

The infraorbital foramen can be visualized by positioning the ultrasound probe horizontally or vertically in the sagittal plane. Fine translational movements from medial to lateral along the lower orbital margin are performed to highlight the disruption of the bone table (Figure 31–6B).

Finally, the mental foramen is localized using a transverse or sagittal plane with dynamic scanning between the upper and lower borders of the mandible (Figure 31–6C).

Clinical Pearls

The following are specific complications associated with Superficial Nerves Blocks of the face:

- Facial artery vasospasm.
- Nerve injury is rare and most cases are transient and resolve completely. However, careful attention is needed

to avoid injection into foramina whose consequences could lead to permanent neurological damage.
- Intravascular injection and systemic toxicity: Generalized seizures may occur with the injection of even small intraarterial volumes of local anesthetic (0.5 mL or less) as the arterial blood flow continues directly from the face arteries to the brain.
- Ecchymosis and Hematoma formation. This complication can be decreased after superficial nerves blocks techniques by using a 25- or 27- gauge needle and applying a manual pressure immediately after injection.
- Needle tract infection is very infrequent complication.

▓ The Maxillary Nerve Block
Anatomy

The maxillary nerve exits the skull through the foramen rotundum before dividing into terminal branches (Table 31–1 and

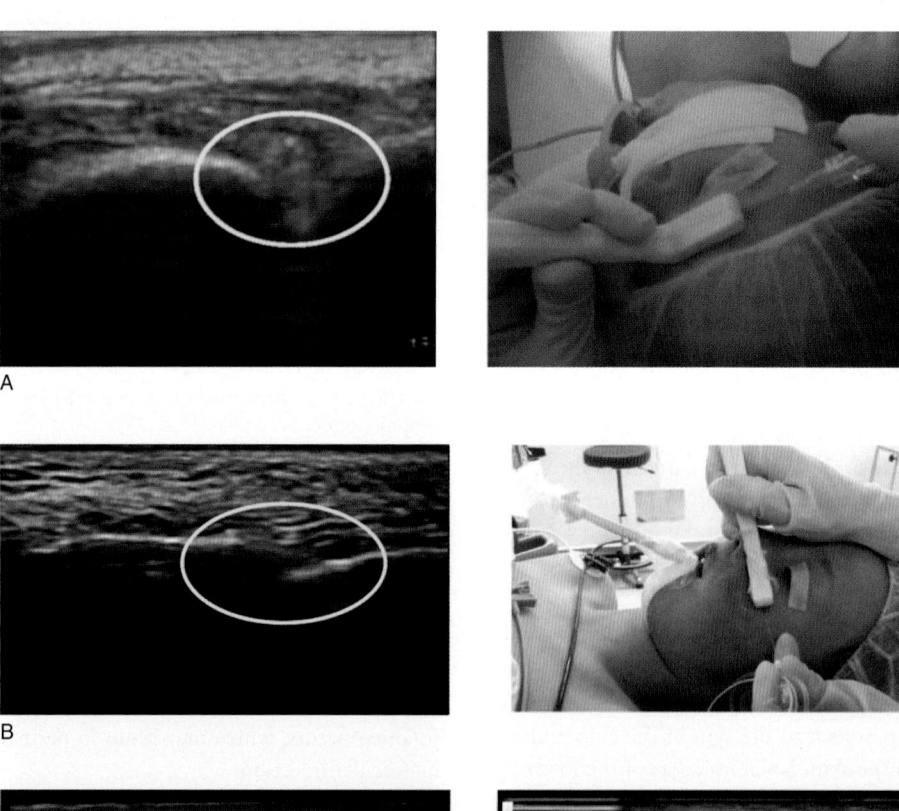

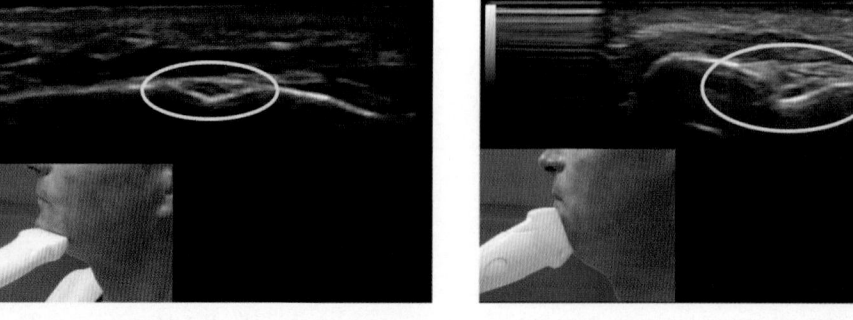

FIGURE 31–6. Ultrasound imaging for superficial trigeminal nerve block. **A:** The supraorbital nerve block under ultrasound guidance. **B:** The infraorbital nerve block under ultrasound guidance. **C:** The mental nerve block under ultrasound guidance.

TABLE 31-1. Branches of the maxillary division.

1. **Middle meningeal nerve**
2. **Pterygopalatine nerve**
   - Sensory fibers to the orbit
   - Nasal branches
   - Nasopalatine nerve
   - Greater palatine nerve
   - Lesser palatine nerve
   - Pharyngeal branch
3. **Zygomatic nerves**
   - Zygomaticofacial
   - Zygomaticotemporal
4. **Posterior superior alveolar nerve**
5. **Infraorbital nerve**
   - Before exits infraorbital canal
     - Middle superior alveolar
     - Anterior superior alveolar
   - After exits infraorbital canal
     - Inferior palpebral
     - Lateral (external) nasal
     - Superior labial

Figure 31–7). Except for the middle meningeal nerve (the intracranial branch that innervates the dura mater), all branches (zygomatic branches, superior alveolar nerve, pterygopalatine and parasympathetic branches, palatine and pharyngeal branches) arise in the pterygopalatine fossa.

Outside the cranial vault, the maxillary nerve supplies sensory branches to

- the skin of the temple and cheek
- the nasal septum and the lateral nasal wall
- the soft and bone palates
- upper teeth and maxillary sinus
- the territory of the infraorbital nerve (previously described)

At the upper part of the pterygopalatine fossa, the maxillary nerve is accessible for a complete maxillary block. The territories supplied by this complete block are the following:

- superficial: lower eyelid, ala of the nose, cheek, upper lip, cutaneous zygomatic, and temporal zone
- deep: superior teeth, palatine zone, maxillary bone

Indications

This block is mainly offered as an adjunct to general anesthesia for major cancer surgery of the maxilla, the ethmoidal sinus, and the pterigomaxillary or infratemporal fossa. In children, bilateral maxillary nerve blocks improve perioperative analgesia and favor the early resumption of feeding following repair of congenital cleft palate.[11] Many other procedures may benefit from a maxillary nerve block, such as maxillary trauma (Lefort I), maxillary osteotomy, or the diagnostic and therapeutic management of trigeminal neuralgias.[12]

Classical Landmark Technique

Many approaches to the classical landmark technique (Figure 31–8) have been described.

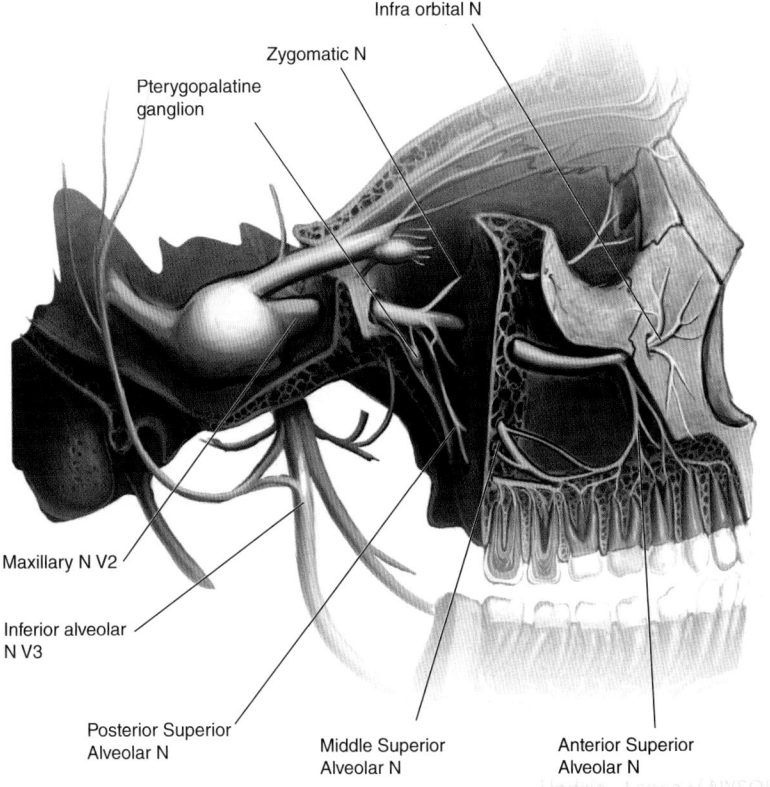

FIGURE 31-7. The maxillary nerve.

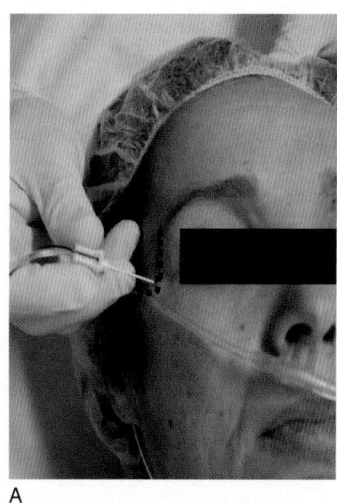
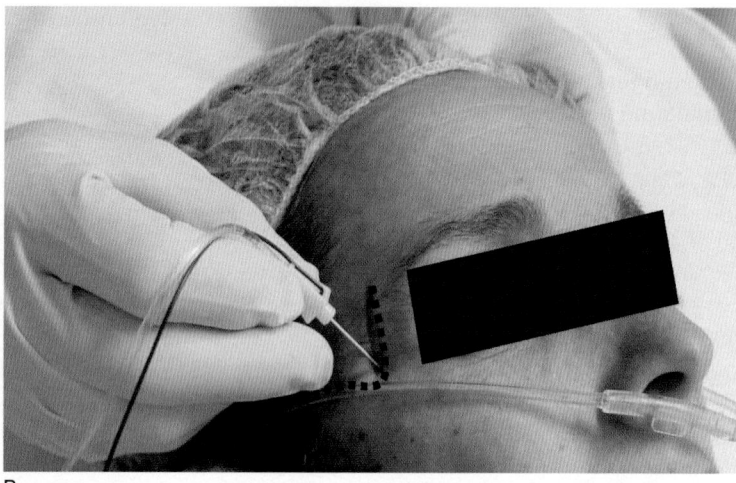

A   B

FIGURE 31–8. A and **B:** Suprazygomatic maxillary nerve block.

- The anterior infrazygomatic approach presents significant risks, including puncture of the maxillary artery, puncture of the posterior pharyngeal wall, submucosal abscess, or intraorbital injection through the superior orbital fissure.

- The suprazygomatic approach seems to be the safest and is easily reproducible in either children or adult patients. The patient is placed supine with the head in a neutral position. The needle entry point is found at the angle formed by the superior edge of the zygomatic arch below and the posterior orbital rim forward. The needle (22 to 25 gauge) is inserted perpendicular to the skin and advanced to reach the greater wing of the sphenoid at a depth of approximately 10–15 mm (Figure 31–8A). The needle is then reoriented in a caudal and posterior direction (Figure 31–8B) and advanced a further 35–45 mm to reach the pterygopalatine fossa. After a negative aspiration test for blood, 0.1 mL kg⁻¹ up to maximum of 5 mL of local anesthetic solution is slowly injected.

Nerve stimulation may help locate the pterygopalatine fossa: Nerve stimulation is associated with paresthesia coinciding with the stimulating frequency of the nerve stimulator. In anesthetized children, stimulation of the temporal muscle that results in a mandibular contraction may be noted. The disappearance of the muscle contraction heralds the passage through the temporal muscle and entrance into the pterygomaxillary fossa.

Ultrasound Guidance Technique

The (Figure 31–9), ultrasound transducer is placed in the infrazygomatic area, over the maxilla, with an inclination of 45° in both the frontal and the horizontal planes. The probe location allows visualization of the pterygopalatine fossa, limited anteriorly by the maxilla and posteriorly by the greater wing of the sphenoid. The needle is advanced using an out-of-plane approach. Real-time ultrasound guidance allows direct localization of the internal maxillary artery, identification of the needle tip, and spread of local anesthetic solution within the pterygopalatine fossa.[13]

Complications

Block failure can occur due to inadequate bony landmarks or inadequate needle tip position external to the pterygomaxillary fossa. Complications include cephalgia, facial paralysis, trismus, and hematoma.

The Mandibular Nerve Block
Anatomy

The mandibular nerve, the largest branch of the trigeminal nerve, exits from the cranium through the foramen ovale of the greater wing of the sphenoid. It divides into an anterior branch, which supplies motor innervation to temporalis, masseter, pterygoids, mylohyoid, tensor tympani, and palati muscles, as well as a sensory branch, the buccal nerve. The large posterior trunk divides into auriculotemporal, lingual, and inferior alveolar nerves (which reach the mental foramen, becoming the mental nerve) (Table 31–2 and Figure 31–10).

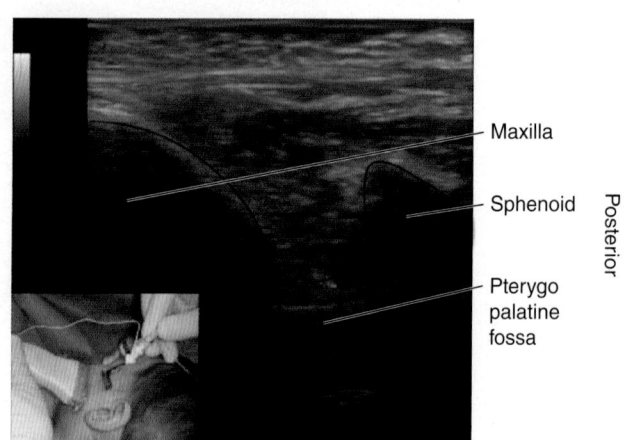

Maxilla

Sphenoid

Pterygo palatine fossa

Posterior

FIGURE 31–9. Ultrasound imaging for the pterygopalatine fossa limited by the maxilla (anterior) and the greater wing of the sphenoid (posterior). The maxillary vessels lie ventral and inferior to the maxillary nerve in the bottom of the pterygopalatine fossa.

TABLE 31–2. Branches of the mandibular division.

1. **Recurrent meningeal nerve**
2. **Motor nerves**
   - Medial pterygoid
   - Masseteric
   - Deep temporal (2)
   - Lateral pterygoid
3. **Buccal nerve**
   - Temporal nerve (upper)
   - Buccinator nerve (lower)
4. **Auriculotemporal nerve**
   - Communication with facial nerve and otic ganglion (to parotid)
   - Articular nerve
5. **Lingual nerve**
   - Via chorda tympani (VII)
     Taste sensations to the anterior third of tongue
6. **Inferior alveolar nerve**
   - Dental
   - Incisive
   - Mental

Mandibular nerve is blocked where the nerve emerges through the foramen ovale. Complete block results in anesthesia of the ipsilateral mandibular bone, lower teeth up to the midline, buccal and lingual hard and soft tissue, anterior two-thirds of the tongue, floor of the mouth, the external acoustic meatus and auricle of the ear in its anterior zone, the skin over the jaw, the posterior part of the cheek, and the temporal area (except the area of the angle of the mandible, which is supplied by the superficial cervical plexus).

Indications

Surgery on the lower lip, the mandible skin or bone (including the lower teeth), and the anterior two-thirds of the tongue can be accomplished with this technique. This block could be useful in patients with cancer or trauma. Nonmalignant chronic pain conditions such as trigeminal, vascular, or postherpetic neuralgia are also good indications for the mandibular block.

Classical Landmark Technique

In the classical landmark technique, the puncture area is bound by the zygomatic arch at the top and the mandibular notch just anterior and below the tragus of the ear. The needle entry point is located between the coronoid and condylar processes of the ramus of the mandible. To avoid the risk of arterial puncture, it is recommended to insert the needle as high as possible in the space between the zygomatic arch and the center of the mandibular notch (Figure 31–11). After perpendicular skin penetration and advancement of 2–4 cm toward the lateral pterygoid plate, the 22- to 25-gauge needle is advanced posteriorly and inferiorly, guided by mandible elevation twitch. Depth required to contact the mandible should not be more than 5–6 cm. The minimal intensity of stimulation (around 0.5 mA)

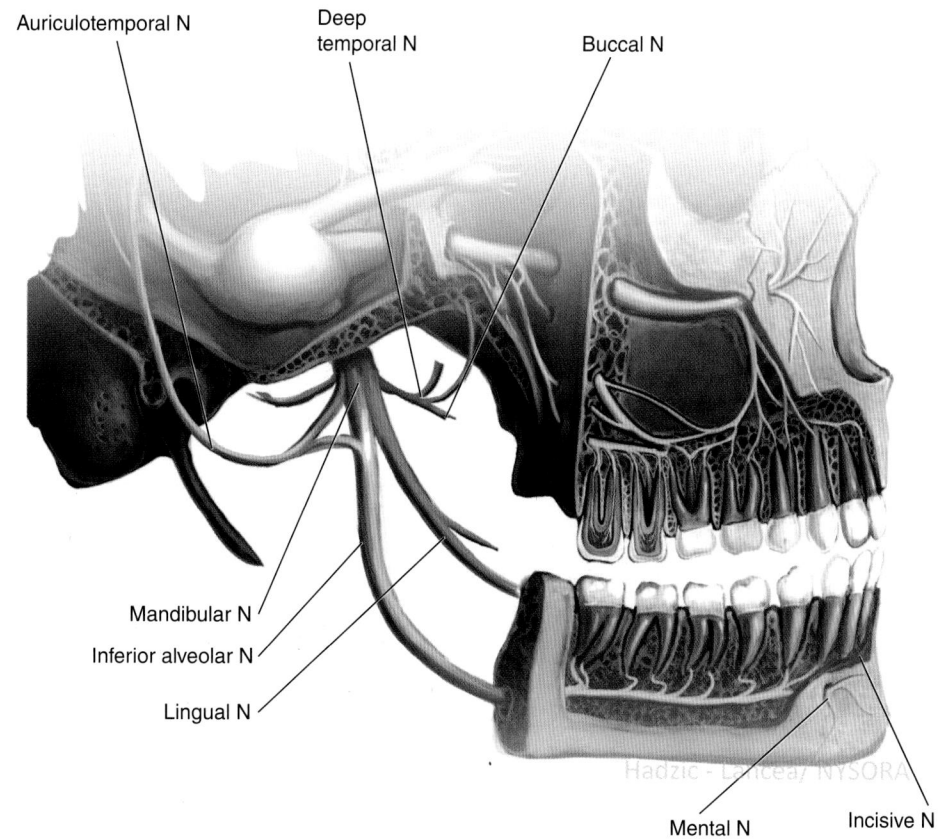

FIGURE 31–10. Mandibular nerve division and its relationship with vascular structures close.

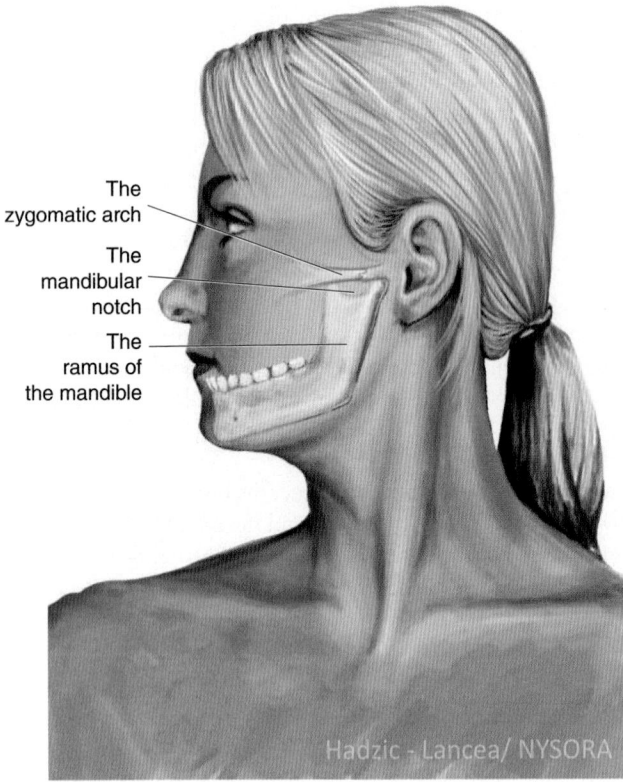

The zygomatic arch

The mandibular notch

The ramus of the mandible

Hadzic - Lancea/ NYSORA

FIGURE 31–11. The mandibular nerve block: classical anatomic landmark.

is determined, and 0.1 mL kg^{-1} to a maximal of 5 mL of local anesthetic solution is slowly injected after negative blood aspiration. This transcutaneous procedure with neurostimulation is associated with a high success rate.

Complications

The risk of puncture of the internal maxillary or middle meningeal arteries (Figure 31–10) can be high when the needle inserted too high in the space between the coronoid and condylar processes. After an injection of a large volume of local anesthetic solution, transient facial nerve block has been reported, which resolved spontaneously without sequelae.

Regional Block of the Nose

Anatomy

The innervation of the nose and nasal cavity is complex and involves both the ophthalmic (V1) and maxillary (V2) branches of the trigeminal nerve (Figures 31–12A and 31–12B)

- The nasociliary nerve (a branch of the ophthalmic nerve, V1) gives off, within the orbital cavity, the following branches: the posterior ethmoidal nerve, long ciliary nerves, communicating branches to the ciliary ganglion, the anterior ethmoidal nerve, and the infratrochlear nerve. The ethmoidal branches supply the superior and anterior half of the nasal cavity and the sphenoidal, ethmoidal, and frontal sinuses. Internal and external nasal branches of the anterior ethmoidal nerve supply the anterior part of the septum, the lateral wall of the nasal cavity, the nasal bone, and skin to the tip of the nose.

- The supratrochlear nerve (terminal branch of the frontal nerve, V1) supplies the root of the nose.
- Nasal and nasopalatine divisions of the maxillary nerve (V2) supply the posterior aspect of the septum and nasal cavity.
- The infraorbital nerve (terminal branch of V2) supplies the wings of the nose and the mobile septum.

Indications

Bilateral nerve blocks are often required. In most cases of intranasal surgery and septoplasty, topical anesthesia or infiltration by surgeons is needed to compliment analgesia and decrease bleeding by vasoconstriction using epinephrine.

Current indications for "nasal" block include rhinoplasty, polyp removal, repair of nasal fracture, and repair of nasal skin laceration.

Classical Technique

In the classical technique, the nasociliary nerve is blocked prior to its division into nasal branches of the anterior ethmoidal nerve and the infratrochlear nerve, close to the ethmoidal foramen. At this location, epinephrine-free solutions should be used to avoid the risk of retinal artery spasm. An intradermal (15–30 mm; 25–27 gauge) needle is inserted 1 cm above the medial canthus, halfway between the posterior palpebral fold and the eyebrow. It is then directed medially and backward to contact the bony roof of the orbit. At a depth of 1.5 cm, the needle should be at the anterior ethmoidal foramen; a maximum of 2 mL of local anesthetic solution is then slowly injected after a negative aspiration test. Continuous injection while removing the needle allows for blockade of the external nasal nerve. Compression of the interior angle of the eye by the finger promotes the diffusion of the solution to the foramen.

The infratrochlear nerve can be blocked by infiltrating at the superomedial border of the orbit and along its medial wall. The external nasal branch of the anterior ethmoidal nerve can also be blocked by infiltration at the junction of the nasal bone and the nasal cartilage.

Accompanied with an infraorbital nerve block and a pterygopalatine ganglion block by topical application of local anesthetic, complete anesthesia of the nasal cavity, septum, and lateral wall of the nose appears effective.

Complications

Most reported complications are minor and transient: palpebral edema, diplopia due to paralysis of the superior obliquus muscle of the eye, ptosis, and ecchymosis at the puncture site or hematoma secondary to ethmoidal vessel puncture. Rare cases of retrobulbar hemorrhage have been described.

REGIONAL BLOCKS OF THE EXTERNAL EAR

Anatomy

The innervation of the pinna of the ear is mainly provided by the trigeminal nerve and the cervical plexus (Figures 31–13A and 31–13B).

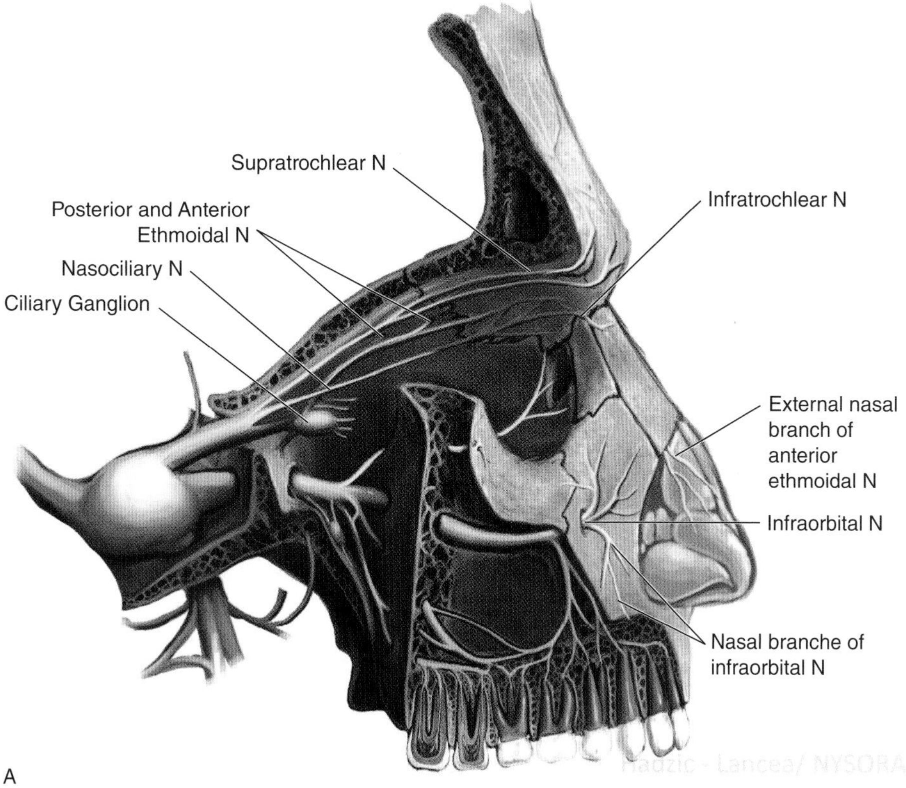

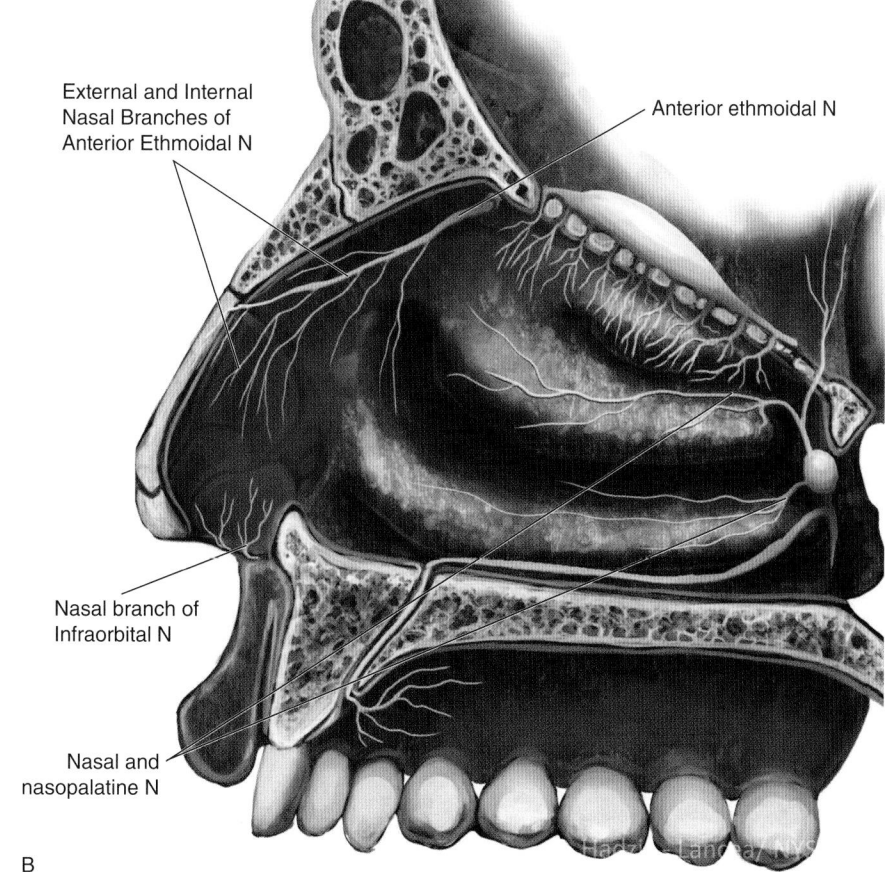

Supratrochlear N
Posterior and Anterior
Ethmoidal N
Nasociliary N
Ciliary Ganglion
Infratrochlear N
External nasal
branch of
anterior
ethmoidal N
Infraorbital N
Nasal branche of
infraorbital N
Hadzic - Lancea/ NYSORA

A

External and Internal
Nasal Branches of
Anterior Ethmoidal N
Anterior ethmoidal N
Nasal branch of
Infraorbital N
Nasal and
nasopalatine N

B

FIGURE 31–12. Innervation of the nose and nasal cavity. **A:** External nose. **B:** Septum and nasal cavity.

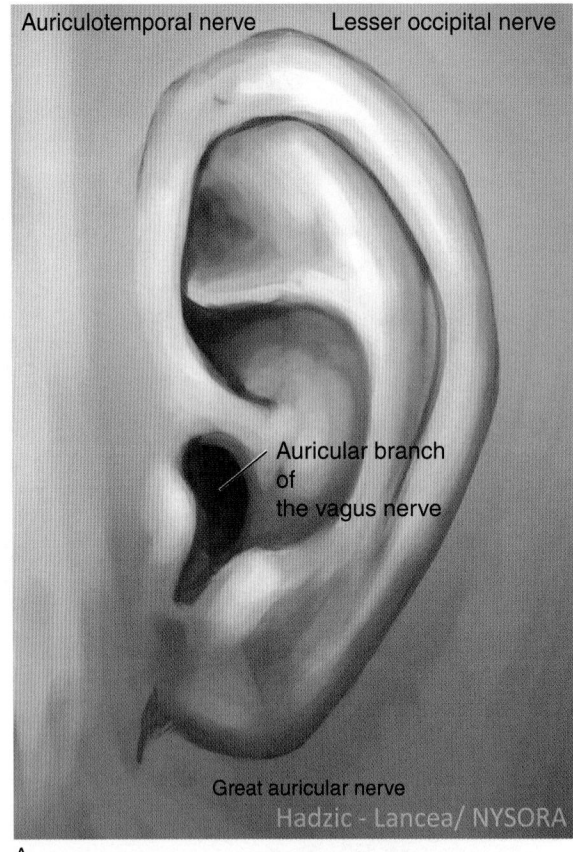

A

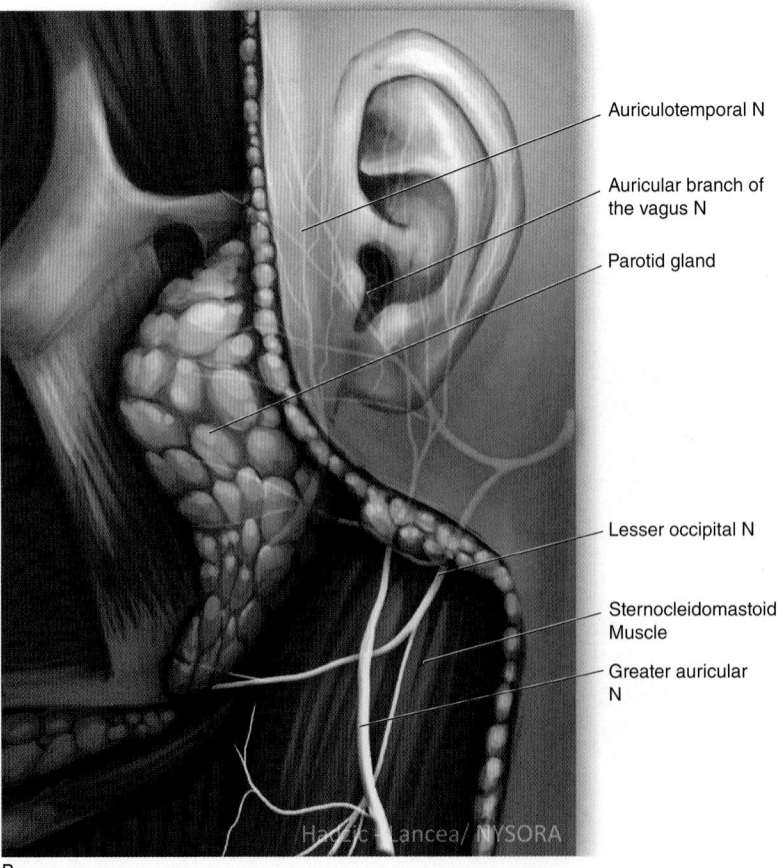

B

FIGURE 31–13. A and **B:** The innervation of the external ear.

- The superior two-thirds of the anterior surface are supplied by the *auriculotemporal branch* of the mandibular division of the trigeminal nerve. The auriculotemporal nerve passes through the parotid gland to ascend anterior to the auditory canal with the superficial temporal artery and passing superiorly superficial to the zygomatic arch.
- The posterior surface of the ear and the lower third of its anterior surface depend on the great auricular nerve and the lesser occipital nerve, two branches of the cervical plexus.
- The *great auricular nerve* arises from the second and third cervical nerve roots, emerges from the posterior border of the sternocleidomastoid muscle, and ascends (dividing into anterior and posterior branches) to the mandible, the parotid gland, and the pinna. It supplies the lower posterior aspect of the auricle, the lobule, and the skin of the angle of the mandible.
- The *lesser occipital nerve* arises from the ventral primary rami of the second and third cervical roots and gives innervation to the upper part of the earlobe and lateral occipital zone.
- The *auricular branch of the vagus nerve* (nerve of Arnold) innervates the concha and most of the posterior wall of the external auditory meatus (zona of Ramsay Hunt) as well as the inferior portion of the tympanic membrane.

Indication

This block is useful for analgesia after several painful procedures such as incision and drainage of an abscess or hematoma,[14] suture of lacerations of the ear or the skin surrounding the ear,[15] postauricular incisions such as tympanomastoid surgery and cochlear implants,[16] otoplasty,[17] or surgical correction of "bat ears."[5]

In children having tympanomastoid surgery, greater auricular nerve block provides analgesia, with lower incidence of postoperative nausea and vomiting secondary to avoidance or reduction in the need for opioids.[16]

Classical Techniques

For classical techniques, regional field block around the auricle allows anesthesia of each nerve branch involved in external ear sensory innervation except the Ramsay Hunt area (Figure 31–14A).

- The auriculotemporal nerve can be blocked by injecting local anesthetic solution above the posterior portion of the zygoma, anterior to the ear and behind the superficial temporal artery. The needle (27 gauge) is inserted anterior and superior to the tragus. Caution is necessary due to the vicinity of the temporal artery.
- The greater auricular nerve and the lesser occipital nerves can be blocked distally over the mastoid process posterior to the ear. The needle is inserted behind the lower lobe of the ear and advanced following the curve of the posterior sulcus.
- Infiltration with the ring block technique also provides additional efficient analgesia of the external ear (Figure 31–14B).

The superficial cervical plexus block is anesthetizes the lesser occipital nerve and the greater auricular nerve, two of its terminal branches. This technique is described elsewhere in this volume.

Recently, a block of the auricular branch of the vagus nerve has been described for pain control following myringotomy and tube placement, tympanoplasty, and paper patch for ruptured tympanic membrane.[14] To perform this block, the tragus is everted, a 30-gauge needle is inserted into the tragus, and after aspiration, 0.2 mL of local anesthetic solution is injected (Figure 31–14C).

Complications

Intravascular injections, hematoma, deep cervical nerve block, potential phrenic nerve block, and transient inability to shrug the shoulder are potential adverse effects of the superficial plexus cervical approach behind the sternocleidomastoid muscle.

Bleeding from the needle entry site is rare, and intravascular injection should be avoided by careful aspiration.

HEAD BLOCKS

Greater Occipital Nerve Block
Anatomy

The greater occipital nerve (GON) arises from the second cervical nerve root that emerges between the atlas and the axis. It ascends between the obliquus capitis inferior and semispinalis capitis before piercing the latter muscle. It then becomes subcutaneous by piercing the trapezius aponeurosis, slightly inferior to the superior nuchal line. At this point, the GON is most often located immediately medial to the occipital artery.

The GON provides cutaneous innervation to the major portion of the posterior scalp from the level of the external occipital protuberance to the vertex.

Indications

This block is useful for pain relief after posterior craniotomies, revision or insertion of a ventriculoperitoneal shunt, as well as for diagnosis and pain treatment secondary to various headache syndromes, such as primary headache, cervicogenic headache, migraine, occipital neuralgia, and tension headache.[18]

Classical Landmark Technique

The GON is located at approximately two-thirds the distance on a line drawn from the center of the mastoid to the external occipital protuberance along the superior nuchal line, where it lies medial to the occipital artery. The pulsation of the occipital artery is easy to palpate. Palpation in this area may elicit a paresthesia or uncomfortable feeling in the distribution of the nerve. A 25- or 27-gauge needle can be used depending on the size of the patient.

The needle is directed at 90° toward the occiput; after aspiration, 1–3 mL of local anesthetic is injected. When the needle is withdrawn, pressure should be maintained over the site of injection to promote soaking the nerve with local anesthetic

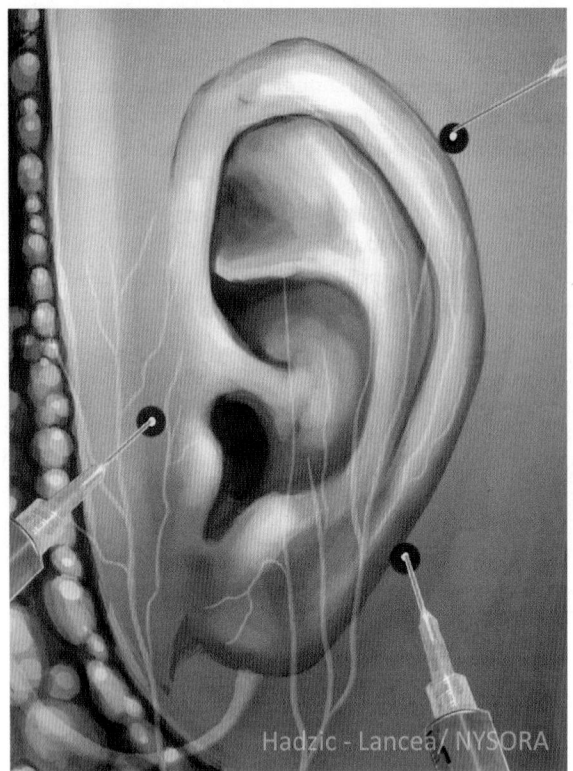

A   Regional field block

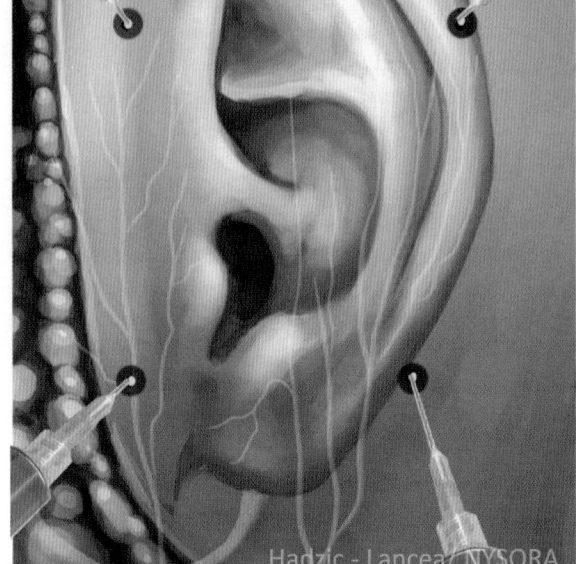

B   Ring block technique

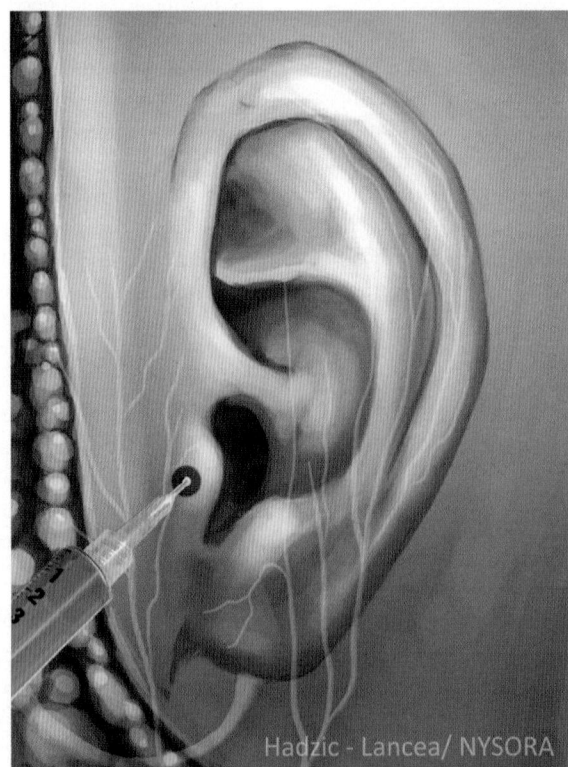

C   The block of the auricular
branch of the vagus nerve

FIGURE 31–14. External ear block techniques. **A:** Regional field block. **B:** Ring block technique. **C:** Auricular block.

and to achieve hemostasis. Numbness over the top of the head is a sign of a successful block.

There is considerable interpatient variability in the nerve location, with high variability (1.5–7.5 cm) of the distance of the GON to the midline at a horizontal level between the external occipital protuberance and the mastoid process.[19] More recently, ultrasound guidance has been described to perform this block.

Ultrasound Guidance Technique

In classical distal block technique, at the level of the superior nuchal line, the ultrasound probe was initially placed in a transverse plane with the center of the probe lateral to the external occipital protuberance (Figure 31–15, area 1).

A more proximal approach at the level of the second cervical vertebra (C2), was developed by Greher and al.[20] At this new site, the GON lies superficial to the obliquus capitis inferior muscle; the relationship of the GON to this muscle appears constant and reliable. The ultrasound transducer is moved down over the atlas (C1) to the location of the spinous process of C2 (that is always bifid). The probe is then moved laterally to identify the obliquus capitis inferior muscle of the neck (Figure 31–15, area 2). The GON can be easily visualized at this level, crossing the obliquus capitis inferior muscle from caudal to rostral and lateral to medial (Figure 31–16).

Complications

There are relatively few complications because of the superficial location of the nerve. Intravascular injection is always possible and prevented by performing careful aspiration prior to injection. Caution needs to be taken because the vertebral artery and the spinal cord are close proximity to the GON. The vertebral artery is lateral to the GON deep to the obliquus capitis inferior muscle and the lamina of the atlas, while the spinal cord is medial and again deep to the muscle.

Scalp Block
Anatomy

The "scalp block" is classically described with potential blockade of seven nerves, including branches from cervical spinal rami and from the trigeminal division (Figure 31–17).

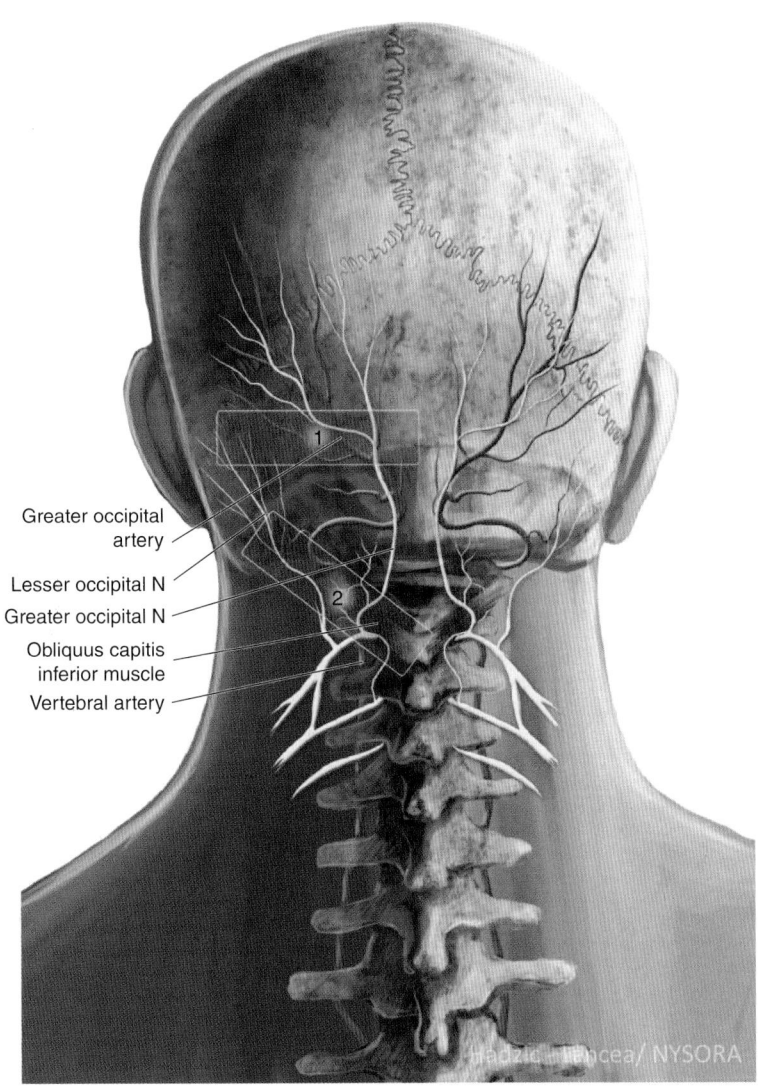

Greater occipital artery
Lesser occipital N
Greater occipital N
Obliquus capitis inferior muscle
Vertebral artery

FIGURE 31–15. Transducer positions for ultrasound-guided blocks of the GON. **1,** Classic block site at the superior nuchal line; **2,** new block site at C2, over the obliquus capitis inferior muscle.

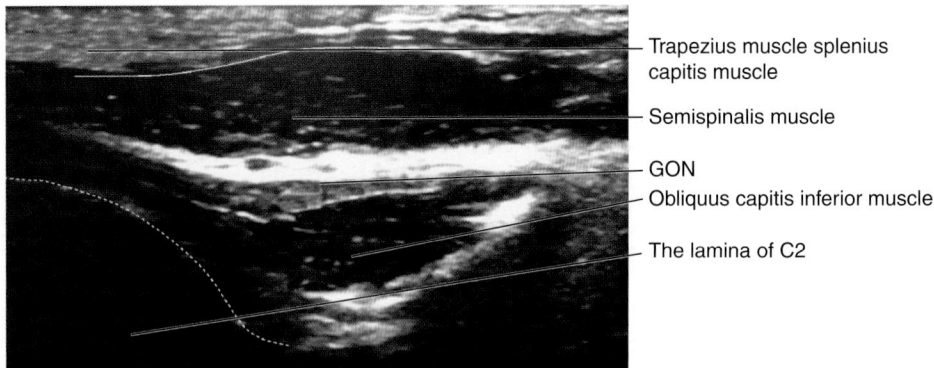

FIGURE 31–16. Sonogram of greater occipital nerve. The probe is placed along the long axis of the obliquus capitis inferior muscle (Figure 31–15, 2).

- Greater occipital, lesser occipital, and great auricular nerves originate from the ventral and the dorsal rami of C2 and C3 spinal nerves. The GON travels up to the vertex, and the lesser occipital nerve innervates skin behind the ear.
- The ophthalmic division of the trigeminal nerve gives off, via the frontal nerve, supraorbital and supratrochlear nerves, which innervate the skin from the forehead to the lamboidal suture.
- The zygomaticotemporal nerve is one of the two branches of the zygomatic nerve that arise from the maxillary division of the trigeminal nerve. It innervates a small area of the forehead and temporal area.
- The auriculotemporal nerve arises from the mandibular division of the trigeminal nerve. It innervates the posterior portion of the skin of the temple.

Indication

Scalp blocks are used in adults and children for a variety of head and neck procedures as well as in neurosurgery or in diagnostic

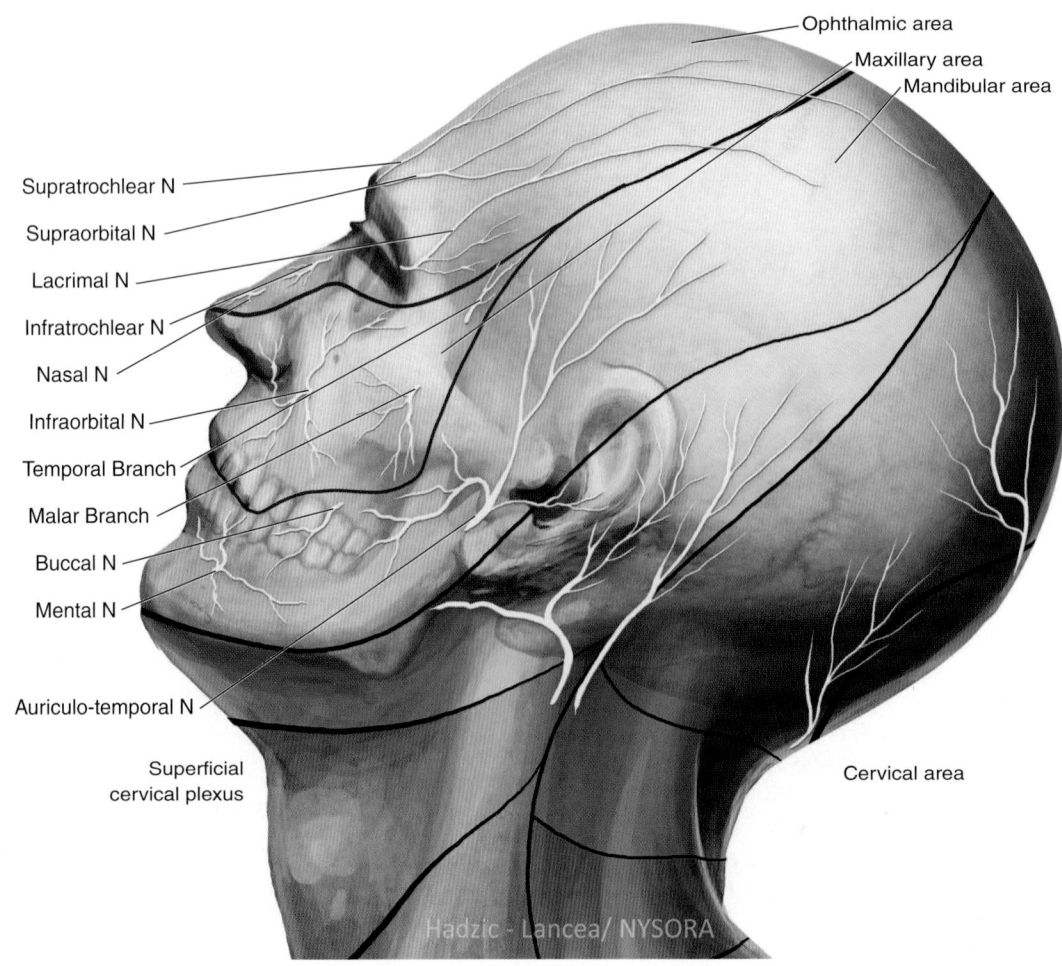

FIGURE 31–17. Innervation of the scalp.

and therapeutic management of chronic pain (eg, headache disorders of muscular and nervous etiology).

Common reasons for providing anesthesia to the scalp are repair of a laceration, foreign body removal, or exploration of scalp wounds and drainage of abscesses or subdural hematomas.

In neurosurgery, adverse hemodynamic reactions can occur during a craniotomy due to algogenic or reflexogenic events (insertion of the cranial pins of the Mayfield head holder, incision of the scalp, craniotomy, and dural incision). These reactions can be modulated by local or regional anesthesia,[21] with the additional benefit of postoperative analgesia.[22]

Local anesthesia for scalp blockad is essential in intraoperative anesthetic management of patients undergoing awake craniotomy Local scalp blocks are particularly useful when the patient's cooperation is needed for functional testing during the neurosurgical procedure, such as during epilepsy surgery and deep brain stimulation for Parkinson's disease, resections of lesions located close to or within functionally essential motor, cognitive, or sensory cortical areas.[23,24]

Infiltrational Anesthesia

All the nerves involved in the sensitivity of the scalp become superficial and accessible to anesthetic. To block the entire scalp, a circumferential infiltration of local anesthetic solution (with 1:200,000 epinephrine) above an imaginary line drawn from the occipital protuberance to the eyebrows, passing along the upper border of the ear, is necessary. Approximately 30 mL are required to perform this ring block around the scalp.

"Regional Blocks" Technique

For the "regional blocks" technique,[21] the supraorbital and supratrochlear nerves are blocked with an intradermic needle as they emerge from the orbit.

- The auriculotemporal nerves are blocked 1.5 cm anterior to the ear at the level of the tragus (see the section on regional blocks of the external ear).
- The postauricular branches of the greater auricular nerves are blocked 1.5 cm posterior to the ear at the level of the tragus (see the section on regional blocks of the external ear).
- Great and lesser occipital nerves are blocked by infiltrating along the superior nuchal line, approximately halfway between the occipital protuberance and the mastoid process (see the section on GON block).

Complications

The most common complication associated with scalp anesthesia is hematoma formation at the site of injection. Careful aspiration is suggested to avoid a potentially intravascular injection; because of the high vascularity of the scalp, the use of a diluted anesthetic solution with 1:100,000 or 1:200,000 epinephrine is usually considered safe to prevent toxic plasma drug levels.

CONCLUSION

A number of nerve block procedures can be used for surgical procedures performed on the face and scalp. The entire face area can be anesthetized using five simple nerve blocks,

providing adequate anesthesia for skin procedures as well as perioperative pain management of orthopedic, craniofacial, and cancer surgery.

REFERENCES

1. Suresh S, Bellig G: Regional anesthesia in a very low-birth-weight neonate for a neurosurgical procedure. Reg Anesth Pain Med 2004;29:58–59.
2. Suresh S, Wagner AM: Scalp excisions: getting "ahead" of pain. Pediatr Dermatol 2001;18:74–76.
3. Dimitriou V, Iatrou C, Malefaki A, Pratsas C, Simopoulos C, Voyagis GS: Blockade of branches of the ophthalmic nerve in the management of acute attack of migraine. Middle East J Anesthesiol 2002;16:499–504.
4. Gain P, Thuret G, Chiquet C, et al: Facial anesthetic blocks in the treatment of acute pain during ophthalmic zoster. J Fr Ophtalmol 2003; 26:7–14.
5. Bosenberg AT: Blocks of the face and neck. Tech Reg Anesth Pain Manag 1999;3:196–203.
6. Bosenberg AT, Kimble FW: Infraorbital nerve block in neonates for cleft lip repair: Anatomical study and clinical application. Br J Anaesth 1995; 74:506–508.
7. Prabhu KP, Wig J, Grewal S: Bilateral infraorbital nerve block is superior to peri-incisional infiltration for analgesia after repair of cleft lip. Scand J Plast Reconstr Surg Hand Surg 1999;33:83–87.
8. Higashizawa T, Koga Y: Effect of infraorbital nerve block under general anesthesia on consumption of isoflurane and postoperative pain in endoscopic endonasal maxillary sinus surgery. J Anesth 2001;15: 136–138.
9. McAdam D, Muro K, Suresh S: The use of infraorbital nerve block for postoperative pain control after transsphenoidal hypophysectomy. Reg Anesth Pain Med 2005;30:572–573.
10. Tsui BC: Ultrasound imaging to localize foramina for superficial trigeminal nerve block. Can J Anaesth 2009;56:704–706.
11. Mesnil M, Dadure C, Captier G, et al: A new approach for peri-operative analgesia of cleft palate repair in infants: the bilateral suprazygomatic maxillary nerve block. Paediatr Anaesth 2010;20:343–349.
12. Han KR, Kim C, Chae YJ, Kim DW: Efficacy and safety of high concentration lidocaine for trigeminal nerve block in patients with trigeminal neuralgia. Int J Clin Pract 2008;62:248–254.
13. Sola C, Raux O, Savath L, Macq C, Capdevila X, Dadure C: Ultrasound guidance characteristics and efficiency of suprazygomatic maxillary nerve blocks in infants: A descriptive prospective study. Paediatr Anaesth 2012; 22:841–846.
14. Giles WC, Iverson KC, King JD, Hill FC, Woody EA, Bouknight AL: Incision and drainage followed by mattress suture repair of auricular hematoma. Laryngoscope 2007;117:2097–2099.
15. Brown DJ, Jaffe JE, Henson JK: Advanced laceration management. Emerg Med Clin North Am 2007;25:83–99.
16. Suresh S, Barcelona SL, Young NM, Seligman I, Heffner CL, Cote CJ: Postoperative pain relief in children undergoing tympanomastoid surgery: Is a regional block better than opioids? Anesth Analg 2002;94:859–862, table of contents.
17. Cregg N, Conway F, Casey W: Analgesia after otoplasty: Regional nerve blockade vs local anaesthetic infiltration of the ear. Can J Anaesth 1996; 43:141–147.
18. Suresh S, Voronov P: Head and neck blocks in infants, children, and adolescents. Paediatr Anaesth 2012;22:81–87.
19. Loukas M, El-Sedfy A, Tubbs RS, et al: Identification of greater occipital nerve landmarks for the treatment of occipital neuralgia. Folia Morphol (Warsz) 2006;65:337–342.
20. Greher M, Moriggl B, Curatolo M, Kirchmair L, Eichenberger U: Sonographic visualization and ultrasound-guided blockade of the greater occipital nerve: A comparison of two selective techniques confirmed by anatomical dissection. Br J Anaesth 2010;104:637–642.
21. Pinosky ML, Fishman RL, Reeves ST, et al: The effect of bupivacaine skull block on the hemodynamic response to craniotomy. Anesth Analg 1996;83:1256–1261.
22. Nguyen A, Girard F, Boudreault D, et al: Scalp nerve blocks decrease the severity of pain after craniotomy. Anesth Analg 2001;93:1272–1276.
23. Bilotta F, Rosa G: "Anesthesia" for awake neurosurgery. Curr Opin Anaesthesiol 2009;22:560–565.
24. Sinha PK, Koshy T, Gayatri P, Smitha V, Abraham M, Rathod RC: Anesthesia for awake craniotomy: A retrospective study. Neurol India 2007;55:376–381.

SECTION 3 Ultrasound-Guided Nerve Blocks for the Upper Extremity

CHAPTER 32A

Ultrasound-Guided Cervical Plexus Block

Thomas F. Bendtsen, Sherif Abbas, and Vincent Chan

CERVICAL PLEXUS BLOCK AT A GLANCE

- Indications: carotid endarterectomy, superficial neck surgery (Figure 32A–1)
- Transducer position: transverse over the midpoint of the sternocleidomastoid muscle (posterior border)
- Goal: local anesthetic spread around the superficial cervical plexus *or* deep to the sternocleidomastoid muscle
- Local anesthetic: 5–15 mL

GENERAL CONSIDERATIONS

The goal of the ultrasound (US)-guided technique of superficial cervical plexus block is to deposit local anesthetic within the vicinity of the sensory branches of the nerve roots C2, C3, and C4 (Figures 32A–2 and 32A–3). Advantages over the landmark-based technique include the ability to visualize the spread of local anesthetic in the correct plane, which therefore increases the success rate, and to avoid a needle insertion that is too deep and the inadvertent puncture of neighboring structures.

Both US-guided superficial and deep cervical plexus blocks have been well described.[1–8] The deep cervical plexus block is an advanced block with a risk of potentially serious complications, such as intrathecal injection or injection into the vertebral artery. For this reason, we will focus primarily on the superficial cervical plexus block technique. It is simpler, safer, and, for most indications, it is equally as suitable as the deep cervical plexus block. An understanding of the fascial planes of the neck and the location of each of these blocks is necessary (see Figure 32A–2). For the superficial cervical plexus block, local anesthetic is injected superficially to the deep cervical fascia. For the superficial (intermediate) cervical plexus block, the injection is made between the investing layer of the deep cervical fascia and the prevertebral fascia, whereas for the deep cervical plexus block, local anesthetic is deposited deep to the prevertebral fascia.

ULTRASOUND ANATOMY

The sternocleidomastoid muscle (SCM) forms a "roof" over the nerves of the superficial cervical plexus (C2–4) (see Figure 32A–2). The roots combine to form the four terminal branches (the lesser occipital, greater auricular, transverse cervical, and supraclavicular nerves) and emerge from behind the posterior border of the SCM (Figures 32A–3, 32A–4, and 32A–5). The plexus can be visualized as a small collection of hypoechoic nodules (honeycomb appearance or hypoechoic [dark] oval structures) immediately deep or lateral to the posterior border of the SCM (see Figure 32A–5), but this is not always apparent. Occasionally, the greater auricular nerve is visualized on the superficial surface of the SCM as a small, round, hypoechoic

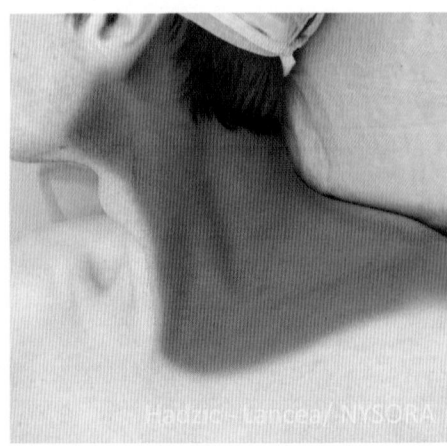

FIGURE 32A–1. Expected sensory distribution of cervical plexus blockade.

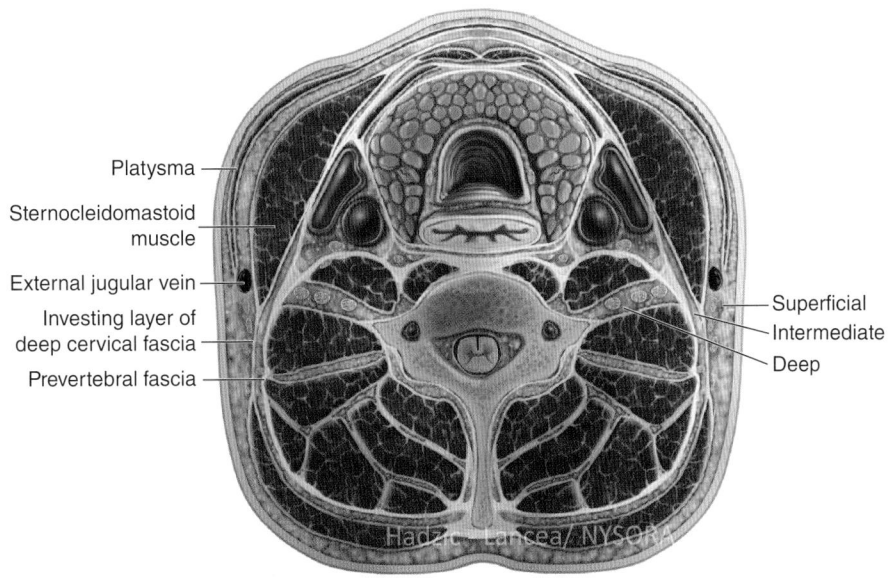

Platysma
Sternocleidomastoid muscle
External jugular vein
Investing layer of deep cervical fascia
Prevertebral fascia

Superficial
Intermediate
Deep

FIGURE 32A–2. Site of injection of local anesthetic for superficial, intermediate, and deep cervical plexus blocks.

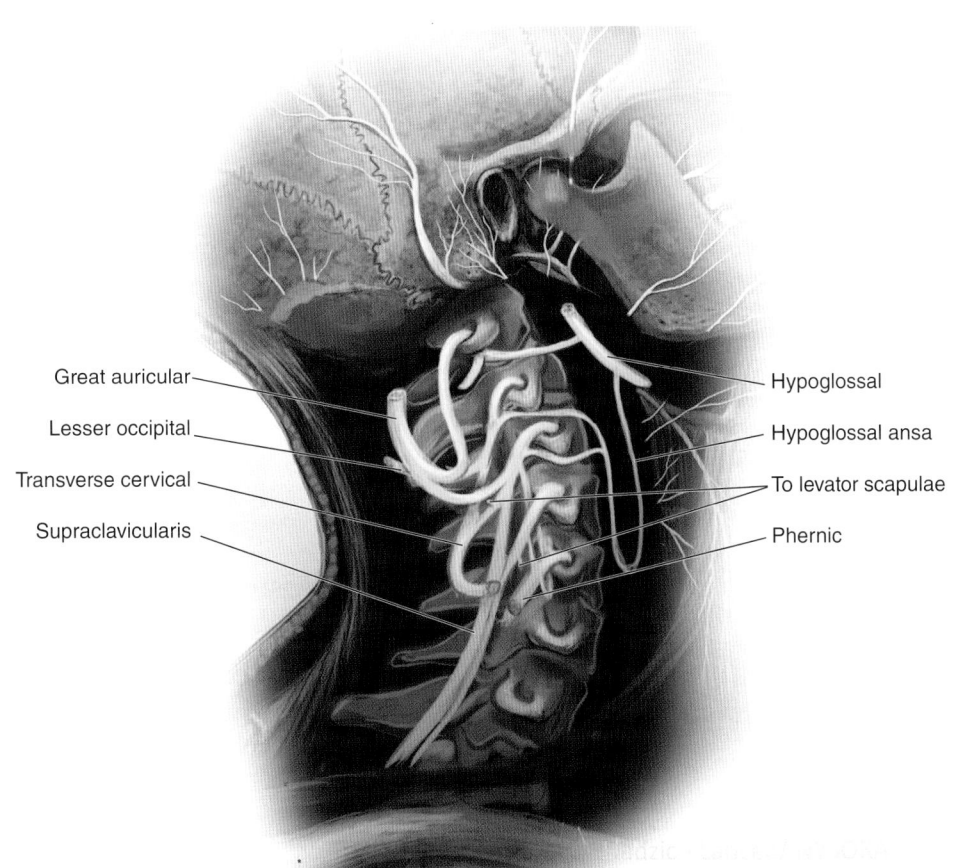

Great auricular
Lesser occipital
Transverse cervical
Supraclavicularis

Hypoglossal
Hypoglossal ansa
To levator scapulae
Phernic

FIGURE 32A–3. Anatomy of the deep cervical plexus and its main branches and anastomoses.

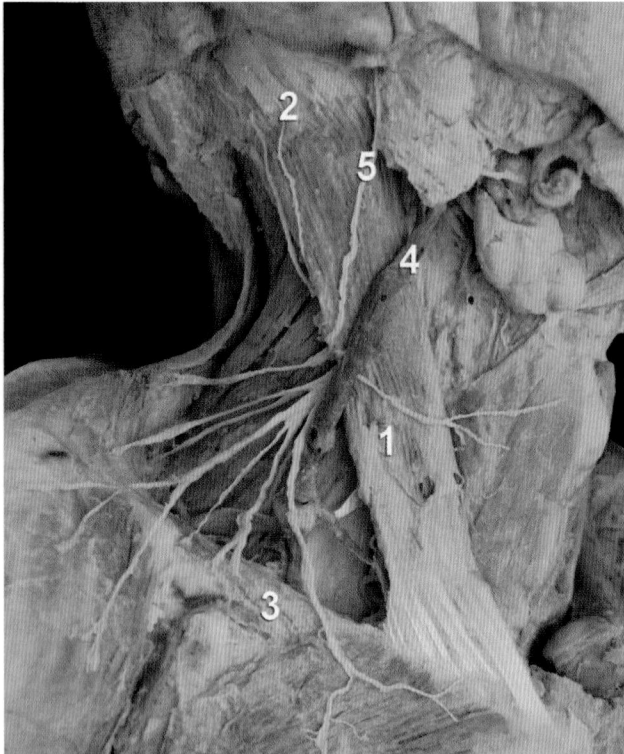

FIGURE 32A–4. Anatomy of the cervical plexus. The cervical plexus is seen emerging behind the posterior border of the sternocleidomastoid muscle at the intersection of the muscle with the external jugular vein. **1:** Sternocleidomastoid muscle. **2:** Mastoid process. **3:** Clavicle. **4:** External jugular vein. **5:** Greater auricular nerve. Supraclavicular nerves are seen crossing the clavicle.

structure. The SCM is separated from the brachial plexus and the scalene muscles by the prevertebral fascia, which can be seen as a hyperechoic linear structure. The cervical plexus lies posterior to the SCM and immediately superficial to the

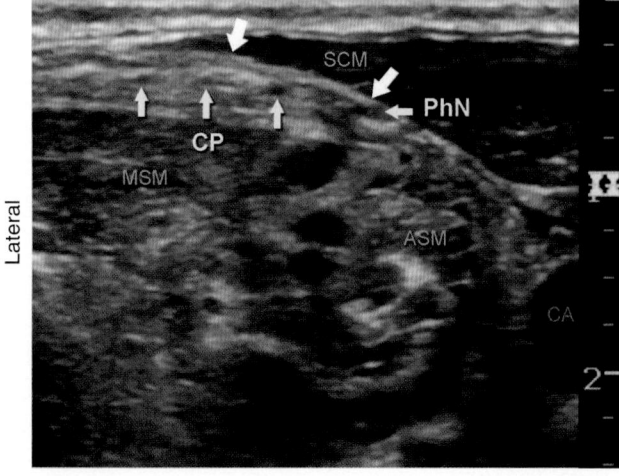

FIGURE 32A–5. Cervical plexus (transverse view). Branches of the cervical plexus (CP) are seen superficial to the prevertebral fascia, which covers the middle (MSM) and anterior (ASM) scalene muscles, and posterior to the sternocleidomastoid muscle (SCM). White arrows, investing fascia of deep cervical fascia; CA, carotid artery; PhN, phrenic nerve.

prevertebral fascia overlying the interscalene groove (see Figure 32A–5). Strictly speaking, the technique we describe, with an injection between the investing layer of the deep cervical fascia and the prevertebral fascia, is thus an intermediate cervical plexus block.

DISTRIBUTION OF ANESTHESIA

The superficial cervical plexus block results in anesthesia of the skin of the anterolateral neck and the ante-auricular and retro-auricular areas, as well as the skin overlying and immediately inferior to the clavicle on the chest wall (Figures 32A-1 and 32A-6). The mental, infraorbital, and supraorbital nerves are branches of the trigeminal nerve and are not blocked with cervical plexus block.

EQUIPMENT

The equipment needed for a cervical plexus block includes the following:

- Ultrasound machine with a linear transducer (8–18 MHz), sterile sleeve, and gel
- Standard nerve block tray
- A 10-mL syringe containing local anesthetic
- A 5 cm, 23- to 25-gauge needle attached to low-volume extension tubing
- Sterile gloves

LANDMARKS AND PATIENT POSITIONING

Any patient position that allows for comfortable placement of the ultrasound transducer and needle advancement is appropriate. This block is typically performed in the supine or semi-sitting position, with the head turned slightly away from the side to be blocked to facilitate operator access (Figure 32A–7). The patient's neck and upper chest should be exposed so that the relative length and position of the SCM can be assessed. The posterior border of the SCM can be difficult to locate, especially in obese patients. Asking the patient to lift his or her head off the bed can facilitate palpation of the posterior border of the SCM.

GOAL

The goal of this block is to place the needle tip in the fascial layer underneath the SCM adjacent to the cervical plexus, which is contained within the tissue space between the cervical fascia and posterior sheath of the SCM. If the elements of the cervical plexus are not easily visualized, the local anesthetic can be deposited in the plane immediately deep to the SCM and superficial investing layer of deep cervical fascia and superficial to the prevertebral fascia. A volume of 5-10 mL of local anesthetic usually suffices.

TECHNIQUE

With the patient in the proper position, the skin is disinfected and the transducer is placed on the lateral neck, overlying the

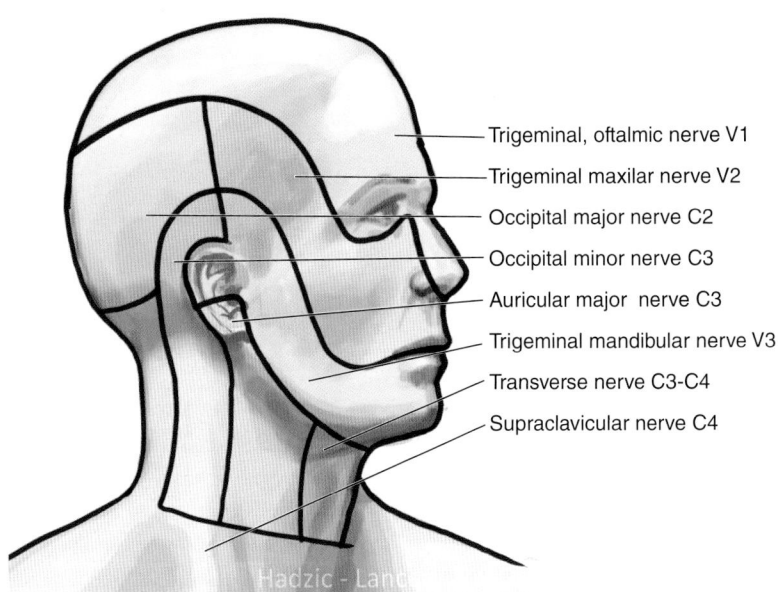

Trigeminal, oftalmic nerve V1
Trigeminal maxilar nerve V2
Occipital major nerve C2
Occipital minor nerve C3
Auricular major nerve C3
Trigeminal mandibular nerve V3
Transverse nerve C3-C4
Supraclavicular nerve C4

FIGURE 32A–6. Innervation of the lateral aspect of the face and neck.

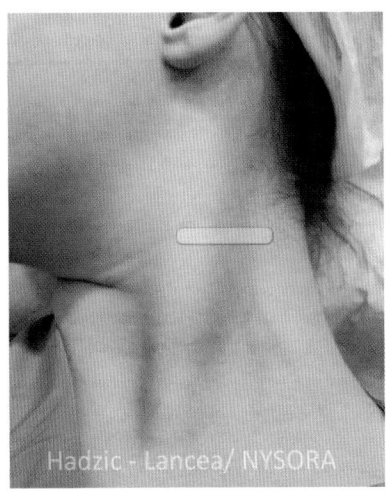

A

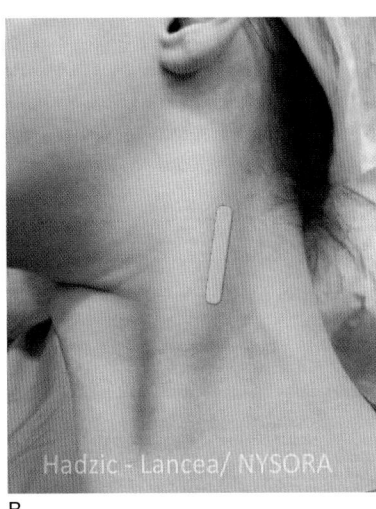

B

FIGURE 32A–7. Cervical plexus block. (**A**) Transverse approach.
(**B**) Longitudinal approach.

SCM at the level of its midpoint (approximately the level of the cricoid cartilage). Once the SCM has been identified, the transducer is moved posteriorly until the tapering posterior edge is positioned in the middle of the screen. At this point, an attempt should be made to identify the brachial plexus and/or the interscalene groove between the anterior and middle scalene muscles. The cervical plexus is visible as a small collection of hypoechoic nodules (honeycomb appearance) immediately superficial to the prevertebral fascia that overlies the interscalene groove (see Figures 32A–2 and 32A–5).

Once the plexus has been identified, the needle is passed through the skin, platysma, and investing layer of the deep cervical fascia, and the tip is placed adjacent to the plexus (Figure 32A–8). Because of the relatively shallow position of the target, both in-plane (from the medial or lateral sides) and out-of-plane approaches may be used. Following negative aspiration, 1–2 mL of local anesthetic is injected to confirm the proper injection site. The remainder of the local anesthetic (5–15 mL) is administered to envelop the plexus (Figure 32A–9).

If the plexus is not visualized, an alternative substernocleidomastoid approach may be used. In this case, the needle is passed behind the SCM, and the tip is directed to lie in the space between the SCM and the prevertebral fascia, close to the posterior border of the SCM (Figures 32A–7b, 32A–10, and 32A–11). Local anesthetic (5–15 mL) is administered and should be visualized layering out between the SCM and the underlying prevertebral fascia (Figure 32A–12). If the injection of local anesthetic does not appear to result in an appropriate spread, needle repositioning and further injections may be necessary. Because the cervical plexus is made up of purely sensory nerves, high concentrations of local anesthetic are usually not required; ropivacaine 0.25–0.5%, bupivacaine 0.25%, or lidocaine 1% is a sufficient.

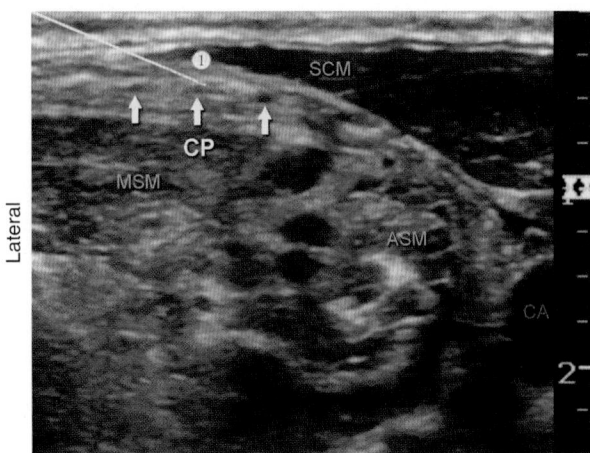

FIGURE 32A–8. Superficial cervical plexus (transverse view): needle path (1) and position to block the cervical plexus (CP). The needle is seen positioned underneath the lateral border of the sternocleidomastoid muscle (SCM) and superficial to the prevertebral fascia with the transducer in a transverse position (see Figure 32A–7a). ASM, anterior scalene muscle; CA, carotid artery; MSM, middle scalene muscle.

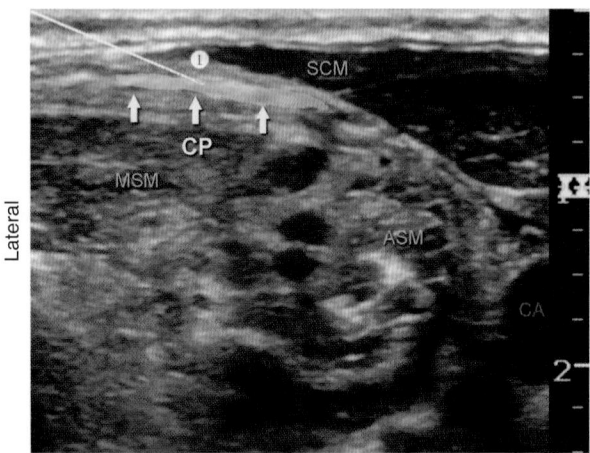

FIGURE 32A–9. Cervical plexus (transverse view): desired distribution of local anesthetic (blue-shaded area) to block the cervical plexus. Needle path: 1. ASM, anterior scalene muscle; CA, carotid artery; CP, cervical plexus; MSM, middle scalene muscle; SCM, sternocleidomastoid muscle.

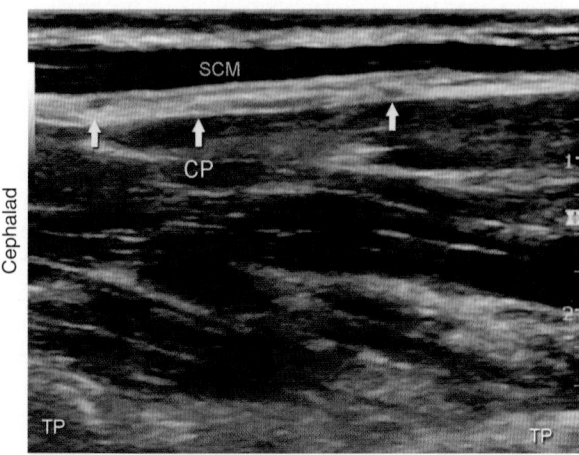

FIGURE 32A–10. Cervical plexus (longitudinal view): Elements of the cervical plexus (CP) underneath the lateral border of the sternocleidomastoid muscle (SCM).

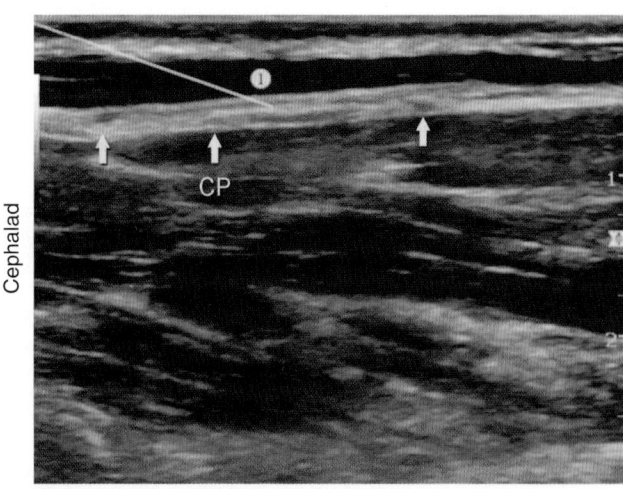

FIGURE 32A–11. Cervical plexus (longitudinal view): needle position to block the cervical plexus (CP).

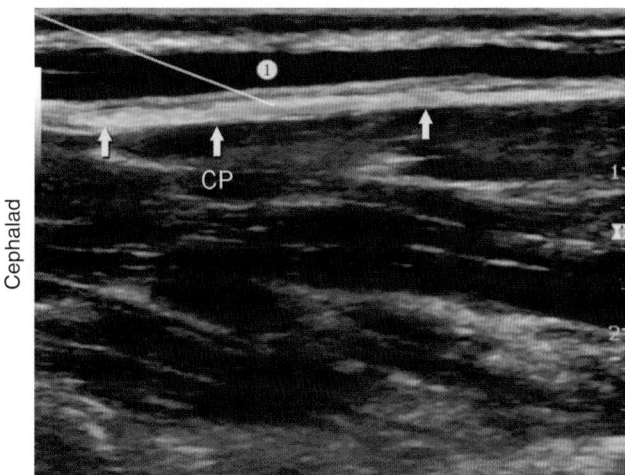

FIGURE 32A–12. Cervical plexus (longitudinal view): desired spread of local anesthetic under the deep cervical fascia to block the cervical plexus (CP).

TIPS

• Visualization of the plexus is *not* necessary to perform this block because the plexus may not always be readily apparent. Administration of 10 mL of local anesthetic deep to the SCM provides a reliable block without the position of the plexus needing to be confirmed.

SUGGESTED READING

Aunac S, Carlier M, Singelyn F, De Kock M: The analgesic efficacy of bilateral combined superficial and deep cervical plexus block administered before thyroid surgery under general anesthesia. *Anesth Analg* 2002;95:746–750.

Christ S, Kaviani R, Rindfleisch F, Friederich P: Brief report: identification of the great auricular nerve by ultrasound imaging and transcutaneous nerve stimulation. *Anesth Analg* 2012;114:1128–1130.

Demondion X, Herbinet P, Boutry N, et al: Sonographic mapping of the normal brachial plexus. *Am J Neuroradiol* 2003;24:1303–1309.

Eti Z, Irmak P, Gulluoglu BM, Manukyan MN, Gogus FY: Does bilateral superficial cervical plexus block decrease analgesic requirement after thyroid surgery? *Anesth Analg* 2006;102:1174–1176.

Flaherty J, Horn JL, Derby R: Regional anesthesia for vascular surgery. *Anesthesiol Clin* 2014;32:639–659.

Guay J: Regional anesthesia for carotid surgery. *Curr Opin Anaesthesiol* 2008; 21:638–644.

Narouze S: Sonoanatomy of the cervical spinal nerve roots: implications for brachial plexus block. *Reg Anesth Pain Med* 2009;34:616.

Roessel T, Wiessner D, Heller AR, et al: High-resolution ultrasound-guided high interscalene plexus block for carotid endarterectomy. *Reg Anesth Pain Med* 2007;32:247–253.

Soeding P, Eizenberg N: Review article: anatomical considerations for ultrasound guidance for regional anesthesia of the neck and upper limb. *Can J Anaesth* 2009;56:518–533.

Tran DQ, Dugani S, Finlayson RJ: A randomized comparison between ultrasound-guided and landmark-based superficial cervical plexus block. *Reg Anesth Pain Med* 2010;35:539–543.

REFERENCES

1. Usui Y, Kobayashi T, Kakinuma H, Watanabe K, Kitajima T, Matsuno K: An anatomical basis for blocking of the deep cervical plexus and cervical sympathetic tract using an ultrasound-guided technique. *Anesth Analg* 2010;110:964–968.

2. Choquet O, Dadure C, Capdevila X: Ultrasound-guided deep or intermediate cervical plexus block: the target should be the posterior cervical space. *Anesth Analg* 2010;111:1563–1564.

3. Dhonneur G, Saidi NE, Merle JC, Asfazadourian H, Ndoko SK, Bloc S: Demonstration of the spread of injectate with deep cervical plexus block: a case series. *Reg Anesth Pain Med* 2007;32:116–119.

4. Seidel R, Schulze M, Zukowski K, Wree A: Ultraschallgesteuerte intermediäre zervikale Plexusanästhesie; Anatomische Untersuchung [Ultrasound-guided intermediate cervical plexus block: Anatomical study]. *Anaesthesist* 2015;64:446–450.

5. Calderon AL, Zetlaoui P, Benatir F, et al. Ultrasound-guided intermediate cervical plexus block for carotid endarterectomy using a new anterior approach: a two-centre prospective observational study. *Anaesthesia* 2015; 70:445–451.

6. Saranteas T, Kostopanagiotou GG, Anagnostopoulou S, Mourouzis K, Sidiropoulou T: A simple method for blocking the deep cervical nerve plexus using an ultrasound-guided technique. *Anaesth Intensive Care* 2011;39:971–972.

7. Perisanidis C, Saranteas T, Kostopanagiotou G: Ultrasound-guided combined intermediate and deep cervical plexus nerve block for regional anaesthesia in oral and maxillofacial surgery. *Dentomaxillofac Radiol* 2013;42:29945724.

8. Sandeman DJ, Griffiths MJ, Lennox AF: Ultrasound guided deep cervical plexus block. *Anaesth Intensive Care* 2006;34:240–244.

Ultrasound-Guided Interscalene Brachial Plexus Block

Philippe E. Gautier, Catherine Vandepitte, and Jeff Gadsden

INTERSCALENE BRACHIAL PLEXUS BLOCK AT A GLANCE

- Indications: shoulder and upper arm surgery, surgery of the clavicle (combined with cervical plexus block)
- Transducer position: transverse on neck, 3–4 cm superior to clavicle, over external jugular vein (Figure 32B–1)
- Goal: local anesthetic spread around superior and middle trunks of brachial plexus, between the anterior and middle scalene muscles
- Local anesthetic: 7–15 mL

GENERAL CONSIDERATIONS

US guidance allows for visualization of the spread of the LA and additional injections around the brachial plexus if needed to ensure adequate spread of local anesthetic, improving block success. The ability to visualize local anesthetic spread and to inject multiple aliquots also allows for a reduction in the volume of local anesthetic required to accomplish the block.[1,2]

ULTRASOUND ANATOMY

The brachial plexus at the interscalene level is seen lateral to the carotid artery and internal jugular vein, between the anterior and middle scalene muscles (Figures 32B–2 and 32B–3). The prevertebral fascia, superficial cervical plexus, and sternocleidomastoid muscle are seen superficial to the plexus. The transducer is moved in the proximal-distal direction until two or more of the brachial plexus elements are seen in the space between the scalene muscles. Depending on the depth of field selected and the level at which scanning is performed, the first

rib and/or the apex of the lung may be seen. The brachial plexus is typically visualized at a depth of 1–3 cm.

BLOCKADE DISTRIBUTION

The interscalene approach to brachial plexus blockade results in reliable anesthesia of the shoulder and upper arm (Figure 32B–4). The supraclavicular branches of the cervical plexus, supplying the skin over the acromion and clavicle, are also blocked due to the proximal and superficial spread of local anesthetic. The inferior trunk (C8-T1) is usually spared, unless the injection occurs at a more distal level of the brachial plexus.

EQUIPMENT

The equipment needed for an interscalene brachial plexus block includes the following:

- Ultrasound machine with linear transducer (8–14 MHz), sterile sleeve, and gel
- Standard nerve block tray
- A 20-mL syringe containing local anesthetic
- A 5-cm, 22-gauge, short-bevel, insulated stimulating needle
- Peripheral nerve stimulator
- Opening injection pressure monitoring system
- Sterile gloves

LANDMARKS AND PATIENT POSITIONING

Any position that allows for comfortable placement of the ultrasound transducer and needle advancement is appropriate. The block is typically performed with the patient in a supine, beach

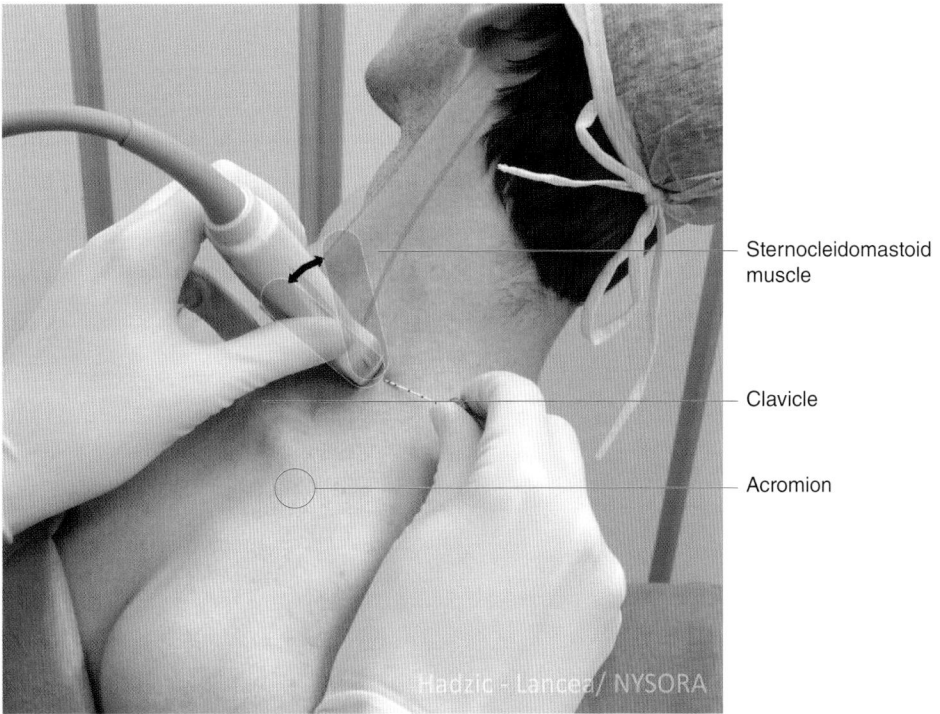

FIGURE 32B–1. Ultrasound-guided interscalene brachial plexus block: transducer and needle position to obtain the desired ultrasound image for an in-plane approach. The knowledge of external landmarks substantially facilitates and shortens the time to obtain the view necessary for block performance. The transducer is positioned behind the clavicular head of the sternocleidomastoid muscle (SCM) and over the external jugular vein (not seen). The patient is in a semi-sitting position. Tilting the transducer in the caudad direction can facilitate recognition of the brachial plexus (arrow).

chair, or semilateral decubitus position, with the patient's head facing away from the side to be blocked. The latter position may prove more ergonomic, especially during an in-plane approach from the lateral side, in which the needle enters the skin at the posterolateral aspect of the neck. A slight elevation of the head of the bed is often more comfortable for the patient and allows for

better drainage and less prominence of the neck veins. The patient should be asked to reach for the ipsilateral knee in order to lower the shoulder and provide more space for the block performance.

Knowledge of the underlying anatomy and the position of the brachial plexus is important to facilitate recognition of the ultrasound anatomy. Scanning usually begins just below the level of the cricoid cartilage and medial to the sternocleidomastoid muscle with the goal of identifying the carotid artery.

FIGURE 32B–2. Relevant anatomy for interscalene brachial block and transducer position to obtain the desired views. The brachial plexus (BP) is seen between middle scalene muscle (MSM) laterally and the anterior scalene muscle (ASM) medially. The ultrasound image often includes a partial view of the lateral border of the sternocleidomastoid muscle (SCM) as well as the internal jugular vein (IJV) and carotid artery (CA). The transverse process of one of the cervical vertebrae is also often seen.

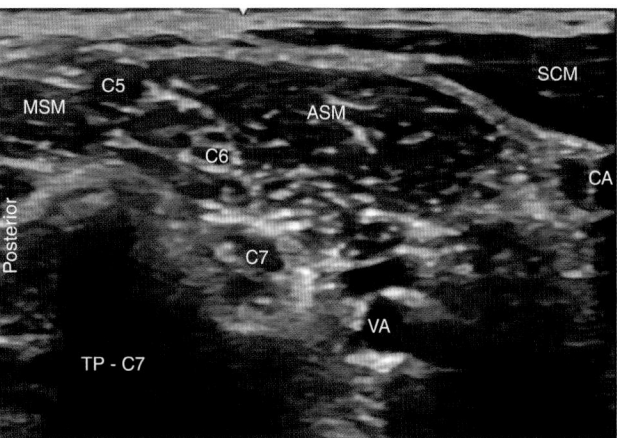

FIGURE 32B–3. Ultrasound image of the brachial plexus at the interscalene groove. The BP is seen positioned between the anterior scalene muscle (ASM) and the middle scalene muscle (MSM). In this particular image, the vertebral artery (VA), carotid artery (CA), and the transverse process of C7 (TP-C7) are also seen.

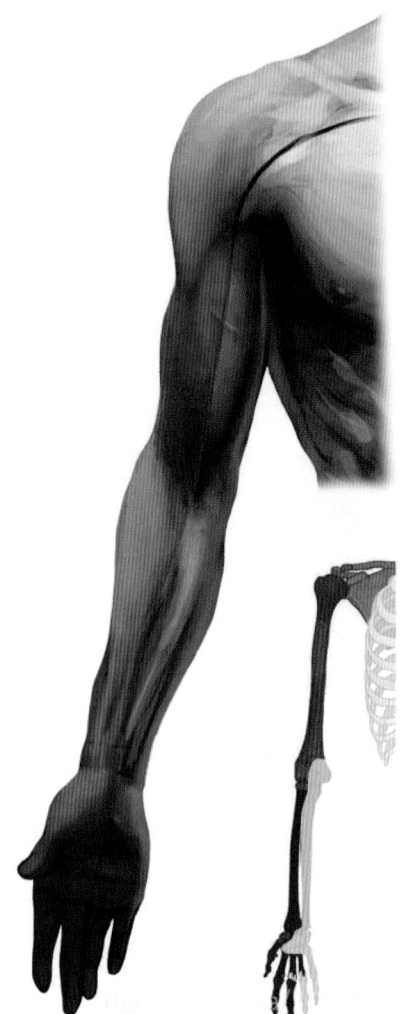

FIGURE 32B–4. Sensory distribution of the interscalene brachial plexus block (in red). Ulnar nerve distribution area (C8-T1) can also be accomplished by using larger volume (e.g. 15-20 ml) and using low interscalene block where the injection occurs between the ISB and supraclavicular block.

GOAL

The goal of this block is to place the needle in the tissue space between the anterior and middle scalene muscles and inject local anesthetic until the spread around the brachial plexus is documented by ultrasound. The volume of the local anesthetic and number of needle insertions are determined during the procedure and depend on the adequacy of the observed spread of local anesthetic.

TECHNIQUE

With the patient in the proper position, the skin is disinfected and the transducer is positioned in the transverse plane to identify the carotid artery (Figure 32B–5). Once the artery has been identified, the transducer is moved slightly laterally across the neck. The goal is to identify the anterior and middle scalene muscles and the elements of the brachial plexus that is located between them.

- When visualization of the brachial plexus between the scalene muscles proves difficult, a "traceback" technique can be used.[3] The transducer is lowered to the supraclavicular fossa. At this position, the brachial plexus is identified posterior and superficial to the subclavian artery (Figure 32B–6). From here, the brachial plexus is traced cranially to the desired level.

It is recommended to use the color Doppler to identify vascular structures and avoid them. The needle is then inserted in plane toward the brachial plexus, typically in a lateral-to-medial direction (Figure 32B–7), although a medial-to-lateral needle orientation can also be used if there is no room for the former. The needle should always be aimed in between the roots instead of directly at them in order to minimize the risk of accidental nerve injury.

As the needle passes through the prevertebral fascia, a certain "pop" is often appreciated. When nerve stimulation is used (0.5 mA, 0.1 msec), the entrance of the needle in the interscalene groove is often associated with a motor response of the shoulder, arm, or forearm as another confirmation of proper needle placement. After careful aspiration to rule out intravascular needle placement, 1–2 mL of local anesthetic is injected to verify proper needle placement (Figure 32B–8a). It is necessary to ensure that high resistance to injection is absent to decrease the risk of intrafascicular injection. Injection of several milliliters of local anesthetic often displaces the brachial plexus away from the needle. An additional advancement of the needle 1–2 mm toward the brachial plexus may be beneficial to ensure proper spread of the local anesthetic (Figure 32B–8b). When injection of the local anesthetic does not appear to result in a spread around the brachial plexus, additional needle repositioning and injections may be necessary.

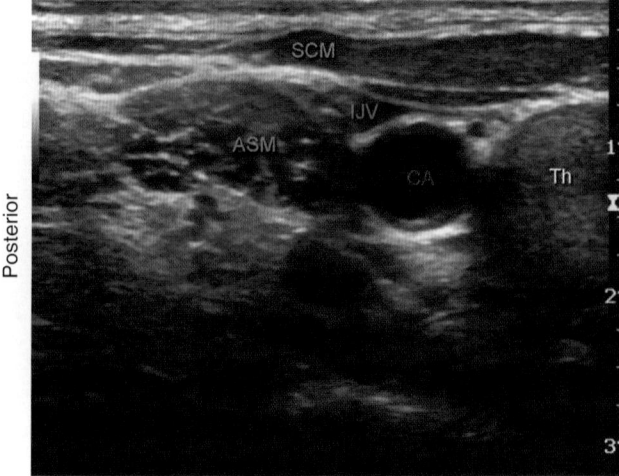

Identifying carotid artery

FIGURE 32B–5. Ultrasound image just below the level of the cricoid cartilage and medial to the sternocleidomastoid muscle (SCM). ASM, anterior scalene muscle; CA, carotid artery; IJV, internal jugular vein; SCM, sternocleidomastoid muscle; Th, thyroid gland.

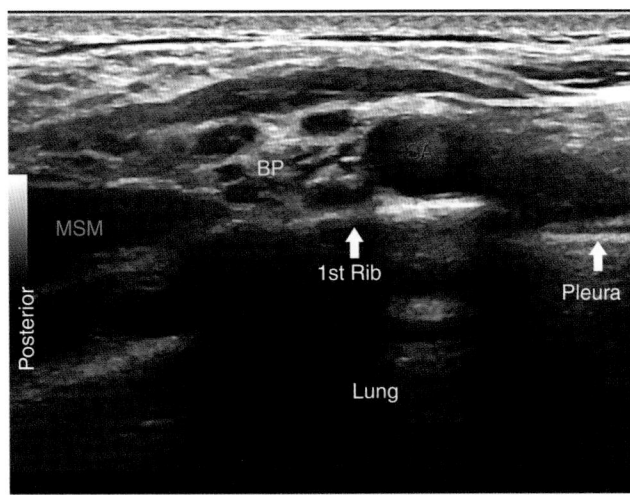

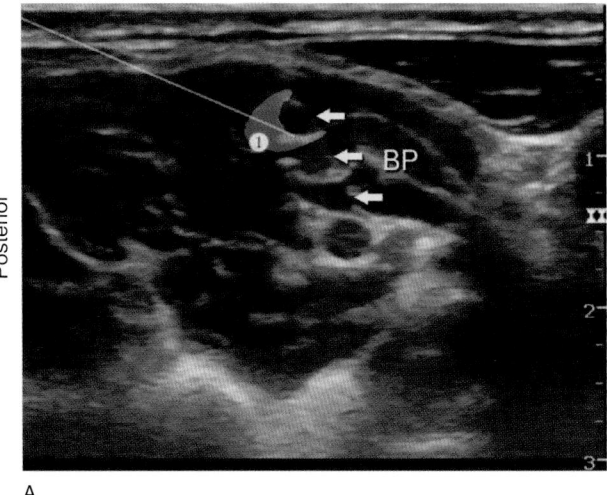

A

FIGURE 32B–6. View of the brachial plexus (BP) at the supraclavicular fossa. When identification of the brachial plexus at the interscalene level proves difficult, the transducer is positioned at the supraclavicular fossa to identify the BP superficial and posterior to the subclavian artery (SA). The transducer is then slowly moved cephalad while continuously visualizing the brachial plexus until the desired level is reached.

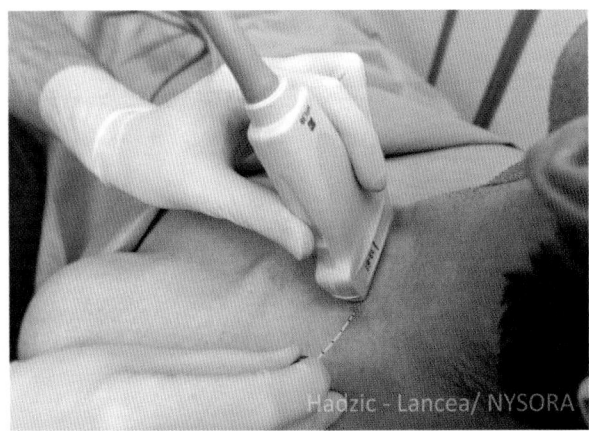

A

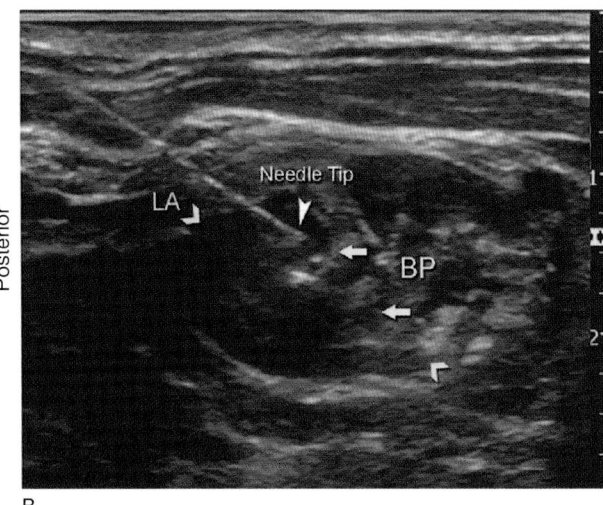

B

FIGURE 32B–8. (**A**) A small volume of local anesthetic (blue-shaded area) is injected through the needle to confirm proper needle placement. A properly placed needle tip will result in distribution of local anesthetic between and/or alongside roots of the brachial plexus (BP). (**B**) An actual needle (white arrowhead) placement in the interscalene groove, with dispersion of local anesthetic (LA) (blue-shaded area or arrows) surrounding the BP.

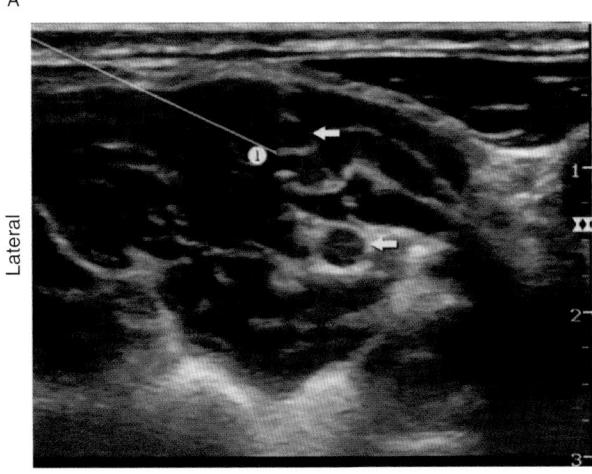

B

FIGURE 32B–7. (**A**) Transducer placement and needle insertion. (**B**) Position of the needle (1) for the interscalene brachial plexus block using an in-plane approach. The needle tip is seen in contact with the elements of the brachial plexus (yellow arrows); this always results in high injection pressure (> 15 psi)—indicating that the needle should be withdrawn slightly away from the trunk.

TIPS

• It is not necessary to elicit a motor response to nerve stimulation; however, when it occurs at intensities < 0.5 mA, the needle should be slightly withdrawn before injecting as it may be intraneural.
• The neck is a highly vascular area, and care must be exercised to avoid needle placement or injection into the vascular structures. Of particular importance is to avoid the vertebral artery and branches of the thyrocervical trunk: the inferior thyroid artery, suprascapular artery, and transverse cervical artery. Use color Doppler imaging at least once before inserting the needle to locate any vessel that might be in the path of the needle. Anatomical variations are common.[4]

- Never inject against high resistance because such resistance may indicate needle–nerve contact or an intrafascicular injection. A high opening injection pressure (> 15 psi) is always present with needle–root contact.[5] Thus, a seemingly extraneural injection may in fact be subepineural.[6] An intraneural injection may spread proximally into the spinal canal.[7]

- One useful maneuver to ensure injection into the proper compartment, after injecting 5–7 mL, is to trace the plexus down to the supraclavicular fossa (while keeping the needle steady to avoid injury). If the injection is performed insede the brachial plexus "sheath," the correct spread can be seen very clearly (Figure 33B–9). The probe can then be moved back until the needle is visualized in order to complete the injection. If the brachial plexus appears unchanged in the supraclavicular area, one must question whether the injection was done outside the correct compartment (see Figure 32B–9).

- The lateral-to-medial insertion is often chosen to prevent injury to the phrenic nerve, which is typically located anteriorly to the anterior scalene, although one should be aware that the dorsal scapular nerve and the long thoracic nerve usually course through the middle scalene and could potentially be injured as well (Figure 32B–10).[8–10]

- It is common for C6 and C7 to split proximally. It is prudent to avoid injecting between the nerves coming from a single root, as this may result in an intraneural injection. Instead, it is safer to inject between C5 and C6, superficial to C5, or deep to C6 (Figure 32B–11).[11]

- Another relatively common anatomical variation involves the C5 root travelling through the anterior scalene for part of its course (Figure 32B–12). To block this anatomical variant, the root should be traced distally until it enters the interscalene groove.

- Multiple injections are best avoided as they are not usually needed to successfully block the brachial plexus and may carry higher risk of nerve injury.

- In an adult patient, 7–15 mL of local anesthetic is usually adequate for a successful and rapid onset of blockade. Smaller volumes of local anesthetic may also be effective;[12,13] however, the rate of success of smaller volumes

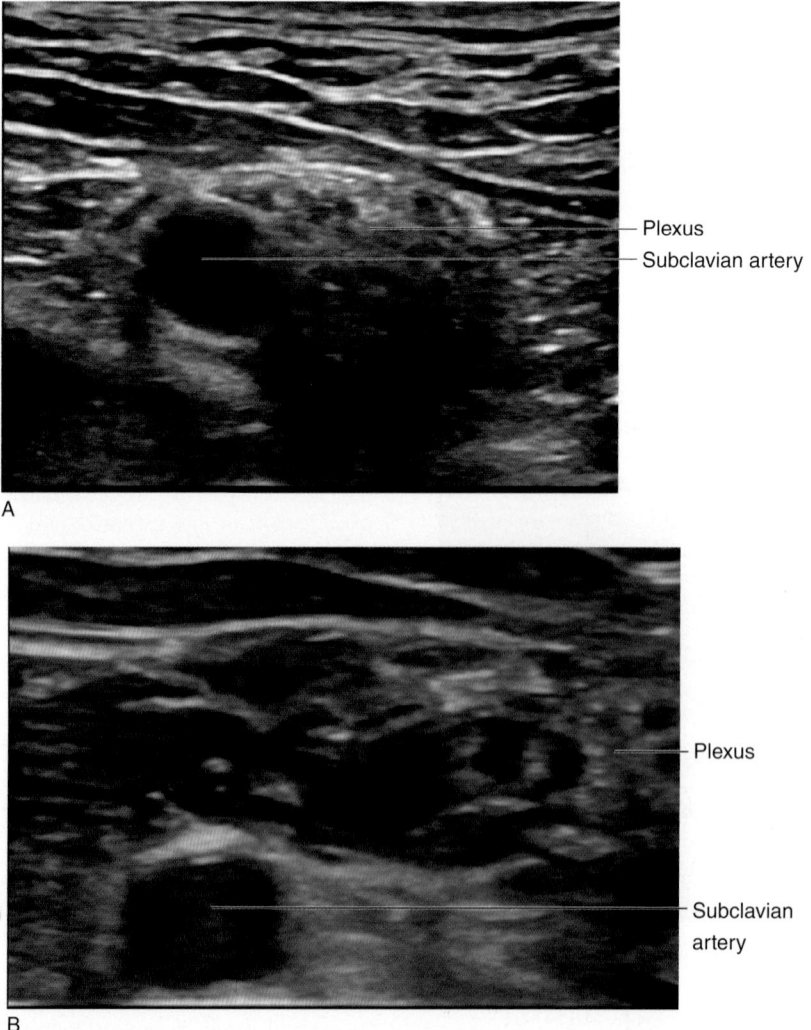

A

B

FIGURE 32B–9. Diffusion of local anesthetic solution to the supraclavicular area during interscalene block performance. (**A**) Before injection. (**B**) After injection of 10 mL at the interscalene level. The nerves lateral to the subclavian artery are surrounded by local anesthetic and appear deeper. This confirms that the injection was performed in the correct space.

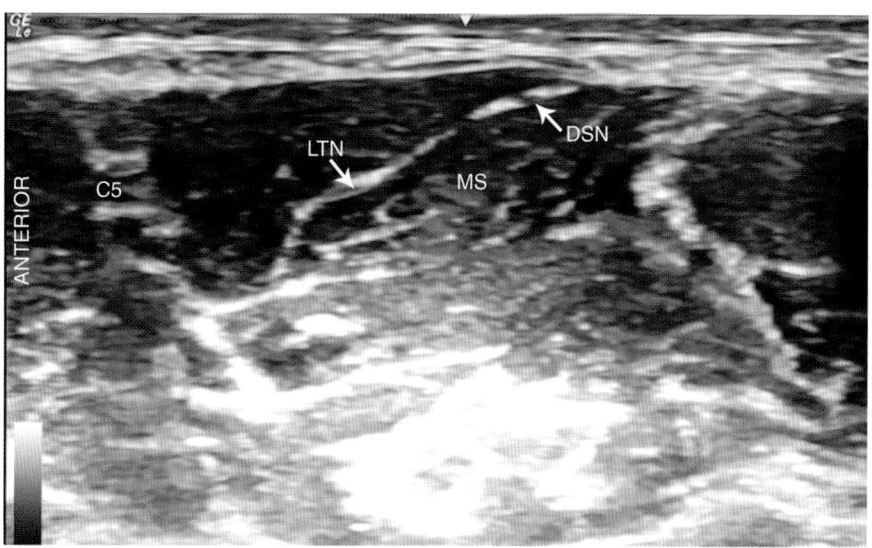

FIGURE 32B-10. Dorsal scapular nerve (DSN) and long thoracic nerve (LTN) visible in the middle scalene muscle (MS).

in everyday clinical practice may be inferior to those reported in meticulously conducted clinical trials.

PHRENIC NERVE BLOCKADE

Phrenic nerve blockade is common following ISB and may compromise respiratory function in patients with pre-existing pulmonary pathology. Four main strategies[14] can be used in such patients to provide analgesia after shoulder surgery while avoiding phrenic blockade: (1) decreasing local anesthetic volume; (2) performing the ISB more caudad in the neck, around

C7; (3) using a supraclavicular block;[15] and (4) using a supra-scapular nerve block (possibly in association with an axillary nerve block).

The phrenic nerve lies just superficially to the interscalene groove at the level of the cricoid cartilage and courses caudad and anteriorly and distally along the superficial aspect of the anterior scalene muscle along the neck.[16]

The use of a low volume of local anesthetic (eg, 5 mL) reduces the incidence of phrenic nerve blockade[17–19] but may also reduce the duration of analgesia[20] and possibly decreases the success rate. Higher volumes (10 mL) injected at the level of the cricoid would cause phrenic nerve blockade.[21]

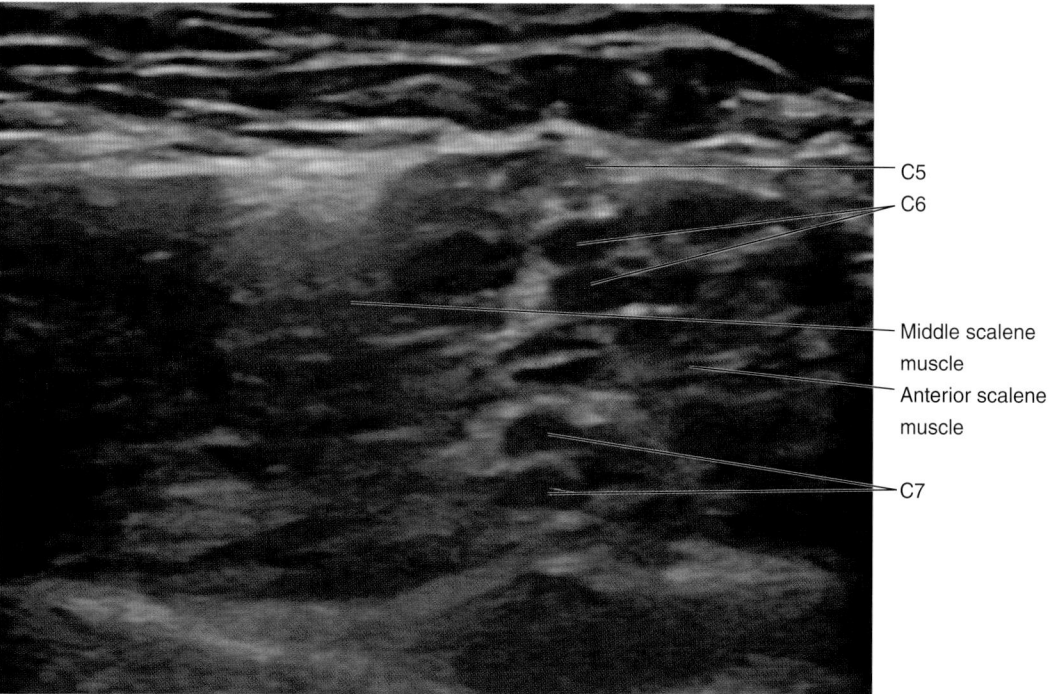

FIGURE 32B-11. Split C6 and C7 roots in the interscalene groove.

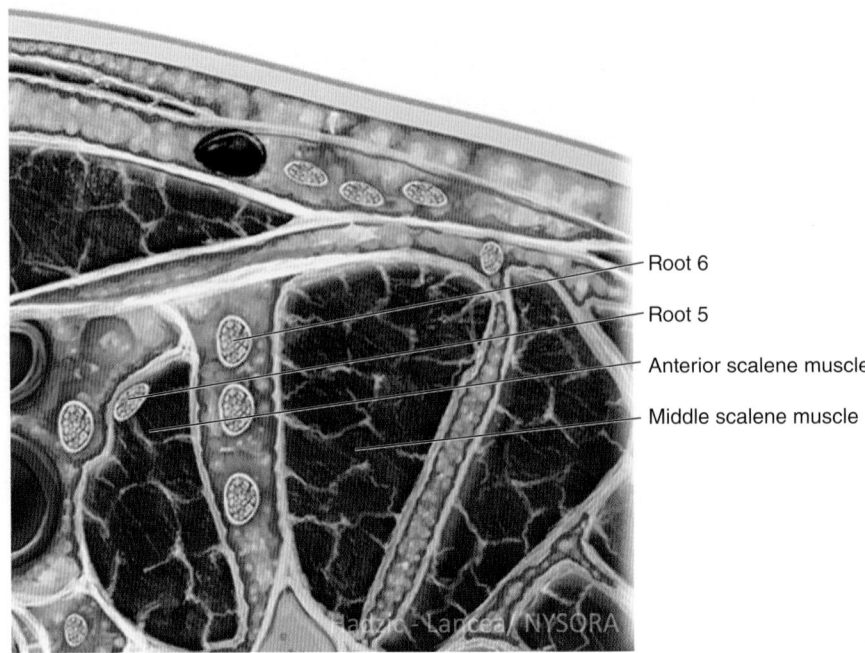

FIGURE 32B–12. Anatomic variation showing the C5 root located in the anterior scalene muscle. To block this anatomical variant, the root should be traced distally until it enters the interscalene groove.

The function of the phrenic nerve can be assessed using ultrasound in M-mode[22] during which a low-frequency curvilinear probe is positioned under the rib cage on the anterior axillary line to evaluate the hemidiaphragm motion (Figure 32B–13).

Of note, some authors have recommended using a combination of suprascapular nerve and axillary nerve blockade to provide postoperative analgesia with minimal motor blockade distal to the shoulder with a lower risk of phrenic nerve blockade and other complications of interscalene block.[23–27] The targeted nerves are small, and may prove difficult to find in obese patient. Moreover, these blocks will not provide surgical anesthesia.

Another issue that must be considered is persistent phrenic nerve palsy. There is little agreement as to what causes persistent phrenic nerve palsy, but it seems to be at least in part related to inflammation and nerve entrapment rather than direct needle trauma.[28] A contribution of cervical spine disease has been suggested.[29] Other factors may be involved, as most patients in published series have been male, overweight or obese, and middle-aged.[30]

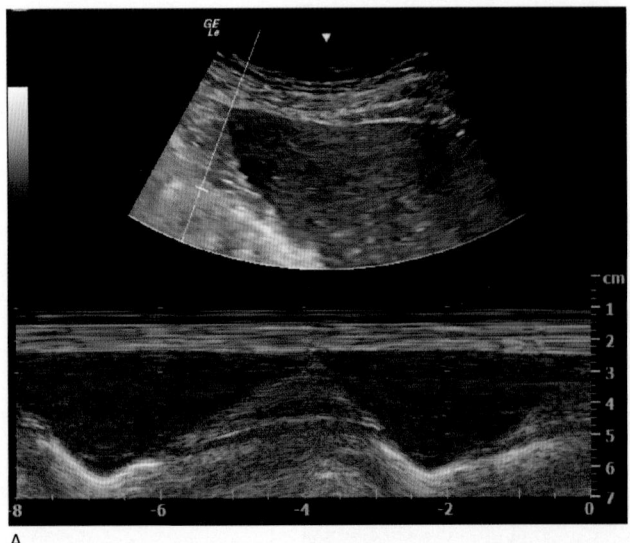
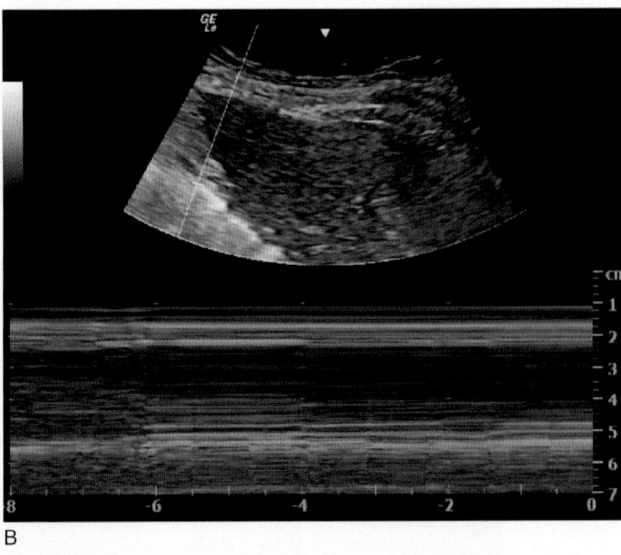

FIGURE 32B–13. Imaging of the right hemidiaphragm under the ribcage on the anterior line. (**A**) Before interscalene block. (**B**) After interscalene block with phrenic nerve block.

CONTINUOUS ULTRASOUND-GUIDED INTERSCALENE BLOCK

The goal of the continuous interscalene block is to place the catheter in the vicinity of the elements of the brachial plexus between the scalene muscles. The procedure consists of: (1) needle placement; (2) LA injection to assure the proper needle tip position and "open up the space" for catheter (3) catheter advancement; (4) Injection through the catheter while monitoring on US to verify its therapeutic position and (5) securing the catheter. For the first two phases of the procedure, ultrasound can be used to ensure accuracy. The needle is typically inserted in plane from the lateral-to-medial direction and underneath the prevertebral fascia to enter the interscalene space (Figure 32B–14), although other needle orientations, such as out-of-plane or aiming caudad, may also be used.

Proper needle placement can also be confirmed by obtaining a motor response of the deltoid muscle, arm, or forearm (0.5 mA, 0.1 msec), at which point 4–5 mL of local anesthetic can be injected. This small dose of local anesthetic serves to ensure adequate distribution of local anesthetic as well as to make the advancement of the catheter more comfortable to the patient. This first phase of the procedure does not significantly differ from the single-injection technique. The second phase of the procedure involves maintaining the needle in the proper position and inserting the catheter 2–3 cm into the interscalene space within the vicinity of the brachial plexus (Figure 32B–15). Catheter insertion can be accomplished by a single operator or with an assistant. Proper catheter location can be confirmed either by visualizing the course of the catheter or by an injection of local anesthetic through the catheter. When this proves difficult, an alternative is to inject a small amount of air (1 mL) to confirm the catheter tip location.

The catheter is secured either by taping to the skin with or without tunneling. Some clinicians prefer one over the other. However, the decision about which method to use can be based on patient age, duration of catheter therapy, and/or anatomy.

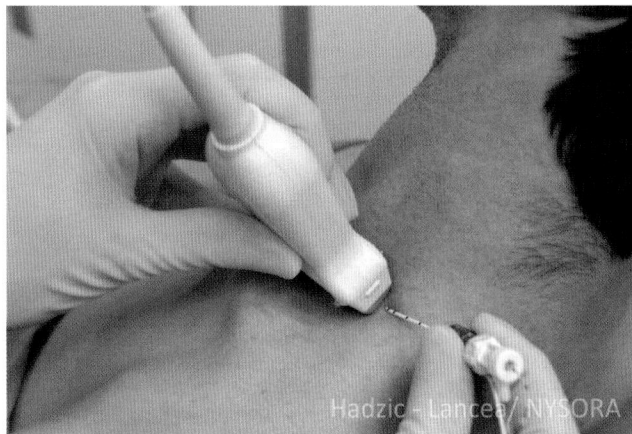

FIGURE 32B–14. Continuous brachial plexus block. The needle is inserted in the interscalene space using an in-plane approach. Note that for didactic purposes, neither sterile drapes nor ultrasound transducer cover are used in this figure.

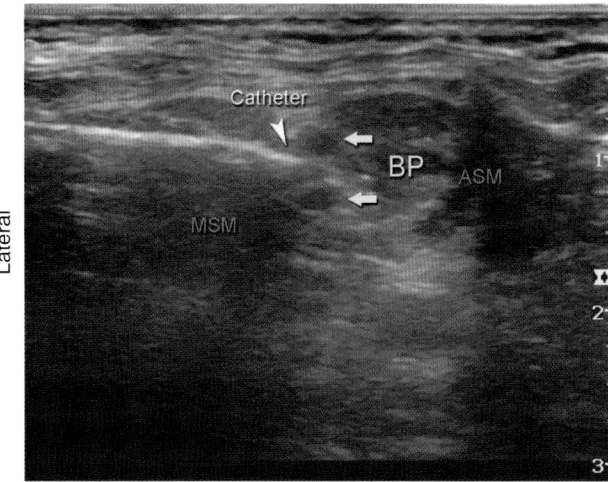

Interscalene block, catheter placement

FIGURE 32B–15. An ultrasound image demonstrating needle and catheter (white arrowhead) inserted in the interscalene space between the anterior (ASM) and middle (MSM) scalene muscles. BP, brachial plexus.

Tunneling may be preferred in older patients with obesity or sagging skin over the neck or when a longer duration of catheter infusion is expected. Two main disadvantages of tunneling are the risk of catheter dislodgement during tunneling and the potential for scar formation. A number of catheter-securing devices are available to help stabilize the catheter.

TIPS

- Both stimulating and nonstimulating catheters can be used. Because motor response on catheter stimulation may be absent even with ideal catheter placement, the use of stimulating catheters may lead to unnecessary needle and catheter manipulation to obtain evoked motor responses.[31]
- The catheter-over-needle technique has recently been reintroduced as an alternative to accomplishing continuous interscalene blockade.[32]

SUGGESTED READINGS

Single-Injection Ultrasound-Guided Interscalene Block

Albrecht E, Kirkham KR, Taffé P, et al: The maximum effective needle-to-nerve distance for ultrasound-guided interscalene block: an exploratory study. *Reg Anesth Pain Med* 2014;39:56–60.

Avellanet M, Sala-Blanch X, Rodrigo L, Gonzalez-Viejo MA: Permanent upper trunk plexopathy after interscalene brachial plexus block. *J Clin Monit Comput* 2016;30:51–54.

Burckett-St Laurent D, Chan V, Chin KJ: Refining the ultrasound-guided interscalene brachial plexus block: the superior trunk approach. *Can J Anaesth* 2014;61:1098–1102.

Errando CL, Muñoz-Devesa L, Soldado MA: Bloqueo interescalénico guiado por ecografía en un paciente con alteraciones anatómicas de la region supraclavicular secundarias a radioterapia y cirugía [Ultrasound-guided interscalene block in a patient with supraclavicular anatomical abnormalities due to radiotherapy and surgery]. *Rev Esp Anestesiol Reanim* 2011;58:312–314.

Falcão LF, Perez MV, de Castro I, Yamashita AM, Tardelli MA, Amaral JL: Minimum effective volume of 0.5% bupivacaine with epinephrine in ultrasound-guided interscalene brachial plexus block. *Br J Anaesth* 2013;110:450–455.

Fredrickson MJ, Kilfoyle DH: Neurological complication analysis of 1000 ultrasound guided peripheral nerve blocks for elective orthopaedic surgery: a prospective study. *Anaesthesia* 2009;64:836–844.

Fritsch G, Hudelmaier M, Danninger T, Brummett C, Bock M, McCoy M: Bilateral loss of neural function after interscalene plexus blockade may be caused by epidural spread of local anesthetics: a cadaveric study. *Reg Anesth Pain Med* 2013;38:64–68.

Gadsden J, Hadzic A, Gandhi K, et al: The effect of mixing 1.5% mepivacaine and 0.5% bupivacaine on duration of analgesia and latency of block onset in ultrasound-guided interscalene block. *Anesth Analg* 2011;112: 471–476.

Ihnatsenka B, Boezaart AP: Applied sonoanatomy of the posterior triangle of the neck. *Int J Shoulder Surg* 2010;4:63–74.

Koff MD, Cohen JA, McIntyre JJ, Carr CF, Sites BD: Severe brachial plexopathy after an ultrasound-guided single-injection nerve block for total shoulder arthroplasty in a patient with multiple sclerosis. *Anesthesiology* 2008;108:325–328.

Lang RS, Kentor ML, Vallejo M, Bigeleisen P, Wisniewski SR, Orebaugh SL: The impact of local anesthetic distribution on block onset in ultrasound-guided interscalene block. *Acta Anaesthesiol Scand* 2012;56:1146–1151.

Liu SS, Gordon MA, Shaw PM, Wilfred S, Shetty T, Yadeau JT: A prospective clinical registry of ultrasound-guided regional anesthesia for ambulatory shoulder surgery. *Anesth Analg* 2010;111:617–623.

Liu SS, YaDeau JT, Shaw PM, Wilfred S, Shetty T, Gordon M: Incidence of unintentional intraneural injection and post-operative neurological complications with ultrasound-guided interscalene and supraclavicular nerve blocks. *Anaesthesia* 2011;66:168–174.

Lu IC, Hsu HT, Soo LY, et al: Ultrasound examination for the optimal head position for interscalene brachial plexus block. *Acta Anaesthesiol Taiwan* 2007;45:73–78.

Madison SJ, Humsi J, Loland VJ, et al: Ultrasound-guided root/trunk (interscalene) block for hand and forearm anesthesia. *Reg Anesth Pain Med* 2013;38:226–232.

Marhofer P, Harrop-Griffiths W, Willschke H, Kirchmair L: Fifteen years of ultrasound guidance in regional anaesthesia: part 2—recent developments in block techniques. *Br J Anaesth* 2010;104:673–683.

McNaught A, McHardy P, Awad IT: Posterior interscalene block: an ultrasound-guided case series and overview of history, anatomy and techniques. *Pain Res Manag* 2010;15:219–223.

McNaught A, Shastri U, Carmichael N, et al: Ultrasound reduces the minimum effective local anaesthetic volume compared with peripheral nerve stimulation for interscalene block. *Br J Anaesth* 2011;106:124–30.

Natsis K, Totlis T, Didagelos M, Tsakotos G, Vlassis K, Skandalakis P: Scalenus minimus muscle: overestimated or not? An anatomical study. *Am Surg* 2013;79:372–374.

Orebaugh SL, McFadden K, Skorupan H, Bigeleisen PE: Subepineurial injection in ultrasound-guided interscalene needle tip placement. *Reg Anesth Pain Med* 2010;35:450–454.

Plante T, Rontes O, Bloc S, Delbos A: Spread of local anesthetic during an ultrasound-guided interscalene block: does the injection site influence diffusion? *Acta Anaesthesiol Scand* 2011;55:664–669.

Renes SH, van Geffen GJ, Rettig HC, Gielen MJ, Scheffer GJ: Minimum effective volume of local anesthetic for shoulder analgesia by ultrasound-guided block at root C7 with assessment of pulmonary function. *Reg Anesth Pain Med* 2010;35:529–534.

Roessel T, Wiessner D, Heller AR, Zimmermann T, Koch T, Litz RJ: High-resolution ultrasound-guided high interscalene plexus block for carotid endarterectomy. *Reg Anesth Pain Med* 2007;32:247–253.

Soeding P, Eizenberg N: Review article: anatomical considerations for ultrasound guidance for regional anesthesia of the neck and upper limb. *Can J Anaesth* 2009;56:518–533.

Spence BC, Beach ML, Gallagher JD, Sites BD: Ultrasound-guided interscalene blocks: understanding where to inject the local anaesthetic. *Anaesthesia* 2011;66:509–514.

Continuous Ultrasound-Guided Interscalene Block

Antonakakis JG, Sites BD, Shiffrin J: Ultrasound-guided posterior approach for the placement of a continuous interscalene catheter. *Reg Anesth Pain Med* 2009;34:64–68.

Fredrickson MJ, Ball CM, Dalgleish AJ: Analgesic effectiveness of a continuous versus single-injection interscalene block for minor arthroscopic shoulder surgery. *Reg Anesth Pain Med* 2010;35:28–33.

Fredrickson MJ, Price DJ: Analgesic effectiveness of ropivacaine 0.2% vs 0.4% via an ultrasound-guided C5–6 root/superior trunk perineural ambulatory catheter. *Br J Anaesth* 2009;103:434–439.

Fredrickson MJ, Ball CM, Dalgleish AJ: Posterior versus anterolateral approach interscalene catheter placement: a prospective randomized trial. *Reg Anesth Pain Med* 2011;36:125–133.

Fredrickson MJ, Ball CM, Dalgleish AJ, Stewart AW, Short TG: A prospective randomized comparison of ultrasound and neurostimulation as needle end points for interscalene catheter placement. *Anesth Analg* 2009;108: 1695–1700.

Mariano ER, Afra R, Loland VJ, et al: Continuous interscalene brachial plexus block via an ultrasound-guided posterior approach: a randomized, triple-masked, placebo-controlled study. *Anesth Analg* 2009;108:1688–1694.

Mariano ER, Loland VJ, Ilfeld BM: Interscalene perineural catheter placement using an ultrasound-guided posterior approach. *Reg Anesth Pain Med* 2009;34:60–63.

Shin HJ, Ahn JH, Jung HI, et al: Feasibility of ultrasound-guided posterior approach for interscalene catheter placement during arthroscopic shoulder surgery. *Korean J Anesthesiol* 2011;61:475–481.

REFERENCES

1. Gautier P, Vandepitte C, Ramquet C, DeCoopman M, Xu D, Hadzic A: The minimum effective anesthetic volume of 0.75% ropivacaine in ultrasound-guided interscalene brachial plexus block. *Anesth Analg* 2011; 113:951–955.

2. Vandepitte C, Gautier P, Xu D, Salviz EA, Hadzic A: Effective volume of ropivacaine 0.75% through a catheter required for interscalene brachial plexus blockade. *Anesthesiology* 2013;118:863–867.

3. Tsui BC, Lou L: Learning the "traceback" approach for interscalene block. *Anaesthesia* 2014;69:83–85.

4. Muhly WT, Orebaugh SL: Sonoanatomy of the vasculature at the supraclavicular and interscalene regions relevant for brachial plexus block. *Acta Anaesthesiol Scand* 2011;55:1247–1253.

5. Moayeri N, Bigeleisen PE, Groen GJ: Quantitative architecture of the brachial plexus and surrounding compartments, and their possible significance for plexus blocks. *Anesthesiology* 2008;108:299–304.

6. Orebaugh SL, McFadden K, Skorupan H, Bigeleisen PE: Subepineurial injection in ultrasound-guided interscalene needle tip placement. *Reg Anesth Pain Med* 2010;35:450–454.

7. Orebaugh SL, Mukalel JJ, Krediet AC, et al: Brachial plexus root injection in a human cadaver model: injectate distribution and effects on the neuraxis. *Reg Anesth Pain Med* 2012;37:525–529.

8. Hanson NA, Auyong DB: Systematic ultrasound identification of the dorsal scapular and long thoracic nerves during interscalene block. *Reg Anesth Pain Med* 2013;38:54–57.

9. Thomas SE, Winchester JB, Hickman G, DeBusk E: A confirmed case of injury to the long thoracic nerve following a posterior approach to an interscalene nerve block. *Reg Anesth Pain Med* 2013;38:370.

10. Saporito A: Dorsal scapular nerve injury: a complication of ultrasound-guided interscalene block. *Br J Anaesth* 2013;111:840–841.

11. Gutton C, Choquet O, Antonini F, Grossi P: Bloc interscalénique échoguidé : variations anatomiques et implication clinique [Ultrasound-guided interscalene block: influence of anatomic variations in clinical practice]. *Ann Fr Anesth Reanim* 2010;29:770–775.

12. Gautier P, Vandepitte C, Ramquet C, DeCoopman M, Xu D, Hadzic A: The minimum effective anesthetic volume of 0.75% ropivacaine in ultrasound-guided interscalene brachial plexus block. *Anesth Analg* 2011;113:951–955.

13. Falcão LF, Perez MV, de Castro I, Yamashita AM, Tardelli MA, Amaral JL: Minimum effective volume of 0.5% bupivacaine with epinephrine in ultrasound-guided interscalene brachial plexus block. *Br J Anaesth* 2013; 110:450–455.

14. Verelst P, van Zundert A: Respiratory impact of analgesic strategies for shoulder surgery. *Reg Anesth Pain Med* 2013;38:50–53.

15. Koscielniak-Nielsen ZJ: Supraclavicular catheter may be an alternative to interscalene catheter in patients at risk for respiratory failure after major shoulder surgery. *Reg Anesth Pain Med* 2013;38:251.

16. Kessler J, Schafhalter-Zoppoth I, Gray AT: An ultrasound study of the phrenic nerve in the posterior cervical triangle: implications for the interscalene brachial plexus block. *Reg Anesth Pain Med* 2008;33: 545–550.

17. Lee JH, Cho SH, Kim SH, et al: Ropivacaine for ultrasound-guided interscalene block: 5 mL provides similar analgesia but less phrenic nerve paralysis than 10 mL. *Can J Anaesth* 2011;58:1001–1006.

18. Smith HM, Duncan CM, Hebl JR: Clinical utility of low-volume ultrasound-guided interscalene blockade: contraindications reconsidered. *J Ultrasound Med* 2009;28:1251–1258.

19. Renes SH, van Geffen GJ, Rettig HC, Gielen MJ, Scheffer GJ: Minimum effective volume of local anesthetic for shoulder analgesia by ultrasound-guided block at root C7 with assessment of pulmonary function. *Reg Anesth Pain Med* 2010;35:529–534.
20. Fredrickson MJ, Abeysekera A, White R: Randomized study of the effect of local anesthetic volume and concentration on the duration of peripheral nerve blockade. *Reg Anesth Pain Med* 2012;37:495–501.
21. Sinha SK, Abrams JH, Barnett JT, et al: Decreasing the local anesthetic volume from 20 to 10 mL for ultrasound-guided interscalene block at the cricoid level does not reduce the incidence of hemidiaphragmatic paresis. *Reg Anesth Pain Med* 2011;36:17–20.
22. Mantuani D, Nagdev A: Sonographic evaluation of a paralyzed hemidiaphragm from ultrasound-guided interscalene brachial plexus nerve block. *Am J Emerg Med* 2012;30:2099.e5–7.
23. Lee SM, Park SE, Nam YS, et al: Analgesic effectiveness of nerve block in shoulder arthroscopy: comparison between interscalene, suprascapular and axillary nerve blocks. *Knee Surg Sports Traumatol Arthrosc* 2012;20:2573–2578.
24. Pitombo PF, Meira Barros R, Matos MA, Pinheiro Módolo NS: Selective suprascapular and axillary nerve block provides adequate analgesia and minimal motor block. Comparison with interscalene block. *Braz J Anesthesiol* 2013;63:45–51.
25. Lee JJ, Kim DY, Hwang JT, et al: Effect of ultrasonographically guided axillary nerve block combined with suprascapular nerve block in arthroscopic rotator cuff repair: a randomized controlled trial. *Arthroscopy* 2014;30:906–914.
26. Rothe C, Steen-Hansen C, Lund J, Jenstrup MT, Lange KH: Ultrasound-guided block of the suprascapular nerve—a volunteer study of a new proximal approach. *Acta Anaesthesiol Scand* 2014;58:1228–1232.
27. Kim YA, Yoon KB, Kwon TD, Kim DH, Yoon DM: Evaluation of anatomic landmarks for axillary nerve block in the quadrilateral space. *Acta Anaesthesiol Scand* 2014;58:567–571.
28. Kaufman MR, Elkwood AI, Rose MI, et al: Surgical treatment of permanent diaphragm paralysis after interscalene nerve block for shoulder surgery. *Anesthesiology* 2013;119:484–487.
29. Pakala SR, Beckman JD, Lyman S, Zayas VM: Cervical spine disease is a risk factor for persistent phrenic nerve paresis following interscalene nerve block. *Reg Anesth Pain Med* 2013;38:239–242.
30. Bellew B, Harrop-Griffiths WA, Bedforth N: Interscalene brachial plexus blocks and phrenic nerve palsy. *Anesthesiology* 2014;120:1056–1057.
31. Birnbaum J, Kip M, Spies CD, et al: The effect of stimulating versus nonstimulating catheters for continuous interscalene plexus blocks in short-term pain management. *J Clin Anesth* 2007;19:434–439.
32. Ip V, Tsui B: The safety of an interscalene catheter-over-needle technique. *Anaesthesia* 2013;68:774–775.

CHAPTER 32C

Ultrasound-Guided Supraclavicular Brachial Plexus Block

Thomas F. Bendtsen, Ana M. Lopez, and Catherine Vandepitte

SUPRACLAVICULAR BRACHIAL PLEXUS BLOCK AT A GLANCE

- Indications: arm, elbow, forearm, hand surgery; anesthesia for shoulder surgery is also possible (Figure 32C–1).[1]
- Transducer position: transverse on neck, just superior to the clavicle at the midpoint (Figure 32C–1)
- Goal: local anesthetic spread around the brachial plexus, posterior and superficial to the subclavian artery
- Local anesthetic: 20–25 mL

GENERAL CONSIDERATIONS

At this location, the proximity of the brachial plexus to the chest cavity and pleura had been of concern (Figure 32C–2) until ultrasound (US) guidance renewed interest in the supraclavicular approach to the brachial plexus block. The ability to image the plexus, rib, pleura, and subclavian artery with US has increased safety due to improved monitoring of anatomy and needle placement. Because the trunks and divisions of the brachial plexus are relatively close as they pass over the first rib, the extension and quality of anesthesia are favorable. For these reasons, the supraclavicular block has become a commonly used technique for surgery of the upper limb distal to the shoulder.

ULTRASOUND ANATOMY

The subclavian artery crosses over the first rib between the insertions of the anterior and middle scalene muscles, posterior to the midpoint of the clavicle. The subclavian artery is readily apparent as an anechoic round structure, whereas the parietal pleura and the first rib can be seen as a linear hyperechoic structure immediately lateral and deep to the subclavian artery (Figure 32C–3). The rib casts an acoustic shadow so that the image field deep to the rib appears anechoic.[2] The brachial plexus can be seen as a bundle of hypoechoic round nodules just posterior and superficial to the artery (Figures 32C–3 and 32C–4). It is often possible to see the fascial sheath of the muscles surrounding the brachial plexus. Adjusting the transducer orientation, the upper, middle and lower trunks of the brachial plexus can be individually identified, as they join together at the costoclavicular space. To visualize the lower trunk, the transducer is oriented in the sagittal plane, until the first rib is seen deep to the plexus and the artery. (Figure 32C-4). Anterior or posterior to the first rib is the hyperechoic pleura, with lung tissue deep to it. This structure can be confirmed by observing a "sliding" motion of the visceral pleura in synchrony with the patient's respiration. The brachial plexus is typically visualized at a 1- to 2-cm depth at this location.

The presence of two separate clusters of elements of the brachial plexus may be more or less obvious, sometimes with a separation by a blood vessel[3] (Figure 32C-4). The dorsal scapular artery commonly passes through or within the vicinity of the brachial plexus. It is important to recognize that the more superficial and lateral branches come from C5–C7 (shoulder, lateral aspect of arm, and forearm) and can be tracked up to the interscalene area, whereas the deeper and more medial contingent are branches of C8 and T1 (hand and medial aspect of forearm). Adequate spread of local anesthetic in both areas is necessary for successful block of the arm and hand.

DISTRIBUTION OF ANESTHESIA

The supraclavicular approach to the brachial plexus blockade results in anesthesia of the upper limb including often the shoulder because all trunks and divisions can be anesthetized from this location. The skin of the proximal part of the medial side of the arm (intercostobrachial nerve, T2), however, is never anesthetized by any technique of the brachial plexus block and, when necessary, can be blocked by an additional subcutaneous injection just distal to the axilla (Figure 32C-1). (For a more

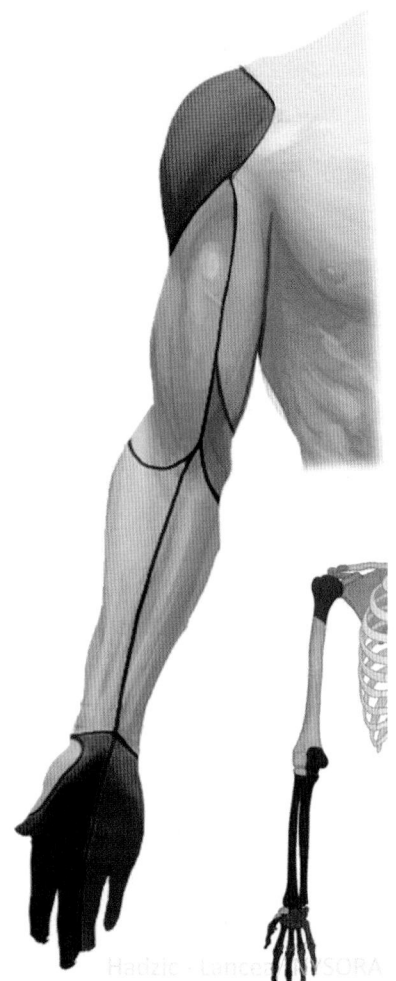

FIGURE 32C–1. Expected sensory distribution of the supraclavicular brachial plexus block.

comprehensive review of the brachial plexus anatomy and distribution, see Chapter 3.)

EQUIPMENT

The equipment needed for a supraclavicular brachial plexus block includes the following:

- Ultrasound machine with linear transducer (8–18 MHz), sterile sleeve, and gel (or other acoustic coupling agent; eg, saline)
- Standard nerve block tray
- 20–25 mL local anesthetic
- 5-cm, 22-gauge, short-bevel, insulated stimulating needle
- Peripheral nerve stimulator
- Opening injection pressure monitoring system
- Sterile gloves

LANDMARKS AND PATIENT POSITIONING

Any position that allows for comfortable placement of the ultrasound transducer and needle advancement is appropriate. This block can be performed with the patient in the supine,

semi-sitting, or slight lateral position, with the patient's head turned away from the side to be blocked. When possible, asking the patient to reach for the ipsilateral knee will depress the clavicle slightly and allow better access to the structures of the anterolateral neck.

Knowledge of the underlying anatomy and the position of the brachial plexus in relation to the subclavian artery, first rib, and pleura is important for the success and safety of the technique. Scanning is usually started just above the clavicle, approximately at its midpoint.

GOAL

The goal of this block is to place the needle within the brachial plexus sheath posterior to the subclavian artery and inject local anesthetic to surround the trunks and divisions of the brachial plexus at this level.

TECHNIQUE

With the patient in the proper position, the skin is disinfected and the transducer is positioned in the transverse plane immediately proximal to the clavicle, slightly posterior to at its midpoint. The transducer is tilted caudally, as if to image the chest contents, to obtain a cross-sectional view of the subclavian artery (Figure 32C–5). The brachial plexus is seen as a collection of hypoechoic oval structures posterior and superficial to the artery. Color Doppler should be routinely used prior to needle insertion to rule out the passage of large vessels (ie, dorsal scapular artery, transverse cervical artery, suprascapular artery) in the anticipated trajectory of the needle.[4]

Clinical Pearl

- To achieve the best possible view, the transducer often must be tilted slightly inferiorly (see arrows in Figure 32C–5). The goal is to see the subclavian artery in the transverse view and the brachial plexus just superficial and posterior to the subclavian artery, enclosed within the brachial plexus sheath. Transducer rotation clockwise often facilitate best imaging of the tissue space (sheath) containing the plexus.

Using a 25- to 27-gauge needle, 1–2 mL of local anesthetic is injected into the skin 1 cm lateral to the transducer to decrease discomfort during needle insertion. To avoid inadvertent puncture of and injection into the brachial plexus, the needle should not be initially inserted deeper than 1 cm. The distribution of local anesthetic via small-volume injections is observed as the needle advances through tissue layers (hydrolocalization); small-volume injections are used to avoid inadvertent needle insertion into the brachial plexus. The block needle is then inserted in plane toward the brachial plexus, in a lateral-to-medial direction (Figures 33C–5 and 33C–6). Nerve stimulation (0.5 mA, 0.1 msec), is often associated with a motor

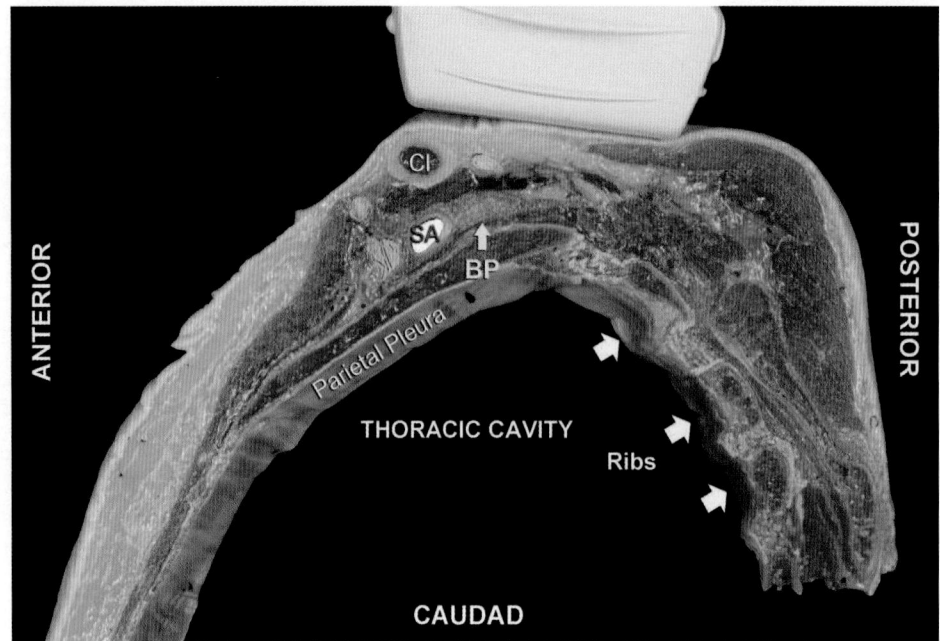

FIGURE 32C–2. Anatomy of the supraclavicular brachial plexus with proper transducer placement slightly oblique above the clavicle (Cl). Yellow arrow: brachial plexus (BP). SA, subclavian artery.

response of the arm, forearm, or hand. Note, however, that motor response may be absent despite accurate needle placement. Insertion of the needle into the sheath is often associated with a palpable "pop." After careful aspiration, 1–2 mL of local anesthetic is injected to confirm proper needle placement. When the injection displaces the brachial plexus away from the needle, an additional advancement of the needle 1–2 mm closer to the plexus may be required to accomplish adequate local anesthetic spread (Figures 32C–7, 32C–8, and 32C–9). When the injection of local anesthetic does not appear to result in a spread around the brachial plexus, needle repositioning may be necessary. Typically, 20–25 mL of local anesthetic is required for adequate block.

It has been suggested that lower volumes can be used in older patients.[5] (see Figure 32C–7).

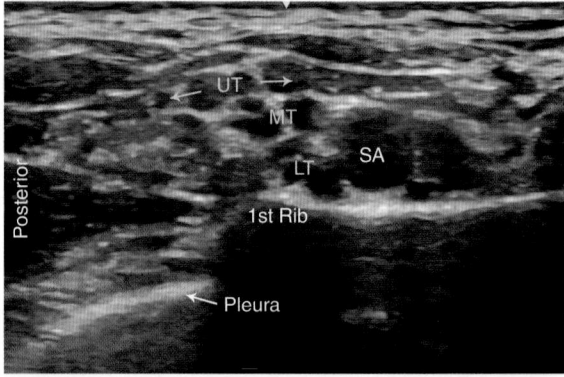

A

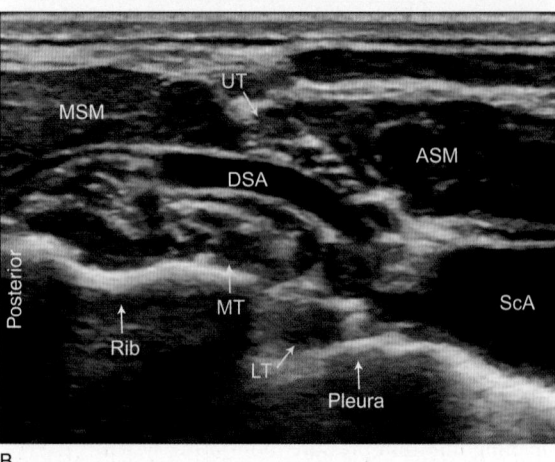

B

FIGURE 32C–4. Ultrasound images of the brachial plexus cephalad to the clavicle. (**A**) Sagittal view: The upper (UT), Middle (MT) and lower (LT) trunks of the brachial plexus are seen posterior to the subclavian artery (SA) and superficial to the first rib. (**B**) Oblique view: The upper trunk (UT) is positioned between the anterior (ASM) and middle (MSM) scalene muscles. The lower trunk (LT) and the subclavian artery are superficial to the pleura.

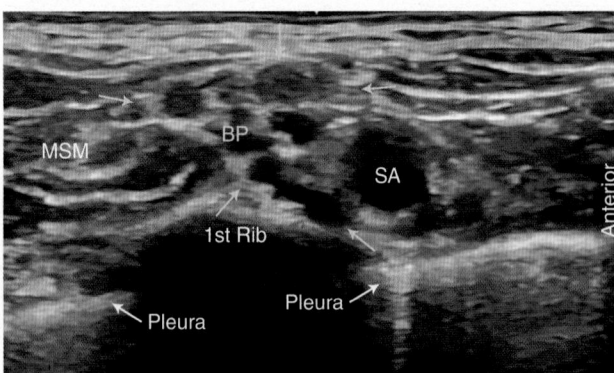

FIGURE 32C–3. Supraclavicular brachial plexus (BP; yellow arrows) seen slightly superficial and posterolateral to the subclavian artery (SA). The brachial plexus is enveloped by a connective tissue sheath. Note the intimate location of the pleura and lung to the brachial plexus and subclavian artery. MSM, middle scalene muscle.

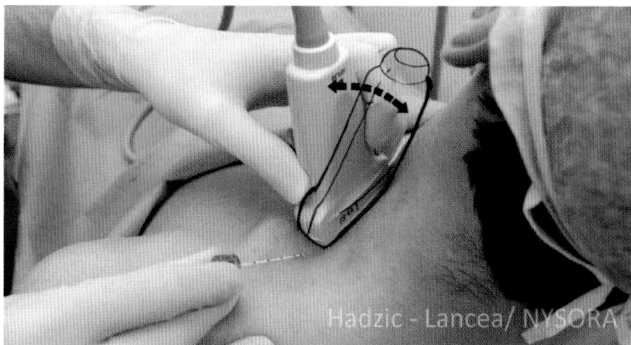

FIGURE 32C–5. Supraclavicular brachial plexus block: transducer position just proximal the clavicle and needle insertion. The brachial plexus is very shallow at this location, typically 1–3 cm; therefore, inclination of the needle should be equally shallow. The image also shows the caudal tilt that is useful in obtaining best image of the plexus.

TIPS

- A motor response to nerve stimulation is not necessary if the plexus, needle, and local anesthetic spread are well visualized.
- The neck is a highly vascular area, and care must be exercised to avoid needle placement or injection into the vascular structures. Of particular importance is to note the intimately located subclavian artery and dorsal scapular artery, which often cross the brachial plexus at this level.[4,6] Other vessels can be found within the vicinity of the brachial plexus, such as the suprascapular artery and the transverse cervical artery.[7] The use of color Doppler before needle placement and injection is highly recommended.
- Pneumothorax is also a rare but possible complication,[9–13] typically delayed rather than immediate, therefore, it is paramount to keep the needle tip visible at all times.
- Never inject against high resistance to injection. The inability to initiate injection with an opening injection pressure of less than 15 psi may signal an intrafascicular injection.

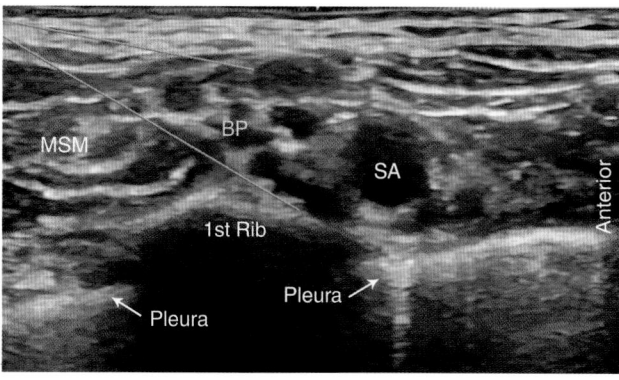

FIGURE 32C–7. The desired spread of local anesthetic (blue-shaded areas) in two different needle positions to accomplish brachial plexus (BP) block. Local anesthetic should spread within the connective tissue sheath resulting in separation of the brachial plexus trunks posterior to the subclavian artery (SCA).

- Multiple injections
  - May increase the speed of onset and the success rate.[14–16]
  - May allow for a reduction in the required volume of local anesthetic.
  - May carry a higher risk of nerve injury.

CONTINUOUS ULTRASOUND-GUIDED SUPRACLAVICULAR BLOCK

The ultrasound-guided continuous supraclavicular block is in many ways similar to the technique used for interscalene catheter placement. The goal is to place the catheter within the vicinity of the trunks and divisions of the brachial plexus adjacent to the subclavian artery. The procedure consists of three phases: (1) needle placement; (2) catheter advancement; and (3) securing the catheter. For the first two steps of the procedure, ultrasound can be used to ensure accuracy in most patients. The needle is typically inserted in plane from the lateral-to-medial direction so that the tip is just posterior to the brachial plexus sheath. The needle is then advanced to pierce the sheath, followed by catheter placement.

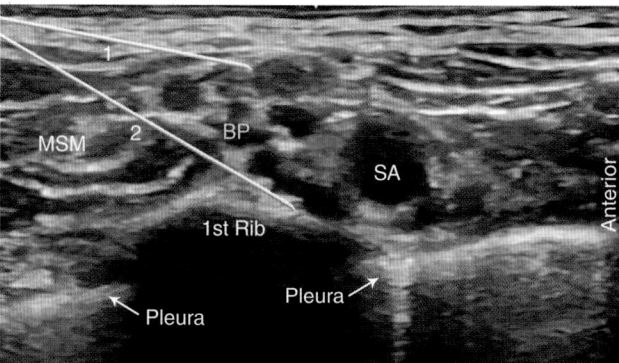

FIGURE 32C–6. Supraclavicular brachial plexus block: needle path and two separate injections required for block of the brachial plexus. Two needle positions (1 and 2) are used to inject local anesthetic within the connective tissue sheath (arrows) containing the brachial plexus (BP).

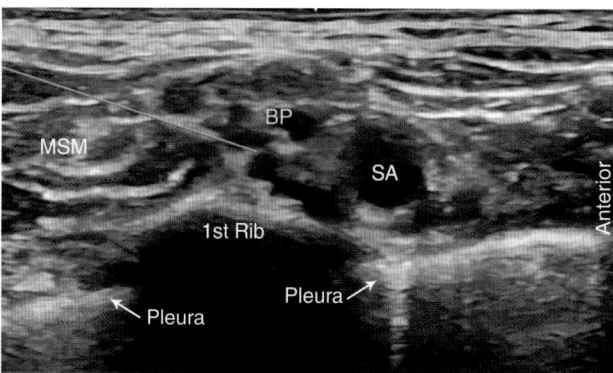

FIGURE 32C–8. Ultrasound image simulating needle path and expected local anesthetic spread after a single injection within the connective tissue sheath surrounding the brachial plexus. Additional monitoring (eg, nerve stimulation and injection pressure) is recommended to decrease the risk of intrafascicular injection.

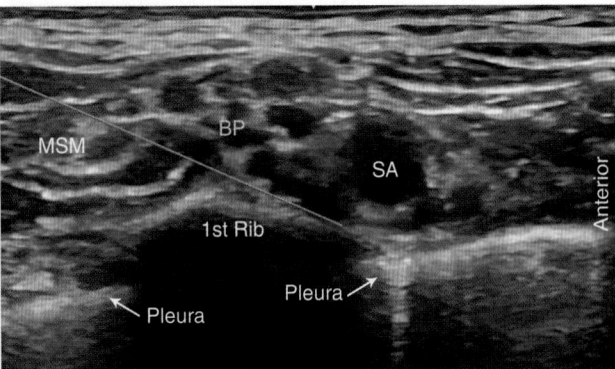

FIGURE 32C–9. Ultrasound-guided supraclavicular brachial plexus block simulating a single injection between the subclavian artery (SA) and the first rib.

Clinical Pearl

- The risk of phrenic nerve palsy is lower than with the interscalene block but cannot be reliably avoided.[8] Therefore, in patients who cannot tolerate a 27–30% decrease in respiratory function with phrenic blockade, an axillary or infraclavicular block is a better choice of anesthesia for upper extremity surgery.

Two main disadvantages of tunneling are the risk of catheter dislodgement during the tunneling and the potential for scar formation. A number of devices are commercially available to help secure the catheter. The starting infusion regimen is typically 5-8 mL/h of 0.2% ropivacaine of bupivacaine 0.125% with 3-5 mL patient-controlled boluses hourly. A catheter-over-needle technique has also been described.[17]

SUGGESTED READINGS

Aguirre J, Ekatodramis G, Ruland P, Borgeat A: Ultrasound-guided supraclavicular block: is it really safer? Reg Anesth Pain Med 2009;34:622.

Arcand G, Williams SR, Chouinard P, et al: Ultrasound-guided infraclavicular versus supraclavicular block. Anesth Analg 2005;101:886–890.

Beach ML, Sites BD, Gallagher JD: Use of a nerve stimulator does not improve the efficacy of ultrasound-guided supraclavicular nerve blocks. J Clin Anesth 2006;18:580–584.

Bigeleisen PE, Moayeri N, Groen GJ: Extraneural versus intraneural stimulation thresholds during ultrasound-guided supraclavicular block. Anesthesiology 2009;110:1235–1243.

Chan VW, Perlas A, Rawson R, Odukoya O: Ultrasound-guided supraclavicular brachial plexus block. Anesth Analg 2003;97:1514–1517.

Chin KJ, Niazi A, Chan V: Anomalous brachial plexus anatomy in the supraclavicular region detected by ultrasound. Anesth Analg 2008;107:729–731.

Chin J, Tsui BC: No change in impedance upon intravascular injection of D5W. Can J Anaesth 2010;57:559–564.

Collins AB, Gray AT, Kessler J: Ultrasound-guided supraclavicular brachial plexus block: a modified Plumb-Bob technique. Reg Anesth Pain Med 2006;31:591–592.

Cornish P: Supraclavicular block—new perspectives. Reg Anesth Pain Med 2009;34:607–608.

Cornish PB, Leaper CJ, Nelson G, Anstis F, McQuillan C, Stienstra R: Avoidance of phrenic nerve paresis during continuous supraclavicular regional anaesthesia. Anaesthesia 2007;62:354–358.

Duggan E, Brull R, Lai J, Abbas S: Ultrasound-guided brachial plexus block in a patient with multiple glomangiomatosis. Reg Anesth Pain Med 2008;33:70–73.

Duggan E, El Beheiry H, Perlas A, et al: Minimum effective volume of local anesthetic for ultrasound-guided supraclavicular brachial plexus block. Reg Anesth Pain Med 2009;34:215–218.

Feigl GC, Dreu M: Important structures to be known for a safe ultrasound-guided supraclavicular plexus block. Reg Anesth Pain Med 2010;35:317–18.

Feigl GC, Pixner T: Combination of variations of the interscalene gap as a pitfall for ultrasound-guided brachial plexus block. Reg Anesth Pain Med 2011;36:523–524.

Fredrickson MJ, Kilfoyle DH: Neurological complication analysis of 1000 ultrasound guided peripheral nerve blocks for elective orthopaedic surgery: a prospective study. Anaesthesia 2009;64:836–844.

Fredrickson MJ, Patel A, Young S, Chinchanwala S: Speed of onset of "corner pocket supraclavicular" and infraclavicular ultrasound guided brachial plexus block: a randomised observer-blinded comparison. Anaesthesia 2009;64:738–744.

Gupta PK, Pace NL, Hopkins PM: Effect of body mass index on the ED50 volume of bupivacaine 0.5% for supraclavicular brachial plexus block. Br J Anaesth 2010;104:490–495.

Hanumanthaiah D, Vaidiyanathan S, Garstka M, Szucs S, Iohom G: Ultrasound guided supraclavicular block. Med Ultrason 2013;15:224–229.

Heil JW, Ilfeld BM, Loland VJ, Mariano ER: Preliminary experience with a novel ultrasound-guided supraclavicular perineural catheter insertion technique for perioperative analgesia of the upper extremity. J Ultrasound Med 2010;29:1481–1485.

Ihnatsenka B, Boezaart AP: Applied sonoanatomy of the posterior triangle of the neck. Int J Shoulder Surg 2010;4:63–74.

Jeon DG, Kim SK, Kang BJ, Kwon MA, Song JG, Jeon SM: Comparison of ultrasound-guided supraclavicular block according to the various volumes of local anesthetic. Korean J Anesthesiol 2013;64:494–499.

Jeon DG, Kim WI. Cases series: ultrasound-guided supraclavicular block in 105 patients. Korean J Anesthesiol 2010;58:267–271.

Kapral S, Krafft P, Eibenberger K, Fitzgerald R, Gosch M, Weinstabl C: Ultrasound-guided supraclavicular approach for regional anesthesia of the brachial plexus. Anesth Analg 1994;78:507–513.

Kinjo S, Frankel A: Failure of supraclavicular block under ultrasound guidance: clinical relevance of anatomical variation of cervical vessels. J Anesth 2012;26:100–102.

Klaastad O, Sauter AR, Dodgson MS: Brachial plexus block with or without ultrasound guidance. Curr Opin Anaesthesiol 2009;22:655–660.

la Grange P, Foster PA, Pretorius LK: Application of the Doppler ultrasound bloodflow detector in supraclavicular brachial plexus block. Br J Anaesth 1978;50:965–967.

Lasserre A, Tran-Van D, Gaertner E, Labadie P, Fontaine B: Ultrasound guided locoregional anaesthesia: realization and diagnosis of complications [in French]. Ann Fr Anesth Reanim 2009;28:584–587.

Macfarlane AJ, Perlas A, Chan V, Brull R: Eight ball, corner pocket ultrasound-guided supraclavicular block: avoiding a scratch. Reg Anesth Pain Med 2008;33:502–503.

Manickam BP, Oosthuysen SA, Parikh MK: Supraclavicular brachial plexus block-variant relation of brachial plexus to subclavian artery on the first rib. Reg Anesth Pain Med 2009;34:383–384.

Marhofer P, Schrogendorfer K, Koinig H, Kapral S, Weinstabl C, Mayer N: Ultrasonographic guidance improves sensory block and onset time of three-in-one blocks. Anesth Analg 1997;85:854–857.

Morfey D, Brull R: Ultrasound-guided supraclavicular block: What is intraneural? Anesthesiology 2010;112:250–251.

Morfey DH, Brull R: Finding the corner pocket: landmarks in ultrasound-guided supraclavicular block. Anaesthesia 2009;64:1381.

Neal JM, Moore JM, Kopacz DJ, Liu SS, Kramer DJ, Plorde JJ: Quantitative analysis of respiratory, motor, and sensory function after supraclavicular block. Anesth Analg 1998;86:1239–1244.

Perlas A, Chan VW, Simons M: Brachial plexus examination and localization using ultrasound and electrical stimulation: a volunteer study. Anesthesiology 2003;99:429–435.

Perlas A, Lobo G, Lo N, Brull R, Chan VW, Karkhanis R: Ultrasound-guided supraclavicular block: outcome of 510 consecutive cases. Reg Anesth Pain Med 2009;34:171–176.

Plunkett AR, Brown DS, Rogers JM, Buckenmaier CC III: Supraclavicular continuous peripheral nerve block in a wounded soldier: when ultrasound is the only option. Br J Anaesth 2006;97:715–717.

Reiss W, Kurapati S, Shariat A, Hadzic A: Nerve injury complicating ultrasound/electrostimulation-guided supraclavicular brachial plexus block. Reg Anesth Pain Med 2010;35:400–401.

Renes SH, Spoormans HH, Gielen MJ, Rettig HC, van Geffen GJ: Hemidiaphragmatic paresis can be avoided in ultrasound-guided supraclavicular brachial plexus block. Reg Anesth Pain Med 2009;34:595–599.

Roy M, Nadeau MJ, Côté D, et al: Comparison of a single- or double-injection technique for ultrasound-guided supraclavicular block: a prospective, randomized, blinded controlled study. Reg Anesth Pain Med 2012;37:55–59.

Samet R, Villamater E: Eight ball, corner pocket for ultrasound-guided supraclavicular block: high risk for a scratch. Reg Anesth Pain Med 2008;33:87.

Shorthouse JR, Danbury CM: Ultrasound-guided supraclavicular brachial plexus block in Klippel-Feil syndrome. Anaesthesia 2009;64:693–694.

Sivashanmugam T, Ray S, Ravishankar M, Jaya V, Selvam E, Karmakar MK: Randomized comparison of extrafascial versus subfascial injection of local anesthetic during ultrasound-guided supraclavicular brachial plexus block. Reg Anesth Pain Med 2015;40:337–343.

Soares LG, Brull R, Lai J, Chan VW: Eight ball, corner pocket: the optimal needle position for ultrasound-guided supraclavicular block. Reg Anesth Pain Med 2007;32:94–95.

Song JG, Jeon DG, Kang BJ, Park KK: Minimum effective volume of mepivacaine for ultrasound-guided supraclavicular block. Korean J Anesthesiol 2013;65:37–41.

Subramanyam R, Vaishnav V, Chan VW, Brown-Shreves D, Brull R: Lateral versus medial needle approach for ultrasound-guided supraclavicular block: a randomized controlled trial. Reg Anesth Pain Med 2011;36:387–392.

Techasuk W, González AP, Bernucci F, Cupido T, Finlayson RJ, Tran DQ: A randomized comparison between double-injection and targeted intracluster-injection ultrasound-guided supraclavicular brachial plexus block. Anesth Analg 2014;118:1363–1369.

Tran DQ, Dugani S, Correa JA, Dyachenko A, Alsenosy N, Finlayson RJ: Minimum effective volume of lidocaine for ultrasound-guided supraclavicular block. Reg Anesth Pain Med 2011;36:466–469.

Tran DQ, Munoz L, Zaouter C, Russo G, Finlayson RJ: A prospective, randomized comparison between single- and double-injection, ultrasound-guided supraclavicular brachial plexus block. Reg Anesth Pain Med 2009;34:420–424.

Tran DQ, Russo G, Munoz L, Zaouter C, Finlayson RJ: A prospective, randomized comparison between ultrasound-guided supraclavicular, infraclavicular, and axillary brachial plexus blocks. Reg Anesth Pain Med 2009;34:366–371.

Tsui BC, Doyle K, Chu K, Pillay J, Dillane D: Case series: ultrasound-guided supraclavicular block using a curvilinear probe in 104 day-case hand surgery patients. Can J Anaesth 2009;56:46–51.

Tsui BC, Twomey C, Finucane BT: Visualization of the brachial plexus in the supraclavicular region using a curved ultrasound probe with a sterile transparent dressing. Reg Anesth Pain Med 2006;31:182–184.

VadeBoncouer TR, Weinberg GL, Oswald S, Angelov F: Early detection of intravascular injection during ultrasound-guided supraclavicular brachial plexus block. Reg Anesth Pain Med 2008;33:278–279.

Vermeylen K, Engelen S, Sermeus L, Soetens F, Van de Velde M: Supraclavicular brachial plexus blocks: review and current practice. Acta Anaesthesiol Belg 2012;63:15–21. Review.

Vernieuwe L, Van de Putte P: Ultrasound-guided supraclavicular block in a patient with no first rib. J Clin Anesth 2015;27:361–362.

Watanabe T, Yanabashi K, Moriya K, Maki Y, Tsubokawa N, Baba H: Ultrasound-guided supraclavicular brachial plexus block in a patient with a cervical rib. Can J Anaesth 2015;62:671–673.

Williams SR, Chouinard P, Arcand G, et al: Ultrasound guidance speeds execution and improves the quality of supraclavicular block. Anesth Analg 2003;97:1518–1523.

Yazer MS, Finlayson RJ, Tran DQ: A randomized comparison between infraclavicular block and targeted intracluster injection supraclavicular block. Reg Anesth Pain Med 2015;40:11–15.

REFERENCES

1. Liu SS, Gordon MA, Shaw PM, Wilfred S, Shetty T, Yadeau JT: A prospective clinical registry of ultrasound-guided regional anesthesia for ambulatory shoulder surgery. Anesth Analg 2010;111:617–623.
2. Hebbard PD: Artifactual mirrored subclavian artery on ultrasound imaging for supraclavicular block. Can J Anaesth 2009;56:537–538.
3. Abrahams MS, Panzer O, Atchabahian A, Horn JL, Brown AR: Case report: limitation of local anesthetic spread during ultrasound-guided interscalene block. Description of an anatomic variant with clinical correlation. Reg Anesth Pain Med 2008;33:357–359.
4. Murata H, Sakai A, Hadzic A, Sumikawa K: The presence of transverse cervical and dorsal scapular arteries at three ultrasound probe positions commonly used in supraclavicular brachial plexus blockade. Anesth Analg 2012;115:470–473.
5. Pavičić Šarić J, Vidjak V, Tomulić K, Zenko J: Effects of age on minimum effective volume of local anesthetic for ultrasound-guided supraclavicular brachial plexus block. Acta Anaesthesiol Scand 2013;57:761–766.
6. Murata H, Sakai A, Sumikawa K: A venous structure anterior to the brachial plexus in the supraclavicular region. Reg Anesth Pain Med 2011;36:412–413.
7. Snaith R, Dolan J: Preprocedural color probe Doppler scanning before ultrasound-guided supraclavicular block. Anesth Pain Med 2010;35:223.
8. Guirguis M, Karroum R, Abd-Elsayed AA, Mounir-Soliman L: Acute respiratory distress following ultrasound-guided supraclavicular block. Ochsner J 2012;12:159–162.
9. Bhatia A, Lai J, Chan VW, Brull R: Case report: pneumothorax as a complication of the ultrasound-guided supraclavicular approach for brachial plexus block. Anesth Analg 2010;111:817–819.
10. Abell DJ, Barrington MJ: Pneumothorax after ultrasound-guided supraclavicular block: presenting features, risk, and related training. Reg Anesth Pain Med 2014;39:164–167.
11. Gauss A, Tugtekin I, Georgieff M, Dinse-Lambracht A, Keipke D, Gorsewski G: Incidence of clinically symptomatic pneumothorax in ultrasound-guided infraclavicular and supraclavicular brachial plexus block. Anaesthesia 2014;69:327–336.
12. Kumari A, Gupta R, Bhardwaj A, Madan D: Delayed pneumothorax after supraclavicular block. J Anaesthesiol Clin Pharmacol 2011;27:121–122.
13. Kakazu C, Tokhner V, Li J, Ou R, Simmons E: In the new era of ultrasound guidance: is pneumothorax from supraclavicular block a rare complication of the past? Br J Anaesth 2014;113:190–191.
14. Tran DQ, Muñoz L, Zaouter C, Russo G, Finlayson RJ: A prospective, randomized comparison between single- and double-injection, ultrasound-guided supraclavicular brachial plexus block. Reg Anesth Pain Med 2009;34:420–424.
15. Techasuk W, González AP, Bernucci F, Cupido T, Finlayson RJ, Tran DQ: A randomized comparison between double-injection and targeted intracluster-injection ultrasound-guided supraclavicular brachial plexus block. Anesth Analg 2014;118:1363–1369.
16. Arab SA, Alharbi MK, Nada EM, Alrefai DA, Mowafi HA: Ultrasound-guided supraclavicular brachial plexus block: single versus triple injection technique for upper limb arteriovenous access surgery. Anesth Analg 2014;118:1120–1125.
17. Ip VH, Tsui BC: The catheter-over-needle assembly facilitates delivery of a second local anesthetic bolus to prolong supraclavicular brachial plexus block without time-consuming catheterization steps: a randomized controlled study. Can J Anaesth 2013;60:692–699.

CHAPTER 32D

Ultrasound-Guided Infraclavicular Brachial Plexus Block

Arthur Atchabahian, Catherine Vandepitte, and Ana M. Lopez

INFRACLAVICULAR BRACHIAL PLEXUS BLOCK AT A GLANCE

- Indications: arm, elbow, forearm, and hand surgery (Figure 32D-1)
- Transducer position: approximately parasagittal, just medial to the coracoid process, inferior to the clavicle
- Goal: local anesthetic spread around axillary artery
- Local anesthetic volume: 20–30 mL

GENERAL CONSIDERATIONS

The ultrasound (US)-guided infraclavicular brachial plexus block is in some ways both simple and challenging. It is simple in that identification of the arterial pulse on the sonographic image is an easy primary goal in establishing the landmark. However, the plexus at this level is situated deeper, and the angle of approach is more acute, making simultaneous visualization of the needle and the relevant anatomy more challenging. Fortunately, although it is not always possible to reliably identify the three cords of the plexus, adequate block can be achieved by simply depositing the local anesthetic in a U shape around the artery. The infraclavicular brachial plexus block is well suited for the catheter technique because the musculature of the chest wall helps stabilize the catheter and prevents its dislodgement compared with the more superficial location used with the interscalene and supraclavicular approaches to brachial plexus blockade.

ULTRASOUND ANATOMY

The axillary artery can be identified deep to the pectoralis major and minor muscles. An effort needs to be made to obtain clear views of both pectoralis muscles and their respective fasciae. This is important because the area of interest lies underneath the fascia of the pectoralis minor muscle. Surrounding the artery are the three cords of the brachial plexus: the lateral, posterior, and medial cords. These are named for their usual position relative to the axillary artery, although there is a great deal of anatomical variation. With the left side of the screen corresponding to the cephalad aspect, the cords can often be seen as round hyperechoic structures at the positions of approximately 9 o'clock (lateral cord), 7 o'clock (posterior cord), and 5 o'clock (medial cord) (Figures 32D–2 and 32D–3). The axillary vein is seen as a compressible hypoechoic structure that lies medially to the axillary artery. Multiple other, smaller vessels (eg, the cephalic vein) are often present as well. The transducer is moved in the cephalad-caudad and medial-lateral direction until the artery is identified in cross-section. Depending on the depth selected and the level at which the scanning is performed, the chest wall and the pleura may be seen in the medial and more caudal aspect of the image. The axillary artery and/or brachial plexus are typically identified at a depth of 3–5 cm in average-size patients.

DISTRIBUTION OF ANESTHESIA

The infraclavicular approach to brachial plexus blockade results in anesthesia of the upper limb below the shoulder. If required, the skin of the medial aspect of the upper arm (intercostobrachial nerve, T2) can be blocked by an additional subcutaneous injection on the medial aspect of the arm just distal to the axilla. A simpler approach is for surgeons to infiltrate the skin with the local anesthetic directly over the incision line as needed. For a more comprehensive review of the brachial plexus distribution, see Chapter 3.

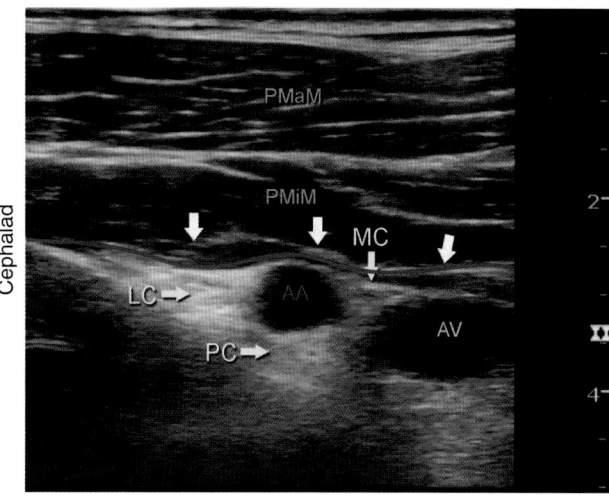

Infraclavicular block

FIGURE 32D-3. Ultrasound image of the brachial plexus (BP) distal to the clavicle. Note that the BP, axillary artery (AA) and axillary vein (AV) are located below the fascia (red line) of the pectoralis minor muscle (PMiM). LC, lateral cord; MC, medial cord; PC, posterior cord; PMaM, pectoralis major muscle.

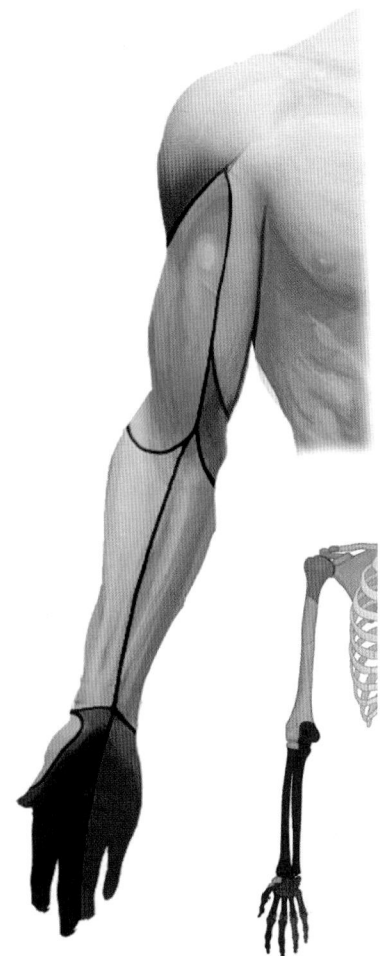

FIGURE 32D-1. Distribution of sensory blockade of the infraclavicular brachial plexus block.

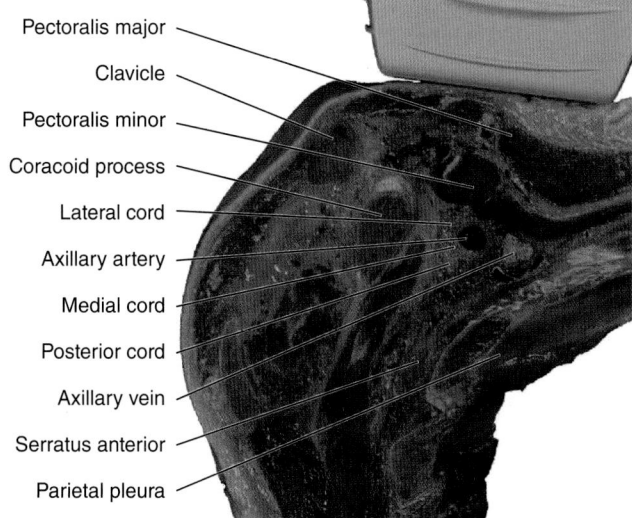

FIGURE 32D-2. Anatomy of the infraclavicular brachial plexus (BP) and the position of the transducer. Paramedian sagittal plane at the level of the coracoid process. The BP is seen surrounding the axillary artery (AA) underneath the coracoid process and pectoralis minor muscle (PMiM). Note that the injection of local anesthetic should take place below the fascia of the PMiM to spread around the AA.

EQUIPMENT

The equipment recommended for an infraclavicular brachial plexus block includes the following:

- Ultrasound machine with linear transducer (8–14 MHz), sterile sleeve, and gel
- Standard nerve block tray
- 20–30 mL of local anesthetic drawn up in syringes
- 8- to 10-cm, 21- to 22-gauge, short-bevel, insulated stimulating needle
- Peripheral nerve stimulator
- Opening injection pressure monitoring system
- Sterile gloves

LANDMARKS AND PATIENT POSITIONING

Any position that allows for the comfortable placement of the ultrasound transducer and needle advancement is appropriate. The block is typically performed with the patient in the supine position with the head turned away from the side to be blocked (Figure 32D–4). The arm is abducted to 90 degrees and the elbow flexed. This maneuver raises the clavicle, reduces the depth from the skin to the plexus,[1] and substantially facilitates visualization of the pectoralis muscles as well as the cords of the brachial plexus and the needle.[2]

The coracoid process is an important landmark and can be easily identified by palpating the bony prominence just medial to the shoulder while the arm is elevated and lowered. As the arm is lowered, the coracoid process meets the fingers of the palpating hand. Scanning usually begins just medial to the coracoid process and inferior to the clavicle.

Keeping the probe in a parasagittal plane, scanning medially and laterally allows the chest wall and pleura to be located (Figure 32D–5). The block should be performed with the

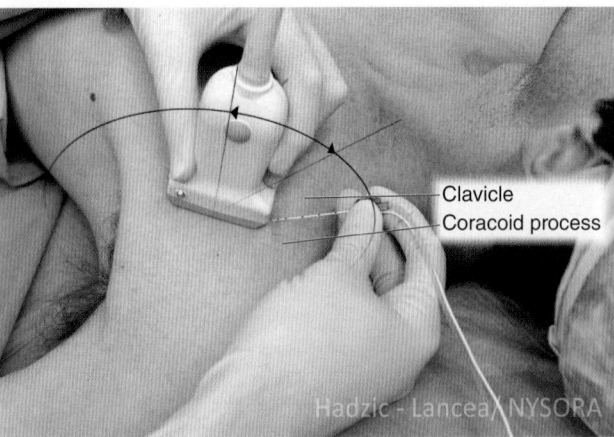

FIGURE 32D–4. Patient position for infraclavicular brachial plexus block needle insertion. The transducer is positioned parasagittally just medial to the coracoid process and inferior to the clavicle.

probe lateral to the pleura in order to minimize the risk of pneumothorax.

GOAL

The goal of the technique is to inject local anesthetic until the spread around the artery is verified by ultrasound. It is not necessary to identify and target individual cords. Instead, injection of local anesthetic to surround the artery in an U-shaped pattern (cephalad, caudad, and posterior) suffices for the block of all three cords.

TECHNIQUE

With the patient in the proper position, the skin is disinfected and the transducer is positioned in the parasagittal plane to identify the axillary artery (see Figures 33D–3 and 33D–4). This may require adjustment of the depth, depending on the thickness of the patient's chest wall musculature. The axillary artery is typically seen between 3 and 5 cm. Once the artery has been identified, an attempt is made to identify the hyperechoic cords of the brachial plexus and their corresponding positions relative to the artery, although these may not always be identifiable. Fortunately, visualization of the cords are not necessary for successful blockade.

The needle is inserted in plane from the cephalad end of the probe, with the insertion point just inferior to the clavicle (see Figure 32D–4). The needle is aimed toward the posterior aspect of the axillary artery and passes through the pectoralis major and minor muscles. If nerve stimulation is used concurrently (0.5–0.8 mA, 0.1 msec), the first motor response is often from the lateral cord (either elbow flexion or finger flexion). As the needle is advanced farther beneath the artery, a posterior cord motor response may appear (finger and wrist extension). After careful aspiration, 1–2 mL of local anesthetic is injected to confirm proper needle placement and spread. The injectate should spread cephalad and caudad to cover the lateral and medial cords, respectively (Figure 32D–6). When a single injection of local anesthetic does not appear to result in adequate spread, additional needle repositioning and injections around the axillary artery may be necessary.

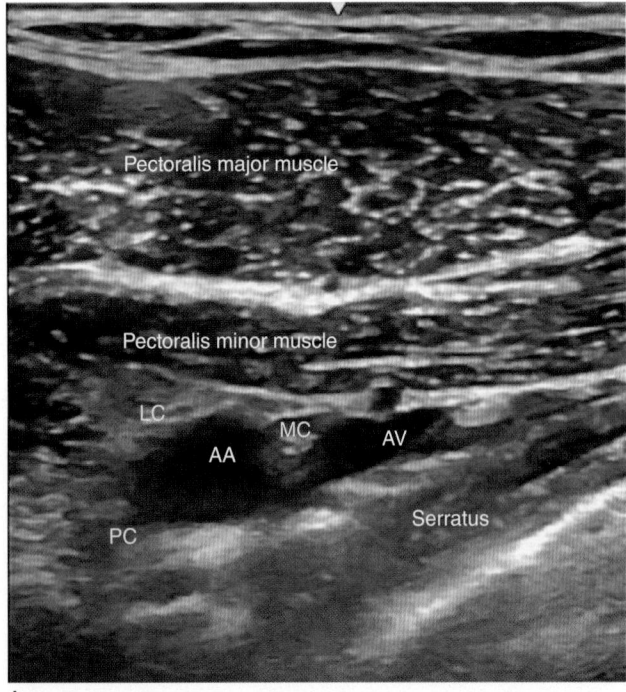

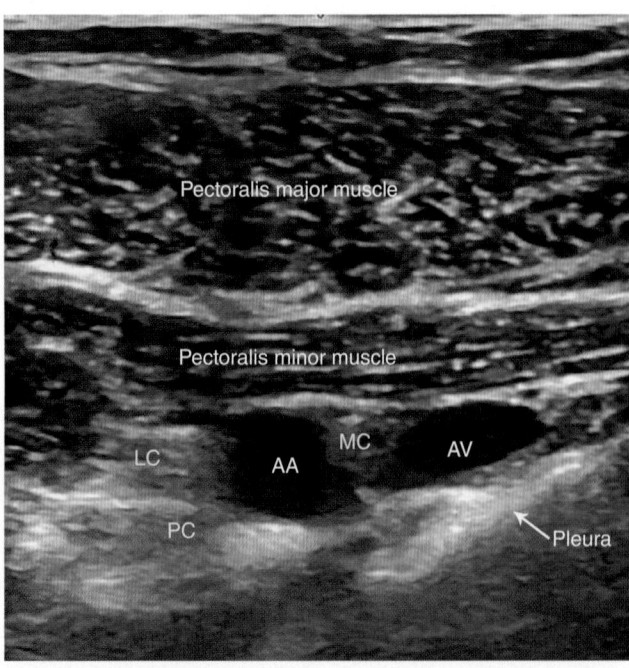

FIGURE 32D–5. Ultrasound-guided infraclavicular block: a medial-to-lateral probe movement is used to avoid the area where the needle advanced in the parasagittal plane could enter the pleura. (**A**) Parasagittal lateral view: the serratus anterior is seen between the neurovascular bundle and the pleura. (**B**) In this probe position, the pleura lies closer to the brachial plexus.

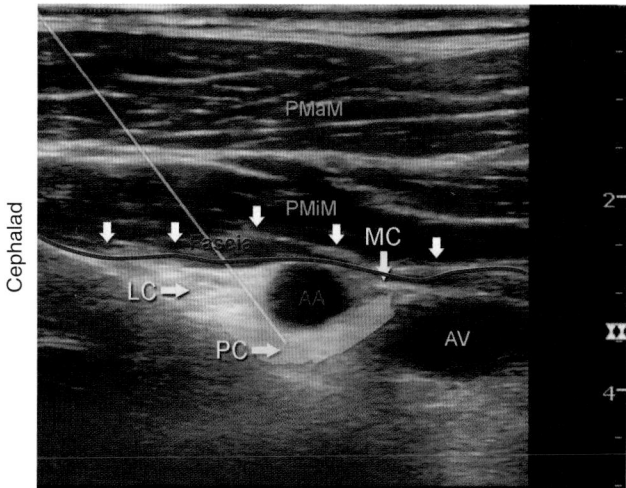

FIGURE 32D-6. Ultrasound image demonstrating an ideal needle path for the infraclavicular brachial plexus block. The blue-shaded area mimics an ideal spread of local anesthetic around the axillary artery (AA) and reaches all three cords of the brachial plexus (the lateral cord [LC], posterior cord [PC], and medial cord [MC]) below the fascia (red line) of the pectoralis minor muscle (PMiM), pectoralis major muscle (PMaM), and axillary vein (AV).

In an adult patient, 20–30 mL of local anesthetic is usually adequate for successful blockade. Although a single injection of such a large volume of local anesthetic often suffices,[3-5] it may be beneficial to inject two to three smaller aliquots at different locations to ensure local anesthetic spread in all planes containing the brachial plexus. There have been reports of septa hindering the diffusion of local anesthetic around the

artery,[6,7] and when that appears to be the case, repositioning the needle tip to achieve a U-shaped spread will ensure block success. Alternative approaches to block the brachial plexus distal to the clavicle have been described. A Single injection in between the cords at a more cephalad level (the coscoclavicular space), where the branchial plexus can be visualized lateral to the artery (Figure 32D-7).

TIPS

- An artifact posterior to the artery is often misinterpreted as the posterior cord. Figure 32D–6.
- A "heel-up" maneuver (rocking the probe toward the patient's head in a parasagittal plane, depressing the tissues caudad to the probe) makes it easier to change the needle's angle as needed (see Figure 32D–4).
- To decrease the risk of complications, adhere to the following guidelines:
  - Aspirate intermittently every 5 mL to decrease the risk of intravascular injection.
  - Do not inject if the injection resistance is high (> 15 psi).

CONTINUOUS ULTRASOUND-GUIDED INFRACLAVICULAR BLOCK

The goal of the continuous infraclavicular block is similar to the non–ultrasound-based techniques: to place the catheter within the vicinity of the cords of the brachial plexus beneath the pectoral muscles. The procedure consists of three phases: (1) needle placement; (2) catheter advancement; and (3) securing the catheter. For the first two phases of the procedure, ultrasound can be used to ensure accuracy in most patients. The needle is typically inserted in plane from the cephalad-to-caudad direction, similar to the single-injection technique (Figure 32D–8).

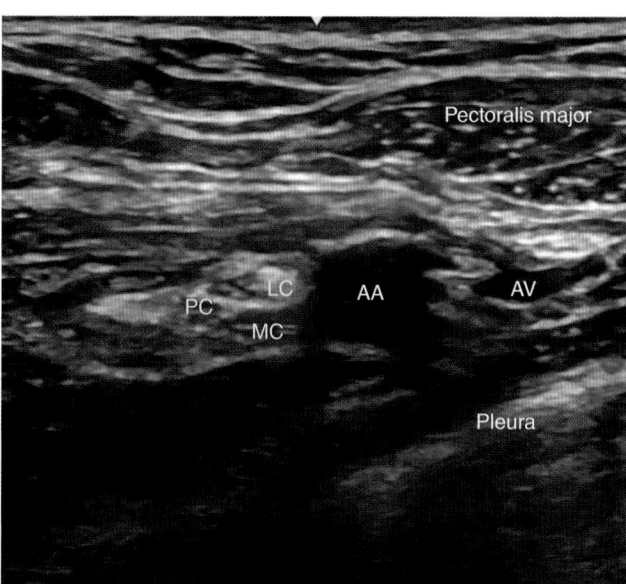

FIGURE 32D-7. Ultrasound view of the brachial plexus at the costoclavicular space. The lateral (LC), medial (MC) and posterior (PC) cords are clustered together lateral to the axillary artery lying more superficial. At this level, the pectoralis minor is not seen deep to the pectoralis mayor.

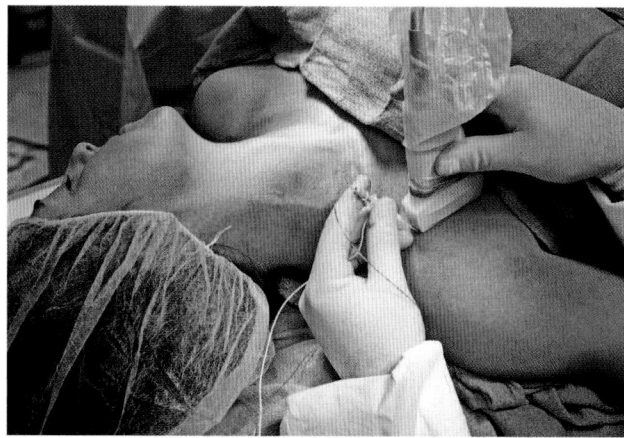

FIGURE 32D-8. The patient position, imaging, and needle placement for continuous infraclavicular brachial plexus block are similar to those for a single-injection technique. Once proper needle tip placement is determined by the injection of a small volume of local anesthetic, the catheter is inserted 2–4 cm beyond the needle tip.

As with the single-injection technique, the needle tip should be placed posterior to the axillary artery prior to injection and catheter advancement. Proper needle placement can also be confirmed by obtaining a motor response of the posterior cord (finger or wrist extension), at which point 1–2 mL of local anesthetic is injected. The rest of the technique, advancing and securing the catheter is the same as previously described (continuous block section, Chapter 32B).

A typical starting infusion regimen is 5 mL/h, followed by 8-mL patient-controlled boluses every hour. The larger bolus volume is necessary for the adequate spread of the injectate around the artery so that all cords of the brachial plexus are reached.

SUGGESTED READINGS

Aguirre J, Baulig B, Borgeat A: Does ultrasound-guided infraclavicular block meet users' expectations? Can J Anaesth 2010;57:176–177.

Akyildiz E, Gurkan Y, Caglayan C, Solak M, Toker K: Single vs. double stimulation during a lateral sagittal infraclavicular block. Acta Anaesthesiol Scand 2009;53:1262–1267.

Arcand G, Williams SR, Chouinard P, et al: Ultrasound-guided infraclavicular versus supraclavicular block. Anesth Analg 2005;101:886–890.

Benkhadra M, Faust A, Fournier R, Aho LS, Girard C, Feigl G: Possible explanation for failures during infraclavicular block: an anatomical observation on Thiel's embalmed cadavers. Br J Anaesth 2012;109: 128–129.

Berry JM: Selective local anesthetic placement using ultrasound guidance and neurostimulation for infraclavicular brachial plexus block. Anesth Analg 2010;110:1480–1485.

Bigeleisen P, Wilson M: A comparison of two techniques for ultrasound guided infraclavicular block. Br J Anaesth 2006;96:502–507.

Bigeleisen PE: Ultrasound-guided infraclavicular block in an anticoagulated and anesthetized patient. Anesth Analg 2007;104:1285–1287.

Bloc S, Garnier T, Komly B, et al: Spread of injectate associated with radial or median nerve-type motor response during infraclavicular brachial-plexus block: an ultrasound evaluation. Reg Anesth Pain Med 2007;32:130–135.

Bowens C Jr, Gupta RK, O'Byrne WT, et al: Selective local anesthetic placement using ultrasound guidance and neurostimulation for infraclavicular brachial plexus block. Anesth Analg 2010;110:1480–1485.

Brull R, Lupu M, Perlas A, Chan VW, McCartney CJ: Compared with dual nerve stimulation, ultrasound guidance shortens the time for infraclavicular block performance. Can J Anaesth 2009;56:812–818.

Brull R, McCartney CJ, Chan VW: A novel approach to infraclavicular brachial plexus block: the ultrasound experience. Anesth Analg 2004;99:950.

Chin KJ, Alakkad H, Adhikary SD, Singh M: Infraclavicular brachial plexus block for regional anaesthesia of the lower arm. Cochrane Database Syst Rev 2013;8:CD005487.

Chin KJ, Singh M, Velayutham V, Chee V: Infraclavicular brachial plexus block for regional anaesthesia of the lower arm. Anesth Analg 2010;111:1072.

Chin KJ, Singh M, Velayutham V, Chee V: Infraclavicular brachial plexus block for regional anaesthesia of the lower arm. Cochrane Database Syst Rev 2010;2:CD005487.

Dhir S, Ganapathy S: Comparative evaluation of ultrasound-guided continuous infraclavicular brachial plexus block with stimulating catheter and traditional technique: a prospective-randomized trial. Acta Anaesthesiol Scand 2008;52:1158–1166.

Dhir S, Ganapathy S: Use of ultrasound guidance and contrast enhancement: a study of continuous infraclavicular brachial plexus approach. Acta Anaesthesiol Scand 2008;52:338–342.

Dhir S, Singh S, Parkin J, Hannouche F, Richards RS: Multiple finger joint replacement and continuous physiotherapy using ultrasound guided, bilateral infraclavicular catheters for continuous bilateral upper extremity analgesia. Can J Anaesth 2008;55:880–881.

Dingemans E, Williams SR, Arcand G, et al: Neurostimulation in ultrasound-guided infraclavicular block: a prospective randomized trial. Anesth Analg 2007;104:1275–1280.

Dolan J: Fascial planes inhibiting the spread of local anesthetic during ultrasound-guided infraclavicular brachial plexus block are not limited to the posterior aspect of the axillary artery. Reg Anesth Pain Med 2009; 34:612–613.

Dolan J: Ultrasound-guided infraclavicular nerve block and the cephalic vein. Reg Anesth Pain Med 2009;34:528–529.

Eren G, Altun E, Pektas Y, et al: To what extent can local anesthetics be reduced for infraclavicular block with ultrasound guidance? Anaesthesist 2014;63: 760–765.

Fredrickson MJ, Patel A, Young S, Chinchanwala S: Speed of onset of "corner pocket supraclavicular" and infraclavicular ultrasound guided brachial plexus block: a randomised observer-blinded comparison. Anaesthesia 2009;64:738–744.

Gleeton D, Levesque S, Trépanier CA, Gariépy JL, Brassard J, Dion N: Symptomatic axillary hematoma after ultrasound-guided infraclavicular block in a patient with undiagnosed upper extremity mycotic aneurysms. Anesth Analg 2010;111:1069–1071.

Gurkan Y, Acar S, Solak M, Toker K: Comparison of nerve stimulation vs. ultrasound-guided lateral sagittal infraclavicular block. Acta Anaesthesiol Scand 2008;52:851–855.

Gurkan Y, Ozdamar D, Hosten T, Solak M, Toker K: Ultrasound guided lateral sagittal infraclavicular block for pectoral flap release. Agri 2009;21: 39–42.

Gurkan Y, Tekin M, Acar S, Solak M, Toker K: Is nerve stimulation needed during an ultrasound-guided lateral sagittal infraclavicular block? Acta Anaesthesiol Scand 2010;54:403–407.

Jiang XB, Zhu SZ, Jiang Y, Chen QH, Xu XZ: Optimal dose of local anesthetic mixture in ultrasound-guided infraclavicular brachial plexus block via coracoid approach: analysis of 160 cases [in Chinese]. Zhonghua Yi Xue Za Zhi 2009;89:449–452.

Kalagara HK, Uppal V, McKinlay S, Macfarlane AJ, Anderson K: Effect of body mass index on angle of needle insertion during ultrasound-guided lateral sagittal infraclavicular brachial plexus block. J Clin Anesth 2015; 27:375–379.

Karmakar MK, Sala-Blanch X, Songthamwat B, Tsui BC: Benefits of the costoclavicular space for ultrasound-guided infraclavicular brachial plexus block: description of a costoclavicular approach. Reg Anesth Pain Med 2015;40:287–288.

Koscielniak-Nielsen ZJ, Frederiksen BS, Rasmussen H, Hesselbjerg L: A comparison of ultrasound-guided supraclavicular and infraclavicular blocks for upper extremity surgery. Acta Anaesthesiol Scand 2009;53: 620–626.

Koscielniak-Nielsen ZJ, Rasmussen H, Hesselbjerg L: Pneumothorax after an ultrasound-guided lateral sagittal infraclavicular block. Acta Anaesthesiol Scand 2008;52:1176–1177.

Lecours M, Lévesque S, Dion N, Nadeau MJ, Dionne A, Turgeon AF: Complications of single-injection ultrasound-guided infraclavicular block: a cohort study. Can J Anaesth 2013;60:244–252.

Levesque S, Dion N, Desgagne MC: Endpoint for successful, ultrasound-guided infraclavicular brachial plexus block. Can J Anaesth 2008;55:308.

Marhofer P, Harrop-Griffiths W, Willschke H, Kirchmair L: Fifteen years of ultrasound guidance in regional anaesthesia: part 2—recent developments in block techniques. Br J Anaesth 2010;104:673–683.

Mariano ER, Loland VJ, Bellars RH, et al: Ultrasound guidance versus electrical stimulation for infraclavicular brachial plexus perineural catheter insertion. J Ultrasound Med 2009;28:1211–1218.

Martinez Navas A, De La Tabla Gonzalez RO: Ultrasound-guided technique allowed early detection of intravascular injection during an infraclavicular brachial plexus block. Acta Anaesthesiol Scand 2009;53:968–970.

Moayeri N, Renes S, van Geffen GJ, Groen GJ: Vertical infraclavicular brachial plexus block: needle redirection after elicitation of elbow flexion. Reg Anesth Pain Med 2009;34:236–241.

Morimoto M, Popovic J, Kim JT, Kiamzon H, Rosenberg AD: Case series: septa can influence local anesthetic spread during infraclavicular brachial plexus blocks. Can J Anaesth 2007;54:1006–1010.

Nadig M, Ekatodramis G, Borgeat A: Ultrasound-guided infraclavicular brachial plexus block. Br J Anaesth 2003;90:107–108.

Ootaki C, Hayashi H, Amano M: Ultrasound-guided infraclavicular brachial plexus block: an alternative technique to anatomical landmark-guided approaches. Reg Anesth Pain Med 2000;25:600–604.

Perlas A, Chan VW, Simons M: Brachial plexus examination and localization using ultrasound and electrical stimulation: a volunteer study. Anesthesiology 2003;99:429–435.

Ponde V, Shah D, Johari A: Confirmation of local anesthetic distribution by radio-opaque contrast spread after ultrasound guided infraclavicular catheters placed along the posterior cord in children: a prospective analysis. Paediatr Anaesth 2015;25:253–257.

Ponde VC, Diwan S: Does ultrasound guidance improve the success rate of infraclavicular brachial plexus block when compared with nerve stimulation in children with radial club hands? Anesth Analg 2009;108: 1967–1970.

Porter JM, McCartney CJ, Chan VW: Needle placement and injection posterior to the axillary artery may predict successful infraclavicular brachial plexus block: a report of three cases. Can J Anaesth 2005;52: 69–73.

Punj J, Joshi A, Darlong V, Pandey R: Ultrasound characteristics of spread during infraclavicular plexus block. Reg Anesth Pain Med 2009;34:73.

Renes S, Clark L, Gielen M, Spoormans H, Giele J, Wadhwa A: A simplified approach to vertical infraclavicular brachial plexus blockade using hand-held Doppler. Anesth Analg 2008;106:1012–1014.

Sahin L, Gul R, Mizrak A, et al: Ultrasound-guided infraclavicular brachial plexus block enhances postoperative blood flow in arteriovenous fistulas. J Vasc Surg 2011;54:749–753.

Sala-Blanch, Reina MA, Pangthipampai P, Karmakar MK. Anatomic Basis for Brachial Plexus Block at the Costoclavicular Space A Cadaver Anatomic Study. Reg Anesth Pain Med 2016;41:387–391.

Sandhu NS, Capan LM: Ultrasound-guided infraclavicular brachial plexus block. Br J Anaesth 2002;89:254–259.

Sandhu NS, Maharlouei B, Patel B, Erkulwater E, Medabalmi P: Simultaneous bilateral infraclavicular brachial plexus blocks with low-dose lidocaine using ultrasound guidance. Anesthesiology 2006;104:199–201.

Sandhu NS, Sidhu DS, Capan LM: The cost comparison of infraclavicular brachial plexus block by nerve stimulator and ultrasound guidance. Anesth Analg 2004;98:267–268.

Sauter AR, Dodgson MS, Stubhaug A, Halstensen AM, Klaastad O: Electrical nerve stimulation or ultrasound guidance for lateral sagittal infraclavicular blocks: a randomized, controlled, observer-blinded, comparative study. Anesth Analg 2008;106:1910–1915.

Sauter AR, Smith HJ, Stubhaug A, Dodgson MS, Klaastad O: Use of magnetic resonance imaging to define the anatomical location closest to all three cords of the infraclavicular brachial plexus. Anesth Analg 2006;103: 1574–1576.

Slater ME, Williams SR, Harris P, et al: Preliminary evaluation of infraclavicular catheters inserted using ultrasound guidance: through-the-catheter anesthesia is not inferior to through-the-needle blocks. Reg Anesth Pain Med 2007;32:296–302.

Taboada M, Rodriguez J, Amor M, et al: Is ultrasound guidance superior to conventional nerve stimulation for coracoid infraclavicular brachial plexus block? Reg Anesth Pain Med 2009;34:357–360.

Tedore TR, YaDeau JT, Maalouf DB, et al: Comparison of the transarterial axillary block and the ultrasound-guided infraclavicular block for upper extremity surgery: a prospective randomized trial. Reg Anesth Pain Med 2009;34:361–365.

Trabelsi W, Amor MB, Lebbi MA, Romdhani C, Dhahri S, Ferjani M: Ultrasound does not shorten the duration of procedure but provides a faster sensory and motor block onset in comparison to nerve stimulator in infraclavicular brachial plexus block. Korean J Anesthesiol 2013;64: 327–333.

Tran DQ, Bertini P, Zaouter C, Muñoz L, Finlayson RJ: A prospective, randomized comparison between single- and double-injection ultrasound-guided infraclavicular brachial plexus block. Reg Anesth Pain Med 2010; 35:16–21.

Tran DQ, Charghi R, Finlayson RJ: The "double bubble" sign for successful infraclavicular brachial plexus blockade. Anesth Analg 2006;103: 1048–1049.

Tran DQ, Clemente A, Tran DQ, Finlayson RJ: A comparison between ultrasound-guided infraclavicular block using the "double bubble" sign and neurostimulation-guided axillary block. Anesth Analg 2008;107: 1075–1078.

Tran DQ, Dugani S, Dyachenko A, Correa JA, Finlayson RJ: Minimum effective volume of lidocaine for ultrasound-guided infraclavicular block. Reg Anesth Pain Med 2011;36:190–194.

Tran DQ, Russo G, Muñoz L, Zaouter C, Finlayson RJ: A prospective, randomized comparison between ultrasound-guided supraclavicular, infraclavicular, and axillary brachial plexus blocks. Reg Anesth Pain Med 2009;34:366–371.

Yazer MS, Finlayson RJ, Tran DQ: A randomized comparison between infraclavicular block and targeted intracluster injection supraclavicular block. Reg Anesth Pain Med 2015;40:11–15.

REFERENCES

1. Ruiz A, Sala X, Bargallo X, Hurtado P, Arguis MJ, Carrera A: The influence of arm abduction on the anatomic relations of infraclavicular brachial plexus: an ultrasound study. Anesth Analg 2009;108: 364–366.

2. Auyong DB, Gonzales J, Benonis JG: The Houdini clavicle: arm abduction and needle insertion site adjustment improves needle visibility for the infraclavicular nerve block. Reg Anesth Pain Med 2010;35: 403–404.

3. Fredrickson MJ, Wolstencroft P, Kejriwal R, Yoon A, Boland MR, Chinchanwala S: Single versus triple injection ultrasound-guided infraclavicular block: confirmation of the effectiveness of the single injection technique. Anesth Analg 2010;111:1325–1327.

4. Tran DQ, Bertini P, Zaouter C, Muñoz L, Finlayson RJ: A prospective, randomized comparison between single- and double-injection ultrasound-guided infraclavicular brachial plexus block. Reg Anesth Pain Med 2010;35:16–21.

5. Desgagnés MC, Lévesque S, Dion N, et al: A comparison of a single or triple injection technique for ultrasound-guided infraclavicular block: a prospective randomized controlled study. Anesth Analg 2009;109: 668–672.

6. Dolan J: Fascial planes inhibiting the spread of local anesthetic during ultrasound-guided infraclavicular brachial plexus block are not limited to the posterior aspect of the axillary artery. Reg Anesth Pain Med 2009; 34:612–613.

7. Morimoto M, Popovic J, Kim JT, Kiamzon H, Rosenberg AD: Case series: septa can influence local anesthetic spread during infraclavicular brachial plexus blocks. Can J Anaesth 2007;54:1006–1010.

CHAPTER 32E

Ultrasound-Guided Axillary Brachial Plexus Block

Catherine Vandepitte, Ana M. Lopez, and Hassanin Jalil

AXILLARY BRACHIAL PLEXUS BLOCK AT A GLANCE

- Indications: elbow, forearm and hand surgery (Figure 32E–1)
- Transducer position: short axis to arm, just distal to the pectoralis major insertion
- Goal: local anesthetic spread around axillary artery
- Local anesthetic: 15–20 mL

GENERAL CONSIDERATIONS

The axillary brachial plexus block is relatively simple to perform and may be associated with a lower risk of complications compared with interscalene (eg, spinal cord or vertebral artery puncture) and supraclavicular brachial plexus blocks (eg, pneumothorax). In clinical scenarios in which access to the upper parts of the brachial plexus is difficult or impossible (eg, local infection, burns, indwelling venous catheters), the ability to anesthetize the plexus at a more distal level may be important. Although individual nerves can usually be identified this is not absolutely necessary because the deposition of local anesthetic around the axillary artery is sufficient for an effective block.

ULTRASOUND ANATOMY

The structures of interest are superficial (1–3 cm below the skin), and the axillary artery is readily identified within a centimeter of the skin surface on the medial aspect of the proximal arm (Figure 32E–2). The artery is accompanied by one or more axillary veins, often located medially to the artery. Importantly, excessive pressure with the transducer during imaging may compress the veins, rendering veins invisible and prone to puncture with the needle. Surrounding the axillary artery, three of the four principal branches of the brachial plexus can be seen: the median (superficial and lateral to the artery), the ulnar (superficial and medial to the artery), and the radial (posterior and lateral or medial to the artery) nerves (see Figure 32E–2). The nerves appear as round hyperechoic structures. Several authors have reported the anatomical variations of the nerves relative to the axillary artery;[1-4] Figure 32E–3 illustrates the most common patterns.

Three muscles surround the neurovascular bundle: the biceps (anterior and superficial), the wedge-shaped coracobrachialis (anterior and deep), and the conjoined tendon of the teres major and latissimus dorsi (medial and posterior). The musculocutaneous nerve is located in the fascial layers between the biceps and coracobrachialis muscles, though its location is variable and can be seen within either muscle. It is usually seen as a hypoechoic flattened oval structure with a bright hyperechoic rim. Moving the transducer proximally and distally along the long axis of the arm, the musculocutaneous nerve appears to move toward or away from the neurovascular bundle in the fascial plane between the two muscles. Variations are determined by the position of the musculocutaneous nerve relative to the median nerve and by the position of the ulnar nerve relative to the axillary vein.

DISTRIBUTION OF ANESTHESIA

The axillary brachial plexus block (including the musculocutaneous nerve) results in anesthesia of the upper limb from the mid-arm down to and including the hand. Importantly, the block lends its name from the approach and not from the

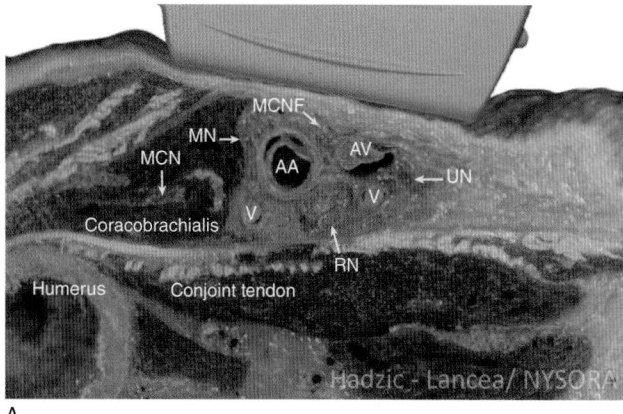

A

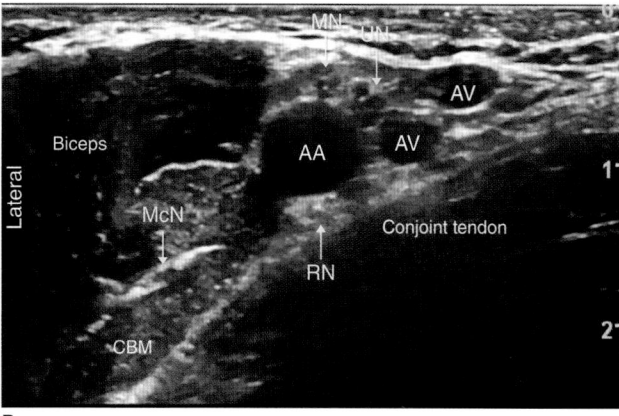

B

FIGURE 32E–2. (**A**) Cross-sectional anatomy of the axillary fossa and ultrasound image (**B**) of the terminal nerves of brachial plexus. The BP is seen scattered around the axillary artery and enclosed within the adipose tissue compartment containing the axillary artery (AA), and axillary veins (AV). MCN, musculocutaneous nerve. MN, median nerve; RN, radial nerve; UN, ulnar nerve; MACN, median antebrachial cutaneous nerve; CBM, corachobrachialis muscle.

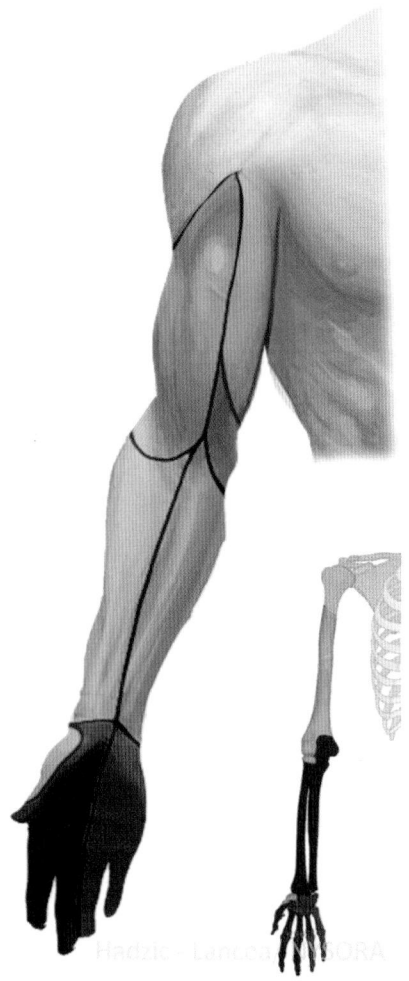

FIGURE 32E–1. Sensory distribution after axillary brachial plexus block.

axillary nerve, which itself is not blocked because it departs from the posterior cord more proximally in the axilla. Therefore, the skin over the deltoid muscle is not anesthetized. With nerve stimulator and landmark-based techniques, the blockade of the musculocutaneous nerve is often unreliable. However, the musculocutaneous nerve is readily visualized and reliably anesthetized by a separate injection using ultrasound guidance. When required, the medial skin of the upper arm (intercostobrachial nerve, T2) can be blocked by an additional subcutaneous injection just distal to the axilla.

EQUIPMENT

- Ultrasound machine with linear transducer (8–14 MHz), sterile sleeve, and gel
- Standard nerve block tray
- Syringes with local anesthetic (20 mL)
- 5-cm, 22-gauge, short-bevel, insulated stimulating needle
- Peripheral nerve stimulator
- Opening injection pressure monitoring system
- Sterile gloves

LANDMARKS AND PATIENT POSITIONING

Abduction of the arm to 90 degrees is necessary to allow for transducer placement and needle advancement, (Figure 32E–4). Care should be taken not to over-abduct the arm, as this may cause patient discomfort as well as traction on the brachial plexus, making it theoretically more vulnerable to injury by needle or injection.

The pectoralis major muscle is palpated as it inserts onto the humerus, and the transducer is placed on the skin immediately distal to that point, perpendicular to the axis of the arm. The starting point should have the transducer overlying both the biceps and triceps muscles (ie, on the medial aspect of the arm). Sliding the transducer proximally will bring the axillary artery, the conjoint tendon and the terminal branches of the brachial plexus into view, if not readily apparent.

GOAL

The goal is to deposit local anesthetic around the axillary artery. Typically, two or three injections are required. In addition,

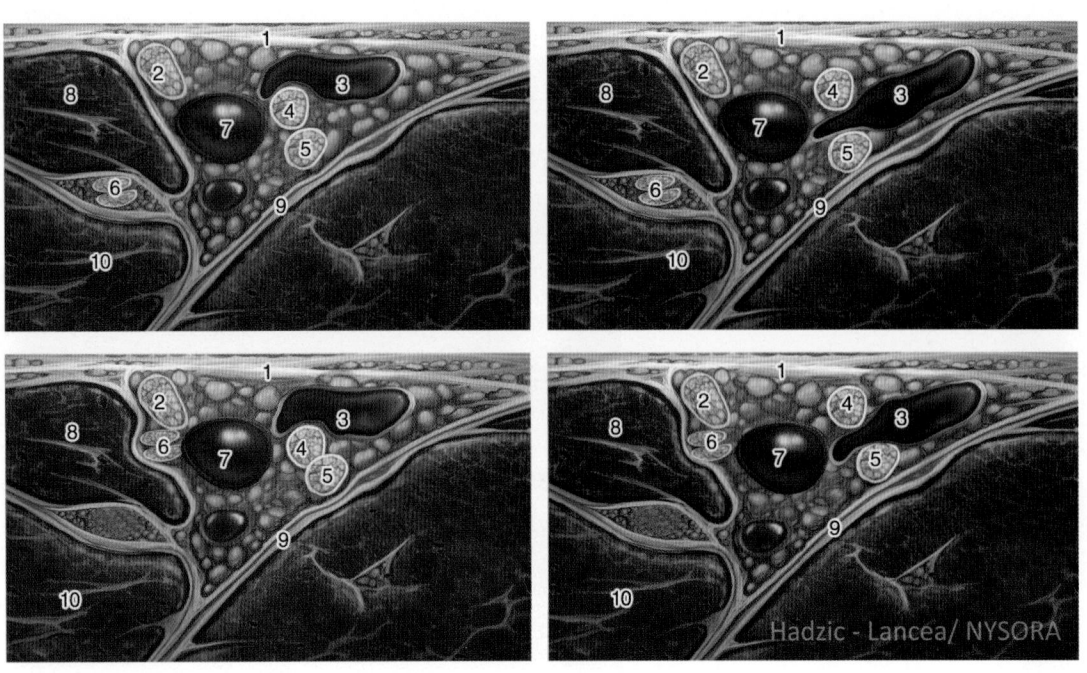

1 Brachial deep
   fascia
2 Median nerve
3 Axillary vein
4 Ulnar nerve
5 Radial nerve
6 Musculocutaneous
   nerve
7 Axillary artery
8 Biceps brachialis m.
9 Conjoint tendon
   (of teres major and
   lat. dorsi mm.)
10 Coracobrachialis m.

FIGURE 32E–3. Most common patterns of nerve location around the axillary artery in ultrasound-guided axillary brachial plexus block.[4]

an aliquot of local anesthetic should be injected around the musculocutaneous nerve.

TECHNIQUE

The skin is disinfected and the transducer is positioned in the short axis orientation to identify the axillary artery about 1–3 cm from the skin surface. Once the artery is identified, an attempt is made to identify the hyperechoic median, ulnar, and radial nerves (Figure 32E–5). However, these may not always be well visualized with ultrasound. Frequently present, an acoustic enhancement artifact deep to the artery is often misinterpreted as the radial nerve. Prescanning should also reveal the position of the musculocutaneous nerve, in the plane between the coracobrachialis and biceps muscles or within either of the muscles (a slight proximal-distal movement of the transducer is often required to bring this nerve into view) (Figure 32E–6). The needle is inserted in plane from the anterior aspect and directed toward the posterior aspect of the axillary artery (Figure 32E–7).

Because nerves and vessels are positioned closely together in the neurovascular bundle by adjacent musculature, advancement of the needle may require careful hydrodissection with a small amount of local anesthetic or other injectate. This technique involves the injection of 0.5–2 mL, indicating the plane in which the needle tip is located. The needle is then carefully advanced stepwise few millimeters at a time. The use of nerve stimulation is recommended to decrease the risk of needle-nerve injury during needle advancement.

Local anesthetic should be deposited posterior to the artery first, to avoid displacing the structures of interest deeper and obscuring the nerves, which may occur if injections for the median or ulnar nerves are carried out first. The posteriorly

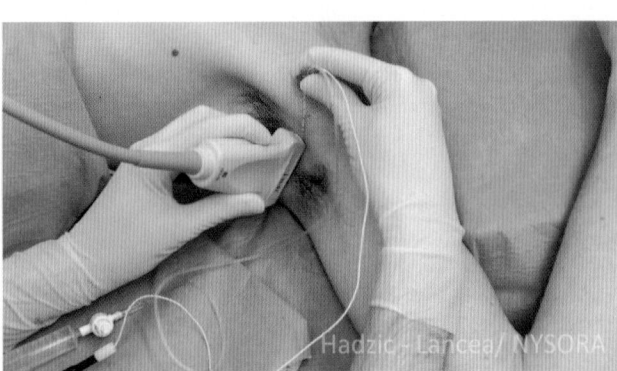

FIGURE 32E–4. Patient position and needle insertion for ultrasound-guided (in-plane) axillary brachial plexus block. All needle redirections are done through the same needle insertion site.

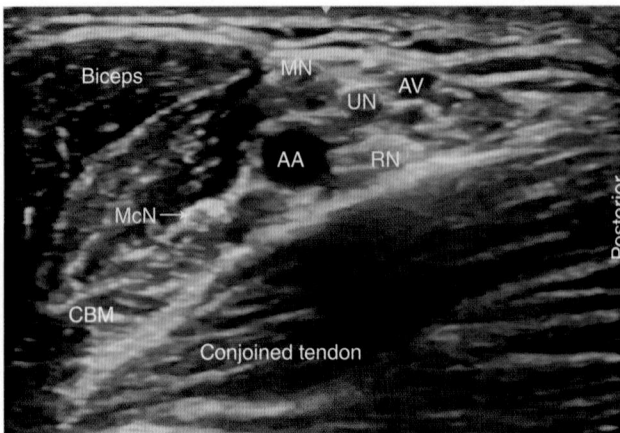

FIGURE 32E–5. The median (MN), ulnar (UN), and radial (RN) nerves are seen scattered around the axillary artery (AA). The musculocutaneous nerve (MCN) is seen between the biceps and coracobrachialis muscle (CBM), away from the rest of the brachial plexus. AV, axillary vein.

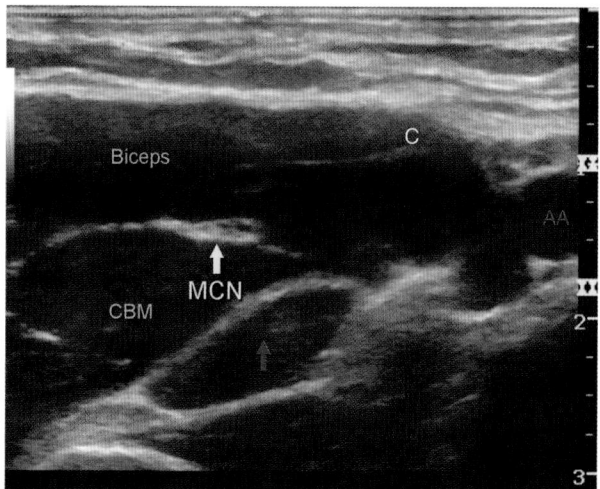

Musculocutaneous nerve at

FIGURE 32E–6. The musculocutaneous nerve (MCN) is located few cm away from the axillary artery (AA) between the biceps and the coracobrachialis muscle. The course of the MCN along the upper arm display frequent anatomic variations. Systematic scanning to identify the nerve and a separate injection of local anesthetic are usually required for a successful axillary brachial plexus block.

located radial nerve is often visualized more clearly once surrounded by local anesthetic. Once 5–7 mL has been administered, the needle is withdrawn almost to the level of the skin, redirected toward the median and ulnar nerves, and a further 7–10 mL is injected in these areas to complete the spread around the nerves. The described sequence of injection is demonstrated in Figure 32E–8.

An alternative, perivascular approach is to simply inject local anesthetic deep to the artery, at the 6 o'clock position, instead of targeting the three nerves individually. This technique may shorten the duration of the block procedure, but also delay

onset time, resulting in no difference in total time from skin puncture to onset of the surgical block.[5]

The last step in the procedure, the needle is withdrawn and redirected toward the musculocutaneous nerve. Once adjacent to the nerve (stimulation will result in elbow flexion), 5–7 mL of local anesthetic is deposited. Occasionally, the musculocutaneous nerve will lie in close proximity to the median nerve, rendering a separate injection unnecessary.

In an adult patient, 20 mL of local anesthetic is usually adequate for successful blockade, although successful blocks have been described with smaller volumes.[6] Adequate spread within the axillary brachial plexus sheath is necessary for success but infrequently seen with a single injection. This is accomplished with two to three redirections and injections of 5-7 mL are usually necessary for reliable blockade, as well as a separate injection to block the musculocutaneous nerve.

TIPS

- Frequent aspiration and slow administration of local anesthetic are critical for decreasing the risk of intravascular injection. Cases of systemic toxicity have been reported after apparently straightforward ultrasound-guided axillary brachial plexus blocks.
- If no spread is seen on the ultrasound image despite local anesthetic injection, the tip of the needle may be located in a vein.[7] If this occurs, injection should be halted immediately and the needle withdrawn slightly. Pressure on the transducer should be eased before reassessing the ultrasound image for the presence of vascular structures.
- Anatomic variations in the position of the musculocutaneous nerve have been described.[8] In 16% of cases, the musculocutaneous nerve splits off of the median nerve distally to the axilla. In this case, a separate injection is not needed to block the musculocutaneous nerve as it will be blocked by the local anesthetic injected around the median nerve.[9]

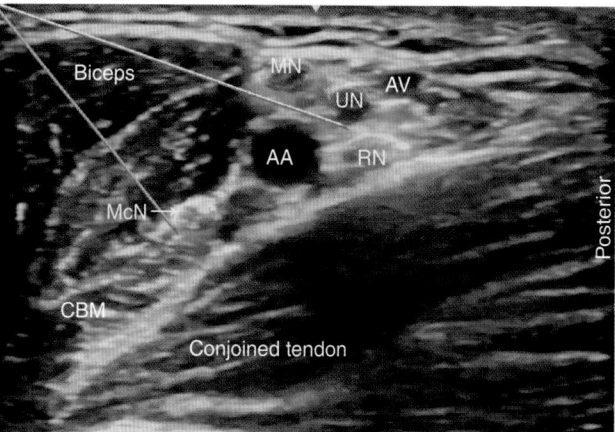

FIGURE 32E–7. Needle insertions for axillary brachial plexus block. Axillary block can be accomplished by two to four separate injections, depending on the disposition of the nerves around the axillary artery (AA) and the quality of the image. MCN, musculocutaneous nerve; MN, median nerve; RN, radial nerve; UN, ulnar nerve. AA, axilary vein, AV, axillary vein.

FIGURE 32E–8. This image demonstrates the ideal distribution pattern of local anesthetic. In this particular disposition of nerves, a single needle pass superficially to the artery allows for two injections: one for the median (MN) and a second one between the ulnar (UN) and radial (RN). The musculocutaneous (MCN) requires a separate injection.

CONTINUOUS ULTRASOUND-GUIDED AXILLARY BLOCK

The indwelling axillary catheter is a useful technique for analgesia and sympathetic block. The goal of the continuous axillary block is to place the catheter within the vicinity of the branches of the brachial plexus (ie, within the "sheath" of the brachial plexus). The procedure is similar to that previously described in Chapter 32B. The needle is typically inserted in plane from the anterior to posterior direction, just as in the single-injection technique).

After an initial injection of local anesthetic to confirm proper needle tip position posterior to the axillary artery, the catheter is inserted 3–5 cm beyond the needle tip. Injection is then repeated through the catheter to document adequate spread of local anesthetic, wrapping the axillary artery. Alternatively, the axillary artery can be visualized in the longitudinal view with the catheter being inserted in the longitudinal plane alongside the axillary artery. The longitudinal approach requires a significantly greater degree of ultrasonographic skill; no data suggesting that one approach is more effective than the other currently exist.

SUGGESTED READINGS

Aguirre J, Blumenthal S, Borgeat A: Ultrasound guidance and success rates of axillary brachial plexus block—I. Can J Anaesth 2007;54:583.

Alakkad H, Chin KJ: The importance of good needling technique in ultrasound-guided axillary block. Reg Anesth Pain Med 2013;38:166.

Aveline C: Ultrasound-guided axillary perivascular approach: efficacy and safety remain to be proved. Reg Anesth Pain Med 2013;38:74.

Baumgarten RK, Thompson GE: Is ultrasound necessary for routine axillary block? Reg Anesth Pain Med 2006;31:88–89.

Berthier F, Lepage D, Henry Y, Vuillier F, et al: Anatomical basis for ultrasound-guided regional anaesthesia at the junction of the axilla and the upper arm. Surg Radiol Anat 2010;32:299–304.

Bigeleisen PE: Nerve puncture and apparent intraneural injection during ultrasound-guided axillary block does not invariably result in neurologic injury. Anesthesiology 2006;105:779–783.

Bloc S, Mercadal L, Garnier T, Komly B, Leclerc P, Morel B, Ecoffey C, Dhonneur G. Comfort of the patient during axillary blocks placement: a randomized comparison of the neurostimulation and the ultrasound guidance techniques. Eur J Anaesthesiol. 2010 Jul;27(7):628-33. [PubMed: 20299995]

Bruhn J, Fitriyadi D, van Geffen GJ: A slide to the radial nerve during ultrasound-guided axillary block. Reg Anesth Pain Med 2009;34:623; author reply 623–624.

Campoy L, Bezuidenhout AJ, Gleed RD, et al: Ultrasound-guided approach for axillary brachial plexus, femoral nerve, and sciatic nerve blocks in dogs. Vet Anaesth Analg 2010;37:144–153.

Casati A, Danelli G, Baciarello M, et al: A prospective, randomized comparison between ultrasound and nerve stimulation guidance for multiple injection axillary brachial plexus block. Anesthesiology 2007;106:992–996.

Chan VW, Perlas A, McCartney CJ, Brull R, Xu D, Abbas S: Ultrasound guidance improves success rate of axillary brachial plexus block. Can J Anaesth 2007;54:176–182.

Chin KJ, Alakkad H, Cubillos JE: Single, double or multiple-injection techniques for non-ultrasound guided axillary brachial plexus block in adults undergoing surgery of the lower arm. Cochrane Database Syst Rev 2013;8:CD003842.

Cho S, Kim YJ, Baik HJ, Kim JH, Woo JH: Comparison of ultrasound-guided axillary brachial plexus block techniques: perineural injection versus single or double perivascular infiltration. Yonsei Med J 2015;56:838–844.

Cho S, Kim YJ, Kim JH, Baik HJ: Double-injection perivascular ultrasound-guided axillary brachial plexus block according to needle positioning: 12 versus 6 o'clock position of the axillary artery. Korean J Anesthesiol 2014;66:112–119.

Clendenen SR, Riutort K, Ladlie BL, Robards C, Franco CD, Greengrass RA: Real-time three-dimensional ultrasound-assisted axillary plexus block defines soft tissue planes. Anesth Analg 2009;108:1347–1350.

Dibiane C, Deruddre S, Zetlaoui PJ: A musculocutaneous nerve variation described during ultrasound-guided axillary nerve block. Reg Anesth Pain Med 2009;34:617–618.

Dolan J, McKinlay S: Early detection of intravascular injection during ultrasound-guided axillary brachial plexus block. Reg Anesth Pain Med 2009;34:182.

Dufour E, Laloe PA, Culty T, Fischler M: Ultrasound and neurostimulation-guided axillary brachial plexus block for resection of a hemodialysis fistula aneurysm. Anesth Analg 2009;108:1981–1983.

Errando CL, Pallardo MA, Herranz A, Peiro CM, de Andres JA: Bilateral axillary brachial plexus block guided by multiple nerve stimulation and ultrasound in a multiple trauma patient [in Spanish]. Rev Esp Anestesiol Reanim 2006;53:383–386.

Ferraro LH, Takeda A, dos Reis Falcão LF, Rezende AH, Sadatsune EJ, Tardelli MA: Determination of the minimum effective volume of 0.5% bupivacaine for ultrasound-guided axillary brachial plexus block. Braz J Anesthesiol 2014;64:49–53.

Forero CM, Gomez Lora CP, Bayegan D: Undetected intravascular injection during an ultrasound-guided axillary block. Can J Anaesth 2013;60:329–30.

Fregnani JH, Macéa MI, Pereira CS, Barros MD, Macéa JR: Absence of the musculocutaneous nerve: a rare anatomical variation with possible clinical-surgical implications. Sao Paulo Med J 2008;126:288–290.

Frkovic V, Ward C, Preckel B, et al: Influence of arm position on ultrasound visibility of the axillary brachial plexus. Eur J Anaesthesiol 2015;32:771–780.

Gelfand HJ, Ouanes JP, Lesley MR, et al: Analgesic efficacy of ultrasound-guided regional anesthesia: meta-analysis. J Clin Anesth 2011;232:90–96.

González AP, Bernucci F, Pham K, Correa JA, Finlayson RJ, Tran DQ: Minimum effective volume of lidocaine for double-injection ultrasound-guided axillary block. Reg Anesth Pain Med 2013;38:16–20.

Gray AT: The conjoint tendon of the latissimus dorsi and teres major: an important landmark for ultrasound-guided axillary block. Reg Anesth Pain Med 2009;34:179–180.

Gray AT, Schafhalter-Zoppoth I: "Bayonet artifact" during ultrasound-guided transarterial axillary block. Anesthesiology 2005;102:1291–1292.

Hadžić A, Dewaele S, Gandhi K, Santos A: Volume and dose of local anesthetic necessary to block the axillary brachial plexus using ultrasound guidance. Anesthesiology 2009;111:8–9.

Harper GK, Stafford MA, Hill DA: Minimum volume of local anaesthetic required to surround each of the constituent nerves of the axillary brachial plexus, using ultrasound guidance: a pilot study. Br J Anaesth 2010;104:633–636.

Imasogie N, Ganapathy S, Singh S, Armstrong K, Armstrong P: A prospective, randomized, double-blind comparison of ultrasound-guided axillary brachial plexus blocks using 2 versus 4 injections. Anesth Analg 2010;110:1222–1226.

Jung MJ, Byun HY, Lee CH, Moon SW, Oh MK, Shin H: Medial antebrachial cutaneous nerve injury after brachial plexus block: two case reports. Ann Rehabil Med 2013;37:913–918.

Kjelstrup T, Courivaud F, Klaastad Ø, Breivik H, Hol PK: High-resolution MRI demonstrates detailed anatomy of the axillary brachial plexus. A pilot study. Acta Anaesthesiol Scand 2012;56:914–919.

Kjelstrup T, Hol PK, Courivaud F, Smith HJ, Røkkum M, Klaastad Ø: MRI of axillary brachial plexus blocks: a randomised controlled study. Eur J Anaesthesiol 2014;31:611–619.

Kokkalis ZT, Mavrogenis AF, Saranteas T, Stavropoulos NA, Anagnostopoulou S: Ultrasound-guided anterior axilla musculocutaneous nerve block. Radiol Med 2014;119:135–141.

Liu FC, Liou JT, Tsai YF, et al: Efficacy of ultrasound-guided axillary brachial plexus block: a comparative study with nerve stimulator-guided method. Chang Gung Med J 2005;28:396–402.

Lo N, Brull R, Perlas A, et al: Evolution of ultrasound guided axillary brachial plexus blockade: retrospective analysis of 662 blocks. Can J Anaesth 2008;55:408–413.

López-Morales S, Moreno-Martín A, Leal del Ojo JD, Rodriguez-Huertas F: Bloqueo axilar ecoguiado frente a bloqueo infraclavicular ecoguiado para la cirugía de miembro superior [Ultrasound-guided axillary block versus ultrasound-guided infraclavicular block for upper extremity surgery]. Rev Esp Anestesiol Reanim 2013;60:313–319.

Luyet C, Constantinescu M, Waltenspül M, Luginbühl M, Vögelin E: Transition from nerve stimulator to sonographically guided axillary brachial plexus anesthesia in hand surgery: block quality and patient satisfaction during the transition period. J Ultrasound Med 2013;32: 779–786.

Luyet C, Schüpfer G, Wipfli M, Greif R, Luginbühl M, Eichenberger U: Different learning curves for axillary brachial plexus block: ultrasound guidance versus nerve stimulation. Anesthesiol Res Pract 2010; 2010:309462.

Mannion S, Capdevila X: Ultrasound guidance and success rates of axillary brachial plexus block—II. Can J Anaesth 2007;54:584.

Marhofer P, Eichenberger U, Stockli S, et al: Ultrasonographic guided axillary plexus blocks with low volumes of local anaesthetics: a crossover volunteer study. Anaesthesia 2010;65:266–271.

Morros C, Pérez-Cuenca MD, Sala-Blanch X, Cedó F: Bloqueo axilar del plexo braquial guiado por ecografía. Curva de aprendizaje y resultados [Ultrasound-guided axillary brachial plexus block: learning curve and results]. Rev Esp Anestesiol Reanim 2011;58:74–79.

Morros C, Perez-Cuenca MD, Sala-Blanch X, Cedo F: Contribution of ultrasound guidance to the performance of the axillary brachial plexus block with multiple nerve stimulation [in Spanish]. Rev Esp Anestesiol Reanim 2009;56:69–74.

O'Donnell BD, Iohom G. An estimation of the minimum effective anesthetic volume of 2% lidocaine in ultrasound-guided axillary brachial plexus block. Anesthesiology 2009;111:25–29.

O'Donnell BD, Ryan H, O'Sullivan O, Iohom G: Ultrasound-guided axillary brachial plexus block with 20 milliliters local anesthetic mixture versus general anesthesia for upper limb trauma surgery: an observer-blinded, prospective, randomized, controlled trial. Anesth Analg 2009;109: 279–283.

O'Sullivan O, Aboulafia A, Iohom G, O'Donnell BD, Shorten GD: Proactive error analysis of ultrasound-guided axillary brachial plexus block performance. Reg Anesth Pain Med 2011;36:502–507.

O'Sullivan O, Shorten GD, Aboulafia A: Determinants of learning ultrasound-guided axillary brachial plexus blockade. Clin Teach 2011;8:236–240.

Orebaugh SL, Williams BA, Vallejo M, Kentor ML: Adverse outcomes associated with stimulator-based peripheral nerve blocks with versus without ultrasound visualization. Reg Anesth Pain Med 2009;34:251–255.

Perlas A, Chan VW, Simons M: Brachial plexus examination and localization using ultrasound and electrical stimulation: a volunteer study. Anesthesiology 2003;99:429–435.

Perlas A, Niazi A, McCartney C, Chan V, Xu D, Abbas S: The sensitivity of motor response to nerve stimulation and paresthesia for nerve localization as evaluated by ultrasound. Reg Anesth Pain Med 2006;31:445–450.

Porter JM, McCartney CJ, Chan VW: Needle placement and injection posterior to the axillary artery may predict successful infraclavicular brachial plexus block: a report of three cases. Can J Anaesth 2005;52: 69–73.

Ranganath A, Srinivasan KK, Iohom G: Ultrasound guided axillary brachial plexus block. Med Ultrason 2014;16:246–251.

Russon K, Blanco R: Accidental intraneural injection into the musculocutaneous nerve visualized with ultrasound. Anesth Analg 2007;105:1504–1505.

Russon K, Pickworth T, Harrop-Griffiths W. Upper limb blocks. Anaesthesia 2010;65(Suppl 1):48–56.

Saranteas T, Anagnostopoulou S, Kostopanagiotou G: Ultrasound imaging in anaesthesia: which is the optimal anatomic point to block the radial nerve in the axilla? Anaesth Intensive Care 2009;37:328–329.

Satapathy AR, Coventry DM: Axillary brachial plexus block. Anesthesiol Res Pract 2011;2011:173796.

Schoenmakers KP, Wegener JT, Stienstra R: Effect of local anesthetic volume (15 vs 40 mL) on the duration of ultrasound-guided single shot axillary brachial plexus block: a prospective randomized, observer-blinded trial. Reg Anesth Pain Med 2012;37:242–247.

Schwemmer U, Schleppers A, Markus C, Kredel M, Kirschner S, Roewer N: Operative management in axillary brachial plexus blocks: comparison of ultrasound and nerve stimulation [in German]. Anaesthesist 2006;55: 451–456.

Sites BD, Beach ML, Spence BC, et al: Ultrasound guidance improves the success rate of a perivascular axillary plexus block. Acta Anaesthesiol Scand 2006;50:678–684.

Spence BC, Sites BD, Beach ML: Ultrasound-guided musculocutaneous nerve block: a description of a novel technique. Reg Anesth Pain Med 2005; 30:198–201.

Strub B, Sonderegger J, Von Campe A, Grünert J, Osterwalder JJ: What benefits does ultrasound-guided axillary block for brachial plexus anaesthesia offer over the conventional blind approach in hand surgery? J Hand Surg Eur Vol 2011;36:778–786.

Sultan SF, Iohom G, Saunders J, Shorten G: A clinical assessment tool for ultrasound-guided axillary brachial plexus block. Acta Anaesthesiol Scand 2012;56:616–623.

Takeda A, Ferraro LH, Rezende AH, Sadatsune EJ, Falcão LF, Tardelli MA: Minimum effective concentration of bupivacaine for axillary brachial plexus block guided by ultrasound. Braz J Anesthesiol 2015;65:163–169.

Tedore TR, YaDeau JT, Maalouf DB, et al: Comparison of the transarterial axillary block and the ultrasound-guided infraclavicular block for upper extremity surgery: a prospective randomized trial. Reg Anesth Pain Med 2009;34:361–365.

Tran DQ, Clemente A, Tran DQ, Finlayson RJ: A comparison between ultrasound-guided infraclavicular block using the "double bubble" sign and neurostimulation-guided axillary block. Anesth Analg 2008;107: 1075–1078.

Tran DQ, Pham K, Dugani S, Finlayson RJ: A prospective, randomized comparison between double-, triple-, and quadruple-injection ultrasound-guided axillary brachial plexus block. Reg Anesth Pain Med 2012;37: 248–253.

Tran DQ, Russo G, Muñoz L, Zaouter C, Finlayson RJ: A prospective, randomized comparison between ultrasound-guided supraclavicular, infraclavicular, and axillary brachial plexus blocks. Reg Anesth Pain Med 2009;34:366–371.

Veneziano GC, Rao VK, Orebaugh SL: Recognition of local anesthetic maldistribution in axillary brachial plexus block guided by ultrasound and nerve stimulation. J Clin Anesth 2012;24:141–144.

Wong DM, Gledhill S, Thomas R, Barrington MJ: Sonographic location of the radial nerve confirmed by nerve stimulation during axillary brachial plexus blockade. Reg Anesth Pain Med 2009;34:503–507.

Wong MH, George A, Varma M: Ultrasound-guided perivascular axillary brachial plexus block: not so simple. Reg Anesth Pain Med 2013;38:167.

Yang ZX, Pho RW, Kour AK, Pereira BP: The musculocutaneous nerve and its branches to the biceps and brachialis muscles. J Hand Surg Am 1995;20: 671–675.

Zetlaoui PJ, Labbe JP, Benhamou D: Ultrasound guidance for axillary plexus block does not prevent intravascular injection. Anesthesiology 2008;108:761.

REFERENCES

1. Conceição DB, Helayel PE, Carvalho FA, Wollmeister J, Oliveira Filho GR: Imagens ultra-sonográficas do plexo braquial na região axilar [Ultrasound images of the brachial plexus in the axillary region]. Rev Bras Anestesiol 2007;57:684–689.

2. Christophe JL, Berthier F, Boillot A, et al: Assessment of topographic brachial plexus nerves variations at the axilla using ultrasonography. Br J Anaesth 2009;103:606–612.

3. Ustuner E, Yılmaz A, Özgencil E, Okten F, Turhan SC: Ultrasound anatomy of the brachial plexus nerves in the neurovascular bundle at the axilla in patients undergoing upper-extremity block anesthesia. Skeletal Radiol 2013;42:707–713.

4. Silva MG, Sala-Blanch X, Marín R, Espinoza X, Arauz A, Morros C: Bloqueo axilar ecoguiado: variaciones anatómicas de la disposición de los 4 nervios terminales del plexo braquial en relación con la arteria humeral [Ultrasound-guided axillary block: anatomical variations of terminal branches of the brachial plexus in relation to the brachial artery]. Rev Esp Anestesiol Reanim 2014;61:15–20.

5. Bernucci F, Gonzalez AP, Finlayson RJ, Tran DQ: A prospective, randomized comparison between perivascular and perineural ultrasound-guided axillary brachial plexus block. Reg Anesth Pain Med 2012;37: 473–477.

6. O'Donnell B, Riordan J, Ahmad I, Iohom G: Brief reports: a clinical evaluation of block characteristics using one milliliter 2% lidocaine in ultrasound-guided axillary brachial plexus block. Anesth Analg 2010;111: 808–810.

7. Robards C, Clendenen S, Greengrass R: Intravascular injection during ultrasound-guided axillary block: negative aspiration can be misleading. Anesth Analg 2008;107:1754–1755.

8. Orebaugh SL, Pennington S: Variant location of the musculocutaneous nerve during axillary nerve block. J Clin Anesth 2006;18:541–544.

9. Remerand F, Laulan J, Couvret C, et al: Is the musculocutaneous nerve really in the coracobrachialis muscle when performing an axillary block? An ultrasound study. Anesth Analg 2010;110:1729–1734.

Ultrasound-Guided Blocks at the Elbow

Jui-An Lin, Thomas F. Bendtsen, Ana M. Lopez, and Hassanin Jalil

FOREARM BLOCKS AT A GLANCE

- Indications: hand and wrist surgery (Figure 32F-1)
- Transducer position: transverse on the elbow
- Goal: injection of local anesthetic within the vicinity of individual nerves (radial, median, and ulnar)
- Local anesthetic: 4–5 mL per nerve

GENERAL CONSIDERATIONS

Ultrasound imaging of individual nerves in the distal upper limb allows for reliable nerve blockade. The two main indications for a forearm block are a standalone technique for hand and/or wrist surgery and as a means of rescuing or supplementing an incomplete or failed proximal brachial plexus block. Advantages of rescue block are the reduction of the risk of vascular puncture and in the overall volume of local anesthetic used. There are a variety of locations where a practitioner could approach each of these nerves, most of which are similar in efficacy. In this chapter, we present the approach for each nerve at the level of the elbow.

Ultrasonographic assessment shows that a median nerve block using nerve stimulation alone is commonly associated with intraneural injection.[1]

Some authors have suggested additional indications for forearm blocks, in combination with a proximal brachial plexus block. Combining proximal and distal blocks allows for a decrease in onset time and improved block consistency.[2] It is possible to use these blocks in the setting of wrist or hand surgery involving the bone to provide long-lasting analgesia without blocking the whole limb for many hours; this is done by combining a short-acting brachial plexus block with distal blocks around the elbow, according to the surgical procedure.[3] If distal blocks are to be performed after a proximal brachial plexus block, it is of paramount importance to clearly visualize the needle tip at all times in order to avoid intraneural injection.

ULTRASOUND ANATOMY

The Radial Nerve

The radial nerve is best visualized above the lateral aspect of the elbow, lying in the interfascial plane between the brachioradialis and the brachialis muscles (Figure 32F–2). The transducer is placed transversely on the anterolateral aspect of the distal arm, 3–4 cm above the elbow crease. The nerve appears as a hyperechoic, triangular or oval structure with the characteristic honeycomb appearance of a distal peripheral nerve. The nerve divides just distal to the elbow crease into the superficial (sensory) and deep (motor) branches. These smaller divisions of the radial nerve are more challenging to identify in the forearm; therefore, a single injection above the elbow is favored because it ensures blockade of both. The transducer can be slid up and down the arm to better visualize the nerve and the musculature surrounding it. As the transducer is moved proximally, the nerve will be seen to travel posteriorly and closer to the humerus, to lie deep to the triceps muscle in the spiral groove (Figure 32F–3).

The Median Nerve

The median nerve is imaged at the level of the elbow crease, as it is located superficially. The transducer is placed just above the crease and adjusted to obtain a clear view of the brachial artery. The median nerve lies on the medial side in close contact to the artery as a hyperechoic oval shaped structure of about the same size of the artery (Figure 32F-4). Scanning proximally, both the nerve and the artery can be easily followed up to the axilla as they course together, although changing the relative position to one another. Scanning distally to the elbow crease, the median

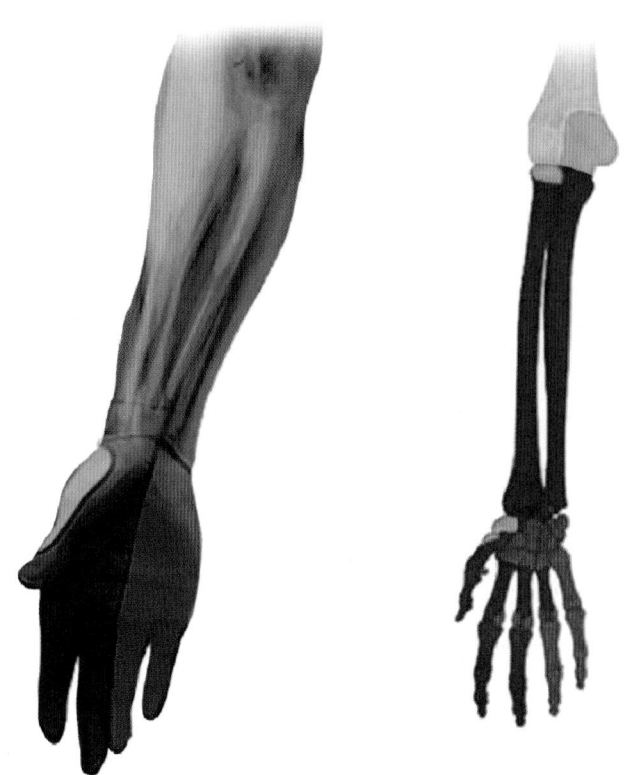

FIGURE 32F–1. Expected sensory distribution of the radial (blue), median (dark blue) and ulnar nerve blocks (red) proximal to the elbow.

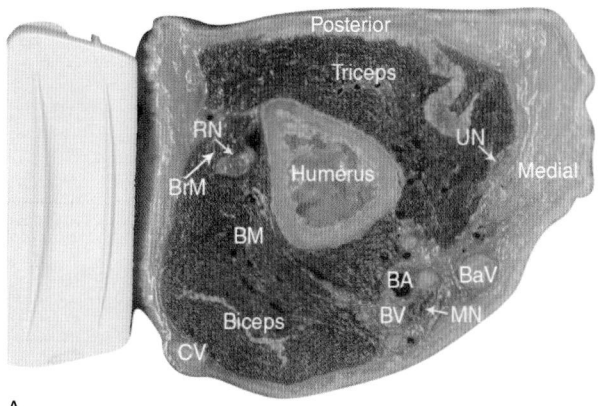

A

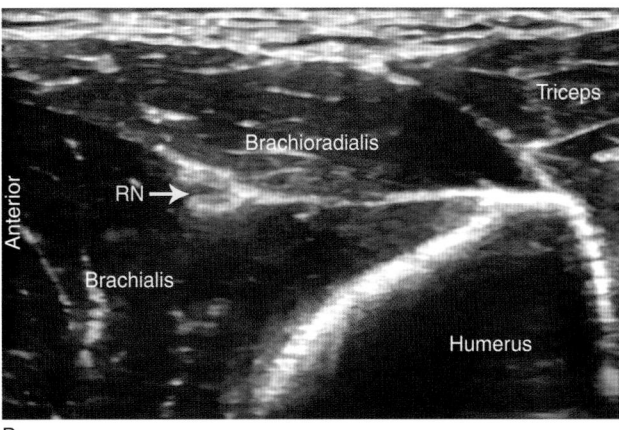

B

FIGURE 32F–2. (A) Radial nerve (RN) anatomy at the distal third of the humerus. BrM, brachioradialis muscle; BM, brachialis muscle; BA, brachial artery; BV, brachial vein, BaV, basilic vein, CV, cephalic vein; UN, ulnar nerve; MN, median nerve. **(B)** Sonoanatomy of the radial nerve at the distal arm. The RN is located between the brachioradialis and the brachialis muscles.

nerve separates from the artery and lies deep to the pronator teres muscle and the flexor digitorum superficialis as it reaches the midforearm.

The Ulnar Nerve

The ulnar nerve is identified at the postero medial aspect of the elbow, few centimeters proximally to the crease, as a hyperechoic oval "honeycomb" structure immediately underneath the brachial fascia and superficial to the triceps muscle (Figure 32F-5). The ulnar nerve can be traced distally toward the ulnar notch, where it appears as a round hypoechoic structure diving into the bony ulnar sulcus before entering the forearm underneath the flexor carpi ulnaris muscle. Sliding the transducer proximally, the nerve can be easily traced back to the axilla along the medial aspect of the arm.

DISTRIBUTION OF ANESTHESIA

Anesthetizing the radial, median, and/or ulnar nerves provides sensory anesthesia and analgesia to the respective territories of the hand, forearm, and wrist. Note that the lateral cutaneous nerve of the forearm (a branch of the musculocutaneous nerve) supplies the lateral aspect of the forearm, and it may need to be blocked separately by a subcutaneous wheal distal to the elbow if lateral wrist surgery is planned. The same applies for the median cutaneous nerve of the forearm (Figure 32E-1). The use of a tourniquet, either on the arm or forearm, usually requires sedation and/or additional analgesia. (For a more

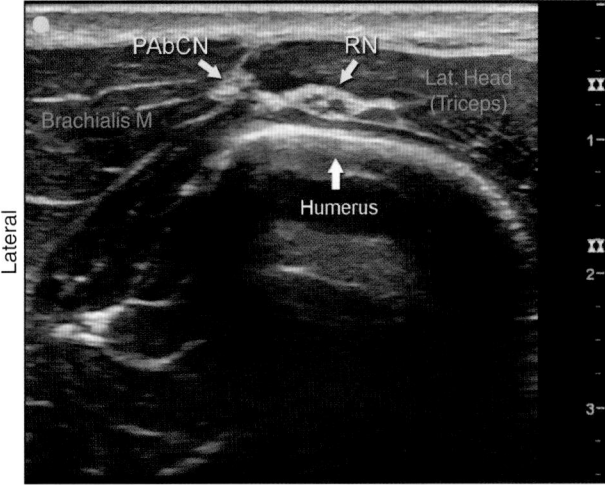

Radial Nerve - Midhumerus

FIGURE 32F–3. Sonoanatomy of the radial nerve (RN) in the spiral groove of the humerus. PAbCN, posterior antebrachial cutaneous nerve.

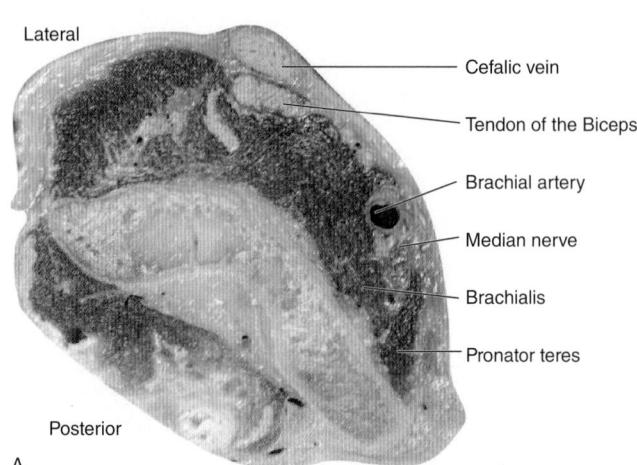

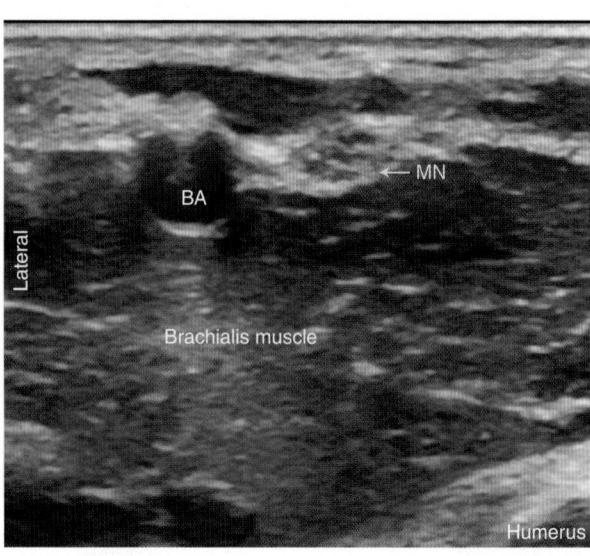

FIGURE 32F–4. (**A**) Anatomy section of the distal arm at the level of the elbow. (**B**) Sonoanatomy of the median nerve proximally to the elbow crease.

comprehensive review of the innervation of the hand, see Chapter 3.)

EQUIPMENT

The equipment recommended for a forearm block includes the following:

- Ultrasound machine with linear transducer (8–14 MHz), sterile sleeve, and gel
- Standard nerve block tray
- Three 5 mL syringes containing local anesthetic
- A 2-in, 22- to 25-gauge, short-bevel, insulated stimulating needle (optional)

- Peripheral nerve stimulator (optional)
- Sterile gloves
- Pressure monitoring

Clinical Pearl

- Because these are superficial blocks of the distal peripheral nerves, some practitioners choose to use a small-gauge (eg, 25-gauge) needle. When using a small-gauge needle, however, meticulous attention should be paid in order to avoid an intraneural injection, which is more likely with a smaller-diameter and sharp-tip design.

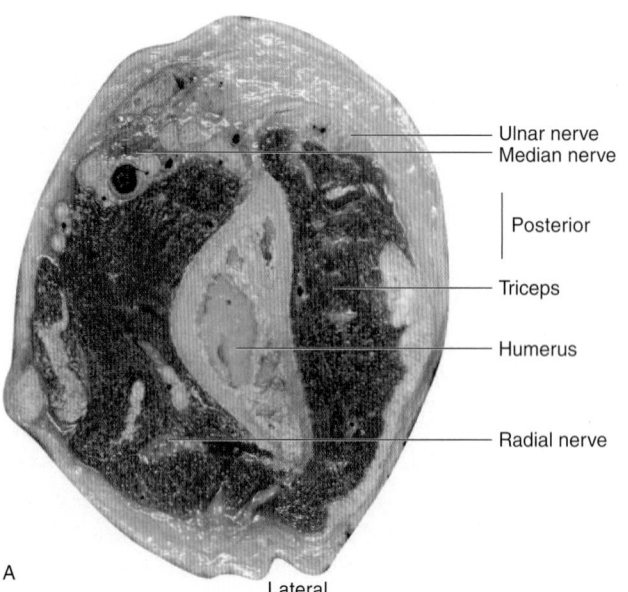

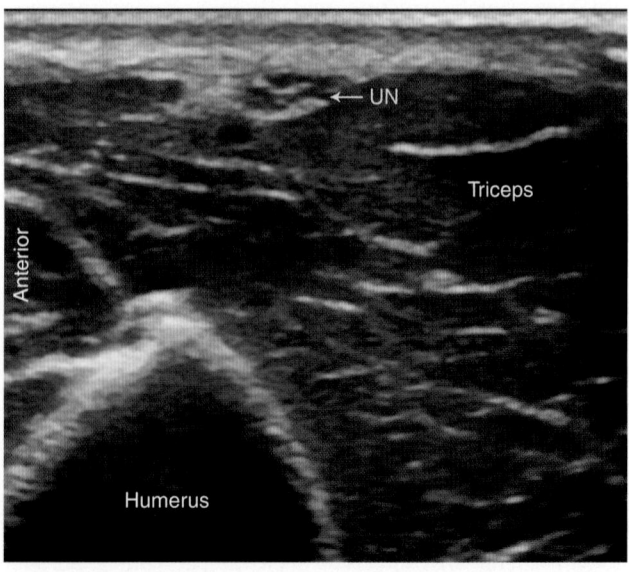

FIGURE 32F–5. (**A**) Anatomy section of the distal arm at the level of the elbow. (**B**) Sonoanatomy of the ulnar nerve proximally to the elbow crease.

LANDMARKS AND PATIENT POSITIONING

Typically, the block is performed with the patient in the supine position. For the radial nerve block, the arm could also be flexed at the elbow, and the hand is placed on the patient's abdomen (see Figure 32F–6a). This position allows for the most practical application of the transducer. The median and ulnar nerves are blocked with the arm abducted. (see Figures 32F-7a and 32F-8a).

GOAL

The goal of a forearm block is to place the needle tip adjacent to the nerve(s) of choice and to deposit 4–5 mL of local anesthetic within the fascial sheath enclosing the nerve. It is unnecessary to completely surround the entire nerve in a circumferencial pattern, although this can enhance the speed of block onset. As with all peripheral blocks, it is imperative to avoid high opening injection pressure in order to decrease the risk of intrafascicular injection.

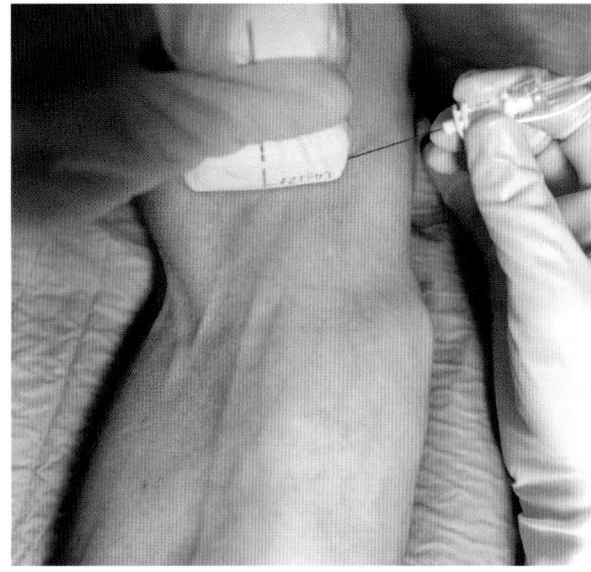

A

B

FIGURE 32F–7. (**A**) Position of the arm, probe and needle for median nerve block proximal to the elbow. (**B**) Distribution of local anesthetic (blue-shaded area) for MN block. BA, brachial artery.

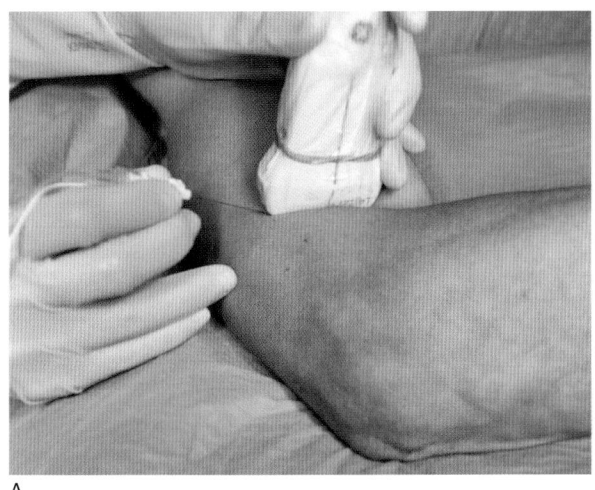

A

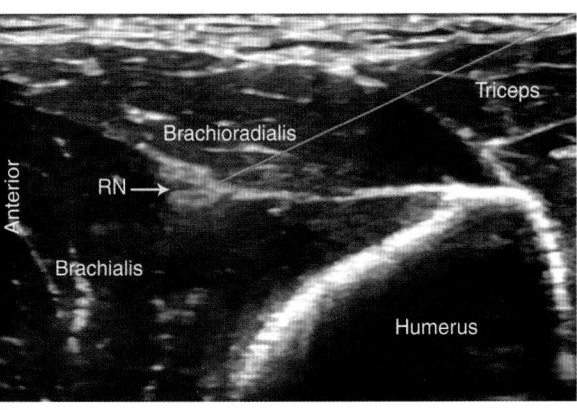

B

FIGURE 32F–6. (**A**) Position of the arm, probe and needle for radial nerve block. (**B**) Distribution of local anesthetic (blue-shaded area) for RN block above the elbow.

TECHNIQUE

The Radial Nerve

The skin is disinfected and the transducer positioned so as to identify the radial nerve. The needle is inserted in plane, with the goal of traversing the brachioradialis muscle and placing the tip next to the radial nerve (Figure 33F–6a). If nerve stimulation is used, a wrist or finger extension response should be elicited when the needle is within proximity of the nerve. After negative aspiration, 4–5 mL of local anesthetic is injected (Figure 32F–6b). If the spread is inadequate, slight adjustments can be made and a further 2–3 mL of local anesthetic administered.

It is also possible to block the branches of the radial nerve in the forearm. Anterior to the elbow joint, the radial nerve can be visualized between the extensor carpi radialis muscles (longus and brevis) and brachioradialis. The superficial branch can then be seen clearly at the proximal forearm covered by the brachioradialis. The deep branch is more difficult to image, as it emerges at the level of the radial neck and passes into the posterior compartment by passing between the two heads of the supinator muscle.[4]

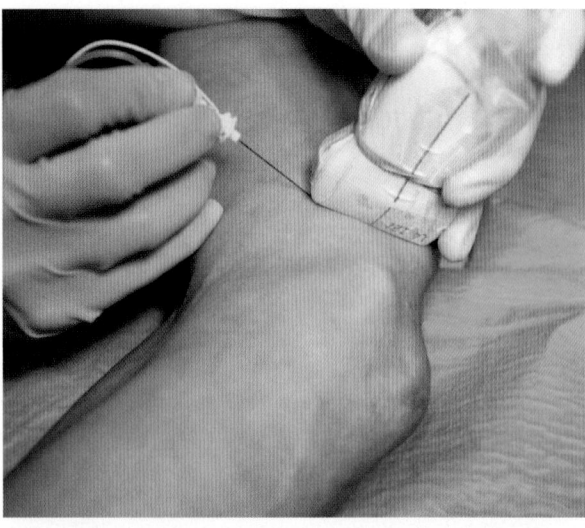

A

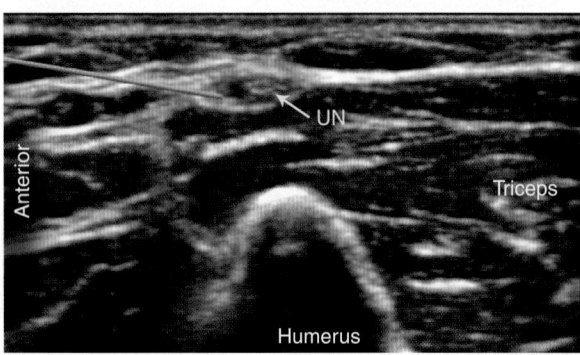

B

FIGURE 32F–8. (**A**) Position of the arm, probe and needle for ulnar nerve block proximal to the elbow. (**B**) Distribution of local anesthetic (blue-shaded area) for UN block.

The Median Nerve

With the arm abducted and the palm facing up, the skin of the anterior and medial side of the elbow is disinfected and the transducer positioned transversely on the antecubital fossa. The median nerve should be identified on the medial side of the artery. If it is not immediately visualized, the transducer should be positioned slightly more medially and the brachial artery identified using color Doppler ultrasound. The needle is inserted in plane from either side of the transducer, although a medial to lateral approach is usually more convenient to avoid the artery that lies lateral to the nerve. (Figure 32F–7a). After negative aspiration, 4–5 mL of local anesthetic is injected (Figure 32F–7b). If the spread is inadequate, slight adjustments can be made and a further 2–3 mL of local anesthetic administered.

The Ulnar Nerve

The transducer is then positioned more medially until the ulnar nerve is identified. The needle is inserted in plane from either side of the transducer (the anterior to posterior side is often more ergonomic) (Figure 32F–8a). After negative aspiration, 4–5 mL of local anesthetic is injected (Figure 32F–8b). If the spread of local anesthetic is inadequate, slight adjustments can be made and a further 2–3 mL administered.

TIPS

- When in doubt, nerve stimulation (0.5–1.0 mA) can be used to confirm localization of the correct nerve.
- The out-of-plane approach can also be used for all three blocks.

SUGGESTED READINGS

Eichenberger U, Stockli S, Marhofer P, et al: Minimal local anesthetic volume for peripheral nerve block: a new ultrasound-guided, nerve dimension-based method. Reg Anesth Pain Med 2009;34:242–246.

Gray AT, Schafhalter-Zoppoth I: Ultrasound guidance for ulnar nerve block in the forearm. Reg Anesth Pain Med 2003;28:335–339.

Lurf M, Leixnering M: Sensory block without a motor block: ultrasound-guided placement if pain catheters in forearm. Acta Anaestbesiol Scand 2010;54:257–258.

McCartney CJ, Xu D, Constantinescu C, Abbas S, Chan VW: Ultrasound examination of peripheral nerves in the forearm. Reg Anesth Pain Med 2007;32:434–439.

Schafhalter-Zoppoth I, Gray AT: The musculocutaneous nerve: ultrasound appearance for peripheral nerve block. Reg Anesth Pain Med 2005;30: 385–390.

Spence BC, Sites BD, Beach ML: Ultrasound-guided musculocutaneous nerve block: a description of a novel technique. Reg Anesth Pain Med 2005;30: 198–201.

REFERENCES

1. Dufour E, Cymerman A, Nourry G, et al: An ultrasonographic assessment of nerve stimulation-guided median nerve block at the elbow: a local anesthetic spread, nerve size, and clinical efficacy study. Anesth Analg 2010;111:561–567.

2. Fredrickson MJ, Ting FS, Chinchanwala S, Boland MR: Concomitant infraclavicular plus distal median, radial, and ulnar nerve blockade accelerates upper extremity anaesthesia and improves block consistency compared with infraclavicular block alone. Br J Anaesth 2011;107: 236–242.

3. Dufeu N, Marchand-Maillet F, Atchabahian A, et al: Efficacy and safety of ultrasound-guided distal blocks for analgesia without motor blockade after ambulatory hand surgery. J Hand Surg Am 2014;39:737–743.

4. Anagnostopoulou S, Saranteas T, Chantzi C, Dimitriou V, Karabinis A, Kostopanagiotou G: Ultrasound identification of the radial nerve and its divisions. Is rescue nerve block at or below the elbow possible? Anaesth Intensive Care 2008;36:457–459.

CHAPTER 32G

Ultrasound-Guided Wrist Block

Ine Leunen, Sofie Louage, Hassanin Jalil, and Xavier Sala-Blanch

WRIST BLOCK AT A GLANCE

- Indications: hand and finger surgery
- Transducer position: transverse at wrist crease or distal third of the forearm (Figure 32G–1)
- Goal: local anesthetic injection next to the median and ulnar nerves and the sensory branch of the radial nerve
- Local anesthetic: 10–15 mL (total volume)

GENERAL CONSIDERATIONS

The wrist block is an effective method to provide anesthesia of the hand and fingers without the arm immobility that occurs with more proximal brachial plexus blocks. Traditional wrist block technique involves advancing needles using surface landmarks toward the three nerves that supply the hand: the median, ulnar, and radial nerves. Since the nerves are located relatively close to the surface, this is a technically easy block to perform, but knowledge of the anatomy of the soft tissues of the wrist is essential for successful blockade with minimum patient discomfort. In addition to providing anesthesia and analgesia, wrist blocks using botulinum toxin to treat hyperhidrosis have been described.[1]

ULTRASOUND ANATOMY

Three individual nerves are involved in a wrist block: the median, ulnar, and radial nerves.

The Median Nerve

The median nerve crosses the elbow medial to the brachial artery and courses toward the wrist deep to the flexor digitorum superficialis in the center of the forearm. As the muscles taper toward tendons near the wrist, the nerve assumes an increasingly superficial position until it is located beneath the flexor retinaculum in the carpal tunnel with the tendons of the flexor digitorum profundus, flexor digitorum superficialis, and flexor pollicis longus. A linear transducer placed transversely at the level of the wrist crease will reveal a cluster of oval hyperechoic structures, one of which is the median nerve. At this location, it is easy to confuse the tendons for the nerve and vice versa; for this reason, it is recommended to slide the transducer 5–10 cm proximally the volar side of the forearm, to confirm the location of the nerve. The tendons will have disappeared on the image, leaving just muscle and the solitary median nerve (Figures 32G-2 and 32G-3), which then can be carefully traced back to the wrist, if desired. In many instances, however, it is much simpler to perform a median nerve block at the midforearm, where the nerve is easier to recognize.

Clinical Pearl

- The median nerve exhibits pronounced anisotropy. Tilting the transducer slightly will make the nerve appear alternately brighter (more contrast) or darker (less contrast) with respect to the background.

The Ulnar Nerve

The ulnar nerve is located medially (ulnar side) to the ulnar artery from the level of the midforearm to the wrist; this provides a useful landmark. A linear transducer placed at the level of the wrist crease will show the hyperechoic anterior surface of the ulna with shadowing behind; just lateral to the bone and very superficial will be the triangular or oval hyperechoic ulnar nerve, with the pulsating ulnar artery immediately next to it

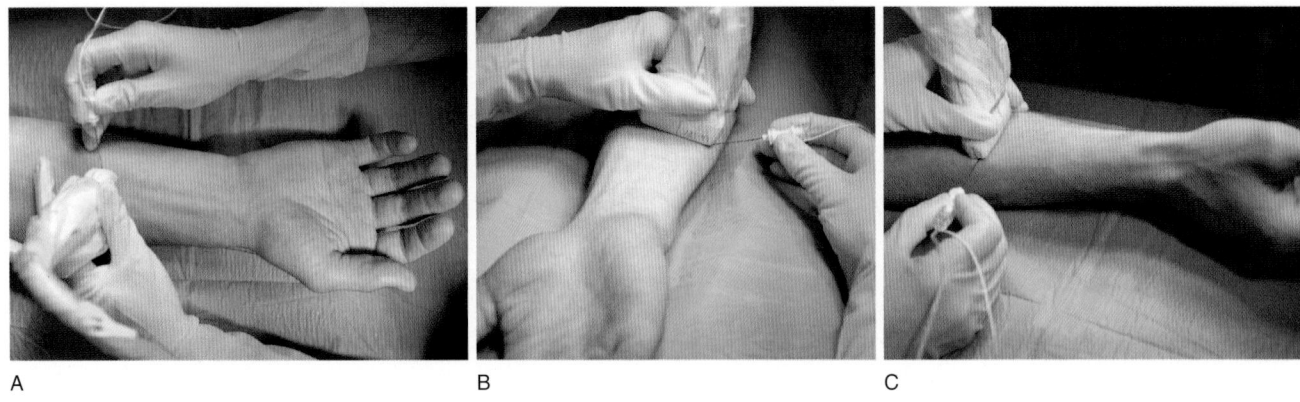

FIGURE 32G–1. Ultrasound-guided wrist block. Transducer and needle positions for (**A**) median nerve block; (**B**) ulnar nerve block; (**C**) radial nerve block.

(Figures 32G–4 and 32G–5). At this location, the tendon of the flexor carpis ulnaris muscle can be seen superficial to the ulnar nerve. Scanning proximally, these two structures can be easily differentiated. Sliding the transducer up and down the forearm helps verify that the structure is the ulnar nerve by following the course of the ulnar artery and looking for the nerve on its ulnar side.

The Radial Nerve

The superficial branch of the radial nerve divides into terminal branches at the level of the wrist; for this reason, ultrasonography is not very useful for block placement guidance at the level of the wrist. A subcutaneous field block around the area of the styloid process of the radius remains an easy method to perform an effective radial nerve block at the level of the wrist. However, ultrasonography can be used at the level of the elbow or in the midforearm. At this level, the nerve is identified as a thin hyperechoic structure lateral to the radial artery and superficial to the radius. The nerve exits the antebrachial fascia between the tendons of the brachioradialis and the extensor carpi radialis muscles (Figures 32–6 and 32–7).

FIGURE 32G–2. (**A**) Cross-sectional anatomy of the distal forearm. (**B**) Sonoanatomy of the median nerve (MN) at the forearm. RA, radial artery; FCRM, flexor carpi radialis muscle; FPLM, flexor pollicis longus muscle; FDSM, flexor digitorum superficialis muscle.

FIGURE 32G–3. Cross-sectional ultrasound image of the median nerve (MN) at the wrist. Needle path to reach the MN at the wrist and spread of local anesthetic to block the MN.

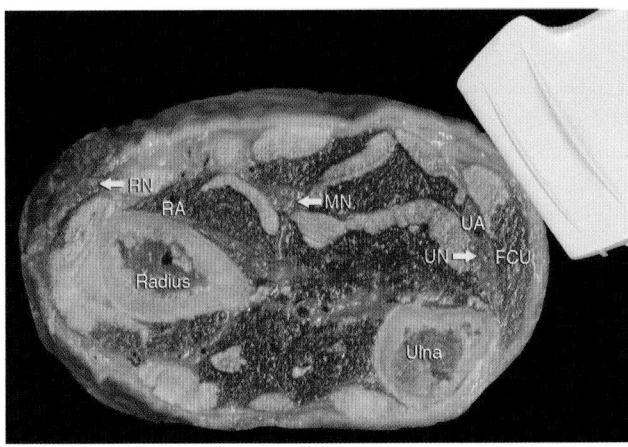

A

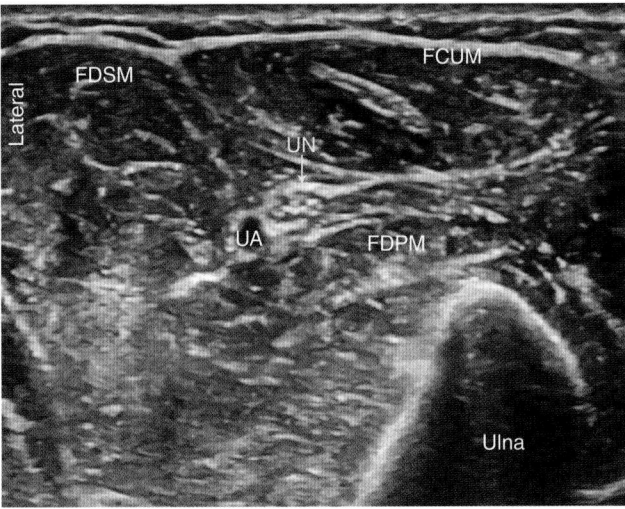

B

FIGURE 32G-4. (**A**) Cross-sectional anatomy of the distal forearm. (**B**) Sonoanatomy of the ulnar nerve (UN) at the forearm. UA, ulnar artery; FCUM, Flexor carpi ulnaris. FDPM, flexor digitorum profundus muscle; FDSM, flexor digitorum superficialis muscle.

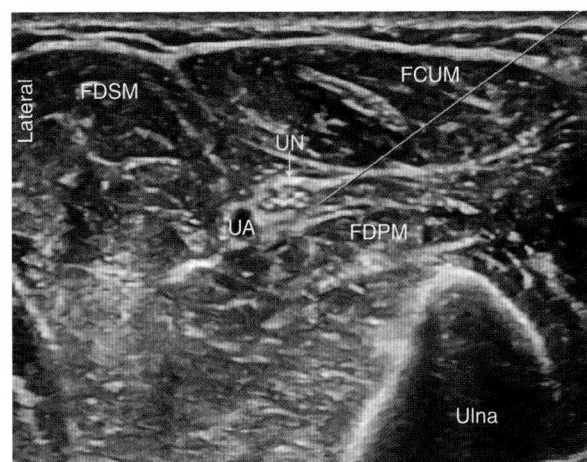

FIGURE 32G-5. Sonoanatomy of the ulnar nerve (UN) at the wrist: needle path to reach the UN at the wrist and approximate spread of local anesthetic (blue-shaded area) to anesthetize the UN. UA, ulnar artery.

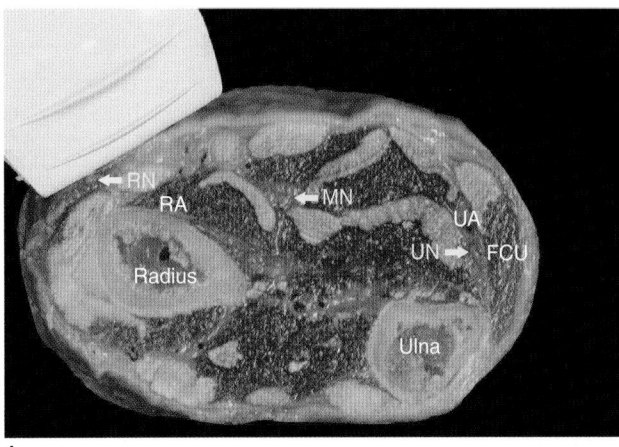

A

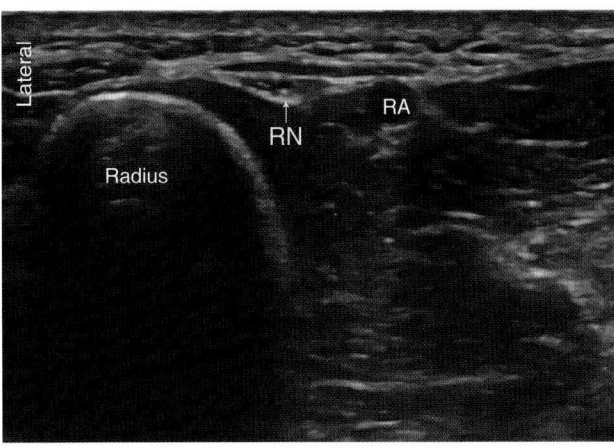

B

FIGURE 32G-6. (**A**) Cross-sectional anatomy of the distal forearm. (**B**) Sonoanatomy of the radial nerve (RN) at the forearm. RA, radial artery.

DISTRIBUTION OF ANESTHESIA

A wrist block results in anesthesia of the entire hand, except the territory of the deep branch of the radial nerve. For a more comprehensive review of the distribution of each terminal nerve, see Chapter 3.

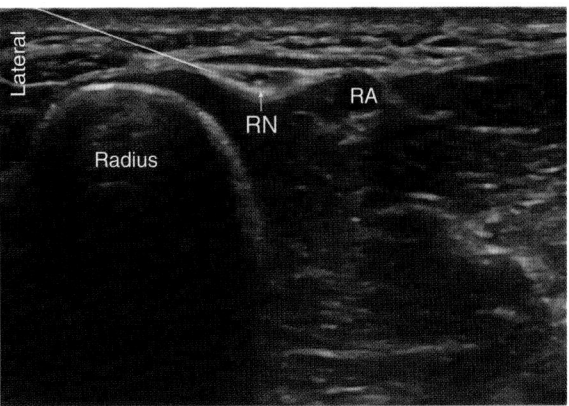

FIGURE 32G-7. Sonoanatomy of the radial nerve (RN) at the level of the wrist. The superficial branch of the RN at the wrist is shown lateral to the radial artery (RA), and the approximate needle path to reach the branch of the radial nerve is shown with an approximate spread of local anesthetic (blue-shaded area) to anesthetize it.

EQUIPMENT

The equipment needed for a wrist block includes the following:

- Ultrasound machine with linear transducer (8–14 MHz), sterile sleeve, and gel
- Standard nerve block tray
- 5 mL syringes containing local anesthetic
- A 2-3 mm 22- to 25-gauge needle with low-volume extension tubing
- Sterile gloves

LANDMARKS AND PATIENT POSITIONING

The wrist block is most easily performed with the patient in the supine position to allow for the volar surface of the wrist to be exposed (Figure 32G-1). It is useful to remove splints and/or bandages on the hand to facilitate placement of the transducer and sterile preparation of the skin surface.

GOAL

The goal of this block is to place the needle tip immediately adjacent to each of the nerves to deposit local anesthetic until its spread around the nerve is documented with ultrasound visualization.

TECHNIQUE

With the arm in the volar side up position, the skin is disinfected. The wrist is a "tightly packed" area that is bounded on three sides by bones. For this reason, a US-guided "wrist" block is often performed 5–10 cm proximally to the wrist crease, where there is more room to maneuver. This location also ensures the blockade of the palmar branches of the median and ulnar nerves, which take off few centimeters proximaly to the

wrist crease. For each of the blocks, the needle may be inserted either in plane or out of plane. Ergonomics often dictates which is most effective. Care must be taken when performing the ulnar and radial nerve blocks since these nerves are intimately associated with arteries. Inadvertent arterial puncture can lead to hematoma. Successful block is predicted by the spread of local anesthetic immediately adjacent to the nerve. Multiple injections to achieve circumferential spread are usually not necessary because these nerves are small and the local anesthetic diffuses quickly into the neural tissue due to the lack of thick epineural tissues. Assuming deposition immediately adjacent to the nerve, 3–4 mL/nerve of local anesthetic is sufficient to ensure an effective block.

SUGGESTED READINGS

Bajaj S, Pattamapaspong N, Middleton W, Teefey S: Ultrasound of the hand and wrist. *J Hand Surg Am* 2009;34:759–760.
Heinemeyer O, Reimers CD: Ultrasound of radial, ulnar, median and sciatic nerves in healthy subjects and patients with hereditary motor and sensory neuropathies. *Ultrasound Med Biol* 1999:25:481–485.
Kiely PD, O'Farrell D, Riordan J, Harmon D: The use of ultrasound-guided hematoma blocks in wrist fractures. *J Clin Anesth* 2009;21:540–542.
Liebmann O, Price D, Mills C, et al: Feasibility of forearm ultrasonography-guided nerve blocks of the radial, ulnar, and median nerves for hand procedures in the emergency department. *Ann Emerg Med* 2006;48:558–562.
Macaire P, Singelyn F, Narchi P, Paqueron X: Ultrasound- or nerve stimulation-guided wrist blocks for carpal tunnel release: a randomized prospective comparative study. *Reg Anesth Pain Med* 2008;33:363–368.
McCartney CJL, Xu D, Constantinescu C, et al: Ultrasound examination of peripheral nerves in the forearm. *Reg Anesth Pain Med* 2007;32:434–439.

REFERENCE

1. Olea E, Fondarella A, Sánchez C, Iriarte I, Almeida MV, Martínez de Salinas A: Bloqueo de los nervios periféricos a nivel de la muñeca guiado por ecografía para el tratamiento de la hiperhidrosis idiopática palmar con toxina botulínica [Ultrasound-guided peripheral nerve block at wrist level for the treatment of idiopathic palmar hyperhidrosis with botulinum toxin]. *Rev Esp Anestesiol Reanim* 2013;60:571–575.

Ultrasound-Guided Nerve Blocks for the Lower Extremity

CHAPTER 33A

Ultrasound-Guided Femoral Nerve Block

Arthur Atchabahian, Ine Leunen, Catherine Vandepitte, and Ana M. Lopez

BLOCK AT A GLANCE

- Indications: femur, patella, quadriceps tendon, and knee sugery; analgesia for hip fracture (Figure 33A–1)
- Transducer position: transverse, femoral crease
- Goal: local anesthetic spread adjacent to the femoral nerve
- Local anesthetic: 10–15 mL

GENERAL CONSIDERATIONS

The ultrasound (US)-guided technique of femoral nerve blockade allows the practitioner to monitor the spread of local anesthetic and needle placement and make appropriate adjustments to accomplish the desirable disposition of the local anesthetic. US also may reduce the risk of femoral artery puncture. Although nerve stimulation is not required for success, motor response observed during nerve stimulation often provides contributory safety information should the needle–nerve relationship be missed by US alone.

ULTRASOUND ANATOMY

Orientation begins with the identification of the femoral artery at the level of the femoral crease. Commonly, the femoral artery and the deep artery of the thigh are both seen. In this case, the transducer should be moved proximal until only the femoral artery is seen (Figure 33A–2a, b). The femoral nerve is lateral to the vessel and covered by the fascia iliaca; it is typically hyperechoic and roughly triangular or oval in shape (Figure 33A–3a, b). The nerve is enveloped within two layers of the fascia iliaca. The femoral nerve typically is visualized at a depth of 2–4 cm.

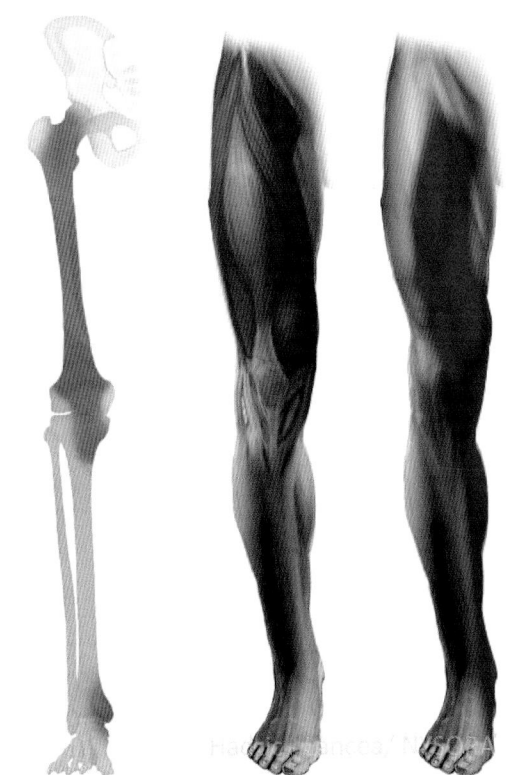

FIGURE 33A–1. Expected distribution of femorar nerve blockade. Left - Osteotomal distribution, Right - Dermatomal distribution.

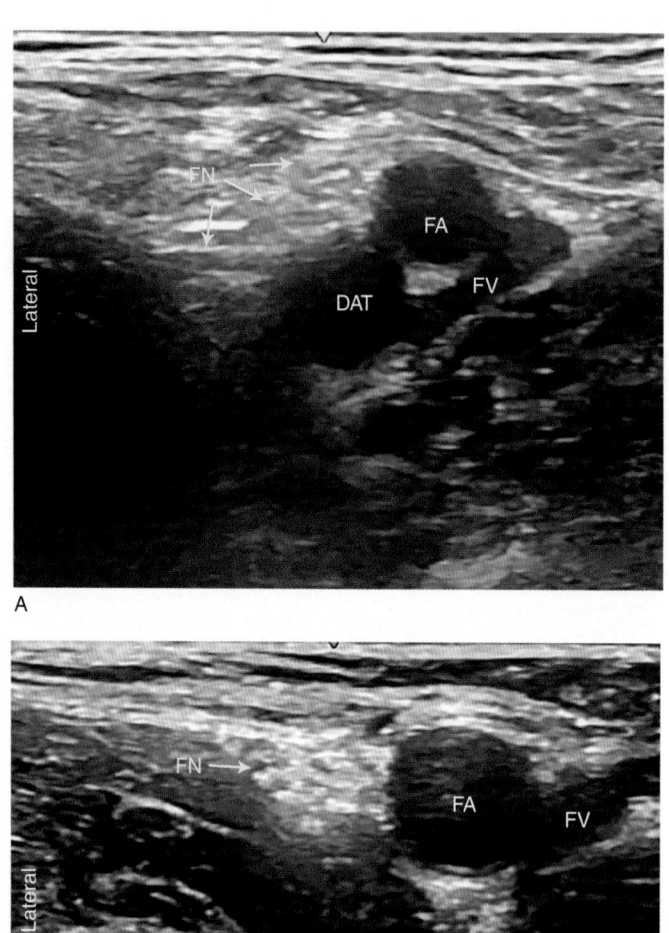

FIGURE 33A–2. Femoral nerve (FN) as seen distally (**A**) and at the femoral crease (**B**). Note that FN is better visualized at B, before the take off the deep artery of the thigh (DAT). Femoral vein (FV) is medial to the artery.

TIPS

- Identification of the femoral nerve often is made easier by slightly tilting the transducer cranially or caudally. This adjustment helps bring out the image of the nerve, making it distinct from the background.

- Applying pressure to the transducer often optimizes the image of the femoral nerve but may collapse veins, obscuring them from the examiner's eye.
  The transducer pressure also may compress the interfascial space and interfere with the adequate spread of the local anesthetic. Therefore, the transducer pressure should be released and vasculature re-ascertained before injection.

DISTRIBUTION OF ANESTHESIA

Femoral nerve block results in anesthesia of the anterior and medial thigh down to and including the knee, as well as a variable strip of skin on the medial leg and foot. It also innervates the hip, knee, and ankle joints.

EQUIPMENT

The equipment recommended for a femoral nerve block includes the following:

- Ultrasound machine with linear transducer (8–18 MHz), sterile sleeve, and gel
- Standard nerve block tray
- One 20-mL syringe containing local anesthetic

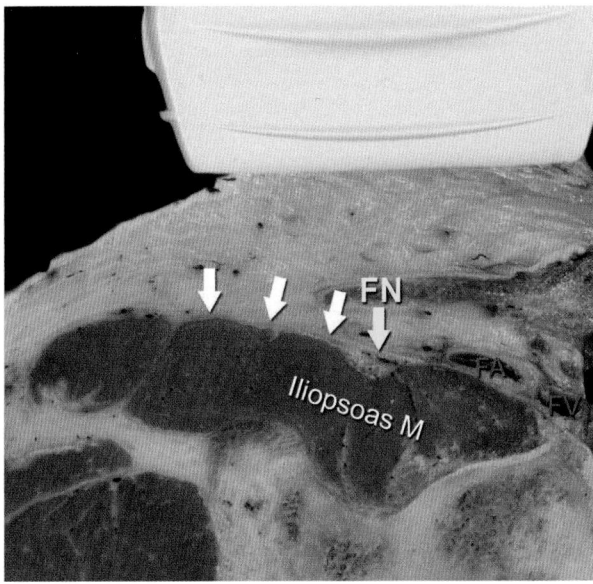

A

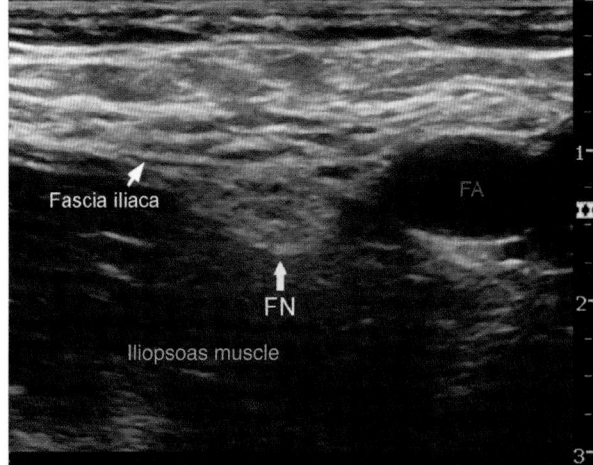

B   Femoral nerve block

FIGURE 33A–3. (**A**) Cross-sectional anatomy of the femoral nerve (FN) at the level of the femoral crease. The FN is seen on the surface of the iliopsoas muscle covered by fascia iliaca (white arrows). The femoral artery (FA) and femoral vein (FV) are seen enveloped within their own vascular fascial sheath created by one of the layers of fascia lata. (**B**) Sonoanatomy of the FN at the femoral triangle. (Reproduced with permission from Hadzic A: *Hadzic's Peripheral Nerve Blocks and Anatomy for Ultrasound-Guided Regional Anesthesia*, 2nd ed. New York: McGraw-Hill, Inc.; 2011.)

- A 50- to 100-mm, 22-gauge, short-bevel, insulated stimulating needle
- Peripheral nerve stimulator
- Injection pressure monitor
- Sterile gloves

LANDMARKS AND PATIENT POSITIONING

This block typically is performed with the patient in the supine position, with the bed or table flattened to maximize operator access to the inguinal area. The transducer is placed transversely

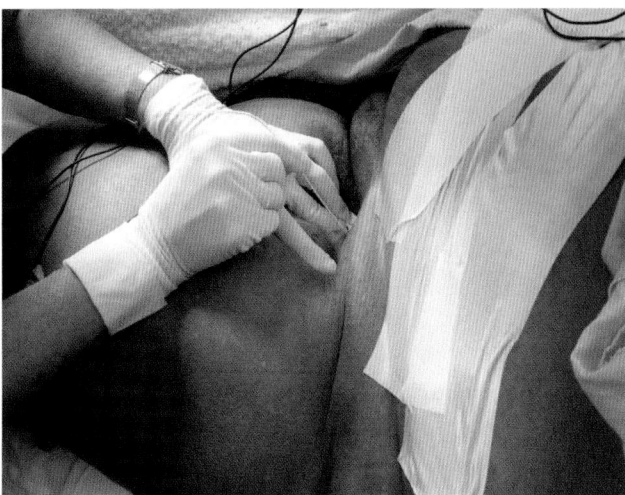

FIGURE 33A–4. Obesity is common in patients who present with an indication for femoral nerve block. Taping the adipose tissue away helps optimize exposure to the femoral crease in patients with morbid obesity.

on the femoral crease, over the pulse of the femoral artery, and moved slowly in a lateral-to-medial direction to identify the artery.

Clinical Pearl

- In such cases, using a wide silk tape to retract the abdomen is a useful maneuver prior to skin preparation and scanning (Figure 33A–4).

GOAL

The goal is to place the needle tip immediately adjacent to the lateral aspect of the femoral nerve, below the fascia iliaca or between the two layers of the fascia iliaca, that surround the femoral nerve. Proper deposition of local anesthetic is confirmed either by observation of the femoral nerve being displaced by the injectate or by the spread of the local anesthetic above or below the nerve, surrounding and separating it from the fascia iliaca layers.

TECHNIQUE

With the patient in the supine position, the skin over the femoral crease is disinfected and the transducer is positioned to identify the femoral artery and nerve. If the nerve is not immediately apparent lateral to the artery, tilting the transducer proximally or distally often helps to image and highlight the nerve from the iliacus muscle and the more superficial adipose tissue. In doing so, an effort should be made to identify the iliacus muscle and its fascia, as well as the fascia lata, because injection underneath a wrong fascial sheath may result in block failure.

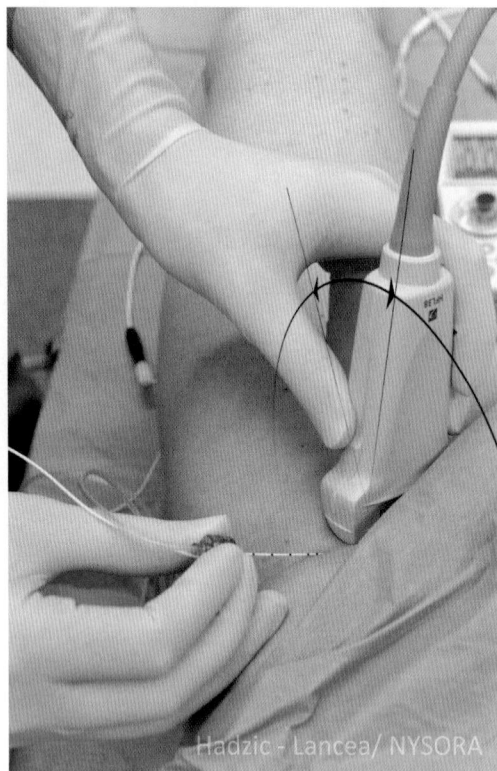

FIGURE 33A–5. Transducer position and needle insertion using an in-plane technique to block the femoral nerve at the femoral crease.

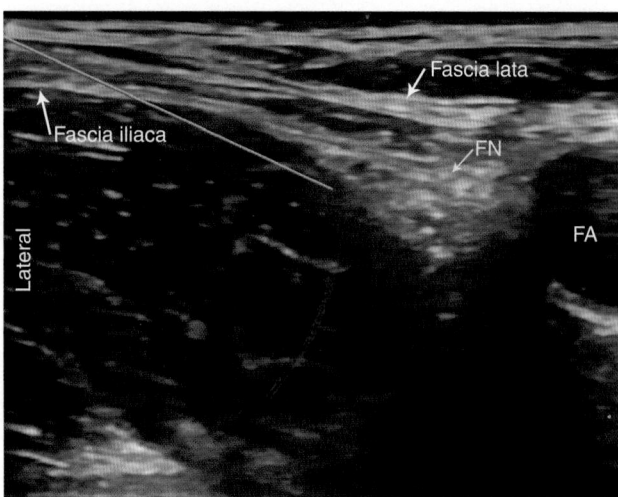

FIGURE 33A–6. Ultrasound image of the needle path to block the femoral nerve. The needle pierces the fascia iliaca lateral to the femoral nerve (FN) and the needle tip is advanced along the deep border of the nerve. FA, femoral artery.

Once the femoral nerve is identified, a skin wheal of local anesthetic is made 1 cm away from the lateral edge of the transducer. The needle is inserted in plane in a lateral-to-medial orientation and advanced toward the femoral nerve (Figure 33A–5). If nerve stimulation is used (0.5 mA, 0.1 msec), the passage of the needle through the fascia iliaca and contact of the needle tip with the femoral nerve usually is associated with a motor response of the quadriceps muscle group. In addition, a needle passage through the fascia iliaca is often felt. Once the needle tip is adjacent (either above, below, or lateral) to the nerve (Figure 33A–6), and after careful aspiration, 1–2 mL of local anesthetic is injected to confirm proper needle placement (Figures 33A–7 and 33A-8). Proper injection will push the femoral nerve away from the injection. Additional needle repositions and injections are done only when necessary. Anatomic variations have been described with aberrant positions of the femoral nerve.[1,2] In an adult patient, 10–15 mL of local anesthetic is adequate for a successful block.

TIPS

- Never inject against high resistance to injection because this may signal an intrafascicular needle placement or needle tip position in a wrong fascial plane.
- Circumferential spread of local anesthetic around the nerve is not necessary for this block. A pool of local anesthetic immediately adjacent to either the posterolateral or the anterior aspects is sufficient.[3]

- Locate the femoral vein, releasing pressure on the transducer, using color Doppler if needed. The femoral vein is typically medial to the artery, but it can occasionally lie deep or even lateral to it.[4,5] It is often compressed by the probe during block performance; being aware of the position of the vein helps decrease the risk of inadvertent intravascular injection.[4,5]
- Applying forceful pressure to the transducer will compress the tissue below it, making injection more difficult and possibly interfering with spread between the fascial layers.
- Following hip arthroscopy, landmarks might be displaced by fluid extravasation, with the artery and the nerve significantly deeper than their preoperative position.[6]

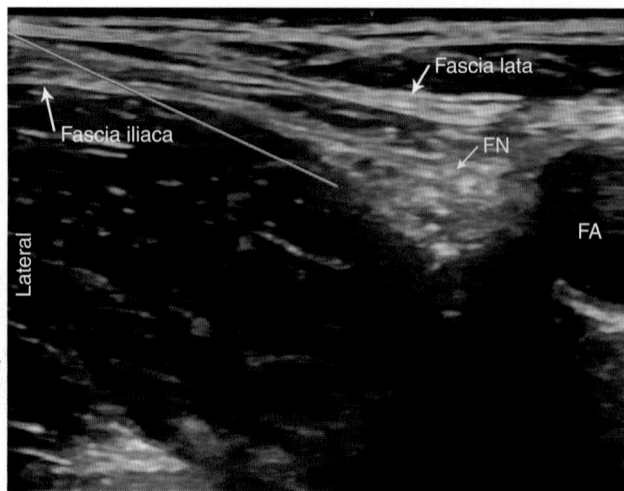

FIGURE 33A–7. Simulated needle path and spread of local anesthetic (blue-shaded area) to block the femoral nerve (FN). FA, femoral artery.

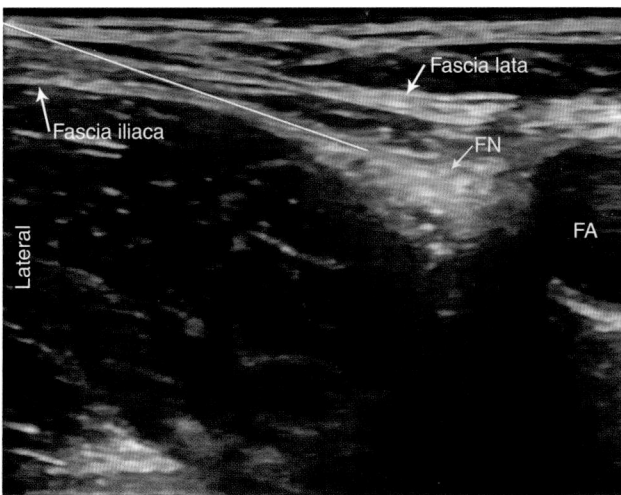

A

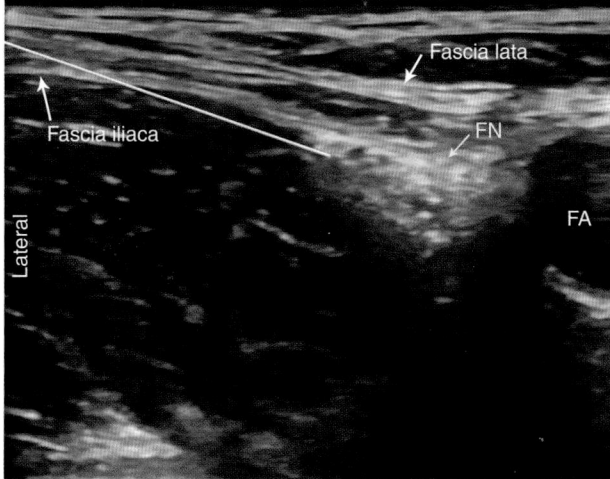

B

FIGURE 33A–8. Simulated needle paths and local anesthetic spread to block the femoral nerve (FN). (**A**) The needle tip is advanced in between the fascia iliaca and the nerve and the local anesthetic deposited superficially to the nerve. (**B**) The tip is located just lateral to the femoral nerve nerve, in between the two layers surrounding the nerve. FA, femoral artery.

CONTINUOUS ULTRASOUND-GUIDED FEMORAL NERVE BLOCK

The goal of the continuous femoral nerve block is placement of the catheter within the vicinity of the femoral nerve just deep to the fascia iliaca. The procedure consists of five steps: (1) needle placement; (2) injection through the needle to confirm needle placement in the proper tissue plane; (3) catheter advancement; (4) injection through the catheter to assure its therapeutic position; (5) securing the catheter. For the first two phases of the procedure, US can be used to ensure accuracy in most patients. The in-line approach from the lateral-to-medial direction is the most common method because the out-of-plane approach holds greater risk for puncture of the femoral nerve if the needle is introduced directly above the nerve (Figure 33A-9).[7,8,9] Alternative approaches, such as the oblique approach, have also been suggested.[10]

- With US guidance, nonstimulating catheters are used for continuous femoral block. Stimulating catheters require a longer insertion time, without improvement in analgesia.[11,12] Stimulating catheters also may lead to unnecessary needle and catheter manipulation to obtain the motor response, when in fact the catheter is often in the proper place even when there is no motor response.
- Adequate catheter placement with US guidance is confirmed by disposition of the local anesthetic in the proper anatomical space rather than by motor stimulation.[13]

For detailed description, please refer to "Continuous US-guided nerve block" in Chapter 32B. In general, the inguinal area is quite mobile, and the femoral nerve is shallow, both of which predispose to catheter dislodgment. The more lateral the starting point for needle insertion for continuous femoral nerve block, the longer the catheter would be within the iliacus muscle, which may help prevent dislodgment because muscle tends to stabilize a catheter better than adipose tissue. A common empirical infusion regimen for femoral nerve block in an adult patient is ropivacaine 0.2% at an infusion rate of 5 mL/h with a 5 mL/h patient-controlled bolus.

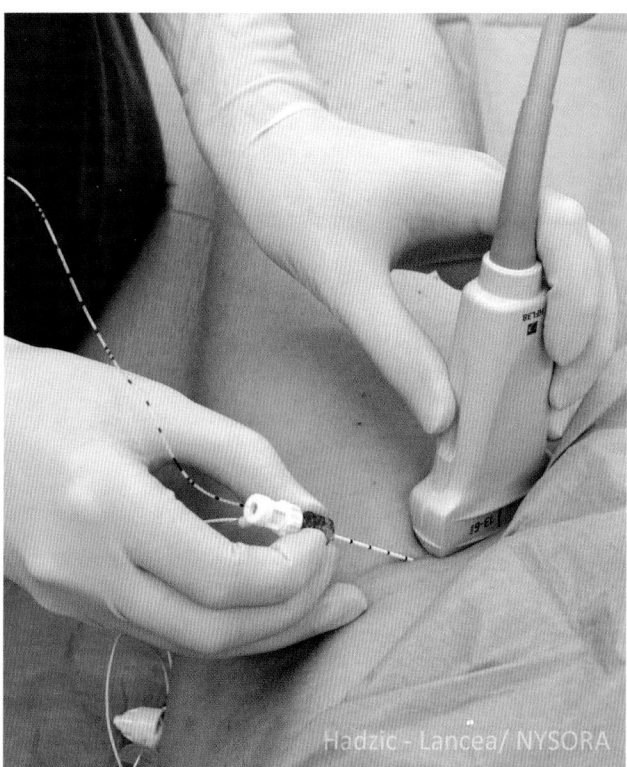

FIGURE 33A–9. Continuous femoral nerve block. The needle is seen inserted in plane approaching the nerve in a lateral-to-medial direction. Although it would seem intuitive that a longitudinal needle insertion would have advantages, the technique demonstrated here is simpler and commonly used. The catheter should be inserted 2–4 cm past the needle tip.

SUGGESTED READINGS

Single-Injection Femoral Nerve Block

Ajmal M, Power S, Smith T, Shorten GD: Ergonomic task analysis of ultrasound-guided femoral nerve block: a pilot study. J Clin Anesth 2011;23:35–41.

Bech B, et al. The successful use of peripheral nerve blocks for femoral amputation. Acta Anaesthesiol Scand 2009;53:257–260.

Brull R, Prasad GA, Gandhi R, Ramlogan R, Khan M, Chan VW: Is a patella motor response necessary for continuous femoral nerve blockade performed in conjunction with ultrasound guidance? Anesth Analg 2011;112:982–986.

Casati A, Baciarello M, Di Cianni S, et al: Effects of ultrasound guidance on the minimum effective anaesthetic volume required to block the femoral nerve. Br J Anaesth 2007;98:823–827.

Dold AP, Murnaghan L, Xing J, Abdallah FW, Brull R, Whelan DB: Preoperative femoral nerve block in hip arthroscopic surgery: a retrospective review of 108 consecutive cases. Am J Sports Med 2014;42:144–149.

Forget P: Bad needles can't do good blocks. Reg Anesth Pain Med 2009;34:603.

Fredrickson MJ, Kilfoyle DH: Neurological complication analysis of 1000 ultrasound guided peripheral nerve blocks for elective orthopaedic surgery: a prospective study. Anaesthesia 2009;64:836–844.

Gupta PK, Chevret S, Zohar S, Hopkins PM: What is the ED95 of prilocaine for femoral nerve block using ultrasound? Br J Anaesth 2013;110:831–836.

Hadzic A, Houle TT, Capdevila X, Ilfeld BM: Femoral nerve block for analgesia in patients having knee arthroplasty. Anesthesiology 2010;113:1014–1015.

Helayel PE, da Conceição DB, Feix C, Boos GL, Nascimento BS, de Oliveira Filho GR: Ultrasound-guided sciatic-femoral block for revision of the amputation stump. Case report. Rev Bras Anestesiol 2008;58:480–482, 482–484.

Hotta K, Sata N, Suzuki H, Takeuchi M, Seo N: Ultrasound-guided combined femoral nerve and lateral femoral cutaneous nerve blocks for femur neck fracture surgery—case report [in Japanese]. Masui 2008;57:892–894.

Ishiguro S, Asano N, Yoshida K, et al: Day zero ambulation under modified femoral nerve block after minimally invasive surgery for total knee arthroplasty: preliminary report. J Anesth 2013;27:132–134.

Ishiguro S, Yokochi A, Yoshioka K, et al: Technical communication: anatomy and clinical implications of ultrasound-guided selective femoral nerve block. Anesth Analg 2012;115:1467–1470.

Ito H, Shibata Y, Fujiwara Y, Komatsu T: Ultrasound-guided femoral nerve block [in Japanese]. Masui 2008;57:575–579.

Lang SA: Ultrasound and the femoral three-in-one nerve block: weak methodology and inappropriate conclusions. Anesth Analg 1998;86:1147–1148.

Marhofer P, Harrop-Griffiths W, Willschke H, Kirchmair L: Fifteen years of ultrasound guidance in regional anaesthesia: part 2—recent developments in block techniques. Br J Anaesth 2010;104:673–683.

Marhofer P, Nasel C, Sitzwohl C, Kapral S: Magnetic resonance imaging of the distribution of local anesthetic during the three-in-one block. Anesth Analg 2000;90:119–124.

Marhofer P, Schrögendorfer K, Koinig H, Kapral S, Weinstabl C, Mayer N: Ultrasonographic guidance improves sensory block and onset time of three-in-one blocks. Anesth Analg 1997;85:854–857.

Mariano ER, Loland VJ, Sandhu NS, et al: Ultrasound guidance versus electrical stimulation for femoral perineural catheter insertion. J Ultrasound Med 2009;28:1453–1460.

Murray JM, Derbyshire S, Shields MO: Lower limb blocks. Anaesthesia 2010;65(Suppl 1):57–66.

Oberndorfer U, Marhofer P, Bösenberg A, et al: Ultrasonographic guidance for sciatic and femoral nerve blocks in children. Br J Anaesth 2007;98:797–801.

O'Donnell BD, Mannion S: Ultrasound-guided femoral nerve block, the safest way to proceed? Reg Anesth Pain Med 2006;31:387–388.

Reid N, Stella J, Ryan M, Ragg M: Use of ultrasound to facilitate accurate femoral nerve block in the emergency department. Emerg Med Australas 2009;21:124–130.

Salinas FV: Ultrasound and review of evidence for lower extremity peripheral nerve blocks. Reg Anesth Pain Med 2010;35(Suppl 2):S16–25.

Schafhalter-Zoppoth I, Moriggl B: Aspects of femoral nerve block. Reg Anesth Pain Med 2006;31:92–93.

Sites BD, Beach M, Gallagher JD, Jarrett RA, Sparks MB, Lundberg CJ: A single injection ultrasound-assisted femoral nerve block provides side effect-sparing analgesia when compared with intrathecal morphine in patients undergoing total knee arthroplasty. Anesth Analg 2004;99:1539–1543.

Sites BD, Beach ML, Chinn CD, Redborg KE, Gallagher JD: A comparison of sensory and motor loss after a femoral nerve block conducted with ultrasound versus ultrasound and nerve stimulation. Reg Anesth Pain Med 2009;34:508–513.

Soong J, Schafhalter-Zoppoth I, Gray AT: The importance of transducer angle to ultrasound visibility of the femoral nerve. Reg Anesth Pain Med 2005;30:505.

Szucs S, Morau D, Iohom G: Femoral nerve blockade. Med Ultrason 2010;12:139–144.

Tran DQ, Muñoz L, Russo G, Finlayson RJ: Ultrasonography and stimulating perineural catheters for nerve blocks: a review of the evidence. Can J Anaesth 2008;55:447–457.

Tsui B, Suresh S: Ultrasound imaging for regional anesthesia in infants, children, and adolescents: a review of current literature and its application in the practice of extremity and trunk blocks. Anesthesiology 2010;112:473–492.

Watson MJ, Walker E, Rowell S, et al: Femoral nerve block for pain relief in hip fracture: a dose finding study. Anaesthesia 2014;69:683–686.

Continuous Femoral Nerve Block

Albrecht E, Morfey D, Chan V, et al: Single-injection or continuous femoral nerve block for total knee arthroplasty? Clin Orthop Relat Res 2014;472:1384–1393.

Aveline C, Le Roux A, Le Hetet H, Vautier P, Cognet F, Bonnet F: Postoperative efficacies of femoral nerve catheters sited using ultrasound combined with neurostimulation compared with neurostimulation alone for total knee arthroplasty. Eur J Anaesthesiol 2010;27:978–984.

Capdevila X, Biboulet P, Morau D, et al: Continuous three-in-one block for postoperative pain after lower limb orthopedic surgery: where do the catheters go? Anesth Analg 2002;94:1001–1006.

Eledjam JJ, Cuvillon P, Capdevila X, et al: Postoperative analgesia by femoral nerve block with ropivacaine 0.2% after major knee surgery: continuous versus patient-controlled techniques. Reg Anesth Pain Med 2002;27:604–611.

Errando CL: Ultrasound-guided femoral nerve block: catheter insertion in a girl with skeletal abnormalities [in Spanish]. Rev Esp Anestesiol Reanim 2009;56:197–198.

Fredrickson MJ, Danesh-Clough TK: Ambulatory continuous femoral analgesia for major knee surgery: a randomised study of ultrasound-guided femoral catheter placement. Anaesth Intensive Care 2009;37:758–766.

Gandhi K, Lindenmuth DM, Hadzic A, et al: The effect of stimulating versus conventional perineural catheters on postoperative analgesia following ultrasound-guided femoral nerve localization. J Clin Anesth 2011;23:626–631.

Koscielniak-Nielsen ZJ, Rasmussen H, Hesselbjerg L: Long-axis ultrasound imaging of the nerves and advancement of perineural catheters under direct vision: a preliminary report of four cases. Reg Anesth Pain Med 2008;33:477–482.

Niazi AU, Prasad A, Ramlogan R, Chan VWS: Methods to ease placement of stimulating catheters during in-plane ultrasound-guided femoral nerve block. Reg Anesth Pain Med 2009;34:380–381.

Villegas Duque A, Ortiz de la Tabla González R, Martínez Navas A, Echevarría Moreno M: Continuous femoral block for postoperative analgesia in a patient with poliomyelitis [in Spanish]. Rev Esp Anestesiol Reanim 2010;57:123–124.

Wasserstein D, Farlinger C, Brull R, Mahomed N, Gandhi R: Advanced age, obesity and continuous femoral nerve blockade are independent risk factors for inpatient falls after primary total knee arthroplasty. J Arthroplasty 2013;28:1121–1124.

REFERENCES

1. Gurnaney H, Kraemer F, Ganesh A: Ultrasound and nerve stimulation to identify an abnormal location of the femoral nerve. Reg Anesth Pain Med 2009;34:615.

2. Chin KJ, Tse C, Chan V: Ultrasonographic identification of an anomalous femoral nerve: the fascia iliaca as a key landmark. Anesthesiology 2011;115:1104.

3. Szdcs S, Morau D, Sultan SF, Iohom G, Shorten G: A comparison of three techniques (local anesthetic deposited circumferential to vs. above vs.

below the nerve) for ultrasound guided femoral nerve block. BMC Anesthesiol 2014;14:6.

4. Muhly WT, Orebaugh SL: Ultrasound evaluation of the anatomy of the vessels in relation to the femoral nerve at the femoral crease. Surg Radiol Anat 2011;33:491–494.

5. Hocking G: Anomalous positioning of femoral artery and vein—even "constant" landmarks can be inconsistent. Anaesth Intensive Care 2011;39: 312–313.

6. Davis JJ, Swenson JD, Kelly S, Abraham CL, Aoki SK: Anatomic changes in the inguinal region after hip arthroscopy: implications for femoral nerve block. J Clin Anesth 2012;24:590–592.

7. Mariano ER, Kim TE, Funck N, et al: A randomized comparison of long- and short-axis imaging for in-plane ultrasound-guided femoral perineural catheter insertion. J Ultrasound Med 2013;32:149–156.

8. Fredrickson MJ, Danesh-Clough TK; Ultrasound-guided femoral catheter placement: a randomised comparison of the in-plane and out-of-plane techniques. Anaesthesia 2013;68:382–390.

9. Wang AZ, Gu L, Zhou QH, Ni WZ, Jiang W: Ultrasound-guided continuous femoral nerve block for analgesia after total knee arthroplasty: catheter perpendicular to the nerve versus catheter parallel to the nerve. Reg Anesth Pain Med 2010;35:127–131.

10. Fredrickson M: "Oblique" needle-probe alignment to facilitate ultrasound-guided femoral catheter placement. Reg Anesth Pain Med 2008;33: 383–384.

11. Farag E, Atim A, Ghosh R, et al: Comparison of three techniques for ultrasound-guided femoral nerve catheter insertion: a randomized, blinded trial. Anesthesiology 2014;121:239–248.

12. Gandhi K, Lindenmuth DM, Hadzic A, et al: The effect of stimulating versus conventional perineural catheters on postoperative analgesia following ultrasound-guided femoral nerve localization. J Clin Anesth 2011;23:626–631.

13. Altermatt FR, Corvetto MA, Venegas C, et al: Brief report: the sensitivity of motor responses for detecting catheter-nerve contact during ultrasound-guided femoral nerve blocks with stimulating catheters. Anesth Analg 2011;113:1276–1278.

CHAPTER 33B

Ultrasound-Guided Fascia Iliaca Block

Arthur Atchabahian, Ine Leunen, Catherine Vandepitte, and Ana M. Lopez

FASCIA ILIACA BLOCK AT A GLANCE

- Indications: anterior thigh and knee surgery, analgesia following hip and knee procedures
- Transducer position: transverse, close to the femoral crease and lateral to the femoral artery (Figure 33B–1)

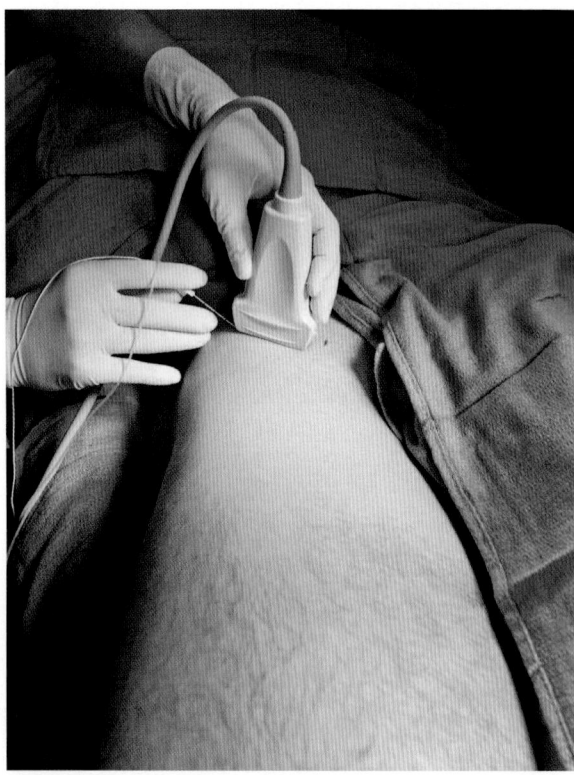

FIGURE 33B–1. Needle insertion for the fascia iliaca block. The blue dot indicates the position of the femoral artery. (Reproduced with permission from Hadzic A: *Hadzic's Peripheral Nerve Blocks and Anatomy for Ultrasound-Guided Regional Anesthesia*, 2nd ed. New York: McGraw-Hill, 2011.)

- Goal: medial–lateral spread of local anesthetic underneath the fascia iliaca
- Local anesthetic: 20–40 mL of dilute local anesthetic (eg, 0.2% ropivacaine)

GENERAL CONSIDERATIONS

The fascia iliaca block (also called the fascia iliaca compartment block) is considered an alternative to a femoral nerve or a lumbar plexus block. Since the femoral nerve and lateral femoral cutaneous nerve (LFCN) lie under the fascia of the iliacus muscle, a sufficient volume of local anesthetic deposited deep to the fascia iliaca may spread underneath the fascia in a medial and lateral direction to reach the femoral nerve and sometimes the LFCN.

Although some authors suggest that the local anesthetic may also spread underneath fascia iliaca proximally toward the lumbosacral plexus, this has not been demonstrated consistently. Before ultrasound (US), the technique involved needle placement at the lateral third of the distance from the anterior superior iliac spine to the pubic tubercle, using a "double-pop" technique as the needle passes through the fascia lata and fascia iliaca. However, block success with this "feel" technique is sporadic because false "pops" can occur. In contrast, the US-guided technique allows monitoring of the needle placement and local anesthetic delivery and ensures delivery of the local anesthetic into the correct plane.[1]

ULTRASOUND ANATOMY

The fascia iliaca is located anterior to the iliacus muscle (on its surface) within the pelvis. It is bound superolaterally by the iliac crest and merges medially with the fascia overlying the psoas muscle. Both the femoral and lateral cutaneous nerves of the thigh lie under the fascia iliaca in their intrapelvic course. Anatomical orientation begins in the same manner as

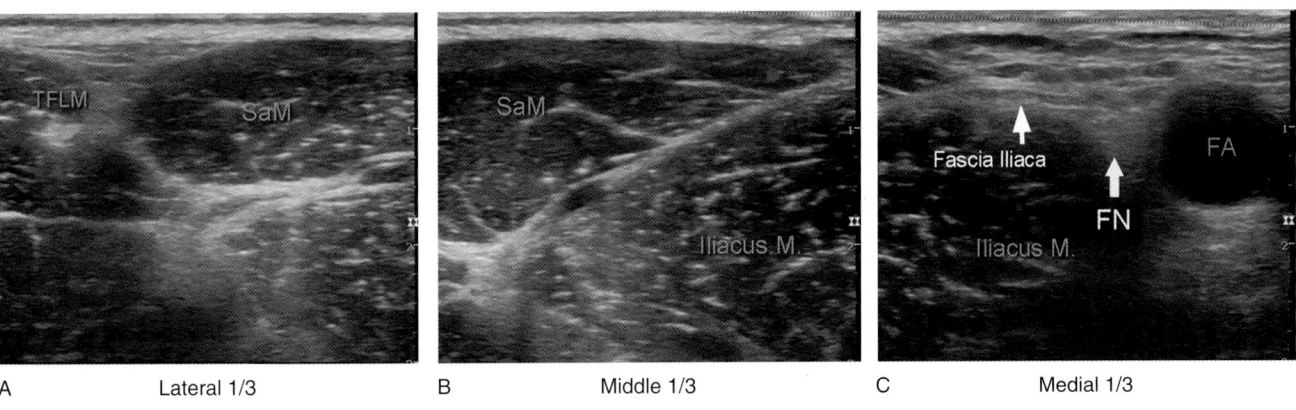

| A | Lateral 1/3 | B | Middle 1/3 | C | Medial 1/3 |

FIGURE 33B–2. A panoramic view of the US anatomy of the femoral (inguinal) crease area. From lateral to medial, shown are the tensor fasciae latae muscle (TFLM), sartorius muscle (SaM), iliac muscle, fascia iliaca, femoral nerve (FN), and femoral artery (FA). The (**A**) lateral, (**B**) middle, and (**C**) medial thirds are derived by dividing the line between the FA and the anterior superior iliac spine in three equal sections. (Reproduced with permission from Hadzic A: *Hadzic's Peripheral Nerve Blocks and Anatomy for Ultrasound-Guided Regional Anesthesia*, 2nd ed. New York: McGraw-Hill, 2011.)

the femoral block: identifying the femoral artery at the level of the inguinal crease. If it is not immediately visible, sliding the transducer medially and laterally will eventually bring the vessel into view. Immediately lateral and deep to the femoral artery and vein is a large hypoechoic structure, the iliopsoas muscle (Figure 33B–2). It is covered by a hyperechoic fascia, which can be seen separating the muscle from the subcutaneous tissue superficial to it.

The hyperechoic femoral nerve should be seen wedged between the iliopsoas muscle and the fascia iliaca, lateral to the femoral artery. The fascia lata (superficial in the subcutaneous layer) is more superficial and may have more than one layer. Moving the transducer laterally several centimeters brings into view the sartorius muscle covered by its own fascia as well as the fascia iliaca. Further lateral movement of the transducer reveals the anterior superior iliac spine (see Figure 33B–2). Additional anatomical detail can be seen in the cross-sectional anatomy presented in Chapter 33A. Since the anatomy is essentially identical to that described for the femoral nerve block, it is not repeated here.

Clinical Pearl

- The transducer can be placed anywhere between the level of the femoral crease and inguinal ligament.

DISTRIBUTION OF ANESTHESIA

The distribution of anesthesia and analgesia depends on the extent of local anesthetic spread and the nerves blocked. Blockade of the femoral nerve results in anesthesia of the anterior and medial thigh (down to and including the knee) and anesthesia of the variable strip of skin on the medial leg and foot (saphenous nerve). The femoral nerve also contributes to articular fibers to both the hip and knee. The lateral femoral cutaneous nerve confers cutaneous innervation to the anterolateral thigh (Figure 33B–3).

For a more comprehensive review of the femoral and lateral femoral cutaneous nerves and lumbar plexus nerve distribution, see Chapter 3.

EQUIPMENT

The equipment needed for a fascia iliaca block includes the following:

- Ultrasound machine with linear transducer (6–14 MHz), sterile sleeve, and gel
- Standard nerve block tray

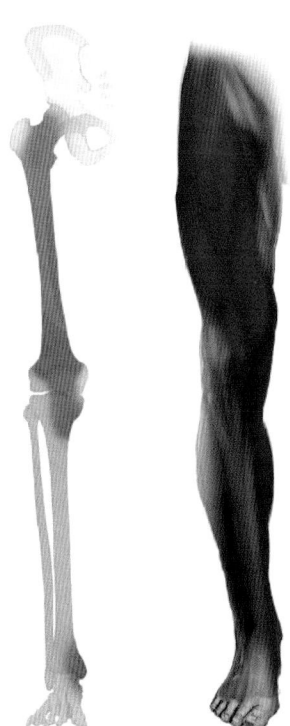

FIGURE 33B–3. Expected distribution of fascia iliaca sensory block (lateral femorocutaneous and femoral nerves blocks).

- Two 20-mL syringes containing local anesthetic
- 80- to 100-mm, 22-gauge needle (a short bevel aids in eliciting the fascial "pop" if desired)
- Sterile gloves

LANDMARKS AND PATIENT POSITIONING

This block is typically performed with the patient in the supine position, with the bed or table flattened to maximize access to the inguinal area (Figure 33B–1). Although palpation of a femoral pulse is a useful landmark, it is not required because the artery is quickly visualized by placement of the transducer transversely on the inguinal crease, followed by slow movement laterally or medially. Tilting the probe while pressing helps to identify the hyperchoic fascia iliaca superficial to the hypoechoic iliopsoas muscle. Medially, the Femoral nerve is visualized deep to the fascia and lateral to the artery (Figure 33B-4). Laterally, the sartorious muscle is identified by its typical triangular shape when compressed by the transducer.

GOAL

The goal is to place the needle tip under the fascia iliaca approximately at a lateral third of the line connecting the anterior superior iliac spine to the pubic tubercle (the injection is made several centimeters lateral to the femoral artery) and to deposit a relatively large volume (20–40 mL) of local anesthetic until its spread laterally toward the iliac spine and medially toward the femoral nerve is observed with US visualization.

TECHNIQUE

With the patient in the proper position, the skin is disinfected and the transducer positioned to identify the femoral artery and the iliopsoas muscle and fascia iliaca. The transducer is moved laterally until the sartorius muscle is identified. After a skin wheal is made, the needle is inserted in plane (see Figure 33B–1). As the needle passes through fascia iliaca, the fascia is first seen

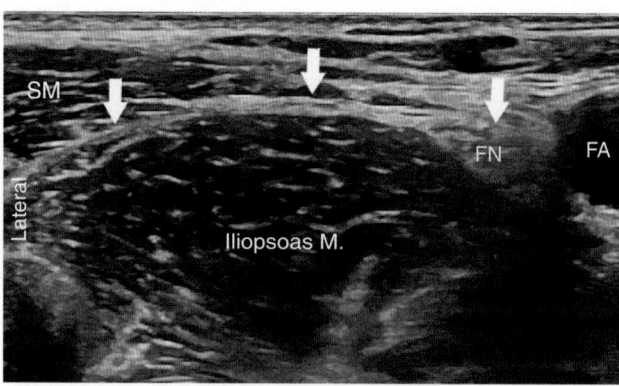

FIGURE 33B–4. Ultrasound image of the fascia iliaca (white line and arrows) at the level of the inguinal ligament. The femoral nerve (FN) and femoral artery (FA) are visualized on the medial side and the sartorious muscle (SM) on the lateral side.

indented by the needle. As the needle eventually pierces the fascia, a "pop" may be felt, and the fascia may be seen to "snap" back on the US image. After negative aspiration, 1–2 mL of local anesthetic is injected to confirm the proper injection plane between the fascia and the iliopsoas muscle (Figure 33B–5a, b). If local anesthetic spread occurs above the fascia or within the substance of the muscle itself, additional needle repositions and injections may be necessary. A proper injection will result in the separation of the fascia iliaca by the local anesthetic in the medial–lateral direction from the point of injection as described. Releasing the pressure of the transducer may reduce the resistance to injection and improve the distribution of local anesthetic. If the spread is deemed inadequate, additional injections laterally or medially to the original needle insertion or injection can be made to facilitate the medial–lateral spread.

In an adult patient, 20–40 mL of local anesthetic is usually required for successful blockade. In children, 0.7 mL/kg is commonly used. The success of the block is best predicted by documenting the spread of local anesthetic toward the femoral nerve medially and underneath the sartorius muscle laterally (Figure 33B-5b). In obese patients, an out-of-plane technique

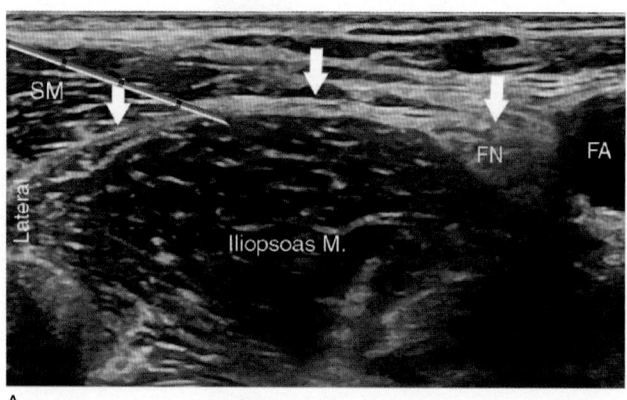

A

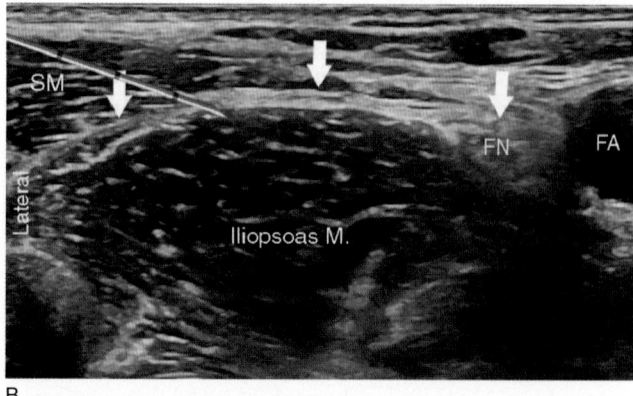

B

FIGURE 33B–5. (**A**) Position of the needle tip for the fascia iliaca block. The needle is shown underneath the fascia iliaca lateral to the femoral artery but not deep enough to be lodged in the iliac muscle. (**B**) A simulated spread (blue-shaded area) of local anesthetic to accomplish a fascia iliaca block.

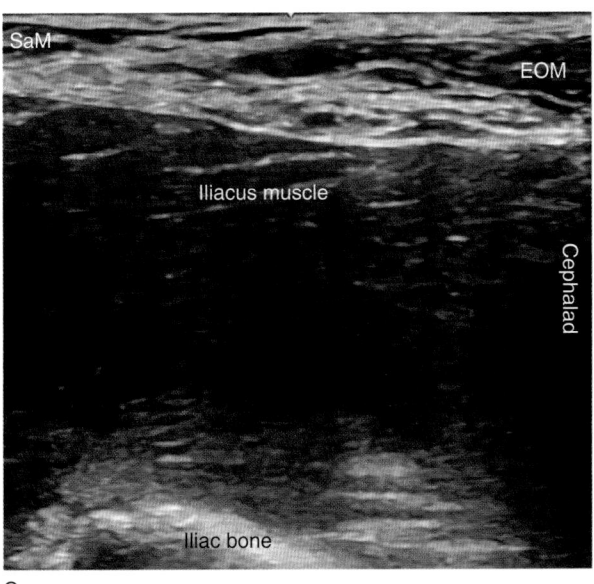
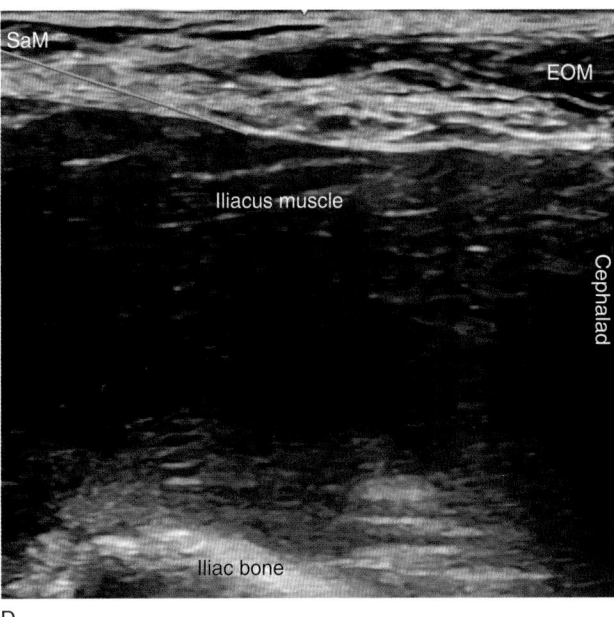

C   D

FIGURE 33B-5. (*Continued*) (**C**) Ultrasound view of the suprainguinal approach with the probe oriented in a sagittal plane along the iliacus muscle. (**D**) Needle path and simulated local anesthetic spread (blue-shaded area) just deep to the fascia iliaca and the external oblique muscle (EOM). SaM, sartorius muscle.

may be favored. The block should result in blockade of the femoral nerve in all instances (100%) and the lateral femoral nerve in most instances (80–100%). Blockade of the anterior branch of the obturator nerve does not occur with the fascia iliaca block.[2,3] When required, this nerve should be blocked as described in Chapter 33D.

An alternative suprainguinal technique may result in a more proximal spread and possibly more efficacious analgesia after hip surgery (Figures 33B-5c, 33B-5d, and 33B-6),[4,5] although there are no data published to support these claims. Likewise, there are no data supporting the use of continuous fascia iliaca block at this time.

TIPS

- The fascia iliaca block is a large-volume block. Its success depends on the spread of local anesthetic underneath the fascia iliaca. A volume of 30–40 mL of injectate is necessary to accomplish the block.
- The spread of local anesthetic is monitored with ultrasonography. If the pattern of spread is not adequate (eg, the local anesthetic is collecting in one location and not "layering out"), the injection is stopped and the needle repositioned before continuing. Additional injections may be made to ensure adequate spread.

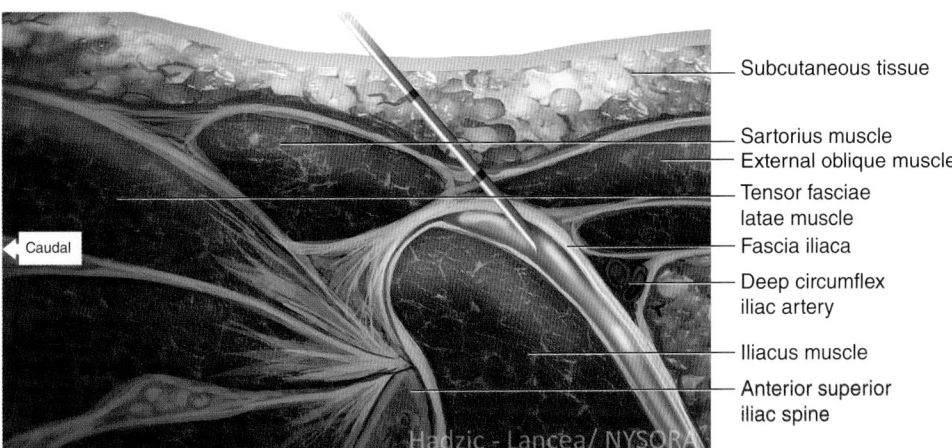

Subcutaneous tissue

Sartorius muscle
External oblique muscle
Tensor fasciae latae muscle
Fascia iliaca
Deep circumflex iliac artery
Iliacus muscle
Anterior superior iliac spine

Caudal

FIGURE 33B-6. Alternative suprainguinal method to perform the fascia iliaca compartment block: anatomical section in the parasagittal plane.

SUGGESTED READINGS

Foss NB, Kristensen BB, Bundgaard M, et al: Fascia iliaca compartment blockade for acute pain control in hip fracture patients: a randomized, placebo-controlled study. Anesthesiology 2007;106:773–778.

Minville V, Gozlan C, Asehnoune K, et al: Fascia-iliaca compartment block for femoral bone fracture in prehospital medicine in a 6-yr-old child. Eur J Anaesthesiol 2006;23:715–716.

Mouzopolous G, Vasiliadis G, Lasanianos N, et al: Fascia iliaca block prophylaxis for hip fracture patients at risk for delirium: a randomized placebo-controlled study. J Orthop Traumatol 2009;10:127–133.

Swenson JD, Bay N, Loose E, et al: Outpatient management of continuous peripheral nerve catheters placed using ultrasound guidance: an experience in 620 patients. Anesth Analg 2006;103:1436–1443.

Wambold D, Carter C, Rosenberg AD: The fascia iliaca block for postoperative pain relief after knee surgery. Pain Pract 2001;1:274–277.

Yun MJ, Kim YH, Han MK, et al: Analgesia before a spinal block for femoral neck fracture: fascia iliaca compartment block. Acta Anaesthesiol Scand 2009;53:1282–1287.

REFERENCES

1. Capdevila X, Biboulet P, Bouregba M, Barthelet Y, Rubenovitch J, d'Athis F: Comparison of the three-in-one and fascia iliaca compartment blocks in adults: clinical and radiographic analysis. Anesth Analg 1998;86: 1039–1044.

2. Dolan J, Williams A, Murney E, Smith M, Kenny GN: Ultrasound guided fascia iliaca block: a comparison with the loss of resistance technique. Reg Anesth Pain Med 2008;33:526–531.

3. Weller RS: Does fascia iliaca block result in obturator block? Reg Anesth Pain Med 2009;34:524.

4. Hebbard P, Ivanusic J, Sha S: Ultrasound-guided supra-inguinal fascia iliaca block: a cadaveric evaluation of a novel approach. Anaesthesia 2011; 66:300–305.

5. Miller BR: Ultrasound-guided fascia iliaca compartment block in pediatric patients using a long-axis, in-plane needle technique: a report of three cases. Paediatr Anaesth 2011;21:1261–1264.

CHAPTER 33C

Ultrasound-Guided Lateral Femoral Cutaneous Nerve Block

Thomas B. Clark, Ana M. Lopez, Daquan Xu, and Catherine Vandepitte

LATERAL FEMORAL CUTANEOUS NERVE BLOCK AT A GLANCE

- Indications: postoperative analgesia for hip surgery, meralgia paresthetica, and muscle biopsy of the proximal lateral thigh
- Transducer position: transverse, inferior to the anterior superior iliac spine; the lateral edge of the sartorius muscle should be visualized with ultrasound
- Goal: local anesthetic spread around LFCN between the tensor fasciae latae and sartorius muscles
- Local anesthetic: 5 mL (adults)

GENERAL CONSIDERATIONS

The lateral femoral cutaneous nerve (LFCN) divides into several branches innervating the lateral and anterior aspects of the thigh. Of note, in 45% of patients, innervation of the LFCN extends even to the anterior thigh.[1] The variable anatomy of the lateral femoral cutaneous nerve makes it challenging to perform an effective landmark-based block. US guidance, however, allows for more accurate needle insertion into the appropriate fascial plane through which the LFCN passes.

ULTRASOUND ANATOMY

The LFCN typically is visualized between the tensor fasciae latae muscle (TFLM) and the sartorius muscle (SaM), 1–2 cm medial and inferior to the anterior superior iliac spine (ASIS) and 0.5–1.0 cm deep to the skin surface (Figure 33C–1). Ultrasound (US) imaging of the LFCN yields an oval hypoechoic small structure with a hyperechoic rim that can be easily seen in the hypoechoic background. The LFCN can be traced proximally, as it runs from the lateral to the medial edge of the superficial fascia of the SaM. The lateral edge of the SaM is a useful landmark, and as such, it can be relied on throughout the procedure. The posterior branch of the LFCN may sometimes be seen across the anterior margin of the TFLM.

DITRIBUTION OF ANESTHESIA

Block of the LFCN provides anesthesia or analgesia in the anterolateral thigh. There is a large variation in the area of sensory coverage among individuals because of the highly variable course of the LFCN and its branches (Figure 33C-2).

EQUIPMENT

The equipment recommended for an LFCN block is as follows:

- Ultrasound machine with linear transducer (18-6 MHz), sterile sleeve, and gel
- Standard nerve block tray
- Syringe(s) with 10 mL of local anesthetic
- 3–5 cm, 22- to 24-gauge needle
- Sterile gloves

LANDMARKS AND PATIENT POSITIONING

Block of the LFCN is performed with the patient in the supine or lateral position. Palpation of the anterior superior spine provides the initial landmark for transducer placement; the transducer is first positioned at 2 cm inferior and medial to the ASIS and adjusted accordingly. Typically, the nerve is identified slightly more distally in its course. Additional confirmation of

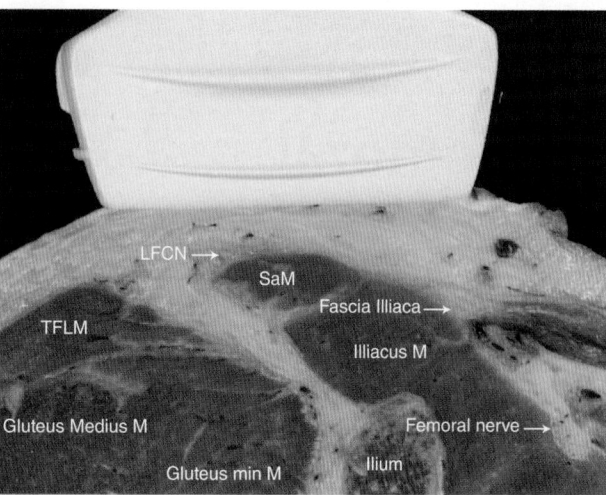

FIGURE 33C–1. Cross-sectional anatomy of the lateral femoral cutaneous nerve (LFCN). Shown are the LFCN, sartorius muscle (SaM), and tensor fasciae latae muscle (TFLM). (Reproduced with permission from Hadzic A: *Hadzic's Peripheral Nerve Blocks and Anatomy for Ultrasound-Guided Regional Anesthesia*, 2nd ed. New York: McGraw-Hill, 2011.)

the correct identification of the LFCN may be made by eliciting a tingling sensation on the lateral side of the thigh using a nerve stimulator.

GOAL

The goal is to inject local anesthetic in the plane between the TFLM and the SaM, typically 1–2 cm medial and inferior to the ASIS.

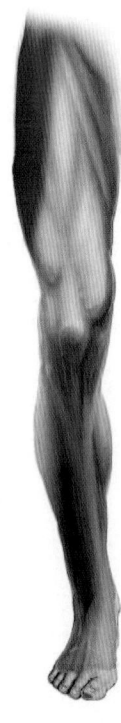

FIGURE 33C–2. Expected distribution of lateral femorocutaneous nerve sensory block.

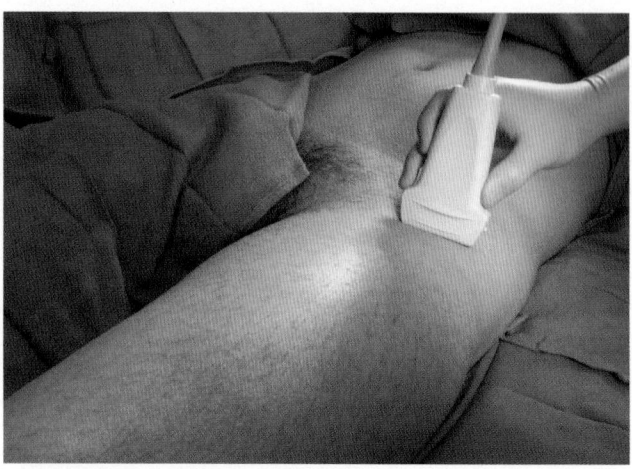

FIGURE 33C–3. Transducer position to accomplish a lateral femoral cutaneous nerve (LFCN) block.

TECHNIQUE

With the patient supine, the skin is disinfected and the transducer placed immediately inferior to the ASIS, parallel to the inguinal ligament (Figure 33C–3). The TFLM and SaM are then identified. The nerve should appear as a small hypoechoic oval structure with a hyperochoic rim between the TFLM and SaM in a short-axis view or superficial to the SaM (Figure 33C-4a).

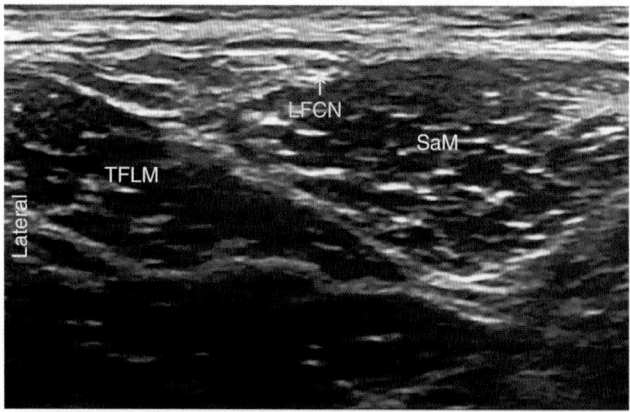

A

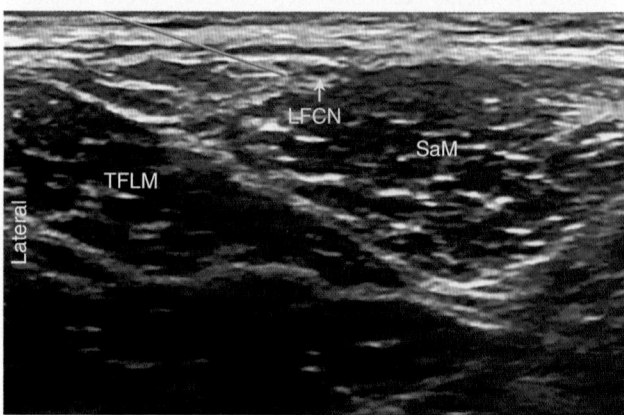

B

FIGURE 33C–4. (**A**) Ultrasound anatomy of the lateral femoral cutaneous nerve (LCFN). (**B**) Simulated needle path and local anesthetic spread (blue-shaded area) to anesthetize the LFCN.

The needle is inserted in plane in a lateral-to-medial orientation, through the subcutaneous tissue. A fascial "pop" or "click" may be felt as the needle tip enters the plane between the TFLM and SaM. A volume of 1–2 mL of local anesthetic is injected to verify the needle tip position. The correct position is achieved by visualizing the spread of local anesthetic in the described plane between the TFLM and SaM or around the LFCN superficial to the SaM (Figure 33C–4b).

TIPS

- A "subinguinal" technique has also been described, in which the US probe straddles the ASIS and the anterior inferior iliac spine (AIIS). Local anesthetic is injected under the inguinal ligament, 1–2 cm medial to the ASIS, without necessarily attempting to visualize the nerve.[3]
- In an adult patient, 5 mL of local anesthetic is usually sufficient. In children, a volume of 0.15 mL/kg per side is adequate for effective analgesia.

SUGGESTED READINGS

Bodner G, Bernathova M, Galiano K, Putz D, Martinoli C, Felfernig M: Ultrasound of the lateral femoral cutaneous nerve: normal findings in a cadaver and in volunteers. Reg Anesth Pain Med 2009;34:265–268.

Carai A, Fenu G, Sechi E, Crotti FM, Montella A: Anatomical variability of the lateral femoral cutaneous nerve: findings from a surgical series. Clin Anat 2009;22:365–370.

Damarey B, Demondion X, Boutry N, Kim HJ, Wavreille G, Cotten A: Sonographic assessment of the lateral femoral cutaneous nerve. J Clin Ultrasound 2009;37:89–95.

Hara K, Sakura S, Shido A: Ultrasound-guided lateral femoral cutaneous nerve block: comparison of two techniques. Anaesth Intensive Care 2011;39: 69–72.

Hebbard P, Ivanusic J, Sha S: Ultrasound-guided supra-inguinal fascia iliaca block: a cadaveric evaluation of a novel approach. Anaesthesia 2011;66: 300–305.

Hurdle MF, Weingarten TN, Crisostomo RA, Psimos C, Smith J: Ultrasound-guided blockade of the lateral femoral cutaneous nerve: technical description and review of 10 cases. Arch Phys Med Rehabil 2007;88: 1362–1364.

Ng I, Vaghadia H, Choi PT, Helmy N: Ultrasound imaging accurately identifies the lateral femoral cutaneous nerve. Anesth Analg 2008;107: 1070–1074.

Ropars M, Morandi X, Huten D, Thomazeau H, Berton E, Darnault P: Anatomical study of the lateral femoral cutaneous nerve with special reference to minimally invasive anterior approach for total hip replacement. Surg Radiol Anat 2009;31:199–204.

Sürücü HS, Tanyeli E, Sargon MF, Karahan ST: An anatomic study of the lateral femoral cutaneous nerve. Surg Radiol Anat 1997;19:307–310.

Tumber PS, Bhatia A, Chan VW: Ultrasound-guided lateral femoral cutaneous nerve block for meralgia paresthetica. Anesth Analg 2008;106:1021–1022.

REFERENCES

1. Corujo A, Franco CD, Williams JM: The sensory territory of the lateral cutaneous nerve of the thigh as determined by anatomic dissections and ultrasound-guided blocks. Reg Anesth Pain Med 2012;37:561–564.

2. Moritz T, Prosch H, Berzaczy D, et al: Common anatomical variation in patients with idiopathic meralgia paresthetica: a high resolution ultrasound case-control study. Pain Physician 2013;16:E287–293.

3. Hara K, Sakura S, Shido A: Ultrasound-guided lateral femoral cutaneous nerve block: comparison of two techniques. Anaesth Intensive Care 2011; 39:69–72.

CHAPTER 33D

Ultrasound-Guided Obturator Nerve Block

Sam Van Boxstael, Catherine Vandepitte, Philippe E. Gautier, and Hassanin Jalil

OBTURATOR NERVE BLOCK AT A GLANCE

- Indications: Relief of painful adductor muscle contractions, to prevent adduction of the thigh during transurethral bladder surgery, additional analgesia after major knee surgery, and may provide postoperative analgesia after hamstring tendon harvest for anterior cruciate ligament (ACL) reconstruction (Figure 33D–1).[1,2]
- Transducer position: medial aspect of the proximal thigh.
- Goal: Local anesthetic spread in the interfascial plane in which the nerves lie or around the anterior and posterior branches of the obturator nerve.
- Local anesthetic: 5 mL into each interfascial space or around the branches of the obturator nerve.

GENERAL CONSIDERATIONS

Ultrasound (US)-guided obturator nerve block is simpler to perform and more reliable than surface landmark–based techniques. There are two approaches to performing a US-guided obturator nerve block. The interfascial injection technique relies on injecting local anesthetic solution into the fascial planes that contain the branches of the obturator nerve. With this technique, it is not important to identify the branches of the obturator nerve on the sonogram, but rather to identify the adductor muscles and the fascial boundaries within which the nerves lie. This is similar in concept to other fascial plane blocks (eg, the transversus abdominis plane [TAP] block in which local anesthetic solution is injected between the internal oblique and transverse abdominis muscles without the need to identify the nerves). Alternatively, the branches of the obturator nerve can be visualized with US imaging and blocked after eliciting a motor response.

ULTRASOUND ANATOMY

The obturator nerve forms in the lumbar plexus from the anterior primary rami of the L2–L4 roots and descends to the pelvis on the medial side of the psoas muscle. In most individuals, the nerve divides into an anterior branch and posterior branch before exiting the pelvis through the obturator foramen. In the thigh, at the level of the femoral crease, the **anterior branch** is located between the fascia of the pectineus and adductor brevis muscles. The anterior branch lies further caudad between the adductor longus and adductor brevis muscles. The anterior branch provides motor fibers to the adductor longus, brevis and gracilis muscles; and cutaneous branches to the medial aspect of the thigh. The anterior branch has a great variability in the extent of sensory innervation of the medial thigh.

The **posterior branch** lies between the fascial planes of the adductor brevis and adductor magnus muscles (Figures 33D–2 and 33D–3). The posterior branch is primarily a motor nerve for the adductors of the thigh; however, it also may provide articular branches to the medial aspect of the knee joint. The articular branches to the hip joint usually arise from the obturator nerve, proximal to its division and only occasionally from the individual branches (Figure 33D–4). In 8–30% of patients, an accessory obturator nerve arises from L3 and L4, travels with the femoral nerve, and gives branches to the hip joint.[2]

A helpful mnemonic to remember the order of the adductor muscles, from anterior to posterior, is as follows: Alabama: Adductor Longus, Adductor Brevis, Adductor MAgnus.

Clinical Pearl

- A psoas compartment (lumbar plexus) block is required to reliably block the articular branches of the obturator nerve to the hip joint because they usually depart proximal to the level at which the obturator nerve block is performed in the proximal thigh.

DISTRIBUTION OF ANESTHESIA

Because there is great variability in the cutaneous innervation to the medial thigh, demonstrated weakness of adductor muscle

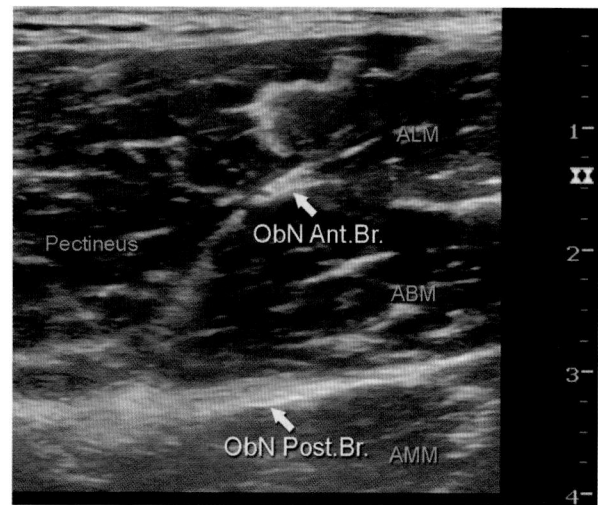

Obturator nerve-transverse view

FIGURE 33D–3. The anterior branch (ant. br.) of the obturator nerve (ObN) is seen between the adductor longus muscle (ALM) and the adductor brevis muscle (ABM), whereas the posterior branch (post. br.) is seen between the ABM and the adductor magnus muscle (AMM). (Reproduced with permission from Hadzic A: *Hadzic's Peripheral Nerve Blocks and Anatomy for Ultrasound-Guided Regional Anesthesia*, 2nd ed. New York: McGraw-Hill, Inc.; 2011.)

magnus). Adductor motor strength is decreased by about 25% following femoral nerve blockade and 11% following sciatic nerve blockade. For this reason, complete loss of adductor muscle strength is uncommon despite a successful obturator nerve block.

Clinical Pearl

- A simple method of assessing adductor muscle strength (motor block) is to instruct the patient to adduct the blocked leg from an abducted position against resistance. Weakness or inability to adduct the leg indicates a successful obturator nerve block.

EQUIPMENT

The equipment recommended for an obturator nerve block includes the following:

- Ultrasound machine with linear (or curved) transducer (5–13 MHz), sterile sleeve, and gel
- Standard block tray
- A 10-mL syringe containing local anesthetic solution
- A 10-cm, 21- to 22-gauge, short-bevel, insulated needle
- Peripheral nerve stimulator (optional)
- Sterile gloves

LANDMARKS AND PATIENT POSITIONING

With the patient supine, the thigh is slightly abducted and laterally rotated. The block can be performed either at the level of femoral (inguinal) crease medial to the femoral vein or 1–3 cm

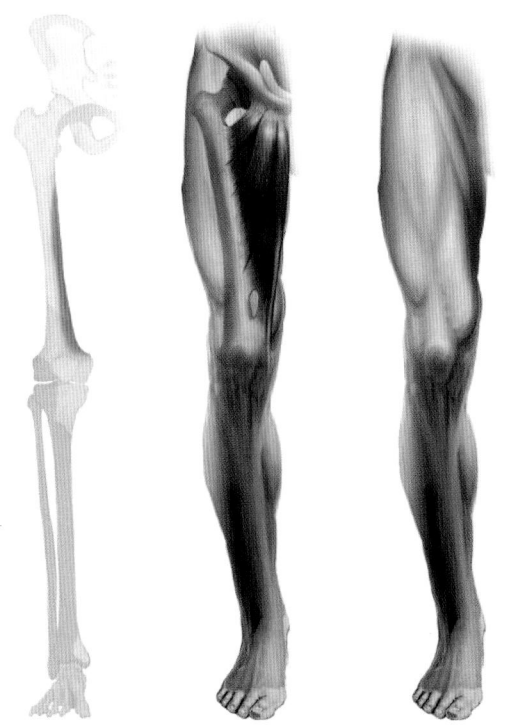

FIGURE 33D–1. Expected distribution of obturator nerve sensory and motor blockade.

strength is the only reliable method of documenting a successful obturator nerve block (Figure 33D-1). However, the adductor muscles of the thigh may have co-innervation from the femoral nerve (pectineus) and the sciatic nerve (adductor

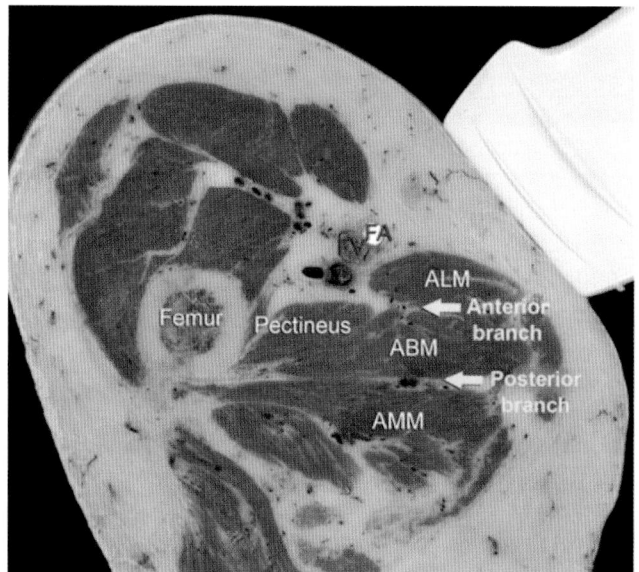

FIGURE 33D–2. Cross-sectional anatomy of relevance to the obturator nerve block. Shown are the femoral vessels (the femoral vein [FV] and femoral artery [FA]), pectineus muscle, adductor longus muscle (ALM), adductor brevis muscle (ABM), and adductor magnus muscle (AMM). The anterior branch of the obturator nerve is seen between the ALM and ABM, whereas the posterior branch is seen between the ABM and AMM. (Reproduced with permission from Hadzic A: *Hadzic's Peripheral Nerve Blocks and Anatomy for Ultrasound-Guided Regional Anesthesia*, 2nd ed. New York: McGraw-Hill, 2011.)

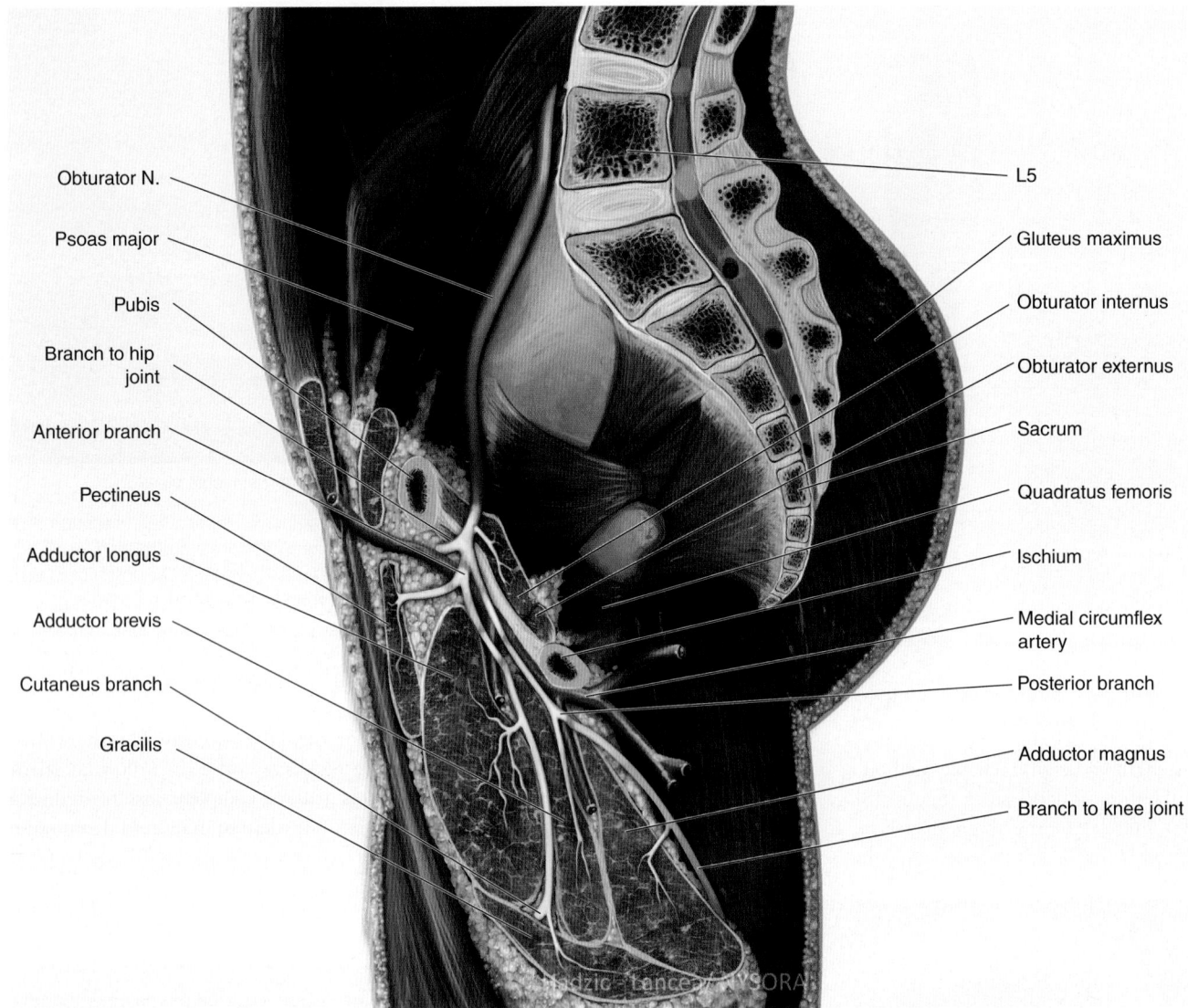

FIGURE 33D-4. The course and divisions of the obturator nerve and its relationship to the adductor muscles.

inferior to the inguinal crease on the medial aspect (adductor compartment) of the thigh (Figure 33D–5).

GOAL

The goal of the interfascial injection technique for blocking the obturator nerve is to inject local anesthetic solution into the interfascial space between the pectineus and adductor brevis muscles to block the *anterior* branch and the adductor brevis and adductor magnus muscles to block the *posterior* branch. When using US guidance with nerve stimulation, the anterior and posterior branches of the obturator nerve are identified and stimulated to elicit a motor response prior to injecting local anesthetic solution around each branch.

TECHNIQUE

The **interfascial approach** is performed at the level of the femoral crease. With this technique, it is important to identify the adductor muscles and the fascial planes in which the individual nerves are enveloped. Color Doppler can be used to visualize the obturator arteries located near the nerve branches in order to avoid puncturing them, although they are not always visible.

The US transducer is placed to visualize the femoral vessels. The transducer is advanced medially along the crease to identify the adductor muscles and their fasciae. The anterior branch is sandwiched between the pectineus and adductor brevis muscles, whereas the posterior branch is located in the fascial plane between the adductor brevis and adductor magnus muscles. The block needle is advanced to initially position the needle tip between the pectineus and adductor brevis (Figure 33D–6a). At this point, 5–10 mL of local anesthetic solution is injected. The needle is advanced farther to position the needle tip between the adductor brevis and adductor magnus muscles, and another 5–10 mL of local anesthetic solution is injected (Figure 33D–6b). It is important for the local anesthetic solution to spread into the interfascial space and not be injected into the muscles. Correct injection of local anesthetic solution into the interfascial space results in an accumulation of the injectate between the

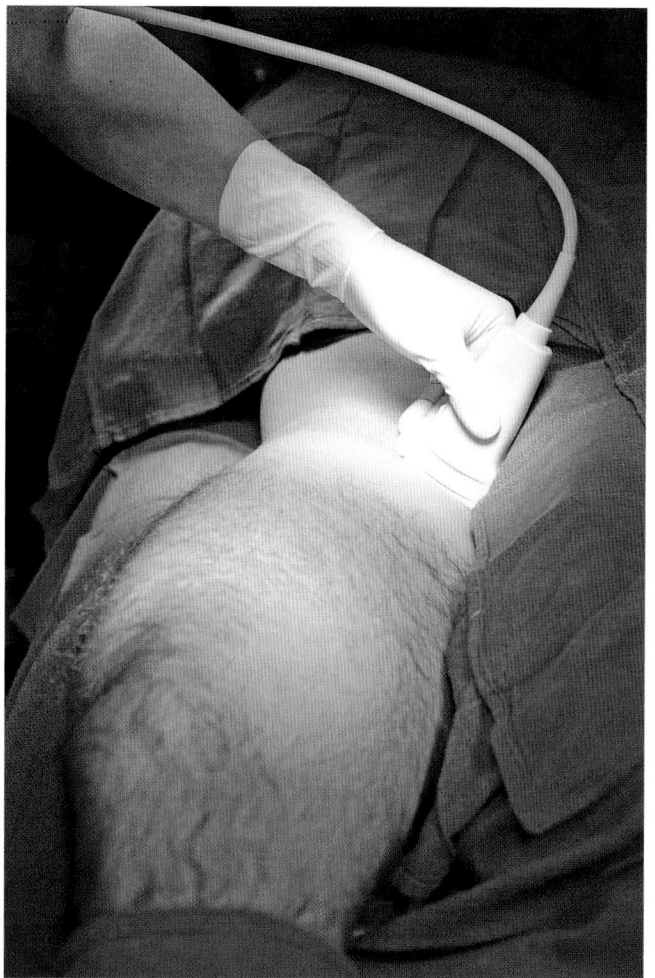

FIGURE 33D-5. Transducer position to image the obturator nerve. The transducer is positioned medial to the femoral artery, slightly below the femoral crease. (Reproduced with permission from Hadzic A: *Hadzic's Peripheral Nerve Blocks and Anatomy for Ultrasound-Guided Regional Anesthesia*, 2nd ed. New York: McGraw-Hill, Inc.; 2011.)

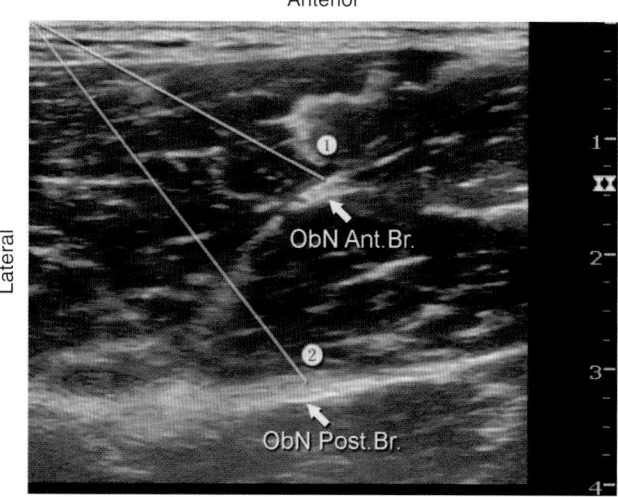

A   Lateral Obturator nerve-transverse view

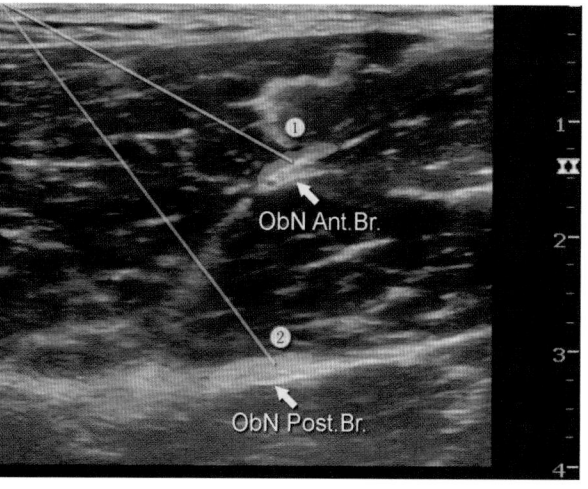

B   Obturator nerve-transverse view

FIGURE 33D-6. (**A**) Needle paths (1, 2) required to reach the anterior branch (ant. br.) and posterior branch (post. br.) of the obturator nerve (ObN). (**B**) Simulated dispersion of local anesthetic (blue-shaded areas) to block the anterior and posterior branches of the obturator nerve. In both examples, an in-plane needle insertion has been used. (Reproduced with permission from Hadzic A: *Hadzic's Peripheral Nerve Blocks and Anatomy for Ultrasound-Guided Regional Anesthesia*, 2nd ed. New York: McGraw-Hill, Inc.; 2011.)

target muscles. The needle may have to be repositioned to allow for precise interfascial injection.

Alternatively, the cross-sectional image of obturator nerve branches can be obtained by scanning 1–3 cm distal to the inguinal crease on the medial aspect of thigh. The nerves appear as hyperechoic, flat, thin, fusiform-shaped structures invested in the fascia of the adductor muscles. The anterior branch is located between the adductor longus and adductor brevis muscles, whereas the posterior branch is located between the adductor brevis and adductor magnus muscles. An insulated block needle attached to the nerve stimulator is advanced toward the nerve with either an out-of-plane or in-plane trajectory. After eliciting contraction of the adductor muscles, 5–7 mL of local anesthetic is injected around each branch of the obturator nerve (see Figure 33D–6b).

SUGGESTED READINGS

Akkaya T, Comert A, Kendir S, et al: Detailed anatomy of accessory obturator nerve blockade. Minerva Anestesiol 2008;74:119–122.

Akkaya T, Ozturk E, Comert A, et al. Ultrasound-guided obturator nerve block: a sonoanatomic study of a new methodologic approach. Anesth Analg 2009;108:1037–1041.

Anagnostopoulou S, Kostopanagiotou G, Paraskeuopoulos T, Chantzi C, Lolis E, Saranteas T: Anatomic variations of the obturator nerve in the inguinal region: implications in conventional and ultrasound regional anesthesia techniques. Reg Anesth Pain Med 2009;34:33–39.

Bouaziz H, Vial F, Jochum D, et al: An evaluation of the cutaneous distribution after obturator nerve block. Anesth Analg 2002;94:445–449.

Macalou D, Trueck S, Meuret P, et al. Postoperative analgesia after total knee replacement: the effect of an obturator nerve block added to the femoral 3-in-1 nerve block. Anesth Analg 2004;99:251–254.

Marhofer P, Harrop-Griffiths W, Willschke H, Kirchmair L: Fifteen years of ultrasound guidance in regional anaesthesia: part 2—recent developments in block techniques. Br J Anaesth 2010;104:673–683.

McNamee DA, Parks L, Milligan KR: Post-operative analgesia following total knee replacement: an evaluation of the addition of an obturator nerve block to combined femoral and sciatic nerve block. Acta Anaesthesiol Scand 2002;46:95–99.

Sakura S, Hara K, Ota J, Tadenuma S: Ultrasound-guided peripheral nerve blocks for anterior cruciate ligament reconstruction: effect of obturator nerve block during and after surgery. J Anesth 2010;24:411–417.

Sinha SK, Abrams JH, Houle T, Weller R: Ultrasound guided obturator nerve block: an interfascial injection approach without nerve stimulation. Reg Anesth Pain Med 2009;34:261–264.

Snaith R, Dolan J: Ultrasound-guided interfascial injection for peripheral obturator nerve block in the thigh. Reg Anesth Pain Med 2010;35: 314–315.

Soong J, Schafhalter-Zoppoth I, Gray AT: Sonographic imaging of the obturator nerve for regional block. Reg Anesth Pain Med 2007;32: 146–151.

Taha AM: Brief reports: ultrasound-guided obturator nerve block: a proximal interfascial technique. Anesth Analg 2012;114:236–239.

REFERENCES

1. Sakura S, Hara K, Ota J, Tadenuma S: Ultrasound-guided peripheral nerve blocks for anterior cruciate ligament reconstruction: effect of obturator nerve block during and after surgery. J Anesth 2010;24: 411–417.
2. Akkaya T, Comert A, Kendir S, et al: Detailed anatomy of accessory obturator nerve blockade. Minerva Anestesiol 2008;74:119–122.

Ultrasound-Guided Saphenous (Subsartorius/Adductor Canal) Nerve Block

Thomas F. Bendtsen, Ana M. Lopez, and Thomas B. Clark

SAPHENOUS NERVE BLOCK AT A GLANCE

- Indications: saphenous vein stripping or harvesting; supplementation for medial foot/ankle surgery in combination with a sciatic nerve block, and analgesia for knee surgery in combination with multimodal analgesia.
- Transducer position: transverse on anteromedial thigh at the junction between the middle and distal third of the thigh or below the knee at the level of the tibial tuberosity, depending on the approach chosen (proximal or distal) (Figure 33E–1)
- Goal: local anesthetic spread lateral to the femoral artery and deep to the sartorius muscle or more distal, below the knee, adjacent to the saphenous vein.
- Local anesthetic: 5–10 mL

GENERAL CONSIDERATIONS

The saphenous nerve is a terminal sensory branch of the femoral nerve. It supplies innervation to the medial aspect of the leg down to the ankle and foot. It also sends infrapatellar branches to the knee joint. A saphenous nerve block is useful as a supplement to sciatic block for foot and ankle procedures that involve the medial aspect of the malleolus and the foot. The block has also been reported as a supplement to multimodal analgesia protocols in patients having knee arthroplasty. Typically, a more proximal (mid-thigh) approach and a larger volume of local anesthetic is used for this "adductor canal block". Several approaches have been described to block the saphenous nerve along its route from the inguinal area to the medial malleolus (Figure 33E–2). The use of ultrasound (US) guidance has improved the success rates of the saphenous blocks compared with field blocks below the knee and blind transsartorial approaches.

ULTRASOUND ANATOMY

The sartorius muscle descends in a lateral to medial direction across the anterior thigh and forms a "roof" over the adductor canal in the lower half of the thigh. The muscle appears as a trapezoid shape beneath the subcutaneous layer of adipose tissue. The sides of the triangular canal are formed by the vastus medialis laterally and the adductor longus or magnus medially (depending on how proximal or distal the scan is). The saphenous nerve is typically imaged by ultrasound as a small, round, hyperechoic structure anterior to the artery. The femoral vein accompanies the artery and saphenous nerve, which all can be identified at a depth of 2–3 cm (Figure 33E-3). When attempting to identify the saphenous nerve on US image, the following anatomical considerations should be kept in mind:

- Above the knee: The saphenous nerve pierces the fascia lata between the tendons of the sartorius and gracilis muscles before becoming a subcutaneous nerve.
- The saphenous nerve lies in close proximity to several vessels along its trajectory: the femoral artery above the knee, the descending genicular artery and its saphenous branch at the knee, and the great saphenous vein in the lower leg and ankle.
- Below the knee, the saphenous nerve passes along the tibial side of the leg, adjacent to the great saphenous vein subcutaneously (Figure 33E–4).

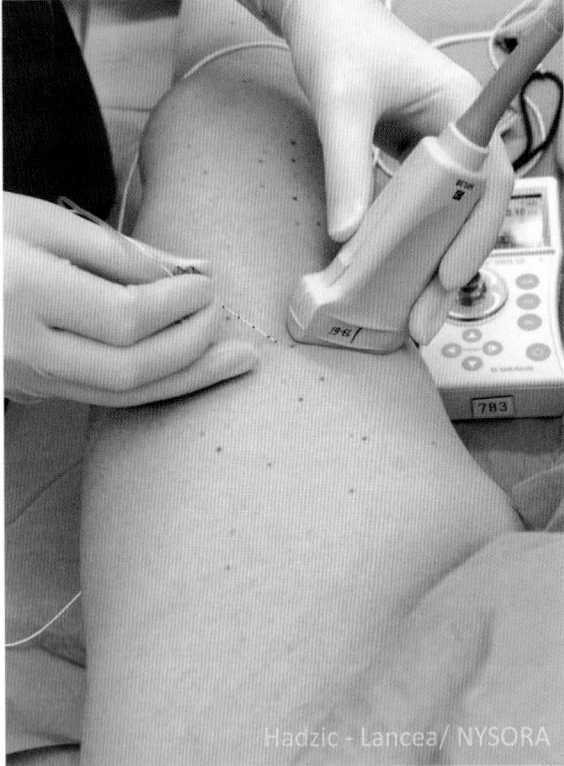

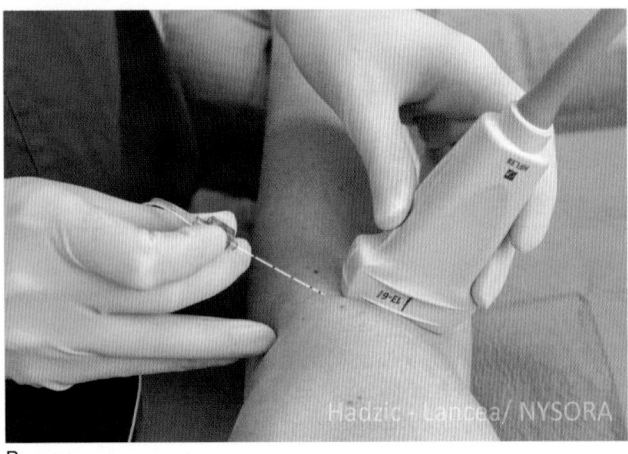

FIGURE 33E–1. Transducer position and needle insertion to block the saphenous nerve (**A**) at the level of the lower third of the thigh and (**B**) below the knee.

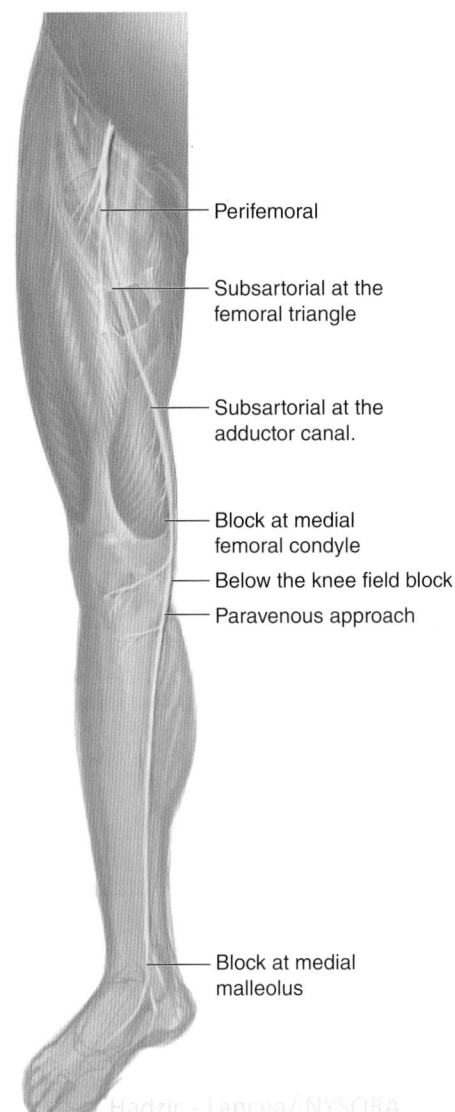

- Perifemoral
- Subsartorial at the femoral triangle
- Subsartorial at the adductor canal.
- Block at medial femoral condyle
- Below the knee field block
- Paravenous approach
- Block at medial malleolus

FIGURE 33E–2. Various approaches to the saphenous nerve block: the perifemoral typically targets the nerve to the vastus medialis muscle with nerve stimulation; the subsartorial at the femoral riangle; subsartorial at the adductor canal; at the medial femoral condyle, between the tendons of the sartorius and the gracilis muscle; once the femoral vessels have crossed the adductor hiatus to become the popliteal vessels; the paravenous approach using the saphenous vein as a landmark at the level of the tibial tuberosity; and at the level of the medial malleolus.[1]

- At the ankle, branches of the saphenous nerve are located medially, next to the subcutaneously positioned saphenous vein.

DISTRIBUTION OF ANESTHESIA

The saphenous nerve block results in anesthesia of the skin on the medial leg and foot (Figure 33E-5). For a more comprehensive review of the femoral and saphenous nerve distributions, see Chapter 3. Of note, although the saphenous nerve block is a sensory block, an injection of a large volume of local anesthetic into the subsartorial space can result in a partial motor block of the vastus medialis due to the block of the femoral nerve branch to this muscle, often contain in the canal. For this reason, caution must be taken when advising patients regarding the safety of unsupported ambulation after undergoing a proximal saphenous block.

EQUIPMENT

- Ultrasound machine with linear transducer (8–14 MHz), sterile sleeve, and gel
- Standard nerve block tray

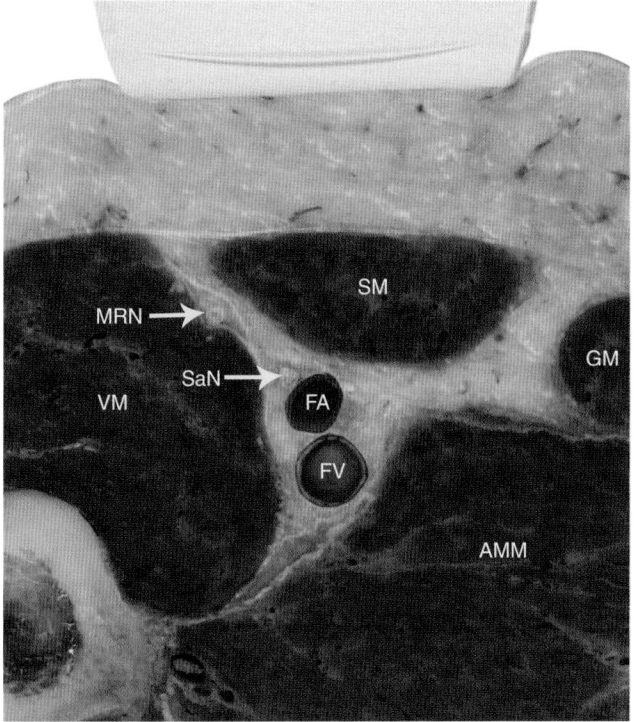

A

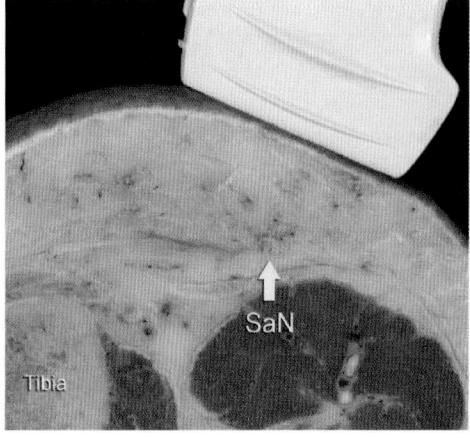

A

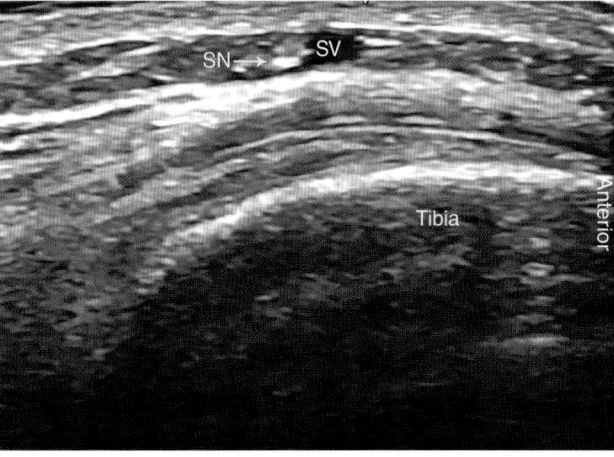

B

FIGURE 33E–4. (**A**) Cross-sectional anatomy of the saphenous nerve (SaN) at the level of the tibial tuberosity. (**B**) US image of the SaN below the knee. The SaN is seen within the immediate vicinity of the great saphenous vein (SV). The transducer should be applied lightly to avoid compression of the SV because the vein serves as an important landmark for the technique.

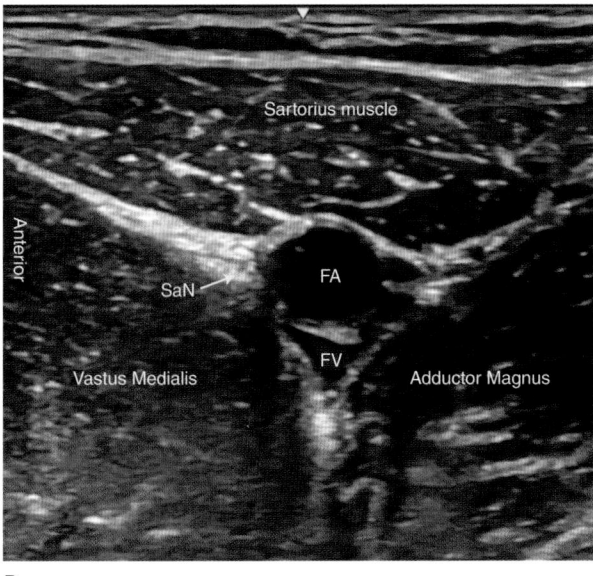

B

FIGURE 33E–3. (**A**) Cross-sectional anatomy of the saphenous nerve at the level of the thigh. The saphenous nerve (SaN) is positioned between the sartorius muscle (SM) and the vastus medialis muscle (VM), anterolateral to the femoral artery (FA) and vein (FV). AMM, adductor magnus muscles; GM, gracilis muscle; MRN, medial retinacular nerve. (**B**) US anatomy of the subsartorial space at the midthigh.

LANDMARKS AND PATIENT POSITIONING FOR THE PROXIMAL APPROACH

The patient is placed in any position that allows for comfortable placement of the US transducer and needle advancement. This block typically is performed with the patient in the supine position, with the thigh abducted and externally rotated to allow access to the medial thigh (see Figure 33E–1a).

GOAL

The goal is to place the needle tip just anterior to the femoral artery, deep to the sartorius muscle, and to deposit 5–10 mL (or up to 20 mL for the adductor canal block) of local anesthetic until its spread around the artery is confirmed with US visualization. Block of the nerve at other, more distal and superficial locations consists of a simple subcutaneous infiltration of the tissues within the immediate vicinity of the nerve under US guidance.

- One 10-mL syringe containing local anesthetic
- A 80 mm 22-25 gauge needle
- Peripheral nerve stimulator to elicit paresthesia
- Sterile gloves

TECHNIQUE

The skin is disinfected and the transducer is placed anteromedially, approximately at the junction between the middle and distal third of the thigh or somewhat lower. If the artery is not immediately obvious, several maneuvers can be used to identify it, including color Doppler scanning to trace the femoral artery caudally from the inguinal crease. Once the femoral artery has been identified, the probe is moved distally to trace the artery until it passes through the adductor hiatus to become the popliteal artery.

The saphenous nerve block should be performed at the most distal level where the artery still lies immediately deep to the sartorius muscle, thus minimizing the amount of motor block of the vastus medialis; an adductor canal block is typically performed more proximally, around the mid-thigh level. The needle is inserted in plane in a lateral-to-medial orientation and advanced toward the femoral artery (Figure 33E-1a and 33E-6). If nerve stimulation is used (1 mA, 1 msec), the passage of the needle through the sartorius and/or adductor muscles and into the adductor canal is usually associated with a paresthesia in the saphenous nerve distribution. Once the needle tip is visualized anterior to the artery and after careful aspiration, 1–2 mL of local anesthetic is injected to confirm the proper injection site (Figure 33E–6). When injection of local anesthetic does not appear to result in its spread around the femoral artery, additional needle repositions and injections may be necessary.

Color Doppler can be used to locate the perisaphenous branch of the descending geniculate artery in order to avoid puncturing it.

Because the saphenous nerve is a purely sensory nerve, high concentrations of local anesthetic are not required and in fact

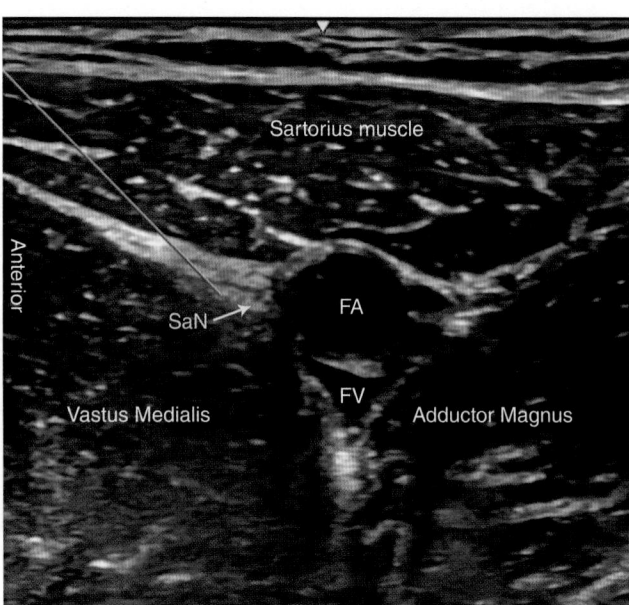

FIGURE 33E-6. Simulated needle path, needle tip position and local anesthetic initial distribution (blue-shaded area) to anesthetize the Saphenous nerve (SaN) at the level of the thigh. FA, femoral artery: FV, femoral vein.

may delay patient ambulation should local anesthetic spread to one of the motor branches of the femoral nerve innervating the quadriceps muscle.

TIPS

- An out-of-plane technique can also be used through the belly of the sartorius muscle. Because the needle tip may not be seen throughout the procedure, small boluses of local anesthetic are administered (0.5–1 mL) as the needle is advanced toward the adductor canal to confirm the location of the needle tip.
- Visualization of the nerve is *not* necessary for this block, as the saphenous nerve is not always well imaged. Administration of 5–10 mL of local anesthetic next to the artery in the plane between the sartorius and vastus medialis muscles should suffice without confirming nerve position.
- Practitioners should be aware of the potential for partial quadriceps weakness following a more proximal approach along the subsartorial space and/or njection of a large volume (20-30 mL) of local anesthetic. Patient education and assistance with ambulation should be encouraged. For that reason, it is recommended to perform this block as distally as practically possible.

SUGGESTED READINGS

Bendtsen TF, Moriggl B, Chan V, Børglum J. Basic Topography of the Saphenous Nerve in the Femoral Triangle and the Adductor Canal. Reg Anesth Pain Med. 2015;40(4):391–2.

Davis JJ, Bond TS, Swenson JD: Adductor canal block: more than just the saphenous nerve? Reg Anesth Pain Med 2009;34:618–619.

Goffin P, Lecoq JP, Ninane V, Brichant JF, Sala-Blanch X, Gautier PE et al. Interfascial Spread of Injectate After Adductor Canal Injection in Fresh Human Cadavers. Anesth Analg. 2016 Aug;123(2):501–3.

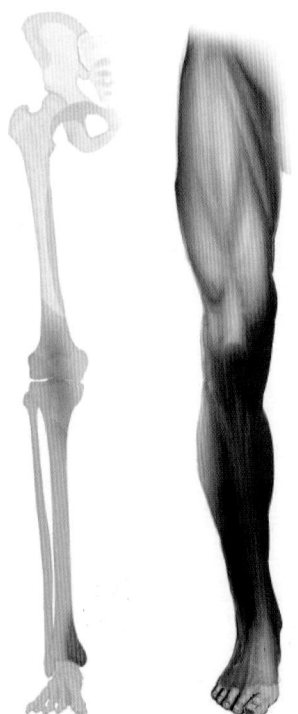

FIGURE 33E–5. Expected distribution of analgesia after saphenous nerve block at the level of midthigh.

Gray AT, Collins AB: Ultrasound-guided saphenous nerve block. Reg Anesth Pain Med 2003;28:148.

Head SJ, Leung RC, Hackman GP, Seib R, Rondi K, Schwarz SK: Ultrasound-guided saphenous nerve block--within versus distal to the adductor canal: a proof-of-principle randomized trial. Can J Anaesth 2015;62: 37–44.

Horn JL, Pitsch T, Salinas F, Benninger B: Anatomic basis to the ultrasound-guided approach for saphenous nerve blockade. Reg Anesth Pain Med 2009;34:486–489.

Kapoor R, Adhikary SD, Siefring C, McQuillan PM: The saphenous nerve and its relationship to the nerve to the vastus medialis in and around the adductor canal: an anatomical study. Acta Anaesthesiol Scand 2012;56: 365–367.

Kirkpatrick JD, Sites BD, Antonakakis JG: Preliminary experience with a new approach to performing an ultrasound-guided saphenous nerve block in the mid- to proximal femur. Reg Anesth Pain Med 2010;35:222–223.

Krombach J, Gray AT: Sonography for saphenous nerve block near the adductor canal. Reg Anesth Pain Med 2007;32:369–370.

Lundblad M, Kapral S, Marhofer P, et al: Ultrasound-guided infrapatellar nerve block in human volunteers: description of a novel technique. Br J Anaesth 2006;97:710–714.

Manickam B, Perlas A, Duggan E, Brull R, Chan VW, Ramlogan R: Feasibility and efficacy of ultrasound-guided block of the saphenous nerve in the adductor canal. Reg Anesth Pain Med 2009;34:578–580.

Marsland D, Dray A, Little NJ, Solan MC: The saphenous nerve in foot and ankle surgery: its variable anatomy and relevance. Foot Ankle Surg 2013;19:76–79.

Miller BR: Ultrasound-guided proximal tibial paravenous saphenous nerve block in pediatric patients. Paediatr Anaesth 2010;20:1059–1060.

Pannell WC, Wisco JJ: A novel saphenous nerve plexus with important clinical correlations. Clin Anat 2011;24:994–996.

Sahin L, Sahin M, Isikay N: A different approach to an ultrasound-guided saphenous nerve block. Acta Anaesthesiol Scand 2011;55:1030–1031.

Saranteas T, Anagnostis G, Paraskeuopoulos T, et al: Anatomy and clinical implications of the ultrasound-guided subsartorial saphenous nerve block. Reg Anesth Pain Med 2011;36:399–402.

Tsai PB, Karnwal A, Kakazu C, Tokhner V, Julka IS: Efficacy of an ultrasound-guided subsartorial approach to saphenous nerve block: a case series. Can J Anaesth 2010;57:683–688.

Tsui BC, Ozelsel T: Ultrasound-guided transsartorial perifemoral artery approach for saphenous nerve block. Reg Anesth Pain Med 2009;34: 177–178.

REFERENCE

1. Sahin L, Sahin M, Isikay N: A different approach to an ultrasound-guided saphenous nerve block. Acta Anaesthesiol Scand 2011;55:1030–1031.

CHAPTER 33F

Ultrasound-Guided Sciatic Nerve Block

Arthur Atchabahian, Catherine Vandepitte, Ana M. Lopez, and Jui-An Lin

SCIATIC NERVE BLOCK AT A GLANCE

- Indications: foot and ankle surgery, below-knee amputation, analgesia following knee surgery involving the posterior compartment (Figure 33F–1)
- Transducer position:
  - Anterior approach: transverse on the proximal medial thigh

- Transgluteal approach: transverse on the posterior buttock, between the ischial tuberosity and greater trochanter
- Subgluteal approach: transverse on the gluteal crease
- Other approaches (eg, parasacral, lateral) have been described but will not be detailed here.
- Goal: local anesthetic spread within the sciatic nerve sheath
- Local anesthetic: 10–20 mL

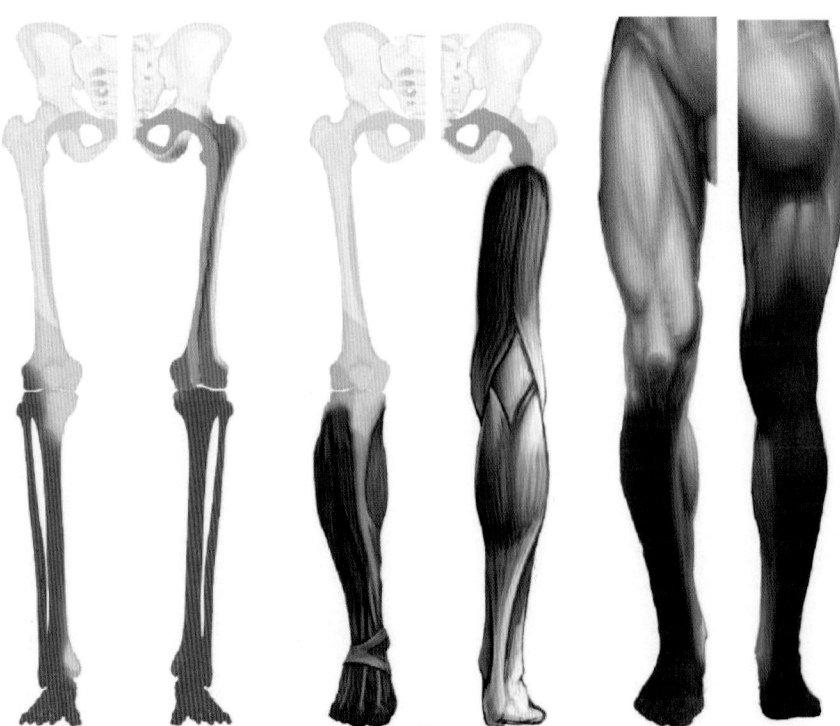

FIGURE 33F–1. Distribution of sensory and motor after sciatic nerve blockade at gluteal and subgluteal level.

PART I: ANTERIOR APPROACH

GENERAL CONSIDERATIONS

The anterior approach to the sciatic nerve block can be useful in patients who cannot be positioned in the lateral position due to pain, trauma, the presence of external fixation devices that interfere with positioning, or other issues. The ultrasound (US)-guided approach may reduce the risk of femoral artery puncture compared with the landmark-based approach. The actual scanning and needle insertion are performed on the anteromedial aspect of the proximal thigh, rather than the anterior surface, and may require a slight abduction and external rotation of the thigh. This block is not well-suited to catheter insertion because a large needle must traverse several muscles (discomfort during procedure and risk of hematoma), it is an awkward catheter location (medial thigh), and catheter insertion at an approximately perpendicular angle to the sciatic nerve is difficult.

ULTRASOUND ANATOMY

The sciatic nerve is imaged approximately at the level of the minor trochanter. At this location, a curved transducer placed over the anteromedial aspect of the thigh will reveal the musculature of all three fascial compartments of the thigh: anterior, medial, and posterior (Figures 33F–2 and 33F–3). Beneath the sartorius muscle is the femoral artery, and deep and medial to this vessel is the deep artery of the thigh. Both can be identified with color Doppler US for orientation. The femur is seen as a

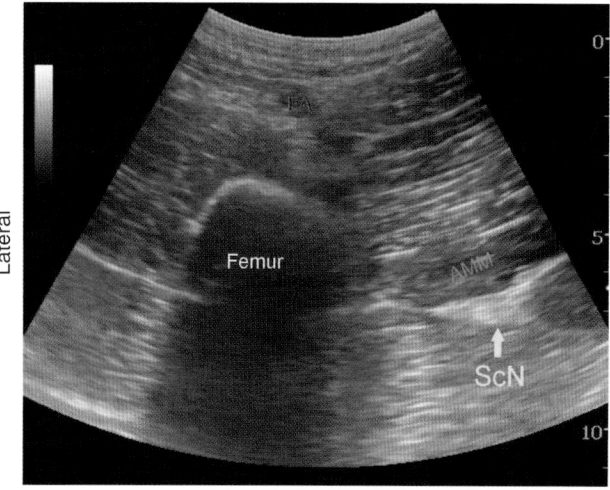

Sciatic nerve block-anterior approach

FIGURE 33F–3. Ultrasound anatomy of the sciatic nerve. From superficial to deep, visualized laterally: femoral artery (FA), femur, adductor magnus muscle (AMM), and sciatic nerve (ScN) laterally. The sciatic nerve is typically located at a depth of 6–8 cm. (Reproduced with permission from Hadzic A: *Hadzic's Peripheral Nerve Blocks and Anatomy for Ultrasound-Guided Regional Anesthesia,* 2nd ed. New York: McGraw-Hill, 2011.)

hyperechoic rim with a corresponding shadow beneath the vastus intermedius. Medial to the femur is the adductor magnus muscle, anterior to the hamstring muscles. The sciatic nerve is visualized as a hyperechoic oval structure sandwiched between these two muscle. The nerve is typically visualized at a depth of 6–8 cm (see Figure 33F–3).

DISTRIBUTION OF ANESTHESIA

The sciatic nerve block results in anesthesia of the posterior aspect of the knee, hamstring muscles, and entire lower limb below the knee, both motor and sensory blockade, with the exception of skin on the medial leg and foot (supplied by the saphenous nerve) (Figure 33F–1). The skin of the posterior aspect of the thigh is supplied by the posterior femoro cutaneous nerve, which deviates away from in the sciatic nerve proximal to the level of the anterior approach, and is therefore not blocked. Unless the surgical incision involves the posterior thigh, the lack of anesthesia in its distribution is of little clinical consequence, as pain caused by a thigh tourniquet, for example, is due more to muscle ischemia than to pressure on the skin.

EQUIPMENT

The equipment recommended for a sciatic nerve block using the anterior approach is as follows:

- Ultrasound machine with curved (phased array) transducer (2–8 MHz), sterile sleeve, and gel
- Standard nerve block tray

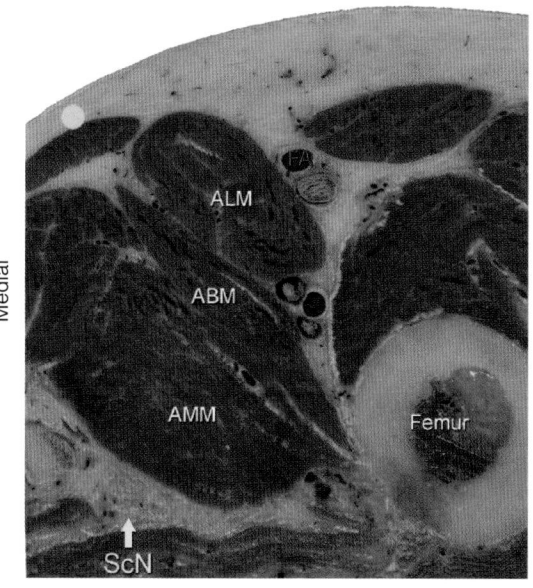

Sciatic Nerve - Anterior Approach, Transverse View

FIGURE 33F–2. Cross-sectional anatomy of the sciatic nerve (ScN). Shown are the femoral artery (FA), adductor longus muscle (ALM), adductor magnus muscle (AMM), adductor brevis muscle (ABM), and femur. The sciatic nerve is seen posterior to the AMM.

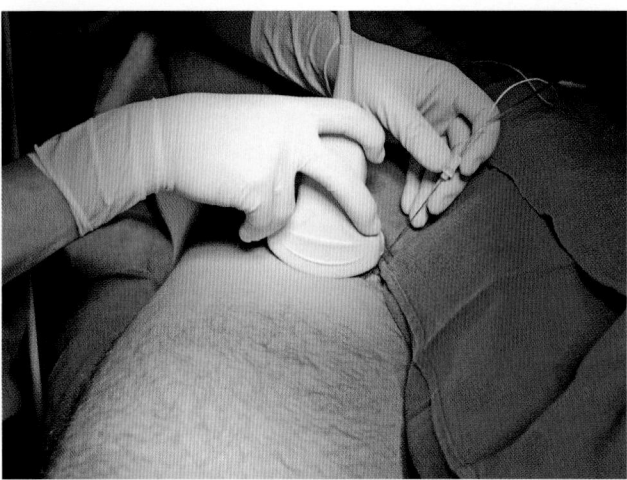

FIGURE 33F–4. Transducer position to visualize the sciatic nerve using the anterior approach. (Reproduced with permission from Hadzic A: *Hadzic's Peripheral Nerve Blocks and Anatomy for Ultrasound-Guided Regional Anesthesia*, 2nd ed. New York: McGraw-Hill, 2011.)

- One 20-mL syringe containing local anesthetic
- A 100- or 120-mm, 21-gauge, short-bevel, insulated stimulating needle
- Peripheral nerve stimulator
- Sterile gloves
- Injection pressure monitor

LANDMARKS AND PATIENT POSITIONING

The anterior approach to the sciatic nerve block is performed with the patient in the supine position. The hip is abducted to facilitate transducer and needle placement (Figures 33F–4 and 33F–5). When feasible, the hip and knee should be somewhat flexed to facilitate exposure. If nerve stimulation is to be used at the same time (this is recommended), exposure of the calf and foot are required to observe motor responses. In either case, it is useful to expose the entire thigh to appreciate the distance from the groin to the knee.

GOAL

The goal is to place the needle tip immediately adjacent to the sciatic nerve, between the adductor magnus muscle and biceps femoris muscle.

TECHNIQUE

With the patient in the proper position, the skin is disinfected and the transducer positioned to identify the sciatic nerve. If the nerve is not immediately apparent, sliding and tilting the transducer proximally or distally can be useful to improve the contrast and bring the nerve "out of the background" from the musculature. If the patient is able to dorsiflex and/or plantar flex the ankle, this maneuver often causes the nerve to move within the intermuscular plane, facilitating identification. The needle is inserted in plane from the medial aspect of the thigh, or out of plane, and advanced toward the sciatic nerve (see Figure 33F–5). An in-plane approach may prove less practical due to the steep angle of the needle and the use of a curved (nonlinear) probe. If nerve stimulation is used (1.0 mA, 0.1 msec), the contact of the needle tip with the sciatic nerve is usually associated with a motor response of the calf or foot. Once the needle tip is in the proper position, 1–2 mL of local anesthetic is injected to confirm the adequate distribution of injectate. Such injection helps delineate the sciatic nerve within its muscular tunnel, and it should displace the sciatic nerve away from the needle. Improper spread of local anesthetic or nerve displacement may require an adjustment of the needle tip position.

In an adult patient, 10–15 mL of local anesthetic is usually adequate for successful blockade (Figure 33F–6). Although a

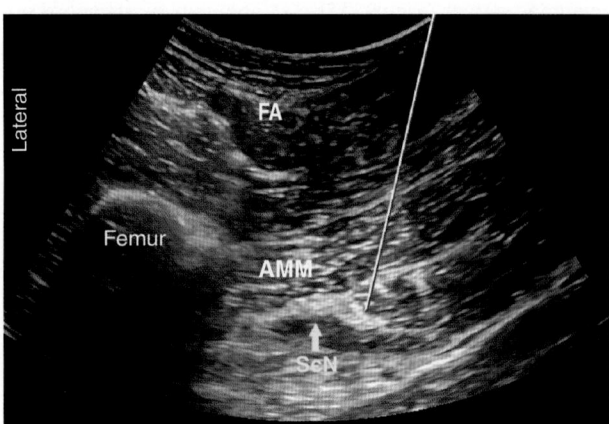

FIGURE 33F–5. Simulated needle path using an out-of-plane technique to reach the sciatic nerve (ScN) using the anterior approach. (Reproduced with permission from Hadzic A: *Hadzic's Peripheral Nerve Blocks and Anatomy for Ultrasound-Guided Regional Anesthesia*, 2nd ed. New York: McGraw-Hill, 2011.)

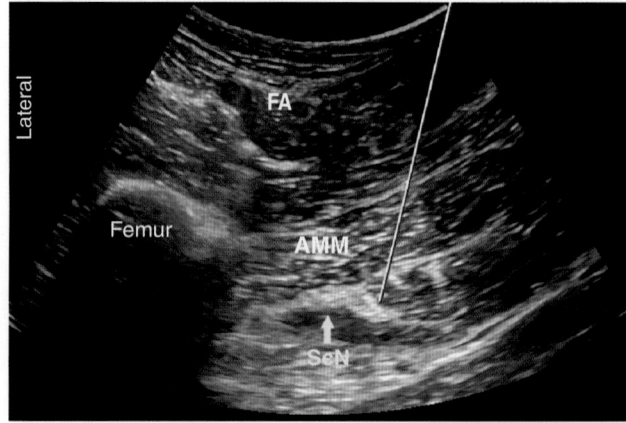

FIGURE 33F–6. Simulated needle path (1) using an out-of-plane technique with proper local anesthetic distribution (blue-shaded area) to anesthetize the sciatic nerve (ScN). (Reproduced with permission from Hadzic A: *Hadzic's Peripheral Nerve Blocks and Anatomy for Ultrasound-Guided Regional Anesthesia*, 2nd ed. New York: McGraw-Hill, 2011.)

single injection of such volume of local anesthetic suffices, it may be beneficial to inject two to three smaller aliquots at different locations to ensure the spread of local anesthetic around the sciatic nerve. The block dynamics and perioperative management are similar to those described in the nerve stimulator technique section.

Clinical Pearl

- Insertion of the needle in an out-of-plane manner using hydrodissection is often a more practical way to accomplish this block compared to an in-plane approach.

SUGGESTED READINGS

Bruhn J, van Geffen GJ, Gielen MJ, Scheffer GJ: Visualization of the course of the sciatic nerve in adult volunteers by ultrasonography. Acta Anaesthesiol Scand 2008;52:1298–1302.

Chan VW, Nova H, Abbas S, McCartney CJ, Perlas A, Xu DQ: Ultrasound examination and localization of the sciatic nerve: a volunteer study. Anesthesiology 2006;104:309–314.

Chantzi C, Saranteas T, Zogogiannis J, Alevizou N, Dimitriou V: Ultrasound examination of the sciatic nerve at the anterior thigh in obese patients. Acta Anaesthesiol Scand 2007;51:132.

Danelli G, Ghisi D, Ortu A: Ultrasound and regional anesthesia technique: are there really ultrasound guidance technical limits in sciatic nerve blocks? Reg Anesth Pain Med 2008;33:281–282.

Dolan J: Ultrasound-guided anterior sciatic nerve block in the proximal thigh: an in-plane approach improving the needle view and respecting fascial planes. Br J Anaesth 2013;110:319–320.

Domingo-Triado V, Selfa S, Martinez F, et al: Ultrasound guidance for lateral midfemoral sciatic nerve block: a prospective, comparative, randomized study. Anesth Analg 2007;104:1270–1274.

Fredrickson MJ, Kilfoyle DH: Neurological complication analysis of 1000 ultrasound guided peripheral nerve blocks for elective orthopaedic surgery: a prospective study. Anaesthesia 2009;64:836–844.

Gnaho A, Eyrieux S, Gentili M: Cardiac arrest during an ultrasound-guided sciatic nerve block combined with nerve stimulation. Reg Anesth Pain Med 2009;34:278.

Gray AT, Collins AB, Schafhalter-Zoppoth I: Sciatic nerve block in a child: a sonographic approach. Anesth Analg 2003;97:1300–1302.

Hamilton PD, Pearce CJ, Pinney SJ, Calder JD: Sciatic nerve blockade: a survey of orthopaedic foot and ankle specialists in North America and the United Kingdom. Foot Ankle Int 2009;30:1196–1201.

Latzke D, Marhofer P, Zeitlinger M, et al: Minimal local anaesthetic volumes for sciatic nerve block: evaluation of ED 99 in volunteers. Br J Anaesth 2010;104:239–244.

Oberndorfer U, Marhofer P, Bosenberg A, et al: Ultrasonographic guidance for sciatic and femoral nerve blocks in children. Br J Anaesth 2007;98:797–801.

Ota J, Sakura S, Hara K, Saito Y: Ultrasound-guided anterior approach to sciatic nerve block: a comparison with the posterior approach. Anesth Analg 2009;108:660–665.

Panhuizen IF, Snoeck MM. van de Blokkade N: Ischiadicus via echogeleide anterieure benadering [Ultrasound-guided anterior approach to sciatic nerve block]. Ned Tijdschr Geneeskd 2011;155:A2372.

Pham Dang C, Gourand D: Ultrasound imaging of the sciatic nerve in the lateral midfemoral approach. Reg Anesth Pain Med 2009;34:281–282.

Saranteas T: Limitations in ultrasound imaging techniques in anesthesia: obesity and muscle atrophy? Anesth Analg 2009;109:993–994.

Saranteas T, Chantzi C, Paraskeuopoulos T, et al: Imaging in anesthesia: the role of 4 MHz to 7 MHz sector array ultrasound probe in the identification of the sciatic nerve at different anatomic locations. Reg Anesth Pain Med 2007;32:537–538.

Saranteas T, Chantzi C, Zogogiannis J, et al: Lateral sciatic nerve examination and localization at the mid-femoral level: an imaging study with ultrasound. Acta Anaesthesiol Scand 2007;51:387–388.

Saranteas T, Kostopanagiotou G, Paraskeuopoulos T, Vamvasakis E, Chantzi C, Anagnostopoulou S: Ultrasound examination of the sciatic nerve at two different locations in the lateral thigh: a new approach of identification validated by anatomic preparation. Acta Anaesthesiol Scand 2007; 51:780–781.

Sites BD, Neal JM, Chan V: Ultrasound in regional anesthesia: where should the "focus" be set? Reg Anesth Pain Med 2009;34:531–533.

Tsui BC, Dillane D, Pillay J, Ramji AK, Walji AH: Cadaveric ultrasound imaging for training in ultrasound-guided peripheral nerve blocks: lower extremity. Can J Anaesth 2007;54:475–480.

Tsui BC, Ozelsel TJ: Ultrasound-guided anterior sciatic nerve block using a longitudinal approach: "expanding the view." Reg Anesth Pain Med 2008;33:275–276.

van Geffen GJ, Bruhn J, Gielen M: Ultrasound-guided continuous sciatic nerve blocks in two children with venous malformations in the lower limb. Can J Anaesth 2007;54:952–953.

PART II: POSTERIOR APPROACH

GENERAL CONSIDERATIONS

With the transgluteal approach, the sciatic nerve is approached deep to the gluteus maximus muscle, where it is identified between two osseous landmarks (the **ischial tuberosity** and the **greater trochanter**). To obtain view of the sciatic nerve and the osseous structures at this level, the curvilinear probe is typically needed.

With the subgluteal approach, the nerve is just below the level of the gluteal crease where the nerve lies more superficial and can be imaged even with a linear probe. The preference of one approach over the other is based on the patient's anatomical characteristics and the operator's personal preference. The subgluteal approach may be a better choice for most patients and indications, including the obese patients.[1]

ULTRASOUND ANATOMY

At the transgluteal level, the sciatic nerve is visualized in the short axis between the two hyperechoic bony prominences of the ischial tuberosity and the greater trochanter of the femur (Figures 33F–7 and 33F–8). The gluteus maximus muscle is seen as the most superficial muscular layer bridging the two osseous structures, typically several centimeters thick. The sciatic nerve is located immediately deep to the gluteus maximus muscle and superficial to the quadratus femoris muscle. Often, it is slightly closer to the ischial tuberosity than to the greater trochanter. At this location in the thigh, it is seen as an oval or roughly triangular hyperechoic structure. At the subgluteal level, the sciatic nerve is positioned between the long head of the biceps femoris muscle and the posterior surface of the adductor magnus.

DISTRIBUTION OF ANESTHESIA

Sciatic nerve block results in anesthesia of the entire lower limb below the knee (both motor and sensory blockade), with the exception of the skin on the medial leg and foot, which is innervated by the saphenous nerve. Both the transgluteal and subgluteal approaches provide motor blockade of the hamstring muscles. The skin of the posterior aspect of the thigh, supplied by the posterior femorocutaneous nerve, is not

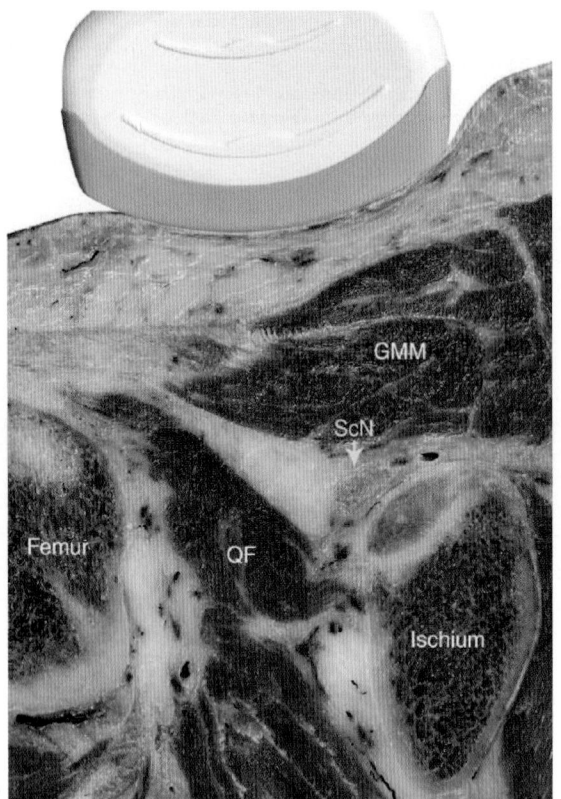

FIGURE 33F–7. Cross-sectional anatomy of the sciatic nerve at the transgluteal level. The sciatic nerve (ScN) is seen between the greater trochanter of the femur and the ischial tuberosity, just deep to the gluteus maximus (GMM) and superficial to the quadratus fermoris (QF) muscles. (Reproduced with permission from Hadzic A: *Hadzic's Peripheral Nerve Blocks and Anatomy for Ultrasound-Guided Regional Anesthesia*, 2nd ed. New York: McGraw-Hill, 2011.)

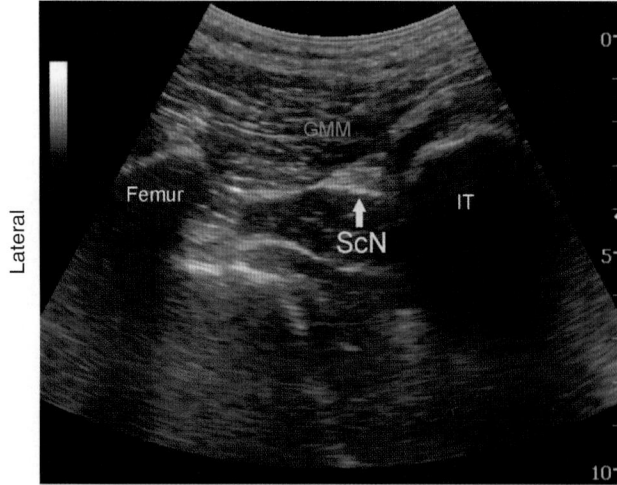

Sciatic nerve block-posterior approach

FIGURE 33F–8. Ultrasound image demonstrating the sonoanatomy of the sciatic nerve (ScN). The ScN often assumes an ovoid or triangular shape and is positioned deep to the gluteus maximus muscle (GMM) between the ischial tuberosity (IT) and femur. (Reproduced with permission from Hadzic A: *Hadzic's Peripheral Nerve Blocks and Anatomy for Ultrasound-Guided Regional Anesthesia*, 2nd ed. New York: McGraw-Hill, 2011.)

anesthetized by the subgluteal, and when indicated, the posterior femoro cutaneous nerve can be anesthetized separately.[2] For a more comprehensive review of the sciatic nerve distribution, see Chapter 3.

EQUIPMENT

The equipment recommended for a sciatic nerve block using the transgluteal or subgluteal approach is as follows:

- Ultrasound machine with curved (phase array) transducer (2–8 MHz), sterile sleeve, and gel
- Standard nerve block tray
- One 20-mL syringe containing local anesthetic
- A 100-mm, 21- to 22-gauge, short-bevel, insulated stimulating needle
- Peripheral nerve stimulator
- Sterile gloves

Clinical Pearl

- Although a linear transducer occasionally can be used for smaller-size patients undergoing transgluteal approach, a curved transducer permits the operator to visualize a wider field, including the osseous landmarks. The ischial tuberosity and greater trochanter are not seen on the same image when using a linear transducer.

LANDMARKS AND PATIENT POSITIONING

For either the transgluteal or subgluteal approach, the patient is placed in a lateral decubitus position (Figures 33F–9 and 33F–10). The limbs are flexed at the hip and knee. When nerve stimulation is used simultaneously (recommended),

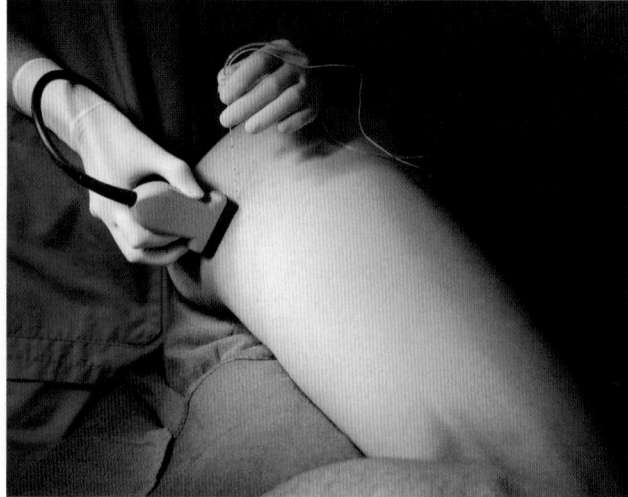

FIGURE 33F–9. Transducer position and needle insertion for subgluteal approach to sciatic nerve block.

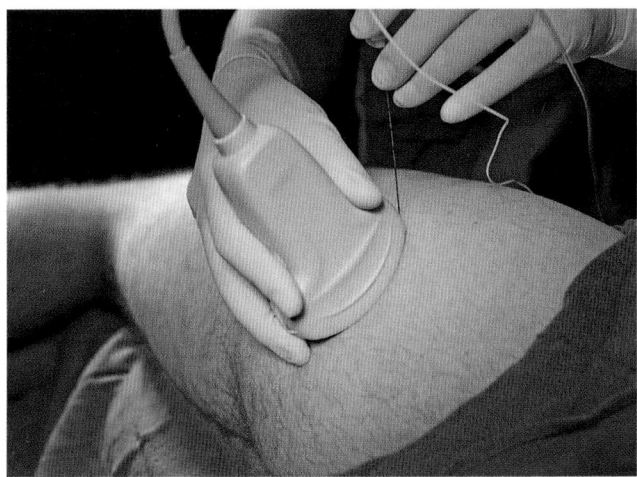

FIGURE 33F–10. Transgluteal approach to sciatic block: patient position, transducer (curved) placement, and needle insertion. (Reproduced with permission from Hadzic A: *Hadzic's Peripheral Nerve Blocks and Anatomy for Ultrasound-Guided Regional Anesthesia*, 2nd ed. New York: McGraw-Hill, 2011.)

FIGURE 33F–11. The sciatic nerve (ScN) as seen in the subgluteal position (using a linear transducer) and simulated needle path to the interfacial plane (white arrows) between the gluteus maximus muscle (GMM) and the adductor magnus. (Reproduced with permission from Hadzic A: *Hadzic's Peripheral Nerve Blocks and Anatomy for Ultrasound-Guided Regional Anesthesia*, 2nd ed. New York: McGraw-Hill, 2011.)

exposure of the hamstrings, calf, and foot is required to detect and interpret motor responses. The osseous prominences of the greater trochanter and ischial tuberosity are palpated and, if desired, marked with a skin marker. The initial transducer position is in the depression between the two bony structures.

GOAL

The goal is to place the needle tip adjacent to the sciatic nerve, deep to the gluteus maximus muscle (the transgluteal technique) and to deposit 15–20 mL of local anesthetic until adequate spread adjacent to the nerve is visualized.

TECHNIQUE

The description of the technique in this chapter will focus primarily on the transgluteal approach. However, since the subgluteal approach is performed just a few centimeters more distally and is technically simpler to perform, the block can be accomplished using either approach by following the general guidelines provided here and by referring to Figures 33F–9 and Figure 33F–11.

The skin is disinfected and the transducer is positioned to identify the sciatic nerve (see Figure 33F–10). Tilting the transducer proximally or distally can help improve the contrast and bring the nerve "out of the background" of the musculature. Often, the nerve is better imaged after the injection of local anesthetic. Alternatively, sliding the transducer slightly proximal or distal can improve the quality of the image and allow for better visualization.

Once identified, the needle is inserted in plane, typically from the lateral aspect of the transducer, and advanced toward the sciatic nerve. If nerve stimulation is used (1.0 mA, 0.1 msec), the

passage of the needle through the fascia on the anterior aspect of the gluteus maximus muscle often is associated with a motor response of the calf or foot. Once the needle tip is positioned adjacent to the nerve (Figure 33F–12), and after careful aspiration to rule out an intravascular needle placement, 1–2 mL of local anesthetic is injected to visualize the proper injection site. Such injection often displaces the sciatic nerve away from the needle; therefore, an additional advancement of the needle 1–2 mm toward the nerve may be necessary to ensure proper local anesthetic spread.

Additional needle repositions and injections may be necessary. Ensuring the absence of high resistance to injection to reduce the risk of intrafascicular injection is of utmost importance because the needle tip is difficult to visualize due to the steep angle and depth of the needle placement.

Although a single injection of 15-20 mL of local anesthetic typically suffices, it may be beneficial to inject two to three smaller aliquots at different locations to ensure the spread of local anesthetic solution around the sciatic nerve.

TIPS

- Never inject against high resistance (> 15 psi) because this may signal an intraneural injection. Even experts may miss signs of intraneural injection.[3]
- While some authors have suggested that intraneural injection is safe for the sciatic nerve, given the high proportion of connective tissue relative to the fascicles,[4,5] it is best avoided since reliable blockade can be obtained by injecting around the nerve. The ability to distinguish the sciatic nerve from its soft tissue surroundings often is improved after the injection of local anesthetic; doing so can be used as a marker to identify the nerve when injection begins.

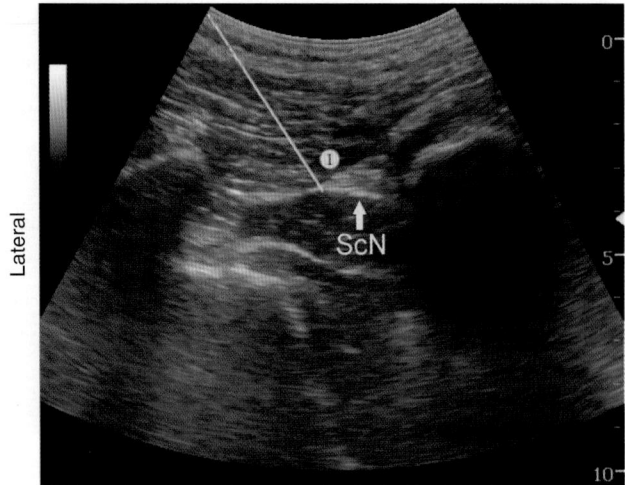

A   Sciatic nerve block-posterior approach

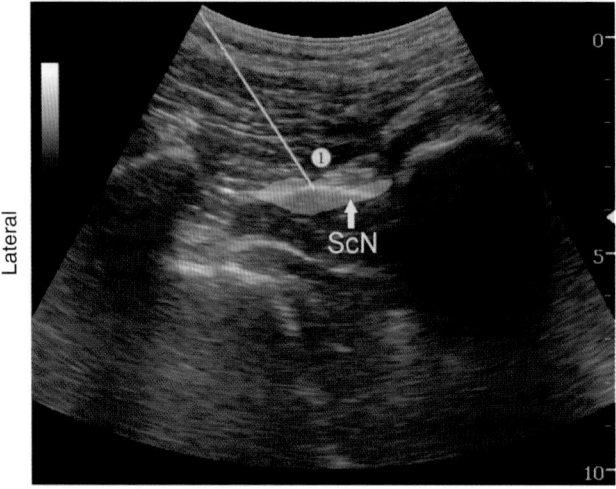

B   Sciatic nerve block-posterior approach

FIGURE 33F–12. (a) Simulated needle path (1) to reach the sciatic nerve (ScN) using an in-plane technique and transgluteal approach. The needle is shown passing through the gluteus muscle with its tip positioned at the lateral aspect of the sciatic nerve. (b) Simulated needle path (1) and local anesthetic distribution (blue-shaded area) to block the ScN with the transgluteal approach. (Reproduced with permission from Hadzic A: *Hadzic's Peripheral Nerve Blocks and Anatomy for Ultrasound-Guided Regional Anesthesia*, 2nd ed. New York: McGraw-Hill, 2011.)

CONTINUOUS ULTRASOUND-GUIDED SUBGLUTEAL SCIATIC BLOCK

The goal of the continuous sciatic nerve block is similar to that of the non–US-based techniques: to place the catheter within the vicinity of the sciatic nerve between the gluteus maximus and quadratus femoris muscles. The procedure is similar to the previously described in the continuous ultrasound-guided block section in Chapter 32A.

Advancement of the needle in plane in a lateral-to- medial direction until the tip is adjacent to the nerve and deep to the gluteus maximus fascia should ensure appropriate catheter location. Proper placement of the needle also can be confirmed by

obtaining a motor response of the calf or foot, at which point 4–5 mL of local anesthetic is injected. This small dose of local anesthetic serves to ensure adequate local anesthetic distribution as well as to make the catheter advancement easier. This first phase of the procedure does not significantly differ from the single-injection technique.

Alternatively, the catheter can be inserted using a longitudinal view. With this approach, after successful imaging of the sciatic nerve in the cross-sectional view, the transducer is rotated 90 degrees so that the sciatic nerve is visualized in the longitudinal view. However, this approach requires significantly greater US imaging skills.

The catheter is secured by either taping it to the skin or tunneling. A common infusion strategy consists of ropivacaine 0.2% at a rate of 5 mL/minute with a patient-controlled bolus of 5 mL/h.

SUGGESTED READINGS

Abbas S, Brull R: Ultrasound-guided sciatic nerve block: description of a new approach at the subgluteal space. Br J Anaesth 2007;99:445–446.

Abdallah FW, Brull R: Is sciatic nerve block advantageous when combined with femoral nerve block for postoperative analgesia following total knee arthroplasty? A systematic review. Reg Anesth Pain Med 2011;36: 493–498.

Abdallah FW, Brull R: Sciatic nerve block for analgesia after total knee arthroplasty: the jury is still out. Reg Anesth Pain Med 2012;37: 122–123.

Abdallah FW, Chan VW, Gandhi R, Koshkin A, Abbas S, Brull R: The analgesic effects of proximal, distal, or no sciatic nerve block on posterior knee pain after total knee arthroplasty: a double-blind placebo-controlled randomized trial. Anesthesiology 2014;121:1302–1310.

Barrington MJ, Lai SL, Briggs CA, Ivanusic JJ, Gledhill SR: Ultrasound-guided midthigh sciatic nerve block—a clinical and anatomical study. Reg Anesth Pain Med 2008;33:369–376.

Benzon HT, Katz JA, Benzon HA, Iqbal MS: Piriformis syndrome: anatomic considerations, a new injection technique, and a review of the literature. Anesthesiology 2003;98:1442–1448.

Bruhn J, Moayeri N, Groen GJ, et al: Soft tissue landmark for ultrasound identification of the sciatic nerve in the infragluteal region: the tendon of the long head of the biceps femoris muscle. Acta Anaesthesiol Scand 2009;53:921–925.

Bruhn J, van Geffen GJ, Gielen MJ, Scheffer GJ: Visualization of the course of the sciatic nerve in adult volunteers by ultrasonography. Acta Anaesthesiol Scand 2008;52:1298–1302.

Cao X, Zhao X, Xu J, Liu Z, Li Q: Ultrasound-guided technology versus neurostimulation for sciatic nerve block: a meta-analysis. Int J Clin Exp Med 2015;8:273–80.

Chan VW, Nova H, Abbas S, McCartney CJ, Perlas A, Xu DQ:. Ultrasound examination and localization of the sciatic nerve: a volunteer study. Anesthesiology 2006;104:309–314.

Chantzi C, Saranteas T, Zogogiannis J, Alevizou N, Dimitriou V: Ultrasound examination of the sciatic nerve at the anterior thigh in obese patients. Acta Anaesthesiol Scand 2007;51:132.

Danelli G, Ghisi D, Fanelli A, et al: The effects of ultrasound guidance and neurostimulation on the minimum effective anesthetic volume of mepivacaine 1.5% required to block the sciatic nerve using the subgluteal approach. Anesth Analg 2009;109:1674–1678.

Danelli G, Ghisi D, Ortu A: Ultrasound and regional anesthesia technique: are there really ultrasound guidance technical limits in sciatic nerve blocks? Reg Anesth Pain Med 2008;33:281–282.

Dillow JM, Rosett RL, Petersen TR, Vagh FS, Hruschka JA, Lam NC: Ultrasound-guided parasacral approach to the sciatic nerve block in children. Paediatr Anaesth 2013;23:1042–1047.

Domingo-Triado V, Selfa S, Martinez F, et al: Ultrasound guidance for lateral midfemoral sciatic nerve block: a prospective, comparative, randomized study. Anesth Analg 2007;104:1270–1274.

Fredrickson MJ, Kilfoyle DH: Neurological complication analysis of 1000 ultrasound guided peripheral nerve blocks for elective orthopaedic surgery: a prospective study. Anaesthesia 2009;64:836–844.

Gnaho A, Eyrieux S, Gentili M: Cardiac arrest during an ultrasound-guided sciatic nerve block combined with nerve stimulation. Reg Anesth Pain Med 2009;34:278.

Gray AT, Collins AB, Schafhalter-Zoppoth I: Sciatic nerve block in a child: a sonographic approach. Anesth Analg 2003;97:1300–1302.

Hamilton PD, Pearce CJ, Pinney SJ, Calder JD: Sciatic nerve blockade: a survey of orthopaedic foot and ankle specialists in North America and the United Kingdom. Foot Ankle Int 2009;30:1196–1201.

Hara K, Sakura S, Yokokawa N: The role of electrical stimulation in ultrasound-guided subgluteal sciatic nerve block: a retrospective study on how response pattern and minimal evoked current affect the resultant blockade. J Anesth 2014;28:524–531.

Karmakar MK, Kwok WH, Ho AM, Tsang K, Chui PT, Gin T: Ultrasound-guided sciatic nerve block: description of a new approach at the subgluteal space. Br J Anaesth 2007;98:390–395.

Keplinger M, Marhofer P, Marhofer D, et al: Effective local anaesthetic volumes for sciatic nerve blockade: a clinical evaluation of the ED99. Anaesthesia 2015;70:585–590.

Krediet AC, Moayeri N, Bleys RL, Groen GJ: Intraneural or extraneural: diagnostic accuracy of ultrasound assessment for localizing low-volume injection. Reg Anesth Pain Med 2014;39:409–413.

Latzke D, Marhofer P, Zeitlinger M, et al: Minimal local anaesthetic volumes for sciatic nerve block: evaluation of ED 99 in volunteers. Br J Anaesth 2010;104:239–244.

Marhofer P, Harrop-Griffiths W, Willschke H, Kirchmair L: Fifteen years of ultrasound guidance in regional anaesthesia: Part 2—recent developments in block techniques. Br J Anaesth 2010;104:673–683.

Meng S, Lieba-Samal D, Reissig LF, et al: High-resolution ultrasound of the posterior femoral cutaneous nerve: visualization and initial experience with patients. Skeletal Radiol 2015;44:1421–1426.

Moayeri N, van Geffen GJ, Bruhn J, Chan VW, Groen GJ: Correlation among ultrasound, cross-sectional anatomy, and histology of the sciatic nerve: a review. Reg Anesth Pain Med 2010;35:442–449.

Murray JM, Derbyshire S, Shields MO: Lower limb blocks. Anaesthesia 2010;65(Suppl 1):57–66.

Oberndorfer U, Marhofer P, Bosenberg A, et al: Ultrasonographic guidance for sciatic and femoral nerve blocks in children. Br J Anaesth 2007;98:797–801.

Osaka Y, Kashiwagi M, Nagatsuka Y, Miwa S: Ultrasound-guided medial mid-thigh approach to sciatic nerve block with a patient in a supine position. J Anesth 2011;25:621–624.

Ota J, Sakura S, Hara K, Saito Y: Ultrasound-guided anterior approach to sciatic nerve block: a comparison with the posterior approach. Anesth Analg 2009;108:660–665.

Pham Dang C, Gourand D: Ultrasound imaging of the sciatic nerve in the lateral midfemoral approach. Reg Anesth Pain Med 2009;34:281–282.

Ponde V, Desai AP, Shah D: Comparison of success rate of ultrasound-guided sciatic and femoral nerve block and neurostimulation in children with arthrogryposis multiplex congenita: a randomized clinical trial. Paediatr Anaesth 2013;23:74–78.

Quah VY, Hocking G, Froehlich K: Influence of leg position on the depth and sonographic appearance of the sciatic nerve in volunteers. Anaesth Intensive Care 2010;38:1034–1037.

Reinoso-Barbero F, Saavedra B, Segura-Grau E, Llamas A: Anatomical comparison of sciatic nerves between adults and newborns: clinical implications for ultrasound guided block. J Anat 2014;224:108–112.

Salinas FV: Ultrasound and review of evidence for lower extremity peripheral nerve blocks. Reg Anesth Pain Med 2010;35:S16–25.

Saranteas T: Limitations in ultrasound imaging techniques in anesthesia: obesity and muscle atrophy? Anesth Analg 2009;109:993–994.

Saranteas T, Chantzi C, Paraskeuopoulos T, et al: Imaging in anesthesia: the role of 4 MHz to 7 MHz sector array ultrasound probe in the identification of the sciatic nerve at different anatomic locations. Reg Anesth Pain Med 2007;32:537–538.

Saranteas T, Chantzi C, Zogogiannis J, et al: Lateral sciatic nerve examination and localization at the mid-femoral level: an imaging study with ultrasound. Acta Anaesthesiol Scand 2007;51:387–388.

Saranteas T, Kostopanagiotou G, Paraskeuopoulos T, Vamvasakis E, Chantzi C, Anagnostopoulou S: Ultrasound examination of the sciatic nerve at two different locations in the lateral thigh: a new approach of identification validated by anatomic preparation. Acta Anaesthesiol Scand 2007;51:780–781.

Sites BD, Neal JM, Chan V: Ultrasound in regional anesthesia: where should the "focus" be set? Reg Anesth Pain Med 2009;34:531–533.

Taha AM: A simple and successful sonographic technique to identify the sciatic nerve in the parasacral area. Can J Anaesth 2012;59:263–267.

Tammam TF: Ultrasound-guided infragluteal sciatic nerve block: a comparison between four different techniques. Acta Anaesthesiol Scand 2013;57:243–248.

Tran DQ, Muñoz L, Russo G, Finlayson RJ: Ultrasonography and stimulating perineural catheters for nerve blocks: a review of the evidence. Can J Anaesth 2008;55:447–457.

Tsui BC, Dillane D, Pillay J, Ramji AK, Walji AH: Cadaveric ultrasound imaging for training in ultrasound-guided peripheral nerve blocks: lower extremity. Can J Anaesth 2007;54:475–480.

Tsui BC, Finucane BT: The importance of ultrasound landmarks: a "traceback" approach using the popliteal blood vessels for identification of the sciatic nerve. Reg Anesth Pain Med 2006;31:481–482.

Tsui BC, Ozelsel TJ: Ultrasound-guided anterior sciatic nerve block using a longitudinal approach: "expanding the view." Reg Anesth Pain Med 2008;33:275–276.

van Geffen GJ, Bruhn J, Gielen M: Ultrasound-guided continuous sciatic nerve blocks in two children with venous malformations in the lower limb. Can J Anaesth 2007;54:952–953.

van Geffen GJ, Gielen M: Ultrasound-guided subgluteal sciatic nerve blocks with stimulating catheters in children: a descriptive study. Anesth Analg 2006;103:328–333.

Young DS, Cota A, Chaytor R: Continuous infragluteal sciatic nerve block for postoperative pain control after total ankle arthroplasty. Foot Ankle Spec 2014;7:271–276.

REFERENCES

1. Abdallah FW, Chan VW, Koshkin A, Abbas S, Brull R: Ultrasound-guided sciatic nerve block in overweight and obese patients: a randomized comparison of performance time between the infragluteal and subgluteal space techniques. Reg Anesth Pain Med 2013;38:547–552.

2. Meng S, Lieba-Samal D, Reissig LF, et al: High-resolution ultrasound of the posterior femoral cutaneous nerve: visualization and initial experience with patients. Skeletal Radiol 2015;44:1421–1426.

3. Krediet AC, Moayeri N, Bleys RL, Groen GJ: Intraneural or extraneural: diagnostic accuracy of ultrasound assessment for localizing low-volume injection. Reg Anesth Pain Med 2014;39:409–413.

4. Hara K, Sakura S, Yokokawa N, Tadenuma S: Incidence and effects of unintentional intraneural injection during ultrasound-guided subgluteal sciatic nerve block. Reg Anesth Pain Med 2012;37:289–293.

5. Sala-Blanch X, López AM, Pomés J, Valls-Sole J, García AI, Hadzic A: No clinical or electrophysiologic evidence of nerve injury after intraneural injection during sciatic popliteal block. Anesthesiology 2011;115:589–595.

Ultrasound-Guided Popliteal Sciatic Block

Admir Hadzic, Ana M. Lopez, Catherine Vandepitte, and Xavier Sala-Blanch

POPLITEAL SCIATIC BLOCK AT A GLANCE

- Indications: foot, ankle and Achilles tendon surgery
- Transducer position: transverse over the popliteal fossa
- Goal: local anesthetic spread surrounding the sciatic nerve within the epineural sheath
- Local anesthetic: 15–20 mL

GENERAL CONSIDERATIONS

The anatomy of the sciatic nerve in the popliteal fossa is variable, and the division into the tibial nerve (TN) and common peroneal nerve (CPN) occurs at an inconstant distance from the popliteal crease (Figure 33G–1). With nerve stimulator–based techniques, larger volumes (eg, > 40 mL) of local anesthetic have been used to increase the chance of block success. However, US guidance reduces the volume required for reliable block because the injection can be halted once adequate spread is observed.

The most common approaches to the popliteal sciatic block are the lateral approach, with the patient in the supine or lateral position, and the posterior approach in the prone or lateral position (Figure 33G–2). While the patient position and needle path differ between the two approaches, the rest of the technique details are similar.

The injection of local anesthetic must occur within the sciatic nerve sheath that contains both components of the nerve.[1–14] The injection is ideally accomplished at the position where both components of the nerve are within the sheath but slightly separated by adipose tissue, allowing for safe placement of the needle between them.[15] Although the sciatic nerve block can be

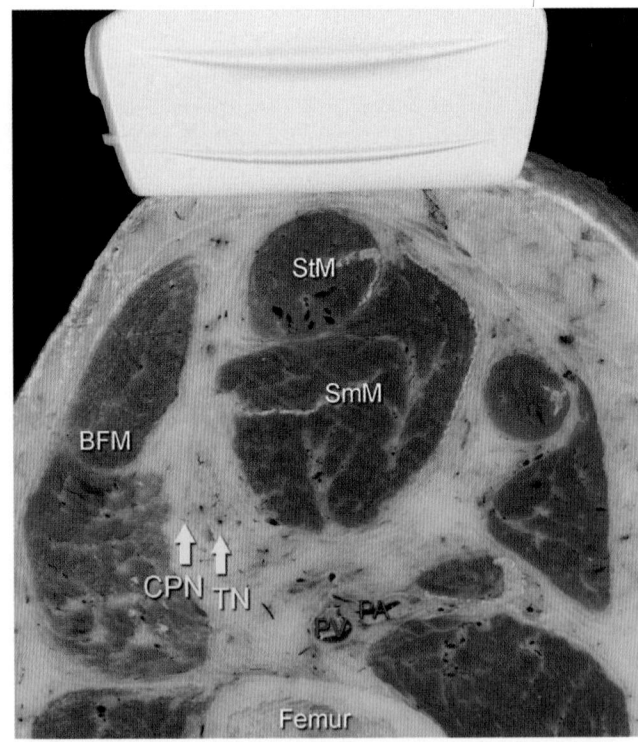

FIGURE 33G–1. Cross-sectional anatomy of the sciatic nerve in the popliteal fossa. Shown are the common peroneal nerve (CPN), tibial nerve (TN), popliteal artery (PA), popliteal vein (PV), femur, biceps femoris muscle (BFM), semimembranosus muscle (SmM), and semitendinosus muscle (StM) muscle. (Reproduced with permission from Hadzic A: *Hadzic's Peripheral Nerve Blocks and Anatomy for Ultrasound-Guided Regional Anesthesia*, 2nd ed. New York: McGraw-Hill, 2011.)

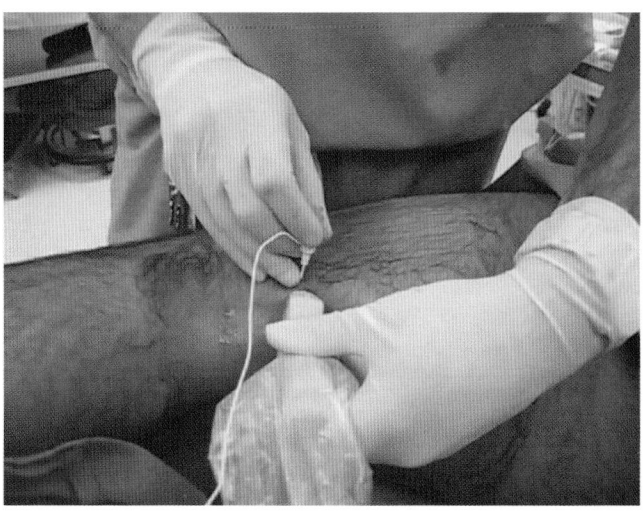
A

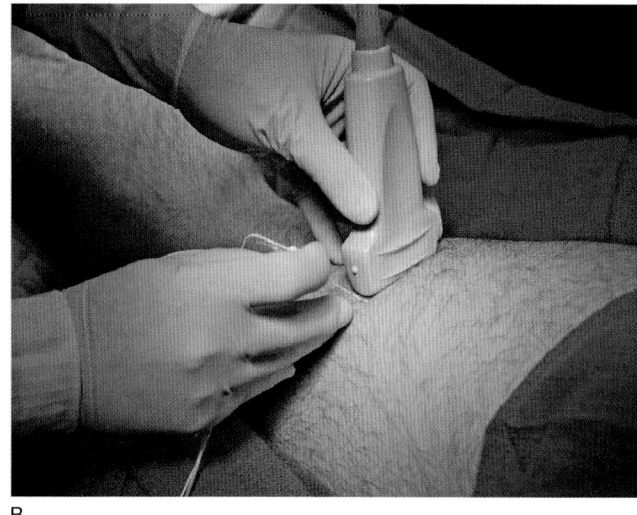
B

FIGURE 33G–2. The posterior approach to the US-guided popliteal sciatic block can be performed (**A**) with the patient in the lateral position, or (**B**) with the patient prone. (Reproduced with permission from Hadzic A: *Hadzic's Peripheral Nerve Blocks and Anatomy for Ultrasound-Guided Regional Anesthesia*, 2nd ed. New York: McGraw-Hill, 2011.)

accomplished with an injection around either nerve component, injecting into the space between both is more common in clinical practice.[16,17]

ULTRASOUND ANATOMY

Beginning with the transducer in the transverse position at the popliteal crease, the popliteal artery is identified, aided with color Doppler US when necessary, at a depth of approximately 3–4 cm. The popliteal vein accompanies the artery at it is positioned just superficial (posterior) to it. On either side of the artery are the biceps femoris muscles (laterally) and the semimembranosus and semitendinosus muscles (medially). The tibial nerve is positioned superficial and lateral to the vein and is seen as a hyperechoic, oval or round structure with a honeycomb pattern (Figure 33G–3). Asking the patient to dorsiflex and plantar flex the ankle makes the two sciatic nerve branches twist or move in relation to each other. Usually, tilting the transducer caudally is necessary to bring out the nerve from the neighboring adipose tissue.

Once the tibial nerve has been identified, the CPN is visualized slightly more superficial and lateral to the tibial nerve. The transducer should be slid proximally until the tibial and peroneal nerves are visualized coming together to form the sciatic nerve before its division (Figure 33G-4). This junction usually occurs at

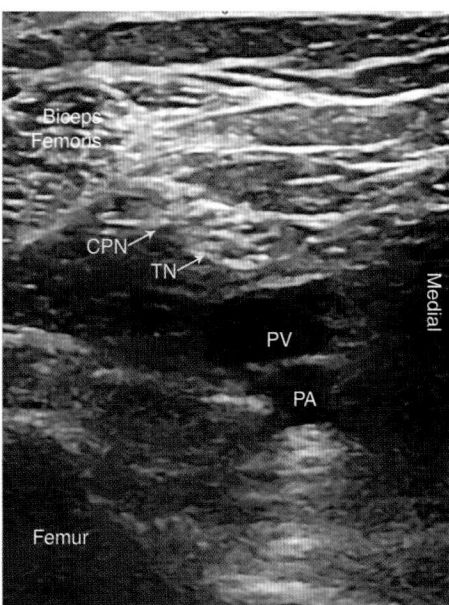

FIGURE 33G–3. Sonoanatomy of the sciatic nerve at the popliteal fossa. The two main divisions of the sciatic nerve, the tibial nerve (TN) and the common peroneal nerve (CPN), are seen immediately lateral and superficial to the popliteal vein (PV) and artery (PA). This image was taken at 5 cm above the popliteal fossa crease, where the TN and CPN have just started diverging.

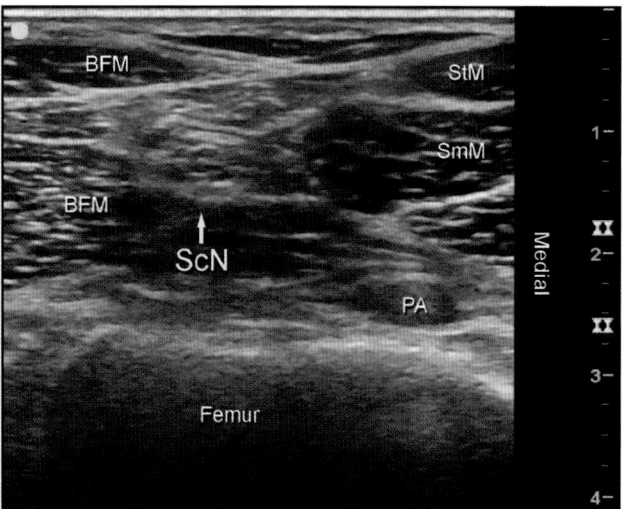

FIGURE 33G–4 Sonoanatomy of the sciatic nerve (ScN) before its division. Shown are the ScN, superior and lateral to the popliteal artery (PA), positioned between the biceps femoris muscle (BFM) the semimembranosus muscle (SmM), and the semitendinosus muscle (StM).

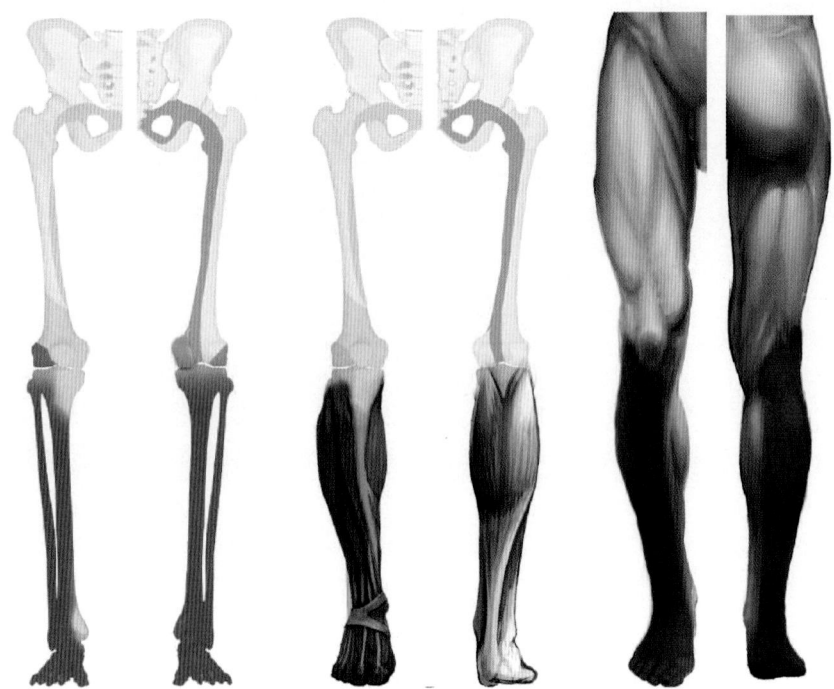

FIGURE 33G–5. Expected distribution of the sciatic nerve sensory blockade at the level of popliteal fossa.

a distance 5–10 cm from the popliteal crease but may occur very close to the crease or, less commonly, more proximally in the thigh. As the transducer is moved proximally, the popliteal vessels move deeper and become more challenging to image. Adjustments in depth, gain, focus, and direction of the US beam should be made to keep the nerve visible at all times. At the popliteal fossa, the sciatic nerve typically is visualized at a depth of 2–4 cm.

Clinical Pearl

- Ultrasound imaging should specifically focus on identifying the sciatic nerve sheath (Vloka's sheath) containing both components of the sciatic nerve (tibial and common peroneal nerves). Successful injection will deposit local anesthetic within the Vloka's sheath

BLOCKADE DISTRIBUTION

Sciatic nerve block results in anesthesia of the lower limb below the knee, both motor and sensory, with the exception of the medial leg and foot, which is the territory of the saphenous nerve, a branch of the femoral nerve. The motor fibers to the hamstring muscles are spared; however, fibers to the posterior aspect of the knee joint are blocked (Figure 33G-5). For a more comprehensive review of the sciatic nerve distribution, see Chapter 3.

EQUIPMENT

The equipment recommended for a popliteal sciatic block includes the following:

- Ultrasound machine with linear transducer (8–12 MHz), sterile sleeve, and gel

- Standard nerve block tray
- A 20-mL syringe containing local anesthetic
- 50- to 100-mm, 21- to 22-gauge, short-bevel, insulated stimulating needle
- Peripheral nerve stimulator
- Injection pressure monitor
- Sterile gloves

LANDMARKS AND PATIENT POSITIONING: LATERAL APPROACH

This block is performed with the patient in the supine or lateral position. This can be accomplished either by resting the foot on an elevated footrest or flexing the knee while an assistant stabilizes the foot and ankle on the bed (Figure 33G–6). If nerve stimulation is used, exposure of the calf and foot is required to observe motor responses.

LANDMARKS AND PATIENT POSITIONING: POSTERIOR APPROACH

This block is performed with the patient in the prone or lateral position (Figure 33G-2). A small footrest is useful to facilitate identification of a motor response if nerve stimulation is used. A footrest also relaxes the hamstring tendons, making transducer placement and manipulation easier.

GOAL

The goal is to inject the local anesthetic within the common connective tissue (Vloka's) sheath that envelops the TN and CPN. Alternatively, separate blocks of TN and CPN can be performed.

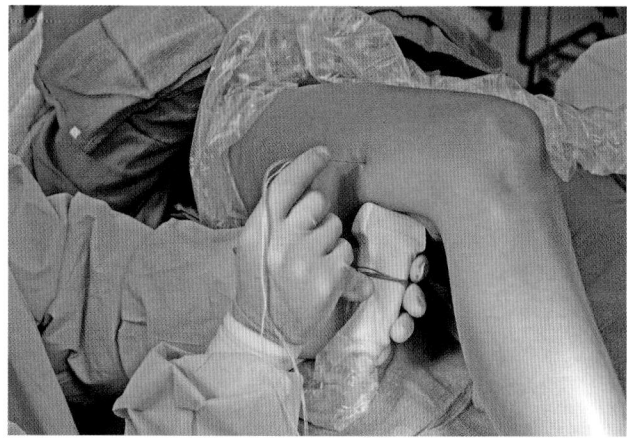

FIGURE 33G–6. Needle insertion technique to block the sciatic nerve in the popliteal fossa using the lateral approach with the patient in the supine position. (Reproduced with permission from Hadzic A: *Hadzic's Peripheral Nerve Blocks and Anatomy for Ultrasound-Guided Regional Anesthesia*, 2nd ed. New York: McGraw-Hill, 2011.)

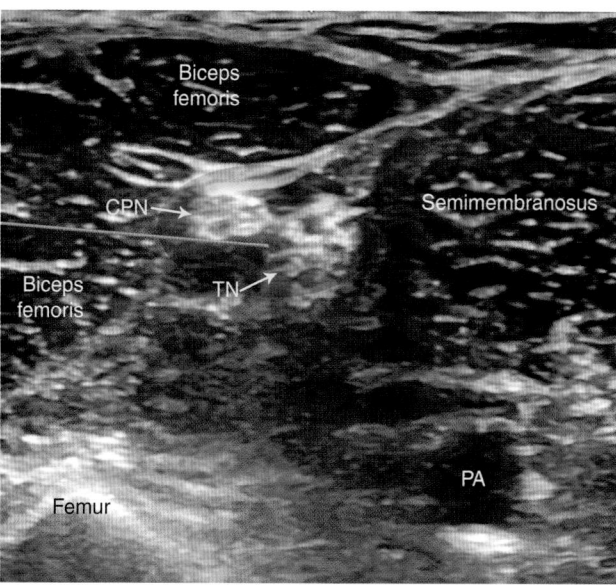

FIGURE 33G–8. Simulated needle path and local anesthetic distribution to block the sciatic nerve (TN and CPN) in the popliteal fossa using the lateral approach. PA, popliteal artery.

TECHNIQUE

The skin is disinfected and the transducer positioned to identify the sciatic nerve. If the nerve is not immediately apparent, tilting the transducer toward the feet can help improve the contrast and bring the nerve "out of the background". Sliding the transducer slightly proximal or distal may improve the quality of the image and allow for better visualization.

It is recommended to perform the block at the level where TN and CPN start diverging but are still in the common sciatic nerve (Vloka's) sheath. For the lateral approach, a skin wheal is made on the lateral aspect of the thigh 2–3 cm above the lateral edge of the transducer, and the needle is inserted in plane in a horizontal orientation from the lateral aspect of the thigh and

advanced toward the sciatic nerve (Figures 33G–7 and 33G-8). For the posterior approach, the needle is inserted in plane from lateral to medial (Figure 33G-9) or out of plane (Figure 33G–10). If nerve stimulation is used (0.5 mA, 0.1 msec), the contact of the needle tip with either branch of the nerve usually is associated with a motor response of the calf or foot. Once the needle tip is placed within the common sciatic nerve sheath, 1–2 mL of local anesthetic is injected to confirm the proper injection site. Such injection should result in a distribution of local anesthetic within the sheath, and separation of the TN and CPN within Vloka's sheath (Figure 33G-11).

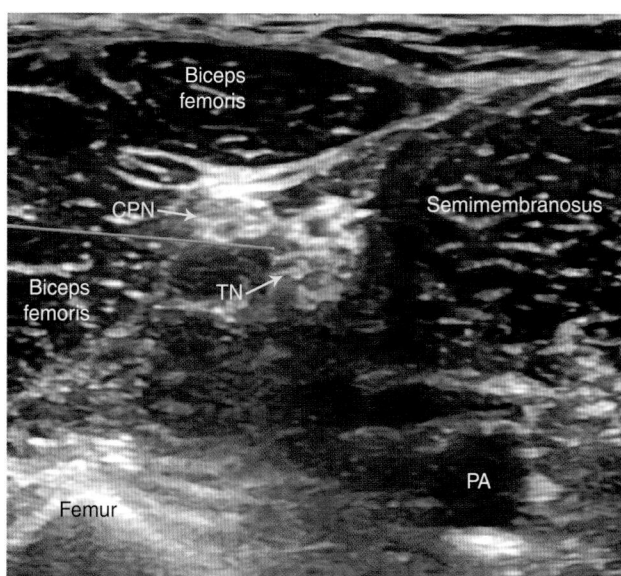

FIGURE 33G–7. Simulated needle path and needle tip placement to block the sciatic nerve (TN and CPN) using the lateral approach. PA, popliteal artery.

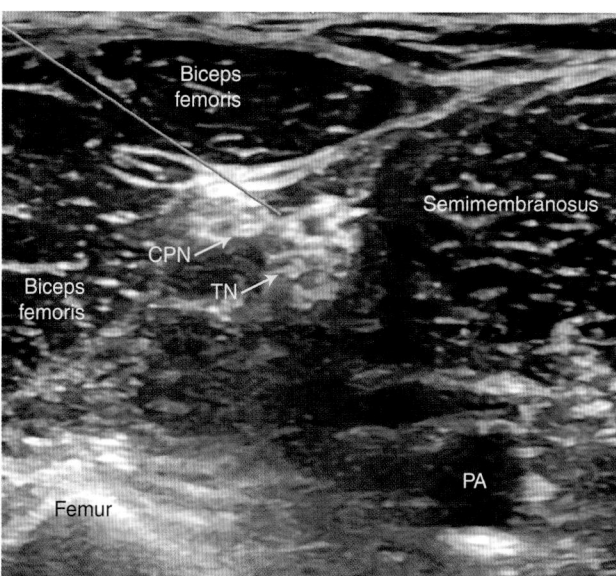

FIGURE 33G–9. Simulated needle path and needle tip placement to block the sciatic nerve (TN and CPN) through the posterior approach, in plane from lateral to medial. PA, popliteal artery.

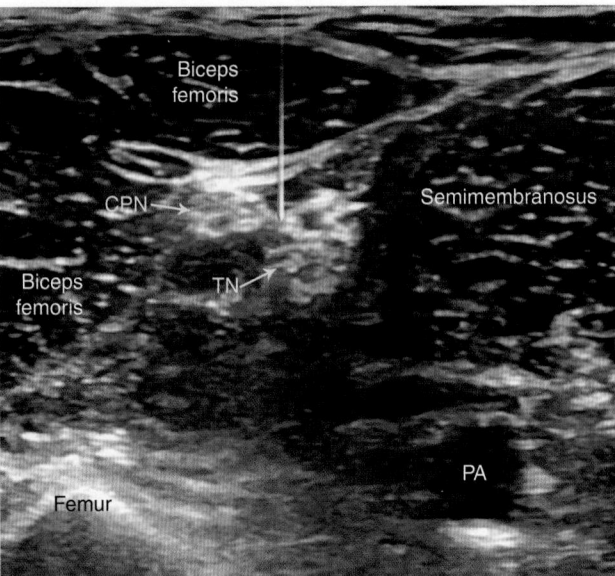

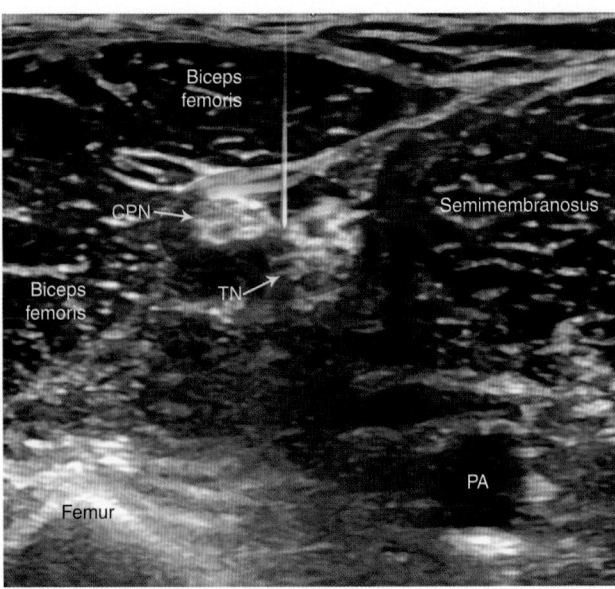

FIGURE 33G–10. Simulated needle path and proper needle tip placement to block the sciatic nerve (TN and CPN) through the posterior approach out of plane. PA, popliteal artery.

FIGURE 33G–11. Simulated needle path, needle tip position and local anesthetic spread (blue-shaded area) to block the sciatic nerve (TN and CPN) through the posterior approach out of plane. PA, popliteal artery.

When local anesthetic injection does not appear to result in a spread inside the sciatic nerve sheath and around the sciatic nerve components, additional needle repositions and injections may be necessary. Correct injection is recognized when local anesthetic spreads proximally and distally to the site of the injection around both divisions of the nerve, which can be documented by observing the spread of the local anesthetic within Vloka's sheath proximal to the site of injection.

A single injection of local anesthetic typically suffices.

TIPS

• To improve needle visualization, a skin puncture site 2–3 cm lateral to the transducer will reduce the angle between the needle and the footprint of the transducer (see Figure 33G–6).

• The presence of a motor response to nerve stimulation is useful but not necessary if the nerve, needle, and local anesthetic spread are well visualized.

• Never inject against high resistance because this may signal an intraneural injection (injection pressure must be < 15 psi).

• In the posterior approach to the popliteal block, either an in-plane (lateral or medial) or out-of-plane technique can be used (Figures 33G-9 through 33G-12). While the in-plane lateral approach is commonly used, the advantage of the out-of-plane approach is that the needle path is through skin and adipose tissue rather than the muscles and thus, less painful.

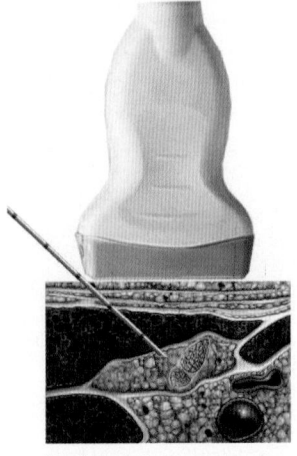
In-plane lateral approach

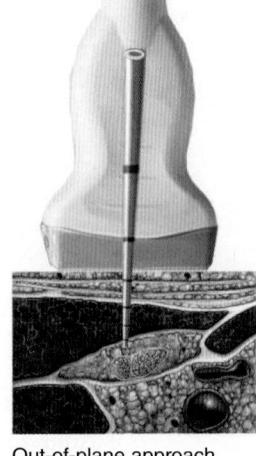
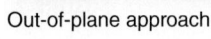
Out-of-plane approach

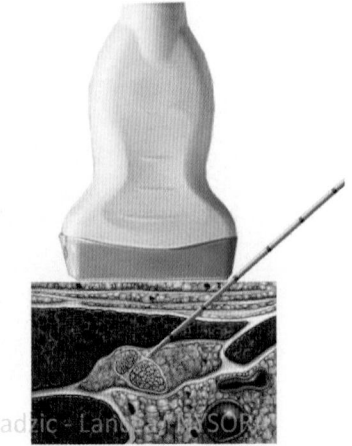
In-plane medial approach

FIGURE 33G–12. In-plane (lateral or medial) or out-of-plane approach are shown - the operator should be able to pick and choose any of these needle orientations, depending on the configuration of tibial and common peroneal branches at the site of injection.

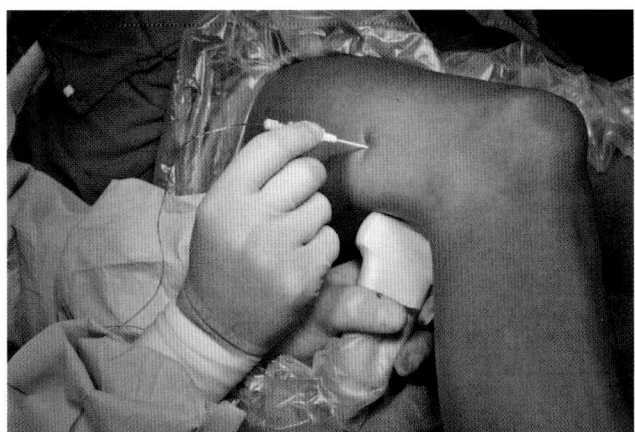

FIGURE 33G–13. Continuous sciatic block in the popliteal fossa using a lateral approach with the patient in the supine position. The needle is positioned within the epineural sheath of the sciatic nerve. After an injection of a small volume of local anesthetic to confirm correct needle position, a catheter is inserted 2–4 cm past the needle tip. Preloading the catheter is useful in facilitating the procedure. (Reproduced with permission from Hadzic A: *Hadzic's Peripheral Nerve Blocks and Anatomy for Ultrasound-Guided Regional Anesthesia*, 2nd ed. New York: McGraw-Hill, 2011.)

CONTINUOUS ULTRASOUND-GUIDED POPLITEAL SCIATIC BLOCK

The goal of the continuous popliteal sciatic block is to place the catheter within the sciatic nerve sheath in the popliteal fossa (Figure 33G-13).

The catheter is inserted 4-5 cm beyond needle tip and its correct placement is documented by observing injection of LA within the sciatic nerve sheath. The catheter is secured either by taping it to the skin or tunneling.

The lateral approach may have some advantage over the prone approach with regard to catheter placement. First, the biceps femoris muscle tends to stabilize the catheter and decrease the chance of dislodgement, compared with the subcutaneous tissue of the popliteal fossa in the prone approach. Second, if the knee is to be flexed and extended, the side of the thigh is less mobile than the back of the knee. Finally, access to the catheter site is more convenient with the lateral approach compared with the prone approach.

A common starting infusion regimen is ropivacaine 0.2% at 5 mL/h with a patient-administered bolus of 5 mL every 60 minutes.

SUGGESTED READINGS

Aguirre J, Perinola L, Borgeat A: Ultrasound-guided evaluation of the local anesthetic spread parameters required for a rapid surgical popliteal sciatic nerve block. Reg Anesth Pain Med 2011;36:308–309.

Aguirre J, Ruland P, Ekatodramis G, Borgeat A: Ultrasound versus neurostimulation for popliteal block: another vain effort to show a nonexisting clinical relevant difference. Anaesth Intensive Care 2009;37:665–666.

Aguirre J, Valentin Neudorfer C, Ekatodramis G, Borgeat A: Ultrasound guidance for sciatic nerve block at the popliteal fossa should be compared with the best motor response and the lowest current clinically used in neurostimulation technique. Reg Anesth Pain Med 2009;34:182–183.

Anderson JG, Bohay DR, Maskill JD, et al: Complications after popliteal block for foot and ankle surgery. Foot Ankle Int 2015;36:1138–1143.

Barbosa FT, Barbosa TR, da Cunha RM, Rodrigues AK, Ramos FW, de Sousa-Rodrigues CF: Bases anatômicas para o bloqueio anestésico do nervo isquiático no nível do joelho. [Anatomical basis for sciatic nerve block at the knee level.] Braz J Anesthesiol 2015;65:177–179.

Barrington MJ, Lai SL, Briggs CA, Ivanusic JJ, Gledhill SR: Ultrasound-guided midthigh sciatic nerve block—a clinical and anatomical study. Reg Anesth Pain Med 2008;33:369–376.

Bendtsen TF, Nielsen TD, Rohde CV, Kibak K, Linde F: Ultrasound guidance improves a continuous popliteal sciatic nerve block when compared with nerve stimulation. Reg Anesth Pain Med 2011;36:181–184.

Birch MD, Matthews JL, Galitzine SV: Patient and needle positioning during popliteal nerve block. Reg Anesth Pain Med 2013;38:253.

Børglum J, Johansen K, Christensen MD, et al: Ultrasound-guided single-penetration dual-injection block for leg and foot surgery: a prospective, randomized, double-blind study. Reg Anesth Pain Med 2014;39:18–25.

Bruhn J, van Geffen GJ, Gielen MJ, Scheffer GJ: Visualization of the course of the sciatic nerve in adult volunteers by ultrasonography. Acta Anaesthesiol Scand 2008;52:1298–1302.

Brull R, Macfarlane AJ, Parrington SJ, Koshkin A, Chan VW: Is circumferential injection advantageous for ultrasound-guided popliteal sciatic nerve block? A proof-of-concept study. Reg Anesth Pain Med 2011;36:266–270.

Buys MJ, Arndt CD, Vagh F, Hoard A, Gerstein N: Ultrasound-guided sciatic nerve block in the popliteal fossa using a lateral approach: onset time comparing separate tibial and common peroneal nerve injections versus injecting proximal to the bifurcation. Anesth Analg 2010;110:635–637.

Cataldo R, Carassiti M, Costa F, et al: Starting with ultrasonography decreases popliteal block performance time in inexperienced hands: a prospective randomized study. BMC Anesthesiol 2012;12:33.

Chin KJ, Perlas A, Brull R, Chan VW: Ultrasound guidance is advantageous in popliteal nerve blockade. Anesth Analg 2008;107:2094–2095.

Clendenen SR, Robards CB, Greengrass RA: Popliteal catheter placement utilizing ultrasound needle guidance system. Local Reg Anesth 2010;3:45–48.

Clendenen SR, York JE, Wang RD, Greengrass RA: Three-dimensional ultrasound-assisted popliteal catheter placement revealing aberrant anatomy: implications for block failure. Acta Anaesthesiol Scand 2008;52:1429–1431.

Compere V, Cornet C, Fourdrinier V, et al: Thigh abscess as a complication of continuous popliteal sciatic nerve block. Br J Anaesth 2005;95:255–256.

Creech C, Meyr AJ: Techniques of popliteal nerve regional anesthesia. J Foot Ankle Surg 2013;52:681–685.

Danelli G, Fanelli A, Ghisi D, et al: Ultrasound vs nerve stimulation multiple injection technique for posterior popliteal sciatic nerve block. Anaesthesia 2009;64:638–642.

Dufour E, Quennesson P, Van Robais AL, et al: Combined ultrasound and neurostimulation guidance for popliteal sciatic nerve block: a prospective, randomized comparison with neurostimulation alone. Anesth Analg 2008; 106:1553–1558.

Eisenberg JA, Calligaro KD, Kolakowski S, et al: Is balloon angioplasty of peri-anastomotic stenoses of failing peripheral arterial bypasses worthwhile? Vasc Endovascular Surg 2009;43:346–351.

Eurin M, Beloeil H, Zetlaoui PJ: A medial approach for a continuous sciatic block in the popliteal fossa [in French]. Can J Anaesth 2006;53: 1165–1166.

Gallardo J, Lagos L, Bastias C, Henríquez H, Carcuro G, Paleo M: Continuous popliteal block for postoperative analgesia in total ankle arthroplasty. Foot Ankle Int 2012;33:208–212.

Gartke K, Portner O, Taljaard M: Neuropathic symptoms following continuous popliteal block after foot and ankle surgery. Foot Ankle Int 2012;33: 267–274.

Germain G, Lévesque S, Dion N, et al: Brief reports: a comparison of an injection cephalad or caudad to the division of the sciatic nerve for ultrasound-guided popliteal block: a prospective randomized study. Anesth Analg 2012;114:233–235.

Gray AT, Huczko EL, Schafhalter-Zoppoth I: Lateral popliteal nerve block with ultrasound guidance. Reg Anesth Pain Med 2004;29:507–509.

Gucev G, Karandikar K, Charlton T: Midcalf continuous peripheral nerve block anesthesia for hallux valgus surgery: case report. Foot Ankle Int 2014;35:175–177.

Gurkan Y, Sarisoy HT, Caglayan C, Solak M, Toker K: "Figure of four" position improves the visibility of the sciatic nerve in the popliteal fossa. Agri 2009;21:149–154.

Harvey S, Corey J, Townley K: A modification of the single-penetration, dual-injection technique for combined sciatic and saphenous nerve blocks. Reg Anesth Pain Med 2014;39:561.

Hegewald K, McCann K, Elizaga A, Hutchinson BL: Popliteal blocks for foot and ankle surgery: success rate and contributing factors. J Foot Ankle Surg 2014;53:176–178.

Huntoon MA, Huntoon EA, Obray JB, Lamer TJ: Feasibility of ultrasound-guided percutaneous placement of peripheral nerve stimulation electrodes in a cadaver model: part one, lower extremity. Reg Anesth Pain Med 2008;33:551–557.

Ilfeld BM, Sandhu NS, Loland VJ, et al: Common peroneal nerve compression by a popliteal venous aneurysm. Am J Phys Med Rehabil 2009;88:947–950.

Jeong JS, Shim JC, Jeong MA, Lee BC, Sung IH: Minimum effective anaesthetic volume of 0.5% ropivacaine for ultrasound-guided popliteal sciatic nerve block in patients undergoing foot and ankle surgery: determination of ED50 and ED95. Anaesth Intensive Care 2015;43:92–97.

Karmakar M, Li X, Li J, Sala-Blanch X, Hadzic A, Gin T: Three-dimensional/four-dimensional volumetric ultrasound imaging of the sciatic nerve. Reg Anesth Pain Med 2012;37:60–66.

Khabiri B, Arbona F, Norton J: "Gapped supine" position for ultrasound guided lateral popliteal fossa block of the sciatic nerve. Anesth Analg 2007;105:1519.

Khabiri B, Hamilton C, Norton J, Arbona F: Ultrasound-guided supine posterior approach for popliteal sciatic nerve block. J Clin Anesth 2012;24:680.

Koscielniak-Nielsen ZJ, Rasmussen H, Hesselbjerg L: Long-axis ultrasound imaging of the nerves and advancement of perineural catheters under direct vision: a preliminary report of four cases. Reg Anesth Pain Med 2008;33:477–482.

Maalouf D, Liu SS, Movahedi R, et al: Nerve stimulator versus ultrasound guidance for placement of popliteal catheters for foot and ankle surgery. J Clin Anesth 2012;24:44–50.

Mariano ER, Cheng GS, Choy LP, et al: Electrical stimulation versus ultrasound guidance for popliteal-sciatic perineural catheter insertion: a randomized controlled trial. Reg Anesth Pain Med 2009;34:480–485.

Mariano ER, Loland VJ, Sandhu NS, et al: Comparative efficacy of ultrasound-guided and stimulating popliteal-sciatic perineural catheters for postoperative analgesia. Can J Anaesth 2010;10:919–926.

Minville V, Zetlaoui PJ, Fessenmeyer C, Benhamou D: Ultrasound guidance for difficult lateral popliteal catheter insertion in a patient with peripheral vascular disease. Reg Anesth Pain Med 2004;29:368–370.

Missair A, Weisman RS, Suarez MR, Yang R, Gebhard RE: A 3-dimensional ultrasound study of local anesthetic spread during lateral popliteal nerve block: what is the ideal end point for needle tip position? Reg Anesth Pain Med 2012;37:627–632.

Morau D, Levy F, Bringuier S, et al: Ultrasound-guided evaluation of the local anesthetic spread parameters required for a rapid surgical popliteal sciatic nerve block. Reg Anesth Pain Med 2010;35:559–564.

Orebaugh SL, Bigeleisen PE, Kentor ML: Impact of a regional anesthesia rotation on ultrasonographic identification of anatomic structures by anesthesiology residents. Acta Anaesthesiol Scand 2009;53:364–368.

Orebaugh SL, Williams BA, Vallejo M, Kentor ML: Adverse outcomes associated with stimulator-based peripheral nerve blocks with versus without ultrasound visualization. Reg Anesth Pain Med 2009;34:251–255.

Perkins JM: Standard varicose vein surgery. Phlebology 2009;24(Suppl 1):34–41.

Perlas A, Brull R, Chan VW, McCartney CJ, Nuica A, Abbas S: Ultrasound guidance improves the success of sciatic nerve block at the popliteal fossa. Reg Anesth Pain Med 2008;33:259–265.

Perlas A, Chan VW, Brull R: Several "correct" approaches to nerve stimulator-guided popliteal fossa block. Reg Anesth Pain Med 2009;34:624–625.

Prakash, Bhardwaj AK, Devi MN, Sridevi NS, Rao PK, Singh G: Sciatic nerve division: a cadaver study in the Indian population and review of the literature. Singapore Med J 2010;51:721–723.

Prasad A, Perlas A, Ramlogan R, Brull R, Chan V: Ultrasound-guided popliteal block distal to sciatic nerve bifurcation shortens onset time: a prospective randomized double-blind study. Re Anesth Pain Med 2010;35:267–271.

Reinoso-Barbero F, Saavedra B, Segura-Grau E, Llamas A: Anatomical comparison of sciatic nerves between adults and newborns: clinical implications for ultrasound guided block. J Anat 2014;224:108–112.

Robards C, Hadžić A, Somasundaram L, et al: Intraneural injection with low-current stimulation during popliteal sciatic nerve block. Anesth Analg 2009;109:673–677.

Robards CB, Porter SB, Logvinov I, Clendenen SR: Success of ultrasound guided popliteal sciatic nerve catheters is not influenced by nerve stimulation. Middle East J Anaesthesiol 2013;22:179–183.

Sala-Blanch X, de Riva N, Carrera A, López AM, Prats A, Hadzic A: Ultrasound-guided popliteal sciatic block with a single injection at the sciatic division results in faster block onset than the classical nerve stimulator technique. Anesth Analg 2012;114:1121–1127.

Sala Blanch X, Lopez AM, Carazo J, et al: Intraneural injection during nerve stimulator-guided sciatic nerve block at the popliteal fossa. Br J Anaesth 2009;102:855–861.

Schwartz AK, Lee DK: Ultrasound-guided (needle-in-plane) perineural catheter insertion: the effect of catheter-insertion distance on postoperative analgesia. Reg Anesth Pain Med 2011;36:261–265.

Sinha A, Chan VW: Ultrasound imaging for popliteal sciatic nerve block. Reg Anesth Pain Med 2004;29:130–134.

Sit M, Higgs JB: Non-popliteal synovial rupture. J Clin Rheumatol 2009;15:185–189.

Sites BD, Gallagher J, Sparks M: Ultrasound-guided popliteal block demonstrates an atypical motor response to nerve stimulation in 2 patients with diabetes mellitus. Reg Anesth Pain Med 2003;28:479–482.

Sites BD, Gallagher JD, Tomek I, Cheung Y, Beach ML: The use of magnetic resonance imaging to evaluate the accuracy of a handheld ultrasound machine in localizing the sciatic nerve in the popliteal fossa. Reg Anesth Pain Med 2004;29:413–416.

Techasuk W, Bernucci F, Cupido T, et al: Minimum effective volume of combined lidocaine-bupivacaine for analgesic subparaneural popliteal sciatic nerve block. Reg Anesth Pain Med 2014;39:108–111.

Tiyaprasertkul W, Bernucci F, González AP, et al: A randomized comparison between single- and triple-injection subparaneural popliteal sciatic nerve block. Reg Anesth Pain Med 2015;40:315–320.

Tran DQ, González AP, Bernucci F, Pham K, Finlayson RJ: A randomized comparison between bifurcation and prebifurcation subparaneural popliteal sciatic nerve blocks. Anesth Analg 2013;116:1170–1175.

Tsui BC, Finucane BT: The importance of ultrasound landmarks: a "traceback" approach using the popliteal blood vessels for identification of the sciatic nerve. Reg Anesth Pain Med 2006;31:481–482.

Tuveri M, Borsezio V, Argiolas R, Medas F, Tuveri A: Ultrasonographic venous anatomy at the popliteal fossa in relation to tibial nerve course in normal and varicose limbs. Chir Ital 2009;61:171–177.

van Geffen GJ, van den Broek E, Braak GJ, Giele JL, Gielen MJ, Scheffer GJ: A prospective randomised controlled trial of ultrasound guided versus nerve stimulation guided distal sciatic nerve block at the popliteal fossa. Anaesth Intensive Care 2009;37:32–37.

Verelst P, van Zundert A: Ultrasound-guided popliteal block shortens onset time compared to prebifurcation sciatic block. Reg Anesth Pain Med 2010;35:565–566.

REFERENCES

1. Sala-Blanch X, López A, Prats-Galino A: Vloka sciatic nerve sheath: a tribute to a visionary. Reg Anesth Pain Med 2015;40:174.

2. Prasad NK, Capek S, de Ruiter GC, Amrami KK, Spinner RJ: The subparaneurial compartment: a new concept in the clinicoanatomic classification of peripheral nerve lesions. Clin Anat 2015;28:925–930.

3. Tiyaprasertkul W, Bernucci F, González AP, et al: A randomized comparison between single- and triple-injection subparaneural popliteal sciatic nerve block. Reg Anesth Pain Med 2015;40:315–320.

4. Choquet O, Noble GB, Abbal B, Morau D, Bringuier S, Capdevila X: Subparaneural versus circumferential extraneural injection at the bifurcation level in ultrasound-guided popliteal sciatic nerve blocks: a prospective, randomized, double-blind study. Reg Anesth Pain Med 2014;39:306–311.

5. Sala-Blanch X, Reina MA, Ribalta T, Prats-Galino A: Sciatic nerve structure and nomenclature: epineurium to paraneurium: is this a new paradigm? Reg Anesth Pain Med 2013;38:463–465.

6. Karmakar MK, Shariat AN, Pangthipampai P, Chen J: High-definition ultrasound imaging defines the paraneural sheath and the fascial compartments surrounding the sciatic nerve at the popliteal fossa. Reg Anesth Pain Med 2013;38:447–451.

7. Lopez AM, Sala-Blanch X, Castillo R, Hadzic A: Ultrasound guided injection inside the common sheath of the sciatic nerve at division level has a higher success rate than an injection outside the sheath. Rev Esp Anestesiol Reanim 2014;61:304–310.

8. Perlas A, Wong P, Abdallah F, Hazrati LN, Tse C, Chan V: Ultrasound-guided popliteal block through a common paraneural sheath versus conventional injection: a prospective, randomized, double-blind study. Reg Anesth Pain Med 2013;38:218–225.

9. Ip V, Tsui B: Injection through the paraneural sheath rather than circumferential spread facilitates safe, effective sciatic nerve block. Reg Anesth Pain Med 2013;38:373.

10. Endersby R, Albrecht E, Perlas A, Chan V: Semantics, misnomer, or uncertainty: where is the epineurium on ultrasound? Reg Anesth Pain Med 2012;37:360–361.

11. Tran DQ, Dugani S, Pham K, Al-Shaafi A, Finlayson RJ: A randomized comparison between subepineural and conventional ultrasound-guided popliteal sciatic nerve block. Reg Anesth Pain Med 2011;36:548–552.

12. Sala-Blanch X, López AM, Pomés J, Valls-Sole J, García AI, Hadzic A: No clinical or electrophysiologic evidence of nerve injury after intraneural injection during sciatic popliteal block. Anesthesiology 2011;115:589–595.

13. Morau D, Levy F, Bringuier S, et al: Ultrasound-guided evaluation of the local anesthetic spread parameters required for a rapid surgical popliteal sciatic nerve block. Reg Anesth Pain Med 2010;35:559–564.

14. Vloka JD, Hadzić A, Lesser JB, et al: A common epineural sheath for the nerves in the popliteal fossa and its possible implications for sciatic nerve block. Anesth Analg 1997;84:387–390.

15. Choquet O, Capdevila X: Ultrasound-guided nerve blocks: the real position of the needle should be defined. Anesth Analg 2012;114:929–930.

16. Sinha SK, Abrams JH, Arumugam S, et al: Femoral nerve block with selective tibial nerve block provides effective analgesia without foot drop after total knee arthroplasty: a prospective, randomized, observer-blinded study. Anesth Analg 2012;115:202–206.

17. Ting PH, Antonakakis JG, Scalzo DC: Ultrasound-guided common peroneal nerve block at the level of the fibular head. J Clin Anesth 2012;24:145–147.

Ultrasound-Guided Ankle Block

Catherine Vandepitte, Ana M. Lopez, Sam Van Boxstael, and Hassanin Jalil

ANKLE BLOCK AT A GLANCE

- Indications: Distal foot and toe surgery
- Transducer position: about the ankle; depends on the nerve to be blocked
- Goal: local anesthetic spread surrounding each individual nerve
- Local anesthetic: 3–5 mL per nerve

GENERAL CONSIDERATIONS

Using an ultrasound (US)-guided technique affords a practitioner the ability to reduce the volume of local anesthetic required for ankle blockade. Because the nerves involved are located relatively close to the surface, ankle blocks are easy to perform; however, knowledge of the anatomy of the ankle is essential to ensure success.[1]

ULTRASOUND ANATOMY

Ankle block involves anesthetizing five separate nerves: two deep nerves and three superficial nerves. The two deep nerves are the tibial nerve and the deep peroneal nerve. The three superficial nerves are the superficial peroneal, sural, and saphenous nerves. All nerves, except the saphenous, are terminal branches of the sciatic nerve; the saphenous nerve is a sensory branch of the femoral nerve.

Tibial Nerve

The tibial nerve is the largest of the five nerves at the ankle level and provides innervation to the heel and sole of the foot. With the linear transducer placed transversely at (or just proximal to) the level of the medial malleolus, the nerve can be seen immediately posterior to the posterior tibial artery

(Figures 33H–1, 33H–2, and 33H–3). Color Doppler can be very useful in locating the posterior tibial artery when it is not readily apparent. The nerve typically appears hyperechoic with honeycomb pattern. A useful mnemonic for the relevant structures in the vicinity is **T**om, **D**ick **AN**d **H**arry, which refers to, from anterior to posterior, the **t**ibialis posterior tendon, flexor **d**igitorum longus tendon, **a**rtery/**n**erve/vein, and flexor **h**allucis longus tendon. These tendons can resemble the nerve in appearance, which can be confusing. The nerve's intimate relationship with the artery should be kept in mind to avoid misidentification. If in doubt, track the structure proximally: tendons will turn into muscle bellies, whereas the nerve will not change in appearance.

Deep Peroneal Nerve

This branch of the common peroneal nerve innervates the ankle extensor muscles, the ankle joint and the web space between the first and second toes. As it approaches the ankle, the nerve crosses the anterior tibial artery from a medial to lateral position. A transducer placed in the transverse orientation at the level of the extensor retinaculum will show the nerve lying immediately lateral to the artery, on the surface of the tibia (Figures 33H–4, 33H–5, and 33H–6). In some individuals the nerve courses along the medial side of the artery. The nerve usually appears hypoechoic with a hyperechoic rim, but it is small and often difficult to distinguish from the surrounding tissue.

Clinical Pearl

- When the deep peroneal nerve is difficult to identify on US, an injection around the artery may help with visualization.

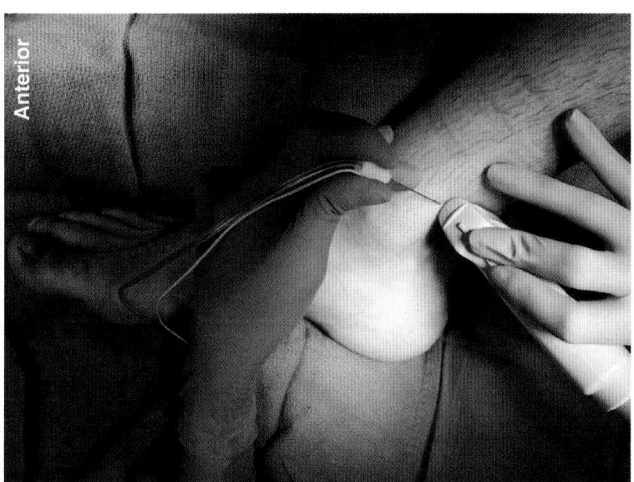

FIGURE 33H–1. Transducer position and needle insertion for a block of the tibial nerve using an in-plane technique.

Superficial Peroneal Nerve

The superficial peroneal nerve innervates the dorsum of the foot. It emerges to lie superficial to the fascia 10–20 cm above the ankle joint on the anterolateral surface of the leg and divides into two or three small branches. A transducer placed transversely on the leg, approximately 5-10 cm proximal and anterior to the lateral malleolus, will identify the hyperechoic nerve branches lying in the subcutaneous tissue immediately superficial to the fascia (Figures 33H–7, 33H–8, and 33H–9). To identify the nerve proximal to its division, the transducer can be traced proximally until, at the lateral aspect, the

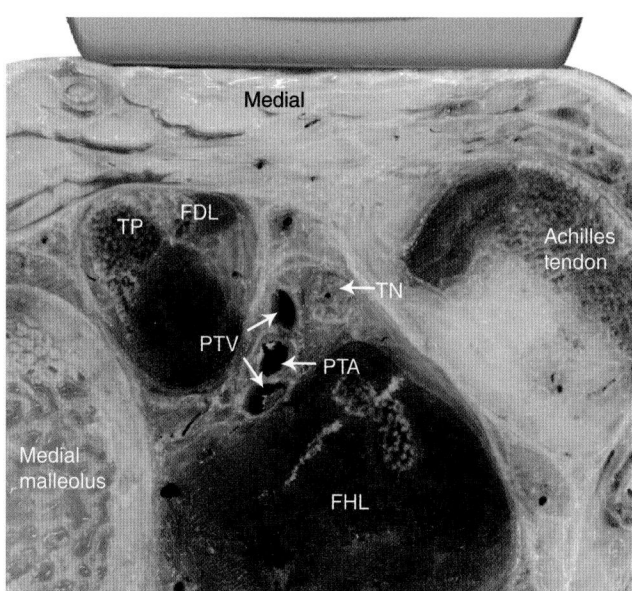

FIGURE 33H–2. Cross-sectional anatomy of the tibial nerve at the level of the ankle. Shown are the posterior tibial artery (PTA) and vein (PTV) behind the medial malleolus , the tibialis posterior (TP) and the flexor digitorum longus (FDL). The tibial nerve (TN) is just posterior to the posterior tibial vessels and superficial to the flexor hallucis longus muscle (FHL). (Reproduced with permission from Hadzic A: *Hadzic's Peripheral Nerve Blocks and Anatomy for Ultrasound-Guided Regional Anesthesia*, 2nd ed. New York: McGraw-Hill, 2011.)

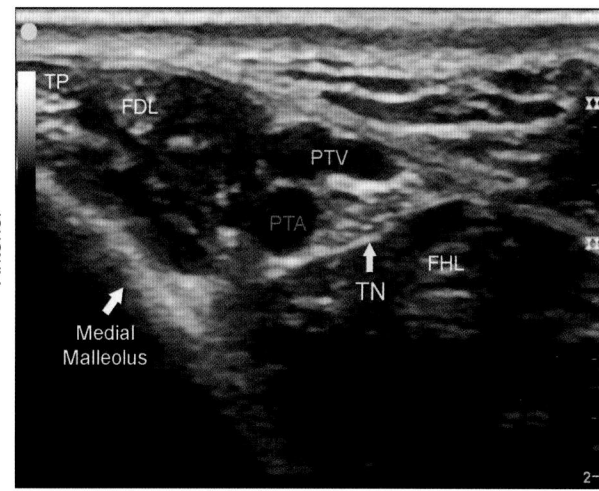

Tibial Nerve - Ankle, Medial Aspect

FIGURE 33H–3. The tibial nerve (TN) is seen posterior and deep to the posterior tibial artery (PTA). TP, tibialis posterior; FDL, flexor digitorum longus; FHL, flexor hallucis longus; PTV, posterior tibial vein.

extensor digitorum longus and peroneus brevis muscle can be seen with a prominent groove between them leading to the fibula (Figure 33H–10). The superficial peroneal nerve is located in this groove, just deep to the fascia. Once it has been identified at this more proximal location, the nerve can be traced distally to the ankle or it can be blocked at this level. Because the superficial nerves are rather small, their identification with US is not always possible.

Clinical Pearl

- The use of a small-gauge needle (25-gauge) is recommended to decrease patient discomfort as needle insertion in this area can be painful.

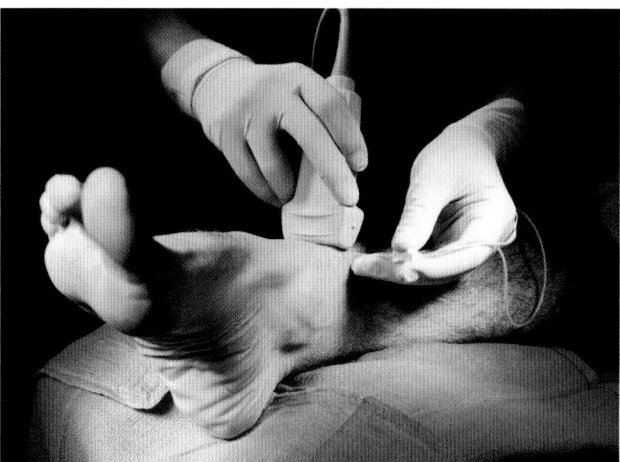

FIGURE 33H–4. Transducer position and needle insertion to block the deep peroneal nerve at the level of the ankle. (Reproduced with permission from Hadzic A: *Hadzic's Peripheral Nerve Blocks and Anatomy for Ultrasound-Guided Regional Anesthesia*, 2nd ed. New York: McGraw-Hill, 2011.)

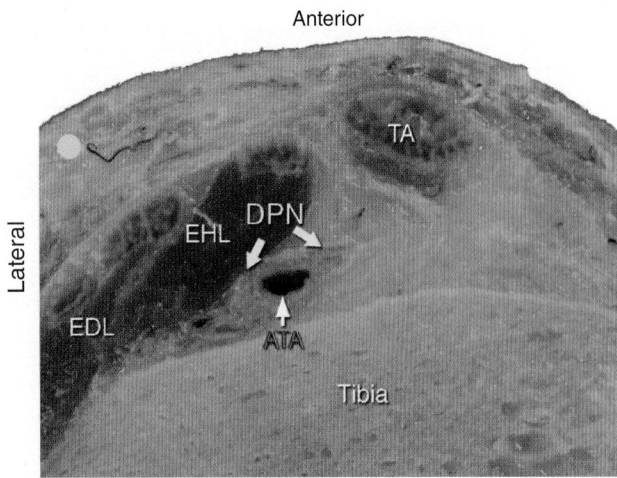

Deep Peroneal Nerve - Ankle

FIGURE 33H–5. Cross-sectional anatomy of the deep peroneal nerve at the level of the ankle. The deep peroneal nerve (DPN) is located just lateral to anterior tibial artery (ATA) and between extensor hallucis longus (EHL) and tibia. Note the proximity of the extensor digitorum longus (EDL) and the tibialis anterior (TA), which can serve as an important landmark; to locate it, flex and extend the patient's great toe manually. The deep peroneal nerve appears divided in this section. (Reproduced with permission from Hadzic A: *Hadzic's Peripheral Nerve Blocks and Anatomy for Ultrasound-Guided Regional Anesthesia*, 2nd ed. New York: McGraw-Hill, 2011.)

Sural Nerve

The sural nerve innervates the lateral margin of the foot and ankle. Proximal to the lateral malleolus, the sural nerve can be visualized as a small hyperechoic structure that is intimately associated with the small saphenous vein superficial to the deep

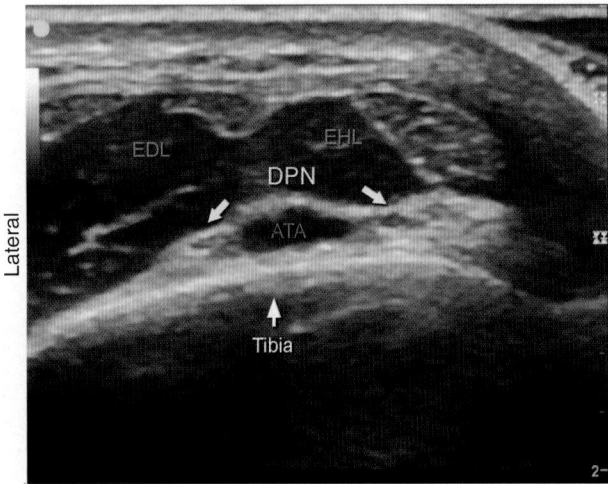

Deep Peroneal Nerve - Ankle, Anterior Aspect

FIGURE 33H–6. US image of the deep peroneal nerve (DPN), seen at the surface of the tibia just lateral to the anterior tibial artery (ATA). The nerve is divided in this image. The surrounding tendons are the extensor hallucis longus (EHL) and the extensor digitorum longus (EDL). (Reproduced with permission from Hadzic A: *Hadzic's Peripheral Nerve Blocks and Anatomy for Ultrasound-Guided Regional Anesthesia*, 2nd ed. New York: McGraw-Hill, 2011.)

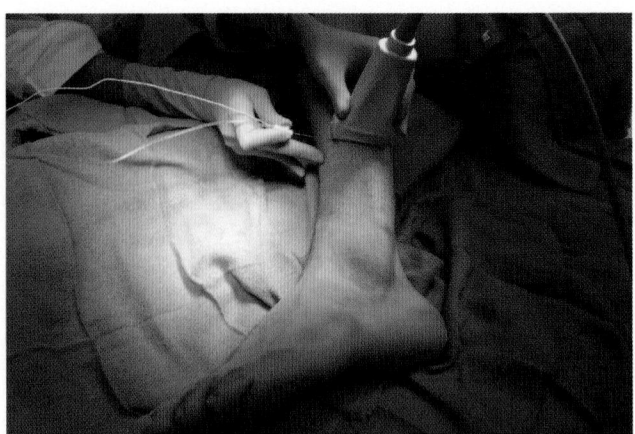

FIGURE 33H–7. Transducer position and needle insertion to block the superficial peroneal nerve.

fascia. The sural nerve, can be traced back along the posterior aspect of the leg, running in the midline superficial to the achiles tendon and gastronemious muscles (Figures 33H–11, 33H–12, and 33H–13). A calf tourniquet can be used to increase the size of the vein and facilitate its imaging; the nerve is often found in the immediate vicinity of the vein.

Saphenous Nerve

The saphenous nerve innervates the medial malleolus and a variable portion of the medial aspect of the leg below the knee. The nerve travels down the medial leg alongside the great saphenous vein. Because it is a small nerve, it is best visualized 10–15 cm proximal to the medial malleolus, using the great saphenous vein as a landmark (Figures 33H–14, 33H–15, and 33H–16). A proximal calf tourniquet can be used to assist in

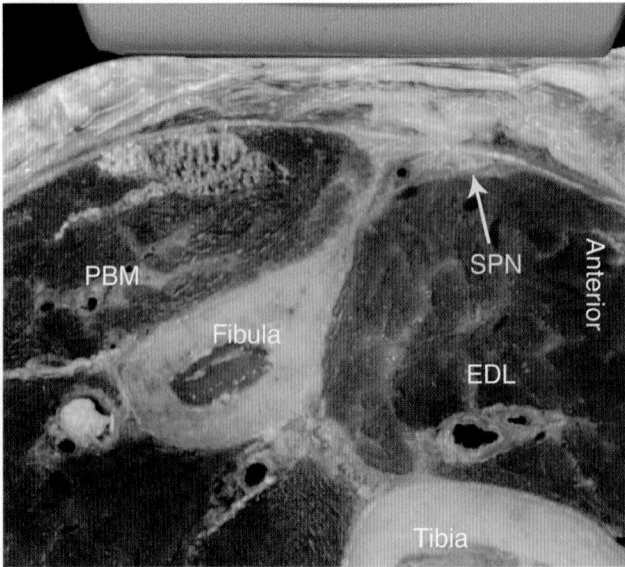

FIGURE 33H–8. Cross-sectional anatomy of the superficial peroneal nerve (SPN). EDL, extensor digitorum longus muscle; PBM, peroneus brevis muscle. (Reproduced with permission from Hadzic A: *Hadzic's Peripheral Nerve Blocks and Anatomy for Ultrasound-Guided Regional Anesthesia*, 2nd ed. New York: McGraw-Hill, 2011.)

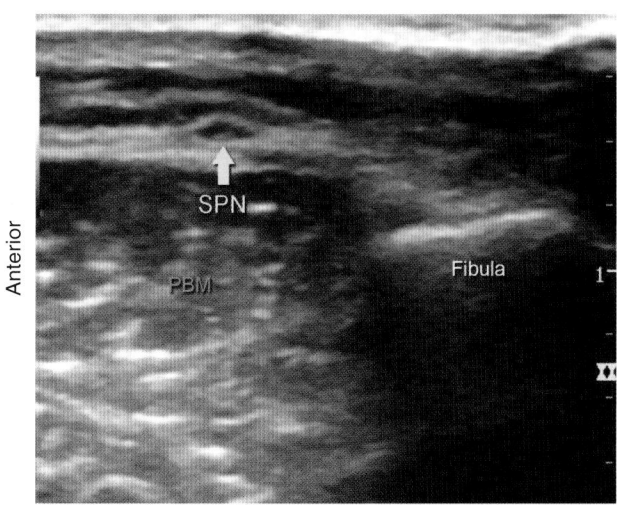

Ankle block-superficial peroneal nerve

FIGURE 33H–9. US anatomy of the superficial peroneal nerve (SPN). PBM, peroneus brevis muscle. (Reproduced with permission from Hadzic A: *Hadzic's Peripheral Nerve Blocks and Anatomy for Ultrasound-Guided Regional Anesthesia*, 2nd ed. New York: McGraw-Hill, 2011.)

increasing the size of the vein. The nerve appears as a small hyperechoic structure, next to the vein. At this level the nerve often has several branches.

Clinical Pearl

- When using veins as landmarks, use as little pressure as possible on the transducer in order to permit the veins to fill.

DISTRIBUTION OF ANESTHESIA

An ankle block results in anesthesia of the entire foot. For a more comprehensive review of the distribution of each nerve, see Chapter 3.

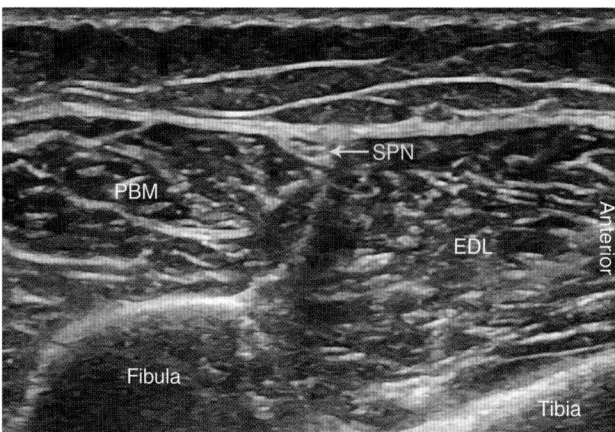

FIGURE 33H–10. US anatomy of the superficial peroneal nerve with structures labeled. EDL, extensor digitorum longus muscle; PBM, peroneus brevis muscle; SPN, superficial peroneal nerve.

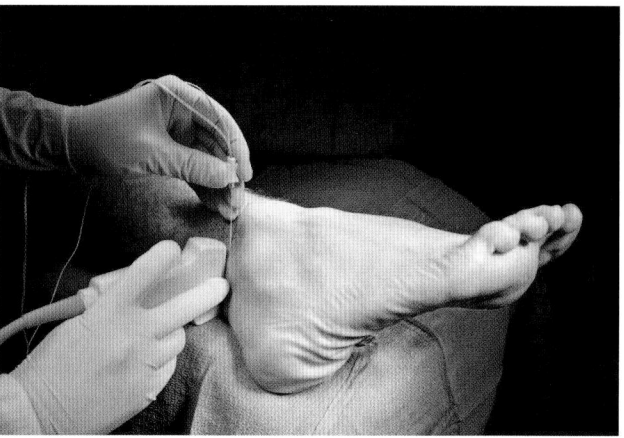

FIGURE 33H–11. Transducer position and needle insertion to block the sural nerve. (Reproduced with permission from Hadzic A: *Hadzic's Peripheral Nerve Blocks and Anatomy for Ultrasound-Guided Regional Anesthesia*, 2nd ed. New York: McGraw-Hill, 2011.)

EQUIPMENT

The equipment recommended for an ankle block is as follows:

- Ultrasound machine with linear transducer (8–18 MHz), sterile sleeve, and gel

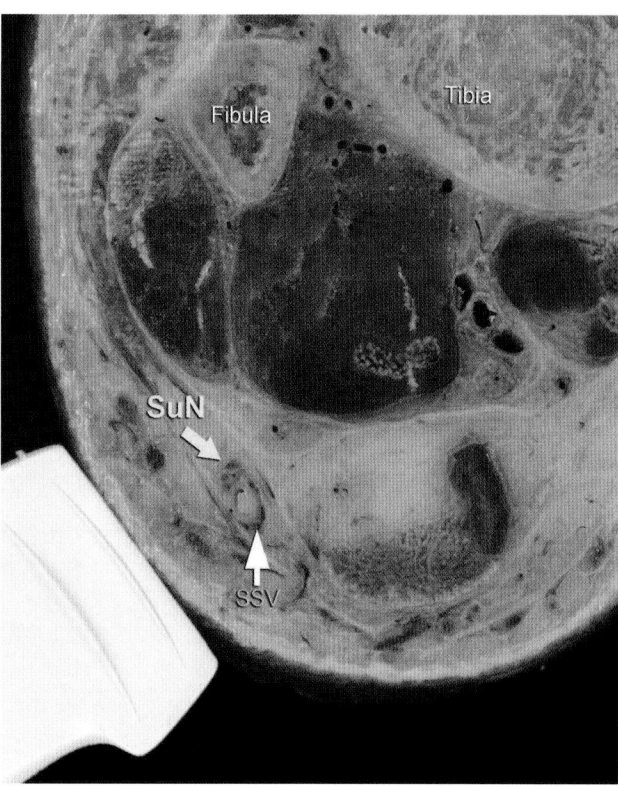

FIGURE 33H–12. Cross-sectional anatomy of the sural nerve at the level of the ankle. Shown is the sural nerve (SuN) in the immediate vicinity of the small saphenous vein (SSV). (Reproduced with permission from Hadzic A: *Hadzic's Peripheral Nerve Blocks and Anatomy for Ultrasound-Guided Regional Anesthesia*, 2nd ed. New York: McGraw-Hill, 2011.)

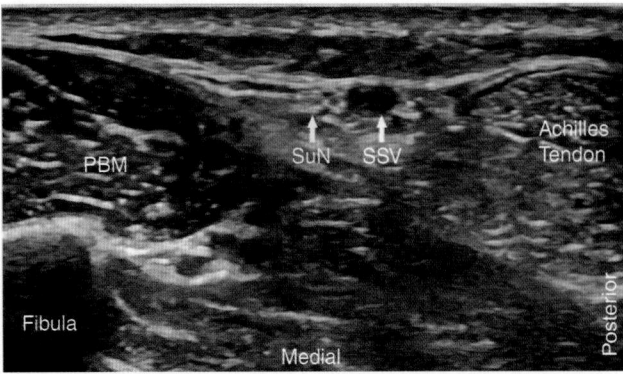

FIGURE 33H–13. US anatomy of the sural nerve (SuN). Shown are the peroneus brevis muscle (PBM) and small saphenous vein (SSV).

- Standard nerve block tray
- Three 10-mL syringes containing local anesthetic
- A 1.5-inch, 22- to 25-gauge needle with low-volume extension tubing
- Sterile gloves

LANDMARKS AND PATIENT POSITIONING

This block is usually performed with the patient in the supine position. A footrest underneath the calf facilitates access to the ankle, especially for the tibial and sural nerve blocks. An assistant is helpful to maintain internal or external rotation of the leg as needed.

GOAL

The goal is to place the needle tip immediately adjacent to each of the five nerves and deposit local anesthetic until the spread around each nerve is accomplished.

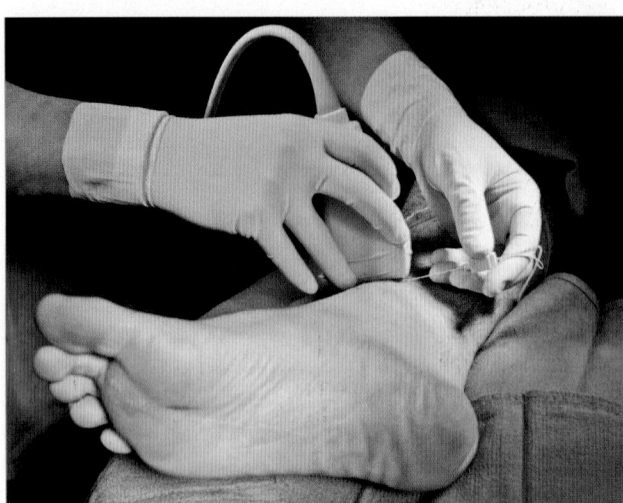

FIGURE 33H–14. Transducer position and needle insertion to block the saphenous nerve. (Reproduced with permission from Hadzic A: *Hadzic's Peripheral Nerve Blocks and Anatomy for Ultrasound-Guided Regional Anesthesia*, 2nd ed. New York: McGraw-Hill, 2011.)

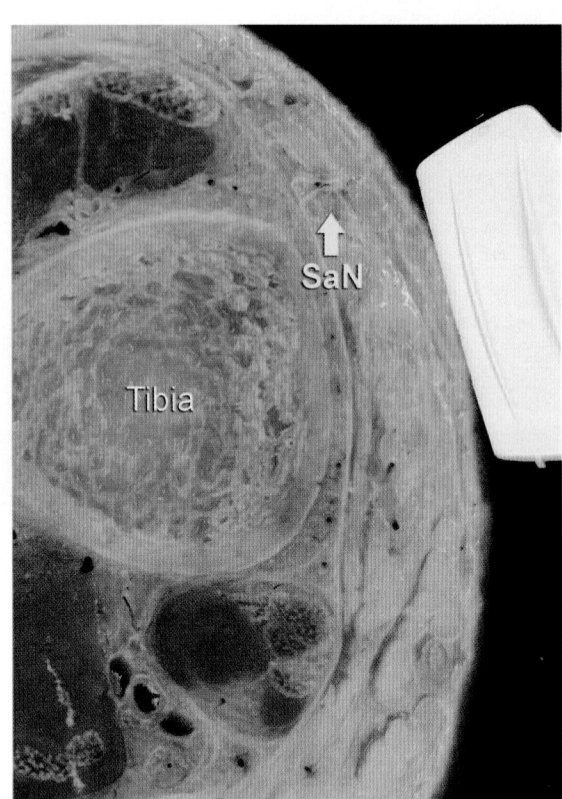

FIGURE 33H–15. Cross-sectional anatomy of the saphenous nerve (SaN) at the level of the ankle. (Reproduced with permission from Hadzic A: *Hadzic's Peripheral Nerve Blocks and Anatomy for Ultrasound-Guided Regional Anesthesia*, 2nd ed. New York: McGraw-Hill, 2011.)

TECHNIQUE

With the patient in the proper position, the skin is disinfected. For each of the blocks, the needle can be inserted either in plane or out of plane. Ergonomics often dictate which approach is

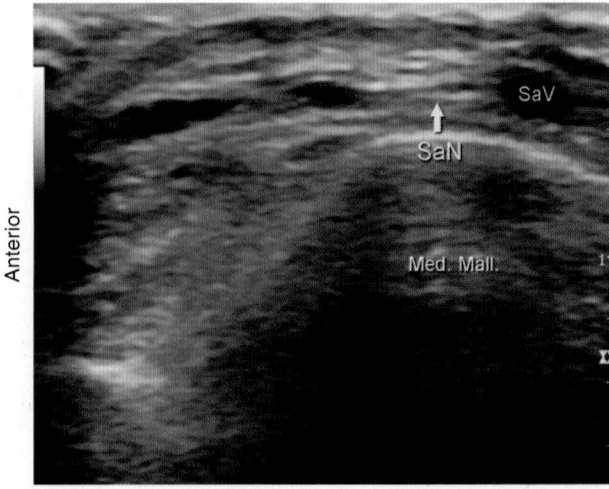

Ankle block-saphenous nerve

FIGURE 33H–16. US anatomy of the saphenous nerve (SaN). Shown are the great saphenous vein (SaV) and the medial malleolus (Med. Mall.). (Reproduced with permission from Hadzic A: *Hadzic's Peripheral Nerve Blocks and Anatomy for Ultrasound-Guided Regional Anesthesia*, 2nd ed. New York: McGraw-Hill, 2011.)

most effective. A successful block is predicted by the spread of local anesthetic immediately adjacent to the nerve; redirection to achieve circumferential spread is not necessary because these nerves are small, and the local anesthetic diffuses quickly into the neural tissue. A 3–5 mL of local anesthetic per nerve is typically sufficient for an effective block.

TIPS

- If the smaller superficial nerves (sural, saphenous and superficial peroneal) are not seen, these nerves can be blocked simply by injecting local anesthetic into the subcutaneous tissue as a "skin wheal"; for the sural nerve, inject from the Achilles tendon to the lateral malleolus; for the superficial peroneal and the saphenous, inject anteriorly from one malleolus to the other, taking care to avoid injuring the great saphenous vein.
- For surgery on the forefoot and toes, the saphenous nerve block may be omitted, as in 97% of patients, the saphenous nerve innervation does not extend beyond the midfoot. However, an anatomical study found branches of the saphenous nerve reaching the first metatarsal in 28% of specimens.[2,3]

SUGGESTED READINGS

Antonakakis JG, Scalzo DC, Jorgenson AS, et al: Ultrasound does not improve the success rate of a deep peroneal nerve block at the ankle. Reg Anesth Pain Med 2010;35:217–221.

Benzon HT, Sekhadia M, Benzon HA, et al: Ultrasound-assisted and evoked motor response stimulation of the deep peroneal nerve. Anesth Analg 2009;109:2022–2024.
Canella C, Demondion X, Guillin R, et al: Anatomic study of the superficial peroneal nerve using sonography. AJR Am J Roentgenol 2009;193:174–179.
Prakash, Bhardwaj AK, Singh DK, Rajini T, Jayanthi V, Singh G: Anatomic variations of superficial peroneal nerve: clinical implications of a cadaver study. Ital J Anat Embryol 2010;115:223–228.
Redborg KE, Antonakakis JG, Beach ML, Chinn CD, Sites BD: Ultrasound improves the success rate of a tibial nerve block at the ankle. Reg Anesth Pain Med 2009;34:256–260.
Redborg KE, Sites BD, Chinn CD, et al: Ultrasound improves the success rate of a sural nerve block at the ankle. Reg Anesth Pain Med 2009;34:24–28.
Russell DF, Pillai A, Kumar CS: Safety and efficacy of forefoot surgery under ankle block anaesthesia. Scott Med J 2014;59:103–107.
Snaith R, Dolan J: Ultrasound-guided superficial peroneal nerve block for foot surgery. AJR Am J Roentgenol 2010;194:W538.

REFERENCES

1. Chin KJ, Wong NW, Macfarlane AJ, Chan VW: Ultrasound-guided versus anatomic landmark-guided ankle blocks: a 6-year retrospective review. Reg Anesth Pain Med 2011;36:611–618.
2. López AM, Sala-Blanch X, Magaldi M, Poggio D, Asuncion J, Franco CD: Ultrasound-guided ankle block for forefoot surgery: the contribution of the saphenous nerve. Reg Anesth Pain Med 2012;37:554–557.
3. Marsland D, Dray A, Little NJ, Solan MC: The saphenous nerve in foot and ankle surgery: its variable anatomy and relevance. Foot Ankle Surg 2013;19:76–79.

CHAPTER 34

Ultrasound-Guided Transversus Abdominis Plane and Quadratus Lumborum Blocks

Hesham Elsharkawy and Thomas F. Bendtsen

INTRODUCTION

Ultrasound-guided transversus abdominis plane (TAP) block has become a common analgesic method after surgery involving the abdominal wall. Because TAP blockade is limited to somatic anesthesia of the abdominal wall and highly dependent on interfascial spread, various newer techniques have been proposed to enhance analgesia, either in addition to TAP block or as a single modality. In particular, variants of quadratus lumborum blocks (QLBs) have been proposed as more consistent methods with an aim to accomplish somatic as well as visceral analgesia of the abdomen. The present evidence, mainly case reports, suggests that different variants of QLB have different analgesic effects and mechanisms of action, although this has not been formally validated. In particular, transmuscular QLB and the so-called QLB2 may result in wider and longer sensory blockade compared to TAP block (T4–L1 for QL block vs. T6–T12 for the TAP blocks) (Figures 34–1 and 34–2). This chapter focuses on underlying principles for TAP blockade and the newer QLB techniques, with an understanding that the information about the latter is based on sparse evidence of limited quality as outcome-based studies are not yet available.

ANATOMY

The **transversus abdominis plane** is the fascial plane superficial to the transversus abdominis muscle, the innermost muscular layer of the anterolateral abdominal wall. The upper fibrous anterior part of the muscle lies posterior to the rectus abdominis muscle and reaches the xiphoid process. The posterior aponeuroses of the transversus abdominis and internal oblique muscles fuse and attach to the thoracolumbar fascia (TLF). In the TAP, the intercostal, subcostal, and L1 segmental nerves communicate to form the upper and lower TAP plexuses, which innervate the anterolateral abdominal wall, including the parietal peritoneum. Therefore, TAP blockade requires anesthesia of the upper (also known as the subcostal or intercostal) TAP plexus, as well as the lower TAP plexus, located in the vicinity of the deep circumflex iliac artery.

The subcostal approach to the TAP block ideally anesthetizes the intercostal nerves T6–T9 between the rectus abdominis sheath and the transversus abdominis muscle. The lateral TAP block in the midaxillary line between the thoracic cage and iliac crest as well as between the internal oblique and transversus abdominis muscles ideally should reach intercostal nerves T10–T11 and the subcostal nerve T12. Of note, the umbilicus is innervated by intercostal nerve T10. The L1 segmental nerves in the TAP are not covered by the lateral TAP block and require an anterior TAP block medial to the anterior superior iliac spine. A posterior approach to block the TAP plexuses via the triangle of Petit has also been described. TAP blocks provide somatic analgesia of the abdominal wall including the parietal peritoneum.

The **quadratus lumborum (QL) muscle** lies in the posterior abdominal wall dorsolateral to the psoas major muscle (Figure 34–3). The QL muscle originates from the posterior part of the iliac crest and the iliolumbar ligament and inserts on the 12th rib and the transverse processes of vertebrae L1–L5. The QL muscle assists in lateral flexion of the lumbar spine.

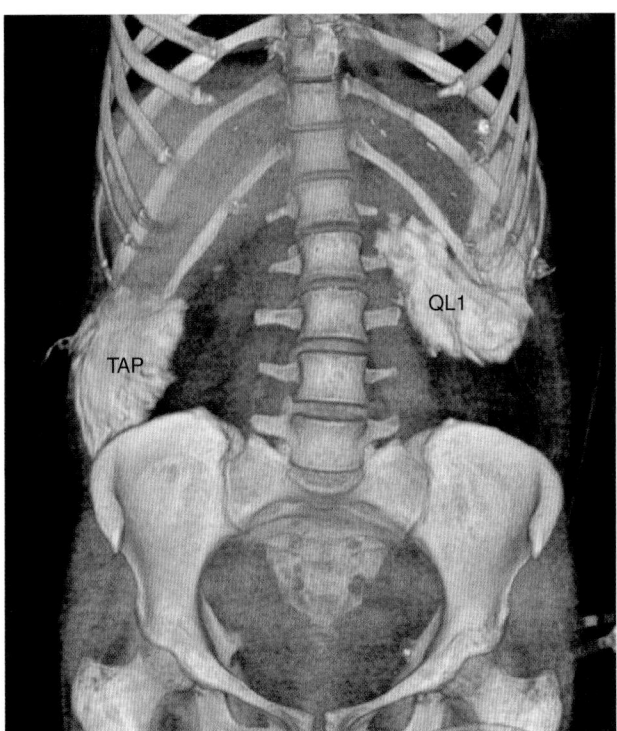

FIGURE 34–1. The transverse abdominis plane (TAP) and quadratus lumborum 1 (QL1) blocks: anterior view. Injection of 20 mL of contrast in the TAP block resulted in the posterolateral spread from the 12th rib to the iliac crest. The QL1 block after injection of 20 mL of contrast resulted in the spread of the contrast toward the transverse process cephalad alongside the thoracolumbar fascia to the 11th and 10th intercostal spaces.

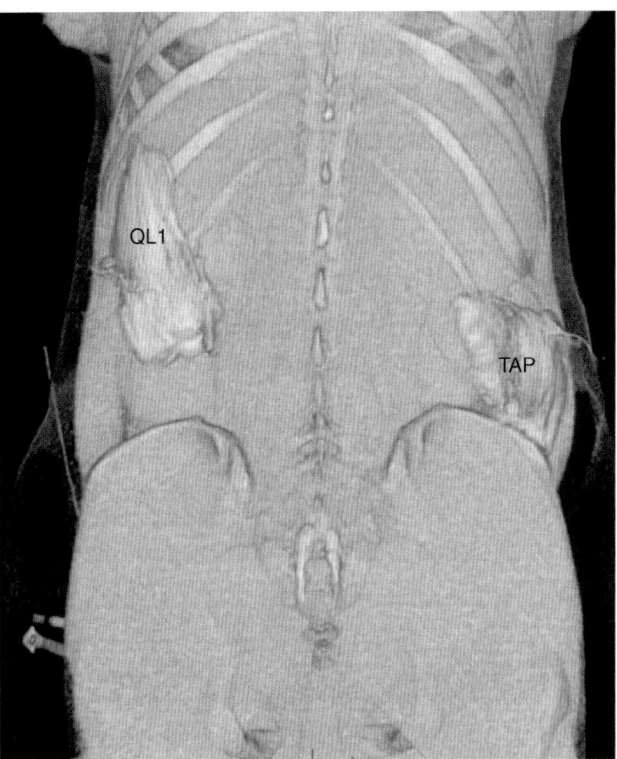

FIGURE 34–2. Transverse abdominis plane (TAP) and quadratus lumborum 1 (QL1) blocks: posterior view. Injection of 20 mL of contrast in the TAP block resulted in the posterolateral spread from the 12th rib to the iliac crest. After injection of 20 mL of contrast, the QL1 block resulted in the spread of the contrast toward the transverse process cephalad alongside the thoracolumbar fascia to the 11th and 10th intercostal spaces.

The **thoracolumbar fascia** consists of anterior, middle, and posterior layers (Figure 34–4). The posterior layer of the TLF forms an attachment to the strong membranous aponeurosis of the latissimus dorsi. The three layers of the TLF are continuous with the fused posterior aponeurosis of the internal oblique and transversus abdominis muscles.

The posterior layer of the TLF covers the superficial side of the erector spinae. In the lumbar region, the posterior layer extends from the spinous processes medially to the lateral margin of the erector spinae, where it fuses with the middle layer of the TLF and forms the so-called lateral raphe, which is a dense connective pillar that extends from the iliac crest to the 12th rib. The deepest lamina of the posterior layer is called the *paraspinal retinacular sheath* (PRS), which encapsulates the erector spinae muscles.[1] The *lateral interfascial triangle* (LIFT)'s is made by the lateral margin of the erector spinae muscle (base), the PRS with overlying posterior and middle layers of the TLF (sides), and the lateral raphe (apex). The middle layer of the TLF separates the QL and erector spinae muscles. The anterior layer of the TLF covers the anterior aspect of the QL muscle.

The **transversalis fascia (TF)** invests the parietal subperitoneal areolar tissue in the abdominal cavity. The outer surface of the TF lines the deep side of the transversus abdominis, QL, and psoas major muscles. The TF communicates with the endothoracic fascia posterior to the diaphragm where the TF is thickened as the medial and lateral arcuate ligaments, with

possibility of spread of injectate from the QL and psoas major muscle compartments to the thoracic paravertebral space (Figure 34–5).[2] Consequently, when local anesthetic is injected into the fascial plane between these muscles in the lumbar region, it could spread cranially to the thoracic paravertebral space. The anterior layer of the TLF is fused with the TF. The iliohypogastric, ilioinguinal, and subcostal nerves that cross the QL muscle lie between this muscle and the TF. The **four lumbar arteries** on each side pass posterior to the psoas major and QL muscles, pierce the aponeurosis of the transversus abdominis muscle, and end up inside the TAP (Figure 34–6).

The lower pole of the kidney lies anterior to the QL muscle and can reach the L4 level with deep inspiration. Therefore, this should be checked when performing QL block as the kidney may be separated from the QL muscle only by perinephric fat, the posterior layer of renal fascia, the TF, and the anterior layer of the TLF. In summary, the kidney should always be visualized with QL blocks to avoid kidney injury.

PATIENT POSITIONING AND EQUIPMENT SELECTION

For QL blocks, the lateral decubitus position is preferred over the supine position as it provides better ergonomics and relevant sono-images of the neuroaxial structures. A low-frequency (5- to 2-MHz) curved array ultrasound transducer in transverse

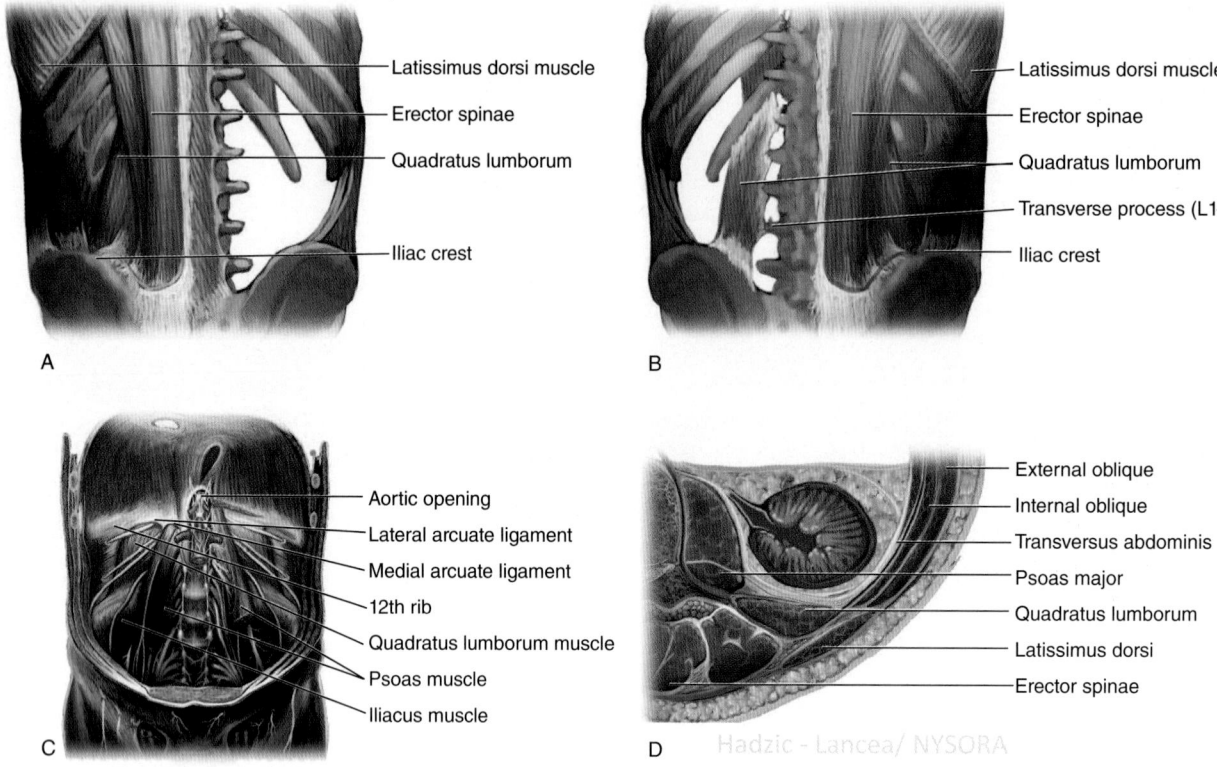

FIGURE 34–3. The quadratus lumborum (QL) muscle in four views: **A:** QL muscle from the back covered by the erector spinae and latissimus dorsi muscles. **B:** QL muscle from the back, with ES and LD muscles removed to show the origin and insertion of the QL muscle. **C:** QL muscle from the front, on the left side the psoas muscle is cut, showing the ventral rami of the spinal nerve roots pass in front of the QL. **D:** QL muscle cross section showing the surrounding muscles and the QL relation to the kidney.

axis is preferred to visualize the three lateral abdominal wall muscle layers and the QL muscle. A 22-gauge, short-bevel needle is recommended for the single-injection technique, whereas an 18- to 21-gauge, 10-cm Tuohy needle with extension tubing is used for catheters. A peripheral nerve stimulator may be useful as a warning sign to prevent further needle advancement should the needle be mistakenly placed too deep and next to the lumbar plexus.

SCANNING AND BLOCK TECHNIQUES

Subcostal TAP Block

A linear transducer is placed alongside the lower margin of the rib cage as medial and cranial as possible for the subcostal TAP block (Figure 34-7a). The rectus abdominis muscle and its posterior rectus sheath are visualized along with the transversus

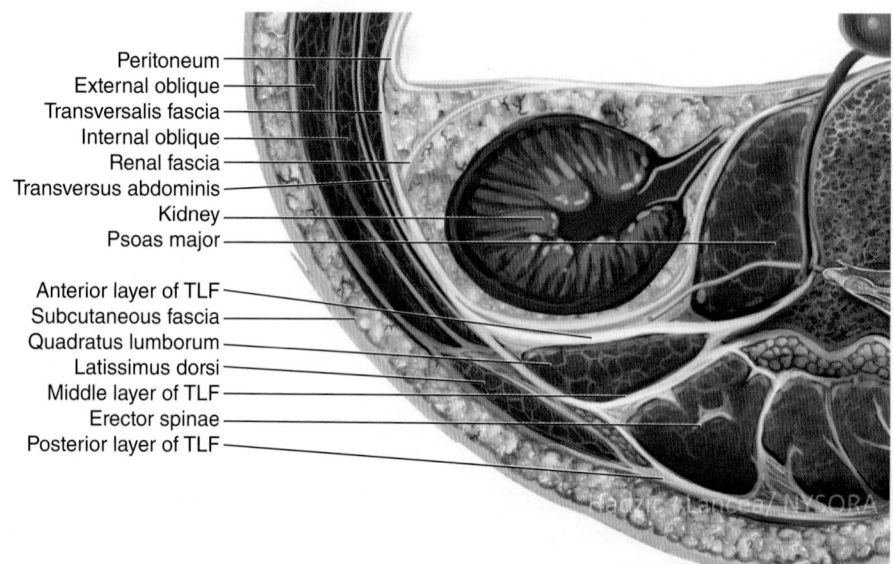

FIGURE 34–4. The different layers of the thoracolumbar fascia (TLF).

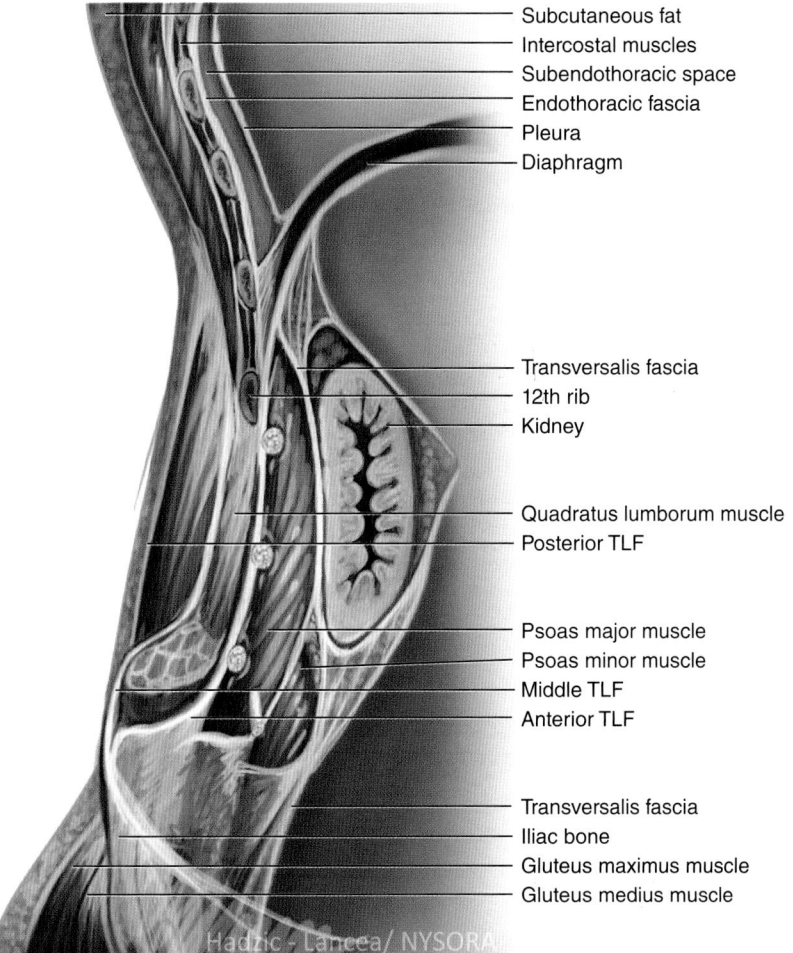

Subcutaneous fat
Intercostal muscles
Subendothoracic space
Endothoracic fascia
Pleura
Diaphragm

Transversalis fascia
12th rib
Kidney

Quadratus lumborum muscle
Posterior TLF

Psoas major muscle
Psoas minor muscle
Middle TLF
Anterior TLF

Transversalis fascia
Iliac bone
Gluteus maximus muscle
Gluteus medius muscle

FIGURE 34–5. A sagittal section showing the fascial relations of the lower thoracic subendothoracic paravertebral space and the retroperitoneal space.

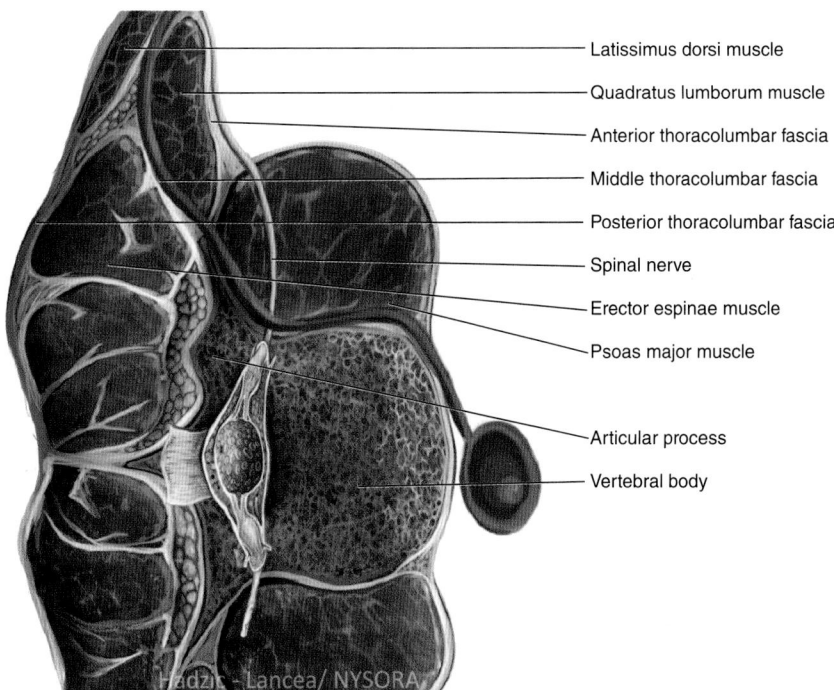

Latissimus dorsi muscle
Quadratus lumborum muscle
Anterior thoracolumbar fascia
Middle thoracolumbar fascia
Posterior thoracolumbar fascia
Spinal nerve
Erector espinae muscle
Psoas major muscle

Articular process
Vertebral body

FIGURE 34–6. Cross section of the quadratus lumborum (QL) muscle and its relation the ventral rami of the spinal nerve roots (yellow) and the abdominal branches of the lumbar arteries (red).

abdominis muscle deep to the posterior rectus sheath. The target is the fascial plane between the posterior rectus sheath and the transversus abdominis muscle. The needle is inserted above the rectus abdominis close to the midline and advanced from medial to lateral (alternatively, lateral to medial). The end point of injection is the spread of local anesthetic between the posterior rectus sheath and the anterior margin of the transversus abdominis muscle.

Lateral TAP Block

For the lateral TAP block, a linear transducer is placed in the axial plane on the midaxillary line between the subcostal margin and the iliac crest (Figure 34-7b). The three layers of abdominal wall muscles are visualized: external and internal oblique as well as the transversus abdominis muscles. The target is the fascial plane between the internal oblique and the transversus abdominis muscles. The needle is inserted in the anterior axillary line, and the needle tip is advanced until it reaches the fascial plane between the internal oblique and transversus abdominis muscles approximately in the midaxillary line.

Anterior TAP Block

A linear transducer is placed medial to the anterior superior iliac spine pointing toward the umbilicus with a caudad tilt for the anterior TAP block (Figure 34-7c). The three abdominal wall muscles are visualized (see discussion for the lateral TAP block). The target is the same fascial plane at the level of the deep circumflex iliac artery. The needle is inserted medial to the anterior superior iliac spine. The needle tip is advanced until it is placed between the internal oblique and transversus abdominis muscles adjacent to the deep circumflex iliac artery.

Posterior TAP Block

For the posterior TAP block, the linear transducer is placed in the axial plane in the midaxillary line and moved posteriorly to the most posterior limit of the TAP between the internal oblique and transversus abdominis muscles (Figure 34-7d). The target is the most posterior end of the TAP. The needle is inserted in the midaxillary line and advanced posteriorly until it reaches the posterior end of the TAP.

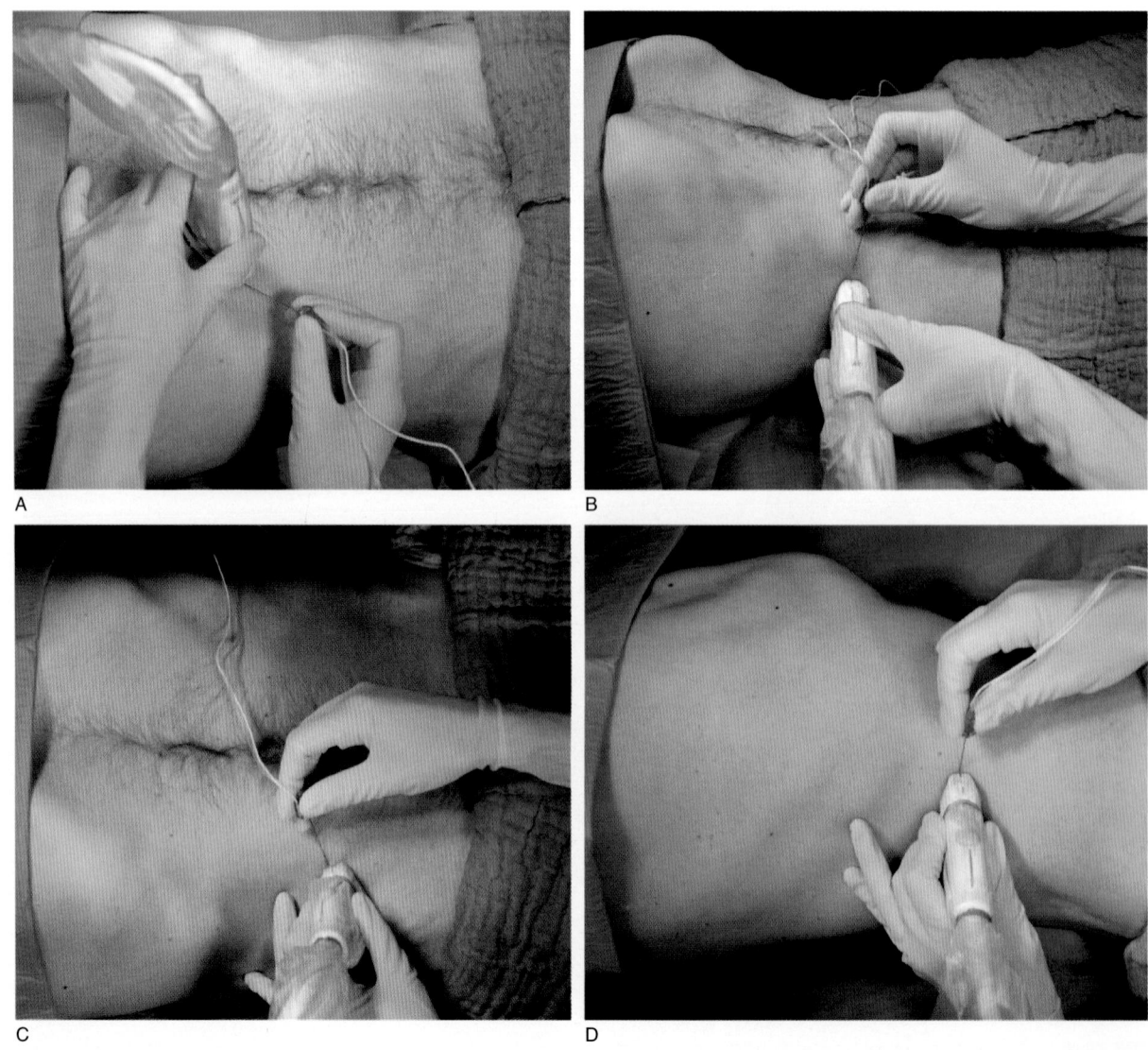

FIGURE 34–7. Patient and transducer position for different TAP block approaches: subcostal (**A**), lateral (**B**), anterior (**C**), and posterior (**D**).

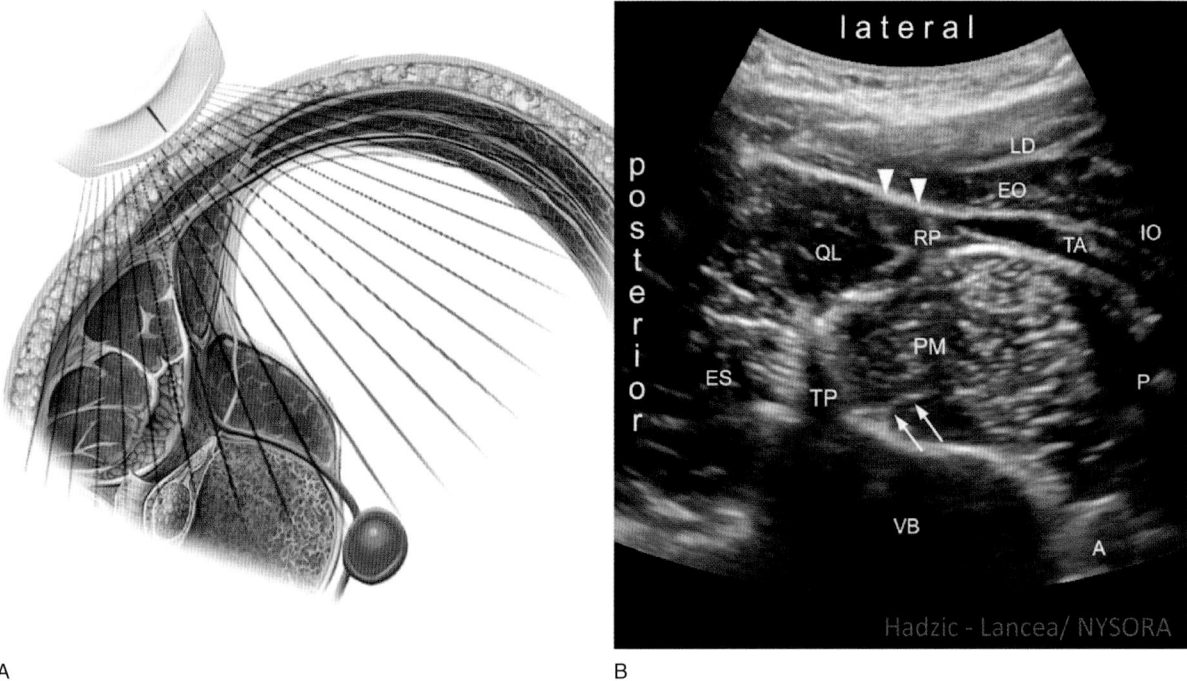

A   B

FIGURE 34–8. Cross section with the ultrasound probe location. B: Ultrasound image of the lateral abdominal wall. QL = quadratus lumborum; PM = psoas major; ES = erector spinae; TP = transverse process; VB = vertebral body (L4); TA = transversus abdominis; IO = internal oblique; EO = external oblique; LD = latissimus dorsi; RP = retroperitoneal space; P = peritoneal space; A = aorta; arrows = lumbar plexus; arrow heads = transversus abdominis aponeurosis.

Transmuscular QL Block

A curved array transducer for the transmuscular QL (TQL) block is placed in the axial plane on the patient's flank just cranial to the iliac crest. The "shamrock sign" is visualized: The transverse process of vertebra L4 is the stem, whereas the erector spinae posteriorly, QL laterally, and psoas major anteriorly represent the three leaves of the trefoil. The target for injection is the fascial plane between the QL and psoas major muscles (Figure 34–8).[3] The needle is inserted using an in-plane technique from the posterior end of the transducer through the QL muscle (Figure 34-9). The injectate should ideally spread from the injection site inside the fascial plane between the QL and psoas major muscles to the thoracic paravertebral space with a goal to accomplish segmental somatic and visceral analgesia from T4 to L1. The needle approaches of the QLBs are shown in Figure 34–10.

Type 1 QL Block

For the type 1 QL (QL1) block, a linear transducer is placed in the axial plane in the midaxillary line and moved posteriorly until the posterior aponeurosis of the transversus abdominis muscle becomes visible as a strong specular reflector. The target is just deep to the aponeurosis but superficial to the TF at the lateral margin of the QL muscle. This is just lateral to the pararenal fat compartment. The QL1 block is identical to the *fascia transversalis plane block*.[4] The needle is inserted from either the anterior or the posterior end of the transducer and advanced until the needle tip just penetrates the posterior aponeurosis of the transversus abdominis muscle. Local anesthetic is injected between the aponeurosis and the TF at the lateral margin of the

QL muscle. The main effect is anesthesia of the lateral cutaneous branches of the iliohypogastric, ilioinguinal, and subcostal nerves (T12–L1).

Type 2 QL Block

In the type 2 QL (QL2) block, a linear transducer is placed in the axial plane in the midaxillary line and moved posteriorly as in the QL1 block, until the LIFT, which encapsulates the paraspinal muscles, becomes visible between the latissimus dorsi and QL muscles. The target is the deep layer (the PRS) of the

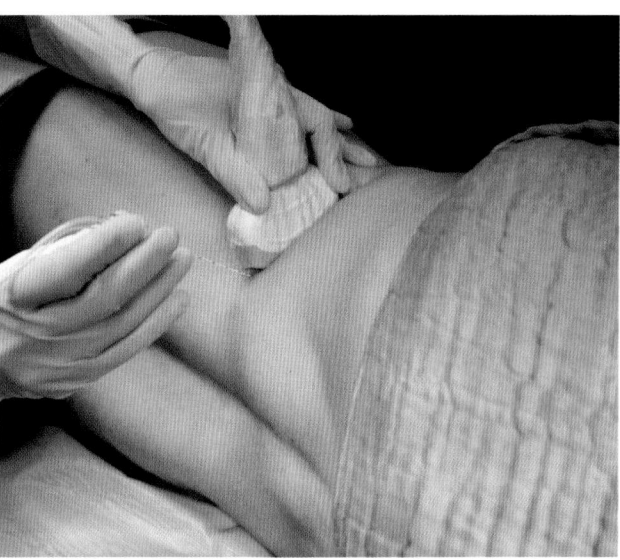

FIGURE 34–9. Patient and transducer position for Transmuscular QLB.

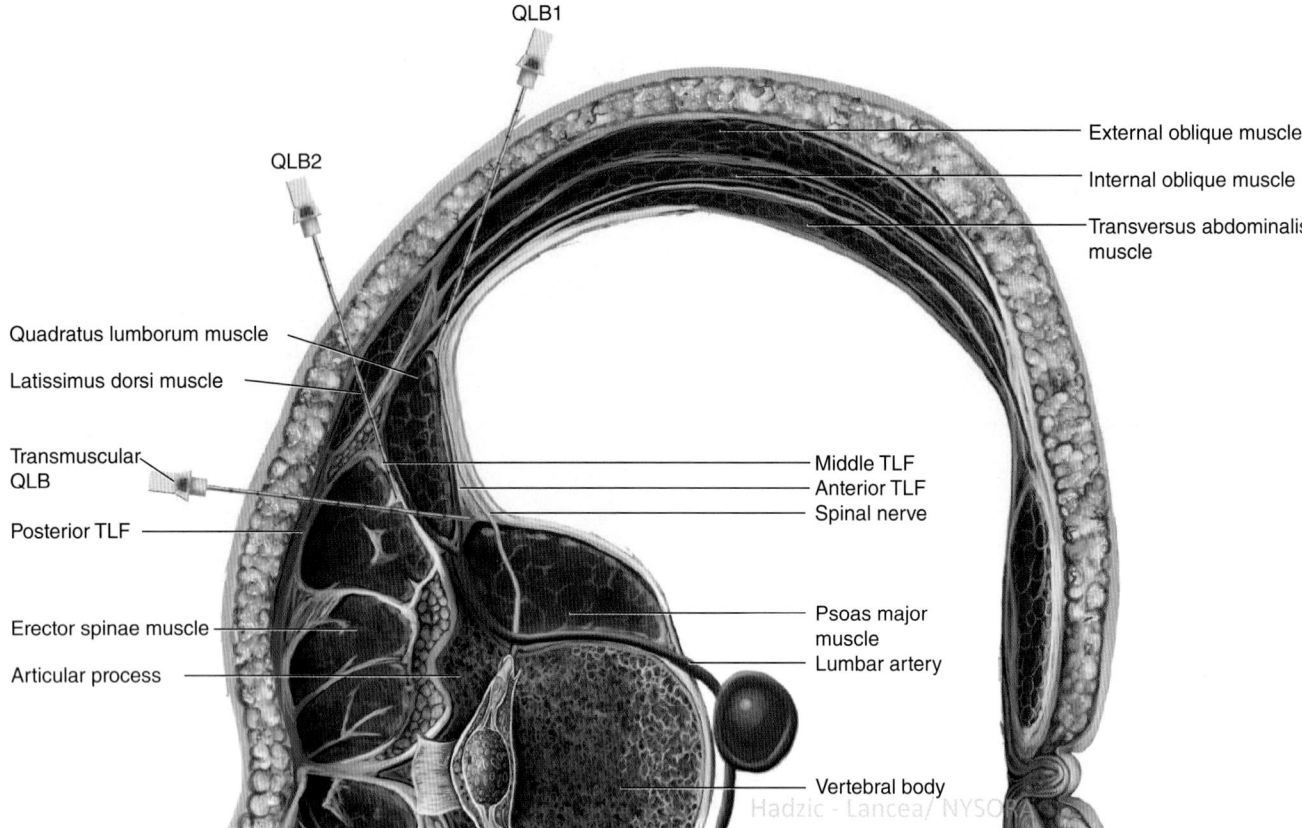

FIGURE 34–10. Trajectory of the needle for all three approaches of the quadratus lumborum (QL) block (QLB1, QLB2, and QLB3).

middle layer of the TLF. The needle is inserted from the lateral end of the transducer. The needle tip is advanced until it is inside the middle layer of the TLF close to the LIFT. The local anesthetic is injected intrafascially and apparently provides analgesia equivalent to TQL block but with faster onset. The mechanism of action is not well understood.

DOSE AND VOLUME OF LOCAL ANESTHETIC

The TAP blocks as well as the TQL block and QLB1 are "tissue plane" blocks and thus require large volumes of local anesthetic to obtain reliable blockade. For each of the TAP blocks, a minimum volume of 15 mL is recommended. The local anesthetic dose needs to be considered for the size of the patient to ensure that a maximum safe dose is not exceeded, especially with dual bilateral TAP blocks. The QL region is relatively vascular as the lumbar arteries lie posterior to the muscle. Absorption of the local anesthetic into the circulation depends primarily on the vascularity of the site of deposition.[14] As the QL muscle is well vascularized and a large volume of local anesthetic is needed, the dose should be calculated accurately to prevent high peak plasma concentrations of local anesthetics in this type of block.

INDICATIONS

Most of the indications for QL blocks are based on case reports and clinical anecdotal experience. There are no studies comparing the safety and efficacy of the three types of QL block. Table 34–1 compares and summarizes the three types of QL

blocks. The various QL blocks share the same indications as the TAP block.[8-13] Some examples are as follows:

- Large-bowel resection, open/laparoscopic appendectomy, and cholecystectomy
- Cesarean section, total abdominal hysterectomy
- Open prostatectomy, renal transplant surgery, nephrectomy, abdominoplasty, iliac crest bone graft
- Ileostomy
- Exploratory laparotomy, bilateral blocks for midline incisions

Clinical Pearls

- Close to the transverse process, the QL muscle appears thin as it is visualized anterior-posterior; visualized from the flank, the muscle looks much broader.
- Use color Doppler before insertion of the needle to detect the lumbar arteries on the posterior aspect of the QL muscle or any other large vessels.
- The QL is identified medial to the transversus abdominis muscle. The latissimus dorsi and erector spinae muscles are superficial and more hyperechoic.

SUMMARY

The various TAP blocks can provide somatic analgesia for abdominal wall surgery. QL blocks can provide somatic as well as visceral analgesia of both the abdominal wall and the lower

TABLE 34–1. Main features of QL blocks.

	QLB1	QLB2	TQLB
Clinical indications	Abdominal surgery below the umbilicus.	Abdominal surgery either above or below the umbilicus (any type of operation that requires intra-abdominal visceral pain coverage and abdominal wall incisions as high as T6)	
Dermatomes covered	L1	T4 to T12-L1; blocks the anterior and the lateral cutaneous branches of the nerves	
Lower extremity weakness	Not reported	Not reported	Potential
Spread to lumbar plexus	Not reported	Not reported	Potential
Needle entry and approach	Lateral abdomen near the posterior axillary line, below the costal margin and above the iliac crest and inserting the needle inplane with the curved array probe oriented axially.		
Potential complications	Complications are related to the lack of anatomical understanding and needle expertise. It is possible to puncture intra-abdominal structures such as the kidney, liver, and spleen.		
Injection site	Potential space medial to the abdominal wall muscles and lateral to QL muscle, anterolateral border of the QL muscle, at the junction with the transversalis fascia, outside the anterior layer of the TLF and fascia transversalis	Posterior to the QL muscle, outside the middle layer of the TLF	Anterior to the QL muscle, between the QL and the psoas major muscles, outside the anterior layer of the TLF and fascia transversalis, close to the intervertebral foramen
Level of difficulty	Intermediate	Intermediate	Advanced

segments of the thoracic wall and therefore could be a useful analgesic modality for selected abdominal surgeries. QL blocks may provide visceral analgesia due to their paravertebral and possibly epidural spread. The information in this chapter is based on the current knowledge, with an understanding that more specific recommendations are pending a stronger evidence base.

REFERENCES

1. Carney J, Finnerty O, Rauf J, et al: Studies on the spread of local anaesthetic solution in transversus abdominis plane blocks. Anaesthesia 2011;66:1023–1030.
2. Elsharkawy H: Quadratus lumborum block with paramedian sagittal oblique (subcostal) approach. Anaesthesia 2016;71:241–242.
3. Skandalakis JE, Colborn GL, Weidman TA, et al: *Skandalakis Surgical Anatomy: The Embryologic and Anatomic Basis of Modern Surgery.* Paschalidis Medical, 2004.
4. Willard FH, Vleeming A, Schuenke MD, Danneels L, Schleip R: The thoracolumbar fascia: Anatomy, function and clinical considerations. J Anat 2012;221:507–536.
5. Karmakar MK, Gin T, Ho AMH. Ipsilateral thoracolumbar anaesthesia and paravertebral spread after low thoracic paravertebral injection. Br J Anaesth 2001;87:312–316.
6. Børglum J, Jensen K, Moriggl B, et al: Ultrasound-guided transmuscular quadratus lumborum blockade. Br J Anesth 2013.
7. Hebbard PD: Transversalis fascia plane block, a novel ultrasound-guided abdominal wall nerve block. Can J Anaesth 2009;56:618–620.
8. Mcdonnell JG, Curley G, Carney J, et al: The analgesic efficacy of transversus abdominis plane block after caesarean delivery: A randomized controlled trial. Anesth Analg 2008;106:186–191.
9. Carney JJ, Mcdonnell JG, Ochana A, Bhinder R, Laffey JG: The transversus abdominis plane block provides effective postoperative analgesia in patients undergoing total abdominal hysterectomy. Anesth Analg 2008;107:2056–2060.
10. Kadam VR: Ultrasound-guided quadratus lumborum block as a postoperative analgesic technique for laparotomy. J Anaesthesiol Clin Pharmacol 2013;29:550–552.
11. Visoiu M, Yakovleva N: Continuous postoperative analgesia via quadratus lumborum block—An alternative to transversus abdominis plane block. Paediatr Anaesth 2013;23:959–961.
12. Chakraborty A, Goswami J, Patro V: Ultrasound-guided continuous quadratus lumborum block for postoperative analgesia in a pediatric patient. A A Case Rep 2015;4:34–36.
13. Blanco R, Ansari T, Girgis E. Quadratus lumborum block for postoperative pain after caesarean section: a randomised controlleds trial. Eur J Anaesthesiol. 2015;32:812–818.
14. Murouchi T, Iwasaki S, Yamakage M. Quadratus Lumborum Block: Analgesic Effects and Chronological Ropivacaine Concentrations After Laparoscopic Surgery. Reg Anesth Pain Med. 2016;41:146–150.

Pectoralis and Serratus Plane Blocks

Rafael Blanco and Michael J. Barrington

INTRODUCTION

Pectoralis nerve (Pecs) and serratus plane blocks are newer ultrasound (US)-guided regional anesthesia techniques of the thorax.[1] The increasing use of ultrasonography to identify tissue layers and, particularly, fascial layers has led to the development of several newer interfascial injection techniques for analgesia of the chest and abdominal wall. For instance, the Pecs I block was devised to anesthetize the medial and lateral pectoral nerves, which innervate the pectoralis muscles.[1] This is accomplished by an injection of local anesthetic in the fascial plane between the pectoralis major and minor muscles. The Pecs II block (which also includes the Pecs I block) is an extension that involves a second injection lateral to the Pecs I injection point in the plane between the pectoralis minor and serratus anterior muscles with the intention of providing blockade of the upper intercostal nerves.[2] A further modification is the serratus plane block, in which local anesthetic is injected between the serratus anterior and latissimus dorsi muscles.[3] These interfascial injections were developed as alternatives to thoracic epidural, paravertebral, intercostal, and intrapleural blocks, primarily for analgesia after surgery on the hemithorax. Initially, Pecs blocks were intended for analgesia after breast surgery; however, case reports have also described the use of Pecs and serratus plane blocks for analgesia following thoracotomy[4] and rib fracture.[5]

Information from the currently published literature on Pecs and serratus plane blocks in peer-reviewed journals is summarized in Table 35–1.[3–8] Pecs blocks have also been proposed in letters to the editor as alternative techniques to anesthetize operative regions such as the axilla, proximal medial upper arm,

and posterior shoulder, which are not innervated by the brachial plexus (Figure 35–1).[9–11]

ANATOMY OF THE PECTORAL AND AXILLARY REGIONS

Pecs blocks are applied in the pectoral and axillary regions, with the muscles in both regions innervated by the brachial plexus. The pectoral region overlies the pectoralis major muscle and is limited by the axillary, mammary, and inframammary regions (Figure 35–2). The axillary region is lateral to the pectoral region and consists of the area of the upper chest that surrounds the axilla. In both regions, there are muscles, nerves, and vessels within the fascial layers (Figure 35–3). In the pectoral region, there are four muscles relevant to Pecs blocks: the pectoralis major, pectoralis minor, serratus anterior, and subclavius muscles. The pectoralis major and minor muscles are innervated by the lateral and medial pectoral nerves; the serratus anterior is innervated by the long thoracic nerve (C5, C6, and C7); and the subclavius is innervated by the upper trunk of the brachial plexus (C5 and C6).

The axillary region is a pyramidal structure with four borders:

1. The apex or axillary inlet, formed by a lateral border of the first rib, superior border of the scapula, and the posterior border of the clavicle
2. The anterior border, formed by the pectoralis major and minor muscles
3. The lateral border, formed by the humerus
4. The posterior border, formed by the teres major, latissimus dorsi, and subscapularis muscles.

TABLE 35–1. Summary of published controlled clinical trials and case reports.

Author, Year	Study Type	Surgery/Indication	Block Type	N	Injectate	Outcome
Blanco et al., 2013	Volunteer study	–	Serratus plane	4	0.4 mL/kg levobupivacaine 0.125% and gadolinium	Mean duration of paresthesia in the intercostal nerve distribution T2–T9, was 752 minutes (injection superficial to serratus anterior)
Wahba and Kamal, 2014	Randomized controlled trial	Mastectomy	Pecs II versus PVB	60	0.25% levobupivacaine: 15–20 mL T4 PVB, 10 mL Pecs I block	Pecs blocks reduced postoperative morphine consumption (first 24 h) and pain scores (first 12 h) in comparison with PVB following mastectomy
Fujiwara et al., 2014	Case report	Insertion of cardiac resynchronization device	Intercostal at first and second interspace, Pecs I block	1	0.375% ropivacaine: 4 mL intercostal block, 10 mL Pecs I block	Surgery performed under intercostal/Pecs I blocks and dexmedetomidine
Kunhabdulla et al., 2014	Case report	Analgesia for rib fracture	Serratus plane	1	20 mL bolus 0.125% bupivacaine, then infusion of 0.0625% bupivacaine at 7–12 mL/h	Effective analgesia to enable physiotherapy and ambulation
Madabushi et al., 2015	Case report	Analgesia for thoracotomy	Serratus plane	1	6 mL bolus 1% lignocaine, then infusion of bupivacaine 0.1% at 7 mL/h	Improvement in pain and ventilation
Murata et al., 2015	Case report	Breast surgery	Pecs II	2	35 mL 0.2% ropivacaine (mastectomy); 45 mL 0.2% ropivacaine (lumpectomy)	Mastectomy performed under Pecs II block and supplemental infiltration
Ueshima, 2015	Case report	Segmental breast resection	TTP combined with Pecs II	1	0.15% levobupivacaine: 15 mL TTP, 10 mL Pecs I, 20 mL Pecs II	Surgery performed under TTP and Pecs II blocks
Bashandy and Abbas, 2015	Randomized controlled trial	Mastectomy	Pecs II	120	0.25% bupivacaine: 10 mL Pecs I, 20 mL Pecs II	Lower visual analog scale pain scores and opioid requirements in the Pecs group compared to control group
Kulhari, 2016	Randomized controlled trial	Radical mastectomy	Pecs II versus PVB	40	25 mL 0.5 % ropivacaine	Duration of analgesia increased in Pec's block compared to PVB group (4.9 versus 3.3 hours)
Hetta, 2016	Randomized controlled trial	Radical mastectomy	Serratus plane	64	30 mL 0.25 % bupivacaine, Serratus plane; 15 mL 0.25% bupivacaine, PVB	Increased opioid consumption in the serratus plane compared to the PVB group

PVB, paravertebral block; TTP, transversus thoracic muscle plane.

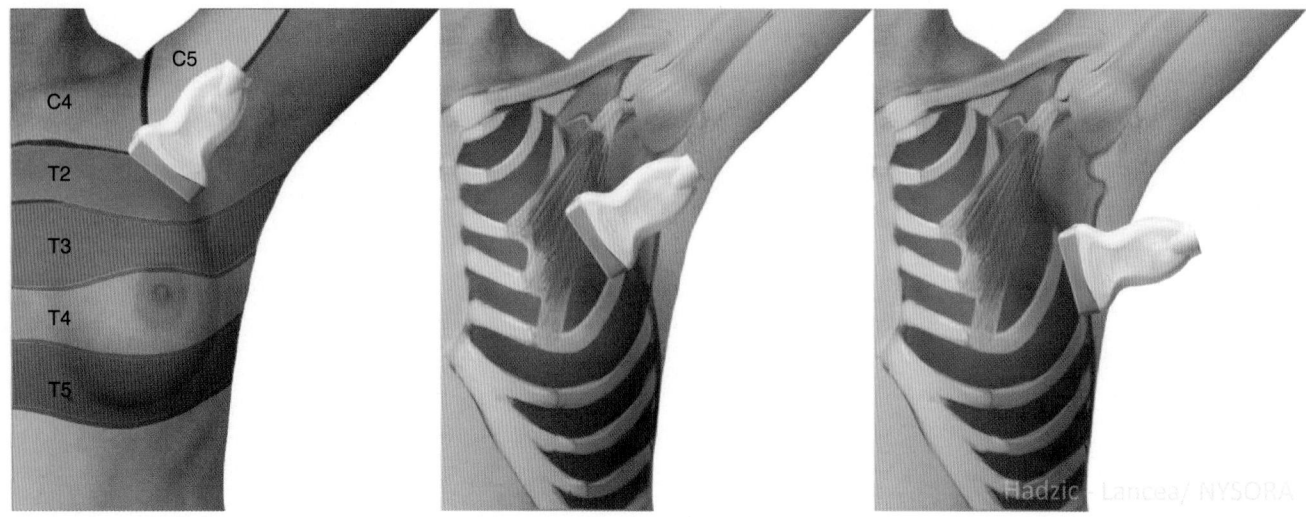

FIGURE 35–1. Transducer position for Pecs blocks. Also refer to Figures 35-9 and 35-11.

Figure 35-2, the muscles, nerves and vessels relevant to Pecs and serratus plane blocks are summarized in Tables 35-2, 35-3 and 35-4 respectively.

The pectoral and axillary regions are separated by fascias. In the pectoral region, there are two main fascias: the superficial fascia and the deep thoracic fascia. The deep thoracic fascia divides into three separate fascias: the pectoral (superficial), clavipectoral (intermediate), and exothoracic (deep). The clavipectoral fascia stretches between the clavicle and the pectoralis minor (Figure 35–4) and encloses the pectoralis minor with a thin layer of fascia. Between the pectoralis minor and subclavius muscles, the two layers of the clavipectoral fascia fuse.

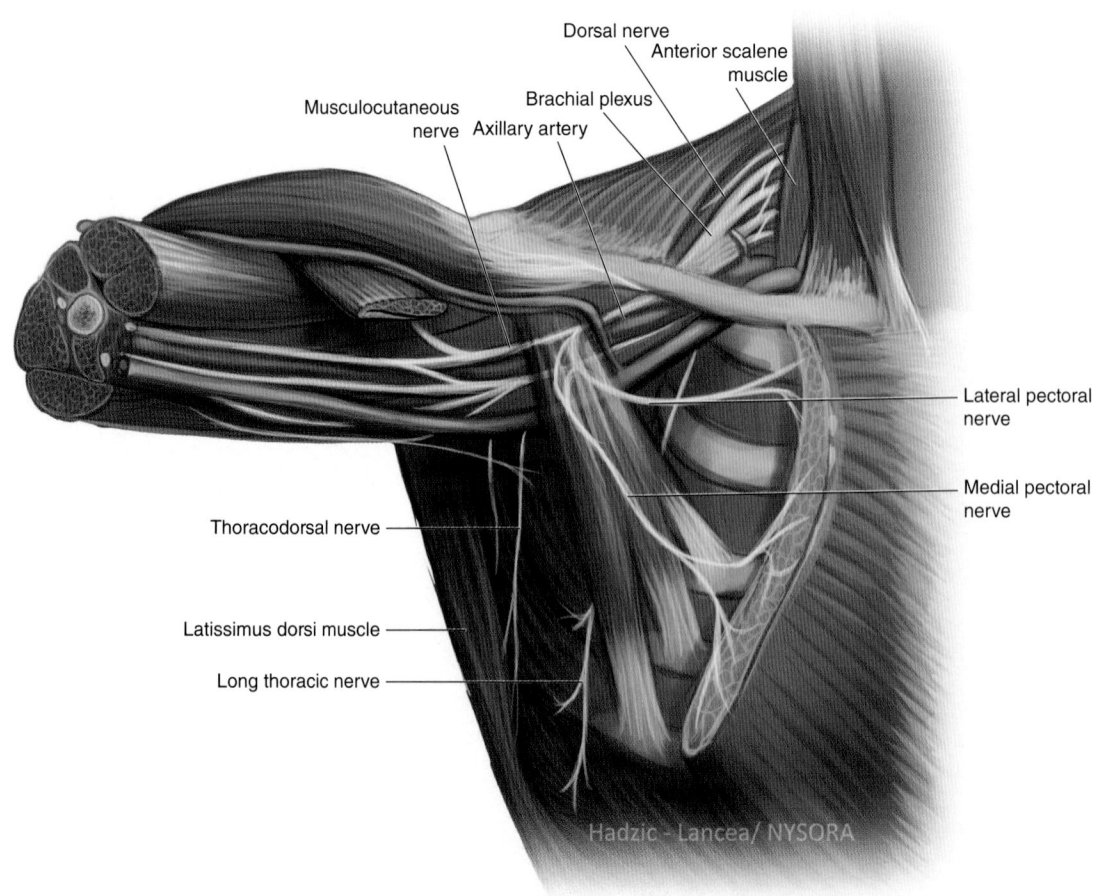

FIGURE 35–2. Pectoral region.

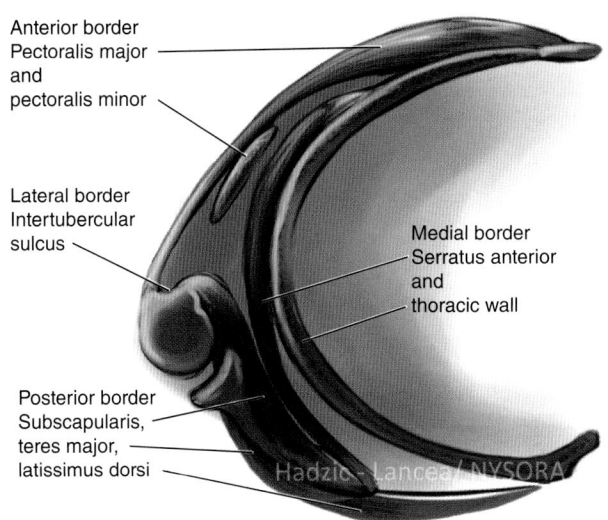

Anterior border
Pectoralis major
and
pectoralis minor

Lateral border
Intertubercular
sulcus

Medial border
Serratus anterior
and
thoracic wall

Posterior border
Subscapularis,
teres major,
latissimus dorsi

Hadzic - Lancea / NYSORA

FIGURE 35–3. Axillary region.

Caudal to the pectoralis minor, the clavipectoral fascial layers rejoin to form the suspensory ligament of the axilla, which is joined to the axillary fascia (Figure 35–5).

At the pectoral level, the fascias create four potential compartments for the injection of local anesthetic:

1. Between the superficial and deep pectoral fascial layers
2. Between the pectoral fascia and the clavipectoral fascia
3. Between the clavipectoral fascia and the superficial border of the serratus anterior muscle
4. Between the serratus anterior muscle and the exothoracic fascia

The first two compartments are in the pectoral region, but the third and fourth communicate with the axillary region. The nerves and vessels in this region create communications by crossing the compartments. The nerves of the pectoral region are mainly the lateral and medial pectoral nerves, but there is also an important innervation from the supraclavicular nerve and from the lateral and anterior branches of the intercostal nerves. The lateral pectoral nerve crosses the axillary artery anteriorly and pierces the clavipectoral fascia in close relationship with the thoracoacromial artery on the undersurface of the upper portion of the pectoralis major muscle, which it supplies with lateral cord fibers from C5–C7 (Figure 35–6). The lateral pectoral nerve is medial to the pectoralis minor before entering the pectoralis major muscle; it communicates across the axillary artery with the medial pectoral nerve and, through this communication (via ansa pectoralis), supplies the pectoralis minor. The medial pectoral nerve arises from the medial cord fibers from C8–T1, behind the axillary artery at the level below the clavicle, and passes through the deep surface of the pectoralis minor, which is perforates and then enters and innervates pectoralis major. Both pectoral nerves enter the deep surface of the pectoralis major, and neither has a cutaneous branch.

The nerves of the axillary region are the intercostobrachialis, intercostal T3–T9, long thoracic, and thoracodorsal. The intercostobrachialis nerve is the lateral cutaneous brnach of the second and third intercostal nerves in 67% and 33% of cases, respectively. It crosses the serratus anterior muscle in the midaxillary line to innervate the axilla. The intercostobrachialis nerve is a vital nerve if regional anesthesia of the axilla is required.

TABLE 35–2. Nerves relevant to pecs and serratus plane blocks.

Nerve	Origin	Innervation	Relevance
Long thoracic	Roots (C5, C6, C7)	Serratus anterior muscle	Known as the nerve to the serratus anterior.
Lateral pectoral	Lateral cord (C5, C6, C7)	Pectoralis major and pectoralis minor muscles	Penetrates the clavipectoral fascia to supply the pectoralis major directly and, through communication with the medial pectoral nerve, the pectoralis minor. There is no cutaneous branch. Can be located on the deep surface of the pectoralis major.
Medial pectoral	Medial cord (C8, T1)	Pectoralis major and pectoralis minor muscles	Penetrates the deep surface of the pectoralis minor to innervate this muscle before penetrating it to supply the pectoralis major muscle.
Intercostal	Anterior rami of thoracic spinal nerves	Segmental somatic sensory innervation to skin	Lateral cutaneous branches of T2-T6 innervate the lateral breast. Accessible in the mid-axillary line.
Thoracodorsal	Posterior cord (C6, C7, C8)	Latissimus dorsi muscle	Large nerve from the posterior cord, which has a course in the posterior axillary wall, crosses the lower border of the teres major to enter the deep surface of the latissimus dorsi muscle. The thoracodorsal nerve is adjacent to the thoracodorsal artery.

TABLE 35–3. Muscles relevant to pecs and serratus plane blocks.

Muscle	Innervation	Relevance
Pectoralis major	Medial (C8, T1) and lateral (C5–C7) pectoral nerves	Sonographic landmark.
Pectoralis minor	Both pectoral nerves (C5–C8)	Sonographic landmark.
Serratus anterior	Long thoracic nerve (C5–C7)	Sonographic landmark for Pecs II and serratus plane blocks. The intercostobrachial, long thoracic, and thoracodorsal nerves lie on this muscle. The thoracodorsal artery is superficial to this muscle.
Teres major	Subscapular nerve (C5–C6) (offspring of subscapularis muscle)	Contributes to the posterior wall of the axilla.
Subscapularis	Upper and lower subscapular nerves (C5–C8)	Contributes to the posterior wall of the axilla.
Latissimus dorsi	Thoracodorsal nerve (C6–C8)	Contributes to the posterior wall of the axilla; sonographic landmark for serratus plane blocks.

The intercostal nerves (T3–T9) provide motor supply to the intercostal muscles and receive sensory information from the skin and parietal pleura. The intercostal nerves have posterior, lateral, and anterior branches and an anterior accessory branch that innervates the sternum. The lateral branches innervate most of the pectoral and axillary regions, together with the posterior hemithorax, back to the scapula. They pierce the external intercostal muscle and exit between the serratus anterior digitations at the level of the midaxillary line. The long thoracic nerve is in the axillary compartment close to the lateral thoracic branch of the thoracoacromial artery and travels down the lateral aspect of the serratus anterior muscle, which it innervates. Arising from the posterior cord, the thoracodorsal nerve, C6–C8 (nerve to the latissimus dorsi), has a course posteriorly in the axillary compartment, in close relationship with the thoracodorsal artery (Tables 35-2 through 35-4). The thoracodorsal nerve becomes prominent when the humerus is abducted and laterally rotated. It is an important and large nerve in

danger during reconstructive surgery and other operations involving the lower axilla (see Table 35–2).

THORACIC WALL BLOCKS

Pecs I Block

The Pecs I block involves a hydrodissection of the plane between the pectoral muscles with local anesthetic to block the lateral and medial pectoral nerves.

The main landmarks to identify the point of injection under US guidance are the pectoralis major and pectoralis minor muscles and the pectoral branch of the thoracoacromial artery. The block is performed with the patient supine, either with the arm next to the chest or abducted 90 degrees. With standard American Society of Anesthesiology (ASA) monitoring and supplemental oxygen, the operator locates the coracoid process on US in the paramedian sagittal plane. The transducer is rotated slightly to

TABLE 35–4. Vessels relevant to pecs and serratus plane blocks.

Vessel	Relevance
Axillary	Is the continuation of the subclavian artery after it passes the lateral border of the first rib. It lies lateral to the axillary vein. It gives of the branches listed below.
Superior thoracic	Branch of the first part of the axillary artery; supplies both pectoral muscles.
Thoracoacromial	Arises from the second part (deep to the pectoralis minor) of the axillary artery, close to the upper border of the pectoralis minor; pierces the clavipectoral fascia in the infraclavicular fossa; has four branches that may arise deep or superficial to the clavipectoral fascia.
Lateral thoracic	Follows the lower border of the pectoralis minor; supplies both pectoral muscles.
Thoracodorsal	Arises from the third part (distal to the pectoralis minor) of the axillary artery; initially known as the subscapular artery, located in the posterior axillary wall (largest branch of the axillary artery), before becoming the thoracodorsal artery; has a course with the thoracodorsal nerve, which innervates the latissimus dorsi.

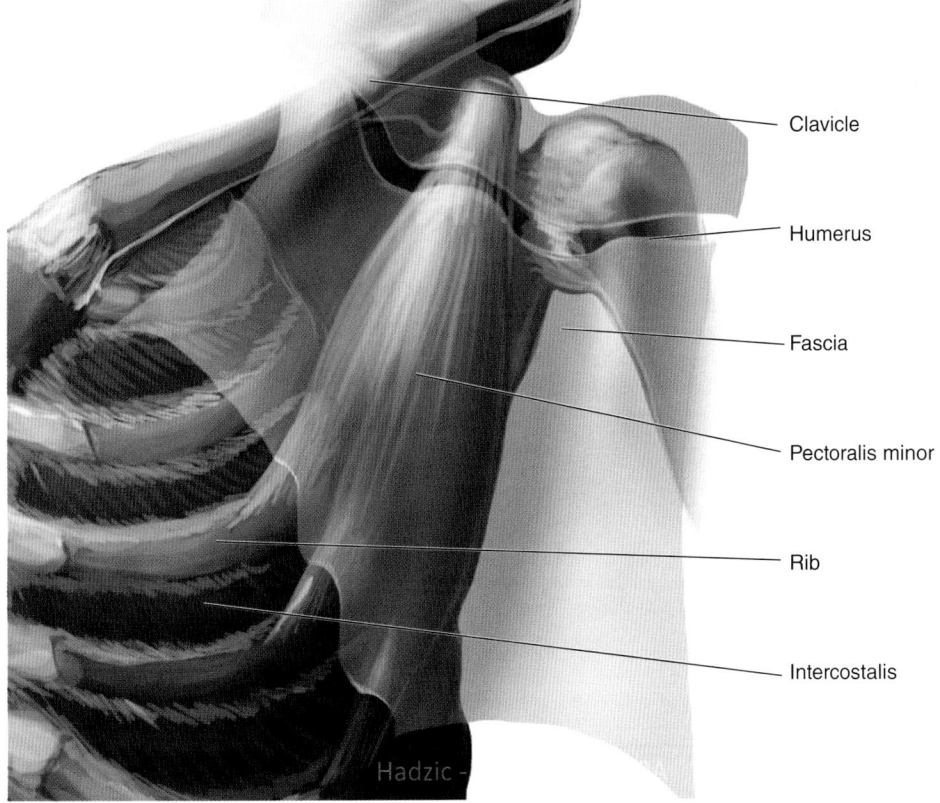

FIGURE 35–4. The clavipectoral fascia and its continuation into the axillary fascia.

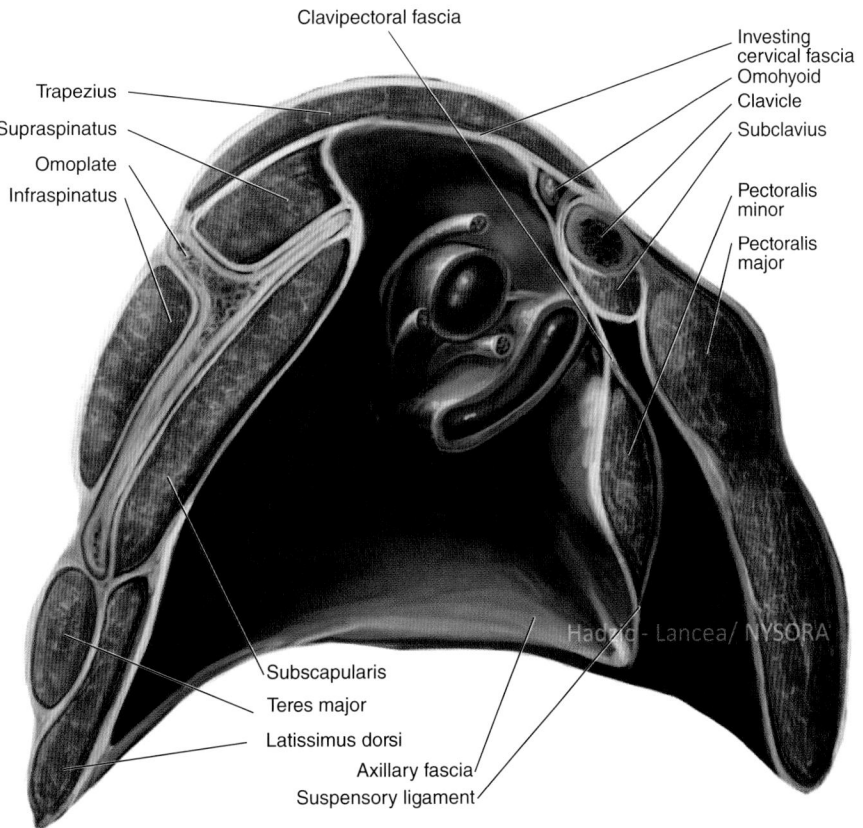

FIGURE 35–5. Section of the axilla showing the clavipectoral fascia enclosing the subclavius and the pectoralis minor muscles. Inferior to the pectoralis minor muscle, the clavipectoral fascia becomes the suspensory ligament.

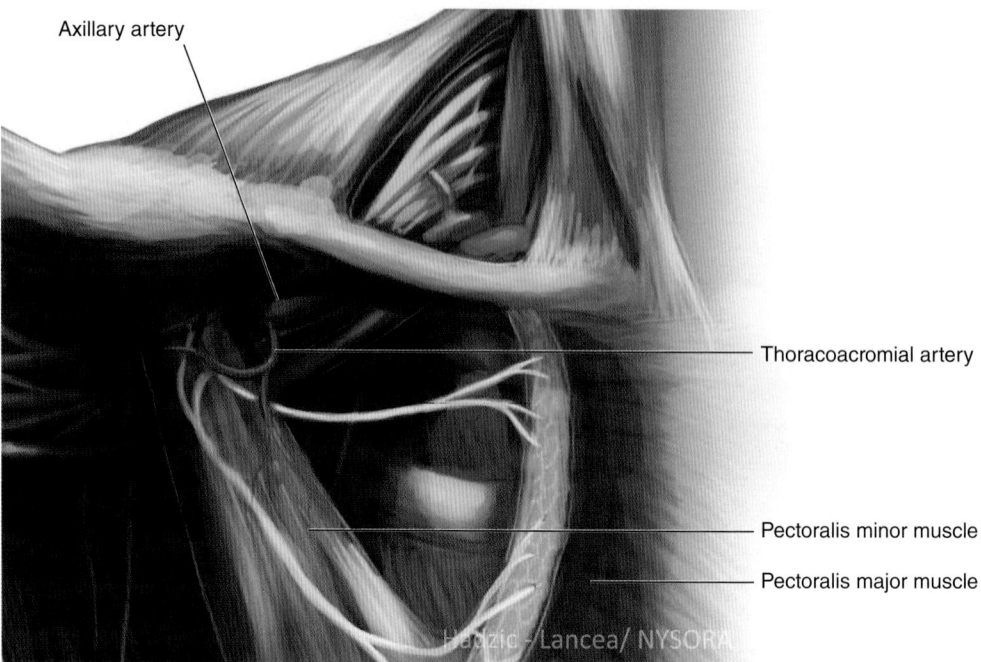

Axillary artery

Thoracoacromial artery

Pectoralis minor muscle

Pectoralis major muscle

FIGURE 35–6. Relationship of the lateral pectoral nerve to the acromiothoracic artery.

allow an in-plane needle trajectory from the proximal and medial side toward the lateral side (ie, the caudal border of the transducer is moved laterally, while the proximal border remains unchanged) (Figure 35–7). This rotation helps image the pectoral branch of the thoracoacromial artery. The proper fascial plane is confirmed by hydrodissection to open the space between the pectoralis muscles. The suggested volume is 0.2 mL/kg of a long-acting local anesthetic (Figure 35–8); however, the reader should be informed that dose-ranging studies have not been conducted at the time of publication, and, therefore, there are no evidence-based recommendations currently available.

Pecs II Block

The goal of the Pecs II block is to infiltrate two fascial compartments by dividing the dose of local anesthetic between the pectoral nerves (the pectoral fascia and clavipectoral fascia) and under the pectoralis minor muscle (between the clavipectoral fascia and the superficial border of the serratus muscle). The local anesthetic should cover two important compartments of the fascias involved: The pectoral compartment with the pectoral nerves and the intercostal branches for the axilla and chest. The block is performed with the patient supine, either with the arm abducted 90 degrees or by his or her side. The first injection is similar to Pecs I, whereas the second is made at the anterior axillary line at the level of the fourth rib. The depth is usually 1–3 cm for the first injection and 3–6 cm for the second injection. With the transducer at the midclavicular level and angled inferolaterally, the axillary artery and vein and the second rib can be identified (Figure 35–9). The transducer is then moved laterally until the pectoralis minor and serratus anterior are identified. With further lateral transducer movement, the third and fourth rib can then be identified. The local anesthetic is injected at two points: A first injection of approximately

0.2 mL/kg long-acting local anesthetic is made between the pectoral major and minor muscles, and a second injection of 0.2 mL/kg is made between the pectoralis minor and serratus anterior muscles. Figure 35–10 illustrates the sonographic anatomy, needle trajectory, and desired spread of injectate.

Serratus Anterior Plane Block

The serratus plane block is performed in the axillary region, at a more lateral and posterior location than the Pecs I and II blocks.[3,4] At the axillary fossa, the intercostobrachialis nerve, lateral cutaneous branches of the intercostal nerves (T3–T9), long thoracic nerve, and thoracodorsal nerve are located in a compartment between the serratus anterior and the latissimus dorsi muscles, between the posterior and midaxillary lines.

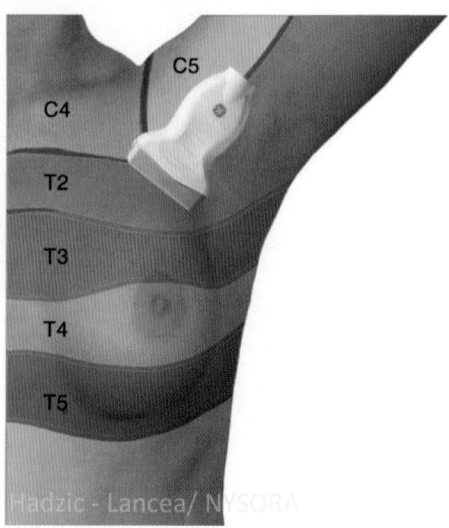

FIGURE 35–7. Transducer position for the Pecs I block.

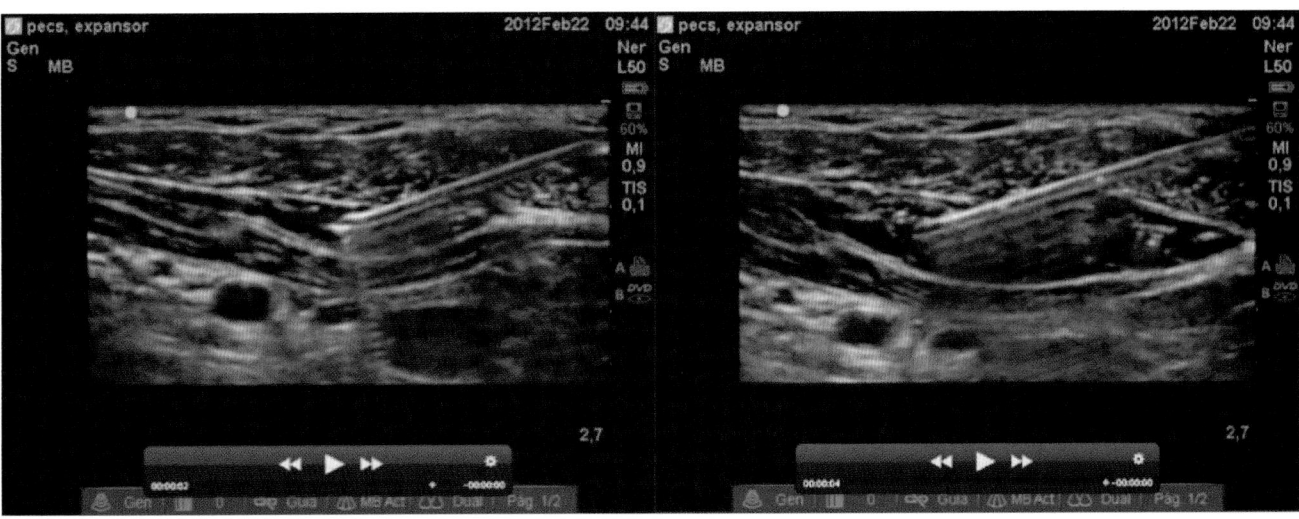

FIGURE 35-8. Sonogram of the Pecs I injection. Left: needle placement; right: desired spread of local anesthetic.

The two main anatomical landmarks are the latissimus dorsi and the serratus anterior muscles. The thoracodorsal artery runs in the fascial plane between the two. The ribs, pleura, and intercostal muscles can also be seen during the procedure.

Lying on the side or supine with the arm brought forward is the preferable patient position. There are two main methods for identifying the plane for the serratus block. The first method requires counting the ribs from the clavicle while moving the transducer laterally and distally until the fourth and fifth ribs are identified (Figure 35–10). The transducer is orientated in the coronal plane and then tilted posteriorly until the latissimus dorsi (a superficial thick muscle) is identified (Figure 35–11). The serratus muscle, a thick, hypoechoic muscle deep to the latissimus dorsi is imaged over the ribs. Translating the transducer posteriorly

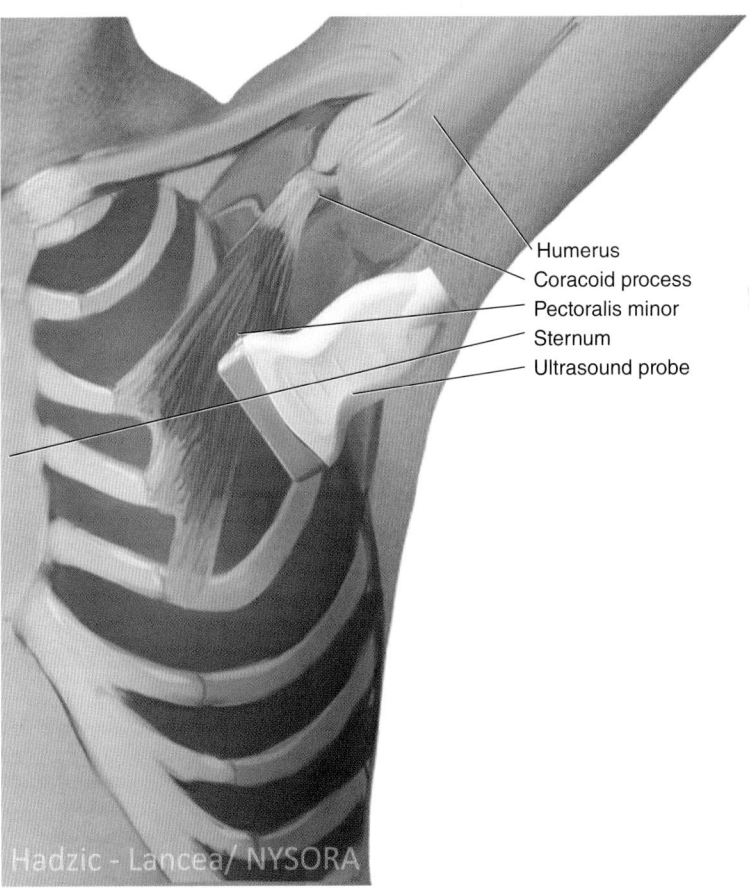

Humerus
Coracoid process
Pectoralis minor
Sternum
Ultrasound probe

Hadzic - Lancea / NYSORA

FIGURE 35-9. Transducer position for the Pecs II block.

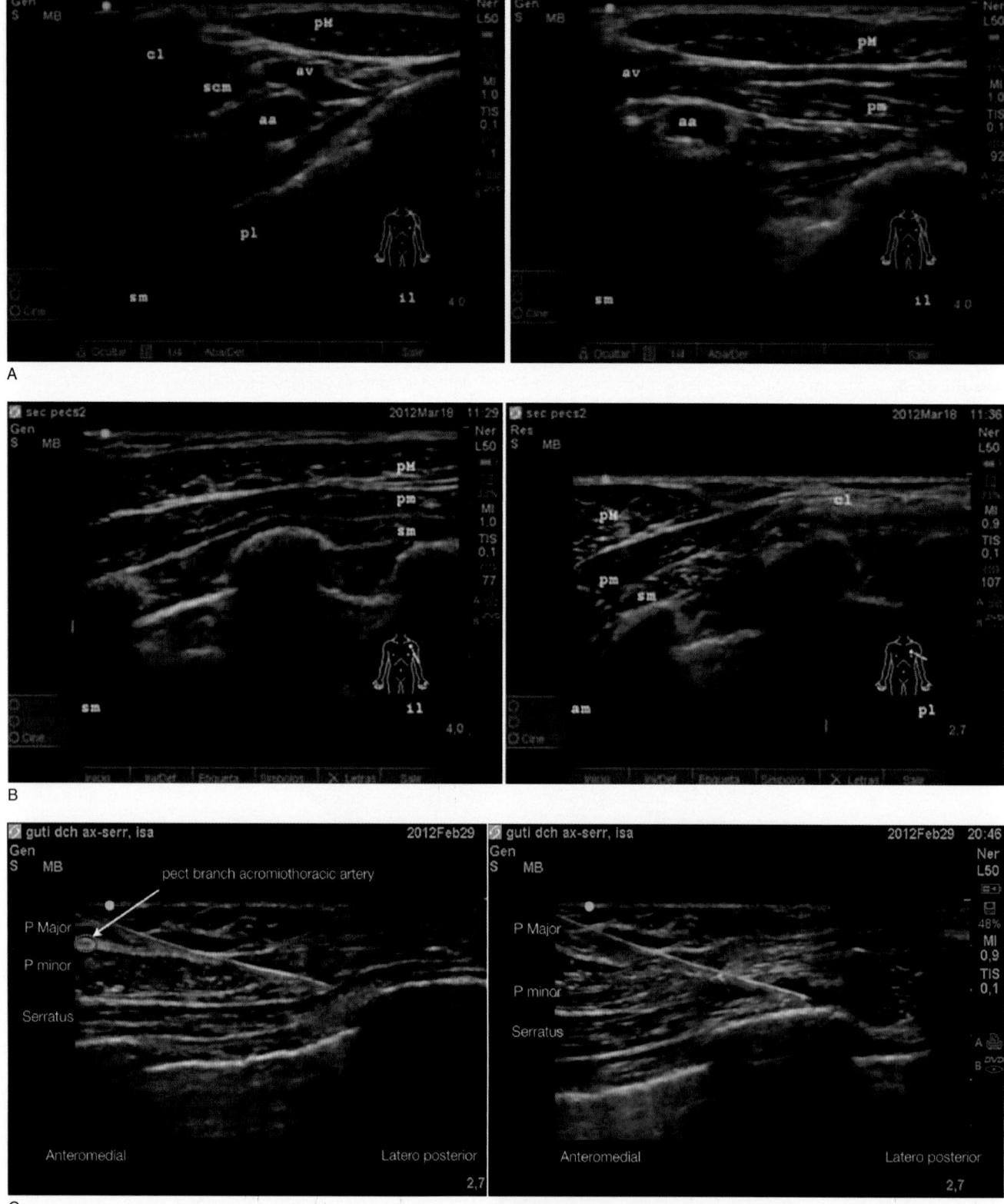

FIGURE 35–10. Pecs II sonogram: steps to locate points of injection. **A:** Left: Start from the clavicle; right: Count ribs down to the axilla. **B:** Left: First injection between the pectoralis major and pectoralis minor; right: Angle probe to locate Gilbert's ligament. **C:** Left: Above the serratus muscle; right: Underneath the serratus muscle; cl, clavicle; scm, subclavius muscle; pM, pectoralis major; pm, pectoralis minor; av, axillary vein; aa, axillary artery; pl, pleura; sm, serratus muscle.

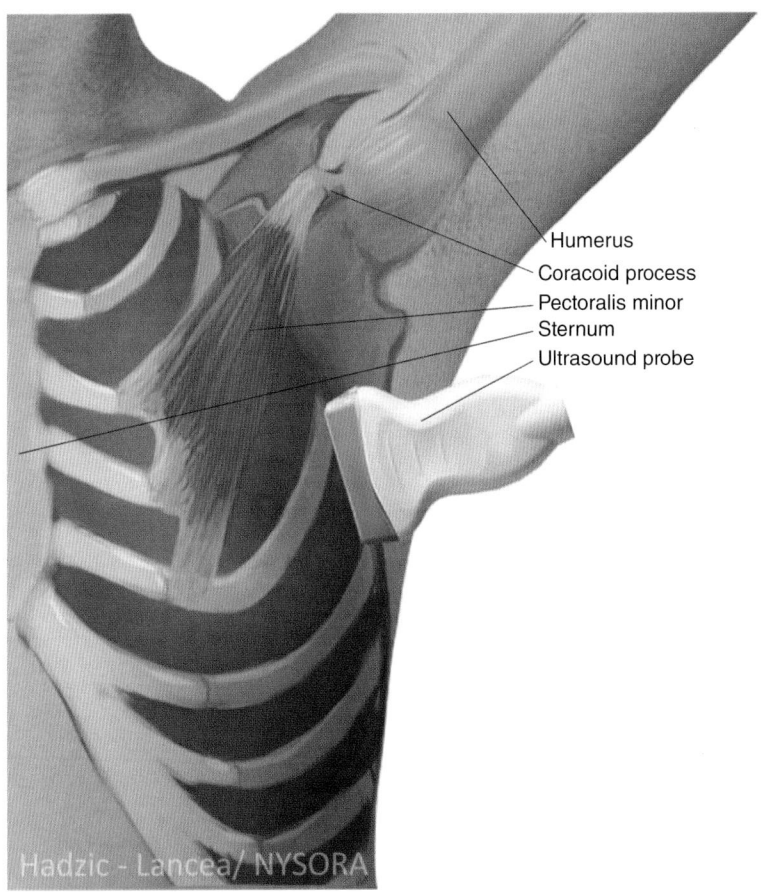

Humerus
Coracoid process
Pectoralis minor
Sternum
Ultrasound probe

Hadzic - Lancea/ NYSORA

FIGURE 35–11. Transducer position required for the serratus plane block.

facilitates identification of the plane between the serratus anterior and latissimus dorsi muscles. An alternative method is to place the transducer across the axilla, where the latissimus dorsi will appear more prominent (Figure 35–12). The location of the thoracodorsal artery is easier to identify this way. Both in-plane and out-of-plane approaches are appropriate.

Following the identification of sonographic landmarks, regional anesthesia can be achieved using a 38-mm, 6–13-MHz, linear transducer set for small parts and a depth of 1–4 cm; a

50–100-mm, 22-gauge regional block needle; and an injectate of 0.4 mL/kg of long-acting local anesthetic.

THE ANALGESIC POTENTIAL OF PECS BLOCKS

A summary of published studies is given in Table 35–1. At the time of writing, there were two randomized controlled trials (180 patients), five case reports (6 patients), and one

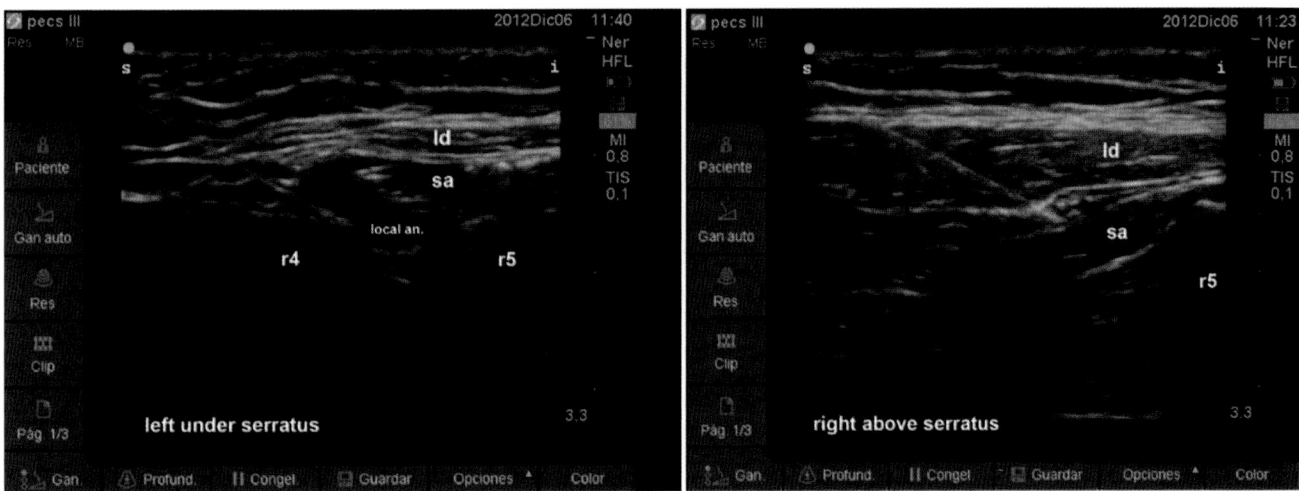

FIGURE 35–12. Sonogram of two possible levels for the serratus plane block below (left) or above the muscle (right).

volunteer study (4 patients, 8 hemithoraces). Bashandy and Abbas reported lower visual analog scale pain scores and opioid requirements in the Pecs group compared to a control group of patients following mastectomy.[12] In this study there was an inadequate description of allocation concealment and blinding of operating room personnel. Wahba and Kamal compared Pecs blocks to paravertebral blocks in 60 patients undergoing mastectomy. They found that Pecs blocks reduced postoperative morphine consumption (in the first 24 hours) and pain scores (in the first 12 hours) in comparison with paravertebral blockade following mastectomy.[13] Pecs blocks have also been used for the insertion of a cardiac resynchronization device.[7] The few remaining reports describe the utility of serratus plane blocks for analgesia following rib fracture[5] and thoracotomy.[4]

SUMMARY

Pecs and serratus plane blocks are newer US-guided blocks for analgesia after breast and lateral thoracic wall surgery. The key sonographic landmarks are the pectoralis major, pectoralis minor, and serratus anterior muscles and the pectoral branch of the acromiothoracic artery. As there are currently few reports on the utility of these US-guided interventional analgesia modalities, data from the imminent randomized controlled trials will be necessary to establish the analgesic benefit, indications, and safety of the Pecs and serratus plane blocks.

REFERENCES

1. Blanco R: The "pecs block": a novel technique for providing analgesia after breast surgery. Anaesthesia 2011;66:847–848.
2. Blanco R, Fajardo M, Parras Maldonado T: Ultrasound description of Pecs II (modified Pecs I): a novel approach to breast surgery. Rev Esp Anestesiol Reanim 2012;59:470–475.
3. Blanco R, Parras T, McDonnell JG, Prats-Galino A: Serratus plane block: a novel ultrasound-guided thoracic wall nerve block. Anaesthesia 2013;68:1107–1113.
4. Womack J, Varma MK: Serratus plane block for shoulder surgery. Anaesthesia 2014;69:395–396.
5. Purcell N, Wu D: Novel use of the PECS II block for upper limb fistula surgery. Anaesthesia 2014;69:1294.
6. Fujiwara A, Komasawa N, Minami T: Pectoral nerves (PECS) and intercostal nerve block for cardiac resynchronization therapy device implantation. Springerplus 2014;3:409.
7. Eid M, Nassr M, Aziz A: Serratus anterior plane block for flail chest injury. Anaesthesia Cases June 18, 2014, 2014-0074.
8. Kunhabdulla NP, Agarwal A, Gaur A, Gautam SK, Gupta R, Agarwal A: Serratus anterior plane block for multiple rib fractures. Pain Physician 2014;17:E651–653.
9. Kiss G, Castillo M: Non-intubated anesthesia in thoracic surgery-technical issues. Ann Transl Med 2015;3:109.
10. Fujiwara S, Komasawa N, Minami T: Pectoral nerve blocks and serratus-intercostal plane block for intractable post thoracotomy syndrome. J Clin Anesth 2015;27:275–276.
11. Madabushi R, Tewari S, Gautam SK, Agarwal A, Agarwal A: Serratus anterior plane block: a new analgesic technique for post-thoracotomy pain. Pain Physician 2015;18:E421–424.
12. Bashandy GM, Abbas DN: Pectoral nerves I and II blocks in multimodal analgesia for breast cancer surgery: a randomized clinical trial. Reg Anesth Pain Med 2015;40:68–74.
13. Wahba SS, Kamal SM: Thoracic paravertebral block versus pectoral nerve block for analgesia after breast surgery. Egyptian J Anaesth 2014; 30:129–135.

LOCAL AND REGIONAL ANESTHESIA FOR ORAL AND MAXILLOFACIAL SURGERY

CHAPTER 36

Oral & Maxillofacial Regional Anesthesia

Benaifer D. Preziosi, Adam T. Hershkin, Paul J. Seider, and Gregory M. Casey

INTRODUCTION

Oral surgical and dental procedures are often performed in an outpatient setting. Regional anesthesia is the most common method of anesthetizing the patient before office-based procedures. Several highly efficacious and practical techniques can be used to achieve anesthesia of the dentition and surrounding the hard and soft tissues of the maxilla and mandible. The type of procedure to be performed as well as the location of the procedure determine the technique of anesthesia to be used. Orofacial anesthetic techniques can be classified into three main categories: local infiltration, field block, and nerve block.

The local infiltration technique anesthetizes the terminal nerve endings of the dental plexus (Figure 36–1). This technique is indicated when an individual tooth or a specific isolated area requires anesthesia. The procedure is performed within the direct vicinity of the site of infiltration.

The field block anesthetizes the terminal nerve branches in the area of treatment. Treatment can then be performed in an area slightly distal to the site of injection. The deposition of local anesthetic at the apex of a tooth for the purposes of achieving pulpal and soft tissue anesthesia is often used by dental and maxillofacial practitioners. Although this is commonly termed "local infiltration," since the terminal. Terminal nerve branches are anesthetized in this technique, such infiltration is more correctly termed as **field block**. In contrast, the nerve block anesthetizes the main branch of a specific nerve, allowing treatment to be performed in the region innervated by the nerve.[1]

This chapter reviews the essential anatomy of orofacial nerves and details the practical approaches to performing nerve blocks and infiltrational anesthesia for a variety of surgical procedures in this region.

ANATOMY OF THE TRIGEMINAL NERVE

General Considerations

Anesthesia of the teeth and the soft and hard tissues of the oral cavity can be achieved with block of the branches of the trigeminal nerve (fifth cranial nerve). In fact, regional, field, and local anesthesia of the maxilla and mandible is accomplished by the deposition of anesthetic solution near terminal nerve branches or a main nerve trunk of the trigeminal nerve.

The largest of all the cranial nerves, the trigeminal nerve gives rise to a small motor root, originating in the motor nucleus within the pons and medulla oblongata, and a larger sensory root, which finds its origin in the anterior aspect of the pons (see Figure 36–1). The nerve travels forward from the posterior cranial fossa to the petrous portion of the temporal bone within the middle cranial fossa. Here, the sensory root forms the trigeminal (semilunar or gasserian) ganglion, situated within Meckel's cavity on the anterior surface of the petrous portion of the temporal bone. The ganglia are paired, with one innervating each side of the face. The sensory root of the trigeminal nerve gives rise to the ophthalmic division (V_1), the maxillary division (V_2), and the mandibular division (V_3) from the trigeminal ganglion (see Figure 36–1).

The motor root travels from the brainstem along with, but separate from, the sensory root. It then leaves the middle cranial fossa through the foramen ovale after passing underneath the trigeminal ganglion in a lateral and inferior direction. The motor root exits the middle cranial fossa along with the third division of the sensory root: the mandibular nerve. It then unites with the mandibular nerve to form a single nerve trunk after exiting the skull. The motor fibers supply the muscles of mastication (masseter, temporalis, medial pterygoid, and lateral pterygoid) and the mylohyoid, anterior belly of the digastric, tensor veli palatine, and tensor tympani muscles.

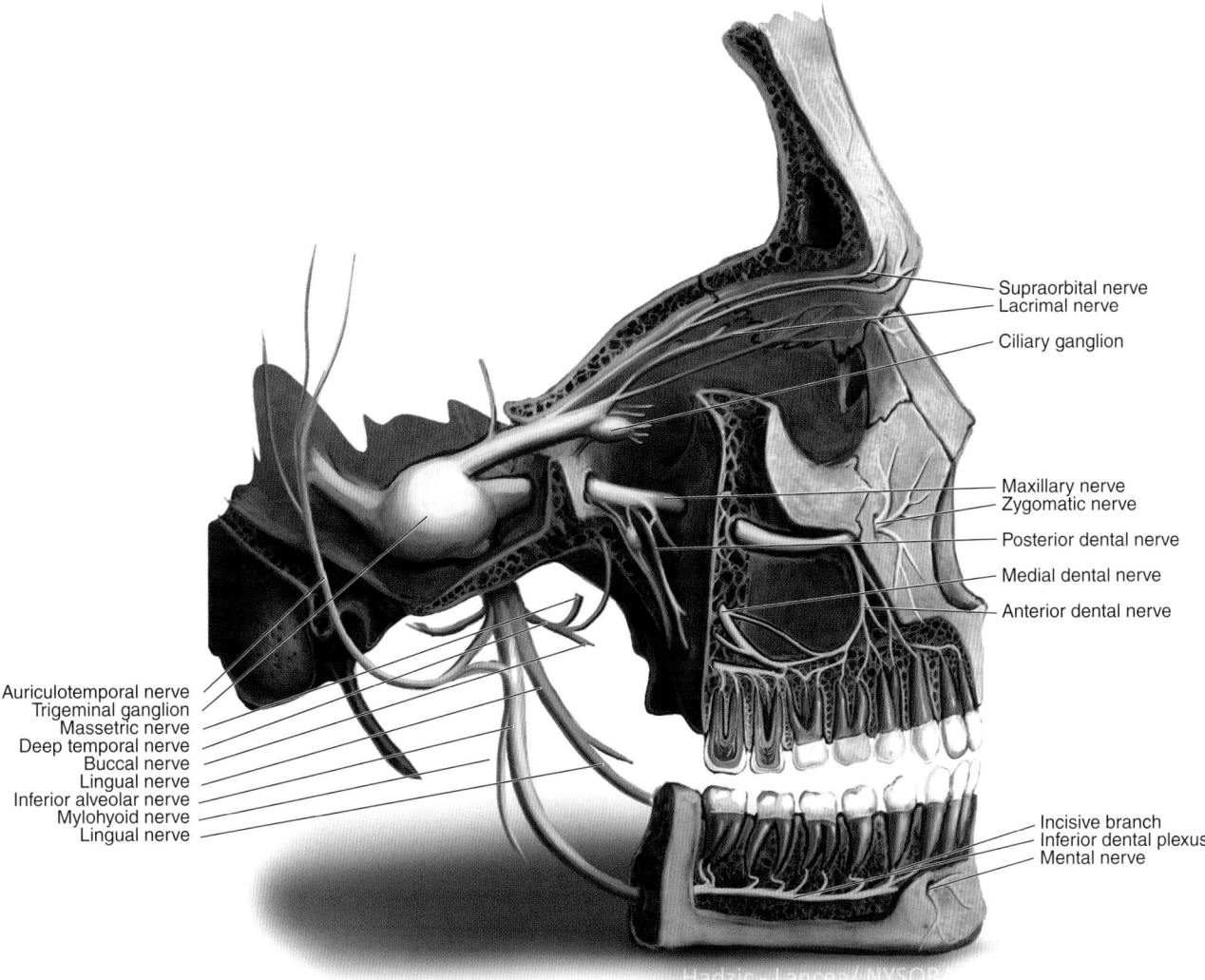

FIGURE 36–1. Anatomy of the trigeminal nerve. The sensory root of the trigeminal nerve gives rise to the ophthalmic division (V_1), maxillary division (V_2), and mandibular division (V_3) from the trigeminal ganglion.

The Ophthalmic Division

The smallest of the three divisions, the ophthalmic division (V_1) is purely sensory and travels anteriorly in the lateral wall of the cavernous sinus in the middle cranial fossa to the medial part of the superior orbital fissure. Before its entrance into the orbit through the superior orbital fissure, the ophthalmic nerve divides into three branches: the frontal, nasociliary, and lacrimal.

The **frontal nerve** is the largest branch of the ophthalmic division and travels anteriorly in the orbit, terminating as the supratrochlear and supraorbital nerves. The supratrochlear nerve lies medial to the supraorbital nerve and supplies the skin and conjunctiva of the medial portion of the upper eyelid and skin over the lower forehead close to the midline. The supraorbital nerve supplies the skin and conjunctiva of the central portion of the upper eyelid, the skin of the forehead, and the scalp as far back as the parietal bone and lambdoid suture.

The **nasociliary branch** travels along the medial aspect of the orbital roof, giving off various branches. The nasal cavity

and the skin at the apex and ala of the nose are innervated by the anterior ethmoid and external nasal nerves. The mucous membrane of the anterior portion of the nasal septum and lateral wall of the nasal cavity are innervated by the internal nasal nerve. The skin of the lacrimal sac, lacrimal caruncle, and adjoining portion of the side of the nose are innervated by the infratrochlear branch. The ethmoid and sphenoid sinuses are supplied by the posterior ethmoidal nerve. The eyeball is innervated by the short and long ciliary nerves.

The **lacrimal nerve** supplies the skin and conjunctiva of the lateral portion of the upper eyelid and is the smallest branch of the ophthalmic division.

The Maxillary Division

The maxillary division (V_2) of the trigeminal nerve is also a purely sensory division. Arising from the trigeminal ganglion in the middle cranial fossa, the maxillary nerve travels forward along the lateral wall of the cavernous sinus. Shortly after stemming from the trigeminal ganglion, the maxillary nerve gives off the only branch within the cranium: the middle meningeal nerve. It then leaves the cranium through the foramen rotundum, located in the greater wing of the sphenoid bone. After exiting the foramen rotundum, the nerve enters a space located behind and below the orbital cavity known as the pterygopalatine fossa. After giving off several branches within the fossa, the nerve enters the orbit through the inferior orbital fissure, at which point it becomes the infraorbital nerve. Coursing along the floor of the orbit in the infraorbital groove, the nerve enters the infraorbital canal and emerges onto the face through the infraorbital foramen.

The **middle meningeal nerve** is the only branch of the maxillary division within the cranium; it provides sensory innervation to the dura mater in the middle cranial fossa.

Within the pterygopalatine fossa, several branches are given off, including the pterygopalatine, zygomatic, and posterior superior alveolar nerves. The **pterygopalatine nerves** are two short nerves that merge within the pterygopalatine ganglion and then give rise to several branches. They contain postganglionic parasympathetic fibers, which pass along the zygomatic nerve to the lacrimal nerve innervating the lacrimal gland, as well as sensory fibers to the orbit, nose, palate, and pharynx. The sensory fibers to the orbit innervate the orbital periosteum.

The posterior aspect of the nasal septum, mucous membrane of the superior and middle conchae, and the posterior ethmoid sinus are innervated by the nasal branches. The anterior nasal septum, floor of the nose, and premaxilla from canine to canine are innervated by a branch known as the nasopalatine nerve. The **nasopalatine nerve** courses downward and forward from the roof of the nasal cavity to the floor to enter the incisive canal. It then enters the oral cavity through the incisive foramen to supply the palatal mucosa of the premaxilla.

The hard and soft palate are innervated by the palatine branches: the greater (anterior) and lesser (middle and posterior) palatine nerves. After descending through the pterygopalatine canal, the greater palatine nerve exits the greater palatine foramen onto the hard palate. The nerve provides sensory innervation to the palatal mucosa and bone of the hard and soft palate. The lesser palatine nerves emerge from the lesser palatine foramen to innervate the soft palate and tonsillar region.

The pharyngeal branch leaves the pterygopalatine ganglion from its posterior aspect to innervate the nasopharynx.

The **zygomatic nerve** gives rise to two branches after passing anteriorly from the pterygopalatine fossa to the orbit. The nerve passes through the inferior orbital fissure and divides into the zygomaticofacial and zygomaticotemporal nerves, supplying the skin over the malar prominence and skin over the side of the forehead, respectively. The zygomatic nerve also communicates with the ophthalmic division via the lacrimal nerve, sending fibers to the lacrimal gland.

The **posterior superior alveolar (PSA) nerve** branches off within the pterygopalatine fossa before the maxillary nerve enters the orbit. The PSA travels downward along the posterior aspect of the maxilla to supply the maxillary molar dentition, including the periodontal ligament and pulpal tissues, as well as the adjacent gingiva and alveolar process. The mucous membrane of the maxillary sinus is also innervated by the PSA. It is

of clinical significance to note that the PSA does not always innervate the mesiobuccal root of the first molar.[1,2] Several dissection studies have been performed tracing the innervation of the first molar back to the parent trunk. These studies have demonstrated the variations in innervation patterns of the first molar, and this is of clinical significance when anesthesia of this tooth is desired.

In a study by Loetscher and Walton,[3] 29 human maxillae were dissected to observe innervation patterns of the first molar. The study evaluated the innervation patterns by the posterior, middle, and anterior superior alveolar nerves on the first molar. The posterior and anterior superior alveolar nerves were found to be present in 100% (29/29) of specimens. The middle superior alveolar (MSA) nerve was found to be present 72% of the time (21/29 specimens). Nerves were traced from the first molar to the parent branches in 18 of the specimens. The PSA nerve was found to provide innervation in 72% (13/18) of specimens. The MSA nerve provided innervation in 28% (5/18) specimens, whereas the anterior superior alveolar nerve did not provide innervation to the first molar in any of the specimens. In the absence of the MSA nerve, the PSA nerve may provide innervation to the premolar region. In a study by McDaniel,[4] 50 maxillae were decalcified and dissected to demonstrate the innervation patterns of maxillary teeth. The PSA nerve was found to innervate the premolar region in 26% of dissections when the MSA nerve was not present. Table 36–1 lists the branches of the ophthalmic, maxillary, and mandibular divisions.

Within the infraorbital canal, the maxillary division is known as the **infraorbital nerve** and gives off the middle and anterior superior alveolar nerves. When present, the MSA nerve descends along the lateral wall of the maxillary sinus to innervate the first and second premolar teeth. It provides sensation to the periodontal ligament, pulpal tissues, gingiva and alveolar process of the premolar region, as well as the mesiobuccal root of the first molar in some cases.[1,2] In a study by Heasman,[5] dissections of 19 human cadaver heads were performed, and the MSA was found to be present in seven specimens. Loetscher and Walton[3] found that the mesial or distal position at which the MSA nerve joins the dental plexus (an anastomosis of the posterior, middle, and anterior superior alveolar nerves described below) determines its contribution to the innervation of the first molar. Specimens in which the MSA joined the plexus mesial to the first molar were found to have innervation of the first molar by the PSA and the premolars by the MSA. Specimens in which the MSA joined the plexus distal to the first molar demonstrated innervation of the first molar by the MSA. In its absence, the premolar region derives its innervation from the PSA and anterior superior alveolar nerves.[4] The anterior superior alveolar nerve descends within the anterior wall of the maxillary sinus. A small terminal branch of the anterior superior alveolar nerve communicates with the MSA to supply a small area of the lateral wall and floor of the nose. It also provides sensory innervation to the periodontal ligament, pulpal tissue, gingiva, and alveolar process of the central and lateral incisor and canine teeth. In the absence of the MSA, the anterior superior alveolar nerve has been shown to provide innervation to the premolar teeth. In the previously mentioned

TABLE 36–1. Branches of three major divisions.

Ophthalmic Division	Maxillary Division	Mandibular Division
1. Frontal • Supratrochlear • Supraorbital 2. Nasociliary • Anterior ethmoid • External nasal • Internal nasal • Infratrochlear • Posterior ethmoid • Short and long ciliary 3. Lacrimal	1. Middle meningeal 2. Pterygopalatine nerves • Sensory fibers to the orbit • Nasal branches • Nasopalatine nerve • Greater palatine nerve • Lesser palatine nerve • Pharyngeal branch 3. Zygomatic • Zygomaticofacial • Zygomaticotemporal 4. Posterior superior alveolar nerve 5. Infraorbital • Middle superior alveolar • Anterior superior alveolar • Inferior palpebral • Lateral nasal • Superior labial	1. Main trunk • Nervous spinosus • Nerve to the pterygoid 2. Anterior division • Masseteric • Deep temporal • Lateral pterygoid • Buccal nerve 3. Posterior division • Auriculotemporal • Lingual • Inferior alveolar • Nerve to the mylohyoid

study by McDaniel, the anterior superior alveolar nerve was shown to provide innervation to the premolar region in 36% of specimens in which no MSA nerve was found.[4]

The three superior alveolar nerves anastomose to form a network known as the dental plexus, which comprises terminal branches coming off the larger nerve trunks. These terminal branches are known as the dental, interdental, and interradicular nerves. The dental nerves innervate each root of each individual tooth in the maxilla by entering the root through the apical foramen and supplying sensation to the pulp. Interdental and interradicular branches provide sensation to the periodontal ligaments, interdental papillae, and buccal gingiva of adjacent teeth.

The infraorbital nerve divides into three terminal branches after emerging through the infraorbital foramen onto the face. The inferior palpebral, external nasal, and superior labial nerves supply sensory innervation to the skin of the lower eyelid, lateral aspect of the nose, and skin and mucous membranes of the upper lip, respectively.

The Mandibular Division

The largest branch of the trigeminal nerve, the mandibular branch (V$_3$), is both sensory and motor (Figure 36–2). The sensory root arises from the trigeminal ganglion, whereas the motor root arises from the motor nucleus of the pons and medulla oblongata. The sensory root passes through the foramen ovale almost immediately after coming off the trigeminal ganglion. The motor root passes underneath the ganglion and through the foramen ovale to unite with the sensory root just outside the cranium, forming the main trunk of the mandibular nerve. The nerve then divides into anterior and posterior divisions. The mandibular nerve gives off branches from its main trunk as well as from the anterior and posterior divisions.

The main trunk gives off two branches known as the **nervus spinosus** (meningeal branch) and the **nerve to the medial**

pterygoid. After branching off the main trunk, the nervus spinosus reenters the cranium, along with the middle meningeal artery, through the foramen spinosum. The nervus spinosus supplies the meninges of the middle cranial fossa as well as the mastoid air cells. The nerve to the medial pterygoid is a small motor branch that supplies the medial (internal) pterygoid muscle. It gives off two branches that supply the tensor tympani and tensor veli palatini muscles.

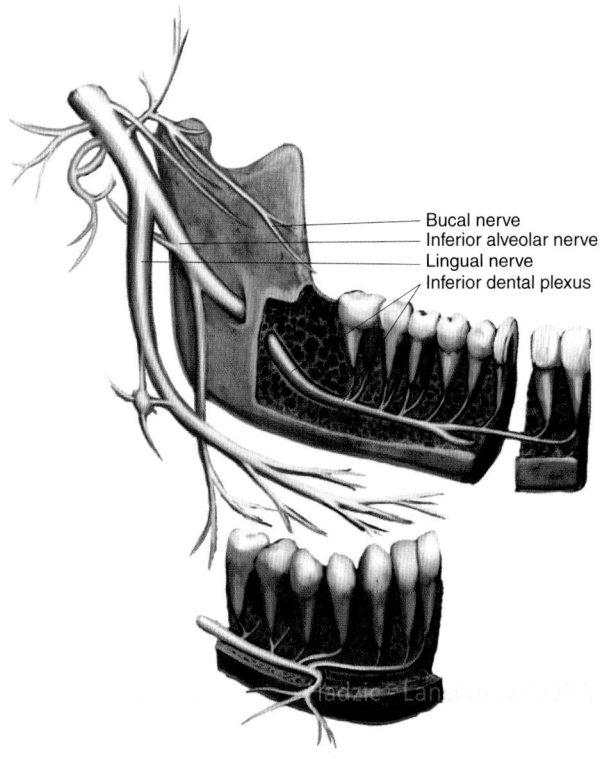

Bucal nerve
Inferior alveolar nerve
Lingual nerve
Inferior dental plexus

FIGURE 36–2. Anatomy of the mandibular nerve.

Three motor branches and one sensory branch are given off by the anterior division of the mandibular nerve. The **masseteric, deep temporal, and lateral pterygoid nerves** supply the masseter, temporalis, and lateral (external) pterygoid muscles, respectively. The sensory division known as the **buccal (buccinator or long buccal) nerve**, runs forward between the two heads of the lateral pterygoid muscle, along the inferior aspect of the temporalis muscle to the anterior border of the masseter muscle. Here, it passes anterolaterally to enter the buccinator muscle; however, *it does not innervate this muscle*. The buccinator muscle is innervated by the buccal branch of the facial nerve. The buccal nerve provides sensory innervation to the skin of the cheek, buccal mucosa, and buccal gingiva in the mandibular molar region.

The posterior division of the mandibular branch gives off two sensory branches (the auriculotemporal and lingual nerves) and one branch made up of both sensory and motor fibers (the inferior alveolar nerve).

The **auriculotemporal nerve** crosses the superior portion of the parotid gland, ascending behind the temporomandibular joint and giving off several sensory branches to the skin of the auricle, external auditory meatus, tympanic membrane, temporal region, temporomandibular joint, and parotid gland via postganglionic parasympathetic secretomotor fibers from the otic ganglion.

The **lingual nerve** travels inferiorly in the pterygomandibular space between the medial aspect of the ramus of the mandible and the lateral aspect of the medial pterygoid muscle. It then travels anteromedially below the inferior border of the superior pharyngeal constrictor muscle deep to the pterygomandibular raphae. The lingual nerve then continues anteriorly in the submandibular region along the hyoglossus muscle, crossing the submandibular duct inferiorly and medially to terminate deep to the sublingual gland. The lingual nerve provides sensory innervation to the anterior two-thirds of the tongue, mucosa of the floor of the mouth, and lingual gingiva.

The **inferior alveolar branch** of the mandibular nerve descends in the region between the lateral aspect of the sphenomandibular ligament and the medial aspect of the ramus of the mandible. It travels along with, but lateral and posterior to, the lingual nerve. While the lingual nerve continues to descend within the pterygomandibular space, the inferior alveolar nerve enters the mandibular canal through the mandibular foramen. Just before entering the mandibular canal, the inferior alveolar nerve gives off a motor branch known as the mylohyoid nerve (discussed below). The nerve accompanies the inferior alveolar artery and vein within the mandibular canal and divides into the mental and incisive nerve branches at the mental foramen. The inferior alveolar nerve provides sensation to the mandibular posterior teeth.

The **incisive nerve** is a branch of the inferior alveolar nerve that continues within the mandibular canal to provide sensory innervation to the mandibular anterior teeth.

The **mental nerve** emerges from the mental foramen to provide sensory innervation to the mucosa in the premolar/canine region, as well as to the skin of the chin and lower lip.

The **mylohyoid nerve** branches off the inferior alveolar nerve before its entry into the mandibular canal. It travels within the mylohyoid groove and along the medial aspect of the

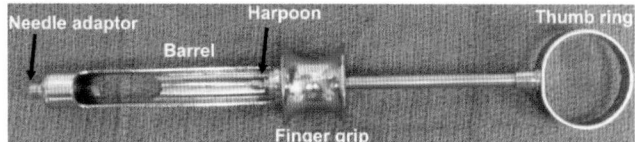

FIGURE 36–3. Breech-loading, metallic, cartridge-type, aspirating syringe.

body of the mandible to supply the mylohyoid muscle as well as the anterior belly of the digastric muscle.[1,2]

EQUIPMENT FOR REGIONAL MAXILLARY & MANDIBULAR ANESTHESIA

Administration of regional anesthesia of the maxilla and mandible is achieved via the use of a dental syringe, needle, and anesthetic cartridge. Several types of dental syringes are available for use. However, the most common is the breech-loading, metallic, cartridge-type, aspirating syringe. The syringe comprises a thumb ring, finger grip, barrel containing the piston with a harpoon, and needle adaptor (Figure 36–3). A needle is attached to the needle adaptor, which engages the rubber diaphragm of the dental cartridge (Figure 36–4). The anesthetic cartridge is placed into the barrel of the syringe from the side (breech-loading). The barrel contains a piston with a harpoon that engages the rubber stopper at the end of the anesthetic cartridge (Figure 36–5). After the needle and cartridge have been attached, a brisk tap is given to the back of the thumb ring to ensure that the harpoon has engaged the rubber stopper at the end of the anesthetic cartridge (Figure 36–6).

Dental needles are referred to in terms of their gauge, which corresponds to the diameter of the lumen of the needle. Increasing gauge corresponds to a smaller lumen diameter. Needles of 25 and 27 gauge are most commonly used for maxillary and mandibular regional anesthesia and are available in long and short lengths. The length of the needle is measured from the tip of the needle to the hub. The conventional long needle is approximately 40 mm in length, whereas the short

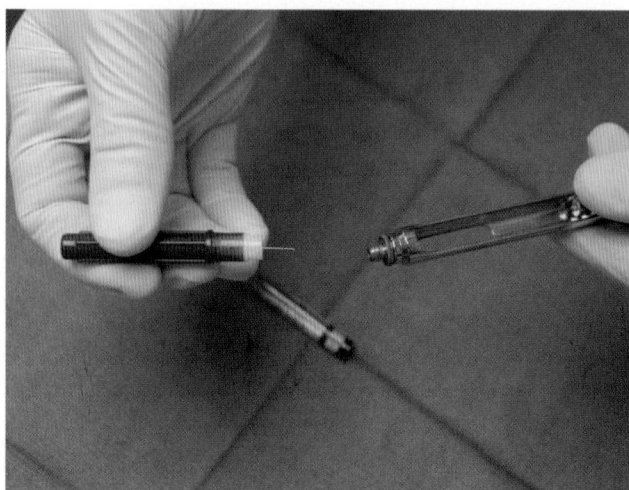

FIGURE 36–4. Needle–syringe assembling. A needle is attached to the needle adaptor.

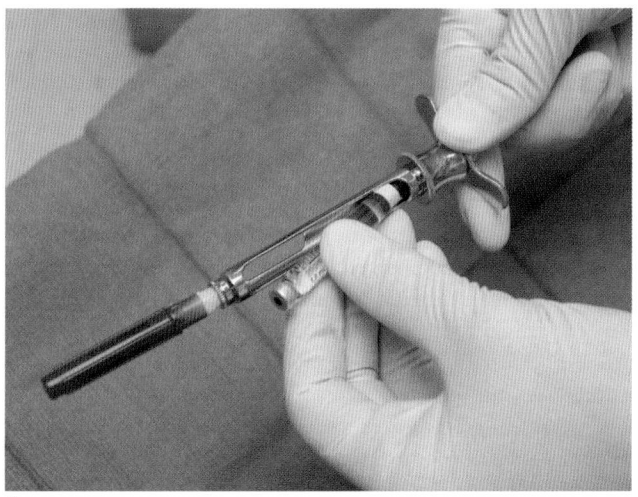

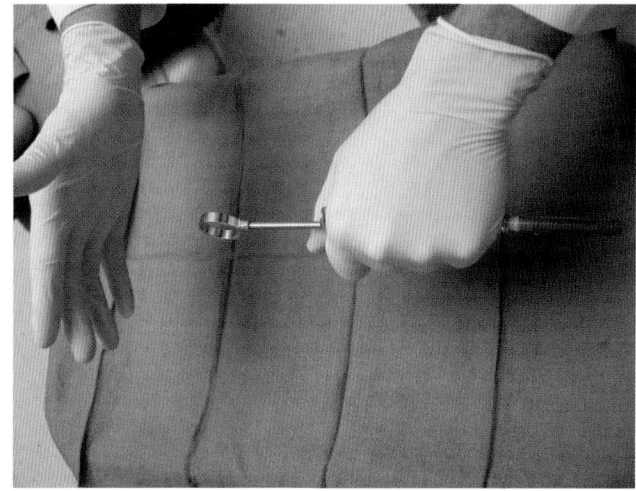

A

A

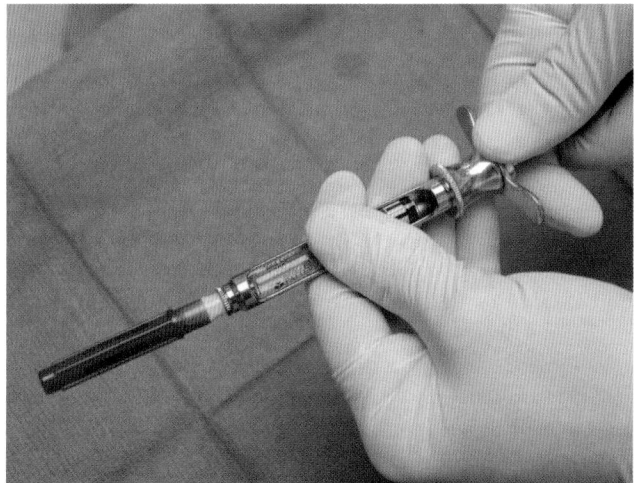

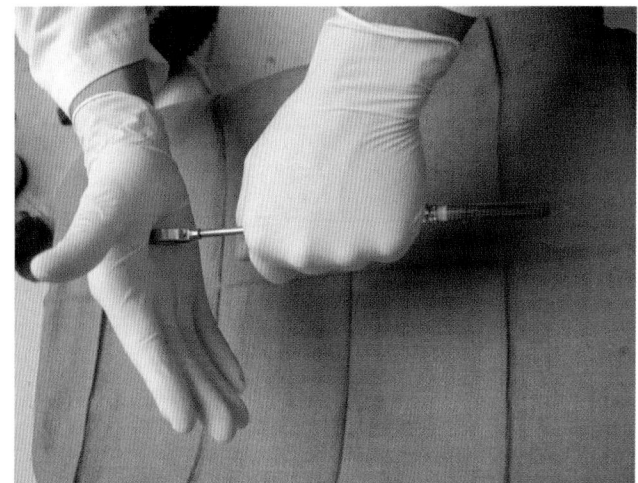

B

B

FIGURE 36–5. **A:** Needle–syringe assembling. The anesthetic cartridge is placed into the barrel of the syringe from the side (breech loading). **B:** A piston with a harpoon engages the rubber stopper at the end of the anesthetic cartridge while the needle adaptor engages the rubber diaphragm of the dental cartridge.

needle is approximately 25 mm. Variations in needle length do exist, depending on the manufacturer.

Anesthetic cartridges are prefilled, 1.8-mL glass cylinders with a rubber stopper at one end and an aluminum cap with a diaphragm at the other end (Figure 36–7). The contents of an anesthetic cartridge are the local anesthetic, vasoconstrictor (anesthetic without vasoconstrictor is also available), preservative for the vasoconstrictor (sodium bisulfite), sodium chloride, and distilled water. The most common anesthetics used in clinical practice are the amide anesthetics: lidocaine and mepivacaine. Other amide anesthetics available for use are prilocaine, articaine, bupivacaine, and etidocaine. Esther anesthetics are not as commonly used but remain available. Procaine, procaine plus propoxycaine, chloroprocaine, and tetracaine are some common esther anesthetics (Table 36-2). Additional armamentaria include dry gauze, topical antiseptic, and anesthetic. The site of injection should be made dry with gauze, and a topical antiseptic should be used to clean

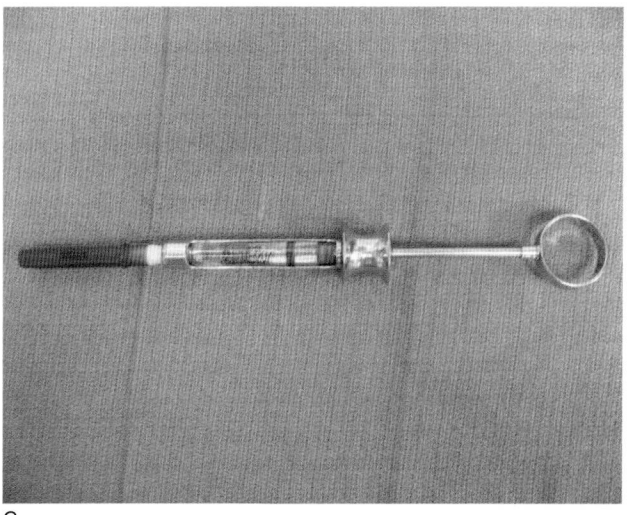

C

FIGURE 36–6. **A** and **B:** Needle–syringe assembling. A brisk tap is given to the back of the thumb ring to ensure that the harpoon has engaged the rubber stopper at the end of the anesthetic cartridge. **C:** A fully loaded anesthetic syringe.

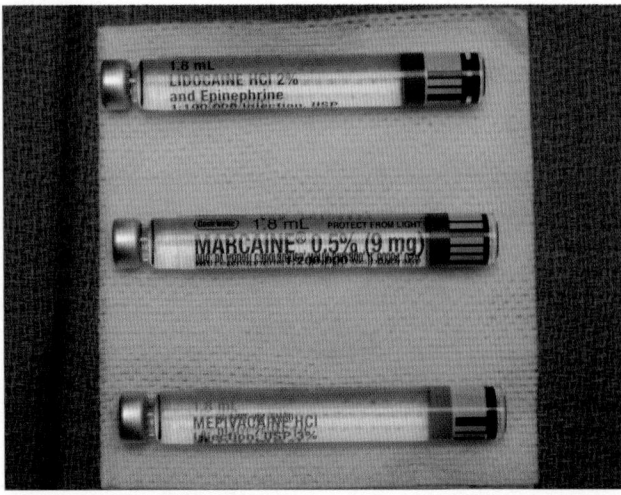

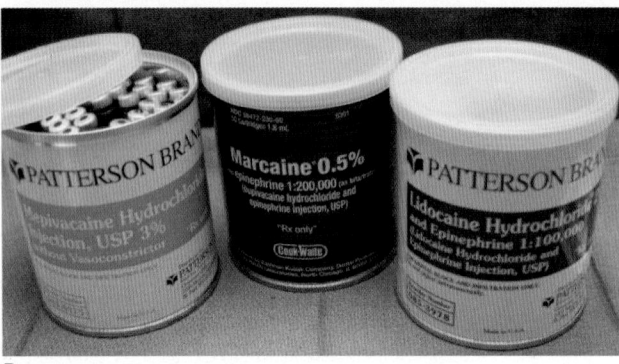

FIGURE 36-7. A: Dental cartridges. The rubber stopper is on the right end of the cartridge while the aluminum cap with the diaphragm is on the left end of the cartridge. **B:** Containers of dental anesthetic.

the area. Topical anesthetic is applied to the area of injection to minimize discomfort during insertion of the needle into the mucous membrane (Figure 36–8). Common topical preparations include benzocaine, butacaine sulfate, cocaine hydrochloride, dyclonine hydrochloride, lidocaine, and tetracaine hydrochloride.

Universal precautions should always be observed by the clinician; these include the use of protective gloves, mask, and eye protection. After withdrawing the needle when a block has been completed, the needle should always be carefully recapped to avoid accidental needle stick injury to the operator.[1]

Retraction of the soft tissue for visualization of the injection site should be performed with the use of a dental mirror or retraction instrument. This is recommended for all maxillary and mandibular regional techniques discussed below. Use of an instrument rather than one's fingers helps to prevent accidental needle-stick injury to the operator.

TECHNIQUES OF REGIONAL MAXILLARY ANESTHESIA

The techniques most commonly used in maxillary anesthesia include supraperiosteal (local) infiltration, periodontal ligament (intraligamentary) injection, PSA nerve block, MSA nerve block,

anterior superior alveolar nerve block, greater palatine nerve block, nasopalatine nerve block, local infiltration of the palate, and intrapulpal injection (Table 36–3). Of less clinical application are the maxillary nerve block and intraseptal injection.

▌ Supraperiosteal (Local) Infiltration

The supraperiosteal, or local, infiltration is one of the simplest and most commonly used techniques for achieving anesthesia of the maxillary dentition. This technique is indicated when any individual tooth or soft tissue in a localized area is to be treated. Contraindications to this technique are the need to anesthetize multiple teeth adjacent to one another (in which case a nerve block is the preferred technique), acute inflammation and infection in the area to be anesthetized, and, less significantly, the density of bone overlying the apices of the teeth. A 25- or 27-gauge short needle is preferred for this technique.

Procedure

Identify the tooth to be anesthetized and the height of the mucobuccal fold over the tooth. This will be the injection site. The right-handed operator should stand at the 9 o'clock to 10 o'clock position, whereas the left-handed operator should stand at the 2 o'clock to 3 o'clock position. Retract the lip, and orient the syringe with the bevel toward bone. This prevents discomfort from the needle coming into contact with the bone and minimizes the risk of tearing the periosteum with the needle tip. Insert the needle at the height of the mucobuccal fold above the tooth to a depth of no more than a few millimeters, and aspirate (Figure 36–9). If aspiration is negative, slowly inject one-third to one-half (0.6–1.2 mL) of a cartridge of anesthetic solution over the course of 30 seconds. Withdraw the syringe, and recap the needle. Successful administration provides anesthesia to the tooth and associated soft tissue within 2–4 minutes. If adequate anesthesia has not been achieved, repeat the procedure, and deposit another one-third to one-half of the cartridge of anesthetic solution.[1]

▌ Periodontal Ligament (Intraligamentary) Injection

The periodontal ligament, or intraligamentary, injection is a useful adjunct to the supraperiosteal injection or a nerve block. Often, it is used to supplement these techniques to achieve profound anesthesia of the area to be treated. Indications for the use of the intraligamentary injection technique are the need to anesthetize an individual tooth or teeth, need for soft tissue anesthesia within the immediate vicinity of a tooth, and partial anesthesia after a field block or nerve block. A 25- or 27-gauge short needle is preferred for this technique.

Procedure

Identify the tooth or area of soft tissue to be anesthetized. The sulcus between the gingiva and the tooth is the injection site for the periodontal ligament injection. Position the patient in the supine position. For the right-handed operator, retract the lip with a retraction instrument held in the left hand, and stand where the tooth and gingiva are clearly visible. The same applies

TABLE 36–2. Commonly used local anesthetics in maxillofacial anesthesia[12,13].

Name	Chemical Structure	Class	Max Adult Dosage (mg/kg)	Max Pediatric Dosage (mg/kg)	Onset of Action (min)	pKa
Articaine (with vasoconstrictor)		Amide	7.0	7.0	1.0–3.0	7.8
Benzocaine		Ester	–	–	0.3–0.5	3.5
Bupivacaine		Amide	1.3	Use not recommended for patients under 12 years of age	6.0–10.0	8.1
Chloroprocaine (with/without epinephrine)		Ester	11.0/14.0	11.0	6.0–12	8.7
Etidocaine (with/without epinephrine)		Amide	8.0/6.0	8.0/6.0	1.5–3.0	7.9

Drug	Structure	Type				
Lidocaine *(with/without epinephrine)*		Amide	4.5/7.0	3.3–4.4	2.0–3.0	7.8
Mepivacaine		Amide	6.6	3.0	1.5–2.0	7.7
Prilocaine		Amide	8.0	6.6–8.0	2.0–4.0	7.8
Procaine		Ester	1000 mg for peripheral nerve blocks	–	6.0–10.0	8.9
Tetracaine		Esther	20 mg for topical application	Safety and effectiveness in children have not been established	0.5	8.5

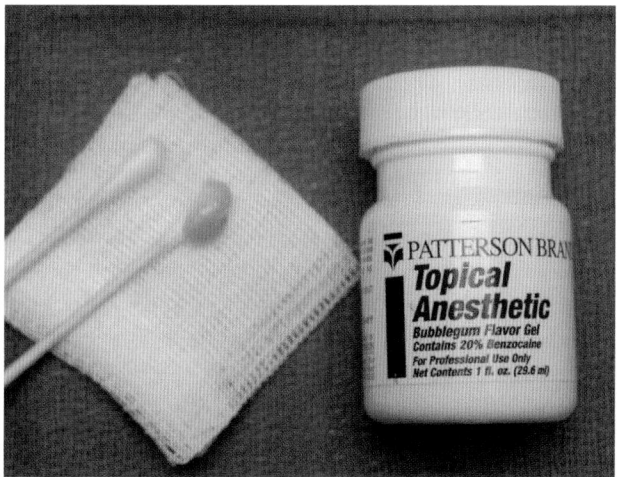

FIGURE 36–8. Topical anesthesia. Before injection, topical anesthetic can be applied on the mucosa in the area of injection to minimize patient discomfort.

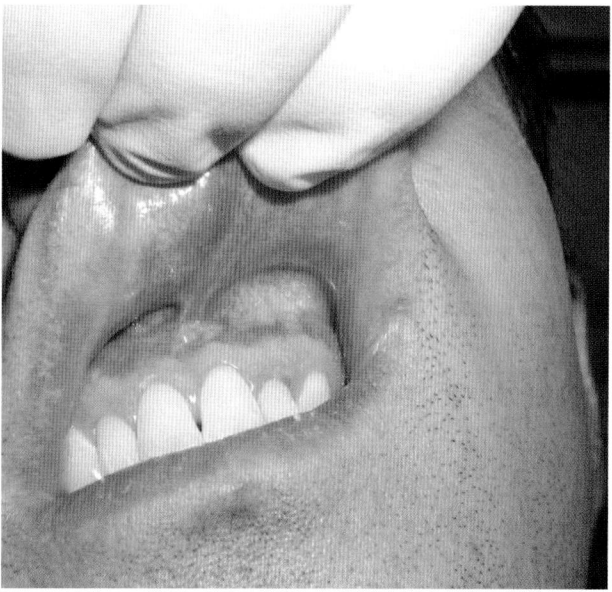

A

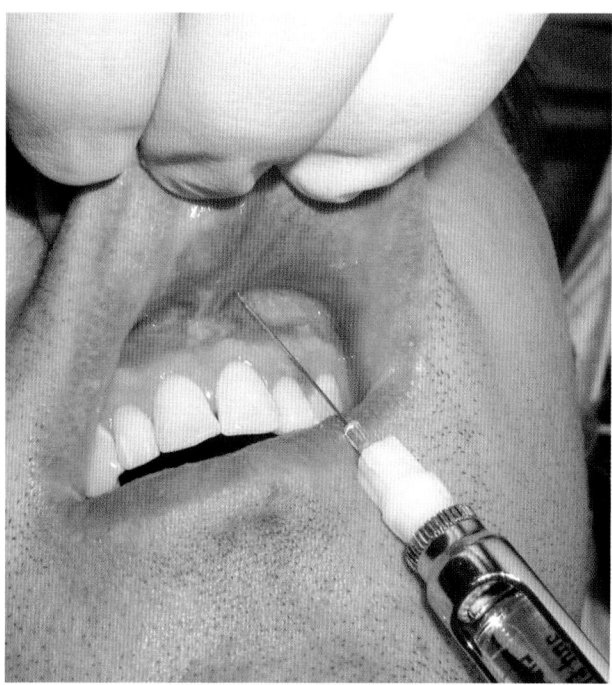

B

FIGURE 36–9. A: Locate the height of the mucobuccal fold over the tooth to be anesthetized. **B:** Clinical picture depicting a local infiltration of the maxillary left central incisor tooth. Note the penetration of the needle at the height of the mucobuccal fold above the maxillary left central incisor.

for the left-handed operator, except that the retraction instrument is held in the right hand. Hold the syringe parallel with the long axis of the tooth on the mesial or distal aspect. Insert the needle (bevel facing the root) to the depth of the gingival sulcus (Figure 36–10). Advance the needle until resistance is met. Then, administer a small amount of anesthetic (0.2 mL) slowly over the course of 20–30 seconds. It is normal to experience resistance to the flow of anesthetic. Successful execution of this technique provides pulpal and soft tissue anesthesia to the individual tooth or teeth to be treated.[1]

Posterior Superior Alveolar Nerve Block

The PSA nerve block, otherwise known as the tuberosity block or the zygomatic block, is used to achieve anesthesia of the maxillary molar teeth up to the first molar, with the exception of its mesiobuccal root in some cases. A possible complication of this technique is the risk of hematoma formation from injection of anesthetic into the pterygoid plexus of veins or from accidental puncture of the maxillary artery. Aspiration before injection is indicated when the PSA block is given. The indications for this technique are the need to anesthetize multiple molar teeth. Anesthesia can be achieved with fewer needle penetrations than with the supraperiosteal technique, providing greater comfort to the patient. The PSA block can be given to provide anesthesia of

the maxillary molars when acute inflammation and infection are present. If inadequate anesthesia is achieved via the supraperiosteal technique, the PSA block can be used to achieve more profound anesthesia of a longer duration. The PSA block also provides anesthesia to the premolar region in a certain percentage of patients in whom the MSA is absent.

Contraindications to the procedure are related to the risk of hematoma formation. In individuals with coagulation disorders, care must be taken to avoid injection into the pterygoid

TABLE 36–3. Techniques of anesthesia for treatment of a localized area or one or two teeth.

Technique	Area Anesthetized
Supraperiosteal injection	Individual teeth and buccal soft tissue
Periodontal ligament injection	Individual teeth and buccal soft tissue
Intraseptal injection	Localized soft tissue
Intrapulpal injection	Individual tooth

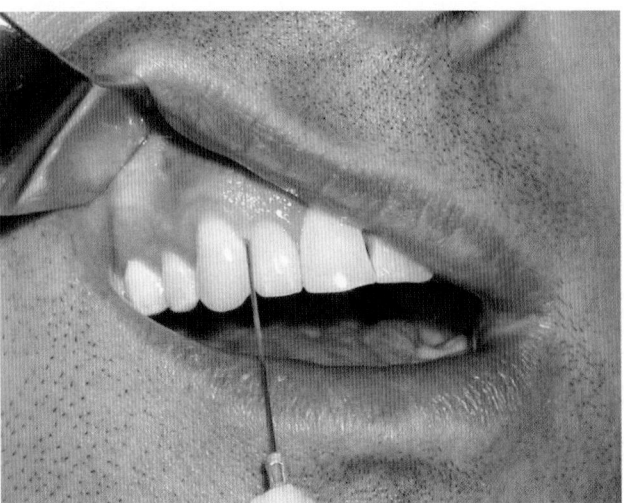

FIGURE 36–10. Clinical picture depicting a periodontal ligament injection. Note the position of the needle between the gingival sulcus and tooth with the needle parallel to the long axis of the tooth.

plexus or puncture of the maxillary artery. A short 25- or 27-gauge needle is preferred for this technique.

Procedure

Identify the height of the mucobuccal fold over the second molar. This is the injection site. The right-handed operator should stand at the 9 o'clock to 10 o'clock position, whereas the left-handed operator should stand at the 2 o'clock to 3 o'clock position. Retract the lip with a retraction instrument. Hold the syringe with the bevel toward the bone. Insert the needle at the height of the mucobuccal fold above the maxillary second molar at a 45-degree angle directed superiorly, medially, and posteriorly (one continuous movement). Advance the needle to a depth of three-fourths of its total length (Figure 36–11). No resistance should be felt while advancing the needle through the

soft tissue. If contact is made with bone, the medial angulation is too great. Slowly retract the needle (without removing it), and bring the syringe barrel toward the occlusal plane. This allows the needle to be angulated slightly more laterally to the posterior aspect of the maxilla. Advance the needle, aspirate, and inject one cartridge of anesthetic solution slowly over the course of 1 minute, aspirating frequently during the administration. Before injecting, one should aspirate in two planes to avoid accidental injection into the pterygoid plexus. After the first aspiration, the needle should be rotated one quarter turn. The operator should then reaspirate. If positive aspiration occurs, slowly retract the needle and re-aspirate in two planes. A successful injection technique results in anesthesia of the maxillary molars (with the exception of the mesiobuccal root of the first molar in some cases) and associated soft tissue on the buccal aspect.[1]

Middle Superior Alveolar Nerve Block

The MSA nerve block is useful for procedures in which the maxillary premolar teeth or the mesiobuccal root of the first molar requires anesthesia. Although not always present it is useful if the posterior or anterior superior alveolar nerve blocks or supraperiosteal infiltration fails to achieve adequate anesthesia. For individuals in whom the MSA nerve is absent, the PSA and anterior superior alveolar nerves provide innervation to the maxillary premolar teeth and the mesiobuccal root of the first molar.

Contraindications to the procedure include acute inflammation and infection in the area of injection or a procedure involving one tooth in which local infiltration will be sufficient. A 25- or 27-gauge short needle is preferred for this technique.

Procedure

Identify the height of the mucobuccal fold above the maxillary second premolar. This is the injection site. The right-handed operator should stand at the 9 o'clock to 10 o'clock position, whereas the left-handed operator should stand at the 2 o'clock

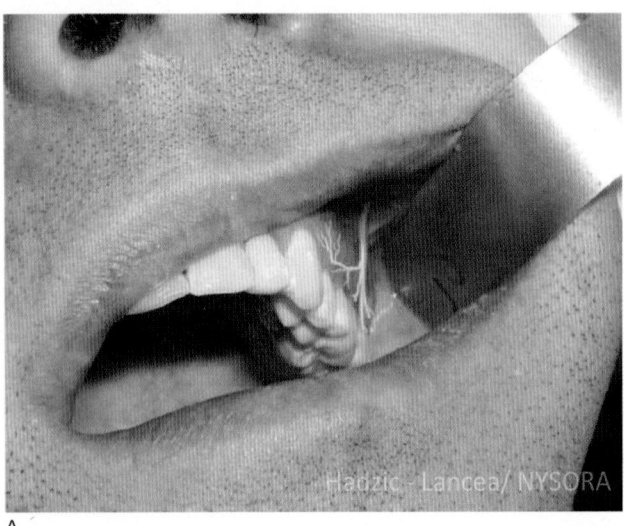

A

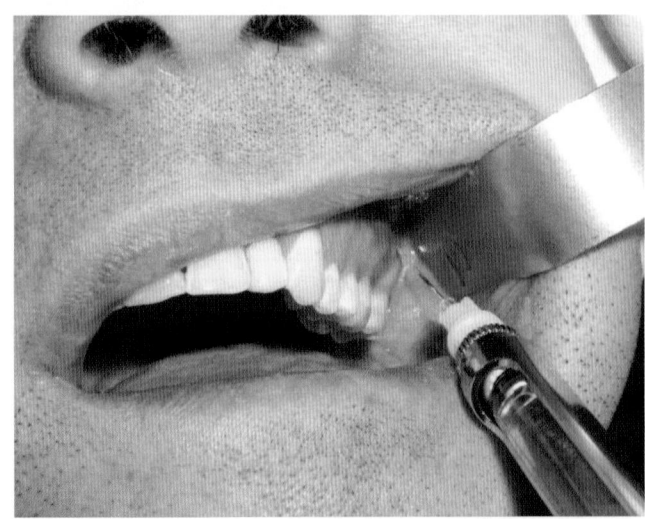

B

FIGURE 36–11. **A:** Location of the posterior superior alveolar (PSA) nerve. **B:** Position of the needle during the PSA nerve block. The needle is inserted at the height of the mucobuccal fold above the maxillary second molar at a 45-degree angle aimed superiorly, medially, and posteriorly.

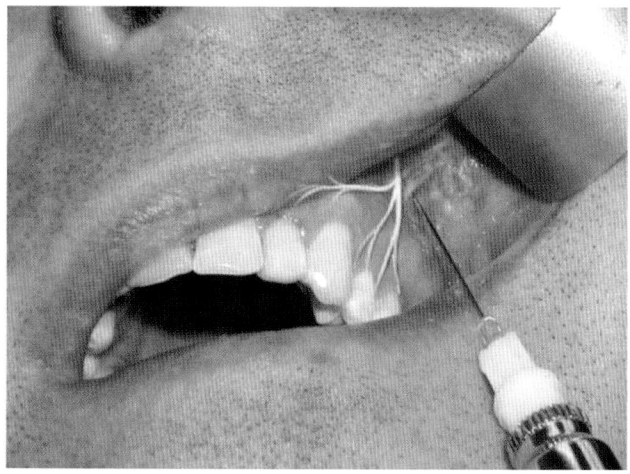

A

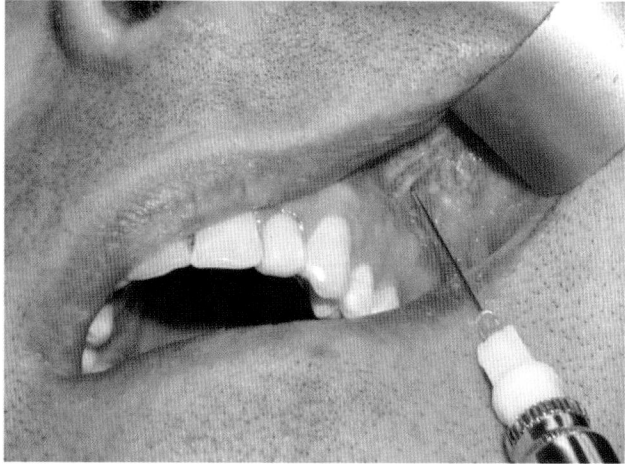

B

FIGURE 36–12. A: Location of the middle superior alveolar nerve. **B:** The needle is inserted at the height of the mucobuccal fold above the maxillary second premolar.

to 3 o'clock position. Retract the lip with a retraction instrument, and insert the needle until the tip is above the apex of the second premolar tooth (Figure 36–12). Aspirate, and inject two-thirds to one cartridge of anesthetic solution slowly over the course of 1 minute. Successful execution of this technique provides anesthesia to the pulp, surrounding soft tissue, and bone of the first and second premolar teeth and the mesiobuccal root of the first molar.[1]

Anterior Superior Alveolar (Infraorbital) Nerve Block

The anterior superior alveolar, or infraorbital, nerve block, is a useful technique for achieving anesthesia of the maxillary central and lateral incisors and canine as well as the surrounding soft tissue on the buccal aspect. In patients who do not have an MSA nerve, the anterior superior alveolar nerve may also innervate the premolar teeth and mesiobuccal root of the first molar. Indications for the use of this technique include procedures involving multiple teeth and inadequate anesthesia from the supraperiosteal technique. A 25-gauge long needle is preferred for this technique.

Procedure

Place the patient in the supine position. Identify the height of the mucobuccal fold above the maxillary first premolar. This is the injection site. The right-handed operator should stand at the 10 o'clock position, whereas the left-handed operator should stand at the 2 o'clock position. Identify the infraorbital notch on the inferior orbital rim (Figure 36–13a). The infraorbital foramen lies just inferior to the notch, usually in line with the second premolar. Slight discomfort is felt by the patient when digital pressure is placed on the foramen. It is helpful but not necessary to mark the position of the infraorbital foramen. Retract the lip with a retraction instrument while noting the location of the foramen. Orient the bevel of the needle toward bone, and insert the needle at the height of the mucobuccal fold above the first premolar (Figure 36–13b).

The syringe should be angled toward the infraorbital foramen and kept parallel with the long axis of the first premolar to avoid hitting the maxillary bone prematurely. The needle is advanced into the soft tissue until contact is made with the bone over the roof of the foramen. This is approximately half the length of the

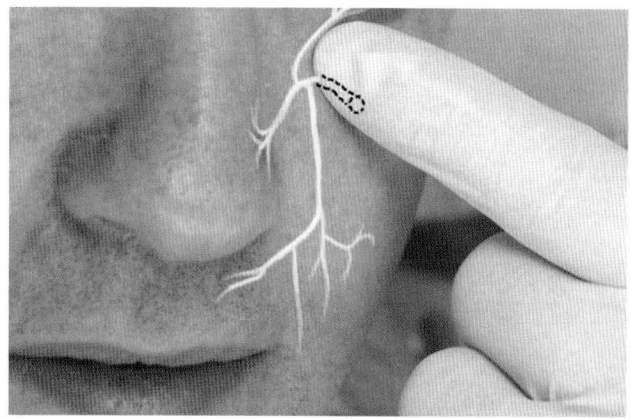

A

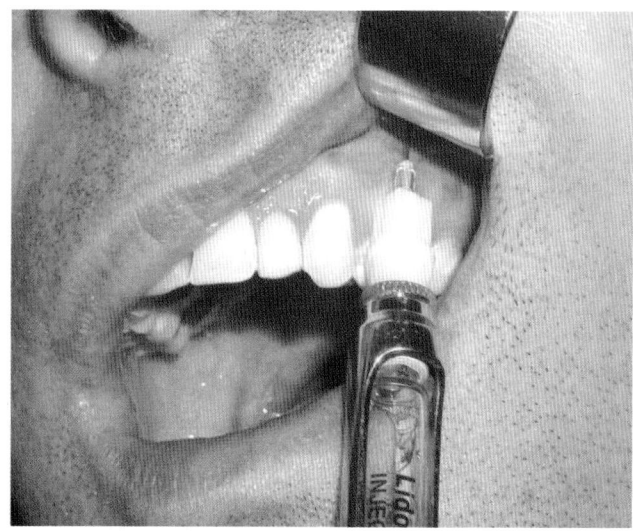

B

FIGURE 36–13. A: Location of the infraorbital nerve. **B:** The needle is kept parallel to the long axis of the maxillary first premolar and inserted at the height of the mucobuccal fold above the first premolar.

needle; however, length varies from individual to individual. After aspiration, approximately one-half to two-thirds (0.9–1.2 mL) of the anesthetic cartridge is deposited slowly over the course of 1 minute. It is recommended that pressure be kept over the site of injection to facilitate the diffusion of anesthetic solution into the foramen. Successful execution of this technique results in anesthesia of the lower eyelid, lateral aspect of the nose, and upper lip. Pulpal anesthesia of the maxillary central and lateral incisors, canine, buccal soft tissue, and bone is also achieved. In a certain percentage of people, the premolar teeth and the mesiobuccal root of the first molar are also anesthetized.[1]

Greater Palatine Nerve Block

The greater palatine nerve block is useful when treatment is necessary on the palatal aspect of the maxillary premolar and molar dentition. This technique targets the area just anterior to the greater palatine canal. The greater palatine nerve exits the canal and travels forward between the bone and soft tissue of the palate.

Contraindications to this technique are acute inflammation and infection at the injection site. A 25- or 27-gauge long needle is preferred for this technique.

Procedure

The patient should be in the supine position with the chin tilted upward for visibility of the area to be anesthetized. The right-handed operator should stand at the 8 o'clock position, whereas the left-handed operator should stand at the 4 o'clock position. Using a cotton swab, locate the greater palatine foramen by placing it on the palatal tissue approximately 1 cm medial to the junction of the second and third molars (Figure 36–14). Although this is the usual position for the foramen, it may be located slightly anterior or posterior to this location. Gently press the swab into the tissue until the depression created by the foramen is felt.

Malamed and Trieger[6] found that the foramen is found medial to the anterior half of the third molar approximately 50%

of the time, medial to the posterior half of the second molar approximately 39% of the time, and medial to the posterior half of the third molar approximately 9% of the time. The area approximately 1–2 mm anterior to the foramen is the target injection site. Using the cotton swab, apply pressure to the area of the foramen until the tissue blanches. Aim the syringe perpendicular to the injection site, which is 1–2 mm anterior to the foramen. While keeping pressure on the foramen, inject small volumes of anesthetic solution as the needle is advanced through the tissue until contact is made with bone. The tissue will blanch in the area surrounding the injection site. Depth of penetration is usually no more than a few millimeters. Once contact is made with bone, aspirate and inject approximately one-fourth (0.45 mL) of the anesthetic solution. Resistance to deposition of anesthetic solution is normally felt by the operator. This technique provides anesthesia to the palatal mucosa and hard palate from the first premolar anteriorly to the posterior aspect of the hard palate and to the midline medially.[1,6]

Nasopalatine Nerve Block

The nasopalatine nerve block, otherwise known as the incisive nerve block or sphenopalatine nerve block, anesthetizes the nasopalatine nerves bilaterally. In this technique, anesthetic solution is deposited in the area of the incisive foramen. This technique is indicated when treatment requires anesthesia of the lingual aspect of multiple anterior teeth. A 25- or 27-gauge short needle is preferred for this technique.

Procedure

The patient should be in the supine position with the chin tilted upward for visibility of the area to be anesthetized. The right-handed operator should be at the 9 o'clock position, whereas the left-handed operator should be at the 3 o'clock position. Identify the incisive papillae. The area directly lateral to the incisive papilla is the injection site. With a cotton swab, hold pressure over the incisive papilla. Insert the needle just lateral to the papilla with the bevel against the tissue

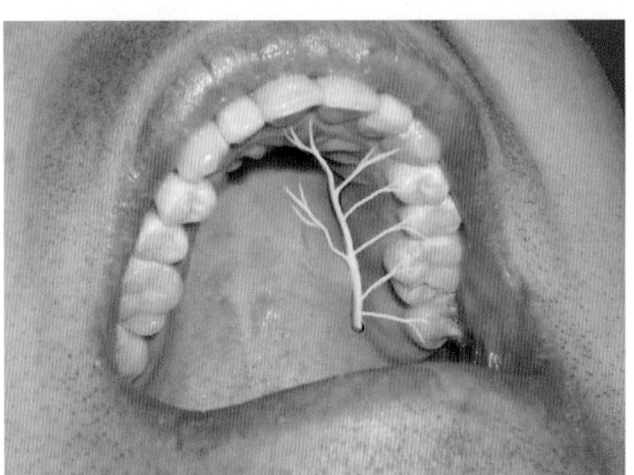
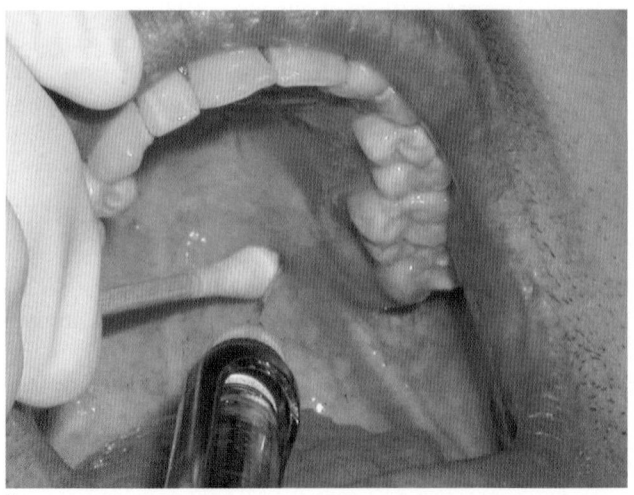

A

B

FIGURE 36–14. A: Location of the greater palatine nerve. **B:** The area of insertion for the greater palatine nerve block is 1 cm medial to the junction of the maxillary second and third molars.

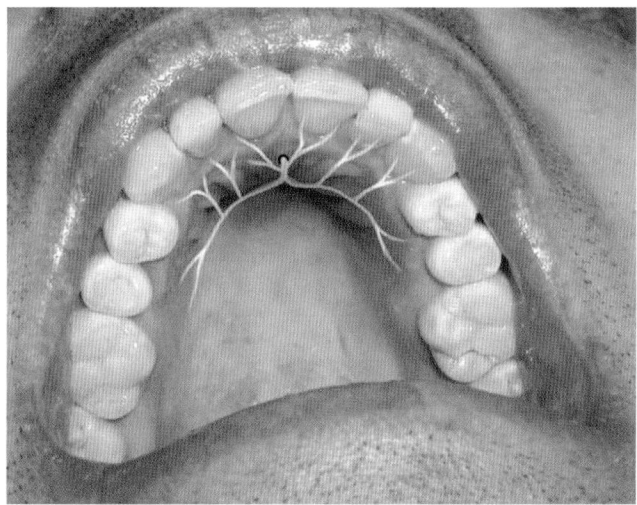

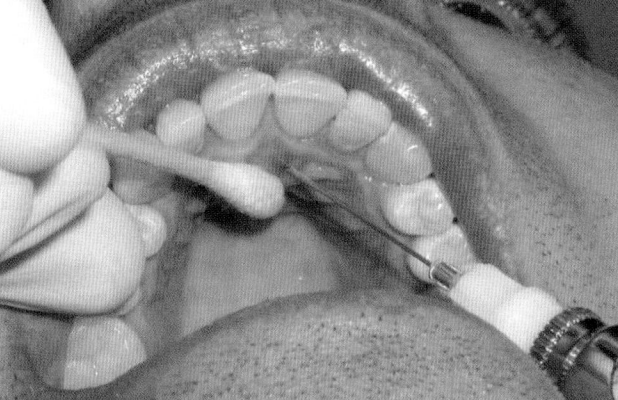

FIGURE 36–15. A: Location of the nasopalatine nerve. **B:** Needle insertion is just lateral to the incisive papilla for the nasopalatine nerve block.

(Figure 36–15). Advance the needle slowly toward the incisive foramen while depositing small volumes of anesthetic and maintaining pressure on the papilla. Once contact is made with bone, retract the needle approximately 1 mm, aspirate, and inject one-fourth (0.45 mL) of a cartridge of anesthetic solution over the course of 30 seconds. Blanching of surrounding tissues and resistance to the deposition of anesthetic solution are normal. Anesthesia is provided to the soft and hard tissue of the lingual aspect of the anterior teeth from the distal of the canine on one side to the distal of the canine on the opposite side.[1]

Local Palatal Infiltration

The administration of local anesthetic for the palatal anesthesia of just one or two teeth is common in clinical practice. When a block is undesirable, local infiltration provides effective palatal anesthesia of the individual teeth to be treated. Contraindications include acute inflammation and infection over the area to be anesthetized. A 25- or 27-gauge short needle is preferred for this technique.

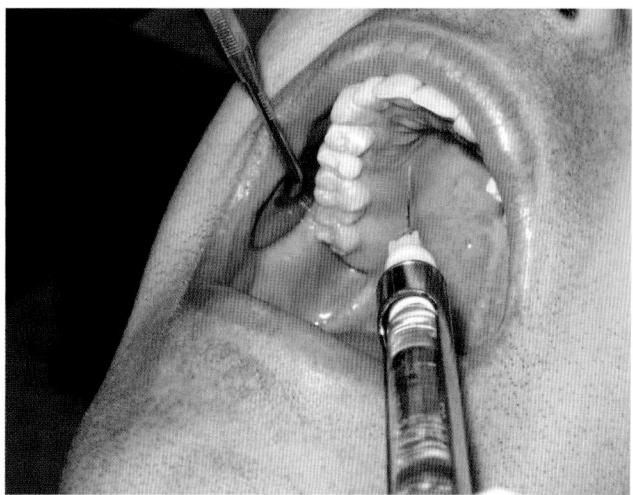

FIGURE 36–16. Local infiltration on the palatal aspect of the maxillary right first premolar. The needle is inserted approximately 5–10 mm palatal to the center of the crown.

Procedure

The patient should be in the supine position with the chin tilted upward for visibility of the area to be anesthetized. Identify the area to be anesthetized. The right-handed operator should be at the 10 o'clock position, whereas the left-handed operator should be at the 2 o'clock position. The area of needle penetration is 5–10 mm palatal to the center of the crown. Apply pressure directly behind the injection site with a cotton swab. Insert the needle at a 45-degree angle to the injection site with the bevel angled toward the soft tissue (Figure 36–16). While maintaining pressure behind the injection site, advance the needle, and slowly deposit anesthetic solution as the soft tissue is penetrated. Advance the needle until contact is made with bone. Depth of penetration is usually no more than a few millimeters. The tissue is very firmly adherent to the underlying periosteum in this region, causing resistance to the deposition of local anesthetic. No more than 0.2–0.4 mL of anesthetic solution is necessary to provide adequate palatal anesthesia. Blanching of the tissue at the injection site immediately follows deposition of local anesthetic. Successful administration of anesthetic using this technique results in hemostasis and anesthesia of the palatal tissue in the area of injection.[1]

Intrapulpal Injection

Intrapulpal injection involves anesthesia of the nerve within the pulp canal of the individual tooth to be treated. When pain control cannot be achieved by any of the aforementioned methods, the intrapulpal method may be used once the pulp chamber is open. There are no contraindications to the use of this technique as it is at times the only effective method of pain control. A 25- or 27-gauge short needle is preferred for this technique.

Procedure

The patient should be in the supine position with the chin tilted upward for visibility of the area to be anesthetized. Identify the tooth to be anesthetized. The right-handed operator should be at the 10 o'clock position, whereas the left-handed operator should be at the 2 o'clock position. Assuming that the pulp chamber has been opened by an experienced dental professional, place the needle into the pulp chamber, and deposit one drop of anesthetic. Advance the needle into the pulp canal, and deposit another 0.2 mL of local anesthetic solution. It may be necessary to bend the needle in order to gain access to the chamber, especially with posterior teeth. The patient usually experiences a brief period of significant pain as the solution enters the canal, followed by immediate pain relief.[1]

Maxillary Nerve Block

Less often used in clinical practice, the maxillary nerve block (second division block) provides anesthesia of a hemimaxilla. This technique is useful for procedures that require anesthesia of multiple teeth and surrounding buccal and palatal soft tissue in one quadrant or when acute inflammation and infection preclude successful administration of anesthesia by the aforementioned methods. There are two techniques one can use to achieve the maxillary nerve block: the high tuberosity approach and the greater palatine canal approach.

The high tuberosity approach carries with it the risk of hematoma formation and is therefore contraindicated in patients with coagulation disorders. The maxillary artery is the vessel of primary concern with the high tuberosity approach. Both techniques are contraindicated when acute inflammation and infection are present over the injection site.

High Tuberosity Approach

A 25-gauge long needle is preferred for this technique. The patient should be in the supine position with the chin tilted upward for visibility of the area to be anesthetized. Identify the area to be anesthetized. The right-handed operator should be at the 10 o'clock position, whereas the left-handed operator should be at the 2 o'clock position. This technique anesthetizes the maxillary nerve as it travels through the pterygopalatine fossa. Identify the height of the mucobuccal fold just distal to the maxillary second molar. This is the injection site. The needle should enter the tissue at a 45-degree angle aimed posteriorly, superiorly, and medially, as in the PSA nerve block (see Figure 36–11b). The bevel should be oriented toward the bone. The needle is advanced to a depth of approximately 30 mm or a few millimeters shy of the hub. At this depth, the needle lies within the pterygopalatine fossa. The operator should then aspirate, rotate the needle one quarter turn, and aspirate again. After negative aspiration in two planes has been established, slowly inject one cartridge of anesthetic solution over the course of 1 minute. The needle is then slowly withdrawn and recapped.

Successful administration of anesthetic using the high tuberosity approach provides anesthesia to the entire hemimaxilla on the ipsilateral side of the block. This includes pulpal anesthesia to the maxillary teeth; the buccal and palatal soft tissue as far medially as the midline; and the skin of the upper lip, lateral aspect of the nose, and lower eyelid.

Greater Palatine Canal Approach

A 25-gauge long needle is preferred for this technique. Place the patient in the supine position. The right-handed operator should be at the 10 o'clock position, whereas the left-handed operator should be at the 2 o'clock position. Identify the greater palatine foramen as described in the technique for the greater palatine nerve block. The tissue directly over the greater palatine foramen is the target for injection. This technique anesthetizes the maxillary nerve as it travels through the pterygopalatine fossa via the greater palatine canal. Apply pressure to the area over the greater palatine foramen with a cotton-tipped applicator. Administer a greater palatine nerve block using the aforementioned technique (see Figure 36–14b). When adequate palatal anesthesia is achieved, gently probe for the greater palatine foramen with the tip of the needle. For this technique, the syringe should be held so that the needle is aimed posteriorly. It may be necessary to change the angulation of the needle to locate the foramen.

In a case study performed by Malamed and Trieger, the majority of canals were angled 45–50 degrees. Once the foramen has been located, advance the needle to a depth of 30 mm. If resistance is met, withdraw the needle a few millimeters, and reenter at a different angle. Malamed and Trieger found bony obstructions preventing needle passage in approximately 5–15% of canals. If resistance is met early and the operator is unable to advance the needle into the canal more than a few millimeters, the procedure should be aborted and the high tuberosity approach should be considered. If no resistance is met and penetration of the canal is successful, aspirate in two planes as described above, and slowly deposit one cartridge of local anesthetic solution. As with the high tuberosity approach, the hemimaxilla on the ipsilateral side as the injection becomes anesthetized with successful execution of this technique.[1,6,7]

Intraseptal Injection

The intraseptal technique is a useful adjunct to the aforementioned techniques (supraperiosteal, PSA, MSA, and anterior superior alveolar). Although not used as often in clinical practice, the technique offers the added advantage of hemostasis in the area of injection. Terminal nerve endings in the surrounding hard and soft tissue of individual teeth are anesthetized with this technique. Contraindications to the procedure include acute inflammation and infection over the site of injection. A 27-gauge short needle is preferred for this technique.

Procedure

Place the patient in the supine position. The target area is the interdental palpillae 2–3 mm apical to the apex of the papillary triangle (Figure 36–17). The right-handed operator should be at the 10 o'clock position, whereas the left-handed operator should be at the 2 o'clock position. The operator may ask the patient to turn his or her head for optimum visibility. The syringe is held at a 45-degree angle to the long axis of the tooth with the bevel facing the apex of the root. The needle is inserted into the soft tissue and is advanced until contact is made with

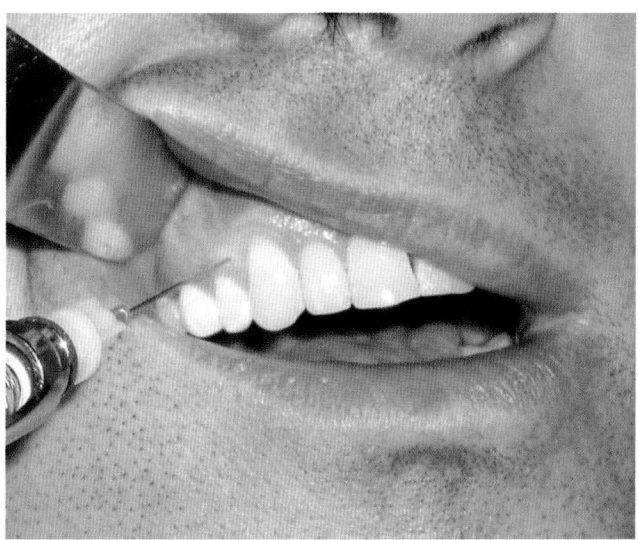

FIGURE 36–17. Intraseptal technique. Note the position of the needle 3 mm apical to the apex of the papillary triangle.

bone. A few drops of anesthetic should be administered at this time. The needle is then advanced into the interdental septum, and 0.2 mL of anesthetic solution is deposited. Resistance to the flow of anesthetic solution is expected, and ischemia of the soft tissue surrounding the injection site ensues shortly after anesthetic solution is administered.[1]

Table 36–4 lists maxillary and mandibular anesthesia techniques for the treatment of a quadrant or multiple teeth.

TECHNIQUES OF MANDIBULAR REGIONAL ANESTHESIA

Techniques used in clinical practice for the anesthesia of the hard and soft tissues of the mandible include the supraperiosteal technique, periodontal ligament injection, intrapulpal anesthesia, intraseptal injection, inferior alveolar nerve block, long buccal nerve block, Gow-Gates technique, Vazirani-Akinosi closed-mouth mandibular block, mental nerve block, and incisive nerve block.

TABLE 36–4. Techniques of anesthesia for treatment of a quadrant or multiple teeth.

Technique	Area Anesthetized
Maxillary	
Posterior superior alveolar nerve block	Maxillary molars (except the mesiobuccal root of the maxillary first molar in some cases), hard and soft tissue on buccal aspect
Middle superior alveolar nerve block	Mesiobuccal root of maxillary first molar (in some cases), premolars, and surrounding hard and soft tissue on buccal aspect
Anterior superior alveolar (infraorbital) nerve block	Maxillary central and lateral incisors and canine, surrounding hard and soft tissue on buccal aspect, mesiobuccal root of maxillary first molar (in some cases)
Greater palatine nerve block	Palatal mucosa and hard palate from first premolar anteriorly to posterior aspect of the hard palate and to midline medially
Nasopalatine nerve block	Hard and soft tissue of lingual aspect of maxillary anterior teeth from distal of canine on one side to distal of canine on the contralateral side
Maxillary nerve block	Hemimaxilla on side of injection (teeth; hard and soft, buccal, and lingual tissue)
Mandibular	
Inferior alveolar nerve block	Mandibular teeth on side of injection, buccal and lingual hard and soft tissue, lower lip
Buccal nerve block	Buccal soft tissue of molar region
Gow-Gates mandibular nerve block	Mandibular teeth to midline; hard and soft tissue of buccal and lingual aspect; anterior two-thirds of tongue; floor of mouth; skin over zygoma, posterior aspect of cheek, and temporal region on side of injection
Vazirani-Akinosi closed-mouth	Mandibular teeth to midline, hard and soft tissue of buccal aspect, anterior two-thirds of tongue, floor of mouth
Mental nerve block	Buccal soft tissue anterior to mental foramen, lower lip, chin
Incisive nerve block	Premolars, canine, incisors, lower lip, skin over chin, buccal soft tissue anterior to mental foramen

The supraperiosteal, periodontal ligament, intrapulpal, and intraseptal techniques are executed in the same manner as described for maxillary anesthesia. When anesthetizing the mandible, the patient should be in the semisupine or reclined position. The right-handed operator should stand at the 9 o'clock to 10 o'clock position, whereas the left-handed operator should stand at the 3 o'clock to 4 o'clock position.

Inferior Alveolar Nerve Block

The inferior alveolar nerve block is one of the most commonly used techniques in mandibular regional anesthesia. It is extremely useful when multiple teeth in one quadrant require treatment. While effective, this technique carries a high failure rate even when strict adherence to protocol is maintained. The target for this technique is the mandibular nerve as it travels along the medial aspect of the ramus before its entry into the mandibular foramen. The lingual, mental, and incisive nerves are also anesthetized. A 25-gauge long needle is preferred for this technique.

Procedure

The patient should be in the semisupine position. The right-handed operator should be in the 8 o'clock position, whereas the left-handed operator should be in the 4 o'clock position. With the patient's mouth open maximally, identify the coronoid notch and the pterygomandibular raphae. Three-fourths of the anteroposterior distance between these two landmarks and approximately 6–10 mm above the occlusal plane is the injection site. Use a retraction instrument to retract the cheek, and bring the needle to the injection site from the contralateral premolar region. As the needle passes through the soft tissue, deposit 1 or 2 drops of anesthetic solution. Advance the needle until contact is made with bone. Then, withdraw the needle 1 mm, and redirect the needle posteriorly by bringing the barrel of the syringe toward the occlusal plane (Figures 36–18a and 36–18b). Advance the needle to three-fourths of its depth, aspirate, and inject three-fourths of a cartridge of anesthetic solution slowly over the course of 1 minute. As the needle is withdrawn, continue to deposit the remaining one-fourth of anesthetic solution so as to anesthetize the lingual nerve (Figure 36–18c). Successful execution of this technique results in anesthesia of the mandibular teeth on the ipsilateral side to the midline, the associated buccal and lingual soft tissue, the lateral aspect of the tongue on the ipsilateral side, and the lower lip on the ipsilateral side.[1]

Buccal Nerve Block

The buccal nerve block, otherwise known as the long buccal or buccinator block, is a useful adjunct to the inferior alveolar nerve block when manipulation of the buccal soft tissue in the mandibular molar region is indicated. The target for this technique is the buccal nerve as it passes over the anterior aspect of the ramus. Contraindications to the procedure include acute inflammation and infection over the site of injection. A 25-gauge long needle is preferred for this technique.

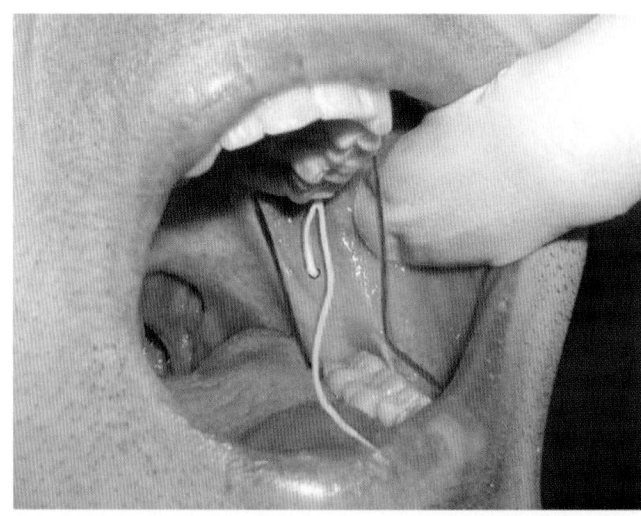

A

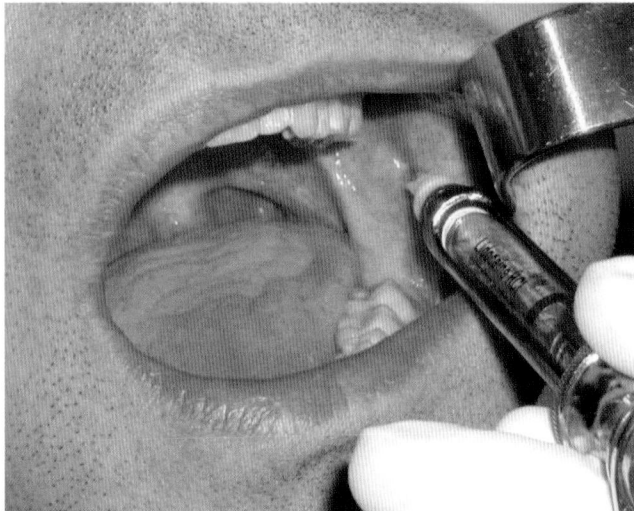

B

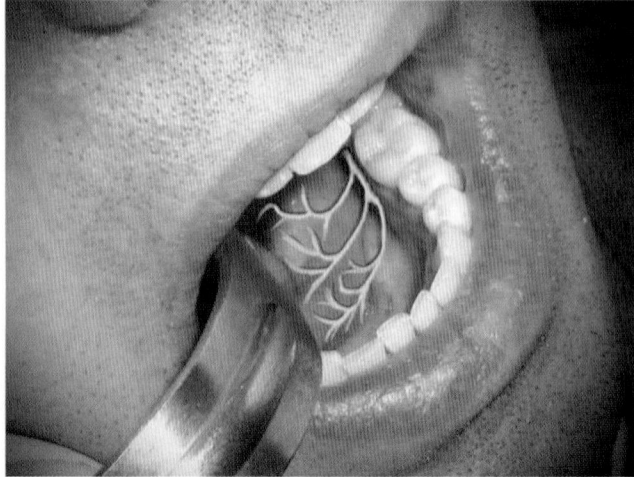

C

FIGURE 36–18. **A:** Location of the inferior alveolar nerve. **B:** After making contact with bone, the needle is redirected posteriorly by bringing the barrel of the syringe toward the occlusal plane. The needle is then advanced to three-fourths of its depth. **C:** Location of the lingual nerve, which is anesthetized during the administration of an inferior alveolar nerve block.

Procedure

The patient should be in the semisupine position. The right-handed operator should be in the 8 o'clock position, whereas the left-handed operator should be in the 4 o'clock position. Identify the most distal molar tooth on the side to be treated. The tissue just distal and buccal to the last molar tooth is the target area for injection (Figure 36–19). Use a retraction instrument to retract the cheek. The bevel of the needle should be toward bone, and the syringe should be held parallel with the occlusal plane on the side of the injection. The needle is inserted into the soft tissue, and a few drops of anesthetic solution are administered. The needle is advanced approximately 1–2 mm until contact is made with bone. Once contact is made with bone and aspiration is negative, 0.2 mL of local anesthetic solution is deposited. The needle is withdrawn and recapped. Successful execution of this technique results in anesthesia of the buccal soft tissue of the mandibular molar region.[1]

Gow-Gates Technique

The Gow-Gates technique, or third division nerve block, is a useful alternative to the inferior alveolar nerve block and is often

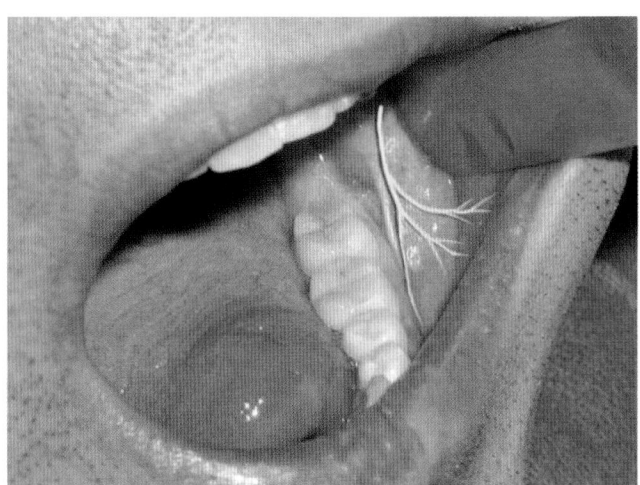

A

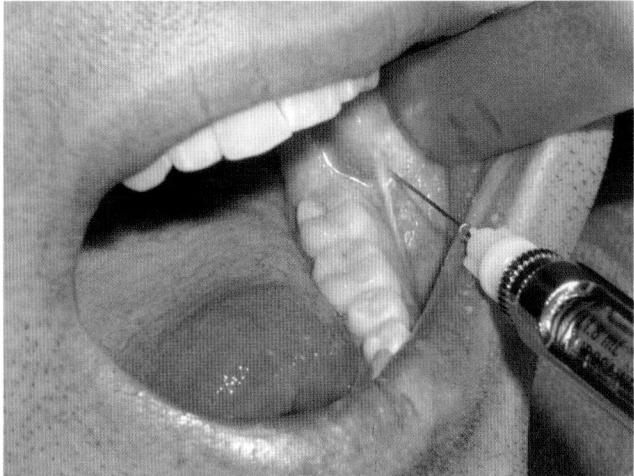

B

FIGURE 36–19. A: Location of the buccal nerve. **B:** The tissue just distal and buccal to the last molar tooth is the target area for injection.

used when the latter fails to provide adequate anesthesia. Advantages of this technique compared with the inferior alveolar technique are its low failure rate and its low incidence of positive aspiration. The Gow-Gates technique anesthetizes the auriculotemporal, inferior alveolar, buccal, mental, incisive, mylohyoid, and lingual nerves. Contraindications include acute inflammation and infection over the site of injection and trismatic patients. A 25-gauge long needle is preferred for this technique.

Procedure

The patient should be in the semisupine position. The right-handed operator should be in the 8 o'clock position, whereas the left-handed operator should be in the 4 o'clock position. The target area for this technique is the neck of the condyle below the area of insertion of the lateral pterygoid muscle. A retraction instrument is used to retract the cheek. The patient is asked to open maximally, and the mesiolingual cusp of the maxillary second molar on the side of desired anesthesia is identified. The insertion site of the needle should be just distal to the maxillary second molar at the level of the mesiolingual cusp. Bring the needle to the insertion site in a plane that is parallel with an imaginary line drawn from the intertragic notch to the corner of the mouth on the same side as the injection (Figure 36–20). The orientation of the bevel of the needle is not important in this technique. Advance the needle through soft tissue approximately 25 mm until contact is made with bone. This is the neck of the condyle. Once contact is made with bone, withdraw the needle 1 mm, and aspirate. Redirect the needle superiorly, and reaspirate. If aspiration in two planes is negative, slowly inject one cartridge of local anesthetic solution over the course of 1 minute. Successful execution of this technique provides anesthesia to the ipsilateral mandibular teeth up to the midline and the associated buccal and lingual hard and soft tissue. The anterior two-thirds of the tongue; the floor of the mouth; and the skin over the zygoma, posterior aspect of the cheek, and temporal region on the ipsilateral side of injection are also anesthetized.[1,8]

Vazirani-Akinosi Closed-Mouth Mandibular Block

The Vazirani-Akinosi closed-mouth mandibular block is a useful technique for patients with limited opening due to trismus or ankylosis of the temporomandibular joint. Limited mandibular opening precludes the administration of the inferior alveolar nerve block or use of the Gow-Gates technique, both of which require the patient to open maximally. Other advantages to this technique are the minimal risk of trauma to the inferior alveolar nerve, artery, and vein and the pterygoid muscle; a low complication rate; and minimal discomfort upon injection. Contraindications to this technique are acute inflammation and infection in the pterygomandibular space, deformity or tumor in the maxillary tuberosity region, and an inability to visualize the medial aspect of the ramus. A 25-gauge long needle is preferred for this technique.

Procedure

The patient should be in the semisupine position. The right-handed operator should be in the 8 o'clock position, whereas

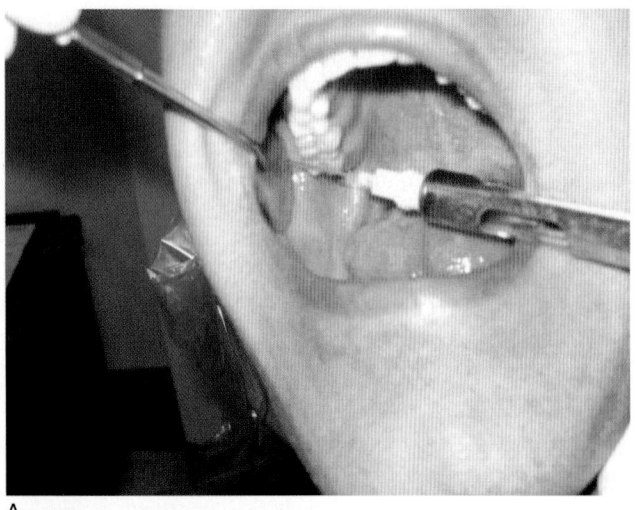

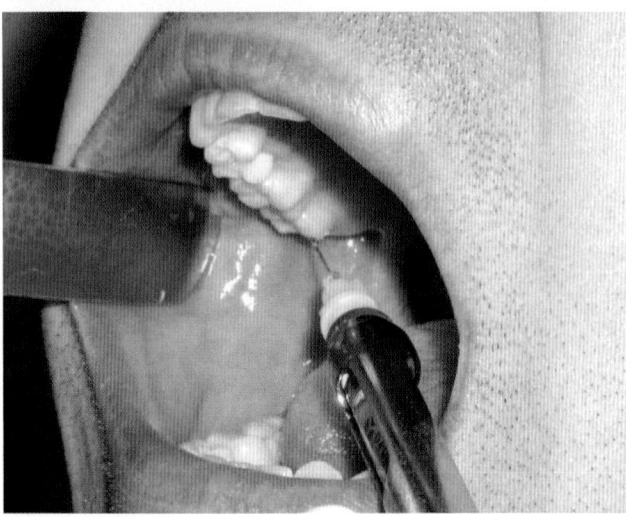

FIGURE 36–20. A: The patient is asked to open his or her mouth maximally. The mesiolingual cusp of the maxillary second molar is the reference point for the height of the injection. **B:** The needle is then moved distally and is held parallel to an imaginary line drawn from the intertragic notch to the corner of the mouth.

the left-handed operator should be in the 4 o'clock position. The gingival margin above the maxillary second and third molars and the pterygomandibular raphae serve as landmarks for this technique. A retraction instrument is used to stretch the cheek laterally. The patient should occlude gently on the posterior teeth. The needle is held parallel with the occlusal plane at the level of the gingival margin of the maxillary second and third molars. The bevel is directed away from the bone facing the midline. The needle is advanced through the mucous membrane and buccinator muscle to enter the pterygomandibular space. The needle is inserted to approximately one-half to three-fourths of its length. At this point, the needle will be in the midsection of the ptyerygomandibular space. Aspirate; if negative, one cartridge of local anesthetic solution is deposited over the course of 1 minute. Diffusion and gravitation of the local anesthetic solution anesthetizes the lingual and long buccal nerves in addition to the inferior alveolar nerve. Successful

execution of this technique provides anesthesia of the ipsilateral mandibular teeth up to the midline and the associated buccal and lingual hard and soft tissue. The anterior two-thirds of the tongue and floor of the mouth are also anesthetized.[9,10]

Mental Nerve Block

The mental nerve block is indicated for procedures in which manipulation of buccal soft tissue anterior to the mental foramen is necessary. Contraindications to this technique are acute inflammation and infection over the injection site. A 25- or 27-gauge short needle is preferred for this technique.

Procedure

The patient should be in the semisupine position. The right-handed operator should be in the 8 o'clock position, whereas the left-handed operator should be in the 4 o'clock position. The target area is the height of the mucobuccal fold over the mental foramen (Figures 36–21a and 36–21b). The foramen

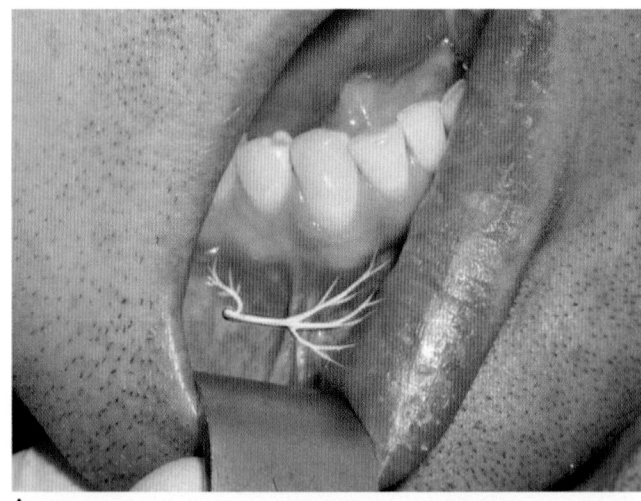

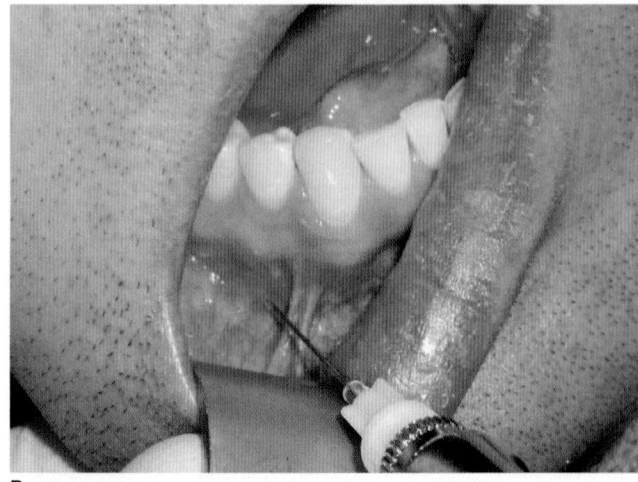

FIGURE 36–21. A: Location of the mental and incisive nerves. **B:** Block of the mental and incisive nerves. The needle is inserted at the height of the mucobuccal fold over the mental foramen for both the mental nerve block and the incisive nerve block.

can be manually palpated by applying gentle finger pressure to the body of the mandible in the area of the premolar apices. The patient will feel slight discomfort upon palpation of the foramen. Use a retraction instrument to retract the soft tissue. The needle is directed toward the mental foramen with the bevel facing the bone. Penetrate the soft tissue to a depth of 5 mm, aspirate, and inject approximately 0.6 mL of anesthetic solution. Successful execution of this technique results in anesthesia of the buccal soft tissue anterior to the foramen, lower lip, and chin on the side of the injection.[1]

Incisive Nerve Block

The incisive nerve block is not as frequently used in clinical practice; however, it proves very useful when treatment is limited to mandibular anterior teeth and full quadrant anesthesia is not necessary. The technique is almost identical to the mental nerve block but with one additional step. Both the mental and incisive nerves are anesthetized using this technique. Contraindications to this technique are acute inflammation and infection at the site of injection. A 25- or 27-gauge short needle is preferred for this technique.

Procedure

The patient should be in the semisupine position. The right-handed operator should be in the 8 o'clock position, whereas the left-handed operator should be in the 4 o'clock position. The target area is the height of the mucobuccal fold over the mental foramen (see Figure 36–21b). Identify the mental foramen as previously described. Give the patient a mental nerve block as described above, and apply digital pressure at the site of injection during administration of anesthetic solution. Continue to apply digital pressure at the site of injection 2–3 minutes after the injection is complete to aid the anesthetic in diffusing into the foramen. Successful implementation of this technique provides anesthesia to the premolars, canine, incisor teeth, lower lip, skin of the chin, and buccal soft tissue anterior to the mental foramen.[1]

REFERENCES

1. Malamed SF: *Handbook of Local Anesthesia*, 4th ed. Maryland Heights, MI: Mosby, 1997.
2. Snell RS: *Clinical Anatomy for Medical Students*, 5th ed. New York: Little, Brown, 1995.
3. Loetscher CA, Walton RE: Patterns of innervation of the maxillary first molar: a dissection study. Oral Surg Oral Med Oral Pathol 1988; 65:86–90.
4. McDaniel WM: Variations in nerve distributions of the maxillary teeth. J Dent Res 1956;35:916–921.
5. Heasman PA: Clinical anatomy of the superior alveolar nerves. Br J Oral Maxillofacial Surg 1884;22:439–447.
6. Malamed SF, Trieger N: Intraoral maxillary nerve block: an anatomical and clinical study. Anesthesia Progr 1983;30:44–48.
7. Poore TE, Carney F: Maxillary nerve block: a useful technique. J Oral Surg 1973;31:749–755.
8. Gow-Gates GAE: Mandibular conduction anesthesia: a new technique using extraoral landmarks. Oral Surg 1973;36:321–328.
9. Akinosi JO: A new approach to the mandibular nerve block. Br J Oral Maxillofacial Surg 1977;15:83–87.
10. Vazirani SJ: Closed mouth mandibular nerve block: a new technique. Dent Digest 1960;66:10–13.

LOCAL AND REGIONAL ANESTHESIA FOR THE EYE

Local and Regional Anesthesia for Ophthalmic Surgery

Stavros Prineas

INTRODUCTION

Ophthalmic surgery is one of the most common surgical procedures requiring anesthesia in developed countries.[1] Ophthalmic anesthesia offers insights into some fundamental principles of good anesthetic practice, especially in the conduct of local and regional blocks.

LOCAL ANESTHESIA IN EYE SURGERY

Clinical strategies to minimize patient movement during eye surgery are essential. Historically, eye surgeons favored general anesthesia (GA), which usually provided akinesia (through neuromuscular blockade) and low intraocular pressure. However, these conditions are not always achieved under GA. A closed-claims analysis by Gild and coworkers[2] found that 30% of eye injury claims associated with anesthesia involved the patient moving during ophthalmic surgery, with most incidents occurring under GA. While perioperative morbidity and mortality rates associated with eye surgery (eg, cataract extraction) are low,[3,4] patients having cataract surgery tend to be older and to have significant comorbidities.[5-10] For this reason, systematic preoperative evaluation should be performed to consider whether a patient is eligible for a GA and surgery.[10]

Appropriate anesthetic management contributes to the success or failure of ophthalmic surgery. Quicker patient rehabilitation and fewer complications in this patient population are the main reasons why many ophthalmic surgeons are now choosing local anesthesia (LA) over GA.[11-13]

Traditionally, the gold standard of eye blocks was retrobulbar anesthesia (RBA), with the surgeon performing the block. However, advances in technology and surgical technique, particularly in cataract surgery, have led to the replacement of the

older wide-incision techniques (eg, extra-capsular cataract extraction) with minimally invasive phacoemulsification (PhE) techniques. Consequently, for new generation of cataract surgeons, total akinesia is no longer necessary for PhE.

Clinical Pearls

- Twenty-first century innovations and trends have revolutionized eye surgery.
- Local and regional anesthetic techniques has largely replaced general anesthesia.
- Understanding functional anatomy and surgical techniques is essential for selection of regional techniques.
- Sub-Tenon's block is one of the most common choices for anesthesia as it can generally achieve akinesia with the favorable safety profile.
- Topical anesthesia, is increasingly becoming most prevalent for cataract surgery.
- Complications of eye blocks are uncommon but can be life- or sight-threatening, emphasizing the need of adequate training.

Innovation has also broadened the anesthetic options for eye surgery. As the conventional RBA carries a greater risk of complications, less invasive techniques have increasingly been used, with a substantial diversity in practice styles around the world. For instance, one Australian study from 2002 reported that peribulbar block was the most popular among an international sample of ophthalmic surgeons.[14] However, a 2006 survey found that 64% of a sample of UK anesthetists favored the sub-Tenon's technique,[15] and, by 2008, a survey of the British Ophthalmic Anaesthesia Society found that over 87% of anesthesiologist members regularly performed sub-Tenon's blocks.[16] On the other hand, an annual survey of the American Society of Cataract and Refractive Surgery reported that its members' preference for using topical anesthesia had risen steadily from 11% in 1995 to 76% in 2012.[17,18] In the same survey, the use of sub-Tenon's blocks appeared to be consistently low over the years (around 1%–3%) despite its growing popularity elsewhere, with the use of retrobulbar and peribulbar blocks seemingly in gradual but sustained decline.

Each anesthetic technique has its strengths and limitations. Knowledge of the relevant anatomy for the various anesthetic techniques is essential to determine the appropriate block for specific clinical situations and to best avoid life- and sight-threatening complications. This chapter reviews the relevant anatomy of the eye, classical needle and non-needle block techniques, and choice of LA and adjuvant agents. With a wider range of options comes a greater burden on the anesthesiologist to discuss individual anesthetic requirements with the surgeon, to be adaptable, and to have excellent communication and team-working skills.

FUNCTIONAL ANATOMY[19]

Orbit

The **orbits** (Figures 37–1 and 37–2) are two symmetrical bony enclosures in the front of the skull, each containing an eyeball (or **globe**) and its associated structures. The cavity of each orbit is a truncated pyramid, with a flattened apex posteriorly and a trapezoidal base facing anterolaterally. The medial (nasal) walls of each orbit are parallel to each other, while the lateral (temporal) walls are perpendicular to each other. The volume of each adult orbit is approximately 30 mL.

Globe

The globe (Figure 37–3) is suspended in the anterosuperior part of the orbit. It is roughly spherical, its contents contained within three outer layers or **tunics**:

- A **fibrous tunic** comprising the translucent **cornea** in front and the opaque **sclera** peripherally and behind
- Deep to the fibrous tunic, a **vascular, pigmented tunic** comprising the **iris** and **ciliary body** in front and the **choroid** peripherally and behind
- Deep to this again, a **neural tunic** overlying the posterior part of the other two tunics internally, comprising the **retina**.

The globe has a large **posterior segment** (comprising the **vitreous humor**, the **retina**, the **macula**, and the root of the **optic nerve**) and a small convex **anterior segment** comprising two **chambers**. The **anterior chamber** immediately behind the cornea is filled with **aqueous humor** produced by the **ciliary body**. The **posterior chamber** contains the **lens**. The two chambers are separated by the **iris** and communicate via the **pupil** of the eye. Externally, the circumferential junction of cornea and sclera (with its overlying **conjunctiva**) is called the **limbus**.

The volume of the globe is approximately 7 mL. The axial (anteroposterior) length of the adult globe is on average about 24 mm; however, this can be considerably longer in myopic individuals (> 26 mm) and shorter in hypermetropia (down to 20 mm). As a rule of thumb, the distance from the front of the globe to its equator is about 12–15 mm, but, where possible, it is better to know the measured axial length of the eye before attempting to inject behind the equator (eg, for patients undergoing cataract surgery, biometric data are routinely found in the surgeon's clinical notes).

The sclera is thinnest at the equator and at the insertion points of the extraocular muscles. However, more myopic eyes (with a longer axial length) have a markedly increased prevalence of posterior staphyloma, an otherwise rare "blow-out" weakness in the fibrous tunic, which poses a major risk for globe perforation with blind needle techniques (see "Complications of Eye Blocks" later).

Muscles of the Eye

The four rectus and two oblique muscles of the eye insert anteriorly near the equator of the globe (see Figure 37–3). Posteriorly, they originate together at the apex from the tendinous **annulus communis of Zinn**. The four rectus muscles, running posteriorly from the equator to the annulus of Zinn, delineate the **retrobulbar cone**. The optic nerve traverses the cone from the posterior part of the globe and enters the orbit through the annulus of Zinn.

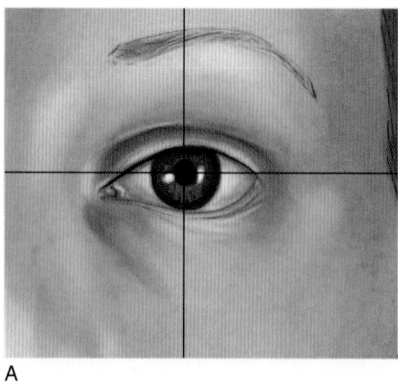

A

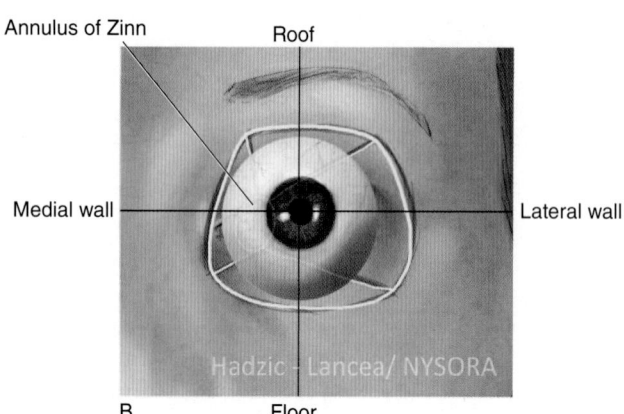

B

FIGURE 37–1. (**A**) The eye. (**B**) Surface anatomy.

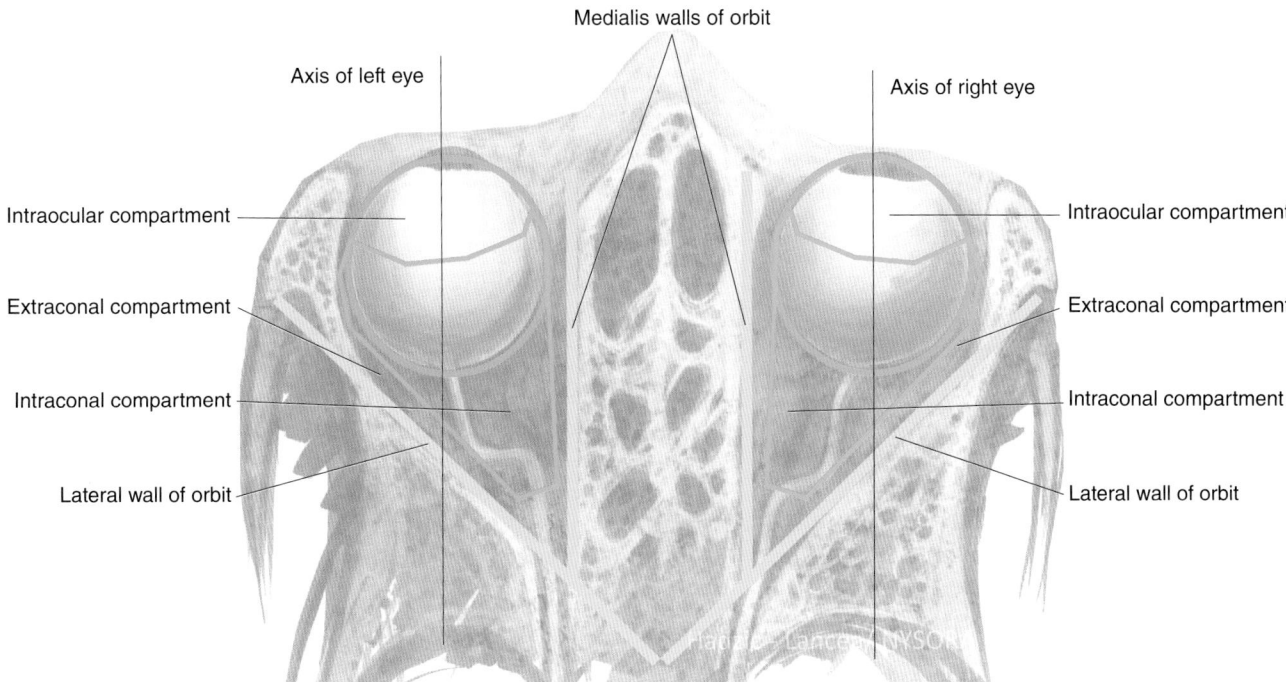

FIGURE 37–2. The orbit: diagrammatic superior view.

Three Intraorbital Compartments

The globe and muscular retrobulbar cone define the three classical anatomical compartments of the orbital cavity: the **intraocular**, **intraconal**, and **extraconal** (see Figure 37–2). However the retrobulbar cone is not sealed by any intermuscular membrane,[20–23] and, in fact, there is free communication between the intraconal and extraconal spaces. Thus, a large-volume peribulbar (extraconal) block can theoretically provide as effective anesthesia and akinesia as a targeted small-volume retrobulbar block.

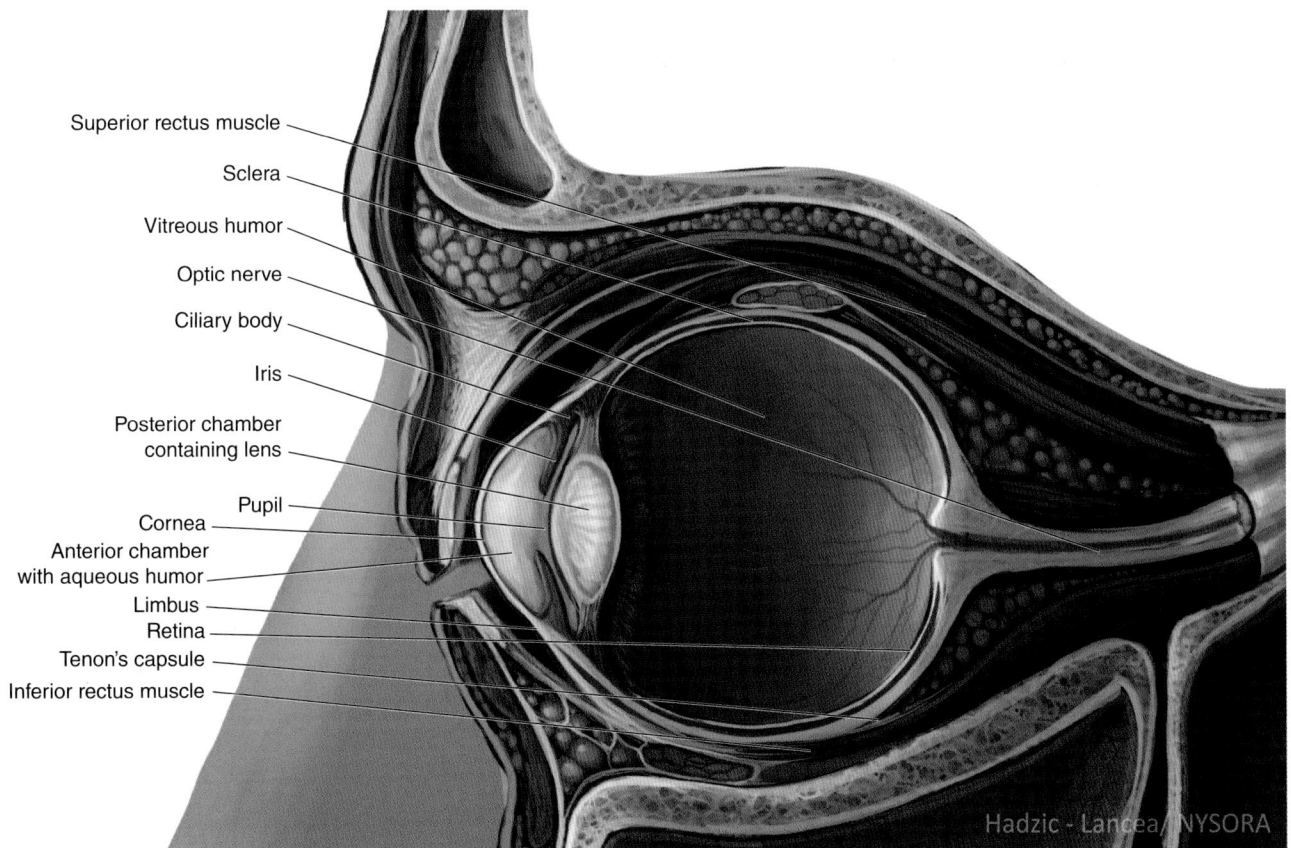

FIGURE 37–3. The globe: sagittal section.

686 CLINICAL PRACTICE OF REGIONAL ANESTHESIA

Innervation of the Orbit

Sensory innervation of the orbit and globe is provided mostly by the frontal and nasociliary branches of the ophthalmic nerve (first branch of the trigeminal nerve, V), which pass through the muscular cone (Figures 37–4 and 37–5), while some of the floor of the orbit is supplied by the infraorbital branch of the maxillary nerve (the second branch of the trigeminal nerve). The trochlear nerve (IV) provides motor control to the superior oblique muscles, the abducens nerve (VI) to the lateral rectus muscle, and the oculomotor nerve (III) to all other extraocular muscles, including the levator muscle. All except the trochlear nerve pass through the muscular conus.

Anatomical Quadrants of the Globe and Orbit

The sphere of the globe can be divided in the three standard perpendicular anatomical planes into eight "quadrants": anterior superomedial, posterior superomedial, and so on. Looking from the front, the corresponding anterior extraocular quadrants of the orbit are often referred to as the superonasal, suprotemporal, inferonasal, and inferotemporal, where *nasal* has the same meaning as *medial*, and *temporal* has the same meaning as

lateral (Figure 37–6). The inferotemporal (or inferolateral) space is usually the largest and least vascular and the preferred quadrant of approach for modern retrobulbar and single-shot peribulbar blocks. The inferonasal (or inferomedial) quadrant is most popular for sub-Tenon's blocks. The superonasal (or superomedial) quadrant is quite vascular but contains the anterior ethmoidal nerve, a useful nerve to block for some oculoplastic procedures (see "Oculoplastic Blocks" below).

Tenon's Capsule and Sub-Tenon's Space

The scleral portion of the globe is surrounded by Tenon's capsule (also known as the fascial sheath of the eyeball), a fibroelastic layer stretching from the corneal limbus anteriorly to the optic nerve posteriorly.[24] Tenon's capsule generally becomes thinner and less adherent to the sclera with age. It delimits a potential space referred to as the episcleral space (sub-Tenon's space), which expands when fluid is injected into it. The conjunctiva overlies the sclera in the anterior part of the eye until it is reflected at the **fornices** of the eye to continue as the mucosal lining of the underside of the eyelids. Note that Tenon's capsule fuses with the sclera about 2 mm from the limbus. Where the sclera is visible, the two layers are easier to pick up

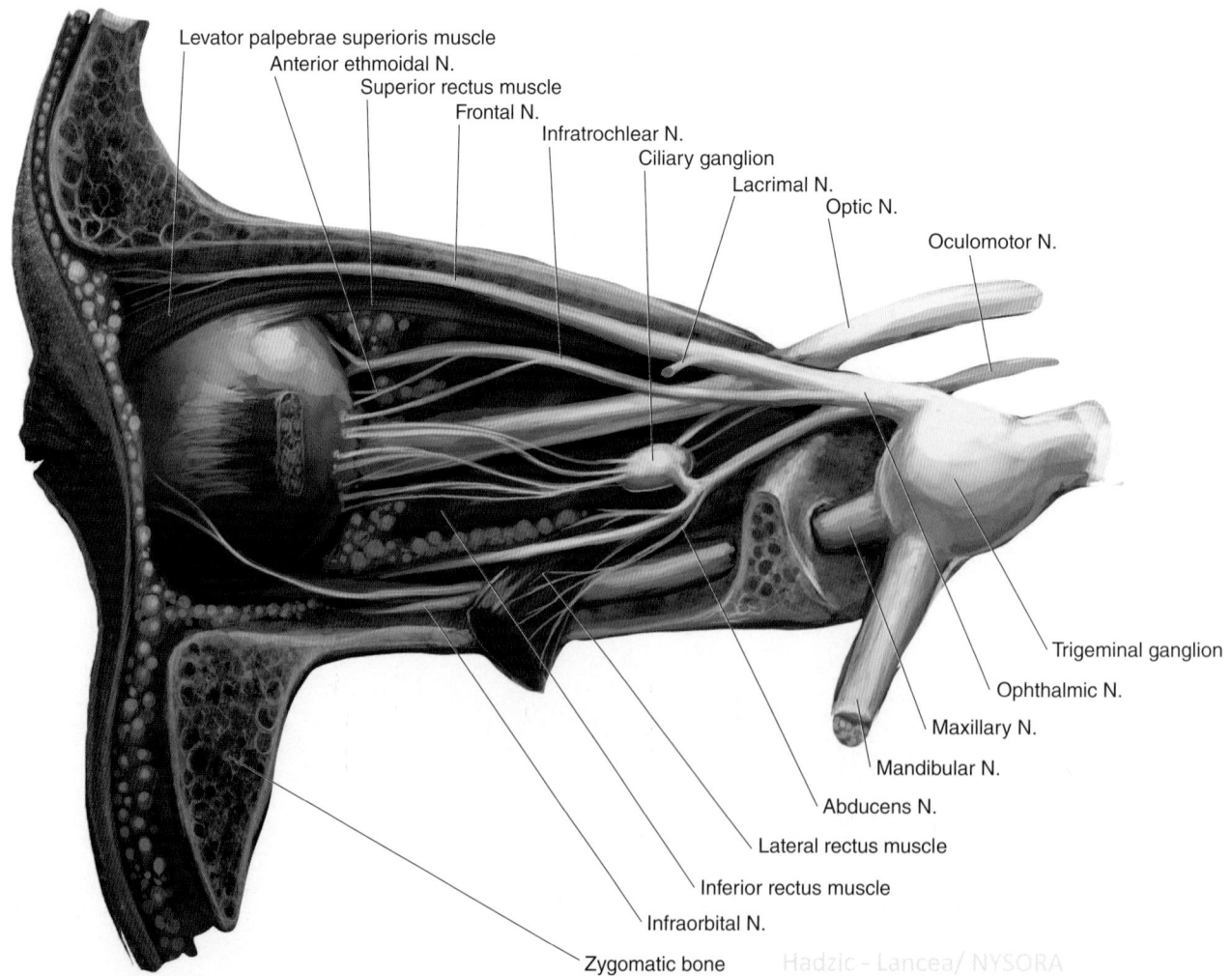

FIGURE 37–4. Left orbit: lateral prosected view. Lateral wall and lacrimal gland removed.

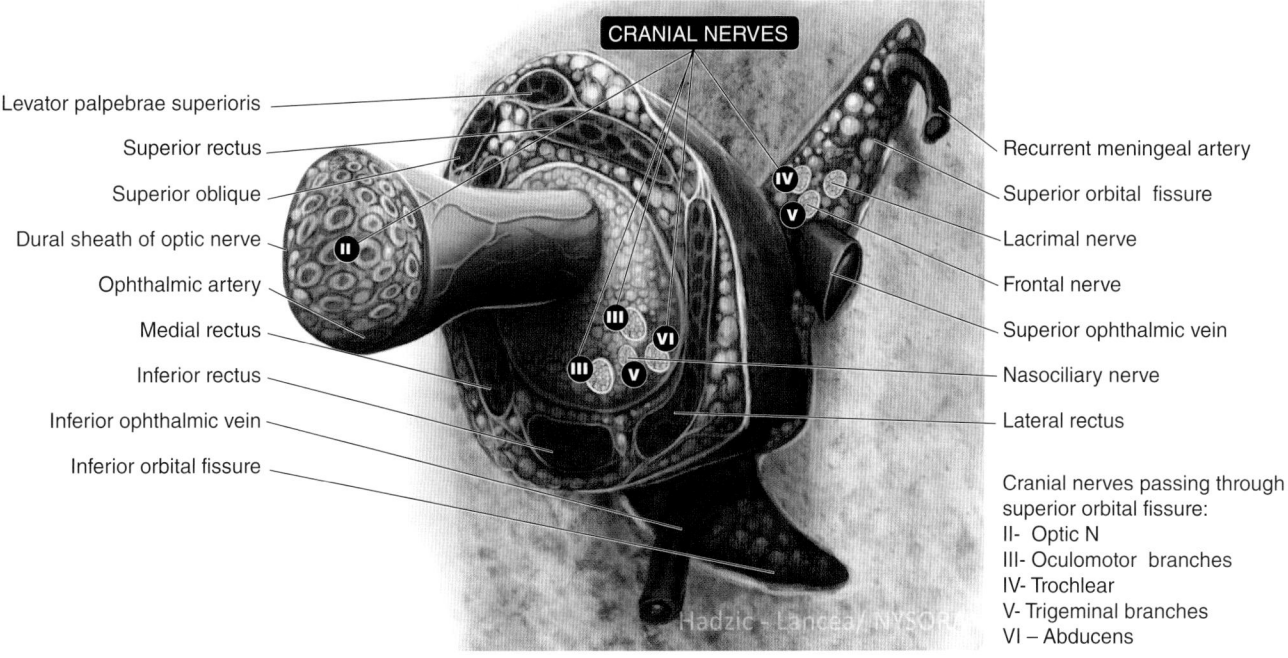

CRANIAL NERVES

Levator palpebrae superioris
Superior rectus
Superior oblique
Dural sheath of optic nerve
Ophthalmic artery
Medial rectus
Inferior rectus
Inferior ophthalmic vein
Inferior orbital fissure

Recurrent meningeal artery
Superior orbital fissure
Lacrimal nerve
Frontal nerve
Superior ophthalmic vein
Nasociliary nerve
Lateral rectus

Cranial nerves passing through superior orbital fissure:
II- Optic N
III- Oculomotor branches
IV- Trochlear
V- Trigeminal branches
VI – Abducens

FIGURE 37–5. Extraocular muscles and innervation of the orbit at the level of the annulus of Zinn. Cranial nerves indicated by Roman numerals.

as one; closer to the fornix, the conjunctivum becomes fleshier and more distinct from the sub-Tenon's layer. This helps identify the ideal breach point for the sub-Tenon's technique (q.v.).

Spread of Local Anesthetic Within the Orbit

Injection of LA solution inside the cone will provide anesthesia and akinesia of the globe and (usually) all extraocular muscles. Only the motor nerve to the orbicularis muscle of the eyelids has an extraorbital course, coming from the superior branch of the facial nerve (VII). Many major structures are located within the

muscular conus and are therefore at risk of needle and injection injury. These include the optic nerve with its meningeal coverings, the blood vessels of the orbit, and the nerves supplying the globe. For this reason, some authors advise that introduction of the needle into the muscular cone be avoided and suggest that needle insertion be limited to the extraconal space.[25,26]

KEY SURGICAL CONSIDERATIONS[27]

It is important to get to know your surgeon. Choosing an appropriate local anesthetic technique requires an understanding

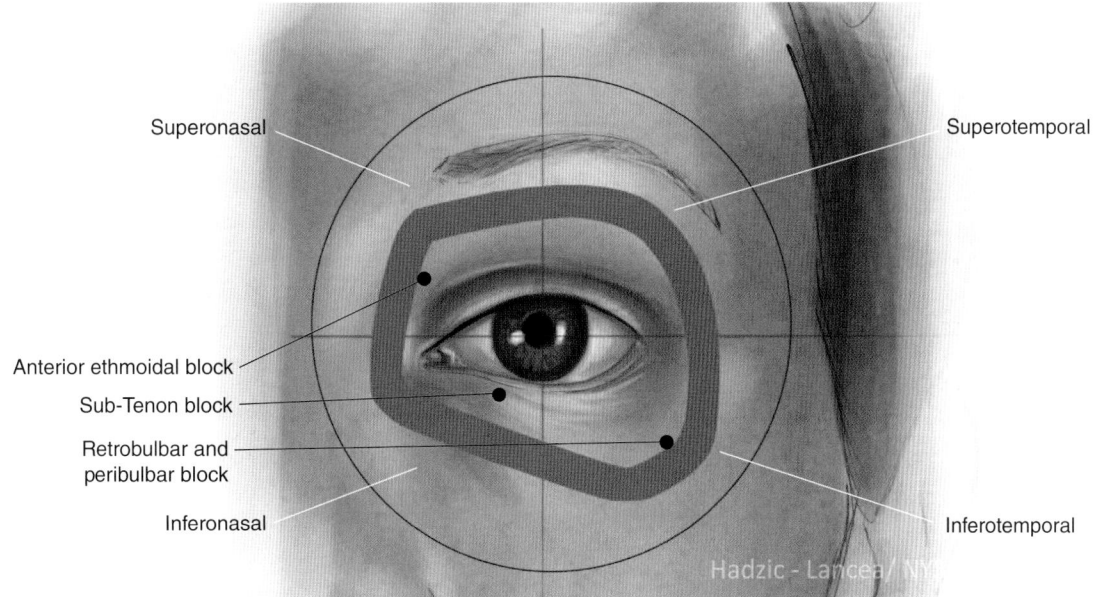

Superonasal
Superotemporal
Anterior ethmoidal block
Sub-Tenon block
Retrobulbar and peribulbar block
Inferonasal
Inferotemporal

FIGURE 37–6. The anterior orbital quadrants.

not only of surgical procedures but also the surgeon's personal preferences.

Akinesia

The requirement for akinesia varies with the procedure (see below) and the surgeon. With blocks behind the equator of the eye, improving the likelihood of akinesia generally requires more volume,[28] more time,[29] or the addition of hyaluronidase[30] (see "Choice of Local Anesthetic and Adjuvant Agents" below).

Primary Position Versus "On-Axis" Position

Complete paresis of all extraocular muscles renders the eye in the "primary" or "neutral" position. Usually, this corresponds with the surgeon having the pupil aligned with the axis of the surgical microscope (ie, the surgeon has an ideal "on-axis" view of the operative field). However, in cases of incomplete motor block, or in patients who have significant spinal curvature or who are unable to lie flat, the "resting" position of the blocked eye may not correspond to an on-axis view. For this reason, many surgeons actually prefer to have a fully mobile eye for certain patients or certain procedures (eg, trabeculectomy, pterygium removal) so that they can ask the patient to look at the light of the microscope, thereby bringing the eye "on axis," or to look away, allowing greater access to more peripheral parts of the globe.

The Volume Effect of Injections Behind the Eye

Any substantial injection (> 3 mL) behind the equator of the eye (a peribulbar, retrobulbar, or posterior sub-Tenon injection) can significantly raise intraocular pressure and push the posterior segment forward, resulting in a crescent-shaped anterior chamber with decreased volume (Figure 37–7). This can make surgical conditions more challenging, and while this can mostly be offset by counter-pressure (through gentle digital pressure or

application of a weight or balloon), some surgeons prefer techniques that retain a "physiological" anterior segment, and most surgeons prefer techniques that avoid large volumes of injectate (> 10 mL) in the orbit. On the other hand, in patients with significant enophthalmos, bringing the globe forward can improve surgical exposure.

"The Only Eye"

In patients who have vision in only one eye—the eye being operated upon—surgeons and anesthetists alike tend to be risk averse and steer away from sharp needle blocks. Techniques that do not involve loss of vision (ie, topical, subconjunctival, "superficial" sub-Tenon's) may be preferable. Techniques that better guarantee akinesia usually cause temporary loss of vision due to anesthesia of the optic nerve. In day-case settings, it may be preferable to use a shorter-duration LA (eg, lidocaine, articaine) over longer-acting agents.

Cataract Surgery

The minimally invasive PhE technique was popularized in the 1990s. The PhE probe is inserted via a small superior, three-plane (self-sealing) incision. The contents of the posterior chamber are manipulated using a needle-width stay probe inserted laterally. After the posterior chamber is voided and cleaned, a foldable or injectable artificial intraocular lens is inserted via the same incision. Anesthesia of the anterior segment is all that is required. Some surgeons require akinesia; others (notably high-turnover surgeons) do not.

Corneal Surgery

The most common operations on the cornea involve trauma, removal of foreign bodies, conjunctival flap and pterygium surgery, corneal transplant surgery, and, increasingly, keratoprosthesis. For these procedures, anesthesia of the anterior segment is typically all that is required. Most surgeons require akinesia for

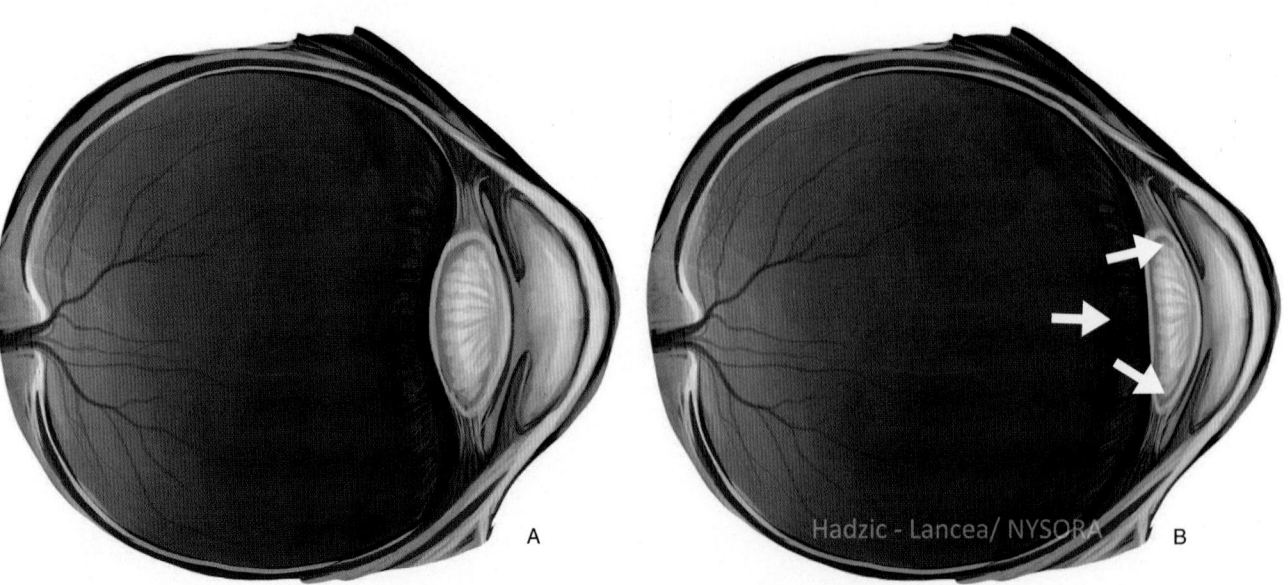

FIGURE 37–7. (**A**) "Physiological" anterior segment. (**B**) The effect of increased retrobulbar volume.

penetrating corneal surgery (eg, trauma, transplant, prosthetic surgery, re-do procedures), while many do not for pterygium surgery, where the fibrous tunic remains essentially intact. Some surgeons find subconjunctival anesthesia useful for separating the conjunctiva from the sclera in pterygium surgery.

Refractive Surgery

Corneal surface ablation, incisional refractive surgery, and intracorneal ring insertion are usually performed under topical anesthesia. Refractive procedures involving the anterior chamber (eg, phakic intraocular lens insertion) are done in a manner similar to cataract surgery.

Glaucoma Surgery

Glaucoma filtration surgery and trabeculectomy both involve creating a fistula between the anterior chamber and the subconjunctival space. Again, anesthesia of only the anterior segment is needed. Depending on the surgeon, there may or may not be a need for akinesia. Some surgeons do not like the disruption of integrity of the conjunctiva that often accompanies the surgical sub-Tenon's (or "snip") technique, particularly in inexperienced hands. Furthermore, conjunctival hematoma can introduce reticuloendothelial cells that interfere with trabeculectomy flaps; consequently, some glaucoma surgeons prefer peribulbar anesthesia for these procedures. Topical anesthesia (with or without intracameral lidocaine) and subconjunctival anesthesia both avoid the potential effect of volume injections behind or around the orbit on pulsatile ocular blood flow in patients with advanced glaucoma. Paradoxically, nonpenetrative glaucoma surgery (eg, deep sclerotomy), being a longer and more difficult procedure, generally requires a technique that guarantees a longer block with akinesia. Procedures involving aqueous tube shunts can be done under topical anesthesia but tend to be more uncomfortable for the patient.

Cyclophotocoagulation is the circumferential ablation of the ciliary body deep to the limbus. Akinesia is not essential for this procedure but may be preferred by some surgeons; however, good analgesia is essential, as the procedure can be very painful. Subconjunctival anesthesia works but needs time; sub-Tenon's or needle blocks usually provide acceptable anesthesia more quickly.

Oculoplastic Surgery

Procedures of the soft tissues of the eye include correction of eyelid malpositions such as entropion and ectropion, eyelash malpositions (districhiasis), ptosis surgery, eyelid tumor surgery, eyelid reconstruction, blepharoplasty, tear duct surgery, orbital decompression (eg, for Grave's disease), and enucleation and evisceration. While many of these procedures can be performed under local infiltration, specific anesthetic techniques are described later in this chapter.

Extraocular Muscle Surgery

Strabismus surgery is most commonly performed in children under general anesthesia. In adults, squint surgery is usually performed in persons under the age of 30, a group which can often be less than stoic, so again GA is usually preferred. However, this surgery can be performed under regional anesthesia. While akinesia is helpful, the main requirement is for deep anesthesia of the muscle cone, as pulling on extraocular muscles is usually quite painful and can induce an oculocardic reflex. Simple suture adjustments can be done under topical anesthesia.[31]

Vitreoretinal Surgery

Vitrectomy and retinal detachment repairs (including scleral buckling) require both anesthesia of the posterior segment and akinesia of the eye; topical and subconjunctival techniques are inadequate for this. Thus, a sub-Tenon's, retrobulbar, or peribulbar block is more appropriate. Prior buckling surgery is a relative contraindication to any regional technique, as both the buckle and scar tissue around it will hamper the spread of local anesthetic. However, if the position of the buckle is known, a deep sub-Tenon's block may be possible via one of the unaffected quadrants. The "tap-and-inject" treatment for endophthalmitis is usually performed using a retrobulbar or peribulbar block.

Open-Globe Injuries

Patients with a known or suspected open-globe injury are most frequently managed under general anesthesia to avoid the risks of infection, retrobulbar hemorrhage, and raised intraocular pressure, which can cause further damage. There are authors who advocate repair under local anesthesia and sedation, arguing that this method avoids the dilemma of using succinylcholine, which can markedly increase intraocular pressure, in patients with both a penetrating eye injury and a full stomach.[32] Rapid-onset nondepolarizing muscle relaxants (NDMRs), such as rocuronium, and the wider availability of the NDMR reversal agent, sugammadex, have largely mitigated this problem. Nevertheless, recent literature appears to suggest that the risk of vitreous extrusion remains very real,[33] and, perhaps in carefully selected situations, local anesthesia should not be discounted as an alternative in cases of eye trauma.

Ophthalmic Oncology

Most procedures for the removal of eye tumors can be performed under local or general anesthesia, according to surgeon and/or patient preference. However, procedures that require stereotactic immobilization or deliberate hypotension should be performed under general anesthesia.

ANESTHETIC TECHNIQUES

Sub-Tenon's (Episcleral) Block
Common Principles

Sub-Tenon's anesthesia, first described in 1884, places the local anesthetic into the potential space between Tenon's capsule and the sclera (Figure 37–8). While this space can theoretically be accessed from any quadrant of the globe, the inferonasal conjunctival fornix is most popular, at approximately the

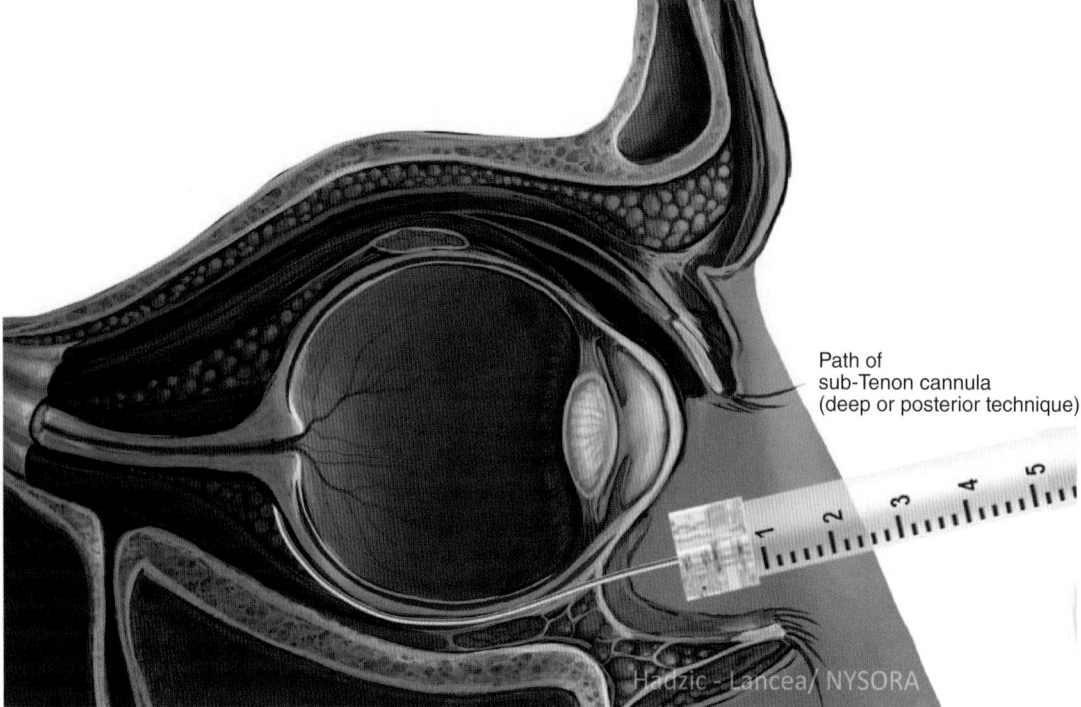

Path of
sub-Tenon cannula
(deep or posterior technique)

FIGURE 37–8. Sub-Tenon block.

4:30 (right eye) or 7:30 (left eye) position to avoid encountering the insertions of the medial rectus and inferior oblique muscles at the equator.

Using either a surgical or nonsurgical approach (see below), a purpose-specific needle or cannula is directed posteriorly following the curve of the globe. A superficial or deep injection of LA solution can then be performed. "Superficial" or more anterior injections (immediately beyond the equator) allow the LA to spread circularly around the scleral portion of the globe, ensuring high-quality analgesia of the whole globe with relatively low injection volumes (usually 3–5 mL).[34,35] Injection of a larger volume (up to 8–11 mL) causes the LA to spread to the extraocular muscle sheaths, ensuring reproducible akinesia.[34-37] However, larger volumes often cause chemosis (a subconjunctival spread of LA), which requires compression to resolve, as well as a significant increase in intraocular pressure.

On the other hand, "deep" or posterior injections direct more injectate into the posterior intra- and extraconal spaces and are more likely to achieve anesthesia at lower volumes and without chemosis, without akinesia (2–3 mL) or with full akinesia (3–5 mL). While the "surgical" deep injection technique is currently the most popular, several approaches have been described.

Surgical ("Snip") Technique with a Blunt Cannula

This technique, first proposed as a supplement to (or rescue block from) retrobulbar anesthesia,[38,39] is probably the most popular variation of the sub-Tenon's approach. After topical anesthesia, the bulbar conjunctiva is grasped with small forceps in the inferonasal quadrant near the fornix. Small scissors are

used to create a small opening into the conjunctiva and Tenon's capsule to gain access to the episcleral space. The same scissors are used to blunt-dissect a passage to the posterior sub-Tenon's space. A blunt metal (eg, Stevens) or plastic (eg, Helica) cannula is then inserted into this space to allow for the injection.[40,41] Some practitioners opt for a superficial passage and then "hydro-dissect" using the local anesthetic injectate; others (particularly for posterior segment surgery) prefer to probe-dissect as close to the intraconal space as possible using closed scissors. It is also possible, particularly in the elderly, to gently push the cannula posteriorly without dissection. The usual LA injection volume is 3–5 mL. Increasing the injection volume (up to 11 mL) results in an increased likelihood of akinesia but is rarely necessary.[37] The main advantage of this technique is its safety, as it avoids the blind introduction of a sharp needle into the orbit. In 6000 cases, no serious complications were reported, with only a 7% rate of subconjunctival hematoma and a 6% rate of subconjunctival edema. Surgery was cancelled because of subconjunctival hematoma in only one patient out of the 6000.[42]

Nonsurgical Technique with a Blunt Cannula

Cutting the conjunctiva can result in long-term scarring and creates a portal for bacteria and occasionally other foreign bodies to enter.[43,44] With practice, a round-tipped blunt cannula (such as a 21-gauge Eagle Laboratories "Tri-Port" sub-Tenon cannula or even a Stevens cannula) can be introduced through the conjunctiva and Tenon's layers without prior incision.[45] This causes less trauma, reduces bleeding, and is preferred particularly where conjunctival damage needs to be minimized (eg, glaucoma surgery).

Nonsurgical Technique with a Sharp Needle

A 25-gauge, 25-mm, short-bevel sharp needle is introduced into the fornix between the semilunaris fold of the conjunctiva and the globe, tangentially to the globe.[34,35] The needle is shifted slightly medially and advanced posteriorly. After a small loss of resistance (click) at 10–15 mm, LA is injected. Using a large volume with this technique (6–11 mL) results in good globe and eyelid akinesia that is more reproducible than classic peribulbar anesthesia;[36] however, note that these are large volumes compared to other techniques, and, as for all sharp-needle techniques, the risk of needle misplacement and its subsequent complications must always be kept in mind. Nevertheless, this technique is associated with a low risk of complications, and it is simple to learn and use. In a series of 2000 cases, no serious complications occurred.[46]

Improvised Cannula Technique

This historical technique was briefly popular before specialized cannulae became widely available. A short intravenous (IV) cannula (18- or 20-gauge) was typically used to inject low volumes of LA (3–5 mL). It provides good globe analgesia but only partial akinesia of the globe and lids.[42] The injection causes only a minor increase in intraocular pressure, and preoperative compression of the globe is typically unnecessary. However, given that it requires introduction of the cannula by piercing the Tenon's capsule, not unlike the technique of IV cannulation, the risk of needle misplacement has reduced the popularity of this technique.

Limitations of the Sub-Tenon's Technique

The sub-Tenon's technique may not be possible where the conjunctival fornices have been obliterated, such as in chronic ocular pemphigus. It should also be avoided where the sclera is known to be thin or frail (eg, the "blue sclerae" of osteogenesis imperfecta or an anterior staphyloma).

Access may be challenging in patients whose inferonasal space is already scarred by multiple previous blocks or in those with a scleral buckle in place, particularly one that is circumferential. In most of these situations, access is possible via an alternative quadrant (most commonly the inferotemporal). Chronic eye inflammation can cause the conjunctiva to become fleshy and painful to touch and to bleed easily. Access through a pterygium should be avoided for the same reasons.

Clinical Pearls

The Surgical "Snip" Technique of the Sub-Tenon's Block According to Guise[47]

- Use half-strength iodine: A substantial body of evidence suggests that this reduces the risk of bacterial endophthalmitis.[48]
- Stay in the "line of longitude" from pole to pole: Keep equally between the medial and inferior recti.
- Keep the Westcott scissors closed: Only one snip at the start is needed.

- Keep the tip of the cannula tight against the sclera: It's easy to overshoot.
- Inject in different directions: Rotating the syringe slightly will aid spread behind the eye.
- Avoid the pterygia: They make access to the sub-Tenon's space more difficult, and they bleed.
- Keep the local anesthetic posterior to the equator: Keep the channel created by the Westcott scissors as narrow as possible to minimize reflux.
- Reduce the rate and force of injection: Too fast and hard is painful for the patient and more likely to cause chemosis.
- Use less than 5mL to minimize chemosis and the increase in intraocular pressure.
- Avoid ocular massage, which can cause dramatic peaks in intraocular pressure and may even cause anterior chamber bleeding. Gentle, steady pressure, if anything, is better.
- Take care with scleral buckles: The inferotemporal quadrant is usually clear, but ask your surgeon. If it is not clear, and you are not comfortable trying a different quadrant, or if you expect or encounter significant scarring, try a different technique.

RETROBULBAR ANESTHESIA

Historically, retrobulbar anesthesia (RBA) was the gold standard for anesthesia of the eye and orbit. This technique generally consists of injecting a small volume of LA solution (3–5 mL) inside the muscular cone (see Figure 38–3). A facial nerve block is occasionally required to prevent blinking (see "Oculoplastic Blocks" below). Because of its extraconal motor control, the superior oblique muscle frequently may remain functional, precluding total akinesia of the globe. The main hazard of RBA is the risk of injury to the globe or to one of the anatomical structures in the muscular cone. Near the apex, these structures are packed in a very small space and are fixed by the tendon of Zinn, which prevents them from moving away from a needle.

Classical Technique (Now Obsolete)

In Atkinson's classical 1936 description,[49] the patient is asked to look in the "up-and-in" direction. The needle is introduced through the skin below the inferior lid at the junction between the lateral third and the medial two-thirds of the inferior orbital edge. The needle is directed toward the apex of the orbit (slightly medially and cephalad) and advanced to a depth of 25–35 mm. A volume of 2–4 mL of LA solution is then injected. An additional facial nerve block may be needed to prevent blinking; the technique most frequently used is the Van Lint block (see "Oculoplastic Blocks").

Modern Techniques

Modern retrobulbar blocks are performed with the eye in the neutral position (Figure 37–9). The Atkinson "up-and-in" gaze position was abandoned when Liu et al.[49] and Unsöld et al.[50] warned that it increased the risk of optic nerve injury, since this

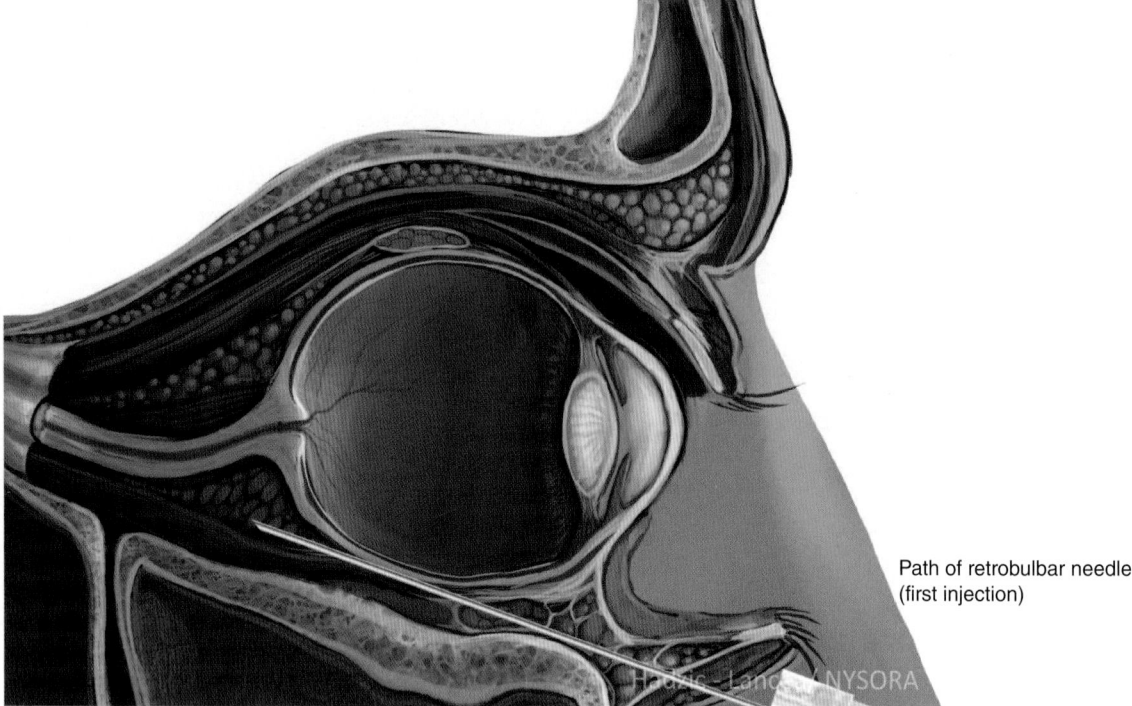

FIGURE 37–9. Retrobulbar block.

position places the optic nerve near the path of the needle. Moreover, the optic nerve is stretched and can be injured easily by the needle, rather than being pushed aside. Alternative puncture sites and specially designed bent or curved needles have been proposed but have not gained popularity.[52,53]

RBA: Is There a Future?

Recently, there has been a growing literature on ultrasound-guided retrobulbar block. The original work in this area was done in human cadavers,[54,55] but there have since been pilot studies in humans.[56] However, concerns have been raised about the ease with which the block may compromise sterility, and questions about the need for this technique have also been asked, given the now-established utility and safety profile of sub-Tenon's blocks, which do not require ultrasonic guidance.[57] It is possible that with future advances in ultrasonic technology this situation may well change. Meanwhile, given the versatility and rising popularity of sub-Tenon's blocks, and given that there is no situation in which a retrobulbar block would be preferred over a peribulbar block, it seems unlikely that retrobulbar blocks will remain part of the repertoire of the modern anesthesiologist.

PERIBULBAR ANESTHESIA

With peribulbar anesthesia (PBA), the needle is introduced into the extraconal space (Figure 37–10).[25,26,58,59] The classical technique involves two injections. The first injection is inferior and temporal, the needle being introduced at the same site as for an RBA injection, but with a lesser up-and-in angle. The second injection is superior and nasal, between the

medial third and lateral two-thirds of the orbital roof edge (see Figure 37–10).

The injected volume of LA (6–12 mL) is larger than that for a retrobulbar injection. This larger volume allows the LA to spread into the whole corpus adiposum of the orbit, including the intraconal space, where the nerves to be blocked are located. Additionally, such a large volume allows for the anterior spread of LA to the lids to provide a block of the orbicularis muscle and to avoid the need for an additional lid block.

Several variations on PBA have been described (Figure 37–11). The most common are (1) medial canthus injection,[60] (2) lacrimal caruncle injection[61,62] and (3) inferior and temporal injections.[25,26]

Principles of Peribulbar Anesthesia

- *Single-injection versus multiple-injection technique:* Increasing the injected volume of LA provides sufficient anesthesia. Additional injections are not needed.[63] In addition, anatomic distortion following the first injection may increase the risk of complications associated with consecutive injections.[64] As a rule of thumb, a second injection should be performed only as a supplement when the first injection has failed to provide effective anesthesia.

- *Needle insertion sites:* Needle insertion through the superior nasal site should be avoided. At this level, the distance between the orbital roof and the globe is reduced, theoretically increasing the risk of globe perforation. Additionally, the needle may injure the superior oblique muscle. The inferonasal approach or an approach through the medial canthus should be used instead.[60] The needle is

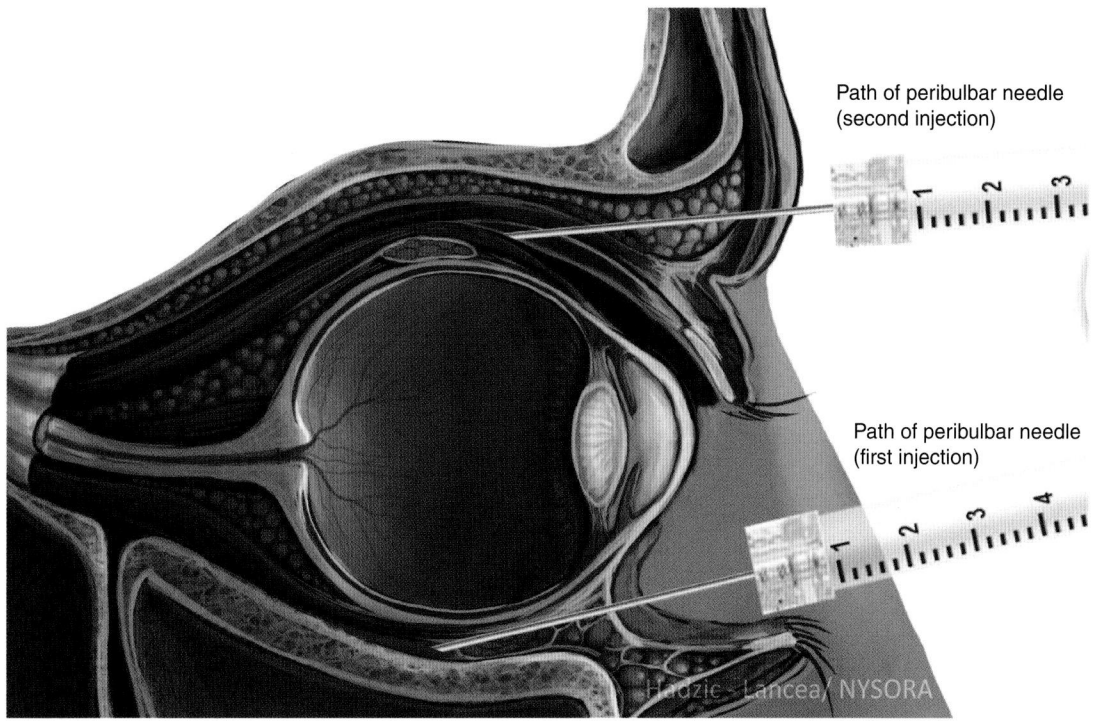

FIGURE 37–10. Peribulbar block: superior second injection technique.

introduced at the medial junction of the lids, nasal to the lacrimal caruncle, in a strictly posterior direction to a depth of 15 mm or less. At this level, the space between the orbital wall and the globe is similar in size to that of the inferior and temporal approach and is free of blood vessels. Moreover, myopic staphyloma, an anatomical anomaly that represents a risk factor for perforation, is infrequently encountered on the nasal side of the globe.

• *Needle insertion depth:* Limit the needle insertion depth to 25 mm. Posterior to the globe, the rectus muscles are in

contact with the orbital walls, so that the extraconal space entirely disappears and becomes virtual. Increasing the needle insertion depth would be expected to cause a peribulbar injection to become a retrobulbar injection.[65] Some posterior peribulbar blocks are in fact unintentional retrobulbar injections. This is a plausible explanation for optic nerve injury after an attempted peribulbar injection. Moreover, a long needle fully introduced into the orbit may reach the apex of the orbit, another hazardous area.[66] Inserting the needle to a depth of 40 mm has led to

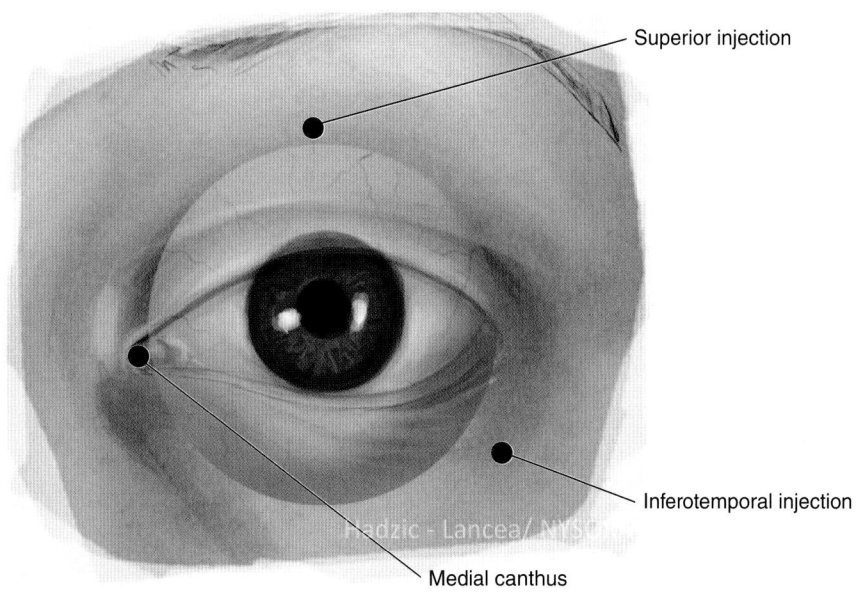

FIGURE 37–11. Peribulbar block: alternative injection sites.

performing the injection directly through the optical foramen in 11% of cases.[67]

- *Fine needles (25-gauge) are suggested for reducing pain on needle insertion:* The use of short-bevel needles may be safer because they may enhance the tactile perception of resistance during needle insertion (intraneural or intramuscular placement). Indeed, on cadavers, more pressure is required with short-bevel needles to perforate the sclera.[68] Nevertheless, these are only theoretical considerations, since the complication rate with peribulbar blocks is low.

- *Use compression to lower intraocular pressure, which increases after injection:* Compression has not been shown to enhance the quality of the block. Applying a pressure of 30 mm Hg for 5–10 minutes is usually sufficient.

- *In all cases, the spread of LA within the corpus adiposum of the orbit remains somewhat unpredictable, leading to the need for more anesthetic to prevent an imperfect block:* Depending on the surgeon's request for akinesia, additional anesthetic is required in up to half of all cases.[58,59] The poor reproducibility in block efficacy is the main disadvantage of peribulbar anesthesia.[26]

Retrobulbar Versus Peribulbar Versus Sub-Tenon's Blocks

RBA has been traditionally assumed to be more effective than PBA. However, when a sufficient volume of LA is injected, both blocks appear to have similar success rates.[69] This is explained by the absence of an intermuscular membrane to separate extra- from intraconal compartments, resulting in a favorable spread of LA (see "Functional Anatomy"). Therefore, if the effectiveness is similar, one should prefer to use the technique with a lower risk of complications. Since RBA theoretically carries a higher risk of complications (eg, optic nerve injury, brainstem anesthesia, retrobulbar hemorrhage; see "Complications of Eye Blocks" below), PBA is deemed preferable to RBA.

However, all other requirements being equal, the sub-Tenon's block offers the best safety profile of the three blocks and can reliably deliver both surgical anesthesia and akinesia if performed by an experienced practitioner with an appropriate volume (with or without adjuvants). However, where chemosis, conjunctival hematoma, or the disruption of the conjunctiva are undesirable, or where the posterior anatomy is seriously abnormal, this technique may not be appropriate.

The diversity of opinion and data suggest, to this author at least, that the individual efficacy of any of these blocks is heavily operator dependent. To a significant extent, the same is true in regard to their safety profiles.

COMPLICATIONS OF EYE BLOCKS

The primary cause of serious complications is needle misplacement. Although some anatomical features may increase the risk of complications, the main risk factor is inadequate knowledge and limited experience on the part of the operator. However, it should be noted that complications such as **retrobulbar hemorrhage** and **oculocardiac reflex** may occur with even the most experienced practitioners. Presenting signs, symptoms, and mechanisms of common complications are summarized in Tables 37–1 and 37–2).

TABLE 37–1. Signs, symptoms, and mechanisms of complications of retrobulbar anesthesia.

Complication	Signs and Symptoms	Mechanism of Complication
Ocular		
Globe perforation	Ocular pain, intraocular hemorrhage, restlessness	Direct trauma: myopic eye, posterior staphyloma, repeated injections
Retrobulbar hemorrhage	Subconjunctival or eyelid ecchymosis, increasing proptosis pain, and/or increased intraocular pressure	Direct trauma (artery or vein)
Optic nerve damage	Visual loss, possible early optic disc swelling, late optic disc pallor	Direct injury to nerve or blood vessels, vascular occlusion
Systemic		
Intra-arterial injection	Cardiopulmonary arrest, convulsions	Retrograde flow to internal carotid and access to midbrain structures
Optic nerve sheath injection	Brainstem anesthesia: agitation, ptosis, mydriasis dysphagia, dizziness, confusion, contralateral ophthalmoplegia, loss of consciousness, respiratory depression/arrest, cardiac arrest	Subdural or subarachnoid injection
Oculocardiac reflex	Bradycardia, other arrhythmias, asystole	Trigeminal nerve (afferent, arc) to floor of fourth ventricle with efferent arc via vagus nerve

TABLE 37–2. Other complications of retrobulbar anesthesia.

Complication	Comment
Chemosis (subconjunctival edema)	Usually of minimal concern; disappears with pressure.
Venous hemorrhage	Usually mild and, while unsightly, is easily controlled.
Arterial hemorrhage	Can be dramatic, causing proptosis, extensive subconjunctival and lid hematoma, and a dramatic increase in intraocular pressure. This is a sight-threatening complication: inform surgeon immediately, as orbital decompression (eg, lateral canthotomy/cantholysis) may be necessary to prevent blindness. Usually causes postponement of surgery.
Globe perforation	Likely more common to occur in long, myopic eyes. A long eye has thinner sclera and may have an irregular outline (staphylomata). The needle should be inserted tangentially to the globe and move freely in the orbital fat without rotating the globe.
Damage to the optic nerve	A result of direct trauma, injection into the nerve sheath, or the ischemic consequences of the pressure on injection.
Decreased visual acuity	Usually resolves with resolution of the block, but beware "wipe-out", especially in patients with advanced glaucoma (see "Choice of Local Anesthetic and Adjuvant Agents").
Myotoxicity	May follow direct injection into a muscle or the use of high concentrations of LA (probably more common than currently recognized; usually resolves during surgical convalescence).
Systemic complications	Subarachnoid injection during retrobulbar block is a possible cause of respiratory arrest.
Grand mal seizures, loss of consciousness, and respiratory depression or cardiac arrest	These complications can result from systemic LA toxicity, injection of LA into the optic nerve sheath (and thence to the brainstem), or retrograde arterial flow.
Pulmonary edema	Rare; mechanism is poorly understood.
Reaction to epinephrine	Often inappropriately referred to as "epinephrine toxicity"; in patients with hypertension, angina, or arrhythmias, the amount of epinephrine injected with the LA should be reduced.
Oculocardiac reflex, vasovagal reaction	See text for presentation and management.
Allergic reactions	Extremely rare with amide-type LAs; more common with animal-derived hyaluronidase.

Central Nervous System Complications

Central nervous system eye block complications may occur following a needle block by two different mechanisms:

1. An unintentional **intra-arterial injection** may reverse the blood flow in the ophthalmic artery up to the anterior cerebral or internal carotid artery,[70] so that an injected volume as small as 4 mL may cause seizures. Symptomatic treatment by maintaining a patent airway; providing oxygenation; and abolishing seizure activity with small doses of benzodiazepam, propofol, or a barbiturate is usually adequate and results in a rapid recovery without sequelae.

2. An unintentional **subarachnoid injection** via puncture of the dura mater sheath of the optic nerve or directly through the optic foramen results in partial or total brainstem anesthesia.[71–73] Katsev et al. have shown that the apex of the orbit may be reached with a 40-mm needle in up to 11% of patients.[67] Depending on the dose and volume of LA spreading toward the brainstem, subarachnoid

injection can lead to bilateral block; cranial nerve palsy with sympathetic activation, confusion, and restlessness; or total spinal anesthesia with tetraparesis, arterial hypotension, bradycardia, and eventually respiratory arrest. Symptomatic treatment (oxygen, vasopressors, and, if required, tracheal intubation and ventilation) should permit complete recovery after the spinal block wears off (a few hours).

Unintentional **globe perforation** and rupture is the most devastating complication of eye blocks. It has a poor prognosis, especially when the diagnosis is delayed. The incidence is between 1 in 350 and 7 in 50,000 cases.[74,75] Main risk factors include inadequate experience of the operator and a highly myopic eye (ie, a long eyeball).[76] In a study of 50,000 cases, Edge and Navon observed that **myopic staphyloma** was a significant risk factor. This suggests that isolated high myopia may not be a risk factor per se but acts as a confounding factor, as staphyloma seems to occur only in myopic eyes.[75] Vohra and

Good[76] observed with B-mode ultrasound that the probability of staphyloma is greater in highly myopic than in slightly myopic eyes. Moreover, staphyloma was more frequently found at the posterior pole of the globe (accounting for perforations after RBA) or in the inferior area of the globe (accounting for perforations after inferior and temporal punctures, both peri- and retrobulbar). As a result, at least in myopic patients, and at best in all patients, ultrasound measurement of the axial length of the globe (biometry) should be available. In cases of a highly myopic eye (axial length greater than 26 mm), a needle block can carry an increased risk of globe perforation, and a sub-Tenon's or topical block is preferable. Unusual causes of globe perforation include misplaced infraorbital nerve blocks (see "Oculoplastic Blocks") and patients sneezing under propofol sedation (see "Sedation").

Extraocular Muscle Injury

Injury to an extraocular muscle may cause diplopia and ptosis. Several mechanisms can be involved, including direct injury by the needle resulting in intramuscular hematoma, high pressure as a result of injection into the muscle sheath, or direct LA myotoxicity.[77]

Direct Extraocular Myotoxicity

It has been known for some time that high concentrations of amide-type local anesthetics, particularly bupivacaine, cause myotoxic changes in skeletal muscle.[78] The extraocular muscles seem particularly susceptible, and numerous case reports of persistent diplopia after cataract surgery have been attributed to this.[79–81] However, to date, no formal clinical evaluation of skeletal muscle function after eye block has been performed. In monkeys, a 0.75% bupivacaine retrobulbar block typically causes a myopathic response that peaks at 14 days and is largely resolved by 27 days.[78] In rabbits, bupivacaine myotoxicity appears to be concentration dependent, with 0.75% solutions producing extensive and longer-lasting damage, whereas 0.19% produces little sign of short- or long-term damage.[82] Lidocaine solutions containing epinephrine cause substantially more damage to skeletal muscle than does plain lidocaine, both in rats and humans.[83] Indeed in humans, bupivicaine toxicity of eye muscles is deliberately induced to treat strabismus.[84] The injury progresses in three steps: first, the muscle is paralyzed; second, the muscle seems to recover; and third, retractile hyperplasia develops.

Given the case reports and the impressive and consistent pathological evidence across species, and with the many thousands of eye blocks being performed each year, it is surprising that the phenomenon is not more clinically apparent. It has been proposed that postoperative pain may mask myopathic changes and that any eye discomfort or dysfunction is readily attributed to the operation rather than other causes.[85] Furthermore, the animal evidence suggests that in most cases there is likely to be rapid recovery with complete tissue regeneration. In another animal study, skeletal muscle damage induced by femoral nerve block was more severe in younger rats than older rats,[86] so perhaps older humans, too, are less susceptible.

Based on the limited available evidence, it would seem that extraocular myotoxicity is probably a more frequent concomitant of volume blocks behind the equator of the eye than is generally recognized and that it is concentration dependent and more likely to occur with bupivacaine, but that any clinically significant adverse effects in the relevant patient population *usually* (but not always) resolve completely within the time frame of healing of the operation.

Clinical Pearls

Retrobulbar Hemorrhage

- Retrobulbar hemorrhage is typically caused by an inadvertent arterial puncture. It may lead to a compressive hematoma, which can threaten retinal perfusion.
- At the time of hemorrhage, it is imperative to have an ophthalmologist present who can monitor intraocular pressure and take the appropriate steps to preserve central retinal artery perfusion. Lack of perfusion for even short periods can lead to permanent, devastating loss of vision.
- Surgical decompression may be required, but in most cases surgery has only to be postponed.[87]
- Venous puncture may occur after both retrobulbar and peribulbar injection. It leads to noncompressive hematoma, the consequences of which are much less severe, so that in most cases surgery can be continued.
- For patients on anticoagulants (including even aspirin and similar medications), consider sub-Tenon's or topical anesthesia to minimize the risk of hemorrhage.

Optic Nerve Trauma

Direct optic nerve trauma by the needle is rare but serious, as it causes blindness. Computed tomography imaging usually shows optic nerve enlargement caused by intraneural hematoma.[88]

Summary

Overall, there is a 1%–3% chance of complications, often necessitating postponement of the planned surgery. Since some complications may be life threatening if patients are not immediately resuscitated, it is recommended that an anesthesiologist be present to monitor the patient perioperatively.[89]

Clinical Pearls

Oculocardiac Reflex

- Bradycardia due to a range of stimuli in or around the orbit, such as traction on the extraocular muscles, pressure on the globe, retrobulbar block, ocular trauma or pressure on residual tissues after enucleation.
- Also causes other arrhythmias including ventricular tachycardia and (rarely) asystole.

- The relevant neural pathways are branches of the trigeminal nerve (afferent) and vagus nerve (efferent). While mainly associated with stimulation of the ophthalmic nerve, it can occur with any branch of the trigeminal nerve.
- The incidence is highest in children (up to 90% without pre-treatment with atropine).
- For prophylaxis in children, atropine 0.02 mg/kg or glycopyrrolate 0.01 mg/kg prior to surgery is indicated.
- Intramuscular atropine is not useful due to delayed onset.
- Prophylaxis in adults is not indicated.
- Treatment of bradycardia includes removal of stimulus or asking the surgeon to stop the stimulation, initiation of intravenous anticholinergics (eg atropine 5-10 mcg/kg or glycopyrrolate 2.5-5 mcg/kg), and checking depth of anaesthesia (where GA is used).

TOPICAL ANESTHESIA

Instillation of LA eye drops provides corneal anesthesia, thus allowing for cataract surgery by PhE (Figure 37–12). This technique is quick and simple to perform and avoids the potential hazards of needle techniques. It has been suggested that the lack of akinesia and intraocular pressure control, associated with the short duration of this technique, may make surgery hazardous;[90] however, this observation does not appear to have dented the growing popularity of the technique. Many US surgeons appear to prefer topical anesthesia for routine PhE in more than 90% of their cases.

Nevertheless, use of topical anesthesia should be limited to uncomplicated procedures performed by experienced surgeons in cooperative patients. In parts of the world where PhE is not technically available, and in some specific indications where PhE is not feasible, total akinesia is still required, and the use of topical anesthesia may be questionable.[91,92]

As to what patients actually prefer, there are conflicting reports. Boezaart has reported that because anesthesia may be incomplete in topical approaches, patients randomly subjected to one of these techniques for one eye and another technique for the other eye preferred the retrobulbar to the topical technique (71% versus 10%).[93] Patients consistently report less intraoperative discomfort under retrobulbar[94,95] or sub-Tenon's [95,96] anesthesia compared to topical anesthesia. On the other hand, a meta-analysis by Zhao et al.[96] reported that patients overwhelmingly preferred topical anesthesia over needle blocks, citing "fear of needles" as a key reason, despite finding that the same population of patients reported more intraoperative discomfort under topical anesthesia compared to needle blocks. In some experienced hands, no anesthesia at all appears to be as effective as topical anesthesia in selected cases.[97]

An intracameral injection of LA appears to substantially enhance analgesia with a topical approach.[98] This consists of injecting small amounts (0.1 mL) of LA into the anterior chamber at the beginning of or during surgery. Intracameral anesthetic agents must be preservative free. Some concerns have been expressed about the toxicity effects of LA on the corneal endothelium, which is unable to regenerate; however, the safety of intracameral injection now seems well established.[99] Some authors have questioned its analgesic benefit when compared with simple topical anesthesia,[98,100,101] and indeed the degree of analgesia does not seem to correlate with intracameral LA concentration.[102] Nevertheless, the combination of topical plus intracameral anesthesia is currently the technique most preferred by US ophthalmic surgeons.

The insertion of sponges soaked in LA into the conjunctival fornices has been proposed.[103] The use of lidocaine jelly instead of eye drops seems to enhance the quality of analgesia of the anterior segment [94,103,104] and is becoming very popular for improving patient comfort under topical anesthesia.

Direct Corneal Epithelial Toxicity of Topical Anesthetics

From animal studies, it has been known for some time that repeated applications of virtually all topical anesthetic agents cause some degree of transient corneal epithelial toxicity that is macroscopically apparent, including reversible corneal thickening and opacification.[105,106] Changes may be evident with even a single topical application, and these may take more than an hour or more to recover.[107] In humans, topical anesthetic abuse is a known cause of severe keratopathy among arc welders and metalworkers,[108] and even in patients who overuse their "comfort drops" after refractive keratectomy.[109,110]

Transient corneal edema has been noted in patients undergoing cataract surgery under topical ropivacaine or lidocaine.[111] Fernandez et al. reviewed the condition of corneal epithelia by slit-lamp examination the day after cataract surgery under topical levobupivacaine or lidocaine.[112] They found mild epithelial changes in 17–22% of patients and signs of significant epithelial damage (punctates) in 2.4–5.8%, respectively; however, no data were provided on how, when, or whether these changes resolved.

Nevertheless, to date, no cases of severe keratopathy associated with the routine administration of topical anesthesia for eye surgery have been reported. The current relative paucity of hard clinical data may in part explain the diversity of practice

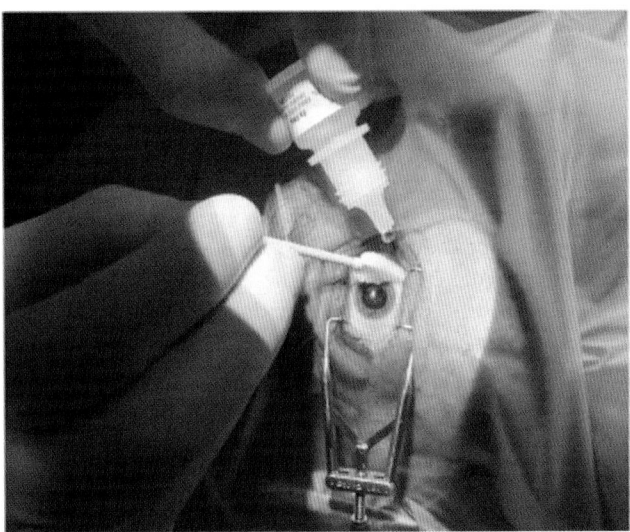

FIGURE 37–12. Topical anesthesia.

across continents, as practitioners may interpret what data there are to affirm their own preferences. Given the growing popularity of the technique (especially in the US), one might assume that, as for extraocular myotoxicity, any clinically significant effect is transient and may be masked by and/or attributed to the effects of surgery during convalescence.

SUBCONJUNCTIVAL ANESTHESIA

Subconjunctival injection of LA, a technique relatively unfamiliar to many anesthesiologists, provides anesthesia of the anterior segment without akinesia.[113] Also known as "perilimbal" anesthesia, it is, in effect, a form of episcleral injection and can also be thought of as a "very anterior" or "very superficial" Sub-tenon's block. This block is useful for cataract, pterygium, and superficial glaucoma surgery. After pretreatment with one drop of topical anesthetic, a fine-bore (27- to 30-gauge) needle is used to lift the superotemporal or inferotemporal conjunctiva at least 5–8 mm from the limbus (Figure 37–13). A surgical microscope or loupes can be used to avoid conjunctival vessels and hematoma. Once the needle is under the conjunctiva, 0.5–0.8 mL of local anesthetic solution will cause chemosis, which is dispersed with gentle, constant pressure, either using fingers or a purpose-specific weight or balloon. Hyaluronidase can be added to assist with the spread of solution and dispersal of chemosis. Compared to retrobulbar injection, this technique is less painful and reduces the need for supplemental anesthesia

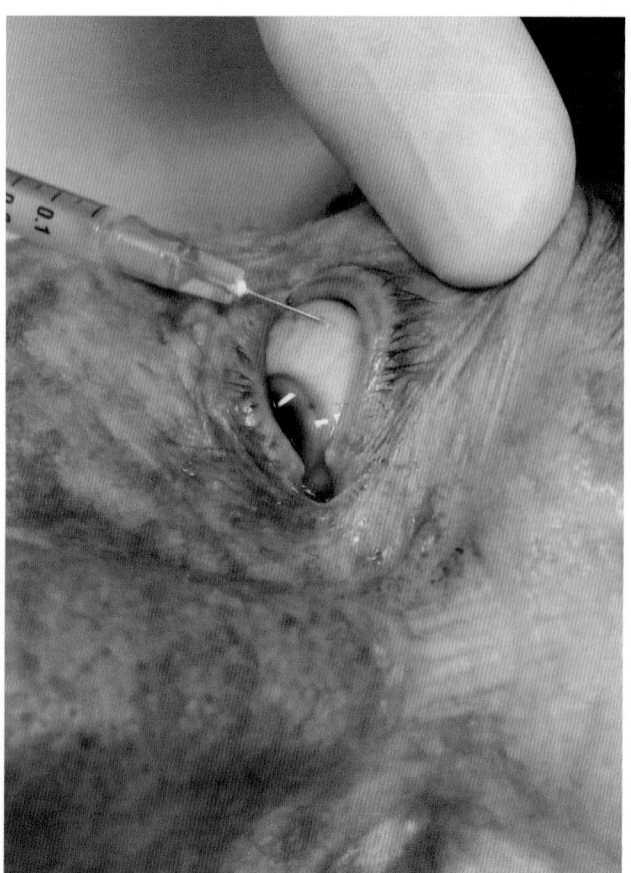

FIGURE 37–13. Subconjunctival block.

during cataract surgery.[114] Injection at the superotemporal conjunctiva appears to be less painful than injection at the inferotemporal conjunctiva.[115] Subconjunctival injection results in reliable and substantial concentrations of local anesthetic in the aqueous humor.[116]

OCULOPLASTIC BLOCKS

Many oculoplastic procedures (Figure 37–14) can be performed under local anesthetic. However, given the sensitive innervation of the face, these blocks are best performed under some form of transient, deep sedation (eg, a small IV dose of propofol), except in the very stoic patient. Note also that, while targeted blockade of individual nerves is useful, there is often significant overlap of sensory supply. Depending on the site and extent of the proposed operative wound, more than one type of block may be required, and supplemental local infiltration may be necessary. Most oculoplastic surgeons are quite accustomed to this.

Upper and Lower Lid blocks

Procedures such as upper and lower blepharoplasty and ectropion repair can be performed under gentle subcutaneous local infiltration of the base of the operative lid. Certain procedures require the surgeon to evert the eyelid under deep sedation and infiltrate distal to the semilunar fold.

Facial Nerve Block

Occasionally, a block of the periocular branches of the facial nerve is required to prevent excessive blinking during eye surgery. Classical approaches include the Van Lint[117] and O'Brien[118] techniques; Atkinson has described a modified technique,[119] variants of which are probably most popular today. A bleb of local anesthetic is raised about 2–3 cm lateral to the lateral rim of the orbit at the level of the lateral canthus, which is somewhere between the locations of the more distal Van Lint and the more proximal O'Brien approaches. Two radii of local infiltration are then injected superiorly and inferiorly from this point forming a "V" that catches the fibers of the facial nerve. A total of 5 mL is typically more than sufficient.

Supratrochlear/Supraorbital Nerve Block

Blocks of the supraorbital and supratrochlear nerves, branches of the ophthalmic nerve, are useful for procedures that involve the upper eyelid area immediately at or above the eyebrow. The supraorbital notch can usually be felt about 2–3 cm from the midline along the medial part of the superior rim of the orbit, usually in line with the patient's pupil. Paresthesia can often be elicited by pressing on this notch. A volume of 2 mL of local anesthetic here should provide some anesthesia to the area immediately around the eyebrow, the upper eyelid, and the lower forehead; however, it is usually also necessary to block the supratrochlear nerve by running a medial band of infiltration (an additional 2–3 mL) from the notch to the midline and approximately 1–2 cm laterally to catch lateral supraorbital fibers that can arise through a separate foramen.

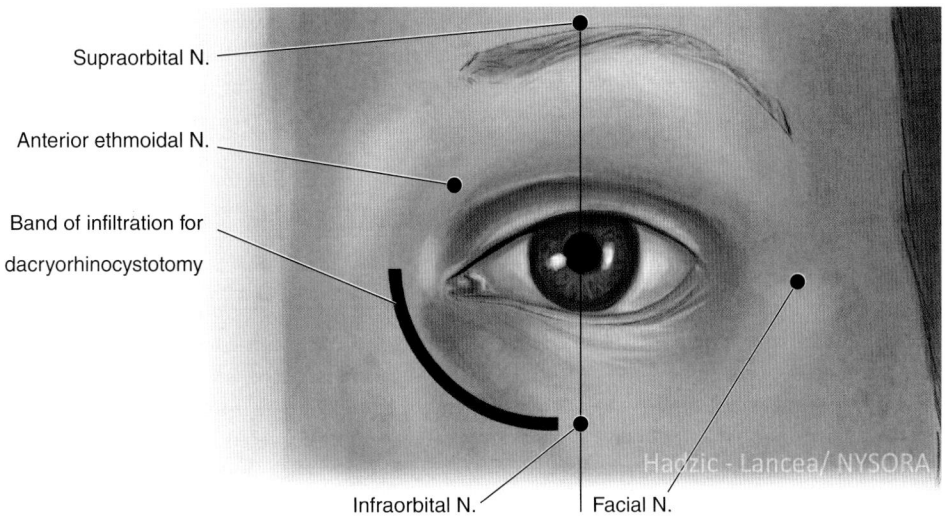

Supraorbital N.

Anterior ethmoidal N.

Band of infiltration for
dacryorhinocystotomy

Infraorbital N.   Facial N.

FIGURE 37–14. Landmarks for oculoplastic blocks.

Infraorbital Nerve Block

The infraorbital nerve, a major branch of the maxillary nerve, supplies sensation to the lower eyelid and the floor of the orbit. It emerges onto the face through the infraorbital foramen, which is reliably found just below the inferior orbital rim, in line with both the pupil and the supraorbital notch. A volume of 2–3 mL of local anesthetic at this point is usually more than enough. In the traditional approach to this block, the needle is directed slightly upward to align with the orientation of the infraorbital canal; however, note that at least two cases of inadvertent globe penetration have been reported with this technique.[120,121]

Nasocilary/Infratrochlear/Anterior Ethmoidal Nerve Block

The nasocilary nerve is a branch of the ophthalmic nerve and supplies, via its intratrochlear and anterior ethmoidal branches, sensation to the medial wall of the orbit, the proximal lacrimal sac, the proximal nasolacrimal duct, the mucosa of the nasal cavity, and much of the skin of the nose. This nerve is blocked via an injection of 2–3 mL of local anesthetic by a vertical insertion of a fine-gauge needle parallel to the medial wall of the orbit approximately in line with the bridge of the nose to a depth of about 25 mm. This corresponds with the foramen through which the anterior ethmoidal nerve exits the orbit. It is important that the needle descend freely to the point of injection, as the orbital wall is thin at this level, and perforation of the ethmoidal and even sphenoidal sinuses is quite possible.

Local Anesthesia for Tear Duct Surgery

Local anesthesia for dacryorhinocystostomy and other procedures involving the lacrimal apparatus is possible using a combination of topical anesthesia of the nasal cavity (for the nasal branches of the anterior and posterior ethmoid, sphenopalatine, and nasopalatine nerves), a nasociliary block, an infraorbital block, and a short band of subcutaneous infiltration along the base of the nose from the level of the medial canthus to the level of the infraorbital foramen.

USE OF EYE BLOCK FOR POSTOPERATIVE ANALGESIA

Regional anesthesia, especially the sub-Tenon's block, has been proposed as a treatment for postoperative pain.[122] However, this is not required for anterior segment surgery, which usually results in minimal or no discomfort postoperatively.

Clinical Pearls

Postoperative Pain

- Significant pain occurring after cataract surgery is unusual and should raise suspicion for increased intraocular pressure, severe inflammation, or infection; the eye should be examined by an ophthalmologist.
- Postoperative pain is more likely after posterior segment surgery. The use of an indwelling retrobulbar, peribulbar, or sub-Tenon's catheter has been proposed to improve intraoperative anesthesia, prolong postoperative regional analgesia, and treat intractable eye pain.[123]

CHOICE OF LOCAL ANESTHETIC AND ADJUVANT AGENTS

All available LAs have been used for eye block, either alone or as a combination of two agents. The injected LAs used most often are lidocaine, bupivacaine, ropivacaine, mepivacaine, or a combination of two of these. The choice of LAs should be based on the pharmacologic properties and availability of the drugs, with the primary consideration being the requirement for quick onset (lidocaine, mepivacaine), prolonged effect, or postoperative residual block for analgesia (ropivacaine, bupivacaine) or akinesia (higher concentration). Because the amount of LA injected is usually small (3–11 mL), systemic toxicity is not a major concern.

Septocaine (articaine) is a relatively novel amide-type LA, commonly used in dentistry, with an emergent use in eye blocks. It has a faster onset than bupivacaine/lidocaine preparations in peribulbar[124] and sub-Tenon's blocks[125] and, because it appears to diffuse through tissues more readily than other LAs, often results in a denser block. There appears to be no clinical advantage of 4% over 2% articaine, at least in dental anesthesia.[126] Despite concerns about its neurotoxic potential in animal studies,[127] there does not seem to any conclusive evidence that it is more toxic than other high-concentration LAs.[128]

Hyaluronidase is an enzyme that has been widely used to facilitate the spread of local anesthetic through connective tissue, thereby improving both the onset and success rate of regional anesthesia for the eye.[129] Another benefit is a reduced incidence of postoperative strabismus connected with its use, possibly by limiting LA myotoxicity owing to its faster spread.[130,131]

Some authors are less confident about the real benefit of hyaluronidase in improving akinesia.[132,133] There are also significant concerns about its allergenic potential;[134–136] however, these may be due to the impurities intrinsic to traditional animal-derived hyaluronidase; newer human recombinant products have been shown to be not only more potent but also to have higher enzyme purity and to be virtually free of hypersensitivity reactions.[137] It would appear that, as the requirement for akinesia relaxes, adjuvants such as hyaluronidase are becoming less popular. Nevertheless, in situations where akinesia is required, hyaluronidase may still have an important role.

α2-adrenergic agonists are well known to ophthalmologists as topical agents that reduce intraocular pressure in glaucoma. **Clonidine** has been shown to enhance intraoperative anesthesia and postoperative analgesia when added to the LA in a range of eye blocks.[138–142] At a dose of 1 mcg/kg, clonidine does not increase the incidence of systemic adverse events such as hypotension or excessive sedation.[143] Moreover, it may help to prevent intraoperative arterial hypertension and lower intraocular pressure. **Dexmedetomidine**, a more highly selective α2 agonist, has been used increasingly as an effective adjuvant in peripheral nerve blocks, including the sub-Tenon's block.[144] It has been proposed that the addition of α2 agonists may allow for surgical anesthesia at lower concentrations of LA, thereby limiting LA-induced myotoxicity. It should be noted that all studies on α2 adjuvants to date have been relatively low-powered, and, while this is a promising area of study, substantially higher sample sizes are required. **Epinephrine** is sometimes used to increase the duration of eye block. However, the availability of long-acting LAs and the fear of vasospasm with subsequent retinal ischemia have decreased its use. "Wipe-out" (a sudden total sight loss not overtly related to ocular pathology) is a rare but serious risk, particularly in glaucoma patients. LA solutions containing epinephrine have been implicated as a contributing factor.[145]

Alkalinization of local anesthetic solutions has been proposed for decreasing pain during injection and accelerating block onset; however, its efficacy remains unproven. Other adjuvant agents have been proposed but have not gained popularity. Small

doses of muscle relaxant may enhance akinesia, but concern has been expressed about their potential risk for systemic effects.[146] Opioids do not appear to be more efficient via a regional ophthalmic route than via systemic administration.[147]

Warming the LA may decrease pain on injection and enhance block efficacy, although these benefits do not appear to be clinically relevant.[148]

WHO SHOULD PERFORM EYE BLOCKS?

Since the 1980s, anesthesiologists have become increasingly involved in eye blocks that previously were performed by surgeons. However, in some countries, anesthesiologists are not available, and surgeons have to manage the block themselves.[149] In other countries, anesthesiologists monitor only the anesthesia care, as the surgeon performs the block.

In many developed countries (eg, France and Australia), anesthesiologists are often responsible for administering eye blocks. The same was true in the United Kingdom; however, recent cost constraints have forced managers to reconsider the role of the anesthesiologist in elective ophthalmic procedures that do not require a general anesthetic. There are currently no hard data to support or refute the idea that having the *anesthesiologist* performing eye blocks, rather than the surgeon, or even having the anesthesiologist in attendance, is *safer* for this patient population. However the available literature does suggest that with proper training, anesthesiologists can perform eye blocks with the same degree of safety as in other regional anesthesia techniques.[42,46,52,60] Having one experienced person performing blocks while another operates is more time efficient, and there is a theoretical benefit to having a person skilled in resuscitation present in the unlikely event of a life-threatening complication[89] (which, unsurprisingly, materializes into an *actual* benefit whenever such a complication occurs).

PERIOPERATIVE MANAGEMENT OF PATIENTS UNDERGOING EYE BLOCK

Patient Selection and Assessment

Older patients undergoing eye surgery frequently have coexisting diseases such as diabetes mellitus, hypertension, coronary artery disease, or cardiac insufficiency. A preoperative assessment should be routinely done to ensure that coexisting medical conditions are reasonably well controlled. Despite the low morbidity and mortality associated with local ophthalmic anesthesia, patients should be carefully screened for their eligibility for surgery. Patients with severe kyphosis or scoliosis pose obvious practical problems for microscopic surgery. Patients who may not be able to lie flat for the requisite period, due to cardiac or respiratory insufficiency, neurological disease, or dementia, are also challenging. Once draped, patients with profound deafness may be unable to respond to intraoperative commands unless carefully briefed preoperatively.

Briefing Patients

Given the potential problems of excessive sedation (see below), an empathic and interactive preoperative briefing is a useful tool for both reducing anxiety and optimizing cooperation during eye surgery. Patients should be given a clear explanation of what will be done to them, what they are likely to experience, and what they may be asked to do during the operation, in language appropriate to their level of understanding.

Monitoring

Intraoperative monitoring should include basic monitoring (ie, electrocardiogram, pulse oximetry, and automated noninvasive blood pressure measurement). Intravascular access is required for any invasive anesthetic technique.

Sedation

Eye surgery (eg, cataract surgery) carries a low risk of perioperative morbidity and mortality. Eye block is associated with lower perioperative morbidity than is general anesthesia used for ophthalmic surgery, provided that heavy sedation is avoided.[150–152] Anxiety and residual pain frequently occur during eye surgery under LA. Perfect immobility is required, and the presence of drapes over the head increases patient anxiety and impairs access to the airway. The patient should be positioned as comfortably as possible, with sufficient space to allow free breathing. Intraoperative sedation with judicious doses of sedatives may be used to limit anxiety and pain. However, an excess of sedation may lead to restlessness, sleeping, snoring, or respiratory depression, which, in the absence of any airway access, pose a significant intraoperative challenge. Maintenance of meaningful patient contact is of paramount importance to avoid disasters that can occur with disoriented or combative patients while the surgery is underway.

Another interesting and dangerous phenomenon associated with ophthalmic needle blocks performed under propofol sedation is involuntary sneezing,[153,154] which may occur in up to one-fifth of patients during injection;[155,156] this reaction is sight threatening, as it can lead to accidental globe perforation.[157] It is more likely to occur in patients who are male, have a history of photic sneezing (sneezing with sudden exposure to bright light or sunshine), are under deeper sedation, or who are given concurrent midazolam.[156] It does not appear to occur in patients undergoing blocks with remifentanil sedation[155] or with no sedation at all.[154] Awareness of this phenomenon should better prepare operators to withdraw the block needle immediately if a sneeze is imminent and possibly reconsider their current sedation practice. Dexmedetomidine, a highly selective α-agonist, is gaining some popularity as a sedative agent in a range of clinical settings, including eye surgery.

Do Patients Undergoing Eye Block Need to Fast?

Fasting practices for patients having procedures under topical, local, or regional block have undergone an evolution in recent years.[158] In the complex machine of public-sector medical practice, the well-intentioned and traditional "NPO from midnight" doctrine often leads to patients fasting well in excess of 12 hours.[159] In addition to an increased likelihood of postoperative nausea and vomiting, inappropriately prolonged fasting

can cause discomfort and distress, as well as dehydration and metabolic derangements, all of which can make patients (especially children and the elderly) restless and uncooperative. Moreover, while there is an obvious theoretical case for fasting prior to any surgical procedure, there have been no reported cases of aspiration under local anesthesia during cataract operations.[160] The joint view of the learned colleges in the United Kingdom is that fasting is generally not required for patients undergoing eye surgery without sedation.[161] Moreover, at least one experienced ophthalmic center has performed blocks under "judicious doses" (0.5–2 mg) of IV midazolam in over 5000 unfasted patients without untoward incident.[162] Nevertheless, where it is anticipated that deep sedation or general anesthesia, however brief, will be needed either to perform the block or during the operation, then standard preoperative fasting remains a sensible prerequisite, and, where needed, systemic measures should be explored to minimize inappropriately prolonged fasting. Where fasting is not routinely required, a small proportion of problematic patients will present for surgery unfasted but for whom the need for deep sedation becomes obvious once they are in the operating room. Individual institutions need to audit the prevalence of this phenomenon and to make cost and risk–benefit decisions accordingly. A comprehensive and compassionate preoperative patient briefing may have an important role in minimizing this issue.

Is Intravenous Access Required in Patients Undergoing Eye Block?

In recent years, many centers, particularly those performing office-based eye procedures, have abandoned the traditional requirement of securing IV access for all surgical procedures, provided that procedures are performed under "needleless" anesthesia (ie, topical anesthesia or sub-Tenon's block). According to a joint statement of the Royal College of Anaesthetists and the Royal College of Ophthalmologists in the UK, "Intravenous access … is essential with peribulbar and retrobulbar blocks and when intraoperative sedation is used" and "recommended for long/complex cases, sub-Tenon's blocks, and patients with poor general health."[161] In relation to this, the author is in agreement with Guise[163] in making the following observations: (1) Sedation may occasionally be required at very short notice by patients even under topical anesthesia, and prior IV access makes timely sedation easier and less stressful; (2) vasovagal and other dysrhythmic reactions, while uncommon, may also occur, in which case IV access already in situ is beneficial for both patient and resuscitator; and (3) it is a prudent clinical precaution, and no real trouble, if a person experienced in IV cannulation (such as an anesthesiologist) is in attendance.

Eye Blocks and the Anticoagulated Patient

Traditionally, anesthesiologists would often make a formulaic decision whether to perform an ophthalmic regional block (which was usually a retrobulbar or peribulbar block) based on results of a blood-clotting profile and by nominating an arbitrary cut-off point (eg, an international normalized ratio [INR] of 1.5–2.0 or a platelet count of 50–100). Nowadays, however, there is not only a diversity of anticoagulant therapies (several of which defy easy assessment), but also a range of anesthetic management options. Moreover, the risks of discontinuing anticoagulant therapy in some patients may outweigh the risks of perioperative bleeding on full anticoagulation. Consequently, there is no clear algorithm for managing "patients undergoing eye surgery who are on anticoagulants."[161,164] It is best to make a balanced benefit-versus-risk decision in each case based on a number of fundamental questions:

- *Which anticogulant(s) is the patient taking?* A variety of agents are now available. While there are established management strategies for drugs such as warfarin and heparin, strategies for others are less straightforward. Dabigatran, for example, is a novel long-acting oral anticoagulant with no direct antidote. The perioperative management of potential bleeding in patients on this drug is currently a matter of much concern, including those undergoing eye surgery. Since there are currently no data on patients on dabigatran undergoing eye block, including sub-Tenon's block, current recommendations are to withhold the drug for two to five days prior to performing the block and surgery.[47,165]

- *Why is the patient being anticoagulated?* Occasionally, patients self-initiate aspirin intake (eg, because they have read about it in a magazine). It is common for patients to be treated with warfarin for acute-onset atrial fibrillation that spontaneously reverts. Such situations make it easier to consider withholding the drug rather than choosing not to perform the block.

- *Is the patient in a high-risk group (eg, with a documented history of thromboembolism)?* Often, there is not only a clear clinical indication for anticoagulation, but also a clear increased risk if perioperative anticoagulation is not managed correctly, and therefore a greater imperative to use a technique that does not require the patient's anticoagulant therapy to be modified. When in doubt, consult with the medical team that started the patient on anticoagulant therapy.

- *What are the relative bleeding risks of the procedure proposed?* Here, the team should consider both the surgical and anesthetic procedures. Oculoplastic and glaucoma surgeries tends to carry a higher bleeding risk, whereas most PhE and vitreoretinal procedures can be done on full anticoagulation (however, discuss individual cases with the surgeon, as the decision is ultimately his or hers). Generally, topical, subconjunctival, and sub-Tenon's blocks are considered low risk, and the limited evidence to date supports going ahead with these techniques without altering the patient's routine anticoagulant therapy. Low-powered studies suggest that, while minor bleeding complications such as subconjunctival hematoma are more frequent with sub-Tenon's blocks performed in patients on aspirin, warfarin, or clopidogrel, major complications such as sight-threatening bleeding are not.[166,167] Retrobulbar and peribulbar blocks are considered high risk.

- *What are the surgical requirements for anesthesia?* Where akinesia is not required for anterior segment surgery, topical or subconjunctival techniques are more attractive. If posterior segment anesthesia and/or akinesia are needed and there are no other contraindications, sub-Tenon's block is now seen to be the safest option.

- *Is it an elective case or a true emergency?* Where there is time to take a more gradual approach that avoids the use of antidotes and prothrombotic agents, this opportunity should be taken.

Working with High-Volume Surgeons

Running a high-turnover cataract list (20 or more patients a day) safely and efficiently is both a science and an art form requiring not only consummate individual technical skill but also good teamwork and communication skills, as well as attention to ergonomic detail. A good surgeon will include all members of his or her theater team in the planning and execution of the list. The anesthesiologist's role is to support the team both technically and tactfully, monitoring the whole team and signaling when the team should slow down or even stop. Standardization wherever possible—from role allocation and patient trolley positioning to the vocabulary used to describe equipment and procedures—helps to streamline activities and to make deviations from routine more salient. The use of a modified World Health Organization (WHO) surgical safety checklist in a fast-paced eye theater[168,169] may also help to detect anomalies and reduce errors. Regular feedback and discussion of individual and team performance helps to promote *kaizen*: the approximation of perfection through small, continuous, incremental improvements over time.

SUMMARY

In developed countries, eye surgery is among the most frequently performed surgical procedures requiring anesthesia. During the past 20 years, anesthesiologists have assumed a growing role in performing eye blocks. The requirement for a deep anesthetic block with total akinesia has been greatly lessened through the use of PhE for cataract surgery, giving a more prominent role to topical anesthesia.

Needle blocks carry a low but real risk of serious complications, mainly the result of needle misplacement. Training and practice are required to minimize such problems. The use of the sub-Tenon's block reduces the risks of needle blocks and is now an established and popular technique, although it does not completely prevent complications. The right anesthetic technique is informed by the anesthesiologist's skill, experience, and understanding of the surgical procedure and the individual surgeon's preferences.

ACKNOWLEDGEMENTS

The author would like to thank Jacques Ripart, Kenneth Mehbridge, and Robert Della Rocca for their first-edition version of this chapter and without whom this revision would not have been possible. Thanks with deep gratitude also to Keith Allman, Tom Eke, Phil Guise, and Chandra Kumar, all of whom devoted substantial time and effort to offer invaluable suggestions and additional references.

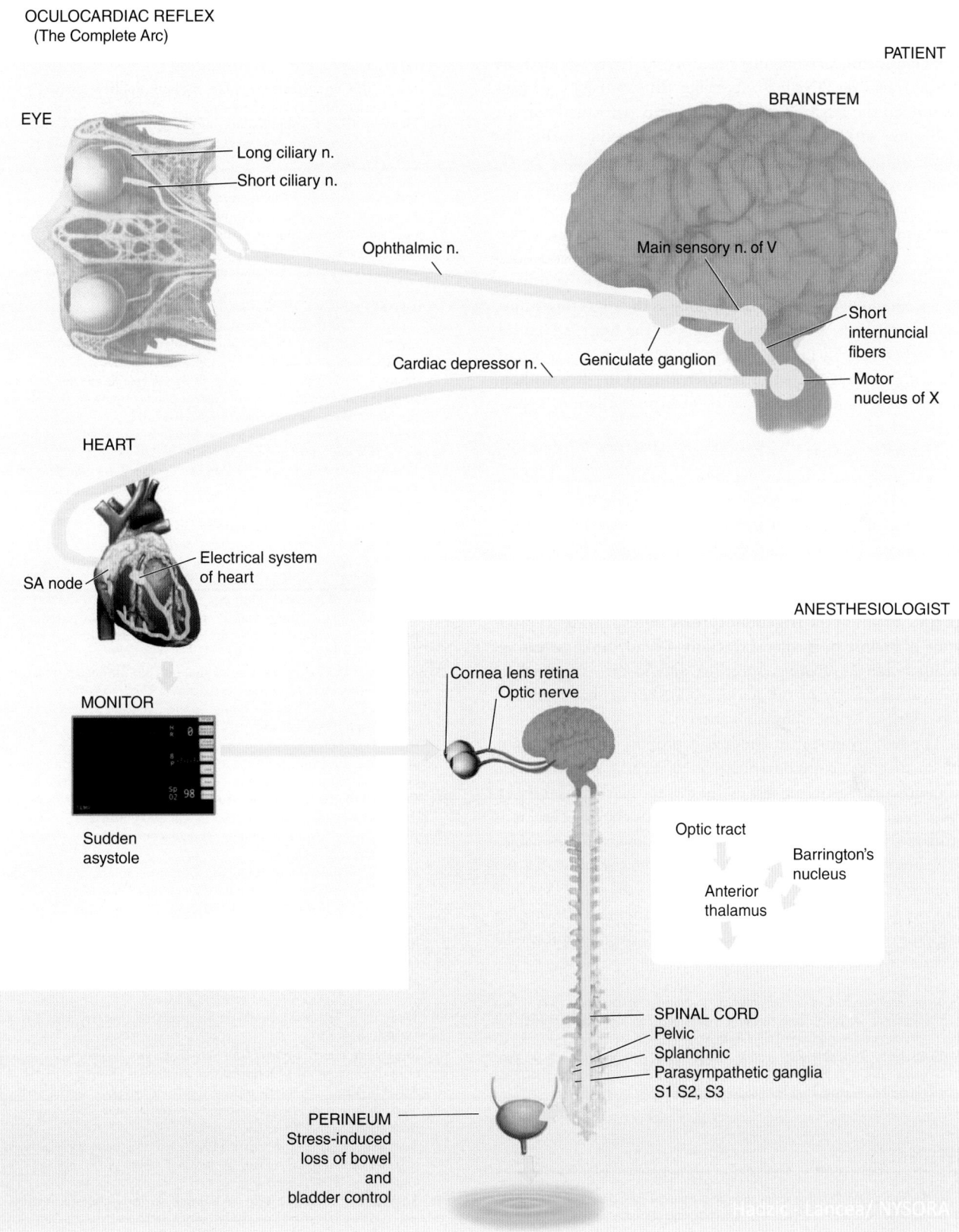

FIGURE 37–15. Oculocardiac reflex arc.

APPENDIX: THE OCULOCARDIAC REFLEX

The **oculocardiac reflex**, first described in 1908; is a decrease in heart rate over 20% below baseline values often seen during traction on the extrinsic muscles of the eye, particularly during strabismus surgery. However, it can also occur during the administration of eye blocks, particularly retrobulbar block. Other triggers include ocular trauma, intraorbital hematoma, acute glaucoma, a sudden increase in intraocular pressure, stretching of the eyelid muscles, and conjunctiva. In unprepared subjects, bradycardia can be quite dramatic, and occasionally leading to asystole in the patient (and tachycardia in the anesthesiologist), which lasts as long as the triggering stimulation is applied. While sinus slowing of the heart is classical, any arrhythmia including ventricular fibrillation may occur. The reflex is exaggerated in children (in up to 90% without pretreatment) and in the presence of hypoventilation, hypoxemia, and acidosis.

The reflex arc has been well described (Figure 37–15), the afferent limb consisting of the long and short branches of the ciliary nerves, the ophthalmic nerve, the geniculate ganglion, and the main sensory nucleus of the trigeminal nerve. Short internuncial fibers then convey the reflex to the efferent limb, consisting of the motor nucleus of the vagus, the vagus nerve, and the cardiac depressor nerve. The oculocardiac reflex is a specific variant of the **trigeminocardiac reflex**, a wider constellation of brainstem-mediated reactions—bradycardia, sweating, breath holding, yawning, sneezing, and so on—triggered by stimulation of any of the sensory branches of the trigeminal nerve (primarily the ophthalmic nerve).

The best treatment in children is prophylaxis: IV atropine 10–20 mcg/kg or glycopyrrolate 5–10 mcg/kg on induction. Intramuscular agents are less useful due to their delayed onset. Prophylaxis in adults is usually not indicated; however, it is prudent to have an IV anticholinergic predrawn and available.

Acute treatment consists of removing the stimulus: Ask the surgeon to stop whatever they are doing. If the pulse does not improve, give an anticholinergic (eg, IV atropine 5–10 mcg/kg or glycopyrrolate 2.5–5 mcg/kg). Check the depth of anesthesia in cases of GA.

*Sources: Aschner B. Ueber einen bisher noch nicht beschrieben Reflex vom Auge auf kreislauf and Atmung. Verschwinden des Radialpulsen bei Druck aut des auge. Wiener Klinische
Wochenschrift 1908;21:1529–1530; Dagnini G. Intemo ad un riflesso provocato in alcuni emiplegici collo stimolo della come e colla pressione sul bulbo oculare. Bull Sci Med 1908;8:380–381.

REFERENCES

1. Leaming DV: Practice styles and preferences of ASCRS members—2003 survey. J Cataract Refract Surg 2004;30:892–900.
2. Gild WM, Posner KL, Caplan RA, et al: Eye injuries associated with anesthesia. A closed claims analysis. Anesthesiology 1992;76:204–208.
3. Quigley HA: Mortality associated with ophthalmic surgery: A 20-year experience at the Wilmer Institute. Am J Ophthalmol 1974;77:517–524.
4. Breslin PP: Mortality in ophthalmic surgery. Int Ophthalmol Clin 1973;13:215–226.
5. McKibbin M: The pre-operative assessment and investigation of ophthalmic patients. Eye 1996;10:138–140.
6. Bass EB, Steinberg EP, Luthra R: Do ophthalmologists, anesthesiologists, and internists agree about preoperative testing in healthy patients undergoing cataract surgery? Arch Ophthalmol 1995;113:1248–1256.
7. Maltzman BA, Cinotti AA, Calderone JP Jr: Preadmission evaluation and elective cataract surgery. J Med Soc N J 1981;78:519–520.
8. Gilvarry A, Eustace P: The medical profile of cataract patients. Trans Ophthalmol Soc UK 1982;102:502–504.
9. Fisher SJ, Cunningham RD: The medical profile of cataract patients. Clin Geriatr Med 1985;1:339–344.
10. Hardesty DC: The ophthalmic surgical patient. In Wolfsthal S (ed): *Medical Perioperative Management.* Norwalk, CT: Appleton & Lange, 1989, pp 417–426.
11. Hodgkins P, Luff A, Morrell A: Current practice of cataract extraction and anaesthesia. Br J Ophthalmol 1992;76:323–326.
12. Hamilton R, Gimble H, Strunin L: Regional anaesthesia for 12,000 cataract extraction and intraocular lens implantation procedures. J Can Anaesth 1988;35:615–623.
13. Eke T, Thompson J: The national survey of local anaesthesia for ocular surgery. II. Survey methodology and current practice. Eye 1999;13:196–204.
14. Eichel R, Goldberg I: Anaesthesia techniques for cataract surgery: a survey of delegates to the Congress of the International Council of Ophthalmology, 2002. Clin Exp Ophth 2005;33:469–472.
15. Thampy R, Hariprasad M, Saha B: Local anaesthesia for ophthalmic surgery: a multicentre survey of current practice amongst anaesthetists in the North West. Anaesthesia 2007;62:101–103.
16. Vohra SB, Murray PI: Sub-tenon's block. a national United Kingdom survey. Ophth Surg Lasers Imag 2008;39:379–385.
17. Leaming DV, Duffey R: Highlights of the 2008 ASCRS Member Practice Style Survey. http://ascrs2009.abstractsnet.com/handouts/000101_Highlights_of_the_2008_ASCRS_member_practice_style.ppt. Accessed June 29, 2013.
18. Leaming DV: Surveys of American Society of Cataract and Refractive Surgery members 1999–2012. www.analeyz.com. Accessed June 29, 2013.
19. Williams PL (ed): Gray's Anatomy, 38th ed. London: Churchill Livingstone, 1995; passim but esp. pp 1225–1241, 1321–1366.
20. Ropo A, Nikki P, Ruusuvaara P, et al: Comparison of retrobulbar and periocular injections of lignocaine by computerized tomography. Br J Ophthalmol 1991;75:417–420.
21. Koornneef L: The architecture of the musculo-fibrous apparatus in the human orbit. Acta Morphol Neerl Scand 1977;15:35–64.
22. Koornneef L: Details of the orbital connective tissue system in the adult. Acta Morphol Neerl Scand 1977;15:1–34.
23. Ripart J, Lefrant J, de La Coussaye J, et al: Peribulbar versus retrobulbar anesthesia for ophthalmic surgery. An anatomical comparison of extraconal and intraconal injections. Anesthesiology 2001;94:56–62.
24. Edward DP, Kaufmann LM: Anatomy, development and pathology of the visual system. Pedatr Clin North Am 2003;50:1–23.
25. Bloomberg L: Administration of periocular anesthesia. J Cataract Refract Surg 1986;12:677–679.
26. Davis D, Mandel M: Posterior peribulbar anesthesia: an alternative to retrobulbar anesthesia. J Cataract Refract Surg 1986;12:182–184.
27. Spaeth GL, Danesh-Meyer H, Goldberg I, Kampik, A (eds): Ophthalmic Surgery: Principles and Practice, 4th ed. Amsterdam, Netherlands: Elsevier, 2012.
28. Ortiz M, Blanco D, Serra J, Vidal F: Peribulbar anaesthesia: the role of local anaesthetic volumes and Thiomucase in motor block and intraocular pressure. Eur J Anaesthesiol 1995;12:603–607.
29. Wong DH: Regional anaesthesia for intraocular surgery. Can J Anaesth 1993;40:635–657.
30. Rowley SA, Hale JE, Finlay RD: Sub-Tenon's local anaesthesia: the effect of hyaluronidase. Br J Ophthmalmol 2000;84:435–436.
31. Aziz ES, Rageh M: Deep topical fornix nerve block versus peribulbar block in one-step adjustable suture horizontal strabismus surgery. Br J Anaesth 2002;88:129–132.
32. Scott IU, McCabe CM, Flynn HW: Local anesthesia with intravenous sedation for surgical repair of selected open globe injuries. Am J Ophthalmol 2002;134:707–711.
33. Amadasun FE, Isele TO: Vitreous humour extrusion after suxamethonium induction of anaesthesia in a polytraumatized patient: a case report. Case Rep Med 2010;2010:913763.
34. Ripart J, Prat-Pradal D, Charavel P, et al: Medial canthus single injection episcleral (sub-Tenon) anesthesia anatomic imaging. Clin Anat 1998;11:390–395.
35. Ripart J, Metge L, Prat-Pradal D, et al: Medial canthus single injection episcleral (sub-Tenon) anesthesia computed tomography imaging. Anesth Analg 1998;87:43–45.
36. Ripart J, Lefrant JY, Vivien B, et al: Ophthalmic regional anesthesia: medial canthus episcleral (sub-tenon) anesthesia is more efficient than peribulbar anesthesia: a double-blind randomized study. Anesthesiology 2000;92:1278–1285.

37. Li H, Abouleish A, Grady J, et al: Sub-Tenon's injection for local anesthesia in posterior segment surgery. Ophthalmology 2000;107:41–47.

38. Mein C, Flynn HW: Augmentation of local anesthesia during retinal detachment surgery [letter]. Arch Ophthalmol 1989;107:1084.

39. Stevens JD: A new local anaesthesia technique for cataract extraction by one quadrant sub-Tenon's infiltration. Br J Ophthalmol 1992;76:670–674.

40. MacNeela BJ, Kumar CM: Sub-Tenon's block using ultrashort cannula. J Cataract Refract Surg 2004;30:858–862.

41. Kumar CM, Mac Neela BJ: Ultrasonic localization of anaesthetic fluids using sub-Tenon's cannulae of three different lengths. Eye 2003;17:1–5.

42. Guise P: Sub-Tenon's anesthesia: a prospective study of 6000 blocks. Anesthesiology 2003;98:964–968.

43. Heatley CJ, Marshall J, Toma M: "A Thrip to eye casualty" an unusual complication of sub-Tenon's anaesthesia. Eye 2006;20:738–739.

44. Costen MT, Bolton K, Boase DL: Lash foreign body complicating sub-Tenon's anaesthesia. Eye 2004;18:192–193.

45. Allman KG, Theron AD, Bayles DB: A new technique of incisionless minimally invasive sub-Tenon's anaesthesia. Anaesthesia 2008;63:782–783.

46. Nouvellon E, L'Hermite J, Chaumeron A, et al: Medial canthus single injection sub-Tenon's anaesthesia: a 2000 case experience. Anesthesiology 2004;100:370–374.

47. Guise P: Sub-Tenon's anesthesia: an update. Local Reg Anesth 2012;5:35–46.

48. Ciulla TA, Starr MB, Masket S: Bacterial endophthalmitis prophylaxis for cataract surgery: an evidence-based update. Ophthalmology 2002;109:13–24.

49. Atkinson W: Retrobulbar injection of anesthetic within the muscular cone (cone injection). Arch Ophthalmol 1936;16:495–503.

50. Liu C, Youl B, Moseley I: Magnetic resonance imaging of the optic nerve in the extremes of gaze. Implications for the positioning of the globe for retrobulbar anaesthesia. Br J Ophthalmol 1992;76:728–733.

51. Unsöld R, Stanley J, Degroot J: The CT-topography of retrobulbar anesthesia. Anatomic-clinical correlation of implications and suggestion of a modified technique. Albrecht Von Graefes Arch Klin Exp Ophthalmol 1981;217:125–136.

52. Hamilton R, Loken R: Modified retrobulbar block. Can J Anaesth 1993;40:1219–1220.

53. Galindo A, Keilson L, Mondshine R, et al: Retro-peribulbar anesthesia: special technique and needle design. Ophthalmol Clin North Am 1990;3:71–81.

54. Chang WM, Stetten GD, Lobes LA Jr, Shelton DM, Tamburo RJ: Guidance of retrobulbar injection with real-time tomographic reflection. J Ultrasound Med 2002;21:1131–1135.

55. Luyet C, Eichenberger U, Moriggl B, Remonda L, Greif R: Real-time visualization of ultrasound-guided retrobulbar blockade: an imaging study. Br J Anaesth 2008;101:855–859.

56. Guyer S, Shaw ES: Ocular ultrasound guided anaesthesia. In Singh AD (ed): Ophthalmic Ultrasonography. Amsterdam, Netherlands: Elsevier, 2012.

57. Kumar C, personal communication, June 23, 2013.

58. Bloomberg L: Anterior periocular anesthesia: five years experience. J Cataract Refract Surg 1991;17:508–511.

59. Davis D, Mandel M: Efficacy and complication rate of 16224 consecutive peribulbar blocks. A prospective multicenter study. J Cataract Refract Surg 1994;20:327–337.

60. Hustead R, Hamilton R, Loken R: Periocular local anesthesia: medial orbital as an alternative to superior nasal injection. J Cataract Refract Surg 1994;20:197–201.

61. Wang BC, Bogart B, Hillman DE, et al: Subarachnoid injection—a potential complication of retrobulbar block. Anesthesiology 1989;71:845–857.

62. Kumar CM, Lawler PG: Pulmonary oedema after peribulbar block. Br J Anaesth 1999;82:777–779.

63. Demirok A, Simsek S, Cinal A, et al: Peribulbar anesthesia: one versus two injections. Ophthalmic Surg Lasers 1997;28:998–1001.

64. Ball JL, Woon WH, Smith S: Globe perforation by the second peribulbar injection. Eye 2002;16:663–665.

65. Sarvela J, Nikki P: Comparison of two needle lengths in regional ophthalmic anesthesia with etidocaine and hyaluronidase. Ophthalmic Surg 1992;23:742–745.

66. Karampatakis V, Natsis K, Gisgis P, Stangos N: The risk of optic nerve injury in retrobulbar anesthesia: a comparative study on 35 and 40 mm retrobulbar needles in 12 cadavers. Eur J Ophthalmol 1998;8:184–187.

67. Katsev D, Drews RC, Rose BT: Anatomic study of retrobulbar needle path length. Ophthalmology 1989;96:1221–1224.

68. Waller S, Taboada J, O'Connor P: Retrobulbar anesthesia risk: do sharp needles really perforate the eye more easily than blunt needles? Ophthalmology 1993;100:506–510.

69. Demediuk O, Dhaliwal R, Papworth D, et al: A comparison of peribulbar and retrobulbar anesthesia for vitreoretinal surgical procedures. Arch Ophthalmol 1995;113:908–913.

70. Aldrete J, Romo-Salas F, Arora S, et al: Reverse arterial blood flow as a pathway for central nervous system toxic responses following injection of local anesthetics. Anesth Analg 1978;57:428–433.

71. Singer SB, Preston R, Hodge WG: Respiratory arrest following peribulbar anesthesia for cataract surgery: case report and review of literature. Can J Ophthalmol 1997;32:450–454.

72. Loken R, Mervyn Kirker GE, Hamilton RC: Respiratory arrest following peribulbar anesthesia for cataract surgery: case report and review of the literature. Can J Ophthalmol 1998;33:225–226.

73. Nicoll J, Acharya P, Ahlen K, et al Central nervous system complication after 6000 retrobulbar blocks. Anesth Analg 1987;66:1298–1302.

74. Duker J, Belmont J, Benson W, et al: Inadvertent globe perforation during retrobulbar and peribulbar anesthesia. Ophthalmology 1991;98:519–526.

75. Edge R, Navon S. Scleral perforation during retrobulbar and peribulbar anesthesia. Risk factor and outcome in 50,000 consecutive injections. J Cataract Refract Surg 1999;25:1237–1244.

76. Vohra S, Good P: Altered globe dimensions of axial myopia as risk factors for penetrating ocular injury during peribulbar anaesthesia. Br J Anaesth 2000;85:242–245.

77. Carlson B, Rainin E: Rat extraocular muscle regeneration. Repair of local anesthetic-induced damage. Arch Ophthalmol 1985;103:1373–1377.

78. Porter JD, Edner DP, et al Extraocular myotoxicity of the retrobulbar anesthetic bupivacaine hydrochloride. Inv Ophth Vis Sci 1988;29:163–174.

79. Gomez-Arnau JI, Yanguela J, Gonzalez A, et al: Anaesthesia-related diplopia after cataract surgery. Br J Anaesth 2003;90:189–193.

80. Han SK, Kim JH, Hwang JM: Persistent diplopia after retrobulbar anesthesia. J Cataract Refract Surg 2004;30:1248–1253.

81. Taylor G, Devys JM, et al: Early exploration of diplopia with magnetic resonance imaging after peribulbar anaesthesia. Br J Anaesth 2004;92:899–901.

82. Zhang C, Phamonvaechavan P, et al: Concentration-dependent bupivacaine myotoxicity in rabbit extraocular muscle. J AAPOS 2010;14:323–327.

83. Yagiela JA, Benoit PW, et al. Comparison of myotoxic effects of lidocaine with epinephrine in rats and humans. Anesth Analg 1981;60:471–480.

84. Scott AB, Alexander DE, Miller JM: Bupivacaine injection of eye muscles to treat strabismus. Br J Ophthalmol 2007;91:146–148.

85. Zink W, Graf BM: Local anesthetic myotoxicity. Reg Anesth Pain Med 2004;29:333–340.

86. Nouette-Gaulain K, Dadure C, et al. Age-dependent bupivacaine-induced muscle toxicity during continuous peripheral nerve block in rats. Anesthesiology 2009;111:1120–1127.

87. Edge K, Nicoll M: Retrobulbar hemorrhage after 12,500 retrobulbar blocks. Anesth Analg 1993;76:1019–1022.

88. Hersch M, Baer G, Diecker JP, et al. Optic nerve enlargement and central retinal-artery occlusion secondary to retrobulbar anesthesia. Ann Ophthalmol 1989;21:195–197.

89. Rubin AP: Complications of local anaesthesia for ophthalmic surgery. Br J Anaesth 1995;75:93–96.

90. Rebolleda G, Munoz-Negrete FJ, Gutierrez-Ortiz C: Topical plus intracameral lidocaine versus retrobulbar anesthesia in phacotrabeculectomy: prospective randomized study. J Cataract Refract Surg 2001;27:1214–1220.

91. Waddell KM, Reeves BC, Johnson GJ: A comparison of anterior and posterior chamber lenses after cataract extraction in rural Africa: a within patient randomized trial. Br J Ophthalmol 2004;88:734–739.

92. Bourne R, Minassian D, et al: Effect of cataract surgery on the corneal endothelium: modern phacoemulsification compared with extracapsular surgery. Ophthalmology 2004;11:679–685.

93. Boezaart A, Berry R, Nell M: Topical anesthesia versus retrobulbar block for cataract surgery: the patient's perspective. J Clin Anesth 2000;12:58–60.

94. Sekundo W, Dick HB, Schmidt JC: Lidocaine-assisted xylocaine jelly anesthesia versus one-quadrant sub-Tenon infiltration for self-sealing sclero-corneal incision routine phacoemulsification. Eur J Ophthalmol 2004;14:111–116.

95. Davison M, Padroni S, Bunce C, Rüschen H: Sub-Tenon's anaesthesia versus topical anaesthesia for cataract surgery. Cochrane Database Syst Rev 2007;3:CD006291.

96. Zhao LQ, Zhu H, et al: Topical anesthesia versus regional anesthesia for cataract surgery: a meta-analysis of randomized controlled trials. Ophthalmology 2012;119:659–667.

97. Pandey S, Werner L, et al: No-anesthesia clear corneal phacoemulsification versus topical and topical plus intracameral anesthesia. Randomized clinical trial. J Cataract Refract Surg 2001;27:1643–1650.

98. Karp CL, Cox TA, et al: Intracameral anesthesia. A report by the American Academy of Ophthalmology. Ophthalmology 2001;108:1704–1710.

99. Heuerman T, Hartman C, Anders N: Long term endothelial cell loss after phacoemulsification: peribulbar anesthesia versus intracameral lidocaine 1%. Prospective randomized study. J Cataract Refract Surg 2002;28:638–643.

100. Pang MP, Fujimoto DK, Wilkens LR: Pain, photophobia, and retinal and optic nerve function after phacoemulsification with intracameral lidocaine. Ophthalmology 2001;108:2018–2025.

101. Roberts T, Boytell K: A comparison of cataract surgery under topical anaesthesia with and without intracameral lignocaine. Clin Experiment Ophthalmol 2002;30:19–22.

102. Boulton J, Lopatazidis A, Luck J, et al: A randomized controlled trial of intracameral lidocaine during phacoemulsification under topical anesthesia. Ophthalmology 2000;107:68–71.

103. Bardocci A, Lofoco G, Perdicaro S, et al: Lidocaine 2% gel versus lidocaine 4% unpreserved drops for topical anesthesia in cataract surgery. A randomized controlled trial. Ophthalmology 2003;110:144–149.

104. Barequet IS, Soriano ES, Green WR, et al: Provision of anesthesia with single application of lidocaine gel. J Cataract Refract Surg 1999;25:626–631.

105. Judge AJ, Najafi K, et al: Corneal endothelial toxicity of topical anesthesia. Ophthalmology 1997;104:1373–1379.

106. Guzey M, Satici A, Dogan Z, Karadede S: The effects of bupivacaine and lidocaine on the corneal endothelium when applied into the anterior chamber at the concentrations supplied commercially. Ophthalmologica 2002;216:113–117.

107. Carney LG, O'Leary DJ, Millodot M: Effect of topical anesthesia on corneal epithelial fragility. Int Ophthalmol 1984;7:71–73.

108. Yagci A, Bozkurt B, Egrilmez S, Palamar M, Ozturk BT, Pekel H: Topical anesthetic abuse keratopathy: a commonly overlooked health care problem. Cornea 2011;30:571–575.

109. Rao SK, Wong VW, Cheng AC, Lam PT, Lam DS: Topical anesthesia-induced keratopathy after laser-assisted subepithelial keratectomy. J Cataract Refract Surg 2007;33:1482–1484.

110. Lee JK, Stark WJ: Anesthetic keratopathy after photorefractive keratectomy. J Cataract Refract Surg 2008;34:1803–1805.

111. Martini E, Cavallini GM, Campi L, Lugli N, Neri G, Molinari P: Lidocaine versus ropivacaine for topical anesthesia in cataract surgery(1). J Cataract Refract Surg 2002;28:1018–1022.

112. Fernandez SA, Dios E, Diz JC: Comparative study of topical anaesthesia with lidocaine 2% vs levobupivacaine 0.75% in cataract surgery. Br J Anaesth 2009;102:216–220.

113. Wood CC, Menon G, Ayliffe W: Subconjunctival block for cataract extraction and keratoplasty. Br J Anaesth 1999;83:969.

114. Kongsap P: Superior subconjunctival anesthesia versus retrobulbar anesthesia for manual small-incision cataract surgery in a residency training program: a randomized controlled trial. Clin Ophthalmol 2012;6:1981–1986.

115. Yuen JS, Prineas S, Pham T, Liu H: Effectiveness of superior versus inferior subconjunctival anaesthesia for cataract surgery. Anaesth Intensive Care 2007;35:945–948.

116. Prineas SN: Unpublished data. Available by contacting the author directly.

117. Van Lint M: Paralysie palpébrale transitoire provoquée dans l'opération de la cataracte. Ann Ocul 1914;151:420–424.

118. O'Brien, CS: Akinesis during cataract extraction. Arch Ophthal 1929;1:447–449.

119. Atkinson WS: Akinesia of the orbicularis. Am J Ophthalmol 1953;36:1255–1258.

120. Saeedi OJ, Wang H, Blomquist PH: Penetrating globe injury during infraorbital nerve block. Arch Otolaryngol Head Neck Surg 2011;137:396–397.

121. Chan BJ, Koushan K, Liszauer A, Martin J: Iatrogenic globe penetration in a case of infraorbital nerve block. Can J Ophthalmol 2011;46: 290–291.

122. Duker J, Nielsen J, Vander JF, Rosenstein RB, Benson WE: Retrobulbar bupivacaine irrigation for postoperative pain after scleral buckling surgery. Ophthalmology 1991;98:514–518.

123. Jonas JB, Jäger M, Hemmerling T: Continuous retrobulbar anesthesia for scleral buckling surgery using an ultra-fine spinal anesthesia catheter. Can J Anesth 2002;49:487–489.

124. Allman KG, Barker LL, Werrett GC, Gouws P, Sturrock GD, Wilson IH: Comparison of articaine and bupivacaine/lidocaine for peribulbar anaesthesia by inferotemporal injection. Br J Anaesth 2002;88:676–678.

125. Gouws P, Galloway P, Jacob J, English W, Allman KG: Comparison of articaine and bupivacaine/lidocaine for sub-Tenon's anaesthesia in cataract extraction. Br J Anaesth 2004;92:228–230.

126. Hintze A, Paessler L: Comparative investigations on the efficacy of articaine 4% (epinephrine 1:200,000) and articaine 2% (epinephrine 1:200,000) in local infiltration anaesthesia in dentistry—a randomised double-blind study. Clin Oral Investig 2006;10:145–150.

127. Hillerup S, Bakke M, Larsen JO, Thomsen CE, Gerds TA: Concentration-dependent neurotoxicity of articaine: an electrophysiological and stereological study of the rat sciatic nerve. Anesth Analg 2011;112:133–138.

128. Snoeck M: Articaine: a review of its use for local and regional anesthesia. Loc Reg Anesth 2012;5:23–33.

129. Guise P, Laurent S: Sub-Tenon's block. The effect of hyaluronidase on speed of onset and block quality. Anaesth Intensive Care 1999;27:179–181.

130. Brown SM, Coats DK, Collins ML, Underdahl JP: Second cluster of strabismus cases after periocular anesthesia without hyaluronidase. J Cataract Refract Surg 2001;27:1872–1875.

131. Strouthidis NG, Sobha S, Lanigan L, Hammond CJ: Vertical diplopia following peribulbar anesthesia: the role of hyaluronidase. J Pediatr Ophthalmol Starbismus 2004;41:25–30.

132. Alwitryy A, Chaudhary S, Gopee K, Butler TK, Holden R: Effect of hyaluronidase on ocular motility in sub-Tenon's anesthesia: randomized controlled trial. J Cataract Refract Surg 2002;28:1420–1423.

133. Dempsey GA, Barrett PJ, Kirby IJ: Hyaluronidase and peribulbar block. Br J Anaesth 1997;78:671–674.

134. Quhill F, Bowling B, Packard RB: Hyaluronidase allergy after peribulbar anaesthesia with orbital inflammation. J Cataract Refract Surg 2004;30:916.

135. Eberhart AH, Weiler CR, Erie JC: Angioedema related to the use of hyaluronidase in cataract surgery. Am J Ophthalmol 2004;138:142.

136. Escolano F, Parés N, Gonzalez I, Castillo J, Valero A, Bartolomé B: Allergic reaction to hyaluronidase in cataract surgery. Eur J Anaesth 2005;22:729–730.

137. Silverstein SM, Greenbaum S, Stern R: Hyaluronidase in ophthalmology. J App Res 2012;12:1–13.

138. Mjahed K, el Harrar N, Hamdani M, Amraoui M, Benaguida M: Lidocaine-clonidine retrobulbar block for cataract surgery in the elderly. Reg Anesth 1996;21:569–575.

139. Baroni MF, Lauretti GR, Lauretti-Fo A, Pereira NL: Clonidine as co-adjuvant in eye surgery: comparison of peribulbar vs oral administration. J Clin Anesth 2002;14:140–145.

140. Madan R, Bharti N, Shende D, Khokhar SK, Kaul HL: A dose response study of clonidine with local anesthetic mixture for peribulbar block: a comparison of three doses. Anesth Analg 2001;93:1593–1597.

141. Khan B, Bajwa SJ, Vohra R, et al: Comparative evaluation of ropivacaine and lignocaine with ropivacaine, lignocaine and clonidine combination during peribulbar anaesthesia for phacoemulsification cataract surgery. Ind J Anaes 2012;56:21–26.

142. Cabral SA, Carraretto AR, Brocco MC, Abreu Baptista JF, Gomez RS: Effect of clonidine added to lidocaine for sub-Tenon's (episcleral) anesthesia in cataract surgery. J Anesth 2014;28:70–75.

143. Bharti N, Madan R, Kaul HL, et al: Effect of addition of clonidine to local anaesthetic mixture for peribulbar block. Anaesth Intensive Care 2002;30:438–441.

144. Eskandr AM, Elbakry AE, Elmorsy OA: Dexmedetomidine is an effective adjuvant to subtenon block in phacoemulsification cataract surgery. Egypt J Anaes 2014;30:261–266.

145. Moster MR, Azura-Blanco A: Wipe-out after glaucoma filtration surgery. J Curr Glauc Prac 2007;1:45–47.

146. Kücükyavuz Z, Arici MK: Effects of atracurium added to local anesthetics on akinesia in peribulbar block. Reg Anesth Pain Med 2002;27:487–490.

147. Hemmerling TM, Budde WM, Koppert W, Jonas JB: Retrobulbar versus systemic application of morphine during titratable regional anesthesia via retrobulbar catheter in intraocular surgery. Anesth Analg 2000;91:585–588.

148. Krause M, Weindler J, Ruprecht KW: Does warming of anesthetic solutions improve analgesia and akinesia in retrobulbar anesthesia? Ophthalmology 1997;104:429–432.

149. Hansen TE: Practice styles and preferences of Danish cataract surgeons—1995 survey. Acta Ophthalmol Scand 1996;74:56–59.

150. Eke T, Thompson JR: Eye: the national survey of local anesthesia for ocular surgery II. Safety profile of local anesthesia techniques. Eye 1999;13:196–204.

151. Glantz L, Drenger B, Gozal Y: Perioperative myocardial ischemia in cataract surgery patients: General vs local anesthesia. Anesth Analg 2000;91:1415–1419.

152. Katz J, Feldman MA, Bass EB, et al. Adverse intraoperative medical events and their association with anesthesia management strategies in cataract surgery. Ophthalmology 2001;108:1721–1726.

153. Abramson DC. Sudden unexpected sneezing during the insertion of peribulbar block under propofol Sedation. Can J Anaesth1995;42(8):740–3.

154. Ahn ES, Mills DM, Meyer DR, Stasior GO: Sneezing reflex associated with intravenous sedation and periocular anesthetic injection. Am J Ophthal 2008;146:31–35.

155. Boezaart AP, Berry RA, Nell MA, van Dyk AL: A comparison of propofol and remifentanil for sedation and limitation of movement during periretrobulbar block. J Clin Anesth 2001;13:422–426.

156. Morley AM, Jazayeri F, Ali S, Malhotra R: Factors prompting sneezing in intravenously sedated patients receiving local anesthetic injections to the eyelids. Ophthalmology 2010;117:1032–1036.

157. Schaack E, Diallo B et al. [Inadvertent globe perforation during peribulbar anaesthesia and sedation with propofol]. Ann Fr Anesth Reanim 2006;25(1):43-5.

158. Steeds C, Mather SJ. Fasting regimens for regional ophthalmic anaesthesia: a survey of members of the British Ophthalmic Anaesthesia Society. Anaesthesia 2001;56:638

159. Crenshaw JT, Winslow EH: Preoperative fasting: old habits die hard. Am J Nurs 2002;102:36–44.

160. The Royal College of Anaesthetists. Guidelines for the Provision of Anaesthetic Services. Chapter 13: Guidance on the Provision of Ophthalmic Anaesthesia Services. London, 2015 weblink http://www.rcoa.ac.uk/system/files/GPAS-2015-13-OPHTHAL.pdf accessed 31 August 2016

161. Royal College of Anaesthetists, Royal College of Ophthalmologists: Local anaesthesia for ophthalmic surgery. Joint guidelines from the Royal College of Anaesthetists and the Royal College of Ophthalmologists. London, 2012. http://www.rcoa.ac.uk/system/files/LA-Ophthalmicsurgery-2012.pdf accessed 31 August 2016

162. Guise P, personal communication, July 16, 2013.

Sonography of the Lumbar Paravertebral Space and Considerations for Ultrasound-Guided Lumbar Plexus Block

Hiroaki Murata, Tatsuo Nakamoto, Takayuki Yoshida, and Manoj K. Karmakar

INTRODUCTION

Traditionally, lumbar plexus block (LPB) is performed using surface anatomical landmarks to identify the site for needle insertion and eliciting quadriceps muscle contraction in response to nerve electrolocalization, as described in the nerve stimulator-guided chapter. The main challenges in accomplishing LPB relate to the depth at which the lumbar plexus is located and the size of the plexus, which requires a large volume of local anesthetic for success.[1] Due to the deep anatomical location of the lumbar plexus, small errors in landmark estimation or angle miscalculations during needle advancement can result in needle placement away from the plexus or at unwanted locations. Therefore, monitoring the needle path and final needle tip placement should increase the precision of the needle placement and the delivery of local anesthetic. Although computed tomography and fluoroscopy can be used to increase precision during LPB, these technologies are impractical in the busy operating room environment, costly, and associated with radiation exposure. It is only logical, then, that ultrasound (US)-guided LPB be of interest because of the ever-increasing availability of portable machines and the improvement in the quality of the images obtained.[2,3]

ANATOMY AND GENERAL CONSIDERATIONS

LPB, also known as psoas compartment block, comprises an injection of local anesthetic in the fascial plane within the posterior aspect of the psoas major muscle, usually at the L3–4

level (occasionally at the L2–3 or L4–5 levels). Because the roots of the lumbar plexus are located in this plane, an injection of a sufficient volume of local anesthetic in the posteromedial compartment of the psoas muscle results in a block of the majority of the plexus (the femoral nerve, lateral femoral cutaneous nerve, and obturator nerve).[1] The anterior boundary of the fascial plane that contains the lumbar plexus is formed by the fascia between the anterior two-thirds of the compartment of the psoas muscle that originates from the anterolateral aspect of the vertebral body and the posterior one-third of the muscle that originates from the anterior aspect of the transverse processes. The lateral and dorsal borders of the psoas major muscle consist of the quadratus lumborum muscle and the erector spinae muscle, respectively. Considering the rich vascularity of the lumbar paravertebral area, such as the dorsal branch of the lumbar artery, the use of smaller-gauge needles and the avoidance of this block in patients on anticoagulants are prudent.[4,5] LPB in patients with obesity can be challenging.

TRANSVERSE IN-PLANE TECHNIQUE

Regardless of technique, the patient is placed in the lateral decubitus position with the side to be blocked uppermost. The operator should identify the transverse processes on a longitudinal sonogram (Figure 38–1a, b, c). One technique involves identifying the flat surface of the sacrum and then scanning proximally until the intervertebral space between L5 and S1 is recognized as an interruption of the sacral line continuity (Figure 38–1b). Once the operator identifies the L5 transverse process, the transverse processes of the other lumbar vertebrae

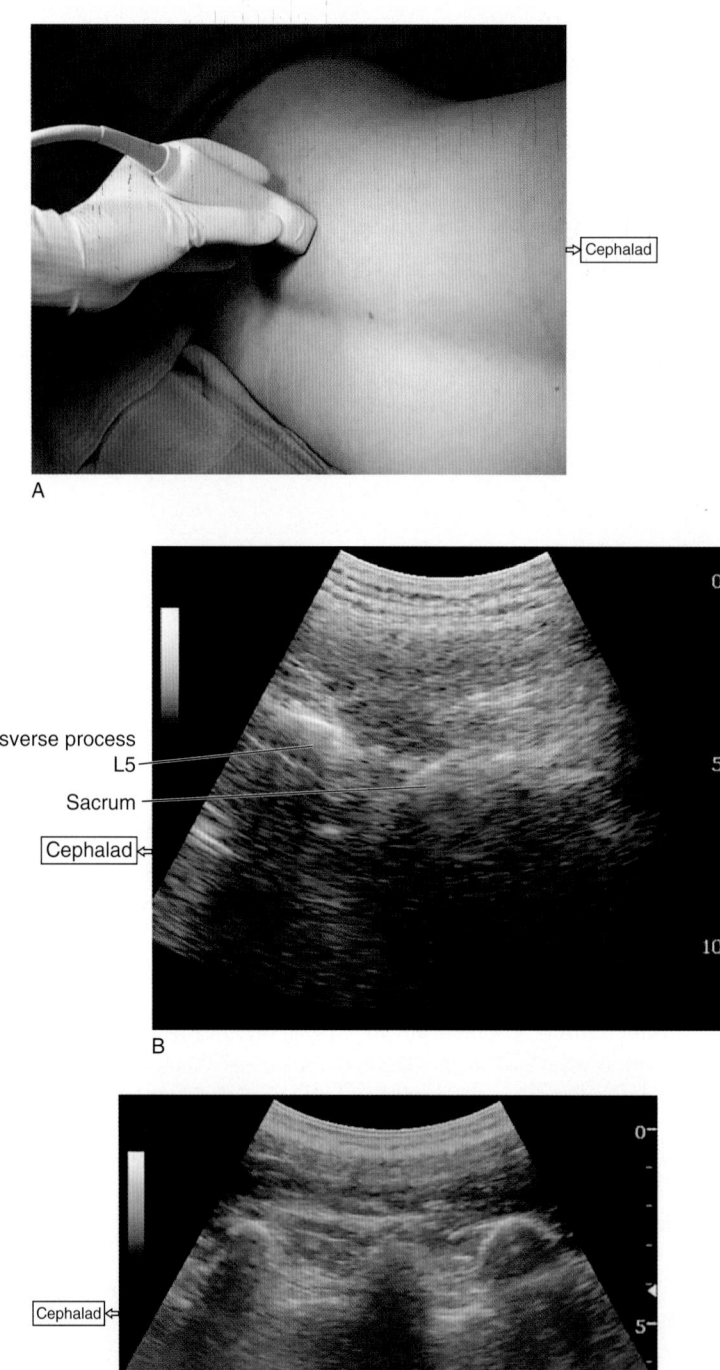

A

Transverse process
L5
Sacrum
Cephalad

B

Cephalad

C

FIGURE 38–1. (**A**) Transducer position to image the longitudinal lumbar paravertebral space including the transverse processes. Lumbar plexus block can be performed with this transducer position using both out-of-plane and in-plane approaches (see also Figure 38–4a). (**B**) Longitudinal US image of the lumbar paravertebral space demonstrating the sacrum and L5 transverse process. When the surface of the sacrum disappears, the next osseous structure is the L5 transverse process. (**C**) US anatomy of the lumbar paravertebral space demonstrating transverse processes at a depth of approximately 3 cm. The acoustic shadows of the transverse processes look like a trident. A lower-frequency, curved array transducer is used to optimize imaging at this deep location and obtain a greater angular view.

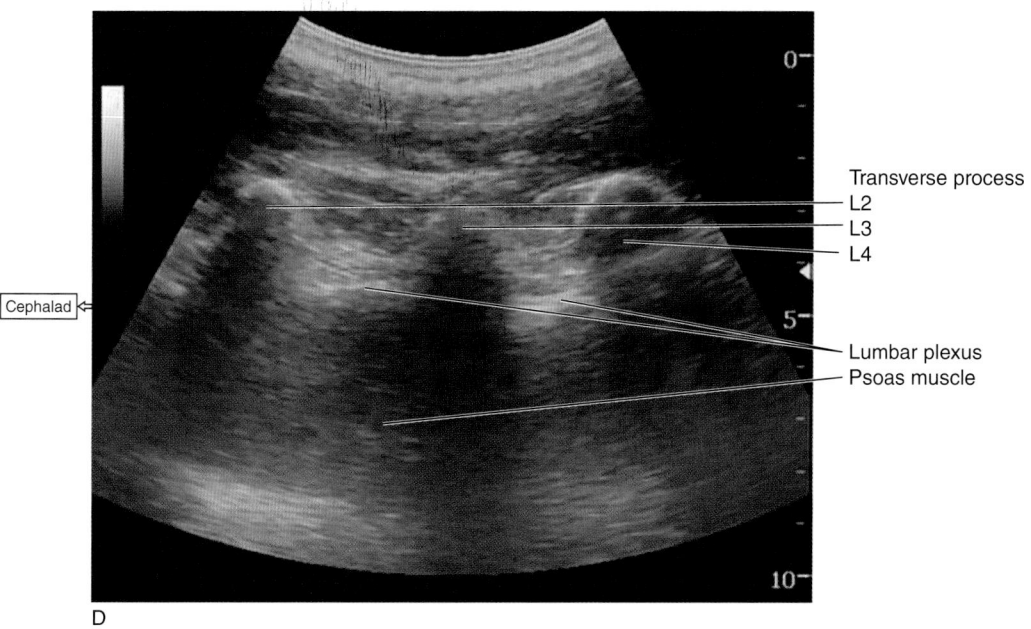

FIGURE 38–1. (*Continued*) (**D**) Labeled US image of Figure 38–1C.

are easily identified by a dynamic cephalad scan in ascending order (Figure 38–1c, d). The following settings are typically used to start the scanning:

- Abdominal preset or nerve preset if available
- Depth: 9–12 cm
- Curved array transducer (4–8 MHz)
- Tissue harmonic imaging and compound imaging functions engaged when available
- Adjustment of the overall gain and time-gain compensation

The transducer is positioned approximately 4 cm lateral from the midline at the level just cephalad to the iliac crest and directed slightly medially to assume a transverse oblique orientation (Figure 38–2a).[6,7] This approach allows imaging of the lumbar paravertebral region with the psoas major, erector spinae, and quadratus lumborum muscles; the vertebral lamina; and the anterolateral surface of the vertebral body (Figure 38–2b, c, d). In this view, the psoas major muscle appears slightly hypoechoic with multiple hyperechoic striations within. The inferior vena cava on the right-sided scan (Figure 38–2e) or the abdominal aorta on the left-sided scan can be seen deep to the psoas major muscle, providing additional information regarding the location of the psoas major muscle, which is positioned superficial to these vessels. When scanning at the L2–L4 level, the lower pole of the kidney can

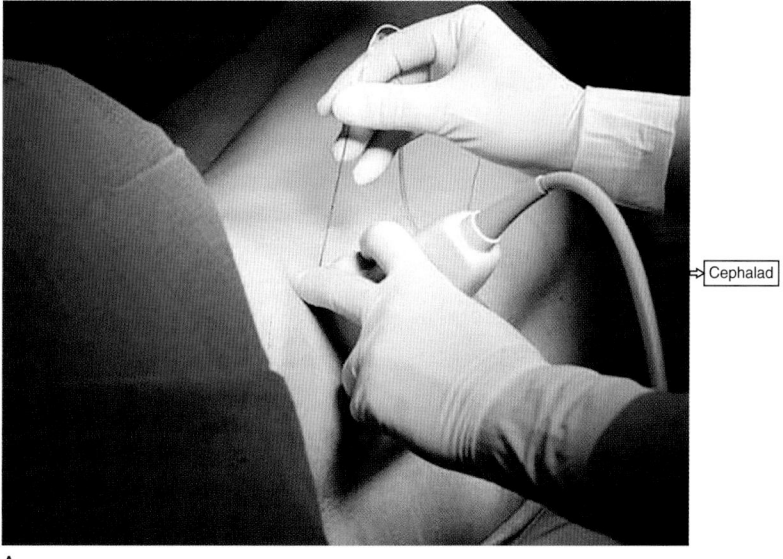

FIGURE 38–2. (**A**) Transducer position and needle insertion point to accomplish US-guided lumbar plexus block in the transverse oblique view using an in-plane approach.

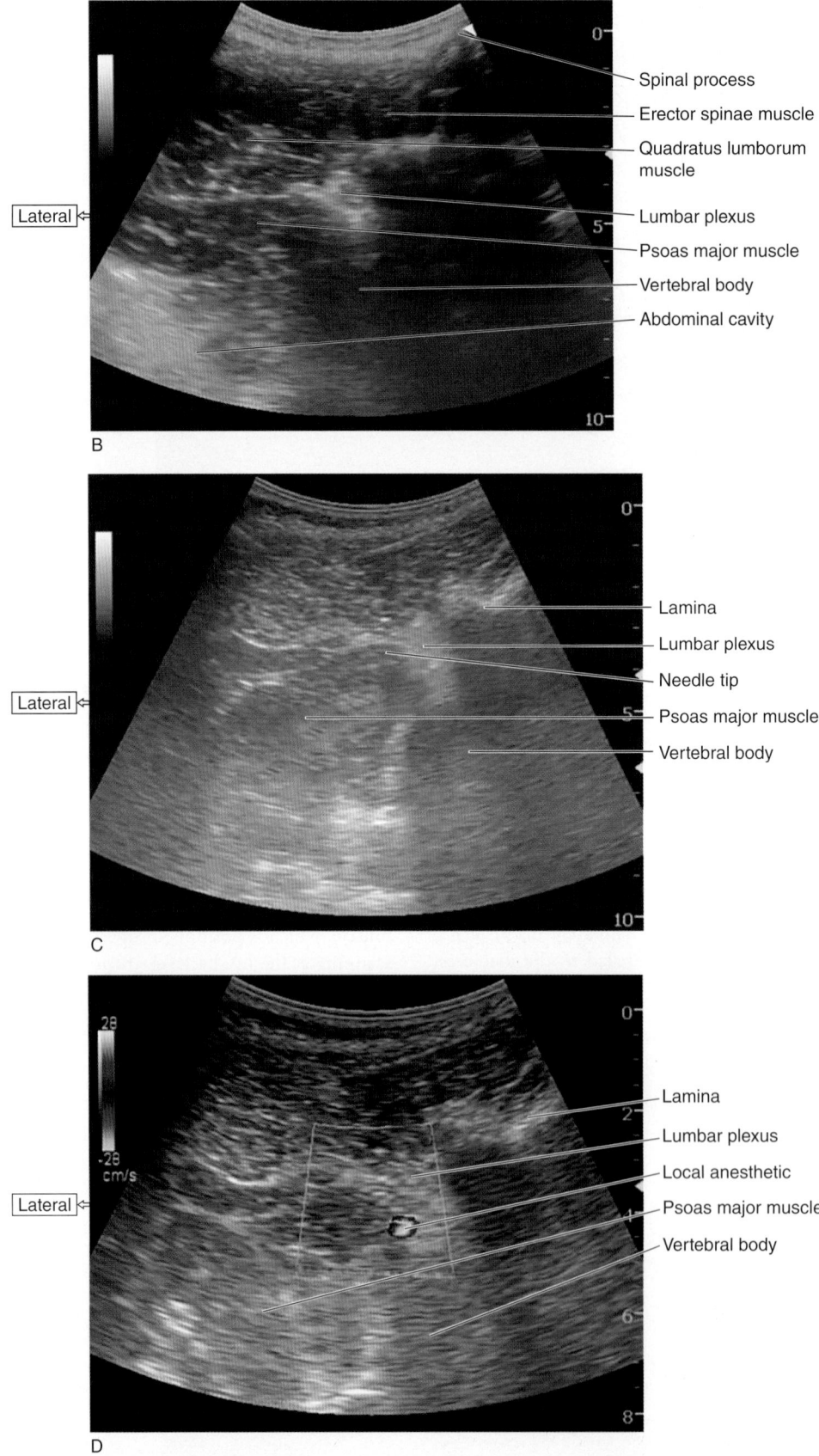

FIGURE 38–2. (*Continued*) (**B**) US anatomy of the lumbar paravertebral space in the transverse oblique view. The lumbar plexus root is seen just below the lamina as it exits the interlaminar space and enters into the posteromedial aspect of the psoas major muscle. (**C**) Needle path in US-guided lumbar plexus block using a transverse oblique view and in-plane approach from the lateral to medial direction. (**D**) Spread of local anesthetic solution with lumbar plexus block injection. Due to the deep location of the plexus, local anesthetic spread may not always be well seen. Color Doppler imaging can be used to help determine the location of the injectate.

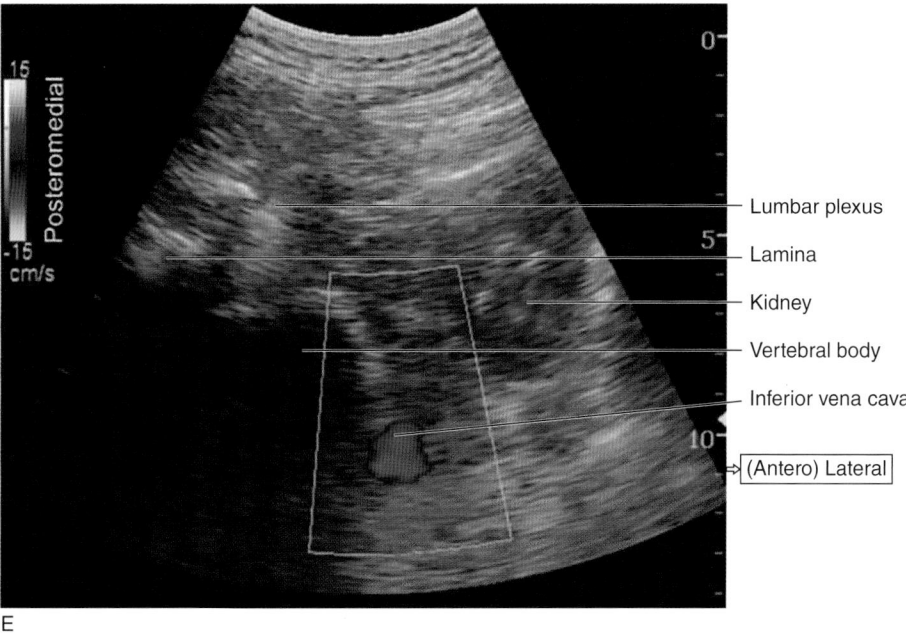

FIGURE 38–2. (*Continued*) (**E**) Transverse image of the right-side lumbar paravertebral space. Color Doppler US captures the flow in the inferior vena cava. The right kidney is also seen.

be seen as an oval structure that ascends and descends with respirations (see Figure 38–2e). The key to obtaining adequate images of the psoas major muscle and lumbar plexus with the transverse oblique scan is to insonate between two adjacent transverse processes (the lumbar intertransverse space).[7] This scanning method avoids the acoustic shadow of the transverse processes, which obscures the underlying psoas major muscle and the intervertebral foramen (angle between the transverse process and vertebral body), and also allows visualization of the articular process of the facet joint. Because the intervertebral foramen is located at the angle between the articular process of the facet joint and vertebral body, lumbar nerve roots can be depicted. The needle can be inserted laterally or medially to the transducer and advanced toward the posterior aspect of the psoas major muscle until either contact of the needle with the lumbar plexus is seen or an ipsilateral quadriceps muscle contraction is elicited.[6] Local anesthetic injection into the lumbar paravertebral area should be performed without excessive force because high injection pressure can lead to unwanted epidural spread and/or rapid intravascular injection.[8]

Recently, the "shamrock method" has become considered one of the standard approaches for US-guided LPB.[9–11] In this method, the transducer is placed transversely in the abdominal flank adjacent to the iliac crest (Figure 38–3a). A shape like a shamrock with three leaves can be seen with the psoas major muscle anteriorly, the erector spinae muscle posteriorly, and the quadratus lumborum muscle at the apex of the transverse process (Figure 38–3b). The lumber plexus can be identified as a hyperechoic oval structure in the posteromedial compartment of the psoas major muscle near the transverse process. By tilting the transducer caudally, the L3 transverse process disappears from the US image, which permits an in-plane posteroanterior

needle approach (Figure 38–3c). The needle insertion point is based on the landmark-guided method; that is, approximately 4 cm lateral to the midline[12] or at the junction of the lateral third and medial two-thirds of a line between the spinous process of L4 and a line parallel to the spinal column passing through the posterior superior iliac spine.[13] The needle insertion point can be decided by an ultrasonographical estimation of the distance from the bottom of the transducer to the posteromedial quadrant of the psoas major muscle, where the lumbar plexus is expected to locate.[10] Then, the needle is advanced anteriorly under US guidance until the needle tip reaches to the lumbar plexus or an appropriate muscle twitch is observed. In this view, the inferior vena cava and abdominal aorta can be seen simultaneously anterior to the vertebral body (Figure 38–3d).

The shamrock method has been reported to have several advantages over US-guided LPB using paramedian transverse scan.[9] First, the needle trajectory is almost the same as in the traditional landmark-guided LPB, which means that this method simply adds ultrasonographical information to the landmark-guided LPB approach. Second, needle can be advanced perpendicularly to the US beam, which allows for a clearer visualization of the needle.

LONGITUDINAL OUT-OF-PLANE AND IN-PLANE TECHNIQUES

In the parasagittal longitudinal US image, the acoustic shadow of the transverse process has a characteristic appearance, referred to as the "trident sign" (see Figure 38–1c, d).[14] Once the transverse processes are recognized at approximately 4 cm lateral and parallel to the lumbar spine, to produce a

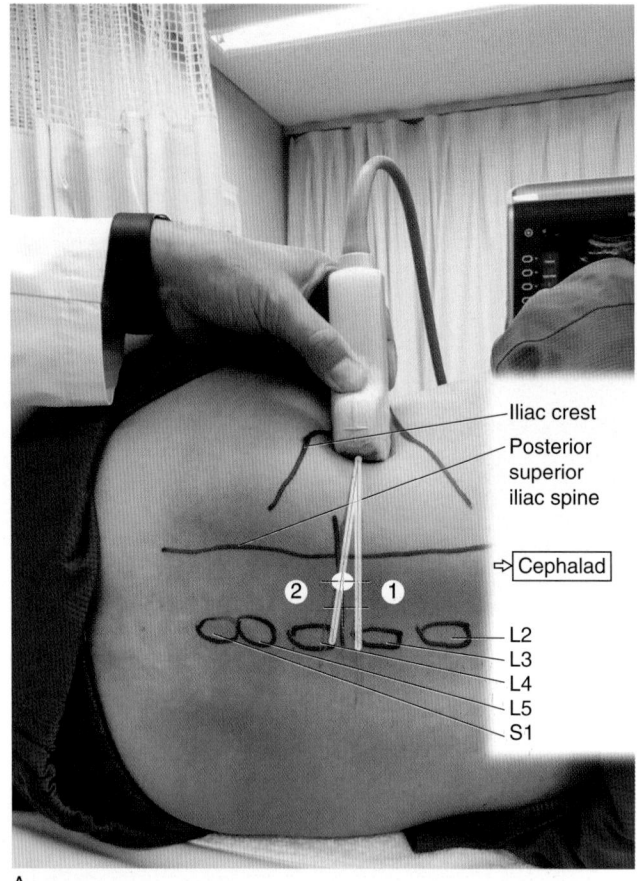

Iliac crest

Posterior superior iliac spine

Cephalad

L2
L3
L4
L5
S1

A

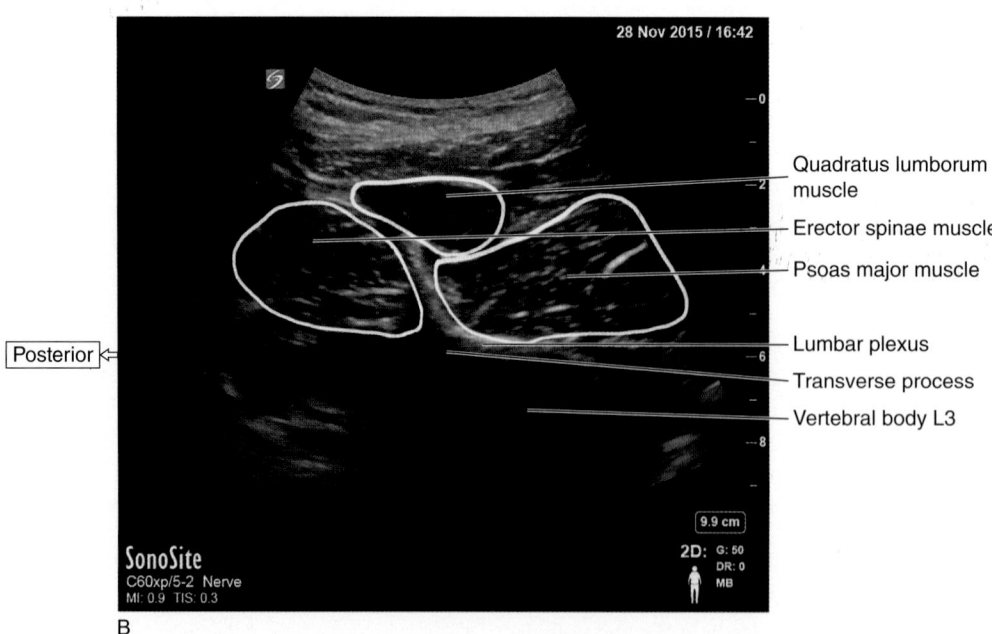

Quadratus lumborum muscle

Erector spinae muscle

Psoas major muscle

Lumbar plexus

Transverse process

Vertebral body L3

Posterior

B

FIGURE 38–3. (**A**) Transducer position and needle insertion point to accomplish US-guided lumbar plexus block with the shamrock method using an in-plane approach. The transducer is placed transversely in the left side of the abdominal flank adjacent to the iliac crest to image the "shamrock" with the transverse process (1). By tilting the transducer (2), the transverse process disappears from the US image, which permits an in-plane posteroanterior needle approach. (**B**) US anatomy of the right lumbar paravertebral region at the level of the L3 transverse process in the shamrock view. A shape that looks like a shamrock with three leaves consists of the erector spinae, quadratus lumborum, and psoas major muscles and the transverse process.

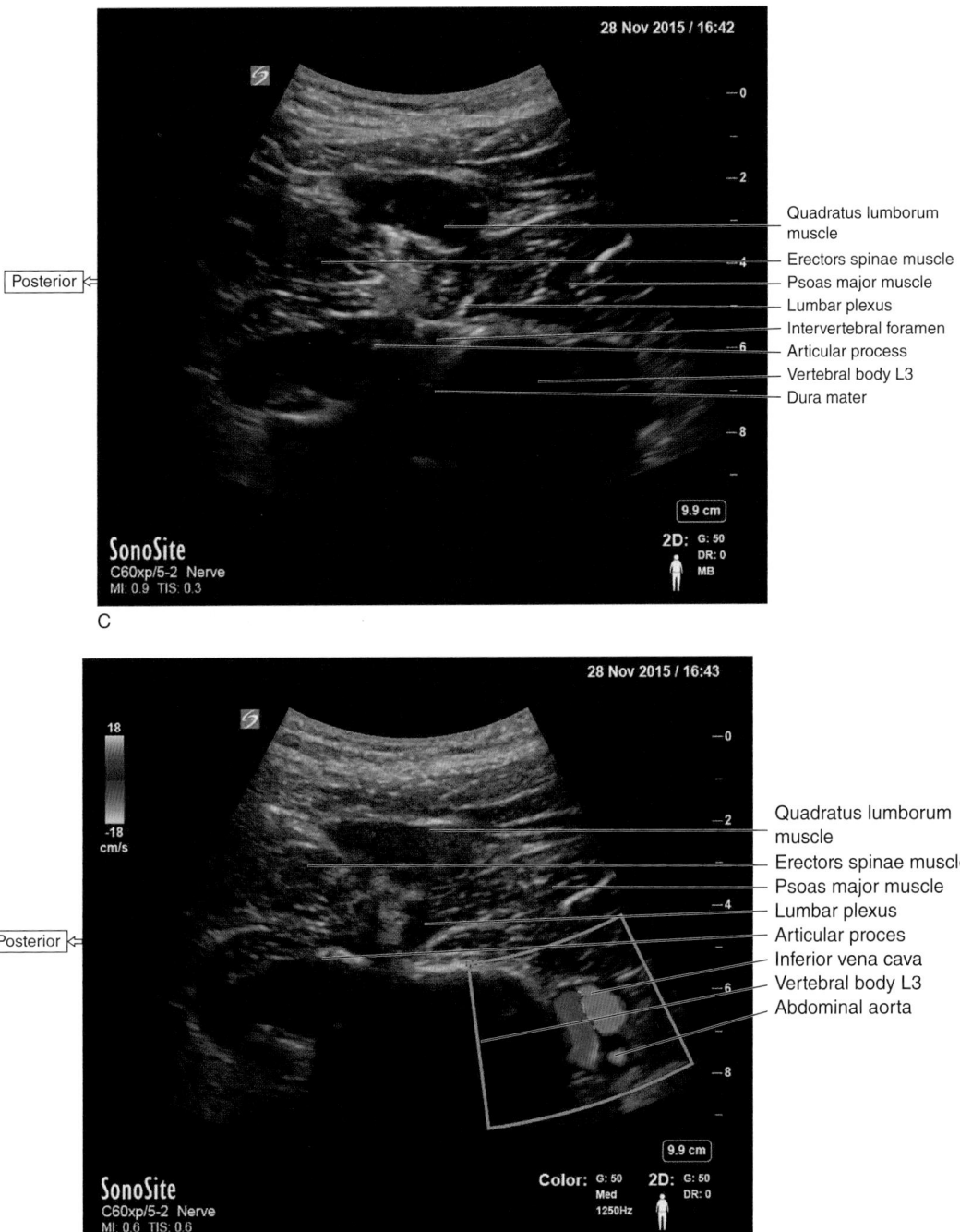

FIGURE 38–3. (*Continued*) (**C**) US anatomy of the right lumbar paravertebral region just caudal to the L3 transvers process (lumbar intertransverse space in the shamrock view). The lumbar plexus root is seen just lateral to the intervertebral foramen. The dura mater is confirmed as a hyperechoic line in the spinal canal through the intervertebral foramen. (**D**) The abdominal aorta and inferior vena cava are confirmed by color Doppler anterior to the vertebral body at the lumbar intertransverse space in the right-side shamrock view.

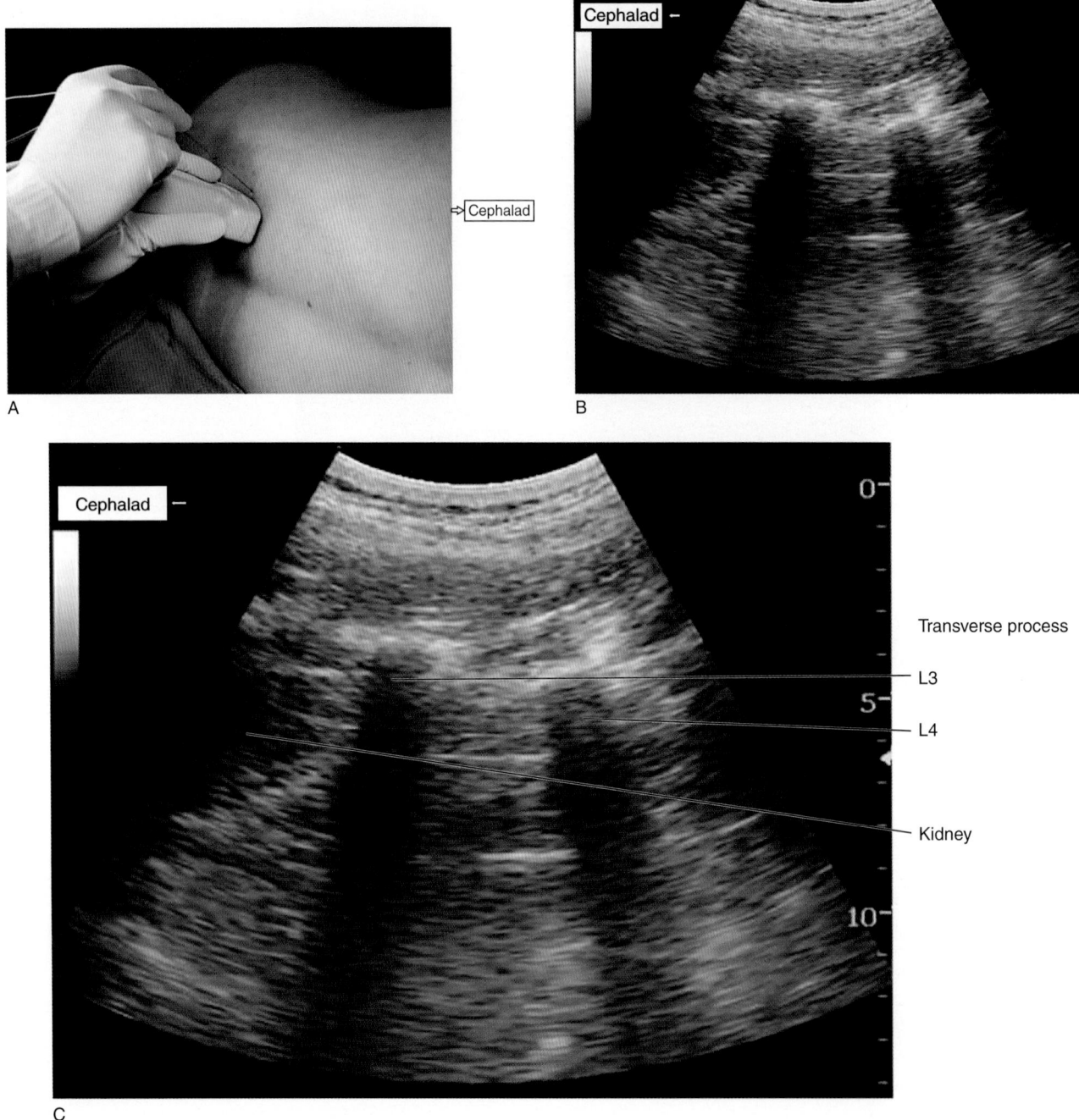

FIGURE 38–4. (**A**) Transducer position and needle insertion point to accomplish US-guided lumbar plexus block in the longitudinal parasagittal view using an out-of-plane approach. (**B**) US anatomy of the longitudinal lumbar paravertebral space at the L2–L3 and L3–L4 levels demonstrating the lower pole of the kidney on the left side of the image at a depth of approximately 5 cm. (**C**) Labeled US image of Figure 38–4b.

longitudinal scan of the lumbar paravertebral region (Figure 38–4a), the psoas major muscle is imaged through the acoustic window of the transverse processes. The psoas muscle appears as a combination of longitudinal hyperechoic striations within a typical hypoechoic muscle appearance just deep to the transverse processes (see Figure 38–1c, d). Some hyperechoic striations may appear particularly intense and may mislead the operator to interpret them as roots of the lumbar

plexus; therefore, the identification of the roots in a longitudinal scan is not reliable without nerve stimulation. This unreliability is partly because intramuscular connective tissues (eg, septa, tendons) within the psoas muscle are thick and may be indistinguishable from the nerve roots at such a deep location. As the transducer is moved progressively cephalad, the lower pole of the kidney often comes into view as low as the level of L2–L4 (Figure 38–4b, c). The goal of the technique

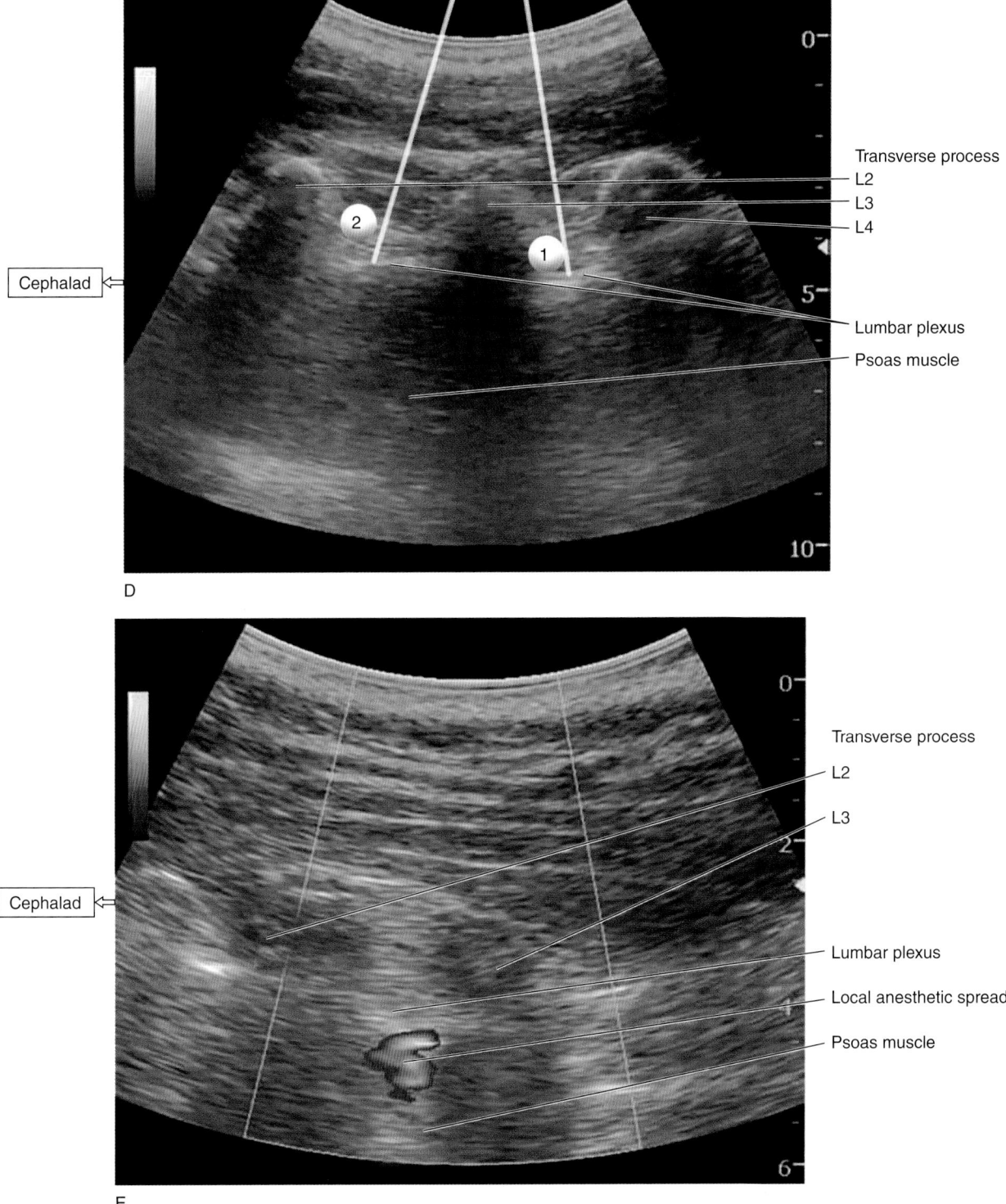

FIGURE 38–4. (*Continued*) (**D**) Simulated needle insertion paths (1, 2) to inject local anesthetic at two different levels to accomplish a lumbar plexus block using an out-of-plane technique. (**E**) Local anesthetic disposition during injection into the psoas muscle and the L2–L3 level. The spread of local anesthetic is often not well visualized using two-dimensional imaging.

is to guide the needle through the acoustic window between the transverse processes (between the "teeth" of the "trident") of L3–L4 or L2–L3 into the posterior part of the psoas major muscle containing the roots of the lumbar plexus. Both out-of-plane (see Figure 38–4a) and in-plane approaches can be employed with the parasagittal longitudinal technique. After obtaining ipsilateral quadriceps muscle contractions, local anesthetic is injected (Figures 38–4d) with a real-time visualization of the injection into the posterior part of the psoas major muscle (Figure 38–4e).

REFERENCES

1. Sauter AR, Ullensvang K, Niemi G, et al: The Shamrock lumbar plexus block: a dose-finding study. Eur J Anaesthesiol 2015;32:764–770.
2. Doi K, Sakura S, Hara K: A modified posterior approach to lumbar plexus block using a transverse ultrasound image and an approach from the lateral border of the transducer. Anaesth Intensive Care 2010;38:213–214.
3. Ilfeld BM, Loland VJ, Mariano ER: Prepuncture ultrasound imaging to predict transverse process and lumbar plexus depth for psoas compartment block and perineural catheter insertion: a prospective, observational study. Anesth Analg 2010;110:1725–1728.
4. Weller RS, Gerancher JC, Crews JC, Wade KL: Extensive retroperitoneal hematoma without neurologic deficit in two patients who underwent lumbar plexus block and were later anticoagulated. Anesthesiology 2003;98:581–585.
5. Narouze S, Benzon HT, Provenzano DA, et al: Interventional spine and pain procedures in patients on antiplatelet and anticoagulant medications: guidelines from the American Society of Regional Anesthesia and Pain Medicine, the European Society of Regional Anaesthesia and Pain Therapy, the American Academy of Pain Medicine, the International Neuromodulation Society, the North American Neuromodulation Society, and the World Institute of Pain. Reg Anesth Pain Med 2015;40:182–212.
6. Karmakar MK, Li JW, Kwok WH, Hadzic A: Ultrasound-guided lumbar plexus block using a transverse scan through the lumbar intertransverse space: a prospective case series. Reg Anesth Pain Med 2015;40:75–81.
7. Karmakar MK, Li JW, Kwok WH, Soh E, Hadzic A: Sonoanatomy relevant for lumbar plexus block in volunteers correlated with cross-sectional anatomic and magnetic resonance images. Reg Anesth Pain Med 2013;38:391–397.
8. Gadsden JC, Lindenmuth DM, Hadzic A, Xu D, Somasundarum L, Flisinski KA: Lumbar plexus block using high-pressure injection leads to contralateral and epidural spread. Anesthesiology 2008;109:683–688.
9. Lin JA, Lu HT, Chen TL: Ultrasound standard for lumbar plexus block. Br J Anaesth 2014;113:188–189.
10. Lin JA, Lu HT: Solution to the challenging part of the Shamrock method during lumbar plexus block. Br J Anaesth 2014;113:516–517.
11. Lin JA, Lee YJ, Lu HT: Finding the bulging edge: a modified shamrock lumbar plexus block in average-weight patients. Br J Anaesth 2014;113:718–720.
12. Parkinson SK, Mueller JB, Little WL, Bailey SL: Extent of blockade with various approaches to the lumbar plexus. Anesth Analg 1989;68:243–248.
13. Capdevila X, Macaire P, Dadure C, et al: Continuous psoas compartment block for postoperative analgesia after total hip arthroplasty: new landmarks, technical guidelines, and clinical evaluation. Anesth Analg 2002;94:1606–1613, table of contents.
14. Karmakar MK, Ho AM, Li X, Kwok WH, Tsang K, Ngan Kee WD: Ultrasound-guided lumbar plexus block through the acoustic window of the lumbar ultrasound trident. Br J Anaesth 2008;100:533–537.

CHAPTER 39

Lumbar Paravertebral Sonography and Considerations for Ultrasound-Guided Lumbar Plexus Block

Manoj K. Karmakar

INTRODUCTION

Lumbar plexus block (LPB) produces anesthesia of the major components of the ipsilateral lumbar plexus, the femoral nerve (FN), lateral femoral cutaneous nerve (LFCN), and the obturator nerve (OBN)[1] LPB is used as a sole technique[2–4] or in combination with a sciatic nerve[5] block for anesthesia or analgesia in patients having hip[2–4] or lower extremity surgery.[2] It is also referred to as psoas compartment block (PCB)[2,6,7] or posterior lumbar plexus block (PLB).[3,7] The term PCB was originally coined by Chayen and colleagues.[6] They believed that branches of the lumbar plexus and parts of the sacral plexus were located close to each other in a "compartment" between the psoas major and quadratus lumborum muscles at the level of the L4 vertebra[6] and could be identified using "loss of resistance."[6] However, the lumbar plexus is located within the substance of the psoas muscle[8–11] and local anesthetic is injected into a fascial plane within the posterior aspect of the psoas muscle during an LPB.[9,10]

LPB is traditionally performed using surface anatomical landmarks and peripheral nerve stimulation.[12] The main challenges with accomplishing LPB with anatomical landmarks and peripheral nerve stimulation relate to the depth at which the lumbar plexus is located.[13] Small errors in estimation of landmark or angle of needle insertion can lead to the block needle being directed away from the plexus, resulting in inadvertent deep needle insertion or renal[12,14] or vascular injury.[12,14–16] Therefore, real-time monitoring of the needle and local anesthetic injection during an LPB is desirable and may improve the accuracy and safety of the technique. While fluoroscopy and computed tomography can be used to improve precision during an LPB, they are impractical in a busy operating room environment, costly, and, more importantly, associated with exposure to radiation. Ultrasound (US) is increasingly being used to guide peripheral nerve blocks, and it is only logical that ultrasound-guided (USG) LPB is of interest because of the ever-increasing availability of US machines, which produce high-quality images, in the operating room. US has been used to preview the relevant anatomy,[7,9,10,13,17] measure the depth to the transverse process, guide the block needle to the posterior aspect of the psoas muscle or the lumbar plexus in real time,[10,13,17–19] and monitor needle–nerve contact[10] or spread of local anesthetic[10,17,19] during an LPB. Understanding of the sonoanatomy of the lumbar paravertebral region is a prerequisite to using US for LPB. This chapter briefly describes the techniques used to perform lumbar paravertebral sonography, the relevant sonoanatomy, and the practical considerations for using US for LPB.

GROSS ANATOMY

The lumbar plexus is formed by the union of the anterior primary rami of L1, L2, and L3 and the greater part of L4 (Figure 39–1) within the substance of the psoas muscle (Figures 39–2, 39–3, 39–4, and 39–5).[8] It also receives variable contribution from T12 (subcostal nerve) and L5 (see Figure 39–1). The lumbar plexus is located in an intramuscular fascial plane or "compartment," also referred to as the psoas compartment, within the posterior one-third of the psoas muscle (Figure 39–6)[8,9] and is very closely related to the lumbar

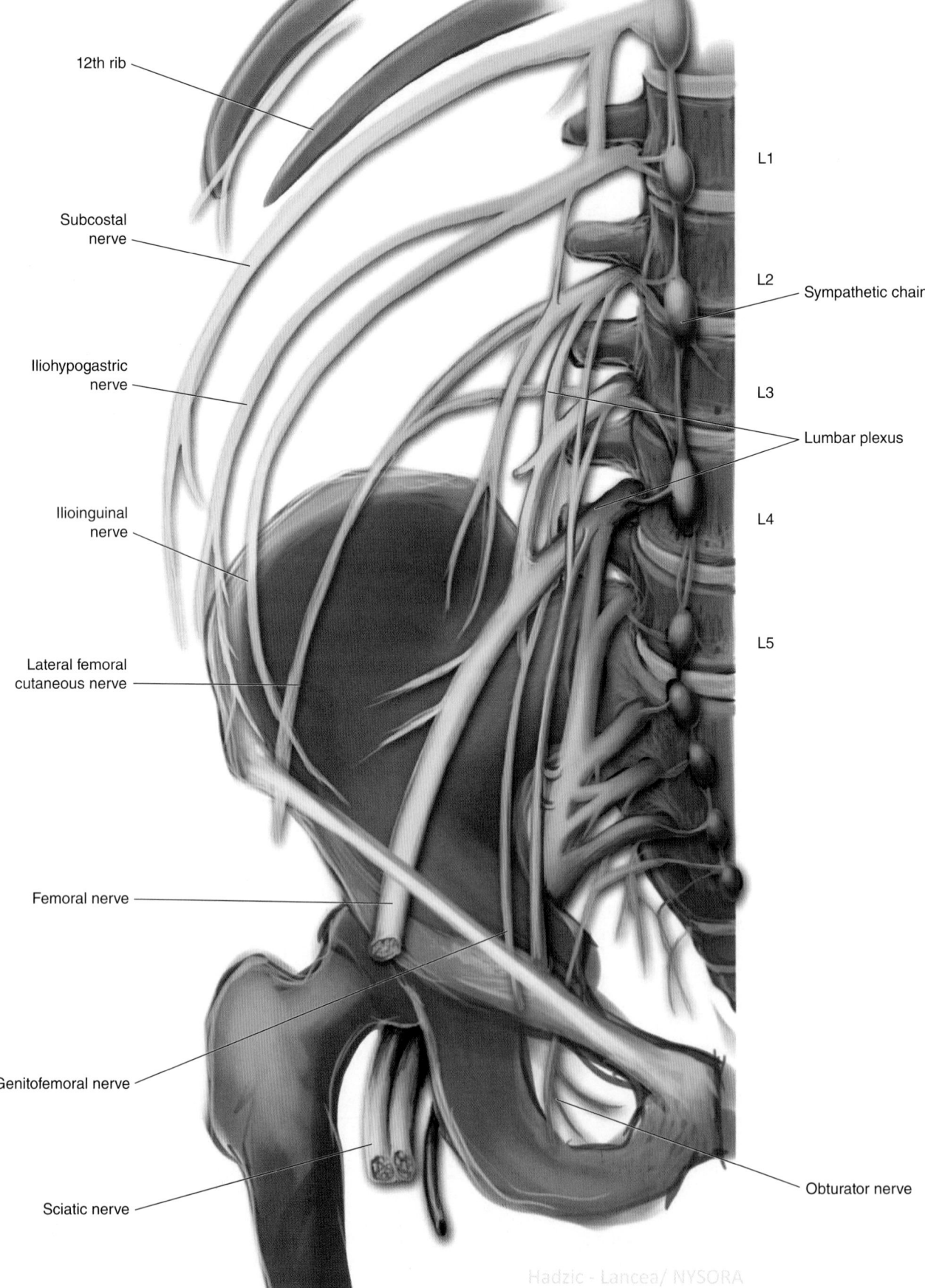

FIGURE 39–1. Lumbar plexus and its three major components: the lateral femoral cutaneous, obturator, and femoral nerves. Note the close anatomical relation of the lumbar plexus to the transverse processes of the vertebra and the lumbar sympathetic chain.

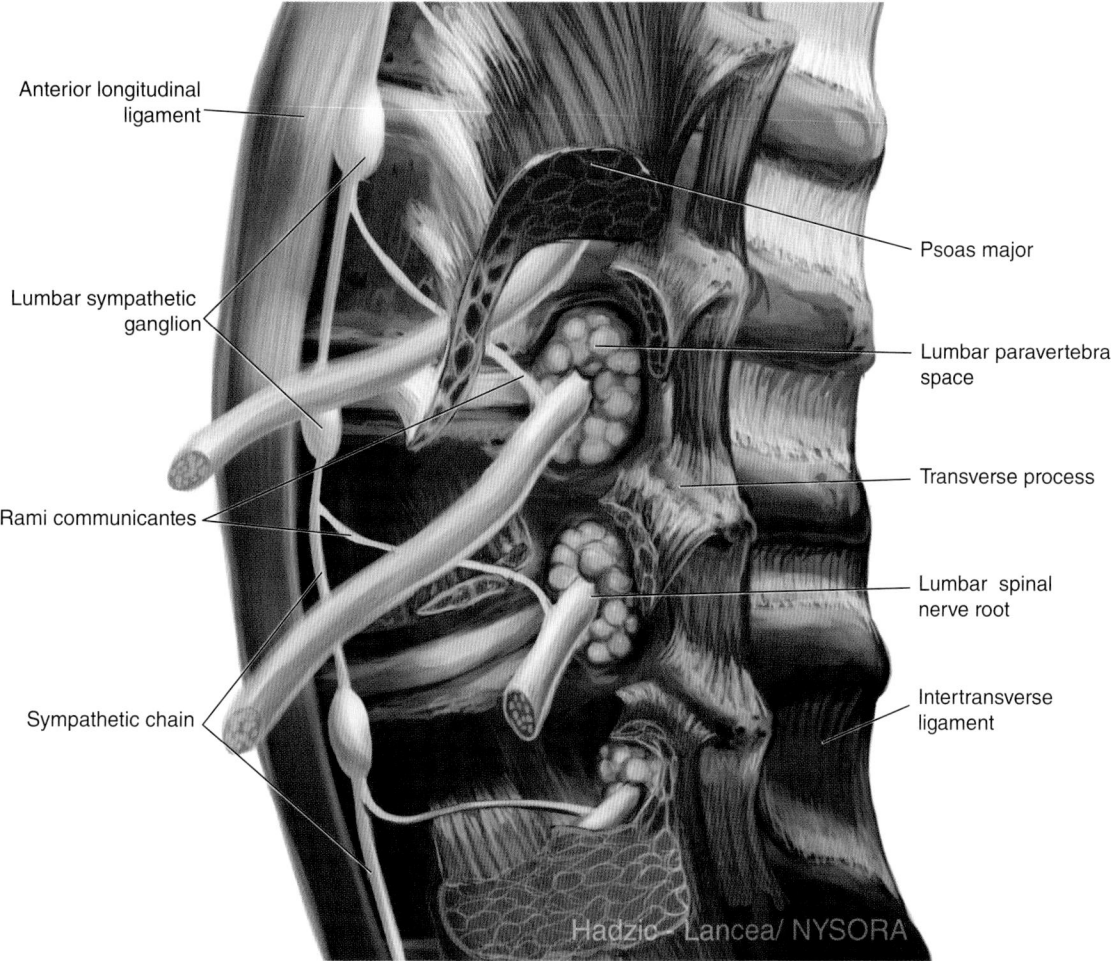

Anterior longitudinal ligament

Lumbar sympathetic ganglion

Rami communicantes

Sympathetic chain

Psoas major

Lumbar paravertebral space

Transverse process

Lumbar spinal nerve root

Intertransverse ligament

Hadzic Lancea/ NYSORA

FIGURE 39–2. Location of the lumbar nerve roots within the substance of the psoas muscle and its relation to the transverse process of the lumbar vertebrae. Also note the formation of the lumbar paravertebral space between the larger (fleshy) anterior part of the psoas muscle, which originates from the anterolateral surface of the vertebral body, and the thinner (accessory) posterior part of the muscle, which originates from the anterior aspect of the transverse processes.

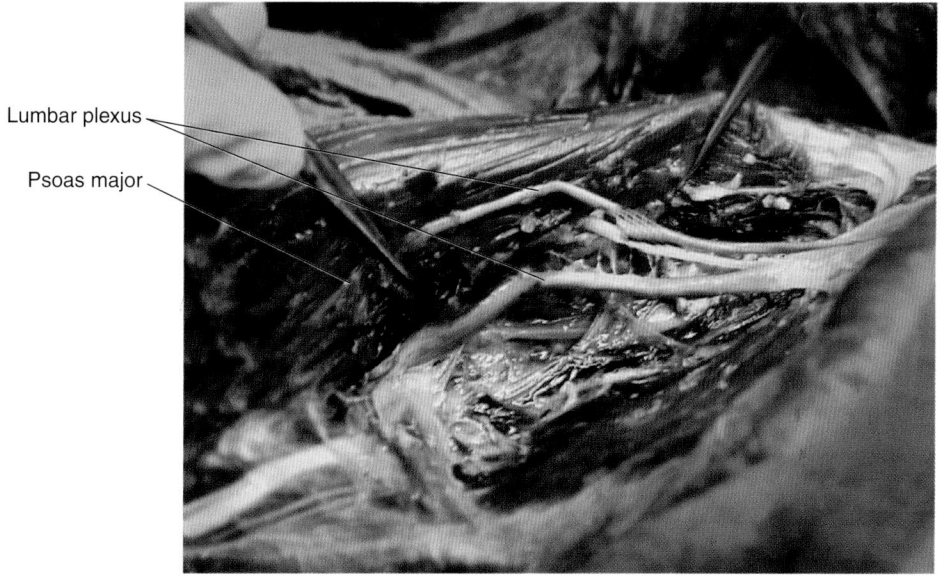

Lumbar plexus

Psoas major

FIGURE 39–3. Human cadaver dissection image showing the lumbar plexus nerves within the substance of the psoas muscle. The psoas muscle has been split longitudinally to expose the lumbar plexus nerves within the posterior aspect of the muscle.

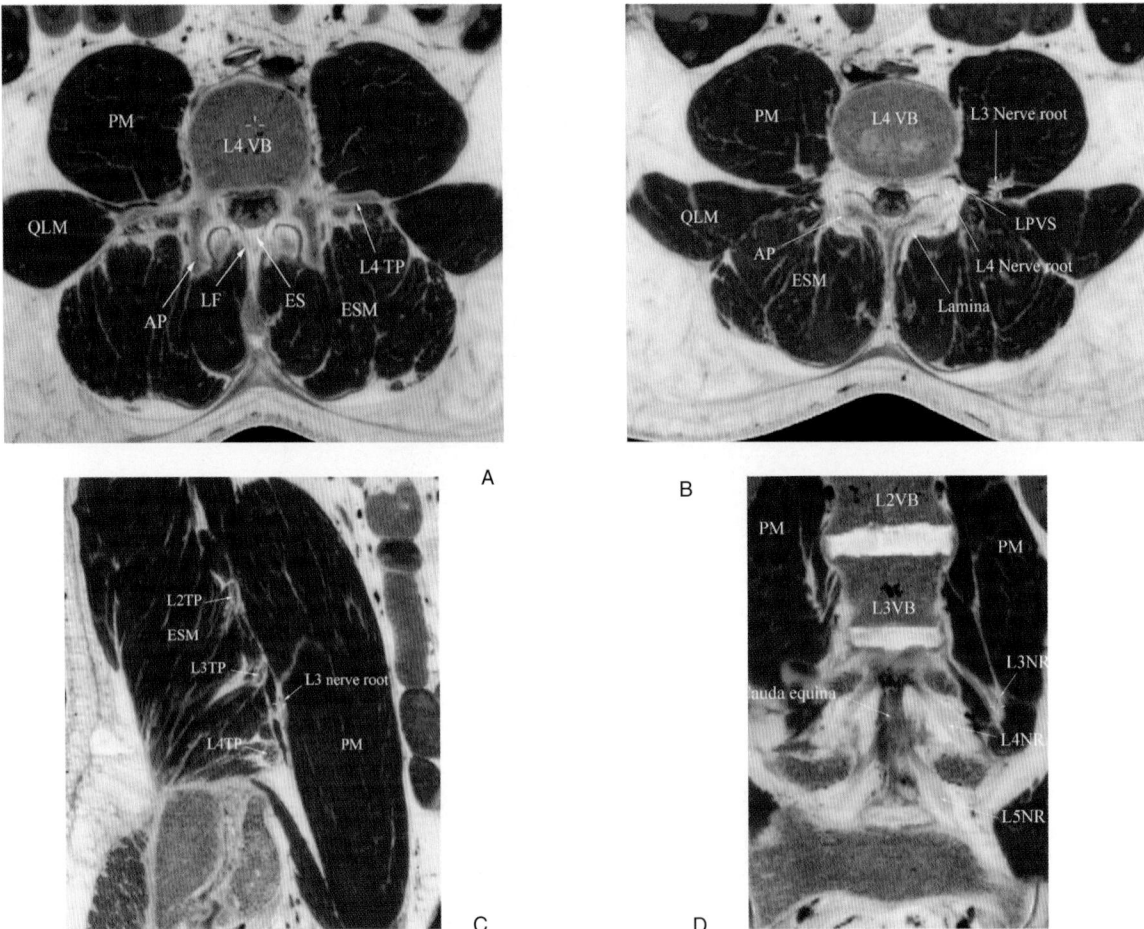

FIGURE 39–4. Multiplanar cadaver anatomical sections showing the anatomical relation of the lumbar nerve root and lumbar plexus to the psoas muscle (PM). (**A**) Cross-section through the L4 vertebral body and transverse process, corresponding to the level at which the paramedian transverse oblique scan at the level of the transverse process (PMOTS-TP) is performed. (**B**) Cross-sectional cadaver anatomical section from just inferior to the L4 transverse process and through the lower part of the L4 vertebral body, corresponding to the level at which the paramedian transverse oblique scan through the intertransverse space and at the level of the articular process (PMOTS-AP) is performed. (**C**) Sagittal cadaver anatomical section showing the relation of the lumbar plexus to the transverse process (TP) and PM. (**D**) Coronal cadaver anatomical section showing how the lumbar nerve roots, after they exit the intervertebral foramen, take a steep caudal course and enter the substance of the PM more caudally. The "reference-marker" of the Java application is seen as a "green cross-hair," which represents the same anatomical point in the multiplanar cadaver anatomical sections. AP, articular process; ES, epidural space; ESM, erector spinae muscle; LF, ligamentum flavum; LPVS, lumbar paravertebral space; NR, nerve root; QLM, quadratus lumborum muscle; TP, transverse process; VB, vertebral body.

transverse processes. The larger anterior (fleshy) part of the psoas muscle originates from the anterolateral surface of the vertebral body and the intervertebral disc, while the thinner posterior (accessory) part of the psoas muscle originates from the anterior aspect of the transverse processes[8] (see Figure 39–2). The two parts of the muscle fuse to form the main bulk of the psoas muscle, but close to the vertebral bodies, they are separated by a fascia or space (see Figure 39–2)[8,9] that contains the lumbar nerve root, branches of the lumbar artery (Figures 39–6 and 39–7), and the ascending lumbar vein.[8,9] This wedge-shaped space close to the intervertebral foramen is called the lumbar paravertebral space (LPVS) (see Figures 39–4, 39–5, and 39–6).[9] After it exits the intervertebral foramen, the lumbar nerve root enters the LPVS (see Figures 39–4, 39–5, and 39–6),[9] after which, instead of entering the psoas muscle at the same vertebral level, it takes a steep caudal course (see

Figures 39–4, 39–5, and 39–6) and enters the psoas compartment at the vertebral level below (see Figures 39–4, 39–5, and 39–6). This explains why the L3 contribution to the lumbar plexus lies opposite the L4 intervertebral foramen and the L4 nerve root (see Figures 39–4 and 39–5). It is not known if the LPVS is continuous with the psoas compartment at the same vertebral level, but the occurrence of epidural spread after a lumbar plexus block[20] suggests that it is. Once the plexus is formed, it is visualized as a triangular shape, narrow cranially and wider at its caudal portion (see Figure 39–5).[8] The nerves that originate from the plexus also exhibit a fanned-out distribution, with the LFC being outermost, the OBN innermost, and the FN in between.[8] The positions of the LFC and FN within the psoas compartment are relatively consistent,[8] but the position of the OBN is variable and may even lie in a fold of the psoas muscle separate from that enclosing the other two

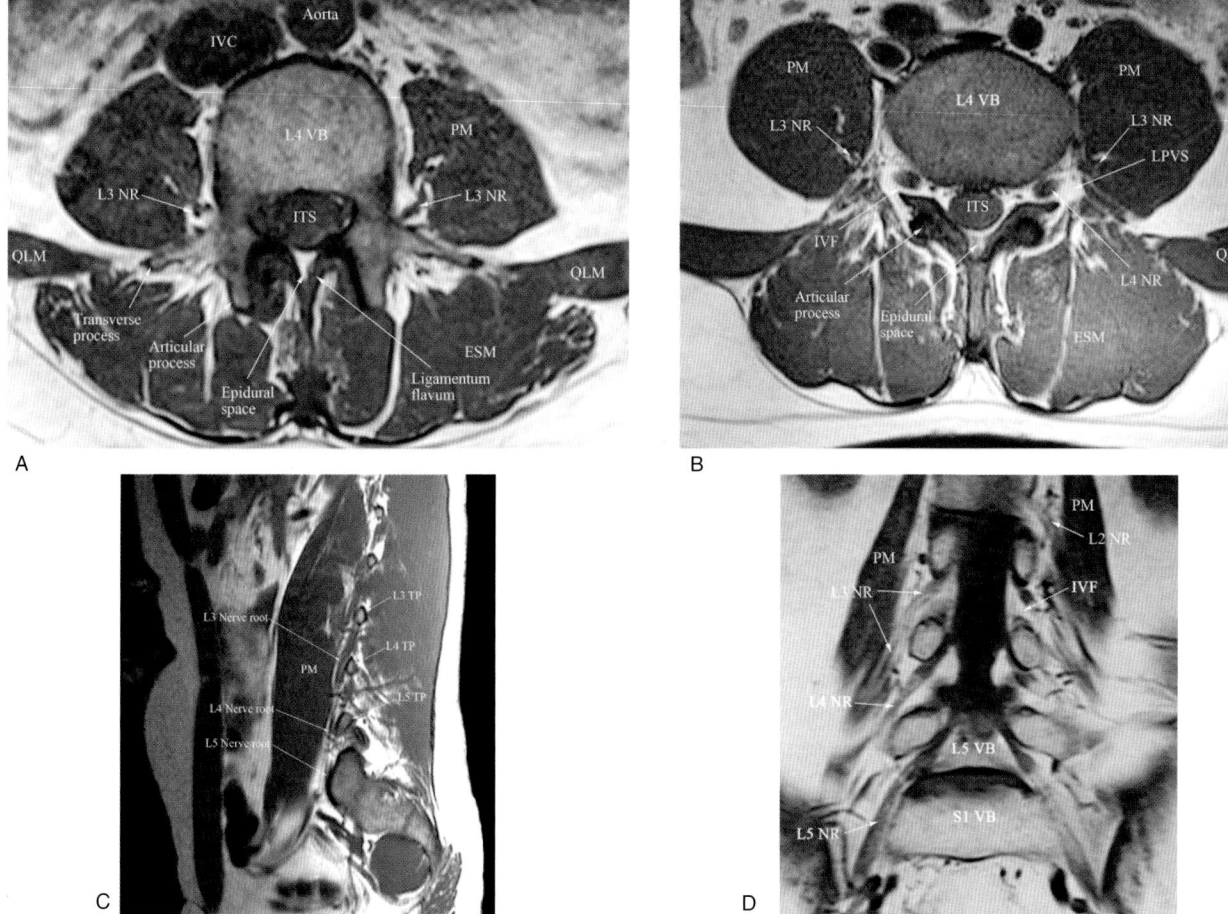

FIGURE 39–5. Multiplanar T1-weighted magnetic resonance imaging (MRI) images showing the anatomical relation of the lumbar nerve root and lumbar plexus to the psoas muscle (PM). (**A**) Transverse view at the level of the L4 vertebral body and the transverse process, corresponding to the level at which the paramedian transverse oblique scan at the level of the transverse process (PMOTS-TP) is performed. (**B**) Transverse view from just below the L4 transverse process and through the lower half of the body of the L4 vertebra and the articular process (inferior), corresponding to the level at which the paramedian transverse oblique scan at the level of the articular process (PMOTS-AP) is performed. Note the hypointense L4 nerve root as it exits the intervertebral foramen (IVF) and enters the hyperintense fat-filled lumbar paravertebral space (LPVS). Also seen in the posterior aspect of the psoas muscle is the L3 nerve of the lumbar plexus, which is surrounded by a layer or hyperintense fat and situated within an intramuscular compartment (the "psoas compartment"). (**C**) Sagittal view of the lumbar paravertebral region at the L3–L5 vertebral level showing the steep caudal course of the lumbar nerve roots. (**D**) Coronal view at the L3–L5 vertebral level showing the steep caudal course of the lumbar spinal nerves after they emerge from the IVF. ESM, erector spinae muscle; ITS, intrathecal space; IVC, inferior vena cava; LPVS, lumbar paravertebral space; NR, nerve root; QLM, quadratus lumborum muscle; VB, vertebral body.

nerves (Figure 39–8).[8] The depth from the skin to the lumbar plexus also varies with gender and body mass index (BMI).

SONOANATOMY FOR LUMBAR PLEXUS BLOCK

General Considerations

The depth of the lumbar plexus necessitates the use of low-frequency US (5–10 MHz) and curved array transducers to image the lumbar paravertebral anatomy. Low-frequency US provides good penetration but lacks spatial resolution at the depths (5–9 cm) at which the anatomy relevant for LPB is located. The lack of spatial resolution often compromises the ability to locate the lumbar plexus nerves within the psoas muscle. However, recent improvements in US technology, the image processing capabilities of US machines, the availability of

compound imaging and tissue harmonic imaging (THI), and the use of new US scan protocols[9,10,19,20] have all contributed to improved imaging of the lumbar paravertebral region.

Ultrasound Scan Techniques

Ultrasound scan for LPB can be performed in the transverse[7,10,13,18,19] or sagittal[17] axis (Figures 39–9 and 39–10) and with the patient in the lateral,[10,17–19,21] sitting, or prone[22] position. A disadvantage of performing LPB with the patient in the prone position is that this position impairs visualization of the quadriceps muscle contraction that is used as an end point for needle placement. The author prefers to perform the US scan with the patient in the lateral decubitus position with the side to be blocked uppermost (see Figure 39–9).[10,17] The following anatomical landmarks are identified and marked on the

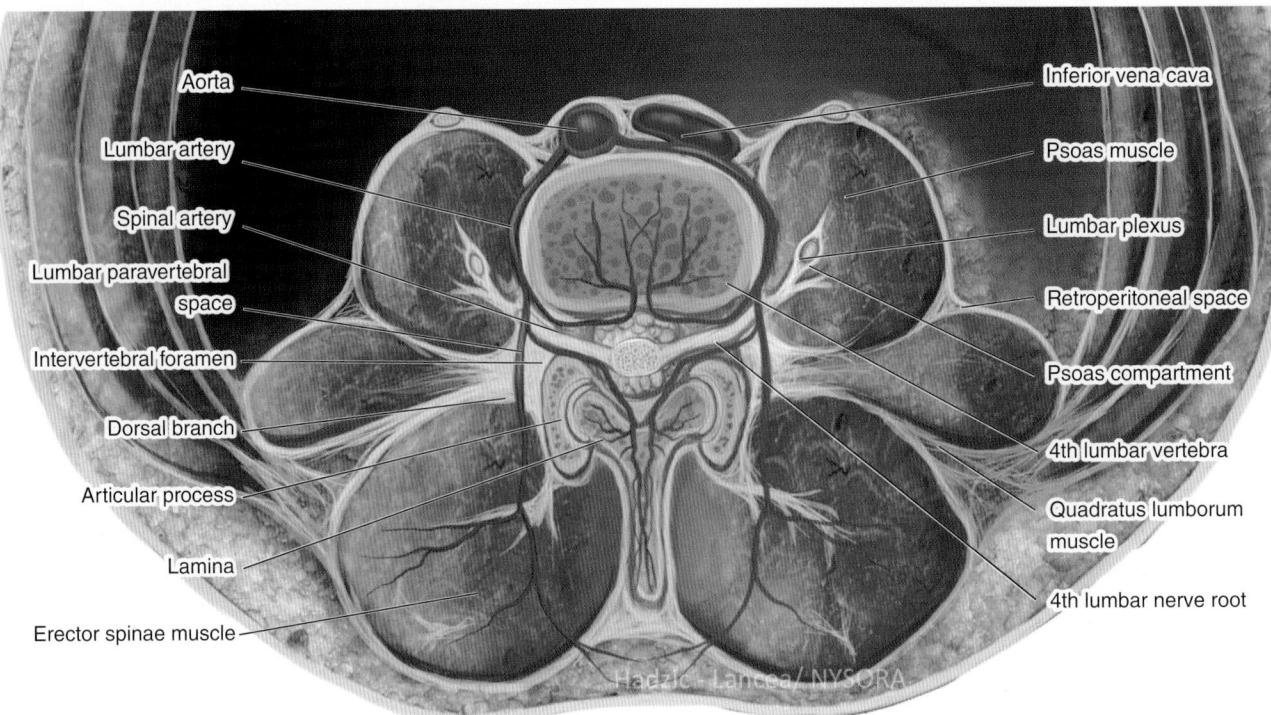

Aorta
Lumbar artery
Spinal artery
Lumbar paravertebral space
Intervertebral foramen
Dorsal branch
Articular process
Lamina
Erector spinae muscle

Inferior vena cava
Psoas muscle
Lumbar plexus
Retroperitoneal space
Psoas compartment
4th lumbar vertebra
Quadratus lumborum muscle
4th lumbar nerve root

FIGURE 39–6. Transverse anatomy of the lumbar paravertebral region at the L4 vertebral level. Note the origin and branching of the lumbar artery.

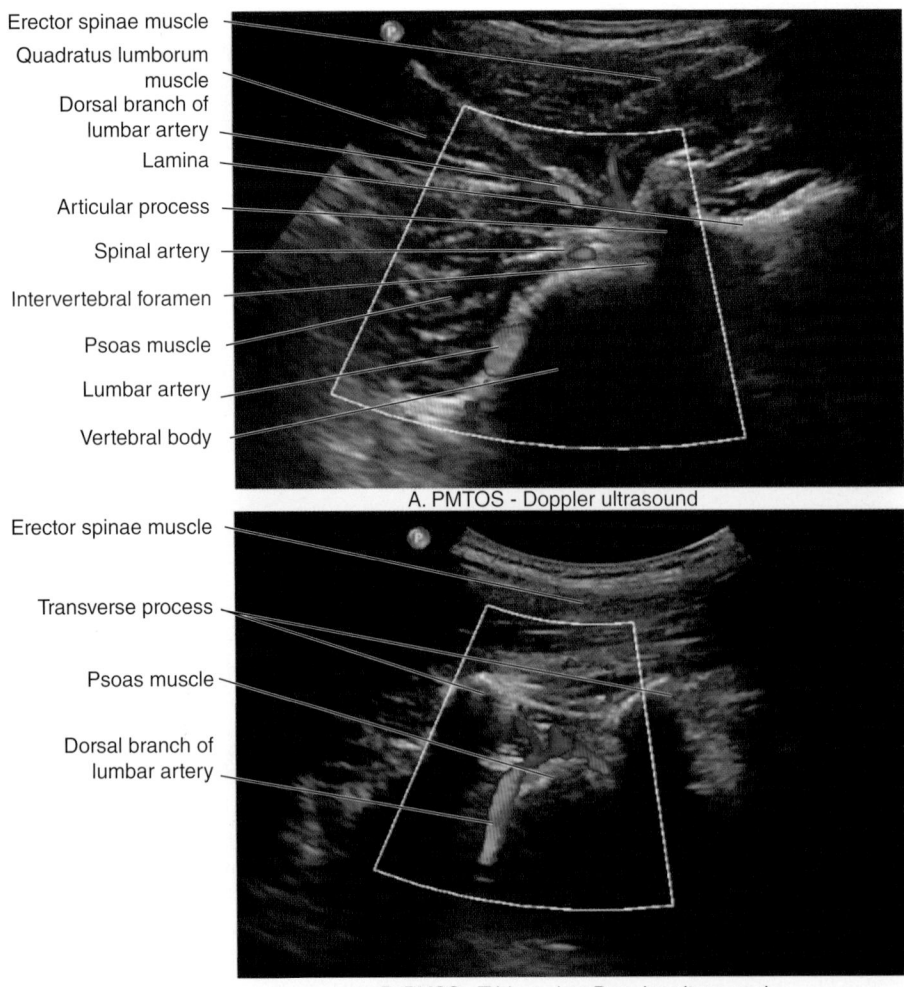

Erector spinae muscle
Quadratus lumborum muscle
Dorsal branch of lumbar artery
Lamina
Articular process
Spinal artery
Intervertebral foramen
Psoas muscle
Lumbar artery
Vertebral body

A. PMTOS - Doppler ultrasound

Erector spinae muscle
Transverse process
Psoas muscle
Dorsal branch of lumbar artery

B. PMSS - Trident view Doppler ultrasound

FIGURE 39–7. Color Doppler US images of the lumbar paravertebral region in the (**A**) transverse and (**B**) sagittal scan planes. Note the dorsal branch of the lumbar artery on the posterior aspect of the psoas muscle in both the transverse and sagittal sonograms and the spinal artery in the transverse sonogram. PMSS, paramedian sagittal scan; PMTOS, paramedian transverse oblique scan.

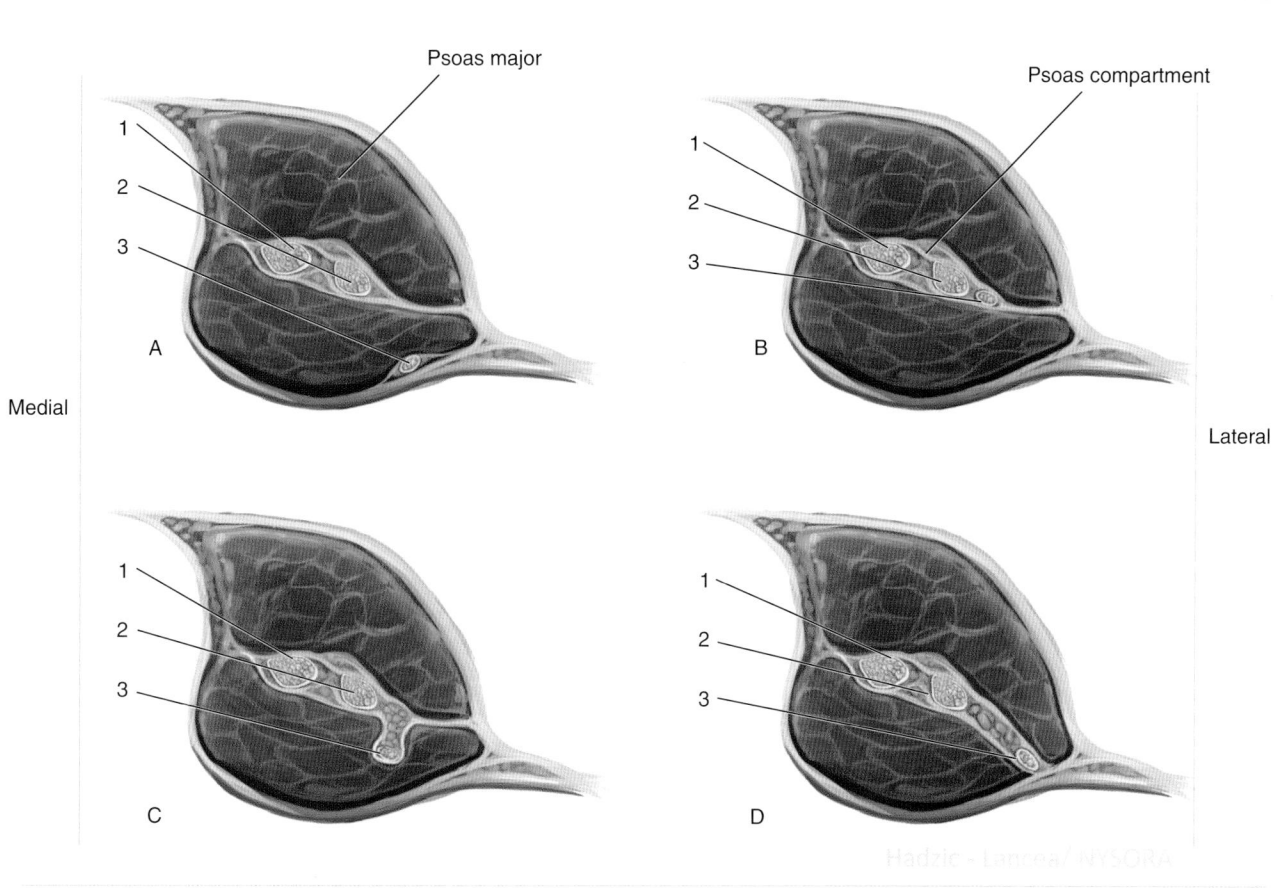

FIGURE 39–8. Position of the (1) lateral femoral cutaneous nerve; (2) femoral nerve; and (3) obturator nerve in the psoas compartment. Note that while the positions of 1 and 2 are fairly consistent, the position of 3 can vary and may even lie in a separate intramuscular fold (c) or compartment separate from the psoas compartment.

skin of the nondependent side of the back: the posterior superior iliac spine, iliac crest, lumbar spinous processes (midline; see Figure 39–9) and intercristal line (see Figure 39–9). Thereafter, a line parallel to the midline, which intersects the intercristal line at a point 4 cm lateral to the midline (paramedian), corresponding to the point at which the block needle is inserted during a landmark-based LPB, is also marked (sagittal scan line; see Figure 39–9). The target vertebral level for the US scan (L3/4/5) is then identified as previously described.[23,24] This involves visualizing the lumbosacral junction (L5–S1 gap) on a sagittal sonogram and then counting cranially to locate the lamina and transverse processes of the L3, L4, and L5 vertebrae.[23,24]

A liberal amount of ultrasound gel is applied to the skin over the lumbar paravertebral region for acoustic coupling. To simplify image orientation, irrespective of the side imaged, the orientation marker of the US transducer is directed cranially during a sagittal scan and laterally (outward) during a transverse scan. For a sagittal scan (Figures 39–9, 39–10, 39–11, and 39–12), the US transducer is positioned over the sagittal scan line (see Figure 39–9a) with its orientation marker directed cranially. For a transverse scan (Figures 39–9, 39–10, 39–13, and 39–14), the US transducer is positioned 4 cm laterally to

the midline along the intercristal line and just above the iliac crest (see Figure 39–9b). The transducer is also directed slightly medially (paramedian transverse oblique scan [PMTOS]; see Figure 39–9b) so as to produce a transverse oblique view of the lumbar paravertebral region (see Figures 39–13 and 39–14).[9] During a PMTOS, the US beam can be insonated either at the level of the transverse process (PMTOS-TP; see Figures 39–10b and 39–13) or through the intertransverse space at the level of the articular process (PMTOS-AP: see Figures 39–10c and 39–14).[9,10] Alternatively, a transverse scan can be performed by placing the US transducer more anteriorly in the flank and above the iliac crest (Figures 39–15, 39–16, 39–17, 39–18, and 39–19), as described by Sauter and colleagues with the "shamrock method."[19]

Sagittal Sonoanatomy

On a sagittal sonogram, the lumbar transverse processes are identified by their hyperechoic reflection and an anterior acoustic shadow (see Figures 39–11 and 39–12), which is typical of bone. The acoustic shadow of the transverse processes produces a sonographic pattern referred to as the "trident sign"[17,25] (see Figures 39–11 and 39–12) because of its similarity in shape to

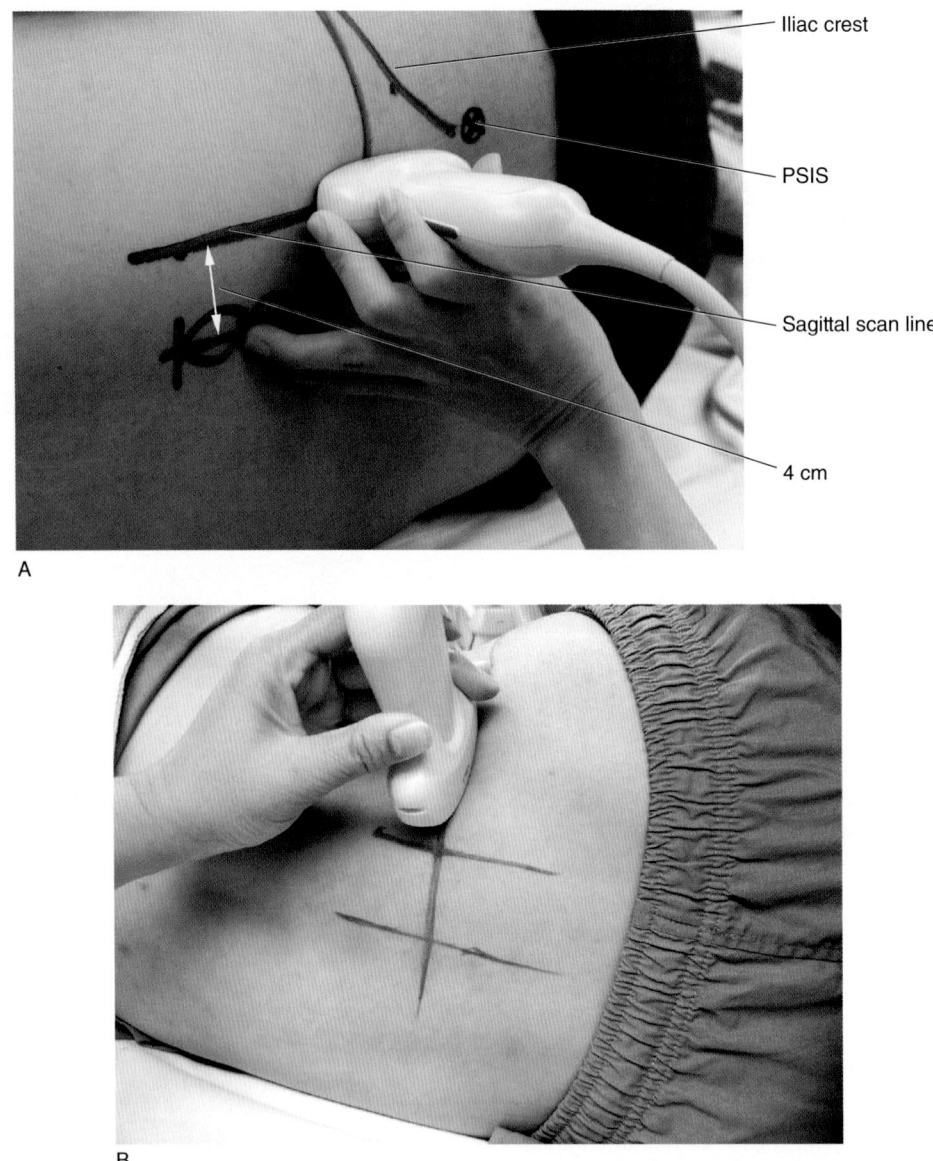

FIGURE 39–9. Position of the patient and US transducer during (**A**) a paramedian sagittal (PMSS) and (**B**) a paramedian transverse oblique (PMTOS) scan of the lumbar paravertebral region. For the PMSS, the US transducer is placed over the "sagittal scan" line, which is a line 4 cm lateral and parallel to the midline (paramedian), at the level of the iliac crest. For the PMTOS, the US transducer is placed laterally to the sagittal scan line and over the intercristal line. Note how the transducer is angled medially for the PMTOS. PSIS, posterior superior iliac spine.

a trident (in Latin, *tridens* or *tridentis*). The psoas muscle is visualized through the acoustic window (see Figures 39–11 and 39–12) of the trident as multiple longitudinal hyperechoic striations against a hypoechoic background typical of muscle (see Figure 39–11). The lumbar plexus nerves are seen as longitudinal hyperechoic structures in the posterior aspect of the psoas muscle (see Figure 39–11) One should note that not all hyperechoic shadows or striations within the psoas muscle are nerves because the psoas muscle contains intramuscular tendons, which also produce hyperechoic shadows (Figure 39–20). Nevertheless, the nerves of the lumbar plexus can be differentiated from the intramuscular tendons as they are thicker than the muscle fibers, take an oblique course through the psoas muscle (see Figure 39–11), and are better visualized after local anesthetic injection.[17] A laterally positioned US transducer will produce a "suboptimal" sagittal sonogram without the US "trident," but with the lower pole of the kidney, which lies anterior to the quadratus lumborum muscle and can reach the L3–L4 level in some patients.

Transverse Sonoanatomy

Kirchmair and colleagues were the first to describe the detailed transverse sonoanatomy of the lumbar paravertebral region relevant for LPB.[7] However, they were unable to delineate the lumbar plexus in the cadavers and volunteers they examined, which they attributed to a loss of spatial resolution due to the use of low-frequency US.[7] The author's group has recently demonstrated that it is possible to accurately delineate the lumbar nerve root, lumbar paravertebral space, lumbar plexus, and

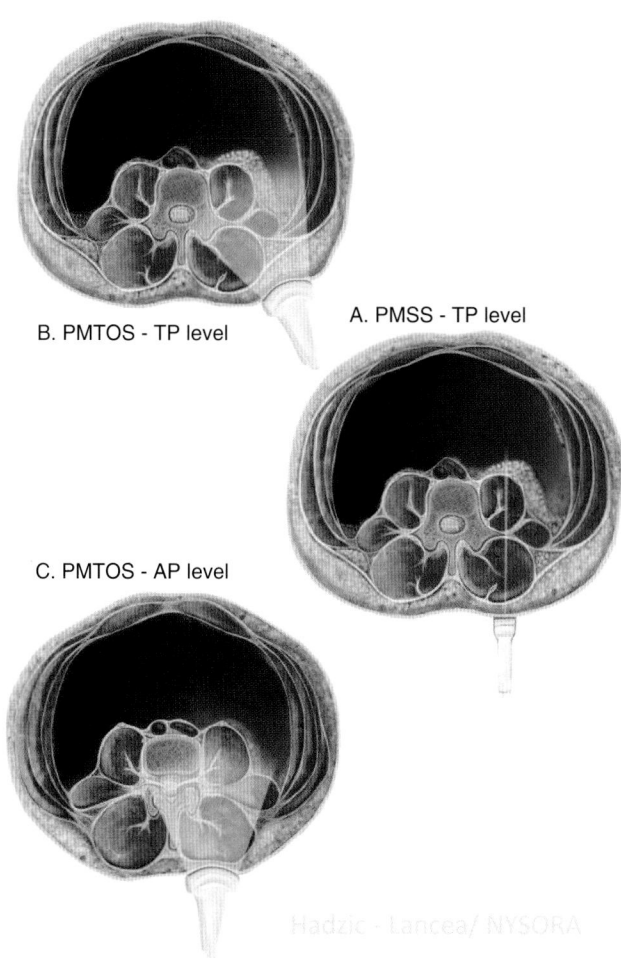

B. PMTOS - TP level

A. PMSS - TP level

C. PMTOS - AP level

FIGURE 39–10. Plane of US imaging during a sagittal and transverse scan of the lumbar paravertebral region for lumbar plexus block. An image of a US transducer and the plane of the US beam has been superimposed onto transverse anatomical sections of the lumbar paravertebral region to illustrate how the US beam is insonated during (**A**) paramedian sagittal scan at the level of the transverse process (PMSS-TP); (**B**) paramedian transverse oblique scan at the level of the transverse process (PMTOS-TP); and (**C**) paramedian transverse oblique scan at the level of the articular process (PMTOS-AP).

psoas compartment using a paramedian transverse oblique scan (describe earlier).[9] On a typical PMTOS-TP (see Figure 39–10b), the erector spinae muscle, transverse process, psoas major muscle, quadratus lumborum muscle, and anterolateral surface of the vertebral body are clearly visualized (see Figure 39–13). The psoas muscle appears hypoechoic, but multiple areas of hyperechogenicity are also interspersed within the central part of the muscle (see Figure 39–13). These hyperechoic speckles represent the intramuscular tendon fibers of the psoas muscle and are more pronounced below the level of the iliac crest. The inferior vena cava (IVC; on the right side) and the aorta (on the left side) are also identified anterior to the vertebral body (see Figure 39–13) and are useful landmarks to look out for while performing a PMTOS. The lower pole of the kidney, which can extend to the L3–L4 level, is closely related to the anterior surfaces of the quadratus lumborum and psoas muscles and frequently seen as an oval structure that moves synchronously with respiration in the retroperitoneal space (Figure 39–21). The acoustic shadow of the transverse process obscures the posterior aspect of the psoas muscle during a PMTOS-TP (see Figure 39–13). Therefore, the lumbar nerve root and lumbar plexus are rarely visualized through the PMTOS-TP scan window. However, the spinal canal, with the dura and the intrathecal space, may be visualized during a PMTOS-TP (see Figure 39–13) due to the US signal entering the spinal canal through the interlaminar space (see Figure 39–13). Being able to visualize the neuraxial structures during a lumbar paravertebral scan may be useful in documenting epidural spread after an LPB.

In contrast, during a PMTOS through the lumbar intertransverse space and at the level of the articular process (PMTOS-AP) (see Figure 39–10c), apart from the erector spinae, psoas, and quadratus lumborum muscles, the intervertebral foramen, articular process, and lumbar nerve root are clearly delineated (see Figure 39–14).[9] The LPVS is also seen as a hypoechoic space adjacent to the intervertebral foramen (see Figure 39–14),[9] and the lumbar nerve root can be seen exiting the foramen to enter the paravertebral space (see Figure 39–14).[9] After it exits the intervertebral foramen, the lumbar nerve root

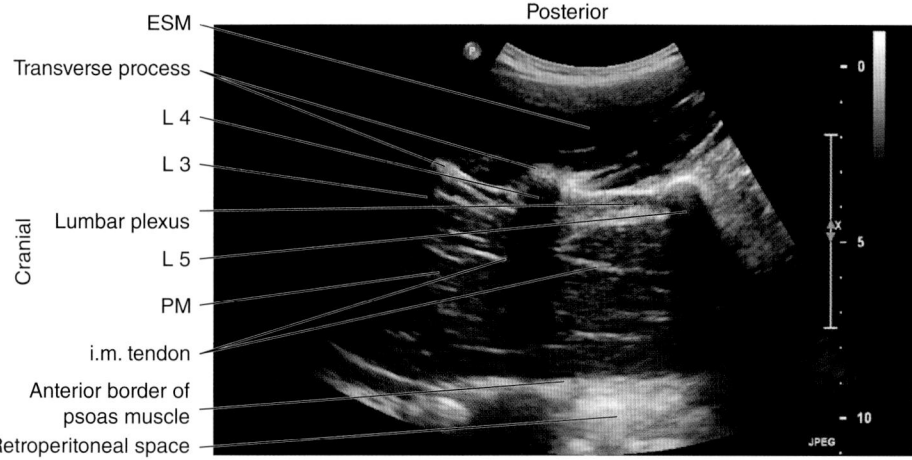

Posterior

ESM
Transverse process
L 4
L 3
Lumbar plexus
L 5
PM
i.m. tendon
Anterior border of psoas muscle
Retroperitoneal space

Cranial

FIGURE 39–11. Sagittal sonogram of the lumbar paravertebral region showing the lumbar plexus as a hyperechoic structure in the posterior aspect of the psoas muscle (PM) between the L4 and L5 transverse processes. Also note the hyperechoic intramuscular tendons within the bulk of the psoas muscle. ESM, erector spinae muscle; i.m. tendon = intramuscular tendon.

Erector spinae muscle

Transverse process
vertebra lumbarum 2

Transverse process
vertebra lumbarum 3

Transverse process
vertebra lumbarum 4

The lumbar
ultrasound trident

Acoustic window

Acoustic shadow
due to
transverse process

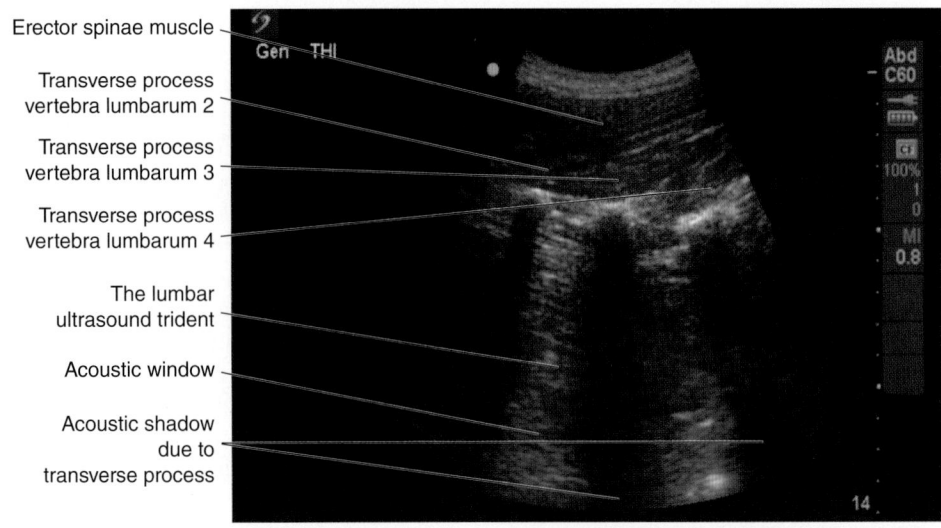

FIGURE 39–12. Sagittal sonogram of the lumbar paravertebral region showing the acoustic shadows of the lumbar transverse processes (L3, L4, and L5), which produce a sonographic pattern called the "trident sign." The psoas muscle is seen in the intervening acoustic window.

Erector spinae muscle

Quadratus lumborum muscle

Transverse process

Articular process

Interlaminar
space

Psoas muscle

Dura

Intrathecal space

Vertebral body

Inferior vena cava

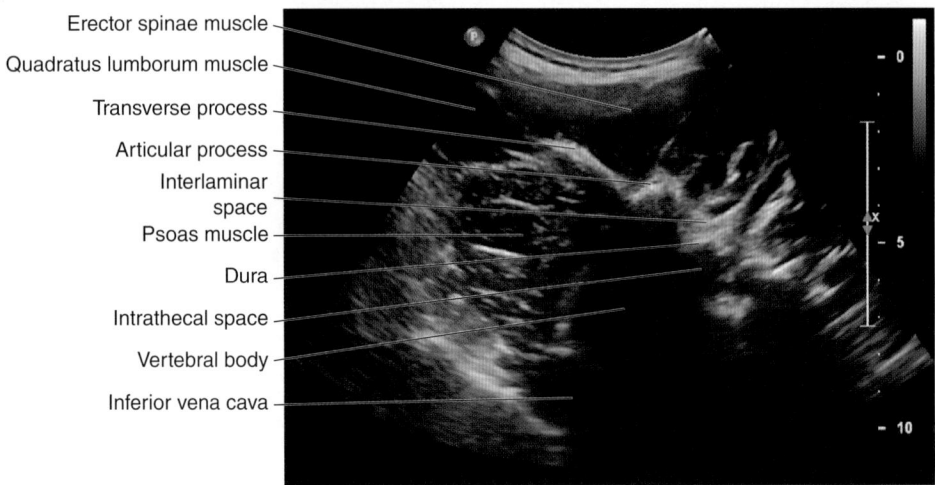

FIGURE 39–13. Paramedian transverse oblique scan of the lumbar paravertebral region at the level of the transverse process (PMTOS-TP). Note how the acoustic shadow of the transverse process obscures the posterior part of the psoas muscle and the intervertebral foramen and how parts of the spinal canal and neuraxial structures (dura and intrathecal space) are seen through the interlaminar space.

Erector spinae muscle

Quadratus lumborum muscle

Articular process

Psoas compartment

Lumbar plexus

Lumbar nerve
root

Lumbar paravertebral space

Inferior vena cava

Psoas muscle

Vertebral body

Retroperitoneal space

Inferior vena cava

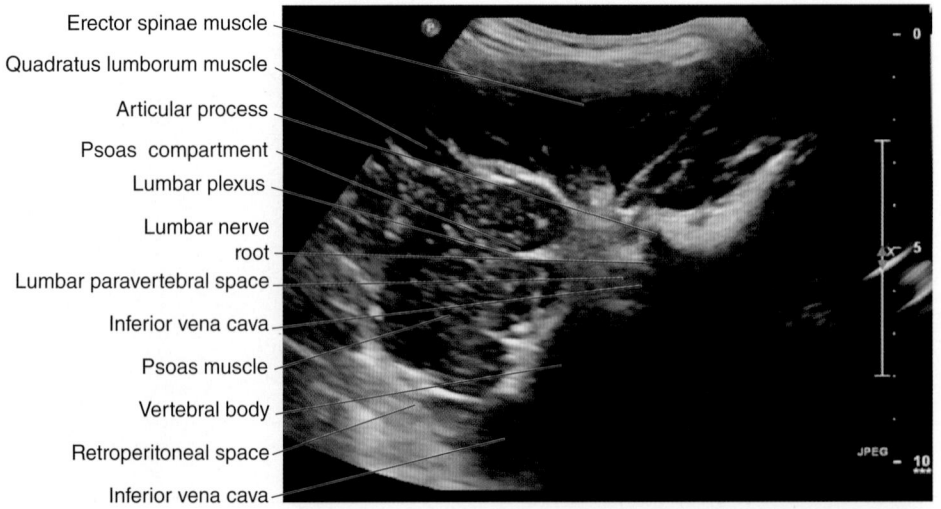

FIGURE 39–14. Paramedian transverse oblique scan of the right lumbar paravertebral region through the lumbar intertransverse space and at the level of the articular process, showing the lumbar plexus as a discrete hyperechoic structure within a hypoechoic intramuscular space (the psoas compartment) in the posteromedial aspect of the psoas muscle.

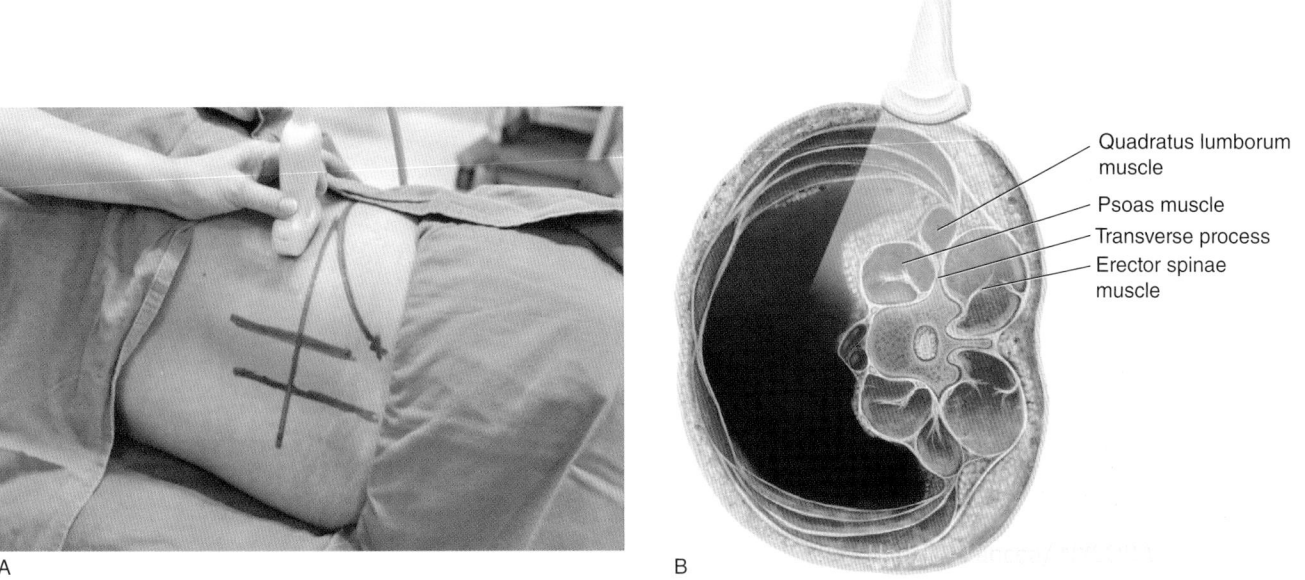

A   B

FIGURE 39–15. (**A**) Position of the patient (lateral decubitus) and US transducer during a transverse scan at the flank for the Shamrock method. (**B**) US transducer and plane of US beam superimposed onto a transverse anatomical section of the lumbar paravertebral region, illustrating how the US beam is insonated (axis of scan) and structures are visualized during the scan.

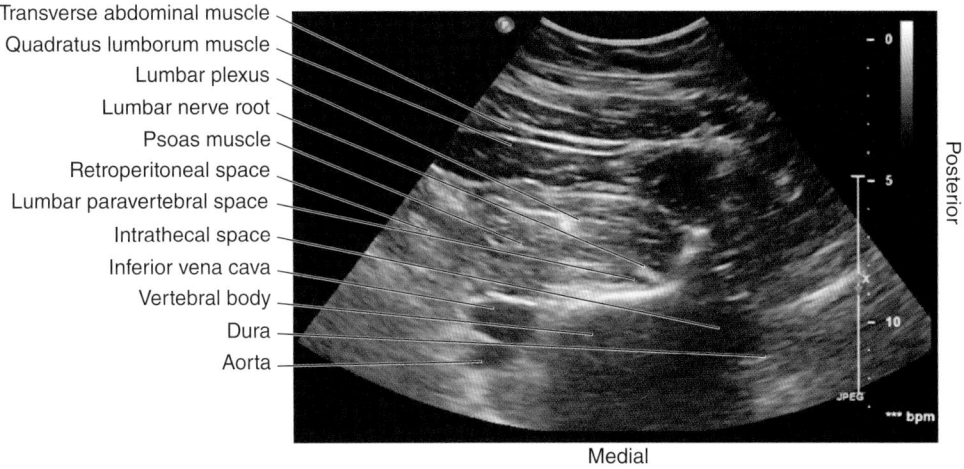

FIGURE 39–16. Transverse sonogram of the lumbar paravertebral region during the Shamrock method, with the US beam insonated at the level of the transverse process.

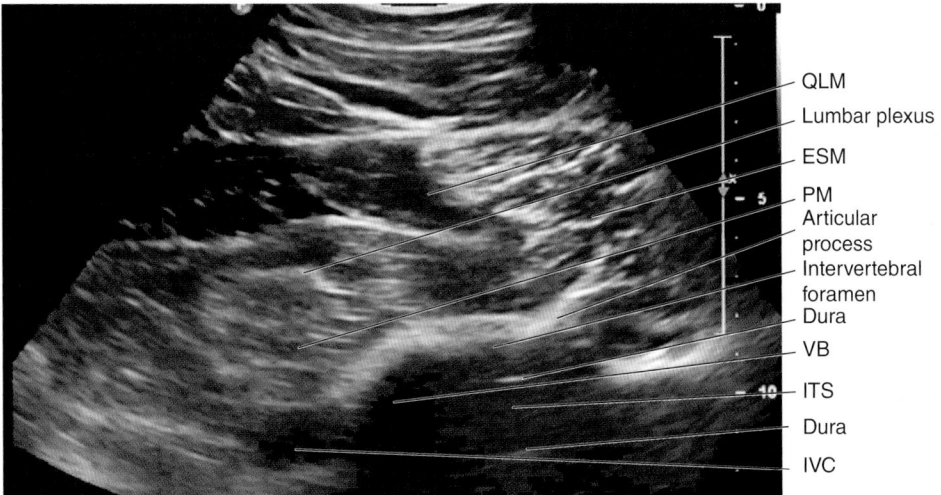

FIGURE 39–17. Transverse sonogram of the lumbar paravertebral region during the shamrock method, with the US beam insonated through the intertransverse space and at the level of the articular process of the vertebra. ESM, erector spine muscle; ITS, intrathecal space; IVC, inferior vena cava; PM, psoas muscle; QLM, quadratus lumborum muscle; VB, vertebral body.

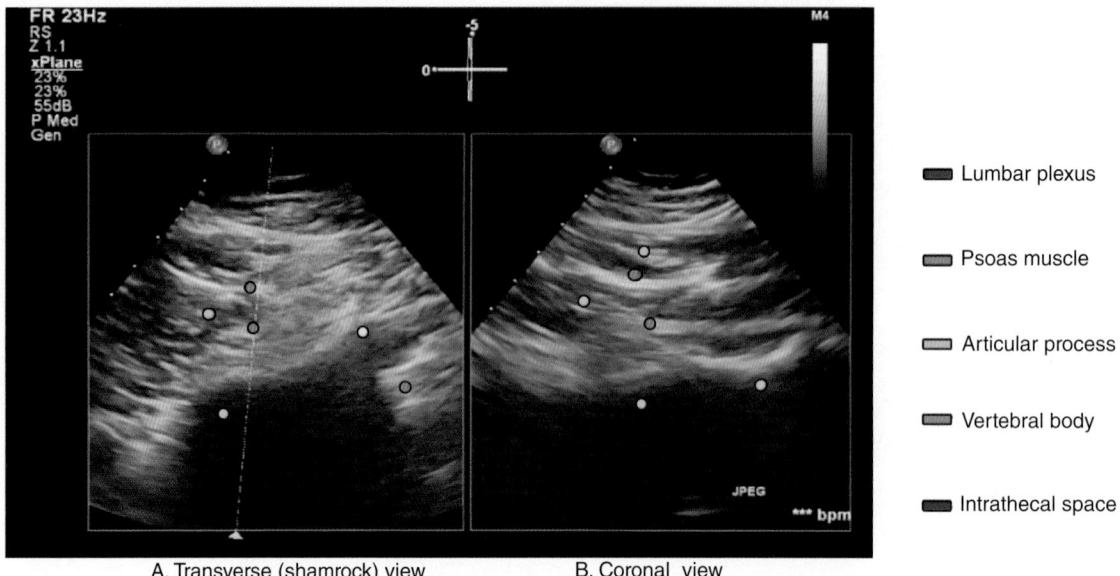

- Lumbar plexus
- Psoas muscle
- Articular process
- Vertebral body
- Intrathecal space

A. Transverse (shamrock) view   B. Coronal view

FIGURE 39–18. Biplanar US image of the lumbar paravertebral region obtained with the shamrock method, with the US beam insonated through the lumbar intertransverse space and at the level of the articular process. Note that the transverse axis (**A**) is the primary data acquisition plane and that the corresponding orthogonal image along the secondary data acquisition plane (dotted line with blue arrowhead in [a]) is a coronal view (**B**) showing the lumbar plexus nerves within the psoas muscle.

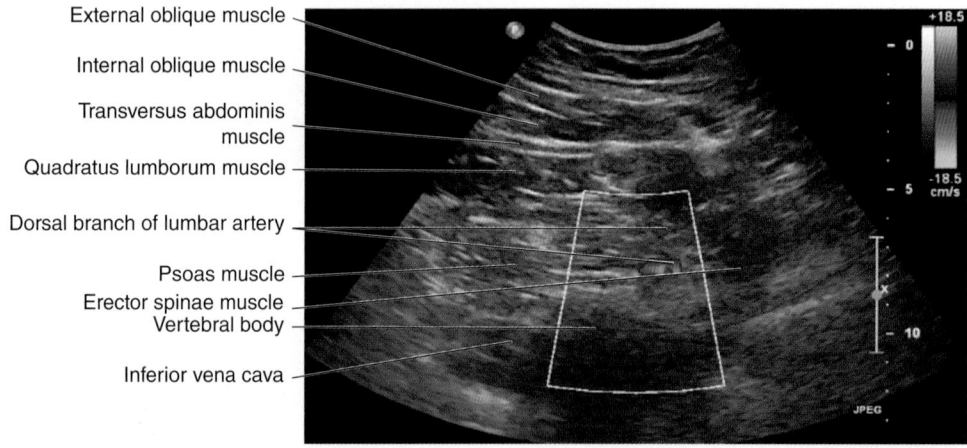

External oblique muscle
Internal oblique muscle
Transversus abdominis muscle
Quadratus lumborum muscle
Dorsal branch of lumbar artery
Psoas muscle
Erector spinae muscle
Vertebral body
Inferior vena cava

FIGURE 39–19. Color Doppler image of the lumbar paravertebral region obtained with the shamrock method. Note the Doppler signal in the posterior aspect of the psoas muscle from the dorsal branch of the lumbar artery.

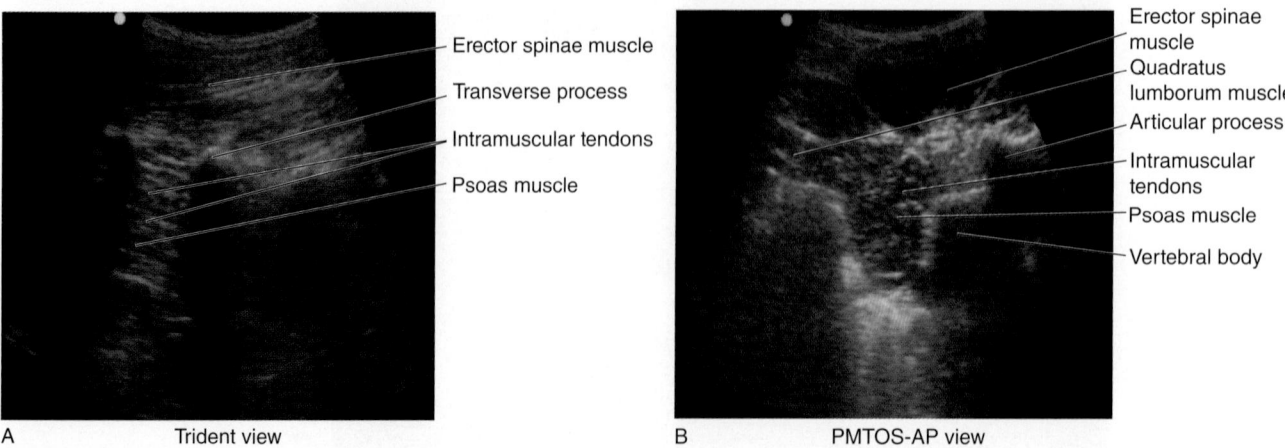

Erector spinae muscle
Transverse process
Intramuscular tendons
Psoas muscle

Erector spinae muscle
Quadratus lumborum muscle
Articular process
Intramuscular tendons
Psoas muscle
Vertebral body

A   Trident view   B   PMTOS-AP view

FIGURE 39–20. Sonograms showing intramuscular tendons within the psoas muscle. They are seen as (**A**) hyperechoic striations in a sagittal sonogram or (**B**) as multiple hyperechoic speckles in a transverse sonogram. PMTOS-AP, paramedian transverse oblique scan at the level of the articular process.

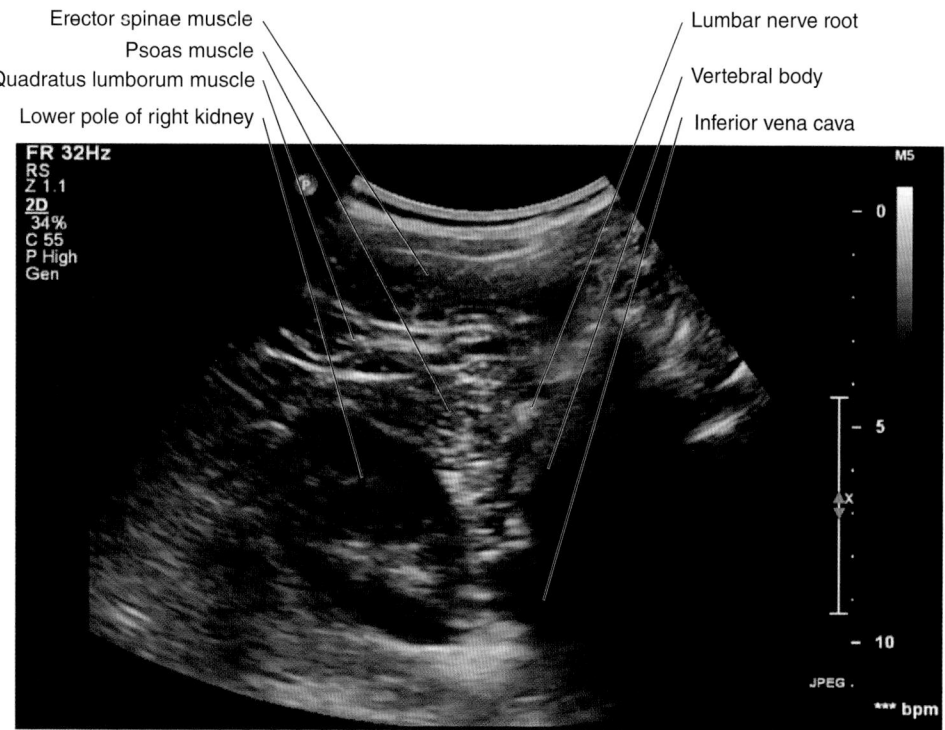

FIGURE 39–21. Paramedian transverse oblique scan of the right lumbar paravertebral region through the intertransverse space and at the level of the articular process (PMTOS-AP). The lumbar nerve root is seen emerging from the intervertebral foramen. Also note that the lower pole of the right kidney is seen anterior to the psoas muscle in this sonogram.

does not enter the psoas muscle directly opposite the intervertebral foramen from which it emerges (see Figure 39–14), but takes a steep caudal course (see Figure 39–14), entering the psoas muscle at the vertebral level below to join the lumbar plexus. The lumbar plexus is seen as a separate hyperechoic structure within a hypoechoic space, the psoas compartment,[9] in the posterior aspect of the psoas muscle (see Figure 39–14).

In a transverse sonogram produced by the shamrock method (see Figure 39–15), the psoas, erector spinae, and quadratus lumborum muscles are also clearly visualized (see Figures 39–16, 39–17, 39–18, and 39–19). The anatomical arrangement of the three muscles around the transverse process—that is, the psoas muscle lying anteriorly, the erector spinae muscle lying posteriorly, and the quadratus lumborum muscle lying at the apex (see Figure 39–16)—produces a sonographic pattern that has been likened to the shape of a "shamrock," with the muscles representing its three leaves.[19] The lumbar nerve root may also be visualized close to the angle between the vertebral body and the transverse process (see Figure 39–16) and the lumbar plexus within the posterior aspect of the psoas muscle, typically about 2 cm anterior to the transverse process (see Figures 39–17 and 39–18).[19] From this position, if the transducer is gently tilted caudally, the acoustic shadow of the L4 transverse process disappears, and the US beam is now insonated through the intertransverse space and at the level of the articular process of the L4 vertebra, similar to that seen with a PMTOS-AP (see Figure 39–17).[9,10,19] As a result, apart from the psoas, erector spinae, and quadratus lumborum muscles, the intervertebral foramen and lumbar plexus may also be visualized (see Figure 39–17).

ULTRASOUND-GUIDED LUMBAR PLEXUS BLOCK

Although it is possible to define the anatomy relevant for LPB with both sagittal[17] and transverse[9] scans, it is not known which approach is best for USG LPB. Therefore, it is not possible to make recommendations of an optimal technique to use for USG LPB. The author believes that the paucity of data on USG LPB reflects only the greater degree of skill required to perform the US scan, interpret the sonograms, and perform the intervention, which is at a depth. Therefore, USG LPB should be considered an advanced-skill-level block and performed only after one has acquired the appropriate level of training and skill. Furthermore, since it is not always possible to accurately delineate the lumbar plexus nerves within the psoas muscle in the US scans, it is prudent to use peripheral nerve stimulation in conjunction with US (dual guidance) for nerve localization during a USG LPB.

Ultrasound-Guided Lumbar Plexus Block Techniques

The following section briefly describes the various techniques used for USG LPB.

1. USG LPB Using the Trident View

As described above, a paramedian sagittal scan is performed with the patient in the lateral decubitus position, with the side to be blocked uppermost (see Figures 39–9 and 39–10). Once an optimal view of the lumbar US trident is obtained

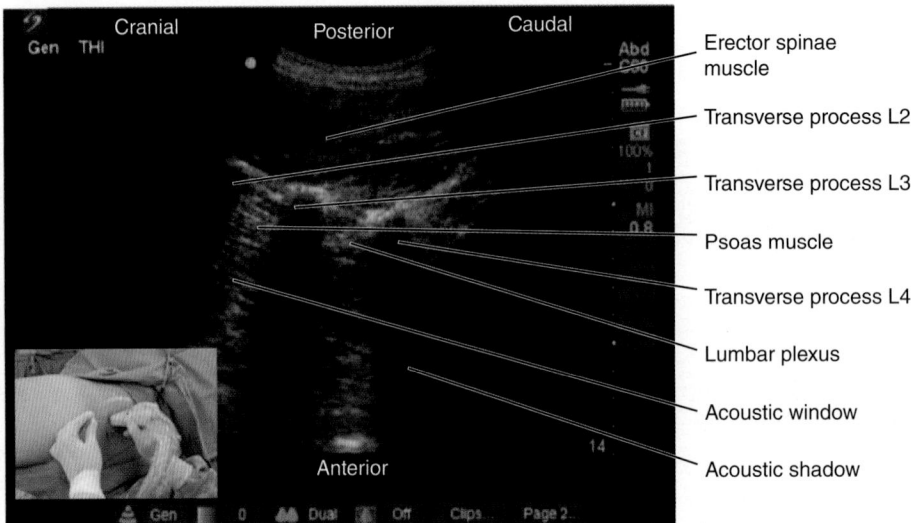

FIGURE 39–22. Sagittal sonogram of the lumbar paravertebral region showing the "trident" view. The psoas muscle is seen in the acoustic window between the transverse processes and is recognized by its typical striated appearance. Part of the lumbar plexus is also seen as a hyperechoic shadow in the posterior aspect of the psoas muscle between the transverse processes of the L3 and L4 vertebrae. The inset photograph shows the orientation of the US transducer and the direction in which the block needle is introduced (in plane) during a USG LPB via the trident view.

(Figure 39–22), an insulated nerve block needle, connected to a nerve stimulator, is inserted in plane from the caudal end of the US transducer (see Figure 39–22).[17] The aim is to guide the block needle through the acoustic window of the lumbar US trident; that is, through the space between the transverse process of L3 and L4 into the posterior aspect of the psoas major muscle until either needle–nerve contact is visualized or an ipsilateral quadriceps muscle contraction is elicited.[17] After negative aspiration, an appropriate dose of local anesthetic (20–25 mL of 0.5% ropivacaine or levobupivacaine) is injected in aliquots over 2–3 minutes and the patient is closely monitored. Spread of local anesthetic within the posterior aspect of the psoas muscle can be visualized in real time, and the nerves of the lumbar plexus are better visualized after the local anesthetic injection (see Figure 39–22).

2. USG LPB Using a Paramedian Transverse Scan

Originally described by Kirchmair and colleagues[13] in cadavers, this technique involves performing a transverse scan of the lumbar paravertebral region to delineate the psoas major muscle (as described above) at the L3–L4 or L4–L5 level. It may be difficult to locate the psoas muscle at the L4–L5 level as the iliac crest interferes with transducer placement, particularly curved array transducers with a large footprint (60 mm). As described above, the author prefers to perform a PMTOS-AP with the patient positioned in the lateral position (Figure 39–23) since it provides better visualization of the anatomy relevant for LPB.[10] Once an optimal PMTOS-AP view is obtained (see Figure 39–14), an insulated block needle, connected to a nerve stimulator, is inserted medially to the US transducer and in the plane of the US beam (in-plane technique) (Figure 23–24a).[10] The point of needle insertion corresponds to a point 4 cm lateral to the midline and at the same location where one would insert the block needle during a landmark-based LPB (see

Figure 39–23).[10] The block needle is slowly advanced under real-time US guidance to the posterior aspect of the psoas muscle, and correct needle tip position is confirmed by observing needle–nerve contact (Figure 39–25) and/or an ipsilateral quadriceps muscle contraction (mostly the latter).[10] There are also reports of the block needle being inserted from the lateral border of the US transducer and being advanced anteromedially in plane toward the psoas muscle from a lateral to medial direction.[18,22] As described above, the lumbar plexus is not sonographically visualized in all patients but, when visualized, is seen as a hyperechoic structure in the posterior part of the psoas muscle (see Figure 39–25). Since the block needle is inserted in the plane of the US beam, it can be visualized and tracked in real time (see Figure 39–25). After negative aspiration, an appropriate dose of local anesthetic (20–25 mL of 0.5% ropivacaine or levobupivacaine) is injected in aliquots over 2–3 minutes and the patient is closely monitored (Figure 39–26). Occasionally, needle–nerve contact can be visualized on the US image during needle insertion or after the local anesthetic injection (see Figure 39–25).[10] Also, the lumbar plexus is better visualized after the local anesthetic injection,[10,17] as the hypoechoic local anesthetic surrounds the lumbar plexus nerves (Figures 39–26 and 39–27).

3. The Shamrock Method

Sauter and colleagues recently described an alternative approach for USG LPB,[19] which they refer to as the "shamrock method (Figure 39-24b)."[19] As described above, a transverse scan is performed at the flank and immediately above the iliac crest, with the patient in the lateral position and with the side to be blocked uppermost (see Figures 39–15a, b and 39-24b). Once the sonographic pattern of the "shamrock" is obtained at the level of the L4 transverse process (see Figure 39–16),[19] the US transducer is tilted slightly caudally until the

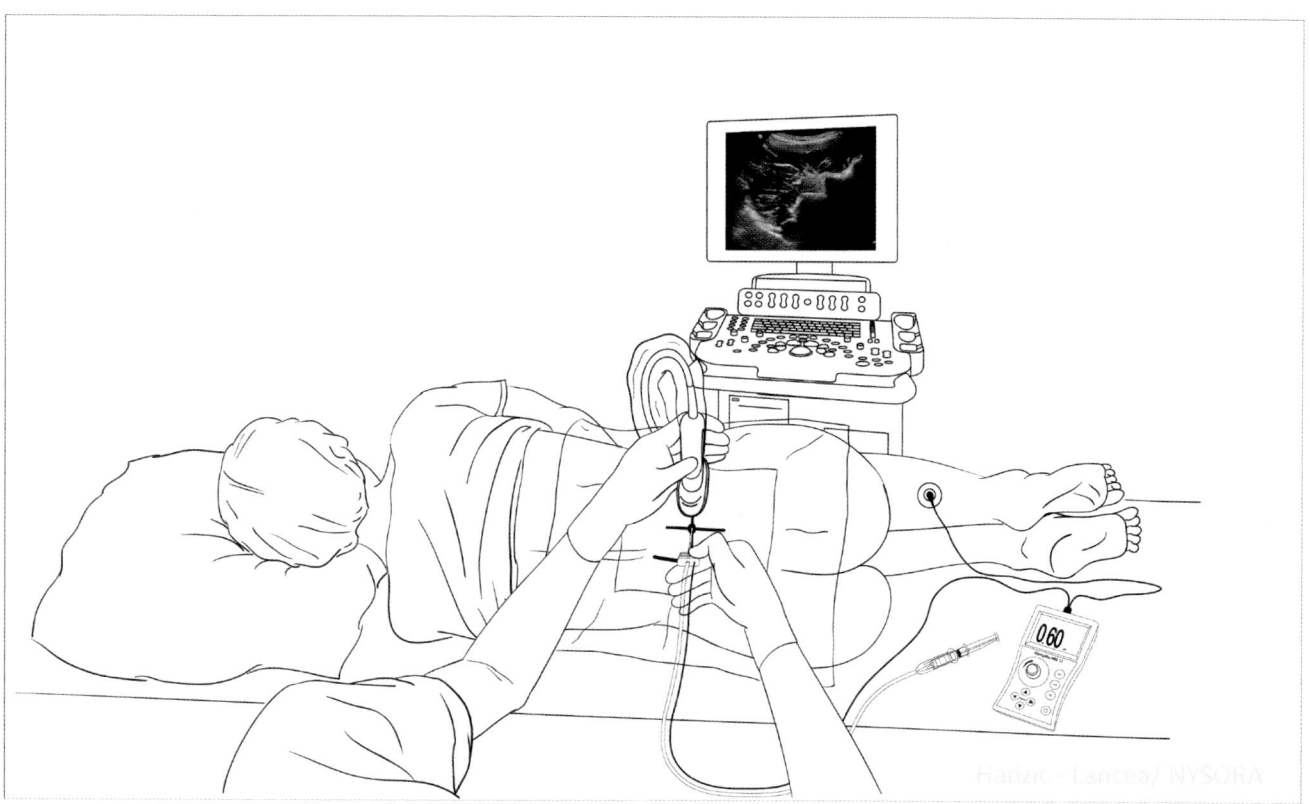

FIGURE 39–23. Position of the patient, anesthesiologist, US system, and US transducer orientation during a paramedian transverse oblique scan through the lumbar intertransverse space and at the level of the articular process.

Ultrasound Guided Lumbar Plexus Block Using a Transverse Scan

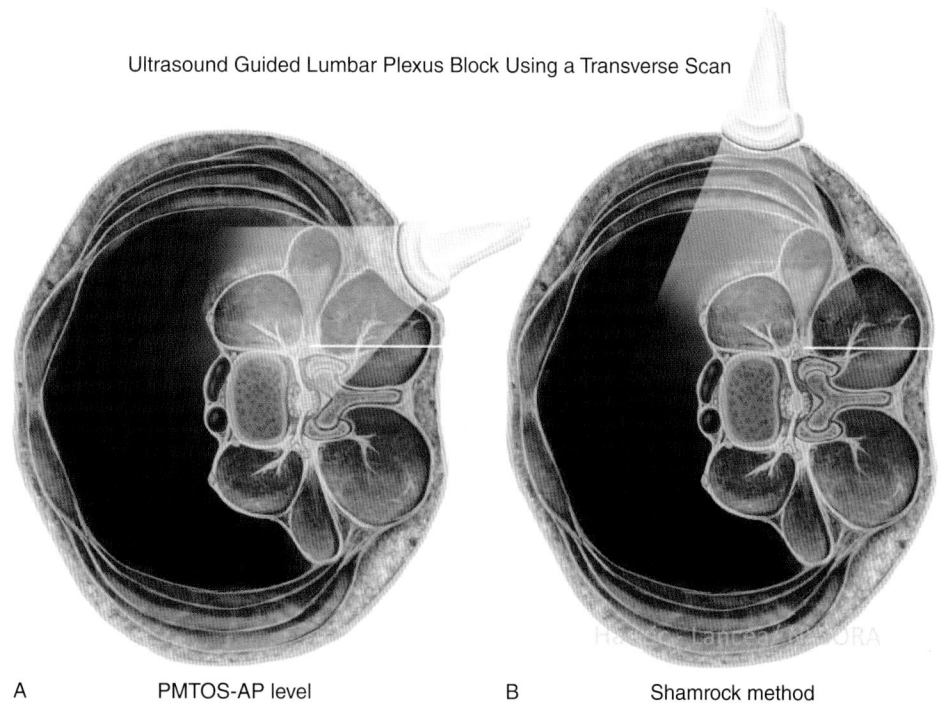

A   PMTOS-AP level   B   Shamrock method

FIGURE 39–24. Position of the US transducer and the plane of the US beam, which has been superimposed on a transverse anatomical section (L4 vertebral level), rendered from the Visible Human Project® male dataset, illustrating the relevant lumbar paravertebral anatomy and how the US beam is insonated during (**A**) the paramedian transverse oblique scan at the level of the articular process (PMTOS-AP) and (**B**) the shamrock method. Note the relationship (in plane) of the nerve block needle to the US beam in both methods.

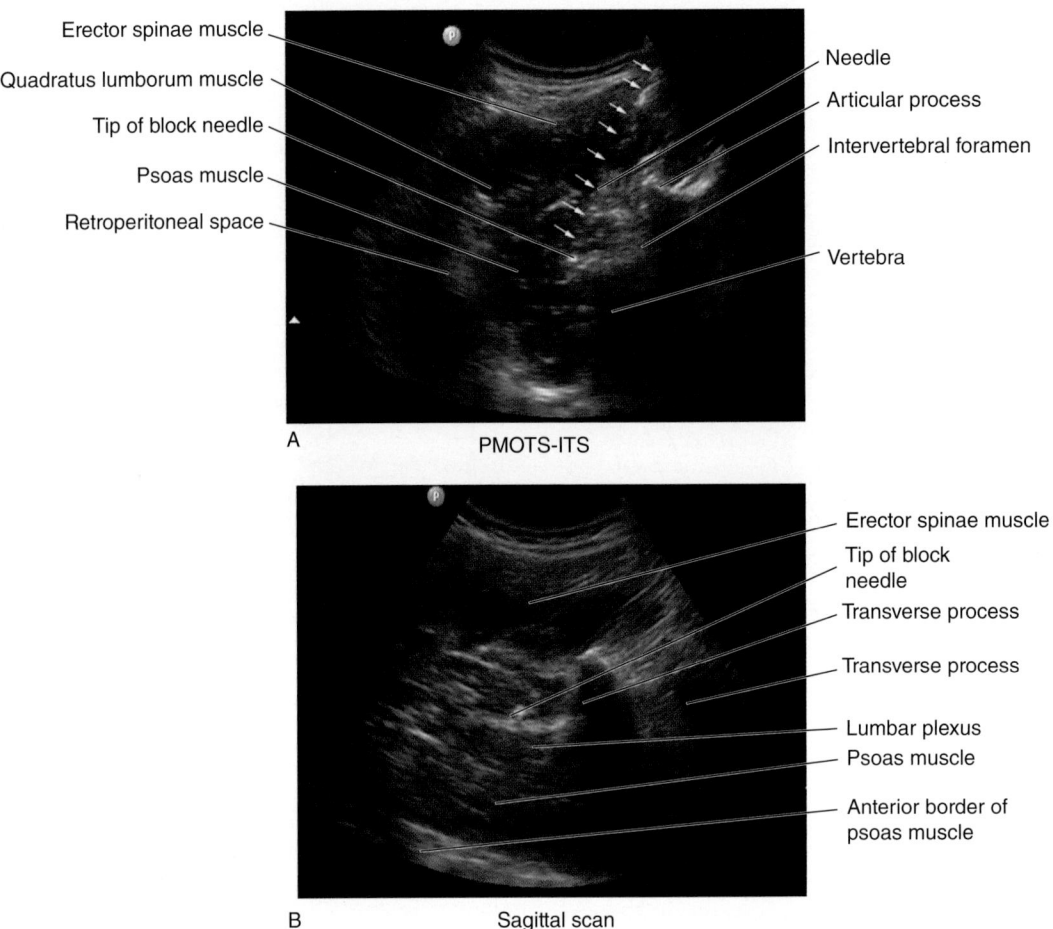

A   PMOTS-ITS

Erector spinae muscle
Quadratus lumborum muscle
Tip of block needle
Psoas muscle
Retroperitoneal space

Needle
Articular process
Intervertebral foramen
Vertebra

Erector spinae muscle
Tip of block needle
Transverse process
Transverse process
Lumbar plexus
Psoas muscle
Anterior border of psoas muscle

B   Sagittal scan

FIGURE 39–25. Sonograms of the lumbar paravertebral region showing the needle–lumbar plexus relationship when an ipsilateral quadriceps muscle contraction is elicited during a USG LPB. (**A**) Paramedian transverse oblique scan at the level of the articular process (PMTS-AP). (**B**) Sagittal sonogram in the same patient, validating the accuracy of the observation. Also note the direction of the in-plane needle insertion.

acoustic shadow of the transverse process is no longer visualized (see Figure 39–17).[19] This view represents the transverse view of the anatomy relevant for LPB through the L4–5 intertransverse space.[19] A line is then drawn on the patient's back extending from the center of the medial end of the IS

transducer to the midline (back). A nerve block needle is inserted 4 cm from the midline along this line (Figure 39–28) and gradually advanced anteriorly under real-time US guidance (in-plane needle insertion; Figure 39–29a) until the needle tip is close to the L3 nerve root.[19] Nerve stimulation

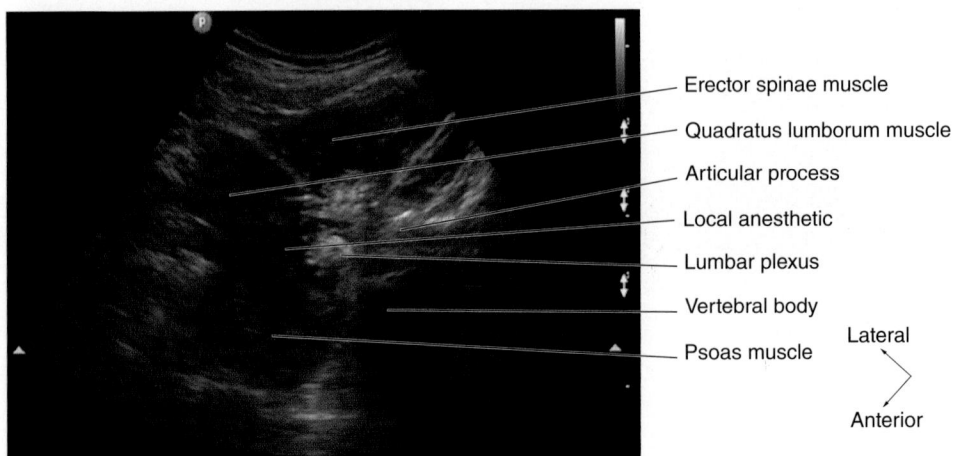

Erector spinae muscle
Quadratus lumborum muscle
Articular process
Local anesthetic
Lumbar plexus
Vertebral body
Psoas muscle

Lateral

Anterior

FIGURE 39–26. Transverse sonogram of the lumbar paravertebral region during a USG LPB and after local anesthetic (LA) injection. Note the spread of the LA relative to the lumbar plexus and the distention of the psoas compartment (short white arrows) by the LA.

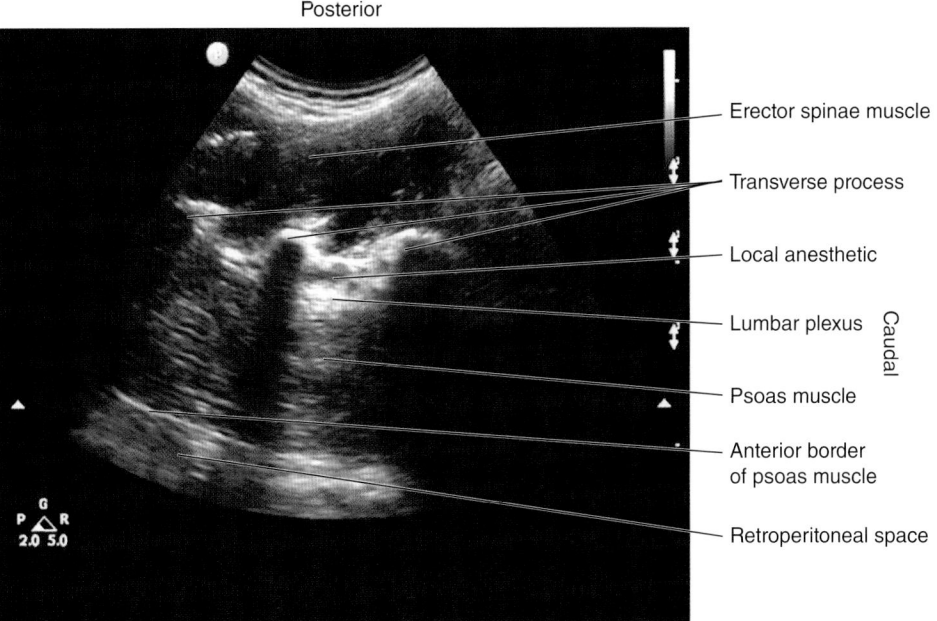

Posterior

Erector spinae muscle

Transverse process

Local anesthetic

Lumbar plexus

Caudal

Psoas muscle

Anterior border
of psoas muscle

Retroperitoneal space

FIGURE 39–27. Sagittal sonogram of the lumbar paravertebral region during a USG LPB using the paramedian transverse oblique scan at the level of the articular process (PMTOS-AP) and after local anesthetic injection. Note the hyperechoic lumbar plexus nerve in the posterior aspect of the psoas muscle and the distribution of LA relative to the nerve (in front, behind, and in a craniocaudal direction) within the psoas compartment.

should be used in conjunction with US to confirm correct needle placement, after which 20–30 mL of ropivacaine or levobupivacaine 0.5% is injected slowly while visualizing the perineural spread of the drug in the posterior aspect of the psoas muscle (Figure 39–29b).[19] The technical challenge with this approach is that although the block needle is inserted in plane, visualizing the needle initially can be very challenging, since the sites for the US scan and needle insertion are separated by a considerable distance (see Figure 39–28).[19] Nevertheless, with experience, needle visualization can be easily accomplished.

THE PEARLS AND PITFALLS OF ULTRASOUND-GUIDED LUMBAR PLEXUS BLOCK

The lumbar paravertebral region is highly vascular and contains the ascending lumbar veins and lumbar arteries, which can be visualized using color and power Doppler US (see Figures 39–7 and 39–19). There is also a rich network of blood vessels (arteries and veins) within the substance of the psoas major muscle including the psoas compartment. The dorsal branch of the lumbar artery is also closely related to the

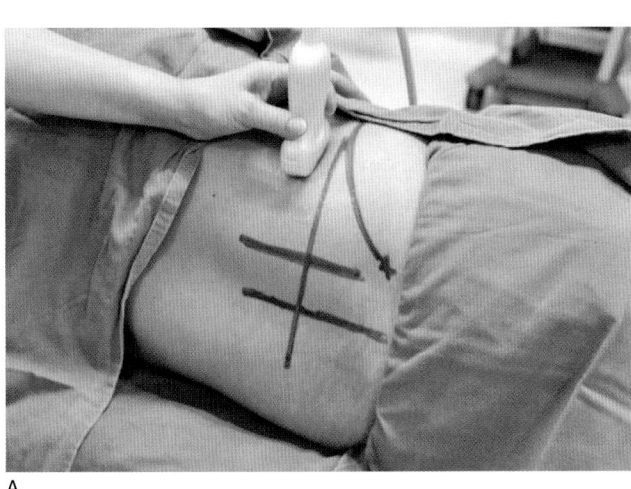

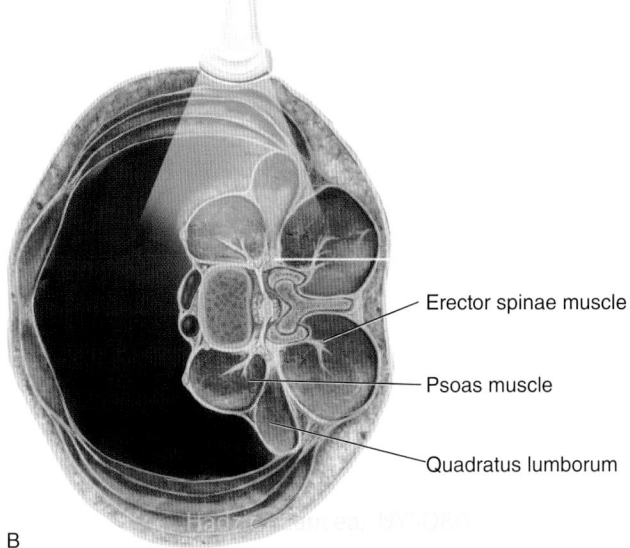

Erector spinae muscle

Psoas muscle

Quadratus lumborum

A

B

FIGURE 39–28. The shamrock method of US LPB. (**A**) Position of the patient (lateral decubitus), anesthesiologist, and US transducer and site and direction of needle insertion. (**B**) Simulated path of the block needle relative to the plane of the US beam (in plane) and paravertebral anatomy.

Lateral

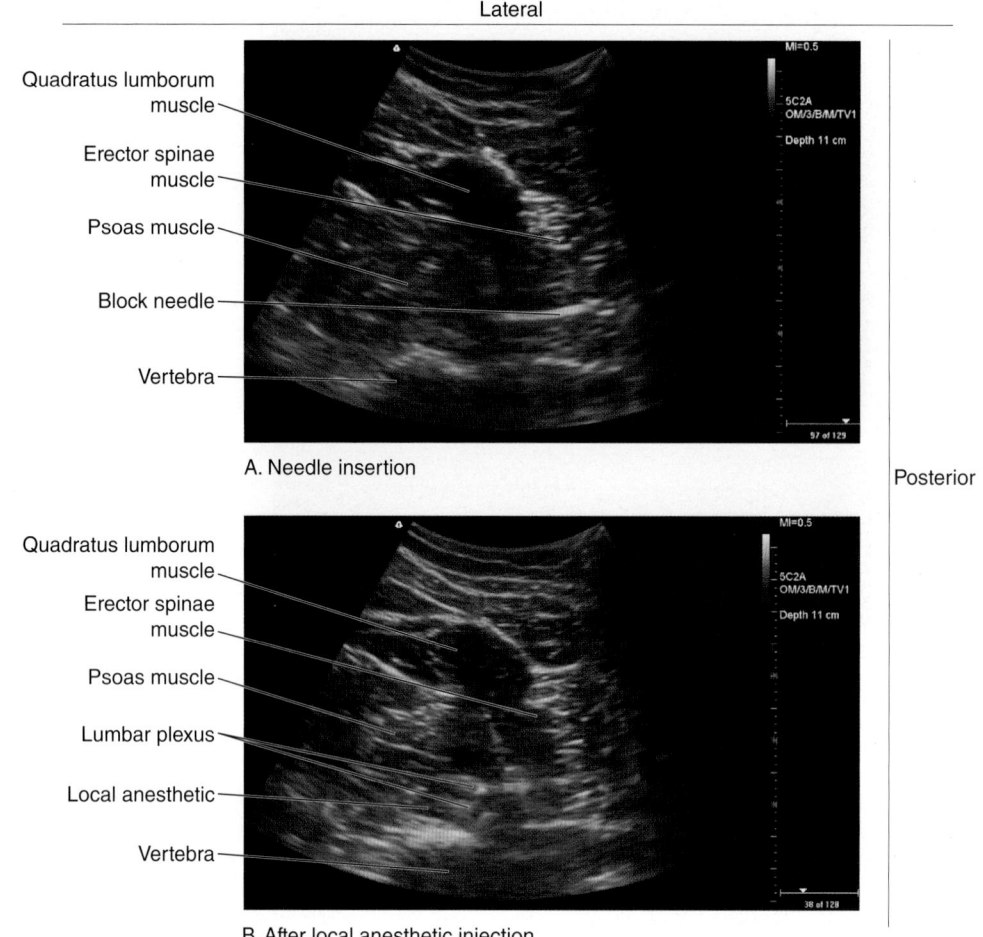

Quadratus lumborum muscle

Erector spinae muscle

Psoas muscle

Block needle

Vertebra

A. Needle insertion

Posterior

Quadratus lumborum muscle

Erector spinae muscle

Psoas muscle

Lumbar plexus

Local anesthetic

Vertebra

B. After local anesthetic injection

FIGURE 39–29. Transverse sonograms showing (**A**) the direction of needle insertion relative to the lumbar paravertebral anatomy and (**B**) the local anesthetic (LA) spread during a USG LPB using the shamrock method.

transverse processes and the posterior aspect of the psoas muscle (see Figure 39–7b), where the lumbar plexus is located. Therefore, this blood vessel may be at risk of needle-related injury during LPB because it is directly in the path of the advancing needle (see Figure 39–7). Considering the vascularity of the lumbar paravertebral region, it is not surprising that inadvertent intravascular injection of local anesthetic and psoas hematoma[26] have been described after LPB. It is for the same reason that one must exercise caution when considering an LPB in patients with mild to moderate coagulopathy or in patients receiving thromboprophylaxis; based on our current understanding, such conditions may be considered a relative contraindication for LPB. That said, there are reports of the safe use of LPB (both the single-injection and continuous techniques) before the initiation of postoperative thromboprophylaxis[27] and the removal of catheters in patients receiving thromboprophylaxis and/or aspirin[27] with an international normalized ratio (INR) of equal to or greater than 1.5.[28] One must exercise caution in interpreting such results, however, because the site at which an LPB is performed is noncompressible, and there are previous reports of retroperitoneal hematoma complicating LPB.[16,26] Moreover, there are currently very few evidence-based indications for LPB.

The echo intensity (EI) of skeletal muscles is significantly increased in the elderly,[29] and there is a strong correlation between the EI of muscles and age. Therefore, in US images, the lumbar paravertebral region in the elderly appears whiter and brighter than in younger patients, and there is also a loss of contrast between the muscle and the adjoining structures, making it more difficult to delineate the lumbar plexus. Therefore, USG LPB in the elderly can be very challenging. The same is also true in the obese, as excessive fat can make US imaging of the lumbar paravertebral anatomy and US guidance during LPB difficult. Gadsden and colleagues[30] have also recently demonstrated that injection of local anesthetic under high pressure (> 20 psi) during a lumbar plexus block results in unwanted bilateral sensory motor blockade and a high incidence of neuraxial block.[30] Therefore, one must ensure that the injection pressure is low (< 15 psi) during USG LPB. Occasionally, one may also find that during USG LPB, the needle tip is in the posterior aspect of the psoas muscle but no motor response is elicited. This may not be an uncommon phenomenon, considering that it is commonly seen during upper extremity blocks. However, one must ensure that the block needle has not been inadvertently inserted in the upper lumbar region because the upper lumbar nerves (L1 and L2) contribute predominantly to sensory nerves, and stimulating these nerves may not elicit a motor response.

SUMMARY

Recent advances in US technology, the image processing capabilities of US machines, and the development of new US scan protocols to image the lumbar paravertebral region have made it possible to image the anatomy relevant for lumbar plexus block. With US, one is able to preview the paravertebral anatomy, determine the safe depth for needle insertion, accurately guide the block needle to the target in real time, and visualize the distribution of the injected local anesthetic. These advantages may translate into improved accuracy, reduced needle-related complications, and improved success. It is also an excellent teaching tool for demonstrating the anatomy of the lumbar paravertebral region. However, the use of US for LPB is still in its infancy, and it is the author's opinion that USG LPB is an advanced-skill-level block that should be performed only after one has acquired the necessary imaging and interventional skills. Published data suggest that it is possible to image the anatomy relevant for LPB, and several USG LPB techniques have been described. Future research is warranted to define the role of US for LPB and to establish evidence-based indications for LPB.

Acknowledgements

Thanks to Dr. Jui-An Lin, M.D., Department of Anesthesiology, Taipei Medical University, Taiwan for sharing sonograms of the "Shamrock technique" from his archive (Figure 29). The cadaver anatomic sections are courtesy of the Visible Human Server at Ecole Polytechnique Fédérale de Lausanne, Visible Human Visualization Software (http://visiblehuman.epfl.ch), and Gold Standard Multimedia (www.gsm.org). The figures were reproduced with kind permission from www.aic.cuhk.edu.hk/usgraweb.

REFERENCES

1. Parkinson SK, Mueller JB, Little WL, Bailey SL: Extent of blockade with various approaches to the lumbar plexus. Anesth Analg 1989;68: 243–248.
2. de Leeuw MA, Zuurmond WW, Perez RS: The psoas compartment block for hip surgery: the past, present, and future. Anesthesiol Res Pract 2011;2011:159541.
3. Ilfeld BM, Mariano ER, Madison SJ, et al: Continuous femoral versus posterior lumbar plexus nerve blocks for analgesia after hip arthroplasty: a randomized, controlled study. Anesth Analg 2011;113: 897–903.
4. Stevens RD, Van GE, Flory N, Fournier R, Gamulin Z: Lumbar plexus block reduces pain and blood loss associated with total hip arthroplasty. Anesthesiology 2000;93:115–121.
5. Ho AM, Karmakar MK: Combined paravertebral lumbar plexus and parasacral sciatic nerve block for reduction of hip fracture in a patient with severe aortic stenosis. Can J Anaesth 2002;49:946–950.
6. Chayen D, Nathan H, Chayen M: The psoas compartment block. Anesthesiology 1976;45:95–99.
7. Kirchmair L, Entner T, Wissel J, Moriggl B, Kapral S, Mitterschiffthaler G: A study of the paravertebral anatomy for ultrasound-guided posterior lumbar plexus block. Anesth Analg 2001;93:477–481.
8. Farny J, Drolet P, Girard M: Anatomy of the posterior approach to the lumbar plexus block. Can J Anaesth 1994;41:480–485.

9. Karmakar MK, Li JW, Kwok WH, Soh E, Hadzic A: Sonoanatomy relevant for lumbar plexus block in volunteers correlated with cross-sectional anatomic and magnetic resonance images. Reg Anesth Pain Med 2013;38:391–397.
10. Karmakar MK, Li JW, Kwok WH, Hadzic A: Ultrasound-guided lumbar plexus block using a transverse scan through the lumbar intertransverse space: a prospective case series. Reg Anesth Pain Med 2015;40:75–81.
11. Kirchmair L, Lirk P, Colvin J, Mitterschiffthaler G, Moriggl B: Lumbar plexus and psoas major muscle: not always as expected. Reg Anesth Pain Med 2008;33:109–114.
12. Capdevila X, Coimbra C, Choquet O: Approaches to the lumbar plexus: success, risks, and outcome. Reg Anesth Pain Med 2005;30: 150–162.
13. Kirchmair L, Entner T, Kapral S, Mitterschiffthaler G: Ultrasound guidance for the psoas compartment block: an imaging study. Anesth Analg 2002;94:706–710.
14. Aida S, Takahashi H, Shimoji K: Renal subcapsular hematoma after lumbar plexus block. Anesthesiology 1996;84:452–455.
15. Aveline C, Bonnet F: Delayed retroperitoneal haematoma after failed lumbar plexus block. Br J Anaesth 2004;93:589–591.
16. Weller RS, Gerancher JC, Crews JC, Wade KL: Extensive retroperitoneal hematoma without neurologic deficit in two patients who underwent lumbar plexus block and were later anticoagulated. Anesthesiology 2003; 98:581–585.
17. Karmakar MK, Ho AM, Li X, Kwok WH, Tsang K, Kee WD: Ultrasound-guided lumbar plexus block through the acoustic window of the lumbar ultrasound trident. Br J Anaesth 2008;100:533–537.
18. Doi K, Sakura S, Hara K: A modified posterior approach to lumbar plexus block using a transverse ultrasound image and an approach from the lateral border of the transducer. Anaesth Intensive Care 2010;38: 213–214.
19. Sauter AR, Ullensvang K, Bendtsen TF, Boerglum J: The "Shamrock Method"—a new and promising technique for ultrasound guided lumbar plexus blocks [letter]. Br J Anaesth February 26, 2013. http://bja.oxfordjournals.org/forum/topic/brjana_el%3B9814. Accessed July 6, 2015.
20. Bendtsen TF, Pedersen EM, Haroutounian S, et al: The suprasacral parallel shift vs lumbar plexus blockade with ultrasound guidance in healthy volunteers—a randomised controlled trial. Anesthesia 2014;69: 1227–1240.
21. Morimoto M, Kim JT, Popovic J, Jain S, Bekker A: Ultrasound-guided lumbar plexus block for open reduction and internal fixation of hip fracture. Pain Pract 2006;6:124–126.
22. Madison SJ, Ilfeld BM, Loland VJ, Mariano ER: Posterior lumbar plexus perineural catheter insertion by ultrasound guidance alone. Acta Anaesthesiol Scand 2011;55:1031–1032.
23. Chin KJ, Karmakar MK, Peng P: Ultrasonography of the adult thoracic and lumbar spine for central neuraxial blockade. Anesthesiology 2011;114:1459–1485.
24. Karmakar MK, Li X, Ho AM, Kwok WH, Chui PT: Real-time ultrasound-guided paramedian epidural access: evaluation of a novel in-plane technique. Br J Anaesth 2009;102:845–854.
25. Karmakar MK, Li X, Kwok WH, Ho AM, Ngan Kee WD: Sonoanatomy relevant for ultrasound-guided central neuraxial blocks via the paramedian approach in the lumbar region. Br J Radiol 2012;85:e262–e269.
26. Klein SM, d'Ercole F, Greengrass RA, Warner DS: Enoxaparin associated with psoas hematoma and lumbar plexopathy after lumbar plexus block. Anesthesiology 1997;87:1576–1579.
27. Chelly JE, Schilling D: Thromboprophylaxis and peripheral nerve blocks in patients undergoing joint arthroplasty. J Arthroplasty 2008;23: 350–354.
28. Chelly JE, Szczodry DM, Neumann KJ: International normalized ratio and prothrombin time values before the removal of a lumbar plexus catheter in patients receiving warfarin after total hip replacement. Br J Anaesth 2008;101:250–254.
29. Li X, Karmakar MK, Lee A, Kwok WH, Critchley LA, Gin T: Quantitative evaluation of the echo intensity of the median nerve and flexor muscles of the forearm in the young and the elderly. Br J Radiol 2012;85:e140–e145.
30. Gadsden JC, Lindenmuth DM, Hadzic A, Xu D, Somasundarum L, Flisinski KA: Lumbar plexus block using high-pressure injection leads to contralateral and epidural spread. Anesthesiology 2008;109: 683–688.

Spinal Sonography and Applications of Ultrasound for Central Neuraxial Blocks

Manoj K. Karmakar and Ki Jinn Chin

INTRODUCTION

Central neuraxial blocks (CNBs), which include spinal, epidural, combined spinal epidural (CSE), and caudal epidural injections, are commonly practiced regional anesthesia techniques and frequently used in the perioperative period for anesthesia and analgesia and for managing chronic pain.[1] Traditionally, CNBs are performed using a combination of surface anatomical landmarks, the operator's perception of tactile sensation (loss of resistance) during needle advancement, and/or visualizing the free flow of cerebrospinal fluid. Although the spinous processes are relatively reliable surface anatomical landmarks in many patients, they are not always easily recognizable in patients with obesity,[2] edema, underlying spinal deformity, or previous back surgery. Tuffier's line, which connects the highest points of the iliac crests, is another surface anatomical landmark that is widely used to estimate the location of the L3–L4 interspace; however, the correlation is inconsistent.[3] Even in the absence of spine abnormalities, estimation of a specific intervertebral level may not be accurate in many patients[4,5] and may result in needle placement one or two spinal levels higher than intended.[4,6,7] The difficulty in identifying the correct spinal level is exaggerated in patients with obesity and in the upper spinal levels.[4,6,8] This inaccuracy has been implicated in cases of injury to the conus medullaris after spinal anesthesia.[6,8] Moreover, surface landmarks alone do not allow the operator to reliably predict the ease or difficulty of needle placement prior to skin puncture. Unanticipated technical difficulty, multiple attempts at needle placement, and failure of CNB are therefore not uncommon.[9,10] Recently, however, ultrasound (US) imaging of the spine has emerged as a useful method of overcoming many of these shortcomings of the surface landmark–guided approach to CNBs.

US imaging offers several advantages when used to guide needle placement during CNBs. It is noninvasive, safe, simple to use, can be performed expeditiously at the point of care, provides real-time images, is devoid of significant adverse effects, and is particularly helpful in delineating abnormal or variant spinal anatomy. When used for chronic pain interventions of the spine, US can reduce or eliminate exposure to ionizing radiation. Presently, US is most frequently used as a preprocedural tool,[11] but it can also be used for real-time needle guidance during CNBs.[12] During the preprocedural scan, one can accurately locate the midline,[13] identify a given lumbar interspace, predict the depth to the epidural space, and identify patients in whom a CNB may be difficult.[11,14] In expert hands, the use of US for epidural needle insertion reduces the number of puncture attempts,[15–20] improves the success rate of epidural access on the first attempt,[16] reduces the need to puncture multiple levels,[16–18] and improves patient comfort during the procedure.[17] However, despite its advantages, the integration of US into clinical practice for CNBs is still in its infancy. A recent survey of anesthesiologists in the United Kingdom showed that more than 90% of respondents were not trained to image the epidural space using US despite national guidelines advocating its use.[21] In this chapter, we describe techniques of spinal sonography, the relevant sonoanatomy, and practical considerations for using US for CNBs.

HISTORICAL BACKGROUND

Bogin and Stulin were probably the first to report the use of US for central neuraxial interventional procedures.[22] In 1971, they described using US for lumbar puncture.[7] Porter and colleagues, in 1978, used US to image the lumbar spine and measure the diameter of the spinal canal in diagnostic radiology.[23] Cork and colleagues were the first group of anesthesiologists to use US to locate the landmarks relevant for epidural anesthesia.[24] Thereafter, US was used mostly to preview the spinal anatomy and measure the distances from the skin to the lamina and epidural space before epidural puncture.[25,26] Between 2001 and 2004, Grau and colleagues, from Heidelberg, Germany, published a series of studies that formed the foundation of the clinical application of US for CNB.[15–18,27–30] Subsequent improvements in US technology and image processing software have allowed for greater image clarity of the spine and neuraxial structures.[12,31,32] Also, the increasing availability of point-of-care US systems has led to further research by other investigators, which has established our current understanding of spinal sonoanatomy.[11]

GROSS ANATOMY OF THE SPINE

The gross anatomy of the spine has been discussed in detail in Chapters 6 and 22. In this section, the anatomy relevant for US imaging of the spine is briefly reviewed. A vertebra is made up of two components: the vertebral body and the vertebral arch (Figure 40–1). The vertebral arch is formed by the supporting pedicles and laminae (Figure 40–2). Seven processes arise from the vertebral arch: one spinous process, two transverse processes, two superior articular processes, and two inferior articular processes (see Figures 40–1 and 40–2). Adjacent vertebrae articulate with each other at the facet joints between the superior and inferior articular processes and the intervertebral disc between the vertebral bodies. This produces two gaps: one between the spinous processes, the "interspinous space" (Figure 40–3), and one between the laminae, the "interlaminar space" (Figure 40–4). It is through these spaces that the US energy enters the spinal canal and makes spinal sonography and CNBs possible.

The three major ligaments of the spine are the ligamentum flavum (Figures 40–3, 40–4, and 40–5), the anterior longitudinal ligament, and the posterior longitudinal ligament (see Figure 40–3). The posterior longitudinal ligament is attached along the length of the anterior wall of the vertebral canal (see Figures 40–3, 40–4, and 40–5). The ligamentum flavum, also referred to as the yellow ligament, is a dense layer of connective tissue that bridges the interlaminar spaces (see Figure 40–4) and connects the laminae of adjacent vertebrae. It is arch-like on cross-section and is widest posteriorly in the midline and in the lumbar region (see Figure 40–5). The ligamentum flavum is attached to the anterior surface of the inferior margin of the

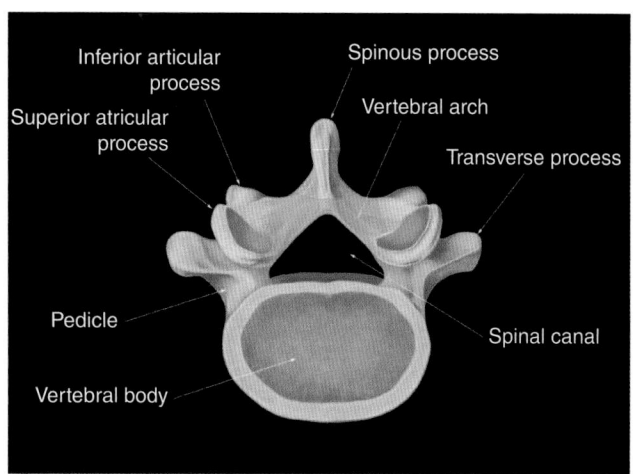

FIGURE 40–2. Vertebral arch of a typical lumbar vertebra. The vertebral arch surrounds the spinal canal and is made up of the posterior surface of the vertebral body, the pedicles, and the laminae.

lamina above but splits inferiorly to attach to both the posterior surface (superficial component) and anterior surface (deep component) of the lamina below. The spinous processes are attached at their tips by the supraspinous ligament, which is thick and cord-like, and along their length by the interspinous ligament, which is thin and membranous (see Figure 40–3).

The spinal (vertebral) canal is formed by the vertebral arch and the posterior surface of the vertebral body (see Figures 40–2 and 40–5). The openings into the spinal canal are through the intervertebral foramen along its lateral wall and the interlaminar space on its posterolateral wall. Within the spinal canal lies the thecal sac (formed by the dura mater and arachnoid mater; see Figure 40–5) and its contents (the spinal cord, cauda equina, and cerebrospinal fluid; see Figures 40–3 and 40–5). The spinal cord extends from the foramen magnum to the conus medullaris, near the lower border of the first lumbar vertebra (see Figure 40–3), finally terminating as the filum terminale. However, there is normal variation in the position of the conus medullaris, and it may extend anywhere from T12 to the upper third of L3.[33] The cauda equina, named after its resemblance to a horse's tail, is made up of lumbar, sacral, and coccygeal nerves that originate in the conus medullaris and descend caudally to exit the spinal canal through their respective intervertebral foramina. Similarly, the dural sac is classically described as ending at the level of the second sacral vertebra (S2) (see Figure 40–3), but this can vary from the upper border of S1 to the lower border of S4.[34] The epidural space is an anatomical space within the spinal canal but outside the dura mater (referred to as extradural; see Figures 40–3 and 40–5). It extends form the level of the foramen magnum cranially to the tip of the sacrum at the sacrococcygeal ligament (see Figure 40–3). The posterior epidural space is of importance for CNBs. The only structure of importance in the anterior epidural space for neuraxial blocks is the internal vertebral venous plexus.

ULTRASOUND IMAGING OF THE SPINE

Foundation

Located at a depth of several centimeters or more in adults, US imaging of the spine typically requires the use of

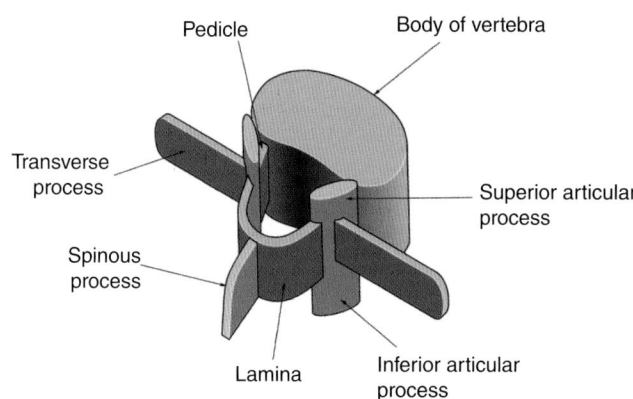

FIGURE 40–1. The components of a typical lumbar vertebra.

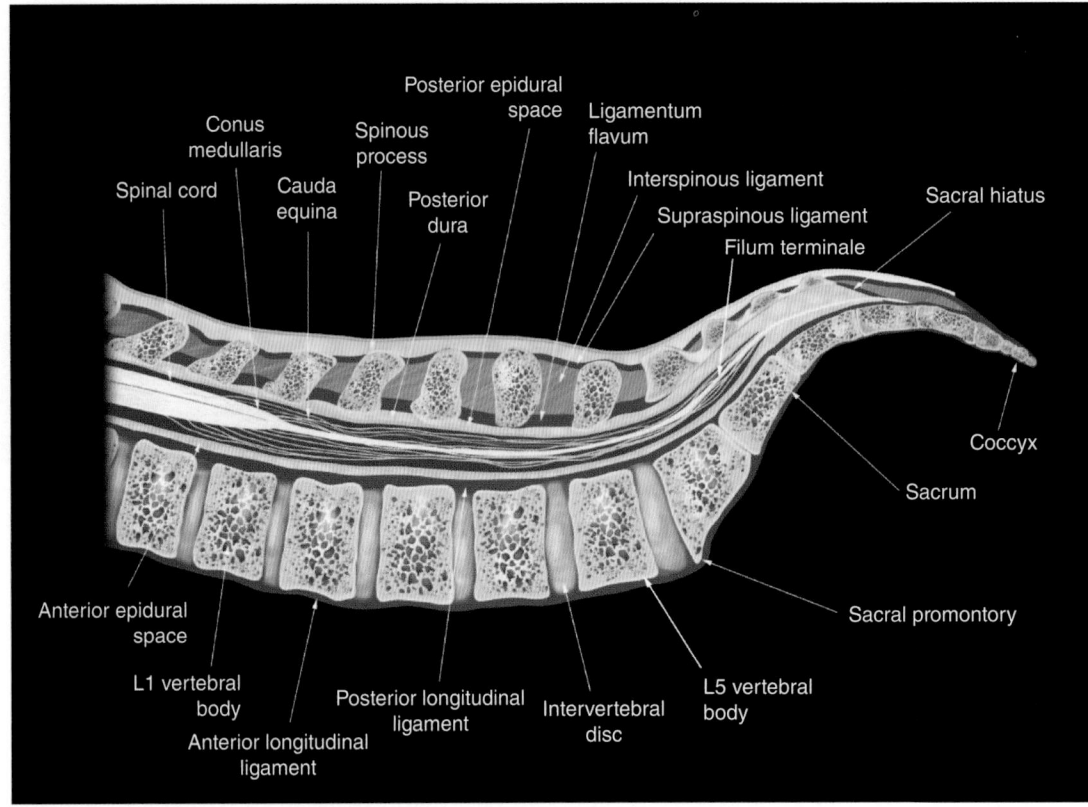

FIGURE 40–3. Sagittal anatomy of the lumbosacral spine in the median plane.

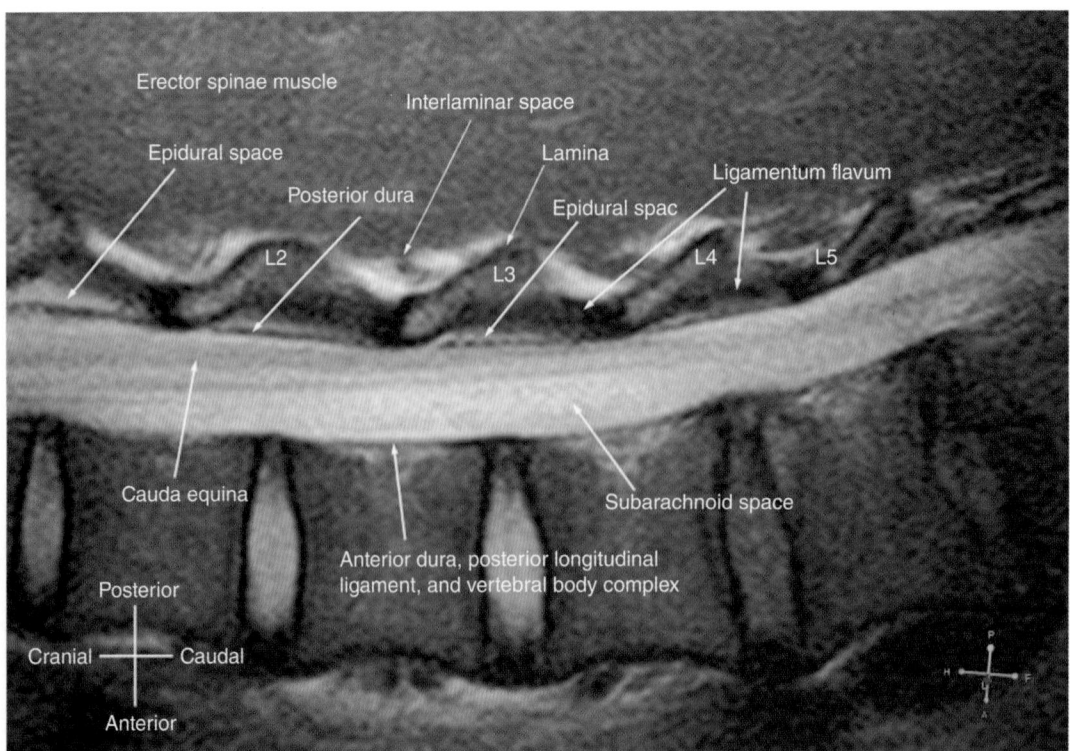

FIGURE 40–4. Paramedian sagittal MRI section of the lumbar spine at the level of the lamina.

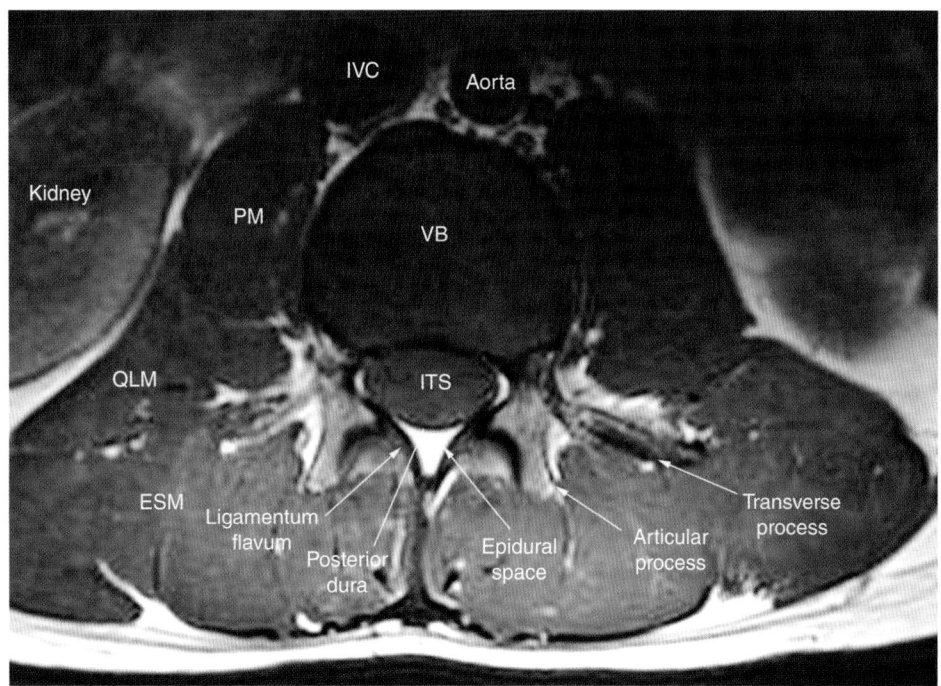

FIGURE 40–5. Transverse MRI section of the lower lumbar spine through the interspinous space. Note the relationship of the articular process to the transverse process and the attachment of the ligamentum flavum to the lamina on either side. Also note that the anterior epidural space is barely seen and that the anterior dura is very closely apposed to the posterior longitudinal ligament of the vertebra. ESM, erector spinae muscle; ITS, intrathecal space; IVC, inferior vena cava; PM, psoas major muscle; QLM, quadratus lumborum muscle; VB, vertebral body.

low-frequency US (2–5 MHz) and curved array transducers. Because of the divergent nature of their US beam, curved array transducers also produce a wide field of view, particularly in the deeper areas, which is useful when using US for CNB. Low-frequency US provides adequate penetration, but unfortunately lacks spatial resolution at the depth (5–7 cm) at which the neuraxial structures are located. The osseous framework of the spine, which envelops the neuraxial structures, reflects much of the incident US signal before it even reaches the spinal canal, presenting additional challenges in acquiring good-quality images. However, this challenge is often offset by improved image processing and advanced image optimization modes in modern US systems, and thus high-quality images of the neuraxis can still be obtained with low-frequency transducers.[32] Also of note is that technology once only available in the high-end cart-based US systems is now available in portable US devices, making US systems even more practical for spinal sonography and US-guided (USG) CNB applications.

Scanning Planes

Although anatomical planes have already been described elsewhere in this text, the importance of understanding them for imaging of the spine dictates a further, more detailed review. There are three anatomical planes: median, transverse, and coronal (Figure 40–6). The **median plane** is a longitudinal plane that passes through the midline, bisecting the body into two equal right and left halves. The **sagittal plane** is a longitudinal plane that is parallel to the median plane and

perpendicular to the ground. Therefore, the median plane can also be defined as the sagittal plane that is exactly in the middle of the body (median sagittal plane). The **transverse plane**, also known as the axial or horizontal plane, is parallel to the ground.

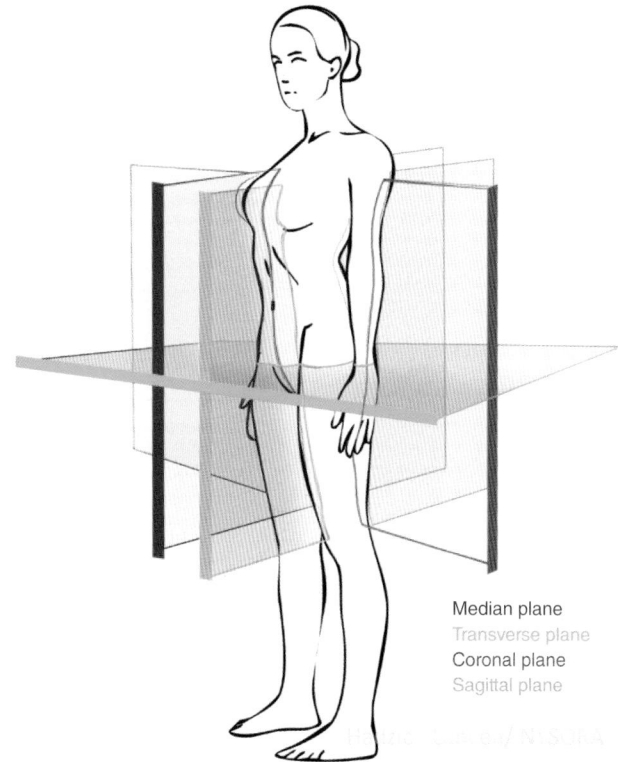

Median plane
Transverse plane
Coronal plane
Sagittal plane

FIGURE 40–6. Anatomical planes of the body.

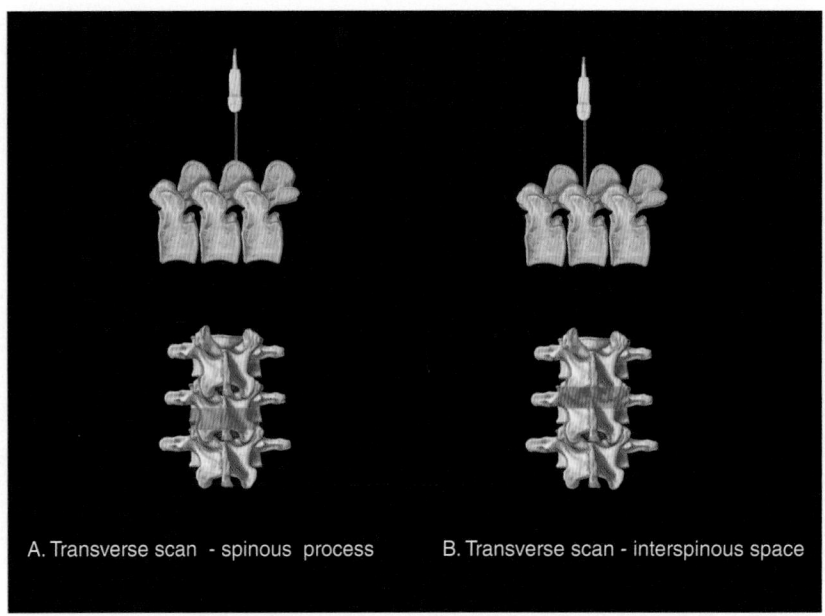

FIGURE 40–7. Axis of scan: transverse scan (**A**) at the level of the spinous process; and (**B**) at the level of the interspinous space.

The **coronal plane**, also known as the frontal plane, is a vertical plane that is perpendicular to the ground and at right angles to the sagittal plane dividing the body into an anterior and a posterior part.

Axis of Scan

US imaging of the spine can be performed in the transverse axis (transverse scan; Figure 40–7) or the longitudinal axis (sagittal scan; Figure 40–8) with the patient in the sitting, lateral decubitus, or prone position. The anatomical information obtained from these two scan planes complement each other during a US examination of the spine. A transverse scan can be performed over the spinous process (see Figure 40–7a) or through the interspinous/interlaminar space (see Figure 40–7b). The former produces the **transverse spinous process view**, whereas the latter produces the **transverse interspinous view** of the spine.[11] Transverse views are relatively easy to acquire in the lumbar region, but the transverse interspinous view is challenging in the midthoracic region (T4–8) due to the acute

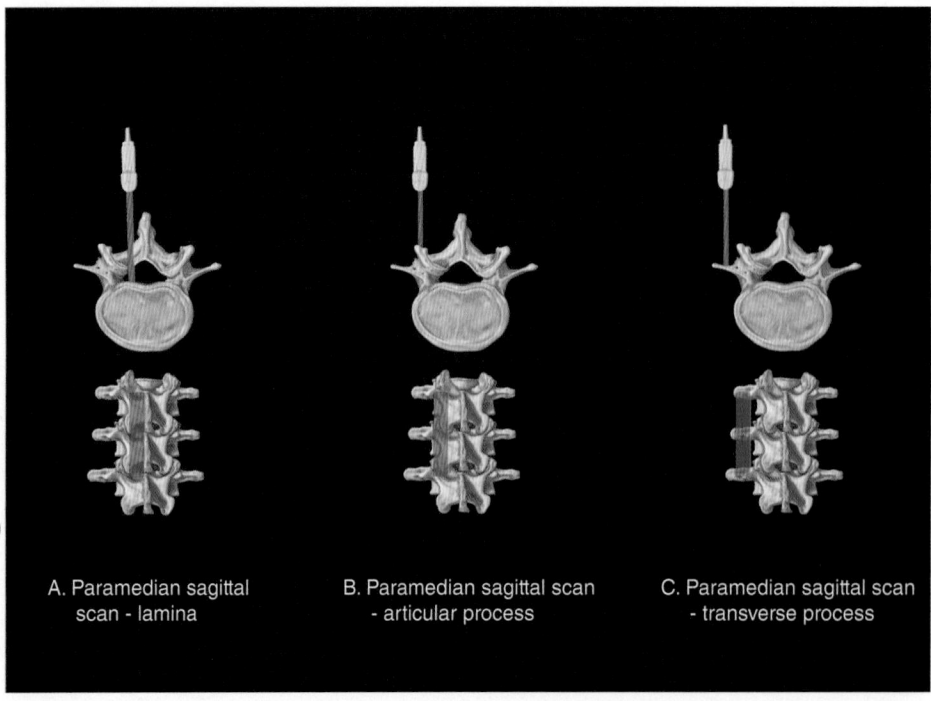

FIGURE 40–8. Axis of scan: paramedian sagittal scan (**A**) at the level of the lamina; (**B**) at the level of the articular process; and (**C**) at the level of the transverse process.

caudal angulation of the spinous processes. Depending on the angle of the spinous processes, the transducer may have to be tilted to produce an optimal interspinous view of the neuraxial structures. A sagittal scan can be performed through the midline (**median sagittal spinous process view**) or through a paramedian plane (Figure 40–8). Overall, three paramedian sagittal views of the spine can be obtained (from medial to lateral): (1) a **paramedian sagittal lamina view** (see Figure 40–8a); (2) a **paramedian sagittal articular process view** (see Figure 40–8b); and (3) a **paramedian sagittal transverse process view** (see Figure 40–8c). Grau et al. have suggested using a paramedian sagittal scan to visualize the neuraxial structures.[27] We have found that the US visibility of neuraxial structures can be further improved when the spine is imaged in the paramedian sagittal oblique plane (Figure 40–9).[12,31] During a paramedian sagittal oblique scan (PMSOS), the transducer is positioned 2–3 cm lateral to the midline (paramedian) and over the laminae in the sagittal axis, tilted slightly medially toward the midline (see Figure 40–9).[12,31] The purpose of the medial tilt is to ensure that the US signal enters the spinal canal through the widest part of the interlaminar space and not the lateral sulcus of the spinal canal.

Sonoanatomy of the Spine

Detailed knowledge of the vertebral anatomy is essential to understand the sonoanatomy of the spine. Unfortunately, cross-sectional anatomy texts describe the anatomy of the spine in traditional orthogonal planes; that is, the transverse, sagittal, and coronal planes. This often results in difficulty interpreting the spinal sonoanatomy because US imaging is generally performed in an arbitrary or intermediary plane by tilting, sliding, and rotating the transducer. Several anatomical models have recently been developed to teach musculoskeletal US imaging techniques (in human volunteers), the sonoanatomy relevant for peripheral nerve blocks (in human volunteers and cadavers), and the required interventional skills (in tissue-mimicking phantoms and fresh cadavers). However, few models or tools are available to learn and practice spinal sonoanatomy or the interventional skills required for USG CNB. Karmakar and colleagues recently described the use of a "water-based spine phantom" (Figure 40–10) to study the osseous anatomy of the lumbosacral spine.[32,35] A gelatin lumbosacral spine phantom,[36] gelatin–agar spine phantom (Figure 40–11), "pig-carcass phantom"[37] (Figure 40–12), and lumbar training phantom (Figure 40–13a; CIRS model 034, CIRS, Inc., Norfolk, VA) have also been described to practice the basic hand–eye coordination skills required to perform USG CNBs. Since three-dimensional (3D) reconstructions of high-definition CT scan data (3D volume datasets) can also be used to study the osseous anatomy (Figure 40–13b, c, d) and validate the structure visualized in multiplanar 3D images (Figure 40–14). Computer-generated anatomical reconstructions from the Visible Human Project dataset that correspond to the US scan planes provide another useful way of studying the sonoanatomy of the spine in vivo[32] (Figure 40–15). Multiplanar 3D reconstructions from archived high-resolution 3D CT datasets of the spine can also be used to study and validate the sonographic appearance of the various osseous elements and neuraxial structures of the spine.

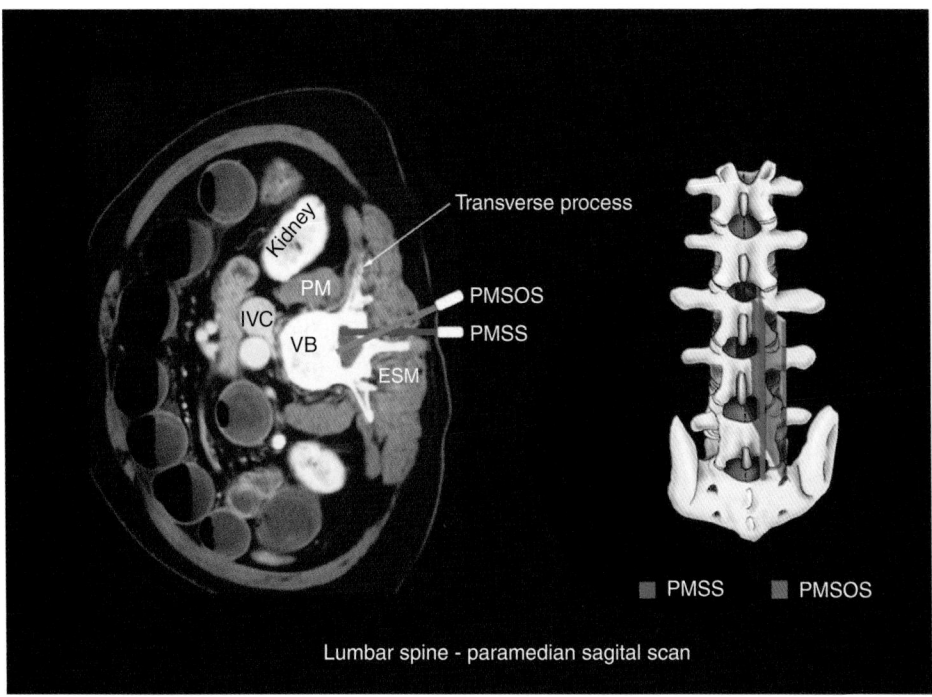

FIGURE 40–9. Axis of scan: paramedian sagittal oblique scan of the lumbar spine. Note the medial direction of the US beam (blue). ESM, erector spinae muscle; IVC, inferior vena cava; PM, psoas major muscle; PMSOS, paramedian sagittal oblique scan; PMSS, paramedian sagittal scan (red); VB, vertebral body.

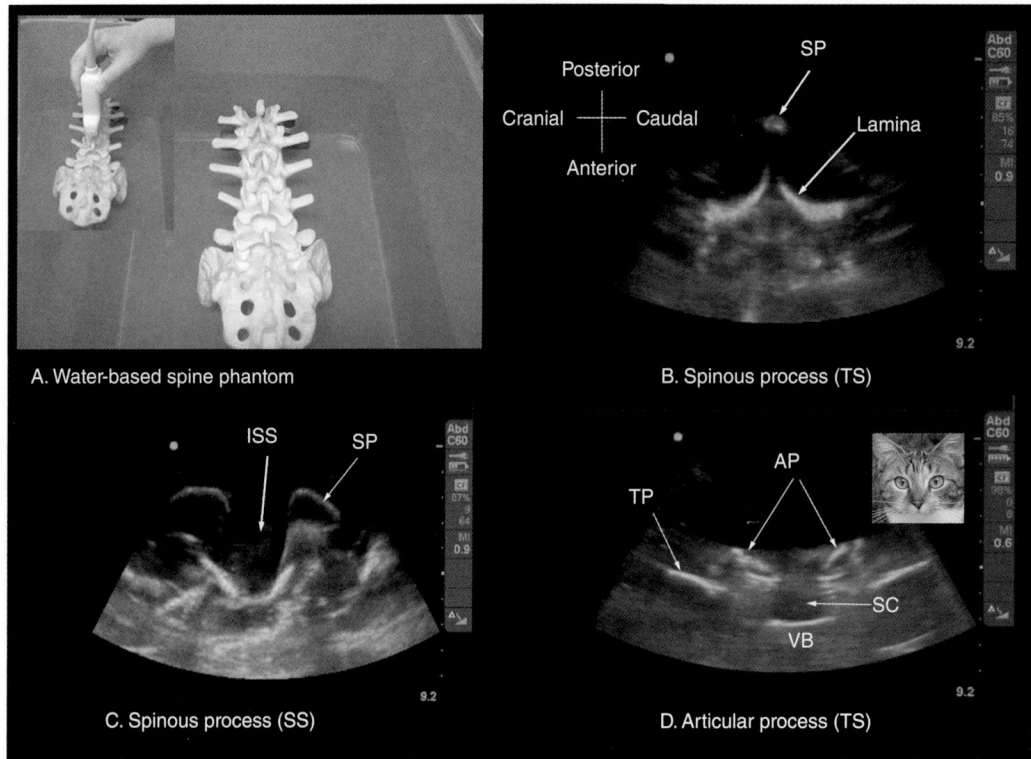

FIGURE 40–10. (A) The water-based spine phantom. The lumbosacral spine is immersed in a water bath and imaged through the water using a curved linear transducer. The other images are sonograms from the water-based lumbosacral spine phantom showing **(B)** the transverse spinous process (SP) view; **(C)** the median sagittal spinous process view; and **(D)** the transverse interspinous view. An inset image has been placed next to figure (d) to illustrate the resemblance of the sonographic appearance of the transverse interspinous view to a cat's head; hence, this is referred to as the "cat's head sign." AP, articular process; ISS, interspinous space; SC, spinal canal; SP, spinous process; SS, sagittal scan; TP, transverse process; TS, transverse scan; VB, vertebral body.

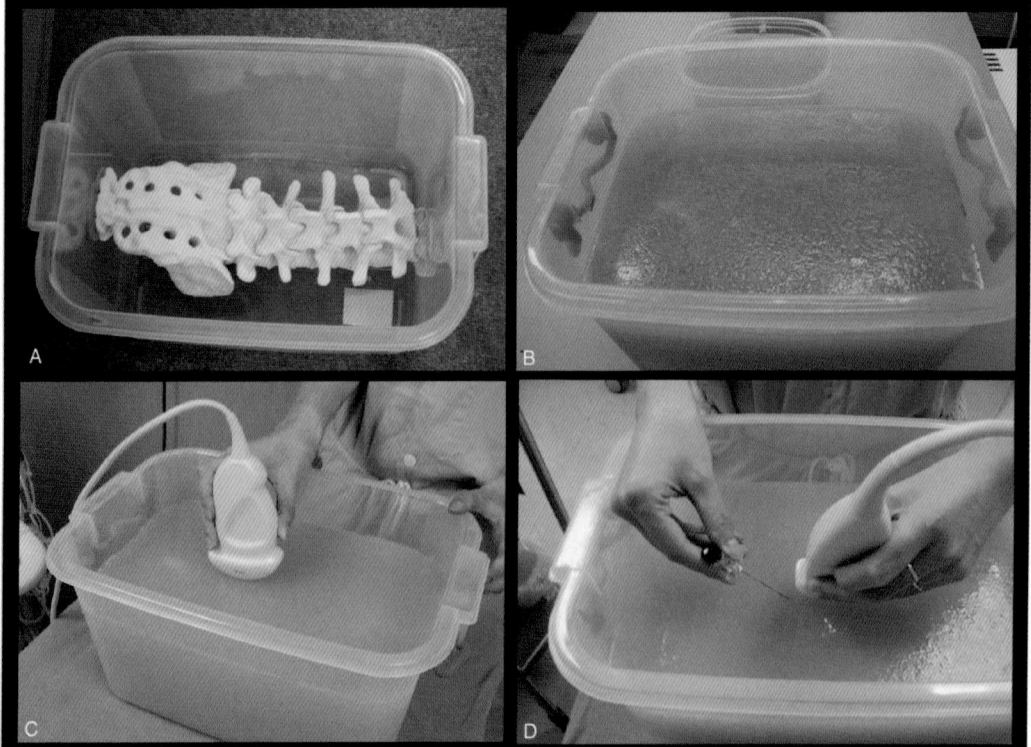

FIGURE 40–11. Gelatin–agar spine phantom. **(A)** Lumbosacral spine model secured to the base of the plastic box. **(B)** Spine phantom after being embedded in the gelatin–agar mixture. **(C)** Performing a US scan of the gelatin–agar spine phantom. **(D)** Simulated in-plane needle insertion in the gelatin–agar spine phantom.

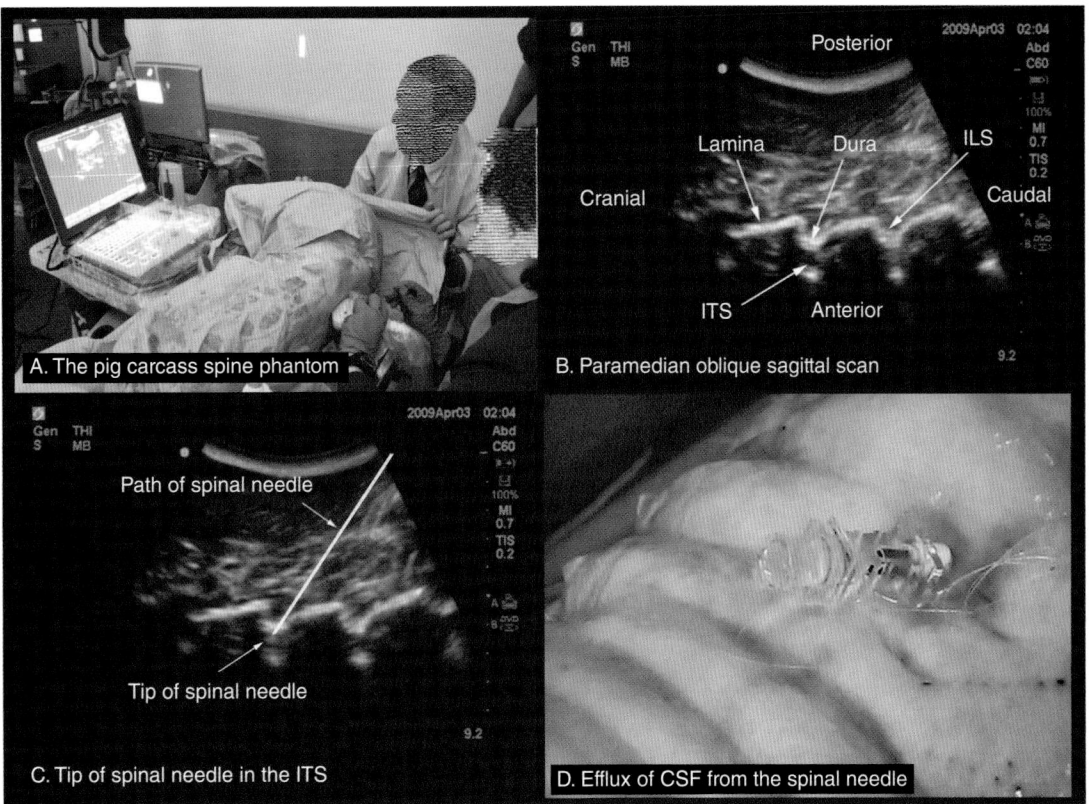

FIGURE 40–12. The pig carcass spine phantom. (**A**) Pig carcass spine phantom being used to practice central neuraxial blocks at a workshop. (**B**) Paramedian sagittal oblique sonogram of the lumbar spine. (**C**) Sonogram showing the tip of a spinal needle in the intrathecal space (ITS). (**D**) Efflux of cerebrospinal fluid (CSF) from the hub of a spinal needle that has been inserted into the ITS. ILS, interlaminar space.

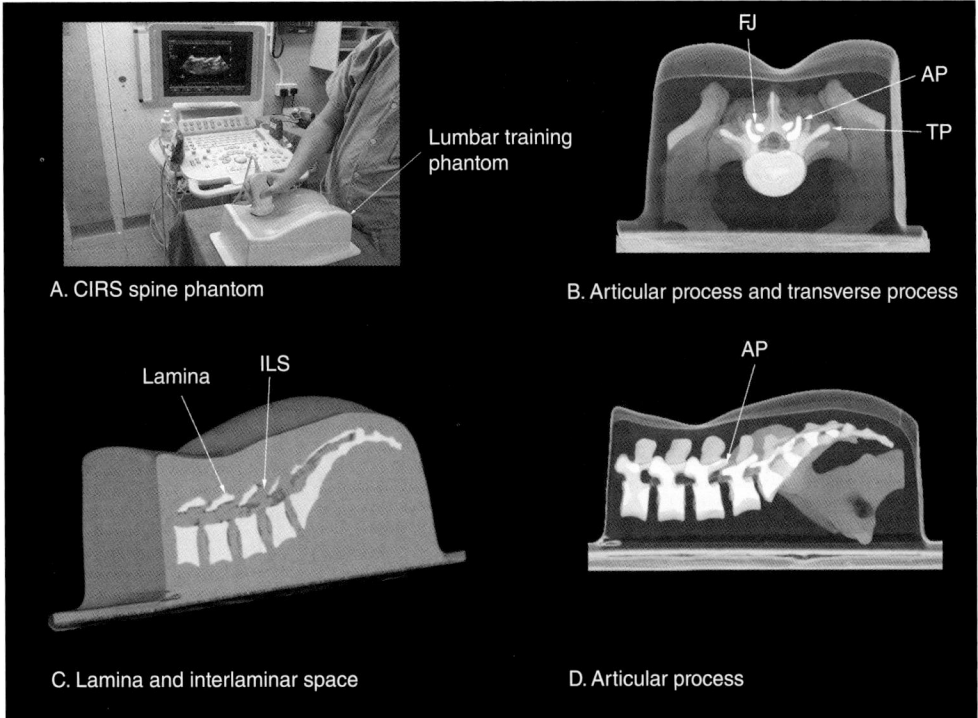

FIGURE 40–13. (**A**) CIRS lumbar training phantom (CIRS model 034, CIRS Inc., Norfolk, VA). The other images illustrate a three-dimensional reconstruction of a high-resolution computed tomography scan dataset from the CIRS phantom showing (**B**) a median transverse interspinous section of the lumbar spine; (**C**) a paramedian sagittal section at the level of the lamina; and (**D**) a paramedian sagittal section at the level of the articular processes (AP). FJ, facet joint; ILS, interlaminar space; TP, transverse process.

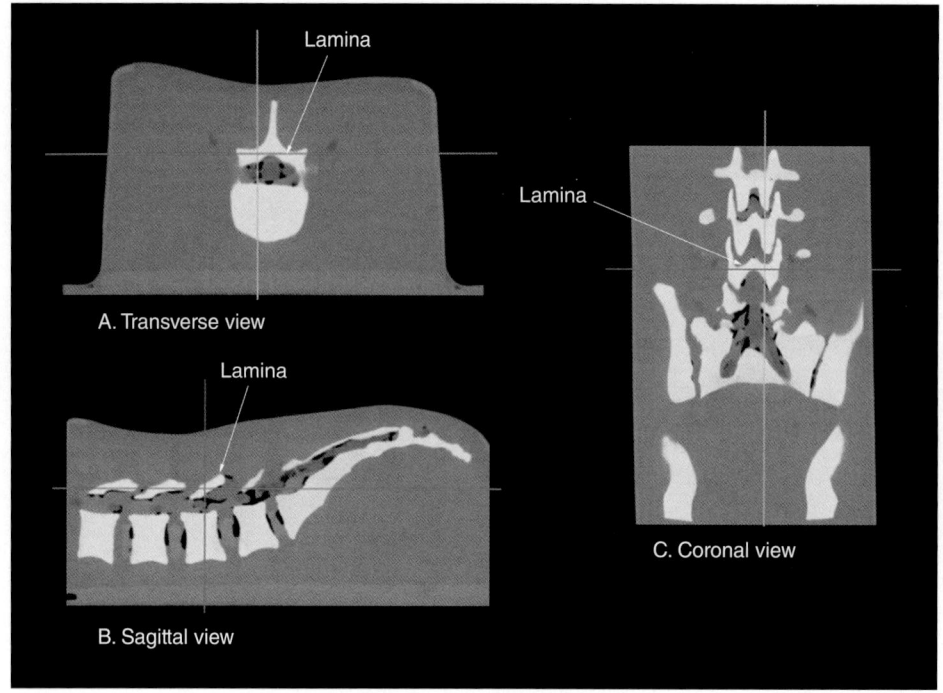

FIGURE 40–14. Multiplanar three-dimensional reconstruction of a high-resolution computed tomography scan dataset from the CIRS phantom. Note that the reference point (where the two orthogonal planes cross) is lying over the lamina. (**A**) Transverse view of the lamina. (**B**) Sagittal view of the lamina. (**C**) Coronal view of the lamina.

Water-Based Spine Phantom

The **water-based spine phantom**[37] simplifies the process of learning the sonoanatomy of the spine in two easy steps: (1) learning the sonoanatomy of the osseous elements of the spine; and (2) learning the sonoanatomy of the soft-tissue structures that make up the spine. The water-based spine phantom[37] is an excellent model to define the osseous anatomy

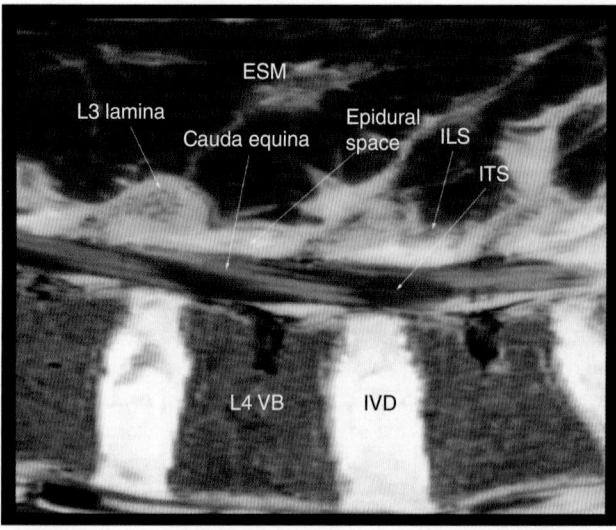

FIGURE 40–15. Sagittal cadaver anatomical section of the lumbar spine through the lamina of the lumbar spine, rendered from the Visible Human Server male dataset. ESM, erector spinae muscle; ILS, interlaminar space; ITS, intrathecal space; IVD, intervertebral disc; VB, vertebral body.

of the spine[32,37] and is based on a model described previously by Greher and colleagues to study the osseous anatomy of relevance to USG lumbar facet nerve block.[38] The model is prepared by immersing a commercially available lumbosacral spine model in a water bath (see Figure 40–10a). A low-frequency curved array transducer is then used to scan the model through the water in the transverse and sagittal axes as one would do in vivo. Each osseous element of the spine produces a characteristic sonographic pattern.[37] The ability to recognize these sonographic patterns is an important step toward understanding the sonoanatomy of the spine. Representative US images of the spinous process, lamina, articular processes, and transverse process from the water-based spine phantom are presented in Figures 10b, c, d and 16a, b, c. The advantage of this water-based spine phantom is that water produces an anechoic (black) background against which the hyperechoic reflections from the bone are clearly visualized. The water-based spine phantom allows a see-through, real-time visual validation of the sonographic appearance of a given osseous element by performing the scan with a marker (eg, a needle) in contact with it (see Figure 40–16a). The described model is also inexpensive, easily prepared, requires little time to set up, and can be used repeatedly without deteriorating or decomposing, as animal tissue-based phantoms do. Once the novice learns to identify the individual osseous elements of the spine in the various US scan planes, it becomes easy to define the gaps between these elements: the interspinous (see Figure 40–10c) and interlaminar spaces (see Figure 40–16a), through which the US energy enters the spinal canal to produce the acoustic window seen on a spinal sonogram. The same gaps or spaces also permit passage of the needle to the neuraxis during USG CNB.

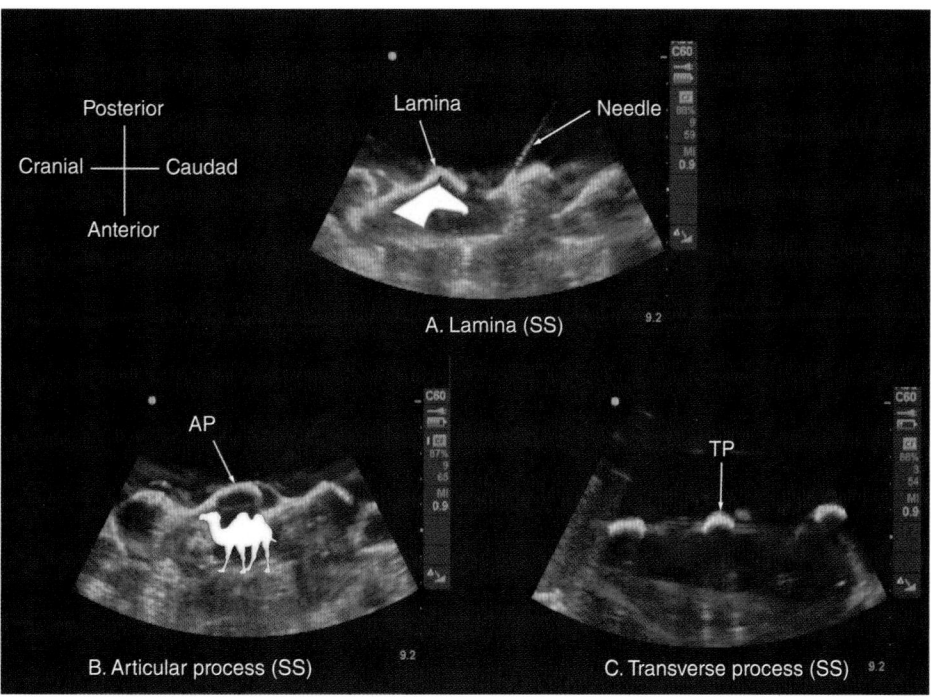

FIGURE 40–16. Paramedian sagittal sonogram of the (**A**) lamina; (**B**) articular process; and (**C**) transverse process from a water-based spine phantom. Note the needle in contact with the lamina in (a), a method that was used to validate the sonographic appearance of the osseous elements in the phantom. The inset image in (a) illustrates the horse-head–like appearance of the laminae, and the inset image in (b) illustrates the camel-hump–like appearance of the articular processes. AP, articular process; SS, sagittal scan; TP, transverse process.

ULTRASOUND IMAGING OF THE LUMBAR SPINE

Sagittal Scan

The patient is positioned in the sitting, lateral, or prone position, with the lumbosacral spine maximally flexed. The transducer is placed 1–2 cm lateral to the spinous process (ie, in the paramedian sagittal plane) at the lower back with its orientation marker directed cranially. A slight medial tilt during the scan insonates the spine in a **paramedian sagittal oblique (PMSO)** plane. First, the sacrum is identified as a flat, hyperechoic structure with a large acoustic shadow anteriorly (Figure 40–17). When the transducer is slid in a cranial direction, a gap is seen between the sacrum and the lamina of the L5 vertebra, which is the L5–S1 interlaminar space, also referred to as the L5–S1gap (Figures 40–17 and 40–18).[32,39] The L3–4 and L4–5 interlaminar spaces can now be located by counting upward (Figure 40–19).[12,32] The erector spinae muscles are hypoechoic and lie superficial to the laminae. The lamina appears hyperechoic and is the first osseous structure visualized (see Figure 40–19). Because bone impedes US penetration, there is an acoustic shadow anterior to each lamina. The sonographic appearance of the lamina produces a pattern that resembles the head and neck of a horse (the "horse head sign") (see Figures 40–16a and 40–19).[32] The interlaminar space is the gap between the adjoining laminae (Figure 40–20) and is the "acoustic window" through which the neuraxial structures are visualized within the spinal canal.

The ligamentum flavum appears as a hyperechoic band across the adjacent laminae (see Figure 40–19). The posterior dura is the next hyperechoic structure anterior to the ligamentum flavum, and the epidural space is the hypoechoic area (a few millimeters wide) between the ligamentum flavum and the posterior dura (see Figure 40–19). The ligamentum flavum and posterior dura may also be seen as a single linear hyperechoic structure, which is referred to as the "posterior complex"[11] or "ligamentum flavum–posterior dura complex."[40] The posterior dura is generally more hyperechoeic than the ligamentum flavum.[32] The thecal sac with the cerebrospinal fluid is the anechoic space anterior to the posterior dura (see Figure 40–19). The cauda equina, which is located within the thecal sac, is often seen as multiple horizontal, hyperechoic shadows within the anechoic thecal sac. Pulsations of the cauda equina are identified in some patients.[12,32] The anterior dura is also hyperechoic, but it is not always easy to differentiate it from the posterior longitudinal ligament and the posterior surface of the vertebral body because they are of similar echogenicity (isoechoic) and closely apposed to each other. What results is a single, composite, hyperechoic reflection anteriorly, which is referred to as the "anterior complex" (see Figures 40–17 and 40–19).[12,32]

If the transducer slides medially, that is, to the median sagittal plane, the **median sagittal spinous process view** is obtained, and the tips of the spinous processes of the L3–L5 vertebrae, which appear as superficial, hyperechoic crescent-shaped structures, are seen (Figures 40–10c, 40–21, and 40–22).[31,32] The acoustic window between the spinous processes in the median plane is narrow and often prevents clear visualization of the neuraxial structures within the spinal canal.

If the transducer is moved laterally from the paramedian sagittal plane at the level of the lamina, the **paramedian**

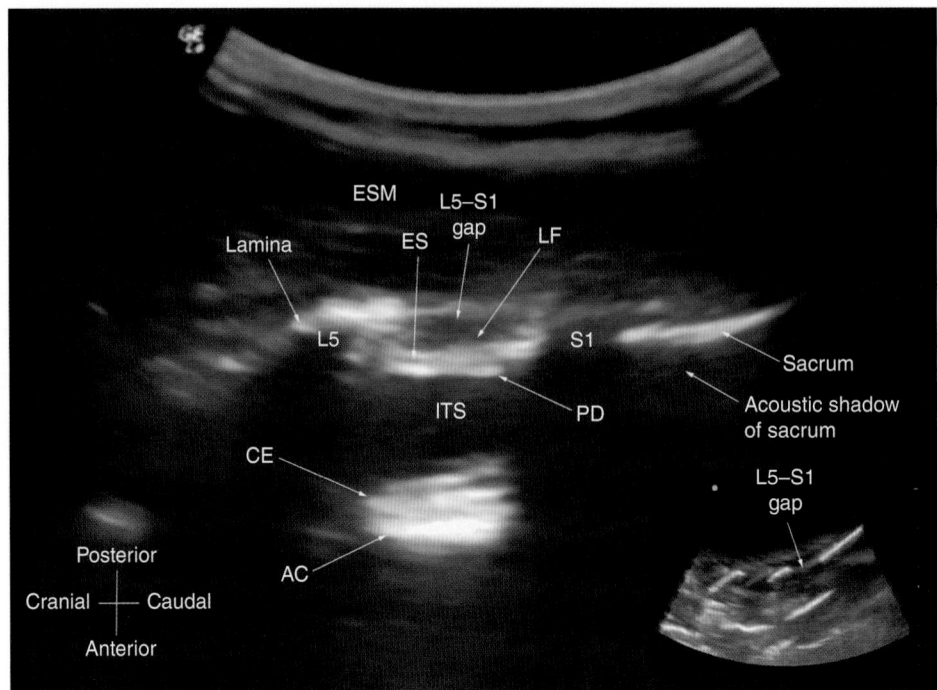

FIGURE 40–17. Paramedian sagittal sonogram of the lumbosacral junction. The posterior surface of the sacrum is identified as a flat hyperechoic structure with a large acoustic shadow anteriorly. The dip or gap between the sacrum and the lamina of L5 is the L5–S1 intervertebral space, or the L5–S1 gap. The inset image is a matching sonogram from a water-based spine phantom showing the L5–S1 gap. AC, anterior complex; CE, cauda equina; ES, epidural space; ESM, erector spinae muscle; ITS, intrathecal space; LF, ligamentum flavum; PD, posterior dura.

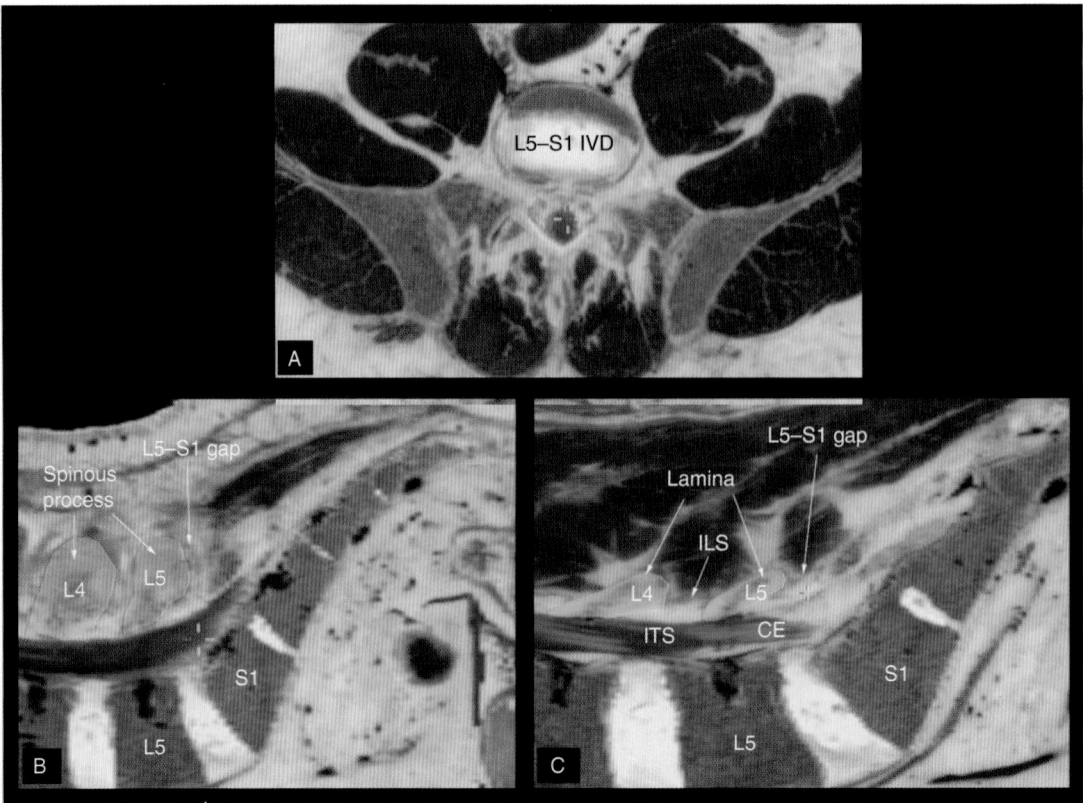

FIGURE 40–18. Cadaver anatomical section showing the lumbosacral junction (L5–S1 gap) in the (**A**) transverse axis; (**B**) median (sagittal) axis and (**C**) paramedian sagittal axis. CE, cauda equina; ILS, interlaminar space; ITS, intrathecal space; IVD, intervertebral disc.

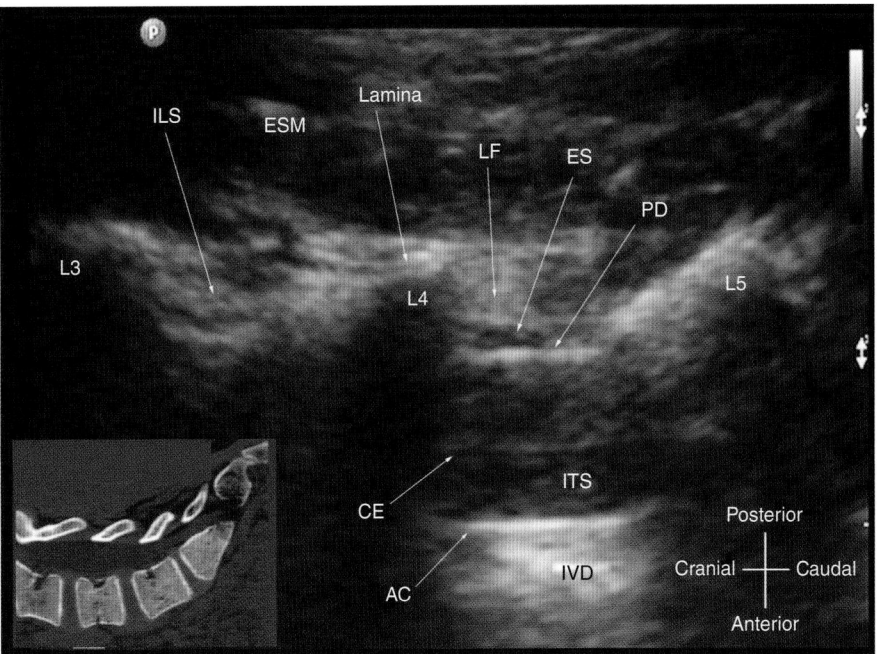

FIGURE 40–19. Paramedian sagittal oblique sonogram of the lumbar spine at the level of the lamina showing the L3–4 and L4–5 interlaminar spaces. Note the hypoechoic epidural space (a few millimeters wide) between the hyperechoic ligamentum flavum and the posterior dura. The intrathecal space is the anechoic space between the posterior dura and the anterior complex. The cauda equina nerve fibers are also seen as hyperechoic longitudinal structures within the thecal sac. The hyperechoic reflections seen in front of the anterior complex are from the intervertebral disc (IVD). The inset image shows a matching computed tomography (CT) scan of the lumbosacral spine in the same anatomical plane as the US scan. The CT slice was reconstructed from a three-dimensional CT dataset from the author's archive. AC, anterior complex; CE, cauda equina; ES, epidural space; ESM, erector spinae muscle; ILS, interlaminar space; ITS, intrathecal space; IVD, intervertebral disc; L3, lamina of L3 vertebra; L4, lamina of L4 vertebra; L5, lamina of L5 vertebra; LF, ligamentum flavum; PD, posterior dura.

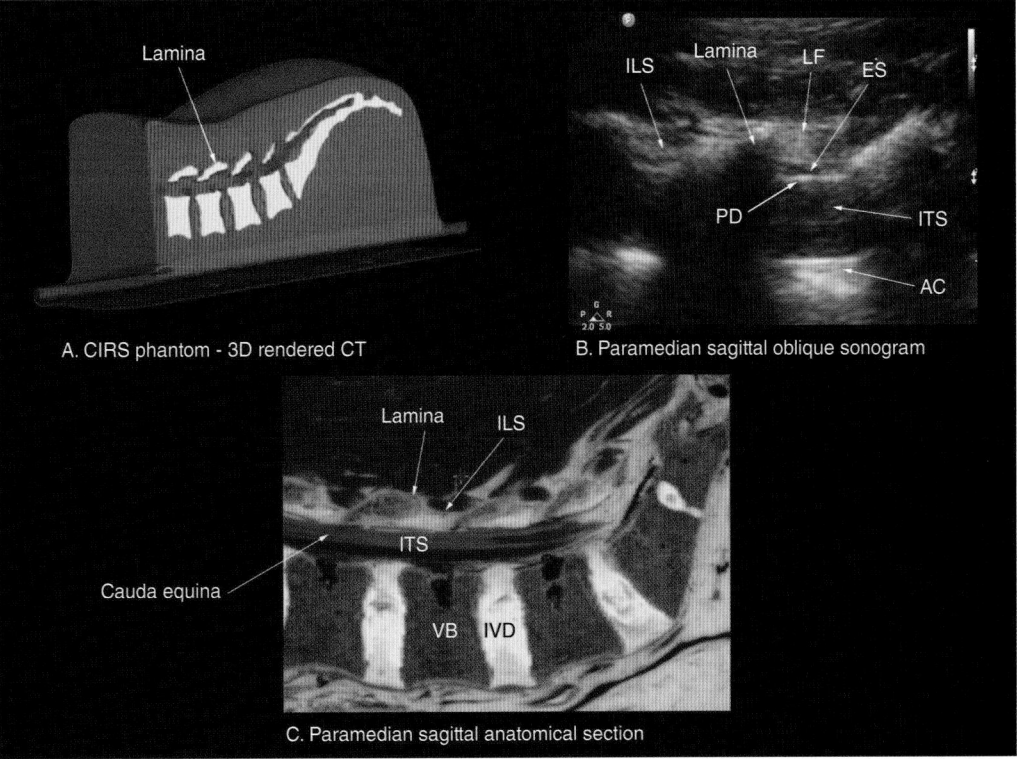

FIGURE 40–20. Paramedian sagittal sections of the lumbosacral spine showing the lamina, interlaminar spaces, and spinal canal. (**A**) Three-dimensional (3D) reconstruction of high-resolution computed tomography (CT) scan dataset from the CIRS phantom. (**B**) Paramedian sagittal oblique sonogram through the L3–5 interlaminar spaces. (**C**) Paramedian sagittal cadaver anatomic section. AC, anterior complex; ES, epidural space; ILS, interlaminar space; ITS, intrathecal space; IVD, intervertebral disc; LF, ligamentum flavum; PD, posterior dura; VB, vertebral body.

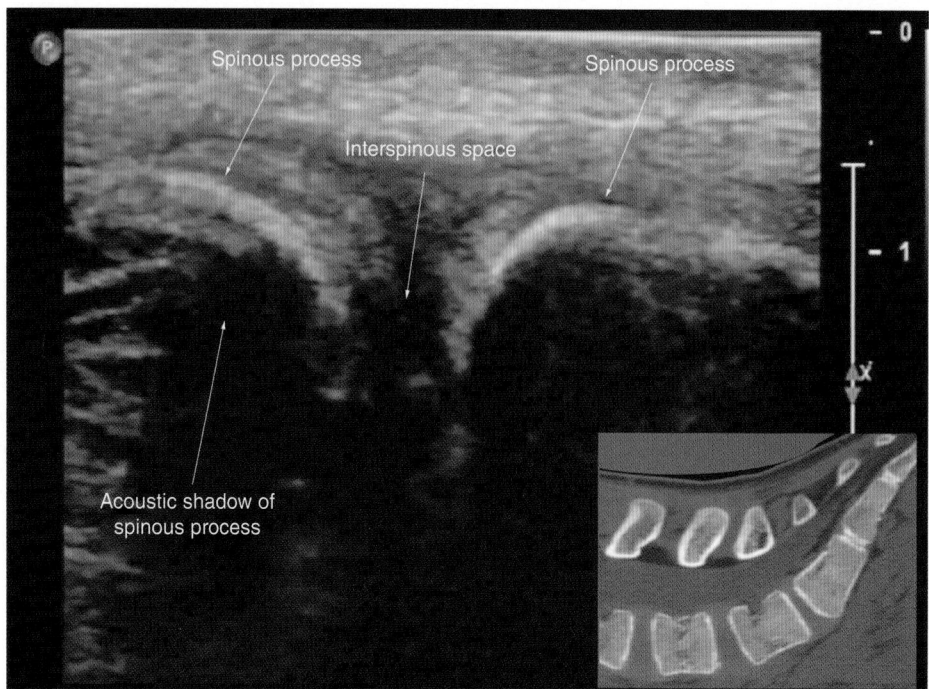

FIGURE 40–21. Median sagittal sonogram of the lumbar spine showing the crescent-shaped hyperechoic reflections of the spinous processes. Note the narrow interspinous space in the midline. The inset image shows a corresponding computed tomography (CT) scan of the lumbosacral spine through the median plane. The CT slice was reconstructed from a three-dimensional CT dataset from the author's archive.

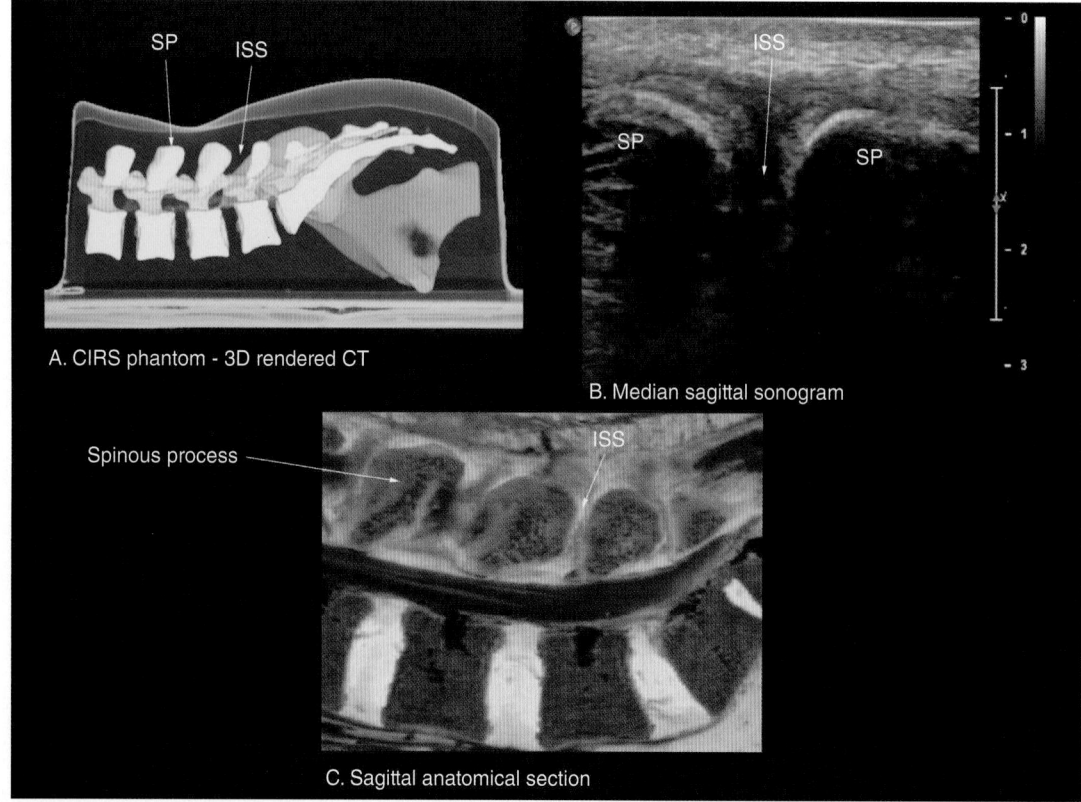

FIGURE 40–22. Median sagittal sections of the lumbosacral spine. (**A**) Three-dimensional (3D) reconstruction of high-resolution computed tomography (CT) scan dataset from the CIRS phantom. (**B**) Median sagittal sonogram showing the spinous process (SP) and interspinous space (ISS). (**C**) Median sagittal cadaver anatomical section.

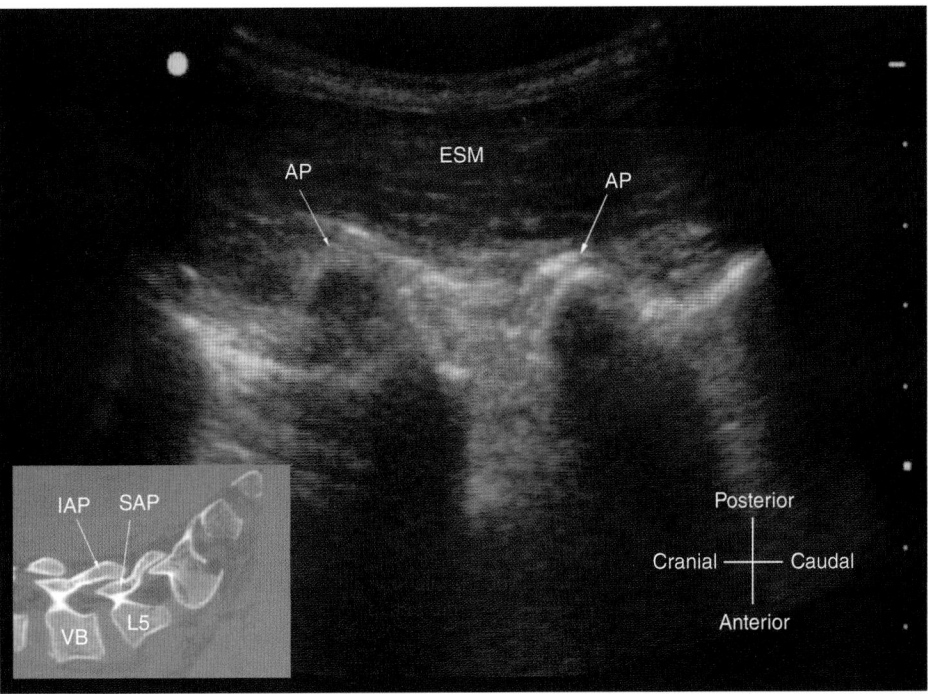

FIGURE 40–23. Paramedian sagittal sonogram of the lumbar spine at the level of the articular processes (APs) of the vertebrae. Note the "camel hump" appearance of the APs. The inset image shows a corresponding computed tomography (CT) scan of the lumbosacral spine at the level of the APs. The CT slice was reconstructed from a three-dimensional CT dataset from the author's archive. ESM, erector spinae muscle; IAP, inferior articular process; SAP, superior articular process; VB, vertebral body.

sagittal articular process view (Figures 40–23 and 40–24) is seen. The articular processes of the vertebrae appear as one continuous, hyperechoic wavy line with no intervening gaps (see Figure 40–23).[31,32] This produces a sonographic pattern that resembles multiple camel humps, which is therefore referred to as the "camel hump sign" (see Figures 40–16b, 40–23, and 40–24).[31,32]

A sagittal scan lateral to the articular processes brings the transverse processes of the L3–L5 vertebrae into view and produces the **paramedian sagittal transverse process view** (Figures 40–25 and 40–26). The transverse processes are recognized by their crescent-shaped, hyperechoic reflections and finger-like acoustic shadows anteriorly (see Figures 40–16c, 40–25, and 40–26).[32,41] These characteristics produce a sonographic pattern that is referred to as the "trident sign" because of its resemblance to the trident (Latin *tridens* or *tridentis*) that is often associated with Poseidon, the god of the sea in Greek mythology, and the trishula of the Hindu god Shiva (Figure 40–25).[41]

Transverse Scan

For a transverse scan of the lumbar spine, the US transducer is positioned over the spinous process (**transverse spinous process view**; see Figure 40–7a), with the patient in the sitting or lateral position. On a transverse sonogram, the spinous process and the lamina on either side are seen as a hyperechoic reflection anterior to which there is a dark acoustic shadow that completely obscures the underlying spinal canal and thus the neuraxial structures (Figures 40–27 and 40–28). Therefore, this view is not suitable for imaging the neuraxial structures but

can be useful for identifying the midline when the spinous processes cannot be palpated (eg, in obese patients).

However, by sliding the transducer slightly cranially or caudally, it is possible to perform a transverse scan through the interspinous or interlaminar space (**transverse interspinous view**; Figures 40–7b, 40–29, and 40–30).[13,31] A slight tilt of the transducer cranially or caudally may be needed to align the US beam with the interspinous space and optimize the US image. In the transverse interspinous view, the posterior dura, thecal sac, and anterior complex are visualized (from a posterior to anterior direction) within the spinal canal in the midline and the articular processes, and the transverse processes are visualized laterally (see Figures 40–29 and 40–30).[13,31] The osseous elements produce a sonographic pattern that resembles a cat's head, with the spinal canal representing the head, the articular processes representing the ears, and the transverse processes representing the whiskers (the "cat's head sign") (see Figure 40–10d).

The ligamentum flavum is rarely visualized in the transverse interspinous view, possibly due to anisotropy caused by the arch-like attachment of the ligamentum flavum to the lamina. The epidural space is also less frequently visualized in the transverse interspinous view than in the PMSOS. The transverse interspinous view can be used to examine for rotational deformities of the vertebrae, such as in scoliosis. Normally, both the laminae and the articular processes on either side should be symmetrically located (see Figures 40–10d, 40–13b, and 40–29). However, if there is asymmetry, a rotational deformity of the vertebral column[42] should be suspected and the needle trajectory altered accordingly.

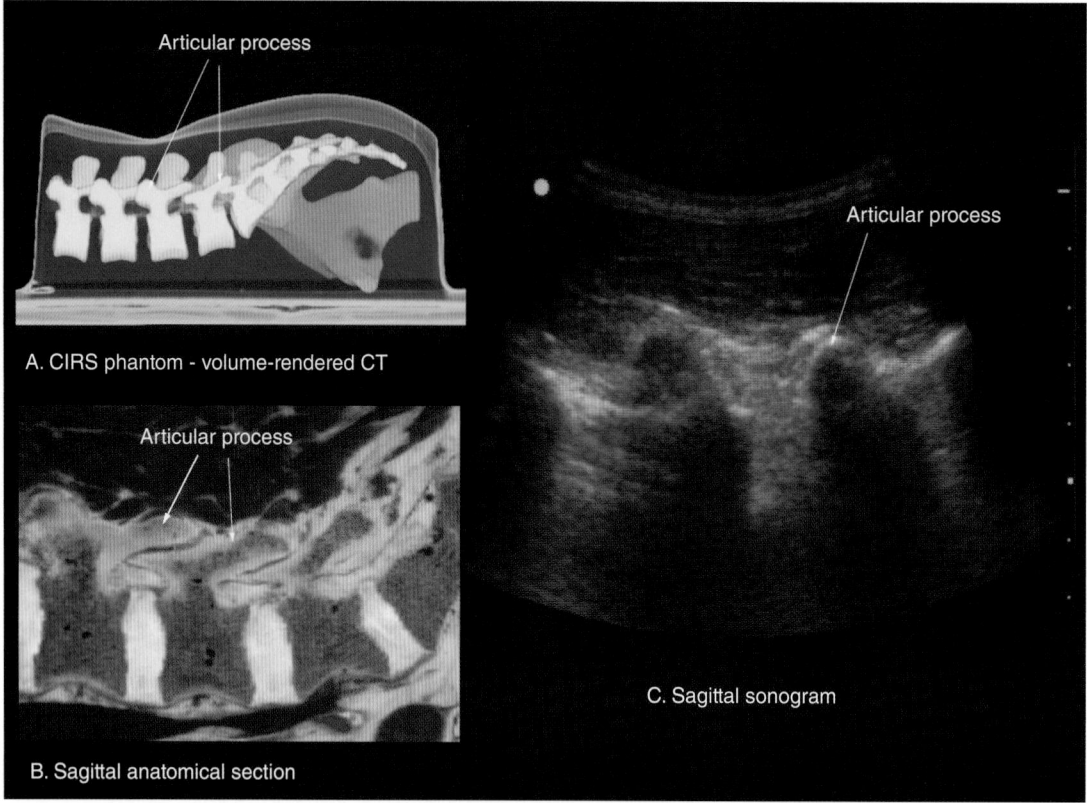

FIGURE 40–24. Paramedian sagittal sections of the lumbar spine at the level of the articular processes (APs). (**A**) Three-dimensional reconstruction of a high-resolution computed tomography (CT) scan dataset from the CIRS phantom. (**B**) Paramedian sagittal cadaver anatomical section. (**C**) Paramedian sagittal sonogram.

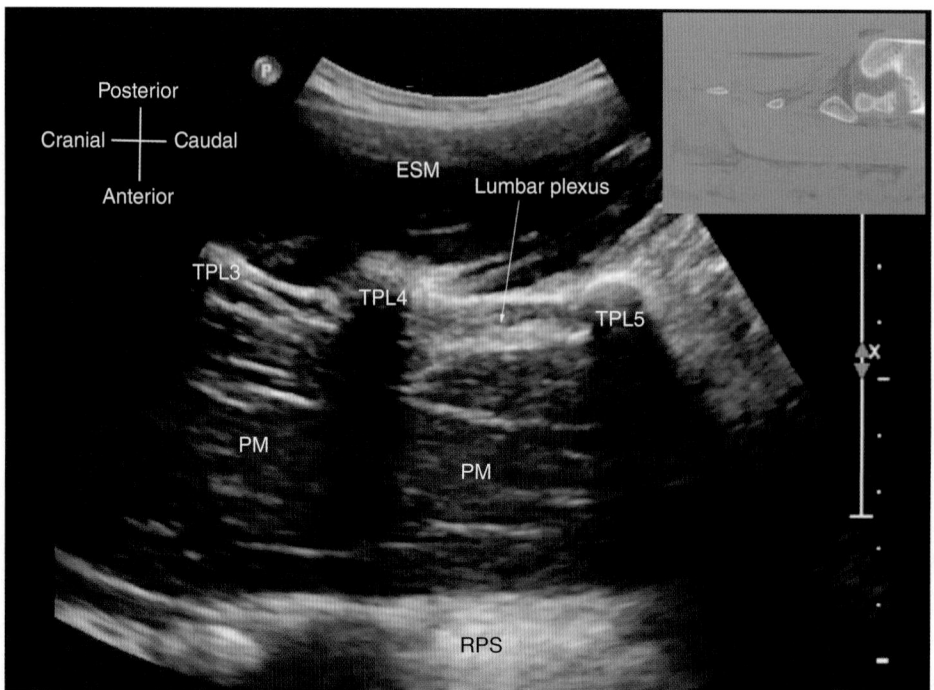

FIGURE 40–25. Paramedian sagittal sonogram of the lumbar spine at the level of the transverse processes (TPs). Note the hyperechoic reflections of the TPs with their acoustic shadow that produces the "trident sign." The psoas muscle (PM) is seen in the acoustic window between the transverse processes and is recognized by its typical hypoechoic and striated appearance. Part of the lumbar plexus is also seen as a hyperechoic shadow in the posterior part of the psoas muscle between the transverse processes of the L4 and L5 vertebrae. The inset image shows a corresponding computed tomography (CT) scan of the lumbosacral spine at the level of the TPs. The CT slice was reconstructed from a three-dimensional CT dataset from the author's archive. ESM, erector spinae muscle; RPS, retroperitoneal space.

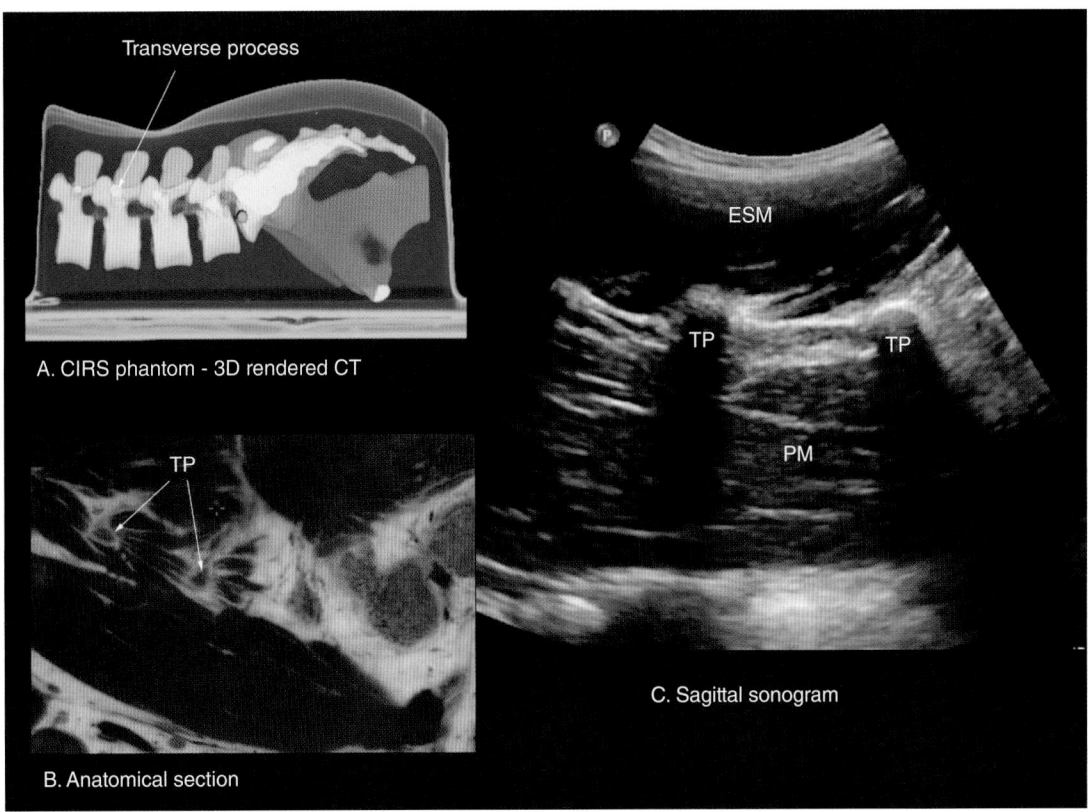

FIGURE 40-26. Paramedian sagittal sections of the lumbar spine at the level of the transverse processes (TPs). (**A**) Three-dimensional (3D) reconstruction of a high-resolution computed tomography (CT) scan dataset from the CIRS phantom. (**B**) Paramedian sagittal cadaver anatomical section. (**C**) Paramedian sagittal sonogram. ESM, erector spinae muscle; PM, psoas major muscle.

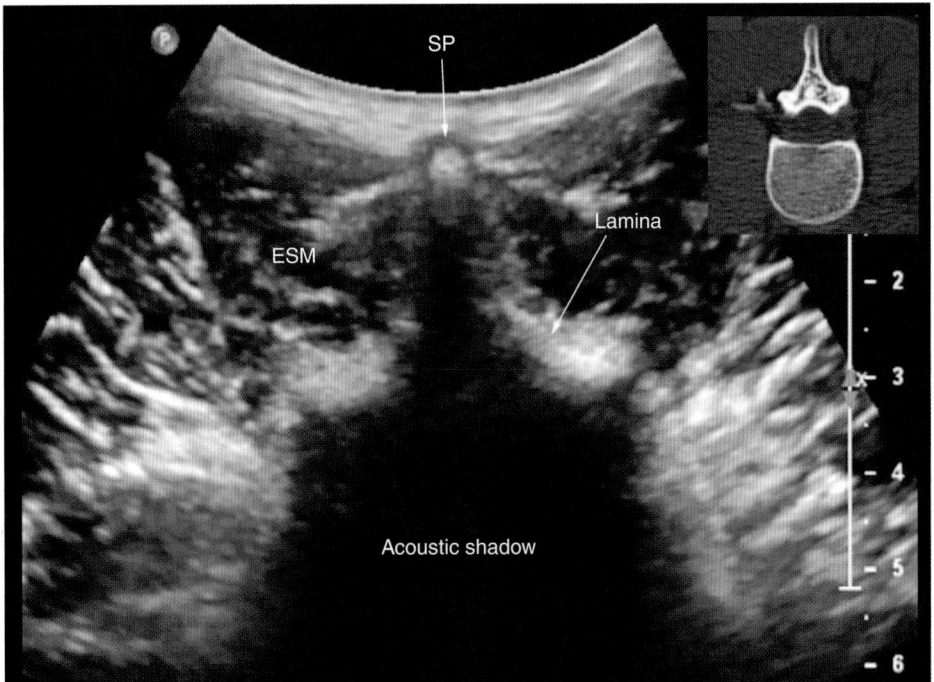

FIGURE 40-27. Transverse sonogram of the lumbar spine with the transducer positioned directly over the L4 spinous process (transverse spinous process view). Note the acoustic shadow of the spinous process and lamina, which completely obscures the spinal canal and the neuraxial structures. The inset image shows a corresponding computed tomography (CT) scan of the lumbar vertebra. The CT slice was reconstructed from a three-dimensional CT dataset from the author's archive. ESM, erector spinae muscle; SP, spinous process.

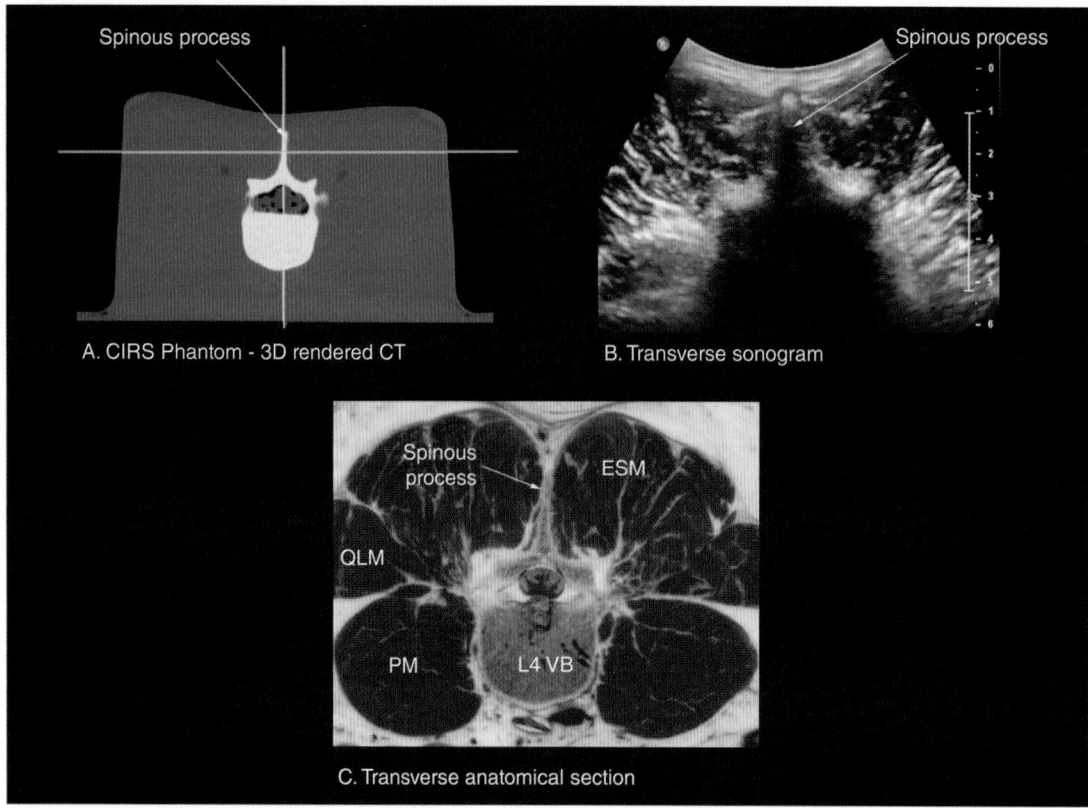

FIGURE 40–28. Transverse sections of the lumbar spine at the level of the L4 spinous process (SP). (**A**) Transverse slice rendered from a high-resolution computed tomography (CT) scan dataset from the CIRS phantom. (**B**) Sonogram: transverse spinous process view. (**B**) Transverse cadaver anatomical section. ESM, erector spinae muscle; PM, psoas major muscle; QLM, quadratus lumborum muscle; VB, vertebral body.

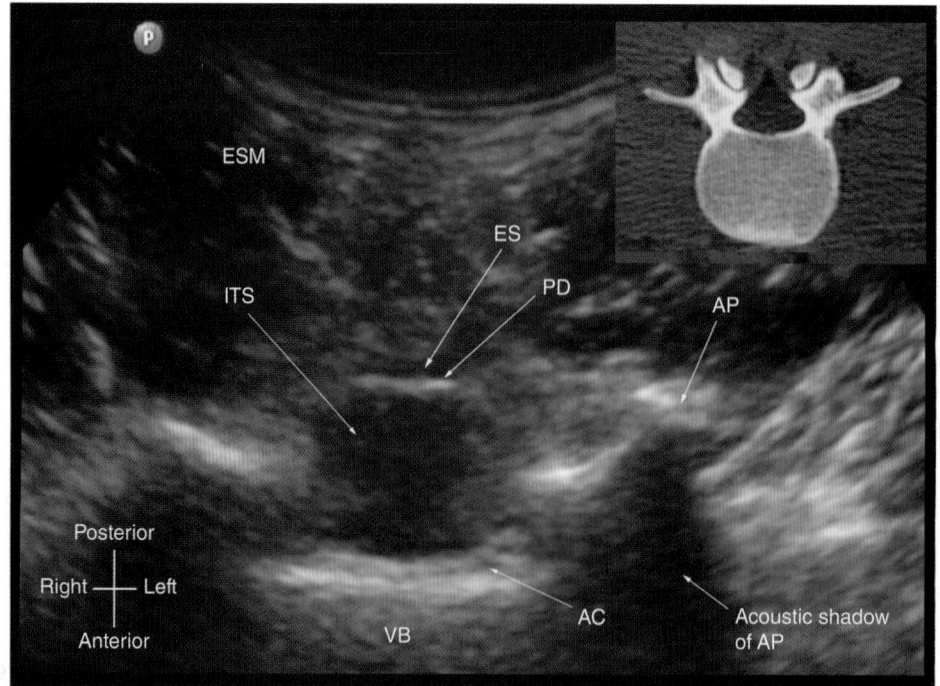

FIGURE 40–29. Transverse sonogram of the lumbar spine with the transducer positioned such that the US beam is insonated through the interspinous space (transverse interspinous view). The epidural space, posterior dura, intrathecal space, and anterior complex are visible in the midline, and the articular process (AP) is visible laterally on either side of the midline. Note how the articular processes on either side are symmetrically located. The inset image shows a corresponding computed tomography (CT) scan of the lumbar vertebra. The CT slice was reconstructed from a three-dimensional CT dataset from the author's archive. AC, anterior complex; ES, epidural space; ESM, erector spinae muscle; ITS, intrathecal space; PD, posterior dura; VB, vertebral body.

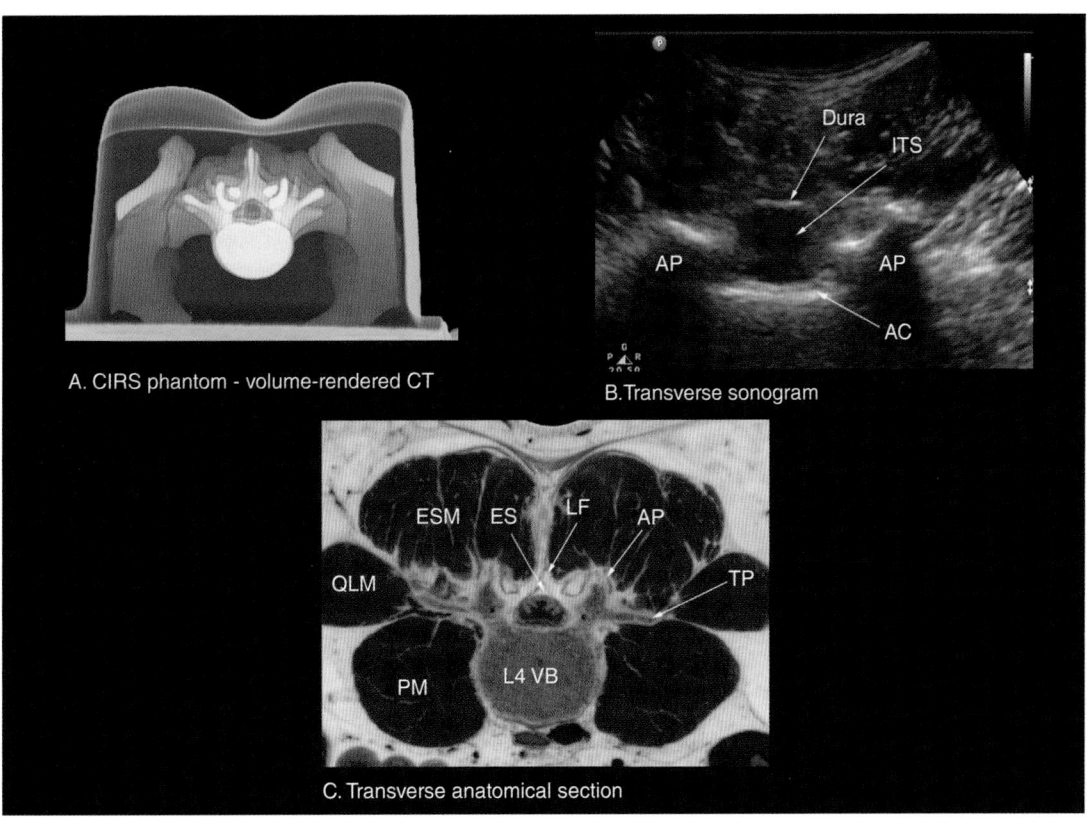

A. CIRS phantom - volume-rendered CT

B. Transverse sonogram

C. Transverse anatomical section

FIGURE 40–30. Transverse sections of the lumbar spine at the level of the L3–4 interspinous space. (**A**) Transverse slice rendered from a high-resolution computed tomography (CT) scan dataset from the CIRS phantom. (**B**) Sonogram: transverse interspinous view. (**C**) Transverse cadaver anatomical section. AC, anterior complex; AP, articular process; ES, epidural space; ESM, erector spinae muscle; ITS, intrathecal sac; LF, ligamentum flavum; PM, psoas major muscle; QLM, quadratus lumborum muscle; TP, transverse process; VB, vertebral body.

ULTRASOUND IMAGING OF THE THORACIC SPINE

US imaging of the thoracic spine is more challenging than the lumbar spine. The ability to visualize the neuraxial structures with US may vary with the level at which the imaging is performed, with poorer visibility of the neuraxis in the upper thoracic levels.[40] Regardless of the level at which the scan is performed, the thoracic spine is probably best imaged with the patient in the sitting position. In the lower thoracic region (T9–T12), the sonographic appearance of the neuraxial structures (Figure 40–31) is comparable to that in the lumbar region because of comparable vertebral anatomy. However, the acute caudal angulation of the spinous processes and the narrow interspinous and interlaminar spaces in the midthoracic region (T4–T8) results in a narrow acoustic window with limited visibility of the underlying neuraxial anatomy (Figures 40–32 and 40–33).

Grau and colleagues[28] performed US imaging of the thoracic spine at the T5–T6 level in young volunteers and correlated findings with matching magnetic resonance imaging (MRI) images.[28] They found that the transverse axis produced the best images of the neuraxial structures.[28] However, the epidural space was best visualized in the paramedian sagittal scans.[28] Regardless, US was limited in its ability to delineate the epidural space or the spinal cord but was better than MRI in demonstrating the posterior dura.[28] The transverse interspinous

view, however, is almost impossible to obtain in the midthoracic region (see Figure 40–33), and, therefore, the transverse scan provides little useful information for CNB other than to help identify the midline.

In contrast, the PMSOS (see Figure 40–32), despite the narrow acoustic window, provides more useful information relevant for CNB.[11,28] The laminae are seen as flat hyperechoic structures with acoustic shadowing anteriorly, and the posterior dura is consistently visualized in the acoustic window (see Figure 40–32). However, the epidural space, spinal cord, central canal, and anterior complex are difficult to delineate and only rarely visualized in the midthoracic region (see Figure 40–32). CNBs are rarely performed in the upper thoracic spine (T1–T4), but US imaging is possible despite the narrow acoustic window (Figures 40–34 and 40–35).

ULTRASOUND IMAGING OF THE SACRUM

US imaging of the sacrum is most commonly performed to identify the sonoanatomy relevant for a caudal epidural injection.[43] Because the sacrum is a superficial structure, a high-frequency linear array transducer can be used for the scan.[43] The patient is positioned in the lateral or prone position, with a pillow under the abdomen to flex the lumbosacral spine. The caudal epidural space is the continuation of the lumbar epidural space and commonly accessed via the sacral hiatus. The sacral hiatus is located at the distal end of the sacrum and is covered by the

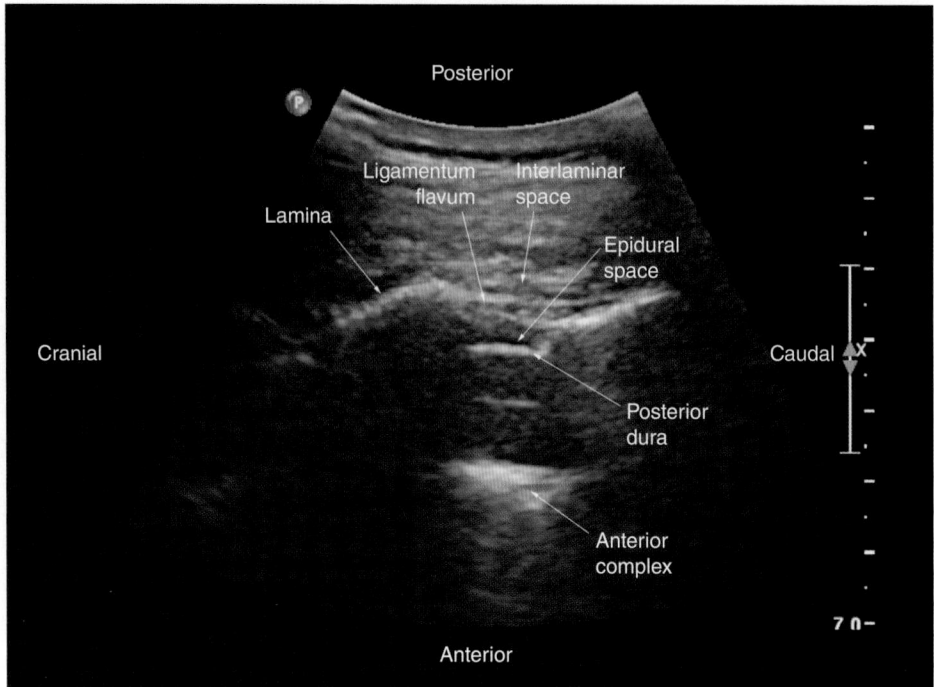

FIGURE 40–31. Paramedian sagittal oblique sonogram of the lower thoracic spine. The acoustic window is relatively large; through it, the ligamentum flavum, posterior dura, epidural space, and anterior complex are clearly visible.

sacrococcygeal ligament. Its lateral margins are formed by the two sacral cornua. On a transverse sonogram of the sacrum at the level of the sacral hiatus, the sacral cornua are seen as two hyperechoic reversed U-shaped structures, one on either side of the midline (Figure 40–36).[43] Connecting the

two sacral cornua, and deep to the skin and subcutaneous tissue, is a hyperechoic band: the sacrococcygeal ligament (see Figure 40–36).[43]

Anterior to the sacrococcygeal ligament is another hyperechoic linear structure, which represents the posterior surface of

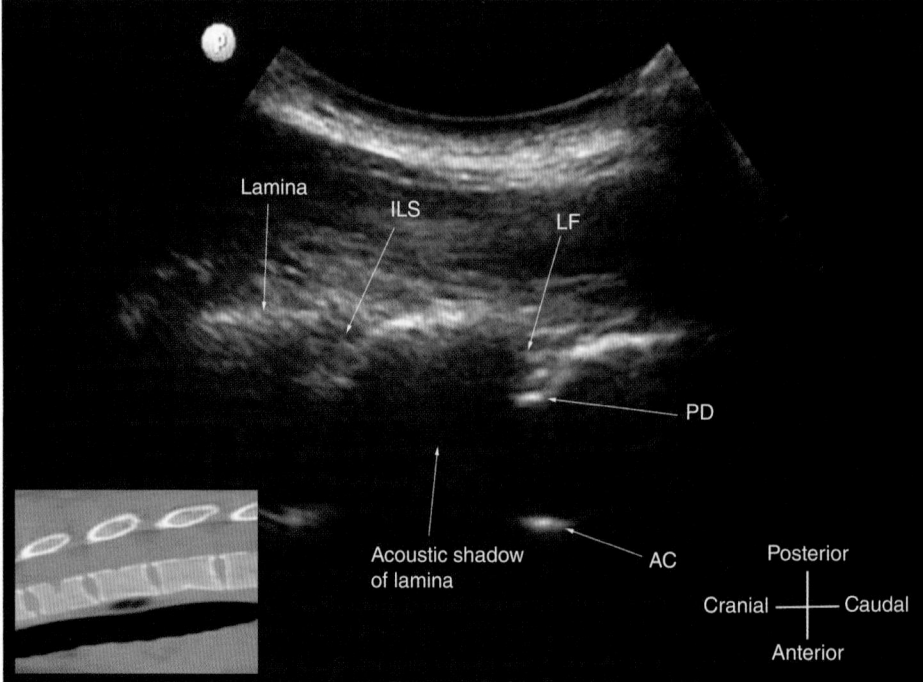

FIGURE 40–32. Paramedian sagittal oblique sonogram of the midthoracic spine. The posterior dura (PD) and the anterior complex (AC) are visible through the narrow acoustic window. The inset image shows a corresponding computed tomography (CT) scan of the midthoracic spine. The CT slice was reconstructed from a three-dimensional CT dataset from the author's archive. ILS, interlaminar space; LF, ligamentum flavum.

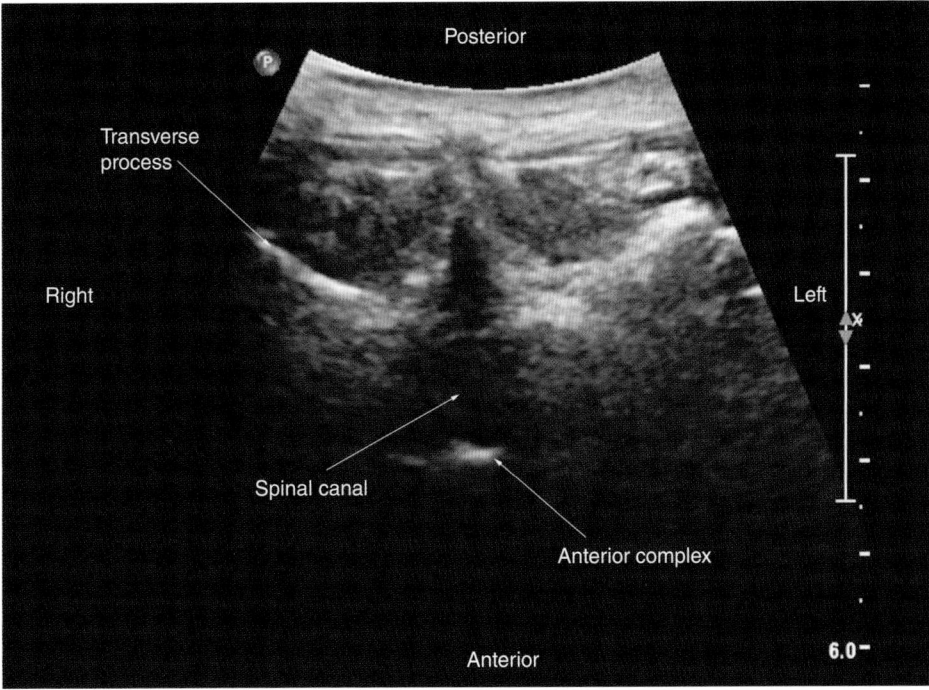

FIGURE 40–33. Transverse interspinous sonogram of the midthoracic region. Visualization of the posterior dura and anterior complex can be very challenging in the midthoracic region due to the acute angulation of the spinous processes and requires cranial angulation of the US transducer.

the sacrum. The hypoechoic space between the sacrococcygeal ligament and the bony posterior surface of the sacrum is the caudal epidural space (see Figure 40–36). The two sacral cornua and the posterior surface of the sacrum produce a pattern on the sonogram that is referred to as the "frog eye sign" because of its resemblance to the eyes of a frog (see Figure 40–36).[31]

On a sagittal sonogram of the sacrum at the level of the sacral cornua, the sacrococcygeal ligament, the base of sacrum, and the caudal canal are also clearly visualized (Figure 40–37).[31] However, due to the acoustic shadow of the posterior surface of the sacrum, only the lower part of the caudal epidural space is seen (see Figure 40–37).

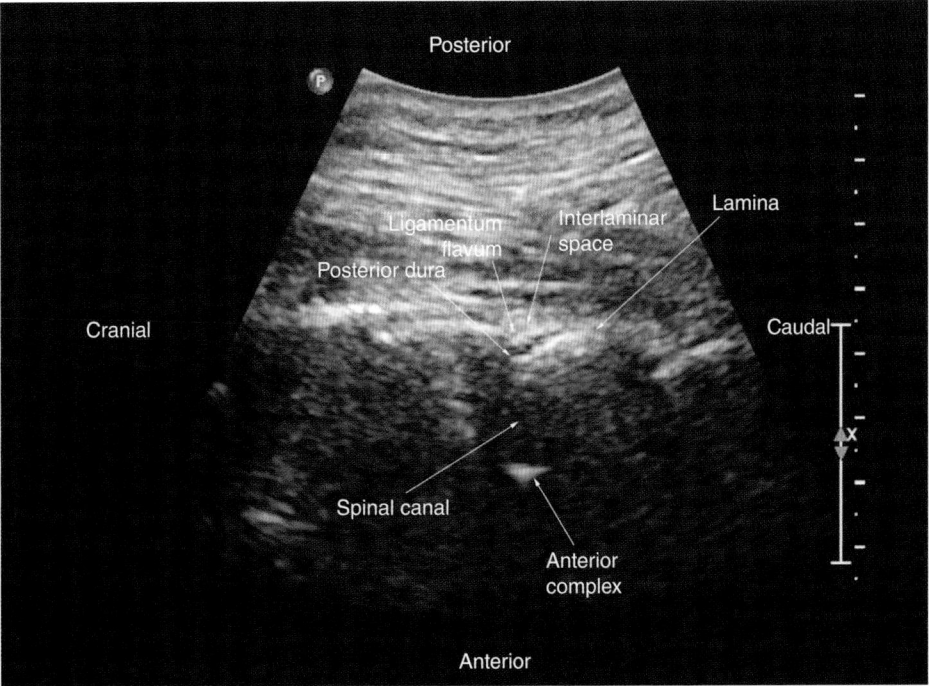

FIGURE 40–34. Paramedian sagittal oblique sonogram of the upper thoracic spine. The posterior dura and the anterior complex are visible through the narrow acoustic window.

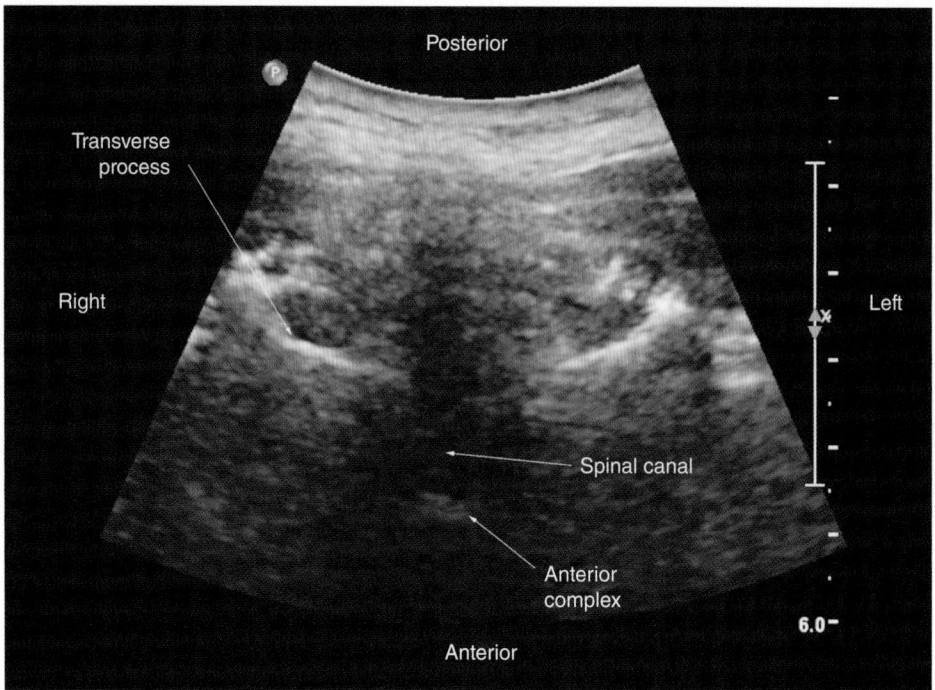

FIGURE 40–35. Transverse interspinous sonogram of the upper thoracic spine.

TECHNICAL ASPECTS OF ULTRASOUND-GUIDED CENTRAL NEURAXIAL BLOCKS

During CNBs, US can be used either as a preprocedural tool or to guide needle insertion in real time. The former involves performing a preprocedural scan (or scout scan) to preview the spinal anatomy and determine the optimal site, depth, and trajectory for needle insertion before performing a traditional spinal or epidural injection.[44,45] In contrast, the latter technique involves performing a real-time USG CNB by one[12] or two[18] operators. Real-time USG CNB demands a high degree of manual dexterity and hand–eye coordination. Therefore, the

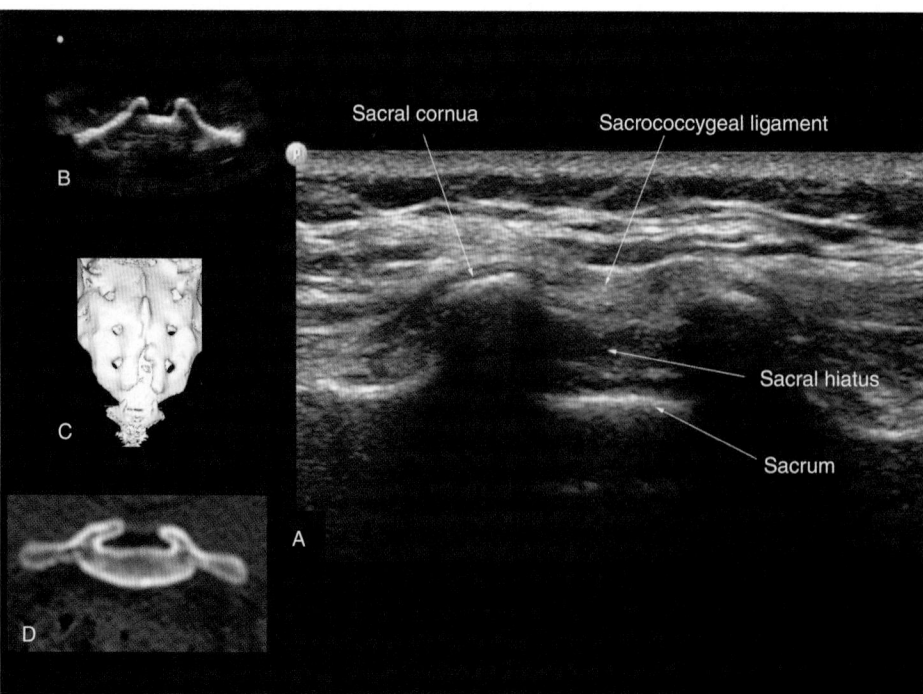

FIGURE 40–36. Transverse sonogram of the sacrum at the level of the sacral hiatus. Note the two sacral cornua and the hyperechoic sacrococcygeal ligament that extends between the two sacral cornua. (**A**) The hypoechoic space between the sacrococcygeal ligament and the posterior surface of the sacrum is the sacral hiatus. The image in (**B**) shows the sacral cornua from the water-based spine phantom; the image in (**C**) shows a three-dimensional (3D) reconstructed image of the sacrum at the level of the sacral hiatus from a 3D CT dataset from the author's archive; and the image in (**D**) shows a transverse CT slice of the sacrum at the level of the sacral cornua.

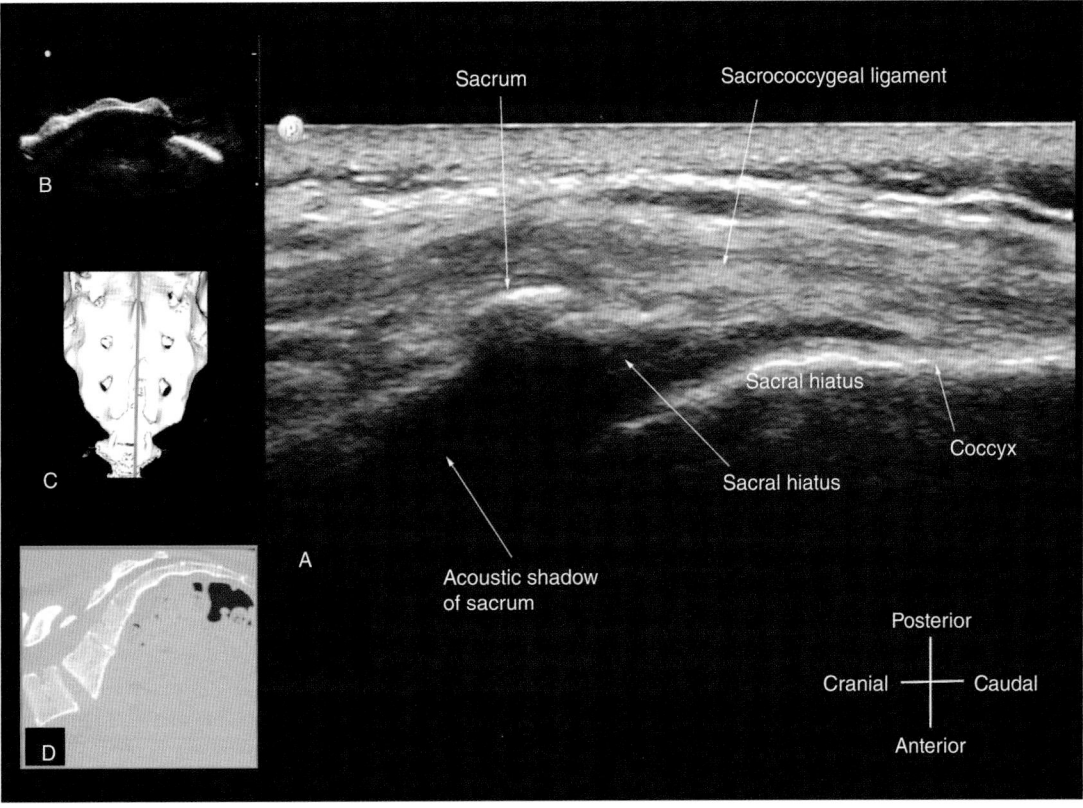

FIGURE 40-37. Sagittal sonogram of the sacrum at the level of the sacral hiatus. Note the hyperechoic sacrococcygeal ligament that extends from the sacrum to the coccyx and the acoustic shadow of the sacrum that completely obscures the sacral canal. The image in (**B**) shows the sacral hiatus from the water-based spine phantom; the image in (**C**) shows a three-dimensional (3D) reconstructed image of the sacrum at the level of the sacral hiatus from a 3D CT dataset from the author's archive; and the image in (**D**) shows a sagittal CT slice of the sacrum at the level of the sacral cornua.

operator should have a sound knowledge of the basics of US, be familiar with the sonoanatomy of the spine and scanning techniques, and have the necessary interventional skills before attempting a real-time USG CNB.

At this time, there are no data on the safety of the US gel if it is introduced into the meninges, subarachnoid space, or nervous tissues during USG CNB. However, data from animal studies in pigs suggests that this results in an inflammatory response within the neuraxial space.[46] Due to the paucity of published data, it is not possible to make recommendations, although some clinicians have resorted to using sterile normal saline solution as an alternative coupling agent to keep the skin moist under the footprint of the transducer during the scan.[12] As a result, there is some degradation in the quality of the US image, but this can be overcome by minor changes in the settings of the US system.

KEY PRINCIPLES

1. The use of US to assist or guide CNBs is an advanced technique that can be helpful in patients with difficult spinal anatomy. It is necessary to gain experience with the use of US for neuraxial blockade before attempting it in patients with difficult anatomy.
2. If the posterior or anterior complex cannot be clearly visualized, the articular and transverse processes identified

in a transverse scan can serve as surrogate markers of the interlaminar space.
3. Asymmetry in the position of the articular processes in a transverse interspinous view of the lumbar spine suggests a rotational defect in the vertebra; for example, as seen in scoliosis.
4. The angle of insonation that provides the best visualization of the posterior dura during a transverse interspinous scan usually reflects the angle (trajectory) at which the needle should be inserted during a midline CNB.
5. When performing a preprocedural scan, meticulous skin marking and keeping the skin from shifting are important.
6. In older patients, the failure to visualize the anterior or posterior complex may indicate narrowed interspaces from degenerative disease. Neuraxial block may still be possible, but difficulty should be anticipated, and there should be a lower threshold for proceeding to alternative methods of anesthesia or analgesia.
7. Strict asepsis must be maintained, and we recommend local protocols be established for USG CNB.
8. Attention to detail with positioning of the patient and ergonomics go a long way in ensuring success during a USG CNB.
9. Needle deviation during insertion may occur, especially with long, thin (25-gauge or less) needles in obese

subjects. This can be avoided by careful needle handling and the use of introducer needles or larger-gauge needles (22-gauge or larger) for the CNB.

10. If bone is encountered during needle insertion, subsequent alterations in trajectory should be small and gradual to avoid overshooting the interlaminar space.

11. The lumbosacral junction (L5–S1 gap) is the largest interlaminar space and must not be overlooked in patients with difficult spines, as it may provide a safe route for access to the neuraxis for CNBs.

TYPES OF INJECTION

Spinal Injection

There are limited data in the published medical literature on the use of US for spinal (intrathecal) injections,[47,48] although US has been reported to guide lumbar punctures by radiologists[49] and emergency physicians.[50] Most available data are anecdotal case reports.[47,48,51–53] Yeo and French, in 1999, were the first to describe the successful use of US to assist spinal injection in a patient with abnormal spinal anatomy.[53] They used US to locate the vertebral midline in a parturient with severe scoliosis with Harrington rods in situ.[53] Yamauchi and colleagues have described using US to preview the neuraxial anatomy and measure the distance from the skin to the dura in a post-laminectomy patient before the intrathecal injection was performed under X-ray guidance.[52] Costello and Balki have described using US to facilitate spinal injection by locating the L5–LS1 gap in a parturient with poliomyelitis and previous Harrington rod instrumentation of the spine.[47] Prasad and colleagues have reported using US to assist spinal injection in a patient with obesity, scoliosis, and multiple previous back surgeries with instrumentation.[48] More recently, Chin and colleagues[51] have described real-time USG spinal anesthesia in two patients with abnormal spinal anatomy (one had lumbar scoliosis, and the other had undergone spinal fusion surgery at the L2–L3 level).

Lumbar Epidural Injection

US imaging can be used to preview the underlying spinal anatomy[16–18] or to guide the Tuohy needle in real time[12] during a lumbar epidural access. Moreover, real-time US guidance for epidural access can be performed by one[12] or two[18] operators. In the latter technique, described by Grau and colleagues[18] for combined spinal epidural anesthesia, one operator performs the US scan via the paramedian axis, while the other carries out the needle insertion through the midline approach using a "loss-of-resistance" technique.[18] Using this approach, Grau and colleagues reported being able to visualize the advancing epidural needle despite different axes of US scan and needle insertion.[18] They were able to visualize the dural puncture in all patients, as well as dural tenting in a few cases, during the needle-through-needle spinal puncture.[18]

Karmakar and colleagues recently described a technique of real-time USG epidural injection in conjunction with loss of resistance (LOR) to saline.[12] The epidural access was performed

by a single operator, and the epidural needle was inserted in the plane of the US beam via the paramedian axis.[12] Generally, it is possible to visualize the advancing epidural needle in real time until it engages in the ligamentum flavum.[12] The need for a second operator to perform the LOR can be circumvented by using a spring-loaded syringe (eg, Episure AutoDetect syringe, Indigo Orb, Inc., Irvine, CA) with an internal compression spring that applies constant pressure on the plunger (Figure 40–38).[12] Anterior displacement of the posterior dura and widening of the posterior epidural space are the most frequently visualized changes within the spinal canal. Compression of the thecal sac can be seen occasionally.[12] These ultrasonographic signs (Figure 40–39) of a correct epidural injection were previously described in children.[54] The neuraxial changes that occur within the spinal canal following the "loss of resistance" to saline may have clinical significance.[12]

Despite the ability to use real-time US for establishing epidural access, visualization of an indwelling epidural catheter in adults has proved more challenging. Occasionally, anterior displacement of the posterior dura and widening of the posterior epidural space after an epidural bolus injection via the catheter can be observed and therefore used as a surrogate marker of the location of the catheter tip. Grau and colleagues postulated that this may be related to the small diameter and poor echogenicity of conventional epidural catheters.[30] It remains to be seen whether the imminent development of echogenic epidural needles and catheters will have an impact on the ability to visualize epidurally placed catheters.

Thoracic Epidural Injection

There are limited published data on the use of US for thoracic epidural blocks.[55] This lack may be due to the poor US visibility of the neuraxial structures in the thoracic region compared with the lumbar region (see above) and the associated technical difficulties. However, despite the narrow acoustic window, the lamina, interlaminar space, and posterior dura are visualized consistently when using the paramedian axis (see Figures 40–31, 40–32, 40–33, 40–34, and 40–35). The epidural space is more difficult to delineate, but it also is best visualized in a paramedian sagittal scan (see Figures 40–31 and 40-32).[28] As a result, US can be used to perform a preprocedural scan[55] or, as we have used it, to assist epidural access via the paramedian window. In the latter approach, the patient is positioned in the sitting position, and a PMSOS is performed at the desired thoracic level with the orientation marker of the transducer directed cranially. Under strict aseptic precautions (described previously), the Tuohy needle is inserted via the paramedian axis in real time and in the plane of the US beam. The needle is advanced steadily until it makes contact with the lamina or enters the interlaminar space. At this point, the US transducer is removed, and a traditional loss-of-resistance-to-saline technique is used to access the epidural space. Because the lamina is relatively superficial in the thoracic region, it is possible to visualize the advancing Tuohy needle in real time. Preliminary experience with this approach indicates that US may improve the likelihood of thoracic epidural access on the first attempt. However, more research to compare the utility of a

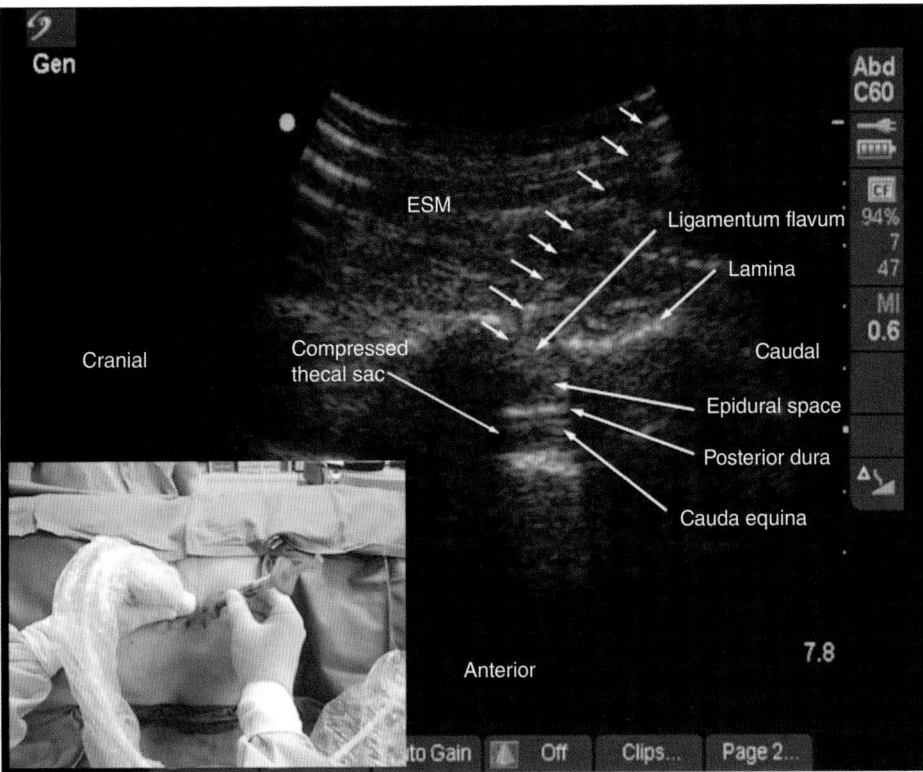

FIGURE 40–38. Paramedian oblique sagittal sonogram of the lumbar spine showing the sonographic changes within the spinal canal after the "loss of resistance" to saline. Note the anterior displacement of the posterior dura, the widening of the posterior epidural space, and the compression of the thecal sac. The cauda equina nerve roots are also now better visualized within the compressed thecal sac in this patient. The inset image shows how the Episure AutoDetect syringe was used to circumvent the need for a third hand for the "loss of resistance."

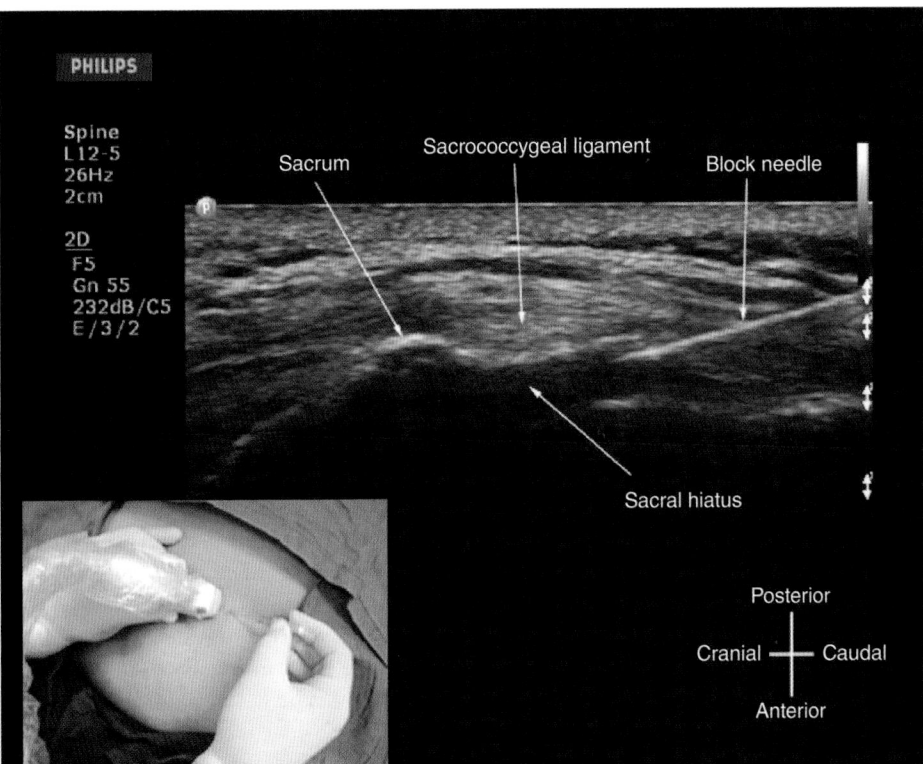

FIGURE 40–39. Sagittal sonogram of the sacrum at the level of the sacral hiatus during a real-time US-guided caudal epidural injection. Note the hyperechoic sacrococcygeal ligament and the block needle that has been inserted in the plane (in-plane) of the US beam. The inset image shows the position and orientation of the transducer and the direction in which the block needle was inserted.

preprocedural scan or the US-assisted technique described above with the traditional approach is necessary before more definitive recommendations on the utility and safety of US for thoracic epidural injections can be made.

Caudal Epidural Injection

For a USG caudal epidural injection, a transverse (see Figure 40–36) or sagittal (see Figure 40–37) scan is performed at the level of the sacral hiatus. Because the sacral hiatus is a superficial structure, a high-frequency (13-6 MHz) linear array transducer is used for the scan as described previously. The needle can be inserted in the short (out-of-plane) or long (in-plane) axis. For a long-axis needle insertion, a sagittal scan is performed, and the passage of the block needle through the sacrococcygeal ligament into the sacral canal is visualized in real time (see Figure 40–39). However, because the sacrum impedes the passage of the US, there is a large acoustic shadow anteriorly, which makes it impossible to visualize the tip of the needle or the spread of the injectate within the sacral canal. An inadvertent intravascular injection, which reportedly occurs in 5%–9% of procedures, may not be detected using US. As a result, the clinician should still factor in traditional clinical signs such as the "pop" or "give" as the needle traverses the sacrococcygeal ligament, ease of injection, absence of subcutaneous swelling, "whoosh test," nerve stimulation, or assessment of the clinical effects of the injected drug to confirm correct needle placement.

Color Doppler US can also be used to confirm spread of the injectate inside the caudal epidural space.[56] This is done by placing the color Doppler interrogation box over the acoustic window of the caudal canal in the sagittal sonogram while the injection is performed. Yoon and colleagues have reported that a correct injection deep to the sacrococcygeal ligament with unidirectional flow produces, in real time, a positive color spectrum change with one predominant color.[56] In contrast, an inadvertent intravascular injection is seen as multicolored spectrum.[56] Chen and colleagues reported a 100% success rate in placing a caudal needle under US guidance as confirmed by contrast fluoroscopy.[43] This report is encouraging, considering that, even in experienced hands, failure to place a needle in the caudal epidural space successfully is as high as 25%.[43,57]

More recently, Chen and colleagues[58] have described using US imaging as a screening tool during caudal epidural injections.[58] In their cohort of patients, the mean diameter of the sacral canal at the sacral hiatus was 5.3 ± 2 mm, and the distance between the sacral cornua (bilateral) was 9.7 ± 1.9 mm.[58] These researchers also identified that the presence of sonographic features such as a closed sacral hiatus and a sacral canal diameter of around 1.5 mm are associated with a greater probability of failure.[58]

Based on the published data, it can be concluded that US guidance, despite its limitation, can be useful as an adjunct tool for caudal epidural needle placement and has the potential to improve technical outcomes, reduce failure rates and accidental intravascular injection, and minimize exposure to radiation in the chronic pain setting and therefore deserves further investigation.

CLINICAL UTILITY OF ULTRASOUND FOR CENTRAL NEURAXIAL BLOCKS

Outcome data on the use of US for CNB have primarily focused on the lumbar region. Most studies to date have evaluated the utility of a preprocedural US scan. A preprocedural scan allows the operator to identify the midline[13] and accurately determine the interspace for needle insertion,[11,12,39] which are useful in patients in whom anatomical landmarks are difficult to palpate, such as in those with obesity,[2,15] edema of the back, or abnormal anatomy (eg, scoliosis,[15,59] postlaminectomy surgery,[52] or spinal instrumentation[47,48,53]). It also allows the operator to preview the neuraxial anatomy,[12,16–18,55,60] identify asymptomatic spinal abnormalities, such as in spina bifida,[61] predict the depth to the epidural space,[16,17,24,25] particularly in obese patients,[44] identify ligamentum flavum defects,[62] and determine the optimal site and trajectory for needle insertion.[17,30] Cumulative evidence suggests that a US examination performed before the epidural puncture improves the success rate of epidural access on the first attempt,[16] reduces the number of puncture attempts[15–20] or the need to puncture multiple levels,[16–18] and also improves patient comfort during the procedure.[17] A preprocedural scan can also be useful in patients presumed to have difficult epidural access, such as those with a history of difficult epidural access, obesity, or kyphosis or scoliosis of the lumbar spine.[15,63] When used for obstetric epidural anesthesia, US guidance was reported to improve the quality of analgesia, reduce side effects, and improve patient satisfaction.[15,18] A preprocedural scan may also improve the learning curve of students for epidural blocks in parturients.[29] Currently, there are limited data on the utility of real-time US guidance for epidural access,[12,18] although preliminary reports indicate that it may improve technical outcomes.[18]

APPLICATIONS IN THE LUMBAR SPINE

Identification of Specific Lumbar Intervertebral Levels

The identification of lumbar intervertebral levels based on surface anatomical landmarks is often imprecise. In one study using MRI as the gold standard, the correct intervertebral level was identified in as few as 29% of patients.[4] Other studies have repeatedly shown significant discordance between US and clinical determinations of lumbar intervertebral level. In an orthopedic population of 50 patients undergoing total joint arthroplasty, the palpated intercristal line corresponded to the L3–L4 level identified by US in 72%, to the L2–L3 level in 26%, and to the L4–L5 level in 2% of patients.[45] In a similar study of 90 parturients, identification of the L3–L4 intervertebral space was concordant in only 53% of nonobese and 49% of obese patients.[64] Of more concern was the fact that in 93% of the cases where there was disagreement, the clinically identified L3–L4 level corresponded to a higher (L1–L2 or L2–L3) level as identified by US. This tendency was confirmed by two other studies of women who had received epidural anesthesia for labor analgesia.[65,66] Both compared the documented epidural insertion level with a postpartum US assessment of the intervertebral level corresponding to the needle insertion scar. Once again, a high rate of discordance (45–63%) was observed between the two assessment methods, and the level of insertion according to US was more likely to be higher (72–76%) than that noted in the clinical record.

The available evidence indicates that US is more accurate than clinical assessment of intervertebral level. In one study comparing clinical assessment, US, and the gold standard of lateral spine X-ray examination,[39] clinical assessment accurately identified the L2–L3 interspace only 30% of the time, with an additional 7% of markings placed over the immediately adjacent spinous processes. US correctly identified the L2–L3 interspace in 60% of cases, with a further 24% of markings placed over the immediately adjacent spinous processes. It should be noted that the margin of error with US was at most either one space above (9%) or below (7%) the intended target. In contrast, clinical assessment showed greater variability, with margins of error up to two spaces higher (9%) or lower (18%). Furthermore, clinical assessment of intervertebral level was deemed impossible in 4% of cases compared to none when US was used.

FACILITATING THE TECHNICAL PERFORMANCE OF SPINAL AND EPIDURAL ANESTHESIA

Measuring Depth to the Epidural and Intrathecal Spaces

Cork et al. provided one of the first reports of the use of US to assist in epidural anesthesia. Despite relatively primitive US equipment, they were able to identify and measure the depth to the ligamentum flavum using a longitudinal neuraxial scan in 33 of 36 patients.[24] They found a high correlation (r = 0.98) between measured depth by US and needle depth to the epidural space. In a subsequent study, Currie et al. also found a high correlation (r = 0.96) between US-measured depth to the lamina in the PMSO view and needle insertion depth to the epidural space.[25] The transverse interspinous view may also be used to measure the depth to the epidural space.

A high correlation between the measured depth to the posterior complex and needle insertion depth has been observed in both obese and nonobese parturients undergoing labor epidural analgesia (r = 0.85–0.88)[44,60] and has been consistently demonstrated in a large number of studies.[15,16,26,67–70] A recent meta-analysis[19] identified 13 studies, involving 875 patients, that specifically addressed the correlation between US-measured depth and actual needle insertion depth. They confirmed that the correlation was high, regardless of which US view was used, with a pooled correlation coefficient of 0.91. The difference between US-measured depth and needle insertion depth in most trials is quite small (approximately 0.5 cm or less), with US usually underestimating needle depth. This difference is commonly attributed to soft-tissue compression by the US transducer during the scan.

Reducing the Number of Needle Passes Required for Block Success

In an early 2001 study of preprocedural US, Grau et al.[15] randomized 72 parturients with difficult anatomy to surface landmark–guided or US-assisted epidural placement. Patients had either a history of difficult epidural, kyphoscoliosis, or a body mass index (BMI) of more than 33 kg/m^2. In this population, needle entry into the epidural space in the surface landmark–guided group required a mean of 2.6 puncture attempts compared to 1.5 in the US-assisted group (p < 0.001).

More recently, Chin et al. evaluated an older population of 120 orthopedic patients with clinical predictors of difficult neuraxial block, including a BMI of more than 35 kg/m^2, scoliosis, and prior lumbar surgery.[63] Patients were randomized to either surface landmark–guided or US-assisted spinal anesthesia. US halved the median number of needle insertions from 2 to 1 and significantly reduced the need for additional needle passes (6 vs. 13).[63]

Improved performance of neuraxial blockade after preprocedural ultrasound imaging is seen even in patients without predictors of technical difficulty. In a randomized controlled trial by Grau et al. of epidural analgesia in 300 parturients, the mean number of needle passes was significantly lower with the use of US compared to surface landmarks alone (1.3 vs. 2.2).[17] These findings were validated in a later study by Vallejo et al., who randomized 15 first-year anesthesia trainees to perform 370 labor epidurals with or without the assistance of preprocedural US imaging.[70] Once again, fewer insertion attempts were required in the US-guided group of patients (median of 1 vs. 2).[70]

Most recently, two separate systematic reviews of the available literature have confirmed these findings. Shaikh et al.[20] compared US-guided and non–US-guided neuraxial procedures, including diagnostic lumbar punctures as well as epidural and spinal anesthetics. They identified 14 publications, involving 1334 patients, that met their inclusion criteria. They found that the use of US significantly reduced both skin punctures and needle redirections required for successful CNB. Perlas et al.[19] performed a similar systematic review of studies involving the use of US for lumbar CNB and lumbar puncture in adults. They identified 14 randomized controlled trials that met inclusion criteria, six of which were newer and had not been included in the previous systematic review. Once again, they found that US significantly reduced the overall number of needle passes required for procedural success.

Improved Block Success and Epidural Efficacy

In addition to reducing the technical difficulty of epidural needle insertion, US may also increase the efficacy of labor epidural analgesia. In two separate randomized controlled trials by Grau et al.,[15,17] there was a significant reduction in the rate of incomplete analgesia (2% vs. 8%) in one study[17] and epidural failure (0% vs. 5.6%) in the other.[15] In addition, a small but statistically significant decrease in post-block pain scores was noted in the US-assisted groups compared to the surface landmark–guided groups. These findings may be partially explained by observed reductions in the incidences of asymmetric and patchy blocks. It is notable that the more recent study by Vallejo et al., involving multiple operators, observed a similarly impressive reduction in the epidural failure rate in the US-assisted group (1.6% vs. 5.5%).[70] Systematic reviews have provided further evidence that US increases block success.[19,20] Shaikh et al. found that the use of US reduced the risk of procedural failure by 79%, with a number needed to treat (NNT) to avoid one failure of 16. A subgroup analysis of intrathecal (relative risk [RR] = 0.19) and epidural (RR = 0.23) procedures confirmed that this effect is similar for both.[20] The findings of Perlas et al. were similar, although more modest in magnitude, with a risk reduction of 49% and an NNT of 34 for procedural failure.[19]

Effect on Procedure Time

In their early evaluations of US-assisted lumbar epidural insertion, Grau et al. reported that US scanning added only 60–75 seconds to the preparation time.[16,17] Similarly, in their large randomized controlled trial of labor epidural insertion by trainees, Vallejo et al. reported that the use of US increased average total procedure time by 60 seconds.[70] The caveat here is that these studies involved a single experienced sonographer and a cohort of healthy obstetric patients with normal anatomy. More time may be required in less-experienced hands or in patients with difficult spinal anatomy. Chin et al.[63] found that in patients with scoliosis, prior lumbar surgery, or a BMI of more than 35 kg/m², preprocedural scanning took 6.7 minutes on average to complete compared to 0.6 minutes for palpation of surface landmarks alone. However, this difference was partially offset by a decrease in time taken to perform the spinal anesthetic (5.0 vs. 7.3 minutes).[63]

Reducing the Risk of Complications

US may potentially reduce adverse effects related to neuraxial anesthesia. Grau et al.[17] observed a significant reduction in the rate of postpartum headache (4.7% vs. 18.7%) and backache (14.7% vs. 22.0%) with US-assisted epidural insertion. The risk of inadvertent dural puncture may also be reduced by the ability to measure the depth to the epidural space.

With regard to more serious complications, although there is no direct supporting evidence, the decreased technical difficulty associated with US suggests that it may theoretically reduce risk in a number of ways. Conus medullaris injuries from spinal needles inserted at a level much higher than intended by the anesthesiologist have been reported.[7,8] Improved accuracy of intervertebral level identification could reduce the risk of this rare but potentially devastating outcome. Spinal hematoma and persistent neurological deficit are similarly rare but important complications. Technical difficulty in performing the block has been identified as an associated risk factor for both these complications;[71,72] thus, preprocedural US has the potential to reduce their incidence. This is supported by the recent meta-analysis by Shaikh et al.[20] of US-guided versus non–US-guided procedures, which found a 73% reduction in the risk of traumatic procedures with the use of US.[20]

Predicting the Feasibility and Ease of Performing Neuraxial Blockade

In addition to assisting the technical performance of neuraxial blockade, US may also be used as a preoperative assessment tool to guide decision making. This has been illustrated in two case reports. The first involved a patient who had a history of L3–L5 spinal decompression and fusion with corresponding hardware in situ and who had experienced two previous failed attempts at a spinal anesthetic. Preprocedural US determined that there was in fact a patent acoustic window at the L3–L4 level, which, due to dense overlying scar tissue, could be penetrated only by a larger-gauge (22-gauge) Quincke-tip spinal needle.[51] The second involved a patient with severe ankylosing spondylitis and a history of failed spinal anesthesia despite persistent efforts by multiple experienced operators. Here, a US scan in the pre-anesthetic clinic identified an acoustic window at L4–L5, which allowed planning for a spinal anesthetic that was successfully performed at that level on the day of surgery.[73]

The potential of using US to predict the ease of performing spinal anesthesia has been evaluated in two cohort studies. These were based on the premise that the ability to visualize the vertebral canal should correspond to the size of the interlaminar space, thus reflecting the ease with which it may be penetrated. Weed et al.[74] performed preprocedural US scans using the PMSO view in 60 orthopedic patients and documented the quality of the images obtained. Clinicians blinded to the results of the imaging performed spinal anesthesia using a surface landmark–guided approach. There was a remarkable difference in block performance between patients in whom the anterior complex was visible on US (a good image) and those in whom it was not (a poor image).[74] When images were poor, the median number of needle passes required was 10 compared to 4 in patients with good images. Spinal anesthesia was classified as difficult by the operator in 9% of patients with good images compared to 50% of patients with poor images of the anterior complex. The positive predictive value of a poor image in the PMSO view for difficult spinal anesthesia was calculated to be 82.3%, with the negative predictive value 67.4%.[74]

In the second study, Chin et al. studied the ability of both the PMSO and transverse interspinous views to predict difficult spinal anesthesia in a cohort of 100 orthopedic patients.[14] As in the study by Weed et al., the anesthesiologists performing the spinal anesthetic were blinded to the results of imaging. If both posterior and anterior complexes were visible (a good-quality view) in the transverse interspinous view, the positive predictive value for absence of technical difficulty at that level was 85%.[14] This discriminative ability was not present, however, with the PMSO view, which may be explained by the fact that a midline needle approach was used in all cases. There were a small number of patients in whom spinal anesthesia was challenging despite a good-quality transverse median (TM) view of the vertebral canal. The authors hypothesized that this could have been avoided if the preprocedure US scan had been used to guide the spinal procedure, as would be the case in the clinical setting.

APPLICATIONS IN THE THORACIC SPINE

Identification of Thoracic Intervertebral Levels

As in the lumbar spine, clinical methods of identifying thoracic intervertebral levels based on surface anatomical landmarks have been shown to be inaccurate when referenced to the gold standard of MRI or X-ray imaging.[6,75,76] In one study, the T7 spinous process was accurately identified only 29% of the time by counting down from the vertebra prominens (C7) and only 10% of the time when the inferior tip of the scapula was used as the primary landmark.[76] The majority of errors tended to be in the caudad direction.[6,76] The accuracy of US in identifying thoracic intervertebral levels has not been verified against a gold-standard imaging modality; however, Arzola et al.[77] have demonstrated a similar lack of agreement between US identification of thoracic intervertebral level (using a counting-up method from the sacrum and twelfth rib) and surface anatomical landmarks. As with the earlier studies, the vertebra prominens was a more accurate landmark for C7 (58% agreement) than the inferior angle of the scapula was for T7 (36% agreement). Errors in identifying T7 were most often in a caudad direction (83% of errors), whereas the errors in identifying C7 were equally distributed in a cephalad and caudad direction.

Determining the Depth to the Thoracic Epidural Space

Rasoulian et al. compared US measurement of the depth to the ligamentum flavum in the PMSO view to actual needle insertion depth in a small cohort of 20 patients receiving thoracic epidural analgesia.[78] There was moderately good correlation ($r^2 = 0.65$) observed between the two measurements, with US tending to underestimate needle insertion depth by a mean of 4.68 mm. It is notable that this correlation was similar to that obtained when CT measurement of the depth to the epidural space was compared to needle insertion depth ($r^2 = 0.69$, mean difference of 4.49 mm). Similar results were reported by Salman et al. in another study of mid-to-lower thoracic epidural insertion in 35 adult patients using a paramedian approach.[55] Correlation between US-measured depth and needle insertion depth was good ($r^2 = 0.75$), and the mean difference was 7.1 mm, with US tending to underestimate the depth. These findings suggest that US is a useful tool for estimating depth to the thoracic epidural space.

Improving the Technical Performance of Thoracic Epidurals

The ability to delineate the underlying anatomy of the thoracic spine can potentially improve the technical performance of thoracic epidurals. However, unlike in the lumbar

spine, there is presently limited evidence supporting the benefit of preprocedural US imaging in this regard. In the aforementioned study by Salman et al.,[55] the PMSO view on US was used to determine the optimal needle insertion point for a paramedian approach to mid-to-lower thoracic epidural insertion.[55] Successful insertion was achieved with only one skin puncture on average and within two or fewer redirections in 88% of cases. In addition, case reports suggest that US is useful in evaluating abnormal anatomy and determining the optimal needle insertion site and trajectory in scoliotic patients.[59,79]

EDUCATION AND TRAINING

Learning USG CNB techniques takes time and patience. Regardless of the technique used, USG CNB and, in particular, real-time USG CNB are advanced techniques and are by far the most difficult USG interventions. They demand a high degree of manual dexterity, hand–eye coordination, and an ability to conceptualize two-dimensional information into a 3D image. Therefore, before attempting to perform a USG CNB, the operator should have a sound knowledge of the basics of US, be familiar with image optimization, understand the sonoanatomy of the spine, and have the necessary interventional skills. It is advisable to start by attending a course or workshop tailored to this purpose where the operator can learn the basic scanning techniques, spinal sonoanatomy, and relevant interventional skills. Further experience in spinal sonography can also be acquired by scanning human volunteers.[80] Currently, there is paucity of data[80,81] on what the minimum training requirement is to attain competence in spinal sonography or USG CNB. Preliminary data suggest that once the basic knowledge on US of the lumbar spine is attained, experience with 40 or more cases may be necessary to attain competence in scanning.

Today, there are several models (phantoms) for learning spinal sonoanatomy and practicing USG central neuraxial interventions. The water-based spine phantom[35] is useful for learning the osseous anatomy of the spine, but it is not a good model for learning USG spinal interventions because it lacks tissue-mimicking properties. Spinal sonography is often taught at workshops, but such workshops are not suitable for practicing actual techniques. Fresh cadaver courses are available, which allow participants to study neuraxial sonoanatomy and practice USG CNB with realistic haptic feedback, but they may be limited by the quality of the US images. Further, such courses are uncommon and conducted in anatomy departments with the cadavers in a position that rarely mimics what is practiced in the operating room. Anesthetized pigs can also be used, but animal ethics approval is required and, for the organizers, a license from the local health department to conduct such workshops. This method entails infectious precautions, and religious beliefs may preclude its use as a model for some. Moreover, such workshops are conducted in designated animal laboratories that are typically small and not suited to accommodate large groups of participants. To circumvent some of these problems, the group at the Chinese University of Hong Kong recently introduced the pig carcass spine phantom (see Figure 40–12),[37] an excellent model that can be used in conference venues, and provides excellent tactile and visual feedback.[37] The limitation of the pig carcass spine phantom is that it is a decapitated model, and there is loss of cerebrospinal fluid during the preparation process. This presentation results in air artifacts and loss of contrast within the spinal canal during spinal sonography unless the thecal sac is cannulated at its cranial end and continuously irrigated with fluid (normal saline), a process that requires surgical dissection to isolate the thecal sac.[82]

Therefore, an "in vitro" model that can facilitate the learning of the scanning techniques and the hand–eye coordination skills required for real-time USG CNB is highly desirable. A low-cost gelatin-based US phantom of the lumbosacral spine has been recently proposed.[36] However, the gelatin phantom is soft in consistency, lacks tissue-mimicking echogenic properties, does not provide haptic feedback, is easily contaminated with mold and bacteria, and is limited in its usefulness by needle track marks,[36] all of which preclude its extended use.

Karmakar and colleagues have recently developed a gelatin–agar spine phantom[83] (see Figure 40–11) that overcomes some of the drawbacks of the gelatin-based spine phantom. It is mechanically stable, has a tissue-like texture and echogenicity, needle track marks are less of a problem, and it can be used over extended periods of time to study the osseous anatomy of the lumbosacral spine and to practice the hand–eye coordination skills required to perform USG CNB.[83] Although a variety of spine phantoms have been described to learn the scanning and needle insertion techniques in the workshop setting, none of these have undergone scrutiny to determine how effective they are for transferring the knowledge and skills necessary for USG CNB.

Once the basic knowledge and skills are attained, it is best to start by performing USG spinal injections, under supervision, before progressing to performing epidural blocks. Real-time USG epidurals can be technically challenging, even for an experienced operator, and it is our opinion that it is not practical in the clinical setting or for everyday use. In contrast, a preprocedural scan is simple to perform and provides valuable information that can translate into improved technical outcomes during a CNB and may be the prudent approach to using US for CNBs. That said, real-time US guidance might be the only way out, for safety, in patients with difficult backs (eg, those with scoliosis, ankylosing spondylitis, or instrumented or operated backs). Therefore, the skills necessary to perform real-time USG CNBs must be developed as part of one's ongoing skill development. If it is not possible to gain experience in USG CNB locally, it is advisable to visit a center where such interventions are practiced.

SUMMARY

USG CNB is a rapidly developing alternative to traditional landmark-based techniques. It is noninvasive, safe, can be quickly performed, does not involve exposure to radiation, provides real-time images, and is free from adverse effects. Experienced sonographers can visualize neuraxial structures with satisfactory clarity using US. A preprocedural scan allows the operator to preview the spinal anatomy, identify the midline, locate a given intervertebral level, accurately predict the

depth to the epidural space, and determine the optimal site and trajectory for needle insertion. A preprocedural scan may also be used to predict the feasibility and ease of performing CNBs. The use of US also improves the success rate of epidural access on the first attempt, reduces the number of puncture attempts or the need to puncture multiple levels, and improves patient comfort during the procedure. US is an excellent teaching tool for demonstrating the anatomy of the spine and improves the learning curve for the performance of epidural blocks in parturients. US guidance also may allow the use of CNB in patients who in the past may have been considered unsuitable for such procedures due to abnormal spinal anatomy.

However, US guidance for CNB is still in its early stages of development; the evidence to support its use is sparse but in favor of its use as a preprocedural imaging tool. Furthermore, initial experience with real-time USG CNB indicates that it is technically demanding and, therefore, unlikely to replace traditional methods of performing CNB in the near future because traditional methods are well established as safe, simple, and effective in most patients. As US technology continues to improve and as skills necessary to perform USG interventions become more widely available, the use of US for CNB may become the standard of care in the future.

REFERENCES

1. Cook TM, Counsell D, Wildsmith JA: Major complications of central neuraxial block: report on the Third National Audit Project of the Royal College of Anaesthetists. Br J Anaesth 2009;102:179–190.
2. Stiffler KA, Jwayyed S, Wilber ST, Robinson A: The use of ultrasound to identify pertinent landmarks for lumbar puncture. Am J Emerg Med 2007;25:331–334.
3. Hogan QH: Tuffier's line: the normal distribution of anatomic parameters. Anesth Analg 1994;78:194–195.
4. Broadbent CR, Maxwell WB, Ferrie R, Wilson DJ, Gawne-Cain M, Russell R: Ability of anaesthetists to identify a marked lumbar interspace. Anaesthesia 2000;55:1122–1126.
5. Furness G, Reilly MP, Kuchi S: An evaluation of ultrasound imaging for identification of lumbar intervertebral level. Anaesthesia 2002;57:277–280.
6. Holmaas G, Frederiksen D, Ulvik A, Vingsnes SO, Ostgaard G, Nordli H: Identification of thoracic intervertebral spaces by means of surface anatomy: a magnetic resonance imaging study. Acta Anaesthesiol Scand 2006;50:368–373.
7. Reynolds F: Damage to the conus medullaris following spinal anaesthesia. Anaesthesia 2001;56:238–247.
8. Hamandi K, Mottershead J, Lewis T, Ormerod IC, Ferguson IT: Irreversible damage to the spinal cord following spinal anesthesia. Neurology 2002;59:624–626.
9. Seeberger MD, Lang ML, Drewe J, Schneider M, Hauser E, Hruby J: Comparison of spinal and epidural anesthesia for patients younger than 50 years of age. Anesth Analg 1994;78:667–673.
10. Tarkkila P, Huhtala J, Salminen U: Difficulties in spinal needle use. Insertion characteristics and failure rates associated with 25-, 27- and 29-gauge Quincke-type spinal needles. Anaesthesia 1994;49:723–725.
11. Chin KJ, Karmakar MK, Peng P: Ultrasonography of the adult thoracic and lumbar spine for central neuraxial blockade. Anesthesiology 2011;114:1459–1485.
12. Karmakar MK, Li X, Ho AM, Kwok WH, Chui PT: Real-time ultrasound-guided paramedian epidural access: evaluation of a novel in-plane technique. Br J Anaesth 2009;102:845–854.
13. Carvalho JC: Ultrasound-facilitated epidurals and spinals in obstetrics. Anesthesiol Clin 2008;26:145–158.
14. Chin KJ, Ramlogan R, Arzola C, Singh M, Chan V: The utility of ultrasound imaging in predicting ease of performance of spinal anesthesia in an orthopedic patient population. Reg Anesth Pain Med 2013;38:34–38.

15. Grau T, Leipold RW, Conradi R, Martin E: Ultrasound control for presumed difficult epidural puncture. Acta Anaesthesiol Scand 2001;45: 766–771.

16. Grau T, Leipold RW, Conradi R, Martin E, Motsch J: Ultrasound imaging facilitates localization of the epidural space during combined spinal and epidural anesthesia. Reg Anesth Pain Med 2001;26:64–67.

17. Grau T, Leipold RW, Conradi R, Martin E, Motsch J: Efficacy of ultrasound imaging in obstetric epidural anesthesia. J Clin Anesth 2002;14:169–175.

18. Grau T, Leipold RW, Fatehi S, Martin E, Motsch J: Real-time ultrasonic observation of combined spinal-epidural anaesthesia. Eur J Anaesthesiol 2004;21:25–31.

19. Perlas A, Chaparro LE, Chin KJ: Lumbar neuraxial ultrasound for spinal and epidural anesthesia: a systematic review and meta-analysis. Reg Anesth Pain Med 2016;41:251–260.

20. Shaikh F, Brzezinski J, Alexander S, et al: Ultrasound imaging for lumbar punctures and epidural catheterisations: systematic review and meta-analysis. BMJ 2013;346:f1720.

21. Mathieu S, Dalgleish DJ: A survey of local opinion of NICE guidance on the use of ultrasound in the insertion of epidural catheters. Anaesthesia 2008;63:1146–1147.

22. Bogin IN, Stulin ID: Application of the method of 2-dimensional echospondylography for determining landmarks in lumbar punctures. Zh Nevropatol Psikhiatr Im S S Korsakova 1971;71:1810–1811.

23. Porter RW, Wicks M, Ottewell D: Measurement of the spinal canal by diagnostic ultrasound. J Bone Joint Surg Br 1978;60-B:481–484.

24. Cork RC, Kryc JJ, Vaughan RW: Ultrasonic localization of the lumbar epidural space. Anesthesiology 1980;52:513–516.

25. Currie JM: Measurement of the depth to the extradural space using ultrasound. Br J Anaesth 1984;56:345–347.

26. Wallace DH, Currie JM, Gilstrap LC, Santos R: Indirect sonographic guidance for epidural anesthesia in obese pregnant patients. Reg Anesth 1992;17:233–236.

27. Grau T, Leipold RW, Horter J, Conradi R, Martin EO, Motsch J: Paramedian access to the epidural space: the optimum window for ultrasound imaging. J Clin Anesth 2001;13:213–217.

28. Grau T, Leipold RW, Delorme S, Martin E, Motsch J: Ultrasound imaging of the thoracic epidural space. Reg Anesth Pain Med 2002;27:200–206.

29. Grau T, Bartusseck E, Conradi R, Martin E, Motsch J: Ultrasound imaging improves learning curves in obstetric epidural anesthesia: a preliminary study. Can J Anaesth 2003;50:1047–1050.

30. Grau T: The evaluation of ultrasound imaging for neuraxial anesthesia. Can J Anaesth 2003;50:R1–R8.

31. Karmakar MK: Ultrasound for central neuraxial blocks. Tech Reg Anesth Pain Manag 2009;13:161–170.

32. Karmakar MK, Li X, Kwok WH, Ho AM, Ngan Kee WD: Sonoanatomy relevant for ultrasound-guided central neuraxial blocks via the paramedian approach in the lumbar region. Br J Radiol 2012;85:e262–e269.

33. Saifuddin A, Burnett SJ, White J: The variation of position of the conus medullaris in an adult population. A magnetic resonance imaging study. Spine (Phila Pa 1976) 1998;23:1452–1456.

34. MacDonald A, Chatrath P, Spector T, Ellis H: Level of termination of the spinal cord and the dural sac: a magnetic resonance study. Clin Anat 1999;12:149–152.

35. Karmakar, MK, Li X, Kwok WH, Ho AM, Ngan Kee WD: The "water-based spine phantom"—a small step towards learning the basics of spinal sonography [letter]. Br J Anaesth March 12, 2009. Available from: http://bja.oxfordjournals.org/forum/topic/brjana_el%3B4114.

36. Bellingham GA, Peng PWH: A low-cost ultrasound phantom of the lumbosacral spine. Reg Anesth Pain Med 2010;35:290–293.

37. Kwok WH, Chui PT, Karmakar MK: The pig carcass spine phantom—a model to learn ultrasound guided neuraxial interventions. Reg Anesth Pain Med 2010;35:472–473.

38. Greher M, Scharbert G, Kamolz LP, et al: Ultrasound-guided lumbar facet nerve block: a sonoanatomic study of a new methodologic approach. Anesthesiology 2004;100:1242–1248.

39. Furness G, Reilly MP, Kuchi S: An evaluation of ultrasound imaging for identification of lumbar intervertebral level. Anaesthesia 2002;57:277–280.

40. Avramescu S, Arzola C, Tharmaratnam U, Chin KJ, Balki M: Sonoanatomy of the thoracic spine in adult volunteers. Reg Anesth Pain Med 2012;37:349–353.

41. Karmakar MK, Ho AM, Li X, Kwok WH, Tsang K, Kee WD: Ultrasound-guided lumbar plexus block through the acoustic window of the lumbar ultrasound trident. Br J Anaesth 2008;100:533–537.

42. Suzuki S, Yamamuro T, Shikata J, Shimizu K, Iida H: Ultrasound measurement of vertebral rotation in idiopathic scoliosis. J Bone Joint Surg Br 1989;71:252–255.

43. Chen CP, Tang SF, Hsu TC, et al: Ultrasound guidance in caudal epidural needle placement. Anesthesiology 2004;101:181–184.

44. Balki M, Lee Y, Halpern S, Carvalho JC: Ultrasound imaging of the lumbar spine in the transverse plane: the correlation between estimated and actual depth to the epidural space in obese parturients. Anesth Analg 2009;108:1876–1881.

45. Chin KJ, Perlas A, Singh M, et al: An ultrasound-assisted approach facilitates spinal anesthesia for total joint arthroplasty. Can J Anaesth 2009;56:643–650.

46. Pintaric TS, Hadzic A, Strbenc M, Podpecan O, Podbregar M, Cvetko E: Inflammatory response after injection of aqueous gel into subarachnoid space in piglets. Reg Anesth Pain Med 2013;38:100–105.

47. Costello JF, Balki M: Cesarean delivery under ultrasound-guided spinal anesthesia [corrected] in a parturient with poliomyelitis and Harrington instrumentation. Can J Anaesth 2008;55:606–611.

48. Prasad GA, Tumber PS, Lupu CM: Ultrasound guided spinal anesthesia. Can J Anaesth 2008;55:716–717.

49. Coley BD, Shiels WE, Hogan MJ: Diagnostic and interventional ultrasonography in neonatal and infant lumbar puncture. Pediatr Radiol 2001;31:399–402.

50. Peterson MA, Abele J: Bedside ultrasound for difficult lumbar puncture. J Emerg Med 2005;28:197–200.

51. Chin KJ, Chan VW, Ramlogan R, Perlas A: Real-time ultrasound-guided spinal anesthesia in patients with a challenging spinal anatomy: two case reports. Acta Anaesthesiol Scand 2010;54:252–255.

52. Yamauchi M, Honma E, Mimura M, Yamamoto H, Takahashi E, Namiki A: Identification of the lumbar intervertebral level using ultrasound imaging in a post-laminectomy patient. J Anesth 2006;20:231–233.

53. Yeo ST, French R: Combined spinal-epidural in the obstetric patient with Harrington rods assisted by ultrasonography. Br J Anaesth 1999;83:670–672.

54. Rapp HJ, Folger A, Grau T: Ultrasound-guided epidural catheter insertion in children. Anesth Analg 2005;101:333–339, table.

55. Salman A, Arzola C, Tharmaratnam U, Balki M: Ultrasound imaging of the thoracic spine in paramedian sagittal oblique plane: the correlation between estimated and actual depth to the epidural space. Reg Anesth Pain Med 2011;36:542–547.

56. Yoon JS, Sim KH, Kim SJ, Kim WS, Koh SB, Kim BJ: The feasibility of color Doppler ultrasonography for caudal epidural steroid injection. Pain 2005;118:210–214.

57. Tsui BC, Tarkkila P, Gupta S, Kearney R: Confirmation of caudal needle placement using nerve stimulation. Anesthesiology 1999;91:374–378.

58. Chen CP, Wong AM, Hsu CC, et al: Ultrasound as a screening tool for proceeding with caudal epidural injections. Arch Phys Med Rehabil 2010;91:358–363.

59. McLeod A, Roche A, Fennelly M: Case series: ultrasonography may assist epidural insertion in scoliosis patients. Can J Anaesth 2005;52:717–720.

60. Arzola C, Davies S, Rofaeel A, Carvalho JC: Ultrasound using the transverse approach to the lumbar spine provides reliable landmarks for labor epidurals. Anesth Analg 2007;104:1188–1192, tables.

61. Asakura Y, Kandatsu N, Hashimoto A, Kamiya M, Akashi M, Komatsu T: Ultrasound-guided neuroaxial anesthesia: accurate diagnosis of spina bifida occulta by ultrasonography. J Anesth 2009;23:312–313.

62. Lee Y, Tanaka M, Carvalho JC: Sonoanatomy of the lumbar spine in patients with previous unintentional dural punctures during labor epidurals. Reg Anesth Pain Med 2008;33:266–270.

63. Chin KJ, Perlas A, Chan V, Brown-Shreves D, Koshkin A, Vaishnav V: Ultrasound imaging facilitates spinal anesthesia in adults with difficult surface anatomic landmarks. Anesthesiology 2011;115:94–101.

64. Locks GF, Almeida MC, Pereira AA: Use of the ultrasound to determine the level of lumbar puncture in pregnant women. Rev Bras Anestesiol 2010;60:13–19.

65. Schlotterbeck H, Schaeffer R, Dow WA, Touret Y, Bailey S, Diemunsch P: Ultrasonographic control of the puncture level for lumbar neuraxial block in obstetric anaesthesia. Br J Anaesth 2008;100:230–234.

66. Whitty R, Moore M, Macarthur A: Identification of the lumbar interspinous spaces: palpation versus ultrasound. Anesth Analg 2008; 106:538–540, table.

67. Gnaho A, Nguyen V, Villevielle T, Frota M, Marret E, Gentili ME: Assessing the depth of the subarachnoid space by ultrasound. Rev Bras Anestesiol 2012;62:520–530.

68. Grau T, Leipold R, Conradi R, Martin E, Motsch J: [Ultrasonography and peridural anesthesia. Technical possibilities and limitations of ultrasonic examination of the epidural space]. Anaesthesist 2001;50:94–101.

69. Tran D, Kamani AA, Lessoway VA, Peterson C, Hor KW, Rohling RN: Preinsertion paramedian ultrasound guidance for epidural anesthesia. Anesth Analg 2009;109:661–667.

70. Vallejo MC, Phelps AL, Singh S, Orebaugh SL, Sah N: Ultrasound decreases the failed labor epidural rate in resident trainees. Int J Obstet Anesth 2010;19:373–378.

71. de Seze MP, Sztark F, Janvier G, Joseph PA: Severe and long-lasting complications of the nerve root and spinal cord after central neuraxial blockade. Anesth Analg 2007;104:975–979.

72. Vandermeulen EP, Van AH, Vermylen J: Anticoagulants and spinal-epidural anesthesia. Anesth Analg 1994;79:1165–1177.

73. Chin KJ, Chan V: Ultrasonography as a preoperative assessment tool: predicting the feasibility of central neuraxial blockade. Anesth Analg 2010;110:252–253.

74. Weed JT, Taenzer AH, Finkel KJ, Sites BD: Evaluation of pre-procedure ultrasound examination as a screening tool for difficult spinal anaesthesia*. Anaesthesia 2011;66:925–930.

75. Stonelake PS, Burwell RG, Webb JK: Variation in vertebral levels of the vertebra prominens and sacral dimples in subjects with scoliosis. J Anat 1988;159:165–172.

76. Teoh DA, Santosham KL, Lydell CC, Smith DF, Beriault MT: Surface anatomy as a guide to vertebral level for thoracic epidural placement. Anesth Analg 2009;108:1705–1707.

77. Arzola C, Avramescu S, Tharmaratnam U, Chin KJ, Balki M: Identification of cervicothoracic intervertebral spaces by surface landmarks and ultrasound. Can J Anaesth 2011;58:1069–1074.

78. Rasoulian A, Lohser J, Najafi M, et al: Utility of prepuncture ultrasound for localization of the thoracic epidural space. Can J Anaesth 2011;58:815–823.

79. Pandin P, Haentjens L, Salengros JC, Quintin J, Barvais L: Combined ultrasound and nerve stimulation-guided thoracic epidural catheter placement for analgesia following anterior spine fusion in scoliosis. Pain Pract 2009;9:230–234.

80. Margarido CB, Arzola C, Balki M, Carvalho JC: Anesthesiologists' learning curves for ultrasound assessment of the lumbar spine. Can J Anaesth 2010;57:120–126.

81. Halpern SH, Banerjee A, Stocche R, Glanc P: The use of ultrasound for lumbar spinous process identification: a pilot study. Can J Anaesth 2010;57:817–822.

82. Chin KJ, Tse CC, Chan V: Practical considerations in preparing the pig carcass spine phantom. Reg Anesth Pain Med 2011;36:91–92.

83. Li JW, Karmakar MK, Li X, Kwok WH, Ngan Kee WD: Gelatin-agar lumbosacral spine phantom: a simple model for learning the basic skills required to perform real-time sonographically guided central neuraxial blocks. J Ultrasound Med 2011;30:263–72.

OBSTETRIC ANESTHESIA

Obstetric Regional Anesthesia

Jason Choi, Liane Germond, and Alan C. Santos

INTRODUCTION

Most women experience moderate to severe pain during labor and delivery, often requiring some form of pharmacologic analgesia.[1] The lack of proper psychological preparation combined with fear and anxiety can greatly enhance the patient's sensitivity to pain and further add to the discomfort during labor and delivery. However, skillfully conducted obstetric analgesia, in addition to relieving pain and anxiety, may benefit the mother in many other ways. This chapter focuses on the management of obstetric patients with a primary focus on regional anesthesia techniques.

Physiologic Changes of Pregnancy

Pregnancy results in significant changes affecting most maternal organ systems (Table 41–1). These changes are initiated by hormones secreted by the corpus luteum and the placenta. Such changes have important implications for the anesthesiologist caring for the pregnant patient. This chapter reviews the most relevant physiologic changes of pregnancy and discusses the approach to obstetric management using regional anesthesia.

Changes in the Cardiovascular System

Oxygen consumption increases during pregnancy, as the maternal cardiovascular system is required to meet the increasing metabolic demands of a growing fetus. The end result of these changes is an increase in heart rate (15%–25%) and cardiac output (up to 50%) compared with values before pregnancy. In addition, lower vascular resistance is found in the uterine, renal, and other vascular beds. These changes result in a lower arterial blood pressure because of a decrease in peripheral resistance, which exceeds the increase in cardiac output. Decreased vascular resistance is mostly due to the secretion of estrogens, progesterone, and prostacyclin.[2] Particularly significant increases in

cardiac output occur during labor and in the immediate postpartum period owing to added blood volume from the contracted uterus.

Clinical Pearls

- Cardiovascular changes and pitfalls in advanced pregnancy include the following:
- Increase in heart rate (15%–25%) and cardiac output (up to 50%).
- Decrease in vascular resistance in the uterine, renal, and other vascular beds.
- Compression of the lower aorta in the supine position may further decrease uteroplacental perfusion and result in fetal asphyxia.
- Significant hypotension is more likely to occur in pregnant versus nonpregnant women undergoing regional anesthesia, necessitating uterine displacement or lateral pelvic tilt maneuvers, intravascular preloading, and vasopressors.

From the second trimester onward, aortocaval compression by the enlarged uterus becomes progressively more important, reaching its maximum effect at 36–38 weeks, after which it may be relieved some as the fetal head descends into the pelvis.[3] Cardiac output may decrease when patients are in the supine position but not in the lateral decubitus position. Venous occlusion by the growing fetus causes supine hypotensive syndrome in 10% of pregnant women and manifests as maternal tachycardia, arterial hypotension, faintness, and pallor.[4]

Compression of the lower aorta in this position may further decrease uteroplacental perfusion and result in fetal asphyxia. Uterine displacement or lateral pelvic tilt should be applied routinely during the anesthetic management of the pregnant

TABLE 41–1. Summary of physiologic changes of pregnancy at term.

Variable	Change	Amount
Total blood volume	Increase	25%–40%
Plasma volume	Increase	40%–50%
Fibrinogen	Increase	50%
Serum cholinesterase activity	Decrease	20%–30%
Cardiac output	Increase	30%–50%
Minute ventilation	Increase	50%
Alveolar ventilation	Increase	70%
Functional residual capacity	Decrease	20%
Oxygen consumption	Increase	20%
Arterial carbon dioxide tension	Decrease	10 mm Hg
Arterial oxygen tension	Increase	10 mm Hg
Minimum alveolar concentration	Decrease	32%–40%

patient. Uterine displacement is best achieved by placing the patient in the left lateral decubitus position. In this position, cardiac vagal activity will be augmented as compared to the supine position.[5] Placing a wedge under the bony pelvis has been used to achieve uterine tilt. However, it has recently been demonstrated that uterine tilt is more effective when the mother is placed in the full left lateral decubitus position and then is turned supine onto the pelvic wedge.[6]

Changes in the electrocardiogram are common in late pregnancy. The QRS axis may initially shift to the right during the first trimester, rotating to left axis by the third trimester as a result of the expanding uterus.[7] A shortening of the PR and QT intervals and an increase in heart rate are also present. The QT interval shortening may have implications for women with long QT syndrome.[8] Indeed, Seth et al. found a reduced risk (risk ratio [RR] = 0.38) of cardiac events during pregnancy in woman with prolonged QT syndrome. However, an increased risk of postpartum cardiac events in the first nine months after delivery was also found, which suggests that the QT interval becomes prolonged again in the early post-delivery period. There is also a tendency toward premature atrial contractions, sinus tachycardia, and paroxysmal supraventricular tachycardia.

Changes in the Respiratory System

Minute ventilation increases from the beginning of pregnancy to a maximum of 50% above normal by term.[9] This is mostly a result of a 40% increase in tidal volume and a small increase in respiratory rate. Dead space does not change significantly during pregnancy; thus, alveolar ventilation is increased by 70% at

term. After delivery, as blood progesterone levels decline, ventilation returns to normal within 1–3 weeks.[10]

Elevation of the diaphragm occurs with an increase in the size of the uterus. Expiratory reserve volume, residual volume, and functional residual capacity (FRC) decrease by the third trimester of pregnancy.[9] However, because there is also an increase in inspiratory reserve volume, total lung capacity remains unchanged. A decreased FRC is typically asymptomatic in healthy parturients. Those with preexisting alterations in closing volume as a result of smoking, obesity, scoliosis, or other pulmonary disease may experience early airway closure with advancing pregnancy, leading to hypoxemia. The Trendelenburg and supine positions also exacerbate the abnormal relationship between closing volume and FRC. The residual volume and FRC return to normal shortly after delivery.

Pregnant women often have difficulty with nasal breathing. Friability of the mucous membranes during pregnancy can cause severe bleeding, especially on airway instrumentation. These changes are caused by increased extracellular fluid and vascular engorgement. It may also be difficult to perform laryngoscopy in obese, short-necked parturients with enlarged breasts. Use of a short-handled laryngoscope has proved helpful.

Clinical Pearl

- Airway edema may be severe in pregnant women, particularly in those with preeclampsia, those in whom the Trendelenburg position is used for prolonged periods, and those in whom tocolytic agents are used.

Metabolic Changes

Oxygen consumption increases during early pregnancy, with an overall increase of 20% by term. Regardless, increased alveolar ventilation occurring during pregnancy actually leads to a reduction in the partial pressure of carbon dioxide in arterial blood ($PaCO_2$) to 32 mm Hg and an increase in the partial pressure of oxygen in arterial blood (PaO_2) to 106 mm Hg. The plasma buffer base decreases from 47 to 42 mEq; consequently, the pH remains practically unchanged. The maternal uptake and elimination of inhalational anesthetics are enhanced because of the increased alveolar ventilation and decreased FRC. However, the decreased FRC and increased metabolic rate predispose the mother to the development of hypoxemia during periods of apnea or hypoventilation.[11]

Changes in the Gastrointestinal System

The effects of pregnancy on the gastrointestinal system are controversial. It has been proposed that enhanced progesterone production causes decreased gastrointestinal motility and slower absorption of food. Gastric secretions are more acidic, and lower esophageal sphincter tone is decreased. However, more recent studies using radiographic, ultrasound, and dye dilution techniques have demonstrated that gastric emptying of liquid and solid materials does not decrease at any time during pregnancy.[12–15]

The risk of regurgitation on induction of general anesthesia depends, in part, on the gradient between the lower esophageal sphincter and intragastric pressures. In parturients with "heartburn," the lower esophageal sphincter tone is greatly reduced.[16] No single routine prophylactic regimen can be recommended with certainty. The efficacy of prophylactic nonparticulate antacids is diminished by inadequate mixing with gastric contents, improper timing of administration, and the tendency for antacids to increase gastric volume. The administration of histamine (H2)-receptor antagonists, such as cimetidine and ranitidine, requires anticipation and careful timing since their onset of action is relatively slow. In those women at greatest risk, an argument can be made for the administration of intravenous (IV) metoclopramide before elective cesarean section delivery. This dopamine antagonist hastens gastric emptying and increases resting lower esophageal sphincter tone in both nonpregnant and pregnant women.[17] However, there have been conflicting data on its efficacy (perhaps due to timing of administration) and the frequency of side effects, such as extrapyramidal reactions and transient neurologic dysfunction.[18,19]

Endocrine Changes Influencing Plasma Volume, Blood Composition, and Glucose Metabolism

Plasma volume and total blood volume begin to increase in early gestation, resulting in an increase of 40%–50% and 25%–40%, respectively, at term. These changes are due to an increased mineralocorticoid activity during pregnancy, which results in sodium retention and increased body water content.[20] The relatively smaller increase in red blood cell volume (20%) accounts for a relative reduction in hemoglobin (to 11–12 g/L) and hematocrit (to 35%); the platelet count, however, remains unchanged. Plasma fibrinogen concentrations increase during normal pregnancy by approximately 50%, whereas clotting factor activity is variable.[21] Coagulation factors I, VII, VIII, IX, X, and XII increase during pregnancy,[22] whereas factor XI and XIII concentrations decrease and factor II and V concentrations remain unchanged during pregnancy.

Serum cholinesterase activity declines to a level of 20% below normal by term and reaches a nadir in the puerperium. The net effect of these changes in the serum cholinesterase is of negligible relevance to the metabolism of clinically used doses of succinylcholine or ester-type local anesthetics (2-choloroprocaine).[23,24] The albumin–globulin ratio declines because of the relatively greater reduction in albumin concentration. A decrease in serum protein concentration may be clinically significant in that the free fractions of protein-bound drugs can be expected to increase.

Human placental lactogen and cortisol increase the tendency toward hyperglycemia and ketosis, which may exacerbate preexisting diabetes mellitus. The patient's ability to handle a glucose load is decreased, and the transplacental passage of glucose may stimulate fetal secretion of insulin, leading, in turn, to neonatal hypoglycemia in the immediate postpartum period.[25]

Altered Drug Responses in Pregnancy

Pregnancy results in a progesterone-mediated increase in neural sensitivity to local anesthetics.[26] Lower doses of local anesthetic are needed per dermatomal segment of epidural or spinal block. This has been attributed to an increased spread of local anesthetic in the epidural and subarachnoid spaces as a result of epidural venous engorgement and enhanced sensitivity to local anesthetic block due to progesterone. The minimum alveolar concentration for inhalational agents is decreased by 8–12 weeks of gestation and may be related to an increase in progesterone levels.[27]

Clinical Pearls

- During pregnancy, there is a progesterone-mediated increase in neural sensitivity to local anesthetics.
- Doses of local anesthetic need to be lowered per dermatomal segment of epidural or spinal block.

PLACENTAL TRANSFER OF LOCAL ANESTHETICS

Local anesthetics readily cross the placenta by simple diffusion. Several factors influence the placental transfer of drugs, including the physicochemical characteristics of the drug itself, maternal drug concentrations in the plasma, properties of the placenta, and hemodynamic events within the fetomaternal unit.

Highly lipid-soluble drugs, such as local anesthetics, cross biologic membranes more readily, and the degree of ionization is important because the nonionized moiety of a drug is more lipophilic than the ionized drug. Local anesthetics are weak bases, with a relatively low degree of ionization and considerable lipid solubility. The relative concentrations of drug existing in the nonionized and ionized forms can be estimated from the Henderson–Hasselbalch equation:

$$pH = pK_a + \log \text{(base)}/\text{(cation)}$$

The ratio of base to cation becomes particularly important with local anesthetics because the nonionized form penetrates tissue barriers, whereas the ionized form is pharmacologically active in blocking nerve conduction. The pK_a (acid dissociation constant) is the pH at which the concentrations of free base and cation are equal. For the amide local anesthetics, the pK_a values (7.7–8.1) are sufficiently close to physiologic pH so that changes in maternal or fetal biochemical status may significantly alter the proportion of ionized and nonionized drug (Figure 41–1). At steady state, the concentrations of nonionized local anesthetics in the fetal and maternal plasma are equal. With fetal acidosis, there is a greater tendency for drug to exist in the ionized form, which cannot diffuse back across the placenta. This causes a larger total amount of local anesthetic to accumulate in the fetal plasma and tissues. This is called ion trapping.[28]

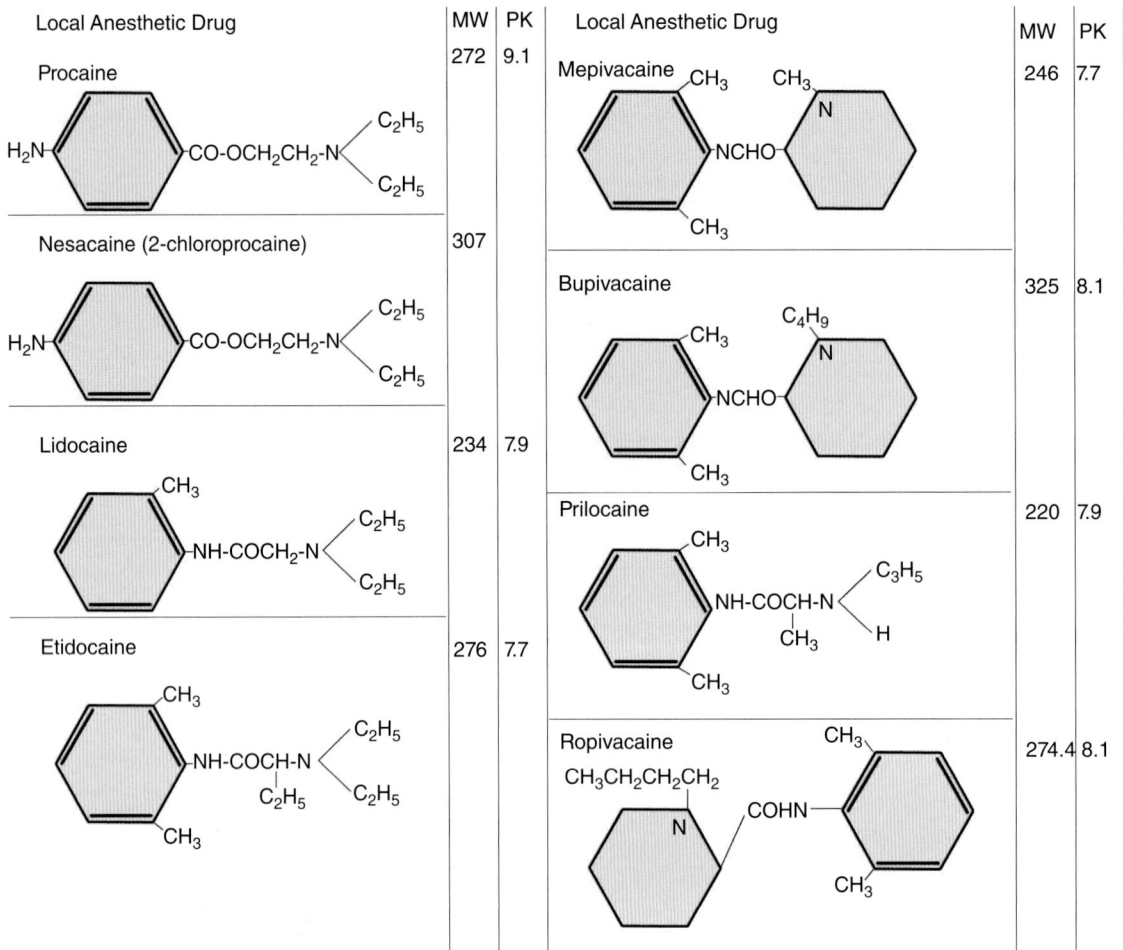

FIGURE 41-1. Chemical structures of local anesthetics. MW = molecular weight; PK = ionizing constant.

Clinical Pearl

- The prolonged administration of highly protein-bound drugs (eg, bupivacaine) may lead to substantial fetal accumulation of the drugs.

The effects of maternal plasma protein binding on the rate and amount of local anesthetic accumulating in the fetus are inadequately understood. Animal studies have shown that the transfer rate is slower for drugs that are extensively bound to maternal plasma proteins, such as bupivacaine.[29,30] However, with the prolonged administration of highly protein-bound drugs, such as bupivacaine, substantial accumulation of drug can occur in the fetus.[31]

The concentration gradient of free drug between the maternal and fetal blood is a significant factor. On the maternal side, the dose administered, the mode and site of administration, and the use of vasoconstrictors can influence fetal exposure. The rates of distribution, metabolism, and excretion of the drug, which may vary, are equally important. Higher doses result in higher maternal blood concentrations. The absorption rate can vary with the site of injection. For instance, an IV bolus results in the highest blood concentration. It was once believed that intrathecal administration resulted in negligible plasma concentrations of local

anesthetics. However, we now know that spinal anesthesia induced with 75 mg lidocaine results in maternal plasma concentrations that are similar to those reported by others after epidural anesthesia.[32] Furthermore, significant levels of the drug can be found in the umbilical vein at birth.

Repeated administration can result in high maternal blood concentrations, depending on the dose and frequency of reinjection, in addition to the kinetic characteristics of the drug. The half-life of amide local anesthetic agents is relatively long, so that repeated injection may lead to accumulation in the maternal plasma (Figure 41–2).[33] In contrast, 2-chloroprocaine, an ester local anesthetic, undergoes rapid enzymatic hydrolysis in the presence of pseudo-cholinesterase. After epidural injection, the mean half-life in the mother is approximately 3 minutes; after reinjection, 2-chloroprocaine can be detected in the maternal plasma for only 5–10 minutes, and no accumulation of this drug has occurred.[34]

Pregnancy is associated with physiologic changes that also may influence maternal pharmacokinetics and the action of anesthetic drugs. These changes may be progressive during the course of gestation and are often difficult to predict for an individual drug. Nonetheless, the elimination half-life of bupivacaine after epidural injection has been shown to be similar in pregnant and nonpregnant women.[35]

Fetal regional blood flow changes can also affect the amount of drug taken up by individual organs. For example, during asphyxia and acidosis, a greater proportion of the fetal cardiac

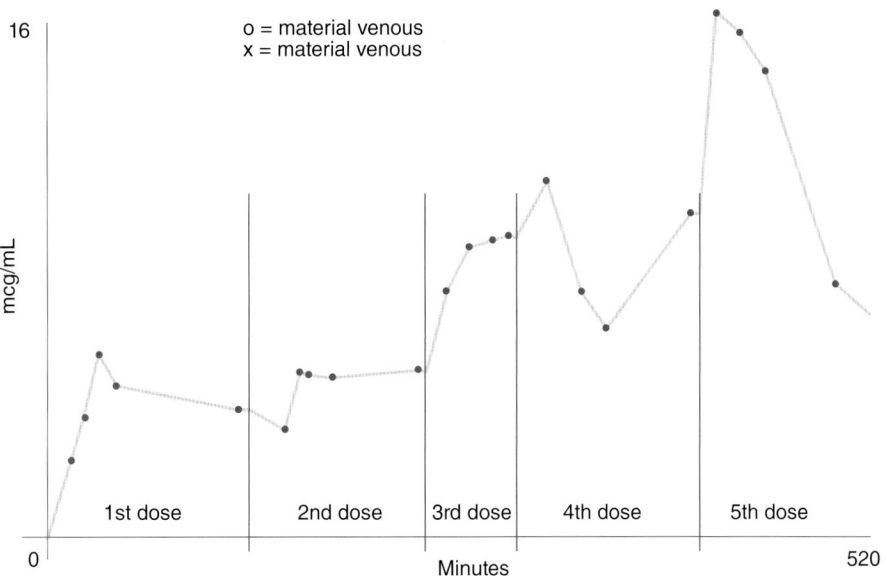

FIGURE 41-2. Increased maternal blood concentration of local anesthetic after repeated doses (300 mg) of mepivacaine.

output perfuses the fetal brain, heart, and placenta. Infusion of lidocaine resulted in increased drug uptake in the heart, brain, and liver of asphyxiated baboon fetuses compared with nonasphyxiated control fetuses.[36]

Risk of Drug Exposure: Fetus Versus Newborn

The fetus can excrete local anesthetics back into the maternal circulation after the concentration gradient of the free drug across the placenta has been reversed. This may occur even if the total plasma drug concentration in the mother exceeds that in the fetus, because there is lower protein binding in fetal plasma.[30] 2-chloroprocaine is the only drug that is metabolized in the fetal blood so quickly that even with acidosis, substantial exposure in the fetus is avoided.[34]

Both term and preterm infants have the hepatic enzymes necessary for the biotransformation of amide local anesthetics. In a comparative study, the pharmacokinetics of lidocaine among adult ewes and fetal/neonatal lambs indicated that the metabolic clearance in the newborn was similar to, and renal clearance greater than, that in the adult.[37] However, the half-life was longer in the newborn; this is related to a greater volume of distribution and tissue uptake, so that, at any given moment, the neonate's liver and kidneys are exposed to a smaller fraction of lidocaine accumulated in the body. Similar results have been reported in another study involving lidocaine administration to human infants in a neonatal intensive care unit.[38]

Neonatal depression occurs at blood concentrations of mepivacaine or lidocaine that are approximately 50% less than those producing systemic toxicity in the adult. However, infants accidentally injected in utero with mepivacaine (intended for maternal caudal anesthesia) stopped convulsing when the mepivacaine level decreased below the threshold for convulsions in the adult.[39] The relative central nervous toxicity and cardiorespiratory toxicity of local anesthetics have been studied in sheep.[40] The doses required

to produce toxicity in the fetal and newborn lamb were greater than those required in the ewe. In the fetus, this difference was attributed to placental clearance of drug into the mother and better maintenance of blood gas tensions during convulsions, whereas in the newborn lamb, a larger volume of distribution was probably responsible for the higher doses needed to induce toxic effects.

It has been suggested that bupivacaine may be implicated as a possible cause of neonatal jaundice because of its high affinity for fetal erythrocyte membranes, resulting in a decrease in filterability and deformability rendering subjects more prone to hemolysis. However, a more recent study has failed to show demonstrable bilirubin production in newborns whose mothers were given bupivacaine for epidural anesthesia during labor and delivery.[41]

Neurobehavioral studies have revealed subtle changes in newborn neurologic and adaptive function with regional anesthesia. In the case of most anesthetic agents, these changes are minor and transient, lasting for only 24–48 hours.[42]

ANESTHESIA FOR LABOR & VAGINAL DELIVERY

In the first stage of labor, pain is caused by uterine contractions related to dilation of the cervix and distention of the lower uterine segment. Pain impulses are carried in visceral afferent type C fibers, which accompany the sympathetic nerves. In early labor, only the lower thoracic dermatomes (T11–T12) are affected. However, with progressive cervical dilation during the transition phase, adjacent dermatomes may be involved and pain referred from T10 to L1. During the second stage, additional pain impulses due to distention of the vaginal vault and perineum are carried in the pudendal nerve, which is composed of lower sacral fibers (S2–S4).

Regional analgesia may benefit the mother in other ways beyond relieving pain and anxiety. In animal studies, pain may cause maternal hypertension and reduced uterine blood flow.[43] Epidural analgesia blunts the increases in maternal cardiac output, heart rate, and blood pressure that occur with painful uterine contractions and "bearing-down" efforts.[44] By reducing the maternal secretion of catecholamines, epidural analgesia may convert a previously dysfunctional labor pattern to a normal one.[45] Regional analgesia can benefit the fetus by eliminating maternal hyperventilation with pain, which often leads to a reduced fetal arterial oxygen tension owing to a leftward shift of the maternal oxygen–hemoglobin dissociation curve.[46]

The most frequently chosen methods for relieving the pain of parturition are psychoprophylaxis, systemic medication, and regional analgesia. Inhalational analgesia, conventional spinal analgesia, and paracervical blockade are less commonly used. General anesthesia is rarely necessary but may be indicated for uterine relaxation in some complicated deliveries.

Systemic Analgesia

The advantages of systemic analgesics include ease of administration and patient acceptability. However, the drug, dose, timing, and method of administration must be chosen carefully to avoid maternal and neonatal depression. Drugs used for systemic analgesia are opioids, tranquilizers, and occasionally ketamine.

Systemic Opioids

In the past, meperidine was the most commonly used systemic analgesic to ameliorate pain during the first stage of labor. It can be administered by IV injection (effective analgesia in 5–10 minutes) or intramuscularly (peak effect in 40–50 minutes). It was also commonly used for postoperative pain in the general population. But with the popularity of its administration, disturbing side effects began to emerge. One of the most serious side effects was the occurrence of seizures both from the primary drug effect and from the drug's metabolite, normeperidine. In the pregnant patient at risk for seizures—that is, with pregnancy-induced hypertension or preeclampsia—confusing the picture by the administration of a drug known to cause seizures complicates patient care.[47,48] Other side effects are nausea and vomiting, dose-related depression of ventilation, orthostatic hypotension, the potential for neonatal depression, and euphoria out of proportion to the analgesic effect, leading to misuse of the drug.[49] Meperidine may also cause transient alterations of the fetal heart rate, such as decreased beat-to-beat variability and tachycardia. Among other factors, the risk of neonatal depression is related to the interval between the last drug injection and delivery.[50] The placental transfer of an active metabolite, normeperidine, which has a long elimination half-life in the neonate (62 hours), has also been implicated in contributing to neonatal depression and subtle neonatal neurobehavioral dysfunction. The effects of systemically administered meperidine on the course of labor are controversial. It has been suggested that meperidine administration may prolong the latent phase of labor but shorten the cumulative length of the first stage of labor. However, a recent study showed no benefit to the administration of meperidine in order to possibly shorten the first stage of labor in women having dystocia.[51]

Experience with the newer synthetic opioids, such as fentanyl and alfentanil, has been limited. Although they are potent, their usefulness during labor is limited by their short duration of action. However, these drugs offer an advantage when analgesia of rapid onset but short duration is necessary (eg, with forceps application). For example, a single IV injection of fentanyl, up to 1 mcg/kg, results in prompt pain relief without severe neonatal depression but for a short period of time.[52] Alfentanil may be associated with greater neonatal depression than equivalent meperidine patient-controlled analgesia (PCA).[53] In another study, alfentanil PCA failed to provide adequate analgesia compared to fentanyl PCA.[54] For more prolonged analgesia, fentanyl can be administered with patient-controlled delivery devices.[55] More commonly, fentanyl (15–25 mcg) and sufentanil (5–10 mcg) have been used with local anesthetics in an initial spinal dose with a local anesthetic during the placement of a continuous spinal–epidural for labor with excellent relief of pain.[56,57]

Remifentanil is an opioid that is rapidly metabolized by serum and tissue cholinesterases, and consequently, has a short (3-minute), context-sensitive half-time.[58] When used in bolus dosing (0.3–0.8 mcg/kg per bolus), remifentanil has been found to have an acceptable level of maternal side effects and a minimal effect on the neonate. Remifentanil crosses the placenta and appears to be either rapidly metabolized or redistributed in the neonate.[59] In one study, Apgar and neurobehavioral scores were good in neonates whose mothers were given an IV infusion of remifentanil, 0.1 mcg/kg/min, during cesarean section delivery under epidural anesthesia.[60] When administered by PCA, remifentanil has been found to provide better pain relief, equivalent hemodynamic stability, less sedation, and less oxygen desaturation compared with meperidine.[59,61] In a recent double-blind trial, remifentanil PCA was compared to lumbar epidural for equivalent analgesia. Twenty-six percent of women in the remifentanil group reported acceptable pain scores compared to 56% of women receiving lumbar epidural analgesia.[62] In countries outside the United States, intermittent nitrous oxide has been used for labor analgesia. When comparing remifentanil with nitrous oxide, remifentanil was found to provide better pain relief with fewer side effects. However, remifentanil can result in hypoventilation and hypoxemia, thus oxygen saturation should be routinely monitored during remifentanil IV PCA.[63]

Opioid agonist-antagonists, such as butorphanol and nalbuphine, have also been used for obstetric analgesia. These drugs have the proposed benefits of a lower incidence of nausea, vomiting, and dysphoria, as well as a "ceiling effect" on depression of ventilation.[64] Intramuscular (IM) nalbuphine has been compared to meperidine in a double-blind study. Analgesia was comparable in both groups; however, nalbuphine was associated with increased maternal sedation compared to meperidine.[65] Butorphanol is probably the most popular of the mixed agonist-antagonists; unlike meperidine, it is metabolized into inactive metabolites and has a ceiling effect on depression of ventilation in doses exceeding 2 mg. Butorphanol results in comparable maternal pain relief to meperidine and no difference in Apgar scores. However, butorphanol use was associated with fewer maternal side effects, such as nausea, vomiting, and dizziness, than meperidine.[66] A potential disadvantage is a high incidence of maternal sedation. The recommended dose is 1–2 mg by IV or IM injection. Nalbuphine 10 mg IV or IM is an alternative to butorphanol.

Naloxone, a pure opioid antagonist, should not be administered to the mother shortly before delivery to prevent neonatal ventilatory depression because it reverses maternal analgesia at a time when it is most needed. In some instances, naloxone has been reported to cause maternal pulmonary edema and even cardiac arrest. If necessary, the drug should be given directly to the newborn IM (0.1 mg/kg).

Ketamine

Ketamine is a potent analgesic. However, it may also induce unacceptable amnesia that may interfere with the mother's recollection of the birth. Nonetheless, ketamine is a useful adjuvant to incomplete regional analgesia during vaginal delivery or for obstetric manipulations. In low doses (0.2–0.4 mg/kg), ketamine provides adequate analgesia without causing neonatal depression.

Regional Analgesia Techniques

Regional techniques provide excellent analgesia with minimal depressant effects in mother and fetus. The techniques most commonly used for labor anesthesia include central neuraxial (spinal, epidural, and combined spinal–epidural), paracervical, and pudendal blocks and, less frequently, lumbar sympathetic blocks. Hypotension resulting from sympathectomy is the most common complication that occurs with central neuraxial blockade. Therefore, maternal blood pressure must be monitored at regular intervals, typically every 2–5 minutes for approximately 15–20 minutes after the initiation of the block and at routine

intervals thereafter. Regional analgesia may be contraindicated in the presence of severe coagulopathy, acute hypovolemia, or infection at the site of needle insertion. Chorioamnionitis without sepsis is not a contraindication to central neuraxial blockade.

Epidural Analgesia

Effective analgesia for the first stage of labor is achieved by blocking the T10–L1 dermatomes with a low concentration of local anesthetic, often in combination with a lipid-soluble opioid. For the second stage of labor, because of pain due to vaginal distention and perineal pressure, the block should be extended to include the pudendal segments, S2–4 (Figures 41–3 and 41–4).

There has been concern that the early initiation of epidural analgesia during the latent phase of labor (2–4 cm cervical dilation) may result in prolongation of the first stage of labor and a higher incidence of dystocia and cesarean section delivery, particularly in nulliparous women.[66–69] Generally speaking, the first stage of labor is not prolonged by epidural analgesia, provided that aortocaval compression is avoided.[66–68,70,71] Chestnut et al.[70,71] demonstrated that the incidence of cesarean section delivery was no different in nulliparous women having epidural analgesia initiated during the latent phase (at 4 cm dilation) compared with women whose analgesia was initiated during the active phase. Others have shown that epidural analgesia is not associated with an increased incidence of cesarean section delivery compared with IV PCA in nulliparous women.[67,68]

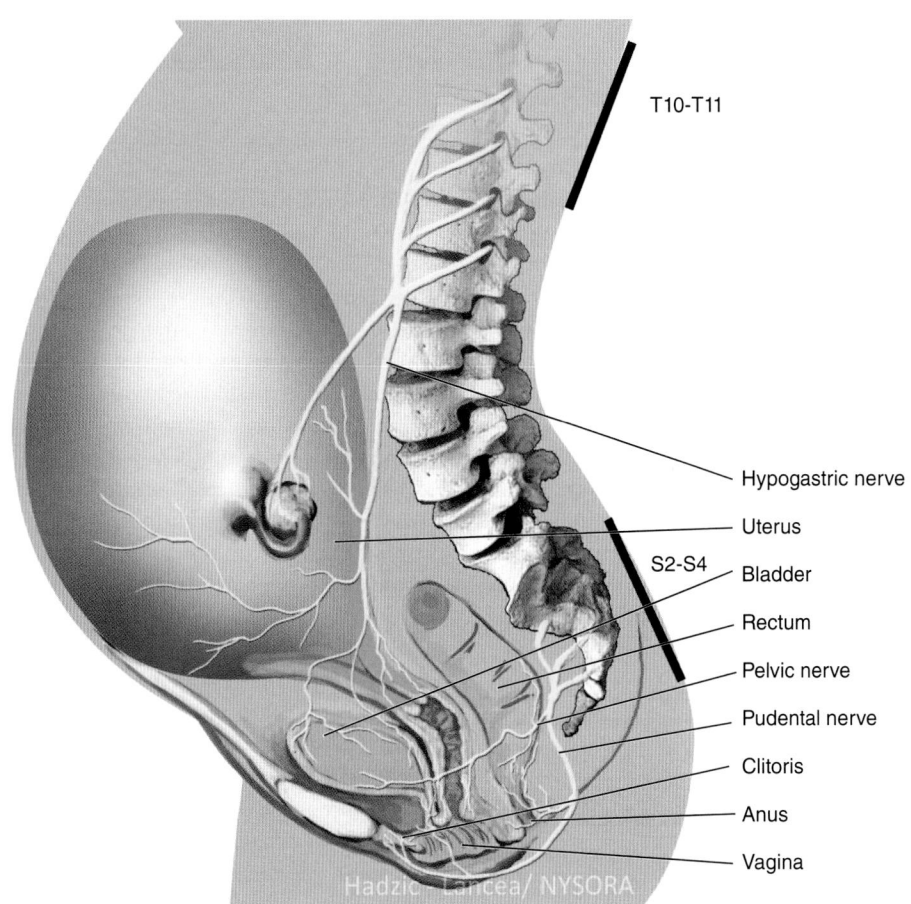

FIGURE 41–3. Pain pathways in a parturient.

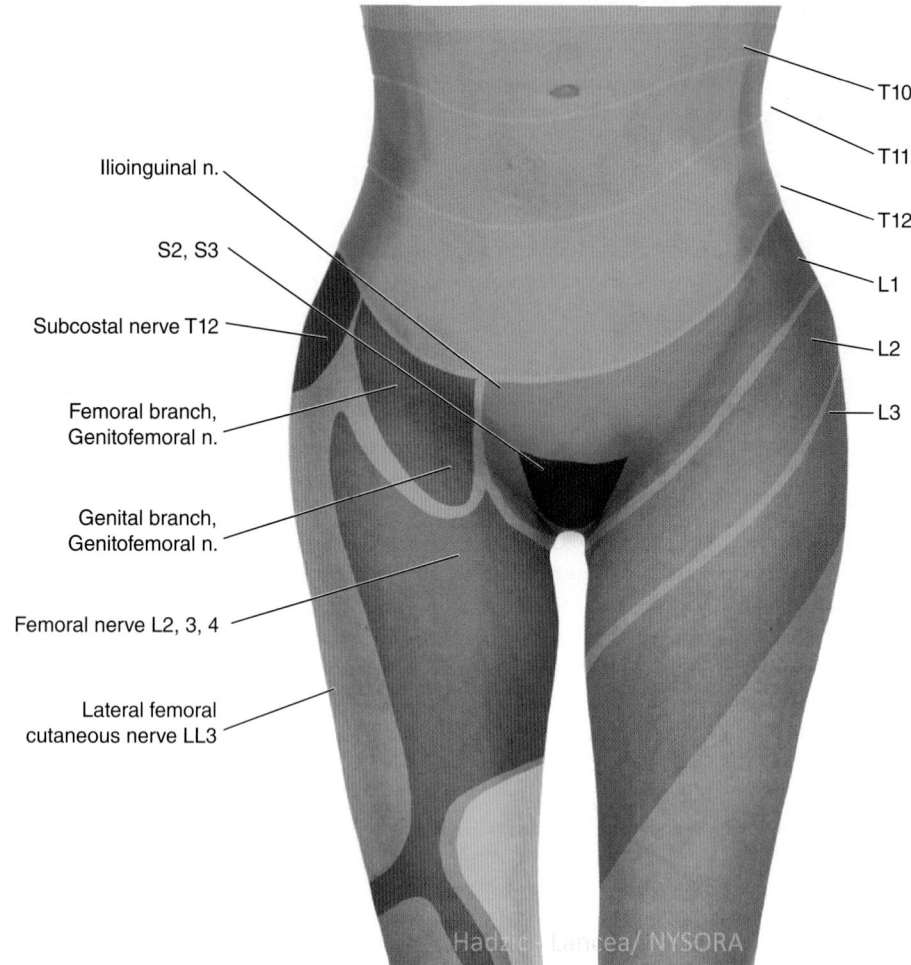

Ilioinguinal n.

S2, S3

Subcostal nerve T12

Femoral branch,
Genitofemoral n.

Genital branch,
Genitofemoral n.

Femoral nerve L2, 3, 4

Lateral femoral
cutaneous nerve LL3

T10

T11

T12

L1

L2

L3

Hadzic Lantea/ NYSORA

FIGURE 41–4. Dermatomal level of the lower abdomen, perineal area, hip, and thigh.

However, a prolongation of the second stage of labor has been reported in nulliparous women, possibly owing to a decrease in expulsive forces or malposition of the fetus.[66,71,72]

Thus, with the use of epidural analgesia, the American College of Obstetricians and Gynecologists (ACOG) has defined an abnormally prolonged second stage of labor as longer than 3 hours in nulliparous women and longer than 2 hours in multiparous women.[73]

A longer second stage of labor may be minimized by the use of an ultra-dilute local anesthetic solution in combination with an opioid.[74] Long-acting amides, such as bupivacaine, ropivacaine, and levobupivacaine, are most frequently used because they produce excellent sensory analgesia while sparing motor function, particularly at the low concentrations used for epidural analgesia.

Clinical Pearls

- Analgesia during the first stage of labor is achieved by blocking the T10–Ll dermatomes with a low concentration of local anesthetic (see Figure 41–3).
- Analgesia for the second stage of labor and delivery requires the block of the S2–4 segments because of pain due to vaginal distention and perineal pressure.

Analgesia for the first stage of labor may be achieved with 5–10 mL of bupivacaine, ropivacaine, or levobupivacaine (0.125%–0.25%), followed by a continuous infusion (8–12 mL/h) of 0.0625% bupivacaine or levobupivacaine, or 0.1% ropivacaine. Fentanyl 1–2 mcg/mL or sufentanil 0.3–0.5 mcg/mL may be added. During the actual delivery, the perineum may be blocked with 10 mL of 0.5% bupivacaine, 1% lidocaine, or, if a rapid effect is required, 2% chloroprocaine in the semirecumbent position.

There is controversy regarding the need for a test dose when using a dilute solution of local anesthetic.[75,77] Catheter aspiration alone is not always diagnostic. For that reason, some authors believe that a test dose should be administered to improve detection of an intrathecally or intravascularly placed epidural catheter. If injected into a blood vessel, 15 mcg epinephrine results in a change in heart rate of 20–30 bpm with a slight increase in blood pressure within 30 seconds of administration. The duration is approximately 30 seconds. The anesthesiologist should observe the pulse oximeter during the first minute after injection to determine whether an accidental intravascular injection has occurred. However, the tachycardia associated with an intravenous test dose of epinephrine is not a reliable indicator of intravascular injection during labor because it may be confounded coincident with a painful uterine contraction. In addition, epinephrine is not reliable in patients who have received a beta-adrenergic receptor antagonist.[77] Other subtle signs of intravascular injection may include a feeling of apprehension or unease or palpitations. It is important to fractionate the total dose of local anesthetic and observe the patient at one-minute intervals.

Patient-controlled epidural analgesia (PCEA) is a safe and effective alternative to conventional bolus or infusion techniques.[78] Maternal acceptance is excellent, and demands on anesthesia manpower may be reduced. Studies have shown that PCEA with a relatively low continuous epidural infusion and top-ups required fewer anesthetic interventions compared to PCEA without a basal rate epidural infusion.[79] Initial analgesia is achieved with bolus doses of local anesthetic. Once the mother is comfortable, PCEA may then be started with a maintenance infusion (8–12 mL/h) of local anesthetic (bupivacaine, levobupivacaine, or ropivacaine 0.0625%–0.125%) with or without an opioid (fentanyl 1–2 mcg/mL or sufentanil 0.3–0.5 mcg/mL). The machine may be programmed to administer an epidural demand bolus of 8 mL with a lockout period of 10 minutes between doses.[78] The caudal, rather than lumbar, approach may result in a faster onset of perineal analgesia and therefore may be preferable to the lumbar epidural approach when an imminent vaginal delivery is anticipated. However, caudal analgesia is no longer popular because of occasionally painful needle placement, a high failure rate, potential contamination at the injection site, and risks of accidental fetal injection. Before caudal injection, a digital rectal examination must be performed to exclude needle placement in the fetal presenting part. Low spinal "saddle block" has virtually eliminated the need for caudal anesthesia in modern practice.

Spinal Analgesia

A single intrathecal injection, usually of an opioid and a small dose of local anesthetic, for labor analgesia has the benefits of a reliable and rapid onset of analgesia for the first stage of labor. However, repeated intrathecal injections may be required for a long labor, thus increasing the risk of postdural puncture headache. In addition, motor block may be uncomfortable for some women and may prolong the second stage of labor. This technique is most useful for multiparous parturients who are rapidly progressing in labor and require analgesia or anesthesia of short duration before complete cervical dilation and anticipated vaginal delivery or in settings in which continuous epidural analgesia is not possible.[80]

Microcatheters were introduced for continuous spinal anesthesia in the 1980s. They were subsequently withdrawn when found to be associated with neurologic deficits, possibly related to maldistribution of local anesthetic in the cauda equina region.[81] Fortunately, in a recent multi-institutional study, no cases of neurologic symptoms occurred after the use of 28-gauge microcatheters for continuous spinal analgesia in laboring women.[82] Spinal anesthesia is also a safe and effective alternative to general anesthesia for instrumental delivery.

Combined Spinal–Epidural Analgesia

Combined spinal–epidural (CSE) analgesia is an ideal analgesic technique for use during labor. It combines the rapid, reliable onset of profound analgesia resulting from spinal injection with the flexibility and longer duration of epidural techniques. In a recent meta-analysis, the onset of analgesia for CSE was significantly faster than with an epidural technique (2–5 minutes vs. 10–15 minutes).[83]

Technique

After identifying the epidural space using a conventional (or specialized) epidural needle, a longer (127-mm), pencil-point spinal needle is advanced into the subarachnoid space through the epidural needle. After intrathecal injection, the spinal needle is removed, and an epidural catheter inserted. Intrathecal injection of fentanyl 10–25 mcg or sufentanil 2.5–5 mcg, alone or in combination with up to 1 mL of isobaric bupivacaine 0.25%, produces profound analgesia lasting for 60–120 minutes with minimal motor block.[84]

It should be noted that the incidence of pruritus is greater with intrathecal opioid administration than with epidural opioid administration.[85] An opioid alone may provide sufficient relief for the early latent phase, but the addition of bupivacaine is almost always necessary for satisfactory analgesia during advanced labor. Other adjuvants have also been used. The addition of adjuvants, such as clonidine and neostigmine, has been disappointing.[85] An epidural infusion of bupivacaine 0.03%–0.0625% with an opioid may be started within 10 minutes of spinal injection. Alternatively, the epidural component may be activated when necessary. Women with hemodynamic stability and preserved motor function who do not require continuous fetal monitoring may ambulate with assistance.[86,87] Before ambulation, women should be observed for 30 minutes after intrathecal or epidural drug administration to assess maternal and fetal well-being. A recent study indicated that the early administration of CSE analgesia to nulliparous women did not increase the cesarean section delivery rate.[88]

Clinical Pearl

- Intrathecal injection of fentanyl 10–25 mcg or sufentanil 5–10 mcg alone or, more commonly, with 1 mL isobaric bupivacaine 0.25% produces profound analgesia lasting for 90–120 minutes with minimal motor block.

The most common side effects of intrathecal opioids are pruritus, nausea, vomiting, and urinary retention. Rostral spread resulting in delayed respiratory depression is rare with fentanyl and sufentanil and usually occurs within 30 minutes of injection.[89] Transient nonreassuring fetal heart rate patterns may occur because of uterine hyperstimulation, presumably as a result of a rapid decrease in maternal catecholamines resulting in the unopposed effects of oxytocin.[90]

A preliminary study by O'Gorman et al.[91] suggests that fetal bradycardia may occur in the absence of uterine hyperstimulation or hypotension and is unrelated to utero-placental insufficiency. The incidence of fetal heart rate abnormalities may be greater in multiparous woman with a rapidly progressing, painful labor.[92] Most studies have demonstrated that the incidence of emergency cesarean section delivery is no greater with CSE analgesia than after conventional epidural analgesia.[93,94] Postdural puncture headache is always a risk after intrathecal injection. However, the incidence of headache is no greater with CSE analgesia compared with standard epidural analgesia.[95]

Unintentional intrathecal catheter placement through the dural puncture site is also rare after use of a 27-gauge spinal needle for CSE analgesia. The potential exists for epidurally administered drug to leak intrathecally through the dural puncture, particularly if large volumes of drug are rapidly injected. In fact, epidural drug requirements are approximately 30% less with CSE analgesia than with standard lumbar epidural techniques for cesarean section delivery.[96] Some clinicians do not advocate the CSE analgesia technique for labor because of the concern for an "unproven" epidural catheter that may need to be used emergently for cesarean section delivery. The patient may have a partial block insufficient for surgery with an epidural that may or may not work. An algorithm for patient management in the event of an incomplete epidural is presented in Figure 41–5.

Paracervical Block

As recently as 2001, only 2%–3% of parturients in the United States received paracervical block during labor.[97] Although

paracervical block effectively relieves pain during the first stage of labor, it is now rarely used in the United States because of its association with a high incidence of fetal bradycardia, particularly with the use of bupivacaine. This may be related to uterine artery constriction or increased uterine tone.[98]

The use of levobupivacaine compared to racemic bupivacaine has been demonstrated to result in fewer fetal bradycardias.[99] Paracervical block is a useful technique to provide analgesia for uterine curettage. The technique is very simple and involves a submucosal injection of local anesthetic at the vaginal fornix near the neural fibers innervating the uterus (Figure 41–6).

Paravertebral Lumbar Sympathetic Block

Paravertebral lumbar sympathetic block is a reasonable alternative to central neuraxial blockade. Lumbar sympathetic block effectively interrupts the painful transmission of cervical and uterine impulses during the first stage of labor.[100] Leighton et al. showed that women who received lumbar sympathetic blocks had a more rapid rate of cervical dilatation during the first two hours of analgesia and a shorter second stage of labor compared to epidural analgesia. However, there was no difference in the rate of dilatation during the active phase of labor.[100] Although there is less risk of fetal bradycardia with lumbar sympathetic block compared with paracervical blockade, technical difficulties associated with the performance of the block and risks of intravascular injection have hampered its routine use. Hypotension may also occur with lumbar sympathetic blocks.

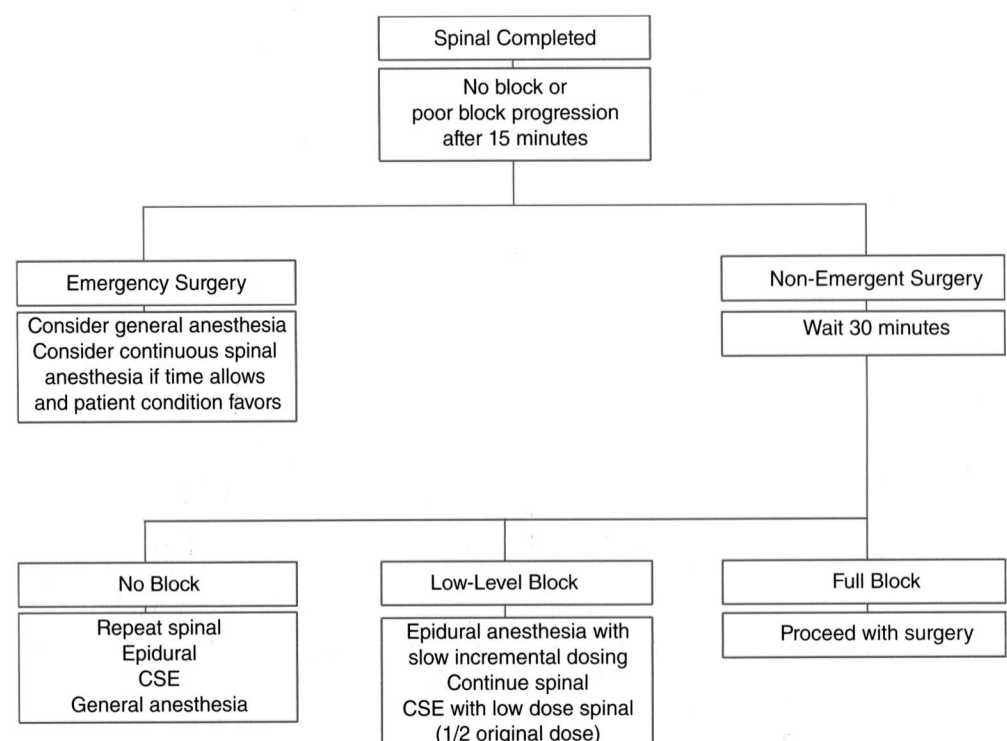

FIGURE 41–5. Management algorithm for an obstetric patient with inadequate neuraxial anesthesia. CSE, combined spinal–epidural.

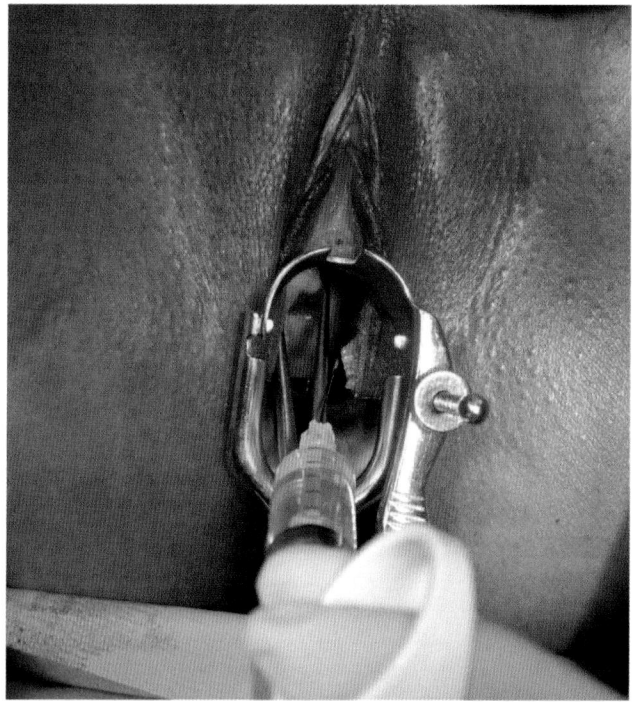

A

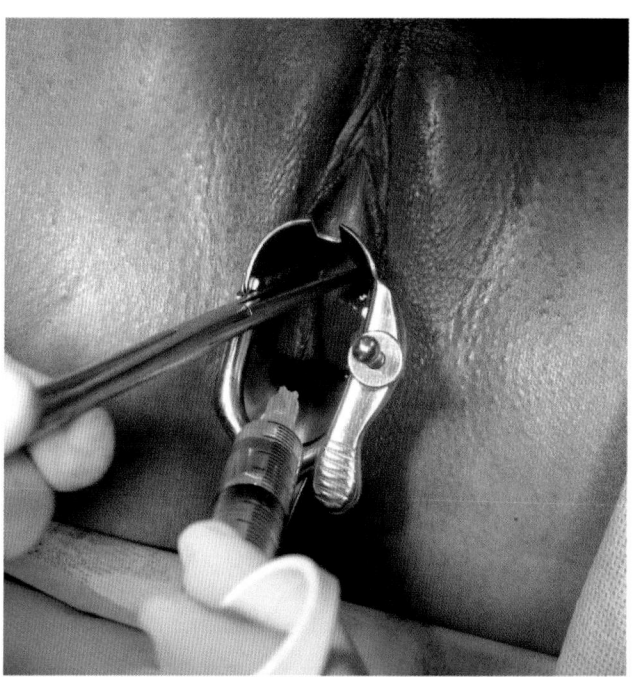

B

FIGURE 41–6. (a) and (b): Paracervical block for uterine curettage. The technique involves a submucosal injection of local anesthetic at the vaginal fornix, near the neural fibers innervating the uterus.

Pudendal Nerve Block

The pudendal nerves are derived from the lower sacral nerve roots (S2–4) and supply the vaginal vault, perineum, rectum, and sections of the bladder. The nerves are easily blocked transvaginally where they loop around the ischial spines.

A recent study demonstrated that a pudendal nerve block does not provide reliable analgesia for the second stage of labor, probably related to the upper vagina being innervated by lumbar, rather than sacral, fibers. However, the block is useful for episiotomy and repair.[101] There may also be postpartum benefits of pudendal nerve block. For instance, a unilateral nerve stimulator–guided pudendal nerve block with ropivacaine was associated with decreased pain and less need for supplemental analgesia during the first 48 hours after the performance of mediolateral episiotomy at vaginal delivery.[102]

ANESTHESIA FOR CESAREAN SECTION DELIVERY

The most common indications for cesarean section delivery include failure to progress, nonreassuring fetal status, cephalopelvic disproportion, malpresentation, prematurity, and prior uterine surgery involving the corpus. The choice of anesthesia should depend on the urgency of the procedure in addition to the condition of the mother and fetus. After a comprehensive discussion of the risks and benefits of all anesthesia options, the mother's desires should be considered. Before the initiation of any anesthetic technique, resuscitation equipment for mother and neonate should be made available (Table 41–2).

TABLE 41–2. Resuscitation equipment in the delivery room.

Radiant warmer

Suction with manometer and suction trap

Suction catheters

Wall oxygen with flow meter

Resuscitation bag-mask positive pressure ventilation device (≤ 750 mL)

Infant face masks

Infant oropharyngeal airways

Endotracheal tubes: 2.5, 3.0, 3.5, and 4.0 mm

Endotracheal tube stylets

Laryngoscope(s) and blade(s)

Sterile umbilical artery catheterization tray

Needles, syringes, three-way stopcocks

Medications and solutions:
- 1:10,000 epinephrine
- Naloxone hydrochloride
- Sodium bicarbonate
- Volume expanders

Advantages of Regional Anesthesia in the Obstetric Patient

Cesarean delivery accounts for more than 30% of all births and is the most common surgical procedure performed in the United States, with more than 1 million performed each year.[103] A 1992 survey of obstetric anesthesia practices in the United States demonstrated that most patients undergoing cesarean section delivery do so under spinal or epidural anesthesia.[104]

Regional techniques have several advantages: They reduce the risk of gastric aspiration, avoid the use of depressant anesthetic drugs, and allow the mother to remain awake during delivery. Operative blood loss may also be reduced with regional compared with general anesthesia. Generally speaking, with regional techniques, the duration of antepartum anesthesia does not affect neonatal outcome, provided that there is no protracted aortocaval compression or hypotension.[105] The risk of hypotension may be greater than during vaginal delivery because the sensory block must extend to at least the T4 dermatome.

Studies have shown preloading with crystalloid does not reliably prevent neuraxial anesthesia–induced hypotension. In fact, recent studies indicate that intravenous co-loading at the time of intrathecal injection is as effective as prehydrating before neuroblockade.[106] If hypotension occurs despite these measures, left uterine displacement should be increased, the rate of IV infusion augmented, and IV ephedrine 5–15 mg (or phenylephrine 25–50 mcg) administered incrementally. The greatest success in preventing hypotension has been found with a continuous low-dose infusion of phenylephrine until delivery.

Spinal Anesthesia

Subarachnoid block is probably the most commonly administered regional anesthetic for cesarean section delivery because of its speed of onset and reliability. It has also become an alternative to general anesthesia for emergency cesarean section.[107]

Hyperbaric solutions of lidocaine 5%, tetracaine 1.0%, or bupivacaine 0.75% have been used. However, bupivacaine has now become the most widely used drug for spinal anesthesia for cesarean delivery. Using 0.75% hyperbaric bupivacaine, Norris[109] has shown that it is not necessary to adjust the dose of drug based on the patient's height. In addition, the patient's age, weight, and vertebral column length do not affect the resulting neuraxial blockade.[109] Recent studies using spinal ropivacaine have shown less hypotension and faster recovery but a slower onset compared to bupivacaine.[110] However, it has been questioned whether ropivacaine produces spinal anesthesia of similar quality to that of bupivacaine. Hemodynamic monitoring during cesarean section should be similar to that used for other surgical procedures, with the exception that blood pressure should be monitored at a minimum of every 3 minutes before the birth of the baby. Before delivery, oxygen should be routinely administered to optimize fetal oxygenation. Reports of transient neurologic syndrome and/or cauda equina syndrome have been associated with lidocaine in doses greater than 60 mg, whether in a 5% or 2% preparation. This has led some clinicians to avoid the use of lidocaine for

TABLE 41–3. Local anesthetics commonly used for cesarean section delivery with subarachnoid block.

Dosage per Height of Patient (cm)	Bupivacaine 0.75% in 8.25% Dextrose (mg)	Bupivacaine 0.5% (Isobaric) (mg)
150–160 cm	8	8
160–180	10	10–12.5
> 180 cm	12	12.5–15
Onset of action	2–4 min	5–10 min

intrathecal administration (see "Systemic Toxicity of Local Anesthetics" below). Table 41–3 lists local anesthetics and the dosages commonly used for cesarean section delivery with subarachnoid block.

Despite an adequate dermatomal level, women may experience varying degrees of visceral discomfort, particularly during exteriorization of the uterus and traction on abdominal viscera. Improved perioperative analgesia can be provided by the addition of fentanyl 20 mcg or preservative-free morphine 0.1 mg to the local anesthetic solution.[111] Preservative-free morphine produces significant analgesia in doses ranging from 0.1 to 0.25 mg.[112] Higher doses of spinal morphine result in greater pruritus. Delayed respiratory depression can occur with spinal morphine but is extremely rare and more often associated with comorbid conditions such as obesity. The respiratory depression is due to the rostral spread of subarachnoid morphine. In a retrospective study of 1915 parturients receiving spinal morphine 0.15 mg for cesarean delivery, five patients (0.26%) experienced bradypnea, and one patient required naloxone.[113] In addition, spinal clonidine, in doses of 60 to 150 mcg, improves intraoperative analgesia and decreases shivering in women undergoing cesarean delivery.[114] However, hypotension and sedation have been reported with spinal clonidine and may limit its routine use. Nausea and vomiting may be alleviated by the administration of ondansetron or metoclopramide. Maternal sedation should be avoided if possible. If the initial block is not adequate, concern exists regarding a repeat spinal injection and the potential for inadvertent high spinal anesthetic. See Figure 41–5 for a range of options available in situations in which spinal anesthesia fails to prove adequate for surgery.

Clinical Pearls

- Even with an adequate dermatomal level for surgery, women undergoing cesarean section may experience discomfort, particularly during exteriorization of the uterus and traction on abdominal viscera.
- Perioperative analgesia may be enhanced by the addition of fentanyl 20 mcg or preservative-free morphine 0.1 mg to the local anesthetic solution.

Lumbar Epidural Anesthesia

Epidural anesthesia has a slower onset of action and a larger drug requirement to establish an adequate sensory block compared with spinal anesthesia. The advantages are a perceived reduced risk of postdural puncture headache and the ability to titrate the local anesthetic through the epidural catheter. However, correct placement of the epidural catheter and avoidance of inadvertent intrathecal or intravascular injection are essential.

Aspiration of the epidural catheter for blood or cerebrospinal fluid is not 100% reliable for detecting catheter misplacement. For this reason, a "test dose" is often used to rule out inadvertent intravascular or intrathecal catheter placement. A small dose of local anesthetic, lidocaine 45 mg or bupivacaine 5 mg, produces a readily identifiable sensory and motor block if injected intrathecally. However, a recent study has suggested that ropivacaine 15 mg was not a useful intrathecal test dose because a slow onset of motor blockade may preclude the timely diagnosis of intrathecal injection.[115] The addition of epinephrine 15 mcg with careful continuous heart rate and blood pressure monitoring may herald intravascular injection with a transient increase in heart rate and blood pressure. However, an epinephrine test dose is not reliable because false-positive results do occur in the form of tachycardia related to painful uterine contractions. In addition, epinephrine may potentially reduce uteroplacental perfusion in some patients. Electrocardiography and the application of a peak-to-peak heart rate criterion may improve detection (10 beats over maximum heart rate preceding epinephrine injection). Rapid injection of 1 mL of air with simultaneous precordial Doppler monitoring appears to be a reliable indicator of intravascular catheter placement.[116] Most important, a negative test, although reassuring, does not eliminate the need for the fractional administration of local anesthetic.

Clinical Pearls

- Aspiration of the epidural catheter for blood or cerebrospinal fluid is not absolutely reliable for detecting catheter misplacement.
- A "test dose" is often used to rule out inadvertent intravascular or intrathecal catheter placement.
- A small dose of local anesthetic, lidocaine 45 mg or bupivacaine 5 mg, produces a readily identifiable sensory and motor block if injected intrathecally.
- The addition of epinephrine 15 mcg with careful hemodynamic monitoring may signal intravascular injection when followed by a transient increase in heart rate and blood pressure.
- However, the use of an epinephrine test dose is controversial because false-positive results do occur in the presence of uterine contractions.

Local Anesthetic Choices

The most commonly used local anesthetic agents are 2-chloroprocaine 3%, bupivacaine 0.5%, and lidocaine 2% with epinephrine 1:200,000.

Adequate anesthesia can be usually achieved with 15–25 mL of local anesthetic given in divided doses. The patient should be monitored as with spinal anesthesia. Because of its extremely high rate of metabolism in maternal and fetal plasma, 2-chloroprocaine provides a rapid-onset, reliable block with minimal risk of systemic toxicity.[34] It is the local anesthetic of choice in the presence of fetal acidosis and when a preexisting epidural block is to be rapidly extended for an urgent cesarean section delivery.[107] Neurologic deficits after massive inadvertent intrathecal administration of the drug have occurred with the formulation containing a relatively high concentration of sodium bisulfite at a low pH.[117]

In a new formulation of 2-chloroprocaine (Nesacaine-MPF), ethylenediaminetetraacetic acid (EDTA) has been substituted for sodium bisulfite. However, severe spasmodic back pain has been described after epidural injection of large volumes of Nesacaine-MPF in surgical patients, but not in parturients.[118] This has been attributed to an EDTA-induced leaching of calcium from paravertebral muscles. The most recent formulation of 2-chloroprocaine contains no additives and is packaged in an amber vial to prevent oxidation.

Bupivacaine 0.5% provides profound anesthesia of slower onset for cesarean section delivery but of longer duration of action. Considerable attention has been focused on the drug because it was reported that unintentional intravascular injection could result not only in convulsions but also in almost simultaneous cardiac arrest, with patients often refractory to resuscitation.[119] The greater cardiotoxicity of bupivacaine (and etidocaine) compared with other amide local anesthetics has been well established.

When using potent long-acting amide local anesthetics, fractioning the induction dose is critical. Lidocaine has an onset and duration intermediate to those of 2-chloroprocaine and bupivacaine. The need to include epinephrine in the local anesthetic solution to ensure adequate lumbosacral anesthesia limits the use of lidocaine in women with maternal hypertension and uteroplacental insufficiency.

Prolonged postoperative pain relief can be provided by the epidural administration of an opioid, such as morphine 4 mg, or the use of PCEA. Delayed respiratory depression may occur with the use of morphine; hence, the patient must be monitored carefully in the postoperative period. Recently, a lipid-encapsulated preparation of morphine (DepoDur) has been approved for post–cesarean section delivery analgesia. It can be used only epidurally, can last up to 48 hours, and the patient must be monitored for delayed respiratory depression. A potential limitation in obstetrics is that once the drug is administered, additional local anesthetic cannot be injected epidurally for a period of up to one hour since the local anesthetic may cause an uncontrolled release of morphine from the lipid. Carvalho et al.[120] evaluated the epidural administration of 5, 10, and 15 mg of extended-release morphine for post–cesarean section analgesia and demonstrated that the 10 mg and 15 mg doses provided good analgesia for up to 48 hours after surgery. No significant side effects were observed. Another study showed lower pain scores and fewer supplemental analgesia requirements for patients receiving extended-release morphine compared to preservative-free morphine.[121] No differences in nausea, pruritus, or sedation scores were observed. In addition, the bolus administration of epidural fentanyl (50–100 mcg) has been found to result in activity at both spinal and supraspinal sites of action and to improve the quality of anesthesia.[122]

ANESTHETIC COMPLICATIONS

Maternal Mortality

A study of anesthesia-related deaths in the United States between 1979 and 1990 showed that the case fatality rate with general anesthesia was 16.7 times greater than that with regional anesthesia. Most anesthesia-related deaths were a result of cardiac arrest due to hypoxemia when difficulties securing the airway were encountered.[104] Pregnancy-induced anatomical and physiological changes, such as reduced FRC, increased oxygen consumption, and oropharyngeal edema may expose the patient to serious risks of desaturation during periods of apnea and hypoventilation.

Pulmonary Aspiration

The risk of the inhalation of gastric contents is increased in pregnant women, particularly if difficulty is encountered establishing an airway or if airway reflexes are obtunded. Measures to decrease the risks of aspiration include comprehensive airway evaluation, prophylactic administration of nonparticulate antacids, and the preferred use of regional anesthesia. If aspiration occurs, management includes immediate treatment of hypoxemia with continuous positive airway pressure (CPAP) and possible rigid bronchoscopy. Recent studies do not support the administration of corticosteroids or lung lavage with saline and bicarbonate to neutralize acidity.[123] Prophylactic antibiotics are not recommended because gastric contents are sterile.

Hypotension

Regional anesthesia may be associated with hypotension, which is related to the degree and rapidity of local anesthetic–induced sympatholysis. Thus, greater hemodynamic stability may be observed with epidural anesthesia, where gradual titration of local anesthetic allows for better control of the block level as well as for adequate time for vasopressor administration in anticipation of blood pressure reduction.

The risk of hypotension is lower in laboring women compared with nonlaboring women.[128] Maternal prehydration with 15 mL/kg of lactated Ringer's solution before the initiation of regional anesthesia and the avoidance of aortocaval compression may decrease the incidence of hypotension. It has been demonstrated that for effective prevention of hypotension, the blood volume increase from preloading must be sufficient to result in a significant increase in cardiac output.[125] This was possible only with the administration of hetastarch 0.5–1 L.[125] Nonetheless, controversy exists regarding the efficacy of volume loading in the prevention of hypotension.[104,126] A recent study using a prophylactic phenylephrine infusion combined with a rapid

crystalloid co-loading given at the time of intrathecal injection markedly reduced the incidence of spinal anesthesia–induced hypotension.[127] If hypotension does occur despite prehydration, therapeutic measures should include increasing the displacement of the uterus, rapid infusion of IV fluids, titration of IV ephedrine (5–10 mg), and oxygen administration. In the presence of maternal tachycardia, phenylephrine 25–50 mcg may be substituted for ephedrine in women with normal uteroplacental function. Continued vigilance and active management of hypotension can prevent serious sequelae in both mother and neonate.[124,128]

High Spinal Anesthesia

High, or total, spinal anesthesia is a rare complication of intrathecal injection in modern-day practice. It occurs with an excessive cephalad spread of local anesthetic in the subarachnoid space. Unintentional intrathecal administration of epidural medication as a result of dural puncture or catheter migration may also result in this complication. Left uterine displacement and continued fluid and vasopressor administration may be necessary to achieve hemodynamic stability. The reverse Trendelenburg position does not prevent cephalad spread and may cause cardiovascular collapse because of venous pooling related to sympathectomy. Rapid control of the airway is essential, and endotracheal intubation may be necessary to ensure oxygenation without aspiration.

Clinical Pearls

- Obstetric patients often complain of difficulty breathing during cesarean section delivery under neuraxial anesthesia.
- Although most common reasons are inability to feel "breathing" as the abdominal and thoracic segments are anesthetized (including the stretch receptors), practitioners must rule out an impending "high spinal" anesthetic by repetitive examinations.
- The following maneuvers are useful to rule out the possibility of high neuraxial anesthesia:
  - The ability of the patient to phonate
  - The ability of the patient to squeeze the practitioner's hand (indicates that the block level is below the level of the brachial plexus (C6–T1)

Systemic Toxicity of Local Anesthetics

Unintended intravascular injection or drug accumulation after repeated epidural injection can result in high serum levels of local anesthetic. Rapid absorption of local anesthetic from highly vascular sites of injection may also occur after paracervical and pudendal blocks.

Resuscitation equipment should always be available when any major nerve block is undertaken. IV access, airway equipment, emergency drugs, and suction equipment should be immediately accessible. To avoid systemic toxicity of local anesthetic agents, strict adherence to recommended dosages and

Obstetric Regional Anesthesia **787**

CHAPTER 41

avoidance of unintentional intravascular injection are essential.

Despite these precautions, life-threatening convulsions and, more rarely, cardiovascular collapse may occur. Seizure activity has been treated with IV thiopental 25–50 mg or diazepam 5–10 mg. In current clinical practice, propofol 20–50 mg or midazolam 2–4 mg is more commonly used.

The airway should be evaluated and oxygenation maintained. If cardiovascular collapse does occur, the Advanced Cardiac Life Support (ACLS) algorithm should be followed. In a 2006 case report, lipid emulsion was used to treat refractory cardiac arrest resulting from bupivacaine toxicity.[129] The mechanism of action is unclear but may result from the greater affinity of bupivacaine for the lipid or because the lipid provides a substrate for a bupivacaine-poisoned mitochondrial energy system. Further study is required to determine the efficacy of this treatment. However, it would seem prudent that treatment of a pregnant woman intoxicated with bupivacaine should include the administration of lipid emulsion early on in the resuscitation. The current recommended protocol for lipid rescue (see http://www.lipidrescue.org) involves a 20% lipid emulsion: a 1.5 mL/kg initial bolus, followed by 0.25 mL/kg/min for 30–60 minutes. The early administration of lipid has also been shown to prevent progression to cardiac arrest when bupivacaine was injected intravascularly.

Whenever there is maternal cardiac arrest, regardless of cause, the fetus should be delivered early on, usually within 5 minutes, if attempts at resuscitation are unsuccessful in relieving aortocaval compression and ensuring the efficiency of cardiac massage.[130]

Postdural Puncture Headache

Pregnant women have a higher risk of developing a postdural puncture headache (PDPH) should an inadvertent dural puncture occur. In a recent meta-analysis, the risk of PDPH was 52.1% (95% confidence interval [CI], 51.4–52.8%) after an accidental dural puncture with an epidural needle.[131] The reduced epidural pressure increases the risk of cerebrospinal fluid leakage through the dural opening. Russell et al. reported that the placement of an intrathecal catheter after an accidental dural puncture did not lower the incidence of headache or the need for blood patch compared to repeating an epidural.[132] The incidence of headache was higher with the use of a 16-gauge compared to an 18-gauge epidural needle. The pathophysiology and management of postdural puncture headache are discussed in greater detail in Chapter 27.

Neurologic Complications

Neurologic sequelae of central neuraxial blockade, although rare, have been reported. Pressure exerted by a needle or catheter on spinal nerve roots produces immediate pain and necessitates repositioning. Infections such as epidural abscess and meningitis are very rare and may be a manifestation of systemic sepsis. In recent years, several cases of epidural

abscess have been reported after epidural catheterization in obstetric patients.[133] Potential risk factors identified from these cases are entry-point infections from usual causative organisms (eg, *Staphylococcus aureus*), possible systemic sources of infection, poor aseptic technique, and prolonged catheterization. Epidural hematoma can also occur, usually in association with coagulation defects. However, epidural hematoma may also occur spontaneously, unrelated to instrumentation.[134] The pathogenesis may be due to a weakened epidural vascular architecture. Nerve root irritation may have a protracted recovery, lasting weeks or months. Peripheral nerve injury as a result of instrumentation, lithotomy position, or compression by the fetal head may occur even in the absence of neuraxial technique.

REGIONAL ANESTHESIA IN COMPLICATED PREGNANCY

Pregnancy and parturition are considered high risk when accompanied by conditions unfavorable to the well-being of the mother or fetus, or both. Maternal problems may be related to the pregnancy; that is, preeclampsia-eclampsia, hypertensive disorders of pregnancy, or antepartum hemorrhage resulting from placenta previa or abruptio placentae. Diabetes mellitus; cardiac, chronic renal, and neurologic problems; sickle cell disease; asthma; obesity; and drug abuse are not related to pregnancy but often are affected by it. Prematurity (gestation of less than 37 weeks), postmaturity (gestation of 42 weeks or longer), intrauterine growth retardation, and multiple gestation are fetal conditions associated with risk. During labor and delivery, fetal malpresentation (eg, breech, transverse lie), placental abruption, compression of the umbilical cord (eg, prolapse, nuchal cord), precipitous labor, or intrauterine infection (eg, prolonged rupture of membranes) may increase the risk to the mother or fetus.

In general, the anesthetic management of the high-risk parturient is based on the same maternal and fetal considerations as for the management of healthy mothers and fetuses. However, there is less room for error because many of these functions may be compromised before the induction of anesthesia.

Preeclampsia-Eclampsia
Pathophysiology and Signs and Symptoms

Hypertensive disorders occur in approximately 7% of all pregnancies and are a major cause of maternal mortality. The most recent diagnostic criterion for preeclampsia is referred to as "proteinaceous increase in blood pressure."[135] The presence or absence of edema is no longer considered one of the required criteria. Rather than a specific blood pressure elevation, a blood pressure that is consistently 15% above baseline is now considered diagnostic. The added appearance of convulsions is diagnostic for eclampsia.[94] Preeclampsia-eclampsia is a disease unique to humans, occurring predominantly in young nulliparous women. Symptoms usually appear after the twentieth week of gestation, occasionally earlier with a hydatidiform mole. Delivery of the infant and placenta is the only effective treatment; as a result, preeclampsia is a leading cause of iatrogenic preterm delivery in developed countries.[136]

The origin of preeclampsia-eclampsia is unknown, but all patients manifest placental ischemia. Decreased placental perfusion occurs in early pregnancy in women destined to become preeclamptic, and there is a failure of the normal trophoblastic invasion.[137] In normal pregnancy, the diameter of spiral arteries increase approximately four-fold to create flaccid tubes that provide a low-resistance pathway to the intervillous space.[138] This angiogenesis is a result of the trophoblast invasion into the decidual and myometrial segments of the spiral arteries. However, in preeclamptic women, the myometrium is not invaded. This causes superficial placental implantation, resulting in decreased placental perfusion and ischemia related to stiff, muscular spiral arteries. Placental ischemia results in a release of uterine renin, an increase in angiotensin activity, and a widespread arteriolar vasoconstriction causing hypertension, tissue hypoxia, and endothelial damage (Figure 41–7). The fixation of platelets at sites of endothelial damage results in coagulopathies, occasionally in disseminated intravascular coagulation. Enhanced angiotensin-mediated aldosterone secretion leads to increased sodium reabsorption and edema. Proteinuria, a sign of preeclampsia, is also attributed to placental ischemia, which leads to local tissue degeneration and a release of thromboplastin with subsequent deposition of fibrin in constricted glomerular vessels. As a result, an increased permeability to albumin and other plasma proteins occurs. Furthermore, there is a decreased production of prostaglandin E, a potent vasodilator secreted in the trophoblast, which normally balances the hypertensive effects of the rennin–angiotensin system.

Many of the symptoms associated with preeclampsia, including placental ischemia, systemic vasoconstriction, and increased platelet aggregation, may result from an imbalance between the placental production of prostacyclin and thromboxane. During normal pregnancy, the placenta produces equal amounts of the two, but in a preeclamptic pregnancy, there is seven times more thromboxane than prostacyclin.[139]

According to the latest theory, endothelial cell injury is central to the development of preeclampsia.[140] This injury occurs as a result of reduced placental perfusion, leading to a production and release of substances (possibly lipid peroxidases) causing endothelial cell injury. Abnormal endothelial cell function contributes to an increase in peripheral resistance and other abnormalities noted in preeclampsia through a release of fibronectin, endothelin, and other substances.

In rodent models, two placental antiangiogenic proteins have been identified and likely play a role in the pathogenesis of preeclampsia.[133] Soluble fms-like tyrosine kinase-1 (sFlt-1) is upregulated in the placenta of preeclamptic women. The elevated sFlt-1 protein levels antagonize and reduce vascular endothelial growth factor (VEGF) and placental growth factor (PlGF).[141] Levine et al. demonstrated that increased sFlt-1 levels and reduced PlGF levels predicted the subsequent development of preeclampsia.[142] Another antiangiogenic protein, soluble endoglin (sEng), is elevated in cases of HELLP syndrome (which consists of hemolysis, elevated liver enzymes, and low platelet count).

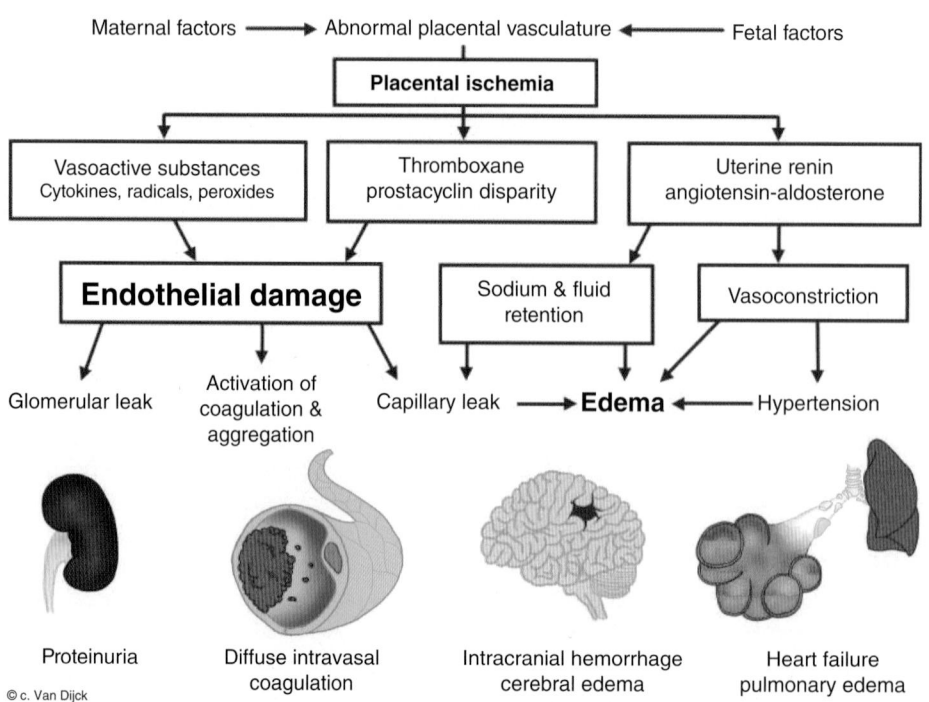

FIGURE 41–7. Pathophysiology of preeclampsia and eclampsia.

In severe preeclampsia-eclampsia, all major organ systems are affected because of widespread vasospasm. Global cerebral blood flow is not diminished, but focal hypoperfusion cannot be ruled out. Postmortem examination has revealed hemorrhagic necrosis in the proximity of thrombosed precapillaries, suggesting intense vasoconstriction. Edema and small foci of degeneration have been attributed to hypoxia. Petechial hemorrhages are common after the onset of convulsions. Symptoms related to the above changes include headache, vertigo, cortical blindness, hyperreflexia, and convulsions. Cerebral hemorrhage and edema are the leading causes of death in preeclampsia-eclampsia, which together account for approximately 50% of deaths. Heart failure may occur in severe cases as a result of peripheral vasoconstriction and increased blood viscosity from hemoconcentration. Decreased blood supply to the liver may lead to periportal necrosis of variable extent and severity. Subcapsular hemorrhages account for the epigastric pain encountered in severe cases.

In the kidneys, there is swelling of glomerular endothelial cells and deposition of fibrin, leading to a constriction of the capillary lumina. Renal blood flow and glomerular filtration rate decrease, resulting in reduced uric acid clearance and, in severe cases, increase in creatinine.[143]

Although preeclampsia is accompanied by exaggerated retention of water and sodium, the shift of fluid and proteins from the intravascular into the extravascular compartment may result in hypovolemia, hypoproteinemia, and hemoconcentration, which may be further aggravated by proteinuria. The risk of uteroplacental hypoperfusion and poor fetal outcome correlates with the degree of maternal plasma and protein depletion.

Platelet adherence at sites of endothelial damage may result in consumption coagulopathy, which develops in approximately 20% of patients with preeclampsia. Mild thrombocytopenia, with a platelet count of 100,000–150,000/mm, is the most common finding. The prolongation of prothrombin and partial thromboplastin times indicates a consumption of procoagulants. Bleeding time, prolonged in approximately 25% of patients with normal platelet counts, is no longer considered a reliable test of clotting.[144] The HELLP syndrome is a particular form of severe preeclampsia characterized by hemolysis, elevated liver enzymes, and low platelets.

The goals of the management of the patient with preeclampsia-eclampsia are to prevent or control convulsions, improve organ perfusion, normalize blood pressure, and correct clotting abnormalities. The mainstay of anticonvulsant therapy in the United States is magnesium sulfate. Its efficacy in preventing seizures has been well substantiated, but its mechanism of action remains controversial. The patient usually receives a loading dose of 4 g in a 20% solution, administered over 5 minutes, followed by a continuous infusion of 1–2 g/h.

Antihypertensive therapy in preeclampsia is used to lessen the risk of cerebral hemorrhage in the mother while maintaining, or even improving, tissue perfusion. There is no evidence to suggest that antihypertensive therapy delays disease progression or improves perinatal outcome.[145] Plasma volume expansion combined with vasodilation fulfills these goals.[146] Hydralazine is the most commonly used vasodilator because it increases uteroplacental and renal blood flows. However, side effects include tachycardia, palpitations, headache, and neonatal thrombocytopenia.[147] Nitroprusside is used during laryngoscopy and intubation to prevent dangerous elevations in blood pressure. Trimethaphan, a ganglion blocking agent, is useful in hypertensive emergencies when cerebral edema and increased intracranial pressure are a concern because it does not cause vasodilation in the brain. Other agents that have been used to control maternal blood pressure include α-methyldopa, nitroglycerine, and, now more frequently, labetalol.[148]

Consumption coagulopathy may require infusion of fresh whole blood, platelet concentrates, fresh frozen plasma, and cryoprecipitate. Delivery is indicated in refractory cases or if the pregnancy is close to term. In severe cases, aggressive management should continue for at least 24–48 hours after delivery.

Anesthesia Management

There are very few contraindications for epidural anesthesia in labor and delivery. In the presence of severe clotting abnormalities or severe plasma volume deficit, the risk–benefit ratio favors other forms of anesthesia.[149] In volume-depleted patients positioned with left uterine displacement, epidural anesthesia does not cause an unacceptable reduction in blood pressure and leads to a significant improvement in placental perfusion.[150] With the use of radioactive xenon, it was shown that the intervillous blood flow increased by approximately 75% after the induction of epidural analgesia (10 mL bupivacaine 0.25%).[151] The total maternal body clearance of amide local anesthetics is prolonged in preeclampsia, and repeated administration of these drugs can lead to higher blood concentrations than in normotensive patients.[152]

For cesarean section delivery, the sensory level of regional anesthesia must extend to T3–4, making adequate fluid therapy and left uterine displacement even more vital.

Epidural anesthesia has been preferred to spinal anesthesia in preeclamptic women because of its slower onset of action and controllability. In the past, the rapid onset of sympathectomy related to spinal anesthesia was associated with hypotension, particularly in volume-depleted patients. However, in two recent studies, the incidence of hypotension, perioperative fluid and ephedrine administration, and neonatal conditions were found to be similar in preeclamptic women who received either epidural or spinal anesthesia for cesarean delivery.[153,154] Aya et al. conducted a prospective cohort study that showed the risk of significant spinal anesthesia–induced hypotension was significantly lower in preeclamptic women compared to normotensive pregnant women.[147] There is an increased sensitivity to vasopressors in preeclampsia; therefore, lower doses of ephedrine and phenylephrine are usually required to correct hypotension.

Antepartum Hemorrhage

Antepartum hemorrhage occurs most commonly in association with placenta previa (abnormal placental implantation on the lower uterine segment and partial to total occlusion of the internal cervical os) and abruptio placentae. Placenta previa occurs in 0.11% of all pregnancies, resulting in up to a 0.9% incidence of maternal and a 17–26% incidence of perinatal mortality. It may be associated with abnormal fetal presentation, such as transverse lie or breech. Placenta previa should be suspected whenever a patient presents with painless, bright red vaginal bleeding, usually after the seventh month of pregnancy. The diagnosis is confirmed by ultrasonography. Unless the lowest placental edge is more than 2 cm from the internal cervical os, an abdominal delivery is usually required.[155] If the bleeding is not profuse and the fetus is immature, obstetric management is conservative to prolong the pregnancy. In severe cases or if the fetus is mature at the onset of symptoms, prompt delivery is indicated, usually by cesarean section. An emergency hysterectomy may be required because of severe hemorrhage, even after the delivery of the placenta, because of uterine atony. In patients who have undergone prior uterine surgery, particularly prior cesarean delivery, the risk of severe hemorrhage is even greater, owing to a higher incidence of placenta accreta (penetration of the myometrium by placental villi).

Abruptio placentae occurs in 0.2–2.4% of pregnant women, usually in the final 10 weeks of gestation and in association with hypertensive diseases. Complications include Couvelaire uterus (which occurs when extravasated blood dissects between the myometrial fibers), renal failure, disseminated intravascular coagulation, and anterior pituitary necrosis (ie, Sheehan syndrome). The maternal mortality is high (1.8–11.0%), and the perinatal mortality rate is even higher (in excess of 50%). The diagnosis of abruptio placentae is based on the presence of uterine tenderness, hypertonus, and vaginal bleeding of dark, clotted blood. Bleeding may be concealed if the placental margins have remained attached to the uterine wall. Changes in maternal blood pressure and pulse rate, indicative of hypovolemia, may occur if the blood loss is severe. Fetal movements may increase during acute hypoxia and decrease if hypoxia is gradual. Fetal bradycardia and death may ensue.

Anesthesia Management

The establishment of invasive monitoring (arterial line, central venous catheter) and blood volume replacement via a 14- or 16-gauge catheter is usually required. If clotting abnormalities exist, blood components and fresh frozen plasma,

cryoprecipitate, and platelet concentrates may be required. The choice of anesthetic for a woman with placental abruption depends on maternal and fetal condition and how urgently the procedure needs to be performed. General anesthesia is indicated in the presence of uncontrolled hemorrhage and coagulation abnormalities.[106,156]

Epidural anesthesia may be used, particularly if there is a functioning epidural in place during labor at the time of abruption and there is no hemodynamic instability. Vincent et al. observed that epidural anesthesia significantly worsened maternal hypotension, uterine blood flow, and fetal PaO_2 and pH during untreated hemorrhage in gravid ewes.[157] However, this was uncorrected hypotension, which, with intravascular fluid replacement hemodynamics, returned to normal even with epidural anesthesia.

Preterm Delivery

Preterm labor and delivery present a significant challenge to the anesthesiologist because both the mother and the infant may be at risk. The definition of prematurity was altered to distinguish between the preterm infant, born before the thirty-seventh week of gestation, and the small-for-gestational-age infant, who may be born at term but whose weight is more than 2 standard deviations below the mean. Although preterm delivery occurs in 8–10% of all births, it accounts for approximately 80% of early neonatal deaths. Severe complications, such as respiratory distress syndrome, intracranial hemorrhage, hypoglycemia, hypocalcemia, and hyperbilirubinemia, are prone to develop in preterm infants.

Obstetricians frequently try to inhibit preterm labor to obtain time for fetal lung maturity. Delaying delivery by even 24–48 hours may be beneficial if glucocorticoids are administered to the mother to enhance fetal lung maturity. Various agents have been used to suppress uterine activity (tocolysis), such as ethanol, magnesium sulfate, prostaglandin inhibitors, β-sympathomimetics, and calcium channel blockers. β-adrenergic drugs, such as ritodrine and terbutaline, are the most commonly used tocolytics. Their predominant effect is β2 receptor stimulation, which results in myometrial inhibition, vasodilation, and bronchodilation. Numerous maternal complications, including hypotension, hypokalemia, hyperglycemia, myocardial ischemia, pulmonary edema, and death, have been reported as a result of these tocolytics.

Anesthesia Management

Complications may occur because of interactions with anesthetic drugs and techniques. With the use of regional anesthesia, peripheral vasodilation caused by β-adrenergic stimulation increases the risk of hemodynamic instability in the presence of preexisting tachycardia, hypotension, and hypokalemia. The premature infant is known to be more vulnerable than the term newborn to the effects of drugs used in obstetric analgesia and anesthesia. However, there have been few systemic studies to determine the maternal and fetal pharmacokinetics and dynamics of drugs throughout gestation.

There are several postulated causes of enhanced drug sensitivity in the preterm newborn: less protein available for drug binding; higher levels of bilirubin, which may compete with the drug for protein binding; greater drug access to the central nervous system because of a poorly developed blood–brain barrier; greater total body water and lower fat content; and a decreased ability to metabolize and excrete drugs. However, most drugs used in anesthesia exhibit low to moderate degrees of binding in the fetal serum: approximately 50% for bupivacaine, 25% for lidocaine, 52% for meperidine, and 75% for thiopental.

In selecting the anesthetic drugs and techniques for delivering a preterm infant, concerns regarding drug effects on the newborn are far less important than preventing asphyxia and trauma to the fetus. For vaginal delivery, well-conducted epidural anesthesia is advantageous in providing good perineal relaxation. Before induction of epidural blockade, the anesthesiologist should ascertain that the fetus is neither hypoxic nor acidotic. Asphyxia results in a redistribution of fetal cardiac output, which increases oxygen delivery to vital organs such as the brain, heart, and adrenals. Regardless, these changes in the preterm fetus may be better preserved with bupivacaine or chloroprocaine than with lidocaine.[158,159] Preterm infants with breech presentation are usually delivered by cesarean section. Regional anesthesia can be successfully used, with nitroglycerin available for uterine relaxation if needed.

Clinical Pearls

- When delivering a preterm infant, concerns about drug effects on the newborn are far less important than preventing asphyxia and trauma to the fetus.
- Before inducing epidural blockade, it should be ascertained that the fetus is neither hypoxic nor acidotic.

Regional analgesia during labor and vaginal delivery has become the preferred technique of pain relief in selected high-risk patients because it prevents obtundation of the mother and depression of the fetus and reduces many of the potential adverse physiologic effects of labor, such as increased oxygen consumption and hemodynamic alterations. For cesarean section delivery, regional anesthesia has emerged as a safe and effective technique in high-risk parturients, partly because of the added ability to provide prolonged postoperative analgesia.

NONOBSTETRIC SURGERY IN THE PREGNANT WOMAN

Approximately 1.6–2.2% of pregnant women undergo surgery for reasons unrelated to parturition. Apart from trauma, the most common emergencies are abdominal, intracranial aneurysms, cardiac valvular disease, and pheochromocytoma.

When the necessity for surgery arises, anesthetic considerations are related to the alterations in maternal physiologic condition with advancing pregnancy, the teratogenicity of anesthetic drugs, the indirect effects of anesthesia on

uteroplacental blood flow, and the potential for abortion or premature delivery. The risks must be balanced to provide the most favorable outcome for mother and child.

Five major studies have attempted to relate surgery and anesthesia during human pregnancy to fetal outcome as determined by anomalies, premature labor, or intrauterine death.[160–162] Although these studies failed to correlate surgery and anesthetic exposure with congenital anomalies, all studies demonstrated an increased incidence of fetal death, particularly after operations performed in the first trimester. No particular anesthetic agent or technique was implicated. The condition that necessitated surgery was the most relevant factor, with fetal mortality greatest following pelvic surgery or procedures performed for obstetric indications; that is, cervical incompetence.

The cytotoxicity of anesthetic agents is closely associated with biodegradation, which, in turn, is influenced by oxygenation and hepatic blood flow. Thus, the complications associated with anesthesia—maternal hypoxia, hypotension, vasopressor administration, hypercarbia, hypocarbia, and electrolyte disturbances—may be greater factors in teratogenesis than the use of the agents themselves.[163–165]

The experimental evidence on exposure to specific drugs and agents is discussed briefly, with the understanding that it is difficult to extrapolate laboratory data to the clinical situation in humans. Very large numbers of patients must be exposed to a suspected teratogen before its safety can be ascertained. Complicating factors include the frequency of maternal exposure to a multiplicity of drugs; the difficulty in separating the effects of the underlying disease process and surgical treatment from those of the drug administered; differing degrees of risk with stage of gestation; and the variety, rather than the consistency, of anomalies that appear in association with one agent. With regard to regional anesthetic agents, local anesthetics have not been shown to be teratogenic in animals or humans.

Caution has been exercised with sedatives before block placement because of several reports describing a specific relationship between diazepam and oral clefts; however, other studies have not confirmed this.[166,167] A prospective study of 854 women who ingested diazepam during the first trimester did not demonstrate a higher risk of cleft palate or cleft lip.[168] Currently, diazepam is not a proven teratogen.[169]

Recently, there has been concern relating to adverse neurocognitive effects in children exposed to anesthetics during fetal life. Indeed, neonatal rats exposed to in utero general anesthesia had a greater degree of neuroadaptive deficits than a control group.[170] Similarly, infants born under general anesthesia for cesarean delivery have also been found to display mild impairment of cognition compared to regional anesthesia.[171] The difficulty with this study is that it was retrospective in nature, and the potential for patient selection bias existed. For instance, the use of general anesthesia is reserved for emergency situations, such as nonreassuring fetal status or placental abruption, which, in our opinion, would affect neurocognition more than the anesthetic. Most worrisome is that infants born via vaginal delivery had similar profiles as children born by cesarean delivery with general anesthesia. Nonetheless, it would seem prudent to avoid general anesthesia in preference for regional techniques during pregnancy because of the maternal and fetal considerations previously discussed. There are few data to guide medical decision making, but altering the type of surgical technique (eg, converting from laparoscopic to open appendectomy) should be entertained in order to facilitate the use of regional anesthesia.[170,171] As maternal pain and apprehension may result in decreased uterine blood flow and deterioration of the fetus (similar to infusions of epinephrine or norepinephrine), early intervention to relieve postoperative pain with regional techniques (ie, peripheral nerve block or epidural infusion) should be considered.[172]

Clinical Pearl

- Local anesthetics have not been shown to be teratogenic in animals or humans.

SUMMARY

Pregnancy results in a number of significant physiologic changes that require adjustment in anesthesia and analgesia techniques for the safe and effective management of the pregnant patient. It is prudent to delay surgery, when possible, until after the birth of the infant. Only emergency surgery should be considered during the first trimester.

Regional techniques have become the most accepted for pain relief during labor and vaginal delivery. Likewise, neuraxial techniques are now the most frequently used techniques to administer anesthetics for cesarean section delivery. Advances in regional anesthesia and its widespread routine use have resulted in significantly enhanced maternal safety compared with that of general anesthesia.

REFERENCES

1. Melzack R, Taenzer P, Feldman P, Kinch RA: Labour is still painful after prepared childbirth training. Can Med Assoc J 1981;125:357.
2. Goodman RP, Killom AP, Brash AR, Branch RA: Prostacyclin production during pregnancy: comparison of production during normal pregnancy and pregnancy complicated by hypertension. Am J Obstet Gynecol 1982; 142:817.
3. Kerr MG, Scott DB, Samuel E: Studies of the inferior vena cava in late pregnancy. BMJ 1964;1:532.
4. Howard BK, Goodson JH, Mengert WE: Supine hypotensive syndrome in late pregnancy. Obstet Gynecol 1953;1:371.
5. Kuo CD, Chen GY, Yang MJ, Tsai YS: The effect of postion on autonomic nervous activity in late pregnancy. Anaesthesia 1997;52:1161–1165.
6. Kundra P, Velraj J, Amirthalingam U, et al: Effect of positioning from supine and left lateral positions to left lateral tilt on maternal blood flow velocities and waveforms in full-term parturients. Anaesthesia 2012;67: 889–893.
7. Carruth JE, Mivis SB, Brogan DR, Wenger NK: The electrocardiogram in normal pregnancy. Am Heart J 1981;102:1075–1078.
8. Seth R, Moss AJ, McNitt S, et al: Long QT syndrome and pregnancy. J Am Coll Cardiol 2007;49:1092–1098.
9. Prowse CM, Gaensler EA: Respiratory and acid-base changes during pregnancy. Anesthesiology 1965;26:381.
10. Moya F, Smith BE: Uptake, distribution and placental transport of drugs and anesthetics. Anesthesiology 1965;26:465.
11. Archer GW, Marx GF: Arterial oxygenation during apnoea in parturient women. Br J Anaesth 1974;46:358.
12. Whitehead EM, Smith M, Dean Y, O'Sullivan G: An evaluation of gastric emptying times in pregnancy and the puerperium. Anaesthesia 1993;48:53–57.
13. La Salvia LA, Steffen EA: Delayed gastric empthling time in labor. Am J Obstet Gynecol 1950;59:1075–1081.
14. Wong CA, Loffredi M, Ganchiff JN, et al: Gastric emptying of water in term pregnancy. Anesthesiology 2002;96:1395–1400.
15. Davison JS, Davison MC, Hay DM: Gastric emptying time in late pregnancy and labour. J Obstet Gynaecol Br Commonw 1970;77: 37–41.
16. Brock-Utne JG, Dow TGB, Dimopoulos GE, et al: Gastric and lower oesophageal sphincter (LOS) pressures in early pregnancy. Br J Anaesth 1981;53:381.
17. Wyner J, Cohen SE: Gastric volume in early pregnancy: Effect of metoclopramide. Anesthesiology 1982;57:209.
18. Cohen SE, Woods WA, Wyner J: Antiemetic efficacy of droperidol and metoclopramide. Anesthesiology 1984;60:67.
19. Scheller MS, Sears KL: Post-operative neurologic dysfunction associated with preoperative administration of metoclopramide. Anesth Analg 1987;66:274.
20. Lund CJ, Donovan JC: Blood volume during pregnancy. Am J Obstet Gynecol 1967;98:393.
21. Pritchard J, MacDonald P: Maternal adaptation to pregnancy. In Williams JW, Pritchard J, MacDonald P (eds), Williams Obstetrics, 16th ed. New York: Appleton-Century-Crofts, 1980, p. 236.
22. Gerbasi FR, Buttoms S, Farag A, Mammen E: Increased intravascular coagulation associated with pregnancy. Obstet Gynecol 1990;75:385–389.
23. Wildsmith JAW: Serum pseudocholinesterase, pregnancy and suxamethonium. Anaesthesia 1972;27:90.
24. Coryell MN, Beach EF, Robinson AR, et al: Metabolism of women during the reproductive cycle: XVII. Changes in electrophoretic patterns of plasma proteins throughout the cycle and following delivery. J Clin Invest 1950;29:1559.
25. Datta S, Kitzmiller JL, Naulty JS, et al: Acid-base status of diabetic mothers and their infants following spinal anesthesia for cesarean section. Anesth Analg 1982;61:662.
26. Datta S, Lambert DH, Gregus J, et al: Differential sensitivities of mammalian nerve fibers during pregnancy. Anesth Analg 1983;62:1070.
27. Gin T, Chan MTV: Decreased minimum alveolar concentration of isoflurane in pregnant humans. Anesthesiology 1994;81:829.
28. Brown WU, Bell GC, Alper MH: Acidosis, local anesthetics and the newborn. Obstet Gynecol 1976;48:27.
29. Hamshaw-Thomas A, Rogerson N, Reynolds F: Transfer of bupivacaine, lignocaine and pethidine across the rabbit placenta: Influence of maternal protein binding and fetal flow. Placenta 1984;5:61.
30. Kennedy RL, Miller RP, Bell JU, et al: Uptake and distribution of bupivacaine in fetal lambs. Anesthesiology 1986;65:247.
31. Kuhnert PM, Kuhnert BR, Stitts JM, Gross TL: The use of a selected ion monitoring technique to study the disposition of bupivacaine in mother, fetus and neonate following epidural anesthesia for cesarean section. Anesthesiology 1981;55:611.
32. Kuhnert BR, Philipson EH, Pimental R, et al: Lidocaine disposition in mother, fetus, and neonate after spinal anesthesia. Anesth Analg 1986;65:139.
33. Morishima HO, Daniel SS, Finster M, et al: Transmission of mepivacaine hydrochloride (Carbocaine) across the human placenta. Anesthesiology 1966;27:147.
34. Kuhnert BR, Kuhnert PM, Prochaska AL, Gross TL: Plasma levels of 2-chloroprocaine in obstetric patients and their neonates after epidural anesthesia. Anesthesiology 1980;53:21.
35. Pihlajamaki K, Kanto J, Lindberg R, et al: Extradural administration of bupivacaine: pharmacokinetics and metabolism in pregnant and non-pregnant women. Br J Anaesth 1990;64:556.
36. Morishima HO, Covino BG: Toxicity and distribution of lidocaine in nonasphyxiated and asphyxiated baboon fetuses. Anesthesiology 1981;54:182.
37. Morishima HO, Finster M, Pedersen H, et al: Pharmacokinetics of lidocaine in fetal and neonatal lambs and adult sheep. Anesthesiology 1979;50:431.
38. Mihaly GW, Moore RG, Thomas J, et al: The pharmacokinetics and metabolism of the anilide local anaesthetics in neonates. Eur J Clin Pharmacol 1978;13:143.
39. Finster M, Poppers PJ, Sinclair JC, et al: Accidental intoxication of the fetus with local anesthetic drug during caudal anesthesia. Am J Obstet Gynecol 1965;92:922.

40. Morishima HO, Pedersen H, Finster M, et al: Toxicity of lidocaine in adult, newborn and fetal sheep. Anesthesiology 1981;55:57.

41. Gale R, Ferguson JE II, Stevenson D: Effect of epidural analgesia with bupivacaine hydrochloride on neonatal bilirubin production. Obstet Gynecol 1987;70:692.

42. Brockhurst NJ, Littleford JA, Halpern SH: The neurological and adaptive capacity score: a systematic review of its use in obstetric anesthesia research. Anesthesiology 2000;92:237.

43. Morishima HO, Yeh M-N, James LS: Reduced uterine blood flow and fetal hypoxemia with acute maternal stress: experimental observation in the pregnant baboon. Am J Obstet Gynecol 1979;134:270.

44. Ueland K, Hansen JM: Maternal cardiovascular dynamics: Ill. Labor and delivery under local and caudal analgesia. Am J Obstet Gynecol 1969;103:8.

45. Moir DD, Willocks J: Management of incoordinate uterine action under continuous epidural analgesia. BMJ 1967;2:396.

46. Miller FC, Petrie RH, Arce JJ, et al: Hyperventilation during labor. Am J Obstet Gynecol 1974;120:489.

47. Beaule PE, Smith MI, Nguyen VN: Meperidine-induced seizure after revision hip arthroplasty. J Arthroplasty 2005;19:516–519.

48. Hagmeyer KO, Mauro LS, Mauro VF: Meperidine-related seizures associated with patient-controlled analgesia pumps. Ann Pharmacother 1993;27:29–32.

49. Kaiko RF, Grabinski PY, Heidrick G, et al: Central nervous system excitatory effects of meperidine in cancer patients. Ann Neurol 1983;13:180–185.

50. Kuhnert BR, Linn PL, Kennard MJ, Kuhnert PM: Effect of low doses of meperidine on neonatal behavior. Anesth Analg 1985;64:335.

51. Sosa CG, Balagueer E, Alonso JG, et al: Meperidine for dystocia during the first stage of labor: a randomized controlled trial. Am J Obstet Gynecol 2004;191:1212–1218.

52. Eisele JH, Wright R, Rogge P: Newborn and maternal fentanyl levels at cesarean section. Anesth Analg 1982;61:179.

53. Shannon KT, Ramanathan S: Systemic medication for labor analgesia. Obstet Pain Manage 1995;2:1–6.

54. Morley-Foster PK, Reid DW, Vandeberghe H: A comparison of patient-controlled analgesia fentanyl and alfentanil for labour analgesia. Can J Anaesth 2000;47:113–119.

55. Muir HA, Breen T, Campbell DC, et al: Is intravenous PCA fentanyl an effective method for providing labor analgesia? Anesthesiology 1999;(Suppl):A28.

56. Vercauteren M, Bettens K, Van Springel G, et al: Intrathecal labor analgesia: Can we use the same mixture as is used epidurally? Int J Obstet Anesth 1997;6:242–246.

57. Breen TW, Giesinger Cm, Halpern SH: Comparison of epidural lidocaine and fentanyl to intrathecal sufentanil for analgesia in early labor. Int J Obstet Anesth 1999;8:226–230.

58. Kapila A, Glass PS, Jacobs JR, et al: Measured context-sensitive half-times of remifentanil and alfentanil. Anesthesiology 1995;83:968–975.

59. Evron S, Glezerman M, Sadan O, et al: Remifentanil: a novel systemic analgesic for labor pain. Anesth Analg 2005;100:233–238.

60. Kan RE, Hughes SC, Rosen M, et al: Intravenous remifentanil: placental transfer, maternal and neonatal effects. Anesthesiology 1998;88:1467.

61. Thurlow JA, Laxton CH, Dick A, et al: Remifentanil by patient-controlled analgesia compared with intramuscular meperidine for pain relief in labor. Br J Anaesth 2002;88:374–378.

62. Volmanen P, Sarvela J, Akural EI, et al: Intravenous remifentanil vs. epidural levobupivacaine with fentanyl for pain relief in early labour: a randomized, controlled, double-blinded study. Acta Anaesthesiol Scand 2008;52:249–255.

63. Volmanen P, Akural E, Raudaskoski T, et al: Comparison of remifentanil and nitrous oxide in labour analgesia. Acta Anaesthesiol Scand 2005;49:453–458.

64. Maduska AL, Hajghassemali M: A double blind comparison of butorphanol and meperidine in labor: Maternal pain relief and effect on newborn. Can Anaesth Soc J 1978;25:398.

65. Wilson CM, McClean E, Moore J, Dundee JW: A double-blind comparison of intramuscular pethidine and nalbuphine in labour. Anaesthesia 1986;41:1207–1213.

66. Hodgkinson R, Huff RW, Hayashi RH, Husain FJ: Double-blind comparison of maternal analgesia and newonatal neurobehaviour following intravenous butorphanol and meperidine. J Int Med Res 1979;7:224–230.

67. Thorp JA, Hu DH, Albin RM, et al: The effect of intrapartum epidural analgesia on nulliparous labor: A randomized, controlled, prospective trial. Am J Obstet Gynecol 1993;169:851.

68. Sharma SK, Sidawi JE, Ramin SM, et al: Cesarean delivery: A randomized trial of epidural versus patient controlled meperidine analgesia during labor. Anesthesiology 1997;87:487.

69. Halpern SH, Leighton BL, Ohlsson A, et al: Effect of epidural vs parenteral opioid analgesia in the progress of labor: A meta-analysis. JAMA 1998;280:2105.

70. Ramin SM, Gambling DR, Lucas MJ, et al: Randomized trial of epidural versus intravenous analgesia in labor. Obstet Gynecol 1995;86:783.

71. Chestnut DH, Vincent RD, McGrath JM, et al: Does early administration of epidural analgesia affect obstetric outcome in nulliparous women who are receiving intravenous oxytocin? Anesthesiology 1994;80:1193.

72. Chestnut DH, McGrath JM, Vincent RD, et al: Does early administration of epidural analgesia affect obstetric outcome in nulliparous women who are in spontaneous labor? Anesthesiology 1994;80:1201.

73. American College of Obstetrics and Gynecology: Obstetric forceps. AGOG Committee on Obstetrics Maternal and Fetal Medicine, Committee Opinion, 1989.

74. Chestnut DH, Laszewski LJ, Pollack RL, et al: Continuous epidural infusion of 0.0625% bupivacaine-0.0002% fentanyl during the second stage of labor. Anesthesiology 1990;72:613.

75. Birnbach DJ, Chestnut DH: The epidural test dose in obstetric practice: Has it outlived its usefulness? Anesth Analg 1999;88:971.

76. Norris MC, Ferrenbach D, Dalman H, et al: Does epinephrine improve the diagnostic accuracy of aspiration during labor epidural analgesia? Anesth Analg 1999;88:1073.

77. Guinard JP, Mulroy MF, Carpenter RL, Knopes KD. Test doses: optimal epinephrine content with and without acute beta-adrenergic blockade. Anesthesiology 1990;73:386–392.

78. Visconti C, Eisenach JC: Patient-controlled epidural analgesia during labor. Obstet Gynecol 1991;77:348.

79. Halpern S: Recent advances in patient-controlled epidural analgesia for labour. Curr Opin Anaesthesiol 2005;18:247–251.

80. Minty RG, Kelly L, Minty A, Hammett DC: Single-dose intrathecal analgesia to control labour pain: is it a useful alternative to epidural analgesia? Can Fam Physician 2007;53:437–442.

81. Rigler ML, Drasner K, Krejcie TC, et al: Cauda equina syndrome after continuous spinal anesthesia. Anesth Analg 1991;72:275.

82. Arkoosh VA, Palmer CM, Van Maren GA, et al: Continuous intrathecal labor analgesia: safety and efficacy. Anesthesiology 1998;(Suppl):A8.

83. Simons SW, Cyna AM, Dennis AT, Hughes D: Combined spinal-epidural versus epidural analgesia in labour. Cochrane Database Syst Rev 2007;3:CD003401.

84. Campbell DC, Camann WR, Datta S: The addition of bupivacaine to intrathecal sufentanil for labor analgesia. Anesth Analg 1995;81:305.

85. Labbene I, Gharsallah H, Abderrahaman A, et al: Effects of 15 mcg intrathecal clonidine added to bupivacaine and sufentanil for labor analgesia. Tunis Med 2011;89:853–859.

86. Collis RE, Davies DWL, Aveling W: Randomized comparison of combined spinal epidural and standard epidural analgesia in labour. Lancet 1995;345:1413.

87. McLeod A, Fernando R, Page F, et al: An assessment of maternal balance and gait using computerized posturography. Anesthesiology 1999;(Suppl):A8.

88. Wong CA, Scavone BM, Peaceman AM, et al: The risk of cesarean delivery with neuraxial analgesia given early versus late labor. N Engl J Med 2005;352:655.

89. Cohen SE, Cherry CM, Holbrook RH, et al: Intrathecal sufentanil for labor analgesia: sensory changes, side-effects and fetal heart rate changes. Anesth Analg 1993;77:1155.

90. Clarke VT, Smiley RM, Finster M: Uterine hyperactivity after intrathecal injection of fentanyl for analgesia during labor: A cause of fetal bradycardia? Anesthesiology 1994;81:1083.

91. O'Gorman DA, Birnbach DJ, Kuczkowski KM, et al: Use of umbilical flow velocimetry in the assessment of the pathogenesis of fetal bradycardia following combined spinal epidural analgesia in parturients. Anesthesiology 2000;(Suppl):A2.

92. Riley ET, Vogel TM, EI-Sayed YY, et al: Patient selection bias contributes to an increased incidence of fetal bradycardia after combined spinal epidural analgesia for labor. Anesthesiology 1999;91:A1054.

93. Nielson PE, Erickson R, Abouleish E, et al: Fetal heart rate changes after intrathecal sufentanil or epidural bupivacaine for labor analgesia: incidence and clinical significance. Anesth Analg 1996;83:742.

94. Albright GA, Forester RM: Does combined epidural analgesia with subarachnoid sufentanil increase the incidence of emergency cesarean section? Reg Anesth 1997;22:400.

95. Norris MC, Grieco WM, Borkowski M, et al: Complications of labor analgesia: epidural versus combined spinal epidural techniques. Anesth Analg 1995;79:529.

96. Leighton BL, Arkoosh VA, Huffnagle S, et al: The dermatomal spread of epidural bupivacaine with and without prior intrathecal sufentanil. Anesth Analg 1996;83:526.

97. Bucklin BA, Hawkins JL, Anderson JR, Ullrich FA: Obstetric anesthesia workforce survey: twenty-year update. Anesthesiology 2005;103:645–653.

98. Baxi LV, Petrie RH, James LS: Human fetal oxygenation following paracervical block. Am J Obstet Gynecol 1979;135:1109.

99. Palomaki O, Huhtala H, Kirkinen P: A comparative study of the safety of 0.25% levobupivacaine and 0.25% racemic bupivacaine for paracervical block in the first stage of labor. Acta Obstet Gynecol Scand 2005;84: 956–961.

100. Leighton BL, Halpern SH, Wilson DB: Lumbar sympathetic blocks speed early and second stage induced labor in nulliparous women. Anesthesiology 1999;90:1039–1046.

101. Pace MC, Aurilio C, Bulletti C, et al: Subarachnoid analgesia in advanced labor: a comparison of subarachnoid analgesia and pudendal block in advanced labor. Analgesic quality and obstetric outcome. Ann NY Acad Sci 2004;1034:356–363.

102. Aissaoui Y, Bruyere R, Mustapha H, et al: A randomized controlled trial of pudendal nerve block for pain relief after episiotomy. Anesth Analg 2008;107:625–629.

103. Berghella V, Baxter JK, Chauhan SP: Evidence-based surgery for cesarean delivery. Am J Obstet Gynecol 2005;193:1607–1617.

104. Hawkins JL, Gibbs CP, Orleans M, et al: Obstetric anesthesia workforce survey 1992 vs 1981. Anesthesiology 1994;81:A1128.

105. Shnider SM, Levinson G: Anesthesia for cesarean section. In Shnider SM, Levinson G (eds): Anesthesia for Obstetrics, 2nd ed. Baltimore: Williams & Wilkins, 1987, p. 159.

106. Dyer RA, Farina Z, Joubert IA, et al: Crystalloid preload versus rapid crystalloid administration after induction of spinal anesthesia for elective caesarean section. Anaesth Intensive Care 2004;32:35–35-7.

107. Marx GF, Luykx WM, Cohen S: Fetal-neonatal status following cesarean section for fetal distress. Br J Anaesth 1984;56:1009.

108. Norris MC: Height, weight and the spread of subarachnoid hyperbaric bupivacaine in the term parturient. Anesth Analg 1988;67:555.

109. Hartwell BL, Aglio LS, Hauch MA, et al: Vertebral column length and spread of hyperbaric subarachnoid bupivacaine in the term parturient. Reg Anesth 1991;16:17–19.

110. Ogun CO, Kirgiz EN, Duman A, et al: Comparison of intrathecal isobaric bupivacaine-morphine and ropivacaine-morphine for Caesarean delivery. Br J Anaesth 2003;90:659–664.

111. Hunt GO, Naulty S, Bader AM, et al: Perioperative analgesia with subarachnoid fentanyl-bupivacaine for cesarean delivery. Anesthesiology 1989;71:535.

112. Palmer CM, Emerson S, Volgoropolous D, et al: Dose-response relationship of intrathecal morphine for postcesarean analgesia. Anesthesiology 1999;90:437–444.

113. Kato R, Shimamoto H, Terui K, et al: Delayed respiratory depression associated with 0.15 mg intrathecal morphine for cesarean section. A review of 1915 cases. J Anesth 2008;22:112–116.

114. Roelants F: The use of neuraxial adjuvant drugs (neostigmine, clonidine) in obstetrics. Curr Opin Anaesthesiol 2006;19:233–237.

115. Ngan Kee WD, Khaw KS, Lee BB, et al: The limitations of ropivacaine with epinephrine as an epidural test dose in parturients. Anesth Analg 2001;92:1529–1531.

116. Leighton BL, Norris MC, Sosis M, et al: Limitations of epinephrine as a marker of intravascular injection in laboring women. Anesthesiology 1987;66:688.

117. Gissen AJ, Datta S, Lambert D: The chloroprocaine controversy: is chloroprocaine neurotoxic? Reg Anaesth 1984;9:135.

118. Hynson JM, Sessler DI, Glosten B: Back pain in volunteers after epidural anesthesia with chloroprocaine. Anesth Analg 1991;72:253.

119. Albright GA: Cardiac arrest following regional anesthesia with etidocaine or bupivacaine. Anesthesiology 1979;51:285.

120. Carvalho B, Riley E, Cohen SE, et al: Single-dose, sustained-release epidural morphine in the management of postoperative pain after elective cesarean delivery: results of a multicenter randomized controlled study. Anesth Analg 2005;100:1150–1158.

121. Carvalho B, Roland LM, Chu FL, et al: Single-dose, extended-release epidural morphine (DepoDur) compared to conventional epidural morphine for post-cesarean pain. Anesth Analg 2007;105:176–183.

122. Ginsar Y, Riley ET, Anst MS: The site of action of epidural fentanyl in humans: the difference between infusion and bolus administration. Anesth Analg 2003;97:1428–1438.

123. Marik PE: Aspiration pneumonitis and aspiration pneumonia. N Engl J Med 2001;344:665–671.

124. Brizgys RV, Dailey PA, Shnider SM, et al: The incidence and neonatal effects of maternal hypotension during epidural anesthesia for cesarean section. Anesthesiology 1987;67:782.

125. Ueyama H, He YL, Tanigami H, et al: Effects of crystalloid and colloid preload or blood volume in the parturient undergoing spinal anesthesia for elective cesarean section. Anesthesiology 1999;91:1571.

126. Rout CC, Roche DA: Spinal hypotension associated with cesarean section: will preload ever work? Anesthesiology 1999;91:1565.

127. Ngan Kee WD, Kaw KS, Ng FF: Prevention of hypotension during spinal anesthesia for cesarean delivery: an effective technique using combination of phenylephrine infusion and crystalloid cohydration. Anesthesiology 2005;103:744–750.

128. Ramanathan S, Grant GJ: Vasopressor therapy for hypotension due to epidural anaesthesia. Acta Anaesthesiol Scand 1988;32:559.

129. Rosenblatt MA, Abel M, Fischer GW, et al: Successful use of a 20% lipid emulsion to resuscitate a patient after a presumed bupivacaine-related cardiac arrest. Anesthesiology 2006;105:217–218.

130. Kasten GW, Martin ST: Resuscitation from bupivacaine-induced cardiovascular toxicity during partial inferior vena cava occlusion. Anesth Analg 1986;65:341.

131. Choi PT, Galinski SE, Takeuchi L, et al: PDPH is a common complication of neuraxial blockade in parturients: a meta-analysis of obstetrical studies. Can J Anaesth 2003;50:460–469.

132. Russell IF: A prospective controlled study of continuous spinal analgesia versus repeat epidural analgesia after accidental dural puncture in labour. Int J Obstet Anesth 2012;21:7–16.

133. Maynard SE, Min J-Y, Merchan J, et al: Excess placental soluble fms-like tyrosine kinase 1 (sFlt1) may contribute to endothelial dysfunction, hypertension, and proteinuria in preeclampsia. J Clin Invest 2003;111: 649–658.

134. Tada S, Yasue A, Nishizawa H, Sekiya T, Hirota Y, Udagawa Y: Spontaneous spinal epidural hematoma during pregnancy: three case reports. J Obstet Gynaecol Res 2011;37:1734–1738.

135. Bodurka D: What's new in gynecology and obstetrics. J Am Coll Surg 2005;201:265–274.

136. Basso O, Rasmussen S, Weinberg CR, et al: Trends in fetal and infant survival following preeclampsia. JAMA 2006;296:1357–1362.

137. Luttun A, Carmeliet P: Soluble VEGF receptor Flt1: the elusive preeclampsia factor discovered? J Clin Invest 2003;111:60–62.

138. Keogh RJ, Harris LK, Freeman A, et al: Fetal-derived trophoblast use the apoptotic cytokine tumor necrosis factor-alpha-related apoptosis-inducing ligand to induce smooth muscle cell death. Circ Res 2007;100:834–841.

139. Walsh S: Preeclampsia: An imbalance in placental prostacyclin and thromboxane production. Am J Obstet Gynecol 1985;152:335.

140. Roberts J, Taylor R, Musci T, et al: Preeclampsia: An endothelial cell disorder. Am J Obstet Gynecol 1989;152:1200.

141. Venkatesha S, Toporsian M, Lam C, et al: Soluble endoglin contributes to the pathogenesis of preeclampsia. Nat Med 2006;12:642.

142. Levine RJ, Karumanchi SA: Circulating angiogenic factors in preeclampsia. Clin Obstet Gynecol 2005;48:372–386.

143. Chesley L: Plasma and red cell volumes during pregnancy. Am J Obstet Gynecol 1972:112:440.

144. Rodgers R, Levin J: A critical reappraisal of the bleeding time. Semin Thromb Hemost 1990:16:1–20.

145. Abalos E, Duley L, Steyn DW, Henderson-Smart DJ: Antihypertensive drug therapy for mild to moderate hypertension during pregnancy. Cochrane Database Syst Rev 207;1:CD002252.

146. Groenendijk R, Trimbos M, Wallenburg H: Hemodynamic measurements in preeclampsia: preliminary observations. Am J Obstet Gynecol 1984; 150:232.

147. Aya AG, Vialles N, Tanoubi I, et al: Spinal anesthesia-induced hypotension: A risk comparison between patients with severe preeclampsia and healthy women undergoing preterm cesarean delivery. Anesth Analg 2005;101: 869–875.

148. Cotton D, Gonik B, Dorman K, Harris R: Cardiovascular alterations in severe pregnancy-induced hypertension: Relationship of central venous pressure to pulmonary capillary wedge pressure. Am J Obstet Gynecol 1985;151:762.

149. Hogg B, Hauth J, Caritis S, et al: Safety of labor epidural anesthesia for women with severe hypertensive disease. Am J Obstet Gynecol 1999;181: 1099.

150. Newsome L, Bramwell R, Curling P: Hemodynamic effects of lumbar epidural anesthesia. Anesth Analg 1986;65:31.

151. Jouppila P, Jouppila R, Hollmen A, Koivula A: Lumbar epidural analgesia to improve intervillous blood flow during labor in severe preeclampsia. Obstet Gynecol 1982;52:158.

152. Ramanathan J, Botorff M, Jeter J, et al: The pharmacokinetics and maternal and neonatal effects of epidural lidocaine in preeclampsia. Anesth Analg 1986;65:120.

153. Wallace D, Leveno KJ, Cunningham F, et al: Randomized comparison of general and regional anesthesia for cesarean delivery in pregnancies complicated by severe preeclampsia. Obstet Gynecol 1995;86:193.

154. Hood D, Curry R: Spinal versus epidural anesthesia for cesarean section in severely preeclamptic patients: a retrospective survey. Anesthesiology 1999;90:1276.

155. Oyelese Y, Smulian JC: Placenta previa, placenta accrete, and vasa previa. Obstet Gynecol 2006;107:927–941.

156. Chestnut DH, Dewan D, Redick L, et al: Anesthetic management for obstetric hysterectomy: a multi-institutional study. Anesthesiology 1989;70:607.

157. Vincent RD Jr, Chestnut DH, Sipes SL, et al: Epidural anesthesia worsens uterine blood flow and fetal oxygenation during hemorrhage in gravid ewes. Anesthesiology 1992;76:799–806.

158. Santos A, Tun E, Bobby P, et al: The effects of bupivacaine, l-nitro-l-arginine-methyl-ester and phenylephrine on cardiovascular adaptations to asphyxia in the preterm fetal lamb. Anesth Analg 1997;84:1299.

159. Morishima HO, Pedersen H, Santos AS, et al: Adverse effects of maternally administered lidocaine on the asphyxiated preterm fetal lamb. Anesthesiology 1989;71:110.

160. Shnider SM, Webster G: Maternal and fetal hazards of surgery during pregnancy. Am J Obstet Gynecol 1965;92:891.

161. Brodsky J, Cohen E, Brown BJ, et al: Surgery during pregnancy and fetal outcome. Am J Obstet Gynecol 1980;138:1165.

162. Smith B: Fetal prognosis after anesthesia during gestation. Anesth Analg 1963;42:521.

163. Duncan P, Pope W, Cohen M, Greer N: Fetal risk of anesthesia and surgery during pregnancy. Anesthesiology 1986;64:790.

164. Heinonen O, Slone O, Shapiro S: Birth defects and drugs in pregnancy. In Birth Defects and Drugs in Pregnancy. Littleton, MA: Publishing Sciences Group, 1977, p. 516.

165. Grabowski C, Paar J: The teratogenic effects of graded doses of hypoxia on the chick embryo. Am J Anat 1958;103:313.

166. Saxen I, Saxen L: Association between maternal intake of diazepam and oral clefts. Lancet 1975;2:498.

167. Safra M, Oakley G: Association between cleft lip with or without cleft palate and prenatal exposure to diazepam. Lancet 1975;2:478.

168. Shiono PH, Mills JL: Oral clefts and diazepam use during pregnancy. N Engl J Med 1984;311:919–920.

169. Shepard TH: Catalog of Teratogenic Agents, 7th ed. Baltimore: Johns Hopkins University Press, 1992.

170. Palanisamy A, Baxter MG, Keel PK, Xie Z, Crosby G, Culley DJ: Rats exposed to isoflurane in utero during early gestation are behaviorally abnormal as adults. Anesthesiology 2011;114:521–528.

171. Sprung J, Fleich RP, Wilder RT, et al: Anesthesia for cesarean delivery and learning disability in a population based birth cohort. Anesthesiology 2009;111:302–310.

172. Adamsons K, Mueller-Heubach E, Myers R: Production of fetal asphyxia in the rhesus monkey by administration of catecholamines to the mother. Am J Obstet Gynecol 1971;109:148.

PEDIATRIC ANESTHESIA

CHAPTER 42

Regional Anesthesia in Pediatric Patients: General Considerations

Steve Roberts

INTRODUCTION

Regional anesthesia is an essential part of modern pediatric anesthetic practice, conveying many significant advantages to the patient and to the hospital (Table 42–1). However, despite a strong body of evidence highlighting the advantages of regional anesthesia, it has been only relatively recently that regional anesthesia has begun to become more common place in anesthetic practice. Large prospective studies by the French-Language Society of Pediatric Anesthesiologists (ADARPEF) have demonstrated no increased risk to children having blocks performed under general anesthesia.[1–2] However, complications were four times greater in children aged less than 6 months compared to those older than 6 months.[2]

Historically, it was thought that neonates required little or no analgesia. However, inadequate analgesia in the neonate can cause biobehavioral changes that may modulate future responses to pain in childhood.[3] As a consequence, advanced regional anesthesia techniques (eg, epidural analgesia) have become increasingly utilized in children of all ages. Interestingly, the ADARPEF studies identified that there is a now a trend away from the central neuraxial blocks toward peripheral nerve catheter techniques. This change may have been influenced by advances in minimally invasive surgery and the more predictable administration of peripheral catheter techniques in modern regional anesthesia practice.[1–2]

All regional anesthetic techniques can be safely performed in the pediatric population with the adequate training and modern equipment.

ANATOMICAL DIFFERENCES BETWEEN CHILDREN & ADULTS

With respect to anatomy, physiology, and pharmacology, adolescents may be considered "little adults"; however, neonates and infants need special consideration.[4–5] Anatomically, the major

difference lies in the spine and its contents; this topic is described in greater detail in Chapter 43. Physiologically, there are a number of differences found in the developing paediatric nervous system when compared to adults. Myelination is incomplete at birth, and the process can take 12 years to complete; consequently, lower concentrations of local anesthetic may be effectively utilized in the pediatric population, thereby also reducing the risk of toxicity. Although the nociceptive pathways are fundamentally the same in children as in adults, there are differences that may result in children experiencing greater pain than adults.[6] In children, the receptive field of a neuron may be greater, leading to poor pain localization. The descending inhibitory pathways are immature, and this may allow unmodulated nociceptive inputs to the ascending spinal pain pathways. The physiological immaturities of the neonatal liver in association with a relatively high cardiac output produce pharmacological differences that combine to increase the risk of local anesthetic toxicity in neonates.

PHARMACOLOGY OF LOCAL ANESTHETICS IN PEDIATRIC PATIENTS

There are two main groups of local anesthetic drugs used in pediatric regional anesthesia: the amino esters and the amino amides. (A detailed discussion of these drugs can be found in Chapter 7.) There are relatively few local anesthetic pharmacokinetics in children, and especially in neonates, is limited; unfortunately, it is this age group that is at the greatest risk of local anesthetic drug toxicity.[7]

Amino Amide–type Local Anesthetics

The most commonly used group of local anesthetics in pediatric practice are the amino amides: lidocaine, bupivacaine, ropivacaine, and levobupivacaine. The amino amide local anesthetics

TABLE 42–1. Advantages of regional anesthesia in children.

Patient benefits	Superior analgesia: Results in calmer patient and parents/caregivers.
	Reduced MAC: Reduced risk of deeper GA, smoother emergence, earlier return of appetite.
	Neurotoxicity: This potential problem is GA dose–dependent; therefore, a reduced MAC exposure may be beneficial.
	Hemodynamic stability: Up to 8 years of age, CNBs rarely cause significant hypotension.
	Reduced requirement for postoperative ventilator support: Particularly in neonates and infants undergoing upper abdominal and thoracic surgery.
	Obtunds the hormonal stress response.
	Reduced intraoperative blood loss: Demonstrated during hypospadias repair, cleft repair, and tonsillectomy.
	Improved GI function: Peristalsis better maintained; improved splanchnic perfusion in cases of NEC and gastroschisis.
	Avoids the need for GA: Premature infants who undergo GA are at risk of postoperative apnea.
Hospital benefits	Easier to nurse: Pain-free children are less labor intensive to care for.
	Reduced MAC: Rapid discharge from first-stage recovery.
	Reduced requirement for postoperative ventilatory support: This is of particular benefit when there is limited PICU support.
	Reduced length of stay.

CNB, central neuraxial block; GA, general anesthesia; GI, gastrointestinal; MAC, minimum alveolar concentration; NEC, necrotizing enterocolitis; PICU, pediatric intensive care unit.

undergo hepatic metabolism. However, the neonatal liver is immature, with the cytochrome systems maturing at varying rates: the CYP3A4 within the first 9 months of life compared to the CYP1A2, which can take until 8 years of age to mature.[8–9] The volume of distribution at steady state in infants is greater than in adults. Fluid compartments change drastically with age, 80% of body weight consisting of water in a premature neonate, 75% in a term neonate, 65% in an infant, and 60% in older children. As age increases, the intracellular fluid increases from 20% of body weight in premature neonates to the 30% seen in adults; within this time frame, extracellular fluids are halved. Local anesthetics are water soluble; therefore, the age-related changes in fluid compartment composition are significant. Infants have lower levels of local anesthetic–binding proteins (eg, alpha-1-acid glycoprotein and albumin), which leads to an increased fraction of unbound local anesthetic and therefore to a greater risk of toxicity. However, in the first 48 hours postoperatively, there is an increase in alpha-1-acid glycoprotein that may act to protect the neonate. The clearance of these drugs is decreased in those less than 3 months of age, gradually reaching adult levels by 8 months of age.[10] Consequently, elimination half-lives of local anesthetics are longer in neonates and infants compared to adults.

Bupivacaine

Bupivacaine is an isomer with both l- and d-enantiomer, the d-enantiomer causing most of the adverse effects that are seen in humans. Given that bupivacaine is the most toxic of the amino amide local anesthetics, consideration should be given to using a safer alternative, particularly for neonates and when continuous infusion techniques through indwelling catheters are administered. The pharmacokinetics and pharmacodynamics of bupivacaine have been well documented in the literature.[11–12] The preferred concentration for children is 0.25% for peripheral nerve blocks and 0.1% for continuous infusions. Older children can tolerate a higher dose of local anesthetic solution (0.4 mg/kg/h) compared with neonates and infants (0.2 mg/kg/h).[13] The dosage of bupivacaine is limited to 2–4 mg/kg for a single-dose injection and 0.2–0.4 mg/kg for a continuous infusion.

Ropivacaine

Ropivacaine is a newer amide local anesthetic that is being used more frequently in pediatric surgery. It is an l-enantiomer with less cardiovascular and central nervous system side effects compared with bupivacaine. Ropivacaine has slight vasoconstrictive properties that may explain the longer T_{max} when administered caudally compared to bupivacaine. Pharmacokinetic data are available in children on the use of ropivacaine in continuous infusions as well as for single-shot injections.[14–18] Pediatric trials have demonstrated a longer duration of action with ropivacaine than with mepivacaine when used for peripheral nerve blockade.[19] Caution should be exercised while using ropivacaine in children as well, as cases of cardiovascular toxicity has been reported.

Levobupivacaine

Levobupivacaine is a newer l-enantiomer with potentially less risk of severe cardiovascular toxicity. Pharmacokinetic data are available in children, and the dosage interval is similar as that of bupivacaine.[20–23] Animal experiments have shown that levobupivacaine causes less myocardial depression and a decreased incidence of inducing fatal dysrhythmias compared with bupivacaine.[24] Although this drug provides the practitioner with the option of a drug that is less cardiotoxic, caution should still be exercised.

Ester-type Local Anesthetics

Due to their short duration of action and propensity to cause allergic reactions, the amino esters (eg, procaine, 2-chloroprocaine, tetracaine) are the least commonly used group of local anesthetics. Unlike amino amide local anesthetics, the amino esters are metabolized by plasma cholinesterases.[25–27] As a result, the metabolism of ester local anesthetics depends on plasma cholinesterase levels.[28–31] Hence, in populations with decreased plasma cholinesterase levels, such as neonates and infants, the plasma level of these drugs may be increased, potentially leading to toxic drug levels. The presence of plasma cholinesterase also limits the duration of action of these drugs, leading to a shortened activity.

The most common ester local anesthetics used in infants and children are chloroprocaine and tetracaine. These drugs are occasionally used in children as an adjuvant to spinal anesthesia in formerly premature infants undergoing spinal anesthesia or as the sole anesthetic solution for caudal analgesia.[32] Tetracaine has been reported in spinal anesthesia, especially in premature infants, as the sole anesthetic for inguinal hernia repair.[33] 2-chloroprocaine has been used extensively in children for analgesia in the central neuraxial space.[34]

DOSING OF LOCAL ANESTHETICS IN PEDIATRIC PATIENTS

Most drug doses in pediatric patients are based on the weight of the patient (Table 42–2), though it is often debated whether total body weight or lean body mass is more appropriate for drug calculations.[35] However, this may not be applicable to local anesthetic considerations; studies done on infants undergoing spinal anesthesia found a larger requirement of local anesthetic solution (weight-scaled) compared with their adult counterparts using bupivacaine or tetracaine.[36]

The concentration of local anesthetic administered should also be carefully considered. A lower concentration of long-acting local anesthetic (eg, 0.25% levobupivacaine) is often used because the child is also receiving a general anesthetic; therefore, the block is used for analgesia only. However, in certain scenarios, lower or higher concentrations of local anesthetic should be administered. Lower concentrations (eg, 0.125% levobupivacaine) are useful in decreasing the risk of toxicity in neonates and are less likely to mask compartment syndrome or delay ambulation. Higher concentrations of local anesthetic(eg, 0.5% levobupivacaine) should be considered where a profound motor block is desirable (eg, lower limb tendon transfer surgery in children with cerebral palsy.

TOXICITY OF LOCAL ANESTHETIC DRUGS

The toxicity of local anesthetics in children include cardiovascular and central nervous system toxicity (Table 42–3) and allergic reactions to ester local anesthetic solutions.[35] The already discussed pharmacokinetic differences, together with the immaturity of the blood–brain barrier, may make central nervous system toxicity more likely in neonates.[37–41] However, the co-administration of general anesthesia may mask early signs and symptoms of systemic toxicity. The local anesthetic dose for children is always calculated on a milligram-per-kilogram basis, rather than predicted volumes as in adult regional anesthesia. While it is recognized that, of pediatric patients, infants are at a higher risk of systemic toxicity, caution should be the norm for children of all ages, as higher concentrations of some local anesthetics have been recorded in adolescents compared to adults. Toxic plasma levels have also been reported following safe doses of local anesthetic used for caudal and ilioinguinal blocks, so the minimum effective dose is recommended.

Interestingly, Weintraud et al. found that US-guided ilioinguinal blocks resulted in higher plasma concentrations when compared to landmark-based techniques.[42] This may be due to

TABLE 42–2. Maximum recommended doses and approximate duration of action of commonly used local anesthetic agents.

Local Anesthetic	Class	Maximum Dose (mg/kg)[a]	Duration of Action (min)	Infusion (mg/kg/h)
Procaine	Ester	10	60–90	–
2-chloroprocaine	Ester	20	30–60	–
Tetracaine	Ester	1.5	180–600	–
Lidocaine	Amide	5	90–200	–
Bupivacaine	Amide	2.5	180–600	0.2–0.4
Ropivacaine	Amide	2.5	180–600	0.2–0.5
Levobupivacaine	Amide	2.5	180–600	0.2–0.5

[a]In neonates, it may be safer to halve the maximum dose.

PART 6

TABLE 42-3. Systemic toxicity of local anesthetic solution.

Central nervous system[a]

Dizziness and lightheadedness

Visual and auditory disturbances

Muscle twitching and tremors

Generalized convulsions

Cardiovascular

Direct cardiac effects

Depressed rapid phase of repolarization of Purkinje fibers

Depressed spontaneous firing of the sinoatrial node

Negative inotropic effect on cardiac muscle

Calcium influx altered, leading to decreased myocardial contractility

Effects on vascular tone

Low concentrations: vasoconstriction

High concentrations: vasodilatation

Increased pulmonary vascular resistance

[a] Particularly in infants and children with special needs, early signs of central nervous system toxicity are often misdiagnosed as a result of poor analgesia; therefore, a high level of suspicion must be maintained at all times in these patients.

a greater surface area of absorption created by placing the local anesthetic precisely in a fascial plane compared to the multiple deposits within muscle that often occur with a landmark-based method.

Clinical Pearls

Preventing Systemic Toxicity in the Pediatric Population

- Choose a less toxic drug (eg, levobupivacaine or ropivacaine).
- Do not exceed the maximum dose (in neonates, it may be prudent to halve the maximum dose).
- Inject small aliquots and aspirate repeatedly.
- US allows for lower doses of drugs to be used and for injection visualization.
- Beware of repeated doses, and limit infusions in neonates to 48 hours.
- An epinephrine-containing test dose may be used to identify intravascular injection but is limited by which general anesthetic is administered.
- No matter which technique is used, all children, given any local anesthetic solution, particularly when given as continuous infusions, should be monitored continuously for adverse effects.

Clinical Pearls

Managing Local Anesthetic Toxicity
In pediatric practice, early warning signs and symptoms of toxicity may be masked by the concurrent administration of general anesthesia. This means the first sign may be arrhythmia or cardiovascular collapse. Consider the following when managing local anesthetic toxicity:

- Stop the local anesthetic injection.
- Institute basic life support, and call for assistance.
- Secure the airway, ventilate with 100% oxygen, and gain intravenous access.
- Seizures can be managed with a benzodiazepine or anesthetic induction agent.
- If cardiac arrest has occurred, commence advanced life support.
- Note that arrhythmias are often refractory, and resuscitation should therefore be prolonged.
- Lipid administration.[43] The Association of Anaesthetists of Great Britain and Ireland has published a simple protocol to follow (Figure 42-1).

TOPICAL ANESTHESIA

It is important to discuss the use of topical anesthesia in children because it is commonly used in clinical practice to provide analgesia for intravenous catheter placement, lumbar puncture, and other invasive procedures (eg, circumcision in neonates). The most common preparations include lidocaine, tetracaine, benzocaine, and prilocaine. The topical anesthetic solution permeates through the skin to provide analgesia. The three most common preparations available include eutectic mixture of local and anesthetics (EMLA), LMX-4 (4% liposomal lidocaine solution), and Ametop (4% amethocaine gel).[44-47] EMLA contains lidocaine and prilocaine and must be applied at least one hour before cannulation. Its duration of action is only 30–60 minutes, though it can be left on for 4–5 hours. LMX-4 requires only 30 minutes to take effect and can also be left on for 4–5 hours. Ametop requires 45 minutes to take effect and must be removed within an hour of application; its duration of effect is up to 3 hours, as it binds to proteins in the stratum corneum. Ametop is vasodilatory, which may aid cannulation. However, Ametop can cause erythema and edema, which may obscure veins.[48]

Clinical Pearls

The following are considerations for children undergoing regional anesthesia:

- Regional anesthesia is mostly commonly performed with the patient under general anesthesia.
- The dose of local anesthetic used is much lower than for adults and is calculated in milligrams per kilogram).
- Use a local anesthetic at the lowest effective concentration.

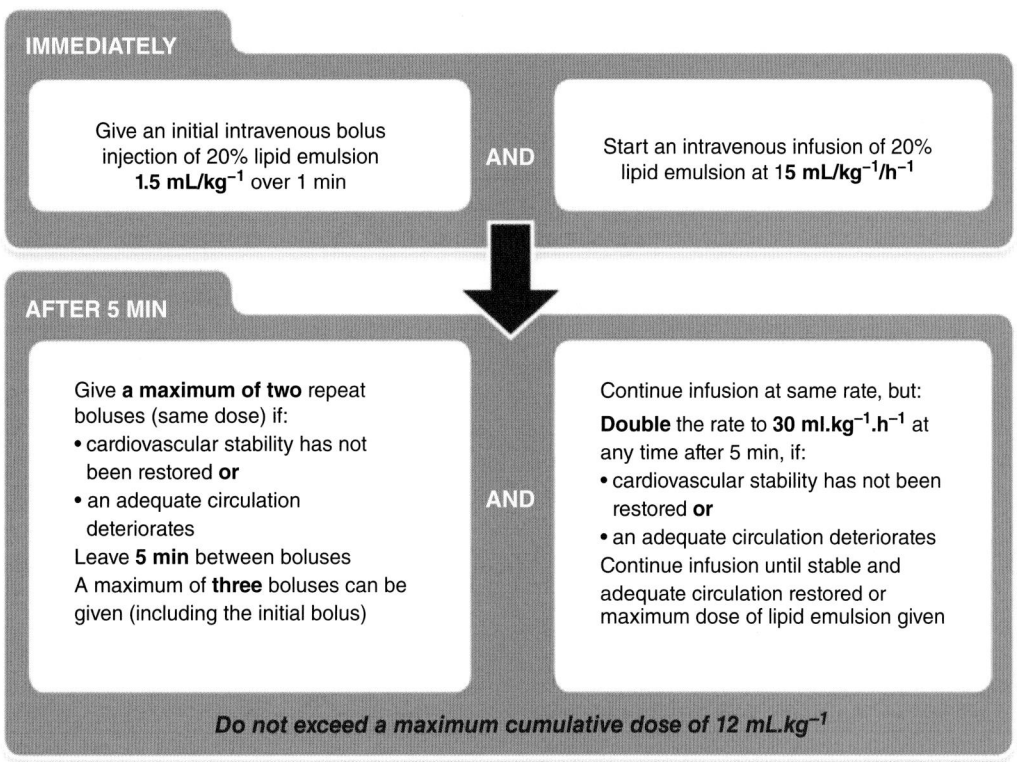

IMMEDIATELY

Give an initial intravenous bolus injection of 20% lipid emulsion **1.5 mL/kg^{-1}** over 1 min

AND

Start an intravenous infusion of 20% lipid emulsion at **15 mL/kg^{-1}/h^{-1}**

AFTER 5 MIN

Give **a maximum of two** repeat boluses (same dose) if:
• cardiovascular stability has not been restored **or**
• an adequate circulation deteriorates
Leave **5 min** between boluses
A maximum of **three** boluses can be given (including the initial bolus)

AND

Continue infusion at same rate, but:
Double the rate to **30 ml.kg^{-1}.h^{-1}** at any time after 5 min, if:
• cardiovascular stability has not been restored **or**
• an adequate circulation deteriorates
Continue infusion until stable and adequate circulation restored or maximum dose of lipid emulsion given

Do not exceed a maximum cumulative dose of 12 mL.kg^{-1}

FIGURE 42–1. Association of Anaesthetists of Great Britain and Ireland (AAGBI) Protocol for Local Anesthetic Toxicity.

• If moderate or severe pain is expected, intense physiotherapy required post operatively, or there is a history of chronic pain, consider using a catheter technique.
• Far fewer regional anesthesia complications are reported in children than in adults.
• Always obtain patient assent or consent if the child is older.
• Always explain postoperative paresthesia to patients.

PREOPERATIVE ASSESSMENT

The preoperative visit is an opportunity to assess and prepare the patient and family for the proposed surgery and anesthetic technique. It is important that the anesthesiologist understand the intended surgery so that a decision can be made to perform either a single-injection or continuous regional anesthetic technique. Generally, the more peripheral block should be chosen, as this typically has the lowest risk and fewest side effects and will therefore have greater acceptability to the patient and parents or caregivers alike. A catheter technique is recommended for moderate to major surgery, procedures that will require prolonged postoperative physiotherapy, and for children with chronic pain. It is also important to ensure there will be nursing staff trained to manage continuous regional anesthetic techniques.

The anesthesiologist should seek potential contraindications (eg, comorbidities) to a given regional anesthetic technique. A thorough pain history should be taken, looking specifically for a history of chronic pain or muscle spasticity. Children with special needs can be particularly challenging, and the anesthesiologist needs to know how the child copes with and expresses pain. The standard preoperative anesthetic examination should include an examination of the proposed block insertion site to identify things such as anatomical difficulties (eg, scoliosis) and local infection. In children with neurological disease, their preoperative neurological deficit should be documented.

The anesthesiologist should explain the advantages, side effects, and potential complications of the proposed anesthetic plan to the child and the parents/caregivers; it is prudent also to discuss a "plan B" should the proposed technique fail. Alternative analgesic strategies should be discussed so that informed consent can be given. In particular, the postoperative paresthesiae of the regional technique should be explained to children in terms they can understand, as this is often an experience they find difficult to cope with. If a continuous regional anesthetic technique will be used, reassure the child that removal of the catheter will not be painful. Parents or caregivers typically provide consent for a procedure for their child. However, if the child has the cognitive ability to discern right from wrong, it is suggested that the child's assent for a regional technique be obtained as well.[49] There is debate as to when or what this age may be. If a child refuses to have a regional procedure despite the parents' or caregivers' insistence, it is important for the anesthesiologist to provide an alternative modality of pain relief.

Analgesic premedication with paracetamol (acetaminophen) and a nonsteroidal anti-inflammatory drug (NSAID) should be considered, especially where it is known that the block will not provide total analgesia (eg, a transverse abdominis plane [TAP] block for appendectomy). Postoperative instructions should be given preoperatively and reinforced postoperatively on discharge.

REGIONAL ANESTHESIA: AWAKE OR ASLEEP?

Whether it is best for the patient to be awake or asleep during regional anesthesia has been a controversial issue in adults, and this debate once permeated the realm of pediatric regional anesthesia practice. Placing a regional block in an awake child is difficult due to the inability of the child to cooperate as well as the cognitive inability of the child to relate to symptoms such as paresthesia or pain. Therefore, the child is best provided with a regional technique under deep sedation or after the induction of general anesthesia; this practice has been the consensus of pediatric anesthesiologists in the U.S. as well as abroad for some time.[50]

However, there are two scenarios in which awake regional techniques are used in children. First, it was thought that by avoiding general anesthesia in premature infants undergoing minor surgery, the incidence of postoperative apnea could be reduced. This is probably less of an issue now that premature neonatal lungs are better protected and with the availability of newer inhalational agents that provide a more rapid emergence.

Second, the more mature child may be considered suitable for an awake regional technique when undergoing a minor surgery if they prefer or when a general anesthetic is considered too risky (eg, lymph node biopsy in a teenager with a mediastinal mass). For older patients, it is essential to prepare the child and parents or caregivers for the whole operating room visit, not just the insertion of the block. The block insertion can be made more comfortable by applying a topical anesthetic cream (EMLA has the best penetration) over the proposed injection site. During the operating room visit, the child should be supported and distracted by a nurse or play specialist. The child may also find the use of a DVD or MP3 player a useful distraction. It may be necessary to use nitrous oxide (Entonox) or anxiolytic doses of propofol or remifentanil to ease proceedings. Marhofer et al. have shown that in the pediatric trauma scenario, brachial plexus blocks are more comfortably inserted with US than with nerve stimulation.[51] In pediatric hospitals, the operating room staff and surgeon must be reminded that the patient will be awake, and the drugs and equipment needed to convert to general anesthesia must be ready.

PERIOPERATIVE BLOCK MANAGEMENT

Some simple rules need to be followed when performing any regional anesthetic technique in children. A skilled assistant should be present at all times, and this individual should understand the basic principles of regional anesthesia, in particular the need to aspirate regularly prior to injection, the need to warn the anesthesiologist about injection resistance. Further, the assistant should be able to make basic adjustments to the peripheral nerve stimulator (PNS) and US machines.

The child should have a secure airway, intravenous access, and full monitoring prior to commencing the block. As part of the World Health Organization (WHO) Surgical Safety Checklist, consent and side of surgery are checked, and just before block insertion, the site should again be confirmed with the anesthesiologist's assistant.

The child, US machine (when used), equipment, and anesthesiologist should be positioned ergonomically.

There is some debate as to the minimal standards for asepsis for regional anesthesia. For single-injection techniques, it is sufficient to scrub one's hands, wear sterile gloves, apply an alcoholic solution to the patient's skin, and cover the US probe. For catheter techniques, a more rigorous aseptic technique is advised. When performing any catheter technique, it is useful when draping the child to have a large area of anatomy visible; this allows the anesthesiologist sufficient room to perform a mapping/scout scan and also a better view, and thus appreciation of, the patient's anatomy (particularly important when placing epidurals in children with scoliosis).

It may be beneficial to tunnel the catheter, as this aids fixation, and in some cases may decrease the risk of infection (eg, with a caudal catheter, the catheter can be tunneled away from the diaper area).

There is no ideal test dose; therefore, repeated, frequent aspiration during injection is suggested.

When the block is not expected to cover all aspects of surgical pain (eg, a rectus sheath block for pyloromyotomy), consideration should be given to the administration of paracetamol intravenously and/or an NSAID per rectum to aid analgesia. Other adjuvants may prove beneficial (eg, intraoperative magnesium sulphate 50 mg/kg may decrease postoperative muscle spasms in cerebral palsy patients undergoing lower-limb surgery).

It is the author's opinion that, where possible, the regional anesthetic technique's efficacy should not be obscured by the administration of opioids or nitrous oxide. It is important in the intraoperative assessment of the block that any changes in heart rate and blood pressure are noted and related to the specific surgical proceedings at the time. This allows for the planning of rescue blocks at the end of the procedure. Even with successful blocks, occasional cardiovascular responses to surgical stimuli may occur, as the blocks are generally performed using a lower concentration of local anesthetic (eg, 0.25% levobupivacaine), and, if a tourniquet is used, a gradual increase in heart rate and blood pressure will occur after the first 30–40 minutes.

The degree of intraoperative cardiovascular stability helps the anesthesiologist decide whether any patient distress during the first stage of recovery is due to pain or another cause (eg, emergence delirium).

In first-stage recovery, if there is doubt as to why a child is upset, then it should be assumed that the patient is in pain, and this should swiftly be dealt with by administering a fast-acting opiate (eg, fentanyl).

POSTOPERATIVE CARE

Postoperative advice pertaining to protecting the anesthetized area should be given verbally preoperatively and repeated postoperatively, and written instructions should also be given to the family. The family and child should be warned of muscle weakness and diminished sensation. Slings should be provided to pediatric patients with upper-limb blocks. Ambulatory children with lower-limb blocks should have the means to mobilize and travel home arranged. Every institution must have guidelines for in-patient nursing care and monitoring of regional anesthetic techniques, and the staff must receive regular education on managing regional blocks postoperatively and care of the anesthetized extremity. It is generally more economical and safer to place patients receiving regional anesthesia and analgesia on specific wards. (For more information on this topic, see Chapter 45.)

TRAINING

The training of anesthesiologists in pediatric regional anesthesia and anatomy is essential for its successful and safe implementation. Where possible, each department should provide a structured approach to teaching the common simple blocks: caudal, penile, femoral, axillary, ilioinguinal, and rectus sheath. Training should include US scanning and needling techniques. Once basic US needling skills have been learned on phantoms and scanning skills developed on adult volunteers, these skills can then be transferred to the clinical setting. Generally, these techniques are easier and more safely performed on older patients first.

Clinical Pearl

- Where possible, each department should provide a structured approach to teaching the common blocks: caudal, penile, femoral, axillary, ilioinguinal, and rectus sheath.

SUMMARY

Regional anesthesia improves the postoperative experience of both children and parents or caregivers and facilitates the efficient use of hospital facilities and it is expected that the use of regional anesthesia in children will continue to grow in popularity. Regional anesthetic techniques should provide the correct balance between risks and benefits for the children and surgery of today. US is allowing a greater array of peripheral blocks to be safer and reliably used in children. Technology is important, but is not a replacement for a solid understanding of anatomy and a high standard of general safe practice.

REFERENCES

1. Giaufre E, Dalens B, Gombert A: Epidemiology and morbidity of regional anesthesia in children: A one-year prospective survey of the French-Language Society of Pediatric Anesthesiologists. Anesth Analg 1996;83:904–912.
2. Ecoffey C, Lacroix F, Giaufre E et al: Epidemiology and morbidity of regional anesthesia in children: a follow-up one-year prospective survey of the French-Language Society of Pediatric Anesthesiologists (ADARPEF). Pediatr Anesth 2010;20:1061–1069.
3. Taddio A, Katz J, Ilersich AL, Koren G: Effect of neonatal circumcision on pain response during subsequent routine vaccination [see comments]. Lancet 1997;349:599–503.
4. Peutrell JM, Mather SJ: Regional Anaesthesia in Babies and Children. Oxford: Oxford University Press, 1997.
5. Suresh S, Wheeler M: Practical pediatric regional anesthesia. Anesthesiol Clin North Am 2002;20:83–113.
6. Fitzgerald M, Walker SM: Infant pain management: a developmental neurobiological approach. Nat Clin Pract Neurol 2009;5:35–50.
7. Mazoit JX, Dalens BJ: Pharmacokinetics of local anaesthetics in infants and children. Clin Pharmacokinet 2004;43:17–32.
8. Besunder JB, Reed MD, Blumer JL: Principles of drug biodisposition in the neonate. A critical evaluation of the pharmacokinetic–pharmacodynamic interface (Part I). Clin Pharmacokinet 1988;14:189–216.
9. Besunder JB, Reed MD, Blumer JL: Principles of drug biodisposition in the neonate. A critical evaluation of the pharmacokinetic–pharmacodynamic interface (Part II). Clin Pharmacokinet 1988;14:261–286.
10. Mazoit JX, Denson DD, Samii K: Pharmacokinetics of bupivacaine following caudal anesthesia in infants. Anesthesiology 1988;68:387–391.
11. Ecoffey C, Desparmet J, Maury M, et al: Bupivacaine in children: pharmacokinetics following caudal anesthesia. Anesthesiology 1985;63:447–448.
12. Murat I, Montay G, Delleur MM, et al: Bupivacaine pharmacokinetics during epidural anaesthesia in children. Eur J Anaesthesiol 1988;5:113–120.
13. Berde CB: Toxicity of local anesthetics in infants and children. [Review]. J Pediatr 1993;122(Pt 2):S14–S20.
14. Petitjeans F, Mion G, Puidupin M, et al: Tachycardia and convulsions induced by accidental intravascular ropivacaine injection during sciatic block. Acta Anaesthesiol Scand 2002;46:616–617.
15. Ivani G, Mereto N, Lampugnani E, et al: Ropivacaine in paediatric surgery: preliminary results. Paediatr Anaesth 1998;8:127–129.
16. Ivani G, Mazzarello G, Lampugnani E, DeNegri P, Torre M, Lonnqvist PA: Ropivacaine for central blocks in children. Anaesthesia 1998;53(Suppl 2):74–76.
17. Ala-Kokko TI, Partanen A, Karinen J, et al: Pharmacokinetics of 0.2% ropivacaine and 0.2% bupivacaine following caudal blocks in children. Acta Anaesthesiol Scand 2000;44:1099–1102.
18. Dalens B, Ecoffey C, Joly A, et al: Pharmacokinetics and analgesic effect of ropivacaine following ilioinguinal/iliohypogastric nerve block in children. Paediatr Anaesth 2001;11:415–420.
19. Fernandez-Guisasola J, Andueza A, Burgos E, et al: A comparison of 0.5% ropivacaine and 1% mepivacaine for sciatic nerve block in the popliteal fossa. Acta Anaesthesiol Scand 2001;45:967–970.
20. Ivani G, DeNegri P, Lonnqvist PA, et al: A comparison of three different concentrations of levobupivacaine for caudal block in children (table). Anesth Analg 2003;97:368–371.
21. Lerman J, Nolan J, Eyres R, et al: Efficacy, safety, and pharmacokinetics of levobupivacaine with and without fentanyl after continuous epidural infusion in children: a multicenter trial. Anesthesiology 2003;99:1166–1174.
22. Ala-Kokko TI, Raiha E, Karinen J, et al: Pharmacokinetics of 0.5% levobupivacaine following ilioinguinal-iliohypogastric nerve blockade in children. Acta Anaesthesiol Scand 2005;49:397–400.
23. Foster RH, Markham A: Levobupivacaine: a review of its pharmacology and use as a local anaesthetic. Drugs 2000;59:551–579.
24. Mather LE, Huang YF, Veering B, Pryor ME: Systemic and regional pharmacokinetics of levobupivacaine and bupivacaine enantiomers in sheep. Anesth Analg 1998;86:805–811.
25. Tobias JD, O'Dell N: Chloroprocaine for epidural anesthesia in infants and children. AANA J 1995;63:131–135.
26. Raj PP, Ohlweiler D, Hitt BA, Denson DD: Kinetics of local anesthetic esters and the effects of adjuvant drugs on 2-chloroprocaine hydrolysis. Anesthesiology 1980;53:307–314.
27. Tobias JD, Rasmussen GE, Holcomb GW III, et al: Continuous caudal anaesthesia with chloroprocaine as an adjunct to general anaesthesia in neonates. Can J Anaesth 1996;43:69–72.
28. Crowhust JA: Cholinesterase deficiency. Anaesth Intensive Care 1983;11:7–9.
29. Kuhnert BR, Philipson EH, Pimental R, Kuhnert PM: A prolonged chloroprocaine epidural block in a postpartum patient with abnormal pseudocholinesterase. Anesthesiology 1982;56:477–478.
30. Monedero P, Hess P: High epidural block with chloroprocaine in a parturient with low pseudocholinesterase activity. Can J Anaesth 2001;48:318–319.

31. Kuhnert BR, Kuhnert PM, Prochaska AL, Gross TL: Plasma levels of 2-chloroprocaine in obstetric patients and their neonates after epidural anesthesia. Anesthesiology 1980;53:21–25.

32. Henderson K, Sethna NF, Berde CB: Continuous caudal anesthesia for inguinal hernia repair in former preterm infants. J Clin Anesth 1993;5:129–133.

33. Krane EJ, Haberkern CM, Jacobson LE: Postoperative apnea, bradycardia, and oxygen desaturation in formerly premature infants: prospective comparison of spinal and general anesthesia. Anesth Analg 1995;80:7–13.

34. Henderson K, Sethna NF, Berde CB: Continuous caudal anesthesia for inguinal hernia repair in former preterm infants. J Clin Anesth 1993;5:129–133.

35. Suresh S, Cote CJ: Local anesthetics for infants and children. In Yaffe SJ, Aranda JV (eds): *Neonatal and Pediatric Pharmacology, Therapeutic Principles in Practice*, 3rd ed. Philadelphia: Lippincott Williams & Wilkins, 2004.

36. Frumiento C, Abajian JC, Vane DW: Spinal anesthesia for preterm infants undergoing inguinal hernia repair. Arch Surg 2000;135:445–451.

37. Kasten GW, Martin ST: Bupivacaine cardiovascular toxicity: comparison of treatment with bretylium and lidocaine. Anesth Analg 1985;64:911–916.

38. Murat I, Esteve C, Montay G, et al: Pharmacokinetics and cardiovascular effects of bupivacaine during epidural anesthesia in children with Duchenne muscular dystrophy. Anesthesiology 1987;67:249–252.

39. Graf BM: The cardiotoxicity of local anesthetics: the place of ropivacaine. Curr Top Med Chem 2001;1:207–214.

40. Bergman BD, Hebl JR, Kent J, Horlocker TT: Neurologic complications of 405 consecutive continuous axillary catheters (table). Anesth Analg 2003;96:247–252.

41. Berde CB: Convulsions associated with pediatric regional anesthesia [editorial comment] [see comments]. Anesth Analg 1992;75:164–166.

42. Weintraud M, Lundblad M, Kettner SC et al: Ultrasound versus landmark-based technique for ilioinguinal-iliohypogastric nerve blockade in children: the implications on plasma levels of ropivacaine. Anesth Analg 2009;108:1488–1492.

43. Ludot H, Tharin JY, Belouadah M, et al: Successful resuscitation after ropivacaine and lidocaine-induced vebtricular arrhythmia following posterior lumbar plexus block in a child. Anesth Analg 2008;106:1572–1574.

44. Acharya AB, Bustani PC, Phillips JD, et al: Randomised controlled trial of eutectic mixture of local anaesthetics cream for venipuncture in healthy preterm infants. Arch Dis Child Fetal Neonatal Ed 1998;78:F138–F142.

45. Benini F, Johnston CC, Faucher D, Aranda JV: Topical anesthesia during circumcision in newborn infants. JAMA 1993;270:850–853.

46. Gourrier E, Karoubi P, el Hanache A, et al: Use of EMLA cream in a department of neonatology. Pain 1996;68:431–434.

47. Eichenfield LF, Funk A, Fallon-Friedlander S, Cunningham BB: A clinical study to evaluate the efficacy of ELA-Max (4% liposomal lidocaine) as compared with eutectic mixture of local anesthetics cream for pain reduction of venipuncture in children. Pediatrics 2002;109:1093–1099.

48. Jain A, Rutter N: Topical amethocaine gel in the newborn infant: how soon does it work and how long does it last? Arch Dis Child Fetal Neonatal Ed 2000;83:F211–214.

49. Tait AR, Voepel-Lewis T, Malviya S: Do they understand? (Part II): assent of children participating in clinical anesthesia and surgery research. Anesthesiology 2003;98:609–614.

50. Krane EJ, Dalens BJ, Murat I, Murrell D: The safety of epidurals placed during general anesthesia. Reg Anesth Pain Med 1998;23:433–438.

51. Marhofer P, Sitzwohl C, GreherM, Kapral S: Ultrasound guidance for infraclavicular brachial plexus anaesthesia in children. Anaesthesia 2004;59:642–646.

Pediatric Epidural and Spinal Anesthesia & Analgesia

Belen De Jose Maria, Luc Tielens, and Steve Roberts

EPIDURAL ANESTHESIA IN CHILDREN

INTRODUCTION

Epidural analgesia is commonly used in addition to general anesthesia and to manage postoperative pain. Effective postoperative pain relief from epidural analgesia has numerous benefits including earlier ambulation, facilitating weaning from ventilators, reducing time spent in a catabolic state, and lowering circulating stress hormone levels.[1] Precise placement of epidural needles for single-injection techniques and catheters for continuous epidural anesthesia ensures that the dermatomes involved in the surgical procedure are selectively blocked, allowing for lower doses of local anesthetics to be used and sparing unnecessary blockade in nondesired regions. The approach to the epidural space can be at the caudal, lumbar, or thoracic level.

ANATOMY AND PHYSIOLOGICAL IMPLICATIONS

There are significant anatomical differences in children compared with adults that should be considered when using neuraxial anesthesia. For instance, in neonates and infants, the conus medullaris is located lower in the spinal column (at approximately the L3 vertebra) compared with that in adults, in whom it is situated at approximately the L1 vertebra. This is a result of different rates of growth between the spinal cord and the bony vertebral column in infants. However, at

approximately 1 year of age, the conus medullaris reaches the L1 level similar to that in an adult.

Clinical Pearls

- In neonates and infants, the conus medullaris ends approximately the L3 level as opposed to adults, where it is located approximately at the L1 vertebra.
- At approximately 1 year of age, the conus medullaris reaches the L1 level, similar to that in an adult.

The sacrum of children is also more flat and narrow compared with the adult population. At birth, the sacral plate, which is formed by five sacral vertebrae, is not completely ossified and continues to fuse until approximately 8 years of age (although it may take until 21 years of age). There is a 6% incidence of sacral atresia. The incomplete fusion of the sacral vertebral arch forms the sacral hiatus. The caudal epidural space can be accessed easily in infants and children through the sacral hiatus. Because of the continuous development of the sacral canal roof, there is considerable variation in the sacral hiatus. In young children, the sacral hiatus is located more cephalad than in older children, and the dural sac may end more caudally: at S4 in infants younger than 1 year and at S2 in older children. Therefore, because of the increased risk of accidental dural puncture, caution is warranted when placing caudal blocks in infants.

- In young children, the sacral hiatus is located more cephalad than in older children, and the dural sac may end more caudally (at S4 in infants younger than 1 year).
- Caution with the use caudal blocks is warranted in infants because of the risk of dural puncture.

Ultrasound (US) assessment of the neuraxial structures is less challenging in younger children because ossification is less developed. In infants, the spinal cord fibers, the cerebrospinal fluid (CSF), and the dura mater are easily identified using linear high-frequency US probes. It has also been suggested that the epidural fat is less densely packed in children than in adults.[2] The loosely packed epidural fat may facilitate the spread of local anesthetic and help achieve a quicker block onset. It may also allow the unimpeded advancement of epidural catheters from the caudal epidural space to the lumbar and thoracic levels. However, the final placement of a catheter's tip is best monitored directly under US guidance or indirectly by identifying the injection of local anesthetic.

The amount of CSF per body weight is higher in neonates and infants (4 mL/kg) compared with adults (2 mL/kg), and the CSF is localized primarily in the spinal canal. In addition, the spinal cord in neonates is still nonmyelinated, meaning that lower concentrations of local anesthetic can be effectively used.

Because children have a higher cardiac output compared to adults, the systemic absorption of local anesthetic occurs faster. This can lead to toxic plasma levels and a shorter duration of block.

Clinical Pearls

- Compared to older children, the sacral hiatus in neonates is located more cephalad, and the dural sac ends lower, increasing the risk of accidental dural puncture.
- US imaging can be used to evaluate the neuraxial anatomy and the approach to the epidural space.

LOCAL ANESTHETICS FOR EPIDURAL ANESTHESIA IN CHILDREN

Since most pediatric patients receive epidural analgesia in conjunction with a general anesthetic, the main purpose of the epidural catheter is to deliver enough local anesthetic solution for effective intraoperative and postoperative analgesia. As with epidural anesthesia in adults, local anesthetic concentration and volume are important factors in determining the density and level of blockade. However, in pediatric patients, knowledge of total drug dose is also important to avoid local anesthetic toxicity. A more detailed description of local anesthetic solutions, their characteristics, and toxicity potential has been described in Chapter 7.

Bupivacaine, ropivacaine, and levobupivacaine are the most commonly used local anesthetics for neuraxial anesthesia in

children.[3-5] Lidocaine is not often used because of its excessive motor block. As a general rule, high concentrations of local anesthetics, such as 0.5% bupivacaine or 0.5% ropivacaine, are seldom used in epidural blocks in children. Instead, larger volumes of more dilute local anesthetic are more commonly used to cover multiple dermatomes. Body weight is usually a better correlation than patient age in predicting spread of local anesthetic after a caudal block. The maximal safe dose of bupivacaine is 2.5 mg/kg. For caudal use, the optimum concentration of bupivacaine is 0.125%–0.175%.[6] Compared with the 0.25% preparation, this concentration provides a similar duration of postoperative analgesia (4–8 hours) but with less motor blockade. Some clinicians prefer administering doses on a volume-per-weight basis. A dose of 1.0 mL/kg of a dilute solution, such as 0.125% bupivacaine, to a maximum volume of 20 mL can sometimes provide T10 sensory block without exceeding the maximum levels recommended in the literature.[7] In infants, higher volumes, such as 1.25 mL/kg or even 1.5 mL/kg, may be administered to provide a more cephalad block without the risk of local anesthetic toxicity.[7] For continuous epidural infusion, a commonly accepted dosage guideline for bupivacaine is 0.2 mg/kg/h for neonates and 0.4 mg/kg/h for older children.[8] Cumulative toxicity is a concern even at lower rates of local anesthetic solution infusions.[9] Therefore, duration of neonatal epidural infusions should be limited to 48 hours.

Ropivacaine has a higher therapeutic index than the older local anesthetic bupivacaine.[10-12] At low concentrations, ropivacaine may produce less motor block and equivalent analgesia compared to bupivacaine with a decreased incidence of cardiac and central nervous system toxicity. Because of its possible vasoconstricting properties, ropivacaine may undergo slower systemic absorption than bupivacaine.[13,14] This may have clinical implications when a prolonged local anesthetic infusion is used in children with impaired hepatic function.[15] For a single-injection caudal block, a bolus of 1 mL/kg of 0.2% ropivacaine is recommended.[16,17] An infusion of 0.1% ropivacaine at 0.2 mg/kg/h in infants and 0.4 mg/kg/h in older children, lasting no longer than 48 hours, has also been shown to be effective and safe.

Levobupivacaine, the S (–)-isomer of bupivacaine, is less likely to cause myocardial depression and fatal arrhythmias and is also less toxic to the central nervous system than racemic bupivacaine. A dose of 0.8 mL/kg of 0.25% levobupivacaine injected caudally provides analgesia in children having penile or groin surgery.[18] For continuous epidural infusion, the dose for levobupivacaine is similar to that for racemic bupivacaine.

Clinical Pearls

- High concentrations of local anesthetic, such as 0.5% bupivacaine or 0.5% ropivacaine, are not recommended in the pediatric population. As the myelination is not complete, lower concentrations of amino amide local anesthetics are effective (eg, 0.125% levobupivacaine).
- Instead, larger volumes of more dilute local anesthetics are more commonly used to cover several dermatomes of interest.

- In the pediatric patients, body weight provides a better correlation than patient age in predicting spread of local anesthetic after a caudal block.
- A simple rule for a caudal single injection in children under 20 kg is to use bupivacaine 0.125%–0.175% or ropivacaine 0.2% and give a bolus of one of the following:
  - 0.5 ml/kg to achieve a sacral surgical level
  - 1.0 ml/kg to achieve a high lumbar surgical level
  - 1.25 ml/kg to achieve a low thoracic surgical level
- For continuous epidural infusion, bupivacaine 0.125% at a rate of 0.2 mg/kg/h for neonates and 0.4 mg/kg/h for older children is often used. Ropivacaine 0.1% at a rate of 0.2 mg/kg/h for neonates and 0.4 mg/kg/h for older children for 48 hours has been shown to be an effective and safe regimen.

ADJUVANTS FOR EPIDURAL ANESTHESIA IN CHILDREN

A single-injection caudal block with local anesthetic is used primarily for minor surgery because of its limited duration of analgesia. Adjuvants may be used to prolong the duration of blockade, and several drugs have been trialed. The most commonly used adjuvant to local anesthetics has been epinephrine. Epinephrine in a concentration of 1:200,000 is used to decrease the absorption rate of local anesthetic and has the added benefit of serving as a possible marker for an inadvertent intravascular injection. Recent research has focused on the use of a multitude of adjuvants. Midazolam and neostigmine have also been studied; however, there is no evidence that these drugs provide any analgesic benefit when administered epidurally.[19] Opioids, clonidine, and ketamine all deserve more consideration and will therefore discussed in greater detail.

Opioids

Epidural opioids may enhance the effect of local anesthetics and prolong analgesia. However, some opioids may not be advisable in an ambulatory setting because of the potential for respiratory depression and other unacceptable side effects (eg, nausea and vomiting, itching, urinary retention).[20] As a result, the use of caudal epidural opioids in children should be restricted to special clinical situations outside the outpatient setting. A dose of 2 mcg/kg of fentanyl for single-injection caudal anesthesia along with the standard local anesthetic solution has been recommended for more extensive or painful procedures and in patients who have a urinary catheter in the postoperative period. The addition of 1–2 mcg/mL fentanyl to 0.1% bupivacaine for continuous epidural infusions has also been used with success in children in a well-monitored inpatient setting. However, fentanyl should *not* be used in neonatal epidural infusions.

Epidural morphine may also be used for inpatients undergoing major abdominal or thoracic surgery. When added to single-injection caudal epidural blocks, it will enhance the level of blockade because of its rostral dispersion (as morphine is a hydrophilic molecule). Doses of caudal morphine vary from 30–90 mcg/kg depending on the type of surgery. Epidural morphine carries a potential risk for respiratory depression; therefore, continuous pulse oximetry is recommended with lower doses of caudal morphine and is mandatory with medium doses. When higher doses of caudal morphine are used, postoperative admission to intensive care must be planned.[21]

Clonidine

Of the various nonopioid adjuncts used in epidural blocks in children, clonidine offers the best profile.[22] Clonidine is an α_1-agonist and acts by stimulating the descending noradrenergic medullospinal pathways, which inhibits the release of nociceptive neurotransmitters in the dorsal horn of the spinal cord. The addition of clonidine (1–5 mcg/kg) can improve the analgesic effect of local anesthetics for single-injection caudal blockade and prolong the local anesthetic duration of action without the unwanted side effects of epidural opioids. For continuous epidural infusions, clonidine 0.1 mcg/kg/h has been used with good effect.[23] It should be cautioned that higher doses have been associated with sedation and hemodynamic instability in the form of hypotension and bradycardia. With bolus doses of 2 mcg/kg, these side effects are unusual. In addition, epidural clonidine blunts the ventilatory response to increasing levels of end-tidal carbon dioxide (PCO_2). Although respiratory depression does not appear to be a common problem,[24] apnea has been reported in a term neonate who received a caudal block consisting of 1 mL/kg of 0.2% ropivacaine with clonidine 2 mcg/kg.[25] Caution should be exercised when using clonidine in very young infants because of the sedation and hypotension that may ensue.

Ketamine

The addition of S-ketamine[23] to a single-injection caudal block prolongs the analgesic effect of local anesthetics. The main disadvantages of ketamine are its psychomimetic effects. However, at small doses (0.25–0.5 mg/kg), ketamine is effective without noticeable behavioral side effects. Ketamine 1 mg/kg can also be used as an effective caudal analgesic solely without the addition of local anesthetic solution.[26] The combination of S (+)-ketamine (0.5–1 mg/kg) and clonidine (1 or 2 mcg/kg) has been shown to provide effective analgesia after inguinal herniotomy in children with a prolonged duration of effect (> 20 hours) without any adverse central nervous system (CNS) effects or motor impairment.[27] One concern regarding the use of ketamine in neonates relates to a controversial series of animal studies suggesting that ketamine can produce apoptotic neurodegeneration in the developing brain.[28] Other infant animal studies have demonstrated that ketamine may have a neuroprotective effect.[29] Nevertheless, many anesthesiologists are hesitant to introduce caudal S-ketamine into their routine clinical practice, and ketamine is unlikely to be widely adopted in countries where preservative-free formulas are unavailable.

COMPLICATIONS ASSOCIATED WITH EPIDURAL ANESTHESIA

Major complications from either single-injection or continuous epidural blocks are rare if proper technique is used.[30]

Neurologic Injury

A large prospective study, which summarized data from over 15,000 central blocks in children, reported no incidence of permanent neurologic injuries and concluded that the incidence of complications is rare.[31] However, three infant deaths and two other incidences of paraplegia and quadriplegia were reported in another large retrospective report published in 1995 with over 24,000 epidural blocks in children.[32] This study also reported two cases of transient paresthesia. Although the overall risk seems low, devastating complications from direct damage to the spinal cord can occur, particularly with thoracic and high lumbar epidural needle placement. In addition, hypotension can compromise spinal perfusion. Because the placement of epidural needles and catheters is usually performed with the patient under sedation or general anesthesia, the fact that unconscious patients are unable to report pain or paresthesia (the currently accepted warning sign of needle encroachment on the spinal cord) raises concern.[33] Keeping the patient spontaneously breathing while performing the neuraxial block has been suggested as a safety measure. Preprocedural US scanning of the neuraxial anatomy where available is highly recommended to assess depth to the epidural space.

A case report of spinal cord injury after placing a single-injection thoracic epidural under general anesthesia for appendectomy[34] highlights the importance of the routine assessment of the risk–benefit ratio of placing a direct thoracic epidural for less extensive surgery. In particular, the use of thoracic and high lumbar epidural catheter placement should be reserved only for extensive thoracic and abdominal procedures and should be performed by anesthesiologists with experience in thoracic epidural placement.

To minimize the risk of spinal cord injury (and the risk of dural puncture), knowledge of the expected depth of the epidural space is important. As a general rule, the epidural space in children weighing more than 10 kg is found at 1 mm/kg of body weight. There are other formulas based on the patient's body weight or age to calculate this depth. However, the best option is to measure the depth by preprocedural US imaging of the neuraxial anatomy (Table 43–1).

Clinical Pearl

- As a general rule, the epidural space in children weighing more than 10 kg is found at a depth of 1 mm/kg of body weight. However, preprocedural US imaging is useful to determine the depth of the epidural space.

TABLE 43–1. Formulas to determine depth of epidural space from skin.

Note: An individual preprocedural ultrasound assessment is the preferred method of determining the depth of epidural space from the skin.

1. Rough estimate: 1 mm/kg body weight
2. Depth (cm) = 1 + (0.15 × age in years)
3. Depth (cm) = 0.8 + (0.05 × weight in kilograms)

Epidural Hematoma

Epidural hematoma associated with epidural analgesia in children is rare. This may be because anticoagulation protocols are rarely indicated during the perioperative period in pediatric patients. Nonetheless, epidural analgesia should be avoided in patients with clinically significant coagulopathy or thrombocytopenia. Guidelines for the use of epidural anesthesia in adult patients should also be applied in pediatric patients receiving antithrombotic or thrombolytic therapy.[35]

Infection

Although the overall infection rate associated with caudal epidural catheters appears to be low, isolated case reports exist of infection related to epidural catheters in children. Compared with lumbar epidural catheters, there is some concern regarding catheter infection with the prolonged use of caudally placed catheters owing to the proximity of the sacral hiatus to the rectum. Although studies have not found clinical evidence of higher infection rates with the caudal approach, bacterial colonization has been reported to be higher. *Staphylococcus epidermidis* is the predominant microorganism colonized on the skin and catheters of lumbar and caudal epidurals.[36] Gram-negative bacteria have also been found on the tips of caudal catheters. Even with widely used single-injection caudal blocks, infections such as sacral osteomyelitis can still occur.[37] To reduce the risk of contamination by stool and urine, techniques such as catheter tunneling and fixing the catheter with occlusive dressing in a cephalad direction can be used.[38] A strict aseptic technique including the use of a sterile closed-infusion system should also be used, and care should be taken to avoid local tissue trauma. Daily inspection of the dressing and entry site is also important, although the dressing should not be changed unless strictly necessary. If the child develops a persistent fever greater than 38°C of unknown origin, the catheter should be removed and sent for culture.

Dural Puncture and Postdural Puncture Headache

Dural puncture during caudal epidural analgesia is uncommon if caution is taken to avoid advancing the needle too far into the sacral canal. The use of real-time US imaging to control needle position makes this risk extremely low. Treatment for postdural puncture headache (PDPH) includes bed rest, oral or intravenous (IV) hydration, analgesia (eg, regular acetaminophen, nonsteroidal anti-inflammatory drugs [NSAIDs]), and antiemetics. Bed rest, although relieving the severity of the headache, has no effect on the incidence or duration of PDPH.

In adults, caffeine has been used for both the prophylaxis and treatment of PDPH. Caffeine causes cerebral vasoconstriction by blocking adenosine receptors, which dilate vessels when activated. Reducing cerebral blood flow decreases the amount of blood in the brain and may lessen the traction on pain-sensitive intracranial structures, thus relieving PDPH.[39] However, caffeine is not frequently used in children for relief of PDPH, and an optimal dose is unknown.

The use of epidural blood patch to treat PDPH has been used with success in adults since 1960. There are now many reports of its successful use in children as well.[40,41] An epidural blood patch is thought to be effective through the formation of a gelatinous cover over the dural hole by the injected blood. In the short term, the epidural blood patch seals the hole and relieves CSF hypotension both by mass effect from CSF cranial displacement and by increasing intracranial volume and pressure. Actual healing takes place over the longer term. In children, it is recommended that approximately 0.3 mL/kg of autologous blood be injected in the awake or mildly sedated patient, if possible, to detect the appearance of radicular symptoms. A more complete discussion on PDPH is presented in Chapter 27.

Hemodynamic Effects and Total Spinal Anesthesia

Significant changes in blood pressure are uncommon in pediatric patients after the accurate administration of epidural analgesia. A high sympathetic single-injection caudal block to T6 has been found to evoke no significant changes in heart rate, cardiac index, or blood pressure in children.[42] Even when thoracic epidural block is combined with general anesthesia, cardiovascular stability is usually maintained in otherwise healthy pediatric patients. Therefore, hypotension should raise the suspicion of total spinal anesthesia and/or an intravascular injection leading to local anesthetic toxicity. After these complications are ruled out, other causes, such as hydration status, intravascular filling pressure, and inotropic state, and the depth of anesthesia should be assessed.

If total spinal anesthesia has occurred, supportive measures must be provided until the effect of the block has dissipated. However, in the event of a life-threatening extension of a total spinal anesthesia, if attempted supportive measures are neither effective nor an option, cerebrospinal lavage may be considered as a last maneuver. A case report has suggested that 20–30 mL of CSF can be withdrawn and replaced with 30–40 mL of preservative-free normal saline, Ringer's lactate, or Plasmalyte via the epidural catheter.[43] This intervention may shorten recovery time, minimize the potential neurotoxic insult, and reduce the incidence of postdural puncture. However, in light of the limited experience and information on cerebrospinal lavage, the potential risks and benefits should be evaluated on a case-by-case basis before using this technique in children.

Clinical Pearls

- Epidural anesthesia and analgesia in otherwise healthy children rarely causes cardiovascular instability.
- The occurrence of hypotension should raise the suspicion of total spinal anesthesia and/or an intravascular injection leading to local anesthetic toxicity.
- After these complications are ruled out, other causes, such as hydration status, intravascular filling pressure, and inotropic state, and the depth of anesthesia should be assessed.

Local Anesthetic Systemic Toxicity

Local anesthetic systemic toxicity (LAST) often stems from accidental intravascular injection into epidural blood vessels. This complication can often be avoided by using careful aspiration and test dosing. Table 43–2 summarizes recommendations for test dosing in epidural blockade. For a single-injection caudal block, vascular puncture and local anesthetic absorption are more likely to occur when sharp-tipped needles are used. For continuous epidural infusion, neonates and very young infants are at greater risk for local anesthetic toxicity than older children. Seizures have been reported in children receiving continuous infusions of local anesthetics. This can be avoided by

---

TABLE 43–2. Test dosing for epidural blockade.

1. Use test dosing routinely, even though test dosing for all available agents is not 100% sensitive. In addition, because the true incidence of intravascular placement is relatively low, most positive tests (ie, heart rate increases) will be false-positives. When there is a borderline response, repeating the test dose increases the specificity and sensitivity of the test.

2. Continuously monitor the ECG, and cycle the blood pressure cuff repeatedly. With epinephrine-containing solutions, if the heart rate does not increase, an increase in blood pressure should raise suspicion of intravascular placement.

3. Avoid performing test dosing when the child is in a very light plane of anesthesia or when there is stimulation (eg, repositioning the patient on the operating table, instrumentation of the airway, incision). Performing the test dose under these conditions increases the likelihood of false-positive, stimulation-induced increases in heart rate or blood pressure.

4. After the test dose, the remainder of the full dose should be administered incrementally. Incremental dosing and continuous monitoring help increase the odds that an intravascular placement will be detected and that further injection will be halted before full cardiodepressant doses are administered.

5. Whenever possible, keep the patient under spontaneous ventilation throughout the placement and initial dosing of the epidural blockade. Any change in the patient's breathing pattern is an alert that an inadvertent intravascular or intrathecal injection may have taken place: tachypnea if pain on injection; respiratory depression if there has been systemic absorption of local anesthetic; or tachypnea followed by bradypnea caused by total spinal anesthesia if local anesthetic has been administerd intrathecally.

ECG, electrocardiogram.

using dilute solutions of local anesthetics ($\leq$ 0.125% bupivacaine) and by following current dosing recommendations (see "Local Anesthetics for Epidural Anesthesia in Children," above).[44] More importantly, vigilant monitoring during the administration of epidural analgesia should be a priority. Guidelines for LAST treatment[45] should be readily accessible in all hospital areas where local anesthetics are used. All personnel of wards where patients undergoing epidural infusion are cared for should be trained in the recognition of symptoms and treatment of LAST. In addition, a complete record of the regional technique and infusion used in each case should be present alongside the patient's observations chart.

Other Adverse Effects

In a retrospective review based on prospective collected data from 286 pediatric patients, pruritus (26.1%), nausea and vomiting (16.9%), and urinary retention (20.8%) were the most common side effects encountered during epidural anesthesia using an infusion of bupivacaine and fentanyl.[46] Sedation and excessive block each occurred in less than 2% of patients. The incidence of respiratory depression was 4.2%, but the administration of naloxone for severe respiratory depression was never necessary. Perforation of the rectum may occur if the caudal needle is angled too steeply. Table 43–3 summarizes the recommended treatments for common adverse effects.

EPIDURAL BLOCKADE FOR PEDIATRIC SURGERY: TECHNIQUES

Epidural analgesia can be delivered via a single-injection or continuous-infusion technique. The needles and catheters can be inserted at the caudal, lumbar, or thoracic level. The main goal of the epidural technique is to accurately position the needle and/or catheter in the epidural space. Aspiration tests and test doses indicate possible inadvertent intravascular or intrathecal drug administration. Epidural stimulation, epidural electrocardiogram (ECG), and US techniques have been developed in addition to conventional X-ray imaging to assist with accurate epidural needle or catheter placement.

Confirmation of Proper Epidural Needle or Catheter Placement

Aspiration and Test Dose

An aspiration test performed before local anesthetic injection is used to avoid total spinal and intravascular injections. However, a negative aspiration of blood or CSF should not be considered an absolute indicator of proper needle and catheter placement. Veins are so small they may collapse easily on aspiration; therefore, it is recommended to use a 2-mL syringe, aspirate slowly, and consider opening to air to look for free flow.

TABLE 43–3. Summary of recommended treatments of effects in epidural blocks.

Itching
1. Exclude and/or correct other remediable causes.
2. Use low-dose naloxone infusions, partial agonist–antagonists (eg, nalbuphine), or antihistamines.
3. If itching persists, remove the opioid from the epidural infusion, and consider clonidine.

Nausea
1. Exclude and/or correct other remediable causes.
2. Use 5-HT antagonists (eg, ondansetron, dolasetron)
3. Use low-dose naloxone infusions or nalbuphine.
4. Avoid opioids in infusions, and consider clonidine.

Ileus and bowel dysfunction
1. Exclude and/or correct other remediable causes.
2. Give laxatives if not otherwise contraindicated.
3. Avoid opioids in infusions, and consider clonidine.
4. Use low-dose naloxone infusions or nalbuphine.
5. Use peripherally or enterally constrained opioid antagonists; for example, methylnaltrexone or alvimopan (currently investigational).

Sedation or hypoventilation
1. Exclude and/or correct other remediable causes.
2. Depending on severity, reduce or hold dosing of opioids or clonidine.
3. Awaken, stimulate, and encourage deep breathing.
4. If severe, consider naloxone or assisted ventilation as needed.

Urinary retention
1. Exclude and/or correct other remediable causes.
2. Avoid using anticholinergics or antihistaminics if alternatives are available.
3. Use low-dose naloxone infusions or nalbuphine.
4. Use bladder catheterization.

The patient's ECG should be continuously monitored while injecting local anesthetic into the caudal space. The ECG specificity changes (ie, > 25% increase in T wave) after the injection of an epinephrine test dose (0.5 mcg/kg) can help predict intravascular injection.[47]

If possible, the patient should be kept under spontaneous ventilation throughout the placement and initial dosing of the epidural blockade. Any change in the patient's breathing pattern is an alert that something might accidentally be happening: respiratory depression if there is systemic absorption of local anesthetic; tachypnea if there is pain on injection; or tachypnea followed by bradypnea if there has been an intratechal administration of local anesthetic (see Table 43–2). Table 43–4 summarizes various methods for confirming epidural catheter placement.

Radiographic Methods

X-ray imaging in conjunction with a contrasting agent precisely identifies the tip of the catheter at a specific spinal level.[47]

TABLE 43–4. Confirmation of epidural catheter position.

Intraoperatively (while the patient is under general anesthesia)

1. Ultrasonography is highly recommended to assess the spread of local anesthetic at the tip of catheter or within the epidural space.
2. Ensure negative aspiration; inject the local anesthetic slowly in small increments through the catheter; and evaluate response to surgery. If possible, maintain spontaneous ventilation.
3. Radiography with contrast.
4. Electrical stimulation and/or ECG technique.

Postoperatively (while the patient is awake, whether or not he or she can give verbal responses)

1. Ultrasonography is the currently recommended method. This is painless and can be done in the PACU without bothering the child too much.
2. If US is not available, the chloroprocaine test can be used. This involves incremental dosing of a chloroprocaine 3% solution to demonstrate analgesia (by self-report or behavioral measures as appropriate) *and* signs of segmental effect:
   a. Lumbar catheter tip:
      • At least partial sensory and motor blockade in both legs
      • Warming of the volar surface of the toes
   b. Lower thoracic catheter tip:
      • Reduced strength in hip flexion
      • Reduced abdominal skin reflexes
      • Some reduction in heart rate and blood pressure
   c. Upper thoracic catheter tip:
      • Some reduction in heart rate and blood pressure
      • Warming of the volar surface of the hands
      • Unilateral or bilateral Horner syndrome

ECG, electrocardiogram; PACU, post-anesthesia care unit.

A radiograph without contrast, however, cannot distinguish inadvertent intrathecal or subdural catheter placement from correct epidural placement. In addition, standard X-ray does not allow the anesthesiologist to adjust the position of the catheter during insertion unless fluoroscopy is used. Although fluoroscopy allows for real-time monitoring and adjustment of advancing catheters, it requires additional set-up, incurs increased expense, and increases the patient's exposure to ionizing radiation. As a result, fluoroscopy is not routinely recommended and is usually limited to difficult and/or special circumstances, such as long-term epidural catheter placement for cancer pain.

Epidural Stimulation Test (Tsui Test) and Epidural ECG Technique

A low-current electrical stimulation test (the Tsui test; Figure 43–1) has been suggested to monitor and guide the position of the epidural catheter during insertion.[48,49] The setup requires the cathode lead (*b*lack for *b*lock) of the nerve stimulator to be connected to the epidural catheter via an electrode adapter while the anode lead is connected to an electrode on the patient's skin as the grounding site. To avoid misinterpretation of the stimulation response (eg, a local muscle contraction may be confused with epidural stimulation), the grounded electrode is placed on the lower extremity for thoracic epidurals and on the upper extremity for lumbar epidurals. Correct placement of the epidural catheter tip (1–2 cm from the nerve roots) is indicated by a motor response elicited with a current between 1 mA and 10 mA. A motor response observed with a significantly lower threshold current (< 1 mA) suggests that the catheter is in the subarachnoid or subdural space or is in close proximity to a nerve root.[50,51] Although chronic spinal cord stimulation is a safe and effective means of pain management, the safety of this epidural stimulation test is not completely known. However, it is anticipated that the risk of a brief intermittent electrical stimulation from this test is minimal. Table 43–5 summarizes the different catheter locations according to motor response and electrical current.

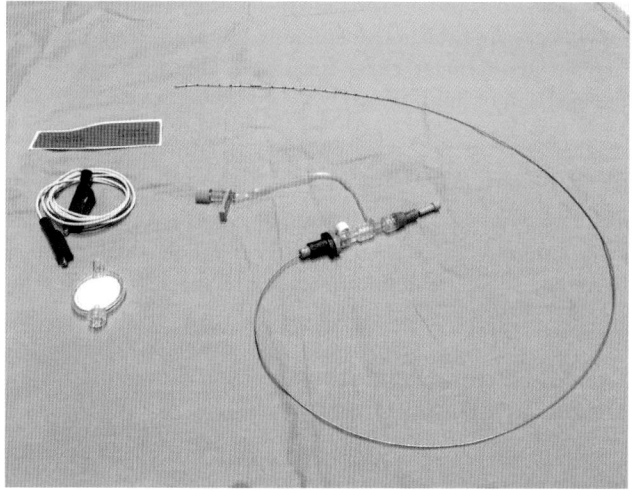

FIGURE 43–1. Tsui stimulating epidural catheter kit.

TABLE 43–5. Electrical stimulation test.

Catheter Location	Motor Response	Current
Subcutaneous	None	> 10 mA
Subdural	Bilateral (many segments)	< 1 mA
Subarachnoid	Unilateral or bilateral	< 1 mA
Epidural space		
Against nerve root	Unilateral	< 1 mA
Nonintravascular	Unilateral or bilateral	1–10 mA (threshold current increase after LA injection)
Intravascular	Unilateral or bilateral	1–10 mA (no change in threshold current after LA injection)

LA, local anesthetic.

One disadvantage of the epidural stimulation technique is that it cannot reliably be performed if any significant clinical neuromuscular blockade is present or if local anesthetics have been administered in the epidural space. To overcome this limitation, an alternative monitoring technique using ECG monitoring has been suggested.[52] A reference ECG is monitored at the required spinal level for surgery; this is then compared to the ECG formed from the epidural catheter tip as it is threaded cephalad. Unfortunately, this technique cannot easily differentiate subtle QRS complexes where the catheter is threaded a short distance; neither does it recognize intravascular or intrathecal catheter positioning.

Ultrasound-Guided Techniques

Since the main goal of an epidural block is to accurately place the needle and/or catheter in the epidural space, knowledge of the expected depth from the skin surface to the epidural space is extremely important. Table 43–1 summarizes some formulas to calculate this depth in children. Where available, US allows for the real-time identification of anatomical landmarks and a much more precise estimation of epidural space depth. It is highly recommended to scan the anatomy with ultrasonography in all children before performing the block and especially in difficult cases, such as patients with scoliosis or sacral dimples. US also allows for needle visualization[53] within the epidural space in neonates. In infants, US can detect epidural catheter advancement, either directly or indirectly by observing the injection of fluid.[54]

Epidural Approaches

The most common types of epidural analgesia are caudal analgesia (which constitutes the most commonly used regional technique in children), lumbar epidural analgesia, and thoracic epidural analgesia.

Caudal Epidural Analgesia: Single-Injection Technique

Single-injection caudal epidural blockade is widely used to provide perioperative analgesia in pediatric practice. As a single injection, it offers a reliable and effective block for patients undergoing urologic, general, and orthopedic surgery involving the lower abdomen and lower limbs. A single-injection caudal epidural may not be suitable for every case because it has a limited dermatomal distribution and a short duration of action. New local anesthetics and adjuvants, as well as continuous catheter approaches, may overcome these limitations.

Choice of Needle for Caudal Analgesia   A variety of needles are available for single-injection caudal blockade. The size or type of needle does not appear to affect the rate of success or the incidence of complications of caudal blockade. Short-bevel Tuohy or Crawford needles (5 cm in length) with stylets offer a better tactile sensation when the sacrococcygeal ligament is punctured. For children aged 1 year or older, a 22-gauge needle is used; for children younger than 1 year of age, a 25-gauge needle may be used. The use of a styletted needle may reduce the risk of introducing a dermal plug into the caudal space,[55] although an epidermal cell graft tumor in the epidural space has yet to be reported. Some authors advocate the use of a 22-gauge angiocath, suggesting that it is easier to detect intravascular placement and intraosseous placement with this needle. The angiocath is used only for the single-injection caudal block and is withdrawn after the dose is administered (ie, it is not intended to be an epidural caudal catheter). To avoid tissue coring with the angiocath, the needle must be removed before any injection is made.

Technique for Performing a Single-Injection Caudal Epidural Block   In all children, it is important to ensure adequate prevention of heat loss during the procedure. In infants, we recommend preventing heat loss with a sterile transparent drape as this will also allow visualization of patient's breathing (Figure 43–2). The patient is placed in a lateral decubitus position with the neck flexed and the knees drawn up to the chest. After proper positioning, the landmarks for caudal epidural block (Figure 43–3) are easily identified in children: Initially the coccyx is identified, and, continuing to palpate in the midline in a cephalad fashion, the sacral cornua can be felt on either side of the midline approximately 1 cm apart. The sacral hiatus is felt as a depression between two bony prominences of the sacral cornua. Under sterile conditions,

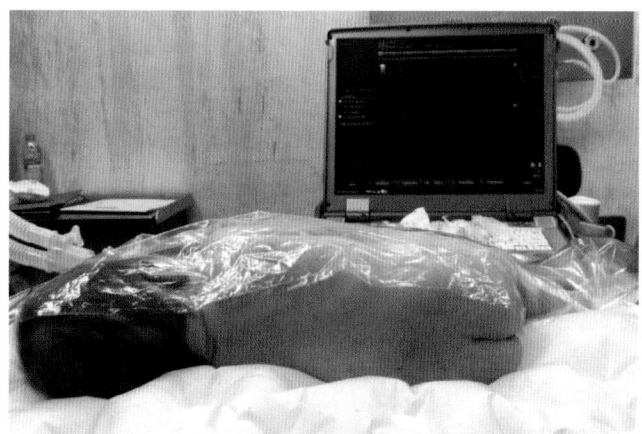

FIGURE 43–2. Transparent cover used in neonates and infants to allow for visualization of the patient and to prevent heat loss. The US machine is placed on the opposite side.

the needle is inserted and advanced into the sacral hiatus at approximately a 70-degree angle to the skin until a distinctive "pop" is felt as the sacrococcygeal ligament is punctured. After this puncture, the angle of the needle should be reduced to approximately 20–30 degrees while the needle is advanced 2–4 mm into the caudal canal. Any advancement past this point is not recommended because the risk of inadvertent dural puncture increases significantly. If an angiocath is used, the plastic catheter should be easily advanced over the needle into the caudal epidural space.

Clinical Pearl

- Care should be taken to ensure the prevention of heat loss during the procedure.

US[56–58] can be used to assess the caudal anatomy prior to the landmark-based technique or to guide needle placement. Pre-assessment is particularly useful in screening children with

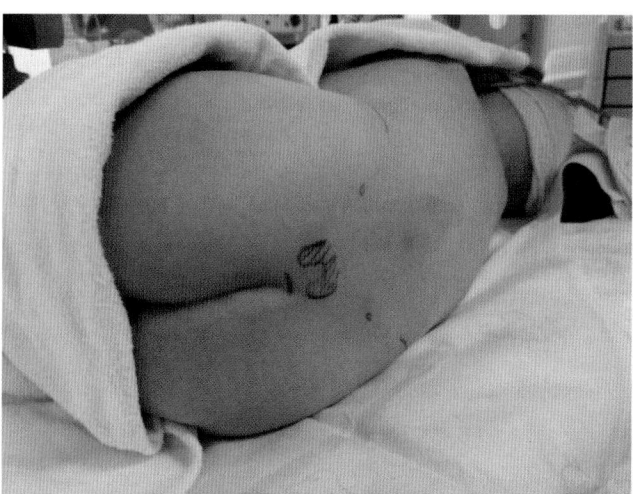

FIGURE 43–3. Patient positioning and landmarks for a caudal block.

cutaneous stigmata of spinal dysraphism. The patient is placed in the lateral decubitus position with the knees flexed toward the chest. The US machine is placed opposite the operator so that he or she can look over his or her hands toward the screen. The patient is prepared, and the US probe is sterilely covered. A high-frequency probe is used: A linear hockey-stick probe is used in infants, whereas a probe with a large footprint is preferable in children weighing more than 10 kg, as it allows more intervertebral spaces to be imaged at a time in the sagittal plane.

The probe is positioned first in a transverse plane at the sacrum level; this is called the short-axis view (SAX). The exact position of the cornua and the sacrococcygeal membrane (SCM) are defined (Figure 43–4). With the sacrococcygeal membrane in the middle of the image (Figure 43–5), the probe is then rotated 90 degrees into a midline sagittal position over the lower sacrum, which is called the long-axis view (LAX; Figure 43–6). The SCM and the ventral and dorsal layer of the os sacrum, with the caudal epidural space in between, are easily identified. In small children, the dural sac may be visible in this position, although in older children you need to scan more in a more cephalad direction (Figure 43–7). These movements can be performed in the opposite order, but a complete exploration of the space in both axes is recommended.

After this preprocedural US assessment of the caudal anatomy, the needle can be introduced into the sacral hiatus with the probe in either axis. If the probe is held in the SAX, the needle insertion will be automatically in the out-of-plane (OOP) approach (Figure 43–8). If the probe is held in the LAX, the needle insertion will then be in the in-plane (IP) approach (Figure 43–9).

The needle insertion angle is noted during the scan. The needle may be advanced 2–4 mm into the caudal space, and the stylet is removed. To ensure optimal caudal placement of the needle, a small bolus of saline or local anesthetic is

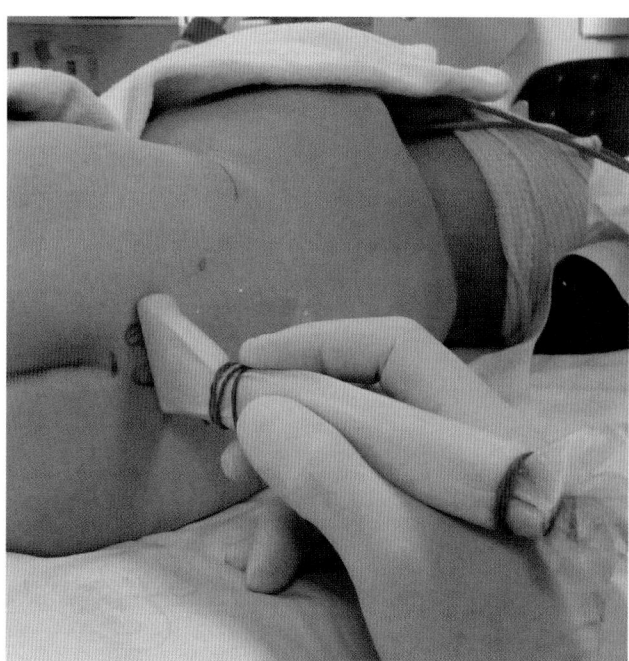

FIGURE 43–4. US probe in the short-axis view.

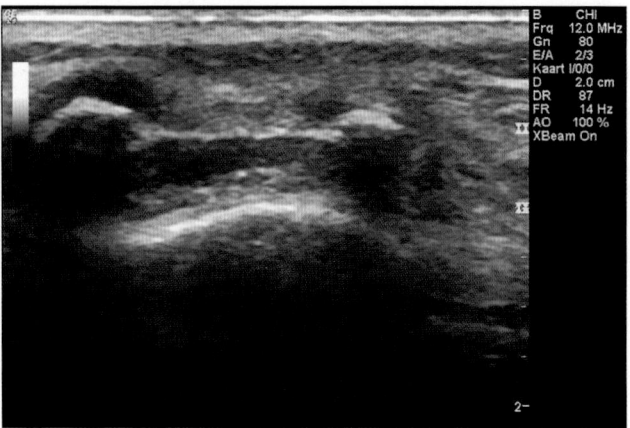

FIGURE 43–5. US image in the short-axis view showing the sacral cornea and sacrococcygeal membrane.

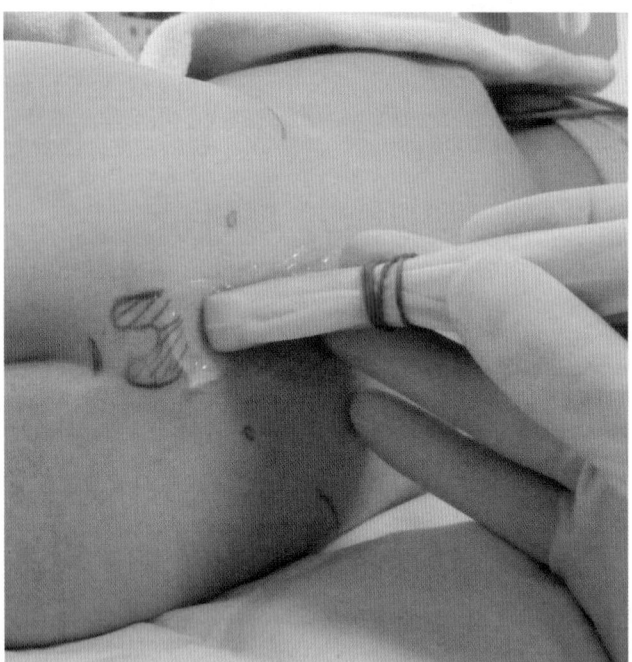

FIGURE 43–6. US probe in the long-axis view.

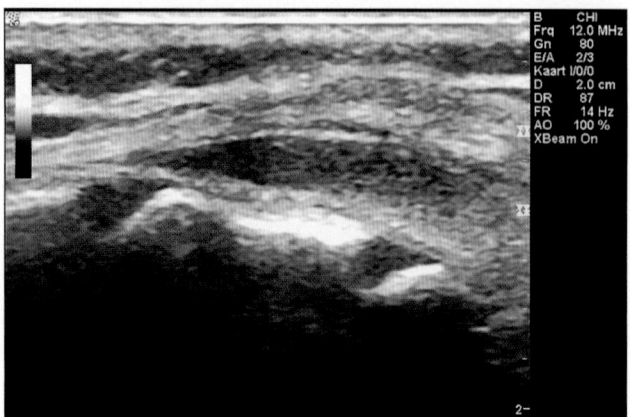

FIGURE 43–7. US image in the long-axis view showing the sacrococcygeal membrane and caudal epidural space in the os sacrum.

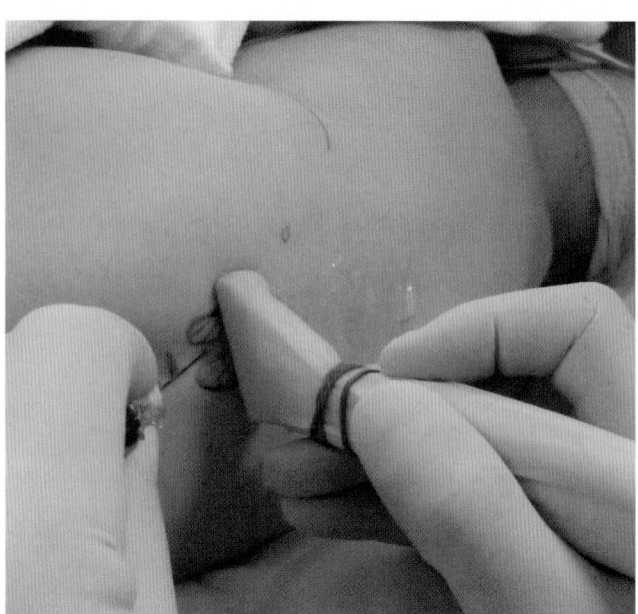

FIGURE 43–8. US probe in the short-axis view and out-of-plane needle insertion.

administered under US guidance with the probe in midline (LAX; Figure 43–10). The probe is positioned as cephalic as needed to visualize the dural sac in the US screen (Figure 43–11). When the injection starts, you will notice the dura being displaced ventrally, especially in younger children. The spread of local anesthetic can be monitored by moving the probe cephalic up the spine in the midline or in a paramedian sagittal axis (Figure 43–12). The same dura movement can be visualized with the probe in the SAX in the more cephalic positions (Figures 43–13 and 43–14).

Confirmation of Correct Local Anesthetic Distribution   The classic "pop" felt as the SCM is pierced is usually sought to confirm proper caudal needle placement.

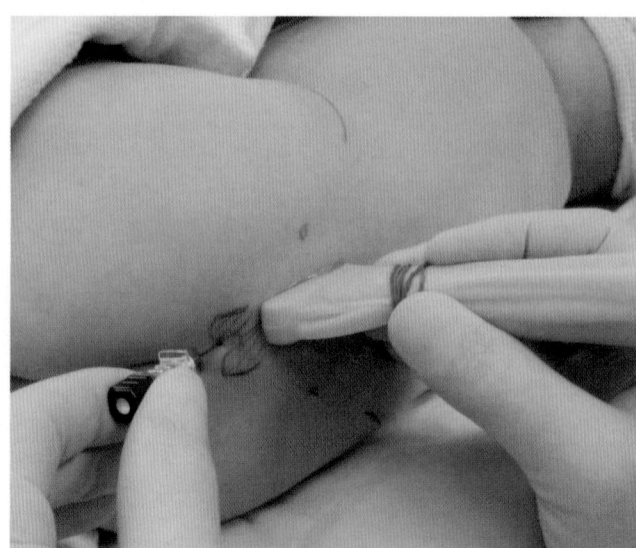

FIGURE 43–9. US probe in the long-axis view and in-plane needle insertion.

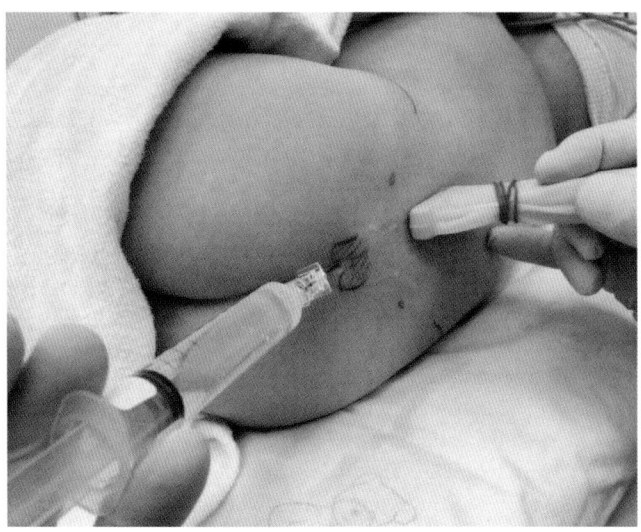

FIGURE 43-10. US-guided injection.

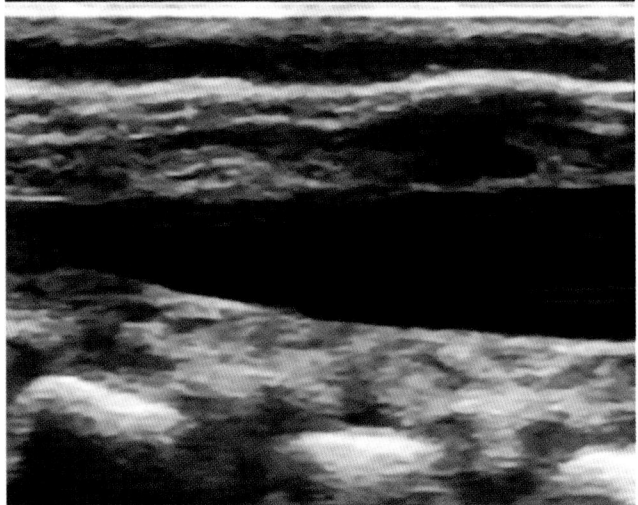

FIGURE 43-11. Dural sac visualized before injection in the long-axis view.

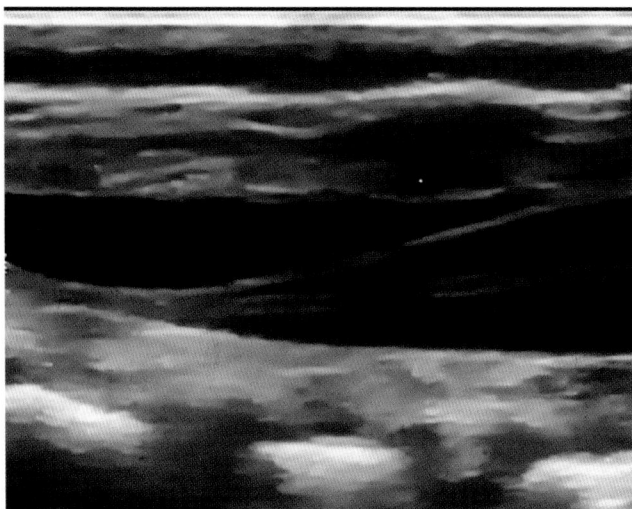

FIGURE 43-12. Dura movement following injection in the long-axis view.

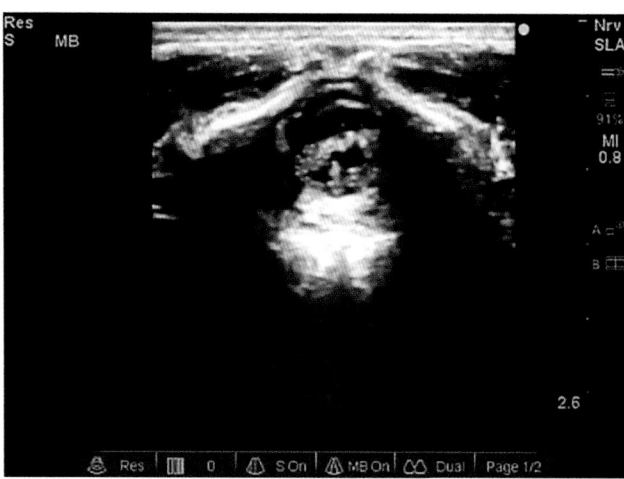

FIGURE 43-13. Dura visualized before injection in the short-axis view.

The absence of subcutaneous bulging and the lack of resistance upon injection are additional signs of correct needle placement and local anesthetic distribution. Aspiration of the needle should be clear of blood and CSF, and a negative response to a test dose of epinephrine should also be used to rule out intravascular placement. US has been used to provide real-time needle guidance into the caudal space and to assess the spread of local anesthetic.[59] Recent US studies have shown that the volume of local anesthetic does not correlate with its cranial spread during caudal blockade in infants and children.[60] Initially, US assessment of the spread of local anesthetic was thought to be a predictor of the dermatome reached, but this proved not to be the case as the majority of caudal blocks are successful despite an immediately monitored lack of spread cephalad. However, it has been found that there is a secondary spread of local anesthetic in the epidural space.[61,62] This occurs in two patterns: a horizontal intrasegmental redistribution from the dorsal to ventral epidural space and a delayed longitudinal cranial spread as the dura returns to its original position, thus pushing the epidural local anesthetic cephalad. The observed

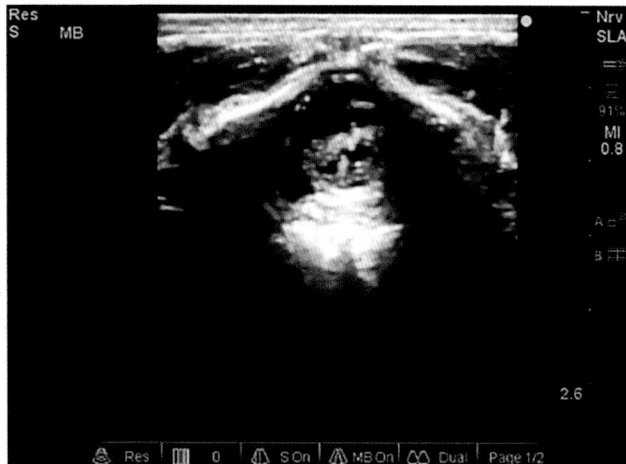

FIGURE 43-14. Dura movement following injection in the short-axis view.

bidirectional movement of CSF (referred to as the "CSF rebound mechanism") also helps explain a component of the difference between the initial US-assessed spread and the final more cephalad effect determined by cutaneous testing. More studies with ultrasonography are needed to determine how best to predict in the spread of local anesthetic.

Caudal Epidural Analgesia: Continuous Technique

Continuous caudal epidural analgesia overcomes the limited duration and segmental effect of a single-injection technique. Caudal catheters can be advanced to the lumbar or thoracic level.[63] The technique for needle insertion for continuous caudal analgesia is very similar to the single-injection caudal approach. It can be done with an IV catheter (an 18-gauge angiocatheter for a 20-gauge epidural catheter or a 16-gauge angiocatheter for a 19-gauge epidural catheter) or with an 18-gauge Crawford or Tuohy needle inserted through the sacrococcygeal membrane, as described for the single-injection technique. The epidural catheter is then advanced carefully from the caudal space to the target level. Minor resistance to the passage of the catheter can usually be overcome by simple flexion or extension of the patient's vertebral column and/or by simultaneously injecting normal saline through the catheter. Some authors[64] use a specialized stimulation epidural catheter (the Epidural Positioning System using the Tsui test, Arrow International Inc., Reading, PA).

It is extremely important to know where the tip of the catheter is finally located: too low a catheter tip level will result in poor analgesia; too high may cause respiratory depression. However, because catheters don't travel linearly in the epidural space, measuring the length of the catheter against the patient's back does not accurately determine the targeted surgical level. Therefore, the location of the catheter tip should be verified using an objective test, as described as in the previous section (ie, radiography, nerve stimulation, electrocardiography, or, preferably, US).

These techniques may be considered cumbersome or redundant, and in children above 1 year of age, the development of a lumbar curve during infancy might prevent easy cephalad advancement of the catheter. Therefore, some have suggested that caudal catheter placement should be limited to patients younger than 1 year of age. It is the opinion of the authors that, at least in children older than 1 year of age, catheters should be placed as close to the surgical dermatome as possible. Appropriate pediatric and ultrasonographic training is therefore recommended in all cases and mandatory prior to performing lumbar or thoracic epidurals in young children.

Lumbar Epidural Anesthesia

Lumbar epidural analgesia is commonly used for continuous infusions and is rarely used as a single-injection technique. A direct lumbar approach is indicated primarily for pain control during and after lower extremity surgery. Lumbar epidural placement, particularly in young children, is performed after the induction of general anesthesia. However, this approach may also be performed awake in a select group of cooperative children and adolescents. Caution should be exercised whenever performing lumbar epidural analgesia above the level of spinal cord end to avoid direct needle trauma.

A midline approach to lumbar epidural needle placement is preferred. Identification of the epidural space is commonly achieved by loss of resistance (LOR) to saline. LOR to air should be avoided due to the risk of introducing a venous air embolism, particularly in neonates and infants. Children should be positioned in the lateral decubitus position for direct lumbar epidural placement. In children over 1 year of age, an 18-gauge, 5-cm Tuohy needle, marked every 0.5 cm, with a 20-gauge epidural catheter is often used. In children under 1 year of age, a 20-gauge, 5-cm Tuohy needle, marked every 0.5 cm, with a 22-gauge catheter should be considered. However, these narrower catheters get kinked, occlude, and leak more often. Although identification of the intervertebral space and ligamentum flavum in most pediatric patients is easy, the ligamentum flavum can be less tensile in children; hence a distinctive "pop" may not be easily felt when penetrating this layer. In addition, the distance from the skin to the epidural space can be very superficial. Formulas for estimating the distance from skin to epidural space have been proposed (see Table 43–1). However, formulas are only a guideline and change according to the angle of epidural needle placement. Today, the best available method to assess the epidural depth is US imaging. With the probe in a paramedian oblique sagittal plane, the distance from the skin to the ligamentum flavum is measured with the US machine's caliper. This measurement provides a good estimate of the depth at which the LOR is going to be felt. Therefore, a preprocedural US assessment of each individual patient is highly recommended.

For an exact description of the lumbar epidural technique, see "Thoracic Epidural Anesthesia," below (figures illustrate a thoracic epidural placement).

Lumbar-to-Thoracic Epidural Approach   Catheters placed via the lumbar route may be advanced cephalad to thoracic vertebral levels. Similar to the problems encountered when advancing catheters in the caudal space in older children, significant resistance also prevents the easy advancement of lumbar epidural catheters to the thoracic levels. Despite favorable results using stimulation via a caudal approach, only one case report[65] has demonstrated the successful placement of a thoracic epidural catheter via the lumbar route with epidural stimulation guidance. Therefore, the authors recommend placing the catheter as close as possible to the surgical site.

Thoracic Epidural Analgesia

Controversy exists concerning the safety of placing thoracic epidurals under heavy sedation or general anesthesia, because unconscious patients are unable to report symptoms that may warn the anesthesiologist of potential neurologic complications.[66] Direct needle trauma to the spinal cord during epidural insertion is rare but can cause devastating complications. Reports have detailed cases of direct needle trauma to the spinal cord during epidural placement in both awake and anesthetized patients.[34,67,68] For thoracic surgery, the catheter should be introduced as close to the dermatomal level of incision as is possible.

The advancement of catheters from the lumbar and caudal epidural spaces to the thoracic level is an alternative only in children upto 1 year of age. However, the advancement of catheters in the epidural space becomes increasingly difficult with advancing age because of the development of the lumbar curvature.

Direct placement of thoracic epidural catheters is more common at tertiary care centers, where well-trained pediatric anesthesiologists perform the blocks on children undergoing major surgery. Preprocedural ultrasonography imaging is strongly recommended.[69] Moreover, the authors believe that training in US-assisted thoracic epidurals should be provided for anesthesiologists willing to perform thoracic epidurals in children.

Clinical Pearls

- Children require a significantly higher volume (dose) of local anesthetic compared with adults to achieve the same dermatomal spread.
- Intended high thoracic catheter advancement from a lumbar insertion site is rarely successful.
- Thoracic epidural catheter insertion should be performed only by practitioners experienced in pediatric thoracic epidural technique.
- Epidural needle insertion in pediatric patients can be performed at any thoracic interspace using either a midline or paramedian approach; however, a midline approach is often preferred.

Thoracic Epidural Analgesia: Midline Approach

The use of the midline approach offers the advantage of being similar to the lumbar approach (with the needle angulated in only one plane). Using the midline approach, insertion of the needle is easier at the lower thoracic level (T10–T12) than at the midthoracic (T4–T7) level. The lower border of the shoulder blade, which is level with the seventh thoracic vertebra, is commonly used as an anatomical landmark. The patient is placed in the lateral decubitus position, and care is taken to prevent heat loss. An assessment of the patient's anatomy may be done in a nonsterile set-up before the block is performed; this is also helpful for teaching purposes. The spinous process of the targeted vertebral level should be identified by counting up from Tuffier's line and by counting down from the most prominent C7 cervical vertebra (Figure 43–15). Preprocedural US imaging is performed with the probe in three planes: transverse (SAX), median sagittal (median LAX), and paramedian oblique sagittal (paramedian oblique LAX). The distance from the patient's skin to the epidural space can thus be measured.

In the SAX (Figure 43–16), the window between two spinous processes must be found, and the anterior complex of the vertebral column (posterior longitudinal ligament, anterior dura, and vertebral body) in the depth of the image will be the first structures to be identified. The posterior complex (ligamentum flavum and posterior dura) may be more difficult to visualize but will be approximately at the level of the lamina (Figure 43–17).

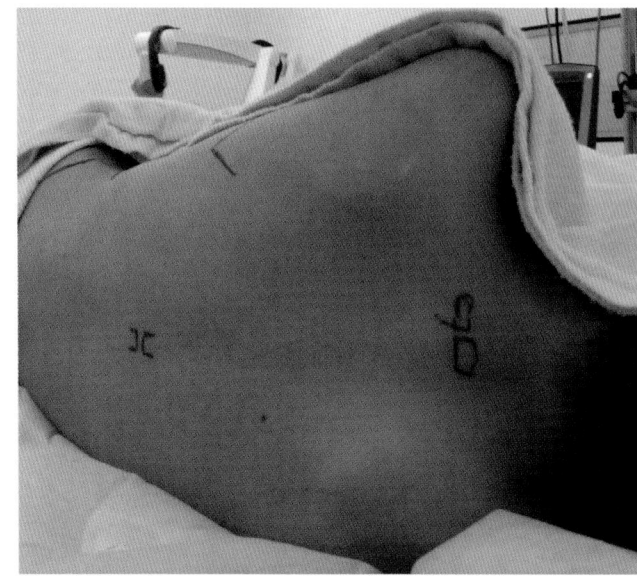

FIGURE 43–15. Thoracic epidural analgesia: patient positioning and landmarks for a midline approach.

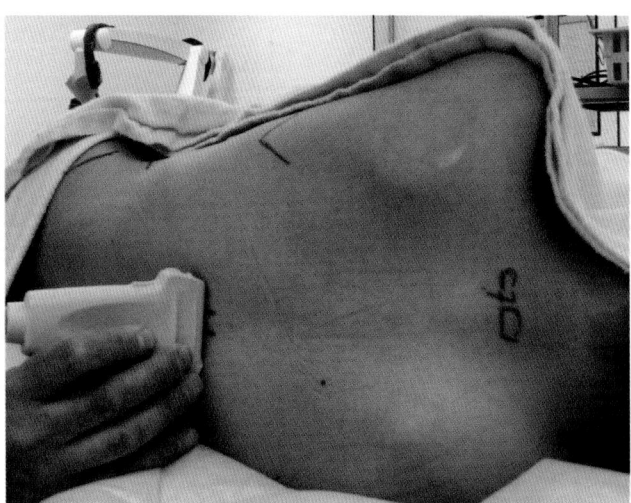

FIGURE 43–16. Preprocedural scanning with nonsterile set-up for teaching purposes; the US probe is in the short-axis view.

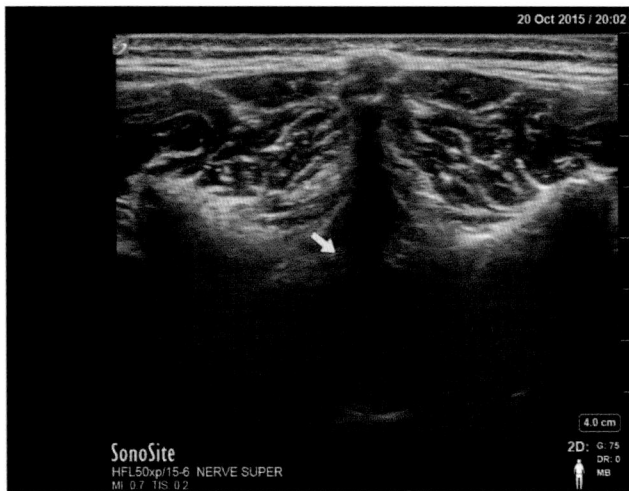

FIGURE 43–17. US image in the short-axis view, showing the posterior complex with the dura (white arrow).

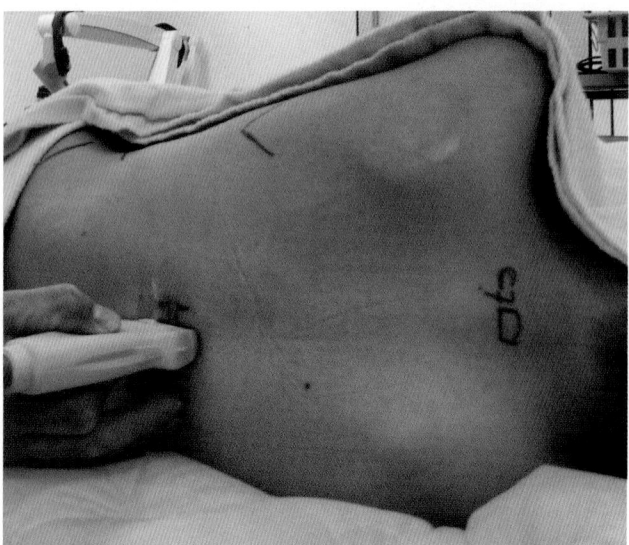

FIGURE 43–18. Preprocedural scanning with nonsterile set-up for teaching purposes; the US probe is in the median long-axis view. The probe must be exactly in the midline, but in this photo, it has been positioned in the paramedian long-axis view to see the direction.

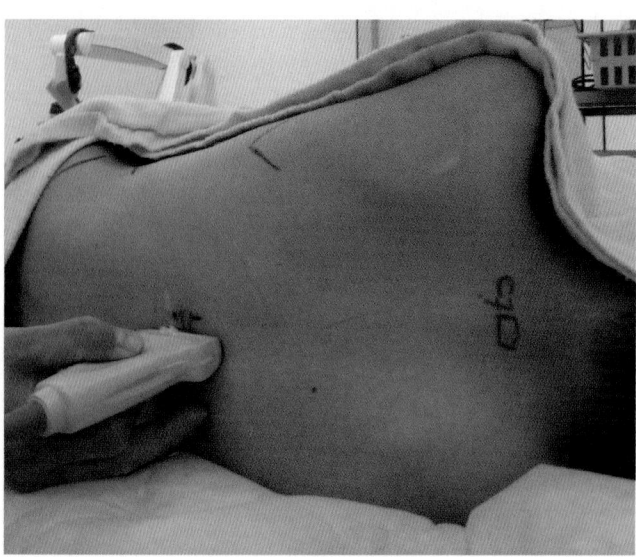

FIGURE 43–20. Preprocedural scanning with nonsterile set-up for teaching purposes; the US probe is in the paramedian oblique long-axis view. The tilting of the probe can be compared to that shown in Figure 43–16.

If the patient is an infant, and the bony structures of the vertebral column are not yet fully ossified, a median LAX (Figure 43–18) provides clear, real-life imaging of the anatomy involved. With this probe position, the spinous process in the image will almost reach the skin (or the top of the US screen). In between the spinous process, the dura mater will be seen as a white double layer; it is found a little less deep than the level at which the posterior complex is found in the SAX (Figure 43–19).

In the paramedian oblique LAX (Figure 43–20), the transverse process and/or the lamina may be visualized, depending on how far lateral and oblique the probe is placed. The anterior complex is again easily visualized, and most of the time the pia mater can be seen in small children. The characteristic "horse heads" may be found in the image, and the dura mater will be seen in between, at a deeper level (Figure 43–21). The depth of

the dura mater will be more or less equal, as in the SAX and median LAX positions.

After the preprocedural imaging to measure the depth at which the epidural space will be reached, the child's skin is prepared and draped (Figure 43–22). An 18-gauge Tuohy epidural needle, 5cm long, with markings every 0.5 cm, is then inserted at the interspace at a cephalad angle of approximately 70 degrees to the longitudinal axis of the spine. A useful maneuver is to insert the needle at a similar angle to that with which the US probe was held when the distance toward the epidural space was measured (Figure 43–23). Continuous resistance should be felt as the needle is inserted through the supraspinous and interspinous ligaments. When the interspinous ligament is reached, the stylet is removed and a saline-filled LOR syringe is connected to the needle. Continuous pressure is placed on the plunger as the needle is farther advanced

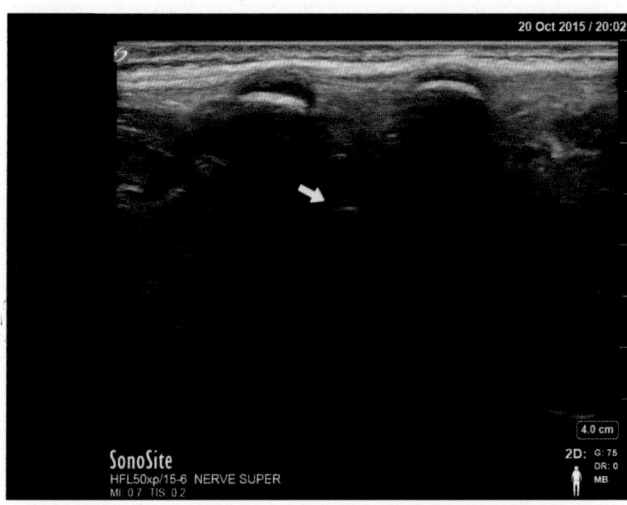

FIGURE 43–19. US image in the median long-axis view, showing the dura (white arrow).

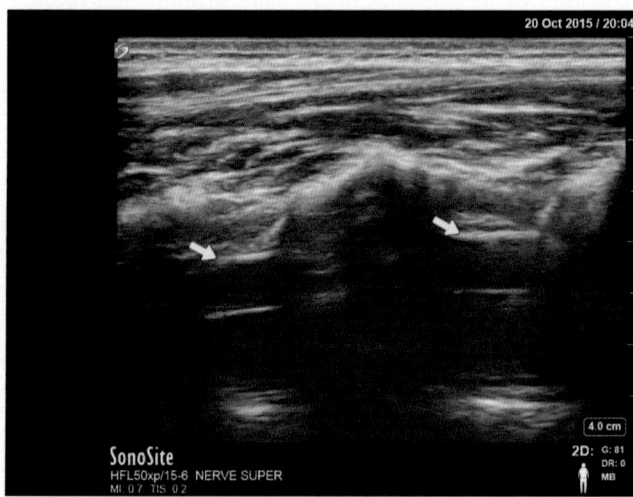

FIGURE 43–21. US image in the paramedian oblique long-axis view, showing the posterior complex with the dura (white arrows).

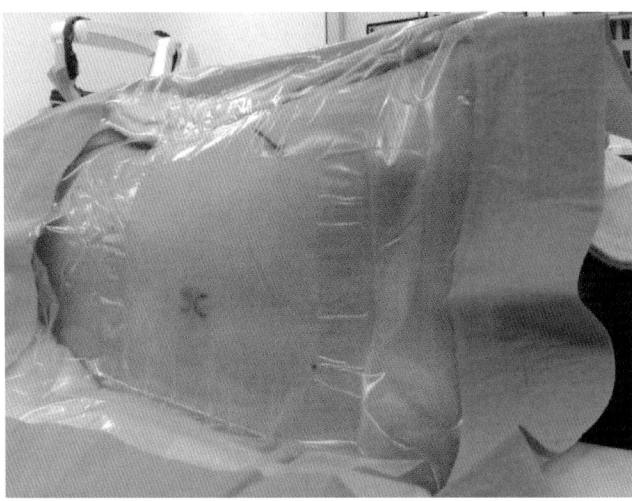

FIGURE 43–22. Sterile, transparent, plastic drape.

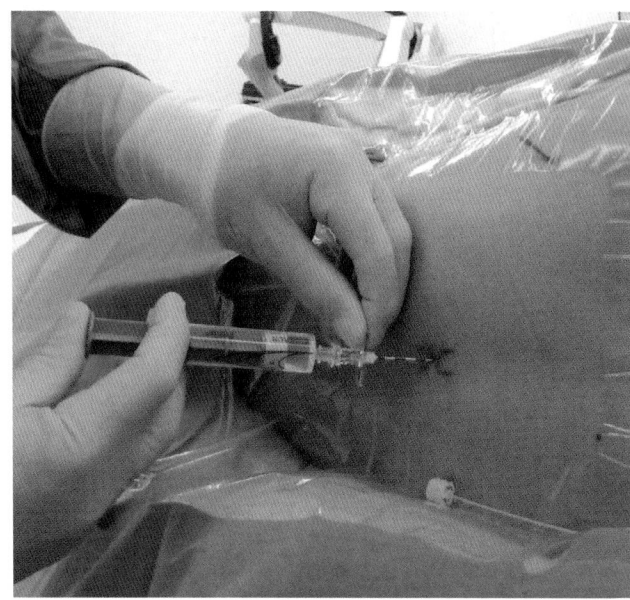

FIGURE 43–24. Needle advancement with continuous pressure placed on the plunger with the right hand as the left hand advances the needle.

(Figure 43–24). In older children, an increase in resistance is initially felt as the ligamentum flavum is entered, just before the LOR is felt. However, in younger children, the resistance met at the ligamentum flavum may not be noticeably different from that of the other ligaments.

The needle must not be inserted to a depth greater than the preprocedural US–estimated depth of the epidural space. The thoracic epidural space is identified with LOR to saline; air is not recommended in children. The syringe is then removed, and, after ruling out dural puncture, the catheter is inserted (Figure 43–25). The length of the catheter inserted should be only about 2 cm beyond the needle tip if the epidural puncture has been performed at the appropriate level. If the puncture has been performed one level beneath, the catheter can be inserted up to 3–4 cm, but it must be kept in mind that in small children, a few centimeters may represent several vertebral segments.

After withdrawing the needle and ensuring that an adequate length of catheter is kept in place, the connector is attached to the catheter. At this point, it is imperative to check for a falling

meniscus and perform slow and careful aspiration through the catheter to check for blood or CSF (Figure 43–26). The filter is then connected, and incremental doses of local anesthetic can be administered with the spread assessed under US imaging.

We recommend tunneling the catheter or using a liquid bandage or the topical skin adhesive Histoacryl to close the entrance hole to prevent leakage. Preventing local anesthetic leakage in pediatric patients is important, as leaked anesthetic may consist of a significant percentage of the total drug delivered. Leaking underneath the fixation device or Tegaderm may present a problem for catheter fixation itself. A transparent epidural fixation device is recommended to allow for observation of any local anesthetic leakage or signs of infection (Figure 43–27).

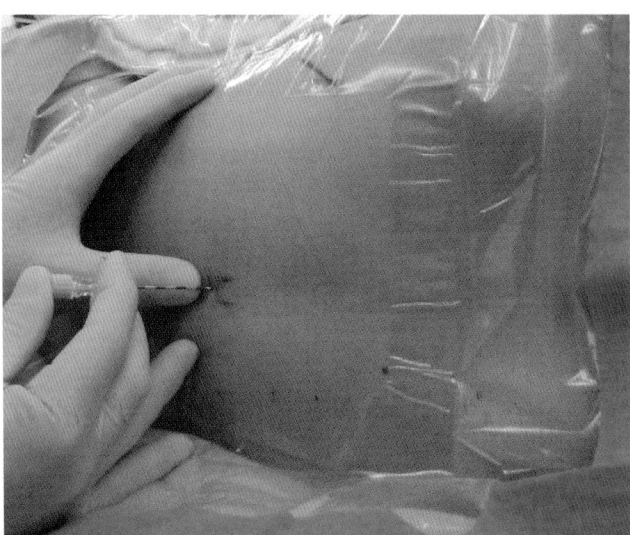

FIGURE 43–23. Needle insertion. Note the direction compared to the probe in Figure 43–14.

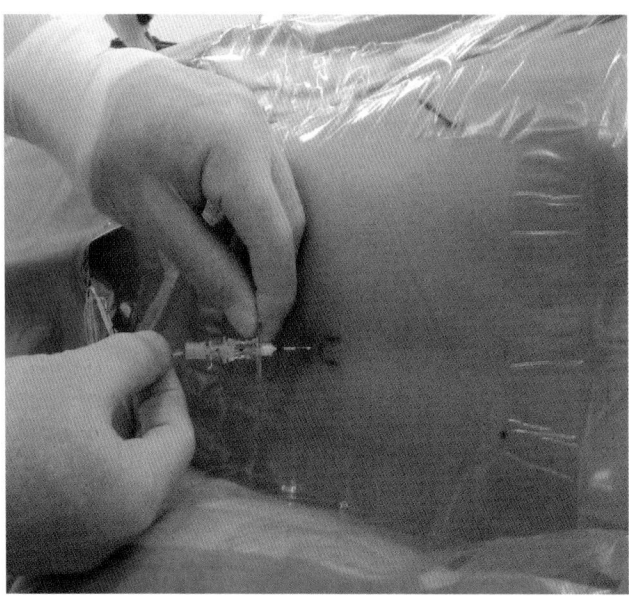

FIGURE 43–25. Catheter insertion.

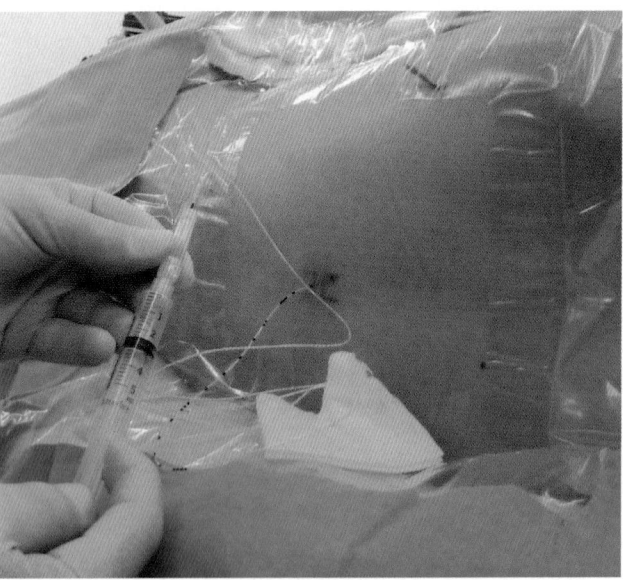

FIGURE 43–26. Aspiration test.

Clinical Pearls

- Various formulas exist for calculating the volume of local anesthetic required to block a given number of segments.
- A bolus of 1.0 mg/kg of 0.25% bupivacaine or 0.2% ropivacaine is administered to establish the block.
- In preschool-aged children and especially infants, irritability or agitation may occur despite an apparently well-functioning epidural analgesia. This is most likely the result of the IV line, nasogastric tube, urinary catheter, or the hospital environment.
- Satisfactory sedation can be achieved with either of the following:
  - IV boluses of morphine 25 mcg/kg as required, or
  - Adding clonidine 0.5 mcg/mL to the epidural mixture

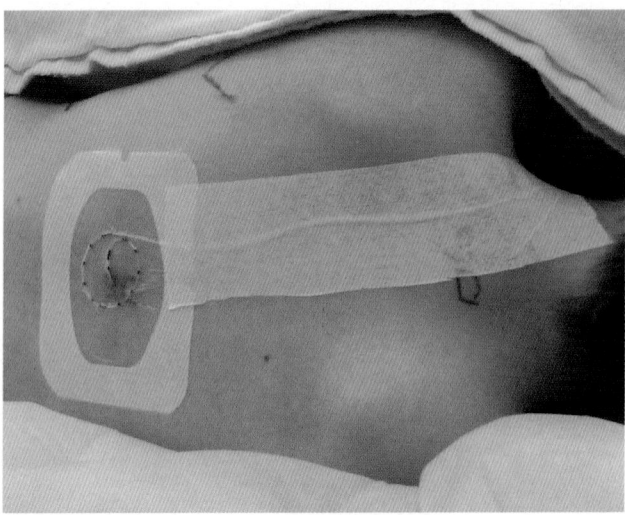

FIGURE 43–27. Catheter securing and fixation.

POSTOPERATIVE EPIDURAL INFUSION MANAGEMENT

For effective and safe epidural analgesia, a systematic and protocol-based approach to patient care is advised. A dedicated pediatric acute pain team, consisting of anesthesiologists and nurses, is vital to ensure standardized assessments of pain, vigilant patient monitoring, and the proper treatment of adverse effects. Precise placement of epidural needles and catheters is the key to successful epidural analgesia. This requires the use of a reliable method to confirm the location of the catheter tip (ie, US, epidural stimulation). The average length of epidural infusion is about 72 hours, although it may be necessary to continue the infusion for longer periods, especially in children with complicated medical histories or a prolonged need for analgesia. In neonates, the length of epidural infusion should be limited to 48 hours due to the risk of systemic toxicity. A team of dedicated personnel with a focus on pain management should care for such patients. When plans to discontinue the epidural infusion are in place, an opioid should be considered to enable adequate analgesia. Finally, the success of the process is based on properly written orders—a crucial part of executing adequate analgesia.

Clinical Pearl

For postoperative analgesia, either bupivacaine 0.125% or ropivacaine 0.1–0.2%, with or without fentanyl 1–2 mcg/mL, is administered at the following rates:

- Age > 3 months: 0.20–0.35 mL/kg/h (< 0.4 mg/kg/h bupivacaine)
- Age < 3 months: 0.1–0.15 mL/kg/h (< 0.2 mg/kg/h bupivacaine)

SPINAL ANESTHESIA IN CHILDREN

INTRODUCTION

Spinal anesthesia is perhaps one of the oldest and most studied modalities for providing pain relief in patients undergoing surgery. J. Leonard Corning[70] is credited with administering the first spinal anesthetic in 1885, and his experience was subsequently published in a medical journal. Although the use of intrathecal anesthesia administration in children was described in the early twentieth century,[71,72] this technique was seldom used in the pediatric population until Melman[73] reported a series of high-risk infants who underwent successful surgery under spinal anesthesia. Reports of apnea following general anesthesia in preterm infants appeared in the literature in the early 1980s,[74–78] and a series from Abajian et al.[79] offered practitioners an impetus to offer an alternative technique with reportedly fewer complications than general anesthesia. A number of series have since been reported in all age groups for a variety of surgical procedures attesting to the safety and efficacy of spinal anesthesia.[80–82]

TABLE 43–6. Anatomic differences between adults and infants in the spinal canal.

Conus medullaris ends at L2–L3 in infants versus L1 in adults.

Infants have a small pelvis, and the sacrum begins more cephalad than in adults.

The dural sac ends more caudad in infants versus adults.

ANATOMY

Understanding the anatomical differences between adults and infants is crucial to safely administer spinal anesthesia in children in a technically proficient manner (Table 43–6).

The spinal cord terminates at a much more caudad level in neonates and infants than in adults. The conus medullaris ends at approximately L1 in adults and at the L2 or L3 level in neonates and infants. To avoid potential injury to the spinal cord, dural puncture should be performed below the level of the spinal cord; that is, below L2–L3 in neonates and infants. In adults, spinal anesthesia is often performed at the interspace nearest an imaginary line stretching across the top of the iliac crests, the intercristal or Tuffier's line, corresponding to the L3–L4 interspace. However, neonates and infants have a proportionally smaller pelvis than adults, and the sacrum is located more cephalad relative to the iliac crests. Therefore, Tuffier's line crosses the midline of the vertebral column at the L4–L5 or L5–S1 interspace, well below the termination of the spinal cord, making this landmark applicable in all pediatric patients.[83–85] The dural sac in neonates and infants also terminates in a more caudad location compared with that in adults, usually at about the level of S3 compared with the adult level of S1. The more caudad termination of the dural sac makes an inadvertent dural puncture more likely during the performance of a single-injection caudal block if the needle is advanced too far into the epidural space.[84]

CSF volume is higher on a milliliter-per-kilogram basis in infants and neonates (4 mL/kg) compared with adults (2 mL/kg). In addition, CSF in infants is distributed relatively more in the spinal canal than in the head, as opposed to the distribution in adults. This may, in part, account for the higher local anesthetic dose requirements and shorter duration of action of spinal anesthesia in infants. The high cardiac output characteristic of the pediatric population shortens the duration of spinal blocks in children still further.

LOCAL ANESTHETICS

A variety of local anesthetics and doses have been described in the literature, including bupivacaine[86] and ropivacaine.[87] Bupivacaine 0.5%, 0.5–1 mg/kg, is generally used for spinal anesthesia in children weighing less than 10 kg. A dose toward the higher end of the range is preferred for smaller children; the risk of total spinal anesthesia is low as long as the procedure is carried out diligently (Table 43–7). An "epinephrine wash" of the

TABLE 43–7. Spinal anesthesia dosage in children.

Local anesthetic solution: ropivacaine or bupivacaine 0.5% 0.5–1 mg/kg.
An easy way to calculate the dose for a single hernia repair in infants is as follows:

Age (mos)	Weight (kg)	Dose bupivacaine 0.5%
1	3	1 mg/kg
2	4	0.8 mg/kg
3	5	0.6 mg/kg
> 4	6	0.4 mg/kg

Possible additives:
- Epinephrine wash
- Clonidine 1 mcg/kg
- Morphine 10 mcg/kg only for cardiac surgery to facilitate earlier extubation)

syringe, rather than a standard dose of epinephrine, is preferred. A hyperbaric bupivacaine solution with glucose 8% provides a block of similar quality and duration than isobaric bupivacaine with glucose 0.9%.[88]

Adjuvants to local anesthetics in spinal blocks have also been described. Clonidine in a dose of 1 mcg/kg added to bupivacaine (1 mg/kg) used in spinal anesthesia for newborn infants has been shown to prolong block duration to almost twice the duration of spinal anesthesia without clonidine.[89] However, the use of 2 mcg/kg of clonidine may cause a transient decrease in blood pressure and greater postoperative sedation. It may be advisable to use a dose of caffeine of 10 mg/kg intravenously to prevent potential postoperative apnea, especially if clonidine is used in the spinal anesthetic solution.[90]

In cases of bilateral hernia repair in former premature infants, the spinal block may be supplemented with a caudal block. The patient is turned on the side of the largest hernia while the block is performed; a spinal injection of 0.8 mg/kg bupivacaine is followed immediately by a caudal injection of 0.1% bupivacaine. This technique prolongs the duration of anesthesia and analgesia. Alternatively, a hypobaric solution of local anesthetic can be injected with the operative side up.

ADVERSE EFFECTS

Adverse effects from spinal anesthesia commonly seen in adults are less common in children. These include hypotension, bradycardia, PDPH, and transient radicular symptoms.

Hypotension and bradycardia are uncommon in children despite the high levels of blockade required. Fluid loading to increase preload is rarely needed in children but, if needed, can be done at a rate of 10 mL/kg.[91] Although some authors obtain venous access in the lower limbs of the patient after the spinal block has been performed (pain-free IV catheter placement), we recommend obtaining venous access before performing the spinal block. Puncuh et al.[86] reported their experience with

1132 consecutive spinal anesthetics in which hypotension was rarely reported: only a mild decrease in blood pressure was reported in 9 of 942 patients younger than 10 years old and in 8 of 190 patients older than 10 years old.

The incidence of PDPH is lower in children than in adults. However, an incidence of 8% has been reported in oncological patients after frequent lumbar punctures for spinal tap.[92] The use of different types of spinal needle was studied in this subgroup of patients, but no difference was found in the incidence of headache (15% Quincke; 9% pencil-point Whitacre; $p = 0.43$).[93] Moreover, the incidence of headache was not different by age group, with 8 of 11 PDPHs occurring in children under 10 years of age and the youngest reported in a 23-month-old. PDPHs have been treated with bed rest and caffeine in adults but are followed by blood patch if the headache doesn't resolve. In children, an optimal dose of caffeine is not known, and an epidural blood patch is performed with 0.3 mL/kg of blood when the headache persists.

Transient radicular symptoms have been reported in children but without long-term adverse effects.[94]

RELATIVE CONTRAINDICATIONS

The major contraindication for a spinal technique in a nonsedated child is a surgery duration of more than 60 minutes. Spinal anesthesia should be avoided in neonates and children who may have increased intracranial pressure. In children with neuromuscular diseases, ventricular shunts (atrial or peritoneal), and poorly controlled seizures, the use of spinal anesthesia is controversial. Other contraindications to spinal anesthesia are similar to those in the adult population and include severe anatomical deformities, systemic infection or at the site of puncture, underlying coagulopathy, and hemodynamic instability (Table 43–8).

When considering spinal anesthesia, special consideration should be given to children with a known difficult airway. Although spinal anesthesia may be a reasonable choice in these patients, the first consideration should be the ability of the practitioner to manage the airway. The need for IV sedation in preschool- and school-aged children poses its own set of risks in pediatric patients with a difficult airway. The surgical site, the anticipated length of the procedure, and the surgical

TABLE 43–8. Relative contraindications to spinal anesthesia in children.

Anatomical abnormalities of the spine
Degenerative neuromuscular disease
Patient and family dissent
Coagulopathy
Bacterial infection
Increased intracranial pressure
Ventriculoperitoneal shunts

position (ie, supine, lateral, or prone) are also important factors to be considered.

Clinical Pearl

Special considerations for infants and children undergoing spinal anesthesia include the following:

- The expertise of the anesthesia provider
- The motivation of the surgeon
- The estimated length of surgery being less than 90 minutes

SPINAL ANESTHESIA FOR PEDIATRIC PATIENTS: TECHNIQUE

Preparation

Eutectic mixture of local anesthetic (EMLA) cream or LMX (4% lidocaine cream) may be applied to the site of insertion, although the risk of methemoglobinemia must be taken into account in very small premature infants. The operating room should be warmed before bringing the patient into the room. Warm blankets and radiant heating lamps help to diminish heat loss in infants. With older children, the room should be quiet and, if possible, surgical instruments covered to minimize patient anxiety. Pediatric operating rooms may be equipped with stereo or video equipment, which may be used to distract older children if the block is performed without sedation. Standard monitoring devices (pulse oximeter, electrocardiogram, and blood pressure cuff) should be applied before performing the block.

A plan should be made regarding the concomitant use of IV sedation or inhalational general anesthesia. The approach should be dictated by the medical condition and age of the patient, the comfort level of the anesthesia provider, and the nature and anticipated length of the surgical procedure. General anesthesia may predispose very preterm infants to apnea and bradycardia.[95] Spinal anesthesia in infants lasts no more than 90 minutes due to their physiological characteristics. Therefore, in former preterm infants undergoing lower abdominal procedures of less than 90 minutes' duration, spinal anesthesia without adjuvant sedation may be performed. However, a short period of inhalational general anesthesia or supplemental IV sedation may sometimes be necessary while the block is being performed, especially if EMLA cream has not been used. Older children may require supplemental sedation or light general anesthesia prior to performing the block. In some cases, spinal anesthesia may be combined with caudal or epidural anesthesia to prolong analgesia.

Patient Position

Spinal anesthesia is customarily administered in the lateral or sitting position in children. If the lateral position is preferred, the patient is positioned at the very border of the surgical table and held firmly by an assistant. Otherwise, the patient can be placed in the middle of the surgical table but on top of several blankets; these will give the necessary height for the anesthesiologist's

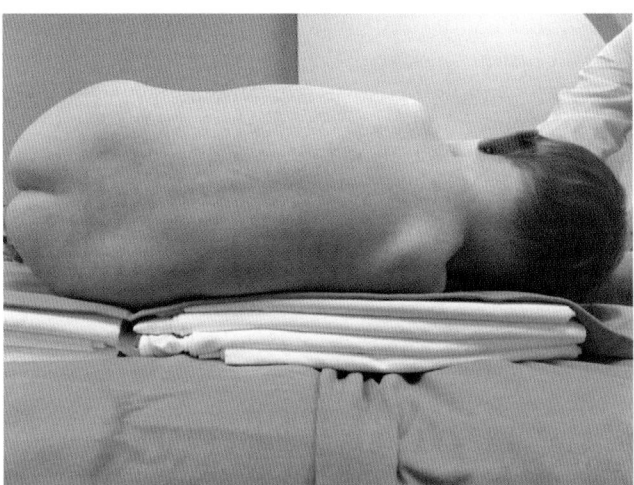

FIGURE 43–28. Spinal anesthesia in the lateral position. The child is placed on top of several blankets to gain height for the anesthesiologist's hands while performing the block.

hands to be placed comfortably while performing the block (Figure 43–28). If the sitting position is preferred, special attention must be paid in infants to ensure that the neck is not flexed, as this could result in airway obstruction (Figure 43–29). It is essential to vigilantly monitor oxygen saturation in infants while performing the spinal to ensure adequacy and patency of the airway. Moreover, neck flexion is not necessary because it does

not facilitate the performance of the block in small children.[96] In older children, an assistant should be present to maintain proper positioning and to reassure and distract the child while the block is being performed. The use of a pacifier while the block is being performed in a nonsedated infant is usually helpful.

Technique

In infants, the L4–L5 or L5–S1 interspace should be identified; the L3–L4 interspace may be used in older children. The area should be prepared and draped in a sterile fashion. If topical anesthetic cream was not applied preoperatively, local anesthesia should be administered before the block in awake or lightly sedated patients. The desired dose of spinal local anesthetic should be calculated and prepared in a syringe before dural puncture to ensure that the correct dose is administered. Because the volume of local anesthetic needed may be small in neonates, it is important to measure the volume corresponding to the hub of the needle and to count this volume, too, in the total dose of local anesthetic. An insulin syringe is helpful to measure the exact dose accurately. A short, 22- or 25-gauge spinal needle is often used (Figure 43–30). A midline approach

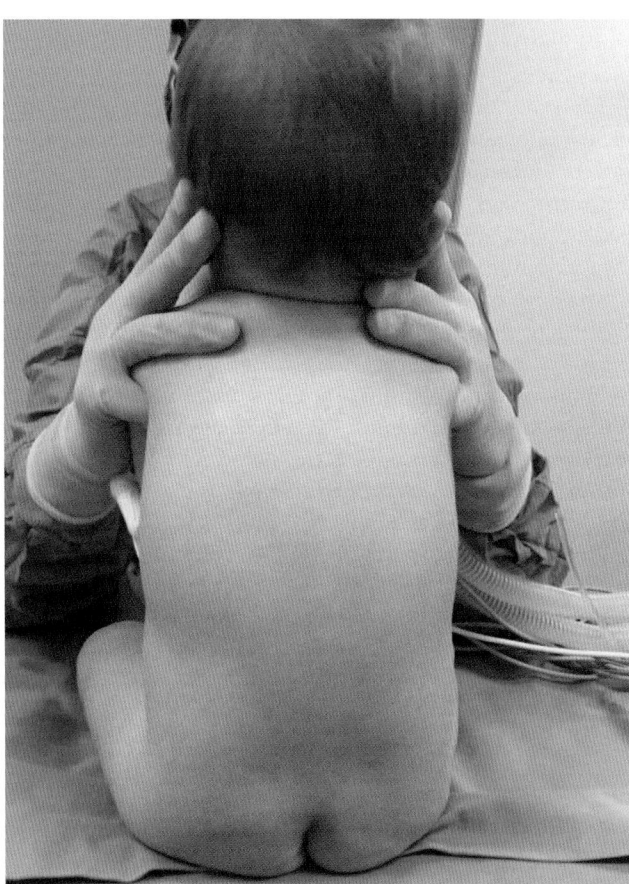

FIGURE 43–29. Spinal anesthesia in the sitting position. Head flexion must be avoided to prevent airway obstruction.

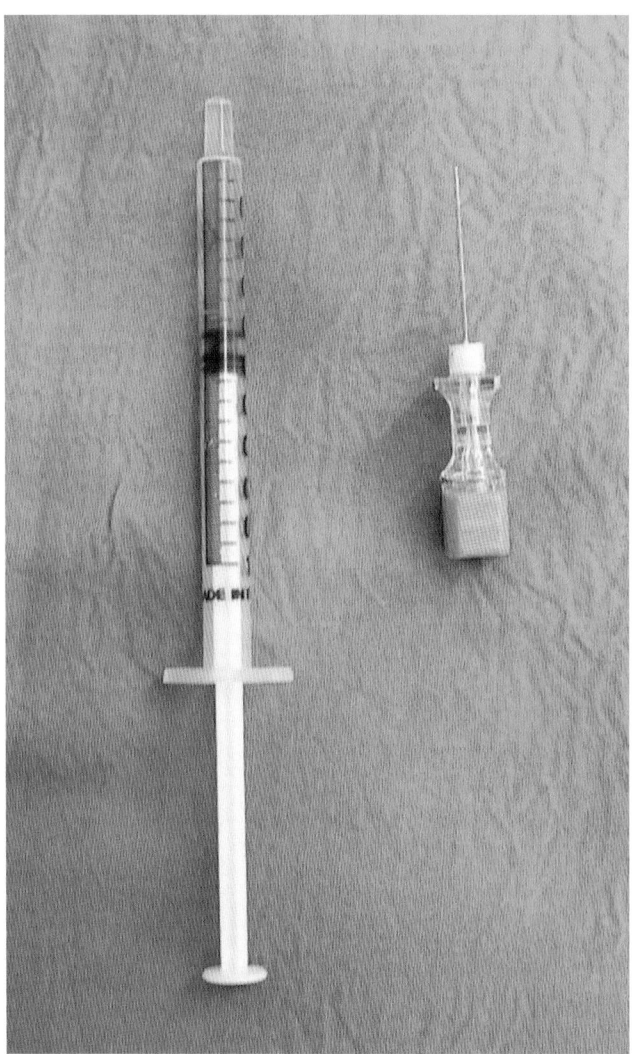

FIGURE 43–30. Equipment used for spinal anesthesia in neonates: spinal needle and syringe with local anesthetic.

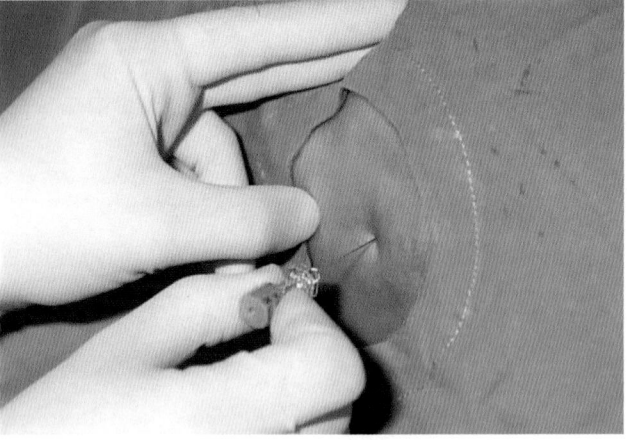

FIGURE 43–31. Spinal anesthesia needle insertion.

is usually recommended over a paramedian approach. The ligamentum flavum is very soft in children, and a distinctive "pop" may not be perceived when the dura is penetrated (Figure 43–31). Once clear CSF is exiting the needle, the drug(s) may be administered and, importantly, must be injected slowly (Figure 43–32).

The barbotage method is not recommended, as it may result in unacceptably high levels of motor blockade and has a potential for total spinal blockade. The patient's lower limbs should not be elevated for the placement of the electrocautery return electrode on the infant's back, as total spinal anesthesia can result from the spread of local anesthetic to a higher spinal level. To prolong the duration of surgical anesthesia in the case of bilateral hernia repair, spinal anesthesia can be supplemented with a caudal block.

Assessing the Block

Assessing the level of blockade may prove difficult in infants and young children, particularly in patients who have received sedation or in those in whom the block is being performed under general anesthesia. In infants, pin prick or response to cold stimuli (eg, an alcohol swab) may be used, as well as observation of ventilation rate and pattern. In children over 2 years

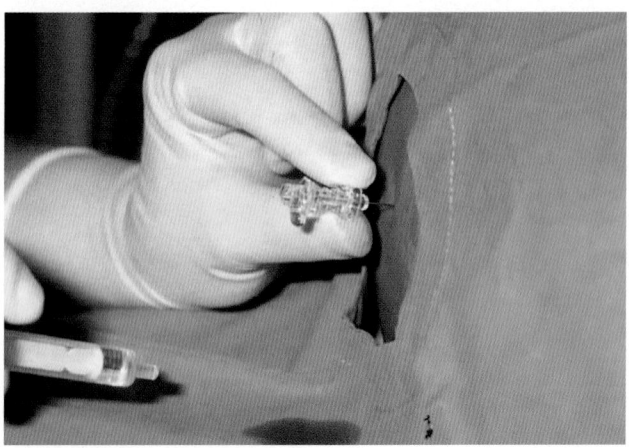

FIGURE 43–32. Spinal anesthesia: Cerebrospinal fluid exits the needle, and local anesthetic is injected.

of age, the Bromage scale is used. Following the block, care should be taken to avoid placing the patient in the Trendelenburg position or lifting the lower limbs; for example, to place an electrocautery pad on the infant's back. In the event of a rapidly rising level of blockade, the patient may be placed in the reverse Trendelenburg position.

Clinical Pearl

Evaluation of Spinal Anesthesia: The Bromage Scale
  I. No block: Free movement of knees and feet is possible
 II. Partial block: Able only to flex knees but free movement of feet still possible
III. Almost complete block: Unable to flex knees but flexion of feet still possible
IV. Complete: Unable to move legs or feet

CLINICAL USES

Apnea and Former Preterm Infants

The most common indication for spinal anesthesia in pediatric patients is in former preterm infants undergoing unilateral inguinal hernia repair (Table 43–9). Apnea can occur in former preterm patients following a general anesthetic.[77,79] Regional anesthesia may decrease, if not eliminate, the risk of postoperative apnea and certainly decreases the risk of desaturation and bradycardia.[97]

However, there is considerable disagreement regarding the incidence of apnea and the conceptual age at which a former preterm infant may safely undergo general anesthesia on an outpatient basis. Lack of uniformity in study design, small patient population sizes, and variations in methodology probably account for the differences noted. Cote at al.[77] performed a meta-analysis of eight studies, comprising 255 patients, investigating postoperative apnea in former preterm infants after general anesthesia. Overall, the risk was independently related to both gestational age and conceptual age. Additional risk factors for postoperative apnea were a hematocrit less than 30% and continued apneic episodes at home. The study stratified infants into two groups: a 5% risk group and a 1% risk group. For patients with a gestational age of 35 weeks, the risk of postoperative apnea did not fall below 5% (with a 95% statistical confidence interval) until patients reached a postconceptual age of 48 weeks and did not decrease below 1% until infants

TABLE 43–9. Indications for spinal anesthesia in children.

Inguinal hernia repair
Myelomeningocele repair
Lower limb and lower abdominal surgery
Early extubation desired after cardiac surgery

reached a postconceptual age of 54 weeks. In more preterm patients, such as those with a gestational age of 32 weeks, the risk of apnea did not fall below 1% (with a 95% statistical confidence interval) until infants reached a postconceptual age of 56 weeks.

The concomitant use of ketamine as a sedative in former preterm infants was also reported to increase the incidence of postoperative apnea above that reported in control patients.

However, these are all somewhat older studies. In the meantime, there have been substantial advances in the ventilatory management of premature neonates and infants, making the risk of apnea controversial at the present day. Moreover, improvements in anesthesia, such as the extended use of sevoflurane instead of halothane and laryngeal masks instead of tracheal intubation, have further decreased the incidence of the deleterious effects of general anesthesia in infants. Craven et al.[98] reviewed several randomized controlled studies and found only a borderline statistical advantage of spinal anesthetic over general anesthesia. In our opinion, administering sevoflurane while spontaneous ventilation for a short period of time may sometimes be useful to aid in performing the spinal block, especially if no EMLA cream is used.

Spinal anesthesia has also been used for a variety of other procedures, including myelomeningocele repair[99] and other abdominal, urological, and orthopedic procedures in children. The early report by Abajian et al.[79] included not only infants undergoing inguinal herniorrhaphy but also other noninfant patients whom the authors felt faced an increased risk for general anesthesia. This study included patients with a variety of medical conditions, including laryngomalacia, macroglossia, micrognathia, congenital heart disease, Down syndrome, adrenogenital syndrome, failure to thrive, and arthrogryposis. Blaise et al.[81] reported 30 patients aged 7 weeks to 13 years old who underwent spinal anesthesia for a variety of surgical procedures. Kokki et al.[88,100] reported satisfactory anesthesia in 92 of 93 children aged 1 to 17 years old undergoing spinal anesthesia with ropivacaine for lower abdominal or lower limb procedures.

Regional techniques have been used in cardiac surgery to facilitate early extubation.[101] This large series investigating spinal anesthesia for cardiac surgery comes from a prospective randomized analysis from Stanford University. The group who received spinal anesthesia for postoperative pain relief had less opioid requirement in the postoperative period after elective cardiac surgery with early extubation in the operating room.

In summary, spinal anesthesia in pediatrics is most commonly used in preterm infants undergoing anesthesia for inguinal hernia repair. Spinal anesthesia can also be used effectively in children for postoperative pain relief in cardiac surgery, especially if opioids are used.

REFERENCES

1. Peutrell JM, Lonnqvist PA: Neuraxial blocks for anaesthesia and analgesia in children. Curr Opin Anaesthesiol 2003;16:461–470.
2. Suresh S, Long J, Birmingham PK, et al: Are caudal blocks for pain control safe in children? An analysis of 18,650 caudal blocks from the Pediatric Regional Anesthesia Network (PRAN) database. Anesth Analg 2015;120:151–156.
3. Gunter JB, Eng C: Thoracic epidural anesthesia via the caudal approach in children. Anesthesiology 1992;76:935–938.
4. Larsson BA, Lonnqvist PA, Olsson GL: Plasma concentrations of bupivacaine in neonates after continuous epidural infusion. Anesth Analg 1997;84:501–505.
5. Luz G, Innerhofer P, Bachmann B, et al: Bupivacaine plasma concentrations during continuous epidural anesthesia in infants and children. Anesth Analg 1996;82:231–234.
6. Berde C: Local anesthetics in infants and children: an update. Paediatr Anaesth 2004;14:387–393.
7. Gunter JB, Dunn CM, Bennie JB, et al: Optimum concentration of bupivacaine for combined caudal–general anesthesia in children. Anesthesiology 1991;75:57–61.
8. Tsui BC, Berde CB: Caudal analgesia and anesthesia techniques in children. Curr Opin Anaesthesiol 2005;18:283–288.
9. Lönnqvist PA: Review article. Toxicity of local anesthetic drugs: a pediatric perspective. Paediatr Anaesth 2012;22:39–43.
10. Da Conceicao MJ, Coelho L, Khalil M: Ropivacaine 0.25% compared with bupivacaine 0.25% by the caudal route. Paediatr Anaesth 1999; 9:229–233.
11. Eledjam JJ, Gros T, Viel E, et al: Ropivacaine overdose and systemic toxicity. Anaesth Intensive Care 2000;28:705–707.
12. Ivani G, Lampugnani E, Torre M, et al: Comparison of ropivacaine with bupivacaine for paediatric caudal block. Br J Anaesth 1998;81: 247–248.
13. Karmakar MK, Aun CS, Wong EL, et al: Ropivacaine undergoes slower systemic absorption from the caudal epidural space in children than bupivacaine (table). Anesth Analg 2002;94:259–265.
14. Kokko TI, Karinen J, Raiha E, et al: Pharmacokinetics of 0.75% ropivacaine and 0.5% bupivacaine after ilioinguinal-iliohypogastric nerve block in children. Br J Anaesth 2002;89:438–441.
15. Gunter JB: Benefit and risks of local anesthetics in infants and children. Paediatr Drugs 2002;4:649–672.
16. Bosenberg A, Thomas J, Lopez T, et al: The efficacy of caudal ropivacaine 1, 2 and 3 mg × l(-1) for postoperative analgesia in children. Paediatr Anaesth 2002;12:53–58.
17. Ivani G. Ropivacaine: is it time for children? Paediatr Anaesth 2002; 12:383–387.
18. Taylor R, Eyres R, Chalkiadis GA, et al: Efficacy and safety of caudal injection of levobupivacaine, 0.25%, in children under 2 years of age undergoing inguinal hernia repair, circumcision or orchidopexy. Paediatr Anaesth 2003;13:114–121.
19. Lonnqvist PA: Adjuncts to caudal block in children—Quo vadis? Br J Anaesth 2005;95:431–433.
20. Lonnqvist PA, Ivani G, Moriarty T: Use of caudal-epidural opioids in children: still state of the art or the beginning of the end? Paediatr Anaesth 2002;12:747–749.
21. Attia J, Ecoffey C, Sandouk P, et al: Epidural morphine in children: pharmacokinetics and CO_2 sensitivity. Anesthesiology 1986;65:590–594.
22. Ansermino M, Basu R, Vandebeek C, et al: Nonopioid additives to local anaesthetics for caudal blockade in children: a systematic review. Paediatr Anaesth 2003;13:561–573.
23. De Negri P, Ivani G, Visconti C, et al: The dose-response relationship for clonidine added to a postoperative continuous epidural infusion of ropivacaine in children. Anesth Analg 2001;93:71–76.
24. Penon C, Ecoffey C, Cohen SE: Ventilatory response to carbon dioxide after epidural clonidine injection. Anesth Analg 1991;72:761–991.
25. Fellmann C, Gerber AC, Weiss M: Apnoea in a former preterm infant after caudal bupivacaine with clonidine for inguinal herniorrhaphy. Paediatr Anaesth 2002;12:637–640.
26. Passariello M, Almenrader N, Canneti A, et al: Caudal analgesia in children: S(+)-ketamine vs S(+)-ketamine plus clonidine. Paediatr Anaesth 2004;14:851–855.
27. Hager H, Marhofer P, Sitzwohl C, et al: Caudal clonidine prolongs analgesia from caudal S (+)-ketamine in children. Anesth Analg 2002; 94:1169–1172.
28. Hayashi H, Dikkes P, Soriano SG: Repeated administration of ketamine may lead to neuronal degeneration in the developing rat brain. Paediatr Anaesth 2002;12:770–774.
29. Proescholdt M, Heimann A, Kempski O: Neuroprotection of S(+) ketamine isomer in global forebrain ischemia. Brain Res 2001; 904: 245–251.
30. Suresh S, Wheeler M: Practical pediatric regional anesthesia. Anesthesiol Clin North Am 2002;20:83–113.
31. Giaufre E, Dalens B, Gombert A: Epidemiology and morbidity of regional anesthesia in children: a one-year prospective survey of the French-Language Society of Pediatric Anesthesiologists. Anesth Analg 1996;83:904–912.

32. Flandin-Blety C, Barrier G: Accidents following extradural analgesia in children. The results of a retrospective study. Paediatr Anaesth 1995;5:41–46.

33. Fischer HB: Performing epidural insertion under general anaesthesia. Anaesthesia 2000;55:288–289.

34. Kasai T, Yaegashi K, Hirose M, et al: Spinal cord injury in a child caused by an accidental dural puncture with a single-shot thoracic epidural needle. Anesth Analg 2003;96:65–67.

35. Horlocker T, Wedel DJ, Rowlingson JC, et al: Regional anesthesia in the patient receiving antithrombotic or thrombolytic therapy. American Society of Regional Anesthesia and Pain Medicine Evidence-Based Guidelines (Third Edition). Reg Anesth Pain Med 2010;35:64–101.

36. Kost-Byerly S, Tobin JR, Greenberg RS, et al: Bacterial colonization and infection rate of continuous epidural catheters in children. Anesth Analg 1998;86:712–716.

37. Wittum S, Hofer CK, Rolli U, et al: Sacral osteomyelitis after single-shot epidural anesthesia via the caudal approach in a child. Anesthesiology 2003;99:503–505.

38. Bubeck J, Boos K, Krause H, Thies KC: Subcutaneous tunneling of caudal catheters reduces the rate of bacterial colonization to that of lumbar epidural catheters. Anesth Analg 2004;99:689–693.

39. Oliver A: Dural punctures in children: what should we do? Paediatr Anaesth 2002;12:473–477.

40. Liley A, Manoharan M, Upadhyay V: The management of a post-dural puncture headache in a child. Paediatr Anaesth 2003;13:534–537.

41. Janssens E, Aerssens P, Alliet P, et al: Post-dural puncture headaches in children. A literature review. Eur J Pediatr 2003;162:117–121.

42. Tsuji MH, Horigome H, Yamashita M: Left ventricular functions are not impaired after lumbar epidural anaesthesia in young children. Paediatr Anaesth 1996;6:405–409.

43. Tsui BC, Malherbe S, Koller J, et al: Reversal of an unintentional spinal anesthetic by cerebrospinal lavage. Anesth Analg 2004;98:434–436.

44. Tobias JD: Caudal epidural block: a review of test dosing and recognition of systemic injection in children. Anesth Analg 2001;93:1156–1161.

45. Neal JM, Mulroy MF, Weinberg GF: American Society of Regional Anesthesia and Pain Medicine. Checklist for Managing Local Anesthetic Systemic Toxicity: 2012 Version. Reg Anesth Pain Med 2012;37:16Y18.

46. Flandin-Blety C, Barrier G: Accidents following extradural analgesia in children. The results of a retrospective study. Paediatr Anaesth 1995; 5:41–46.

47. Valairucha S, Seefelder C, Houck CS: Thoracic epidural catheters placed by the caudal route in infants: the importance of radiographic confirmation. Paediatr Anaesth 2002;12:424–428.

48. Tsui BC, Gupta S, Finucane B: Confirmation of epidural catheter placement using nerve stimulation. Can J Anaesth 1998;45:640–644.

49. Tsui BC, Seal R, Koller J, et al: Thoracic epidural analgesia via the caudal approach in pediatric patients undergoing fundoplication using nerve stimulation guidance. Anesth Analg 2001;93:1152–1155.

50. Tsui BC, Gupta S, Finucane B: Detection of subarachnoid and intravascular epidural catheter placement. Can J Anaesth 1999;46:675–678.

51. Tsui BC, Gupta S, Emery D, Finucane B: Detection of subdural placement of epidural catheter using nerve stimulation. Can J Anaesth 2000;47:471–473.

52. Tsui BC: Thoracic epidural catheter placement in infants via the caudal approach under electrocardiographic guidance: simplification of the original technique. Anesth Analg 2004;98:273.

53. Chen CP, Tang SF, Hsu TC, et al: Ultrasound guidance in caudal epidural needle placement. Anesthesiology 2004;101:181–184.

54. Chawathe MS, Jones RM, Gildersleve CD, et al: Detection of epidural catheters with ultrasound in children. Paediatr Anaesth 2003;13: 681–684.

55. Baris S, Guldogus F, Baris YS, et al: Is tissue coring a real problem after caudal injection in children? Paediatr Anaesth 2004;14:755–758.

56. Lam DK, Corry GN, Tsui BC: Evidence for the use of ultrasound imaging in pediatric regional anesthesia: a systematic review. Reg Anesth Pain Med 2016;41:229–241.

57. Rubin K, Sullivan D, Sadhasivam S: Are peripheral and neuraxial blocks with ultrasound guidance more effective and safe in children? Paediatr Anaesth 2009;19:92–96.

58. Perlas A: Evidence for the use of ultrasound in neuraxial blocks. Reg Anesth Pain Med 2010;35(2 Suppl):S43–46.

59. Triffterer L, Machata AM, Latzke D, et al: Ultrasound assessment of cranial spread during caudal blockade in children: effect of the speed of injection of local anaesthetics. Br J Anaesth 2012;108:670–674.

60. Brenner L, Marhofer P, Kettner SC, et al: Ultrasound assessment of cranial spread during caudal blockade in children: the effect of different volumes of local anaesthetics. Br J Anaesth 2011;107:229–235.

61. Lundblad M, Lönnqvist PA, Eksborg S, et al: Segmental distribution of high-volume caudal anesthesia in neonates, infants, and toddlers as assessed by ultrasonography. Paediatr Anaesth 2010;21:121–127.

62. Lundblad M, Eksborg S, Lönnqvist PA: Secondary spread of caudal block as assessed by ultrasonography. Br J Anaesth 2012;108:675–681.

63. Tamai H, Sawamura S, Kanamori Y, et al: Thoracic epidural catheter insertion using the caudal approach assisted with an electrical nerve stimulator in young children. Reg Anesth Pain Med 2004;29:92–95.

64. Tsui BC, Wagner A, Cave D, et al: Thoracic and lumbar epidural analgesia via the caudal approach using electrical stimulation guidance in pediatric patients: a review of 289 patients. Anesthesiology 2004;100:683–689.

65. Tsui BC, Entwistle L: Thoracic epidural analgesia via the lumbar approach using nerve stimulation in a pediatric patient with Down syndrome. Acta Anaesthesiol Scand 2005;49:712–714.

66. Fischer HB: Performing epidural insertion under general anaesthesia. Anaesthesia 2000;55:288–289.

67. Kasai T, Yaegashi K, Hirose M, et al: Spinal cord injury in a child caused by an accidental dural puncture with a single-shot thoracic epidural needle. Anesth Analg 2003;96:65–67.

68. Bromage PR, Benumof JL: Paraplegia following intracord injection during attempted epidural anesthesia under general anesthesia. Reg Anesth Pain Med 1998;23:104–107.

69. Chawathe MS, Jones RM, Gildersleve CD, et al: Detection of epidural catheters with ultrasound in children. Paediatr Anaesth 2003;13: 681–684.

70. Corning JL: Spinal anesthesia and local medication of the cord. NY J Med 1885;42:483–485.

71. Gray H: A study of spinal anaesthesia in children and infants: from a series of 200 cases. Lancet 1909;2:913–917.

72. Bainbridge W: Analgesia in children by spinal injection with a report of a new method of sterilization of the injection fluid. Med Rec 1900;58:937–940.

73. Melman E, Penuelas JA, Marrufo J: Regional anesthesia in children. Anesth Analg 1975;54:387–390.

74. Gregory GA, Steward DJ: Life-threatening perioperative apnea in the ex-"premie." Anesthesiology 1983;59:495–498.

75. Steward DJ: Postoperative apnea syndrome in premature infants. West J Med 1992;157:567.

76. Steward DJ: Preterm infants are more prone to complications following minor surgery than are term infants. Anesthesiology 1982;56:304–306.

77. Cote CJ, Zaslavsky A, Downes JJ, et al: Postoperative apnea in former preterm infants after inguinal herniorrhaphy. A combined analysis [see comments]. Anesthesiology 1995;82:809–822.

78. Liu LM, Cote CJ, Goudsouzian NG, et al: Life-threatening apnea in infants recovering from anesthesia. Anesthesiology 1983;59:506–510.

79. Abajian JC, Mellish RW, Browne AF, et al: Spinal anesthesia for surgery in the high-risk infant. Anesth Analg 1984;63:359–362.

80. Frumiento C, Abajian JC, Vane DW: Spinal anesthesia for preterm infants undergoing inguinal hernia repair. Arch Surg 2000;135:445–451.

81. Blaise GA, Roy WL: Spinal anaesthesia for minor paediatric surgery. Can Anaesth Soc J 1986;33:227–230.

82. Kokki H, Tuovinen K, Hendolin H: Spinal anaesthesia for paediatric day-case surgery: a double-blind, randomized, parallel group, prospective comparison of isobaric and hyperbaric bupivacaine. Br J Anaesth 1998;81:502–506.

83. Busoni P, Messeri A: Spinal anesthesia in children: surface anatomy. Anesth Analg 1989;68:418–419.

84. Busoni P, Messeri A: Spinal anesthesia in infants: could a L5-S1 approach be safer? Anesthesiology 1991;75:168–169.

85. Gray H: *Anatomy of the Human Body: Gray's Anatomy*, 30th ed. Philadelphia: Lippincott Williams & Wilkins, 1985.

86. Puncuh F, Lampugnani E, Kokki H: Use of spinal anaesthesia in paediatric patients: a single centre experience with 1132 cases. Paediatr Anaesth 2004;14:564–567.

87. Kokki H, Ylonen P, Laisalmi M, et al: Isobaric ropivacaine 5 mg/mL for spinal anesthesia in children. Anesth Analg 2005;100:66–70.

88. Kokki H, Hendolin H: Hyperbaric bupivacaine for spinal anaesthesia in 7–18 yr old children: comparison of bupivacaine 5 mg mL-1 in 0.9% and 8% glucose solutions. Br J Anaesth 2000;84:59–62.

89. Rochette A, Raux O, Troncin R, et al: Clonidine prolongs spinal anesthesia in newborns: a prospective dose-ranging study. Anesth Analg 2004;98:56–59.

90. Welborn LG, de Soto H, Hannallah RS, et al: The use of caffeine in the control of post-anesthetic apnea in former premature infants. Anesthesiology 1988;68:796–798.

91. Oberlander TF, Berde CB, Lam KH, et al: Infants tolerate spinal anesthesia with minimal overall autonomic changes: analysis of heart rate variability in former premature infants undergoing hernia repair. Anesth Analg 1995;80:20–27.

92. Ramamoorthy C, Geiduschek JM, Bratton SL, et al: Postdural puncture headache in pediatric oncology patients. Clin Pediatr 1998;37:247–251.

93. Kokki H, Salonvaara M, Herrgard E, Onen P: Postdural puncture headache is not an age-related symptom in children: s prospective, open-randomized, parallel group study comparing a 22-gauge Quincke with a 22-gauge Whitacre needle. Paediatr Anaesth 1999;9:429–434.

94. Salmela L, Aromaa U: Transient radicular irritation after spinal anesthesia induced with hyperbaric solutions of cerebrospinal fluiddiluted lidocaine 50 mg/mL or mepivacaine 40 mg/mL or bupivacaine 5 mg/mL. Acta Anaesthesiol Scand 1998;42:765–769.

95. Welborn LG, Rice LJ, Hannallah RS, et al: Postoperative apnea in former preterm infants: prospective comparison of spinal and general anesthesia. Anesthesiology 1990;72:838–842.

96. Gleason CA, Martin RJ, Anderson JV, et al: Optimal position for a spinal tap in preterm infants. Pediatrics 1983;71:31–35.

97. Krane EJ, Haberkern CM, Jacobson LE: Postoperative apnea, bradycardia, and oxygen desaturation in formerly premature infants: prospective comparison of spinal and general anesthesia. Anesth Analg 1995;80:7–13.

98. Craven PD, Badawi M, Henderson-Smart DJ, O'Brien M: Regional (spinal, epidural, caudal) versus general anaesthesia in preterm infants undergoing inguinal herniorrhaphy in early infancy. Cochrane Database Syst Rev 2003;(3):CD003669.

99. Viscomi CM, Abajian JC, Wald SL, et al: Spinal anesthesia for repair of meningomyelocele in neonates. Anesth Analg 1995;81:492–495.

100. Kokki H, Hendolin H. Comparison of spinal anaesthesia with epidural anaesthesia in paediatric surgery. Acta Anaesthesiol Scand 1995;39:896–900.

101. Hammer GB, Ramamoorthy C, Cao H, et al: Postoperative analgesia after spinal blockade in infants and children undergoing cardiac surgery. Anesth Analg 2005;100:1283–1288.

Peripheral Nerve Blocks for Children

Steve Roberts

INTRODUCTION

Peripheral nerve blocks have been gaining significant popularity in the daily practice among pediatric anesthesiologists. Nerve blocks in children have an excellent risk–benefit ratio and are readily acceptable by both parents and children. Although the performance of peripheral nerve blocks in anesthetized adults is often debated, such practice is well accepted in pediatric patients. Successive large prospective studies performed by the French-Language Society of Pediatric Anesthesiologists (ADARPEF) have demonstrated no increased incidence of complications when regional anesthesia techniques were performed under general anesthesia.[1,2] The overall incidence of regional anesthesia–related complications was less than 0.9 of 1000 anesthetic procedures performed. Interestingly, a six-fold increase in the complication rate for central versus peripheral techniques was demonstrated, which should further persuade pediatric anesthesiologists to modify their practice toward more peripherally based regional anesthetic strategies. The complication rate was four times higher in children under 6 months of age; as such, these patients should be managed only by suitably trained specialist pediatric anesthesiologists. Because of the concomitant use of general anesthesia in children, the intraoperative efficacy of nerve blocks is often assessed indirectly using hemodynamic parameters and required depth of anesthesia. Most regional techniques used in children are primarily used for the purpose of providing postoperative pain control rather than surgical anesthesia.

Although most peripheral nerve blocks in children are performed in an operating room environment, their application extends to the emergency department as well as the intensive care unit (ICU) setting.[3,4] Peripheral nerve blocks are also used in children with chronic pain conditions, such as chronic headache or chronic regional pain syndrome type 1 (CRPS-1). All adult regional anesthetic techniques are possible in children (Table 44–1); when these procedures are performed with skill and knowledge, their success rates and safety should not significantly differ from those in adults. This chapter will concentrate on the commonly performed pediatric blocks. For each technique, a short description of the relevant anatomy will be followed by descriptions of both landmark-based and ultrasound (US)-guided methods where appropriate. It is assumed for all blocks that appropriate monitoring, intravenous (IV) access, trained assistance, resuscitation equipment, and aseptic precautions are taken.

EQUIPMENT

Regional anesthesia in children must be performed only with the appropriate equipment. To this end, a selection of 18-gauge, short-beveled needles must be available; lengths of 40–50 mm and 90–100 mm will cover all patient ages. A short bevel is used as it improves the sensation of passing through tissues. The needle should be connected to a short extension tube to which a syringe can be attached; this prevents the needle being displaced as the injection is being made. Some anesthesiologists prefer to nick the skin with a sharp beveled needle to allow easy passage through the skin and ensure no superficial fascial clicks are missed.

A reliable nerve stimulator can be used to help locate mixed nerves for blockade. A nerve stimulator with adequate current output capable of eliciting percutaneous stimulation (eg, 5 mA/1 msec) for surface mapping is suggested. Once a needle is placed close to a nerve or plexus and proper stimulation is obtained, the current output is decreased to maintain the motor response at 0.4–0.2 mA to ensure intimate needle–nerve relationship. However, a number of recent human and animal studies have provided compelling evidence that peripheral nerve stimulation is not a specific determinate of the needle–nerve distance; indeed, it is possible for the needle to be placed intraneurally but have no motor response.[5,6]

TABLE 44–1. Pediatric regional anesthetic techniques: common indications and suggested volume of local anesthetic.

Block	Indication	Local Anesthetic Volume (mL/kg)[a]
Greater auricular	Otoplasty Mastoidectomy	1.0–3.0
Infraorbital	Cleft lip repair Endoscopic sinus surgery	Infants: 0.5–1.0 Children: 1.0–2.0
Supraorbital and supratrochlear	Frontal scalp incisions; eg, simple minor plastic surgery, frontal craniotomy	1.0–2.0
Superficial cervical plexus	Otoplasty Tympanomastoid surgery Cochlear implant	1.0–3.0
Greater occipital	Posterior fossa surgery Occipital neuralgia, migraine headaches	1.0–2.0
Nerve of Arnold	Myringotomy	0.5–1.0
Interscalene	Shoulder surgery	0.3–0.5
Supraclavicular	Upper arm surgery	0.3–0.5
Infraclavicular	Upper arm surgery	0.3–0.5
Axillary	Elbow and forearm surgery	0.3–0.5
Median, ulna, and radial	Syndactyly surgery	0.1–0.3
TAP, unilateral[b] TAP, bilateral[b]	Open appendectomy Inguinal herniorrhaphy Colostomy formation Subumbilical midline laparotomy	0.3–0.5 per side
Subcostal TAP	Cholecystectomy PEG	0.3–0.5 per side
Rectus sheath[c]	Umbilical herniotomy Pyloromyotomy[b]	0.2-0.3 per side
Ilioinguinal	Inguinal herniotomy	0.2–0.3
Penile	Circumcision Distal hypospadias	0.1 per side
Unilateral paravertebral Bilateral Paravertebral	Thoracotomy; eg, TOF Renal surgery Sternotomy Pectus surgery	0.3–0.5 per side
Intercostal	Chest drain insertion Thoroscopy	0.5
Lumbar plexus	Hip surgery	0.5
Femoral	Femoral fracture Slipped upper femoral epiphysis (combined with LFC)	0.2–0.4
Fascia iliaca	Femoral fracture Slipped upper femoral epiphysis	0.5
Lateral femoral cutaneous	Thigh muscle biopsy	0.1

(continued)

TABLE 44–1. Pediatric regional anesthetic techniques: common indications and suggested volume of local anesthetic. (*Continued*)

Block	Indication	Local Anesthetic Volume (mL/kg)[a]
Proximal sciatic[d]	Cruciate ligament repair	0.3–0.5
Popliteal[d]	Tendon transfers/lengthening	0.3–0.5
Ankle	Syndactyly surgery	0.1–0.2
Digital nerve	Distal finger/toe surgery	0.05–0.1

[a]No volumes have been quoted for US-guided techniques, as the end point should be when the nerve is surrounded by local anesthetic solution. For US-guided fascial plane blocks, the volumes are the same as for the landmark-based techniques.
[b]Systemic analgesia for visceral pain is essential.
[c]Always bilateral.
[d]Depending on the operation, a femoral or saphenous nerve block may be required for complete analgesia.

LFC, lateral femoral cutaneous; PEG, percutaneous endoscopic gastrostomy; TAP, transverse abdominis plane; TOF, tracheoesophageal fistula.

As an adjunct to peripheral nerve stimulation, objective injection pressure monitoring during local anesthetic injection may decrease the risk of intraneural injection.[7]

The introduction of US to guide nerve blocks has significantly increased the efficacy of these techniques and may decrease the risk of neurologic and systemic complications (see Chapter 60). Due to the superficiality of the structures in children, a US machine with a high frequency probe (> 13 MHz) should be available. When scanning children with very superficial structures, a 5-mm sterile US gel pad may allow better focusing of the US beam. Linear probes with a small footprint approximately 25 mm in length are a necessity to allow blocks to be performed on infants and children weighing less than 15 kg, as larger footprints tend to be too cumbersome in such patients. Because of the wide range of ages cared for in pediatric anesthesiology, a curvilinear probe will still need to be purchased to facilitate deep blocks (eg, lumbar plexus blocks in adolescents).

LOCAL ANESTHETICS

This chapter describes the use of local anesthetic solutions in children. It is imperative, however, to remember that the dosage of local anesthetic solutions should be on a *milligram-per-kilogram basis* and *not* based on total volume used (see Chapter 42, Table 42–2), as is often the practice in regional anesthesia in adult population. Consideration should be given to using a more modern amino amide local anesthetic (eg, levobupivacaine or ropivacaine), particularly in neonates and infants and when infusions are planned. The dosage should be adjusted downward in infants and neonates owing to the decrease in protein binding and α_1-acid glycoprotein, allowing for a greater amount of the free fraction of the drug in the systemic circulation. The addition of epinephrine to the local anesthetic solution may offer additional advantages by revealing intravascular placement, particularly in children under general anesthesia, and by prolonging local anesthetic action when used for peripheral nerve blockade.[8]

Choosing the most appropriate concentration of local anesthetic for a given situation is imperative. In children, successful blocks can be provided using a medium concentration of amino amide (eg, 0.25% levobupivacaine). However, a weaker solution (eg, 0.125%) is more appropriate for neonates, when ambulation is important, and when there is a significant risk of compartment syndrome. In some circumstances, the administration of stronger concentrations of local anesthetic (eg, 0.5%) may be indicated; for example, when postoperative muscle spasms are a major issue.

NERVE LOCALIZATION METHODS

To assist standard landmark-based methods, a variety of techniques have been developed, including nerve stimulation, surface mapping, and ultrasonography. All techniques require a sound knowledge of anatomy.

Surface Mapping and Percutaneous Peripheral Nerve Stimulation

The most common method of nerve localization involves using a stimulating needle (sheathed needle). Mixed nerves can be identified percutaneously (surface mapping) and/or subcutaneously using a nerve stimulator. Surface mapping may decrease the number of needle insertions required.[9] To elicit stimulation percutaneously, the nerve stimulator must have an adequate current output (eg, 5 mA/1 msec). The negative electrode is attached to the needle (*b*lack to *b*lock), and the positive electrode is attached to the patient (*p*ositive to *p*atient). Prior to inserting the stimulating needle, it is possible to percutaneously stimulate and thus identify a superficial nerve's position using a higher current and/or duration. To provide effective contact, the skin should be covered with a lubricating jelly or wiped with an alcohol swab. Once the needle is inserted, the nerve is located by trying to position the needle such that a current of 0.5 mA produces an appropriate muscle group response. The disadvantages of nerve stimulation are that it is a "blind" technique, is insensitive to intraneural injection, cannot be used in conjunction with muscle relaxants, is unreliable in children with neuromuscular conditions, and is painful if an awake block is being performed in the trauma setting. For these reasons, neurostimulation is being superseded by ultrasonography.

Ultrasonography

US-guided regional anesthesia has been with us for more than a decade; interest in this technology to aid in nerve localization has significantly increased, coinciding with increasing worldwide experience and the advances made in portable US equipment.[10-12] US has been shown to reliably identify nerves and fascial planes in children, plan the safest needle trajectory, and visualize the dispersion of local anesthetic within the desired tissue planes.

This technology, however, requires significant training and skill for its successful implementation; the success of US techniques is highly operator dependent. The key to the successful use of US is a specific training module and mentorship from a skilled practitioner. Although children are generally easier subjects to scan due to the superficial nature of their nerves, there are challenging morbidities (eg, cerebral palsy; Figure 44–1). To succeed with these difficult patients, the operator must have

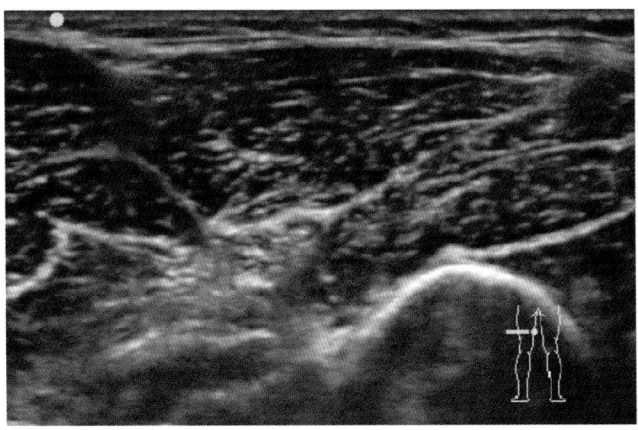

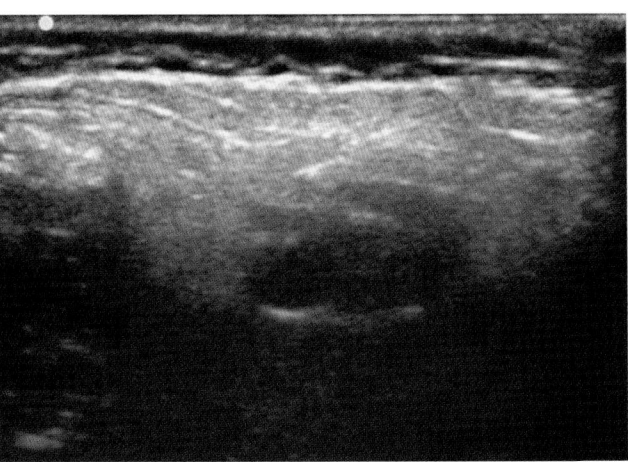

FIGURE 44–1. Comparison of US images of the popliteal fossae in (**A**) a healthy child and (**B**) a child with cerebral palsy.

TABLE 44–2. Specific advantages of pediatric ultrasound-guided regional anesthesia.

No ionizing radiation.

Because of the lower levels of ossification in pediatric patients, there are larger echo windows that can be used to visualize inside the spinal column.

Ultrasound allows for far lower doses of local anesthetic to be used, thereby reducing the risk of local anesthetic toxicity.

A lower volume of local anesthetic allows for multiple blocks to be performed within the maximum dose of local anesthetic.

In infants, the anatomy is compact and the risk of damage is greater; therefore, visualization of the nerve and adjacent structures makes for an inherently safer technique.

an established routine for each block, such that similar scanning conditions are used each time so that the expected US pattern is easily recognized.

For very superficial nerves, it may be beneficial to use a 5-mm sterile US gel pad to allow the US beam to better focus on the target nerve. When learning, and particularly with small children, it is useful to initially use saline to identify correct needle placement; in this way, no local anesthetic is wasted. (See Chapter 30 for a detailed discussion of general US techniques.) Table 44–2 summarizes the advantages of US-guided regional anesthesia in children.

Peripheral Nerve Catheter Techniques

Peripheral catheters are becoming increasingly popular in pediatric anesthesia, providing prolonged analgesia for surgery associated with moderate to severe postoperative pain.[13] They are predominantly used for limb surgery, though they can be inserted for abdominal fascial plane blocks or indeed for simple wound irrigation. Other indications for the use of peripheral nerve catheters include the following:

- To facilitate intensive physiotherapy post–limb surgery
- To potentiate perfusion following reimplantation surgery
- To treat CRPS-1
- To manage nonsurgical pain (eg, epidermolysis bullosa)
- For palliative care (if the catheter is fixed correctly, it is the author's experience that patients can be managed at home for as many months as is required)

Infective complications are rare and also less common than in adults; nevertheless, a strict aseptic technique should be used when placing peripheral nerve catheters. It is debatable whether it is helpful to make a space around the nerve for the catheter to be inserted into. With US, an advantage of making a space with local anesthetic is that the anesthesiologist knows that he or she has at least provided a reliable single injection of local anesthetic. The position of the catheter is confirmed by using a neurostimulating catheter or US. However, neurostimulating catheters are expensive, and their advantages are insignificant. When using US, it is often helpful to identify the catheter tip by scanning in both the transverse and longitudinal planes; local anesthetic or saline can then be injected and the spread assessed. Generally, no more than 2–3 cm of the catheter is inserted beyond the needle tip.

To ensure catheter security, tunneling should be performed for the majority of techniques (Figure 44–2). In addition, tissue glue should be applied to the original and secondary puncture sites to stop local anesthetic solution from leaking during infusion. Leakage of infusion causes the dressing to become wet and lift off the skin, leading to catheter dislodgement. Indermil or Dermabond glue can be used; the advantage of the latter is that it can be easily removed with yellow paraffin. It is usually a good idea to flush the catheter once it is tunneled and secured to ensure no kink has formed under the skin. The local anesthetic pump should be run intraoperatively so that any occlusion is detected prior to the patient being recovered.

As confidence has grown with nerve catheter techniques, their use in older children at home is being increasingly described; this has been aided by the development of disposable elastomeric pumps. A typical infusion prescription of 0.125% levobupivacaine or ropivacaine runs at 0.1–0.3 mL/kg/h. For fascial plane blocks that require volume to work, a local anesthetic bolus regime may be preferable to running an infusion. The postoperative analgesia management should be clearly documented and verbally handed over to the ward staff and parents or caregivers. It should include rescue analgesia (eg, Oramorph or diazepam 0.1mg/kg to a maximum of 5 mg) for muscle spasms, an antiemetic, and a proposed time and date to stop the peripheral nerve catheter infusion. When the peripheral nerve catheter infusion is stopped, the patient should be loaded with simple analgesics. If the patient is managing their pain 4–6 hours later, the catheter can be removed.

Clinical Pearls

- Children under 6 months of age should undergo regional anesthetic techniques only by anesthesiologists with specific training in pediatric regional anesthesia.
- Always use the most peripheral technique possible.
- When learning catheter techniques, begin with easier sites for catheter insertion, such as the femoral nerve.
- When learning US-guided techniques, and particularly with small children, it is useful to initially use saline to identify correct needle placement; in this way, no local anesthetic is wasted and overdose is prevented.
- For the best US images of very superficial structures, a 5-mm jelly pad is useful.
- Local anesthetic absorption may be greater with US-guided fascial blocks.

ANATOMICAL DIVISIONS

Head & Neck Blocks

The use of nerve blocks for various head and neck procedures is gaining in popularity, particularly in the pediatric population. Most of these blocks are sensory nerve blocks, which are easy to administer (field blocks) and virtually devoid of complications. They can, however, provide quality analgesia in the postoperative period, facilitating immediate postoperative recovery and pain management. Most of the innervation for the face and scalp is derived from the trigeminal nerve (cranial nerve V) and the cervical plexus (C2–C4).

V1 Division of the Trigeminal Nerve

The supraorbital and supratrochlear nerves are branches of the first division of the trigeminal nerve that exit from the supraorbital foramen. The supraorbital nerve provides sensory innervation to the anterior portion of the scalp, except for the midportion of the forehead, which is innervated by the supratrochlear nerve. This block can be used for frontal craniotomies as well as for minor surgical procedures, including excision of scalp nevi.[14,15]

Technique　The supraorbital nerve can be easily blocked as it exits the supraorbital foramen; the block location is easily correlated to the midpoint of the pupil. When the foramen is located, a subcutaneous injection of local anesthetic solution (1–2 mL 0.25% bupivacaine with 1:200,000 epinephrine) is performed. Once the local anesthetic solution is injected, gentle pressure is maintained to decrease the risk of hematoma formation. Complications with this block are rare.

V2 Branch of the Trigeminal Nerve

The second division of the trigeminal nerve is also referred to as the maxillary division of the trigeminal nerve. It exits from the maxillary foramen or the infraorbital foramen, which is located about 2 cm from the midline, and is usually aligned with the midpoint of the pupils. This nerve provides sensory supply to the upper lip, choana, maxillary sinus, part of the nasal septum, and tip of the nose. This block can be used to provide analgesia for cleft lip surgery, nasal septal repair, and endoscopic sinus surgery.[16–20]

Technique　There are two approaches to the maxillary division of the trigeminal nerve:

1. *Extraoral route:* The needle is directed into the infraorbital foramen from an external location of the nerve. The foramen is located externally, and a 27-gauge needle is inserted into the foramen. After aspiration to rule out intravascular injection, 1–2 mL of local anesthetic solution is injected.

2. *Intraoral route:* The nerve is accessed through the subsulcal area in the buccal mucosa. This is our preferred modality for blocking the infraorbital nerve. The upper incisor or the second bicuspid on the side to be blocked is located; a needle is passed via a subsulcal route toward the location of the infraorbital foramen. After careful

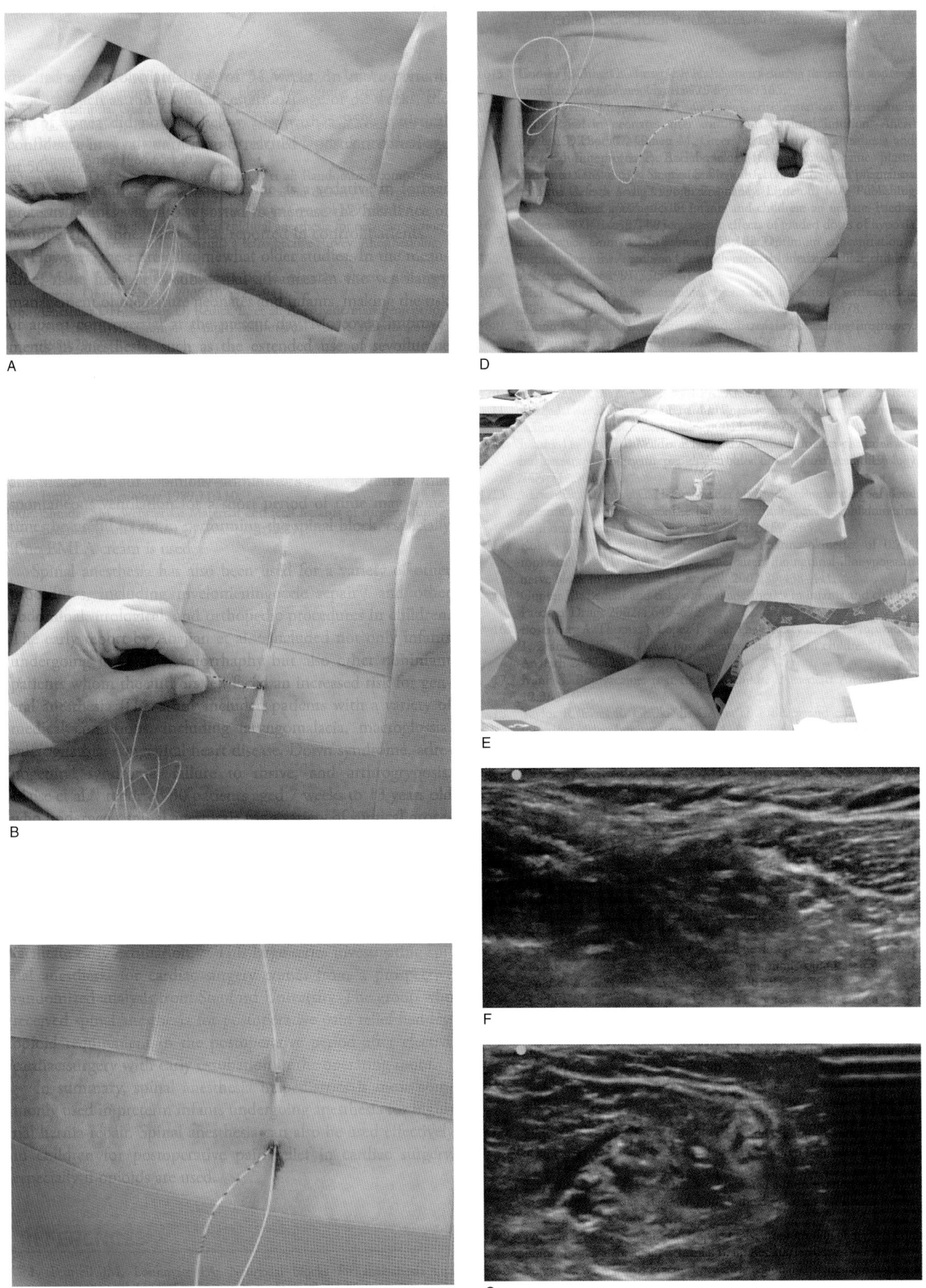

FIGURE 44–2. Tunneling of the popliteal catheter. The image in (**F**) illustrates an in-plane approach, whereas (**G**) illustrates an out-of-plane approach.

aspiration, local anesthetic solution is injected. For infants scheduled for cleft lip repairs, we use 0.5 mL of local anesthetic solution for each side; for older children and adolescents, we use 1.5–2 mL of local anesthetic solution. The upper lip is likely to remain numb for several hours after the block, which can be disconcerting to patients. Care should be provided to prevent biting of the upper lip during the period of emergence from anesthesia.

V3 Mandibular Division of the Trigeminal Nerve

The mandibular division of the trigeminal nerve provides analgesia for the lower jaw, lower lip, and portions of the temporoparietal portions of the scalp. The most common nerve targeted in children is the mental nerve, which exits from the mental foramen located at the level of the midline in line with the pupil and the supraorbital and infraorbital foramina.

Technique   An intraoral route is again preferred for placement of the mental nerve block. The needle is directed at the level of the lower incisor toward the infraorbital foramen; 1.5 mL of local anesthetic solution is then injected after careful aspiration. Gentle massage of the area is carried out after the injection.

The auriculotemporal nerve supplies the lateral scalp and is blocked at the midpoint between the pinna and the angle of the eye. A block of this nerve involves a subcutaneous injection of 1–2 mL of local anesthetic solution.

Greater Occipital Nerve   The greater occipital nerve is a branch of cervical root C2. The nerve pierces the aponeurosis and traverses medially to the occipital artery inferiorly and crosses over to the lateral aspect of the artery superiorly by the nuchal line as it innervates the posterior portions of the scalp. A greater occipital nerve block can be used for providing adequate block of the scalp for posterior fossa craniotomies as well as for patients with chronic occipital neuralgia.[14]

Technique   The occipital protuberance is palpated. The midline is identified, and the occipital artery is palpated. A 27-gauge needle is inserted, and a subcutaneous injection of local anesthetic solution is performed (1.5–2 mL of 0.25% bupivacaine with 1:200,000 epinephrine). The area is massaged gently after the injection. Complications are rare with this technique.

Ultrasound-Guided Technique   The US-guided technique is the same as that used for adults (see Chapter 31). A linear probe of 10 MHz or more is used to identify the obliquus capitis, and the nerve can be found superficial to the muscle.

Superficial Cervical Plexus

The superficial cervical plexus is a pure sensory nerve derived from the C2–C4 nerve roots. It wraps around the belly of the sternocleidomastoid at the level of the cricoid and divides into four branches: the lesser occipital supplying the posterior

auricular area; the great auricular supplying the mastoid area and the pinna; the transverse cervical supplying the anterior portion of the neck; and the superficial cervical supplying the skin over the shoulder in a cape-like distribution over the shoulder joint. Blockade of the superficial cervical plexus can provide good postoperative analgesia for tympanomastoid surgery, otoplasty, thyroid surgery, and for procedures performed on the anterior portion of the neck.[21–24] The use of this nerve block decreases the use of opioids in the perioperative period, thereby decreasing the incidence of nausea and vomiting.[21]

Technique   The technique is essentially identical to that used in the adult patient. The clavicular head of the sternocleidomastoid is identified, and a line drawn from the cricoid cartilage to intersect the posterior border of the sternocleidomastoid is identified. A subcutaneous injection of local anesthetic solution (1–3 mL of 0.25% bupivacaine with epinephrine 1:200,000) is performed. Caution must be exercised during injection because of the close proximity of the nerve to the external jugular vein. Deep injections should be avoided to prevent potential injection into the deep cervical plexus, which is associated with adverse effects including recurrent laryngeal nerve paralysis, paralysis of the hemidiaphragm, and Horner syndrome as a result of unilateral sympathetic ganglion blockade. Complications, though rare, are related to deep cervical plexus blockade and intravascular injection. (See Chapter 80A for a more detailed description of this technique.)

Ultrasound-Guided Technique   The US-guided is the same as that used for adults (see Chapter 32A).

Nerve of Arnold

The nerve of Arnold is the auricular branch of the vagus nerve; it supplies sensory innervation to the auditory canal and the lower half of the tympanic membrane. A block of this nerve provides analgesia for myringotomy. Using a fine needle, 0.5–1 mL of local anesthetic is injected into the cartilage of the posterior tragus.

Upper Extremity Blocks

A complete review of the anatomy of the brachial plexus is provided in Chapters 3 and 32B–E. There are multiple approaches to the brachial plexus in children. Although the interscalene block is often used in adults for surgical procedures of the shoulder, this approach is used infrequently in children. This is due to the limited indications and increased incidence of complications associated with the use of the interscalene approach in children. The most common approaches to the brachial plexus in children include the supraclavicular, infraclavicular, and axillary approaches. The complications described include hematoma, intravascular injection, intraneural injection, and pneumothorax for the periclavicular blocks. Except for the axillary approach, all approaches should always be performed under US guidance. Often, these blocks are being performed on children with severe musculoskeletal complaints (eg, fixed contractures, muscles absent or fibrosed); in these patients, US is superior to neurostimulation in terms of its ability to define individual anatomy. For prolonged analgesia, peripheral catheters can be easily fixed in the supraclavicular or infraclavicular region.

Supraclavicular Approach

In the close anatomical relationships of children, only small probe movements are required to change from an interscalene view to a supraclavicular view. Prior to US, this block had been underused in children due to the close proximity of the cervical pleura. However, with appropriate training and mentorship, the sonoanatomy (Figure 44–3) becomes easy to understand, and the block generally becomes technically easy to perform. It is recommended that this block be performed only with the use of US.

Ultrasound-Guided Technique In the US-guided supraclavicular approach, the child is placed supine with a head ring and shoulder roll; this arrangement creates enough room for the anesthesiologist's needling hand to approach from the posterior aspect. In the younger child, the first rib may not be fully ossified. Always use Doppler to identify potentially dangerous vessels in the proposed needle trajectory. The probe is positioned parallel to and touching the clavicle and is angled caudad, aiming into the thorax. An in-plane needling technique from the posterolateral to anteromedial direction is employed (see Figure 44–3).[25]

Infraclavicular Approach

The US-guided infraclavicular approach is second choice to the supraclavicular approach as the brachial plexus is generally deeper at this point and an out-of-plane technique is employed.[10, 25] However, an infraclavicular approach is indicated if the supraclavicular fossa is inaccessible or there is local infection. US guidance is recommended for this approach (see Chapter 32D for more detail).

Axillary Approach

The axillary approach to the brachial plexus is the most commonly used landmark-based approach in children and adolescents and is used for procedures on the arm and hand. The primary advantage of the axillary approach is the relatively lower risk of complications. However, there is a 40–50% chance of missing the musculocutaneous nerve with this approach, owing to the proximal exit of this nerve from the axillary sheath. Hence, while performing a block using this approach, the musculocutaneous nerve should be blocked separately when analgesia of the biceps and anterior forearm is sought. Peripheral nerve catheters in the axilla are difficult to immobilize and protect from bacterial colonization. A US-guided technique has been described but differs little from the adult technique described in Chapter 32E.[26]

Technique There are several techniques for placing an axillary block. The commonly used approaches include the transarterial approach and the nerve stimulation approach. Although greater success with the transarterial approach has been reported in adults, this approach is not often used in children,[27] due to the higher incidence of vessel spasm and increased potential for ischemia in children versus adults. Although many methods have been reported in adults, the simple, common single-injection technique seems to be effective in children.[28]

For this technique, the patient is positioned with the arm abducted 90 degrees. The elbow is flexed, and the arm is placed above the head. A stimulating needle is inserted superior to the axillary artery at an angle of 30 degrees, with the tip pointed toward the midpoint of the clavicle. A "pop" may be felt as the needle enters the axillary sheath. After eliciting a response to nerve stimulation at 0.5 mA, local anesthetic solution is injected. A volume of 0.3–0.5 mL/kg is recommended, to a maximum of 20 mL. When anesthesia of the musculocutaneous nerve is required to augment this block, the needle is directed above the pulse of the axillary artery and toward the belly of the coracobrachialis muscle. Contraction of the biceps confirms placement of the needle close to the musculocutaneous nerve.

Nerve Block at the Wrist Blockade of the radial, ulnar, and median nerves can be accomplished at the level of the wrist. The advantage of these peripheral blocks is the absence of motor blockade. They are used primarily for surgery on the hand, such as syndactyly repair. These blocks are performed in conjunction with general anesthesia, since tourniquet pain cannot be eliminated with this block alone. (See Chapters 32G and 80F for more information on the US-guided and landmark-based techniques, respectively; these techniques are essentially identical to those used in adults.) With US, the nerves can be blocked at any point along their path. The following discussion outlines some specific issues that relate to the landmark application of wrist blocks in pediatric patients.

Radial Nerve The radial nerve is a superficial sensory nerve proximal to the radial head. The radial nerve divides into two branches: the thenar branch and the dorsal branch. This division takes place proximal to the distal end of the radius. This block is performed for children undergoing trigger thumb release or minor surgical procedures involving the thumb and index finger.

Technique The anatomical "snuff box" is identified, and local anesthetic is infiltrated subcutaneously approximately 2 cm proximal to the this location. A volume of 2 mL is adequate to provide good analgesia in the postoperative period.

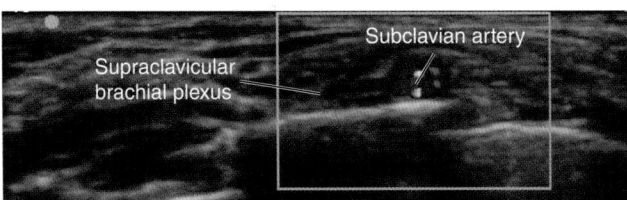

FIGURE 44–3. Supraclavicular block in a child: probe position and relevant sonoanatomy.

Median Nerve   The median nerve is located between the tendons of the palmaris longus and the flexor carpi radialis. The nerve can be blocked at the level of the flexor retinaculum or at midforearm level. One of the important anatomical advantages of blocking the median nerve at the wrist is the presence of a bursa at the level of the flexor retinaculum. This bursa encompasses the median nerve; hence, blockade of this nerve can be carried out without damage to the nerve.

Technique   The tendons of the flexor carpi radialis and the palmaris longus are identified. Flexion of the wrist identifies the tendons. A 27-gauge needle is inserted at the medial border of the palmaris longus tendon. A "pop" is felt as the bursa is entered. An injection of 2 mL of local anesthetic solution is made. Smaller quantities are used in younger children and infants.

Ulnar Nerve   The palmar cutaneous branch of the ulnar nerve accompanies the ulnar artery to the wrist. It perforates the flexor retinaculum and ends in the palm, communicating with the median nerve.

Technique   The nerve is easily blocked at the wrist. The flexor carpi ulnaris tendon is identified. The nerve is blocked under the flexor carpi ulnaris tendon, just proximal to the pisiform bone. A 27-gauge needle is passed under the flexor carpi ulnaris, proximal to the pisiform bone, about 0.5 cm. After aspiration, 2 mL of local anesthetic solution is injected.

Lower Extremity Blocks

The lumbar plexus and sacral plexus supply the lower extremity. The lumbar plexus is contained in the psoas compartment and consists of a small portion of T12 and lumbar nerves L1–L4. The femoral, lateral femoral cutaneous, and obturator nerves are branches of the lumbar plexus and supply most of the thigh and upper leg. The lower leg is innervated by the sacral plexus, which is derived from the anterior rami of L4, L5, S1, S2, and S3. The sacral plexus gives rise to the sciatic nerve, which is the largest nerve in the body. The complications of lower extremity blocks described include hematoma, intravascular injection, and intraneural injection. The landmark/nerve stimulation method is made difficult in cerebral palsy patients in whom there are limb contractures and absent or hypoplastic or fibrosed muscles. The contractures are occasionally so severe that it is nearly impossible to gain access to perform the block.

Femoral Nerve

The femoral nerve block is the most commonly performed lower extremity peripheral nerve block in children. It is used to provide pain relief after femoral fractures, Ilizarov frame placement, patellar ligament realignment, and slipped upper femoral epiphysis fixation.[29–32] The femoral nerve is located at the level of the crease at the groin, lateral to the pulsation of the femoral artery.

Technique   The technique for this block is similar to that used in adults (see Chapter 82C). The femoral artery pulse is located, and the needle is inserted immediately lateral to

the pulse to elicit a quadriceps muscle contraction. The nerve stimulator is initially set at 1 mA and then reduced to 0.5 mA while observing the quadriceps contraction. The location of the needle is stabilized and aspiration performed repeatedly as 0.2–0.4 mL/kg of local anesthetic is injected.

Ultrasound-Guided Technique   The patient is positioned supine, with the anesthesiologist on the side of the intended nerve block, facing the US machine opposite. The linear probe is placed just below and parallel to the inguinal ligament. Using minimal transducer pressure to avoid collapsing vessels, Doppler is used to identify the superficial circumflex iliac artery, as this artery frequently passes superficially to the femoral nerve (Figure 44–4). The needle is introduced in plane from a lateral to medial direction, aiming to just "pop" the fascia iliaca as it spreads over the femoral nerve. Note that more than two "pops" are often felt and that repeated test injections of 0.5 mL may be required to ensure that the correct plane has been located.[33] If required, the needle can then be rotated 180 degrees to block the lateral femoral cutaneous nerve.

Lateral Femoral Cutaneous Nerve   The lateral femoral cutaneous nerve is derived from L3 and L4 segments of the lumbar plexus. It is a pure sensory nerve and passes superficially along the lateral border of the iliac crest. It appears from beneath the inguinal ligament medial to the anterior superior iliac spine, travelling between the fascia lata and the fascia iliaca. It supplies the skin of the lateral aspect of the buttock and the anterolateral aspect of the thigh below the greater trochanter. A lateral femoral cutaneous nerve is useful for providing analgesia for surgery on the lateral aspect of the thigh, including muscle biopsies and graft excisions.[34]

Note that the lateral femoral cutaneous nerve does not supply the skin of the thigh above the greater trochanter; this area is supplied by branches of the L1 and T12 nerve roots. If the incision is to extend this cephalad, a superficial infiltration around the upper lateral aspect of the thigh or a transverse abdominis plane (TAP) (T12–L1) block may be required. Where children have undergone previous hip surgery, scarring can make both the landmark- and US-based techniques difficult. The technique for this block is similar to that used in adults (see Chapter 33C).

Technique   The anterior superior iliac spine is identified. A point 1–2 cm below and medial to the anterior superior iliac spine is identified. After careful aseptic preparation of the area, a blunt needle is introduced into the marked site. Once the

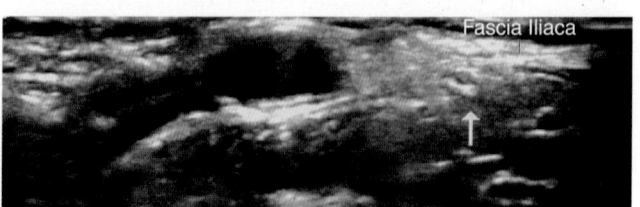

FIGURE 44–4. Femoral nerve block in a child: probe position and relevant sonoanatomy.

needle is through the skin, a "pop" is felt as the needle pierces the fascia lata. Once the needle is lodged within this space, loss of resistance may be felt as the local anesthetic solution is injected. A total volume of 0.1 mL/kg (to a maximum of 5 mL) of local anesthetic solution is injected.

Ultrasound-Guided Technique

A reliable location to identify the nerve is 10–20 mm below the anterior superior iliac spine, in the groove between the sartorius muscle and the tensor fascia lata.[33] The lateral femoral cutaneous nerve is a small hyperechoic nerve (Figure 44–5). Note that the nerve may pass through the ligament or laterally to the anterior superior iliac spine.

Sciatic Nerve

The sacral plexus comprises the sciatic nerve and provides innervation to the posterior thigh, leg, and most of the foot, except the medial portion, which is innervated by the femoral nerve. A number of techniques are used in children for a sciatic nerve block. When choosing which level to block the nerve, it is essential that the most distal approach be chosen. Tourniquet pain is rarely a problem in children, as they are under general anesthesia. Further, distal nerve components are more likely to be missed if a proximal block is performed, thus creating a "patchy" block. We will address two techniques: the subgluteal and the popliteal fossa approaches. However, with US, the sciatic nerve can essentially be blocked at whichever level is appropriate to the surgery and where the nerve is easiest to visualize.

Subgluteal Approach

This approach is indicated for hamstring releases and anterior cruciate ligament repairs. Catheter placement is straightforward; it is helpful to tunnel the catheter laterally subcutaneously 30–40 mm. Placing a tourniquet over the catheter is not problematic, though care should be taken on removal of the tourniquet to prevent catheter dislodgement by the surgeon.

Technique

The subgluteal sciatic nerve block can be performed either in the lateral (operative side uppermost) or supine position with the limb elevated. The subgluteal line where the gluteal crease is present is marked. The biceps femoris tendon is identified, and a point inferior to the gluteal crease, just medial to the biceps femoris tendon, is delineated. A sheathed needle connected to a nerve stimulator is introduced in an anterior plane and cephalad at an angle of 60–70 degrees. Inversion of the foot indicates blockade of the tibial nerve.[35]

The current is then reduced to 0.4 mA, and if inversion is still present, the local anesthetic solution is injected. If eversion is noted, the needle is withdrawn to the skin and inserted medially. If the biceps femoris tendon is contracting, the needle is drawn back to the skin and inserted medially, away from the muscle belly of the biceps femoris tendon. Plantar flexion is also an indicator of adequate block placement, although this yields a potential for failed blockade.[35] A volume of 0.3–0.5 mL/kg (to a maximum of 20 mL) is injected into the space. On initial injection of 1 mL of local anesthetic solution, the twitch disappears, confirming correct needle placement.

Ultrasound-Guided Technique

A linear probe suffices in all but the largest adolescent. Applying probe pressure improves the US image, as this brings the sciatic nerve closer to the probe (Figure 44–6). Visualizing the nerve may be difficult in arthrogryptotic children, in whom it may be obscured by fibrosis. Where there is difficulty identifying the nerve, a longitudinal scan from medial to lateral and back may be attempted, looking for a band of hyperechogenicity (Figure 44–7). Once the sciatic nerve identified, rotate the probe back into the transverse plane. Alternatively, track down distally to the popliteal fossa, and identify the nerve before retracing your steps. With US, it is often possible to see the posterior cutaneous branch of the thigh, medial and superficial to the sciatic nerve, and it is important to ensure the local anesthetic covers it. An in-plane technique is advisable for single injections, whereas an out-of-plane technique is often better for catheter placement.[33] When placing catheters, first inject one-third of the available local anesthetic by the lateral aspect of the nerve; the remaining two-thirds is used medially to make space for the catheter. This technique ensures the nerve is surrounded.

Popliteal Fossa Block

The indications for popliteal block include trauma surgery and correction of congenital abnormalities. In conjunction with a saphenous nerve block, the lower limb below the knee can be completely anesthetized.

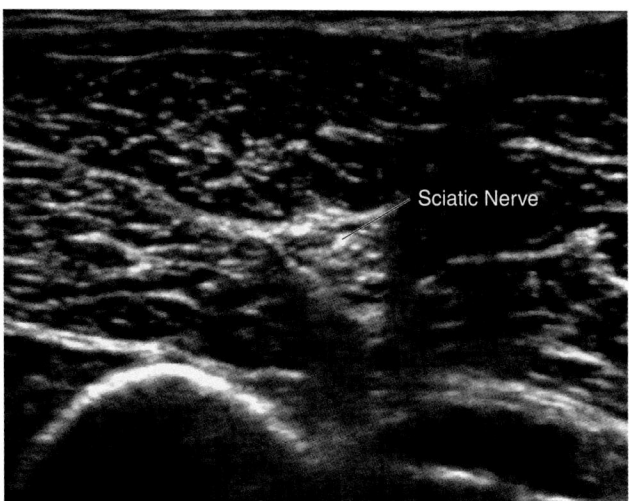

FIGURE 44–6. Probe position and sonoanatomy at the subgluteal level.

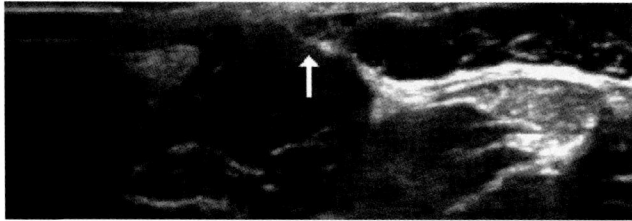

FIGURE 44–5. Lateral cutaneous nerve of the thigh in a 6-year-old: probe position and relevant sonoanatomy.

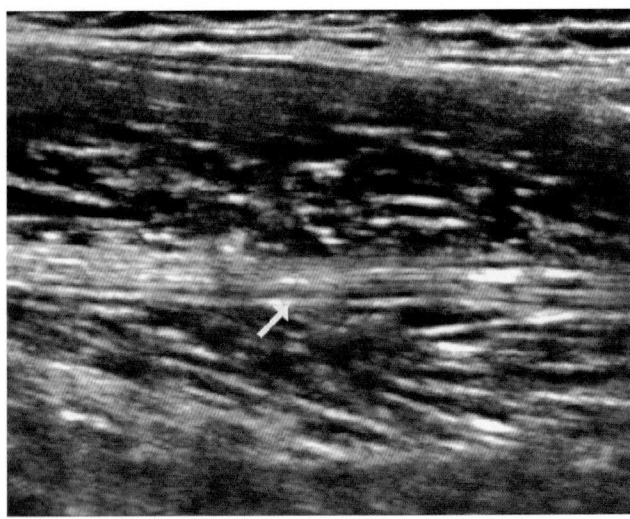

FIGURE 44–7. Longitudinal scan of the thigh highlighting the sciatic nerve in a 6-year-old.

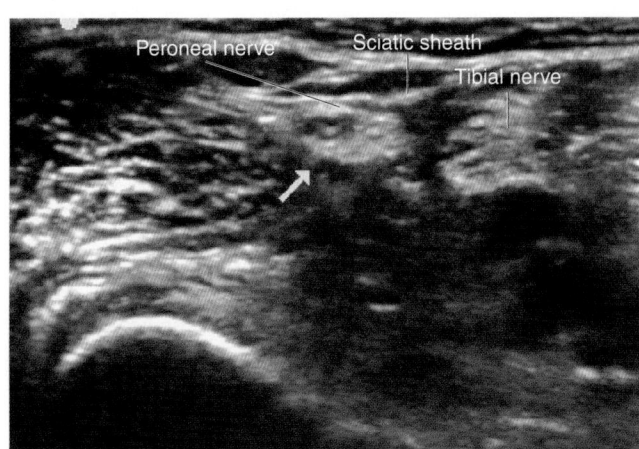

FIGURE 44–8. Popliteal block: probe position and sonoanatomy.

The popliteal fossa is a diamond-shaped area with the superior triangle formed by the tendons of the semitendinosus and semimembranosus medially and the biceps femoris tendon laterally.[36] The sciatic nerve divides into the common peroneal nerve and the tibial nerve. The common peroneal nerve exits the popliteal fossa laterally, and the tibial nerve exits medially. The branching of the sciatic nerve takes place at varying levels above the popliteal crease. A common epineural sheath is present that envelops both the tibial and common peroneal nerve; as a result, complete blockade of both branches may result.[37]

Technique   The patient is positioned laterally (operative side uppermost to allow for better needle access), with the lower knee flexed or prone. The needle is inserted at the apex of the popliteal fossa, lateral to the artery. A response to nerve stimulation at 0.4 mA confirms the position of the needle and its proximity to the sciatic nerve. The tibial nerve is localized by the presence of inversion and plantar flexion (*i*nternal nerve = *i*nversion); the common peroneal nerve is localized by the presence of eversion and dorsiflexion (*e*xternal nerve = *e*version). After aspiration to rule out intravascular placement, local anesthetic solution is injected. A volume of 0.5 mL/kg is injected (to a maximum volume of 20 mL).

Ultrasound-Guided Technique   The patient is positioned as described above, though, when supine, in many children with cerebral palsy, the leg will rotate externally sufficiently to allow the nerves to be approached medially. Children with flexed flexion deformities will not display the "see-saw" sign. For a single injection, an in-plane technique is recommended, from either the medial or lateral aspect of the leg.[33] With US, the exact level of sciatic nerve branching can be identified; at this point, the combined circumference of the two nerves will be greater than the circumference of the "sciatic" nerve; a block at this location provides greater local anesthetic–nerve contact (Figure 44–8).[38] For catheter insertion, an out-of-plane approach is preferred by the author; with a view to threading

the catheter along the axis of the nerve, position can be checked in the longitudinal view. The catheter should be inserted at the level of sciatic nerve division.

Ankle

The ankle block is a very common and easy block to perform in children undergoing foot surgery. There are five main nerves to be blocked: the posterior tibial, deep peroneal, superficial peroneal, saphenous, and sural (Figure 44–9). All these nerves are distal branches of the sciatic nerve, except for the saphenous nerve, which is a branch of the femoral nerve. The nerves are superficial and therefore do not require much volume. Epinephrine should not be added to the local anesthetic solution because end arteries are present at the site of injection (see Chapter 82F for illustrations and a detailed description of the ankle block).

A US-guided approach is also possible (see Chapter 32H). Ideally, a probe with a small footprint and a frequency of 15 MHz or more should be readily available, but unfortunately, many of the highest-frequency probes have large footprints and do not readily sit on a small ankle. Once again, a sterile US gel pad may aid visualization.

Tibial Nerve   The tibial nerve is the largest nerve supplying the plantar aspect of the foot and is an important nerve to be blocked for any foot surgery. We routinely use surface mapping with a current of 5 mA to locate the tibial nerve before injection. The nerve is located behind the posterior tibial pulsation, below the medial malleolus. A 27-gauge needle is advanced to the bone and slightly withdrawn to avoid injection into the periosteum; 2–5 mL of local anesthetic solution is then injected. Alternatively, a sheathed needle can be used, and plantar flexion or inversion can be elicited before injection.

Saphenous Nerve   The saphenous nerve is the distal cutaneous branch of the femoral nerve. It is located superficially, anterior to the medial malleolus. A superficial ring is injected along the medial malleolus, and 2–5 mL of local anesthetic solution is injected. Caution must be exercised to

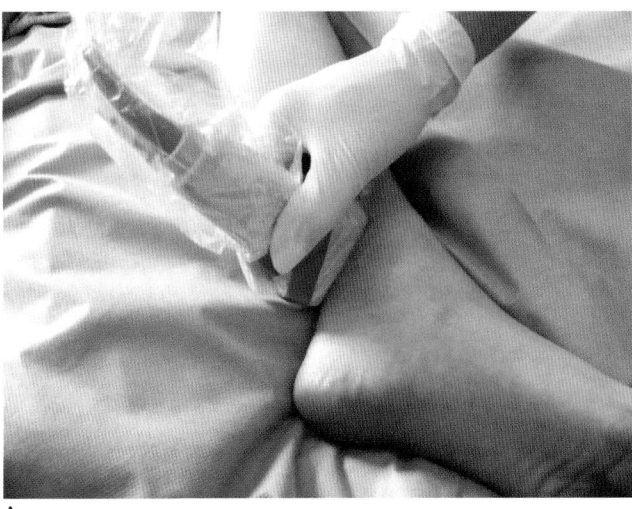

A

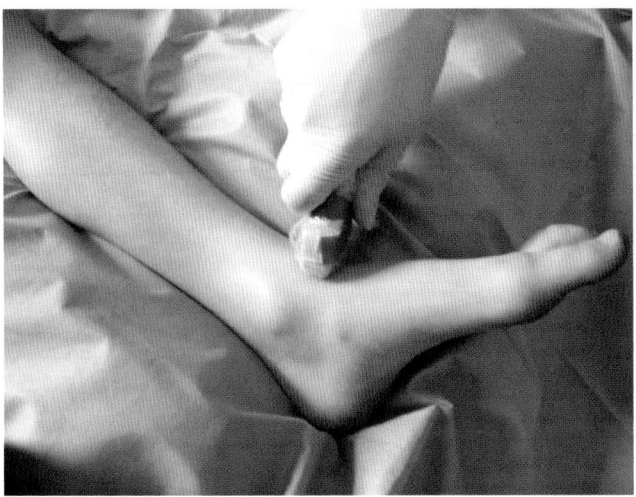

B

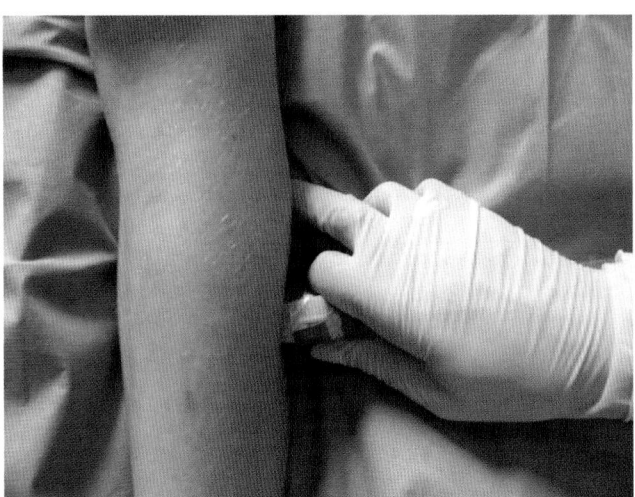

C

FIGURE 44–9. Transducer position for a block of the (**A**) posterior tibial nerve; (**B**) superficial peroneal nerve; and (**C**) deep peroneal nerve.

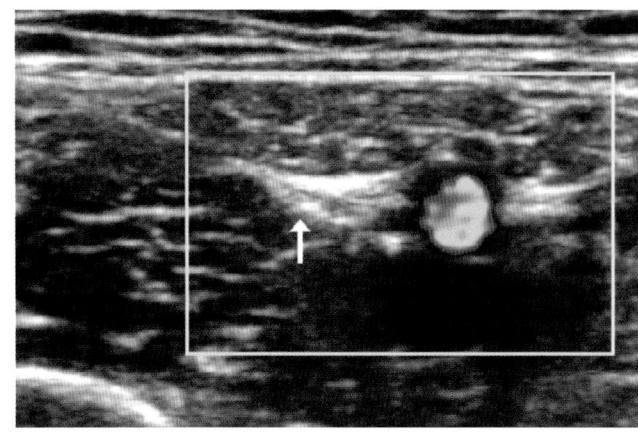

FIGURE 44–10. Subsartorial saphenous nerve block.

avoid intravascular injection, as the saphenous vein courses alongside the nerve. The saphenous nerve supplies the skin over the medial aspect of the leg below the knee and ankle. When performing a US-guided saphenous nerve block, it may be easier to find the nerve lateral to the artery, at the level of the adductor canal in the thigh, just before the vessels enter the posterior compartment (Figure 44–10). At this level, the nerve to the vastus medialis will also be blocked.

Deep Peroneal Nerve   The peroneal nerve innervates the first web space of the foot. It can be blocked by depositing local anesthetic solution lateral to the extensor hallucis longus tendon. The needle is advanced until the periosteum of the tibia is encountered, then drawn back slightly. A volume of 2–3 mL of local anesthetic solution is then injected. When using US, the nerve is more easily found by identifying the dorsalis pedis artery and tracking the artery proximally until it lies on the distal tibia; at this point, the nerve can be seen travelling over the artery.

Superficial Peroneal Nerve   The superficial peroneal nerve supplies sensory supply to the dorsum of the foot. It is superficial and can be easily blocked by injecting a superficial ring of local anesthesia between the lateral malleolus and the extensor hallucis longus tendon. This nerve is more easily visualized with US at the midcalf level, where it lies subcutaneously; it can be readily tracked back into the popliteal fossa, where it joins to form the common peroneal nerve.

Sural Nerve   The sural nerve supplies sensory innervation to the lateral aspect of the foot. It can be easily blocked by injecting local anesthetic solution between the lateral malleolus and the calcaneus. This nerve is very difficult to visualize with US.

Digital Nerve Blocks

A digital nerve block is provided for analgesia of the fingers and toes. It is an ideal block for simple procedures such as trigger finger release and ingrown toenail excision and for foreign body removal and minor lacerations requiring suturing. We have used these blocks successfully for analgesia after laser therapy for warts in children. The digital nerve block technique is addressed in Chapter 80G.

Hand

Anatomy   The common digital nerves of the hand are derived from the median and ulnar nerves and divide in the palm to supply the fingers. All digital nerves are accompanied by digital vessels. The median nerve provides three digital nerves. The first common palmar digital nerve divides into the three palmar digital nerves that supply the side of the thumb; the second common palmar digital nerve supplies the web space between the index and middle fingers, and the third common palmar digital nerve communicates with the ulnar nerve to supply the web space between the middle and ring fingers. These nerves then become the proper digital nerves that supply the skin of the distal phalanx. There are also smaller digital nerves derived from the radial and ulnar nerves that supply the dorsum of the fingers. The four dorsal digital nerves are located on the ulnar side of the thumb and the radial side of the index finger, adjacent to the index and middle fingers. All digital nerves terminate in two main branches: one supplying the skin under the fingertips, and the other supplying the pulp under the nail.

Technique   The digital nerves are blocked using non–epinephrine-containing solution on each side of the finger at the bifurcation between the metacarpal heads. A dorsal or volar injection accomplishes similar results. A needle is inserted into the web space between the thumb and index finger to a distance of about 1 cm. A second needle is inserted into the thenar eminence on the radial aspect of the thumb. For the other fingers, the needle is inserted between the metacarpal heads. A needle is inserted proximal to the thenar web space at the distal palmar crease. After aspiration, 1 mL of local anesthetic solution (without epinephrine) is injected.

Complications   A large volume of local anesthetic solution is contraindicated as it can cause vascular compromise.

Feet

Anatomy   The digital nerves to the feet are derived from the plantar cutaneous branch of the tibial nerve. The proper digital nerve of the toe supplies the medial aspect of the great toe. The three common digital nerves split into two proper digital nerves each. The first supplies the adjacent areas of the great and second toes, the second supplies the adjacent sides of the second and third toes, and the third supplies the adjacent sides of the third and fourth toes. Each of these terminates at the tip of the toe. A branch from the superficial peroneal nerve supplies the dorsum of the foot. This is derived from two nerves: (1) the dorsal cutaneous nerve, which divides into two branches, a medial branch supplying the great toe and a lateral branch supplying the adjacent sides of the second and third toes; and (2) the intermediate dorsal cutaneous nerve, which passes along the lateral part of the foot, supplying the lateral

aspect of the foot and communicating with the sural nerve. The two dorsal digital terminal branches supply the adjacent parts of the third and fourth toes and another branch supplying the adjacent sides of the fourth and fifth toes.

Technique   It is easy to block the digital nerves by accessing the web space on the dorsolateral aspect of the foot. It is best to avoid these blocks in children who may have compromised blood flow to the toes. Vasoconstrictors are to be avoided for all these blocks.

Trunk Blocks

For most surgery involving truncal blocks, there will be an element of visceral pain that is not covered. Therefore, all children should receive some systemic analgesic adjuncts (eg, paracetamol and ibuprofen). Remember that with US-guided fascial blocks, local anesthetic absorption may be greater than with standard landmark-based techniques.

Ilioinguinal/Iliohypogastric Nerve

The ilioinguinal/iliohypogastric nerve block is indicated for inguinal hernia, orchidopexy, and varicocele surgery.

Anatomy   The ilioinguinal and iliohypogastric nerves originate from the T12 (subcostal nerve) and L1 (ilioinguinal, iliohypogastric) nerve roots of the lumbar plexus. These nerves pierce the internal oblique aponeurosis 2–3 cm medial to the anterior superior iliac spine. The ilioinguinal nerve travels between the internal oblique and the external oblique aponeuroses. Here, it accompanies the spermatic cord and is part of the neurovascular bundle to the genital area.[39] US studies have shown that there is no relationship between a child's weight and the depth or position of the nerves.

Technique   A line is drawn between the umbilicus and anterior superior iliac spine. A point is marked 2 mm medial from the anterior superior iliac spine. The needle is advanced toward the inguinal canal and passed in until a "pop" is felt. Local anesthetic solution is then injected into the area after aspiration. US studies have shown that blind administration usually does not inject the local anesthetic into the correct fascial plane between the internal oblique and transversus abdominis muscles; yet, clinically, the majority of blocks work, presumably due to the diffusion of the local anesthetic.[40] Alternatively, an ilioinguinal nerve block can be performed by the surgeon; the disadvantage of this is the need for a deeper plane of general anesthesia intraoperatively.

Ultrasound-Guided Technique   The probe is placed on a line from the anterior superior iliac spine to the umbilicus, with the lateral end of the probe resting on the bone (Figures 44–11). With practice, the nerves can be tracked more proximally toward the midaxillary line, which prevents the local anesthetic spreading too far into the surgeon's field and disrupting their tissue planes.[41] Experts in this field have managed to

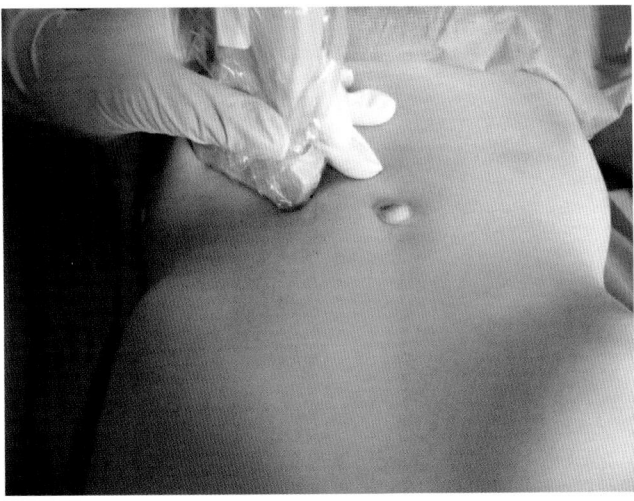

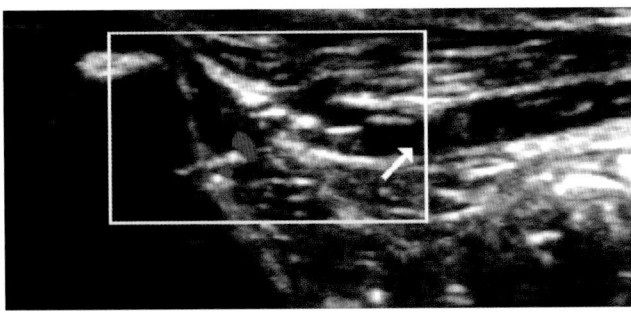

FIGURE 44–11. Ilioinguinal/iliohypogastric nerve block: (**A**) probe position; (**B**) US image.

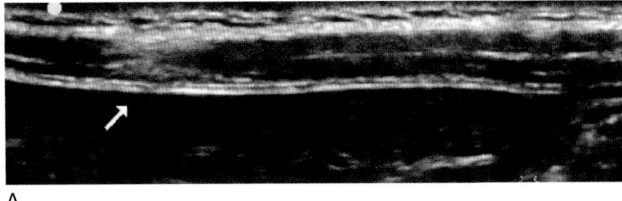

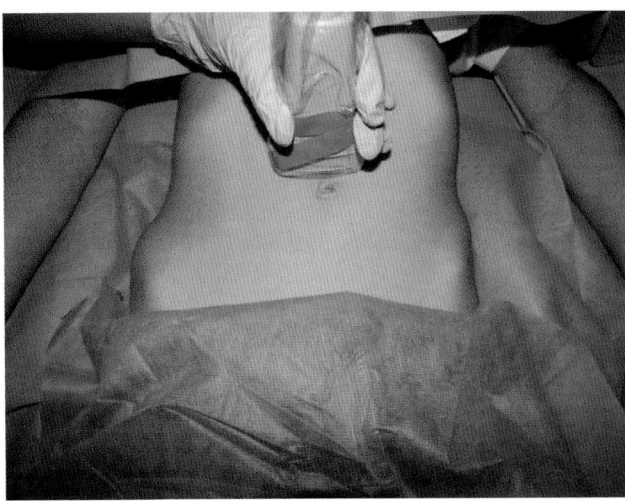

FIGURE 44–12. Neonatal rectus sheath block: (**A**) sonoanatomy; (**B**) probe position.

successfully block these nerves with a volume of local anesthetic as little as 0.075 mL/kg.[42]

Complications An ilioinguinal/iliohypogastric nerve block is relatively safe. Perforation of the bowel wall can occur, however, and has been reported.[43] Femoral nerve blockade may occur in up to 11% of cases; therefore, all ambulant children should be tested for weight bearing prior to discharge.[44]

Rectus Sheath

A rectus sheath block (Figure 44–12) is useful in children for umbilical area surgery (eg, umbilical hernia, pyloromyotomy, duodenal atresia). It must be performed bilaterally, as the nerves cross over the midline from each side. The technique is essentially the same as that used in adults (see Chapter 81) but requires a greater degree of finesse when performed in neonates, in whom muscle thickness may be as little as 2 mm.

Anatomy The umbilical area is innervated by the tenth thoracoabdominal intercostal nerves from the right and left sides. Each nerve passes behind the costal cartilage and between the transverse abdominis and the internal oblique muscles. The nerve runs between the sheath and the posterior wall of the rectus abdominis muscle and ends at the anterior cutaneous branch, supplying the skin of the umbilical area. The rectus muscle is attached anteriorly to the sheath at three intertendinous intersections; however, posteriorly there are no attachments, and it is this which allows the spread of local anesthetic.

Technique The aim of this block is to deposit local anesthetic solution between the muscle and the posterior aspect of the sheath. The technique has been well described by Ferguson et al.[45] A 23-gauge needle is inserted above or below the umbilicus, 0.5 cm medial to the linea semilunaris in a perpendicular plane. The anterior rectus sheath is identified by moving the needle in a back-and-forth motion until a scratching sensation is felt and the rectus sheath is identified and entered. After the belly of the muscle is entered, the needle is farther advanced until the posterior aspect of the rectus sheath is appreciated with a scratching sensation as the needle is moved again in a back-and-forth motion. Once the sheath is felt, it is entered, and local anesthetic solution is deposited posterior to the sheath. The usual depth of needle entry is about 5–15 mm. After aspiration, 0.2–0.3 mL/kg of bupivacaine 0.25%–0.5% is injected on each side.

If resistance to injection is felt, the needle is advanced deeper, as resistance may indicate that the needle is within the body of the muscle. Caution should be taken, as US studies have shown that the depth from the skin to the posterior sheath is independent of age and weight. Indeed, the distance is rarely greater than 10 mm in children under 10 years of age.

Ultrasound-Guided Technique This block can be performed with a greater degree of precision with the assistance of US.[46] The anatomy is easy to understand, and the sonoanatomy is simple, with no anisotropy to contend with. As such, this block is an ideal one to teach a beginner, though initially older children should be practiced on. With practice, the anesthesiologist should be able to block both sides without having to swap his or her position or that of the US machine. An in-plane technique is ideally suited to this block, aiming from lateral to medial. Care should be taken when choosing the needle insertion point; it should be sufficiently lateral to allow a shallow needle trajectory. In this way, the needle tip can be slid into the potential space between muscle and sheath and avoid a trajectory down toward the abdominal cavity. Prior to needling, Doppler should be used to assess the position of the inferior epigastric artery; this is easily found lying deep to the muscle at the level of the arcuate line. It can then be tracked cephalad into the muscle belly. A volume of 0.1 mL/kg is sufficient to provide analgesia for an umbilical hernia; more extensive midline incisions will require greater volume. Holding the probe in a paramedian longitudinal plane, the local anesthetic spread can be readily assessed passing beneath the intertendinous intersections caudad and cephalad.

Transversus Abdominis Plane

The TAP block is a relative newcomer to regional anesthesia. It may be performed unilaterally (eg, for procedures such as stoma formation and open appendectomy) or bilaterally (eg, for vesicostomy).[47] Though single injections are generally employed, catheters may also be used. The block may be performed at a level midway between the iliac crest and costal margin for sub-umbilical surgery or higher as a subcostal approach (eg, for cholecystectomy).[48] Either way, the block must be performed using US guidance. This is an easy block to learn, as the sono-anatomy is simple and there is no anisotropy for the novice to contend with. As with all abdominal blocks, there is no visceral analgesia, and systemic analgesia must be given. The block is performed as in adults (see Chapter 34).

Anatomy   The lateral abdominal wall consists of three muscles. From the peritoneum outward are the fascia transversalis and then the transversus abdominis, internal oblique, and external oblique muscles. The neurovascular plexus is fixed to the outer surface of transversus abdominis by a thick fascial sheet. It is unclear whether this must be breached for the block to be successful. Local anesthetic injected into the TAP will usually cover the T11–L1 segmental nerves and will also cover T10 50% of the time.[49]

Ultrasound-Guided Technique   The patient is positioned supine, with the anesthesiologist standing on the side to be blocked and the US machine placed opposite. For bilateral blocks, it is unnecessary to change positions. The probe is placed over the midaxillary line, between the iliac crest and costal margin in a transverse plane. Count the muscle layers from inside out; if the layers are identified from out to in, it is easy to mistake a subcutaneous layer for a muscle layer, particularly in obese patients. An in-plane technique is used (Figure 44–13). If it is difficult to place the needle tip within the correct plane, insert the needle carefully into the transversus abdominis muscle; as you withdraw, have an assistant inject. As the needle tip enters the correct plane, loss of resistance will be felt.

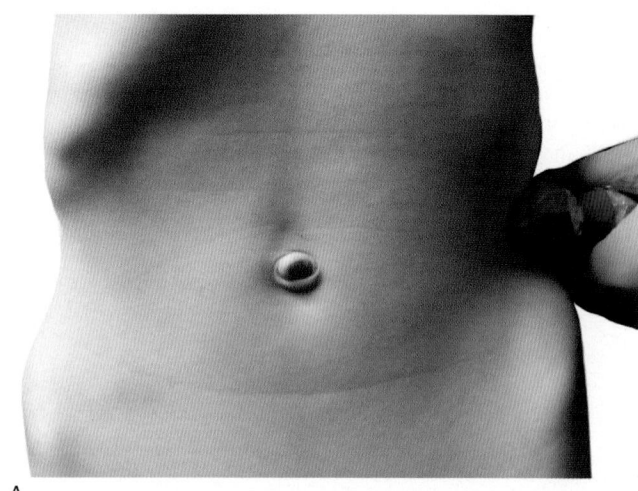

A

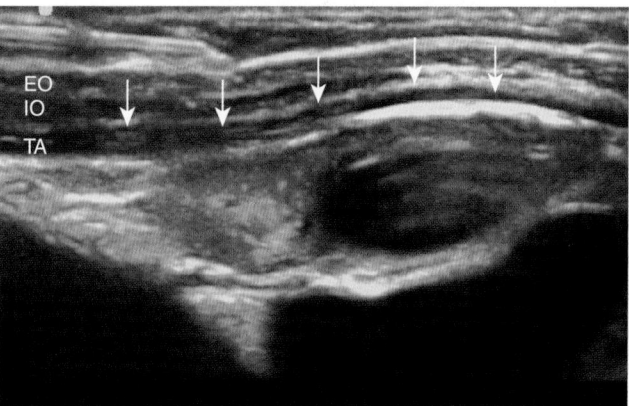

B

FIGURE 44–13. Transverse abdominis plane block: (**A**) probe position; (**B**) sonoanatomy. Arrows indicate TAP plane between transverse abdominis (TA); internal oblique muscles (IO); and external oblique (EO).

Penile Nerve

A penile nerve block is indicated for circumcision and distal hypospadias repair (where a caudal block is contraindicated). The sensory innervation of the penis is derived from the pudendal nerve. The pudendal nerve give rise to the dorsal nerves of the penis; these are accompanied by vessels medially as they enter the subpubic space at the level of the symphysis pubis before travelling distally to supply sensation to the shaft of the penis. The two nerves and their accompanying vessels are separated from one another by the suspensory ligament of the penis, hence the requirement for a bilateral approach. The subpubic space is roofed by Scarpa's fascia, a deep membranous continuation of the superficial abdominal fascia. A US-guided technique has been described but did not improve on the efficacy of the landmark-based technique. Epinephrine-containing solutions and ropivacaine, with its intrinsic vasoconstrictive properties, should not be used for penile nerve blocks.

Technique   The subpubic approach requires the penis to be gently retracted downward to make the Scarpa's fascia taut. Just below the symphysis pubis, a needle is inserted 5–10 mm lateral to the midline and advanced slightly caudally until a "pop" is felt as the needle enters the fascial compartment bounded superficially by Scarpa's fascia. Depth varies from 5–30 mm and is independent of both the age and weight of the child. After careful aspiration, 0.1 mL/kg of plain local anesthetic is injected (to a maximum of 5 mL). The injection is then repeated on the other side of the midline. Some anesthesiologists recommend infiltrating the ventral aspect of the shaft of the penis for a more reliable block.

An alternative approach is to place a subcutaneous ring block around the base of the penile shaft. Although a simpler technique, it is associated with a higher incidence of inadequate postoperative pain relief.[50]

Complications The most feared complication associated with penile nerve block is hematoma formation.

Thoracic Paravertebral Space

Thoracic paravertebral blocks should be performed only by specialist pediatric regional anesthesiologists. Both single-injection and catheter techniques have been described.[51] Indications for this block include postoperative thoracotomy pain, sternotomy, and unilateral abdominal surgery (eg, open splenectomy, nephrectomy).[52] Contraindications for this technique include severe coagulopathy, local infection, previous ipsilateral thoracic surgery (a relative contraindication), and previous total pleurectomy, as local anesthetic will not stay within the paravertebral space. Empyema or localized tumor near the injection site should be carefully considered to avoid seeding malignant cells or infection. An 18-gauge pediatric (50-mm length with 5-mm markings) epidural kit is suitable for all pediatric patients, except for infants and neonates, for whom a 19-gauge kit is preferred.

Anatomy The thoracic paravertebral space is wedge shaped. The base of the wedge is formed by the vertebral body and intervertebral discs. Posteriorly, it is bound by the costotransverse ligament; anterolaterally, it is bordered by parietal pleura. The costotransverse ligament is attached from the inferior edge of the transverse process to the superior edge of the rib tubercle. Laterally, it is continuous with the internal intercostal membrane (the aponeurosis of the internal intercostal muscle). The paravertebral space is filled with fatty tissue, through which the intercostal nerves and vessels, dorsal rami, rami communicantes, and sympathetic chain pass. The paravertebral space is connected laterally to the intercostal space and medially to the epidural space. The paravertebral space is limited inferiorly at T12 by the origin of the psoas major muscle.

Technique The patient is positioned in the lateral decubitus position in the neutral position, with the operative side uppermost; for bilateral blocks, the patient is positioned prone. Needle insertion should be at the level of T4 for sternotomy (a bilateral block is required), T6 for thoracotomy, T9 for renal surgery, and T12 and L1 for inguinal surgery. The needle point is typically positioned 1–2 cm lateral to the midline or equivalent to the interspinous process distance of the patient. The depth to the paravertebral space is estimated as 20 + (0.5 × weight in kg) mm. The needle is inserted through the skin,

and the stylet is removed. A syringe of saline is attached for assessment of loss of resistance. The needle is advanced until the transverse process is contacted. At this point, the needle is advanced 1 cm past the transverse process. Alternatively, the syringe is advanced until the loss of resistance is appreciated. A bolus of 0.3–0.5 mL/kg of 0.25% bupivacaine is injected. The same technique can be used to insert a paravertebral catheter for continuous infusion.

Ultrasound-Guided Technique The patient is positioned as for the landmark-based technique. The probe is placed in a transverse plane over the spinous process at the desired level of needle insertion. The level is easily determined by counting down from C7 (the vertebra prominens). The probe is slid laterally to identify the transverse process and then moved caudad, between the transverse processes, to visualize the paravertebral space. The pleura is readily identifiable moving with respiration; superficial to this, forming the posterior border of the paravertebral space, is the internal intercostal membrane (Figure 44–14).

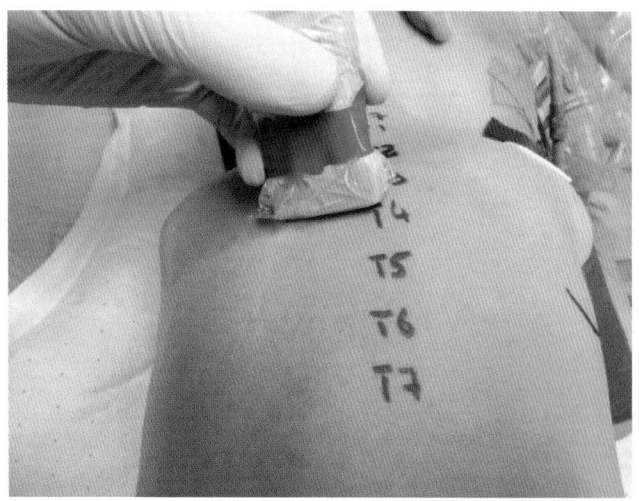

A

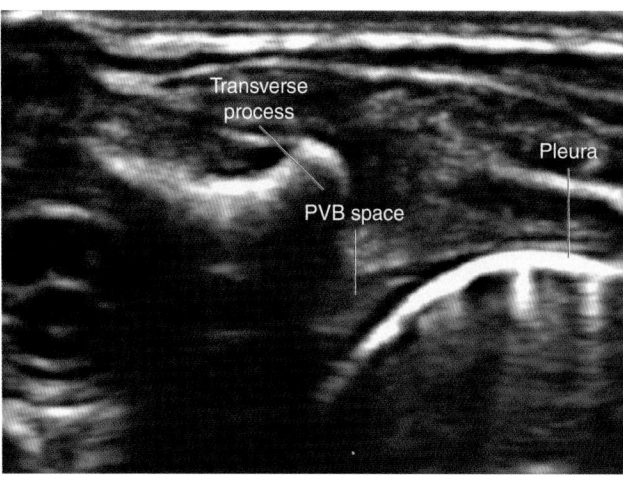

B

FIGURE 44–14. Thoracic paravertebral block: (**A**) probe position; (**B**) sonoanatomy.

An in-plane lateral-to-medial needling technique is employed, which requires excellent needle visualization skills, as the needle is being directed toward the spinal cord. A "pop" is seen and felt as the needle penetrates the membrane.[53,54] Local anesthetic spread caudad and cephalad can be assessed by scanning in a paramedian longitudinal plane. In neonates, it may be possible to see spread into the epidural space.

Complications　The potential complications of this block are serious and include pneumothorax. As such, this block should be performed only by or under the supervision of a pediatric regional anesthesiologist. Other complications include hypotension (4.6% of cases), vascular puncture, and inadvertent epidural or intrathecal injection.

SUMMARY

Peripheral nerve blocks can be performed with ease in children and adolescents. Adequate knowledge of the anatomy of the area along with appropriate indications and knowledge of complications facilitate the use of peripheral nerve blocks in children. The fear of the use of peripheral nerve blocks in children under general anesthesia is not unfounded, but US guidance may make complications even less frequent than reported with current methods. With time, US-guided approaches will become the gold standard of regional anesthesia techniques.

REFERENCES

1. Giaufre E, Dalens B, Gombert A: Epidemiology and morbidity of regional anesthesia in children: A one-year prospective survey of the French-LanguageSociety of Pediatric Anesthesiologists. Anesth Analg 1996;83:904–912.
2. Ecoffey C, Lacroix F, Giaufre E et al. Epidemiology and morbidity of regional anesthesia in children: a follow-up one year prospective survey ofthe French-Language Society of Pediatric Anaesthesiologists (ADARPEF). Pediatr Anesth 2010; 20:1061–1069.
3. Berde CB, Sethna NF, Levin L, et al: Regional analgesia on pediatric medical and surgical wards. Intensive Care Med 1989;15(Suppl 1):S40–S43.
4. Tobias JD: Continuous femoral nerve block to provide analgesia following femur fracture in a paediatric ICU population. Anaesth Intensive Care 1994;22:616–618.
5. Urmey WF, Stanton J. Inability to consistently elicit a motor response following sensory paresthesia during interscalene block administration. Anesthesiology 2002; 96: 5.
6. Chan VW, Brull R, McCartney CJL et al. An Ultrasonographic and Histological Study of Intraneural Injection and Electrical Stimulation in Pigs. Anesth Analg 2007;104:1281-4 52–4.
7. Hadzic A, Dilberovic F, Shah S, et al: Combination of intraneural injection and high injection pressure leads to fascicular injury and neurologicdeficits in dogs. Reg Anesth Pain Med 2004;29:417–423.
8. Freid EB, Bailey A, Valley R: Electrocardiographic and hemodynamic changes associated with unintentional intravascular injection of bupivacainewith epinephrine in infants. Anesthesiology 1993;79:394–398.
9. Bosenberg AT, Raw R, Boezaart AP: Surface mapping of peripheral nerves in children with a nerve stimulator. Paediatr Anaesth 2002;12:398–403.
10. Marhofer P, Sitzwohl C, Greher M, Kapral S: Ultrasound guidance for infraclavicular brachial plexus anaesthesia in children. Anaesthesia 2004;59:642–646.
11. Tsui B and Suresh S. Ultrasound Imaging for Regional Anaesthesia in Infants, Children and Adolescents. Anaesthesiology 2010;112: 473–492.
12. Kirchmair L, Enna B, Mitterschiffthaler G, et al: Lumbar plexus in children. A sonographic study and its relevance to pediatric regionalanesthesia. Anesthesiology 2004;101:445–450.
13. Dadure C and Capdevila X. Peripheral catheter techniques. Paediatric Anaesthesia 2012; 22: 93–101.
14. Suresh S, Bellig G: Regional anesthesia in a very low-birth-weight neonate for a neurosurgical procedure. Reg Anesth Pain Med 2004;29:58–59.
15. Suresh S, Wagner AM: Scalp excisions: Getting "ahead" of pain. Pe-diatr Dermatol 2001;18:74–76.
16. Prabhu KP, Wig J, Grewal S: Bilateral infraorbital nerve block is superior to peri-incisional infiltration for analgesia after repair of cleft lip. Scand J Plastic Reconst Surg Hand Surg 1999;33:83–87.
17. Molliex S Navez M, Baylot D, et al: Regional anesthesia for outpatient nasal surgery. Br J Anaesth 1996;76:151–153.
18. Suresh S, Patel AS, Dunham, ME, et al. A randomized double-blind controlled trial of infraorbital nerve block versus intravenous morphine sulfatefor children undergoing endoscopic sinus surgery: Are postoperative outcomes different? Anesthesiology 2002;97:A-1292.
19. Yasan H, Dogru H: Effect of infraorbital nerve block under general anesthesia on consumption of isoflurane and postoperative pain in endoscopicendonasal maxillary sinus surgery by Higashizawa and Koga. J Anesth 2003;17:68.
20. Higashizawa T, Koga Y: Effect of infraorbital nerve block under general anesthesia on consumption of isoflurane and postoperative pain inendoscopic endonasal maxillary sinus surgery. J Anesth 2001;15:136–138.
21. Suresh S, Barcelona SL, Young NM, et al: Postoperative pain relief in children undergoing tympanomastoid surgery: Is a regional block better thanopioids? Anesth Analg 2002;94:859–862.
22. Cregg N, Conway F, Casey W: Analgesia after otoplasty: Regional nerve blockade vs local anaesthetic infiltration of the ear. Can J Anaesth 1996;43(2):141–147.
23. Dieudonne N, Gomola A, Bonnichon P, Ozier YM: Prevention of postoperative pain after thyroid surgery: Adouble-blind randomized study of bilateralsuperficial cervical plexus blocks. Anesth Analg 2001;92:1538–1542.
24. Suresh S, Templeton L: Superficial cervical plexus block for vocal cord surgery in an awake pediatric patient. Anesth Analg 2004;98:1656–1657.
25. De Jose Maria B, Banus E, Navarro Egea M et al. Ultrasound-guided supraclavicular vs infraclavicular brachial plexus blocks in children. Pediatr Anesth 2008; 18: 838–844.
26. Ting PL, Sivagnanaratnam V: Ultrasonographic study of the spread of local anaestheticduring axillary brachial plexus block. Br J Anaesth 1989;63:326–329.
27. Aantaa R, Kirvela O, Lahdenpera A, Nieminen S: Transarterial brachial plexus anesthesia for hand surgery: A retrospective analysis of 346 cases. JClin Anesth 1994;6:189–192.
28. Carre P, Joly A, Cluzel FB, et al: Axillary block in children: Single or multiple injection? Paediatr Anaesth 2000;10:35–39.
29. Dalens B, Tanguy A, Vanneuville G: Lumbar plexus block in children: A comparison of two procedures in 50 patients. Anesth Analg 1988;67:750–758.
30. Grossbard GD, Love BR: Femoral nerve block: A simple and safe method of instant analgesia for femoral shaft fractures in children. Aust N Z J Surg 1979;49:592–594.
31. Johnson CM: Continuous femoral nerve blockade for analgesia in children with femoral fractures. Anaesth Intensive Care 1994;22:281–283.
32. Ronchi L, Rosenbaum D, Athouel A, et al: Femoral nerve blockade in children using bupivacaine. Anesthesiology 1989;70:622–624.
33. Flack S, Anderson C. Ultrasound guided lower extremity blocks. Pediatr Anesth 2012; 22:72–80.
34. Maccani RM, Wedel DJ, Melton A, Gronert GA: Femoral and lateral femoral cutaneous nerve block for muscle biopsies in children. Paediatr Anaesth 1995;5:223–227.
35. Sukhani R, Candido KD, Doty R Jr, et al: Infragluteal-parabiceps sciatic nerve block: An evaluation of a novel approach using a single-injectiontechnique. Anesth Analg 2003;96:868–873.
36. Vloka JD, Hadzic A, April E, Thys DM: The division of the sciatic nerve in the popliteal fossa: Anatomical implications for popliteal nerveblockade. Anesth Analg 2001;92:215–217.
37. Vloka JD, Hadzic A, Lesser JB, et al: A common epineural sheath for the nerves in the popliteal fossa and its possible implications for sciaticnerve block. Anesth Analg 1997;84:387–390.
38. Schwemmer U, Markus CK, Greim CA et al. Sonographic imaging of the sciatic nerve and its division in the popliteal fossa in children. PaediatrAnaesth 2004; 14(12):1005–1008.
39. van Schoor A-N, Bosman MC, Bosenberg AT. Revisiting the anatomy of the ilio-inguinal/iliohypogastric nerve block. Paediatr Anaesth 2013;23(5):390–394.
40. Weintraud M, Marhofer P, Bosenberg A et al. Ilioinguinal/iliohypogastric blocks in children: where do we administer the local anesthetic withoutdirect visualization? Anesth Analg 2008; 106:89–93.

41. Willschke H, Marhofer P, Bosenberg AT et al. Ultrasonography for ilioinguinal/iliohypogastric nerve blocks in children. Br J Anaesth 2005; 95:226–30.

42. Willschke H, Bosenberg AT, P. Marhofer, et al. Ultrasonographic-Guided Ilioinguinal/Iliohypogastric Nerve Block in Pediatric Anesthesia: What isthe Optimal Volume? Anesth Analg 2006;102:1680–4.

43. Amory C, Mariscal A, Guyot E, et al: Is ilioinguinal/iliohypogastric nerve block always totally safe in children? Paediatr Anaesth 2003;13:164–136.

44. Leng SA: Transient femoral nerve palsy after ilioinguinal nerve block. Anaesth Intensive Care 1997;25:92.

45. Ferguson S, Thomas V, Lewis I: The rectus sheath block in paediatric anaesthesia: New indications for an old technique? Paediatr Anaesth 1996;6:463–466.

46. De Jose Maria B, Gotzens V, Mabrok M. Ultrasound-guided umbilical nerve blocks in children: a brief description of a new technique. Pediatr Anesth 2007; 17:44–50.

47. Carney J, Finnerty O, Rau J et al. Ipsilateral transversus abdominis plane block provides effective analgesia after appendicectomy in children: arandomised controlled trial. Anesth Analg 2010;111(4):998–1003.

48. Hebbard P. Subcostal Transversus Abdominis Plane Block Under Ultrasound Guidance. Anesth Analg 2008;106(2):673–674.

49. Carney J, Finnerty O, Rauf J et al. Studies on the spread of local anaesthetic solution in transversus abdominis plane blocks. Anaesthesia. 2011; 66:1023–1030.

50. Holder KJ, Peutrell JM, Weir PM: Regional anaesthesia for circumcision. Subcutaneous ring block of the penis and subpubic penile block compared. Eur J Anaesthesiol 1997;14:495–498.

51. Richardson J and Lonnqvist PA. Thoracic Paravertebral Block. Br J Anaesth 1998; 81: 230–238.

52. Lönnqvist PA. Continuous paravertebral block in children. Initial experience. Anaesthesia 1992 Jul;47(7):607–9.

53. Riain SC, Donnell BO, Harmon DC et al. Thoracic Paravertebral Block Using Real-Time Ultrasound Guidance. Anesth Analg 2010; 110 (1): 248–251.

54. Marhofer P, Kettner SC, Hajbok L et al. Lateral ultrasound-guided paravertebral blockade: an anatomical-based description of a new technique. Br JAnaesth 2010; 105 (4): 526–32.

Acute and Chronic Pain Management in Children

Rishi M. Diwan

1. ACUTE PAIN MANAGEMENT

INTRODUCTION

The treatment and alleviation of pain constitute a basic human right that exists regardless of age.[1,2] Pain is defined as an unpleasant sensory and emotional experience associated with actual or potential tissue damage.[3] Previous experience and management of pain, even from very early stages in life, alter the responses and behavior toward further "painful" experiences and events. Hence, no two people experience pain the same way, which adds to the complexity of the management of pain.

Unfortunately, even when pain is obvious, children frequently receive no or inadequate treatment for pain and painful procedures. The newborn and critically ill child are especially vulnerable to receiving no treatment or undertreatment.[4,5] The conventional notion that children neither respond to nor remember painful experiences to the same degree that adults do is inaccurate. Many of the nerve pathways essential for the transmission and perception of pain are present and functioning by 24–29 weeks of gestation.[6,7] Research in newborn animals has revealed that failure to provide analgesia for pain results in "rewiring" of the nerve pathways responsible for pain transmission in the dorsal horn of the spinal cord, resulting in increased pain perception of *future* painful insults. This confirms human newborn research that found that the failure to provide anesthesia or analgesia for newborn circumcision resulted not only in short-term physiologic perturbations but also in longer-term behavioral changes.[8,9]

Nurses are traditionally taught or cautioned to be wary of physicians' orders and patients' requests for pain management, as well. The most common prescription order for potent analgesics, "to give as needed" (*pro re nata*, PRN), in reality means "to give as infrequently as possible." The PRN order also means that either the patient must know or remember to ask for pain medication or the nurse must be able to identify when a patient is in pain. Neither requirement may be met by children in pain. Children less than 3 years of age and critically ill children may be unable to adequately verbalize when they are in pain or where they hurt. Moreover, they may be afraid to report their pain. Several studies have documented the inability of nurses, physicians, and parents/guardians to correctly identify and treat pain, even in postoperative pediatric patients.

Societal fears of opioid addiction and lack of advocacy are also causal factors in the undertreatment of pediatric pain. Unlike adult patients, pain management in children is often dependent on the ability of parents/guardians to recognize and assess pain and on their decision whether to treat or not. Parental misconceptions concerning pain assessment and pain management may therefore also result in inadequate pain treatment. Even in hospitalized patients, most of the pain that children experience is managed by their parents/guardians. Parents/guardians may fail to report pain either because they are unable to assess it or are afraid of the consequences of pain therapy. In one study, false beliefs about addiction and the proper use of acetaminophen and other analgesics resulted in the failure to provide analgesia to children.[10] In another, the belief that pain was useful or that repeated doses of analgesics lead to medication underperformance resulted in the failure of the parents/guardians to provide or ask for prescribed analgesics to treat their children's pain.[11] Parental/guardian education is therefore essential if children are to be adequately treated for pain.

All of these factors make children an extremely vulnerable group. Fortunately, the past 25 years have seen substantial advances in research and interest in pediatric pain management and in the development of pediatric pain services, primarily under the direction of pediatric anesthesiologists. Pain service teams provide pain management for acute, postoperative, terminal, neuropathic, and chronic pain. Nevertheless, the assessment and treatment of pain in children are important aspects of pediatric care, regardless of who provides it. Failure to provide adequate control of pain amounts to substandard and unethical medical practice.

PAIN ASSESSMENT

The perception of pain is a subjective, conscious experience; operationally, it can be defined as "what the patient says hurts" and existing "when the patient says it does." Infants, preverbal children, and children between the ages of 2 and 7 years may be unable to describe their pain or their subjective experiences. This has led many to conclude incorrectly that children do not experience pain in the same way that adults do. Clearly, children do not have to know (or be able to express) the meaning of an experience to have an experience. Therefore, because pain is essentially a subjective experience, it is becoming increasingly clear that the child's perspective of pain is an indispensable facet of pediatric pain management and an essential element in the specialized study of childhood pain. Sometimes there is an overreliance on objective assessments of pain, whether from a healthcare professional or parental/guardian assessment. This objective assessment, though sometimes important, should remain only a minor partner in the assessment and management of pain, as objective assessments are also subject to bias and preconceived notions. Indeed, pain assessment and management are interdependent, and one is essentially useless without the other.

The goal of pain assessment is to provide accurate data about the location and intensity of pain, as well as the effectiveness of measures used to alleviate or eradicate it.

Instruments currently exist to assess pain in children of all ages.[8,12–18] Indeed, the sensitivity and specificity of these instruments have been widely debated and have resulted in a plethora of studies to validate their reliability and validity. The most commonly used instruments measure the quality and intensity of pain and are "self-report measures" that make use of pictures or word descriptors to describe pain. Pain intensity or severity can be measured in children as young as 3 years of age by using either the Oucher scale (developed by Judith E. Beyer, RN, PhD; Antonia M. Villarreal, RN, PhD; and Mary J. Denyes, RN, PhD)—a two-part scale including both a numeric scale (from 0 to 100) and a photographic scale of six photographs of a young child's face expressing increasing degrees of discomfort—or a visual analog scale—a 10-cm line with a distraught, crying face at one end and a smiling face at the other. The visual analog scale has been validated by both sex and race. In our practice, we use the six-face Wong-Baker FACES Pain Rating Scale (developed by Dr. Donna Wong and Connie M. Baker), primarily because of its simplicity (Figure 45–1).[16] This scale is attached to the vital sign record, and nurses are instructed to use it or a more age-appropriate self-report measure whenever vital signs are taken.

Clinical Pearl

- Regular assessment using appropriate pain assessment tools, involving the patient and carers in decision making, and being as flexible as possible to the patient's needs all play a vital role in achieving a successful outcome.

Pain assessment in preverbal children poses challenges as they are unable to self-report. There are many pain assessment tools available in this age group, but none are ideal. The CRIES[19]

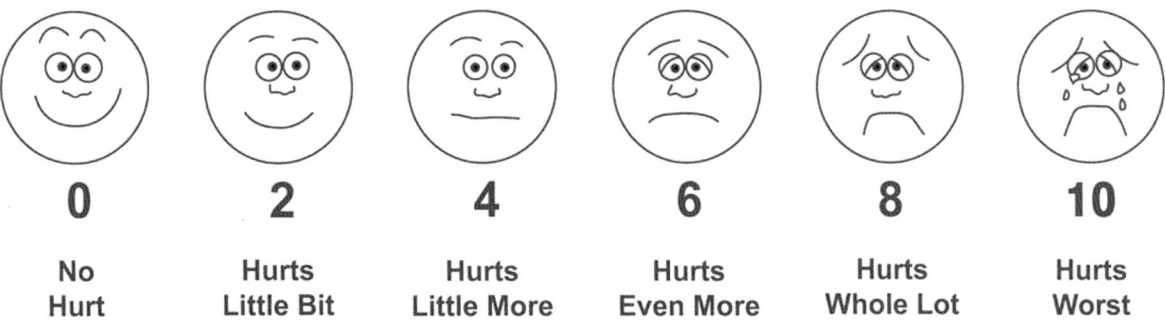

FIGURE 45–1. The six-face Wong-Baker FACES Pain Rating Scale. (Wong-Baker FACES Foundation (2015). Wong-Baker FACES® Pain Rating Scale. Retrieved January 28, 2017 with permission from http://www.WongBakerFACES.or.)

TABLE 45–1. CRIES pain scale for babies from 32 weeks' gestational age.

	0	1	2
Crying Characteristic cry of pain is high pitched	No cry or cry that is not high pitched	High-pitched cry but infant is consolable	High-pitched cry and infant is inconsolable
Requires O₂ to maintain SaO₂ > 95 Consider other changes in oxygenation	No	Requires O_2 < 30%	Requires O_2 > 30%
Increased vital signs Take BP last as this may cause difficulty with other assessments	HR and BP +/– 10% of baseline	10%–20% increase in BP or HR	> 20% increase in HR or BP
Expression Grimace characterized by brow bulge, eyes shut, open mouth, deepening nasolabial furrow	Neutral	Grimace	Grimace/grunt
Sleeplessness Based on state during the hour preceding the assessment	No	Wakes frequently	Constantly awake

Instructions: Each of the five categories is scored 0, 1, or 2, resulting in total score between 0 and 10.

pain score is frequently used to score pain in neonates (Table 45–1). Children with developmental delay, complex needs, and or in intensive care need special pain assessment tools to monitor pain. Most such tools incorporate physiological parameters for stress (cardiac, respiratory, and endocrine) with behavioral changes associated with pain (facial expressions, crying, body and limb movements).[20] A separate pain assessment scale called the Paediatric Pain Profile (PPP)[21] is available at our institution for use in children with complex needs. It is used primarily by parents/guardians to measure their child's pain and incorporates scoring of the aforementioned behavioral changes. Irrespective of the pain assessment tool used in these patient groups, it is important that healthcare professionals understand what causes pain, appreciate that pediatric patients perceive pain, and have a variety of assessment methods and treatments in their armamentarium to achieve effective pain control.

PAIN MANAGEMENT

Acute pediatric pain management is increasingly characterized by a multimodal or "balanced" approach in which smaller doses of opioid and nonopioid analgesics, such as nonsteroidal anti-inflammatory drugs (NSAIDs), local anesthetics, N-methyl-D-aspartate (NMDA) antagonists, and α_2-adrenergic agonists, are combined to maximize pain control and minimize drug-induced adverse side effects. Pain management also includes management of both patient and parental/guardian expectations and being knowledgeable, open, and frank about what to expect during the course of the postoperative and rehabilitation periods. It should be recognized that certain procedures "hurt" more than others and that, in spite of our best efforts, it is not always possible to achieve "no pain," although that should always be the aim. At the same time, preoperative discussion of the various analgesic strategies available and reassurance that

the patient "will be looked after" go a long way to achieving a satisfactory outcome for all concerned. In addition, a multimodal approach utilizes nonpharmacological, complementary, and alternative medicine therapies, as well. These techniques include distraction, guided imagery, transcutaneous nerve stimulation, acupuncture, therapeutic massage, among others.[22]

Clinical Pearls

- The aim of acute pain management is providing a comfortable/pain-free perioperative period in order to facilitate early ambulation and rehabilitation.
- Preoperative discussions with the patient and his or her parents/guardians detailing the achievable outcome, expected course, and various available pain management modalities play an important role in achieving a satisfactory outcome for all concerned.
- A multimodal approach to pain management achieves the best results.
- If possible, regional anesthesia/analgesia should be part and parcel of any multimodal analgesia regime.

Clinical Pearl

Alternative medicine pain therapy:

- Distraction
- Guided imagery
- Transcutaneous nerve stimulation
- Acupuncture
- Therapeutic massage

Procedural pain is often a forgotten and ignored aspect of pain management in children admitted to hospital. Various interventions and procedures, some of which are done repeatedly, may inflict pain or are perceived as painful by an anxious child (eg, cannulation, phlebotomy, lumbar puncture, and wound dressing and cleaning). It is essential to practice how to explain procedures and how to prepare and reassure the child and parents/guardians. Simple techniques such as local anesthetic creams and play/distraction therapy can help in many situations. Some patients may also need formal psychological intervention and support or pharmacological aids such as sedation or nitrous oxide (N_2O), all of which require time and planning. Lastly, if conscious sedation or N_2O is required, adequate monitoring and emergency equipment, including oxygen, suction, and appropriate personnel, should be immediately available.

Pain management strategies for day case surgery should include local anesthetic infiltration, regional blocks, simple analgesics (eg, acetaminophen/paracetamol, NSAIDS, and "milder" opioids such as codeine or tramadol, if necessary). "Strong" opioids should be avoided, although they are not contraindicated. Ultrasound-guided regional anesthesia is increasing in popularity, providing safer and more effective regional anesthesia.

Clinical Pearl

Pain management strategies for day case surgery:

- Local anesthetic infiltration
- Regional anesthesia
- Nonopioid analgesics (acetaminophen, NSAIDs)
- Mild opioids (codeine, tramadol) when necessary
- More potent opioids should be avoided when possible but are not contraindicated

Anesthesiologists must work closely with surgical colleagues to identify appropriate day case surgeries and develop patient care pathways with standard analgesia management plans for specific procedures.

For major surgery, in addition to all the above mentioned analgesics, opioid and/or local anesthetic infusions may be necessary. These can be complemented by other treatment modalities including ketamine, clonidine, or diazepam for muscle spasm after orthopedic surgeries; gabapentin for acute pain; intraoperative magnesium; and the addition of dexamethasone systemically or to a local anesthetic for nerve blocks.

Analgesics with Antipyretic Activity or Nonopioid ("Weaker") Analgesics

The "weaker" or milder analgesics with antipyretic activity, of which acetaminophen, ibuprofen, naproxen, and diclofenac are the classic examples, make up a heterogeneous group of NSAIDs that are nonopioid analgesics (Table 45–2).[23–25]

They provide pain relief primarily by blocking peripheral and central prostaglandin production by inhibiting cyclooxygenase types I and II. These analgesic agents are primarily administered enterally via the oral or rectal route and are particularly useful for inflammatory, bone, and rheumatic pain. Parenterally administered acetaminophen and NSAIDs, such as ketorolac, are available for use in children in whom the oral or rectal routes of administration are not possible.[26] Unfortunately, regardless of dose, the nonopioid analgesics reach a "ceiling effect," above which pain cannot be relieved by these drugs alone. Because of this, these weaker analgesics are considered the basic building blocks in a multimodal therapeutic approach and are often administered in combination forms with opioids such as codeine, oxycodone, hydrocodone, or tramadol. Aspirin has been largely abandoned in pediatric practice because of its possible role in Reye syndrome, its effects on platelet function, and its gastric irritant properties.

Clinical Pearls

- The nonopioid analgesics have a "ceiling effect," above which pain cannot be relieved by these drugs alone, regardless of dose.
- Nonopioid analgesics are considered the basic building blocks in a multimodal therapeutic approach and are often administered in combination forms with opioids such as codeine, oxycodone, hydrocodone, or tramadol.

The most commonly used nonopioid analgesic in pediatric practice remains acetaminophen. Unlike NSAIDs, acetaminophen works primarily centrally and has minimal, if any, anti-inflammatory activity. When administered in normal doses ($10–15$ mg · kg^{-1}, PO), acetaminophen is extremely safe and has very few serious side effects. It is an antipyretic and, like all enterally administered NSAIDs, takes about 30 minutes to provide effective analgesia. Several investigators have reported that when administered rectally, acetaminophen should be given in significantly higher doses than previous recommendations had suggested.[27,28] However this author does not use acetaminophen loading doses when the drug is administered rectally. Regardless of route of delivery, to prevent hepatotoxicity, the daily maximum acetaminophen dose in the preterm neonate, term neonate, and older child is 30, 60, and 80 mg/kg, respectively (Table 45–3). The maximum adult dose is 4 g/day.

The discovery of at least two cyclooxygenase (COX) isoenzymes, referred to as COX-1 and COX-2, has increased our knowledge of NSAIDs.[29–32] These two COX isoenzymes share structural and enzymatic similarities but are uniquely regulated at the molecular level and may be distinguished by their functions. Protective prostaglandins, which preserve the integrity of the stomach lining and maintain normal renal function in a compromised kidney, are synthesized by COX-1.[29,30,33] COX-2 is an inducible isoform. The inducing stimuli include proinflammatory cytokines and growth factors, implying a role for COX-2 in both inflammation and control of cell growth. In

TABLE 45–2. Dosing guidelines for commonly used nonopioid analgesics *(Institutional or national guidelines may vary.)*

	Premature Neonates (32–36 weeks Postmenstrual Age[a])	Term Neonates (> 36–44 weeks Postmenstrual Age[a])	Infants and Children (> 44 weeks Postmenstrual Age[a] and up to 50 kg)	> 12 Years (and Weight > 50 kg[b])
Acetaminophen (Paracetamol)				
Acetaminophen (Paracetamol)	15 mg/kg PO/PR every 8 hours (max 60 mg/kg/day)	15 mg/kg PO/PR every 6 hours (max 60 mg/kg/day)	15–20 mg/kg PO/PR[bc] every 4–6 hours (max 90 mg/kg/day)	1g PO/PR every 4–6 hours (max 4 g/day)
IV acetaminophen	7.5 mg/kg IV every 8 hours (max 25 mg/kg/day)	7.5 mg/kg IV every 6 hours (max 30 mg/kg/day)	15 mg/kg IV[b] every 6 hours (max 60mg/kg/day)	15 mg/kg IV (maximum 1 g) every 6 hours
Nonsteroidal anti-inflammatory drugs (NSAIDs) Prescribe one drug only.				
Ibuprofen	Not recommended	Not recommended	Less than 3 months of age: 5 mg/kg PO every 8 hours From 3 months of age: 10 mg/kg PO (maximum 400 mg) every 8 hours (max 30 mg/kg/day)	400 mg PO every 8 hours
Diclofenac	Not recommended	Not recommended	From 6 months of age: 1 mg/kg PO/PR every 8 hours	50 mg PO/PR every 8 hours
Naproxen	Not recommended	Not recommended	5 mg/kg every 12 hours	5mg/kg every 12 hours (max 1g/day)

[a]Postmenstrual age in weeks is the gestational age plus the postnatal age (time elapsed after birth).

[b]Doses based on weight in obese patients or based on age in underweight patients may need to be reduced to avoid overdosage.

[c]A higher dose of acetaminophen 20 mg/kg PO/PR every 6 hours may be used when pain is not controlled with the standard dose (15 mg/kg) when no contraindications exist. This dose should be reviewed every 24 hours. Loading doses are not recommended in order to minimize the potential for error.

addition to the induction of COX-2 in inflammatory lesions, COX-2 is present constitutively in the brain and spinal cord, where it may be involved in nerve transmission, particularly for pain and fever. Prostaglandins made by COX-2 are also important in ovulation and in the birth process.[28,29,31] The discovery of COX-2 has made possible the design of drugs that reduce inflammation without removing the protective prostaglandins in the stomach and kidney made by COX-1. In fact, developing a more specific COX-2 inhibitor has been an important goal of much drug research because this class of drug has all of the anti-inflammatory and analgesic properties that one desires in a

drug with none of the gastrointestinal and antiplatelet side effects. Unfortunately, the growing controversy regarding the potential adverse cardiovascular risks of the prolonged use of COX-2 inhibitors has dampened much of the enthusiasm for these drugs and has led to the removal of rofecoxib from the market by its manufacturer.[34,35] Other NSAIDs, especially diclofenac, are now facing similar scrutiny. Many orthopedic surgeons are also concerned about the negative effect of all NSAIDs on bone growth and healing.[36–38] While some pediatric orthopedic surgeons have recommended that these drugs not be used in their patients in the postoperative period, it is this

TABLE 45–3. Opioid analgesic initial dosage guidelines *(institutional or national guidelines may vary.)*

Drug	Equianalgesic Dose (mg)		Usual Starting IV Dose and Interval		IV/Oral Ratio	Usual Starting Oral Dose and Interval	
	IV, IM, SC	Oral	< 50 kg	> 50 kg		< 50 kg	> 50 kg
Codeine	120	200	NR	NR	1:2	0.5–1[a] mg/kg every 4-6 hours	0.5–1[a] mg/kg every 4–6 hours
Fentanyl	0.1	NA[b]	Bolus: 0.5–1 mcg/kg, 0.5–2 h (max 50 mcg) *NCA/PCA (drug concentration: 1 mcg/kg/mL, max 50 mcg/mL)* NCA: Bolus: 0.5–1 mcg/kg, 30 min–1 h; infusion: 0.5–1 mcg/kg/h PCA: Bolus: 0.5 mcg/kg, 10 min–1 h; infusion: 0.5–1 mcg/kg/h	NA	NA	NA	NA
Hydrocodone	NA	10–20	NA	NA	NA	0.1 mg/kg every 3–4 hours	5–10 mg every 3–4 hours
Hydromorphone	1.5–2	3–5[c]	Bolus: 0.02 mg/kg, 0.5–2 h; infusion: 0.004 mg/kg/h	Bolus: 1 mg, 0.5–2 h; infusion: 0.3 mg/h	1:2	0.03–0.08 mg/kg every 4 hours	2–4 mg every 4 hours
Methadone	10	10–20	0.1 mg/kg every 4–8 hours	5–10 mg every 4–8 hours	1:2	0.2 mg/kg every 4–8 hours	10 mg every 4–8 hours
Morphine	10	30–50	Bolus: 0.03–0.1 mg/kg, 0.5–2 h (max 10 mg) *NCA/PCA (drug concentration 20mcg/kg/mL, max 1mg/mL)*[d] NCA: Bolus: 20 mcg/kg, 15 min–1 h; infusion: 20 mcg/kg/h PCA: Bolus: 20 mcg/kg (max 1 mg), 5min; infusion: 4 mcg/kg/h	Bolus: 5–10 mg every 4–8 hours	1:2–3	0.2–0.3 mg/kg every 4–6 hours Sustained release: 0.4–0.5 mg/kg every 8–12 hours	15 mg/kg every 4–6 hours Sustained release: 30 mg every 8–12 hours
Oxycodone	NA	10–20	NA	NA	NA	0.1 mg/kg every 3–4 hours	5–10 mg every 3–4 hours[e]

[a]Due to the highlighted problem with "ultra-rapid metabolizers," it is best to start with a dose of 0.5 mg/kg.

[b]Oral transmucosal route available: dose 10–15 mcg/kg.

[c]The equianalgesic oral dose and parenteral/oral dose ratio are not well established.

[d]For neonates and infants younger than 13 weeks, the drug concentration is to be halved: bolus 5 mcg/kg,1 h; infusion 5–10 mcg/kg/h.

[e]A sustained-release preparation is available.

author's view that in spite of the controversies, NSAIDs remain effective and useful drugs in pediatric acute pain management when used wisely and for short duration.

Opioid Drug Selection

Many factors are considered when deciding which is the appropriate opioid analgesic to administer to a pediatric patient in pain. These include pain intensity, patient age, coexisting disease, potential drug interactions, treatment history, physician preference, patient preference, and route of administration. Some opioids are preferred over others, and some may be unavailable depending on institution, country, or continent, for reasons not entirely understood. The idea that some opioids are "weak" (eg, codeine) and others "strong" (eg, morphine) is outdated. All are capable of treating pain regardless of intensity if the dose is adjusted appropriately (Table 45–4). At equipotent doses, most opioids have similar effects and side effects. Meperidine (pethidine) at an equianalgesic dose has the same side effect profile as morphine;[39] however, it is no longer commonly prescribed.

Commonly Used Oral Opioids: Codeine, Oxycodone, Hydrocodone, Morphine, and Tramadol

Codeine, oxycodone, and hydrocodone are opioids that are frequently used to treat pain in children and adults, particularly less severe pain and when patients are being converted from parenteral to enteral opioids (see Table 45–3). Morphine is commonly used in regimens for chronic pain (eg, cancer). Codeine, oxycodone, and hydrocodone are most commonly administered in oral form, usually in combination with acetaminophen or aspirin.[40] Unfortunately, very few, if any, pharmacokinetic or dynamic studies have been performed in children, and most dosing guidelines are anecdotally based. In equipotent doses, codeine, oxycodone, hydrocodone, and morphine are equal both as analgesics and respiratory depressants (see Table 45–3). In addition, these drugs share common effects on the central nervous system with other opioids, including sedation, respiratory depression, and stimulation of the chemoreceptor trigger zone in the brain stem, the latter

particularly the case for codeine. There are fewer nausea and vomiting side effects with oxycodone and hydrocodone. Codeine, hydrocodone, and oxycodone have a bioavailability of approximately 60% after oral ingestion. The analgesic effects occur as early as 20 minutes after ingestion and reach a maximum after 60–120 minutes. The plasma half-life of elimination is 2.5–4 hours. Codeine undergoes nearly complete metabolism in the liver before its final excretion in urine. Approximately 10% of codeine is metabolized into morphine (CYP2D6), and it is this 10% that is responsible for codeine's analgesic effect. Interestingly, approximately 10% of the population and most newborn infants cannot metabolize codeine into morphine, and in these patients, codeine produces little, if any, analgesia.

Codeine needs special mention, as its use has come under increased scrutiny at the time of writing this chapter. A few instances of fatalities and life-threatening episodes of respiratory depression have been reported in children who are cytochrome P450 CYP2D6 "ultra-rapid metabolizers" and were given codeine after tonsillectomy or adenoidectomy in the treatment of obstructive sleep apnea.[41,42] The CYP2D6 enzyme is subject to genetic polymorphism. Having multiple gene copies, some patients metabolize codeine more rapidly (and are thus termed "ultra-rapid metabolizers") and therefore have an increased risk of experiencing morphine toxicity, ie, respiratory depression. The prevalence of this varies with ethnicity, from as low as 0%–2% in Asians to as high as 10%–16% in Ethiopians and Saudi Arabians.[43]

The current position on codeine use is as follows. The U.S. Federal Drug Administration (FDA),[44] the Pharmacovigilance Risk Assessment Committee (PRAC) of the European Medicines Agency (EMA),[45] and the U.K. Medicines and Healthcare Products Regulatory Agency (MHRA) have recommended restrictions on the use of codeine in children. These include the following:

- Restrict the use of codeine to children over 12 years of age (EMA and MHRA).
- Avoid codeine use in patients under 18 years of age who are undergoing tonsillectomy or adenoidectomy, especially for obstructive sleep apnea (EMA and FDA).

TABLE 45–4. Maximum local anesthetic dosing guidelines.

Drug	Dose mg/kg Without Epinephrine	Dose mg/kg with Epinephrine	Duration in Hours	Contra-Indications	Comments
Bupivacaine[a]	2.5	3	3–6		Reduce dose by 50% in neonates
Chloroprocaine[b]	8	10	1	Plasma cholinesterase deficiency	Short-acting, rapid metabolism, useful in neonates and possibly patients with seizures or liver disease
Lidocaine	5	7	1		
Ropivacaine[c]	3	never mixed	3–6		Less cardiotoxicity than bupivacaine

[a]When given by epidural continuous infusion: 0.2–0.4 mg/kg/h.
[b]In neonatal epidural continuous infusion: 10–15 mg/kg/h.
[c]Infusion rates is 0.5 mg/kg for pediatric patients older than 4-6 months of age.

- In all other cases, use codeine only if required. It should be prescribed on an "as-needed basis" only, with the dose restricted to 0.5 mg/kg (maximum 30 mg) every 6 hours, and limited in treatment duration.
- Patient receiving codeine should be closely monitored for respiratory depression; nurses and parents/guardians should be advised to watch for signs of morphine overdose.

For many years codeine has been more or less universally used in pediatric practice for the relief of moderate pain, as a step-down medication, and as a take-home medication on discharge. Possible dilemmas include the following:

- Due to its widespread use, various "child-friendly" preparations and formulations exist to provide versatile delivery systems for all ages. However, recent developments may have led to discouraging the development of versatile formulations of other similar-"strength" opioids. Thus, many countries are left with limited or no suitable alternatives to codeine.
- Licensing and use of alternative drugs is lagging in certain countries. For instance, tramadol is not licensed in the U.K. for patients below 12 years of age.
- There are few data to determine if any the available alternatives are as effective as codeine.[46]
- Although morphine is the most logical alternative to codeine, issues of concern include controlled drug regulations in certain countries, institutional and local practices, and the reluctance of some healthcare professionals to prescribe oral morphine due to social concerns and the perceived potential for abuse.
- For institutions and countries where other safe, effective, and versatile formulations of codeine alternatives, such as tramadol, oxycodone, and buprenorphine, are available, local interim guidelines may need to be agreed upon (with or without the continued use of codeine) in order to continue to provide safe and effective analgesia to the pediatric population.
- These issues may encourage pharmaceutical companies to develop more "child-friendly" analgesic products and encourage similar research of other opioids to validate their efficacy in children.
- These concerns may also lead to the development of commercially viable patient genotyping.

Like codeine and oxycodone, morphine is very effective when given orally, but only about 40% of an oral dose of morphine reaches the systemic circulation. In the past, this led many to inappropriately conclude that morphine is ineffective when administered orally; instead, the lack of efficacy was simply the result of inadequate PO dosing. Therefore, when converting a patient's required intravenous morphine dose to an oral maintenance dose, one must multiply the intravenous dose by a factor of 2 to 3.

Clinical Pearl

- When converting a patient's required intravenous morphine dose to an oral maintenance dose, multiply the intravenous dose by a factor of 2 to 3.

Whereas oral morphine is prescribed alone, oral codeine, hydrocodone, oxycodone, and tramadol are usually prescribed in combination with either acetaminophen or aspirin. Acetaminophen potentiates the analgesia produced by codeine (and other opioids) and allows the use of a smaller dose of the opioid with satisfactory analgesia. In all "combination preparations," beware of inadvertently administering a hepatotoxic dose of acetaminophen when increasing opioid doses for uncontrolled pain.[47] Because of this concern, it is preferred to prescribe the opioid and acetaminophen (or ibuprofen) separately.

Although it is an effective analgesic when administered parenterally, intramuscular codeine has no advantage over morphine or any other opioid; hence, its use is discouraged. Similar to codeine, tramadol is used to treat moderate to severe pain. Although tramadol is often categorized as a μ-receptor agonist, it has multiple proposed mechanisms of action. It is also a serotonin releaser, a norepinephrine reuptake inhibitor, and an NMDA receptor antagonist. The licensing age of tramadol varies by country, but it has been studied in children as young as 1 year.[48] Tramadol is prescribed in a dose of 1–2 mg/kg every 6 hours to a maximum of 400 mg/day (in 4 divided doses for patients over 50 kg).

Hydrocodone is prescribed in a dose of 0.05–0.1 mg/kg. An elixir is available as 2.5 mg/5 mL combined with acetaminophen 167 mg/5 mL. As a tablet, it is available in hydrocodone doses between 2.5 mg and 10 mg, combined with 500–650 mg acetaminophen. Oxycodone is prescribed in a dose of 0.05–0.1 mg/kg. Unfortunately, an elixir is not available in most pharmacies. When it is, it is prepared as either 1 mg/mL *or* 20 mg/mL. This can obviously result in catastrophic dispensing errors. In tablet form, oxycodone is commonly available as a 5-mg tablet or as Tylox (500 mg acetaminophen and 5 mg oxycodone) or Percocet (325 mg acetaminophen and 5 mg oxycodone).

Oxycodone is also available without acetaminophen in a sustained-release tablet for use in chronic pain. Like many other timed-release tablets, it must *not* be crushed and therefore cannot be administered through a gastric tube. Breaking the tablet results in the immediate release of a huge amount of oxycodone. Like sustained-release morphine (see below), sustained-release oxycodone is only for use in opioid-tolerant patients with chronic pain, *not* for routine postoperative pain. Also, note that in patients with rapid gastrointestinal transit, sustained-release preparations may not be absorbed at all (liquid methadone may be an alternative).

Oral morphine is available as a liquid in various concentrations (as much as 20 mg/mL), a tablet (eg, MSIR [**m**orphine **s**ulfate **i**mmediate **r**elease], available in 15- and 30-mg tablets), and in a sustained-release preparation. Because it is so concentrated, the liquid is particularly easy to administer to children and severely debilitated patients. Indeed, in terminal patients who cannot swallow, liquid morphine provides analgesia when simply dropped into the patient's mouth.[40]

Patient- and Parent/Nurse-Controlled Analgesia

Among the many reasons for the undertreatment of pediatric pain is the lack of familiarity of physicians (and nurses) with appropriate drugs, drug dosing, and routes of administration. When drugs are given on demand (PRN), there is a lag between the time of the patient's request and the nurse's response and the preparation and administration of analgesia. In moderate to severe pain, around-the-clock administration interval administration (eg, q4h) is not always the answer either, however, because of the great individual variation in pain perception and opioid metabolism. Indeed, fixed doses and time intervals make little sense. Based on the pharmacokinetics of opioids, it should be clear that intravenous boluses of morphine may need to be given at intervals of 1–2 hours to avoid marked fluctuations in plasma drug levels.

Continuous intravenous infusions may provide steady analgesic levels, are preferable to intramuscular injections, and have been used with great safety and effectiveness in children. However, they are not a panacea because the perception and intensity of pain are not constant. For example, a postoperative patient may be very comfortable resting in bed and require little adjustment in pain management. But this same patient may experience excruciating pain when coughing, voiding, or getting out of bed. Thus, rational pain management requires some form of titration to effect whenever any opioid is administered. To give patients (in some cases nurses and, rarely, parents/guardians) some measure of control over pain therapy, demand analgesia, or patient-controlled analgesia (PCA), devices have been developed.[49,50] These devices are microprocessor-driven pumps with a button that the patient presses to self-administer a small dose of opioid.

PCA devices allow patients to administer small amounts of an analgesic whenever they feel a need for more pain relief. The opioid, usually morphine, hydromorphone, or fentanyl, is administered either intravenously or subcutaneously. The dosage of opioid (with or without background infusion), number of boluses per hour, and the time interval between boluses (the "lockout period") are programmed into the equipment by the pain service physician or nurse to allow maximum patient flexibility and a sense of control with minimal risk of overdosage. Generally, when older patients know that if they have severe pain, they can obtain relief immediately, many prefer dosing regimens that result in mild to moderate pain in exchange for fewer side effects such as nausea or pruritus. Typically, morphine is prescribed, 20 mcg/kg per bolus (or hydromorphone 3–4 mcg/kg/h or fentanyl 0.5 mcg/kg/h), with a 5- to 15-minute lockout interval between each bolus. Variations include larger or smaller boluses, shorter or longer time intervals, and varying background infusion; these tend to be based on institutional practice and preferences.

The PCA pump computer stores within its memory the number of boluses the patient has received as well as the number of attempts the patient has made to receive boluses. This allows the physician to evaluate how well the patient understands the use of the pump and provides information to program the pump more efficiently. Most PCA units allow low "background" continuous infusions (eg, morphine 2–30 mcg/kg/h, hydromorphone 3–4 mcg/kg/h, fentanyl 0.5-1 mcg/kg/h) in addition to self-administered boluses. A continuous background infusion is particularly useful at night and often provides more restful sleep by preventing the patient from awakening in pain. However, it also increases the potential for overdosage.[49–51] Although the adult literature on pain does not support the use of continuous background infusions, our experience has been that continuous infusions are essential for good pain management in the pediatric patient. Indeed, in our practice, we almost always use continuous background infusions when we prescribe PCAs or nurse-controlled analgesia (NCA).

PCA requires a patient with enough intelligence, manual dexterity, and strength to operate the pump. Thus, these devices were initially limited to adolescents, but the lower age limit in whom this treatment modality can be used continues to fall (currently around age 5–6 years). Contraindications to the use of PCA include inability to push the bolus button, inability to understand how to use the machine, and patient desire not to assume responsibility for his or her care.

In patients considered below "competent" age, neonates, toddlers, and patients with complex needs, the practice of allowing surrogates such as nurses to initiate a PCA bolus is called nurse-controlled analgesia (NCA). This is standard practice in our institution. It has been demonstrated that nurses and, in rare cases, parents can be empowered to initiate PCA boluses and to use this technology safely in children, even in those younger than 1 year of age, the incidence of common opioid-induced side effects being similar to that observed in older patients.[51] NCAs tend to have a slightly higher background infusion rate and longer lockout period than PCAs. For neonates and infants 1–3 months old, we use NCA morphine: a background infusion of 5 or 10 mcg/kg/h, respectively, with a bolus of 5 mcg/kg and a lockout of 60 minutes.

Interestingly, respiratory depression is very rare, but does occur, reinforcing the need for close monitoring and established nursing protocols. Difficulties with PCA include its increased cost, patient age limitations, and the bureaucratic obstacles (protocols, nurse education, storage arrangements) that must be overcome before its implementation.

Transmucosal, Intranasal, and Transdermal Fentanyl

Because fentanyl is extremely lipophilic, it can be readily absorbed across any biologic membrane, including the skin. Thus, it can be given painlessly by new, nonintravenous routes of drug administration, including the transmucosal (nose and mouth) and transdermal routes. The transmucosal route of fentanyl administration is extremely effective for acute pain relief. When given intranasally (2 mcg/kg), it produces rapid analgesia that is equivalent to intravenously administered fentanyl.[52]

Alternatively, fentanyl has been manufactured in a candy matrix (Actiq) attached to a plastic applicator (it looks like a lollipop) for transoral/transmucosal absorption. As the child sucks on the candy, fentanyl is absorbed across the buccal mucosa and is rapidly (over 10–20 minutes) absorbed into the systemic circulation.[53–58] If excessive sedation occurs, the fentanyl is removed from the child's mouth by the applicator. This method is more efficient than ordinary oral–gastric intestinal administration because transmucosal absorption bypasses the efficient first-pass hepatic metabolism of fentanyl that occurs after enteral absorption into the portal circulation. Actiq has been approved by the FDA for use in children for premedication before surgery and for procedure-related pain (eg, lumbar puncture, bone marrow aspiration).[59] It is also useful in the treatment of cancer pain and as a supplement to transdermal fentanyl.[60] When administered transmucosally, fentanyl is given in doses of 10–15 mcg/kg, is effective within 20 minutes, and lasts approximately 2 hours. Approximately 25%–33% of the given dose is absorbed. Thus, when administered in doses of 10–15 mcg/kg, blood levels equivalent to 3–5 mcg/kg IV fentanyl are achieved. The major side effect, nausea and vomiting, occurs in approximately 20%–33% of patients who receive it.[61]

The transdermal route is frequently used to administer chronically administered drugs, including scopolamine, clonidine, and nitroglycerin. Many factors, such as body site, skin temperature, skin damage, ethnic group, and age, affect the absorption of transdermally administered drugs. Placed in a selective semipermeable membrane patch, a reservoir of drug provides slow, steady-state absorption of drug across the skin. The patch is attached to the skin by a contact adhesive, which often causes skin irritation.

The use of transdermal fentanyl has revolutionized adult cancer pain management. As fentanyl is painlessly absorbed across the skin, a substantial amount is stored in the upper skin layers, which then acts as a secondary reservoir. The presence of a skin depot has several implications: it dampens the fluctuations of fentanyl effect, it needs to be reasonably filled before significant vascular absorption occurs, and it contributes to a prolonged residual fentanyl plasma concentration after patch removal. Indeed, the amount of fentanyl remaining within the system and skin depot after patch removal is substantial. At the end of a 24-hour period, approximately 30% of the total delivered dose from the patch remains in the skin depot. Thus, removing the patch does not stop the continued absorption of fentanyl into the body.[62]

Because of the long onset time, inability to rapidly adjust drug delivery, and long elimination half-life, the use of transdermal fentanyl for *acute* pain management is controversial. As stated above, the safety of this drug delivery system is compromised even further because fentanyl continues to be absorbed from the subcutaneous fat for almost 24 hours after the patch is removed. In fact, the use of this drug delivery system for acute pain has resulted in the death of an otherwise healthy patient. Transdermal fentanyl is generally reserved for patients with chronic pain (eg, cancer) and those who are opioid tolerant. Even when transdermal fentanyl is appropriate, the vehicle imposes its own constraints. The lowest-dose fentanyl "patch" delivers 25 mcg fentanyl per hour; the others deliver 50, 75, and 100 mcg of fentanyl per hour. Patches *cannot* be physically cut into smaller pieces to deliver less fentanyl. This often limits usefulness in patients with lower body weights, and, as with other opioids, this drug delivery system has neither been tested nor approved for use in children.

A new noninvasive method of transdermal PCA is on the horizon. Using iontophoresis (electrotransport), small doses of fentanyl (40 mcg) can be self-administered across the skin (E-Trans, Alza Corporation).[63] Transdermal PCA may offer logistic advantages for patients and nursing staff by eliminating the need for venous access, IV tubing, and specialized pumps.

Complications

Regardless of method of administration, all opioids produce common unwanted side effects, such as pruritus, nausea and vomiting, constipation, urinary retention, cognitive impairment, tolerance, and dependence.[64] Indeed, many patients suffer needlessly from agonizing pain because they would rather suffer pain than experience these opioid-induced side effects.[65] In addition, physicians are often reluctant to prescribe opioids because of these side effects and because of their fear of other less common, but more serious, side effects such as respiratory depression. Several clinical and laboratory studies have demonstrated that low-dose naloxone infusions (0.25–1 mcg/kg/h) can treat or prevent opioid-induced side effects without affecting the quality of analgesia or opioid requirements.[66,67]

Some opioids, when given concomitantly with selective serotonin reuptake inhibitors (SSRIs), monoamine oxidase inhibitors (MAOIs), or serotonin–norepinephrine reuptake inhibitors (SNRIs), have been associated with serotonin syndrome; these include fentanyl, oxycodone, hydrocodone, and tramadol.

Transition to Oral Medication

Successful transition from intravenous (or epidural) analgesics to oral medication depends on the clinician's ability to provide alternative therapy that is palatable, acceptable, and above all, equally effective in treating pain. There are many advantages in providing pain medication by the oral route. Enteral therapy consists of a less invasive route of drug administration and enables children to more rapidly return to their normal lives. Moreover, oral medications are easier and less expensive to deliver than IV and epidural drugs.

Certain criteria are essential for the successful transition to oral medication. Normal gastrointestinal function must be present before attempting enteral therapy. Thus, the child must be able to drink and/or eat (or have a functioning gastric tube). A child who is nauseated or vomits after eating will simply not tolerate oral analgesics. Second, severe pain is difficult, if not impossible, to control with oral analgesics alone. Therefore, oral analgesics should be reserved for the treatment of mild to moderate pain during the latter part of the recovery process. Assessment of the degree of pain and existing treatment modalities are steps that aid the transition process. Third, an oral formulation that is palatable and appropriate must be available. Finally, one must convert the current parenteral opioid dosing to a roughly equianalgesic oral dose.

This conversion is fairly straightforward even when patients are receiving multiple forms and doses of parenteral opioids. As a first step, convert the entire daily dose of administered opioids into IV morphine equivalents (Example 1). Then, convert that morphine dose to an equianalgesic dose of oral morphine (1:2) or other oral opioid, if desired. This formula actually underestimates the bioequivalence of the drugs but is used to minimize the risk of overdose during the transition.

Example 1

A 5-year-old, 20-kg boy was the victim of a motor vehicle accident and sustained a pelvic fracture. He has been on IV PCA morphine for 2 weeks and will be discharged home for further outpatient therapy and recovery. He receives morphine 2 mg/h and averages one bolus of 0.5 mg morphine every hour. He cannot swallow pills.

> Step 1: 2 mg/h for 24 hours = 48 mg morphine/24 hours
> Step 2: 0.5 mg/bolus for 24 boluses/day = 12 mg morphine
> Step 3: Total 24-hour morphine = 48 mg + 12 mg = 60 mg
> Step 4: 60 mg IV morphine = 120 mg PO morphine (actually, this represents a 25%–40% decrease in bioequivalence)
> Step 5: Prescribe oral morphine 20 mg every 4 hours and an analgesic with antipyretic activity (eg, acetaminophen or ibuprofen).
> Step 6: Stop the basal opioid infusion (PCA) immediately or concomitantly with oral dose; increase oral dose by 20%–25% if pain relief is deemed inadequate. If the opioid requirement is high, PCA can be used to provide "rescue" boluses only for the period of transition or to wean the background infusion/PCA doses to more manageable oral doses.

Local Anesthetics

Over the past 25 years, the use of local anesthetics and regional anesthetic techniques in pediatric practice has undergone a dramatic change. Unlike most drugs used in medical practice, local anesthetics must be physically deposited at their site of action by direct application. This requires patient cooperation and the use of specialized needles and equipment; because of this, children were long considered poor candidates for regional anesthetic techniques because of their overwhelming fear of needles. However, once it was recognized that regional anesthesia could be used as an adjunct, and not as a replacement for general anesthesia, its use has increased exponentially. Regional anesthesia offers the anesthesiologist and pain specialist many benefits. It modifies the neuroendocrine stress response, provides profound postoperative pain relief, ensures a more rapid recovery, and may shorten the hospital stay. Furthermore, because catheters placed in the epidural, upper or lower extremity, or lumbar plexi can be used for days or months, local anesthetics are increasingly being used not only for postoperative pain relief but also for medical (eg, sickle cell vaso-occlusive crisis), neuropathic, and terminal pain relief.[68–72] These techniques range from simple infiltration of local anesthetics to neuraxial blocks (eg, spinal and epidural analgesia). With the use of ultrasound guidance, regional anesthesia in the pediatric population has gained further popularity. Peripheral nerve blocks can also provide significant pain relief following many common pediatric procedures and have the potential to replace or provide an alternative to "gold standard" epidural treatment. This is particularly true in the neonatal population where paravertebral block for a thoracotomy or a transverse abdominis plane (TAP) block for a laparotomy can replace an epidural for effective pain relief and avoid the risks associated with neuroaxial blockade. To be used safely, a working knowledge of anatomy, limitations of technique, and differences in how local anesthetics are metabolized in infants and children is necessary. All aspects of local anesthetics are discussed in detail in previous chapters.

Other Adjutants in a Multimodal Analgesia Regime

Gabapentin

Gabapentin is well established in chronic pain management. A few studies have shown that perioperative gabapentin reduces acute postoperative opioid consumption[73] in patients undergoing a variety of surgeries, including coronary artery bypass[74] and knee arthroplasty.[75] In one study, gabapentin was shown to reduce perioperative opioid use but not opioid-related side effects in pediatric patients undergoing posterior spinal fusion.[76] Dosing varies from a single perioperative dose to treatment for 1–2 weeks. At our institution, we use gabapentin for spinal fusion surgeries and selected surgeries where postoperative pain relief is deemed challenging. We normally administer gabapentin at a dose of 5–10 mg/kg every 8 hours for 5 days. For patients with complex needs, doses may need to be revised down, as in some cases, gabapentin can produce noticeable sedation or drowsiness.

Ketamine

Ketamine is a well-known anesthetic that produces dissociative anesthesia but also provides a very good-quality analgesia at very low doses via its NMDA receptor antagonist activity. Healthcare professionals remain wary of ketamine, however, due to its unpleasant side effect of hallucinations and its recent implication in neuroapoptosis in the developing brain.[77,78] These concerns have now led to the avoidance of ketamine use in patients under 1 year of age and has also decreased the popularity of ketamine as an additive in caudal and epidural blocks.

However, in older children and adolescents, ketamine is still widely used with good effect. Ketamine can also be added to morphine PCA in a 1:1 ratio. At our institution, a single low dose of ketamine (0.1–0.25 mg/kg) forms part of a balanced intraoperative analgesic regime for adenotonsillectomy and major surgeries. Ketamine infusion is also used as a second-line IV analgesic for complex and painful conditions and in cases of acute or chronic pain where other treatments have failed to produce effective analgesia. The infusion dose of ketamine used is 0.05–0.2 mg/kg/h (using a drug concentration of 0.1 mg/kg/mL, up to a maximum of 250 mg in 50 mL).

Magnesium

Magnesium is used in variety of medical emergencies and treatments. The intravenous use of magnesium has been reported to improve postoperative analgesia. Though the mechanism of action is not yet fully understood, the analgesic properties of magnesium are believed be due to the regulation of calcium influx into the cell and NMDA receptor antagonist activity.[79,80] Evidence has been equivocal, however, and although relatively safe, magnesium is not without side effects. A recent meta-analysis concluded that perioperative intravenous magnesium reduces opioid consumption, and to a lesser extent pain scores, in the first 24 hours postoperatively without any reported serious adverse effects.[81] The use of magnesium, either as a bolus or infusion (at a dose of 30–50 mg/kg), for major surgeries, particularly spinal fusions, and for other major orthopedic and general surgeries, is standard practice at our institution.

2. CHRONIC PAIN MANAGEMENT

THE TRANSITION FROM ACUTE TO CHRONIC PAIN

Acute pain has evolved as a vital defense mechanism, alerting the animal to injury and physical harm in order to stop the exposure to injury, such as with the pain reflex or to signal the need for rest to allow healing to occur. Chronic pain, however, serves no protective function. Chronic pain is considered to be pain that extends beyond the expected period of healing.[82] There are increasing studies in the adult literature demonstrating the development of postoperative chronic pain, which is then associated with significant negative consequences for the individual, in terms of both physical and mental health, and for the wider society, in terms of both economic and healthcare resource burdens. The incidence of chronic postoperative pain varies depending on surgery type, with estimates between 5% and 50% in the most common surgical procedures,[83] including hernia repair, hip replacement, and cholecystectomy, versus up to 85% in amputations. Although the literature for the development of chronic pain postoperatively is sparse in pediatric age ranges, studies are beginning to indicate that it does occur, although its incidence may be lower than in the adult population.

Fortier[83] studied 113 children between the ages of 2 and 17 years who had undergone general urological or orthopedic surgery and found that 13.3% reported chronic pain resulting from surgery. The surgeries most related to the development of chronic pain were orthopedic. Over one-quarter reported interference in sleep patterns and extracurricular activities, and 1 in 6 reported interference in school activities. Chronic pain in adults after inguinal surgery has a reported incidence of 5%–35%; however, in children, studies suggest the incidence may be lower. One particular surgery in adolescents associated with a high incidence of persistent pain is scoliosis, where estimates of 50% are reported.[84] A study by Wong demonstrated a trend for those who experienced more severe postoperative pain to have a greater tendency toward developing persistent pain; only 39% of those with mild postoperative pain developed persistent pain compared with 74% of those with severe postoperative pain. Studies have indicated that persistent pain can be a complication for as long as 12 months after surgery; however, thoracotomy in childhood has been associated with pain persisting into adulthood up to 30 years later. This risk appears less when surgery takes place at a younger age and increases with the age at which surgery is

performed. Although the mechanisms for the transition from acute to chronic pain are complex, some risk factors identified in the adult literature (in the absence of many studies in children) may also be relevant to the pediatric population. These include the presence of preoperative pain, the severity of acute postoperative pain, and open versus laparoscopic surgery. Good postoperative multimodal pain management therefore plays an important role in efforts to prevent the subsequent development of persistent pain in children.

Clinical Pearls

- Chronic pain can be a postoperative complication in the pediatric population.
- Chronic pain has a negative impact on sleep, activities, school attendance, and school achievement.
- Risks for the development of chronic pain include preoperative pain, the severity of acute postoperative pain, and open versus laparoscopic surgery.

THE MANAGEMENT OF ACUTE-ON-CHRONIC PAIN

The management of patients undergoing surgery with preoperative chronic pain can be problematic, and the presence of preoperative pain increases pain perception postoperatively. Good preoperative preparation and planning are important, incorporating education for both the child and parents/guardians and involving them in decision making. Psychological interventions, such as cognitive behavioral therapy and decatastrophization can be beneficial preparation. Patients experiencing preoperative pain may be taking adjuvant analgesia medications, some of which should not be stopped abruptly, such as anticonvulsants (eg, gabapentin). Other medications may have significant interactions with commonly used analgesic medications; for example, the combination of amitriptyline and tramadol has resulted in serotonin syndrome. There are a small number of pediatric patients who present for surgery on long-term opioids, and not all of these patients will be palliative. The prolonged administrations of opioids may occur in children in intensive care units, those requiring frequent and repeated surgery (eg, for burns), those with frequent disease exacerbations (eg, sickle cell), adolescents using opioids illicitly, and in a small number of children with medically unexplained pain. Recommendations for the management of such patients are primarily extrapolated from the adult literature due to a lack of evidence in children (Table 45–5).

SUMMARY

The past 25 years have seen an explosion in research and interest in pediatric pain management. In this brief review, we have tried to consolidate in a comprehensive manner some of the most commonly used agents and techniques in current practice.

TABLE 45–5. Considerations for the perioperative management of children on long-term opioids.

Educate and involve the child and his or her parents/guardians in preoperative planning.

Continue maintenance opioids or consider conversion to parenteral opioids.

Supplementation with systemic opioid (oral or intravenous) may be necessary if a neuroaxial technique is used.

Titrate opioids postoperatively.

The dose may need to be 30%–100% higher than for opioid-naïve patients.

Use multimodal therapy, including adjuvant medications (eg, ketamine) and nonpharmacologic techniques.

Use regional anesthesia techniques where possible.

When transitioning from parenteral opioids to oral delivery calculate total dose requirement over 24 hours. Deliver 50% of the estimated oral dose as long-acting and the remainder as breakthrough.

Taper oral opioids to preoperative doses slowly, over a period of 2-4 weeks.

In the first 24 postoperative hours, reduce the dose by 20–40%.

Following the first 24 postoperative hours, reduce the dose by 5–20% (use a slower rate in the presence of withdrawal signs).

Ensure chronic pain service is involved in the transition to long-term pain management.

Source: Reproduced with permissions from Geary T, Negus A, Anderson BJ, et al: Perioperative management of the child on long-term opioids. *Paediatr Anaesth.* 2012 Mar;22(3):189-202.

REFERENCES

1. Schechter NL, Berde CB, Yaster M: *Pain in Infants, Children, and Adolescents*, 2nd ed. Philadelphia: Lippincott Williams & Wilkins; 2003.
2. Yaster M, Krane EJ, Kaplan RF, et al: *Pediatric Pain Management and Sedation Handbook*. Maryland Heights, MI: Mosby; 1997.
3. Merskey H, Albe-Fessard DG, Bonica JJ: Pain terms: A list with definitions and notes on usage. Recommended by the IASP Subcommittee on Taxonomy. *Pain* 1979;6:249–252.
4. Anand KJ, Hickey PR: Pain and its effects in the human neonate and fetus. *N Engl J Med* 1987;317:1321–1329.
5. Stevens B, Gibbins S, Franck LS: Treatment of pain in the neonatal intensive care unit. *Pediatr Clin North Am* 2000;47:633–650.
6. Fitzgerald M: Neurobiology of fetal and neonatal pain. In: Wall PD, Melzack R (eds): *Textbook of Pain*, 3rd ed. London: Churchill Livingstone; 1994:153–164.
7. Lee SJ, Ralston HJ, Drey EA, et al: Fetal pain: a systematic multidisciplinary review of the evidence. *JAMA* 2005;294:947–954.
8. Taddio A, Katz J, Ilersich AL, Koren G: Effect of neonatal circumcision on pain response during subsequent routine vaccination. *Lancet* 1997;349:599–603.
9. Taddio A, Katz J: The effects of early pain experience in neonates on pain responses in infancy and childhood. *Paediatr Drugs* 2005;7:245–257.
10. Forward SP, Brown TL, McGrath PJ: Mothers' attitudes and behavior toward medicating children's pain. *Pain* 1996;67:469–474.
11. Finley GA, McGrath PJ, Forward SP, et al: Parents' management of children's pain following 'minor' surgery. *Pain* 1996;64:83–87.
12. Varni JW, Thompson KL, Hanson V: The Varni/Thompson Pediatric Pain Questionnaire. I. Chronic musculoskeletal pain in juvenile rheumatoid arthritis. *Pain* 1987;28:27–38.
13. Thompson KL, Varni JW: A developmental cognitive-biobehavioral approach to pediatric pain assessment. *Pain* 1986;25:283–296.
14. Beyer JE, Wells N: The assessment of pain in children. *Pediatr Clin North Am* 1989;36:837–854.
15. Beyer JE, Denyes MJ, Villarruel AM: The creation, validation, and continuing development of the Oucher: a measure of pain intensity in children. *J Pediatr Nurs* 1992;7:335–346.
16. Wong DL, Baker CM: Pain in children: comparison of assessment scales. *Pediatr Nurs* 1988;14:9–17.
17. Franck LS, Greenberg CS, Stevens B: Pain assessment in infants and children. *Pediatr Clin North Am* 2000;47:487–512.
18. Anthony KK, Schanberg LE: Pediatric pain syndromes and management of pain in children and adolescents with rheumatic disease. *Pediatr Clin North Am* 2005;52:611–639, vii.
19. Krecher SW, Bildner J: CRIES: a neonatal postoperative pain measurement score. Initial testing of validity & reliability. *Paediatr Anaesth* 1995;5:53–65.
20. Cunliffe M, Roberts SA: Pain management in children. *Curr Anaesth Crit Care* 2004;15:272–283.
21. Hunt A, Goldman A, Seers K, et al: Clinical validation of the paediatric pain profile. *Dev Med Child Neurol* 2004;46(1):9–18.
22. Rusy LM, Weisman SJ: Complementary therapies for acute pediatric pain management. *Pediatr Clin North Am* 2000;47:589–599.
23. Berde CB, Sethna NF: Analgesics for the treatment of pain in children. *N Engl J Med* 2002;347:1094–1103.
24. Yaster M: Non-steroidal anti-inflammatory drugs. In: Yaster M, Krane EJ, Kaplan RF (eds): *Pediatric Pain Management and Sedation Handbook*. Maryland Heights, MI: Mosby; 1997:19–28.
25. Tobias JD: Weak analgesics and nonsteroidal anti-inflammatory agents in the management of children with acute pain. *Pediatr Clin North Am* 2000;47:527–543.
26. Maunuksela EL, Kokki H, Bullingham RE: Comparison of intravenous ketorolac with morphine for postoperative pain in children. *Clin Pharmacol Ther* 1992;52:436–443.
27. Birmingham PK, Tobin MJ, Henthorn TK, et al: Twenty-four-hour pharmacokinetics of rectal acetaminophen in children: an old drug with new recommendations. *Anesthesiology* 1997;87:244–252.
28. Rusy LM, Houck CS, Sullivan LJ, et al: A double-blind evaluation of ketorolac tromethamine versus acetaminophen in pediatric tonsillectomy: Analgesia and bleeding. *Anesth Analg* 1995;80:226–229.
29. Vane JR, Botting RM: Mechanism of action of nonsteroidal anti-inflammatory drugs. *Am J Med* 1998;104:2S–8S; discussion 21S–2.
30. Vane JR, Botting RM: Mechanism of action of aspirin-like drugs. *Semin Arthritis Rheum* 1997;26:2–10.
31. Jouzeau JY, Terlain B, Abid A, et al: Cyclo-oxygenase isoenzymes. How recent findings affect thinking about nonsteroidal anti-inflammatory drugs. *Drugs* 1997;53:563–582.
32. Cashman JN: The mechanisms of action of NSAIDs in analgesia. *Drugs* 1996;52(Suppl 5):13–23.
33. Vane JR, Bakhle YS, Botting RM: Cyclooxygenases 1 and 2. *Annu Rev Pharmacol Toxicol* 1998;38:97–120.
34. Johnsen SP, Larsson H, Tarone RE, et al: Risk of hospitalization for myocardial infarction among users of rofecoxib, celecoxib, and other NSAIDs: a population-based case-control study. *Arch Intern Med* 2005;165:978–984.
35. Levesque LE, Brophy JM, Zhang B: The risk for myocardial infarction with cyclooxygenase-2 inhibitors: a population study of elderly adults. *Ann Intern Med* 2005;142:481–489.
36. Dahners LE, Mullis BH: Effects of nonsteroidal anti-inflammatory drugs on bone formation and soft-tissue healing. *J Am Acad Orthop Surg* 2004;12:139–143.
37. Simon AM, Manigrasso MB, O'Connor JP: Cyclo-oxygenase 2 function is essential for bone fracture healing. *J Bone Miner Res* 2002;17:963–976.
38. Einhorn TA: Cox-2: Where are we in 2003? The role of cyclooxygenase-2 in bone repair. *Arthritis Res Ther* 2003;5:5–7.
39. Radnay PA, Duncalf D, Novakovic M, Lesser ML: Common bile duct pressure changes after fentanyl, morphine, meperidine, butorphanol, and naloxone. *Anesth Analg* 1984;63:441–444.
40. Krane EJ, Yaster M: Transition to less invasive therapy. In: Yaster M, Krane EJ, Kaplan RF, et al (eds): *Pediatric Pain Management and Sedation Handbook*. Maryland Heights, MI: Mosby; 1997:147–162.
41. Ciszkowski C, Madadi P. Codeine, ultrarapid-metabolism genotype and postoperative death. *N Engl J Med* 2009;361(8):827–828.

42. Kelly LE, Rieder M, van den Anker J, et al. More codeine fatalities after tonsillectomy in North American children. *Pediatrics* 2012;129(5): e1343–1347. doi: 10.1542/peds.2011-2538.

43. Ingelman-Sundberg M, Oscarson M, McLellan RA. Polymorphic human cytochrome P450 enzymes: an opportunity for individualized drug treatment. *Trends Pharmacol Sci* 1999;20(8):342–349.

44. U.S. Food and Drug Administration (FDA). Drug safety communications: safety review update of codeine use in children; new boxed warning and contraindication on use after tonsillectomy and/or adenoidectomy. http://www.fda.gov/downloads/Drugs/DrugSafety/UCM339116.pdf. Published February 20, 2013. Accessed February 26, 2013.

45. European Medicines Agency (EMA). PRAC recommends restricting the use of codeine when used for pain relief in children. http://www.ema.europa.eu/docs/en_GB/document_library/Press_release/2013/06/WC500144444.pdf. Published June 14, 2013. Accessed June 18, 2013.

46. Tremlett M, Anderson BJ, Wolf A. Pro-con debate: is codeine a drug that still has a useful role in pediatric practice? *Paediatr Anaesth* 2010;20(2):183–194.

47. Heubi JE, Barbacci MB, Zimmerman HJ: Therapeutic misadventures with acetaminophen: hepatotoxicity after multiple doses in children. *J Pediatr* 1998;132:22–27.

48. Viitanen H, Annila P: Analgesic efficacy of tramadol 2 mg kg⁻¹ for paediatric day-case adenoidectomy. *Br J Anaesth* 2001;86(4):572–575.

49. Berde CB, Lehn BM, Yee JD, Sethna NF, Russo D: Patient-controlled analgesia in children and adolescents: A randomized, prospective comparison with intramuscular administration of morphine for postoperative analgesia. *J Pediatr* 1991;118:460–466.

50. Yaster M, Billett C, Monitto C: Intravenous patient controlled analgesia. In: Yaster M, Krane EJ, Kaplan RF, et al (eds): *Pediatric Pain Management and Sedation Handbook*. Maryland Heights, MI: Mosby; 1997: 89–112.

51. Monitto CL, Greenberg RS, Kost-Byerly S, et al: The safety and efficacy of parent-/nurse-controlled analgesia in patients less than six years of age. *Anesth Analg* 2000;91:573–579.

52. Galinkin JL, Fazi LM, Cuy RM, et al: Use of intranasal fentanyl in children undergoing myringotomy and tube placement during halothane and sevoflurane anesthesia. *Anesthesiology* 2000;93:137–383.

53. Schechter NL, Weisman SJ, Rosenblum M, et al: The use of oral transmucosal fentanyl citrate for painful procedures in children. *Pediatrics* 1995;95:335–339.

54. Goldstein-Dresner MC, Davis PJ, Kretchman E, et al: Double-blind comparison of oral transmucosal fentanyl citrate with oral meperidine, diazepam, and atropine as preanesthetic medication in children with congenital heart disease. *Anesthesiology* 1991;74:28–33.

55. Streisand JB, Stanley TH, Hague B, et al: Oral transmucosal fentanyl citrate premedication in children. *Anesth Analg* 1989;69:28–34.

56. Stanley TH, Hague B, Mock DL, et al: Oral transmucosal fentanyl citrate (lollipop) premedication in human volunteers. *Anesth Analg* 1989;69:21–27.

57. Ashburn MA, Lind GH, Gillie MH, et al: Oral transmucosal fentanyl citrate (OTFC) for the treatment of postoperative pain. *Anesth Analg* 1993;76:377–381.

58. Streisand JB, Varvel JR, Stanski DR, et al: Absorption and bioavailability of oral transmucosal fentanyl citrate. *Anesthesiology* 1991;75:223–229.

59. Dsida RM, Wheeler M, Birmingham PK, et al: Premedication of pediatric tonsillectomy patients with oral transmucosal fentanyl citrate. *Anesth Analg* 1998;86:66–70.

60. Portenoy RK, Payne R, Coluzzi P, et al: Oral transmucosal fentanyl citrate (OTFC) for the treatment of breakthrough pain in cancer patients: A controlled dose titration study. *Pain* 1999;79:303–312.

61. Epstein RH, Mendel HG, Witkowski TA, et al: The safety and efficacy of oral transmucosal fentanyl citrate for preoperative sedation in young children. *Anesth Analg* 1996;83:1200–1205.

62. Grond S, Radbruch L, Lehmann KA: Clinical pharmacokinetics of transdermal opioids: Focus on transdermal fentanyl. *Clin Pharmacokinet* 2000;38:59–89.

63. Chelly JE, Grass J, Houseman TW, et al: The safety and efficacy of a fentanyl patient-controlled transdermal system for acute postoperative analgesia: A multicenter, placebo-controlled trial (table). *Anesth Analg* 2004;98:427–433.

64. Yaster M, Kost-Byerly S, Maxwell LG: Opioid agonists and antagonists. In: Schechter NL, Berde CB, Yaster M (eds: *Pain in Infants, Children, and Adolescents*, 2nd ed. Philadelphia: Lippincott Williams & Wilkins; 2003:181–224.

65. Watcha MF, White PF: Postoperative nausea and vomiting. Its etiology, treatment, and prevention. *Anesthesiology* 1992;77:162–184.

66. Gan TJ, Ginsberg B, Glass PS, et al: Opioid-sparing effects of a low-dose infusion of naloxone in patient-administered morphine sulfate. *Anesthesiology* 1997;87:1075–1081.

67. Maxwell LG, Kaufmann SC, Bitzer S, et al: The effects of a small-dose naloxone infusion on opioid-induced side effects and analgesia in children and adolescents treated with intravenous patient-controlled analgesia: A double-blind, prospective, randomized, controlled study. *Anesth Analg* 2005;100:953–958.

68. Dalens B: Regional anesthesia in children. Anesth Analg 1989;68:654–672.

69. Giaufre E, Dalens B, Gombert A: Epidemiology and morbidity of regional anesthesia in children: A one-year prospective survey of the French-Language Society of Pediatric Anesthesiologists. *Anesth Analg* 1996;83:904–912.

70. Yaster M, Maxwell LG: Pediatric regional anesthesia. *Anesthesiology* 1989;70:324–338.

71. Ross AK, Eck JB, Tobias JD: Pediatric regional anesthesia: beyond the caudal. *Anesth Analg* 2000;91:16–26.

72. Golianu B, Krane EJ, Galloway KS, Yaster M: Pediatric acute pain management. *Pediatr Clin North Am* 2000;47:559–587.

73. Dauri M, Faria S, Gatti A, et al: Gabapentin and pregabalin for the acute post-operative pain management. A systemic-narrative review of recent clinical evidences. *Curr Drug Targets* 2009;10:716–733.

74. Ucak A, Onan B, Sen H, Selcuk I, Turan A, Yilmaz AT: The effects of gabapentin on acute and chronic post-operative pain after coronary artery bypass graft surgery. *J Cardiothorac Vasc Anaesth* 2011;25:824–829.

75. Clarke H, Pereira S, Kennedy D, et al: Gabapentin decreases morphine consumption and improves functional recovery following total knee arthroplasty. *Pain Res Manag* 2009;14:217–222.

76. Rusy LM, Hainswork KR, Nelson TJ, et al. Gabapentin use in pediatric spinal fusion patients: a randomized, double-blind, controlled trial. *Anesth Analg* 2010;110:1393–1398.

77. Green SM, Cote CJ: Ketamine and neurotoxicity: clinical perspective and implications for emergency medicine. *Ann Emerg Med* 2009;54:181–190.

78. Bambrink AM, Evers AS, Avidan MS, et al: Ketamine induced neuroapoptosis in the fetal and neonatal rhesus macaque brain. *Anaesthesialogy* 2012;116: 372–384.

79. Iseri LT, French JH. Magnesium: nature's physiologic calcium blocker. *Am Heart J* 1984;108:188–193.

80. Woolf CJ, Thompson SW. The induction and maintenance of central sensitization is dependent on N-methyl-D-aspartic acid receptor activation: implications for the treatment of post-injury pain hypersensitivity states. *Pain* 1991;44:293–299.

81. Albrecht E, Kirkham KR, Liu SS, Brull R: Peri-operative intravenous administration of magnesium sulphate and post-operative pain: a meta-analysis. *Anaesthesia* 2013;68:79–90.

82. Turk, DC, Okifuji A. Pain and terms and taxonomies. In: Loeser D, Butler SH, Chapman JJ, et al. *Bonica's Management of Pain*, 3rd ed. Philadelphia: Lippincott Williams & Wilkins; 2001:18–25.

83. Fortier MA, Chou J, Muarer EL, Kain ZN. Acute to chronic postoperative pain in children: preliminary findings. *J Ped Surg* 2011;46:1700–1705.

84. Wong GTC, Yuen VMY, Chow BFM, Irwin MG. Persistent pain in patients following scoliosis surgery. *Eur Spine* J 2007;18:1551–1556.

PART 7

ANESTHESIA IN PATIENTS WITH SPECIFIC CONSIDERATIONS

CHAPTER 46

Perioperative Regional Anesthesia in the Elderly

Jennifer E. Dominguez and Thomas M. Halaszynski

INTRODUCTION AND DEFINITION OF ELDERLY

Healthcare providers have become increasingly focused on providing effective management of acute perioperative pain in all patients, but especially older adults, as the size of this patient population has steadily increased in recent years.[1] Advances in anesthetic and surgical techniques, an improved understanding of the pathophysiology of pain, the development of new opioid and nonopioid analgesic drugs, the incorporation of regional techniques that reduce or eliminate reliance on traditional opioid analgesics, and novel methods of drug delivery have all led to greater numbers of older patients undergoing major surgery.[2,3] An increased prevalence of chronic medical conditions among older individuals may also lead to higher degrees of acute and chronic pain (including acute-on-chronic pain). For instance, acute exacerbations of arthritis, osteoporotic fractures of the spine, cancer pain, and pain from acute medical conditions (eg, ischemic heart disease, herpes zoster, peripheral vascular disease) must be properly addressed in order to maximize multimodal perioperative pain management.[4] In addition, older individuals are adopting more active lifestyles that can predispose them to trauma and orthopedic injuries that require surgery.

The term *elderly* encompasses both chronologic and physiologic factors. Chronologic age is the actual number of years an individual has lived, whereas physiologic age refers to functional capacity or reserve within organ systems defined in pathophysiologic parameters. The chronologic component can be divided into two separate groups: the "young old" (65 to 80 years of age) and the "older old" (greater than 80 years of age).[5] Physiologic reserve describes the functional capacity of organ systems to compensate for acute stress and traumatic derangements. When present, comorbid disease states such as diabetes mellitus, arthritis, renal insufficiency, ischemic heart disease, and chronic obstructive pulmonary disease (COPD) can all decrease a patient's physiologic reserve making it difficult for him or her to recover from traumatic or surgical injury.

There are a host of additional factors that may compromise the ability to provide optimal and effective acute pain management to older patients. A consequence of the comorbid diseases that afflict this patient population with increased frequency is the medications used in treatments for such diseased conditions, along with a subsequent increased risk of drug-to-drug and disease-to-drug interactions. An improved understanding of age-related changes in physiology, pharmacodynamics, and pharmacokinetics must be incorporated into any acute pain medicine care plan for older individuals. Altered responses to pain among the elderly population along with difficulties in pain assessment for certain individuals with cognitive dysfunction are potential problems that must also be considered.

Several theories have been advocated to describe the multidimensional aspects and consequences of aging that underscore the complexities and difficulties encountered in developing optimal regional anesthetic and analgesic choices for elderly patients. Therefore, the focus of this chapter is to outline the physiologic and pharmacologic implications of aging on surgical anesthesia and acute pain management, as well as the potential risks and benefits of neuraxial blockade along with peripheral nerve/nerve plexus blockade in geriatric patients.

PHYSIOLOGIC CHANGES ASSOCIATED WITH AGING AND CONSIDERATIONS FOR REGIONAL ANESTHESIA/ANALGESIA

Aging is characterized by progressive reductions in the homeostatic reserves of nearly every organ system.[6] Declining organ function, often referred to as *homeostenosis*, may be gradual or progressive and becomes evident by the third decade of life. The compromised function of each organ system generally occurs independent of changes to other organ systems and may be influenced by a host of factors, including diet, environment, habits, and genetic predisposition. Optimal anesthetic management using regional techniques in elderly patients depends upon a knowledge and understanding of normal age-related changes in anatomy, physiology, and response to pharmacologic agents. It is also important to distinguish normal physiologic alterations of the central nervous system (CNS), cardiovascular, pulmonary, and hepatorenal systems from disease-related pathophysiologic changes.

Clinical Pearls

- The pain thresholds to a variety of noxious stimuli are altered in older individuals.
- Older patients have a reduction in pain tolerance.
- Patient-controlled analgesia (PCA) and epidural analgesia are more effective in elderly patients than most other conventional (PO and IM) opioid analgesic regimens.
- Physiologic changes associated with aging vary markedly among individuals. The administration of pain medications warrants a decrease in dose (maintenance and/or bolus) of drug required for analgesia to avoid the risk of increased plasma drug accumulation and accumulation of active metabolites.

Nervous System Function

Aging results in anatomical and biochemical changes of the brain, spinal cord, and peripheral nervous system (PNS) that result in qualitative and quantitative alterations in function (Table 46–1). In addition, advanced age can be associated with decreased brain volume, a manifestation of the loss of neurons, as well as a reduction in cerebral white matter nerve fibers. Specifically, the number of cholinergic and dopaminergic neurons declines, and morphologic changes in neuronal fibers occur that result in fewer synaptic contacts and neuroreceptors.

Levels of acetylcholine, dopamine, and other neurotransmitters also decline, and there may be an extraneuronal accumulation of amyloid, which underlies neurocognitive dysfunction. Alterations in brain phospholipid chemistry associated with changes in second messengers, such as diacylglycerol, are also evident in the elderly.[7] Overall, both cerebral electrical and metabolic activity are decreased in elderly compared to younger individuals and may be a result of the multitude of anatomic, structural, and biochemical changes that accompany aging. It is possible that degenerative changes in the myelin sheaths of nerve fibers in the CNS and PNS can also lead to changes in nerve conduction velocity and disrupt the normal timing of neuronal circuits. Additional anatomical changes occur that affect nervous system function, including decreased spinal cord volume and degeneration of the bony spinal canal.

Changes in the somatic nervous system of the PNS associated with aging include (1) peripheral nerve deterioration; (2) dysfunction of genes responsible for myelin sheath protein components; (3) decreased myelinated nerve fiber conduction velocity; (4) motor and sensory discriminatory changes in the feet; and (5) changes in sensation (eg, pain, touch).[8] The autonomic nervous system (ANS) of the PNS also experiences age-related changes that dictate most of the involuntary physiological functions of the body through the parasympathetic and sympathetic divisions. Aging of the ANS is characterized by (1) limited adaptability to stress; (2) decreased basal activity of the parasympathetic nervous system and overall net activation of the sympathetic nervous system; (3) decreased baroreflex sensitivity; and (4) slowing and weakening of homeostatic functions.[9] The increase in sympathetic tone in older patients should also be considered when choosing an anesthetic with sympathomimetic properties, as such anesthetics may be poorly tolerated by some individuals with cardiovascular disease.

Clinical Pearl

- Aging is associated with a shift in balance within the autonomic nervous system toward a predominance of sympathetic tone.

TABLE 46–1. Physiologic central nervous system changes associated with aging and effects on pharmacokinetic variables.

Physiologic Process	Magnitude of Change	Variable Kinetic/Dynamic Consequences	General Dosing Strategy
Cerebral blood flow, metabolism, and volume	↓ 20% ↓ 20%	↓ distribution to the CNS ↓ apparent volume in the CNS	Little net effect on drug dose
Active blood–brain barrier transport (efflux)	Drug-specific ↓	↑ apparent volume in the CNS	↓ bolus dose during drug titration ↓ maintenance dose
Pain threshold sensitivity	Little change	↑ apparent sensitivity of the CNS	Need for titration is unchanged
Concentration response (opioids)	↑ 50% for some opioids	↑ response to opioids	↓ bolus dose during titration ↓ maintenance dose

Aging affects peripheral nerves, resulting in deterioration and decreases in the number of myelinated nerve fibers. Large myelinated fibers are particularly affected by aging, resulting in atrophy along with degenerative changes to the myelin.[10] Levels of expression for key genes that encode major protein components of the myelin sheath, such as proteolipid protein and myelin basic protein, may influence this process.[11,12] Maintenance of myelin sheath integrity involves continued expression of genes specifically associated with myelin protein production. Restoration of myelin sheaths to demyelinated axons occurs spontaneously in the adult nervous system, but aging has a detrimental effect on this process. Spontaneous remyelination efforts and the rate of reappearance of proteolipids and myelin basic proteins are slowed. In the CNS, oligodendrocyte progenitor recruitment and differentiation are also impaired by age-related decline in remyelination.[11,12]

Changes in both the PNS and CNS may affect functional outcomes during the recovery phase following surgery and anesthesia and should be considered in the perioperative evaluation. The neurologic dysfunction of aging can produce altered pharmacodynamics, resulting in increased sensitivity to anesthetic medications with signs and symptoms of altered reflexes, deterioration of gait and mobility, altered sleep patterns, impairment of memory and intellect, and decrements of the senses. Perioperative delirium, a common form of acute cognitive impairment in elderly patients, can increase postoperative morbidity, present with difficult pain management scenarios, impair postoperative rehabilitation and prolong hospital stays.[13-17] Delirium can occur in up to 80% of elderly postoperative patients depending upon the type and extent of surgery, perioperative anesthesia and analgesic needs of the patient, and type of pain therapy administered. It is more common with emergency, trauma, and major surgery. Risk factors associated with the development of delirium are numerous and include increased age, level of patient education, preexisting pain, and use of preoperative medications such as opioids, ketamine, and benzodiazepines.[14-16,18-20] Subsequent to the negative effects of delirium, some patients may go on to experience postoperative cognitive dysfunction (POCD). A systematic review has confirmed that POCD is very common and that older patients are at a higher risk of POCD after major noncardiac surgery than are younger patients.[21]

Clinical Pearl

- Advancing age, level of patient education, and evidence of preexisting cerebral vascular disease are strong predictors of perioperative delirium.

Cardiovascular Function

There are a variety of morphological and functional changes in the cardiovascular system associated with aging, including a reduction in left ventricular compliance, generalized hypertrophy of the left ventricular wall, fibrotic changes of the heart, and decreased myocardial compliance. These changes can result in increased stroke volume and elevated diastolic and systolic

blood pressure (Table 46–2).[22] Many elderly patients present with cardiac pathology, including moderate to severe coronary artery disease, valvular heart disease, and conduction defects that increase the risk of postsurgical morbidity and death. The effects of aging on cardiac output in the absence of coexisting disease may have minimal influence on the resting individual, but functional changes can become evident with stress and effort-dependent stress.[23] Anesthetics and anesthesia technique may also interact with the patient's preexisting cardiovascular disease in a manner that may be unfavorable. For example, patients with a fixed cardiac output (as in aortic stenosis) may not tolerate a decrease in systemic vascular resistance associated with neuraxial anesthesia well. Acute/extreme hemodynamic variability in the setting of regional anesthesia, however, can be overcome with careful titration of neuraxial anesthesia with an epidural or spinal catheter and skillful use of vasopressors.

Age-related influences on the cardiovascular system may have important clinical implications for the treatment of elderly surgical patients and for postoperative pain management, especially for those patients receiving regional anesthesia/analgesia. Several recent studies have demonstrated benefits of regional techniques on cardiac morbidity, intensive care unit (ICU) admissions and short-term survival.[24,25] Although there are sparse data to indicate evidence-based and statistically significant differences in the impact of anesthetic technique on mortality or major complications, regional analgesia can positively influence pain management and lead to better outcomes when the type of surgery being performed is considered. Regional anesthesia/analgesia may have positive implications for perioperative cardiac function. For example, ischemic heart disease and hypertension are more common among elderly than younger patients, and coronary blood flow in such patients could be compromised in response to the sympathetic stimulation of surgery, perioperative stress, pain, and anesthesia. In a study by Park et al, researchers investigated the use of epidural anesthesia/analgesia combined with general anesthesia for abdominal aortic aneurysm repair. They showed that the duration of postoperative tracheal intubation, mechanical ventilation, and total ICU stay were reduced. In addition, the quality of postoperative analgesia improved, whereas the incidence of major complications and death were reduced.[26] Research has also shown that placement of thoracic epidural analgesia can improve left ventricular function[27,28] and increase myocardial oxygen availability.[29] In addition, patients with ischemic heart disease treated with a high thoracic epidural injection of bupivacaine showed improved myocardial blood flow in response to sympathetic stimulation.[30] However, neuraxial anesthesia with an epidural in older patients undergoing coronary artery bypass grafting surgery has not been shown to improve perioperative outcomes.[31] Therefore, to permit physicians to development preliminary guidelines and anesthesia protocols that could positively affect the cardiovascular outcomes of elderly surgical patients, studies investigating regional techniques should be tailored to match the planned surgery and adjusted for comorbid diseases and perioperative patient management needs (ie, procedure- and patient-specific anesthesia/analgesia).

In addition to the mounting evidence of the regional anesthesia (with or without continuous local anesthetic infusion) on

TABLE 46–2. Physiologic cardiovascular changes associated with aging and effects on pharmacokinetic variables.

Physiologic Process	Magnitude	Variable Kinetic/Dynamic Consequences	General Dosing Strategy
Cardiac output	↓ 0–20%	↓ central compartment volume ↑ peak concentration of drug after bolus	Use smaller initial bolus dose Use slower injection rate *Potential for change in clearance and oral bioavailability* *Potential for change in cerebral effects*
Fat	↑ 10–50%, then ↓	Drug-specific changes are seen in distribution volume	Drug-specific (dose based on total body weight and/or lean body weight)
Muscle mass and blood flow	↓ 20%		
Plasma volume	Little change		
Total body water	↓ 10%	↓ distribution volume (water-soluble drugs)	
Plasma albumin	↓ 20%	↑ free fraction of drug	Potential for change in clearance and oral bioavailability Potential for change in cerebral effects
Alpha-1 glycoprotein	↑ 30–50%	Variable hepatic clearance of high-extraction drugs ↑ hepatic clearance of low-extraction drugs ↑ cerebral uptake of drugs	
Drug binding	Drug specific		

perioperative cardiac morbidity and mortality[32] effectively managed postoperative pain could mitigate myocardial dysfunction if catecholamine levels associated with stress and pain are reduced. Regional anesthesia can also may provide superior analgesia compared to systemic opioids. Peripheral nerve blocks and neuraxial anesthesia the elderly can provide preemptive analgesia, reduce the side-effects or eliminate the need for general anesthesia (or completely avoid it in certain surgical settings), reduce sympathetic stimulation and stress responses associated with surgery, and directly inhibit transduction, transmission, and conduction of nociception from the surgical trauma site(s). Regional techniques that complement multimodal analgesic therapies have been demonstrated to have beneficial effects on acute pain and may lead to a reduction in cardiac morbidity and mortality.[33] Another factor to consider is the duration of postoperative analgesic needs because pain from surgery, surgical stress, and effects on the cardiovascular system often do not subside until several days following surgery. Therefore, the use of an effective regional technique (eg, continuous catheter) may provide sustained benefits by reducing postsurgical pain and its associated sympathetic and neuroendocrine stress responses. However, patients with coexisting cardiovascular disease may be treated with anticoagulants or antiplatelet medications, or both, and careful attention should be paid to

this issue prior to the administration of certain regional peripheral or neuraxial techniques.

Pulmonary Function

Respiratory compromise and complications among the elderly in the perioperative period can often be explained by functional and structural changes within the pulmonary system. Such alterations are commonly associated with aging as well as physiologic changes in response to hypoxemia and hypercarbia and increased sensitivity to the respiratory depressant effects of anesthetic agents and opioids. With aging, the elastic recoil of the lung parenchyma decreases in a fashion that functionally resembles emphysema, with less efficient alveolar gas exchange due to a loss of alveolar surface area and collapse of small airways. In addition, compliance of the chest wall decreases, which can lead to an increased work of breathing and increased risk for respiratory failure in the postoperative period for older patients.[34] In all patients, there are reductions in functional residual capacity (FRC) created by assuming the supine position, being under the influence of general anesthesia, and experiencing surgery. These negative effects on FRC may persist for 7 to 10 days following surgery.[35] FRC and closing volume gradually increase with age, and by age 45, closing volume exceeds FRC in the supine position.[33] Vital capacity can be reduced by 25% to 50% from inadequate postoperative pain management (ie, splinting), along with the administration of systemic opioid analgesics that also contribute to alterations in tidal volume and respiratory rate and that can impair clearing of secretions (via altered cough mechanics). Elderly also have decreased responsivity to hypoxia and hypercapnia, as well as a greater incidence of COPD and obstructive sleep apnea (OSA).[35] All of the above factors make opioid-sparing approaches to postoperative pain control desirable. However, while regional techniques may be beneficial in providing superior postoperative pain control with opioid-sparing effects, these modalities should be selected carefully given that patients with underlying pulmonary disease may poorly tolerate phrenic nerve dysfunction that can be associated with upper (interscalene and supraclavicular) brachial plexus blockade approaches.[36] Therefore, patients should be assessed frequently for evidence of any adverse side effects, respiratory dysfunction, and adequate pain control throughout the perioperative period regardless of chosen analgesic methods.

Airway manipulation can be avoided, and respiratory parameters of lung function, respiration rate, tidal volume, respiratory drive (effort), and end-tidal carbon dioxide concentration can be preserved if surgical anesthesia can be achieved with regional modalities. Careful attention to the type of sedation used as an adjunct during these regional block placement procedures should be considered given the potential for increased sensitivity to opioids and benzodiazepines in the elderly, as well as the decreased responses to hypoxemia and hypercapnia and the increased incidence of OSA in this population. Unchanged FRC from baseline has been observed during spinal and lumbar epidural anesthesia. However, intercostal blocks and cervical, thoracic paravertebral, and high thoracic epidural blockade can be associated with lung volume reductions secondary to intercostal muscle relaxation. Therefore, choice of anesthesia may affect the degree of pulmonary dysfunction. Studies comparing regional versus general anesthesia/analgesia in elderly patients undergoing lower extremity orthopedic and major abdominal surgical procedures have shown that (1) older patients experience fewer hypoxic events with epidural and regional anesthesia (using local alone) compared to systemic opioids; (2) general anesthesia in older patients results in lower PaO_2 levels (on postoperative day 1) compared to epidural and regional anesthesia; and (3) respiratory complications are less frequent when comparing general anesthesia with postoperative intravenous morphine analgesia versus general anesthesia with postoperative epidural analgesia.[37-39] However, the elderly have increased sensitivity to the respiratory depressant effects of neuraxial opiates, and therefore these should be used with caution.[40]

Pharmacokinetic and Pharmacodynamic Changes in the Elderly

Aging affects the pharmacokinetics and pharmacodynamics of medications (eg, sedative/hypnotics, opiates, nonopioid analgesics, local anesthetics), the physiologic functions of the body, and the composition/characteristics of organs and tissues within the body to variable degrees. The physiologic changes

and effects on pharmacokinetics and pharmacodynamics in older patients, as well as some alterations that may be required for drug regimens in older patients, are listed in Tables 46–1, 46–2, and 46–3. Information in these tables addresses a number of issues related to local anesthetics and opioid analgesics in view of their widespread use and importance in perioperative pain management for older patients. The altered response to drugs associated with aging can be highly variable and somewhat unpredictable among individuals and are generally attributable to aging alone, but such responses may be compounded by a higher incidence of degenerative and other coexisting diseases in this patient population.[41]

Multimodal Drug Therapy and the Elderly

A perioperative plan of care that includes a regional technique in an elderly patient must consider the inherent risk of sedation/hypnosis, multimodal drug regimens, and local anesthetic medications. Safety principles of treatment with analgesic and sedative medications for pain management in older patients, specific to regional and regional peripheral nerve blockade, are discussed and listed in Tables 46–1, 46–2, and 46–3. Sedative drugs (eg, midazolam, propofol) used during block placement should be easy to administer, short-acting, have a high safety margin, and limited adverse effects. Epinephrine can prolong peripheral nerve blockade duration, but caution must be exercised as epinephrine may cause an ischemic neurotoxicity in peripheral nerves with preexisting neuropathy (eg, in patients with diabetes).[42,43]

There are several pharmacodynamic changes associated with aging.[44] Understanding of how medications may affect older patients can be complex and unpredictable. Studies that have examined opioid pain management have been somewhat arbitrary, and surrogate measurements of effect other than clinical pain relief have not been adequately studied. An animal study by Piva et al, identified fewer mu-opioid receptors in the hypothalami of older rats, and, in contrast, greater concentrations of kappa-opioid receptors in the thalamus and amygdala of these animals.[45] They also found that concentrations of delta-opioid receptors were not significantly different in young versus old rats. Scott et al. conducted a study of the pharmacokinetics and pharmacodynamics of fentanyl and alfentanil in older men by examining blood samples with a radioimmunoassay and found that the pharmacokinetics of these drugs were unaffected by age.[46] However, the sensitivity of the brain to these opioids as measured by electroencephalogram (EEG) proved to be increased by 50% in these older subjects. Whether this finding can be attributed to a change in the number or function of opioid receptors in the CNS that is associated with aging or due to an increased penetration of opioids in the CNS remains unclear.

There is no literature to support the need to alter ketamine doses in older patients. However, in aged animals, changes in composition of the N-methyl-D-aspartate (NMDA) receptor site and function have been reported.[44,47,48] If one can extrapolate from these earlier animal studies, older patients may be more sensitive to the effects of ketamine, and doses may need to be decreased in this patient population. Clearance of tricyclic antidepressant (TCA) drugs and their active metabolites by

TABLE 46–3. Physiologic hepatic and renal changes associated with aging and effects on pharmacokinetic variables.

Physiological Process	Magnitude	Variable Kinetic/Dynamic Consequences	General Dosing Strategy
Liver			
Liver size	↓ 25–40%	↓ hepatic clearance of high-extraction drugs Equivocal hepatic clearance of low-extraction drugs ↓ hepatic clearance of some low-extraction drugs	Minimal effect on drug IV bolus dose ↓ maintenance dose Potential for changes in oral bioavailability
Hepatic blood flow	↓ 25–40%		
Phase I (eg, oxidation)	↓ 25%		
Phase II	Little change		
Kidney			
Nephron mass	↓ 30%	↓ clearance of drugs Little effect on opioids (parent compound) ↓ clearance of some active metabolites (eg, M6G)	↓ maintenance dose (renally cleared drugs for renal clearance) Assume and monitor for accelerated accumulation of polar active (M6G) or toxic (M3G, norpethidine) metabolites
Renal blood flow	↓ 10% per 10 years		
Plasma flow at 80 years	↓ 50%		
Glomerular filtration rate	↓ 30–50%		
Creatinine clearance	↓ 50–70%		

The net effect of these changes in drug disposition may be minimal; M6G: morphine-6-glucuronide; M3G: morphine-3-glucuronide.

hepatic cytochrome P450 and the kidney, respectively, decreases with increasing patient age, and lower initial doses are recommended in older patients.[49,50] In addition, elderly patients may be particularly prone to the side effects of TCAs, including sedation, confusion, orthostatic hypotension, dry mouth, constipation, urinary retention, and gait disturbances (eg, increased risk of falls).[50] As with TCAs, initial doses of anticonvulsant agents used for pain management (pregabalin, gabapentin, and topiramate) should be lower than for younger patients, and increases in dose should be titrated carefully.[49] Adverse side effects such as somnolence and dizziness, especially with pregabalin, may be a problem in this group of patients.[51,52] As renal function declines with increasing age, elimination of gabapentin and pregabalin may be reduced, and lower doses may be required.[53]

Age-related changes in the body are responsible for alterations seen with systemic absorption, distribution, and clearance of local anesthetics that may result in an increased sensitivity, decreased dose requirement, and change in the onset and duration of action in elderly patients. For example, decreases in neural cell population, nerve conduction velocity, and inter-Schwann cell distance can produce an increased sensitivity to local anesthetics in the elderly. Advancing age also results in a decrease in the clearance of bupivacaine[54-56] and ropivacaine.[57] Older patients are more sensitive to the effects of local anesthetic agents secondary to a slowing of the conduction velocity (in the spinal cord and peripheral nerves) and a decrease in the number of neurons in the spinal cord.[58]

Clinical Pearls

- The administration of nonsteroidal anti-inflammatory drugs (NSAIDs) and cyclooxygenase-2 (COX-2) inhibitors in elderly patients requires caution; acetaminophen may be the preferred nonopioid analgesic.
- The age-related decrease in opioid requirements in the elderly patient is related to the changes in pharmacodynamics that accompany aging.

Physiology and the Perception of Pain in the Elderly and Clinical Implications

Several review articles have summarized the many age-related changes that occur in pain perception and the neurophysiology of nociception in elderly surgical patients.[59-61] There are extensive alterations in the structure, neurochemistry, and function of both the PNS and CNS of older patients. Included among these changes is the neurochemical deterioration of opioid and serotonergic systems. Therefore, there may be changes in nociceptive processing, including impairment of the pain inhibitory system, and pain intensity after surgery may be greater or less than otherwise expected from the severity of surgical trauma induced. In one study, older patients matched for surgical procedure reported less pain in the postoperative period, and pain intensity decreased by 10% to 20% for each decade after 60 years of age.[62]

The structural and neurochemical changes that have been described in the PNS and CNS of the elderly continue to compromise optimal pain medicine protocols for these patients. Studies of the elderly nervous systems show a decrease in the density of myelinated and, particularly, unmyelinated peripheral nerve fibers.[63] In addition, there is an increase in the number of nerve tissue fibers with evidence of degeneration and a slowing of nerve conduction velocity in older individuals.[64] Gagliese et al reviewed animal and human experimental evidence on the neurobiology of aging and reported the following findings: (1) reductions in level of the neuropeptide substance P; (2) lowered concentrations of calcitonin gene-related peptide (a vasodilator neuropeptide expressed in a subgroup of small neurons in the dorsal root); and (3) reduced somatostatin levels within the circulatory system.[65,66] Sensory neuron degenerative changes, loss of myelin in the dorsal horn of the spinal cord, and reductions in neurochemical mediators (substance P, somatostatin, and calcitonin gene-related peptide) have been noted.[67,68] Once again, the clinical implications of these degenerative changes in many older individuals translate into pain being expressed as less severe along with evidence of increased pain thresholds in older patients.[61,69]

A decrease in pain tolerance sometimes seen in elderly patients could also be secondary to decreases in noradrenergic and serotonergic neurons that contribute to the impairment of descending inhibitory mechanisms.[70,71] Age-related loss of neurons and dendritic connections, along with changes in neurotransmitter synthesis, axonal transport, and receptor binding seen in the human brain are particularly evident in the cerebral cortex, including areas of the brain involved in nociceptive processing.[11,72] The density of opioid receptors in the brain is decreased (although not evident in the spinal cord), and there may also be decreases in concentrations of circulating endogenous opioids.[11] Therefore, compared to younger patients having the same type of surgery performed, older patients may report less pain or atypical pain, complain of pain at a later time during recovery, or report no pain from a surgical insult that generally produces at least mild-to-moderate pain scores in younger patients.[73]

Clinical Pearl

- There is an age-related decrease in opioid requirements and significant interpatient variability in pain tolerance in elderly surgical patients.

Functional MRI (fMRI) studies performed on older individuals show more similarities than differences in the magnitude of activation in the brain response to acute noxious stimulation.[74] However, the functional consequences of age-related changes in the brain still remain a subject of debate. For example, studies investigating the effects of experimental pain stimuli (short periods of noxious stimuli not resulting in tissue injury) on pain thresholds are conflicting and appear to depend on the type of stimulus used.[75,76] In addition, elderly individuals tend to have higher pain thresholds for thermal stimuli, but results from mechanical stimulation appear equivocal, and there is evidence that no change is seen in response to electrical stimuli across all age groups.[61] However, in the clinical setting (where pain is often associated with tissue injury), these observations may explain the deficits seen in the early warning function of pain in older patients. For example, in elderly patients experiencing an acute myocardial infarction, a greater intensity of symptoms of chest discomfort and pain was inversely correlated with a lower pain threshold.[77] There also appears to be a gap between identification of pain stimulus and recognition of the stimulus as being capable of causing tissue injury.[69] Therefore, differences in the perception and reporting of pain by older surgical patients may result in pain therapy, medications, and regional analgesic interventions being delayed or deemed unnecessary.

A review of studies on age-related changes in pain tolerance (involving a variety of experimental pain stimuli) has shown a reduced ability of older individuals to endure or tolerate strong painful stimuli.[61] This may have deleterious effects in the more vulnerable elderly patient and could mean that severe pain may have a greater negative impact if not effectively treated. In addition, elderly individuals show smaller increases in pain thresholds following prolonged noxious stimulation and evidence of prolonged recovery from hyperalgesia.[69,78]

Clinical Pearl

- The assessment of pain and evaluation of pain management therapies in older patients present problems arising from differences in (1) reporting mechanisms; (2) cognitive dysfunction; (3) end-organ impairment/compromise (affecting medication metabolism and excretion); (4) variations in medication tolerance and abuse; and (5) inherent difficulties in the assessment of pain.

Assessment of Pain in Older Cognitively Impaired Patients

Inadequate treatment of acute pain is more likely to occur in older patients, especially those that are cognitively impaired.[79-82] Even though cognitively impaired patients are just as likely as others of the same age and younger to experience painful conditions, the number of pain complaints, along with reported pain intensity, has been shown to be inversely related to the degree of cognitive impairment (due to diminished memory, impairment of capacity to report, or because less pain is experienced).[83,84] However, studies in patients with dementia suggest that pain perception and processing are not diminished, and it would be false to assume that these patients experience less pain with surgery.[85-87] Therefore, careful consideration must be given to the ways in which pain is assessed in older cognitively impaired individuals. While cognitively intact elderly patients can use a range of unidimensional pain scales (visual analog scale [VAS], verbal rating scale [VRS], numeric rating scale [NRS], or facial pain scale [FPS]), in patients with mild to moderate or severe cognitive impairment, a VRS or behavioral scale (eg, Doloplus-2 or Algoplus) may prove to be better pain assessment tools.[88,89]

Clinical Pearls

- Elderly patients often describe pain as being less intense and often provide atypical descriptions of perioperative pain.
- The reported frequency and description of intensity of acute pain in clinical situations may often be reduced in older patients.
- Unidimensional measurements of pain can be used in older patients in the acute pain setting; in the clinical setting, VRS and NRS measurements provide the best validity in older adults.
- The undertreatment of acute pain is more likely to occur in cognitively impaired older patients than in those who are cognitively intact.
- Obtaining a history regarding past experiences with pain can be challenging in patients with cognitive impairment; the observations of caregivers may be helpful in these situations.

Considerations for the Use of Peripheral Regional and Neural Blockade in Elderly Patients

There are limited evidence-based guidelines regarding the use of specific regional analgesic modalities in older patients due to a host of secondary concerns, such as patient age, comorbidities, safety profile issues, and concurrent medications, which often exclude elderly individuals from clinical trials. However, many of these factors, along with several other concerns related to advanced age, need to be taken into consideration when choosing a procedure-specific analgesic regimen that may prove more advantageous than other more conventional pain management options, such as unimodal opioid analgesics. Decisions regarding regional options and peripheral nerve blockade choice should take into account the health status of the older patient, the operation being performed, and the expertise of the perioperative pain management healthcare providers. Therefore, to ensure safe use and conduct evidence-based research on regional and peripheral nerve blockade techniques in the elderly, needs should be assessed on a patient-to-type-of-surgery basis and geared toward regional pain medicine options that target the surgical site.

The number of elderly patients that present for anesthesia and surgery has increased exponentially in recent years, and neuraxial and peripheral nerve blockade techniques are frequently used in this patient population. Elderly patients can benefit from regional modalities of perioperative pain management. One important clinical observation that has emerged from the literature on regional anesthesia/analgesia is evidence that the use of regional techniques allows for the minimization or elimination of the negative side effect profiles of other systemic pain management options, such as bowel and bladder dysfunction, hemodynamic derangements, and cognitive effects often experienced with opiates and other analgesic adjuncts and sedative/hypnotics, to which older patients are often more sensitive.

A multitude of factors can influence surgical outcomes in older patients, such as the type, duration, and invasiveness of an operation, coexisting medical or mental status dysfunction, and the skill and expertise of both the anesthesiologist and surgeon.[41,90] These factors and others often make it difficult to decide if and when one regional analgesic technique is unequivocally better than another. Therefore, until evidence-based research can provide conclusive guidelines on regional anesthesia/analgesia in the elderly, it is important to focus on optimizing the overall perioperative pain management choices for elderly patients by implementing patient- and procedure-specific modes of regional anesthesia.

Anatomic changes associated with aging may make performing neuraxial and regional peripheral nerve anesthesia/analgesia more technically difficult in the geriatric population. Elderly individuals may have dorsal kyphosis, a tendency to flex their hips and knees because of osteoarthritic changes, decreased range of motion in the extremities, issues associated with advanced osteoporosis and rheumatoid arthritis, and calcification of cartilage. All of these issues may make positioning elderly patients for regional block placement more challenging. Neuraxial techniques may be complicated not only by difficulty with positioning patients, but also by degenerative disk and vertebral joint changes, along with the distortion and compression of intervertebral and epidural spaces associated with aging. The ligamentum flavum often becomes more calcified with age, such that attempts to accomplish an epidural block or dural puncture may be more challenging due to difficult needle placement and advancement through such dense, calcified ligaments. The presence of osteophytes may also decrease the size of the intervertebral space, which limits access to the subarachnoid space. A lateral (paramedian) needle approach to the epidural or subarachnoid space may avoid issues caused by vertebral midline ligament calcification and distortion of dorsal vertebrae. In addition, access to the epidural or subarachnoid space in patients with severe osteoarthritis and ossified ligaments may be more easily achieved by approaching the L5–S1 interspace, which is typically the largest intervertebral space.

Clinical Pearl

- A paramedian approach may facilitate needle placement to the epidural or subarachnoid space in patients with age-related changes to the vertebral anatomy.

Epidural Anesthesia and Analgesia

Epidural anesthesia/analgesia can provide an effective modality for pain management in a host of perioperative settings. The heterogeneity of studies regarding the use of epidural anesthesia/analgesia makes it difficult to draw conclusive evidence for optimal use in elderly patients. However, the consistent efficacy of epidural analgesia in the elderly has been well demonstrated, regardless of analgesic agent, location of catheter (if used), type of surgery, and type or time of pain assessment, and has been shown to provide superior pain relief compared to parenteral opioid administration.[37,91-94]

A host of additional outcome studies have noted reductions in morbidity with regional techniques provided to elderly patients undergoing certain surgical procedures. For example, following hip fracture surgery, a continuous epidural infusion (local anesthetic and opioid) provided better pain relief, both at rest and with movement, but did not lead to improved rehabilitation.[95] A meta-analysis reviewed studies that included a wide variety of epidural regimens and surgical procedures and examined the benefits of combining epidural analgesia with general anesthesia.[91] The author reported a reduction in a range of adverse outcomes with epidural analgesia, including a reduced incidence of arrhythmias, earlier extubation times, a reduced need for and time spent in the ICU, reduced stress hormone levels, lower cortisol and glucose concentrations, and a reduced incidence of renal failure, when local anesthetics were used in thoracic epidurals. Another meta-analysis compared systemic opioids delivered via PCA versus epidural analgesia (both patient-controlled epidural analgesia [PCEA] and continuous infusion) and concluded that epidural analgesia provided superior pain relief at rest and with movement and was superior in terms of overall pain management. Further, a lower incidence of nausea and vomiting and sedation following all types of surgery was found with epidural analgesia. However, this meta-analysis also revealed that epidural analgesia was associated with a higher incidence of pruritus and motor blockade.[96] Other studies have also supported the finding that older patients treated with neuraxial versus general anesthesia had lower pain scores at rest and with movement, higher satisfaction scores, improved mental status, more rapid recovery of bowel function, and a decreased risk of deep vein thrombosis and pulmonary embolism.[94,97,98]

Epidural opioid requirements can be decreased as patient age increases.[99-101] Some studies have revealed that older patients require a lower dose of opioid than younger patients to achieve the same degree of pain relief.[102-105] However, a large degree of interpatient variability remains, and doses should be titrated cautiously and to effect in all elderly patients. The decreased need for epidural opioids in elderly patients appears greater than would be predicted by age-related alterations in physiology alone and may also have pharmacodynamic components.[101] A comparison of fentanyl PCEA in patients over 65 years of age versus patients 20–64 years of age showed no difference in fentanyl PCEA requirements, pain scores at rest, or incidence of pruritus. However, dynamic pain (coughing) experienced from the abdominal surgery being performed was significantly better controlled in patients over age 65.[106]

Decreased glomerular filtration rate (GFR) in older patients can result in a more rapid accumulation of active opioid metabolites (eg, M6G, M3G, hydromorphone-3-glucuronide, nordextropropoxyphene, norpethidine, desmethyl-tramadol) following continuous epidural administration. In addition, concerns for respiratory depression in elderly patients, particularly those with obesity, OSA, or other respiratory disease, can sometimes lead to inadequate neuraxial opioid doses being administered. However, respiratory depression is rare if appropriate concentration guidelines are followed and appropriate monitoring is implemented. In addition, the incidence of nausea and vomiting and pruritus in the postoperative period seems to lessen with increasing age.[100,107] Some additional evidence shows that neuraxial fentanyl may cause less POCD than morphine,[94,108] along with less potential for confusion.[109] While the elderly may be more sensitive to the effects of opiates and require lower doses for analgesia, adequate postoperative pain control is also important to prevent delirium and maintain preoperative levels of cognitive function.[81,110,111]

Age is a factor when determining spread of injected local anesthetic into the neuraxial space and the subsequent sensory level and degree of motor blockade achieved.[57,112,113] Thus, the systemic absorption and disposition of long-acting local anesthetics dictate that smaller volumes are needed to cover the same number of dermatomes than in younger patients. The same bolus volume of epidural local anesthetic administered to all patients revealed that the concentration required to achieve an effective motor blockade decreased as patient age increased.[114] Therefore, older patients may be more susceptible to some of the adverse effects of epidural analgesia, including hypotension, if patient age and local anesthetic concentration/volume are not taken into consideration.[112,115,116] In addition, combinations of local anesthetic and opioid are commonly used for epidural analgesia and may provide an additive/synergistic effect, so it is reasonable to use lower infusion rates in older patients.[101]

Clinical Pearl

- The L5–S1 vertebral interspace is typically the largest intervertebral location to target for neuraxial techniques.

Intrathecal Opioid Analgesia

Subarachnoid administration of opioids (at varying doses) combined with local anesthetics during neuraxial techniques can provide effective anesthesia and perioperative analgesia, can create a synergistic effect with the local anesthetic, may prolong analgesic effects without associated motor blockade, and often provides for more effective targeted pain relief than with other routes (eg, intramuscular, PCA) of opioid administration. In addition, when used in combination with general anesthesia for major surgery, a spinal injection of opioid and local anesthetic can reduce the intraoperative requirement for inhalational anesthetic agents. However, caution must be exercised as the additional systemic administration (intravenous bolus or PCA) of opioid medications can create a risk of respiratory depression and pruritus.[40] Therefore, secondary to advanced patient age, the potential for respiratory depression effects can be considered a serious enough risk factor to warrant consideration of postoperative admission and recovery in a monitored environment or ICU setting for patients over the age of 70 years.[117] However, it has been reported that the subarachnoid administration of up to 200 mcg of intrathecal morphine with a local anesthetic for peripheral vascular surgery in older patients (average age 69 years) can be safely performed with minimal adverse respiratory sequelea.[118] In addition, it has also been shown that respiratory depression can be minimized through the implementation of respiratory safety protocols, education of nursing and other healthcare providers on general wards, and postoperative management by an acute pain medicine service following strict respiratory parameter guidelines.[118]

Intrathecal morphine provides excellent postoperative analgesia but may cause side effects such as postoperative nausea and vomiting, pruritus, and respiratory depression, particularly at larger doses; older patients may be at an increased risk of such side effects. The ideal or optimal dose of intrathecal opioid that should be mixed with local anesthetic during spinal anesthesia procedures for elderly patients is currently unknown. Despite a lack of evidence-based data, a subarachnoid morphine dose of 200 mcg has been suggested. Intrathecal morphine (200 mcg mixed with a local anesthetic) administration during spinal anesthesia in addition to general anesthesia in older patients (average age 70 years) undergoing abdominal aortic surgery resulted in improved postoperative analgesia along with a reduced need for postoperative analgesics when compared to elderly patients given general anesthesia alone.[119] In a dose-response study by Murphy et al, three different doses of intrathecal morphine for elective hip arthroplasty surgery in elderly patients (patients aged > 65 years) were studied. Patients received either 50, 100, or 200 mcg of subarachnoid morphine, along with 15 mg of bupivacaine hydrochloride. The investigators concluded that 100 mcg of morphine added to the spinal anesthetic during hip surgery provided the most optimal balance between analgesia, pain relief, and pruritus. In addition, they observed that there was no difference in the incidence of nausea and vomiting or respiratory depression among the three groups of patients.[120]

Evidence has shown that the strategic use of a low-dose opioid as an adjunct to local anesthetics during spinal anesthesia can reduce the concentration of inhalation agents required during general anesthesia. In addition, intrathecal morphine is a widely used method for postoperative pain relief after major abdominal and lower extremity orthopedic surgery. In many cases, it provides more effective perioperative analgesia with fewer side effects than intravenous opioid analgesics.[121-123] In a randomized study of patients over age 70 who underwent colorectal surgery, Beaussier et al. compared preoperative intrathecal morphine (300 mcg) in addition to postoperative PCA with morphine (study group) with PCA morphine alone (control group). The investigation concluded that intrathecal morphine plus intravenous PCA, as compared with intravenous PCA morphine alone, improves immediate postoperative pain intensity and significantly reduces daily parenteral morphine consumption following surgery.[124]

Clinical Pearl

- Intrathecal morphine at a dose below 200 mcg can be a useful adjunct for pain management following surgery with acceptable risk of respiratory depression.

Regional Anesthesia and Analgesia Using Peripheral Nerve and Nerve Plexus Blockade

One approach to perioperative pain management in geriatric patients is to consider the postoperative complications commonly associated with routine surgical procedures and then evaluate how one might mitigate these complications using peripheral nerve and nerve plexus blockade. Elderly patients are more likely to have underlying neurologic, pulmonary, and cardiovascular disease, all of which can lead to serious complications in any surgical setting. While there are established clinical practices and theoretical indications regarding the use of safe and effective regional techniques for elderly patients, a lack of consistency among studies has prevented the development of firm recommendations to guide which regional anesthetics and analgesia techniques offer the greatest advantages for elderly patients undergoing particular surgical procedures.

Peripheral nerve blockade can be a supplemental analgesic technique for medical interventions and satisfactory analgesia for a host of surgical procedures on the upper and lower extremities, abdomen, groin, and chest wall. Definitions and descriptions of regional peripheral nerve block techniques are variable, as are the definitions of the various techniques of analgesia and anesthesia (Table 46–4). Clinical investigations often use neuraxial anesthesia (with or without analgesia) in the definition of regional anesthesia. However, other studies include only peripheral nerve and nerve plexus blockade, local anesthetic infiltration, and local anesthetic injection in the definition of regional anesthesia. When strategically applied (ie, procedure- and patient-specific) and with effective results, regional peripheral nerve and nerve plexus block techniques may offer distinct advantages in the care of older surgical and medical patients. In particular, regional peripheral nerve and nerve plexus block techniques may allow for a reduction in the incidence of adverse side effects compared to other conventional pain management therapies (intramuscular, oral, and parenteral analgesics and central neuraxial blockade).[125]

Some clinicians feel that epidural analgesia remains the standard of care for pain relief for a host of surgical procedures in the elderly, but peripheral nerve and nerve plexus blockade have proven to be as effective and are gaining popularity since the incidence of potential side effects associated with neuraxial techniques may be less. Systematic reviews and meta-analyses of randomized trials comparing epidural analgesia with peripheral nerve blockade for major knee surgery have shown similar relative analgesic efficacy between both pain management strategies (neuraxial versus peripheral nerve block).[126,127] And, although pain profiles from peripheral nerve blockade techniques compared favorably with lumbar epidural analgesia for major knee surgery with no significant difference in pain scores at rest,

TABLE 46–4. Analgesia and anesthesia techniques.

Local Monitored Anesthesia Care (LMAC) (LMAC)	LMAC with or without Intravenous and Oral Sedatives, Hypnotics, Analgesics (Opioid and Nonopioid)
General Anesthesia and analgesia Anesthesia Analgesia	With or without perioperative medications Inhalation agents, intravenous agents, and/or total intravenous anesthesia (TIVA) Systemically administered analgesia with opioids, nonopioids, and other adjuncts • Intramuscular injections • Intravenous boluses • Patient-controlled analgesia (PCA) • Transdermal, mucous membrane, and oral routes
Regional Anesthesia and Analgesia Neuraxial Peripheral nerve/nerve plexus blockade Infiltration/field block	With or without other intravenous perioperative medications (analgesics, sedation) Spinal (subarachnoid) and/or epidural anesthesia and/or analgesia • Single injection, with or without catheters • Local anesthetic (type, concentration) with or without opioids and other adjuncts • Vertebral level of block placement/initiation • Level of blockade achieved • Length or duration of postoperative anesthesia and analgesia Peripheral nerve block • Local anesthetic with or without additives • Single injection or continuous catheter technique Brachial plexus blockade • Femoral block • Sciatic/popliteal blockade • Paravertebral block • Transverse abdominis plane block, etc. Local anesthetic infiltration/injection (diffusion blockade) • With or without indwelling catheters

complications such as hemodynamic variability, nausea and vomiting, urinary retention and bowel dysfunction, increased dynamic (ie, movement, rehabilitation) pain scores and an increased need for supplemental opioid analgesics for breakthrough pain occurred more frequently in the epidural group. Rehabilitation indices were similar between groups, but patient satisfaction was higher in the groups that received peripheral nerve blocks, and these modalities are not likely to cause neuraxial complications.

In an investigation by Zaric et al, epidural analgesia was compared to combined femoral and sciatic peripheral nerve blockade following total knee replacement surgery.[125] Primary outcome measures included the incidence of side effects, including urinary retention, moderate to severe degrees of dizziness, pruritus, sedation, and nausea and vomiting during the postoperative period. Intensity of motor blockade, pain at rest and on mobilization, and rehabilitation indices were also registered for three days after surgery. Side effects in the epidural group were present in 87% of patients (one or more side effects), whereas only 35% of patients in the femoral and sciatic block group were affected. In addition, motor blockade was more intense (operated and nonoperated limb) on the day of surgery and the first postoperative day in the epidural group. Pain on mobilization was well controlled in both groups, rehabilitation indices were similar, and there were no differences in

the length of hospital stay between groups. The results demonstrate a reduced incidence of side effects in the femoral and sciatic nerve block group compared to the epidural group.

Similarly, epidural analgesia is considered to be a superior method of pain relief after major thoracic surgery. However, placement of a paravertebral blockade (PVB) using a PVB catheter can offer comparable analgesic effectiveness and a better side effect profile than neuraxial options with an epidural catheter.[128-130] In addition to there being no significant difference between each group in terms of pain relief, these systematic reviews and meta-analyses of relevant randomized trials comparing PVB with epidural analgesia for thoracic surgery revealed that hemodynamic variability, urinary retention, increased plasma cortisol concentrations (as a marker of postoperative stress), nausea, pruritus, respiratory depression (atelectasis, pneumonia), prolonged operative time, reports of incomplete (or failed) epidural, and paraplegia (in rare cases) were reported far more frequently in the epidural groups when compared to those in the paravertebral groups. The most common and often serious compromising side effect profiles of respiratory complications, nausea and vomiting, and hypotension were less common with PVBs, as were a lower rate of failed blocks and a reduced incidence of urinary retention.

Elderly patients may also benefit when they receive procedure-specific regional techniques for postoperative pain management as doses of intravenous opioid drugs may be reduced. In addition, optimal target-specific perioperative analgesic management and the potential to reduce negative cognitive effects[131] is possible by incorporating regional anesthesia procedure-specific pain therapy.[132] POCD can be a common complication after cardiac and major noncardiac surgery with general anesthesia in the elderly, and it has been hypothesized that POCD may occur less often with regional anesthesia.[133,134] The incidence of cognitive dysfunction after general or regional anesthesia in elderly patients raises the questions of whether a causative relationship exists between certain types of anesthesia and long-term POCD and whether regional anesthesia may decrease mortality and the incidence of POCD early after surgery.[135] In another study of older hip fracture patients, those who received a femoral nerve block for perioperative analgesia, in addition to regularly scheduled nonopioid analgesics, were less likely to develop postoperative delirium, were able to sit up at the bedside sooner, and required no supplemental opioid analgesics compared to patients administered only nonopioid analgesics (28% of whom required supplemental morphine analgesia).[136]

Proper patient selection and surgery-specific peripheral nerve and nerve plexus blockade when effectively administered (timed correctly and matched with appropriate type of surgical intervention) can provide excellent perioperative pain management in all patient populations.[137] However, there is some evidence to suggest that the effects of peripheral nerve blockade can be prolonged in some elderly patients, thereby reducing or eliminating the need for opioid medications for breakthrough pain following hospital discharge.[135] In addition, when considering prolonged duration of peripheral nerve blockade effects, elderly patients should be counseled appropriately regarding such effects prior to block placement, and care should be taken to ensure that older patients have appropriate assistance in their home if peripheral nerve blocks are to be placed for outpatient surgery.[138] With these safeguards in place, efficacious administration of regional analgesic modalities can result in a reduction or elimination of opioid analgesics for breakthrough pain in the postoperative period. For example, two studies showed a prolonged duration of effective analgesia in older patients following (1) a sciatic nerve block for lower extremity surgery;[139] and (2) brachial plexus blockade for upper extremity surgery.[140]

As mentioned previously, there are factors affecting the spread of both local anesthetics and adjuncts when placed into the epidural space. Therefore, could a paravertebral approach provide effective anesthesia or analgesia without unwanted spread of local anesthetics when placed in the neuraxial space of older patients? In a study by Akin et al, patients older than 65 years of age who underwent urological surgery following administration of a paravertebral lumbar plexus blockade (using ropivacaine or bupivacaine) showed improved pain scores, reduced incidence of cognitive dysfunction, and a stable heart rate and blood pressure.[141] Cheema et al. investigated patients undergoing paravertebral nerve block procedures for the treatment of chronic pain conditions. Findings from this study revealed that, unlike the variable spread of local anesthetics administered for epidural analgesia, the age of the patient did

not influence the spread of bupivacaine when placed in the thoracic paravertebral space.[142]

An additional important factor to consider in all patients is the contraindication to regional anesthesia in anesthetized patients. Unlike neuraxial anesthesia, it may be safe to perform paravertebral blocks in heavily sedated or anesthetized patients without any apparent increased risk of neurological injury.[143] Therefore, in elderly patients who experience pain or discomfort during positioning for neuraxial or paravertebral blockade techniques, paravertebral blocks may be placed under heavy sedation or general anesthesia without concern for significant compromise of neurologic injury. Studies have also addressed whether a paravertebral block is as effective as epidural analgesia for pain management in elderly patients undergoing thoracic surgery. In a review of the literature (184 papers found with seven representing the best evidence), all studies agreed that a paravertebral block was at least as effective as epidural analgesia for post-thoracotomy pain control but with a more favorable side effect profile and lower complication rates.[125] Pain assessed via VAS at rest and with coughing was significantly lower in the paravertebral groups compared to the epidural groups ($P = 0.02$ and $P = 0.0001$, respectively). Pulmonary function assessed by peak expiratory flow rate (PEFR) was better preserved in the paravertebral groups; the lowest PEFR as a fraction of preoperative control was 0.73 in the paravertebral groups in contrast with 0.54 in the epidural groups ($P < 0.004$), and oxygen saturation was better in the paravertebral groups of patients compared to the epidural groups ($P = 0.0001$). Plasma concentrations of cortisol (marker of postoperative stress) increased markedly in both groups, but the increments were statistically different and more favorable in the paravertebral groups of patients ($P = 0.003$). Patients in the epidural block groups were associated with more frequent side effects such as (1) urinary retention (42%); (2) nausea (22%); (3) itching (22%); and (4) hypotension (3%). The epidural block groups experienced prolonged operative times and were associated with more technical failures and epidural displacement (8%) compared to the paravertebral groups. In addition, the epidural groups also experienced a higher complication of atelectasis and pneumonia compared to the paravertebral block groups, and the paravertebral block groups were found to experience a quicker return to normal pulmonary function.[130]

The incidence of cancer and cancer surgery is significantly greater in the elderly patient population.[144] Some evidence from animal and retrospective human studies has emerged indicating that regional analgesia may attenuate the immunosuppressive effects of surgery, anesthesia, and perioperative pain and may therefore improve patient outcomes.[145,146] Metastatic disease remains an important cause of cancer-related death, and the likelihood of tumor metastases depends on the balance between antimetastatic host defenses (eg, cell-mediated immunity, natural killer cell function) and the metastatic potential of any given tumor. Snyder et al suspected anesthetic technique along with other perioperative factors could have the potential to affect the long-term outcome after cancer surgery since surgery can inhibit important host defenses, thus increasing the likelihood of the development of metastases. The investigators questioned whether anesthetic technique and medication choices (eg, intravenous anesthetics, volatile agents) could interact with the cellular immune system and affect long-term outcome. The investigators had a particular interest in whether there was any beneficial effect from regional anesthesia and whether regional anesthesia may play a role in pain and stress reduction, along with other potentially important perioperative risk factors that might impact cancer recurrence.[146] In addition, opioid analgesia is suspected to induce some degree of suppression of cell-mediated immunity (notably natural killer cell activity). Therefore, using opioid-sparing anesthetic and analgesic techniques during the perioperative period could potentially have a positive effect on long-term survival and cancer disease recurrence.[147] Data regarding anesthetic technique and cancer survival or recurrence has been mixed, and further prospective studies are still needed to further elucidate these relationships.

SUMMARY

People over 65 years of age represent a fast-growing segment of society, and these older individuals have surgery more frequently than younger age-group populations. Effective postoperative analgesia remains essential in older patients because inadequate pain control after surgery is often associated with a host of well-documented adverse outcomes. Management of postoperative pain in older patients can be complicated by a number of variables, including a higher risk of age- and disease-related changes in physiology and anatomy, disease–drug and drug–drug interactions, altered cognitive baseline, potential negative effects from acute trauma (surgical or accidental), and lack of evidence-based, procedure-specific regional anesthesia and analgesia techniques for elderly individuals. Therefore, the concept of "diligence, start low, and go slow" should be adopted for any chosen analgesic strategy in the elderly surgical population.

With knowledge, skill, and comprehension of limitations, postoperative analgesic treatment using most medications (acetaminophen, NSAIDs, opioids, local anesthetics), analgesic techniques (intravenous or epidural PCA, intrathecal opioid, peripheral nerve and nerve plexus blockade), and pain management strategies (pre-emptive or multimodal analgesia) can be used effectively for acute perioperative pain management in older patients. The physiologic changes of aging need to be carefully considered because mammalian aging is often individualized and progressive. Proper assessment of pain management in the elderly must take into account chronological age, biological age, individual profiles of pathology, and prescribed medications, along with regard to organ system function and compromise. Methods of assessing pain in older individuals must also be carefully considered, particularly in those with cognitive impairment. Treatment options must be carefully adjusted and tailored to each patient in view of the pharmacokinetic and pharmacodynamic changes that occur in older individuals. In addition, since there is often a higher incidence of comorbidities and a greater use of concurrent medications in elderly versus younger populations, careful selection from among the multitude of analgesic options must be considered. Therefore, consistent and frequent evaluation of treatment

efficacy of any selected regional technique along with monitoring and adjusting for incidence and severity of any adverse events should be thoughtfully and vigilantly controlled in the elderly.

REFERENCES

1. White PF, White LM, Monk T, et al: Perioperative care for the older outpatient undergoing ambulatory surgery. Anesth Analg 2012;114:1190–1215.
2. Konttinen N, Rosenberg PH: Outcome after anaesthesia and emergency surgery in patients over 100 years old. Acta Anaesthesiol Scand 2006; 50:283–289.
3. Kojima Y, Narita M: Postoperative outcome among elderly patients after general anesthesia. Acta Anaesthesiol Scand 2006;50:19–25.
4. Soltow QA, Jones DP, Promislow DE: A network perspective on metabolism and aging. Integr Comparative Biol 2010;50:844–854.
5. Schwab CW, Kauder DR: Trauma in the geriatric patient. Arch Surg 1992;127:701–706.
6. Troncale JA: The aging process. Physiologic changes and pharmacologic implications. Postgrad Med 1996;99:111–114, 120–112.
7. Turnheim K: When drug therapy gets old: pharmacokinetics and pharmacodynamics in the elderly. Exp Gerontol 2003;38:843–853.
8. Morrison JH, Hof PR: Life and death of neurons in the aging brain. Science 1997;278:412–419.
9. Collins KJ, Exton-Smith AN, James MH, Oliver DJ: Functional changes in autonomic nervous responses with ageing. Age and ageing. 1980;9: 17–24.
10. Meier-Ruge W, Ulrich J, Bruhlmann M, Meier E: Age-related white matter atrophy in the human brain. Ann N Y Acad Sci 1992;673:260–269.
11. Salat DH: The declining infrastructure of the aging brain. Brain Connect 2011;1:279–293.
12. Madden DJ, Bennett IJ, Song AW: Cerebral white matter integrity and cognitive aging: contributions from diffusion tensor imaging. Neuropsychol Rev 2009;19:415–435.
13. Bekker AY, Weeks EJ: Cognitive function after anaesthesia in the elderly. Best Pract Res Clin Anaesthesiol 2003;17:259–272.
14. Bitsch MS, Foss NB, Kristensen BB, Kehlet H: Acute cognitive dysfunction after hip fracture: frequency and risk factors in an optimized, multimodal, rehabilitation program. Acta Anaesthesiol Scand 2006;50: 428–436.
15. Fong HK, Sands LP, Leung JM: The role of postoperative analgesia in delirium and cognitive decline in elderly patients: a systematic review. Anesth Analg 2006;102:1255–1266.
16. Greene NH, Attix DK, Weldon BC, Smith PJ, McDonagh DL, Monk TG: Measures of executive function and depression identify patients at risk for postoperative delirium. Anesthesiology 2009;110:788–795.
17. Hovens IB, Schoemaker RG, van der Zee EA, Heineman E, Izaks GJ, van Leeuwen BL: Thinking through postoperative cognitive dysfunction: How to bridge the gap between clinical and pre-clinical perspectives. Brain Behav Immun 2012;26:1169–1179.
18. Vaurio LE, Sands LP, Wang Y, Mullen EA, Leung JM: Postoperative delirium: the importance of pain and pain management. Anesth Analg 2006;102:1267–1273.
19. Casati A, Fanelli G, Pietropaoli P, et al: Monitoring cerebral oxygen saturation in elderly patients undergoing general abdominal surgery: a prospective cohort study. Eur J Anaesthesiol 2007;24:59–65.
20. Morimoto Y, Yoshimura M, Utada K, Setoyama K, Matsumoto M, Sakabe T: Prediction of postoperative delirium after abdominal surgery in the elderly. J Anesth 2009;23:51–56.
21. Newman S, Stygall J, Hirani S, Shaefi S, Maze M: Postoperative cognitive dysfunction after noncardiac surgery: a systematic review. Anesthesiology 2007;106:572–590.
22. North BJ, Sinclair DA: The intersection between aging and cardiovascular disease. Circ Res 2012;110:1097–1108.
23. Taddei S, Virdis A, Ghiadoni L, Versari D, Salvetti A: Endothelium, aging, and hypertension. Curr Hypertens Rep 2006;8:84–89.
24. Atanassoff PG: Effects of regional anesthesia on perioperative outcome. J Clin Anesth 1996;8:446–455.
25. Roy RC: Choosing general versus regional anesthesia for the elderly. Anesthesiol Clin North America 2000;18:91–104, vii.
26. Park WY, Thompson JS, Lee KK: Effect of epidural anesthesia and analgesia on perioperative outcome: a randomized, controlled Veterans Affairs cooperative study. Ann Surg 2001;234:560–569; discussion 569–571.

27. Schmidt C, Hinder F, Van Aken H, et al: The effect of high thoracic epidural anesthesia on systolic and diastolic left ventricular function in patients with coronary artery disease. Anesth Analg 2005;100:1561–1569.

28. Jakobsen CJ, Nygaard E, Norrild K, et al: High thoracic epidural analgesia improves left ventricular function in patients with ischemic heart. Acta Anaesthesiol Scand 2009;53:559–564.

29. Lagunilla J, Garcia-Bengochea JB, Fernandez AL, et al: High thoracic epidural blockade increases myocardial oxygen availability in coronary surgery patients. Acta Anaesthesiol Scand 2006;50:780–786.

30. Nygard E, Kofoed KF, Freiberg J, et al: Effects of high thoracic epidural analgesia on myocardial blood flow in patients with ischemic heart disease. Circulation 2005;111:2165–2170.

31. Barrington MJ, Kluger R, Watson R, Scott DA, Harris KJ: Epidural anesthesia for coronary artery bypass surgery compared with general anesthesia alone does not reduce biochemical markers of myocardial damage. Anesth Analg 2005;100:921–928.

32. Perlas A, Chan VW, Beattie S. Anesthesia Technique and Mortality after Total Hip or Knee Arthroplasty: A Retrospective, Propensity Score-matched Cohort Study. Anesthesiology. 2016 Oct;125(4):724–31.

33. Richman JM, Liu SS, Courpas G, et al: Does continuous peripheral nerve block provide superior pain control to opioids? A meta-analysis. Anesth Analg 2006;102:248–257.

34. Sprung J, Gajic O, Warner DO: Review article: age-related alterations in respiratory function - anesthetic considerations. Can J Anaesth 2006;53:1244–1257.

35. Don HF, Wahba M, Cuadrado L, Kelkar K: The effects of anesthesia and 100 per cent oxygen on the functional residual capacity of the lungs. Anesthesiology 1970;32:521–529.

36. Corcoran TB, Hillyard S: Cardiopulmonary aspects of anaesthesia for the elderly. Best Pract Res Clin Anaesthesiol 2011;25:329–354.

37. Urmey WF, Talts KH, Sharrock NE: One hundred percent incidence of hemidiaphragmatic paresis associated with interscalene brachial plexus anesthesia as diagnosed by ultrasonography. Anesth Analg 1991;72:498–503.

38. Werawatganon T, Charuluxanun S: Patient-controlled intravenous opioid analgesia versus continuous epidural analgesia for pain after intra-abdominal surgery. Cochrane Database Syst Rev 2005:CD004088.

39. Hudcova J, McNicol E, Quah C, Lau J, Carr DB: Patient-controlled opioid analgesia versus conventional opioid analgesia for postoperative pain. Cochrane Database Syst Rev 2006:CD003348.

40. Rigg JR, Jamrozik K, Myles PS, et al: Epidural anaesthesia and analgesia and outcome of major surgery: a randomised trial. Lancet 2002;359:1276–1282.

41. Meylan N, Elia N, Lysakowski C, Tramer MR: Benefit and risk of intrathecal morphine without local anaesthetic in patients undergoing major surgery: meta-analysis of randomized trials. Br J Anaesth 2009;102:156–167.

42. Snoeck MM, Vree TB, Gielen MJ, Lagerwert AJ: Steady state bupivacaine plasma concentrations and safety of a femoral "13-in-1" nerve block with bupivacaine in patients over 80 years of age. Int J Clin Pharmacol Ther 2003;41:107–113.

43. Hebl JR, Kopp SL, Schroeder DR, Horlocker TT: Neurologic complications after neuraxial anesthesia or analgesia in patients with preexisting peripheral sensorimotor neuropathy or diabetic polyneuropathy. Anesth Analg 2006;103:1294–1299.

44. Hogikyan RV, Wald JJ, Feldman EL, Greene DA, Halter JB, Supiano MA: Acute effects of adrenergic-mediated ischemia on nerve conduction in subjects with type 2 diabetes. Metabolism 1999;48:495–500.

45. Vuyk J: Pharmacodynamics in the elderly. Best Pract Res Clin Anaesthesiol 2003;17:207–218.

46. Piva F, Celotti F, Dondi D, et al: Ageing of the neuroendocrine system in the brain of male rats: receptor mechanisms and steroid metabolism. J Reprod Fertil Suppl 1993;46:47–59.

47. Scott JC, Stanski DR: Decreased fentanyl and alfentanil dose requirements with age. A simultaneous pharmacokinetic and pharmacodynamic evaluation. J Pharmacol Exp Ther 1987;240:159–166.

48. Clayton DA, Grosshans DR, Browning MD: Aging and surface expression of hippocampal NMDA receptors. J Biol Chem 2002;277:14367–14369.

49. Fu L, Mao YH, Gao Y, Liu L, Wang ZP, Li LC: [Expression of NR1 mRNA of NMDA receptor by gastrodine on hypoxia injury in cultured rat cerebral cortical neurons]. Zhongguo Zhong Yao Za Zhi [China Journal of Chinese Materia Medica] 2008;33:1049–1052.

50. Ahmad M, Goucke CR: Management strategies for the treatment of neuropathic pain in the elderly. Drugs & Aging 2002;19:929–945.

51. Fine PG: Pharmacological management of persistent pain in older patients. Clin J Pain 2004;20:220–226.

52. Argoff CE: Pharmacotherapeutic options in pain management. Geriatrics 2005;Suppl:3–9.

53. Guay DR: Pregabalin in neuropathic pain: a more "pharmaceutically elegant" gabapentin? American J Geriatr Pharmacother 2005;3:274–287.

54. McGeeney BE: Pharmacological management of neuropathic pain in older adults: an update on peripherally and centrally acting agents. J Pain Symptom Manage 2009;38:S15–27.

55. Veering BT, Burm AG, van Kleef JW, Hennis PJ, Spierdijk J: Epidural anesthesia with bupivacaine: effects of age on neural blockade and pharmacokinetics. Anesth Analg 1987;66:589–593.

56. Veering BT, Burm AG, Vletter AA, van den Hoeven RA, Spierdijk J: The effect of age on systemic absorption and systemic disposition of bupivacaine after subarachnoid administration. Anesthesiology 1991;74:250–257.

57. Olofsen E, Burm AG, Simon MJ, Veering BT, van Kleef JW, Dahan A: Population pharmacokinetic-pharmacodynamic modeling of epidural anesthesia. Anesthesiology 2008;109:664–674.

58. Simon MJ, Veering BT, Vletter AA, Stienstra R, van Kleef JW, Burm AG: The effect of age on the systemic absorption and systemic disposition of ropivacaine after epidural administration. Anesth Analg 2006;102:276–282.

59. Sadean MR, Glass PS: Pharmacokinetics in the elderly. Best Pract Res Clin Anaesthesiol 2003;17:191–205.

60. Gibson SJ, Farrell M: A review of age differences in the neurophysiology of nociception and the perceptual experience of pain. Clin J Pain 2004;20:227–239.

61. Gagliese L, Weizblit N, Ellis W, Chan VW: The measurement of postoperative pain: a comparison of intensity scales in younger and older surgical patients. Pain 2005;117:412–420.

62. Gibson SJ, ed: Pain and Aging: The Pain Experience Over the Adult Life Span. Seattle: IASP, 2003; Dostrovsky JO, Carr DB, Koltzenburg M, eds. Proceedings of the 10th World Congress on Pain. Progress in Pain Research and Management 24.

63. Thomas T, Robinson C, Champion D, McKell M, Pell M: Prediction and assessment of the severity of post-operative pain and of satisfaction with management. Pain 1998;75:177–185.

64. Sato A, Sato Y, Suzuki H: Aging effects on conduction velocities of myelinated and unmyelinated fibers of peripheral nerves. Neurosci Lett 1985;53:15–20.

65. Rivner MH, Swift TR, Malik K: Influence of age and height on nerve conduction. Muscle Nerve 2001;24:1134–1141.

66. Gagliese L, Ferrell M: The neurobiology of ageing, nociception and pain: an integration of animal and human experimental evidence. In: Gibson SJ, Weiner DK (eds): *Progress in Pain Research and Management: Pain in the Older Person*. Seattle: IASP, 2005, pp 25–44.

67. Gagliese L, Gauthier LR, Macpherson AK, Jovellanos M, Chan VW: Correlates of postoperative pain and intravenous patient-controlled analgesia use in younger and older surgical patients. Pain Med 2008;9:299–314.

68. Long X, Liao W, Jiang C, Liang D, Qiu B, Zhang L: Healthy aging: an automatic analysis of global and regional morphological alterations of human brain. Acad Radiol 2012;19:785–793.

69. Fjell AM, Walhovd KB: Structural brain changes in aging: courses, causes and cognitive consequences. Rev Neurosci 2010;21:187–221.

70. Gibson SJ: Older people's pain. In Pain: Clinical Updates. Volume 14. Seattle: IASP, 2006, pp 147–164.

71. Ralston HJ, 3rd: Pain and the primate thalamus. Prog Brain Res 2005;149:1–10.

72. Knyihar E, Csillik B: Plasticity of nociception: recent advances in function-oriented structural pain research. Ideggyogy Sz 2006;59:87–97.

73. Onur OA, Piefke M, Lie CH, Thiel CM, Fink GR: Modulatory effects of levodopa on cognitive control in young but not in older subjects: a pharmacological fMRI study. *J Cog Neurosci* 2011;23:2797–2810.

74. Pickering G: Age differences in clinical pain states. In: Gibson SJ, Weiner DK (eds): *Progress in Pain Research and Management: Pain in the Older Person*. Seattle: IASP Press, 2005.

75. Cole LJ, Farrell MJ, Gibson SJ, Egan GF: Age-related differences in pain sensitivity and regional brain activity evoked by noxious pressure. Neurobiol Aging 2010;31:494–503.

76. Peyron R, Laurent B, Garcia-Larrea L: Functional imaging of brain responses to pain. A review and meta-analysis (2000). Neurophysiol Clin 2000;30:263–288.

77. Seifert F, Maihofner C: Representation of cold allodynia in the human brain—a functional MRI study. Neuroimage 2007;35:1168–1180.

78. Granot M, Khoury R, Berger G, et al: Clinical and experimental pain perception is attenuated in patients with painless myocardial infarction. Pain 2007;133:120–127.

79. Zheng Z, Gibson SJ, Khalil Z, Helme RD, McMeeken JM: Age-related differences in the time course of capsaicin-induced hyperalgesia. Pain 2000;85:51–58.

80. Feldt KS, Ryden MB, Miles S: Treatment of pain in cognitively impaired compared with cognitively intact older patients with hip-fracture. J Am Geriatr Soc 1998;46:1079–1085.

81. Forster MC, Pardiwala A, Calthorpe D: Analgesia requirements following hip fracture in the cognitively impaired. Injury 2000;31:435–436.

82. Morrison RS, Siu AL: A comparison of pain and its treatment in advanced dementia and cognitively intact patients with hip fracture. J Pain Symptom Manage 2000;19:240–248.

83. Ardery G, Herr K, Hannon BJ, Titler MG: Lack of opioid administration in older hip fracture patients (CE). Geriatr Nurs 2003;24:353–360.

84. Farrell MJ, Katz B, Helme RD: The impact of dementia on the pain experience. Pain 1996;67:7–15.

85. Herr K, Bjoro K, Decker S: Tools for assessment of pain in nonverbal older adults with dementia: a state-of-the-science review. J Pain Symptom Manage 2006;31:170–192.

86. Cole LJ, Farrell MJ, Duff EP, Barber JB, Egan GF, Gibson SJ: Pain sensitivity and fMRI pain-related brain activity in Alzheimer's disease. Brain 2006;129:2957–2965.

87. Benedetti F, Arduino C, Costa S, et al: Loss of expectation-related mechanisms in Alzheimer's disease makes analgesic therapies less effective. Pain 2006;121:133–144.

88. Day A, Fawcett WJ, Scott MJ, Rockall TA: Fast-track surgery and the elderly. Br J Anaesth 2012;109():124; author reply 124.

89. Zwakhalen SM, Hamers JP, Abu-Saad HH, Berger MP: Pain in elderly people with severe dementia: a systematic review of behavioural pain assessment tools. BMC Geriatr 2006;6:3.

90. While C, Jocelyn A: Observational pain assessment scales for people with dementia: a review. Br J Community Nurs 2009;14:438–442.

91. Tsui BC, Wagner A, Finucane B: Regional anaesthesia in the elderly: a clinical guide. Drugs Aging 2004;21:895–910.

92. Guay J: The benefits of adding epidural analgesia to general anesthesia: a meta-analysis. J Anesth 2006;20:335–340.

93. Nishimori M, Low JH, Zheng H, Ballantyne JC: Epidural pain relief versus systemic opioid-based pain relief for abdominal aortic surgery. Cochrane Database Syst Rev 2012;7:CD005059.

94. Marret E, Remy C, Bonnet F: Meta-analysis of epidural analgesia versus parenteral opioid analgesia after colorectal surgery. Br J Surg 2007;94: 665–673.

95. Falzone E, Hoffmann C, Keita H: Postoperative analgesia in elderly patients. Drugs Aging 2013;30:81–90.

96. Foss NB, Kristensen MT, Kristensen BB, Jensen PS, Kehlet H: Effect of postoperative epidural analgesia on rehabilitation and pain after hip fracture surgery: a randomized, double-blind, placebo-controlled trial. Anesthesiology 2005;102:1197–1204.

97. Wu CL, Cohen SR, Richman JM, et al: Efficacy of postoperative patient-controlled and continuous infusion epidural analgesia versus intravenous patient-controlled analgesia with opioids: a meta-analysis. Anesthesiology 2005;103:1079–1088; quiz 1109–1010.

98. Mann C, Pouzeratte Y, Boccara G, et al: Comparison of intravenous or epidural patient-controlled analgesia in the elderly after major abdominal surgery. Anesthesiology 2000;92:433–441.

99. Luger TJ, Kammerlander C, Gosch M, et al: Neuroaxial versus general anaesthesia in geriatric patients for hip fracture surgery: does it matter? Osteoporosis Int 2010;21:S555–572.

100. Ready LB, Chadwick HS, Ross B: Age predicts effective epidural morphine dose after abdominal hysterectomy. Anesth Analg 1987; 66:1215–1218.

101. McLachlan AJ, Bath S, Naganathan V, et al: Clinical pharmacology of analgesic medicines in older people: impact of frailty and cognitive impairment. Br J Clin Pharmacol 2011;71:351–364.

102. Macintyre PE, Upton R: Acute pain management in the elderly patient. In: Macintyre PE, Walker, SM, Rowbotham, DJ (eds): Clinical Pain Management: Acute Pain, 2nd ed. London: Hodder Arnold; 2008.

103. Macintyre PE, Jarvis DA: Age is the best predictor of postoperative morphine requirements. Pain 1996;64:357–364.

104. Woodhouse A, Mather LE: The influence of age upon opioid analgesic use in the patient-controlled analgesia (PCA) environment. Anaesthesia 1997;52:949–955.

105. Gagliese L, Jackson M, Ritvo P, Wowk A, Katz J: Age is not an impediment to effective use of patient-controlled analgesia by surgical patients. Anesthesiology 2000;93:601–610.

106. Upton RN, Semple TJ, Macintyre PE, Foster DJR: Population pharmacokinetic modelling of subcutaneous morphine in the elderly. Acute Pain 2006;8:109–116.

107. Ishiyama T, Iijima T, Sugawara T, et al: The use of patient-controlled epidural fentanyl in elderly patients. Anaesthesia 2007;62:1246–1250.

108. Coldrey JC, Upton RN, Macintyre PE: Advances in analgesia in the older patient. Best Pract Res Clin Anaesthesiol 2011;25:367–378.

109. Herrick IA, Ganapathy S, Komar W, et al: Postoperative cognitive impairment in the elderly. Choice of patient-controlled analgesia opioid. Anaesthesia 1996;51:356–360.

110. Narayanaswamy M, Smith J, Spralja A: Choice of opiate and incidence of confusion in elderly postoperative patients. Paper presented at: Annual Scientific Meeting of the Australian and New Zealand Society of Anaesthetists 2006; Adelaide, Australia.

111. Lynch EP, Lazor MA, Gellis JE, Orav J, Goldman L, Marcantonio ER: The impact of postoperative pain on the development of postoperative delirium. Anesth Analg 1998;86:781–785.

112. Aubrun F, Marmion F: The elderly patient and postoperative pain treatment. Best Pract Res Clin Anaesthesiol 2007;21:109–127.

113. Simon MJ, Veering BT, Stienstra R, van Kleef JW, Burm AG: The effects of age on neural blockade and hemodynamic changes after epidural anesthesia with ropivacaine. Anesth Analg 2002;94:1325–1330, table of contents.

114. Simon MJ, Veering BT, Stienstra R, van Kleef JW, Burm AG: Effect of age on the clinical profile and systemic absorption and disposition of levobupivacaine after epidural administration. Br J Anaesth 2004;93: 512–520.

115. Li Y, Zhu S, Bao F, Xu J, Yan X, Jin X: The effects of age on the median effective concentration of ropivacaine for motor blockade after epidural anesthesia with ropivacaine. Anesth Analg 2006;102:1847–1850.

116. Crawford ME, Moiniche S, Orbaek J, Bjerrum H, Kehlet H: Orthostatic hypotension during postoperative continuous thoracic epidural bupivacaine-morphine in patients undergoing abdominal surgery. Anesth Analg 1996;83:1028–1032.

117. Veering BT: Hemodynamic effects of central neural blockade in elderly patients. Can J Anaesth 2006;53:117–121.

118. Gwirtz KH, Young JV, Byers RS, et al: The safety and efficacy of intrathecal opioid analgesia for acute postoperative pain: seven years' experience with 5969 surgical patients at Indiana University Hospital. Anesth Analg 1999;88:599–604.

119. Lim PC, Macintyre PE: An audit of intrathecal morphine analgesia for non-obstetric postsurgical patients in an adult tertiary hospital. Anaesth Intensive Care 2006;34:776–781.

120. Blay M, Orban JC, Rami L, et al: Efficacy of low-dose intrathecal morphine for postoperative analgesia after abdominal aortic surgery: a double-blind randomized study. Reg Anesth Pain Med 2006;31: 127–133.

121. Murphy PM, Stack D, Kinirons B, Laffey JG: Optimizing the dose of intrathecal morphine in older patients undergoing hip arthroplasty. Anesth Analg 2003;97:1709–1715.

122. Rebel A, Sloan P, Andrykowski M: Retrospective analysis of high-dose intrathecal morphine for analgesia after pelvic surgery. Pain Res Manag 2011;16:19–26.

123. Bujedo BM, Santos SG, Azpiazu AU: A review of epidural and intrathecal opioids used in the management of postoperative pain. J Opioid Manag 2012;8:177–192.

124. Sultan P, Gutierrez MC, Carvalho B: Neuraxial morphine and respiratory depression: finding the right balance. Drugs 2011;71:1807–1819.

125. Beaussier M, Weickmans H, Parc Y, et al: Postoperative analgesia and recovery course after major colorectal surgery in elderly patients: a randomized comparison between intrathecal morphine and intravenous PCA morphine. Reg Anesth Pain Med 2006;31:531–538.

126. Zaric D, Boysen K, Christiansen C, Christiansen J, Stephensen S, Christensen B: A comparison of epidural analgesia with combined continuous femoral-sciatic nerve blocks after total knee replacement. Anesth Analg 2006;102:1240–1246.

127. Fowler SJ, Symons J, Sabato S, Myles PS: Epidural analgesia compared with peripheral nerve blockade after major knee surgery: a systematic review and meta-analysis of randomized trials. Br J Anaesth 2008;100: 154–164.

128. Paul JE, Arya A, Hurlburt L, et al: Femoral nerve block improves analgesia outcomes after total knee arthroplasty: a meta-analysis of randomized controlled trials. Anesthesiology 2010;113:1144–1162.

129. Helms O, Mariano J, Hentz JG, et al: Intra-operative paravertebral block for postoperative analgesia in thoracotomy patients: a randomized, double-blind, placebo-controlled study. Eur J Cardiothorac Surg 2011;40: 902–906.

130. Davies RG, Myles PS, Graham JM: A comparison of the analgesic efficacy and side-effects of paravertebral vs epidural blockade for thoracotomy—a systematic review and meta-analysis of randomized trials. Br J Anaesth 2006;96:418–426.

131. Scarci M, Joshi A, Attia R: In patients undergoing thoracic surgery is paravertebral block as effective as epidural analgesia for pain management? Interact Cardiovasc Thorac Surg 2010;10:92–96.

132. Anwer HM, Swelem SE, el-Sheshai A, Moustafa AA: Postoperative cognitive dysfunction in adult and elderly patients-general anesthesia vs subarachnoid or epidural analgesia. Middle East J Anesthesiol 2006;18:1123–1138.

133. Gerbershagen HJ, Aduckathil S, van Wijck AJ, Peelen LM, Kalkman CJ, Meissner W: Pain intensity on the first day after surgery: a prospective cohort study comparing 179 surgical procedures. Anesthesiology 2013;118:934–944.

134. Papaioannou A, Fraidakis O, Michaloudis D, Balalis C, Askitopoulou H: The impact of the type of anaesthesia on cognitive status and delirium during the first postoperative days in elderly patients. Eur J Anaesthesiol 2005;22:492–499.

135. Rasmussen LS, Johnson T, Kuipers HM, et al: Does anaesthesia cause postoperative cognitive dysfunction? A randomised study of regional versus general anaesthesia in 438 elderly patients. Acta Anaesthesiol Scand 2003;47:260–266.

136. Mason SE, Noel-Storr A, Ritchie CW: The impact of general and regional anesthesia on the incidence of post-operative cognitive dysfunction and post-operative delirium: a systematic review with meta-analysis. J Alzheimers Dis 2010;22:67–79.

137. Del Rosario E, Esteve N, Sernandez MJ, Batet C, Aguilar JL: Does femoral nerve analgesia impact the development of postoperative delirium in the elderly? A retrospective investigation. Acute Pain 2008;10:59–64.

138. White PF, Kehlet H: Improving postoperative pain management: what are the unresolved issues? Anesthesiology 2010;112:220–225.

139. Ilfeld BM: Continuous peripheral nerve blocks: a review of the published evidence. Anesth Analg 2011;113:904–925.

140. Hanks RK, Pietrobon R, Nielsen KC, et al: The effect of age on sciatic nerve block duration. Anesth Analg 2006;102:588–592.

141. Paqueron X, Boccara G, Bendahou M, Coriat P, Riou B: Brachial plexus nerve block exhibits prolonged duration in the elderly. Anesthesiology 2002;97:1245–1249.

142. Akin S, Aribogan A, Turunc T, Aridogan A: Lumbar plexus blockade with ropivacaine for postoperative pain management in elderly patients undergoing urologic surgeries. Urol Int 2005;75:345–349.

143. Cheema S, Richardson J, McGurgan P: Factors affecting the spread of bupivacaine in the adult thoracic paravertebral space. Anaesthesia 2003;58:684–687.

144. Daly DJ, Myles PS: Update on the role of paravertebral blocks for thoracic surgery: are they worth it? Curr Opin Anaesthesiol 2009; 22:38–43.

145. Gao W, Ho YK, Verne J, Glickman M, Higginson IJ: Changing patterns in place of cancer death in England: a population-based study. PLoS Med 2013;10:e1001410.

146. Snyder GL, Greenberg S: Effect of anaesthetic technique and other perioperative factors on cancer recurrence. Br J Anaesth 2010;105:106–115.

147. Heaney A, Buggy DJ: Can anaesthetic and analgesic techniques affect cancer recurrence or metastasis? Br J Anaesth 2012;109:i17–i28.

148. Forget P, De Kock M: [Could anaesthesia, analgesia and sympathetic modulation affect neoplasic recurrence after surgery? A systematic review centred over the modulation of natural killer cells activity]. Ann Fr Anesth Reanim 2009;28:751–768.

CHAPTER 47

Regional Anesthesia & Cardiovascular Disease

Christiana C. Burt, Sanford M. Littwin, Jolaade Adebayo, Navin A. Mallavaram, and Daniel M. Thys

INTRODUCTION

The decision to utilize regional anesthesia is dependent on many factors. Patient characteristics, the type of surgery proposed, and the potential anesthetic risks will all have an impact on anesthetic choice and perioperative management. In patients with cardiovascular disease, regional anesthesia techniques (either alone or in conjunction with general anesthesia) can offer the potential perioperative benefits of stress response attenuation, cardiac sympathectomy, earlier extubation, shorter hospital stay, and intense postoperative analgesia. However, the decision to utilize regional anesthesia should be made with caution in some circumstances. The aim of this chapter is to provide an overview of the physiological effects of different regional anesthesia techniques on the cardiovascular system, to examine the role of regional anesthesia in cardiac surgery and noncardiac surgery and to provide an overview of the physiological requirements of patients with different types of cardiac and vascular disease.

THE CARDIOVASCULAR EFFECTS OF REGIONAL ANESTHESIA

Thoracic Epidural Anesthesia

High thoracic epidural anesthesia (TEA) from T1–T5 blocks the cardiac afferent and efferent sympathetic fibers with a loss of chronotropic and inotropic drive to the myocardium[1] and reduced perception of cardiac pain.

In healthy volunteers, there is some evidence that thoracic epidural blockade reduces left ventricular contractility as measured by transesophageal echocardiography[2] and that this effect is present in high thoracic epidural blockade but not in low thoracic epidural blockade,[3] which is consistent with a loss of inotropic drive to the myocardium with high epidural blockade. During exercise, it has been reported that TEA does not affect oxygen consumption (VO_2) but does reduce systemic

arterial blood pressure compared to control subjects.[4] Another study compared the cardiovascular effects of 0.5% bupivacaine administered via the thoracic epidural route against the effects when administered via the intramuscular route and found no significant difference and postulated whether the effects of epidural anesthesia may in part be due to systemic effects. However, their conclusions are limited by the low number (9) of subjects enrolled.[5]

Several studies have documented the effects of TEA on cardiovascular function in patients with heart disease. In a small study of 10 patients scheduled for thoracotomy, a TEA with a mean analgesic level of C7 to T5 had only minor effects on the cardiovascular system.[6] In patients with severe coronary artery disease and unstable angina pectoris, Blomberg et al observed that TEA relieved chest pain.[7] It also significantly decreased heart rate and systolic arterial, pulmonary arterial, and pulmonary capillary wedge pressures without any significant changes in coronary perfusion pressure, cardiac output, stroke volume, or systemic or pulmonary vascular resistances. The investigators also found that TEA may increase the diameter of stenotic epicardial coronary arteries in patients with coronary artery disease without causing a dilation of coronary arterioles.[8]

Intraoperatively, during abdominal aortic aneurysm surgery, Reinhart et al observed a lower cardiac index and O_2 delivery (QO_2) in patients receiving TEA and general anesthesia (GA) than in those receiving GA alone; VO_2 was similar.[9] They also reported that the oxygen supply–demand ratio (QO_2/VO_2) was less in the TEA group throughout the perioperative period and about 30% below baseline values during early recovery. The authors attributed the reduced adaptation of cardiac output to tissue O_2 needs during TEA to negative inotropic and chronotropic effects of sympathetic blockade. In patients on chronic β-adrenergic blocking medication, TEA has been reported to induce a moderate decrease in mean arterial pressure and coronary perfusion pressure, but without producing clinically significant cardiovascular effects.[10]

Conversely, improvements in parameters of cardiac function have been reported, specifically in improved regional left ventricular function during coronary artery bypass surgery.[11] This was attributed to the cardiac sympathectomy effect of the thoracic epidural. A separate study evaluating left ventricular systolic and diastolic function in patients with coronary artery disease found that TEA induced a significant improvement in left ventricular diastolic function, whereas indices of systolic function did not change (Figure 47–1).[12]

Hemodynamic changes during laryngoscopy and intubation can increase the risk of ischemia in some patients with cardiac disease. Licker et al. reported that patients who received TEA in addition to GA had smaller increases in mean arterial pressure and heart rate during laryngoscopy and tracheal intubation than those who received GA only; this would suggest that TEA affords hemodynamic protection during these maneuvers.[13]

The effect of TEA on hemodynamic stability during open abdominal aortic surgery has been investigated, with findings of minimal effects on cardiac index (CI) and pulmonary capillary wedge pressure (PCWP) reported during aortic cross-clamping in a group who received GA with TEA as opposed to detrimental effects (decrease in CI and increase in PCWP) seen in the group who received GA only.[14] Whether this outcome results in a difference in morbidity or mortality is unclear, though, with some groups reporting no difference in outcome,[15,16] and one reporting detrimental effects in the epidural group with rebound myocardial ischemia seen on termination of the epidural.[17]

TEA has been reported to be beneficial in morbidly obese patients undergoing gastric bypass surgery with better postoperative pain relief but no firm conclusions regarding cardiovascular function other than a significant reduction in SVR and intrapulmonary shunt compared to GA.[18]

The clinical effect of cardiac sympathectomy and peripheral vasodilation caused by TEA appears to vary between populations of patients. The level of sympathetic blockade that follows a TEA depends in part on the degree of sympathetic tone before the block, which may explain some of the different effects on the cardiovascular system reported by different studies. In addition, the effect on cardiac function will depend on the exact nature of the patient's cardiovascular disease. This is explored in more detail later in this chapter.

Lumbar Epidural Anesthesia

Lumbar epidural anesthesia (LEA) predominantly results in a drop in systemic vascular resistance via peripheral vasodilation, without the effects of cardiac sympathectomy that occur with high TEA. The influence of LEA without cardiac sympathectomy on global and regional left ventricular function was investigated prior to surgery in healthy subjects and in patients suffering from stable mild, effort-related angina.[19] In both groups, epidural blockade was performed with 10 mL of 0.5% bupivacaine. Radionuclide angiography was used to determine cardiac output, left ventricular ejection fraction, and end-systolic and end-diastolic volumes and to analyze left ventricular wall motion. Throughout the procedure, patients with a history of angina exhibited neither chest pain nor electrocardiographic evidence of myocardial ischemia. At control, left ventricular ejection fraction (LVEF) and systolic pressure–volume ratio (SPVR) were lower in the patients with angina. These patients also had evidence of regional left ventricular dysfunction. Epidural blockade without volume loading resulted in slight improvements in LVEF and regional function. Such changes were not observed in normal patients. After volume loading, the improvements in ventricular function subsided. These observations led the authors to conclude that lumbar epidural anesthesia may improve global and regional ventricular function in patients with angina provided volume loading is limited.

In hypertensive patients, LEA has been shown to cause decreases in mean arterial pressure with associated decreases in systemic vascular resistance and cardiac output.[20]

The importance of good pain relief in reducing ischemic episodes has been studied in elderly patients undergoing surgery for hip fracture with a reduction in ischemic episodes shown in the groups that received continuous epidural analgesia preoperatively.[21,22] In addition, lumbar epidural anesthesia may reduce the risk of arterial thrombotic complications in patients undergoing lower extremity revascularization,[23,24] and this may be as a result of prevention of the postoperative inhibition of fibrinolysis.[25] However, other studies report no

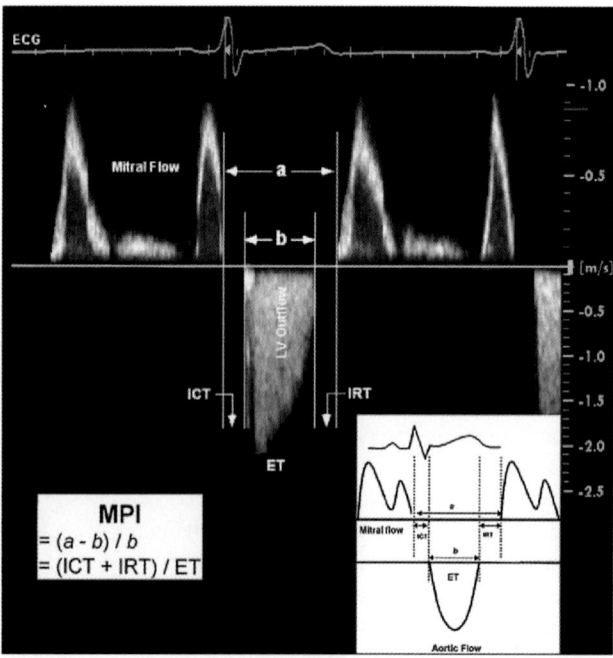

FIGURE 47–1. Estimation of the myocardial performance index (MPI; Tei index). MPI is calculated from two time intervals as a–b/b. Interval a: from cessation to next onset of mitral flow. Interval b: from onset to cessation of aortic flow. Time intervals a and b are indicated in milliseconds. A typical example of measuring the MPI using Doppler ECG registration of mitral and aortic flow velocity profiles is demonstrated. For illustrative purposes, the original Doppler tracings of mitral inflow and left ventricular (LV) outflow are plotted together. ET, ejection time of LV outflow; ICT, isovolumic contraction time; IRT, isovolumic relaxation time. (Reproduced with permission from Schmidt C, Hinder F, Van Aken H, et al: The effect of high thoracic epidural anesthesia on systolic and diastolic left ventricular function in patients with coronary artery disease. *Anesth Analg.* 2005 Jun;100(6):1561–1569.)

difference in major morbidity and mortality in patients with high cardiac risk undergoing peripheral vascular surgery with or without lumbar epidural anesthesia.[26,27]

The successful use of lumbar epidural anesthesia has been reported in obstetric patients with a variety of types of cardiac disease.[28]

Intrathecal Anesthesia

Intrathecal anesthesia using local anesthetic agents and/or opioids has been investigated in the context of cardiac and noncardiac surgery. Intrathecal anesthesia can be expected to produce profound vasodilation as well as motor and sensory blockade below the level of action.

The hemodynamic response to lumbar spinal anesthesia using single-shot hyperbaric bupivacaine or lidocaine with morphine has been evaluated in cardiac surgical patients.[29] It was observed that the induction of GA produced a decrease in mean arterial pressure and that the addition of spinal anesthesia produced a decrease in heart rate. Heart rate and mean arterial pressure did not change with sternotomy (suggesting good-quality analgesia).

In mixed populations (some with documented ischemic heart disease, some without), there has been no difference found in episodes of myocardial ischemia between patients receiving general anesthesia and patients receiving spinal anesthesia for transurethral surgery,[30,31] although there was a relatively high rate of silent ischemia in both groups in both studies. An interesting study looking at hemodynamics and markers of myocardial ischemia in patients with coronary artery disease undergoing elective hip surgery[32] found that while the number of patients who experienced episodes of ST segment depression did not differ between those who received incremental spinal anesthesia, single-shot spinal anesthesia, or general anesthesia, 56% of hypotensive patients developed ST-segment depression compared to only 10% of normotensive patients ($P < 0.003$). The incidence of hypotension and myocardial ischemia was lowest in the group receiving incremental spinal anesthesia.

Various investigators have reported on the effects of different doses of intrathecal local anesthetic as a single-shot spinal. A dose of 7.5 mg hyperbaric bupivacaine in combination with 5 mcg sufentanil has been reported to produce reliable anesthesia for repair of hip fractures in elderly patients with few episodes of hypotension and little need for vasopressor support of blood pressure.[33] Other investigators have reported 4 mg bupivacaine with 20 mcg fentanyl to be effective in the same population.[34]

Intrathecal anesthesia has not been reliably shown to have an effect on the stress response to surgery in terms of levels of serum catecholamines and serum cortisol. Some studies have reported a lower stress response during coronary artery bypass grafting (CABG) surgery in patients who received intrathecal bupivacaine in addition to general anesthesia compared to those who received general anesthesia and intravenous opioid (Figure 47–2),[35] whereas other authors have reported no attenuation of the stress response.[36,37]

Intrathecal opioid in addition to GA has been studied for elective abdominal aortic surgery.[38] The addition of intrathecal opioid provided more intense analgesia compared to PCA during the first 24 hours postoperatively, but there was no difference between the groups in the incidence of combined major cardiovascular, respiratory, and renal complications or mortality.

A group of patients judged to be at high risk for postoperative myocardial ischemia undergoing either elective hip arthroplasty or peripheral vascular surgery were randomized to receive either spinal anesthesia or general anesthesia.[39] There was no significant difference between the groups in the incidence of myocardial ischemia during or after surgery.

A number of case reports have reported on the usefulness of spinal anesthesia in obstetric patients with a variety of cardiac diseases. Velickovic et al. successfully used continuous spinal anesthesia for two patients with recurrent peripartum cardiomyopathy presenting in congestive heart failure for emergent cesarean section.[40] In one patient, a continuous spinal not only provided adequate anesthesia but also markedly reduced the patient's symptoms.[41] Others have reported similar success with spinal anesthesia in obstetric patients with hypertrophic obstructive cardiomyopathy,[42] severe pulmonary stenosis,[43] and coronary artery disease.[44]

Thoracic Blocks (Paravertebral and Intercostal)

The extent of a single percutaneous paravertebral injection was studied in 6 patients with chronic chest wall pain.[45] It was shown that a large unilateral somatic and sympathetic block was obtainable. No significant postural changes in blood pressure were seen, but there was a small but significant decrease in supine heart rate. While it has been shown that paravertebral blocks can spread to the epidural space,[46] a systematic review and meta-analysis concluded that paravertebral block causes less hypotension than epidural blockade after thoracotomy.[47]

There is anecdotal evidence that paravertebral blocks can be beneficial in patients with ischemic heart disease. Ho et al. reported on the intraoperative resolution of ST-segment depression after a right thoracic PVB,[48] although it is possible that this would have resolved spontaneously without PVB.

Intercostal nerve blocks have similarly been reported to be safe with no adverse hemodynamic consequences[49] with an ultrasound-assisted approach to blocking the intercostal nerves in the midaxillary line for nonreconstructive breast and axilla surgery.

Upper Extremity Regional Anesthesia and Cardiac Disease
Cervical Plexus Blockade

Several studies have investigated the difference in outcome after carotid endarterectomy (CEA) between general anesthesia (GA) and regional anesthesia (RA) in the form of deep and/or superficial cervical plexus blockade. As with other types of vascular surgery, CEA patients are more likely to be hypertensive, diabetic, and at increased risk for cardiac morbidity. In the context of this surgery, however, there are other causes of hemodynamic instability in addition to the effects of pain, specifically

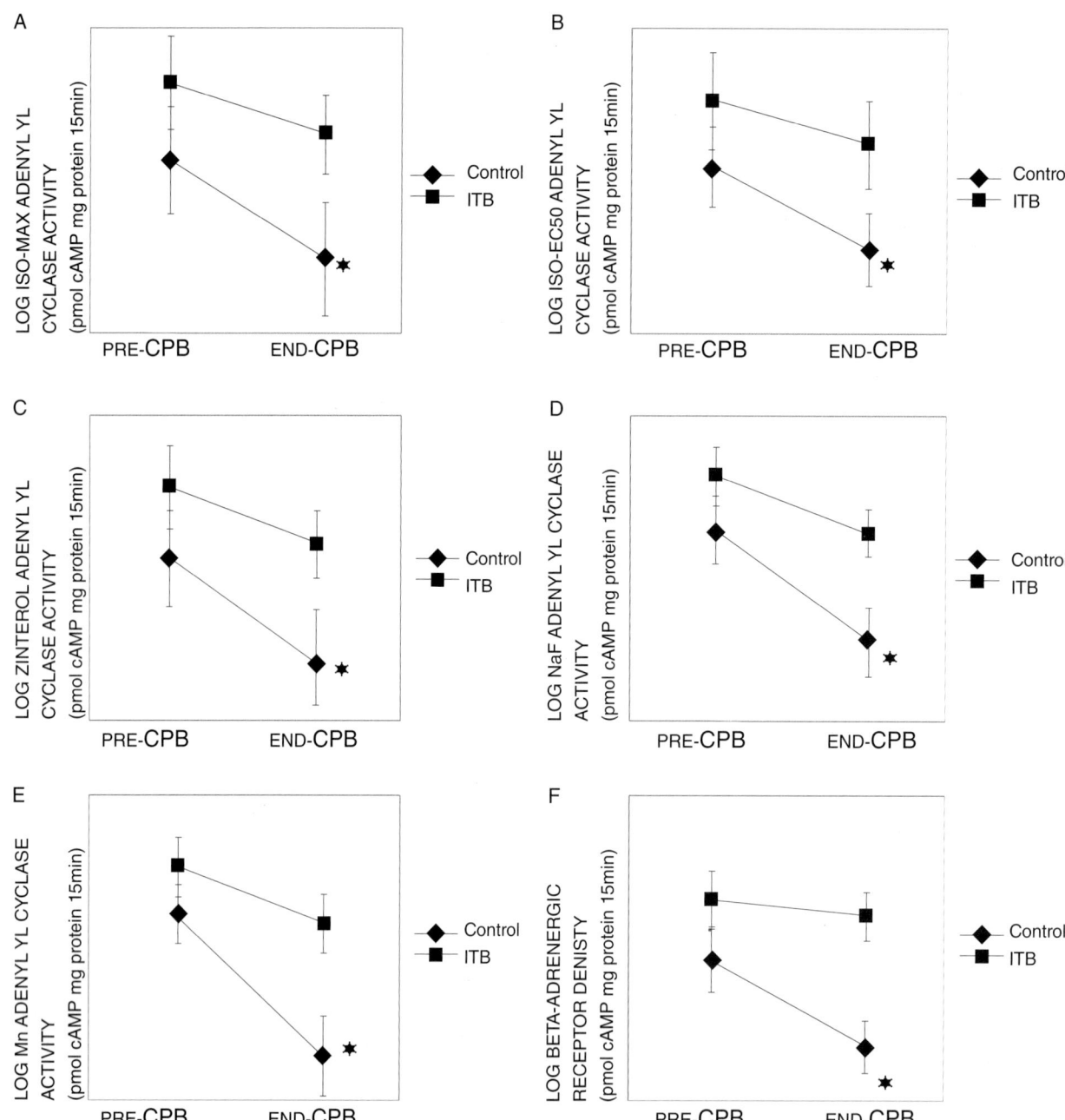

FIGURE 47-2. A: Maximal isproterenol (ISO MAX), **B:** 50% maximal isoproterenol (ISO EC₅₀), **C:** zinterol, **D:** sodium fluoride (NaF)-stimulated, and **E:** manganese (Mn)-stimulated -adrenergic receptor (AR) responsiveness, as measured by adenylyl cyclase activity in control and intrathecal bupivacaine (ITB) groups with cardiopulmonary bypass (CPB) times from 61–120 min. The control group shows a significant decline in adenylyl cyclase activity in each of these measures, whereas the ITB group does not. **F:** AR density in control and ITB groups with CPB times from 61–120 min. The control group shows a significant decline in AR density at P 0.02. Adenylyl cyclase activity and AR density (AR Bmax) are reported as picomoles of cyclic adenosine monophosphate per milligram of protein per 15 min and femtomoles per milligram of protein, respectively. The data were log-transformed. Results are expressed as mean SEM (*$P < 0.05$, ‡$P < 0.005$).

baroreceptor stimulation and sensitivity and impaired arterial pressure regulation following cerebrovascular accident (CVA).

Although greater hemodynamic stability and reduced cardiovascular complications have been reported with the use of cervical plexus blockade compared to GA alone,[50] and a meta-analysis including prospective and retrospective studies[51] reported reduced incidences of stroke, myocardial infarction (MI), and death with the use of cervical plexus block without

GA, these findings were potentially confounded by bias relating to the use of GA in higher-risk patients. A recent multicenter, randomized, prospective, controlled trial (General Anaesthetic versus Local Anaesthetic for Carotid Surgery [GALA]),[52] which included over 3500 patients randomly assigned to surgery under GA or RA, showed no difference in stroke, MI, or death in the first 30 days after surgery (among other outcomes). It is possible, though, that the highest-risk patients may not have been included in the study and that the study did not address whether there is any difference between GA or RA in higher-risk groups of patients.

Brachial Plexus Blockade

Most of the literature investigating the physiological consequences of interscalene brachial plexus blockade (BPB) has focused on its effect on the phrenic nerve and ventilatory function. A reasonable conclusion from the literature on hemodynamic effects would appear to be that significant hemodynamic effects occur as a result of intravascular absorption of local anesthetic rather than from the block itself. Continuous interscalene BPB performed with 1.25 mg/kg of 0.5% bupivacaine in 24 patients followed by an infusion of 0.25% bupivacaine at a dose of 0.25 mg/kg/h was reported to result in no hemodynamic problems after 30 minutes and in an undetectable concentration of free plasma bupivacaine after 24 hours of infusion.[53] Interscalene BPB alone for shoulder surgery was found to be more hemodynamically stable than interscalene BPB combined with GA, with a significant decrease in mean arterial pressure (MAP) when the patient was moved into the sitting position with block and GA; heart rate remained stable in both groups.[54] The addition of clonidine to interscalene BPB appears to have haemodynamic effects, with Culebras reporting that a dose of 150 mcg added to 40 mL of 0.5% bupivacaine resulted in a reduction in heart rate and blood pressure but did not prolong the duration of analgesia.[55] Hypotension and bradycardia were also reported to be more common with a dose of 2 mcg/kg clonidine compared to a dose of 1 mcg/kg clonidine added to 30 mL 0.5% bupivacaine.[56]

Lower Extremity Regional Anesthesia and Cardiac Disease

Lower extremity peripheral nerve blocks are associated with minimal hemodynamic disturbances. Fanelli et al. compared the hemodynamic changes induced by unilateral spinal anesthesia to the changes induced by combined sciatic–femoral nerve block in 20 ASA I–II patients undergoing elective orthopedic surgery with tourniquet.[57] Both groups had adequate anesthesia for the surgery. The combined sciatic–femoral nerve block group (obtained with 7 mg/kg of 2% mepivacaine) resulted in no significant hemodynamic changes, whereas the spinal anesthesia group (8 mg of hyperbaric 0.5% bupivacaine administered intrathecally) experienced small but significant differences in MAP, cardiac index, and stroke volume.

There are several case reports detailing the successful use of lower extremity peripheral nerve blocks in high-risk patients. Chia et al. presented the practical benefits of a combined sciatic–femoral nerve block on a 56-year-old man with severe sepsis and recent myocardial infarction requiring an urgent above-knee amputation.[58] Ho et al. have reported on the use of a combined paravertebral lumbar plexus and parasacral sciatic nerve block for the reduction of a hip fracture in an elderly patient with severe aortic stenosis.[59] Tanaka et al. have described the use of a psoas compartment block (PCB) in a 72-year-old female with severe heart failure due to rheumatoid myocarditis

who required an open reduction of a left femoral neck (trochanteric) fracture.[60] With the patient in the lateral position with the fractured side up, the block was performed at L3/4' using a 22-gauge Tuohy needle to inject 10 mL of normal saline and 20 mL of 2% mepivacaine. No complications were reported. Rizzo et al. used regional anesthesia to anesthetize a 32-year-old male patient suffering from Eisenmenger's syndrome with left-type-only ventricle, who needed an extirpation of meniscus by arthroscopic surgery.[61] The investigators used sciatic, femoral, and lateral cutaneous thigh nerves blocks with ropivacaine without complications.

REGIONAL ANESTHESIA AND CARDIAC SURGERY

Several authors have examined the relationship between regional anesthesia and outcome in cardiac surgery. A selection of the literature looking at thoracic epidural anesthesia is summarized in Table 47–1, and a summary of the literature looking at intrathecal anesthesia is summarized in Table 47–2. One consistent conclusion from the literature is that the quality of pain relief overall appears to be better with regional anesthesia compared to intravenous morphine. Some studies also report a reduction in the incidence of atrial fibrillation and other supraventricular dysrhythmias with regional anesthesia versus intravenous morphine. Further conclusions regarding outcome in terms of patient morbidity and mortality with or without regional anesthesia are unclear, which is likely related to the nature of the surgery itself and the greater influence of this on parameters such as cardiac function and dysrhythmias.

Many studies examining the time to extubation after cardiac surgery did so in the days before fast-tracking protocols became widespread and as such are less applicable to the majority of practice today. Having said that, regional anesthesia undoubtedly had a role to play in the early days of cardiac fast-tracking and still does in many centers, with a seemingly low risk of complications. It is, however, the potential risk of neuraxial complications in the face of full systemic heparinization and the lack of conclusive data on hard patient outcome measures that has resulted in continued debate and differing practices across centers with regard to the use of neuraxial anesthesia in cardiac surgery. This is illustrated by a survey of 892 cardiac anesthesiologists, in which only 68 (7.6%) reported the use of spinal techniques.[62]

The timing of insertion and removal of the epidural catheter in cardiac surgery is still controversial. Some clinicians will insert the epidural 60–90 minutes before heparinization in off-pump coronary artery bypass (OPCAB) but will insert it a day before surgery in planned cardiopulmonary bypass cases.[63] This method presumably relies on a high success of OPCAB and a low conversion rate to cardiopulmonary bypass intraoperatively. However, it also raises a question regarding the efficient use of resources, as the insertion of an epidural the day before surgery will, in most cases, necessitate admission to hospital the day before surgery. Insertion in the operating room without reported epidural hematomas has also been described.[64] Removal of the epidural catheter after surgery requires normalization of coagulation for a period of time. In patients requiring

TABLE 47–1. Studies investigating thoracic epidural anesthesia in cardiac surgery.

Author	Year	Population Studied	Type of Technique	Conclusion
Richter et al[75]	2002	37 patients with refractory angina	TEA	Decreased frequency of angina attacks and nitroglycerin intake. Increased self-rated quality of life.
Olausson et al[76]	1997	40 patients with severe refractory unstable angina	TEA vs standard anti-anginal therapy	Lower incidence of myocardial ischemia. Shorter duration of ischemic episodes in TEA group.
Salvi et al[77]	2004	106 patients undergoing OPCAB	TEA + GA	TEA with GA is a feasible technique for OPCAB with intense postoperative analgesia.
Kessler et al[78]	2005	90 patients undergoing OPCAB	TEA (30) vs TEA + GA (30) vs GA (30)	GA + TEA was the most comprehensive technique, providing good hemodynamic stability and reliable postoperative analgesia.
Stritesky et al[79]	2004	129 patients undergoing awake on-and-off pump cardiac surgery	TEA	10 conversions to GA intraoperatively. TEA provided rapid recovery from cardiac surgery.
Hansdottir et al[68]	2006	97 patients undergoing elective cardiac surgery	GA + TEA (48) vs GA + IV morphine (49)	Shorter time to extubation (2.3 h vs 7.3 h) in the TEA group. No differences in postoperative analgesia, lung volume, degree of ambulation, cardiac morbidity, neurologic outcome, length of ICU stay, or length of hospital stay (LOS).
Kessler et al[80]	2002	20 patients undergoing OPCAB	TEA	3 required conversion to GA. High degree of reported patient satisfaction.
Anderson et al[81]	2002	10 patients undergoing OPCAB via left anterior thoracotomy	TEA	1 required conversion to GA; 2 required brief periods of assisted ventilation. High degree of patient satisfaction.
Noiseaux et al[82]	2008	15 patients undergoing OPCAB	TEA + femoral NB	3 required conversion to GA; 5 experienced postoperative AF.
Barrington et al[83]	2005	120 patients undergoing CABG	GA vs GA + TEA	No difference in troponin T postoperatively. The TEA group had better analgesia and reduced time to extubation.
Kendall et al[84]	2004	30 patients undergoing OPCAB	Propofol vs isoflurane vs isoflurane + TEA	No difference in mean troponin T at 24 hours postoperatively.
Loick et al[85]	1999	70 patients undergoing CABG	GA + TEA vs GA + IV clonidine vs control group	TEA + GA had a beneficial effect on perioperative stress response and decreased postoperative myocardial ischemia as measured by troponin T.
Fillinger et al[86]	2002	60 patients undergoing cardiac surgery with bypass (prospective RCT)	GA + IV opioid vs GA + TEA	No differences in time to extubation, duration of ICU stay, length of hospital stay, pain control, urinary free cortisol, cardiopulmonary complication rate, or total hospital charges.

(continued)

TABLE 47–1. Studies investigating thoracic epidural anesthesia in cardiac surgery. (*Continued*)

Author	Year	Population Studied	Type of Technique	Conclusion
Scott et al[87]	2001	420 patients undergoing CABG (prospective RCT)	GA vs GA + TEA	The TEA group experienced less supraventricular dysrhythmia, better maximal inspiratory lung volume, earlier extubation, less respiratory tract infection, less acute confusion, less acute renal failure, and no neurological complications associated with TEA.
Turfrey et al[88]	1997	218 patients undergoing CABG (retrospective)	GA vs GA + TEA	The TEA group experienced less dysrhythmia, a trend toward reduced respiratory complications, reduced time to extubation, and no serious neurological complications from the use of TEA.
Karagoz et al[89]	2003	137 patients undergoing CABG	TEA alone	5 converted to GA; no mortality; mean LOS in hospital 1 day.
Liu SS et al[90]	2004	Meta-analysis: TEA: 15 trials, 1178 patients undergoing CABG; IT: 17 trials, 668 patients undergoing CABG and CABG-valve.	TEA vs GA IT morphine vs GA	No difference in mortality or MI with central neuraxial analgesia vs GA, but faster tracheal extubation and decreased respiratory complications, cardiac dysrhythmias, and pain scores with neuraxial analgesia.
Hemmerling et al[91]	2004	30 patients undergoing AVR, AVR + CABG, ascending aorta repair, and PFO repair	TEA + GA	All patients extubated within 15 minutes of end of surgery; no complications related to TEA.
Klokocovnik et al[92]	2004	Case report: 1 patient undergoing awake minimally invasive AVR	TEA alone	Operation proceeded uneventfully; discharge on day 2; no complications within 30 days.
Slin'ko[93]	2000	55 children aged 1–14 years undergoing cardiac surgery using cardiopulmonary bypass	TEA using lidocaine and fentanyl + GA vs TEA using lidocaine and clonidine + GA	Endocrine stress response decreased in lidocaine–clonidine group compared to lidocaine–fentanyl group.
Peterson et al[94]	2000	220 children undergoing cardiac surgery (retrospective review)	GA + TEA vs GA + LEA vs GA + caudal vs GA + IT	Extubation in operating room achieved for 89% patients. Lower rate of adverse events following use of TEA compared to others.
Hammer et al[95]	2000	50 children undergoing open heart surgery (retrospective)	GA + TEA vs GA + IT	No significant differences in incidence of clinically significant changes in vital signs, O_2 desaturation, hypercarbia, or vomiting.
Royse et al[96]	2003	76 patients undergoing CABG with cardiopulmonary bypass (prospective)	GA + TEA (37) vs GA + IV morphine (39)	The TEA group experienced significantly less pain on days 1–2 postoperatively, earlier extubation, improved cooperation with physiotherapy, and a reduced risk of depression and posttraumatic stress.
Liem et al[97]	1992	54 patients undergoing uncomplicated CABG (retrospective)	GA + TEA (27) vs GA + IV opioid	The TEA group experienced better intraoperative and postoperative pain management and earlier waking and extubation.

(*continued*)

TABLE 47–1. Studies investigating thoracic epidural anesthesia in cardiac surgery. (*Continued*)

Author	Year	Population Studied	Type of Technique	Conclusion
Hemmerling et al[98]	2004	100 patients undergoing OPCAB (prospective audit)	GA + TEA vs GA + IV opioid	Immediate extubation is possible using either TEA or IV opioid for pain relief. TEA results in lower pain scores compared to morphine PCA.
Bois et al[99]	1997	124 patients undergoing aortic surgery (prospective)	GA + TEA vs GA + IV opioid	The TEA group experienced better postoperative pain control. No difference in incidence of early myocardial ischemia.
Ho et al[100]	2002	244 patients undergoing CABG (retrospective survey on persistent pain)	GA + TEA vs GA + IV opioid	No difference in frequency or intensity of persistent pain postoperatively.
Jensen et al[101]	2004	49 patients undergoing cardiac valve surgery	GA + TEA (35) vs GA + IV opioid (14)	TEA provided excellent analgesia in the peri- and postoperative periods. No protective effect on chronic poststernotomy pain.
Pastor et al[64]	2003	714 patients undergoing CABG with cardiopulmonary bypass (prospective observational)	GA + TEA	TEA inserted in operating room just before surgery. Protocol for management followed. No epidural hematomas detected.
Sanchez et al[102]	1998	558 patients undergoing CABG	GA + TEA	TEA inserted the day before surgery and left in for 5 days. No documented neuraxial hematomas.

AF: atrial fibrillation; AVR: aortic valve replacement; CABG: coronary artery bypass grafting; GA: general anesthesia; ICU: intensive care unit; IT: intrathecal; IV: intravenous; LOS: length of stay; NB: nerve block; OPCAB: off-pump coronary artery bypass; PCA: patient-controlled analgesia; PFO: patent foramen ovale; RCT: randomized controlled trial; TEA: thoracic epidural anesthesia.

anticoagulation post–cardiac surgery, this practice increases the risk of thromboembolic consequences.

A systematic review and meta-analysis from 12 published cohorts, including over 14,000 patients, suggested the maximum risk for transient neurological injury following the use of thoracic epidural to be 1 in 1700 for cardiac and vascular surgery.[65] There were no reported cases of epidural hematoma or permanent neurological injury in this analysis, although there are case reports in the literature.[66,67]

As with all regional techniques, there is the possibility of failure. Hansdottir et al. reported a 5.2% (3 out of 52) failure rate of insertion and a 12.7% (7 out of 55) failure rate of placed catheters.[68]

The use of neuraxial anesthesia in the form of epidural and spinal anesthesia in cardiac surgery is controversial. An interesting analysis suggested that for each episode of neurologic complication, the use of neuraxial anesthesia would prevent 20 myocardial infarctions and 76 episodes of atrial fibrillation.[69] Whether this is an acceptable trade-off is the key question. Paravertebral and intercostal blockade, however, do not carry

the same risks as neuraxial anesthesia and may be useful additions to postoperative analgesia (Table 47–3).

THE PATIENT WITH CARDIAC DISEASE PRESENTING FOR NONCARDIAC SURGERY

Cardiac disease is a blanket term that covers a wide range of pathology. In deciding whether to utilize regional anesthesia, a consideration of the type and severity of cardiac disease is essential in predicting the likely or possible response to a regional anesthetic. Table 47–4 lists the recommendations for active cardiac conditions for which it is recommended that the patient undergo evaluation and treatment before noncardiac surgery.

The Patient with Hypertension/Left Ventricular Hypertrophy

Severe long-standing hypertension is not only associated with a shift in the autoregulatory curve for many vascular beds but also commonly results in concentric left ventricular (LV)

TABLE 47–2. Studies investigating intrathecal anesthesia in cardiac surgery.

Author	Year	Population Studied	Type of Technique	Conclusion
Vanstrum et al[103]	1988	30 patients undergoing CABG (prospective, randomized)	GA + 0.5 mg IT morphine (16) vs GA + placebo (14)	The IT morphine group required less IV morphine and less sodium nitroprusside. No difference in pain scores.
Kowalewski et al[29]	1994	18 patients undergoing CABG (case series)	GA + IT bupivacaine and morphine	No change in heart rate or MAP with sternotomy. Postoperative analgesic requirements were minimal.
Bettex et al[104]	2002	24 patients undergoing elective cardiac surgery (prospective, randomized)	GA + IT sufentanil and morphine vs GA + IV sufentanil	The IT sufentanil and morphine group experienced earlier extubation, a reduced need for IV opioids postoperatively, and improved postoperative maximal inspiratory capacity.
Mehta et al[105]	2004	100 patients undergoing elective OPCAB (prospective, randomized)	GA + IT morphine 8 mcg/kg vs GA + placebo	The IT morphine group experienced better postoperative analgesia, better lung function as measured by spirometry, and earlier extubation.
Fitzpatrick et al[106]	1988	44 patients undergoing CABG	GA + IT morphine 1 mg (15), GA + IT morphine 2 mg (15) vs GA + IV morphine	The IT morphine groups reported lower pain scores, required less supplementary IV morphine, and had better PEFRs. Mean $PaCO_2$ was significantly higher in patients given 2 mg IT morphine.
Latham et al[107]	2000	40 patients undergoing elective CABG or valve surgery	GA + IV remifentanil + IT morphine vs GA + IV sufentanil	No difference between regimens in hemodynamic stability or recovery profile.
Alhashemi et al[108]	2000	50 patients undergoing elective CABG (prospective)	GA + 250 mcg IT morphine vs GA + 500 mcg IT morphine vs GA + placebo	The IT morphine group experienced decreased postoperative IV morphine requirements and no clinically relevant effect on extubation time. The study suggests 250 mcg IT morphine is the optimal dose to provide significant analgesia without delaying extubation.
Chaney et al[109]	1997	40 patients undergoing cardiac surgery (prospective, randomized)	GA + IT morphine 10 mcg/kg (19) vs GA + IT placebo (21)	No significant difference in postoperative IV morphine use. 3 IT morphine patients experienced prolonged ventilatory depression and delayed extubation.
Finkel et al[110]	2003	30 children aged 7 months to 13 years undergoing open heart surgery	GA + IT hyperbaric tetracaine with morphine	All age groups tolerated the technique well hemodynamically.
Pirat et al[111]	2002	30 children aged 6 months to 6 years undergoing cardiac surgery (prospective, randomized)	GA + IT fentanyl (10) vs GA + IV fentanyl (10) vs GA + combined IT and IV fentanyl	The combined group was the only group to experience nonsignificant rises in HR and MAP from presurgery to poststernotomy. A single IT injection of fentanyl 2 mcg/kg offered no benefit over IV fentanyl with regard to hemodynamic stability and reduced stress response.

TABLE 47–2. Studies investigating intrathecal anesthesia in cardiac surgery. (*Continued*)

Author	Year	Population Studied	Type of Technique	Conclusion
Williams et al[112]	1997	15 children undergoing PDA repair (series)	IT tetracaine	2 patients required supplemental isoflurane. Minimal changes in blood pressure noted.
Chaney et al[36]	1996	60 patients undergoing CABG (prospective, randomized)	GA + IT morphine vs GA + IT placebo	No significant differences in perioperative epinephrine and norepinephrine levels. The IT morphine group required significantly less postoperative IV morphine.
Hall et al[37]	2000	25 patients undergoing CABG (prospective)	GA + IT morphine vs GA + IV morphine	IT morphine partially attenuated the postsurgical stress response (measured via cortisol and plasma epinephrine levels).
Zarate et al[113]	2000	20 patients undergoing elective CABG or valve replacement	GA + IT morphine + remifentanil vs GA + sufentanil	Remifentanil combined with IT morphine provided superior pain control after cardiac surgery compared to a sufentanil-based technique.
Boulanger et al[114]	2002	62 patients undergoing elective cardiac surgery	GA + IT morphine + PCA vs GA + IT placebo + PCA vs GA + SC morphine	The IT group experienced a tendency toward longer extubation times. Comparable pain scores in all 3 groups.

CABG: coronary artery bypass grafting; GA: general anesthesia; HR: heart rate; IT: intrathecal; IV: intravenous; MAP: mean arterial pressure; OPCAB: off-pump coronary artery bypass; $PaCO_2$: partial pressure of carbon dioxide; PCA: patient-controlled analgesia; PDA: patent ductus arteriosus; PEFR: peak expiratory flow rate; SC: subcutaneous.

hypertrophy as a result of long-standing increased systemic vascular resistance (SVR) and pressure overload of the LV. Sudden drops in SVR must be avoided in these patients as such drops may not only compromise coronary perfusion and LV subendocardial perfusion but may also precipitate LV outflow tract obstruction as a result of systolic anterior motion (SAM) of the mitral valve or midcavity ventricular obstruction.

Diastole is the period of the cardiac cycle when the LV is perfused via the coronary arteries and when the LV chamber relaxes and fills. In general, tachycardia is poorly tolerated by hypertrophied hearts due to increased myocardial work, oxygen requirement, and a reduced diastolic time, which reduces both cardiac output via LV filling and coronary perfusion, further increasing the risk of myocardial ischemia. In addition, LV hypertrophy is usually associated with a degree of diastolic dysfunction, making the maintenance of sinus rhythm (if possible) and avoidance of tachycardia even more important.

A regional technique may be very helpful in the avoidance of tachycardia due to pain. A localized technique that minimizes vasodilation may be preferable to central neuraxial techniques, although careful titration of these can avoid hemodynamic instability.

▉ The Patient with Ischemic Heart Disease

Ischemic heart disease is synonymous with coronary artery disease. The American College of Cardiology Foundation

(ACCF) has published guidelines on the diagnosis and management of patients with known stable ischemic heart disease, including indications for investigation and revascularization.[70] There is also, however, a significant proportion of the population with undiagnosed, asymptomatic coronary artery disease. In 2010, the ACCF and the American Heart Association (AHA) published guidelines on how best to estimate cardiovascular risk in asymptomatic adults using a combination of history, examination, and investigation.[71] Guidance is also available on the perioperative management of patients with ischemic heart disease presenting for noncardiac surgery.[72,73]

Patients with ischemic heart disease may experience a range of complications, including myocardial infarction, dysrhythmias, heart failure, deteriorating ventricular function, and sudden death. Ischemic heart disease may also coexist with other cardiac pathologies, including valvular lesions and cardiomyopathies. The management of an individual patient will depend on the combination of these problems and the predominant lesion.

The relationship between hypotension and an increase in myocardial ischemia in patients with known coronary artery disease has been demonstrated in a population of elderly patients undergoing hip surgery.[32] In general terms, a patient with known coronary artery stenoses who has an otherwise normal, well-functioning heart will benefit from efforts to maintain preload (filling), prevent excessive vasodilation (causing a reduction in SVR), and prevent tachycardia, which would

TABLE 47–3. Studies investigating paravertebal and intercostal blockade in cardiac surgery.

Author	Year	Population Studied	Type of Technique	Conclusion
Canto et al[115]	2003	111 patients undergoing elective cardiac surgery using CP bypass (case series)	GA + 2 paravertebral catheters	Good hemodynamic stability, good postoperative analgesia, short times to tracheal extubation.
Exadaktylos et al[116]	2004	9 patients undergoing MIDCAB (case series)	GA + preoperative ipsilateral intercostal nerve blocks	All were extubated within 15 minutes and experienced good analgesia.
McDonald et al[117]	2005	17 patients undergoing cardiac surgery via midline sternotomy (prospective, randomized)	GA + parasternal block vs GA + placebo	The parasternal block with levobupicaine group used significantly less morphine in the first 4 hours postoperative; no patients needed rescue pain medication.
Behnke et al[118]	2002	43 patients undergoing MIDCAB (prospective, randomized)	GA + ICB vs GA + PCA	The ICB group experienced better pain relief.
Dowling et al[119]	2003	35 patients undergoing CABG (prospective, randomized)	GA + bilateral ICB with ropivacaine (16) vs GA + bilateral ICB with saline (19)	The ICB with ropivacaine group reported significantly lower pain scores and experienced a decrease in hospital LOS.
Dhole et al[120]	2001	41 patients undergoing MIDCAB (prospective, randomized)	GA + TEA vs GA + left-sided paravertebral catheter	No significant differences in pain scores or supplemental analgesia requirement. CI was higher in the TEA group. The PVB group had lower respiratory rates.

CABG: coronary artery bypass grafting; CI: cardiac index; CP: cardiopulmonary; GA: general anesthesia; ICB: intercostal blockade; LOS: length of stay; MIDCAB: minimally invasive direct coronary artery bypass; PCA: patient-controlled analgesia; PVB: paravertebral blockade; TEA: thoracic epidural anesthesia.

increase oxygen requirement by the myocardium while reducing the time available for coronary perfusion. A patient with coronary artery disease and poor LV systolic function (defined as an ejection fraction < 30%) can be challenging, as reducing systemic vascular resistance will reduce resistance to outflow and increase ejection fraction, but this must not done at the expense of coronary artery perfusion pressure. In this circumstance, careful titration of central neuraxial anesthesia and a reduced volume of total local anesthetic is advisable.

The Patient with Valvular Heart Disease
Regurgitant Valvular Disease

In general, regurgitant valvular disease is improved symptomatically by peripheral vasodilation and worsened by peripheral vasoconstriction. Central neuraxial block and peripheral neuraxial block therefore tend to be well tolerated cardiovascularly and are ideal for preventing a worsening in regurgitant fraction as a result of peripheral vasoconstriction caused by pain and anxiety. Care needs to be taken, however, in patients with concomitant coronary artery disease or stenotic valvular disease.

Stenotic Valvular Disease

Aortic and mitral valve stenoses are much more prevalent in the adult population than tricuspid or pulmonary valve stenosis. Although it is recommended that a patient with severe aortic stenosis or symptomatic mitral stenosis be referred for investigation and management before undergoing noncardiac surgery,[73] there may be emergency situations when this is not possible.

Aortic valve stenosis results in a fixed obstruction to LV systolic outflow and usually results in concentric LV hypertrophy. Sudden decreases in SVR need to be avoided as such decreases may compromise coronary perfusion. As with patients with LV hypertrophy from other causes, maintenance of filling status and avoidance of tachycardia and fast dysrhythmias is desirable.

Mitral stenosis results in a fixed obstruction to LV inflow. Particular care needs to be taken to maintain filling status and preload, but not excessively, as large boluses of fluid may result in pulmonary edema. Careful titration of regional anesthesia with a low threshold for invasive monitoring is desirable.

TABLE 47–4. Active cardiac conditions for which the patient should undergo evaluation and treatment before noncardiac surgery (class 1, level of evidence: B).

Condition	Examples
Unstable coronary syndromes	Unstable or severe angina (CCS class III or IV) Recent MI (7–30 days)
Decompensated heart failure	NYHA class IV Worsening or new-onset heart failure
Significant dysrhythmias	High-grade atrioventricular block Mobitz II atrioventricular block Third-degree atrioventricular block Symptomatic ventricular dysrhythmias Supraventricular dysrhythmias with uncontrolled ventricular rate (HR > 100 at rest) Symptomatic bradycardia Newly recognized ventricular tachycardia
Severe valvular disease	Severe aortic stenosis (mean pressure gradient > 40 mm Hg, aortic valve area < 1cm^2 or symptomatic) Symptomatic mitral stenosis (progressive dyspnea on exertion, exertional presyncope or heart failure)

CCS: Canadian Cardiovascular Society; HR: heart rate; MI: myocardial infarction; NYHA: New York Heart Association.

Source: Adapted with permission from Fleisher LA, Beckman JA, Brown KA, et al: 2009 ACCF/AHA focused update on perioperative beta blockade incorporated into the ACC/AHA 2007 guidelines on perioperative cardiovascular evaluation and care for noncardiac surgery: a report of the American college of cardiology foundation/American heart association task force on practice guidelines. *Circulation.* 2009 Nov 24;120(21):e169-e276.

The Adult Patient with Congenital Heart Disease

The term *congenital heart disease* covers an extremely broad range of conditions, from relatively simple acyanotic lesions to complex cyanotic pathology requiring complex surgery. As pediatric congenital cardiac surgical techniques have advanced over the past few decades, more children with congenital heart disease are surviving into adulthood and presenting for noncardiac surgery where the use of regional anesthesia may be employed. Ideally, a patient with complex congenital heart disease should be managed in a specialist facility with support from clinicians and staff who are familiar with the patient, his or her condition, and his or her current medical status.

While it is not the aim of this chapter to provide a comprehensive review of every type of congenital heart disease, there are a number of general issues that should be taken into consideration when planning the use of regional anesthesia in these patients:

- Abnormal anatomy, including alterations as a result of previous surgery (Table 47–5)
- The presence of anticoagulation
- Cardiac function, including the presence of dysrhythmias
- Dependence of the pulmonary circulation on passive venous return without right ventricular assistance (Fontan or hemi-Fontan physiology)
- The likely effect on cardiovascular stability of a reduction in systemic vascular resistance
- The need for additional monitoring intraoperatively and postoperatively (the site of insertion of invasive monitoring will require knowledge of abnormal anatomy, including thrombosed veins and arterial shunts)

The most common causes of low cardiac output in a patient with Fontan physiology are inadequate preload, elevated pulmonary vascular resistance, ventricular dysfunction, and dysrhythmias.[74] The use of regional anesthesia may be very useful in these patients, as general anesthesia with positive pressure ventilation carries its own risks. Poorly controlled postoperative pain and poor respiratory effort may lead to life-threatening complications.

TABLE 47–5. Anesthetic relevance of previous surgical intervention in adult congenital heart disease.

Anatomic Lesion/Surgical Correction	Brief Description of Lesion	Anesthetic Relevance
Blalock–Taussig shunt	Subclavian artery to pulmonary artery	Avoid blood pressure measurement (invasive and noninvasive) in affected arm.
Bidirectional Glenn (hemi-Fontan)	Surgical connection of superior vena cava (SVC) to pulmonary artery	Blood flow through pulmonary circulation dependent on venous return and pulmonary vascular resistance.
Total cavopulmonary connection (Fontan type)	Surgical connection of SVC and inferior vena cava (IVC) to pulmonary artery	Blood flow through pulmonary circulation totally dependent on venous return and pulmonary vascular resistance.

Modifications to regional anesthetic technique in patients with complex congenital heart disease include the following:

- Consider a reduction in the total dose of local anesthetic administered, particularly in patients with poor cardiac function or a history of dysrhythmias.
- Use a slow titration of or avoid narcotic or anxiolytic sedation in patients with Fontan or hemi-Fontan physiology. Avoidance of hypoxia and hypercarbia is imperative due to the risk of precipitating an acute rise in pulmonary vascular resistance and the corresponding reduction in cardiac output.
- Avoid a sudden reduction in systemic vascular resistance in the patient with Fontan or hemi-Fontan physiology. Carefully titrate the central neuraxial block with appropriate fluid administration and close monitoring.

SUMMARY

Regional anesthesia, by virtue of its ability to provide intense analgesia and in some circumstances avoid general anesthesia, plays an essential role in the management of patients with cardiovascular disease undergoing surgery. The method proposed should take into account not only the type of surgery being undertaken but also the combination of issues present in the individual patient. In general terms, patients with a poor ejection fraction and regurgitant valvular lesions respond well to peripheral vasodilation, as long as adequate preload and coronary artery perfusion are maintained. Patients with stenotic valvular lesions, severe coronary artery stenosis not amenable (or practical in an emergency) to revascularization preoperatively, and/or left ventricular hypertrophy can still benefit greatly from regional anesthesia in terms of avoiding an increase in myocardial work and oxygen demand caused by pain and tachycardia. However, caution is required in these patients, as a sudden or excessive reduction in peripheral vascular resistance, particularly with central neuraxial blockade, may precipitate a drop in myocardial perfusion and/or a drop in preload and cardiac output with severe consequences. In these patients, the decision to utilize regional anesthesia should be made with caution and undertaken with appropriate monitoring. As in all other circumstances in which regional anesthesia is proposed, attention should be paid to anticoagulation, weighing the potential thromboembolic risks of stopping anticoagulation against the potential benefits. Skillfully performed major peripheral blocks for distal extremity (e.g. amputation, extremity debridement, etc), can be life-saving in patients with severe cardiovascular disease, such.

REFERENCES

1. Veering BT, Cousins MJ: Cardiovascular and pulmonary effects of epidural anaesthesia. Anaesth Intensive Care 2000;28:620–635.
2. Goertz AW et al: Influence of high thoracic epidural anesthesia on left ventricular contractility assessed using the end-systolic pressure-length relationship. Acta Anaesthesiol Scand 1993;37:38–44.
3. Niimi Y et al: Echocardiographic evaluation of global left ventricular function during high thoracic epidural anesthesia. J Clin Anesth 1997;9:118–124.
4. Ottesen S: The influence of thoracic epidural analgesia on the circulation at rest and during physical exercise in man. Acta Anaesthesiol Scand 1978;22:537–547.
5. Wattwil M et al: Circulatory changes during high thoracic epidural anaesthesia—influence of sympathetic block and of systemic effect of the local anaesthetic. Acta Anaesthesiol Scand 1985;29:849–855.
6. Hasenbos M et al: The influence of high thoracic epidural analgesia on the cardiovascular system. Acta Anaesthesiol Belg 1988;39:49–54.
7. Blomberg S, Emanuelsson H, Ricksten SE: Thoracic epidural anesthesia and central hemodynamics in patients with unstable angina pectoris. Anesth Analg 1989;69:558–562.
8. Blomberg S et al: Effects of thoracic epidural anesthesia on coronary arteries and arterioles in patients with coronary artery disease. Anesthesiology 1990;73:840–847.
9. Reinhart K et al: Effects of thoracic epidural anesthesia on systemic hemodynamic function and systemic oxygen supply-demand relationship. Anesth Analg 1989;69:360–369.
10. Stenseth R et al: The influence of thoracic epidural analgesia alone and in combination with general anesthesia on cardiovascular function and myocardial metabolism in patients receiving beta-adrenergic blockers. Anesth Analg 1993;77:463–468.
11. Berendes E et al: Reversible cardiac sympathectomy by high thoracic epidural anesthesia improves regional left ventricular function in patients undergoing coronary artery bypass grafting: a randomized trial. Arch Surg 2003;138:1283–1290; discussion 1291.
12. Schmidt C et al: The effect of high thoracic epidural anesthesia on systolic and diastolic left ventricular function in patients with coronary artery disease. Anesth Analg 2005;100:1561–1569.
13. Licker M, Farinelli C, Klopfenstein CE: Cardiovascular reflexes during anesthesia induction and tracheal intubation in elderly patients: the influence of thoracic epidural anesthesia. J Clin Anesth 1995;7:281–287.
14. Her C et al: Combined epidural and general anesthesia for abdominal aortic surgery. J Cardiothorac Anesth 1990;4:552–557.
15. Norris EJ et al: Double-masked randomized trial comparing alternate combinations of intraoperative anesthesia and postoperative analgesia in abdominal aortic surgery. Anesthesiology 2001;95:1054–1067.
16. Davies MJ et al: Combined epidural and general anaesthesia versus general anaesthesia for abdominal aortic surgery: a prospective randomised trial. Anaesth Intensive Care 1993;21:790–794.
17. Garnett RL et al: Perioperative ischaemia in aortic surgery: combined epidural/general anaesthesia and epidural analgesia vs general anaesthesia and i.v. analgesia. Can J Anaesth 1996;43:769–777.
18. Gelman S et al: Thoracic epidural vs balanced anesthesia in morbid obesity: an intraoperative and postoperative hemodynamic study. Anesth Analg 1980;59:902–908.
19. Baron JF et al: Left ventricular global and regional function during lumbar epidural anesthesia in patients with and without angina pectoris. Influence of volume loading. Anesthesiology 1987;66:621–627.
20. Dagnino J, Prys-Roberts C: Studies of anaesthesia in relation to hypertension. VI: Cardiovascular responses to extradural blockade of treated and untreated hypertensive patients. Br J Anaesth 1984;56:1065–1073.
21. Scheinin H et al: Epidural infusion of bupivacaine and fentanyl reduces perioperative myocardial ischaemia in elderly patients with hip fracture—a randomized controlled trial. Acta Anaesthesiol Scand 2000;44:1061–1070.
22. Matot I et al: Preoperative cardiac events in elderly patients with hip fracture randomized to epidural or conventional analgesia. Anesthesiology 2003;98:156–163.
23. Perler BA et al: The influence of anesthetic method on infrainguinal bypass graft patency: a closer look. Am Surg 1995;61:784–789.
24. Christopherson R et al: Perioperative morbidity in patients randomized to epidural or general anesthesia for lower extremity vascular surgery. Perioperative Ischemia Randomized Anesthesia Trial Study Group. Anesthesiology 1993;79:422–434.
25. Rosenfeld BA et al: The effects of different anesthetic regimens on fibrinolysis and the development of postoperative arterial thrombosis. Perioperative Ischemia Randomized Anesthesia Trial Study Group. Anesthesiology 1993;79:435–443.
26. Bode RH Jr et al: Cardiac outcome after peripheral vascular surgery. Comparison of general and regional anesthesia. Anesthesiology 1996;84:3–13.
27. Cohen MC et al: Types of anesthesia and cardiovascular outcomes in patients with congestive heart failure undergoing vascular surgery. Congest Heart Fail 1999;5:248–253.
28. Goldszmidt E et al: Anesthetic management of a consecutive cohort of women with heart disease for labor and delivery. Int J Obstet Anesth 2010;19:266–272.

29. Kowalewski RJ et al: Anaesthesia for coronary artery bypass surgery supplemented with subarachnoid bupivacaine and morphine: a report of 18 cases. Can J Anaesth 1994;41:1189–1195.

30. Windsor A et al: Silent myocardial ischaemia in patients undergoing transurethral prostatectomy. A study to evaluate risk scoring and anaesthetic technique with outcome. Anaesthesia 1996;51:728–732.

31. Edwards ND et al: Perioperative myocardial ischaemia in patients undergoing transurethral surgery: a pilot study comparing general with spinal anaesthesia. Br J Anaesth 1995;74:368–372.

32. Juelsgaard P et al: Perioperative myocardial ischaemia in patients undergoing surgery for fractured hip randomized to incremental spinal, single-dose spinal or general anaesthesia. Eur J Anaesthesiol 1998;15:656–663.

33. Olofsson C et al: Low-dose bupivacaine with sufentanil prevents hypotension after spinal anesthesia for hip repair in elderly patients. Acta Anaesthesiol Scand 2004;48:1240–1244.

34. Ben-David B et al: Minidose bupivacaine-fentanyl spinal anesthesia for surgical repair of hip fracture in the aged. Anesthesiology 2000;92:6–10.

35. Lee TW et al: High spinal anesthesia for cardiac surgery: effects on beta-adrenergic receptor function, stress response, and hemodynamics. Anesthesiology 2003;98:499–510.

36. Chaney MA et al: Large-dose intrathecal morphine for coronary artery bypass grafting. Anesth Analg 1996;83:215–222.

37. Hall R et al: Does intrathecal morphine alter the stress response following coronary artery bypass grafting surgery? Can J Anaesth 2000;47:463–466.

38. Fleron MH et al: A comparison of intrathecal opioid and intravenous analgesia for the incidence of cardiovascular, respiratory, and renal complications after abdominal aortic surgery. Anesth Analg 2003;97:2–12, table of contents.

39. Backlund M et al: Factors associated with post-operative myocardial ischaemia in elderly patients undergoing major non-cardiac surgery. Eur J Anaesthesiol 1999;16:826–833.

40. Velickovic IA, Leicht CH: Peripartum cardiomyopathy and cesarean section: report of two cases and literature review. Arch Gynecol Obstet 2004;270:307–310.

41. Velickovic IA, Leicht CH: Continuous spinal anesthesia for cesarean section in a parturient with severe recurrent peripartum cardiomyopathy. Int J Obstet Anesth 2004;13:40–43.

42. Okutomi T et al: Continuous spinal analgesia for labor and delivery in a parturient with hypertrophic obstructive cardiomyopathy. Acta Anaesthesiol Scand 2002;46:329–331.

43. Ransom DM, Leicht CH: Continuous spinal analgesia with sufentanil for labor and delivery in a parturient with severe pulmonary stenosis. Anesth Analg 1995;80:418–421.

44. Honig O et al: [Cesarean section with continuous spinal anesthesia in a cardiopulmonary high-risk patient]. Anaesthesist 1998;47:685–689.

45. Cheema SP et al: A thermographic study of paravertebral analgesia. Anaesthesia 1995;50:118–121.

46. Purcell-Jones G, Pither CE, Justins DM: Paravertebral somatic nerve block: a clinical, radiographic, and computed tomographic study in chronic pain patients. Anesth Analg 1989;68:32–39.

47. Davies RG, Myles PS, Graham JM: A comparison of the analgesic efficacy and side-effects of paravertebral vs epidural blockade for thoracotomy—a systematic review and meta-analysis of randomized trials. Br J Anaesth 2006;96:418–426.

48. Ho AM et al: The resolution of ST segment depressions after high right thoracic paravertebral block during general anesthesia. Anesth Analg 2002;95:227–228, table of contents.

49. Dieguez Garcia P et al: [Ultrasound-assisted approach to blocking the intercostal nerves in the mid-axillary line for non-reconstructive breast and axilla surgery]. Rev Esp Anestesiol Reanim 2013;60:365–370.

50. Sternbach Y et al: Hemodynamic benefits of regional anesthesia for carotid endarterectomy. J Vasc Surg 2002;35:333–339.

51. Guay J: Regional or general anesthesia for carotid endarterectomy? Evidence from published prospective and retrospective studies. J Cardiothorac Vasc Anesth 2007;21:127–132.

52. Group, GTC et al: General anaesthesia versus local anaesthesia for carotid surgery (GALA): a multicentre, randomised controlled trial. Lancet 2008;372:2132–2142.

53. Tuominen M et al: Continuous interscalene brachial plexus block: clinical efficacy, technical problems and bupivacaine plasma concentrations. Acta Anaesthesiol Scand 1989;33:84–88.

54. Ozzeybek D et al: Comparison of the haemodynamic effects of interscalene block combined with general anaesthesia and interscalene block alone for shoulder surgery. J Int Med Res 2003;31:428–433.

55. Culebras X et al: Clonidine combined with a long acting local anesthetic does not prolong postoperative analgesia after brachial plexus block but does induce hemodynamic changes. Anesth Analg 2001;92:199–204.

56. Kohli S et al: Brachial plexus block: Comparison of two different doses of clonidine added to bupivacaine. J Anaesthesiol Clin Pharmacol 2013;29:491–495.

57. Fanelli G et al: Cardiovascular effects of two different regional anaesthetic techniques for unilateral leg surgery. Acta Anaesthesiol Scand 1998;42:80–84.

58. Chia N, Low TC, Poon KH: Peripheral nerve blocks for lower limb surgery—a choice anaesthetic technique for patients with a recent myocardial infarction? Singapore Med J 2002;43:583–586.

59. Ho AM, Karmakar MK: Combined paravertebral lumbar plexus and parasacral sciatic nerve block for reduction of hip fracture in a patient with severe aortic stenosis. Can J Anaesth 2002;49:946–950.

60. Tanaka Y, Negoro T: [Psoas compartment block for surgery of the femoral neck (trochanteric) fracture in a patient with severe heart failure due to rheumatoid myocarditis]. Masui 2000;49:1133–1135.

61. Rizzo D et al: [Sciatic, femoral and cutaneous nerve block for arthroscopic meniscectomy in a patient with Eisenmerger's syndrome. Case report]. Minerva Anestesiol 1999;65:733–736.

62. Goldstein S et al: A survey of spinal and epidural techniques in adult cardiac surgery. J Cardiothorac Vasc Anesth 2001;15:158–168.

63. Mehta Y, Arora D: Benefits and Risks of Epidural Analgesia in Cardiac Surgery. J Cardiothorac Vasc Anesth 2014;28:1057–1063.

64. Pastor MC et al: Thoracic epidural analgesia in coronary artery bypass graft surgery: seven years' experience. J Cardiothorac Vasc Anesth 2003;17:154–159.

65. Ruppen W et al: Incidence of epidural haematoma and neurological injury in cardiovascular patients with epidural analgesia/anaesthesia: systematic review and meta-analysis. BMC Anesthesiol 2006;6:10.

66. Rosen DA et al: An epidural hematoma in an adolescent patient after cardiac surgery. Anesth Analg 2004;98:966–969, table of contents.

67. Berman M et al: Safety and efficacy of aprotinin and tranexamic acid in pulmonary endarterectomy surgery with hypothermia: review of 200 patients. Ann Thorac Surg 2010;90:1432–1436.

68. Hansdottir V et al: Thoracic epidural versus intravenous patient-controlled analgesia after cardiac surgery: a randomized controlled trial on length of hospital stay and patient-perceived quality of recovery. Anesthesiology 2006;104:142–151.

69. Djaiani G, Fedorko L, Beattie WS: Regional anesthesia in cardiac surgery: a friend or a foe? Semin Cardiothorac Vasc Anesth 2005;9: 87–104.

70. Fihn SD et al: 2012 ACCF/AHA/ACP/AATS/PCNA/SCAI/STS Guideline for the diagnosis and management of patients with stable ischemic heart disease: a report of the American College of Cardiology Foundation/American Heart Association Task Force on Practice Guidelines, and the American College of Physicians, American Association for Thoracic Surgery, Preventive Cardiovascular Nurses Association, Society for Cardiovascular Angiography and Interventions, and Society of Thoracic Surgeons. J Am Coll Cardiol 2012;60: e44–e164.

71. Greenland P et al: 2010 ACCF/AHA guideline for assessment of cardiovascular risk in asymptomatic adults: a report of the American College of Cardiology Foundation/American Heart Association Task Force on Practice Guidelines. J Am Coll Cardiol 2010;56:e50–103.

72. Fleisher LA et al: ACC/AHA 2006 guideline update on perioperative cardiovascular evaluation for noncardiac surgery: focused update on perioperative beta-blocker therapy—a report of the American College of Cardiology/American Heart Association Task Force on Practice Guidelines (Writing Committee to Update the 2002 Guidelines on Perioperative Cardiovascular Evaluation for Noncardiac Surgery). Anesth Analg 2007;104:15–26.

73. Fleisher LA et al: 2009 ACCF/AHA focused update on perioperative beta blockade incorporated into the ACC/AHA 2007 guidelines on perioperative cardiovascular evaluation and care for noncardiac surgery: a report of the American college of cardiology foundation/American heart association task force on practice guidelines. Circulation 2009; 120:e169–e276.

74. Eagle SS, Daves SM: The adult with Fontan physiology: systematic approach to perioperative management for noncardiac surgery. J Cardiothorac Vasc Anesth 2011;25:320–334.

75. Richter A et al: Effect of thoracic epidural analgesia on refractory angina pectoris: long-term home self-treatment. J Cardiothorac Vasc Anesth 2002;16:679–684.

76. Olausson K et al: Anti-ischemic and anti-anginal effects of thoracic epidural anesthesia versus those of conventional medical therapy in the treatment of severe refractory unstable angina pectoris. Circulation 1997;96:2178–2182.

77. Salvi L et al: High thoracic epidural anesthesia for off-pump coronary artery bypass surgery. J Cardiothorac Vasc Anesth 2004;18:256–262.

78. Kessler P et al: Comparison of three anesthetic techniques for off-pump coronary artery bypass grafting: general anesthesia, combined general and high thoracic epidural anesthesia, or high thoracic epidural anesthesia alone. J Cardiothorac Vasc Anesth 2005;19:32–39.

79. Stritesky M et al: On-pump cardiac surgery in a conscious patient using a thoracic epidural anesthesia—an ultra fast track method. Bratisl Lek Listy 2004;105:51–55.

80. Kessler P et al: High thoracic epidural anesthesia for coronary artery bypass grafting using two different surgical approaches in conscious patients. Anesth Analg 2002;95:791–797, table of contents.

81. Anderson MB et al: Thoracic epidural anesthesia for cardiac surgery via left anterior thoracotomy in the conscious patient. Heart Surg Forum 2002;5:105–108.

82. Noiseux N et al: Coronary artery bypass grafting in the awake patient combining high thoracic epidural and femoral nerve block: first series of 15 patients. Br J Anaesth 2008;100:184–189.

83. Barrington MJ et al: Epidural anesthesia for coronary artery bypass surgery compared with general anesthesia alone does not reduce biochemical markers of myocardial damage. Anesth Analg 2005;100:921–928.

84. Kendall JB et al: A prospective, randomised, single-blind pilot study to determine the effect of anaesthetic technique on troponin T release after off-pump coronary artery surgery. Anaesthesia 2004;59:545–549.

85. Loick HM et al: High thoracic epidural anesthesia, but not clonidine, attenuates the perioperative stress response via sympatholysis and reduces the release of troponin T in patients undergoing coronary artery bypass grafting. Anesth Analg 1999;88:701–709.

86. Fillinger MP et al: Epidural anesthesia and analgesia: effects on recovery from cardiac surgery. J Cardiothorac Vasc Anesth 2002;16:15–20.

87. Scott NB et al: A prospective randomized study of the potential benefits of thoracic epidural anesthesia and analgesia in patients undergoing coronary artery bypass grafting. Anesth Analg 2001;93:528–535.

88. Turfrey DJ et al: Thoracic epidural anaesthesia for coronary artery bypass graft surgery. Effects on postoperative complications. Anaesthesia 1997;52:1090–1095.

89. Karagoz HY et al: Coronary artery bypass grafting in the awake patient: three years' experience in 137 patients. J Thorac Cardiovasc Surg 2003;125:1401–1404.

90. Liu SS, Block BM, Wu CL: Effects of perioperative central neuraxial analgesia on outcome after coronary artery bypass surgery: a meta-analysis. Anesthesiology 2004;101:153–161.

91. Hemmerling TM et al: Immediate extubation after aortic valve surgery using high thoracic epidural anesthesia. Heart Surg Forum 2004; 7:16–20.

92. Klokocovnik T et al: Minimally invasive aortic valve replacement under thoracic epidural anesthesia in a conscious patient: case report. Heart Surg Forum 2004;7:E196–E197.

93. Slin'ko SK: [State of the sympathoadrenal system and hemodynamics in children during congenital heart defect surgery with high thoracic epidural anesthesia using lidocaine-clofelin]. Anesteziol Reanimatol 2000; 1:10–13.

94. Peterson KL et al: A report of two hundred twenty cases of regional anesthesia in pediatric cardiac surgery. Anesth Analg 2000;90:1014–1019.

95. Hammer GB, Ngo K, Macario A: A retrospective examination of regional plus general anesthesia in children undergoing open heart surgery. Anesth Analg 2000;90:1020–1024.

96. Royse C et al: Prospective randomized trial of high thoracic epidural analgesia for coronary artery bypass surgery. Ann Thorac Surg 2003;75: 93–100.

97. Liem TH et al: Coronary artery bypass grafting using two different anesthetic techniques: Part 2: Postoperative outcome. J Cardiothorac Vasc Anesth 1992;6:156–161.

98. Hemmerling TM et al: Ultra-fast-track anesthesia in off-pump coronary artery bypass grafting: a prospective audit comparing opioid-based anesthesia vs thoracic epidural-based anesthesia. Can J Anaesth 2004;51: 163–168.

99. Bois S et al: Epidural analgesia and intravenous patient-controlled analgesia result in similar rates of postoperative myocardial ischemia after aortic surgery. Anesth Analg 1997;85:1233–1239.

100. Ho SC et al: Persistent pain after cardiac surgery: an audit of high thoracic epidural and primary opioid analgesia therapies. Anesth Analg 2002;95:820–823, table of contents.

101. Jensen, MK, Andersen C: Can chronic poststernotomy pain after cardiac valve replacement be reduced using thoracic epidural analgesia? Acta Anaesthesiol Scand 2004;48:871–874.

102. Sanchez R, Nygard E: Epidural anesthesia in cardiac surgery: is there an increased risk? J Cardiothorac Vasc Anesth 1998;12:170–173.

103. Vanstrum GS, Bjornson KM, Ilko R: Postoperative effects of intrathecal morphine in coronary artery bypass surgery. Anesth Analg 1988;67: 261–267.

104. Bettex DA et al: Intrathecal sufentanil-morphine shortens the duration of intubation and improves analgesia in fast-track cardiac surgery. Can J Anaesth 2002;49:711–717.

105. Mehta Y et al: Spinal (subarachnoid) morphine for off-pump coronary artery bypass surgery. Heart Surg Forum 2004;7:E205–E210.

106. Fitzpatrick GJ, Moriarty DC: Intrathecal morphine in the management of pain following cardiac surgery. A comparison with morphine i.v. Br J Anaesth 1988;60:639–644.

107. Latham P et al: Fast-track cardiac anesthesia: a comparison of remifentanil plus intrathecal morphine with sufentanil in a desflurane-based anesthetic. J Cardiothorac Vasc Anesth 2000;14:645–651.

108. Alhashemi JA et al: Effect of subarachnoid morphine administration on extubation time after coronary artery bypass graft surgery. J Cardiothorac Vasc Anesth 2000;14:639–644.

109. Chaney MA et al: Intrathecal morphine for coronary artery bypass grafting and early extubation. Anesth Analg 1997;84:241–248.

110. Finkel JC, Boltz MG, Conran AM: Haemodynamic changes during high spinal anaesthesia in children having open heart surgery. Paediatr Anaesth 2003;13:48–52.

111. Pirat A, Akpek E, Arslan G: Intrathecal versus IV fentanyl in pediatric cardiac anesthesia. Anesth Analg 2002;95:1207–1214, table of contents.

112. Williams RK, Abajian JC: High spinal anaesthesia for repair of patent ductus arteriosus in neonates. Paediatr Anaesth 1997;7:205–209.

113. Zarate E et al: Fast-track cardiac anesthesia: use of remifentanil combined with intrathecal morphine as an alternative to sufentanil during desflurane anesthesia. Anesth Analg 2000;91:283–287.

114. Boulanger A et al: Intrathecal morphine after cardiac surgery. Ann Pharmacother 2002;36:1337–1343.

115. Canto M et al: Bilateral paravertebral blockade for conventional cardiac surgery. Anaesthesia 2003;58:365–370.

116. Exadaktylos AK et al: Pre-operative intercostal nerve blockade for minimally invasive coronary bypass surgery: a standardised anaesthetic regimen for rapid emergence and early extubation. Cardiovasc J S Afr 2004;15:178–181.

117. McDonald SB et al: Parasternal block and local anesthetic infiltration with levobupivacaine after cardiac surgery with desflurane: the effect on postoperative pain, pulmonary function, and tracheal extubation times. Anesth Analg 2005;100:25–32.

118. Behnke H et al: [Postoperative pain therapy in minimally invasive direct coronary arterial bypass surgery. I.v. opioid patient-controlled analgesia versus intercostal block]. Anaesthesist 2002;51:175–179.

119. Dowling R et al: Improved pain control after cardiac surgery: results of a randomized, double-blind, clinical trial. J Thorac Cardiovasc Surg 2003; 126:1271–1278.

120. Dhole S et al: Comparison of continuous thoracic epidural and paravertebral blocks for postoperative analgesia after minimally invasive direct coronary artery bypass surgery. J Cardiothorac Vasc Anesth 2001; 15:288–292.

Regional Anesthesia & Systemic Disease

Malikah Latmore, Matthew Levine, and Jeff Gadsden

INTRODUCTION

Patients with coexisting systemic disease may be at a higher risk for specific perioperative complications related to surgery and anesthesia. Regional anesthesia is often thought of as being particularly beneficial in patients. However, the physiologic changes that occur with some regional anesthesia techniques must be understood and viewed within the context of an individual patient's pathophysiology so that the technique used provides maximum patient benefit and reduces the risk of complications. This chapter focuses on the pathophysiology of systemic diseases frequently encountered by the regional anesthesiologist and discusses the interplay between common regional anesthesia techniques and patient disease.

PULMONARY DISEASE

Surgical patients with coexisting pulmonary impairment are at risk for intraoperative or postoperative pulmonary complications, regardless of anesthetic technique.[1] A growing body of evidence suggests that regional anesthesia may be associated with improved pulmonary outcomes compared with general anesthesia.[2–6] However, regional anesthetic blockade may carry risks in some patients. A thorough understanding of respiratory physiology and the implications of regional anesthetic techniques is crucial to the safe and effective use of regional anesthesia in these patients.

Epidural & Spinal Anesthesia

Most of the pulmonary effects of neuraxial anesthesia are due to motor block of the intercostal and abdominal musculature. If significant systemic uptake of local anesthetic occurs, some central and direct myoneural respiratory depression can also be seen, although this plays a minor role overall.[7] Since neuraxial anesthesia produces a "differential" blockade of motor, sensory,

and autonomic fibers, the degree to which respiratory function is impaired depends on the relative extent of segmental motor blockade. Using dilute concentrations of epidural local anesthetic may provide adequate sensory block as high as the cervical levels, while sparing the motor function of the respiratory muscles in the lower somatic segments.[8] Diaphragmatic paralysis (phrenic nerve block, C3–C5) in the absence of total spinal anesthesia does not occur with neuraxial blockade, since even a sensory block as high as C3 will only produce a motor block at approximately T1 through T3.[7] Apnea following high neuraxial anesthesia is most likely precipitated by brainstem hypoperfusion as a result of hypotension and unlikely to be related to phrenic nerve blockade. Spontaneous respiration returns following adequate volume resuscitation and/or vasopressor therapy.

Clinical Pearls

- Apnea associated with a high spinal anesthetic is most often related to hypotension and hypoperfusion of the brainstem, rather than motor blockade of the nerve roots supplying the phrenic nerve (C3–5).
- Supporting ventilation while maintaining the blood pressure with fluids and vasopressor therapy is the key resuscitative strategy.

With a high level of epidural or spinal anesthesia, the chest wall musculature and intercostal muscles may become impaired. This may even result in altered chest wall motion during spontaneous respiration. During high neuraxial anesthesia, the more compliant chest wall is retracted during inspiration and may actually display paradoxical rib cage motion.[9,10] Some, however, have found that epidural blockade to sensory levels of T6 or even T1 may increase the contribution that chest wall expansion makes to tidal volume.[11,12] This may be explained by an incomplete motor block of high intercostal muscles or the compensatory role played by the "accessory" muscles of respiration, such as the anterior and middle scalene muscles.[13]

Lumbar epidural anesthesia does not affect resting minute ventilation, tidal volume, or respiratory rate.[14–16] Likewise, functional residual capacity (FRC) and closing capacity appear to be relatively unchanged during lumbar epidural anesthesia.[17–19] Effort-dependent tests of respiratory function, such as forced expiratory volume in one second (FEV_1), forced vital capacity, and peak expiratory flow, do exhibit modest decreases in the setting of lumbar epidural blockade, reflecting the reliance of these indices on intercostal and abdominal musculature.[20] This decrease in pulmonary function increases proportionally as the block progresses in a cephalad fashion from lower to upper lumbar regions.

Thoracic epidural anesthesia has no effect on minute ventilation, tidal volume, or respiratory rate but does result in a modest decrease in vital capacity (VC), FEV_1, total lung capacity, and maximal midexpiratory flow rate (Table 48–1).[17] Even low cervical/high thoracic epidural anesthesia (C4–T9) in patients with severe chronic obstructive pulmonary disease (COPD) undergoing breast surgery produces only a very mild decrease in FEV_1.[21] One volunteer study found that high thoracic epidural anesthesia (T1 sensory level) led to an increase in FRC of approximately 15% with no change in tidal volume or respiratory rate.[12] This somewhat surprising finding may be explained by two mechanisms offered by the investigators. First, most volunteers exhibited a decrease in intrathoracic blood volume, a physiologic phenomenon confirmed by Arndt and colleagues.[22] Second, the study also found that the end-expiratory position of the diaphragm was shifted caudally, which may be related to a relative increase in diaphragmatic tonic activity or a reduction in intra-abdominal pressure.

Cervical epidural anesthesia reduces the VC and FEV_1 to a degree similar to that of high thoracic epidurals that extend to lower cervical levels. Studies on healthy patients have demonstrated a 15–30% reduction in VC and FEV_1 with cervical epidurals (sensory block to C2) that varied by level and local anesthetic concentration.[8,23]

The ventilatory response to hypercarbia and hypoxia is preserved with neuraxial anesthesia.[11,16] Partial pressures of both oxygen (Po_2) and carbon dioxide (Pco_2) are essentially unchanged during epidural or spinal anesthesia.[11,12] In addition, bronchomotor tone is not altered to any significant degree, despite theoretical concerns of bronchoconstriction secondary to sympatholysis.[22] Indeed, epidural anesthesia has

been used successfully in high-risk patients with COPD and asthma undergoing abdominal operations.[21,24]

Neuraxial anesthesia has been shown in a number of settings to lead to reduced postoperative pulmonary complications compared with general anesthesia. Perlas and colleagues reported an association between spinal anesthesia and lower 30-day mortality.[7] The reasons behind this are probably multifactorial, owing in part to superior analgesia, reduced diaphragmatic impairment, altered stress response, and a decreased incidence of postoperative hypoxemia.[25,26] Epidural anesthesia provides superior pain control over general anesthesia with postoperative opioids for abdominal and thoracic surgery, which leads to reduced splinting, a more effective cough mechanism, and preserved postoperative lung volumes, including FRC and VC.[27] One study directly comparing epidural and general anesthesia in high-risk patients concluded that overall outcomes, including the need for prolonged postoperative ventilation, were improved with the regional technique.[28] Another trial in patients undergoing lower limb vascular surgery reported a greater than 50% reduction in the incidence of respiratory failure in the group randomized to epidural anesthesia.[29]

Patients undergoing repair of hip fractures also benefits from regional anesthesia. Neuman et al. compared neuraxial versus general anesthesia for hip fracture repair in over 18,000 patients and found a 25% reduction in pulmonary complications in those who received neuraxial techniques.[6] A meta-analysis of 141 randomized trials (including over 9000 patients) comparing regional and general anesthesia for hip surgery showed a risk reduction for pulmonary embolism, pneumonia, and respiratory depression of 55%, 39%, and 59%, respectively, with the regional anesthesia.[26] Interestingly, these outcomes were unchanged regardless of whether neuraxial anesthesia was continued into the postoperative period, illustrating that the beneficial effect of epidural and spinal anesthesia on pulmonary physiology occurs, at least in part, at the time of surgical insult.

Brachial Plexus Block

In the absence of rare complications such as pneumothorax, any alterations in respiratory mechanics seen with brachial plexus block are due primarily to phrenic nerve blockade and hemidiaphragmatic paralysis (Figure 48–1). This has been shown to occur in 100% of patients receiving interscalene block when performed without ultrasound guidance and using between 34 and 52 mL of local anesthetic.[30] When diaphragmatic paresis occurs, there is an associated 27% reduction in

TABLE 48–1. The effect of epidural anesthesia on respirator volumes and mechanics.

	VC	TLC	FRC	VT	RR	MV	FEV_1	FVC	PEF
LEA	↔	↔	↔	↔	↔	↔	↓	↓	↓
TEA	↓	↓	↑	↔	↔	↔	↓	↓	↓

LEA: lumbar epidural anesthesia; TEA: thoracic epidural anesthesia; VC: vital capacity; TLC: total lung capacity; FRC: functional residual capacity; VT: tidal volume; RR: respiratory rate; MV: minute volume; FEV_1: forced expiratory volume in 1 second; FVC: forced vital capacity; PEF: peak expiratory flow. ↓ = decrease; ↑ = increase; ↔ = no change.

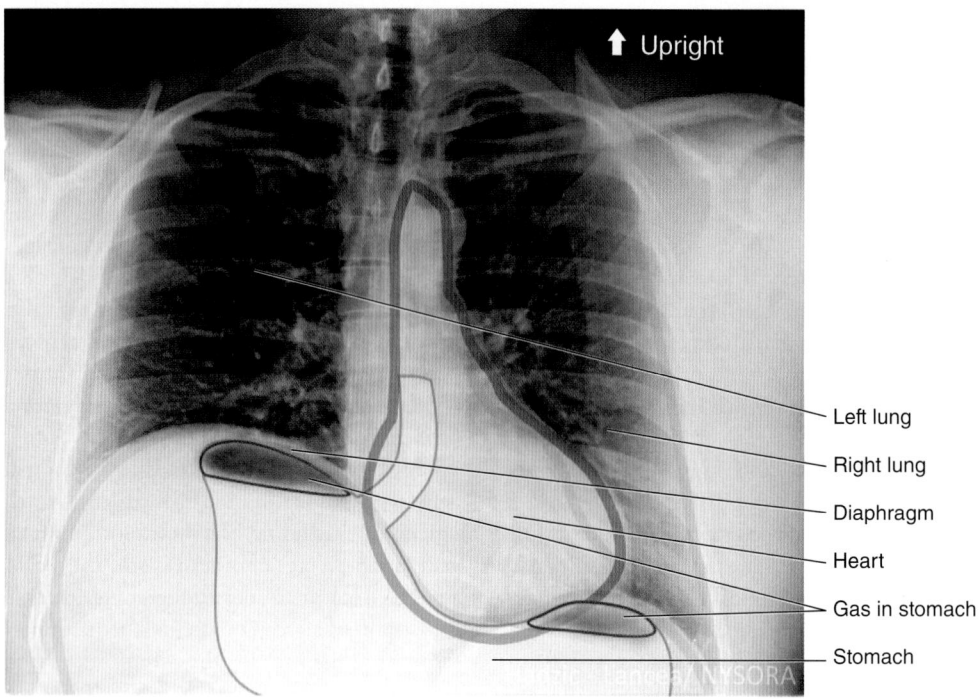

FIGURE 48–1. Upright chest radiograph of a patient who underwent a right interscalene brachial plexus block. Note the elevated right hemidiaphragm.

both FVC and FEV$_1$.[31] While the clinical significance of this reduction in healthy patients is not entirely clear, it may be useful to risk-stratify patients about to undergo interscalene blocks as one would a patient undergoing lung resection. In other words, ask the question, "Will this patient tolerate a perioperative FEV$_1$ reduction of 27%?"

Some investigators have attempted to reduce the incidence of phrenic nerve palsy by decreasing the volume of local anesthetic. However, Sinha et al. found no reduction in the incidence of hemidiaphragmatic paresis (as measured by ultrasound) when the volume of ropivacaine 0.5% was reduced from 20 mL to 10 mL.[32] Others have reported that reducing volume to 5 mL decreases the incidence by 45%–50% and results in a significantly reduced impairment of FEV$_1$ and peak expiratory flow (PEF).[33,34] Low volumes of local anesthetic are no guarantee of preservation of phrenic nerve function. Clinically significant respiratory compromise requiring tracheal intubation has been reported following an interscalene brachial plexus block using a volume of 3 mL of 2% mepivacaine.[35]

Clinical Pearls

- Interscalene block with low (≤ 5 mL) volumes of local anesthetic may reduce but not eliminate the risk of phrenic block and diaphragmatic paresis.
- Therefore, interscalene brachial plexus block should be avoided in patients who could not tolerated a 25% decrease in respiratory function.

The risk of phrenic nerve blockade decreases as one moves more distally along the plexus. The axillary approach to the brachial plexus has no effect on diaphragm function

and presents a good choice for those patients with marginal pulmonary reserve (ie, cannot tolerate a 27% reduction in lung function). On the other hand, the supraclavicular block has been traditionally associated with a 50%–67% incidence of hemidiaphragmatic paralysis, although recent studies have shown that with ultrasound guidance the incidence can be as low as zero.[36–39] The infraclavicular approach is probably sufficiently distant from the course of the phrenic nerve so as to spare the diaphragm,[40,41] although there are case reports of phrenic nerve involvement.[42,43] These discrepancies probably relate to the different approaches to the infraclavicular block—for instance the "coracoid block" is performed with a relatively lateral or distal puncture site, whereas the vertical infraclavicular block begins at a more medial location. There may also be some anatomic variations in the course of the phrenic nerve, such as an accessory phrenic nerve, which would make it more susceptible to blockade at more distal levels of the brachial plexus.[44] Although the infraclavicular or axillary blocks may be desirable for their relative pulmonary-sparing profiles, they carry the disadvantage of providing incomplete anesthesia for the shoulder and require higher degree of expertise to perform. However, creative solutions have been employed to get around this issue. Martinez and colleagues combined an infraclavicular block with a suprascapular nerve block for emergent humeral head surgery in a patient with acute asthma and a baseline FEV$_1$ of 1.13 L (32% predicted). The combination of axillary and suprascapular blocks has also been suggested as an alternative to interscalene block.[45] Therefore, a carefully considered selection of peripheral nerve blocks can provide complete anesthesia of the upper limb while avoiding respiratory complications in patients with pulmonary disease.[46]

Continuous brachial plexus blocks with perineural catheters can extend the benefits of plexus blockade into the postoperative period and reduce postoperative pain, oral opioid requirements and their side effects, and sleep disturbances after shoulder surgery.[47,48] However, there have been reports of complications attributed to the prolonged phrenic nerve paresis that can occur with this technique. These have included chest pain, atelectasis, pleural effusion, and dyspnea.[49–51] This is of particular concern because many patients are being discharged home with catheters and may not have access to timely intervention should these complications arise. On the other hand, the degree of clinically significant respiratory impairment with continuous interscalene blockade varies among patients, and, in fact, interscalene blockade may be well tolerated, especially if using relatively dilute concentrations of local anesthetic that provide only a partial phrenic nerve block.[52,53] Maurer and associates reported a case of a patient with no preexisting pulmonary disease who underwent bilateral shoulder arthroplasty under combined bilateral continuous interscalene blockade and general anesthesia.[54] Postoperative analgesia was maintained in the hospital for 72 hours via the catheters using infusions of 7 mL/h of 0.2% ropivacaine for each side (total 14 mL/h). Despite a marked postoperative reduction in FVC (60%) from baseline as well as sonographic evidence of diaphragmatic impairment, the patient had an uneventful postoperative course (with excellent analgesia) and good recovery. This anecdotal example illustrates that the clinical significance of phrenic paresis in patients with good respiratory function is questionable. Regardless, the use of continuous brachial plexus techniques should be carefully considered in patients with preexisting pulmonary disease, especially if they are to be discharged home with the catheters in situ. Other complications that may have pulmonary implications include interpleural, epidural, or even intrathecal catheter migration and irritation of the phrenic nerve.[55–57]

Clinical Pearls

- The clinical consequences of phrenic in patients with normal respiratory function are typically asymptomatic or mild.
- The use of continuous brachial plexus techniques should be carefully considered in patients with preexisting significant pulmonary disease.
- When indicated, catheter can be bolus with a small amount of short-acting local anesthetic (eg, 2% chloroprocaine 5 ml) to evaluate the effect on the respiratory function before using long-acting local anesthetics.
- In symptomatic patients with indwelling catheter, an injection of 0.9% NaCl can shorten the duration of phrenic (and brachial plexus) block ("washout").

Paravertebral & Intercostal Nerve Blocks

Several studies have investigated the effects of paravertebral and intercostal blocks on pulmonary function in patients with rib fractures or those undergoing thoracotomy. Intercostal blockade has been shown to improve arterial oxygen saturation (Sao_2) and peak expiratory flow rate (PEFR) in patients with traumatic rib fractures associated with severe pain.[58] In addition to

improved pulmonary function, some studies found significantly improved pain control and shortened hospital length of stay following intercostal catheter placement.[59] Likewise, Karmakar and co-investigators found that continuous paravertebral blockade over a period of four days in patients with multiple fractured ribs led to significant improvement in respiratory rate, FVC, PEFR, Sao_2, and the ratio of partial pressure of oxygen to fraction of inspired oxygen (Pao_2:Fio_2).[60] These findings are probably related to the favorable effect of analgesia on respiratory efforts by the patient and improved respiratory mechanics, facilitating weaning from ventilator support and return to activities of daily living in patients who were otherwise in distress from their injuries.[61,62]

Paravertebral blocks are effective for the management of pain following thoracotomy and can significantly improve postoperative spirometry. One review of 55 randomized, controlled trials of analgesic techniques following posterolateral thoracotomy revealed that paravertebral blockade was the method that best preserved pulmonary function compared with either intercostal or epidural analgesia.[63] The combined results showed an average preservation of approximately 75% of preoperative pulmonary function when paravertebral analgesia was used versus 55% for both intercostal and epidural analgesia. In addition, Davies et al showed that even when comparable analgesia was obtained with paravertebral block and thoracic epidural, the side effect profile with paravertebral blockade was significantly better, resulting in fewer pulmonary complications and less hypotension, nausea, and urinary retention.[64] It is unclear why paravertebral blockade might result in improved PEFR and SaO_2 compared with epidural analgesia in this and other studies, but it may be related to the increased utilization of opioids, a higher incidence of nausea and vomiting, and the presence of bilateral intercostal muscle blockade (and therefore diminished chest wall mobility) in the epidural cohorts.[65]

Clinical Pearls

- Paravertebral or intercostal blockade provides excellent analgesia following both rib fracture and thoracotomy.
- These blocks also result in improved spirometry and pulmonary outcomes.

Pulmonary Complications Not Related to Conduction Blockade

Pulmonary complications related to the use of regional anesthetic techniques fall into two categories. The first is those related directly or indirectly to the physiologic changes that occur with the blockade itself. Examples include atelectasis and pneumonia resulting from an inability to mobilize secretions. The second category comprises those that are independent of the effect of blockade, and although there are sporadic reports of rare complications such as pulmonary hemorrhage[66] and chylothorax,[67] the most common of these is pneumothorax. Not surprisingly, pneumothoraces occur most frequently when the puncture site overlies the pleura, and especially when performing supraclavicular and intercostal blocks. The overall reported incidence is low, but the actual numbers are likely to be underreported, since many pleural punctures will result in small pneumothoraces that resolve spontaneously.[68–72] Refinements of previously published infraclavicular techniques based on MRI studies and the widespread use of ultrasound guidance may confer additional safety to these procedures,[73–75] although is important to note that pneumothoraces have been reported with ultrasound-guided techniques, highlighting the fact that ultrasound guidance is an imperfect means of preventing adverse events.[76]

RENAL DISEASE

Renal dysfunction is commonly present in the surgical population. Perioperative acute kidney injury accounts for approximately 50% of all patients requiring acute hemodialysis in the United States. Patients with chronic renal insufficiency frequently present for procedures such as the creation of vascular shunts and revascularization of the lower limbs. Regional anesthetic techniques are frequently ideal options to provide anesthesia for these patients and procedures.

Effect of Regional Anesthesia on Renal Function

The treatment of patients at risk for perioperative renal dysfunction should focus on two principles: avoiding nephrotoxic agents and maintaining kidney perfusion. Local anesthetics do not possess any nephrotoxic properties per se, and in fact the coadministration of procaine has been shown to mitigate some of the nephrotoxic effects of cisplatin in rats.[77] Of greater relevance is the effect of anesthetic-induced hypotension on renal blood flow. The kidneys are capable of autoregulation over a wide variety of mean arterial pressures (approximately 80–180 mmHg) and maintain the glomerular filtration rate (GFR) by autonomous changes in renal vascular resistance.[78] Below the so-called lower limit of autoregulation, the kidney begins to shut down its energy-dependent physiologic processes, and the GFR and urinary output fall as a result. Ultimately, if left unchecked, renal ischemia develops, especially in the sensitive renal medulla. Although neuraxial anesthesia and the concurrent sympathectomy can reduce mean arterial pressure (MAP), renal blood flow is often preserved.[79] This is believed to reflect an increase in left ventricular stroke volume in response to the drop in systemic vascular resistance (SVR). Rooke and colleagues studied hemodynamic responses and abdominal organ perfusion (as measured by scintigraphy) in 15 patients undergoing lidocaine spinal anesthesia with a sensory block ranging from T1 to T10.[80] Whereas the MAP and SVR fell on average by 33% and 26%, respectively, blood volume in the kidneys increased by approximately 10%. There may be limits to the degree of compensation afforded by cardiac output, however. One study using a primate model showed that although renal blood flow was minimally affected by T10 spinal anesthesia, it was significantly reduced by a T1 sensory block.[81] This finding illustrates again that lumbar and low-thoracic levels of neuraxial anesthesia in patients with renal disease are well tolerated physiologically and that significant changes do not begin to manifest until higher levels are achieved.

The renin–angiotensin system, which is initiated in the kidney in response to a reduction in renal perfusion, plays an important role in blood pressure homeostasis. It serves as a complementary humoral mechanism to the sympathetic nervous systems. Hopf and colleagues conducted a study to determine if thoracic epidural anesthesia suppressed the renin response to induced hypotension.[82] Plasma renin and vasopressin concentrations were measured before, during, and after a hypotensive challenge with nitroprusside in patients with and without thoracic epidural anesthesia (sensory levels T1 through T11). With an intact sympathetic nervous system (ie, no epidural), plasma renin levels doubled in response to the hypotensive challenge lasting 15 minutes. In contrast, there was no change in the renin concentration when hypotension was induced to the same MAP in the epidural cohort. This suggests that sympathetic fibers play a key role in the renin–angiotensin system and that thoracic epidural anesthesia interferes with the functional integrity of that system.

Clinical Pearl

- Lumbar and low-thoracic levels of neuraxial anesthesia significantly renal hemodynamics.

For obvious reasons, postoperative renal function is of foremost concern when administering anesthesia for recipients of renal transplantation. Several studies have looked at the effect of general versus regional (or combined epidural/general) anesthesia on postoperative renal function in this setting. While regional anesthesia has been shown to reduce the stress response to renal transplant surgery and improve postoperative pain control, anesthetic technique was not shown to have an effect on graft outcome in either adult or pediatric populations.[83,84] Also, the choice of anesthetic technique for living donors was shown to be independent of recipient graft outcome.[85] Other nontransplant outcomes data, including those from the large meta-analysis by Rodgers et al., indicate that regional anesthesia is associated with a lower risk of postoperative renal failure than general anesthesia. However, the authors cautioned that the confidence intervals were wide and were compatible with both no effect and a two-thirds risk reduction.[26] Overall, it appears that a well-conducted regional anesthetic does not negatively affect perioperative kidney function or renal outcome compared with general anesthesia.

Considerations for Regional Anesthesia in Chronic Renal Failure

Patients with chronic renal failure often manifest a large number of pathophysiologic changes that may influence regional anesthetic care. These may include the presence of an anion-gap metabolic acidosis, electrolyte disturbances such as hyperkalemia, and coagulopathies due to uremia-induced platelet dysfunction. Plasma concentrations of local anesthetic following peripheral nerve blocks are often high enough to cause central nervous system (CNS) or cardiac toxicity in any patient, even when no obvious intravascular injection has occurred. This is probably dose-related when performing "high-volume blocks" such as plexus blocks. Some authors have recommended that dosages be adjusted in patients with chronic renal insufficiency based on observations of toxicity presumed to be related to concurrent acidosis or hyperkalemia.[86,87] Indeed, experimental evidence suggests that acidemia decreases the protein binding of bupivacaine, thereby increasing the free fraction and risk of toxicity.[88] In addition, it has been shown that hyperkalemia (5.4 vs 2.7 mEq/L) in dogs results in just half the dose of bupivacaine being required to induce cardiotoxicity.[89] Interestingly, the potassium level had no effect on in the same animals. This is an ominous finding, as it suggests that the so-called safety margin of plasma levels between CNS and cardiac toxicity, which is already relatively narrow with bupivacaine, is even less reliable in the presence of hyperkalemia.

Clinical Pearls

- Acidemia and hyperkalemia decrease the protein binding of bupivacaine, thereby increasing the free fraction and the risk of toxicity.
- Patients with uremia may have higher plasma levels of local anesthetic following peripheral nerve block.

Even in the absence of acid–base or electrolyte disturbances, plasma levels of local anesthetics following peripheral nerve block are often higher in patients with chronic renal failure.[90,91] The reason for this is not entirely clear but may relate to increased blood flow (and hence uptake at the injection site) due to the hyperdynamic circulation often seen in uremic patients.[92] On the other hand, a$_1$-acid glycoprotein (AAG) levels are increased in uremia and may lend a protective effect by binding more local anesthetic in the blood stream.[93,94] The increased levels of AAG also result in both a reduced free fraction available for hepatic metabolism and in a reduced volume of distribution. These two pharmacokinetic consequences appear to balance each other so that the serum half-life is not significantly changed.[90] Hemodialysis is ineffective in removing lidocaine from plasma and therefore cannot be relied on to treat toxicity.[95] However, lipid emulsion has been used successfully to treat both cardiovascular and neurologic systemic toxicity in patients with renal failure.[96,97]

No significant difference exists between patients with chronic renal failure and healthy patients with respect to peripheral nerve block latency, duration, or quality.[90,98,99] In one study of spinal anesthesia in patients with chronic renal failure versus healthy patients, Orko and associates found that block quality was similar but that both onset time and duration of the block were reduced in patients with uremia.[100] The authors postulated a volume-contracted intrathecal space in uremic patients as a mechanism for the quicker onset, but the actual cause remains unclear. The shorter duration of sensory block may again be related to enhanced uptake in the setting of a hyperdynamic circulation.

Uremic coagulopathy is characterized by a defect of platelet aggregation that is probably due to a toxic effect by uremic substances on the binding of fibrinogen to the platelet glycoprotein IIb/IIIa receptor.[101] This often manifests in clinically appreciable bleeding, and at least one case of subarachnoid hematoma leading to paraplegia after a spinal anesthetic in a chronic renal failure patient has been published.[102] Patients undergoing hemodialysis require intermittent anticoagulation and may present to the operating room with an unclear coagulation status. Care must be taken to delineate heparin or other anticoagulant regimens. Despite this platelet dysfunction, uremic patients are at higher risk for thrombotic events.[103] One case of hypoxia following a brachial plexus block in a uremic patient was later found to be secondary to pulmonary embolism.[104] The authors of the report suggested that a likely mechanism was the dislodgment of a preexisting thrombus from the proximal arm, facilitated by block-related manipulation and vasodilation of the upper extremity.

Several studies have compared anesthetic techniques for the creation of arteriovenous fistulae, a procedure that is common in patients with end-stage renal disease and is well suited to brachial plexus block.[105] Some investigators have concluded that little difference exists in outcome among general, local, and brachial plexus anesthesia for this operation.[106,107] Mouquet and colleagues specifically studied the effects of these three techniques on brachial artery blood flow and concluded that both general anesthesia and brachial plexus block improved blood flow through the fistula during surgery, whereas local infiltration did not.[108] Several subsequent studies have shown increased vein diameter, increased rates of native fistula formation, increased fistula blood flow, and shorter maturation time when regional anesthesia is used, compared to either general or local anesthesia.[109–111]

HEPATIC DISEASE

Liver injury or dysfunction can range from a mild, asymptomatic "transaminitis" to frank hepatic failure. There are many causes of liver disease, both acquired and congenital, but all manifest as either failure of parenchymal cell function (ie, acute and chronic hepatitis, cirrhosis) or cholestasis.[112] Considerations for regional anesthesia in patients with liver disease include the potential for altered disposition and metabolism of local anesthetics, the effect of regional anesthesia on hepatic perfusion, and possible coagulopathy related to liver dysfunction.

Pharmacokinetics of Local Anesthetics in Liver Disease

Amide local anesthetics are metabolized in liver microsomes by the cytochrome P450 system.[113] A decrease in microsomal function, as may be seen in acute or chronic liver disease, can lead to a reduction in biotransformation and clearance of these drugs, putting the patient at risk for local anesthetic toxicity. As with other drugs that are metabolized in the liver, the hepatic extraction ratio determines the relative importance of hepatic perfusion versus intrinsic enzyme activity in the overall clearance of the drug. For example, bupivacaine has a low extraction ratio (ie, its clearance is more sensitive to alterations in hepatic enzyme activity), whereas etidocaine exhibits a relatively high extraction ratio and depends on adequate liver perfusion for clearance.[114] Lidocaine has an intermediate hepatic extraction ratio and therefore relies on both perfusion and enzymatic activity. Severe hepatic disease such as cirrhosis can affect both liver perfusion and intrinsic enzyme function. In this scenario, the clearance of all amide local anesthetics, regardless of their extraction ratio, is likely to be reduced. Because the volume of distribution of local anesthetics (and many other drugs) is increased in hepatic disease, the actual plasma levels may not differ significantly from healthy patients with a single dose, despite the diminished clearance.[115–118] The altered distribution may be related to decreased levels of plasma AAG, which are reduced in proportion to the severity of liver disease.[119] Clinically, it appears that single-dose peripheral nerve blocks with amide local anesthetics probably do not require a dosage adjustment in this population, whereas continuous infusions or repeated boluses have the potential to accumulate to toxic levels.[118,120] This is supported by a study comparing plasma levels of levobupivacaine in patients undergoing hepatic resection or colorectal surgery who received epidural levobupivacaine by repeated bolus. Patients in the hepatic resection group were found to have significantly higher plasma levels, which correlated with indocyanine green clearance (a measure of hepatic function) and plasma bilirubin concentration.[121]

The cytochrome P450 enzyme system is subject to induction or inhibition by a variety of drugs and dietary nutrients. This may play a role in the subsequent metabolism of amide local anesthetics. For example, substances that inhibit microsomal enzymes, such as cimetidine or grapefruit juice, may lead to an accumulation of local anesthetic, augmenting the risk of toxicity, especially in the setting of preexisting hepatic dysfunction.[122]

Ester local anesthetics are cleared by plasma cholinesterases in the blood and liver. Severe hepatic disease may result in decreased levels of cholinesterase and result in prolonged plasma half-lives of esters such as procaine.[123] On the other hand, red cell esterases remain intact during liver disease and are able to provide some hydrolytic function.[124] Because plasma cholinesterase is extremely efficient, it is unlikely that an enzyme deficiency secondary to hepatic disease could impair the hydrolysis of ester-type local anesthetics to a degree sufficient to cause toxicity.[114]

Clinical Pearls

- The pharmacokinetics of local anesthetics in patients with liver disease can be complex due to the decrease in protein production and drug metabolism.
- Single injection-dose peripheral nerve blocks with amide local anesthetics probably do *not* require a dosage adjustment in patients with hepatic disease.

Effect of Regional Anesthesia on Hepatic Blood Flow

The hepatic blood supply is unique in that it relies on both portal venous return and hepatic artery blood flow, which make up approximately 75% and 25% of the total flow, respectively.

The regulation of hepatic blood flow is complex. The portal system is passive and not subject to autoregulation, whereas the hepatic artery can increase or decrease its contribution to flow in response to alterations in portal venous flow.[125] The hepatic artery also autoregulates in response to MAP, in much the same way that cerebral or renal vessels do, but may rely on an intact sympathetic response.[126]

General anesthesia has been shown to cause a decrease in hepatic blood flow, which may lead to ischemia and postoperative liver dysfunction.[127] Less is known about the effects of regional anesthesia on hepatic perfusion. Grietz et al. performed a high epidural (block level T1 through T4) in 16 dogs and examined the effect on systemic and hepatic hemodynamics.[128] MAP and portal venous flow were both reduced compared with control values, by 52% and 26%, respectively. In contrast, hepatic artery flow was unchanged, probably relating to a reduction in hepatic artery resistance of 51%. In addition, hepatic oxygen uptake was preserved through an increased oxygen extraction. Another study by Vagts and colleagues found that thoracic epidural anesthesia in anesthetized pigs was associated with decreased mean arterial blood pressure and hepatic artery blood flow but no change in hepatic oxygen delivery or uptake or tissue oxygen partial pressure compared with pigs receiving general anesthesia alone.[129] Taken together, these findings should reassure the clinician that high neuraxial anesthesia may be well tolerated with respect to hepatic oxygenation, despite a modest reduction in MAP. Care should be taken to maintain cardiac output and perfusion pressure during anesthesia to ensure the adequate perfusion of all the vital organs.

Hepatic Coagulopathy

Severe hepatic disease is associated with abnormalities of the coagulation system. The cause is multifactorial and may include the decreased synthesis of procoagulant proteins, impaired clearance of activated coagulation factors, nutritional deficiency (eg, vitamin K, folate), the synthesis of functionally abnormal fibrinogen, splenomegaly secondary to portal hypertension (sequestrational thrombocytopenia), qualitative platelet defects, and bone marrow suppression of thrombopoiesis (eg, by alcohol, hepatitis virus infection).[130] Because of the potential complexity of the coagulopathy, it may be necessary to perform additional laboratory tests such as clotting factor and fibrinogen assays to completely delineate the nature of the problem. Clotting factor deficiencies can be treated with vitamin K supplementation fresh frozen plasma transfusion, or both. Platelet transfusion maybe necessary in the case of thrombocytopenia. Other therapies such as recombinant factor VIIa have also been used to correct bleeding associated with liver failure.[131]

Since the vitamin K–dependent clotting factors are more susceptible to hepatocellular disease, the prothrombin time (PT) and international normalized ratio (INR) are often used as markers of coagulation system integrity. However, the predictive value of PT/INR on hemorrhage during bedside procedures such as lumbar puncture or central line placement has been shown to be poor.[132] As such, it is important to carefully weigh the risks and benefits of a neuraxial anesthetic technique in a patient with suspected hepatic-induced coagulopathy.

Although an INR of less than 1.5 "should be associated with normal hemostasis" according to the American Society of Regional Anesthesia and Pain Medicine (ASRA) consensus guidelines on anticoagulation,[133] this statement applies primarily to warfarin-induced anticoagulation and may not be a reliable indicator of the likelihood of problematic bleeding in liver failure. Epidural analgesia is frequently used during and following major liver resection, although there are some safety concerns as postoperative derangement of coagulation parameters is common; however, there are no reports of epidural hematoma in this setting.[134] The risks associated with performing peripheral nerve blocks in patients with abnormal coagulation parameters are less clear. Obviously, the risk of bleeding is increased with techniques in which the needle is placed in the vicinity of a major blood vessel. Careful consideration of risks and benefits should be performed when considering lumbar plexus block in coagulopathic patients, as a retroperitoneal hemorrhage in this space may be extensive and not obvious until the patient is in shock. Likewise, care should be taken when performing blocks in the vicinity of noncompressible blood vessels (eg, the subclavian artery in the case of infraclavicular block) in patients who have a coagulation abnormality. The risks of regional anesthesia in the setting of a disorder are elaborated on in Chapter 53.

> ### Clinical Pearls
>
> - Deep blocks, such as anterior sciatic or lumbar plexus blocks, should be practiced with special care in patients with coagulopathy.
> - Similarly, blocks in the vicinity of noncompressible blood vessels, such as the artery in the fossa, should be carefully considered.

DIABETES MELLITUS

Diabetes is a multisystem disease characterized by carbohydrate intolerance and insulin dysregulation that has many implications for the regional anesthesiologist.[135] Besides the usual anesthetic concerns, such as the presence of coronary artery, cerebrovascular, and renal disease, diabetics have a high incidence of preexisting peripheral neuropathy, which has implications for block performance and success and poses a risk for neurologic complications. Other considerations are the effect of regional anesthesia on glucose homeostasis and the increased risk of infection in diabetic patients.

Peripheral Neuropathy in Diabetics

Diabetic neuropathy is one of the most common neurologic diseases, affecting up to 100% of diabetic patients with long-standing disease.[136] Patients can be asymptomatic, but in affected patients, symptoms are typically described as paresthesias, sensory loss, or neuropathic pain. The mechanism of diabetic neuropathy is thought to be related to either a direct metabolic and osmotic effect of chronic hyperglycemia on neurons or a microvascular insult leading to nerve ischemia.[137]

Performing nerve blocks in patients with peripheral neuropathy is controversial. Kalichman and Calcutt studied sciatic nerve histology in rats following blockade with lidocaine and found significantly more nerve edema in the nerves of the rats with diabetes versus healthy controls.[138] The reason for the edema is probably multifactorial and may include the presence of an altered blood–nerve barrier or decreased uptake of local anesthetic, leading to a longer duration of nerve bathing. An increase in endoneural fluid pressure due to edema may constrict small transperineural vessels, precipitating ischemia in an already compromised nerve. This may translate to an increased incidence of postoperative paresthesias following nerve blocks, including neuraxial blocks, in diabetics. Al-Nasser reported a case of prolonged (> 8 weeks) bilateral lower limb paresthesias and pain following lumbar epidural analgesia with 0.2% ropivacaine in a diabetic patient undergoing radical prostatectomy.[139] Postoperative electromyographic studies showed widespread sensory neuropathy of both upper and lower limbs, indicating that the patient, although asymptomatic, had preexisting neuropathy that may have predisposed him to this rare complication. Studies have demonstrated a prolonged duration of sensory and motor blockade following sciatic nerve block in diabetics when compared to nondiabetics and that the duration of blockade increases as glycemic control worsens (as measured by glycosylated hemoglobin levels).[140,141] A study in diabetic rats showed a similar prolongation of local anesthetic effect which was reversed by 2 weeks of insulin treatment but unaffected by 6 hours of insulin, suggesting that the increased sensitivity to local anesthetics is mediated by chronic changes in the nervous system as opposed to the current blood glucose level.[142] It is unclear whether this increased sensitivity to local anesthetics represents an increased risk of neurological complications. The actual prevalence of neurologic complications in diabetics receiving nerve blocks is unknown but is probably quite low. Diabetes is a common disease, and reports of neurologic complications in the literature are sparse, suggesting that in the vast majority of cases, recovery from peripheral nerve blocks is uneventful.

Patients with diabetes should also be considered at increased risk for infectious complications of regional anesthesia due to the immune suppression that occurs as a result of the disease. Diabetes has been implicated as a risk factor for infection following both peripheral and neuraxial blockade.[143] Although it is unclear to what extent diabetes truly increases the risk of infection, it seems wise to be extra vigilant with infection control precautions in these patients.

The effect of diabetic neuropathy on electrolocation of nerves while using a nerve stimulator is another matter of controversy. Patients with long-standing diabetes may require somewhat higher current intensity in order to produce a motor response.[144,145] While nerve conduction studies in diabetics with neuropathy consistently show a reduction in conduction velocity and amplitude for both motor and sensory nerves, this does not tend to be the case in actual clinical practice, as most patients with diabetes have similar current intensity thresholds as non-diabetic patients without neuropathy.[146]

Clinical Pearls

- Patients with diabetes are prone to a metabolic neuropathy that impairs nerve conduction.
- A stimulating current of greater intensity is only occasionally needed to obtain visible muscle twitches when using a nerve stimulator to electrolocate nerves.

Effect of Regional Anesthesia on Glucose Homeostasis

It is well known that surgery performed in combination with general anesthesia provokes a counterregulatory response that significantly increases plasma levels of glucose, as well as levels of cortisol and catecholamines. This so-called stress response has long been considered a homeostatic defense mechanism that is important in an organism's adaptation to harmful stimuli, providing substrates for energy in times of need. However, prolonged periods of hyperglycemia may have deleterious effects on patients, with evidence supporting an increase in mortality rates, hospital length of stay, and incidence of nosocomial infection.[147,148] Hyperglycemia may be particularly hazardous in patients who have incurred trauma.[149]

Regional anesthesia has been shown to ameliorate the hyperglycemic response to surgery and therefore may play a role in this protective phenomenon. An intraoperative glucose tolerance test resulted in markedly elevated plasma glucose levels in patients receiving general versus epidural anesthesia for such procedures as inguinal herniorrhaphy and hysterectomy.[150,151] Likewise, abdominal hysterectomy performed under spinal anesthesia is associated with lower intra- and postoperative glucose levels compared with neuroleptanesthesia.[152] Retrobulbar block reduces the hyperglycemic stress response to both cataract[153] and scleral buckle[154] surgery.

Glucose homeostasis is complex, and several factors likely contribute to the salutary action of regional anesthesia on glycemic control. These may include the inhibition of hepatic gluconeogenesis as well as the inhibition of catecholamine and cortisol responses to surgery.[155] In addition, the "absence of general anesthesia" may be a causative factor in glycemic control, as volatile agents such as halothane and enflurane have been shown to impair glucose tolerance in dogs.[156] It seems clear from the available data that to improve outcomes from major surgery, anesthesiologists must prevent as much nociceptive input from reaching the central nervous and neuroendocrine systems as possible.[157] The use of regional anesthesia can easily facilitate this goal and may be especially pertinent for "brittle" diabetics in whom tight glycemic control is difficult at the best of times.

THYROID NEUROPATHY

Diabetes and uremia are the most common metabolic neuropathies; however, several other less common neuropathies also have implications for the regional anesthesiologist. These include those neuropathies that result from the use of certain medications or exposure to toxins and those related to connective tissue, autoimmune, and vascular diseases.[158] One of the most prevalent causes of metabolic neuropathy is that associated with overt hypothyroidism. Thyroid neuropathy is a largely sensory phenomenon that is poorly understood but present in approximately 40% of patients diagnosed with hypothyroidism.[159] It is most obvious in frank myxedema, but nerve conduction studies have shown evidence of velocity impairment in subclinical hypothyroidism.[160] Thyroid neuropathy is most likely to present as peripheral nerve entrapment, particularly of the median nerve, and these patients are frequently referred for carpal tunnel decompression.[161] Entrapment of the eighth cranial nerve leading to deafness is also common. Patients may complain of dysesthesias in a glove-and-stocking pattern, as well as lancinating pains suggestive of nerve root compression. "Hung" deep tendon reflexes (brisk reflex response with a delayed return to normal tone) are a hallmark of hypothyroidism and probably relate to both neuropathy and myopathy. Pathologically, affected nerves exhibit mucinous deposition and, in advanced cases, segmental demyelination with loss of large myelinated nerve fibers.[162]

Few data exist on the effect preexisting thyroid neuropathy may have on the management of regional anesthesia in this population. A potential consequence of performing regional anesthesia in patients with nerve entrapment is what has been termed the "double-crush syndrome."[163] This refers to the enhanced susceptibility of nerves to injury or impairment at one anatomic location when already compressed or otherwise injured at another, separate location. A classic example is the patient with symptoms of carpal tunnel syndrome after seemingly minor trauma or injury to the median nerve, who is later found to have compression of the C6 nerve root. Although originally described in terms of mechanical injury, it has been recognized that metabolic and pharmacologic factors can contribute to the double-crush syndrome,[164] including hypothyroidism. Thus, it may be that patients with thyroid neuropathy are at increased risk for neurologic injury when receiving regional anesthesia blocks, as minor needle trauma to a susceptible nerve may produce functional neurologic deficits. Although this remains speculative at present, this possibility reinforces the need for a detailed history and documentation of preexisting neurologic deficit in patients with hypothyroidism and the careful consideration of techniques in these patients. Finally, if suspected, thyroid neuropathy has been shown to be correctable in many cases by prompt treatment with thyroid replacement therapy, which may this complication.[165,166]

OBESITY

Obesity is an increasingly prevalent problem, with worldwide obesity rates having doubled since 1980.[167] Over the last 20 years, there has been a dramatic rise in obesity in the U.S., with 35% of adults and 17% of children and adolescents meeting the criteria for obesity in 2012.[168] In addition to the usual anesthetic considerations for morbidly obese patients, such as the presence of various cardiopulmonary, gastrointestinal, and endocrine comorbidities, the abundance of extra tissue can present a challenge to regional anesthesiologists. Obesity has been shown to impair the ability of anesthesiologists to correctly identify lumbar spinal interspaces.[169] Outcomes are similarly affected in overweight patients. In a study of over 9000 mixed blocks at a single institution, patients with a body mass index (BMI) greater than 30 kg/m² were 1.62 times more likely to experience a failed regional block than were those with a BMI less than 25 kg/m².[170] Not surprisingly, the investigators cited difficulty in landmark identification, patient positioning, and insufficient length of needle used as the main impediments to successful block placement. These findings are supported by a study of axillary blocks using nerve stimulator guidance, where obesity was associated with longer block performance time, decreased success rate, increased complication rate, and decreased patient satisfaction.[171] Despite these relative difficulties, block success rates in obese patients were high, and rates of serious complications were low. Regional anesthesia remains an attractive option for obese patients because it may reduce the incidence of cardiopulmonary and airway complications compared with those experienced during general anesthesia.

Clinical Pearls

- Obese patients are more likely to experience a failed regional block than patients with a BMI within the normal range.
- Reasons for this include difficult surface or sonographic landmarks, difficulty in patient positioning.

Obese patients seem to benefit from image-guided regional anesthetic blocks. Fluoroscopy has been used in the placement of axillary brachial plexus catheters,[172] in the performance of sciatic nerve blocks,[173] and as an aid in facilitating spinal anesthesia in morbidly obese patients.[174] However, its use is limited by the need to relate neural anatomy to structures that appear radiodense, such as bones, needles, or contrast-injected vessels.

Ultrasound may be especially useful in obese patients with obscured surface landmarks, although excess adipose tissue can make ultrasound examination itself more difficult due to attenuation of the ultrasound beam.[175,176] This difficulty can be partly overcome by decreasing the frequency of the transducer to increase penetration depth, although image resolution will be reduced (Figure 48–2). When median and sciatic nerves were scanned in normal-weight and obese volunteers, Marhofer et al. concluded that visualization of superficial peripheral nerves is independent of BMI, whereas deeper nerves are more difficult to visualize in obese subjects.[177] Studies conducted in obese parturients and in nonobstetric patients with difficult surface anatomic landmarks have verified the utility of ultrasound in identifying the epidural space and other spinal structures prior to the performance of a neuraxial block.[178–180] To date, few studies have compared ultrasound-guided peripheral nerve blocks with landmark or nerve stimulator–guided techniques in the obese population; however, ultrasound seems to be a useful modality for this potentially challenging group of patients.

Obesity may have an effect on the dosing of spinal medications, although the issue is somewhat controversial. A common notion is that increased abdominal mass leads to compression of intrathecal volume by engorgement of epidural plexuses, leading to an increased, and potentially dangerous, block height during spinal anesthesia. This is supported by data correlating block height with patient weight during standardized spinal anesthesia for cystoscopy.[181] Indeed, some authors have advocated the consideration of "low-dose" spinal anesthesia in the morbidly obese, due to wide variations in their dosing requirements. In one extremely overweight parturient (BMI = 66 kg/m²), cesarean section was completed successfully with a 5-mg spinal dose of bupivacaine as the sole anesthetic agent.[182] However, patient weight does not necessarily correlate with the degree of

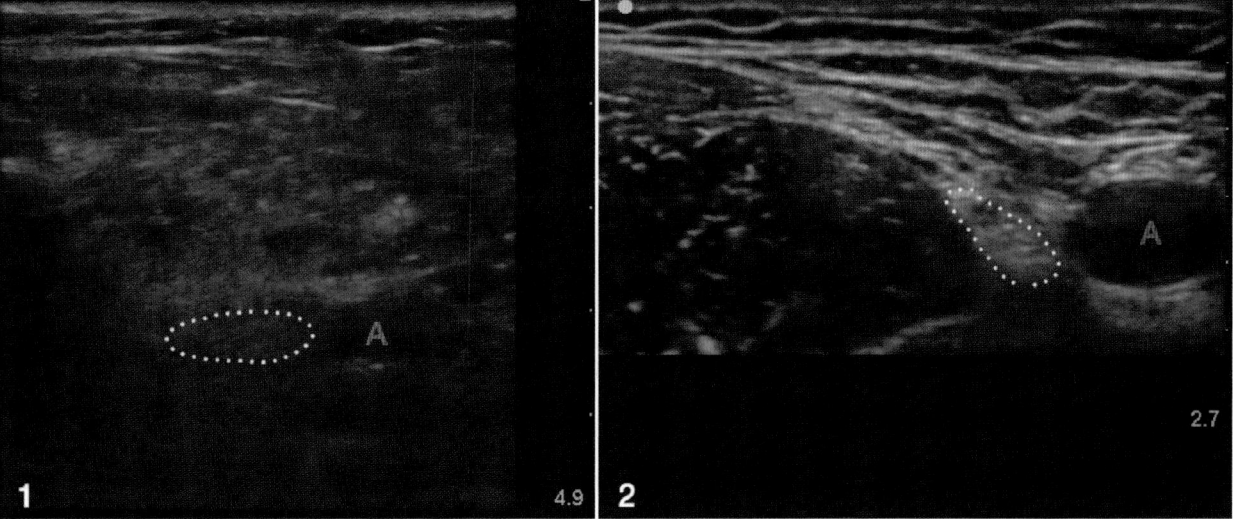

FIGURE 48–2. Ultrasound scans of the femoral regions in an obese (**1**) patient and a slim (**2**) patient. Note the increased depth required to image the artery (A) and nerve (dotted outline) in the obese example, as well as the overall poor resolution quality due to the excess adipose tissue. In contrast, the nerve, artery, muscles, and fascial planes in the slim patient are crisp and well defined.

compression of the thecal sac, and many investigators have argued that weight alone is not a reliable predictor of block height during spinal anesthesia.[183–185] A dose-finding study of hyperbaric bupivacaine in patients undergoing knee replacement found no difference in the dose required to achieve a block to T12 between obese and nonobese patients but did find a slightly longer duration of block and reduced incidence of tourniquet pain in the obese group.[186] However, no patients in the obese group had a BMI over 40, so these findings may not be reflective of the morbidly obese population. It is probably reasonable to approach the spinal dosing of morbidly obese patients with a degree of caution, and when practical, to incrementally adjust the anesthetic dose.

REFERENCES

1. Duggan M, Kavanagh BP: Perioperative modifications of respiratory function. Best Pract Res Clin Anaesthesiol 2010;24:145–155.
2. Cuschieri RJ, Morran CG, Howie JC, McArdle CS: Postoperative pain and pulmonary complications: comparison of three analgesic regimens. Br J Surg 1985;72:495–498.
3. Ballantyne JC, Carr DB, deFerranti S, Suarez T, Lau J, Chalmers TC, Angelillo IF, Mosteller F: The comparative effects of postoperative analgesic therapies on pulmonary outcome: cumulative meta-analyses of randomized, controlled trials. Anesth Analg 1998;86:598–612.
4. Slinger P, Shennib H, Wilson S: Postthoracotomy pulmonary function: a comparison of epidural versus intravenous meperidine infusions. J Cardiothorac Vasc Anesth 1995;9:128–134.
5. Lier F van, Geest PJ van der, Hoeks SE, et al: Epidural analgesia is associated with improved health outcomes of surgical patients with chronic obstructive pulmonary disease. Anesthesiology 2011;115:315–321.
6. Neuman MD, Silber JH, Elkassabany NM, Ludwig JM, Fleisher LA: Comparative effectiveness of regional versus general anesthesia for hip fracture surgery in adults. Anesthesiology 2012;117:72–92.
7. Cousins MJ, Veering B. Epidural neural blockade. In: Cousins MJ, Bridenbaugh PO, Carr DB, Horlocker TT (eds), Cousins and Bridenbaugh's Neural Blockade in Clinical Anesthesia and Pain Medicine, 4th ed. Philadelphia: Lippincott Williams & Wilkins, 2008.
8. Michalek P, David I, Adamec M, Janousek L: Cervical epidural anesthesia for combined neck and upper extremity procedure: a pilot study. Anesth Analg 2004;99:1833–1836, table of contents.
9. Eisele J, Trenchard D, Burki N, Guz A: The effect of chest wall block on respiratory sensation and control in man. Clin Sci 1968;35:23–33.
10. Kochi T, Sako S, Nishino T, Mizuguchi T: Effect of high thoracic extradural anaesthesia on ventilatory response to hypercapnia in normal volunteers. Br J Anaesth 1989;62:362–367.
11. Yamakage M, Namiki A, Tsuchida H, Iwasaki H: Changes in ventilatory pattern and arterial oxygen saturation during spinal anaesthesia in man. Acta Anaesthesiol Scand 1992;36:569–571.
12. Warner DO, Warner MA, Ritman EL: Human chest wall function during epidural anesthesia. Anesthesiology 1996;85:761–773.
13. Troyer A De, Kelly S: Action of neck accessory muscles on rib cage in dogs. J Appl Physiol Respir Environ Exerc Physiol 1984;56:326–332.
14. Labaille T, Clergue F, Samii K, Ecoffey C, Berdeaux A: Ventilatory response to CO2 following intravenous and epidural lidocaine. Anesthesiology 1985;63:179–183.
15. Sakura S, Saito Y, Kosaka Y: Effect of lumbar epidural anesthesia on ventilatory response to hypercapnia in young and elderly patients. J Clin Anesth 1993;5:109–113.
16. Sakura S, Saito Y, Kosaka Y: The effects of epidural anesthesia on ventilatory response to hypercapnia and hypoxia in elderly patients. Anesth Analg 1996;82:306–311.
17. McCarthy GS: The effect of thoracic extradural analgesia on pulmonary gas distribution, functional residual capacity and airway closure. Br J Anaesth 1976;48:243–248.
18. Lundh R, Hedenstierna G, Johansson H: Ventilation-perfusion relationships during epidural analgesia. Acta Anaesthesiol Scand 1983;27: 410–416.
19. Reber A, Bein T, Högman M, Khan ZP, Nilsson S, Hedenstierna G: Lung aeration and pulmonary gas exchange during lumbar epidural anaesthesia and in the lithotomy position in elderly patients. Anaesthesia 1998;53:854–861.
20. Moir DD: Ventilatory function during epidural analgesia. Br J Anaesth 1963;35:3–7.
21. Groeben H, Schäfer B, Pavlakovic G, Silvanus M-T, Peters J: Lung function under high thoracic segmental epidural anesthesia with ropivacaine or bupivacaine in patients with severe obstructive pulmonary disease undergoing breast surgery. Anesthesiology 2002;96: 536–541.
22. Arndt JO, Höck A, Stanton-Hicks M, Stühmeier KD: Peridural anesthesia and the distribution of blood in supine humans. Anesthesiology 1985;63:616–623.
23. Capdevila X, Biboulet P, Rubenovitch J, Serre-Cousine O, Peray P, Deschodt J, Athis F d': The effects of cervical epidural anesthesia with bupivacaine on pulmonary function in conscious patients. Anesth Analg 1998;86:1033–1038.
24. Kolker AR, Hirsch CJ, Gingold BS, Stamatos JM, Wallack MK: Use of epidural anesthesia and spontaneous ventilation during transabdominal colon and rectal procedures in selected high-risk patient groups. Dis Colon Rectum 1997;40:339–343. Anesthesia Technique and Mortality after Total Hip or Knee Arthroplasty: A Retrospective, Propensity Score-matched Cohort Study. Perlas A, Chan VW, Beattie S. Anesthesiology. 2016 Oct;125(4):724–31.
25. Liu S, Carpenter RL, Neal JM: Epidural anesthesia and analgesia. Their role in postoperative outcome. Anesthesiology 1995;82: 1474–1506.
26. Rodgers A, Walker N, Schug S, et al: Reduction of postoperative mortality and morbidity with epidural or spinal anaesthesia: results from overview of randomised trials. BMJ 2000;321:1493.
27. Wahba WM, Don HF, Craig DB: Post-operative epidural analgesia: effects on lung volumes. Can Anaesth Soc J 1975;22:519–527.
28. Yeager MP, Glass DD, Neff RK, Brinck-Johnsen T: Epidural anesthesia and analgesia in high-risk surgical patients. Anesthesiology 1987;66: 729–736.
29. Christopherson R, Beattie C, Frank SM, et al: Perioperative morbidity in patients randomized to epidural or general anesthesia for lower extremity vascular surgery. Perioperative Ischemia Randomized Anesthesia Trial Study Group. Anesthesiology 1993;79:422–434.
30. Urmey WF, Talts KH, Sharrock NE: One hundred percent incidence of hemidiaphragmatic paresis associated with interscalene brachial plexus anesthesia as diagnosed by ultrasonography. Anesth Analg 1991;72: 498–503.
31. Urmey WF, McDonald M: Hemidiaphragmatic paresis during interscalene brachial plexus block: effects on pulmonary function and chest wall mechanics. Anesth Analg 1992;74:352–357.
32. Sinha SK, Abrams JH, Barnett JT, et al: Decreasing the local anesthetic volume from 20 to 10 mL for ultrasound-guided interscalene block at the cricoid level does not reduce the incidence of hemidiaphragmatic paresis. Reg Anesth Pain Med 2011;36:17–20.
33. Lee J-H, Cho S-H, Kim S-H, et al: Ropivacaine for ultrasound-guided interscalene block: 5 mL provides similar analgesia but less phrenic nerve paralysis than 10 mL. Can J Anaesth 2011;58:1001–1006.
34. Riazi S, Carmichael N, Awad I, Holtby RM, McCartney CJL: Effect of local anaesthetic volume (20 vs 5 ml) on the efficacy and respiratory consequences of ultrasound-guided interscalene brachial plexus block. Br J Anaesth 2008;101:549–556.
35. Koscielniak-Nielsen ZJ: Hemidiaphragmatic paresis after interscalene supplementation of insufficient axillary block with 3 mL of 2% mepivacaine. Acta Anaesthesiol Scand 2000;44:1160–1162.
36. Knoblanche GE: The incidence and aetiology of phrenic nerve blockade associated with supraclavicular brachial plexus block. Anaesth Intensive Care 1979;7:346–349.
37. Mak PH, Irwin MG, Ooi CG, Chow BF: Incidence of diaphragmatic paralysis following supraclavicular brachial plexus block and its effect on pulmonary function. Anaesthesia 2001;56:352–356.
38. Neal JM, Moore JM, Kopacz DJ, Liu SS, Kramer DJ, Plorde JJ: Quantitative analysis of respiratory, motor, and sensory function after supraclavicular block. Anesth Analg 1998;86:1239–1244.
39. Renes SH, Spoormans HH, Gielen MJ, Rettig HC, Geffen GJ van: Hemidiaphragmatic paresis can be avoided in ultrasound-guided supraclavicular brachial plexus block. Reg Anesth Pain Med 2009;34: 595–599.
40. Rodríguez J, Bárcena M, Rodríguez V, Aneiros F, Alvarez J: Infraclavicular brachial plexus block effects on respiratory function and extent of the block. Reg Anesth Pain Med 1998;23:564–568.
41. Dullenkopf A, Blumenthal S, Theodorou P, Roos J, Perschak H, Borgeat A: Diaphragmatic excursion and respiratory function after the modified Raj technique of the infraclavicular plexus block. Reg Anesth Pain Med 2004;29:110–114.

42. Gentili ME, Deleuze A, Estèbe J-P, Lebourg M, Ecoffey C: Severe respiratory failure after infraclavicular block with 0.75% ropivacaine: a case report. J Clin Anesth 2002;14:459–461.

43. Yang CW, Jung SM, Kwon HU, Kang PS, Cho CK, Choi HJ: Transient hemidiaphragmatic paresis after ultrasound-guided lateral sagittal infraclavicular block. J Clin Anesth 2013;25:496–498.

44. Bigeleisen PE: Anatomical variations of the phrenic nerve and its clinical implication for supraclavicular block. Br J Anaesth 2003; 91:916–917.

45. Verelst P, Zundert A van: Respiratory impact of analgesic strategies for shoulder surgery. Reg Anesth Pain Med 2013;38:50–53.

46. Martínez J, Sala-Blanch X, Ramos I, Gomar C: Combined infraclavicular plexus block with suprascapular nerve block for humeral head surgery in a patient with respiratory failure: an alternative approach. Anesthesiology 2003;98:784–785.

47. Ilfeld BM, Morey TE, Wright TW, Chidgey LK, Enneking FK: Continuous interscalene brachial plexus block for postoperative pain control at home: a randomized, double-blinded, placebo-controlled study. Anesth. Analg. 2003; 96:1089–1095, table of contents

48. Mariano ER, Afra R, Loland VJ, et al: Continuous interscalene brachial plexus block via an ultrasound-guided posterior approach: a randomized, triple-masked, placebo-controlled study. Anesth Analg 2009;108:1688–1694.

49. Souron V, Reiland Y, Delaunay L: Pleural effusion and chest pain after continuous interscalene brachial plexus block. Reg Anesth Pain Med 2003;28:535–538.

50. Sardesai AM, Chakrabarti AJ, Denny NM: Lower lobe collapse during continuous interscalene brachial plexus local anesthesia at home. Reg Anesth Pain Med 2004;29:65–68.

51. Ilfeld BM, Morey TE, Wright TW, Chidgey LK, Enneking FK: Interscalene perineural ropivacaine infusion: a comparison of two dosing regimens for postoperative analgesia. Reg Anesth Pain Med 2004;29: 9–16.

52. Borgeat A, Perschak H, Bird P, Hodler J, Gerber C: Patient-controlled interscalene analgesia with ropivacaine 0.2% versus patient-controlled intravenous analgesia after major shoulder surgery: effects on diaphragmatic and respiratory function. Anesthesiology 2000;92: 102–108.

53. Ilfeld BM, Le LT, Ramjohn J, et al: The effects of local anesthetic concentration and dose on continuous infraclavicular nerve blocks: a multicenter, randomized, observer-masked, controlled study. Anesth Analg 2009;108:345–350.

54. Maurer K, Ekatodramis G, Hodler J, Rentsch K, Perschak H, Borgeat A: Bilateral continuous interscalene block of brachial plexus for analgesia after bilateral shoulder arthroplasty. Anesthesiology 2002;96:762–764.

55. Salinas FV: Location, location, location: Continuous peripheral nerve blocks and stimulating catheters. Reg Anesth Pain Med 2003;28:79–82.

56. Souron V, Reiland Y, Traverse A De, Delaunay L, Lafosse L: Interpleural migration of an interscalene catheter. Anesth Analg 2003;97:1200–1201.

57. Faust A, Fournier R, Hagon O, Hoffmeyer P, Gamulin Z: Partial sensory and motor deficit of ipsilateral lower limb after continuous interscalene brachial plexus block. Anesth Analg 2006;102:288–290.

58. Osinowo OA, Zahrani M, Softah A: Effect of intercostal nerve block with 0.5% bupivacaine on peak expiratory flow rate and arterial oxygen saturation in rib fractures. J Trauma 2004;56:345–347.

59. Truitt MS, Murry J, Amos J, et al: Continuous intercostal nerve blockade for rib fractures: ready for primetime? J Trauma 2011;71:1548–1552; discussion 1552.

60. Karmakar MK, Critchley LAH, Ho AM-H, Gin T, Lee TW, Yim APC: Continuous thoracic paravertebral infusion of bupivacaine for pain management in patients with multiple fractured ribs. Chest 2003;123: 424–431.

61. Murata H, Salviz EA, Chen S, Vandepitte C, Hadzic A: Case report: ultrasound-guided continuous thoracic paravertebral block for outpatient acute pain management of multilevel unilateral rib fractures. Anesth Analg 2013;116:255–257.

62. Buckley M, Edwards H, Buckenmaier CC 3rd, Plunkett AR: Continuous thoracic paravertebral nerve block in a working anesthesia resident-when opioids are not an option. Mil Med 2011;176:578–580.

63. Richardson J, Sabanathan S, Shah R: Post-thoracotomy spirometric lung function: the effect of analgesia. A review. J Cardiovasc Surg (Torino) 1999;40:445–456.

64. Davies RG, Myles PS, Graham JM: A comparison of the analgesic efficacy and side-effects of paravertebral vs epidural blockade for thoracotomy—a systematic review and meta-analysis of randomized trials. Br J Anaesth 2006;96:418–426.

65. Richardson J, Sabanathan S, Jones J, Shah RD, Cheema S, Mearns AJ: A prospective, randomized comparison of preoperative and continuous balanced epidural or paravertebral bupivacaine on post-thoracotomy pain, pulmonary function and stress responses. Br J Anaesth 1999;83: 387–392.

66. Thomas PW, Sanders DJ, Berrisford RG: Pulmonary haemorrhage after percutaneous paravertebral block. Br J Anaesth 1999; 83:668–669.

67. Fine PG, Bubela C: Chylothorax following celiac plexus block. Anesthesiology 1985;63:454–456.

68. Shanti CM, Carlin AM, Tyburski JG: Incidence of pneumothorax from intercostal nerve block for analgesia in rib fractures. J Trauma 2001;51: 536–539.

69. Naja Z, Lönnqvist PA: Somatic paravertebral nerve blockade. Incidence of failed block and complications. Anaesthesia 2001;56:1184–1188.

70. Borgeat A, Ekatodramis G, Kalberer F, Benz C: Acute and nonacute complications associated with interscalene block and shoulder surgery: a prospective study. Anesthesiology 2001;95:875–880.

71. Brown DL, Cahill DR, Bridenbaugh LD: Supraclavicular nerve block: anatomic analysis of a method to prevent pneumothorax. Anesth Analg 1993;76:530–534.

72. Bhatia A, Lai J, Chan VWS, Brull R: Case report: pneumothorax as a complication of the ultrasound-guided supraclavicular approach for brachial plexus block. Anesth Analg 2010;111:817–819.

73. Klaastad Ø, Smith H-J, Smedby O, et al: A novel infraclavicular brachial plexus block: the lateral and sagittal technique, developed by magnetic resonance imaging studies. Anesth Analg 2004;98:252–256, table of contents.

74. Chan VWS, Perlas A, Rawson R, Odukoya O: Ultrasound-guided supraclavicular brachial plexus block. Anesth Analg 2003;97:1514–1517.

75. Perlas A, Lobo G, Lo N, Brull R, Chan VWS, Karkhanis R: Ultrasound-guided supraclavicular block: outcome of 510 consecutive cases. Reg Anesth Pain Med 2009;34:171–176.

76. Gauss A, Tugtekin I, Georgieff M, Dinse-Lambracht A, Keipke D, Gorsewski G: Incidence of clinically symptomatic pneumothorax in ultrasound-guided infraclavicular and supraclavicular brachial plexus block. Anaesthesia 2014;69:327–336.

77. Fenoglio C, Boicelli CA, Ottone M, Addario C, Chiari P, Viale M: Protective effect of procaine hydrochloride on cisplatin-induced alterations in rat kidney. Anticancer Drugs 2002;13:1043–1054.

78. Navar LG: Renal autoregulation: perspectives from whole kidney and single nephron studies. Am J Physiol 1978;234:F357–F370.

79. Suleiman MY, Passannante AN, Onder RL, Greene-Helms WF, Perretta SG: Alteration of renal blood flow during epidural anesthesia in normal subjects. Anesth Analg 1997;84:1076–1080.

80. Rooke GA, Freund PR, Jacobson AF: Hemodynamic response and change in organ blood volume during spinal anesthesia in elderly men with cardiac disease. Anesth Analg 1997;85:99–105.

81. Sivarajan M, Amory DW, Lindbloom LE, Schwettmann RS: Systemic and regional blood-flow changes during spinal anesthesia in the rhesus monkey. Anesthesiology 1975;43:78–88.

82. Hopf HB, Schlaghecke R, Peters J: Sympathetic neural blockade by thoracic epidural anesthesia suppresses renin release in response to arterial hypotension. Anesthesiology 1994;80:992–999; discussion 27A–28A.

83. Hadimioglu N, Ulugol H, Akbas H, Coskunfirat N, Ertug Z, Dinckan A: Combination of epidural anesthesia and general anesthesia attenuates stress response to renal transplantation surgery. Transplant Proc 2012;44: 2949–2954.

84. Ricaurte L, Vargas J, Lozano E, Díaz L, Organ Transplant Group: Anesthesia and kidney transplantation. Transplant Proc 2013;45:1386–1391.

85. Sener M, Torgay A, Akpek E, et al: Regional versus general anesthesia for donor nephrectomy: effects on graft function. Transplant Proc 2004; 36:2954–2958.

86. Gould DB, Aldrete JA: Bupivacaine cardiotoxicity in a patient with renal failure. Acta Anaesthesiol Scand 1983; 27:18–21.

87. Lucas LF, Tsueda K: Cardiovascular depression after brachial plexus block in two diabetic patients with renal failure. Anesthesiology 1990;73: 1032–1035.

88. Coyle DE, Denson DD, Thompson GA, Myers JA, Arthur GR, Bridenbaugh PO: The influence of lactic acid on the serum protein binding of bupivacaine: species differences. Anesthesiology 1984;61:127–133.

89. Avery P, Redon D, Schaenzer G, Rusy B: The influence of serum potassium on the cerebral and cardiac toxicity of bupivacaine and lidocaine. Anesthesiology 1984;61:134–138.

90. Pere P, Salonen M, Jokinen M, Rosenberg PH, Neuvonen PJ, Haasio J: Pharmacokinetics of ropivacaine in uremic and nonuremic patients after axillary brachial plexus block. Anesth Analg 2003;96:563–569, table of contents.

91. Rodríguez J, Quintela O, López-Rivadulla M, Bárcena M, Diz C, Alvarez J: High doses of mepivacaine for brachial plexus block in patients with end-stage chronic renal failure. A pilot study. Eur J Anaesthesiol 2001;18:171–176.

92. Mostert JW, Evers JL, Hobika GH, Moore RH, Kenny GM, Murphy GP: The haemodynamic response to chronic renal failure as studied in the azotaemic state. Br J Anaesth 1970;42:397–411.

93. Vasson MP, Baguet JC, Arveiller MR, Bargnoux PJ, Giroud JP, Raichvarg D: Serum and urinary alpha-1 acid glycoprotein in chronic renal failure. Nephron 1993;65:299–303.

94. Mather LE, Thomas J: Bupivacaine binding to plasma protein fractions. J Pharm Pharmacol 1978;30:653–654.

95. Vaziri ND, Saiki JK, Hughes W: Clearance of lidocaine by hemodialysis. South Med J 1979;72:1567–1568.

96. Shih Y-H, Chen C-H, Wang Y-M, Liu K: Successful reversal of bupivacaine and lidocaine-induced severe junctional bradycardia by lipid emulsion following infraclavicular brachial plexus block in a uremic patient. Acta Anaesthesiol Taiwan 2011;49:72–74.

97. Lange DB, Schwartz D, DaRoza G, Gair R: Use of intravenous lipid emulsion to reverse central nervous system toxicity of an iatrogenic local anesthetic overdose in a patient on peritoneal dialysis. Ann Pharmacother 2012;46:e37.

98. Rice AS, Pither CE, Tucker GT: Plasma concentrations of bupivacaine after supraclavicular brachial plexus blockade in patients with chronic renal failure. Anaesthesia 1991;46:354–357.

99. McEllistrem RF, Schell J, O'Malley K, O'Toole D, Cunningham AJ: Interscalene brachial plexus blockade with lidocaine in chronic renal failure-a pharmacokinetic study. Can J Anaesth 1989;36:59–63.

100. Orko R, Pitkänen M, Rosenberg PH: Subarachnoid anaesthesia with 0.75% bupivacaine in patients with chronic renal failure. Br J Anaesth 1986;58:605–609.

101. Gawaz MP, Dobos G, Späth M, Schollmeyer P, Gurland HJ, Mujais SK: Impaired function of platelet membrane glycoprotein IIb-IIIa in end-stage renal disease. J Am Soc Nephrol 1994;5:36–46.

102. Grejda S, Ellis K, Arino P: Paraplegia following spinal anesthesia in a patient with chronic renal failure. Reg Anesth 1989;14:155–157.

103. Boccardo P, Remuzzi G, Galbusera M: Platelet dysfunction in renal failure. Semin Thromb Hemost 2004;30:579–589.

104. Rose M, Ness TJ: Hypoxia following interscalene block. Reg Anesth Pain Med 2002;27:94–96.

105. Alsalti RA, el-Dawlatly AA, al-Salman M, et al: Arteriovenous fistula in chronic renal failure patients: comparison between three different anesthetic techniques. Middle East J Anaesthesiol 1999;15:305–314.

106. Solomonson MD, Johnson ME, Ilstrup D: Risk factors in patients having surgery to create an arteriovenous fistula. Anesth Analg 1994;79:694–700.

107. Elsharawy MA, Al-Metwalli R: Does regional anesthesia influence early outcome of upper arm arteriovenous fistula? Saudi J Kidney Dis Transpl 2010;21:1048–1052.

108. Mouquet C, Bitker MO, Bailliart O, et al: Anesthesia for creation of a forearm fistula in patients with endstage renal failure. Anesthesiology 1989;70:909–914.

109. Malinzak EB, Gan TJ: Regional anesthesia for vascular access surgery. Anesth Analg 2009;109:976–980.

110. Schenk WG: Improving dialysis access: regional anesthesia improves arteriovenous fistula prevalence. Am Surg 2010;76:938–942.

111. Sahin L, Gul R, Mizrak A, et al: Ultrasound-guided infraclavicular brachial plexus block enhances postoperative blood flow in arteriovenous fistulas. J Vasc Surg 2011;54:749–753.

112. Rahimzadeh P, Safari S, Faiz SHR, Alavian SM: Anesthesia for patients with liver disease. Hepat Mon 2014;14:e19881.

113. Tucker GT, Mather LE: Clinical pharmacokinetics of local anaesthetics. Clin Pharmacokinet 1979;4:241–278.

114. Tucker GT, Mather LE: Pharmacology of local anaesthetic agents. Pharmacokinetics of local anaesthetic agents. Br J Anaesth 1975;47suppl: 213–224.

115. Rosenberg PH, Veering BT, Urmey WF: Maximum recommended doses of local anesthetics: a multifactorial concept. Reg Anesth Pain Med 2004; 29:564–575; discussion 524.

116. Magorian T, Wood P, Caldwell J, et al: The pharmacokinetics and neuromuscular effects of rocuronium bromide in patients with liver disease. Anesth Analg 1995;80:754–759.

117. Servin F, Cockshott ID, Farinotti R, Haberer JP, Winckler C, Desmonts JM: Pharmacokinetics of propofol infusions in patients with cirrhosis. Br J Anaesth 1990;65:177–183.

118. Jokinen MJ, Neuvonen PJ, Lindgren L, et al: Pharmacokinetics of ropivacaine in patients with chronic end-stage liver disease. Anesthesiology 2007;106:43–55.

119. Barry M, Keeling PW, Weir D, Feely J: Severity of cirrhosis and the relationship of alpha 1-acid glycoprotein concentration to plasma protein binding of lidocaine. Clin Pharmacol Ther 1990;47:366–370.

120. Thomson PD, Melmon KL, Richardson JA, et al: Lidocaine pharmacokinetics in advanced heart failure, liver disease, and renal failure in humans. Ann Intern Med 1973;78:499–508.

121. Lauprecht A-E, Wenger FA, El Fadil O, Walz MK, Groeben H: Levobupivacaine plasma concentrations following major liver resection. J Anesth 2011;25:369–375.

122. Naguib M, Magboul MM, Samarkandi AH, Attia M: Adverse effects and drug interactions associated with local and regional anaesthesia. Drug Saf 1998;18:221–250.

123. Reidenberg MM, James M, Dring LG: The rate of procaine hydrolysis in serum of normal subjects and diseased patients. Clin Pharmacol Ther 1972;13:279–284.

124. Calvo R, Carlos R, Erill S: Effects of disease and acetazolamide on procaine hydrolysis by red blood cell enzymes. Clin Pharmacol Ther 1980;27:179–183.

125. Lautt WW, Greenway CV: Conceptual review of the hepatic vascular bed. Hepatology 1987;7:952–963.

126. Lautt WW, Macedo MP: Hepatic circulation and toxicology. Drug Metab Rev 1997;29:369–395.

127. Gelman S: General anesthesia and hepatic circulation. Can J Physiol Pharmacol 1987;65:1762–1779.

128. Greitz T, Andreen M, Irestedt L: Haemodynamics and oxygen consumption in the dog during high epidural block with special reference to the splanchnic region. Acta Anaesthesiol Scand 1983;27:211–217.

129. Vagts DA, Iber T, Puccini M, et al: The effects of thoracic epidural anesthesia on hepatic perfusion and oxygenation in healthy pigs during general anesthesia and surgical stress. Anesth Analg 2003;97:1824–1832.

130. Kelly DA, Tuddenham EG: Haemostatic problems in liver disease. Gut 1986;27:339–349.

131. Shami VM, Caldwell SH, Hespenheide EE, Arseneau KO, Bickston SJ, Macik BG: Recombinant activated factor VII for coagulopathy in fulminant hepatic failure compared with conventional therapy. Liver Transpl 2003;9:138–143.

132. Dzik WH: Predicting hemorrhage using preoperative coagulation screening assays. Curr Hematol Rep 2004;3:324–330.

133. Horlocker TT, Wedel DJ, Rowlingson JC, et al: Regional anesthesia in the patient receiving antithrombotic or thrombolytic therapy: American Society of Regional Anesthesia and Pain Medicine Evidence-Based Guidelines (Third Edition). Reg Anesth Pain Med 2010;35:64–101.

134. Tzimas P, Prout J, Papadopoulos G, Mallett SV: Epidural anaesthesia and analgesia for liver resection. Anaesthesia 2013;68:628–635.

135. Coursin DB, Connery LE, Ketzler JT: Perioperative diabetic and hyperglycemic management issues. Crit Care Med 2004;32:S116–S125.

136. Greene DA, Stevens MJ, Feldman EL: Diabetic neuropathy: scope of the syndrome. Am J Med 1999;107:2S–8S.

137. Downs CA, Faulkner MS: Toxic stress, inflammation and symptomatology of chronic complications in diabetes. World J Diabetes 2015;6: 554–565.

138. Kalichman MW, Calcutt NA: Local anesthetic-induced conduction block and nerve fiber injury in streptozotocin-diabetic rats. Anesthesiology 1992;77:941–947.

139. Al-Nasser B: Toxic effects of epidural analgesia with ropivacaine 0.2% in a diabetic patient. J Clin Anesth 2004;16:220–223.

140. Cuvillon P, Reubrecht V, Zoric L, et al: Comparison of subgluteal sciatic nerve block duration in type 2 diabetic and non-diabetic patients. Br J Anaesth 2013;110:823–830.

141. Sertoz N, Deniz MN, Ayanoglu HO: Relationship between glycosylated hemoglobin level and sciatic nerve block performance in diabetic patients. Foot Ankle Int 2013;34:85–90.

142. Kroin JS, Buvanendran A, Tuman KJ, Kerns JM: Effect of acute versus continuous glycemic control on duration of local anesthetic sciatic nerve block in diabetic rats. Reg Anesth Pain Med 2012;37:595–600.

143. Gronwald C, Vowinkel T, Hahnenkamp K: Regional anesthetic procedures in immunosuppressed patients: risk of infection. Curr Opin Anaesthesiol 2011;24:698–704.

144. Sites BD, Gallagher J, Sparks M: Ultrasound-guided popliteal block demonstrates an atypical motor response to nerve stimulation in 2 patients with diabetes mellitus. Reg Anesth Pain Med 2003;28:479–482.

145. Keyl C, Held T, Albiez G, Schmack A, Wiesenack C: Increased electrical nerve stimulation threshold of the sciatic nerve in patients with diabetic foot gangrene: a prospective parallel cohort study. Eur J Anaesthesiol 2013;30:435–440.

146. Partanen J, Niskanen L, Lehtinen J, Mervaala E, Siitonen O, Uusitupa M: Natural history of peripheral neuropathy in patients with non-insulin-dependent diabetes mellitus. N Engl J Med 1995;333:89–94.

147. Krinsley JS: Effect of an intensive glucose management protocol on the mortality of critically ill adult patients. Mayo Clin Proc 2004;79: 992–1000.

148. Falciglia M, Freyberg RW, Almenoff PL, D'Alessio DA, Render ML: Hyperglycemia-related mortality in critically ill patients varies with admission diagnosis. Crit Care Med 2009;37:3001–3009.

149. Sung J, Bochicchio GV, Joshi M, Bochicchio K, Tracy K, Scalea TM: Admission hyperglycemia is predictive of outcome in critically ill trauma patients. J Trauma 2005;59:80–83.

150. Jensen CH, Berthelsen P, Kühl C, Kehlet H: Effect of epidural analgesia on glucose tolerance during surgery. Acta Anaesthesiol Scand 1980;24: 472–474.

151. Houghton A, Hickey JB, Ross SA, Dupre J: Glucose tolerance during anaesthesia and surgery. Comparison of general and extradural anaesthesia. Br J Anaesth 1978;50:495–499.

152. Møller IW, Hjortsø E, Krantz T, Wandall E, Kehlet H: The modifying effect of spinal anaesthesia on intra- and postoperative adrenocortical and hyperglycaemic response to surgery. Acta Anaesthesiol Scand 1984;28:266–269.

153. Barker JP, Robinson PN, Vafidis GC, Hart GR, Sapsed-Byrne S, Hall GM: Local analgesia prevents the cortisol and glycaemic responses to cataract surgery. Br J Anaesth 1990;64:442–445.

154. Vogt G, Heiden M, Lösche CC, Lipfert P: A preoperative retrobulbar block in patients undergoing scleral buckling reduces pain, endogenous stress response, and improves vigilance. Reg Anesth Pain Med 2003;28: 521–527.

155. Milosavljevic SB, Pavlovic AP, Trpkovic SV, Ilić AN, Sekulic AD: Influence of spinal and general anesthesia on the metabolic, hormonal, and hemodynamic response in elective surgical patients. Med Sci Monit 2014;20:1833–1840.

156. Camu F: Carbohydrate intolerance during halothane anesthesia in dogs. Acta Anaesthesiol Belg 1973;24:177–188.

157. Richardson J, Jones J, Atkinson R: The effect of thoracic paravertebral blockade on intercostal somatosensory evoked potentials. Anesth Analg 1998;87:373–376.

158. Mendell JR, Sahenk Z: Clinical practice. Painful sensory neuropathy. N Engl J Med 2003;348:1243–1255.

159. Duyff RF, Bosch J Van den, Laman DM, Loon BJ van, Linssen WH: Neuromuscular findings in thyroid dysfunction: a prospective clinical and electrodiagnostic study. J Neurol Neurosurg Psychiatr 2000;68: 750–755.

160. Misiunas A, Niepomniszcze H, Ravera B, Faraj G, Faure E: Peripheral neuropathy in subclinical hypothyroidism. Thyroid 1995;5:283–286.

161. Khedr EM, El Toony LF, Tarkhan MN, Abdella G: Peripheral and central nervous system alterations in hypothyroidism: electrophysiological findings. Neuropsychobiology 2000;41:88–94.

162. Shirabe T, Tawara S, Terao A, Araki S: Myxoedematous polyneuropathy: a light and electron microscopic study of the peripheral nerve and muscle. J Neurol Neurosurg Psychiatr 1975;38:241–247.

163. Upton AR, McComas AJ: The double crush in nerve entrapment syndromes. Lancet 1973;2:359–362.

164. Hebl JR, Horlocker TT, Pritchard DJ: Diffuse brachial plexopathy after interscalene blockade in a patient receiving cisplatin chemotherapy: the pharmacologic double crush syndrome. Anesth Analg 2001;92:249–251.

165. Schenker M, Kraftsik R, Glauser L, Kuntzer T, Bogousslavsky J, Barakat-Walter I: Thyroid hormone reduces the loss of axotomized sensory neurons in dorsal root ganglia after sciatic nerve transection in adult rat. Exp Neurol 2003;184:225–236.

166. Norcross-Nechay K, Richards GE, Cavallo A: Evoked potentials show early and delayed abnormalities in children with congenital hypothyroidism. Neuropediatrics 1989;20:158–163.

167. World Health Organization. Obesity and overweight. Updated January 2015. http://www.who.int/mediacentre/factsheets/fs311/en/.

168. Centers for Disease Control and Prevention. Obesity and overweight for professionals: data and statistics; facts. Updated September 14, 2015. http://www.cdc.gov/obesity/data/facts.html.

169. Broadbent CR, Maxwell WB, Ferrie R, Wilson DJ, Gawne-Cain M, Russell R: Ability of anaesthetists to identify a marked lumbar interspace. Anaesthesia 2000;55:1122–1126.

170. Nielsen KC, Guller U, Steele SM, Klein SM, Greengrass RA, Pietrobon R: Influence of obesity on surgical regional anesthesia in the ambulatory setting: an analysis of 9,038 blocks. Anesthesiology 2005;102:181–187.

171. Hanouz J-L, Grandin W, Lesage A, Oriot G, Bonnieux D, Gérard J-L: Multiple injection axillary brachial plexus block: influence of obesity on failure rate and incidence of acute complications. Anesth Analg 2010; 111:230–233.

172. Pham-Dang C, Meunier JF, Poirier P, et al: A new axillary approach for continuous brachial plexus block. A clinical and anatomic study. Anesth Analg 1995;81:686–693.

173. Tan WS, Spigos DG: Sciatic nerve block under fluoroscopic guidance. Cardiovasc Intervent Radiol 1986; 9:59–60.

174. Eidelman A, Shulman MS, Novak GM: Fluoroscopic imaging for technically difficult spinal anesthesia. J Clin Anesth 2005;17:69–71.

175. Brodsky JB, Mariano ER: Regional anaesthesia in the obese patient: lost landmarks and evolving ultrasound guidance. Best Pract Res Clin Anaesthesiol 2011;25:61–72.

176. Al-Nasser B: Review of interscalene block for postoperative analgesia after shoulder surgery in obese patients. Acta Anaesthesiol Taiwan 2012; 50:29–34.

177. Marhofer P, Pilz-Lubsczyk B, Lönnqvist P-A, Fleischmann E: Ultrasound-guided peripheral regional anaesthesia: a feasibility study in obese versus normal-weight women. Int J Obes (Lond) 2014;38:451–455.

178. Wallace DH, Currie JM, Gilstrap LC, Santos R: Indirect sonographic guidance for epidural anesthesia in obese pregnant patients. Reg Anesth 1992;17:233–236.

179. Grau T, Leipold RW, Horter J, Conradi R, Martin E, Motsch J: The lumbar epidural space in pregnancy: visualization by ultrasonography. Br J Anaesth 2001;86:798–804.

180. Chin KJ, Perlas A, Chan V, Brown-Shreves D, Koshkin A, Vaishnav V: Ultrasound imaging facilitates spinal anesthesia in adults with difficult surface anatomic landmarks. Anesthesiology 2011;115:94–101.

181. McCulloch WJ, Littlewood DG: Influence of obesity on spinal analgesia with isobaric 0.5% bupivacaine. Br J Anaesth 1986;58:610–614.

182. Reyes M, Pan PH: Very low-dose spinal anesthesia for cesarean section in a morbidly obese preeclamptic patient and its potential implications. Int J Obstet Anesth 2004;13:99–102.

183. Norris MC: Patient variables and the subarachnoid spread of hyperbaric bupivacaine in the term parturient. Anesthesiology 1990;72:478–482.

184. Greene NM: Distribution of local anesthetic solutions within the subarachnoid space. Anesth Analg 1985;64:715–730.

185. Stienstra R, Greene NM: Factors affecting the subarachnoid spread of local anesthetic solutions. Reg Anesth 1991;16:1–6.

186. Kim WH, Lee JH, Ko JS, et al: The effect of body mass index on spinal anaesthesia for total knee replacement arthroplasty: a dose-response study. Anaesth Intensive Care 2012;40:410–416.

CHAPTER 49

Regional Anesthesia in the Patient with Preexisting Neurologic Disease

Adam K. Jacob, Sandra L. Kopp, and James R. Hebl

INTRODUCTION

Preexisting disorders of the peripheral nervous system, central nervous system, and spinal canal present a unique challenge to both patients and anesthesiologists who desire to use regional anesthetic techniques. Because each of these clinical conditions involves compromise to neural structures, the concern is that further insult from surgical (eg, intraoperative stretch or compression, tourniquet ischemia, hemorrhage) or anesthetic (eg, mechanical trauma, vasoconstrictor-induced ischemia, local anesthetic toxicity) causes may result in new or worsening postoperative neurologic deficits.

Regardless of the underlying etiology, the presence of chronic neural compromise secondary to mechanical (eg, spinal stenosis or compressive radiculopathy), ischemic (eg, peripheral vascular disease), toxic (eg, vincristine or cisplatin chemotherapy), metabolic (eg, diabetes mellitus), or autoimmune (eg, multiple sclerosis) derangements may place patients at increased risk of further neurologic injury.[1-3] Upton and McComas[1] were the first to describe the "double-crush phenomenon," which suggests that patients with preexisting neural compromise may be more susceptible to injury at another site when exposed to a secondary insult (Figure 49–1). Secondary insults may include a variety of acute surgical or anesthetic risk factors, including those of regional anesthetic techniques. Osterman[2] emphasized that not only are two low-grade insults along a peripheral nerve trunk worse than just one at a single site, but that the damage of the dual injury far exceeds the expected additive damage caused by each isolated insult. It may be further postulated that the second insult need not be along the peripheral nerve trunk itself, but rather at any point along the neural transmission pathway. Therefore, the performance of peripheral or neuraxial regional techniques in patients with preexisting neurologic disorders may place them at increased risk of the double-crush phenomenon.

Unfortunately, the data available regarding any association of pre-existing neurologic disease and post-regional anesthesia dysfunction often conflicting in terms of outcomes and conclusions. As a result, definitive recommendations can rarely be made from the existing scientific literature. However, the following discussion provides a comprehensive review of the available literature on the topic so that patients and clinicians can make an informed decision regarding the potential neurologic risk of performing regional anesthesia in the presence of preexisting neurologic disorders.

PERIPHERAL NERVOUS SYSTEM DISORDERS

The peripheral nervous system is composed of numerous cell types that serve diverse sensory, motor, and autonomic functions. Signs and symptoms of impaired function depend on the distribution and severity of the injury, in addition to the specific element of the nerve that is affected. More than 100 peripheral neuropathies have been identified, each with its own pathophysiology, symptoms, and prognosis.[4]

Hereditary Peripheral Neuropathy

Inherited neuropathies represent a heterogeneous group of diseases that often share the features of an insidious onset and indolent course over years to decades. A wide range of genotypes results in phenotypes ranging from mild symptoms and subclinical disease to severe, debilitating conditions. The most common inherited neuropathies are a group of disorders collectively referred to as Charcot–Marie–Tooth (CMT) disease. CMT affects approximately 1 in 2500 people, often beginning in childhood or adolescence.[5] CMT neuropathies are caused

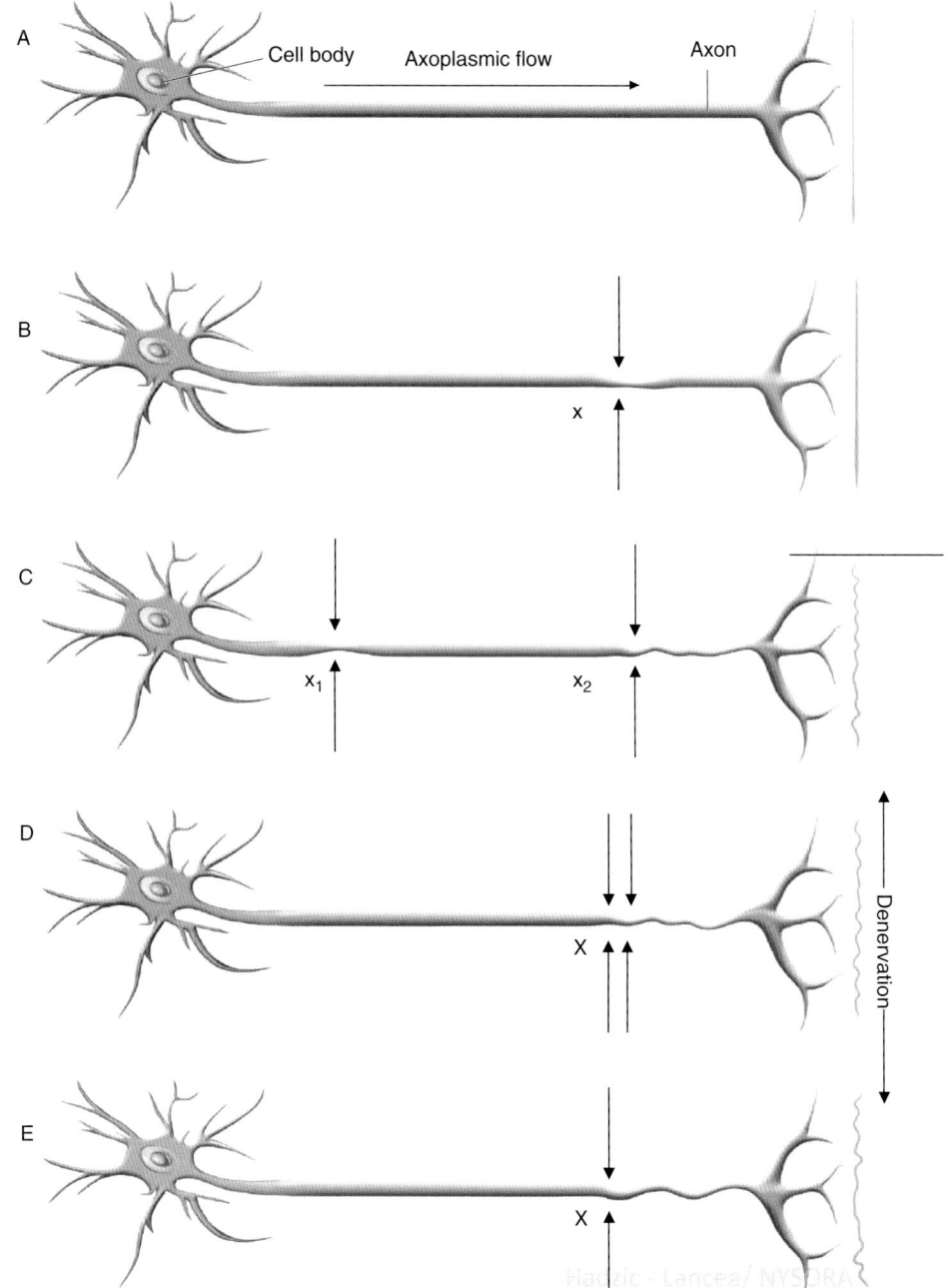

FIGURE 49-1. Neural lesions resulting in denervation. Axoplasmic flow is indicated by the degree of shading. Complete loss of axoplasmic flow results in denervation (C, D, E). **A:** Normal neuron. **B:** Mild neuronal injury at a single site (x) is insufficient to cause denervation distal to the insult. **C:** Mild neuronal injury at two separate sites (x₁ and x₂) may cause distal denervation (ie, "double crush"). **D:** Severe neuronal injury at a single site (X) may also cause distal denervation. **E:** Axon with a diffuse, preexisting underlying disease process (toxic, metabolic, ischemic) may have impaired axonal flow throughout the neuron, which may or may not be symptomatic but predisposes the axon to distal denervation following a single minor neural insult at x (ie, "double crush"). (Reproduced with permission from Mayo Foundation for Medical Education and Research.)

from mutations in more than 30 genes responsible for manufacturing neurons or the myelin sheath.[6] Typical signs and symptoms include extreme motor weakness and muscle wasting within the distal lower extremities and feet, gait abnormalities, loss of tendon reflexes, and numbness within the lower limbs.

The reported use of peripheral[7,8] or central[9–12] regional anesthetic techniques in patients with CMT has been limited to small case series and anecdotal case reports. All patients made

uneventful recoveries without worsening of their neurologic conditions. Of note, two cases involving single-injection regional techniques (epidural anesthesia using 18 mL 0.75% ropivacaine[10] and supraclavicular analgesia using 30 mL 0.5% bupivacaine[7]) reported a prolonged effect (12 hours and 30 hours, respectively) of the regional technique compared to the anticipated duration. In both cases, the use of higher local anesthetic concentrations may have contributed to the delayed recovery.

Hereditary neuropathy with liability to pressure palsy (HNPP) is another rare inherited demyelinating peripheral neuropathy in which individuals suffer from repeated motor and sensory neuropathies following brief nerve compression or mild trauma (ie, pressure palsies). First described in the early 1990s, HNPP has been linked to a mutation on the PMP-22 gene resulting in reduced myelin production. Evidence of the use of a regional technique in the setting of HNPP has been limited to a single case report. Lepski and Alderson[13] reported the successful use of an epidural for labor analgesia in a 24-year-old parturient with HNPP. The patient made an uneventful recovery without a worsening of her neurologic condition.

Based upon the lack of clinical evidence, definitive recommendations cannot be made about the safety and use of regional anesthesia in patients with preexisting inherited peripheral neuropathies. However, isolated case reports suggest that peripheral and central regional techniques *may* be used without worsening a patient's stable neurologic condition. However, caution should be used to minimize other surgical (eg, tourniquet use) and anesthetic (eg, reduced concentration or dose of local anesthetic) risk factors for perioperative nerve injury when considering the use of regional anesthesia within this patient population.

Acquired Peripheral Neuropathy
Diabetic Polyneuropathy

The increasing prevalence of diabetes mellitus (DM) and its associated comorbidities will likely translate to a larger number of diabetic patients presenting for surgery. Despite the clinical benefits and widespread use of regional anesthesia (peripheral and neuraxial blockade), there remains concern regarding its use in patients with DM.[14–17] It has been suggested that patients with a history of chronic neural compromise secondary to metabolic conditions such as diabetes may be at an increased risk of worsening neurologic injury following neuraxial or peripheral nerve blockade.[16–18]

Diabetes mellitus is currently the most common cause of systemic polyneuropathy. There are several types of neuropathy associated with DM, but distal symmetric sensorimotor polyneuropathy is the most common form and is generally synonymous with the term *diabetic polyneuropathy* (DPN). The frequency of DPN ranges from 4%–8% at the time of diagnosis to more than 50% in patients with long-standing diabetes. Despite the fact that patients may be asymptomatic, nearly all will have evidence of abnormal nerve conduction.[19,20] Furthermore, it is relatively common for patients to present for surgery with either undiagnosed diabetes mellitus or known diabetes with uncontrolled hyperglycemia.[21]

The pathophysiology of DPN is poorly understood and likely multifactorial. Early symptoms, such as numbness, pain, and autonomic dysfunction, are caused by damage to small nerve fibers, which occurs before damage to large fibers becomes apparent.[22] There is pathophysiologic evidence of abnormalities in both large and small neural blood vessels, ultimately contributing to multifocal fiber loss. Axonal degeneration is the most prominent feature of DPN and occurs secondary to the reduced delivery of essential nutrients and other components (oxygen, blood, adenosine triphosphate, glucose) to the axon. Proposed mechanisms include (1) sorbitol deposition in the nerve due to glucose accumulation; (2) local tissue ischemia in sensory and autonomic fibers secondary to endoneurial hypoxia; (3) abnormal tissue repair mechanisms caused by excess glucose; and (4) mitochondrial dysfunction within the dorsal root ganglia.[23–26]

Currently, there is an abundance of animal data that suggests diabetic nerves may have an increased risk of neurologic injury following regional anesthesia compared to nondiabetic nerves.[27–29] Kalichman and Calcutt[18] were the first to hypothesize that diabetic nerve fibers may be more susceptible to local anesthetic neurotoxicity for two reasons: (1) the nerve is already stressed due to chronic ischemic hypoxia; and (2) the nerves are exposed to larger concentrations of local anesthetics due to decreased perineural blood flow. More recently, these findings have been supported with both animal and clinical data. Lirk and colleagues[30] used Zucker diabetic fatty rats exposed to hyperglycemia to demonstrate that although the overall neuronal survival difference was low, in vitro local anesthetic neurotoxicity was more pronounced in neurons from diabetic animals. The authors also reported that preexisting subclinical neuropathy led to substantial prolongation of the block duration in vivo. Kroin and colleagues[28] also reported that the duration of sciatic nerve block with lidocaine 1% or ropivacaine 0.5% was longer in streptozotocin-induced diabetic rats compared with nondiabetic rats and that block duration correlated with nerve fiber degeneration. In a subsequent study, the same authors also concluded that, with continuous glycemic control, diabetic rats had a block duration that was similar to nondiabetic rats and 40 minutes shorter than in diabetic rats without glycemic control.[27] Interestingly, acute glycemic control did not lessen the nerve block duration, suggesting that diabetic neuropathy is not rapidly reversed within this animal model. Currently, it is unclear whether the results from animal studies using experimentally induced hyperglycemia can be used to make recommendations for patients with long-standing diabetes mellitus.[31]

Although animal studies have consistently found that diabetic nerves are more sensitive to local anesthetics and potentially more susceptible to neural injury, it is unclear whether diabetic patients experience a higher incidence of neurologic injury after regional anesthesia.[18,27,28,32] There are limited clinical data suggesting that the success of peripheral nerve blockade (supraclavicular brachial plexus) may be higher in diabetic patients independent of other predictors of success (eg, body mass index) compared to nondiabetic patients.[32] Gebhard and colleagues[32] have proposed several theories for this finding, including (1) a higher sensitivity of diabetic nerve fibers to local anesthetics; (2) possible unknown intraneural penetration before injection; and (3) preexisting DPN with accompanying decreased sensation. Preexisting pathology has long been reported to play a role in the development of postoperative neurologic dysfunction.[33–35] A recent case report described a persistent postoperative femoral neuropathy after discontinuing a femoral nerve catheter in a patient with a preexisting subclinical diabetic neuropathy that had been undiagnosed preoperatively.[15]

In patients with diabetes mellitus, a decreased sensitivity to electrical stimulation combined with diminished sensory function and an increased sensitivity to local anesthetic toxicity may increase the risk of intraneural injection during peripheral nerve blockade using a peripheral nerve stimulator.[36–38] Currently, there is a lack of clinical evidence suggesting that the use of ultrasound guidance is safer than peripheral nerve stimulation within the general population.[39,40] However, this lack of established clinical benefit is less clear for diabetic patients. For example, there are a limited number of animal and clinical studies that suggest that ultrasound guidance may be a more desirable method of neural localization in diabetic patients. Animal studies have shown that low-threshold electrical stimulation may not offer protection from intraneural injection in the presence of hyperglycemia. Rigaud and colleagues[41] demonstrated that all needle insertions within a hyperglycemic dog model resulted in intraneural injection (6/6), whereas only one (1/18) intraneural injection occurred in control dogs. Sites and colleagues[38] also concluded that ultrasound guidance may be a preferred method of neural localization in diabetic patients after failing to elicit a motor response or paresthesia in two patients undergoing sciatic nerve blockade using peripheral nerve stimulation. The authors described a very weak motor response in both diabetic patients with a stimulating current of more than 2.4 mA despite perineural placement of the stimulating needle using ultrasound guidance. Another potential application of ultrasound technology is the ability to use the cross-sectional area of a peripheral nerve to identify a clinical or subclinical peripheral neuropathy: a diagnosis that historically would have required complex nerve conduction studies.[42,43]

Findings of spinal cord involvement in diabetic patients suggest that the same or similar mechanism of injury may affect not only peripheral nerves but neural elements within the central neuraxis as well.[44,45] Using magnetic resonance imaging, Selvarahah and colleagues[46] described early central nervous system involvement consisting of a significant reduction in the spinal cord cross-sectional area in patients with both subclinical and clinically detectable diabetic peripheral neuropathy. A case report of a diabetic patient experiencing a persistent lower extremity neuropathy after what appeared to be uneventful epidural analgesia reinforces concerns that diabetic patients may be at an increased risk of neurologic injury following neuraxial anesthesia.[14] A retrospective review also evaluated neurologic complications in patients with preexisting peripheral sensorimotor neuropathy or diabetic polyneuropathy who subsequently underwent neuraxial anesthesia or analgesia.[23] Of the 567 patients studied, two (0.4%; 95% CI 0.1%–1.3%) experienced new or progressive postoperative neurologic deficits when compared to preoperative findings. The authors concluded that although the risk of severe postoperative neurologic injury among diabetic patients is rare, it appears to be higher than that reported in the general population. Although the neuraxial technique could not be definitively implicated as the primary cause of the neurologic insult, it may have been a contributing factor among patients with preexisting neural compromise.

In summary, patients with DPN likely have neural elements that are more sensitive to the effects of local anesthetic. As a result, diabetic peripheral nerves may be more susceptible to subsequent injury from local anesthetic toxicity or ischemic insults. Ultimately, the decision to use regional anesthesia in diabetic patients should be made on an individual basis after a thorough discussion with the patient regarding the potential risks and benefits of the technique. Consideration should be given to decreasing the concentration or total dose of local anesthetic for both peripheral and neuraxial techniques[47]— particularly in profoundly symptomatic patients. Furthermore, the use of ultrasound guidance may facilitate perineural needle placement and the use of lower local anesthetic volumes in diabetic patients, although definitive data ensuring increased safety with ultrasound guidance are currently lacking.[48] Decreasing the concentration or dose of local anesthetic and eliminating epinephrine additives should also be considered given that diabetic nerves are already at risk of neural ischemia and infarction due to changes within the endoneural microvasculature.[26]

Chemotherapy-Induced Neuropathy

Chemotherapy-induced peripheral neuropathy (CIPN) is a frequent side effect of several commonly used chemotherapeutic agents. It is a dose-limiting side effect that occurs in approximately 30%–40% of patients.[49] The exact mechanism of injury is unclear, although damage to microtubules, interference with microtubule-based axonal transport, mitochondrial disruption, and cytotoxic effects on DNA are all possible mechanisms.[49,50] The degree of neurotoxicity depends on the agent used, the duration of administration, and the cumulative dose received. Cisplatin, oxaliplatin, and carboplatin characteristically induce a pure sensory, painful peripheral neuropathy, whereas vincristine, paclitaxel, and suramin tend to induce a mixed sensorimotor neuropathy with or without involvement of the autonomic nervous system.[51] Symptoms are often in the "glove-and-stocking" distribution and consist of pain or paresthesias. Patients at risk of developing CIPN include those with preexisting neural damage secondary to diabetes mellitus, excessive alcohol use, or inherited peripheral neuropathy. In general, a prolonged period of regeneration is required to restore neurologic function with incomplete recovery being the most common outcome.[50–52] However, patients who recover from CIPN have an increased risk of developing progressive neuropathic symptoms if exposed to additional neurotoxic agents.[53] Local anesthetics are potentially neurotoxic, and caution should be used when deciding whether to perform regional anesthesia in patients who have received chemotherapeutic agents known to cause CIPN. It is common for patients to have a subclinical neuropathy that presents only following a second neurologic insult, such as a peripheral or neuraxial block.[54]

Entrapment Neuropathy

Entrapment neuropathy, one of the most prevalent disorders of the peripheral nervous system, occurs when a single nerve is chronically compressed or mechanically injured at a specific location. Ulnar nerve entrapment at the elbow, referred to as "cubital entrapment syndrome," is the second most frequent upper extremity compression neuropathy.[55] The ulnar nerve is at increased risk because of its superficial location in the region of the medial elbow. Injury to the nerve may occur as a result of acute trauma, compression, repetitive traction, subluxation of the nerve, osteoarthritis, or gout or following an upper extremity surgical procedure. Initial symptoms include hyperesthesia in the ulnar nerve distribution, elbow pain, and paresthesias in the ring and small fingers. These symptoms are often intermittent and may progress over the course of months to years. In the later stages of the disease, weakness of the intrinsic muscles of the hand with or without visible atrophy may be observed. At present, the most common practice is to conservatively treat patients with mild symptoms without weakness or atrophy, whereas surgery is indicated for patients who do not improve after conservative management or present with severe neurological signs and symptoms (eg, persistent paraesthesia, objective weakness, muscular atrophy).[55]

General, regional, or local anesthesia can be used for surgical decompression of an entrapped ulnar nerve. The choice of anesthetic depends on the surgical procedure, whether nerve function will be tested intraoperatively, and the extent of damage accompanying the nerve injury. In a 2001 cohort study of 360 patients with preexisting ulnar neuropathy undergoing ulnar nerve transposition, Hebl and colleagues[56] found that anesthetic technique (general anesthesia versus regional anesthesia) did not affect the neurologic outcome immediately after surgery or two to six weeks postoperatively. A preoperative discussion with the surgeon to determine the intraoperative plan and address specific concerns related to the patient's disease process will assist the anesthesiologist in choosing the most appropriate anesthetic technique.

Inflammatory Neuropathy
Guillain–Barré Syndrome

Guillain–Barré syndrome (GBS) is an acute, inflammatory demyelinating polyneuropathy characterized by areflexia and diffuse ascending neuromuscular paralysis. The etiology of GBS is unclear, although infection, pregnancy, vaccinations, immunosuppression, systemic illnesses, and transfusion have all been proposed as potential triggers.[57] The degree and distribution of paralysis is variable and can include sensory nerve, cranial nerve, and autonomic nervous system involvement. Symptoms peak approximately two to four weeks after the initial onset with most patients experiencing a prolonged recovery. Unfortunately, many patients experience moderate to severe neurological impairment for years after the initial diagnosis.

There are several reports of GBS occurring in the postoperative period following a variety of surgical procedures using various types of anesthetic.[58–60] However, case reports of regional anesthesia use in patients with GBS are generally limited to the obstetric population.[61–64] Some patients with GBS may have autonomic instability and will subsequently experience an exaggerated response to neuraxial blockade,[63] whereas other GBS patients will exhibit a normal response to neuraxial anesthesia.[61,64] Although there have been reports of successful neuraxial anesthesia in parturients with GBS, the potential for local anesthetics to interact with peripheral myelin or cause direct nerve trauma cannot be ignored.[22] There is some evidence to

suggest that epidural anesthesia may precipitate or reactivate GBS hours to weeks following surgery.[58,65,66] However, it is difficult to determine if this is due to the effects of the epidural, the natural progression of the disease, the surgical procedure, or the stress response related to surgery.

Although it has been suggested that acute neuronal inflammation may be a relative contraindication to regional anesthesia, existing data provide little information regarding the safety of neuraxial anesthesia or peripheral nerve blockade in patients with GBS.[22] Ultimately, the decision to perform regional anesthesia should be made on an individual basis after a thorough discussion with the patient regarding the potential risks and benefits.

Postsurgical Inflammatory Neuropathy

Postsurgical inflammatory neuropathy (PSIN) is a recently described autoimmune or inflammatory process that may be the cause of severe postoperative neurologic deficits. Staff and colleagues[67] recently described a series of 33 patients who developed PSIN within 30 days of surgery. The diagnosis was confirmed in most patients following a peripheral nerve biopsy. PSIN is believed to be an idiopathic, immune-mediated response to a physiologic stress such as an infectious process, a vaccination, or a surgical procedure.[67] The condition may present as focal, multifocal, or diffuse neurologic deficits in the setting of negative radiographic imaging. Complicating the diagnosis, the onset of neurologic deficits may not be apparent during the immediate postoperative period, and the deficits may be in an anatomic distribution remote from the surgical site or regional anesthetic technique. Risk factors or potential triggers for PSIN include malignancy, diabetes mellitus, tobacco use, systemic infection, volatile anesthetic use, and recent blood transfusion.[67] Suppression of the immune response with prolonged high-dose corticosteroids or intravenous immunoglobulin is the current treatment of choice. The goal of treatment is to sufficiently blunt the inflammatory response to allow for axonal regeneration. Fortunately, most patients improve with current treatment recommendations, with pain and sensory deficits improving before the resolution of motor deficits.[67]

The degree to which inflammatory mechanisms play a role in postoperative neurologic dysfunction is unknown and poorly characterized, particularly within the anesthesia literature.[68] As a result, anesthesia providers and surgeons rarely consider this potential etiology of nerve injury when evaluating patients with postoperative deficits. This is problematic, as the common approach of watchful waiting and conservative management will not be effective in patients with PSIN. Rather, PSIN is a clinical condition that must be suspected early in the disease process so that a definitive diagnosis can be obtained (via nerve biopsy) and aggressive immunotherapy initiated to attempt to improve neurologic outcome.[67]

CENTRAL NERVOUS SYSTEM DISORDERS

Historically, neuraxial anesthesia techniques have not been offered to patients with preexisting neurologic disorders of the central nervous system (eg, multiple sclerosis, postpolio syndrome, amyotrophic lateral sclerosis) for fear of worsening neurologic outcome.[69–72] In fact, many historians believe that the recommendation of Dripps and Vandam[70] in 1956 to avoid regional anesthesia in patients with preexisting neurologic disorders has impacted clinical management for nearly half a century. Several theoretical mechanisms have been proposed based upon the double-crush phenomenon, including neurologic injury from needle or catheter-induced trauma, local anesthetic neurotoxicity, and neural ischemia due to local anesthetic additives. However, the avoidance of regional anesthesia within this patient population may also be due to physician and patient biases or potential medicolegal concerns. There are several confounding factors (age, body habitus, surgical trauma, tourniquet times and pressures, positioning, anesthetic technique) that make it difficult to determine the etiology of worsening postoperative neurologic deficits.

A recent review evaluated 139 patients with a history of one or more central nervous system disorders who subsequently underwent a neuraxial anesthetic technique.[71] Preoperative neurologic disorders primarily included postpolio syndrome (PPS), multiple sclerosis (MS), amyotrophic lateral sclerosis (ALS), and chronic spinal cord injury (SCI). In contrast to the findings of Vandam and Dripps several decades ago, the authors identified no new or worsening postoperative neurologic deficits (0.0%; 95% CI, 0.0%–0.3%) within their patient cohort. This was despite the fact that 74% of the patients reported active neurologic symptoms (paresthesias, dysesthesias, hyperreflexia) or sensorimotor deficits during the immediate preoperative period and subsequently received standard doses of local anesthetics. Two smaller reviews in parturients receiving smaller doses of local anesthetic for labor analgesia have reported similar results.[73,74]

Clearly, further investigations with a larger number of patients are needed to make definitive recommendations. However, the current data suggest that the decision to perform neuraxial anesthesia in patients with preexisting central nervous system disorders be based on the risks and benefits for each individual patient. Some authors have postulated that the neurologic risk may be higher in patients who have progressive neurologic deficits compared to those with chronic, stable sensorimotor symptoms that have not changed over the course of several months or years.

Multiple Sclerosis

Multiple sclerosis is an inflammatory autoimmune disorder of the central nervous system with a lifetime risk of 1 in 400, making it the most common debilitating neurologic disease in young adults.[75] It is a chronic, degenerative disease characterized by focal demyelination within the spinal cord and brain. This demyelination results in a fluctuating conduction block that causes a classic "waxing and waning" of symptoms that is characteristic of the disease. Signs and symptoms include sensory or motor deficits, diplopia or vision loss, bowel or bladder dysfunction, and ataxia. The precise etiology is unclear; however, a combination of genetic risk factors and environmental factors likely play a role. Twenty-five percent of MS patients are essentially asymptomatic, and their activities of daily living are unaffected. However, up to 15% of patients may become severely disabled with significant sensorimotor deficits within a short period of time.[76]

Several factors common to surgery can negatively impact the disease process, including hyperpyrexia, emotional stress, and infection.[77] The mechanism of worsening neurologic function in patients with MS is unclear and may occur coincidentally within the postoperative period independent of anesthetic technique. Evidence regarding the risk of regional anesthesia in patients with MS is limited. Despite some evidence for demyelination of the peripheral nerves in MS, peripheral nerve blockade has traditionally been considered safe.[78] However, a recent report of severe brachial plexopathy following an ultrasound-guided interscalene block has raised the concern that a segment of MS patients may have subclinical peripheral neuropathy.[79] Several investigators have demonstrated evidence of axonal demyelinating peripheral lesions (sensory more than motor) in patients with MS.[80–82] Misawa and colleagues[81] demonstrated that peripheral demyelination may occur in 5% of MS patients, whereas Pogorzelski and colleagues[80] have reported peripheral demyelination may occur in up to 47% of patients. Similarly, Sarova-Pinhas and colleagues[82] have described nerve conduction abnormalities in up to 14.7% of peripheral nerves within MS patients compared to only 2.4% of nerves within the general population. Despite this evidence, the overall incidence and clinical relevance of this underlying peripheral neuropathy remains undefined in the setting of performing peripheral nerve blockade in patients with MS.

In contrast to peripheral nerve blockade, the potential risk of new or progressive neurologic deficits in MS patients after spinal anesthesia was first described in 1937. Critchley and colleagues[83] described three patients with [disseminated (multiple) sclerosis] who experienced a worsening of symptoms after spinal anesthesia. The authors concluded that [spinal anesthesia may be a precipitating agent in the evolution of disseminated (multiple) sclerosis.] Several subsequent studies demonstrated similar outcomes with the development of new or worsening neurologic deficits or a higher likelihood of symptom exacerbation after spinal anesthesia.[69,84–86] In contrast, a more recent study demonstrated no new or worsening neurologic symptoms after spinal anesthesia in 35 MS patients undergoing a variety of surgical procedures.[71]

The safety of epidural anesthesia and analgesia in MS patients has been focused almost exclusively within the obstetric population, which may not accurately represent the nonpregnant MS patient. Pregnancy is frequently associated with a decrease in disease relapse, whereas the postpartum period is often associated with an increased risk of relapse. The transition from cellular immunity to humoral immunity required for the mother's immune system to tolerate the fetus is thought to be protective during pregnancy.[73] However, as cell-mediated immunity rebounds during the postpartum period, patients will often experience a transient worsening of neurologic symptoms that could be falsely attributed to recent regional anesthetic techniques.

Confavreux and colleagues[73] have performed one of the few prospective studies evaluating risk factors associated with disease relapse during the postpartum period. They concluded that epidural analgesia during labor and delivery did not contribute to a higher risk of relapse compared to patients who did not receive neuraxial techniques. Similarly, Kuczkowski[87] found no association between any form of obstetric regional analgesia and the worsening of MS symptoms among obstetric patients. Epidural anesthesia and analgesia have traditionally been recommended over spinal anesthesia in MS patients because the concentration of local anesthetic in the white matter of the spinal cord is one-fourth the level after epidural injection compared to intrathecal injection.[88] It is believed that the lack of myelin may leave the spinal cord susceptible to the neurotoxic effects of local anesthetics.[88] Although definitive studies on the pharmacological effects of local anesthetic concentrations and doses are lacking, many recommend limiting neuraxial local anesthetic doses and concentrations to the lowest level possible. There is some evidence that lidocaine can reversibly worsen symptoms of MS by blocking sodium channels in demyelinated areas enough to cause symptoms compared to healthy myelinated areas that remain unaffected.[89] With regard to the obstetric patient, the risk of neuraxial anesthesia or analgesia needs to be weighed against the increased risk of general anesthesia. A recent survey from the United Kingdom demonstrated that 90% of obstetric anesthesiologists would perform spinal anesthesia for an emergency cesarean section in an MS patient after carefully weighing the potential risks and benefits.[90]

In summary, there remains little conclusive evidence to support or refute the use of regional anesthesia in patients with MS. Peripheral nerve blockade has not been definitively shown to be harmful in the setting of MS, and therefore MS should not be considered an absolute contraindication to this regional technique. In contrast, given that demyelinated fibers may be more prone to the toxic effects of local anesthetics, epidural anesthesia and analgesia may be considered safer than spinal techniques. However, reducing the local anesthetic concentration and total dose to the lowest effective levels may be prudent for both peripheral and neuraxial blockade. All decisions regarding the use of regional anesthesia and analgesia in patients with MS need to be made after careful consideration of the potential risks and benefits. Regardless of the anesthetic technique chosen, patients should be informed of the risk of new or worsening neurologic symptoms during the postoperative period because of exposure to multiple exacerbating factors.

Postpolio Syndrome

Postpolio syndrome refers to new-onset neurologic symptoms that develop several years after an acute poliomyelitis infection. The onset of new or progressive symptoms may occur up to 30 years after the initial episode of poliomyelitis. PPS affects anterior horn cells within the anterior portion of the spinal cord and is therefore considered a lower motor neuron disorder.[91] Initial symptoms include muscle weakness, fatigue, gait instability, joint pain, and muscle atrophy within muscle groups that were previously affected by the disease. Sensory deficits are generally not characteristic of the syndrome and are only observed if a secondary disorder is present (eg, compressive radiculopathy or disk herniation). The motor effects of PPS are thought to be related to an ongoing process of denervation and

reinnervation that ultimately ends when denervation is no longer compensated for by reinnervation.[91]

Postpolio syndrome is the most prevalent motor neuron disease in North America. Furthermore, because acute poliomyelitis continues to occur in developing countries, PPS will likely remain an anesthetic concern for years to come.[22] It is not uncommon for patients with PPS to require orthopedic procedures; therefore, it is important to determine the safety of regional anesthetic techniques under these clinical circumstances. Although patients with PPS have fewer motor neurons than normal, it is difficult to know whether the remaining motor neurons are more susceptible to the toxic effects of local anesthetics. There have been no reports of worsening neurologic status following neuraxial anesthesia with normal doses of tetracaine and bupivacaine in patients with PPS.[92,93] However, this finding does not imply that regional anesthetic techniques are without risk.[94] As with all patients, the potential risk of regional anesthesia must be balanced against the disadvantages of general anesthesia, including a hypersensitivity to sedative or opioid medications, the risk of muscle relaxant use, and the risk of hypoventilation and aspiration. The largest series of patients with PPS (*n* = 79) undergoing neuraxial anesthesia or analgesia demonstrated no worsening of neurologic symptoms during the postoperative period.[71] However, the paucity of clinical data on this topic prevents clear recommendations from being made regarding the safety of neuraxial anesthesia or peripheral nerve blockade in patients with PPS. Ultimately, the decision to use regional anesthesia should be made on an individual basis after a thorough discussion of the potential risks and benefits with each patient. Given the increased sensitivity to opioid and sedative medications within this patient subgroup, these medications should always be used with caution.

Amyotrophic Lateral Sclerosis

Amyotrophic lateral sclerosis is a progressive degenerative disease of upper and lower motor neurons. The cause is unknown, but theories include glutamate excitotoxicity, oxidative stress, mitochondrial dysfunction, paraneoplastic tumors, autoimmune disease, and viral infection.[92] Initially, ALS presents as atrophy, weakness, and fasciculations in the intrinsic hand muscles. As it progresses, atrophy and weakness develop in all skeletal muscles including those of the tongue, pharynx, larynx, and respiratory muscles of the chest. Patients lose the ability to cough, increasing the risk of aspiration. Autonomic dysfunction may be evident and is manifested by orthostatic hypotension and an increased resting heart rate. Unfortunately, in the majority of patients, death from respiratory failure occurs within a few years of disease onset.[95]

The existing evidence, albeit limited, has not supported the fear that neuraxial or peripheral blockade will exacerbate preexisting symptoms in ALS patients.[65,96–100] However, given the potential for worsening respiratory failure following general anesthesia due to the use of muscle relaxants and opioid medications, the ability to avoid airway manipulation may be considered a benefit within this high-risk patient population. Regardless of anesthetic technique, the possibility of postoperative respiratory or neurologic deterioration is quite high in patients with

ALS. Ultimately, the decision to use regional anesthesia should be made on an individual basis after a thorough discussion of the potential risks and benefits with each patient.

Spinal Stenosis and Lumbar Disk Disease

Spinal canal pathology has been proposed as a potential risk factor for neurologic complications following neuraxial blockade. Several mechanisms of injury have been proposed, including an ischemic or compressive effect after the injection of large volumes of local anesthetic into a relatively confined space (ie, epidural anesthesia) and local anesthetic neurotoxicity (ie, spinal anesthesia). Although the precise mechanism(s) of injury remain unclear, there are several isolated case reports and large case series that are believed to support these hypotheses.

Spinal stenosis occurs as age-related changes within the intervertebral disks and facet joints resulting in a narrowing of the spinal canal or neural foramina. Changes include disk degeneration, facet joint hypertrophy, osteophyte formation, and an infolding of the ligamentum flavum. The precise mechanism by which spinal nerve root compression results in signs or symptoms of spinal stenosis is not completely understood.[101] Classic symptoms include back and leg radicular pain that significantly worsens with extension and is alleviated with flexion. Preexisting spinal stenosis or compressive lumbar disk disease has been proposed as a potential risk factor for neurologic complications following a neuraxial (spinal or epidural) technique. Proposed mechanisms of injury include mechanical trauma,[102,103] local anesthetic neurotoxicity,[104,105] ischemia,[106–108] or a multifactorial etiology.[109,110] Pathophysiologically, patients with spinal stenosis have a reduction in the diameter of the spinal canal resulting in less anatomic space for fluid collections such as blood or local anesthetic. As a result, small quantities of fluid may result in significant increases in pressure around the neuraxis that would have no clinical effect in a widely patent spinal canal.

Two relatively large case series and several case reports have been published that suggest undiagnosed spinal stenosis may be a risk factor for neurologic complications following neuraxial blockade.[102,104,106,109,111] The majority of cauda equina cases involved epidural analgesia, which may suggest an ischemic etiology (mechanical compression of the cord by the infusing local anesthetic) to the injury.[110] Hebl and colleagues[109] performed a retrospective review of 937 patients with preexisting spinal stenosis or lumbar disk disease with and without a history of prior spinal surgery and concluded that this cohort of patients were at an increased risk for the development or worsening of neurologic deficits when compared to the general population undergoing a neuraxial technique. In addition, patients with more than one neurologic diagnosis (eg, spinal stenosis, compressive radiculopathy, preexisting peripheral neuropathy) appeared to have an even higher risk of injury. Similarly, Moen and colleagues[104] performed a large epidemiologic survey in Sweden that revealed similar trends. During a 10-year study period, 1,260,000 spinal anesthetics and 450,000 epidural blocks were evaluated. Overall, the authors identified 127 serious complications, including 85 (67%) patients with permanent injuries. Although 14 patients had preexisting spinal stenosis, 13 (93%) of these were diagnosed in the postoperative period during the evaluation of the neurologic deficit. The

authors concluded that the incidence of severe anesthesia-related complications may not be as low as previously reported and that preexisting spinal canal pathology may be a "neglected risk factor." Finally, although patients with prior spine surgery may have an increased risk of paraplegia following transforaminal epidural steroid injections,[112,113] no similar risk has been found in patients after neuraxial anesthesia or analgesia.

In summary, although it appears that patients with spinal stenosis or compressive lumbar disk disease may be at increased risk of neurologic complications following neuraxial blockade, the existing literature fails to provide a direct comparison of surgical patients with similar spinal pathology undergoing general anesthesia. Therefore, it is unclear whether the higher incidence of neurologic complications in this patient population is due to surgical factors, anesthetic technique, the natural progression of disease process, or a combination of these factors.

Spinal Cord Injury

Spinal cord injury affects over 10,000 Americans each year.[114] Of these, approximately 50% of injuries occur at the cervical level.[114] Most SCI cases are secondary to motor vehicle accidents, with a smaller percentage resulting from sports injuries, falls, or penetrating trauma. The ratio of complete to incomplete neurologic deficits in the United States appears to be decreasing over the past decade, reflecting a greater proportion of incomplete deficits.[114] A potentially dangerous condition that may develop in the month(s) after the resolution of acute spinal shock is autonomic dysreflexia (AD). AD is a life-threatening syndrome resulting from cutaneous or visceral stimulation below the level of the spinal cord injury, leading to extreme vascular instability. The lifetime prevalence of AD has been estimated to range from 17% to 70%, with most episodes occurring in SCI cases if the level of injury is at or above T6.[115]

General anesthesia with low-concentration volatile anesthetic does not offer protection against AD. Although higher concentrations of volatile anesthetic may be effective, anesthesia-related hemodynamic instability may not be well tolerated within this patient population. Therefore, neuraxial (spinal or epidural) regional anesthesia techniques can be valuable adjuncts in the management of patients with chronic SCI undergoing lower extremity, abdominal, obstetric, gynecologic, and urologic procedures. Numerous case reports and case series have demonstrated that neuraxial techniques are safe and effective in preventing episodes of AD in SCI patients, even those with high cord lesions.[87,116–118] At this point, there is no clear evidence to suggest that use of regional techniques may potentially worsen preexisting neurologic deficits in patients with SCI. However, difficulty in determining appropriate anesthetic level, the potential for hemodynamic instability and respiratory difficulty, and challenging block placement are important considerations when evaluating patients with SCI for a neuraxial technique.

SUMMARY

Patients with preexisting neurologic disease present a unique challenge to the anesthesiologist who is contemplating a regional anesthetic technique. A thorough preoperative assessment is vital in order to establish the patient's baseline neurologic status. Anesthesia providers should be aware of the risk factors for postoperative neurologic complications during their selection of suitable candidates for a central or peripheral block and adapt their technique to minimize these risks as much as possible. While most preexisting neurologic disorders are not absolute contraindications to regional anesthesia, the decision to proceed with a regional technique should be made on an individual, case-by-case basis as select patients may benefit from a regional anesthetic technique compared to other anesthetic or analgesic options.

REFERENCES

1. Upton AR, McComas AJ: The double crush in nerve entrapment syndromes. Lancet 1973;2:359–362.
2. Osterman AL: The double crush syndrome. Orthop Clin North Am 1988; 19:147–155.
3. Neal JM, Bernards CM, Hadzic A, et al: ASRA practice advisory on neurologic complications in regional anesthesia and pain medicine. Reg Anesth Pain Med 2008;33:404–415.
4. Jacob AK, Kopp, SL: Regional anesthesia in the patient with preexisting neurologic disorders. Advances in Anesthesia 2011;29:1–18.
5. Skre H: Genetic and clinical aspects of Charcot-Marie-Tooth's disease. Clin Genet 1974;6:98–118.
6. Saporta AS, Sottile SL, Miller LJ, Feely SM, Siskind CE, Shy ME: Charcot-Marie-Tooth disease subtypes and genetic testing strategies. Ann Neurol 2011;69:22–33.
7. Bui AH, Marco AP: Peripheral nerve blockade in a patient with Charcot-Marie-Tooth disease. Can J Anaesth 2008;55:718–719.
8. Dhir S, Balasubramanian S, Ross D: Ultrasound-guided peripheral regional blockade in patients with Charcot-Marie-Tooth disease: a review of three cases. Can J Anaesth 2008;55:515–520.
9. Fernandez Perez AB, Quesada Garcia C, Rodriguez Gonzalez O, Besada Estevez JC: [Obstetric epidural analgesia, a safe choice in a patient with Charcot-Marie-Tooth disease]. Rev Esp Anestesiol Reanim 2011;58: 255–256.
10. Schmitt HJ, Muenster T, Schmidt J: Central neural blockade in Charcot-Marie-Tooth disease. Can J Anaesth 2004;51:1049–1050.
11. Sugai K, Sugai Y: [Epidural anesthesia for a patient with Charcot-Marie-Tooth disease, bronchial asthma and hypothyroidism]. Masui 1989;38: 688–691.
12. Tanaka S, Tsuchida H, Namiki A: [Epidural anesthesia for a patient with Charcot-Marie-Tooth disease, mitral valve prolapse syndrome and IInd degree AV block]. Masui 1994;43:931–933.
13. Lepski GR, Alderson JD: Epidural analgesia in labour for a patient with hereditary neuropathy with liability to pressure palsy. Int J Obstet Anesth 2001;10:198–201.
14. Al-Nasser B: Toxic effects of epidural analgesia with ropivacaine 0.2% in a diabetic patient. J Clin Anesth 2004;16:220–223.
15. Blumenthal S, Borgeat A, Maurer K, et al: Preexisting subclinical neuropathy as a risk factor for nerve injury after continuous ropivacaine administration through a femoral nerve catheter. Anesthesiology 2006; 105:1053–1056.
16. Horlocker TT, O'Driscoll SW, Dinapoli RP: Recurring brachial plexus neuropathy in a diabetic patient after shoulder surgery and continuous interscalene block. Anesth Analg 2000;91:688–690.
17. Waters JH, Watson TB, Ward MG: Conus medullaris injury following both tetracaine and lidocaine spinal anesthesia. J Clin Anesth 1996;8: 656–658.
18. Kalichman MW, Calcutt NA: Local anesthetic-induced conduction block and nerve fiber injury in streptozotocin-diabetic rats. Anesthesiology 1992;77:941–947.
19. Dyck PJ, Kratz KM, Karnes JL, et al: The prevalence by staged severity of various types of diabetic neuropathy, retinopathy, and nephropathy in a population-based cohort: the Rochester Diabetic Neuropathy Study. Neurology 1993;43:817–824.
20. Ross MA: Neuropathies associated with diabetes. Med Clin North Am 1993;77:111–124.
21. Centers for Disease Control and Prevention: *National Diabetes Fact Sheet: National Estimates and General Information on Diabetes and Prediabetes in the United States.* Atlanta, GA: Centers for Disease Control and Prevention, U.S. Department of Health and Human Services; 2011.
22. Lirk P, Birmingham B, Hogan Q: Regional anesthesia in patients with preexisting neuropathy. Int Anesthesiol Clin 2011;49:144–165.
23. Hebl JR, Kopp SL, Schroeder DR, Horlocker TT: Neurologic complications after neuraxial anesthesia or analgesia in patients with preexisting peripheral sensorimotor neuropathy or diabetic polyneuropathy. Anesth Analg 2006;103:1294–1299.
24. Krishnan AV, Kiernan MC: Altered nerve excitability properties in established diabetic neuropathy. Brain 2005;128:1178–1187.
25. Sinnreich M, Taylor BV, Dyck PJ: Diabetic neuropathies. Classification, clinical features, and pathophysiological basis. Neurologist 2005;11: 63–79.
26. Williams BA, Murinson BB, Grable BR, Orebaugh SL: Future considerations for pharmacologic adjuvants in single-injection peripheral nerve blocks for patients with diabetes mellitus. Reg Anesth Pain Med 2009;34:445–457.
27. Kroin JS, Buvanendran A, Tuman KJ, Kerns JM: Safety of local anesthetics administered intrathecally in diabetic rats. Pain Med 2012; 13:802–807.
28. Kroin JS, Buvanendran A, Williams DK, et al: Local anesthetic sciatic nerve block and nerve fiber damage in diabetic rats. Reg Anesth Pain Med 2010;35:343–350.
29. Williams BA: Toward a potential paradigm shift for the clinical care of diabetic patients requiring perineural analgesia: strategies for using the diabetic rodent model. Reg Anesth Pain Med 2010;35:329–332.
30. Lirk P, Flatz M, Haller I, et al: In Zucker diabetic fatty rats, subclinical diabetic neuropathy increases in vivo lidocaine block duration but not in vitro neurotoxicity. Reg Anesth Pain Med 2012;37:601–606.
31. Williams BA, Murinson BB: Diabetes mellitus and subclinical neuropathy: a call for new paths in peripheral nerve block research. Anesthesiology 2008;109:361–362.
32. Gebhard RE, Nielsen KC, Pietrobon R, Missair A, Williams BA: Diabetes mellitus, independent of body mass index, is associated with a "higher success" rate for supraclavicular brachial plexus blocks. Reg Anesth Pain Med 2009;34:404–407.
33. Alvine FG, Schurrer ME: Postoperative ulnar-nerve palsy. Are there predisposing factors? J Bone Joint Surg Am 1987;69:255–259.
34. Chaudhry V, Glass JD, Griffin JW: Wallerian degeneration in peripheral nerve disease. Neurol Clin 1992;10:613–627.
35. Selander D, Edshage S, Wolff T: Paresthesiae or no paresthesiae? Nerve lesions after axillary blocks. Acta Anaesthesiol Scand 1979;23: 27–33.
36. Bigeleisen PE: Nerve puncture and apparent intraneural injection during ultrasound-guided axillary block does not invariably result in neurologic injury. Anesthesiology 2006;105:779–783.
37. Lok C, Kirk P: Problems performing a sciatic nerve block in an amputee. Anaesthesia 2003;58:289–290.
38. Sites BD, Gallagher J, Sparks M: Ultrasound-guided popliteal block demonstrates an atypical motor response to nerve stimulation in 2 patients with diabetes mellitus. Reg Anesth Pain Med 2003;28:479–482.
39. Liu SS, Ngeow JE, Yadeau JT: Ultrasound-guided regional anesthesia and analgesia: a qualitative systematic review. Reg Anesth Pain Med 2009; 34:47–59.
40. Sites BD, Taenzer AH, Herrick MD, et al: Incidence of local anesthetic systemic toxicity and postoperative neurologic symptoms associated with 12,668 ultrasound-guided nerve blocks: an analysis from a prospective clinical registry. Reg Anesth Pain Med 2012;37:478–482.
41. Rigaud M, Filip P, Lirk P, Fuchs A, Gemes G, Hogan Q: Guidance of block needle insertion by electrical nerve stimulation: a pilot study of the resulting distribution of injected solution in dogs. Anesthesiology 2008; 109:473–478.
42. Lucchetta M, Pazzaglia C, Granata G, Briani C, Padua L: Ultrasound evaluation of peripheral neuropathy in POEMS syndrome. Muscle Nerve 2011;44:868–872.
43. Riazi S, Bril V, Perkins BA, et al: Can ultrasound of the tibial nerve detect diabetic peripheral neuropathy? A cross-sectional study. Diabetes Care 2012;35:2575–2579.
44. Eaton SE, Harris ND, Rajbhandari SM, et al: Spinal-cord involvement in diabetic peripheral neuropathy. Lancet 2001;358:35–36.
45. Varsik P, Kucera P, Buranova D, Balaz M: Is the spinal cord lesion rare in diabetes mellitus? Somatosensory evoked potentials and central conduction time in diabetes mellitus. Med Sci Monit 2001;7:712–715.
46. Selvarajah D, Wilkinson ID, Emery CJ, et al: Early involvement of the spinal cord in diabetic peripheral neuropathy. Diabetes Care 2006; 29:2664–2669.
47. Drasner K: Local anesthetic neurotoxicity: clinical injury and strategies that may minimize risk. Reg Anesth Pain Med 2002;27:576–580.
48. Koscielniak-Nielsen ZJ: Ultrasound-guided peripheral nerve blocks: what are the benefits? Acta Anaesthesiol Scand 2008;52:727–737.

49. Pachman DR, Barton DL, Watson JC, Loprinzi CL: Chemotherapy-induced peripheral neuropathy: prevention and treatment. Clin Pharmacol Ther 2011;90:377–387.
50. Peters CM, Jimenez-Andrade JM, Kuskowski MA, Ghilardi JR, Mantyh PW: An evolving cellular pathology occurs in dorsal root ganglia, peripheral nerve and spinal cord following intravenous administration of paclitaxel in the rat. Brain Res 2007;1168:46–59.
51. Quasthoff S, Hartung HP: Chemotherapy-induced peripheral neuropathy. J Neurol 2002;249:9–17.
52. Pignata S, De Placido S, Biamonte R, et al: Residual neurotoxicity in ovarian cancer patients in clinical remission after first-line chemotherapy with carboplatin and paclitaxel: the Multicenter Italian Trial in Ovarian cancer (MITO-4) retrospective study. BMC Cancer 2006;6:5.
53. Kaley TJ, Deangelis LM: Therapy of chemotherapy-induced peripheral neuropathy. Br J Haematol 2009;145:3–14.
54. Hebl JR, Horlocker TT, Pritchard DJ: Diffuse brachial plexopathy after interscalene blockade in a patient receiving cisplatin chemotherapy: the pharmacologic double crush syndrome. Anesth Analg 2001;92:249–251.
55. Caliandro P, La Torre G, Padua R, Giannini F, Padua L: Treatment for ulnar neuropathy at the elbow. Cochrane Database Syst Rev 2012;7:CD006839.
56. Hebl JR, Horlocker TT, Sorenson EJ, Schroeder DR: Regional anesthesia does not increase the risk of postoperative neuropathy in patients undergoing ulnar nerve transposition. Anesth Analg 2001;93:1606–1611, table of contents.
57. Pithadia AB, Kakadia N: Guillain-Barré syndrome (GBS). Pharmacol Rep 2010;62:220–232.
58. Bamberger PD, Thys DM: Guillain-Barré syndrome in a patient with pancreatic cancer after an epidural-general anesthetic. Anesthes Analg 2005;100:1197–1199.
59. Gautier PE, Pierre PA, Van Obbergh LJ, Van Steenberge A: Guillain-Barre syndrome after obstetrical epidural analgesia. Reg Anesth 1989;14:251–252.
60. Heyworth BE, Fabricant PD, Pizzurro MM, Beksac B, Salvati EA: Guillain-Barré syndrome mimicking nerve injury after total hip arthroplasty. HSS J 2011;7:286–289.
61. Alici HA, Cesur M, Erdem AF, Gursac M: Repeated use of epidural anaesthesia for caesarean delivery in a patient with Guillain-Barré syndrome. Int J Obstet Anesth 2005;14:269–270.
62. McGrady EM: Management of labour and delivery in a patient with Guillain-Barré syndrome. Anaesthesia 1987;42:899.
63. Perel A, Reches A, Davidson JT: Anaesthesia in the Guillain-Barré syndrome. A case report and recommendations. Anaesthesia 1977;32:257–260.
64. Vassiliev DV, Nystrom EU, Leicht CH: Combined spinal and epidural anesthesia for labor and cesarean delivery in a patient with Guillain-Barre syndrome. Reg Anesth Pain Med 2001;26:174–176.
65. Otsuka N, Igarashi M, Shimodate Y, Nakabayashi K, Asano M, Namiki A: [Anesthetic management of two patients with amyotrophic lateral sclerosis (ALS)]. Masui 2004;53:1279–1281.
66. Steiner I, Argov Z, Cahan C, Abramsky O: Guillain-Barré syndrome after epidural anesthesia: direct nerve root damage may trigger disease. Neurology 1985;35:1473–1475.
67. Staff NP, Engelstad J, Klein CJ, et al: Post-surgical inflammatory neuropathy. Brain 2010;133:2866–2880.
68. Ahn KS, Kopp SL, Watson JC, Scott KP, Trousdale RT, Hebl JR: Postsurgical inflammatory neuropathy. Reg Anesth Pain Med 2011;36:403–405.
69. Bamford C, Sibley W, Laguna J: Anesthesia in multiple sclerosis. Can J Neurol Sci 1978;5:41–44.
70. Dripps RD, Vandam LD: Exacerbation of pre-existing neurologic disease after spinal anesthesia. N Engl J Med 1956;255:843–849.
71. Hebl JR, Horlocker TT, Schroeder DR: Neuraxial anesthesia and analgesia in patients with preexisting central nervous system disorders. Anesth Analg 2006;103:223–228, table of contents.
72. Keschner M: The effect of injuries and illness on the course of multiple sclerosis. Res Publ Assoc Res Nerv Ment Dis 1950;28:533–547.
73. Confavreux C, Hutchinson M, Hours MM, Cortinovis-Tourniaire P, Moreau T: Rate of pregnancy-related relapse in multiple sclerosis. Pregnancy in Multiple Sclerosis Group. N Engl J Med 1998;339:285–291.
74. Crawford JS: Epidural analgesia for patients with chronic neurological disease. Anesth Analg 1983;62:621–622.
75. Noseworthy JH, Lucchinetti C, Rodriguez M, Weinshenker BG: Multiple sclerosis. N Engl J Med 2000;343:938–952.
76. Compston A, Coles A: Multiple sclerosis. Lancet 2002;359:1221–1231.
77. Korn-Lubetzki I, Kahana E, Cooper G, Abramsky O: Activity of multiple sclerosis during pregnancy and puerperium. Ann Neurol 1984;16:229–231.
78. Pollock M, Calder C, Allpress S: Peripheral nerve abnormality in multiple sclerosis. Ann Neurol 1977;2:41–48.
79. Koff MD, Cohen JA, McIntyre JJ, Carr CF, Sites BD: Severe brachial plexopathy after an ultrasound-guided single-injection nerve block for total shoulder arthroplasty in a patient with multiple sclerosis. Anesthesiology 2008;108:325–328.
80. Pogorzelski R, Baniukiewicz E, Drozdowski W: [Subclinical lesions of peripheral nervous system in multiple sclerosis patients]. Neurol Neurochir Pol 2004;38:257–264.
81. Misawa S, Kuwabara S, Mori M, Hayakawa S, Sawai S, Hattori T: Peripheral nerve demyelination in multiple sclerosis. Clinical Neurophysiol 2008;119:1829–1833.
82. Sarova-Pinhas I, Achiron A, Gilad R, Lampl Y: Peripheral neuropathy in multiple sclerosis: a clinical and electrophysiologic study. Acta Neurol Scand 1995;91:234–238.
83. Critchley EP: Multiple sclerosis initially presenting as facial palsy. Aviat Space Environ Med 2004;75:1001–1004.
84. Hammes E: Neurological complications associated with spinal anesthesia (eight cases). Minn Med 1943;36:339–345.
85. Keschner M: The effect of injuries and illness on the course of multiple sclerosis. Res Publ Assoc Res Nerv Ment Dis 1950;28:533–547.
86. Stenuit J, Marchand P: [Sequelae of spinal anesthesia]. Acta Neurol Psychiatr Belg 1968;68:626–635.
87. Kuczkowski KM: Labor analgesia for the parturient with neurological disease: what does an obstetrician need to know? Arch Gynecol Obstet 2006;274:41–46.
88. Warren TM, Datta S, Ostheimer GW: Lumbar epidural anesthesia in a patient with multiple sclerosis. Anesth Analg 1982;61:1022–1023.
89. Sakurai M, Mannen T, Kanazawa I, Tanabe H: Lidocaine unmasks silent demyelinative lesions in multiple sclerosis. Neurology 1992;42:2088–2093.
90. Drake E, Drake M, Bird J, Russell R: Obstetric regional blocks for women with multiple sclerosis: a survey of UK experience. Int J Obstet Anesth 2006;15:115–123.
91. Gonzalez H, Olsson T, Borg K: Management of postpolio syndrome. Lancet Neurol 2010;9:634–642.
92. Bordes J, Gaillard PE, Lacroix G, Palmier B: Spinal anaesthesia guided by computed tomography scan in a patient with severe post-polio sequelae. Br J Anaesth 2010;105:702–703.
93. Higashizawa T, Sugiura J, Takasugi Y: [Spinal anesthesia in a patient with hemiparesis after poliomyelitis]. Masui 2003;52:1335–1337.
94. Lambert DA, Giannouli E, Schmidt BJ: Postpolio syndrome and anesthesia. Anesthesiology 2005;103:638–644.
95. Pratt AJ, Getzoff ED, Perry JJ: Amyotrophic lateral sclerosis: update and new developments. Degener Neurol Neuromuscul Dis 2012;2012:1–14.
96. Chen LK, Chang Y, Liu CC, Hou WY: Epidural anesthesia combined with propofol sedation for abdominal hysterectomy in a patient with amyotrophic lateral sclerosis—a case report. Acta Anaesthesiol Sin 1998;36:103–106.
97. Hara K, Sakura S, Saito Y, Maeda M, Kosaka Y: Epidural anesthesia and pulmonary function in a patient with amyotrophic lateral sclerosis. Anesth Analg 1996;83:878–879.
98. Hobaika AB, Neves BS: Combined spinal-epidural block in a patient with amyotrophic lateral sclerosis: case report. Rev Bras Anestesiol 2009;59:206–209.
99. Kitoh T, Kobayashi K, Ina H, et al: Effects of lumbar sympathetic ganglion block for a patient with amyotrophic lateral sclerosis (ALS). J Anesth 2006;20:109–112.
100. Kochi T, Oka T, Mizuguchi T: Epidural anesthesia for patients with amyotrophic lateral sclerosis. Anesth Analg 1989;68:410–412.
101. Katz JN, Harris MB: Clinical practice. Lumbar spinal stenosis. N Engl J Med 2008;358:818–825.
102. Stambough JL, Stambough JB, Evans S: Acute cauda equina syndrome after total knee arthroplasty as a result of epidural anesthesia and spinal stenosis. J Arthroplasty 2000;15:375–379.
103. Tetzlaff JE, Dilger JA, Wu C, Smith MP, Bell G: Influence of lumbar spine pathology on the incidence of paresthesia during spinal anesthesia. Reg Anesth Pain Med 1998;23:560–563.
104. Moen V, Dahlgren N, Irestedt L: Severe neurological complications after central neuraxial blockades in Sweden 1990–1999. Anesthesiology 2004;101:950–959.
105. Yuen EC, Layzer RB, Weitz SR, Olney RK: Neurologic complications of lumbar epidural anesthesia and analgesia. Neurology 1995;45:1795–1801.

106. de Seze MP, Sztark F, Janvier G, Joseph PA: Severe and long-lasting complications of the nerve root and spinal cord after central neuraxial blockade. Anesth Analg 2007;104:975–979.

107. Hooten WM, Hogan MS, Sanemann TC, Maus TJ: Acute spinal pain during an attempted lumbar epidural blood patch in congenital lumbar spinal stenosis and epidural lipomatosis. Pain Physician 2008;11: 87–90.

108. Usubiaga JE, Wikinski JA, Usubiaga LE: Epidural pressure and its relation to spread of anesthetic solutions in epidural space. Anesth Analg 1967;46:440–446.

109. Hebl JR, Horlocker TT, Kopp SL, Schroeder DR: Neuraxial blockade in patients with preexisting spinal stenosis, lumbar disk disease, or prior spine surgery: efficacy and neurologic complications. Anesth Analg 2010; 111:1511–1519.

110. Horlocker TT: Neuraxial blockade in patients with spinal stenosis: between a rock and a hard place. Anesth Analg 2010;110:13–15.

111. Kubina P, Gupta A, Oscarsson A, Axelsson K, Bengtsson M: Two cases of cauda equina syndrome following spinal-epidural anesthesia. Reg Anesth 1997;22:447–450.

112. Houten JK, Errico TJ: Paraplegia after lumbosacral nerve root block: report of three cases. Spine J 2002;2:70–75.

113. Huntoon MA, Martin DP: Paralysis after transforaminal epidural injection and previous spinal surgery. Reg Anesth Pain Med 2004;29: 494–495.

114. Devivo MJ: Epidemiology of traumatic spinal cord injury: trends and future implications. Spinal Cord 2012;50:365–372.

115. Hagen EM, Faerestrand S, Hoff JM, Rekand T, Gronning M: Cardiovascular and urological dysfunction in spinal cord injury. Acta Neurol Scand Suppl 2011:71–78.

116. Crosby E, St-Jean B, Reid D, Elliott RD: Obstetrical anaesthesia and analgesia in chronic spinal cord-injured women. Can J Anaesth 1992;39: 487–494.

117. Hambly PR, Martin B: Anaesthesia for chronic spinal cord lesions. Anaesth 1998;53:273–289.

118. Agostoni M, Giorgi E, Beccaria P, Zangrillo A, Valentini G: Combined spinal-epidural anaesthesia for Caesarean section in a paraplegic woman: difficulty in obtaining the expected level of block. Eur J Anaesthesiol 2000;17:329–331.

Acute Compartment Syndrome of the Limb: Implications for Regional Anesthesia

Xavier Sala-Blanch, Jose A de Andrés, and Steven Dewaele

INTRODUCTION

Compartment syndrome is an orthopedic emergency. It is an acute condition of the limbs in which the pressure of isolated or groups of poorly compliant muscle compartments increases dramatically and limits local soft tissue perfusion to the point of motor and sensory impairment and neuronal and tissue ischemic necrosis. Although regional anesthesia is often thought to delay diagnosis and treatment of acute compartment syndrome (ACS), there are only isolated case reports and a lack of evidence-based information to guide the clinical practice. Regardless, practitioners should be aware of the patient risk factors, clinical presentation, and management of this potentially limb-threatening condition. The musculoskeletal structures of the limbs are enclosed within compartments created by investing fascial layers with a limited ability to stretch. These compartments enclose skeletal muscles along with the neurovascular structures that pass through the compartments. If missed, compartment syndrome[1] can be a limb- and life-threatening condition.

Compartment syndrome is most common in the lower leg and forearm, although it can also occur in the hand, foot, thigh, and upper arm. In theory, the upper leg muscles are at a lower risk for injury than are the smaller muscles of the lower leg, because the muscles of the thigh can dissipate the large forces of direct trauma, causing less muscle injury and resultant edema.[2] Acute compartment syndrome occurs more commonly in one of the four smaller compartments of the lower leg.

The consequences of persistently elevated intracompartmental pressures were first described by Richard von Volkmann,[3] who documented nerve injury and late muscle contracture from compartment syndrome after supracondylar fracture of the distal humerus. Jepson[4] described ischemic contractures in dog hind legs, resulting from limb hypertension after experimentally induced venous obstruction. Only after about 40 years (since the 1970s) has the importance of measuring compartmental pressures become apparent.

Etiology

Any condition that can reduce the volume of the compartment or increase the size of the contents of the compartment can lead to an acute compartment syndrome. Examples of factors leading to these changes are presented in Table 50–1.

Pathophysiology

Compartment syndrome is essentially soft tissue ischemia, generally associated with trauma, fracture with subsequent casting, prolonged malpositioning during surgery, or reperfusion injury. However, the entire mechanism of compartment syndrome is unclear. Because various osseofascial compartments have a relatively fixed volume, introduction of excess fluid or external constriction increases pressure within the compartment and decreases tissue perfusion (Figure 50–1). As the compartmental pressure increases, the tissue hypoperfusion results in tissue hypoxia impeding cellular metabolism. If prolonged, permanent myoneural tissue damage occurs.[5–7] Under physiologic circumstances, the venous pressure exceeds that of the interstitial tissue pressure, sustaining venous outflow.[5] However, as tissue pressure increases, extrinsic venous luminal pressure is exceeded, resulting in vein collapse. The pressure at which this occurs is not known; however, it is generally agreed that compartmental pressures greater than 30 mm Hg require emergent intervention because ischemia is imminent.

Hypoxic injury causes cells to release free radicals, which increases endothelial permeability. This, in turn, leads to a vicious cycle of continued fluid loss, further increasing tissue pressure and injury. Diminished blood flow to local nerves first

TABLE 50-1. Factors leading to compartment syndrome.

Conditions that Increase the Compartment Volume
- Direct soft tissue trauma with or without long bone fracture (10%–20% incidence after closed fracture)
- Closed tibial shaft fractures (40%) and closed forearm fractures (12%)
- Soft tissue crush injuries without fractures in 23% of cases of compartment syndrome[5,6]
- Open fractures, which should theoretically decompress the adjacent compartments, may lead to compartment syndrome[7]
- Hemorrhage: Vascular injury, coagulopathy
- Anticoagulation therapy[8]
- Revascularization of limb after ischemia
- High-energy trauma, as from high-speed motor vehicle accident or crush injury
- Increased capillary permeability after burns (especially circumferential)
- Infusions or high-pressure injections (eg, regional blocks, paint guns)
- Extravasations of arthroscopic fluid (eg, after routine knee arthroscopy[9])
- Reperfusion after prolonged periods of ischemia
- Anabolic steroid use, resulting in muscle hypertrophy[10]
- Decreased serum osmolarity (eg, nephritic syndrome[11])
- Strenuous exercise, especially in previously sedentary people

Conditions that Lead to a Reduction in Volume of Tissue Compartments
- Tight circumferential dressings (eg, can occur with cotton cast padding alone)
- Closure of fascial defects[12]
- Cast or splint, especially if placed before removal of surgical tourniquet
- Prolonged limb compression, as in Trendelenburg and lateral decubitus positions[6,13] or in patients obtunded from alcohol or drug abuse
- Excessive traction to fractured limbs[14]

manifests as sensory changes. Paresthesias develop within 30 minutes of onset of ischemia. Irreversible nerve damage begins after 12–24 hours of total ischemia.[5] Irreversible changes in the muscles begin after only 4–8 hours, leading to muscle fiber death and late myocontracture.[8]

DIAGNOSIS OF COMPARTMENT SYNDROME

Compartment syndrome is often a diagnosis based primarily on variation in the patient's clinical signs and symptoms in sequential examinations. Pain out of proportion to the injury, especially with passive stretch of the muscles in the suspicious compartment or limb, is one of the most significant indicators. A palpably tense extremity compared with the uninjured limb

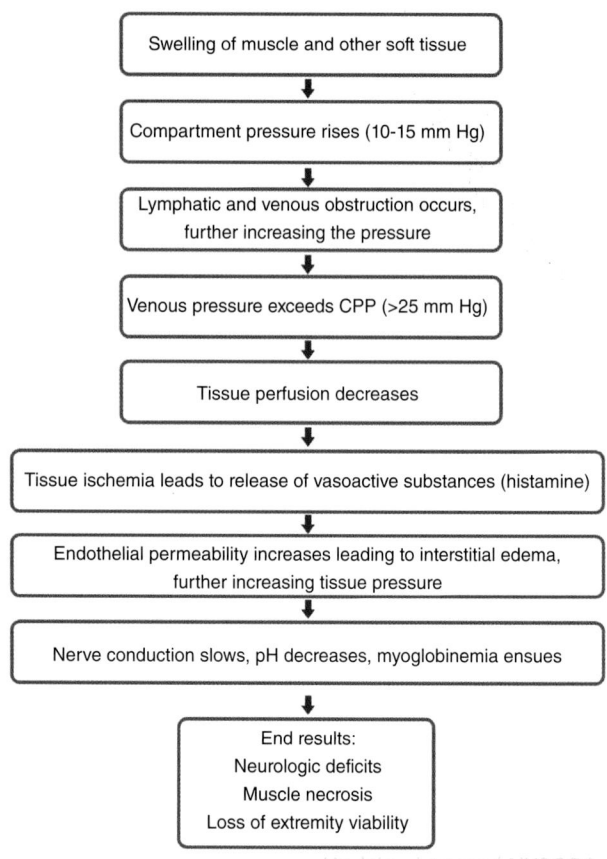

FIGURE 50-1. Pathophysiology of acute compartment syndrome. CPP, capillary perfusion pressure.

is also an important finding. However, none of these warning signs has proven to be reliable.[9] The other classic Ps of pallor, pulselessness, and paresis have very poor predictive value. In fact, pallor and pulselessness are rarely present in compartment syndrome, and by the time paresis manifests, the damage is largely irreversible. On the other hand, breakthrough pain in a patient with a previously well-functioning continuous block may be an early warning sign of ACS.

Clinical Pearl

- Pain out of proportion to the injury is an important symptom.

In general, establishment of the diagnosis based on clinical judgment alone can be difficult.[10–12] Instead, diagnosis should be supported by objective measurement of compartmental pressures with a needle and arterial line transducer or other pressure-measuring device(s). Assuming that the correct compartment is identified, measurement of interstitial tissue pressures remains the only objective reference method for the diagnosis of ACS and is particularly useful in the unresponsive, obtunded, or anesthetized patient (Figures 50–2 and 50–3). An absolute value above 30 mm Hg in the normotensive patient is consistent with compartment syndrome. This value is

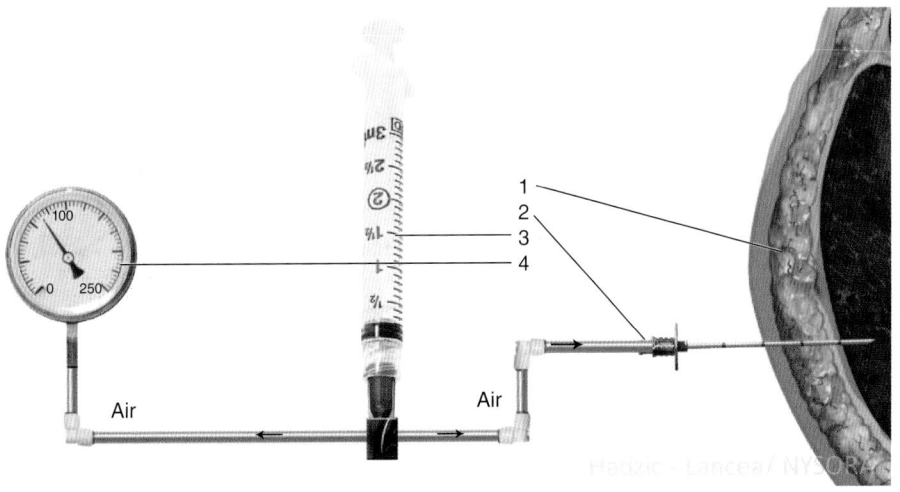

FIGURE 50-2. Intramuscular pressure measurement by the Whiteside technique. (1) Intramuscular needle, 18 gauge. (2) Perfusion line. (3) 20-mL syringe. (4) Mercury manometer.

diminished in the hypotensive patient as the lower arterial pressure renders the limbs even more susceptible to ischemic injury. Near-infrared spectroscopy is another noninvasive method suggested for monitoring the oxygen saturation of hemoglobin and myoglobulin in the tissue at risk (Figure 50–4).[13] More recently, intramuscular pH monitoring has been introduced as an additional diagnostic tool in order to accurately identify ACS.[14]

The Upper Limb

There are several compartments of the upper extremity that, when injured, may result in compartment syndrome requiring fasciotomy in the arm, forearm, or hand.

The arm has two compartments: anterior and posterior (Figure 50–5).

The forearm has three compartments: the volar and dorsal compartments and the compartment containing the muscles of the mobile wad. Mubarak et al.[15] have demonstrated that these compartments are interconnected, unlike the compartments of the leg (Figures 50–6 and 50–7). Consequently, decompression of the volar compartment alone may decrease the pressure in the other two compartments. Regardless, dorsal compartment fasciotomy should still be performed if the dorsal compartment remains tight after volar decompression.[16] The muscles of the volar compartment of the forearm include the digital and wrist flexors and the forearm pronators. These muscles are tested by passive extension of the digits and wrist and by supination of the forearm.

The dorsal forearm compartment contains the thumb and finger metacarpophalangeal joint extensors, the ulnar wrist extensors, and the forearm supinators and is tested by passive finger, thumb, and wrist flexion and by forearm pronation. The mobile wad includes the brachioradialis and the two radial wrist extensors and is tested by passive wrist flexion.

There are 10 compartments in the hand, the most prominent being the dorsal and palmar interosseous compartments, of which there are four and three, respectively (Figure 50–8). The other compartments are the hypothenar, thenar, and adductor. The compartment containing the adductor muscle of the thumb is often overlooked when doing fasciotomies. Studies using Renografin dye have shown no connection between the dorsal interossei and the other compartments, showing that each compartment must be decompressed separately.

The finger is enclosed in a tight investing fascia and is compartmentalized by the fascia and the volar skin at the flexor crease. Although no muscle bellies are distal from the metacarpophalangeal joints, ischemia and engorgement can lead to tissue loss (Figure 50–9).

The Lower Limb

Thigh

The thigh muscles are divided into three compartments invested by thick fascia: the anterior, medial, and posterior (Figures 50–10 and 50–11). Because thigh compartment syndrome is uncommon, it may go unrecognized. A history of anticoagulant use is common in patients with thigh

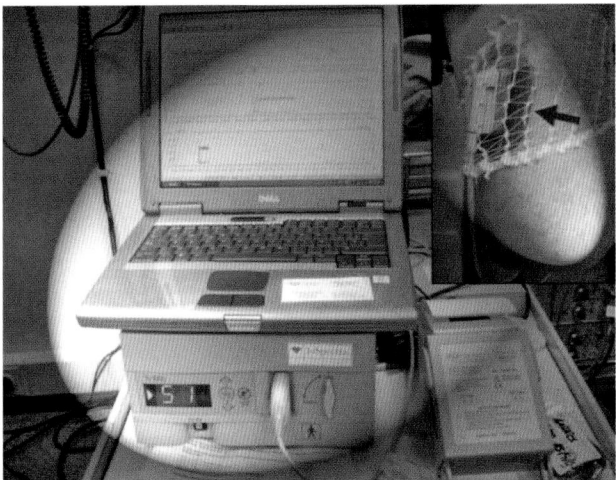

FIGURE 50-3. Near-infrared spectroscopy is a noninvasive method for monitoring the oxygen saturation of hemoglobin and myoglobulin.

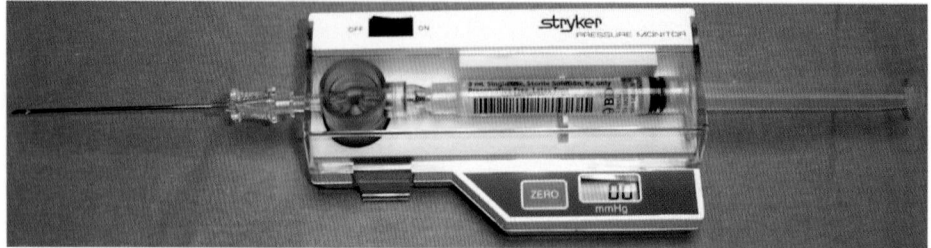

FIGURE 50–4. Intracompartmental pressure monitoring device with digital display.

compartment syndrome. Signs and symptoms include a history of thigh swelling and/or hematoma and pain after a minor injury in a patient who is anticoagulated.[17,18] Although rare, the thigh syndrome can also occur in patients after joint replacement surgery. The combination of minor trauma and anticoagulation produces bleeding into muscle and tissue spaces, leading to increased compartment pressure. Pain ranges from mild to severe and may be elicited only when the hip and knee are flexed and extended. Other findings of vascular occlusion—loss of pulse, pallor, paresthesias, and paralysis—are frequently absent.

Lower Leg

The lower leg contains four compartments, each invested by inelastic fascia (Figures 50–12 and 50–13). Each compartment contains a major nerve: the deep peroneal in the anterior compartment, the superficial peroneal in the lateral compartment, the saphenous in the superficial posterior compartment, and the tibial in the deep posterior compartment. Swelling in the lateral or anterior compartment can compress both the deep and superficial peroneal nerves against the neck of the fibula. The superficial peroneal nerve usually lies in the interval between the two peroneal muscles for a short distance and then emerges anterior to the peroneus brevis. It pierces the lateral compartment fascia at the junction of the middle and distal third of the leg. The anatomy of the superficial and

deep posterior compartments is somewhat variable, but both compartments, and especially the deep compartment, are frequently involved in compartment syndrome.

Foot

The foot has numerous rigidly bound compartments, and even mild bleeding into these spaces can elevate the pressures dramatically (Figure 50–14). According to Manoli and Weber,[19] there are nine compartments in the foot. Three compartments run the entire length of the foot (medial, lateral, and superficial). Five compartments are contained within the forefoot (adductor and four interossei). The calcaneal compartment is confined to the hind foot but communicates with the posterior compartment of the leg. This compartment contains the quadratus muscle and the lateral plantar neurovascular bundle. The clinically most relevant compartments are the medial, central, lateral, and interossei.[20,21]

A wide spectrum of injuries can result in compartment syndrome of the foot, the most likely ones being crush injuries, especially those associated with multiple metatarsal fractures. Often, the only reliable method of diagnosis is by clinical suspicion and measurement of the intracompartmental pressures. Loss of posterior tibial or dorsalis pedis pulse is notoriously unreliable in the early diagnosis of compartment syndrome. The earliest clinical findings are muscle and nerve ischemia and pain. Although this pain might be confused with the pain of the injury itself, it may be exacerbated by gentle, passive dorsiflexion of the toes, which stretches the intrinsic muscles of the foot. Lack of sensation is generally accepted as an important

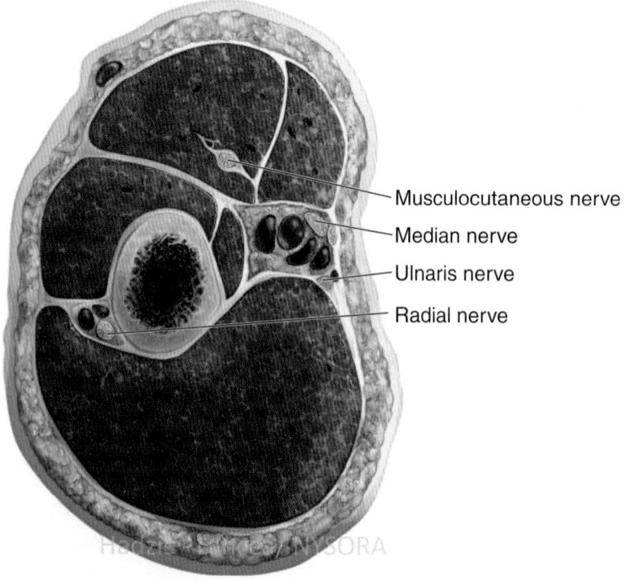

Musculocutaneous nerve
Median nerve
Ulnaris nerve
Radial nerve

FIGURE 50–5. Tissue compartments of the arm.

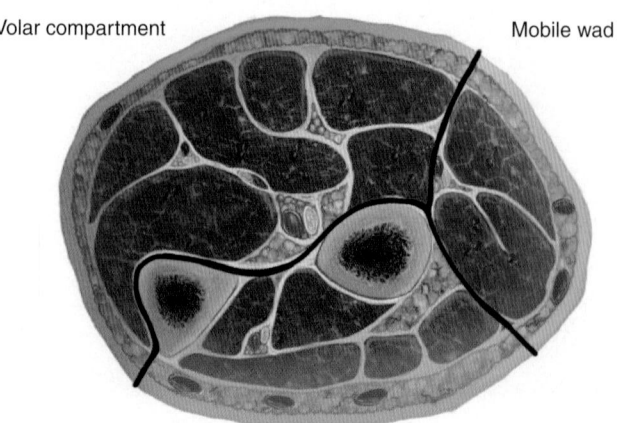

Volar compartment

Mobile wad

Dorsal compartment

FIGURE 50–6. Tissue compartments of the forearm.

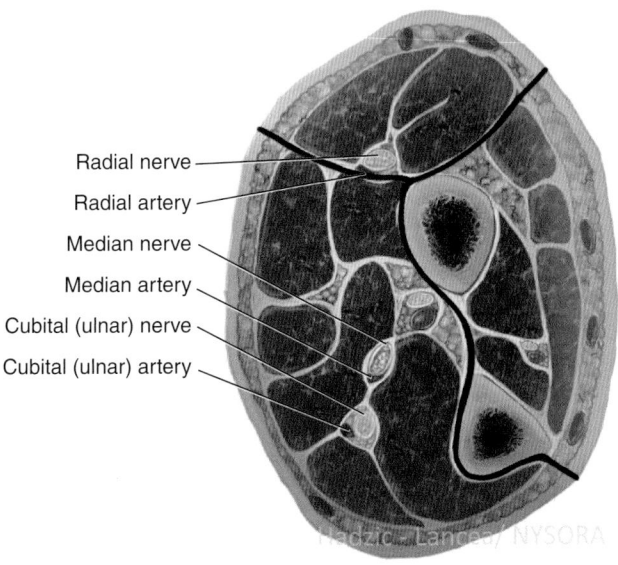

Radial nerve
Radial artery
Median nerve
Median artery
Cubital (ulnar) nerve
Cubital (ulnar) artery

FIGURE 50–7. Forearm compartments.

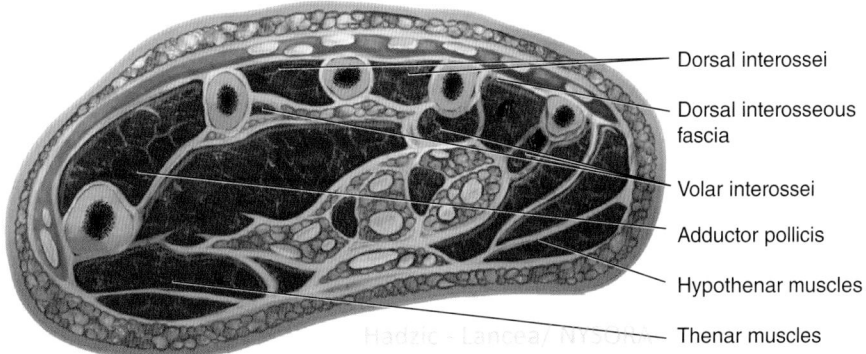

Dorsal interossei
Dorsal interosseous fascia
Volar interossei
Adductor pollicis
Hypothenar muscles
Thenar muscles

FIGURE 50–8. Cross-section through the palm showing the compartments of the hand.

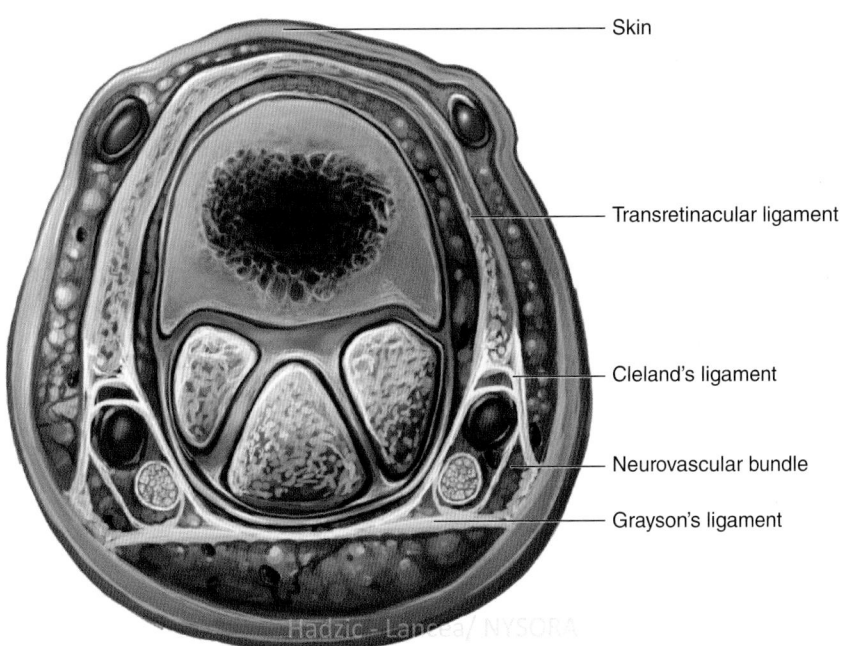

Skin
Transretinacular ligament
Cleland's ligament
Neurovascular bundle
Grayson's ligament

FIGURE 50–9. Cross-section through the finger.

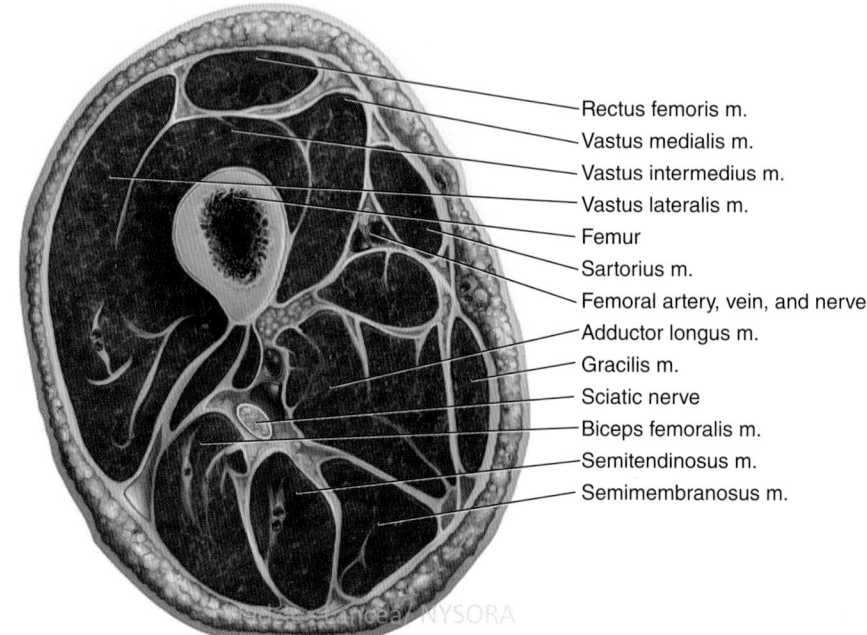

Rectus femoris m.
Vastus medialis m.
Vastus intermedius m.
Vastus lateralis m.
Femur
Sartorius m.
Femoral artery, vein, and nerve
Adductor longus m.
Gracilis m.
Sciatic nerve
Biceps femoralis m.
Semitendinosus m.
Semimembranosus m.

FIGURE 50–10. Compartments of the upper thigh.

sign of nerve ischemia, but it is not reliable when compared with a two-point discrimination and light touch over the plantar aspect of the foot and toes.

Clinical Pearl

- Compartment pressure measurement is the only objective and accurate test to diagnose and monitor compartment syndrome.

Compartment pressure measurement is the only objective and accurate test to diagnose and record compartment syndrome, particularly because changes in compartment pressures can precede the clinical signs of compartment syndrome.

The central compartment can be measured by passing a needle between the metatarsal and abductor hallucis muscle at the base of the first metatarsal. The interossei compartment is measured in two positions by introducing the needle through the intermetatarsal spaces, preferably between the second and forth web spaces to avoid punctures to the dorsalis pedis within the first intermetatarsal region.

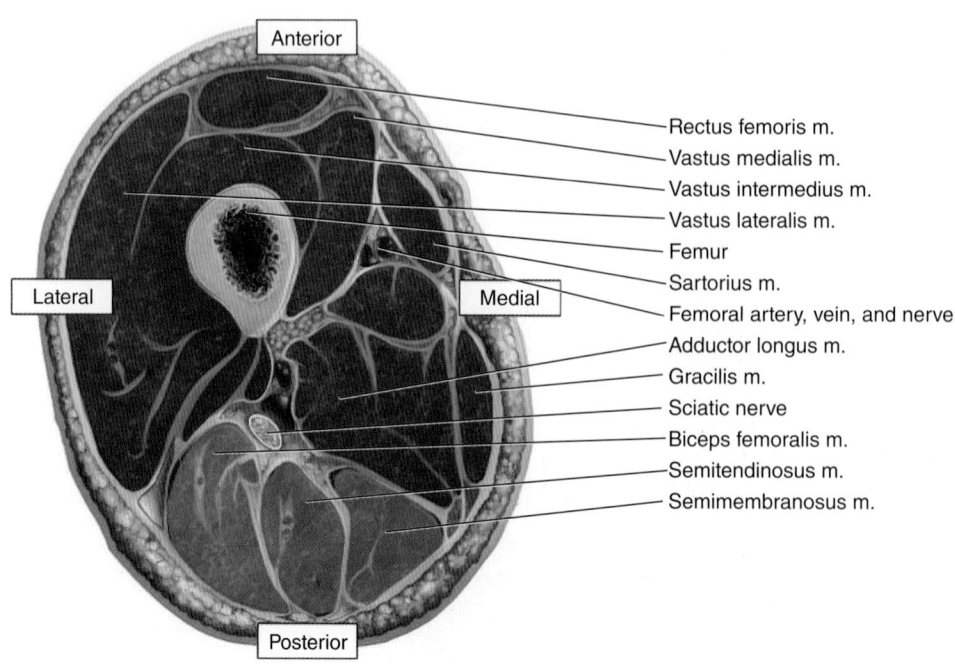

Anterior
Lateral
Medial
Posterior

Rectus femoris m.
Vastus medialis m.
Vastus intermedius m.
Vastus lateralis m.
Femur
Sartorius m.
Femoral artery, vein, and nerve
Adductor longus m.
Gracilis m.
Sciatic nerve
Biceps femoralis m.
Semitendinosus m.
Semimembranosus m.

FIGURE 50–11. Compartments of the thigh.

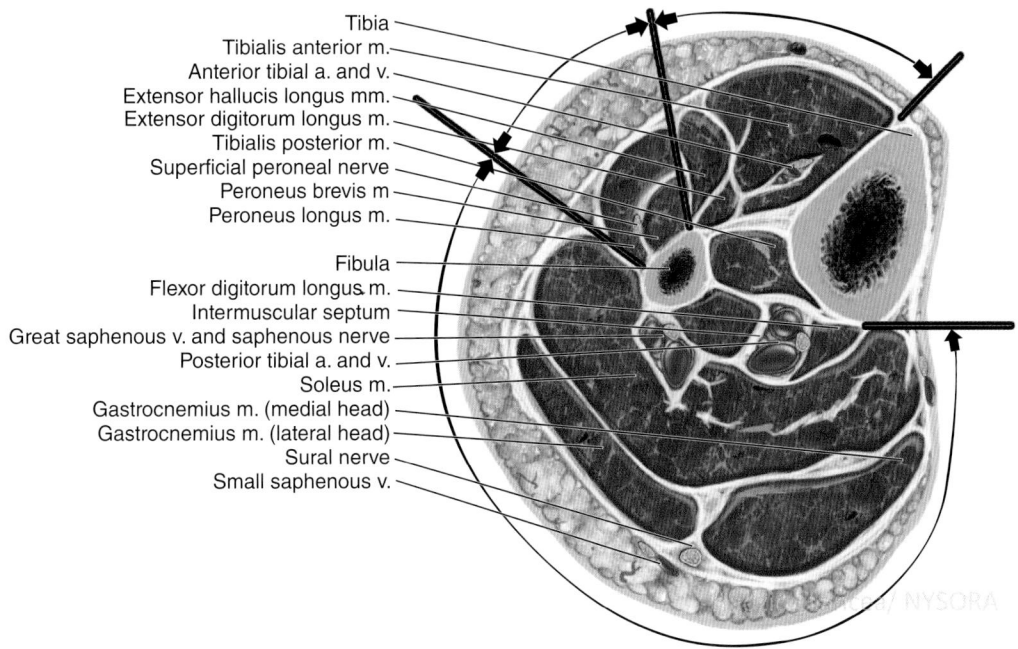

FIGURE 50–12. Contents of the four compartments of the lower leg.

The calcaneal or quadratus compartment is measured by inserting the needle 5 cm distal and 2 cm inferior to the medial malleolus and advancing through the abductor muscle.

Acute Compartment Syndrome and Regional Anesthesia

There is a significant medicolegal aspect of ACS and its outcome in clinical practice; in 50% of all cases and claims related to ACS, data show that decisions are ruled in favor of the plaintiff (the patient). Several case reports and case series suggest that regional anesthesia may have delayed diagnosis of ACS.[22–24] In contrast, there are also a number of cases and reviews suggesting that regional anesthesia may not mask timely diagnosis[25–30] and, in fact, may even facilitate detection of ACS.[31] Consequently, the use of a regional anesthesia technique in the face of risk factors for ACS remains controversial.

In recent literature, "best practice rules" have been suggested to reduce the risk of missing a compartment syndrome in children

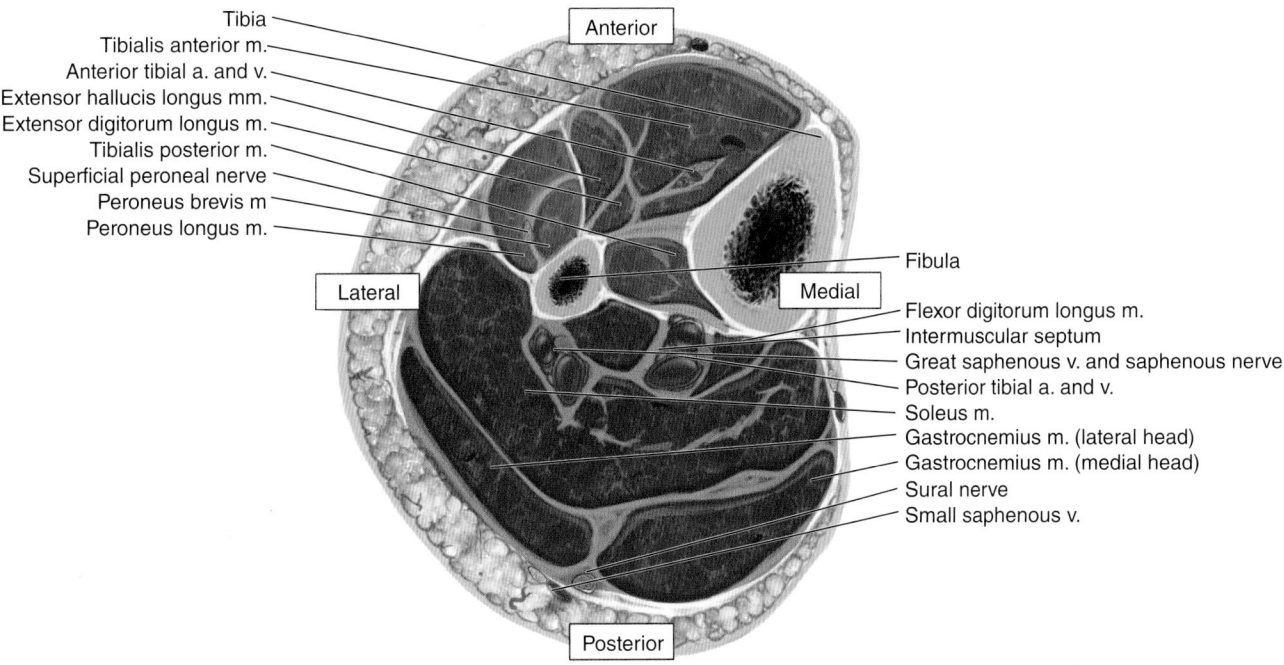

FIGURE 50–13. Lower leg compartments: Spatial distribution.

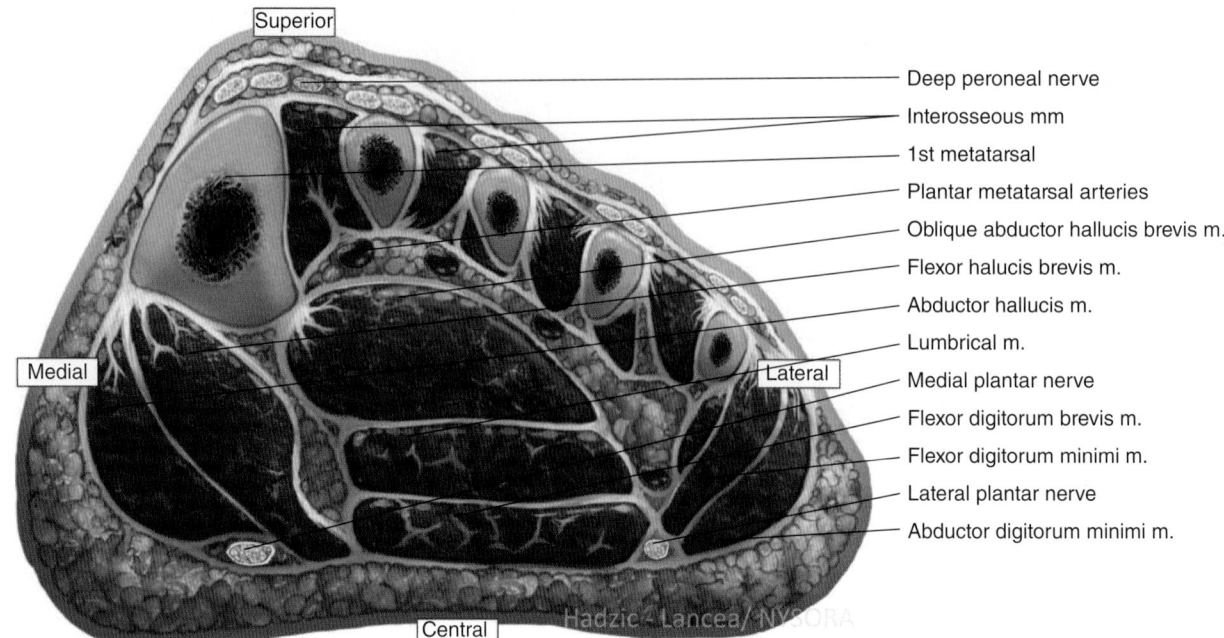

Superior

— Deep peroneal nerve
— Interosseous mm
— 1st metatarsal
— Plantar metatarsal arteries
— Oblique abductor hallucis brevis m.
— Flexor halucis brevis m.
— Abductor hallucis m.
— Lumbrical m.
— Medial plantar nerve
— Flexor digitorum brevis m.
— Flexor digitorum minimi m.
— Lateral plantar nerve
— Abductor digitorum minimi m.

Medial

Lateral

Central

FIGURE 50–14. Coronal section of the foot through the base of the metatarsals depicting the medial, central, lateral, and interosseous compartments.

undergoing surgery with perioperative regional anesthesia; these rules may be also be applicable to adults.[32] It should be noted that although these recommendations appear succinct, they are largely theoretical considerations to help guide the clinical decision making; they have not been put to test in clinical practice.

Clinical Pearls

When regional analgesia is planned to treat intractable pain in patients with risk of compartment syndrome:

- Reduce the concentration of local anesthetics (0.1% to 0.25% bupivacaine, levobupivacaine, or ropivacaine) as lower concentrations are less likely to mask ischemic pain.
- For continuous infusions of bupivacaine, levobupivacaine, or ropivacaine, concentrations should be limited to 0.1%.
- In high-risk surgeries for compartment syndrome (eg, tibial compartment surgery), restricting both volume and concentration is advisable.
- Patients should have careful follow-up by acute pain services to allow for early detection of potential signs and symptoms (h).
- If ACS is clinically suspected, compartment pressure measurement without delay is mandatory.

TREATMENT OF COMPARTMENT SYNDROME

Emergency fasciotomy remains the definitive treatment for a diagnosis of compartment syndrome because of its well-documented, limb-saving results. It is universally accepted as being the best chance for complete recovery and for prevention of further tissue necrosis. Treatment is based primarily on the

clinical picture together with corroborative compartmental pressure measurements (Figure 50–15). The surgeon should proceed emergently with a decompression fasciotomy when clinically indicated because the exact pressure at which fasciotomy should be performed remains controversial. Most studies have shown that fasciotomy is indicated when the compartment pressure reaches 30 mm Hg.[21,33–35] Fasciotomy is also recommended when the compartmental pressure is within 30 mm Hg of the patient's diastolic pressure.[34]

After a complete fasciotomy, there is rarely a need for additional releases. The fasciotomy incisions are always left open with wound closure delayed for a minimum of 5 days. The patient is followed up clinically unless anesthetized or obtunded, in which case regular compartment pressure measurements should be made.

Clinical Pearls

- Emergency fasciotomy remains the definitive treatment for compartment syndrome.
- Its limb-saving results make it universally accepted as the best chance for complete recovery and for prevention of further tissue necrosis.
- Fasciotomy is indicated when compartment pressure reaches 30 mm Hg.
- After a complete fasciotomy is performed, additional release is rarely needed.

SUMMARY

Prolonged surgery, especially in patients undergoing procedures in the Trendelenburg or lateral decubitus positions, poses a risk of compartment syndrome. The Trendelenburg position requires

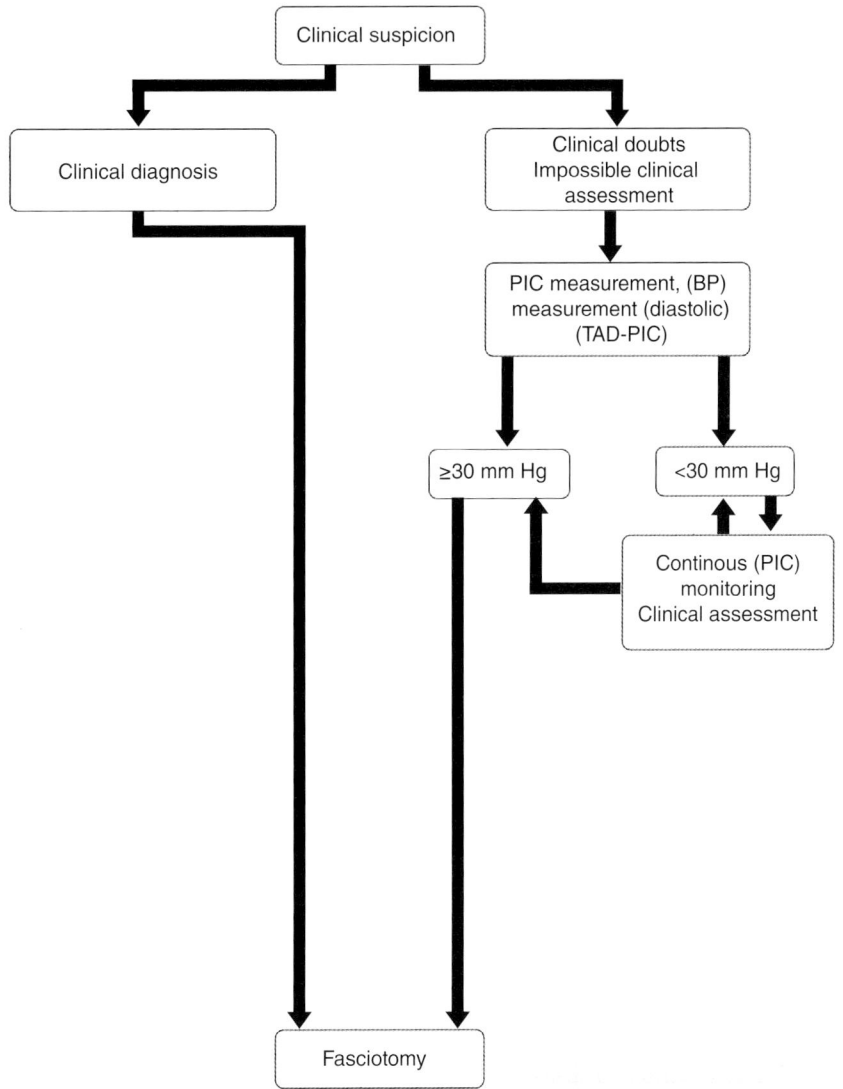

FIGURE 50-15. Diagnosis and management of compartment syndrome. BP, blood pressure; PIC, pressure within the compartment; TAD-PIC, diastolic blood pressure.

that the legs are strapped at a higher level than the heart. This can be avoided by repositioning and redraping the legs, or, if this is not possible, the head-down tilt position should be reversed every 2 hours so that reperfusion of the lower limbs can occur. In the lateral decubitus position, the down arm and the down leg must be well padded to avoid excessive compression.

On recent analysis of risk factors, age appeared to be a strong predictor of developing ACS (P < 0.001), with the highest prevalence between 12–19 years and 20–29 years. Occupation and implant type were the only other factors that remained significant after adjusting for age.[36]

Patients on anticoagulation medication tend to have a high risk of thigh compartment syndrome, even with relatively minor trauma or surgical interventions. This clinical scenario must be approached with a high index of suspicion.

In conclusion, the use of regional anesthesia in patients with risk of compartment syndrome is controversial. Therefore, regional blocks should be performed in consultation with the patient and with the surgical team. When deemed beneficial to patient care, regional anesthesia can be used when indicated to alleviate severe pain; however, astute management, compartment tissue monitoring, and perhaps lower concentrations and volumes of local anesthetics should be considered.

REFERENCES

1. Matsen F, Winquist R, Krugmire R: Diagnosis and management of compartment syndromes. J Bone Joint Surg 1980;62A:286.
2. Schwartz J, Brumback R, Lakatos R: Acute compartment syndrome of the thigh: A spectrum of injury. J Bone Joint Surg 1989;71:392–400.
3. von Volkmann R: Die ischamischen Kontakturen. Zentralbl Chir 1881; 8:801.
4. Jepson P: Ischemic contracture, experimental study. Ann Surg 1926; 68A:820.
5. Matsen F: Compartmental syndrome. A unified concept. Clin Orthop 1975;113:8–14.
6. Botte M, Santi M, Prestianni C, Abrams R: Ischemic contracture of the foot and ankle: Principles of management and prevention. Orthopedics 1996;19:235–244.
7. Ziv I, Mosheiff R, Zeligowski A, et al: Crush injuries of the foot with compartment syndrome: Immediate one-stage management. Foot Ankle 1989;9:185–189.
8. Whitesides T, Harada H, Morimoto K: The response of skeletal muscle to temporary ischemia: An experimental study. J Bone Joint Surg 1971;53A: 1027–1028.

9. McQueen M, Gaston P, Court-Brown C: Acute compartment syndrome: Who is at risk? J Bone Joint Surg 2000;82B:200–203.

10. Ulmer T: The clinical diagnosis of compartment syndrome of the lower leg: Are clinical findings predictive of the disorder? J Orthop Trauma 2002;16:572–577.

11. Shuler FD, Dietz MJ: Physician's ability to manually detect isolated elevations in leg intracompartmental pressure. J Bone Joint Surg Am 2010; 92:361-367.

12. McQueen MM. Acute compartment syndrome. In: Bucholz RW, Court-Brown CM, Heckman JD, Tornetta P 3rd (eds): Rockwood and Green's Fractures in Adults, 7th ed. Philadelphia: Lippincott Williams & Wilkins; 2010:689–708.

13. Tighe PJ, Elliott CE, Lucas SD, et al: Noninvasive tissue oxygen saturation determined by near-infrared spectroscopy following peripheral nerve block. Acta Anesth Scand 2011;55:1239–1246.

14. Elliott KG: Intramuscular pH as a novel diagnostic tool for acute compartment syndrome: A prospective clinical study [dissertation]. Aberdeen, Scotland: University of Aberdeen; 2007. uk.bl.ethos.485671.

15. Gelberman R, Zakaib G, Mubarak S, et al: Decompression of the forearm compartments. Clin Orthop 1978;134:225–229.

16. Allen M, Steingold R, Kotecha M: The importance of volar compartment in crush injuries in the forearm. Injury 1985;16:173–175.

17. Choyce A, Chan V, Middleton W, et al: What is the relationship between paresthesia and nerve stimulation for axillary brachial plexus block? Reg Anesth Pain Med 2001;26:100–104.

18. An H, Simpson M, Gale S, Jackson W: Acute anterior compartment syndrome in the thigh: A case report and review of the literature. J Orthop Trauma 1987;1:180–183.

19. Manoli A II, Weber T: Fasciotomy of the foot: An anatomical study with special reference to release of the calcaneal compartment. Foot Ankle 1990;10(6):267–275.

20. Sarraffian S: Anatomy of the Foot and Ankle. Philadelphia: J. B. Lippincott, 1983.

21. Myerson M: Experimental decompression of the fascial compartment of the foot: The basis for fasciotomy in an acute compartment syndromes. Foot Ankle 1988;8:308–314.

22. Dunwoody J, Reichert CC, Brown KL: Compartment syndrome associated with bupivacaine and fentanyl epidural analgesia in pediatric orthopaedics. J Pediatr Orthop 1997;17:285–328.

23. Hyder N, Kessler S, Jennings A, et al: Compartment syndrome in tibial shaft fracture missed because of local nerve block. J Bone Joint Surg 1996;78-B:499–500.

24. Tang W, Chiu K: Silent compartment syndrome complicating total knee arthroplasty. J Arthroplasty 2000;15:241–243.

25. Walker BJ, Noonan KJ, Bosenberg AT: Evolving compartment syndrome not masked by a continuous nerve block. Reg Anesth Pain Med 2012;3:393–397.

26. Mar GJ, Barrington MJ, McGuirk BR: Acute compartment syndrome of the lower limb and the effect of postoperative analgesia on diagnosis. Br J Anaesth 2009;102:3–11.

27. Cometa MA, Esch AT, Boezaart AP: Did continuous femoral and sciatic nerve block obscure the diagnosis or delay the treatment of acute lower leg compartment syndrome? A case report. Pain Med 2011;12:823–828.

28. Kucera TJ, Boezaart AP: Regional anesthesia does not consistently block ischemic pain: Two further cases and review of the literature. Pain Med 2014;15:316–319.

29. Rauf J, Iohom G, O'Donnell B: Acute compartment syndrome and regional anaesthesia—a case report. Rom J Anaesth Int Care 2015;22: 51–54.

30. Sermeus L, Boeckx S, Camerlynck HP, et al: Postsurgical compartment syndrome of the forearm in a child. Acta Anaesthesiol Belg 2015;66: 29–32.

31. Aguirre JA, Gresch D, Ropovici A, et al: Case scenario: Compartment syndrome of the forearm in patient with infraclavicular catheter. Anesthesiology 2013;118:1198–1205.

32. Ivani G, Suresh S, Ecoffey C, et al: The European Society of Regional Anaesthesia and Pain Therapy and the American Society of Regional Anesthesia and Pain Medicine Joint Committee Practice Advisory on Controversial Topics in Pediatric Regional Anesthesia. Reg Anesth Pain Med 2015;40:526–532.

33. Mubarak S, Owen C: Compartment syndrome and its relationship to the crush syndrome: A spectrum of disease—a review of 11 cases of prolonged limb compression. Clin Orthop 1975;113:81– 89.

34. Whitesides T, Haney T, Morimoto K: Tissue pressure measurements as a determinant for the need of fasciotomy. Clin Orthop 1975;113:43–51.

35. Staudt JM, Smeulders MJ, van der Horst CM: Normal compartment pressures of the lower leg in children. J Bone Joint Surg Br 2008;90: 215–219.

36. McQueen MM, Duckworth AD, Aitken SA, et al: Predictors of compartment syndrome after tibial fracture. J Orthop Trauma 2015;29: 451–455.

Peripheral Nerve Blocks for Outpatient Surgery

Christina M. Spofford, Peter Foldes, and John Laur

INTRODUCTION

An increasing number of patients are undergoing surgical procedures in hospital outpatient departments (HOPDs) or ambulatory surgery centers (ASCs).[1] Outpatient surgical procedures have become more complex, and patients are presenting for surgery with a greater number of comorbid conditions than in the past.[2] Regional anesthesia (RA) and peripheral nerve blocks (PNBs) can help meet the goals of caring for these patients in the outpatient setting.

In 1976, there were 67 Medicare-certified ASCs in the United States, and in 2011, there were 5,344.[3] In 1982, 30 ambulatory surgical procedures were covered by Medicare; today there are hundreds.[4] In an analysis of National Survey of Ambulatory Surgery (NSAS) data, Tighe et al. found that 15% of an estimated 4 million orthopedic outpatient cases implemented a "regional block" as part of the anesthetic used.[6,7] Over 580,000 PNBs were performed in HOPDs or ASCs in 2006.[5]

From 2006 to 2010, outpatient services per Medicare enrollee increased by 5.7% annually. In 2011, the rate increased by 1.9%, accounting for $3.4 billion in charges, a 2.2% increase from 2010.[3,4] Currently, about 57 million outpatient procedures (surgical and nonsurgical) are performed in the United States at a cost of $3.2 billion.[4,8] In 2014, over 3 million of these cases are estimated to be orthopedic procedures.[5] At some institutions, including the authors', most PNBs are performed for orthopedic cases.[9] Based on NSAS data from 1996 through 2006, arthroscopic knee procedures in the U.S. increased by 49%.[10] As minimally invasive surgery becomes available for surgeries that require an inpatient stay due to the severity of postoperative pain, RA can allow for safe same-day discharge.[11] A study by Koenig and Gu indicated that the growth of ASCs may reduce Medicare spending due to lower reimbursements relative to number of hospitals.[12] There is

preliminary evidence that outcomes at ASCs are better than those at in-hospital settings for similar otolaryngologic surgical cases.[13] Future research in this area needs to be completed for other services.

With the growth in both complex outpatient surgeries and ASCs, there is a need for more anesthesiologists with specific training in the use of acute pain medicine with integrated RA and PNB techniques. With the use of these techniques, the first priority should be on safety, the second on reducing patient pain and minimizing opioid and general anesthesia (GA) side effects, the third on economics, and the fourth on efficiency.[14,15]

Outpatient Surgery Stakeholders

Patients, providers, payers, and "internal customers," including anesthesiologists, nurses, and support staff,[16] may have differing views on the value on the various outpatient operational and clinical outcomes. In healthcare, value is defined as patient outcome per costs used to achieve those outcomes.[17,18] For payers, value consists of providing a service with good outcome at a lower cost than competitors.[4,5,16] Typically, a standalone outpatient surgery center can provide patient care with greater patient convenience and lower overhead costs than a hospital outpatient surgery department.[1] Busy surgeons focus on ASC efficiency[19] and understand the value of RA and PNBs, but they may object to additional procedures that could delay surgery.[20] The available data, however, point out that greater than half of surgery-start delays are caused by the surgeon rather than nerve block placement.[21] Factors that contribute to delays include the need for surgical consent, updating the patient's medical history and performing the physical examination, the patient's desire to speak with the surgeon prior to going to the operating room (OR), and the need for additional preoperative testing.[20]

Anesthesiologists work to provide safe high-quality care by applying methods that reduce or prevent adverse events and side-effects. Minimizing or eliminating nausea, vomiting, and pain are important for maintaining patient satisfaction. Secondary goals for anesthesiologists include accurate and fast RA placement and nerve block onset, sufficient duration of analgesia, avoidance of "rebound pain" when the nerve block resolves, post-anesthesia care unit (PACU) bypass, and rapid patient discharge from the facility.[15,18] Avoiding side effects, hence bypassing the PACU, can reduce hospital costs by an estimated 12% while still meeting the goals of the surgeons, anesthesiologists, payers, and patients.[18,20,22]

Patients fear nausea, vomiting, gagging on the endotracheal tube, surgical pain, recall, residual weakness, shivering, sore throat, and somnolence. They wish to experience restful sleep and then return to work and physical function with little pain or motor blockade.[23] Most of these patient-centric goals can be achieved by designing an appropriate anesthesia regimen tailored to the patient and surgical procedure(s). In many cases, the use of RA achieves these goals.

Clinical Pearls

- The anesthesiologist's priorities are (1) safety; (2) reducing patient pain and minimizing opioid and GA side effects; (3) economics; and (4) efficiency.
- Factors that contribute to surgery-start delays include the need for surgical consent, updating the patient's medical history and performing the physical examination, the patient's desire to speak with the surgeon prior to going to the OR, and the need for additional preoperative testing.
- Hospital costs can be reduced by bypassing the PACU while meeting the goals of the surgeon, anesthesiologist, payers, and patient through the avoidance of side effects.
- Most patient-centric goals can be achieved by designing an appropriate anesthesia regimen tailored to the patient and surgical procedure(s).

Defining Outpatient Regional Anesthesia Success

There are multiple, and possibly overlapping, metrics defining outpatient RA success.[18] A single set of outcomes may not please all stakeholders. In randomized, controlled trials (RCTs), success is determined by avoiding the following: conversion to GA, loss of sensation to pin-prick or cold, loss of motor function, and time to first pain medication request.[18] Many RCTs ask about patient satisfaction with RA, and it is important to understand what patients prefer with respect to outcomes after RA.[22] Recently, a validated, multidimensional, self-reported questionnaire was created to assess RA in the outpatient surgery setting.[24] Factors included avoiding RA-related delays and complications, providing anesthesia during the surgical procedure and continuing adequate postoperative analgesia, reducing the costs of drugs and equipment, reducing patient time spent in the healthcare

facility, avoiding unplanned hospital admissions, ensuring patient satisfaction, maintaining postoperative function (particularly with a partially or wholly insensate body region), safety at home, and other clinical and economic outcomes.

Motor weakness can be desirable for surgery yet is often undesirable afterward when physical therapy is necessary or patients want to walk or hold an object.[25] While acknowledging that RA is superior to GA in terms of pain control and reduction of postoperative nausea and vomiting, orthopedic surgeons often report avoiding RA due to case-start delays and unpredictable RA success.[26]

Clinical Pearl

- Numerous factors must be taken into account in the outpatient surgery setting, including avoiding RA-related delays and complications, providing anesthesia during the surgical procedure and continuing adequate postoperative analgesia, reducing the costs of drugs and equipment, reducing patient time spent in the health-care facility, avoiding unplanned hospital admissions, ensuring patient satisfaction, maintaining postoperative function (particularly with a partially or wholly insensate body region), safety at home, and other clinical and economic outcomes.

Peripheral Nerve Blocks and Multimodal Analgesia

Managing postoperative pain with minimal side effects is an important factor in determining if a surgical case can proceed in an outpatient setting. An anesthesiologist has an armamentarium of agents and methods to provide multimodal analgesic therapy. Boezaart and Tighe contend that PNBs are an inherent part of the rapidly developing field of acute pain medicine that they remark should focus on the patient and his or her pain control.[13] In an outpatient setting, RA with PNBs is a cornerstones of multimodal analgesia and opioid-sparing strategies. High-dose opioids can cause hyperalgesia by activating neurons and glial cells.[27] Furthermore, potent opioids, such as remifentanil and fentanyl, can cause hyperalgesia and rapid tolerance in humans.[28] Other undesirable side effects are nausea, somnolence, and respiratory depression, all which are highly undesirable in the outpatient setting.

Well-planned multimodal analgesia is important in the ambulatory surgery setting for several reasons. First, *patients* prefer to avoid side effects such as nausea, vomiting, and somnolence.[22,29] Second, uncontrolled side effects can result in unplanned hospital admission, which is costly and inconvenient for all parties. Third, the use of multimodal analgesia has the potential for real synergistic positive effects while also reducing the likelihood of serious side effects.[2] Lastly, multimodal analgesic regimens improve the likelihood of early recovery.[30] One example is the same-day discharge of patients undergoing unicompartment knee replacement surgery. By utilizing a continuous femoral nerve block and minimizing opioids as part of a multimodal analgesia regimen, these patients can safely undergo surgery in an ASC.[10]

Used in a multimodal analgesic regimen, gabapentinoids, nonsteroidal anti-inflammatory drugs (NSAIDs), acyclooxygenase-1 and -2 (COX-1 and COX-2) inhibitors, glucocorticoids, ketamine, clonidine, and lidocaine infusions can reduce postoperative opioid use by 20%–60%.[31-34] Intravenous lidocaine infusions have demonstrated a preventive analgesic effect lasting from 8.5 to 72 hours, which is greater than 5.5 lidocaine half-lives.[35] Local anesthetics may reduce pain scores and opioid consumption when administered via PNB *or* the intravenous route (using lidocaine), although the evidence for this is sometimes contradictory.[34,36]

Some facilities are performing "fast-track" total hip and knee replacement surgeries in an outpatient setting with 23-hour observation. The American Academy of Orthopaedic Surgeons guidelines on preventing venous thromboembolism recommend neuraxial anesthesia during hip and knee replacement procedures to reduce blood loss.[37] In fact, due to its superior analgesia in joint replacement surgery, RA is the centerpiece of a multimodal analgesia algorithm in such surgeries.[38]

Clinical Pearls

- PNBs have progressed to become a component of the larger field of acute pain medicine that focuses on the patients and their pain control.
- In the outpatient setting, RA with PNBs is the cornerstone of multimodal analgesia.

Nerve Blocks in Outpatients

A wide variety of PNBs can be used in the ambulatory setting, including upper and lower extremity blocks, truncal blocks, and head-and-neck PNBs (Table 51–1). Moreover, neuraxial RA techniques can achieve outpatient anesthesia goals.[39] In an ambulatory setting, surgeon-performed blocks can also be timely, cost effective, and remarkably safe. Done at the time of the procedure, they often include rapidly acting local anesthetics. Some of the most commonly used peripheral nerve blocks are listed in Table 51–2.[40-43]

TABLE 51–1. Peripheral nerve blocks.

Upper Extremity PNBs	Lower Extremity PNBs	Truncal Blocks
Cervical paravertebral	Subgluteal sciatic	Thoracic paravertebral
Interscalene	Femoral	Transverse abdominis plane
Interscalene	Popliteal	Ilioinguinal
Infraclavicular	Saphenous	
Axillary	Ankle	

TABLE 51–2. Commonly used regional anesthesia blocks.

Service	Type of Block
Ophthalmology	Retrobulbar, peribulbar
General surgery	Ilioinguinal
Urology	Penile
Orthopedics	Joint injections, local infiltration
Vascular surgery	Cervical plexus blocks
Gynecology	Paracervical block

Block Latency

One strategy to decrease onset time is to add mepivacaine to the longer-acting local anesthetics that are traditionally used (eg, ropivacaine, bupivacaine), albeit at the cost of shortening the duration of the blockade.[44,45] The best strategy is to have one provider perform the nerve block in the block room and have the other providers remain in the operating room. This procedure prevents delays in turnover, optimizes care by having a dedicated person providing specialized care, and creates a team atmosphere. This model can either be expensive or pay for itself, depending on the system and methods of reimbursement for care.[46] For example, it can be cost prohibitive in practices where there are too few blocks placed in a single day or too few personnel trained in peripheral nerve blockade.[20]

Peripheral Nerve Blocks and Adjuvants

Regional anesthesiologists combine local anesthetics with adjuvant drugs to achieve prolonged analgesia, reduce local anesthetic dose to avoid toxicity, and potentially reduce motor blockade.[34,47,48] Clinical doses of clonidine, buprenorphine, dexamethasone, and midazolam have no neurotoxicity in vitro.[46,49,50] These drugs are thought to act through an indirect mechanism without influencing the potency or duration of the local anesthetic, specifically ropivacaine or lidocaine.[49]

Providing surgical anesthesia and then maintaining the patient's motor strength while achieving postoperative analgesia may be difficult with single local injections. Adjuvants can prolong analgesia duration with single-injection PNBs.[34,51,52] This application reduces the mechanical, logistical, billing, and clinical management hurdles associated with outpatient indwelling PNB catheters and improves patient convenience.[53] While clonidine and dexmedetomidine may prolong analgesic duration in some blocks, these agents may not have the same benefit in other blocks (eg, sciatic) when combined with a long-acting local anesthetic.[54-56] The undesirable side effects of clonidine (and other alpha-2 blockers) include hypotension, bradycardia, orthostatic hypotension, and sedation.[53] Clonidine increases the duration of motor blockade, which may or may not be desirable depending on the type of surgery.[55]

Dexamethasone is an adjuvant that can enhance or prolong the duration of analgesia when injected perineurally *or intravenously*.[57-62] Recent work suggests that perineural adjuvants can control post-surgical pain while sparing motor strength.[15] However, safety data on perineural injections in animals are limited, and human safety data are also lacking.[46] Most PNB adjuvant drugs are used off label in the U.S.

Clinical Pearls

- Clinical doses of clonidine, buprenorphine, dexamethasone, and midazolam have been shown to have no neurotoxicity in vitro.
- Adjuvants may prolong analgesia duration with single-injection PNBs. Dexamethasone enhances and prolongs analgesia injected perineurally *or intravenously*.

Sedation for Ambulatory Peripheral Nerve Blocks

Patients having surgery on an outpatient basis are typically healthier than patients having surgery as inpatients and may have limited or no previous experience with surgery.[63] Many patients undergoing surgical procedures experience preoperative anxiety.[64-66] In an effort to improve the perioperative experience, short-acting anxiolytic agents and/or other medications (eg, midazolam, opioids, ketamine, gabapentinoids) are often given before a PNB is placed.[67,68] Historically, the placement of a PNB using anatomical landmarks has led to multiple attempts at nerve location (ie, seeking a specific motor response to electrical nerve stimulation). Adding nerve stimulation can help confirm proper needle location but may cause considerable discomfort to the patient.[69] Even with ultrasound guidance and the use of local anesthetics to anesthetize the needle pathway, many patients benefit from judicious premedication before undergoing PNB. Heavy premedication, however, may lead to loss of airway tone and subsequent hypoxia and hypercapnia.[70] Premedicating patients judiciously while maintaining a meaningful patient contact may improve the patient's experience and allow for beneficial patient feedback during the procedure. From a cost perspective, premedicated patients require bedside monitoring, and more personnel may be required depending on the physical layout, surgical case workload, and current staffing levels. Furthermore, heavily premedicated patients may take longer to recover and need to remain within the surgical center longer,[71] resulting in patient dissatisfaction. Lastly, from a patient satisfaction perspective, patients may appreciate ongoing dialogue and reassurance as the block is being placed and the opportunity of being an active participant in their care.

In an effort to reduce patient wait times, patients are instructed to arrive close to the time of surgical start based on mathematical principles.[72]

The Block Team and Block Nurse

In academic training centers, residents and fellows can be organized into block teams.[19,20,73] These teams can provide safe and efficient RA while allowing trainees to focus on a single aspect of their education. A multidisciplinary group at Duke University initiated a "block nurse" team in 2010. Block nurses completed a focused training program that emphasized patient flow,

educating and preparing patients, assisting anesthesiologists, monitoring patients, and enhancing safety during the pre-, intra- and post-procedure periods. Within a year, rapid OR turnover time increased by 26%, OR on-time starts increased by 7%, orthopedic cases receiving preoperative blocks increased by 19%, and patient safety (eg, no wrong-sided blocks) improved.[8] While resources are lean at free-standing ASCs, the block nurse concept could perhaps be incorporated into an existing nursing team, thus potentially improving a facility's processes by increasing the number of patients who can benefit from preoperative PNB, increasing PACU bypass rates, and improving patient satisfaction.

PACU Bypass Criteria

Fast-tracking patients is an important goal of ambulatory anesthesia strategy.[74] In a meta-analysis by Liu et al. of 15 trials including 1003 patients given central neuraxial block (CNB) and 7 trials of 359 patients given PNB, for RA versus GA, induction time was increased 9 minutes.[75] There was a greater PACU bypass with PNB versus CNB, perhaps due to lack of a formal PACU bypass criteria for CNB patients. The odds of bypassing PACU using PNB was 14 times greater compared to GA. Both PNB and CNB patients reported an increased satisfaction level compared to GA patients, though PNB patient satisfaction was much higher than those having CNB. Patients receiving regional anesthesia reported lower pain scores, had less need of analgesics, and experienced less nausea and vomiting.[76] Williams et al. and others who matched interventional technique to surgical pain[15,72] have remarked on the possibility of "rebound pain," that is, pain above baseline that patients experience after a nerve block resolves.[77,78]

Breast surgery on an outpatient basis using thoracic paravertebral blocks is another good example of the benefits of PNBs.[79] A review article by Thavaneswaran et al. has shown that length of stay was reduced for breast surgery when using paravertebral block versus GA alone. Length of hospital stay, postoperative nausea and vomiting, and patient satisfaction were improved over GA (relative risk 0.25; 95% CI 0.13–0.50).[80]

Clinical Pearl

- In the fast-paced outpatient setting, assistance in setting up equipment, preparing and positioning patients, monitoring patients after blockade, and educating patients regarding safety and protection of insensate body regions are important.

Outcomes

Through 2007, most literature reports on RA outcomes were based on neuraxial techniques.[81] Since 2007, more literature has been published focusing on PNBs in outpatient surgery settings.[82]

Improved outcomes from neuraxial use in the outpatient surgery setting include improved short-term and long-term pain control, reduced surgical stress, improved gastrointestinal function, lower rates of postoperative nausea and vomiting, and fewer unplanned admissions or readmissions.[73–75,78] More physiologically significant outcomes include reductions in perioperative myocardial infarction, pulmonary complications, and mortality.[83,84] However, a systematic study of these outcomes in ambulatory patients has not been published, and it is unclear whether outpatient surgical patients would achieve the same benefit.

In an effort to improve care after colorectal surgery, a working group analyzed outcomes from randomized controlled trials published through 2007 for colorectal surgeries and created recommendations for the use of thoracic epidural catheters, avoiding long-acting opioids, reducing the amount of time under GA, and preventing gut paralysis.[85,86] Epidurals provide efficient analgesia, reduce surgical stress responses, and minimize the side effects of systemic opioid administration (pulmonary, gastrointestinal, and cognitive dysfunction). Once RA methods are discontinued, the use of NSAIDs further reduces or avoids the need for opioid administration and their side effects. RA has been demonstrated to improve outcomes such as mortality, major morbidity, and rehabilitation.[87]

Since superior pain control has been shown with the use of RA, focus on functional outcome improvement has become paramount.[88] This requires the ability to measure outcomes accurately. For outpatient RA outcomes, some measures include electromechanical dynamometer, which measures motor contraction; the 36-item Short Form Health Survey (SF-36), which measures physical and mental status before and after surgery; and the Western Ontario and McMaster Universities Osteoarthritis Index (WOMAC), which assesses pain and stiffness in the hips and knees. The recently validated Patient Reported Outcome Measurement Information System (PROMIS) is a computerized, adaptive test that provides an excellent method for assessing outcomes in patients who have had foot or ankle surgery.[89]

In recent years, functional outcome studies comparing RA to GA have shown a tendency toward improved early outcomes with RA.[90,91] Patients undergoing stable fixation of distal radius fracture under brachial plexus block demonstrated improved pain scores and better wrist and finger motion at all time points during follow-up compared to GA. Disabilities of the Arm, Shoulder and Hand (DASH) scores also demonstrated higher function at both 3 and 6 months (P = 0.04 and P = 0.02, respectively).[88]

Spinal anesthesia is used for outpatient lower extremity surgery. Compared to GA, patients undergoing ankle fracture fixation under spinal anesthesia reported improved early pain scores and function as measured by the American Orthopaedic Foot and Ankle Society Clinical Rating Scale at 3 months (mean [SD] 81.7 [11.9] vs 78.1 [15.2], P = 0.02).[92] At 6 months, spinal patients had lower pain scores (P = 0.04). Functional outcomes for the spinal group were not statistically significant by 6 and 12 months.

Clinical Pearl

- RA has been demonstrated to improve outcomes such as mortality, major morbidity, and rehabilitation.

Complications in the Ambulatory Setting

Complications of regional anesthesia range from minor sensory deficits that resolve within weeks to devastating injuries that result in permanent nerve injury, strokes, and on occasion, death.[93–95] Cardiac dysrhythmias can occur as late as 30–75 minutes after the injection of local anesthetics and may be intractable despite adherence to advanced cardiac life support guidelines.[96] This delayed response highlights the need for continuous monitoring of patients in the block area as well as the operating room. Although uncommon, local anesthetic systemic toxicity (LAST) can be a life-threatening complication for patients. Guidelines on the care of patients with LAST include airway management, prevent hyperventilation (to avoid increase in seizure threshold), and treating a seizure if it occurs, intravenous lipid emulsion therapy, and transfer to a tertiary care setting with cardiopulmonary bypass capability.[97] Ambulatory facilities should consider creating LAST kits with checklists that are housed in the areas where blocks are performed.[95] Fortunately, ultrasound guidance coupled with decreasing doses and volumes of local anesthetics required for successful nerve blockade have resulted in a substantial decrease in the risk of LAST, a trend likely to continue as ultrasound-guided techniques become more refined.[98]

Other complications, such as wrong-sided blocks, can be greatly reduced by adherence to established time-out policies. Block site marking, as well as encouraging patients to engage in dialogue during block placement, can reinforce a culture of safety.[99] Permanent nerve injuries, with subsequent long-term morbidity and/or disability are uncommon.[100] The development of more objective methods of monitoring needle placement and administering local anesthetics, such as ultrasound guidance, low-current nerve stimulation, and opening injection pressure monitoring are likely to even further decrease the risk of intrafascicular injection and neurologic injury.[101–103] When present, however, intrafascicular injections and neurologic injuries require a thorough evaluation, and expert consultation by a neurologist should be considered.

When an RA complication occurs, prompt and well-planned disclosure is warranted. When possible, a quiet, private area is required for patient and family disclosure. Anesthesiologists should have another member of the healthcare team present during the disclosure. The provider should investigate how much is known about the adverse event and how much detail the patient and family require. With empathy, knowledge of the event needs to be conveyed in a manner that is clear and understandable. This often requires planned pauses, repetition of information, reassurance, and open body language. Saying "I'm sorry this event happened to you" does not imply fault; rather, it is a statement of empathy about the adverse event and the subsequent pain, suffering, or other inconvenience that may have been experienced. Lastly, all disclosure discussions need to be documented and patients and/or family need to have a mechanism for further follow-up.[104] Several studies suggest that thoughtful and prompt disclosure of adverse events or complications results in less legal action and possibly less emotional impact on the provider.[105,106]

Clinical Pearls

- Guidelines on the care of patients who experience toxic reactions from local anesthetics include airway management, hyperventilation on prevention, seizure control, intravenous lipid emulsion therapy, and consideration of transfer to a tertiary care setting with cardiopulmonary bypass capability.
- Ambulatory facilities should develop LAST kits with checklists that are housed in the area where blocks are performed.
- Thoughtful and prompt disclosure of adverse events or complications may prevent or lessen the legal action and diminish the emotional impact on all parties.

Objective monitoring of the needle–nerve relationship and injection process during PNB, such as via ultrasound guidance, low-current intensity nerve stimulation, and avoidance of high opening injection pressures (> 15 psi), can further decrease the risk of already uncommon neurologic complications.

■ Peripheral Nerve Blocks and Outpatient Surgery Economics

Patient satisfaction, while perhaps intuitive in some ways, is not easily measured in a scientifically valid manner. In the United States, patient satisfaction and whether patients would recommend their family or friends to have surgery at a facility or institution are correlated with improved operating revenue margins.[14,107] A new patient-centered assessment by Szamburski et al. is the first psychometrically evaluated, internally and externally validated patient satisfaction instrument developed to date.[108] This new measure may prove useful in future work investigating linkages between RA and outcomes or economic indicators.

Physician-owned free-standing ASCs, through a profit motive, may be an incentive for physicians to divert cases from hospital operating rooms to their own centers.[1] ASCs have lower overhead than hospitals but are paid less by Medicare.[1] Physicians may also choose to steer their patients toward ASCs based on nonfinancial factors, such as convenience, enhanced patient experience, ease of scheduling, and the ability to complete more cases per day than in a hospital environment. An analysis of the 1996 and 2006 NSAS data found that a 10% increase in profit (facility fees, not professional fees) was associated with a 1.2%–1.4% increase in the probability that a surgery would be performed at an ASC.[1]

The presence and type of insurance also influence the choice to provide a PNB. When compared with self-pay patients or those receiving charity care, patients with government-paid care or private insurance were roughly 2.5 times more likely to receive a nerve block.[5] However, this association is not necessarily causal, and other confounding factors are likely to be involved. Hospital revenue streams may be reduced as patients are recruited to have surgery at nonhospital ASCs.[5] This may lower societal healthcare costs since ASCs are reimbursed at lower rates and have lower overhead costs than hospitals for a given procedure.[4,5,11]

By implementing RA techniques, facilities can potentially lower costs and enhance efficiency. One report demonstrated that when RA is used in a hospital at a rate higher than the median of its competing hospitals, that hospital can reduce patient length of stay and increase profit per diagnosis-related group (DRG) while also increasing patient satisfaction and reducing complications.[109]

Clinical Pearls

- By implementing RA techniques, facilities may be able to lower costs and enhance efficiency.
- Hospitals that use RA at a rate higher than the median of competing hospitals may reduce patient length of stay and increase profit per DRG while increasing patient satisfaction and reducing complications.

SUMMARY

Outpatient surgical cases are increasing, and regional anesthetic techniques, including PNB, are amenable to the types of cases performed in the outpatient setting. RA and PNBs can benefit patients by avoiding the side effects of GA and opioids. RA techniques and the use of local anesthetics are a major component of a multimodal analgesia and anesthesia plan. RA techniques offer improved patient outcomes, do not disproportionately delay case start time, can improve fast-tracking of patients, and may enhance economic outcomes for a facility. Complications may occur, however, and providers should be prepared to handle these situations appropriately, particularly in a standalone ASC with fewer resources than hospitals.

REFERENCES

1. Plotzke MR, Courtemanche C: Does procedure profitability impact whether an outpatient surgery is performed at an ambulatory surgery center or hospital? Health Econ 2011;20:817–830.
2. Joshi GP: Multimodal analgesia techniques for ambulatory surgery. Int Anesthesiol Clin 2005;43:197–204.
3. Medicare Payment Advisory Commission: Report to Congress: Medicare Payment Policy Published March, 2013. Accessed June 28, 2013. http://www.medpac.gov.
4. Manchikanti L, Parr AT, Singh V, Fellows B: Ambulatory surgery centers and interventional techniques: A look at long-term survival. Pain Physician 2011;14:E177–E215.
5. Medicare Payment Advisory Commission. Report to Congress: Medicare Payment Policy. Published March 2013. Accessed June 28, 2013. http://www.medpac.gov.
6. Tighe, PJ, Brennan M, Moser M, et al: Primary payer status is associated with the use of nerve block placement for ambulatory orthopedic surgery. Reg Anesth Pain Med 2012;37:254–261.
7. Centers for Disease Control and Prevention. National Survey of Ambulatory Surgery. Page last updated May 4, 2010. Accessed June 27, 2013. http://www.cdc.gov/nchs/nsas.htm.
8. Cullen KA, Hall MJ, Golosinskiy A: Ambulatory surgery in the United States, 2006. Natl Health Stat Report 2009;28:1–25.

9. Russell RA, Burke K, Gattis K: Implementing a regional anesthesia block nurse team in the perianesthesia care unit increases patient safety and perioperative efficiency. J Perianesth Nurs 2013;28:3–10.

10. Kim S, Bosque J, Meehan JP, et al: Increase in outpatient knee arthroscopy in the United States: a comparison of National Surveys of Ambulatory Surgery, 1996 and 2006. J Bone Joint Surg Am 2011;93: 994–1000.

11. Dervin GF, Madden SM, Crawford-Newton BA, et al: Outpatient unicompartment knee arthroplasty with indwelling femoral nerve catheter. J Arthroplasty 2012;27:1159–1165.e1.

12. Koenig L, Gu Q: Growth of ambulatory surgery centers, surgery volume, and savings to Medicare. Am J Gastroenterol 2013;108:10–15.

13. Grisel J, Arjmand, E: Comparing quality at an ambulatory surgery center and a hospital-based facility: Preliminary findings. Otolaryngol Head Neck Surg 2009;141:701–709.

14. Boezaart AP, Tighe PJ: The progression of regional anesthesia into acute and perioperative pain medicine. Int Anesthesiol Clin 2011;49:104–109.

15. Lee F. If Disney ran your hospital: 9-1/2 things you would do differently. Swanson G, ed. Bozeman, MT: Second River Healthcare; 2004:28.

16. Williams BA: Forecast for perineural analgesia procedures for ambulatory surgery of the knee, foot, and ankle: applying patient-centered paradigm shifts. Int Anesthesiol Clin 2011;50:126–142.

17. Porter ME: What is value in health care? N Engl J Med 2010;363: 2477–2481.

18. Porter ME, Teisberg EO. *Redefining Health Care: Creating Value-Based Competition on Results.* Boston: Harvard Business School; 2006.

19. Faraj WA, Brull R: Making sense of block "success" in ambulatory anesthesia practice. Int Anesthesiol Clin 2011;49:1–9.

20. Eappen S, Flanagan H, Lithman R, et al: The addition of a regional block team to the orthopedic operating rooms does not improve anesthesia-controlled times and turnover time in the setting of long turnover times. J Clin Anesth 2007;19:85–91.

21. Chelly JE, Horne JL, Hudson ME: Factors impacting on-time transfer to the operating room in patients undergoing peripheral nerve blocks in the preoperative area. J Clin Anesth 2010;22:115–121.

22. Williams BA, Kentor ML, Vogt MT, et al: Potential hospital cost savings via associated postanesthesia care unit bypass and same-day discharge. Anesthesiology 2004;100:697–706.

23. Macario AA, Weinger MM, Carney SS, et al: Which clinical anesthesia outcomes are important to avoid? The perspective of patients. Anesth Analg 1999;89:652–658.

24. Maurice-Szamburski A, Bruder N, Loundou, A, et al: Development and validation of a perioperative satisfaction questionnaire in regional anesthesia. Anesthesiology 2013;118:78–87.

25. Fredrickson MJ, Smith KR, Wong AC: Importance of volume and concentration for ropivacaine interscalene block in preventing recovery room pain and minimizing motor block after shoulder surgery. Anesthesiology 2010;112:1374–1381.

26. Oldman M, McCartney CJ, Leung A, et al: A survey of orthopedic surgeons' attitudes and knowledge regarding regional anesthesia. Anesth Analg 2004;98:1486–1490.

27. Richebé P, Rivat C, Laulin JP, et al: Ketamine improves the management of exaggerated postoperative pain observed in perioperative fentanyl-treated rats. Anesthesiology 2005;102:421–428.

28. Chia YY, Liu K, Wang, JJ, et al: Intraoperative high dose fentanyl induces postoperative fentanyl tolerance. Can J Anaesth 1999;46: 872–877.

29. Macario A, Weinger M, Truong P, et al: Which clinical anesthesia outcomes are both common and important to avoid? The perspective of a panel of expert anesthesiologists. Anesth Analg 1999;88:1085–1091.

30. Young A, Buvanendran A: Multimodal systemic and intra-articular analgesics. Int Anesthesiol Clin 2011;49:117–133.

31. Tiippana EM, Hamunen K, Kontinen VK, et al: Do surgical patients benefit from perioperative gabapentin/pregabalin? A systematic review of efficacy and safety. Anesth Analg 2007;10:1545–1556.

32. White PF, Sacan O, Tufanogullari B, et al: Effect of short-term postoperative celecoxib administration on patient outcome after outpatient laparoscopic surgery. Can J Anesth 2007;54:342–348.

33. Salerno A, Hermann R: Efficacy and safety of steroid use for postoperative pain relief. J Bone Joint Surg Am 2006;88A:1361–1372.

34. Oliveira GS de, Agarwal D, Benzon HT: Perioperative single dose ketorolac to prevent postoperative pain. Anesth Analg 2012;114: 424–433.

35. Barreveld, A, Witte J, Chahal H, et al: Preventive analgesia by local anesthetics. Anesth Analg 2013;116:1141–1161.

36. McKay A, Gottschalk A, Ploppa A, et al: Systemic lidocaine decreased the perioperative opioid analgesic requirements but failed to reduce discharge time after ambulatory surgery. Anesth Analg 2009;109: 1805–1808.

37. Mont MA, Jacobs JJ, Boggio LN, et al: Preventing venous thromboembolic disease in patients undergoing elective hip and knee arthroplasty. J Am Acad Orthop Surg 2011;19:786–776.

38. Kettner SC, Willschke H, Marhofer P: Does regional anaesthesia really improve outcome? Br J Anaesth 2011;107(Suppl 1):i90–i95.

39. Hurford WE: Updates in head-to-toe applications of regional anesthesia for ambulatory surgery. Int Anesthesiol Clin 2012;50:x–xi.

40. Mercier RJ, Zerden ML: Intrauterine anesthesia for gynecologic procedures: A systematic review. Obstet Gynecol 2012;120:669–677.

41. Lee E, Khandwala M, Jones C: A randomised controlled trial to compare patient satisfaction with two different types of local anaesthesia in ptosis surgery. Orbit 2009;28:388–391.

42. Varitimidis S, Venouziou A, Dailiana Z, et al: Triple nerve block at the knee for foot and ankle surgery performed by the surgeon: Difficulties and efficiency. Foot Ankle Int 2009;30:854–859.

43. Cyna A, Middleton P: Caudal epidural block versus other methods of postoperative pain relief for circumcision in boys. Cochrane Database of Syst Rev 2008;4:CD003005.

44. Laur JJ, Bayman EO, Foldes PJ, et al: Triple-blind randomized clinical trial of time until sensory change using 1.5% mepivacaine with epinephrine, 0.5% bupivacaine, or an equal mixture of both for infraclavicular block. Reg Anesth Pain Med 2012;37:28–33.

45. Gadsden J, Hadzic A, Gandhi K, et al: The effect of mixing 1.5% mepivacaine and 0.5% bupivacaine on duration of analgesia and latency of block onset in ultrasound-guided interscalene block. Anesth Analg 2011;112:471–476.

46. Hudson ME, Chelly JE, Williams BA: Economics: projecting costs and revenue for an interventional pain service in the ambulatory setting. Int Anesthesiol Clin 2011;49:68–83.

47. Williams BA, Hough KA, Tsui BYK, et al: Neurotoxicity of adjuvants used in perineural anesthesia and analgesia in comparison with ropivacaine. Reg Anesth Pain Med 2011;36:225–230.

48. Hogan Q: Pathophysiology of peripheral nerve injury during regional anesthesia. Reg Anesth Pain Med 2008;33:435–441.

49. Ibinson JW, Mangione MP, Williams, BA: Local anesthetics in diabetic rats (and patients). Reg Anesth Pain Med 2012;37:574–576.

50. Yilmaz-Rastoder E, Gold MS, Hough KA, et al: Effect of adjuvant drugs on the action of local anesthetics in isolated rat sciatic nerves. Reg Anesth Pain Med 2012;37:403–409.

51. Jarbo K, Batra YK, Panda NB: Brachial plexus block with midazolam and bupivacaine improves analgesia. Can J Anaesth 2005;52:822–826.

52. Neal J, Gerancher J, Hebl J, et al: Upper extremity regional anesthesia: essentials of our current understanding, 2008. Reg Anesth Pain Med 2009;34:134–170.

53. Goravanchi F, Kee SS, Kowalski AM, Berger, et al: A case series of thoracic paravertebral blocks using a combination of ropivacaine, clonidine, epinephrine, and dexamethasone. J Clin Anesth 2012;24: 664–667.

54. Fournier R, Faust A, Chassot O, et al: Perineural clonidine does not prolong levobupivacaine 0.5% after sciatic nerve block using the Labat approach in foot and ankle surgery. Reg Anesth Pain Med 2012;37: 521–524.

55. Marhofer D, Kettner SC, Marhofer P, et al: Dexmedetomidine as an adjuvant to ropivacaine prolongs peripheral nerve block: a volunteer study. Br J Anaesth 2013;110:438–442.

56. Pöpping DM, Elia N, Marret E, et al: Clonidine as an adjuvant to local anesthetics for peripheral nerve and plexus blocks: a meta-analysis of randomized trials. Anesthesiology 2009;111:406–415.

57. Rasmussen SB, Saied NN, Bowens C, et al: Duration of upper and lower extremity peripheral nerve blockade is prolonged with dexamethasone when added to ropivacaine: A retrospective database analysis. Pain Med 2013;14:1239–1247.

58. Desmet M, Braems H, Reynvoet M, et al: I.V. and perineural dexamethasone are equivalent in increasing the analgesic duration of a single-shot interscalene block with ropivacaine for shoulder surgery: a prospective, randomized, placebo-controlled study. Br J Anaesth 2013;111:445–452.

59. Parrington SJ, O'Donnell D, Chan VW, et al: Dexamethasone added to mepivacaine prolongs the duration of analgesia after supraclavicular brachial plexus blockade. Reg Anesth Pain Med 2010;35:422–426.

60. Vieira PA, Pulai I, Tsao GC, et al: Dexamethasone with bupivacaine increases duration of analgesia in ultrasound-guided interscalene brachial plexus blockade. Eur J Anaesthesiol 2010;27:285–288.

61. Cummings KC III, Napierkowski DE, Parra-Sanchez I, et al: Effect of dexamethasone on the duration of interscalene nerve blocks with ropivacaine or bupivacaine. Br J Anaesth 2011;107:446–453.

62. Abdallah FW, Johnson J, Chan V, et al: Intravenous dexamethasone and perineural dexamethasone similarly prolong the duration of analgesia

after supraclavicular brachial plexus block: a randomized, triple-arm, double-blind, placebo-controlled trial. Reg Anesth Pain Med 2015;40: 125–132.

63. Bryson G, Chung F, Finegan B, et al: Patient selection in ambulatory anesthesia—An evidence-based review: Part I. Can J Anaesth 2004;51: 768–781.

64. Lichtor JL, Johanson CE, Mhoon D, et al: Preoperative anxiety: Does anxiety level the afternoon before surgery predict anxiety level just before surgery? Anesthesiology 1987;67:595–598.

65. Brand LR, Munroe DJ, Gavin J: The effect of hand massage on preoperative anxiety in ambulatory surgery patients. AORN J 2013; 97:708–717.

66. Norris W, Baird WLM: Pre-operative anxiety: A study of the incidence and aetiology. Br J Anaesth 1967;39:503–509.

67. White PF, Tufanogullari B, Taylor J, et al: The effect of pregabalin on preoperative anxiety and sedation levels: A dose-ranging study. Anesth Analg 2009;108:1140–1145.

68. Shafer A, White PF, Urquhart ML, et al: Outpatient premedication: Use of midazolam and opioid analgesics. Anesthesiology 1989;71:495–501.

69. Bloc S, Mercadal L, Garnier T, et al: Comfort of the patient during axillary blocks placement: A randomized comparison of the neurostimulation and the ultrasound guidance techniques. Eur J Anaesthesiol 2010;27:628–633.

70. Eichhorn V, Henzler D, Murphy MF: Standardizing care and monitoring for anesthesia or procedural sedation delivered outside the operating room. Curr Opin Anaesthesiol 2010;23:494–499.

71. Viitanen H, Annila P, Viitanen M, et al: Premedication with midazolam delays recovery after ambulatory sevoflurane anesthesia in children. Anesth Analg 1999;89:75.

72. Dexter F, Epstein R: Scheduling of cases in an ambulatory center. Anesthesiol Clin North America 2003;21:387–402.

73. Williams BA, Kentor ML, Williams JP, et al: PACU bypass after outpatient knee surgery is associated with fewer unplanned hospital admissions but more phase II nursing interventions. Anesthesiology 2002;97:981–988.

74. Carli F, Kehlet H, Baldini G, et al: Evidence basis for regional anesthesia in multidisciplinary fast-track surgical care pathways. Reg Anesth Pain Med 2011;36:63–72.

75. Liu SS, Strodtbeck WM, Richman JM, et al: A comparison of regional versus general anesthesia for ambulatory anesthesia: A meta-analysis of randomized controlled trials. *Anesth Analg* 2005;101:1634–1642.

76. Fischer, B: Benefits, risks, and best practice in regional anesthesia. Reg Anesth Pain Med 2010;35:545–548.

77. DeMarco JR, Componovo R, Barfield WR, et al: Efficacy of augmenting a subacromial continuous-infusion pump with a preoperative interscalene block in outpatient arthroscopic shoulder surgery: A prospective, randomized, blinded, and placebo-controlled study. Arthroscopy 2011; 27:603–610.

78. Williams B, Bottegal M, Kentor M, et al: Rebound pain scores as a function of femoral nerve block duration after anterior cruciate ligament reconstruction: Retrospective analysis of a prospective, randomized clinical trial. Reg Anesth Pain Med 2007;32:186–192.

79. Kitowski NJ, Landercasper J, Gundrum JD, et al: Local and paravertebral block anesthesia for outpatient elective breast cancer surgery. Arch Surg 2010;145:592–594.

80. Thavaneswaran P, Rudkin GE, Cooter RD, et al: Paravertebral block for anesthesia. Anesth Analg 2010;110:1740–1744.

81. Wu CL, Williams BA: Effects of regional anesthesia and analgesia on perioperative outcome. In Hadzic A (ed): *NYSORA Textbook of Regional Anesthesia and Acute Pain Management*. New York: McGraw Hill; 2007, p 1076.

82. Bernucci F, Carli F: Functional outcome after major orthopedic surgery. Curr Opin Anaesthesiol 2012;25:621–628.

83. Rodgers A, Walker N, Schug S, et al: Reduction of postoperative mortality and morbidity with epidural or spinal anaesthesia: results from overview of randomised trials. BMJ 2000;321:1493–1504.

84. Bonnet F, Maret E: Influence of anaesthetic and analgesic techniques on outcome after surgery. Br J Anaesth 2005;95:52–58.

85. Gustafsson UO, Scott MJ, Schwenk W, et al: Guidelines for perioperative care in elective colonic surgery: Enhanced Recovery After Surgery (ERAS®) Society recommendations. Clin Nutr 2012;31:783–800.

86. Lassen K, Soop M, Nygren J, et al. Consensus review of optimal perioperative care in colorectal surgery: Enhanced Recovery After Surgery (ERAS) Group recommendations. Arch Surg 2009;144: 961–969.

87. Hanna MN, Murphy JD, Kumar K, et al: Regional techniques and outcome: what is the evidence? Curr Opin in Anaesthesiol 2009;22: 672–677.

88. Bernucci F, Carli F: Functional outcome after major orthopedic surgery. Curr Opin Anaesthesiol 2012;25:621–628.

89. Man H, Baumhauer JF, Latt LD, et al: Validation of the PROMIS® physical function computerized adaptive tests for orthopaedic foot and ankle outcome research. Clin Orthop Relat Res 2013;471:3466–3474.

90. Egol KAK, Soojian MGM, Walsh MM, et al: Regional anesthesia improves outcome after distal radius fracture fixation over general anesthesia. J Orthop Trauma 2012;26:545–549.

91. Jordan C, Davidovitch RI, Walsh M, et al: Spinal anesthesia mediates improved early function and pain relief following surgical repair of ankle fractures. J Bone Joint Surg Am 2010;92:368–374.

92. Jordan C, Davidovitch RI, Walsh M, et al: Spinal anesthesia mediates improved early function and pain relief following surgical repair of ankle fractures. J Bone Joint Surg Am 2010;92(2):368–374.

93. Lee L, Posner K, Cheney F, et al: Complications associated with eye blocks and peripheral nerve blocks: An American Society of Anesthesiologists closed claims analysis. Reg Anesth Pain Med 2008;33: 416–422.

94. Lee LA, Posner KL, Kent CD, Domino KB: Complications associated with peripheral nerve blocks: lessons from the ASA Closed Claims Project. Int Anesthesiol Clin 2011;49:56–67.

95. Ben-David B: Complications of regional anesthesia: an overview. Anesthesiol Clin North America 2002;20:665–667.

96. Dix SK, Rosner GF, Nayar M, et al: Intractable cardiac arrest due to lidocaine toxicity successfully resuscitated with lipid emulsion. Crit Care Med 2011;39:872–874.

97. Neal JM, Mulroy MF, Weinberg GL: American Society of Regional Anesthesia and Pain Medicine checklist for managing local anesthetic systemic toxicity: 2012 version. Reg Anesth Pain Med 2012;37:16–18.

98. Sites BD, Taenzer AH, Herrick MD, et al: Incidence of local anesthetic systemic toxicity and postoperative neurologic symptoms associated with 12,668 ultrasound-guided nerve blocks: an analysis from a prospective clinical registry. Reg Anesth Pain Med 2012;37:478–482.

99. Watson DS: Implementing the universal protocol. *AORN J* 2009; 90:283–287.

100. Lee L, Posner K, Cheney F, et al: Complications associated with eye blocks and peripheral nerve blocks: An American Society of Anesthesiologists closed claims analysis. Reg Anesth Pain Med 2008;3: 416–422.

101. Ip VH, Tsui BC: Practical concepts in the monitoring of injection pressures during peripheral nerve blocks. Int Anesthesiol Clin 2011; 49:67–80.

102. Tsui BC, Knezevich MP, Pillay JJ: Reduced injection pressures using a compressed air injection technique (CAIT): an in vitro study. Reg Anesth Pain Med 2008;33:168–173.

103. Gadsden JC, Choi JJ, Lin E, Robinson A: Opening injection pressure consistently detects needle-nerve contact during ultrasound-guided interscalene brachial plexus block. Anesthesiology 2014;120:1246–1253.

104. Baile WF, Buckman R, Lenzi R, et al: SPIKES-A six-step protocol for delivering bad news: application to the patient with cancer. Oncologist 205;5:302–311.

105. Boothman R, Imhoff S, Campbell DJ: Nurturing a culture of patient safety and achieving lower malpractice risk through disclosure: lessons learned and future directions. Front Health Serv Manage 2012;28:13–28.

106. Gazoni FM, Amato PE, Malik ZM, et al: The impact of perioperative catastrophes on anesthesiologists: results of a national survey. Anesth Analg 2012;114:598–603.

107. American Hospital Directory: Higher hospital margins distinguished by higher patient satisfaction. Healthc Financ Manage 2010;64:136.

108. Maurice-Szamburski A, Bruder N, Loundou A, et al: Development and validation of a perioperative satisfaction questionnaire in regional anesthesia. Anesthesiology 2013;118:78–87.

109. Heller AR, Bauer KR, Eberlein-Gonska M, et al: [Regional anaesthesia as advantage in competition between hospitals. Strategic market analysis]. Der Anaesthesist 2009;58:459–468.

Neuraxial Anesthesia & Peripheral Nerve Blocks in Patients on Anticoagulants

Honorio T. Benzon, Rasha S. Jabri, and Tom C. Van Zundert

INTRODUCTION

Intraspinal hematoma is a relatively rare condition resulting from a variety of causes. Traumatic causes include lumbar puncture and neuraxial anesthesia. It is more likely to occur in anticoagulated or thrombocytopenic patients, patients with neoplastic disease, or in those with liver disease or alcoholism. Approximately one-quarter to one-third of all cases are associated with anticoagulation therapy. The risk of intraspinal hematoma formation after administration of neuraxial anesthesia and analgesia is increased in patients who have received anticoagulant therapy or have a coagulation disorder.[1] For this reason, neuraxial anesthesia is often contraindicated in the presence of a coagulopathy. Other risk factors for the development of epidural or spinal hematoma include technical difficulty (multiple attempts) in the performance of the neuraxial procedures due to anatomic abnormalities of the spine and multiple or bloody punctures.

The incidence of spinal hematoma was originally reported to be one in 150,000 epidurals and one in 220,000 spinal anesthetics.[2] Recent epidemiologic studies have shown the incidence of spinal hematoma to be more frequent, ranging from one in 2700 to one in 19,505 epidurals.[3–6] The most recent study showed an overall risk of 1 in 21,643 epidural injections.[7] The elderly (one in 3800)[4] are at increased risk due to degenerative spine abnormalities, osteoporosis, and peripheral vascular disease.[8,9] Obstetric populations seems to have a lower incidence of spinal hematoma (one in 200,000),[4] probably secondary to the hypercoagulable state of pregnancy, the wider capacity of the epidural space in younger parturients, and higher intra-epidural pressure. Based on a recent large retrospective study, the incidence of epidural hematoma in patients with abnormal coagulation may be as low as one in 315 patients.[10]

The introduction of low-molecular-weight heparin (LMWH) was associated with a spike in the incidence of spinal hematoma, resulting in a warning by the Food and Drug Administration (FDA) and the introduction of the first consensus statement on regional anesthesia in patients on anticoagulants by the American Society of Regional Anesthesia and Pain Medicine (ASRA) in 1998.[11] The guidelines were based on an extensive review of the literature and of the pharmacology of the different anticoagulants. Recommendations were made on the timing of the neuraxial block, removal of the epidural catheter, and the subsequent administration of anticoagulants. In particular, the use of low concentrations of local anesthetics for epidural infusion (to preserve motor strength for easier monitoring) and subsequent neurologic monitoring were recommended by the ASRA. The consensus guidelines, published in 1998 and updated in 2003 and 2010,[12,13] have greatly assisted clinicians in decision making with regard to the use of neuraxial procedures in the setting of anticoagulation therapy. Two other sets of guidelines, published by the European Society of Anaesthesiology and the Scandinavian Society of Anaesthesiology and Intensive Care Medicine, are influential in Europe.[14,15]

In this chapter, we discuss the significance of common anticoagulants and hope to offer the reader a guide in decision making about the use of neuraxial anesthesia and peripheral nerve blocks (PNBs) in clinical practice. We will also discuss the new anticoagulants, drugs that were not adequately covered in the latest ASRA guidelines and only partly covered by the European and Scandinavian guidelines.

ANTIPLATELET THERAPY

Antiplatelet medications inhibit the platelet cyclooxygenase enzyme and prevent the synthesis of thromboxane A_2. Thromboxane A_2 is a potent vasoconstrictor that facilitates secondary platelet aggregation and release reactions. The role of platelets in coagulation and hemostasis is shown in Figures 52–1 and 52–2. Platelets from patients on these medications have normal platelet adherence to subendothelium and normal primary hemostatic plug formation. An adequate, although potentially fragile, clot may form. Although such plugs may be satisfactory hemostatic barriers for smaller vascular lesions, they may not ensure adequate perioperative hemostatic clot formation. Platelet function in patients receiving antiplatelet medications should be assumed to be decreased for 1 week with aspirin and 1–6 days with nonsteroidal anti-inflammatory drugs (NSAIDs).[16] This assumption does not take into consideration the continuous formation of new, functional platelets. The continuous production of fresh, normally functioning platelets, combined with the residual function of already circulating platelets, may explain the relative safety of performing neuraxial procedures in these patients.

The risk of epidural and spinal hematoma in patients on antiplatelet therapy has been raised by a case report of spontaneous epidural hematoma formation in the absence of spinal or epidural anesthesia in a patient with a history of aspirin ingestion.[17] Vandermeulen and colleagues implicated antiplatelet therapy in 3 of the 61 cases of spinal hematoma occurring after spinal or epidural anesthesia.[18] Other studies have shown a relatively low risk of spinal hematoma in patients on aspirin or NSAIDs undergoing a neuraxial procedure. The Collaborative Low-dose Aspirin Study in Pregnancy (CLASP) Group[19] included 1422 high-risk obstetric patients who were administered 60 mg of aspirin daily and underwent epidural anesthesia without any neurologic sequelae. In a retrospective study of 1013 spinal and epidural anesthetics in which antiplatelet drugs were taken by 39% of the patients, including 11% of patients who were on multiple antiplatelet medications, no patient developed signs of spinal hematoma.[20] The patients on antiplatelet medications, however, showed a higher incidence of blood aspiration through the spinal or epidural needle or the catheter. A subsequent prospective study in 1000 patients, 39% of whom reported preoperative antiplatelet therapy, noted the absence of hemorrhagic complications.[21] Therefore, preoperative antiplatelet therapy was not a risk factor for bloody needle or catheter placement. Female gender, increased age, history of excessive bruising or bleeding, continuous catheter technique, large needle gauge, multiple attempts, and difficult needle placement were noted to be significant risk factors. Clinical studies in pain clinic patients are similar to those undergoing surgery. Patients on aspirin[22] or NSAIDs[23] who underwent epidural steroid injections did not develop signs or symptoms of intraspinal hematoma.

The lack of correlation between antiplatelet medication and bloody needle or catheter placement provides some evidence that preoperative antiplatelet therapy does not represent a significant risk factor for the development of neurologic dysfunction from spinal hematoma in patients on antiplatelet therapy. It should be noted that there have been case reports of intraspinal hematoma in patients on aspirin or NSAIDs, although there were complicating factors in these case reports. These included concomitant heparin administration, coexisting epidural venous angioma, and technical difficulty in performing the procedure.[24] More recently, more case reports of spinal hematoma have been published in relation to pain interventional procedures, specifically spinal cord stimulation placements.[25]

Based on the available evidence, the ASRA has made several recommendations concerning antiplatelet medications.[12,13] Preoperative antiplatelet therapy does not represent a significant risk factor for the development of neurologic dysfunction from spinal hematoma in patients on antiplatelet therapy. The risk of bleeding complications, however, may be increased in patients on several antiplatelet medications and concurrent use of other medications affecting clotting mechanisms, such as oral anticoagulants, standard heparin, and LMWH.[24]

Clinical Pearls

- It is probably safe to do neuraxial and regional anesthesia procedures in patients on aspirin and NSAIDs.
- The risk factors for increased bleeding and spinal hematoma include the patient's intake of several antiplatelet drugs and making multiple attempts.

Aspirin and Interventional Pain Procedures

There have been several case reports of spinal hematoma after epidural steroid injection or placement or removal of a spinal cord stimulator in patients who were on aspirin alone, NSAIDs alone, or when the ASRA guidelines were followed.[26–30] These occurrences may be related to the frequent spine abnormalities found in these patients, the presence of fibrosis following spine surgery, larger needles used in spinal cord stimulator placement, or the frequent manipulations (advancements and retractions) of the electrodes. Medications used in pain managements also cause bleeding; these include oxcarbazepine and the selective serotonin reuptake inhibitors.[31,32] For these reasons, the ASRA liaised with the European Society of Regional Anaesthesia and Pain Therapy, the American Academy of Pain Medicine, the International Neuromodulation Society, the North American Neuromodulation Society, and the World Institute of Pain to formulate specific guidelines for interventional pain procedures.[33] In contrast to the ASRA regional anesthesia guidelines, the multisociety guidelines recommended that aspirin be stopped for 4–6 days before interventional pain procedures.

Clinical Pearl

- The guidelines on interventional pain procedures in patients on antiplatelet and anticoagulant medications are more restrictive than the ones on regional anesthesia.

COX-2 Inhibitors and P2Y12 Inhibitors

Cyclooxygenase-2 (COX-2) inhibitors gained popularity because of their analgesic properties and lack of platelet and gastrointestinal effects, and studies have shown their analgesic

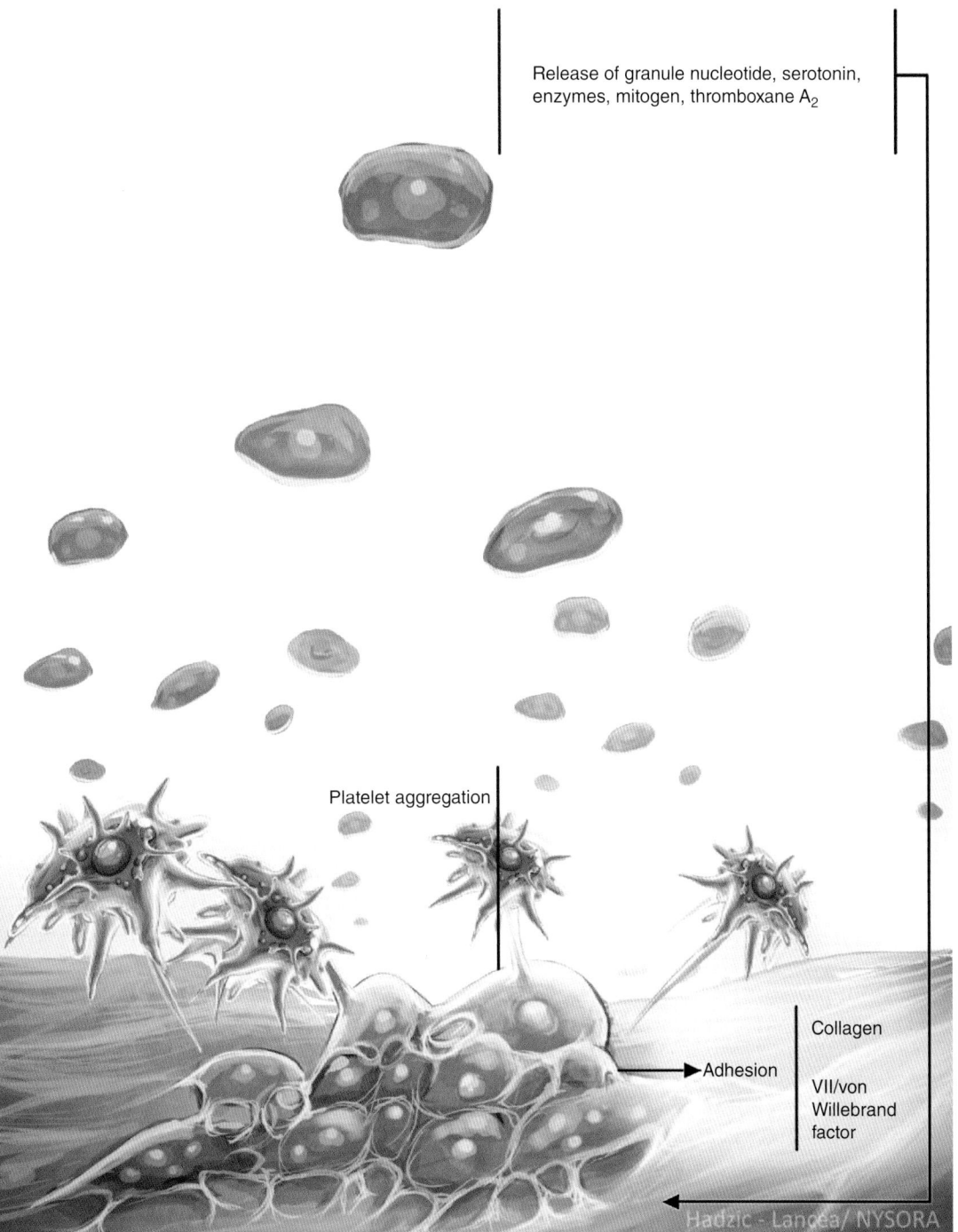

Release of granule nucleotide, serotonin, enzymes, mitogen, thromboxane A_2

Platelet aggregation

Collagen

Adhesion

VII/von Willebrand factor

Hadzic - Langea/ NYSORA

FIGURE 52–1. Role of platelets in coagulation. Platelets carry out their role in hemostasis through three basic reactions: adhesion, activation (and secretion), and aggregation. When vascular endothelium is damaged, platelets rapidly bind to the subendothelium by a process termed *adhesion*.

property in a variety of perioperative settings.[34–38] The drugs have minimal gastrointestinal (GI) toxicity and are ideal for patients who are at increased risk for serious upper GI adverse events. Compared with aspirin or NSAIDs, the effect of COX-2 inhibitors on platelet aggregation and bleeding times were not different from placebo.[39–41] Blood loss does not increase during spinal fusion surgery when COX-2 inhibitors are given preoperatively. The platelet properties of these drugs make them ideal for perioperative use when neuraxial anesthetic is planned. Unfortunately, rofecoxib and valdecoxib have

been withdrawn from the market because of their cardiovascular side effects,[42] leaving only celecoxib available, but at dosages lower than previously recommendeded.

The thienopyridine drugs ticlopidine and clopidogrel have no direct effect on arachidonic acid metabolism. These drugs prevent platelet aggregation by inhibiting adenosine diphosphate (ADP) receptor–mediated platelet activation.[24,43] They also modulate vascular smooth muscle, reducing vascular contraction.[44] Ticlopidine is rarely used because it causes neutropenia, thrombocytopenic purpura, and hypercholesterolemia.

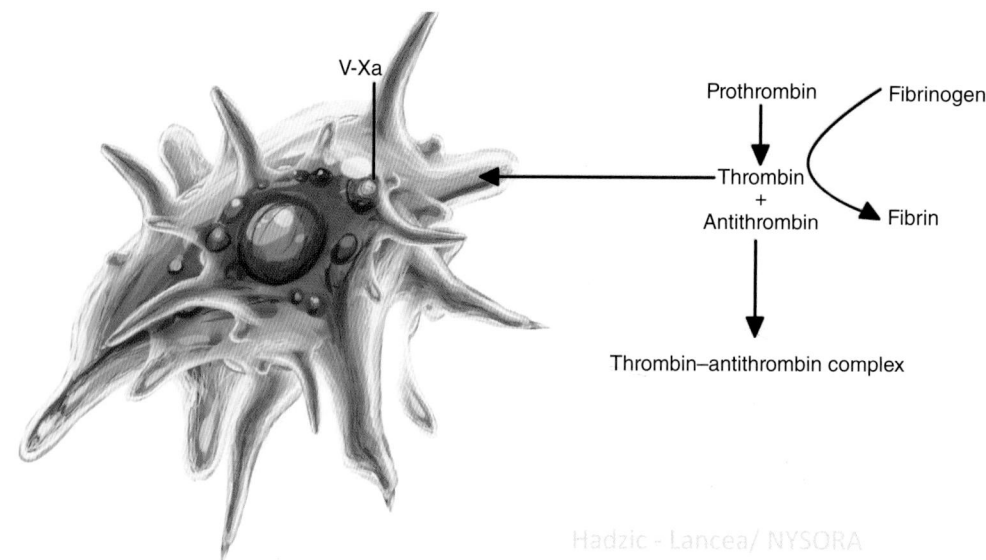

FIGURE 52–2. Role of platelets in coagulation: Platelets support plasma coagulation reactions. When activated, platelets bind several plasma protein complexes and secrete an activated form of factor V (factor Va), which binds to the platelet surface and binds factor Xa. Platelet-bound factor Xa then accelerates the conversion of prothrombin to thrombin.

Clopidogrel is preferred because of its improved safety profile and proven efficacy. It was noted to be better than aspirin in patients with peripheral vascular disease.[45] The maximal inhibition of ADP-induced platelet aggregation with clopidogrel occurs 3–5 days after initiation of a standard dose (75 mg) but within 4 to 6 hours after the administration of a large loading dose of 300–600 mg.[46] A large loading dose is usually given to patients before they undergo percutaneous coronary intervention (PCI). There has been a case report of spinal hematoma in a patient on ticlopidine.[47] Although there has been no case of intraspinal hematoma in a patient on clopidogrel alone, a case of quadriplegia in a patient on clopidogrel, diclofenac, and aspirin has been reported.[24]

For the thienopyridine drugs, it is recommended that ticlopidine be discontinued for 10–14 days and clopidogrel for 7 days before neuraxial injection. There have been case reports on the safety of spinal anesthesia 5 days after stoppage of clopidogrel. A study showed that most patients had minimal platelet inhibition 5 days after clopidogrel was stopped.[48] If a neuraxial procedure must be performed 5–6 days after discontinuation of clopidogrel, then a P2Y12 assay,[48] or another appropriate test, should be performed to ensure minimal or no inhibition of platelet activity.

Clinical Pearls

- The ASRA guidelines recommend a 7-day interval between discontinuation of clopidogrel and a neuraxial procedure.
- If a spinal or epidural must be performed is indicated, a test of platelet function is recommended to ensure that the residual platelet inhibition is gone or negligible.

For a spinal cord stimulation trial, a 5-day discontinuation may be observed since the patient will be off clopidogrel during the trial. A test of platelet function (eg, the VerifyNow P2Y12 assay or the platelet mapping portion of the Thrombelastograph [TEG]) must be performed to ensure adequate platelet activity.

Newer Antiplatelet Drugs

Clopidogrel is the commonly used antiplatelet drug in dual antiplatelet therapy, wherein aspirin is combined with a P2Y12 receptor inhibitor, in patients with acute coronary syndromes. Prasugrel is a pro-drug similar to clopidogrel but with salutary features over clopidogrel, and ticagrelor is a direct-acting P2Y12 receptor inhibitor.[49–51] The median time to peak effect is 1 hour with prasugrel and 4 hours with clopidogrel.[52] The mean time to peak plasma concentration with prasugrel is 30 minutes,[53] and its median half-life is 3.7 hours. These values do not reflect the duration of platelet inhibition because the inhibition of the P2Y12 receptor is irreversible. It takes 7 days for platelet activity to normalize after stopping prasugrel.[54]

Prasugrel and ticagrelor cause 90% inhibition of platelet function compared to 60%–70% for clopidogrel.[52] Patients with a low body mass index (BMI), those over 75 years of age, and those with a history of stroke are at risk for bleeding.[55,56] Unlike clopidogrel, prasugrel is reliably converted to its active metabolite and has no drug interactions. Also, it is not susceptible to genetic polymorphisms.[57,58]

Ticagrelor reversibly binds to the P2Y12 receptor, blocking ADP-mediated receptor activation. In contrast to the thienopyridines, the active metabolite and the parent drug exhibit antiplatelet activity with the parent drug responsible for the majority of the in vivo platelet inhibition.[59,60] The antiplatelet effect of ticagrelor is rapid; peak platelet inhibition occurs at 2 to 4 hours after intake compared to 24 hours with clopidogrel.[61] Mean platelet inhibition by ticagrelor is 93% compared to 58% for clopidogrel.[62] Platelet recovery is rapid with ticagrelor; platelet activity is normal at 5 days after the last dose.[62]

Time Between Discontinuation/Resumption of an Antiplatelet Drug and Neuraxial Injection

The interval between discontinuation of an antiplatelet drug and neuraxial injection is based on the percent platelet inhibition and percent platelet turnover. Prasugrel and ticagrelor cause 90% inhibition. Ten to 15 percent of the circulating platelet pool is formed every day,[63] resulting in new platelets comprising 50–75% of the circulating platelet pool 5–7 days after discontinuation of the drug.[48] An interval of 5–7 days has been recommended for ticagrelor and an interval of 7–10 days for prasugrel.[14,15] These recommendations are appropriate as platelet aggregation normalizes 7 days after stopping prasugrel[54] and 5 days after ticagrelor.[62,64]

The Scandinavian guidelines note that it is acceptable to restart antiplatelet drugs at the time of catheter removal,[15] whereas the European Society of Anaesthesiology guidelines recommended an interval of 6 hours between removal of epidural catheter and resumption of prasugrel or ticagrelor.[14] Other reviews have recommended caution in restarting prasugrel and ticagrelor because of their rapid effect and potent antiplatelet inhibition.[65] A 24-hour interval may be more appropriate for these agents.

Clinical Pearls

- Prasugrel and ticagrelor should be stopped 7 and 5 days, respectively, before a spinal or epidural.
- Antiplatelet drugs can be restarted 6–24 hours after a neuraxial procedure or catheter removal.

Monitoring Platelet Function

The Ivy bleeding time was considered to be a reliable predictor of abnormal bleeding in patients receiving antiplatelet drugs.[22] However, the post-aspirin bleeding time is not a reliable indicator of platelet function.[66] There is large intra- and interpatient variability in the results of the test, and there is no evidence to suggest that bleeding time can predict hemostatic function, as studies have failed to show a correlation between aspirin-induced prolongation of bleeding time and surgical blood loss.[67]

Special platelet function assays are now available to monitor platelet aggregation and degranulation. The platelet function analyzer (PFA) is a test of in vitro platelet function. It is a good screening test for von Willebrand disease and monitors the effect of desmopressin administration. The PFA is prolonged after antiplatelet therapy.[68] Unfortunately, the PFA-100 is not a sensitive test for monitoring the antiplatelet function of the P2Y12 inhibitors clopidogrel, prasugrel, and ticagrelor. However, the PFA-200, a recent update of the PFA-100,[69] appears to be sensitive to the effects of the P2Y12 inhibitors. However, point-of-care studies on this new PFA test are still lacking.

Newer tests that monitor P2Y12 receptor activity include the vasodilator-stimulated phosphoprotein (VASP) assay,[70,71] the VerifyNow assay,[72] the multiple-platelet aggregometry test (Multiplate),[73] and the platelet mapping component of the Thromboelastograph (TEG).[74] The VerifyNow assay can monitor the antiplatelet effects of aspirin and the P2Y12 inhibitors.[75] The platelet mapping component of the TEG is commonly used in surgery and anesthesiology, whereas VerifyNow is the predominant assay in clinical cardiology. A review on the monitoring of platelet function has been discussed by several reviews and is beyond the scope of this chapter.[48,76]

ORAL ANTICOAGULANTS

Warfarin exerts its anticoagulant effect by interfering with the synthesis of the vitamin K–dependent clotting factors (VII, IX, X, and thrombin)[77] (Figure 52–3). It also inhibits anticoagulant proteins C and S. Factor VII has a relatively short half-life (6–8 h), and the prothrombin time (PT) may be prolonged into the therapeutic range (1.5–2 times normal) within 24–36 hours. Anticoagulant protein C also has a short half-life (6–7 h). The initial prolongation of the international normalized ratio (INR) is the result of competing effects of reduced factor VII and protein C and the washout of existing clotting factors. Because of this, the INR is unpredictable during the initial stage of treatment with warfarin.[78,79] Factor VII participates only in the extrinsic pathway, and adequate anticoagulation is not achieved until the levels of biologically active factors II (half-life of 50 h) and X are sufficiently depressed. This requires 4–5 days. High loading doses of warfarin (15 mg) are occasionally employed for the first 2–3 days of therapy, and the desired anticoagulant effect is achieved within 48–72 hours.[80] The anticoagulant effect of warfarin persists for 4–6 days after termination of therapy while new biologically active vitamin K factors are synthesized. The drawbacks of warfarin therapy include the necessity of monitoring its effect with serial monitoring of INR, its interaction with other drugs, and the need for it to be discontinued a few days before surgery.[81] The effect of warfarin can be reversed by the transfusion of fresh frozen plasma and vitamin K injections. The 3-factor or 4-factor prothrombin complex concentrate (PCC) can be used to antagonize warfarin in emergency situations.

Few data exist regarding the risk of spinal hematoma in patients with indwelling spinal or epidural catheters who are subsequently anticoagulated with warfarin. Odoom and Sih[82] performed 1000 continuous lumbar epidural anesthetics in 950 patients who underwent vascular procedures and received preoperative oral anticoagulants. The thrombotest (a test of factor IX activity) was decreased and the activated partial thromboplastin time (aPTT) was prolonged in all the patients prior to epidural placement. Heparin was also administered intraoperatively. The epidural catheters remained in place for 48 hours postoperatively, and there were no neurologic complications. Unfortunately, the coagulation status of the patients at the time of catheter removal was not described. Although the results of this study are reassuring, the antiquated nature of the thrombotest as a measure of anticoagulation combined with the unknown coagulation status of the patients at the time of catheter removal limits the usefulness of the study.

The use of an indwelling epidural or intrathecal catheter and the timing of its removal in an anticoagulated patient are controversial. Although the trauma of needle placement occurs with both single-dose and continuous catheter techniques, the

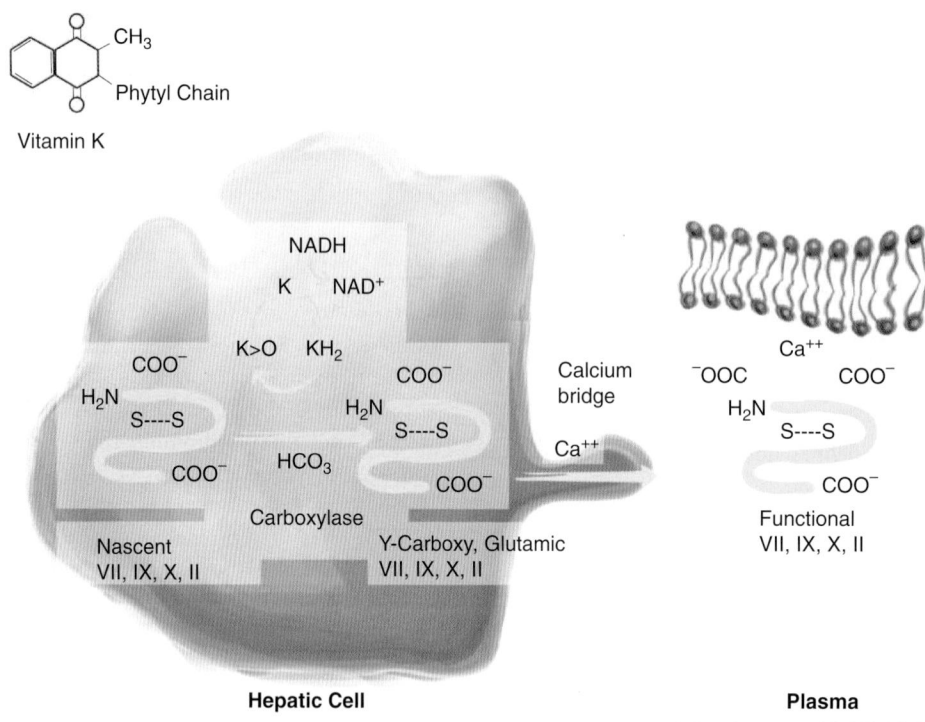

FIGURE 52–3. Vitamin K–dependent coagulation factor synthesis. Vitamin K is necessary for posttranslational modification of prothrombin; proteins C and S; and factors VII, IX, and X. Vitamin K is stored in hepatocytes.

presence of an indwelling catheter may result additional injury to tissues and vascular structures. Since intraspinal hematomas have occurred after catheter removal,[18] it is recommended that the same laboratory values apply to placement and removal of the epidural catheter.[83] No spinal hematomas were reported in 192 patients receiving postoperative epidural analgesia in conjunction with low-dose warfarin after total knee arthroplasty.[84] In this study, the patients received warfarin to prolong their PT to 15.0–17.3 seconds. The epidural catheters were left indwelling for 37 ± 15 hours (range 13–96 h). The mean PT at the time of epidural catheter removal was 13.4 ± 2 seconds (range 10.6–25.8 s). This and several subsequent studies have documented the relative safety of low-dose warfarin anticoagulation in patients with an indwelling epidural catheter.[85] Another study showed higher INR levels (up to 1.9) are acceptable for the removal of epidural catheters as long as it is done within 12–14 hours after warfarin intake.[79] A study showed the absence of spinal hematoma when the epidural catheters were removed 2–3 days after warfarin intake, even with markedly elevated INRs.[86] The practice of pulling the epidural catheter out 3 days after initiation of warfarin, when the levels of clotting factors VII, IX, and X are low (factor II levels may still be acceptable) needs to be studied. This is especially the case since patients vary greatly in their response to warfarin,[79] prompting some authors to recommend close monitoring of coagulation status to avoid excessive PT prolongation. Factors responsible for a prolonged PT and PTT are illustrated in Figures 52–4 and 52–5.

The ASRA recommended an INR value of 1.4 or less as acceptable for the performance of neuraxial blocks.[12,13,77] This value is based on studies that showed excellent perioperative hemostasis when the INR value was ≤1.5.[78] Studies on the levels of clotting factors at different INR values have shown that the decline of these factors may not be significant at an INR of 1.5. At INR values of 1.5–2.0, the concentrations of

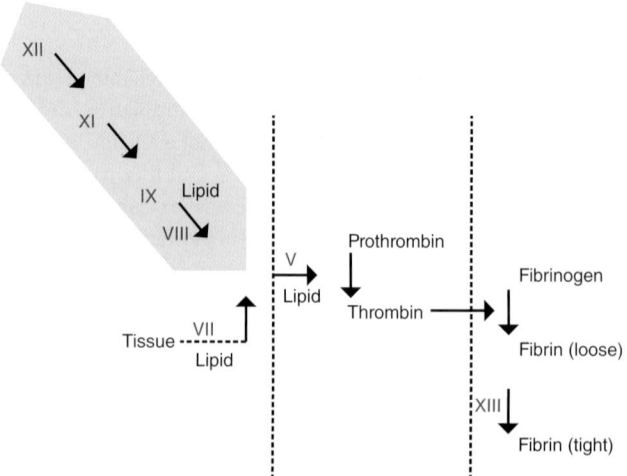

FIGURE 52–4. Coagulation reaction. Factors responsible for a prolonged PTT are in the shaded area. Patients who have an abnormal PTT but whose PT and other tests are normal can be divided into 2 groups: those who are prone to bleeding and those who are not. The patients who do not bleed may have an extremely prolonged PTT (90 seconds or more) but do not have a history of bleeding. They will have a deficiency in factor XII, prekalikrein, or high-molecular-weight kininogen. These patients should not be denied surgery or epidural anesthesia. The other group, patients who bleed, have both prolonged PTT and a history of bleeding. They will have a deficiency of factor VIII (hemophilia A), factor IX (hemophilia B or Christmas disease), or factor XI.

PT: The Test of the Extrinsic Pathway

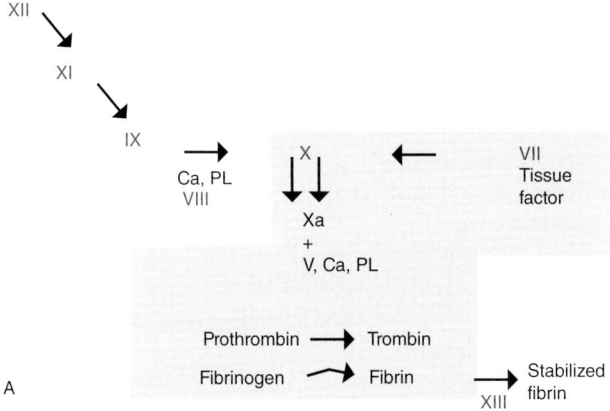

FIGURE 52–5A. Coagulation reaction. Factors involved in PT are in the shaded area. The PT is carried out by adding a source of tissue factor to the patient's plasma along with calcium or phospholipid. Tissue factor forms a complex with and activates factor VII. (Ca, calcium; PL, phospholipid.)

PTT: The Test of the Intrinsic Pathway

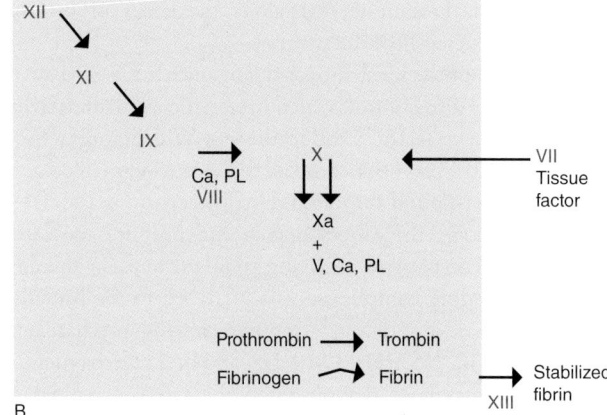

FIGURE 52–5B. Coagulation reaction. Factors involved in PTT are in the shaded area. In assessing PTT, coagulation is initiated by an agent that activates the Hageman factor–kininogen–prekalikrein complex. Most coagulation factors are screened by PTT, except factors VII and XIII, the protein that stabilizes fibrin clots by cross-linking them, and components of the fibrinolytic system. (Ca, calcium; PL, phospholipid.)

factor II were noted to be 74%–82% of baseline, whereas factor VII levels were 27%–54% of baseline values.[79] At INR values of 2.1 ± 1 during the initial phase of warfarin administration, factors II and VII were 65 ± 28% and 25 ± 20% of control values.[87] Activities of 40% are considered adequate for normal hemostasis at the time of major surgery. Another study[88] found that at INRs of 1.3–2, under stable anticoagulation with warfarin, the concentrations of clotting factors VII, IX, and X were within normal limits.

The clinician should be aware of the effect of warfarin on the coagulation cascade and the role of the INR in monitoring this effect. To minimize the risk of complications, the ASRA recommends several precautions.[12,13] Chronic oral warfarin therapy should be stopped and the INR measured before a neuraxial block is performed. The concurrent use of other medications, such as aspirin, NSAIDs, and heparins, which affect the clotting mechanism, increases the risk of bleeding complications without affecting the INR. If an initial dose of warfarin is given prior to surgery, the INR should be checked if the dose was given more than 24 hours earlier. If patients are on low-dose warfarin treatment (mean daily dose approximately 5 mg) during epidural analgesia, the INR should be checked daily and before catheter removal if the initial dose was given more than 36 hours previously. Higher daily doses may need more intensive monitoring. The warfarin dose should be held or reduced when the INR is >3 in patients with indwelling neuraxial catheters to prevent epidural hematoma and hemarthroma. While on warfarin therapy, the patient's neurologic status should be checked routinely during epidural analgesic infusion, as well as 24 hours after the catheter has been removed. Dilute concentrations of local anesthetic should be utilized to minimize the degree of sensory and motor blockade. Clinical judgment must be exercised in making decisions about removing or maintaining neuraxial catheters in patients with therapeutic levels of anticoagulation during neuraxial catheter infusion. The warfarin dose should be reduced for patients who are likely to have an enhanced response to the drug, especially

the elderly. For patients on chronic oral anticoagulation, the warfarin must be stopped and the INR measured.

Clinical Pearls

- An INR of 1.4, in the absence of easy bruisability and normal liver function is acceptable before neuraxial injection in patients planned for neuraxial blocks.
- The INR should be checked if the patient took warfarin more than 24 hours earlier.
- The INR should be normal 5 days after warfarin is stopped before a neuraxial procedure.

HEPARIN

Intravenous Heparin

Heparin is a complex polysaccharide that exerts its anticoagulant effect by binding to antithrombin. The conformational change in antithrombin accelerates its ability to inactivate thrombin factors Xa and IXa.[89]

Unfractionated heparin releases tissue factor pathway inhibitor from endothelium, enhancing its activity against factor Xa.[89] The anticoagulant effect of subcutaneous heparin takes 1–2 hours, but the effect of intravenous heparin is immediate. In fact, the coagulation time is prolonged 2–4 times the baseline level 5 minutes after the intravenous injection of 10,000 units of heparin. Heparin has a half-life is 1.5–2 hours. The therapeutic dose of heparin ceases 4–6 hours after its administration. The aPTT is used to monitor the effect of heparin; therapeutic anticoagulation is achieved with a prolongation of the aPTT greater than 1.5 times the baseline value or a heparin level of 0.2–0.4 U/mL.[90] The aPTT is usually not prolonged by the subcutaneous administration of low doses of heparin and is not monitored. Protamine neutralizes the effect of intravenously administered heparin.

Heparin is not the ideal anticoagulant since it is a mixture of molecules, only a fraction of which have anticoagulant activity. It binds to platelet factor 4 and to the von Willebrand factor.[91] The heparin–antithrombin complex is also not very effective in neutralizing clot-bound thrombin. Finally, heparin is associated with immunologic thrombocytopenia and immune-mediated thrombosis.[91] For patients receiving standard heparin therapy, the risk of bleeding complications is increased in the presence of other medications that affect other clotting mechanisms, including aspirin, NSAIDs, LMWHs, and oral anticoagulants.

Several studies have demonstrated the safety of spinal or epidural anesthesia followed by systemic heparinization if certain precautions are observed. Rao and El-Etr[92] reported no spinal hematomas in over 4000 patients who underwent lower extremity vascular surgery under continuous spinal or epidural anesthesia. In their study, patients with preexisting coagulation disorders were excluded, heparinization occurred at least 60 minutes after catheter placement, the level of anticoagulation was carefully monitored, and the indwelling catheters were removed at a time when heparin activity was low. Surgery was canceled in patients when frank blood was noted in the needle and performed the following day under general anesthesia. The same findings were noted in a subsequent report in the neurologic literature. Ruff and Dougherty[93] noted spinal hematomas in 7 of 342 (2%) patients who underwent lumbar puncture and subsequent heparinization for evaluation of cerebral ischemia. The presence of blood during the procedure, concomitant aspirin therapy, and heparinization within 1 hour were identified as risk factors in the development of spinal hematoma.

The ASRA has made several recommendations for when a neuraxial technique is used in the presence of intraoperative anticoagulation.[12,13,94] The ASRA advises that technique should be avoided in patients with other coagulopathies. There should be at least a 1-hour delay between needle placement and heparin administration. The catheter should be removed 2–4 hours after the last heparin dose and 1 hour before subsequent heparin administration. The aPTT or activated clotting time (ACT) should be monitored to avoid excessive heparin effect. The patient should followed postoperatively for early detection of reoccurrence of motor blockade. Dilute concentrations of local anesthetics are recommended to minimize motor blockade. Although there may be an increased risk in the event of a traumatic (bloody) or difficult needle placement, there are no data to support mandatory cancellation of surgery. The decision to proceed should be based on appropriate clinical judgment and full discussion with the surgeon and patient.

Clinical Pearls

- There should be at least a 1-hour delay between a neuraxial procedure and heparin readministration.
- The catheter can be removed 2–4 hours after the last heparin dose.

Neuraxial procedures are occasionally performed in patients who undergo cardiopulmonary bypass. The following precautions have been recommended to prevent the development of intraspinal hematoma in these patients:[95]

1. Neuraxial procedures should be avoided in patients with known coagulopathy.
2. Surgery should be delayed 24 hours in patients with a traumatic tap.
3. The time from the neuraxial procedure to the systemic heparinization should exceed 1 hour.
4. Heparinization and reversal should be monitored and controlled tightly.
5. The epidural catheter should be removed when normal coagulation is restored, and the patient should be monitored closely for signs of spinal hematoma.

Subcutaneous Heparin

The therapeutic basis of low-dose twice-daily subcutaneous heparin (5000 units every 8–12 hours) is the heparin-mediated inhibition of activated factor X. Smaller doses of heparin are required when administered as prophylaxis rather than as treatment for thromboembolic disease. Following the intramuscular or subcutaneous injection of 5000 units of heparin, maximum anticoagulation effect is observed in 40–50 minutes and returns to baseline within 4 to 6 hours. The aPTT may remain in the normal range and often is not monitored. However, wide variations in individual patient responses to subcutaneous heparin have been reported. Neuraxial techniques are not contraindicated during subcutaneous (mini-dose) prophylaxis, but the risk of bleeding may be reduced by delaying heparin administration until after the block. Bleeding may be increased in debilitated patients or after prolonged therapy. The safety of major neuraxial anesthesia in the presence of anticoagulation with twice-daily subcutaneous doses of unfractionated heparin has been documented by several studies.[94] The twice-daily subcutaneous heparin regimen has been replaced by a thrice-daily regimen in most hospitals to decrease the incidence of postoperative venous thromboembolism.[96] However, this practice has been associated with spontaneous hematomas.[97] For this reason, the latest ASRA guidelines recommend against neuraxial procedures in patients on a thrice-daily regimen until more data become available.[13]

Clinical Pearls

- Neuraxial procedures can be performed in patients on twice-daily subcutaneous heparin.
- Because of the lack of adequate data, the ASRA recommends that neuraxial procedures not be performed in patients on thrice-daily subcutaneous heparin.

Low-Molecular-Weight Heparin

Unfractionated heparin is a heterogeneous mixture of polysaccharide chains that can be separated into fragments of various molecular weights.[98,99] The anticoagulant effect of LMWH is similar to that for unfractionated heparin; it activates antithrombin, accelerating antithrombin's interaction with thrombin and factor Xa. LMWH has a greater activity against factor Xa, whereas unfractionated heparin has equivalent activity against thrombin and factor Xa. The plasma half-life of the LMWHs ranges from 2–4 hours after an intravenous injection and 3–6 hours after a subcutaneous injection; the half-life of an LMWH is 2–4 times that of standard heparin. It has a low affinity for plasma protein, resulting in a greater bioavailability. The advantages of LMWH over unfractionated heparin include a higher and more predictable bioavailability after subcutaneous administration and a longer biological half-life. Also, laboratory monitoring of the anticoagulant response of LMWH is not required, and dose adjustment for weight is not necessary (although an overdose may occur in patients with a low BMI). LMWH exhibits a dose-dependent antithrombotic effect that is accurately assessed by measuring the anti-Xa activity level. The recovery of anti-factor Xa activity after a subcutaneous injection of LMWH approaches 100%,[100] making laboratory monitoring unnecessary except in patients with renal insufficiency or those with body weight less than 50 kg or more than 80 kg.[98] The reaction time from the thrombelastogram appears to correlate with the serum anti-Xa concentration.[101]

The three commercially available LMWHs in the United States are enoxaparin (Lovenox), dalteparin (Fragmin), and tinzaparin (Innohep), although the latter has been discontinued because of low usage. Enoxaparin is given either once daily or every 12 hours when used as prophylaxis, and dalteparin and tinzaparin are given once daily. The three drugs appear to have comparable efficacy in the treatment and prevention of venous thromboembolism.[102] Enoxaparin and dalteparin have comparable efficacy in the prevention of death or myocardial infarction among patients with unstable angina.[102]

The recommended thromboprophylactic dose in the United States is 30 mg enoxaparin twice daily, although some clinicians increase the dose in patients who are obese (1.5 mg/kg daily or 1 mg/kg every 12 hours). The European dosing schedule is enoxaparin 20–40 mg once daily, and patients receive their starting dose 12 hours before surgery, a practice not observed in the United States.

Numerous cases of neuraxial hematoma occurred in the United States, prompting the FDA to issue a health advisory in December 1997 and the convening of the first ASRA consensus conference on anticoagulation and neuraxial anesthesia.[103] The ASRA guidelines recommend the smallest effective dose of LMWH should be administered. The postoperative administration of LMWH therapy should be delayed as long as possible, for a minimum of 12 hours and ideally 24 hours postoperatively. A single-dose spinal anesthetic may be the safest neuraxial technique in patients receiving preoperative LMWH. Waiting for at least 12 hours after the prophylactic LMWH dose is recommended before performing a neuraxial technique. Patients who receive higher doses of LMWH (eg, enoxaparin 1 mg/kg twice daily) require longer delays (24 h). The catheter should be removed when anticoagulation activity is low, at least 12 hours after prophylactic LMWH administration and 4 hours before the next dose.[104] Extreme vigilance of

the patient's neurologic status must be observed if LMWH thromboprophylaxis is implemented while an indwelling catheter is infusing. Dilute local anesthetic solution is recommended so that neurologic function can be better monitored. The use of other medications affecting hemostasis, such as antiplatelet drugs, standard heparin, dextran, or oral anticoagulants, in combination with LMWH creates an additional risk of bleeding complications.

Clinical Pearls

- In patients on a prophylactic dose of LMWH, a 12-hour interval is recommended before a neuraxial injection.
- For patients on a therapeutic dose of LMWH, a 24-hour interval is appropriate.
- A 4-hour delay following epidural catheter removal before LMWH is resumed has been recommended by the FDA.

THROMBOLYTIC THERAPY

Thrombolytic agents actively dissolve fibrin clots that have already formed. Exogenous plasminogen activators such as streptokinase and urokinase not only dissolve thrombus but also affect circulating plasminogen, leading to decreased levels of both plasminogen and fibrin. Recombinant tissue-type plasminogen activator (r-TPA), an endogenous agent, is more fibrin selective and has less effect on circulating plasminogen levels. Clot lysis leads to an elevation of fibrin degradation products, which have an anticoagulant effect by inhibiting platelet aggregation.

Although epidural or spinal needle and catheter placement with subsequent heparinization appears relatively safe, the risk of spinal hematoma in patients who receive thrombolytic therapy is not well defined. Cases of spinal hematoma in patients who had epidural or indwelling epidural catheters and who received thrombolytic agents have been reported in the literature.[105]

The ASRA guidelines make recommendations with respect to neuraxial procedures after thrombolytic or fibrinolytic therapy.[12,13,105] The concurrent use of heparin with fibrinolytic or thrombolytic drugs places patients at high risk of adverse neuraxial bleeding during spinal or epidural anesthesia. Except in highly unusual circumstances, patients receiving fibrinolytic or thrombolytic therapy should be cautioned against receiving spinal or epidural anesthesia. There are no available data to clearly determine the appropriate length of time after discontinuation of these drugs and the safe performance of a neuraxial technique. The European guidelines recommend leaving the epidural catheter in place when a patient is given a thrombolytic drug, removing it only once effect of the drug is gone.[14] The Scandinavian guidelines recommend a 24-hour interval between discontinuation of the drug and neuraxial procedure.[15] Frequent neurologic monitoring is recommended for an appropriate length of time in patients who have had neuraxial blocks after fibrinolytic or thrombolytic therapy. If a patient has a continuous epidural infusion and has received fibrinolytic or thrombolytic therapy, drugs that minimize sensory and motor blockade should be used. There has been no definitive recommendation on the timing of removal of neuraxial catheters in patients who unexpectedly receive fibrinolytic or thrombolytic therapy. Measurement of fibrinogen levels may be helpful in guiding a decision about catheter removal or maintenance.

Herbal Therapy

The most commonly used herbal medications are garlic, ginkgo, and ginseng. Garlic inhibits platelet aggregation, and its effect on hemostasis appears to last 7 days. Ginkgo inhibits platelet-activating factor, and its effect lasts 36 hours. Ginseng has a variety of effects: it inhibits platelet aggregation in vitro and prolongs both thrombin time (TT) and aPTT in laboratory animals; its effect lasts 24 hours.[12,13] In spite of their effect on platelet function, herbal drugs by themselves appear to present no added significant risk in the development of spinal hematoma in patients having epidural or spinal anesthesia. Mandatory discontinuation of these medications, or cancellation of surgery in patients in whom these medications have been continued, is not supported by available clinical data. However, the concurrent use of other medications that affect clotting mechanisms, such as oral anticoagulants or heparin, may increase the risk of bleeding complications in these patients. There is no accepted test to assess adequacy of hemostasis in the patient who has taken herbal medications. At this time, there appear to be no specific concerns as to the timing of neuraxial block in relationship to the dosing of herbal therapy, postoperative monitoring, or the timing of neuraxial catheter removal.[12,13]

Thrombin Inhibitors

Recombinant hirudin derivatives, including desirudin, and bivalirudin, inhibit both free and clot-bound thrombin.[12,13] Argatroban, an L-arginine derivative, has a similar mechanism of action. These drugs are primarily used in the treatment of heparin-induced thrombocytopenia. There is no pharmacologic reversal to the effect of these drugs. There have been no case reports of spinal hematoma related to neuraxial anesthesia in patients who have received a thrombin inhibitor. However, spontaneous intracranial bleeding has been reported.[12] According to the ASRA guidelines, no statement regarding risk assessment and patient management can be made.

Fondaparinux

Fondaparinux is a synthetic anticoagulant that produces its antithrombotic effect through selective inhibition of factor Xa.[106] The drug exhibits consistency in its anticoagulant effect since it is chemically synthesized. It is 100% bioavailable. Rapidly absorbed, it attains maximum concentration within 1.7 hours of administration. Its half-life is 17–21 hours.[106] Fondaparinux is recommended as an antithrombotic agent after major orthopedic surgery[107] and as initial treatment for

pulmonary embolism.[108] The extended half-life (approximately 20 hours) allows once-daily dosing. The FDA has issued a black box warning for fondaparinux similar to that for the LMWHs and heparin.

The actual risk of spinal hematoma with fondaparinux is unknown. A study showed no complications in patients who received neuraxial injections.[109] In this study, the catheters were removed 36 hours after the last dose of fondaparinux, and dosing was delayed for 12 hours after catheter removal. Patients were excluded from the study if difficulties were encountered in performing the neuraxial procedure (more than 3 attempts required), the procedure was complicated by bleeding, they required antiplatelet drugs, or the plan was to withdraw the epidural catheter the day after surgery. Because of the unrealistic requirements in clinical practice, the ASRA[12,13] recommends against the use of fondaparinux in the presence of an indwelling epidural catheter. Their recommendations are based on the sustained and irreversible antithrombotic effect of fondaparinux, early postoperative dosing, and the spinal hematoma reported during the initial clinical trials of the drug. Close monitoring of the literature for risk factors associated with surgical bleeding may be helpful in risk assessment and patient treatment. Performance of neuraxial techniques should occur under conditions used in clinical trials (single needle pass, atraumatic needle placement, avoidance of indwelling neuraxial catheters).[12,13] If this is not feasible, an alternative method of prophylaxis should be considered.

Summary

The time interval between discontinuation of the anticoagulant and neuraxial procedure and between epidural catheter removal and resumption of the drug are summarized in Table 52–1.

NEW ANTICOAGULANTS

A discussion of the new anticoagulants dabigatran, rivaroxaban, and apixaban involves a review of certain background information.

The Interval Between Anticoagulant Discontinuation and Neuraxial Injection and Between Neuraxial Procedure or Epidural Catheter Removal and Resumption of Anticoagulant

It has been recommended that two half-lives is an adequate compromise between the risk of venous thromboembolism (VTE) and the prevention of spinal hematoma.[110] The European and Scandinavian guidelines recommended a 2-half-life interval between discontinuation of anticoagulant and neuraxial injection. This decision was like made because subclinical VTE occurs in a fair percentage of patients immediately after surgery and having residual anticoagulation might prevent this occurrence. The presence of residual anticoagulation facilitates the transition to full anticoagulation after a neuraxial procedure.

After 1, 2, 3, 4, 5, and 6 half-lives, the following percentages of drug remain in the circulation: 50%, 25%, 12.5%, 6.25%,

TABLE 52-1. Recommended time intervals before or after neuraxial procedure and epidural catheter removal.

Drug	Time Before Neuraxial Procedure or Catheter Removal	Time After Neuraxial Procedure or Catheter Removal	Comments
Aspirin	None	None	
NSAIDs	None	None	
Clopidogrel	7 days*	After catheter removal	Per European & & Scandinavian guidelines
Prasugrel	7-10 days	6h	Per European Guidelines
Ticagrelor	5 days	6h	(As above)
Warfarin	5 days (normal INR)	After catheter removal	
Heparin (IV)	4-6 h	1-2h	
Heparin			
(Sc, BID)	None	None	
(Sc, TID)	Not applicable		Neuraxial procedure
			Not recommended
LMWH			
Prophylactic	12 hours	4 hours	FDA recommendation
Therapeutic	24 hours	4 hours	
Fondaparinux	36-42 hours	6-12 hours	Per European guidelines. ASRA recommended against neuraxial procedures in patients on the drug.

*If neuraxial procedure has to be performed at 5 days, a test of platelet function is recommended (see text).

3.125%, and 1.5625%, respectively (Table 52–2).[111] However, these findings are based on studies in young healthy volunteers in single-dosing pharmacokinetic studies in the absence of other anticoagulants. By contrast, in clinical practice, patients are usually older and have concomitant comorbidities.

In patients who are at risk for VTE, such as those with a previous history of stroke,[112] a 2- or 3-half-life interval might be appropriate, recognizing that adequate hemostasis is not assured.

For patients without thrombotic risk factors, an interval of 4–6 half-lives between the last dose of anticoagulant and neuraxial injection ensures a more complete elimination of the drug and less risk of bleeding.[113,114] A compromise between the conservative recommendations of 4–6 half-lives and 2–3 half-lives[14,15] is an interval of 5 half-lives with LMWH bridge therapy.

Regarding the resumption of the anticoagulant after neuraxial injection or removal of epidural catheter, the Scandinavian

TABLE 52-2. Recommended time intervals before or after neuraxial procedure and epidural catheter for the new anticoagulants.

Drug	Half-life	European Guidelines	Scandinavian Guidelines	Five Half-lives
Dabigatran	12-17h 28 hours (renal disease)	(Contraindicated per manufacturer)	Data not available	85h (4d) 6d (renal patients)
Rivaroxaban	9-13h	22-26h	18h	65h (3d)
Apixaban	15.2 +/-8.5h	26-30h	Data not available	75h (3-4d)

At 5 half-lives, 96.8% of the drug is eliminated. The upper limit of the half-life was used to calculate the 5 half-lives of the drug.

The European and Scandinavian guidelines used a 2 half-life interval when data is available.

guidelines are based on the recommendation of Rosencher et al. of 8 hours minus the time it takes for the anticoagulant to reach peak effect.[110] Eight hours was presumed to be adequate for the clot to stabilize, a presumption supported by the efficacy of thrombolytic agents to lyze a clot if given within 6 hours of clot formation.[115] Tertri and colleagues also noted that giving enoxaparin within 24–48 hours after intracerebral hemorrhage did not enlarge the size of hematoma,[116] so a 24-hour interval is probably safer. Other authors recommend a more conservative approach because the reinstitution of antithrombotic therapy within 24 hours after a major procedure might increase the risk of periprocedural bleeding.[65] Liew and Douketis[117] recommend a minimum of 24 hours in patients with low bleeding risk and 48 hours in those with a high bleeding risk before resuming dabigatran, rivaroxaban, or apixaban. The options therefore are either 8 hours or 24 hours minus the peak effect of the drug. There is probably little difference between these two options since the risks of VTE, stroke, or acute coronary syndrome are probably the same. In addition, the onset and times to peak effect of the new anticoagulants are short.

Dabigatran

Dabigatran etexilate is a prodrug that is hydrolyzed by esterases in the stomach to the active drug. Dabigatran etexilate has a bioavailability of 7.2%.[118] Dabigatran is a direct thrombin inhibitor that blocks the interaction of thrombin with various substrates.[76,119,120] Peak plasma concentrations are attained 1.5–3 hours after intake of the prodrug.[121] It has a half-life of 14–17 hours.[121–123] Renal clearance accounts for 80% of the total clearance of dabigatran.[124] In cases of end-stage renal disease, the elimination half-life doubles from 14 hours to 28 hours.[124,125]

Dabigatran is effective in the treatment of acute VTE and in the prevention of recurrent VTE. In patients with atrial fibrillation, dabigatran reduces the rates of stroke and systemic embolism to a degree similar to that of warfarin. Dabigatran was not shown to be consistent in preventing VTE after total joint surgery. Studies have shown it to be either more effective,[126] noninferior,[127,128] or inferior to enoxaparin.[129] A meta-analysis of the trials noted no differences between dabigatran and enoxaparin in any of the endpoints analyzed.[130]

The manufacturer states that epidural catheters should not be placed in patients receiving dabigatran.[14] A 2-hour minimum interval between indwelling catheter removal and dabigatran administration has been recommended by Levy and colleagues.[120] This interval appears to be shorter than 6 hours, that is, the difference between 8 hours minus the 2-hour time to reach peak effect of the drug. There have been reports of increased bleeding after taking dabigatran. The Haematology Society of Australia and New Zealand identified 78 bleeding episodes in approximately 7000 patients over a 2-month period.[131] An audit by the FDA, however, concluded that there was not an absolute increase of bleeding with dabigatran compared to warfarin.

The aPTT is prolonged after dabigatran, but the relationship is curvilinear.[113,132] The thrombin time (TT), also known as thrombin clotting time (TCT), is highly sensitive to the effects of dabigatran[113,133] and is more appropriately used for

detecting the presence of the anticoagulant effect of dabigatran than quantifying the effect of the drug.[134] A dilute TT has linearity across pharmacologically relevant plasma dabigatran concentrations.[113,132] The ecarin clotting time (ECT), which directly measures thrombin generation, is dose-dependent prolonged by dabigatran.[134] It is the most sensitive assay for dabigatran, but few institutions have the test available. The prothrombin time (PT) is the least sensitive test. The dilute TT and the ECT are the tests of choice for dabigatran.[132]

To date, there is no antidote to reverse the effect of dabigatran or the other new oral anticoagulants.[135–137] Activated charcoal prevents absorption of the drug, but it needs to be given within 2 hours of dabigatran ingestion. Dialysis might speed drug elimination. Plasma complex concentrates (PCCs) that contain either 3 (factors II, IX, and X) or 4 (factors II, VII, IX, and X) clotting factors have been suggested,[133,134] but their efficacy has not been proven. Idarucizumab, a monoclonal antibody fragment that binds with free and thrombin-bound dabigatran, was recently approved by the FDA.

Clinical Pearls

- Dabigatran is primarily dependent on the kidneys for elimination, and its half-life is doubled in patients with kidney disease.
- A longer interval between stoppage of the drug and neuraxial procedure, probably 6 days, is recommended in these patients.

Rivaroxaban

Rivaroxaban is a direct factor Xa inhibitor. Peak plasma concentrations are observed within 2.5–4 hours,[138,139] and the maximum inhibition of factor Xa (up to 68%) occurs 3 hours after dosing and is maintained for at least 12 hours,[139] or 24–48 hours when higher doses are given in elderly patients.[140] Rivaroxaban has a terminal half-life of 5.7–9.2 hours,[138,139] but this can be as long as 11–13 hours in elderly patients due to age-related decline in renal function.[141,142] One-third of the drug is eliminated by the kidneys, one-third by the fecal/biliary route, and one-third is changed to inactive metabolites.[139,143] The maximum concentration is not affected by obesity (patients weighing ≥120 kg) but is increased by 24% in patients weighing ≤50 kg. The renal clearance of rivaroxaban decreases with increasing renal impairment.[144]

Rivaroxaban is effective in the treatment of symptomatic VTE[142] and noninferior to warfarin in the prevention of embolic stroke during atrial fibrillation.[145] The addition of rivaroxaban to standard antiplatelet therapy reduces the composite endpoint of death from cardiovascular causes, myocardial infarction, or stroke in patients with a recent acute coronary syndrome.[76]

Rivaroxaban was reported to be as effective or superior to enoxaparin in preventing VTE after total joint surgery[146–150] In the RECORD1, 2, 3, and 4 studies,[146–149] rivaroxaban was a more effective thromboprophylactic agent than enoxaparin, with a similar safety profile. Rosencher et al. stated that epidural catheters were not removed until at least 2 half-lives after the last dose of rivaroxaban, and the next rivaroxaban dose was given 4-6 hours after catheter removal.[151] None of the 1141 patients who were given rivaroxaban and had neuraxial anesthesia developed spinal hematoma. However, this small number of patients is not adequate to make a firm conclusion on the perioperative safety of this regimen.

The European and Scandinavian guidelines recommend a 2-half-life interval between rivaroxaban discontinuation and epidural catheter placement or removal (18 hours in the Scandinavian guidelines and 22–26 hours in the European guidelines).[14,15] These guidelines also recommend a 4–6-hour interval before resumption of the next dose, as rivaroxaban takes 2.5–4 hours to reach peak effect.

A linear correlation was observed between the effects of rivaroxaban and PT.[114,134] However, there is marked variability in the sensitivity of PT reagents to rivaroxaban, so it is recommended that each laboratory should calibrate their PT specifically for rivaroxaban. The aPTT lacks sufficient sensitivity to determine the effect of rivaroxaban.[114,134] The inhibition of factor Xa may also be a surrogate for the plasma concentrations of rivaroxaban.[152] The PT and anti-Xa are the recommended tests for monitoring the effects of rivaroxaban.[132]

The use of activated charcoal has been recommended to remove rivaroxaban, but it must be given within 8 hours of rivaroxaban intake. A 4-factor PCC has been shown to reverse the in vitro anticoagulant activity of rivaroxaban in healthy volunteers.[134] Because of their high protein binding, rivaroxaban and apixaban may not be dialyzable.

Apixaban

Apixaban is a highly specific factor Xa inhibitor. It is rapidly absorbed and attains peak concentrations in 1–2 hours. Studies have shown the terminal half-life of apixaban to be 13.5 +/- 9.9 hours, or 15.2 +/- 8.5 hours after a single 5 mg dose and 11.7 +/- 3.3 after multiple 5 mg doses.[153–155] Maximum plasma concentration is affected by body weight, with higher concentrations of apixaban in subjects with low body weight. Plasma anti–factor Xa activity has shown a direct linear relationship with apixaban plasma concentration.[155]

Apixaban has an oral bioavailability of more than 45%.[153] After oral administration, it is eliminated via multiple elimination pathways as well as direct renal and intestinal excretion.[156] Twenty-four to 29 percent of the dose is excreted via the kidneys, and 56% of the dose is recovered in the feces.[153] More than half of apixaban is excreted unchanged, lessening the risk of metabolic drug–drug interactions.

Apixaban is effective in reducing stroke or systemic embolism without increasing the risk of bleeding. Apixaban is superior to warfarin in preventing stroke or systemic embolism in patients with atrial fibrillation.[76] Apixaban provides effective thromboprophylaxis in total knee arthroplasty, comparable to enoxaparin or warfarin.[157] Apixaban is equally efficacious with enoxaparin in preventing VTE after total knee replacement (TKR) while having a lower[158] or similar[159] rate of major bleeding. Apixaban is more effective than enoxaparin in preventing VTE after total hip replacement (THR) without increased bleeding.[160] In this trial, "devices in connection with intrathecal or epidural anesthesia were removed at least 5 hours before the first dose" of apixaban. In all studies of apixaban, the drug was started 12–24 hours after surgery.

Compared to rivaroxaban, apixaban has little effect on PT when given in approved doses.[114] The dilute PT assay has improved sensitivity over conventional PT. There appears to be a linear correlation between anti-Xa activity and the plasma concentrations of apixaban. The anti-Xa assay was noted to be more sensitive than the PT and as sensitive as the dilute PT assay[161] and appears to be the best choice for clinical monitoring of the anticoagulant effect of apixaban.[132] Activated charcoal, given within 3 hours of ingestion, reduces the absorption of apixaban.

Andexanet is a recombinant modified human factor Xa decoy protein that binds and sequesters factor Xa inhibitors. Studies in volunteers and in patients showed andexanet to reveres the anticoagulant activity of rivaroxaban and apixaban.[162] As of 2016, andexanet is not yet clinically available in the United States.

Summary of Recommendations for the New Anticoagulants

While a 2–3-half-life interval may be acceptable in patients who are at high risk for VTE or stroke, an interval of 4–6 half-lives between stoppage of the drug and neuraxial injection is probably safer in most patients at low risk of thrombosis. A 5-half-life interval in conjunction with an LMWH bridge therapy is an alternative in most patients, as shown in Table 52–2. After a neuraxial procedure or removal of an epidural catheter, the anticoagulant can be resumed 6 hours (8 hours minus the onset/peak effect of the drug, which is usually 2 hours) later. Anticoagulants are typically resumed within 24–48 hours in most patients, but they can be resumed sooner in patients who are at higher risk for VTE or stroke; that is, 24 hours minus the time to peak effect of the drug. Others recommended a 24-houir interval (Table 52–3).

TABLE 52-3. Recommended time intervals for resumption of drug after neuraxial procedure or catheter removal.

Drug	European Guidelines	Scandinavian Guidelines	Liew & Douketis (102); Connolly and Spyropoulos (98)
Dabigatran	6h	6h	24h
Rivaroxaban	4-6h	6h	24h
Apixaban	4-6h	6h	24h

The interval from the European and Scandinavian guidelines was based on 8 hours (time for the clot to stabilize) minus the time to peak onset of the drug.

Laboratory monitoring of the anticoagulant effect is appropriate in some situations, and reversal agents are suggested when there is a need to rapidly restore hemostatic function.

Clinical Pearls

- For the new anticoagulants, a 5-half-life interval between discontinuation of the drug and neuraxial procedure is recommended until there is more experience with these agents.
- An interval of either 8 or 24 hours-time to peak effect of the drug is recommended before the drug is resumed after catheter removal; a 24-hour interval is probably the safest.

CLINICAL FEATURES, DIAGNOSIS & MANAGEMENT OF EPIDURAL HEMATOMA

Patients who develop spinal hematoma usually present with sudden, severe, constant back pain with or without a radicular component. Percussion over the spine aggravates the pain as do maneuvers that increase intraspinal pressure, including coughing, sneezing, or straining. In addition, the return of the motor weakness and/or sensory deficit after the apparent resolution of the epidural or spinal blockade is highly suggestive of epidural or spinal hematoma formation. Motor and sensory findings depend entirely on the level and size of the hematoma but may include weakness, paresis, loss of bowel or bladder function, and virtually any sensory deficit. Magnetic resonance imaging (MRI) is the diagnostic study of choice. The differential diagnosis includes spinal abscess, epidural neoplasm, acute disk herniation, and spinal subarachnoid hemorrhage. Recovery without surgery is rare, and neurosurgical consultation for consideration of emergent decompressive laminectomy should be obtained as soon as spinal hematoma is suspected. Functional recovery is related primarily to the length of time the symptoms are present before surgery. The clinical features, diagnosis, differential diagnosis, and treatment of a patient with a spinal hematoma are discussed in more detail in Chapter 65.

SUMMARY

Practitioners should periodically update their knowledge base on new anticoagulant medications, anticoagulation protocols, current guideline recommendations, and FDA alerts. Since spinal hematoma may occur even in the absence of identifiable risk factors, vigilance in monitoring is critical for early evaluation of neurologic dysfunction and prompt intervention. The decision to perform neuraxial blockade and the timing of catheter removal in a patient receiving anticoagulant therapy should be made on an individual basis, weighing the benefits of regional anesthesia against the small, though definite, risk of spinal hematoma.

Anticoagulation & Peripheral Nerve Blocks

If appropriate, peripheral nerve blocks can be performed in patients taking anticoagulants. In contrast to neuraxial procedures in the presence of anticoagulants, there have been no prospective studies on peripheral nerve blocks in the presence of anticoagulants. The ASRA recommends the same guidelines for peripheral nerve blocks as for neuraxial procedures. Cases of psoas and retroperitoneal hematomas have been reported after lumbar plexus blocks and psoas compartment blocks.[13] These patients were either on enoxaparin, ticlopidine, or clopidogrel. In some cases, the hematoma occurred in spite of adherence to the ASRA guidelines.

The symptoms of hematoma formation after peripheral nerve block may include pain (flank or paravertebral pain, or groin pain in psoas bleeding), tenderness in the area, a steady decline in hemoglobin/hematocrit, hypotension due to hypovolemia, and sensory–motor deficit. Definite diagnosis is made by computerized tomography (CT); ultrasound can also be used to detect the presence of renal subcapsular hematoma after psoas compartment block. Treatment may include surgical consultation, reversal of anticoagulation, blood transfusion as necessary, and watchful waiting versus surgical drainage.

It is probably too restrictive to adapt the ASRA guidelines on neuraxial blocks to patients undergoing peripheral nerve blocks. The European Society of Anaesthesiology has noted that the guidelines for neuraxial block do not routinely apply to peripheral nerve blocks. The Austrian Society for Anesthesiology, Resuscitation and Intensive Care, on the other hand, has suggested that superficial nerve blocks can be safely performed in the presence of anticoagulants.[161] Because of the possibility of retroperitoneal hematoma, lumbar plexus and paravertebral blocks merit the same recommendations as for neuraxial injections. The same guidelines should also apply to visceral sympathetic blocks. The ASRA guidelines may therefore be applicable to blocks in vascular and noncompressible areas, such as celiac plexus blocks, superior hypogastric plexus blocks, and lumbar plexus blocks. Clinicians should individualize their decision and discuss the risks and benefits of the block with the patient and the surgeon. Most importantly, the clinician should follow the patient closely after the block placement.

Clinical Pearls

- The guidelines on neuraxial injections should also apply to lumbar plexus blocks and visceral sympathetic blocks.
- For superficial nerve blocks, ultrasound-guided regional nerve blocks can probably be performed in the presence of residual anticoagulation.

REFERENCES

1. Horlocker TT, Wedel DJ: Anticoagulation and neuraxial block: historical perspective, anesthetic implications, and risk management. Reg Anesth Pain Med 1998;23:129–134.
2. Tryba M: [Epidural regional anesthesia and low molecular heparin: Pro]. Anasthesiol Intensivmed Notfallmed Schmerzther 1993;28:179–181.

3. Pöpping DM, Zahn PK, Van Aken HK, Dasch B, Boche R, Pogatzki-Zahn EM: Effectiveness and safety of postoperative pain management: a survey of 18 925 consecutive patients between 1998 and 2006 (2nd revision): a database analysis of prospectively raised data. Br J Anaesth 2008;101:832–840.

4. Moen V, Dahlgren N, Irestedt L: Severe neurological complications after central neuraxial blockades in Sweden 1990–1999. Anesthesiology 2004;101:950–959.

5. Volk T, Wolf A, Van Aken H, Bürkle H, Wiebalck A, Steinfeldt T: Incidence of spinal haematoma after epidural puncture: analysis from the German network for safety in regional anaesthesia. Eur J Anaesthesiol 2012;29:170–176.

6. Ehrenfeld JM, Agarwal AK, Henneman JP, Sandberg WS: Estimating the incidence of suspected epidural hematoma and the hidden imaging cost of epidural catheterization: a retrospective review of 43,200 cases. Reg Anesth Pain Med 2013;38:409–414.

7. Bateman BT, Mhyre JM, Ehrenfeld J, et al: The risk and outcomes of epidural hematomas after perioperative and obstetric epidural catheterization: a report from the multicenter perioperative outcomes group research consortium. Anesth Analg 2013:116:1380–1385.

8. Horlocker T, Kopp S: Epidural hematoma after epidural blockade in the United States: It's not just low molecular weight heparin following orthopedic surgery anymore. Anesth Analg 2013;116:1195–1197.

9. Horlocker T: Neuraxial blockade in patients with spinal stenosis: between a rock and a hard place. Anesth Analg 2010;110:1305.

10. Gulur P, Tsui B, Pathak R, Koury KM, Lee H: Retrospective analysis of the incidence of epidural haematoma in patients with epidural catheters and abnormal coagulation parameters. Br J Anaesth 2015;114:808–811.

11. Heit JA, Horlocker TT (eds): Neuraxial anesthesia and anticoagulation. Reg Anesth Pain Med 1998;23:S129–S193.

12. Horlocker TT, Wedel DJ, Benzon HT, et al: Regional anesthesia in the anticoagulated patient: Defining the risks (The second ASRA consensus conference on neuraxial anesthesia and anticoagulation). Reg Anesth Pain Med 2003;28:171–197.

13. Horlocker TT, Wedel DJ, Rowlingson JC, et al: Regional anesthesia in the patient receiving antithrombotic therapy or thrombolytic therapy: American Society of Regional Anesthesia and Pain Medicine evidence-based guidelines (third edition). Reg Anesth Pain Med 2010;35:64–101.

14. Gogarten W, Vandermeulen E, Van Aken H, Kozek S, Llau JV, Samama CM: European Society of Anaesthesiology. Regional anaesthesia and antithrombotic agents: recommendations of the European Society of Anaesthesiology. Eur J Anaesthesiol 2010;27:999–1015.

15. Breivik H, Bang U, Jalonen J, Vigfusson G, Alahuhta S, Lagerkranser M: Nordic guidelines for neuraxial blocks in disturbed haemostasis from the Scandinavian Society of Anaesthesiology and Intensive Care Medicine. Acta Anaesthesiol Scand 2010;54:16–41.

16. Cronberg S, Wallmark E, Söderberg I: Effect on platelet aggregation of oral administration of 10 non-steroidal analgesics to humans. Scand J Haematol 1984;33:155–159.

17. Locke GE, Giorgio AJ, Biggers SL Jr, et al: Acute spinal epidural hematoma secondary to aspirin-induced prolonged bleeding. Surg Neurol 1976;5:293–296.

18. Vandermeulen EP, Van Aken H, Vermylen J: Anticoagulants and spinal–epidural anesthesia. Anesth Analg 1994;79:1165–1177.

19. CLASP (Collaborative Low-Dose Aspirin Study in Pregnancy) Collaborative Group. CLASP: a randomized trial of low-dose aspirin for the prevention and treatment of pre-eclampsia among 9364 pregnant women. Lancet 1994;343:619–629.

20. Horlocker TT, Wedel DJ, Offord KP: Does preoperative antiplatelet therapy increase the risk of hemorrhagic complications associated with regional anesthesia? Anesth Analg 1990;70:631–634.

21. Horlocker TT, Wedel DJ, Schroeder DR, et al: Preoperative antiplatelet therapy does not increase the risk of spinal hematoma associated with regional anesthesia. Anesth Analg 1995;80:303–309.

22. Benzon HT, Brunner EA, Vaisrub N: Bleeding time and nerve blocks after aspirin. Reg Anesth 1984;9:86–90.

23. Horlocker TT, Bajwa ZH, Ashraft Z, et al: Risk assessment of hemorrhagic complications associated with nonsteroidal antiinflammatory medications in ambulatory pain clinic patients undergoing epidural steroid injection. Anesth Analg 2002;95:1691–1697.

24. Benzon HT, Wong HY, Siddiqui T, et al: Caution in performing epidural injections in patients on several antiplatelet drugs. Anesthesiology 1999;91:1558–1559.

25. Benzon HT, Huntoon M: Do we need new guidelines for interventional pain procedures in patients on anticoagulants? Reg Anesth Pain Med 2014;39:1–3.

26. Giberson CE, Barbosa J, Brooks ES, et al: Epidural hematomas following removal of percutaneous spinal cord stimulator trial leads: two case reports. Reg Anesth Pain Med 2014;39:73–77.

27. Williams KN, Jackowski A, Evans PJD: Epidural haematoma requiring surgical decompression following repeated cervical epidural steroid injections for chronic pain. Pain 1990;42:197–199.

28. Ain RJ, Vance MB: Epidural hematoma after epidural steroid injection in a patient withholding enoxaparin per guidelines. Anesthesiology 2005;102:701–703.

29. Buvanendran A, Young A: Spinal epidural hematoma after spinal cord stimulator trial lead placement in a patient taking aspirin. Reg Anesth Pain Med 2014;39:70–72.

30. Desai MJ, Dua S: Perineural hematoma following lumbar transforaminal steroid injection causing acute-on-chronic lumbar radiculopathy: a case report. Pain Pract 2014;14:271–277.

31. Mahmoud J, Mathews M, Verna S, Basil B: Oxcarbazepine-induced thrombocytopenia. Psychosomatics 2006;47:73–74.

32. Meijer WEE, Heerdink ER, Nolen WA, Herings RMC, Leufkens HGM, Egberts ACG. Association of risk of abnormal bleeding with degree of serotonin reuptake inhibition by antidepressants. Arch Intern Med 2004;164:2367–2370.

33. Narouze S, Benzon HT, Provenzano DA, et al: Interventional spine and pain procedures in patients on antiplatelet and anticoagulant medications: guidelines from the American Society of Regional Anesthesia and Pain Medicine, the European Society of Regional Anaesthesia and Pain Therapy, the American Academy of Pain Medicine, the International Neuromodulation Society, the North American Neuromodulation Society, and the World Institute of Pain. Reg Anesth Pain Med 2015;40:182–212.

34. Gajraj NM: Cyclooxygenase-2 inhibitors. Anesth Analg 2003;96:1720–1738.

35. Buvanendran A, Kroin JS, Tuman KJ, et al: Effects of perioperative administration of a selective cyclooxygenase 2 inhibitor on pain management and recovery of function after knee replacement: a randomized controlled trial. JAMA 2003;290:2411–2418.

36. Gajraj NM, Joshi GP: Role of cyclooxygenase-2 inhibitors in postoperative pain management. Anesthesiol Clin North America 2005;23:49–72.

37. Desjardins PJ, Shu VS, Recker DP, et al: A single preoperative dose of valdecoxib, a new cyclooxygenase-2 specific inhibitor, relieves post-oral surgery or bunionectomy pain. Anesthesiology 2002;97:565–573.

38. Sinatra RS, Shen QJ, Halaszynski T, et al: Preoperative rofecoxib oral suspension as an analgesic adjunct after lower abdominal surgery: the effects of an effect-dependent pain and pulmonary function. Anesth Analg 2003;98:135–140.

39. Lessee PT, Hubbard RC, Karim A, et al: Effects of celecoxib, a novel, cyclooxygenase-2-inhibitor, on platelet function in healthy adults: a randomized, clinical trial. J Clin Pharmacol 2000;40:124–132.

40. van Heeken H, Schwartz JI, Depre M, et al: Comparative inhibitory activity of rofecoxib, meloxicam, diclofenac, ibuprofen and naproxen on COX-2 versus COX-1 in healthy volunteers. J Clin Pharmacol 2000;40:1109–1120.

41. Greenberg H, Gottesdiener K, Huntington M, et al: A new cyclooxygenase-2-inhibitor, rofecoxib (VIOXX) did not alter the antiplatelet effects of low-dose aspirin in healthy volunteers. J Clin Pharmacol 2000;40:1509–1515.

42. Psaty BM, Furberg CD: Cox-2 inhibitors—Lessons in drug safety. N Engl J Med 2005;352:1133–1135.

43. Schror K: Antiplatelet drugs: a comparative review. Drugs 1995;50:7–28.

44. Yang LH, Fareed J: Vasomodulatory action of clopidogrel and ticlopidine. Thromb Res 1997;86:479–491.

45. CAPRIE Steering Committee: A randomized blind trial of clopidogrel versus aspirin in patients at risk of ischaemic stroke (CAPRIE). Lancet 1996;348:1329–1339.

46. Helft G, Osende JI, Worthley SG, et al: Acute antithrombotic effect of a front-loaded regimen of clopidogrel in patients with atherosclerosis on aspirin. Arterioscler Thromb Vasc Biol 2000;29:2316–2321.

47. Mayumi T, Dohi S: Spinal subarachnoid hematoma after lumbar puncture in a patient receiving antiplatelet therapy. Anesth Analg 1983;62:777–779.

48. Benzon HT, McCarthy R, Benzon HA, et al: Determination of the residual antiplatelet activity of clopidogrel. Br J Anaesth 2011;107:966–971.

49. Hall R, Mazer CD: Antiplatelet drugs: a review of their pharmacology and management in the perioperative period. Anesth Analg 2011;112:292–318.

CHAPTER 52

50. Wallentin L: P2Y(12) inhibitors: differences in properties and mechanisms of action and potential consequences for clinical use. Eur Heart J 2009;30:1964–1977.

51. Capodanno D, Ferreiro JL, Angiolillo DJ: Antiplatelet therapy: new pharmacological agents and changing paradigms. J Thromb Haemost 2013;11(Suppl 1):316–329.

52. Brandt JT, Payne CD, Wiviott SD, et al: A comparison of prasugrel and clopidogrel loading doses on platelet function: magnitude of platelet inhibition is related to active metabolite formation. Am Heart J 2007;153:66.e9–16.

53. Dobesh PP: Pharmacokinetics and pharmacodynamics of prasugrel, a thienopyridine P2Y12 inhibitor. Pharmacotherapy 2009;29:1089–1102.

54. Asai F, Jacubowski JA, Nagamura H, et al: Platelet inhibitory activity and pharmacokinetics of prasugrel (CS-747) a novel thienopyridine P2Y12 inhibitor: a single ascending dose study in healthy humans. Platelets 2006;17:209–217.

55. Wiviott SD, Trenk D, Frelinger AL, et al: Prasugrel compared with high loading- and maintenance-dose clopidogrel in patients with planned percutaneous coronary intervention: the Prasugrel in Comparison to Clopidogrel for Inhibition of Platelet Activation and Aggregation-Thrombolysis in Myocardial Infarction 44 trial. Circulation 2007;116: 2923–2932.

56. Wiviott SD, Antman EM, Winters KJ, et al: Randomized comparison of prasugrel (CS-747, LY640315), a novel thienopyridine P2Y12 antagonist, with clopidogrel in percutaneous coronary intervention: results of the Joint Utilization of Medications to Block Platelets Optimally (JUMBO)-TIMI 26 trial. Circulation 2005;111:3366–3373.

57. Brandt JT, Close SL, Iturria SJ, et al: Common polymorphisms of CYP2C19 and CYP2C9 affect the pharmacokinetic and pharmacodynamic response to clopidogrel but not prasugrel. J Thromb Haemost 2007;5:2429–2436.

58. Mega JL, Close SL, Wiviott SD, et al: Cytochrome P450 genetic polymorphisms and the response to prasugrel: relationship to pharmacokinetic, pharmacodynamic, and clinical outcomes. Circulation 2009;119:2553–2560.

59. Teng R, Butler K: Pharmacokinetics, pharmacodynamics, tolerability and safety of single ascending doses of ticagrelor, a reversibly binding oral P2Y(12) receptor antagonist, in healthy subjects. Eur J Clin Pharmacol 2010;66:487–496.

60. Teng R, Oliver S, Hayes MA, Butler K: Absorption, distribution, metabolism, and excretion of ticagrelor in healthy subjects. Drug Metab Dispos 2010;38:1514–1521.

61. Husted S, Emanuelsson H, Heptinstall S, Sandset PM, Wickens M, Peters G: Pharmacodynamics, pharmacokinetics, and safety of the oral reversible P2Y12 antagonist AZD6140 with aspirin in patients with atherosclerosis: a double-blind comparison to clopidogrel with aspirin. Eur Heart J 2006;27:1038–1047.

62. Gurbel PA, Bliden KP, Butler K, et al: Randomized double-blind assessment of the ONSET and OFFSET of the antiplatelet effects of ticagrelor versus clopidogrel in patients with stable coronary artery disease: the ONSET/OFFSET study. Circulation 2009;120:2577–2585.

63. George JN: Platelets. Lancet 2000;355:1531–1539.

64. van Giezen J, Nilsson L, Berntsson P, et al: Ticagrelor binds to human P2Y(12) independently from ADP but antagonizes ADP-induced receptor signaling and platelet aggregation. J Thromb Haemost 2009;7:1556–1565.

65. Baron TH, Kamath PS, McBane RD: Management of antithrombotic therapy in patients undergoing invasive procedures. N Engl J Med 2013;368:2113–2124.

66. Rodgers RPC, Levin J: A critical reappraisal of the bleeding time. Semin Thromb Hemost 1990;16:1–20.

67. Ferraris VA, Swanson E: Aspirin usage and perioperative blood loss in patients undergoing unexpected operations. Surg Gynecol Obstet 1983;156:439–442.

68. Mammen EF, Comp PC, Gosselin R, et al: PFA-100 system. A new method for assessment of platelet dysfunction. Semin Thromb Hemost 1998;24:195–202.

69. Edwards A, Jakubowski JA, Rechner AR, Sugidachi A, Harrison P: Evaluation of the INNOVANCE PFA P2Y test cartridge: sensitivity to P2Y(12) blockade and influence of anticoagulant. Platelets 2012;23: 106–115.

70. Gorog DA, Fuster V: Platelet function tests in clinical cardiology. J Am Coll Cardiol 2013;61:2115–2129.

71. Bouman HJ, Parlak E, van Werkum JW, et al: Which platelet function test is suitable to monitor clopidogrel responsiveness? A pharmacokinetic analysis on the active metabolite of clopidogrel. J Thromb Haemost 2010;8:482–488.

72. van Werkum JW, Harmsze AM, Elsenberg EH, Bouman HJ, ten Berg JM, Hackeng CM: The use of the VerifyNow system to monitor antiplatelet therapy: a review of the current evidence. Platelets 2008;19:479–488.

73. Mueller T, Dieplinger B, Poelz W, Haltmayer M: Utility of the PFA-100 insturment and the novel multiplate analyzer for the assessment of aspirin and clopidogrel effects on platelet functionin patients with cardiovascular disease. Clin Appl Thromb Hemost 2009;15:652–659.

74. Scharbert G, Auer A, Kozek-Langenecker S: Evaluation of the Platelet Mapping Assay on rotational thromboelastometry ROTEM. Platelets 2009;20:125–130.

75. Malinin A, Pokov A, Swaim L, Kotob M, Serebruany V: Validation of a VerifyNow-P2Y12 cartridge for monitoring platelet inhibition with clopidogrel. Methods Find Exp Clin Pharmacol 2006;28:315.

76. Benzon HT, Avram J, Green D, Bonow RO: New oral anticoagulants and regional anaesthesia. Br J Anaesth 2013;111(Suppl 1):i96–i113.

77. Kearon C, Hirsh J: Management of anticoagulation before and after elective surgery. N Engl J Med 1997;336:1506–1511.

78. Harrison L, Johnston M, Massicote MP, et al: Comparison of 5-mg and 10-mg doses in initiation of warfarin therapy. Ann Intern Med 1997;126:133–136.

79. Benzon HT, Benzon HA, Kirby-Nolan M, Avram MJ, Nader A: Factor VII levels and risk factors for increased international normalized ratio in the early phase of warfarin therapy. Anesthesiology 2010;112:298–304.

80. Schulman S, Lockner D, Bergstrom K, Blomback M: Intensive initial oral anticoagulation and shorter heparin treatment in deep vein thrombosis. Thromb Haemost 10984;52:276–280.

81. Enneking FK, Benzon HT: Oral anticoagulants and regional anesthesia: a perspective. Reg Anesth Pain Med 1998;23:140–145.

82. Odoom JA, Sih IL: Epidural analgesia and anticoagulant therapy. Anesthesia 1983;38:254–259.

83. Horlocker TT: When to remove a spinal or epidural catheter in an anticoagulated patient. Reg Anesth 1993;18:264–265.

84. Horlocker TT, Wedel DJ, Schlichting JL: Postoperative epidural analgesia and oral anticoagulant therapy. Anesth Analg 1994;79:89–93.

85. Wu CL, Perkins FM: Oral anticoagulant prophylaxis and epidural catheter removal. Reg Anesth 1996;21:517–524.

86. Liu SS, Buvanendran A, Viscusi ER, et al: Uncomplicated removal of epidural catheters in 4365 patients with international normalized ratio greater than 1.4 during initiation of warfarin therapy. Reg Anesth Pain Med 2011;36:231–235.

87. Weinstock DM, Chang P, Aronson DL, et al: Comparison of plasma prothrombin and factor VII and urine prothrombin F1 concentrations in patients on long-term warfarin therapy and those in initial phase. Am J Hematol 1998;57:193–199.

88. Jerkeman A, Astermark J, Hedner U, et al: Correlation between different intensities of anti-vitamin K treatment and coagulation parameters. Thromb Res 2000;98:467–471.

89. Abildgaard U, Lindahl AK, Sandset PM: Heparin requires both antithrombin and extrinsic pathway inhibitor for its anticoagulant effect in human blood. Haemostasis 1991;21:254–257.

90. Murray DJ, Brodsnahan WJ, Pennell B, et al: Heparin detection by the activated coagulation time: A comparison of the sensitivity of coagulation tests and heparin assays. J Cardiothorac Vasc Anesth 1997; 11:24–28.

91. Shapiro SS: Treating thrombosis in the 21st century. N Engl J Med 2003;349:1762–1764.

92. Rao TL, El-Etr AA: Anticoagulation following placement of epidural and subarachnoid catheters: an evaluation of neurologic sequelae. Anesthesisology 1981;55:618–620.

93. Ruff DL, Dougherty JH: Complications of anticoagulation followed by anticoagulation. Stroke 1981;12:879–881.

94. Liu SS, Mulroy MF: Neuraxial anesthesia and analgesia in the presence of standard heparin. Reg Anesth Pain Med 1998;23:157–163.

95. Chaney MA: Intrathecal and epidural anesthesia and analgesia for cardiac surgery. Anesth Analg 1997;84:1211–1221.

96. Geerts WH, Bergqvist D, Pineo GF, et al: Prevention of venous thromboembolism. American College of Chest Physicians Evidence-Based Clinical Practice Guidelines (8th edition). Chest 2008;133: 381S–453S.

97. King CS, Holley AB, Jackson JL, et al: Twice versus three times daily heparin dosing for thromboembolism prophylaxis in the general population: a metaanalysis. Chest 2007;131:507–516.

98. Weitz JI. Drug therapy: low-molecular-weight heparins. N Engl J Med 1997;337:688–698.

99. Horlocker TT, Heit JA: Low molecular weight heparin: biochemistry, pharmacology, perioperative prophylaxis regimens, and guidelines for regional anesthetic management. Anesth Analg 1997;85:874–885.

100. Bara L, Billaud E, Gramond G, et al: Comparative pharmacokinetics of a low molecular weight heparin (PK 10 169) and unfractionated heparin after intravenous and subcutaneous administration. Thromb Res 1985;39:631–636.

101. Klein S, Slaughter T, Vail PT, et al: Thrombelastography as a perioperative measure of anticoagulation resulting from low molecular weight heparin: a comparison with anti-Xa concentrations. Anesth Analg 2000;91:1091–1095.

102. White RH: Low-molecular-weight heparins: are they all the same? Br J Haematol 2003;121:12–20.

103. Horlocker TT, Wedel DJ: Neuraxial block and low molecular weight heparin: balancing perioperative analgesia and thromboprophylaxis. Reg Anesth Pain Med 1998;23:164–177.

104. U.S. Food and Drug Administration. FDA Drug Safety Communication: updated recommendations to decrease risk of spinal column bleeding and paralysis in patients on low molecular weight heparins. http://www.fda.gov/drugs/drugsafety/ucm373595.htm. Updated January 19, 2016. Accessed September 9, 2015.

105. Rosenquist RW, Brown DL: Neuraxial bleeding: Fibrinolytics/thrombolytics. Reg Anesth Pain Med 1998;23S:152–156.

106. Bauer KA: Fondaparinux: basic properties and efficacy and safety in venous thromboembolism prophylaxis. Am J Orthop 2002;31:4–10.

107. Turpie AG, Bauer KA, Eriksson BL, et al: Fondaparinux vs enoxaparin for the prevention of venous thromboembolism in major orthopedic surgery: a meta-analysis of 4 randomized double-blind studies. Arch Intern Med 2002;162:1833–1840.

108. The Matisse Investigators: Subcutaneous fondaparinux versus intravenous unfractionated heparin in the initial treatment of pulmonary embolism. N Engl J Med 2003;349:1695–1702.

109. Singelyn FJ, Verheyen CC, Piovella F, Van Aken HK, Rosenceher N, EXPERT Study Investigators: The safety and efficacy of extended thromboprophylaxis with fondaparinux after major orthopedic surgery of the lower limb with or without a neuraxial or deep peripheral nerve catheter: the EXPERT Study. Anesth Analg 2007;105:1540–1547.

110. Rosencher N, Bonnet MP, Sessler DI: Selected new antithrombotic agents and neuraxial anaesthesia for major orthopedic surgery: management strategies. Anaesthesia 2007;62:1154–1160.

111. Greenblatt DJ: Elimination half-life of drugs: value and limitations. Ann Rev Med 985;36:421–427.

112. Olesen JB, Lip GY, Hansen ML, et al: Validation of risk stratification schemes for predicting stroke and thromboembolism in patients with atrial fibrillation: nationwide cohort study. BMJ 2011;342:d124.

113. Connolly G, Spyropoulos AC: Practical issues, limitations, and periprocedural management of the NOACs. J Thromb Thrombolysis 2013;36:212–222.

114. Garcia D, Barrett YC, Ramaciotti E, Weitz JI: Laboratory assessment of the anticoagulant effects of the next generation of oral anticoagulants. J Thromb Haemost 2013;11:245–252.

115. IST-3 Collaborative Group: The benefits and harms of intravenous thrombolysis with recombinant tissue plasminogen activator within 6 h of acute ischaemic stroke (the third international stroke trial [IST-3]): a randomized trial. Lancet 2012;379:2352–2363.

116. Tertri S, Hakal J, Juvela S, et al: Safety of low-dose subcutaneous enoxaparin for the prevention of venous thromboembolism after primary intracerebral haemorrhage. Thromb Res 2008;123:206–212.

117. Liew A, Douketis J: Perioperative management of patients who are receiving a novel oral anticoagulant. Intern Emerg Med 2013;8:477–484.

118. Blech S, Ebner T, Ludwig-Schwellinger E, Stangier J, Roth W: The metabolism and disposition of the oral direct thrombin inhibitor, dabigatran, in humans. Drug Metab Disposition 2008;36:386–399.

119. Di Nisio M, Middeldorp S, Buller HR. Direct thrombin inhibitors. N Engl J Med 2005;353:1028–1040.

120. Levy JH, Faraoni D, Spring JL, Douketis JD, Samana CM: Managing new oral anticoagulants in the perioperative and intensive care unit setting. Anesthesiology 2013;118:1466–1474.

121. Stangier J, Clemens A: Pharmacology, pharmacokinetics, and pharmacodynamics of dabigatran etexilate, an oral direct thrombin inhibitor. Clin Appl Thromb Hemost 2009;15(S1):9S–16S.

122. Stangier J, Stahle H, Rathgen K, Fuhr R: Pharmacokinetics and pharmacodynamics of the direct oral thrombin inhibitor dabigatran in healthy elderly subjects. Clin Pharmacokinet 2008;47:47–59.

123. Eisert WG, Hauel N, Stangier J, Wienen W, Clemens A, Van Ryn J: Dabigatran: an oral novel potent reversible nonpeptide inhibitor of thrombin. Arterioscler Thromb Vasc Biol 2010;30:1885–1889.

124. Stangier J, Rathgen K, Stahle H, Mazur D: Influence of renal impairment on the pharmacokinetics and pharmacodynamics of oral dabigatran etexilate. An open label, parallel-group, single-centre study. Clin Pharmacokinet 2010;49:259–268.

125. Ezekowitz MD, Reilly PA, Nehmiz G, et al. Dabigatran with or without concomitant aspirin comparedwithwarfarin alone in patients with nonvalvular atrial fibrillation (PETRO Study). Am J Cardiol 2007;100:1419–1426.

126. Eriksson BI, Dahl OE, Buller HR, et al; BISTRO II Study Group: A new oral direct thrombin inhibitor, dabigatran etexilate, compared with enoxaparin for prevention of thromboembolic events following total hip or knee replacement: the BISTRO II randomized trial. J Thromb Haemost 2005;3:103–111.

127. Eriksson BI, Dahl OE, Rosencher N, et al; RE-MODEL Study group: Oral dabigatran etexilate vs. subcutaneous enoxaparin for the prevention of venous thromboembolism after total knee replacement: the RE-MODEL randomized trial. J Thromb Haemost 2007;5:2178–2185.

128. Eriksson BI, Dahl OE, Rosencher N, et al; RE-NOVATE Study Group. Dabigatran etexilate versus enoxaparin for prevention of venous thromboembolism after total hip replacement: a randomized, double-blind, non-inferiority trial. Lancet 2007;370:949–956.

129. RE-MOBILIZE Writing Committee, Ginsberg JS, Davidson BL, Comp PC, et al: Oral thrombin inhibitor dabigatran etexilate vs North American enoxaparin regimen for prevention of venous thromboembolism after knee arthroplasty surgery. J Arthroplasty 2009;24:1–9.

130. Wolowacz SE, Roskell NS, Plumb JM, Caprini JA, Eriksson BI: Efficacy and safety of dabigatran etaxilate for the prevention of venous thromboembolism following hip or knee arthroplasty. A meta-analysis. Thromb Haemost 2009;101:77–85.

131. Harper P, Young L, Merriman E: Bleeding risk with dabigatran in the frail elderly. N Engl J Med 2012;366:864–866.

132. Tripodi A: The laboratory and the direct oral anticoagulants. Blood 2013;121:4032–4035.

133. Siegal DM, Cuker A: Reversal of novel oral anticoagulants in patients with major bleeding. J Thromb Thrombolysis 2013;35:391–398.

134. Miyares MA, Davis K: Newer oral anticoagulants: a review of laboratory monitoring options and reversal agents in the hemorrhagic patient. Am J Health Syst Pharm 2012;69:1473–1484.

135. Baron TH, Kamath PS, McBane RD: Management of antithrombotic therapy in patients undergoing invasive procedures. N Engl J Med 2013;368:2113–2124.

136. Breuer G, Weiss DR, Ringwald J: 'New' direct oral anticoagulants in the perioperative setting. Curr Opin Anaesthesiol 2014;27:409–419.

137. Lévy S: Newer clinically available antithrombotics and their antidotes. J Interv Card Electrophysiol 2014;40:269–275.

138. Laux V, Perzborn E, Kubitza D, Misselwitz F: Preclinical and clinical characteristics of rivaroxaban: a novel, oral, direct factor Xa inhibitor. Sem Thromb Hemost 2007;33:515–523.

139. Kubitza D, Becka M, Wensing G, Voith B, Zuehlsdorf M: Safety, pharmacodynamics, and pharmacokinetics of BAY 59-7939-an oral, direct factor Xa inhibitor-after multiple dosing in healthy male subjects. Eur J Clin Pharmacol 2005;61:873–880.

140. Jiang J, Hu Y, Zhang J, et al: Safety, pharmacokinetics and pharmacodynamics of single doses of rivaroxaban—an oral, direct factor Xa inhibitor—in elderly Chinese subjects. Thromb Haemost 2010;103:234–241.

141. Kubitza D, Becka M, Roth A, Mueck W: Dose-escalation study of the pharmacokinetics and pharmacodynamics of rivaroxaban in healthy elderly subjects. Curr Med Res Opin 2008;24:2757–2765.

142. Eriksson BI, Quinlan DJ, Weitz JI: Comparative pharmacodynamics and pharmacokinetics of oral direct thrombin and factor Xa inhibitors in development. Clin Pharmacokinet 2009;48:1–22.

143. Weitz JI, Eikelboom JW, Samama MM: New antithrombotic drugs. Chest 2012;141S:e120S–e151S.

144. Kubitza D, Becka M, Mueck W, et al: Effects of renal impairment on the pharmacokinetics, pharmacodynamics and safety of rivaroxaban, an oral, direct factor Xa inhibitor. Br J Clin Pharmacol 2010;70:703–712.

145. Patel MR, Mahaffey KW, Garg J, et al; ROCKET AF Investigators: Rivaroxaban versus warfarin in nonvalvular atrial fibrillation. N Engl J Med 2011;365:883–891.

146. Eriksson BI, Borris LC, Friedman RJ, et al; RECORD1 Study Group: Rivaroxaban versus enoxaparin for thromboprophylaxis after hip arthroplasty. N Engl J Med 2008;358:2765–2775.

147. Kakkar AK, Brenner B, Dahl O, et al; RECORD2 Investigators: Extended duration rivaroxaban versus short-term enoxaparin for the prevention of venous thromboembolism after total hip arthroplasty: a double-blind, randomized controlled trial. Lancet 2008;372:31–39.

148. Lassen MR, Ageno W, Borris LC, et al; RECORD3 Investigators: Rivaroxaban versus enoxaparin for thromboprophylaxis after total knee arthroplasty. N Eng J Med 2008;358:2776–2786.

149. Turpie AG, Lassen MR, Davidson BL, et al; RECORD4 Investigators: Rivaroxaban versus enoxaparin for thromboprophylaxis after total knee arthroplasty (RECORD4): a randomized trial. Lancet 2009;373:1673–1680.

150. Ericksson BI, Kakkar AK, Turpie AG, et al: Oral rivaroxaban for the prevention of symptomatic venous thromboembolism after elective hip and knee replacement. J Bone Joint Surg Br 2009;91:636–644.

151. Rosencher N, Liau JV, Mueck W, Loewe A, Berkowitz SD, Homering M: Incidence of neuraxial haematoma after total hip or knee surgery: RECORD programme (rivaroxaban vs, enoxaparin). Acta Anaesthesiol Scand 2013;57:565–572.

152. Samama MM: Which test to use to measure the anticoagulant effect of rivaroxaban: the anti-factor Xa assay. J Thromb Haemost 2013;11:579–580.

153. Raghavan N, Frost CE, Yu Z, et al: Apixaban metabolism and pharmacokinetics after oral administration to humans. Drug Metab Dispos 2009;37:74–81.

154. Frost C, Wang J, Nepal S, et al: Apixaban, an oral, direct factor Xa inhibitor: single dose safety, pharmacokinetics, pharmacodynamics and food effect in healthy subjects. Br J Pharmacol 2013;75:476–487.

155. Frost C, Nepal S, Wang J, et al: Safety, pharmacokinetics and pharmacodynamics of multiple oral doses of apixaban, a factor Xa inhibitor, in healthy subjects. Br J Clin Pharmacol 2013;76:776–786.

156. Zhang D, He K, Raghavan N, et al: Comparative metabolism of 14C-labeled apixaban in mice, rats, rabbits, dogs, and humans. Drug Metab Dispos 2009;37:1738–1748.

157. Lassen MR, Davidson BL, Gallus A, Pineo G, Ansell J, Deitchman D: The efficacy and safety of apixaban, an oral, direct factor Xa inhibitor, as thromboprophylaxis in patients following total knee replacement. J Thromb Haemost 2007;5:2368–2375.

158. Lassen MR, Rasskob GE, Gallus A, Pineo G, Chen D, Portman RJ: Apixaban or enoxaparin for thromboprophylaxis after knee replacement. N Engl J Med 2009;361:594–604.

159. Lassen MR, Raskob GE, Gallus A, Pineo G, Chen D, Hornick P; ADVANCE-2 Investigators: Apixaban versus enoxaparin for thromboprophylaxis after knee replacement (ADVANCE-2): a randomized double-blind trial. Lancet 2010;375:807–815.

160. Lassen MR, Gallus A, Raskob GE, Pineo G, Chen D, Ramirez LM; ADVANCE-3 Investigators: Apixaban versus enoxaparin for thromboprophylaxis after hip replacement. N Engl J Med 2010;363:2487–2498.

160. Barrett YC, Wang Z, Frost C, Shenker A: Clinical laboratory measurement of direct factor Xa inhibitors: anti Xa assay is preferable to prothrombin time assay. Thromb Haemost 2010;104:1263–1271.

161. Kozek-Langenecker SA, Fries D, Gutl M, et al: Locoregional anesthesia and coagulation inhibitors. Recommendations of the Task Force on Perioperative Coagulation of the Austrian Society for Anesthesiology and Intensive Care Medicine. Anaesthesist 2005;54:476–484.

162. Siegal DM, Curnutte JT, Connolly SJ, et al. Andexanet alfa for the reversal of factor Xa inhibitor activity. N Engl J Med 2015;373:2413–2424.

Regional Analgesia in the Critically Ill

Sebastian Schulz-Stübner

INTRODUCTION

Intensive care specialists play increasingly greater role in the prevention and treatment of physiologic and psychological stress in critically ill patients[1-3] in order to prevent detrimental consequences ranging from systemic inflammatory response syndrome,[4] to cardiac complications,[5,6] to posttraumatic stress disorder.[7-9] Studies have addressed the questions of an optimal sedation regimen, and several evidence-based guidelines and strategies have been published but are frequently not followed.[10-14] The analgesic component for sufficient stress relief, however, has not been addressed extensively, and few recommendations, primarily based on individual clinical practices, are currently available.[15-17]

In view of the side effects of opioids, especially respiratory depression, altered mental status, and reduced bowel function, regional analgesia utilizing neuraxial and peripheral nerve blocks offer significant advantages. The lack of a universally reliable pain assessment tool ("analgesiometer") in the critically ill contributes to the dilemma of adequate analgesia. Many patients in the critical care unit are not able to communicate or use a conventional visual or numeric analog scale to quantify pain. Alternative assessment tools derived from pediatric[18-20] or geriatric[21] practice that rely on grimacing and other physiologic responses to painful stimuli might be useful but have been inadequately studied in the intensive care unit (ICU). Changes in heart rate and blood pressure in response to nursing activities, dressing changes, or wound care can also serve as indirect measurements of pain,[22] and sedation measures like the Ramsay Sedation Scale or the Riker Sedation-Agitation Scale[23,24] scale might be helpful although not specifically designed for pain assessment.

The objective of this chapter is to describe the indications, limitations, and practical aspects of continuous regional analgesic techniques in the critically ill based on the available evidence, which at the moment is limited to case reports, cohort studies, expert opinion, and extrapolation from studies looking primarily at the intraoperative use of regional anesthesia extending into the postoperative ICU stay as summarized in a 2012 systematic review in *Regional Anesthesia Pain Medicine* by Stundner and Memtsoudis who conclude, "Regional anesthesia can be useful in the management of a large variety of conditions and procedures in critically ill patients. Although the attributes of regional anesthetic techniques could feasibly affect outcomes, no conclusive evidence supporting this assumption exists to date, and further research is needed to elucidate this entity."[25]

EPIDURAL ANALGESIA

Epidural analgesia is probably the most commonly used regional analgesic technique in the ICU setting.[26] Some indications in which epidural analgesia may not improve mortality rates but may facilitate management and improve patient comfort in the ICU include chest trauma,[27-30] thoracic[31,32] and abdominal surgery,[5,33,34] major vascular surgery,[35,36] major orthopedic surgery,[37] acute pancreatits,[38] paralytic ileus,[39-42] cardiac surgery,[43,44] and intractable angina pain.[45,46] Although high-risk patients seem to profit most from epidural analgesia,[47,48] the current literature does not address the specific circumstances of the critically ill patient with multiple comorbidities and organ failure. For that reason, an individual approach is necessary when considering the application of epidural analgesia in this population.[49]

In a survey of 216 general ICUs in England, Low[50] found that 89% of the responding units used epidural analgesia, but only 32% had a written policy governing its use. Although 68% of the responding units would not place an epidural catheter in a patient with positive blood cultures, only 52% considered culture-negative sepsis or systemic inflammatory response syndrome (SIRS) to be a contraindication. The majority of respondents did not list lack of consent or the need for anticoagulation after catheter placement as contraindications to the insertion an epidural catheter. Although the issues of consent, possible coagulopathy, and infection can be addressed rather easily in elective procedures, they become major problems in newly admitted patients; for example, those with multiple trauma or painful intraabdominal processes, especially acute pancreatitis. There is also controversy regarding the safety of placing epidural catheters in sedated patients,[51,52] and confirmation of a good catheter position can be difficult in the critically ill patient if sensory level testing is not reliable.

Positioning the patient for the procedure may be difficult depending on the underlying injury, the number and position of drains and catheters, and the presence of external fixation devices. Table 53–1 summarizes the indications, contraindications, and practical problems involved with the placement of epidural catheters.

The help of trained nursing staff is essential for good positioning and safe handling of tubes and catheters during the procedure. Maximum barrier precautions, similar to those used in the placement of central lines, should also be considered when placing epidural catheters in the critically ill. Tunneling the catheter should be considered to prevent dislocation and reduce the risk of catheter site infection.[53] To confirm the correct position of the epidural catheter, electrical stimulation during placement or a postplacement radiograph with a small amount of nonneurotoxic contrast medium may be beneficial.[54,55]

Bolus injections of long-acting local anesthetics, such as bupivacaine, ropivacaine, or levobupivacaine, or the discontinuation of continuous infusion as needed will allow neurologic assessment when necessary. Monitoring of motor-evoked potentials (MEPs) to the lower extremities and somatosensory-evoked potentials (SSEPs) of the tibial nerve may serve as indicators when the neurologic examination is doubtful due to the patient's altered mental status. Although routinely used in the operating room for monitoring spinal cord integrity and for the diagnosis and prognosis of spinal cord injury, the use of this technology in the ICU in the context of epidural analgesia has not been adequately assessed.

The most common side effects of epidural blocks are bradycardia and hypotension related to sympathetic block. Hemodynamic changes can be more pronounced with intermittent

TABLE 53–1. Epidural analgesia in the critically Ill.

Indications	Contraindications	Practical Problems	Dose Suggestions
Thoracic epidurals:			
Chest trauma	Coagulopathy or current use of anticoagulants during catheter placement and removal[61,62]	Positioning of patient	*Bolus regimen:*
Thoracic surgery		Monitoring of neurologic function (consider MEP/SSEP)	5–10 mL 0.125–0.25% bupivacaine or 0.1–0.2% ropivacaine q 8–12 h
Abdominal surgery			
Paralytic ileus			Consider addition of 1–2 meg clonidine in hemodynamically stable patients
Pancreatitis	Sepsis/bacteremia		
Intractable angina	Local infection at puncture site		
Lumbar epidurals:			
Orthopedic surgery or trauma of lower extremities	Severe hypovolemia		*Continuous infusion:*
	Acute hemodynamic instability		0.0625% bupivacaine or 0.1% ropivacaine at 5 mL/h
Peripheral vascular disease of lower extremities	Obstructive ileus		Consider addition of opioids (eg, hydromorphone, sufentanil) or clonidine if high systemic opioid demands persist

MEP, motor-evoked potentials; SSEP, somatosensory-evoked potentials.

Source: Reproduced with permission from Schulz-Stübner S1, Boezaart A, Hata JS: Regional analgesia in the critically ill. *Crit Care Med.* 2005 Jun;33(6):1400–1407.

bolus dosing, in patients with hypovolemia, and in those with reduced venous return secondary to high positive end-expiratory pressure (PEEP) ventilation. Based on data from lumbar punctures and meningitis from the beginning of the twentieth century,[56] current sepsis and bacteremia are considered contraindications for intrathecal opioid applications and, by analogy, for the placement of an epidural catheter. However, many ICU patients, especially after trauma or major surgery, present with a clinical picture of SIRS. Fever and increased white blood cell counts alone, that is, in the absence of positive blood cultures, do not provide a reliable diagnosis of bacteremia. The combination of the serum markers C-reactive protein (CRP), procalcitonin, and interleukin-6, on the other hand, have been shown to indicate bacterial sepsis with a high degree of sensitivity and specificity[57-60] and can guide the decision to place an epidural catheter. Regarding the patient's coagulation status, the current recommendations of the American Society of Regional Anesthesia and Pain Medicine (ASRA)[61] should be followed. Adequate safety intervals during the administration of anticoagulant drugs are equally important for the placement and removal of epidural catheters.[62,63] Although there is no compelling evidence of an increased risk of epidural bleeding with developing coagulopathy or therapeutic anticoagulation while an epidural catheter is in place, the benefits of epidural analgesia should be weighed against this potential, highly detrimental complication. This risk might lead to an increasing utilization of paravertebral blocks, as described in a U.K. survey of elective thoracic surgery.[64] However, Luvet and colleagues have described a high misplacement rate of paravertebral catheters using the landmark technique and a discrepancy between contrast medium spread and loss of sensation,[65] which makes an assessment of the effectiveness of this technique in the sedated critically ill patient very difficult.

In a small cohort study of 153 thoracic and 4 lumbar epidurals in critically ill patients, we could not identify an increased complication risk compared to the reference databank. However, the duration of catheter use was significantly longer (mean 5 days, range 1–21 days) in the critically ill group.[66]

Clinical Pearls

- The most common side effects of epidural blocks are bradycardia and hypotension related to sympathetic block.
- Hemodynamic changes can be more pronounced with intermittent bolus dosing, in patients with hypovolemia, or in patients with reduced venous return secondary to high positive end-expiratory pressure ventilation.
- Discontinuation of continuous infusion allows neurologic assessment when necessary.
- There is no hard evidence that there is increased risks of epidural bleeding with developing coagulopathy or therapeutic anticoagulation while an epidural catheter is in place. Nevertheless, the benefits of epidural analgesia should be weighed against the risk of this serious complication.

PERIPHERAL NERVE BLOCKS FOR THE UPPER EXTREMITIES

There are currently no randomized, controlled trials or large prospective trials evaluating the use of peripheral nerve blocks for the upper extremity in critically ill patients. Nevertheless, severe trauma to the shoulder or arm is often part of multiple injuries due to traffic or workplace accidents, often in combination with blunt chest trauma requiring mechanical ventilation. These injuries can contribute to severe pain, especially during positioning of the patient. If the orthopedic injury is part of complex trauma including brain injury in which the mental status of the patient is altered and opioid-based analgesic regimens might mask the neurologic situation, sufficient analgesia can be achieved for the shoulder or upper limb with either continuous interscalene,[65-69] continuous cervical paravertebral,[69-72] or infraclavicular[73] approaches to the brachial plexus.

Particular concerns arise concerning the placement of regional blocks in ICU patients with impaired mental status due to neurologic injury or therapeutic sedation. Benumof reported a small series of serious complications, including spinal cord injury related to the interscalene approach, which may have been associated with sedation or general anesthesia.[74] His case descriptions relate to spinal cord injury in heavily sedated or anesthetized patients and not to injury of the peripheral nerves. Despite this, the performance of blocks anatomically close to the centroneuraxis can indeed carry a higher risk of spinal cord needle or injection injury. In sedated critically ill patients, a combination of ultrasound and nerve stimulation for the placement of interscalene catheters and a technique with a less medial needle direction[75,76] should help to minimize the risk of complications. Perhaps most importantly, such blocks should be performed only by clinicians with adequate experience. The unavoidable blocking of the phrenic nerve and the loss of hemidiaphragmatic function[77] should be considered while planning the intervention. Although phrenic nerve blockade has negligible effects in mechanically ventilated patients, it may impair weaning from mechanical ventilation in high-risk patients. Furthermore, the proximity of the insertion site of the interscalene catheter to a tracheostomy tube might increase the risk of infection, and careful, standardized monitoring of the puncture site is therefore needed. Positioning problems might limit the use of the cervical paravertebral approach, which provides good analgesia for the shoulder, arm, and hand.

The continuous infraclavicular[69,73,78-80] and axillary[69,81-83] approaches provide good analgesia for most of the arm, elbow, and hand. A bolus injection of local anesthetic through the catheter should be considered especially in patients who need surgical anesthesia for procedures such as painful dressing changes or debridements for burns or large soft tissue wounds in the affected area. A lateral infraclavicular approach[84-86] avoids the pneumothorax and allows better securing of the catheter, compared to more proximal approaches to brachial plexus block where the catheter is placed more superficially and the soft tissue is more movable.

Clinical Pearls

- In patients with altered mental status in whom opioid-based analgesic regimens might make neurologic evaluation difficult, excellent analgesia can be achieved for the shoulder or upper limb with continuous interscalene, cervical paravertebral, or infraclavicular approaches to the brachial plexus.
- Performance of blocks anatomically close to the centroneuraxis can carry a higher risk of spinal cord needle or injection injury. In heavily sedated critically ill patients, such blocks should be performed only by clinicians with adequate experience.
- An interscalene brachial plexus block results in the loss of hemidiaphragmatic function. Although phrenic nerve blockade has negligible effects in mechanically ventilated patients, it may impair weaning from mechanical ventilation in high-risk patients.
- Real-time ultrasound guidance for peripheral catheter placement might be especially beneficial in the sedated critically ill patient.

PERIPHERAL NERVE BLOCKS FOR THE LOWER EXTREMITIES

Femoral nerve catheters are helpful in the management of acute pain from femoral neck fractures in the period between injury to shortly after surgical stabilization of the fracture.[87,88] Skilled use of ultrasound[89] might limit the unavoidable pain associated with nerve stimulation in this situation, which otherwise can be treated with small doses of intravenous remifentanil (0.3–0.5 mcg/kg) or ketamine (0.2–0.4 mg/kg). A fascia iliaca compartment block[90,91] might be a technical alternative.

A continuous femoral catheter in combination with a sciatic block provides excellent pain relief for the whole leg and even surgical anesthesia for procedures like external fixation.[92] Whether an anterior[93] or posterior approach (midgluteal[94] or subgluteal[95] classical Labat approach with one or two injections[96]) to the sciatic nerve is chosen depends largely on the skills of the operator and the ability to adequately position the patient for the procedure. If a combination of catheter techniques is used, as is often needed for the lower extremity, the total daily dose of local anesthetic should be adjusted based on catheter location, admixtures like epinephrine, drug interactions, and disease states as summarized in a recent review by Rosenberg and coworkers.[97]

A bolus injection of long-lasting local anesthetics in combination with clonidine[98] or buprenorphine[99] may help to reduce the overall amount of local anesthetic needed and minimize the effects of local anesthetic toxicity, although research results on these adjuvants are equivocal at present.[100,101]

OTHER REGIONAL ANALGESIC TECHNIQUES

Celiac plexus blocks may provide excellent analgesia for pancreatitis and cancer-related upper abdominal pain, but technical difficulties in the critically ill (computed tomography [CT]

guidance, fluoroscopy, or transgastric ultrasound) and the need for repeated injections limit their value for acutely critically ill patients.

Intrapleural catheters for pain control after chest trauma are of limited value secondary to concurrent drainage from chest tubes. The risk of pneumothorax limits their benefits for the management of pain after conventional cholecystectomy compared with the epidural or paravertebral technique in ventilated patients. Thoracic paravertebral catheters can be a valuable alternative to epidural catheters for the management of unilateral pain restricted to a few dermatomes (eg, rib fractures[102] or zoster neuralgia). Table 53–2 provides a summary of the most utilized continuous peripheral catheters.

Single-injection nerve blocks (eg, intercostal blocks for the placement of chest tubes), scalp blocks[103] for the placement of halo fixation, and sufficient local infiltration anesthesia for typical ICU procedures (eg, placement of arterial and central venous catheters, lumbar punctures, and ventriculostomies) are often forgotten, although they are easy and safe to perform. If EMLA cream is used for topical anesthesia, it needs to be applied 30–45 minutes before the procedure to achieve optimal effect.

Intrathecal morphine[104-107] injections as a single shot or via spinal catheter (microcatheters are currently not approved in the United States but are available in Europe) can be an alternative to epidural catheters, especially if only short-term use after surgery is anticipated.

SYSTEMIC EFFECTS & COMPLICATIONS OF LOCAL ANESTHETICS IN THE CRITICALLY ILL PATIENT

Local anesthetics have been shown to have several positive systemic effects (including analgesic, bronchodilatory, neuroprotective, anti-inflammatory, antiarrhythmic, and antithrombotic properties)[108] when given or absorbed in adequate quantities (the exact dose–response relationships are widely unknown). They also have negative effects, such as neurotoxicity (dose dependent), myotoxicity,[109,110] inhibition of wound healing, cardiotoxicity (dose dependent), and central nervous excitation or depression (dose dependent).[111]

To prevent local anesthetic systemic toxicity from accidental intravascular injection, a test dose of local anesthetic or saline with 1:200,000 epinephrine can be used with catheter placement, but the sensitivity of heart rate, blood pressure increase, and T-wave changes[108] might be altered in ICU patients, especially those treated with beta-blockade and α_2-agonists or catecholamines. Careful aspiration to check for blood return should be performed before each bolus injection.

Most studies examining plasma levels of local anesthetics were not performed in critically ill patients. Scott and colleagues described the safe use of epidural ropivacaine 0.2% for 72 hours with plasma levels far below the toxic threshold,[112] and Gottschalk and associates observed safe plasma levels after 96 hours in patients treated with thoracic epidural ropivacaine 0.375%, indicating no significant accumulation over time.[113]

A lipid resuscitation protocol[114] should be in place and part of the regular resuscitation drills in the ICU, where

TABLE 53–2. Continuous peripheral nerve blocks in the critically Ill.

Block	Indications	Contraindications	Practical Problems	Dose Suggestions
Interscalene	Shoulder/arm pain	Untreated contralateral pneumothorax	Horner syndrome may obscure neurologic assessment	*Bolus regimen:*[a]
				10 mL 0.25% bupivacaine or 0.2% ropivacaine q 8–12 h and on demand
		Dependence on diaphragmatic breathing	Block of ipsilateral phrenic nerve	
		Contralateral vocal cord palsy	Close proximity to tracheostomy and jugular vein line sites	*Continuous infusion:*
				0.125% bupivacaine or 0.1–0.2% ropivacaine at 5 mL/h
		Local infection at puncture site		
Cervical paravertebral	Shoulder/elbow/ wrist pain	Severe coagulopathy	Horner syndrome may obscure neurologic assessment	*Bolus regimen:*[a]
		Dependence on diaphragmatic breathing		10 mL 0.25% bupivacaine or 0.2% ropivacaine q 8–12 h and on demand
		Contralateral vocal cord palsy	Block of ipsilateral phrenic nerve	*Continuous infusion:*
		Local infection at puncture site	Patient positioning	0.125% bupivacaine or 0.1–0.2% ropivacaine at 5 mL/h
Infraclavicular	Arm/hand pain	Severe coagulopathy	Pneumothorax risk	*Bolus regimen:*[a]
		Untreated contralateral pneumothorax	Steep angle for catheter placement	10–20 mL 0.25% bupivacaine or 0.2% ropivacaine q 8–12 h and on demand
		Local infection at puncture site	Interference with subclavian lines	*Continuous infusion:*
				0.125% bupivacaine or 0.1–0.2% ropivacaine at 5–10 mL/h
Axillary	Arm/hand pain	Local infection at puncture site	Arm positioning	*Bolus regimen:*[a]
			Catheter maintenance	10–20 mL 0.25% bupivacaine or 0.2% ropivacaine q 8–12 h and on demand
				Continuous infusion:
				0.125% bupivacaine or 0.1–0.2% ropivacaine at 5–10 mL/h

(continued)

CHAPTER 53

TABLE 53–2. Continuous peripheral nerve blocks in the critically Ill. *(Continued)*

Block	Indications	Contraindications	Practical Problems	Dose Suggestions
Paravertebral Thoracic Lumbar	Unilateral chest or abdominal pain restricted to few dermatomes	Severe coagulopathy	Patient positioning	*Bolus regimen:*[a]
		Untreated contralateral pneumothorax	Stimulation success sometimes hard to visualize	10–20 mL 0.25% bupivacaine or 0.2% ropivacaine q 8–12 h and on demand
		Local infection at puncture site		
				Continuous infusion:
				0.125% bupivacaine or 0.1–0.2% ropivacaine at 5–10 mL/h
Femoral or sciatic	Unilateral leg pain	Severe coagulopathy	Patient positioning	*Bolus regimen:*[a]
		Local infection at puncture site	Interference of femoral nerve catheters with femoral lines	10 mL 0.25% bupivacaine or 0.2% ropivacaine q 8–12 h and on demand
				Continuous infusion:
				0.125% bupivacaine or 0.1–0.2% ropivacaine at 5 mL/h

[a]Consider addition of 50–100 mcg clonidine in hemodynamically stable patient or 150–300 mcg buprenorphine[99,125] to each bolus dose q 12–24 h to prolong duration of action.

Source: Adapted with permission from Schulz-Stübner S1, Boezaart A, Hata JS: Regional analgesia in the critically ill. *Crit Care Med.* 2005 Jun;33(6):1400–1407.

practitioners are often not as familiar with this topic as are operating room (OR) anesthesiologists but have easy access to the required quantities of lipid emulsion.

GENERAL MANAGEMENT ASPECTS OF CONTINUOUS REGIONAL ANALGESIA CATHETERS IN CRITICALLY ILL PATIENTS

In general, given the lack of cooperation and communication in many ICU patients, regional analgesia techniques using continuous catheters in the ICU require a higher level of vigilance than needed for regular ward patients. Close cooperation between the ICU team and the acute pain or anesthesia service of the hospital is required.

Critical care nursing personnel should be specifically trained in handling regional analgesia catheters and must be aware of the potential complications and their early warning signs. Because of the frequently large and confusing numbers of various infusion catheters in critically ill patients, the risk of drug errors and incorrect administration of drugs through continuous regional analgesia catheters may be higher in these patients. Well-trained and highly qualified personnel are the best safeguard against these complications aside from eye-catching

labels, standardized care protocols, and perhaps specially designed connectors for those catheters.

Comprehensive diagnostic approaches, including magnetic resonance imaging (MRI) or CT, should be undertaken when there are clinical signs of possible bleeding complications (eg, suspected epidural or retroperitoneal hematoma). Structured observations of catheters for infectious complications and careful adherence to aseptic technique during catheter placement and tunneling, as well as the possible use of antibiotic-coated catheters in the future, may reduce possible infectious complications. Catheters should not be removed routinely after certain time intervals but only when clinical signs of infection appear.

A study by Langevin[115] suggests that if catheters become disconnected when the fluid in the catheter is static, the proximal 25 centimeters of the catheter may be immersed in a disinfectant, cut, and reconnected to a sterile connector. This technique is feasible only for catheters in which the fluid column can be observed. Stimulating catheters should never be cut because of the danger of unwinding the internal metal spiral wire, which conducts electrical current. No study has examined the risk of reconnecting these catheters after thorough disinfection of the outer surface, which is likely a common practice in many institutions. Cuvillon and colleagues[116] reported a high overall incidence of colonization (57%) of femoral catheters without septic complications. Therefore, the decision to reconnect or remove the catheter must be made on a case-by-case basis and based on the specific clinical circumstances. The overall risk of permanent neurologic damage (from direct trauma, bleeding, or serious infection) or death from regional anesthesia and analgesia seems to be low in the perioperative setting, as shown by large surveys by Auroy and coworkers[117,118] and Moen and associates.[119] Although both studies certainly include critically ill patients, there are no specific subgroup data available.

If the patient is cooperative enough, a patient-controlled regional anesthesia (PCRA) regimen is preferable,[120] and such systems can also be used in a nurse-controlled fashion for intermittent bolus application without the need for additional manipulation of the infusion system.

While the evidence for the overall improvement of patient safety using ultrasound-guided regional anesthesia (UGRA) placement techniques is limited[121] and a certain level of training necessary,[122] the use of ultrasound seems to be especially beneficial in the critically ill patient. In a semiquantitative review, Morin and coworkers demonstrated better analgesia with the use of stimulating catheters, which seem to be another instrument to improve the effectiveness of regional analgesia in the critically ill.[123]

The complexity of individual clinical situations can be demonstrated by the following case example:[124]

A 55-year-old male patient with polycythemia vera, treated with periodic phlebotomy and a history of lower extremity DVTs [deep venous thromboses], was admitted to the hospital with acute ischemia of all 5 fingers of his right hand. His INR [international normalized ratio] on admission was 2.5. His fingers were cold and painful and showed bluish discoloration. The patient was evaluated by vascular surgeons and an angiogram showed arterial thrombosis of the right hand and rtPA [recombinant tissue plasminogen activator] thrombolysis was started by an indwelling catheter from the right femoral artery to the right subclavian artery. The patient was admitted to the Surgical Intensive Care Unit for monitoring during TPA [tissue plasminogen activator]-thrombolysis. Overnight, no significant improvement in limb perfusion could be seen and the patient underwent re-angiography on postoperative day 1. Given the amount of residual thrombosis, rtPA-treatment was continued. Overnight, on postoperative day 1, the patient became disoriented after receiving a single dose of meperidine in addition to his morphine PCA [patient-controlled analgesia] for worsening pain in his arm. A CT scan performed at that time to exclude an acute bleeding complication was read as normal and his neurologic status returned to baseline. rtPA treatment was discontinued after 48 hours on postoperative day 2, and the catheter was removed. A heparin infusion was titrated to a PTT [partial thromboplastin time] around 70 seconds. Around midnight the patient became agitated and disoriented. Another head CT was

performed which showed left cerebellum hypodensity and the patient became more and more unresponsive. Brain MRI revealed multiple infarcts involving the left cerebellum, the right cerebellum, the bilateral thalami and the left medial temporal occipital region. MRA [magnetic resonance angiogram] showed left vertebral artery thrombosis. The patient was treated symptomatically with small doses of haloperidol and the heparin infusion was discontinued by the neurologist's recommendation to prevent hemorrhagic transformation of the cerebellar infarcts. In the morning, the patient was still somnolent but complained about severe pain in his right arm when aroused. Also, the discoloration of his fingers was slowly progressing proximally and the distal parts were cold and numb. The patient also described a burning sensation in addition to the sharp and shooting pain. Morphine PCA and systemic narcotics had been discontinued secondary to his worsened neurostatus. 18 hours after discontinuation of rtPA and 9 hours after discontinuation of the heparin infusion his fibrinogen levels were still markedly elevated but his INR and PTT had returned to high normal values. An axillary brachial plexus catheter was placed using the stimulating catheter (Stimucath®, Arrow International, Reading, USA) and a good motor response with hand extension and thumb adduction at 0.44 mA was elicited via the indwelling catheter after ultrasound guided advancement of the catheter. A bolus of 20 mL of mepivacaine 1.5 percent and 20 mL of ropivacaine 0.75 percent were injected through the catheter and resulted in pain relief after 10 minutes. The skin temperature in the affected hand rose from 34.5 degrees Celsius to 36 degrees Celsius 30 minutes after injection of the local anesthetic. Ultrasound guidance was used for the placement of the axillary catheter to avoid accidental puncture of the axillary artery or vein 4. The catheter was tunneled to prevent dislocation and there was mild oozing at the tunnel site but no hematoma formation. A cerebral angiogram was performed and showed left vertebral artery thrombosis and a patent right vertebral artery. Lower extremity duplex sonography showed extensive subacute deep venous thrombosis bilaterally and an inferior vena cava filter was placed. Transthoracic echo and transesophageal echo showed a small PFO [patent foramen ovale] with minimal right to left shunt with Valsalva maneuver. The axillary catheter was bolused with 10 mL of 0.5 percent ropivacaine every 8 hours. This regimen allowed consistent pain relief and sympathetic block. Finger cyanosis was improving rapidly. With improved neurostatus, the patient was also started on gabapentin 900 mg every 8 hours, 325 mg of aspirin and codeine tablets PRN. The hematologist recommended enoxaparin 100 mg sc q 12 hours for the treatment of his hypercoagulable state. The axillary catheter was removed after 5 days immediately before his evening dose of enoxaparin. No bleeding complications were observed. His neurological status as well as the finger ischemia continued to improve.

SUMMARY

Regional analgesia, whether utilizing single-injection regional blocks or continuous neuraxial or peripheral catheters, can play a valuable role in a multimodal approach to pain management in the critically ill patient to achieve optimum patient comfort and to reduce physiologic and psychological stress. By avoiding high systemic doses of opioids, several complications, such as withdrawal syndrome, delirium, mental status changes, and gastrointestinal dysfunction, can be reduced or minimized. Because of the limited patient cooperation that is common during the placement and monitoring of continuous regional analgesia in the critically ill, indications for its use must be carefully based on anatomy, clinical features of pain, coagulation status, and logistic circumstances. Highly trained nursing personnel and well-trained physicians are essential prerequisites for the safe use of these techniques in the critical care environment. These recommendations are based on small series, uncontrolled trials, and extrapolations from controlled trials in the perioperative setting; further research on the use of regional analgesia techniques in the critically ill is needed before definitive guidelines can be established.

REFERENCES

1. Brodner G, Pogatzki E, Van Aken H, et al: A multimodal approach to control postoperative pathophysiology and rehabilitation in patients undergoing abdominothoracic esophagectomy. Anesth Analg 1998;86:228–234.
2. Brodner G, Mertes N, Buerkle H, et al: Acute pain management: Analysis, implications and consequences after prospective experience with 6349 surgical patients. Eur J Anaesthesiol 2000;17:566–575.
3. Herridge MS: Long-term outcomes after critical illness. Curr Opin Crit Care 2002;8:331–336.
4. Afessa B, Green B, Delke I, et al: Systemic inflammatory response syndrome, organ failure, and outcome in critically ill obstetric patients treated in an ICU. Chest 2001;120:1271–1277.
5. Peyton PJ, Myles PS, Silbert BS, et al: Perioperative epidural analgesia and outcome after major abdominal surgery in high-risk patients. Anesth Analg 2003;96:548.
6. De Leon-Casasola OA, Lema MJ, Karabella D, et al: Postoperative myocardial ischemia: Epidural versus intravenous patient-controlled analgesia. A pilot project. Reg Anesth 1995;20:105–112.
7. Jones C, Skirrow P, Griffiths RD, et al: Rehabilitation after critical illness: A randomized, controlled trial. Crit Care Med 2003;31:2456–2461.
8. Cuthbertson BH, Hull A, Strachan M, et al: Post-traumatic stress disorder after critical illness requiring general intensive care. Intensive Care Med 2004;30:450–455.
9. Campbell AS: Recognising post-traumatic stress in intensive care patients. Intensive Crit Care Nurs 1995;11:60–65.
10. Dellinger RP, Levy MM, Rhodes A, et al: Surviving sepsis campaign: international guidelines for management of severe sepsis and septic shock, 2012. Crit Care Med 2013;39:165–228.
11. Mehta S, McCullagh I, Burry L: Current sedation practices: lessons learned from international surveys. Anesthesiol Clin 2011;29:607–624.
12. Barr J, Fraser GL, Puntillo K et al: Clinical practice guidelines for the management of pain, agitation and delirium in adult patients in the intensive care unit. Crit Care Med 2013;41:263–306.
13. Lütz A, Goldmann A, Weber-Carstens S et al: Weaning from mechanical ventilation and sedation. Curr Opinion Anaesthesiol 2012;25:164–169.
14. Degrado JR, Anger KE, Szumita PM, et al: Evaluation of a local ICU sedation guideline on goal directed administration of sedatives and analgesics. J Pain Res 2011;4:127–134.
15. Pasero C, McCaffery M: Multimodal balanced analgesia in the critically ill. Crit Care Nurs Clin North Am 2001;13:195–206.
16. Schulz-Stübner S, Boezaart A, Hata J: Regional Analgesia in the Critically Ill. Crit Care Med 2005;33:1400–1407.
17. Schulz-Stübner S: The critically ill patient and regional anesthesia. Curr Opin Anaesthesiol 2006;19:538–544.
18. Dilworth NM, MacKellar A: Pain relief for the pediatric surgical patient. J Pediatr Surg 1987;22:264–266.
19. Manworren RC, Hynan LS: Clinical validation of FLACC: preverbal patient pain scale. Pediatr Nurs 2003;29:140–146.
20. Breau LM, Finley GA, McGrath PJ, et al: Validation of the Noncommunicating Children's Pain Checklist-Postoperative Version. Anesthesiology 2002;96:528–535.
21. Feldt KS: The checklist of nonverbal pain indicators (CNPI). Pain Manag Nurs 2000;1:13–21.
22. Blenkharn A, Faughnan S, Morgan A: Developing a pain assessment tool for use by nurses in an adult intensive care unit. Intensive Crit Care Nurs 2002;18:332–341.
23. Riker RR, Picard JT, Fraser GL: Prospective evaluation of the Sedation-Agitation Scale for adult critically ill patients. Crit Care Med 1999;27:1325–1329.
24. Riker RR, Fraser GL: Sedation in the intensive care unit: refining the models and defining the questions. Crit Care Med 2002;30:1661–1663.
25. Stundner O, Memtsoudis SG: Regional anesthesia in critically ill patients. Reg Anesth Pain Med 2012;37:537–544.
26. Naber L, Jones G, Halm M: Epidural analgesia for effective pain control. Crit Care Nurse 1994;14:69–72, 77–83; quiz 84–85.
27. Holcomb JB, McMullin NR, Kozar RA, et al: Morbidity from rib fractures increases after age 45. J Am Coll Surg 2003;196:549–555.
28. Karmakar MK, Ho AM: Acute pain management of patients with multiple fractured ribs. J Trauma 2003;54:615–625.
29. Luchette FA, Radafshar SM, Kaiser R, et al: Prospective evaluation of epidural versus intrapleural catheters for analgesia in chest wall trauma. J Trauma 1994;36:865–9; discussion 869–870.
30. Catoire P, Bonnet F: [Locoregional analgesia in thoracic injuries]. Can Anesthesiol 1994;42:809–814.
31. Asantila R, Rosenberg PH, Scheinin B: Comparison of different methods of postoperative analgesia after thoracotomy. Acta Anaesthesiol Scand 1986;30:421–425.
32. Licker M, Spiliopoulos A, Frey JG, et al: Risk factors for early mortality and major complications following pneumonectomy for non-small cell carcinoma of the lung. Chest 2002;121:1890–1897.
33. Carli F, Trudel JL, Belliveau P: The effect of intraoperative thoracic epidural anesthesia and postoperative analgesia on bowel function after colorectal surgery: a prospective, randomized trial. Dis Colon Rectum 2001;44:1083–1089.
34. Jorgensen H, Wetterslev J, Moiniche S, et al: Epidural local anaesthetics versus opioid-based analgesic regimens on postoperative gastrointestinal paralysis, PONV and pain after abdominal surgery. Cochrane Database Syst Rev 2000:CD001893.
35. Albani A, Renghi A, Gramaglia L, et al: Regional anaesthesia in vascular surgery: a multidisciplinary approach to accelerate recovery and postoperative discharge. Minerva Anestesiol 2001;67:151–154.
36. Bush RL, Lin PH, Reddy PP, et al: Epidural analgesia in patients with chronic obstructive pulmonary disease undergoing transperitoneal abdominal aortic aneurysmorraphy—a multi-institutional analysis. Cardiovasc Surg 2003;11:179–184.
37. Wu CL, Anderson GF, Herbert R, et al: Effect of postoperative epidural analgesia on morbidity and mortality after total hip replacement surgery in Medicare patients. Reg Anesth Pain Med 2003;28:271–278.
38. Niesel HC, Klimpel L, Kaiser H, et al: [Epidural blockade for analgesia and treatment of acute pancreatitis]. Reg Anaesth 1991;14:97–100.
39. Baig MK, Wexner SD: Postoperative ileus: a review. Dis Colon Rectum 2004;47:516–526.
40. Kreis ME, Kasparek MS, Becker HD, et al: [Postoperative ileus: part II (Clinical therapy)]. Zentralbl Chir 2003;128:320–328.
41. Holte K, Kehlet H: Postoperative ileus: progress towards effective management. Drugs 2002;62:2603–2615.
42. Kehlet H, Holte K: Review of postoperative ileus. Am J Surg 2001;182:3S–10S.
43. Peterson KL, DeCampli WM, Pike NA, et al: A report of two hundred twenty cases of regional anesthesia in pediatric cardiac surgery. Anesth Analg 2000;90:1014–1019.
44. Aybek T, Kessler P, Dogan S, et al: Awake coronary artery bypass grafting: utopia or reality? Ann Thorac Surg 2003;75:1165–1170.
45. Svorkdal N: Pro: anesthesiologists' role in treating refractory angina: spinal cord stimulators, thoracic epidurals, therapeutic angiogenesis, and other emerging options. J Cardiothorac Vasc Anesth 2003;17:536–545.
46. Marchertiene I: [Regional anesthesia for patients with cardiac diseases]. Medicina (Kaunas) 2003;39:721–729.
47. Thompson JS: The role of epidural analgesia and anesthesia in surgical outcomes. Adv Surg 2002;36:297–307.

48. Rodgers A, Walker N, Schug S, et al: Reduction of postoperative mortality and morbidity with epidural or spinal anaesthesia: results from overview of randomised trials. BMJ 2000;321:1493.

49. Burton AW, Eappen S: Regional anesthesia techniques for pain control in the intensive care unit. Crit Care Clin 1999;15:77–88, vi.

50. Low JH: Survey of epidural analgesia management in general intensive care units in England. Acta Anaesthesiol Scand 2002;46:799–805.

51. Bromage PR, Benumof JL: Paraplegia following intracord injection during attempted epidural anesthesia under general anesthesia. Reg Anesth Pain Med 1998;23:104–107.

52. Krane EJ, Dalens BJ, Murat I, et al: The safety of epidurals placed during general anesthesia. Reg Anesth Pain Med 1998;23:433–438.

53. Herwaldt LA PJ, Coffin SA, Schulz-Stübner S: Nosocomial infections associated with anesthesia. In Mayhall CG (ed): *Hospital Epidemiology and Infection Control*, 3rd ed. Philadelphia: Lippincott Williams & Wilkins, 2004, pp 1073–1117.

54. Tsui BC, Gupta S, Finucane B: Confirmation of epidural catheter placement using nerve stimulation. Can J Anaesth 1998;45:640–644.

55. Tsui BC, Guenther C, Emery D, et al: Determining epidural catheter location using nerve stimulation with radiological confirmation. Reg Anesth Pain Med 2000;25:306–309.

56. Wegeforth PLJ: Lumbar puncture as a factor in the pathogenesis of meningitis. Am J Med Sci 1919;158:183–202.

57. Bell K, Wattie M, Byth K, et al: Procalcitonin: a marker of bacteraemia in SIRS. Anaesth Intensive Care 2003;31:629–636.

58. Du B, Pan J, Chen D, et al: Serum procalcitonin and interleukin-6 levels may help to differentiate systemic inflammatory response of infectious and non-infectious origin. Chin Med J (Engl) 2003;116:538–542.

59. Luzzani A, Polati E, Dorizzi R, et al: Comparison of procalcitonin and C-reactive protein as markers of sepsis. Crit Care Med 2003;31:1737–1741.

60. Delevaux I, Andre M, Colombier M, et al: Can procalcitonin measurement help in differentiating between bacterial infection and other kinds of inflammatory processes? Ann Rheum Dis 2003;62:337–340.

61. Horlocker TT, Wedel DJ, Rowlingson JC, et al: Regional anesthesia in the patient receiving antithrombotic or thrombolytic therapy. American Society of Regional Anesthesia and Pain Medicine Evidence-Based Guidelines (Third Edition). Reg Anesth Pain Med 2010;35:64–101.

62. Gogarten W, Van Aken H, Büttner J, et al: Regional anesthesia and thromboembolism prophylaxis/anticoagulation. Revised guidelines of the German Society of Anesthesiology and Intensive Care Medicine. Anaesth Intesivmed 2003;44:218–230.

63. Vandermeulen E, Gogarten W, Van Aken H: [Risks and complications following peridural anesthesia]. Anaesthesist 1997;46(Suppl 3):S179–S186.

64. Kotemane C, Gopinath N, Vaja R: Analgesic techniques following thoracic surgery: a survey of United Kingdom practice. Eur J Anesthesiol 2010;27:897–899.

65. Luvet C, Siegenthaler A, Szucs-Farkas Z et al: The location of paravertebral catheters placed using the landmark technique. Anesthesia 2012;67:1321–1326.

66. Schulz-Stübner S, Czaplik M: Quality management in regional anesthesia using the example of the Regional Anesthesia Surveillance System (RASS). Schmerz 2013;27:56–66.

67. Boezaart AP, de Beer JF, du Toit C, et al: A new technique of continuous interscalene nerve block. Can J Anaesth 1999;46:275–281.

68. Brown DL: Brachial plexus anesthesia: An analysis of options. Yale J Biol Med 1993;66:415–431.

69. Schulz-Stübner S: [Brachial plexus. Anesthesia and analgesia]. Anaesthesist 2003;52:643–657.

70. Boezaart AP, De Beer JF, Ncll ML: Early experience with continuous cervical paravertebral block using a stimulating catheter. Reg Anesth Pain Med 2003;28:406–413.

71. Boezaart AP, Koorn R, Borene S, et al: Continuous brachial plexus block using the posterior approach. Reg Anesth Pain Med 2003;28:70–71.

72. Boezaart AP, Koorn R, Rosenquist RW: Paravertebral approach to the brachial plexus: an anatomic improvement in technique. Reg Anesth Pain Med 2003;28:241–244.

73. Ilfeld BM, Enneking FK: Brachial plexus infraclavicular block success rate and appropriate endpoints. Anesth Analg 2002;95:784.

74. Benumof JL: Permanent loss of cervical spinal cord function associated with interscalene block performed under general anesthesia. Anesthesiology 2000;93:1541–1544.

75. Meier G, Bauereis C, Maurer H, et al: [Interscalene plexus block. Anatomic requirements—Anesthesiologic and operative aspects]. Anaesthesist 2001;50:333–341.

76. Meier G, Bauereis C, Heinrich C: [Interscalene brachial plexus catheter for anesthesia and postoperative pain therapy. Experience with a modified technique]. Anaesthesist 1997;46:715–719.

77. Sala-Blanch X, Lazaro JR, Correa J, et al: Phrenic nerve block caused by interscalene brachial plexus block: Effects of digital pressure and a low volume of local anesthetic. Reg Anesth Pain Med 1999;24:231–235.

78. Neuburger M, Kaiser H, Rembold-Schuster I, et al: [Vertical infraclavicular brachial-plexus blockade. A clinical study of reliability of a new method for plexus anesthesia of the upper extremity]. Anaesthesist 1998;47:595–599.

79. Borene SC, Edwards JN, Boezaart AP: At the cords, the pinkie towards: Interpreting infraclavicular motor responses to neurostimulation. Reg Anesth Pain Med 2004;29:125–129.

80. Sandhu NS, Capan LM: Ultrasound-guided infraclavicular brachial plexus block. Br J Anaesth 2002;89:254–259.

81. Ang ET, Lassale B, Goldfarb G: Continuous axillary brachial plexus block—a clinical and anatomical study. Anesth Analg 1984;63:680–684.

82. Sia S, Lepri A, Campolo MC, et al: Four-injection brachial plexus block using peripheral nerve stimulator: a comparison between axillary and humeral approaches. Anesth Analg 2002;95:1075–1079, table of contents.

83. Retzl G, Kapral S, Greher M, et al: Ultrasonographic findings of the axillary part of the brachial plexus. Anesth Analg 2001;92:1271–1275.

84. Kapral S, Jandrasits O, Schabernig C, et al: Lateral infraclavicular plexus block vs. axillary block for hand and forearm surgery. Acta Anaesthesiol Scand 1999;43:1047–1052.

85. Greher M, Retzl G, Niel P, et al: Ultrasonographic assessment of topographic anatomy in volunteers suggests a modification of the infraclavicular vertical brachial plexus block. Br J Anaesth 2002;88:632–636.

86. Jandard C, Gentili ME, Girard F, et al: Infraclavicular block with lateral approach and nerve stimulation: extent of anesthesia and adverse effects. Reg Anesth Pain Med 2002;27:37–42.

87. Finlayson BJ, Underhill TJ: Femoral nerve block for analgesia in fractures of the femoral neck. Arch Emerg Med 1988;5:173–176.

88. Tan TT, Coleman MM: Femoral blockade for fractured neck of femur in the emergency department. Ann Emerg Med 2003;42:596–597; author reply 597.

89. Marhofer P, Schrogendorfer K, Koinig H, et al: Ultrasonographic guidance improves sensory block and onset time of three-in-one blocks. Anesth Analg 1997;85:854–857.

90. Lopez S, Gros T, Bernard N, et al: Fascia iliaca compartment block for femoral bone fractures in prehospital care. Reg Anesth Pain Med 2003;28:203–207.

91. Cuignet O, Pirson J, Boughrouph J, et al: The efficacy of continuous fascia iliaca compartment block for pain management in burn patients undergoing skin grafting procedures. Anesth Analg 2004;98:1077–1081, table of contents.

92. Kaden V, Wolfel H, Kirsch W: [Experiences with a combined sciatic and femoral block in surgery of injuries of the lower leg]. Anaesthesiol Reanim 1989;14:299–303.

93. Barbero C, Fuzier R, Samii K: Anterior approach to the sciatic nerve block: Adaptation to the patient's height. Anesth Analg 2004;98:1785–1788, table of contents.

94. Franco CD: Posterior approach to the sciatic nerve in adults: is euclidean geometry still necessary? Anesthesiology 2003;98:723–728.

95. Di Benedetto P, Casati A, Bertini L, et al: Posterior subgluteal approach to block the sciatic nerve: Description of the technique and initial clinical experiences. Eur J Anaesthesiol 2002;19:682–686.

96. Bailey SL, Parkinson SK, Little WL, et al: Sciatic nerve block. A comparison of single versus double injection technique. Reg Anesth 1994;19:9–13.

97. Rosenberg PH, Veering BT, Urmey WF: Maximum recommended doses of local anesthetics: A multifactorial concept. Reg Anesth Pain Med 2004;29:564–575.

98. Casati A, Magistris L, Fanelli G, et al: Small-dose clonidine prolongs postoperative analgesia after sciatic-femoral nerve block with 0.75% ropivacaine for foot surgery. Anesth Analg 2000;91:388–392.

99. Gao F, Waters B, Seager J, et al: Comparison of bupivacaine plus buprenorphine with bupivacaine alone by caudal blockade for postoperative pain relief after hip and knee arthroplasty. Eur J Anaesthesiol 1995;12:471–476.

100. Culebras X, Van Gessel E, Hoffmeyer P, et al: Clonidine combined with a long acting local anesthetic does not prolong postoperative analgesia after brachial plexus block but does induce hemodynamic changes. Anesth Analg 2001;92:199–204.

101. Picard PR, Tramer MR, McQuay HJ, et al: Analgesic efficacy of peripheral opioids (all except intra-articular): a qualitative systematic review of randomised controlled trials. Pain 1997;72:309–318.

102. Wehling MJ, Koorn R, Leddell C, et al: Electrical nerve stimulation using a stimulating catheter: What is the lower limit? Reg Anesth Pain Med 2004;29:230–233.

103. Costello TG, Cormack JR, Hoy C, et al: Plasma ropivacaine levels following scalp block for awake craniotomy. J Neurosurg Anesthesiol 2004;16:147–150.

104. Rawal N, Tandon B: Epidural and intrathecal morphine in intensive care units. Intensive Care Med 1985;11:129–133.

105. Shroff A, Rooke GA, Bishop MJ: Effects of intrathecal opioid on extubation time, analgesia, and intensive care unit stay following coronary artery bypass grafting. J Clin Anesth 1997;9:415–419.

106. Hall R, Adderley N, MacLaren C, et al: Does intrathecal morphine alter the stress response following coronary artery bypass grafting surgery? Can J Anaesth 2000;47:463–466.

107. Bowler I, Djaiani G, Abel R, et al: A combination of intrathecal morphine and remifentanil anesthesia for fast-track cardiac anesthesia and surgery. J Cardiothorac Vasc Anesth 2002;16:709–714.

108. Schulz-Stübner S: Regionalanästhesie und -analgesie: Techniken und Therapieschemata für die Praxis. Stuttgart: Schattauer, 2003.

109. Zink W, Seif C, Bohl JR, et al: The acute myotoxic effects of bupivacaine and ropivacaine after continuous peripheral nerve blockades. Anesth Analg 2003;97:1173–1179, table of contents.

110. Zink W, Graf BM: Local anesthetic myotoxicity. Reg Anesth Pain Med 2004;29:333–340.

111. Zink W, Graf BM: [Toxicology of local anesthetics. Clinical, therapeutic and pathological mechanisms]. Anaesthesist 2003;52:1102–1123.

112. Scott DA, Emanuelsson BM, Mooney PH, et al: Pharmacokinetics and efficacy of long-term epidural ropivacaine infusion for postoperative analgesia. Anesth Analg 1997;85:1322–1330.

113. Gottschalk A, Burmeister MA, Freitag M, et al: [Plasma levels of ropivacaine and bupivacaine during postoperative patient controlled thoracic epidural analgesia]. Anasthesiol Intensivmed Notfallmed Schmerzther 2003;38:705–709.

114. Weinberg GL: Lipid emulsion infusion: resuscitation for local anesthetic and other drug overdose. Anesthesiology 2012;117:180–187.

115. Langevin PB, Gravenstein N, Langevin SO, et al: Epidural catheter reconnection. Safe and unsafe practice. Anesthesiology 1996;85:883–888.

116. Cuvillon P, Ripart J, Lalourcey L, et al: The continuous femoral nerve block catheter for postoperative analgesia: bacterial colonization, infectious rate and adverse effects. Anesth Analg 2001;93:1045–1049.

117. Auroy Y, Benhamou D, Bargues L, et al: Major complications of regional anesthesia in France: the SOS Regional Anesthesia Hotline Service. Anesthesiology 2002;97:1274–1280.

118. Auroy Y, Narchi P, Messiah A, et al: Serious complications related to regional anesthesia: Results of a prospective survey in France. Anesthesiology 1997;87:479–486.

119. Moen V, Dahlgren N, Irestedt L: Severe neurological complications after central neuraxial blockades in Sweden 1990–1999. Anesthesiology 2004;101:950–959.

120. Savoia G, Alampi D, Amantea B, et al: Postoperative pain treatment SIAARTI recommendations 2010. Short version. Minerva Anestesiol 2010;76:657–667.

121. Neal JM, Brull R, Chan VW, et al: The ASRA evidence-based assessment of ultrasound guided regional anesthesia and pain medicine: executive summary. Reg Anesth Pain Med 2010;35:S1–S9.

122. Sites BD, Chan VW, Neal JM, et al: The American Society of Regional Anesthesia and Pain Medicine, the European Society of Regional Anesthesia and Pain Therapy and joint committee recommendations for education and training in ultrasound-guided regional anesthesia. Reg Anesth Pain Med 2010;35:S74–S80.

123. Morin AM, Kranke P, Wulf H: The effect of stimulating versus nonstimulating catheter techniques for continuous regional anesthesia: a semiquantitative systematic review. Reg Anesth Pain Med 2010;35:194–199.

124. Schulz-Stübner S, Martin C: Axillary catheter with intermittent boluses of local anesthetic for ischemic upper limb pain 18 hours after failed rtPA thrombolysis. Eur J Anaesthesiol 2007;24:722–724.

125. Candido KD, Franco CD, Khan MA, et al: Buprenorphine added to the local anesthetic for brachial plexus block to provide postoperative analgesia in outpatients. Reg Anesth Pain Med 2001; 26:352–356.

Acute Pain Management in the Opioid-Dependent Patient

Lisa Doan, Joseph Largi, Lynn Choi, and Christopher Gharibo

INTRODUCTION

Opioid use is increasing worldwide leading to an increasing amount of opioid-tolerant patients who may require acute pain management. Pain in this patient population is often poorly understood and therefore may be inadequately treated. The main goals in treating acute pain in opioid-tolerant patients are providing effective pain relief and minimizing withdrawal symptoms. Other challenges include assisting with social issues, poor coping, and psychiatric issues. This chapter discusses important factors to consider when treating acute pain in opioid-dependent patients.

DEFINITIONS

Tolerance

Tolerance is a physiologic adaptation in which increasing amount of a drug is required to achieve the same pharmacologic effects after prolonged use. Tolerance develops to most effects of opioids, including analgesia, euphoria, sedation, respiratory depression, and nausea; however, tolerance does not develop to miosis or constipation.[1]

Withdrawal

Withdrawal refers to physiologic symptoms resulting from the abrupt discontinuation of chronically administered opioids. Although withdrawal from opioids is rarely life threatening, it can be very uncomfortable. The symptoms of opioid withdrawal include abdominal cramps, anxiety, diarrhea, disturbed sleep, irritability, dysphoria, nausea and vomiting, rhinorrhea, urinary frequency, twitching, lacrimation, and increased muscle spasms.

Clinical Pearl

- The symptoms of opioid withdrawal include abdominal cramps, anxiety, diarrhea, disturbed sleep, irritability, dysphoria, nausea and vomiting, rhinorrhea, urinary frequency, twitching, lacrimation, and increased muscle spasms.

The onset and time course of opioid withdrawal are determined by the half-life of the drug (Figure 54–1). Withdrawal symptoms of short-acting opioids such as heroin and morphine typically begin more rapidly than long-acting agonist opioids such as methadone. Symptoms of withdrawal with short-acting opioids start 6–24 hours after the last dose, peak at 24–48 hours, and resolve within 5–10 days. Methadone is a long-acting opioid agonist; its withdrawal symptoms emerge 36–48 hours after the last dose. Some low-grade symptoms of withdrawal may linger for 3–6 weeks after last use due to its long half-life.[2]

Clinical Pearls

- Withdrawal symptoms may develop in opioid-tolerant patients if their usual dose of opioids is stopped, reduced too quickly, or the effect of the opioid is reversed by an antagonist such as naloxone.
- Withdrawal symptoms can occur even with small decreases (10%–15%) in opioid dosing and can manifest as myalgias and arthralgias in addition to return of the pain.

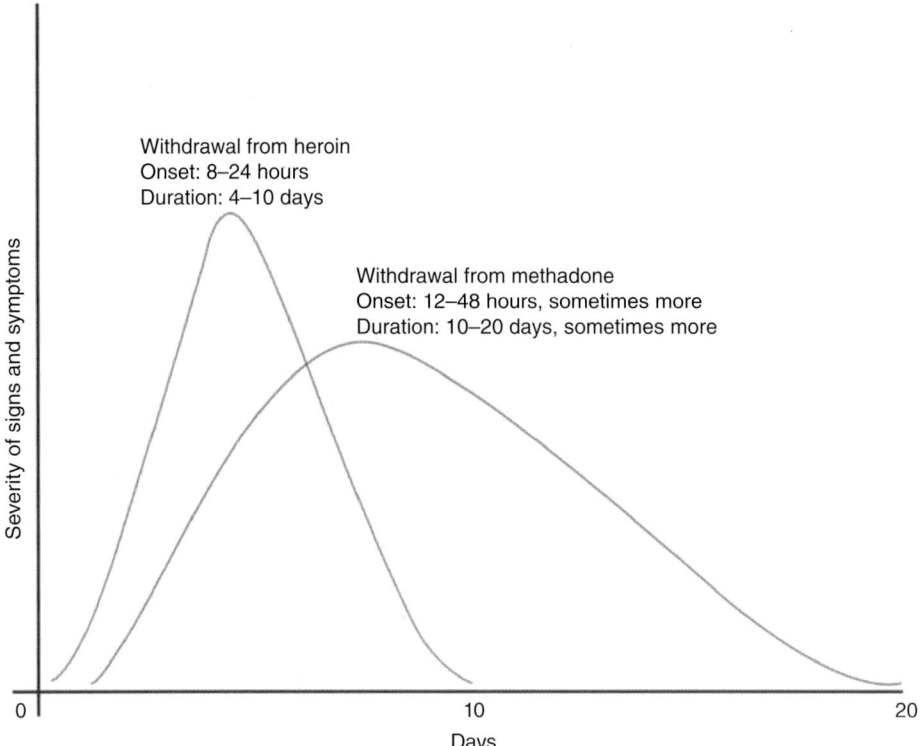

FIGURE 54–1. Symptoms and duration of heroin and methadone withdrawal.

Substance Abuse and Dependence

Before the release of the fifth edition of the Diagnostic and Statistical Manual of Mental Disorders in 2013, substance abuse and dependence were considered two separate disorders. They are now considered to be a single disorder measured on a continuum from mild to severe. Substance abuse and dependence are now recognized as the recurrent maladaptive use of a substance that leads to clinically significant impairment or distress personally, professionally, or socially.[3] Physical dependence is recognized as a state of adaption manifested by withdrawal symptoms that can be elicited by abrupt discontinuation, rapid dose reduction, or the administration of an antagonist.[4]

Addiction

Addiction is defined as the continued use of a substance despite adverse consequences. It is a behavioral syndrome characterized by evidence of psychological dependence or craving, use despite harmful adverse effects, and other drug-related aberrant behavior (eg, altering prescriptions, drug hoarding or sales, unsanctioned dose escalation).

Maintenance

Maintenance therapy aims to prevent the craving and withdrawal symptoms of opioid-dependent individuals by substituting substances with long-acting and less euphoric opioids such as methadone and buprenorphine.[5] The goals of treatment are to achieve a stable maintenance dose of opioid agonist and mitigate withdrawal symptoms.

TYPES OF OPIOID-TOLERANT PATIENTS

Anesthesiologists and pain medicine specialists often encounter patients who are opioid dependent. The majority of this patient population have chronic pain conditions and have been using opioid analgesics for a prolonged period of time. The chronic pain can be a result of cancer or a nonmalignant process. The use of opioids in the management of cancer pain has been widely accepted.[6] The estimated cancer prevalence in the United States was over 12 million in 2009.[7] It is estimated that 20%–50% of cancer patients experience pain as a presenting symptom and that up to 90% experience pain in the advanced stages of disease.[8] The estimated prevalence of chronic noncancer pain is predicted to increase as the population ages. The use of opioids in chronic noncancer pain has become increasingly common, and guidelines have been set forth by the American Pain Society, the American Academy of Pain Medicine, and the American Society of Interventional Pain Physicians for this purpose.[9,10] However, evidence for the efficacy of long-term opioid use in noncancer pain has been inconclusive. With the increasing awareness of the potential adverse consequences of long-term opioid use, a "universal precautions" approach with appropriate risk assessment and management has been recommended. This approach includes proper diagnosis for the etiology of pain; informed consent; the use of treatment agreements; assessment of analgesia, activity, adverse effects, and aberrant behavior; and careful documentation.[11]

The smaller portion of the opioid-dependent population includes opioid abusers. Heroin is the most common illicit opioid that is abused, although its use has plateaued over the past 10 years. However, prescription opioids are increasingly being abused. Prescription opioid sales quadrupled between 1999 and 2010.[12] In 2010, the number of Americans reporting nonmedical use of prescription opioids reached 12 million.[13] Since 2003, more deaths due to opioid overdose have involved prescription opioid analgesics than heroin and cocaine combined.[14] Further complicating the picture is that opioid abuse and misuse may also be seen in patients prescribed opioids for chronic pain. In a review examining the prevalence of addiction in chronic pain patients, prevalence varied from 0%–31%.[15] Patients with a past history of opioid abuse in methadone or buprenorphine opioid treatment programs compose another subpopulation of opioid-dependent patients who may need acute pain management.

Pain is prevalent in patients with a history of opioid abuse. In studies of patients receiving methadone maintenance treatment, 61% report chronic pain, and 37% report severe chronic pain.[16,17] Increased reports of pain may occur as a result of opioid-induced hyperalgesia (OIH), which occurs when the long-term use of opioids causes a hypersensitivity to painful stimuli.[18]

TOLERANCE AND OPIOID-INDUCED HYPERALGESIA MECHANISMS

Tolerance can develop after the prolonged use of opioids. It is a phenomenon that is described as a decrease in the effect of a drug after repeated administration, which can be overcome by increasing the dose of the drug. OIH is a mechanism by which the analgesic properties of a drug are decreased secondary to increased pain sensitivity. As a result of OIH and tolerance, opioid-dependent patients may have a lower pain threshold and require higher doses of opioids to achieve adequate pain relief. It is important to recognize that while OIH and tolerance are distinctly different processes, they are related and have overlapping mechanisms. While tolerance causes a rightward shift in the dose-response curve, OIH leads to a downward shift in the dose-response curve (Figure 54–2).

Clinical Pearl

• The initial clinical strategy for the treatment of tolerance and OIH are similar: regional anesthesia techniques, optimize nonopioids, control withdrawal, and adjust opioid doses.

OIH should be suspected when the effect of opioids seems to decrease in the absence of disease progression, especially if found in the context of diffuse allodynia unrelated to the original pain or increased levels of pain with increasing opioid requirements.[19] The precise molecular mechanisms underlying tolerance and OIH are not fully understood and are still being

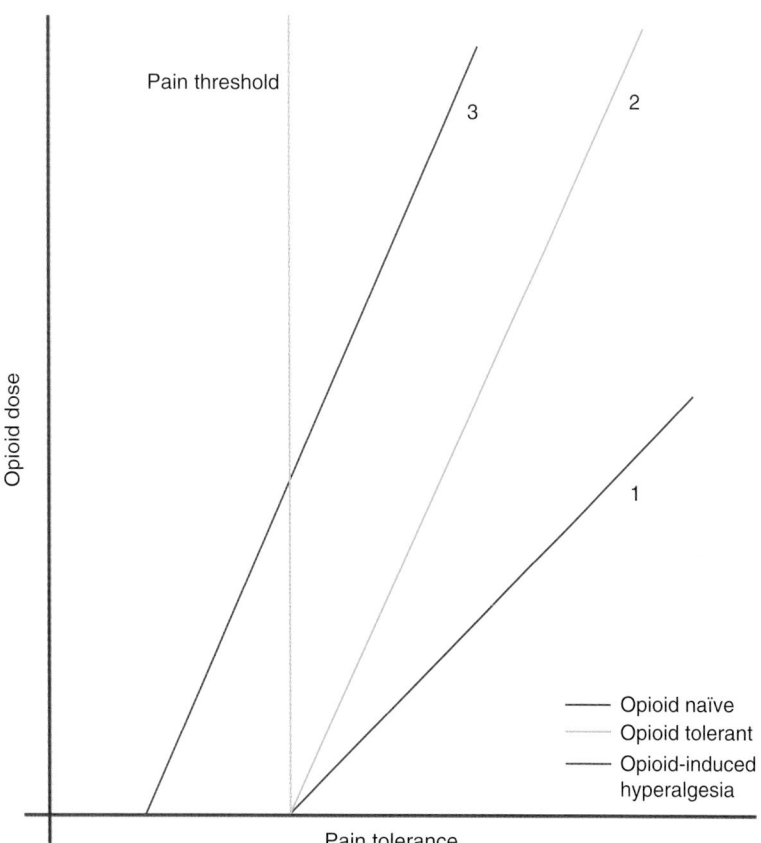

Pain threshold

Opioid dose

3

2

1

—— Opioid naïve
—— Opioid tolerant
—— Opioid-induced hyperalgesia

Pain tolerance

FIGURE 54–2. In opioid-naïve patients, increasing the opioid dose results in increased analgesia (1). In opioid-tolerant patients, the baseline threshold remains the same, but an increased dose of opioid is required to reach the same analgesic effect (2). Note that in opioid-induced hyperalgesia, maximal analgesic effect is not reached, baseline pain tolerance is reduced, and there is a downward shift from the opioid-tolerant patient (3).

investigated. Tolerance is classically thought to be due to the downregulation of opioid receptors. However, other mechanisms likely play a role, as well, such as adaptations downstream of receptor activation.[20] OIH has many proposed mechanisms, including those involving the central glutaminergic system, spinal dynorphins, descending facilitation, genetic mechanisms, and enhanced nociceptive responses.[21]

The Glutaminergic System

Current data suggest that the most likely molecular mechanism of OIH involves the central glutaminergic system. The main mechanisms by which opioids trigger the glutaminergic system involve the activation of N-methyl-D-aspartate (NMDA) receptors, which are glutamate receptors; the inhibition of glutamate reuptake; and the activation of protein kinase C.[22] Animal studies have shown that the coadministration of ketamine, an NMDA receptor antagonist, with morphine reduces analgesic tolerance as well as the development of OIH after the cessation of systemic or intrathecal morphine administration.[23] Similarly, human studies have found that the administration of ketamine attenuated remifentanil induced OIH as measured by intradermal electrical stimulation. Low-dose ketamine has been reported to prevent remifentanil-induced postoperative hyperalgesia in humans.[24]

Spinal Dynorphins

Spinal dynorphins are endogenous opioid peptides that are modulators of the pain response. It has been shown that levels of spinal dynorphin are increased with continuous infusions of opioids.[25] These increases are associated with hyperalgesia that can be reversed with dynorphin antiserum.

Descending Facilitation

Another proposed mechanism of the development of OIH is the facilitation of descending pathways from the rostral ventromedial medulla. The rostral ventromedial medulla has both descending inhibitory and excitatory projections to the spinal cord. The subset of excitatory neurons that facilitate nociceptive processing has been shown to be involved in OIH.[26]

Enhanced Nociceptive Responses

Another proposed mechanism of OIH is a decrease in the reuptake of neurotransmitters from the primary afferent fibers and enhanced responsiveness of spinal neurons to nociceptive neurotransmitters, such as substance P and glutamate. Morphine administration over several days has been shown to increase substance P and the expression of its receptor, the NK-1 receptor, in the spinal cord.[27]

Genetic Contributions

Many studies have supported the conclusion that genetic influences play a crucial role in pain sensitivity and analgesic response and therefore also in OIH.

ACUTE PAIN MANAGEMENT OF THE OPIOID-DEPENDENT PATIENT

Despite opioid tolerance and/or dependence, effective pain management during the perioperative period is an achievable goal by treating acute pain aggressively with nonopioid and opioid medications and by using nonpharmacological modalities and early mobilization.

Preoperative Assessment and Management

Clinical Pearls

- Opioid-tolerant patients can often be identified during preoperative assessment.
- In some patients, tolerance may not become evident until a diminished response to intraoperative opioids is noted or when postoperative pain control becomes challenging.
- Patients with chronic pain on opioids and other centrally acting analgesics should be advised to continue taking their medications as prescribed, including on the morning of surgery.

A crucial first step in the management of the perioperative pain in opioid-dependent patients is identifying the extent of opioid tolerance in a given patient. In some patients, the diagnosis can be made by the preoperative assessment, whereas in others, tolerance may not become evident until a diminished response to intraoperative opioids is noted or when postoperative pain control is found to be difficult. Some patients may be willing to divulge their opioid use or abuse history, whereas others may be reluctant due to a distrust of the medical community and concern of discrimination by being labeled a drug seeker by medical staff. Therefore, it is important that the provider begin to gain the patient's trust from the first meeting with the patient. A clue in the patient's history that may indicate possible opioid tolerance and dependence is the abuse of nonopioid substances. Patients who abuse other substances, such as alcohol, marijuana, or nicotine, are more likely to have opioid dependence than the general population.[28] When deception is suspected, the provider can administer a urine toxicology screen, which, in addition to screening for opioids, will also screen for other drugs of abuse, which can aid in the management of the patient.[29] The provider should provide reassurance that acute pain management is realistic and to make sure that both the patient and the medical team are working towards a common goal. The provider should also be careful to maintain privacy and confidentiality in an attempt to build trust. The plan for the patient should be discussed in a nonjudgmental manner. In addition to the usual preoperative assessment, certain additional information should be obtained from the opioid-dependent patient. This includes the documentation of all medications and their doses. This is especially important when trying to provide adequate postoperative analgesia and to prevent withdrawal from opioids or other medications. These medications and doses should be confirmed with the original provider of the prescriptions, the patient's pharmacy, and, when applicable, the patient's methadone clinic.

Clinical Pearls

- Provide reassurance that acute pain management is realistic.
- Maintain privacy and confidentiality, and build trust.
- Discuss the plan in a nonjudgmental manner.
- Document all medications the patient is taking, along with the medication doses
- Confirm medications and doses with the original provider.
- Keep in mind the psychosocial aspect of pain; pain is often compounded by anxiety and depression.
- Continue antidepressant and anti-anxiety medications perioperatively.
- Avoid naltrexone and naloxone in the perioperative period.
- Advise continuation of pain medications as prescribed, including the morning of surgery.

It is important to remember that patients who are being treated for chronic pain often exhibit poor coping and have a psychosocial aspect to their pain that is compounded by anxiety and depression. For this reason, antidepressants and anti-anxiety medications should be continued during the perioperative period. In patients with opioid abuse, it is also important to note that the perioperative period is not an optimal time to detoxify the patient. Opioid antagonists such as naltrexone and naloxone are not advised in the perioperative period for an opioid-dependent patient. The postoperative administration of these drugs can bring upon withdrawal symptoms in this patient population, which may place the patient at medical risk, especially in the presence of comorbidities. If the administration of an opioid antagonist is needed for respiratory depression, it should be administered carefully in titrated doses.

Patients with chronic pain on opioids should be advised to continue taking their medications as prescribed, including on the morning of surgery. Strong consideration can be given to preoperative dosing with nonsteroidal anti-inflammatory drugs (NSAIDs) such as celecoxib, intravenous acetaminophen, or anticonvulsants on the morning of surgery.

Patients with a history of opioid abuse may be in opioid treatment programs using methadone or buprenorphine. It is important for providers to understand that maintenance opioids typically have no analgesic effect at their prescribed dosages, likely because of tolerance or OIH; therefore, in most cases, the maintenance dose should be continued. Methadone and buprenorphine, in addition to being used for the treatment of opioid abuse, may also be used in the treatment of pain and are discussed below.

Clinical Pearls

- Patients on methadone maintenance should continue their verified methadone dose throughout hospitalization.
- The treatment of acute pain can be challenging in patients treated for opioid dependence with buprenorphine. Because of its long half-life and high affinity for the mu-opioid receptor, buprenorphine competes with other opioids attempting to bind to opioid receptors, thus preventing appropriate analgesia. Therefore, options include stopping buprenorphine or switching to another opioid before surgery.

Methadone

Methadone is a long-acting opioid agonist that also has activity as an NMDA antagonist. Methadone is the most commonly used medication to treat opioid addiction. The half-life of methadone is long and variable, ranging from 12–28 hours.[30] Methadone has a biphasic elimination curve with a rapid alpha-elimination phase followed by a much longer beta-elimination phase. Thus, for maintenance treatment of opioid addiction, the use of methadone once daily prevents withdrawal. However, the analgesic effects of methadone require more frequent dosing.[31] Due to methadone's properties as an NMDA antagonist, it may reduce opioid tolerance and OIH.

Methadone has certain pharmacological characteristics that require precautions with its use. Methadone is metabolized by the cytochrome P450 enzyme, primarily CYP3A4 and CYP2B6, in the liver. Because of its P450 metabolism, methadone has many drug interactions. For example, the use of P450 inducers (eg, phenytoin, rifampin), antiretrovirals (eg, efavirenz), and P450 inhibitors (eg, azole-based antifungals) will each result in a different methadone metabolism, thus affecting plasma levels and therapeutic effect. With inhibitors of methadone metabolism, side effects such as sedation and respiratory depression can also occur.[30]

Clinical Pearls

- Methadone is metabolized by the cytochrome P450 enzyme.
- Because of its P450 metabolism, methadone has many drug interactions.
- The use of P450-inducing medications such as phenytoin, rifampin, and antiretrovirals (eg, efavirenz or P450 inhibitors such as azole-based antifungals) affect the plasma level and therapeutic effect of methadone.

Methadone may prolong the QT interval, which can lead to fatal cardiac arrhythmias. Caution should be used when methadone is combined with other drugs that may also prolong the QT interval. Caution should be exercised when switching from one opioid to methadone, because the pharmacokinetics of methadone can vary greatly from person to person, potentially leading to overdose if the conversion results in greater than expected potency of methadone. Patients being switched from higher doses of opioids to methadone seem to be at greater risk for toxicity.[32] Due to the variable pharmacokinetics of methadone, consultation with a pain medicine specialist should be considered when the use of methadone is contemplated.

Patients on methadone maintenance with acute pain should continue their verified methadone dose and be prescribed multimodal analgesia, likely including short-acting opioids to treat the incident pain.

Buprenorphine

Buprenorphine is a partial mu-opioid agonist. For the treatment of opioid addiction, buprenorphine comes in tablets that are taken sublingually, formulated either with buprenorphine alone or combined with naloxone. Transdermal buprenorphine is indicated for the management of moderate to severe chronic pain. Buprenorphine has a long half-life of approximately 37 hours. Thus, for the treatment of addiction it can be used once daily. The transdermal formulation offered in the U.S. is meant to be changed every 7 days. Buprenorphine is also metabolized by the hepatic cytochrome P450 system, primarily CYP3A4 and CYP2B6. It may also be associated with a prolongation of the QT interval.[30] Buprenorphine has great affinity for the mu-opioid receptor, approximately 1000 times that of morphine.[33] For that reason, it may precipitate withdrawal in patients already on opioids because its high receptor affinity displaces other opioids. However, in a patient who has stopped using opioids and is in withdrawal, buprenorphine will ease symptoms of withdrawal through its partial agonist effect.[30] In the U.S., buprenorphine can be prescribed at a physician's office for opioid addiction treatment, which differs from methadone, which requires a specific methadone clinic to oversee prescription and distribution.

The treatment of acute pain can be challenging in a patient on buprenorphine with a history of opioid dependence. Because of its long half-life and high affinity for the mu-opioid receptor, buprenorphine competes with other opioids attempting to bind to opioid receptors, thus interfering with analgesia. For patients on buprenorphine maintenance, there are several treatment options to consider. One option is to continue buprenorphine and add additional short-acting opioids for the acute pain. It may take larger than normal doses of short-acting opioids to provide adequate analgesia. Another option is to divide the dose of buprenorphine and administer it every 6–8 hours in an attempt to utilize its analgesic properties; additional opioids may still be required to provide adequate analgesia. A further option is to discontinue the buprenorphine altogether several days before the surgery and then restart it when the patient no longer requires opioid management for acute pain. Alternatively, buprenorphine can be converted to methadone, and short-acting opioids can be titrated for the treatment of the acute pain.[34]

Clinical Pearl

Treatment options for patients on buprenorphine maintenance:

- Continue buprenorphine maintenance, and add a short-acting opioid for acute pain.
- Larger-than-normal doses of a short-acting opioid may be required for adequate analgesia.
- Consider dividing buprenorphine doses q6–8 h to optimize its analgesic properties and adding a short-acting opioid as needed.
- Consider discontinuing buprenorphine several days preoperatively and restarting postoperatively.
- Consider switching from buprenorphine to methadone perioperatively.

INTRAOPERATIVE MANAGEMENT

Clinical Pearls

- Respiratory rate can be used as a guide for titrating opioids intraoperatively.
- Opioid tolerant patients may be at an increased risk of awareness.

A multimodal approach for pain control including regional techniques and nonopioid analgesics should be considered for opioid-dependent patients. This plan ideally should be initiated preoperatively and followed throughout the perioperative period. Regional techniques and nonopioid analgesics are described in further detail in the section on postoperative care.

Patients who are opioid dependent should continue their baseline opioid dose during the perioperative period prior to the induction of anesthesia with additional analgesics provided as needed. Baseline opioids include sustained-release opioids, methadone maintenance, buprenorphine maintenance, transdermal fentanyl patches, and epidural or intrathecal opioid infusions. If a fentanyl patch is removed prior to surgery, a fentanyl infusion can be used during surgery as a substitute to provide maintenance opioid therapy. Patients who abuse illicit opioids such as heroin can be given either intravenous or oral doses of methadone and morphine as their baseline.[35] However, determination of a baseline dose can be difficult for illicit drugs, as their formulations are variable.

Opioid-dependent patients may require larger intraoperative opioid doses than opioid-naïve patients. Respiratory rate can be used as a method to appropriately dose opioids intraoperatively. If the patient is spontaneously breathing either throughout the case or at the end after reversal of muscle relaxant, the opioid dose may be titrated to a respiratory rate of 8–12 breaths per minute. Opioid effects can also occur in the opioid-tolerant patient, including nausea, vomiting, pruritus, and respiratory depression. Therefore, it is essential to monitor vital signs and sedation level in the perioperative period while opioids are being administered even in this group of patients. If remifentanil is being used for intraoperative analgesia, a long-acting opioid at the end of the surgery can be administered to ensure analgesia after the remifentanil infusion is discontinued.

Caution is warranted if a warming blanket is used with a patient who has been administered a transdermal fentanyl or buprenorphine patch, as the application of heat over the patch may lead to an increase in medication release.

Anesthesiologists should be aware that opioid-tolerant patients under anesthesia are at an increased risk of awareness intraoperatively.[36]

THE POSTOPERATIVE PERIOD

A multimodal analgesic plan should be continued into the postoperative period for opioid-dependent patients.

Opioids

Clinical Pearls

- PCA is an effective option for postoperative analgesia. Carefully consider the basal rate dosing to decrease the probability of opioid-related side effects and complications.
- Not all patients will need their preoperative opioid dose postoperatively. The pain generators may be different postoperatively, and the patient may require a decreased or increased dose of opioids.
- Opioid rotation may be useful in improving efficacy, decreasing daily opioid requirements, and reducing opioid-related side effects.

A patient's usual baseline dose of opioid is typically continued perioperatively. Intravenous patient-controlled analgesia (PCA) is an effective option for postsurgical analgesia especially in the opioid-dependent patient. PCA allows the patient to administer pain medication almost instantly on an as-needed basis, decreasing the risk of under-medication and breakthrough pain and increasing patient satisfaction. By allowing patients to administer their own pain medication, demands on nursing staff are also reduced. Though not recommended for opioid-naïve patients, a basal rate of opioid may be administered to opioid-dependent patients to supply baseline requirements in patients not able to take oral medications. The provider should be prepared to prescribe higher bolus doses in opioid-dependent patients compared to opioid-naïve patients and should shorten the lock-out interval for opioid-dependent patients using a PCA.

Once a patient can tolerate oral medications after surgery and the pain is well controlled with PCA, the patient may be switched to oral opioids. An equianalgesic table for conversion to oral opioids is featured in Table 54–1. Generally, the calculated equianalgesic amount of opioid medication is reduced by 50%–75% to account for incomplete cross-tolerance.

Opioid rotation or switching between different opioids is an option to improve analgesia while decreasing the overall daily opioid dose and opioid-related side effects for individual compound failures despite titration. Proposed mechanisms for the efficacy of opioid rotation include incomplete opioid cross-tolerance, active metabolites, and different opioid and nonopioid receptor affinity.[8] When rotating opioids, the equianalgesic dose should be reduced to account for incomplete cross-tolerance.

Clinical Pearl

- Regional anesthesia should be considered for opioid-dependent patients when appropriate.

Neuraxial Anesthesia

Neuraxial anesthesia with local anesthetics and opioids can provide effective pain control while minimizing the need to administer systemic analgesics. However, neuraxially administered opioids may not effectively prevent withdrawal if systemic opioids are not given as baseline. This is due to the fact that plasma concentrations and supraspinal binding of the opioid will decrease, resulting in withdrawal symptoms.[5]

Regional Anesthesia

Regional anesthesia should be considered for opioid-dependent patients where appropriate, especially for surgery on the extremities. Local anesthetic infiltration, specific nerve blocks, or plexus blocks all can provide complete or adjunct analgesia. The goal of regional anesthesia in the opioid-dependent patient is to provide adequate analgesia while also lowering or potentially eliminating the need to administer additional opioids.

Clinical Pearl

- Nonopioid adjuvants, including acetaminophen, NSAIDs, anticonvulsants, antidepressants, and ketamine, should be considered as part of a multimodal approach to pain control.

Ketamine

Ketamine, an NMDA receptor antagonist, can be used perioperatively as an infusion for adjunct analgesia. A ketamine infusion has been found to reduce pain intensity and opioid consumption at 48 hours postoperatively as well as at 6 months postoperatively following spinal surgery in opioid-dependent patients.[37] A low-dose ketamine infusion used intraoperatively and postoperatively may also enhance the effects of opioids, reduce opioid tolerance, and reduce opioid-induced hyperalgesia.[38,39]

TABLE 54–1. Opioid dose equivalence table.

Drug	mg PO	mg IV	Half-life (h)	Duration (h)
Morphine	30	10	2–3	3–4
MS Contin	30	—	2–3	8–12
Oxycodone	20	—	2–3	3–4
Oxycontin	20	—	2–3	8–12
Hydrocodone	30	—	3–4	4
Hydromorphone	7.5	1.5	2–3	2–4

Methadone	• 2
	• 24 h oral morphine/methodone ratio
	  • < 30 mg 2:1
	  • 31–99 mg 4:1
	  • 100–299 mg 8:1
	  • 300–499 mg 12:1
	  • 500–999 mg 15:1
	  • 1000–1200 mg 20:1
	  • > 1200 mg, *consider consult*
		1	12–100	4–12

Fentanyl	—	• 100 µg single dose IM/IV
		• 80 µg buccal
		• 24 h oral morphine dose/patch
		  • 30–59 mg = 12.5 µg/h
		  • 60–134 mg = 25 µg/h
		  • 135–224 mg = 50 µg/h
		  • 225–314 mg = 75 µg/h
		  • 315–404 mg = 100 µg/h
			10-20 min	48–72 per patch

Oxymorphone	10	1	3–14	4–24
Tapentadol	100	—	4	4–6
Tramadol	200	—	5.5–7	6–8
Buprenorphine	0.4 (sublingual only)	0.3	20–70	

IM, intramuscular; IV, intravenous; PO, *per os* (oral).

Source: Reproduced with permission from Atchabahian A, Gupta R: *The Anesthesia Guide.* New York: McGraw-Hill; 2013.

Acetaminophen

A single dose of intravenous acetaminophen has been found to provide 4–6 hours of effective analgesia for patients in variety of postoperative pain models with a decrease in overall opioid consumption and an increase in patient satisfaction.[40] In a review of the use of intravenous acetaminophen perioperatively, the majority of studies examined showed improved analgesia and decreased opioid requirements.[41] Dosing is usually 1 g intravenously every 6–8 hours, not to exceed the daily maximum dose of 4 g in an average-size adult patient. An oral combination opioid containing acetaminophen can be given 4 hours after intravenous acetaminophen. Care should be taken when using opioid–acetaminophen combination products to not exceed the maximum recommended daily dose of 4 g due to the risk of hepatotoxicity.

NSAIDs and Cyclooxygenase-2 Inhibitors

NSAIDs should be considered for all patients with mild or moderate acute pain unless contraindicated.[42] Examples of NSAIDs include ketorolac, ibuprofen, naproxen, and the newer cyclooxygenase-2 inhibitors (COXIBs). NSAIDs provide analgesia by inhibiting prostaglandin synthesis, which results in an anti-inflammatory effect. The prostaglandin synthesis inhibition results in NSAID side effects, however, including gastritis and platelet and renal dysfunction. Because of these side effects, NSAIDs are contraindicated in patients with renal dysfunction, gastritis, and peptic ulcer disease. The COXIBs do not affect platelets and have fewer effects on the gastrointestinal system.

Ketorolac is an intravenous NSAID approved for use in the United States for the indication of acute pain. A dose of 30 mg of intravenous ketorolac is equipotent to approximately 6–10 mg of intravenous morphine. Ketorolac has been shown to have an opioid-sparing effect, and its use has resulted in reduced opioid-related side effects.[43] The maximum recommended duration of use of intravenous ketorolac is 5 days.

Tramadol

Tramadol is a synthetic analog of codeine that is a weak mu-opioid receptor agonist. In addition to its effect on opioid receptors, tramadol has an additional analgesic effect by inhibiting the reuptake of norepinephrine and serotonin. Though not particularly effective in the treatment of severe pain alone, it can be used to treat mild to moderate pain in the postoperative period and has a lower abuse potential than other opioids.

Gabapentinoids

The gabapentinoids gabapentin and pregabalin are another option for the multimodal treatment of acute pain when they are administered in the perioperative period. The gabapentinoids are anticonvulsants that bind to voltage-gated calcium channels, reducing the release of excitatory neurotransmitters and producing an analgesic effect. In a systematic review of the literature, a single preoperative dose of gabapentin 1200 mg improved postoperative analgesia and decreased postoperative opioid consumption. The efficacy of multiple doses of gabapentin perioperatively was less conclusive due to a limited number of trials.[44] Based on a meta-analysis, pregabalin for postoperative pain appears to decrease opioid consumption and lower the incidence of opioid-related adverse effects postoperatively; most studies used preoperative dosing.[45] Side effects of both gabapentin and pregabalin include dizziness, ataxia, and somnolence. Table 54–2 presents suggested dosing regimens for these agents.

A Multidisciplinary Approach

The multimodal analgesic plan should be communicated with the patient and other members of the care team. Patients with chronic pain may have anxiety or depression that may benefit from the input of psychology or psychiatry services. Consultation with addiction specialists should be considered in patients with substance abuse.

DISCHARGE PLANNING

The multimodal plan should be continued with suggestions for dose reductions as the acute pain episode resolves. In patients with a history of opioid abuse, consideration should be given to limiting the amount of opioid prescribed and providing for early and frequent follow-up. Referrals to pain medicine specialists or addiction specialists may be considered.

REFERENCES

1. Gustin HB, Alik H: Opioid analgesics. In Hardman JG, Limbird LE (eds): *Goodman and Gilman's The Pharmacological Basis of Therapeutics*. New York: McGraw-Hill, 2001, pp 569–619.
2. Farrell M: Opiate withdrawal. Addiction 1994;89:1471–1475.
3. American Psychiatric Association: *Diagnostic and Statistical Manual of Mental Disorders*, 5th ed. Arlington, VA: American Psychiatric Publishing, 2013.
4. Stein C, Kopf A: Anesthesia and treatment of chronic pain. In Miller RD, Eriksson LI, Fleisher LA, Wiener-Kronish JP, Young WL (eds): *Miller's Anesthesia*, 7th ed. Philadelphia: Churchill Livingstone, 2009, pp 1803–1804.
5. Mitra S, Sinatra RS: Perioperative management of acute pain in the opioid-dependent patient. Anesthesiology 2004;101:212–227.
6. Miaskowski C, Cleary J, Buryney R, et al; The American Pain Society: Guideline for the management of cancer pain in adults and children. Glenview, IL: American Pain Society, 2005.
7. Centers for Disease Control and Prevention. United States Cancer Statistics. http://apps.nccd.cdc.gov/uscs/. Accessed June 10, 2013.
8. Huxtable CA, Roberts LJ, Somogyi AA, et al: Acute pain management in opioid-tolerant patients: a growing challenge. Anaesth Intensive Care 2011;39:804–823.
9. Chou R, Fanciullo GJ, Fine PG, et al: Clinical guidelines for the use of chronic opioid therapy in chronic noncancer pain. J Pain 2009;10:113–130.
10. Manchikanti L, Salahadin A, Atluri S, et al: American Society of Interventional Pain Physicians (ASIPP) guidelines for responsible opioid prescribing in chronic non-cancer pain: part 2—guidance. Pain Physician 2012;15:S67–S116.
11. Gourlay DL, Heit HA, Almahrezi A: Universal precautions in pain medicine: a rational approach to the treatment of chronic pain. Pain Med 2005;6:107–112.
12. Substance Abuse and Mental Health Services Administration. Results from the 2010 National Survey on Drug Use and Health: detailed table, table 7.1.a. http://www.samhsa.gov/data/NSDUH/2k10NSDUH/tabs/Sect7peTabs1to45.htm#Tab7.1A. Accessed June 11, 2013.
13. Centers for Disease Control and Prevention. Prescription painkiller overdose in the U.S. http://www.cdc.gov/features/vitalsigns/painkilleroverdoses/. Accessed June 1, 2013.
14. Centers for Disease Control and Prevention. Vital signs: overdoses of prescription opioid pain relievers. http://www.cdc.gov/mmwr/preview/mmwrhtml/mm6043a4.htm. Accessed June 30, 2013.
15. Minozzi S, Amato L, Davoli M, et al: Development of dependence following treatment with opioid analgesics for pain relief: a systematic review. Addiction 108:688–698, 2013.
16. Jamison RN, Kauffman J, Katz NP: Characteristics of methadone maintenance patients with chronic pain. J Pain Symptom Manage 2000;19:53–62.
17. Rosenblum A, Joseph H, Fong C, et al: Prevalence and characteristics of chronic pain among chemically dependent patients in methadone maintenance and residential treatment facilities. JAMA 2003;289:2370–2378.
18. Compton P, Athanasos P, Elashoff D: Withdrawal hyperalgesia after acute opioid physical dependence in nonaddicted humans: a preliminary study. J Pain 2003;4:511–19.
19. Angst MS, Clark JD: Opioid-induced hyperalgesia: a qualitative systematic review. Anesthesiology 2006;104:570–587.

TABLE 54–2. Dosing of perioperative gabapentin and pregabalin.

Drug	Dosing Recommendations
Gabapentin	Single preoperative dose of 1200 mg by mouth.[44]
Pregabalin	300 mg or 600 mg by mouth 1 hour prior to or after surgery. Consider repeating dose 12 hours after first dose.[45]

20. Bailey CP, Connor M: Opioids: cellular mechanisms of tolerance and physical dependence. Curr Opin Pharmacol 2005;5:60–68.

21. Lee M, Silverman SM, Hansen H, et al: A comprehensive review of opioid-induced hyperalgesia. Pain Physician 2011;14:145–165.

22. Silverman S: Opioid-induced hyperalgesia: clinical implications for the pain practitioner. Pain Physician 2009;12:679–684.

23. Li X, Angst MS, Clark JD: A murine model of opioid-induced hyperalgesia. Brain Res Mol Brain Res 2001;86:56–62.

24. Joly V, Richebe P, Guignard B, et al: Remifentanil-induced postoperative hyperalgesia and its prevention with small-dose ketamine. Anesthesiology 2005;103:147–155.

25. Gardell LR, Wang R, Burgess SE, et al: Sustained morphine exposure induces a spinal dynorphin-dependent enhancement of excitatory transmitter release from primary afferent fibers. J Neurosci 2002;22:6747–6755.

26. Vanderah TW, Suenaga NM, Ossipov MH, et al: Tonic descending facilitation from the rostral ventromedial medulla mediates opioid-induced abnormal pain and antinociceptive tolerance. J Neurosci 2001; 121:279–286.

27. King T, Gardell LR, Wang R, et al: Role of NK-1 neurotransmission in opioid-induced hyperalgesia. Pain 2005;116:276–288.

28. O'Brien CP: Drug addiction and drug abuse. In Hardman JG, Limbrid LE (eds): Goodman and Gilman's The Pharmacological Basis of Therapeutics, 10th ed. New York: McGraw-Hill, 2001, pp 621–642.

29. Moeller K, Lee K, Kissack J: Urine drug screening: practical guide for clinicians. Mayo Clin Proc 2008;83:66–76.

30. Bart G: Maintenance medication for opiate addiction: the foundation of recovery. J Addict Dis 2012;31:207–225.

31. Ferrari A, Coccia CP, Bertolini A, et al: Methadone—metabolism, pharmacokinetics and interactions. Pharmacol Res 2004;50:551–559.

32. Trafton JA, Ramani A: Methadone: a new old drug with promises and pitfalls. Curr Pain Headache Rep 2009;13:24–30.

33. Bryson EO, Lipson A, Gevirtz C: Anesthesia for patients on buprenorphine. Anesthesiol Clin 2010;28:611–617.

34. Alford DP, Compton P, Samet JH: Acute pain management for patients receiving maintenance methadone or buprenorphine therapy. Ann Intern Med 2006;144:127–134.

35. Rubenstein RB, Spira I, Wolff WI: Management of surgical problems in patients on methadone maintenance. Am J Surgery 1976;131:566–569.

36. Myles PS, Leslie K, McNeil J, et al: Bispectral index monitoring to prevent awareness during anaesthesia: the B-Aware randomized controlled trial. Lancet 2004;363:1757–1763.

37. Loftus RW, Yeager MP, Clark JA, et al: Intraoperative ketamine reduces perioperative opiate consumption in opiate-dependent patients with chronic back pain undergoing back surgery. Anesthesiology 2010;113:639–646.

38. Suzuki M, Tseuda K, Lansing PS, et al: Small-dose ketamine enhances morphine-induced analgesia for the management of pain in an opioid addict. Anesthesiology 2002;96:1265–1266.

39. Himmelseher S, Durieux ME: Ketamine for perioperative pain management. Anesthesiology 2005;102:211–220.

40. Tzortzopoulou A, McNicol ED, Cepeda MS, et al: Single dose intravenous propacetamol or intravenous parecetamol for postoperative pain. Cochrane Database Syst Rev 2011;10:CD007126. DOI: 10.1002/14651858. CD007126.pub2.

41. Macario A, Royal MA: A literature review of randomized clinical trials of intravenous acetaminophen (paracetamol) for acute postoperative pain. Pain Pract 2011;11:290–296.

42. American Society of Anesthesiologists Task Force on Acute Pain Management: Practice guidelines for acute pain management in the perioperative setting: an updated report by the American Society of Anesthesiologists Task Force on Acute Pain Management. Anesthesiology 2012;116:248–273.

43. Cepeda MS, Carr DB, Miranda N, et al: Comparison of morphine, ketorolac, and their combination for postoperative pain: results from a large, randomized, double-blind trial. Anesthesiology 2005;103:1225–1232.

44. Ho KY, Gan TJ, Habib AS: Gabapentin and postoperative pain: a systematic review of randomized controlled trials. Pain 2006;126:91–101.

45. Zhang J, Ho KY, Wang Y: Efficacy of pregabalin in acute postoperative pain: a meta-analysis. Br J Anaesth 2011;106:454–462.

CHAPTER 55

Regional Anesthesia in Patients with Trauma

Jeff Gadsden, Emily Lin, and Alicia L. Warlick

INTRODUCTION

Trauma is the leading cause of death in those aged 1–44 years and the third leading cause of death for all age groups.[1] Trauma accounts for 30% of all life years lost in the United States—more than cancer, heart disease, and HIV combined.[1] The economic burden of trauma exceeds $400 billion in the United States annually. This chapter aims to discuss the role of regional anesthesia within the overall framework of pain management in trauma, explore several examples of where regional anesthesia may affect outcomes in specific injuries, and briefly address the issue of acute compartment syndrome in the context of neuraxial and peripheral nerve blockade.

MANAGEMENT OF ACUTE PAIN IN PATIENT WITH TRAUMA

The management of pain in the acutely injured patient can be challenging. Resuscitation and the assessment and treatment of life-threatening injuries are the first priorities in the trauma patient, and provision of adequate analgesia must frequently be delayed until the patient is stable. However, there is mounting evidence that the pain associated with injury is often undertreated (oligoanalgesia).[2] There are several barriers to effective analgesia for trauma patients. Physicians are often hesitant to administer pain medications (especially systemic opioids) to trauma patients for fear of causing hemodynamic instability or respiratory depression and airway compromise. Patients with head and/or spinal cord injury require frequent reassessments, which may be impaired or obscured with systemic opioids. Opioid-induced delirium is also a concern, particularly in the elderly population. Trauma patients are frequently unable to communicate their pain intensity due to the need for sedation and mechanical ventilation, among other considerations, which can impair adequate pain assessment.

Analgesia is often unjustifiably delayed, even in patients with injuries that are not life threatening. In a study of 36 Australian emergency departments, patients who presented with hip fracture (n = 645) were found to have a mean time to first treatment of their fracture-related pain of 126 minutes.[2] Reported barriers included confusion/dementia, comorbidities such as head injury or hypotension, patient refusal, and language or communication problems. Notably, only 7% of these patients received a femoral nerve block. Another study of patients presenting to the emergency department predominantly with injuries of the extremities showed that while 91% had pain on admission (mean numeric rating scale rating 5.9), 86% still had pain upon discharge (mean numeric rating scale rating 5.0), and pain actually *increased* in 17% at the time of discharge.[3] Of the 450 patients in this study, only 19% received any type of pharmacologic pain therapy.

Intravenous opioids are the most common approach to treating pain in trauma patients. While opioids are potent analgesics and a rational choice in patients with multiple injuries, they carry a significant burden of potential adverse effects, including the following:[4]

- Nausea and vomiting
- Constipation
- Delirium
- Vasodilation and hypotension (especially in hypovolemia)
- Respiratory depression
- Pruritus
- Immunosuppression
- Increased staffing requirements to monitor the patient (primarily due to the risk of respiratory depression)
- Increased length of stay in emergency department or recovery room

Rather than single-drug therapy with opioids, a multimodal approach is increasingly becoming a standard approach for treating pain in a wide variety of elective surgical patients, where it has been shown to lead to a reduction in both opioid requirements and opioid-related adverse effects.[5,6] Examples include nonsteroidal anti-inflammatory drugs (NSAIDs), acetaminophen, gabapentinoids, ketamine, and corticosteroids, as well as locoregional analgesia. One difference between the trauma and elective surgical populations is the frequent inability to utilize the oral route for medications in trauma patients due to sedation, neurologic impairment, or the presence of an airway device. Fortunately, many of the standard multimodal classes of drugs are available in parenteral form, including ketamine, acetaminophen, ketorolac, clonidine, and dexmedetomidine.

THE ROLE OF REGIONAL ANESTHESIA IN TRAUMA

Musculoskeletal injury is common in the trauma patient. While skeletal fractures and muscular injuries can occur anywhere on the body, the extremities are disproportionately affected. Approximately 60% of multiple-trauma patients with an injury severity score of ≥ 16 have an extremity injury of some type, and 18% have both lower and upper extremity injuries.[7] Over 30% of the same population will have 2 or more extremity fractures. Since the majority of regional anesthesia procedures involve the extremities, its role in analgesia for trauma patients is particularly well suited.

Mechanism of injury is an important epidemiologic factor—for example, those in motor vehicle crashes (MVCs) have a significantly higher prevalence of extremity injury; similarly, due to improvements in battlefield medicine and body armor, modern military combatants have a dramatically reduced rate of fatal torso injury. As a result, more trauma victims are surviving with higher rates of extremity injury. While patients with isolated extremity injuries tend to have favorable outcomes, it has been shown that orthopedic and general health outcomes are significantly poorer if the same injury is present in a polytrauma patient.[8]

Regional anesthetic techniques, and peripheral nerve blocks in particular, provide high-quality analgesia that is site specific and devoid of any systemic (especially opioid-related) side effects. Regional anesthesia may also confer several other advantages over systemic analgesic therapies for trauma patients, including decreased length of stay in the emergency department and critical care unit,[9,10] improved ability to perform neurologic assessments,[11] improved comfort and safety for transport,[11,12] and cost savings compared to procedural sedation.[13]

The persistence of pain well beyond the time of injury and the development of chronic pain is a significant problem following acute injury. Up to 77% of patients who incur severe musculoskeletal trauma will report posttraumatic chronic pain, defined as pain lasting greater than 3 months from the time of injury.[14] There are multiple risk factors that contribute to the likelihood of transitioning from acute to chronic pain. These include age, comorbid medical conditions, depression or anxiety states, and alcohol and tobacco consumption. The risk factor that appears to be most predictive of eventual chronic pain is the intensity of acute pain at the time of injury (odds ratio

between 2.4 and 11.2).[15,16] Regional anesthesia has been shown to significantly reduce acute pain intensity in traumatic injury.[17] Despite this, the evidence supporting the preventive role of regional anesthesia in the development of chronic pain in trauma is very weak at present, and properly powered, randomized, controlled studies are needed.[14] Regardless, there are multiple other benefits in providing high-quality analgesia in the acute setting with regional anesthesia and analgesia.

Clinical Pearls

- Up to 77% of patients with severe musculoskeletal trauma may develop chronic posttraumatic pain.
- The severity of the acute pain is predictive of development of chronic pain after trauma.

CONTINUOUS PERIPHERAL NERVE BLOCKS IN PATIENTS WITH TRAUMA

Single-injection techniques with bupivacaine or ropivacaine can be expected to provide 16–24 hours of analgesia, whereas continuous peripheral nerve block (CPNB) techniques can significantly prolong the duration of analgesia. The pain intensity associated with trauma is often severe and longstanding, making CPNBs useful. Catheters can be left in for days to weeks. Patients with complex injuries that require repeated debridement, fracture fixation, and/or skin grafting may benefit from indwelling catheters (Figure 55–1). The pumps can be programmed to deliver a background infusion of a low-concentration, long-acting local anesthetic (eg, 0.1%–0.2% ropivacaine) while on the ward or intensive care unit. The catheters can be manually bolused with a higher-concentration solution upon return to the operating room to provide surgical anesthesia. Buckenmaier et al. described a series of 187 patients injured in combat who were treated with CPNBs for a median of

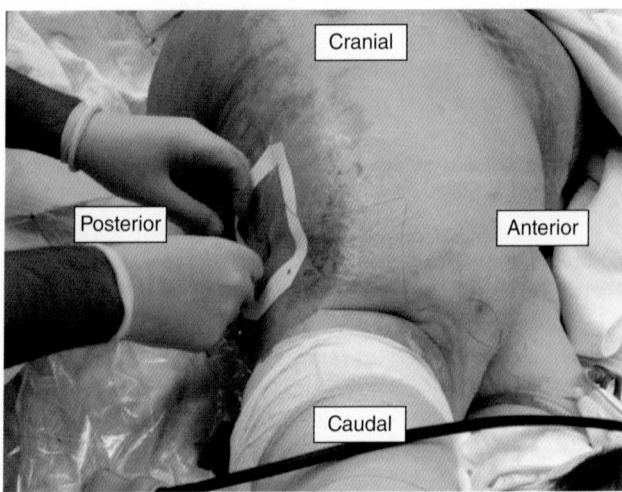

FIGURE 55–1. A popliteal catheter being placed for the management of pain following a traumatic amputation of the foot.

8 days (range 1–33 days); catheter-specific complications were rare (3.7%) and included kinking, dislodgement, and superficial infection.[18] It should be noted that these data reflect a specific patient population: healthy, fit, young soldiers. Catheter techniques in the elderly and unhealthy civilian trauma victims may have additional challenges, although there are limited data to suggest that these techniques have a lower safety profile in certain age or physical status subpopulations.

Colonization and infection of the catheter site is a concern when using an indwelling catheter in the trauma population, since these patients are at risk for bacteremia and sepsis, and procedures are often performed in less than ideal environments, such as the emergency room or intensive care unit (ICU). Capdevila et al. demonstrated that injured patients admitted to a trauma ICU were 5 times more likely to develop a CPNB catheter infection than elective surgical patients.[19] Other factors reported to increase the risk of catheter infection include duration of catheter use greater than 48 hours, the use of prophylactic antibiotics, insertion at the femoral or axillary location, and frequent dressing changes.[19–23] Catheter type may also play a role in the development of infection. Lai et al. reported a case series of 2 superficial and 4 deep infections, in which the deep infections requiring operative incision and drainage were associated with stimulating catheter use.[24] The authors hypothesized that repetitive movements of a catheter with an internal metal coil could result in microhematoma formation, providing a rich culture medium for hematogenously spread bacteria. Despite these data, the overall incidence is still low, with only 0%–3% of all catheters showing evidence of infection.

Approximately 20% of polytrauma patients have both upper and lower extremity injuries; thus, the opportunity to use multiple catheters arises frequently. Plunkett and Buckenmaier placed bilateral sciatic nerve catheters and a single femoral nerve catheter in a patient with bilateral leg injuries who was receiving treatment doses of enoxaparin that precluded epidural analgesia.[25] Care must be taken to consider the dose of local anesthetic that is being delivered in order to prevent toxic plasma levels; however, this is rarely an issue since the concentrations that are used clinically for catheters are low (eg, 0.1%–0.2% ropivacaine). One prospective study of 13 combat trauma patients receiving 0.2% ropivacaine infusions at 6–14 mL/h for a period of 4–25 days showed a median unbound plasma ropivacaine level over the duration of the study of 0.11 mg/L (range: undetectable–0.63 mg/L) with no reports of toxic events.[26] The toxic unbound plasma concentration of ropivacaine is approximately 0.6 mg/L.[27] However, two patients' plasma levels neared this threshold after a large dose (60 mL bolus of 0.5% ropivacaine) prior to the determination of the plasma level. Taken together, these data suggest that long-term infusions of ropivacaine at low concentrations are safe in the trauma population. Notwithstanding, polytrauma patients frequently have two catheters infusing simultaneously, which may increase the risk of toxic plasma levels of local anesthetic. Common strategies to mitigate this risk include lowering the concentration of the local anesthetic infusate (eg, ropivacaine 0.1% or 0.15% rather than 0.2%) and/or relying more on periodic intermittent boluses than on a high-rate continuous background infusion.

REGIONAL ANALGESIA IN THE EMERGENCY DEPARTMENT AND PREHOSPITAL SETTINGS

Regional anesthesia has been used effectively in the emergency department for injured patients requiring analgesia for a variety of indications, including hip fracture, as well as during procedures such as reductions of fractures or dislocated joints and repair of lacerations. Compared to procedural sedation, upper extremity blocks confer several advantages. Interscalene block for shoulder reduction has been shown to reduce emergency department length of stay and the requirement for one-to-one monitoring.[10] Patients with upper extremity fractures, dislocations, and/or abscesses who received supraclavicular block for their procedure experienced a shorter length of stay without any impact on patient safety or satisfaction.[9] Ultrasound-guided intercostal blocks have been effective for chest drain placement following traumatic pneumothorax.[28]

Clinical Pearl

- Peripheral nerve blocks improve clinical flow and decrease the length of stay in the ED compared to procedural sedation for selected procedures.

Anesthesiologists are typically the physicians most qualified to perform nerve blocks. However, due to work demands and time constraints, anesthesiologists may not be able to attend to patients in the emergency department or critical care unit in a prompt manner, leading to significant delays in providing quality analgesia. Randall et al. reported the results of a successful initiative to train orthopedic nurses in the performance of fascia iliaca blockade.[29] This creation of a "physician extender" improved patient access to effective pain control with the use of a simple and safe procedure that is easily taught. (The topic of regional and local anesthesia in the emergency department is covered in more detail in Chapter 60.)

It may also be safe and appropriate to provide regional analgesia in the field or during transport to hospital. This decision has to be made in the context of the skill and experience of the doctors or medics attending to the patient, as well as the nature and severity of the injuries. In North America, where emergency medical services (EMS) teams are largely staffed by paramedics, emergency medical technicians (EMTs), or firefighters as first responders, there is a limited set of interventions available. In some parts of the world, physicians (eg, anesthesiologists in western Europe) highly trained in resuscitative and trauma medicine are dispatched by ambulance and helicopter to perform retrievals; these tend to be systems that benefit most from on-scene triaging, evaluation, and intervention.

Several studies have shown the fascia iliaca block to significantly reduce pain associated with femoral shaft or neck fractures when performed at the scene of the accident or injury.[30–33] Advantages to the fascia iliaca block include minimal equipment required (a syringe and needle), a simple approach that does not rely on ultrasound or nerve stimulation, and a good safety profile with little chance of puncturing a vessel or nerve. Femoral block has also been reported to be effective in prehospital care, but its success depends more on the experience and skill level of the operator.

Additional block techniques that have been reported to successfully reduce pain intensity prior to arriving at hospital include sciatic nerve block,[34] interscalene nerve block,[35] multiple nerve blocks about the elbow,[36] and digital nerve block.[37]

SPECIFIC INJURIES: HIP FRACTURES

Fracture of the femur at the hip joint is a very common injury and is associated with significant morbidity and mortality. Patients with hip fracture tend to be older and have multiple medical comorbidities, placing them at higher risk for complications, especially chest infection, delirium, and heart failure.[38] Over 95% of hip fractures are fall related.[1] Falls are the leading cause of death in adults over 64 years of age, with hip fracture being the most serious and costly injury resulting from a fall.[39]

The reported pain intensity from a fractured hip can be moderate to severe. The pain resulting from these fractures is well suited to regional techniques due to the anatomical location of the fractures. In a systematic review of 83 studies addressing various analgesic options for hip fracture (including systemic analgesia, traction, multimodal pain management, and neurostimulation), the only intervention that was found to be effective at reducing acute pain was peripheral nerve blockade.[40]

An understanding of the osteotomal innervation of the femur and hip joint is important in block planning. (Figure 55–2). Several studies have demonstrated that a femoral nerve block reduces pain intensity following hip fracture and is a valuable adjunct in this population, allowing patients to sit up, move in bed, breathe deeply, and cough with reduced pain while awaiting surgery.[41–43] A Cochrane collaboration review of nerve blocks in patients with hip fracture concluded that femoral nerve block resulted in significant reductions in both pain

intensity and opioid requirements both preoperatively and during surgery.[44]

Several studies have found that fascia iliaca block reduced pain scores and opioid requirements in patients with hip fracture. Fascia iliaca block aims to block the femoral and lateral femoral cutaneous nerve (and possibly the obturator nerve) with one injection. The technique is less technically demanding than femoral nerve block, but when compared to femoral block, fascia iliaca may not provide the same degree of pain relief.[43,45] This may be due to imprecise placement of the local anesthetic during what is traditionally a landmark technique, relying on the spread of a large (30–40 mL) volume for efficacy.[33,46] Ultrasound guidance increases the frequency of sensory loss of all three nerves compared to the landmark technique.[46] Obturator nerve block appears to also be an effective analgesic technique following hip fracture, which is not surprising given the proportion of the proximal femur and hip joint innervated by this nerve.[47] However, this technique is not as widely practiced as femoral blockade and even with ultrasound guidance is an intermediate-level technique, limiting its widespread use.

Patients with hip fracture benefit from regional analgesia immediately on admission to hospital, both to improve comfort and reduce the side effects of opioids. An increasing number of hospitals have a hip fracture clinical pathway that includes femoral nerve block placement in the emergency department. Catheter techniques are particularly valuable in this situation since patients with hip fracture may not receive their operative fixation for 48 hours or longer for various medical or logistical reasons. Pedersen et al. introduced a care pathway for hip fracture that replaced parenteral opioids with a continuous femoral nerve block in a retrospective cohort study; the nerve block group had a significantly reduced incidence of in-hospital complication (odds ratio 0.61, 95% CI 0.4–0.9, P = 0.002), as well as significantly reduced rates of confusion and pneumonia.[48] Mortality was also decreased from 23% to 12%, although this trend was not present in patients who were admitted from nursing homes.

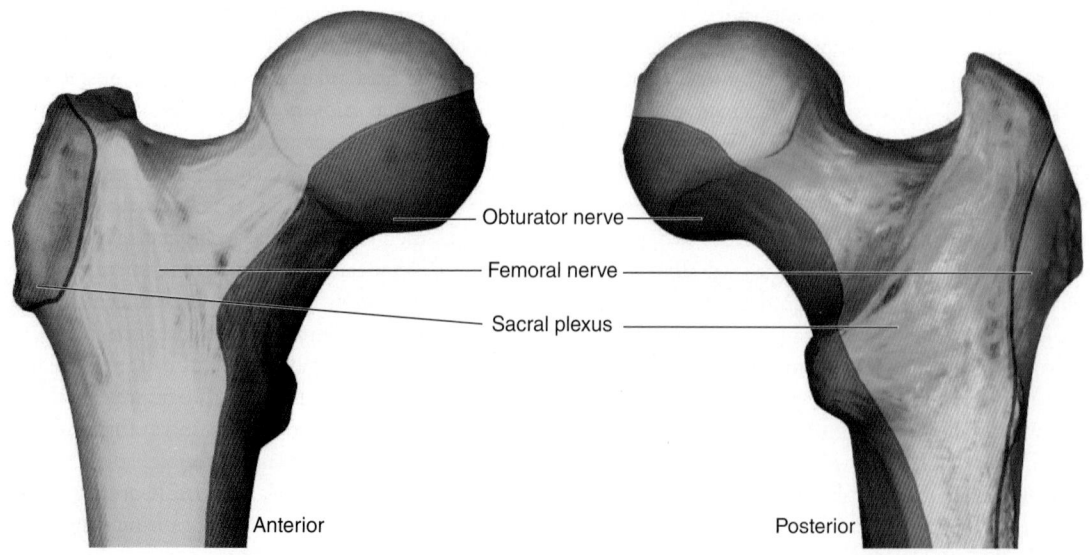

FIGURE 55–2. Osteotomal innervation of the proximal femur.

Confusion and delirium are common in the hospitalized elderly patient. Delirium is an independent risk factor for death, institutionalization, and dementia after hip fracture.[49] Two factors that are known to substantially increase the likelihood of delirium are moderate to severe pain and opioids, both of which can be minimized with regional techniques. The impact of regional analgesia on the risk for developing perioperative delirium is unclear, and the absence of effect in some studies likely relates to the complex pathophysiology of delirium. However, there may be specific subpopulations of hip fracture patients who benefit from nerve blocks. Mouzopolous et al. risk-stratified hip fracture patients for delirium on admission using a validated instrument and investigated the effect of daily fascia iliaca block on delirium in intermediate- and high-risk patients.[50] No difference was seen between high-risk patients who received the block with bupivacaine versus a sham block. However, intermediate-risk patients in the fascia iliaca block with bupivacaine group were significantly less likely (2%) to become delirious versus those in the sham block group (17%). Data from these studies support the idea that regional analgesic techniques should be initiated timely in hip fracture patients and continued until pain intensity is sufficiently low that oral nonopioid analgesics are all that are required for pain management.

Clinical Pearl

- A clinical pathway including a femoral nerve block and/or catheter may reduce the incidence of confusion, delirium, pneumonia and opioid requirements for patients with hip fracture.

The best choice of *anesthetic* technique for operative fixation of hip fracture is still a matter of some controversy. Several recent large studies have focused on this question. Luger and colleagues conducted a meta-analysis of 34 randomized, controlled trials, 14 observational studies, and 8 reviews/meta-analysis publications (n = 18,715) and demonstrated that neuraxial anesthesia was associated with significantly reduced early mortality, fewer incidents of deep venous thrombosis, less postoperative confusion, and fewer overall pulmonary complications, including postoperative hypoxia, pneumonia, and fatal pulmonary embolism.[51] There were no differences between groups in the rates of arrhythmias, myocardial events, congestive heart failure, intraoperative blood loss, renal failure, or stroke. Hypotension seemed to occur independent of anesthetic technique, although continuous spinal appeared to have an advantage over single-injection spinal in this regard. Geriatric patients are typically at low risk for postdural puncture headache, and the placement of a spinal catheter is usually free of side effects.

In 2012, Neuman and colleagues published a retrospective analysis of a prospectively collected database collected over 2 years from 126 New York State hospitals.[52] Over 18,000 patients admitted for hip fracture from 126 hospitals were identified and the association between type of anesthesia and patient outcomes tested. Regional anesthesia in this study reduced the risk of in-hospital mortality relative to general anesthesia by 29% and the risk of pulmonary complications by 25%. There was no difference between groups with regard to cardiovascular morbidity.

More recently, White et al. reported the results of an observational audit of over 65,000 patients from the National Hip Fracture Database in the United Kingdom.[53] The authors specifically looked at early mortality and found no difference between groups receiving general versus neuraxial anesthesia in terms of either 5-day or 30-day mortality. The authors suggest that with modern advances in pharmacotherapy and monitoring, as well as improved methods for optimizing patients prior to surgery, may have diminished any difference in this metric. They also suggest that our research efforts should now be focused on postoperative confusion, hypotension, pain, mobility, and respiratory complications.

On balance, it appears that data tend to show that there are morbidity advantages to regional anesthesia techniques, if not mortality advantages. Although regional anesthesia is not yet a standard of care, the burden of proof is increasingly on the anesthesia provider to demonstrate why it would be more appropriate to proceed with a general rather than regional anesthetic in this group of patients.

SPECIFIC INJURIES: FRACTURED RIBS

Rib fractures are the most common injury associated with chest trauma, with an incidence of 12% of all trauma admissions.[54] The number of rib fractures is directly related to the associated mortality: 5% for 1–2 ribs, 15% for 3–5 ribs, and 34% for 6 or more ribs fractured.[54] The cause of mortality is related primarily to pulmonary injury, such as lung contusion and pneumothorax, and delayed pulmonary processes, such as pneumonia and acute respiratory distress syndrome.[55] Fractured ribs are a marker of injury severity, especially in young patients with compliant ribs cages where this injury is associated with more impact energy.

Fractured ribs and significant pain may limit the patient's ability to breathe adequately. The lack of deep inspiratory sighs and shallow tidal breathing promote atelectasis, V/Q mismatching, and hypoxemia, increasing the risk of pneumonia and respiratory failure. Chest physiotherapy is usually either contraindicated or ineffective due to the chest wall pain. Effective analgesia for patients with rib fractures is the primary management goal for these patients, since operative fixation is not performed in most cases. There are several options available for pain management, and the management plan should be individualized, as there is no one best modality for all patients. The goal of therapy should be to minimize respiratory depression and optimize respiratory excursion, while minimizing the possible side effects and complications of the technical procedure, such as local anesthetic systemic toxicity (LAST) or iatrogenic pneumothorax.

Intravenous opioids are a common analgesic option but have the downside of causing sedation and respiratory depression; because of this, opioids may in fact promote respiratory complications at the same time that they reduce pain. NSAIDs can be effective for mild rib fracture pain but may potentiate bleeding in patients who have vascular injury or are taking anticoagulant medications. Acetaminophen is a fairly safe mild analgesic with few side effects, but its effect is limited in multiple rib fractures when pain intensity is high.

There are several regional analgesic options for relief of rib fracture pain. Thoracic epidural analgesia (TEA) is a very effective regional anesthetic technique for broken ribs, especially when injuries are bilateral. The Eastern Association for the Surgery of Trauma (EAST) has stated that epidural analgesia may improve clinically significant outcomes (Grade B recommendation) and that it should be considered the preferred analgesic modality (Grade A recommendation).[56] Several studies have evaluated the effect of TEA on outcomes. Bulger et al. randomized 46 patients with 3 or more rib fractures to receive either TEA with bupivacaine or intravenous opioid therapy.[57] Despite a higher severity of pulmonary injury in the epidural group, the incidence of pneumonia was significantly higher in the opioid group (38% vs. 18%). When adjusted for the presence of direct pulmonary injury, the relative risk of pneumonia in the opioid group was 6-fold higher. In addition, randomization to epidural analgesia decreased the number of days requiring mechanical ventilation by half. This reduction in ventilator-dependent days has also been shown in other randomized, controlled studies.[58,59] TEA also reduces the pain associated with coughing or deep breathing compared with intravenous opioids or intrapleural bupivacaine.[60-62] In contrast, a retrospective review of 64 patients with rib fractures demonstrated that while TEA provided superior analgesia to intravenous patient-controlled morphine, hospital or ICU length of stay and major morbidity were unaffected.[63] Furthermore, a meta-analysis of 8 studies (n = 232) also failed to show a difference in major outcomes such as mortality, hospital/ICU length of stay, and duration of mechanical ventilation with epidural analgesia, although the studies chosen were heterogeneous, with both lumbar and thoracic epidural sites included and various combinations of local anesthetic and/or epidural opioid in the infusate.[64]

Although TEA may be effective at reducing morbidity and other outcomes in the setting of rib fractures, it is not appropriate for all patients. Contraindications include hypovolemia and hypotension, coagulopathy, head or spinal injury, and sepsis, conditions that are all relatively common in the trauma population. Thoracic epidural analgesia is performed infrequently in patients who are heavily sedated or under general anesthesia because of the traditional belief that the absence of patient feedback may put the patient at risk for a needle-related spinal cord injury. For this reason, the actual impact of TEA on the reduction in ventilator-dependent days may be limited, since these patients are likely to be sedated and mechanically ventilated prior to consultation for pain management.

Paravertebral nerve block (PVB) is an alternative regional anesthetic procedure that provides excellent unilateral (or bilateral, if performed on both sides) analgesia.[65] A catheter technique is typically employed for fractured ribs, with the needle insertion at the midpoint of the rib levels. The block can then be manipulated to the desired level by the administration of increasing volumes of local anesthetic. In a randomized study

of TEA versus thoracic PVB for unilateral multiple fractured ribs, both techniques were found to be equivalent with respect to pain relief, improvement in respiratory function, and incidence of pulmonary complications.[66] The risks of the technique are generally small and include contralateral spread via the epidural space (1%), pneumothorax (0.5%), hypotension (5%), and vascular puncture (4%).[67]

One unique advantage to PVB catheters over TEA is the ability to provide long-duration analgesia in the ambulatory setting. Murata and colleagues reported a case of a patient with multiple (T3–T8) unilateral rib fractures who was experiencing intense pain and respiratory distress.[68] A paravertebral catheter provided rapid and long-lasting (60 h) relief and facilitated discharge home from the critical care unit the day after the block. In another example, Buckley et al. reported that an anesthesiology resident who was experiencing debilitating pain from multiple fractured ribs was able to continue clinical work opioid-free while receiving an infusion of local anesthetic through a paravertebral catheter for a total of 18 days.[69]

Clinical Pearls

- Continuous paravertebral analgesia provides excellent relief from pain associated with rib fractures and facilitates improved respiratory mechanics.
- Selected patients can be safely discharged home with paravertebral catheters for days to weeks in order to prolong the high-quality analgesia.

Alternative regional techniques have been used but have not been shown to be as effective as either TEA or PVB. Intercostal blocks provide good initial relief but suffer from a limited duration of action and the need to repeat the procedure.[70] In addition, the risk of pneumothorax with each level attempted is additive and thus increases the risk of this complication. Intrapleural block with local anesthetic is similarly limited in efficacy and carries a high risk for rapid systemic absorption of local anesthetic.[71] Transdermal lidocaine patches placed over rib fracture sites have not been shown to significantly improve pain control in patients with traumatic rib fractures.[72]

SPECIFIC INJURIES: DIGITAL REPLANTATION

Long-term graft function after digital replantation (Figure 55–3) is contingent on the grafted digits receiving an optimal blood supply and the avoidance of vasospasm and thrombosis. Continuous nerve blocks of the limbs facilitate these goals first and foremost by providing sympathetic blockade, which interrupts injury-induced vasospasm and allows maximal vasodilation. The profound reduction in afferent input reduces the stress response, which both reduces the tendency toward hypercoagulability and potential thrombotic events and reduces circulating catecholamines, thereby promoting maximal vasodilation. Acral systolic blood pressure and flow are improved, and the muscle relaxation associated with a continuous nerve block

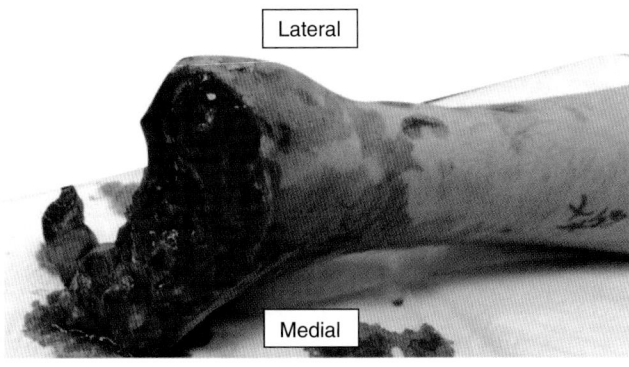

Lateral

Medial

FIGURE 55–3. Multiple digital amputations resulting from an industrial accident. An infraclavicular catheter was placed preoperatively and local anesthetic infused for 6 days. All four fingers that were replanted survived with good function.

helps to prevent inadvertent movement-related mishaps with the delicate anastomoses.[73]

Improvements in outcomes with continuous brachial plexus blockade have been demonstrated in several studies. In one study that randomized patients to continuous supraclavicular block versus parenteral opioids for digit transfer and/or replantation, reoperation rates due to vascular insufficiency were 0% vs. 29%, respectively.[74] Skin temperature, a marker of tissue perfusion, is consistently elevated in patients with brachial plexus blocks.[75–77] Pain scores have also been shown to be improved, as well as the incidence of vasospasm.[74,77] On the other hand, one study failed to show a difference in overall graft survival at 6 months when continuous brachial plexus block was used.[78] However, the retrospective nature of this study limits the strength of its conclusions. Additional prospective, randomized studies are needed to clarify the extent of the impact of these techniques on outcomes.

REGIONAL ANESTHESIA FOR SHOULDER REDUCTION

Reduction of a dislocated shoulder is a common procedure performed in the emergency department. Intravenous procedural sedation using propofol, ketamine, or etomidate is commonly employed to produce sufficient muscle relaxation to reduce the joint.[79] However, procedural sedation is often not ideal for such short and limited procedures. Approximately 6 hours of fasting is required to reduce the risk of gastric aspiration, a condition not commonly met in trauma patients presenting to the emergency room. Hypotension and respiratory compromise are real risks, especially with the use of such potent cardiopulmonary depressive agents as propofol. These risks mandate close monitoring and one-on-one care in the emergency room that can occupy nursing resources.

Regional anesthesia, particularly interscalene brachial plexus block (ISB), offers an attractive alternative that eases the requirements for performing shoulder dislocation reduction. ISB provides profound shoulder girdle muscle relaxation by anesthetizing the superior trunk of the brachial plexus. ISB does not require sedation, and, although cardiorespiratory monitoring is still required, the risk of apnea or hypotension is

virtually nonexistent. Blaivas et al. demonstrated that length of stay in the emergency department and the need for one-on-one care are reduced in patients receiving ISB versus procedural sedation for shoulder reduction.[10]

REGIONAL ANESTHESIA FOR BURNS

Early management of burn injuries should focus on (1) an airway with a low threshold for intubation; (2) breathing with the availability of high-flow 100% oxygen administration; and (3) aggressive fluid resuscitation. Standard protocols suggest 2-4 mL/kg of crystalloid for each 1% body surface area (BSA) affected. This applies to large burns only (ie >20% total BSA) given this population's increased vascular permeability and fluid requirement.[80]

Pain related to burn injuries can range from mild to debilitating, depending on the area involved and the depth of the burn. Skin nociceptors that are not destroyed transmit pain immediately after injury, and the perception of pain is complicated by both primary and secondary hyperalgesia, which occur at the wound and spinal level, respectively. Patients with extensive burns often experience more postoperative pain at the split-thickness skin donor site than in the grafted wound itself. Single-injection nerve blocks have provided much success in the harvesting of these donor sites.[81,82] Burn patients, however, commonly require repeated visits to the operating room and painful procedures such as physical therapy and dressing changes in the burn unit. This pattern of brief, intense painful procedures superimposed on moderate background pain makes effective analgesia challenging in these patients. Such procedures can occasionally be severe enough to require general anesthesia or deep sedation in the ICU or operating room. This is disadvantageous for a number of reasons, not least of which is the frequent interruption of enteral nutrition to keep patients fasted at a time when anything by mouth (*nil per os*, NPO) at a time when their metabolic demand is supranormal.

Therefore, the use of continuous peripheral or neuraxial catheter may be favored over single-injection techniques whenever appropriate.[83] Given the greater risk of infection from the loss of a protective barrier and altered immune response in burn patients, the decision to use catheters should be made carefully. Catheters should not be placed through burned skin. Burns result in a hypercoagulable state, and deep blocks or neuraxial analgesic techniques are generally safe, unless the patient develops coagulation abnormalities from sepsis or profound blood loss without factor replacement.

Multiple peripheral nerve catheters can aid in covering extensive burn injuries. While the principal concern with continuous infusions is systemic toxicity, evidence has shown this to be rare with clinically relevant dosing regimens and primarily a theoretical concern (see discussion above under heading "Continuous Peripheral Nerve Blockade in Patients with Trauma").[26] Moreover, plasma levels of alpha-1 acid glycoprotein (AAG), the plasma protein and acute phase reactant that binds local anesthetics, are known to be significantly elevated in burns (and trauma in general) for at least 20 days, which may help to provide an increased margin of safety in these patients.

Much of the morbidity in burn patients is due to the significant stress response that results, with its attendant effects on metabolism, wound healing, and immune function. Neural blockade of a burned area can substantially reduce this profound stress response via its inhibition of nociceptive input to the central nervous system. It has been demonstrated that neural blockade reduces the incidence of hyperalgesia following thermal injury.[84] Moreover, regional anesthesia results in reduced vasospasm and local thrombosis during skin grafting procedures, effects that are detrimental to graft function.

ACUTE COMPARTMENT SYNDROME CONSIDERATIONS

Acute compartment syndrome (ACS) is a serious soft tissue injury of an extremity that can occur following trauma. This pathologic syndrome arises when the pressure within a closed compartment rises above a capillary perfusion pressure, compromising the circulation and tissue function within that space. This is typically the result of a high-energy injury to soft tissue but has also been reported with crush or reperfusion injury, exercise, arterial puncture, circumferential dressings, burns, and snake bites. Over one-third of all cases of ACS are associated with tibial fracture, particularly the proximal and middle thirds of the diaphysis (due to the bulkier muscle mass compared with the ankle). Fractures of the forearm are also common injuries that may lead to ACS.

Clinical Pearls

- ACS occurs in areas packed with muscles, such as the proximal leg or forearm.
- The risk of ACS is highest in proximal tibial fractures, occurring at a rate of approximately 6%–10%.

Following capillary collapse, flow into the venous system ceases, leading to tissue hypoxia and the release of vascular mediators. The resultant leakage of fluid through capillary and muscle membranes increases edema and worsens the intracompartmental pressure, leading to a vicious cycle of increased pressure → ischemia → leakage → increased pressure. Tissue pressure in muscular compartments is usually 0–10 mm Hg, and capillary filling pressure is equivalent to diastolic arterial pressure. When the gradient between tissue pressure and diastolic blood pressure falls to within 30 mm Hg, the risk for capillary collapse and the development of ACS rises significantly. Emergent fasciotomy is required to release the tense muscles from the inelastic osteofascial compartments (Figure 55–4); if not performed within 3–6 hours of the onset of ischemia, myonecrosis occurs, followed by rhabdomyolysis, myoglobinuria, acute tubular necrosis, and hyperkalemia. ACS can be a fatal complication.

Regional anesthesia and analgesia in the presence of injuries at high risk for ACS remain controversial. Many anesthesiologists and orthopedic surgeons agree to avoid regional techniques for fear that the neural blockade may mask the

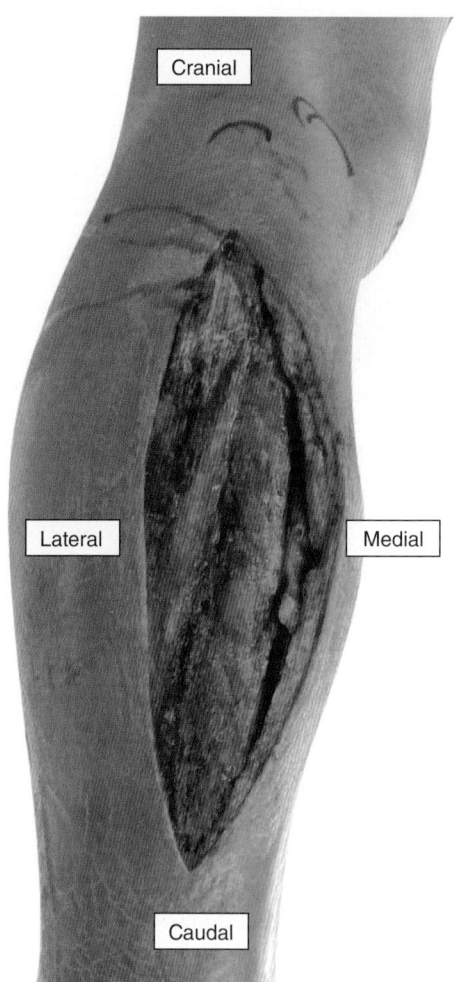

FIGURE 55–4. Fasciotomy of the anterior and lateral compartments of the leg to relieve acute compartment syndrome following a tibial fracture.

developing syndrome, since ACS is traditionally diagnosed on the basis of pain out of proportion to the injury (especially on passive stretch) and paresthesia.[85] However, these clinical signs and symptoms appear to have a sensitivity and positive predictive value of only 11%–19%, whereas the specificity and negative predictive value for lower leg injuries are 97%–98%.[86] In other words, the classic clinical findings are more likely to be present in an injured patient without ACS than in a patient with the syndrome. While the absence of clinical signs and symptoms appears to be a reassuring sign, it is unlikely that a patient who has a sufficiently serious injury to be at risk for ACS would be free of pain, therefore calling into question the utility of the high negative predictive value. In addition, these signs are probably even less useful in the sedated or neurologically impaired patient.

A handful of case reports have been published relating specifically to peripheral nerve blocks and ACS. However, in all but one of these cases, a nerve block actually *facilitated* the early detection and prompt treatment of the ischemic limb by the development of new-onset breakthrough pain, alerting the clinicians to a change in the status.[87–91] One case report did assert that a femoral block was responsible for a missed anterior compartment syndrome of the leg following intramedullary nailing.

However, the anterior compartment is supplied by the deep peroneal nerve, making femoral block a very unlikely contributing factor.[92] In contrast to peripheral nerve blockade, epidural analgesia has been implicated in at least 3 reports of ACS when dense motor block has been present.[85] This finding highlights the need to use dilute solutions of local anesthetics when placing peripheral nerve blocks in trauma patients. Catheter techniques are particularly effective and safe, as the concentration of the local anesthetic can be adjusted to match the intervention (surgical procedure vs. postoperative pain), and the infusion can be stopped entirely if required. Catheters can be placed at any time during the hospital course and left "dry" (or with a small infusion of saline to prevent clotting) and bolused when appropriate.

Clinical Pearl

- To date, there are no published cases of regional anesthesia delaying the diagnosis of ACS. In contrast, there are several reports of pain breaking through a block, which has facilitated the early diagnosis of a developing ACS.

Since randomized controlled trials are unlikely to be forthcoming due to ethical issues, hard data on the safety of nerve blocks is unavailable. Furthermore, it is possible that the diagnosis of ACS in the setting of peripheral nerve blocks is underreported or simply avoided in high-risk patients. Rather than focusing on whether or not to perform a PNB, our attention might better be directed toward careful monitoring of analgesic consumption and breakthrough pain and the use of compartment pressure monitoring for high-risk patients. Vigilance by both surgical and anesthetic teams involved in the patient's care is the key to the early detection of ACS. More information on the pathophysiology of acute compartment syndrome can be found in Chapter 51.

SUMMARY

Patients with acute trauma frequently require complex management, with coexisting, often competing, priorities. High-quality analgesia in this population must also be addressed. In addition to improving patient comfort, peripheral nerve and neuraxial blockade significantly reduce the requirement for systemic opioid analgesia and the adverse effects associated with opioid use. This is often critical in the multiply injured patient who suffers from neurologic, cardiovascular, and/or pulmonary impairment. In addition, the early use of regional anesthetic techniques in selected trauma patients appears to improve outcomes such as pulmonary morbidity, delirium, and mortality and facilitates reductions in length of stay in both the emergency room and hospital overall.

Additional research is required to clarify the impact of peripheral nerve blocks and neuraxial analgesia on outcomes such as the development of delirium, mobility, chronic posttraumatic pain and posttraumatic stress disorder. While peripheral nerve blocks may not delay the diagnosis of acute compartment syndrome, prudent use of regional techniques in trauma patients should be combined with a multidisciplinary approach, astute clinical judgment, and vigilance.

REFERENCES

1. Centers for Disease Control and Prevention. FastStats: All Injuries. http://www.cdc.gov/nchs/fastats/injury.htm. Accessed March 16, 2015.
2. Holdgate A, Shepherd SA, Huckson S: Patterns of analgesia for fractured neck of femur in Australian emergency departments. Emerg Med Australas 2010;22:3–8. doi: 10.1111/j.1742-6723.2009.01246.x.
3. Berben SAA, Meijs THJM, van Dongen RTM, et al: Pain prevalence and pain relief in trauma patients in the accident & emergency department. Injury 2008;39:578–585. doi: 10.1016/j.injury.2007.04.013.
4. Choi JJ, Lin E, Gadsden J: Regional anesthesia for trauma outside the operating theatre. Curr Opin Anaesthesiol 2013;26:495–500. doi: 10.1097/ACO.0b013e3283625ce3.
5. Elvir-Lazo OL, White PF: The role of multimodal analgesia in pain management after ambulatory surgery. 2010;23:697–703. doi: 10.1097/ACO.0b013e32833fad0a.
6. Kehlet H, Dahl JB: The value of "multimodal" or "balanced analgesia" in postoperative pain treatment. Anesth Analg 1993;77:1048–1056.
7. Banerjee M, Bouillon B, Shafizadeh S, et al: Epidemiology of extremity injuries in multiple trauma patients. Injury 2013;44:1015–1021. doi: 10.1016/j.injury.2012.12.007.
8. Gallay SH, Hupel TM, Beaton DE, Schemitsch EH, McKee MD: Functional outcome of acromioclavicular joint injury in polytrauma patients. J Orthop Trauma 1998;12:159–163.
9. Stone MB, Wang R, Price DD: Ultrasound-guided supraclavicular brachial plexus nerve block vs procedural sedation for the treatment of upper extremity emergencies. Am J Emerg Med 2008;26:706–710. doi: 10.1016/j.ajem.2007.09.011.
10. Blaivas M, Adhikari S, Lander L: A prospective comparison of procedural sedation and ultrasound-guided interscalene nerve block for shoulder reduction in the emergency department. Acad Emerg Med 2011;18:922–927. doi: 10.1111/j.1553-2712.2011.01140.x.
11. Edwards D, Bowden M, Aldington DJ: Pain management at role 4. J R Army Med Corps 2009;155:58–61.
12. Hughes S, Birt D: Continuous peripheral nerve blockade on OP HERRICK 9. J R Army Med Corps 2009;155:57–58.
13. Miller SL, Cleeman E, Auerbach J, Flatow EL: Comparison of intra-articular lidocaine and intravenous sedation for reduction of shoulder dislocations: a randomized, prospective study. J Bone Joint Surg Am 2002; 84A:2135–2139.
14. Radresa O, Chauny J-M, Lavigne G, Piette E, Paquet J, Daoust R: Current views on acute to chronic pain transition in post-traumatic patients: risk factors and potential for pre-emptive treatments. J Trauma Acute Care Surg 2014;76:1142–1150. doi: 10.1097/TA.0000000000000188.
15. Clay FJ, Watson WL, Newstead SV, McClure RJ: A systematic review of early prognostic factors for persisting pain following acute orthopedic trauma. Pain Res Manag 2012;17:35–44.
16. Macrae WA: Chronic post-surgical pain: 10 years on. Br J Anaesth 2008; 101:77–86. doi: 10.1093/bja/aen099.
17. Buckenmaier CC3 rd, Rupprecht C, McKnight G, et al: Pain following battlefield injury and evacuation: a survey of 110 casualties from the wars in Iraq and Afghanistan. Pain Med 2009;10:1487–1496. doi: 10.1111/j.1526-4637.2009.00731.x.
18. Buckenmaier CC 3rd, Shields CH, Auton AA, et al: Continuous peripheral nerve block in combat casualties receiving low-molecular weight heparin. Br J Anaesth 2006;97:874–877. doi: 10.1093/bja/ael269.
19. Capdevila X, Bringuier S, Borgeat A: Infectious risk of continuous peripheral nerve blocks. Anesthesiology 2009;110:182–188. doi: 10.1097/ALN.0b013e318190bd5b.
20. Neuburger M, Büttner J, Blumenthal S, Breitbarth J, Borgeat A: Inflammation and infection complications of 2285 perineural catheters: a prospective study. Acta Anaesthesiol Scand 2007;51:108–114. doi: 10.1111/j.1399-6576.2006.01173.x.
21. Morin AM, Kerwat KM, Klotz M, et al: Risk factors for bacterial catheter colonization in regional anaesthesia. BMC Anesthesiol 2005;5:1. doi: 10.1186/1471-2253-5-1.
22. Cuvillon P, Ripart J, Lalourcey L, et al: The continuous femoral nerve block catheter for postoperative analgesia: bacterial colonization, infectious rate and adverse effects. Anesth Analg 2001;93:1045–1049.

23. Capdevila X, Pirat P, Bringuier S, et al: Continuous peripheral nerve blocks in hospital wards after orthopedic surgery: a multicenter prospective analysis of the quality of postoperative analgesia and complications in 1,416 patients. Anesthesiology 2005;103:1035–1045.

24. Lai TT, Jaeger L, Jones BL, Kaderbek EW, Malchow RJ: Continuous peripheral nerve block catheter infections in combat-related injuries: a case report of five soldiers from Operation Enduring Freedom/Operation Iraqi Freedom. Pain Med 2011;12:1676–1681. doi: 10.1111/j.1526-4637.2011.01251.x.

25. Plunkett AR, Buckenmaier CC 3rd: Safety of multiple, simultaneous continuous peripheral nerve block catheters in a patient receiving therapeutic low-molecular-weight heparin. Pain Med 2008;9:624–627. doi: 10.1111/j.1526-4637.2008.00418.x.

26. Bleckner LL, Bina S, Kwon KH, McKnight G, Dragovich A, Buckenmaier CC 3rd: Serum ropivacaine concentrations and systemic local anesthetic toxicity in trauma patients receiving long-term continuous peripheral nerve block catheters. Anesth Analg 2010;110:630–634. doi: 10.1213/ANE.0b013e3181c76a33.

27. Knudsen K, Beckman Suurküla M, Blomberg S, Sjövall J, Edvardsson N: Central nervous and cardiovascular effects of i.v. infusions of ropivacaine, bupivacaine and placebo in volunteers. Br J Anaesth 1997;78:507–514.

28. Stone MB, Carnell J, Fischer JWJ, Herring AA, Nagdev A: Ultrasound-guided intercostal nerve block for traumatic pneumothorax requiring tube thoracostomy. Am J Emerg Med 2011;29:697.e1–2. doi: 10.1016/j.ajem.2010.06.014.

29. Randall A, Grigg L, Obideyi A, Srikantharajah I: Fascia iliaca compartment block: a nurse-led initiative for preoperative pain management in patients with a fractured neck of femur. J Orthop Nurs 2008;12:69–74.

30. Minville V, Gozlan C, Asehnoune K, Zetlaoui P, Chassery C, Benhamou D: Fascia-iliaca compartment block for femoral bone fracture in prehospital medicine in a 6-yr-old child. Eur J Anaesthesiol 2006;23:715–716. doi: 10.1017/S0265021506271126.

31. Gozlan C, Minville V, Asehnoune K, Raynal P, Zetlaoui P, Benhamou D: [Fascia iliaca block for femoral bone fractures in prehospital medicine]. Ann Fr Anesth Reanim 2005;24:617–620. doi: 10.1016/j.annfar.2005.03.030.

32. Lopez S, Gros T, Bernard N, Plasse C, Capdevila X: Fascia iliaca compartment block for femoral bone fractures in prehospital care. Reg Anesth Pain Med 2003;28:203–207. doi: 10.1053/rapm.2003.50134.

33. McRae PJ, Bendall JC, Madigan V, Middleton PM: Paramedic-performed fascia iliaca compartment block for femoral fractures: a controlled trial. J Emerg Med 2015;48:581–589. doi: 10.1016/j.jemermed.2014.12.016.

34. Gros T, Amaru P, Basuko C, Dareau S, Eledjam JJ: [Sciatic nerve block in prehospital care]. Ann Fr Anesth Reanim 2010;29:162–164. doi: 10.1016/j.annfar.2009.11.006.

35. Gros T, Delire V, Dareau S, Sebbane M, Eledjam JJ: [Interscalene brachial plexus block in prehospital medicine]. Ann Fr Anesth Reanim 2008;27:859–860. doi: 10.1016/j.annfar.2008.09.002.

36. Lopez S, Gros T, Deblock N, Capdevila X, Eledjam JJ: [Multitruncular block at the elbow for a major hand trauma for prehospital care]. Ann Fr Anesth Reanim. 2002;21(10):816-819.

37. Simpson PM, McCabe B, Bendall JC, Cone DC, Middleton PM: Paramedic-performed digital nerve block to facilitate field reduction of a dislocated finger. Prehosp Emerg Care 2012;16:415–417. doi: 10.3109/10903127.2012.670690.

38. Roche JJW, Wenn RT, Sahota O, Moran CG: Effect of comorbidities and postoperative complications on mortality after hip fracture in elderly people: prospective observational cohort study. BMJ 2005;331:1374. doi: 10.1136/bmj.38643.663843.55.

39. Roudsari BS, Ebel BE, Corso PS, Molinari N-AM, Koepsell TD: The acute medical care costs of fall-related injuries among the U.S. older adults. Injury 2005;36:1316–1322. doi: 10.1016/j.injury.2005.05.024.

40. Abou-Setta AM, Beaupre LA, Rashiq S, et al: Comparative effectiveness of pain management interventions for hip fracture: a systematic review. Ann Intern Med 2011;155:234–245. doi: 10.7326/0003-4819-155-4-201108160-00346.

41. Beaudoin FL, Nagdev A, Merchant RC, Becker BM: Ultrasound-guided femoral nerve blocks in elderly patients with hip fractures. Am J Emerg Med 2010;28:76–81. doi: 10.1016/j.ajem.2008.09.015.

42. Watson MJ, Walker E, Rowell S, et al: Femoral nerve block for pain relief in hip fracture: a dose finding study. Anaesthesia 2014;69:683–686. doi: 10.1111/anae.12683.

43. Temelkovska-Stevanovska M, Durnev V, Jovanovski-Srceva M, Mojsova-Mijovska M, Trpeski S: Continuous femoral nerve block versus fascia iliaca compartment block as postoperative analgesia in patients with hip fracture. Prilozi 2014;35:85–94.

44. Parker MJ, Handoll HHG, Griffiths R: Anaesthesia for hip fracture surgery in adults. Cochrane Database Syst Rev. 2004;(4):CD000521. doi: 10.1002/14651858.CD000521.pub2.

45. Newman B, McCarthy L, Thomas PW, May P, Layzell M, Horn K: A comparison of pre-operative nerve stimulator-guided femoral nerve block and fascia iliaca compartment block in patients with a femoral neck fracture. Anaesthesia 2013;68:899–903. doi: 10.1111/anae.12321.

46. Dolan J, Williams A, Murney E, Smith M, Kenny GNC: Ultrasound guided fascia iliaca block: a comparison with the loss of resistance technique. Reg Anesth Pain Med 2008;33:526–531.

47. Rashiq S, Vandermeer B, Abou-Setta AM, Beaupre LA, Jones CA, Dryden DM: Efficacy of supplemental peripheral nerve blockade for hip fracture surgery: multiple treatment comparison. Can J Anaesth 2013;60:230–243. doi: 10.1007/s12630-012-9880-8.

48. Pedersen SJ, Borgbjerg FM, Schousboe B, et al: A comprehensive hip fracture program reduces complication rates and mortality. J Am Geriatr Soc 2008;56:1831–1838. doi: 10.1111/j.1532-5415.2008.01945.x.

49. Marcantonio ER, Flacker JM, Michaels M, Resnick NM: Delirium is independently associated with poor functional recovery after hip fracture. J Am Geriatr Soc 2000;48:618–624.

50. Mouzopoulos G, Vasiliadis G, Lasanianos N, Nikolaras G, Morakis E, Kaminaris M: Fascia iliaca block prophylaxis for hip fracture patients at risk for delirium: a randomized placebo-controlled study. J Orthop Traumatol 2009;10:127–133. doi: 10.1007/s10195-009-0062-6.

51. Luger TJ, Kammerlander C, Gosch M, et al: Neuroaxial versus general anaesthesia in geriatric patients for hip fracture surgery: does it matter? Osteoporos Int 2010;21(Suppl 4):S555–S572. doi: 10.1007/s00198-010-1399-7.

52. Neuman MD, Silber JH, Elkassabany NM, Ludwig JM, Fleisher LA: Comparative effectiveness of regional versus general anesthesia for hip fracture surgery in adults. Anesthesiology 2012;117:72–92. doi: 10.1097/ALN.0b013e3182545e7c.

53. White SM, Moppett IK, Griffiths R: Outcome by mode of anaesthesia for hip fracture surgery. An observational audit of 65 535 patients in a national dataset. Anaesthesia 2014;69:224–230. doi: 10.1111/anae.12542.

54. Sharma OP, Oswanski MF, Jolly S, Lauer SK, Dressel R, Stombaugh HA: Perils of rib fractures. Am Surg 2008;74:310–314.

55. Flagel BT, Luchette FA, Reed RL, et al: Half-a-dozen ribs: the breakpoint for mortality. Surgery 2005;138:717–723; discussion 723–725. doi: 10.1016/j.surg.2005.07.022.

56. Simon BJ, Cushman J, Barraco R, et al: Pain management guidelines for blunt thoracic trauma. J Trauma 2005;59:1256–1267.

57. Bulger EM, Edwards T, Klotz P, Jurkovich GJ: Epidural analgesia improves outcome after multiple rib fractures. Surgery 2004;136:426–430. doi: 10.1016/j.surg.2004.05.019.

58. Ullman DA, Fortune JB, Greenhouse BB, Wimpy RE, Kennedy TM: The treatment of patients with multiple rib fractures using continuous thoracic epidural narcotic infusion. Reg Anesth 1989;14:43–47.

59. Sahin S, Uckunkaya N, Soyal S, et al: The role of epidural continuous pain treatment on duration of intubation, ventilation and ICU stay in flail chest patients. Agri Dergisi 1993;5:18–20.

60. Pierre E, Martin P, Frohock J, et al: Lumbar epidural morphine versus. Patient-controlled analgesia morphine in patients with multiple rib fractures. Anesthesiology 2005;103:A289.

61. Luchette FA, Radafshar SM, Kaiser R, Flynn W, Hassett JM: Prospective evaluation of epidural versus intrapleural catheters for analgesia in chest wall trauma. J Trauma 1994;36:865–869; discussion 869–870.

62. Moon MR, Luchette FA, Gibson SW, et al: Prospective, randomized comparison of epidural versus parenteral opioid analgesia in thoracic trauma. Ann Surg 1999;229:684–691; discussion 691–692.

63. Wu CL, Jani ND, Perkins FM, Barquist E: Thoracic epidural analgesia versus intravenous patient-controlled analgesia for the treatment of rib fracture pain after motor vehicle crash. J Trauma 1999;47:564–567.

64. Carrier FM, Turgeon AF, Nicole PC, et al: Effect of epidural analgesia in patients with traumatic rib fractures: a systematic review and meta-analysis of randomized controlled trials. Can J Anaesth 2009;56:230–242. doi: 10.1007/s12630-009-9052-7.

65. Gadsden J, Kwofie K, Shastri U: Continuous intercostal versus paravertebral blockade for multiple fractured ribs. J Trauma Acute Care Surg 2012;73:293–294; author reply 294. doi: 10.1097/TA.0b013e31825aaeb5.

66. Mohta M, Verma P, Saxena AK, Sethi AK, Tyagi A, Girotra G: Prospective, randomized comparison of continuous thoracic epidural and thoracic paravertebral infusion in patients with unilateral multiple fractured ribs—a pilot study. J Trauma 2009;66:1096–1101. doi: 10.1097/TA.0b013e318166d76d.

67. Karmakar MK: Thoracic paravertebral block. Anesthesiology 2001;95:771–780.

68. Murata H, Salviz EA, Chen S, Vandepitte C, Hadzic A: Case report: ultrasound-guided continuous thoracic paravertebral block for outpatient acute pain management of multilevel unilateral rib fractures. Anesth Analg 2013;116:255–257. doi: 10.1213/ANE.0b013e31826f5e25.

69. Buckley M, Edwards H, Buckenmaier CC 3rd, Plunkett AR: Continuous thoracic paravertebral nerve block in a working anesthesia resident-when opioids are not an option. Mil Med 2011;176:578–580.

70. Hwang EG, Lee Y: Effectiveness of intercostal nerve block for management of pain in rib fracture patients. J Exerc Rehabil 2014;10:241–244. doi: 10.12965/jer.140137.

71. Ho AM-H, Karmakar MK, Critchley LAH. Acute pain management of patients with multiple fractured ribs: a focus on regional techniques. Curr Opin Crit Care 2011;17:323–327. doi:10.1097/MCC.0b013e328348bf6f.

72. Ingalls NK, Horton ZA, Bettendorf M, Frye I, Rodriguez C: Randomized, double-blind, placebo-controlled trial using lidocaine patch 5% in traumatic rib fractures. J Am Coll Surg 2010;210:205–209. doi: 10.1016/j.jamcollsurg.2009.10.020.

73. Shanahan PT: Replantation anesthesia. *Anesth Analg* 1984;63:785–786.

74. Kurt E, Ozturk S, Isik S, Zor F: Continuous brachial plexus blockade for digital replantations and toe-to-hand transfers. Ann Plast Surg 2005;54:24–27.

75. Berger A, Tizian C, Zenz M: Continuous plexus blockade for improved circulation in microvascular surgery. Ann Plast Surg 1985;14:16–19.

76. Su H-H, Lui P-W, Yu C-L, et al: The effects of continuous axillary brachial plexus block with ropivacaine infusion on skin temperature and survival of crushed fingers after microsurgical replantation. Chang Gung Med J 2005;28:567–574.

77. Taras JS, Behrman MJ: Continuous peripheral nerve block in replantation and revascularization. J Reconstr Microsurg 1998;14:17–21. doi: 10.1055/s-2007-1006896.

78. Niazi AU, El-Beheiry H, Ramlogan R, Graham B, von Schroeder HP, Tumber PS: Continuous infraclavicular brachial plexus blockade: effect on survival of replanted digits. Hand Surg 2013;18:325–330. doi: 10.1142/S0218810413500342.

79. Vinson DR, Hoehn CL: Sedation-assisted orthopedic reduction in emergency medicine: the safety and success of a one physician/one nurse model. West J Emerg Med 2013;14:47–54. doi: 10.5811/westjem.2012.4.12455.

80. Gadsden J: Regional Anesthesia in Trauma. Cambridge: Cambridge University Press, 2012.

81. Shteynberg A, Riina LH, Glickman LT, Meringolo JN, Simpson RL: Ultrasound guided lateral femoral cutaneous nerve (LFCN) block: safe and simple anesthesia for harvesting skin grafts. Burns 2013;39:146–149. doi:10.1016/j.burns.2012.02.015.

82. Gupta A, Bhandari PS, Shrivastava P: A study of regional nerve blocks and local anesthetic creams (Prilox) for donor sites in burn patients. Burns 2007;33:87–91. doi: 10.1016/j.burns.2006.04.019.

83. Cuignet O, Pirson J, Boughrouph J, Duville D: The efficacy of continuous fascia iliaca compartment block for pain management in burn patients undergoing skin grafting procedures. Anesth Analg 2004;98:1077–1081, table of contents.

84. Pedersen JL, Crawford ME, Dahl JB, Brennum J, Kehlet H: Effect of preemptive nerve block on inflammation and hyperalgesia after human thermal injury. Anesthesiology 1996;84:1020–1026.

85. Mar GJ, Barrington MJ, McGuirk BR: Acute compartment syndrome of the lower limb and the effect of postoperative analgesia on diagnosis. Br J Anaesth 2009;102:3–11. doi: 10.1093/bja/aen330.

86. Ulmer T: The clinical diagnosis of compartment syndrome of the lower leg: are clinical findings predictive of the disorder? J Orthop Trauma 2002;16:572–577.

87. Walker BJ, Noonan KJ, Bosenberg AT: Evolving compartment syndrome not masked by a continuous peripheral nerve block: evidence-based case management. Reg Anesth Pain Med 2012;37:393–397. doi: 10.1097/AAP.0b013e31824df1ac.

88. Cometa MA, Esch AT, Boezaart AP: Did continuous femoral and sciatic nerve block obscure the diagnosis or delay the treatment of acute lower leg compartment syndrome? A case report. Pain Med 2011;12:823–828. doi: 10.1111/j.1526-4637.2011.01109.x.

89. Uzel A-P, Steinmann G: Thigh compartment syndrome after intramedullary femoral nailing: possible femoral nerve block influence on diagnosis timing. Orthop Traumatol Surg Res 2009;95:309–313. doi: 10.1016/j.otsr.2009.03.014.

90. Noorpuri BS, Shahane SA, Getty CJ: Acute compartment syndrome following revisional arthroplasty of the forefoot: the dangers of ankle-block. Foot Ankle Int 2000;21:680–682.

91. Kucera TJ, Boezaart AP: Regional anesthesia does not consistently block ischemic pain: two further cases and a review of the literature. Pain Med 2014;15:316–319. doi: 10.1111/pme.12235.

92. Hyder N, Kessler S, Jennings AG, De Boer PG: Compartment syndrome in tibial shaft fracture missed because of a local nerve block. J Bone Joint Surg Br 1996;78:499–500.

Regional Anesthesia for Cardiac and Thoracic Anesthesia

Paul Kessler

REGIONAL ANESTHESIA FOR CARDIAC SURGERY

General anesthesia is the most commonly used anesthetic technique for cardiac surgery, both for valvular procedures and for coronary artery bypass grafting (CABG) performed either on pump or off pump. However, there are several reports from the 1970s and 1980s describing improved postoperative analgesia through the intrathecal and epidural application of opiates in cardiac surgery.[1,2] Faster extubation of patients is another benefit of the neuroaxial application of opiates.[3] Local anesthetics are also routinely applied as they suppress the stress hormone response in addition to having analgesic properties, resulting in improved outcomes.[4]

For intrathecal application, two procedures have been reported: opiates or the "high spinal technique," achieved with large doses of local anesthetic. In contrast to a single-shot intrathecal technique, epidural opiates and local anesthetics can be applied continuously. As a result, the intraoperative benefits of a neuraxial procedure can be continued beyond the postoperative phase. Intrathecal and epidural procedures are typically combined with a general anesthetic, although segmental pain elimination allows for cardiac procedures through the sole use of a high thoracic epidural anesthesia.[5]

Paravertebral blockade (PVB) is another reported regional anesthetic procedure in cardiac surgery (Table 56–1).[6] Varying techniques are used: single-shot or continuous application; unilateral for thoracotomy or bilateral for sternotomy.[6,7] Due to the limited number of published cases, the importance of PVB in cardiac surgery currently cannot be assessed.

Techniques
High Thoracic Epidural Anesthesia

Despite some beneficial effects of regional anesthesia, especially the neuraxial techniques, its use is not yet widely accepted in cardiac surgery. This is due to the ongoing discussion regarding the potential risks of epidural hematoma formation and subsequent adverse neurological sequelae related to perioperative anticoagulation, which thus discourages the use of epidurals in these patients by many anesthesiologists. There is a great deal of controversy in the cardiac literature concerning neuraxial techniques in cardiac surgery.[8,9]

Physiological Effects High thoracic epidural anesthesia (hTEA) results in excellent analgesia achieved throughout the epidural application of opiates and/or local anesthetics, allowing for faster recovery and extubation after surgery.[10,11] This is due to the superior analgesia of hTEA after CABG surgery, which may improve respiratory muscles strength.[12]

Beyond its analgesic properties, hTEA's beneficial effects on the postoperative neurohumoral stress response and cardiovascular pathophysiology have been demonstrated in both clinical and experimental investigations. hTEA results in a segmental thoracic sympathectomy; at a level between T1 and T5, this sympatholysis dilates the coronary arteries and the internal mammary arteries and thus improves perfusion of the respective vessels.[13–15] Heart rate is reduced,[16] cardiac arrhythmia is less frequent, and intraoperative hemodynamic stability can be significantly improved.[16–18] In addition, hTEA lowers the incidence of intraoperative myocardial ischemia,[18,19] reduces the endogenous stress response to surgical manipulation,[4,20] and decreases stress hyperglycemia and the need for insulin in cardiac surgery patients.[21] Reductions in both tachycardia and ischemic events have also been demonstrated with hTEA in the postoperative period. Improved pulmonary function without affecting the ventilation–perfusion ratio allows for earlier and smoother weaning of mechanical ventilation and a decreased incidence of postoperative pulmonary dysfunction.[12,16–19] There is also evidence of a reduction in postoperative neurologic complications when hTEA is used.[22]

TABLE 56–1. Techniques of regional anesthesia and analgesia for cardiac surgery.

Epidural
Spinal
Paravertebral

Clinical Pearls

- High thoracic epidural analgesia (hTEA) has beneficial effects on the postoperative neurohumoral stress response and cardiovascular pathophysiology.
- Addition of hTEA and general anesthesia may reduce postoperative morbidity (postoperative arrhythmias, pulmonary complications, renal failure) in addition to providing analgesia.

High Thoracic Epidural Anesthesia and General Anesthesia

In the past two decades, hTEA as an adjunct to general anesthesia has become more prevalent and has been demonstrated to be potentially beneficial in patients with coronary artery disease (Table 56–2).[17,23]

Case series regarding the use of hTEA in valvular surgery have been published.[24,25] hTEA has been shown to provide superior analgesia and to be associated with a lower incidence of pulmonary and cardiac events and a reduced median time on mechanical ventilation. A randomized, controlled study demonstrated that hTEA improves cardiac performance in low-to-moderate-risk patients undergoing elective coronary artery bypass graft surgery with or without aortic valve replacement. Time spent in the intensive care unit (ICU) and quality of recovery, however, remained unchanged.[26,27]

The combination of hTEA with general anesthesia remains controversial among cardiac anesthesiologists.[8,9,28] The results of the existing studies are contradictory: some studies show a reduction in postoperative morbidity (postoperative arrhythmias, pulmonary complications, renal failure) and an improvement in pain control, allowing for earlier extubation and hospital discharge.[17,29–31] Others have shown no improved outcome.[32,33]

There are also conflicting data from meta-analyses on this topic. Whereas one analysis suggested that epidural analgesia

TABLE 56–2. Possible benefits of epidural anesthesia in cardiac surgery.

Decreased myocardial ischemia
Reduced cardiac arrhythmia
Improved ventricular function
Increased hemodynamic stability
Improved pulmonary function
Earlier extubation and ambulation, shorter ICU stay
Reduction in overall cost

ICU, intensive care unit.

combined with general anesthesia reduces the incidence of perioperative acute renal failure and time on mechanical ventilation and improves outcomes on the composite endpoints of mortality and myocardial infarction in patients undergoing cardiac surgery,[34] other meta-analyses, including more than 1000 patients, have found no difference in mortality rate or incidence of myocardial infarction between general versus regional anesthetic techniques.[35,36] However, patients undergoing cardiac surgery with hTEA have a reduced risk of postoperative supraventricular arrhythmias and respiratory complications.[35,36] In addition, patients receiving regional analgesia seem to benefit from superior postoperative analgesia and shorter postoperative ventilation.[37] These are the main reasons why epidural anesthesia plays an integral part of fast-track anesthesia protocols in cardiac surgery that utilize hTEA. In addition to improvements in short-term recovery, hTEA may also have positive psychological effects.[38]

Clinical Application

Patient Selection A concomitant hTEA can be used in different types of cardiac surgery: CABG with cardiopulmonary bypass (CPB), off-pump coronary artery bypass (OPCAB), and valve replacement.

In principle, hTEA can be used in all cardiac surgery procedures. Contraindications for hTEA should be taken into account, however, and include patient refusal, past surgery on the cervical or upper thoracic spine, infection at the local site of injection, and continued use of antithrombotic and antiplatelet drugs. According to the American Society of Anesthesiologists and European Society of Anaesthesiology guidelines, strict adherence to the recommended time intervals between the administration of anticoagulants, neuraxial blockade, and the removal of catheters is thought to improve patient safety.[39,40] Patients with abnormal coagulation (thromboplastin time < 80%, prothrombin time > 40 sec, platelets < 100/nL) or a bleeding disorder should be excluded.

Epidural Technique The question regarding the optimal time interval between placement of hTEA and surgery remains unanswered. In the early days, catheters for hTEA were placed a day before surgery to ensure safe timing from placement to intraoperative heparinization. This practice also ensured that surgery would not have to be postponed in case of a "bloody tap" (blood in the epidural catheter). Many centers now place the catheter on the day of surgery. This procedure offers organizational advantages and apparently does not increase the risk of epidural bleeding if a gap of less than 1 hour between catheter placement and application of heparin is avoided. Currently, there is no evidence-based guidance regarding the safe minimum time interval between catheter placement and heparinization.[39–41]

Catheter placement is performed while the patient is sitting or lying on his or her side with a midline approach and is usually located at T1–2 or T2–3. Using a 16- or 18 gauge Tuohy needle, the epidural space is identified either by loss of resistance or using the hanging drop technique. The catheter is advanced 2–3 centimeters beyond the needle tip, and correct placement is verified with a test dose of, for example, 2 mL of lidocaine 2%.[42]

The literature discusses many regimes concerning when and how the epidural catheter is used and which substances are applied. Most studies start with a loading dose before surgery and then use either a continuous application or intermittent boluses during the procedure.

The continuous administration of local anesthetic via TEA is preferable as it seems to provide very stable hemodynamic conditions compared to intermittent bolus application.

Local anesthetics, preferably bupivacaine, ropivacaine, or levobupivacaine, in concentrations from 0.2%–0.5% are used either exclusively or in combination with opiates (eg, fentanyl or sufentanil).[41,43–45] After surgery, local anesthetics in low concentrations from 0.1%–0.2%, with or without opiates, are administered continuously, intermittently, or via patient-controlled analgesia (PCA). Since the maximum pain after cardiac surgery occurs within the first 48 hours, hTEA is typically used for up to 3 days.[46]

Postoperative Management   Removing the catheter requires exact synchronization with postoperative anticoagulation to reduce the risk of complications due to bleeding. The timing and type of anticoagulation is important and is discussed in more detail in Chapter 53. The safest route is to remove the epidural catheter prior to commencing anticoagulation.[39,40] Unfortunately, this complicates the management and decreases the utility of TEA, as the immediate use of anticoagulation post-surgery has become more common, making safe catheter removal without pausing the medication difficult. As an alternative, a single-shot technique, either spinal anesthesia or paravertebral blockade, can be used. Prior to removal of the catheter, current lab results with regard to clotting are mandatory.

Complications of High Thoracic Epidural Anesthesia

Transient Neurological Symptoms
There are no reports in the literature of permanent neurological symptoms following hTEA in cardiac surgery. In a review publication, Ruppen et al. found 4 cases out of 4971 patients in 9 studies reporting neurological symptoms, and Jack and Scott reported on 12 cases out of 2837 patients.[17,44,47] All patients fully recovered. From these data, the reported incidence of transient neurological complications in patients undergoing cardiac surgery with TEA is 0.20%.

Severe Infectious Complications
To date, no reports of epidural abscess or meningitis after hTEA in patients undergoing cardiac surgery have been published. The incidence of epidural abscess or meningitis after hTEA in patients in non-cardiac surgery patients varies from 0.04%–0.6%.[48]

Epidural Hematoma
The risk of bleeding complications after hTEA is not known. Nevertheless, the possibility of developing an epidural hematoma is the main cause for concern regarding hTEA among cardiac anesthesiologists, and the risk–benefit ratio of hTEA in cardiac surgery remains controversial.[28,49] Under the conditions of an off-pump procedure, with considerably less heparinization in comparison to CPB, most anesthesiologists consider the associated risk to

TABLE 56–3. Epidural safety issues.

Strict adherence to the recommended time intervals of antiplatelet drugs

Insertion of the catheter the night before or at least 1 hour prior to heparinization

Normal clotting at the time of insertion

Antagonize heparin at the end of operation (ACT)

Removal of the catheter after coagulation is normalized

Withholding of heparin (s/c) prior to catheter removal

ACT, activated clotting time.

be reduced. However, there is no definitive evidence for this. The removal of the catheter and postoperative anticoagulation remain unresolved problems when considering hTEA for cardiac surgery. If the catheter must be removed, then, according to the guidelines, anticoagulation must be stopped.[39,40] This, however, introduces a risk of coronary ischemia or thromboembolic event (Table 56–3).[50]

Until now, only very few epidural hematomas have been described in cardiac surgery patients in the context of hTEA, but all associated with intraoperative hepatinization or postoperative catheter issues.[51–54] Regardless, meticulous monitoring of cardiac patients with hTEA in the postoperative period is essential. It is also important to coordinate the postoperative course and drug therapy (particularly anticoagulant therapies) with the timing of catheter removal and monitor for new sensory and/or motor deficits for the entire postoperative period and at least 12 hours after catheter removal. If patients are not extubated in the operating room, close neurological surveillance is often delayed. Undetected cord compression reduces the chance of early hematoma evacuation and the chance of full neurological recovery.[55]

The first risk calculation of blockade-induced hematoma with a 95% confidence interval was from 1:150,000 to 1:1,500 for epidurals;[56] the most recently published risk estimation was 1:12,000.[45] The actual number of epidural hematomas is likely higher, but so is the actual number of performed, but unpublished, thoracic epidurals. The 1:12,000 incidence of hematoma is similar to that described with epidural in noncardiac surgery.

Summary

To this day, no randomized controlled trial or meta-analysis has demonstrated that hTEA decreases mortality after cardiac surgery. However, it is well-documented that hTEA reduces postoperative morbidity (postoperative arrhythmias and pulmonary complications) and improves pain control, allowing for earlier extubation and hospital discharge. The accepted benefits of hTEA in cardiac surgery need to be carefully weighed against the potentially catastrophic outcome of high thoracic epidural hematoma.

High Thoracic Epidural Anesthesia and Awake Cardiac Surgery

Awake cardiac surgery was first performed in 1998 as coronary artery graft surgery by the Turkish cardiac surgeon Karagoz.[5]

With thoracic epidural anesthesia as the sole anesthetic modality, the author reported that 5 patients successfully underwent OPCAB surgery.

Minimal surgical access (eg, partial lower sternotomy or thoracotomy) and operation techniques on the beating heart (OPCAB) avoiding CPB and full heparinization were the requirements for the first set of awake cardiac surgeries. The majority of published awake cardiac surgeries have been performed on OPCAB patients,[42,49,57–60] but there are also case reports of OPCAB technique for total revascularization via a full median sternotomy.[49,61] Recently, small case series including valve replacements with CPB on awake high-risk patients have been published.[62–66]

Clinical Application

Patient Selection   Patients undergoing awake cardiac surgery need to be extensively and thoroughly informed about the anesthetic technique used, potential adverse events, and the pre- and intraoperative routines. An awake OPCAB procedure is not applicable to all kinds of coronary artery stenoses. Revascularization of the left circumflex artery requires Trendelenburg positioning and luxation of the heart and is therefore difficult to perform awake. In addition, patients with highly impaired left ventricular function dependent on a certain cardiac sympathetic tone should be excluded from this new technique. Further exclusion criteria arise from the common contraindications of epidural puncture, such as compromised coagulation, bleeding disorders, and the use of any antiplatelet drugs.

Anesthetic Technique   The process of epidural puncture does not differ from the technique described earlier. Regarding intraoperative catheter use, various regimens have been described. Commonly, a loading dose of local anesthetic, with or without opiates, is given until the desired level is achieved after verification of correct positioning. Thereafter, the infusion rate is reduced to maintenance dosage. During wound closure, the epidural infusion is stopped and restarted with a lower concentration of local anesthetic, with or without opiates, for analgesia postsurgery (Table 56–4).[67]

After commencing the loading infusion, the level of anesthesia is checked every 5 minutes via pinprick and warm–cold discrimination. The motor blockade is estimated by observing intercostal breathing or arm movement. For full median sternotomy, the level of sensory and motor blockade must be at C7–C8; for partial or lower sternotomy and thoracotomy, the level is adjusted according to the required surgical access.[49,67] Extending regional anesthesia with other techniques (eg, femoral nerve block[58,68] or lumbar spinal anesthesia[59]) allows for additional removal of veins from the legs for grafting.[68] Furthermore, a case report has been published in which coronary artery bypass graft surgery with TEA was followed by disobliteration of the carotid artery using a cervical plexus block.[69]

After onset of sensorimotor blockade, cannulation of the radial artery and siting of the central venous catheter is performed. Patient monitoring includes arterial blood pressure, 5-lead electrocardiogram (ECG) with continuous ST-segment analysis, and saturation and ventilation via pulse oximetry and capnography. All patients receive oxygen continuously via

TABLE 56–4. Local anesthetics and opioids for high thoracic epidural anesthesia in awake cardiac surgeries.

Study	Drugs and Concentrations	Administered Dose
Karagoz et al.[5,71]	Bupivacaine 2 mg/mL Lidocaine 8 mg/mL Fentanyl 5 μg/mL	Initial bolus of 10 mL; additional boluses when necessary
Kessler et al.[67,70]	Ropivacaine 5 mg/mL Sufentanil 1.66 μg/mL	Initial bolus infusion of 10–12 mg over 15–20 min; maintenance with 2–5 mL/h
Lucchetti et al.[59]	Ropivacaine 5 mg/mL Clonidine 7.5 g/mL Fentanyl 5 μg/mL	Initial bolus of 12mL; maintenance with bolus of 4 mL
Hemmerling et al.[58]	Bupivacaine 5 mg/mL Sufentanil 2 μg/mL	Initial bolus of 12 mL over 25 min; maintenance with 4–7 mL/h
Gerosa et al.[69]	*Initial:* Ropivacaine 6 mg/mL Lidocaine 6 mg/mL Fentanyl 5 μg/mL *Maintenance:* Bupivacaine 2.5 mg/mL	Bolus of 10 mL; additional boluses when necessary
Noiseux et al.[68]	Bupivacaine 5 mg/mL Sufentanil 1.66 μg/mL	Initial bolus of 20 mL over 60 min; maintenance with 2–14 mL/h
Watanabe et al.[49]	Lidocaine 10 mg/mL Bupivacaine[a] Morphine 50 μg/mL	Maintenance with 20 mL/h

[a]Concentration not given in publication.

mask. As long as the application of larger amounts of sedatives is avoided, appropriate ventilation and oxygenation of awake patients is guaranteed during surgery.[70] Additional intraoperative IV sedation is not mandatory since the epidural opioids result in a sedative effect. A low-dose infusion of propofol or midazolam boluses can be beneficial to allay anxiety.[70]

TABLE 56–5. Potential benefits of awake cardiac surgery.

Excellent postoperative pain relief
Bypass of ICU or short-term ICU stay
Avoidance of endotracheal intubation
No weaning
Faster mobilization
Shorter hospital stay
Decreased costs
High patient acceptance

ICU, intensive care unit.

TABLE 56–6. Side effects and disadvantages of awake cardiac surgery.

Insufficient analgesia
High motor block
Phrenic nerve palsy
Permanent neurologic symptoms resulting from the TEA
Hemodynamic changes
Unprotected airway
Inability to perform a TEE

TEA, thoracic epidural anesthesia; TEE, transesophageal echocardiography.

Awake Cardiac Surgery

The hypothetical benefits of awake cardiac surgery may result from the avoidance of endotracheal intubation and from the use of hTEA (Table 56–5). The following advantages of awake cardiac surgery with hTEA have been described: stable intraoperative hemodynamics;[70] faster mobilization (some activities of daily living may be performed) within a few hours after surgery;[67,71] shorter-term ICU stay or even complete avoidance of the ICU;[57,70] shorter hospitalization; and, overall, a modern fast-tracking technique for cardiac patients[57,71] with significant cost reduction potential and high patient acceptance.[70] Furthermore, case reports have demonstrated advantages for patients with significant pulmonary risk factors, such as chronic obstructive pulmonary disease (COPD) or post-tracheal reconstruction, due to the avoidance of endotracheal intubation and, consequently, potential weaning difficulties postoperatively.[72,73] In addition, awake CABG allows for verbal intraoperative monitoring of patients with compromised cerebrovascular function (eg, severe carotid artery stenosis) (Figure 56-1).[69]

Clinical Pearl

- Awake cardiac surgery is described primarily in coronary artery graft surgery on the beating heart (OPCAB).

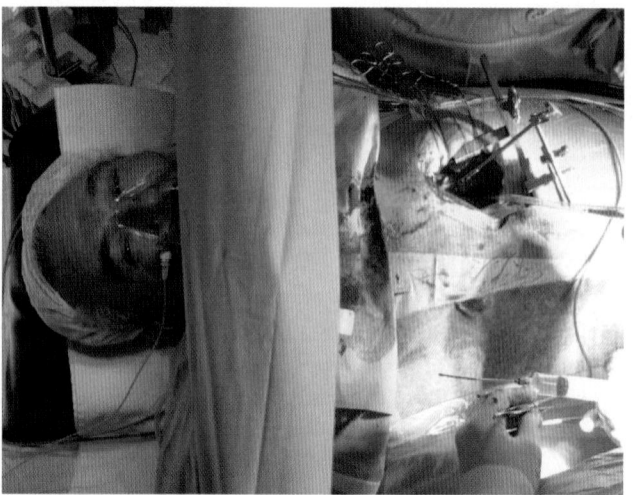

FIGURE 56–1. Awake off-pump coronary artery bypass surgery.

Awake Cardiac Surgery Risks

The side effects and complications of awake cardiac surgery may result from the use of epidural anesthesia and from the avoidance of general anesthesia (Table 56–6). Uncontrolled spreading of epidural anesthesia toward the cranium can result in cardiovascular changes (hypotension, bradycardia), requiring a supportive increase of heart rate or the use of vasopressors.

A unilateral or bilateral paresis of the phrenic nerve and thus paralysis of the diaphragm is possible should the hTEA spread to C5/6, in which case the patient must be intubated and ventilated. Extubation is usually not a problem if the administration of local anesthetic is stopped toward the end of surgery.[70]

Accidental perforation of the pleura during surgery is no rare incident while preparing the internal thoracic artery but usually remains without clinical relevance in intubated and ventilated patients. However, if the patient is breathing spontaneously and mechanics are compromised due to other factors (eg, complete discontinuity of the bony thorax structure through sternotomy or loss of intercostal muscle function), a perforation can result in lung collapse and acute respiratory insufficiency requiring controlled ventilation.[70,71,74] While maintaining spontaneous breathing, it is possible to seal the lesion. This is followed by the insertion of a pleural drainage.[71]

Further reasons for conversion to general anesthesia include insufficiency of the hTEA and the surgical necessity to use CPB (Table 56–7).

Awake cardiac surgery may be associated with significant patient anxiety. However, to date, there has been no study focusing on the psychological impact of awake cardiac surgery on patients. In contrast to presumptions,[28] compared to general anesthesia, the patient's stress response does not seem to be increased in awake surgery, and postoperative surveys have shown very high levels of patient acceptance.[70,71,74] One report compared the experiences of patients who underwent awake surgery who had previously undergone cardiac surgery with general surgery; all of these patients reported preferring the experience of awake cardiac surgery.[75]

There are no differences between patients undergoing awake cardiac surgery and those undergoing such surgery with combined TEA and general anesthesia in terms of the risks of epidural bleeding, transient neurologic symptoms, or epidural infection.

TABLE 56-7. Surgical and anesthetic complications of awake cardiac procedures.

Study	Patients	Horner-Syndrome	Phrenic Nerve Palsy	Insufficient Anesthesia	Pneumothorax	Start of CPB	Conversion to GA
Karagoz et al.[71]	137	71 (51.8%)	0	11 (8.0%)	39 (28.4%)	1 (0.7%)	5 (3.6%)
Kessler et al.[70]	30	N/A	1 (3.3%)	1 (3.3%)	2 (6.7%)	0	4 (13.3%)
Chakravarthy et al.[75]	151	N/A	N/A	N/A	29 (19.2%)	1 (0.6%)	3 (2.0%)
Aybek et al.[74]	34	2 (5.9%)	0	1 (2.9%)	2 (5.9%)	0	3 (8.8%)
Noiseux et al.[68]	15	N/A	N/A	1 (6.7%)	N/A	1 (6.7%)	3 (20.0%)

Data are given as number (percentage).

CPB, cardiopulmonary bypass; GA, general anesthesia; N/A, not available.

Summary

For over 15 years, awake cardiac surgery has been performed and results have been published by a few specialist centers. This technique is used mainly in coronary artery graft surgery on the beating heart (OPCAB) based on the reduced heparinization and therefore the lower possible risk of epidural hematoma. Most of the published accounts of awake cardiac surgeries are case reports or observational studies that simply describe the feasibility of this method. Only a few studies have had control groups comparing awake cardiac surgery using hTEA alone with hTEA plus general anesthesia and cardiac surgery with general anesthesia only. These studies showed no advantage in the awake cardiac surgery group versus the hTEA with additional general anesthesia group.[49,70,76,77]

The future of hTEA and awake cardiac surgery is not known. There may be selected centers with experienced teams of anesthesiologists and cardiac surgeons with clearly defined perioperative protocols who will continue to use hTEA. However, many patients are now treated interventional by cardiologists, thus avoiding surgery altogether. Patients scheduled for bypass surgery these days are usually high-risk patients with compromised myocardial function or patients requiring additional valve surgery. In addition, intraoperative transesophageal echocardiography (TEE) is now a standard procedure and cannot be performed on the awake patient. Finally, the feasibility of performing cardiac surgery with hTEA in patients with coronary artery disease and the current anticoagulation strategy should always be considered in terms of the risk–benefit ratio.

Spinal Anesthesia

Indication

Spinal anesthesia (SPA) has been used in combination with general anesthesia for various cardiac surgery procedures for several decades, most frequently in patients undergoing CABG. The primary rationale for the use of SPA is to provide prolonged, profound postoperative analgesia. In most studies, intrathecal morphine was used.[78–80] Lipophilic opiates are of little use due to their short duration of action. Other benefits of SPA are reduced perioperative attenuation of sympathetic autonomic activity and the realization of so-called "fast-track"

targets, such as rapid extubation and patient transfer. Although SPA has excellent analgesic properties, the technique is not in widespread use in cardiac surgery, at least partly due to risk of spinal hematoma as a result of systemic anticoagulation.

Clinical Application

The intrathecal application of morphine has been well studied with dosages of ranging from 0.25–4.0 mg;[81–84] most studies have reported improved postoperative analgesia with this technique as compared to an IV technique. However, the optimal dose for striking a balance between optimal analgesia and a minimal side effects remains undetermined. An increased dose of morphine improves and prolongs postoperative analgesia, although at the cost of increased levels of side effects (ie, pruritus, nausea, vomiting, and urine retention).[78] Additionally, higher doses of intrathecal morphine prevent early extubation after surgery.[46] On the other hand, the absence of local anesthetic infusion lacks the titratability of analgesia and significantly limits the benefits up to 24 hours postoperatively.

Of note, intrathecal opioids alone do not alter the sympathetic response to cardiac surgery and cardiopulmonary bypass; this benefit is seen only with local anesthetic.[85] Subsequent studies have investigated the sole application of high-dose intrathecal local anesthetic as a "high spinal" anesthesia or in combination with intrathecal opiates.[86,87] Both treatments efficiently suppress the stress response during surgery, although with a higher incidence of bradycardia and hypotension with increased amounts of vasoconstrictors required as compared to a technique without intrathecal application of local anesthetics and/or opioids.

Complications

Spinal analgesia has not acquired widespread acceptance in cardiac surgery; this is mainly because of the potentially increased risk of neuraxial hematoma in patients receiving heparin during surgery. The concerns are founded; many of these patients receive antiplatelet drugs, receive intraoperative high-dose heparin for CPB, and continue anticoagulation after valve surgery. However, there is still a lack of sufficient data and experience to determine if the risk of epidural hematoma is increased when combining neuraxial techniques with anticoagulation in cardiac surgery.

It is important to observe the relevant guidelines issued by the anesthesiology societies[39,40] regarding perioperative anticoagulation and neuraxial procedures. In addition to adhering to recommendations regarding the timing of the procedure and anticoagulation, postoperative monitoring of neurologic function and selection of a neuraxial procedure that minimizes postoperative sensory and motor block in order to facilitate the detection of new or progressive neurodeficits are required.

In contrast to TEA, thus far no case reports of hematoma-related permanent spinal cord damage after SPA in cardiac surgery patients have been reported. However, this may be because SPA is performed less frequently than TEA in cardiac surgery. The potentially lower risk of neuraxial hematoma with spinal anesthesia is probably due to the small-gauge needles used with spinal anesthesia and the avoidance of catheter insertion and removal. Based on reports, almost 50% of epidural hematomas occur after catheter removal.[88]

Outcomes Data

Reviews and meta-analyses have evaluated the existing studies of the use of SPA in cardiac surgery.[8,35,37,89] The critical question is whether spinal analgesia might influence patients' outcomes after cardiac surgery. The meta-analysis performed by Liu and colleagues on spinal analgesia in coronary artery bypass graft surgery including 17 randomized, controlled trials (RCTs) showed no improvement in major clinical endpoints.[35] Two observed benefits of spinal analgesia were modestly decreased systemic morphine use and pain scores.[25] A meta-analysis from Zangrillo et al. including 25 randomized studies on spinal analgesia confirmed no reduced perioperative mortality, myocardial infarction, or arrhythmia but an increased rate of postoperative pruritus.[89]

Summary

The intrathecal administration of opiates or local anesthetics can provide effective postoperative analgesia with decreased intravenous analgesic requirements. However, studies of intrathecal analgesia in cardiac surgery have not demonstrated a significant positive effect on morbidity and mortality.

Paravertebral Blockade

The effectiveness of thoracic paravertebral blockade (tPVB) in thoracic surgery has been well-documented.[90] For thoracic surgery, tPVB is considered equivalent in its analgesic properties to hTEA but with a more favorable side effect profile.[91] The application of local anesthetic into the paravertebral compartment generates an ipsilateral somatic and sympathetic nerve blockade across several thoracic dermatomes.[92]

The use of tPVB in cardiac surgery is limited to a few case series and individual case reports.[6,7,93–95] A tPVB with continuous application of local anesthetic has been used in minimally invasive procedures with thoracoscopic access[6] and was found to be as effective as hTEA for analgesia.[93] Other authors have reported the use of a bilateral tPVB using a bilateral single-shot or continuous-catheter technique for conventional cardiac

surgery with complete sternotomy.[7,94] Side effects included hypotension, blood vessel puncture with an incidence of around 5%,[96] a failure rate of between 6.1% and 10.7%, and a rate of pneumothorax of between 0.4% for unilateral technique and 4% for bilateral technique.[97] As the location of puncture in tPVB is close to the spinal canal, which may cause complications if bleeding occurs, the same safety time intervals regarding application of anticoagulants as for neuraxial procedures are required for puncture and catheter removal.[39,40] The few data available concerning tPVB and cardiac surgery do not allow for a definitive recommendation.

REGIONAL ANESTHESIA FOR THORACIC SURGERY

Surgeries on the chest wall are among the most painful procedures performed[98] and carry a high risk of chronic pain.[99] Splinting of the wound or immobilization is near impossible, whereas postoperative pain reduces pulmonary function and impairs effective cough and clearing of secretions. Combined, these factors predispose patients for the development of atelectasis and pneumonia.[100] Surgical access (minimal vs. open) and incision technique (posterolateral vs. muscle sparing vs. sternotomy) have a significant effect on postoperative pain intensity. The increasingly used technique of video-assisted thoracoscopic surgery (VATS) results in less postoperative pain compared to open thoracotomies.[101]

Several clinical studies indicate that effective intra- and postoperative analgesia management reduces the number and severity of complications encountered after surgery, especially pulmonary complications.[100,102] Systemic analgesics (opiates and nonopiates) and regional analgesia procedures (intercostal, paravertebral, interpleural, and epidural blockades with local anesthesia and opiates) have all been used with success for pain management after thoracic surgery. Comparative studies, meta-analyses, and systemic reviews consistently demonstrate that regional analgesic techniques (TEA or PVB) are superior to systemic analgesia.[91,103–105] Used intraoperatively, regional anesthesia reduces the need for intraoperative opioids and their side effects.

Techniques
Thoracic Epidural Anesthesia

TEA is typically used in combination with general anesthesia, making use of its excellent analgesic properties. It is currently considered the gold standard in the treatment of thoracotomy pain.[103,105] In many comparative studies of the use of systemic opiates, TEA was proven superior.[106–107] TEA has also been used exclusively in selected surgical procedures.[108]

Physiological Effects

Along with the excellent analgesic properties of TEA, the sympathetic blockade of local anesthetics has significant beneficial effects on several organ systems: increased gastrointestinal motility and perfusion and decreased myocardial ischemia and systemic stress response. However, the effective analgesia must be balanced against the possible alteration of lung function

TABLE 56–8. Pulmonary effects of thoracic epidural anesthesia.[114,116,117]

Decreased bronchial reactivity as a result of systemic effect of local anesthetic

No increased airway resistance in patients with severe obstructive pulmonary disease

No influence on hypoxic pulmonary vasoconstriction (HPV)

through the epidural motor blockade of respiratory muscles and the potentially detrimental effects of sympathicolysis, leaving an unopposed vagal tone with a potentially increased bronchial tone and reactivity.

Data show that in healthy volunteers, TEA with sensory blockade up to the cervicothoracic region decreases vital capacity (VC) and forced expiratory volume in one second (FEV_1) significantly.[109] This is mainly due to a motor blockade of the intercostal muscles. The effect is more pronounced when local anesthetics in high concentrations are used. In patients undergoing thoracic or abdominal surgery with general anesthesia exclusively, though, TEA improves the reduced VC postsurgery.[110] Two effects of TEA contribute to this improvement: improved diaphragmatic function and better postoperative analgesia than systemic opioids. Higher values of functional residual capacity (FRC), FVC, and FEV_1 in patients treated with TEA show that the analgesic effect outweighs the potential negative effects on relaxation of the intercostal muscles.[111] Postoperative FEV_1 seems to be a useful predictor of postoperative outcome. A low predicted postoperative value of FEV_1 has been shown to correlate significantly with a complicated postoperative course and poor surgical outcome.[112] By increasing lung volume, TEA may help reduce the incidence of pulmonary complications post-thoracotomy.[113]

A further caveat against the use of TEA, especially in patients with COPD, however, stems from thoracic sympathicolysis and its effects on bronchial muscle and vascular tone.

Since the pulmonary vasculature is innervated by the autonomic nervous system, hypoxic pulmonary vasoconstriction (HPV) may be influenced by sympathetic neural blockade. Prospective clinical observations demonstrated that TEA in combination with general anesthesia did not affect arterial oxygenation or shunt fraction during one-lung ventilation. TEA therefore seems to be suitable for analgesia during thoracic surgery.[114,115] TEA does not increase airway obstruction in patients with COPD or severe obstructive pulmonary disease (Table 56–8).[116,117]

Thoracic Epidural Anesthesia and General Anesthesia

Several studies have shown a reduction in pulmonary complications when general anesthesia was combined with intra- and postoperative epidural anesthesia and analgesia. This reduction was a result of early extubation, better analgesia during mobilization and coughing, attenuation of bronchial reactivity, and improved diaphragmatic function.[107,111,118]

Meta-analyses of pulmonary outcomes have confirmed that TEA in combination with general anesthesia decreases the incidence of atelectasis, reduces the incidence of pulmonary infection, increases arterial oxygen tension, and decreases pulmonary complications overall.[119,120] TEA in combination with general anesthesia can also be recommended for patients with severe COPD and asthma undergoing lung resection surgery.[113,121,122]

Clinical Application

The epidural catheter should be inserted between level T3 and T8 in a midline or paramedian approach using the "loss of resistance" or "hanging drop" technique. Typically, a combination of dilute concentration of local anesthetic (bupivacaine or ropivacaine) with a lipophilic opiate (fentanyl or sufentanil) is used pre- and intraoperatively.[91,123] This combination allows for a reduced dose and side effects of both components.

The epidural application of bupivacaine 0.1% in addition to a concentration of fentanyl 5 μg/ml is a common mixture used with success by many.[124] Combinations of ropivacaine with sufentanil (ropivacaine 0.2%, 0.5–0.75 μg/mL sufentanil) are also common place.[125–127]

The TEA catheter usually remains in situ for 3–4 days after surgery and is usually discontinued after removal of the thorax drainage. During this period, the epidural medication is given in the same combination as during surgery: a low concentration of local anesthetic (0.5–1 mg/mL bupivacaine or 1–2 mg/mL ropivacaine) with a lipophilic opiate (5 μg/mL fentanyl or 0.5 μg/mL sufentanil).

Complications

TEA can be technically challenging and is associated with a failure rate of over 10%. It may cause hypotension or difficulty in voiding and poses a risk of epidural hematoma.[128] More considerations on this topic can be found in Chapter 48.

Thoracic Epidural Anesthesia and Awake Thoracic Surgery

Several case reports and small case series have been published regarding the successful use of TEA in awake cardiac surgery.[108,129,130] The overriding benefit of TEA, in addition to effective analgesia, is the avoidance of intubation and mechanical ventilation required with general anesthesia, as this carries a risk of complications in patients with decreased respiratory function and in patients with comorbidities undergoing cardiac surgery. A few examples of the risks involved with intubation and mechanical ventilation include delayed extubation, increased risk of pneumonia, impaired cardiac performance, neuromuscular problems due to neuromuscular blocking agents, airway pressure–induced injury (barotrauma), lung inflation–induced injury (volutrauma), and the release of a variety of proinflammatory mediators (biotrauma) (Table 56–9).[131]

Clinical Application

A wide variety of thoracic surgical procedures have been performed under TEA as the sole anesthetic modality: resection of pulmonary nodules[108] and solitary metastases,[132] management

TABLE 56–9. Adverse effects of general anesthesia with one-lung ventilation.

Difficult airway

Impaired cardiac performance

Pressure-induced lung injury (barotrauma)

Lung inflation–induced injury (volutrauma)

Atelectasis in the nondependent lung favored by exclusion from ventilation

Bronchospasm and airway traumatism elicited by instrumental tracheal intubation

TABLE 56–10. Potential advantages of awake thoracic surgery over conventional surgery.

Easier acceptance of surgery

Reduced need for high-dependency stay postoperatively

Better respiratory function in the early postoperative period

Reduced operative mortality

Reduced morbidity

Shorter hospital stay

Lower procedure-related costs

Attenuated stress hormone response

Attenuated impairment of immune response

Better survival in oncological surgery

of pneumothorax,[133,134] lung volume reduction surgery,[129] transsternal thymectomy,[135] and even major thoracic procedures such as thoracotomy and median sternotomy (Figure 56–2).[136]

Several randomized studies on awake thoracoscopic operations demonstrated beneficial effects in a wide variety of procedures, such as a lower incidence of postoperative respiratory complications, less nursing care required, shorter in-hospital stay, and higher patient satisfaction than with procedures performed under general anesthesia.[89,132,137–139] In addition, the perioperative surgical stress response may be attenuated in awake VATS as a result of reduced postoperative stress hormones (Table 56–10).[140]

Whether thoracic surgery can be performed on the awake patient under TEA depends on the planned surgery and patient-specific factors. The duration of surgery is a considerable criterion. In the majority of cases, patients considered for awake surgery are high-risk and have several comorbidities. Avoiding general anesthesia in these cases, theoretically at least, can be beneficial. The patient's acceptance, coordination, and close cooperation are mandatory prerequisites for awake procedures.

Contraindications for awake surgery are the same as those for TEA and procedures requiring lung isolation to protect the contralateral lung from contamination: pus, alveolar proteinosis, bronchopleural fistula, and massive bleeding.

Anesthetic Technique

Standard perioperative monitoring includes ECG, peripheral oxygen saturation, noninvasive blood pressure, and end-tidal carbon dioxide to monitor spontaneous ventilation. Invasive monitoring, such as direct arterial pressure and central venous pressure, should be based on the individual patient's general condition and the type of procedure.

TEA is usually performed at level T4–T6 using a median or paramedian access, allowing for a sensorimotor blockade from level T1–T9 depending on the surgical proceeding. Verification of successful puncture and adequate level is performed using warm–cold discrimination. Intraoperative medication via TEA consists of higher-concentrated local anesthetics (bupivacaine 0.5% or ropivacaine 0.75%, with or without opiates [fentanyl or sufentanil]). Sedation during surgery is not usually necessary but should be considered depending on the patient, as it may reduce anxiety and discomfort during awake procedures. However, sedation may also increase the risks of hypercapnia and hypoxemia. Low-dose propofol infusion or small boluses of midazolam have been used.

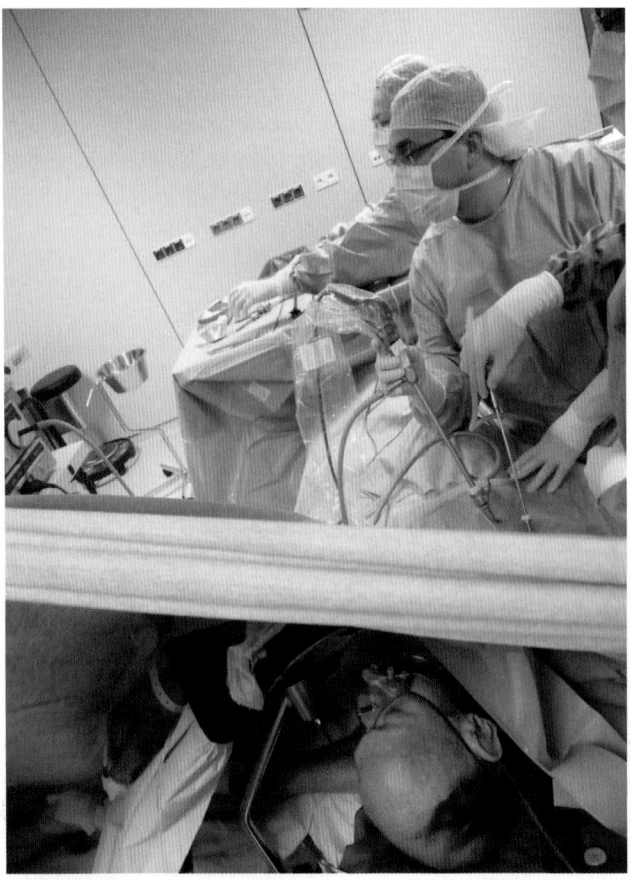

FIGURE 56–2. Video-assisted thoracoscopic surgery in the awake patient.

Clinical Pearl

- Available studies have demonstrated that TEA and PVB are superior to systemic analgesia in treatment of thoracotomy pain.

Side Effects and Complications of Awake Thoracic Surgery

The overall incidence of side effects and complications with awake thoracic surgery is low. Incomplete analgesia of TEA requires immediate conversion to general anesthesia. Spontaneous breathing may become difficult due to the open pneumothorax resulting in mediastinal shift and compression of the dependent lung. However, maintenance of diaphragmatic tone will tend to reduce compromised breathing. Therefore, in most cases, no additional management in awake patients with spontaneous ventilation and lung collapse is necessary.[129]

Nevertheless, hypoxemia and hypercapnia may occur during awake thoracic surgery, mainly due to increased intrapulmonary shunt and paradoxical respiration. Hypoxemia can be treated with oxygen. Hypercapnia may occur for several reasons. First, the sustained hypoventilation of the collapsed lung increases carbon dioxide levels in the respiratory system, which is rebreathed in the contralateral lung. Second, blocking of the intercostal muscles or the diaphragm may occur due to high TEA with phrenic nerve palsy (C3–C5). The conversion rate ranges from 0%–10%.[136,138,141]

Postoperative Management

Adequate postoperative analgesia is essential after thoracic surgery. Analgesia is necessary to allow effective chest physiotherapy, in addition to the administration of bronchodilators and early mobilization. Effective postoperative analgesia can be successfully implemented with TEA by continuously administering local anesthetics in low concentration with or without opioids, via intermittent boluses, or via PCA. As part of a multimodal pain management regimen, TEA should be combined with nonsteroidal anti-inflammatory drugs (NSAIDs).

Summary

Awake thoracic surgery under TEA is feasible, and several studies have demonstrated benefit, especially in thoracoscopic procedures. However, this technique is currently used only in a few specialized centers.

Paravertebral Blockade

In addition to TEA, tPVB plays a significant role in the treatment of intra- and postoperative pain in thoracic surgery (91). tPVB allows for unilateral, effective analgesia across several thoracic segments. It is applied as a single shot or as a continuous, intermittent or PCA infusion of local anesthetic via catheter. Adding adjuvants (eg, opiates) provides no additional benefit.[142] Bilateral use of tPVB has also been reported.[143] tPVB is typically combined with general anesthesia during surgery, though there are reports of tPVB being used exclusively on awake patients for VATS.[144]

Clinical Application and Anatomy

The paravertebral space lies on both sides of the spinal column. It is delimited ventrally by the pleura, medially by the vertebrae, and dorsally by the costotransversal processus. The spinal nerves are embedded in paravertebral adipose tissue and are not surrounded by a thick fascia. The thoracic paravertebral space continues laterally into the intercostal space and medially into the epidural space.

A local anesthetic is injected at the site where the spinal nerve emerges from the intervertebral foramen, resulting in a blockade of the anterior and posterior rami of the intercostal nerve, sympathetic chain, and rami communicantes. Placement of local anesthetic within the paravertebral space produces unilateral somatic and sympathetic block. Spreading of the local anesthetic occurs laterally along the intercostal nerve and medially through the intervertebral foramen. The craniocaudal spread occurs ipsilaterally and depends on the amount of anesthetic administered and the level of puncture.[145]

Technique

Standard techniques use surface landmarks and can be combined with either nerve stimulation or loss of resistance.[92,146] The patient is placed in the sitting or lateral position. At a position 2.5 centimeters lateral of the spinous processes, corresponding to the required level of block, a Touhy needle is advanced until the transverse process is located. The needle is then withdrawn and redirected superiorly or inferiorly to "walk off" 1–1.5 centimeters past the transverse process. For thoracic surgery, a block between T3 and T9 is required. A catheter may be placed but should not be advanced more than 2–3 centimeters past the cannula, as the catheter tip may be inadvertently placed in the pleura, epidural space, or prevertebral space (Figures 56–3 and 56–4).[147]

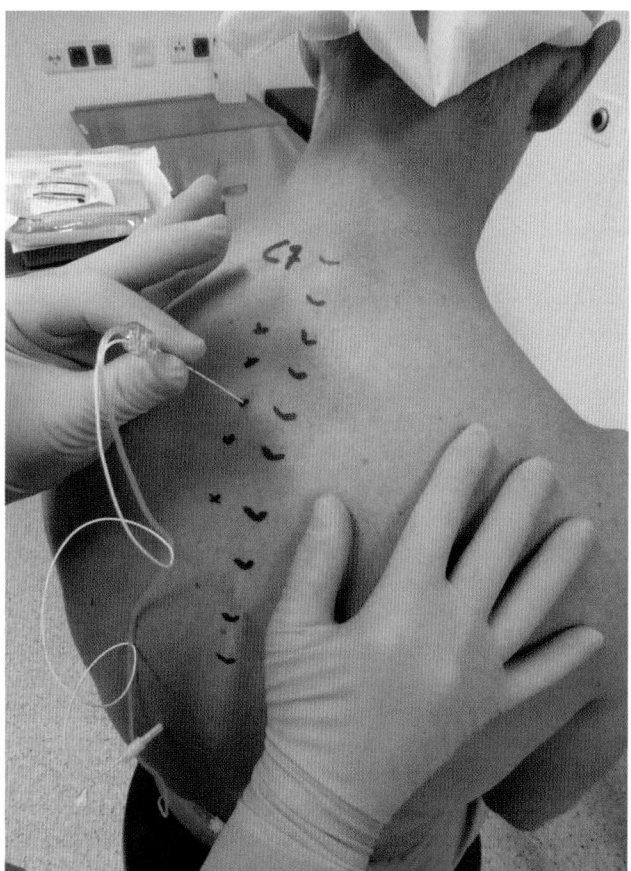

FIGURE 56–3. Surface landmark technique of tPVB. Skin puncture sites are 2.5 cm lateral to the spinous processes.

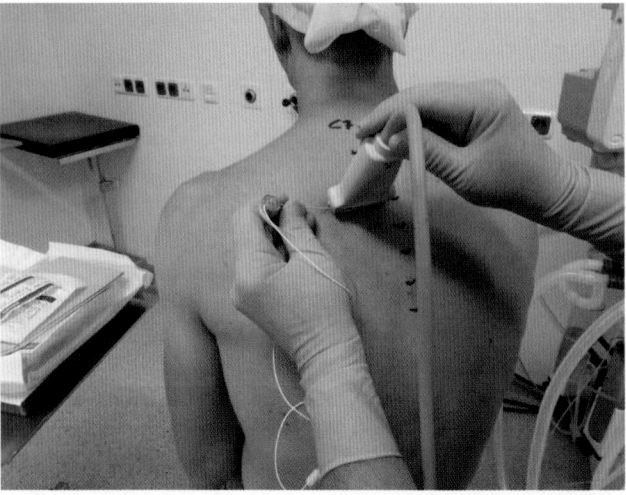

A

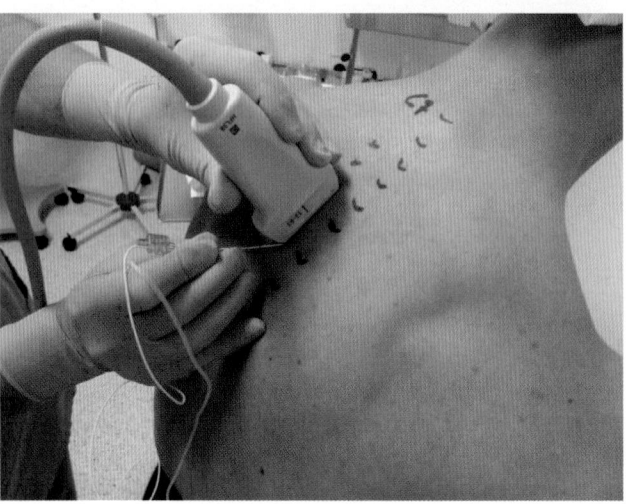

B

FIGURE 56–4. Different ultrasound-guided approaches to perform tPVB. **A:** transversal approach; **B:** parasagittal approach.

As an alternative, paravertebral catheters can be inserted under direct vision by the surgeon during thoracotomy. The success rate is much higher if tears and incisions in the medial parietal pleura are sutured before closure. The insertion of paravertebral catheters during VATS has also been described.

In the last few years, tPVB has increasingly been successfully performed using ultrasound (US).[148] Various positions for probe alignment and angles of approach for needle insertion have been suggested (eg, parasagittal, transversal), but no approach has been described as superior to the others.[149,150] The available literature suggests that tPVB may be performed with a high probability of success using US guidance as an adjunct to traditional techniques. At this time, there is insufficient evidence to show that US guidance improves block success rates or reduces the risk of complications compared to traditional techniques for performing single-shot or continuous paravertebral blocks.[151]

Levobupivacaine and ropivacaine are the most widely used local anesthetic agents for tPVB in current practice. No reliable relationship between the extent of spread and the volume injected has yet been established. A single injection of 15 mL of local anesthetic produces a somatic block over a median of

3 dermatomes and a sympathetic block over 8 dermatomes.[92] For continuous local anesthetic infusions, a rate of 0.1 mL/kg per hour in adults is recommended.[92]

Contraindications

The contraindications for tPVB include infection at the site of puncture, tumor in the paravertebral space, and allergy to local anesthetic drugs. Coagulation disorders and anticoagulation are relative contraindications. Due to the paravertebral space being in close vicinity to the spinal column, the same recommendations that are used for neuraxial blockades, regarding safety intervals between puncture and thromboprophylaxis should be observed.[39,40] To date, no case concerning hematoma-related damage to the spinal column in association with a tPVB has been published.

Clinical Pearls

- A meta-analysis and 2 systemic reviews have shown that tPVB can be at least as effective as epidural analgesia with a better side effect profile and a reduced rate of complications versus epidural analgesia.
- Due to the paravertebral space being in close vicinity to the spinal column, the same recommendations regarding safety intervals between puncture and thromboprophylaxis should be observed.

Complications

The overall incidence of reported complications with tPVBs is low, between 2.6% and 5%.[152] The failure rate varies between 6.8% and 10%.[96] Other specific complications include hypotension (4.6%), vascular puncture (3.8%), pleural puncture (1.1%), pneumothorax (0.5%), epidural or intrathecal spread of anesthetic, and hemothorax or pneumothorax (Table 56–11).[151]

Comparison of TEA and tPVB

Several prospective randomized studies have compared the efficacy of tPVB versus TEA in thoracic surgery. The various studies were re-examined in a meta-analysis and 2 systemic reviews, which reached the conclusion that tPVB is at least as effective as epidural analgesia but has a better side effect profile and a

TABLE 56–11. Complications of tPVB as described in the literature.

Sympathetic blockade, hypotension (< 4.6%)
Horner syndrome (5%–20%)
Vascular puncture (< 3.86%)
Hematoma
Pneumothorax (0.01%–1.2%)
Hemothorax

tPVB, thoracic paravertebral blockade.

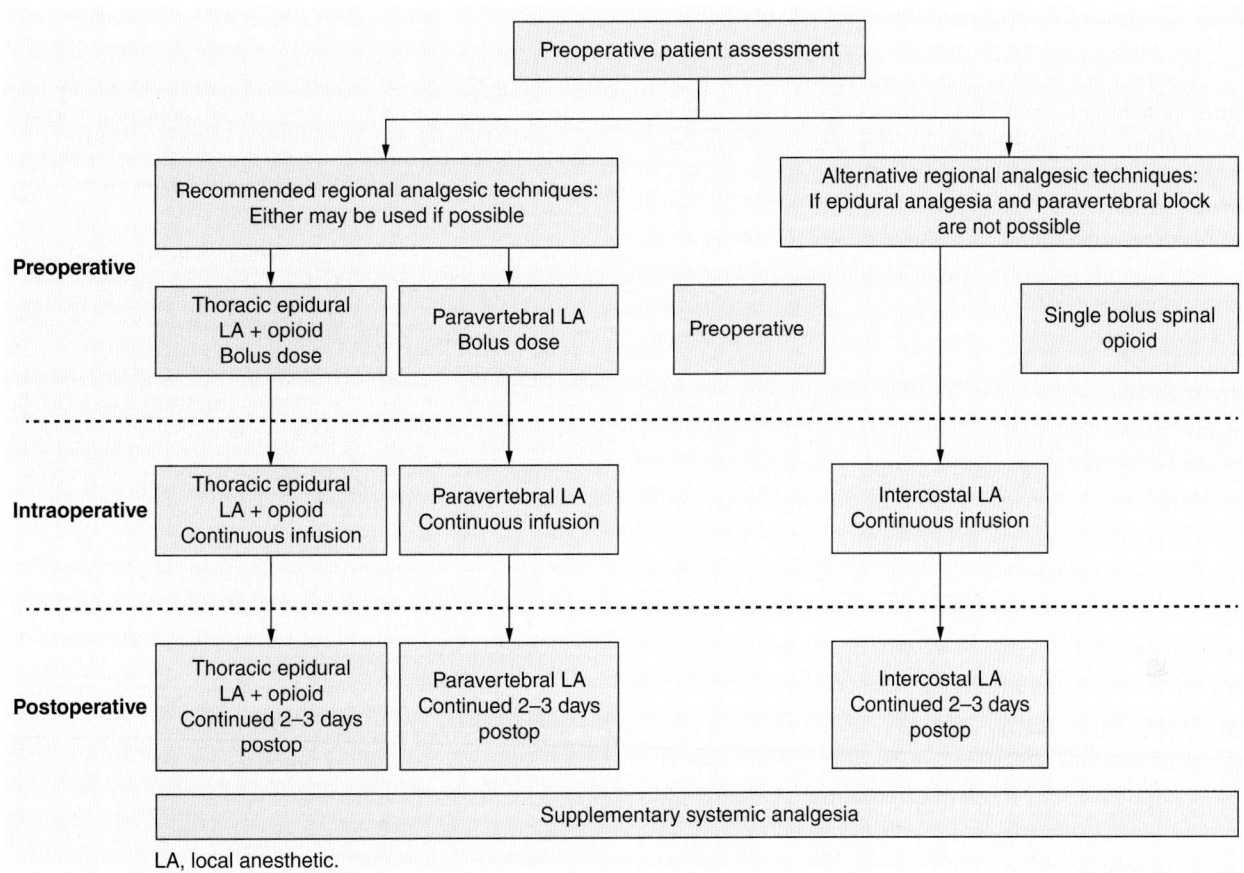

FIGURE 56–5. Recommendations regarding regional techniques for post-thoracotomy analgesia.

reduced rate of complications.[91,90,153] Experts rated both procedures equally in a treatment algorithm for pain management after thoracic surgery,[91] though there have been objections regarding these conclusions due to weaknesses in methodology in the comparative studies.[152] Optimally conducted epidural analgesia has not been compared with tPVB. The current literature indicates that tPVB may be an alternative for post-thoracotomy pain when TEA is not feasible. Severe coagulation abnormalities constitute a contraindication for both tPVB and TEA.[39,40] Higher concentrations of local anesthetics are needed to obtain intercostal nerve blocks and epidural analgesia with tPVB, thus introducing a risk of local anesthetic systemic toxicity (Figure 56–5).

Other Techniques
Intercostal Nerve Blockade

Intercostal nerve block (ICNB) seems to be the most frequently used technique worldwide for post-thoracotomy pain control.[153,154] It is easier, less time-consuming, and, perhaps, a safer technique when ICNB is performed by the surgeon under direct vision before closure of the thoracotomy.[155] ICNB can be performed as a single shot or continuously via catheter.[156] Due to the limited number of comparative studies available, an evaluation of whether US-guided ICNB is superior to the surface landmark technique is currently not possible. Perioperative ICNB reduces pain and the required opiates after thoracic surgery but has

been found to be markedly inferior in terms of analgesia to TEA in comparative studies.[157–159] ICNB in combination with systemic analgesia remains an alternative if contraindications preclude the use of TEA or tPVB or if the puncture has been unsuccessful.

Clinical Pearl

- ICNB in combination with systemic analgesia remains an alternative if contraindications preclude the use of TEA or tPVB.

Intrathecal Opioids

The effectiveness of the intrathecal application of opiates for analgesia after thoracic surgery has been demonstrated in several clinical trials.[80,160,161] Its use decreased the amount of systemic morphine required, although this effect was limited to the first 24 hours postoperatively. Morphine (100–1000 μg) is used either exclusively or in combination with sufentanil as a single bolus before surgery.

One of the side effects of intrathecal opioids found during an investigation was an increased rate of urinary retention.[80] Additionally, depending on the dose, an increased incidence of postoperative respiratory complications was observed, and thus appropriate monitoring is required.[162]

1000   ANESTHESIA IN PATIENTS WITH SPECIFIC CONSIDERATIONS

PART 7

Based on the available studies, a single preoperative bolus of intrathecal opioid is a recommended alternative if epidural analgesia or paravertebral block techniques cannot be used. The application of intrathecal opioids should be part of a multianalgesic regimen and preferred to intravenous opioids via PCA, based on this method's greater pain reduction for up to 24 hours. However, it is important to note that the intrathecal administration of an opioid as a single shot is insufficient for most thoracotomy patients, as it does not provide analgesia beyond 24 hours.[91]

SUMMARY

Several regional techniques can be used for analgesia after for thoracic surgery. Optimal analgesia in thoracic surgery should not be limited to a single technique or medication. It requires early application of a multimodal therapeutic regimen combining the systemic application of nonopiates with a central regional technique (TEA or tPVB) and intensive physiotherapy including mobilization of the patient.

TEA with continuous application of a local anesthetic and opioids is currently considered the standard by most experts. In addition to its analgesia effect, additional cardiovascular, gastrointestinal, and neuroendocrine system benefits may be attained, although the effect of TEA on postoperative mortality and severe morbidity is unclear. Reductions in morbidity postsurgery and in 30-day mortality could be demonstrated only in high-risk patients with obstructive pulmonary disease. Treatment with anticoagulants and antiplatelet drugs presents limitations for the use of TEA. tPVB is an effective analgesic alternative to TEA in thoracic surgery, and both should be considered standard analgesic modalities in thoracic surgical interventions.

REFERENCES

1. Mathews ET, Abrams LD, et al: Intrathecal morphine in open heart surgery. Lancet 1980;2:543–544.
2. El-Baz, Goldin M, et al: Continuous epidural infusion of morphine for pain relief after cardiac operations. J Thorac Cardiovasc Surg 1987;93:878–883.
3. Fitzpatrick GJ, Moriarty DC, et al: Intrathecal morphine in the management of pain following cardiac surgery. Br J Anaesth 1988;60:639–644.
4. Kirno K, Friberg P, Grzegorczyk A, et al: Thoracic epidural anesthesia during coronary artery bypass surgery: Effects on cardiac sympathetic activity, myocardial blood flow and metabolism, and central hemodynamics. Anesth Analg 1994;79:1075–1081.
5. Karagoz HY, Sönmez B, Bakkaloglu B, et al: Coronary artery bypass grafting in the conscious patient without endotracheal general anesthesia. Ann Thorac Surg 2000;70:91–96.
6. Ganapathy S, Murkin JM, Boyd DW, et al: Continuous percutaneous paravertebral block for minimally invasive cardiac surgery. J Cardiothorac Vasc Anesth 1999;13:594–596.
7. Canto M, Sanchez MJ, Casas MA, et al: Bilateral paravertebral blockade for conventional cardiac surgery. Anaesthesia 2003;58:365–370.
8. Chaney MA: Intrathecal and epidural anesthesia and analgesia for cardiac surgery. Anesth Analg 2006;102:45–64.
9. Hemmerling TM, Djaiani G, Babb P, et al: The use of epidural analgesia in cardiac surgery should be encouraged. Anesth Analg 2006;103:1592.
10. Djaiani GN, Ali M, Heinrich L, et al: Ultra-fast-track anesthetic technique facilitates operating room extubation in patients undergoing off-pump coronary revascularization surgery. J Cardiothorac Vasc Anesth 2001;15:152–157.
11. Horswell JL, Herbert MA, Prince SL, et al: Routine immediate extubation after off-pump coronary artery bypass surgery: 514 consecutive patients. J Cardiothorac Vasc Anesth 2005;19:282–287.
12. Tenling A, Joachimsson P-O, Tydén H, et al: Thoracic epidural analgesia as an adjunct to general anaesthesia for cardiac surgery. Effects on pulmonary mechanics. Acta Anaesthesiol Scand 2000;44:1071–1076.
13. Blomberg S, Emanuelsson H, Kvist H, et al: Effects of thoracic epidural anesthesia on coronary arteries and arterioles in patients with coronary artery disease. Anesthesiology 1990;73:840–847.
14. Nabel EG, Ganz P, Gordon JB, et al: Dilation of normal and constriction of artherosclerotic coronary arteries caused by the cold pressure test. Circulation 1988;77:43–52.
15. Nygård E, Kofoed KF, Freiberg J, et al: Effects of high thoracic epidural analgesia on myocardial blood flow in patients with ischemic heart disease. Circulation 2005;111:2165–2170.
16. Liem TH, Booij LH, Hasenbos MA, et al: Coronary artery bypass grafting using two different anesthetic techniques. Part 1: hemodynamic results. J Cardiothorac Vasc Anesth 1992;6:148–155.
17. Scott NB, Turfrey DJ, Ray DA, et al: A prospective randomized study of the potential benefits of thoracic epidural anesthesia and analgesia in patients undergoing coronary artery bypass grafting. Anesth Analg 2001;93:528–535.
18. Fawcett WJ, Edwards RE, Quinn AC, et al: Thoracic epidural analgesia started after cardiopulmonary bypass. Adrenergic, cardiovascular and respiratory sequelae. Anaesthesia 1997;52:294–299.
19. Stenseth R, Bjella L, Berg EM, et al: Effects of thoracic epidural analgesia on pulmonary function after coronary artery bypass surgery. Eur J Cardiothorac Surg 1996;10:859–865.
20. Loick HM, Schmidt C, Van Aken H, et al: High thoracic epidural anesthesia, but not clonidine, attenuates the perioperative stress response via sympatholysis and reduces the release of troponin T in patients undergoing coronary artery bypass grafting. Anesth Analg 1999;88:701–709.
21. Greisen J, Nielsen DV, Sloth E, et al: High thoracic epidural analgesia decreases stress hyperglycemia and insulin need in cardiac surgery patients. Acta Anaesthesiol Scand 2013;57:171–177.
22. Tenling A, Joachimsson PO, Tyden H, et al: Thoracic epidural anesthesia as an adjunct to general anesthesia for cardiac surgery: effects on ventilation-perfusion relationships. J Cardiothorac Vasc Anesth 1999;13:258–264.
23. Djaiani G, et al: Thoracic epidural anesthesia as an adjunct to general anesthesia for cardiac surgery: effects on ventilation-perfusion relationships. J Cardiothorac Vasc Anesth 2000;14:359–360.
24. Monaco F, Biselli C, Landoni G, et al: Thoracic epidural anesthesia improves early outcome in patients undergoing cardiac surgery for mitral regurgitation: a propensity-matched study. J Cardiothorac Vasc Anesth 2013;27:445–450.
25. Hemmerling TM, Le N, Olivier JF, et al: Immediate extubation after aortic valve surgery using high thoracic epidural analgesia or opioid-based analgesia. J Cardiothorac Vasc Anesth 2005;19:176–181.
26. Jakobsen CJ, Bhavsar R, Nielsen DV, et al: High thoracic epidural analgesia in cardiac surgery: part 1-high thoracic epidural analgesia improves cardiac performance in cardiac surgery patients. J Cardiothorac Vasc Anesth 2012;26:1039–1047.
27. Nielsen DV, Bhavsar R, Greisen J, et al: High thoracic epidural analgesia in cardiac surgery: part 2-high thoracic epidural analgesia does not reduce time in or improve quality of recovery in the intensive care unit. J Cardiothorac Vasc Anesth 2012;26:1048–1054.
28. Mangano CM, et al: Risky business. J Thorac Cardiovasc Surg 2003;125:1204–1207.
29. Royse C, Royse A, Soeding P, et al: Prospective randomized trial of high thoracic epidural analgesia for coronary artery bypass surgery. Ann Thorac Surg 2003;75:93–100.
30. Caputo M, Alwair H, Rogers C, et al: Thoracic epidural anesthesia improves early outcomes in patients undergoing off-pump coronary artery bypass surgery: A prospective randomized controlled trial. Anesthesiology 2011;114:380–390.
31. Priestley MC, Cope L, Halliwell R, et al: Thoracic epidural anesthesia for cardiac surgery: the effects on tracheal intubation time and length of hospital stay. Anesth Analg 2002;94:275–282.
32. Svircevic V, Nierich AP, Moons KG, et al: Thoracic epidural anesthesia for cardiac surgery: a randomized trial. Anesthesiology 2011;114:262–270.
33. Gu WJ, Wei CY, Huang DQ, et al: Meta-analysis of randomized controlled trials on the efficacy of thoracic epidural anesthesia in preventing atrial fibrillation after coronary artery bypass grafting. BMC Cardiovasc Disord 2012;19:12–67.

34. Bignami E, Landoni G, Biondi-Zoccai GG, et al: Epidural analgesia improves outcome in cardiac surgery: a meta-analysis of randomized controlled trials. J Cardiothorac Vasc Anesth 2009;23:594–599.

35. Liu SS, Block BM, Wu CL, et al: Effects of perioperative central neuraxial analgesia on outcome after coronary artery bypass surgery: a meta-analysis. Anesthesiology 2004;101:153–163.

36. Svircevic V, van Dijk D, Nierich AP, et al: Meta-analysis of thoracic epidural anesthesia versus general anesthesia for cardiac surgery. Anesthesiology 2011;114:271–282.

37. Djaiani G, Fedorko L, Beattie WS, et al: Regional anesthesia in cardiac surgery: a friend or a foe? Semin Cardiothorac Vasc Anesth 2005;9: 87–104.

38. Royse C, Remedios C, Royse A, et al: High thoracic epidural analgesia reduces the risk of long-term depression in patients undergoing coronary artery bypass surgery. Ann Thorac Cardiovasc Surg 2007;13:32–35.

39. Horlocker TT, Wedel DJ, Rowlingson JC, et al: Regional anesthesia in the patient receiving antithrombotic or thrombolytic therapy: American Society of Regional Anesthesia and Pain Medicine evidence-based guidelines (third edition). Reg Anesth Pain Med 2010;35:64–101.

40. Gogarten W, Vandermeulen E, Van Aken H, et al; European Society of Anaesthesiology. Regional anaesthesia and antithrombotic agents: recommendations of the European Society of Anaesthesiology. Eur J Anaesthesiol 2010;27:999–1015.

41. Royse CF, Soeding PF, Royse AG, et al: High thoracic epidural analgesia for cardiac surgery: an audit of 874 cases. Anaesth Intensive Care 2007;35:374–377.

42. Kessler P, Neidhart G, Bremerich DH, et al: High thoracic epidural anesthesia for coronary artery bypass grafting using two different surgical approaches in conscious patients. Anesth Analg 2002;95:791–797.

43. Chakravarthy M, Thimmangowda P, Krishnamurthy J, et al: Thoracic epidural anesthesia in cardiac surgical patients: a prospective audit of 2,113 cases. J Cardiothorac Vasc Anesth 2005;19:44–48.

44. Jack ES, Scott NB, et al: The risk of vertebral canal complications in 2837 cardiac surgery patients with thoracic epidurals. Acta Anaesthesiol Scand 2007;51:722–725.

45. Bracco D, Hemmerling T: Epidural analgesia in cardiac surgery: an updated risk assessment. Heart Surg Forum 2007;10:E334–E337.

46. Roediger L, Larbuisson R, Lamy M, et al: New approaches and old controversies to postoperative pain control following cardiac surgery. Eur J Anaesthesiol 2006;23:539–550.

47. Ruppen W, Derry S, McQuay HJ, et al: Incidence of epidural haematoma and neurological injury in cardiovascular patients with epidural analgesia/anaesthesia: systematic review and meta-analysis. BMC Anesthesiol 2006;6:10.

48. Grewal S, Hocking G, Wildsmith JA, et al: Epidural abscesses. Br J Anaesth 2006;96:292–302.

49. Watanabe G, Tomita S, Yamaguchi S, et al: Awake coronary artery bypass grafting under thoracic epidural anesthesia: great impact on off-pump coronary revascularization and fast-track recovery. Eur J Cardiothorac Surg 2011;40:788–793.

50. Oscarsson A, Gupta A, Fredrikson M, et al: To continue or discontinue aspirin in the perioperative period: a randomized, controlled clinical trial. Br J Anaesth 2010;104:305–312.

51. Sharma S, Kapoor MC, Sharma VK, et al: Epidural hematoma complicating high thoracic epidural catheter placement intended for cardiac surgery. J Cardiothorac Vasc Anesth 2004;18:759–762.

52. Rosen DA, Hawkinberry DW 2nd, Rosen KR, et al: An epidural hematoma in an adolescent patient after cardiac surgery. Anesth Analg 2004;98:966–969.

53. Yoshida S, Nitta Y, Oda K, et al: Anterior spinal artery syndrome after minimally invasive direct coronary artery bypass grafting under general combined epidural anesthesia. Jap J Thorac Cardiovasc Surg 2005;53: 230–233.

54. Bang J, Kim JU, Lee YM, et al: Spinal epidural hematoma related to an epidural catheter in a cardiac surgery patient: a case report. Korean J Anesthesiol 2011;61:524–527.

55. Perlas A, et al: Management of a suspected spinal-epidural hematoma. Tech Reg Anesth Pain Manage 2006;10:62–65.

56. Ho AM, Chung DC, Joynt GM, et al: Neuraxial blockade and hematoma in cardiac surgery: estimating the risk of a rare adverse event that has not (yet) occurred. Chest 2000;117:551–555.

57. Chakravarthy M, Jawali V, Patil TA, et al: High thoracic epidural anesthesia as the sole anesthetic for performing multiple grafts in off-pump coronary artery bypass surgery. J Cardiothorac Vasc Anesth 2003;17: 160–164.

58. Hemmerling TM, Noiseux N, Basile F, et al: Awake cardiac surgery using a novel anesthetic technique. Can J Anaesth 2005;52:1088–1092.

59. Lucchetti V, Moscariello C, Catapano D, et al: Coronary artery bypass grafting in the awake patient: combined thoracic epidural and lumbar subarachnoid block. Eur J Cardiothorac Surg 2004;26:658–659.

60. Kirali K, Kocak T, Guzelmeric F, et al: Off-pump awake coronary revascularization using bilateral internal thoracic arteries. Ann Thorac Surg 2004;78:1598–1602.

61. Meininger D, Neidhart G, Bremerich DH, et al: Coronary artery bypass grafting via sternotomy in conscious patients. World J Surg 2003;27: 534–538.

62. Schachner T, Bonatti J, Balogh D, et al: Aortic valve replacement in the conscious patient under regional anesthesia without endotracheal intubation. J Thorac Cardiovasc Surg 2003;125:1526–1527.

63. Stritesky M, Semrad M, Kunstyr J, et al: On-pump cardiac surgery in a conscious patient using a thoracic epidural anesthesia—an ultra fast track method. Bratisl Lek Listy 2004;105:51–55.

64. Bottio T, Bisleri G, Piccoli P et al: Heart valve surgery in a very high-risk population: a preliminary experience in awake patients. J Heart Valve Dis 2007;16:187–194.

65. Chakravarthy M, Jawali V, Manohar MV, et al: Conscious cardiac surgery with cardiopulmonary bypass using thoracic epidural anesthesia without endotracheal GA. J Cardiothorac Vasc Anesth 2005;19: 300–305.

66. Picozzi P, Lappa A, Menichetti A, et al: Mitral valve replacement under thoracic epidural anesthesia in an awake patient suffering from systemic sclerosis. Acta Anaesthesiol Scand 2007;51:644.

67. Kessler P, Neidhart G, Lischke V, et al: Coronary bypass operation with complete median sternotomy in awake patients with high thoracic peridural anesthesia. Anaesthesist 2002;51:533–538.

68. Noiseux N, Prieto I, Bracco D, et al: Coronary artery bypass grafting in the awake patient combining high thoracic epidural and femoral nerve block: first series of 15 patients. Br J Anaesth 2008;100:184–189.

69. Gerosa G, Grego F, Falasco G, et al: Simultaneous coronary artery bypass grafting and carotid endarterectomy in an awake Jehova's witness patient without endotracheal intubation. Eur J Cardiothorac Surg 2005;27: 168–170.

70. Kessler P, Aybek T, Neidhart G, et al: Comparison of three anesthetic techniques for off-pump coronary artery bypass grafting: general anesthesia, combined general and high thoracic epidural anesthesia, or high thoracic epidural anesthesia alone. J Cardiothorac Vasc Anesth 2005;19:32–39.

71. Karagoz HY, Kurtoglu M, Bakkaloglu B, et al: Coronary artery bypass grafting in the awake patient: three years' experience in 137 cases. J Thorac Cardiovasc Surg 2003;125:1401–1404.

72. Chakravarthy M, Jawali V, Manohar MV, et al: Conscious off-pump coronary artery bypass surgery in a patient with a reconstructed trachea with high thoracic epidural as the sole anesthetic. J Cardiothorac Vasc Anesth 2004;18:392–394.

73. Knapik P, Przybylski R, Nadziakiewicz P et al: Awake heart valve surgery in a patient with severe pulmonary disease. Ann Thorac Surg 2008; 86:293–295.

74. Aybek T, Kessler P, Khan MF et al: Operative techniques in awake coronary artery bypass grafting. J Thorac Cardiovasc Surg 2003;125: 1394–1400.

75. Chakravarthy M, Jawali V, Manohar M, et al: Conscious off pump coronary artery bypass surgery-an audit of our first 151 cases. Ann Thorac Cardiovasc Surg 2005;11:93–97.

76. Kurtoglu M, Ates S, Bakkaloglu B, et al: Epidural anesthesia versus general anesthesia in patients undergoing minimally invasive direct coronary artery bypass surgery. Anadolu Kardiyol Derg 2009;9: 54–58.

77. Porizka M, Stritesky M, Semrad M, et al: Postoperative outcome in awake, on-pump, cardiac surgery patients. J Anesth 2011;25:500–508.

78. Chaney MA, Smith KR, Barclay JC, et al: Large-dose intrathecal morphine for coronary artery bypass grafting. Anesth Analg 1996;83: 215–222.

79. Lena P, Balarac N, Arnulf JJ, et al: Intrathecal morphine and clonidine for coronary artery bypass grafting. Br J Anaesth 2003;90:300–303.

80. Liu N, Kuhlman G, Dalibon N, et al: A randomized, double-blinded comparison of intrathecal morphine, sufentanil and their combination versus IV morphine patient-controlled analgesia for postthoracotomy pain. Anesth Analg 2001;92:31–36.

81. Bowler I, Djaiani G, Abel R, et al: A combination of intrathecal morphine and remifentanil anesthesia for fast-track cardiac anesthesia and surgery. J Cardiothorac Vasc Anesth 2002;16:709–714.

82. Alhashemi JA, Sharpe MD, Harris CL, et al: Effect of subarachnoid morphine administration on extubation time after coronary artery bypass graft surgery. J Cardiothorac Vasc Anesth 2000;14:639–644.

83. Latham P, Zarate E, White PF, et al: Fast-track cardiac anesthesia: a comparison of remifentanil plus intrathecal morphine with sufentanil in a desflurane-based anesthetic. J Cardiothorac Vasc Anesth 2000;14: 645–651.

84. Zarate E, Latham P, White PF, et al: Fast-track cardiac anesthesia: use of remifentanil combined with intrathecal morphine as an alternative to sufentanil during desflurane anesthesia. Anesth Analg 2000;91: 283–287.

85. Lee TW, Grocott HP, Schwinn D, et al: High spinal anesthesia for cardiac surgery: effects on beta-adrenergic receptor function, stress response, and hemodynamics. Anesthesiology 2003;98:499–510.

86. Kowalewski RJ, MacAdams CL, Eagle CJ, et al: Anaesthesia for coronary artery bypass surgery supplemented with subarachnoid bupivacaine and morphine: a report of 18 cases. Can J Anaesth 1994;41:1189–1195.

87. Bettex DA, Schmidlin D, Chassot PG, et al: Intrathecal sufentanil-morphine shortens the duration of intubation and improves analgesia in fast-track cardiac surgery. Can J Anaesth 2002;49:711–717.

88. Vandermeulen EP, Van Aken H, Vermylen J, et al: Anticoagulants and spinal epidural anesthesia. Anesth Analg 1994;79:1165–1177.

89. Zangrillo A, Bignami E, Biondi-Zoccai GG, et al: Spinal analgesia in cardiac surgery: a meta-analysis of randomized controlled trials. J Cardiothorac Vasc Anesth 2009;23:813–821.

90. Davies RG, Myles PS, Graham JM, et al: A comparison of analgesic efficacy and side-effects of paravertebral vs epidural blockade for thoracotomy. A systematic review and meta-analysis of randomised trials. Br J Anaesth 2006;96:418–426.

91. Joshi GP, Bonnet F, Shah R et al: A systematic review of randomized trials evaluating regional techniques for postthoracotomy analgesia. Anesth Analg 2008;107:1026–1040.

92. Karmakar MK, et al: Thoracic paravertebral block. Anesthesiology 2001;95:771–780.

93. Dhole S, Mehta Y, Saxena H, et al: Comparison of continuous thoracic epidural and paravertebral blocks for postoperative analgesia after minimally invasive direct coronary artery bypass surgery. J Cardiothorac Vasc Anesth 2001;15:288–292.

94. Olivier J-F, Bracco D, Nguyen P, et al: A novel approach for pain management in cardiac surgery via median sternotomy: bilateral single-shot paravertebral blocks. Heart Surg Forum 2007;10:E357–E362.

95. Lynch JJ, Mauermann WJ, Pulido JN, et al: Use of paravertebral blockade to facilitate early extubation after minimally invasive cardiac surgery. Semin Cardiothorac Vasc Anesth 2010;14:47–48.

96. Lonnqvist PA, MacKenzie J, Soni AK, et al: Paravertebral blockade: failure rate and complications. Anaesthesia 1995;50:813–815.

97. Naja Z, Lonnqvist PA, et al: Somatic paravertebral nerve blockade. Incidence of failed block and complications. Anaesthesia 2001;56: 1184–1188.

98. Loan WB, Morrison JD, et al: The incidence and severity of postoperative pain. Br J Anaesth 1967;39:695–698.

99. Kehlet H, Jensen TS, Woolf CJ, et al: Persistent postsurgical pain: risk factors and prevention. Lancet 2006;367:1618–1625.

100. Muehling BM, Halter GL, Schelzig H, et al: Reduction of postoperative pulmonary complications after lung surgery using a fast track clinical pathway. Eur J Cardiothorac Surg 2008;34:174–180.

101. Forster R, Storck M, Schafer JR, et al: Thoracoscopy versus thoracotomy: A prospective comparison of trauma and quality of life. Langenbecks Arch Surg 2002;387:32–36.

102. Wijeysundera DN, Beattie WS, Austin PC, et al: Epidural anaesthesia and survival after intermediate-to-high risk non-cardiac surgery: a population-based cohort study. Lancet 2008;372:562–569.

103. Block BM, Liu SS, Rowlingson AJ et al: Efficacy of postoperative epidural analgesia: a meta-analysis. JAMA 2003;290:2455–2463.

104. Liu SS, Wu CL, et al: The effect of analgesic technique on postoperative patient–reported outcomes including analgesia: a systematic review. Anesth Analg 2007;105:789–808.

105. Wu CL, Cohen SR, Richman JM, et al: Efficacy of postoperative patient-controlled and continuous infusion epidural analgesia versus intravenous patient-controlled analgesia with opioids. A meta-analysis. Anesthesiology 2005;103:1079–1088.

106. Behera BK, Puri GD, Ghai B. Patient-controlled epidural analgesia with fentanyl and bupivacaine provides better analgesia than intravenous morphine patient–controlled analgesia for early thoracotomy pain. J Postgrad Med 2008;54:86–90.

107. Ali M, Winter DC, Hanly AM et al: Prospective, randomized, controlled trial of thoracic epidural or patient–controlled opiate analgesia on perioperative quality of life. Br J Anaesth 2010;104:292–297.

108. Pompeo E, Mineo D, Rogliani P, et al: Feasibility and results of awake thoracoscopic resection of solitary pulmonary nodules. Ann Thorac Surg 2004;78:1761–1768.

109. Sundberg A, Wattwil M, Arvill A, et al: Respiratory effects of high thoracic epidural anaesthesia. Acta Anaesthesiol Scand 1986;30: 215–217.

110. Mankikian B, Cantineau JP, Bertrand M, et al: Improvement of diaphragmatic function by a thoracic extradural block after abdominal surgery. Anesthesiology 1988;68:379–386.

111. Bauer C, Hentz JG, Ducrocq X, et al: Lung function after lobectomy: a randomized, double-blinded trial comparing thoracic epidural ropivacaine/sufentanil and intravenous morphine for patient-controlled analgesia. Anesth Analg 2007;105:238–244.

112. Win T, Jackson A, Sharples L, et al: Relationship between pulmonary function and lung cancer surgical outcome. Eur Respir J 2005;25: 594–599.

113. Licker MJ, Widikker I, Robert J, et al: Operative mortality and respiratory complications after lung resection for cancer: impact of chronic obstructive pulmonary disease and time trends. Ann Thorac Surg 2006;81:1830–1837.

114. Chow MY, Goh MH, Boey SK, et al: The effects of remifentanil and thoracic epidural on oxygenation and pulmonary shunt fraction during one-lung ventilation. J Cardiothorac Vasc Anesth 2003;17:69–72.

115. Garutti I, Cruz P, Olmedilla L, et al: Effects of thoracic epidural meperidine on arterial oxygenation during one-lung ventilation in thoracic surgery. J Cardiothorac Vasc Anesth 2003;17:302–305.

116. Groeben H, Schäfer B, Pavlakovic G, et al: Lung function under high thoracic segmental epidural anesthesia with ropivacaine or bupivacaine in patients with severe obstructive pulmonary disease undergoing breast surgery. Anesthesiology 2002;96:536–541.

117. Groeben H, Schwalen A, Irsfeld S, et al: High thoracic epidural anesthesia does not alter airway resistance and attenuates the response to an inhalational provocation test in patients with bronchial hyperreactivity. Anesthesiology 1994;81:868–874.

118. Cywinski JB, Xu M, Sessler DI, et al: Predictors of prolonged postoperative endotracheal intubation in patients undergoing thoracotomy for lung resection. J Cardiothorac Vasc Anesth 2009;23:766–769.

119. Ballantyne JC, Carr DB, deFerranti S, et al: The comparative effect of postoperative analgesic therapies on pulmonary outcome: cumulative meta-analyses of randomized, controlled trials. Anesth Analg 1998;86: 598–612.

120. Popping DM, Elia N, Marret E, et al: Protective effects of epidural analgesia on pulmonary complications after abdominal and thoracic surgery: a meta-analysis. Arch Surg 2008;143:990–999.

121. Hirshman CA et al: Perioperative management of the asthmatic patient. Can J Anaesth 1991;38:R26–R32.

122. Gruber EM, Tschernko EM, Kritzinger M, et al: The effects of thoracic epidural analgesia with bupivacaine 0.25% on ventilatory mechanics I. Patients with severe chronic obstructive pulmonary disease. Anesth Analg 2001;92:1015–1019.

123. Senturk M, Ozcan PE, Talu GK, et al: The effects of three different analgesia techniques on long–term postthoracotomy pain. Anesth Analg 2002;94:11–15.

124. Tan CN, Guha A, Scawn ND, et al: Optimal concentration of epidural fentanyl in bupivacaine 0.1% after thoracotomy. Br J Anaesth 2004;92: 670–674.

125. Manion SC, Brennan TJ, et al: Thoracic epidural analgesia and acute pain management. Anesthesiology 2011;115:181–188.

126. Tuncel G, Ozalp G, Savli S, et al: Epidural ropivacaine or sufentanil-ropivacaine infusions for post-thoracotomy pain. Eur J Cardiothorac Surg 2005;28:375–379.

127. De Cosmo G, Congedo E, Lai C et al: Ropivacaine vs. levobupivacaine combined with sufentanil for epidural analgesia after lung surgery. Eur J Anaesthesiol 2008;25:1020–1025.

128. McLeod G, Davies H, Munnoch N, et al: Postoperative pain relief using thoracic epidural analgesia: outstanding success and disappointing failures. Anaesthesia 2001;56:75–81.

129. Mineo TC, Pompeo E, Mineo D, et al: Awake nonresectional lung volume reduction surgery. Ann Surg 2006;243:131–136.

130. Kaseda S, Aoki T, Hangai N, et al: Better pulmonary function and prognosis with video-assisted thoracic surgery than with thoracotomy. Ann Thorac Surg 2000;70:1644–1646.

131. Whitehead T, Slutsky AS, et al: The pulmonary physician in critical care. 7: ventilator induced lung injury. Thorax 2002;57:635–642.

132. Pompeo E, Tacconi F, Mineo D, et al: The role of awake video-assisted thoracoscopic surgery in spontaneous pneumothorax. J Thorac Cardiovasc Surg 2007;133:786–790.

133. Mukaida T, Andou A, Date H, et al: Thoracoscopic operation for secondary pneumothorax under local and epidural anesthesia in high-risk patients. Ann Thorac Surg 1998;65:924–926.

134. Sugimoto S, Date H, Sugimoto R, et al: Thoracoscopic operation with local and epidural anesthesia in the treatment of penumothorax after lung transplantation. J Thorac Cardiovasc Surg 2005;130:1219–1220.

135. Tsunezuka Y, Oda M, Matsumoto I, Tamura et al: Extended thymectomy in patients with myasthenia gravis with high thoracic epidural anesthesia alone. World J Surg 2004;28:962–965.

136. Al-Abdullatief M, Wahood A, Al-Shirawi N, et al: Awake anaesthesia for major thoracic surgical procedures: an observational study. Eur J Cardiothorac Surg 2007;32:346–350.

137. Pompeo E, Rogliani P, Tacconi F, et al: Randomized comparison of awake nonresectional versus nonawake resectional lung volume reduction surgery. J Thorac Cardiovasc Surg 2012;143:47–54.

138. Chen JS, Cheng YJ, Hung MH, et al: Nonintubated thoracoscopic lobectomy for lung cancer. Ann Surg 2011;254:1038–1043.

139. Noda M, Okada Y, Maeda S, et al: Is there a benefit of awake thoracoscopic surgery in patients with secondary spontaneous pneumothorax? J Thorac Cardiovasc Surg 2012;143:613–616.

140. Tacconi F, Pompeo E, Fabbi E, et al: Awake video-assisted pleural decortication for empyema thoracis. Eur J Cardiothorac Surg 2010;37: 594–601.

141. Tseng YD, Cheng YJ, Hung MH, et al: Nonintubated needlescopic video-assisted thoracic surgery for management of peripheral lung nodules. Ann Thorac Surg 2012;93:1049–1054.

142. Kotze A, Scally A, Howell S, et al: Efficacy and safety of different techniques of paravertebral block for analgesia after thoracotomy: a systemic review and metaregression. Br JAnaesth 2009;103:626–636.

143. Karmakar MK, Booker PD, Franks, et al: Bilateral continuous paravertebral block used for postoperative analgesia in an infant having bilateral thoracotomy. Paediatr Anaesth 1997;7:469–471.

144. Piccioni F, Langer M, Fumagalli L, et al: Thoracic paravertebral anaesthesia for awake video-assisted thoracoscopic surgery daily. Anaesthesia 2010;65:1221–1224.

145. Richardson J, Lönnqvist PA, Naja Z, et al: Bilateral thoracic paravertebral block: potential and practice. Br J Anaesth 2011;106:164–171.

146. Wheeler LJ, et al: Peripheral nerve stimulation end-point for thoracic paravertebral block. Br J Anaesth 2001;86:598–599.

147. Luyet C, Eichenberger U, Greif R, et al: Ultrasound-guided paravertebral puncture and placement of catheters in human cadavers: an imaging study. Br J Anaesth 2009;102:534–539.

148. Hara K, Sakura S, Nomura T, et al: Use of ultrasound for thoracic paravertebral block. Masui 2012;56:925–931.

149. Ben-Ari A, Moreno M, Chelly JE, et al: Ultrasound-guided paravertebral block using an intercostal approach. Anesth Analg 2009;109: 1691–1694.

150. Chelly JE: Paravertebral blocks. Anesthesiol Clin 2012;30:75–90.

151. Abrahams MS, Horn JL, Noles LM, et al: Evidence-based medicine: ultrasound guidance for truncal blocks. Reg Anesth Pain Med 2010;35: S36–S42.

152. Norum HM, Breivik H, et al: A systematic review of comparative studies indicates that paravertebral block is neither superior nor safer than epidural analgesia for pain after thoracotomy. Scand J Pain 2010;1:12–23.

153. Detterbeck FC, et al: Efficacy of methods of intercostal nerve blockade for pain relief after thoracotomy. Ann Thorac Surg 2005;80:1550–1559.

154. Concha M, Dagnino J, Cariaga M, et al: Analgesia after thoracotomy: epidural fentanyl/bupivacaine compared with intercostal nerve block plus intravenous morphine. J Cardiothorac Vasc Anesth 2004;18:322–326.

155. Takamori S, Yoshida S, Hayashi A, et al: Intraoperative intercostal nerve blockade for postthoracotomy pain. Ann Thorac Surg 2002;74: 338–341.

156. Chan VW, Chung F, Cheng DC et al: Analgesic and pulmonary effects of continuous intercostal nerve block following thoracotomy. Can J Anaesth 1991;38:733–739.

157. Wurnig PN, Lackner H, Teiner C, et al: Is intercostal block for pain management in thoracic surgery more successful than epidural anaesthesia? Eur J Cardiothorac Surg 2002;21:1115–1119.

158. Debreceni G, Molnar Z, Szelig L et al: Continuous epidural or intercostal analgesia following thoracotomy: a prospective randomized double-blind clinical trial. Acta Anaesthesiol Scand 2003;47:1091–1095.

159. Meierhenrich R, Hock D, Kühn S, et al: Analgesia and pulmonary function after lung surgery: is a single intercostal nerve block plus patient-controlled intravenous morphine as effective as patient-controlled epidural anaesthesia? A randomized non-inferiority clinical trial. Br J Anaesth 2011;106:580–589.

160. Askar FZ, Kocabas S, Yucel S et al: The efficacy of intrathecal morphine in post–thoracotomy pain management. J Int Med Res 2007;35:314–322.

161. Mason N, Gondret R, Junca A, et al: Intrathecal sufentanil and morphine for post–thoracotomy pain relief. Br J Anaesth 2001;86: 236–240.

162. Meylan N, Elia N, Lysakowski C, et al: Benefit and risk of intrathecal morphine without local anaesthetic in patients undergoing major surgery: meta-analysis of randomized trials. Br J Anaesth 2009;102:156–167.

CHAPTER 57

Regional Anesthesia in Austere Environment Medicine

Chester C. Buckenmaier III

INTRODUCTION

Regional anesthesia has played a pivotal role in the development of anesthesiology as a medical specialty since the discovery of the local anesthetic properties of cocaine by Carl Köller in 1884. In the decades since this landmark discovery, surgeons and anesthesia providers have appreciated the advantages of regional anesthesia in their patients, particularly in surgical situations complicated by limited resources and austere environmental conditions. War, more than any other human endeavor, has driven the need to provide effective anesthesia for surgery in austere environments. Indeed, the development of anesthesiology as a distinct specialty has been attributed to the medical experience obtained in World War II.[1] The physician-anesthetists of that era quickly recognized that regional anesthesia imparted the least physiologic insult to the wounded soldier and allowed a more awake patient to be returned to the recovery ward, thus reducing the burden on limited wartime medical resources.[1] As anesthesiology matured as a medical specialty and departments of anesthesiology began to break away from departments of surgery in academic centers, regional anesthesia continued to evolve. During the Vietnam War, the value of regional anesthesia in harsh medical conditions was reestablished. In one series of 1000 battle casualties, nerve block, spinal, or local anesthesia was used in 49% of cases: "This allowed increased anesthesia coverage of more surgical procedures at any one time as well as decreasing the demands on postoperative ward personnel in a multiple casualty situation."[2] The role of regional anesthesia in combat casualty care continues to expand in modern conflicts. Consequently, military medical planners are understandably interested in austere environment anesthesia due to the realities of military wartime missions. Civilian anesthesiologists are also interested in the advantages of regional anesthesia in austere environments for disasters, civil defense, and missions to medically underserved regions of the world.

In the last 20 years, regional anesthesia has undergone a renaissance. New equipment, such as peripheral nerve stimulators and ultrasound technology, has facilitated block placement and enhanced resident training in regional anesthesia. Continuous peripheral nerve block (CPNB) catheters and peripheral nerve infusion pumps have extended the benefits of regional block techniques beyond the immediate perioperative period to days after an operation and even into the home.[3] Additionally, the practice of regional anesthesia has evolved into an important subspecialty of anesthesiology termed *acute* or *perioperative pain medicine*. Acute pain services are now an integral component of quality healthcare in the United States.[4] In this chapter, the advantages and application of advanced regional anesthesia in austere environment medicine will be examined. The role of recent advances in regional anesthesia equipment and techniques for facilitating anesthesia in less-than-ideal conditions will also be discussed.

AUSTERE ENVIRONMENT ANESTHESIOLOGY

The practice of medicine in an austere environment requires a significantly different approach than that used for medicine practiced in major medical centers and in developed countries in general. This is especially true for the practice of anesthesiology. In developed countries, the anesthesiologist has a tremendous resource base that is readily available and largely transparent to the production of an anesthetic plan. The utilities, roads, computers, and other wonders of modern infrastructure common to developed nations are rarely noticed by anesthesiologists, but they impart a tremendous advantage in ensuring a successful anesthetic outcome. In contrast, the anesthesiologist practicing austere environment anesthesiology (AEA) becomes very aware of the effect limited resources can have on anesthetic decisions. In AEA, the anesthesiologist must factor

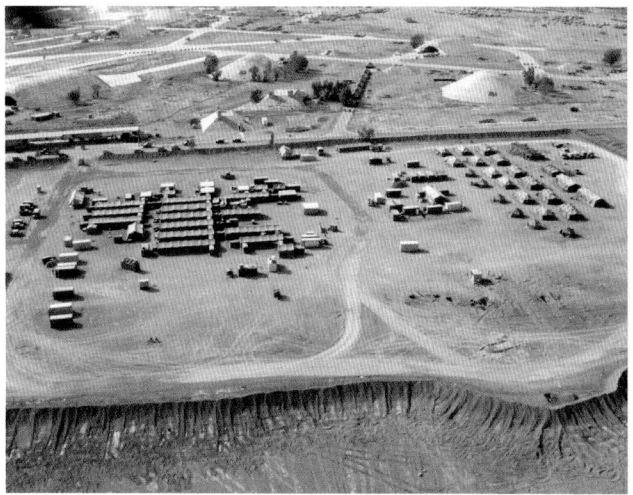

FIGURE 57–1. Twenty-first Combat Support Hospital, Balad, Iraq, 2003. The hospital is on the left with living quarters on the right.

TABLE 57-1. Advantages of regional anesthesia in austere environmental conditions.

Excellent operating conditions

Profound perioperative analgesia

Stable hemodynamics

Limb-specific anesthesia

Reduced need for other anesthetics

Improved postoperative alertness

Minimal side effects

Rapid recovery from anesthesia

Simple, easily transported equipment needed

Source: Reproduced with permission from Buckenmaier CC, Lee EH, Shields CH, et al: Regional anesthesia in austere environments. *Reg Anesth Pain Med.* 2003 Jul-Aug;28(4):321–327.

local infrastructure and logistic realities into anesthetic plans. Anesthetic choices and plans that work well in state-of-the-art operating rooms can have disastrous consequences if applied to austere environments without due consideration of local resources and conditions. The available roads; electrical, sanitation, medical, and gas services; climatic conditions; and operating room facilities, among other issues, will greatly affect the anesthetic plan in AEA.

The influence of local environmental and weather conditions on AEA is a particularly important consideration, especially during medical missions following natural disasters. Temperature and terrain extremes, along with dangerous faunae and disease, must be included in any successful anesthetic plan in these environments. Temperature extremes can affect patient health directly and degrade equipment, medication, and anesthesiologist function. Rough terrain can affect practitioner and patient travel, impede communication, and limit resupply of consumable medical supplies. Finally, local geopolitics, in its most extreme form, war, can have a tremendous influence on AEA.

One approach to overcoming the realities of AEA is to surmount local resource limitations by transporting the modern anesthesia infrastructure to the AEA location, thus freeing the anesthesiologist from many if not all of these considerations. This approach is best illustrated by the U.S. military in caring for wounded soldiers on the battlefields of Iraq and Afghanistan through the fielding of combat support hospitals (CSHs) that have capabilities similar to civilian hospitals in developed countries (Figure 57–1). While the CSH is a successful approach to caring for injured patients anywhere in the world, the logistics required to place and support such a facility are well beyond the capability of most humanitarian medical mission planners or disaster medicine planners.

ADVANTAGES OF REGIONAL ANESTHESIA IN AUSTERE ENVIRONMENTS

Because of the logistical constraints and the environmental realities inherent to AEA, anesthesiologists involved in these types of missions must find anesthetic and analgesic techniques that require minimal logistical support, provide adequate surgical conditions, afford postoperative pain control, and result in a patient that is alert in the postoperative recovery room. Modern advanced regional anesthesia has many characteristics that make it an attractive choice for AEA missions (Table 57–1).

Compared with general anesthesia using a volatile anesthetic, regional anesthesia is particularly suited for AEA because of its small logistics footprint. The equipment for regional anesthesia (peripheral nerve stimulator and/or ultrasound machine, single-injection or continuous peripheral nerve block needle and tubing, local anesthetic, and infusion pump) is compact, lightweight, and easily transported. In contrast, the equipment used to deliver volatile anesthetics does not possess these attributes (Figure 57–2a). Though general anesthesia remains the gold standard for AEA, this capability must be planned for and surgical cases that demand general anesthesia carefully triaged. The availability of compressed oxygen can often dictate the number and types of cases that can be managed in austere environments. Many anesthetic ventilators are pneumatically driven and can consume significant quantities of compressed oxygen during a typical general anesthetic. Oxygen cylinders or oxygen generation equipment (eg, the portable oxygen generation system [POGS], shown in Figure 57–2b, which required 6 men to lift into place) can represent a significant logistics challenge to any AEA mission. Possible alternatives to pneumatically driven volatile anesthetics include draw-over anesthesia or total intravenous anesthesia (TIVA) using target-controlled infusion (TCI) pumps. These alternatives remain in development and may not be available to many anesthesiologists. Whenever possible, regional anesthesia is the preferred technique for most cases during an AEA mission because it allows conservation of resources that may be required for more complicated surgeries or emergencies.[5]

Regional anesthesia provides excellent operating conditions for the surgeon. With the establishment of a surgical block, motor, sensory, and sympathetic nerves to a body region are blocked. This provides muscle relaxation,[6] preemptive analgesia,[7]

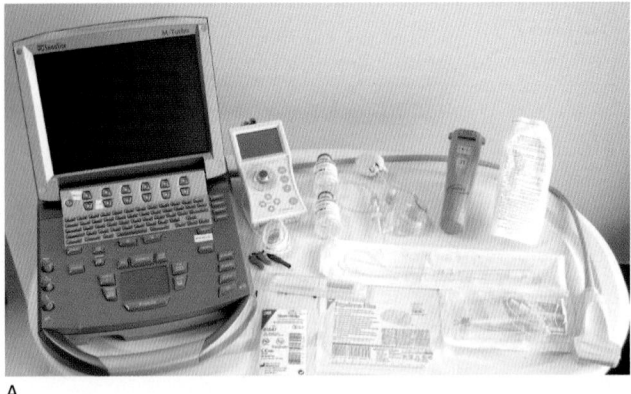

A

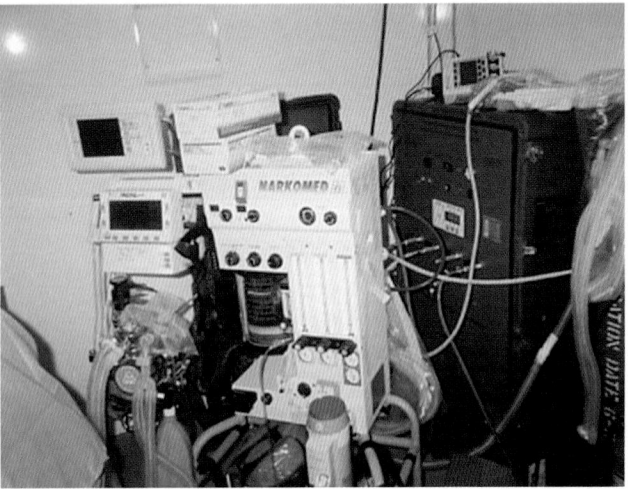

B

FIGURE 57–2. Equipment for regional anesthesia and equipment for general inhalational anesthesia. **A:** SonoSite Micromaxx (SonoSite, Inc, Bothell, WA), Stimuplex HNS-11 nerve stimulator (B. Braun Medical Inc., Bethlehem, PA), Naropin 0.5% (ropivacaine HCL, AstraZeneca, Wilmington, DE), AmbIT infusion pump (Sorenson Medical, Inc., West Jordan, UT), Chloraprep (Medi-Flex Hospital Products, Inc., Overland Park, KS), Dermabond (Ethicon Inc., Cornelia, GA), Steri-Strip (3M Health Care, St. Paul, MN), CarraSmart (Carrington Laboratories, Inc., Irving, TX), StimuQuick insulated peripheral block needle (Arrow International Inc., Reading, PA), and Contiplex Tuohy continuous nerve block set (B. Braun Medical Inc., Bethlehem, PA). **B:** Equipment for general inhalational anesthesia used at the Twenty-eighth Combat Support Hospital, Iraq. Items include Narcomed M (Dräger Medical Inc., Lübeck, Germany) connected to a portable oxygen generation system (POGS On Site Gas Systems, Inc., Newington, CT).

reduced overall stress response to surgery,[8] a reduction in thromboembolic complications,[9] and reduced blood loss.[10,11] Because afferent nociceptive stimulation from the surgical site is greatly attenuated or eliminated during the operative procedure, stable hemodynamics are characteristic of regional anesthesia. In AEA, when monitoring capability is often constrained, intraoperative hemodynamic stability is important. Regional anesthetic techniques allow the procedure to be performed on an awake or lightly sedated patient who can communicate with the anesthesiologist, providing the best monitor of patient well-being.

Postoperatively, the advantages of regional anesthesia in AEA become even more apparent. Unlike general anesthesia, which provides for little to no postoperative analgesia, regional techniques with long-acting local anesthetics can provide analgesia for hours after surgery. If CPNB techniques are employed, analgesia can be extended for days postoperatively. Another important benefit of regional anesthesia in the postsurgical recovery area is the mental acuity and reduced nausea and vomiting associated with these techniques. In the modern ambulatory surgery setting, the increased incidence of postoperative nausea and vomiting, drowsiness, and pain are the most frequent causes of prolonged postoperative stay.[12,13] Although these issues have economic significance in developed countries, in the resource-limited practice of AEA, difficult recovery can have a profoundly negative effect on mission success. Recovery area personnel and monitoring capability are usually limited in AEA. Anesthesiologists working in this environment favor techniques, like regional anesthesia, that facilitate discharging alert patients, free of pain and nausea, who can be active proponents in their recovery despite limited resources. Rapid recovery of the patient's own airway protective reflexes is a significant advantage of regional compared with general anesthesia in AEA.

There is also a growing body of evidence that aggressive acute pain management can prevent "chronification," that is, the development of chronic pain following surgery or trauma.[14] Continuous peripheral nerve block procedures are particularly well suited for managing acute pain as part of a multimodal pain plan that is designed to reduce the patient's stress response to surgery and mitigate the unwanted cascade of events associated with poorly managed perioperative pain that leads to a risk of neuropathy, psychopathology, and eventual disability (Figure 57–3).

ACCEPTANCE OF ADVANCED REGIONAL ANESTHESIA IN AEA

Effective perioperative pain management is an important consideration following any operative procedure regardless of the location and conditions under which it is performed. Since Sertürner, a German pharmacist, first identified and isolated morphine from opium in 1803, morphine and other opioid drugs have played a major role in pain management in austere environments, especially in the military. Although the preeminence and success of opioid medications in pain management is well established, their use is not without significant side effects that are undesirable in the best medical environments but can be potentially devastating in AEA. International regulations concerning the transportation of opioids and limited monitoring capability can further complicate the use of these drugs in AEA. Studies have demonstrated a reduced requirement for opioid pain medication following surgery when regional anesthesia techniques are used.[3,15,16] Using CPNB techniques, pain relief can be extended for days, further reducing the need for opioid pain medications. The efficacy of CPNB infusions has been demonstrated in the ambulatory surgery setting, allowing anesthesiologists to extend the benefits of peripheral nerve block following surgery well into the patient's recovery at home.[17–20]

Despite the benefits of regional anesthesia techniques, information regarding the use of CPNB in AEA is limited.

Chronification Pain

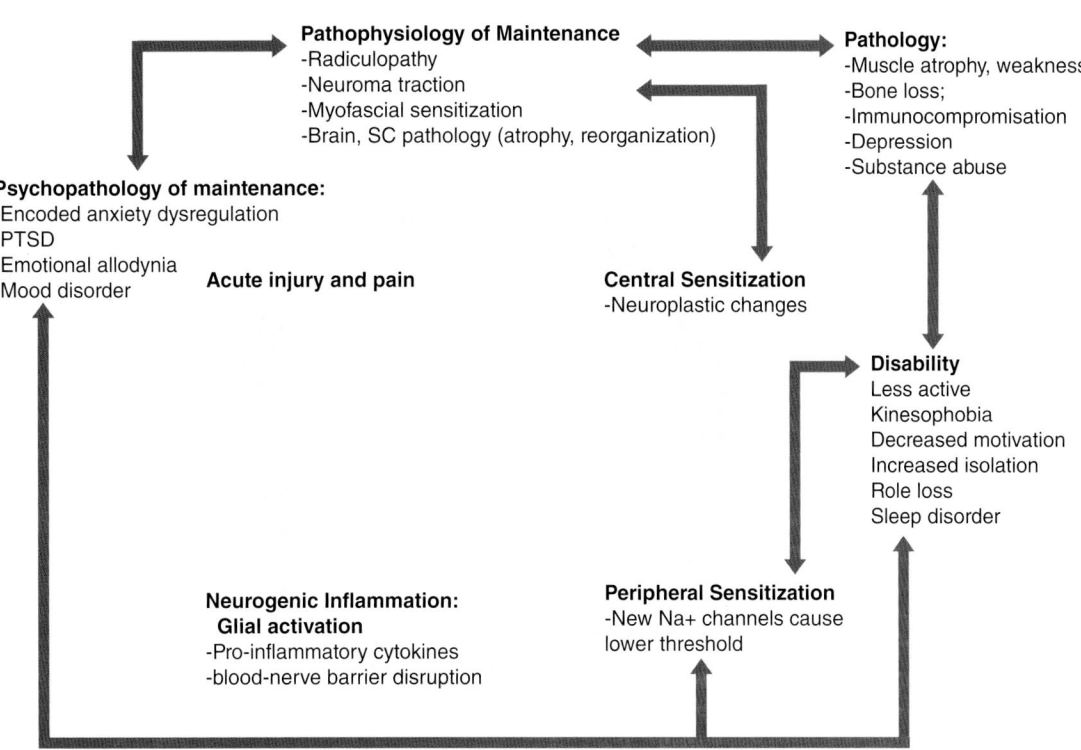

FIGURE 57–3. Chronification: The Chronic Pain Cycle. (Modified with permission from Ebert M and Kerns R: *Behavioral and Psychopharmacological Pain Management.* New York: Cambridge University Press; 2011.)

Recently, the use of CPNB for surgical anesthesia and analgesia on the modern battlefield and throughout the evacuation chain back to the United States has been demonstrated successfully.[21] Since this first success, CPNB catheters have been increasingly used to treat a number of patients within the Iraq combat theater. In 2009, the first deployment of an acute pain medicine service (APS) at a CSH occurred at Camp Bastion, Afghanistan. In general, the wounded treated by the APS had a significant decrease in pain scores immediately following wounding, and, overall, the perceived quality of pain control provided by the APS was high.[22] During this deployment, military healthcare providers at Camp Bastion were surveyed regarding their perceptions of the APS as part of the trauma team. The survey sample (*n*=70, of which 61.4% were male) included 50% nursing staff, 15.8% surgeons, and 10% anesthesiologists who completed the survey following the 3-month APS implementation period. Overall, the majority of providers surveyed indicated support for the APS within the CSH system and confirmed its contribution to improved trauma care.[23] This pilot project has led to formal military doctrine, the Joint Theater Trauma System Clinical Practice Guideline—Management of Pain, Anxiety, and Delirium in Injured Warfighters, that supports the establishment of APS assets within theater CSHs and military treatment facilities throughout the evacuation chain.

The application of regional anesthesia, CPNB in particular, has been one of the medical success stories from the military's experience in the Iraq war. Although the technology remains new to the modern battlefield and is far from being universally accepted, many soldiers have enjoyed the benefits of advanced regional anesthesia and CPNB in the management of their combat wounds in the austere battlefield environments of Iraq and Afghanistan. Advances in soldier body armor and improvised explosive devices have resulted in a preponderance of extremity wounds and traumatic amputations. The application of CPNB catheters in many of these patients has facilitated the multiple operative procedures that these patients often undergo, since reestablishment of a surgical block can be easily accomplished via the existing catheter(s). Additionally, the analgesic block provided by CPNB allows for far superior pain control on the long, evacuation flights to Germany and the United States compared with morphine alone, which until relatively recently was the only option for pain control on an evacuation aircraft.

Regardless of this initial success, the military has been slow to embrace advanced regional anesthesia as a viable battlefield medicine standard of care. The reasons are not easily defined but worth exploring since the military medical community's concerns over advanced regional anesthesia will also provide insight into why, despite its many advantages, advance regional anesthesia is not the predominate anesthetic for AEA. First, general anesthesia with volatile anesthetics is the "gold standard" anesthetic in developed countries. The safety and efficacy of general anesthesia has been established over the decades with countless successful applications. Anesthesiology training programs focus on general anesthesia techniques, and most practitioners are very comfortable with its use for all surgical indications. Unfortunately, the technology and personnel support needed to employ general anesthesia successfully can quickly exhaust the resources available during AEA as previously noted. In the U.S. military, a tremendous investment has been made in technology to safely provide general anesthesia to war casualties, regardless of the environment. Additional requirements on the military medical supply system, such as advanced regional anesthesia, are less attractive to medical logistical planners when so much effort has already been directed toward volatile-anesthetic-based general anesthesia. Although the capability to perform general anesthesia in AEA is vital, general anesthesia is not necessarily the best choice for every clinical situation encountered on the mission. The availability of other options is a key to AEA mission success.

Lack of training in advanced regional anesthesia has also hampered the development of this anesthetic in the AEA environment.[24,25] Advanced regional anesthesia training, at least in U.S. anesthesiology residency programs, is far from what it needs to be for these techniques to become ubiquitous within the anesthesia community and not just the domain of a select few regional anesthesia specialists. A considerable investment is required by the anesthesiologist to learn block techniques and detailed human anatomy before advanced regional anesthesia can become part of routine anesthesia practice. This investment includes system and facility enhancements, such as establishing an APS, that will allow full realization of the benefits of regional anesthesia when offered as part of a multimodal perioperative acute pain medicine plan. The increased availability of regional anesthesia courses, the development of acute pain medicine and regional anesthesia fellowship training programs, and the expansion of interest in the medical literature suggests that this will change in the near future. The Defense & Veterans Center for Integrative Pain Management (DVCIPM; www.dvcipm.org), a congressionally sponsored program established in 2003, has done much to establish advanced regional anesthesia and other modern pain management techniques on the modern battlefield.

With the resurgence of interest in regional anesthesia, there has been a number of advances in technology to support and enhance the practice of advanced regional anesthesia. The new technologies, such as peripheral nerve stimulators, stimulating catheters, portable infusion pumps, and ultrasound, to name just a few, have revolutionized the practice of regional anesthesia However, the plethora of equipment and the lack of consensus among regional anesthesiologists as to which technologies and practices are best for physician and patient alike often make standardization and training difficult. Stimulating versus non-stimulating catheters, ultrasound-guided versus stimulating needle placement, local anesthetic selection and adjuncts, needle sharpness and design, CPNB catheter infusion rates, and bolus parameters are just a few of the topics that often pervade regional anesthesia conference floor discussions. Unlike general anesthesia, modern regional anesthesia (particularly CPNB) does not have a track record of decades of standardized application and ubiquitous expertise. Considerable effort is needed to take the "art" out of regional anesthesia and establish its "science" before these techniques can become generally accepted.

Perhaps the most unusual reason for the slow acceptance of regional anesthesia in AEA and in the military is our professional and social attitudes toward pain. The science of understanding pain and its management is a relatively new. Before the advent of modern anesthesia practice, surgeons were instructed to not display excessive concern over a patient's discomfort during surgery and to operate fast, since a speedy surgery limited suffering.[26] Even after the development of anesthesiology as a medical specialty, pain has been, and still is, considered an unfortunate and unavoidable consequence of surgical intervention. In the AEA environment, expending limited medical resources on the management of pain can seem a luxury. As evidence mounts on the destructive aspects of pain, particularly as it contributes to the overall surgical stress response and postoperative morbidity, effective pain control is fast becoming less a luxury and more a necessary component of successful surgical care.[27,28] Though compassion and the relief of suffering are reason enough to provide good pain control, in the twenty-first century it an inherent aspect of good medicine.

PERIOPERATIVE MEDICINE & ACUTE PAIN CONTROL

The successful application of regional anesthesia in austere environments requires anesthesiologists to embrace their role as physicians of perioperative medicine. The anesthesia practitioners must accept responsibility for the patient's operative care before, during, and long after his or her surgical procedure. Although this extended role for the anesthesiologist beyond the operating room and recovery area is nontraditional, the anesthesiologist is uniquely trained to manage perioperative pain and enhance recovery using a multimodal approach that includes advanced regional anesthesia techniques and technologies. The anesthesiologist's perioperative role is enhanced through the establishment of an APS. The anesthesiologist working outside of the operating room in the APS facilitates the introduction of advanced regional anesthesia both in modern hospitals and in AEA. This location is equipped with regional anesthesia supplies and should have basic monitors, oxygen, suction, airway, and resuscitation equipment and medications in the event of an emergency. This investment in resources has advantages in the AEA environment. The regional anesthesia area facilitates patient preparation for surgery, and, if appropriate, blocks with long-acting local anesthetics or CPNB can be established before previous surgery patients are out of the operating room, thus improving efficiency. The APS practitioner is also available to serve as a perioperative medical consultant, critical care provider, and acute pain specialist for recovering patients. Additionally, the APS provides a framework for establishing an interdisciplinary acute pain management team of physicians, pain nurses, integrative medicine providers, and other specialists working with patients in a coordinated fashion.

The need for this expanded role of anesthesiologists in perioperative analgesia is exemplified by the austere military medical environment that currently exists in Afghanistan and existed in Iraq. In previous conflicts, wounded American soldiers often spent days recovering from combat wounds before they were deemed fit to be evacuated to higher levels of medical care outside the war theater. In the current conflicts, a soldier's evacuation from point of injury to a major medical facility outside the combat theater is often measured in hours. This aggressive evacuation policy has contributed significantly to the salvage of many soldiers who likely would have died in previous conflicts. Traditional opioid-based pain management techniques alone are not well suited to the challenging air evacuation environment that makes rapid removal of casualties to distant major medical facilities. Medical personnel on evacuation flights are often faced with a number of wounded patients in significant pain. In the low-light, high-noise, high-vibration, and difficult-monitoring environment of evacuation aircraft, the side effects associated with opioid-only pain control become magnified. The advantage of CPNB and modern peripheral nerve infusion pumps that allow patients to manage their own pain control is obvious. These catheters also facilitate repeated operations and dressing changes by allowing reestablishment of surgical blocks through bolus administration of local anesthetic via established CPNB catheters. Military anesthesiologists are actively pursuing this technology.

PEARLS & PITFALLS OF REGIONAL ANESTHESIA IN AN AUSTERE ENVIRONMENT

Patients receiving regional anesthesia as part of their care should be warned to avoid weight bearing on blocked extremities. They should also be advised to take special precautions to avoid further injury to the blocked region of the body since normal protective sensations and proprioception will be diminished or absent. Patients should also be cautioned about possible side effects that may be associated with specific block procedures. For example, patients receiving an interscalene block should be warned of the possibility of developing Horner syndrome and a hoarse voice. They should be reassured that these conditions are temporary and will resolve completely with resolution of the block. These warnings are especially important in AEA where cultural differences can heighten patient fears and negatively affect the patient's perception of their anesthetic care. Planning for adequate translator resources is vital for any medical mission in which language differences exist between caregivers and patients.

CPNB, can extend the benefits of regional anesthesia for days into a patient's recovery from surgery. This can have a profoundly positive influence on the care of patients who require evacuation over long distances or have injuries that necessitate frequent surgical interventions or dressing changes. Although this technique has important advantages in AEA, it also presents the medical team with unique management challenges that are best addressed by the APS anesthesiologist working outside the operating room. The decision to use CPNB on AEA patients must be individualized to each patient's clinical situation. During the clinical evaluation of the patient for anesthesia, the anesthesiologist will be able to ascertain if the patient is a suitable candidate for CPNB. Not all patients are willing or

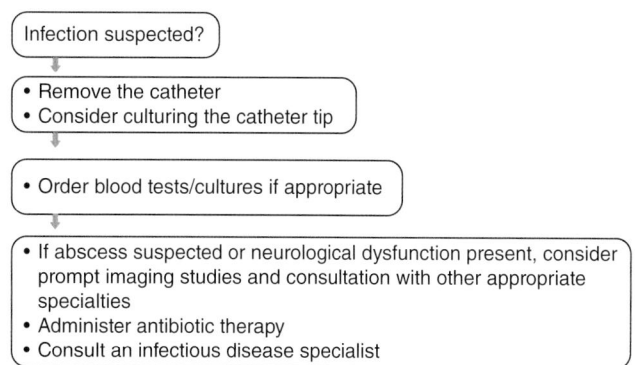

FIGURE 57–4. Algorithm for suspicion of infection at catheter site.

able to tolerate CPNB infusions despite the relative simplicity of the technology. If a patient remains resistant to CPNB therapy after thoughtful discussion with a physician, then the technique should be abandoned in favor of more traditional anesthetic and pain management techniques. Additionally, personnel resources must be available to monitor and appropriately manage any development of local anesthetic toxicity following a block. The anesthesiologist must also weigh the benefits of applying CPNB for each surgical situation against the risks of the technique. In the author's practice, all patients are warned, "The use of a block needle can result in injury or infection (Figure 57–4), and, because we are working near nerves, the possibility of nerve damage does exist, though these complications are rare." The least invasive intervention that can adequately control a patient's pain should always be sought for each clinical situation. In polytrauma situations, the patient is often unable to have a meaningful conversation about the risks and benefits of CPNB. Implied consent is often applied in trauma management to justify the use of invasive treatments that the trauma team has determined are in the patient's best interest. With the introduction of ultrasound technology to regional anesthesia in Afghanistan, CPNB catheters have been placed in anesthetized trauma patients when the surgical team determined the benefits of the catheter exceeded the risk of placement in an unconscious patient. The author, utilizing ultrasound guidance, performed over 50 CPNB catheters in anesthetized trauma patients with no complications. This practice should be reserved for serious trauma situations and only in consultation with the trauma team leader. Finally, the anesthesiologist must have an established plan for a follow-up of CPNB patients. Follow-up can be as simple as a telephone call, but CPNB patients and their catheters should be evaluated daily. Patients treated with CPNB catheters should also be educated on signs and symptoms of local anesthetic toxicity. The patient must have 24-hour access to an anesthesia provider should problems occur during the infusion. Fortunately, the answer for any CPNB infusion problem is the same: stop the infusion, resort to back-up pain medications or therapies, and seek medical help. The U.S. Air Force has developed a series of infusion pump labels to provide CPNB patients and their caregivers basic instructions during air evacuation to manage infusion problems when an anesthesiologist may not be immediately available (Figure 57–5). Email is also a valuable

- Will be placed on the pump at initial catheter insertion

> **TURN THE PUMP OFF**
> For signs of local anesthetic toxicity (**metallic taste in mouth, jittery feeling, eye or muscle twitching, tongue extension or seizure**) or the patient wants the pump off. The patient had been educated on these signs and symptoms.

> **DO NOT ASSESS CATHETER INSERTION SITE, REMOVE THE CATHETER OR DISCONNECT THE PUMP WHILE EN ROUTE**
> Catheters should NOT be removed during periods of defective anticoagulation.

Patient Name_____
SSN_____
Insertion site_____
Insertion date/time_____
Medication_____
Flow rate _____cc/hr   Bolus dose_____cc
Lockout time_____
Initial medication volume_____cc

FIGURE 57–5. Military and U.S. Air Force AeroEvacuation-specific labels for continuous peripheral nerve block infusions.

communication tool when physicians and nurses are required to treat CPNB patients that are being transferred to medical facilities separated by great distance. Email can often be accessed in the most remote areas where other forms of long-distance communication are unavailable. Although these CPNB management principles may seem burdensome to apply in the AEA environment, the advantages in pain relief for patients are clear and consistent with compassionate anesthetic care. With proper planning, CPNB works well in austere environments.

One of the frequent complaints concerning CPNB infusions is catheter dislodgement. Poorly secured catheters can migrate or fall out, reducing the effectiveness of the technique, especially when patients require evacuation to other medical facilities. Although many devices and procedures are available to secure catheters, in the military evacuation environment and in military hospitals, the following CPNB catheter-securing procedures seem to work best. After placement, all catheters are gently aspirated for blood and 5 mL of local anesthetic containing epinephrine 1:400,000 is injected to diagnose possible intravascular placement. Catheters are tunneled 3–5 cm under the skin in any CPNB patient who will be evacuated or is expected to maintain the catheter for more than 72 hours (this includes epidural catheters). Whether tunneled or not, all catheters are secured with cyanoacrylate glue at the skin puncture site,[29] followed by a medical spray adhesive. The catheter is looped at the puncture site and further secured with Steri-Strips and a transparent dressing. All catheters are labeled with the site of the block and the date and time of catheter placement.

A variety of excellent peripheral nerve infusion pumps are available. A discussion of infusion pump technology is beyond the scope of this chapter, but more information comparing and contrasting the devices can be found in Chapter 13.[30,31] The ambIT (Summit Medical products, Inc., Sandy, Utah) is a multiuse, adjustable electronic infusion pump that is currently being used throughout the casualty evacuation care continuum.

These devices were selected because of their consistent infusion performance in temperature extremes and at altitude, light weight, simplicity of function, and patient-controlled bolus function, among other parameters. The device also has a unique shape and color (international orange) that distinguishes it from other infusion devices as a safety precaution.

A variety of local anesthetics are available for use in AEA regional anesthesia. Ropivacaine is the long-acting local anesthetic preferred by the author for single-injection blocks and CPNB catheter infusions. Compared with other long-acting local anesthetics such as bupivacaine and levobupivacaine, ropivacaine is the safest long-acting local anesthetic available.[32,33] Mepivacaine is the intermediate-acting local anesthetic often selected when a shorter-duration block is desirable or when catheters are bolused to reestablish a surgical-level block for dressing changes or surgery. Table 57–2 provides some examples of effective single-injection and CPNB infusion rates for a variety of regional anesthetic blocks.

SUMMARY

Regional anesthesia is uniquely suitable in AEA. The obvious advantages, such as improved postoperative alertness, pain control, and possibly enhanced recovery are apparent, these benefits are only realized through a significant investment by anesthesiologists in the education and increased effort to apply advanced regional anesthesia requires under difficult circumstances. Anesthesiologists who embrace the challenge of advanced regional anesthesia, particularly as part of an APS, become more versatile anesthesia providers whether their practice is in a modern, high-technology hospital or an isolated, austere tent. As recent events involving terrorism and natural disasters have demonstrated, the ability to provide safe anesthesia and effective analgesia regardless of environmental circumstances is a paramount skill in twenty-first century.

TABLE 57-2. Standard adult ropivacaine dosages for single-injection and continuous regional anesthesia at Walter Reed army medical center.[a]

Regional Anesthesia Technique	Adult Single-Injection Dose of Ropivacaine (mL 0.5% ropivacaine, except as noted)	Continuous Infusion of 0.2% Ropivacaine (mL)	Patient-Controlled Bolus Rate of 0.2% Ropivacaine[b] (mL bolus/20 min lockout)	Notes
Interscalene	20-30	8-10	2	Often supplemented with an intercostal brachial nerve block
Supraclavicular	20-30	8-10	2	Shortest-latency block of the brachial plexus
Infraclavicular	20-30	10-12	2	Catheter techniques less effective than supraclavicular catheters
Axillary	30	10-12	2	Catheter techniques less common
Paravertebral	3-5 per hadel blocked	8-10	2	Catheters effective in thoracic region only
Transversus abdominis plane (TAP)	10-20 per side	8-12	2	Alternative when epidural is not an option for abdominal analgesia
Lumbar plexus (posterior approach)	35-40	8-10	2	Epidural spread is a concern
Femoral	20-30	8-10	2	Catheter techniques less effective than lumbar plexus catheters
Sciatic (anterior or posterior approach)	20-30	8-10	2	Proximal approaches to the sciatic nerve preferable Not conducive to catheters
Sciatic (lateral or popliteal approach)	35-40	10-12	2	Catheter techniques less common
Lumbar plexus or femoral + sciatic	40-50 mL between both sites	5-10 for both catheters	2 mL on one catheter	Infusion rates divided between catheters based on distribution of patient's pain
Epidural	20-25	6-10	2	Opioids often added to infusions
Spinal	5-15 mg of 1.0% ropivacaine	N/A	N/A	Opioids often added to injections

[a]Information is based on the authors' experience with ropivacaine in a successful and busy regional anesthesia practice. Ultrasound guidance is assumed. Mepivacaine 1.5% can be used in place of ropivacaine at the volumes noted when a shorter-duration block is desirable.

[b]Occasionally, a 5 mL bolus/30-min lockout is used in selected patients. Generally, total infusions (continuous plus bolus) >20 mL/h are avoided.

REFERENCES

1. Waisel DB: The role of World War II and the European theater of operations in the development of anesthesiology as a physician specialty in the USA. Anesthesiology 2001;94:907–914.
2. Thompson GE: Anesthesia for battle casualties in Vietnam. JAMA 1967; 201:215–219.
3. Klein SM, Buckenmaier CC III: Ambulatory surgery with long acting regional anesthesia. Minerva Anestesiol 2002;68:833–841.
4. Upp J, Kent M, Tighe P: The Evolution and Practice of Acute Pain Medicine. Pain Medicine 2013;14:124–144.
5. Buckenmaier CC III, Lee EH, Shields CH, et al: Regional anesthesia in austere environments. Reg Anesth Pain Med 2003;28:321–327.
6. Brown AR, Weiss R, Greenberg C, et al: Interscalene block for shoulder arthroscopy: comparison with general anesthesia. Arthroscopy 1993;9: 295–300.
7. Kelly DJ, Ahmad M, Brull SJ: Preemptive analgesia I: physiological pathways and pharmacological modalities. Can J Anaesth 2001;48:1000–1010.

8. Greengrass RA: Regional anesthesia for ambulatory surgery. Anesthesiol Clin North Am 2000;18:341–353, vii.

9. Tuman KJ, McCarthy RJ, March RJ, et al: Effects of epidural anesthesia and analgesia on coagulation and outcome after major vascular surgery. Anesth Analg 1991;73:696–704.

10. Buckenmaier CC III, Xenos JS, Nilsen SM: Lumbar plexus block with perineural catheter and sciatic nerve block for total hip arthroplasty. J Arthroplasty 2002;17:499–502.

11. Twyman R, Kirwan T, Fennelly M: Blood loss reduced during hip arthroplasty by lumbar plexus block. J Bone Joint Surg Br 1990;72:770–771.

12. Chung F, Mezei G: Factors contributing to a prolonged stay after ambulatory surgery. Anesth Analg 1999;89:1352–1359.

13. Pavlin DJ, Rapp SE, Polissar NL, et al: Factors affecting discharge time in adult outpatients. Anesth Analg 1998;87:816–826.

14. Kehlet H, Jensen TS, Woolf CJ. Persistent postsurgical pain: risk factors and prevention. Lancet 2006;367:1618–1625.

15. Wang H, Boctor B, Verner J: The effect of single-injection femoral nerve block on rehabilitation and length of hospital stay after total knee replacement. Reg Anesth Pain Med 2002;27:139–144.

16. Richman JM, Liu SS, Courpas G, et al: Does continuous peripheral nerve block provide superior pain control to opioids? A meta-analysis. Anesth Analg 2006;102:248–257.

17. Buckenmaier CC III, Klein SM, Nielsen KC, et al: Continuous paravertebral catheter and outpatient infusion for breast surgery. Anesth Analg 2003;97:715–717.

18. Klein SM, Buckenmaier CC III: Ambulatory continuous inter-scalene brachial plexus blockade. Tech Reg Anesth Pain Manage 2004;8:58–62.

19. Nielsen KC, Greengrass RA, Pietrobon R, et al: Continuous inter-scalene brachial plexus blockade provides good analgesia at home after major shoulder surgery—report of four cases. Can J Anaesth 2003;50:57–61.

20. Ilfeld BM, Enneking FK: Continuous peripheral nerve blocks at home: a review. Anesth Analg 2005;100:1822–1833.

21. Buckenmaier CC, McKnight GM, Winkley JV, et al: Continuous peripheral nerve block for battlefield anesthesia and evacuation. Reg Anesth Pain Med 2005;30:202–205.

22. Buckenmaier C, III, Mahoney PF, Anton T, Kwon N, Polomano RC: Impact of an acute pain service on pain outcomes with combat-injured soldiers at Camp Bastion, Afghanistan. Pain Med 2012;13:919–926.

23. Polomano RC, Chisholm E, Anton TM, Kwon N, Mahoney PF, Buckenmaier C, III: A survey of military health professionals' perceptions of an acute pain service at Camp Bastion, Afghanistan. Pain Med 2012; 13:927–936.

24. Brown DL, Boezaart A: Regional training circa 2000: what's really new. Reg Anesth Pain Med 2002;27:1–2.

25. Kopacz DJ, Neal JM: Regional anesthesia and pain medicine: residency training—the year 2000. Reg Anesth Pain Med 2002;27:9–14.

26. Condon-Rall ME: A brief history of military anesthesia. In Zajtchuk R, Grande CM (eds): *Part IV: Anesthesia and Perioperative Care of the Combat Casualty.* Washington DC: Office of the Surgeon General, 1995, pp 855–896.

27. Kehlet H: Multimodal approach to control postoperative pathophysiology and rehabilitation. Br J Anaesth 1997;78:606–617.

28. Kelly DJ, Ahmad M, Brull SJ: Preemptive analgesia II: recent advances and current trends. Can J Anaesth 2001;48:1091–1101.

29. Klein SM, Nielsen KC, Buckenmaier CC III, et al: 2-Octyl cyanoacrylate glue for the fixation of continuous peripheral nerve catheters. Anesthesiology 2003;98:590–591.

30. Ilfeld BM, Morey TE, Enneking FK: The delivery rate accuracy of portable infusion pumps used for continuous regional analgesia. Anesth Analg 2002;95:1331–1336, table.

31. Ilfeld BM, Morey TE, Enneking FK: Portable infusion pumps used for continuous regional analgesia: delivery rate accuracy and consistency. Reg Anesth Pain Med 2003;28:424–432.

32. Graf BM: The cardiotoxicity of local anesthetics: the place of ropivacaine. Curr Top Med Chem 2001;1:207–214.

33. Wang RD, Dangler LA, Greengrass RA: Update on ropivacaine. Expert Opin Pharmacother 2001;2:2051–2063.

CHAPTER 58

Anesthesia for Humanitarian Relief Operations

Andres Missair

INTRODUCTION

The World Health Organization (WHO) Centre for Research on the Epidemiology of Disasters (CRED) defines a disaster as "a situation or event which overwhelms local capacity, necessitating a request to a national or international level for external assistance; an unforeseen and often sudden event that causes great damage, destruction and human suffering." Specific criteria include the following:

- 10 or more people reported killed
- 100 or more people reported affected
- Declaration of a state of emergency
- Call for international assistance

While natural disasters are categorized according to causality (tectonic events, flood, plague, etc.), many share similar patterns of increasing frequency, severity, and humanitarian impact (Figure 58–1).[1] Whether this is a result of improved data reporting or growing population and increased urbanization in susceptible areas, the result is a growing need for rapid and effective strategies to provide anesthetic care for trauma victims treated during the emergency medical relief scenarios of a collapsed medical infrastructure.

Much of the published data from medical humanitarian relief efforts comes from seismic events. Over 500,000 earthquakes are documented yearly, of which 3000 are perceptible. In the last 30 years, an annual average of 21 major earthquakes has been reported. Since 2005, however, this average has increased to more than 30 major events.[2] Since 1975, over 1.2 million deaths have been reported due to seismic events as per the U.S. Geologic Survey (USGS), with nearly half of all fatalities occurring within the last 10 years as a result of growing urban population density.[3] According to the United Nations

Environment Programme Global Resource Information Database (UNEP GRID), humanitarian disasters resulting from climatic and tectonic events demonstrate the greatest and most rapid impact on human health (Figure 58–2).[4] Consequently, anesthetic strategies designed for these specific scenarios are of utmost importance from a healthcare perspective.

ANESTHESIA FOR DISASTER RELIEF FOLLOWING MAJOR NATURAL DISASTERS: EARTHQUAKES

Patient Injury Patterns: Presentation

In order for anesthetic medical relief to be effective, it must address the needs of the predominant injury pattern of those patients who are considered "salvageable." Malish et al. conclude that the consideration of typical injury patterns helps establish early diagnosis and predict treatment requirements with the goal of stabilizing patients in the mass-casualty scenario.[5] Based on various studies, early disaster surgical intervention focuses on surviving patients with limb injuries. In the proceedings of the WHO Symposium on Earthquakes and People's Health,[6] a global incidence of 51.2% was reported for limb injury based on earthquake data from 11 separate epidemiologic studies. In another study by Missair et al., the average incidence of traumatic limb injury per seismic event was 63.01% for the 16 studies analyzed, totaling 30,822 patients. In those studies that identified upper versus lower extremity injury, lower limb involvement invariably exceeded 60% of cases. Conversely, cranial, thoracic, and abdominal injuries combined represented less than 36% of all cases across earthquake survivors (Figure 58–3).[7] Ganjouei et al. report strong intracluster correlations between skull, thorax, and spine fractures versus a weak link between lower extremity fracture and

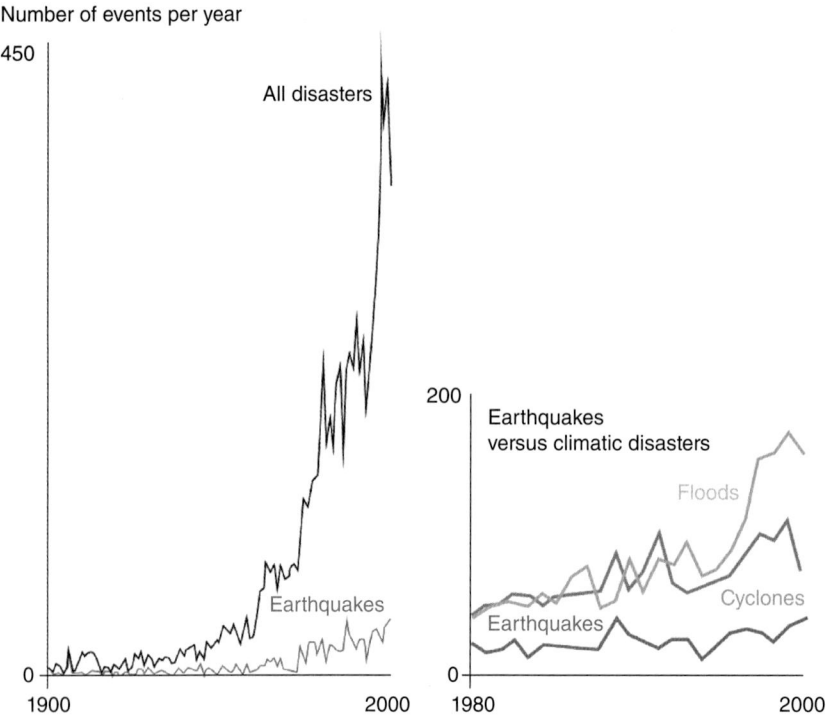

FIGURE 58-1. Natural disaster trends over time. United Nations Environmental Programme/GRID-Arendal.

any other fractures following the 2003 Bam earthquake in Iran that left more than 30,000 injured.[8] This finding supports recommendations regarding the focus of anesthetic management during the acute phase of earthquake medical relief on limb injury (Table 58–1) versus all other anatomic locations.

Patient Injury Patterns: Evolution

Anesthetic relief efforts must respond to the evolving needs of the overall medical disaster relief mission. Over the short course

of a humanitarian aid operation, the acuity and chronicity of patient morbidity can change dramatically. Consequently, the phases of medical relief are divided as follows (Figure 58–4).

During the emergent phase, medical relief teams face complete infrastructure collapse: electrical power, clean water, telecommunications, and transportation are either critically limited or nonexistent. Hospitals and buildings have collapsed or are structurally unsafe for occupation. Aftershocks continue to destabilize the field, and victims and relief teams are exposed to the

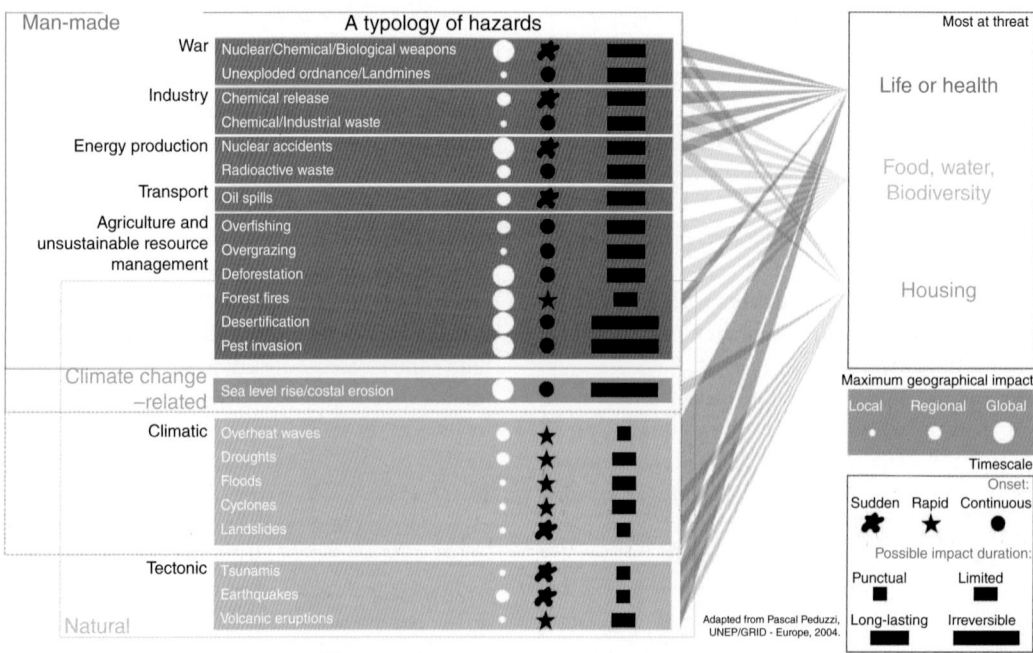

FIGURE 58-2. Epidemiology of disasters by type and impacted humanitarian area. United Nations Environmental Programme/GRID-Arendal.

limb and superficial soft tissue) are presented for emergency treatment. The majority of surgical interventions at this stage are for hemodynamic stabilization and infection mitigation. As a result, most surgical efforts focus on limb amputation and soft tissue incision and drainage. During the major earthquakes in Armenia (1988), Japan (1995), Pakistan (2003), and Haiti (2010), field hospitals could not be established for the first 4–14 days following the disaster despite intact local medical facilities, equipment, and personnel only 30–40 kilometers away.[9–11] Regardless of the socioeconomic status and geographic location of the affected region and population, field hospitals remain an unattainable goal during the emergency and acute phases of disaster medical relief (Figure 58–6).

During the chronic phase, field hospitals are created, and limited ancillary surgical services are available, such as ventilators, oxygen, suction, and electrical cautery. Supply chains are now established and largely dependable. Emergency transportation begins to improve, although other aspects of basic infrastructure remain collapsed. Patients from the emergent and acute phases are evacuated to intact neighboring medical facilities; those who remain may begin to present with medical complications such as infection, sepsis, phantom limb pain, pneumonia, and thromboembolic events. Surgical efforts begin to encompass a broader range of services, including open reduction internal fixations (ORIFs), cesarean sections, intra-abdominal procedures, and ongoing care of the critically ill (Figure 58–7). New patients now present with infectious disease, dehydration, malnutrition, and exacerbations of predisaster chronic ailments (eg, diabetes, hypertension).

Logistical Obstacles

After the 2010 Haiti earthquake that killed over 200,000 people, CNN reported the headline, "Expect Gettysburg: Civil War Anesthesia During the Haiti Earthquake."[12] Importantly, what we learned from this event was that time equals lives and that a surgical team staffed and equipped to provide regional anesthesia could be dispatched rapidly to serve as a bridge to more advanced field surgical care, which takes longer to deploy and set up (on average 2–3 weeks). During the emergent and acute phases of natural disasters, or on the battlefield, the ability to access an established medical infrastructure is often compromised, and complete operational autonomy is fundamental to ensure safe and effective anesthetic care by the first-response team. The numerous advantages of regional anesthesia in the modern battlefield include excellent operating conditions, profound perioperative analgesia, stable hemodynamics, minimal side effects, and simple portable equipment requirements.[13] These characteristics are paramount when anesthetic delivery faces the logistical obstacles of manmade and natural disasters resulting in the total collapse of medical infrastructure.

In order to design an effective anesthesia disaster response plan, certain goals and obstacles must be considered, as illustrated in Table 58–2.

Interestingly, certain obstacles encountered during field operations are created by the relief effort itself: medical provider nutrition, hydration, hygiene, and rotation must be addressed prior to deployment so that volunteers do not become victims

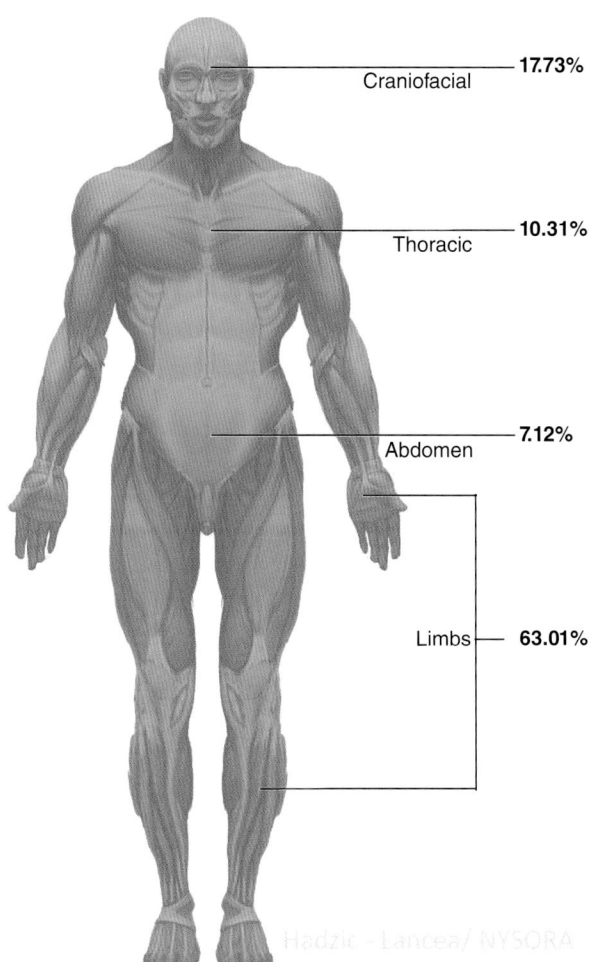

FIGURE 58–3. Anatomic distribution pattern of traumatic injuries immediately following major earthquakes.

elements. Local emergency services personnel are overwhelmed or absent. Access to the disaster zone can be extremely limited and only possible on foot or by helicopter (Figure 58–5).

During the acute phase, international disaster relief teams composed of medical volunteers and professional rescue personnel begin to appear in the field. Portable infrastructure support is established, such as tents, electricity generators, and basic supplies. Compressed gases are either critically limited or absent. The supply chain remains precarious and undependable such that extreme rationing continues. At this stage, patients who have sustained cranial or thoracic trauma have already expired, and those with salvageable injuries (predominantly

TABLE 58–1. Typical limb injuries.
Long-bone fractures
Crush injury
Contusion
Laceration
Wound infection
Hemorrhage

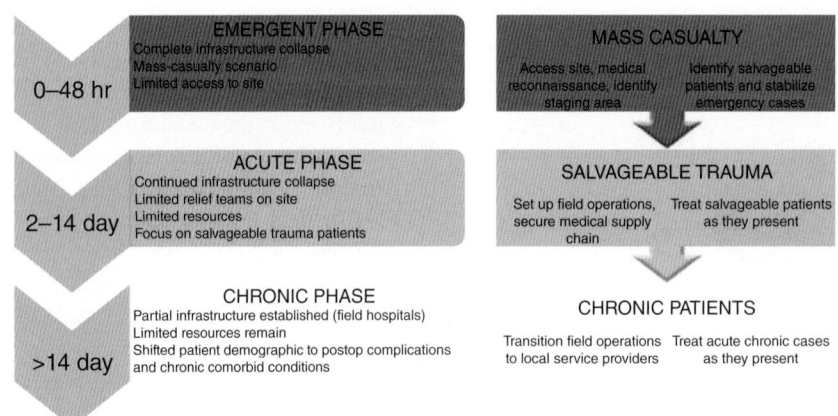

FIGURE 58–4. Phases of medical relief during humanitarian natural disasters.

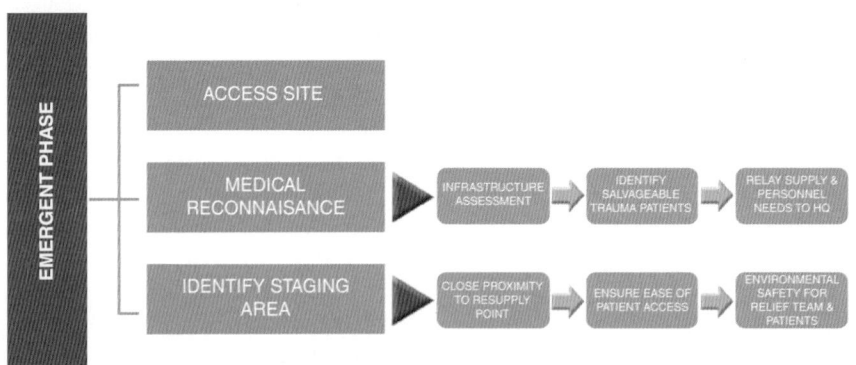

FIGURE 58–5. Anesthesia medical relief objectives during the emergent phase.

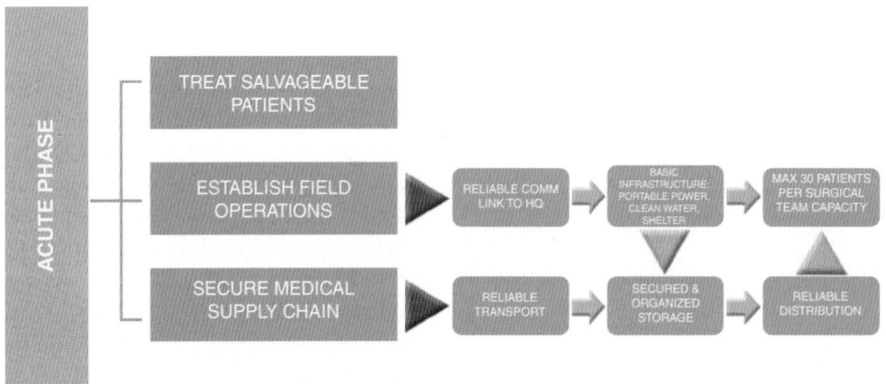

FIGURE 58–6. Anesthesia medical relief objectives during the acute phase.

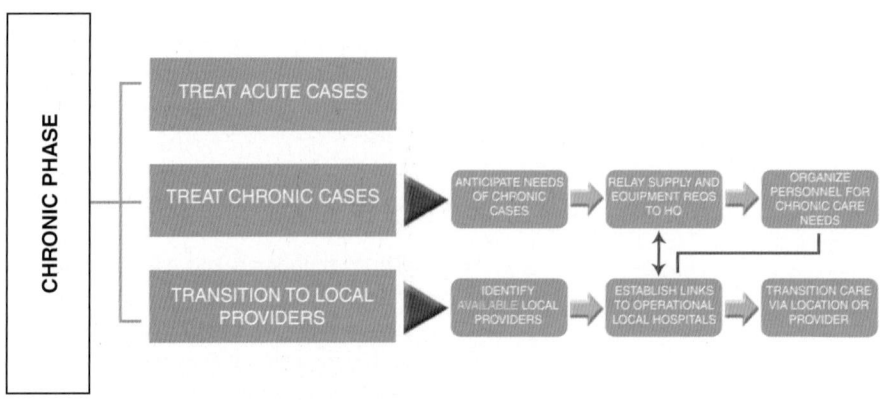

FIGURE 58–7. Anesthesia medical relief objectives during the chronic phase.

TABLE 58-2. Effective anesthesia disaster response plans: goals and obstacles.

Goals
- Rapid field deployment within 24 hours
- Complete autonomy
- Patient safety
- 30-patient capacity per day per provider
- Guaranteed communication link to headquarters
- Provider safety in the field
- Sustainability

Obstacles
- Limited access to field
- Absent medical infrastructure
- Austere, unstable environment
- Provider fatigue
- Supply chain integrity
- Mass-casualty scenario
- Evolving patient presentations
- Transition

themselves. Staff turnover can become a logistical nightmare in the context of compromised access to the field and can lead to complete operational collapse within 72 hours. For this reason, the WHO recommends that the majority of medical relief efforts be conducted locally or by neighboring countries with rapid access to the affected disaster zone.

Anesthetic Solutions
Ketamine Monitored Anesthesia Care/Local Anesthesia

There are both pros and cons to the use of ketamine in monitored anesthesia care (MAC), as shown in Table 58–3.

Ketamine MAC with unsecured airways has been used extensively during medical relief operations. The safety and efficacy of ketamine as the primary anesthetic drug under disaster conditions has been well described by Mulvey et al.[14,15]

TABLE 58-3. Pros and cons of ketamine monitored anesthesia care in disaster situations.

Pros
- Stable hemodynamics
- IV and IM routes
- Spontaneous ventilation maintained
- Anesthetic and analgesic
- Proven use in the mass-casualty scenario following earthquakes and tsunamis
- Inexpensive

Cons
- <5% incidence of nausea and vomiting reported
- Risk of intraoperative hallucinations

IM, intramuscular; IV, intravenous.

After the 2005 7.8-magnitude earthquake in Kashmir that resulted in 86,000 deaths and more than 80,000 severe injuries, the authors reported on the use of ketamine as the sole anesthetic for 149 patients (adult and pediatric) undergoing emergency surgery within a completely devastated hospital infrastructure. The conditions reported by the authors (absence of mechanical ventilation, vital sign monitors, and supplemental oxygen) are similar to those encountered during the 2010 Haiti earthquake, where Missair et al.[10] reported more than 500 surgeries performed with combined ketamine MAC anesthesia and single-shot peripheral nerve block. Both studies describe the use of ketamine with an unsecured airway and reported a rate of less than 5% complications following its use, comparable to results found by Paix et al.[16] during the 2004 Banda Aceh tsunami.

REGIONAL ANESTHESIA

The pros and cons of regional anesthesia in disaster scenarios are described in Table 58–4.

Regional anesthetic techniques can be divided into neuraxial approaches and peripheral nerve blocks. The intravascular volume status of the natural disaster patient population is typically compromised and must be considered before the use of neuraxial techniques in light of the induced sympathectomy and the potential for severe intraoperative hypotension. In fact, Jiang et al.[17] report significant hypotension requiring resuscitation after spinal anesthetics in 80% of patients treated in the field. It is prudent, therefore, to fluid resuscitate any patient before placing a neuraxial block under these conditions. The time required to safely accomplish this goal, however, is often limited by the emergent nature of surgery performed during mass casualties.

In our experience in the battlefield, peripheral nerve blocks provide "excellent operating conditions, profound perioperative analgesia, stable hemodynamics, minimal side effects, and simple portable equipment requirements."[13] These attributes have since been confirmed in the civilian scenario, following the 2010 Haiti earthquake medical relief effort by Project

TABLE 58-4. Pros and cons of regional anesthesia via single-shot nerve block in disaster situations.

Pros
- Stable hemodynamics
- Proven use in the battlefield and in disaster medical relief scenarios
- Minimal side effects
- Rapid establishment of surgical conditions
- Analgesic coverage extended to the postoperative period
- Minimal, portable equipment requirements
- No reliance on ventilator equipment, compressed gas, or electrical power

Cons
- Requires specialty training
- Limited anatomic coverage
- Specialized equipment requirements

TABLE 58–5. Pros and cons of continuous peripheral nerve blocks in disaster situations.

Pros
- Prolonged analgesia
- Simplified and rapid reestablishment of surgical conditions
- Decreased postoperative opioid consumption and associated side effects

Cons
- Increased risk of infection
- Increased equipment and supply requirements (especially if pumps are used)
- Increased personnel demands for care and monitoring

Medishare, where hundreds of patients received single-shot nerve blocks for emergency limb surgeries. Operating conditions are rapidly established with single-shot neural blockade, and postoperative analgesia is provided by the use of long-acting local anesthetic drugs.[7,13] The prolongation of analgesia may help reduce field post-anesthesia care unit (PACU) complications such as opioid-induced emesis and respiratory depression and decrease the burden on limited drug supplies and the already limited and overextended medical personnel caring for postoperative patients.

For the earthquake trauma patient in the austere medical environment, the placement of indwelling catheters such as epidurals or continuous peripheral nerve blocks has been reported in a few studies. For example, Buckenmaier et al. report on the safe use of continuous peripheral nerve blocks (CPNBs) during military field operations;[13] however, it must be emphasized that these patients were either rapidly evacuated to hospitals in military bases abroad or cared for in military field hospitals. In mass-casualty scenarios, such as earthquakes, the feasibility and necessary manpower for the subsequent care and monitoring of patients with indwelling catheters must be taken into consideration. In addition, the environmental conditions of the field hospital (if one exists) may present an infection risk

for these particular anesthetic techniques. Finally, the additional equipment and supply requirements, such as infusion pumps, intravenous (IV) fluids, tubing, and available resuscitation drugs may preclude the safe and effective implementation of indwelling catheters for anesthesia and postoperative pain management. On the other hand, it can be argued that the benefits of prolonged analgesic coverage and the possibility of quickly reestablishing surgical conditions of the injured limb requiring serial wound debridements or procedures may justify the additional resources and risks inherent to the use of CPNBs in austere environments. In these scenarios, therefore, it might be prudent to consider using *bolus-only* catheter techniques without infusion pumps, thereby reducing demands on limited resources and personnel (Table 58–5).

Interestingly, no short-term complications specific to regional anesthetic management have been reported in the literature. Nevertheless, it is important to emphasize that patient safety must always be ensured, as per the WHO guidelines for disaster relief operations. This goal is easily achieved with minimal but specific portable ancillary monitoring equipment:

1. Manual manometer
2. Portable finger pulse oximeter (eg, Lifebox)
3. Injection pressure monitor (eg, B-Smart)

These three monitoring tools support the goal of autonomous and safe anesthetic delivery while minimizing energy requirements and being lightweight enough to be portable.

Rapid and streamlined deployment is crucial in order to respond during the first 24 hours. For this reason, portability is a critical design consideration when developing a regional anesthesia kit for disaster response. Access to the impact zone is often via helicopter, horseback, or on foot once relief personnel reach the nearest airport, seaport, or available mass-transit point. All relevant equipment and supplies must, therefore, be carried by hand via carry-on bags or backpacks (Figure 58–8).[7] In addition to size and weight restrictions, kits must ensure adequate protection of supplies and equipment from the elements since shelter from the environment is seldom guaranteed and often limited or structurally unsafe. During the initial 72 hours

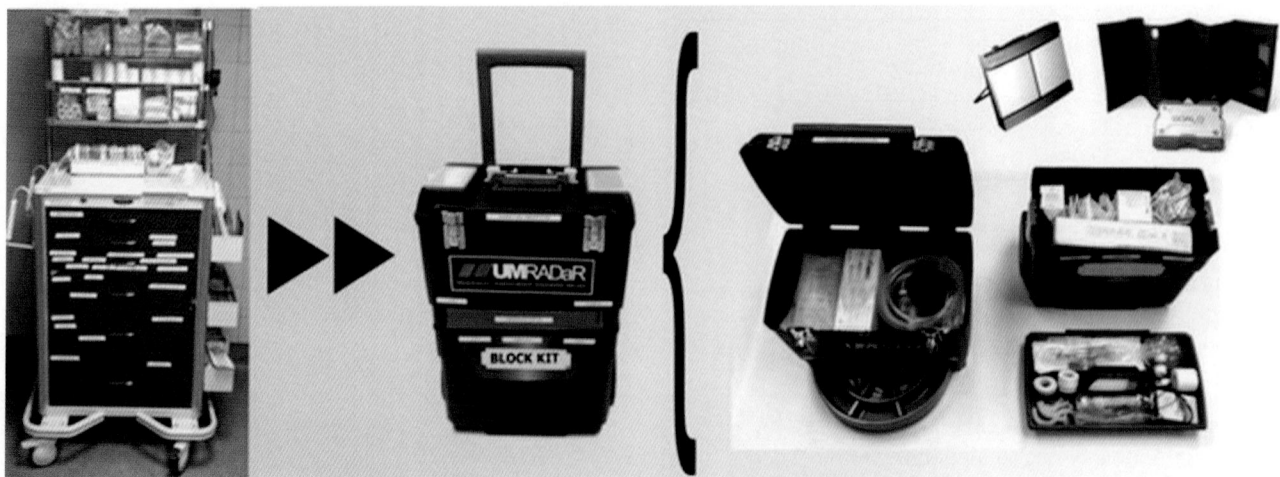

FIGURE 58–8. Portable regional anesthesia kit (RADAR™ Kit) developed by A. Missair, MD.

TABLE 58–6. Contents of a portable regional anesthesia disaster response kit.

REGIONAL ANESTHESIA DISASTER RELIEF BLOCK KIT/AIRPLANE CARRY-ON

BASIC INFRASTRUCTURE	AIRWAY EQUIPMENT	MED ID/SAFETY	IV ACCESS (for 30 pt)	RESUS DRUGS
	LMA sz 4(reusable)	Syringe lables × 1 roll (blank)	18G IV needles × 15	Epinephrine 1:1000 × 3 vials
	LMA sz 2 (reusable)	Pt ID bracelets × 48 (blank)	20G IV needles × 15	Atropine 0.4mg × 2 vials
	Laryngoscope handle	Nitrile gloves × 1 box (150 gloves)	IV bags (NS 250mL) × 4	Ephedrine 50mg × 2 vials
	MAC 3 blade	Permanent markers × 2	Toumiquets × 2	Phenylephrine 10mg × 2 vials
	Miller 2 blade	Surgical masks × 4	Tegaderms (small) × 30	Midazolam 5mg × 3 vials
	ADULT FM for AMBU	DEET insect repellent × 1 bottle	IVT-piece hubs × 30	Intralipid 20% × 250mL
	PEDI FM for AMBU	Chlorine tablets × 1 box	40IB fishing line × 1 roll	
	PEDI AMBU (can deliver up to 600mL TV)		Paper dips × 1 box (30)	
	Oral airways (60, 70, 80, 90mm)	**MONITORING**	Silk tape × 1 roll	
	Tongue depressors × 5	Finger pulseoximeter × 2	doth tape (2-inch) × 1 roll	
	ETT sz 7.0 and sz 4.0 (cuffed)	Manual BP cuff × 1	hytape × 1 roll	
		injection pressure nerve block monitor × 30	dear tape × 1 roll	

REGIONAL ANESTHETIC	NERVE BLOCK EQUIPMENT (for 60 blocks max)	LOCAL ANESTHETICS SEDATIVES		
	Nerve Stimulator × 1	IA Capacity = 30 mL bottles × 60		
	9V battery × 1	Ketamine Capacity = 30 mL bottles × 40		
	18G blunt needles × 1 box (=100)			
	2 Inch stimupelx needles × 20			
	4 Inch Stimuplex needles × 20			
	20 mL syringes (for LA) × 30			
	5 mL syringes (for ketamine) × 30			
	Alcohol prep pads × 1 box (=100)			
	Marking pens × 5			

LOGISTIC SUPPORT	COMMUNICATION			MISCELLANEOUS
	Satellite phone (or)			Swiss Army knife × 1
	Cell phone with international service and camera			LG plastic bag × 2
	Universal SOLAR battery charger			
	Phone number list for Disaster Response HQ			
	Dedicated cell phone text line at HQ			
	Portable SAT WiFi			

of the Haiti earthquake, for example, the medical team from the University of Miami treated patients outdoors due to the danger of aftershocks causing subsequent collapse of remaining buildings.[10]

The emphasis for regional anesthesia kit supply should be placed on airway management, basic monitoring, IV access, resuscitation, and single-shot nerve-stimulated blockade (Table 58–6).[7] Due to space and weight limitations, a portable finger pulse oximeter and a manual manometer with stethoscope are the most relevant and appropriate equipment for perioperative monitoring. It must be emphasized that field conditions during the acute phase of perioperative medical care will preclude any capacity for mechanical ventilation during extended periods of time. As a result, any airway equipment selected for inclusion in these kits is based on the need for temporary intraoperative airway control only.

Disaster response kits should implement a modular design, maximizing resource efficiency by separating reusable supplies (eg, monitors, nerve stimulators) from single-use items and medications. Each kit should then be equipped with the capacity to treat 30 patients, which is the average surgical case load per anesthesiologist over 48 hours during disaster relief efforts. This model simplifies field logistics and prevents redundancy and waste, while providing a capacity that is both portable, in terms of weight and volume, and compatible with average resupply chain times (48 hours).

SUMMARY

In the context of predominant limb injury requiring urgent surgical intervention, all anesthesia techniques may be safe, but single-shot peripheral nerve blocks may provide the necessary safety, patient comfort, portability, and efficiency to support mass casualties in the face of a collapsed medical infrastructure.[7,8,10,18] Regardless of the socioeconomic status and geographic location of the affected region and population, field hospitals remain an unattainable goal during the emergent and acute phases of disaster medical relief. Based on study findings, a well-equipped portable nerve block kit (see Figure 58–8), designed to provide basic monitoring and ketamine MAC capabilities, can serve as the first critical step in effective and safe anesthetic care during the acute phase of medical relief and act as a bridge to the subsequent establishment of field hospitals.

The solution proposed herein to address the acute perioperative anesthetic needs of a displaced patient population without medical facilities is consistent with the recommendations of the WHO Interagency Emergency Health Kit (IEHK) manual which states, "In situations of war, earthquakes or epidemics, specialized teams with medicines and medical devices will be required."[19] In fact, the WHO and its partner agencies intentionally excluded equipment for resuscitation and major

surgery from the IEHK. Regional anesthesia, therefore, directly complements the primary care and first aid provided by the interagency IEHK and affords the emergency anesthetic capabilities required during the acute phase of medical relief.

REFERENCES

1. Bournay E, United Nations Environmental Programme/GRID-Arendal: Trends in natural disasters. http://www.grida.no/graphicslib/detail/trends-in-natural-disasters_a899. Accessed March 3, 2014.
2. Ramirez M, Peek-Asa C: Epidemiology of traumatic injuries from earthquakes. Epidemiol Rev 2005;27:47–55.
3. United States Geologic Survey Earthquake Hazards Program: Earthquakes with 1,000 or more deaths since 1900. http://earthquake.usgs.gov/earthquakes/world/world_deaths.php. Accessed March 6, 2011.
4. Bournay E, United Nations Environmental Programme/GRID-Arendal: Typology of hazards. http://www.grida.no/graphicslib/detail/typology-of-hazards_1457. Accessed March 3, 2014.
5. Malish R, Oliver DE, Rush RM Jr, et al: Potential roles of military-specific response to natural disasters—analysis of the rapid deployment of a mobile surgical team to the 2007 Peruvian earthquake. Prehosp Disaster Med 2009;24:3–8.
6. Goncharov SF: Medical consequences of earthquake disasters in Russia. In World Health Organization Centre for Health Development: Earthquakes and people's health: proceedings of a WHO symposium, part 2. Kobe, Japan, January 27–30, 1997.
7. Missair A, Pretto EA, Visan A, et al: A matter of life or limb? A review of traumatic injury patterns and anesthesia techniques for disaster relief after major earthquakes. Anesth Analg 2013;117:934–941.
8. Ganjouei KA, Ekhlaspour L, Iranmanesh E, et al: The pattern of injuries among the victims of the Bam earthquake. Iranian J Publ Health 2008; 37:70–76.
9. Tanaka K: The Kobe earthquake: the system response. A disaster report from Japan. Eur J Emerg Med 1996;3:263–269.
10. Missair A, Gebhard R, Pierre E, et al. Surgery under extreme conditions in the aftermath of the 2010 Haiti earthquake: the importance of regional anesthesia. Prehosp Disaster Med 2010;25:487–493.
11. Mohebbi HA, Mehrvarz S, Saghafinia M, et al: Earthquake related injuries: assessment of 854 victims of the 2003 Bam disaster transported to tertiary referral hospitals. Prehosp Disaster Med 2008;23:510–515.
12. Cohen E: Expect Gettysburg. http://thechart.blogs.cnn.com/2010/01/15/expect-gettysburg/. Accessed March 2010.
13. Buckenmaier CC 3rd, Lee EH, Shields CH, Sampson JB, Chiles JH: Regional anesthesia in austere environments. Reg Anesth Pain Med 2003;28:321–327.
14. Mulvey JM, Qadri AA, Maqsood MA: Earthquake injuries and the use of ketamine for surgical procedures: the Kashmir experience. Anaesth Intensive Care 2006;34:489–494.
15. Mulvey JM, Awan SU, Qadri AA, Maqsood MA: Profile of injuries arising from the 2005 Kashmir earthquake: the first 72 h. Injury 2008;39: 554–560.
16. Paix BR, Capps R, Neumeister G, Semple T: Anaesthesia in a disaster zone: a report on the experience of an Australian medical team in Banda Aceh following the 'Boxing Day Tsunami'. Anaesth Intensive Care 2005; 33:629–634.
17. Jiang J, Xu H, Liu H, et al: Anaesthetic management under field conditions after the 12 May 2008 earthquake in Wenchuan, China. Injury 2010;41:1–3.
18. Qiu J, Liu GD, Wang SX, et al: Analysis of injuries and treatment of 3,401 inpatients in 2008 Wenchuan earthquake—based on Chinese Trauma Databank. Chin J Traumatol 2010;13:297–303.
19. World Health Organization: The Interagency Emergency Health Kit 2006—Medicines and Medical Devices for 10,000 People for Approximately 3 Months, 3rd ed. Geneva, Switzerland: World Health Organization, 2006, pp 11–49.

CHAPTER 59

Regional Anesthesia and Acute Pain Management in the Emergency Department

Andrew A. Herring, Sam Van Boxstael, Pascal Vanelderen, and Knox H. Todd

INTRODUCTION

Emergency physicians are called upon to provide care for a variety of acute and life threatening conditions. Often patients present with pain as the primary symptom of their illness or require diagnostic and/or therapeutic interventions that are inherently painful to perform. As a result, the management of pain in the emergency department (ED) is a critical skill and an important element in the overall care of patients in emergency settings. This chapter provides an overview of acute pain in the ED as well as potential therapies, including regional anesthetic techniques for the emergency physician.

EMERGENCY MULTIMODAL ANALGESIA

Systems-Based Multimodal Approach

The management of acute pain relies on providers and systems of care that are motivated, trained, organized, and equipped to rapidly treat acute pain. Without a clear organizational initiative and focus, pain treatment easily reverts to the low priority it has traditionally held in the emergency setting. Current understanding of the pathophysiology of pain suggests that opioids should preferentially be used only within a multimodal analgesic strategy tailored to the individual patient and his or her specific needs. Integrated use of complementary pharmacologic, interventional, and nonpharmacologic approaches enables the use of opioids that maximizes their beneficial properties while minimizing risk.

Nonpharmacologic Interventions

Effective treatment of the dislocated glenohumeral joint is prompt relocation. The underlying principle is that the ED should be organized so that simple, nonpharmacologic interventions such as elevation, icing, and immobilization of an acutely injured limb are prioritized from the point of triage. A humanistic approach with an outward expression of empathy and kindness can help to alleviate patient anxiety and fear.

Identify Injuries and Conditions Appropriate for Regional Anesthesia at Triage

Regional blocks should be placed as close to the time of initial injury as possible to maximize the potential of the block to limit the cascade of adverse physiologic events triggered by uncontrolled pain. Minimizing "door-to-block time" should be made a priority through collaborative systems development between emergency physicians and consultants.

Nonsteroidal Anti-inflammatory Drugs

Patients with severe acute pain should receive a nonsteroidal anti-inflammatory drug (NSAID) *and* acetaminophen unless contraindicated. Unfortunately, impaired platelet function and the risk of associated bleeding are of relative concern whereas nonselective NSAIDs should be avoided in the setting of acute trauma. An alternative strategy is the use of a selective cyclooxygenase-2 (COX-2) inhibitor such as celecoxib in combination with acetaminophen. Acetaminophen, although a relatively weak analgesic on its own, significantly enhances the analgesic effects of NSAIDs and opioids.

Avoid a "One Size Fits All" Individual

The dose response to opioids is notoriously variable. Rapid titration of relatively small doses every 10-15 minutes helps to both avoid overshooting the analgesic target and prevent oligoanalgesia.

Ketamine

Ketamine is an *N*-methyl-D-aspartate (NMDA) receptor antagonist that has a well-established track record in acute pain management and profound analgesic properties at low doses. Its stimulating cardiovascular and bronchodilatory activity has made it particularly popular in prehospital and austere settings. In the ED, ketamine is particularly useful to rapidly establish analgesia in the hypotensive severely injured trauma patient. Opioid-tolerant patients may particularly benefit from the addition of subdissociative-dose ketamine as a bolus or infusion. Finally, in our experience, the quality of multimodal analgesia incorporating is more profound and may help establish a degree of comfort with extremely painful injuries, such as an unstable fracture, that is not possible with opioids alone.

Anticonvulsants

Pregabalin and gabapentin are analgesic, anxiolytic, and antihyperalgesic agents that have been shown to reduce anxiety, improve pain control, and reduce opioid consumption in the perioperative setting. In the acute setting, a single oral dose of 600–1200 mg is preferred, and its primary side effect is somnolence without hemodynamic depression. Its role in acute injury has yet to be clearly established.

Adjuvant Analgesics

Alpha-antagonists, such as clonidine and dexmedetomidine, have analgesic properties. Clonidine can be administered intravenously, intramuscularly, intra-articularly, or as an adjuvant to peripheral nerve blocks. Dexmedetomidine has similar analgesic properties but is profoundly sedating. Tricyclic antidepressants, adenosine, droperidol, naloxone, corticosteroids, and magnesium have also all been used for acute pain management, but there is limited available evidence to clearly define their role in emergency pain medicine.

OLIGOANALGESIA IS A PROBLEM IN THE ED

Pain is the single most common reason patients seek care in the ED, and it accounts for up to 79% of visits.[1] Given the prevalence of pain as a presenting complaint, there is an increasing focus within emergency medicine to assign a high priority to analgesia. However, in the fast-paced, high acuity setting of the ED, pain can all-to-often be overlooked by providers of emergency medical care. The resulting inadequate use of methods to relieve pain was termed Oligoanalgesia by Wilson and Pendleton[2] in 1989. Several studies have established that oligoanalgesia is a common and complex problem in emergency medicine.[3] Notwithstanding the goal of providing compassionate care, pain that is not acknowledged and managed appropriately causes anxiety, depression, sleep disturbances, increased oxygen demands with the potential for end-organ ischemia, and decreased movement with an increased risk of venous thrombosis.[4,5] Failure to recognize and treat pain may also result in patients' dissatisfaction with medical care, unscheduled returns to the ED, delayed return to full function, and an increased risk of litigation (Table 59–1).[6]

Several studies have defined the prevalence of pain and oligoanalgesia in ED settings. For instance, Johnston and

TABLE 59–1. Adverse consequences of inadequate analgesia.

Patient Experience	• Decreased patient satisfaction, needless suffering
Physiologic	• Metabolic stress response • Hyperglycemia • Protein catabolism • Increased free fatty acids (decreased myocardial contractility, increased myocardial oxygen demand, impaired vasodilation) • Hypercoagulability • Thromboembolic events • Pulmonary complications • Immunosuppression • Delirium • Development of chronic pain states • Complex regional pain syndrome
Long-term psychologic	• Posttraumatic stress disorder • Insomnia
Logistic	• Increased duration of intensive care unit and hospital stay • Decreased participation in rehabilitation

colleagues[7] investigated the incidence and severity of pain among patients presenting to noncritical treatment areas within the EDs of 2 urban hospitals in Canada. They found that 58% of adults and 47% of children reported pain on ED arrival. Approximately 50% of these patients described their pain as moderate to severe. At the time of discharge, one-third of both groups reported persistent pain of moderate to severe. In fact, 11% of children and adults in this study reported clinically significant increases in pain intensity during their stay in the ED.

Another prospective study showed that among adults treated at one Chicago ED, 78% presented with pain as a chief complaint.[8] Of all patients, 58% received analgesics or nonpharmacologic interventions, but only 15% received opioids, despite high levels of pain intensity. Guru and Dubinsky[9] found that 50% of patients who were treated for acutely painful conditions did not receive prescriptions for pain management at discharge. Data from a review of urban, university-based EDs revealed that 69% of patients with painful conditions, including thermal burns, long-bone fractures, and vaso-occlusive crises, received no pain medication at all and that 55% were discharged with no analgesic prescription.[10]

A study by Brown and colleagues[11] revealed that pain medications were frequently not part of ED treatment for fractures, even for patients with documented moderate or severe pain.

Yet, in spite of the tendency to undertreat pain in the ED, patients appear to expect better analgesia. As an example, Fosnocht and colleagues[12] used a 100-mm visual analog scale

(VAS) to gauge patients' expectations of pain relief in the ED (0 mm = no relief; 100 mm = complete relief). Patients with pain reported a mean expectation for pain relief of 72%, and 18% of patients expected complete relief of their pain. Interestingly, this value was seemingly independent of the initial pain severity, so that those with mild pain expected the same degree of relief as those with severe pain. Other studies have suggested that patients' expectations are very influential on both their experience of pain and satisfaction with their care.[13,14]

Several factors conspire to result in under treatment of pain in ED. Difficulty in accurately assessing pain is a well-known problem to providers of emergency medical care. Data from several studies indicated that caregivers underestimate pain when their assessment of pain is compared with those reported by the patients themselves.[9,15] The assessment may also be hindered by the limitations of commonly used verbal scales. For example, Rupp and Delaney[3] pointed out that asking a patient to describe his or her pain in relation to the "worst pain imaginable" obviously yields different answers, depending on the patient's particular frame of reference. Other factors leading to oligoanalgesia may include apprehension (on the part of both the patient and the physician) about opioid dependence,[16] concern regarding side effects such as respiratory depression,[17] the desire to withhold pain medication until informed consent for a procedure has been obtained, and concern about the risk of adequate pain management obscuring a diagnosis (eg, in patients with an acute abdomen). However, there is mounting evidence that adequate analgesia may actually diminish involuntary guarding as a confounding factor and allow for a more precise evaluation of localized sensitivity.[3,18–20] Suitable treatment of pain is not only a necessity from a ethical point of view; better analgesia can also prevent delayed complications of certain injuries. For instance, an intervention as simple as the early administration of ketorolac reduces the risk of pneumonia after rib fractures and increases intensive care unit- and ventilator- free days without increasing the risk for acute kidney injury, gastrointestinal hemorrhage, or non-union of the fractures.[21]

Some patient populations are at a higher risk of oligoanalgesia (Figure 59–1). For example, several studies have documented lower rates of analgesic administration for both young children and the elderly when compared with other patients in pain.[10,22,23] Kozlowski and colleagues[24] reported that in patients with isolated lower extremity injuries, those with fractures were twice as likely to receive pain medication as those without fractures, even when controlling for the severity of pain. Patients' gender does not appear to influence the quality of analgesia in ED, according to one prospective study.[25]

Patients' ethnicity is perhaps the best-studied risk factor for oligoanalgesia in the ED. In 1993, Todd and colleagues[26] examined the medical records of all patients with acute, isolated, long-bone fractures seen at the UCLA Emergency Medicine Center in 1991 and 1992. Hispanic patients in this study were twice as likely as non-Hispanic white patients to receive no pain medications during their ED stay (RR 2.1; 95% CI 1.4–3.3). This relative risk for Hispanic patients to receive no analgesia remained significant after controlling for covariates related to characteristics of the patient (gender, language, and insurance coverage), injury (open versus closed fracture, admittance versus discharge, and need for reduction), and physician (ethnicity, sex, and specialty). After multiple logistic regression analyses, patients' ethnicity remained the strongest predictor of ED analgesic administration. In a follow-up study at a large university-affiliated community ED in urban Atlanta, Todd and colleagues[27] found similar disparities in analgesic treatment between white and African American patients with isolated long-bone fractures despite similar documentation of pain complaints.

The solution to these disparities may involve more than simply addressing cultural biases, however. Research into the genomic basis of pain sensation is beginning to show that different individuals, as well as groups of individuals, process pain signals differently.[28] This may help guide providers of analgesia as to which individuals may be experiencing more intense pain from the same injury or illness. In addition, response to analgesics may also be attributable in part to gene expression, just as cytochrome P450 receptor differences determine a patient's ability to metabolize codeine.[29]

PAIN ASSESSMENT IN THE ED

Recognizing that pain is a major public health problem, the Joint Commission on Accreditation of Healthcare Organizations (JCAHO) has placed a great deal of emphasis on the

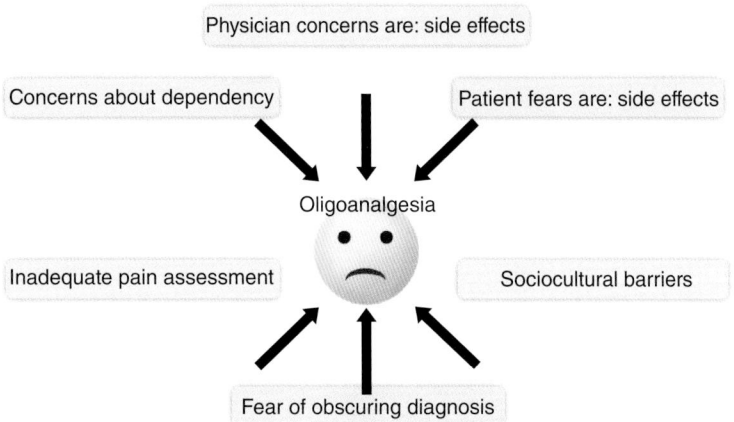

FIGURE 59–1. Factors leading to under treatment of pain.

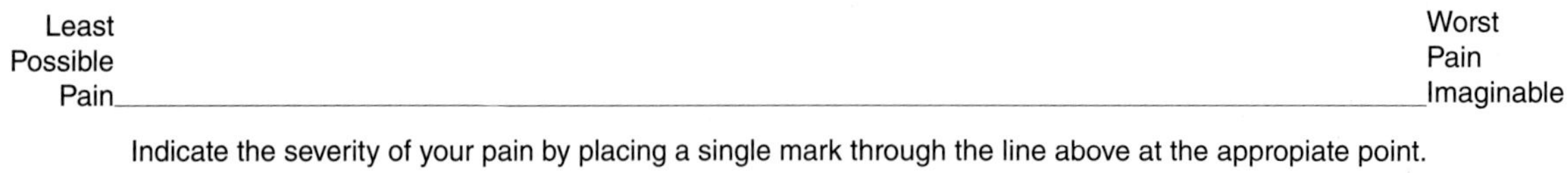

```
Least                                                                    Worst
Possible                                                                 Pain
Pain_____Imaginable
```

Indicate the severity of your pain by placing a single mark through the line above at the appropiate point.

FIGURE 59–2. Visual analog scale.

importance of pain management, in part by implementing standards that create new expectations for the assessment and management of pain.[30] These standards have been endorsed by the American Pain Society.

One of the key JCAHO's recommendations focuses on the use of standardized tools for frequent assessment of pain, documentation, and treatment. Indeed, many hospital EDs have begun to include pain as the "fifth vital sign" to encourage frequent and standardized reassessment.

Several pain assessment tools are available for use in the ED. One of the most common is the VAS, which is easy to use and convenient for statistical analysis. Patients are asked to make a mark on a horizontal line that corresponds to the intensity of their pain (Figure 59–2). This scale is attractive for acute care settings in which short-term changes in VAS scores can be used to guide the titration of analgesic therapy. Todd and colleagues[30] conducted serial interviews with patients reporting acute pain and concluded that a change of less than 13 mm in the VAS score is clinically insignificant. A similar tool is the 11-point numeric rating scale (NRS), which asks the patient to verbally rate his or her pain on a numerical scale, usually from 1 to 10. Both the VAS and NRS have been shown to be reliable and valid tools for assessing acute pain.[31-33] However, the numeric rating scale is becoming the pain scale of choice because of its ease of use, broader range of

applications, and consistent results across a wide range of languages and cultures.[34,35] A reduction of 2 points or 30% in NRS was deemed clinically important by Farrar et al.[36] Moreover, the relationship between the percent change in NRS and the patïent's global impression of change is more consistent regardless of baseline pain scores. Finally, mandated reporting of pain scores has been shown to result in improved frequency of analgesic administration for ED patients presenting with acute pain.[37]

MONITORING DURING SEDATION AND ANALGESIA

Urgent procedures in the ED are common and often require some level of sedation for optimal patient comfort. This may range from light sedation via a small dose of midazolam and fentanyl before the placement of a regional block to deep sedation via propofol for a complex abscess incision and drainage or etomidate for cardioversion. An overview of the many options for ED sedation is presented in Table 59–2. The recommendations regarding sedative use in the ED should be based on the indication and resulting sedation state, not the specific pharmacologic agent involved. Therefore, ED staff should apply monitoring standards solely on the basis of the anticipated depth of sedation. For example, low dose of midazolam or ketamine in

TABLE 59–2. Emergency sedation.

Drug	Emergency Dosing	Comments
Midazolam	1–2 mg IV titrated to effect; more than 5 mg IV cumulative should be avoided.	Sedative only with dose-dependent cardiovascular respiratory depression.
Propofol	0.5–1.0 mg/kg IV loading dose titrated to effect.	Sedative only with dose-dependent cardiovascular respiratory depression; very quick onset and rapid recovery.
Ketamine	Broad range from as low as 5 mg IV (<0.1 mg/kg) for analgesia to 150 mg IV (2–3 mg/kg) for dissociative anesthesia; rapid onset within 3–4 min allows rapid titration.	Powerful analgesic at low doses; at higher doses results in a surgical dissociative anesthesia; dose-dependent dissociative effects are bothersome to some patients. Addition of an opioid or benzodiazepine tends to increase patient tolerability of the dissociative effects.
"Ketofol" (1:1 mixture of ketamine and propofol combined in a single syringe)	0.5 mg/kg ketamine + 0.5 mg/kg propofol delivered together.	Potentially balancing side effect profile.
Etomidate	0.1–0.2 mg/kg slow IV push.	Myoclonus and adrenal suppression are considerations; clinically, most commonly used for cardioversion and endotracheal intubation.

Abbreviation: IV, intravenous.

young, healthy subjects may not always require full monitoring as such could lead to the underutilization of sedation and oligoanalgesia.

The classification of sedation proposed by the American Society of Anesthesiologists comprises 4 categories: minimal-moderate-deep sedation and general anesthesia with clear definitions of these categories in terms of responsiveness, airway, cardiovascular and spontaneous ventilation.[38] Any patient who is treated with moderate or deep sedation requires the presence of an physician at the bedside with appropriate nursing assistance to allow for continuous monitoring of cardiac function and oxygenation. Oxygen, suction, reversal agents, and advanced life support medications and airway equipment should be available. Continuous capnography may help in the early identification of hypoventilation.

PHARMACOLOGIC STRATEGIES FOR TREATING ACUTE PAIN

Analgesic protocols that involve standing orders for the nursing staff with mandatory and frequent pain assessments are particularly effective in the ED setting where the emergency physician may not be able remain at the bedside to titrate analgesia. The cornerstone analgesics are acetaminophen and NSAIDs. In general, patients should receive both in combination unless there are specific contraindications.

Clinical Pearls

Acetaminophen and NSAIDs are the foundation of emergency analgesia.

- Any patient considered for opioid analgesics should also be given acetaminophen in combination with an NSAID unless there are specific contraindications.
- Acetaminophen should be given in combination with an NSAID unless contraindicated.
- Trauma patients should receive a selective COX-2 NSAID (such as celecoxib) because non-selective NSAIDs are associated with increased bleeding risk.
- IV formulations of both acetaminophen and NSAIDs are available for patients who are unable to take medications by mouth.

Acetaminophen

Acetaminophen has both analgesic and antipyretic, but no anti-inflammatory, properties. Although acetaminophen's precise mechanism of action is unclear, it likely involves some inhibition of prostaglandin synthesis. It is an appropriate first-line analgesic option for mild to moderate pain, such as, musculoskeletal pain, headache, earache, and dysmenorrhea. The most serious adverse effect is hepatotoxicity, most commonly seen in the setting of accidental overdose with combined opioid–acetaminophen preparations. Another point of attention is the dose-dependent interaction between acetaminophen and vitamine K antagonists, leading to clinically relevant increases in INR of 0.17 per gram

of ingested acetaminophen.[39] Because of its long safety record and low incidence of adverse effects, acetaminophen is the most frequently used analgesic in North America. In combination with NSAIDs it is the base on which to build a multimodal analgesic regimen. A parenteral formulation of acetaminophen is now available potentially increasing its applicability in the ED setting.[40,41] With regard to pain related to soft tissue injuries (sprain, strain or contusion of a joint, ligament, tendon or muscle), a recent Cochrane review could not identify superiority of acetaminophen or NSAID's when used in monotherapy. Similar conclusions applied to swelling and return to function. There was low-quality evidence of more gastrointestinal adverse effects with non-selective NSAID compared with acetamoniphen.[42] However, in the setting of postoperative pain relief, a combination of NSAID's and acetaminiphen was more proficient than either drug in monotherapy.[43]

NSAIDs

In addition to their analgesic and antipyretic properties, NSAIDs function by inhibiting cyclooxygenase (COX), an enzyme responsible for prostaglandin synthesis. This property renders NSAIDs useful for treating inflammatory and prostaglandin-related pain, such as rheumatoid arthritis and dysmenorrhea, as well as renal and biliary colic, headache, and musculoskeletal injuries. The inhibition of COX is also responsible for the side effects of NSAIDs, which include nephrotoxicity via decreased renal perfusion and an increased risk of gastroduodenal ulcer formation. These side effects are dose dependent and are more likely to occur in the elderly and those with preexisting renal or peptic ulcer disease.[44] Other adverse effects include hypersensitivity, platelet dysfunction, and asthmatic exacerbation in sensitive individuals.[45]

There are many NSAIDs to choose from, and they appear to be relatively interchangeable as a class. In other words, with the correct dosing, ibuprofen is as effective as indomethacin or diclofenac. Ketorolac is unique in that it may be used parenterally, thereby ensuring a rapid onset, which is an attractive attribute in the ED. Ketorolac has been used favorably in emergency medicine for various types of acute pain.[46] Topical NSAID's are effective for analgesia in patients with acute sprains, strains and overuse injuries, probably similar to that provided by oral formulations and with few systemic side effects.[47] Mainly gel formulations of diclofenac, ibuprofen, and ketoprofen provide the best results with NNT of 1.8, 3.9 and, 2.5, respectively for 50% pain relief. Selective COX-2 inhibitors are associated with adverse cardiovascular outcomes with long-term use; however, they have shown promise as part of a multimodal approach to patients with major trauma in whom non-selective NSAIDs, such as ketorolac, are contraindicated due to bleeding risk. (ref:48).

Opioids

Despite being a mainstay of acute pain management in the ED, opioids are often associated with widely divergent attitudes toward dosing and application in the ED. Both under-dosing for fear of opioid-associated adverse events resulting in under-treated pain and excessive dosing resulting in sedation, respiratory depression, nausea, and delirium are common in the ED. routine use of a multimodal approach—combining opioids with adjuvant analgesics whenever possible—with rapid titration can help avoid both of these undesirable outcomes (Table 59–3).[49–51]

Clinical Pearls

Protocolized, rapid titration of morphine to improve analgesia and reduce the incidence of adverse events.

- Opioids are often the best agent for acute severe pain in the ED.
- Potentially life-threatening adverse events attributable to opioids are largely preventable.
- Individual dose response is highly variable. Response cannot be accurately predicted based on pain score and weight alone.
- Relatively small doses can be surprisingly effective, just as large doses may not provide substantial relief.
- CNS concentrations of morphine peak within 20-30 minutes.
- Avoid large (ie > 0.15 mg/kg) single-dose orders without close observation of clinical effect.
- In opioid-naïve patients, start with a lower dose (eg, <0.1 mg/kg IV).
- Titrate rapidly with repeat doses every 10-20 minutes based on clinical response
- Instruct patients about safe use and opioid addiction whenever prescribing these drugs for out-of-hospital use.

Opioids however, carry a risk of dependency and addiction for both ED personnel and patients. A recent study showed that patients in the ED often have misconceptions about opioid addiction and under- as well as overestimate their personal risk for addiction.[52] As such, ED physicians should discuss opioid addiction with patients whenever they prescribe these drugs. A simple educational intervention consisting of verbal instructions and a one-page information sheath has shown to improve the patient's knowledge concerning safe use of opioids.[53] A realistic appreciation of this reality in a setting of nonjudgmental and empathetic care is warranted whenever opioids are used.[54] Additionally, chronic opioid use poses unique challenges for acute ED pain management such as opioid tolerance and opioid-induced hyperalgesia. In particular some opioid tolerance patients will demonstrate a very narrow therapeutic window, special care is often needed to avoid fluctuating between undertreated pain and opioid toxicity in these patients. The use of adjuvant acetaminophen, NSAIDs, and low-dose ketamine in conjunction with the rapid titration of an intravenous (IV) opioid is the best available strategy for this challenging clinical situation.[55]

In addition to morphine, a wide spectrum of opioids, such as fentanyl and sufentanil, are suitable because of their rapid onset and limited duration of action during procedural sedation and analgesia.[56] Other commonly used parenteral opioids are meperidine and hydromorphone, although the use of meperidine is declining owing to its neurotoxic and anticholinergic side effects. Major side effects common to all opioids include dose-dependent respiratory depression, nausea, constipation, pruritus, and urinary retention (Tables 59-3 and 59-4).

In Europe, tramadol is often used in the ED for its analgesic properties, particularly in children and the elderly. It poses less risk for of side effects of such as respiratory depression or altered consciousness. Another advantage of Tramadol is the spinal re-uptake inhibition of noradrenaline and serotonin, which makes the drug suitable for patients with neuropathic pain syndromes. It is administered typically in combination with an anti-emetic to reduce the risk of nausea and vomiting.

The use of opioids in combination with acetaminophen or an NSAID has increased dramatically in recent decades, and combinations of hydrocodone and acetaminophen are the most commonly prescribed medications in the United States by a large margin. There is little evidence to support such a large role for this class of medicine in moderate, non-malignant pain. Conversely, there is no high-quality evidence that this practice is harmful. As a result, community practice is widely divergent, as are expectations for ED-based opioid prescribing. A consistent approach coordinated with inpatient and outpatient services is ideal when possible.

Ketamine

Ketamine, an NMDA receptor antagonist, is a potent analgesic at low doses (0.1–0.3 mg/kg IV) and has a unique dissociative anesthetic effect at higher doses (1–2 mg/kg IV). Ketamine has several unique applications in emergency care.[57,58]

Clinical Pearls

Ketamine Analgesia in Emergency Care
Monitoring
- Ketamine at doses less than 0.3 mg/kg IV does not produce more than mild sedation, and additional monitoring beyond typical or IV opioids is not necessary.
- Reconsider the use or reduce the dose of ketamine in patients with suspected intracranialtraumatic brain injury hypertension because the effect of ketamine on intracranial pressure is still uncertain.[59] Care should also be taken or in patients with myocardial ischemia due to increases in myocardial oxygen consumption associated with ketamine.

Psychomimetic effects
- Ketamine can produce fleeting, difficult-to-describe alterations in perception and sensation that for most patients are not unpleasant. Is important to obtain informed consent and advise patients beforehand so these experiences do not come as a surprise.
- Emergence reactions do not occur at low doses. While not available in the USA, the racemic ketmaine (ketmaine-S) is uniquely suitable in the ED because of the substantially reduced psychotropic side-effects.

Important ED applications
- Ketamine is recommended for agitated, hypotensive trauma patients; brief, painful procedures such as the infiltration of local anesthetic around a laceration or abscess; opioid-dependent patients presenting with complex pain crises; and intractable cancer pain.

TABLE 59–3. Example of multimodal analgesia for an injured 70-kg opioid-naive patient.

1. Rapid identification of patients with acute pain and immediate intervention
Prompt relocation, proper splinting, wound protection, cooling, and positioning using a humanistic approach that maximizes the beneficial psychologic effects of provider attention, empathy, and kindness.

2. Evaluation for regional anesthesia
The preparation for regional anesthesia can begin in parallel with the other components of a multimodal approach.

3. Early initiation of anti-inflammatory regimen
+ an NSAID or selective COX-2 inhibitor should be administered.

Medication	Emergency Dose	Comments
Acetaminophen	15 mg/kg orally, rectally, or IV every 6 h 60 mg/kg maximum per day	Few contraindications which should not be overlooked, as it has potent effects when used in combination with other analgesics.
Celecoxib (selective COX-2 inhibitor)	400 mg oral loading dose then 200 mg daily, 4 mg/kg daily	

Consider risk/benefits ration of using ibuprofen, ketorolac, naproxen, and other nonselective COX inhibitors in the acute trauma setting because of bleeding risk or in patients with acute kidney injury and GI disease (eg, peptic ulcer).

Ibuprofen	400–800 mg orally every 8 h (5-10 mg/kg oral every 4-8 h)	
Ketorolac	0.5 mg/kg IV every 6 h	May cause severe bronchospasm in asthmatic patients.

4. Rapid titration of IV opioid (fentanyl) every 3–5 minutes and transition to longer-acting opioids (morphine or hydromorphone) as needed

Medication	Emergency Dose for Acute Pain	Comments
Fentanyl	25–100 mcg every 5 min titrated at bedside (1-2 μ/kg)	Synthetic opioid; rapid action; relatively limited cardiovascular impact.
Hydromorphone	1–3 mg every 3–4 h IV (0.05-0.1 mg/kg)	Can titrate as quickly as every 5–10 min with caution.
Morphine	5–15 mg every 3–4 h IV (0.1-0.2 mg/kg)	Most commonly used opioid.

Protocolized pain assessment and drug administration may help achieve rapid titration. For prolonged stays in the ED, consider patient-controlled analgesia and /or the addition of long-acting oral opioids such as oxycodone, tramadol, or oral morphine.

5. Ketamine
Consider ketamine as a coanalgesic for intractable severe pain, opioid tolerance, or hypotension. Ketamine can also be used to rapidly establish deep analgesia or as rescue bolus followed by infusion for refractory pain and may be a first-line agent in patients with hypovolemia, hypotension and/or agitation. Where available, consider using racemic ketamine (S).

Drug	Emergency Dose	Comments
Ketamine	0.1–0.3 mg IV bolus every 5 min titrated at bedside; 10–30 mg/h IV continuous infusion	Rapid acting; can result in profound analgesia; unpleasant "drugged" feeling is decreased at lower doses; true dissociation uncommon at lower doses.

6. Consideration of a gabapentinoid

Drug	Emergency Dose	Comments
Gabapentin	300–600 mg orally every 8 h Initial dose as high as 1200 mg orally	Used routinely in the U.S. military for acutely injured; side effects include somnolence.
Pregabalin	75–150 mg orally every 12 h	Similar to gabapentin.

Abbreviations: COX-2, cyclooxygenase-2; ED:, emergency department; NSAID, nonsteroidal anti-inflammatory drug.

TABLE 59–4. Limitations of opioid analgesics.

Acute side effects	Respiratory depression, nausea and vomiting, pruritus, vasodilation and hypotension, immunosuppression
Logistic	Most common source of dosing errors
	Prolonged recovery and increased duration of stay
	Resource-intensive monitoring at higher doses
Pharmacologic	Opioid-induced hyperalgesia and tolerance that limit effectiveness
	Risk for abuse and dependence that affects both patients and providers

The Agitated, Hypotensive Trauma Patient

Agonal patients in hypovolemic shock from hemorrhage can become confused and thrash wildly, delaying full evaluation and potentially life-saving administration of blood products. Small doses of ketamine (0.1–0.2 mg/kg IV) can have a profound calming and analgesic effect with a lower risk of hypotension than that associated with opioids (including fentanyl).

Brief, Painful Procedures

Examples of these procedures include infiltration of local anesthetic around a laceration or abscess, followed by suturing or evacuation, respectively. The patient should first receive an NSAID and acetaminophen. Next, an IV opioid is given, and then 5 minutes before the expected maximum intensity of pain, low-dose ketamine is administered (0.1–0.2 mg IV). We find that high-quality analgesia greater than that normally achieved with an opioid alone occurs rapidly with only a light sedative effect and mild psychomimetic effects that are not unpleasant.[57,58]

Clinical Pearls

Reducing the pain of local infiltration
- Use small needles (ie, 27- to 30-gauge).
- Inject the anesthetic slowly (1 mL over 30 s).
- Buffer local anesthetics with sodium bicarbonate.
- Inject anesthetics from within lacerations rather than through intact skin.
- Use some type of topical anesthesia beforehand.

Opioid-Dependent Patients Presenting with Complex Pain Crises

In this setting, NMDA receptor–mediated pro-nociceptive pathways may play a substantial role in the suffering of the patient. Small doses (0.1–0.2 mg IV or 0.2–0.4 mg intramuscularly) of ketamine can be very effective.[58] Intractable cancer pain is increasingly common in the ED setting. These patients are often receiving long-term opioid therapy and may benefit from the addition of a ketamine bolus (0.1–0.2 mg IV) followed by an infusion of 0.3 mg/kg IV per hour.[57,58,60]

Other Adjuvants

There is a wide variety of patients presenting with severe pain in ED that may respond favorably to additional adjuvants. This is an area in need of further study, and the role of agents such as gabapentin, clonidine, and lidocaine has not yet been clarified.

Topical Anesthetics

Topical anesthesia involves the application of a local anesthetic directly to a mucosal or skin surface. The application of a topical local anesthetic mixture before the injection of a local anesthetic can significantly reduce the severity of pain on injection for patients with lacerations or abscesses.[61,62]

Oropharyngeal anesthesia is most commonly used for peritonsillar abscess incision and drainage and endotracheal intubation in awake patients. Lidocaine 1–4% can be administered several different ways: viscous lidocaine jelly can be swished around the mouth; liquid lidocaine can be nebulized for anesthesia of the oropharynx and airway; and lidocaine-soaked pledgets can be applied directly to a mucosal area in the nose or oral cavity. Pretreatment with an antisialagogue such as glycopyrrolate (0.2 mg IV) 10 minutes before the application of lidocaine can promote better tissue penetration. Because relatively higher concentrations (eg, 4%) of lidocaine are used and system uptake from mucosal surfaces can be rapid, safe dosages should be calculated in advance and adhered to. Common options for topical anesthesia for venipuncture, wound repair, or use prior to local anesthetic injection are presented in Table 59–5.

Nitrous oxide

Nitrous oxide is mainly used for sedation of children that require minor surgical procedures or painful interventions in the ED. Appropriate equipment for airway management, intravenous access and hemodynamic and respiratory monitoring must be available in case of too deep sedation. Provisions for scavenging of gases must be present in the ED since N2O can have deleterious effect on the fetus and chronic exposure may lead to infertility, and adverse effects on bone marrow and the central nervous system.[63,64] In a prospective trial, the effect of a N2O/O2 (50:50 mixture) sedation was evaluated in 210 children (mean age 9y, range 2.7-16y).[65] In 137 cases nitrous oxide was used to facilitate administration of local anesthetic, other indications were skin sutures, reduction of fractures and dislocations, venapunctures, abcess and hemotoma drainage. The average duration of N2O administration was 10 min (range 5-30 min). Patients were calm and pain free in 73.8% of the procedures. Failure defined as any event necessitating the termination of N2O administration occurred in 1.4%. Compared to intravenous ketamine, nitrous oxide sedation allows for a more controlled depth of sedation with faster recovery times.[66] Frequently observed side effects with nitrous oxide sedation are nausea and vomiting, euphoria, dizziness which occur in 5 to 16% of patients. The odds of vomiting increase with concomitant administration of opioids or when clear fluids were

TABLE 59–5. Emergency topical anesthesia[a].

Agent	Action
Intact Skin	
Eutectic 1:1 mixture of 2.5% lidocaine and 2.5% prilocaine (EMLA)	Onset is 60 min; occlusive dressing is required; methemoglobinemia is a rare complication of prilocaine.
4% lidocaine cream in a liposomal matrix (LMX)	Onset 30 min, and no occlusive dressing is required.
Vapocoolant spray	Ethyl chloride is the most commonly used agent. Spray until skin blanches for up to 10 s 3–9 in. from skin surface; duration is approximately 1 min after blanching.
Nonintact Skin	
Lidocaine 4%, epinephrine 0.1%, and tetracaine 0.5% (LET)	Onset 30 min after direct application to open wound.

[a]Other techniques for delivering lidocaine topical anesthesia such as iontophoresis and needle-free jet delivery remain uncommon in the emergency department and are under study. Agents containing cocaine and benzocaine are less commonly used owing to concerns about systemic toxicity (cocaine) and methemoglobinemia (benzocaine).

ingested <2 h before N2O administration.[67] More serious complications consist of oxygen desaturation and generalized tonic-clonic seizures which are increasingly seen with N2O concentrations >50% and prolonged administration of N2O >15 min. The use of a face mask with a patient demand valve can be helpful to prevent oversedation. Recently, a case of laryngospasm, pulmonary aspiration and desaturation associated with nitrous oxide (70%) sedation was described in a 16 month old child which was fasted for 4 h. This case once more highlights the need for adequately monitoring in sedated patients and the presence of ED staff skilled in emergency airway management.

Overview

A wide variety of regional anesthetic techniques are used in the ED setting (Table 59–6). Nerve blocks placed as close to the time of injury as logistically feasible are one of the most important recent advances in emergency pain management. Widespread adoption of early regional anesthesia has proven revolutionary in the contemporary military trauma setting.[68] Nerve blocks have multiple important advantages. First, they reduce or eliminate the need for opioids. Moreover, by halting the nociception from of an acute injury, nerve blocks reduce central nervous system (CNS) sensitization or "wind-up." Finally, nerve blocks offer improved analgesia and a decreased metabolic stress response to acute injury (see Table 59–7).[68-71]

Traumatic injury results in a catabolic stress response that is directly proportional to the degree of tissue injury and may be attenuated by regional anesthesia, that blocks peripheral afferent noxious stimuli from reaching the CNS. The barrage of noxious stimuli to the CNS after traumatic injury triggers a cascade of metabolic, neurohormonal, and inflammatory events leading to detrimental physiologic changes such as hyperglycemia, hypercoagulability, and immunosuppression. Although, the stress response is an adaptive "fight or flight" mechanism to promote survival, but in the medical context, it may be associated with delayed recovery, delayed healing, and increased morbidity.[71]

Tailoring Multimodal Analgesia in ED

Mastery of emergency pain management requires matching the best agent or modality to the tremendous variety of individual clinical circumstances and patient types that present to a busy ED (see Table 59–6). For example, there is evidence to support preferentially using NSAIDs for ureteral colic and vascular headaches, whereas some anterior shoulder dislocations may be best treated with manual muscle massage.

TABLE 59–6. Types of emergency regional anesthesia.

Regional Anesthesia Technique	Comments
Tissue infiltration	Simple; but can be painful and anesthesia may be incomplete, particularly with fractures.
Field blocks	Can be very effective in select anatomic locations.
Intra-articular injection	Analgesia is limited to joint surface relatively of short duration.
Fracture hematoma injection	Can be rapidly placed once fracture is identified; limited duration and scope of analgesia.
Regional nerve block	Superior analgesia for extremity trauma.
Neuraxial and IV techniques	ED applications are currently limited; somewhat higher risk profile and unclear benefit compared with regional nerve blocks.

Abbreviations: ED, emergency department; IV, intravenous.

TABLE 59-7. Benefits of regional anesthesia.

- Targets effective analgesia to a specific anatomic area.
- Reduces the need for opioids and the incidence/severity of opioid-related side effects.
- Reduces the need for sedatives and the incidence/severity of sedative-related side effects.
- In hypovolemic patients, may reduce the incidence of hypotension compared with traditional sedation and analgesia.
- May reduce the stress response to injury.
- Improves the quality of pain control.
- Decreases the need for close medical supervision of awake and alert patients with well-controlled pain.

TABLE 59-8. Nerve blocks suitable for use in ED.

Head and face
- Infraorbital
- Mental
- Supraorbital, supratrochlear, and infratrochlear
- Dorsal nasal nerve
- Zygomaticotemporal
- Zygomaticofacial
- Mandibular

Neck and upper extremity
- Superficial cervical plexus
- Suprascapular nerve
- Brachial plexus
- Cutaneous blocks of the forearm
- Peripheral radial, median, and ulnar nerves

Trunk
- Intercostal and paravertebral
- Abdominal wall

Lower extremity
- Femoral nerve block
- Lateral femoral cutaneous nerve
- Popliteal sciatic nerve
- Common peroneal nerve
- Posterior tibial nerve

Low-dose ketamine may be a good analgesic choice for an elderly patient with cancer-related pain already taking opioids or for a heroin user undergoing procedural sedation with propofol. The skillful emergency physician will also recognize that pain is not simply nociceptive and is often accompanied by other unpleasant sensory and emotional experiences. The liberal use of adjunctive benzodiazepines and antiemetics is a well-established practice for maximizing patient comfort and satisfaction. Small details, such as the use of topical anesthesia prior to local anesthetic infiltration may have a large impact on the patient's satisfaction and overall pain experience (Table 59–7). Finally, organizational protocols and structures can have a significant impact on common ED barriers to quality pain management. Objective, protocolized, pain assessment that begins at triage and is linked to an immediate and simple analgesia protocol is likely the best approach ref 50. Perhaps above all, mastery of emergency pain management requires the accumulation of experience using the entire pain management armamentarium (see Table 68-6).

In summary, the best approach to acute ED pain management is generally one that (1) includes immediate pain assessment and treatment at the point of triage, followed by multimodal analgesia that is tailored to the patient and the diagnosis; (2) combines complementary analgesic agents; (3) incorporates loco-regional anesthesia when appropriate; and (4) addresses associated problems like nausea and anxiety.

PERIPHERAL NERVE BLOCKS IN ED

A wide variety of peripheral nerve blocks are applicable to emergency care (see Table 68-8).[72,73] ED staff are becoming increasingly more accustomed to performing loco-regional anesthesia procedures in a timely manner and provide close nursing observation. Optimizing the capacity of an ED to implement peripheral nerve blocks involves several steps: (1) patient selection and care coordination; (2) technique standardization; (3) local anesthetic toxicity (LAST); and (4) long-term complication management (Table 59-8).

Patient Selection and Care Coordination

Establishing close partnerships with consultants in orthopedic surgery, trauma, general surgery, and anesthesia services to develop consensus protocols that detail the specific use of peripheral nerve blocks in the emergency setting is necessary. Treatment protocols can be particularly effective in reducing delays and confusion about which injuries are appropriate for use of loco-regional anesthesia in the ED. Clear and logical protocols for block administration, documentation, and continued management of the block in the inpatient or outpatient setting are essential for safety and efficacy.

Standardization of Techniques

Safe and effective use of peripheral nerve blocks in the ED requires a well-developed staff training program and standardized techniques that maximize efficiency and consistency, and minimize the risk of complications such as LAST, nerve injury, and delayed diagnosis of compartment syndrome. Additionally, a well-organized and stocked "block cart" can promote the efficiency and standardization of the consenting process, materials used, and technical aspects of the procedures.[74]

Local Anesthetic Toxicity (Last)

Any ED where regional nerve blocks are performed should have guidelines for the recognition and treatment of LAST and should be equipped with readily available IV lipid infusions.

A recent study identified 67 reports of LAST over a 4 year period.[75] LAST most frequently occurred with single injections of LA (50/67 cases), followed by continuous infusions (8/67 cases) and topical administrations (7/67cases). Two reports concerned the unintentional injection of LA through an intravenous cannula. In the group of single injections associated with LAST, interscalene block (23%) is the most often reported technique followed by local field infiltration anesthesia (22%), epidural/caudal block (16%) and dorsal penile block (13%). 78% of LAST symptoms appear within the first 30 min with only 10% occurring after 60 min. Toxicity associated with topical LA mostly occurs in pediatric patients. LAST symptoms have a tendency to progress from central nervous system to cardiovascular manifestations in 83% of the patients. The most common sign of central nervous system toxicity was seizure (54%). Other symptoms included confusion, dizziness, tinnitus, dysgeusia, hallucinations, slurred speech, gait problems, limb twitching, extremity paresthesia, intention tremor, hypotonia, and facial sensorimotor and eye movement abnormalities. The most common cardiovascular expressions of LAST were bradycardia, hypotension and shock (41%) followed by tachycardia, hypertension, ventricular fibrillation (15%) and cardiac arrest (7%). Treatment of LAST is discussed in another chapter in this volume.

Long-Term Complication Management

All patients who receive a nerve block in the ED should have a developed pathway for the evaluation and management of delayed complications such as nerve injury that is coordinated with neurology and the chronic pain medicine service.

Ultrasound

Ultrasound has become an essential part of emergency care, and nearly all U.S. EDs have ready access to a modern ultrasound machine. Given the clear advantages of ultrasound guidance, we see few reasons not to use an ultrasound-guided technique for regional nerve blocks in the ED.

Matching the Peripheral Block to the Clinical Need

The most challenging aspect of administering emergency regional anesthesia is matching the correct peripheral nerve block to the clinical injury or procedure in the most site-specific and effective manner. Given the unpredictability of injuries in the ED, a well-established knowledge of the peripheral innervation patterns and a broad armamentarium of peripheral blocks is required (Table 59–9).

Emergency Regional Anesthesia by Area of Injury

Neck and Shoulder Girdle

The superficial cervical plexus block is a particularly useful block in the ED owing to its technical ease of implementation and relatively large area of innervation. The greater auricular nerve, although quite small, can frequently be found on the superficial surface of the sternocleidomastoid and blocked selectively (Table 59–10 and Figure 59–3). Clavicle fractures are common in the ED and generally excellent analgesia can be obtained with a low dose interscalane plexus block.[76]

Emergency Regional Anesthesia for the Shoulder

Shoulder dislocations are very common in the ED and are an excellent indication for a low-volume interscalene brachial plexus block. Compared with etomidate sedation, ultrasound guided interscalene block resulted in comparable pain scores and patient satisfaction. Reduction is possible in most patients.[77] In contrast, reduction was not possible in 4/30 patients after a interscalene block in a study by Underhill and colleagues.[78] The use of a surface landmark technique without the use of a nerve stimulator is probably the main reason for the 4 failed reductions in the latter study. The key component of a successful shoulder reduction is muscle relaxation, which is generally very consistently achieved with an interscalene brachial plexus block. A short-acting local anesthetic such as 3% 2-chloroprocaine or 1% lidocaine is ideal. A retrospective study with 224 patients in France reported a complication rate of 8% associated when with sedations for repositioning of shoulder dislocations mainly because standard guidelines concerning fasting and sedation are not followed. The authors reported no complications with the use of an was used for reposition of the shoulder dislocations versus no complications when interscalene block.[79] Moreover the use of regional anesthesia can significantly shorten the time care providers spend on monitoring patients as well as shorten the time patients spend in the ED and hereby allowing for a more efficient deployment ED resources k was used.[77,80]

Intra-articular lidocaine is a valuable alternative to interscalene block for the reduction of schoulder dislocation. In a recent meta-analysis of 9 randomized, controlled studies, intra-articular lidocaine was associated with equal success rates but less complications (vomiting, respiratory depression, thrombophlebitis) than intravenous sedation. Among injection drug users, deltoid abscesses are common, and brachial plexus blockade (interscalene or supraclavicular) or a selective axillary nerve block provides excellent anesthesia for incision and drainage in these cases (Table 59–11 and Figure 59–4).[81,82]

Emergency Regional Anesthesia for the Arm

Elbow dislocation is also common in the ED and can be well managed with a supraclavicular brachial plexus block (Figure 59–5). Although blockade of the C8–T1 innervation of the elbow may not always be complete, in most cases, anesthesia is sufficient to permit closed relocation.

Proximal humerus fractures are quite common in the elderly and notoriously painful. These fractures are generally very unstable and do not immobilize well with splinting. In this setting, developing a consensus plan with the orthopedic service is particularly important given the risk of a "double crush" nerve injury (Table 59–12).[83]

Below the elbow, superficial injuries of the forearm require blockade of the radial nerve and the lateral and medial

TABLE 59–9. Emergency peripheral nerve blocks: applications.

Block	Emergency Indication	Comments
Head and Face		
Infraorbital		
Mental	Facial lacerations	
Supraorbital, supratrochlea/infratrochlear		
Zygomaticotemporal		
Zygomaticofacial		
Greater auricular	Lacerations to the ear lobe	Blocked as part of the superficial cervical plexus or alone.
Greater occipital	Intractable migraine	
Dorsal nasal	Nasal laceration, abscess I&D	Normally combined with infraorbital block.
Neck		
Superficial cervical plexus	Ear lobe laceration repair, neck abscess I&D or laceration repair, IJ cannulation, clavicle fracture analgesia	Wide area of anesthesia from blockade of the supraclavicular, transverse cervical, lesser occipital, and greater auricular nerves.
Shoulder		
Suprascapular nerve	"Frozen shoulder"/adhesive capsulitis	Provides partial analgesia and relaxation to glenohumeral joint and can be used for shoulder reduction.
Axillary nerve	Deltoid abscess I&D Deltoid laceration repair	May provide significant analgesia for proximal humerus fractures if a full brachial plexus block is contraindicated.
Upper Extremity: Brachial Plexus		
Interscalene	Injury to the upper extremity above the mid-humerus	Typically misses the C8, T1 roots and elbow, wrist, and hand are incompletely blocked. Low volumes are effective for shoulder applications.
Supraclavicular	"Spinal of the arm" covers the entire arm	Most reliable block for anesthesia to elbow and distally.
Axillary and infraclavicular	Elbow, forearm, wrist, and hand injuries	Misses the medial antebrachial cutaneous nerve. Blocked with musculocutaneous nerve.
Radial nerve	Wrist, thumb, and hand injuries	Posterior interosseous nerve contributes to wrist.
Median nerve	Wrist and hand injuries	Anterior interosseous nerve contributes innervation to the wrist.
Ulnar nerve	Elbow, wrist, hand, and small finger injuries	An isolated boxer's fracture can usually be reduced with an ulnar block alone. However, significant injuries to the wrist and hand typically require blocking all three terminal nerves—radial, ulnar, and median.
Musculocutaneous nerve and its terminal branch nerve, the lateral antebrachial cutaneous	Lateral aspect of the skin of the forearm	Can be blocked in the upper arm with ultrasound guidance or as a cutaneous field block.
Medial antebrachial cutaneous nerves	Medial aspect of the skin of the forearm	Small cutaneous nerve; can be visualized and blocked with ultrasound or with field infiltration. When combined with blocks of the radial nerve and musculocutaneous nerve, a complete cutaneous forearm anesthesia results.

(continued)

TABLE 59–9. Emergency peripheral nerve blocks: applications. (*Continued*)

Block	Emergency Indication	Comments
Intra-artiuclar injection and fracture hematoma injection	Shoulder, elbow, and wrist fracture dislocations	Analgesia is somewhat unpredictable and short lived; however, can be placed rapidly at bedside as long-term analgesic plan is established.
Trunk		
Intercostal and paravertebral	Thoracic wall trauma such as rib fractures, lacerations, or placement of thoracostomy tubes.	The anesthesia includes the parietal pleura itself. Thoracostomy tubes can be placed painlessly with well-placed, posterior intercostal blocks. Area of high local anesthetic absorption and concomitant toxicity risk.
Rib fracture hematoma injection	Rib fractures can be visualized well with ultrasound.	Likely lower risk for pneumothorax and technically less challenging than paravertebral blocks; however, a shorter duration and less complete analgesia is found.
Anterior Abdomen		
Transversus abdominis plane block	Anterior abdominal wall injury or abscess I&D	Target a contiguous anatomic space and the interconnected plexus of nerves that innervate the anterior abdominal wall from the pubis symphysis to T8.
Rectus sheath		
Ilioinguinal and iliohypogastric nerves	Inguinal injury, abscess I&D, or hernia repair wound complications	
Superior cluneal nerves	Superficial buttock abscess I&D	The superior cluneal nerves innervate the skin overlying the superior buttocks but not the underlying muscle.
Lower Extremity		
Femoral nerve	Hip fracture, hip dislocation, femoral shaft fracture, tibial plateau fracture, patellar fractures, lacerations or abscess I&D to the anterior thigh	Effective for analgesia. Owing to mixed innervation, complete pain control for hip fracture requires both a sciatic and obturator blockade.
Saphenous nerve	Lacerations or abscess I&D to the medial lower leg, ankle fracture dislocations in combination with sciatic nerve blocks	Terminal branch of the femoral nerve.
Lateral femoral cutaneous nerve	Hip abscess I&D as is common among patients who "skin pop" heroin in this area.	Superficial nerve does not innervate the deep muscle layers.
Popliteal sciatic nerve	Ankle dislocation and fracture	Always consider more selective blocks. Combine with a saphenous block for ankle fracture reductions.
Common peroneal and sural nerves	Injury or abscess I&D to the dorsum of the foot	Deeper structures innervated by the posterior tibial nerve.
Posterior tibial nerve	Closed calcaneal fracture, foreign body removal, or laceration to the sole of the foot	When blocking for calcaneal fracture, always be vigilant for concomitant lumbar vertebral fractures.
Intra-articular hip injection	Acetabular fracture	Relatively brief duration of action; can be very effective in acute period to establish analgesia.

Abbreviations: ED, emergency department; I&D, incision and drainage; IJ

TABLE 59–10. Peripheral nerve blocks for the neck and shoulder girdle.

Emergency Indication	Regional Block
Laceration to the auricle of the ear including the helix, lobule, and antitragus. The antihelix, concha, tragus, and most superior portions of the helix are not blocked.	SCP, greater auricular nerve or selective greater auricular nerve
Laceration or abscess I&D on the neck from the submandibular region to shoulder "cape"	SCP, transverse cervical nerves, and supraclavicular nerves
Internal jugular cannulation	SCP, transverse cervical nerves
Clavicle fracture analgesia	SCP, supraclavicular nerves

Abbreviations: SCP, superficial cervical plexus; I&D, incision and drainage.

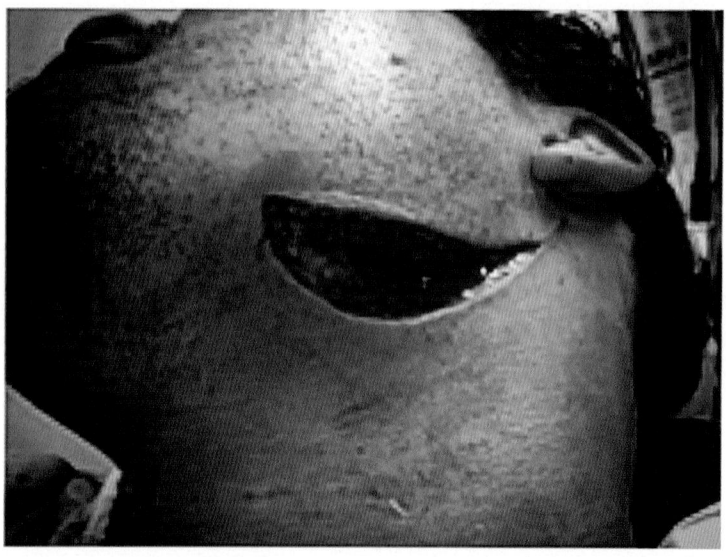

FIGURE 59–3. Large neck laceration repaired in the ED with anesthesia provided by a superficial cervical plexus block.

TABLE 59–11. Peripheral nerve blocks for the shoulder.

Emergency Indication	Regional Block
Acromioclavicular separation	Interscalene brachial plexus block or direct infiltration.
Shoulder dislocation	Interscalene brachial plexus block. We prefer a low volume of a short-acting local anesthetic such as 2-choloroprocaine. Provides analgesia and deep muscle relaxation. Intra-articular infiltration under ultrasound guidance is also successful in some patients, although the level of anesthesia and analgesia is far lower. Selective suprascapular block provides partial analgesia that is adequate for some patients.
Deltoid abscess	Common in drug abusers. A selective axillary nerve block if there is no overlying cellulitis is the most selective approach but can miss the most superior/proximal aspect of the shoulder (augment with local infiltration). The interscalene or supraclavicular approaches provide excellent anesthesia for even large abscesses. Premedication is particularly important in these patients who are often hyperesthetic and in opioid withdrawal.
"Frozen shoulder"	Suprascapular block. For some patients, pain relief is dramatic; corticosteroid is typically added. Low dose interscalene block.

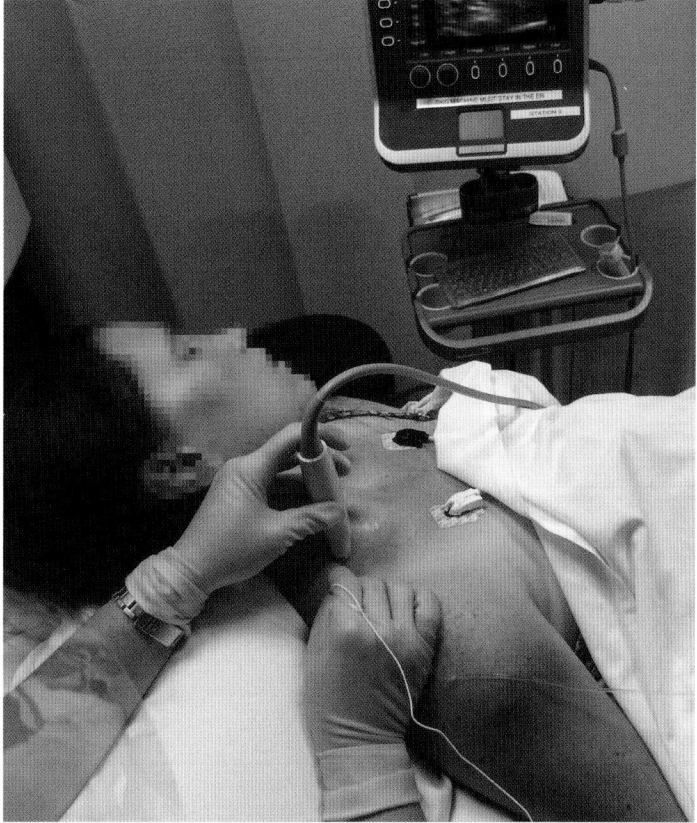

FIGURE 59–4. Deltoid abscesses are common in patients who "skin pop" heroin. This abscess was drained in the ED after an interscalene brachial plexus block.

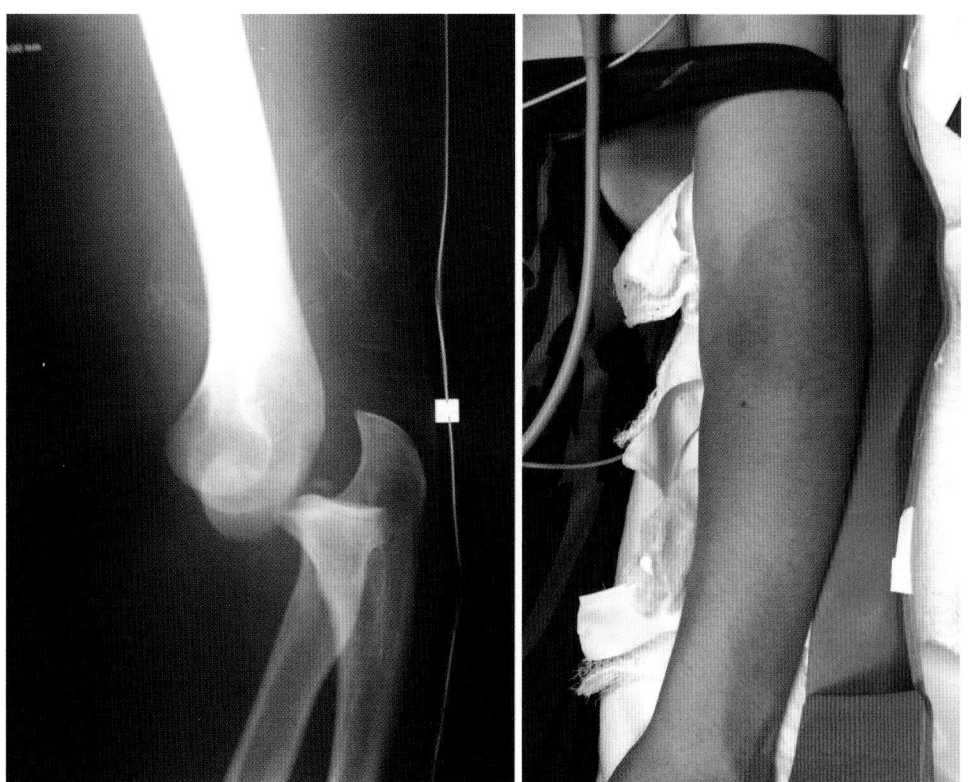

FIGURE 59–5. Elbow dislocation successfully reduced in the ED with a supraclavicular brachial plexus block.

TABLE 59–12. Peripheral nerve blocks for the upper arm.

Emergency Indication	Regional Block
Proximal humerus fracture	Interscalene or supraclavicular brachial plexus block.
Mid and distal humerus fracture	Supraclavicular or infraclavicular brachial plexus block.
Elbow fracture/dislocation	Supraclavicular or infraclavicular brachial plexus block.
Superficial lacerations or injury on lateral aspect of upper arm	The cutaneous innervation most superior aspect of the shoulder is primarily via the supraclavicular nerves. Moving distally, the deltoid (or "regimental patch") area is primarily axillary, and the area below the deltoid is innervated primarily by the radial nerve. Local infiltration or field block can be particularly suitable/effective.
Superficial lacerations on medial aspect of upper arm	Medial antebrachial cutaneous. Not a common area for injury. Blocked with a field block in the axilla.

antebrachial cutaneous nerves depending on the injury location (Figures 59–6 and 59–7).

Radial and ulnar fractures such as the common Colles' fracture are best treated with a supraclavicular brachial plexus block. Although some patients receive excellent anesthesia from a fracture hematoma block, the results are inconsistent (Table 59–13).[84]

Recently, proximal periosteal nerve blocks were advocated for distal ulna and radius fracture manipulations.[85] This technique consists of LA injection in and around the lateral (in case of the radius) or medial (in case of the ulna), ventral, and dorsal periosteum 6 cm proximal to the wrist via a skin entry on the radial and medial side. In a prospective study with 40 patients, this technique resulted in successful fracture relocation in 95%. The relocation was described as painless in 85% of the cases.

Emergency Regional Anesthesia for the Hand

The hand is well anesthetized with distal blocks of the radial, median, and ulnar nerves in combination or selectively depending on the injury. These superficial nerves are generally very well visualized with ultrasound (Table 59–14 and Figure 59–8).[86]

Emergency Regional Anesthesia for the Thorax and Abdominal Wall

Rib fractures are quite common in the ED and are associated with severe pain. The major issue that arises with ED

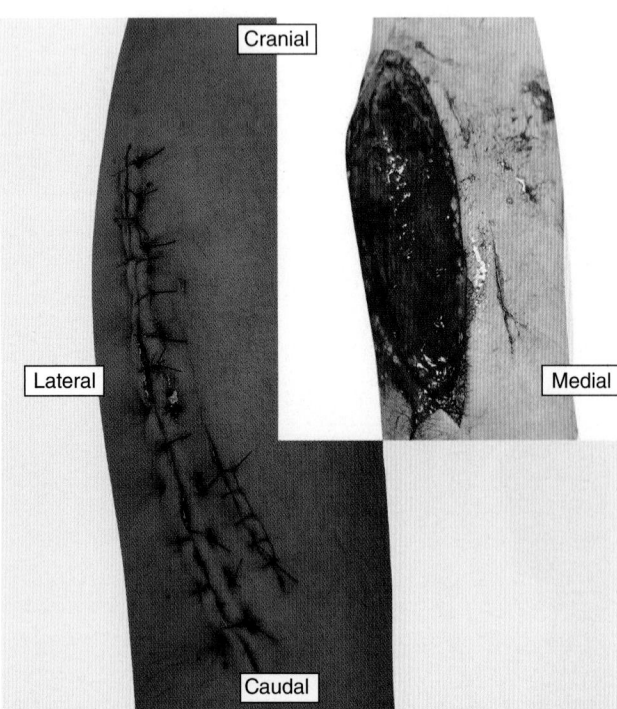

FIGURE 59–6. This volar forearm injury (A) was large but superficial and was repaired using anesthesia from a medial and lateral antebrachial field blocks placed just above the elbow.

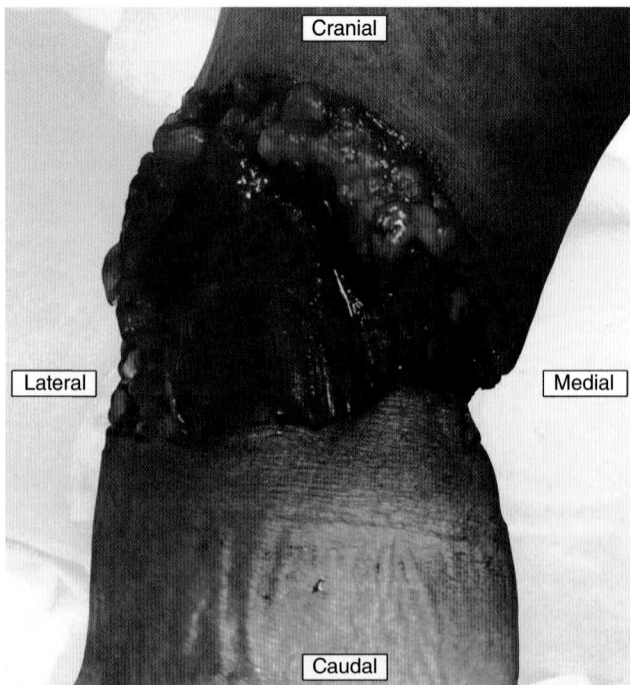

FIGURE 59–7. This forearm injury involved deeper structures and a supraclavicular brachial plexus block was used for anesthesia with excellent results.

TABLE 59–13. Peripheral nerve blocks for the forearm.

Emergency Indication	Regional Block
Forearm laceration or injury	The superficial innervation of the forearm is supplied by the lateral antebrachial cutaneous nerve (a terminal branch of the musculocutaneous nerve), the medial antebrachial cutaneous nerve, and branches of the radial nerve. The emergency provider has three options: (1) supraclavicular brachial plexus block, (2) selective ultrasound-guided block of the component nerves based on the injury location, and (3) landmark-based field blocks.
Anterior forearm	Medial and lateral antebrachial cutaneous nerves. (It is important to note the underlying muscle and bones of forearm have separate innervations.) These blocks can be accomplished either with a landmark-based skin wheal or selective blockade. The musculocutaneous nerve is quite easy to locate and block; the medial antebrachial cutaneous nerve is quite small and superficial, and the relative of advantage of ultrasound guidance is less clear.
Posterior forearm	Radial nerve and medial and lateral antebrachial cuntaneous nerves.
Forearm fractures	Supraclavicular or axillary brachial plexus block.
Wrist fracture or dislocation, distal ulna radius fractures, and carpal bone dislocations	Axillary, infraclavicular, or supraclavicular blocks. The wrist has a complex innervation that includes the radial, medial, ulnar, and musculocutaneous nerves. Distal radius fractures are very common, and the degree and pattern of pain associated with reduction is variable. For some patients, fracture hematoma injection may suffice, although rarely without some degree of discomfort, and is generally inferior to a brachial plexus block. Below-the-elbow radial, ulnar, and median blocks will not address innervation via the posterior interosseous, anterior interosseous, and musculocutaneous nerves.

placement of intercostal blocks is the time required to place the block at multiple levels. Particular vigilance for signs of LAST is needed given the high systemic intake of local anesthetic at this location. A paravertebral approach is less time consuming, as multiple levels can be blocked with a single injection, but requires more technical skill. Tube thoracostomy is often performed at the bedside in the ED, and the analgesia for the procedure can be accomplished by either intercostal or paravertebral block. A key strategy is to carefully identify the thoracic levels to match the injury with the appropriate block; one level above and one below the level of insertion is necessary (Table 59–15 and Figure 59–9). In patients with multiple level s or bilateral rib fractures, an epidural analgesia may provide more consistent, extendable analgesia with catheter placement and requires lower volumes of LA's. In a retrospective study with 64 patients sustaining rib fractures after motor vehicle accidents, Wu et al. found thoracic epidural analgesia to be superior to patient-controlled intravenous analgesia.[87] Epidural analgesia for thoracic trauma also proves to be superior with regard to mortality and mobidity. In an elderly population (mean age 70 y) with thoracic trauma, epidural analgesia with opioids reduced mortality and

TABLE–59-14. Peripheral nerve blocks for the hand.

Emergency Indication	Regional Block
Major hand injury	Radial, median, and ulnar blocks at the mid-forearm. Given the degree of overlap, any major injury should have all three nerves blocked. Radial block below the elbow avoids a wrist drop. Axillary and supraclavicular brachial plexus blocks are also options. In principle, choosing the most distal feasible block for a given injury is preferable.
Localized hand injuries	
Thumb and index finger	Radial and median nerve blocks at the forearm for any significant thumb injury.
Thumb cutaneous only	Dorsum blocked with a radial nerve block, palmar aspect with a median nerve block.
Superficial palm	Median and ulnar blocks at the forearm.
Superficial dorsum	Radial and ulnar blocks at the forearm.
Small finger	Ulnar block at the forearm.

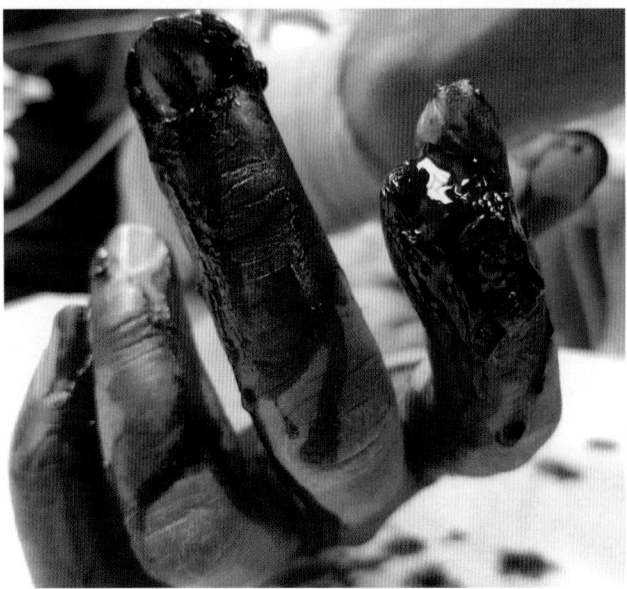

FIGURE 59–8. Median and radial nerve blocks were used as anesthesia method for partial index finger amputation in ED.

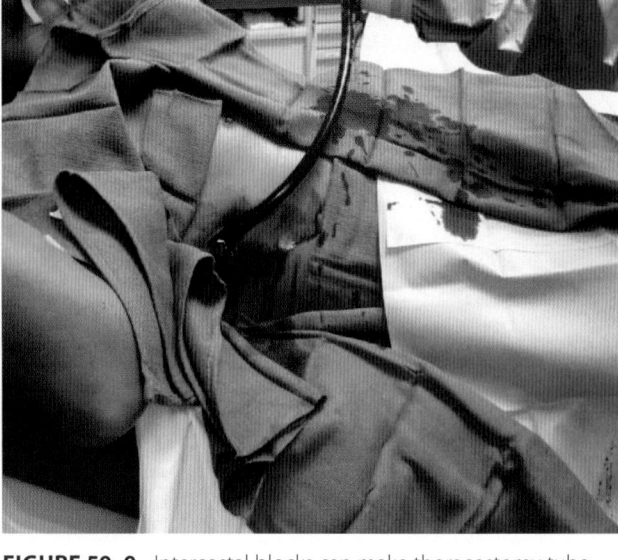

FIGURE 59–9. Intercostal blocks can make thoracostomy tube placement in the ED much more comfortable procedure.

pulmonary complications compared with parenteral analgetics. There were no procedure related complications in the epidural group *vs.* 9% in patients that received intercostal nerve blocks (pneumothorax and intravascular injection).[88] Similar results were noted in a younger population (mean age 49 y) with ≥ 3 rib fractures: systemic opioid analgesia was associated with a 6-fold increase in the risk of pneumonia and

TABLE 59–15. Peripheral nerve blocks for the thorax.

Emergency Indication	Regional Block
Rib fracture or other thoracic wall trauma	Intercostal or paravertebral blocks. Isolated rib fractures can be treated with direct infiltration of local anesthetic into the fracture site.
Thoracostomy tube insertion	
Abdominal wall injuries and abscess I&D.	The rectus sheath, transversus abdominis plane, and ilioinguinal/iliohypogastric nerve blocks all target contiguous anatomic space that contains the arborbized plexus of thoracic nerves innervating the anterior abdominal wall and parietal peritoneum.
• Central, periumbilical	Rectus sheath block.
• Periumbilical level to inguinal region	Transversus abdominis plane block.
• Inguinal region	Ilioinguinal/iliohypogastric block.

a 2-fold increase in ventilator days compared with epidural analgesia notwithstanding the fact that patients in the epidural group tended to have more flail segments and lung contusions. The reported complication rate with epidural analgesia was higher than in the former study (27%) but consisted mainly of minor adverse events: pruritus, transient motor block, catheter site inflammation and allergic reaction.[89] Finally, epidural analgesia can favorably alter myocardial oxygen supply/demand, reduce thromboembolic complications, and shorten the duration of gastrointestinal ileus.[90] However, epidural analgesia is not suitable for all patients. Contraindications include hypotension, hypovolemia, coagulopathy, raised intracranial pressure, sepsis and aortic valve stenosis. Paravertebral nerve block may be an alternative for patients with contraindications for epidural analgesia and provides similar pain relief and improvements in respiratory function.[91] Abdominal wall abscesses can become large and require emergency incision and drainage for which abdominal fascial plane blocks can be quite effective.[92]

Clinical Pearl

• Meticulously marking the rib levels can help avoid inadvertently skipping a level when placing multiple blocks.

Emergency Regional Anesthesia for the Lower Extremity

Emergency regional anesthesia for the proximal lower extremity involves blockade of the femoral, lateral femoral cutaneous, and sciatic nerves. Hip fractures are common and painful injuries in the elderly that are associated with significant morbidity and mortality. Since the femoral nerve innervates a large part of the hip joint and the femur, targeting this nerve either individually with a femoral nerve block or combined with the lateral femoral and obturator nerve as with a fascia iliaca block (FIB) provides good pain relief. Femoral nerve blocks also provide adequate pain relief for diaphyseal or distal femur fractures.[93] A femoral nerve block for femoral fractures is the most widely used nerve block in emergency medicine.[94–97] Although administering this block is technically easy, the challenge lies in developing the capacity of the ED to consistently provide the block in a timely manner. A prospective study in 137 patients with hip fractures, showed a significant improvement of 3 points on a NRS in 77.4% of the patients 60min after a FIB with a surface landmark technique.[98] Compared to intravenous morfine, femoral nerve block significant shortened the time to lowest pain score and significantly reduced opioid consumption.[99] Surface landmark FIB has also proven to be useful in children

TABLE 59–16. Peripheral nerve blocks for the lower extremity.

Emergency Indication	Regional Block
Hip fracture or dislocation	Femoral or Fascia Iliaca block. There are obturator and sciatic nerve afferents to the hip joint that are not blocked by a femoral block, resulting in analgesia, but not surgical anesthesia.
Acetabular fracture	Intra-articular injection. Quick, rapid relief but short lived. Best for initial presentation to establish analgesia.
Femoral shaft fracture	Femoral nerve block. Very effective for mid and distal fractures.
Patellar fracture	Femoral nerve block.
Tibial plateau fracture	Given the concern for compartment syndrome, must establish a collaborative consensus with orthopedic surgeon.
Lateral thigh laceration or abscess I&D	Lateral femoral cutaneous block.
Anterior thigh laceration or abscess I&D	Femoral nerve block.
Patellar laceration or abscess I&D	Femoral nerve or femoral triangle block.
Medial calf laceration or abscess I&D	Saphenous nerve block at mid-thigh.
Tibia and fibula fractures	Popliteal sciatic block. The notorious vulnerability of traumatic tibial fractures to develop compartment syndrome demands a well-developed census plan with surgical services for patient selection and monitoring.
Lateral lower leg injury	Common peroneal block. The skin of the lateral lower leg is innervated via the peroneal nerve; medially it is supplied by the saphenous nerve.
Ankle fracture/dislocation	Popliteal sciatic and saphenous blocks. The majority of innervation is supplied via the sciatic nerve; however, there is potentially significant contribution to the joint from the femoral (via saphenous) nerve.
Calcaneal fracture	Posterior tibial block. Isolated calcaneal fractures respond very well to selective posterior tibial block. However, high-energy injuries with extensive soft-tissue injury or additional fractures will require a popliteal sciatic block.
Extensive foot injury	Popliteal sciatic block. Diabetic patients with large abscesses are a common ED presentation.
Dorsum of the foot	Common peroneal block.
Sole of the foot	Posterior tibial block. Very effective for foreign body removal as the deeper structures of the sole of the foot are well anesthetized, allowing for deep exploration.

Abbreviations: ED, emergency department; I&D, incision and drainage.

for analgesia of lower limb fractures. In a retrospective study, 158 pediatric patients that received a FIB were compared with 101 patients that received IV analgetics for femur fractures.[100] The FLACC and Bieri pain scores were 1.5 points lower in the FIB group. One patient in the FIB group developed seizures due to LA toxicity that required treatment with intravenous lipid emulsion. A prospective randomized controlled trial comparing FIB with IV morphine in comparable settings yielded similar findings.[101] In a prospective feasibility study, ultrasound guidance was used to perform FIB in 20 patients with hip fractures. The investigators reported significant reductions (over 50% improvement) in VAS scores up to 8 hours after an ultrasound guided FIB with 30ml of 0.25% bupivacaine.[102] However, a confounding factor in this study could be the administration of morphine 2h before the administration of the FIB. Since the observed pain relief lasted longer than the clinical effect of morphine, the authors attributed this analgesia to the FIB. Similar outcomes were noted after ultrasound guided femoral nerve block for patients with hip fractures.[103] The latter studies outline the important aspect that outcomes and safety of regional anesthetic techniques in the ED could be improved by the use of ultrasound guidance. These findings are confirmed in a randomized controlled trial that compared ultrasound guided femoral nerve block with a landmark technique.[104] Ultrasound guidance resulted in significant more complete blocks and shorter times to complete block than the landmark technique. Additionally, the role of the placement of continuous catheters in the ED is evolving and may have a significant role in the future.[87,88] Selective saphenous or lateral femoral cutaneous blocks can be an elegant way to provide anesthesia for large skin lacerations. The popliteal approach to the distal sciatic nerve combined with a saphenous nerve block is ideal for complex ankle fracture dislocations. Selective posterior tibial blocks are particularly useful for common ED presentations such as plantar foreign body removal and calcaneal fracture analgesia (Table 59–16 and Figure 59–10).[105] Regional anesthesia techniques must be used judiciously in injuries that

lead to an acute compartment syndrome since early signs can be masked.

SUMMARY

Acute pain is well recognized as a problem in the ED. Emergency departments must develop an approach to caring for acutely ill patients that includes the assessment and treatment of pain as well as the treatment of the underlying illness. Multimodal analgesia with a combination of oral, parenteral, and nerve block techniques is the most effective way to provide quality pain relief in the ED while minimizing the risk of adverse effects. Regional anesthesia is a powerful adjunct to acute pain management that has been gaining popularity in the ED, particularly with the advent of the point-of-care ultrasound.

REFERENCES

1. Cordell WH, Keene KK, Giles BK, et al: The high prevalence of pain in emergency medical care. Am J Emerg Med 2002;20:165–169.
2. Wilson JE, Pendleton JM: Oligoanalgesia in the emergency department. Am J Emerg Med 1989;7:620–623.
3. Rupp T, Delaney KA: Inadequate analgesia in emergency medicine. Ann Emerg Med 2004;43:494–503.
4. Gureje O, Von Korff M, Simon Ge, et al: Persistent pain and well-being: A World Health Organization study in primary care. JAMA 1998;280:147–151.
5. Anderson FA Jr, Spencer FA: Risk factors for venous thromboembolism. Circulation 2003;107(23 Suppl 1):I9–I16.
6. Furrow BR: Pain management and provider liability: No more excuses. J Law Med Ethics 2001;29:28–51.
7. Johnston CC, Gagnon AJ, Fullerton L, et al: One-week survey of pain intensity on admission to and discharge from the emergency department; a pilot study. J Emerg Med 1998;16:377–382.
8. Tanabe P, Buschmann M: A prospective study of ED pain management practices and the patient's perspective. J Emerg Nurs 1999;25:171–177.
9. Guru V, Dubinsky I: The patient versus caregiver perception of acute pain in the emergency department. J Emerg Med 2000;18:7–12.
10. Selbst SM, Clark M: Analgesic use in the emergency department. Ann Emerg Med 1990;19:1010–1013.
11. Brown JC, Klein EJ, Lewis CW, et al: Emergency department analgesia for fracture pain. Ann Emerg Med 2003;42:197–205.
12. Fosnocht DE, Heaps ND, Swanson ER: Patient expectations for pain relief in the ED. Am J Emerg Med 2004;22:286–288.
13. Afilalo M, Tselios C: Pain relief versus patient satisfaction. Ann Emerg Med 1996;27:436–438.
14. Carragee EJ, Vittom D, Truong TP, et al: Pain control and cultural norms and expectations after closed femoral shaft fractures. Am J Orthop 1999;28:97–102.
15. Choiniere M, Melzack R, Girard N, et al: Comparisons between patients' and nurses' assessment of pain and medication efficacy in severe burn injuries. Pain 1990;40:143–152.
16. Potter M, Schafer S, Gonzalez-Mendez E, et al: Opioids for chronic nonmalignant pain: Attitudes and practices of primary care. J Fam Pract 2001;50:145–151.
17. Bailey PL, Pace NL, Ashburn MA: Frequent hypoxemia and apnea after sedation with midazolam and fentanyl. Anesthesiology 1990;73:826–830.
18. Attard AR, Corlett MJ, Kidner NJ, et al: Safety of early pain relief for acute abdominal pain. BMJ 1992;305:554–556.
19. LoVecchio F, Oster N, Sturmann K, et al: The use of analgesics in patients with acute abdominal pain. J Emerg Med 1997;15:775–779.
20. Silen W: Cope's Early Diagnosis of the Acute Abdomen, 20th ed. Oxford University Press, 2000.
21. Yang Y, Young JB, Schermer CR, Utter GH: Use of ketorolac is associated with decreased pneumonia following rib fractures. Am J Surg 2014;207:566–572.

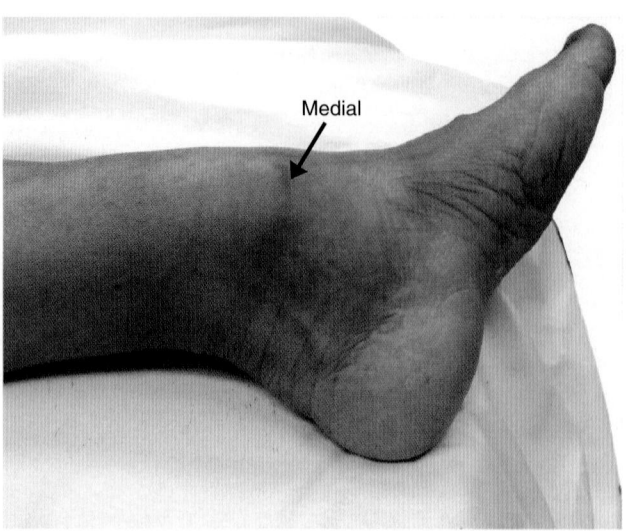

FIGURE 59–10. A popliteal sciatic block was used to reduce and splint this patients ankle fracture dislocation.

22. Friedland LR, Kulick RM: Emergency department analgesic use in pediatric trauma victims with fractures. Ann Emerg Med 1994;23: 203–207.
23. Jones JS, Johnson K, McNinch M: Age as a risk factor for inadequate emergency department analgesia. Am J Emerg Med 1996;14:157–160.
24. Kozlowski MJ, Wiater JG, Pasaqual RG, et al: Painful discrimination: The differential use of analgesia in isolated lower limb injuries. Am J Emerg Med 2002;20:502–505.
25. Raftery KA, Smith-Coggins R, Chen AH: Gender-associated differences in emergency department pain management. Ann Emerg Med 1995;26: 313–321.
26. Todd KH, Samaroo N, Hoffman JR: Ethnicity as a risk factor for inadequate emergency department analgesia. JAMA 1993;269:1537–1539.
27. Todd KH, Deaton C, D'Adamo AP, Goe L: Ethnicity and analgesic practice. Ann Emerg Med 2000;35:11–16.
28. Carpenter KJ, Dickenson AH: Molecular aspects of pain research. Pharacogenomics J 2002;2:87–95.
29. Dresser GK, Bailey DG: A basic conceptual and practical overview of interactions with highly prescribed drugs. Can J Clin Pharmacol 2002;9:191–198.
30. Joint Commission on Accreditation of Healthcare Organizations: Pain Management Standards for 2001: Joint Commission on Accreditation of Healthcare Organizations. 2001:1.2.7–1.2.8.
31. Todd KH, Funk KG, Funk JP, Bonacci R: Clinical significance of reported changes in pain severity. Ann Emerg Med 1996;27:485–489.
32. Bijur PE, Silver W, Gallagher EJ: Reliability of the visual analog scale for measurement of acute pain. Acad Emerg Med 2001;8:1153–1157.
33. Bijur PE, Latimer CT, Gallagher EJ: Validation of a verbally administered numerical rating scale of acute pain for use in the emergency department. Acad Emerg Med 2003;10:390–392.
34. Keller S, Bann CM, Dodd SL, et al: Validity of the brief pain inventory for use in documenting the outcomes of patients with noncancer pain. Clin J Pain 2004;20:309–318.
35. Farrar JT, Polomano RC, Berlin JA, Strom BL: A comparison of change in the 0–10 numeric rating scale to a pain relief scale and global medication performance scale in a short-term clinical trial of breakthrough pain intensity. Anesthesiology 2010;112:1464–1472.
36. Farrar JT, Young JP Jr, LaMoreaux L, Werth JL, Poole RM: Clinical importance of changes in chronic pain intensity measured on an 11-point numerical pain rating scale. Pain 2001;94:149–158.
37. Nelson BP, Cohen D, Lander O, et al: Mandated pain scales improve frequency of ED analgesic administration. Am J Emerg Med 2004;22: 582–585.
38. American Society of Anesthesiologists Task Force on Sedation and Analgesia by Non-Anesthesiologists; Gross JB, Bailey PL, Connis RT et al: Practice guidelines for sedation and analgesia by non-anesthesiologists. Anesthesiology 2002;96:1004–1017.
39. Caldeira D, Costa J, Barra M, Pinto FJ, Ferreira JJ: How safe is acetaminophen use in patients treated with vitamin K antagonists? A systematic review and meta-analysis. Thromb Res 2015;135:58–61.
40. Sinatra RS, Jahr JS, Reynolds LW, Viscusi ER, Groudine SB, Payen-Champenois C: Efficacy and safety of single and repeated administration of 1 gram intravenous acetaminophen injection (paracetamol) for pain management after major orthopedic surgery. Anesthesiology 2005;102: 822–831.
41. Craig M, Jeavons R, Probert J, Benger J: Randomised comparison of intravenous paracetamol and intravenous morphine for acute traumatic limb pain in the emergency department. Emerg Med J2012;29:37–39.
42. Jones P, Dalziel SR, Lamdin R, Miles-Chan JL, Frampton C: Oral non-steroidal anti-inflammatory drugs versus other oral analgesic agents for acute soft tissue injury. Cochrane Database Syst Rev 2015;7:CD007789.
43. Derry CJ, Derry S, Moore RA: Single dose oral ibuprofen plus paracetamol (acetaminophen) for acute postoperative pain. Cochrane Database Syst Rev 2013;6:CD010210.
44. Gutthann SP: Nonsteroidal anti-inflammatory drugs and the risk of hospitalization for acute renal failure. Arch Intern Med 1996;156: 2433–2439.
45. Berges-Gimeno MP, Stevenson DD: Nonsteroidal anti-inflammatory drug-induced reactions and desensitization. J Asthma 2004;41:375–384.
46. Yealy DM: Ketorolac in the treatment of acute pain. Ann Emerg Med 1992;21:985–986.
47. Derry S, Moore RA, Gaskell H, McIntyre M, Wiffen PJ: Topical NSAIDs for acute musculoskeletal pain in adults. Cochrane Database Syst Rev. 2015;6:CD007402.
48. Slappendel R, Weber EW, Benraad B, Dirksen R, Bugter ML: Does ibuprofen increase perioperative blood loss during hip arthroplasty? Eur J Anaesthesiol 2002;19:829–831.
49. O'Connor AB, Zwemer FL, Hays DP: Outcomes after intravenous opioids in emergency patients: a prospective cohort analysis. Acad Emerg Med 2009;16:477–487.
50. Chang AK, Bijur PE, Campbell CM, Murphy MK: Safety and efficacy of rapid titration using 1 mg doses of intravenous hydromorphone in emergency department patients with acute severe pain: the "1 + 1" protocol. Ann Emerg Med 2009;54:221–225.
51. Lvovschi V, Aubrun F, Bonnet P: Intravenous morphine titration to treat severe pain in the ED. Am J Emerg Med 2009;26:676–682.
52. Conrardy M, Lank P, Cameron KA, et al: Emergency department patient perspectives on the risk of addiction to prescription opioids. Pain Med 2016;17:114–121.
53. McCarthy DM, Wolf MS, McConnell R, et al: Improving patient knowledge and safe use of opioids: A randomized controlled trial. Acad Emerg Med 2015;22:331–339.
54. McQuay H, Moore A, Justins D: Treating acute pain in hospital. BMJ 1997;314:1531–1535.
55. Mitra S, Sinatra RS: Perioperative management of acute pain in the opioid-dependent patient. Anesthesiology 2004;101:212–227.
56. Walsh M, Smith GA, Yount RA: Continuous intravenous infusion fentanyl for sedation and analgesia of the multiple trauma patient. Ann Emerg Med 1991;20:913–915.
57. Herring AA, Ahern T, Frazee B: Emerging applications of low-dose ketamine for pain management in the ED. Am J Emerg Med 2013;31:416–419.
58. Ahern T, Herring AA, Frazee B: Effective analgesia with low-dose ketamine and reduced dose hydromorphone in ED patients with severe pain. Am J Emerg Med 2013;31:847–851.
59. Cohen L, Athaide V, Wickham ME, Doyle-Waters MM, Rose NG, Hoh CM. The effect of ketamine on intracranial and cerebral perfusion pressure and health outcomes: a systematic review. Ann Emerg Med 2015;65:43–51.e2.
60. Jackson K, Ashby M, Martin P: "Burst" ketamine for refractory cancer pain: An open-label audit of 39 patients. J Pain Symptom Manage 2001;22:834–842.
61. Singer AJ, Stark MJ: Pretreatment of lacerations with lidocaine, epinephrine, and tetracaine at triage: A randomized double-blind trial. Acad Emerg Med 2002;7:751–756.
62. Priestly S, Kelly AM, Chow L: Application of topical local anesthetic at triage reduces treatment time for children with lacerations: A randomized controlled trial. Ann Emerg Med 2003;42:34–40.
63. Tobias JD. Applications of nitrous oxide for procedural sedation in the pediatric population. Pediatr Emerg Care 2013;29:245–265.
64. Olfert SM: Reproductive outcomes among dental personnel: A review of selected exposures. J Can Dent Assoc 2006;72:821–825.
65. Heinrich M, Menzel C, Hoffmann F, Berger M, Schweinitz DV: Self-administered procedural analgesia using nitrous oxide/oxygen (50:50) in the pediatric surgery emergency room: Effectiveness and limitations. Eur J Pediatr Surg 2015;25:250–256.
66. Lee JH, Kim K, Kim TY, et al: A randomized comparison of nitrous oxide versus intravenous ketamine for laceration repair in children. Pediatr Emerg Care 2012;28:1297–1301.
67. Tsze DS, Mallory MD, Cravero JP: Practice patterns and adverse events of nitrous oxide sedation and analgesia: A report from the Pediatric Sedation Research Consortium. J Pediatr 2016;169:260–265.e2.
68. Stojadinovic A, Auton A, Peoples GE: Responding to challenges in modern combat casualty care: Innovative use of advanced regional anesthesia. Pain Med 2006;7:330–338.
69. De Buck F, Devroe S, Missant C: Regional anesthesia outside the operating room: Indications and techniques. Curr Opin Anesthesiol 2012;25:501–507.
70. Neuman MD, Silber JH, Elkassabany NM: Comparative effectiveness of regional versus general anesthesia for hip fracture surgery in adults. Anesthesiology 2012;117:72–92.
71. Wolf AR: Effects of regional analgesia on stress responses to pediatric surgery. Pediatr Anesth 2012;22:19–24.
72. Grabinsky AS, Sam RS: Regional anesthesia for acute traumatic injuries in the emergency room. Expert Rev Neurother 2009;9:1677–1690.
73. Bhoi S, Tej PS, Mahaveer R: Feasibility and safety of ultrasound-guided nerve block for management of limb injuries by emergency care physicians. J Emerg Trauma Shock 2012;5:28.
74. Jeng CL, Toni MT, Anderson MR: Development of a mobile ultrasound-guided peripheral nerve block and catheter service. J Ultrasound Med 2011;30:1139–1144.
75. Vasques F, Behr AU, Weinberg G, Ori C, Di Gregorio G. A review of local anesthetic systemic toxicity cases since publication of the American Society of Regional Anesthesia Recommendations: To whom it may concern. Reg Anesth Pain Med 2015;40:698–705.

76. Herring AA, Stone BS, Frenkel O: The ultrasound-guided superficial cervical plexus block for anesthesia and analgesia in emergency care settings. Am J Emerg Med 2012;30:1263–1267.

77. Blaivas M, Adhikari S, Lander L: A prospective comparison of procedural sedation and ultrasound-guided interscalene nerve block for shoulder reduction in the emergency department. Acad Emerg Med 2011;18:922–927.

78. Underhill TJ, Wan A, Morrice M: Interscalene brachial plexus blocks in the management of shoulder dislocations. Arch Emerg Med 1989;6:199–204.

79. Minville V, Plante B, Eychenne, Colombani A, Fourcade O: Retrospective study on six years of anaesthesia for reduction of shoulder dislocation in emergency. Ann Fr Anesth Reanim 2009;28:949–953.

80. Tezel O, Kaldirim U, Bilgic S, et al: A comparison of suprascapular nerve block and procedural sedation analgesia in shoulder dislocation reduction. Am J Emerg Med 2014;32:549–552.

81. Stone MB, Wang R, Price DD: Ultrasound-guided supraclavicular brachial plexus nerve block vs procedural sedation for the treatment of upper extremity emergencies. Am J Emerg Med 2008;26:706–710.

82. Blaivas M, Srikar A, Lina L: A prospective comparison of procedural sedation and ultrasound-guided interscalene nerve block for shoulder reduction in the emergency department. Acad Emerg Med 2011;18:922–927.

83. Prielipp RC, Warner MA. Perioperative nerve injury: a silent scream? Anesthesiology 2009;111:464–466.

84. Kendall JM, Allen P, Younge S: Haematoma block or Bier's block for Colles' fracture reduction in the accident and emergency department—which is best? J Accid Emerg Med 1997;14:352–356.

85. Tageldin ME, Alrashid M, Khoriati AA, Gadikoppula S, Atkinson HD: Periosteal nerve blocks for distal radius and ulna fracture manipulation—the technique and early results. J Orthop Surg Res 2015;10:134.

86. Liebmann Otto, Price DD, Mills C: Feasibility of forearm ultrasonography-guided nerve blocks of the radial, ulnar, and median nerves for hand procedures in the emergency department. Ann Emerg Med 2006;48:558–562.

87. Wu CL, Jani ND, Perkins FM, Barquist E: Thoracic epidural analgesia versus intravenous patient-controlled analgesia for the treatment of rib fracture pain after motor vehicle crash. J Trauma 1999;47:564–567.

88. Wisner DH: A stepwise logistic regression analysis of factors affecting morbidity and mortality after thoracic trauma: effect of epidural analgesia. J Trauma 1990;30:799–804.

89. Bulger EM, Edwards T, Klotz P, Jurkovich GJ: Epidural analgesia improves outcome after multiple rib fractures. Surgery 2004;136:426–430.

90. Liu S, Carpenter RL, Neal JM: Epidural anesthesia and analgesia: Their role in postoperative outcome. Anesthesiology 1995;82:1474–1506.

91. Mohta M, Verma P, Saxena AK, Sethi AK, Tyagi A, Girotra G: Prospective, randomized comparison of continuous thoracic epidural and thoracic paravertebral infusion in patients with unilateral multiple fractured ribs—a pilot study. J Trauma 2009;66:1096–1101.

92. Herring AA, Michael BS, Nagdev AD: Ultrasound-guided abdominal wall nerve blocks in the ED. Am J Emerg Med 2012;30:759–764.

93. Mutty CE. Femoral nerve block for diaphyseal and distal femoral fractures in the emergency department. Surgical technique. J Bone Joint Surg Am 2008;90(suppl 2, pt 2):218–226.

94. Fletcher AK, Rigby AS, Heyes LP: Three-in-one femoral nerve block as analgesia for fractured neck of femur in the emergency department: A randomized, controlled trial. Ann Emerg Med 2003;41:227–233.

95. Mutty CE, Jensen EJ, Manka MA Jr, Anders MJ, Bone LB: Femoral nerve block for diaphyseal and distal femoral fractures in the emergency department. J Bone Joint Surg 2007;89:2599–2603.

96. Beaudoin FL, Nagdev A, Merchant RC, Becker BM: Ultrasound-guided femoral nerve blocks in elderly patients with hip fractures. Am J Emerg Med 2010;28:76–81.

97. Beaudoin FL, Haran JP, Liebmann O: A comparison of ultrasound-guided three-in-one femoral nerve block versus parenteral opioids alone for analgesia in emergency department patients with hip fractures: A randomized controlled trial. Acad Emerg Med 2013;20:584–591.

98. Elkhodair S, Mortazavi J, Chester A, Pereira M. Single fascia iliaca compartment block for pain relief in patients with fractured neck of femur in the emergency department: A pilot study. Eur J Emerg Med 2011;18:340–343.

99. Fletcher AK, Rigby AS, Heyes FL: Three-in-one femoral nerve block as analgesia for fractured neck of femur in the emergency department: a randomized, controlled trial. Ann Emerg Med 2003;41:227–233.

100. Neubrand TL, Roswell K, Deakyne S, Kocher K, Wathen J: Fascia iliaca compartment nerve block versus systemic pain control for acute femur fractures in the pediatric emergency department. Pediatr Emerg Care 2014;30:469–473.

101. Wathen JE, Gao D, Merritt G, Georgopoulos G, Battan FK: A randomized controlled trial comparing a fascia iliaca compartment nerve block to a traditional systemic analgesic for femur fractures in a pediatric emergency department. Ann Emerg Med 2007;50:162–171.

102. Haines L, Dickman E, Ayvazyan S, et al: Ultrasound-guided fascia iliaca compartment block for hip fractures in the emergency department. J Emerg Med 2012;43:692–697.

103. Beaudoin FL, Nagdev A, Merchant RC, Becker BM: Ultrasound-guided femoral nerve blocks in elderly patients with hip fractures. Am J Emerg Med. 2010;28:76–81.

104. Reid N, Stella J, Ryan M, Ragg M: Use of ultrasound to facilitate accurate femoral nerve block in the emergency department. Emerg Med Australas 2009;21:124–130.

105. Herring AA, Stone MB, Fischer J: Ultrasound-guided distal popliteal sciatic nerve block for ED anesthesia. Am J Emerg Med 2011;29:697–698.

Complications and Prevention of Neurologic Injury with Peripheral Nerve Blocks

Michael J. Barrington, Richard Brull, Miguel A. Reina, and Admir Hadzic

INTRODUCTION

This chapter reviews various factors that may contribute to neurologic complications after peripheral nerve blocks (PNBs) and suggests principles of practice and implications of monitoring modalities to mitigate the risk of neurologic complications.

ANATOMY CONSIDERATIONS OF PERIPHERAL NERVE BLOCK–RELATED NERVE INJURY

A nerve is a distinct organ comprising neural tissue, a specific connective tissue stroma, and a designated blood supply (Figure 60–1). Nerve cells, or neurons, are composed of a cell

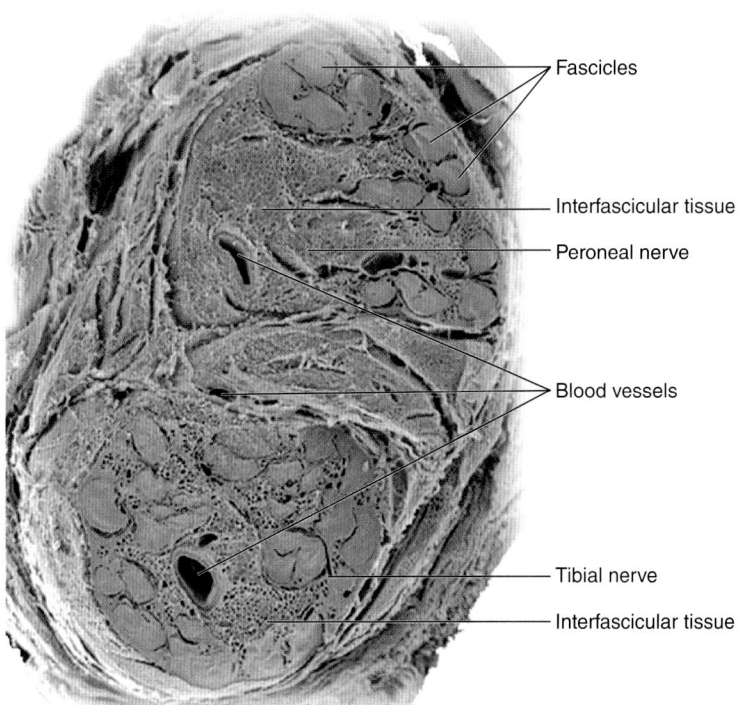

FIGURE 60–1. Human sciatic nerve. Scanning electron microscopy. (Reproduced with permission from Reina MA: *Atlas of Functional Anatomy for Regional Anesthesia and Pain Medicine*. Heidelberg: Springer; 2015.)

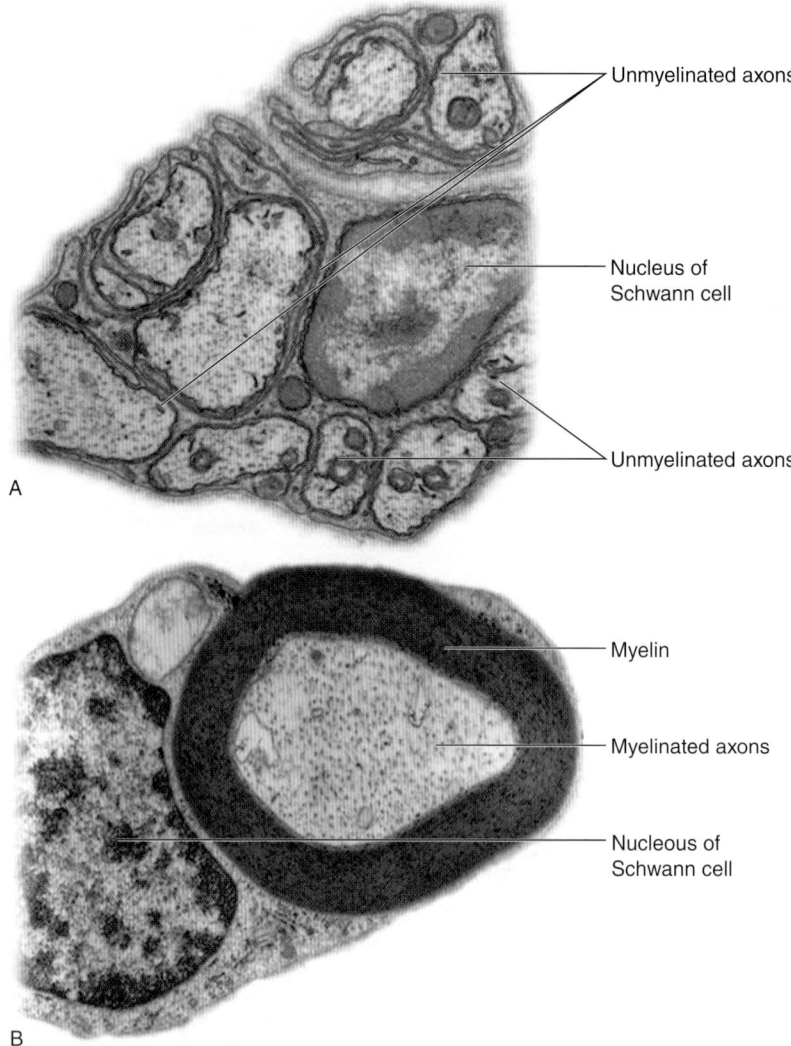

FIGURE 60–2. A: Unmyelinated axon of a human nerve rootlet. **B:** Myelinated axon of a human sciatic nerve. Transmission electron microscopy. (Reproduced with permission from Reina MA: *Atlas of Functional Anatomy for Regional Anesthesia and Pain Medicine*. Heidelberg: Springer; 2015.)

body, dendrites, and an axon. The axon is a cytoplasmic extension of the neuron that transmits electrical signals along its length from the cell body proximally to anywhere from just a few millimeters up to nearly 1 m distally. Most peripheral nerves can transmit both afferent motor and efferent sensory signals.

In the peripheral nervous system, the vast majority of axons are myelinated, characterized by a sheath of Schwann cells that encase the axon in a layer of myelin (Figure 60–2). The Schwann cells are interrupted at interposed spaces, known as the nodes of Ranvier, where the process of depolarization and repolarization occurs during the saltatory propagation of the action potential. Together with its myelin sheath, each axon is bound by a thin layer of connective tissue called an endoneurium (Figure 60–3) and then termed a nerve fiber.

Nerve fibers are organized into groups called fascicles (Figure 60–4). Within each fascicle, the nerve fibers form an intraneural plexus in which the axons take different positions along their path (Figure 60–5). In the vicinity of joints, the fascicles are thinner and more numerous and tend to be

surrounded by a greater amount of connective tissue, which reduces the vulnerability of the fascicles to insults such as pressure and stretching.

Each fascicle is surrounded by perineurium consisting of continuous and concentric layers of 8 to 18 cells (Figure 60–6). The thickness of the perineurium is typically 7 to 20 μm. The layers of perineurial cells provide a barrier for diffusion of substances into and out of the fascicles. The space between perineurial cells is composed of fundamental amorphous substances, collagen fibers, and fibroblasts. These collagen fibers can be aligned in different directions, but predominantly along the longitudinal axis of the fascicle (Figure 60–6). The perineurium allows for some movement of axons within a fascicle and maintains intrafascicular pressure while serving as an effective physical barrier against mechanical and chemical injury. Likewise, the perineurium serves as an important diffusion barrier, preventing exposure of the axons to potentially noxious substances, such as local anesthetics.

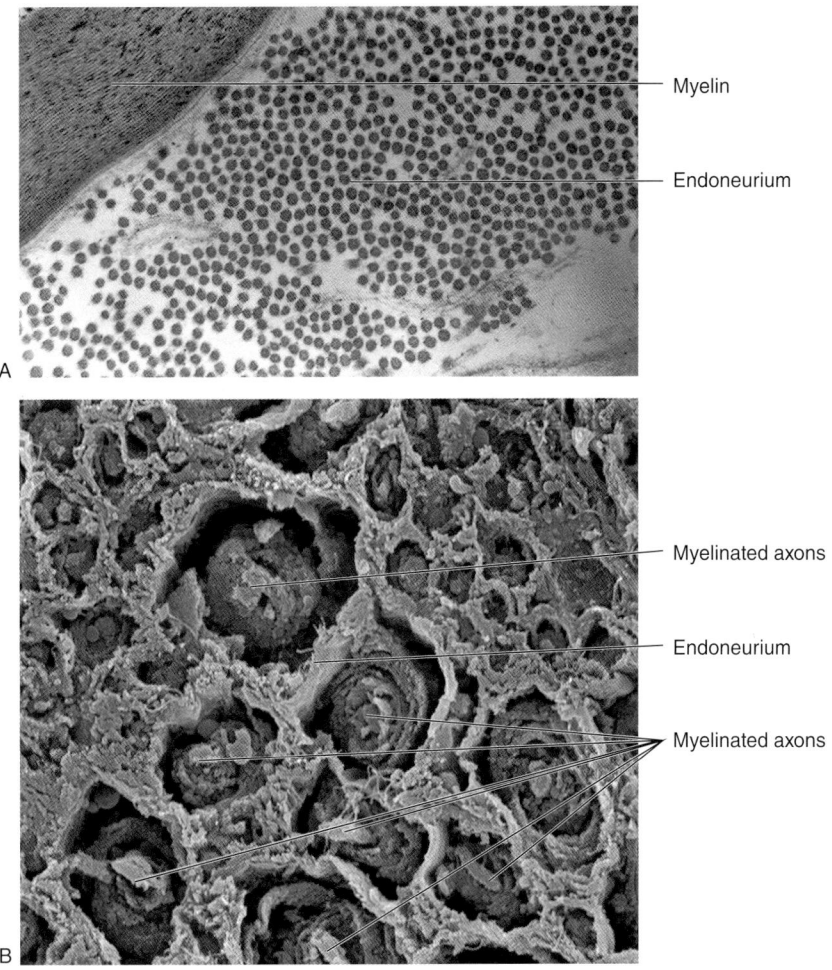

FIGURE 60–3. Endoneurium. Myelinated axons enveloped by endoneurium obtained from a human sciatic nerve. **A:** Transmission electron microscopy. (Reproduced with permission from Reina MA: *Atlas of Functional Anatomy for Regional Anesthesia and Pain Medicine.* Heidelberg: Springer; 2015.) **B:** Scanning electron microscopy. (Reproduced with permission from Reina MA: *Atlas of Functional Anatomy for Regional Anesthesia and Pain Medicine.* Heidelberg: Springer; 2015.)

Groups of fascicles are bound together by an epineurium, the thickest of the three connective tissue layers that encases groups of fascicles along with their interfascicular supporting tissue and adipocytes (Figure 60–1). The epineurium is composed mainly of collagen fibers and a small number of blood vessels (Figure 60–7). The collagen fibers of the epineurium are similar in size and appearance to collagen fibers of the dura or dural sleeves. The epineurium gives the nerve its characteristic external appearance on ultrasound imaging (ie, it appears as a discrete structure.

Peripheral nerves have two independent, yet interconnecting, vascular systems. The extrinsic system consists of arteries, arterioles, and veins that lie within the epineurium, while the intrinsic vascular system comprises a group of longitudinal capillaries that run within the fascicles and endoneurium (Figure 60–8). Anastomosis between the two vascular systems is formed by vessels (Figure 60–1) that originate in the epineurium and traverse the perineurium. Injury to these vessels can lead to a range of complications, from ischemia to inflammation due to hematoma.

Nerve roots have less tensile strength and elasticity compared to the axons and their supporting elements in peripheral nerve trunks.[1] Axons included within the spinal nerve roots are not surrounded by a perineurium or other structure with a barrier effect. More distally (eg, spinal nerves and plexus trunks/divisions), fascicles have their own protective perineurium[2] (Figures 60–9, 60–10, and 60–11) and have a plexiform arrangement that contributes to their tensile strength. Nerve trunks within tissue beds, fascicles within nerve trunks, and axons within fascicles have a slight undulating course, resulting in relative excess length. In addition, nerves are often attached loosely by their epineurium to adjacent structures. There is a nonspecialized network of areolar (deep fascial) connective tissue that fills the space between specialized structures such as nerves, muscles, and vessels (Figure 60–12). This tissue loosely connects these structures so that movement of one on another is permitted.[1] This movement is reduced when nerves are tethered by entering blood vessels, branches, or other landmarks.[2]

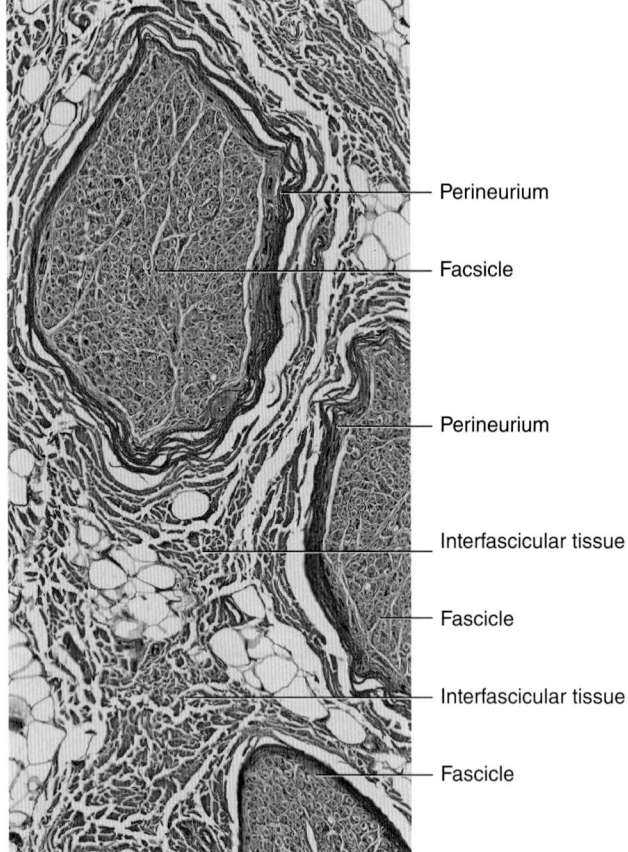

Perineurium

Facsicle

Perineurium

Interfascicular tissue

Fascicle

Interfascicular tissue

Fascicle

FIGURE 60–4. Fascicles of human median nerve. (Used with permission from M.A. Reina.)

PATHOPHYSIOLOGY OF PERIPHERAL NERVE INJURY

Severity of Peripheral Nerve Injury

The primary determinants of prognosis of peripheral nerve injury (PNI) are the severity of the injury and the residual integrity of the axons. PNI severity is typically classified according to the relative degree of axonal disruption. Proximal axonal lesions (ie, close to the cell body) are traditionally

believed to be more severe than distal axonal lesions (ie, closer to the innervation target) as the likelihood for reinnervation and recovery appears to vary indirectly with the distance between the location of the axonal lesion and the target tissue.

The two most commonly used anatomical classifications are the Seddon[3] and Sunderland[4] classifications (Table 60–1). The more commonly used classification in clinical practice is the three-tier Seddon classification, which includes (from mild to severe) neuropraxia, axonotmesis, and neurotmesis. *Neuropraxia* refers to damage to the myelin sheath typically associated with nerve stretching or compression where the axons and supporting elements (endoneurium, perineurium, and epineurium) remain intact. The prognosis for a neuropraxic injury is favorable, with complete recovery of function occurring within weeks to months.

Axonotmesis refers to axonal injury associated with fascicular impalement, nerve crush, or toxic injury, with damage to the endoneurium and possibly to the perineurium (Figure 60–13). Recovery following axonal loss may be prolonged and variable, depending on the extent (partial or complete) of disruption to the perineurium and on the distance from the injury site to the corresponding muscle.

Finally, *neurotmesis* refers to complete transection of the nerve, including the axons, endoneurium, perineurium, and epineurial connective tissue. It typically requires surgical intervention. The prognosis is often poor.

Mechanisms of Injury

The mechanism of PNI related to the use of PNBs falls into one of three broad categories: mechanical and injection injury (traumatic), vascular (ischemic), and chemical (neurotoxicity). Most information on peripheral nerve injection injury are obtained from experimental research in animal models. Because such research is not possible in humans, mechanisms of PNI are not fully understood.[6] This is because animal models significantly vary in species used, nerves injected, and study protocols, making it difficult to readily extrapolate such data to actual clinical practice.

Mechanical and Injection Injury

Mechanical or traumatic injury includes compression, stretch, laceration, or injection injury. Nerve compression or entrapment may produce a conduction block and, if prolonged, a focal demyelination of some axons. Needle trauma and other mechanical insults to nerves result in an increase in neuropeptide production and dorsal horn activity.[6,7] Needle-related nerve compression can result from forceful needle-nerve contact from

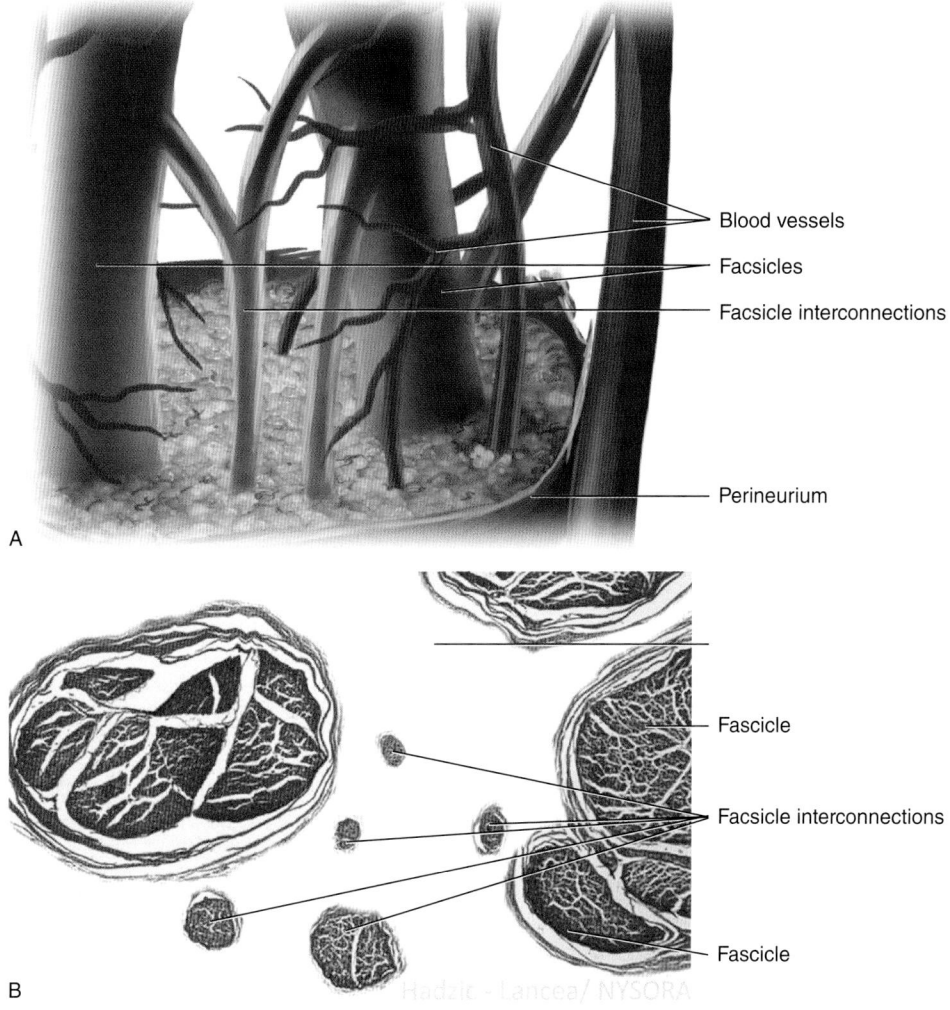

Blood vessels

Facsicles

Facsicle interconnections

Perineurium

A

Fascicle

Facsicle interconnections

Fascicle

B

FIGURE 60–5. Intraneural plexus. **A:** Diagram. **B:** Fascicles and interconnection fascicles. (B, Reproduced with permission from Reina MA: *Atlas of Functional Anatomy for Regional Anesthesia and Pain Medicine.* Heidelberg: Springer; 2015.)

an approaching needle[8] or injection inside the nerve itself. It has been postulated that an intraneural injection may lead to sustained high intraneural pressure,[9] which, when exceeding capillary occlusion pressure, may lead to nerve ischemia and potentially injury. Inadvertent injections of antibiotics, steroids, bovine collagen, botulinum toxin, and local anesthetics into peripheral nerves have all been associated with deleterious neurologic deficits.[1,10–13] In a cadaveric model of deliberate intraneural injection of the sciatic nerve, the needle tip disrupted 3% of axons.[14] Although some degree of axonal injury may potentially occur even in the absence of injury to the perineurium, the actual anatomical site of injury (eg, injection) is critical prognostically.[15] One of the main causes of block-related PNI is injection of local anesthetic into a fascicle, causing direct needle and injection trauma, rupture of perineurium, and loss of the protective environment within the fascicle with consequent myelin and axonal degeneration.[6,11,15–18] Stretch injuries

to the nerves may result when nerves or plexi are placed in a nonphysiologic or exaggerated physiologic position. Finally, mechanical injury from laceration results when the nerve is injured by a needle, with the potential for spontaneous recovery most unlikely following complete transection. Table 60–2 indicates the evidence-based recommendations to reduce the risk of block-related PNIs.

Vascular Injury

Damage to the nerve vasculature during nerve blocks can result in local or diffuse ischemia and occurs when there is direct vascular injury, acute occlusion of the arteries from which the vasa nervorum are derived, or from a hemorrhage within a nerve sheath. The epineurial circulation is a critical component of the overall neural circulation, and its removal reduces nerve blood supply by 50%.[19] In most circumstances, no single vessel dominates the pattern over an entire length of nerve; however,

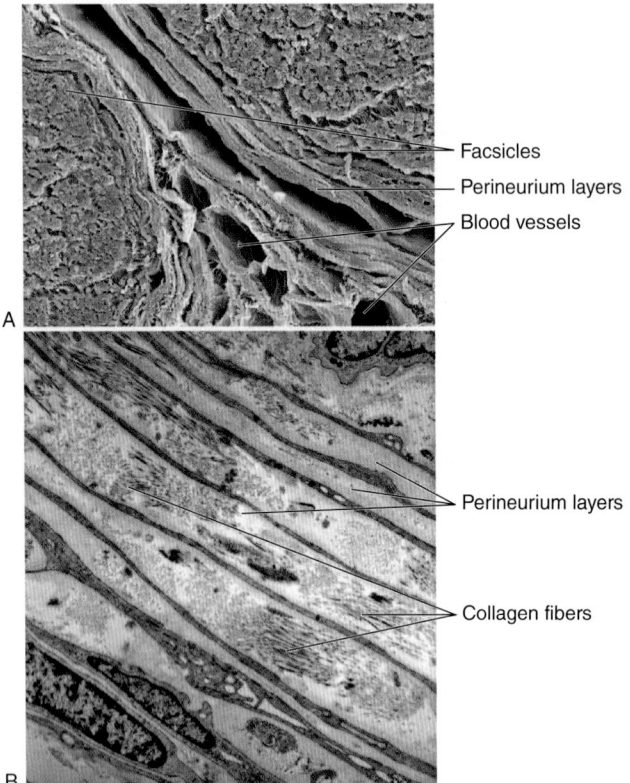

FIGURE 60–6. Perineurium. Perineural layers of human sciatic nerve. **A:** Transmission electron microscopy. (Reproduced with permission from Reina MA, López A, Villanueva MC, et al: The blood-nerve barrier in peripheral nerves. *Rev Esp Anestesiol Reanim.* 2003 Feb;50(2):80-86.) **B:** Scanning electron microscopy. (Reproduced with permission from Reina MA: *Atlas of Functional Anatomy for Regional Anesthesia and Pain Medicine.* Heidelberg: Springer; 2015.)

the sciatic nerve is an exception to this rule, receiving its major arterial supply in the gluteal region from the arteria comitans nervi ischiadici.[1]

Clinical Pearl

• Vascular supply of the sciatic nerve is less abundant than the supply of most other peripheral nerves. This may explain the clinical observation regarding why addition of epinephrine to local anesthetic appears to prolong sciatic block significantly longer than for most other PNBs.

Nerves with an abundance of connective tissue may be less susceptible to compression because external forces are not transmitted directly to epineurial vessels. Local anesthetics and adjuncts potentially reduce neural blood flow in an agent- and concentration-dependent manner.[19,20] Epinephrine has the potential to cause local vasoconstriction, but its role in causing nerve ischemia and injury is controversial.[20] Trauma from injection may compromise blood flow further. Neural ischemia may also occur following disruption of the intrafascicular

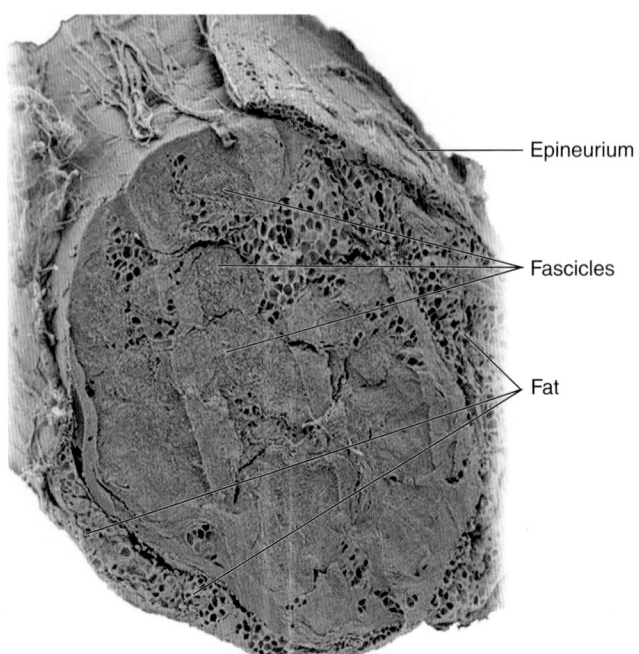

FIGURE 60–7. Epineurium. Human tibial nerve: detail of fascicles, interfascicular tissue, and epineurium. Scanning electron microscopy. (Reproduced with permission from Reina MA, Arriazu R, Collier CB, et al: Electron microscopy of human peripheral nerves of clinical relevance to the practice of nerve blocks. A structural and ultrastructural review based on original experimental and laboratory data. *Rev Esp Anestesiol Reanim.* 2013 Dec;60(10):552–562.)

microvasculature, high injection pressures, tourniquets, and other compressive insults. Factors regarding inadvertent vessel puncture, resulting in the formation of an internal or external hematoma that can mechanically compress the fascicles from within or outside the nerve sheath and cause nerve inflammation, have been implicated in neurologic injury.[21,22]

Chemical Injury

Chemical nerve injury results from tissue toxicity of injected solutions (eg, local anesthetics, alcohol, or phenol) or its additives. The toxic solution may be injected directly into the nerve or into adjacent tissues, causing an acute inflammatory reaction or chronic fibrosis that indirectly involves the nerve. Much of the research on neurotoxicity of local anesthetics has been done in in vitro models, particularly with intrathecal application. There is evidence that nearly all local anesthetics can have myotoxic, neurotoxic, and cytotoxic effects in various tissues under certain conditions[23–33]; however, local anesthetics vary in their neurotoxic potential.[34–36] Several studies have demonstrated that local anesthetics can lead to fragmentation of DNA and disrupt the membrane potential in mitochondria, resulting in the uncoupling of oxidative phosphorylation, which may result in apoptosis.[37] There is also a direct correlation between concentration of the local anesthetic and duration of exposure to the nerve, with death of Schwann cells, infiltration with macrophages, and myelin damage.[34,38] Some local anesthetics have an intrinsic vasoconstrictive effect that can decrease blood flow to the nerves, potentially resulting in ischemia and injury.[39] However, the inherent difficulty in extrapolating these

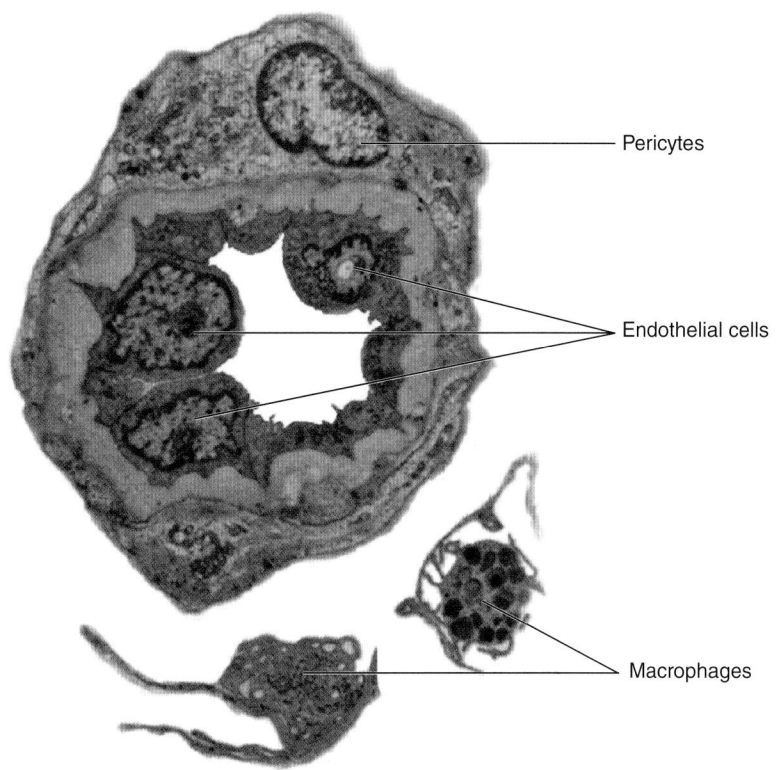

FIGURE 60–8. Endoneural continuous capillaries. Transmission electron microscopy. (Reproduced with permission from Reina MA: *Atlas of Functional Anatomy for Regional Anesthesia and Pain Medicine.* Heidelberg: Springer; 2015.)

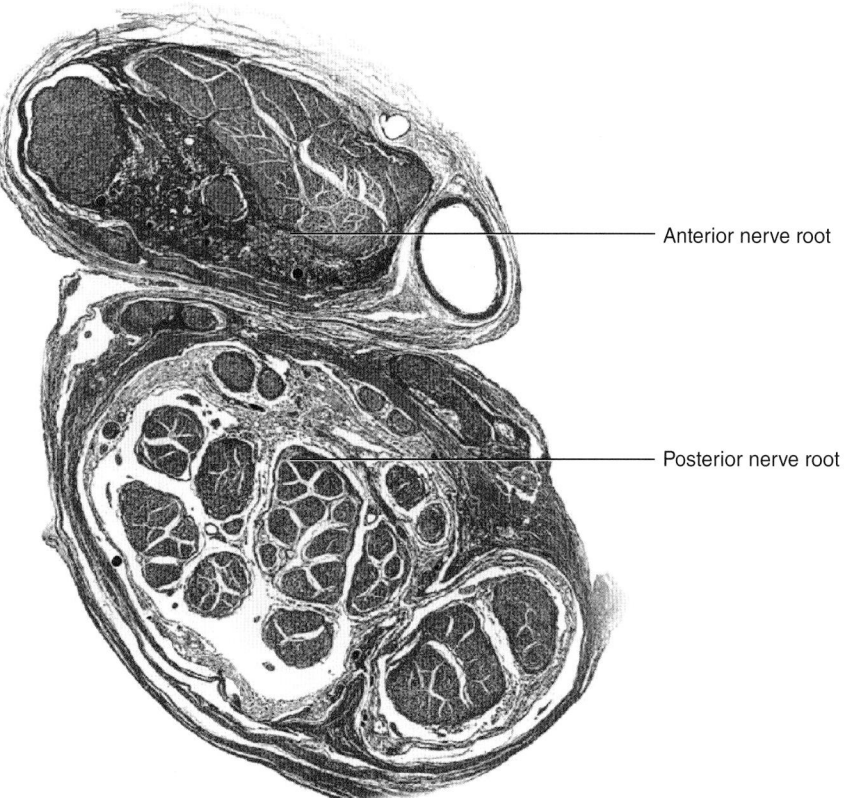

FIGURE 60–9. Ventral and dorsal nerve root. Transversal section at seventh nerve root cuff between dural sac and dorsal root ganglion. (Used with permission from M.A. Reina.)

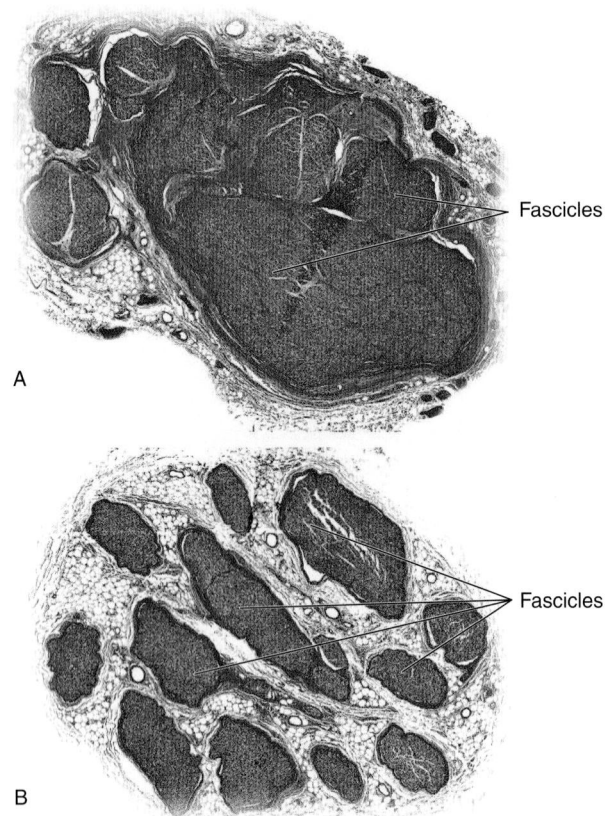

FIGURE 60–10. Nerve root. Transversal section at seventh nerve root cuff outer dorsal root ganglion. **A:** Outer to 2 mm. **B:** Outer to 5 mm. (Used with permission from M.A. Reina.)

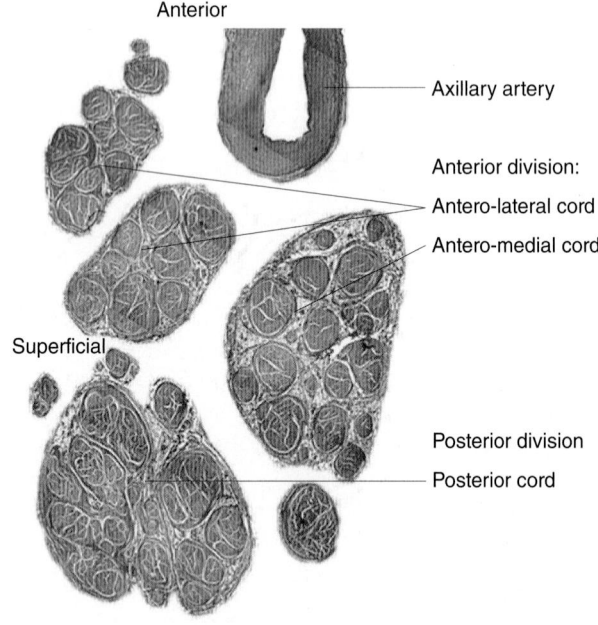

FIGURE 60–11. Brachial plexus cords. Anteromedial cord, anterolateral cord, and posterior cord. Details of fascicles and interfascicular tissue within the cords. (Reproduced with permission from Reina MA: *Atlas of Functional Anatomy for Regional Anesthesia and Pain Medicine.* Heidelberg: Springer; 2015.)

laboratory studies to the clinical practice of modern PNBs is that there is a substantial decrease in the concentration of local anesthetics by the time it reaches the axons.

The site of local anesthetic application (extraneural, intraneural, interfascicular, intrafascicular) (Figures 60–12, 60–14, and 60–15) may be the primary determinant of whether neurotoxicity will occur, especially if the concentration is high and duration of exposure prolonged.[11] Most chemical substances, including all local anesthetics, injected intrafascicularly lead to severe fascicular injury, whereas the same substances injected intraneurally but interfascicularly cause less injury or no detectable injury at all.[40] Indeed, needle penetration of a nerve may result in minimal damage if it is not combined with local anesthetic injection within the nerve fascicle.[6,15]

In a rodent model, Whitlock demonstrated that intrafascicular injection of 0.75% ropivacaine resulted in severe histological abnormalities, including demyelination, axonal degeneration, and Wallerian degeneration.[11] However, extrafascicular injection of 0.75% ropivacaine also resulted in axonal injury, although reduced in severity.

Farber and colleagues recently reported that all commonly used local anesthetics (bupivacaine, lidocaine, and ropivacaine) produced nerve injury when injected intrafascicularly.[41] In their study, the degree of injury decreased with increasing distance from site of injection. Of note, even administration of saline intrafascicularly resulted in intermediate damage to nerves, indicating a baseline level of injury associated with injecting any agent into a nerve.

Clinical Pearl

- While the clinical importance of neurotoxicity remains controversial,[33] the location of the needle tip during injection of the local anesthetic plays a crucial role in determining the likelihood and severity of nerve injury.

Inflammatory Injury

Inflammatory mechanisms of PNI are being increasingly recognized as an important mechanism in post-PNBs neurologic deficit.[42,43] Nonspecific inflammatory responses targeting peripheral nerves can occur either remote from the site of surgery or within the operative limb, where it may be difficult to distinguish from other causes of PNI. Inflammatory mechanisms have been proposed as responsible for persistent phrenic nerve injury following interscalene block for shoulder surgery (Figure 60–12).

Kaufman and colleagues reported a series of 14 patients with chronic diaphragmatic paralysis following interscalene block.[44] During surgical exploration, adhesions, fascial thickening, vascular changes, and scar tissue (present in 10 of 14 patients) involving the phrenic nerve suggested chronic inflammation and were consistent with compression neuropathy. Recent research suggested that intrathecal and intraneural injection of ultrasound gel can also lead to inflammation in the subarachnoidal and peripheral nerves, respectively.[45,46]

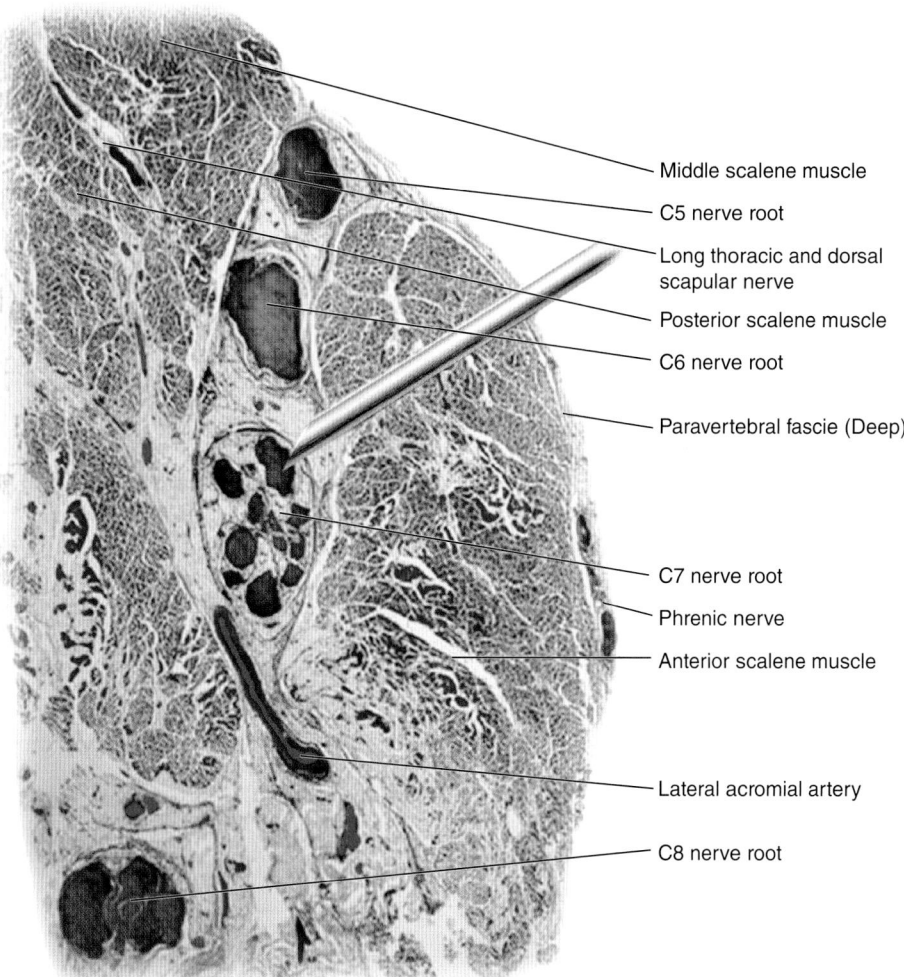

Middle scalene muscle

C5 nerve root

Long thoracic and dorsal scapular nerve

Posterior scalene muscle

C6 nerve root

Paravertebral fascie (Deep)

C7 nerve root

Phrenic nerve

Anterior scalene muscle

Lateral acromial artery

C8 nerve root

FIGURE 60–12. Interaction of the block needle and the interscalene brachial plexus. Placement of the needle into fascicles (as shown here) results in fascicular injury. Additional injury can be committed when an injection is being made through an intrafascicularly placed needle. Observe the difference in size between the needle and fascicles. (Reproduced with permission from Reina MA: *Atlas of Functional Anatomy for Regional Anesthesia and Pain Medicine*. Heidelberg: Springer; 2015.)

ETIOLOGY OF NERVE INJURY FOLLOWING PERIPHERAL NERVE BLOCKADE

Anesthetic Factors

Several studies have reported that the type of anesthesia (regional vs general) does not appear to influence the incidence of PNI. The University of Michigan performed a retrospective analysis of PNI and did not identify PNB as an independent risk factor for PNI in their series.[47] Three epidemiologic studies from the Mayo Clinic reported that regional anesthesia does not increase the risk of PNI following total knee arthoplasty (TKA),[48] total hip arthroplasty (THA),[49] and total shoulder arthroplasty.[50] Recent surgical literature suggested that the risk of postoperative neurologic injury associated with PNB may be higher than that reported in anesthesia literature.[44,51–53] We discuss several technical factors related to PNB that may increase the risk of PNI.

Intraneural Injection

Avoidance of deliberate trauma to nerves, including intraneural injection, is probably a key safety principle of regional anesthesia.[54]

However, intraneural injection may occur in clinical practice without resulting in overt signs of nerve injury.[55–57] In fact, unintentional intraneural (but probably extrafascicular) epineurial injection may be more common than previously recognized.[58] The presumed risks of intraneural injection have been challenged by Bigeleisen and colleagues,[56] who reported that nerve puncture and apparent intraneural injection during axillary brachial plexus block in healthy patients did not lead to neurologic injury. A larger study by Liu recruited 257 young, healthy patients having ultrasound-guided interscalene or supraclavicular block for shoulder surgery.[55] The incidence of unintentional intraneural injection was 17% without any occurrence of PNI. However, clinical experience is limited, and the sample sizes of current studies are inadequate to capture infrequent events, such as nerve injury. In contrast, in a case report by Cohen, PNI occurred following intraneural injection during ultrasound-guided interscalene block.[59]

Unfortunately, reports of intraneural injection do not inform us regarding sites of injection in relation to fascicles. Distinguishing the outer epineurium of a peripheral nerve

TABLE 60–1. Classification of nerve injury.

Seddon[3]	Sunderland[4]	Processes	Prognosis
Neuropraxia	1	Myelin damage Conduction slowing and blocking	Good
Axonotmesis	2	Loss of axonal continuity; endoneurium intact No conduction	Fair
Neurotmesis	3	Loss of axonal and endoneurial continuity; perineurium intact No conduction	Poor
	4	Loss of axonal, endoneurial, and perineurial continuity; epineurium intact No conduction	
	5	Complete nerve transection No conduction	

from surrounding tissues using ultrasound imaging is challenging. Orebaugh performed mock interscalene injections (albeit with small volumes) in a cadaver model.[60] Ultrasound imaging cannot differentiate extrafascicular and intrafascicular

neural components over the range of locations that PNB is performed.[61] Furthermore, an injection adjacent to the outer epineurium may generate a halo similar in appearance to an intraneural injection, making it difficult to discern hazardous from nonhazardous needle placement. Importantly, only a small amount of local anesthetic (eg, 0.1–0.5 mL) is sufficient to rupture the fascicle and its perineurium.

Clinical Pearl

- Relying on observation of nerve swelling on ultrasound during PNBs as a monitoring method is inadequate for detection of intrafascicular injection and injury prevention. Most recent experimental and clinical data suggest that PNI from local anesthetic injection into the nerve occurs and remains a real clinical danger.[41] The sequelae from such an injury may be long lasting and require surgical intervention.[41,44]

Proximal Versus Distal PNBs and Risk of Neurologic Injury

The PNB injections at more proximal sites (ie, roots of brachial plexus vs peripheral nerves of the brachial plexus) (Figures 60–9, 60–10, and 60–11) may be at higher risk of nerve injury compared to distal sites of PNB. This is likely due to differences in neural architecture, primarily the ratio of neural versus nonneural (connective) tissue[62,63] (Figure 60–16). Clinically, intraneural injection into the extrafascicular connective tissue within the epineurium may not result in nerve injury.[62] This is consistent with experimental work that has correlated intrafascicular injection to peripheral nerve injection injury.[15]

The structural organization of the peripheral nerve provides insight into the relative risk for mechanical injury among different nerves or even at different locations within the same nerve (Figure 60–16). Because the epineurium is typically a tougher layer than the surrounding adipose tissue, nerves tend to be "pushed away" by an advancing needle, rather than penetrated.

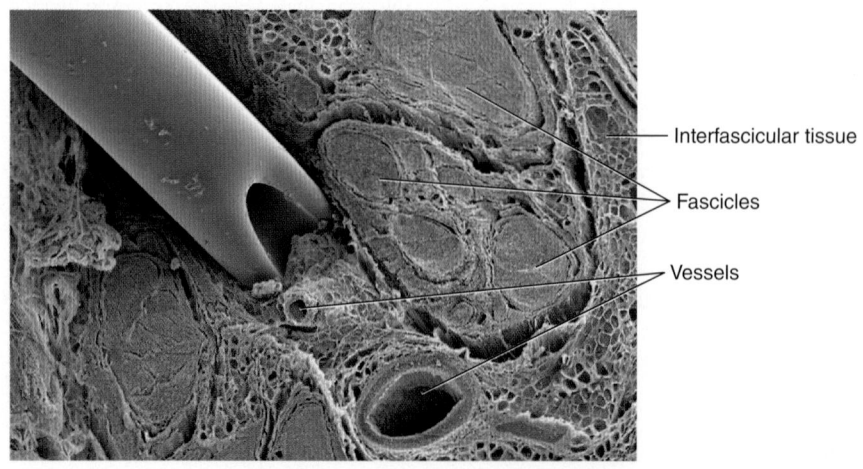

FIGURE 60–13. Human tibial nerve. In vitro puncture of nerve with neurostimulation needle. Scanning electron microscopy. (Reproduced with permission from Reina MA: *Atlas of Functional Anatomy for Regional Anesthesia and Pain Medicine.* Heidelberg: Springer; 2015.)

TABLE 60–2. Evidence-based recommendations to reduce the risk of block-related PNI.

- Intraneural needle insertion may not always lead to nerve injury.

- Intrafascicular needle placement and injection should be avoided.

- Neither the presence nor the absence of a paresthesia during needle advancement or on injection of local anesthetic is entirely predictive of nerve injury.

- Elicitation of severe pain during needle advancement or on injection of local anesthetic should prompt cessation of injection.

- Presence of an evoked motor response at a current of less than 0.5 (0.1 ms) indicates intimate needle-nerve relationship, needle-nerve contact, or intraneural needle placement. This information is useful in clinical decision-making.

- Injection pressure monitoring can detect injection into a poorly compliant tissue space, such as a nerve fascicle.

- Ultrasound can detect intraneural injection, although such detection may occur too late to prevent injury as a small quantity of injectate is sufficient to rupture the fascicle.

- Current ultrasound technology does not have adequate resolution to discern between an interfascicular and an intrafascicular injection.

- Adequate images of needle-nerve interface are not consistently obtained by all operators and in all patients.

Similarly, when the epineurium is penetrated by a needle, the needle tip and injection are much more likely to enter the interfascicular adipose tissue than the fascicles (Figure 60–15). The adipose tissue within the epineurium allows the fascicles to escape the advancing needle; however, this protection may be undermined by abrupt needle advancement needle or forceful needle-nerve contact.[8] The nerves characterized by tightly packed fascicles and high fascicular-to-connective tissue content may be at greater risk of mechanical nerve injury than those characterized by lower fascicular-to-connective tissue content.[62,63]

Relatively high incidences of transient neurologic sequelae are reported following interscalene block, where there is a 1:1 ratio of neural to nonneural tissue[62] (Figure 60–12). Several studies documented a rather high incidence of neurologic symptoms after brachial plexus block, but without severe sequelae.[64–66] In other studies, there were low absolute numbers of upper extremity PNB-related neurologic complications, rendering any comparison of outcomes at proximal sites with distal sites problematic.[67–69]

Injury rates following lower extremity PNB have been reported as 0.41% (95% confidence interval [CI], 0.02–9.96) in the gluteal region, compared with 0.24% (95% CI,

0.10–0.61) in the popliteal region,[5] indicating no significant difference. It is possible that many of the neurologic symptoms reported by the patients postoperatively after PNBs are inflammatory and due to needle-nerve contact or forceful injection, leading to intraneural inflammation, leading to symptoms, as demonstrated by Steinfeldt.[8,72] Therefore, the wisdom in Selander's teaching that "nerves should be handled with care" remains relevant.

Needle Type

Needle-tip characteristics influence the likelihood of fascicular penetration and nerve injury.[70] Long-bevel needles are more likely to puncture and enter the fascicle compared with short-bevel needles[14]; however, short-bevel needles appear to cause more damage in case of fascicular penetration[70] (Figure 60–17). The severity of nerve injury after needle-nerve perforation is also linked to the needle diameter[71]; however, no such difference exists with regard to extent of inflammation after needle-nerve trauma.[71,72]

The effect of needle design on the likelihood and severity of mechanical nerve injury has been extensively debated.[24,29,32] It is not surprising that mechanical needle trauma and intraneural injection are key mechanisms in iatrogenic nerve injury, such as with regional anesthesia. For example, in the setting for neuraxial anesthesia, the dural lesions produced by different needle types vary greatly in morphology; a Whitacre needle produces a more traumatic opening, with tearing and severe disruption of the collagen fibers, than a Quincke-style needle.[73] Similarly, the likelihood and extent of mechanical injury to nerve fascicles following intraneural injection during PNB also depend on needle-tip design. It seems intuitive that short-bevel needle types are less likely to penetrate the protective connective tissue layers of the peripheral nerves (epineurium, perineurium). Indeed, Selander and colleagues documented that a needle with a 45° bevel is much less likely to penetrate perineurium and inflict fascicular injury than a needle with a 15° bevel.[70,74,75] However, should a nerve fascicle become accidentally impaled during a nerve block procedure, the lesions induced by short-bevel needles may be more severe and take longer to repair than those induced by long-bevel needles.[23]

Surgical Factors
Surgical Positioning Requirements

Neurologic complications can occur following positioning for surgical requirements. Mechanisms of nerve injury related to surgery include traction, transection, compression, contusion, ischemia, and stretch. Regardless of mechanism, the final pathway of nerve injury may include the following factors: physical disruption of intraneural blood vessels causing patchy ischemia or hemorrhage; elevated intraneural venous pressures; endoneurial edema; impairment of axoplasmic flow; Schwann cell damage; myelin displacement; axonal degeneration; and Wallerian degeneration.[76] During surgery, patients are placed in positions they would not otherwise tolerate unless anesthetized. In addition, the physical forces required during surgery (eg, placement of prostheses) can be excessive, potentially stressing anatomical

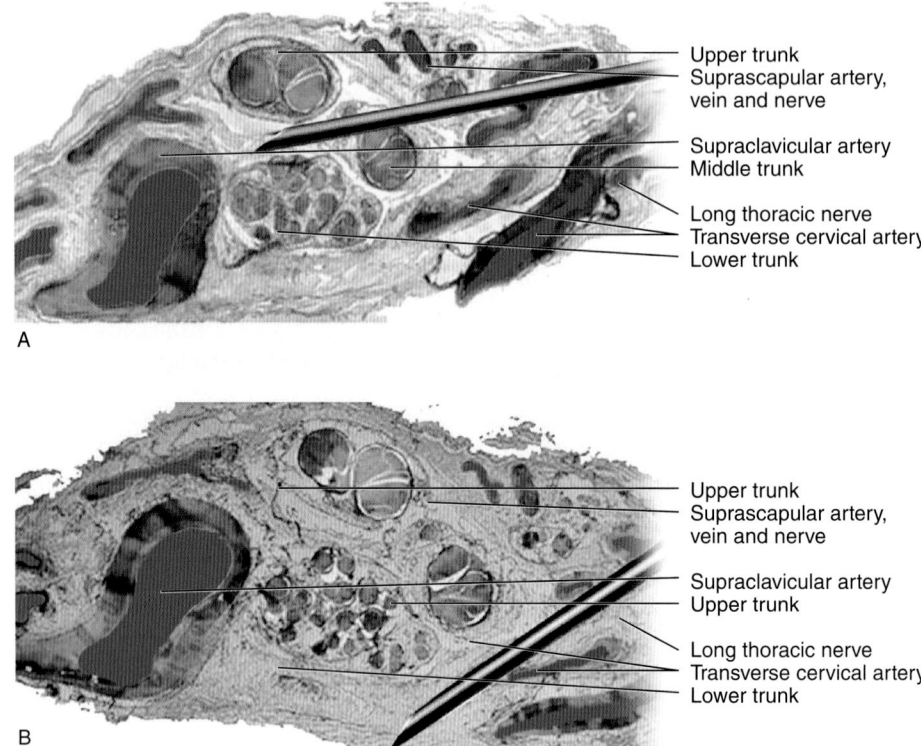

Upper trunk
Suprascapular artery,
vein and nerve

Supraclavicular artery
Middle trunk

Long thoracic nerve
Transverse cervical artery
Lower trunk

A

Upper trunk
Suprascapular artery,
vein and nerve

Supraclavicular artery
Upper trunk

Long thoracic nerve
Transverse cervical artery
Lower trunk

B

FIGURE 60–14. Overlap of the needle in the supraclavicular brachial plexus. If the neurostimulation needle pierces the nerve, as compared with the static images, the needle injures the fascicles. Different approaches are shown in **A.** and **B.** (Reproduced with permission from Reina MA: *Atlas of Functional Anatomy for Regional Anesthesia and Pain Medicine.* Heidelberg: Springer; 2015.)

structures remote from the surgical site, including the vertebral column. In a closed-claims analysis, 9 of 53 anesthetic-related brachial plexus injuries were related to intraoperative positioning (shoulder braces in the head-down position [three claims], patient's arm suspended on a bar [two claims], and other malpositions [four claims]). Only two claims were related to a regional anesthesia technique.[77]

Effects of the Pneumatic Tourniquet

Tourniquet inflation causes nerve damage by mechanical deformation or ischemia.[7,78,79] The main features of tourniquet neuropathy include weakness or paralysis, diminished touch, vibration and position sense, and preserved senses of heat, cold, and pain.[80] In an experimental model, tourniquet compression

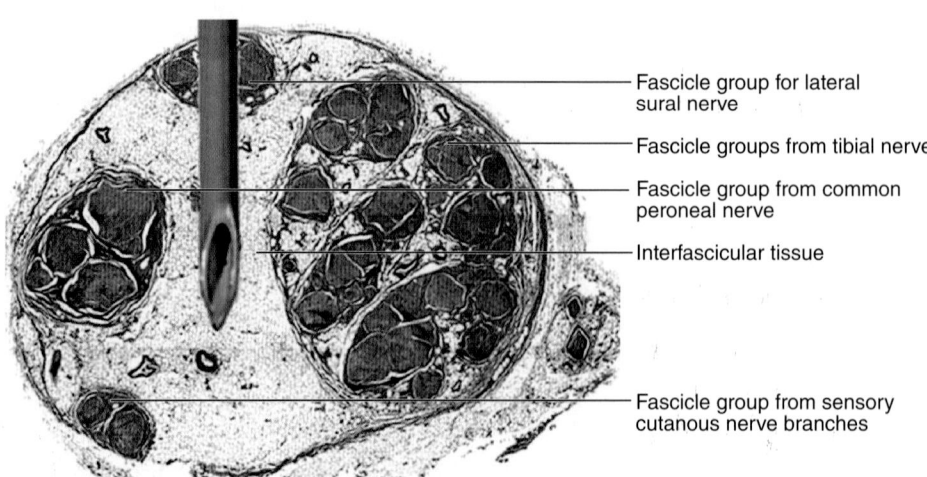

Fascicle group for lateral sural nerve

Fascicle groups from tibial nerve

Fascicle group from common peroneal nerve

Interfascicular tissue

Fascicle group from sensory cutaneous nerve branches

FIGURE 60–15. Overlap of the needle in the sciatic nerve, posterior approach. If the neurostimulation needle pierces the nerve, based on the static images, the needle injures the fascicles. Observe the difference in size between the needle and fascicles. If there is a large amount of interfascicular tissue, as occurs within the sciatic nerve, the risk of fascicular injury is reduced. (Reproduced with permission from Reina MA: *Atlas of Functional Anatomy for Regional Anesthesia and Pain Medicine.* Heidelberg: Springer; 2015.)

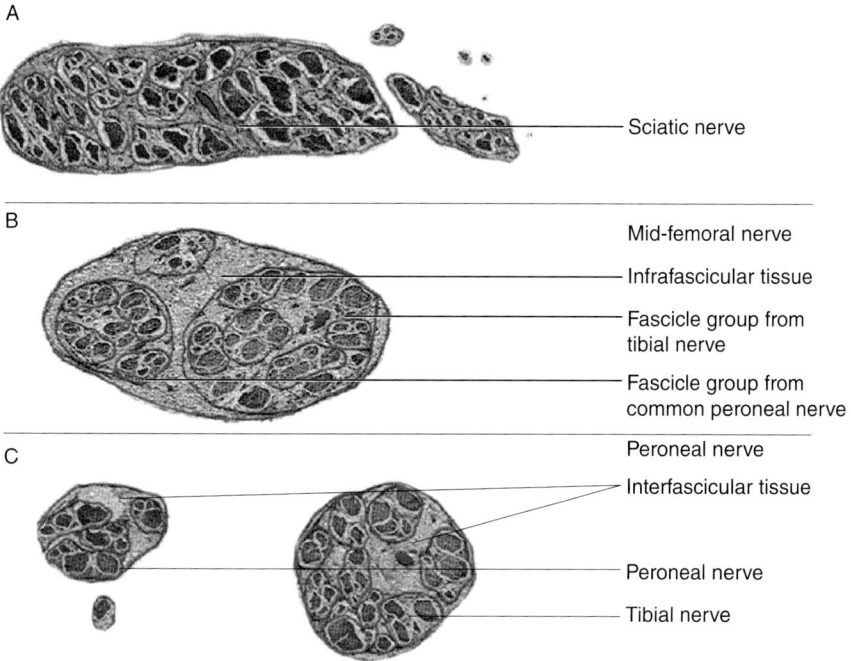

FIGURE 60–16. Transversal section of sciatic nerve at subgluteal region (**A**), mid-femoral region (**B**), and tibial and peroneal nerves at popliteal region (**C**). (Reproduced with permission from Reina MA: *Atlas of Functional Anatomy for Regional Anesthesia and Pain Medicine.* Heidelberg: Springer; 2015.)

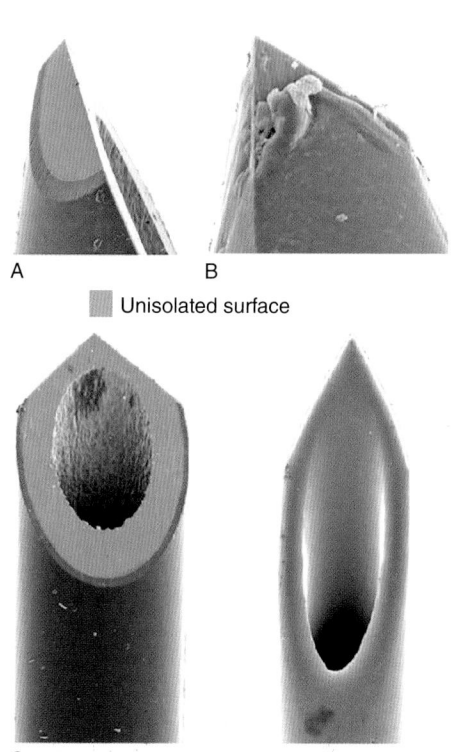

FIGURE 60–17. Presented is 21-gauge neurostimulation, peripheral needle type A (**A** and **B**) and type D (**C** and **D**). Scanning electron microscopy. (Reproduced with permission from Reina MA: *Atlas of Functional Anatomy for Regional Anesthesia and Pain Medicine.* Heidelberg: Springer; 2015.)

resulted in increased vascular permeability, intraneural edema, and sciatic nerve degeneration.[82] For instance, tourniquet compression during meniscectomy surgery can lead to femoral nerve denervation and delayedfunctional recovery.[83,84] Wider tourniquets, using lower cuff pressures, and limiting the duration of inflation have been proposed as methods to prevent tourniquet neuropathy.[81]

Postsurgical Inflammatory Neuropathy

Patients with postsurgical inflammatory neuropathy typically present with a neuropathy that is delayed in onset and remote from the surgery. The neuropathies are focal and multifocal with pain and weakness. An inflammatory-immune mechanism is responsible, and there is evidence of axonal degeneration and lymphocytic-mediated inflammation.

Clinical Pearl

• Not all episodes of PNI are mechanical in origin.[43]

Patient Factors
Preexisting Neuropathy

A preoperative neurologic deficit or neural compromise, whether from nerve entrapment or metabolic, ischemic, toxic, hereditary, and demyelination reasons, may be present in patients presenting for surgery. Many of these preexisting neurologic conditions are subclinical, yet they may be associated with increased risk of PNI postoperatively.[85] For instance, often-overlooked, but common, cervical spondylosis may result in rough and irregular opening of the intervertebral foramen. The spinal nerve–nerve root complex becomes subject to repeated trauma, resulting in fibrosis reducing its mobility. The spinal nerve–nerve root complex is consequently at increased risk of traction injury during upper extremity movement and positioning.[1] The ulnar nerve may become entrapped in the cubital tunnel at the elbow or at the wrist. Risk factors for perioperative ulnar neuropathy include male gender, extremes of body habitus, and prolonged admission.[86,87]

Diabetic neuropathies are common and represent a wide range of clinical entities commonly resulting in distal symmetric sensory polyneuropathy. Asymmetric diabetic neuropathies comprise acute or subacute proximal motor neuropathy (often painful), cranial neuropathy, truncal or thoracoabdominal neuropathy (often painful), and entrapment neuropathy in the limbs.[88] Diabetic lumbar radiculopathy can present with pain radiating from the back to the lower limbs and mild weakness. There may be diffuse neuropathy with abnormal electromyography of paraspinal muscles and muscles innervated by the sacral plexus, gluteal, femoral, and sciatic nerves. Elderly patients with diabetes may have combined proximal and distal involvement, placing these patients at increased risk of PNI. Diabetic nerve fibers may be more susceptible to toxic effects of local anesthetics because of chronic ischemic hypoxia and because nerves are exposed to larger concentrations of local anesthetics related to decreased blood flow.[89] The occurrence of PNI following neuraxial blockade in patients with diabetic neuropathy has been reported as being higher (0.4%; 95% CI, 0.1%–1.3%) than the general population; however, its true clinical relevance is controversial as many of these patients are among the greatest beneficiaries of PNBs.[90]

Similarly, the actual risk of PNBs in the setting of severe peripheral vascular disease, vasculitis, cigarette smoking, and hypertension is not known.[47,91] Regardless, patients with these conditions could be more vulnerable to further ischemic insults during the perioperative period, similar to patients with alcohol-[92] and cisplatin-induced neuropathies.[93] Patients with multiple sclerosis and hereditary neuropathy may have subclinical preoperative neural compromise within the peripheral nervous system.[94]

Lumbar Spinal Canal Stenosis

Lumbar spinal canal stenosis may exaggerate a peripheral injury, adversely affecting physical recovery.[95] Spinal canal stenosis is a risk factor for common peroneal palsy following THA and may be significant in cases of paraplegia or cauda equina syndrome following epidural anesthesia.[96,97] Hebl documented new or progressive neurologic deficits following neuraxial anesthesia in patients with preexisting spinal canal stenosis or lumbar disk disease.[98] Overall, 10 (1.1%, 95% CI 0.5%–2.0%) patients developed new deficits or worsening of preexisting symptoms. The frequency of complications was higher in patients who had compressive radiculopathy or multiple central neuraxial diagnoses. However, it is likely that there were multiple etiological factors because deficits often correlated with the side of preexisting pathology or surgical procedure. A summary of anatomical, anesthetic, surgical, and patient factors contributing to PNI is listed in Table 60–3.

MONITORING NEEDLE-NERVE DISTANCE DURING PNBS AND PREVENTION OF COMPLICATIONS

While the risk of needle-nerve contact, intraneural needle placement, and intraneural injection has recently been questioned in small clinical series where overt injuries did not occur,[55–57,105] PNB-related nerve injuries continue to be reported. Susan MacKinnon's team has recently sternly warned against intentional intraneural injection based on their results of neurotoxicity following intrafascicular injections of local anesthetics.[36] This publication in one of the premier journals in the specialty (*Anesthesia and Analgesia*) specifically warned against the recent recommendations by some providers that intraneural injection is without risk and, in fact, can be beneficial for block quality.[106] It is important to note that MacKinnon's team's warning stems from decades of clinical practice of peripheral nerve repair surgery and over 350 scientific publications on the subject. Although the incidence of PNB-related nerve injuries is relatively uncommon, they are among the most common disabling complications related to administration of anesthesia and are likely underreported in the literature due to medicolegal and institutional reputation-related implications.[28] The potentially devastating impact of a severe nerve injury on the patient's quality of life mandates a systematic approach to mitigating the risk through standardization of injection techniques.

Mechanical Elicitation of Paresthesias

The association between the mechanical elicitation of paresthesias and consequent PNI has been the subject of debate for a long time.[17,57,107] While some large observational trials[17,108] have indeed implicated the elicitation of paresthesias as a risk factor for PNI, such an association has not been supported by others.[109–111] Moreover, the occurrence of paresthesias is not a sensitive sign of needle-nerve contact, as only 38% of patients experienced paresthesias during real-time visualization of needle-nerve contact.[112] Therefore, the absence of paresthesias during the performance of a nerve block does not reliably exclude needle-nerve contact, and nerve injury has been reported both in patients who have experienced severe paresthesias *and* in those experiencing no paresthesias during the PNB procedure. Regardless, a severe paresthesia, or pain on needle advancement or injection, may indicate intraneural needle placement and, when present, should prompt cessation of injection and needle repositioning.

If and how the use of deep sedation influences patients' perception and interpretation of the paresthesia as a symptom has not been studied. Likewise, ultrasound-guided PNBs often involved multiple injections of aliquots of local anesthetic in several different anatomical areas. It is not known how the spread of the local anesthetic during multiple-injection techniques and the incipient sensory blockade that occurs during the procedure may have an impact on the value of paresthesia as a safety monitor.

Peripheral Nerve Stimulation

Motor response to peripheral nerve stimulation relies on Coulomb's law, whereby a smaller current intensity (mA; or, more correctly, electrical energy) is required to elicit a motor or sensory response as the needle tip approaches the nerve.[113]

TABLE 60–3. Summary of anatomical, anesthetic, surgical, and patient factors contributing to perioperative nerve injury.

	Factor Potentially Contributing to or Relevant to PNI	Comment
Anatomical	Internal morphology of nerve, including connective tissue supporting fascicles and axons[1,63]	Epineurial tissue may offer protection from direct trauma and external compression
	Gross anatomical factors: location, course, relations, attachments, and relative mobility of nerves[1]	—
	Specific structures are at risk	Examples: ulnar nerve at elbow,[76,99] CPN [81,100,101]
Anesthetic	Type of anesthesia	EA and GA but not PNB were associated with PNI.[47] PNB not associated with PNI following TKA,[48] THA,[49] or TSA.[50]
	Insensate limb	Places nerves at risk from compression or stretching[76]
	Site of PNB: proximal at increased risk versus distal PNB	Not supported by clinical evidence
	Level of sedation during nerve blockade	Continues to be controversial. However, with objective monitoring of needle-nerve relationship and disposition of injectate (US, nerve stimulation, opening injection pressure monitoring), this issue is likely to become mute. For latest published recommendation, consult ASRA practice Advisory
	Mechanical trauma from needle, catheter, or injectate	—
	Direct local anesthetic toxicity	Time and concentration dependent; risk with intrafascicular greater than extrafascicular exposure[6,15]
	Neural ischemia	Secondary to compression,[76] vasoconstrictors,[19,20] intrafascicular injection,[54] tourniquet[82,103]
Surgical	Trauma: contusion, compression, retraction, traction, transection	
	Perioperative positioning[76]	
	Tourniquet: duration of inflation and pressure[81,104]	Associated with marked clinical deficits[80] and
	Swelling, plaster casts	pathological changes on EMG[84]
	Specific procedures have unique risk profile[95]	Risks of PNI following TKA,[48] THA,[49] and TSA[50] were 0.79%, 0.72%, and 2.2%, respectively
Patients	Preoperative neural compromise theoretically increases risk of PNI	Etiology includes entrapment, metabolic, ischemic, toxic,[93] hereditary, and demyelination causes[94]
	Lumbar canal stenosis	May be significant risk factor following neuraxial blockade[96,98]
Other	Inflammatory mechanism	Nonmechanical cause physically and temporally remote from PNB[43]

ASRA, American Society of Regional Anesthesia and Pain Medicine; CPN = common peroneal nerve; EA = epidural analgesia; EMG = electromyography; GA = general anesthesia; PNB = peripheral nerve block; PNI = peripheral nerve injury; THA = total hip arthroplasty; TKA = total knee arthroplasty; TSA = total shoulder arthroplasty.

The importance of avoiding injection when motor response is obtained by very low current intensity (<0.2 mA) and risk of nerve injury was first reported by Voelckel and colleagues.[114] Histological nerve injury occurred in 50% of the pigs when motor response was obtained at less than 0.2 mA, compared to no histological changes at 0.3–0.5 mA. Presence of motor response at less than 0.2 mA has been shown to be a specific but not sensitive indicator of intraneural needle placement in both animals[59,115,116] and humans.[55,117,118]

Peripheral nerve stimulation as a nerve localization technique is characterized by relatively low sensitivity but high specificity for predicting relative needle-nerve proximity, suggesting that such a response actually reflects needle-axon distance.[116] Both experimental data and clinical reports have shown that an evoked motor response may not be reliably elicited when the needle is placed in the immediate vicinity of the nerve or even intraneurally.[117,119] However, the same research indicated that when a motor response is elicited at low current intensity (eg,

< 0.5 mA, 0.1 ms), the needle tip is invariably positioned on the nerve or within the nerve. Importantly, peripheral nerve stimulation has withstood the test of time, as evidenced by the largest published data sets related to PNI,[67,68,108,120,121] all of which relied primarily on peripheral nerve stimulation to achieve safe and successful PNB.

Opening Injection Pressure Monitoring

The association between high injection pressures and intrafascicular injection was first described in 1979 by Selander[122] and subsequently studied in several animal models. In a dog model, an intentional intrafascicular injection was associated with both high opening injection pressure (≥25 psi) and corresponding clinical and histological nerve injury.[16] In contrast, extrafascicular injections were not associated with high injection pressures or with nerve injury. In another study in a dog model,[123] high injection pressure (≥20 psi) was also associated with intrafascicular injection as well as clinical and histological nerve injury, while intraneural but interfascicular injection was associated with low injection pressure (<10 psi) and no neurologic or histologic consequences.

During intraneural injection into the median nerves of pigs, Lupu and colleagues were unable to detect a significant correlation between the maximum pressure generated and clinical or histological nerve injury.[124] In this study, peak injection pressures were well below 25 psi, yet 7 of 10 nerve specimens had evidence of axonal damage on histological examination. In one case, axonal damage ensued following a maximum injection pressure of only 2.2 psi. Importantly, functional deficits measured up to 7 days postinsult were absent in all 10 pigs studied. More recently, in the first such study in human tissue, Orebaugh and colleagues reported that 100% of injections directly into the roots of the brachial plexus of fresh human cadavers resulted in high injection pressures (>30 psi), with one occurrence of injectate spread into the epidural space.[125] Importantly, analysis of the attained injection pressure curves indicated that all injections into the brachial plexus roots were associated with pressures greater than 15 psi.

Similar data on the injection pressure–nerve relationship were reported by Krol et al[126] in the peripheral nerves. In a study on pressure monitoring during injections for median, radial, and ulnar nerve PNBs in fresh human cadavers, the authors reported significant differences between intraneural and perineural injection pressures. Intraneural injection pressures showed low specificity but high sensitivity with intraneural needle placement.

Several studies have utilized injection pressure as a monitoring tool for intraneural (intraepineurial) injection during sciatic nerve block without complications.[117,127,128] Robards and colleagues studied 24 patients, who each received an injection inside their sciatic nerve at the level of the popliteal fossa. Injection pressures of less than 20 psi were recorded in 20 patients, while injection pressures greater than 20 psi were observed in the remaining 4 patients, prompting cessation of the injection; none of the patients suffered any neurologic dysfunction, suggesting that injections that occurred intraneurally were extrafascicular.[117]

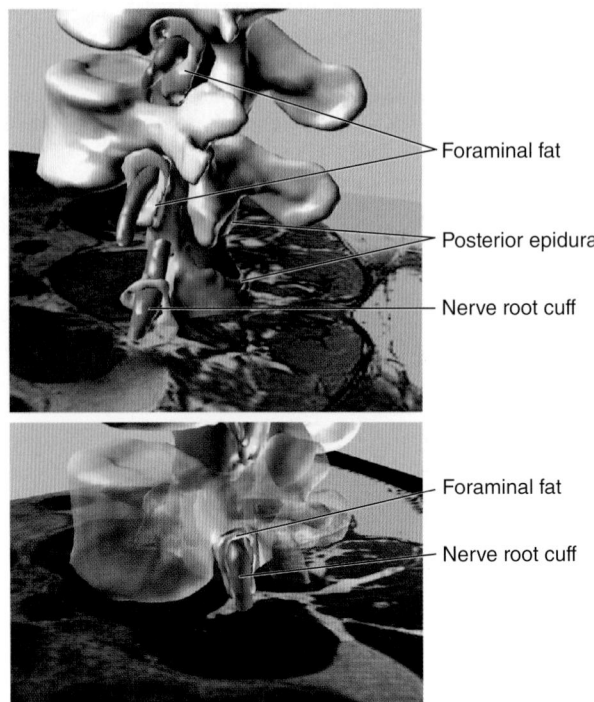

FIGURE 60–18. Three-dimensional reconstruction of MRI image of vertebrae, dural sac, epidural fat and foraminal adipose tissue. The yellow painted areas represent interconnections between the adipose tissues which can serve as potential paths for spread for injected solutions. (Used with permission from M.A. Reina.)

In a study of intraneural stimulation thresholds during ultrasound-guided supraclavicular brachial plexus blocks, Bigeleisen and colleagues reported a combination of high resistance to injection, low current stimulation, and pain on injection coincided in two patients with an intraneural needle placement that necessitated needle repositioning before completing the injection without complications.[57]

Beyond the risk of neurologic injury, high injection pressures can lead to several other unwanted effects or serious complications. For instance, Gadsden and colleagues reported that high injection pressure during lumbar plexus block carries a risk for epidural spread[129] (Figures 60–18 and 60–19). In this study, injection pressures greater than 20 psi during lumbar plexus block led to unacceptable risk of high-level epidural block, in some patients as high as the T3 level, necessitating early termination of the study for safety reasons.

More recently, Gautier et al reported that high injection pressure during interscalene injection can lead to substantial epidural spread of the injectate. Gautier's report offered an explanation for the precipitous respiratory and cardiovascular demise occasionally reported immediately following interscalane block, as well as suggested that injection force/pressure should be monitored during the injection process.

Assessment of injection pressure (resistance) during PNB is of increasing interest to clinicians and researchers.[130,131] This is not surprising, given that injection into densely packed nerve fascicles requires more force to initiate an injection (opening pressure) than perineural or intraneural-interfascicular injections into the loose perineural or perifascicular connective

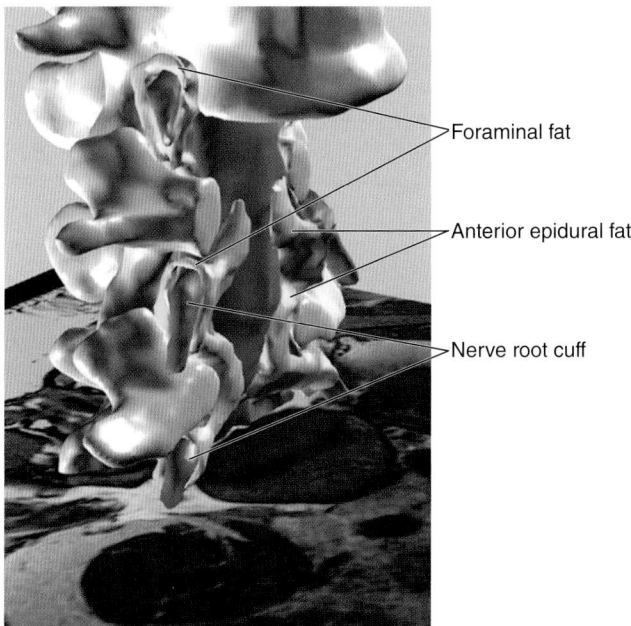

FIGURE 60–19. Three-dimensional reconstruction of vertebrae, dural sac, epidural fat, and foraminal fat from magnetic resonance images of a patient. We can see the potential pathway through the fat from epidural fat, foraminal fat, to other fat compartments, as the fat envelops the nerve roots outer the foraminal canal of the spine or the fat found among the muscular fascias. Two vertebral bodies were removed, allowing visualization of epidural fat in the anterior epidural space. (Used with permission from M.A. Reina.)

tissue (Figures 60–12, 60–14, and 60–15). In an attempt to standardize monitoring and documentation of nerve block procedures, a group of North American experts suggested documenting the resistance to injection as one of the elements of the standard clinical note.[132] However, two independent groups found that the clinician's accuracy in gauging injection pressure or the tissue being injected is limited when using a subjective, syringe feel technique, thus questioning the reliability of subjective assessments.[133,134] In the meantime, several means of monitoring injection pressures have been recommended.[131,135]

Taken together, the data to date suggest that high opening injection pressure can detect an intrafascicular injection, but not an intraneural interfascicular injection.[123,125] In the first study in patients, Gadsden and colleagues demonstrated that opening injection pressure with the needle tip at 1 mm away from the nerve roots of the interscalene brachial plexus was consistently lower than 15 psi (mean peak pressure 8.2 ± 2.4 psi). In contrast, opening injection pressure during needle-nerve contact was 15 psi or more (mean peak pressure 20.9 ± 3.7 psi) in 35 of 36 injections. In this study, aborting the injection when opening injection pressure reached 15 psi reliably prevented commencement of injection in 97% cases of needle-nerve contacts.[136] In addition, high opening injection may correlate well with other indices of needle-nerve contact, such as low current stimulation and paresthesia on injection.[57,117]

In a follow-up study, Gadsden et al used similar methodology to determine whether high opening pressure can also detect needle-nerve contact in peripheral nerves, such as the femoral nerve. The researchers reported that high opening injection

pressure consistently detected (97%) needle-nerve contact and prevented an injection against the femoral nerve or fascicles. Moreover, their research suggested that high opening injection pressure can detect insertion of the needle into a wrong tissue plane. In this report, inability to inject local anesthetic with opening injection pressure below 15 psi detected 100% of instances of the needle placement on the wrong aspect of the fascia iliaca.

Further research is needed to determine the clinical benefits of routine injection pressure monitoring and actual "safe" opening injection pressure values for various nerve block procedures. Regardless, sufficient data exist to suggest that monitoring opening injection pressure during interscalene and femoral nerve blocks adds additional critical safety information that can influence clinical decision-making. Injection pressure monitoring may prove to be most useful for its negative predictive value for functional nerve injury, as no cases of clinically significant neuropathy have been reported in the literature with low injection pressures. Based on the available data, avoidance of high resistance and opening injection pressure greater than 15 psi appears to be a prudent strategy. At the very least, this is because during nerve block injections, the injections into the loose perineural connective tissue should never require more than 15 psi; therefore, when opening pressure of 15 psi is reached before injection actually occurs, the operator has an opportunity to reposition the needle away from the nerve before injection into possibly the wrong tissue space or vulnerable parts of the nerve (fascicles, needle-nerve contact).

Electrical Impedance

Electrical impedance monitoring measures the resistance to flow of an alternating current in an electrical circuit and could be added to the existing nerve stimulators. Electrical impedance is sensitive to changes in tissue composition, particularly water content. In a pig sciatic nerve model, Tsui and colleagues demonstrated that nerves have greater electrical impedance than the surrounding muscle and interstitial fluid due to their low water and high lipid content.[137] They found that the electrical impedance increased abruptly on entrance into the intraneural compartment relative to the extraneural compartment. The absolute value at which intraneural needle placement occurred could not be determined because of substantial variance within the data.

While electrical impedance monitoring appears promising to detect intraneural needle tip placement, it necessarily implies that nerve puncture must occur before a change in impedance is detected. There is also reasonably strong evidence that measurement of electrical impedance can differentiate intravascular from perineural placement of a needle when 5% dextrose in water is injected before performance of the block.[138] Based on the currently available data, impedance monitoring can differentiate between certain tissues, such as muscle and adipose/connective tissue. However, the variability of impedance measurements among different nerves or even the same nerves at different locations requires further research before any recommendations regarding the potential clinical applicability of this modality can be made.[139]

Ultrasound

Although ultrasound can detect intraneural injection, the widespread use of ultrasound guidance has not decreased the rate of PNI. In animals, ultrasound is sensitive enough to detect as little as 1 mL of injectate[61,115]; however, a much smaller amount of injectate is sufficient to injure the fascicles.[41] Regardless, no animal or human study to date has definitively demonstrated an association between real-time sonographic visualization of intraneural injection of local anesthetic and consequent functional (or otherwise clinically important) nerve injury.[56,57,105]

One reason may be that the resolution of the current ultrasound machines produced is not high enough to differentiate potentially hazardous intrafascicular injection from injection into the potentially more forgiving extrafascicular compartment. In addition, the ability to interpret such images is highly user dependent, and the ability to obtain high-definition, quality images varies among patients.[140] The use of ultrasound guidance has substantially facilitated the teaching and popularized the utilization of PNBs while decreasing the incidence of systemic toxicity of local anesthetics.[141] However, in studies to date, ultrasound has not decreased the incidence of PNI.[68,121,141] More information about ultrasound and monitoring is covered in Chapter 63.

Clinical Pearl

- The main mechanisms of PNB-mediated injury include mechanical trauma, ischemia, local anesthetic toxicity, and inflammation. The main source of PNB-mediated neurologic complications is likely mechanical fascicular injury or injection of local anesthetic into a fascicle, causing myelin and axonal degeneration.

SUMMARY

Neurological complications associated with PNB are multifactorial and associated with a range of perioperative processes and patient, anesthetic, and surgical factors, The anatomy of peripheral nerves is variable in location, structure, and susceptibility to injury. The main mechanisms of PNB-mediated injury include mechanical trauma, ischemia, local anesthetic toxicity, and inflammation. The main source of PNB-mediated neurologic complications is likely mechanical fascicular injury or injection of local anesthetic into a fascicle, causing myelin and axonal degeneration. The reported incidences of neurologic complications following PNB vary significantly, and interpreting the literature is difficult because of varied study methodologies, including differences in the neurological outcomes captured. Fortunately, most postoperative neurological deficits appear to resolve with time, and the incidence of serious long-term neurologic complications attributable to PNB is relatively uncommon.

Avoidance of deliberate trauma to nerves, including intraneural injection, is a key safety principle of regional anesthesia. At this time, there is evidence that objective monitoring of needle placement and injection, such as ultrasound, nerve stimulation, and opening injection pressure, can help detect needle-nerve contact and intraneural needle placement. Although, as with many other monitors in clinical practice (eg, pulse oximetry), there is no evidence these monitors can reduce incidence of neurologic complications, there are data suggesting that their combination should confer additional safety during PNBs. Careful patient selection, combined use of more than one nerve localization technique or monitor, avoiding injection with opening injection pressure, and limiting the number of needle passes and injections where appropriate will further decrease the risk and make the practice of PNBs less of an art than a science.

REFERENCES

1. Sunderland S: *Nerve Injuries and Their Repair: A Critical Appraisal.* Churchill Livingstone, 1991.
2. Boezaart AP: That which we call a rose by any other name would smell as sweet—and its thorns would hurt as much. Reg Anesth Pain Med 2009;34:3–7.
3. Seddon HJ: A classification of nerve injuries. Br Med J 1942;2: 237–239.
4. Sunderland S: A classification of peripheral nerve injuries producing loss of function. Brain 1951;74:491–516.
5. Brull R, McCartney CJ, Chan VW, El-Beheiry H: Neurological complications after regional anesthesia: contemporary estimates of risk. Anesth Analg 2007;104:965–974.
6. Hogan QH: Pathophysiology of peripheral nerve injury during regional anesthesia. Reg Anesth Pain Med 2008;33:435–441.
7. Burnett MG, Zager EL: Pathophysiology of peripheral nerve injury: a brief review. Neurosurg Focus 2004;16:E1.
8. Steinfeldt T, Poeschl S, Nimphius W, et al: Forced needle advancement during needle-nerve contact in a porcine model: histological outcome. Anesth Analg 2011;113:417–420.
9. Kerns JM: The microstructure of peripheral nerves. Techn Reg Anesth Pain Manag 2008;12:127–133.
10. Gentili F, Hudson AR, Kline D, Hunter D: Early changes following injection injury of peripheral nerves. Can J Surg 1980;23:177–182.
11. Whitlock EL, Brenner MJ, Fox IK, Moradzadeh A, Hunter DA, Mackinnon SE: Ropivacaine-induced peripheral nerve injection injury in the rodent model. Anesth Analg 2010;111:214–220.
12. Mackinnon SE, Hudson AR, Gentili F, Kline DG, Hunter D: Peripheral nerve injection injury with steroid agents. Plast Reconstr Surg 1982; 69:482–490.
13. Gentili F, Hudson AR, Hunter D: Clinical and experimental aspects of injection injuries of peripheral nerves. Can J Neurol Sci 1980;7:143–151.
14. Sala-Blanch X, Ribalta T, Rivas E, et al: Structural injury to the human sciatic nerve after intraneural needle insertion. Reg Anesth Pain Med 2009;34:201–205.
15. Gentili F, Hudson A, Kline DG, Hunter D: Peripheral nerve injection injury: an experimental study. Neurosurgery 1979;4:244–253.
16. Hadzic A, Dilberovic F, Shah S, et al: Combination of intraneural injection and high injection pressure leads to fascicular injury and neurologic deficits in dogs. Reg Anesth Pain Med 2004;29:417–423.
17. Selander D, Edshage S, Wolff T: Paresthesiae or no paresthesiae? Nerve lesions after axillary blocks. Acta Anaesthesiol Scand 1979;23:27–33.
18. Selander D, Sjostrand J: Longitudinal spread of intraneurally injected local anesthetics. An experimental study of the initial neural distribution following intraneural injections. Acta Anaesthesiol Scand 1978;22: 622–634.
19. Myers RR, Heckman HM: Effects of local anesthesia on nerve blood flow: studies using lidocaine with and without epinephrine. Anesthesiology 1989;71:757–762.
20. Partridge BL: The effects of local anesthetics and epinephrine on rat sciatic nerve blood flow. Anesthesiology 1991;75:243–250.
21. Rodriguez J, Taboada M, Garcia F, Bermudez M, Amor M, Alvarez J: Intraneural hematoma after nerve stimulation-guided femoral block in a patient with factor XI deficiency: case report. J Clin Anesth 2011;23: 234–237.
22. Ben-David B, Stahl S: Axillary block complicated by hematoma and radial nerve injury. Reg Anesth Pain Med 1999;24:264–266.

23. Mackinnon SE, Hudson AR, Llamas F, Dellon AL, Kline DG, Hunter DA: Peripheral nerve injury by chymopapain injection. J Neurosurg 1984;61:1–8.
24. Topuz K, Kutlay M, Simsek H, Atabey C, Demircan M, Senol Guney M: Early surgical treatment protocol for sciatic nerve injury due to injection—a retrospective study. Br J Neurosurg 2011;25:509–515.
25. Amaniti E, Drampa F, Kouzi-Koliakos K, et al: Ropivacaine myotoxicity after single intramuscular injection in rats. Eur J Anaesthesiol 2006;23:130–135.
26. Beyzadeoglu T, Torun Kose G, Ekinci ID, Bekler H, Yilmaz C: Cytotoxicity of local anesthetics to rats' articular cartilage: an experimental study. Acta Orthop Traumatol Turc 2012;46:201–207.
27. Cereda CM, Tofoli GR, Maturana LG, et al: Local neurotoxicity and myotoxicity evaluation of cyclodextrin complexes of bupivacaine and ropivacaine. Anesth Analg 2012;115:1234–1241.
28. Dragoo JL, Braun HJ, Kim HJ, Phan HD, Golish SR: The in vitro chondrotoxicity of single-dose local anesthetics. Am J Sports Med 2012;40:794–799.
29. Mishra P, Stringer MD: Sciatic nerve injury from intramuscular injection: a persistent and global problem. Int J Clin Pract 2010;64:1573–1579.
30. Nouette-Gaulain K, Dadure C, Morau D, et al: Age-dependent bupivacaine-induced muscle toxicity during continuous peripheral nerve block in rats. Anesthesiology 2009;111:1120–1127.
31. Padera R, Bellas E, Tse JY, Hao D, Kohane DS: Local myotoxicity from sustained release of bupivacaine from microparticles. Anesthesiology 2008;108:921–928.
32. Small SP: Preventing sciatic nerve injury from intramuscular injections: literature review. J Adv Nurs 2004;47:287–296.
33. Zink W, Sinner B, Zausig Y, Graf BM: [Myotoxicity of local anaesthetics: experimental myth or clinical truth?]. Anaesthesist 2007;56:118–127.
34. Perez-Castro R, Patel S, Garavito-Aguilar ZV et al: Cytotoxicity of local anesthetics in human neuronal cells. Anesth Analg 2009;108:997–1007.
35. Radwan IA, Saito S, Goto F: The neurotoxicity of local anesthetics on growing neurons: a comparative study of lidocaine, bupivacaine, mepivacaine, and ropivacaine. Anesth Analg 2002;94:319–324, table of contents.
36. Farber SJ, Saheb-Al-Zamani M, Zieske L, et al: Peripheral nerve injury after local anesthetic injection. Anesth Analg 2013;117:731–739.
37. Lirk P, Haller I, Myers RR, et al: Mitigation of direct neurotoxic effects of lidocaine and amitriptyline by inhibition of p38 mitogen-activated protein kinase in vitro and in vivo. Anesthesiology 2006;104:1266–1273.
38. Yang S, Abrahams MS, Hurn PD, Grafe MR, Kirsch JR: Local anesthetic Schwann cell toxicity is time and concentration dependent. Reg Anesth Pain Med 2011;36:444–451.
39. Kalichman MW: Physiologic mechanisms by which local anesthetics may cause injury to nerve and spinal cord. Reg Anesth 1993;18:448–452.
40. Gentili F, Hudson AR, Hunter D, Kline DG: Nerve injection injury with local anesthetic agents: a light and electron microscopic, fluorescent microscopic, and horseradish peroxidase study. Neurosurgery 1980;6:263–272.
41. Farber SJ, Saheb-Al-Zamani M, Zieske L, et al: Peripheral nerve injury after local anesthetic injection. Anesth Analg 2013;117:731–739.
42. Ahn KS, Kopp SL, Watson JC, Scott KP, Trousdale RT, Hebl JR: Postsurgical inflammatory neuropathy. Reg Anesth Pain Med 2011;36:403–405.
43. Staff NP, Engelstad J, Klein CJ, et al: Post-surgical inflammatory neuropathy. Brain 2010;133:2866–2880.
44. Kaufman MR, Elkwood AI, Rose MI, et al: Surgical treatment of permanent diaphragm paralysis after interscalene nerve block for shoulder surgery. Anesthesiology 2013;119:484–487.
45. Pintaric TS, Cvetko E, Strbenc M, Mis K, Podpecan O, Mars T, Hadzic A. Intraneural and perineural inflammatory changes in piglets after injection of ultrasound gel, endotoxin, 0.9% NaCl, or needle insertion without injection. Anesth Analg 2014;118(4):869–873.
46. Pintaric TS, Hadzic A, Strbenc M, Podpecan O, Podbregar M, Cvetko E. Inflammatory response after injection of aqueous gel into subarachnoid space in piglets. Reg Anesth Pain Med 2013;38(2):100–105.
47. Welch MB, Brummett CM, Welch TD, et al: Perioperative peripheral nerve injuries: a retrospective study of 380,680 cases during a 10-year period at a single institution. Anesthesiology 2009;111:490–497.
48. Jacob AK, Mantilla CB, Sviggum HP, Schroeder DR, Pagnano MW, Hebl JR: Perioperative nerve injury after total knee arthroplasty: regional anesthesia risk during a 20-year cohort study. Anesthesiology 2011;114:311–317.
49. Jacob AK, Mantilla CB, Sviggum HP, Schroeder DR, Pagnano MW, Hebl JR: Perioperative nerve injury after total hip arthroplasty: regional anesthesia risk during a 20-year cohort study. Anesthesiology 2011;115:1172–1178.
50. Sviggum HP, Jacob AK, Mantilla CB, Schroeder DR, Sperling JW, Hebl JR: Perioperative nerve injury after total shoulder arthroplasty: assessment of risk after regional anesthesia. Reg Anesth Pain Med 2012;37:490–494.
51. Lenters TR, Davies J, Matsen FA 3rd: The types and severity of complications associated with interscalene brachial plexus block anesthesia: local and national evidence. J Shoulder Elbow Surg 2007;16:379–387.
52. Widmer B, Lustig S, Scholes CJ, et al: Incidence and severity of complications due to femoral nerve blocks performed for knee surgery. Knee 2013;20:181–185.
53. Hogan QH: Phrenic nerve function after interscalene block revisited: now, the long view. Anesthesiology 2013;119:250–252.
54. Gadsden J, Gratenstein K, Hadzic A: Intraneural injection and peripheral nerve injury. Int Anesthesiol Clin 2010;48:107–115.
55. Liu SS, YaDeau JT, Shaw PM, Wilfred S, Shetty T, Gordon M: Incidence of unintentional intraneural injection and postoperative neurological complications with ultrasound-guided interscalene and supraclavicular nerve blocks. Anaesthesia 2011;66:168–174.
56. Bigeleisen PE: Nerve puncture and apparent intraneural injection during ultrasound-guided axillary block does not invariably result in neurologic injury. Anesthesiology 2006;105:779–783.
57. Bigeleisen PE, Moayeri N, Groen GJ: Extraneural versus intraneural stimulation thresholds during ultrasound-guided supraclavicular block. Anesthesiology 2009;110:1235–1243.
58. Sala Blanch X, Lopez AM, Carazo J, et al: Intraneural injection during nerve stimulator-guided sciatic nerve block at the popliteal fossa. Br J Anaesth 2009;102:855–861.
59. Cohen JM, Gray AT: Functional deficits after intraneural injection during interscalene block. Reg Anesth Pain Med 2010;35:397–399.
60. Orebaugh SL, McFadden K, Skorupan H, Bigeleisen PE: Subepineurial injection in ultrasound-guided interscalene needle tip placement. Reg Anesth Pain Med 2010;35:450–454.
61. Altermatt FR, Cummings TJ, Auten KM, Baldwin MF, Belknap SW, Reynolds JD: Ultrasonographic appearance of intraneural injections in the porcine model. Reg Anesth Pain Med 2010;35:203–206.
62. Moayeri N, Bigeleisen PE, Groen GJ: Quantitative architecture of the brachial plexus and surrounding compartments, and their possible significance for plexus blocks. Anesthesiology 2008;108:299–304.
63. Moayeri N, Groen GJ: Differences in quantitative architecture of sciatic nerve may explain differences in potential vulnerability to nerve injury, onset time, and minimum effective anesthetic volume. Anesthesiology 2009;111:1128–1134.
64. Borgeat A, Ekatodramis G, Kalberer F, Benz C: Acute and nonacute complications associated with interscalene block and shoulder surgery: a prospective study. Anesthesiology 2001;95:875–880.
65. Candido KD, Sukhani R, Doty R Jr, et al: Neurologic sequelae after interscalene brachial plexus block for shoulder/upper arm surgery: the association of patient, anesthetic, and surgical factors to the incidence and clinical course. Anesth Analg 2005;100:1489–1495, table of contents.
66. Bilbao Ares A, Sabate A, Porteiro L, Ibanez B, Koo M, Pi A: [Neurological complications associated with ultrasound-guided interscalene and supraclavicular block in elective surgery of the shoulder and arm. Prospective observational study in a university hospital.]. Rev Esp Anestesiol Reanim 2013;60:384–391.
67. Auroy Y, Benhamou D, Bargues L, et al: Major complications of regional anesthesia in France: The SOS Regional Anesthesia Hotline Service. Anesthesiology 2002;97:1274–1280.
68. Barrington MJ, Watts SA, Gledhill SR, et al: Preliminary results of the Australasian Regional Anaesthesia Collaboration: a prospective audit of more than 7000 peripheral nerve and plexus blocks for neurologic and other complications. Reg Anesth Pain Med 2009;34:534–541.
69. Fanelli G, Casati A, Garancini P, Torri G: Nerve stimulator and multiple injection technique for upper and lower limb blockade: failure rate, patient acceptance, and neurologic complications. Study Group on Regional Anesthesia. Anesth Analg 1999;88:847–852.
70. Selander D, Dhuner KG, Lundborg G: Peripheral nerve injury due to injection needles used for regional anesthesia. An experimental study of the acute effects of needle point trauma. Acta Anaesthesiol Scand 1977;21:182–188.
71. Steinfeldt T, Nimphius W, Werner T, et al: Nerve injury by needle nerve perforation in regional anaesthesia: does size matter? Br J Anaesth 2010;104:245–253.
72. Steinfeldt T, Werner T, Nimphius W, et al: Histological analysis after peripheral nerve puncture with pencil-point or Tuohy needletip. Anesth Analg 2011;112:465–470.

73. Reina MA, de Leon-Casasola OA, Lopez A, De Andres J, Martin S, Mora M: An in vitro study of dural lesions produced by 25-gauge Quincke and Whitacre needles evaluated by scanning electron microscopy. Reg Anesth Pain Med 2000;25:393–402.

74. Selander D: Peripheral nerve injury caused by injection needles. Br J Anaesth 1993;71:323–325.

75. Selander DE: Labat lecture 2006. Regional anesthesia: aspects, thoughts, and some honest ethics; about needle bevels and nerve lesions, and back pain after spinal anesthesia. Reg Anesth Pain Med 2007;32:341–350.

76. Winfree CJ, Kline DG: Intraoperative positioning nerve injuries. Surg Neurol 2005;63:5–18; discussion 18.

77. Kroll DA, Caplan RA, Posner K, Ward RJ, Cheney FW: Nerve injury associated with anesthesia. Anesthesiology 1990;73:202–207.

78. Jankowski CJ, Keegan MT, Bolton CF, Harrison BA: Neuropathy following axillary brachial plexus block: is it the tourniquet? Anesthesiology 2003;99:1230–1232.

79. Kornbluth ID, Freedman MK, Sher L, Frederick RW: Femoral, saphenous nerve palsy after tourniquet use: a case report. Arch Phys Med Rehabil 2003;84:909–911.

80. Maguina P, Jean-Pierre F, Grevious MA, Malk AS: Posterior interosseous branch palsy following pneumatic tourniquet application for hand surgery. Plast Reconstr Surg 2008;122:97e–99e.

81. Barner KC, Landau ME, Campbell WW: A review of perioperative nerve injury to the lower extremities: part I. J Clin Neuromuscul Dis 2002;4: 95–99.

82. Nitz AJ, Dobner JJ, Matulionis DH: Structural assessment of rat sciatic nerve following tourniquet compression and vascular manipulation. Anat Rec 1989;225:67–76.

83. Dobner JJ, Nitz AJ: Postmeniscectomy tourniquet palsy and functional sequelae. Am J Sports Med 1982;10:211–214.

84. Weingarden SI, Louis DL, Waylonis GW: Electromyographic changes in postmeniscectomy patients. Role of the pneumatic tourniquet. JAMA 1979;241:1248–1250.

85. Fabre T, Piton C, Andre D, Lasseur E, Durandeau A: Peroneal nerve entrapment. J Bone Joint Surg Am 1998;80:47–53.

86. Prielipp RC, Warner MA: Perioperative nerve injury: a silent scream? Anesthesiology 2009;111:464–466.

87. Warner MA, Warner ME, Martin JT: Ulnar neuropathy. Incidence, outcome, and risk factors in sedated or anesthetized patients. Anesthesiology 1994;81:1332–1340.

88. Morales-Vidal S, Morgan C, McCoyd M, Hornik A: Diabetic peripheral neuropathy and the management of diabetic peripheral neuropathic pain. Postgrad Med 2012;124:145–153.

89. Kalichman MW, Calcutt NA: Local anesthetic-induced conduction block and nerve fiber injury in streptozotocin-diabetic rats. Anesthesiology 1992;77:941–947.

90. Hebl JR, Kopp SL, Schroeder DR, Horlocker TT: Neurologic complications after neuraxial anesthesia or analgesia in patients with preexisting peripheral sensorimotor neuropathy or diabetic polyneuropathy. Anesth Analg 2006;103:1294–1299.

91. Neal JM, Bernards CM, Hadzic A, et al: ASRA Practice Advisory on Neurologic Complications in Regional Anesthesia and Pain Medicine. Reg Anesth Pain Med 2008;33:404–415.

92. Mellion M, Gilchrist JM, de la Monte S: Alcohol-related peripheral neuropathy: nutritional, toxic, or both? Muscle Nerve 2011;43: 309–316.

93. Hebl JR, Horlocker TT, Pritchard DJ: Diffuse brachial plexopathy after interscalene blockade in a patient receiving cisplatin chemotherapy: the pharmacologic double crush syndrome. Anesth Analg 2001;92:249–251.

94. Hebl JR: Ultrasound-guided regional anesthesia and the prevention of neurologic injury: fact or fiction? Anesthesiology 2008;108:186–188.

95. Uskova AA, Plakseychuk A, Chelly JE: The role of surgery in postoperative nerve injuries following total hip replacement. J Clin Anesth 2010;22: 285–293.

96. Moen V, Dahlgren N, Irestedt L: Severe neurological complications after central neuraxial blockades in Sweden 1990–1999. Anesthesiology 2004;101:950–959.

97. Kubina P, Gupta A, Oscarsson A, Axelsson K, Bengtsson M: Two cases of cauda equina syndrome following spinal-epidural anesthesia. Reg Anesth 1997;22:447–450.

98. Hebl JR, Horlocker TT, Kopp SL, Schroeder DR: Neuraxial blockade in patients with preexisting spinal stenosis, lumbar disk disease, or prior spine surgery: efficacy and neurologic complications. Anesth Analg 2010;111:1511–1519.

99. Barner KC, Landau ME, Campbell WW: A review of perioperative nerve injury to the upper extremities. J Clin Neuromuscul Dis 2003;4: 117–123.

100. Sunderland S: The relative susceptibility to injury of the medial and lateral popliteal divisions of the sciatic nerve. Br J Surg 1953;41:300–302.

101. Sunderland S: The sciatic nerve and its tibial and common peroneal divisions. Anatomical and physiological features. Nerves and Nerve Injuries, Churchill Livingstone, 1978, pp 924–966.

102. Bernards CM, Hadzic A, Suresh S, Neal JM: Regional anesthesia in anesthetized or heavily sedated patients. Reg Anesth Pain Med 2008;33: 449–460.

103. Nitz AJ, Dobner JJ, Matulionis DH: Pneumatic tourniquet application and nerve integrity: motor function and electrophysiology. Exp Neurol 1986;94:264–279.

104. Horlocker TT, Cabanela ME, Wedel DJ: Does postoperative epidural analgesia increase the risk of peroneal nerve palsy after total knee arthroplasty? Anesth Analg 1994;79:495–500.

105. Sala-Blanch X, Lopez AM, Carazo J, et al: Intraneural injection during nerve stimulator-guided sciatic nerve block at the popliteal fossa. Br J Anaesth 2009;102:855–861.

106. Jeng CL, Rosenblatt MA: Intraneural injections and regional anesthesia: the known and the unknown. Minerva Anestesiol 2011;77:54–58.

107. Moore DC: "No paresthesias-no anesthesia," the nerve stimulator or neither? Reg Anesth 1997;22:388–390.

108. Auroy Y, Narchi P, Messiah A, Litt L, Rouvier B, Samii K: Serious complications related to regional anesthesia: results of a prospective survey in France. Anesthesiology 1997;87:479–486.

109. Winchell SW, Wolfe R: The incidence of neuropathy following upper extremity nerve blocks. Reg Anesth Pain Med 1985;10:12–15.

110. Urban MK, Urquhart B: Evaluation of brachial plexus anesthesia for upper extremity surgery. Reg Anesth 1994;19:175–182.

111. Liguori GA, Zayas VM, YaDeau JT, et al: Nerve localization techniques for interscalene brachial plexus blockade: a prospective, randomized comparison of mechanical paresthesia versus electrical stimulation. Anesth Analg 2006;103:761–767.

112. Perlas A, Niazi A, McCartney C, Chan V, Xu D, Abbas S: The sensitivity of motor response to nerve stimulation and paresthesia for nerve localization as evaluated by ultrasound. Reg Anesth Pain Med 2006;31:445–450.

113. Klein SM, Melton MS, Grill WM, Nielsen KC: Peripheral nerve stimulation in regional anesthesia. Reg Anesth Pain Med 2012;37: 383–392.

114. Voelckel WG, Klima G, Krismer AC, et al: Signs of inflammation after sciatic nerve block in pigs. Anesth Analg 2005;101:1844–1846.

115. Chan VW, Brull R, McCartney CJ, Xu D, Abbas S, Shannon P: An ultrasonographic and histological study of intraneural injection and electrical stimulation in pigs. Anesth Analg 2007;104:1281–1284, table of contents.

116. Tsai TP, Vuckovic I, Dilberovic F, et al: Intensity of the stimulating current may not be a reliable indicator of intraneural needle placement. Reg Anesth Pain Med 2008;33:207–210.

117. Robards C, Hadzic A, Somasundaram L, et al: Intraneural injection with low-current stimulation during popliteal sciatic nerve block. Anesth Analg 2009;109:673–677.

118. Reiss W, Kurapati S, Shariat A, Hadzic A: Nerve injury complicating ultrasound/electrostimulation-guided supraclavicular brachial plexus block. Reg Anesth Pain Med 2010;35:400–401.

119. Urmey WF, Stanton J: Inability to consistently elicit a motor response following sensory paresthesia during interscalene block administration. Anesthesiology 2002;96:552–554.

120. Watts SA: Long-term neurological complications associated with surgery and peripheral nerve blockade: outcomes after 1065 consecutive blocks. Anaesth Intensive Care 2007;35:24–31.

121. Orebaugh SL, Williams BA, Vallejo M, Kentor ML: Adverse outcomes associated with stimulator-based peripheral nerve blocks with versus without ultrasound visualization. Reg Anesth Pain Med 2009;34: 251–255.

122. Selander D, Brattsand R, Lundborg G, Nordborg C, Olsson Y: Local anesthetics: importance of mode of application, concentration and adrenaline for the appearance of nerve lesions. An experimental study of axonal degeneration and barrier damage after intrafascicular injection or topical application of bupivacaine (Marcain). Acta Anaesthesiol Scand 1979;23:127–136.

123. Kapur E, Vuckovic I, Dilberovic F, et al: Neurologic and histologic outcome after intraneural injections of lidocaine in canine sciatic nerves. Acta Anaesthesiol Scand 2007;51:101–107.

124. Lupu CM, Kiehl TR, Chan VW, El-Beheiry H, Madden M, Brull R: Nerve expansion seen on ultrasound predicts histologic but not functional nerve injury after intraneural injection in pigs. Reg Anesth Pain Med 2010;35:132–139.

125. Orebaugh SL, Mukalel JJ, Krediet AC, et al: Brachial plexus root injection in a human cadaver model: injectate distribution and effects on the neuraxis. Reg Anesth Pain Med 2012;37:525–529.

126. Andrzej Krol, Matthew Szarko, Arber Vala, Jose De Andres: Pressure Monitoring of Intraneural an Perineural Injections Into the Median, Radial, and Ulnar Nerves; Lessons From a Cadaveric Study. Anesth Pain Med. 2015 June;5(3):e22723. DOI: 10.5812/aapm.22723.

127. Sala-Blanch X, de Riva N, Carrera A, Lopez AM, Prats A, Hadzic A: Ultrasound-guided popliteal sciatic block with a single injection at the sciatic division results in faster block onset than the classical nerve stimulator technique. Anesth Analg 2012;114:1121–1127.

128. Sala-Blanch X, Lopez AM, Pomes J, Valls-Sole J, Garcia AI, Hadzic A: No clinical or electrophysiologic evidence of nerve injury after intraneural injection during sciatic popliteal block. Anesthesiology 2011;115:589–595.

129. Gadsden JC, Lindenmuth DM, Hadzic A, Xu D, Somasundarum L, Flisinski KA: Lumbar plexus block using high-pressure injection leads to contralateral and epidural spread. Anesthesiology 2008;109:683–688.

130. Tsui BC, Li LX, Pillay JJ: Compressed air injection technique to standardize block injection pressures. Can J Anaesth 2006;53:1098–1102.

131. Siegmueller C, Ramessur S: A simple low-cost way of measuring injection pressure during peripheral nerve block. Anaesthesia 2011;66:956.

132. Gerancher JC, Viscusi ER, Liguori GA, et al: Development of a standardized peripheral nerve block procedure note form. Reg Anesth Pain Med 2005;30:67–71.

133. Claudio R, Hadzic A, Shih H, et al: Injection pressures by anesthesiologists during simulated peripheral nerve block. Reg Anesth Pain Med 2004;29:201–205.

134. Theron PS, Mackay Z, Gonzalez JG, Donaldson N, Blanco R: An animal model of "syringe feel" during peripheral nerve block. Reg Anesth Pain Med 2009;34:330–332.

135. Ip VH, Tsui BC: Practical concepts in the monitoring of injection pressures during peripheral nerve blocks. Int Anesthesiol Clin 2011;49:67–80.

136. Gadsden JC, Choi JJ, Lin E, Robinson A: Opening injection pressure consistently detects needle-nerve contact during ultrasound-guided interscalene brachial plexus block. Anesthesiology 2014;120:1246–1253.

137. Tsui BC, Pillay JJ, Chu KT, Dillane D: Electrical impedance to distinguish intraneural from extraneural needle placement in porcine nerves during direct exposure and ultrasound guidance. Anesthesiology 2008;109:479–483.

138. Byrne K, Tsui BC: Practical concepts in nerve stimulation: impedance and other recent advances. Int Anesthesiol Clin 2011;49:81–90.

139. Sauter AR, Dodgson MS, Kalvoy H, Grimnes S, Stubhaug A, Klaastad Ø: Current threshold for nerve stimulation depends on electrical impedance of the tissue: a study of ultrasound-guided electrical nerve stimulation of the median nerve. Anesth Analg 2009;108:1338–1343.

140. Sites BD, Spence BC, Gallagher JD, Wiley CW, Bertrand ML, Blike GT: Characterizing novice behavior associated with learning ultrasound-guided peripheral regional anesthesia. Reg Anesth Pain Med 2007;32:107–115.

141. Sites BD, Taenzer AH, Herrick MD, et al: Incidence of local anesthetic systemic toxicity and postoperative neurologic symptoms associated with 12,668 ultrasound-guided nerve blocks: an analysis from a prospective clinical registry. Reg Anesth Pain Med 2012;37:478–482.

CHAPTER 61

Assessment of Neurologic Complications of Regional Anesthesia

James C. Watson

INTRODUCTION

Neurologic injury following regional anesthesia is an uncommon, but dreaded, complication that creates high levels of anxiety in the patient and anesthesiologist.[1-3] Most deficits will be sensory predominant and limited in duration and severity and can be handled with reassurance and appropriate follow-up. Discerning these cases from the rare complications that require emergent imaging, neurologic or neurosurgical consultation, or treatment is vital. This chapter focuses on recognition of postoperative neurologic complications, recognition of barriers to their recognition and evaluations, and an efficient, structured clinical approach to postanesthesia neurologic complications.

BARRIERS TO RECOGNITION OF POSTOPERATIVE NEUROLOGIC INJURY

Neurologic deficits in the postoperative setting may result from perioperative anesthetic procedures, surgical factors or iatrogenic injury, nerve compression occurring in the operative theater or during postoperative recuperation, or recognition of preexisting, but previously unappreciated, neurologic disease. While recognizing a neurologic complication immediately postoperatively would strongly implicate a perioperative complication (surgical, anesthetic, or positioning), there are many barriers to early recognition of perioperative neurologic complications. Postoperative sedation or analgesia may mask the complication.

Given expected neurologic symptoms postoperatively after regional anesthesia, patients and caregivers may presume that the patient's symptoms are block related. Patients therefore fail to complain of symptoms that may be unrelated to the block, and caregivers may fail to pursue reported symptoms because they presume they are block related, when in fact they may be

distinct in distribution from the expected neurologic deficit. Patients also are unaware of what to expect postoperatively and may presume that postoperative symptoms are normal. Surgical dressings, drains, castings, and postoperative activity restrictions limit a patient's activity level postoperatively such that a postoperative neurologic deficit may be unrecognized until more normal activity levels can be resumed. Finally, patients often see the postoperative period as a single time epoch (the perioperative blur) instead of individual days where precise recognition of symptom onset would have been useful in fine-tuning the differential diagnosis regarding the cause of a postoperative neurologic complication. In a prospective study of postoperative ulnar neuropathy, some patients in follow-up reported that their symptoms were noted "immediately" following surgery, while the prospective evaluations had clearly documented an onset of signs and symptoms more than 48 hours after surgery, hence exonerating the surgical and anesthesia operative teams and implicating a postoperative convalescence complication.[4]

Given these barriers, only 77%–90% of sensorimotor and 20% of sensory nerve injury complications following total hip and knee arthroplasties were recorded during the procedural hospitalization.[5,6] Studies that only include early neurologic injury (less than 48 hours postoperatively) likely underestimate risk.[7]

Conversely, injuries recognized late often have (or perhaps more likely have) nonanesthetic/operative-related causes, including infection, postoperative inflammation, and consequences of immobilization or compression in the recovery period. The frequency of ulnar neuropathy in surgical cohorts more than 2 days postoperatively, for example, is similar to the frequency in medical patients hospitalized for the same duration.[8] These nonanesthetic/operative complications are often obvious as they occur in a distribution distinct from the surgical or anesthetic site, but when they do not, they further confuse the clinical picture.[5,6,9]

BARRIERS TO NEUROLOGIC EVALUATION OF A POSTOPERATIVE NEUROLOGIC COMPLICATION

Neurologic evaluation of an identified postoperative neurologic complication is limited by many of the same factors that interfere with recognition. Dressings, casting, drains, and activity restrictions limit the ability to perform a comprehensive neurologic examination and hence the ability to localize a nerve injury. Electrophysiologic testing has the same limitations in being able to adequately access muscles and nerves that may be discriminatory for localization. The operating room and specifically regional anesthetic and surgical approaches to various problems are generally foreign to most neurologists, and as such they may be unaware of which structures were most at risk or which mechanism of injury may be most probable from a given surgical or anesthetic technique. In many institutions, the anesthetic record may be unavailable to the consulting neurologist or when available formatted in a way that makes extracting usable information challenging for the nonanesthesiologist. Useful neurologic consultation is facilitated by direct and frank discussion between the anesthesia, surgical, and neurologic services.

Mechanisms of Injury

The potential mechanisms of anesthesia-related neurologic injury have been previously articulated[10]; however, the mechanism of injury is pertinent to workup and prognosis. Documentation and recognition of preexisting neurologic disease is important, as it may explain falsely localizing neurologic signs evident during the assessment of an apparent postoperative nerve injury. For example, hyperreflexia and a Babinski sign from preexisting cervical spinal stenosis may falsely suggest a central nervous system etiology in a patient with a peripheral nerve injury (PNI). Preexisting neurologic disease, while sometimes insufficient alone to cause clinical symptoms, limits the neurologic reserve of a nerve, meaning that it is more susceptible to developing clinical deficits from a second injury. This has been shown to be particularly relevant in postanesthesia nerve injuries, which are more common in at-risk nerves (the double-crush phenomenon).[11,12]

Similarly metabolic derangements that are frequently associated with peripheral neuropathy, such as diabetes mellitus, may have caused unrecognized PNI previously insufficient to have caused clinical symptoms, but sufficient to decrease the neurologic reserve and put a peripheral nerve at risk from a second hit. This likely explains the frequent association of diabetes as a risk factor for post–regional anesthesia neurologic complications. Preexisting systemic diseases associated with neurogenic impairment (diabetes with neuropathy, for example) likely also impair the potential for recovery following a PNI.

Vascular injuries are the most catastrophic of possible postanesthesia complications. Ischemic vascular injuries may be related to an embolic phenomenon, direct trauma, or vasoconstriction

of the artery of Adamkiewicz causing an anterior spinal artery syndrome (ASAS) or from watershed ischemia related to hypotension or vasoconstriction. Notably, spinal cord blood flow is autoregulated, and hypotension would need to be extreme (mean arterial pressure < 50 mmHg) or occur in the setting of impaired autoregulation to cause a watershed spinal cord ischemic event.[10] Hematoma formation is critical to recognize, as it is treatable; it is devastating if unrecognized. Anticoagulation or a bleeding diathesis predispose to hematoma risk, and consensus recommendations exist for antiplatelet and anticoagulation use in the setting of regional anesthesia.[1]

Infectious processes can cause neurologic impairment from diffuse involvement (meningitis or a polyradiculopathy) or from abscess formation and compression (epidural abscess). Infectious processes are obviously treatable, but potentially devastating when unrecognized.

Direct neurogenic injury (spinal cord or peripheral nerve) from needle or catheter trauma, local anesthetic toxicity, or surgical trauma is variable in its severity and prognosis. Unfortunately, once it has occurred, there is little that can be done to intervene on or improve its natural history and likelihood of recovery.

Some peripheral nerve injuries are unrelated to the anesthetic or surgical intervention, although the anesthesiologist or surgeon are often erroneously blamed. For example, there would be appropriate concern for a neuraxial complication in a patient with an epidural catheter who awoke with a foot drop, but careful evaluation may show a simple peroneal compressive neuropathy at the fibular head unrelated to the epidural catheter. In addition, while compressive neuropathies can occur in the operative theater, they commonly occur during postoperative hospitalization and the period of convalescence.[4] Similarly, there has been increasing recognition that some postsurgical neuropathies are related to an inappropriate inflammatory response directed at the peripheral nervous system.[13] These are important to recognize as they are unrelated to a specific anesthetic or surgical intervention and are potentially treatable.

Neuraxial Complications

Neuraxial complications from anesthetic techniques include epidural hematoma (EH), spinal epidural abscess (SEA), ASAS, and direct cord trauma. Fortunately, these are very rare (EH, 2 per 100,000 to 1 per 140,000–220,000 neuraxial techniques[14–16]; SEA, 1 in 40,000 to 1 in 100,000 neuraxial anesthetics[2,3,17–19]), but they can be neurologically devastating if unrecognized. With all neuraxial complications, the longer it takes to diagnose and treat, the worse the prognosis is. As such, unless the neurologic deficit is distinctly limited to the distribution of a peripheral nerve susceptible to compression (ulnar or peroneal nerve), in the setting of a postoperative neurologic complication occurring following neuraxial anesthesia, the patient needs emergent advanced spine neuroimaging.

Magnetic resonance imaging (MRI) is the imaging modality of choice given its ability to localize the catheter (if an epidural catheter intervention), differentiate soft tissue structures, define neurogenic impingement of adjacent structures (cord or root[s]), and identify preexisting, but pertinent, comorbidities (such as spinal stenosis).[20-23] Computed tomography (CT) of the spine is sufficient to identify space-occupying lesions such as EHs or abscesses that require emergent neurosurgical intervention but lacks the soft tissue discriminatory sensitivity of MRI.[24] As such, CT would not be able to identify an intrinsic spinal cord injury such as ASAS or direct needle trauma. If MRI is not immediately available on recognition of a postanesthetic complication following neuraxial intervention, CT of the spine should be pursued. It will exclude a neurosurgical emergency (SEA or EH), but if the CT is negative without resolving neurologic deficits, MRI should be arranged as soon as possible to assess for an intrinsic cord process even if it requires transfer to a facility with more immediate resources.

Clinical Pearls

- In the setting of neuraxial anesthesia, any concern for spinal cord dysfunction requires emergent neuroimaging.
- MRI is the preferred imaging modality. However, imaging should not be delayed to arrange MRI or to obtain neurologic consultation. CT or CT myelography is acceptable as initial imaging to exclude a compressive lesion.

Epidural hematoma in the setting of neuraxial anesthesia generally presents more fulminantly (75% present with deficits maximizing over 24 hours) than when EH is related to anticoagulation or unknown causes.[25] However, 25% present with a slower evolution of symptoms, and, as such, the absence of a fulminant presentation should not reassure the anesthesia team. Emergent imaging should be pursued for any unexplained neurologic deficit following neuraxial intervention.

Typically, EH is heralded by localized spinal pain at the time of bleeding onset; however, anesthesia or analgesics frequently mask this. Patients progress from vague sensory symptoms below the site of the hematoma to a dense sensory loss below this level (a sensory level) that can be identified with cold (alcohol swab) or pinprick. A flaccid lower extremity paralysis develops concomitantly as the sensory deficits become more severe, and two-thirds of patients develop neurogenic bowel and bladder as a late complication.[25] Risk factors include anticoagulation (most common), antiplatelet usage, bleeding diathesis, an emergency operation, technically challenging epidural or spinal anesthesia, and older age.[14,25,26]

Spinal epidural abscess risk factors include diabetes, immunosuppression, systemic cancer, preexisting infection, intravenous drug abuse, alcoholism, trauma, and prolonged duration of epidural catheter maintenance.[27,28] Like EH, localized spinal pain is frequently the first sign for SEA, but this is often masked by postoperative analgesia. Fevers and elevated serologic inflammatory markers follow, but in patients who are immunosuppressed, these signs may not develop. The first neurologic sign is usually root irritation in a distinct radicular pain pattern. Neurologic deficits, including sensory level, paraparesis, and neurogenic bowel and bladder, develop below

the level of the SEA with time, although a smaller percentage than with EH progress to frank paralysis before diagnosis.[29] SEA may also seed the leptomeninges, causing frank meningitis, with such patients showing signs of sedation, confusion, headache, nuchal rigidity, light sensitivity, and possibly seizure.

Anterior spinal artery syndrome results from a complication involving the anterior spinal artery causing ischemia to the anterior two-thirds of the spinal cord. This has been reported most commonly with neuraxial pain interventions, particularly transforaminal epidural steroid injections, but could conceivably occur with paravertebral procedures or neuraxial anesthetic procedures during which the needle is placed laterally in the interlaminar space. Mechanisms include embolization (particulate steroid, vertebroplasty cement, or atherosclerotic debris), dissection, vasospasm, or direct trauma to the artery of Adamkiewicz in the thoracolumbar spine or to the vertebral, ascending, or deep cervical arteries in the cervical spine.[10,30-35] Patients present fulminantly and progress rapidly to para- or tetraplegia, with a sensory level limited to pain and temperature modalities (spinothalamic tract dysfunction) with relative sparing of the posterior columns (proprioception). Hyperreflexia and spasticity will eventually develop, but in the hyperacute phase, spinal shock causes areflexia and a flaccid tone.

Direct needle trauma to the spinal cord with neuraxial anesthesia may be the most difficult of neuraxial complications to recognize. Needle insertion into the cord without injection may not cause pain. While pain would be expected with increased intramedullary pressure with injection into the cord, this may not be evident in a sedated patient. In addition, paresthesias are not uncommon with properly performed epidural anesthetics, so their presence alone does not indicate cord trauma.[36] ASA closed-claim data indicate these are most common in cervical spine procedures (including pain interventions) and are commonly associated with major morbidity or mortality.[37] The clinical manifestations and prognosis of direct needle trauma to the cord are variable depending on the site of injury and whether an injection was performed.

A diagnostic algorithm for the evaluation of postneuraxial anesthesia neurologic complications is presented in Figure 61–1.

TREATMENT AND PROGNOSIS OF NEUROLOGIC COMPLICATIONS OF NEURAXIAL PROCEDURES

The prognosis following a neurologic complication of neuraxial anesthesia can be dire: 5.5% of patients with EH and 15% with SEA die.[25,26,28,29,38] For EH and SEA, early recognition and intervention improve neurologic functional outcome. For EH, of those evacuated within 8–12 hours, 40%–66% make a complete recovery, whereas when evacuation occurs more than 12 hours after presentation more than half of patients are left with no improvement or severe residual neurologic deficits.[25,26,38] For SEA, functional recovery is significantly improved in those treated definitively before paralysis or in those with paralysis for less than 36 hours. Patients with paralysis for more than 48 hours at the time of

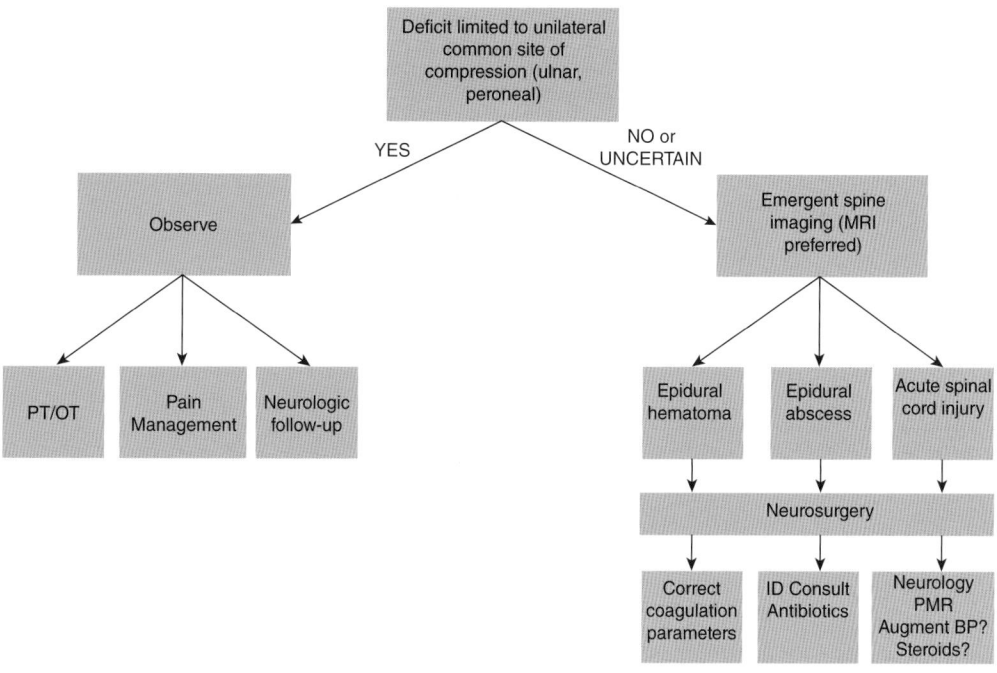

FIGURE 61-1. Diagnostic algorithm for neurologic deficit following neuraxial anesthesia. BP = blood pressure; MRI = magnetic resonance imaging; OT = occupational therapy; PT = physical therapy; ID = infectious disease, PMR = polymyalgia rheumatica.

evacuation are unlikely to recover.[28,29] Of all patients with SEA, almost one-third remain paralyzed.[29] The severity of the neurologic deficit at the time of evacuation predicts outcome, with more severe deficits at evacuation having a lower likelihood of a good recovery.[14,38] As such, for EH or SEA, the goal should be surgical evacuation as soon as possible after diagnosis, and neurosurgical consultation should be obtained immediately even if it requires transfer to a facility with more immediate access to neurosurgical services.

Clinical Pearls

- Diagnosis of a compressive lesion (EH or SEA) within or near the neuraxis demands emergent neurosurgical consultation for consideration of decompression.
- Outcomes for compressive lesions (EH or SEA) are dependent on the severity of neurologic impairment and the duration of symptoms at the time of neurosurgical decompression. Neurologic recovery is improved with early decompression (<8–12 hours from symptom onset in EH and < 36 hours from symptom onset for SEA) and with milder preoperative neurologic deficits.

Unlike EH and SEA, for which early intervention can improve neurologic outcome, there is no proven treatment for ASAS or for direct cord trauma. Almost two-thirds with ASAS do not improve, minimally improve, or die. Those that survive often require gait aides or a wheelchair for motor and sensory deficits and are left with neurogenic bowel and bladder functional deficits.[39-41]

Corticosteroids are frequently used in the setting of acute traumatic spinal cord injury. Treatment is with methylprednisolone at a dosage of 30 mg/kg over 15 minutes within 8 hours of the injury, followed by a maintenance infusion of 5.4 mg/kg/h for an additional 23 hours, having been shown in meta-analysis and Cochrane review to improve motor outcomes at 1 year postinjury.[42-44] Others have questioned the validity of this practice or the assertion that it has a benign side effect profile and thus concluded that the evidence is insufficient to recommend corticosteroids as a standard guideline to treat acute spinal cord injury.[45-48] Steroids are commonly empirically given intraoperatively with variable dosing in the setting of presumed neurologic injury. The role of corticosteroids in the setting of neuraxial complications of regional anesthesia is unknown. Considerations to their unproven use in this setting include that the postoperative neurologic complication may have been delayed in recognition, whereas the supportive data for traumatic spinal cord injury are in the hyperacute phase immediately following the injury. In addition, corticosteroids may increase the risk of postoperative infection or impaired wound healing.

Peripheral Nerve Injury

There are multiple risk factors for PNI in the setting of regional anesthesia (Table 61-1).[7,12,49-52] These include patient characteristics that make regional anesthetic procedures more challenging (body mass index) or lead to limited neurogenic reserve, putting nerves at risk from a second perioperative insult (double-crush syndrome), as well as perioperative factors.

There are three steps to evaluating a postanesthetic or operative peripheral nerve injury (PNI). (1) Is there an active process (hematoma or compartment syndrome) causing neurologic

TABLE 61-1. Risk factors associated with perioperative peripheral nerve injury.

Patient Characteristics	Perioperative Characteristics
- reexisting neurologic disease[a]	- Paresthesia with needle placement
- Diabetes[a]	- Pain with injection
- Smoker	- Prolonged tourniquet time
- Body mass index (BMI) extremes	- Positioning: compression or stretch
- Elderly	- Sedated patient during regional block
	- Prolonged hospitalization

[a]Double-crush syndrome.

impairment that can be treated? (2) Is the PNI surgically related? (3) Localize the neurologic deficit.

Similar to neuraxial complications, a bleeding complication (perineural or retroperitoneal hematoma) should be considered in patients whose perioperative interventions were performed or maintained while on anticoagulation or antiplatelet agents, in the setting of thrombocytopenia or bleeding diathesis, or if the procedure was performed in close proximity to vascular structures (particularly if the regional anesthetic was performed without ultrasound guidance). When considered, urgent imaging (CT or ultrasound) should be pursued. If identified, coagulation parameters should be corrected and, if severe, surgical evacuation to be considered.

The second issue to be considered is whether the deficit is iatrogenic, but surgically related. In a study of 1614 axillary blocks, surgical variables were thought responsible for 89% of the identified PNIs, most commonly related to direct trauma or stretch.[53] Of PNIs serious and lasting enough to require peripheral nerve exploration, 17% were for iatrogenically induced neuropathies, of which 94% of these were originally injured intraoperatively.[54] The surgical team would be aware of suspicious sutures, clips, or instrumentation placed intraoperatively, whether any nerve relevant to the patient's symptoms was directly at risk intraoperatively from direct trauma or transection, whether excessive traction was necessary, or whether there were intraoperative concerns raised regarding vascular structures, hemodynamics, or intraoperative monitoring. Cases with severe neurologic deficits and a concern for a potential surgical complication may require urgent surgical exploration. Patient care is facilitated by direct, nonincriminatory discussion between the anesthesia and surgical teams.

The final step in evaluation is localization and characterization of the PNI. This will help stratify which patients can be reassured and simply followed and which patients deserve early neurologic consultation and further workup. Localization is important as PNI is often in a distribution distinct from where the peripheral regional anesthetic was performed.[5,6,9] While this may exonerate the anesthesiologist, it still requires further assessment and arrangements for appropriate follow-up. If the clinical symptoms are sensory in nature (two-thirds of PNIs)

and limited to the distribution in which the block or infusion was performed, the prognosis is excellent, and patients can be reassured that these symptoms should resolve over days to weeks.[12,55-57] Appropriate follow-up should be arranged to ensure symptom resolution. In the rare case where symptoms persist at follow-up several weeks after symptom onset, further neurologic and electrophysiologic assessment should be considered.

If symptoms are in a territory distinct from the distribution of the block, it should be determined if the clinical findings are limited to a nerve that is vulnerable to compression in the operative theater (most commonly, ulnar nerve at the elbow and peroneal nerve at the fibular head). If the symptoms are limited to this distribution, then the presumed mechanism of injury is neurapraxia, whereby there is localized myelin sheath dysfunction, usually from compression. Even if associated with weakness, these usually improve over a period of days to weeks and can be managed with reassurance and scheduled follow-up to direct further assessment if symptoms or deficits persist. Nerve conduction studies (NCSs) can identify conduction block indicating neurapraxia at a common site of compression in the acute postoperative period and can be useful to confirm compressive mononeuropathy if there is clinical uncertainty in the immediate postoperative period. Beyond this, electrophysiology is of limited utility in the immediate postoperative period (see the section on the role of electrophysiology).

If clinical signs and symptoms are limited to a single nerve distribution (mononeuropathy) but severe (defined as a neurologic deficit causing functional limitations), motor predominant, or progressing, then early (in-hospital) neurologic assessment is appropriate, as is consideration of active treatable causes (hematoma, compartment syndrome, inflammatory neuropathy) or of a surgical complication. If the PNI cannot be localized to an individual nerve territory and is diffuse or multifocal (or simply challenging to localize), then early neurologic assessment is appropriate, especially if associated with functional impairment or progressive signs and symptoms (Table 61-2).

TABLE 61-2. Indications for early neurologic consultation for PNI.

- Deficit(s) are
  - Severe
  - Functionally limiting
  - Progressive[a]
  - Multifocal of difficult to localize[a]
- Unexplained neurologic impairment outside the block region or region of common compression
- Associated severe pain (disproportionate to typical postoperative course)[a]
- Intervening return to neurologic baseline after surgery before development of PNI[a]

[a]These features may suggest an inflammatory cause of the postoperative nerve injury.

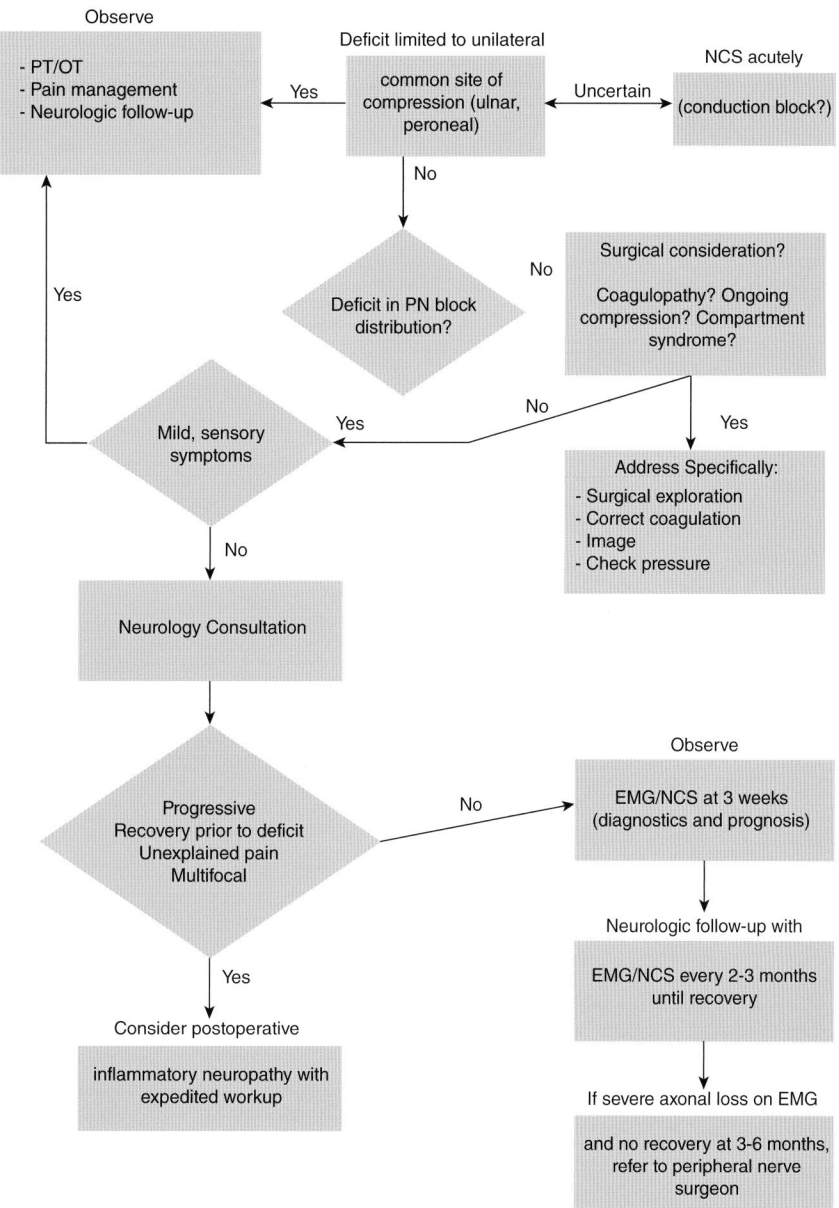

FIGURE 61–2. Diagnostic algorithm for peripheral nerve injury following regional anesthesia. EMG = electromyography; NCS = nerve conduction studies; OT = occupational therapy; PN = peripheral nerve; PT = physical therapy.

Clinical Pearl

- Once an active process that requires urgent intervention to remove something causing ongoing damage has been excluded, unfortunately there is nothing further that can be done that will materially affect the patient's neurologic functional outcome.

Figure 61–2 outlines an algorithmic approach to peripheral nerve injuries following regional anesthesia.

Postsurgical Inflammatory Neuropathies

There is an evolving literature on postoperative peripheral nerve deficits arising from an inflammatory-immune response triggered by the stressor of surgery or anesthesia that inappropriately targets the nerves of the peripheral nervous system.[13,58,59] Postsurgical inflammatory neuropathies are most often multifocal or diffuse within a limb, but mononeuropathies have been reported as well. Most commonly, they are recognized in a distribution distinct from the surgery or regional anesthetic, but they can occur within the same distribution, which makes discerning them from a direct surgical or regional anesthetic complication challenging. The temporal onset of the neurologic symptoms can be useful in distinguishing a postsurgical inflammatory neuropathy from other causes of PNI.

Classically, inflammatory neuropathies such as Parsonage-Turner syndrome (idiopathic brachial plexopathy),[60] diabetic or nondiabetic lumbosacral radiculoplexus neuropathy,[61] or postsurgical inflammatory neuropathies[13] have severe pain at their onset, developing hours to weeks after a stressor (surgery, anesthesia, vaccination, illness). The pain is usually poorly localized but often affects the proximal more than the distal limb. While it can be confused for a radiculopathy, back or neck pain is absent or limited and, in the context of a postoperative complication, mechanistically unlikely. Weakness will develop subsequently, although sometimes is not appreciated until pain has started to improve. The weakness is variable in distribution but usually multifocal within the limb. Sensory deficits accompany the motor weakness, but clinically the pain and weakness predominate the clinical picture, and there are notable functional limitations related to both.

In cases occurring during the postoperative hospitalization, perioperative analgesia and regional anesthesia (particularly infusion catheters) make recognition of the painful onset of an inflammatory neuropathy challenging. A contextual cue of an inflammatory cause of PNI in the immediate perioperative period would be unexplained, refractory severe postoperative pain distinct from that typically expected or a period of good pain control followed by the emergence of severe, unexplained limb pain. Similarly, severe pain in a region distinct from the surgery or regional anesthetic that progresses to neurologic deficits would suggest the possibility of an inflammatory postsurgical neuropathy, as would neurologic symptoms emerging, in a painful limb, after a period of documented return to baseline neurologic function postoperatively. When clinical features raise the possibility of an inflammatory postsurgical neuropathy, early neurologic consultation is appropriate (Table 61-2).

Clinical Pearl

- Clinical cues of a possible postoperative inflammatory neuropathy include atypical, unexplained, refractory postoperative pain; severe limb pain and emerging neurologic dysfunction after a period of documented return to baseline neurologic function postoperatively; and multifocal or difficult-to-localize, progressive postoperative neurologic deficits.

The cause of postsurgical inflammatory neuropathies is unknown, but biopsy of affected nerves in postoperative cases demonstrated perivascular lymphocytic inflammation consistent with a microvasculitis.[13] There is significant axonal loss with this form of PNI, and as such the recovery is protracted. The process is usually monophasic, and functional prognosis has been reported to be good (90% have good functional recovery within 3 years in Parsonage-Turner syndrome).[60] However, patients whose peak deficits are severe or located distally may have incomplete recovery. Given the pathologically proven inflammatory etiology, corticosteroids are mechanistically a rationale as a potential treatment (and often used in practice) but have not been evaluated in randomized controlled trials.

The Role of Electrophysiology in Evaluating Postoperative Nerve Injuries

Electrophysiologic studies consist of NCSs and electromyography (EMG). NCSs are electrophysiologic tests whereby a peripheral motor, sensory, or mixed sensorimotor nerve is stimulated and a recording made of the motor or sensory response. Normal values have been established using standard techniques to define abnormalities of the response amplitude (corresponding with axonal loss) and speed of transmission along a nerve (conduction velocity and distal latency, corresponding to demyelination). EMG is an electrophysiologic test whereby a small (commonly 26-gauge) concentric recording needle is placed into muscles innervated by different spinal roots, pathways through the plexus, and peripheral nerves to identify characteristic electrical changes of neurogenic, myopathic, or neuromuscular transmission disorders. Pertinent to PNI, by evaluating different muscles innervated by different peripheral nerves, EMG can help localize the site of a nerve injury as well as assess the severity of the injury and whether recovery is occurring. EMG and NCS are complementary to one another and are almost always performed together and in common practice are referred to collectively simply as EMG.

Nerve injury (from any source) can be categorized, and these categories are important prognostically (Table 61-3).[62] Most perioperative PNIs are related to compression or transient dysfunction of the myelin in a focal area of the nerve (neurapraxia)

TABLE 61-3. Classification of nerve injury.[62]

	Pathology	Electrophysiology	Prognosis

Neurapraxia	Localized myelin derangement
	  - Axons intact
	    Sensory > motor
		Conduction block or focal slowing	Excellent

Axonotmesis	Axonal integrity and transport impaired
	  → Wallerian degeneration
	  - Endoneurial tube intact
		NCS: low amplitude/absent motor
		  and sensory responses
		EMG: denervation
			Slow recovery

Neurotmesis	Axonal and connective tissue strata (neural tube) destroyed	Similar to axonotmesis, but no reinnervation on serial studies	No recovery

without any underlying damage to the nerve axon. Neurapraxia is evident on NCS, almost immediately after injury and symptom onset, as conduction block: There is normal nerve conduction distal to the site of injury and abnormal conduction proximal and through the site of injury. As such, NCS can be used in the acute perioperative period to identify patients with a common compression neuropathy (usually ulnar or peroneal) by identifying conduction block at a common site of compression. Because sensory fascicles of nerves are more susceptible to injury than motor fascicles, most perioperative compression neuropathies are sensory predominant. Patients with predominantly sensory symptoms or evidence of neurapraxia (conduction block) on NCS have an excellent prognosis, with expected complete recovery over days to a couple of months.

When the PNI results from more severe or longer duration compression, from direct trauma to the nerve (needle, scalpel, suture, staple, or cautery), or from ischemia, the injury affects not only the myelin sheath but also the axons within the nerve. When the axon is injured, axonoplasmic flow is disrupted such that the axon cannot be maintained and will degenerate (Wallerian degeneration). Because Wallerian degeneration occurs over a few weeks following axonal nerve injury, its effects on electrophysiologic testing are not evident in the acute perioperative period, and the extent (severity) of axonal injury cannot be determined acutely with electrodiagnostic testing. As such, in cases of functionally significant PNIs that are not purely sensory or localized to a single nerve territory, the role of electrophysiologic testing in the acute perioperative period is limited. It could be used to identify preexisting neurogenic injury, but the electrophysiologic effects of the acute axonal injury from the PNI will not be definitively identifiable until approximately 2 to 3 weeks following the injury.[63-65] Therefore, definitive electrophysiologic localization of a PNI and determination of injury severity cannot be determined electrophysiologically in the immediate perioperative period and can be done only 2 to 3 weeks postinjury. Importantly, while electrophysiologic testing localizes a lesion, defines its severity, and provides prognostic information, it does not elucidate the cause of the injury.

Clinical Pearls

- Electrodiagnostic studies (EMG and NCSs) may help confirm neurapraxia with conduction block or define preexisting disease when performed acutely.
- Axonal loss (prognostic) and the extent of a perioperative neurogenic injury will be better clarified by electrodiagnostic studies performed 3 weeks after injury.

The prognosis is much less favorable when there is significant axonal injury and degeneration compared to when there is only evidence of neurapraxia. Axonal injury can be classified depending on whether the injury is only to the axon (axonotmesis) or whether the connective tissue strata around the axon (the neural tube) has been damaged as well (neurotmesis), such as in transection.[62] Peripheral nerve axons will regenerate back

through the neural tube to their original targets of innervation if the neural tube is intact (axonotmesis), but not in neurotmesis. A single EMG (here used collectively to refer to NCS and EMG) study cannot differentiate these categorizations of axonal injury (any other clinical or imaging test also cannot). However, in axonotmesis, serial studies performed every 2–3 months will show axonal regeneration and reinnervation into muscles adjacent to the area of injury initially and proceeding distally with time. Electrodiagnostic evidence of reinnervation and recovery will be evident before clinical recovery. In cases of more severe axonal injury (neurotmesis), no recovery will be seen on serial studies. When this occurs, patients should be referred to a peripheral nerve neurosurgeon for surgical options. Functional improvement is improved if surgical intervention occurs before 6 to 9 months following the time of injury.[54,63,66]

Clinical Pearl

- Nerve lesions that fail to resolve 3–5 months after initial neurologic evaluation should prompt consideration of consultation with a peripheral nerve neurosurgeon.

CONCLUSION

Perioperative central or peripheral nervous system injuries from anesthetic or surgical factors are fortunately rare, and most are sensory predominant and transient. Neurologic complications in the setting of neuraxial anesthesia require urgent evaluation as delay in the diagnosis of EH, epidural abscess, or spinal cord injury contributes to long-term morbidity. In the setting of peripheral nerve injuries, early neurologic evaluation should be considered when deficits are severe, progressive, or difficult to localize.

Unfortunately, once an active process has been excluded as the cause of a perioperative neurologic injury, there is nothing that can be done to improve the neurologic outcome. However, patient perceptions of a perioperative neurologic injury can be managed by providing adequate patient education, pain management, functional assistance through physical and occupational therapy, and scheduled follow-up with neurologic and electrophysiologic consultation if appropriate. All of these should be in place before dismissal for a patient with a significant perioperative nerve injury. For patients with only sensory symptoms, clinical follow-up to ensure symptom resolution should be arranged.

REFERENCES

1. Horlocker TT, Wedel DJ, Rowlingson JC, et al: Regional anesthesia in the patient receiving antithrombotic or thrombolytic therapy: American Society of Regional Anesthesia and Pain Medicine Evidence-Based Guidelines (third edition). Reg Anesth Pain Med 2010;35(1):64–101.
2. Brull R, McCartney CJ, Chan VW, El-Beheiry H: Neurological complications after regional anesthesia: contemporary estimates of risk. Anesth Analg 2007;104(4):965–974.
3. Moen V, Dahlgren N, Irestedt L: Severe neurological complications after central neuraxial blockades in Sweden 1990–1999. Anesthesiology 2004;101(4):950–959.

4. Warner MA, Warner DO, Matsumoto JY, Harper CM, Schroeder DR, Maxson PM: Ulnar neuropathy in surgical patients. Anesthesiology 1999;90(1):54–59.

5. Jacob AK, Mantilla CB, Sviggum HP, Schroeder DR, Pagnano MW, Hebl JR: Perioperative nerve injury after total hip arthroplasty: regional anesthesia risk during a 20-year cohort study. Anesthesiology 2011;115(6):1172–1178.

6. Jacob AK, Mantilla CB, Sviggum HP, Schroeder DR, Pagnano MW, Hebl JR: Perioperative nerve injury after total knee arthroplasty: regional anesthesia risk during a 20-year cohort study. Anesthesiology 2011;114(2):311–317.

7. Welch MB, Brummett CM, Welch TD, et al: Perioperative peripheral nerve injuries: a retrospective study of 380,680 cases during a 10-year period at a single institution. Anesthesiology 2009;111(3):490–497.

8. Warner MA, Warner DO, Harper CM, Schroeder DR, Maxson PM: Ulnar neuropathy in medical patients. Anesthesiology 2000;92(2): 613–615.

9. Fredrickson MJ, Kilfoyle DH: Neurological complication analysis of 1000 ultrasound guided peripheral nerve blocks for elective orthopaedic surgery: a prospective study. Anaesthesia 2009;64(8):836–844.

10. Neal JM: Anatomy and pathophysiology of spinal cord injury associated with regional anesthesia and pain medicine. Reg Anesth Pain Med 2008;33(5):423–434.

11. Hebl JR, Horlocker TT, Sorenson EJ, Schroeder DR: Regional anesthesia does not increase the risk of postoperative neuropathy in patients undergoing ulnar nerve transposition. Anesth Analg 2001;93(6): 1606–1611, table of contents.

12. Neal JM, Bernards CM, Hadzic A, et al: ASRA practice advisory on neurologic complications in regional anesthesia and pain medicine. Reg Anesth Pain Med 2008;33(5):404–415.

13. Staff NP, Engelstad J, Klein CJ, et al: Post-surgical inflammatory neuropathy. Brain 2010;133(10):2866–2880.

14. Li SL, Wang DX, Ma D: Epidural hematoma after neuraxial blockade: a retrospective report from China. Anesth Analg 2010;111(5):1322–1324.

15. Ruppen W, Derry S, McQuay H, Moore RA: Incidence of epidural hematoma, infection, and neurologic injury in obstetric patients with epidural analgesia/anesthesia. Anesthesiology 2006;105(2):394–399.

16. Renck H: Neurological complications of central nerve blocks. Acta Anaesthesiol Scand 1995;39(7):859–868.

17. Aromaa U, Lahdensuu M, Cozanitis DA: Severe complications associated with epidural and spinal anaesthesias in Finland 1987–1993. A study based on patient insurance claims [see comment]. Acta Anaesthesiol Scand 1997;41(4):445–452.

18. Cook TM, Counsell D, Wildsmith JA: Major complications of central neuraxial block: report on the Third National Audit Project of the Royal College of Anaesthetists. Br J Anaesth 2009;102(2):179–190.

19. Hebl JR, Niesen AD: Infectious complications of regional anesthesia. Curr Opin Anaesthesiol 2011;24(5):573–580.

20. Boukobza M, Haddar D, Boissonet M, Merland JJ: Spinal subdural haematoma: a study of three cases. Clin Radiol 2001;56(6):475–480.

21. Boukobza M, Guichard JP, Boissonet M, et al: Spinal epidural haematoma: report of 11 cases and review of the literature. Neuroradiology 1994;36(6):456–459.

22. Braun P, Kazmi K, Nogues-Melendez P, Mas-Estelles F, Aparici-Robles F: MRI findings in spinal subdural and epidural hematomas. Eur J Radiol 2007;64(1):119–125.

23. Ackland HM, Cameron PA, Varma DK, et al: Cervical spine magnetic resonance imaging in alert, neurologically intact trauma patients with persistent midline tenderness and negative computed tomography results. Ann Emerg Med 2011;58(6):521–530.

24. Boye S, Schumacher J: Diagnosis of vertebral canal haematoma by myelography and spiral computer tomography in a patient with an implantable cardioverter-defibrillator contraindicating magnetic resonance imaging. Br J Anaesth 2009;103(1):137–138.

25. Kreppel D, Antoniadis G, Seeling W: Spinal hematoma: a literature survey with meta-analysis of 613 patients. Neurosurg Rev 2003;26(1):1–49.

26. Vandermeulen EP, Van Aken H, Vermylen J: Anticoagulants and spinal-epidural anesthesia. Anesth Analg 1994;79(6):1165–1177.

27. Practice advisory for the prevention, diagnosis, and management of infectious complications associated with neuraxial techniques: a report by the American Society of Anesthesiologists Task Force on Infectious Complications Associated With Neuraxial Techniques. Anesthesiology 2010;112(3):530–545.

28. Rigamonti D, Liem L, Wolf AL, et al: Epidural abscess in the cervical spine. Mt Sinai J Med 1994;61(4):357–362.

29. Reihsaus E, Waldbaur H, Seeling W: Spinal epidural abscess: a meta-analysis of 915 patients. Neurosurg Rev 2000;23(4):175–204; discussion 205.

30. Silver JR, Buxton PH: Spinal stroke. Brain 1974;97(3):539–550.

31. Mutch JA, Johansson JE: Occlusion of the artery of Adamkiewicz after hip and knee arthroplasty. J Arthroplasty 2011;26(3):e505–e508.

32. Charles YP, Barbe B, Beaujeux R, Boujan F, Steib JP: Relevance of the anatomical location of the Adamkiewicz artery in spine surgery. Surg Radiol Anat 2011;33(1):3–9.

33. Singh U, Silver JR, Welply NC: Hypotensive infarction of the spinal cord. Paraplegia 1994;32(5):314–322.

34. Tsai YD, Liliang PC, Chen HJ, Lu K, Liang CL, Wang KW: Anterior spinal artery syndrome following vertebroplasty: a case report. Spine (Phila Pa 1976) 2010;35(4):E134–E136.

35. Huntoon MA: Anatomy of the cervical intervertebral foramina: vulnerable arteries and ischemic neurologic injuries after transforaminal epidural injections. Pain 2005;117(1–2):104–111.

36. Horlocker TT, McGregor DG, Matsushige DK, Schroeder DR, Besse JA: A retrospective review of 4767 consecutive spinal anesthetics: central nervous system complications. Perioperative Outcomes Group. Anesth Analg 1997;84(3):578–584.

37. Rathmell JP, Michna E, Fitzgibbon DR, Stephens LS, Posner KL, Domino KB: Injury and liability associated with cervical procedures for chronic pain. Anesthesiology 2011;114(4):918–926.

38. Lawton MT, Porter RW, Heiserman JE, Jacobowitz R, Sonntag VK, Dickman CA: Surgical management of spinal epidural hematoma: relationship between surgical timing and neurological outcome. J Neurosurg 1995;83(1):1–7.

39. Cheshire WP, Santos CC, Massey EW, Howard JF Jr: Spinal cord infarction: etiology and outcome. Neurology 1996;47(2):321–330.

40. Salvador de la Barrera S, Barca-Buyo A, Montoto-Marques A, Ferreiro-Velasco ME, Cidoncha-Dans M, Rodriguez-Sotillo A: Spinal cord infarction: prognosis and recovery in a series of 36 patients. Spinal Cord 2001;39(10):520–525.

41. Kumral E, Polat F, Gulluoglu H, Uzunkopru C, Tuncel R, Alpaydin S: Spinal ischaemic stroke: clinical and radiological findings and short-term outcome. Eur J Neurol 2011;18(2):232–239.

42. Bracken MB: Steroids for acute spinal cord injury. Cochrane Database Syst Rev 2012;1:CD001046.

43. Bracken MB, Shepard MJ, Collins WF, et al: A randomized, controlled trial of methylprednisolone or naloxone in the treatment of acute spinal-cord injury. Results of the Second National Acute Spinal Cord Injury Study. N Engl J Med 1990;322(20):1405–1411.

44. Bracken MB, Shepard MJ, Holford TR, et al: Administration of methylprednisolone for 24 or 48 hours or tirilazad mesylate for 48 hours in the treatment of acute spinal cord injury. Results of the Third National Acute Spinal Cord Injury Randomized Controlled Trial. National Acute Spinal Cord Injury Study. JAMA 1997;277(20):1597–1604.

45. Markandaya M, Stein DM, Menaker J: Acute treatment options for spinal cord injury. Curr Treat Options Neurol 2012 Feb 3. [Epub ahead of print]

46. Pharmacological therapy after acute cervical spinal cord injury. Neurosurgery 2002;50(3 Suppl):S63–S72.

47. Sayer FT, Kronvall E, Nilsson OG: Methylprednisolone treatment in acute spinal cord injury: the myth challenged through a structured analysis of published literature. Spine J 2006;6(3):335–343.

48. Short DJ, El Masry WS, Jones PW: High dose methylprednisolone in the management of acute spinal cord injury—a systematic review from a clinical perspective. Spinal Cord 2000;38(5):273–286.

49. Selander D, Brattsand R, Lundborg G, Nordborg C, Olsson Y: Local anesthetics: importance of mode of application, concentration and adrenaline for the appearance of nerve lesions. An experimental study of axonal degeneration and barrier damage after intrafascicular injection or topical application of bupivacaine (Marcain). Acta Anaesthesiol Scand 1979;23(2):127–136.

50. Lundborg G, Dahlin LB: Anatomy, function, and pathophysiology of peripheral nerves and nerve compression. Hand Clin 1996;12(2): 185–193.

51. Kalichman MW, Calcutt NA: Local anesthetic-induced conduction block and nerve fiber injury in streptozotocin-diabetic rats. Anesthesiology 1992;77(5):941–947.

52. Winfree CJ, Kline DG: Intraoperative positioning nerve injuries. Surg Neurol 2005;63(1):5–18; discussion 18.

53. Horlocker TT, Kufner RP, Bishop AT, Maxson PM, Schroeder DR: The risk of persistent paresthesia is not increased with repeated axillary block. Anesth Analg 1999;88(2):382–387.

54. Kretschmer T, Heinen CW, Antoniadis G, Richter HP, Konig RW: Iatrogenic nerve injuries. Neurosurg Clin N Am 2009;20(1):73–90, vii.

55. Borgeat A, Ekatodramis G, Kalberer F, Benz C: Acute and nonacute complications associated with interscalene block and shoulder surgery: a prospective study. Anesthesiology 2001;95(4):875–880.

56. Urban MK, Urquhart B: Evaluation of brachial plexus anesthesia for upper extremity surgery. Reg Anesth 1994;19(3):175–182.
57. Ben-David B: Complications of peripheral blockade. Anesthesiol Clin North America 2002;20(3):695–707.
58. Ahn KS, Kopp SL, Watson JC, Scott KP, Trousdale RT, Hebl JR: Postsurgical inflammatory neuropathy. Reg Anesth Pain Med 2011;36(4): 403–405.
59. Laughlin RS, Dyck PJ, Watson JC, et al: Ipsilateral inflammatory neuropathy after hip surgery. Mayo Clin Proc 2014;89:454–461.
60. van Alfen N, van Engelen BG: The clinical spectrum of neuralgic amyotrophy in 246 cases. Brain 2006;129(Pt 2):438–450.
61. Dyck PJ, Windebank AJ: Diabetic and nondiabetic lumbosacral radiculoplexus neuropathies: new insights into pathophysiology and treatment. Muscle Nerve 2002;25(4):477–491.
62. Sunderland S: The anatomy and physiology of nerve injury. Muscle Nerve 1990;13(9):771–784.
63. Robinson LR: Traumatic injury to peripheral nerves. Muscle Nerve 2000;23(6):863–873.
64. Aminoff MJ: Electrophysiologic testing for the diagnosis of peripheral nerve injuries. Anesthesiology 2004;100(5):1298–1303.
65. Gilchrist JM, Sachs GM: Electrodiagnostic studies in the management and prognosis of neuromuscular disorders. Muscle Nerve 2004;29(2): 165–190.
66. Kandenwein JA, Kretschmer T, Engelhardt M, Richter HP, Antoniadis G: Surgical interventions for traumatic lesions of the brachial plexus: a retrospective study of 134 cases. J Neurosurg 2005;103(4): 614–621.

CHAPTER 61

CHAPTER 62

Perioperative Nerve Injury Unrelated to Nerve Blockade

Steven L. Orebaugh

INTRODUCTION

Injury to the peripheral nerve is a relatively uncommon but potentially serious complication of regional anesthesia. The fear of neurologic injury with nerve blocks may influence some practitioners as well as patients to avoid peripheral nerve blocks. The mechanisms by which nerve blocks may cause neural injury, along with evaluation and management, are discussed in separate chapters. Instead, this chapter discusses other potential causes of nerve injury as a number of possible factors may result in neurologic symptoms in the perioperative period.

To understand how the perioperative period may adversely influence nerves in extremities, even in subtle ways, ulnar nerve injuries reported in the anesthesiology literature over a decade ago are discussed.[1,2] Injury to the ulnar nerve may be the most common nerve injury associated with general anesthesia and a significant source of litigation.[3] These injuries appear to occur in the absence of obvious trauma to the involved extremity and are often delayed in their clinical presentation. The compression, pressure, and stretch at the level of the elbow all likely play a role in the pathophysiology,[4,5] and preexisting neural compromise may also be a consideration.[6] The deleterious effects of stretching or pressure on the ulnar nerve in an anesthetized patient can be prevented by simple maneuvers; for example, placing the extended forearm in supination, rather than pronation, was found to protect an unconscious patient against ulnar nerve injury.[7]

However, when an extremity is itself the site of surgical intervention, many more additional factors may conspire to result in a nerve injury. Initially, the skin is subjected to harsh antimicrobial solutions after clipping or shaving. A pneumatic tourniquet is often placed for these surgeries, with resultant distal ischemia and high pressures on the nerves of the proximal extremity. The surgery itself offers potential for sharp, blunt, or thermal trauma, which could adversely affect nerves, both at the level of small, local cutaneous branches near the incisions and at the level of peripheral nerve trunks. Non-physiologic body position may occur and held for long periods, typically involving the surgical extremity, but sometimes the nonsurgical ones as well. In the postoperative phase, long periods of immobilization in nonphysiologic positions have the potential to cause nerve stretch or compression, as do the immobilizing devices, especially in the presence of unavoidable dependent, posttraumatic edema. Combined with the lack of perception due to general anesthesia or postoperative opioid analgesics, as well as any loss of sensation caused by local anesthetics, there is risk for neural dysfunction or injury or alterations in sensory function (Tables 62–1 and 62–2).

SURGICAL TOURNIQUETS

Use of the pneumatic tourniquet for extremity surgery has several benefits, including control of blood loss and improved operating conditions for surgeons (Figure 62–1). However, the pressure created by these devices may result in muscle or nerve injury, and recommendations for safe use (and safe technology) continue to evolve. The reported incidence of complications related to the use of a tourniquet in one report was as high as 0.15%.[8] However, other large databases have reported a lower risk of injury.[9,10] If electrophysiologic, subclinical abnormalities are used as a criterion for incidence of neurologic disturbances, incidence could be much higher, especially with high tourniquet pressures. For instance, Saunders et al noted electromyography (EMG) changes, lasting on average 51 days, in 62.5% of knee arthrotomy patients subjected to tourniquet pressures set at 350 to 450 mm Hg.[11] In a randomized, controlled study of 48 patients undergoing knee arthroscopy, Dobner et al noted denervation on EMG in 71% of cases with tourniquets, which

TABLE 62–1. Potential intraoperative causes of nerve injury.

Surgical tourniquet (pressure, duration, cuff size/fit)
Positioning of operative extremity
Positioning of extremities
Incision/sharp dissection
Retraction/stretch/pressure on nerves
Electrocautery thermal injury
Insertion of fixators or other sharp instrumentation
Limb/joint over-extension or malposition

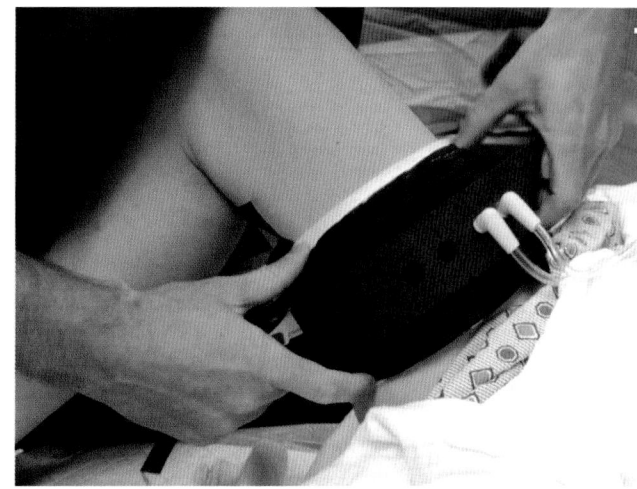

FIGURE 62–1. Application and use of a surgical tourniquet should take into account limb size, cuff size and shape, and arterial pressure. If possible, a limb occlusion pressure should be obtained, which allows for lower intraoperative cuff pressures while maintaining a bloodless field.

had a mean cuff pressure of 393 mm Hg,[12] versus no such changes in the control group, which had no tourniquet for the surgery. These electrophysiologic abnormalities correlated with delayed return of function and lasted several months.

While ischemia may contribute to nerve injury with tourniquets, actual physical compression of tissue beneath the cuff may be the dominant insult.[13,14] In primate studies, the injury to the nerve was primarily found deep to, and at the edges of, the cuff. Such nerve injuries are characterized by microvascular injury, edema formation, disruption of myelin, and axonal degeneration.[14,15]

The inflation pressure, the duration of cuff inflation, and the shape and size of the cuff are all significant variables related to tissue trauma with pneumatic tourniquets.[16] Existing evidence is insufficient to establish exact recommendations for duration of inflation to ensure that no nerve damage will occur. In general, longer durations of inflation seem to predispose to a higher frequency of nerve injury; most animal studies suggested that 2 hours is a threshold beyond which cellular injury may become irreversible.[17–21] Beyond this time, periodic deflation and reinflation is recommended, although there is no clinical evidence linking this to improved outcomes.[22]

Tourniquet cuff pressures are frequently set at 150 mm Hg above systolic pressure for the lower extremity and 100 above systolic pressure for the upper extremity. However, absolute safe levels are difficult to determine. Simple prescriptions to inflate to 250 mm Hg for the lower extremity, with a somewhat lower level for the upper extremity, for up to 2 hours fail to take into account all of the potential hazards of these devices. If incorrectly incorrectly applied, inappropriate size, or utilization

for prolonged duration are used, tourniquets can lead to neuropraxia.

The recognition that higher pressures cause more tissue damage and increase the risk of nerve injury[12,22,23] has led to a recommendation for use of lower tourniquet pressures in the past two decades, as well as an interest in finding ways to diminish blood flow to the surgical site while keeping cuff pressures low. Cessation of blood flow to an extremity is actually a function of the limb occlusion pressure (LOP), rather than simply of the systolic arterial pressure; the LOP is determined by the shape and size of the extremity and the site and conformation of the tourniquet, together with the arterial inflow pressure.[22] Interestingly, LOP does not vary directly with the arterial pressure. As such, it is unique for each patient and extremity, suggesting that it is difficult to prescribe universal recommendations for setting cuff pressure based on systolic blood pressure.

Existing pneumatic tourniquets may be modified to determine LOP.[24] Some newer tourniquet systems also feature an integrated means of determining LOP, as well as recommendations, based on this parameter, for setting the optimal tourniquet cuff pressure. Wider, contoured cuffs allow lower pressures as well, which may contribute to patient safety.[16,24]

While there are no specific guidelines suggested by orthopedic specialty societies for tourniquet management, other specialty societies have issued recommendations for safe use of these devices. Table 62–3 summarizes existing guidelines and recommendations from the literature. The Association of Surgical Technicians recommends that tourniquets on the lower extremity not be inflated higher than 100 mm Hg above the systolic arterial pressure for the lower extremity and 50 mm Hg above systolic pressure for the upper extremity—significantly lower than the prevailing wisdom might suggest.[25]

Some guidelines for tourniquet management rely specifically on the determination of the LOP. Setting the tourniquet at this level of pressure, with the addition of a safety factor (in case of

TABLE 62–2. Potential postoperative causes of nerve injury.

Inflammatory changes/postsurgical inflammatory neuropathy
Immobilization devices, such as casts/braces, with direct compression
Prolonged immobilization in nonphysiologic extremity position
Edema of extremity, within an immobilizing device
Lack of pain or pressure perception due to opioids or numb extremity

TABLE 62–3. Recommendations for tourniquet inflation pressures.

AST[25] UE: 50 mm Hg above the systolic pressure
LE: 100 mm Hg above the systolic pressure
AORN[27] Determine LOP; 40 mm Hg above LOP for an LOP less than 130 mm Hg, 60 mm Hg above LOP for LOP between 130 and 190 mm Hg, 80 mm Hg above LOP if LOP more than 190 mm Hg
Crenshaw[57] 50-75 mm Hg above systolic pressure for UE 100-150 mm Hg above systolic pressure for LE
Noordin[22] Determine LOP; base the cuff pressure on level of LOP
Estersohn[58] 90-100 mm Hg above systolic pressure for LE

AORN = Association of periOperative Nurses; AST = Association of Surgical Technicians; LE = lower extremity; LOP = limb occlusion pressure; UE = upper extremity.

blood pressure elevation during the case), allows for an overall lower cuff pressure to control blood flow, with a potentially beneficial effect on patient safety. In one series, when LOP was utilized in patients undergoing anterior cruciate ligament reconstruction, tourniquet cuff pressures were dropped by over half compared to the use of standard inflation pressures based solely on systolic blood pressures.[26] The American Society of Operating Room Nurses (AORN) recommends determination of LOP, with addition of a variable degree of pressure, depending on the patient's systolic blood pressure (greater pressures are added for higher patient blood pressures).[27] Some authors in the orthopedic literature have suggested the use of LOPs as well to favorably affect patient outcomes[22] (Table 62–3).

Since transmission of pressure to deep tissues is related to the quantity of tissue located directly beneath the cuff,[28] the pressure/shearing effect of the tourniquet is mitigated by a greater thickness of tissue between the cuff and the nerve. This explains the need for higher cuff pressures in larger extremities to control blood flow into the surgical field and the recommendation for use of lower cuff pressures in the arm of adults (as compared to the leg) and in pediatric patients.[29] In general, the lowest pressures that are effective for control of blood flow, coupled with the shortest duration possible, are likely to be safest for the patient.[23] The use of LOPs, which take into account limb size and shape, as well as prevailing arterial inflow pressures, allows for this.

Tourniquet-related nerve injury due to the pressure imparted directly by the cuff on the underlying nerve (as opposed to the distal ischemic insult) frequently results in a greater degree of motor loss than sensory loss, hence the historic term *tourniquet paralysis*.[10] In the lower extremity, tourniquet injury most commonly affects the sciatic nerve, while in the arm, the radial nerve appears to be most vulnerable.[23] Fortunately, many of these injuries resolve over time,[30] and permanent injury is uncommon. It should also be noted that, while pneumatic tourniquet use has been the subject of much research, the combination of shear stress and ischemia from the tourniquet, coupled with temporary disruption of normal

nerve physiology by local anesthetic administration, has not been sufficiently studied.

POSTSURGICAL INFLAMMATORY NEUROPATHY

Another potential cause of nerve injury that may occur in the wake of surgery, with no apparent relationship to peripheral nerve block, is postsurgical inflammatory neuropathy (PSIN). In this pathologic entity, surgical trauma with tissue damage results in immune stimulation, which is primarily expressed as inflammation of neural tissue.[31,32] This inflammatory nerve dysfunction may occur in the region of the surgery, at a distant site in the same extremity, or at a completely remote site in the body. PSIN may even develop diffusely at multiple sites. Affected nerves show evidence of edema, microvascular derangements, myelin injury and loss, and axonal injury, with influx of acute inflammatory cells.[31] Biopsy is required for definitive diagnosis of PSIN; however, magnetic resonance imaging is supportive of the diagnosis and, together with clinical evidence, may allow for presumptive diagnosis and therapy[31] (Figures 62–2 and 62–3). Treatment with corticosteroids is helpful in many cases, and while most episodes of PSIN improve gradually over time, permanent sequelae have been reported.[33]

In 2011, Staff et al. summarized the most extensive database of cases of PSIN to date.[31] A variety of different surgical types were involved, including orthopedic procedures, general surgery, and even dental cases. None of the 33 patients had received peripheral nerve blockade. The typical presentation was pain and weakness in the territory of the affected nerves; sensory changes were common as well. Twenty-one of the cases were confirmed by biopsy. The authors noted that nerve injuries may sometimes be inappropriately ascribed to mechanical causes during surgery, when immune mechanisms are actually the unsuspected cause, and that PSINs may underlie such symptoms of neural compromise much more commonly than is recognized.[31,32] Given this potential, serious nerve injuries should likely be evaluated, not only with EMG and nerve conduction studies, which are relatively nonspecific unless a level of injury can be clearly established, but also with magnetic resonance neurography, which may provide additional information regarding the severity, extent, and location of the neural insult(s).[34] If a diagnosis cannot be established, nerve biopsy should be considered.

SURGICAL CAUSES OF NERVE INJURY

Given the invasive nature of surgical procedures, unintended injuries to anatomic structures are not surprising. Injury to nerves from surgical trauma, whether by sharp dissection or insertion of surgical or fixation devices, is a potential risk of many types of procedures. For instance, in shoulder surgery, injuries may occur to the suprascapular, axillary, musculocutaneous, subscapular, or spinal accessory nerves from either open or arthroscopic procedures.[35–38] Femoral nerve injuries in the perioperative period are commonly related to ischemia from stretch or retraction occurring during abdominal or pelvic procedures.[39] During hip arthroscopy, sciatic nerve injury may occur and is

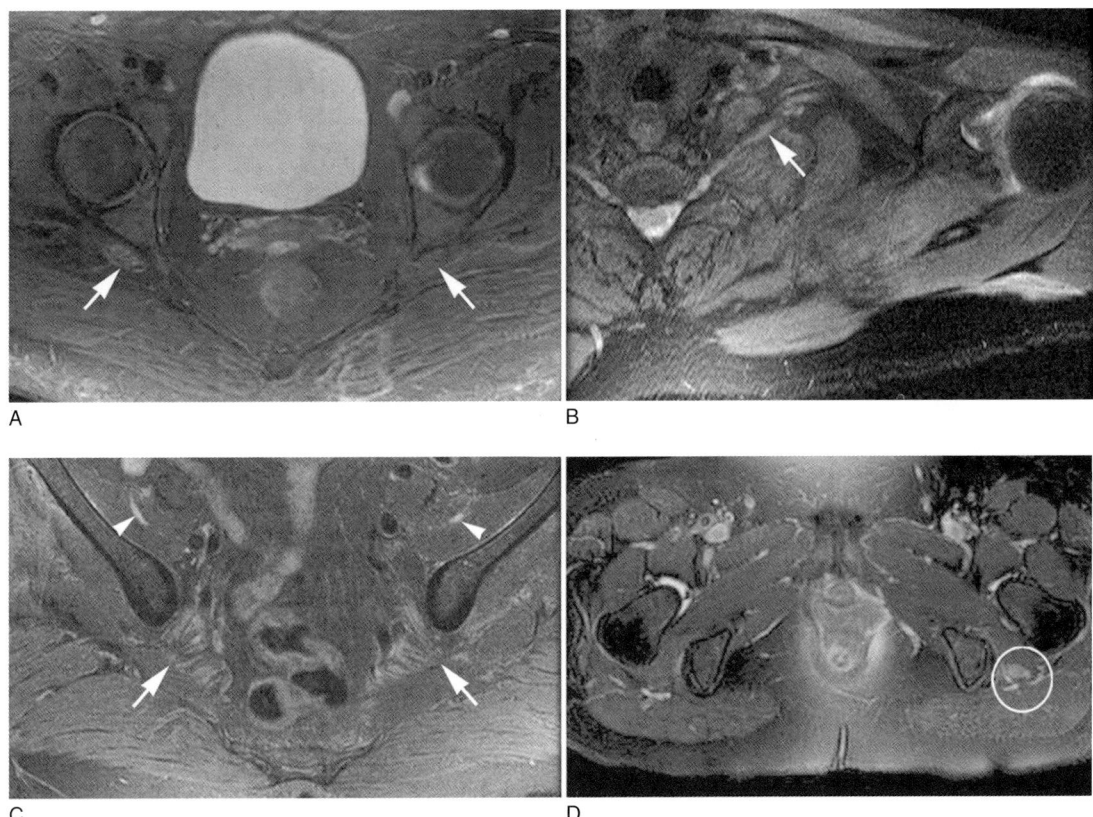

FIGURE 62–2. Magnetic resonance imaging characteristics of postsurgical inflammatory neuropathy. **A:** T_2 hyperintensity and mild enlargement of bilateral sciatic nerves, right more than left (arrows). **B:** T_2 hyperintensity and mild enlargement of left C8 root and lower trunk (arrow). **C:** T_2 hyperintensity and moderate enlargement of the bilateral femoral nerves (arrowheads) and mild enlargement of the sciatic nerves (arrows). **D:** T_2 hyperintensity and severe enlargement of left sciatic nerve (circled).

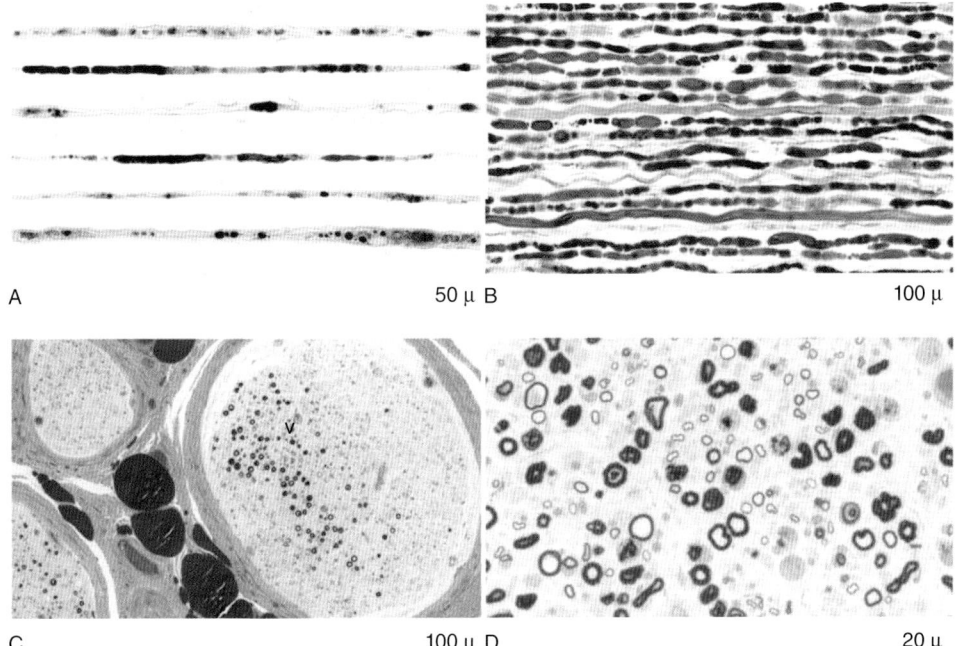

FIGURE 62–3. Axonal degeneration and focal fiber loss in postsurgical inflammatory neuropathy. **A:** Teased fiber preparation showing multiple strands with fulminant late axonal degeneration. **B:** Teased fiber preparation showing multiple closely aligned strands of fulminant early axonal degeneration. **C:** Low-power methylene blue epoxy section of nerve illustrating multifocal fiber loss. **D:** High-power methylene blue epoxy sections showing prominent axonal degeneration of large myelinated fibers.

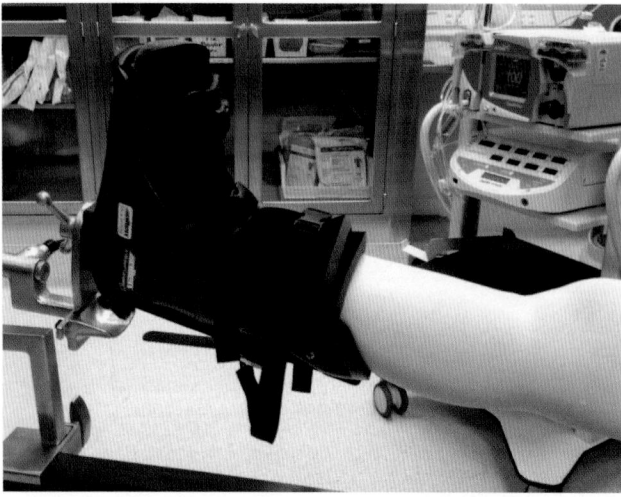

FIGURE 62–4. Hip arthroscopy surgery requires forceful distraction of the operative leg, which poses a risk for sciatic nerve injury.

most closely related to the force of distraction on the operative leg[40] (Figure 62–4). During hamstring tendon harvest for autograft anterior cruciate ligament reconstruction, injury to the infrapatellar or sartorial branch of the saphenous nerve, with consequent sensory deficits, occurs in as many as 74% of patients.[41] Fixation devices, such as K wires, may inadvertently cause trauma to nerves as well.[42,43] Aberrant anatomy may result in unpredictable positions of nerves, putting them at risk during otherwise-routine procedures.[44]

Positioning for Surgery

Surgical positioning in the operating room may play a crucial role in nerve injury and should be considered when new nerve symptoms are reported, especially when positions other than supine are utilized. Prone position, lithotomy, and severe degrees of Trendelenburg are all known to predispose to nerve injury.[45] In addition, the lateral position is more likely to result in brachial plexus nerve injury than beach-chair position for shoulder procedures[46] (Figure 62–5). In the sitting position,

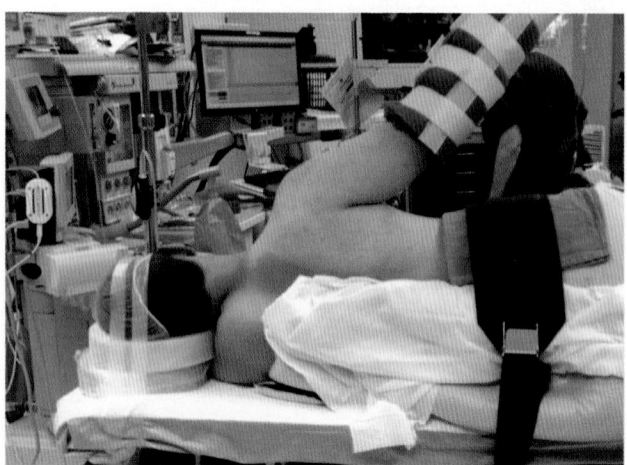

FIGURE 62–5. Lateral position for shoulder surgery is associated with a higher incidence of nerve injury.

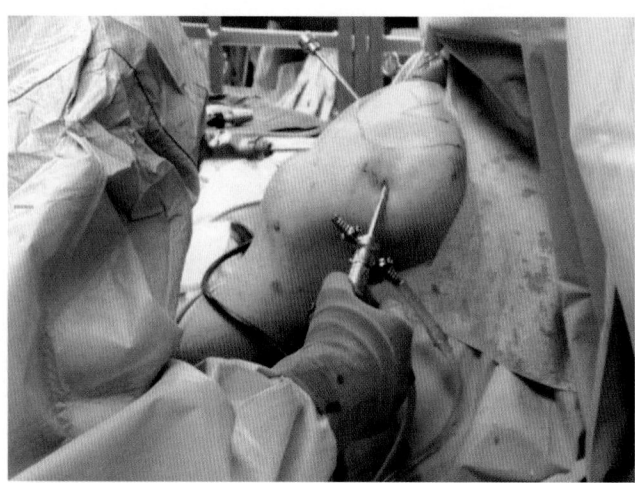

FIGURE 62–6. The beach-chair position, when adopted for prolonged periods, may result in sciatic nerve compression injury.

prolonged cases have resulted in neuropraxia to either or both sciatic nerves, including sensory loss and disabling motor weakness[47] (Figure 62–6). Lateral tilting of the head in the sitting position may result in stretch of the brachial plexus, with the potential for nerve compromise as well.[48,49]

Postoperative Immobilization

The positioning of the extremity after an operation may also contribute to nerve compromise. While immobilization in a relatively neutral position at the hip, knee, and ankle is usual for lower extremity procedures, this is not the case for the upper extremity. In orthopedic procedures for hand, wrist, shoulder, and some elbow conditions, holding the extremity in flexion at the elbow for long periods, in a sling or shoulder immobilizer, helps to protect the injured extremity and reduce the severity of postoperative edema. However, prolonged immobilization in flexion, sometimes for weeks, may be deleterious to the ulnar nerve, which is placed in a degree of stretch[5] (Figure 62–7). The combination of this position with relative immobility and the inevitable postoperative edema that occurs may predispose to ulnar entrapment, compression, and sulcus ulnaris syndrome.[50]

Another concern in the postoperative period is the immobilizing device itself. Splints, casts, and braces, if applied without regard to underlying nerves, may present a hazard.[51] Even when placed with care for potential pressure or constriction, the unavoidable edema that occurs in the aftermath of surgical trauma, especially with dependency, may serve to make a comfortable device quite tight (Figure 62–8). Compartment syndrome may result when such appliances completely extinguish blood flow to the underlying tissues,[52] and this is discussed more fully in Chapter 50.

However, even in the absence of such severe circulatory embarrassment, pressure over a nerve, with resultant palsy, may occur.[51] One example is the potential for a knee brace, placed after anterior cruciate ligament reconstruction, to impinge on the peroneal nerve over the neck of the fibula, with resultant numbness over the top of the foot and weakness of dorsiflexion[53] (Figure 62–9). Shoulder immobilization devices, with snug

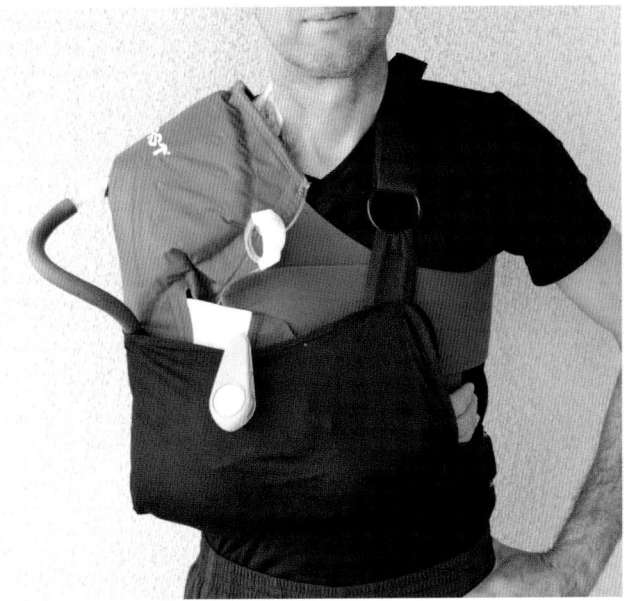

FIGURE 62–7. Shoulder surgeries and other upper extremity procedures usually require a prolonged period of immobilization in flexion at the elbow, in slings or other devices. This may result in ulnar nerve dysfunction or injury.

straps over the distal extremity or circular cutouts that lie at the base of the thumb, may lead to sensory changes in the tip of a digit, which typically resolve rapidly when this constriction is addressed, as experienced in my own practice.

Prolonged Skin Pressure

Pressure over a digital or more substantial nerve may lead to sensory or motor deficits in the territory of that nerve. However, prolonged contact with a patch of underlying skin caused by an immobilizing splint, brace, or cast may lead to sensory deficits in that region, simply as a result of long-term compression of sensory

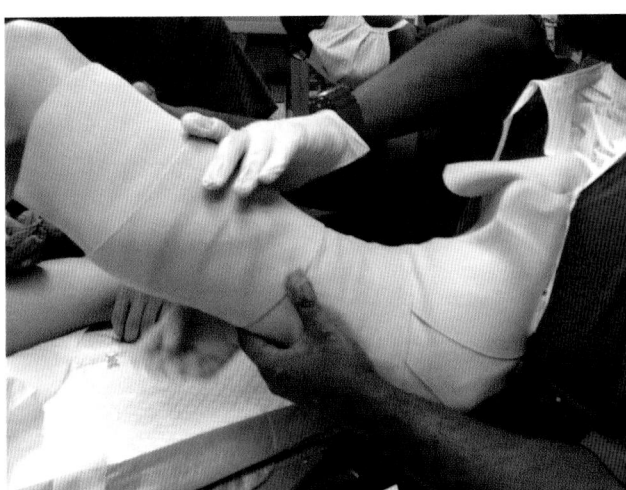

FIGURE 62–8. Postoperative casts or splints should be placed with care to avoid firm apposition against skin or pressure over bony prominences or superficial nerves, with consideration of likely edema of the affected extremity.

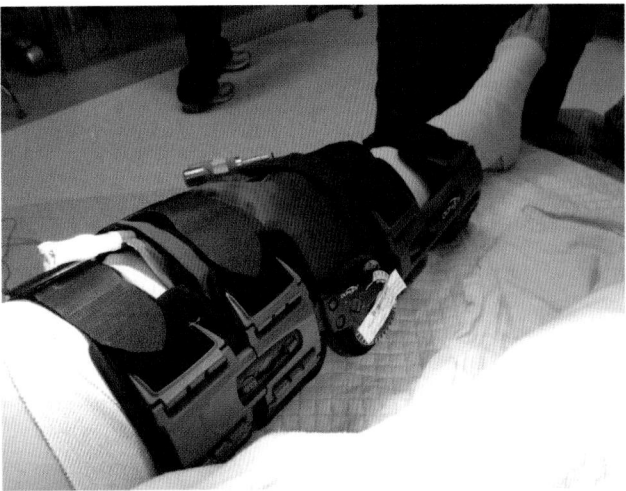

FIGURE 62–9. During placement of a knee brace after surgery, care should be taken to avoid a tight fit or pressure directly over the common peroneal nerve, which may result in sensory or motor loss in the foot.

receptors in the skin.[54] Such abnormalities of sensation would not be expected to cause changes in either EMG or nerve conduction studies. While these effects on nerve function are not, of themselves, related to anesthesia interventions, the mere presence of a protracted period of sensory alteration due to peripheral nerve blockade (whether applied by the anesthesiologist or the surgeon) may make it difficult for the patient to perceive the pressure caused over skin or a subcutaneous nerve, contributing to the potential for injury or temporary dysfunction of these tiny nerves. Of particular concern is heel ischemia and ulceration after prolonged heel rest in patients who have received sciatic nerve block.[55] Thus, careful home-going instructions and follow-up of such patients is essential.

Complex Regional Pain Syndrome

Complex regional pain syndrome (CRPS) after surgery is usually the result of the traumatic event itself, although it may also occur as a result of nerve injury, so called type 2 CRPS.[56] While this entity usually manifests with pain and limb dysfunction, sensory disturbances may be primary symptoms early in its course.[50] Severe cases may result in atrophy and weakness as well.[56] Distinguishing early CRPS from nerve injury can be accomplished with careful neurologic exam, quantitative sensory testing, the quantitative sudomotor axon reflex test (QSART), and appreciation of other changes that come with this disease. Sensory disturbances in CRPS will not likely be limited to the territory of a single peripheral nerve, as is expected with peripheral nerve injury.[57]

POSTOPERATIVE EVALUATION

Determining the etiology of a nerve injury requires integration of the physical examination, electrophysiology or imaging. When all diagnostic modalities are carefully scrutinized, the majority of postoperative nerve injuries in fact are caused by factors other than regional technique.[58] The utility of EMG as a test depends on both patient tolerance of the procedure and the skill and experience of the examiner.[59] Physical findings may add further specific information about the level of the actual nerve lesion.

For instance, in femoral nerve injury, the level of the lesion may be reliably determined to be above or below the inguinal ligament by assessing whether the hip flexor muscles (iliacus and psoas muscles), which are innervated high in the pelvis, are affected, along with the knee extensors, which are innervated in the thigh itself, below the level of arborization of the nerve.[60] A lesion that occurs proximally, in the pelvis—such as an inflammatory lumbar plexopathy[61]—with weakness of hip flexion as well as knee extension cannot be related to structural damage to the femoral nerve caused by a peripheral block at the level of the femoral crease. Similarly, a sciatic nerve injury with loss of hamstring innervation could not be attributable to trauma from a popliteal/sciatic block, which occurs at a significant distance below the release of branches to these muscles.

SUMMARY

There are numerous potential causes of neurologic injury or dysfunction in the perioperative period. Anesthesiologists should assume the leading role in establishing the cause of postoperative neurologic injury to guide therapy as well as for medicolegal reasons. This requires a multidisciplinary approach with detailed motor and sensory examination, neurology or physical medicine referral, appropriate electrophysiologic testing, as well as imaging, as detailed in Chapter 61.

REFERENCES

1. Warner MA, Warner ME, Martin JT: Ulnar neuropathy: incidence, outcome, risk factors in sedated or anesthetized patients. Anesthesiology 1994;81:1332–1340.
2. Warner MA, Warner DO, Matsumoto JY, et al: Ulnar neuropathy in surgical patients. Anesthesiology 1999;90:54.
3. Cheney FW, Domino KB, Caplan RA, et al: Nerve injury associated with anesthesia. Anesthesiology 1999;90:1062.
4. O'Driscoll SW, Horii E, Carmichael SW, et al: The cubital tunnel and ulnar neuropathy. J Bone Joint Surg Am 1991;73:613.
5. Macnicol MF. Extraneural pressures affecting the ulnar nerve at the elbow. J Hand Surg Eur 1982;14:5.
6. Alvine FG, Schurrer ME. Posoperative ulnar nerve palsy: are there predisposing factors? J Bone Joint Surg Am 1987;69:255.
7. Prielipp RC, Morell RC, Walker FO, et al: Ulnar nerve pressure: influence of arm position and relationship to somatosensory evoked potentials. Anesthesiology 1999;91:345.
8. McEwen JA: Complications of and improvements in pneumatic tourniquet used in surgery. Med Instrum 1981;15:253.
9. Odinsson A, Finson V: Tourniquet use and its complications in Norway. J Bone Joint Surg Br 2006;88:1090.
10. Middleton RWD, Varian JPW: Tourniquet paralysis. Aust N Z J Surg 1974;44:124.
11. Saunders KC, Louis DL, Weingarden SI, et al: Effect of tourniquet time on postoperative quadriceps function. Clin Orthoped Relat Res 1979;143:194.
12. Dobner JJ, Nitz AJ: Postmeniscectomy tourniquent palsy and functional sequelae. Am J Sports Med 1982;10:211.
13. Ochoa J, Danta G, Fowler TJ, et al: Nature of the nerve lesion caused by a pneumatic tourniquet. Nature 1971;233:265.
14. Ochoa J, Fowler TJ, Rudge P, et al: Anatomic changes in peripheral nerves compressed by a pneumatic tourniquet. J Anat 1972;113 (pt 3):433.
15. Rydevik B, Lundborg G, Bagge U: Effects of graded compression on intraneural blood flow. J Hand Surg Am 1981;6:3.
16. Wakai A, Winter DC, Street JT, et al: Pneumatic tourniquets in extremity surgery. J Am Acad Orthop Surg 2001;9:345.
17. Heppenstall RB, Balderston R, Goodwin C: Pathophysiologic effects distal to a tourniquet in the dog. J Trauma 1979;19:234.
18. Klenerman L, Biswas M, Hulands GH, et al: Systemic and local effects of application of a tourniquet. J Bone Joint Surg Br 1980;62:385.
19. Nitz AJ, Dobner JJ, Matulionis DH. Pneumatic tourniquet application and nerve integrity: motor function and electrophysiology. Exp Neurol 1986;94:264.
20. Rorabeck CH: Tourniquet-induced nerve ischemia. An experimental investigation. J Trauma 1980;20:280.
21. Pedowitz RA. Tourniquet-induced neuromuscular injury: a review of rabbit and clinical experiments. Acta Orthoped Scand 1991;Suppl 245:1.
22. Noordin S, McEwen JA, Kragh JF Jr, et al: Surgical tourniquets in orthopaedics. J Bone Joint Surg Am 2009;91:2958.
23. Kam PCA, Kavanaugh R, Yoong FFY: The tourniquet: pathophysiological consequences and anaesthetic implications. Anaesthesia 2001;56:534.
24. Ishii Y, Noguchi H, Matsuda Y, et al: A new tourniquet system that determines pressure in synchrony with systolic blood pressure. Arch Orthop Traum Surg 2008;128:297.
25. Association of Surgical Technologists: Recommended standards of practice for safe use of pneumatic tourniquets. 2007. http://www.ast.org//pdf/Standards_of_Practice/RSOP_Pneumatic_Tourniquets.pdf. Accessed June 28, 2015.
26. Reilly CW, McEwen JA, Leveille L, et al: Minimizing tourniquet pressure in pediatric anterior cruciate ligament reconstructive surgery. J Pediatr Orthop 2009;29:275.
27. Conner R, Blanchard J, Burlingame B, Chard R, Denholm B, Downing D: AORN. Recommended practices for the use of the pneumatic tourniquet. In Perioperative Standards and Recommended Practices. AORN, 2009, p. 373.
28. Shaw JA, Murray DG: The relationship between tourniquet pressure and underlying soft-tissue pressure in the thigh. J Bone Joint Surg Am 1982;64:1148.
29. Lieberman JR, Staneli CT, Dales MC: Tourniquet pressures on pediatric patients: a clinical study. Orthopedics 1997;20:1143.
30. Horlocker TT, Hebl JR, Gali B, et al: Anesthetic, patient and surgical risk factors for neurologic complications after prolonged total tourniquet time during total knee arthroplasty. Anesth Analg 2006;102:950.
31. Staff NP, Engelstad J, Klein CJ, et al: Post-surgical inflammatory neuropathy. Brain 2010;133:2866.
32. Malamut RI, Marques W, England JD, et al: Postsurgical idiopathic brachial neuritis. Muscle Nerve 1994;17:320.
33. Ahn KS, Kopp SL, Watson JC, et al: Postsurgical inflammatory neuropathy. Reg Anesth Pain Med 2011;36:403.
34. Barrington MJ, Morrison W, Sutherland T, et al: Case scenario: postoperative brachial plexopathy associated with infraclavicular brachial plexus blockade. Anesthesiology 2014;121:383.
35. Sully WF, Wilson DJ, Parada SA, et al: Iatrogenic nerve injuries in shoulder surgery. J Am Acad Orthop Surg 2013;21:717.
36. Rhee PC, Spinner RJ, Bishop AT, et al. Iatrogenic brachial plexus injuries assocaiated with open subpectoral biceps tenodesis. Am J Sports Med 2013;41:2048.
37. Carofino BC, Brogan DM, Kircher MF, et al: Iatrogenic nerve injuries during shoulder surgery. J Bone Joint Surg 2013;95:1667.
38. Yoo JC, Lee YS, Ahn JH, et al: Isolated suprascapular nerve injury below the spinoglenoid notch after SLAP repair. J Shoulder Elbow Surg 2009;18:e27.
39. Moore AE, Stringer MD: Iatrogenic femoral nerve injury. Surg Radiol Anat 2011;33:649.
40. Telleria JJ, Safran MR, Harris AH, et al: Risk of sciatic nerve traction injury during hip arthroscopy—is it the amount or duration? J Bone Joint Surg Am 2012;94:2025.
41. Sanders B, Rolf R, McClelland W, et al: Prevalence of saphenous nerve injury after autogenous hamstring harvest. Arthroscopy 2007;23:956.
42. Glanvill R, Boon JM, Birkholtz F, et al: Superficial radial nerve injury during standard K-wire fixation of uncomplicated distal radius fracture. Orthopedics 2006;29:639.
43. Jou IM, Lai KA. Acute median nerve injury due to migration of a Kirschner wire. J Hand Surg Br 1998;23:112.
44. Jeon IH, Kim PT, Park IH, et al: High bifurcation of median nerve at the wrist causing common digital nerve injury in endoscopic carpal tunnel release. J Hand Surg Br 2002;27:580.
45. Warner ME: Patient positioning. In Barash PG, Cullen BF, Stoelting RK (eds): Clinical Anesthesia, 7th ed. Lipincott, Williams and Wilkins, 2013, p 803.

46. Rains DD, Rooke GA, Wahl CJ: Pathomechanisms and complications related to patient positioning and anesthesia during shoulder arthroscopy. Arthroscopy 2011;27:532.

47. Wang J-C, Wong T-T, Chen H-H, et al: Bilateral sciatic neuropathy as a complication of craniotomy in the sitting position. Childs Nerv Syst 2012;28:159.

48. Lowdon IMR: Neurocirculatory disturbances of the extremities. In Duthie RB, Bentley G (eds): *Mercer's Orthopedic Surgery*. Oxford University Press, 1996, p 881.

49. Coppieters MW, Van De Velde M, Stappaerts KH: Positioning in anesthesiology. Anesthesiology 2002;97:75.

50. Borgeat A, Ekatodramis G, Kalberer F, et al: Acute and nonacute complications associated with interscalene block and shoulder surgery. Anesthesiology 2001;97:1274.

51. Arnold WD, Elsheikh BH: Entrapment neuropathies. Neurol Clin 2013;31:405.

52. Mauser N, Gissel H, Henderson C, et al: Acute lower-leg compartment syndrome. Orthopedics 2013;36:619.

53. Flanigan RM, DiGiovanni BF: Peripheral nerve entrapments of the lower leg, ankle, and foot. Foot Ankle Clin N Am 2011;16:255.

54. Guzelkucuk U, Skempes D, Kumnerddee W: Common peroneal nerve palsy caused by compression stockings after surgery. Am J Phys Med Rehab 2014;93:609.

55. Todkar M: Sciatic nerve block causing heel ulcer after total knee replacement in 36 patients. Acta Orthop Belg 2005;71(6):724–725.

56. Rockett M: Diagnosis, mechanisms and treatment of complex regional pain syndrome. Curr Opin Anesthesiol 2014;27:494–500.

57. Gierthmuhlen J, Maier C, Baron R, et al: Sensory signs in complex regional pain syndrome and peripheral nerve injury. Pain 2012;153:765.

58. Barrington MJ, Watts SA, Gledhill SR, et al: Preliminary report of the Australasian Regional Anesthesia Collaboration. Reg Anesth Pain Med 2009;34:534.

59. Preston DC, Shapiro BE: *Electromyography and Neuromuscular Disorders*, 2nd ed. Elsevier, 2005, p 3.

60. Preston DC, Shapiro BE: *Electromyography and Neuromuscular Disorders*, 2nd ed. Elsevier, 2005, p 355.

61. Laughlin RS, Dyck P: Electrodiagnostic testing in lumbosacral plexopathies. Phys Med Rehab Clin N Am 2013;24:93, 2013.

CHAPTER 63

Monitoring, Documentation, and Consent for Regional Anesthesia Procedures

Jeff Gadsden

INTRODUCTION

The incidence of complications from general anesthesia has diminished substantially in recent decades, largely due to advances in monitoring of the respiratory and cardiovascular function during administration of anesthesia.[1] The use of objective monitors such as pulse oximetry, capnography, electrocardiography, etc., allow practitioners to timely identify changing physiologic parameters, intervene rapidly and appropriately, and guide their therapeutic decisions.

The practice of regional anesthesia has traditionally suffered from a lack of objective monitors that aid the practitioner in more objectively monitoring the needle-nerve relationship and preventing neurologic injury. The practice of peripheral nerve blocks traditionally relied on subjective end points to gauge the potential risk to the patient. This is changing, however, with the introduction and adoption of standardized methods by which to safely perform peripheral nerve blocks with the minimal possible risk to the patient. For example, instead of relying on feeling "clicks," "pops," and "scratches" to identify needle-tip position, practitioners can now monitor the interaction at the needle–fascial layers using ultrasonography. Likewise, quantifying the minimal current intensity and resistance to injection can be used to gather additional data useful in clinical decision-making to minimize the risk of needle placement into an unwanted tissue plane, intravascularly, or into vulnerable anatomical structures intraneurally. Recent advances in monitoring therefore may reduce the three most feared complications of peripheral nerve blockade: nerve injury, local anesthetic toxicity, and inadvertent damage to adjacent structures ("needle misadventure").

Objective monitoring, and the rationale for its use, is discussed in the first part of this chapter. The latter section focuses on documentation of nerve block procedures, which is logical record keeping of the objective information obtained by the monitors. Objective and robust documentation of *how* a nerve block was performed has obvious medicolegal implications and provides a useful database to guide advances in safety and efficacy.

MONITORING

Available Means for Monitoring Needle-Nerve Relationships

Monitors, as used in the medical practice, are devices that assess a specific physiologic state and warn the clinician of impending harm. The monitors discussed in this chapter include those for nerve stimulation, ultrasonography, and monitoring injection pressure. Each of these has its own distinct set of both advantages and limitations and each is best used in an additive, complementary fashion (Figure 63–1) to minimize the potential for patient injury, rather than just relying on the information provided by one monitor alone. There is sufficient evidence-based information that the combination of all three monitors is likely to produce the safest possible process during the practice of peripheral nerve blocks.

Another, pharmacologic monitor, that many clinicians utilize regularly is the use of epinephrine in the local anesthetic. There is some evidence to support this practice as a means of improving safety for most patients during peripheral nerve blocks. First, it acts as a marker of intravascular absorption. Intravenous injection of 10 to 15 μg epinephrine reliably increases the systolic blood pressure more than 15 mm Hg, even in sedated patients or patients treated with β-blockers.[2,3] The recognition of this increase may allow for early detection of intravascular injection and permits the clinician to promptly halt the injection and sharpen vigilance for signs of systemic toxicity. Second, epinephrine decreases the peak plasma level of

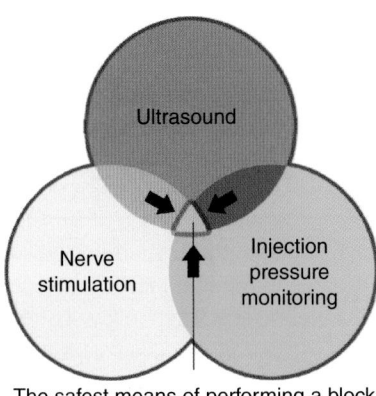

The safest means of performing a block

FIGURE 63–1. Three modes of monitoring peripheral nerve blocks for patient injury. The overlapping area of all three (blue area) represents the safest means of performing a block.

local anesthetic, resulting in a lower risk for systemic toxicity.[4,5] Concerns regarding the vascular effects of epinephrine, vasoconstriction and nerve ischemia have not been substantiated, and in fact concentrations of 2.5 μg/mL (1:400,000) have been associated with an increase in nerve blood flow, likely due to the predominance of the β-effect of the drug.[6] Therefore, epinephrine can enhance safety during administration of larger doses of local anesthetics without docummented risk of limb ischemia and neurologic demise.

Of note, the use of ultrasound guidance during peripheral nerve blocks has significantly decreased the risk of severe systemic toxicity of local anesthetics for several reasons. This is most likely because ultrasound guidance has allowed for decreased volume and dose of local anesthetic to accomplish most nerve block procedures by monitoring its spread. In addition, observation of the needle path on ultrasound, avoidance of intravascular placement, and confirmation of the spread of local anesthetic in the tissues all add to greater safety with ultrasound-guided regional anesthesia.[7]

Nerve Stimulation

Neurostimulation largely replaced paresthesia as the primary means of nerve localization in the 1980s. However, its utility as a method of precisely locating nerves has been recently challenged by data of several studies that demonstrated that evoked motor response (EMR) may be absent despite intimate needle-nerve contact as confirmed by ultrasonography. Indeed, in a number of needle-nerve contacts or even intraneural needle placement, unexpectedly high current intensity may be required to elicit an EMR.[8–10] For instance, in some instances an EMR could be obtained only with a relative current intensity of more than 1 mA even with intraneural needle placement as seen on ultrasound.

There are probably multiple factors that contribute to the explanation for this phenomenon. The most important factor is most likely the shunting of the electrical current alongside the path of least resistance (impedance). In other words, even when the needle is in the immediate vicinity of the nerve, the electrical current may not necessary chose to travel toward the nerve but rather travels alongside the path of least resistance to exit

via the skin electrode. An additional factor may include the nonuniform distribution of motor and sensory fibers in the compound nerve.

This, however, does not mean that electrical stimulation of peripheral nerves is obsolete in an era of ultrasound guidance. For instance, data from several animal and human studies suggested that the presence of a motor response at a very low current (ie, < 0.2 mA) is associated with intraneural needle-tip placement and intraneural inflammation after an injection in this condition (Table 63–1). Voelckel et al. reported that when local anesthetic was injected at currents between 0.3 and 0.5 mA, the resulting nerve tissue showed no signs of an inflammatory process, whereas injections at less than 0.2 mA resulted in lymphocytic and granulocytic infiltration in 50% of the nerves.[11] Tsai et al. performed a similar study investigating the effect of distance to the nerve on current required; while a range of currents were recorded for a variety of distances, the only instances in which the motor response was obtained at less than 0.2 mA were when the needle tip was placed intraneurally.[12]

Bigeleisen et al. studied 55 patients scheduled for upper limb surgery who received ultrasound-guided supraclavicular brachial plexus blocks. The authors set out to determine the minimum current threshold for motor response both inside and outside the first trunk encountered.[13] They reported that the median minimum stimulation threshold was 0.60 mA outside the nerve and 0.3 mA inside the nerve. However, EMR was not observed with stimulation currents of 0.2 mA or less outside the nerve, whereas 36% of patients had an EMR twitch at currents less than 0.2 mA with the intraneural needle placement.

To further refine this relationship, Wiesmann and colleagues applied an electrical current to the brachial plexus of pigs at three different positions (intraneural, with the needle contacting the epineurium, and at 1 mm from the nerve) while varying the pulse duration (0.1, 0.3, and 1.0 ms).[14] The minimum threshold current to elicit a motor response was identical between the intraneural and needle-nerve contact positions, and both were significantly lower than the position 1 mm away. Pulse duration had no effect on the minimal threshold current. These authors concluded that a motor response at less than 0.2 mA (irrespective of pulse duration) indicated *either* intraneural or needle-nerve contact. This is important because it has been established that, even in the absence of puncture of the epineurium, even forceful needle-nerve (epineurium) contact results in inflammation and potential for nerve injury.[15,16]

Taken together, the available data suggest that the sensitivity of a "low current" to elicit an EMR in a potentially dangerous needle-nerve relationship (intraneural/epineurial placement) is about 75%.[17] However, the specificity of the EMR when present at less than 0.5 mA nears 100%. In other words, a motor response is elicited by a low-intensity stimulating current (eg, < 0.2 mA according to Voelckel et al[11]), the tip is always intraneural or intimately related to the epineurium. Therefore, the utility of the nerve stimulator is obvious: Unexpected appearance of an EMR at 0.5 mA indicates a dangerous needle-nerve relationship (eg, needle-nerve contact) and may allow the operator to stop the needle advancement before the needle enters the nerve.

TABLE 63-1. Summary of recent studies of nerve stimulation current and needle-tip position.

Study	Subject	Method	Findings

Voelckel et al (2005)[11]	Pigs (n = 10)	• Posterior sciatic nerve blocks performed bilaterally
		• Two groups
		  - Injection after EMR at 0.3–0.5 mA
		  - Injection after EMR at < 0.2 mA
		• 6 hours postinjection, sciatic nerves harvested for histologic analysis
			• Normal, healthy appearance of nerves in high-current group
			• 50% of nerves in low-current group showed evidence of lymphocyte and polymorphic granulocyte sub-, peri-. and intraneurally
			• One specimen in low-current group showed gross disruption of perineurium and multiple nerve fibers

Tsai et al (2008)[12]	Pigs (n = 20)	• General anesthesia • Sciatic nerves exposed bilaterally • Current applied with needle at various distances from 2 cm away to intraneural • Two blinded observers agreed on minimal current required to obtain hoof twitch • 40 attempts at each distance	• Sciatic nerve twitches only obtainable 0.1 cm or closer • Wide range of currents required to elicit motor response • Only when intraneural did a motor response result from current < 0.2 mA

Bigeleisen et al (2009)[13]	Patients for hand/wrist surgery (n = 55)	• Supraclavicular block
		• Minimum current (mA) recorded
		  - With needle outside nerve trunk (but contacting nerve)
		  - Inside trunk
		• "Intraneural" position sonographically confirmed with 5-mL injection of local anesthetic
			• Median minimal current threshold outside nerve 0.60 mA ± 0.37 mA
			• Median minimal current threshold outside nerve was 0.30 ± 0.19 mA
			• No EMR observed at any time with < 0.2 mA when needle placed outside nerve

Wiesmann et al (2014)[14]	Pigs (n = 6)	• Open brachial plexus model • Stimulation at three positions: intraneural, needle-nerve contact, and 1 mm away from nerve • 3 pulse durations tested (0.1, 0.3, and 1 ms)	• Current intensity cannot distinguish between intraneural and needle-nerve contact • Motor response < 0.2 mA (irrespective of pulse duration) indicated intraneural or needle-nerve contact

It is universally accepted that injection of local anesthetic into the nerve carries a a risk factor for nerve injury; therefore, extraneural deposition of local anesthetic constitutes safer practice.[18,19] While unquestionably useful, ultrasonography is far from an infallible monitor of the needle-nerve relationship.[20] Because injection into a fascicle carries a high risk of injury,[21] addition of electrical monitoring of the needle-tip position is useful for safety, particularly in patients with challenging ultrasound anatomy when imaging proves to be difficult or the quality of an image is poor. If an EMR is elicited at currents below 0.5 mA, this indicates an intimate needle-nerve relationship that should prompt slight withdrawal of the needle and careful injection while avoiding an opening injection pressure greater than 15 psi. Overall, nerve stimulation adds little to the cost of a nerve block procedure, in terms of time or cost and can also serve as a useful functional confirmation of the anatomical image shown on the ultrasound screen (eg, "Is that the median or ulnar nerve?"). For these reasons, nerve stimulation should be used routinely in conjunction with ultrasound as a valuable additional monitor of the needle-tip position.

Ultrasonography

Ultrasound has revolutionized the practice of regional anesthesia and allowed a substantial evolution of the subspecialty from an art practiced by a few to a science that is more reproducible. The advantages are that ultrasound makes it possible to see the needle in real time and therefore quickly and more accurately guide the needle toward the target. Ultrasound also allows for additional injection when the first attempt is not adequate and accurately depositing the injectate into tissue spaces for reproducible nerve blockade. Also, ultrasound allows nerve blockade to be performed even in patients who are paralyzed, amputees who do not have a limb for an EMR, and so on.

Ultrasound has the potential to improve the safety of peripheral nerve blocks for a number of reasons. Adjacent structures of importance can be seen and avoided. The resurgence in popularity of the supraclavicular block is a testament to this. Prior to ultrasound, this highly effective block was relatively unpopular as a means of anesthetizing the brachial plexus for fear of causing a pneumothorax, due to the proximity of the plexus and sight of needle placement to the pleura and chest cavity. However, because the brachial plexus, and more importantly the rib, pleura, and subclavian artery can be identified on ultrasound, supraclavicular block has become commonplace in clinical practice. Regardless, ultrasound should not be thought of as fail-safe because complications, including pneumothorax, still do occur with ultrasound guidance.[22] Similarly, there are reports of intravascular and intraneural needle placement witnessed by (and despite the use of) ultrasound.[23-25]

An important advantage of ultrasound screening is the ability to determine the distance from skin to target. This, coupled with needles that have depth markings etched on the side, confers an additional safety margin by warning the clinician of a "stop distance," or a depth beyond which the clinician should stop advancing the needle to deeper tissue and reassess.

Another important advantage that ultrasound is the ability to see the local anesthetic distribution in real time. (Figure 63–2). If corresponding tissue expansion is not seen when injection begins, then the needle tip may not be *not* where it is thought to be, and the clinician can halt injection and reassess the location of the needle tip. This is particularly important in vascular areas, as the lack of local anesthetic spread can signal intravascular needle placement. On the other hand, ultrasound monitoring can be used to diagnose intra-arterial needle-tip placement when an echogenic "blush" is noted in the lumen of the artery, decreasing the risk of systemic toxicity.[26,27]

Ultrasonography appears to decrease the risk of local anesthetic systemic toxicity (LAST).[28,29] In one analysis of a large, multicenter registry of peripheral nerve blocks (>25,000 peripheral nerve blocks), the risk of LAST was reduced by greater than 65% with the use of ultrasound guidance.[28] The mechanism proposed by the authors was the ability to substantially reduce the volumes and doses of local anesthetic required to accomplish regional block. Indeed, decreasing the dose and volume of local anesthetic needed for success of regional anesthesia has been a consistent trend over the last decade. Numerous reports have documented substantial reductions in the volume required to effect an equivalent block as compared to pre-ultrasound–guided regional anesthesia techniques.[30,31] For instance, brachial plexus blocks can be performed with as little as less than 10 mL of local anesthetic, without sacrifice in effectiveness of anesthesia or analgesia.[32-34] Even if the entire volume of injectate is administered intravenously by accident, severe LAST resulting from, for example, a volume of 7 mL of 0.5% ropivacaine in an adult of average size is unlikely.

In contrast, the use of ultrasound guidance during peripheral nerve blocks has not decreased the risk or incidence of nerve injury. This disappointing observation was documented in several reports and is likely multifactorial. Ability to discern the needle-nerve relationship is user and anatomy dependent. In fact, studies have demonstrated that practitioners may miss approximately as much as one in six intraneural injections.[35-37] Second, the current resolution of the ultrasound machine may not be adequate to discern between an intra- versus

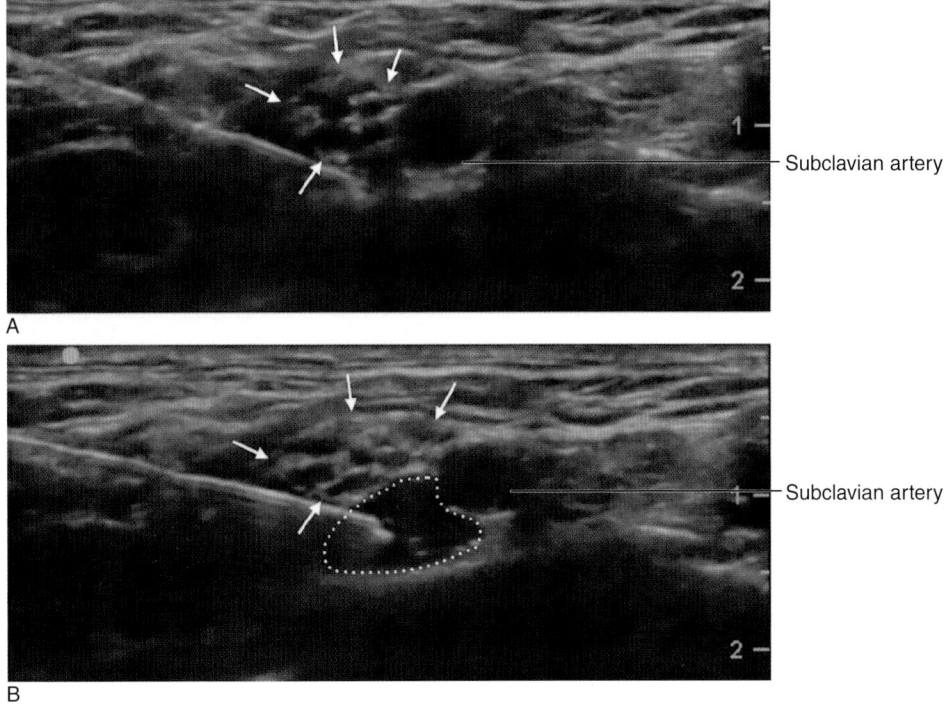

A

B

FIGURE 63–2. Supraclavicular brachial plexus block showing plexus (arrows) adjacent to subclavian artery (SA). **A** Before and **B** after deposition of 10 mL of local anesthetic (dotted outline).

extrafascicular needle-tip location. This difference is crucial, as an intraneural (but extrafascicular) injection is likely not associated with injury, whereas injection inside the fascicles themselves produces clinical and histological damage.[21,38] Importantly, one cannot rely on the nerve swelling as warning of an intraneural injection because once this is noted on ultrasound, it may be too late to prevent injury. This is because even a miniscule amount of local anesthetic will produce damage if injected into the fascicule, yet such small quantities of local anesthetic (eg, 0.1–0.5 mL) may not be detected by ultrasound.[39] Therefore, reliance on the visual confirmation of tissue expansion may result in damage before expansion is detected on the screen.

Injection Pressure Monitoring

An injection of lidocaine while the needle tip was in an intrafascicular position in canine sciatic nerves was associated with high opening pressure (>20 psi), followed by a return of injection pressure tracing to normal (ie, < 5 psi) after fascicular rupture. In contrast, perineural and intraneural extrafascicular injections yielded low opening and injection pressures.[21] The limbs in which sciatic nerve injections were associated high opening injection pressures experienced clinical signs of neuropathy (muscle wasting, weakness) as well as histological evidence of neurologic injury (inflammation, disruption of the nerve architecture). The implication is that injection into a low-compliance compartment, such as within perineurium-bound fascicles, requires high opening injection pressure before the injection can be initiated.

The intraneural needle-tip position is also associated with high opening injection pressures in human cadavers. Orebaugh et al placed needles into cadaveric cervical roots using ultrasound and quantified the pressure over the course of a 5-mL injection of ropivacaine and ink over 15 s.[40] In contrast to the control needles placed outside the roots (peak pressure < 20 psi), the intraneural injections resulted in a mean peak pressure of 49 psi (range 37–66 psi). Similarly, Krol et al performed ultrasound-guided injections intraneurally and perineurally in more distal nerves in fresh human cadavers (median, ulnar, and radial nerves) and also reported that the opening injection pressure was more than 15 psi intraneurally, while extraneural opening injection pressures were less than 10 psi.[41]

In a clinical study of 16 patients undergoing shoulder surgery, needle-nerve contact during interscalene brachial plexus block was associated with an opening injection greater than 15 psi.[42] In fact, at the needle-nerve contact and just before needle entry into the roots of the brachial plexus, the flow of injectate was not able to commence at pressures less than 15 psi. Halting an injection when the required opening injection pressure to commence an injection reached 15 psi allowed avoidance of injection in this hazardous position in 97% of subjects. In contrast, a needle position 1 mm away from the nerve was associated with the initiation of flow at opening pressures less than 15 psi. Therefore, as a monitor of needle-nerve contact, an opening injection pressure greater than 15 psi was far more sensitive than a minimum threshold current of either 0.5 or 0.2 mA or occurrence of paresthesia.

These data suggest that when the pressure in the system approaches 15 psi without the ability to commence flow of injectate, this high opening injection pressure may signal a dangerous needle-nerve relationship or needle placement in wrong tissue plane. Therefore, the injection should be halted and needle position reevaluated.

How should injection pressure be monitored? The use of "hand feel" to avoid high injection pressure is unfortunately not reliable. Studies of experienced practitioners blinded to the injection pressure and asked to perform a mock injection using standard equipment revealed wide variations in applied pressure, some grossly exceeding the established thresholds for safety.[43] Similarly, anesthesiologists performed poorly when asked to distinguish between intraneural injection and injection into other tissues, such as muscle or tendon, in an animal model.[44] Therefore, the only meaningful and reproducible monitoring is by using an objective and quantifiable method of monitoring opening injection pressure.

While the practice of injection pressure monitoring during peripheral nerve blocks is relatively new, there are several monitoring options. Tsui et al described a "compressed air injection technique" by which 10 mL of air is drawn into the syringe along with the local anesthetic.[45] Holding the syringe upright, a maximum threshold of 1 atm (or 14.7 psi) can be avoided by allowing only the gas portion of the syringe contents to compress to half of its original volume, or 5 mL (Figure 63–3). This is based on Boyle's law, which states that pressure × volume must be constant. A pressure of 20 psi or less is considered to be a safe threshold for initiating injection during peripheral nerve blocks. Boyle's law has also been employed in another simple apparatus using a four-way stopcock and a 1-mL syringe filled with air.[46] If, during the initiation of injection, the fluid meniscus reaches the halfway point in the 1-mL syringe (ie, 0.5 mL), this is indicative of doubling of the pressure in the system (ie, another atmosphere or 14.7 psi). These are both inexpensive and ubiquitously

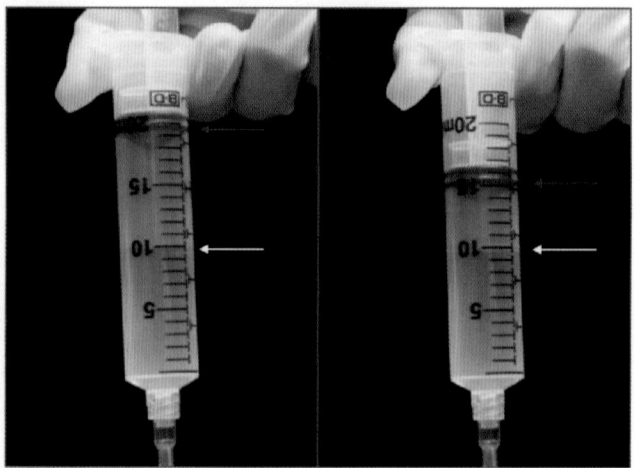

FIGURE 63–3. The compressed air injection technique. A 10-mL bubble of air is placed in the syringe of local anesthetic, which is then inverted. Compression of that bubble in a closed system to half of its original volume (ie, 5 mL) will increase the pressure in the system by 1 atm (14.7 psi).

available ways to limit injection pressure during peripheral nerve blocks. Practical limitations include the need either to hold the syringe upright or to periodically turn the stopcock to the 1-mL syringe off when aspirating so air is not allowed to enter the injection tubing.

Another option to monitor injection pressure is the use of in-line, disposable pressure manometers specifically manufactured for this purpose. These devices bridge the syringe and needle tubing and, via a spring-loaded piston, allow the clinician to continuously monitoring the pressure in the syringe-tubing-needle system. On the shaft of the piston are markings delineating three different pressure thresholds: less than 15 psi, 15–20 psi, and more than 20 psi (Figure 63–4). An advantage of this method is the ease with which an assistant who is performing the injection can read and communicate the attained pressures. This method also allows objective documentation of the injection pressure during a peripheral nerve block procedure. Importantly, the opening pressure (pressure at which the flow begins) is independent of the size of the syringe, tubing, and needle or injection speed (Pascal's law) (Figure 63–5). While greater pressure can be generated by a smaller syringe and higher injection pressure can be attained by fast injection, the opening pressure at which the flow begins is the same and independent of these variables for common syringe-tubing-needle sizes (ie, 18–25 gauge). When the injection begins, however, these factors will influence the attained injection pressure. Therefore, a slow, steady injection speed is suggested with all nerve block procedures (10–15 mL/min). The opening injection pressure becomes relevant with every needle reposition and consequent injection.

Pressure monitoring may be a useful safety monitor in several other aspects of peripheral nerve blocks. In a study of patients receiving lumbar plexus blocks randomized to low (<15 psi) versus high (>20 psi) pressures, Gadsden et al demonstrated that 60% of patients in the high-pressure group experienced a bilateral epidural block.[47] Furthermore, 50% of the patients in the same group developed an epidural block in the thoracic distribution, whereas no patient in the low-pressure group experienced bilateral or epidural blockade. Similarly, Gautier et al demonstrated that when volunteers were randomized to low (<15 psi) versus high (>20 psi) pressures during interscalene brachial plexus block, cervical epidural spread occurred in 11% of high-pressure injections (vs 0% in the low-pressure group).[48] In addition, all subjects requested that the injection be halted in the high-pressure condition due to discomfort, but not during the low-pressure injection. These data suggest that monitoring opening injection pressure is important for several aspects of safety and patient comfort during the practice of peripheral nerve blocks.

Summary

Regional anesthesia has been making a transition from art to science, as more rigorous and precise means of locating nerves are developed. The same process should be expected for monitoring peripheral blockade. The use of neurostimulation, ultrasonography, and injection pressure monitoring

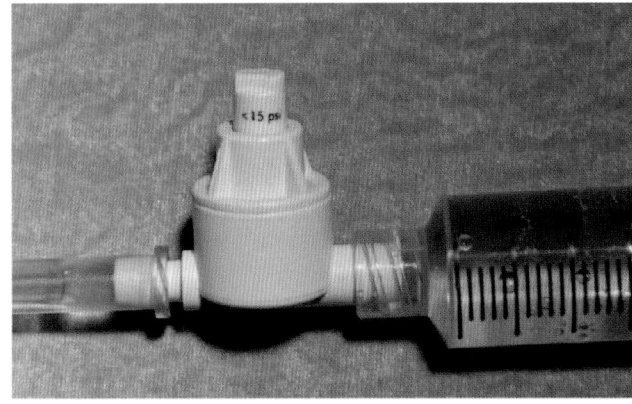

A

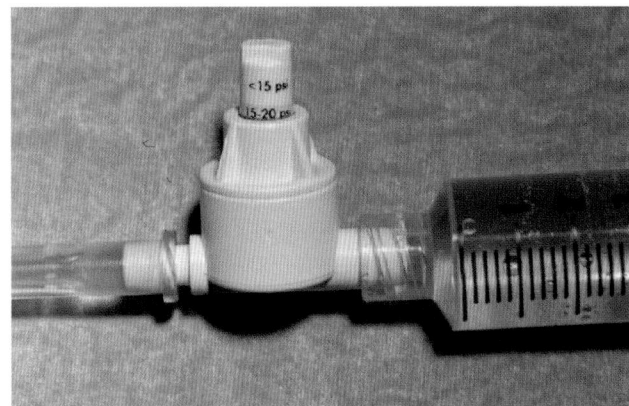

B

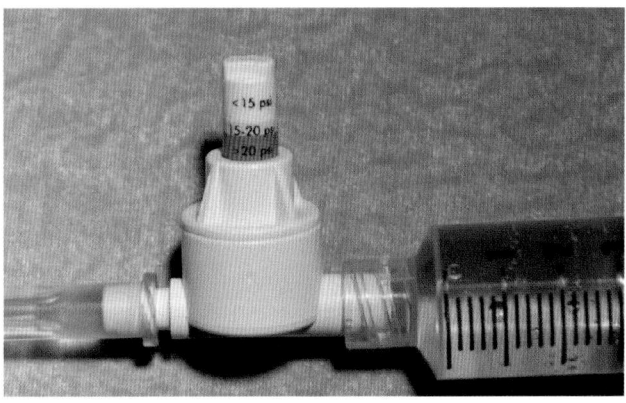

C

FIGURE 63–4. An example of a commercially available in-line pressure manometer (B-Smart, B. Braun Medical, Bethlehem, PA). As seen in **A–C**, respectively, the monitor displays pressure ranges in color on the movable piston: 0–15 psi (white), 15–20 psi (yellow), and more than 20 psi (orange). In clinical use, the exact opening injection pressure (OIP) is less important than prevention of exceeding the range of OIP associated with fascicular injury (>15 psi). Practically, this is avoided by aborting the injection with appearance of *any* color on the piston throughout the injection cycle (>15 psi). Importantly, opening pressure (pressure at which the flow begins) is independent of the size of the syringe, tubing, and needle or injection speed (Pascal's law).

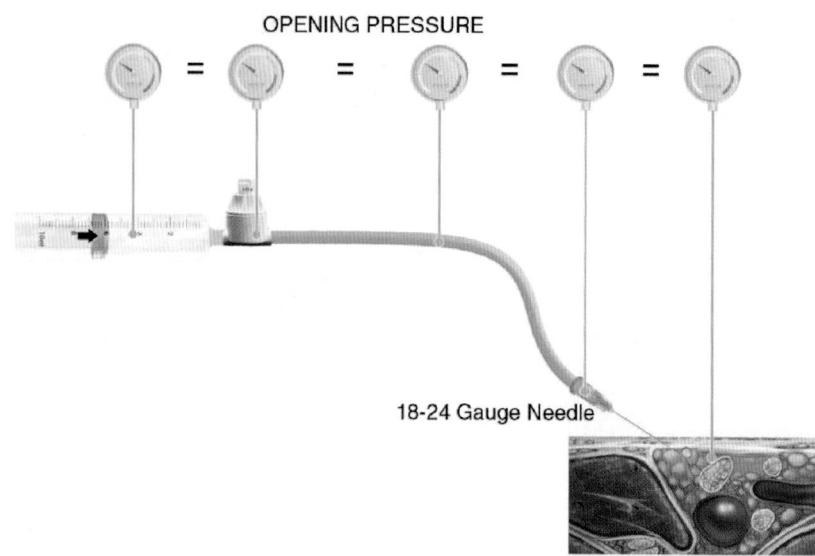

OPENING PRESSURE

18-24 Gauge Needle

FIGURE 63–5. Opening injection pressure (pressure at which the flow begins) is independent of the size of the syringe, tubing, and needle or injection speed, and it is equal throughout the injection system (Pascal's law).

together provides a complementary package of objective data that can guide clinicians to perform the safest blocks possible.

Figure 63–6 is a flowchart outlining how these monitors are used in our practice.

DOCUMENTATION

Block Procedure Notes

Documentation of nerve block procedures has, lagged behind the documentation of general anesthesia, and it is often relegated to a few scribbled lines in the corner of the anesthetic record. Increasing pressure from legal, billing, and regulatory sources has provoked an effort to improve the documentation for peripheral nerve blocks. Samples of a peripheral nerve block documentation form that incorporates all of the monitoring elements mentioned previously in this chapter are shown in Figures 63–7 and 63–8. These can be adopted and modified to suit individual practices. The forms have a number of features that should be considered by institutions attempting to formulate their own procedure note. These include the following:

Paper records are increasingly being replaced with electronic medical record-keeping systems. Block documentation

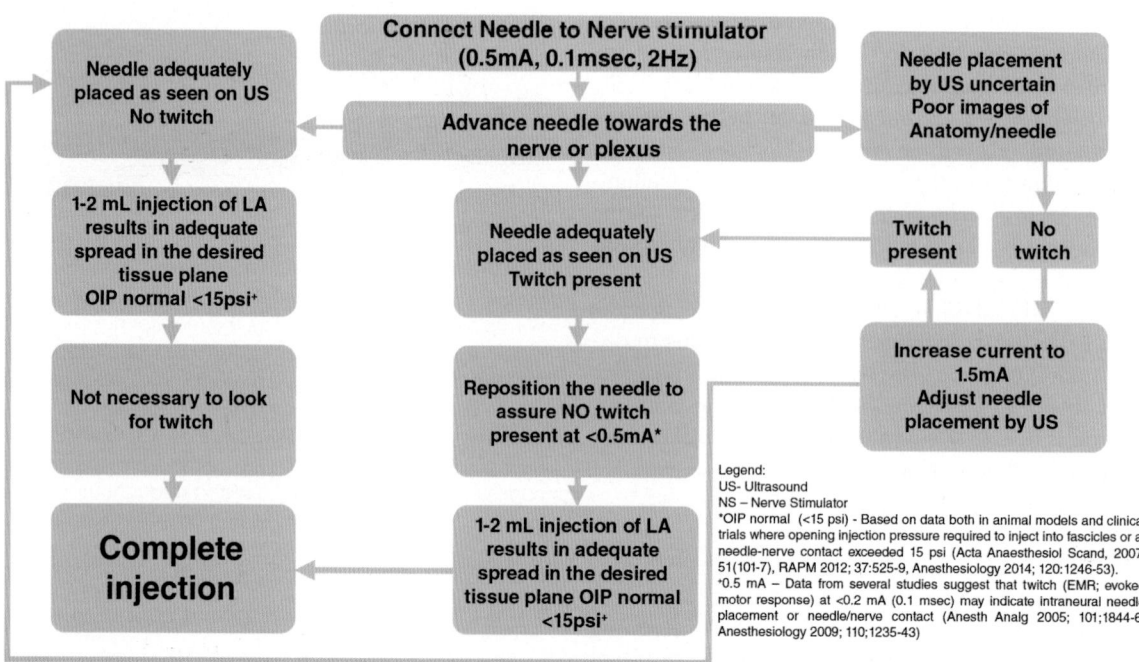

FIGURE 63–6. Flowchart depicting the order of correctly monitoring nerve block procedures by combining ultrasound (US), nerve stimulation (NS), and injection pressure monitoring. LA = local anesthetic.

Regional Anesthesia Procedure Form

Date		Time Out (time)	
Consult/Block Requested By		
Pre-op Diagnosis		
Surgical Procedure		
Purpose of Block	☐ Surgical ☐ Postop Pain	
Block Procedure Location		

Patient Identification Sticker

Side:

Monitors	Premedication	Level of Sedation/Anesthesia
Full ASA monitoring: ☐	Midazolam (mg)	No sedation ☐
Oxygen by:	Fentanyl (mcg)	Sedated, easily arousable, conversant ☐
Other:	Alfentanil (mcg)	Deep sedation/general anesthesia ☐
	Other:	Neuraxial Anesthesia in situ ☐

Block Procedure: _____ Ultrasound Guidance ☐ **[76942]**

Technique: ☐ single injection   ☐ continuous   ☐ nerve-stimulator guided   ☐ landmark-based

Needle/Catheter	Sterility
Type/Size:	☐ Aseptic skin prep ☐ Sterile drape(s) ☐ Sterile gloves ☐ Sterile transducer cover

Local Anesthetic & Additives

Type/Concentration: _____   ☐ Epinephrine (concentration: _____)

Volume: _____ mL   ☐ Bicarbonate (0.1 mEq/ml) ☐ _____

Procedure Notes

☐ Skin anesthetized with local anesthetic   Patient Position:

Needle depth: ____ cm   Minimal current: ____ mA   Motor response: _____ ☐ No response <0.2 mA

If ultrasound guided: ☐ In-plane   ☐ Out-of-plane   ☐ Local anesthetic directly observed spreading adjacent to nerve

Catheter tip location confirmed by: ☐ Ultrasound   ☐ Motor stimulation   Depth at skin: _____ cm

Blood aspirated: _____   Action taken: _____

Pain on injection: _____   Action taken: _____

Injection pressure <15 psi: _____   Action taken: _____

Other notes:

Resident/Fellow:	Signature:		
Attending:	Signature:	Date:	Time:

FIGURE 63–7. Example of a block documentation form.

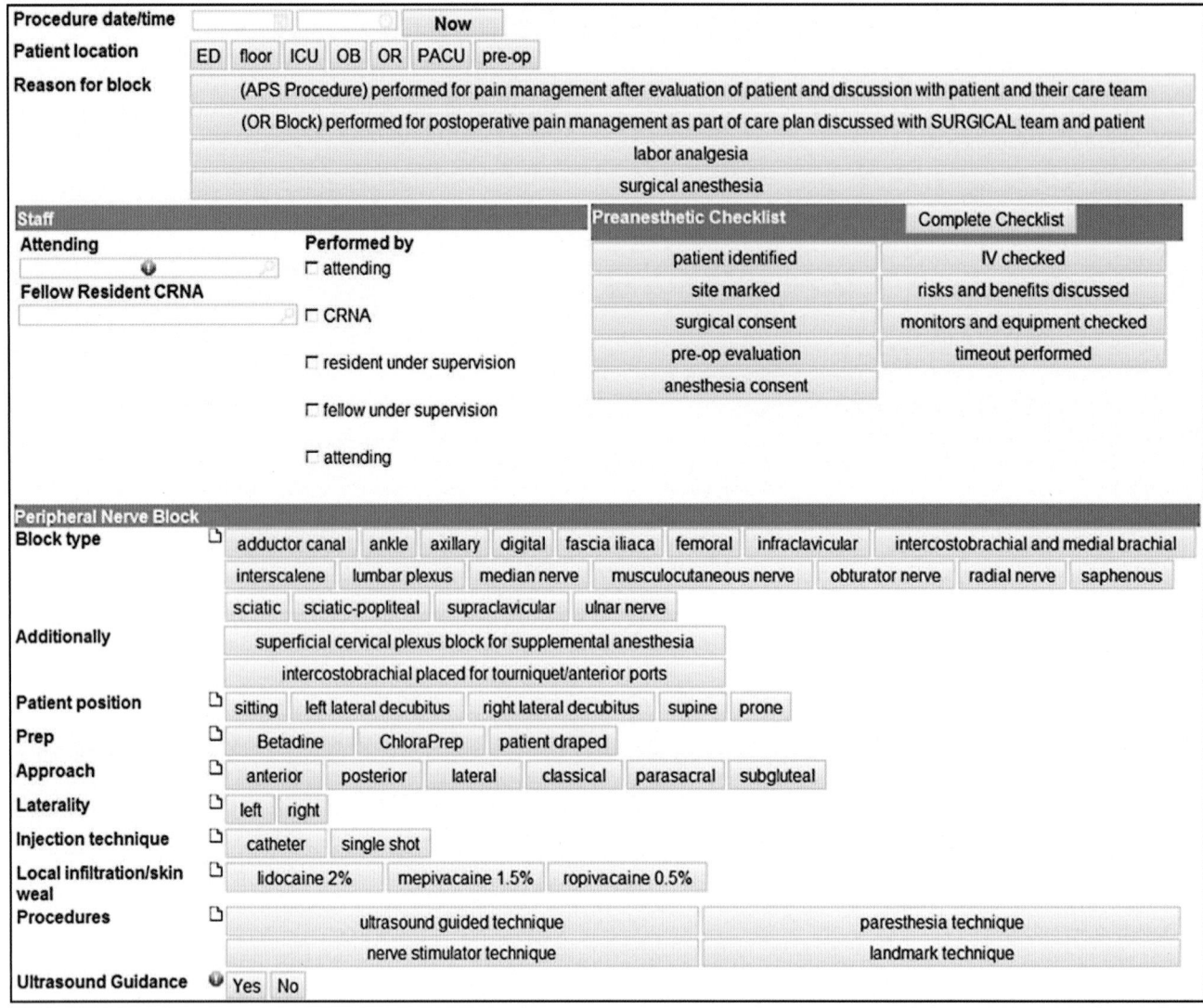

FIGURE 63–8. Screenshot from a block documentation page taken from an electronic medical record.

Useful Features of a Peripheral Nerve Block Procedure Note	Example
Elements that guide the practitioner to meet a given standard of care	A space to indicate the use of epinephrine in the local anesthetic solution or if none was used, why not
A compromise between efficiency and ability to individualize	Information recorded using both tick boxes and blank line spaces
Documentation to safeguard against common medicolegal challenges	Practitioner must indicate patient's level of consciousness
Documentation of compliance with regulatory agencies (eg, Joint Commission)	Tick boxes indicate laterality
Elements to facilitate successful billing	Language required by many insurance companies indicating block specifically requested by surgeon
Documentation of clinicians involved and in what capacity	Was the attending the individual performing the block, or was he or she medically directing a resident?

is simple with computerized systems such as these, as the block variables can be selected quickly from a list by indicating relevant documentation items, whereas any narrative elements can be rapidly typed using a keyboard (Figure 63–8). Legibility and ability to correct errors are advantages to the e-block note.

Another useful aspect of peripheral nerve block documentation is the recording of an ultrasound image or video clip, to be stored either as a hard copy in the patient's chart or as a digital copy in the electronic health record (EHR) or separate secure hard drive. This not only is good practice from a medicolegal point of view but also is a required step that must be taken if the clinician wishes to bill for the use of ultrasound guidance. Any hard copies should have a patient identification sticker attached, the date recorded, and any pertinent findings highlighted with a marker, such as local anesthetic spreading around nerve. Additional examples of highly practical documentation of essential nerve block and spinal anesthesia procedures are shown in Figures 63–9 and 63–10, respectively.

Informed Consent

Documentation of informed consent is an important aspect of regional anesthesia practice. Practice patterns vary widely on this issue, and specific written consent for nerve block procedures is often not obtained. However, the written documentation of this process can be important for a number of reasons:

- Patients are often distracted and anxious on the day of surgery (when many consents are obtained) and may not remember the details of a discussion with their anesthesiologist. Studies have shown that a written record of the informed consent process improves patient recall of risks and benefits.[49]
- A written consent establishes that a discussion of risks and benefits occurred between the patient and the physician.
- A specific document for regional anesthesia can be tailored to include all the common and serious risks; this allows the physician to explain them to the patient as a matter of routine and reduce the chance of omitting important risks.

The following tips can be utilized to maximize the consent process:

Suggestions for improving the consent process.

Be brief. A simple, short explanation helps recall of the risks and benefits more than lengthy paragraphs.

Include not only serious and major risks but also benefits and expected results of the proposed regional anesthetic procedure. It is difficult for patients to make an informed choice if only risks are discussed.

Use the consent process as a means to educate the patient simultaneously.

Offer a copy of the form to the patient. This has been shown to aid in recall of consent-related information.

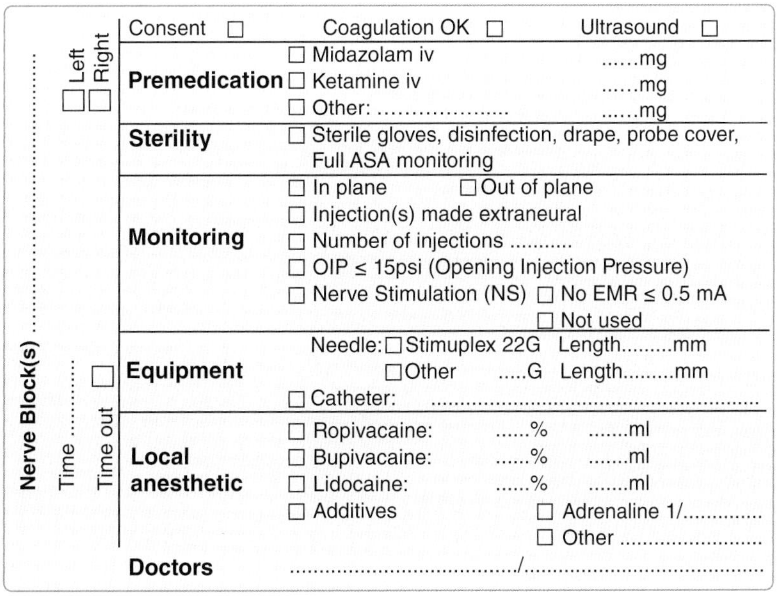

Nerve Block(s) ....
Time ....
Time out ☐
☐ Left ☐ Right

Consent ☐ Coagulation OK ☐ Ultrasound ☐

Premedication ☐ Midazolam iv ......mg
☐ Ketamine iv ......mg
☐ Other: ....mg

Sterility ☐ Sterile gloves, disinfection, drape, probe cover, Full ASA monitoring

Monitoring ☐ In plane ☐ Out of plane
☐ Injection(s) made extraneural
☐ Number of injections ....
☐ OIP ≤ 15psi (Opening Injection Pressure)
☐ Nerve Stimulation (NS) ☐ No EMR ≤ 0.5 mA
☐ Not used

Equipment Needle: ☐ Stimuplex 22G Length.........mm
☐ Other .....G Length.........mm
☐ Catheter: ....

Local anesthetic ☐ Ropivacaine: ......% ....ml
☐ Bupivacaine: ......% ....ml
☐ Lidocaine: ......% ....ml
☐ Additives ☐ Adrenaline 1/.............
☐ Other ....

Doctors ..../..................................

FIGURE 63–9. Essential elements of documentation of peripheral nerve block procedures used at NYSORA-Europe CREER (Center for Research, Education, and Enhanced Recovery From Orthopedic Surgery) at ZOL (Ziekenhuis Oost-Limburg), Genk, Belgium.

Spinal Anesthesia		
Time............ / Time out ☐ / ☐ Level ☐ Other / L3 / L4 L.../ L...	Consent ☐	Coagulation OK ☐
Position	☐ Sitting	☐ Lateral decubitus R / L
Premedication	☐ Midazolam iv ☐ Ketamine iv ☐ Other:	......mg ......mg ......mg
Sterility	☐ Sterile gloves, disinfection, drape, full ASA monitoring	
Technique	☐ Number of attempts......... ☐ No pain/paresthesia on needle insertion and injection, easy procedure, clear CSF, atraumatic ☐ Midline	 ☐ Paramedian R / L
Equipment	Needle: ☐Pencan 27G Length 88 mm ☐Other ....G Length ....mm	
Local anesthetic	☐ Bupivacaine: ☐ Other....................	0.5% ....ml .....% ....ml
Doctors	................................/...	

FIGURE 63–10. Essential elements of documentation of spinal anesthesia procedures used at NYSORA-Europe CREER (Center for Research, Education, and Enhanced Recovery From Orthopedic Surgery) at ZOL (Ziekenhuis Oost-Limburg), Genk, Belgium.

REFERENCES

1. Buhre W, Rossaint R: Perioperative management and monitoring in anaesthesia. Lancet 2003;362:1839–1846.
2. Guinard JP, Mulroy MF, Carpenter RL, Knopes KD: Test doses: optimal epinephrine content with and without acute beta-adrenergic blockade. Anesthesiology 1990;73:386–392.
3. Tanaka M, Sato M, Kimura T, Nishikawa T: The efficacy of simulated intravascular test dose in sedated patients. Anesth Analg 2001;93: 1612–1617, table of contents.
4. Karmakar MK, Ho AM-H, Law BK, Wong ASY, Shafer SL, Gin T: Arterial and venous pharmacokinetics of ropivacaine with and without epinephrine after thoracic paravertebral block. Anesthesiology 2005;103:704–711.
5. Van Obbergh LJ, Roelants FA, Veyckemans F, Verbeeck RK: In children, the addition of epinephrine modifies the pharmacokinetics of ropivacaine injected caudally. Can J Anaesth 2003;50:593–598.
6. Neal JM: Effects of epinephrine in local anesthetics on the central and peripheral nervous systems: neurotoxicity and neural blood flow. Reg Anesth Pain Med 2003;28:124–134.
7. Sites BD, Taenzer AH, Herrick MD, et al: Incidence of local anesthetic systemic toxicity and postoperative neurologic symptoms associated with 12,668 ultrasound-guided nerve blocks: an analysis from a prospective clinical registry. Reg Anesth Pain Med 2012;37(5):478–482.
8. Perlas A, Niazi A, McCartney C, Chan V, Xu D, Abbas S: The sensitivity of motor response to nerve stimulation and paresthesia for nerve localization as evaluated by ultrasound. Reg Anesth Pain Med 2006;31:445–450.
9. Chan VWS, Brull R, McCartney CJL, Xu D, Abbas S, Shannon P: An ultrasonographic and histological study of intraneural injection and electrical stimulation in pigs. Anesth Analg 2007;104:1281–1284, table of contents.
10. Robards C, Hadzic A, Somasundaram L, et al: Intraneural injection with low-current stimulation during popliteal sciatic nerve block. Anesth Analg 2009;109:673–677.
11. Voelckel WG, Klima G, Krismer AC, et al: Signs of inflammation after sciatic nerve block in pigs. Anesth Analg 2005;101:1844–1846.
12. Tsai TP, Vuckovic I, Dilberovic F, et al: Intensity of the stimulating current may not be a reliable indicator of intraneural needle placement. Reg Anesth Pain Med 2008;33:207–210.
13. Bigeleisen PE, Moayeri N, Groen GJ: Extraneural versus intraneural stimulation thresholds during ultrasound-guided supraclavicular block. Anesthesiology 2009;110:1235–1243.
14. Wiesmann T, Bornträger A, Vassiliou T, et al: Minimal current intensity to elicit an evoked motor response cannot discern between needle-nerve contact and intraneural needle insertion. Anesth Analg 2014;118:681–686.
15. Steinfeldt T, Graf J, Schneider J, et al: Histological consequences of needle-nerve contact following nerve stimulation in a pig model. Anesthesiol Res Pract 2011;2011:591851.
16. Steinfeldt T, Poeschl S, Nimphius W, et al: Forced needle advancement during needle-nerve contact in a porcine model: histological outcome. Anesth Analg 2011;113:417–420.
17. Gadsden J, Latmore M, Levine DM, Robinson A: High opening injection pressure is associated with needle-nerve and needle-fascia contact during femoral nerve block. Reg Anesth Pain Med 2016;41(1):50–55.
18. Hogan QH: Pathophysiology of peripheral nerve injury during regional anesthesia. Reg Anesth Pain Med 2008;33:435–441.
19. Whitlock EL, Brenner MJ, Fox IK, Moradzadeh A, Hunter DA, Mackinnon SE: Ropivacaine-induced peripheral nerve injection injury in the rodent model. Anesth Analg 2010;111(1):214–220.
20. Sala-Blanch X, Ribalta T, Rivas E, et al: Structural injury to the human sciatic nerve after intraneural needle insertion. Reg Anesth Pain Med 2009;34:201–205.
21. Hadzic A, Dilberovic F, Shah S, et al: Combination of intraneural injection and high injection pressure leads to fascicular injury and neurologic deficits in dogs. Reg Anesth Pain Med 2004;29:417–423.
22. Gauss A, Tugtekin I, Georgieff M, Dinse-Lambracht A, Keipke D, Gorsewski G: Incidence of clinically symptomatic pneumothorax in ultrasound-guided infraclavicular and supraclavicular brachial plexus block. Anaesthesia 2014;69:327–336.
23. Russon K, Blanco R: Accidental intraneural injection into the musculocutaneous nerve visualized with ultrasound. Anesth Analg 2007;105:1504–1505, table of contents.
24. Schafhalter-Zoppoth I, Zeitz ID, Gray AT: Inadvertent femoral nerve impalement and intraneural injection visualized by ultrasound. Anesth Analg 2004;99:627–628.
25. Loubert C, Williams SR, Hélie F, Arcand G: Complication during ultrasound-guided regional block: accidental intravascular injection of local anesthetic. Anesthesiology 2008;108:759–760.
26. Vadeboncouer T, Weinberg G, Oswald S, Angelov F: Early detection of intravascular injection during ultrasound-guided supraclavicular brachial plexus block. Reg Anesth Pain Med 2008;33:278–279.
27. Martínez Navas A, DE LA Tabla González RO: Ultrasound-guided technique allowed early detection of intravascular injection during an infraclavicular brachial plexus block. Acta Anaesthesiol Scand 2009;53:968–970.
28. Barrington MJ, Kluger R: Ultrasound guidance reduces the risk of local anesthetic systemic toxicity following peripheral nerve blockade. Reg Anesth Pain Med 2013;38:289–297.
29. Orebaugh SL, Kentor ML, Williams BA: Adverse outcomes associated with nerve stimulator-guided and ultrasound-guided peripheral nerve blocks by supervised trainees: update of a single-site database. Reg Anesth Pain Med 2012;37:577–582.
30. Casati A, Baciarello M, Di Cianni S, et al: Effects of ultrasound guidance on the minimum effective anaesthetic volume required to block the femoral nerve. Br J Anaesth 2007;98:823–827.
31. Sandhu NS, Bahniwal CS, Capan LM: Feasibility of an infraclavicular block with a reduced volume of lidocaine with sonographic guidance. J Ultrasound Med 2006;25:51–56.

32. Vandepitte C, Gautier P, Xu D, Salviz EA, Hadzic A: Effective volume of ropivacaine 0.75% through a catheter required for interscalene brachial plexus blockade. Anesthesiology 2013;118:863–867.

33. Riazi S, Carmichael N, Awad I, Holtby RM, McCartney CJL: Effect of local anaesthetic volume (20 vs 5 ml) on the efficacy and respiratory consequences of ultrasound-guided interscalene brachial plexus block. Br J Anaesth 2008;101:549–556.

34. O'Donnell B, Riordan J, Ahmad I, Iohom G: Brief reports: a clinical evaluation of block characteristics using one milliliter 2% lidocaine in ultrasound-guided axillary brachial plexus block. Anesth Analg 2010;111:808–810.

35. Krediet AC, Moayeri N, Bleys RLAW, Groen GJ: Intraneural or extraneural: diagnostic accuracy of ultrasound assessment for localizing low-volume injection. Reg Anesth Pain Med 2014;39:409–413.

36. Liu SS, YaDeau JT, Shaw PM, Wilfred S, Shetty T, Gordon M: Incidence of unintentional intraneural injection and postoperative neurological complications with ultrasound-guided interscalene and supraclavicular nerve blocks. Anaesthesia 2011;66:168–174.

37. Hara K, Sakura S, Yokokawa N, Tadenuma S: Incidence and effects of unintentional intraneural injection during ultrasound-guided subgluteal sciatic nerve block. Reg Anesth Pain Med 2012;37:289–293.

38. Bigeleisen PE: Nerve puncture and apparent intraneural injection during ultrasound-guided axillary block does not invariably result in neurologic injury. Anesthesiology 2006;105:779–783.

39. Selander D, Dhunér KG, Lundborg G: Peripheral nerve injury due to injection needles used for regional anesthesia. An experimental study of the acute effects of needle point trauma. Acta Anaesthesiol Scand 1977;21:182–188.

40. Orebaugh SL, Mukalel JJ, Krediet AC, et al: Brachial plexus root injection in a human cadaver model: injectate distribution and effects on the neuraxis. Reg Anesth Pain Med 2012;37:525–529.

41. Krol A, Szarko M, Vala A, De Andres J: Pressure monitoring of intraneural and perineural injections into the median, radial and ulnar nerves: lessons from a cadaveric study. Anesth Pain Med 2015;5:e22723.

42. Gadsden JC, Choi JJ, Lin E, Robinson A: Opening injection pressure consistently detects needle–nerve contact during ultrasound-guided interscalene brachial plexus block. Anesthesiology 2014;120:1246–1253.

43. Claudio R, Hadzic A, Shih H, et al: Injection pressures by anesthesiologists during simulated peripheral nerve block. Reg Anesth Pain Med 2004;29:201–205.

44. Theron PS, Mackay Z, Gonzalez JG, Donaldson N, Blanco R: An animal model of "syringe feel" during peripheral nerve block. Reg Anesth Pain Med 2009;34:330–332.

45. Tsui BCH, Knezevich MP, Pillay JJ: Reduced injection pressures using a compressed air injection technique (CAIT): an in vitro study. Reg Anesth Pain Med 2008;33:168–173.

46. Patil J, Ankireddy H, Wilkes A, Williams D, Lim M: An improvised pressure gauge for regional nerve blockade/anesthesia injections: an initial study. J Clin Monit Comput 2015. doi:10.1007/s10877-015-9701-z.

47. Gadsden JC, Lindenmuth DM, Hadzic A, Xu D, Somasundarum L, Flisinski KA: Lumbar plexus block using high-pressure injection leads to contralateral and epidural spread. Anesthesiology 2008;109:683–688.

48. Gautier P, Vandepitte C, Schaub I, et al: The disposition of radiocontrast in the interscalene space in healthy volunteers. Anesth Analg 2015;120:1138–1141.

49. Gerancher JC, Grice SC, Dewan DM, Eisenach J: An evaluation of informed consent prior to epidural analgesia for labor and delivery. Int J Obstet Anesth 2000;9:168–173.

CHAPTER 64

Diagnosis and Management of Spinal and Peripheral Nerve Hematoma

Ariana Nelson, Honorio T. Benzon, and Rasha S. Jabri

INTRODUCTION

Spinal epidural hematoma (SEH) is an accumulation of blood in the loose areolar tissue between the vertebrae and the dura of the spinal canal. Typically, the hematoma is asymptomatic, but in rare cases it will compress the spinal cord, with potentially devastating neurological consequences. These symptoms include sensory disruption, bowel and bladder incontinence, motor weakness, or, in severe cases, complete paralysis of the affected limbs. This clinical entity was first described in the medical literature in 1682 as spinal hematoma with spinal apoplexy in the *Histoire de l'Academie Royale des Science* (Volume 2; G.J. Duverney).[1] Nearly 200 years later, in 1869, a report of the first clinical diagnosis of SEH was published in the *Lancet*.[2]

The SEHs can be spontaneous in nature or may occur in the setting of an invasive procedure, such as lumbar puncture, neuraxial anesthesia, or spine surgery. Hematoma is more likely to be symptomatic in the cervical and thoracic regions, given the constricted spinal canal in this area compared to the greater space available for volume compensation in the lumbar and particularly the cauda equina region.[3]

SPINAL EPIDURAL HEMATOMA

Incidence

Symptomatic SEH accounts for less than 1% of all spinal space-occupying lesions[4] and affects only 1 per 1 million people annually.[5,6] SEHs arise from myriad etiologies but most often from a procedure performed in or near the epidural space. For example, the presence of SEH can be found on postoperative imaging in 33% to 100% of patients after spinal surgery,[7] but patients will rarely show any neurologic deficit. A 2010 systematic review found an overall calculated incidence of symptomatic SEH after spine surgery of 0.2%, with individual study calculations ranging between 0% and 1.0%.[8] Therefore, the incidence of SEH is routinely quoted as the incidence of *symptomatic* SEH; henceforth in this chapter, the qualifying term *symptomatic* is implied.

The incidence of SEH after neuraxial anesthesia has historically been approximated to be less than 1 in 150,000 epidural placements and less than 1 in 220,000 spinal anesthetics.[9] However, according to recent epidemiologic studies, the incidence may be increasing.[10] This estimation was confirmed by a large-scale Swedish study that found an incidence of SEH after epidural blockade of 1:18,000, a figure that results from the average of an obstetric incidence of 1:200,000 and a remarkably high incidence of 1:3600 calculated in a population of elderly female patients undergoing knee arthroplasty.[11] Another study showed an overall SEH incidence of 1:4741 that increased to 1:1000 if the population assessed was narrowed to include only elderly women undergoing lower extremity surgery.[12] This large disparity can be attributed to the presence or absence of risk factors in these incongruent patient populations. Pregnancy induces a relatively hypercoagulable state and obstetric patients are also younger with a larger and more compliant epidural space than elderly patients.[13] The lower incidence of SEH in obstetric patients was confirmed in a recent study wherein there were no recognized cases of SEH in 709,837 patients evaluated in the peripartum period.[14] This study noted an incidence of 1:9000 (95% confidence interval [CI]: 1:20,189–1:4330) in patients who received perioperative epidural placements.

Risk Factors

Increasing age carries with it an increased risk of SEH. The reduction in the size of the epidural space with age was first reported in 1967 in a study of local anesthetic spread.[15] This can be extrapolated to account for the higher incidence of SEH in the elderly because an equivalent volume of blood will cause increased pressure in the smaller epidural space of an elderly patient compared to a younger counterpart. No racial prediction has been reported, but SEH is more frequent in females. This could potentially be explained by the higher prevalence of osteoporosis in female patients,[16] which causes vertebral deformities or fractures and enlargement of the vertebral bodies, resulting in narrowing of the spinal canal.[17] Osteoporotic narrowing of the epidural space therefore could account for both the gender and the age predilections of SEH and may contribute to the greater than 50-fold increased likelihood of SEH after epidural anesthesia for knee arthroplasty as compared to epidural labor analgesia. However, thromboprophylaxis is a necessity in the orthopedic surgical population, which also may contribute to their relatively higher incidence of SEH compared to obstetric patients, who do not require routine prophylaxis against deep vein thrombosis.[11]

Indeed, the most important risk factor for SEH is the presence of a physiologic or iatrogenic disorder of the coagulation system, such as liver disease, alcoholism, thrombocytopenia, or pharmacologic anticoagulation.[7] A recent retrospective study also identified a significant increase in SEH after spine surgery in patients with Rh⁺ blood types, intraoperative blood loss greater than 1 L, hemoglobin level less than 10 g/dL, and an international normalized ratio greater than 2.0 in the first 48 hours.[18] Anticoagulant therapy in association with neuraxial analgesia as well as the length and intensity of anticoagulation have been identified as the most significant risk factors for epidural hematoma.[19] Approximately one-quarter to one-third of all SEH cases are associated with anticoagulation therapy.[20,21] In an extensive review of every case of SEH associated with neuraxial anesthesia, 87% of patients had either a hematologic abnormality or a procedure complicated by technical difficulty.[22] Cases of spontaneous hematoma are rare, but when they do occur are often associated with anticoagulation, thrombolysis, blood dyscrasias, coagulopathies, thrombocytopenia, neoplasms, vascular malformations, or vertebral hemangioma.[23,24]

Decreased patient weight, which may exaggerate the anticoagulant response, represents a theoretical concern for bleeding tendency and has been suggested as the explanation for the increased risk in women and the elderly. However, in Sweden, a gender-specific reduced dose of low molecular weight heparin for prophylaxis against deep vein thrombosis has not been shown to improve the well-described increased incidence of SEH in women.[11] Thrombolytic therapy imposes the greatest risk of bleeding complications, and neuraxial procedures should be diligently avoided in patients who have recently undergone thrombolysis.[25]

Etiology and Location of Hematoma

The proposed factors that cause SEH include trauma, anticoagulation, thrombolysis, lumbar puncture, epidural or spinal anesthesia, interventional spine procedures or surgeries, coagulopathy or bleeding diathesis, hepatic disease with portal hypertension, vascular malformation, disk herniation, Paget disease of the vertebral bones, Valsalva maneuver, and hypertension.[26] The most important causes of spontaneous SEH are clotting disorders, which may be acquired (eg, anticoagulant therapy, malignancies) or congenital (eg, hemophilia).[27,28] Vascular malformations are rarely responsible for spontaneous epidural hematomas; only 4% in a series of 158 cases and 6.5% in a series of 199 cases were reported to be due to vascular malformation.[29,30] Less-common predisposing factors include systemic lupus erythematosus, ankylosing spondylitis, rheumatoid arthritis, Paget disease, disk herniation, and hypertension.[31–33]

The dorsal venous plexus is the most commonly implicated source of hemorrhage because this plexus lacks valves and permits reversal in blood flow during increased intravascular pressure from physical activity.[34,35] These veins lack protection as they are surrounded only by loose areolar tissue and are therefore vulnerable to sudden increases in intra-abdominal or intrathoracic pressure, leading to rupture and hemorrhage.[36,37] The epidural venous plexus is most prominent in the thoracic spine,[23] and spontaneous SEH most often occurs in the thoracic and cervicothoracic region, followed by the thoracolumbar area.[4,30,38,39] SEH is typically posterior or posterolateral to the thecal sac (Figure 64–1) because the firm adherence of the dural sac to the posterior longitudinal ligament in the ventral aspect of the spinal canal prevents the accumulation of hematoma. The dorsal aspect of the thoracic or lumbar region is commonly involved, and expansion is typically limited to only a few vertebral levels.

In pregnant women, it has been proposed that increased venous pressure due to uterine enlargement, in association with the hemodynamic changes of pregnancy, may predispose to rupture of a preexisting pathologic epidural venous plexus wall.[40,41] Although a venous source is the most widely accepted, debate continues regarding a potential arterial source of SEH, with proponents of this theory stating that venous blood pressure is less than intrathecal pressure; therefore, although forward flow is possible into the low-pressure epidural space, venous blood could not cause compression of the spinal cord.[42]

Clinical Pearl

- Recent studies on the incidence of the risk of spinal hematoma in patients without overt risk factors showed an increase to 1:18,000 after epidural and 1:3600, even 1:1000, in elderly patients undergoing lower extremity surgery.

Clinical Pearls

- Hemorrhage into the spinal canal most commonly occurs in the epidural space because of the prominent epidural venous plexus.
- SEH may be spontaneous or may follow minor trauma, such as lumbar puncture or neuraxial anesthesia.
- SEH occurs primarily in anticoagulated or thrombocytopenic patients.

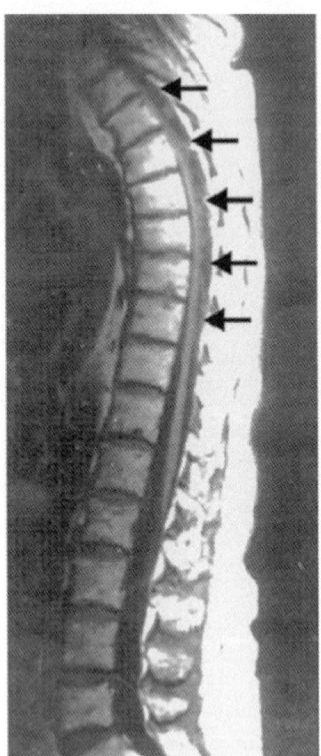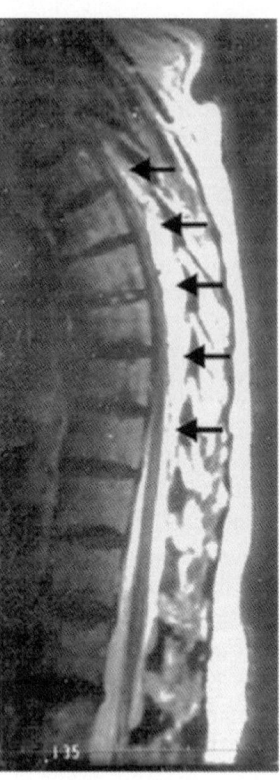

FIGURE 64–1. Sagittal magnetic resonance images of the thoracolumbar spine. A large complex epidural hematoma extending from T3 to T10 through T11 is seen with hypo- and isodense signal characteristics on a T1-weighted image (left; arrows) and hyperintense signal characteristics on a T2-weighted image (right; arrows). At the center of the hematoma, the spinal cord abuts the posterior aspect of the thoracic vertebral bodies (left). No signal abnormalities of the cord itself are seen. (Reproduced with permission from Schwarz SK, Wong CL, McDonald WN: Spontaneous recovery from a spinal epidural hematoma with atypical presentation in a nonagenarian. *Can J Anaesth.* 2004 Jun-Jul;51(6):557–561.)

History and Physical Examination

Classically, the presenting symptom of SEH is acute axial back pain that radiates to corresponding dermatomes and evolves to focal neurologic deficit with signs of nerve root or spinal cord compression.[43] The pain is generally described as a severe, localized constant back pain with or without a radicular component that may mimic disk herniation, especially in the lumbar spine. Back pain is amplified by percussion over the spine, as well as maneuvers that increase intraspinal pressure, such as coughing, sneezing, or straining. However, a 2010 analysis demonstrated that lower extremity weakness is the most common presenting sign, although back pain is still a common early symptom.[44] Associated symptoms may include numbness, weakness, and urinary or fecal incontinence.[38,45]

The onset of pain is occasionally related to minor strain, such as with lifting, coughing, sneezing, or Valsalva maneuvers, although in the majority of cases the onset of pain is spontaneous.[31,39] Depending on the level and the size of the hematoma, physical findings may include unilateral or bilateral weakness, sensory deficits with unilateral or bilateral radicular paresthesias, various

alterations in deep tendon reflexes, and alterations of bladder or anal sphincter tone.[46] Signs of spinal cord and nerve root dysfunction appear rapidly and may progress to paraparesis or, in high thoracic or cervical locations, quadriparesis. In cases of SEH related to neuraxial anesthesia or lumbar puncture, the presence of new or progressive postoperative neurologic symptoms should alert the physician to a possible epidural hematoma.[47]

Clinical Pearls

- The patient may present with a severe, localized, constant back pain with or without a radicular component that may mimic disk herniation.
- Associated symptoms may include weakness, numbness, and urinary or fecal incontinence.
- Return of sensory or motor deficit several hours after spinal or epidural block has worn off (with or without back pain) is highly pathognomonic and should be considered and treated as spinal or epidural hematoma until proven otherwise.
- Neurologic recovery after conservative management has been reported in patients with back pain and leg weakness without paralysis.
- Neurologic recovery can occur if surgery and decompression is performed within 36 hours of a complete motor deficit and within 48 hours of a partial deficit.

Diagnosis

As noted previously, the clinical findings of SEH usually include back pain and motor/sensory deficits that may rapidly progress to paraplegia, quadriplegia, or autonomic dysfunction. An epidural hematoma ordinarily presents within the first 24–48 hours after a procedure. Any new or progressive neurologic symptoms warrant immediate clinical evaluation and diagnostic workup to rule out any space-occupying lesion, including epidural hematoma. A neurologic deficit occurring in the presence of epidural analgesia mandates immediate discontinuation of the infusion, with the catheter left in place, to rule out any contribution from the local anesthetic. If the epidural infusion is the cause of the neurologic manifestation, a return of sensory and motor function will be noted. Otherwise, an immediate workup and radiographic imaging studies should be obtained and a consultation with a spine surgeon sought to rule out an evolving epidural lesion.

In a patient presenting with acute axial back pain with progression of neurologic deficits, immediate assessment for the presence of pathologic entities associated with nerve root and spinal cord compression is required to differentiate miscellaneous lesions simulating SEH. The clinical presentation of a patient with suspected epidural hematoma may resemble presentation for epidural abscess, spinal cord disease, neoplasm, or acute disk herniation.[47] The differential diagnosis of new or progressive postoperative neurologic symptoms includes surgical neuropraxia, prolonged or exaggerated neuraxial block, anterior spinal artery syndrome, exacerbation of a preexisting neurologic disorder, and presentation of a previously undiagnosed neurologic condition.

A complete blood cell count with platelets should be ordered to assess the extent of bleeding and to determine the presence of infection. Prothrombin time and activated partial thromboplastin time determine the presence of bleeding diathesis.

Rapid radiologic evaluation is essential to minimize delay in treatment of SEH. Currently, magnetic resonance imaging (MRI) is the diagnostic imaging method of choice for spinal emergencies because it allows rapid, noninvasive evaluation of the vertebral column and the spinal cord in all planes. Spinal MRI may delineate the location of an epidural hematoma and identify an associated vascular malformation; it will also provide information regarding the extent of the hematoma as well as the degree of cord compression. MRI can also aid in assessment of the age of the hematoma (Figure 64–1).[31,48,49]

The chronologic characteristics of an MRI of SEH are similar to those seen with intracranial hemorrhage. In the hyperacute stage (first 6 hours), the SEH appears isointense compared to the spinal cord on T1-weighted images and mildly hyperintense and heterogeneous on T2-weighted images, as a result of the presence of intracellular oxyhemoglobin. In the acute stage (7–72 hours), the hematoma is still isointense on T1-weighted images and becomes hypointense on T2-weighted images.[49] This is due to the presence of intracellular deoxyhemoglobin, which causes T2 shortening. As the concentration of methemoglobin increases, the hematoma becomes hyperintense and homogeneous on T1- and T2-weighted images. Gadolinium-enhanced magnetic resonance arteriography (MRA) may further define the extent of an arteriovenous malformation.

Conventional computed tomography (CT) has the potential to diagnose an epidural hematoma but may give false-negative results if the hematoma is isodense to the thecal sac or spinal cord and the image quality is affected by artifacts often seen in the upper thoracic region.[49] Spinal CT scanning may be nondiagnostic in the thoracic spine, where resolution is poorer than in the lumbar and cervical spine because of the high contrast between the lung parenchyma and vertebral bone. Conventional angiography may be required to definitively demonstrate the presence of a vascular malformation.[31,37]

Myelography, and later CT myelography, were previously the main modalities for diagnosis of epidural hematoma.[50] Combined with spinal CT scanning, myelography will display SEH as an intraspinal biconvex and hyperdense lesion with a density equivalent to blood.[51] Although this may demonstrate an epidural lesion with partial or complete spinal block, the findings are not specific. Moreover, myelography is invasive and may worsen the patient's clinical status. In addition, although it can demonstrate signs of compression with visualization of nonspecific contrast blockade or extradural convex compression, myelography cannot determine the nature and the true extent of the lesion.[52] These techniques are now rarely used in the United States as MRI has become the gold standard diagnostic measure.[53]

Prevention, Treatment, and Prognosis

Lumbar puncture or epidural anesthesia should be avoided in individuals who are on anticoagulant therapy, have received thrombolytic therapy, or are suspected to have a bleeding diathesis. Anesthesiologists are urged to be up to date on their knowledge of anticoagulation protocols, new anticoagulant medications, and current guideline recommendations. The decision to perform neuraxial blockade and the timing of catheter removal in a patient receiving antithrombotic therapy should be made on an individual basis, weighing the risks of spinal hematoma with the benefits of regional anesthesia for a specific patient. The American Society of Regional Anesthesia and the European and Scandinavian Society of Anaesthesiologists have published consensus statements on neuraxial anesthesia and anticoagulation, which provide an up-to-date source for guidelines in the decision-making process in performing neuraxial anesthesia in a patient with risk factors (see Chapter 52, Neuraxial Anesthesia and Peripheral Nerve Blocks in Patients on Anticoagulants).[44,54,55]

In contrast, no guidelines exist regarding anticoagulation in surgical patients. Recent retrospective studies regarding the incidence of postoperative hematoma after spine surgery concluded that perhaps patients should receive deep vein thrombosis prophylaxis as this does not appear to have an impact on the likelihood of SEH formation.[8,18,56] However, further prospective studies are needed prior to widespread institution of thromboprophylaxis after spine surgery given the devastating consequences of SEH.

Case reports have described successful conservative management of epidural hematoma.[57,58] Nonoperative treatment with good outcome was mainly reported in hematomas localized at the cauda equina level and those with mild neurologic deficit.[20] It appears that complete recovery can occur with conservative management when the patient reports back pain and leg weakness or numbness but does not exhibit leg paralysis.[59,60] Reversal of clotting abnormalities, close observation of neurologic deficits, and, in rare cases, steroid administration may achieve a good outcome without surgery.[61,62] A practical approach to management of suspected epidural hematoma is displayed in Figure 64–2.

Urgent surgical decompression is the treatment of choice for SEH causing acute compromise of cord function. Laminectomy is followed by evacuation of the hematoma, coagulation of bleeding sites, and inspection of the dura. The dura is then tented to the bone, and, occasionally, epidural drains are employed for as long as 24 hours. Although historically the efficacy of drains has been controversial, recent data suggest that subfascial drains significantly decrease SEH formation.[63] Recovery after prolonged paralysis without surgery is rare, and surgical consultation for consideration of emergent decompressive laminectomy must be obtained as soon as possible. The overall mortality rate is 8%.[64]

Ultimately, the surgery team must decide to observe or operate on a case-by-case basis. The critical factors for recovery after SEH are the level of preoperative neurologic deficit and the operative interval.[27,65] Prognosis for neurologic recovery primarily depends on the patient's preoperative neurologic status and

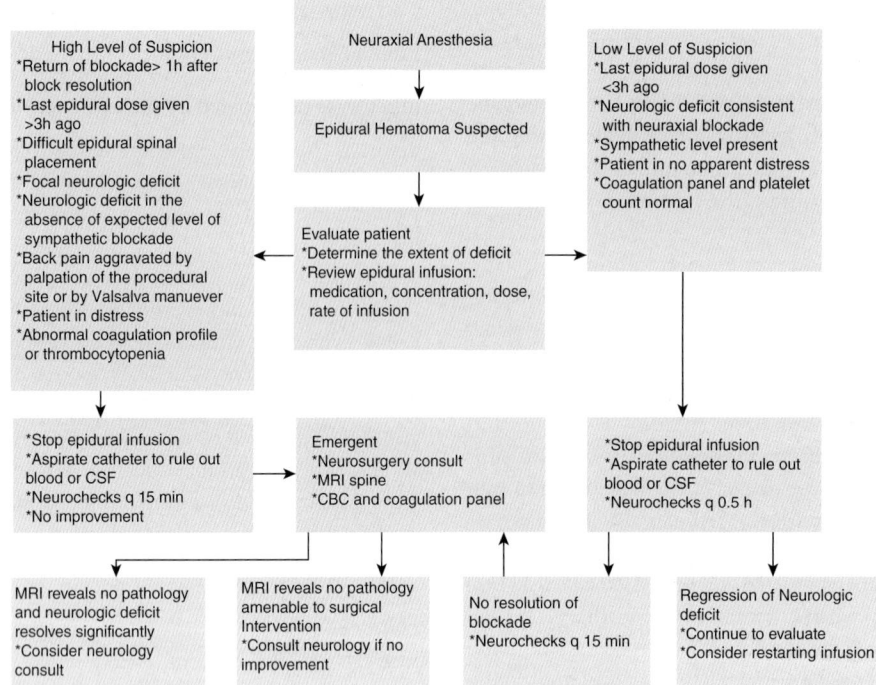

FIGURE 64–2. Practical approach to decision-making in workup and treatment of a patient with suspected epidural hematoma. CBC = complete blood cell count; CSF = cerebrospinal fluid; MRI = magnetic resonance imaging; q = every.

duration of neurologic dysfunction.[36,66] The prognosis is worse when there is a delay between the injury and surgical intervention. Previously, complete neurologic recovery was considered to be unlikely if more than 8 hours had elapsed between the development of paralysis and surgical intervention.[67] However, other authors have noted recovery when surgery is performed within 12 hours of paralysis.[48,68]

This recommended time frame for intervention has been further delineated by the recent finding that recovery can be achieved when surgery is performed within 48 hours of an incomplete motor deficit and within 36 hours of a complete motor deficit (Table 64–1).[69] It is interesting to note that functional recovery after 72 hours of symptoms has been reported.[70] While it is reassuring that functional recovery may occur after such intervals, appraisal of the patient's symptoms and emergency MRI take time. Therefore, consultation with a spine surgeon regarding potential emergent evacuation of the hematoma should be obtained as soon as possible.

Spinal Epidural Hematoma: Summary

Spinal epidural hematoma is a rare source of neurologic deterioration and can result in autonomic, sensory, and motor disturbance of varying degrees depending on the location and size of the hemorrhage. SEH may be acute or chronic, spontaneous, post-traumatic, or iatrogenic. Known risk factors include technically difficult neuraxial procedure, presence of intrinsic or acquired coagulopathy, female gender, and advanced age. Potential risk factors as evidenced by inconsistent data in the literature include low hemoglobin level, presence of Rh⁺ antibody, and anatomical abnormalities of the spinal cord.

Given that SEH is a rare but potentially reversible cause of spinal cord compression, it is essential that the diagnosis be made without delay to enable full recovery. Spinal hematoma may occur even in the absence of identifiable risk factors; therefore, health care providers must maintain a high index of suspicion and vigilance in monitoring for new neurologic symptoms. Although MRI cannot be conducted with the rapidity of a CT scan, it is the diagnostic modality of choice because it is both sensitive and specific. Swift detection of neurologic deterioration is critical to early diagnostic imaging and prompt intervention.

It is reassuring to note that recovery can occur without surgery in the absence of paralysis. When paralysis occurs, surgical decompression of the spinal cord and nerve roots can result in full functional recovery when accomplished within a reasonably rapid interval. If intervention is delayed, permanent sequelae of SEH can include sensory deficits, paraplegia, spasticity, neuropathic pain, and urinary or anal sphincter dysfunction.

TABLE 64-1. Neurologic recovery in relation to timing of surgery.

Author	Interval between paralysis and recovery	
Wulf[68]	8 hours	36 hours of a complete motor deficit
Lawton et al[48]	12 hours	48 hours of an incomplete motor deficit
Groen and Van Alphen[69]		

PERIPHERAL HEMATOMA AFTER NERVE BLOCKS

Hematoma in the epidural space is certainly the most devastating hemorrhagic sequelae of neuraxial or peripheral regional anesthesia, but hematoma may also occur in the periphery after single-shot[71–75] or continuous nerve blocks.[76–79] The most common risk factors appear to be procedural difficulty and concomitant anticoagulation or antiplatelet therapy.[80] This complication is exceedingly rare, with fewer than 30 cases of hematoma after peripheral nerve block (PNB) reported in the literature to date,[44] and the consequences are also less dire as compared to SEH given that hemorrhage occurs in a compressible peripheral space.

In contrast to SEH, the presenting symptom of hematoma after PNB is rarely neurologic dysfunction but more typically visible bruising (Figure 64–3), local tenderness, decrease in hemoglobin/hematocrit, or relative hypotension due to blood loss. This is not to say that that the compliant nature of the peripheral space precludes significant morbidity and mortality, as there is one reported case of a patient fatality secondary to retroperitoneal hemorrhage after lumbar sympathetic block in the setting of antiplatelet therapy.[73] The patient was found on autopsy to have lost 3 L of blood in his retroperitoneal space, which speaks to the occult threat presented by the compliant periphery. Indeed, several other cases have been reported where patients suffered significant morbidity due to PNB hematoma, including lengthened hospital stay, requirement for transfusion, or acute renal failure.[54]

Given that in every case reported in the literature, the neurologic deficit, if present, had resolved by 1 year, it appears that the more concerning source of morbidity is blood loss into the

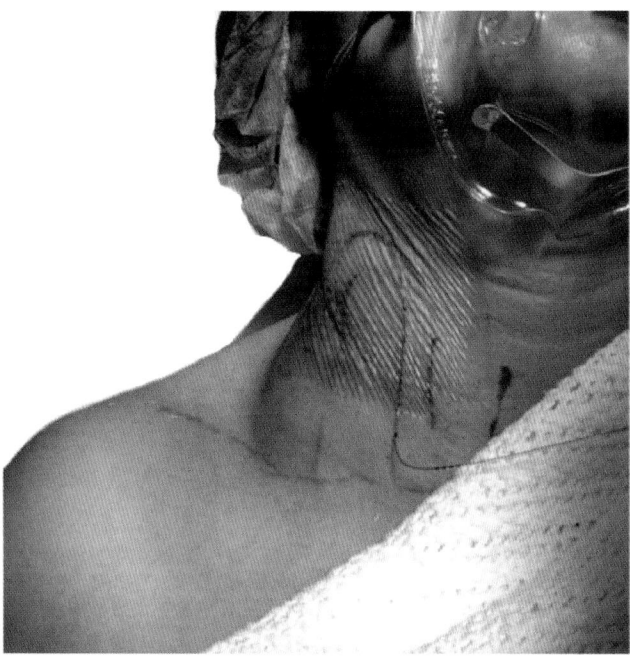

FIGURE 64–3. Neck hematoma in a patient in whom the external jugular vein was punctured with an 18-gauge Tuohy-style needle during insertion of a catheter in the interscalene groove. The hematoma shown was self-contained and was treated conservatively with local compression.

hematoma. However, due to the rare nature of this complication, it is difficult for experts to make recommendations regarding this procedure in the setting of anticoagulation. This difficulty is exacerbated by the existence of case reports wherein a hematoma occurred despite the practitioners following American Society of Regional Anesthesia and Pain Medicine (ASRA) guidelines.[71] In addition, there are reported cases of spontaneous hematomas that have occurred in patients on enoxaparin or thrice-daily heparin.[81–85] Taken together, these facts have led to somewhat-contrasting guidelines in different countries. For example, the German Society of Anaesthesiology and Intensive Care has issued recommendations regarding cessation of anticoagulation prior to PNB, but the Austrian Society states that distal PNBs, such as sciatic or axillary blocks, may be performed in an anticoagulated patient.[86]

The ASRA guidelines state that the recommendations regarding neuraxial techniques should be applied to deep plexus blocks and PNBs.[44] Therefore, patients receiving anticoagulation are not candidates for these anesthetic techniques, but some researchers suggested that with the advent of ultrasound guidance, these anticoagulated patients could safely undergo blockade of peripheral nerves.[75] In addition, studies showed not only a reduced incidence of vascular puncture with the use of ultrasound[87,88] but also a decreased rate of local anesthetic toxicity.[89–91] This option has the potential to improve patient safety, given that patients on anticoagulation often have risk factors for general anesthesia and would benefit from avoiding the resultant fluctuations in hemodynamics and fluid status.

A CT scan is currently the most common imaging technique for diagnosis of blood in peripheral tissues, especially the retroperitoneal space.[92] However, ultrasound has been used to demonstrate the presence of renal subcapsular hematoma[93] and could potentially be a more easily accessible diagnostic technique than CT in regions of the body amenable to this method of visualization. The increased use of ultrasound in initial placement of PNBs could facilitate diagnosis of suspected cases of post-block hematoma as the ultrasound equipment will be readily available.

Although timely diagnosis is ideal, subsequent treatment of hematoma after PNBs is typically expectant management. A surgical team is ordinarily consulted, blood transfusions are ordered as necessary, and surgical drainage is considered only in critical or rapidly deteriorating patients. Certain case reports of psoas hematoma have resolved without surgical evacuation of the hematoma,[71,93] and the patients regained their sensory and motor status a few days to 4 months after the diagnosis. As for hematoma concomitant with peripheral nerve catheter, these also are often self-limiting, but there are reports where surgical drainage was performed.[77]

Given the dearth of data available regarding hemorrhage after PNB or continuous nerve block, it may be difficult to accurately determine superiority of a certain anesthetic technique for a specific patient. Anesthesiologists should individualize their decision based on the suitability of PNBs in patients on anticoagulants and, as always, discuss in detail the risks and benefits of the block with the patient and the surgeon. If a block is performed, the patient should be observed closely in the perioperative period for signs and symptoms of peripheral hematoma.

PART 9

REFERENCES

1. Plagne R: L'hematoma extra-dural rachidien non traumatique (hematoma epidural spontane) [dissertation]. Clermont-Ferrand, France: University of Clermont-Ferrand, 1961.
2. Jackson R: Case of spinal apoplexy. Lancet 1869;2:538–539.
3. Holtas S, Heiling M, Lonntoft M: Spontaneous spinal epidural hematoma: findings at MR imaging and clinical correlation. Radiology 1996;199:409–413.
4. Alexiadou-Rudolf C, Ernestus R, Nanassis K, et al: Acute nontraumatic spinal epidural hematomas. Spine 1998;23:1810–1813.
5. Tekkok IH, Cataltepe O, Tata K, et al: Extradural hematoma after continuous extradural anaesthesia. Br J Anaesth 1991;67:112–115.
6. Hejazi N, Thaper PY, Hassler W: Nine cases of nontraumatic spinal epidural hematoma. Neurol Med Chir 1998;38:718–723.
7. Sokolowski MJ, Garvey TA, Perl J, et al: Prospective study of postoperative lumbar epidural hematoma. Spine 2008;33:108–113.
8. Glotzbecker MP, Bono CM, Wood KB, Harris M: Postoperative spinal epidural hematoma: a systematic review. Spine 2010;35:E413–E420.
9. Tryba M: Epidural regional anesthesia and low molecular heparin: pro [in German]. Anasthesiol Intensivmed Notfallmed Schmerzther 1993;28:179–181.
10. Horlocker T: Complications of regional anesthesia and acute pain management. Anesthesiol Clin 2011;29:257–278.
11. Moen V, Dahlgren N, Irestedt L: Severe neurological complications after central neuraxial blockades in Sweden in 1990–1999. Anesthesiology 2004;101:950–959.
12. Popping DM, Zahn PK, Van Aken HK, Dasch B, Boche R, Pogatzki-Zahn EM: Effectivenes and safety of postoperative pain management: a survey of 18,925 consecutive patients between 1998 and 2006 (2nd revision): a database analysis of prospectively raised data. Br J Anaesth 2008;101:832–840.
13. Horlocker T, Kopp S: Epidural hematoma after epidural blockade in the United States: it's not just low molecular weight heparin following orthopedic surgery anymore. Anesth Analg 2013;116:1195–1197.
14. Bateman BT, Mhyre JM, Ehrenfeld J, et al: The risk and outcomes of epidural hematomas after perioperative and obstetric epidural catheterization: a report from the multicenter perioperative outcomes group research consortium. Anesth Analg 2013;116:1380–1385.
15. Usubiaga JE, WJ, Usabiaga LE: Epidural pressure and its relation to spread of anesthetic solutions in epidural space. Anesth Analg 1967;46:440–446.
16. Cummings SR, Nevitt MC, Browner WS, et al: The study of osteoporotic fractures research group: risk factors for hip fracture in white women. N Engl J Med 1995;332:767–773.
17. Hasserius R, Johnell O, Nilsson BE, et al: Hip fracture patients have more vertebral deformities than subjects in population based studies. Bone 2003;32:180–184.
18. Awad JK, Kebaish KM, Donigan J, Cohen DB, Kostuik JP: Analysis of risk factors for the development of post-operative spinal epidural hematoma. J Bone Joint Surg Br 2005;87:1248–1252.
19. Horlocker TT, Wedel DJ: Neuraxial blockade and low molecular weight heparin: balancing perioperative analgesia and thromboprophylaxis. Reg Anesth 1998;23:164–177.
20. Johnston RA: The management of acute spinal cord compression. J Neurol Neurosurg Psychiatr 1993;56:1046–1054.
21. Wysowski DK, Talarico L, Bacsanyi J, et al: Spinal and epidural hematoma and low-molecular-weight heparin. N Engl J Med 1998;338:1774–1775.
22. Vandermeulen E, Van Aken H, Vermylen J: Anticoagulants and spinal-epidural anesthesia. Anesth Analg 1994;79:1165–1177.
23. Dickman CA, Shedd SA, Spetzler RF: Spinal epidural hematoma associated with epidural anesthesia: complications of systemic heparinization in patients receiving peripheral vascular thrombolytic therapy. Anesthesiology 1990;72:947–950.
24. Mattle H, Sieb JP, Rohner M, et al: Nontraumatic spinal epidural and subdural hematomas. Neurology 1987;37:1351–1356.
25. Levine MN, Goldhaber SZ, Gore JM, et al: Hemorrhagic complications of thrombolytic therapy in the treatment of myocardial infarction and venous thromboembolism. Chest 1995;108(Suppl 4):291S–301S.
26. Graziani N, Bouillot P, Figarella-Bragner D, et al: Cavernous angiomas and arteriovenous malformations of the spinal epidural space: report of 11 cases. Neurosurgery 1994;35:856–864.
27. Harik S, Raichle M, Reis D: Spontaneously remitting spinal epidural hematoma in a patient on anticoagulants. N Engl J Med 1971;284:1355–1357.
28. Zuccarello M, Scanarini M, D'Avella, et al: Spontaneous spinal extradural hematoma during anticoagulant therapy. Surg Neurol 1980;14:411–413.
29. Chen C, Fang W, Chen C, et al: Spontaneous spinal epidural hematomas with repeated remission and relapse. Neuroradiology 1997;39:737–740.
30. Groen R, Ponssen H: The spontaneous spinal epidural hematoma: a study of the etiology. J Neurolog Sci 1990;98:121–138.
31. Packer N, Cummins B: Spontaneous epidural hemorrhage: a surgical emergency. Lancet 1978;1:356–358.
32. Hebl JR, Horlocker TT, Kopp SL, Schroeder DR: Neuraxial blockade in patients with preexisting spinal stenosis, lumbar disk disease, or prior spine surgery: efficacy and neurologic complications. Anesth Analg 2010;111:1511–1519.
33. Joseph A, Vinen J: Acute spinal epidural hematoma. J Emerg Med 1993;11:437–441.
34. Beatty RM, Winston KR: Spontaneous cervical epidural hematoma. A consideration of etiology. J Neurosurg 1984;61:143–148.
35. Pan G, Kulkarni M, MacDougall DJ, et al: Traumatic epidural hematoma of the cervical spine: diagnosis with magnetic resonance imaging. J Neurosurg 1988;68:798–801.
36. Foo D, Rossier A: Preoperative neurological status in predicting surgical outcome of spinal epidural hematomas. Surg Neurol 1981;15:389–340.
37. David S, Salluzzo RF, Bartfield JM, et al: Spontaneous cervicothoracic epidural hamatoma following prolonged Valsalva secondary to trumpet playing. Am J Emerg Med 1997;15:73–75.
38. Fukui M, Swarnkar A, Williams R: Acute spontaneous spinal epidural hematomas. Am J Neuroradiol 1999;20:1365–1372.
39. Joseph A, Vinen J: Acute spinal epidural hematoma. J Emerg Med 1993;11:437–441.
40. Bidzinski J: Spontaneous spinal epidural hematoma during pregnancy. J Neurosurg 1966;24:1017–1018.
41. Carroll S, Malhotra R, Eustace D, et al: Spontaneous spinal extradural hematoma during pregnancy. J Matern Fetal Med 1997;6:218–219.
42. Stoll AS, Sanchez M: Epidural hematoma after epidural block: implications for its use in pain management. Surg Neurol 2002;57:235–240.
43. Bruyn GW, Bosma NJ: Spinal extradural hematoma. In Vinken PJ, Bruyn GW (eds): Handbook of Clinical Neurology. North-Holland, 1976, pp 1–30.
44. Horlocker T, Wedel DJ, Rowlingson JC, et al: Regional anesthesia in the patient receiving antithrombotic or thrombolytic therapy: American Society of Regional Anesthesia and Pain Medicine evidence-based guidelines (third edition). Reg Anesth Pain Med 2010;35:64–101.
45. Matsume M, Shimoda M, Shibuya N: Spontaneous cervical epidural hematoma. Surg Neurol 1987;28:381–384.
46. Lonjon M, Paquis P, Chanalet S, et al: Nontraumatic spinal epidural hematoma: report of four cases and review of the literature. Neurosurgery 1997;41:483–487.
47. Cwik J: Postoperative considerations of neuraxial anesthesia. Anesthesiol Clin 2012;30;433–443.
48. Lawton M, Porter R, Heiserman J, et al: Surgical management of spinal epidural hematoma: relationship between surgical timing and neurological outcome. J Neurosurg 1995;83:1–7.
49. Avrahami E, Tadmor R, Ram Z, et al: MR demonstration of spontaneous acute epidural hematoma of thoracic spine. Neuroradiology 1989;31:89–92.
50. Mattle H, Sieb J, Rohner M, et al: Nontraumatic spinal epidural and subdural hematomas. Neurology 1987;37:1351–1356.
51. Beatty RM, Winston KR: Spontaneous cervical epidural hematoma. A consideration of etiology. J Neurosurg 1984;61:143–148.
52. Cooper DW: Spontaneous spinal epidural hematoma. Case report. J Neurosurg 1967;26:343–345.
53. Uribe JM, Moza K, Jimenez O, Green B, Levi AD: Delayed postoperative spinal epidural hematomas. Spine J 2003;3:125–129.
54. Gogarten W, Vandermeulen E, Van Aken H, Kozek S, Llau JV, Samama CM; European Society of Anaesthesiology: Regional anaesthesia and antithrombotic agents: recommendations of the European Society of Anaesthesiology. Eur J Anaesthesiol 2010;27:999–1015.
55. Breivik H, Bang U, Jalonen J, Vigfusson G, Alahuhta S, Lagerkranser M: Nordic guidelines for neuraxial blocks in disturbed haemostasis from the Scandinavian Society of Anaesthesiology and Intensive Care Medicine. Acta Anaesthesiol Scand 2010;54:16–41.
56. Jacobs LJ, Woods BI, Chen AF, Lunardini DJ, Holh JB, Lee JY: The safety of thromboembolic chemoprophylaxis in spinal trauma patient requiring surgical stabilization. Spine 2013;38:E1041–7.
57. Pahapill PA, Lownie SP: Conservative treatment of acute spontaneous spinal epidural hematoma. Can J Anaesth 1998;25:159–163.

58. Schwarz SK, Wong CL, McDonald WN: Spontaneous recovery from a spinal epidural hematoma with atypical presentation in a nonagenarian. Can J Anesth 2004;51:557–561.

59. Benzon HT, Snitzer J, Hoxie S, Pollina R, Nelson A: Review of case reports of spinal hematoma. Presented at the American Society of Anesthesiologists annual meeting, Washington, DC, October 16, 2012.

60. Tailor J, Dunn IF, Smith E: Conservative management of spontaneous spinal epidural hematoma associated with oral anticoagulant therapy in a child. Childs Nerv Syst 2006;22:1643–1645.

61. Connoly SE, Winfree CJ, McCormick PC: Management of spinal epidural hematoma after tissue plasminogen activator. A case report. Spine 1996;21:1694–1698.

62. Lopez AG, Lara JMP, Hidalgo RH, Gonzalo PE; Spinal epidural hematoma following thrombolytic therapy for acute myocardial infarction. Orthopedics 1999;22:987–988.

63. Marzai H, Eminoglu M, Orguc S: Are drains useful for lumbar disc surgery? A prospective randomized clinical study. J Spinal Disord Tech 2006;19:171–177.

64. Hejazi N, Thaper PY, Hassler W: Nine cases of nontraumatic spinal epidural hematoma. Neurol Med Chir 1998;38:718–723.

65. Wolfgang P, Klaus M: Spinal hematoma unrelated to previous surgery: analysis of 15 consecutive cases treated in a single institution within a 10-year period. Spine 2004;24:555–561.

66. Rohde V, Küker W, Reinges MHT, et al: Microsurgical treatment of spontaneous and non-spontaneous spinal epidural hematomas: neurological outcome in relation to aetiology. Acta Neurochir 2000;142: 787–793.

67. Wulf H: Epidural anaesthesia and spinal hematoma. Can J Anaesth 1996;43:1260–1271.

68. Mukerji N, Todd N. Spinal epidural haematoma; factors influencing outcome. Br J Neurosurg 2013;27:712–717.

69. Groen RT, Van Alphen HA: Operative treatment of spontaneous spinal epidural hematomas: a study of the factors determining postoperative outcome. Neurosurgery 1996;39:494–508.

70. Enomato T, Maki Y, Nakagawa K, et al: Spontaneous spinal epidural hematoma: report of a case. Neurol Surg 1980;8:875–880.

71. Klein SM, D'Ercole F, Greengrass RA, et al: Enoxaparin associated with psoas hematoma and lumbar plexopathy after lumbar plexus block. Anesthesiology 1997;87:1576–1579.

72. Weller RS, Gerancher JC, Crews JC, et al: Extensive retroperitoneal hematoma without neurologic deficit in two patients who underwent lumbar plexus block and were later anticoagulated. Anesthesiology 2003;98:581–583.

73. Maier C, Gleim M, Weiss T, Stachetzki U, Nicolas V, Zenz M: Severe bleeding following lumbar sympathetc blockade in two patients under medication with irreversible platelet aggregation inhibitors. Anesthesiology 2002;97:740–743.

74. Poivert C, Malinovsky JM: Thigh haematoma after sciatic nerve block and fondaparinux. Ann Fr Anesth Reanim 2012;31:484–485.

75. Ferraro LH, Tardelli MA, Yamashita AM, Cardone JD, Kishi JM: Ultrasound-guided femoral and sciatic nerve blocks in an anticoagulated patient. Case reports. Rev Bras Anestesiol 2010;60:422–428.

76. Clendenen SR, Robards CB, Wang RD, Greengrass RA: Continuous interscalene block associated with neck hematoma and postoperative sepsis. Anesth Analg 2010;110:1236–1238.

77. Johr M: A complication of continuous blockade of the femoral nerve. Reg Anaesth (German) 1987;10:37–38.

78. Neuberger M, Breithbarth J, Reisig F, Lang D, Buttner J: Complications and adverse events in continuous peripheral regional anesthesia. Results of investigations on 3,491 catheters [in German]. Anaesthesist 2006;55: 33–40.

79. Wiegel M, Gottschaldt U, Hennebach R, Hirschberg T, Reske A: Complications and adverse effects associated with continuous peripheral nerve blocks in orthopedic patients. Anesth Analg 2007;104: 1578–1582.

80. Enneking FK, Chan V, Greger J, Hadzic A, Lang SA, Horlocker TT: Lower-extremity peripheral nerve blockade: essentials of our current understanding. Reg Anesth Pain Med 2005;30:4–35.

81. Antonelli D, Fares L, Anene C: Enoxaparin associated with huge abdominal wall hematomas: a report of two cases. Am Surgeon 2000;66:797–800.

82. Dickinson LD, Miller L, Patel CP, et al: Enoxaparin increases the incidence of postoperative intracranial hemorrhage when initiated preoperatively for deep vein thrombosis prophylaxis with brain tumors. Neurosurgery 1998;43:1074–1081.

83. Ho KJ, Gawley SD, Young MR: Psoas hematoma and femoral neuropathy associated with enoxaparin therapy. Int J Clin Pract 2003;57:553–554.

84. Houde JP, Steinberg G: Intrahepatic hemorrhage after use of low-molecular-weight heparin for total hip arthroplasty. J Arthroplasty 1999;14:372–374.

85. King CS, Holley AB, Jackson JL, et al: Twice versus three times daily heparin dosing for thromboembolism prophylaxis in the general population: a metaanalysis. Chest 2007;131:507–516.

86. Kozek-Langenecker SA, Fries D, Gutl M, et al: Locoregional anesthesia and coagulation in inhibitors. Recommendations of the Task Force on Perioperative Coagulation of the Austrian Society of Anesthesiology and Intensive Care Medicine [in German]. Anaesthesist 2005;54:476–484.

87. Abrahams MS, Aziz MF, Fu RF, Horn J-L: Ultrasound guidance compared with electrical neurostimulation for peripheral nerve block: a systematic review and meta-analysis of randomized controlled trials. Br J Anaesth 2009;102:408–417.

88. Barrington MJ, Watts SA, Gledhill RA, et al: Preliminary results of the Australasian Regional Anaesthesia Collaboration: a prospective audit of more than 7000 peripheral nerve and plexus blocks for neurologic and other complications. Reg Anesth Pain Med 2009;34:534–541.

89. Sites BD, Taenzer AH, Herrick MD, et al: Incidence of local systemic toxicity and postoperative neurologic symptoms associated with 12,668 ultrasound-guided nerve blocks. An analysis froma prospective clinical registry. Reg Anesth Pain Med 2012;37:478–482.

90. Orebaugh SL, Mentor ML, Williams BA: Adverse outcomes associated with nerve stimulator-guided and ultrasound-guided peripheral nerve blocks by supervised trainees: update of a single-site database. Reg Anesth Pain Med 2012;37:577–582.

91. Barrington MJ, Kluger R: Ultrasound guidance reduces the risk of local anaesthetic toxicity following peripheral nerve block. Reg Anesth Pain Med 2013;38:289–299.

92. Monib S, Ritchie A, Thabet E: Idiopathic retroperitoneal hematoma. J Surg Tech Case Rep 2011;3:49–51.

93. Aida S, Takahashi H, Shimoji K: Renal subcapsular hematoma after lumbar plexus block. Anesthesiology 1996;84:452–455.

PART 10

LAST: LOCAL ANESTHETIC SYSTEMIC TOXICITY

CHAPTER 65

Local Anesthetic Systemic Toxicity

Marina Gitman, Michael Fettiplace, and Guy Weinberg

INTRODUCTION

The introduction of cocaine as the first local anesthetic (LA) in the late nineteenth century was soon accompanied by reports of its systemic toxicity. The symptoms of toxicity were frequently described as seizures or respiratory failure, but some cases also included accounts of adverse cardiac effects. Often lethal, local anesthetic systemic toxicity (LAST) was treated with caffeine, ammonia, or even hypodermic ether.[1] The development of procaine in 1904 did not solve the problem of systemic toxicity, and the Committee for the Study of Toxic Effects of Local Anesthetics published a report of 43 fatal cases linked to the use of LAs.[2] Identification of contributing factors, emphasis on prevention and the almost-complete elimination of cocaine from clinical practice helped decrease the incidence of LAST for nearly 50 years.

However, the synthesis of long-acting, lipid-soluble LAs such as bupivacaine in the late 1950s with subsequent associated reports of LAST resulted in return of lethal LAST. These included multiple cases of fetal demise associated with paracervical blocks, ventricular fibrillation after an interscalene block, and what is considered to be the "sentinel" case of a young man who suffered a cardiac arrest after a caudal block.[1,3,4] The following several decades were plagued by isolated accounts describing a common problem: cardiovascular (CV) demise associated with LAST that was particularly resistant to available resuscitative measures, such as vasopressors (eg, epinephrine) and defibrillation.

MECHANISM OF LOCAL ANESTHETIC TOXICITY

Local anesthetics are generally safe and effective when limited to the site of therapy, such as tissue infiltration, near a nerve or a plexus of nerves. However, if large amount of LA reaches the systemic circulation, supratherapeutic blood and tissue levels can cause toxicity. This transit into the blood may be due to inadvertent intravascular injection or vascular uptake from local spread. At the target site, LAs reduce the sodium ion flux through voltage-gated sodium channels by a combination of an increased energy barrier and steric hindrance. This block occurs from the intracellular side and requires LAs to move across the lipid bilayer first.[5] LAs also block calcium channels and other channels at similar concentrations.[6] At lower concentrations, LAs block protein kinase signaling induced by tumor necrosis factor α.[7] At higher concentrations, LAs can inhibit other channels, enzymes, and receptors, including the carnitine-acylcarnitine translocase in mitochondria.[8]

Although there is no clear consensus, cardiac toxicity is likely caused by the combination of electrophysiologic and contractile dysfunction. Compared with other LAs *in common clinical use*, bupivacaine is more lipophilic and has a greater affinity for the voltage-gated sodium channels. These qualities may contribute to its cardiotoxic profile.[9–11] Of note, toxicity can occur at serum concentrations that are lower than expected because LAs accumulate in mitochondria[12] and cardiac tissue[13] at a ratio of about 6:1 (or greater) relative to plasma.

DIAGNOSIS AND CONTRIBUTING FACTORS

The typical presentation of LAST usually begins with prodromal symptoms and signs, such as perioral numbness, tinnitus, agitation, dysarthria, and confusion. These may be followed by more severe central nervous system (CNS) derangements such as seizures and coma. CV derangements can occur as well, initially presenting with hypertension and tachycardia, then bradycardia and hypotension, with progression to more serious complications, including ventricular arrhythmias and asystole. The majority of adverse events occur within 1 minute after injection of LA, but not all cases follow this pattern. Toxicity can have a delayed onset of greater than 1 hour after injection and can manifest as isolated CV dysfunction or as a combination of CNS and CV signs without the classical progression.[14]

Variables that increase the risk of toxicity include the type of LA and dose, site of injection, the patient's comorbidities, extremes of age, and small size or limited muscle mass. The lipophilicity of a LA is associated with toxicity. More lipophilic LAs like bupivacaine have an increased risk of toxicity relative to the less-lipophilic LAs like mepivacaine and lidocaine.

Higher total dose and the dose-to-weight ratio of the drug can potentially increase the possibility of LAST.[15,16] In particular, skeletal muscle acts as a depot for systemically absorbed LA,[13] which may account for the clinical risk of LAST in diminutive patients whose muscle mass is substantially less than normal. Accordingly, nerve blocks and epidural anesthetics that require larger doses carry an inherent risk for such patients. For example, bilateral transversus abdominus plane blocks performed with as much as 40 mL of 0.5% ropivacaine can result in an increased incidence of local toxicity.[17]

Last, but not least, the site of injection also contributes to the risk of vascular spread of the drug. The classical teaching that the vascular absorption of LAs is highest with intercostal blocks followed by epidural and brachial plexus injections corresponds to the clinical data demonstrating that the highest incidence of LAST occurs with paravertebral blocks, followed by upper extremity and trunk/lower extremity blocks.[16]

Patient-dependent risk factors include organ dysfunction, the serum level of the binding proteins, and age. Preexisting cardiac disease can make patients more prone to the arrhythmogenic and myocardial depressant effects of LAs. Extreme caution is advised for those with decompensated heart failure, severe valvular pathology, or depressed ventricular function. Hepatic or renal dysfunction can result in decreased metabolism and clearance and a higher level of circulating drug. In addition, liver/kidney failure, malnutrition, or any other disease process that results in a decreased serum level of albumin can indirectly increase the level of the free drug for a given dose.[18,19]

Patients at the extremes of age are more susceptible to toxicity, a finding that may be related to a number of factors. The elderly are more likely to have organ dysfunction, which will contribute to toxicity. Further, both elderly and pediatric patients may have diminished muscle mass and, as such, are more likely to receive a higher dose of drug for their weight. Most children are anesthetized when a block is placed, so the early symptoms will be missed, and more serious CNS/cardiac derangement could be the first sign of toxicity.[20]

OCCURRENCE OF TOXICITY

Neuraxial anesthesia and peripheral nerve blocks (PNBs) are the most commonly performed procedures requiring the use of LAs. The low volume of drug required for intrathecal dosing rarely poses a problem. However, the high volume required for epidural anesthesia and PNBs increases the risk of LAST. Currently available data indicate that the incidence of LAST associated with PNBs has decreased from 1.6–2/1000 in the 1990s to 0.08–0.98/1000 between 2003 and 2013.[16,21–25] In fact, one recent study observed no cases of LAST with more than 9000

PNBs over a period of 6 years.[26] Likewise, the incidence of LAST with epidural anesthesia decreased from 9.75/1000 in the early 1980s to 0.1–1.2/1000 in the 1990s and stayed at 0.1/1000 in 2003.[23,27,28]

While large population studies are mostly limited to epidurals and PNBs, there are numerous reports describing LAST with other types of local anesthesia. For example, with the recent popularity of a transversus abdominus plane block for abdominal procedures, there have been several cases of LAST after these blocks were performed for cesarean sections.[29,30] Neurologic toxicity has also been described after the topical use of LAs, which anesthesia providers frequently use prior to airway instrumentation for awake intubation.[31] This is likely underreported because the neurological symptoms may be mild (perioral numbness, tinnitus, agitation) and masked by preoperative sedation that precedes the induction of general anesthesia that immediately follows awake intubation.

Occasional causes of LAST outside the usual scope of an anesthesiologist include retrobulbar blocks for ophthalmologic surgery and inferior alveolar nerve blocks for dental procedures. Toxicity from a retrobulbar block is caused by subarachnoid spread of the anesthetic causing brainstem anesthesia; which can be manifest as altered mental status, apnea, and seizures.[32–34] Specific reports of LAST after inferior alveolar blocks are rare, but it is clearly a potential risk. The richly vascular area of the pterygomandibular space increases the risk for intravascular needle placement, which can be as high as 15.3% even among experienced oral surgeons.[35] Finally, there is a recent increase in utilization of regional blocks in emergency room settings[36] and corresponding reports of LAST in the emergency room,[37,38] but the scope of this problem is currently unknown.

TREATMENT

Presently, the three pillars of LAST treatment consist of seizure management, advanced cardiac life support (ACLS), and prompt administration of a 20% lipid emulsion. For hemodynamically stable patients with isolated seizure activity, intravenous benzodiazepines may be used. Small doses of propofol are considered by some an acceptable alternative for seizure control but can worsen cardiac dysfunction that may develop with LAST. Supplemental oxygen is appropriate for any patient exhibiting signs of LAST, but for patients with apnea, hemodynamically unstable arrhythmias, or cardiac arrest, immediate, more aggressive airway management or circulatory support is required. The goals are to maintain pulmonary ventilation and adequate organ perfusion with well oxygenated blood and to avoid further acidosis until initiation of lipid emulsion therapy.[39]

Before the introduction of lipid emulsion resuscitation, the treatment of severe cardiac toxicity was limited to ACLS and cardiopulmonary bypass. The use of vasopressors during resuscitation potentially worsened acidosis and arrhythmias. Cardiopulmonary bypass had been used in some cases; unfortunately, not all hospitals have that capability.[40] The idea that a lipid-rich substance has the potential to reverse the effects of certain drugs began in the 1960s, when several animal experiments demonstrated that intravenous administration of an oil emulsion decreased the duration of action of thiopental or decreased the free fraction of chlorpromazine in blood.[41,42] Serendipitously, in 1997, the case of LAST in a young woman with isovaleric acidemia and carnitine deficiency inspired a series of animal experiments. Carnitine is required for the transport of fatty acids into the mitochondria for β-oxidation, and accumulation of cytoplasmic acylcarnitines (eg, during myocardial ischemia) is associated with arrhythmias.[43] So, Weinberg et al hypothesized that overloading cells with exogenous fatty acids by infusing a lipid emulsion would exacerbate LA toxicity.[44] Surprisingly, the opposite was seen. Infusing a fat emulsion decreased and even reversed LA toxicity.[45]

In 2006, the first successful resuscitation of a human patient with a lipid emulsion was reported.[46] Since then, there have been many clinical reports describing effective reversal of LAST in adults and children.[47,48] Treatment of toxicity with an intravenous lipid emulsion has been termed *lipid resuscitation therapy* (LRT). The mechanism of LRT is multimodel in action, with lipid exerting both a scavenging effect (previously known as the "lipid sink") and a direct cardiotonic effect.[49,50] The scavenging effect is moderated by the lipid emulsion's ability to take up lipophilic moieties[51] and transfer them around the blood to sites of storage and detoxification. This provides a "lipid shuttle" effect. However, the scavenging effect is not sufficient to explain the rapid recovery.[52] A second effect occurs whereby in laboratory models infusing the lipid emulsion increases cardiac output through a combination of volume and direct cardiotonic effects to improve cardiac output once the cardiac concentration of drug drops below ion channel–blocking thresholds.[53,54] A 20% lipid emulsion is efficacious in the treatment of LAST caused by bupivacaine as well as other less-soluble LAs, such as ropivacaine, mepivacaine, and lidocaine.[55]

The lipid emulsion LD_{50} (median lethal dose) tested in a rat model was found to be much higher than the doses used for lipid rescue in humans.[56] Potential side effects include interference with clinical laboratory measurements (hemoglobin, methemoglobin, electrolytes, base excess); allergic reactions; nausea/emesis; dyspnea; and chest pain. Nonetheless, actual reported side effects are limited to bronchospasm, hyperamylasemia, and laboratory measurement interference. Transaminitis, hepatosplenomegaly, and bacterial contamination are typically associated with prolonged use of a lipid emulsion and do not play a role in the short-term administration for LAST. Although the use of high volumes of lipid emulsion (especially 30%) in premature and low birth weight neonates has been associated with death from fat accumulation in the lungs, there are case reports in neonates, toddlers, and older children of successful reversal of drug overdose (bupivacaine and non-LAs) using standard recommended regimes of 20% lipid.[55,57,58]

Last, as mentioned, one should exercise caution with the use of propofol in this setting: It is not a substitute for a lipid emulsion. There is insufficient lipid content in standard sedating or antiseizure doses of propofol to exert a benefit in the overdose setting; however, propofol can compromise CV stability.

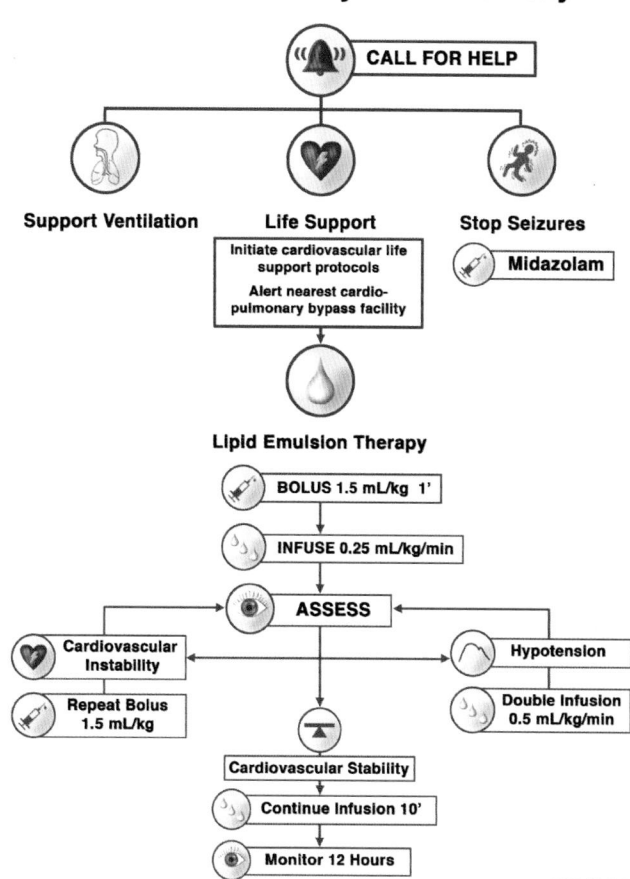

FIGURE 65-1. Checklist for management of local anesthetic systemic toxicity.

After numerous case reports validated the role of LRT as an effective treatment of LAST, the American Society of Regional Anesthesia and Pain Medicine (ASRA) issued a practice advisory in 2010 followed in 2012 by a checklist for managing LAST (Figure 65-1). The guidelines stress the importance of immediate cardiopulmonary resuscitation and provide a detailed algorithm for the dosing and administration of the lipid emulsion.[59,60] Timely use of the LRT, at the earliest signs of toxicity, can improve resuscitative efforts and decrease the amount of vasopressors used. As with any life-threatening emergency, securing intravenous access is essential; however, intraosseous administration of lipid emulsion is a possible alternative if intravenous access proves problematic.[61]

PREVENTION

As always, the best treatment is prevention. This is especially true for LAST. The efficacy and availability of LRT does not decrease the potential morbidity even in cases of successful treatment. The presence of a "silver bullet" does not remove the need for caution. For that reason, the use of ultrasound, intravascular markers, incremental injection with aspiration, less-toxic drugs, and the lowest effective dose is recommended.

Clinical Pearls

- There is a greater likelihood for LA systemic toxicity in petite patients (small muscle mass), those at the extremes of age, and patients with preexisting heart disease or carnitine deficiency.
- Roughly half the cases of LAST are atypical, with no seizures (other CNS symptoms), only CV toxicity or delayed onset.
- The incidence of toxicity increases with injections near richly vascular areas. It is highest with paravertebral injections, followed by upper and lower extremity PNBs.
- Prevention of LAST-related morbidity requires optimizing a complete system for regional anesthesia: patient selection, block choice, drug and dose, complete monitoring and use of USGRA when possible, and preparing for LAST by having a kit available and practicing with simulation.
- Prevention also includes raising awareness and educating our nonanesthesiology colleagues about proper use of LAs and risks, including management of LAST.

Ultrasound offers several potential advantages. It allows for direct visualization of injectable spread of drug, detection of unintended intravascular injection, and the use of smaller volumes of LAs.[26,62-64] Moreover, there is evidence that the use of ultrasound for PNBs can reduce the incidence of LAST.[16,25,26] An intravascular marker such as 10–15 μg of epinephrine has reasonable (albeit imperfect) sensitivity and positive predictive value and can be administered with a test dose. An increase in heart rate of 10 beats/minute or greater or an increase in systolic blood pressure of 15 mm Hg or greater suggests an intravascular injection. Incremental injection of LAs (usually 3–5 mL) and frequent aspiration have been regularly recommended and, together with the use of the test dose, may have contributed to the decrease in the incidence of LAST seen with epidurals. Finally, the use of the lowest effective dose provides an additional margin of safety.[65] It is also reasonable to adjust a dose downward for patients recognized to have a condition that could increase their susceptibility to LAST. This seems somewhat redundant if one always uses the least dose necessary for any block.

Prudence is the point. None of these measures is in itself precise or perfect; hence, it is vital not to rely on a single prevention step, but to incorporate several plus common sense to put patient safety first.[66]

AWARENESS AND EDUCATION

Anesthesiologists use LAs every day in various practice locations and for a wide variety of procedures. Thus, every site where LAs are used in potentially toxic doses should be equipped with basic resuscitation equipment and a 20% lipid emulsion. In addition, the ASRA checklist for the treatment of LAST can help guide the treatment process.[67] An electronic decision support tool was shown to improve adherence to guidelines during simulation of management of LAST and may be of benefit during actual cases.[68] Finally, education of nonanesthesia providers is crucial to raise their awareness of both the risk of LAST and its treatment. Patients could be saved if such very rare events are properly diagnosed and managed by nonanesthesiologists or others among the uninitiated who will otherwise remain ignorant of the risk. Education differs among institutions and departments, but there is suboptimal knowledge of LA dosing, safety precautions, and treatment of LAST among other specialties.[69] For that reason, the ASRA checklist and the electronic decision support tool can be invaluable for physicians in the event of LA toxicity.

REFERENCES

1. Drasner K: Local anesthetic systemic toxicity. A historical perspective. Reg Anesth Pain Med 2010;35:162–166.
2. Mayer E: The toxic effects following the use of local anesthetics: an analysis of the reports of forty-three deaths submitted to the Committee for the Study of Toxic Effects of Local Anesthetics of the American Medical Association, and the recommendations of the committee. JAMA 1924;82:875–876.
3. Edde RR, Deutsch S: Cardiac arrest after interscalene brachial-plexus block. Anesth Analg 1977;56:446–447.
4. Prentiss JE: Cardiac arrest following caudal anesthesia. Anesthesiology 1979;50:51–53.
5. Clarkson CW, Hondeghem LM: Mechanism for bupivacaine depression of cardiac conduction: fast block of sodium channels during the action potential with slow recovery from block during diastole. Anesthesiology 1985;62:396–405.
6. Coyle DE, Sperelakis N: Bupivacaine and lidocaine blockade of calcium-mediated slow action potentials in guinea pig ventricular muscle. J Pharmacol Exp Ther 1987;242:1001–1005.
7. Piegeler T, Votta-Velis, Bakhshi FR, et al: Endothelial barrier protection by local anesthetics: ropivacaine and lidocaine block tumor necrosis factor-a-induced endothelial cell Src activation. Anesthesiology 2014;120:1414–1428.
8. Weinberg GL, Palmer JW, VadeBoncouer, et al: Bupivacaine inhibits acylcarnitine exchange in cardiac mitochondria. Anesthesiology 2000;92:523–528.
9. Wolfe JW, Butterworth JF: Local anesthetic systemic toxicity: update on mechanisms and treatment. Curr Opin Anesthesiol 2011;24:561–566.
10. Albright EA: Cardiac arrest following regional anesthesia with etidocaine or bupivacaine. Anesthesiology 1979;51:285–287.
11. Heavner JE: Cardiac toxicity of local anesthetics in the intact isolated heart model: a review. Reg Anesth Pain Med 2002;27:545–555.
12. Hiller N, Mirtschink P, Merkel C, et al: Myocardial accumulation of bupivacaine and ropivacaine is associated with reversible effects on mitochondria and reduced myocardial function. Anesth Analg 2013;116:83–92.
13. Fettiplace MR, Pichurko A, Ripper R, et al: Cardiac depression induced by cocaine or cocaethylene is alleviated by lipid emulsion more effectively than by sulfobutylether-B-cyclodextrin. Acad Emerg Med 2015;22:508–517.
14. Di Gregorio, Neal JM, Rosenquist RW, et al: Clinical presentation of local anesthetic systemic toxicity. A review of published cases, 1979–2009. Reg Anesth Pain Med 2010;35:181–187.
15. Pertrar S: Total local anesthetic administered is integral to the syndrome of local anesthetic systemic toxicity. Anesthesiology 2014;121:1130–1131.
16. Barrington MJ, Kluger R: Ultrasound guidance reduces the risk of local anesthetic systemic toxicity following peripheral nerve blockade. Reg Anesth Pain Med 2013;38:289–299.
17. Eng HC, Ghosh SM, Chin KJ: Practical use of local anesthetics in regional anesthesia. Curr Opin Anesthesiol 2015;27:382–387.
18. Calenda E, Baste JM, Hajjej R, et al: Toxic plasma concentration of ropivacaine after a paravertebral block in a patient suffering from severe hypoalbuminemia. J Clin Anesth 2014;26:149–151.
19. Fagenholz PJ, Bowler GM, Carnochan FM, et al: Systemic local anaesthetic toxicity from continuous thoracic paravertebral block. Br J Anaesth 2012;109:260–262.

20. Lonnqvist PA: Toxicity of local anesthetic drugs: a pediatric perspective. Paediatr Anaesth 2012;22:39–43.

21. Auroy Y, Narchi P, Messiah A, et al: Serious complications related to regional anesthesia: results of a prospective survey in France. Anesthesiology 1997;87:447–486.

22. Auroy Y, Benhamou D, Barques L, et al: Major complications of regional anesthesia in France: the SOS Regional Anesthesia Hotline Service. Anesthesiology 2002;97:1274–1280.

23. Brown, Ransom DM, Hall JA, et al: Regional anesthesia and local anesthetic-induced systemic toxicity: seizure frequency and accompanying cardiovascular changes. Anesth Analg 1995;81:321–328.

24. Barrington MJ, Watts SA, Gledhill SR, et al: Preliminary results of the Australian Regional Anaesthesia Collaboration. A prospective audit of more than 7000 peripheral nerve and plexus blocks for neurologic and other complications. Reg Anesth Pain Med 2009;34:534–541.

25. Sites BD, Taenzer AH, Herrick MD, et al: Incidence of local anesthetic systemic toxicity and postoperative neurologic symptoms associated with 12,668 ultrasound-guided nerve blocks. An analysis from a prospective clinical registry. Reg Anesth Pain Med 2012;37:478–482.

26. Orebaugh SL, Kentor ML, Williams BA: Adverse outcomes associated with nerve stimulator-guided and ultrasound-guided peripheral nerve blocks by supervised trainees: update of a single-site database. Reg Anesth Pain Med 2012;37:577–582.

27. Tanaka K, Watanabe R, Harada T, et al: Extensive application of epidural anesthesia and analgesia in a university hospital: incidence of complications related to technique. Reg Anesth 1993;18:34–38.

28. Kenepp NB, Gutsche BB: Inadvertent intravascular injections during lumbar epidural anesthesia. Anesthesiology 1981;54:172–173.

29. Griffiths JD, Le NV, Grant S, et al: Symptomatic local anaesthetic toxicity and plasma ropivacaine concentrations after transversus abdominis plane block for caesarean section. Br J Anaesth 2013;110:996–1000.

30. Weiss E, Jolly C, Dumoulin JL, et al: Convulsions in 2 patients after bilateral ultrasound-guided transversus abdominis plane blocks for cesarean section. Reg Anesth Pain Med 2014;39:248–251.

31. Giordano D, Panini A, Pernice C, et al: Neurologic toxicity of lidocaine during awake intubation in a patient with tongue base abscess. Case report. Am J Otolaryngol 2014;35:62–65.

32. Gunja N, Varshney K: Brainstem anaesthesia after retrobulbar block: a rare cause of coma presenting to the emergency department. Emerg Med Australas 2006;18:83–85.

33. Dahle JM, Iserson KV: ED treatment of brainstem anesthesia after retrobulbar block. Am J Emerg Med 2007;25:105–106.

34. Tatum PL, Defalque RJ: Subarachnoid injection during retrobulbar block: a case report. Am Assoc Nurse Anesth J 1994;62:49–52.

35. Zenous AT, Ebrahimi H, Mahdipour M, et al: The incidence of intravascular needle entrance during inferior alveolar nerve block injection. J Dent Res Dent Clin Dent Prospects 2008;2:38–41.

36. Hahn C, Nagdev A: Color Doppler ultrasound-guided supraclavicular brachial plexus block to prevent vascular injection. West J Emerg Med 2014;15:703–705.

37. Monti M, Monti A, Borgognoni F, et al: Treatment with lipid therapy to resuscitate a patient suffering from toxicity due to local anesthetics. Emerg Care J 2014;10:41–44.

38. Harvey M, Cave G, Chanwai G, et al: Successful resuscitation from bupivacaine-induced cardiovascular collapse with intravenous lipid emulsion following femoral nerve block in an emergency department. Emerg Med Australas 2014;23:209–214.

39. Weinberg GL: Treatment of local anesthetic systemic toxicity. Reg Anesth Pain Med 2010;35:188–193.

40. Soltesz EG, van Pelt F, Byrne JG, et al: Emergent cardiopulmonary bypass for bupivacaine cardiotoxicity. J Cardiothorc Vasc Anesth 2003;17:357–358.

41. Russell RL, Westfall BA: Alleviation of barbiturate depression. Anesth Analg 1962;41:582–585.

42. Krieglstein J, Meffert A, Niemeyer DH: Influence of emulsified fat on chlorpromazine availability in rabbit blood. Experientia 1974;30:924–926.

43. Corr PB, Yamada KA: Selected metabolic alterations in the ischemic heart and their contributions to arrhythmogenesis. Herz 1995;20:156–168.

44. Weinberg GL, Laurito CE, Geldner P, et al: Malignant ventricular dysrhythmias in a patient with isovaleric academia receiving general and local anesthesia for suction lipectomy. J Clin Anesth 1997;9:668–670.

45. Weinberg GL, Ripper R, Murphy P, et al: Lipid infusion accelerates removal of bupivacaine and recovery from bupivacaine toxicity in the isolated rat heart. Reg Anesth Pain Med 2006;31:296–303.

46. Rosenblatt MA, Abel M, Fischer GW, et al: Successful use of a 20% lipid emulsion to resuscitate a patient after a presumed bupivacaine-related cardiac arrest. Anesthesiology 2006;105:217–218.

47. Cave G, Harvey M, Willers J, et al: LIPAEMIC report: results of clinical use of intravenous lipid emulsion in drug toxicity reported to an online lipid registry. J Med Toxicol 2014;10:133–142.

48. Presley JD, Chyka PA: Intravenous lipid emulsion to reverse acute drug toxicity in pediatric patients. Ann Pharmacother 2013;47:735–743.

49. Fettiplace MR, Weinberg G: Past, present, and future of lipid resuscitation therapy. JPEN J Parent Enteral Nutr 2015;39(1 Suppl):72S–83S, 2015.

50. Wagner M, Zausiq YA, Ruf S, et al: Lipid rescue reverses the bupivacaine-induced block of the fast Na^+ current (I_{Na}) in cardiomyocytes of the rat left ventricle. Anesthesiology 2014;120:724–736.

51. Mazoit JX, Le Guen R, Beloeil H, et al: Binding of long-lasting local anesthetics to lipid emulsions. Anesthesiology 2009;110:380–386.

52. Kuo IK, Akpa BS: Validity of the lipid sink as a mechanism for the reversal of local anesthetic systemic toxicity. Anesthesiology 2013;118:1350–1361.

53. Fettiplace MR, Ripper R, Lis K, et al: Rapid cardiotonic effects of lipid emulsion infusion. Crit Care Med 2013;41:e156–e162.

54. Fettiplace MR, Akpa BS, Ripper R, et al: Resuscitation with lipid emulsion: dose-dependent recovery from cardiac pharmacotoxicity requires a cardiotonic effect. Anesthesiology 2014;120:915–925.

55. Ozcan MS, Weinberg G: Update on the use of lipid emulsions in local anesthetic systemic toxicity: a focus on differential efficacy and lipid emulsion as part of advanced cardiac life support. Int Anesthesiol Clin 2011;49:91–103.

56. Hiller DB, DiGrigorio G, Kelly K, et al: Safety of high volume lipid emulsion infusion. A first approximation of LD_{50} in rats. Reg Anesth Pain Med 2010;35:140–144.

57. Ozcan MS, Weinberg G: Intravenous lipid emulsion for the treatment of drug toxicity. J Intensive Care Med 2014;29:59–70.

58. Brull SJ: Lipid emulsion for the treatment of local anesthetic toxicity: patient safety implications. Anesth Analg 2008;106:1337–1339.

59. Neal JM, Bernards CM, Butterworth JF 4th, et al: ASRA practice advisory on local anesthetic systemic toxicity. Reg Anesth Pain Med 2010;35:152–161.

60. Neal JM, Mulroy MF, Weinberg GL: American Society of Regional Anesthesia and Pain Medicine checklist for managing local anesthetic systemic toxicity: 2012 version. Reg Anesth Pain Med 2012;37:16–18.

61. Fettiplace MR, Ripper R, Lis K, et al: Intraosseous lipid emulsion: an effective alternative to IV delivery in emergency situation. Crit Care Med 2014;42:157–160.

62. Neal JM: Ultrasound-guided regional anesthesia and patient safety. Reg Anesth Pain Med 2010;35:S59–S67.

63. Orebaugh SL, Williams BA, Vallejo M, et al: Adverse outcomes associated with stimulator-based peripheral nerve blocks with versus without ultrasound visualization. Reg Anesth Pain Med 2009;34:251–255.

64. Salinas FV, Hanson NA: Evidence-based medicine for ultrasound-guided regional anesthesia. Anesthesiol Clin 2014;32:771–787.

65. Mulroy MF, Hejtmanek MR: Prevention of local anesthetic systemic toxicity. Reg Anesth Pain Med 2010;35:177–180.

66. Neal JM: Local anesthetic systemic toxicity. Improving patient safety one step at a time. Reg Anesth Pain Med 2013;38:259–261.

67. Neal JM, Hsiung Rl, Mulroy MF, et al: ASRA checklist improves trainee performance during a simulated episode of local anesthetic systemic toxicity. Reg Anesth Pain Med 212;37:8–15.

68. McEvoy MD, Hand WR, Stoll WD, et al: Adherence to guidelines for the management of local anesthetic systemic toxicity is improved by an electronic decision support tool and designated "reader." Reg Anesth Pain Med 2014;392:299–305.

69. Sagir A, Goyal R: An assessment of awareness of local anesthetic systemic toxicity among multi-specialty postgraduate residents. J Anesth 2015;29:299–302.

PART 11

PERIOPERATIVE OUTCOME AND ECONOMICS OF REGIONAL ANESTHESIA

Pharmacoeconomics of Regional Anesthesia: Implications in Ambulatory Orthopedic Surgery, Hospital Admission, and Early Rehabilitation

Brian A. Williams, Patrick J. Hackett, Pulsar Li, and Andrew J. Gentilin

INTRODUCTION

The analysis of the relationship of pharmaceutical and device costs to health care systems has been termed *pharmacoeconomics*, and four types of analytical techniques are commonly used for this purpose: cost-minimization, cost-benefit, cost-effectiveness, and cost-utility analyses.[1] With changing payments from private and government-based health insurance programs worldwide, physicians and administrators are forced to focus attention toward cost containment to maintain a profitable (or at least "break-even") enterprise. Cost analysis is an emerging tool in health care economics that can help physicians and administrators meet these new challenges.

TYPES OF COST ANALYSES

Cost analysis examines health care expenditures, and the subtypes of cost analysis also examine factors that are inserted into a denominator of a cost equation. Such factors include monetary benefits (eg, cost-benefit analysis, or CBA), incremental changes of health status variables (eg, cost-effectiveness analysis, or CEA), and patient-reported quality of life (eg, cost-utility analysis, or CUA).[2] If outcomes are determined to be equivalent regardless of the treatment program implemented, then a basic cost-minimization analysis is all that is required because the denominators are equal and the only relevant comparison is between the cost numerators of the compared programs.[3]

Cost-effectiveness analysis is applicable when the effects of comparable health treatments or services share the same therapeutic goals but have different degrees of effectiveness.[4] With CEA, the analyst can compare alternative treatment strategies so that results can be expressed in identical effectiveness units. CEA accounts for the effect of a treatment plan on all clinical outcomes and its economic implications, rather than considering only the cost of devices, supplies, and pharmaceuticals.[4] Effectiveness indicators, such as the number of adverse effects avoided or hospital stay reductions, are useful for comparing the different therapeutic alternatives considered. For this reason, CEA is one way of comparing treatment plans with the same desired effect but different outcome profiles, thus producing results expressed in terms of the number of adverse effects avoided. This approach implies weighing all adverse effects alike or weighing the different adverse effects in the way deemed most suitable by the analyst.[4]

With respect to anesthesia selection, it is highly unlikely that comparing regional anesthesia (RA) with general anesthesia/volatile agent (GAVA) techniques would show equal benefits or equal effectiveness (ie, life-years gained, days of disability avoided). RA significantly differs from GAVA, and the relevant side-effect profiles and risks are quite different as well. In fact, in the past few years, it has become clear in ambulatory procedures, for example, that the choices of the anesthetic and postoperative analgesic techniques have significant consequences for both the length of hospital stay and the frequency of unplanned hospitalization[5,6] and, consequently, the overall cost of the surgery. As a result, comparisons between RA and GAVA would require a CBA, CUA, or CEA.

Clinical Pearls

The four types of analytical techniques used in pharmacoeconomics are
- Cost minimization
- Cost-benefit analysis
- Cost-effectiveness analysis
- Cost-utility analysis

As physicians caring for individual patients, it is important to note that basing a clinical practice strictly on cost analysis is not well advised because individual patients have individual needs. However, in the setting of identifiable patient and hospital benefits when RA is used instead of GAVA, proper patient education regarding the benefits of RA is a most necessary step before any patient or health system benefits can be enjoyed.

It is also important to note that the literature is not replete with conclusive evidence addressing the cost-effectiveness of RA versus GAVA for surgical procedures in which both options are viable alternatives for patient care. Limited studies available can be used to apply cost analysis estimations for other studies that did not specifically address costs, but such approaches must be interpreted with caution.

ANESTHESIOLOGY INTERVENTIONS APPLIED TO COST ANALYSES

Selection of Techniques, Drugs, and Agents

Rationale for Avoiding General Anesthesia With Volatile Agents in Outpatients

When considering invasive outpatient orthopedic surgery, the routine use of GAVA without peripheral nerve blocks (PNBs) as the centerpiece of a multimodal analgesic plan is commonly associated with the following costly outcomes:(1) postanesthesia care unit (PACU) admission; (2) multiple nursing interventions for pain and postoperative nausea or vomiting (PONV); (3) PACU and same-day surgery discharge delays; and (4) unplanned hospital admission.[7–11] However, most hospital pharmacy and therapeutics committees are primarily focused on the pharmacy budget. Six percent or less of all hospital costs related to surgical care are attributed to pharmacy drug costs,[12] and examining drug costs in isolation without regard to patient outcomes is ill advised. The "least-expensive" outpatient GAVA technique, from the standpoint of drug acquisition for line items used for anesthetic maintenance, would probably include volatile agents, opioids, and muscle relaxants.

Postoperative Nausea and Vomiting and Comprehensive Multimodal Analgesia in Outpatient Regional Anesthesia Practice

Clinical Pearls

- General anesthesia with volatile agents causes PONV.
- Opioids (including patient-controlled intravenous analgesia) cause PONV.
- Propofol and multimodal antiemetics prevent PONV.
- Multimodal analgesia minimizes opioid requirements.

A traditional GAVA plan (volatile agents, opioids, and muscle relaxants) is traditionally favored for these specific line-item budgets of the anesthesia department and the hospital pharmacy, but the technique is fraught with "downstream" expenses for the hospital and presents a common basis for patient dissatisfaction. It has been well documented that GA techniques that exclusively use propofol for induction *and* maintenance (or as an intravenous sedative technique combined with RA) has a significantly lower PONV rate than do GAVA techniques,[10,13,14] and volatile agents and opioids are considered to be the leading causes of PONV.[15] Exclusive use of propofol instead of volatile agents is considered to provide an important but incomplete method of prevention of PONV.[15]

Three antiemetics of differing mechanisms are required to prevent equivalent PONV outcomes in GAVA patients versus propofol total intravenous technique patients.[16] RA techniques (without GA) are historically considered to be protective against PONV,[17] but research has indicated that there can be significant differences in PONV incidence when differing RA techniques are compared for the same type of surgical procedure.[18] In fact, patients undergoing single-injection PNB techniques that are later prescribed intravenous patient-controlled analgesia (IVPCA) do not appear to have significant benefit of PONV prevention versus similar patients undergoing GAVA with IVPCA[17], whereas patients receiving sustained analgesia primarily with continuous PNBs obtain additional PONV prevention benefits.[17]

For simple knee arthroscopy (mean procedure time < 30 minutes), GA with desflurane was compared with ipsilateral hyperbaric bupivacaine spinal anesthesia (4 mg) to assess PONV and myriad other outcomes.[19] Desflurane patients received PONV prophylaxis with dexamethasone and ondansetron if at least two risk factors were present (female, nonsmoker, PONV history, or motion sickness). Despite PONV prophylaxis in at-risk desflurane patients, all desflurane patients encountered significantly more PONV (6/32, 19%) than did patients receiving selective spinal anesthesia (zero PONV, $P = .024$).[19] In addition, desflurane patients encountered significantly more pain in both phases of postoperative recovery and more "extreme tiredness" in phase II recovery than did patients receiving selective spinal anesthesia.[19]

Generally, the following hold for outpatient orthopedic anesthesia routinely incorporating RA techniques: (1) GAVA should be avoided; (2) opioids should be minimized; and (3) at least two, if not three, antiemetics of differing mechanisms of antiemetic prophylaxis should be used. Our suggested criteria for multimodal antiemetics in outpatient orthopedics is all inclusive, primarily because all patients are likely to have at least one dose of an opioid at some point perioperatively. In outpatient orthopedics, use of a volatile agent alone is a sufficient sole risk factor for routine multimodal antiemetic prophylaxis, regardless of other risk factors, and volatile agents are frankly most logically avoided in the presence of other options (such as propofol total intravenous anesthesia [TIVA]). We suggest (1)[1] oral perphenazine[18,20–22] (8 mg preoperatively, but avoided in patients with Parkinson disease or a history of adverse extrapyramidal reactions to phenothiazines); (2) dexamethasone[18,22–27] (4 mg intravenously, perhaps avoided in patients with diabetes); and (3) a serotonin receptor 5-HT$_3$ serotoninergic antagonist. The combination of dexamethasone and a 5-HT$_3$ antagonist is more effective in preventing nausea and vomiting after discharge than is a 5-HT$_3$ antagonist used alone.[28]

In addition to their emetogenic potential, it is now known that volatile anesthetics possess hyperalgesic properties.[29,30] In a recent prospective randomized clinical trial, Cheng and colleagues reported significantly less pain and less morphine use in women undergoing uterine surgery ($P < .01$ and $P < .01$) with propofol TIVA versus GAVA. This transient hyperalgesia is believed to be due to inhibition of neuronal nicotinic acetylcholine receptors.[31]

It should be understood that opioids are commonly going to be used for RA procedure premedication, intraoperative management of nerve block onset latency, and postoperative analgesic rescue of symptomatic pain not covered by the peripheral block's nerve distribution. In addition, multimodal analgesic techniques, such as low-dose intravenous ketamine,[32–35] pre- and postoperative inhibitors of the cyclooxygenase type 2 (COX-2) enzyme,[36,37] and intra-articular injections by the surgeon to cover myriad mechanisms of the acute pain inflammatory cascade, also have the potential to be useful.[38–44] While COX-2 inhibitors valdecoxib and rofecoxib have been previously withdrawn from the market due to their cardiac side effects, studies are reassuring that the single-dose preoperative use of celecoxib remains safe.[36]

Minimizing Anesthesia-Controlled Time in the Operating Room

The potential value of the RA induction room should not be underestimated from the pharmacoeconomic perspective. Performing PNB techniques before operating room (OR) entry has been shown to be associated with a time savings of approximately 4–9 minutes of OR time per case compared with using GAVA without blocks.[9,45] In general, when the patient enters the OR ready for surgical preparation and has a faster emergence (and exit) due to the use of sedation versus GAVA, an OR with five cases can save 20–45 minutes each day. If the cost of a minute of OR time is estimated to be $30, then 1 day of this amount of time savings for five cases carries a potential cost reduction of $600–$1350. A portion of this theoretical savings is likely "real" in centers operating at or above 80% capacity, in which forced overtime (of preoperative, intraoperative, and postoperative nursing/ancillary staff) is a major budgetary

expenditure. The cost savings becomes even more significant when cases later in the day (eg, after 3 PM or 5 PM) are commonly "stacked" into fewer available staffed ORs, further lengthening already-long clinical days. Dexter and colleagues estimated that emergence that is 6 minutes faster than baseline likely translates to a per case overtime reduction ranging from 1.3 to 2.6 minutes.[46] In a 50-case surgical pavilion, this translates to 65 to 130 minutes of overtime saved.

How the reduction of anesthesia-controlled time influences OR staff retention is unknown. Repeated episodes of forced overtime for OR staff may lead to a loss of staff morale, which may translate to staff turnover. Staff turnover implies the replacement of departed, experienced staff with less-experienced staff, associated training, and possible surgical process inefficiencies until training is complete and posttraining experience is sufficient to resume an optimally efficient surgical process. Prolonged anesthesia-controlled time may also adversely affect staff morale in both phase I and phase II PACUs. While no studies to date have correlated reduced anesthesia-controlled time and perioperative nursing or OR staff retention, a recent study inferred an increase in several adverse events and errors with increased nursing work hours.[47]

Clinical Pearl

- Performing RA procedures in induction rooms decreases both induction time and emergence time in the OR.

Operating room time savings for outpatient shoulder surgery, via shorter induction time and emergence time values, has also been substantiated when interscalene nerve block was used alone without GAVA.[48] In this study, recovery room times and unplanned hospital admissions were also reduced in the patients treated with the interscalene block versus GAVA.[48]

Bypass of the Postanesthesia Care Unit in Ambulatory Surgery

In outpatient surgery, PACU bypass has been shown to be achievable in nearly 90% of patients receiving exclusively RA techniques (including neuraxial techniques if hemodynamic criteria are met).[10] To achieve PACU bypass in an institution where RA techniques are used in high volume, it is important to use tested criteria that incorporate both physiologic parameters and immediate symptomatic outcomes to determine PACU bypass eligibility and to use criteria that incorporate specific outcomes for both RA patients and GA patients.[49] The WAKE score[50] entails criteria that incorporate the original regional anesthesia PACU bypass criteria,[10] the traditional Modified Aldrete score,[51] the White-Song fast-tracking criteria,[52] and the Mayo Modified Discharge Scoring System[49,50] (Table 66–1).[49,53] Appropriately adjusting legacy criteria to the modern practice of ambulatory anesthesia and RA while incorporating "zero-tolerance criteria,"[50] which are applicable to all anesthetic types, appears to allow for "maximal return on investment" from the routine use of RA.

TABLE 66–1. Parameter-scored and zero-tolerance criteria for phase I PACU bypass (outpatient surgery) or phase I PACU discharge (inpatient or outpatient surgery) and likely effects of anesthetic drug/technique selection on meeting the described criteria for fast-tracking purposes.

Movement (LE: Lower Extremity; UE: Upper Extremity)	Scores
Purposeful movement of (at least) 1 LE and 1 UE	2
Purposeful movement of at least 1 UE (and neither LE)	1
No purposeful movement	0

Clinical correlations:
1. An isobaric spinal anesthesia would decrease the likelihood of achieving a score of 2 compared to an ipsilateral hyperbaric spinal anesthesia.
2. Prolonged emergence time from GA with volatile anesthetic (± neuromuscular blocking drugs) would increase the likelihood of achieving a score of 0 as opposed to a 1 or 2.
3. Interscalene block patients with blocks designed to provide overnight anesthesia-analgesia would not achieve an Aldrete parameter score of 2 because only three of four extremities would achieve purposeful movement.

Blood Pressure (Sitting and Supine)	Scores
Within 20% of preoperative baseline, not orthostatic	2
Within 20%–40% of preoperative baseline, not orthostatic	1
Less than 40% of preoperative baseline and/or orthostatic	0

Clinical correlations:
4. Isobaric bilateral spinal would likely cause a greater sympathectomy and hypotension than would an ipsilateral hyperbaric spinal.
5. Vasodilatory effects of propofol sedation would likely dissipate equal to or faster than the vasodilatory effects of volatile anesthetics.
6. Low-dose ketamine sedation would not typically cause vasodilation and subsequent hypotension.

Level of Consciousness	Scores
Awake and/or easily aroused by single stimulus, follows commands	2
Arouses to repeated or continuous stimuli, protective reflexes, follows commands	1
Obtunded or persistently somnolent; ± protective reflexes	0

Clinical correlations:
7. Avoidance of airway instrumentation, mechanical ventilation, volatile agents, and systemic opioids allows faster emergence from anesthesia and return of a level of consciousness consistent with a score of 2.
8. Perphenazine, ondansetron, and dexamethasone are all off-patent nonsedating antiemetics.

Respiratory Effort	Scores
Coughs and deep breathes freely and/or on command	2
Involuntarily cough only; unsupported airway	1
Tachypnea, dyspnea, or apnea and/or requiring airway support	0

Clinical correlations:
9. Avoidance of airway instrumentation, mechanical ventilation, volatile agents, and neuromuscular blocking drugs all favor a more timely score of 2.

Oxygen Saturation	Scores
≥95% or (preoperative reading minus 2) without supplemental O_2	2
≥95% or (preoperative reading minus 2) with supplemental O_2	1
<95% or (preoperative reading minus 2) ± supplemental O_2	0

(continued)

TABLE 66–1. Parameter-scored and zero-tolerance criteria for phase I PACU bypass (outpatient surgery) or phase I PACU discharge (inpatient or outpatient surgery) and likely effects of anesthetic drug/technique selection on meeting the described criteria for fast-tracking purposes. (*Continued*)

Clinical correlations:

10. Systemic opioids and neuromuscular blocking drugs can cause hypoventilation-induced desaturation; ipsilateral hyperbaric spinal anesthesia and/or peripheral nerve blocks would be unlikely to do so.

A score of 8 or higher, along with meeting all the zero-tolerance criteria (see next section), is sufficient to qualify for phase I PACU bypass after outpatient surgery or to fast-track phase I PACU discharge when transfer to an inpatient nonmonitored bed is planned after surgery. For patients with diagnosed obstructive sleep apnea (OSA), a score of 9 is recommended, along with the same zero-tolerance criteria (next section), and after 30–60 minutes of no episodes of witnessed apnea in an otherwise-nonstimulating PACU environment. The authors will send OSA patients to a postoperative monitored bed (eg, continuous pulse oximetry with or without capnography) if these OSA-specific WAKE criteria are not met.

Zero-tolerance criteria for WAKE score PACU bypass (outpatient surgery) or fast-track PACU discharge (inpatient or outpatient surgery) and the likely effects of anesthetic drug/technique selection on meeting the described criteria for fast-tracking purposes.

(1) Pain as appropriately adjusted to patients' baseline pain scores (with movement) at the surgical site

Clinical correlations:

1. Multimodal analgesia is logically employed on a routine basis, emphasizing nonsedative analgesics such as acetaminophen, type 2 cyclooxygenase inhibitors or nonsteroidal anti-inflammatory drugs, and N-methyl-D-aspartate antagonists (low-dose intravenous ketamine, and/or perioperative oral dextromethorphan, and/or intravenous magnesium).
   - Preoperative PNBs render patients as more likely to meet this criterion than would postoperative systemic opioids for rescue analgesia.
   - If a patient has a preoperative baseline pain score with movement of 8 of 10, in the absence of a PNB, it is highly likely that the patient will meet PACU bypass/discharge criteria on all other parameters and be successfully discharged with a postoperative pain score with movement of 10 of 10, by the nature of the limited analog scale available to choose from given the high preoperative pain score. However, in the presence of PNBs covering all relevant nerve distributions (eg, femoral and sciatic for total knee replacement), this would seem much less likely.
2. Buprenorphine added to peripheral nerve blocks will likely carry much greater analgesic duration than would an equivalent systemic dose of morphine or other opioid.
3. Maintenance anesthesia with propofol avoids the hyperalgesic effects of volatile anesthetics.
4. Spinal/regional anesthesia is likely far less hyperalgesic than is anesthesia with volatile anesthetics and short-acting opioids.

(2) PONV as a "yes-no" assessment

Clinical correlations:

5. Preoperative oral perphenazine is less sedating than intraoperative prochlorperazine and is similarly nonsedating as ondansetron and dexamethasone.
6. Systemic clonidine (eg, as a nerve block adjuvant) may have antiemetic benefits.
7. Volatile anesthetics and systemic opioids are emetogenic.

(3) Shivering, pruritus, and/or orthostatic symptoms (light-headedness and/or hypotension in the sitting position)

Clinical correlations:

8. Ipsilateral hyperbaric spinal (comprising a lower overall total intrathecal dose than would an isobaric bilateral spinal) may be less likely to create light-headedness in the sitting position when compared with isobaric spinal anesthesia by the time surgery is finished.
9. Systemic clonidine (eg, added to peripheral nerve blocks) and phenylephrine infusions (commonly coadministered during spinal anesthesia) have favorable antishivering and/or thermoregulatory benefits.
10. Volatile anesthetics disrupt thermoregulation more so than does regional anesthesia.
11. Systemic opioids commonly cause pruritus.

GA = general anesthesia; PNBs = peripheral nerve blocks; PONV = postoperative nausea and vomiting.

Source: Modified with permission from Moore JG, Ross SM, Williams BA: Regional anesthesia and ambulatory surgery. *Curr Opin Anaesthesiol.* 2013 Dec;26(6):652–660.

In surgical pavilions with large caseloads (eg, 50 cases/day), an 80% PACU bypass rate (compared with no PACU bypass) can lead to a PACU nurse full-time-equivalent (FTE) staffing reduction of up to four FTEs if the PACU nurses are full-time employees or by 20 nursing hours if the PACU nurses are part-time employees.[46,54] When combined with forced overtime of OR staff and step-down (phase II) recovery staff, OR time savings and PACU bypass (documented to be achievable with exclusive use of RA) can present important cost-saving opportunities for the hospital. In addition, a reduction in medical errors from reduced mandatory nursing hours previously noted could lead to additional decreases in hospital costs, as well as improved patient outcomes.[47]

In a patient population undergoing anterior cruciate ligament (ACL) reconstruction, PACU bypass using criteria resembling the described WAKE score was associated with a $420 hospital cost reduction (in year 2000 inflation).[55] The cost-savings component from the initial amount of $420 per PACU bypass patient (which excluded savings associated with nurse staffing reductions highlighted by Dexter and colleagues detailed previously) were likely attributable to RA patients experiencing fewer symptoms than those receiving GAVA. Williams and coworkers also reported that throughout the multi-pavilion university hospital during peak use of PACU bypass (3000 outpatient orthopedics procedures per year), PACU nurse staffing requirements for 25,000 surgical patients per year (throughout all pavilions) consisted of 28 FTE PACU nurses.[55] When the main campus multipavilion hospital relocated outpatient orthopedics to another off-site hospital in the health system, PACU bypass was used on the main campus for monitored anesthesia care cases only. Soon after, PACU nurse staffing requirements increased to 36 FTE (from 28 FTE) for the same annual caseload.[55] When nerve blocks are routinely used, PACU bypass is a potentially powerful cost management tool in ambulatory orthopedic anesthesia not only from a staffing standpoint, but also with respect to overall symptom reduction and return to wakefulness during same-day recovery.

Successful Same-Day Discharge in Ambulatory Surgery

Woolhandler and Himmelstein estimated that the cost of hospital admission (for all types of diagnoses and procedures, in 1997 inflationary dollars) is $1050.[56] Williams and coworkers found that the hospital cost increment associated with an overnight admission after ACL reconstruction was $385.[55] The likely cost differences in the findings of Williams and coworkers versus those of Woolhandler and Himmelstein are likely related to the generally healthy status of outpatients presenting for ACL reconstruction. The key point is that it will always be less expensive to the hospital administrator for a patient to go home immediately after outpatient surgery than to be admitted overnight for observation.[57] That said, precautions are required to ensure that costs are not incurred later in the form of requiring hospital readmission for complications improperly managed during the initial admission, especially because these readmissions are often ineligible for third-party reimbursement. Indeed, refractory pain is the most common cause of hospital readmission after discharge, accounting for over one-third of such readmissions.[58]

It is important to understand that the associated hospital cost reductions of $420 for PACU bypass and $385 for successful same-day discharge were calculated using standard econometric techniques of multivariate regression analysis.[55] These are not necessarily nursing cost reductions. Further detailed cost center study methodology would be required to determine if cost reductions were traced to nursing costs in particular, versus via another cost center. Thus, the associated cost savings captured in these values incorporate any and all expenditures related to OR time, additional RA equipment and medications used, prophylactic antiemetics, and postoperative parenteral nursing interventions required for symptoms. When specific time-resource and symptomatic outcomes were incorporated into the stated multivariate regression analysis, these covariates were not independent predictors of hospital costs; only PACU bypass and successful same-day discharge were independent predictors of hospital cost reductions. Thus, when deriving any cost analysis equation using these cost-saving values, it is important to use these values only for such analyses, pending the results of future, more detailed, economic studies. It would not be methodologically correct to simultaneously incorporate cost values from myriad other studies that calculate various itemized costs of events such as "minutes of PACU time," "minutes of phase II recovery time," or individual drug costs or labor costs. The use of cost estimate values from multiple studies is methodologically incorrect because "double counting" would occur, which may artificially elevate incremental differences in cost, cost-benefit, cost-effectiveness, and cost-utility analyses.

Successful Resource Management of Well-Trained RA Practitioners in the Ambulatory Surgery Setting

In ambulatory surgery, well-trained RA practitioners may be tempted to implement a comprehensive nerve block care algorithm for all surgical patients. This enthusiasm should be tempered by the consideration of the "opportunity cost" of providing labor-intensive nerve block anesthesia for patients who may not necessarily benefit from these procedures. For instance, in the study by Williams and colleagues,[11] 543 patients underwent "relatively noninvasive" outpatient knee surgery, while the remainder underwent "more invasive" knee surgery. Forty-seven percent (253/543) of the patients undergoing the noninvasive procedure received femoral (with or without sciatic) nerve blocks, but the use of nerve blocks (with local anesthetics) in these patients was not associated with a reduction in symptoms, nursing interventions, or unplanned hospital admissions.[11] As a result, these authors concluded that, based on this retrospective review of a significant clinical caseload of noninvasive knee surgery outpatients, nerve blocks with local anesthetics should be reserved for patients who have significant refractory postoperative pain or in other special situations, such as a complicated pain history or intolerance to traditional oral analgesic techniques. Whether future efforts of motor-sparing perineural analgesia with avoidance of motor block (via avoidance of local anesthetics in nerve blocks to avoid the risk of patient falls) have the potential of proving cost-benefit advantage or cost-effectiveness requires further study.

Clinical Pearls

- Hospital admission and readmission are costly.
- Additional material costs for an RA program for outpatients are likely offset by significant overall hospital cost savings when reliably achieving PACU bypass and same-day discharge.

In the same review of 1200 consecutive knee surgery outpatients, 657 underwent more invasive knee surgery, and 527 of these 657 (80%) received femoral with or without sciatic nerve blocks.[11] In these patients, nerve block anesthesia and analgesia were significantly associated with reduced pain symptoms during recovery (therefore, fewer nursing interventions for pain management) and fewer unplanned hospital admissions. It is important to note that the selection of nerve block anesthesia-analgesia appears to be necessary but not sufficient to comprehensively reduce postoperative nursing interventions and unplanned hospital admissions: Whenever GAVA was used (in the presence or the absence of nerve block anesthesia/analgesia), the odds ratio of more associated symptoms after GAVA was 2.1 ($P < .001$), whereas the odds ratio of more associated unplanned hospital admissions after GAVA was 3.3 ($P = .001$).[11] Thus, nerve block anesthesia and analgesia for indicated (more invasive) procedures (ideally in the setting of a comprehensive multimodal analgesic care plan) and the avoidance of GAVA (for all procedures) would likely provide the anesthesia care team (and the hospital) with the fewest possible side effects and the greatest facilitation of successful same-day discharge. However, routine sensorimotor blocks (ie, with local anesthetics) for non-invasive knee surgery may be an investment of RA practitioners' time (and risk) that may provide relatively little benefit and that takes away the opportunity for RA practitioners to engage in other value-adding activities. Such value-adding activity may include the placement of continuous nerve block (CNB) catheters for select patients, when time may have been only available previously to administer a single-injection nerve block (SINB).

Pain Risk Stratification

Clinical Pearls

- Routine use of PNBs in outpatient surgery is most efficient when patients are likely to encounter sufficient postoperative pain to justify their use.
- It is important to categorize surgery as "sufficiently non-invasive" versus "sufficiently invasive" to justify nerve block use on a per patient basis.

Upper Extremity Surgery

Shoulder For outpatient shoulder or upper extremity surgery, there have been few substantiated, comprehensive recommendations for allocating nerve blocks (single injection vs continuous infusion) based on anticipated postoperative pain, postoperative nursing interventions (with vs without), or unplanned hospital admissions.

In shoulder surgery, the comparison of single-injection blocks with GAVA has shown predictable findings. For arthroscopic acromioplasty of the shoulder performed under GAVA, Singelyn and colleagues showed that interscalene nerve block provided definitive recovery advantages over suprascapular nerve block, single-injection intra-articular local anesthetic, and controls.[59] For outpatient open surgery of the rotator cuff, Hadzic and coworkers reported that GAVA use (vs single-injection brachial plexus block with ropivacaine) led to increased PACU admissions (vs phase I recovery bypass), higher reports of postoperative pain, longer time to ambulation, longer time to same-day discharge, and higher risk of unplanned hospital admission.[60] In this study, no outcome differences occurred in follow-up from 24 hours to 2 weeks after surgery, but this study was underpowered.

In addition to the potential for cost savings mentioned, recent studies have shown data supportive for the use of RA with sedation (instead of GA) when the beach-chair position is used for shoulder surgery.[61] A recent study by Koh et al. found a significantly higher incidence of cerebral deoxygenation with GA versus interscalene block and monitored sedation, 56.7% versus 0%, respectively.[62]

Past literature has shown favorable analgesic outcomes with the use of intra-articular analgesic infusions for postoperative analgesia in less-invasive shoulder surgery.[63] But, many case reports have shown that this practice, especially continuous infusions of local anesthetic, can lead to chondrotoxicity. This devastating but rare complication can lead to irreversible cartilage breakdown, at times necessitating total joint arthroplasty.[64] While it seems likely that using only single injections with lower concentrations of local anesthetics in fact may attenuate chondrotoxicity risk, intra-articular anesthesia is no longer recommended.[65,66]

A review by Chelly and associates[67] provides an overview that may guide practitioners for categories of postoperative shoulder pain until more definitive evidence is available. In this review, shoulder procedures are clustered into a catheter-eligible category if the following procedures are involved: shoulder arthroplasty, rotator cuff repair, Bankart repair, and open reduction/internal fixation of the humerus.

The benefit of continuous interscalene catheters for shoulder arthroplasty and rotator cuff repair is well documented.[68-74] Although logic would indicate similar effectiveness for less-invasive procedures, there is little evidence at this time to indicate that interscalene brachial plexus catheters would be similarly useful for patients undergoing less-invasive shoulder operations (eg, shoulder stabilization procedures, distal clavicle resection or acromioplasty, subacromial decompression, biceps tenodesis or tenotomy, or even routine debridement inside the glenohumeral joint) when compared with SINBs and perioperative multimodal oral analgesia. Thus, studies are needed to show the benefit of CNBs (vs single injection) and single-injection blocks (vs no blocks) for a wide variety of shoulder procedures that produce an uncertain magnitude of postoperative pain.

Upper Extremity Distal to Shoulder

For outpatient wrist and hand surgery, Hadzic and coworkers addressed this patient population comparing chloroprocaine infraclavicular nerve block against GAVA, showing that GAVA use led to more PACU admissions (vs phase I recovery bypass), higher reports of postoperative pain, longer time to ambulation, and longer time to same-day discharge.[75] However, there were no outcome differences in follow-up from 24 hours to 2 weeks after surgery. This last finding was underpowered and did not show statistical equivalence.[75]

Chan and associates prospectively studied nonrandomized hand surgery patients ($n = 126$) undergoing GAVA ($n = 39$), axillary block ($n = 42$), or Bier block ($n = 45$).[76] GAVA was associated with the most postoperative symptoms and nursing labor intensity, as well as the longest discharge times. Bier block patients not only had the fastest recovery times and lowest associated total perioperative costs but also were at small risk for conversion of the anesthesia plan (2/45) to GAVA due to tourniquet pain.

Gebhard and colleagues retrospectively studied hand surgery patients ($n = 62$) receiving GAVA ($n = 20$), Bier block ($n = 21$), or wrist block ($n = 21$).[77] They found that wrist block patients were discharged home soonest and encountered (1) less hypertension than did Bier block patients and (2) less hypotension than did GAVA patients.[77]

McCartney and coworkers prospectively studied 100 hand surgery outpatients randomized to receive GAVA ($n = 50$) or brachial plexus block with lidocaine ($n = 50$). These authors found essentially similar, if not identical, findings to those reported by Hadzic (prospectively) and Chan (retrospectively) as mentioned previously. McCartney and coworkers also concluded that there were no long-term (2-week) pain outcome differences, although the brachial plexus block group only received the short-acting local anesthetic lidocaine.[78]

For other (distal) upper extremity surgery, Chelly and associates stated that PNB catheters are likely indicated for implantation procedures after trauma, as well as for open reduction/internal fixation of the hand or digits,[67] although a prospective randomized trial to definitively verify this intuitive concept may be difficult to achieve. Ilfeld and colleagues have shown that a continuous infraclavicular brachial plexus catheter (vs placebo catheter infusion) resulted in less postoperative dynamic pain and opioid consumption and fewer sleep disturbances.[79]

Less-invasive upper extremity procedures (typically applicable to outpatients) have not been comprehensively studied with respect to the potential value of continuous catheters versus single-injection blocks. However, Rawal and coworkers[80] showed that an axillary CNB catheter with intermittent-bolus dosing provided excellent wrist and hand analgesia for patients undergoing surgical procedures that may have been somewhat less invasive than those described earlier by Ilfeld and colleagues.[79] Rawal and coworkers' study included 60 patients who received a mepivacaine axillary block bolus and concomitant nerve block

catheter placement and were undergoing carpal tunnel release ($n = 11$), finger fracture repair ($n = 11$), tendon repair ($n = 10$), finger joint arthrodesis ($n = 10$), wrist arthroscopy ($n = 8$), and tumor resection or other procedures ($n = 10$). This study studied neither a control group of patients undergoing no nerve block nor a treatment group undergoing SINB only. In fact, 3 of the 60 patients studied did not use the bolus dose function postoperatively. However, almost every bolus treatment was prompted by patients achieving a verbal pain score of at least 5 (of 10), and bolus treatments returned pain scores to around 3 (of 10), thus providing clinically significant analgesia.[80] Patients in this study used all of their allotted boluses by the 12th hour after surgery; as such, the reader may speculate that patients may simply benefit from a long-acting, SINB designed to provide 18 hours or more of postoperative analgesia, instead of the technical complexity of a nerve block catheter.

While Rawal and coworkers found that the most common cause of patient dissatisfaction with the continuous-catheter, intermittent-bolus technique was hand numbness, a recent randomized-observer blinded study by Fredrickson et al showed that motor block related to a long-acting brachial plexus block did not appear to cause patient dissatisfaction.[80,81] Therefore, patient uncertainty and potential dissatisfaction associated with prominent numbness or motor block should likely be factored into the decision of which nerve block technique is selected when a single-injection versus a continuous-catheter technique is considered.

Recent literature has also pointed toward an increase in OR efficiency with the use of RA for upper extremity surgery. Mariano et al. (2009) showed reduced anesthesia-controlled time with both intravenous RA and RA for upper extremity procedures when a nerve block induction room was utilized preoperatively.[45] In this study, anesthesia-controlled time was reduced from an average of 32 minutes with GA to 28 and 25 minutes with PNB and intravenous RA, respectively.

Clinical Pearls

- Arthroscopic debridement and subacromial decompression of the shoulder are likely among the "least-invasive" procedures with respect to postoperative pain, but this does not translate to "no pain" after least-invasive shoulder surgery.
- Rotator cuff repair and arthroplasty of the shoulder are likely among the "most invasive" procedures with respect to postoperative pain.
- Wrist and hand surgery can generate significant postoperative pain; however, the pragmatic value of catheter techniques for these same-day discharge procedures requires further evaluation.

To summarize, outpatient hand surgery often results in significant postoperative pain, with patient pain scores often reaching or exceeding a 5 (of 10) on a visual analog scale.[82] Retrospective reviews and prospective studies have demonstrated uniformly that patients receiving PNBs have significantly improved outcomes on the day of surgery compared with patients receiving GAVA. For shoulder surgery, the use of continuous brachial plexus catheters is sufficiently substantiated to recommend their routine placement (by trained practitioners) for invasive shoulder surgery, pending other economic considerations (eg, reimbursement from third-party or government entities). Perineural catheters and associated CNBs provide incremental benefits, but not without higher technical difficulty of percutaneous catheter placement. Ambulatory CNBs have been shown to be effective with a relatively low complication rate in postoperative pain management.[83] Because of difficulty in follow-up and reimbursement as well as lack of incremental pay, it may be more beneficial to consider use of perineural adjuvant medication to prolong the patient-perceived effectiveness of a SINB.[84] These findings also encourage the routine use (by trained practitioners) of all peripheral/regional techniques for upper extremity surgery, although further research is needed to determine outcome benefits of continuous blocks versus SINBs in the days and weeks following mildly to moderately invasive shoulder and distal upper extremity surgery. The usefulness of intra-articular and incisional infusions after simple arthroscopic procedures of the shoulder has been documented, but due to the risk of chondrotoxicity, they are no longer recommended.

Knee Surgery

Recommendations for rational nerve block selection (SINB vs CNB vs none) in outpatient knee surgery have previously been suggested.[85] This guideline incorporates the resource management principles described previously and creates three major categories: (1) noninvasive, (2) more invasive, and (3) most invasive (Table 66–2). *Noninvasive* implies that routine use of nerve block analgesia is probably not necessary, as described previously.[11] *More invasive* implies that a routine femoral nerve block would be recommended, but that a sciatic nerve block is probably not necessary because the vast majority of the postoperative pain is likely attributable to femoral nerve distribution. *Most invasive* implies that the postoperative pain will likely be attributable to both femoral and sciatic nerve distributions, and both nerves would likely benefit from routine blockade. The more invasive and most invasive knee surgery categories are based on clustering moderate and severe into one category of surgical invasiveness.[11]

This algorithm[85] also describes when a single-injection block would likely be sufficient versus when a CNB catheter would likely be of greater benefit than a single injection. If multimodal perineural analgesia applied to SINB provides meaningful extensions of patient-perceived analgesic duration, this may lead to a significant paradigm shift away from the more labor-intensive CNB care plan.

Foot and Ankle Surgery

For outpatient foot and ankle surgery, few, if any, substantiated, comprehensive recommendations are available for allocating nerve blocks (single injection vs continuous infusion) based on anticipated postoperative pain, postoperative nursing interventions (with vs without), or unplanned hospital admissions. Interestingly, few studies compared SINBs against GAVA for

surgery below the knee. In addition, few studies have categorized postoperative foot and ankle pain as sufficiently manageable with SINB versus CNB. Most studies evaluating the use of various approaches to the sciatic nerve block for foot and ankle surgery have simply evaluated block success rate (with no comparative treatment group), compared varying popliteal/sciatic nerve block approaches (sometimes with neuraxial techniques), or compared continuous-infusion strategies.

Singelyn and colleagues provided one of the first studies describing the efficacy of the popliteal fossa block placed with nerve stimulator guidance and reported a low 3% (15/507) rate of conversion to GAVA,[86] whereas Provenzano and coworkers reported an 18% conversion rate to GAVA (84/467).[87] In the same study, Provenzano and coworkers reported a significant reduction in postoperative opioid requirements in patients with a successful popliteal fossa block compared with 367 patients who did not receive the block.[87]

When neuraxial techniques are being considered, Curatolo and associates provides important insight that epidural anesthesia for foot and ankle procedures is associated with a high (4.4%, 7/160) conversion rate to GAVA, although epidural success was correlated with larger per-segment doses.[88] Several studies have compared the efficacy of spinal anesthesia with popliteal fossa block. All have shown the intraoperative efficacy of both techniques, although the in-hospital recovery after spinal anesthesia was more lengthy,[89,90] with an additional risk of urinary retention after spinal.[90] Protić and colleagues showed faster onset of time until surgical anesthesia was achieved with spinal, but with significantly shorter duration of analgesia.[91]

Generally, meaningful postoperative analgesia should not be expected after neuraxial techniques, and analgesia after popliteal fossa block will depend on the local anesthetic agent (and additives) used. In addition, when the analgesic duration of the popliteal sciatic block (with long-acting local anesthetics) is compared with the durations of ankle block, foot block, or subcutaneous infiltration, one should expect doubling or tripling the analgesic duration with a sciatic-specific depot injection.[92]

Continuous sciatic nerve catheters have gained popularity in recent years. After being introduced by Singelyn and colleagues, who described a complex Seldinger (catheter-over-guide-wire) technique for catheter placement (achieving a 92% success rate),[93] authors have repeatedly found that CNB techniques lead to excellent analgesic outcomes when compared with SINB techniques (or placebo catheters).[94-96] At this time, there are no definitive guidelines for the selection of SINB versus CNB techniques based on anticipated surgery, with the exception of recommendations implied by the myriad findings reported previously. Others have suggested that for hardware removal from the foot and ankle, a single-injection block is sufficient, whereas for most other foot-ankle procedures, CNB use may have additional benefits.[67]

A recent prospective randomized trial by Elliot and colleagues showed a significant difference in pain scores and oral opioid usage in postoperative days 2–3 after major ankle surgery when given a sciatic CNB local anesthetic bolus, with saline infusion or with bupivacaine infusion, for 3 days postoperatively. The authors, however, questioned the clinical

TABLE 66–2. Algorithm for recommended nerve block analgesia for knee surgery.

Category I (Noninvasive)

Types of Procedures: Knee arthroscopy with debridement, lateral release, meniscal surgery, simple meniscal repair, removal of superficial hardware, dropout cast application

Care Plan: No blocks unless unanticipated postoperative pain occurs

Category II (More Invasive)—Femoral Nerve-Distributed Pain

Category IIA: Less Painful Category II

Types of Procedures: Arthrotomy, deep hardware removal, microfracture, mosaicplasty/chondroplasty or cartilage transplant, complex meniscal surgery, ACL with single-bundle allograft

Care Plan: Single-injection femoral nerve block recommended: no sciatic block unless unanticipated pain refractory to femoral block

Category IIB: More Painful Category II

Types of Procedures: ACL with patellar tendon autograft or double-bundle allograft

Care Plan: Continuous catheter recommended: no sciatic block unless unanticipated pain refractory to femoral block

Category III (Most Invasive)—Femoral and Sciatic Nerve-Distributed Pain

Category IIIA: Least-Painful Category III

Types of Procedures: Distal patella realignment, some complex meniscal repairs involving the posterior knee

Care Plan: Single-injection femoral and sciatic nerve blocks

Category IIIB: More Painful Category III

Types of Procedures: ACL hamstring autograft, meniscal reconstruction, unicompartmental knee arthroplasty

Care Plan: Continuous femoral catheter and single-injection sciatic nerve block

Category IIIC: Most Painful Category III

Types of Procedures: Total knee replacement ACL double-bundle autograft, meniscal reconstruction, high tibial osteotomy, multiligament reconstruction (including PCL, LCL, MCL, POL), posterolateral corner reconstruction, management of knee trauma involving multiple incisions affecting anterior and posterior knee

Care Plan: Continuous femoral and sciatic nerve block catheters; caution with block of sciatic nerve via bolus or catheter infusion dose until dorsiflexion of the foot is documented postoperatively; consider perineural analgesics without local anesthetics (eg, clonidine-buprenorphine) until common peroneal nerve function is confirmed, before use of perisciatic local anesthetics

ACL = anterior cruciate ligament; LCL = lateral collateral ligament; MCL = medial collateral ligament; PCL = posterior cruciate ligament; POL = posterior oblique ligament.

Source: Adapted with permission from Williams BA, Spratt D, Kentor ML: Continuous nerve blocks for outpatient knee surgery. *Tech Reg Anesth Pain Manage.* Apr 2004;8(2):76–84.

significance of their study given the highest pain levels were 3.5/10, in addition to the added cost and inherent risks of CNB catheters in outpatients.[97]

The ultimate decision about the use of SINB versus sciatic CNB may depend on realistic expectations by the surgeon regarding return to weight-bearing status. In this situation, the surgeon may not have an accurate impression of weight-bearing success rates in the setting of uncontrolled pain, but full weight bearing in the setting of a partially anesthetized sciatic nerve (via a continuous sciatic catheter) may be ill advised. Evolving work with multimodal perineural anesthesia may lead to increasing analgesia with decreased risk of motor block.[98]

Summary Statement Regarding Nerve Block Technique Allocation

The rational use of SINB versus CNB in ambulatory surgery, that is, allocating the "scarce resource" of the well-trained RA practitioner and avoiding routine nerve blocks for patients who probably do not need them (or providing SINBs when a continuous catheter is not likely needed) will free time to perform catheter techniques for patients undergoing indicated procedures. Again, because of continued decreases in reimbursement and difficulties arranging follow-up for perineural catheters in the outpatient setting, SINB (perhaps with multimodal perineural analgesia, pending further study) with concomitant use of multimodal oral/systemic analgesics may be a reasonable and more cost-effective approach in the ambulatory surgery setting.[84] In OR settings that care for both outpatients and inpatients, this strategy allows the skilled RA practitioner to also dedicate time to CNB placement, where the incremental workload and cost would seem to be more beneficial.

EFFECTS OF PNB TECHNIQUES ON POSTOPERATIVE LENGTH-OF-STAY AND REHABILITATION OUTCOMES

The Need for Training and the Importance of Multimodal Analgesia

Despite the evolution of multimodal analgesia and nerve block analgesia, little progress has been made with respect to patient perceptions of quality improvements in analgesia care. This has been documented in two studies almost a decade apart, with Warfield and Kahn[99] and Apfelbaum and coworkers[100] using similar methodologies. Warfield and Kahn surveyed hospital patients from 300 hospitals (42% of which had acute pain management programs) and found that 77% of patients experienced pain after surgery, with 80% of these respondents categorizing their pain as moderate to severe. In the study by Apfelbaum and coworkers 8 years later, 80% of surveyed adults (n = 250) experienced pain after surgery, with 86% of these respondents characterizing the pain as moderate, severe, or extreme.[100] This latter study did not characterize the hospital-based acute pain management infrastructure where respondents underwent surgery.[100] Thus, the time between the first development in 1992 of federal recommendations for acute pain management[101] and pain management mandates in 2001 by the US Joint Commission[102] did not show perceptions of improvement in pain management after surgery in the general population.

Clinical Pearls

- Pain is often undermanaged in the opinion of the general public.
- Many health care professionals feel they need more training in understanding analgesic methods and means to implement them.

One approach to making significant progress toward improving postoperative pain management is to properly educate clinical staff. One study by Loder and colleagues described the surveying of the clinical staff of a rehabilitation hospital about their knowledge and attitudes regarding effective pain management.[103] This study showed that rehabilitation hospital staff held generally progressive attitudes toward the treatment of pain, but with a substantial degree of ambivalence about the use of opioids in that treatment.[103] The same staff rated their own lack of education about pain management as one of the chief barriers to effective pain management, and a large percentage reported feeling uncomfortable with various technical aspects of pain care.[103] As pain management techniques

continue to increase in both effectiveness and complexity, detailed planning and education are required for all health care providers, patients, and families (surgical hospital, rehabilitation hospital, outpatient rehabilitation facilities, and outpatients at home) to help make meaningful analgesia a successful endeavor.

Opioid protocols have been successfully implemented in rehabilitation hospital settings. Cheville and associates reported on the successful implementation in a randomized controlled trial of the use of controlled-release oxycodone for rehabilitation inpatients after unilateral total knee replacement surgery.[104] In this study (n = 59), patients were randomized to receive controlled-release oxycodone versus placebo every 12 hours, with the opportunity to receive immediate-release oxycodone every 4 hours as needed for breakthrough pain. Patients in the treatment group had lower pain scores, significantly better range of motion of the knee, and improved quadriceps strength than did the placebo group.[104] In addition, treatment group patients were discharged home from the inpatient rehabilitation facility 2.3 days sooner than placebo patients.[104] To summarize, a straightforward treatment intervention of a regularly scheduled controlled-release oral opioid led to significant outcome improvements and lower use of health care resources compared with the likely typical care plan of analgesics only as needed. However, such an approach has kindled (or substantiated) fears of opioid dependence and diversion. In addition, escalating doses of oral opioids are well associated with increasing side effects.

Dose-dependent opioid-related side effects were well described in a study showing that the increase of daily opioid dosing by the equivalent of 4 mg of morphine was associated with one additional clinically meaningful opioid-related symptom or one additional patient-day with an opioid-related clinically meaningful event.[105] These symptoms and events specifically included nausea, vomiting, constipation, urinary difficulty, difficulty with concentration, drowsiness, light-headedness, confusion, fatigue or weakness, pruritus, dry mouth, and headache.[105]

Logic would dictate that using multimodal analgesia, with a PNB technique as an integral component, will likely help improve patient perceptions of pain relief after surgery, especially when the patients are no longer in a surgical hospital (eg, inpatient rehabilitation or discharged to home). Kehlet has reviewed important principles of multimodal analgesia on postsurgical physiology.[106] However, neuraxial (epidural) analgesic techniques are unlikely to be a meaningful contributor to postoperative analgesia out of the surgical hospital setting, for obvious reasons. PNB anesthesia, including CNB, may provide a useful component of multimodal analgesia outside the surgical hospital setting in the years to come, but these prospects will likely disappear in settings where such services had been reimbursed but are no longer reimbursed (as in the United States). Even though significant progress has been made with respect to infusion technology; dose-response curve derivation; and education of clinical staff, patients, and family members when an anesthesiologist is not in immediate attendance, it would be difficult to economically justify the continuation of this costly subspecialty service for outpatients in the absence of payment to offset the costs and risks of delivering this service.

Decreasing Role for Epidural Techniques

For many years, neuraxial anesthesia was highly recommended as a technique of first choice for patients undergoing lower extremity total joint replacement or hip fracture repair. Much of this enthusiasm was based on the classic meta-analysis by Sorenson and Pace, which reported that the use of neuraxial anesthesia versus GA was associated with a significant reduction in mortality (odds ratio = 0.67), and a 31% reduction in deep venous thrombosis, for the repair of fractures of the femoral head.[107] Years later, the meta-analysis of several types of surgery (including orthopedics) by Rodgers and coworkers reported significant reductions in mortality (odds ratio = 0.70), pulmonary embolism (odds ratio = 0.45), deep vein thrombosis (DVT; odds ratio = 0.56), myocardial infarction (odds ratio = 0.67), renal failure (odds ratio = 0.57), pneumonia (odds ratio = 0.61), respiratory depression (odds ratio = 0.41), and transfusion requirements (odds ratio = 0.45 to 0.50) when neuraxial anesthesia was used instead of GAVA with postoperative intravenous patient-controlled opioid analgesia.[108] As discussed in the next section, it is unlikely that neuraxial epidural anesthetic-analgesic techniques will be sustainable and practical, but there are no apparent restrictions to the ongoing preferential use of spinal anesthesia combined with PNBs as a routine replacement for GAVA/opioid techniques.

Regional Anesthesia Techniques in the Setting of Modern Anticoagulants

Although the aforementioned studies would logically serve as landmarks for change in clinical practice, enthusiasm for epidural techniques has significantly decreased with the introduction of more potent and effective anticoagulants in routine clinical practice. Guidelines for neuraxial anesthetic use in the setting of systemic anticoagulation have been well publicized,[109,110] and the risks have been more accurately defined.[111] However, it seems less likely that patients will have epidural anesthesia-analgesia available to them in these clinical settings in the near future, pending a long-term outcome study that describes the frequency of adverse events created (eg, hemorrhagic cerebral infarction[112]) versus adverse events prevented (eg, pulmonary embolism and death) by the use of newer antithrombotics and anticoagulant agents.

Clinical Pearls

- Regional anesthesia techniques have been traditionally associated with fewer thromboembolic complications.
- Newer anticoagulants have offset previous thromboembolic differences seen between RA and GA.
- Indwelling perineural catheters have emerged as a valuable anesthetic technique for postoperative analgesia, but have led to some theoretical concerns regarding bleeding complications in anticoagulated patients.

In a meta-analysis of outcomes after the use of fondaparinux versus enoxaparin,[113] fondaparinux was shown to reduce the odds of venous thromboembolism by 55% compared with enoxaparin. Although fondaparinux was associated with higher "major bleeding," this did not translate to a clinically adverse outcome, such as risk of reoperation or death. In addition, the use of fondaparinux appeared to offset any outcome benefits achieved by neuraxial anesthesia versus GAVA, specifically for the avoidance of venous thromboembolism. The likely loss of the availability of epidural techniques as surgeons focus on the prevention of venous thromboembolism, without regard for the other documented benefits of neuraxial anesthesia/analgesia (eg, on the cardiac, pulmonary, and renal organ systems), forces the well-trained RA practitioner to incorporate SINB or CNB to give patients any chance for meaningful postoperative analgesia after lower extremity joint replacement or fracture repair. Therefore, the RA practitioner should actively ensure that patients' doses of the described anticoagulants are stopped in advance appropriately to render spinal anesthesia as the routine anesthetic of choice, supplementing spinal instead with ipsilateral PNBs (acknowledging the limited usefulness of continuous epidurals in current care, as described).

Horlocker and colleagues have documented the popularity of PNBs due to improved surgical outcomes. However, they also cited or speculated regarding block-related morbidity and mortality from serious hemorrhagic complications occurring in blocks given to anticoagulated patients. This underscores the importance of a firm understanding about anticoagulation as its popularity continues to increase regardless of nerve block technique.[114] We forecast that single-injection spinal anesthesia and SINB (especially in the form of multimodal perineural analgesia) will dominate clinical practice in the near future as decreasing reimbursements and added inconveniences of coordinating catheter placement and removal render "coordinated care" impracticable.

Evolving Role for Continuous PNB in Lower Extremity Surgery

Clinical Pearls

- Knee surgery has two tiers of postoperative pain considerations.
    1. For least-invasive procedures, blocks are probably not required.
    2. For moderately invasive procedures, a femoral nerve block is likely required.
    3. For the most invasive procedures, femoral and sciatic blocks are likely required.
- The other tier is **likely pain duration**: short duration (likely manageable with SINBs) versus longer duration (manageable with continuous-infusion blocks).

The use of PNBs for joint replacement has been examined during the past 20 years. Early on, outcomes were equivocal, but many studies primarily focused on SINB techniques. One exception is a study by Hirst and colleagues, where patients receiving GA did not gain additional analgesic benefit from a femoral perineural infusion compared with patients who received a SINB, although both groups required less postoperative opioid analgesia than did controls who received no block.[115] A study by J. G. Allen and associates showed that patients receiving femoral-sciatic single-injection blocks had better short-term (24-hour) pain outcomes than did patients only receiving spinal.[116] Another single-injection block study for total knee replacement patients by H. W. Allen and colleagues showed that the addition of single-injection sciatic nerve block did not confer any additional benefit versus the use of femoral nerve block alone.[117] This latter finding has not been reproduced in any study with similar methodology.

The late 1990s produced two important studies from Europe examining rehabilitation outcomes after total knee replacement when a continuous femoral catheter was used (vs epidural catheter or active control IVPCA device). These studies were predicated on the notion that continuous femoral nerve block analgesia (vs IVPCA) leads not only to better pain relief but also to significantly better knee flexion, faster achievement of ambulation goals, and overall faster convalescence. Studies by Capdevila and coworkers[118] and Singelyn and associates[119] showed that patients for total knee replacement undergoing GA with either continuous epidural analgesia or continuous femoral nerve block analgesia made faster progress in meeting rehabilitation objectives and were discharged from the inpatient rehabilitation unit sooner than were patients receiving IVPCA. Patients receiving femoral nerve catheter infusions experienced fewer side effects than did patients receiving epidurals in both studies, and patients with a continuous femoral catheter were discharged home from inpatient rehabilitation units sooner by 20% (40 vs 50 days[118] and 17 vs 21 days[119] in the femoral catheter vs IVPCA groups, respectively).

In the United States, a similar anesthetic treatment method was applied by Chelly and colleagues to patients receiving total knee replacement.[120] All patients received GAVA and were randomized to receive IVPCA, epidural infusion, or single-injection femoral-sciatic blocks followed by a continuous femoral infusion. Patients with continuous femoral blocks (vs patients with IVPCA) had an associated reduction of postoperative bleeding by 72% ($P < .05$), achieved better performance on continuous passive motion, had a 90% decrease in serious complications (including less blood loss), ambulated sooner (2.5 vs 3.5 days), and had a 20% decrease in the length of hospitalization (4 vs 5.5 days).[120] Duration of hospitalization did not include postoperative long-term rehabilitation (which is usually done on an outpatient basis in the United States),[120] as did the two previously listed European studies,[118,119] although early postoperative rehabilitation was aggressive.

Additional studies have supported the findings of Chelly and colleagues associating femoral nerve blocks with less opioid requirement, superior range of motion, and shorter hospital stay.[121,122] However, none of the aforementioned reports examined the benefits of sciatic CPNB, given the concern for "foot drop" and loss of proprioception/weight bearing below the knee from L4–S3 nerve block by local anesthetics. Future research is needed to examine the use of multimodal perineural analgesia excluding local anesthetics in relation to analgesia in the L4–S3 distribution.

The question of the need for a continuous sciatic catheter after total knee replacement was addressed in a prospective pilot study by Ben-David and coworkers.[123] In this study, 12 consecutive patients had continuous femoral and sciatic catheters placed preoperatively, but only the femoral catheters were dosed to allow for postoperative evaluation of sciatic nerve function (specifically aiming to produce dorsiflexion). Sciatic catheters were dosed only if dorsiflexion was intact and postoperative knee pain was refractory to additional boluses through the femoral nerve catheter. Ten of these 12 patients required dosing of the sciatic catheters, with median pain scores of 7.5 (of 10) before dosing and 2.0 after dosing. This pilot study refutes the earlier finding by H. W. Allen and colleagues[117] with respect to the value of sciatic nerve block for total knee replacement.

For hip fracture surgery, there has been less-convincing evidence with respect to PNBs, pain management, and rehabilitation outcomes. From the Cochrane Database of Systematic Reviews in 2002, lacking an update since, Parker and associates reported that:

> Because of the small number of patients included in this review and the differing type of nerve blocks and timing of insertion, it is not possible to determine if nerve blocks confer any significant benefit when compared with other analgesic methods as part of the treatment of a hip fracture. They do reduce the degree of pain experienced by the patient from hip fracture and subsequent surgeries. Further trials with larger numbers of patients and full reporting of clinical outcomes would be justified (p. 2, verbatim from the abstract).[124]

However, this systematic review of hip fracture surgery would not have included subsequent studies that addressed either hip fractures or other hip procedures.

Fournier and coworkers reported that patients receiving single-injection femoral nerve block versus sham block had a 4-hour delay in requests for first parenteral analgesic after prosthetic hip surgery, although pain outcomes were no different at 24 and 48 hours.[125] Stevens and colleagues reported that patients undergoing total hip arthroplasty receiving lumbar plexus single-injection blocks had less pain for up to 6 hours after surgery and less blood loss during and for up to 48 hours after surgery.[126]

Naja and associates reported (retrospectively) that elderly patients with hip fracture receiving lumbar plexus and parasacral blocks (vs GAVA) (1) encountered significantly less hypotension during surgery, (2) were less likely to be admitted to the intensive care unit after surgery (0/30 vs 11/30), and (3) had a shorter length of hospital stay (7 vs 14 days).[127] De Visme and colleagues ($n = 15$)[128] and Buckenmaier and coworkers ($n = 10$)[129] provided the first two reports of lumbar plexus and parasacral plexus blocks as the sole anesthetic for hip surgery (ie, coadministered GAVA or spinal anesthesia were not deemed necessary).

Souron and associates found that patients receiving intrathecal morphine (0.1 mg) versus single-injection lumbar plexus block with ropivacaine had better overall analgesic outcomes with intrathecal morphine after primary hip arthroplasty, although patients receiving intrathecal morphine had a 37% incidence of urinary retention (vs 11% for lumbar plexus block; $P < .05$).[130] Biboulet and colleagues compared single-injection femoral and lumbar plexus blocks with intravenous opioid patient-controlled analgesia (PCA) for patients undergoing total hip arthroplasty and found that PCA was as efficient as the single-injection blocks used in overall outcome, even though the pain scores and opioid requirements were lowest in the lumbar plexus single-injection group during the first 4 hours after surgery.[131]

Kullenberg and coworkers prospectively studied 80 patients who underwent hip fracture repair and were randomized to receive single-injection femoral nerve block (*n* = 40, block placed postoperatively) or no block (*n* = 40).[132] This study found that patients receiving nerve block had 15 hours of meaningful pain relief and ambulated 13 hours sooner (23 vs 36 hours) than did patients who received no block.[132]

The aforementioned studies particularly addressed SINBs for hip surgery and did not address CNB catheters. The following three studies did specifically address perineural infusions for such patients: Singelyn and Gouverneur prospectively evaluated 1338 patients undergoing total hip arthroplasty who chose IVPCA, continuous femoral block, or patient-controlled epidural analgesia.[133] These authors reported that patients who received continuous femoral infusion had the highest satisfaction, fewest side effects, the lowest request rate for supplemental opioids, and the fewest technical problems, but pain scores themselves did not significantly differ.[133] In a randomized clinical trial, Turker and coworkers compared patients receiving continuous lumbar plexus catheter (*n* = 15) with others receiving epidural catheter (*n* = 15) for hip hemiarthroplasty under GAVA and found that patients with the lumbar plexus catheter (1) had less motor block, (2) ambulated sooner, and (3) had significantly fewer overall complications.[134]

However, there have also been data showing an association between CPNB for hip arthroplasty and patient falls. Ilfeld et al examined three previously published, randomized, placebo-controlled trials involving femoral CPNB, with one arm receiving saline (*n* = 86) and another ropivacaine 0.2% (*n* = 85). None of the patients in the saline group fell, while the ropivacaine group showed seven falls among six patients (7%; 95% confidence interval [CI] = 3%–15%; *P* = .013). They concluded by stating a causal association between femoral CPNB and a risk of falling, with the caveat that four of the seven falls occurred after hospital discharge, with these patients not properly using a knee immobilizer.[135]

Based on the available evidence, femoral or lumbar plexus single-injection blocks have the potential to improve immediate postoperative analgesic outcome and possibly reduce hospital resource utilization in patients having invasive hip surgery. Unlike single-injection femoral nerve blocks, single-injection lumbar plexus blocks can be associated with a risk of bilateral spread, which carries a risk of perioperative implications in a frail elderly patient with limited cardiovascular reserve. One theoretical strategy to avoid precipitous hypotension (from bilateral spread with a single-injection lumbar plexus block) is to provide slow incremental doses via a continuous lumbar plexus catheter. In this setting, the incremental doses can be stopped as soon as it appears that surgical anesthesia/analgesia seems to be in place, but still keeping the catheter injection port available to the anesthesia team during surgery in the event additional boluses are needed intraoperatively.

Other than bilateral spread, a potential concern for lumbar plexus blocks (specifically continuous catheters) is the risk of

hematoma in an anticoagulated patient. Technically more challenging, continuous lumbar plexus blocks have been associated with hematoma-related complications in four patients documented in three case reports.[136–138] In one patient who was fully anticoagulated and receiving aspirin (325 mg daily), three serial single-injection lumbar plexus blocks were given, the last of which was considered "difficult," and a retroperitoneal hematoma was diagnosed a few days later.[137] A second patient developed a retroperitoneal hematoma in which significant vascular trauma was noted at the time the block was performed and the catheter placed.[136] A third patient developed a retroperitoneal hematoma 2 days after the single-injection psoas compartment block was placed, and this patient was rendered supratherapeutic on intravenous heparin throughout the 2 days after surgery.[136] The final patient had a history of factor 5 Leiden mutation treated with phenylindanedione; further details are described in the case report.[138] In each of these four cases, the clinical situations could not be reasonably considered routine, and all of these cases resolved without sequelae and without requiring surgical evacuation.

Other than these four cases, there have been no reports of hemorrhagic complications in patients receiving lumbar plexus catheters or fascia iliaca compartment blocks in the setting of modern anticoagulation practice.[139] There have been no published data regarding the estimated risk of retroperitoneal hematoma associated with lumbar plexus catheter removal in patients receiving effective postoperative anticoagulant therapy for the prevention of deep venous thrombosis. More cases are required to establish the safety of such a protocol. When considering the risk of bleeding associated with the removal of a lumbar plexus catheter in patients who are anticoagulated for the prevention of DVT, it is also important to acknowledge that the consequences of such bleeding are less serious than the bleeding that may result from the placement or removal of an epidural catheter. Epidural hematoma has been associated with serious neurologic complications in over 50% of cases, whereas no serious neurologic complications have been associated with the development of a retroperitoneal hematoma. Nevertheless, many clinicians who often utilize lumbar plexus and other CNB techniques tend not to address removal of CNB catheters with the same detailed scrutiny that has been deemed appropriate for epidural catheters.

Role of CNB Catheters and Effects on Rehabilitation in Upper Extremity Surgery

Data addressing physical therapy outcomes after major shoulder surgery performed with nerve block anesthesia are limited. Two studies addressed in more detail the recovery of motor function, comparing different CNB infusion drugs and concentrations. Borgeat and colleagues studied hand motor function and the presence of paresthesias in the fingers after open-shoulder surgery, when pain was managed via a brachial plexus CNB. Two infusion drugs were compared: bupivacaine 0.15% and ropivacaine 0.2%.[71] Infusions were run via an electronic device at 5 mL/h, with a 4-mL bolus available with a 20-minute lockout. Although both treatment groups' patients had equal analgesia and were equally satisfied, patients receiving bupivacaine CNB had more hand weakness at 24, 48, and

54 hours while reporting more finger paresthesias up to 48 hours after the initial nerve block than did patients receiving ropivacaine.[71]

Another study addressing motor function was conducted by Casati and coworkers.[140] Patients who underwent open-shoulder surgery were assigned to one of two CNB infusion drugs: ropivacaine 0.2% or levobupivacaine 0.125%. The infusion was run at 6 mL/h and allowed for a 2-mL bolus with a lockout of 15 minutes. There were no clinical differences in pain relief quality or motor function during the 24-hour infusion period. Thus, it appears that ropivacaine 0.2% and bupivacaine/levobupivacaine 0.125% are equipotent in providing CNB analgesia in the brachial plexus. The infusion rate of 5 to 6 mL/h while allowing for intermittent boluses of 2 to 4 mL with a 15- to 20-minute lockout provided an optimal balance of analgesia and preserved motor function.

One important safety feature to consider in the postoperative recovery of patients receiving continuous interscalene analgesia is adequate ventilatory function. It is generally accepted that most patients undergoing brachial plexus nerve blocks for shoulder surgery will encounter simultaneous block of the phrenic nerve, which is responsible for proper function of the diaphragm.[141–144] Borgeat and associates measured respiratory function during use of a CNB dosing technique that used both a continuous infusion (ropivacaine 0.2%, 5 mL/h) and a CNB bolus function (3–4 mL with a 20-minute lockout).[145] In this study, all patients received a preoperative bolus injection of ropivacaine 0.75%, 30 mL, and all patients underwent major shoulder surgery (rotator cuff repair, $n = 26$; arthroplasty, $n = 7$). The control group consisted of patients receiving IVPCA with opioids. Patients in the CNB group had better pain relief for up to 24 hours after surgery than the patients who were randomized to the opioid IVPCA. An important new finding was that overall respiratory function was better in the CNB group than in the IVPCA group. Forced respiration (ie, movement in the diaphragm on the nonoperative side) was better in the CNB group at 24 and 48 hours than in the IVPCA group. The rationale for this finding was that the pain control was better in the CNB group, and that there were fewer opioid-related side effects (eg, respiratory depression) in the CNB group, facilitating patients' forced respiratory efforts. Interestingly, forced diaphragmatic excursion on the side of surgery was not significantly different between the CNB and IVPCA groups at 24 and 48 hours after surgery. This study showed that forced respiratory effort was improved up to 48 hours after surgery in the CNB group, which when combined with better analgesia in the CNB group, provided an important safety validation in the evolution of same-day discharge of patients with CNB catheters and appropriate infusion devices after shoulder surgery.

Clinical Pearls

- More studies are needed to delineate define the severity of postoperative pain.
- Postoperative physical therapy and range-of-motion goals should be considered when deciding on the use of PNBs for postoperative pain management.

To date, there is limited research regarding the role of CNBs and the achievement of physical therapy milestones. One such study was performed by Ilfeld and colleagues, who retrospectively examined the charts of 50 patients having total shoulder arthroplasty (TSA), one-half who received an interscalene CNB with 0.2% ropivacaine infusing at a rate of at least 7 mL/h and the other half that did not receive a block. The cohort treatment arms were matched for age, gender, and type of TSA (primary vs revision). The results showed the CNB group achieved superior maximum shoulder elevation and external rotation. Ilfeld et al also showed median numeric pain scores for the CNB group of 2 versus 8.5 for the controls ($P < .001$).[146] These data imply improved physical therapy outcomes with interscalene CNB for TSA most likely from improved pain scores; however, more work is required, including more prospective, randomized trials to solidify the role of RA for upper extremity surgery.

Cost Analysis Illustrations Based on Available Data

Cost-Minimization Analysis

For this cost-minimization analysis, we compare three anesthesia treatments for a traumatic, closed patellar fracture in one patient. The mathematical formulas described here can be applied to actual incidences of compared outcomes using weighted-average techniques derived from larger surgical population data.[147] For the individual patient in this example, GAVA is compared with two spinal anesthesia techniques, one of which uses a single-injection femoral nerve block (two-needle technique), and the other that uses a femoral perineural catheter with single-injection sciatic nerve block (three-needle technique). Assumptions are as follows: (1) The patient receiving GAVA will encounter a routine recovery room stay, then hospital admission for 2 days (pain management, antiemesis, and resolution of somnolence); (2) the two-needle patient will encounter an unplanned hospital admission to "23-hour observation" after experiencing posterior knee pain treated with opioids and leading to PONV; and (3) the three-needle patient will be discharged home the same day with a disposable continuous-infusion device after successfully bypassing the PACU. Based on cost assumptions (Table 66–3) described in previous reports,[8,55] the sole task of cost minimization shows the incremental cost savings is roughly $800 for using the two-needle technique and an additional $200 when the added cost of equipment and medication for the three-needle technique is offset by the cost savings of PACU bypass and the avoided hospital admission.

Cost-Effectiveness Analysis

For a hypothetical CEA from the patient's (and the societal) perspective, we assume that patients are most interested in returning to nonstrenuous work as soon as possible, with sufficient cognitive function and pain control. In what should be interpreted as a strictly speculative illustration, the GAVA patient is assumed to require 10 days to return to work due to lingering effects of volatile agents, cumulative dose of opioids, and sedative effects of antiemetics. The two-needle patient

TABLE 66–3. Cost analysis illustration: ORIF patellar fracture.

Cost item	Anesthesia Care Plan for 3 Individual Patients			Incremental		
	(1) GAVA	**(2) Spi-Fem ("2-Needle")**	**(3) Spi-Fem Cath-Sci Single-Injection ("3-Needle")**	**2 vs 1**	**3 vs 2**	**3 vs 1**
Base	$50	$60	$90			
Infusion device and drug	0	0	$200			
PACU admission	$400	0	0			
Hospital admission	$800 (2d)	$400 (23 hr)	0			
Total cost	$1250	$460	$290			
Effectiveness parameter: *lost workdays (nonstrenuous work)*	10	8	2			
Incremental Cost Savings				$790	$170	$960
<u>Cost-effectiveness analysis:</u> *ratio of incremental hospital costs to workdays preserved*						
Incremental Workdays Preserved				2	6	8
Incremental cost-effectiveness ratios (hospital costs per day of work preserved for the patient)				790/2 → $395: 1 day	170/6 → $28: 1 day	960/8 → $120: 1 day
Benefit parameter: *lost wages at $200/day (strenuous work)*	$2000	$1600	$400			
Incremental Wages Preserved				$400	$1200	$1600
<u>Cost-benefit analysis:</u> *ratio of incremental hospital costs to wages preserved*						
Incremental cost-benefit ratios (hospital costs per dollar of wage preserved for the patient)				790/400 → 1.98	170/1200 → 0.14	960/1600 → 0.6
Utility parameter: *Outcome units on QoR-40 anesthesia outcome survey on postoperative day 2 (maximum score = 200)*	170	175	180			
Incremental Utility Units Preserved				5	5	10
<u>Cost-utility analysis:</u> *ratio of incremental hospital costs to patient utility units preserved*						
Incremental cost-utility ratios (hospital costs per preserved utility unit)				790/5 → 158	170/5 → 34	960/10 → 96

Cath = perineural catheter; GAVA = general anesthesia with volatile agents; ORIF = open reduction and internal fixation; QoR-40 = Quality of Recovery 40-item scale, as reported in 2000 by Myles et al[148]. Sci single-injection = single-injection sciatic nerve block; Spi-Fem = spinal anesthesia with single-injection femoral nerve block.

All values in dollars.

Base costs for GAVA and Spi-Fem based on Williams et al.[8]

PACU and hospital admission costs based on Williams et al.[55]

would probably have less cognitive dysfunction from (1) avoiding volatile agents and (2) encountering less cumulative effects of opioids and antiemetics, whereas the three-needle patient is pain free with the clearest cognition and is able to return to work on postoperative day 3 (with an infusing perineural catheter).

The increments of improvement in the return-to-work parameter are calculated by determining the difference in days to return to work from the reference value of 10 days (for the GAVA patient). Then, the incremental differences are inserted in the denominator, and the incremental hospital costs comprise the numerator. The ratio of incremental hospital cost savings to days of work saved for the patient (Table 66–3) was most cost effective (ie, the lowest cost-effectiveness ratio) when the decision was made to use a femoral catheter and sciatic single-injection block (three-needle technique) instead of just a femoral block (two-needle technique). It should be understood that an isolated cost-effectiveness ratio is only meaningful in the context of comparative methods being evaluated. In addition, hospital costs for each anesthetic technique do not clearly reflect the costs associated with anesthesiologist labor because the incremental workload is increased from GAVA, to the two-needle technique, to the three-needle technique, respectively. One would hope that well-trained RA practitioners recognize the value of their services and compassionately care for patients in such a way that gives the patient the best chance for immediate return to work in a health care system that is otherwise optimized.

With respect to using more population-based return-to-work data for a given procedure in an institution, certainly, Gaussian curves illustrating the 95% confidence intervals of actual return-to-work outcomes could be incorporated into the calculation, and similarly 95% confidence intervals of the cost-effectiveness ratio can be determined to evaluate the extent of overlap between techniques for the desired parameter of effectiveness. However, population-based return-to-work data after the wide variety of orthopedic procedures performed are scarce, and available population data are likely based currently only on a vast preponderance of cases being performed under GAVA without any PNB techniques.

Cost-Benefit Analysis

Using the design for the CEA example discussed, the effectiveness variable for CBA analysis now takes on a monetary value in the denominator. In this analysis, we assume the patient requires reasonable ambulation capabilities at work as a factory foreman paid an hourly wage who is not paid for time off for medical leave. The return-to-work benefit outcome takes the form of achieved wages. The return-to-work timeline remains the same as that described in the previous CEA example (Table 66–3).

In this example, the reference value for 10 days of lost wages is $2000 (after receiving GAVA with no blocks). Patients receiving spinal anesthesia with a femoral nerve block are assumed to return to work on postoperative day 8, incrementally reclaiming $400 of the lost $2000 in wages. Patients receiving spinal, femoral nerve block catheter, and single-injection sciatic block are assumed to return to work on postoperative day 3, thus

reclaiming $1600 of the lost $2000 in wages. These reclaimed wages are inserted into the denominator of the incremental cost-benefit equations, with the respective hospital cost increments inserted into the numerator. The cost-benefit ratios (CBRs; Table 66–3) indicate that the selection of the three-needle technique provides a better (lower) CBR than does the two-needle technique when the reference GAVA technique is considered as the standard for comparison.

Cost-utility analysis involves the insertion of a patient-reported effectiveness variable into the denominator of the cost analysis. We use the QoR-40 of Myles and colleagues[148] as a measure of utility from the patient's perspective, again comparing the hospital costs of the GAVA patient ($1250 cost) versus $460 and $290 for spinal anesthesia patients receiving single-injection femoral nerve block versus continuous femoral and single-injection sciatic nerve blocks, respectively. The achieved utility scores based on the QoR-40 by Myles and colleagues (with possible highest score of 200) are assumed to be 170 (GAVA), 175 (two needle), and 180 (three needle), respectively. These QoR-40 scores were validated by our published data of 154 patients undergoing ACL reconstruction standardized with spinal anesthesia and then randomized to receive perineural catheter injection-infusion with either normal saline or 0.25% levobupivacaine.[149] The incremental cost-utility ratios would be described as "hospital costs per preserved QoR-40 score unit" (Table 66–3). The two-needle technique shows an incremental cost-utility ratio of 158:1 versus GAVA, and the three-needle technique cost-utility ratio is 96:1 versus GAVA.

In both the cost-benefit and cost-utility illustrations, as with the cost-effectiveness illustration, the decision to use the three-needle technique instead of the two-needle technique provided the most impressive incremental pharmacoeconomic benefit. For the CEA and CBA, the analyses showed that the selection of the three-needle technique versus the two-needle technique provided a magnitude of "patient/societal benefit" by a factor of 14 (in comparison with the selection of the two-needle technique vs GAVA), whereas for the cost-utility benefit, the magnitude of benefit was a factor of almost 5 when comparing the same increments per technique. Indeed, it is conceivable that a win-win anesthetic technique (eg, total RA incorporating select nerve block catheters) may provide much greater societal benefit than the patient may be able to recognize if using only symptom-specific patient satisfaction surveys.

Obviously, the examples provided are simplistic and do not account for the significant variability in the care of many patients. However, the core structure of the analyses, including multiple variables that are important contributors to costs and outcomes, can be analyzed using decision analysis trees and weighted-average techniques to provide meaningful comparisons of anesthesia care techniques.

SUMMARY AND CONCLUSION

In the pharmacoeconomic analysis of the value of RA, several considerations are important. The first is to distinguish the objectives of outpatient surgery from the objectives for inpatient care. The second is to recognize that almost every decision made by the anesthesiologist may have a crucial influence on patient outcome not only in the short term but also potentially in the long term. The third is for the skilled RA practitioner to rationally allocate his or her own labor-related resources to ensure that patient-specific and procedure-specific criteria are met for each and every patient being considered for RA techniques to minimize wasted effort on patients unlikely to benefit from these labor-intensive interventions. The fourth is that the anesthesiologist is likely the primary patient advocate with respect to analgesic outcome, due to less likelihood of expertise or even interest among surgical colleagues and other health care personnel with respect to subspecialized pain management and its cost-related patient-centered benefits. The fifth is that a coordinated effort is required to gain the surgeon's and patient's confidence in the anesthesia team while simultaneously guiding all other related health care personnel with education efforts to redefine policies and procedures. Finally, awareness of overall cost implications, to both the hospital and society at large, is required to justify the expansion of (and reimbursement for) RA services to hospital administrators (and third-party payers or legislative entities).

REFERENCES

1. White PF, Watcha MF: Pharmacoeconomics in anaesthesia: what are the issues? Eur J Anaesthesiol 2001;23:10–15.
2. Drummond MF, O'Brien B, Stoddart GL, et al: *Methods for the Economic Evaluation of Health Care Programmes*, 2nd ed. Oxford University Press, 1997.
3. Williams BA, Kentor ML, Chelly JE: Cost-benefit and cost-utility analyses: outpatient implications. In Steele SM, Nielsen KC, Klein SM (eds): *Ambulatory Anesthesia and Perioperative Analgesia*. McGraw-Hill, 2004; Chapter 14.
4. Rodriguez-Monguio R, Otero MJ, Rovira J: Assessing the economic impact of adverse drug effects. Pharmacoeconomics 2003;21(9):623–650.
5. Pavlin DJ, Rapp SE, Polissar NL, Malmgren JA, Koerschgen M, Keyes H: Factors affecting discharge time in adult outpatients. Anesth Analg 1998;87(4):816–826.
6. Pavlin DJ, Chen C, Penaloza DA, Polissar NL, Buckley FP: Pain as a factor complicating recovery and discharge after ambulatory surgery. Anesth Analg 2002;95(3):627–634.
7. Williams BA, DeRiso BM, Engel LB, et al: Benchmarking the perioperative process: II. Introducing anesthesia clinical pathways to improve processes and outcomes, and reduce nursing labor intensity in ambulatory orthopedic surgery. J Clin Anesth 1998;10(7):561–569.
8. Williams BA, DeRiso BM, Figallo CM, et al: Benchmarking the perioperative process: III. Effects of regional anesthesia clinical pathway techniques on process efficiency and recovery profiles in ambulatory orthopedic surgery. J Clin Anesth 1998;10(7):570–578.
9. Williams BA, Kentor ML, Williams JP, et al: Process analysis in outpatient knee surgery: effects of regional and general anesthesia on anesthesia-controlled time. Anesthesiology 2000;93(2):529–538.
10. Williams BA, Kentor ML, Williams JP, et al: PACU bypass after outpatient knee surgery is associated with fewer unplanned hospital admissions but more phase II nursing interventions. Anesthesiology 2002;97(4):981–988.
11. Williams BA, Kentor ML, Vogt MT, et al: Femoral-sciatic nerve blocks for complex outpatient knee surgery are associated with less postoperative pain before same-day discharge: a review of 1,200 consecutive cases from the period 1996–1999. Anesthesiology 2003;98(5):1206–1213.
12. Macario A, Vitez TS, Dunn B, McDonald T: Where are the costs in perioperative care? Analysis of hospital costs and charges for inpatient surgical care. Anesthesiology 1995;83(6):1138–1144.
13. Sneyd JR, Carr A, Byrom WD, Bilski AJ: A meta-analysis of nausea and vomiting following maintenance of anaesthesia with propofol or inhalational agents. Eur J Anaesthesiol 1998;15(4):433–445.
14. Sinclair DR, Chung F, Mezei G: Can postoperative nausea and vomiting be predicted? Anesthesiology 1999;91(1):109–118.
15. Apfel CC, Roewer N: Postoperative nausea and vomiting [in German]. Anaesthesist 2004;53(4):377–389.
16. Apfel CC, Korttila K, Abdalla M, et al: A factorial trial of six interventions for the prevention of postoperative nausea and vomiting. N Engl J Med 2004;350(24):2441–2451.
17. Borgeat A, Ekatodramis G, Schenker CA: Postoperative nausea and vomiting in regional anesthesia: a review. Anesthesiology 2003;98(2):530–547.
18. Williams BA, Vogt MT, Kentor ML, Figallo CM, Kelly MD, Williams JP: Nausea and vomiting after outpatient ACL reconstruction with regional anesthesia: are lumbar plexus blocks a risk factor? J Clin Anesth 2004;16(4):276–281.
19. Korhonen A-M, Valanne JV, Jokela RM, Ravaska P, Korttila KT: A comparison of selective spinal anesthesia with hyperbaric bupivacaine and general anesthesia with desflurane for outpatient knee arthroscopy. Anesth Analg 2004;99(6):1668–1673.
20. Desilva PH, Darvish AH, McDonald SM, Cronin MK, Clark K: The efficacy of prophylactic ondansetron, droperidol, perphenazine, and metoclopramide in the prevention of nausea and vomiting after major gynecologic surgery. Anesth Analg 1995;81(1):139–143.
21. Chestnutt WN, Dundee JW: The influence of cyclizine and perphenazine on the emetic effect of meptazinol. Eur J Anaesthesiol. 1986;3:27–32.
22. Kentor ML, Williams BA: Antiemetics in outpatient regional anesthesia for invasive orthopedic surgery. Int Anesthesiol Clin 2005;43(3):205–213.
23. Splinter W, Roberts DJ: Prophylaxis for vomiting by children after tonsillectomy: dexamethasone versus perphenazine. Anesth Analg 1997;85(3):534–537.
24. Coloma M, Duffy LL, White PF, Kendall Tongier W, Huber PJ: Dexamethasone facilitates discharge after outpatient anorectal surgery. Anesth Analg 2001;92(1):85–88.
25. Wang JJ, Ho ST, Lee SC, Liu YC, Ho CM: The use of dexamethasone for preventing postoperative nausea and vomiting in females undergoing thyroidectomy: a dose-ranging study. Anesth Analg 2000;91(6):1404–1407.
26. Wang JJ, Ho ST, Lee SC, Liu YC, Liu YH, Liao YC: The prophylactic effect of dexamethasone on postoperative nausea and vomiting in women undergoing thyroidectomy: a comparison of droperidol with saline. Anesth Analg 1999;89(1):200–203.
27. Coloma M, White PF, Markowitz SD, et al: Dexamethasone in combination with dolasetron for prophylaxis in the ambulatory setting: effect on outcome after laparoscopic cholecystectomy. Anesthesiology 2002;96(6):1346–1350.
28. Gupta A, Wu CL, Elkassabany N, Krug CE, Parker SD, Fleisher LA: Does the routine prophylactic use of antiemetics affect the incidence of postdischarge nausea and vomiting following ambulatory surgery? A systematic review of randomized controlled trials. Anesthesiology 2003;99(2):488–495.
29. Cheng SS, Yeh J, Flood P: Anesthesia matters: patients anesthetized with propofol have less postoperative pain than those anesthetized with isoflurane. Anesth Analg 2008;106(1):264–269.
30. Tan T, Bhinder R, Carey M, Briggs L: Day-surgery patients anesthetized with propofol have less postoperative pain than those anesthetized with sevoflurane. Anesth Analg 2010;111(1):83–85.
31. Flood P, Sonner JM, Gong D, Coates KM: Isoflurane hyperalgesia is modulated by nicotinic inhibition. Anesthesiology 2002;97(1):192–198.
32. Frizelle HP, Duranteau J, Samii K: A comparison of propofol with a propofol-ketamine combination for sedation during spinal anesthesia. Anesth Analg 1997;84(6):1318–1322.
33. Menigaux C, Fletcher D, Dupont X, Guignard B, Guirimand F, Chauvin M: The benefits of intraoperative small-dose ketamine on postoperative pain after anterior cruciate ligament repair. Anesth Analg 2000;90(1):129.
34. Menigaux C, Guignard B, Fletcher D, Sessler DI, Dupont X, Chauvin M: Intraoperative small-dose ketamine enhances analgesia after outpatient knee arthroscopy. Anesth Analg 2001;93(3):606–612.
35. Mortero RF, Clark LD, Tolan MM, Metz RJ, Tsueda K, Sheppard RA: The effects of small-dose ketamine on propofol sedation: respiration, postoperative mood, perception, cognition, and pain. Anesth Analg 2001;92(6):1465–1469.
36. Sun T, Sacan O, White PF, Coleman J, Rohrich RJ, Kenkel JM: Perioperative versus postoperative celecoxib on patient outcomes after major plastic surgery procedures. Anesth Analg 2008;106(3):950–958.
37. White PF, Sacan O, Tufanogullari B, Eng M, Nuangchamnong N, Ogunnaike B: Effect of short-term postoperative celecoxib administration

on patient outcome after outpatient laparoscopic surgery. Can J Anaesth 2007;54(5):342–348.

38. Cepeda MS, Uribe C, Betancourt J, Rugeles J, Carr DB: Pain relief after knee arthroscopy: intra-articular morphine, intra-articular bupivacaine, or subcutaneous morphine? Reg Anesth 1997;22(3):233–238.

39. Soderlund A, Westman L, Ersmark H, Eriksson E, Valentin A, Ekblom A: Analgesia following arthroscopy—a comparison of intra-articular morphine, pethidine and fentanyl. Acta Anaesthesiol Scand 1997;41(1 Pt 1):6–11.

40. Yang LC, Chen LM, Wang CJ, Buerkle H: Postoperative analgesia by intra-articular neostigmine in patients undergoing knee arthroscopy. Anesthesiology 1998;88(2):334–339.

41. Buerkle H, Boschin M, Marcus MA, Brodner G, Wusten R, Van Aken H: Central and peripheral analgesia mediated by the acetylcholinesterase-inhibitor neostigmine in the rat inflamed knee joint model. Anesth Analg 1998;86(5):1027–1032.

42. Gupta A, Axelsson K, Allvin R, et al: Postoperative pain following knee arthroscopy: the effects of intra-articular ketorolac and/or morphine. Reg Anesth Pain Med 1999;24(3):225–230.

43. Reuben SS, Connelly NR: Postoperative analgesia for outpatient arthroscopic knee sugery with intraarticular bupivacaine and ketorolac. Anesth Analg 1995;80(6):1154–1157.

44. Soderlund A, Boreus LO, Westman L, Engstrom B, Valentin A, Ekblom A: A comparison of 50, 100 and 200 mg of intra-articular pethidine during knee joint surgery, a controlled study with evidence for local demethylation to norpethidine. Pain 1999;80(1–2):229–238.

45. Mariano ER, Chu LF, Peinado CR, Mazzei WJ: Anesthesia-controlled time and turnover time for ambulatory upper extremity surgery performed with regional versus general anesthesia. J Clin Anesth 2009; 21(4):253–257.

46. Dexter F, Macario A, Manberg PJ, Lubarsky DA: Computer simulation to determine how rapid anesthetic recovery protocols to decrease the time for emergence or increase the phase I postanesthesia care unit bypass rate affect staffing of an ambulatory surgery center. Anesth Analg 1999;88(5):1053–1063.

47. Olds DM, Clarke SP: The effect of work hours on adverse events and errors in health care. J Safety Res 2010;41(2):153–162.

48. Chelly JE, Greger J, Al Samsam T, et al: Reduction of operating and recovery room times and overnight hospital stays with interscalene blocks as sole anesthetic technique for rotator cuff surgery. Minerva Anestesiol 2001;67(9):613–619.

49. Williams BA: For outpatients, does regional anesthesia truly shorten the hospital stay, and how should we define postanesthesia care unit bypass eligibility? Anesthesiology 2004;101(1):3–6.

50. Williams BA: The WAKE© score: patient-centered ambulatory anesthesia and fast-tracking outcomes criteria. Int Anesthesiol Clin 2011;49(3): 33–43.

51. Aldrete JA: The post-anesthesia recovery score revisited. J Clin Anesth 1995;7(1):89–91.

52. White PF, Song D: New criteria for fast-tracking after outpatient anesthesia: a comparison with the modified Aldrete's scoring system. Anesth Analg 1999;88(5):1069–1072.

53. Jankowski CJ, Hebl JR, Stuart MJ, et al: A comparison of psoas compartment block and spinal and general anesthesia for outpatient knee arthroscopy. Anesth Analg 2003;97(4):1003–1009.

54. Williams BA, Kentor ML: Fast-track ambulatory anesthesia: impact on nursing workload when analgesia and antiemetic prophylaxis are near-optimal. Can J Anaesth 2007;54(3):243–244.

55. Williams BA, Kentor ML, Vogt MT, et al: Economics of nerve block pain management after anterior cruciate ligament reconstruction: potential hospital cost savings via associated postanesthesia care unit bypass and same-day discharge. Anesthesiology 2004;100(3):697–706.

56. Woolhandler S, Himmelstein DU: Costs of care and administration at for-profit and other hospitals in the United States. N Engl J Med 1997; 336(11):769–774.

57. Kitz DS, Slusarz-Ladden C, Lecky JH: Hospital resources used for inpatient and ambulatory surgery. Anesthesiology 1988;69(3):383–386.

58. Coley KC, Williams BA, DaPos SV, Chen C, Smith RB: Retrospective evaluation of unanticipated admissions and readmissions after same day surgery and associated costs. J Clin Anesth 2002;14(5):349–353.

59. Singelyn FJ, Lhotel L, Fabre B: Pain relief after arthroscopic shoulder surgery: a comparison of intraarticular analgesia, suprascapular nerve block, and interscalene brachial plexus block. Anesth Analg 2004; 99(2):589–592.

60. Hadzic A, Williams BA, Karaca PE, et al: For outpatient rotator cuff surgery, nerve block anesthesia provides superior same-day recovery over general anesthesia. Anesthesiology 2005;102(5):1001–1007.

61. Rohrbaugh M, Kentor ML, Orebaugh SL, Williams B: Outcomes of shoulder surgery in the sitting position with interscalene nerve block: a single-center series. Reg Anesth Pain Med 2013;38(1):28–33.

62. Koh JL, Levin SD, Chehab EL, Murphy GS: Neer Award 2012: cerebral oxygenation in the beach chair position: a prospective study on the effect of general anesthesia compared with regional anesthesia and sedation. J Shoulder Elbow Surg 2013;22:1325–1331.

63. Harvey GP, Chelly JE, AlSamsam T, Coupe K: Patient-controlled ropivacaine analgesia after arthroscopic subacromial decompression. Arthroscopy 2004;20(5):451–455.

64. Webb ST, Ghosh S: Intra-articular bupivacaine: potentially chondrotoxic? Br J Anaesth 2009;102(4):439–441.

65. Fredrickson MJ, Krishnan S, Chen CY: Postoperative analgesia for shoulder surgery: a critical appraisal and review of current techniques. Anaesthesia 2010;65(6):608–624.

66. Sripada R, Bowens C: Regional anesthesia procedures for shoulder and upper arm surgery upper extremity update—2005 to present. Int Anesthesiol Clin 2012;50(1):26–46.

67. Chelly JE, Ben-David B, Williams BA, Kentor ML: Anesthesia and postoperative analgesia: outcomes following orthopedic surgery. Orthopedics 2003;26(8 Suppl):865–871.

68. Klein SM, Grant SA, Greengrass RA, et al: Interscalene brachial plexus block with a continuous catheter insertion system and a disposable infusion pump. Anesth Analg 2000;91(6):1473–1478.

69. Borgeat A, Schappi B, Biasca N, Gerber C: Patient-controlled analgesia after major shoulder surgery: patient-controlled interscalene analgesia versus patient-controlled analgesia. Anesthesiology 1997;87(6): 1343–1347.

70. Borgeat A, Tewes E, Biasca N, Gerber C: Patient-controlled interscalene analgesia with ropivacaine after major shoulder surgery: PCIA vs PCA. Br J Anaesth 1998;81(4):603–605.

71. Borgeat A, Kalberer F, Jacob H, Ruetsch YA, Gerber C: Patient-controlled interscalene analgesia with ropivacaine 0.2% versus bupivacaine 0.15% after major open shoulder surgery: the effects on hand motor function. Anesth Analg 2001;92(1):218–223.

72. Ilfeld BM, Morey TE, Wright TW, Chidgey LK, Enneking FK: Continuous interscalene brachial plexus block for postoperative pain control at home: a randomized, double-blinded, placebo-controlled study. Anesth Analg 2003;96(4):1089–1095.

73. Ilfeld BM, Morey TE, Wright TW, Chidgey LK, Enneking FK: Interscalene perineural ropivacaine infusion: a comparison of two dosing regimens for postoperative analgesia. Reg Anesth Pain Med 2004;29(1): 9–16.

74. Singelyn FJ, Seguy S, Gouverneur JM: Interscalene brachial plexus analgesia after open shoulder surgery: continuous versus patient-controlled infusion. Anesth Analg 1999;89(5):1216–1220.

75. Hadzic A, Arliss J, Kerimoglu B, et al: A comparison of infraclavicular nerve block versus general anesthesia for hand and wrist day-case surgeries. Anesthesiology 2004;101(1):127–132.

76. Chan VW, Peng PW, Kaszas Z, et al: A comparative study of general anesthesia, intravenous regional anesthesia, and axillary block for outpatient hand surgery: clinical outcome and cost analysis. Anesth Analg 2001;93(5):1181–1184.

77. Gebhard RE, Al-Samsam T, Greger J, Khan A, Chelly JE: Distal nerve blocks at the wrist for outpatient carpal tunnel surgery offer intraoperative cardiovascular stability and reduce discharge time. Anesth Analg 2002; 95(2):351–355.

78. McCartney CJ, Brull R, Chan VW, et al: Early but no long-term benefit of regional compared with general anesthesia for ambulatory hand surgery. Anesthesiology 2004;101(2):461–467.

79. Ilfeld BM, Morey TE, Enneking FK: Continuous infraclavicular brachial plexus block for postoperative pain control at home: a randomized, double-blinded, placebo-controlled study. Anesthesiology 2002;96(6): 1297–1304.

80. Rawal N, Allvin R, Axelsson K, et al: Patient-controlled regional analgesia (PCRA) at home: controlled comparison between bupivacaine and ropivacaine brachial plexus analgesia. Anesthesiology 2002;96(6): 1290–1296.

81. Fredrickson MJ, Wolstencroft PJ, Chinchanwala S, Boland MR: Does motor block related to long-acting brachial plexus block cause patient dissatisfaction after minor wrist and hand surgery? A randomized observer-blinded trial. Br J Anaesth 2012;109(5):809–815.

82. Rawal N, Axelsson K, Hylander J, et al: Postoperative patient-controlled local anesthetic administration at home. Anesth Analg 1998;86(1): 86–89.

83. Swenson JD, Bay N, Loose E, et al: Outpatient management of continuous peripheral nerve catheters placed using ultrasound guidance: an experience in 620 patients. Anesth Analg 2006;103(6):1436–1443.

84. Hudson ME, Chelly JE, Williams BA: Economics: projecting costs and revenue for an interventional pain service in the ambulatory setting. Int Anesthesiol Clin 2011;49(3):68–83.

85. Williams BA, Spratt D, Kentor ML: Continuous nerve blocks for outpatient knee surgery. Tech Reg Anesth Pain Manage 2004;(8):76.

86. Singelyn FJ, Gouverneur JM, Gribomont BF: Popliteal sciatic nerve block aided by a nerve stimulator: a reliable technique for foot and ankle surgery. Reg Anesth 1991;16(5):278–281.

87. Provenzano DA, Viscusi ER, Adams SB, Kerner MB, Torjman MC, Abidi NA: Safety and efficacy of the popliteal fossa nerve block when utilized for foot and ankle surgery. Foot Ankle Int 2002;23(5): 394–399.

88. Curatolo M, Orlando A, Zbinden A, Venuti FS: Failure rate of epidural anaesthesia for foot and ankle surgery. A comparison with other surgical procedures. Eur J Anaesthesiol 1995;12(4):363–367.

89. Vloka JD, Hadzic A, Mulcare R, Lesser JB, Koorn R, Thys DM: Combined popliteal and posterior cutaneous nerve of the thigh blocks for short saphenous vein stripping in outpatients: an alternative to spinal anesthesia. J Clin Anesth 1997;9(8):618–622.

90. Casati A GC, Aldegheri G, et al: Peripheral or central nerve blocks for foot surgery: a prospective, randomized clinical comparison. Foot Ankle Surg 2002;8:95.

91. Protic A, Horvat M, Komen-Usljebrka H, et al: Benefit of the minimal invasive ultrasound-guided single shot femoro-popliteal block for ankle surgery in comparison with spinal anesthesia. Wien Klin Wochenschr 2010;122(19–20):584–587.

92. McLeod DH, Wong DH, Claridge RJ, Merrick PM: Lateral popliteal sciatic nerve block compared with subcutaneous infiltration for analgesia following foot surgery. Can J Anaesth 1994;41(8):673–676.

93. Singelyn FJ, Aye F, Gouverneur JM: Continuous popliteal sciatic nerve block: an original technique to provide postoperative analgesia after foot surgery. Anesth Analg 1997;84(2):383–386.

94. White PF, Issioui T, Skrivanek GD, Early JS, Wakefield C: The use of a continuous popliteal sciatic nerve block after surgery involving the foot and ankle: does it improve the quality of recovery? Anesth Analg 2003;97(5):1303–1309.

95. Ilfeld BM, Morey TE, Wang RD, Enneking FK: Continuous popliteal sciatic nerve block for postoperative pain control at home: a randomized, double-blinded, placebo-controlled study. Anesthesiology 2002;97(4): 959–965.

96. Chelly JE, Greger J, Casati A, Al-Samsam T, McGarvey W, Clanton T: Continuous lateral sciatic blocks for acute postoperative pain management after major ankle and foot surgery. Foot Ankle Int 2002; 23(8):749–752.

97. Elliot R, Pearce CJ, Seifert C, Calder JD: Continuous infusion versus single bolus popliteal block following major ankle and hindfoot surgery: a prospective, randomized trial. Foot Ankle Int 2010;31(12): 1043–1047.

98. Williams BA: Forecast for perineural analgesia procedures for ambulatory surgery of the knee, foot, and ankle: applying patient-centered paradigm shifts. Int Anesthesiol Clin 2012;50(1):126–142.

99. Warfield CA, Kahn CH: Acute pain management. Programs in US hospitals and experiences and attitudes among US adults. Anesthesiology 1995;83(5):1090–1094.

100. Apfelbaum JL, Chen C, Mehta SS, Gan TJ: Postoperative pain experience: results from a national survey suggest postoperative pain continues to be undermanaged. Anesth Analg 2003;97(2):534–540.

101. AHCPR. Acute Pain Management Guideline Panel: *Acute Pain Management: Operative or Medical Procedures and Trauma.* Agency for Health Care Policy and Research, Public Health Service, US Department of Health and Human Services, February 1992. Clinical Practice Guideline. AHCPR publication no. 92–0032.

102. *Joint Commission Pain Management Standards.* 2001. https://www.jointcommission.org/joint_commission_statement_on_pain_management/ Accessed August 20, 2016.

103. Loder E, Witkower A, McAlary P, Huhta M, Matarrazzo J: Rehabilitation hospital staff knowledge and attitudes regarding pain. Am J Phys Med Rehabil 2003;82(1):65–68.

104. Cheville A, Chen A, Oster G, McGarry L, Narcessian E: A randomized trial of controlled-release oxycodone during inpatient rehabilitation following unilateral total knee arthroplasty. J Bone Joint Surg Am 2001;83-A(4):572–576.

105. Zhao SZ, Chung F, Hanna DB, Raymundo AL, Cheung RY, Chen C: Dose-response relationship between opioid use and adverse effects after ambulatory surgery. J Pain Symptom Manage 2004;28(1):35–46.

106. Kehlet H. Multimodal approach to control postoperative pathophysiology and rehabilitation. Br J Anaesth 1997;78(5):606–617.

107. Sorenson RM, Pace NL: Anesthetic techniques during surgical repair of femoral neck fractures. A meta-analysis. Anesthesiology 1992;77(6): 1095–1104.

108. Rodgers A, Walker N, Schug S, et al: Reduction of postoperative mortality and morbidity with epidural or spinal anaesthesia: results from overview of randomised trials. BMJ 2000;321(7275):1493–1493.

109. Horlocker TT, Wedel DJ, Benzon H, et al: Regional anesthesia in the anticoagulated patient: defining the risks. Reg Anesth Pain Med. 2004;29(2 Suppl):1.

110. Horlocker TT, Wedel DJ, Benzon H, et al: Regional anesthesia in the anticoagulated patient: defining the risks (the second ASRA Consensus Conference on Neuraxial Anesthesia and Anticoagulation). Reg Anesth Pain Med 2003;28(3):172–197.

111. Mantilla CB, Horlocker TT, Schroeder DR, Berry DJ, Brown DL: Risk factors for clinically relevant pulmonary embolism and deep venous thrombosis in patients undergoing primary hip or knee arthroplasty. Anesthesiology 2003;99(3):552–560.

112. Dickinson LD, Miller LD, Patel CP, Gupta SK: Enoxaparin increases the incidence of postoperative intracranial hemorrhage when initiated preoperatively for deep venous thrombosis prophylaxis in patients with brain tumors. Neurosurgery 1998;43(5):1074–1081.

113. Turpie AGG, Bauer KA, Eriksson BI, Lassen MR: Fondaparinux versus enoxaparin for the prevention of venous thromboembolism in major orthopedic surgery: a meta-analysis of 4 randomized double-blind studies. Arch Intern Med 2002;162(16):1833–1840.

114. Horlocker TT, Wedel DJ, Rowlingson JC, et al: Regional anesthesia in the patient receiving antithrombotic or thrombolytic therapy: American Society of Regional Anesthesia and Pain Medicine evidence-based guidelines (third edition). Reg Anesth Pain Med 2010;35(1):64–101.

115. Hirst GC, Lang SA, Dust WN, Cassidy JD, Yip RW: Femoral nerve block. Single injection versus continuous infusion for total knee arthroplasty. Reg Anesth 1996;21(4):292–297.

116. Allen JG, Denny NM, Oakman N: Postoperative analgesia following total knee arthroplasty: a study comparing spinal anesthesia and combined sciatic femoral 3-in-1 block. Reg Anesth Pain Med 1998;23(2): 142–146.

117. Allen HW, Liu SS, Ware PD, Nairn CS, Owens BD: Peripheral nerve blocks improve analgesia after total knee replacement surgery. Anesth Analg 1998;87(1):93–97.

118. Capdevila X, Barthelet Y, Biboulet P, Ryckwaert Y, Rubenovitch J, d'Athis F: Effects of perioperative analgesic technique on the surgical outcome and duration of rehabilitation after major knee surgery. Anesthesiology 1999;91(1):8–15.

119. Singelyn FJ, Deyaert M, Joris D, Pendeville E, Gouverneur JM: Effects of intravenous patient-controlled analgesia with morphine, continuous epidural analgesia, and continuous three-in-one block on postoperative pain and knee rehabilitation after unilateral total knee arthroplasty. Anesth Analg 1998;87(1):88–92.

120. Chelly JE, Greger J, Gebhard R, et al: Continuous femoral blocks improve recovery and outcome of patients undergoing total knee arthroplasty. J Arthroplasty 2001;16(4):436–445.

121. De Ruyter ML, Brueilly KE, Harrison BA, Greengrass RA, Putzke JD, Brodersen MP: A pilot study on continuous femoral perineural catheter for analgesia after total knee arthroplasty: the effect on physical rehabilitation and outcomes. J Arthroplasty 2006;21(8):1111–1117.

122. Kadic L, Boonstra MC, De Waal Malefijt MC, Lako SJ, Van Egmond J, Driessen JJ: Continuous femoral nerve block after total knee arthroplasty? Acta Anaesthesiol Scand 2009;53(7):914–920.

123. Ben-David B, Schmalenberger K, Chelly JE: Analgesia after total knee arthroplasty: is continuous sciatic blockade needed in addition to continuous femoral blockade? Anesth Analg 2004;98(3):747–749.

124. Parker MJ, Griffiths R, Appadu BN: Nerve blocks (subcostal, lateral cutaneous, femoral, triple, psoas) for hip fractures. Cochrane Database Syst Rev 2002;(1):CD001159.

125. Fournier R, Van Gessel E, Gaggero G, Boccovi S, Forster A, Gamulin Z: Postoperative analgesia with "3-in-1" femoral nerve block after prosthetic hip surgery. Can J Anaesth 1998;45(1):34–38.

126. Stevens RD, Van Gessel E, Flory N, Fournier R, Gamulin Z: Lumbar plexus block reduces pain and blood loss associated with total hip arthroplasty. Anesthesiology 2000;93(1):115–121.

127. Naja Z, el Hassan MJ, Khatib H, Ziade MF, Lonnqvist PA: Combined sciatic-paravertebral nerve block versus general anaesthesia for fractured hip of the elderly. Middle East J Anesthesiol 2000;15(5):559–568.

128. de Visme V, Picart F, Le Jouan R, Legrand A, Savry C, Morin V: Combined lumbar and sacral plexus block compared with plain bupivacaine spinal anesthesia for hip fractures in the elderly. Reg Anesth Pain Med 2000;25(2):158–162.

129. Buckenmaier CC, Xenos JS, Nilsen SM: Lumbar plexus block with perineural catheter and sciatic nerve block for total hip arthroplasty. J Arthroplasty 2002;17(4):499–502.

130. Souron V, Delaunay L, Schifrine P: Intrathecal morphine provides better postoperative analgesia than psoas compartment block after primary hip arthroplasty. Can J Anaesth 2003;50(6):574–579.

131. Biboulet P, Morau D, Aubas P, Bringuier-Branchereau S, Capdevila X: Postoperative analgesia after total-hip arthroplasty: comparison of intravenous patient-controlled analgesia with morphine and single injection of femoral nerve or psoas compartment block. A prospective, randomized, double-blind study. Reg Anesth Pain Med 2004;29(2):102–109.

132. Kullenberg B, Ysberg B, Heilman M, Resch S: Femoral nerve block as pain relief in hip fracture. A good alternative in perioperative treatment proved by a prospective study [in Swedish]. Lakartidningen 2004;101(24):2104–2107.

133. Singelyn FJ, Gouverneur JM: Postoperative analgesia after total hip arthroplasty: i.v. PCA with morphine, patient-controlled epidural analgesia, or continuous "3-in-1" block? A prospective evaluation by our acute pain service in more than 1300 patients. J Clin Anesth 1999;11(7):550–554.

134. Turker G, Uckunkaya N, Yavascaoglu B, Yilmazlar A, Ozcelik S: Comparison of the catheter-technique psoas compartment block and the epidural block for analgesia in partial hip replacement surgery. Acta Anaesthesiol Scand 2003;47(1):30–36.

135. Ilfeld BM, Duke KB, Donohue MC: The association between lower extremity continuous peripheral nerve blocks and patient falls after knee and hip arthroplasty. Anesth Analg 2010;111(6):1552–1554.

136. Weller RS, Gerancher JC, Crews JC, Wade KL: Extensive retroperitoneal hematoma without neurologic deficit in two patients who underwent lumbar plexus block and were later anticoagulated. Anesthesiology 2003;98(2):581–585.

137. Klein SM, D'Ercole F, Greengrass RA, Warner DS: Enoxaparin associated with psoas hematoma and lumbar plexopathy after lumbar plexus block. Anesthesiology 1997;87(6):1576–1579.

138. Aveline C, Bonnet F: Delayed retroperitoneal haematoma after failed lumbar plexus block. Br J Anaesth 2004;93(4):589–591.

139. Hantler C, Despotis GJ, Sinha R, Chelly JE: Guidelines and alternatives for neuraxial anesthesia and venous thromboembolism prophylaxis in major orthopedic surgery. J Arthroplasty 2004;19(8):1004–1016.

140. Casati A, Borghi B, Fanelli G, et al: Interscalene brachial plexus anesthesia and analgesia for open shoulder surgery: a randomized, double-blinded comparison between levobupivacaine and ropivacaine. Anesth Analg 2003;96(1):253–259.

141. Urmey WF, McDonald M: Hemidiaphragmatic paresis during interscalene brachial plexus block: effects on pulmonary function and chest wall mechanics. Anesth Analg 1992;74(3):352–357.

142. Urmey WF, Talts KH, Sharrock NE: One hundred percent incidence of hemidiaphragmatic paresis associated with interscalene brachial plexus anesthesia as diagnosed by ultrasonography. Anesth Analg 1991;72(4):498–503.

143. Urmey WF, Gloeggler PJ: Pulmonary function changes during interscalene brachial plexus block: effects of decreasing local anesthetic injection volume. Reg Anesth 1993;18(4):244–249.

144. Urmey WF, Grossi P, Sharrock NE, Stanton J, Gloeggler PJ: Digital pressure during interscalene block is clinically ineffective in preventing anesthetic spread to the cervical plexus. Anesth Analg 1996;83(2):366–370.

145. Borgeat A, Perschak H, Bird P, Hodler J, Gerber C: Patient-controlled interscalene analgesia with ropivacaine 0.2% versus patient-controlled intravenous analgesia after major shoulder surgery: effects on diaphragmatic and respiratory function. Anesthesiology 2000;92(1):102–108.

146. Ilfeld BM, Wright TW, Enneking FK, Morey TE: Joint range of motion after total shoulder arthroplasty with and without a continuous interscalene nerve block: a retrospective, case-control study. Reg Anesth Pain Med 2005;30(5):429–433.

147. Williams BA, Kentor ML: Making an ambulatory surgery centre suitable for regional anaesthesia. Best Pract Res Clin Anaesthesiol 2002;16(2):175–194.

148. Myles PS, Weitkamp B, Jones K, Melick J, Hensen S: Validity and reliability of a postoperative quality of recovery score: the QoR-40. Br J Anaesth 2000;84(1):11–15.

149. Bost JE, Williams BA, Bottegal MT, Dang Q, Rubio DM: The 8-item Short-Form Health Survey and the physical comfort composite score of the quality of recovery 40-item scale provide the most responsive assessments of pain, physical function, and mental function during the first 4 days after ambulatory knee surgery with regional anesthesia. Anesth Analg 2007;105(6):1693–1700.

CHAPTER 67

Regional Anesthesia, Cost, Operating Room, and Personnel Management

John Laur and Franklin Dexter

INTRODUCTION

Whether in a private practice anesthesia group, academic institution, hospital organization, or some hybrid of these, understanding how regional anesthesia (RA) affects your budget and costs, as well as the perceptions and outcomes of patients, is important for planning and conducting economic discussions with health care administrators and surgeons. This chapter reviews the costs and economics of RA and describes the concepts that apply to anesthesia providers and groups across the globe. Billing is not included as each country chooses how it bills and is paid for RA procedures. Moreover, we focus on outpatient anesthesia, for which cost savings can be better defined. While facilities may benefit financially from RA applied in inpatient settings, such billing and cost issues are local. The economics of heterogeneity in bringing down costs for measured reductions in length of stay (LOS) were reviewed recently.[1-4] In brief, although RA can reduce patient LOS, Taheri et al demonstrated that for patients with an average LOS of 4 days or more, the majority of costs occur in the initial days of the hospital stay, and only 3% of costs are incurred in the concluding hospital days.[1]

Clinical Pearl

- Understanding how RA and analgesia affects budget and costs, as well as the perceptions and outcomes of patients, is important for planning and conducting economic discussions with health care administrators and surgeons.

OPERATING ROOM EFFICIENCY

Perhaps the most basic and important management decision is to increase the efficiency of use of operating room (OR) time. Maximizing OR efficiency is a major cost reduction strategy that is implemented by reducing the hours of over- and underutilized OR time. Allocated OR times are assigned by the institution to its surgical services. On days of the week that a service has allocated time, their cases are scheduled within the specified start and stop times of the service.[5-7]

Overutilized time is the positive difference between the total duration of cases (including all turnover times) and the allocated OR time interval, when the allocated time has been calculated as that which maximizes the efficiency of use of OR time. For example, cases and turnover times have a total duration of 10 hours, yet 8 hours of time are allocated—this yields 2 hours of overutilized time. Importantly, referring to time as overutilized implicitly assumes that the time allocated has been calculated to maximize the efficiency of use of OR time (ie, minimizing the weighted combination of overutilized and underutilized time).

Underutilized time is the positive difference between total case duration, including turnover time, and the time allocated for that day. An example would be having 8 hours allocated and cases completed in 6 hours, including all turnover time, resulting in 2 hours of underutilized time. If a surgical services committee sets the policy that all ORs are planned for 10 hours, then there are not 4 hours of underutilized time, just the 2 hours. That is because referring to time as underutilized implicitly assumes that the time allocated was calculated based on maximizing the efficiency of use of OR time.

Due to an improved side-effects profile and the excellent pain control provided by RA techniques compared to general anesthesia (GA) with volatile anesthetic agents and opioids, RA may reduce total OR case time (*case duration*, defined as patient in OR to patient out of OR), patient recovery duration, and time until discharge. However, to reduce the inefficiency of use of OR time, the technique has to help reduce the hours of overutilized OR time and/or the allocated hours of OR time (same amount of work done in less time).[8]

The cost of an hour of underutilized time is negligible relative to the cost of an hour of overutilized time. Consequently, the decision to use RA on the day of surgery will often have a negligible effect on OR efficiency. In other words, working faster generally does not increase OR efficiency; it is just "working faster." Because RA use is based on reducing undesirable side effects for patients, lowering incidence of unplanned admissions, and reducing patient and surgeon waiting times, appropriate OR allocation has a far greater impact on OR efficiency and economics than it does on RA use.[7]

The following narrative explains how use of RA can influence OR efficiency[5,6,9]:

Today, the allocated times for OR5 and OR6 are from 7 AM to 7 PM and for OR7 from 7 AM to 3 PM. OR5 will complete its present case at 3:30 PM and begin its last case (of 2.5-hours duration) at 4 PM. *Case duration* here refers to the time period from patient in to patient out of the OR, not surgical time. OR6 is expected to finish its present case at 4:30 PM and begin its last case (of 1.5-hours duration) at 5 PM. OR7 is estimated to complete its last case at 2:30 PM.

The same surgeon has requested a peripheral nerve block (PNB) for the last two cases in OR5 and OR6.

- *Scenario 1*: For the cases to *start on time*, the medical director plans to ask the OR nurses and the anesthesiologist in OR7 to stay late to place the nerve blocks, monitor the patients, and make them ready for OR5 and OR6. Each PNB procedure requires 20 minutes to complete.

If the staff from OR7 stay late and prepare the patient going to OR5, that patient will go into OR5 at 4 PM, incision can be made at 4:10 PM, and surgery will be finished at 6:30 PM. There would be no overutilized OR time in OR5. The patient scheduled to start next in OR6 would instead start in OR7 and would enter OR7 at 5 PM. Incision would be made by 5:10 PM, and the patient would be out by 6:30 PM. By 5:00 PM, the current OR6 case has exited, handoff can occur, and the team from OR7 can leave. *Alternatively*, the anesthesiologist out of OR7 could sequentially cover anesthesiologists in OR5 and OR6, allowing them to provide PNBs to their own patients while the OR7 nurse monitors them in a preoperative area (Figure 67–1). Either way, after those two nerve block procedures are completed and the last two patients for those rooms are brought to the respective ORs,

the OR7 team who stayed late could go home. The net effect is 2 hours of overutilized time (from 3:00 to 5:00 PM with OR7).

- *Scenario 2*: Suppose that the OR7 team leaves after OR7 work is completed (by 3:00 PM). The OR5 staff would then bring their patient to OR5 by 4 PM, perform the PNB, make incision at 4:30 PM (20 minutes to place the block, 10 minutes for positioning and preparation). The surgery then finishes by 6:50 PM (total duration 2.5 hours). The OR6 team escorts their patient to OR6 by 5 PM and proceeds with PNB placement. At 5:30 PM, incision is made, and surgery is finished by 6:50 PM. Both OR5 and OR6 end 20 minutes *later* than originally scheduled but still within the allocated OR time (7:00 PM). Thus, the OR7 surgery is finished before 3 PM, and OR5 and OR6 complete their cases by 7:00 PM (Figure 67–2). There is no overutilized OR time.

When OR time is *properly allocated*, RA use will have no effect on OR efficiency for the greater portion of management decisions made on the day of surgery. To help drive this home, the scenarios exaggerated the consequences that the day of surgery OR management decisions would have on OR efficiency. Still, the point remains that the most important factor influencing how RA affects OR efficiency is use of good statistical forecasting, done months in advance, to plan allocated OR time (also known as OR staffing).

Other opportunities for labor cost reduction are often limited. Dexter et al analyzed data obtained from the 2006 National Survey of Ambulatory Surgery for determining the amount of OR time used for sedation or monitored anesthesia care (MAC) alone after PNB. This data set sampled all ambulatory surgical procedures from all licensed freestanding ambulatory surgery centers and nonfederal hospitals performing ambulatory surgery within the United States in 2006. MAC with a PNB or PNB alone accounted for approximately one-third of ambulatory center OR time with an anesthesiologist or certified registered nurse anesthetist (CRNA). In short, PNB cases accounted for a large portion of total ambulatory care in the United States. The consequence is that, faced with economic constraints, payers may consider reducing payments for RA, and groups may want to prepare for the impact on their facilities.

For example, if there are two ORs on a given day with hand surgery cases and some are performed by RA only and others under GA, an OR manager may consider resequencing the cases so that one room (surgeon A) has GA cases for the first half of the day and another room (surgeon B) has GA cases during the second half of the day. A CRNA or anesthesiologist assistant (AA) could work one room at a time, performing all the GA cases, and a nurse, certified in moderate sedation, could provide light-to-moderate sedation for the RA cases. Managing such an OR schedule would require no overlap of cases needing a CRNA or AA. Certain statistical methods can be used to minimize the probability of overlap accounting for built-in

Scenario 1 Timeline					
Time		Pre-Op/Block Room	OR7	OR6	OR5
2:30			Last case out	2nd to last case out	2nd to last case out of OR5
3:00	OR7 Staff work 2 hours over utilized time (3 to 5 pm)	OR7 staff handoff patient in PACU, then stay to help prepare OR5 and OR6 cases	OR cleaned		
3:30		OR7 covers for OR5 staff in order to place nerve block and also monitor OR5 patient			
4:00					Turnover time
4:30		OR7 staff covers OR6 staff to place nerve block and also monitor OR6 patient			Last OR5 case (2.5-h duration) enters
5:00		OR7 staff handoff patient and leave for the day		Turnover time	
5:30				Last OR6 case in (1.5-h duration)	
6:00					
6:30				Last case out	Last case out

FIGURE 67–1. Graphical timeline of scenario 1.

uncertainty. If no time buffer was used, surgeons and patients could expect delays. Also, patient requests for or denial of RA would create delays and increase costs.[10]

Clinical Pearls

- Increasing the efficiency of use of OR time is implemented by reducing the hours of over- and underutilized OR time.
- Appropriate OR allocation has a far greater impact on OR efficiency and economics than RA use.
- The most important factor influencing how RA affects OR efficiency is use of good statistical to plan allocated OR time.

ON-TIME STARTS

In a prospective time-motion study on first cases of the day, Chelly et al described an academic setting with the use of an acute interventional pain service team consisting of two anesthesiologists, two nurses, and four anesthesia residents or fellows performing the procedures in a preoperative area. They succeeded in having only four to six patients receive their nerve blocks and enter the OR on time. During the study, up to nine patients were indicated to have PNBs placed preoperatively, indicating a mismatch of pain service personnel to demand. This conclusion was based in part on the amount of time required for an advanced trainee (postgraduate year 4 anesthesia resident or postgraduate year 5 regional anesthesia and acute pain medicine fellow) to place a nerve block (20–30 minutes) under constant supervision of the attending physician. The study included landmarks or nerve stimulator–based techniques; no ultrasound guidance was used.[11] Mean time to place a block was 21 minutes (95% confidence interval [CI], 20–22 minutes). Duration of the PNB procedure varied by block type, and placing two catheters required the most time (mean, 30 minutes; 95% CI, 28–33 minutes).[11]

Mean time from patient arrival until transfer to the OR was 11 minutes longer for PNB patients than for controls (2:03, 95% CI 1:59, 2:07 h:min vs 1:51, 95% CI 1:42, 2:01 h:min, respectively) (P = .0019). For controls, 49% left on time for the OR compared to 40% of those in the PNB group (P = .067 one sided). More than half of the delays transferring patients to the OR were caused by surgical issues (control group 52%, PNB group 54%). Of delays in the PNB group, 15% were related to performing the nerve blocks, with 13% of that time being due to a lack of personnel. In fact, there was an average of 5.4 patients in the PNB group compared with 4.2 patients in the

Scenario 2 Timeline			
Time	OR7	OR6	OR5
2:30	Last case out	2nd-to-last case out	2nd-to-last case out of OR5
3:00	OR cleaned		
3:30			
4:00			Turnover time
4:30			Last OR5 case (2.5-h duration) enters, block performed, patient prep, incision at 4:30
5:00		Turnover time	
5:30		Last OR6 case (1.5-h duration) enters, block performed, patient prep, incision at 6:00 Last case out at 6:50	
6:00			Last case out at 6:50
6:30			
7:00			
7:30		OR cleaned	OR cleaned

FIGURE 67–2. Graphical timeline of scenario 2.

control group (P = .0007). The specific values are likely sensitive to the characteristics of the facilities. The RA team should arrive on time and early enough based on prior data to place successful blocks so surgery is not delayed. In many hospitals policy states that the surgeons must arrive early enough to consent patients and mark the surgical site before a nerve block is allowed to be placed. Also, when possible, the team should first perform block procedures for patients in the ORs with expected hours of overutilized time. When feasible, the team should next perform block procedures for patients in rooms where there is a single surgeon and more than 8 hours of cases. Further, months in advance when staff scheduling is calculated, more anesthesia providers who perform PNB cases should be planned for those days of the week when more PNB cases are expected.[6,9]

Clinical Pearls

- When possible, the team should prioritize block procedures for patients in the ORs with expected hours of overutilized time. When feasible, the team should next perform block procedures for patients in rooms where there is a single surgeon and more than 8 hours of cases.
- Months in advance, when staff scheduling is calculated, plan for more anesthesia providers who perform PNB cases on days of the week when more PNB cases are expected.

BLOCK TEAM AND SURGEON PERCEPTION

The most common complaints among surgeons about implementing RA are delays in induction of anesthesia and unpredictability of success.[12,13] However, other factors can be involved. In a study by Eappen et al, the addition of an RA team with dedicated space to place blocks did not reduce anesthesia-controlled times (ACTs) or turnover times.[14] A "block team" was created to shorten turnover times in an institution that was experiencing long turnover times of greater than 60 minutes. The team identified potential RA patients, transported them to a block room about 1 hour before the intended start time, and placed the block while the OR was performing the preceding case. Nerve blocks consisted of PNBs and epidurals (spinal anesthetics were placed in the OR by the OR anesthesia team). Patients with nerve blocks placed in the block room were "ready for incision" as they entered the OR. Anesthetic care was handed over to the OR anesthesia team once the patient was brought to the OR. It was up to the discretion of the OR anesthesia team whether to use GA.

Anesthesia emergence time was reduced by 1 minute among cases where regional block was used. There were no improvements in other segments of total OR time. Of note, there were only 0.7 turnovers per day on average; hence, there were less than two cases per room per day on average. In this academic hospital setting, having an impact on turnover time or on other OR times would not have significant clinical or economic impact. These time-motion results were probably specific to that hospital. More important, 10 orthopedic surgeons who collectively performed 80% of the cases completed a survey as part of the Eappen et al study. The surgeons indicated that the block team was effective, had changed the quality of their day for the better, and should be available every day. The surgeons may have had a positive perception originating from actually seeing their patients' readiness to go to the OR. Later studies showed that surgeon perceptions of nonoperative times are based on a mental model of workflow, not on actual time to place PNBs.[15] Consequently, even though the time to place PNBs is the major source of criticism, it does not explain the use or nonuse of PNBs.[12,13]

Surgeons were surveyed whether they would choose a block for themselves if they were undergoing the same surgical procedure.[12,13] The concordance between surgeon choice of a nerve block and his or her recommendation for a patient was high.[12,13] The concordance rates between surgeons' wanting a block for themselves and what they preferred for their own patients were 89% for arthroscopic shoulder surgery, 87% for arthroscopic anterior cruciate ligament reconstruction, and 93% for total knee replacement (Cohen's κ, $P < .001$ for each). Surgeon perceptions of time to place the PNB ($P \geq .27$) and PNB success rate ($P \geq .30$) were not correlated with whether they would recommend PNBs to their patients.

It is important to define block team members and have a plan for expected tasks, required skills, training, and the costs and benefits of hiring block team personnel. This can be part of a business plan when bringing the concept of a block team to hospital or group administrators and decision-makers.[16] A block team model often includes some type of assistant for the practitioner performing the procedure. Literature describing the concept of a RA "block nurse" is available.[17,18] This team member assists with preparation, performs a time-out, confirms medication labeling, assists with injections, monitors the patients after the block, and can be certified in moderate sedation and other tasks. Some procedures can be done in the preoperative holding area or in a block/induction room, thereby reducing time spent completing these procedures in the OR.

Clinical Pearl

- The concordance is high between a surgeon's preference of a nerve block for him- or herself and the surgeon's recommendation of a nerve block for his or her patient. Concordance is not with perceptions of time to place the PNB and PNB success rate.

BLOCK ROOM MODEL

Armstrong et al described a block room model for which upper extremity plastics or orthopedic surgical procedures were performed by nine surgeons. The anesthetic method was chosen at the discretion of the attending anesthesiologist and included brachial plexus blocks.[19] Intravenous and local anesthetic infiltration methods were excluded. Brachial plexus blockade was

performed in the block room or in the OR at the discretion of the anesthesiologist. There was no standardization of technique.

Placing a PNB in a block room significantly reduced presurgical OR time compared to GA alone or to PNB placed in the OR (mean 11.4 vs 17.8 vs 32.9 minutes, respectively; $P < .05$). Compared to GA alone, postsurgical OR time was significantly reduced using either PNB alone or combined with GA. ACT was longer when the PNB was performed in the OR than in a block room (mean 37.1 vs 15.1 minutes, respectively; $P < .05$). The surgical procedure time was shorter with PNB than with GA alone (mean 75.3 vs 99.4 minutes; $P < .05$).[19]

An editorial on the Armstrong-Cherry study noted that less than half of the PNBs were performed in a block room. This may be due to multiple factors involved in a busy practice environment, suggesting that perhaps the block room could be used more systematically.[20] Using the block room no more than twice a day would not make much sense from a cost-effectiveness perspective unless the area also doubled as a surveillance area.[17,20] In the Armstrong-Cherry study, the block room did, in fact, serve as a monitoring area for ophthalmology patients, whose nerve blocks were also placed there.

Findings such as the number of nerve blocks performed per day and additional uses of block areas imply that there is no single economic value to PNBs. Instead, the science shows which factors are important to the local business plan.[16]

SWING ROOM MODEL

The use of two ORs for performing hand and wrist surgeries under PNB alone was studied by Head et al. The anesthesia model consisted of one anesthesiologist and two AAs monitoring patients in the OR. The "swing-room" patients (RA-SR group) received a brachial plexus block, the non–swing-room control patients received GA (GA-OR).[21]

The RA-SR group had shorter turnover times than the GA-OR group.[21] The surgeon was able to proceed with the procedure on the next case in one room while an assistant closed and dressed the incision of the case just completed in another room. A "negative" turnover time was created for 10% of cases with that surgeon (not with the individual OR). This was not applicable in the GA-OR group because personnel were held to one room.[21] The swing-room system can be costly, and if an institution is considering this, it should be determined that more surgeries per OR per day will be performed using this dual-room model for one surgeon compared to a single-room model.

ANESTHESIA-CONTROLLED TIME

Williams et al demonstrated that ACT in the OR can be shortened by using RA instead of GA with volatile anesthetics.[22] Blocks for anterior cruciate ligament reconstruction procedures performed by one surgeon were placed in the preoperative holding area with an anesthesiologist and an RA resident. Patients were monitored by a preoperative nurse or an anesthesia resident. When the OR was available, the patient was brought into the OR, monitors were applied, and the patient was prepared and positioned. Patients with planned GA were prepared and positioned before GA was induced.[22]

Anesthesia-controlled time for RA patients was shifted from inside the OR (costly time) to the preoperative holding area (less-costly time). ACT was lowest when RA was performed in the holding area (mean, 11.4 ± 1.3 minutes, ± 2 SEM). Patients having GA combined with PNB also had shorter ACT (mean, 15.7 ± 1.0 minutes) than GA alone (mean, 20.3 ± 1.2 minutes).[22] In a stepwise regression model, using the preoperative holding area to induce RA predicted lower ACT than inducing GA in the OR. In-OR induction time (for GA) increased ACT when compared to RA performed in the preoperative holding area or local anesthetic infiltration/Bier block administered in the OR.[22]

Mariano et al demonstrated that upper extremity surgery ACT was significantly reduced by placing PNBs in the preoperative holding area or by performing a Bier block or certain local anesthetic infiltration procedures in the OR compared with GA. That is, the median ACT was 28 minutes (interquartile range, IQR [15]) compared to the median ACT of 32 minutes (IQR [12]) for RA versus GA, respectively (P = .039). Mean ACT in the nerve block group may have been 4.5 minutes shorter than in the GA group, although the difference did not reach statistical significance (95% CI, −9.4 to 0.4 minutes).[23]

The OR intervals (minutes) have been analyzed by Shuster et al.[24] Mean ACT was similar for GA and spinal anesthesia (mean, 30.4 ± 15.1 minutes and 31.7 ± 13.6 minutes, respectively). Mean ACT was statistically significantly greater for PNB and epidural anesthesia placed in the OR (mean, 44.8 ± 17.9 minutes and 46.4 ± 21.7 minutes, respectively) than compared to GA (P < .05).[20] RA care pathway patients had shorter OR duration (from surgery end until patient out of room) than patients with GA alone.[25]

INDUCTION AND SURGICAL TIME

Liu et al compared RA and GA in a meta-analysis of randomized controlled trials.[26] "Anesthesia induction time" described the interval from "beginning of induction until the patient was ready for surgery," that is, when the patient's level of anesthesia allowed the surgical procedure to begin. Central neuraxial block (odds ratio, 8.1; 95% CI, 4.1 to 12.1) and PNB (odds ratio, 8.1; 95% CI, 2.6 to 13.7) were both associated with an increased time until anesthesia ready compared to GA.

Dexter et al performed a meta-analysis of studies that used RA and compared nerve block methods with GA. The intent was to evaluate the effect of increased use of RA on overall performance of the surgical suite. Retrobulbar, local anesthetic infiltration (2 studies, 163 patients); spinal (10 studies, 812 patients); and epidural (11 studies, 702 patients) techniques were included. There were no significant differences in surgical times for the regional techniques compared with GA (mean difference, 1.7 minutes; 95% CI, −0.05 to 3.9 minutes).[27]

TURNOVER TIMES

Preoperative RA procedures and activation of anesthesia start times associated with the RA procedure significantly lengthened the time from anesthesia start to patient-in-room time compared to the GA care pathway group or to all historical controls.[25] However, turnover times were not significantly different between GA (median 24 minutes, IQR [12]) and either the nerve block (median 25 minutes, IQR [20]) (P = .88 vs GA) or local anesthetic infiltration (including Bier block) (median 21 minutes, IQR [20]) groups (P = .948 vs GA).[23]

Williams et al showed that nerve blocks often do not increase turnover time.[22] Instead, turnover time must be thought of as a product of a multidisciplinary team, not simply as part of an anesthesia-limited process. This finding adds more data that indicate turnover times are influenced by multiple factors and not solely by RA procedures.[11,22,28,29]

PACU COSTS

Compared with personnel costs, drugs and materials represent only a small (2%) portion of PACU charges. Dexter et al created simple simulations to quantify the degree to which three interventions can reduce postanesthesia care unit (PACU) costs: (1) use of short-acting anesthetic agents, (2) elimination of nausea and vomiting by any means, and (3) adjustments to OR scheduling practices. For a brief workday in their ambulatory surgery center, the number of admissions per hour rose linearly to a peak and then linearly declined to zero. This triangular distribution was used to determine how admission rates to the PACU would affect the peak PACU patient census by hour of the day. Changes in the peak patient admission rates were simulated. The OR schedule had far greater impact on the number of PACU nurses needed than eliminating nausea and vomiting entirely or using short-acting anesthetic agents only. The distribution of patient admissions to the PACU throughout the day was the main factor determining PACU costs.[30] Varying the time of day of the last patient admission to the PACU had a smaller effect than altering the arrival times.

Minor differences in patient PACU durations that have full-time nursing staff are unlikely to create lower labor costs. In contrast, depending on the number of patients admitted daily, the use of RA to increase the PACU bypass rate can decrease staff and associated labor expenses. Table 67–1 is a resource for managers wishing to estimate the number of PACU nurses that could be reduced by bypassing the PACU at various rates and at different quantities of patients per day. The top eight rows of the original table are reproduced here. The table is designed to be used as a screening tool for facilities to decide whether to perform their own detailed analyses.

For example, hypothetically every ambulatory surgery center patient is brought into the PACU by 4:00 PM at the latest. Care is provided for 40 patients per day on average (5 patients per OR with eight ORs), where there is an average of a 30-minute stay in the phase I PACU and 60 minutes in the second-stage recovery. An initial starting point is that 20% of MAC or RA patients bypass the phase I PACU. By increasing the PACU

TABLE 67–1. Example of what to reproduce from the original (the top eight rows).

Time in Phase II (minutes)	Time in Phase I (minutes)	Time of Last Admit (PM)	Mean Number of Patients Each Day	Full-Time PACU Nurses at Specified Phase I Bypass Rates						
				0%	20%	30%	40%	50%	60%	80%
60	30	2	20	7	6	6	6	6	5	5
60	30	2	30	9	8	8	8	7	7	6
60	30	2	40	11	10	10	9	9	8	8
60	30	2	50	12	12	11	11	11	10	9
60	30	4	20	6	5	5	5	5	5	4
60	30	4	30	7	7	7	7	6	6	6
60	30	4	40	9	9	8	8	8	7	7
60	30	4	50	11	10	10	9	9	8	8

Source: Adapted with permission from Dexter F, Macario A, Manberg PJ, et al: Computer simulation to determine how rapid anesthetic recovery protocols to decrease the time for emergence or increase the phase I postanesthesia care unit bypass rate affect staffing of an ambulatory surgery center. *Anesth Analg.* 1999 May;88(5):1053–1063.

bypass rate from 20% to 30%, a facility can reduce the need for one PACU nurse (from 9 to 8) and save on labor costs.[31]

Clinical Pearl

- The distribution of PACU admissions throughout the day is the main factor determining PACU costs. Altering this distribution by using RA to increase PACU bypass rates can reduce PACU labor costs.

PACU BYPASS

Using a multivariable linear regression model to predict the determinants of discharge times for patients following outpatient lower extremity surgery, Williams et al found that time to patient discharge can be reduced by using an RA PACU bypass criteria (RAPBC) scoring system. The anesthetic plans consisted of GA alone, an anesthetic lower extremity PNB alone, an analgesic PNB combined with either a GA or neuraxial anesthetic, or neuraxial anesthetic alone. GA was maintained with nitrous oxide and oxygen with either sevoflurane or desflurane. Anesthetic methods were categorized into "GA" versus "no GA," and "recommended blocks used" versus "not used." Surgical invasiveness was categorized into "mild" (e.g., arthroscopic knee meniscus repair), where short-term anesthetic blocks with or without GA or spinal, but no long-acting PNBs, were used; or "invasive" (eg, arthroscopic anterior cruciate ligament reconstruction), where long-lasting PNBs were provided based on the observed surgical pain patterns prior to the study.[32]

The RAPBC scoring system allowed an 87% PACU bypass rate. After mild surgery, the linear regression showed an 18%

reduction in time until discharge for GA-alone cases and a 14% reduction when the PACU was bypassed. Invasive surgery showed an 18% reduction in discharge time when the PACU was bypassed. Any nursing interventions in the phase II recovery unit had a 45-minute (18%) or 47-minute (32%) increase in discharge time with mild or invasive surgery, respectively. Age, gender, GA, or the use of PNBs were not associated with mean differences in discharge times after invasive surgery.

The RAPBC was later modified and called the "WAKE© score," published in 2011 by Williams and Kentor.[33] This score targeted patients having MAC, GA, or RA, whereas prior scoring systems were focused on patients having GA. Some important differences in the WAKE (C) score from the RAPBC are the modification of the requirement to move a blocked limb, the measurement of blood pressure in a sitting or head-elevated position (checking orthostatic symptoms) before leaving the OR after any neuraxial blockade, and the addition of a "zero-tolerance criteria," which includes an adjustment of the patient's PACU pain score to their baseline pain score and inclusion of any postoperative nausea and vomiting symptoms.

As described by Armstrong and Cherry, the PACU bypass rate was 53% among patients with PNB only. Their PACU stay before going to phase II recovery was shorter than that of GA-only patients (mean difference = 26 minutes, *P* = .02). Phase II recovery times may also have been shorter in patients with PNB compared to patients with GA; the difference was not statistically significant.[19]

Patients who received only regional anesthetics were more likely to bypass the PACU than were patients who received GA with volatile anesthetics. RA patients bypassed the PACU at a greater rate than GA patients (86% vs 62%; odds ratio, 3.85; 95% CI 2.70 to 5.56; *P* < .001).[34] Given that PACU bypass can be achieved in 87% of RA patients, work by Dexter et al showed that with 50 cases/day, an institution can achieve staffing reductions of as many as 4 full-time equivalents in PACU staffing compared to *no* PACU bypass.[31] Thus, the appropriate PACU bypass criteria used in combination with RA can result in substantial savings.

Patients who bypassed the PACU exhibited no sequelae that necessitated nursing interventions at a PACU level of care. In the Williams et al study, the GA and RA historical control groups did not bypass the PACU, while the RA care pathway groups that had femoral nerve block or epidural anesthesia both experienced a 91% PACU bypass rate ($P < .001$). The historical control patient group and the GA care pathway group exhibited unexpected hospital admissions with a frequency of 20%, while the GA with femoral nerve block and epidural anesthesia care pathway groups had a 4% and 6% ($P = .002$) unexpected admissions rate, respectively.[25]

In the meta-analysis conducted by Liu et al, PACU bypass occurred with greater frequency using PNB (odds ratio, 14; 95% CI, 7.5 to 27.4) and was associated with shorter PACU time in minutes (odds ratio, –24.3; 95% CI, –36.3 to –12); decreased nausea (odds ratio, 0.17; 95% CI, 0.08 to 0.33); and increased patient satisfaction rating of excellent (odds ratio, 4.7; 95% CI, 1.8 to 12).[26] PACU bypass patients have been shown to have a reduced time until discharge.[32] Thus, the question remains regarding why the meta-analysis did *not* demonstrate shortened time until discharge with PNB. Possible explanations include the lack of discharge criteria (eg, the WAKE (C) score) during the time the studies were analyzed, the wait until a long-acting block has worn off until discharging patients, or other medical practice differences.

In the Head et al swing-room study for wrist and hand procedures, the RA group demonstrated shorter time for discharge (median 28 minutes and 95% CI 20–46 vs 156 minutes and 95% CI 118–215); shorter total time in facility (median 186 minutes and 95% CI 153–224 vs 345 minutes and 95% CI 290–430); fewer postoperative antiemetics (2% vs 17%; $P < .0001$); and less need for rescue opioids (0.6% vs 80%; $P < .0001$) compared to the GA-OR group.[21]

SUPPLIES, ULTRASOUND, BILLING, AND PAYMENTS

Liu and John performed a sensitivity analysis for the costs of using ultrasound during PNB.[35] If billed and revenue is obtained, ultrasound guidance can become profitable regardless of clinical setting (ie, ambulatory vs inpatient hospital). If billing procedures are not in place, then the clinical setting predominates. For example, in the ambulatory surgery center, nerve stimulator–guided nerve blocks would require a 96% success rate to compete with ultrasound guidance. The factors with the biggest cost impact for ultrasound were billing revenue (85% of variability), proportion of patients on whom the device is used (10% of variability), and success rate of the ultrasound-guided nerve block (2.6% of variability). In contrast, the factors with the biggest cost impact for the peripheral nerve stimulation model were block success rate (89% of

variability) and liability paid out in a failed airway situation (9% of variability). Individual facilities should consider these factors when making important purchasing decisions.

Supplies, direct costs, and process time intervals were analyzed by Shuster et al according to anesthesia techniques used for trauma and orthopedic services, including spinal, brachial plexus, epidural anesthesia, and GA.[24] The study showed that 11% of costs were related to drugs and supplies, suggesting that opportunities for cost savings are small. However, as almost 78% of the costs were due to personnel, labor savings could make a significant economic impact.

A best-fit regression line of anesthesia-related costs estimated a statistically significant but small cost advantage of spinal over GA, which was shown to be 13% for a 50-minute case, 9% for a 100-minute case, and 5% for a 200-minute case.[24] Anesthesia-related costs of PNB using brachial plexus blocks were statistically significantly greater than GA costs but were still small. The cost difference for brachial plexus block over GA was much greater for shorter cases and estimated at 19%, 8%, and 1% higher for a 50-, 100-, and 200-minute cases, respectively. There was no difference in costs between GA and epidural anesthesia.

The publications that discussed supply costs and use of ultrasound consider a US perspective.[16,36,37] These concepts may apply to countries outside the United States that have similar private and governmental insurance billing payment structures, but the actual revenue quantities and ratios are likely to be different. Further, economic circumstances are known to change over time, and specific details may no longer apply. Payment source can affect patients' access to RA methods, and further research on the factors that affect patient access to RA is needed.[38]

Clinical Pearl

- Payment sources affect patient access to RA and analgesia methods, and further research on the factors that affect patient access to RA is needed.

SUMMARY

The majority of OR costs are due to personnel. The ability to reduce these costs often has limitations.[2] A large and important consideration in how RA influences OR economics lies in the use of statistical forecasting to plan allocated OR time months ahead of time. Consequently, on the day of surgery, the decision regarding whether to use RA methods will not affect OR economics by a large factor; instead, decisions should be made based on improved patient outcomes and reducing patient and surgeon waiting. Another consequence is that sequencing cases for blocks (eg, among first cases of the day) can have economic benefit.

Avoiding the side effects of GA can reduce unplanned admissions, reduce length of hospital stay, and shorten surgical unit stay when proper bypass and discharge criteria are implemented. RA has demonstrated the ability to allow patients to bypass the PACU and move directly to the second-stage recovery or "step-down" unit. PACU and recovery times can be affected by the use of RA techniques. PACU costs are less affected by reducing postoperative nausea and vomiting or using faster-acting anesthetic agents to speed anesthesia emergence. Rather, PACU costs can be determined to a large degree by the distribution of patient admissions to the PACU.

Practitioners should understand the literature and apply the findings to their own facilities or institutions in order to determine what specific cost savings could be realized. Science has demonstrated that RA procedures that are properly planned and executed do not increase OR time and can decrease PACU time, thereby potentially reducing costs.

REFERENCES

1. Taheri PA, Butz, DA, Greenfield LJ: Length of stay has minimal impact on the cost of hospital admission. J Am Coll Surg 2000;191:123–130.
2. Dexter F, Wachtel R: Strategies for net cost reductions with the expanded role and expertise of anesthesiologists in the perioperative surgical home. Anesth Analg 2014;118:1062–1071.
3. Krenk L, Kehlet H, Hansen TB, Solgaard S, Soballe K, Rasmussen LS: Cognitive dysfunction after fast-track hip and knee replacement. Anesth Analg 2014;118:1034–1040.
4. Crosby G, Culley DJ, Dexter F: Cognitive outcome of surgery: is there no place like home? Anesth Analg 2014;118:898–900.
5. Dexter F, Traub RD: How to schedule elective surgical cases into specific operating rooms to maximize the efficiency of use of operating room time. Anesth Analg 2002;94:933–942.
6. Dexter F, Epstein RH, Traub RD, et al: Making management decisions on the day of surgery based on operating room efficiency and patient waiting times. Anesthesiology 2004;101:1444–1453.
7. O'Sullivan CTC, Dexter F: Assigning surgical cases with regional anesthetic blocks to anesthetists and operating room based on operating room efficiency. AANA J 2006;74:213–218.
8. McIntosh C, Dexter F, Epstein RH: The impact of service-specific staffing, case scheduling, turnovers, and first-case starts on anesthesia group and operating room productivity: a tutorial using data from an Australian hospital. Anesth Analg 2006;103:1499–1516.
9. Dexter F, Wachtel RE, Epstein RH: Event-based knowledge elicitation of operating room management decision-making using scenarios adapted from information systems data. BMC Med Inform Decis Mak 2011;11:2.
10. Bayman EO, Dexter F, Laur JJ, et al: National incidence of use of monitored anesthesia care. Anesth Analg 2011;113:165–169.
11. Chelly JE, Horne JL, Hudson ME, et al: Factors impacting on-time transfer to the operating room in patients undergoing peripheral nerve blocks in the preoperative area. J Clin Anesth 2010;22:115–121.
12. Masursky D, Dexter F, McCartney CJL, et al: Predicting orthopedic surgeons' preferences for peripheral nerve blocks for their patients. Anesth Analg 2008;106:561–567.
13. Oldman M, McCartney CJL, Leung A, et al: A survey of orthopedic surgeons' attitudes and knowledge regarding regional anesthesia. Anesth Analg 2004;98:1486–1490.
14. Eappen S, Flanagan H, Lithman R, et al: The addition of a regional block team to the orthopedic operating rooms does not improve anesthesia-controlled times and turnover time in the setting of long turnover times. J Clin Anes 2007;19:85–91.
15. Masursky D, Dexter F, Isaacson SA, et al: Surgeons' and anesthesiologists' perceptions of turnover times. Anesth Analg 2011;112:440–444.
16. Hudson ME, Chelly JE, Williams, BA: Economics: projecting costs and revenue for an interventional pain service in the ambulatory setting. Int Anesthesiol Clin 2011;49:68–83.
17. Russell RA, Burke K, Gattis K: Implementing a regional anesthesia block nurse team in the perianesthesia care unit increases patient safety and perioperative efficiency. J Perianesth Nurs 2013;28:3–10.
18. Mathias JM: A new role for RNs: assisting in regional blocks. OR Manager 2011;27:29–30.
19. Armstrong KP, Cherry RAR: Brachial plexus anesthesia compared to general anesthesia when a block room is available. Can J Anaesth 2004;51:41–44.
20. Drolet P, Girard M: Regional anesthesia, block room and efficiency: putting things in perspective. Can J Anaesth 2004;51:1–5.
21. Head SJ, Seib R, Osborn JA et al: A "swing room" model based on regional anesthesia reduces turnover time and increases case throughput. Can J Anaesth 2011;58:725–732.
22. Williams BA, Kentor ML, Williams JP, et al: Process analysis in outpatient knee surgery: effects of regional and general anesthesia on anesthesia-controlled time. Anesthesiology 2000;93:529–538.
23. Mariano ER, Chu LF, Peinado CR, et al: Anesthesia-controlled time and turnover time for ambulatory upper extremity surgery performed with regional versus general anesthesia. J Clin Anesth 2009;21:253–257.
24. Schuster M, Gottschalk A, Berger JR, et al: A retrospective comparison of costs for regional and general anesthesia techniques. Anesth Analg 2005;100:786–794.
25. Williams BA, DeRiso BM, Figallo CM, et al: Benchmarking the perioperative process: III. Effects of regional anesthesia clinical pathway techniques on process efficiency and recovery profiles in ambulatory orthopedic surgery. J Clin Anesth 1998;10:570–578.
26. Liu SS, Strodtbeck WM, Richman JM, et al: A comparison of regional versus general anesthesia for ambulatory anesthesia: a meta-analysis of randomized controlled trials. Anesth Analg 2005;101:1634–1642.
27. Dexter F: Regional anesthesia does not significantly change surgical time versus general anesthesia—a meta-analysis of randomized studies. Reg Anesth Pain Med 1998;23:439–443.
28. Mazzei WJ: Operating room start times and turnover times in a university hospital. J Clin Anesth 1994;6:405–8.
29. Eappen S, Flanagan H, Lithman R, et al: The addition of a regional block team to the orthopedic operating rooms does not improve anesthesia-controlled times and turnover time in the setting of long turnover times. J Clin Anesth 2007;19:85–91.
30. Dexter F, Tinker JH: Analysis of strategies to decrease postanesthesia care unit costs. Anesthesiology 1995;82:94–101.
31. Dexter F, Macario A, Manberg PJ, et al: Computer simulation to determine how rapid anesthetic recovery protocols to decrease the time for emergence or increase the phase I postanesthesia care unit bypass rate affect staffing of an ambulatory surgery center. Anesth Analg 1999;88:1053–1063.
32. Williams BA, Kentor ML, Williams JP, et al: PACU bypass after outpatient knee surgery is associated with fewer unplanned hospital admissions but more phase II nursing interventions. Anesthesiology 2002;97:981–988.
33. Williams BA, Kentor ML: The WAKE© score: patient-centered ambulatory anesthesia and fast-tracking outcomes criteria. Int Anesthesiol Clin 2011;49:33–43.
34. Williams BA, Kentor ML, Vogt MT, et al: Economics of nerve block pain management after anterior cruciate ligament reconstruction: potential hospital cost savings via associated postanesthesia care unit bypass and same-day discharge. Anesthesiology 2004;100:697–706.
35. Liu SS, John RS: Modeling cost of ultrasound versus nerve stimulator guidance for nerve blocks with sensitivity analysis. Reg Anesth Pain Med 2010;35:57–63.
36. Swenson JD, Davis JJ: Getting the best value for consumable supplies in regional anesthesia. Int Anesthesiol Clin 2011;49:94–103.
37. Kim TW, Mariano ER: Updated guide to billing for regional anesthesia (United States). Int Anesthesiol Clin 2011;49:84–93.
38. Tighe PJ, Brennan M, Moser M, et al: Primary payer status is associated with the use of nerve block placement for ambulatory orthopedic surgery. Reg Anesth Pain Med 2012;37:254–261.

CHAPTER 68

Regional Anesthesia and Perioperative Outcome

Ottokar Stundner, Suzuko Suzuki, and Stavros G. Memtsoudis

INTRODUCTION

The focus of anesthesiologists on patient safety has led to advancements in anesthetic techniques and perioperative pain management, as well as profoundly affected patient care in the entire perioperative period. However, studies of the contributions of anesthesia and advances in analgesic approaches as well as their effects on measurable outcomes have only recently gained momentum and widespread recognition. The increasing realization that anesthesia-related factors and choices made by anesthesiologists can influence perioperative events and patient safety has thus sparked interest in a variety of outcomes previously thought beyond our control.

As the patient population seeking surgical care presents with serious comorbidity more commonly, the perioperative challenges will demand that anesthetic considerations assumes a major part of the care plan for patients to ensure the best possible outcomes. Utilizing regional anesthesia provides a significant benefit in achieving this goal.

In the past, the scope of neuraxial anesthesia and peripheral nerve blocks has primarily encompassed their use for intraoperative anesthesia and postoperative analgesia, respectively. However, the choice of anesthesia may positively influence the risk of perioperative cardiopulmonary complications, infections, and mortality.[1,2] The pathophysiologic reasons for these findings remain incompletely understood. Attempts to explain these associations depend on a number of observations made in small clinical or preclinical studies. The effects seen, however, might feasibly represent a composite result of avoidance of general anesthesia on the one hand and intrinsic positive effects brought about by regional anesthesia on the other hand. General anesthesia, systemic analgesia, and mechanical ventilation often prove problematic in patients with comorbidity,[3] especially those with pulmonary pathologies. Regarding the latter, neuraxial anesthesia was associated with lower blood loss, shorter surgical time, and a lower incidence of thromboembolism,[4,5] possibly conferred by its sympatholytic action and beneficial effects on the coagulation system.[6] In orthopedic patients, earlier mobilization and discharge readiness may contribute to a lower complication incidence. Advances in perioperative pain control have also been associated with better medical and economic outcomes as well as improved patient satisfaction.[7,8] Moreover, recent research suggested that regional anesthesia may have long-term outcome benefits from reduction of cancer recurrence and prevention of chronic postsurgical pain.

However, there is little quantitative evidence on these beneficial effects of regional anesthesia, particularly for peripheral nerve blocks. Available studies are mostly limited by their small sample sizes and scope. Nonetheless, data gained from large-scale, population-based studies show promising results.

This chapter summarizes currently available data on outcomes pertaining to the use of regional anesthesia. The discussion focuses on its use in the context of specific surgical interventions. Regional anesthetic techniques and their impact on perioperative outcomes in selected types of surgeries, long-term medical outcomes, and finally economic outcomes and cost-effectiveness issues are reviewed.

SHORT-TERM OUTCOME: MORBIDITY AND MORTALITY

With the advent of advanced preoperative evaluation, perioperative monitoring, and treatment modalities, the incidence of many major perioperative complications, including mortality, has substantially declined over the last century. Anesthesia-related mortality was reported to be as low as 1.1 deaths for a population of 1 million per year.[9] Surgical mortality, on the other hand, largely depends on the type of surgery and associated patient demographics, with mortality rates ranging from 0.07% for low-risk breast surgery to almost one-fifth of patients undergoing liver transplantation.[10] Anesthesia has long been thought to play a secondary role with regard to major perioperative complications and mortality, not least because it has been difficult to reliably assess its impact in the setting of low-incidence outcomes. Only recently, advanced techniques for data aggregation were introduced, including pooling of studies in meta-analyses, database-driven population-based approaches, and assembly of dedicated, prospective adverse event registries.

Most available data on morbidity and mortality in the perioperative setting focuses on the differential impact of general and neuraxial anesthesia. For peripheral nerve blocks and other techniques of lower invasiveness (like local anesthetic wound instillation), conclusive data on perioperative outcome are still scarce.

General Noncardiac Surgery Populations

Rodgers and colleagues integrated 141 randomized controlled studies, including 9559 patients receiving neuraxial versus general anesthesia for noncardiac surgery into a meta-analysis.[1] The primary outcome was defined as differential mortality. The authors reported a reduction in overall mortality by 30% in patients receiving neuraxial blockade compared to general anesthesia (odds ratio [OR] = 0.70; confidence interval [CI], 0.54–0.90), along with reductions in complications, including deep vein thrombosis, pulmonary embolism, blood product transfusion, pneumonia, respiratory depression, myocardial infarction, and renal failure (Figures 68–1 and 68–2). However, in a subgroup analysis, no clear difference was apparent between different types of surgery. The authors conceded that the study was underpowered to reliably detect differences across surgical specialties. Another limitation of the meta-analysis approach is that individual studies with largely different research questions, protocols, and time of origin are pooled, representing the introduction of cofounders that cannot entirely be accounted for. Moreover, although individual randomized controlled trials are thought to be of high scientific validity, they may feasibly introduce bias by restricting the patient population to a tightly controlled academic environment.

Thus, for the purpose of risk assessment on a public health level, administrative or billing databases are increasingly

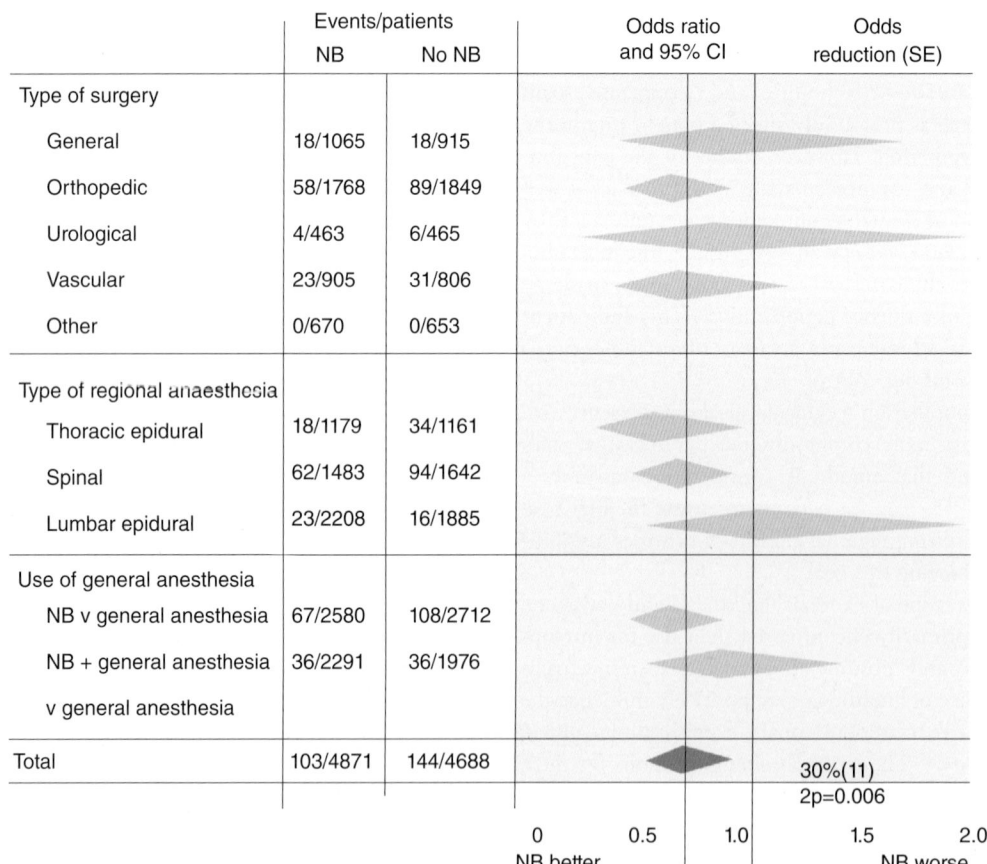

FIGURE 68–1. Effect of neuraxial blockade (NB) on postoperative mortality, by surgical group, type of neuraxial blockade, and use of general anesthesia. Obstetrics and gynecology trials are included with other surgery. One trial with unknown details of anesthesia was grouped with lumbar epidural and neuraxial blockade plus general anesthesia versus general anesthesia comparisons. Diamonds denote 95% confidence intervals for odds ratios of combined trial results. The left vertical line represents the overall pooled result. Size of shaded boxes is proportional to number of events. χ^2 test for heterogeneity between different surgical groups, $P = .9$. (Reproduced with permission from Rodgers A, Walker N, Schug S, et al: Reduction of postoperative mortality and morbidity with epidural or spinal anaesthesia: results from overview of randomised trials. *BMJ*. 2000 Dec 16;321(7275):1493.)

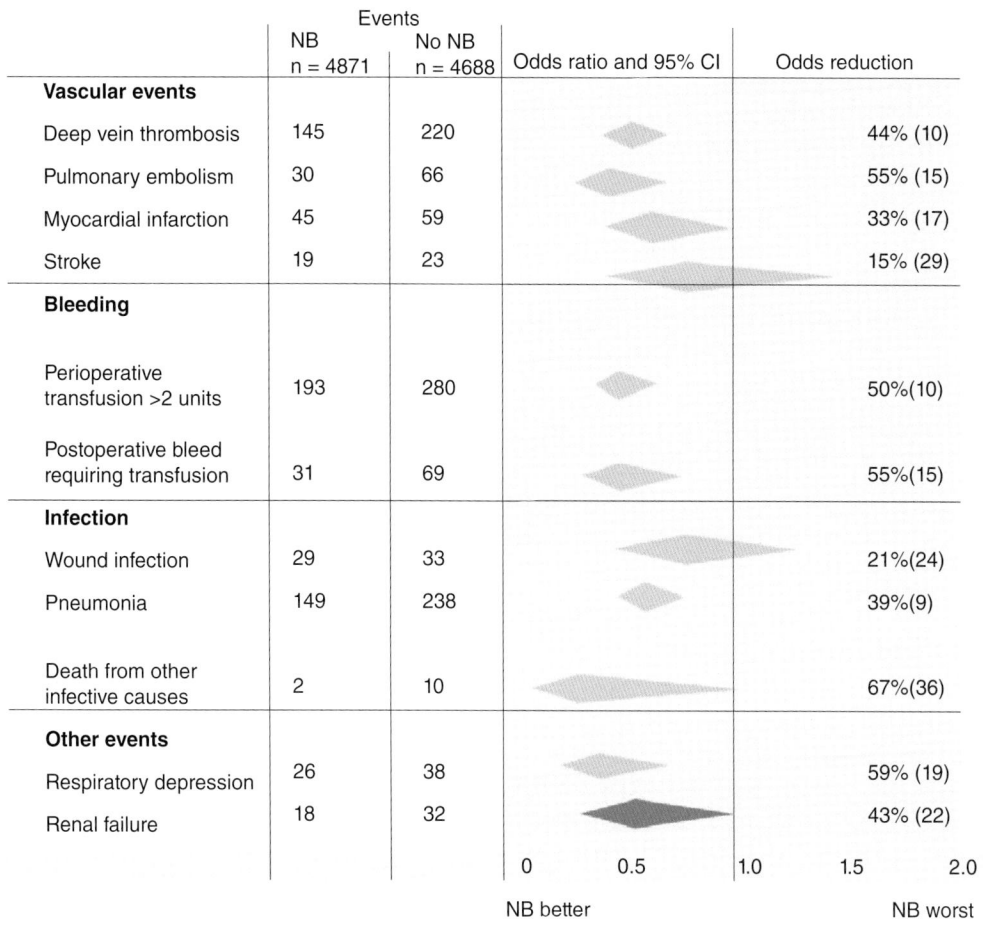

	Events			
	NB n = 4871	No NB n = 4688	Odds ratio and 95% CI	Odds reduction
Vascular events				
Deep vein thrombosis	145	220		44% (10)
Pulmonary embolism	30	66		55% (15)
Myocardial infarction	45	59		33% (17)
Stroke	19	23		15% (29)
Bleeding				
Perioperative transfusion >2 units	193	280		50%(10)
Postoperative bleed requiring transfusion	31	69		55%(15)
Infection				
Wound infection	29	33		21%(24)
Pneumonia	149	238		39%(9)
Death from other infective causes	2	10		67%(36)
Other events				
Respiratory depression	26	38		59% (19)
Renal failure	18	32		43% (22)

0   0.5   1.0   1.5   2.0

NB better   NB worst

FIGURE 68–2. Effects of neuraxial blockade (NB) on postoperative complications. Diamonds denote 95% confidence intervals for odds ratios of combined trial results. The vertical dashed line represents the overall pooled result. Size of shaded boxes is proportional to number of events. (Reproduced with permission from Rodgers A, Walker N, Schug S, et al: Reduction of postoperative mortality and morbidity with epidural or spinal anaesthesia: results from overview of randomised trials. *BMJ*. 2000 Dec 16;321(7275):1493.)

utilized for comparative effectiveness research. Wijeysundera and colleagues queried population-based administrative databases originating from Ontario, Canada.[11] They studied more than a quarter of a million patients aged 40 or older undergoing elective, medium- to high-risk noncardiac surgery during a 10-year period. Within a matched-pairs cohort generated using propensity scoring, 30-day mortality was compared between patients receiving epidural versus general anesthesia. The 22% of patients receiving epidural anesthesia had a slightly lower rate (1.7% vs 2.0%) and relative risk (RR) (0.89 [CI, 0.81–0.98], P = .02) of mortality than those undergoing surgery under general anesthesia (Figure 68–3). The effect was more pronounced in thoracic and orthopedic surgery compared to abdominal or vascular surgery. While the authors acknowledged that their findings were not as convincing in terms of mortality reduction as earlier results, they emphasized the relative safety of epidural anesthesia for indications other than reduction of mortality. However, it must be kept in mind that the data used here only represent a geographically restricted region and might not be fully applicable to other areas.

In contrast, Wu et al used a random sample from the Medicare database.[12] Differential outcomes of patients undergoing intermediate- to high-risk noncardiac surgery with or without epidural anesthesia were compared with regard to death within 7 or 30 days. Regression analysis controlling for race, gender, age, comorbidities, hospital size, hospital teaching status, and hospital technology status were performed. Epidural anesthesia was associated with lower adjusted odds ratios for mortality at 7 days (OR = 0.52 [CI, 0.38–0.73], P = .0001) and 30 days (OR = 0.74 [CI, 0.63–0.89], P = .0005), but no difference in major complications was apparent except for pneumonia, which was, oddly, higher in the epidural group.

Limitations of most database studies revolve around the reliability of the data source, in terms of adequate coding of events and the propensity to readily identify complications. For statistical adjustment, the granularity of available information on preexisting morbidity is important, as this is known to be a prime determinant of postoperative outcome. Finally, there is considerable heterogeneity not only within the individuals undergoing surgery, but also across various types of procedures. All previously discussed studies attempted to specify differences between surgical subspecialties from the overall cohort. However, their sample sizes were likely too small to provide adequate power to answer specific related questions.

PART 11

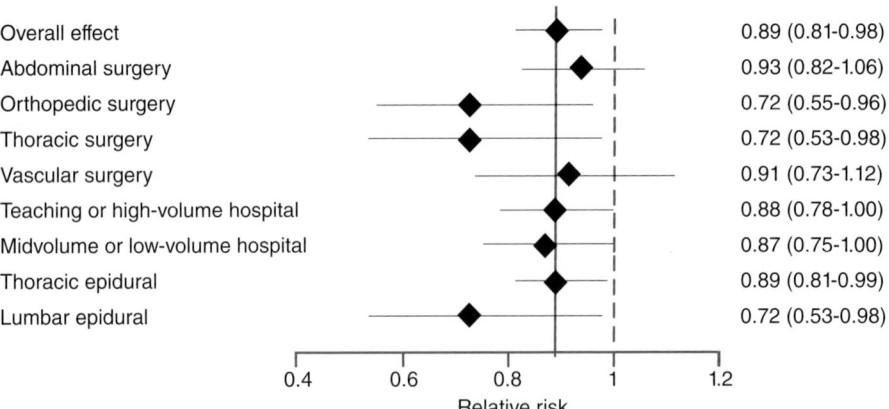

Overall effect	0.89 (0.81-0.98)
Abdominal surgery	0.93 (0.82-1.06)
Orthopedic surgery	0.72 (0.55-0.96)
Thoracic surgery	0.72 (0.53-0.98)
Vascular surgery	0.91 (0.73-1.12)
Teaching or high-volume hospital	0.88 (0.78-1.00)
Midvolume or low-volume hospital	0.87 (0.75-1.00)
Thoracic epidural	0.89 (0.81-0.99)
Lumbar epidural	0.72 (0.53-0.98)

FIGURE 68–3. Association of epidural anesthesia or analgesia with 30-day mortality in the subgroup analyses. Diamonds represent relative risks for 30-day mortality within each subgroup. Error bars are 95% CI. The corresponding numerical values for these point estimates and confidence intervals are presented on the right. The solid vertical line represents the overall treatment effect (relative risk 0.89). The dashed vertical line represents a null effect (relative risk 1). (Reproduced with permission from Wijeysundera DN, Beattie WS, Austin PC, et al: Epidural anaesthesia and survival after intermediate-to-high risk non-cardiac surgery: a population-based cohort study. *Lancet.* 2008 Aug 16;372(9638):562–569.)

Orthopedics and Trauma Surgery

A number of studies have focused on orthopedics and trauma surgery, predominantly when utilized for lower extremity joint surgery. Regional anesthesia lends itself to the management of these procedures, as it does provide complete coverage of the entire operative field along with sustained analgesia, thus allowing for the avoidance of general anesthesia and mechanical ventilation. Pugely and colleagues queried the American College of Surgeons National Surgical Quality Improvement Program (ACS NSQIP) database for patients undergoing primary total knee arthroplasty between 2005 and 2010 and evaluated 30-day complication rates and mortality, according to type of anesthesia (spinal vs general anesthesia).[13] Of the 14,052 patients identified, 57.1% of surgeries were performed using spinal anesthesia. Compared to the group receiving general anesthesia, patients receiving regional anesthesia had lower unadjusted rates of overall complications, shorter duration of surgery, and shorter length of hospital stay. Adjustment for covariates yielded a significantly higher likelihood of complications in the general anesthesia group (OR, 1.129 [CI, 1.004–1.269]). Patients with a high comorbidity load were most likely to incur complications.

Unlike other large studies, a study by Memtsoudis et al managed to discriminate between the use of sole neuraxial anesthesia versus the addition of neuraxial to general anesthesia.[2] The authors utilized a commercial administrative discharge database containing data from approximately 400 US hospitals to examine the impact of the type of anesthesia in over half a million patients undergoing primary hip or knee arthroplasty between 2006 and 2010. Three groups were established: patients receiving neuraxial anesthesia alone (11%), general anesthesia alone (74.8%), or a combination of both (14.2%). The unadjusted incidence of 30-day mortality was significantly lower in the first two groups (0.10%, 0.10%), compared to the last (0.18%; *P* < .0001). After adjustment for demographic and health care–related variables, type of surgery, and preexisting comorbidities, the multivariate regression yielded 30-day mortality odds ratios of 1.83 (CI, 1.08–3.1;

P = .0211) for general versus neuraxial anesthesia and 1.70 (CI, 1.06–2.74; *P* = .0228) for general versus combined general-neuraxial anesthesia and thus a substantially lower risk for the regional techniques. The same observation held true for numerous in-hospital complications, including cerebrovascular events, pulmonary compromise, cardiac complications, pneumonia, infectious complications, mechanical ventilation, and blood product transfusion, all of which exhibited higher odds ratios in the general-only group. Interestingly, the beneficial effects of neuraxial anesthesia appeared to be most pronounced when it was used as the sole anesthetic (Tables 68–1 and 68–2); in combination with general anesthesia, the odds ratios often ranged in between those of neuraxial and general anesthesia as the sole technique. The authors concluded from this finding that the benefits seen in this cohort not only might stem from avoidance of general anesthesia but also might imply a positive modifiable effect conferred by neuraxial anesthesia itself.

Very similar results to those gained in elective orthopedic surgery were recently published in the field of acute trauma surgery. A retrospective study of 18,158 patients undergoing surgery for hip fracture in 126 hospitals in the New York State area found no difference in unadjusted mortality whether neuraxial or general anesthesia was used.[14] However, after adjustment for covariates, regional anesthesia was associated with significantly lower odds of mortality (OR, 0.71 [CI, 0.54–0.93]; *P* = .014) and pulmonary complications (OR, 0.75 [CI, 0.64-0.89]; *P* < .0001) compared to general anesthesia. Patients with intertrochanteric fractures benefitted more than those with femoral neck fractures.

Thoracic and Cardiac Surgery

Pulmonary mechanics were reported to be better in patients receiving regional anesthesia, which is of particular importance for spontaneous ventilation and fast rehabilitation after intrathoracic procedures.[15] This improvement is likely associated with better pain relief achieved with regional anesthesia compared to systemic opioid administration.[16] Paravertebral block

TABLE 68-1. Multivariable regression analysis results for total hip arthroplasty.

	General vs Neuraxial		General vs Neuraxial/General	
	Odds Ratio (Adjusted 95% CI)	Adjusted P Value	Odds Ratio (Adjusted 95% CI)	Adjusted P Value
Systemic Complications				
Pulmonary embolism	1.26 (0.68–2.31)	.8079	1.29 (0.78–2.15)	.5252
Cerebrovascular event	3.15 (1.11–8.92)	.0271	1.27 (0.69–2.33)	.7513
Pulmonary compromise	3.34 (2.10–5.32)	<.0001	1.41 (1.07–1.86)	.0105
Cardiac complications (non–myocardial infarction)	1.13 (1.02–1.25)	.0171	1.01 (0.92–1.11)	>.9999
Pneumonia	1.51 (1.13–2.01)	.0029	1.14 (0.90–1.43)	.4221
All infections	1.45 (1.27–1.65)	<.0001	1.17 (1.05–1.30)	.0028
Acute renal failure	1.70 (1.35–2.13)	<.0001	1.31 (1.10–1.57)	.0014
Gastrointestinal complication	1.22 (0.93–1.60)	.1939	1.28 (1.01–1.64)	.0439
Acute myocardial infarction	1.11 (0.71–1.73)	1.0000	1.27 (0.81–1.97)	.4623
Resource Utilization				
Mechanical ventilation	1.57 (1.10–2.22)	.0085	1.49 (1.09–2.04)	.0091
Blood product transfusion	1.14 (1.07–1.22)	<.0001	1.40 (1.33–1.49)	<.0001
Mortality				
30-day mortality	1.28 (0.70–2.37)	.7192	1.55 (0.88–2.70)	.1609

was reported to be as effective as epidural anesthesia for intrathoracic surgery, with potentially lower risk of neuraxial bleeding complications but higher risk of pneumothorax.[17] In cardiac surgery, the addition of thoracic epidural anesthesia to general anesthesia was associated with improved coronary perfusion and myocardial oxygen supply as well as reduced incidence of arrhythmias, probably evoked by sympatholysis at the thoracic level. Moreover, relief of sternotomy pain may allow for early tracheal extubation and faster initiation of respiratory therapy. However, epidural anesthesia for cardiac surgery is subject to intense controversy, as high-dose systemic anticoagulation necessary for cardiopulmonary bypass might increase the risk for epidural hematoma and its potentially devastating consequences. In addition, pronounced hypotension as a result of sympatholysis may be problematic and difficult to counteract in these patients.

Svircevic and colleagues' recent meta-analysis including 2731 patients from 28 randomized controlled studies yielded a better risk profile for patients receiving epidural in addition to general anesthesia[18]: fewer respiratory complications (RR, 0.53 [CI, 0.40–0.69]); supraventricular arrhythmias (RR, 0.68 [CI, 0.50–0.093]); lower risk of mortality (RR, 0.81 [CI, 0.40–1.64]); perioperative myocardial infarction (RR, 0.80 [CI, 0.52–1.24]); and stroke (RR, 0.59 [CI, 0.24–1.46]). Given the potential risks, further research is necessary to clarify the potential of the use of regional anesthesia with

regard to major morbidity and mortality outcomes, most of which did not reach statistical significance in this and earlier studies.

Abdominal Surgery

The scope of abdominal surgery ranges widely from ventral herniorrhaphy and appendectomy to liver resection and abdominal thoracic aneurysm repair. Despite the advent of laparoscopic procedures and minimally invasive surgical techniques, there continues to be a need for open and major abdominal surgeries. The ramifications of abdominal surgeries may include, but are not limited to, multiple-organ involvement, large fluid shifts and blood loss, need for blood transfusions, intensive care unit admissions, need for specialty consultations, pain control, infections, prolonged hospital stay, malnutrition, and deconditioning.

Regional anesthesia is frequently utilized in major abdominal surgeries, most commonly in the form of epidural anesthesia. The use of epidural anesthesia in addition to general anesthesia for abdominal surgeries is associated with a number of conceivably beneficial effects that could address many of the potential perioperative challenges.

First and foremost, epidural anesthesia can provide excellent analgesia for large abdominal incisions. Adequate pain control leads to reduced opioid consumption and its

TABLE 68–2. Multivariable regression analysis results for total knee arthroplasty.

	General vs Neuraxial		General vs Neuraxial/General	
	Odds Ratio (Adjusted 95% CI)	Adjusted P Value	Odds Ratio (Adjusted 95% CI)	Adjusted P Value
Systemic Complications				
Pulmonary embolism	1.24 (0.97–1.59)	.1029	1.28 (1.02–1.6)	.0281
Cerebrovascular event[a]	1.58 (0.90–2.78)	.1397	1.09 (0.71–1.66)	>.9999
Pulmonary compromise	1.83 (1.43–2.35)	<.0001	1.23 (1.02–1.48)	.0248
Cardiac complications (non–myocardial infarction)	1.09 (1.02–1.16)	.0086	1.00 (0.95–1.07)	>.9999
Pneumonia[a]	1.27 (1.05–1.53)	.0083	1.05 (0.90–1.23)	.9761
All infections[a]	1.38 (1.26–1.52)	<.0001	1.12 (1.04–1.21)	.0017
Acute renal failure	1.44 (1.24–1.67)	<.0001	1.11 (0.98–1.25)	.1342
Gastrointestinal complication[a]	1.04 (0.86–1.27)	>.9999	0.96 (0.80–1.15)	>.9999
Acute myocardial infarction	1.10 (0.78–1.54)	>.9999	0.93 (0.70–1.23)	>.9999
Resource Utilization				
Mechanical ventilation	1.72 (1.35–2.18)	<.0001	1.32 (1.09–1.60)	.0021
Blood product transfusion[a]	1.23 (1.17–1.28)	<.0001	1.01 (0.97–1.05)	>.9999
Mortality				
30-day mortality	1.83 (1.08–3.1)	.0211	1.70 (1.06–2.74)	.0228

associated side effects, earlier ambulation, and increased patient satisfaction. Thoracic epidural analgesia is also known to improve functional residual capacity (FRC) and vital capacity (VC) after abdominal surgeries,[19] possibly due to better pain control and prevention of atelectasis. In addition, the associated sympathectomy at the thoracic level may blunt the cascades of neuroendocrine responses to the surgical insults. The use of epidural blockade is shown to attenuate the rise of cortisol and proinflammatory cytokines in response to surgical stimulation.[20–22] Attenuation of the stress response and cardiovascular stability are obviously desirable and may lead to decreased perioperative cardiovascular complications, wound infection, and better healing. It also has been observed that thoracic epidural anesthesia increases the gastrointestinal and hepatic blood flow and improves tissue oxygenation during surgery.[23] Furthermore, postoperative ileus was significantly reduced by epidural analgesia, although the risk of postoperative nausea and vomiting was not shown to be affected.[24] The implication of these findings may include better nutritional support, reduced risk of infectious complications, earlier hospital discharge, and improved patient satisfaction.

Some of the effects mentioned may be reflected in the data from the study by Rodgers et al, which included abdominal surgeries.[1] In this study, the use of regional anesthesia was associated with a reduction in the risk of pulmonary embolism by 55%, pneumonia by 39%, myocardial infarction by 33%, bleeding by 50%, blood transfusion by 55%, renal failure by 43%, and 30-day mortality by 30%.

In conclusion, the available data on outcome measures and regional anesthesia in abdominal surgeries are positive but limited. Further and more definitive conclusions await additional studies and analysis.

Obstetrics

Owing to the reported benefits for mother and newborn, regional anesthesia is widely used in obstetrics for both cesarean section and vaginal delivery. For the former, general anesthesia is usually only chosen when contraindications for the regional technique prevail or in highly time-critical situations. For this reason, large-scale data on comparative perioperative outcomes and mortality in parturients are scarce. In a meta-analysis of 16 studies comparing neuraxial to general anesthesia for uncomplicated cesarean delivery, no significant difference was seen in the incidence of neonatal Apgar scores of 6 or less or 4 or less at 1 and 5 minutes, respectively, and the requirement of neonatal resuscitation.[25] The primary advantages of neuraxial anesthesia for cesarean section include avoidance of general anesthesia, airway manipulation, and systemic administration of anesthetic drugs. Induction of general anesthesia and intubation is associated with a considerably higher risk for the mother due to the possible presence of a difficult airway and higher risk of aspiration. Moreover, the fetus is only exposed to a very small dose of systemically absorbed local anesthetics when neuraxial anesthesia is used, thus reducing the direct impact of anesthesia on its physiology. However, spinal and epidural anesthesia can still affect the fetus through indirect effects, including pronounced maternal blood pressure drops evoked by sympathicolysis. While, untreated, this can have detrimental effects on the neonate's circulation and acid-base status, it can usually be readily counteracted with vasopressors.[26]

Low-dose ("walking") epidural anesthesia is often applied for pain relief in women during labor. While systemic administration of analgesics can be avoided with this approach, it was suspected to potentially delay the birthing process and increase rates of vaginal instrumentation and cesarean section. In a meta-analysis by Liu et al including seven trials of nulliparous women comparing epidural anesthesia to systemic opioid administration, epidural anesthesia was not associated with an increased risk of cesarean section (OR, 1.03 [CI, 0.71–1.48]) but with a nonsignificantly increased risk for instrumental vaginal delivery (OR, 2.11 [CI, 0.95–4.65]).[27]

Interest in the effects of anesthesia on long-term cognitive development is growing. Sprung et al reviewed medical and educational records of 5320 children in Minnesota who were delivered vaginally, via Cesarean section under general anesthesia, or under regional anesthesia.[28] The risk of learning disabilities was significantly lower in those receiving regional anesthesia for cesarean section compared to standard vaginal delivery (hazard ratio, 0.64 [CI, 0.44–0.92], P = .017).

LONG-TERM OUTCOME

The anesthesiologists' role as perioperative clinicians has been constantly redefined in the context of the rapid expansion of research. The fields of anesthesiology and perioperative medicine have started to have an impact beyond the traditional, acute perioperative period with the realization that what happens at and around the time of surgery may have measurable effects months and even years later.

Regional Anesthesia and Cancer Recurrence

The time of tumor resection is a critical period in cancer cell survival and proliferation. A growing body of literature has suggested that various aspects of anesthetic care may have significant effects on the rate of cancer metastasis and recurrence. Stress and surgical tumor resection have long been known to promote cancer metastasis.[29] The body's major defenses against such pathophysiology are the neuroendocrine and anti-inflammatory responses. In simplistic terms, factors that increase the stress and inflammatory response or conversely weaken the immune systems will likely promote cancer metastasis and growth. In theory, interventions opposing the stress response may therefore have beneficial effects. The choice of anesthetic types and medications may significantly influence this cascade.

General anesthesia is suggested to suppress the immune response by direct effects or by activation of the hypothalamic-pituitary-adrenal axis and the sympathetic nervous system.[30] Several anesthetic agents, including ketamine, thiopental, and volatile agents, have been shown to reduce the function of natural killer (NK) cells, which carry out the body's major antineoplastic activity. Opioids also suppress the immune system, and it has been suggested that morphine may promote angiogenesis. In addition, pain itself is known to suppress NK cell function.[31]

The use of regional anesthesia has been suggested to reduce cancer recurrence after prostatectomy and mastectomy. A retrospective study compared the use of epidural analgesia to opioid analgesia in addition to general anesthesia and suggested a 57% reduction in cancer recurrence rate,[32] while another showed reduced cancer progression after prostatectomy (hazard ratio, 0.45).[33] Exadaktylos et al. reported that postmastectomy recurrence- and metastasis-free survival was significantly higher in patients who received paravertebral catheter analgesia compared to those who received morphine patient-controlled anesthesia (94% vs 77% at 36 months).[34] In addition, the serum from patients who received propofol and a paravertebral block has been shown to inhibit cancer cell proliferation compared to that of patients who received sevoflurane and opioids. Furthermore, the use of spinal in addition to general anesthesia was associated with 70% reduction in metastatic progression of lung cancer after unrelated surgery (laparotomy) in a rat model.

The effect of regional anesthesia on cancer recurrence, if substantiated by further trials, is likely multifactorial and may include the prevention or blunting of neuroendocrine response to surgical insults, reduction of the dose of anesthetic agents and opioid consumption and their related effects, as well as the reduction of pain. In addition, local anesthetics themselves have been suggested to possess antineoplastic and even cytotoxic properties.[35]

Regional Anesthesia and Postsurgical Chronic Pain

Patients may undergo successful surgery and can still be burdened by lingering postsurgical pain many months or years after the operation. Certain types of surgeries have been associated with a higher incidence of postsurgical pain; these include thoracotomies, coronary artery bypass grafting (CABG), breast surgeries, and inguinal herniorrhaphies with an individual incidence of 30%–60%, 30%–50%, 20%–30%, and 10%, respectively (Table 68–3).[36] For instance, the rate of postthoracotomy pain was reported as 30%–60% but could be as high as 80%. In one study, 40% of patients with pain reported that the pain limited their daily activities and 46% thought that pain was their worst problem.[37]

The prevention of such postsurgical pain is of interest for anesthesiologists, and the possible influence of preemptive analgesia using regional anesthesia has been investigated. Although data are limited, positive influences on this outcome have been suggested. A meta-analysis based on a pool of 250 patients showed that epidural analgesia was associated with decreased rates of postthoracotomy pain at 6 months (OR, 0.33).[38] In the same analysis, 89 patients from two studies favored paravertebral block for the outcome of decreased postmastectomy pain at 5 to 6 months (OR, 0.37). Nonetheless, further studies are needed to draw any firm conclusions.

TABLE 68–3. Surgeries associated with higher incidence of postsurgical pain.

Surgery Type	Rate of Chronic Pain (%)	Rate of Chronic Severe Pain (VAS >5) (%)
Amputation	30–50	5–10
Thoracotomy	30–40	10
CABG	30–50	5–10
Breast surgery (mastectomy, lumpectomy)	20–30	5–10
Inguinal hernia repair	10	2–4

Source: Modified with permission from Kehlet H, Jensen TS, Woolf CJ: Persistent postsurgical pain: risk factors and prevention. *Lancet.* 2006 May 13;367(9522):1618–1625.

The mechanism of chronic postsurgical pain is complex and includes inflammatory and neuropathic components.[36] Therefore, the use of regional anesthesia for this purpose is likely most effective in combination with improved surgical techniques and optimization of multimodal analgesic approaches containing neuropathic pain medication such as ketamine, gabapentin, pregabalin, acetaminophen, cyclooxygenase (COX) inhibitors, and steroids.

ECONOMIC OUTCOMES

Performance of regional anesthetic procedures is frequently suspected to be more complex and time consuming than other modes of anesthesia and analgesia (eg, induction of general anesthesia or systemic opioid administration). In this context, regional anesthesia is sometimes thought to prolong turnover time. However, Mariano and colleagues recently reported that anesthesia-controlled time was in fact shorter when nerve blocks were applied for upper extremity surgery, compared to general anesthesia (28 minutes vs 32 minutes, $P = .0392$).[39] Turnover time did not differ between groups. When complex techniques (eg, multiple nerve blocks, thoracic epidural anesthesia) are applied, anesthesia-controlled time and turnover time might also be decreased by usage of dedicated block rooms or swing rooms.[40]

Moreover, numerous reports exist evidencing economic benefits of regional anesthesia in terms of shorter length of hospital stay and lower resource utilization.[41] The previously mentioned study by Memtsoudis et al found significant differences in the median number of days patients stayed in the hospital after major lower extremity joint replacement. The incidence of prolonged length of stay (exceeding the 75th percentile) was lower in the neuraxial and neuraxial plus general groups, compared to the general-only group (28.7%, 27.4%, and 35.4%, respectively; $P < .001$), as well as the adjusted odds ratios for this outcome. Similarly, odds ratios for mechanical ventilation

and blood product transfusion, which considerably add to perioperative cost, were significantly higher in patients receiving general, compared to regional, anesthesia.[2]

These direct and indirect economic benefits could outweigh the increased amount of time and trained personnel required for the performance of regional anesthetic techniques. Additional benefits could arise from circumvention of complications and their treatment. However, because of vastly different settings, modes of compensation, and other costs associated with either technique, it is difficult to quantify the direct economic difference between regional and general anesthesia.

CONCLUSION

Regional anesthesia is increasingly recognized as anesthesia modality associated with improved perioperative outcomes beyond better pain management. As many interventions have been introduced over the last decades to reduce severe complications in patients undergoing surgery, it remains challenging to reliably identify new ways that are capable of further reducing the risk. Regional anesthesia may emerge as one such intervention. Large multiinstitutional registries with a high volume of granular data could help gain better insight into many outstanding questions on this topic.

REFERENCES

1. Rodgers A, Walker N, Schug S, et al: Reduction of postoperative mortality and morbidity with epidural or spinal anaesthesia: results from overview of randomised trials. BMJ 2000;321:1493.
2. Memtsoudis SG, Sun X, Chiu Y-L, et al: Perioperative comparative effectiveness of anesthetic technique in orthopedic patients. Anesthesiology 2013;118:1046–1058.
3. Stundner O, Danninger T, Memtsoudis SG: Regional anesthesia in patients with significant comorbid disease. Minerva Anestesiol 2013;79:1281–1290.
4. Mauermann WJ, Shilling AM, Zuo Z: A comparison of neuraxial block versus general anesthesia for elective total hip replacement: a meta-analysis. Anesth Analg 2006;103:1018–1025.
5. Hu S, Zhang ZY, Hua YQ, et al: A comparison of regional and general anaesthesia for total replacement of the hip or knee: a meta-analysis. J Bone Joint sSurg Br 2009;91:935–942.
6. Delis KT, Knaggs AL, Mason P, et al: Effects of epidural-and-general anesthesia combined versus general anesthesia alone on the venous hemodynamics of the lower limb. A randomized study. Thromb Haemost 2004;92:1003–1011.
7. Royse CF, Chung F, Newman S, et al: Predictors of patient satisfaction with anaesthesia and surgery care: a cohort study using the Postoperative Quality of Recovery Scale. Eur J Anaesthesiol 2013;30:106–110.
8. Husted H, Holm G, Jacobsen S: Predictors of length of stay and patient satisfaction after hip and knee replacement surgery: fast-track experience in 712 patients. Acta Orthop 2008;79:168–173.
9. Li G, Warner M, Lang BH, et al: Epidemiology of anesthesia-related mortality in the United States, 1999–2005. Anesthesiology 2009;110:759–765.
10. Noordzij PG, Poldermans D, Schouten O, et al: Postoperative mortality in the Netherlands: a population-based analysis of surgery-specific risk in adults. Anesthesiology 2010;112:1105–1115.
11. Wijeysundera DN, Beattie WS, Austin PC, et al: Epidural anaesthesia and survival after intermediate-to-high risk non-cardiac surgery: a population-based cohort study. Lancet 2008;372:562–569.
12. Wu CL, Hurley RW, Anderson GF, et al: Effect of postoperative epidural analgesia on morbidity and mortality following surgery in medicare patients. Reg Anesth Pain Med 29:525–33; discussion 515–519.
13. Pugely AJ, Martin CT, Gao Y, et al: Differences in short-term complications between spinal and general anesthesia for primary total knee arthroplasty. J Bone Joint Surg Am 2013;95:193–199.

14. Neuman MD, Silber JH, Elkassabany NM, et al: Comparative effectiveness of regional versus general anesthesia for hip fracture surgery in adults. Anesthesiology 2012;117:72–92.

15. Ballantyne JC, Carr DB, deFerranti S, et al: The comparative effects of postoperative analgesic therapies on pulmonary outcome: cumulative meta-analyses of randomized, controlled trials. Anesth Analg 1998;86:598–612.

16. Bauer C, Hentz J-G, Ducrocq X, et al: Lung function after lobectomy: a randomized, double-blinded trial comparing thoracic epidural ropivacaine/sufentanil and intravenous morphine for patient-controlled analgesia. Anesth Analg 2007;105:238–244.

17. Davies RG, Myles PS, Graham JM: A comparison of the analgesic efficacy and side-effects of paravertebral versus epidural blockade for thoracotomy—a systematic review and meta-analysis of randomized trials. Br J Anaesth 2006;96:418–426.

18. Svircevic V, Van Dijk D, Nierich AP, et al: Meta-analysis of thoracic epidural anesthesia versus general anesthesia for cardiac surgery. Anesthesiology 2011;114:271–282.

19. Wahba WM, Don HF, Craig DB: Post-operative epidural analgesia: effects on lung volumes. Can Anaesth Soc J 1975;22:519–527.

20. Li Y, Zhu S, Yan M: Combined general/epidural anesthesia (ropivacaine 0.375%) versus general anesthesia for upper abdominal surgery. Anesth Analg 2008;106:1562–1565, table of contents.

21. Moore CM, Desborough JP, Powell H, et al: Effects of extradural anaesthesia on interleukin-6 and acute phase response to surgery. Br J Anaesth 1994;72:272–279.

22. Aono H, Takeda A, Tarver SD, et al: Stress responses in three different anesthetic techniques for carbon dioxide laparoscopic cholecystectomy. J Clin Anesth 1998;10:546–550.

23. Kabon B, Fleischmann E, Treschan T, et al: Thoracic epidural anesthesia increases tissue oxygenation during major abdominal surgery. Anesth Analg 2003;97:1812–1817.

24. Jorgensen H, Wetterslev J, Moiniche S, et al: Epidural local anaesthetics versus opioid-based analgesic regimens on postoperative gastrointestinal paralysis, PONV and pain after abdominal surgery. Cochrane Database Syst Rev 2000;(4):CD001893.

25. Afolabi BB, Lesi FEA, Merah NA: Regional versus general anaesthesia for caesarean section. Cochrane Database Syst Rev 2006;CD004350.

26. Lee A, Ngan Kee WD, Gin T: A quantitative, systematic review of randomized controlled trials of ephedrine versus phenylephrine for the management of hypotension during spinal anesthesia for cesarean delivery. Anesth Analg 2002;94:920–926, table of contents.

27. Liu EHC, Sia ATH: Rates of caesarean section and instrumental vaginal delivery in nulliparous women after low concentration epidural infusions or opioid analgesia: systematic review. BMJ 2004;328:1410.

28. Sprung J, Flick RP, Wilder RT, et al: Anesthesia for cesarean delivery and learning disabilities in a population-based birth cohort. Anesthesiology 2009;111:302–310.

29. Gottschalk A, Sharma S, Ford J, et al: Review article: the role of the perioperative period in recurrence after cancer surgery. Anesth Analg 2010;110:1636–1643.

30. Kurosawa S, Kato M: Anesthetics, immune cells, and immune responses. J Anesth 2008;22:263–277.

31. Shavit Y, Martin FC, Yirmiya R, et al: Effects of a single administration of morphine or footshock stress on natural killer cell cytotoxicity. Brain Behav Immun 1987;1:318–328.

32. Biki B, Mascha E, Moriarty DC, et al: Anesthetic technique for radical prostatectomy surgery affects cancer recurrence: a retrospective analysis. Anesthesiology 2008;109:180–187.

33. Wuethrich PY, Hsu Schmitz S-F, Kessler TM, et al: Potential influence of the anesthetic technique used during open radical prostatectomy on prostate cancer-related outcome: a retrospective study. Anesthesiology 2010;113:570–576.

34. Exadaktylos AK, Buggy DJ, Moriarty DC, et al: Can anesthetic technique for primary breast cancer surgery affect recurrence or metastasis? Anesthesiology 2006;105:660–664.

35. Snyder GL, Greenberg S: Effect of anaesthetic technique and other perioperative factors on cancer recurrence. Br J Anaesth 2010;105:106–115.

36. Kehlet H, Jensen TS, Woolf CJ: Persistent postsurgical pain: risk factors and prevention. Lancet 2006;367:1618–1625.

37. Maguire MF, Ravenscroft A, Beggs D, et al: A questionnaire study investigating the prevalence of the neuropathic component of chronic pain after thoracic surgery. Eur J Cardiothorac Surg 2006;29:800–805.

38. Andreae MH, Andreae DA: Local anaesthetics and regional anaesthesia for preventing chronic pain after surgery. Cochrane Database Syst Rev 2012;10:CD007105.

39. Mariano ER, Chu LF, Peinado CR, et al: Anesthesia-controlled time and turnover time for ambulatory upper extremity surgery performed with regional versus general anesthesia. J Clin Anesth 2009;21:253–257.

40. Head SJ, Seib R, Osborn JA, et al: A "swing room" model based on regional anesthesia reduces turnover time and increases case throughput. Can J Anaesth 2011;58:725–732.

41. Lenart MJ, Wong K, Gupta RK, et al: The impact of peripheral nerve techniques on hospital stay following major orthopedic surgery. Pain Med 2012;13:828–834.

CHAPTER 69

The Effects of Regional Anesthesia on Functional Outcome After Surgery

Arthur Atchabahian and Michael H. Andreae

INTRODUCTION

The goal of this chapter is to additionally discuss the benefits of regional anesthesia with beyond the immediate perioperative period. While there are several other outcomes of interest, such as morbidity and mortality or cancer recurrence, our focus is on three long-term outcomes after elective surgery because of their particular importance: (1) chronic pain, (2) joint function, and (3) cognitive outcomes.

These outcomes were selected because their importance is understandable and easy to communicate to surgical colleagues, patients or health consumers, hospital administrators, and lawmakers.

REGIONAL ANESTHESIA FOR THE PREVENTION OF CHRONIC PAIN AFTER SURGERY

Chronic or persistent pain (defined as pain beyond 6 months after surgery) is often severe and frequent, condition.[1] Table 69–1 details the risk of chronic pain after several common surgical procedures.[2] Because there are only a few effective treatments to date,[1] prevention wherever possible is paramount. Even mild chronic pain can significantly diminish quality of life and impair daily functioning.[3] Between 25% and 40% of patients undergoing thoracotomy, amputation, or breast surgery suffer from persistent pain lasting for months afterward.[4] Even for procedures with a low risk of persistent postsurgical pain, such as hernia repair or cesarean section, prevention is equally important.[5] Some 5% of patients suffer from persistent pain after minor surgery, and around 40% of patients do so after limb amputation or thoracotomy.[6] About 10% of patients will develop persistent pain following cesarean section.[5]

Mechanism

Figure 69–1 graphically represents how regional anesthesia, by interrupting the development of central sensitization, may prevent chronic pain from arising after surgery. In Figure 69–1A, pain impulses are transmitted from the primary nociceptor via a synapse in the dorsal horn of the spinal cord to the secondary neuron and from there to the brain. During surgery, the high nociceptive input from the surgical site may induce central sensitization—a permanent change in synaptic strength leading to perception of pain disproportionate to the stimulus (Figure 69–1B); this causes hyperalgesia (exaggerated perception of painful stimuli); allodynia (painful perception of nonpainful stimuli, such as touch); and persistent pain after surgery.[7] Regional anesthesia, by blocking nociceptive transmission, prevents sensitization and thus the development of chronic pain (Figure 69–1C).

Summary of the Evidence

A systematic review and meta-analysis for the Cochrane Collaboration included 23 randomized controlled trials (RCTs) investigating regional anesthesia or local anesthetics for the prevention of chronic pain after surgery.[8,9] Pooled data from 250 patients in four RCTs with contrasting outcomes at 6 months after thoracotomy strongly favored epidural anesthesia with an odds ratio (OR) of 0.34 and a 95% confidence interval (CI) of 0.19–0.60. Data from 89 participants in two RCTs with outcomes at 5 or 6 months favored paravertebral block after breast cancer surgery, with an OR of 0.37 and 95% CI of 0.14–0.94. Pooled results are shown in Figure 69–2 as forest plots. When studies of cosmetic breast surgery and a study using multimodal topical analgesia were added, the strength of the evidence was increased. However, the intermediate methodological quality of the included studies weakened the conclusions.

TABLE 69–1. Risk[a] for persistent postoperative pain (PPP) after various types of surgery, with estimated surgical volumes per year in the United States.[b]

Type of Surgery	Risk of Persistent Postoperative Pain (%)	Risk of Severe Persistent Postoperative Pain (%)	Approximate Number of Cases per Year in the United States in 2003
Amputation	40	10	130,000
Breast surgery	25	10	110,000
Thoracotomy	40	10	70,000
Hernia repair	10	4	250,000
Cesarean section	10	4	1,200,000

Although the risk may seem low for some interventions, the sheer number of cases leads to a significant number of previously healthy patients having severe, disabling pain after surgery.

[a]Risk values adapted from Kehlet et al.[1]

[b]Number of surgical cases adapted from Merrill and Elixhauser.[2]

The currently available evidence supports the use of epidural anesthesia to reduce the risk of persistent pain 6 months after surgery for patients undergoing thoracotomy and the use of paravertebral blocks for women undergoing breast cancer surgery, shown in Table 69–2. Persistent postsurgical pain may be devastating, yet possibly preventable in one of four patients by using an effective perioperative regional nerve blockade. The different RCTs, conducted in diverse settings,

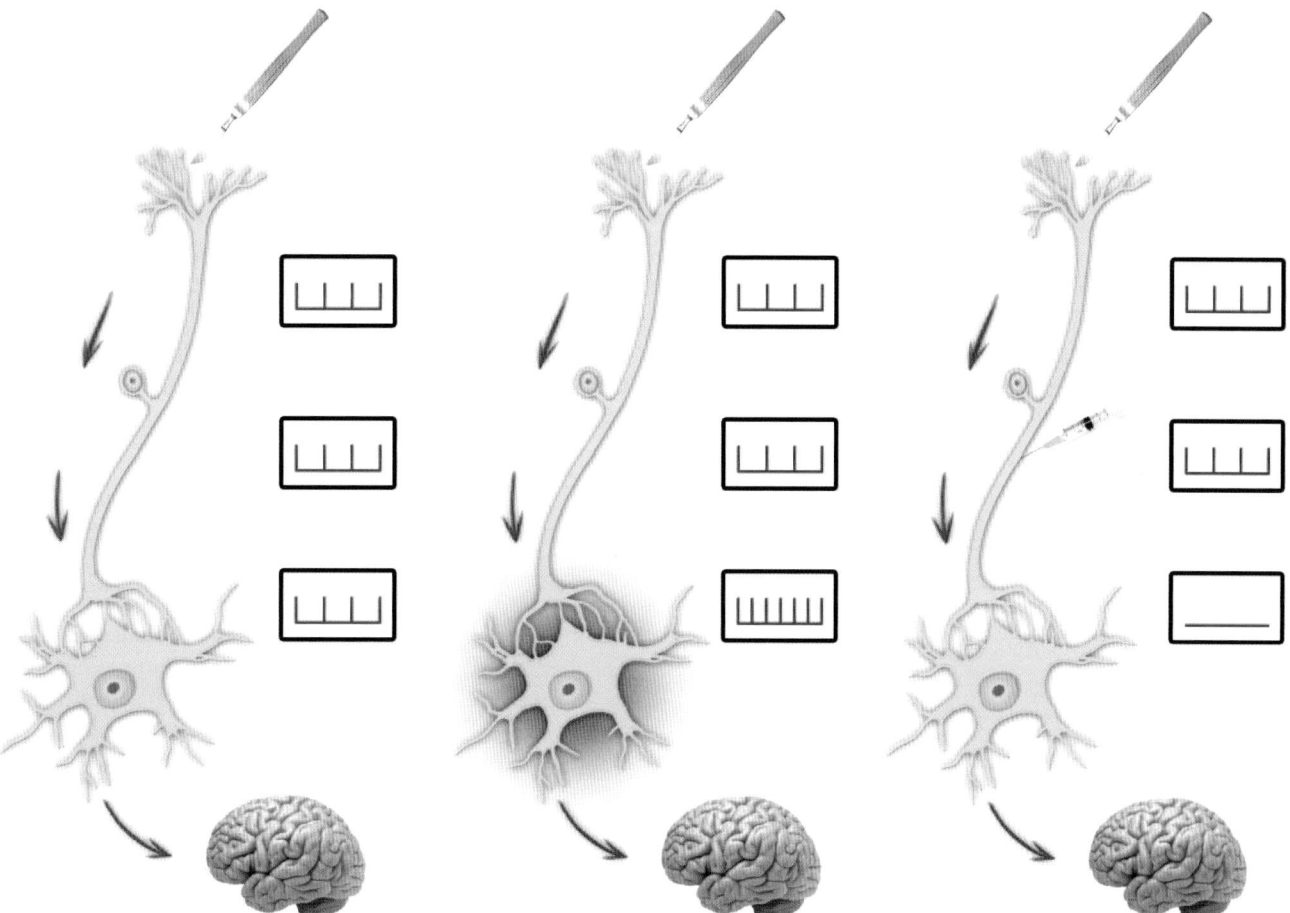

FIGURE 69–1. Site of action of local and regional anesthesia techniques in the signal pathway relevant to the development of chronic post-surgical pain.

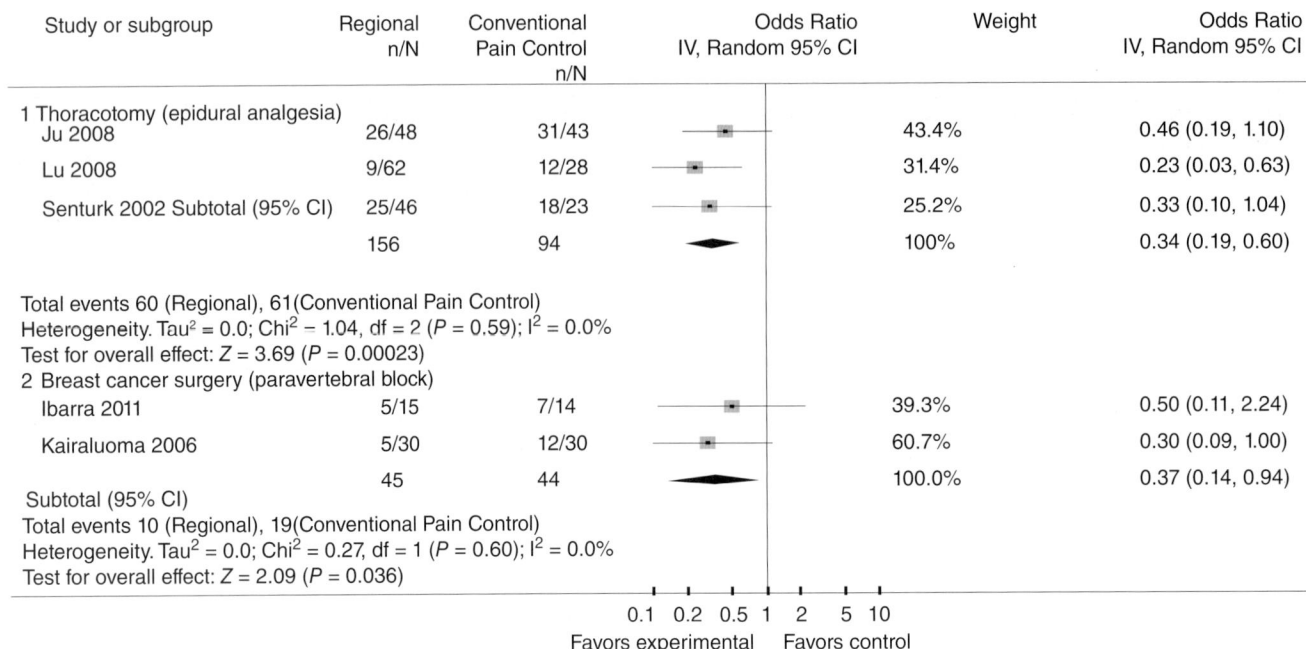

Study or subgroup	Regional n/N	Conventional Pain Control n/N	Odds Ratio IV, Random 95% CI	Weight	Odds Ratio IV, Random 95% CI
1 Thoracotomy (epidural analgesia)					
Ju 2008	26/48	31/43		43.4%	0.46 (0.19, 1.10)
Lu 2008	9/62	12/28		31.4%	0.23 (0.03, 0.63)
Senturk 2002 Subtotal (95% CI)	25/46	18/23		25.2%	0.33 (0.10, 1.04)
	156	94		100%	0.34 (0.19, 0.60)

Total events 60 (Regional), 61(Conventional Pain Control)
Heterogeneity. Tau^2 = 0.0; Chi^2 = 1.04, df = 2 (P = 0.59); I^2 = 0.0%
Test for overall effect: Z = 3.69 (P = 0.00023)

2 Breast cancer surgery (paravertebral block)					
Ibarra 2011	5/15	7/14		39.3%	0.50 (0.11, 2.24)
Kairaluoma 2006	5/30	12/30		60.7%	0.30 (0.09, 1.00)
	45	44		100.0%	0.37 (0.14, 0.94)

Subtotal (95% CI)
Total events 10 (Regional), 19(Conventional Pain Control)
Heterogeneity. Tau^2 = 0.0; Chi^2 = 0.27, df = 1 (P = 0.60); I^2 = 0.0%
Test for overall effect: Z = 2.09 (P = 0.036)

0.1 0.2 0.5 1 2 5 10
Favors experimental   Favors control

FIGURE 69–2. Pooled results for the Cochrane Collaboration included 23 randomized controlled trials (RCTs) investigating regional anesthesia or local anesthetics for the prevention of chronic pain after surgery.

were remarkably homogeneous and consistent in their estimates of the long-term effect. It is important to remember that effects of one specific block for one specific surgical intervention may not translate to other regional anesthesia techniques or surgical procedures.

Perioperative regional anesthesia and analgesia may reduce the risk of developing chronic pain after surgery. Outside the scope of this chapter, there is additional evidence suggesting that the avoidance of general anesthesia and opioids along with the use of regional anesthesia and analgesia could also reduce the risk of cancer recurrence.[19] These are compelling arguments in favor of the use of regional anesthesia and analgesia.

REGIONAL ANESTHESIA TO IMPROVE JOINT FUNCTION AFTER MAJOR JOINT REPLACEMENT

As the population in developed countries ages, severe arthritis has become more prevalent, leading to increased demand for total joint replacements (shoulder, hip, knee). Improved function over the long term, rather than immediately postoperatively, is the main outcome of these interventions. Improved functionality and mobility dictate the activity and independence of the patients and are linked to secondary comorbidities, such as diabetes mellitus, obesity, and possibly even cognitive decline.

Mechanism

Severe postoperative pain can hinder effective rehabilitation through reflex inhibition of muscle fibers, limiting strength and muscle building, as well as decreasing joint range of motion. Optimal pain control enables patients to participate more actively in physical therapy. Single injection, continuous

administration through catheters, or sustained-release preparations of local anesthetics block the conduction of pain impulses from the operated joint to the central nervous system. They offer excellent analgesia, especially in combination with acetaminophen/paracetamol, nonsteroidal anti-inflammatory drugs (NSAIDs), gabapentinoids, and opioids. Better pain control may allow more effective rehabilitation.[20] Early mobilization and range-of-motion exercises are the key factors for optimal long-term joint function—the outcome of interest. Therapy facilitated by regional analgesia can increase passive joint range of motion, with sustained gains lasting for at least a few months after surgery.[21]

Summary of the Evidence

Reported findings are derived from a systematic review and meta-analysis for the Cochrane Collaboration.[22] In Table 69–3, eight RCTs reporting functional outcomes at or after 3 months following major joint replacement are listed. Results from the pooled data from 140 participants from three studies suggest no significant improvement in range of motion (improvement of 4° with 95% CI ranging from –2.23 to 10.21). Of note, two of the studies included in Table 69–3 were not included in the Cochrane review as they compared short-term (24-hour) versus longer-term (4-day) regional analgesia.

In the results from this meta-analysis, short-term improvements in function were not sustained in the long run. However, there are important limitations in the quality of evidence, starting with the heterogeneity of patients, interventions, and agents used. In addition, no study detailed the rehabilitation protocol used. No studies were found demonstrating long-term shoulder function, and only one study of patients following hip replacement was identified in this search.

TABLE 69–2. Randomized controlled trials investigating the effect of regional anesthesia/analgesia versus general anesthesia or conventional analgesia for persistent postoperative pain after breast surgery and thoracotomy.

Study	Intervention vs. Control	Other Analgesic Modalities	Outcome Studies	Follow-up (Months)
Breast Surgery				
Baudry et al[10]	Single-injection postoperative local infiltration vs. none	None	Pain/no pain Allodynia/hyperalgesia	12
Bell et al[11]	Single-injection preincision local infiltration vs. none	None	Pain/no pain	6
Ibarra et al[12]	Single-injection preincision paravertebral block vs. none	None	Myofascial, phantom, or neuropathic pain	4–5
Kairaluoma et al[13]	Single-injection preincision paravertebral block vs. none	None	NRS > 3 Analgesic consumption	12
Fassoulaki et al[14]	Single-injection blocks + continuous postoperative topical application vs. none	Gabapentin vs. none	Pain/no pain Analgesic consumption	6
Thoracotomy				
Ju et al[15]	Continuous preincision and postoperative epidural analgesia vs. none	None	Pain/no pain Allodynia	12
Sentürk et al[16]	Continuous preincision and postoperative epidural analgesia vs. none	None	Pain/no pain NRS Pain affecting daily living	6
Lu et al[17]	Continuous preincision and postoperative epidural analgesia vs. none	None	Pain/no pain	6
Katz et al[18]	Single-injection preincision intercostal blocks vs. none	Morphine, perphenazine, and indomethacin vs. midazolam and placebo	Pain/no pain VRS Analgesic consumption	18

NRS = numeric rating scale; VRS = verbal rating scale.

Source: Data from Andreae MH, Andreae DA: Local anaesthetics and regional anaesthesia for preventing chronic pain after surgery. *Cochrane Database Syst Rev.* 2012 Oct 17;10.

An absence of evidence is not evidence of absence of effect; the jury is still out regarding whether regional anesthesia and analgesia lead to improved long-term function after total knee surgery. Although there is little evidence to support periarticular infiltration, many surgeons have been using it, often with extended-release local anesthetics. At this time, however, there is no convincing level 1 evidence of long-term benefits.

REGIONAL ANESTHESIA FOR IMPROVED COGNITIVE OUTCOMES AFTER NONCARDIAC SURGERY

Long-term cognitive outcomes are important to an aging surgical population; postoperative cognitive dysfunction (POCD) has a major impact on quality of life and independence of the elderly even after a successful surgical procedure.[30] Three months after surgery, POCD[31] is still present in 1 of 10 high-risk (elderly) patients.[32] POCD and delirium independently predict other adverse outcomes, such as increased morbidity and mortality, higher associated health care costs, long-term cognitive impairment, and further decline beyond 12 months.[33]

Mechanism

The pathophysiology of POCD after surgery is unclear.[30] Microemboli can reach the brain during orthopedic and cardiac surgery. Perioperative imbalances in neurotransmitters and inflammatory mediators have been implicated. Regional anesthesia may improve cognitive outcomes after surgery by attenuating the inflammatory response. Benzodiazepines,

TABLE 69–3. Randomized controlled trials investigating the effect of regional anesthesia/analgesia versus general anesthesia or conventional analgesia for long-term functional outcomes after major joint replacement.

Study Blinding	Intervention	Control	Outcomes
Primary Total Hip Replacement			
Ilfeld et al[23] Triple	CLPB until POD 4	CLPB until POD 1	WOMAC at 1, 2, 3, 6, and 12 months
Primary Total Knee Replacement			
Ilfeld et al[24] Triple	CFNB until POD 4	CFNB until POD 1	WOMAC at 1, 2, 3, 6, and 12 months
Kadic et al[25] Single	CFNB	No block	Knee function after 3 months (knee range of motion, KSS), WOMAC
Nader et al[26] Unblinded	CFNB Epidural infusion until POD 1	No block Epidural infusion until morning of POD 1	Knee flexion and functional outcomes at 1, 6, and 12 months
Singelyn et al[20] Unblinded	CFNB Epidural analgesia	No block	Knee flexion at 6 weeks and 3 months postoperatively
Tammachote et al[27] Single	Periarticular infiltration	Intrathecal morphine	Knee flexion and Thai version of the WOMAC at 6 and 12 weeks
Wu and Wong[28] Unblinded	CFNB until POD 3	No block	KSS (difference with preoperative value) at discharge, 6 weeks, 3 months, and 6 months postoperatively
Zhang et al[29] Double	Periarticular infiltration, then ropivacaine/ketorolac infusion	Saline intra-articular infusion	Maximum knee flexion at 90 days

CFNB = continuous femoral nerve block; CLPB = continuous lumbar plexus block; KSS = Knee Society Score; POD = postoperative day; WOMAC = Western Ontario and McMaster Osteoarthritis Index.

opioids, and other psychoactive medications are associated with POCD and may trigger a vicious cycle of POCD, leading to more medication and therefore leading to more POCD. Regional anesthesia, by controlling pain and eliminating the need for opioids, may improve cognitive outcomes; however, it is unclear whether these mechanisms would lead to sustained improvement over conventional general anesthesia.

Summary of the Evidence

A meta-analysis[34] of 26 RCTs with over 1100 patients in each group combining both long-term and short-term studies failed to support the concern that general anesthesia contributed to long-term POCD in adults (standardized difference in means −0.08; 95% CI −0.17–0.01; P = .094). The weakness of this meta-analysis is in pooling heterogeneous cognitive outcome measurements and patient populations. Certain published systematic reviews of short-term cognitive dysfunction suggest a

clear benefit of regional anesthesia in the elderly,[35] while others do not.[36,37]

The few clinical RCTs with long-term cognitive outcomes comparing a regional anesthesia intervention versus a conventional general anesthesia approach are tabulated in Table 69–4. These studies do not seem to support the hypothesis that regional anesthesia versus general anesthesia, or regional analgesia versus conventional analgesia, improves long-term cognitive function.

These conclusions are mostly based on older small studies (in Guay's review,[34] 18 of 26 studies were published in 1995 or earlier) with significant attrition, while most recent RCTs did not follow patients long enough to assess long-term cognitive outcomes. Many confounders can muddle the results. Patients with worse POCD may have selectively dropped out to avoid the embarrassment of failure in cognitive tests, biasing the studies toward the null hypothesis. Many patients in the regional anesthesia groups received midazolam, which may offset the potential benefit of regional anesthesia.[44] Most important, the focus of

TABLE 69–4. Randomized controlled trials comparing regional versus general anesthesia with cognitive outcome evaluation beyond 90 days.

Study	Surgery	Intervention vs Control	Outcomes Evaluated
Jones et al[38]	Total hip or knee replacement	Spinal anesthesia vs. general anesthesia	National Adult Reading Test Choice Reaction Time Critical flicker fusion threshold Objective learning test Digit copying test Functional life scale Cognitive difficulties test
Nielson et al[39]	Total knee replacement	Spinal anesthesia vs. general anesthesia	Wechsler Adult Intelligence Scale–Revised Trail Making Test Controlled Oral Word Association Test Finger Oscillation Test Two-point discrimination Hand preference questionnaire Sickness impact profile
Bigler et al[40]	Hip fracture	Spinal anesthesia vs. general anesthesia	Abbreviated Mental Test
Williams-Russo et al[41]	Total knee replacement	Epidural anesthesia (followed in over 95% of the cases by epidural analgesia) vs. general anesthesia (followed by intravenous patient-controlled anesthesia)	Boston Naming Test Controlled word association Digit symbol Trail Making Tests A Trail Making Tests B Digit span test Benton Visual Retention Test Benton Visual Recognition Test Mattis-Kovner Verbal Recall Mattis-Kovner Verbal Recognition
Rasmussen et al[42]	Major noncardiac surgery	Regional (spinal or epidural) anesthesia vs. general anesthesia	Part of the Visual Verbal Learning Test Part of the Concept Shifting Test Part of the Stroop Color Word Interference Test Part of the Letter Digit Coding Test Geriatric Depression Scale Subjective cognitive functioning questionnaire (patients and relatives) Instrument for activities of daily living (patients and relatives)
Campbell et al[43]	Cataract	Regional (topical + retrobulbar or peribulbar) anesthesia vs. general anesthesia	Part of the Rivermead Behavioral Memory Test 2 parts of the Fuld Object Memory Test Part of the Wechsler Adult Intelligence Scale–Revised Digit copying test Felix post unit questionnaire Holbrook activity index National Adult Reading Test

these studies was on intraoperative management, not on extended postoperative regional analgesia, where opioid sparing might have the strongest effect in preventing cognitive dysfunction.

While there is evidence that short-term cognitive impairment might be more likely after general rather than regional anesthesia, long-term differential effects have not been demonstrated. Especially in elderly patients, preferring regional anesthesia when the procedure is amenable and there are no medical contraindications is reasonable and may avoid the confusion sometimes induced by opioids.

CONCLUSION

In the ever changing health care system, patients, payers, providers, and the public must be convinced that regional anesthesia is worth the investment. Pointing to its obvious benefits immediately after surgery may not be sufficient. Rather, sustained effects on long-term outcomes, among them chronic pain after surgery, long-term function after joint replacement, and sustained cognitive outcomes in the elderly, must be studied.

The effects of regional anesthesia on the prevention of persistent postsurgical pain are robust. They are supported by many RCTs and a Cochrane review and are based on a well-founded molecular mechanism. At this time, there is insufficient evidence for improvement of long-term function after major joint repair, but because the rationale is compelling, further studies are warranted. For long-term cognitive outcomes, the benefit of regional anesthesia is unclear at present.

More research is needed on the sustained benefits of patient-centered extended perioperative nociceptive blockade and its effects on the rehabilitation.

REFERENCES

1. Kehlet H, Jensen TS, Woolf CJ: Persistent postsurgical pain: risk factors and prevention. Lancet 2006;367(9522):1618–1625.
2. Merrill C, Elixhauser A: *Procedures in US Hospitals, 2003*. Rockville, MD: Agency for Healthcare Research and Quality, 2005. HCUP Fact Book No. 7. AHRQ Publication No. 06-0039.
3. Gottschalk A, Cohen SP, Yang S, Ochroch EA: Preventing and treating pain after thoracic surgery. Anesthesiology 2006;104(3):594–600.
4. Macrae WA: Chronic post-surgical pain: 10 years on. Br J Anaesth 2008;101(1):77–86.
5. Sng BL, Sia AT, Quek K, Woo D, Lim Y: Incidence and risk factors for chronic pain after caesarean section under spinal anaesthesia. Anaesth Intensive Care 2009;37(5):748–752.
6. Jung BF, Ahrendt GM, Oaklander AL, Dworkin RH: Neuropathic pain following breast cancer surgery: proposed classification and research update. Pain 2003;104(1–2):1–13.
7. Woolf CJ, Salter MW: Neuronal plasticity: increasing the gain in pain. Science 2000;288(5472):1765–1769.
8. Andreae MH, Andreae DA: Local anaesthetics and regional anaesthesia for preventing chronic pain after surgery. Cochrane Database Syst Rev 2012;10:CD007105.
9. Andreae MH, Andreae DA: Regional anaesthesia to prevent chronic pain after surgery: a Cochrane systematic review and meta-analysis. Br J Anaesth 2013;111(5):711–720.
10. Baudry G, Steghens A, Laplaza D, et al: Infiltration de ropivacaïne en chirurgie carcinologique du sein: effet sur la douleur postopératoire aiguë et chronique [Ropivacaine infiltration during breast cancer surgery: postoperative acute and chronic pain effect]. Ann Fr Anesth Reanim 2008;27(12):979–986.
11. Bell RF, Sivertsen A, Mowinkel P, Vindenes H: A bilateral clinical model for the study of acute and chronic pain after breast-reduction surgery. Acta Anaesthesiol Scand 2001;45(5):576–582.
12. Ibarra MM, S-Carralero GC, Vicente GU, Cuartero del Pozo A, López Rincón R, Fajardo del Castillo MJ: Chronic postoperative pain after general anesthesia with or without a single-dose preincisional paravertebral nerve block in radical breast cancer surgery [in Spanish]. Rev Esp Anestesiol Reanim 2011;58(5):290–294.
13. Kairaluoma PM, Bachmann MS, Rosenberg PH, Pere PJ: Preincisional paravertebral block reduces the prevalence of chronic pain after breast surgery. Anesth Analg 2006;103(3):703–708.
14. Fassoulaki A, Triga A, Melemeni A, Sarantopoulos C: Multimodal analgesia with gabapentin and local anesthetics prevents acute and chronic pain after breast surgery for cancer. Anesth Analg 2005;101(5):1427–1432.
15. Ju H, Feng Y, Yang BX, Wang J: Comparison of epidural analgesia and intercostal nerve cryoanalgesia for post-thoracotomy pain control. Eur J Pain 2008;12(3):378–384.
16. Sentürk M, Ozcan PE, Talu GK, et al: The effects of three different analgesia techniques on long-term postthoracotomy pain. Anesth Analg 2002;94(1):11–15.
17. Lu YL, Wang XD, Lai RC: Correlation of acute pain treatment to occurrence of chronic pain in tumor patients after thoracotomy [in Chinese]. Ai Zheng 2008;27(2):206–209.
18. Katz J, Jackson M, Kavanagh BP, Sandler AN: Acute pain after thoracic surgery predicts long-term post-thoracotomy pain. Clin J Pain 1996;12(1):50–55.
19. Vaghari BA, Ahmed OI, Wu CL: Regional anesthesia-analgesia: relationship to cancer recurrence and infection. Anesthesiol Clin 2014;32(4):841–851.
20. Singelyn FJ, Deyaert M, Joris D, Pendeville E, Gouverneur JM: Effects of intravenous patient-controlled analgesia with morphine, continuous epidural analgesia, and continuous three-in-one block on postoperative pain and knee rehabilitation after unilateral total knee arthroplasty. Anesth Analg 1998;87(1):88–92.
21. Capdevila X, Barthelet Y, Biboulet P, Ryckwaert Y, Rubenovitch J, d'Athis F: Effects of perioperative analgesic technique on the surgical outcome and duration of rehabilitation after major knee surgery. Anesthesiology 1999;91(1):8–15.
22. Atchabahian A, Schwartz G, Hall CB, Lajam CM, Andreae MH: Regional analgesia for improvement of long-term functional outcome after elective large joint replacement. Cochrane Database Syst Rev 2015;8:CD010278.
23. Ilfeld BM, Ball ST, Gearen PF, et al: Health-related quality of life after hip arthroplasty with and without an extended-duration continuous posterior lumbar plexus nerve block: a prospective, 1-year follow-up of a randomized, triple-masked, placebo-controlled study. Anesth Analg 2009;109(2):586–591.
24. Ilfeld BM, Shuster JJ, Theriaque DW, et al: Long-term pain, stiffness, and functional disability after total knee arthroplasty with and without an extended ambulatory continuous femoral nerve block: a prospective, 1-year follow-up of a multicenter, randomized, triple-masked, placebo-controlled trial. Reg Anesth Pain Med 2011;36(2):116–120.
25. Kadic L, Boonstra MC, De Waal Malefijt MC, Lako SJ, Van Egmond J, Driessen JJ: Continuous femoral nerve block after total knee arthroplasty? Acta Anaesthesiol Scand 2009;53(7):914–920.
26. Nader A, Kendall MC, Wixson RL, Chung B, Polakow LM, McCarthy RJ: A randomized trial of epidural analgesia followed by continuous femoral analgesia compared with oral opioid analgesia on short- and long-term functional recovery after total knee replacement. Pain Med 2012;13(7):937–947.
27. Tammachote N, Kanitnate S, Manuwong S, Yakumpor T, Panichkul P: Is pain after TKA better with periarticular injection or intrathecal morphine? Clin Orthop Rel Res 2013;471(6):1992–1999.
28. Wu JW, Wong YC: Elective unilateral total knee replacement using continuous femoral nerve blockade versus conventional patient-controlled analgesia: perioperative patient management based on a multidisciplinary pathway. Hong Kong Med J 2014;20(1):45–51.
29. Zhang S, Wang F, Lu ZD, Zhang L, Jin QH: Effect of single-injection versus continuous local infiltration analgesia after total knee arthroplasty: a randomized, double-blind, placebo-controlled study. J Int Med Res 2011;39(4):1369–1380.
30. Wu CL, Hsu W, Richman JM, Raja SN: Postoperative cognitive function as an outcome of regional anesthesia and analgesia. Reg Anesth Pain Med 2004;29(3):257–268.
31. Sanders RD, Pandharipande PP, Davidson AJ, Ma D, Maze M: Anticipating and managing postoperative delirium and cognitive decline in adults. BMJ 2011;343:d4331.
32. Moller JT, Cluitmans P, Rasmussen LS, et al: Long-term postoperative cognitive dysfunction in the elderly ISPOCD1 study. ISPOCD investigators. International Study of Post-Operative Cognitive Dysfunction. Lancet 1998;351(9106):857–861.
33. Marcantonio ER, Flacker JM, Michaels M, Resnick NM: Delirium is independently associated with poor functional recovery after hip fracture. J Am Geriatr Soc 2000;48(6):618–624.
34. Guay J: General anaesthesia does not contribute to long-term postoperative cognitive dysfunction in adults: a meta-analysis. Indian J Anaesth 2011;55(4):358–363.
35. Parker MJ, Handoll HH, Griffiths R: Anaesthesia for hip fracture surgery in adults. Cochrane Database Syst Rev 2004;4:CD000521.

36. Barbosa FT, Jucá MJ, Castro AA, Cavalcante JC: Neuraxial anaesthesia for lower-limb revascularization. Cochrane Database Syst Rev 2013;7:CD007083.

37. Mason SE, Noel-Storr A, Ritchie CW: The impact of general and regional anesthesia on the incidence of post-operative cognitive dysfunction and post-operative delirium: a systematic review with meta-analysis. J Alzheimers Dis 2010;22(Suppl 3):67–79.

38. Jones MJ, Piggott SE, Vaughan RS, et al: Cognitive and functional competence after anaesthesia in patients aged over 60: controlled trial of general and regional anaesthesia for elective hip or knee replacement. BMJ 1990;300(6741):1683–1687.

39. Nielson WR, Gelb AW, Casey JE, Penny FJ, Merchant RN, Manninen PH: Long-term cognitive and social sequelae of general versus regional anesthesia during arthroplasty in the elderly. Anesthesiology 1990;73(6): 1103–1109.

40. Bigler D, Adelhøj B, Petring OU, Pederson NO, Busch P, Kalhke P: Mental function and morbidity after acute hip surgery during spinal and general anaesthesia. Anaesthesia 1985;40(7):672–676.

41. Williams-Russo P, Sharrock NE, Mattis S, Szatrowski TP, Charlson ME: Cognitive effects after epidural vs general anesthesia in older adults. A randomized trial. JAMA 1995;274(1):44–50.

42. Rasmussen LS, Johnson T, Kuipers HM, et al; ISPOCD2 (International Study of Postoperative Cognitive Dysfunction) Investigators: Does anaesthesia cause postoperative cognitive dysfunction? A randomised study of regional versus general anaesthesia in 438 elderly patients. Acta Anaesthesiol Scand 2003;47(3):260–266.

43. Campbell DN, Lim M, Muir MK, et al: A prospective randomised study of local versus general anaesthesia for cataract surgery. Anaesthesia 1993;48(5):422–428.

44. Sieber FE, Zakriya KJ, Gottschalk A, et al: Sedation depth during spinal anesthesia and the development of postoperative delirium in elderly patients undergoing hip fracture repair. Mayo Clin Proc 2010;85(1): 18–26.

ACUTE PAIN MANAGEMENT

CHAPTER 70

Intravenous Patient-Controlled Analgesia

Marie N. Hanna, Omar Ahmed, and Sarah Hall

INTRODUCTION

Management of postoperative pain has improved in the last few decades. In 2000, the Joint Commission on Accreditation of Healthcare Organizations (JCAHO) officially recognized patients' rights in pain management and implemented standards for assessment, monitoring, and treatment of pain[1]; in 2004, the American Society of Anesthesiologists established the Pain Task Force and published clinical practice guidelines to promote standardization of procedures and the use of multimodal analgesia[2]; and in 2010, the Department of Health and Human Services and the Institute of Medicine agreed to promote the recognition of pain as a significant public health problem. Now, pain management has become a focus of the healthcare system and an important ethical responsibility of the medical profession. Opioids remain the primary analgesic agent for treating moderate and severe pain after surgery; however, opioid-related side effects may compromise quality of recovery.

Preventive analgesia is a method of attenuating the central sensitization that results from a painful insult and the inflammatory reaction that develops after the insult.[3] For effective prevention of central sensitization and reduction of postoperative and chronic pain,[4,5] aggressive multimodal analgesic interventions should be used during the perioperative period. Maximum benefit occurs when pain interventions are extended into the postoperative phase.[6]

Multimodal analgesia (Figure 70–1) involves the administration of two or more analgesic agents by one or more routes. The different agents should exert their effects via different analgesic mechanisms and ideally act synergistically at different sites in the nervous system, thereby providing superior analgesia with fewer side effects. Multimodal analgesia can include regional analgesia with local anesthetics, acetaminophen, nonsteroidal anti-inflammatory drugs (NSAIDs), and opioids.[7] The combination of several nonopioid analgesics with opioids delivered by patient-controlled analgesia (PCA) offers advantages over opioids alone.[8,9] Multimodal pain-control strategies for certain procedures could become an integral part of clinical pathways to provide effective postoperative analgesia and rehabilitation.[8,9]

The broader concept of PCA is not restricted to intravenous opioid use. In fact, any analgesic delivered by any route (epidural, peripheral nerve catheter, subcutaneous, or transdermal) can be administered under patient control (with or without a continuous background infusion). This technique is based on delivering a preprogrammed dose of drug when the patient pushes a demand button through a microprocessor-controlled infusion pump.[10]

HISTORY OF INTRAVENOUS ANALGESIA

In 1963, Roe[11] was the first to demonstrate that postoperative narcotics are necessary and that small intravenous (IV) doses of opioids provide more effective pain relief than do conventional intramuscular (IM) injections. In 1968, Sechzer,[12] the true pioneer of PCA, evaluated the analgesic response to small IV doses of opioid administered by a nurse at the patient's request. In 1971, the first apparatus for delivering opioid on demand was introduced and marked the initial development of PCA technologies.[13] Forrest et al.[14] and Keeri-Szanto[15] initiated the concept of a demand mode. In 1976, the Cardiff Palliator, the first commercially available PCA pump, was developed at the Welsh National School of Medicine.[16] Since then, PCA devices have evolved in technologic sophistication.

In the 1970s, Marks and Sachar[17] started the revolution of pain management. Their study demonstrated that pain was undertreated in a large proportion of hospitalized patients, and that healthcare providers lack adequate experience and knowledge in the use of opioids.

In 1990, Ferrante and Covino[18] described the essential components of effective opioid analgesia that cannot be achieved

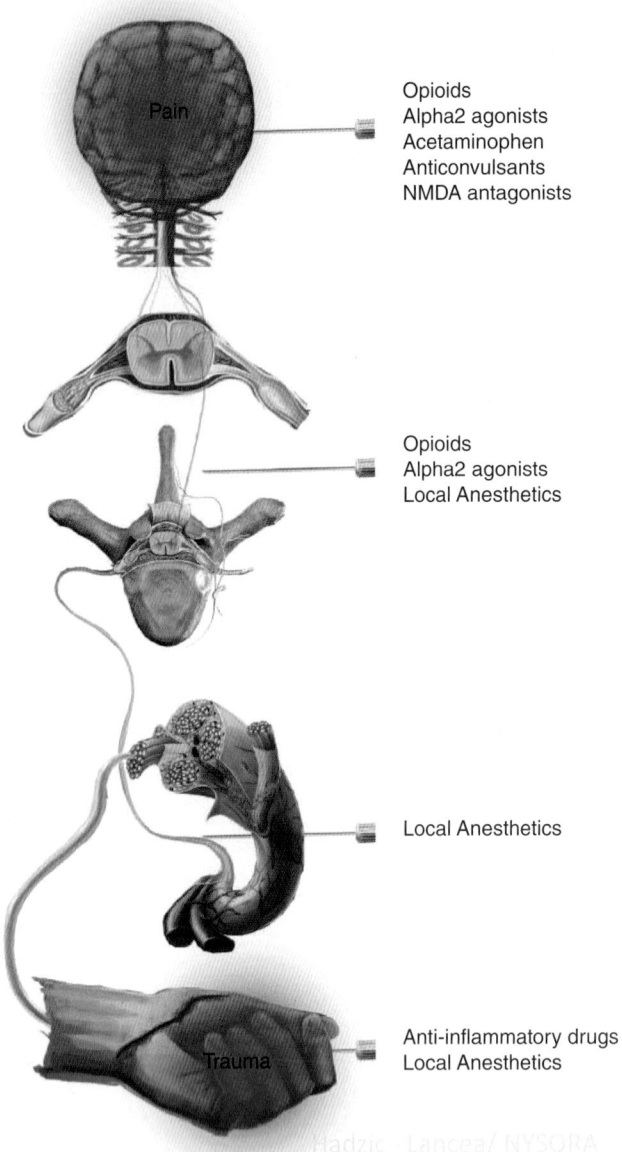

Pain

Opioids
Alpha2 agonists
Acetaminophen
Anticonvulsants
NMDA antagonists

Opioids
Alpha2 agonists
Local Anesthetics

Local Anesthetics

Anti-inflammatory drugs
Local Anesthetics

Trauma

FIGURE 70–1. Possible sites for intervention.

stem from numerous and sometimes profound adverse effects.[19–21] These include somnolence, respiratory depression, hypotension, urinary retention, and emesis due to chemoreceptor trigger zone activation. Slowed gastrointestinal transmit often results in constipation and ileus as well. Opioids as a class have few absolute contraindications, aside from hypersensitivity to a specific opioid. Relative contraindications relate especially to metabolism. For instance, the half-lives of hydromorphone and morphine are prolonged in renal insufficiency.

The mechanism of action for opioids is via mu-receptors in the central nervous system, with some evidence of peripheral opioid receptor activity as well.[22] There are three classes of mu opioid–receptor binding: pure agonists, agonist-antagonists, and partial agonists.[23] The pure agonists are obviously the most useful for acute pain management because of their complete mu-receptor binding. In equianalgesic doses, all of the common parenteral opioids are equally effective for pain control and do not differ in side-effect profiles (Table 70–1). Patients receiving mu-agonists have a risk of acute withdrawal.

Agonist-antagonist opioids act as kappa-receptor agonists and mu-receptor antagonists. These drugs were marketed as having a better safety profile owing to the ceiling effect they have on respiratory depression. However, this effect also translates to having a ceiling effect on their analgesic properties, limiting their effective usage in acute pain control. Similarly, partial agonists have limited clinical application for pain control because they exhibit only partial mu- receptor binding.

Clinical Pearls

- Common opioid side effects include somnolence, respiratory depression, hypotension, urinary retention, emesis, and constipation.
- There are three classes of mu opioid–receptor binding: pure agonists, agonist-antagonists, and partial agonists.
- Agonist-antagonist opioids act as a kappa-receptor agonist and a mu-receptor antagonist.

with PRN (as needed) or scheduled IM injections. These essentials were mainly to maintain constant plasma opioid concentrations, avoid peaks and troughs, and titrate the opioid dose to achieve the most effective analgesia with the minimum effective analgesic concentration. In contrast, patients who receive IM bolus injections experience frequent periods of severe pain, as plasma opioid concentrations fall below their individual minimum effective analgesic concentration, followed by periods of "overshoot," when higher-than-optimal plasma concentrations cause excessive sedation, possible respiratory depression, and poor analgesia.

OPIOID ANALGESIA

Opium and its derivatives are the most commonly used medications for the treatment of acute and chronic pain. Although opioids have no analgesic ceiling effect, their main limitations

TABLE 70–1. Opioid agonist equianalgesic dosing.

Drug	Parenteral IV/IM (mg)
Morphine	10
Hydromorphone	1.5-2.0
Fentanyl	0.1-0.2
Sufentanil	0.01-0.04
Remifentanil	0.05
Tramadol	100
Meperidine	75-100
Methadone	10

Abbreviations: IV, intravenous; IM, intramuscular.

ROLE OF IV ANALGESIA IN PAIN MANAGEMENT

Intravenous (IV) PCA is considered the "gold standard" by which systemic opioids are delivered postoperatively. Unlike traditional PRN analgesic regimens, IV PCA allows the clinician to compensate for several factors, including the wide inter-patient and intrapatient variability in analgesic needs, variability in serum drug levels, and administrative delays, which might result in inadequate postoperative analgesia. When compared with traditional PRN analgesic regimens, use of IV PCA may be associated with improved patient outcomes, including superior postoperative analgesia, improved patient satisfaction,[22,23] and possibly decreased risk for pulmonary complications.[24,25] Although IV PCA provides no apparent decrease in cost or length of hospital stay, it does reduce demand on the nursing staff, who are required for delivery of IV or IM PRN analgesics. This reduced workload of the nursing staff may indeed have a cost benefit.[26]

The incidence of opioid-related side effects, including respiratory depression (0.5%), from IV PCA does not appear to differ significantly from that of other administration routes (e.g., IV, IM, or subcutaneous).[24,27–29] Similarly, all of the mu-agonists, when used in common IV-PCA dosages, have similar effects on gut motility.[30]

The occurrence of respiratory depression with IV PCA is relatively low. It is no higher than with PRN systemic or neur-axial administration.[31,32] Many factors could contribute to the occurrence of respiratory depression with IV PCA, including the use of a background infusion, concomitant use of a sedative or hypnotic agent, advanced age, and the presence of pulmonary disease or sleep apnea.[24,27,28,33]

Clinical studies have shown iontophoretic patient-controlled transdermal fentanyl to be superior to placebo and comparable to IV PCA with morphine for the treatment of acute postoperative pain.[34,35] Transdermal delivery of fentanyl, a continuous passive dose, is not indicated for the treatment of acute pain but could be an option for the treatment of chronic cancer pain; it could also be an alternative to oral opioids when patients cannot tolerate oral intake for an extended time. A recent technologic development has added the process of iontophoresis to substantially increase dermal penetration capacity and thereby allow in essence a "PCA fentanyl patch."[36]

In general, there is no standard opioid that should be considered first-line. However, individual patient characteristics may steer the practitioner toward choosing one opioid over another. Variability in individual patient responses to specific opioids will ultimately guide practice.[21] A basic understanding of each specific IV-PCA opioid's pharmacology is, therefore, necessary.

Clinical Pearls

- When compared with traditional PRN analgesic regimens, use of IV PCA may be associated with improved patient outcomes, including superior postoperative analgesia, and improved patient satisfaction.

- Factors that could contribute to the occurrence of respiratory depression with IV PCA, include the use of a background infusion, concomitant use of a sedative or hypnotic agent, advanced age, and the presence of pulmonary disease or sleep apnea.
- Transdermal fentanyl usage should be reserved for chronic cancer pain, or as an alternative for patients who are NPO.

DOSAGE PARAMETERS OF IV-CONTROLLED ANALGESIA

The programmable components of IV PCA include the demand dose, a lockout interval, background or basal infusions, and dosing limitations. Each of these variables allows for substantial versatility in delivering IV opioids. The flexibility of IV PCA helps account for the variability in individual patient pain-control requirements. The effectiveness of IV PCA does, however, require regular and frequent assessment of the patient's needs by his or her healthcare provider.[37]

Demand Dose

The demand dose is the amount of drug that is delivered when the patient pushes the PCA delivery button. It may also be referred to as the incremental, PCA, or bolus dose. Ideally, the dose should produce noticeable pain relief without causing toxicity.[38] It should be noted that this bolus or demand dose is separate from the initial loading dose, which is used at the initiation of PCA usage.[23] The initial loading dose is used to titrate opioid to the minimum plasma concentration required for analgesia. Alternatively, large loading doses like this may be used for severe breakthrough pain.

Lockout Interval

The lockout interval is the minimum amount of time that must elapse before the PCA will deliver more drug on demand. This restriction will ignore demand attempts within a certain time and thereby prevents overdosage. The lockout time should account for the minimum amount of time for the drug to reach an effective plasma concentration (i.e., the opioid's onset time). After the minimum effective analgesic concentration has been reached, onset times among common PCA opioids do not appear to differ greatly.[23,39]

The number of demand attempts during lockout intervals, hourly, and over 24 hours may be a valuable piece of information for practitioners who are assessing the patient's opioid requirements. However, adjusting lockout times for variable patient pain may be less useful than initially thought. It has been suggested that decreasing the lockout time to allow for more than three demand doses per hour may be an ineffective way to improve pain relief.[28,40] Patients who require more than three demand doses per hour may in fact benefit more from an increase in the demand dose.

Basal Infusions

Basal, or background, infusions continuously deliver a low dose of drug to the patient regardless of demand attempts. Initially, background infusions were thought to help with patient pain satisfaction and sleep. However, numerous studies have shown that there is no improvement in pain or sleep scores, but a significant increase in respiratory depression.[41,42] A recent meta-analysis determined that use of continuous infusions with demand dosing was associated with a higher incidence of respiratory events in adult, but not pediatric, populations.[43] Generally, continuous infusions are not recommended for routine use with IV PCA, except for a few select patient populations and with appropriate monitoring.

Dosing Limits

Dose delivery can be restricted over a certain period as an added safety measure against overuse, most commonly over 1 or 4 hours. However, routine use of these dosing limits is controversial because of the unpredictable amount of opioid needed for analgesia or adverse effects.

Clinical Pearls

- IV PCA glossary: Demand dose is the amount of drug delivered when the patient pushes the PCA button.
- Lockout interval is the minimum time that must elapse before the next demand dose can be initiated.
- Basal infusions continuously deliver a low dose of drug.
- Dosing limits set a maximum dose delivery over a set period of time.

WAYS TO IMPROVE EFFICACY OF OPIOID IV PCA

IV PCA should not be considered the only therapy for postoperative pain management. Multimodal analgesia has been shown to decrease opioid consumption, sedation, and narcotic side effects.[44] Scheduled doses of NSAIDs clearly improve analgesia and reduce IV-PCA opioid requirements. Peripheral nerve blocks and continuous catheter techniques can all be used effectively in conjunction with IV PCA.

Several meta-analyses suggest that the use of NSAIDs, cyclooxygenase (COX)-2 inhibitors, or acetaminophen in combination with IV PCA produces an opioid-sparing effect. However, acetaminophen and COX-2 inhibitors do not appear to decrease the relative risk for opioid-related side effects (e.g., postoperative nausea and vomiting [PONV], sedation, pruritus, urinary retention) or adverse events (respiratory depression), whereas nonspecific NSAIDs appear to decrease the relative risk only for some opioid-related side effects (e.g., PONV, sedation).[44-46] In terms of pain control, the addition of NSAIDs (multiple dose or infusion only) and COX-2 inhibitors, but not acetaminophen or single-dose NSAIDs, produces significantly lower pain scores postoperatively.[44-46]

A systematic review revealed that perioperative administration of ketamine (vs control) resulted in lower pain scores

and significantly decreased morphine consumption over a 24-hour period, with no difference in morphine-related adverse effects between the groups.[47] However, use of ketamine as an adjunct to IV PCA may not improve postoperative analgesia.[48] Low-dose ketamine infusions do not appear to cause hallucinations or cognitive impairment, and in patients undergoing general anesthesia, the incidence of hallucinations appears to be low and may be independent of benzodiazepine premedication.[47,49,50] A study that evaluated adding small doses of ketamine to morphine IV PCA[51] showed no differences in pain scores, morphine consumption, patient satisfaction, or nausea scores. The ketamine group had an increased incidence of side effects, including dysphoria, resulting in early withdrawal from the study.

Similar studies evaluated the addition of 16 mg IV lidocaine to IV-PCA morphine and concluded that adding lidocaine 10 or 20 mg/mL to morphine 1 mg/mL produced no differences in opioid use, pain levels, side effects, or speed of recovery.[52,53]

MONITORING PATIENTS ON IV PCA

One of the most concerning adverse effects of IV PCA is oversedation culminating in respiratory depression and cardiac arrest. Therefore, it is recommended that patients on IV PCA receive either continuous monitoring (possibly in an intensive care unit [ICU] setting) or periodic monitoring in a nonacute setting. The level of monitoring should be based on a patient's comorbidities and risk factors for respiratory depression (e.g., obstructive sleep apnea [OSA] or other pulmonary disease, advance age, morbid obesity, concomitant administration of sedative or hypnotics). Monitoring should be frequent in the early postoperative period and during times of opioid dose adjustments.

Usually, a respiratory rate of less than 10 breaths per minute is a sign of respiratory depression. However, this may be a late sign and is not a sensitive indicator when used alone.[54] Monitoring end tidal carbon dioxide ($EtCO_2$) is a more effective way to detect respiratory depression than using standard monitors, such as pulse oximetry,[54,55] and respiratory rate. Technically advanced IV-PCA pumps have $EtCO_2$ modules that monitor a patient's $EtCO_2$ value and provide a capnograph.[56] The $EtCO_2$ module can be used in intubated and nonintubated patients and is. Therefore, not limited to an ICU setting. The Alaris Pump (CareFusion, San Diego, CA) also pauses the IV-PCA infusion if a patient's respiratory status falls below a set limit determined by the clinician. This added safety feature is especially beneficial for patients at risk for respiratory depression.

In addition to monitoring the patient, members of the acute pain service and nursing staff should also routinely check the PCA pump and its settings. Detrimental adverse events have occurred more commonly as a result of operator error than as a result of pump malfunction.[27,28]

CHOICE OF IV-PCA OPIOID

IV PCA with opioids is ideally used for acute postoperative pain, cancer pain, and sometimes chronic pain. The choice of a specific opioid for IV PCA depends on numerous factors, including patient characteristics, clinical setting, and

TABLE 70–2. Common dosing parameters for intravenous patient-controlled analgesia in adults.

Drug/Concentration	Demand Dose	Lockout Interval (min)	Background Infusion
Agonist			
Morphine	0.5-2.5 mg	5-10	0.5-2.5 mg/hr
Hydromorphone	0.05-0.25 mg	5-10	0.05-0.25 mg/hr
Fentanyl	10-20 mcg	4-10	20-100 mcg/hr
Sufentanil	2-5 mcg	4-10	2-5 mcg/hr
Remifentanil	0.2-0.7 mcg/kg/min	1-3	0.025-0.1 mcg/kg/min
Tramadol	10-20 mg	5-10	
Methadone	0.5-2.5 mg	8-20	0.5-2.5 mg/hr
Meperidine	5-25 mg	5-10	5-10 mg/hr
Agonist-Antagonist			
Nalbuphine	1-5 mg	5-15	
Buprenorphine	0.03-0.1 mg	8-20	
Pentazocine	5-30 mg	5-15	

practitioner preference.[40] In essence, nearly all of the most common opioids have been used effectively (Table 70–2).[57–59] Unless the patient is opioid tolerant, continuous settings should be avoided because their use can increase the risk of respiratory depression.[28]

Fentanyl PCA

Fentanyl's fast onset, owing to its lipophilicity, makes it a good choice for IV PCA. Common dosing parameters include a bolus of 10–40 mcg and a lockout of 4–10 minutes. When fentanyl is given in single doses, it can be considered to be 80–100 times as potent as morphine. However, because of its shorter duration of action, in a IV-PCA format, it is usually considered to be only 30–40 times as potent.[23,60]

When compared to morphine and hydromorphone, patients on fentanyl IV PCA may report less nausea/vomiting, pruritus, urinary retention, and sedation. However, the rate of respiratory depression does not differ significantly among these three agents when administered as IV PCA. In a multicenter, retrospective analysis, patients receiving fentanyl IV PCA had a lower median pain score on postoperative days 1 and 2 of orthopedic surgeries than did receiving morphine or hydromorphone IV PCA.[61]

Fentanyl undergoes hepatic metabolism via CYP3A4 and is a good choice for patients with renal failure. Furthermore, it has no active metabolites and a wider therapeutic index than morphine.[62] However, because of its rapid onset and rapid offset, patients on a fentanyl IV PCA may actually have higher requirements for the drug. There is also a marked increase in context-sensitive half-time with fentanyl, even after a few hours of infusion, owing to its high volume of distribution and long elimination half-life.[63]

Fentanyl Analogue PCA

Of the fentanyl analogues, sufentanil and remifentanil have been studied the most. Alfentanil has been used much less frequently and may have questionable or limited clinical applicability.[64]

Common dosing parameters for sufentanil are a bolus of 2–5 mcg with a lockout of 4–10 minutes. Sufentanil is generally considered to be 5–10 times more potent than fentanyl.[62] Biotransformation occurs mainly in the liver and small intestine. It has a relatively immediate onset of action, limited accumulation, and rapid elimination from body storage sites.

With the highest therapeutic index, sufentanil may be associated with less incidence of respiratory depression, less oxygen desaturation, and more effective analgesia.[65] Because of its extremely short-acting nature, a basal infusion may also be necessary. However, unlike fentanyl, sufentanil does not exhibit a dramatic increase in the context-sensitive half-time with prolonged infusions. Despite these characteristics, the rapid redistribution of this drug makes it an unpopular choice for IV PCA.

Remifentanil is considered an ultra–short-acting fentanyl analogue. Remifentanil has approximately double the potency of fentanyl and 100–200 times the potency of morphine. It undergoes hydrolysis of its ester linkage by nonspecific blood and tissue esterases to form inactive metabolites. Its analgesic effect occurs within 30–60 seconds, peaking at 2.5 minutes, and it has a half-life of 6 minutes.[66–68] In 1-minute infusions, patients may experience a dose-dependent drop in blood pressure and heart rate.

Remifentanil has been tried in situations where there is severe but brief pain, such as in labor.[69] In a recent study comparing remifentanil to fentanyl and meperidine PCA for labor analgesia, remifentanil was found to provide better pain control for patients, but only during the first hour of treatment.[70] Remifentanil also was noted to produce greater sedation scores and cause a greater decrease in oxygen saturation compared to meperidine and fentanyl. Despite these drawbacks, in this and previous studies, patients' overall satisfaction scores were best for remifentanil and worse for meperidine.[71,72]

The use of background infusions with ultra–short-acting opioids is controversial. It would seem intuitive that, owing to their inability to reach a steady-state plasma concentration, a continuous infusion would be necessary. However, studies have shown more frequent decreases in oxygen saturations with a background remifentanil infusion. Furthermore, when used in the correct setting, e.g., labor analgesia, remifentanil PCA without a background infusion has been shown to be more effective than with a background infusion.[73]

Hydromorphone PCA

Because of its alternate route of metabolism, hydromorphone is considered by many to be a reasonable alternative to morphine.[23] Extensively metabolized via glucuronidation in the liver, more than 95% of the dose will be metabolized to hydromorphone-3-glucuronide along with minor amounts of 6-hydroxy reduction metabolites.

Hydromorphone is approximately 5–6 times as potent as morphine. Common dosing parameters will, therefore, have a bolus range of 0.05 mg to upward of 0.5 mg, with a lockout of 5–10 minutes. This higher potency may have the added practical benefit of increasing the interval between reservoir refills, as most PCA concentrations are 0.5 mg/mL or 1.0 mg/mL. This characteristic may be helpful in the opioid-tolerant population.

The adverse-event profile is relatively similar to that of morphine. In a systematic review of common opioids and their associated adverse events, Wheeler et al.[19] found that hydromorphone was second only to meperidine in central nervous system side effects. While this was attributed. mainly to somnolence, hydromorphone's metabolites may also have an excitatory effect as well.[19,62] Interestingly, Wheeler et al.[19] found that hydromorphone caused more pruritus but less urinary retention than did morphine. However, a multicenter comparison of morphine and hydromorphone did not show a difference in any of the most common adverse reactions when used in IV-PCA form.[61]

Morphine PCA

As one of the oldest and most studied parenteral opioids, morphine is still one of the most common opioids used in IV PCA. Common dosing parameters include a bolus range of 0.5–2.5 mg and a lockout interval between 5 and 10 minutes.

Morphine is primarily metabolized in the liver, with approximately 87% of a dose being excreted in the urine within 72 hours. Although morphine itself undergoes glucuronidation, its metabolites are primarily excreted in the kidney. Morphine's active metabolites, morphine-3-glurcuronide (M3G) and morphine-6-glucuronide (M6G), have been shown also to produce analgesia, sedation, and respiratory depression.[74,75] These effects are especially evident and prolonged in patients with impaired renal function.[76,77]

Histamine is released after morphine administration and may produce flushing, tachycardia, hypotension, pruritus, and bronchospasm. Furthermore, IV-PCA morphine may cause higher rates of adverse side effects such as nausea, pruritus, and somnolence than does IV-PCA fentanyl.[61] Morphine's low therapeutic index also implies that it may not be the best postoperative analgesic for many patients.[62,78]

Sam et al.[79] recently measured mean plasma concentrations of morphine, M3G, and M6G in patients receiving IV-PCA morphine with and without increasing levels of background infusion. They found that background infusions up to 1 mg/hour did not offer any distinct advantages over PCA alone. Moreover, background infusions of 2 mg/hour conferred the greatest risk of respiratory depression. This evidence suggests that morphine, like other forms of IV PCA, should not routinely be used with a background infusion, both from an efficacy and safety perspective.

Tramadol PCA

Tramadol has been used safely in injectable and IV-PCA forms in a few European countries for many years, but in the United States, it has been used most commonly in oral form.[23] Tramadol is a racemic mixture and controls pain through both opioid and nonopioid centrally acting mechanisms. In addition to its weak mu-receptor activity, which is approximately 6000 times less potent than that of morphine, tramadol inhibits both serotonin and norepinephrine reuptake.[80] Tramadol is also known to have weak kappa and delta affinity.

Tramadol undergoes cytochrome P450 metabolism, and its metabolites are excreted in the kidney. One of its major active metabolites, O-desmethyltramadol, has a greater mu affinity and longer elimination half-life than does tramadol itself. This metabolite has been cited as one of the reasons for tramadol's effective analgesic properties. Seizures have also been reported when tramadol is used in high doses or with monoamine oxidase inhibitors, selective serotonin reuptake inhibitors, or tricyclic antidepressants.

Tramadol has been recommended in patients with poor cardiopulmonary function and when a pure nonopioid is contraindicated.[81] It also appears to cause less dependence than equipotent doses of stronger mu-agonists.

In equipotent doses, tramadol has been shown to have analgesic and sedative effects that are similar to those of morphine IV PCA. However, tramadol IV PCA may be associated with more gastrointestinal side effects, such as nausea and vomiting, which can lower overall patient satisfaction.[82–85] The usage of metoclopramide has been suggested not only to decrease the nausea and vomiting, but also to enhance the multimodal feature of tramadol.[86]

Methadone PCA

Methadone is rarely used in IV-PCA form, but it may be well suited for highly opioid-tolerant patients, such as those with cancer pain.[87] In addition to being a mu-opioid agonist, methadone also binds to the glutamatergic N-methyl-D-aspartate (NMDA) receptor, and thus acts as a glutamate receptor antagonist.[88] This NMDA antagonism is thought to aid in the reversal of morphine tolerance. Common IV-PCA dosing will have a bolus range of 0.5–2.5 mg and a lockout interval of 8–20 minutes.

Side effects of many of the common opioid agonists may limit their usage. When these side effects precede the analgesic effects of the opioid agonist, or when there is tolerance to a certain opioid agonist, patients may benefit from trials of other agonists.[87,89] Methadone has been cited in particular as an alternative to other opioids because of its NMDA antagonistic properties, which allow for incomplete cross-tolerance, reversal of tolerance, and possible reduction in dose requirements.[88,90]

Methadone is metabolized in the liver, but the rate of metabolism varies greatly among individuals. Compared to most other opioids, it has a large initial volume of distribution and high bioavailability. Generally speaking, it also has a longer, but inconsistent, elimination half-life than do other opioids, which could increase risk for toxicity secondary to accumulation.

When given IV, methadone has a faster onset of action than morphine.[91] This quick onset, coupled with its long elimination half-life, could be advantageous in IV-PCA format. The long elimination half-life can be useful in patients with chronic, intractable pain, such as those with cancer. However, the marked variability in elimination half-life makes routine use of methadone IV PCA challenging. Dosage should be titrated carefully and determined on an individual basis.

Meperidine PCA

Meperidine was historically one of the most commonly used opioids for IV PCA. However, it has largely fallen out of favor for routine use. Dosing parameters included a bolus size between 5 and 25 mg with a lockout of 5–10 minutes. Meperidine is approximately one-tenth as potent as morphine.

The Institute of Safe Medication Practices and the American Pain Society currently do not recommend meperidine for pain control.[92,93] In general, it should be avoided because of the accumulation of its toxic metabolite, normeperidine, and its central nervous system excitation effects, which include delirium, irritability, tremors, myoclonus, and generalized seizures.[94] These symptoms are to be considered irreversible and may actually be exacerbated by opioid antagonists. Overdose is usually handled with supportive treatment.

Because normeperidine relies on renal excretion for elimination, meperidine is contraindicated in patients with renal dysfunction. It is also contraindicated in patients with seizure disorders and in patients taking monoamine oxidase inhibitors. Patients using meperidine PCA have been shown to be at particularly high risk for adverse drug reactions caused by overall cumulative dose and duration.[95]

Meperidine may not offer any better analgesic effect than that provided by morphine or hydromorphone, but it does carry significantly more risk.[96,97] When meperidine is used, patients may require up to 10 mg/kg or more per day for adequate analgesia. This high dosage requirement can lead to normeperidine accumulation with extended usage, even in patients without renal dysfunction. It has previously been suggested that a maximum dose of 10 mg/kg per day for a 3-day period can be considered to be safe.[94] Extreme caution should

be exercised, especially when meperidine is used for longer durations. Because meperidine has no advantage over morphine or other opioids, its use is generally reserved as a last resort when all other mu-agonists have failed.[40,98]

Clinical Pearls

- Fentanyl's lipophilicity allows for fast onset and offset, but over prolonged periods of time there will be a marked increase in context-sensitive half-time.
- Fentanyl may have less nausea/vomiting, pruritus, urinary retention, and sedation compared to morphine and hydromorphone.
- Sufentanil has a fast onset with no increase in context-sensitive half-time.
- Remifentanil is useful in situations of severe, but brief pain, such as labor.
- Hydromorphone undergoes metabolism in the liver and can be considered to be a reasonable alternative to morphine in renal insufficiency.
- Morphine has active metabolites that may accumulate in kidney failure.
- Morphine releases histamine, which may produce flushing, tachycardia, hypotension, pruritus, and bronchospasm.
- Tramadol is a racemic mixture that works via opioid and nonopioid mechanisms; i.e., inhibition of serotonin and norepinephrine reuptake.

IV PCA IN THE OPIOID-TOLERANT PATIENT

Patients may become opioid tolerant from use of chronic opioid therapy for cancer pain or other chronic pain conditions or from illicit narcotic use, including heroin abuse or methadone maintenance.[99] Pain control with opioids can be challenging in such patients. Standard IV-PCA settings used for opioid-naïve patients will likely provide inadequate pain control in the opioid-tolerant patient[23] and lead to withdrawal symptoms as a result of physical dependence. On the other side of this spectrum, when conventional IV-PCA settings are used, these patients can develop high rates of adverse effects as opioid doses are escalated in an attempt to achieve pain control. This situation occurs because over time, patients develop tolerance to the analgesic effects of opioids but remain sensitive to the untoward effects, such as somnolence and respiratory depression. To further complicate the problem, opioid requirements and clinical responses may vary widely between patients.[100–102]

A baseline pain score should be assessed and the goals of pain management should be discussed with the patient and healthcare care team, ideally before the commencement of pain management. The patient and members of the acute pain service should actively participate in formulating a plan for pain management. Providing pain relief adequate for patient functionality (i.e., ambulation, use of an incentive spirometer, physical therapy exercises, and performing appropriate activities of daily living) is paramount to obtaining a pain score of zero. However, undertreatment of pain is a violation of a patient's rights and may lead to drug-seeking behavior known as pseudoaddiction.[99,103] Regardless of why a patient is opioid tolerant, it is important from both a patients' rights perspective and an ethical perspective to treat pain adequately.

Higher than normal opioid doses are often required to provide adequate pain relief in opioid-tolerant patients.[40] To achieve this goal, it may be necessary to allow increased opioid IV-PCA boluses and use a background opioid infusion.[23,104] However, the risk of developing respiratory depression also increases. To prevent withdrawal, the total 24-hour opioid dose should be maintained and may be given via background infusion over 24 hours with IV-PCA boluses for breakthrough pain. Although opioid IV PCA can be used safely and effectively in this population, it is also recommended that clinicians institute a multimodal approach to pain management, including nonopioid IV or oral adjuvants and regional anesthesia techniques, to avoid excessive use of opioids.[99] When patients become refractory to the analgesic effects of one opioid, switching to another opioid may be effective; however, the dose of opioid must be appropriately adjusted, owing to cross-tolerance. There have also been reports of switching IV-PCA medications from high-dose morphine to methadone in refractory cases.[87] Opioid agonists-antagonists may lead to acute withdrawal and, therefore, should be avoided in this patient population.[99,105,106]

Notably, high pain scores have been reported in opioid-tolerant patients.[23,100,107] To gain further insight into the adequacy of pain control, objective techniques such as behavioral pain assessment may be helpful. Behavioral scoring includes assessing for signs of discomfort, such as facial grimacing, increased muscle tone, groaning, crying, inconsolability, and restlessness. During this assessment, members of the healthcare team should also note signs of increasing sedation and respiratory depression.

Clinical Pearls

- Standard IV-PCA settings used for opioid-naïve patients will likely provide inadequate pain control in the opioid-tolerant patient and lead to withdrawal symptoms. It may be necessary to allow increased opioid IV-PCA boluses and use a background opioid infusion.
- Although opioid IV-PCA can be used safely and effectively in this population, it is also recommended that clinicians institute a multimodal approach to pain management, including nonopioid IV or oral adjuvants and regional anesthesia techniques, to avoid excessive use of opioids.
- To gain further insight into the adequacy of pain control, objective techniques such as behavioral pain assessment may be helpful.

IV PCA IN OBSTRUCTIVE SLEEP APNEA/OBESITY

Obstructive sleep apnea (OSA) affects up to 20% of the general population, and a significant number (75%) of those who could benefit from treatment remain undiagnosed.[32,108] OSA is defined as five or more episodes of apnea per hour.[109] Moderate to severe OSA varies from 15 to >30 apneic-hyponeic episodes per hour.[109]

The clinical suspicion for OSA should be raised in patients with risk factors for OSA. One study[110] revealed that preoperatively, anesthesiologists and surgeons failed to identify a significant number of patients with diagnosed OSA and symptomatic undiagnosed OSA. This study included 819 patients, of which 111 had preexisting OSA. Sixty-four (58%) of those were not diagnosed by the surgeons and 17 (15%) were not diagnosed by the anesthesia practitioners. Preoperatively, of the 267 patients with moderate to severe OSA, 245 (92%) and 159 (60%) were not diagnosed by the surgeons and anesthesiologists, respectively.

Obesity is frequently associated with OSA.[111] Patients with OSA commonly have a higher mean body mass index and a higher frequency of comorbidities than do patients without OSA.[112] In general, postoperative complications, most commonly oxygen desaturation, in OSA patients may be significant.[112] According to one study, the highest rate of postoperative complications was seen in patients who did not use a continuous positive airway pressure (CPAP) device preoperatively, but required one in the postoperative period.

Multimodal pain management is recommended in patients with OSA,[113] but depending on the clinical scenario, the use of IV PCA may be warranted. The concomitant use of sedatives or hypnotics should be avoided while patients are on IV PCA. The use of a background infusion with IV PCA increases the risk of respiratory depression, especially in patients with OSA. Progressive sedation, not a decrease in respiratory rate, is the best early clinical indicator of opioid-induced respiratory depression; use of respiratory rate is unreliable.[114–116] The progression from sedation to respiratory depression or cardiac arrest that is attributed to opioids administered by IV PCA is usually a gradual process. If sedation is noted at an early stage, the opioid can be discontinued and later implemented at a lower dose, when concern for sedation has abated.[108] In addition to receiving standard monitoring (pulse oximetry, respiratory rate), OSA patients on IV PCA should receive $EtCO_2$ monitoring with capnography. Providing adequate supplemental oxygen (e.g., O_2 face mask, CPAP) to OSA patients in the perioperative period is important. Oxygen therapy does not alter the number of apneic-hyponeic episodes, but it can reduce the occurrence of significant hypoxemia in these patients.[108,117,118]

There is no evidence that supports modifying the IV-PCA dose based on patient's weight in the adult population.[23] In fact, morbid obesity is common in patients with OSA, and the same considerations in OSA patients should be made in patients with morbid obesity.[32,109]

Clinical Pearls

- Multimodal pain management is recommended in patients with OSA, and the concomitant use of sedatives or hypnotics should be avoided while patients are on IV PCA.

- Progressive sedation, not a decrease in respiratory rate, is the best early clinical indicator of opioid-induced respiratory depression; use of respiratory rate is unreliable.
- In addition to receiving standard monitoring (pulse oximetry, respiratory rate), OSA patients on IV PCA should receive $EtCO_2$ monitoring with capnography.

IV PCA IN THE ELDERLY

The elderly population (age >65) is vastly expanding and is projected to more than double between 2012 and 2060, from 43.1 million to 92.0 million according to the US Census Bureau. Therefore, knowledge of the interaction between elderly patients and pain management is important. Pain in the elderly may be overlooked and undermanaged[119] by healthcare workers for fear of untoward adverse effects of opioids.[120,121]

Elderly patients may have age-related decreases in physiologic reserves and should be assessed for comorbidities such as cardiac, pulmonary, hepatic, and renal dysfunction, which would affect the choice and dose of opioid used for IV PCA. For example, a patient with chronic kidney disease would not be given morphine IV PCA.[122] Because of comorbidities, elderly patients have a higher incidence of postoperative complications, especially in the presence of poor pain control. Polypharmacy is also common in this patient population[122,123] and may complicate the multimodal approach to pain management.

Pain perception can change with age. The elderly may have decreased pain perception, possibly from decreased Aδ-fiber and C-fiber function and delays in central sensitization.[124,125] In general, elderly patients exhibit increased tolerance to low-intensity and short noxious stimuli, but they may have increased perception of pain from high-intensity and persistent stimuli.[126,127] This phenomenon may involve a decrease in descending modulation subsequent to intense stimuli.[125,127] Over time, such alterations may contribute to the development of chronic pain in elderly patients.[125,127]

Because of an age-related decline in physiologic reserves and changes in pharmacokinetics, elderly patients are particularly sensitive to opioids. Diminished first-pass metabolism of opioids leads to increases in its bioavailability. In addition, analgesic requirements decrease with age. Opioids should be titrated slowly to produce the desired level of analgesia while limiting adverse effects. Although the incidence of pulmonary complications does not differ between PCA and conventional boluses,[121] the use of IV PCA will compensate for the wide interpatient Variability.[128,129]

Elderly patients are also prone to develop delirium and postoperative cognitive dysfunction, especially with poor pain control.[130–132] Patients with baseline cognitive dysfunction or delirium are generally not candidates for IV PCA. It may be challenging to assess pain score via visual analogue scales in this patient population owing to cognitive dysfunction, poor communication, debilitating depression, or cultural and social barriers.[133–136] Behavioral assessments[124] in conjunction with neurologic and pulmonary assessments play a vital role in this scenario.

IV PCA has been used effectively in elderly patients. It is associated with high patient satisfaction and provides better analgesia than conventional intermittent IV opioids.[121,128,137–139] However, because elderly patients are at risk for developing respiratory depression, a background infusion of opioid via PCA is not recommended. Supplemental oxygen may also be of benefit www.census.gov/newsroom/releases/archives/population/cb12-243.html.

Clinical Pearls

- Because of an age-related decline in physiologic reserves and changes in pharmacokinetics, elderly patients are particularly sensitive to opioids.
- In general, elderly patients exhibit increased tolerance to low-intensity and short noxious stimuli, but they may have increased perception of pain from high-intensity and persistent stimuli.
- Elderly patients are also prone to develop delirium and postoperative cognitive dysfunction, especially with poor pain control.

IV PCA IN OBSTETRIC ANALGESIA

IV PCA also has a place in providing labor analgesia. It is most commonly used when access to neuraxial anesthesia is not readily available. IV PCA may also be an option for labor analgesia in patients with contraindications to epidural analgesia.[140]

Miyakoshi et al.[141] compared the effects IV PCA and no analgesia on nulliparous women in labor. The study revealed that the women who received IV-PCA fentanyl had longer labor and a greater need for augmentation of labor with oxytocin than did nulliparous women without analgesia. Additionally, the rate of cesarean section was less frequent in the IV PCA group. Vacuum-assisted delivery rate and neonatal outcomes (i.e., Apgar score <7 at 1 or 5 minutes, umbilical artery pH <7.20) were comparable between groups, irrespective of mode of delivery. In a subset of women who were asked about their satisfaction, 72% (48/67) rated their satisfaction as "excellent" or "good" for IV PCA use.

Remifentanil IV PCA is considered for use in labor analgesia because it has an extremely fast onset of action (30–60 seconds) and peak analgesic effect (2.5 minutes),[142,143] its metabolism is independent of organ function, and it has rapid maternal and fetal clearance.[144–146] Tveit et al.[147] reported that remifentanil IV PCA provided adequate pain relief and high maternal satisfaction during the first and second stages of labor. However, moderate maternal sedation and respiratory depression occurred. Multiple studies have found that women in labor are at risk for sedation, especially during the time between uterine contractions.[72,144,148–150] Therefore, continuous monitoring is necessary. No serious neonatal side effects have been recorded.

Marwah et al.[146] compared the analgesic efficacy of remifentanil and fentanyl IV PCA during labor and their effects on neonatal outcomes. Both remifentanil and fentanyl IV PCA provided moderate labor analgesia. However, transient maternal oxygen desaturation occurred more commonly with remifentanil, and fentanyl was associated with increased need for neonatal resuscitation. The cumulative effects of fentanyl can be seen with continuous infusions, owing to redistribution from inactive tissue sites.[146,151,152] As a result, the context-sensitive halftime increases[146,152,153] in neonates, in whom the elimination half-life varies from 75 to 440 minutes.[153]

Douma et al.[70] compared IV PCA with remifentanil, fentanyl, and meperidine during labor. The pain scores differed during the first hour of labor, but subsequently they were comparable. Within 3 hours, pain scores returned to values that were similar to those reported before the implementation of IV PCA. There were no differences in neonatal outcomes,[70] and the drugs were apparently safe for use during labor analgesia, as reported in other studies.[66,69,72,73,144–146,148–150,154–160] However, there have been conflicting reports of fentanyl IV PCA causing neonatal respiratory depression.[146,153,161–165]

Clinical Pearls

- IV PCA for labor analgesia may be used when access to neuraxial anesthesia is not readily available or in patients with contraindications to neuraxial analgesia.
- IV PCA for labor analgesia may cause longer labor, a greater need for augmentation of labor with oxytocin, moderate maternal sedation, and respiratory depression. Therefore, continuous monitoring is necessary.
- Remifentanil IV PCA is considered for use in labor analgesia because it has an extremely fast onset of action (30–60 seconds) and peak analgesic effect (2.5 minutes), its metabolism is independent of organ function, and it has rapid maternal and fetal clearance.

REFERENCES

1. Phillips DM: JCAHO pain management standards are unveiled. Joint Commission on Accreditation of Healthcare Organizations. 2000;JAMA 284:428.
2. American Society of Anesthesiologists Task Force on Acute Pain Management: practice guidelines for acute pain management in the perioperative setting: an updated report by the American Society of Anesthesiologists Task Force on Acute Pain Management. Anesthesiology 2004;100:1573.
3. Kissin I: Preemptive analgesia. Anesthesiology 2000;93:1138.
4. Obata H, Saito S, Fujita N, et al: Epidural block with mepivacaine before surgery reduces long-term post-thoracotomy pain. Can J Anaesth 1999;46:1127.
5. Perkins FM, Kehlet H: Chronic pain as an outcome of surgery. A review of predictive factors. Anesthesiology 2000;93:1123.
6. Kissin I, Lee SS, Bradley EL, Jr: Effect of prolonged nerve block on inflammatory hyperalgesia in rats: prevention of late hyperalgesia. Anesthesiology 1998;88:224.
7. Elvir-Lazo OL, White PF: The role of multimodal analgesia in pain management after ambulatory surgery. Curr Opin Anaesthesiol 2010;23:697.
8. Rajpal S, Gordon DB, Pellino TA, et al: Comparison of perioperative oral multimodal analgesia versus IV PCA for spine surgery. J Spinal Disord Tech 2010;23:139.
9. Kehlet H, Wilmore DW: Multimodal strategies to improve surgical outcome. Am J Surg 2001;183:630.
10. Ferrante FM: Patient-controlled analgesia: a conceptual framework for analgesic administration. In Ferrante FM, Vadeboncouer TR (eds):
11. ROE BB: Are postoperative narcotics necessary? Arch Surg 1963;87:912.
12. Sechzer PH: Objective measurement of pain (abstract). Anesthesiology 1968;50:209.
13. Sechzer PH: Studies in pain with the analgesic-demand system. Anesth Analg 1971;50:1.
14. Forrest WH, Jr., Smethurst PW, Kienitz ME: Self-administration of intravenous analgesics. Anesthesiology 1970;33:363.
15. Keeri-Szanto M: Apparatus for demand analgesia. Can Anaesth Soc J 1971;18:581.
16. Evans JM, Rosen M, MacCarthy J, et al: Apparatus for patient-controlled administration of intravenous narcotics during labour. Lancet 1976;1:17.
17. Marks RM, Sachar EJ: Undertreatment of medical inpatients with narcotic analgesics. Ann Intern Med 1973;78:173.
18. Ferrante FM, Covino BG: Patient-controlled analgesia: a historical perspective. In Ferrante FM, Ostheimer GW, Covino BG (eds): Patient-Controlled Analgesia. Boston, MA, Blackwell Scientific Publications, 1990, p 3.
19. Wheeler M, Oderda GM, Ashburn MA, et al: Adverse events associated with postoperative opioid analgesia: a systematic review. J Pain 2002;3:159.
20. Cashman JN, Dolin SJ: Respiratory and haemodynamic effects of acute postoperative pain management: evidence from published data. Br J Anaesth 2004;93:212.
21. Dolin SJ, Cashman JN: Tolerability of acute postoperative pain management: nausea, vomiting, sedation, pruritus, and urinary retention. Evidence from published data. Br J Anaesth 2005;95:584.
22. Stein C: The control of pain in peripheral tissue by opioids. N Engl J Med 1995;332:1685.
23. Grass JA: Patient-controlled analgesia. Anesth Analg 2005;101:S44-S61.
24. Hudcova J, McNicol E, Quah C, et al: Patient controlled opioid analgesia versus conventional opioid analgesia for postoperative pain. Cochrane Database Syst RevCD003348, 2006.
25. Walder B, Schafer M, Henzi I, et al: Efficacy and safety of patient-controlled opioid analgesia for acute postoperative pain. A quantitative systematic review. Acta Anaesthesiol Scand 2001;45:795.
26. Chan VW, Chung F, McQuestion M, et al: Impact of patient-controlled analgesia on required nursing time and duration of postoperative recovery. Reg Anesth 1995;20:506.
27. Hankin CS, Schein J, Clark JA, et al: Adverse events involving intravenous patient-controlled analgesia. Am J Health Syst Pharm 2007;64:1492.
28. Macintyre PE: Safety and efficacy of patient-controlled analgesia. Br J Anaesth 2001;87:36.
29. Sidebotham D, Dijkhuizen MR, Schug SA: The safety and utilization of patient-controlled analgesia. J Pain Symptom Manage 1997;14.202.
30. Radnay PA, Duncalf D, Novakovic M, et al: Common bile duct pressure changes after fentanyl, morphine, meperidine, butorphanol, and naloxone. Anesth Analg 1994;63:441.
31. Looi-Lyons LC, Chung FF, Chan VW, et al: Respiratory depression: an adverse outcome during patient controlled analgesia therapy. J Clin Anesth 1996;8:151.
32. Etches RC: Respiratory depression associated with patient-controlled analgesia: a review of eight cases. Can J Anaesth 1994;41:125.
33. Thomas V, Heath M, Rose D, et al: Psychological characteristics and the effectiveness of patient-controlled analgesia. Br J Anaesth 1995;74:271.
34. Chelly JE, Grass J, Houseman TW, et al: The safety and efficacy of a fentanyl patient-controlled transdermal system for acute postoperative analgesia: a multicenter, placebo-controlled trial. Anesth Analg 2004;98:427, table.
35. Viscusi ER, Witkowski TA: Iontophoresis: the process behind noninvasive drug delivery. Reg Anesth Pain Med 2005;30:292.
36. Viscusi ER, Reynolds L, Chung F, et al: Patient-controlled transdermal fentanyl hydrochloride vs intravenous morphine pump for postoperative pain: a randomized controlled trial. JAMA 2004;291:1333.
37. Etches RC: Patient-controlled analgesia. Surg Clin North Am 1999;79:297.
38. Owen H, Plummer JL, Armstrong I, et al: Variables of patient-controlled analgesia. 1. Bolus size. Anaesthesia 1989;44:7.
39. Mather LE, Owen H: The pharmacology of patient-administered opioids. In Ferrante FM, Ostheimer GW, Covino BG (eds): Patient-Controlled Analgesia. Boston, MA, Blackwell Scientific Publications, 2013, p 27.

Postoperative Pain Management. New York, NY, Churchill Livingston, 1993, p 255.

40. Macintyre PE: Intravenous patient-controlled analgesia: one size does not fit all. Anesthesiol Clin North Am 2005;23:109.

41. Parker RK, Holtmann B, White PF: Patient-controlled analgesia. Does a concurrent opioid infusion improve pain management after surgery? JAMA 1991;266:1947.

42. Dal D, Kanbak M, Caglar M, et al: A background infusion of morphine does not enhance postoperative analgesia after cardiac surgery. Can J Anaesth 2003;50:476, 2003.

43. George JA, Lin EE, Hanna MN, et al: The effect of intravenous opioid patient-controlled analgesia with and without background infusion on respiratory depression: a meta-analysis. J Opioid Manag 2010;6:47.

44. Elia N, Lysakowski C, Tramer MR: Does multimodal analgesia with acetaminophen, nonsteroidal antiinflammatory drugs, or selective cyclooxygenase-2 inhibitors and patient-controlled analgesia morphine offer advantages over morphine alone? Meta-analyses of randomized trials. Anesthesiology 2005;103:1296.

45. Kranke P, Morin AM, Roewer N, et al: Patients' global evaluation of analgesia and safety of injected parecoxib for postoperative pain: a quantitative systematic review. Anesth Analg 2004;99:797, table.

46. Marret E, Kurdi O, Zufferey P, et al: Effects of nonsteroidal antiinflammatory drugs on patient-controlled analgesia morphine side effects: meta-analysis of randomized controlled trials. Anesthesiology 2005;102:1249.

47. Elia N, Tramer MR: Ketamine and postoperative pain—a quantitative systematic review of randomised trials. Pain 2005;113:61.

48. Subramaniam K, Subramaniam B, Steinbrook RA: Ketamine as adjuvant analgesic to opioids: a quantitative and qualitative systematic review. Anesth Analg 2004;99:482, table.

49. Krystal JH, Karper LP, Bennett A, et al: Interactive effects of subanesthetic ketamine and subhypnotic lorazepam in humans. Psychopharmacology (Berl) 1998;135:213.

50. Sethna NF, Liu M, Gracely R, et al: Analgesic and cognitive effects of intravenous ketamine-alfentanil combinations versus either drug alone after intradermal capsaicin in normal subjects. Anesth Analg 1998; 86:1250.

51. Burstal R, Danjoux G, Hayes C, et al: PCA ketamine and morphine after abdominal hysterectomy. Anaesth Intensive Care 2001;29:246.

52. Cepeda MS, Delgado M, Ponce M, et al: Equivalent outcomes during postoperative patient-controlled intravenous analgesia with lidocaine plus morphine versus morphine alone. Anesth Analg 1996;83:102.

53. Chia YY, Tan PH, Wang KY, et al: Lignocaine plus morphine in bolus patient-controlled intravenous analgesia lacks post-operative morphine-sparing effect. Eur J Anaesthesiol 1998;15:664.

54. Campbell L, Plummer J: Guidelines for the implementation of patient-controlled analgesia. Dis Manag Health Outcomes 1998;4:27.

55. Miner JR, Heegaard W, Plummer D: End-tidal carbon dioxide monitoring during procedural sedation. Acad Emerg Med 2002;9:275.

56. CareFusion: Alaris EtCO$_2$ Module. http://www.carefusion.com/medical-products/infusion/devices/alaris-etco2-module.aspx.

57. Ferrante FM, Ostheimer GW, Covino BG: Patient-Controlled Analgesia. Boston, MA, Blackwell Scientific Publications, 1990.

58. White PF: Patient-controlled analgesia: an update on its use in the treatment of postoperative pain. Anesthesiol Clin North Am 1989;7:63.

59. Carr DB, Jacox A, Chapman CR: Acute pain management: operative or medical procedures and trauma. Clinical Practice Guideline. AHCDPR Pub. No. 92-0032. Rockville, MD, Agency for Health Care Policy and Research, Public Health Service, U.S. Department of Health and Human Services, 1992.

60. Parab PV, Ritschel WA, Coyle DE, et al: Pharmacokinetics of hydromorphone after intravenous, peroral and rectal administration to human subjects. Biopharm Drug Dispos 1988;9:187.

61. Hutchison RW, Chon EH, Tucker WF, et al: A comparison of a fentanyl, morphine, and hydromorphone patient-controlled intravenous delivery for acute postoperative analgesia: a multicenter study of opioid-induced adverse reactions. Hosp Pharm 2006;41:659.

62. Palmer PP, Miller RD: Current and developing methods of patient-controlled analgesia. Anesthesiol Clin 2010;28:587.

63. Hughes MA, Glass PS, Jacobs JR: Context-sensitive half-time in multicompartment pharmacokinetic models for intravenous anesthetic drugs. Anesthesiology 1992;76:334.

64. Owen H, Brose WG, Plummer JL, et al: Variables of patient-controlled analgesia. 3: Test of an infusion-demand system using alfentanil. Anaesthesia 1990;45:452.

65. Savoia G, Loreto M, Gravino E: Sufentanil: an overview of its use for acute pain management. Minerva Anestesiol 2001;67:206.

66. Hinova A, Fernando R: Systemic remifentanil for labor analgesia. Anesth Analg 2009;109:1925.

67. Egan TD: Pharmacokinetics and pharmacodynamics of remifentanil: an update in the year 2000. Curr Opin Anaesthesiol 2000;13:449.

68. Glass PS, Hardman D, Kamiyama Y, et al: Preliminary pharmacokinetics and pharmacodynamics of an ultra–short-acting opioid: remifentanil (GI87084B). Anesth Analg 1993;77:1031.

69. Thurlow JA, Laxton CH, Dick A, et al: Remifentanil by patient-controlled analgesia compared with intramuscular meperidine for pain relief in labour. Br J Anaesth 2002;88:374.

70. Douma MR, Verwey RA, Kam-Endtz CE, et al: Obstetric analgesia: a comparison of patient-controlled meperidine, remifentanil, and fentanyl in labour. Br J Anaesth 2010;104:209.

71. Volikas I, Male D: A comparison of pethidine and remifentanil patient-controlled analgesia in labour. Int J Obstet Anesth 2001;10:86.

72. Volmanen P, Akural EI, Raudaskoski T, et al: Remifentanil in obstetric analgesia: a dose-finding study. Anesth Analg 2002;94:913, table.

73. Blair JM, Hill DA, Fee JP: Patient-controlled analgesia for labour using remifentanil: a feasibility study. Br J Anaesth 2001;87:415.

74. Ratka A, Wittwer E, Baker L, et al: Pharmacokinetics of morphine, morphine-3-glucuronide, and morphine-6-glucuronide in healthy older men and women. Am J Pain Manage 2004;14:45.

75. Baker L, Hyrien O, Ratka A: Contributions of morphhine-3-glucuronide and morphine-6-glucuronide to differences in morphine analgesia in humans. Am J Pain Manage 2003;13:28.

76. Osborne RJ, Joel SP, Slevin ML: Morphine intoxication in renal failure: the role of morphine-6-glucuronide. Br Med J (Clin Res Ed) 1986 292:1548.

77. Sear JW, Hand CW, Moore RA, et al: Studies on morphine disposition: influence of renal failure on the kinetics of morphine and its metabolites. Br J Anaesth 1989;62:28.

78. Mather LE: Opioids: a pharmacologist's delight! Clin Exp Pharmacol Physiol 1995;22:833.

79. Sam WJ, MacKey SC, Lotsch J, et al: Morphine and its metabolites after patient-controlled analgesia: considerations for respiratory depression. J Clin Anesth 2011;23:102.

80. Grond S, Sablotzki A: Clinical pharmacology of tramadol. Clin Pharmacokinet 2004;43:879.

81. Scott LJ, Perry CM: Tramadol: a review of its use in perioperative pain. Drugs 2000;60:139.

82. Ng KF, Tsui SL, Yang JC, et al: Increased nausea and dizziness when using tramadol for post-operative patient-controlled analgesia (PCA) compared with morphine after intraoperative loading with morphine. Eur J Anaesthesiol 1998;15:565.

83. Silvasti M, Svartling N, Pitkanen M, et al: Comparison of intravenous patient-controlled analgesia with tramadol versus morphine after microvascular breast reconstruction. Eur J Anaesthesiol 2000;17:448.

84. Erolcay H, Yuceyar L: Intravenous patient-controlled analgesia after thoracotomy: a comparison of morphine with tramadol. Eur J Anaesthesiol 2003;20:141.

85. Pang WW, Mok MS, Lin CH, et al: Comparison of patient-controlled analgesia (PCA) with tramadol or morphine. Can J Anaesth 1999; 46:1030.

86. Pang W, Liu YC, Maboudou E, et al: Metoclopramide improves the quality of tramadol PCA indistinguishable to morphine PCA: a prospective, randomized, double blind clinical comparison. Pain Med 2013;14:1426.

87. Fitzgibbon DR, Ready LB: Intravenous high-dose methadone administered by patient controlled analgesia and continuous infusion for the treatment of cancer pain refractory to high-dose morphine. Pain 1997;73:259.

88. Gorman AL, Elliott KJ, Inturrisi CE: The d- and l-isomers of methadone bind to the non-competitive site on the N-methyl-D-aspartate (NMDA) receptor in rat forebrain and spinal cord. Neurosci Lett 1997; 223:5.

89. Galer BS, Coyle N, Pasternak GW, et al: Individual variability in the response to different opioids: report of five cases. Pain 1992;49:87.

90. Bruera E, Pereira J, Watanabe S, et al: Opioid rotation in patients with cancer pain. A retrospective comparison of dose ratios between methadone, hydromorphone, and morphine. Cancer 1996;78:852.

91. Inturrisi CE, Colburn WA, Kaiko RF, et al: Pharmacokinetics and pharmacodynamics of methadone in patients with chronic pain. Clin Pharmacol Ther 1987;41:392.

92. Institute for Safe Medication Practices: Medication safety alert. High alert medication feature: reducing patient harm from opiates. http://www.ismp.org/Newsletters/acutecare/articles/20070222.asp. 2012. Last accessed on September 16, 2013.

93. American Pain Society: Principles of Analgesic Use in the Treatment of Acute Pain and Cancer Pain, 6th ed. Glenview, IL, 2008.

94. Simopoulos TT, Smith HS, Peeters-Asdourian C, et al: Use of meperidine in patient-controlled analgesia and the development of a normeperidine toxic reaction. Arch Surg 2002;137:84.

95. Seifert CF, Kennedy S: Meperidine is alive and well in the new millennium: evaluation of meperidine usage patterns and frequency of adverse drug reactions. Pharmacotherapy 2004;24:776.

96. O'Connor A, Schug SA, Cardwell H: A comparison of the efficacy and safety of morphine and pethidine as analgesia for suspected renal colic in the emergency setting. J Accid Emerg Med 2000;17:261.

97. Jasani NB, O'Conner RE, Bouzoukis JK: Comparison of hydromorphone and meperidine for ureteral colic. Acad Emerg Med 1994;1:539.

98. Latta KS, Ginsberg B, Barkin RL: Meperidine: a critical review. Am J Ther 9:53, 2002.

99. Hanna MN, Ouanes JP, Tomas VG: Postoperative pain and other acute pain syndromes. In Benzon HT, Rathmell JP, Wu CL, et al (eds): Practical Management of Pain. 5th ed. Philadelphia, PA, Elsevier, 2013, p 271.

100. Rapp SE, Ready LB, Nessly ML: Acute pain management in patients with prior opioid consumption: a case-controlled retrospective review. Pain 1995;61:195.

101. Gourlay GK, Kowalski SR, Plummer JL, et al: Fentanyl blood concentration-analgesic response relationship in the treatment of postoperative pain. Anesth Analg 1988;67:329.

102. Davis JJ, Johnson KB, Egan TD, et al: Preoperative fentanyl infusion with pharmacokinetic simulation for anesthetic and perioperative management of an opioid-tolerant patient. Anesth Analg 2003;97:1661.

103. Weissman DE, Haddox JD: Opioid pseudoaddiction—an iatrogenic syndrome. Pain 1989;36:363.

104. Baird MB, Schug SA: Safety aspects of postoperative pain relief. Pain Digest 1996;6:225.

105. Hartree C: Caution with nalbuphine in patients on long-term opioids. Palliat Med 2005;19:168.

106. Jacobs EA, Bickel WK: Precipitated withdrawal in an opioid-dependent outpatient receiving alternate-day buprenorphine dosing. Addiction 1999;94:140.

107. Magnani B, Johnson LR, Ferrante FM: Modifiers of patient-controlled analgesia efficacy. II. Chronic pain. Pain 1989;39:23.

108. Young T, Skatrud J, Peppard PE: Risk factors for obstructive sleep apnea in adults. JAMA 2004;291:2013.

109. Practice parameters for the indications for polysomnography and related procedures. Polysomnography Task Force, American Sleep Disorders Association Standards of Practice Committee. Sleep 1997;20:406.

110. Parikh SN, Stuchin SA, Maca C, et al: Sleep apnea syndrome in patients undergoing total joint arthroplasty. J Arthroplasty 2002;17:635.

111. Benumof JL: Obstructive sleep apnea in the adult obese patient: implications for airway management. J Clin Anesth 2001;13:144.

112. Liao P, Yegneswaran B, Vairavanathan S, et al: Postoperative complications in patients with obstructive sleep apnea: a retrospective matched cohort study. Can J Anaesth 2009;56:819.

113. Wiesel S, Fox GS: Anaesthesia for a patient with central alveolar hypoventilation syndrome (Ondine's curse). Can J Anaesth 1990;37:122.

114. Phillips BA, Schmitt FA, Berry DT, et al: Treatment of obstructive sleep apnea. A preliminary report comparing nasal CPAP to nasal oxygen in patients with mild OSA. Chest 1990;98:325.

115. Landsberg R, Friedman M, Ascher-Landsberg J: Treatment of hypoxemia in obstructive sleep apnea. Am J Rhinol 2001;15:311.

116. Blake DW, Yew CY, Donnan GB, et al: Postoperative analgesia and respiratory events in patients with symptoms of obstructive sleep apnoea. Anaesth Intensive Care 2009;37:720.

117. Young T, Shahar E, Nieto FJ, et al: Predictors of sleep-disordered breathing in community-dwelling adults: the Sleep Heart Health Study. Arch Intern Med 2002;162:893.

118. Peppard PE, Young T, Palta M, et al: Longitudinal study of moderate weight change and sleep-disordered breathing. JAMA 2000;284:3015.

119. Karani R, Meier DE: Systemic pharmacologic postoperative pain management in the geriatric orthopaedic patient. Clin Orthop Relat Res 2004;26–34.

120. Bettelli G: Anaesthesia for the elderly outpatient: preoperative assessment and evaluation, anaesthetic technique and postoperative pain management. Curr Opin Anaesthesiol 2010;23:726.

121. Aubrun F, Marmion F: The elderly patient and postoperative pain treatment. Best Pract Res Clin Anaesthesiol 2007;21:109.

122. Smith H, Bruckenthal P: Implications of opioid analgesia for medically complicated patients. Drugs Aging 2010;27:417.

123. Montamat SC, Cusack BJ, Vestal RE: Management of drug therapy in the elderly. N Engl J Med 1989;321:303.

124. Herr KA, Garand L: Assessment and measurement of pain in older adults. Clin Geriatr Med 2001;17:457, vi.

125. Gloth FM, III: Geriatric pain. Factors that limit pain relief and increase complications. Geriatrics 2000;55:46.

126. Gibson SJ, Farrell M: A review of age differences in the neurophysiology of nociception and the perceptual experience of pain. Clin J Pain 2004;20:227.

127. Gibson SJ, Helme RD: Age-related differences in pain perception and report. Clin Geriatr Med 2001;17:433.

128. Macintyre PE, Jarvis DA: Age is the best predictor of postoperative morphine requirements. Pain 1996;64:357.

129. Aubrun F, Monsel S, Langeron O, et al: Postoperative titration of intravenous morphine in the elderly patient. Anesthesiology 2002;96:17.

130. Ramaiah R, Lam AM: Postoperative cognitive dysfunction in the elderly. Anesthesiol Clin 2009;27:485, table.

131. Vaurio LE, Sands LP, Wang Y, et al: Postoperative delirium: the importance of pain and pain management. Anesth Analg 2006;102:1267.

132. Halaszynski TM: Pain management in the elderly and cognitively impaired patient: the role of regional anesthesia and analgesia. Curr Opin Anaesthesiol 2009;22:594.

133. Kaasalainen S, Crook J: An exploration of seniors' ability to report pain. Clin Nurs Res 2004;13:199.

134. Landi F, Onder G, Cesari M, et al: Pain and its relation to depressive symptoms in frail older people living in the community: an observational study. J Pain Symptom Manage 2005;29:255.

135. Tsai YF, Wei SL, Lin YP, et al: Depressive symptoms, pain experiences, and pain management strategies among residents of Taiwanese public elder care homes. J Pain Symptom Manage 2005;30:63.

136. Coldrey JC, Upton RN, Macintyre PE: Advances in analgesia in the older patient. Best Pract Res Clin Anaesthesiol 2011;5:367.

137. Gagliese L, Jackson M, Ritvo P, et al: Age is not an impediment to effective use of patient-controlled analgesia by surgical patients. Anesthesiology 2000;93:601.

138. Keita H, Geachan N, Dahmani S, et al: Comparison between patient-controlled analgesia and subcutaneous morphine in elderly patients after total hip replacement. Br J Anaesth 2003;90:53.

139. Falzone E, Hoffmann C, Keita H: Postoperative analgesia in elderly patients. Drugs Aging 2013;30:81.

140. El-Kerdawy H, Farouk A: Labor analgesia in preeclampsia: remifentanil patient controlled intravenous analgesia versus epidural analgesia. Middle East J Anesthesiol 2010;20:539.

141. Miyakoshi K, Tanaka M, Morisaki H, et al: Perinatal outcomes: intravenous patient-controlled fentanyl versus no analgesia in labor. J Obstet Gynaecol Res 2013;39:783.

142. Glass PS: Remifentanil: a new opioid. J Clin Anesth 1995;7:558.

143. Babenco HD, Conard PF, Gross JB: The pharmacodynamic effect of a remifentanil bolus on ventilatory control. Anesthesiology 2000;92:393.

144. Volikas I, Butwick A, Wilkinson C, et al: Maternal and neonatal side-effects of remifentanil patient-controlled analgesia in labour. Br J Anaesth 2005;95:504.

145. Kan RE, Hughes SC, Rosen MA, et al: Intravenous remifentanil: placental transfer, maternal and neonatal effects. Anesthesiology 1998;88:1467.

146. Marwah R, Hassan S, Carvalho JC, et al: Remifentanil versus fentanyl for intravenous patient-controlled labour analgesia: an observational study. Can J Anaesth 2012;59:246.

147. Tveit TO, Halvorsen A, Seiler S, et al: Efficacy and side effects of intravenous remifentanil patient-controlled analgesia used in a stepwise approach for labour: an observational study. Int J Obstet Anesth 2013;22:19.

148. Balki M, Kasodekar S, Dhumne S, et al: Remifentanil patient-controlled analgesia for labour: optimizing drug delivery regimens. Can J Anaesth 2007;54:626.

149. Evron S, Glezerman M, Sadan O, et al: Remifentanil: a novel systemic analgesic for labor pain. Anesth Analg 2005;100:233.

150. Blair JM, Dobson GT, Hill DA, et al: Patient controlled analgesia for labour: a comparison of remifentanil with pethidine. Anaesthesia 2005;60:22.

151. Egan TD, Lemmens HJ, Fiset P, et al: The pharmacokinetics of the new short-acting opioid remifentanil (GI87084B) in healthy adult male volunteers. Anesthesiology 1993;79:881.

152. Kapila A, Glass PS, Jacobs JR, et al: Measured context-sensitive half-times of remifentanil and alfentanil. Anesthesiology 1995;83:968.

153. Koehntop DE, Rodman JH, Brundage DM, et al: Pharmacokinetics of fentanyl in neonates. Anesth Analg 1986;65:227.

154. D'Onofrio P, Novelli AM, Mecacci F, et al: The efficacy and safety of continuous intravenous administration of remifentanil for birth pain relief: an open study of 205 parturients. Anesth Analg 2009;109:1922.

155. Balcioglu O, Akin S, Demir S, et al: Patient-controlled intravenous analgesia with remifentanil in nulliparous subjects in labor. Expert Opin Pharmacother 2007;8:3089.

156. Roelants F, De FE, Veyckemans F, et al: Patient-controlled intravenous analgesia using remifentanil in the parturient. Can J Anaesth 2001; 48:175.

157. Owen MD, Poss MJ, Dean LS, et al: Prolonged intravenous remifentanil infusion for labor analgesia. Anesth Analg 2002;94:918, table.

158. Olufolabi AJ, Booth JV, Wakeling HG, et al: A preliminary investigation of remifentanil as a labor analgesic. Anesth Analg 2000;91:606.

159. Dhileepan S, Stacey RG: A preliminary investigation of remifentanil as a labor analgesic. Anesth Analg 2001;92:1358.

160. Hill D: The use of remifentanil in obstetrics. Anesthesiol Clin 2008;26:169, viii.

161. Rayburn WF, Smith CV, Parriott JE, et al: Randomized comparison of meperidine and fentanyl during labor. Obstet Gynecol 1989;74:604.

162. Nikkola EM, Ekblad UU, Kero PO, et al: Intravenous fentanyl PCA during labour. Can J Anaesth 1997;44:1248.

163. Morley-Forster PK, Reid DW, Vandeberghe H: A comparison of patient-controlled analgesia fentanyl and alfentanil for labour analgesia. Can J Anaesth 2000;47:113.

164. Morley-Forster PK, Weberpals J: Neonatal effects of patient-controlled analgesia using fentanyl in labor. Int J Obstet Anesth 1998;7:103.

165. Halpern SH, Muir H, Breen TW, et al: A multicenter randomized controlled trial comparing patient-controlled epidural with intravenous analgesia for pain relief in labor. Anesth Analg 2004;99:1532.

CHAPTER 71

Continuous Peripheral Nerve Blocks

Amanda M. Monahan and Brian M. Ilfeld

INTRODUCTION

The maximum duration of a single-injection peripheral nerve block is approximately 8–24 hours.[1] Prolonging a peripheral nerve block may be desirable, and can be achieved with a continuous local anesthetic infusion via a perineural catheter. A continuous peripheral nerve block (CPNB) requires placement of a perineural catheter in the vicinity of a targeted peripheral nerve for the purpose of subsequently administering local anesthetic. Another term for this practice is *perineural local anesthetic infusion*. CPNBs are utilized for a wide variety of indications, most typically for anesthesia or analgesia in a peripheral nerve distribution. While not every application of CPNB has been exhaustively validated by randomized trials, continuous blocks have been reported for over 20 anatomic locations. The majority of described applications of CPNBs relate to the treatment of perioperative surgery-related pain.

HISTORY AND BACKGROUND OF CPNBS

The practice of continuous perineural analgesia has developed in parallel with technologic advances over nearly 70 years' time. Methods for identification of the catheter target have included anatomic landmarks, paresthesias, electrical stimulation, fluoroscopy, and ultrasound.[1] Continuous peripheral nerve blockade was described as early as 1946 by Ansbro.[2] A series of patients undergoing upper extremity surgeries as long as 4 hours in duration received a cork-stabilized needle at the supraclavicular level of the brachial plexus.[2] Other early reports include a similar practice in 1950 by Humphries.[3] In 1951, Sarnoff and colleagues reported placement of a polyethylene tube advanced through an insulated needle placed adjacent to a peripheral nerve using electrical stimulation.[4] By 1995, continuous perineural catheters were being inserted using multiple modalities. Pham-Dang and colleagues described fluoroscope-guided catheter placement adjacent to the brachial plexus within the axilla.[5]

In that same year, Guzeldemir reported using ultrasound to place an axillary brachial plexus catheter.[6] By the late 1990s, ambulatory continuous peripheral nerve blocks gained popularity.[7,8] Relatively small, light, and inexpensive portable infusion pumps permitted outpatient infusion.[9]

Equipment providing a continuous infusion has evolved from a simple cork stabilizing a delivery needle,[2] to a catheter sheath advanced over a needle stylet,[5] to epidural-type catheters threaded through stimulating needles.[10–12] Stimulating catheters were introduced in an attempt to improve perineural location of the catheter tip,[13] although they are being reported far less frequently due to the evolution of ultrasound-guided (nonstimulating) catheter insertion techniques.[14] Whatever the technique or method of insertion, catheters are always placed within a tissue space that contains the plexus or nerve(s) of interest. (Figure 71–1) Patient selection for perineural catheters has also evolved from a solely hospital-based practice to inclusion of outpatient infusions.[15] While adhering to patient selection criteria, continuous techniques can be applied to pediatric, pregnant, and geriatric patients, as well as healthy ambulatory patients and the critically ill. Reported locations for continuous nerve blocks span a multitude of anatomic sites in the upper extremities, trunk, and lower extremities.

Klein and colleagues were some of the first investigators to objectively quantify the benefits of local anesthetic infusion in a randomized double-blind placebo-controlled manner.[16] Patients undergoing open shoulder surgery were randomized and underwent interscalene catheter placement using electrical stimulation. They received a postoperative infusion of either ropivacaine 0.2% or normal saline at 10 mL/hour via a disposable elastomeric pump for up to 23 hours. Pain scores were lower in the ropivacaine infusion group, averaging 1 (of 10) compared with 3 for subjects receiving perineural saline. These results suggested a significant benefit for continuous perineural infusion in the postoperative setting with the use of a portable pump. However, the possible advantages for use in the outpatient

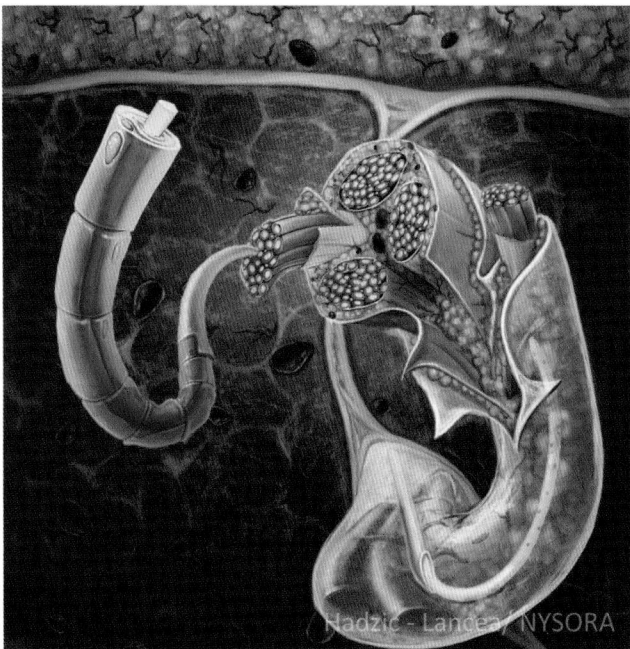

FIGURE 71–1. An illustration depicting the general concept of catheter insertion. After successful needle placement into the tissue plane that contains the nerve, the catheter is inserted beyond the needle tip to provide access to the tissue plane for infusion and/or boluses of local anesthetic.

setting remained in question. A series of 70 outpatient catheter infusions was described by Rawal and colleagues in 1998.[9] Data from randomized, controlled studies involving CPNBs in the outpatient setting were subsequently published.[15]

PATIENT SELECTION FOR CPNB

Indications

Most reports of CPNBs involve management of acute perioperative pain of greater than 12–24 hours' duration that is expected to be difficult to control by traditional methods such as systemic analgesics.[17] This is one of the few indications that has been evaluated with randomized controlled trials.[18] A catheter may also be advantageous in a patient who does not tolerate other analgesic regimens due to adverse effects.[19] Other reported indications include sympathectomy/vasodilation after vascular accidents or embolism,[20,21] digit replantation,[22,23] limb salvage,[24] and treatment of Raynaud phenomenon.[25] In the combat trauma setting, continuous perineural infusions have been utilized during transport to a treatment center.[26] Continuous infusions have also been described for chronic painful conditions such as phantom limb pain,[27,28] complex regional pain syndrome,[29] cancer pain,[30] preoperative pain control,[31] and

trigeminal neuralgia.[32] Both pediatric and adult CPNBs have been described.[1,24,29,33–38]

Contraindications

While most contraindications to CPNB are relative in nature, commonly described absolute contraindications include infection at the catheter-insertion site,[39] allergy to local anesthetics,[40] and patient refusal/inability to cooperate. Many relative contraindications have been described, including coagulopathy/anticoagulation,[40] systemic infection/bacteremia, preexisting neuropathy, desire for postoperative neurovascular examinations, and elevated fall risk/inability to comply with activity restrictions.[1] For ambulatory infusions, inability to care for the infusion at home may also be a relative contraindication.[15] Additional relative contraindications are unique to the proposed catheter location. Certain infusions may affect ipsilateral phrenic nerve and diaphragm functions, such as interscalene, supraclavicular, or cervical paravertebral catheters. While the effects of ipsilateral diaphragmatic paralysis may be minimal in relatively healthy patients,[41] this may not hold true for those with significant pulmonary morbidity, such as chronic obstructive pulmonary disease or preexisting contralateral diaphragmatic paralysis.

Catheter Insertion

Whatever the technique or method of insertion, catheters are always placed within a tissue space that contains the plexus or nerve(s) of interest (see Figure 71–1). Early catheters were inserted by inducing a paresthesia, seeking the tactile feedback of a tactile "pop" or "click," or using fluoroscopy.[1] From the time period of the 1970s to 1990s, most reported perineural catheters were inserted using electrical nerve stimulation.[1]

Ultrasound-guided catheter insertion has been compared to nerve stimulation techniques in multiple randomized controlled trials.[1] Insertion time and insertion discomfort are often reduced with ultrasound techniques, and the quality of analgesia is similar.[1] Ultrasound guidance can allow for catheter placement that would not otherwise be feasible with electrical stimulation techniques, such as patients with amputated limbs or those unable to elicit a muscle response.[42] Real-time

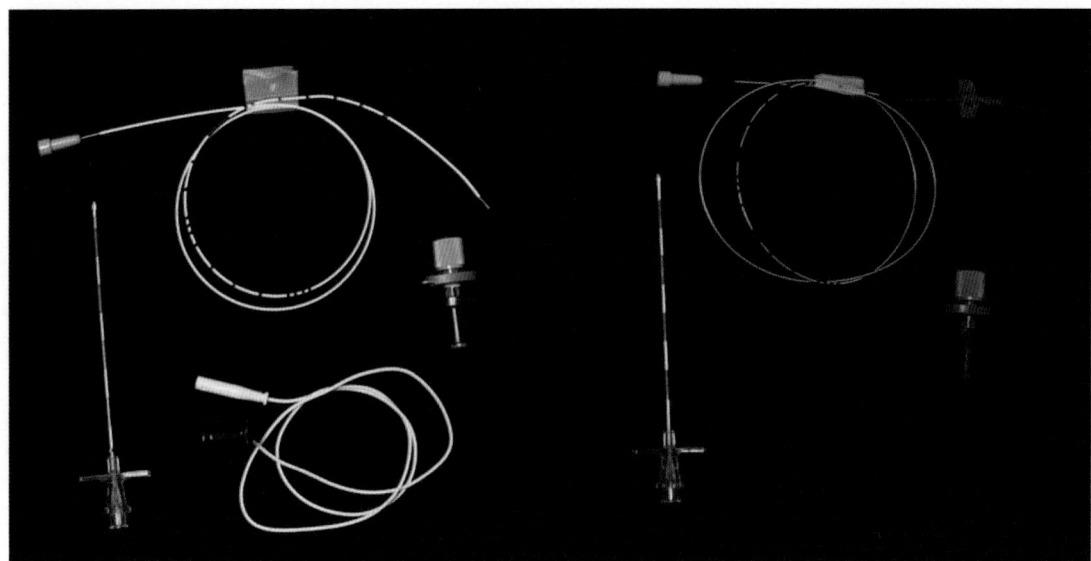

FIGURE 71–2. Examples of two perineural catheter designs: (**A**) an insulated needle and stimulating catheter (StimuCath, Teleflex/Arrow, Reading, PA); and, (**B**) an uninsulated needle and nonstimulating catheter (FlexBlock, Teleflex/Arrow, Reading, PA).

ultrasound allows for identification of vessels, which may make it an attractive modality when abnormal coagulation status is encountered.[43] Numerous methods for ultrasound-guided perineural catheter placement have been described.[14] Combining ultrasound and nerve stimulation has not demonstrated significant benefit—and it sometimes introduced new difficulties—in the majority of studies.[44–46]

Several types of catheters are available for perineural use. Some are specifically marketed for perineural infusions, and others are designed and approved for epidural infusions, and thus are used off-label when inserted adjacent to a peripheral nerve. Two broad design categories are stimulating and non-stimulating catheters (Figure 71–2). A stimulating catheter conducts electrical current to its distal end.[47] Elicited muscle movement is monitored as the catheter is advanced as an approximation of the distance between the catheter tip and target nerve. Nonstimulating catheters are typically advanced either "blindly" or under ultrasound visualization (unfortunately, the latter is technically challenging since flexible catheters do not remain within a two-dimensional plane).[14]

Optimal catheter insertion distance will allow for minimal dislodgements while also avoiding catheter knotting. Catheter knots have been reported with insertion greater than 5 cm.[48–50]

Clinical Pearl

- Optimal perineural catheter insertion distance will allow for minimal dislodgements while also avoiding catheter knotting; catheter knots have been reported with insertion greater than 5 cm.

Benefits

While case reports describe numerous potential benefits for continuous peripheral nerve blocks, available randomized

controlled trials (RCTs) focus on benefits in the postoperative setting.[1] Postoperative pain relief is the primary benefit for performing a CPNB, and other benefits appear to derive from the improved analgesia.[18] Additional benefits demonstrated by RCTs include decreased opioid analgesic requirements and opioid-related adverse effects such as nausea/vomiting,[51,52] pruritus,[53,54] sedation, dizziness, and bowel dysfunction.[53,55] Non–opioid-related benefits include earlier achievement of physical therapy goals,[51,56] less sleep disturbance,[57] decreased pain upon coughing,[58] higher patient satisfaction scores,[52] and earlier readiness for and decreased time until hospital discharge.[53,59–61]

A small number of studies have explored the benefits of CPNB extending beyond the time of catheter removal. Currently, there are little data suggesting that a perioperative CPNB decreases subsequent chronic pain or disability following the perineural infusion.[1]

The location of the catheter and surgical site will influence the degree of benefit. Coverage of the entire surgical site within the sensory distribution of the target nerve typically provides the most complete analgesia. For this reason, shoulder (interscalene catheter) and foot procedures (sciatic catheter) are particularly amenable to regional anesthesia.[11,12,16,59,62,63] Infraclavicular catheters have also been validated by RCT.[10] However, to provide adequate analgesia often requires a relatively high dose of local anesthetic at this location, which may lead to an insensate arm or fingers.[64,65]

Surgical sites such as the knee or hip are innervated by multiple nerves, thus even with a functional CPNB, additional analgesics are typically required.[60,66] Femoral catheters have been studied extensively in the setting of knee arthroplasty, and continuous femoral infusions have been validated with multiple documented in-hospital benefits including improved analgesia and earlier attainment of range-of-motion. Short-term postinfusion benefits include continued improved knee range-of-motion at 1 month postoperatively.[67] One study reported improved physical therapy endpoints 6 weeks postoperatively in patients receiving a continuous femoral nerve block[68]; however, multiple other trials detected no such prolonged benefit.[69–72] The value of adding a sciatic perineural catheter in addition to the femoral catheter for total knee arthroplasty has also been evaluated by randomized controlled trials. Pain control until the second postoperative day is superior with combined catheters.[73] However, discharge readiness remains unaffected. In a review of four randomized and three observational trials, no benefit beyond 24 hours postoperatively was found by the addition of a sciatic single block or continuous block.[74] Efforts to minimize motor block while providing femoral nerve-distribution analgesia have led to placement of perineural catheters near the femoral nerve at the mid-thigh "adductor canal" region.[75,76] Decreased quadriceps weakness, relative to an inguinal-level block, has been demonstrated in a volunteer study.[77] While decreased opioid requirements and earlier ambulation have been demonstrated with adductor canal infusion versus placebo,[78] it remains unknown if this relatively new modality provides equivalent analgesia compared with continuous femoral nerve blocks.[75]

Popliteal-sciatic catheters provide significant improvements in analgesia, opioid consumption, sleep disturbance, patient satisfaction, and same-day hospital discharge following foot and ankle surgery.[11,61] Paravertebral catheters have been validated by RCTs to demonstrate the benefits of pain relief and tissue oxygenation. In one study when compared to intravenous (IV) opioids, a continuous thoracic paravertebral technique for breast reconstruction has been associated with improved analgesia as well as superior latissimus flap tissue oxygen tension.[79] Following open lung surgery, paravertebral catheters provide similar analgesia with superior cardiovascular stability as thoracic epidural infusion.[80] Case series suggest improved spirometry performance after paravertebral infusion for rib fractures.[81] RCTs documenting benefits are sparse for other locations, such as axillary,[82] supraclavicular,[83,84] transversus abdominis plane,[85,86] and intercostal catheters.[87]

Clinical Pearls

- The majority of Benefits are derived from decreasing pain, and include avoiding opioid-related adverse effects, earlier achievement of physical therapy goals, less sleep disturbance, higher patient satisfaction scores, and earlier readiness for and decreased time until hospital discharge.
- To provide adequate analgesia with an infraclavicular catheter often requires a relatively high dose of local anesthetic at this location, which may lead to an insensate arm or fingers.
- Surgical sites such as the knee or hip are innervated by multiple nerves, thus even with a functional CPNB, additional analgesics are typically required.
- There are little data suggesting significant benefits from catheters in the axillary, supraclavicular, transversus abdominis plane, and intercostal anatomic locations.

Risks

All medical procedures carry some degree of risk, which must be carefully balanced with the potential benefits. Known risks common to any regional anesthetic include bleeding, infection, or neurologic injury. When compared to single-injection blocks, continuous techniques appear to have a similar frequency of complications, most of which are relatively minor.[88]

Catheters may be unintentionally inserted into the intravascular, epidural,[89–91] intrathecal,[92–94] or intraneural spaces.[95] Infectious risks specific to perineural catheters have been investigated in multiple studies. A range of data has been reported; recent studies report up to 29%–58% catheter colonization, 3%–4% local inflammation, and 2%–3% clinically relevant infection rates.[96–98] Within these studies, 0.8%–0.9% of patients required incision and drainage. Neurologic complications are a rare but serious complication of any regional technique. It is difficult to attribute the contribution of the surgical procedure, patient positioning, the single-injection block, or the catheter/infusion. Despite these limitations, the incidence of transient neurologic symptoms after a continuous technique has been reported from 0%–1.4%.[1] Long-lasting (greater than 6 weeks) neurologic symptoms have been reported at a rate of 0.2% in one large study of 3500 catheters.[96] Catheters may unintentionally dislodge, occlude, break, or be retained.[1] A recent study in healthy volunteers reported that up to 25% of femoral catheters may dislodge from their original intended location.[97]

The third edition of the American Society of Regional Anesthesia and Pain Medicine guidelines regarding regional anesthesia in the patient receiving antithrombotic or thrombolytic therapy outlined a 26-patient case series of bleeding complications with plexus or peripheral blockade.[98] All patients with neurologic deficits experienced a resolution within 6–12 months. Serious blood loss appeared to be the most morbid complication associated with the bleeding.

In addition, site-specific risks have been identified. For example, the incidental phrenic or recurrent laryngeal nerve blockade with an interscalene catheter may not be tolerated in patients with limited pulmonary reserve or contralateral vocal cord lesion.[99] Falls are a concerning risk, especially with CPNBs of the lower extremity. A pooled analysis of several studies suggests an increased association of falls with continuous femoral/psoas compartment blocks after knee or hip arthrolasty.[100]

Clinical Pearls

Perineural infusions that affect the femoral nerve have been associated with an increased risk of falling.

- Adductor canal perineural infusion may provide similar analgesia to femoral infusions while decreasing induced quadriceps weakness; however, further research is required to draw conclusions.
- CPNB's risk of complications is relatively low, but includes infection, bleeding, and neurologic injury. When compared to single-injection blocks, continuous techniques appear to have a similar frequency of complications, most of which are relatively minor.

SUMMARY

A CPNB, or perineural local anesthetic infusion, is a method to extend the effects of a single-injection technique by placement of a perineural catheter and subsequent local anesthetic infusion. Precatheter patient selection and counseling are crucial for both inpatient and ambulatory cases. Numerous techniques are used for accurate catheter tip placement. Multiple benefits have been documented by randomized controlled trials, most of which result from improving analgesia. Finally, most related adverse effects are minor and easily remedied; however, rare serious complications have also been reported.

REFERENCES

1. Ilfeld BM: Continuous peripheral nerve blocks: a review of the published evidence. Anesth Analg 2011;113:904–925.
2. Ansbro FP: A method of continuous brachial plexus block. Am J Surg 1946;71:716–722.
3. Humphries S: Brachial plexus block; report on 350 cases. BMJ 1950;21:163.
4. Sarnoff SJ, Sarnoff LC: Prolonged peripheral nerve block by means of indwelling plastic catheter. Treatment of hiccup. Anesthesiology 1951;12:270–275.
5. Pham-Dang C, Meunier JF, Poirier P, et al: A new axillary approach for continuous brachial plexus block. A clinical and anatomic study. Anesth Analg 1995;81:686–693.
6. Guzeldemir ME, Ustunsoz B: Ultrasonographic guidance in placing a catheter for continuous axillary brachial plexus block. Anesth Analg 1995;81:882–883.
7. Rawal N, Hylander J, Nydahl PA, Olofsson I, Gupta A: Survey of postoperative analgesia following ambulatory surgery. Acta Anaesthesiol Scand 1997;41:1017–1022.
8. Klein SM, Greengrass RA, Gleason DH: Major ambulatory surgery with continuous regional anesthesia and a disposable infusion pump. Anesthesiology 1999;91:563–565.
9. Rawal N, Axelsson K, Hylander J, et al: Postoperative patient-controlled local anesthetic administration at home. Anesth.Analg 1998;86:86–89.
10. Ilfeld BM, Morey TE, Enneking FK: Continuous infraclavicular brachial plexus block for postoperative pain control at home: a randomized, double-blinded, placebo-controlled study. Anesthesiology 2002;96:1297–1304.
11. Ilfeld BM, Morey TE, Wang RD, Enneking FK: Continuous popliteal sciatic nerve block for postoperative pain control at home:a randomized, double-blinded, placebo-controlled study. Anesthesiology 2002;97:959–965.
12. Ilfeld BM, Morey TE, Wright TW, et al: Continuous interscalene brachial plexus block for postoperative pain control at home: a randomized, double-blinded, placebo-controlled study. Anesth Analg 2003;96:1089–1095.
13. Boezaart AP, de Beer JF, du TC, van Rooyen K: A new technique of continuous interscalene nerve block. Can.J.Anaesth 1999;46:275–281.
14. Ilfeld BM, Fredrickson MJ, Mariano ER: Ultrasound-guided perineural catheter insertion: three approaches but few illuminating data. Reg Anesth Pain Med 2010;35:123–126.
15. Ilfeld BM, Enneking FK: Continuous peripheral nerve blocks at home: a review. Anesth Analg 2005;100:1822–1833.
16. Klein SM, Grant SA, Greengrass RA, et al: Interscalene brachial plexus block with a continuous catheter insertion system and a disposable infusion pump. Anesth Analg 2000;91:1473–1478.
17. Boezaart AP: Perineural infusion of local anesthetics. Anesthesiology 2006;104:872–880.
18. Richman JM, Liu SS, Courpas G, et al: Does continuous peripheral nerve block provide superior pain control to opioids? A meta-analysis. Anesth Analg 2006;102:248–257.
19. Rawal N, Allvin R, Axelsson K, et al: Patient-controlled regional analgesia (PCRA) at home: controlled comparison between bupivacaine and ropivacaine brachial plexus analgesia. Anesthesiology 2002;96:1290–1296.
20. Manriquez RG, Pallares V: Continuous brachial plexus block for prolonged sympathectomy and control of pain. Anesth Analg 1978;57:128–130.
21. Cheeley LN: Treatment of peripheral embolism by continuous sciatic nerve block. Curr Res Anesth Analg 1952;31:211–212.
22. Berger A, Tizian C, Zenz M: Continuous plexus blockade for improved circulation in microvascular surgery. Ann Plast Surg 1985;14:16–19.
23. Mezzatesta JP, Scott DA, Schweitzer SA, Selander DE: Continuous axillary brachial plexus block for postoperative pain relief. Intermittent bolus versus continuous infusion. Reg Anesth 1997;22:357–362.
24. Loland VJ, Ilfeld BM, Abrams RA, Mariano ER: Ultrasound-guided perineural catheter and local anesthetic infusion in the perioperative management of pediatric limb salvage: a case report. Paediatr Anaesth 2009;19:905–907.
25. Greengrass RA, Feinglass NG, Murray PM, Trigg SD: Continuous regional anesthesia before surgical peripheral sympathectomy in a patient with severe digital necrosis associated with Raynaud's phenomenon and scleroderma. Reg Anesth Pain Med 2003;28:354–358.
26. Buckenmaier CC, III, Rupprecht C, McKnight G, McMillan B, White RL, Gallagher RM, Polomano R: Pain following battlefield injury and evacuation: a survey of 110 casualties from the wars in Iraq and Afghanistan. Pain Med 2009;10:1487–1496.
27. Lierz P, Schroegendorfer K, Choi S, et al: Continuous blockade of both brachial plexus with ropivacaine in phantom pain: a case report. Pain 1998;78:135–137.
28. Ilfeld BM, Moeller-Bertram T, Hanling SR, et al: Treating intractable phantom limb pain with ambulatory continuous peripheral nerve blocks: a pilot study. Pain Med 2013;14(6):935–942.
29. Dadure C, Motais F, Ricard C, et al: Continuous peripheral nerve blocks at home for treatment of recurrent complex regional pain syndrome I in children. Anesthesiology 2005;102:387–391.
30. Fischer HB, Peters TM, Fleming IM, Else TA: Peripheral nerve catheterization in the management of terminal cancer pain. Reg Anesth 1996;21:482–485.
31. Burgoyne LL, Bertani LA, Kaddoum RN, et al: Long-term use of nerve block catheters in paediatric patients with cancer related pathologic fractures. Anaesth Intensive Care 2012;40(4):710.
32. Umino M, Kohase H, Ideguchi S, Sakurai N: Long-term pain control in trigeminal neuralgia with local anesthetics using an indwelling catheter in the mandibular nerve. Clin J Pain 2002;18:196–199.
33. Dadure C, Raux O, Gaudard P, et al: Continuous psoas compartment blocks after major orthopedic surgery in children: a prospective computed tomographic scan and clinical studies. Anesth Analg 2004;98:623–628.
34. Dadure C, Bringuier S, Nicolas F, et al: Continuous epidural block versus continuous popliteal nerve block for postoperative pain relief after major podiatric surgery in children: a prospective, comparative randomized study. Anesth Analg 2006;102:744–749.
35. Ludot H, Berger J, Pichenot V, et al: Continuous peripheral nerve block for postoperative pain control at home: a prospective feasibility study in children. Reg Anesth Pain Med 2008;33:52–56.
36. Ilfeld BM, Smith DW, Enneking FK: Continuous regional analgesia following ambulatory pediatric orthopedic surgery. Am J Orthop 2004;33:405–408.
37. Ganesh A, Rose JB, Wells L, et al: Continuous peripheral nerve blockade for inpatient and outpatient postoperative analgesia in children. Anesth Analg 2007;105:1234–1242.
38. Mariano ER, Ilfeld BM, Cheng GS, et al: Feasibility of ultrasound-guided peripheral nerve block catheters for pain control on pediatric medical missions in developing countries. Paediatr Anaesth 2008;18:598–601.
39. Capdevila X, Bringuier S, Borgeat A: Infectious risk of continuous peripheral nerve blocks. Anesthesiology 2009;110:182–188.
40. Liu SS, Salinas FV: Continuous plexus and peripheral nerve blocks for postoperative analgesia. Anesth.Analg 2003;96:263–272.
41. Borgeat A, Perschak H, Bird P, et al: Patient-controlled interscalene analgesia with ropivacaine 0.2% versus patient-controlled intravenous analgesia after major shoulder surgery: effects on diaphragmatic and respiratory function. Anesthesiology 2000;92:102–108.
42. Plunkett AR, Brown DS, Rogers JM, Buckenmaier CC, III: Supraclavicular continuous peripheral nerve block in a wounded soldier: when ultrasound is the only option. Br J Anaesth 2006;97:715–717.
43. Klein SM, D'Ercole F, Greengrass RA, Warner DS: Enoxaparin associated with psoas hematoma and lumbar plexopathy after lumbar plexus block. Anesthesiology 1997;87:1576–1579.
44. Dhir S, Ganapathy S: Comparative evaluation of ultrasound-guided continuous infraclavicular brachial plexus block with stimulating catheter and traditional technique: a prospective-randomized trial. Acta Anaesthesiol.Scand 2008;52:1158–1166.
45. Walker A, Roberts S: Stimulating catheters: a thing of the past? Anesth Anal. 2007;104:1001–1002.

46. Fredrickson MJ: The sensitivity of motor response to needle nerve stimulation during ultrasound guided interscalene catheter placement. Reg Anesth Pain Med 2008;33:291–296.

47. Mariano ER, Loland VJ, Sandhu NS, et al: Comparative efficacy of ultrasound-guided and stimulating popliteal-sciatic perineural catheters for postoperative analgesia. Can J Anaesth 2010;57:919–926.

48. Offerdahl MR, Lennon RL, Horlocker TT: Successful removal of a knotted fascia iliaca catheter: principles of patient positioning for peripheral nerve catheter extraction. Anesth Analg 2004;99:1550–1552.

49. Burgher AH, Hebl JR: Minimally invasive retrieval of knotted nonstimulating peripheral nerve catheters. Reg Anesth Pain Med 2007;32:162–166.

50. Motamed C, Bouaziz H, Mercier FJ, Benhamou D: Knotting of a femoral catheter. Reg Anesth 1997;22:486–487.

51. Chan EY FM, Sathappan S, Chua NH, Chan YH, Chua N.: Comparing the analgesia effects of single-injection and continuous femoral nerve blocks with patient controlled analgesia after total knee arthroplasty. J Arthroplasty 2013;28:6.

52. Bingham AE, FU R, Horn JL, Abrahams MS: Continuous peripheral nerve block compared with single-injection peripheral nerve block: a systematic review and meta-analysis of randomized controlled trials. Reg Anesth Pain Med 2012;37(6):583–594.

53. Capdevila X, Dadure C, Bringuier S, et al: Effect of patient-controlled perineural analgesia on rehabilitation and pain after ambulatory orthopedic surgery: a multicenter randomized trial. Anesthesiology 2006;105:566–573.

54. Marino J, Russo J, Kenny M, et al: Continuous lumbar plexus block for postoperative pain control after total hip arthroplasty. A randomized controlled trial. J Bone Joint Surg Am 2009;91:29–37.

55. Mistraletti G, De La Cuadra-Fontaine JC, Asenjo FJ, et al: Comparison of analgesic methods for total knee arthroplasty: metabolic effect of exogenous glucose. Reg Anesth Pain Med 2006;31:260–269.

56. Sakai N IT, Kunugiza Y, Tomita T, Mashimo T: Continuous femoral versus epidural block for attainment of 120° knee flexion after total knee arthroplasty: a randomized controlled trial. J Arthroplasty 2013;28:8.

57. Andersen HL GJ, Møller L, Christensen B, Zaric D: Continuous saphenous nerve block as supplement to single-dose local infiltration analgesia for postoperative pain management after total knee arthroplasty. Reg Anesth Pain Med 2013;38:6.

58. Fortier S HH, Bernard A, Girard C: Comparison between systemic analgesia, continuous wound catheter analgesia and continuous thoracic paravertebral block: a randomised, controlled trial of postthoracotomy pain management. Eur J Anaesthesiol 2012;29:7.

59. Ilfeld BM, Vandenborne K, Duncan PW, et al: Ambulatory continuous interscalene nerve blocks decrease the time to discharge readiness after total shoulder arthroplasty: a randomized, triple-masked, placebo-controlled study. Anesthesiology 2006;105:999–1007.

60. Ilfeld BM, Le LT, Meyer RS, et al: Ambulatory continuous femoral nerve blocks decrease time to discharge readiness after tricompartment total knee arthroplasty: a randomized, triple-masked, placebo-controlled study. Anesthesiology 2008;108:703–713.

61. White PF, Issioui T, Skrivanek GD, .et al: The use of a continuous popliteal sciatic nerve block after surgery involving the foot and ankle: does it improve the quality of recovery? Anesth Analg 2003;97:1303–1309.

62. Mariano ER, Afra R, Loland VJ, et al: Continuous interscalene brachial plexus block via an ultrasound-guided posterior approach: a randomized, triple-masked, placebo-controlled study. Anesth Analg 2009;108:1688–1694.

63. Zaric D, Boysen K, Christiansen J, et al: Continuous popliteal sciatic nerve block for outpatient foot surgery—a randomized, controlled trial. Acta Anaesthesiol Scand 2004;48:337–341.

64. Ilfeld BM, Morey TE, Enneking FK: Infraclavicular perineural local anesthetic infusion: A comparison of three dosing regimens for postoperative analgesia. Anesthesiology 2004;100:395–402.

65. Ilfeld BM, Le LT, Ramjohn J, et al: The effects of local anesthetic concentration and dose on continuous infraclavicular nerve blocks: a multicenter, randomized, observer-masked, controlled study. Anesth Analg 2009;108:345–350.

66. Ilfeld BM, Ball ST, Gearen PF, et al: Ambulatory continuous posterior lumbar plexus nerve blocks after hip arthroplasty: a dual-center, randomized, triple-masked, placebo-controlled trial. Anesthesiology 2008;109:491–501.

67. Nader A KM, Wixson RL, Chung B, et al: A randomized trial of epidural analgesia followed by continuous femoral analgesia compared with oral opioid analgesia on short- and long-term functional recovery after total knee replacement. Pain Med 2012;13:10.

68. Carli F, Clemente A, Asenjo JF, et al: Analgesia and functional outcome after total knee arthroplasty: periarticular infiltration vs continuous femoral nerve block. Br J anaesth 2010;105:185–195.

69. Wegener JT, van Ooij B, van Dijk CN, et al: Long-term pain and functional disability after total knee arthroplasty with and without single-injection or continuous sciatic nerve block in addition to continuous femoral nerve block: a prospective, 1-year follow-up of a randomized controlled trial. Reg Anesth Pain Med 2013;38:5.

70. Ilfeld BM, Meyer RS, Le LT, et al: Health-related quality of life after tricompartment knee arthroplasty with and without an extended-duration continuous femoral nerve block: a prospective, 1-year follow-up of a randomized, triple-masked, placebo-controlled study. Anesth Analg 2009;108:1320–1325.

71. Ilfeld BM, Shuster JJ, Theriaque DW, et al: Long-term pain, stiffness, and functional disability after total knee arthroplasty with and without an extended ambulatory continuous femoral nerve block: a prospective, 1-year follow-up of a multicenter, randomized, triple-masked, placebo-controlled trial. Reg Anesth Pain Med 2011;36:116–120.

72. Ilfeld BM, Ball ST, Gearen PF, et al: Health-related quality of life after hip arthroplasty with and without an extended-duration continuous posterior lumbar plexus nerve block: a prospective, 1-year follow-up of a randomized, triple-masked, placebo-controlled study. Anesth Analg 2009;109:586–591.

73. Wegener JT, van Ooij B, van Dijk CN, et al: Value of single-injection or continuous sciatic nerve block in addition to a continuous femoral nerve block in patients undergoing total knee arthroplasty: a prospective, randomized, controlled trial. Reg Anesth Pain Med 2011;36:481–488.

74. Abdallah FW, Brull R: Is sciatic nerve block advantageous when combined with femoral nerve block for postoperative analgesia following total knee arthroplasty? A systematic review. Reg Anesth Pain Med 2011;36:6.

75. Ilfeld BM, Hadzic A: Walking the tightrope after knee surgery: optimizing postoperative analgesia while minimizing quadriceps weakness. Anesthesiology 2013;118:248–250.

76. Lund J, Jenstrup MT, Jaeger P, et al: Continuous adductor-canal-blockade for adjuvant post-operative analgesia after major knee surgery: preliminary results. Acta anaesthesiol Scand 2011;55:14–19.

77. Jaeger P, Nielsen ZJ, Henningsen MH, et al: Adductor canal block versus femoral nerve block and quadriceps strength: a randomized, double-blind, placebo-controlled, crossover study in healthy volunteers. Anesthesiology 2013;118:7.

78. Jenstrup MT, Jaeger P, Lund J, et al: Effects of adductor-canal-blockade on pain and ambulation after total knee arthroplasty: a randomized study. Acta Anaesthesiol Scand 2012;56:357–364.

79. Buggy DJ, Kerin MJ: Paravertebral analgesia with levobupivacaine increases postoperative flap tissue oxygen tension after immediate latissimus dorsi breast reconstruction compared with intravenous opioid analgesia. Anesthesiology 2004;100:375–380.

80. Pintaric TS, Potocnik I, Hadzic A, et al: Comparison of continuous thoracic epidural with paravertebral block on perioperative analgesia and hemodynamic stability in patients having open lung surgery. Regional anesthesia and pain medicine 2011;36:256–260.

81. Karmakar MK CL, Ho AM, Gin T, Lee TW: Continuous thoracic paravertebral infusion of bupivacaine for pain management in patients with multiple fractured ribs. Chest 2003;424–431.

82. Salonen MH, Haasio J, Bachmann M, et al: Evaluation of efficacy and plasma concentrations of ropivacaine in continuous axillary brachial plexus block: High dose for surgical anesthesia and low dose for postoperative analgesia. Reg Anesth Pain Med 2000;25:47–51.

83. Mariano ER, Sandhu NS, Loland VJ, et al: A randomized comparison of infraclavicular and supraclavicular continuous peripheral nerve blocks for postoperative analgesia. Reg Anesth Pain Med 2011;36: 26–31.

84. Cornish PB, Leaper CJ, Nelson G, et al:: Avoidance of phrenic nerve paresis during continuous supraclavicular regional anaesthesia. Anaesthesia 2007;62:354–358.

85. Heil JW, Ilfeld BM, Loland VJ, et al:: Ultrasound-guided transversus abdominis plane catheters and ambulatory perineural infusions for outpatient inguinal hernia repair. Reg Anesth Pain Med 2010;35: 556–558.

86. Niraj G, Kelkar A, Jeyapalan I, et al: Comparison of analgesic efficacy of subcostal transversus abdominis plane blocks with epidural analgesia following upper abdominal surgery. Anaesthesia 2011;66:465–461.

87. Wildgaard K, Petersen RH, Hansen HJ, et al: Multimodal analgesic treatment in video-assisted thoracic surgery lobectomy using an

intraoperative intercostal catheter. Eur J Cardiothorac Surg 2012;41: 1072–1077.

88. Borgeat A, Ekatodramis G, Kalberer F, Benz C: Acute and nonacute complications associated with interscalene block and shoulder surgery:a prospective study. Anesthesiology 2001;95:875–880.

89. Cook LB: Unsuspected extradural catheterization in an interscalene block. Br J Anaesth 1991;67:473–475.

90. Mahoudeau G, Gaertner E, Launoy A, et al: [Interscalenic block: accidental catheterization of the epidural space.] Ann Fr Anesth Reanim 1995;14:438–441.

91. Faust A, Fournier R, Hagon O, et al: Partial sensory and motor deficit of ipsilateral lower limb after continuous interscalene brachial plexus block. Anesth Analg 2006;102:288–290.

92. Litz RJ, Vicent O, Wiessner D, Heller AR: Misplacement of a psoas compartment catheter in the subarachnoid space. Reg Anesth Pain Med 2004;29:60–64.

93. Pousman RM, Mansoor Z, Sciard D: Total spinal anesthetic after continuous posterior lumbar plexus block. Anesthesiology 2003;98: 1281–1282.

94. Lekhak B, Bartley C, Conacher ID, Nouraei SM: Total spinal anaesthesia in association with insertion of a paravertebral catheter. Br.J Anaesth. 2001;86:280–282.

95. Rodriguez J, Taboada M, Blanco M, et al: Intraneural catheterization of the sciatic nerve in humans: a pilot study. Reg Anesth Pain Med 2008;33:285–290.

96. Neuburger M, Breitbarth J, Reisig F, et al: [Complications and adverse events in continuous peripheral regional anesthesia Results of investigations on 3,491 catheters.] Anaesthesist 2006;55:33–40.

97. Marhofer D, Marhofer P, Triffterer L, et al: Dislocation of perineural catheters: a volunteer study. Br J Anaeth 2013;111(5):800–8006.

98. Horlocker TT, Wedel DJ, Rowlingson JC, et al: Regional anesthesia in the patient receiving antithrombotic or thrombolytic therapy. In *American Society of Regional Anesthesia and Pain Medicine Evidence-Based Guidelines*, 3rd ed. Reg Anesth Pain Med 2010;35:64–101.

99. Sardesai AM, Chakrabarti AJ, Denny NM: Lower lobe collapse during continuous interscalene brachial plexus local anesthesia at home. Reg Anesth Pain Med 2004;29:65 68.

100. Ilfeld BM, Duke KB, Donohue MC: The association between lower extremity continuous peripheral nerve blocks and patient falls after knee and hip arthroplasty. Anesth Analg 2010;111:1552–1554.

Organization of an Acute Pain Management Service Incorporating Regional Anesthesia Techniques

Amanda Lukof, Eugene R. Viscusi, Leslie Schechter, Suzanne Lenart, Kathleen Colfer, and Thomas Witkowski

INTRODUCTION

Acute pain management is constantly evolving, especially in recent years. In the past, acute pain management consisted primarily of opioids given intermittently by intramuscular injection. In addition to pain on injection, this led to undesirable "analgesic gaps," or periods of inadequate pain control between peak and trough opioid levels. Consequently, patients were often reluctant to request pain medications that were ordered "as needed."

To provide more consistent analgesia, intravenous patient-controlled analgesia (IV-PCA) was introduced in the 1980s, leading to the development of specialized pain management teams, most often under the direction of anesthesiologists. The additional advancement intrathecal opioids and epidural analgesia for postoperative pain management heralded the first pain service in the United States.[1] In Europe, Narinder Rawal promoted the role of nurses as valued members of the acute pain management team.[2] By the early 1990s, 40% of US hospitals had acute pain services.[3]

In recent years, regional anesthesia has gained popularity because if its contribution to postoperative pain management. Single-injection and continuous peripheral neural blockade are increasingly practiced in both the inpatient and outpatient settings. This provides another key component of multimodal therapy, in which pain is targeted with a variety of techniques and medication classes.[4] However, effective application of these techniques requires adequate expertise, surveillance, and organization.

A dedicated acute pain management team is the pivotal component in managing these procedures and techniques to optimize pain control. The primary goals of the team are to offer a wide variety of services, provide a high level of patient surveillance, and integrate these services into the overall hospital setting. Optimal analgesia requires judicious dose adjustments to maximize the benefits and minimize the side effects of therapy. This can only occur if the patient is adequately monitored.

The American Society of Anesthesiologists (ASA) Task Force first established practice guidelines for acute pain management in 1995.[5] The most recent revision was in 2012; please refer to this document for details.[6] The Joint Commission on Accreditation of Healthcare Organizations (JCAHO) established standards (Table 72–1) for pain management in January 2001 that are still practiced today.[7] These standards provided an impetus for hospitals to have an institutionwide commitment for policies and procedures to support effective pain management. This effort promoted the concept of pain as the "fifth vital sign" and established the patient's right to pain management. It also became evident that an effective pain management program can only be achieved with a strong institutional commitment. The revised ASA guidelines of 2012 highlighted the importance of multidisciplinary collaboration among anesthesiologists, surgeons, nurses, pharmacists, and other members of the healthcare team.

The purpose of this chapter is to provide strategies for effective postoperative pain management while enhancing safety and facilitating delivery of services. An organizational model for

TABLE 72–1. Key points from JCAHO pain management standards.

- Patient has a right to pain management.
- Pain must be assessed at regular intervals. Pain should be reassessed soon following an intervention to treat pain to ensure a response.
- Institutions are required to have policies and procedures for pain assessment and treatment.
- Patient education for pain management is mandated.
- Staff education concerning pain management is required.
- Pain assessments are required as a discharge criteria.

JCAHO, Joint Commission on Accreditation of Healthcare Organizations.

TABLE 72–2. Pasero opioid-induced sedation score.

S = **Sleeping, easy to arouse**
  Acceptable; no action necessary; may increase opioid dose if needed.
1 = **Awake and alert**
  Acceptable; no action necessary; may increase opioid dose if needed.
2 = **Slightly drowsy, easily aroused**
  Acceptable; no action necessary; may increase opioid dose if needed.
3 = **Frequently drowsy, arousable, drifts off to sleep during conversation**
  Unacceptable; monitor respiratory status and sedation level closely until sedation level is stable at less than 3 and respiratory status is satisfactory; decrease opioid dose 25%–50% (1) or notify prescriber (2) or anesthesiologist for orders; consider administering a nonsedating, opioid-sparing nonopioid, such as acetaminophen or an NSAID, if not contraindicated.
4 = **Somnolent, minimal or no response to verbal and physical stimulation**
  Unacceptable, stop opioid; consider administering naloxone[3,4]; notify prescriber or anesthesiologist; monitor respiratory status and sedation level closely until sedation level is stable at less than 3 and respiratory status is satisfactory.

NSAID, nonsteroidal anti-inflammatory drug.

a nursing-based acute pain service is presented. Standard orders and protocols are also provided to facilitate implementation of the suggested principles and approaches. Finally, we provide many of the organizational tools and concepts we have found useful in the organizational design of our acute pain service.

ROLE IN PATIENT SAFETY

The acute pain management team should focus not only on effective pain management, but delivery in the safest way possible. Many advisory organizations have released guidelines on the safe use of opioids. In 2012, the Joint Commission released their Sentinel Event Alert #49: *Safe Use of Opioids in Hospitals*.[8] The Joint Commission's Sentinel Events are a review and recommendations on unexpected occurrences that result in death or serious injury in medical settings in the United States.

In the case of Sentinel Event #49, the unexpected occurrences were adverse events caused by opioid administration. In their review, 47% of these events were associated with the erroneous dose of opioid being administered; this can be from human error in ordering or dosing, or a lack of adequate knowledge regarding the medications. Interestingly, 29% were due to inadequate monitoring. There were a variety of suggestions made to reduce these events with the strongest focus on development of policies and procedures regarding use of opioids, and having a group of practitioners with appropriate training not only to use opioids safely, but troubleshoot when problems do arise. They also encourage use of nonnarcotics either with or even before opioids to decrease side effects. All of these recommendations can be met by the implementation of an acute pain management team.

Adverse events related to opioids often occur in a "high-risk" patient. Acute Pain Management Service (APMS) teams can identify these patients, particularly those who are opioid tolerant, and implement individualized strategies that go beyond dose escalation (see below section on opioid tolerance). Multimodal therapy can be used not only for patient comfort, but to increase safety as well.[9] Many of the recommendations are in widespread use already, such as the avoidance of arbitrary pain ratings in favor of standardized tools such as Posero Opioid-Induced Sedation Score (POSS) scoring (Table 72–2).[10]

INTRAVENOUS PATIENT-CONTROLLED ANALGESIA

IV-PCA is commonly used as part of a multimodal approach to postoperative pain control. Sechzer[11] and Forrest[12] popularized the concept of PCA. Patients self-administer small doses of intravenous opioid at predetermined intervals (lockout), to maintain a minimum effective analgesic concentration (MEAC). This titration of the opioid provides a more constant plasma level of analgesic[13] and more consistent analgesia.[14] Maintaining opioid plasma levels within a tight range improves analgesia while reducing unwanted side effects that can occur with larger boluses. PCA pumps can be programmed to deliver opioids either by intermittent patient-controlled bolus doses alone or with a continuous background (or basal) infusion. PCA pumps are programmed to set the demand dose, lockout interval, hourly total dose, and basal infusion. Importantly, before starting PCA, analgesia must be established with an initial loading dose of opioid.[15] Without front loading, MEAC is not achieved for at least three elimination half-lives.[16] PCA is intended to *maintain* a level of pain control, not to initiate satisfactory analgesia. Therefore, if the PCA process is interrupted by pump failure, a faulty intravenous line, or inadequate patient dosing, the patient will require bolus titration to achieve comfort before reinitiating PCA. PCA advantages over intermittent injections include fewer analgesic gaps, maintaining analgesia with less total opioid consumption (thus with fewer side effects), less use of nursing staff time, and improved patient satisfaction. Patients can anticipate and proactively manage their pain, particularly before moving or coughing. There is also a psychologic advantage because of the shortened interval between perception of pain and administration of medication.

Clinical Pearl

- PCA advantages over intermittent injections include fewer analgesic gaps, maintenance of analgesia with less total opioid comsumption, fewer side effects, less use of nursing time, and greater patient satisfaction.

In the opioid-naïve patient, the addition of a basal infusion to IV-PCA has been shown not to improve analgesia, but increases the risks of this technique.[17] Without a basal infusion, the risk of clinically significant respiratory depression is generally low. Patients maintain normal levels of arterial CO_2 in the early postoperative period while receiving PCA therapy. Postoperative respiratory functions (forced expiratory volume, functional residual capacity, and peak flow rates) are not significantly different from those in patients receiving intramuscular injections of opioids.[18,19] Basal infusions are not recommended except in a very limited subset of patients. Studies have demonstrated they have a higher risk of respiratory depression and may not provide any improvement in pain scores.[20] The most common problem associated with IV-PCA use is operator error, the most common cause of which is programming error and incorrect drug concentration.[21] When a medication error involves a PCA pump, the risk of patient harm increases 3.5 times.[22] The Food and Drug Administration's (FDA's) Manufacturer and User Facility Device Experience (MAUDE) Database for 2004 identified 21 deaths involving IV-PCA pumps; 16 deaths were related to large-volume infusion pumps (LVPs). Given that there are approximately 10 times as many LVPs as PCA pumps, it appears that the risk of a severe respiratory event from a PCA pump is at least 10 times greater than with an LVP.[23] To avoid these errors, the nursing staff must understand the basis for therapy and be knowledgeable about the operational aspects of PCA pumps. Patient-related PCA problems include failure to understand PCA therapy, intentional analgesic abuse, underutilization because of unwarranted fears of addiction, and PCA by proxy (operation by an individual other than the patient). Patients should be educated about PCA before surgery; the education should be frequently reinforced throughout treatment.

Clinical Pearl

- The addition of a basal infusion to PCA increases the risk of respiratory depression without the benefit of improving analgesia. Without a basal infusion, the risk of clinically significant respiratory depression is low.

Morphine is the most commonly used PCA opioid. Hydromorphone and fentanyl are also favored because of their favorable metabolite profile. Meperidine has little place as an analgesic because of its neurotoxic metabolite, normeperidine. Table 72–3 summarizes the commonly used IV-PCA equianalgesic opioid solutions.

When converting the equivalent dose of opioids, calculated dose should be considered as an approximation because of incomplete cross tolerance. Patient responses may vary when converting from one opioid to another. Similar rules apply when converting the IV opioid therapy to the oral opioid analgesic therapy. Clinicians must have a thorough understanding of equianalgesic opioid doses. However, they must also appreciate that these dose conversions are simply guidelines and can vary patient to patient. There should be room to titrate in safe conversions.

Clinical Pearl

- Before starting PCA, analgesia must be established with loading doses of opioid.

Safe and effective use of PCA requires institutionwide protocols and standard orders. These protocols allow primary floor nursing and medical staff to utilize these systems without constant direct supervision from the acute pain management team.

There are a number of nonintravenous PCA alternatives. An iontophoretic, transdermal drug-delivery system (ITS) has demonstrated the ability to provide needle-free patient-controlled delivery of fentanyl. This patient-controlled transdermal analgesia (PCTA) system is a preprogrammed and self-contained

TABLE 72–3. Common IV-PCA equianalgesic opioid solutions.

	Concentration (mg/mL)	Dose (mL)[a]	Lockout Interval (min)	Max Hourly Dose (mL)
Morphine sulfate	1	1–2	6	10–20
Hydromorphone (Dilaudid)	0.2	0.5–2	6–8	8–10
Fentanyl (Sublimaze)	0.01–0.02	1–2	6	10–20

Abbreviation: IV-PCA, intravenous patient-controlled analgesia

[a]Intended for opioid-naïve patients.

device about the size of a credit card. Clinical trials have demonstrated analgesic efficacy similar to that from standard morphine IV-PCA.[24]

Another form of PCA currently under evaluation by the FDA is the Sufentanil NanoTab. This is a noninvasive, sublingual delivery of sufentanil using new PCA technology that may become an option in the United States in the future. Thus far, clinical trials have demonstrated safety and efficacy of this system.[25]

PERIPHERAL NERVE BLOCKS

Peripheral nerve blocks are useful in providing surgical anesthesia and postoperative analgesia[26] with an acceptable side-effect profile.[26,27] Single-injection techniques are limited in duration but can be extremely useful in the immediate postoperative period. Continuous catheter techniques can extend the duration of analgesia to the desired length of time. There are commercially available catheter insertion kits and drug-delivery systems that are small, portable, lightweight, and frequently disposable. There is a large variety of commercially available PCA pumps with different characteristics.[28] The introduction of these lightweight, portable infusion pumps has made home infusion possible, and it has been shown to be effective in randomized, double-blind, placebo-controlled studies.[29–31]

Numerous approaches have been described to the lumbar, sacral, and brachial plexuses and in the paravertebral space. The planned surgical procedure will determine the peripheral nerve block needed for postoperative analgesia. The reader should refer to the respective chapters on individual nerve block techniques for in-depth discussion on indications and technical aspects of their use. In general, the peripheral nerve block techniques are indicated in patients expected to have moderate-to-severe postoperative pain that is not easily controlled with opioids or when opioid side effects are problematic.

Possible modes of local anesthetic infusion through these catheters include intermittent bolus, continuous infusion, or continuous infusion with PCA boluses. Infusion mode is often a matter of clinician preference. Continuous infusions and continuous infusion with PCA have been shown to be superior to the intermittent bolus technique.[32] Successful use of infusions requires a solid infrastructure consisting of anesthesiologists with additional training in regional techniques who can provide coverage around the clock, supportive surgeons, pharmacists familiar with local anesthetic dosing, and specially trained nurses who can manage catheters and educate patients. There must also be an institutional commitment to provide these services and organizational tools to implement them including standardized procedure note, order sets, and documentation records. Recommendations for local anesthetic injection volume and catheter infusion rates are provided in the respective chapters. The reader should note that the suggested doses, volumes, concentrations, and infusion rates are only general guidelines and must be adjusted for individual patients. More in-depth discussion on these variables can be found in Chapters 10 (Local Anesthetic Solutions for Continuous Nerve Blocks) and 71 (Continuous Peripheral Nerve Blocks in Outpatients).

In an ambulatory setting, patient selection is critical when considering continuous infusion techniques. Only patients who are capable of accepting the additional responsibility of the catheter and infusion pump should be selected. Since some degree of cognitive dysfunction may occur in the early postoperative period, patients will benefit from a caregiver at home for the first 24–48 hours who can participate in patient care. To decrease the risk of local anesthetic toxicity, patients with hepatic or renal insufficiency should not be sent home with continuous catheters if they do not have a caregiver at home. Hence, patients without a caregiver, with baseline cognitive difficulties, with certain underlying medical problems, or patients living a distance from the medical facility may be poor candidates for ambulatory infusion techniques.

The successful use of peripheral catheters in the ambulatory setting requires patient education that should start in the preoperative area and extend into the postoperative period. Both patients and their caregivers must be involved. Instructions should be both verbal and written and include pager numbers and telephone numbers of responsible healthcare providers who will be available around the clock if problems occur. Although the surgeon is responsible for the overall care of the patient, the anesthesiologist providing the continuous regional technique must be responsible and available for catheter-related problems.

Key elements of patient instructions include:

- Protect the operative limb for the duration of the block.
- Keep the catheter site clean and dry.
- Do not operate machinery or drive a vehicle for the duration of the block.
- Approximate duration/resolution of the surgical block.
- Use of supplemental oral analgesics/opioids.
- Portable pump instructions.
- When and how to remove the catheter.
- Look for signs of catheter/local anesthetic infusion complications.
- Observe catheter site for swelling, tenderness, and drainage.

Clinical Pearl

- Successful use of peripheral catheters in the ambulatory setting requires thorough patient education, including written and verbal instructions.

Careful follow-up is necessary with any continuous catheter technique. Visiting nurses may be helpful. Patients may benefit from daily telephone contact with specific questions about quality of analgesia, local anesthetic side effects, and possible catheter site infection. Documentation of these patient contacts should be made. Patients may remove their peripheral infusion catheters at home, may return to the medical facility to have them removed, or a visiting nurse may remove the catheter. This may depend on the patients' abilities, the distance they must travel from the hospital, and their degree of mobility. In the ambulatory setting, disposable elastomeric pumps are utilized. With proper selection and education of patients, the incidence of injury to the blocked limb is very low.[33]

Complications of Continuous Catheter Techniques

1. Local anesthetic toxicity is a potential complication that can occur when large volumes or high concentrations of local anesthetics are used. Intravascular placement of catheters can be detected with epinephrine-containing local anesthetic test doses. Low concentrations of a long-acting local anesthetic with an acceptable safety profile are advisable. Ropivacaine, in 2 mg/mL concentration, infused in a continuous interscalene (brachial plexus) catheter at 6–9 mL/h has demonstrated safety.[34, 35]

2. Patients should be instructed to look for signs of local infection at the catheter site, local tenderness, redness, and fever. These should be immediately reported to the healthcare providers. Even though infection at catheter sites is uncommon, one study reported 57% of femoral catheters showed bacterial colonization at 48 h.[36]

3. Although a rare occurrence, catheter migration must always be considered. Catheter failure is the most common sign of migration. Since the actual location of the local anesthetic infusion cannot be determined, failed catheters should always be removed promptly. Catheters may migrate into the intravascular compartment. Patients should be provided with a list of signs of intravascular infusion of local anesthetics: tinnitus, metallic taste in the mouth, and anxiety. Intramuscular migration of the catheter will result in either a decrease or complete cessation of analgesia. The infusion should be stopped since there is a theoretic risk of myositis.[37]

4. Careful dressing of the catheter site and use of surgical tape can reduce catheter dislodgment. Clear dressings are advantageous since they permit visualization of the insertion site. Commercially available skin preparations (similar to ostomy site skin preparations) may increase adhesion while reducing skin breakdown. Adhesive surgical strips may be beneficial in regions that are difficult to secure. Catheters can also be secured by suturing or tunneling. This may be helpful for longer term placement.

5. Many varieties of infusion pumps are available for either continuous infusion or patient-controlled boluses. Use of LVPs (250–400 mL) will provide longer periods of analgesia. However, larger volumes of local anesthetic may increase the risk of systemic toxicity.

MULTIMODAL APPROACH TO ACUTE PAIN MANAGEMENT

Multimodal analgesia produces optimal pain relief by targeting pain at multiple pathways.[38] Combining analgesic techniques and drugs has a synergistic or additive effect and decreases the requirement for individual medication, thereby reducing the incidence of side effects.[39] One of the strongest recommendations from the revised 2012 ASA guidelines on acute pain was for

providers to use at least two nonopioid therapies around the clock for baseline pain. Opioids should be employed as rescue therapy in this management plan.

Clinical Pearl

- All patients should be approached with a suitable multimodal analgesia regimen. Opioids should not be used as the sole agent.

The surgical stress response produces endocrine and metabolic responses in the body. These pathways can be targeted pharmacologically at specific levels by adopting a multimodal approach to pain control.[40] The focus of the multimodal approach to acute postoperative pain management is to facilitate the patient's rehabilitation. Multimodal approaches combined with accelerated recovery protocols can reduce length of hospital stay.[41] This has been shown to work when the surgical team, anesthesiologists, nurses, and patients work together within established clinical pathways.[42]

Chronic pain has been identified as a consequence of surgery and poorly controlled acute pain.[43] Multimodal techniques may reduce central sensitization, improve pain control, and ultimately reduce long-term sequelae. Local anesthetics and regional anesthesia techniques are critical components of multimodal analgesia. These methods reduce the need for systemic pain medications and allow patients to get out of bed sooner, which decreases hospital stay and hastens recovery.

Ketamine, an N-methyl-D-aspartate (NMDA) receptor antagonist, when used in small doses (0.5–0.15 mg/kg IV) has been shown to improve pain relief if administered with opioids intravenously or epidurally.[44,45] This is discussed in further detail later in the chapter in the section on opioid tolerance.

With appropriate patient selection, nonsteroidal anti-inflammatory drugs (NSAIDs) can be very effective in multimodal pain plans. However, in some patients and situations NSAIDs can exert an antiplatelet effect that can cause surgical bleeding. They may also cause renal dysfunction. NSAIDs have an opioid-sparing effect[46] and can be administered orally or parentally. Cyclooxygenase-2 (COX-2) inhibitors, such as celecoxib, do not have an antiplatelet effect, making them desirable for postoperative pain management. Concern for cardiovascular problems has led to the withdrawal of other COX-2 inhibitors from the market. However, this risk is associated with duration of use longer than is indicated for most acute pain situations.

Acetaminophen is also used commonly in the multimodal scheme. It is particularly effective in conjunction with opioids. Dosed appropriately, it is equally effective both orally and intravenously (both 1000 mg q6h) to improve pain scores and lessen opioid requirements.[47] IV acetaminophen is preferred when the patient is unable to take medications by mouth, as during the immediate preoperative or postoperative period. This was approved for use in the United States in 2010.

Neuropathic pain is often the most difficult pain to control, particularly since the drugs previously mentioned do not target this pain pathway as effectively. Gabapentin, a gamma-amino-butyric acid (GABA) analogue that was developed originally as an antiseizure medication, has been found to be effective to help treat this pain type. Pregabalin, another medication for this modality, has a higher bioavailability than gabapentin, making it more useful in the acute pain setting as patients can get an effect with lower doses. This helps keep side effects, most notably sedation, at a minimum. Both medications also can decrease narcotic use in the postoperative period.[48] These are the most commonly used antiepileptics for pain control, although others are available and may be used in certain patient populations.

CONTINUOUS EPIDURAL ANALGESIA

Use of continuous epidural infusions of local anesthetic with or without opioids has become a cornerstone of multimodal analgesia.[49] The use of dilute local anesthetic solutions has been shown to decrease the incidence of deep venous thrombosis in the postoperative period.[50] It is an effective weapon in attenuating the endocrine metabolic response to surgical stress and to provide dynamic pain relief.[51] The epidural catheter must be functional and cover the dermatomal distribution of the surgical incision to be effective. Epidural catheters are best inserted at the mid-dermatome of anticipated surgical trauma. Care must also be taken to advance between 3 and 5 cm of epidural catheter into the epidural space. A shallower insertion results in greater incidence of catheter dislodgement, whereas an excessive length of catheter reduces efficacy and increases risk of catheter knotting. The routinely used nylon epidural catheters are difficult to direct in the epidural space, regardless of the direction of the epidural needle bevel. Hence, it is best to target a short length of catheter at the precise spinal cord level to cover surgical pain.

Clinical Pearl

- Use of continuous epidural infusions of local anesthetic with or without opioids is a cornerstone of multimodal analgesia.

In a meta-analysis comparing epidural analgesia with parenteral opioids, epidural analgesia was found to provide more effective pain control.[52] Epidural opioids or local anesthetics either alone or in combination demonstrated superiority. Hence, when surgical pain is of high intensity and likely to last at least 48 hours, epidural analgesia deserves consideration. Side effects of epidural analgesia include motor block, nausea and vomiting, pruritus, urinary retention, sedation, and respiratory depression. Epidural catheters in the presence of anticoagulation may increase the risk of epidural hematoma. The American Society of Regional Anesthesia & Pain Medicine (ASRA) has established specific guidelines for neuraxial anesthetic techniques in the presence of anticoagulants that is important for all members of an acute pain team to know and understand.[53]

A number of other agents have demonstrated analgesic efficacy when administered by the epidural route either alone or in combination with other agents. These agents include anticholinergic agents, NMDA receptor antagonists (e.g., ketamine) and α_2-adrenergic agonists. Epidural epinephrine, clonidine,[54]

and dexmedetomidine[55] have demonstrated analgesic efficacy. However, these agents are seldom used, perhaps due to varied side effects.

Clinical Pearls

- Check coagulation status before placement and removal of epidural catheters.
- Insert epidural needle at mid-dermatome of surgical trauma.
- Obtain an anesthetic level and ensure epidural is functioning BEFORE surgery.
- If breakthrough pain, always establish a level before dosing. This can be determined with ice (cold sensation).

A standard epidural order form and an epidural procedure note (both seen in Figures 72–1 and 72–2) enhance documentation and reduce medication errors. Commonly used solutions for epidural infusion and rates of administration are detailed in Tables 72–4 and 72–5.

Infiltration With Local Anesthetics

Infiltrating the operative site with local anesthetic is a simple way to enhance pain control.[56] Local anesthetics can be injected or infused into joint spaces, surgical wounds, or in the vicinity of nerves near the surgical site. Local anesthetics are relatively inexpensive and remain the most useful and safe component of multimodal analgesia. With introduction of delayed-release local anesthetic on the market, the utility of infiltration has substantially increased along with the increased duration of analgesic action.

Acute Pain in the Patient With Chronic Pain

Patients with chronic pain present special challenges in the perioperative period. Their pain is typically poorly controlled by the routine administration of opioids alone. It is critical that such patients are identified in the preoperative period and an analgesia plan established before surgery[57] to avoid unnecessary prolonged periods of severe uncontrolled postoperative pain. Evidence from the literature supports that the opioid requirement in these patients can be much higher than in opioid-naïve patients.[58] These patients may present with a history of chronic opioid use, often at high doses and perhaps in conjunction with a variety of other pain medications. Following identification, these patients require careful assessment in the preoperative phase to fully describe the nature of their chronic pain, to quantify opioid requirements, and to document all current medications. Then, an analgesic plan must be formulated with the patient as an active participant.[59] Table 72–6 details practical approach to postoperative pain management in the patient with history of chronic pain.

Opioid-Tolerant Patients

Opioid-tolerant patients may include patients with chronic pain,[60] active opioid abusers, or former addicts enrolled in

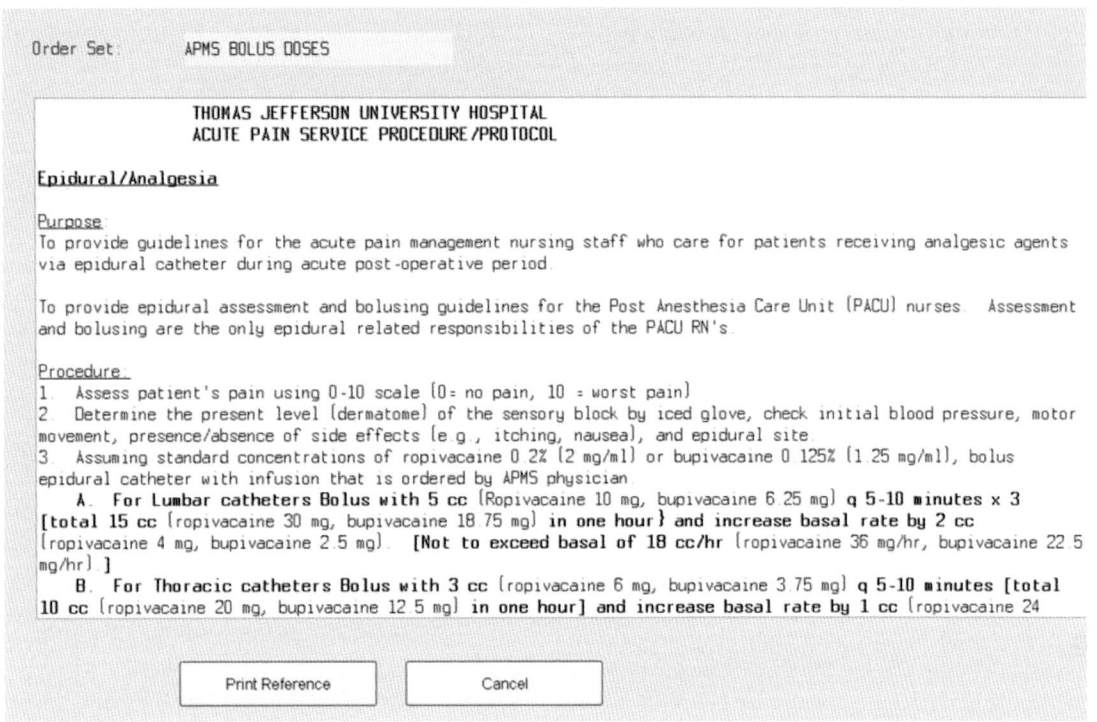

FIGURE 72–1. A standard epidural order form.

long-term methadone maintenance programs. All of these patients have a high tolerance to the antinociceptive effects of opioids,[61] are pain-intolerant,[62] and can have opioid-induced hyperalgesia.[63]

It is important to identify these patients in the preoperative period and establish a sound pain management strategy before surgery. In the postoperative period these patients will often require more than twice their stable opioid dose. This rapid increase in opioid requirement has been termed *acute tolerance.* Patients should receive their daily maintenance opioid dose on the morning of surgery. Even if regional anesthesia techniques are used, these patients must receive their minimum opioid requirement to prevent opioid withdrawal symptoms. In the immediate postoperative period, consider higher than routine

```
Order Set:      APMS BOLUS DOSES

     B.  For Thoracic catheters Bolus with 3 cc [ropivacaine 6 mg, bupivacaine 3.75 mg] q 5-10 minutes [total
10 cc [ropivacaine 20 mg, bupivacaine 12.5 mg] in one hour] and increase basal rate by 1 cc [ropivacaine 24
mg/hr, bupivacaine 15 mg/hr].]
     C.  It is necessary to check the patient's vital signs every 5 minutes for a 15-minute period after bolusing.
4   Document therapy and outcome on epidural/PCA flow sheet. When an epidural bolus is administered the following
information is recorded on the epidural/PCA flow sheet.
     a.  Date/Time
     b.  Medication [dose and concentration]
     c.  Physical assessment findings [HR, BP, RR] q 5 minutes x 3
     d.  Initials of individual performing patient assessment
     e.  Patient response to therapy should be documented on flow sheets [post bolus pain score]
5   When no pain relief is achieved after 2 boluses:
     A.  Check site for fluids and kinks in epidural tubing
     B.  Offer comfort measures
     C.  check connections
     D.  Check patient positioning. passive motion device may need to stop temporarily until patient's pain is
controlled.
6   For Hypotension:
     A.  Have floor RN call primary service to address fluid status
     B.  May need to decrease rate of epidural drip or shut drip off until fluid status is addressed
     C.  If patient has significant side effects of epidural opioid [nausea, vomiting, pruritus, sedation], may
discontinue opioid in epidural infusion.


                        Print Reference              Cancel
```

FIGURE 72–2. An epidural procedure note.

TABLE 72–4. Common epidural analgesia LA solutions.

Lower extremity (Lumbar Catheters)
- Ropivacaine 0.2%/morphine 0.025 mg/mL
- Ropivacaine 0.15%/morphine 0.025 mg/mL
- Ropivacaine 0.2% (plus patient-controlled analgesia)

Thoracic/Abdominal Surgery (Thoracic Catheters)
- Bupivacaine 0.125%/morphine 0.05 mg/mL
- Bupivacaine 0.125%/morphine 0.025 mg/mL

Labor and Delivery (Lumbar Catheters)
- Bupivacaine 0.1%/fentanyl 1.5 mcg/mL

doses of IV-PCA with morphine or hydromorphone. Hydromorphone and sufentanil are regarded as higher efficacy opioids and may be more helpful in opioid-tolerant patients.

Regional analgesia with local anesthetic and systemic opioid is a more efficient way of providing pain control than parenteral opioids alone. Use of an opioids with high intrinsic efficacy, such as sufentanil, is more effective[64] in the setting of opioid receptor downregulation.[65] These patients may benefit from the regional anesthesia, epidural, or parenteral opioids for a longer period of time than opioid-naïve patients.

Clinical Pearls

- Regional anesthesia with local anesthetic and systemic opioid is a particularly efficient tool in opioid-tolerant patient.
- Opioid with high intrinsic efficacy, such as sufentanil, is more effective.
- Before and after hospital discharge, referral to a pain specialist can be helpful in optimizing management and facilitate dose tapering.

In the postoperative period, converting opioid-tolerant patients to oral opioids can be quite challenging. One approach is to calculate the patient's 24-hour opioid requirement from IV-PCA and give two thirds that amount in the form of a long-acting oral opioid and one third in the form of a short-acting oral opioid to be used as needed. Baseline opioid doses should be tapered slowly to prevent withdrawal. Addition of other adjuncts such as α_2-adrenergic receptor agonists like clonidine, dexmedetomidine, NMDA receptor antagonists, and COX-2 inhibitors all help to decrease opioid need and improve analgesia. Tricyclic antidepressants may help with neuropathic pain, although these agents usually require several weeks to achieve efficacy. Membrane-stabilizing agents (e.g., gabapentin) can be

TABLE 72–5. Recommended epidural infusion rate.

Thoracic catheter: 3–6 mL/h

Lumbar catheter: 6–10 mL/h

TABLE 72–6. Management of acute pain in the patient with chronic pain.

Preoperative Phase
1. Identify the patient with chronic pain preoperatively.
2. Assure the patient that pain control is a priority.
3. Evaluate the location and character of chronic pain.
4. Accurately determine the preoperative opioid requirement and identify all other pain medications.
5. Formulate a multimodal analgesic plan (as part of the anesthetic plan) that incorporates the patient's preferences and cooperation.
6. Communicate this plan to the primary anesthesia team and surgeon.

Operative Phase
1. Ensure that patient has received morning doses of opioids and other pain medications and adequate preoperative sedation.
2. Communicate with members of the surgical team the specific considerations for this patient.
3. Incorporate a multimodal approach to the anesthetic (preoperative NSAID or COX-2 inhibitor, possible dose of membrane-stabilizing agents, local anesthetics wherever practical, adequate intraoperative doses of opioids).
4. Ensure that patient is reasonably comfortable before leaving the operating room.

Postoperative Phase
1. Inform recovery room nurse of plan and ensure that patient is comfortable prior to discharge from recovery room.
2. Inform floor staff nurse of plan and provide individual or service to contact for pain issues.
3. Maintain patient's routine pain medications throughout the perioperative period.
4. Consider acute pain plan as an "overlay" on the patient's chronic pain management.
5. Initiate oral therapy as soon as is practical.
6. Utilize extended-release oral opioids to reduce the analgesic "gap" between doses of short- acting opioids.
7. Evaluate patient daily and adjust plan as needed.
8. Pain medication requirements may change drastically during the weeks following discharge, so plan early for outpatient pain management.

Abbreviations: COX-2, cyclooxygenase-2; NSAID, nonsteroidal anti-inflammatory drug.

very helpful during the perioperative period in the presence of neurogenic or neuropathic pain. Routine doses of these agents should be continued.

Ketamine is being used more frequently in recent years to help treat opioid-tolerant patients both intraoperatively and postoperatively. Ketamine has been used for decades but fell out of favor for a time due to its psychotropic side effects. These include vivid dreams, hallucinations, confusion, and an out-of-body sensation. At high doses, ketamine causes a dissociative anesthetic state. Lower doses (a continuous infusion of up to 1 mg/kg/min) can be used to effectively treat pain in the opioid -tolerant population. The side effects at these doses are minimal and can be improved with benzodiazepines. Where available (Europe), the racemic ketamine (S) can be used to minimize the psychotropic side-effects. Ketamine is effective both in the perioperative period and also in select groups of nonoperative patients, such as those with cancer or sickle-cell disease.[66,67] These nonoperative patients are often on very high doses of opioids and develop remarkable tolerance to those medications.

Many institutions, including our own, have restricted the titration and management of ketamine to the Acute Pain Management Service. Because this drug is an anesthetic, only trained anesthesia providers should manage it. This management should be driven by an APMS-developed protocol.

Regardless of the inpatient therapy selected, referral to a pain specialist can be very helpful in treating the opioid-dependent patient to help optimize pain management during rehabilitation and facilitate opioid dose tapering. Whenever possible, the pain specialist familiar with the patient's history should be involved in the postdischarge pain management. This is best accomplished when the visit occurs prior to surgery or hospitalization to formulate a clear plan. With patients chronically treated with opioids, patients may be better served by having a single opioid prescriber.

Clinical Pearl

- Converting opioid-tolerant patients to oral opioids can be challenging. One approach is to calculate the patients 24-hour requirement from IV-PCA and give two thirds that amount as long-acting medication and one third as short-acting medication as needed.

ACUTE PAIN MANAGEMENT FROM A NURSING PERSPECTIVE

Nurses are a key component of an acute pain service. The pain nursing team may be composed of acute pain management nurses, pain resource nurses, and floor nurses. Acute pain management nurses are dedicated to promoting and providing care for patients in pain. In most settings, acute pain nurses work in collaboration with the department of anesthesiology. Acute pain management nurses operate best within an established framework of hospital-approved protocols and guidelines and through decision trees. Guidelines and protocols are intended to establish the basic standard of care and provide consistency in management.[68] Protocols prescribe methods of care in a less flexible way then guidelines,[69] but neither is a substitute for personal knowledge. Thoughtful application is essential if guidelines and protocols are to be safe and effective.

A nurse-driven acute pain service consists of a physician director and the nursing team. The physician determines the appropriate analgesic technique. The care team, consisting of

an attending physician, resident, and an acute pain nurse, assesses patients on morning rounds and develops a comprehensive management plan. A standard daily clinical note will facilitate documentation. The pain management plan is communicated and coordinated by the acute pain nurse to the other members of the patient care team. The pain resource nurse is a floor nurse with special training in the assessment of pain and technical expertise in the various infusion devices. Optimally, every nursing unit has a pain resource nurse to provide peer support to other floor nurses and provide basic troubleshooting and assessment. Standard documentation sheets for pain assessment, epidural, and PCA are helpful. The roles of the various team members are discribed in Table 72–7.

A very specific process is followed so that protocols can be considered, approved, and eventually become part of a standard order set. The proposed protocols are then reviewed by the pharmacy and therapeutics (P&T) committee that makes recommendations resulting from evidence-based practice. The P&T committee is a multidisciplinary group composed of physicians, pharmacists, administrators, and nurses. Standard order sets then typically require the approval of a medical executive committee. Where computer physician order entry is employed (CPOE), standard order sets must be configured to maintain all necessary order details of the protocol. Thus, physicians are able to order a protocol of decision trees that allow the acute pain nurses to follow a defined path in the management of specific pain management scenarios.

With a nurse-driven acute pain service, the pain nurse is the first to respond to calls for the patient's pain issues. Pain nurses must possess astute assessment and critical thinking skills. This requires a background in critical care or postanesthesia care. Utilizing decision trees and critical thinking, pain nurses are called on to manage pain and side effects of pain therapies, troubleshoot epidural and peripheral block catheters, titrating and bolusing as needed, and removing catheters when indicated. Pain nurses must be well trained at assessing hypotension, motor block, and excessive sedation. All actions and interventions of the pain nurse are entirely within the scope of institutional protocols.

Pain management is truly a specialty in nursing. It is recommended that pain nurses become board certified. Attaining certification confirms that the pain nurse has the necessary skills to practice safely and effectively.

Although pain management teams strive to provide an opioid-sparing multimodal pain management regimen, opioids are frequently the primary pharmacologic choice, often necessitated by the increasing numbers of opioid-tolerant patients being admitted to hospitals, as discussed above. In an effort to provide superior care, pain teams may institute plans of care that are quite complex, often including opioids in very high doses. It is for this reason that acute pain nurses must be clinically astute in their assessment and monitoring of sedation and respiratory depression in all patients who are receiving opioids.

Pain management nurses should be familiar with the American Society for Pain Management Nursing Guidelines on Monitoring for Opioid-Induced Sedation and Respiratory Depression.[70] This position paper offers recommendations

TABLE 72–7. Description of roles on an acute pain management service (APMS)[a].

Director
- Determines direction of service
- Defines and coordinates clinical, educational, and research goals
- Develops protocols and policies for pain assessment and treatment
- Reviews quality assurance indicators

Attending Staff
- Conducts daily patient rounds
- Performs and supervises regional anesthesia procedures
- Performs and supervises consultations
- Participates in education and research

Residents and Fellows
- Daily patient rounds
- Responds to APMS consults
- Performs various regional anesthesia techniques both preoperatively and postoperatively
- When "on-call": rounds with pain nurse late in the day to discuss management issues; available by pager for questions and/or consults throughout the night
- Participates in research and education

Clinical Nurse Specialist (Advanced Practice Nurse)
- Coordinator of services providing continuity of care to APMS patients
- Designs and implements educational programs for the department of nursing and patient observation
- Responsible for data collection and quality assurance activity
- Assists director in development of goals, policies, protocols, and standards

Acute Pain Nurse
- Holds service pager and responds to calls for pain-related problems
- Conducts frequent proactive assessments of analgesia and its side effects
- Adjusts pain therapy according to algorithms in coordination with residents and staff
- Employs complementary techniques (i.e., relaxation, imaging, distraction)
- Point-of-care peer support to staff nurses

[a]All members work together by staying in communication regarding all issues. Frequent discussion about specific patients, especially where therapy is actively being modified.

for analgesic pharmacotherapy, education, and monitoring. It is often the acute pain management nurses who are responsible for disseminating these evidence- based guidelines throughout their facility. This task can be accomplished by establishing hospitalwide, policies and procedures, and educational programs.

In an effort to provide effective and safe pain management, it is imperative to have in place an easy and reliable as well as valid assessment tool for opioid-induced sedation, as opposed to sedation tools that assess purposeful, goal-directed, sedation for procedures or for ventilated critical care patients. In a descriptive survey-based study the POSS (see Table 72–2) scored highest in combined measures of ease of use, nursing confidence, and usefulness of information provided to make clinical decisions. The POSS has been considered to be a superior scale and is recommended for the assessment of sedation in adult patients during opioid administration for pain management in noncritical care settings.[71] In addition, the POSS scale includes directed nursing interventions when advancing sedation is present. Again, acute pain nurses can be instrumental in having this scale added to their facility's nursing assessment tools. The addition of this tool can only facilitate better assessment and, likely, better patient outcomes.

Clinical Pearl

- Pain should always be assessed using a validated pain assessment tool.

Pain nurses are the critical link in providing education and peer support to the various members of the nursing service. Nurse-driven acute pain services function proactively, closely monitoring and anticipating problems. The visible presence of pain nurses increases patient satisfaction, improves pain control and safety, and may improve patient outcome. Busy acute pain services utilizing aggressive regional anesthesia/analgesia techniques and opioid therapies may benefit from an organizational design that places nurses in key patient management positions. A nurse-driven acute pain service integrates the treatment of these patients into the overall hospital milieu, and helps facility institutional consistency in the management of all pain issues within the facility.

PHARMACIST CONSIDERATIONS IN ACUTE PAIN MANAGEMENT

A pharmacist offers a unique perspective when establishing or expanding an acute pain service using regional anesthesia/analgesia techniques. Pharmacists have extensive training in pharmacology, pharmacokinetics, and pharmacoeconomics. In addition to the traditional role of the pharmacist in compounding and dispensing medications, a pharmacist can be a valued team member who provides clinical services in the areas of safe, rationale, and cost-effective drug therapy. Pharmacists may provide patient education and instruction, drug information, and alternative therapy options. Pharmacists may also be included in quality assurance data collection, proper pump selection, proper medication labeling, safety considerations, and the development of policies and procedures. Pharmacists can also be involved in hospital formulary medication decisions and have an important role in evaluating new products for formulary addition.

Pharmacy Considerations With Epidural Delivery

When the technique of epidural and intrathecal administration was developed, it was standard practice to administer medication as a single bolus or multiple as-needed bolus injections. Anesthesiologists generally prepared and administered the doses. This technique, however, may result in periods of inadequate pain control and has been associated with a higher frequency of adverse effects resulting from temporary peak levels of medications creating unwanted side effects.[72] Development of protocols for initial bolus doses followed by continuous infusions with or without patient-controlled epidural analgesia (PCEA) has revolutionized pain management. Continuous infusions of epidural opioids or local anesthetics (or both) avoid the peaks and valleys of pain control and the need for multiple bolus injections.[72–74] Studies comparing continuous infusions and intermittent bolus administration have shown that continuous administration provides better analgesia with lower total doses administered.[73]

Pharmacists should be involved in the procurement and preparation of the epidural continuous infusion solutions. The preparation of epidural infusions must follow strict aseptic techniques outlined by the standard of practice for compounding sterile preparations, published in Chapter 797 in *The United States Pharmacopeia* (USP).[75] Epidural solutions are considered a "moderate risk level" for microbial contamination based on the fact that the solution contains no preservatives. Appropriate labeling of epidural solutions is detailed in Table 72–8.

Peripheral Nerve Blocks and Catheters

Peripheral anesthetic techniques have increased in popularity for the management of acute and chronic pain conditions. Studies have shown that patients who receive peripheral nerve blocks experience reduced postoperative pain and analgesia

---

TABLE 72–8. Suggestions for appropriate epidural labeling.

1. All solution ingredients
   a. Drug names
   b. Volumes
   c. Strength
2. Final concentration
3. Total volume
4. Rate of administration (mL/h)
5. Diluent used
6. Date of preparation
7. Expiration date
8. Unique and prominent label stating "For Epidural Use Only"

---

requirements and report more satisfaction with their pain management.[76] These techniques involve either bolus or intermittent doses, or continuous infusions of local anesthetics through a catheter near or around the nerve or nerve plexus that supplies the surgical area.[77,78]

A perineural placement of catheters for continuous local anesthetic is growing in popularity.[79–81] This technique of continuous peripheral nerve blocks or perineural local anesthetic infusions involves the percutaneous insertion of a catheter directly adjacent to the peripheral nerves or plexuses supplying an affected surgical site.[82] In the hospital setting, local anesthetic infusions can be prepared by the pharmacy, and the continuous infusion can be accomplished with an infusion pump. In recent years, smaller electronic infusion pumps, syringe pumps, elastomeric pumps, and spring-powered pumps have been designed for use in the ambulatory setting. Because of the inherent risks of sending a patient home with an infusion device, most published studies limit ambulatory use of the pumps to patients expected to have moderate to severe postoperative pain of a duration of more than 24 hours and who will have difficulty managing the pain with oral opioids.[82] In addition, special consideration must be given to the caregiver's capability for managing the pump or the need for home care or visiting nurses to monitor, regulate, or discontinue the infusion.

An alternative to continuous regional blocks is continuous infusion of local anesthetic directly into the wound site.[83] A pump is attached to a catheter inserted near an incision site. The pump infuses a continuous flow of local anesthetic and may include the capability for patient control. For wound instillation devices, the local anesthetic may be added to the device in the sterile environment of the operating room or added into the device by pharmacy personnel using aseptic technique.

With the capability of infusing local anesthetics epidurally, intrathecally, peripherally, and topically, guidelines must be established for all healthcare providers to be aware of the type and route of local anesthetic administration. Unintentional administration of local anesthetic via two different routes may increase the risk for systemic toxicity. To prevent double administration, all local anesthetic administration should be documented in the patient chart. If CPOE is available, all orders should be entered into the computer. A warning screen should appear if duplicate local anesthetic orders are entered for a patient.

With the evolution of multimodal therapy, anesthesiologists and surgeons must communicate regarding all pain management therapy. In addition, pharmacists must review medication profiles and be aware of all local anesthetics dispensed and administered to patients. Pharmacists play a crucial role in monitoring the overall pharmacologic management of the patient.

Infusion Devices

Pharmacist involvement in the selection of infusion devices will offer a unique perspective on the advantages and disadvantages of various pumps. Many factors must be considered to determine the optimal device for a given clinical situation. Infusion devices should be safe, accurate, reliable, easy to use, and compatible with the drug-delivery systems available.[74] For the management of acute pain, an external pump is standard. Several external devices are available on the market, including syringe pumps, peristaltic devices, and elastomeric reservoir pumps. When selecting a pump, several factors should be considered, including the acceptable infusion rate accuracy, PCA bolus capability, and total local anesthetic volume required.

Syringe pumps are used to deliver the contents of a syringe over a given period.[74] These devices can be programmed to deliver the contents of a syringe over several hours to several days. These pumps are commonly used for the delivery of opioids for IV-PCA. Prefilled morphine and meperidine syringes are commercially available. Pharmacy personnel or pharmacy outsourced compounding companies must compound other opioids or differing concentrations of commercially available products. Most of these devices must be locked to prevent patient manipulation and to prevent diversion of a controlled substance.

Peristaltic devices deliver a drug from a flexible reservoir via administration tubing that is mechanically squeezed.[74] These pumps are traditionally used to administer intravenous fluids. Some peristaltic devices have locked chambers to secure solutions. This would be of benefit for opioid infusions. Peristaltic pumps can accommodate larger volumes of solution. Flow rate capabilities range from 0.1 to 999 mL/h. Newer pumps have more sophisticated programming, allowing for minimum and maximum rates of any drug programmed into the device. Some programs also calculate infusion rates based on the patient's weight and the amount of drug to be administered per minute or hour. This new technology was developed to help prevent potential medication errors.

Elastomeric reservoir pumps force fluid through a flow regulator via elastomeric pressure of a balloon reservoir.[74] Depending on the brand, the reservoir volume varies, allowing for varying rates and length of therapy. This technology is used for continuous delivery of local anesthetics for continuous peripheral blocks or instillation directly into the wound.

Regardless of the type of infusion pump used, the maximum reservoir volume must be considered when establishing the use of epidural solutions or continuous nerve infiltrations. In addition, the range of administration rates is a critical factor in epidural delivery of medications.[74] Epidural infusion rates vary depending on the location of the epidural catheter and the drugs administered into the epidural space. Rates greater than 20 mL/h are generally not indicated.

When choosing an infusion device, consideration should be given to devices that allow for safe and secure administration of solutions while maximizing the time between refills or the interval between bag, syringe, or cassette changes. Smart infusion technology now allows for increasingly sophisticated programming features including close error reduction software, commonly known as drug libraries.[84] This technology allows infusion pumps to perform functions that assist healthcare providers with accurate programming. However, while smart pump technology helps reduce medication error, it is not intended to replace clinical judgment. The potential for pump misidentification or confusion is ever-present, leading to medication errors or error in route of deliver. From a systems standpoint, rigorous policies are needed to prevent medication errors. This may include special labeling, route-specific tubing, and dedicated pumps for specific techniques, color-coding of labels and tubing, and two practitioner pump set-up checks. Representatives from the departments of biomedical engineering, nursing, anesthesiology, and pharmacy should all be involved in pump selection.

Solution Preparation, Stability, and Sterility

As described previously, pharmacists offer many valuable services to all areas of patient care. In regard to regional anesthesia, the most important contributions include accurate preparation and assurance of sterility and stability for all solutions prepared.

Any drug administered into the epidural or intrathecal space must be free of neurotoxic preservatives.[73,85] Agents containing preservatives such as methylparaben, benzyl alcohol, methylhydroxybenzoate, propylhydroxybenzoate, phenol, and formaldehyde must be avoided.[73,85] Standard epidural preparations guidelines call for the use of preservative-free solutions.

Although infection of the epidural or intrathecal space is rare, it can be fatal, as evidenced by the outbreak of fungal meningitis from contaminated lots of methylprednisolone acetate compounded by the New England Compounding Center, Framingham, MA. As of May 6, 2013, 741 reported cases of fungal meningitis and other fungal infections had been reported with 55 deaths in 20 states attributed to the contaminated methylprednisolone product.[86] Preparation of all epidural solutions must be performed with strict adherence to sterile aseptic technique. As of January 1, 2004, the Joint Commission officially surveys accredited organizations for compliance with the USP general Chapter 797, Pharmaceutical compounding—sterile preparations.[75] USP Chapter 797 details the procedures and requirements for compounding sterile preparations and sets standards that are applicable to all practice settings in which sterile preparations are compounded. Based on these guidelines, because epidural solutions contain no preservatives, they are considered to be a medium risk for microbial contamination. Certified pharmacy personnel using a laminar flow hood should prepare epidural, intrathecal solutions as well as solutions for continuous peripheral neural blockade.

The stability of morphine, fentanyl, hydromorphone, and fentanyl mixed with various local anesthetics in a variety of syringes and reservoirs has been studied.[87–90] Solutions studied maintained potency for at least 12 days. However, the risk of microbial contamination in preservative-free solutions is problematic. Current guidelines from the Centers for Disease Control and Prevention (CDC) recommend that preservative-free infusion solutions be completely used or discarded within 24 hours of preparation when not refrigerated.[73,91,92] CDC guidelines also recommend that preservative-free solutions be stored under refrigeration for no more than 7 days.[91] Refrigeration must be continuous and occur immediately after mixing the solution. After the product is dispensed for patient use, a 24-hour expiration date must be applied. USP Chapter 797 gives a medium risk level to preparations 30 hours at room temperature and 7 days under refrigeration.[75] According to

USP Chapter 797, if the product is not made in a laminar flow hood, it will be considered high risk and should be used within 24 hours.[75] It would be prudent for institutions administering epidural, intrathecal, and continuous peripheral local anesthetic solutions to have the solutions prepared in accordance with USP Chapter 797.

Standardization of Regional Anesthesia Continuous Solutions

Standardizing epidural solution volumes, medications used, and drug concentrations is important consideration when establishing an epidural program. Consistency in prescribing and preparing epidural, intrathecal, and continuous peripheral local anesthetic solutions helps to reduce the potential for medication errors and simplifies the preparation process.[93–95] Having a limited number of concentrations for epidural solutions will prevent medication errors in prescribing, preparing, and administering epidurals. Pharmacists should work with anesthesiologists to determine dosing ranges for epidural drugs. Pharmacists should be familiar with the dosing ranges and should question orders that deviate from established guidelines. It would be beneficial to minimize the size of the solution bag for epidurals. If the rate of an epidural is mistakenly increased, a limited amount of epidural solution would be infused at the incorrect rate.

When initially establishing standard epidural solutions, physician preference and stability considerations should be assessed.[95] Decisions regarding standard epidural preparations must also take into consideration safety, cost, time, narcotic accountability, and reservoir volume of the infusion device.[93–95] When possible, using whole rather than partial ampules and vials and using available package sizes of the drugs will help to minimize waste.[95] This is beneficial in helping to keep narcotic inventories as simple as possible. Although standard epidural solutions are usually adequate for most patients, it should be noted that these standard preparations might not be suitable for every patient. There may be instances when a patient requires a specialized preparation. The patient may have an allergy to one of the standard epidural components, or the patient may have a history of opioid tolerance and will require higher concentrations. If a nonstandard epidural is ordered, highlighting the concentrations may help to prevent confusion and errors.

Standardization of epidural solutions may allow for batch preparation. Batch preparation helps to prevent a delay in starting an epidural. In addition, depending on the infusion rate, more than one infusion bag may be needed per day. If an infusion is running dry, having batched solutions available prevents the possibility of interrupting continuous pain therapy. Batching puts less stress on pharmacy personnel preparing solutions and on nurses in a need of a new solution bag. However, maintenance of continuous pain relief therapy for the patient is the most important benefit. To provide the maximum expiration dating, certified individuals should do batch preparation of epidural solutions without preservative under strict aseptic conditions. Storage should be in accordance with the CDC and USP Chapter 797.[75]

Compounding pharmacies offer a wide range of sterile pharmaceutical products, including epidural infusions, PCA syringes, and prefilled elastomeric pain devices in various volumes and drug concentrations. Currently, compounding pharmacies are not regulated by the FDA, although legislation has been proposed for federal regulation. If an institution purchases sterile compounded products from a compounding pharmacy, appropriate quality assurance measures must be ensured. Expiration dating is extended beyond 7 days based on USP Chapter 797 guidelines. Institutions handling a large number of surgical and obstetric cases may find this service of use because compounding large amounts of epidurals requires additional staffing, supplies, and time. Therefore, the cost of the compounded products should be weighed against pharmacy considerations associated with preparing the solutions.[95]

Safety Considerations

Medication errors related to the use of opioid infusions and epidurals are among the most frequently reported.[93] To help prevent medication errors, it is imperative that all epidural solutions be labeled in a clear, concise, consistent manner. Labels should be legible and permanently affixed to the infusion bag or syringe in a manner that makes it easily readable.[92] The patient's name, date of preparation, and solution expiration should be clearly stated. The medication contents should be distinctly labeled with the name of the drugs and volumes used to prepare the solution. In addition, the final concentration and total volume should be clearly marked on the bag in bold lettering. Last, a bright auxiliary label reading *For Epidural Use Only* should be affixed to the bag or syringe.

Drugs intended for intravenous administration have been accidentally administered into the epidural or intrathecal space.[73,93–94] An error in the route of administration could have catastrophic consequences. The route of administration must be clearly noted on all order forms. Drug concentrations vary dramatically between intravenous, continuous peripheral block, epidural, and intrathecal routes. If an intravenous solution of morphine 1 mg/mL is administered epidurally, respiratory depression and death may result. In addition to anesthesiologists and nurses, pharmacists should be familiar with dosing ranges and standard concentrations for epidural and intrathecal preparations.

Proper labeling of the epidural tubing is also imperative. It is recommended that the distal ends of epidural and intravenous lines be labeled to clearly differentiate them.[93] A line dedicated to the administration of epidurals with port-free tubing should always be used to prevent accidental epidural administration of drugs intended for intravenous use.[93–94] It is also helpful to use single-chamber pumps dedicated to epidural infusions. Infusion pumps should also be labeled *For Epidural Use Only.* If a multiple-chamber pump must be used for epidural administration, the other chambers should not be used for the infusion of any other medications. If an adjustment in rate or another medication is administered to the patient, nurses should always trace the tubing from the insertion site to a pump. If more than one pump is being used, placing the IV pump on the opposite side of the patient's bed from the epidural pump may help to prevent mistakes.[93]

TABLE 72–9. Important elements of epidural analgesia preprinted orders.

1. Drugs with concentrations
2. Instructions for administration
   a. If boluses
      i. Drug dose
      ii. Interval between injections
   b. If infusion
      i. Loading dose
      ii. Infusion dose
3. Instructions for treating breakthrough pain
4. Maintain intravenous route and access for emergency administration of drugs
5. A statement or warning that other central nervous system depressants should not be ordered on this patient unless approved by an anesthesiologist
6. Monitoring instructions
   a. Opioids
      i. Respiratory rate
      ii. Sedation level
      iii. Pain score
   b. Local anesthetics
      i. Bradycardia
      ii. Hypotension
      iii. Extensive sensory or motor block
7. Instructions for treatment of side effects
   a. Respiratory depression
   b. Nausea and/or vomiting
   c. Pruritus
   d. Urinary retention
8. Observations that should be communicated to the anesthesiologist
   a. Hypotension
   b. Uncontrolled nausea and vomiting
   c. Uncontrolled pruritus
9. Instructions for whom to contact if problems occur
10. Date, time, and signature of prescribing anesthesiologist

Healthcare practitioners should be aware of the potential for error with handwritten orders. Only proper abbreviations should be accepted, and clarification of any order should be completed prior to processing. The use of preprinted order forms has helped to reduce these types of errors. The ASA Task Force on Pain Management has established guidelines for the use of preprinted order forms in acute pain management.[96] The key elements for epidural analgesia preprinted order forms are listed in Table 72–9.

Clinical Pearl

- The service or anesthesiologist managing the epidural should be the only service or anesthesiologist prescribing additional sedatives or opioids.

If a patient is receiving an epidural opioid, prescribing other sedative agents should be done with extreme caution. The service or anesthesiologist managing the epidural should be the only service or anesthesiologist prescribing other sedatives. If another service prescribes another sedative, the pharmacist should intervene and notify the service managing the opioid epidural. If CPOE is available, a warning screen should be displayed if a sedative is ordered. The pharmacist's role in regional anesthesia may include reviewing patients' drug therapy, optimizing medication selection, and developing policies and procedures. Pharmacists also supervise and evaluate solution preparation, stability, storage, and safety issues. Additionally, the pharmacist can provide information on the cost of different mediation modalities, offering suggestions for the most cost-effective choices.

CONSIDERATIONS FOR THE FUTURE: POLICIES IN THE UNITED STATES

A recent strategy in improving patient care has focused on patient satisfaction. In 2008, a new initiative, the Hospital Consumer Assessment of Healthcare Providers and Systems (HCAHPS), was launched to measure how hospitals are meeting patient needs.[97] Hospitals self-administer questionnaires that address six main issues related to patient experience: Communication with Nurses, Communication with Doctors, Staff Responsiveness, Pain Management, Communication about Medicines, and Discharge Information, in addition to one composite that combines the hospital Cleanliness and Quietness survey items; and one Global item, Overall Score of hospital. It is designed to allow patients to "make 'apples to apples' comparisons to support consumer choice"[97] by having a standardized measurement tool. However, it is also being used by the Center for Medicare and Medicaid (CMS) to modulate payment to hospital and physician groups, starting in Fiscal Year 2013. The Hospital Value-Based Purchasing (Hospital VBP) program links a portion of hospital pay to performance on a set of quality measures with two parts, the Clinical Process of Care and the Patient Experience of Care; the latter part is based on HCAHPS. Put another way, patient experience will determine up to 30% of reimbursement for services the medical team provides.[98]

Anesthesiologists have a unique and important role in this new framework because of their input regarding inpatient pain control. Their interactions with patients can significantly alter patient experience, and downstream alter compensation. Studies have demonstrated that a high level of pain control is strongly correlated with overall satisfaction and higher HCAHPS scores.[99] Implementation of an APMS helps to facilitate this interaction by helping patients achieve improved pain scores, particularly in the population where standard treatments are not adequate. Having a team available with specialized expertise may make the difference in how a patient perceives their experience.

While patient satisfaction is obviously an important part of why patients choose a particular healthcare system, certain members of the medical community have started to question whether such strong focus on making patients happy is actually improving outcomes. An interesting study published in the *Archives of Internal Medicine* systematically addresses this question. A prospective cohort study was performed on a large population across the United States comparing patients' satisfaction scores with mortality and healthcare utilization measures over a 7-year period. The results of the study were surprising. Patients in the highest quartile of patient satisfaction scores had statistically significant increased mortality when adjusted for various socioeconomic and environmental factors.[100] As the practice of medicine evolves we must decide where is the line between patient happiness and good medicine? And when, or should, we have to sacrifice one to achieve the other? The answers to these questions are not simple, and it is not within the scope of this chapter to discuss them. However, these considerations are important for pain providers to bear in mind in striving to care for patients.

SUMMARY

Anesthesiologists, surgeons, pharmacists, and various members of the nursing team all have important roles when considering the organization of an acute pain service. Acute pain management requires a multimodal and multidisciplinary approach with a clear organizational framework. Regional anesthesia techniques for surgical anesthesia are a highly effective component of acute pain management. Maximizing the contributions of regional anesthesia to acute pain management requires integrating these techniques into the larger framework of patient care. This requires an organizational framework that includes all members of the healthcare team, standard order sets, assessment and documentation forms, and institutionwide policies and procedures for the management of aggressive pain techniques.

Clinicians comprising of acute pain team must regard their efforts as extending beyond the operating room and postanesthesia care unit. The team improves not only the experience of the patients they directly care for, but also the entire healthcare system by instituting protocols and safety measures that impact all patients. These specially trained clinicians are uniquely positioned to assist and lead efforts to make these broader changes, which are vital to optimizing patient experiences. Unwavering institutional commitment to these measures is imperative.

REFERENCES

1. Ready LB, Oden R, Chadwick HS, et al: Development of an anesthesiology-based postoperative pain management service. Anesthesiology 1988;68:100–106.
2. Rawal N, Berggren L: Organization of acute pain services: A low-cost model. Pain 1994;57(1):117–123.
3. Warfield CA, Kahn CH: Acute pain management. Anesthesiology 1995;83:1090–1094.
4. Kehlet H, Morgensen T: Hospital stay of 2 days after open sigmoidectomy with a multimodal rehabilitation programme. Br J Surg 1999;86: 227–230.
5. Anonymous: Practice guidelines for acute pain management in the perioperative setting. A report by the American Society of Anesthesiologists Task Force on Pain Management, Acute Pain Section. Anesthesiology 1995;82:1071–1081.
6. An Updated Report by the American Society of Anesthesiologists Task Force on Acute Pain Management. Anesthesiology 2012;116:248–273.

7. Joint Commission on the Accreditation of Healthcare Organizations: *Accreditation Manual for Hospitals*. Oakbrook Terrace, IL: JCAHO, 2001.
8. The Joint Commission Sentinel Event Alert. *Safe Use of Opioids in Hospitals*. Issue 49; August 8, 2012. http://www.jointcommission.org/assets/1/18/SEA-49-opioids-8-2-12-final.pdf
9. Garcia RM, Cassinelli GH, Messerschmitt PJ: a multimodal approach for postoperative pain management after lumbar decompression surgery: a prospective randomized study. J Spinal Disord Tech 2013;26(6): 291–297.
10. Pasero, C: Assessment of sedation during opioid administration for pain management. J PeriAnesth Nurs 2009;3(3):187.
11. Sechzer PH: Studies in pain with analgesic demand system. Anesth Analg 1971;50:1–10.
12. Forrest WH, Jr. Smithurst PW, Kienitz ME: Self-administration of intravenous analgesics. Anesthesiology 1970;33:363–365.
13. Dahlstrom B, Tamser A, Paalzow L, et al: Patient controlled analgesic therapy. Part IV. Pharmacokinetics and analgesic plasma concentration of morphine. Clin Pharmacokinet 1982;7:266–279.
14. Ferrante FM, Orav EJ, Rocco AG, et al: A statistical model for pain in patient- controlled analgesia and conventional intramuscular opioid regimens. Anesth Analg 1988;67:457–461.
15. White PF: Use of PCA for management of acute pain. JAMA 1988; 259:243–247.
16. Gibaldi M, Perrier D: *Pharmacokinetics*. Marcel Dekker, 1975.
17. Parker RK, Holtmann B, White PF: Patient-controlled analgesia. Does a concurrent opioid infusion improve pain management after surgery? JAMA 1991;266(14):1947–1952.
18. Ellis R, Haines D, Shah R: Pain relief after abdominal surgery, comparison of IM morphine sublingual buprenorphine and self-administered IV pethidine. Br J Anaesth 1982;54:421–428.
19. Welcher EA: On demand analgesia a double-blind comparison of on demand IV fentanyl with IM morphine. Anesthesia 1983;38;19–25.
20. Parker RK, Holtmann B, White PF: Patient-controlled analgesia. Does a concurrent opioid infusion improve pain management after surgery? JAMA 1991;266(14):1947–1952.
21. White PF: Mishaps with PCA. Anesthesiology 1987;66:81–83.
22. Sullivan M, Phillips MS: Patient-controlled analgesia pumps. USP Q R 2004;81:1–3.
23. Manufacturer and User Facility Device Experience Database (MAUDE): U.S. Food and Drug Administration, Center for Devices and Radiologic Health, Department of Health and Human Services. Available on the web at: www.fda.gov/cdrh/maude.html.
24. Viscusi ER, Reynolds L, Chung F, et al: Patient-controlled transdermal fentanyl hydrochloride vs intravenous morphine pump for postoperative pain: a randomized controlled trial. JAMA 2004;291(11): 1333–1141.
25. Royal M, Ringold F, Minkowitz H: A randomized, double-blind trial to evaluate the efficacy and safety of the Sufentanil NanoTab® PCA System/15mcg plus rescue morphine vs. placebo plus rescue morphine in patients with moderate-to-severe pain after open abdominal surgery. http://www.acelrx.com/pipeline/arx-01.html.
26. Klein SM, Grant SA, Greengrass RA, et al: Interscalene brachial plexus block with continuous catheter insertion system and a disposable infusion pump. Anesth Analg 2000;91:1473–1478.
27. Ilfeld BM, Morey TE, Wang RD: Continuous popliteal sciatic nerve block for postop pain control at home. A double-blinded placebo controlled study. Anesthesiology 2000;97:959–965.
28. Ilfeld BM: Ambulatory perineural local anesthetic infusions: Portable pumps and dosing regimen selection. Tech Reg Anesth Pain Manag 2004;8(2):90–98.
29. Rawal N, Allvin R, Axelsson K: Patient-controlled regional anesthesia (PCRA) at home. Controlled comparison between bupivacaine and ropivacaine brachial plexus analgesia. Anesthesiology 2000;96: 1290–1296.
30. Ilfeld BM, Morey TE, Enneking FK: Outpatient use of patient-controlled local anesthetic administration via a PSOAS compartment catheter to improve pain control and patient satisfaction after ACL reconstruction. Anesthesiology 2001;95:A38 (abstract).
31. Klein SM: Beyond the hospital, continuous peripheral nerve blocks at home. Anesthesiology 2002;96:1283–1285.
32. Singelyn FJ, Seguy S, Gouverneur JM: Interscalene brachial plexus analgesia after open shoulder surgery: Continuous versus patient-controlled infusion. Anesth Analg 1999;89:1216–1220.
33. Klein SM, Nielsen KC, Greengrass RA, et al: Ambulatory discharge after long-acting peripheral nerve blockade: 2382 blocks with ropivacaine. Anesth Analg 2002;94:65–70.

34. Ekatodramis G, Borgeat A, Huledel G, et al: Continuous interscalene analgesia with ropivacaine 2 mg/ml after major shoulder surgery. Anesthesiology 2003;98:143–150.

35. Klein SM, Nielsen KC: Brachial plexus blocks: nfusion and other mechanisms to provide prolonged analgesia. Curr Opin Anaesth 2003; 16:393–399.

36. Cuvillon P, Ripart J, Lalourcey L, et al: The continuous femoral nerve block catheter for postop analgesia: bacterial colonization infusion rate and adverse effects. Anesth Analg 2001;93:1045–1049.

37. Hogan Q, Dotson R, Erickson S, et al: Local anesthetics myotoxicity: a case and review. Anesthesiology 1994;80:942–947.

38. Kehlet H, Dahl JB: The value of multimodal or balanced analgesia in postoperative pain treatment. Anesth Analg 1993;77:1048–1056.

39. Gillies GWA, Kenny GNC, Bullingham RES: The morphine sparing effect of ketorolac tromethamine. Anesthesia 1987;42:727–731.

40. Kehlet H, Werner M, Perkins F: Balanced analgesia: what is it and what are its advantages in postoperative pain? Drugs 1999;58:793–797.

41. Kehlet H, Morgensen T: Hospital stay of 2 days after open sigmoidectomy with a multimodal rehabilitation programme. Br J Surg 1999;86: 227–230.

42. Bradshaw BG, Liu S, Thirlby RC: Standardized perioperative care protocols and reduced length of stay after colon surgery. J Am Coll Surg 1998;186:501–506.

43. Perkins FM, Kehlet H: Chronic pain as an outcome of surgery. Anesthesiology 2000;93:1123–1133.

44. Lash V, Anderson K, Asenjo JF, et al: Low dose ketamine reduces morphine use after total knee arthroplasty. Can J Anaesth 2003;50:A5.

45. Taura P, Fuster J, Blasi A, et al: Postoperative pain relief after hepatic resection in cirrhotic patients: the efficacy of a single small dose of ketamine plus morphine epidurally. Anesth Analg 2003;96:475–580.

46. McCrory C, Lindahl S: Cyclooxygenase inhabitation for postoperative analgesia. Anesth Analg 2002;95:169–176.

47. Khalili G, Janghorbani M, Saryazdi H, Emaminejad A: Effect of preemptive and preventive acetaminophen on postoperative pain score: a randomized, double-blind trial of patients undergoing lower extremity surgery. J Clin Anesth 2013;25(3):188–192.

48. Finnerup NB, Sindrup SH, Jensen TS: The evidence for pharmacological treatment of neuropathic pain. Pain 2010;150(3):573–581.

49. Brodner G, Van Aken H, Hertle L, et al: Multimodal perioperative management—combining thoracic epidural analgesia, forced mobilization, and oral nutrition—reduces hormonal and metabolic stress and improves convalescence after major urologic surgery. Anesth Analg 2001;2:1594–1600.

50. Hahnenkamp K, Theilmeier G, Van Aken H: The effects of local anesthetics in perioperative coagulation, inflammation and micro-circulation. Anesth Analg 2002;94:1441–1447.

51. Kehlet H: Modification of responses to surgery by neural blockade. Clinical implications. In Cousins MJ, Brindenbaugh PO (eds): *Neural Blockade in Clinical Anesthesia and Management of Pain.* Lippincott Williams & Wilkins, pp 129–175.

52. Block BM, Liu SS, Rowlingson AJ, et al: Efficacy of postoperative epidural analgesia. JAMA 2003;290(18):2455–2463.

53. Horlocker TT, Wedel DJ, Rowlingson JC, et al: Regional anesthesia in the patient receiving antithrombotic or thrombolytic therapy: American Society of Regional Anesthesia and Pain Medicine Evidence-Based Guidelines (Third Edition). Reg Anesth Pain Med 2010; 35(1): 64–101.

54. Sites B, Beech M, Biggs R: Intrathecal clonidine added to bupivacaine-morphine spinal anesthesia improves postoperative analgesia for total knee arthroplasty. Anesth Analg 2003;96:1083–1088.

55. Arain SR, Richlow RM, Uhrich TD: The efficacy of dexmedetomidine versus morphine for postoperative analgesia after major inpatient surgery. Anesth Analg 2004;98:153–158.

56. Pettersson N, Berggren P, Larsson N, et al: Pain relief by wound infiltration with bupivacaine or high-dose ropivacaine after inguinal hernia repair. Reg Anesth Pain Med 1999;24:569–575.

57. Carroll IR, Augst MS, Clark D: Management of perioperative pain in patients chronically consuming opioids. Reg Anesth Pain Med 2004;29:576–591.

58. de Leon-Casasola OA, Myers DP, Donaparthi S, et al: A comparison of postoperative epidural analgesia between patients with chronic cancer taking high doses of oral opioids versus opioid naïve patients. Anesth Analg 1993;76:302–307.

59. Mitra S, Sinatra RS: Perioperative management of acute pain in the opioid-dependent patient. Anesthesiology 2004;101:212–227.

60. Fishbain DA, Rosomoff HL, Rosomoff RS: Drug abuse, dependence, and addiction in chronic pain patients. Clin J Pain 1992;8:77–85.

61. Doverty M, Somogyi AA, White JM, et al: Methadone maintenance patients are cross-tolerant to the antinociceptive effects of morphine. Pain 2001;93:155–163.

62. Compton P, Charuvastra VC, Kintaudi K, et al: Pain responses in methadone-maintained opioid abusers. J Pain Symptom Manage 2000; 20:237–245.

63. Angst MS, Koppert W. Pabh I, et al: Short-term infusion of the mu-opioid agonist remifentanil in humans causes hyperalgesia during withdrawal. Pain 2003;106:49–57.

64. deLeon-Casasola OA, Lema MJ: Epidural sufentanil for acute pain control in a patient with extreme opioid dependency. Anesthesiology 1992;76:853–856.

65. Sosnowski M, Yaksh TL: Differential cross-tolerance between intrathecal morphine and sufentanil in the rat. Anesthesiology 1990;73: 1141–1147.

66. Tawfic QA, Faris AS, Kausalya R: The role of a low-dose ketamine-midazolam regimen in the management of severe painful crisis in patients with sickle-cell disease. J Pain Symptom Manage 12 Jul 2013.

67. Bredlau AL, Thakur R, Korones DN, Dworkin RH: Ketamine for pain in adults and children with cancer: a systematic review and synthesis of literature. Pain Med 5 Aug 2013.

68. www.worldwidewounds.com

69. Fletcher J: Framework guidelines for wound care. Prof Nurse 2000;17(2): 917–921.

70. Jarzyna D, Jungquist CR, Pasero C, et al: American Society of Pain Management Nursing Guidelines on Monitoring for Opioid-Induced Sedation and Respiratory Depression. Pain Manag Nurs 2011;12:118–145.

71. Nisbet, A, Mooney-Cotter, F. Comparison of selected sedation scales for reporting opioid-induced sedation assessment. Pain Manag Nurs 2009; 10:154–164.

72. Mulroy MF: Epidural opioid delivery methods: Bolus, continuous infusion, and patient-controlled epidural analgesia. Reg Anesth 1996;21:100–104.

73. Littrell RA: Epidural analgesia. Am J Hosp Pharm 1991;48: 2460–2474.

74. Kwan JW: Use of infusion devices for epidural or intrathecal administration of spinal opioids. Am J Hosp Pharm 1990;47:S18–S23.

75. Pharmaceutical considerations—sterile preparations (general information Chapter 797). In *The United States Pharmacopeia,* 27th rev, and *The National Formulary,* 22nd ed. Rockville, MD: The United States Pharmacopeial Convention, 2004, pp 2350–2370.

76. Murauski JD, Gonzalez, KR: Peripheral nerve blocks for postoperative analgesia. AORN J 2002;75(1):136–147.

77. Holder KA, Dougherty TB, Porche VH, et al: Postoperative pain management. Int Anesthesiol Clin 1998;36:71–86.

78. Peng PWH, Chan VWS. Local and regional block in postoperative pain control. Surg Clin North Am 1999;79:345–370.

79. Liu SS, Salinas FV: Continuous plexus and peripheral nerve blocks for postoperative analgesia. Anesth Analg 2003;96:263–272.

80. Rawal N, Axelsson K, Hylander J, et al: Postoperative patient-controlled local anesthetic administration at home. Anesth Analg 1998;86:86–89.

81. Ilfeld, BM, Enneking FK: Continuous peripheral nerve blocks at home: a review. Anesth Analg 2005;100(6):1822–1833.

82. Zohar E, Fredman B, Phillipov A, et al: The analgesic efficacy of patient-controlled bupivacaine wound instillation after total abdominal hysterectomy with bilateral salpingo-oophorectomy. Anesth Analg 2002;93(2):482–487.

83. Carfagno ML, Schechter LN: Regional anesthesia and acute pain management: a pharmacist's perspective. Tech Reg Anesth Pain Manag 2002;6(2):77–86.

84. Wilson K, Sullivan M. Preventing medication errors with smart infusion technology. Am J Health Syst Pharm 2004;61(2):177–183.

85. Shafer AL, Donnelly AJ: Management of postoperative pain by continuous epidural infusions of analgesics. Clin Pharm 1991;10:745–764.

86. Centers for Disease Control and Prevention: Spinal and paraspinal infections associated with contaminated methylprednisolone acetate injections —Michigan 2012–2013. MMWR 2013;62:377–381.

87. Stiles ML, Tu YH, Allen LV: Stability of morphine sulfate in portable pump reservoirs during storage and simulated administration. Am J Hosp Pharm 1989;46:1404–1407.

88. Tu YH, Stiles ML, Allen LV: Stability of fentanyl citrate and bupivacaine hydrochloride in portable pump reservoirs. Am J Hosp Pharm 1990;40: 2037–2040.

89. Altman L, Hopkins RJ, Bolton S: Stability of morphine sulfate in Cormed III (Kalex) intravenous bags. Am J Hosp Pharm 1990;47: 2040–2042.

90. Duafala ME, Kleinberg MI, Nacov C, et al: Stability of morphine sulfate in infusion devices and containers for intravenous administration. Am J Hosp Pharm 1990;47:143–146.
91. Centers for Disease Control and Prevention: Guideline for the prevention of intravascular device-related infections. Am J Infect Control 1996;24:262–293.
92. American Society of Health-System Pharmacists: ASHP guideline on quality assurance for pharmacy-based sterile products. Am J Health Sys Pharm 2000;57:1150–1169.
93. ISMP Canada Safety Bulletin: Reports of epidural infusion errors. ISMP Medication Safety Alert 2003;3(1):1.
94. Wheeler SJ, Wheeler DW: Medication errors in anaesthesia and critical care. Anaesthesia 2005;60:257–273.
95. Dollard JV, Python JP: Standardization of epidural preparations for postoperative analgesia. Am J Health-Sys Pharm 1995;52:2565–2567.
96. American Society of Anesthesiologists Task Force on Pain Management: Practice guidelines for acute pain management in the perioperative setting. Anesthesiology 1995;82:1071–1081.
97. *HCAHPS Fact Sheet*. Agency for Healthcare Research and Quality, a U.S. Government agency. Updated 28 Aug 2013. http://www.hcahpsonline.org/files/August%202013%20HCAHPS%20Fact%20Sheet.pdf
98. HCAHPS Project Team. *A Step-by-Step Guide to Calculating the Patient Experience of Care Domain Score in the Hospital Value-Based Purchasing FY 2013 Actual Percentage Payment Summary Report*. Agency for Healthcare Research and Quality, a U.S. Government agency. 26 Oct 2012. http://www.hcahpsonline.org/Files/Hospital%20VBP%20Domain%20Score%20Calculation%20Step-by-Step%20Guide_V2.pdf
99. Gupta A, Dagle S, Molica J, Hurley RW: Patient perception of pain care in hopsitals in the United States. J Pain Res 2008;2:157–164.
100. Fenton JJ, Jerant JF, Bertakis KD, Franks P: The cost of satisfaction: a national study of patient satisfaction, health care utilization, expenditures, and mortality. Arch Intern Med 2012;172(5):405–411.

CHAPTER 73

Neurobiologic Mechanisms of Nociception

Qing Liu and Michael S. Gold

INTRODUCTION

Optimal postoperative pain management is a clinical priority because poorly managed pain may delay functional recovery from surgery and /or lead to chronic pain.[1] Nevertheless, despite considerable effort to improve postoperative pain management, one third of patients continue to suffer from moderate to severe pain.[2] The lack of consistently effective analgesics devoid of deleterious consequences remains one of the main causes of the inadequacy of postoperative pain management. Therefore, identification of novel therapeutic targets and more effective management strategies remain high priorities in pain research.

To provide a framework to facilitate understanding of the mechanisms underlying the efficacy of currently available pain management strategies, at least some of the reasons for the failure to achieve adequate pain relief, as well as identify viable targets for future interventions, this chapter covers fundamental neurobiologic mechanisms of the nociceptive system. Given space constraints, and the fact the functional alterations of the nociceptive system in the context of chronic pain are addressed in more detail in subsequent chapters, this issue will be not be discussed at length here.

NEUROBIOLOGIC MECHANISMS OF PAIN

Overview of Nociceptive/Pain Pathway

The simplest depiction of the neural circuit underlying the perception of pain in response to noxious or potentially tissue damaging stimulation of peripheral tissue involves three neurons. The first is a nociceptor, a specialized primary afferent neuron with a peripheral terminal innervating the site of stimulation, a cell body in a spinal or dorsal root ganglia or trigeminal ganglia, and a central terminal in the spinal cord or brainstem dorsal horn. The second is an "output," or projection, neuron in the spinal cord/trigeminal dorsal horn that

receives input from the nociceptor and projects to the thalamus. And the third neuron projects from the thalamus to the sensory cortex. But as a sensory and emotional experience that is highly motivational (i.e., withdrawal/escape), pain necessarily involves far more than three neurons. This point is further underscored when one considers the heterogeneity of the pain experience which varies in intensity, quality, duration, location, emotional valence, whether it is evoked or ongoing, and so on.

The integration of nociceptive information in supraspinal regions leads to complex sensory, emotional, and motivational components that make up the perception of pain. Ascending sensory information reaches many cortical sites via parallel pathways. Along the way, however, this information also impinges upon subcortical and brainstem sites that underlie coordinated physiologic responses required for "fight or flight" as well as the modulation of the ascending nociceptive signal. Projections from the brainstem to the spinal cord are referred to as descending modulations. These sites may also be accessed via therapeutic interventions to block or attenuate pain (Figure 73–1, Table 73–1).

PERIPHERAL MECHANISMS

Nociceptors and Signal Transduction

In contrast to other afferent subtypes responsible for signaling low-threshold mechanical stimuli (touch, vibration, stretch), the peripheral terminals of nociceptors, sensory neurons that encode noxious, or potentially tissue-damaging stimuli, are not associated with a particular cell type or structure. Rather, they are said to terminate in "free" nerve endings. Consequently, while there is increasing evidence indicating that other cells in the periphery, such as the urothelial cells that line the bladder[3] or the keratinocytes that make up skin,[4] contribute to the afferent response to noxious stimuli, as predicted, there is also evidence the nociceptors express proteins that enable them to respond to noxious thermal (heat and cold), mechanical, and chemical stimuli.[5]

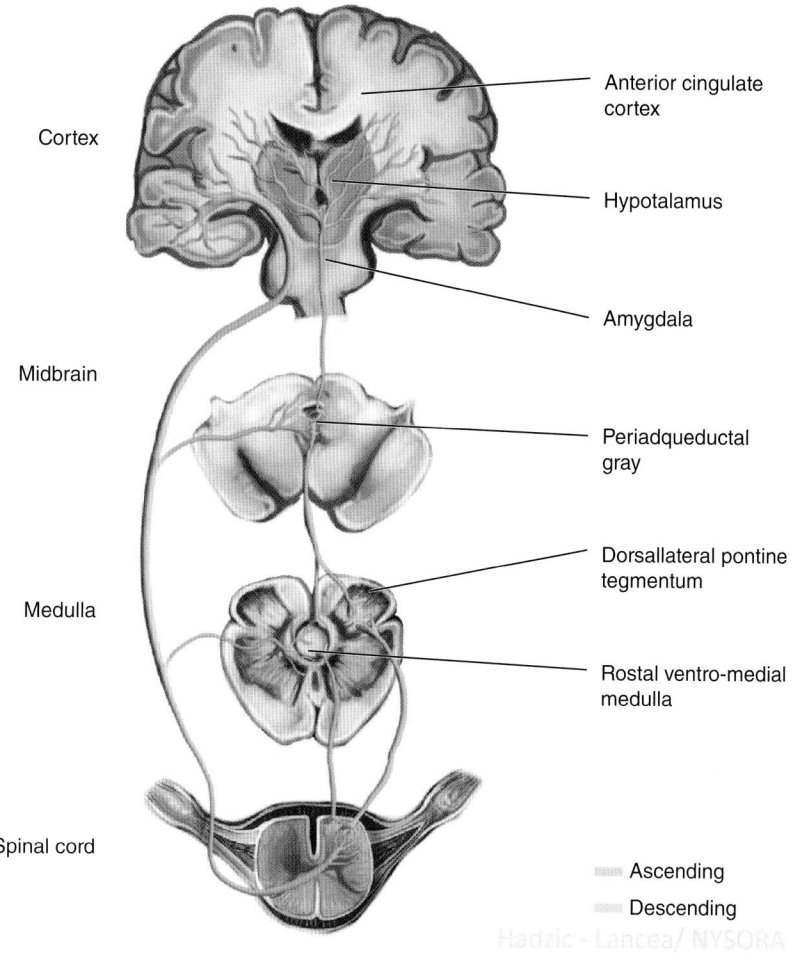

Cortex

Anterior cingulate
cortex

Hypotalamus

Amygdala

Midbrain

Periadqueductal
gray

Dorsallateral pontine
tegmentum

Medulla

Rostal ventro-medial
medulla

Spinal cord

Ascending
Descending

FIGURE 73–1. Overview of nociceptive pain pathway. Major structures in ascending and descending nociceptive pathway. Ascending: primary afferent fibers provide nociceptive input to the spinal cord, which projects to brainstem (spinomedullar tract) and thalamus (spinothalamic tract). The projections ultimately target the hypothalamus, amygdala, and somatosensory cortex to process the sensory, affective, and cognitive components of pain. Descending: Brain structures relevant for the affective and cognitive components of pain (Insulate cortex, amygdala, and hypothalamus) exert descending nociceptive control. The PAG and RVM are to integrate input from cerebral structures and relay processed information to the spinal dorsal horn. Nuclei at the dorsolateral pontine constitute a second most important structure projecting to the dorsal horn. PAG: periaqueductal gray; RVM: rostral ventromedial medulla.

Thus, nociception typically starts when noxious mechanical, thermal, and/or chemical stimuli act on these specialized proteins or receptors. To enable the energy of the noxious stimulus to be converted, or transduced, into an electrical signal, these receptors either contain an ion channel, or are coupled to an ion channel, such that receptor activation results in a change in membrane conductance and, consequently, membrane depolarization. Such a depolarization is referred to as a generator potential, which passively spreads through the peripheral terminal. If the generator potential is large enough and/or spreads far enough to drive activation of enough voltage-gated Na^+ channels, an action potential is generated. This process is referred to as transformation. The action potential is propagated along slowly conducting unmyelinated (C fibers), or more rapidly conducting thinly myelinated (A delta fibers) axons of the nociceptors to the central terminals in the superficial layers of the spinal cord dorsal horn. As the action potential invades the central terminals of nociceptive afferents, voltage-gated Ca^{2+} channels are activated, enabling Ca^{2+} influx necessary for transmitter release. While subpopulations of nociceptive afferents

contain neuropeptides that can act within the dorsal horn, all nociceptive afferents use the excitatory amino acid, glutamate, as a transmitter for fast excitatory signaling via ionotropic glutamate receptors on postsynaptic neurons.

The majority of cell surface proteins studied in detail for the process of nociceptive signal transduction, transformation, propagation, and transmitter release fall into two major classes: ion channels and metabotropic receptors. The former are further subdivided into voltage-dependent or voltage-independent channels, Ca^{2+}–activated/modulated channels, and ligand-gated channels. The latter are subdivided into G protein–coupled receptors (GPCRs), and receptor tyrosine kinases and non–tyrosine kinase receptors. A detailed review of these proteins has been provided elsewhere.[5] The following is a brief description of the channels, at each phase of the process, that serve as targets for the currently available therapeutics.

Ion Channels

While many ion channels have been identified that are involved in signal transduction, transformation, and propagation, very

TABLE 73-1. Glossary.

- **Action potential,** electrical signal propagated along neuronal processes that enables communication to postsynaptic neurons in the pain pathway
- **Allodynia,** pain evoked by a normally innocuous stimulus
- **Central sensitization,** increased synaptic efficacy in central (spinal dorsal horn) neurons leading to increased pain perception
- Generator potential
- **Hyperalgesia,** increased pain perception elicited by a noxious stimulus; **primary hyperalgesia,** hyperalgesia in the area of injury or exposure to noxious stimulus; **secondary hyperalgesia,** hyperalgesia in the region surrounding the area exposed to a noxious stimulus. Reflecting a decrease in threshold and/or increase in suprathreshold response.
- **Inflammatory pain,** pain associated with tissue injury and inflammation
- **Nociception,** neural process of encoding the processing noxious stimuli
- **Nociceptors,** peripherally localized primary afferent nerve fibers capable of encoding noxious stimuli
- **Noxious stimuli,** damaging or potentially damaging stimuli (mechanical, thermal and chemical) that provoke and avoidance response
- **Plasticity,** a dynamic modulation of signaling
- **Sensitization,** increased excitability of nociceptors, which usually develops as a

few are currently targets for therapeutic interventions. These include several members of the transient receptor potential (TRP) family, voltage-gated Na⁺ channels, and voltage-gated Ca²⁺ channels. However, because an antiepileptic compound approved for use in Europe targets a K⁺ channels, we have included a brief discussion of this channel as well.

TRP Channels

Long before the discovery of the TRP vanilloid type 1 (TRPV1) as the receptor for capsaicin, the pungent compound in chili peppers, there was evidence that this compound had efficacy for the treatment of pain. Applied cutaneously via a variety of vehicles, this compound was shown to block pain by "desensitizing" cutaneous tissue to thermal, mechanical, and chemical stimulation. This appeared to be due Ca^{2+} influx and the subsequent retraction of afferent terminals from the sight of the capsaicin application.[6] This phenomena serves as the basis for the therapeutic efficacy of the various preparations of capsaicin currently in use today, which includes the capsaicin patch (Qutenza) for the topical treatment of pain for postherpetic neuralgia.[7] Most recently, in this regard, is the use of intrathecal administration of the ultrapotent TRPV1 agonist, resiniferatoxin, as a way to selectively "ablate" the central terminals of nociceptive afferents as an effective way of blocking pain from even deeper peripheral structures.[8]

The identification of TRPV1 as the target for capsaicin has proven to be a watershed in the pain field for the number of additional observations that have arisen from its discovery. First, it was shown that TRPV1 is not only a receptor for capsaicin, but functions as a "heat" receptor, playing a major role in the heat hypersensitivity observed in the presence of inflammation. It is also activated by a number of endogenous mediators associated with tissue injury and/or inflammation, such as protons, and a variety of lipids. And it serves as a common target for a variety of second-messenger cascades activated with tissue injury, resulting in the sensitization of the receptor (such that it is activated with lower intensities of stimulation), and increases in receptor density as a result of altered trafficking, translation, and expression. Consequently, a number of antagonists of TRPV1 have been developed, at least one of which made it into clinical trials.[9] Unfortunately, because this channel also functions in the neural circuits controlling core body temperature, hyperthermia was the side effect that stopped the further development of these compounds (although there is some evidence that it may be possible to avoid this side effect with a properly targeted compound.[10] Finally, because the TRPV1 channel dilates with prolonged activation, there is evidence that the channel can be used to enable a nociceptor-specific nerve block.[11]

Other members of the TRP family have also been studied. Most notable are the TRPM8 (sensing coldness and menthol) and TRPA1 (sensing noxious coldness, pungent chemicals, such as cinnamon and wasabi, and acrolein) receptors. Low concentrations of menthol (0.01%–1.0%) have been used in over-the-counter analgesics.[12]

Voltage-Gated Ion Channels

Voltage-gated Na⁺ channels (NaVs) play an essential role in the initiation and propagation of action potentials. NaV channels are composed of α- and β-subunits. Nine isoforms of the α-subunit (NaV1.1 –1.9) have been identified, with three (NaV1.7, 1.8, and 1.9) preferentially expressed in nociceptors. Compelling lines of evidence have implicated each of these subunits in the pain and hypersensitivity of inflammation and/or nerve injury, and, consequently, all three subunits remain activity targets of drug development. However, because of the high homology between α-subunits in both the voltage sensor and pore domains of the channel, subtype-selective antagonists have remained elusive. Nevertheless, even nonselective Na⁺ channel blockers, such as local anesthetics, antiepileptics, and even tricyclic antidepressants, have therapeutic efficacy for the treatment of pain. The most widely used of these, of course, are the local anesthetics, that have remained the mainstay of regional anesthetic techniques, and enable complete pain relief with an appropriately placed peripheral nerve block.

The high-voltage–activated (HVA) Ca²⁺ channels are essential for the transmitter release at the central terminal of the primary afferents.[13] Consequently, they are a primary mechanism underlying presynaptic inhibition via endogenous signaling mechanisms involving adrenergic, gababergic, and opioidergic receptors. Thus, HVA channels are a primary target for exogenous agonists of these receptors such as clonidine and

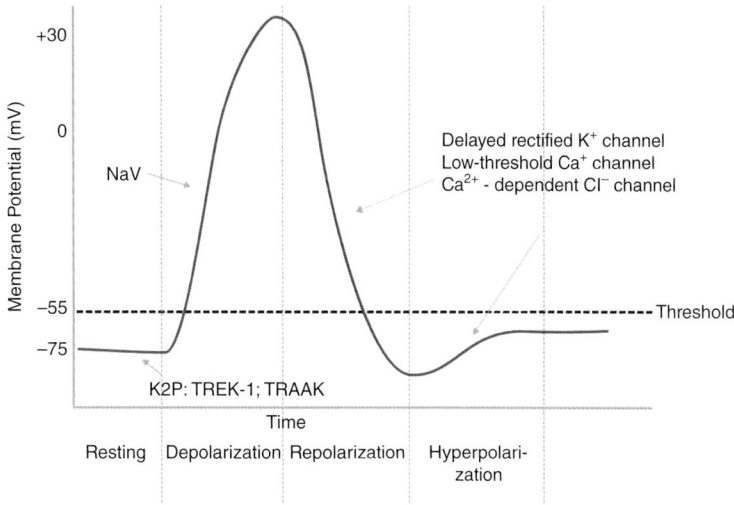

FIGURE 73-2. Schematic diagram of neuronal membrane and action potential showing typical ion channels for each of the phases (resting, depolarization, repolarization, and hyperpolarization). K2P: two-pore domain potassium channel; TREK1: TWIK-related potassium channel 1; TRAAK: TWIK-activated arachidonic acid potassium channel; NaV: voltage-gated sodium channel. Each of the ion channels could serve as a novel therapeutic target.

morphine. Direct inhibition of these channels is also useful for the treatment of pain, as has been demonstrated for ziconotide.[14] Furthermore, because tissue injury may result in the upregulation of the alpha2delta subunit, which is critical for trafficking HVA channels to the afferent terminals, and this subunit is the primary binding site for gabapentin and pregabalin, the available evidence suggests that the analgesic efficacy of these compounds is ultimately due to the inhibition of HVA channels.[15]

K+ channels are crucial to maintain the membrane potential and the repolarization of the action potential. K+ channel openers effectively decrease the membrane excitability, making them potentially powerful therapeutic targets. Consistent with this suggestion, retigabine, a K+ channel opener, may hold a promise for the treatment of inflammatory pain[16] (Figure 73–2).

G Protein–Coupled Receptors

GPCRs are a large family of receptors that underlie both pronociceptive pathways, such as those associated with inflammatory mediators (CGRP [calcitonin gene–related peptides, bradykinin and prostaglandin), as well as antinociceptive pathways, such as opioids and adrenergic receptors. While many targets have been explored for therapeutic use, currently available analgesics appear to focus on the three major pathways: (1) the inhibition of HVA channels as noted above, (2) the activation of K+ channels, most commonly G protein–gated inwardly rectifying K+ (GIRK) channels,[17] and (3) the inhibition of pronociceptive second-messenger cascades via the inhibition of adenylate cyclase.[18] While the activation of GIRK channels is a common mechanism of inhibition in the central nervous system, there are only indirect lines of evidence suggesting that such a mechanism contributes to the GPCR-induced inhibition of nociceptor signaling. In contrast, the inhibition of adenylate cyclase appears to be particularly important for the antinociceptive actions of peripherally administered opioid agonists.[18] It is important to note that there are GPCRs that appear to be uniquely engaged, enabling the therapeutic

specificity of triptans (5-HT$_1$ subtype–selective agonists); e.g., for the treatment of migraine.[19] More recently, a biologic approach has been developed to block pronociceptive GPCR signaling, with antibodies against CGRP or the CGRP receptor showing efficacy in initial trials for the treatment of migraine.[20] It is interesting in this regard as to why antagonists for the receptors of major proinflammatory mediators such as prostaglandin and bradykinin have not done better in clinical trials, but this may be a reflection of the parallel pathways activated in the presence of inflammation, as well as crosstalk between pathways. The extent of the crosstalk is illustrated by considering modulation of TRPV1 (Figure 73–3).

Neurotrophin Receptors

Neurotrophic factors are not only essential for survival and axon guidance during development, but are also important for maintaining afferent phenotype and, more relevantly, pain in adults. The best studied of these in the peripheral nervous system is nerve growth factor (NGF), which is dramatically upregulated in the presence of inflammation,[21] and has been shown both to acutely sensitize TRPV1 and NaV channels as well as drive longer term changes in gene expression that appear to contribute to the manifestation of inflammatory pain.[22] However, while preclinical data are all very promising, the phase 3 clinical trial of an NGF antibody for the treatment of osteoarthritis was stopped because of unexplained joint damage.[23] Another neurotrophic factor that also appears to contribute to inflammatory hypersensitivity is artemin, a member of the glial cell line–derived family of trophic factors. Artemin is also increased in the presence of inflammation and appears to act synergistically with NGF to prolong the sensitization of nociceptor afferents.[24] However, there is evidence that under certain conditions, artemin may also attenuate nociceptive signaling, particularly in the presence of nerve injury.[25] There are ongoing clinical trials with artemin, also called neublastin, for the treatment of neuropathic pain.

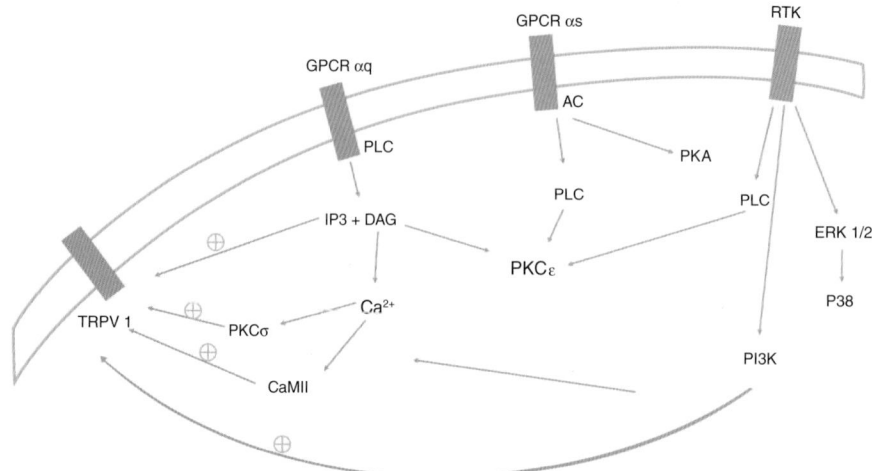

FIGURE 73–3. TRPV1 as a common target of multiple-second messenger signaling pathways after nociceptor activation. There are multiple other points of interaction between each pathway, including at the level of signaling molecules such as Ca^{2+}, and effector molecules such as PKCε. CaM: calmodulin; PLC: phospholipase C; DAG: diacyglycerol; IP3: inositol triphosphate; AC: adenylate cyclase; PI3K: phosphoinositide 3-kinase; ERK 1/2: extracellular signal-regulated kinases 1 and 2; RTK: receptor tyrosine kinase.

SPINAL MECHANISMS

While the nociceptive signal is subject to a considerable degree of modulation from the site of its initiation in the periphery, this modulation pales in comparison to the degree that it occurs in the spinal cord dorsal horn. Organized in cytoarchitecturally distinct parallel laminae, the major components of the spinal cord dorsal horn include the central terminals of primary afferents, the terminals of axons from neurons located at other segments, the brainstem or higher brain structures, interneurons, projection neurons, and glia. Nociceptive afferents terminate predominantly in the superficial layers of the spinal cord (lamina I and II), as well in lamina V, while nonnociceptive input largely terminates in laminae III and IV (Figure 73–4). While there is evidence of monosynaptic connections between nociceptive afferents and projection neurons, the majority of input and output from the dorsal horn is organized in microcircuits with both inhibitory and excitatory interneurons that serve to

sculpt both the temporal and spatial features of the sensory input.[26] Emerging evidence suggests that this circuitry is also critical for defining the sensory features of the input, such as would be needed to distinguish itch from pain.[27] Importantly, these microcircuits appear to be the substrate upon which descending input from the supraspinal and intrasegmental sites acts to modulate sensory signals. Glutamate is the major neurotransmitter released by excitatory primary afferents and interneurons, which binds to ionotropic glutamatergic receptors, such as N-methyl-D-aspartate (NMDA) receptors. Gamma-aminobutyric acid (GABA) and glycine are the main neurotransmitters released by inhibitory interneurons and descending inputs (Figure 73–5).

Both tissue inflammation and nerve injury can result in abnormal pain sensations, including hyperalgesia, allodynia, and spontaneous pain. Several changes in the spinal cord that could underlie these phenomena have been reviewed.[28] They include intrinsic plasticity of dorsal horn neurons, changes in

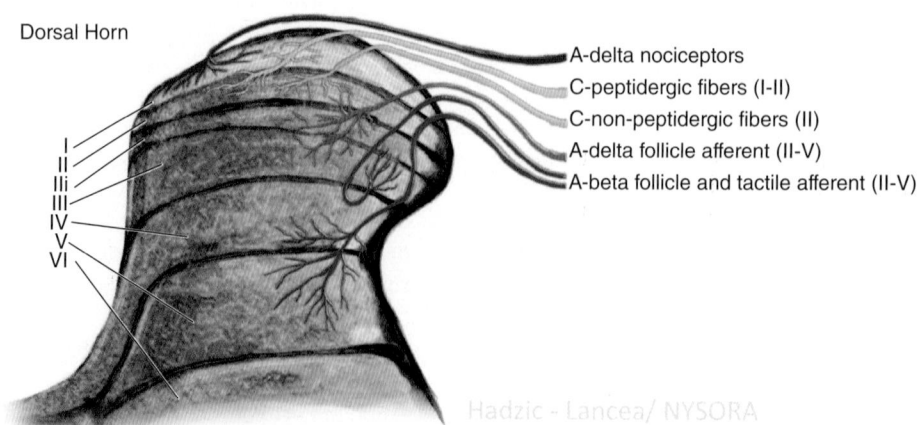

FIGURE 73–4. Schematic example of laminar organization (I–V) of spinal dorsal horn and the termination sites of primary afferents. Abeta tactile afferents mainly end in laminae II–V. A delta nociceptors predominately terminate in lamina I. C-peptidergic primary afferents end in lamina I and the outer portion of lamina II. C-nonpeptidergic afferents terminate in lamina II. (Modified with permission from Todd AJ: Neuronal circuitry for pain processing in the dorsal horn. *Nat Rev Neurosci.* 2010 Dec;11(12):823–836.)

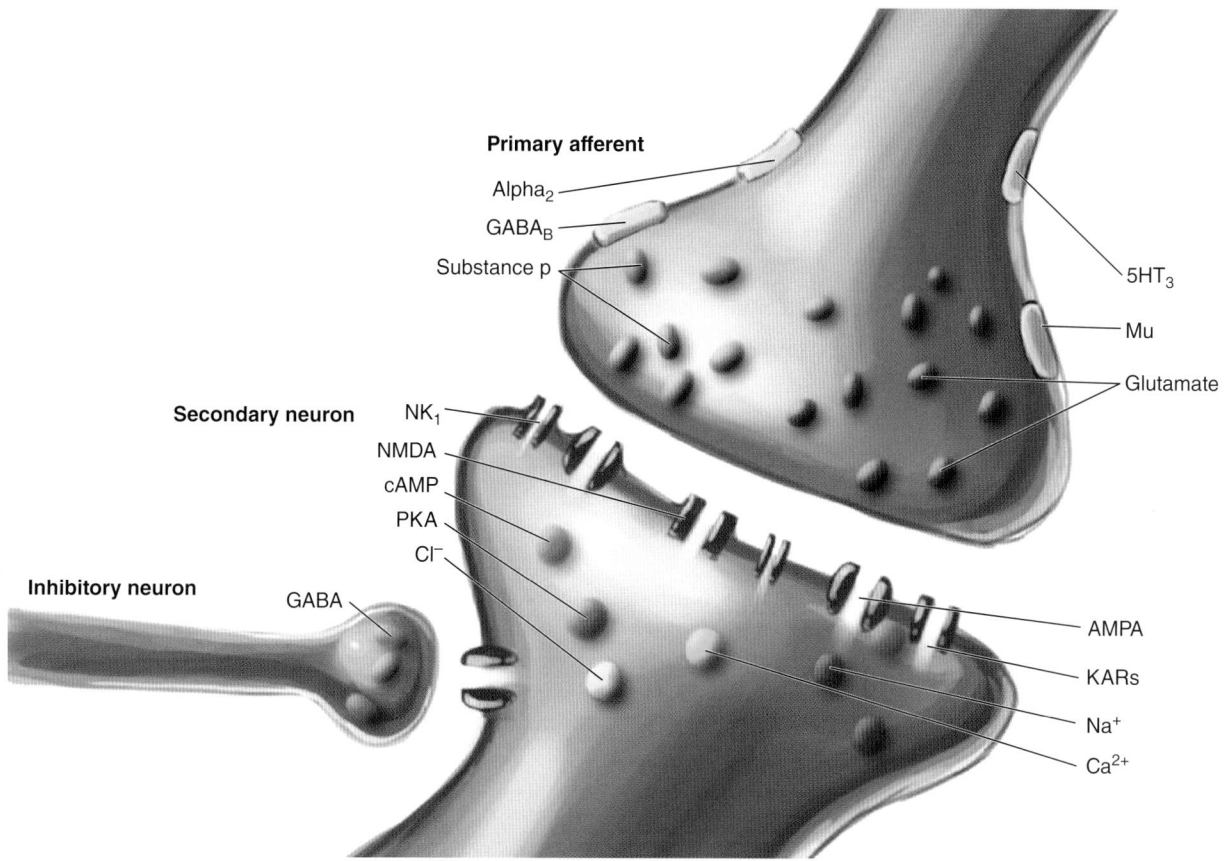

FIGURE 73–5. Schematic diagram of spinal dorsal horn synapse. The central terminal of the primary afferent contains neurotransmitters such as substance P and glutamate and neuromodulators such as BDNF. Release glutamate activates AMPA /kainate receptors leading to fast Na^+ influx and depolarization of the postsynaptic membrane. Sustained synaptic input can depolarize the postsynaptic membrane sufficiently to activate the voltage gated NMDA receptor leading to Ca^{2+} influx, underlying the hyperalgesic states. This process is modulated by activities of many presynaptic (e.g., 5-HT$_3$, α_2- adrenergic, opioid mu, GABA$_B$) and postsynaptic (e.g., GABA$_A$) receptor systems. For example, activation of postsynaptic NK1 receptors via substance P activates cAMP-PKA signaling pathway, which facilitates NMDA receptor activation, whereas release of presynaptic GABA enhances Cl influx, which hyperpolarizes postsynaptic membranes and inhibits activity. BDNF: brain-derived neurogenic factor; AMPA:; cAMP: cyclic adenosine monophosphate; GABA: gamma-aminobutyric acid; NK1: neurokinin; NMDA: N-methyl-D-aspartate; PKA: protein kinase A.

spinal microcircuits, changes in descending inputs, and changes in glial cells.

Intrinsic plasticity of dorsal horn neurons refers to the changes in the properties of the neurons themselves that influence excitability. This generally includes the same types of ion channels as those impacting excitability and transmitter release in nociceptive afferents. The net result is a change in the output (action potentials) of a dorsal horn neuron in response to a given input (synaptic transmission). There is, of course, synaptic plasticity (presynaptic or postsynaptic), that can underlie changes in the stimulus-response function of a dorsal horn neuron, where changes in receptor density and/or functional synapses have both been described. Mechanisms underlying changes in synaptic strength are analogous to the long-term potentiation and depression[29] described in the hippocampus in association with learning and memory, but do not appear to involve the mechanisms enabling the changes to persist indefinitely.

Importantly, it is the changes in spinal microcircuits that appear to underlie the emergence of the phenomena of mechanical allodynia, where low-threshold Abeta afferent activation can produce the sensation of pain.[30] While

there is evidence to suggest several changes contribute to this phenomena, the most compelling evidence to date suggests that changes in microcircuits involving both a decrease in inhibitory interneuron signaling[31] and a change in excitatory interneuron signaling[32] enable the low-threshold input to deeper layers of the dorsal horn to gain access to nociceptive circuits in the superficial layers.[33] The role of NDMA receptors in the initiation and/or maintenance of these changes is thought to account for the therapeutic efficacy of NMDA receptor antagonists such as ketamine.[34,35]

Changes in descending inputs include a shift from inhibitory to facilitatory influences on the spinal processes in pronociceptive states associated with inflammation and injury.[36]

Finally, changes in glial cells (microglia and astrocytes) in response to nerve injury and inflammation include the release of inflammatory mediators (brain-derived neurogenic factor [BDNF], prostaglandin, interleukins IL-1β and IL-6, and tumor necrosis factor-α [TNF-α]) through the purinergic (P2X$_4$, P2X$_7$, P2Y$_{12}$) signaling mechanisms.[37,38]

Findings from these studies have provided many therapeutic targets for analgesia in yhe spinal cord in addition to the

NMDA receptor. For example, nonsteroidal anti-inflammatory drugs (NSAIDs) produce the analgesic effects by inhibiting the cyclooxygenase (COX) enzyme, consequently the generation of prostaglandins in the dorsal horn.[39] Since the loss of inhibition is an important mechanism underlying many spinal changes, research has recently focused on the restoration of the normal inhibition.[40,41] Drugs that modulate the glial cell activation have also been introduced to treat pain. For example, methotrexate has been shown to attenuate osteoarthritis pain.[42] However, the failure of propentofylline, a nonspecific glial inhibitor to treat postherpetic pain[43] highlights the need for further research.

SUPRASPINAL MECHANISMS

Neurons of spinal dorsal horn (laminae I and V) project along the spinothalamic and spinoreticulothalamic tracts to supraspinal sites (brainstem, thalamus, amygdale, and cortex), where pain signals are processed, integrated, and modulated. Neuroimaging studies have now identified several important supraspinal regions in humans that appear to play a critical role in the processing of ascending nociceptive signaling, including brainstem periaqueductal gray (PAG), hypothalamus, amygdala, the S1 and S2 cortices, the insular and anterior cingulate, and the prefrontal cortices (PFCs). The relatively large number of brain regions activated by noxious stimuli is often referred as the "pain matrix," which together appear to account for the sensory, emotional, and motivational aspects of pain.[44] It should be noted that none of the brain regions included in the pain matrix are exclusively activated by noxious stimuli, and, in fact, many of the same brain regions have been implicated in a variety of physiologic and pathophysiologic States.[45] More recently, researchers have attempted to understand how the pain is encoded in the brain by studying dynamic changes in brain function. This includes the assessment of how well activity in different brain areas is correlated, which used to infer "functional connectivity," where pain states are associated with changes in functional connectivity. Similarly, researchers have identified a pattern of activity when the brain is at "rest," referred to as the default mode network, where again the presence of pain has been shown to result in disruption in this network.[46] As with all brain imaging, distinguishing cause from effect remains an elusive goal. Even more elusive is the "signature" of the chronic pain brain, despite the fact that is it is now possible to determine not just whether an individual is experiencing acute pain but how much acute pain an individual may be experiencing.[47]

Descending Modulation Pathways

Structures at the midbrain, such as the PA, and the rostral ventromedial medulla (RVM) are the gateway through which cortical and subcortical sites can influence nociception. It is now well established that the PAG is a source of descending opioid-mediated inhibition of nociceptive inputs. This region receives inputs from cortical sites and has reciprocal connections with the amygdala[48] and receives ascending nociceptive inputs from the spinal dorsal horns by way of the parabrachial nuclei. The inputs from the rostral anterior cingulated nucleus (rACC) (rACC) to the PAG likely mediates the placebo analgesia.[49] The PAG influences descending pain modulation primarily through its reciprocal connections with the RVM, which in turn projects to superficial and deep laminae in the dorsal horn (see Figure 73–1). While both excitatory and inhibitory modulation can occur, the best-studied mechanism related to pain is descending inhibition, which involves the action of a number of endogenous neurotransmitters, such as opioids, serotonin, norepinephrine, cannabinoids, GABA and glycine. Many traditional pain-management strategies act at least partially via these inhibitory mechanisms.

Other brainstem sites appear to work in concert with the PAG and RVM and include the noradrenergic projection of the pontine locus coeruleus to the dorsal horn via the ventrolateral funiculus[50] and the subnucleus reticularis dorsalis (SRD) at the caudal medulla for the diffuse noxious inhibitory controls (DNIC).[51]

Descending pain modulation is the underlying mechanism for many surgical, psychologic, and pharmacologic interventions for pain treatment. The surgical interventions include deep brain and spinal cord stimulation.[52] The psychologic interventions include biofeedback, cognitive-behavioral therapy (CBT), and conditioned pain modulation (CPM).[53] The pharmacologic interventions include the traditional opioids, antidepressants, and anticonvulsants as well as newly developed strategies, such as intranasal oxytocin.[54]

Challenges for Analgesic Discovery

Pain is a complex process by which the specific mechanisms as well as the severity and duration can be influenced by many factors. These include (1) type of injury (inflammation vs nerve injury); (2) the site of injury; (3) timing, in terms of the trajectory of the response to injury, chronologic age, and previous history; (4) sex; and (5) genetic background. With respect to the type of injury, inflammatory and neuropathic pain may share some common mechanisms but are also fundamentally distinct, and as a result, they require different treatments.[55] Similarly, the neurons and circuits underlying pain arising from somatic structures (skin, muscle, joints, and bone) appear to be very different from each other as well as those underlying visceral and trigeminal structures. Time-dependent changes in the mechanisms underlying pain after injury have been well documented.[56] There are some pain syndromes such as migraine and temporomandibular disorder that are far more common in young adults, while others, such as trigeminal neuralgia and postherpetic neuropathy, are more common in the elderly.[57] Similarly, nerves with a preexisting injury (diabetic and/or chemotherapeutic neuropathies) are at much greater risk of a second, possibly subclinical, insult. This "double crush syndrome" highlights the impact of the history of injury on the choice of treatment.[58] Despite the relatively small sexual differences described in the laboratory in association with either pain or analgesia, it remains a fact that the incidence and severity of chronic pain is higher in women than in men.[59] Finally, it has now been well documented that genetic differences contribute to differences in pain susceptibility and in responses to analgesics.[60]

TABLE 73–2. Neurobiologic mechanisms for nociception.

Site of Actions	Mechanisms	Analgesics
Peripheral	Block signal transduction	Inflammatory factor release inhibition: NSAIDs
		TRPV1 agonist: capsaicin
		TRPV1 antagonist: resiniferotoxin
		TRPM8 agonist: menthol, peppermint oil
	Block action potential initiation/propagation	NaV blockers: local anesthetics, antiepileptics, TCAs
		HVA Ca^{2+} channel blockers: clonidine, opioids, gabapentin, ziconotide
		K$^+$ channel blocker: retigabine
		GPCR blocker: triptans, peripheral opioids
		NGF inhibitor: Fasinumab, Neublastin
Spinal	Prevent intrinsic plasticity	NMDA receptor antagonist: ketamine, dextromethorphan
	Block hypersensitivity	Inflammatory factor release inhibition: NSAIDs
	Restore normal inhibition	GABA receptor agonist: baclofen, benzodiazepine
	Glial cell modulation	Glial cell modulator: methotrexate, propentofylline
Supraspinal	Modulate descending pain pathways	Surgical: DBS/SCS
		Psychologic: biofeedback, CPM
		Pharmacologic: opioids, TCAs, oxytocin

Abbreviations: CPM: conditioned pain modulation; deep brain stimulation; GABA: gamma-aminobutyric acid; GPCR: G protein-coupled receptor; HVA: high voltage activated; NaV: voltage-gated Na$^+$ channel; NGF: nerve growth factor; NMDA: N-methyl-D-aspartate; NSAIDs: nonsteroidal anti-inflammatory drugs; SCS: spinal cord stimulation; TCAs: tricyclic antidepressants; TRPV: transient receptor potential cation channel.

SUMMARY

Both the existing and future therapeutic interventions for the treatment of pain are grounded in the neurobiologic mechanisms of nociception (Table 73–2). While it may not be possible to identify the ultimate, "silver bullet" for pain treatment, with an increased understanding of the multitude of variables that influence both the development of pain and the response to interventions, the promise of personalized medicine with interventions tailored to the specific needs of the patient appears to be a possibility in foreseeable future. Given the specific needs of the patient in the perioperative setting, we may be even closer to providing optimal pain management for all patients with the tools and approaches already available.

REFERENCES

1. Joshi GP, Ogunnaike BO: Consequences of inadequate postoperative pain relief and chronic persistent postoperative pain. Anesthesiol Clin North America 2005;23(1):21–36.
2. Maroney CL, et al: Acceptability of severe pain among hospitalized adults. J Palliat Med 2004;7(3):443–450.
3. Charrua A, et al: Transient receptor potential vanilloid subfamily 1 is essential for the generation of noxious bladder input and bladder overactivity in cystitis. J Urol 2007;177(4):1537–1541.
4. Peier AM, et al: A heat-sensitive TRP channel expressed in keratinocytes. Science 2002;296(5575):2046–2049.
5. Gold MS, Gebhart GF: Nociceptor sensitization in pain pathogenesis. Nat Med 2010;16(11):1248–1257.
6. Anand P, Bley K: Topical capsaicin for pain management: therapeutic potential and mechanisms of action of the new high-concentration capsaicin 8% patch. Br J Anaesth 2011;107(4):490–502.
7. Burness CB, McCormack PL: Capsaicin 8 % patch: a review in peripheral neuropathic pain. Drugs 2016:76(1)123–134.
8. Iadarola M, Mannes AJ: The vanilloid agonist resiniferatoxin for interventional-based pain control. Curr Top Med Chem 2011;11(17):2171–2179.
9. Chizh BA, et al: The effects of the TRPV1 antagonist SB-705498 on TRPV1 receptor-mediated activity and inflammatory hyperalgesia in humans. Pain 2007;132(1–2):132–141.
10. Lazar J, et al: Screening TRPV1 antagonists for the treatment of pain: lessons learned over a decade. Exp Opin Drug Discov 2009;4(2):159–180.
11. Binshtok AM, Bean BO, Woolf CJ: Inhibition of nociceptors by TRPV1-mediated entry of impermeant sodium channel blockers. Nature 2007;449(7162):607–610.
12. Patel T, Ishiuji Y, Yosipovitch G;, Menthol: a refreshing look at this ancient compound. J Am Acad Dermatol 2007;57(5):873–878.
13. Todorovic SM, Jevtovic-Todorovic V: T-type voltage-gated calcium channels as targets for the development of novel pain therapies. Br J Pharmacol 2011;163(3):484–495.
14. Zamponi GW, et al: The physiology, pathology, and pharmacology of voltage-gated calcium channels and their future therapeutic potential. Pharmacol Rev 2015;67(4):821–870.
15. Kukkar A, et al: Implications and mechanism of action of gabapentin in neuropathic pain. Arch Pharm Res 2013;36(3):237–251.
16. Hayashi H, et al: Activation of peripheral KCNQ channels attenuates inflammatory pain. Mol Pain 2014:10:15.

17. Luscher C, Slesinger PA:, Emerging roles for G protein-gated inwardly rectifying potassium (GIRK) channels in health and disease. Nat Rev Neurosci 2010;11(5):301–315.

18. Pierre S, et al: Capturing adenylyl cyclases as potential drug targets. Nat Rev Drug Discov 2009;8(4):321–335.

19. Hamel E: The biology of serotonin receptors: focus on migraine pathophysiology and treatment. Can J Neurol Sci, 1999;26(Suppl 3):S2–S6.

20. Bell IM: Calcitonin gene-related peptide receptor antagonists: new therapeutic agents for migraine. J Med Chem 2014;57(19):7838–7858.

21. McMahon SB: NGF as a mediator of inflammatory pain. Philos Trans R Soc Lond B Biol Sci 1996;351(1338):431–440.

22. Mizumura K, Murase S:, Role of nerve growth factor in pain. Handb Exp Pharmacol 2015;227:57–77.

23. Tiseo PJ, et al: Fasinumab (REGN475), an antibody against nerve growth factor for the treatment of pain: results from a double-blind, placebo-controlled exploratory study in osteoarthritis of the knee. Pain 2014; 155(7):1245–1252.

24. Malin SA, et al: Glial cell line-derived neurotrophic factor family members sensitize nociceptors in vitro and produce thermal hyperalgesia in vivo. J Neurosci 2006;26(33):8588–8599.

25. Wang R, et al: Artemin induced functional recovery and reinnervation after partial nerve injury. Pain 2014;155(3):476–484.

26. Yasaka T, et al: Populations of inhibitory and excitatory interneurons in lamina II of the adult rat spinal dorsal horn revealed by a combined electrophysiological and anatomical approach. Pain 2010;151(2):475–488.

27. Braz J, et al: Transmitting pain and itch messages: a contemporary view of the spinal cord circuits that generate gate control. Neuron 2014;82(3): 522–536.

28. Todd AJ: Neuronal circuitry for pain processing in the dorsal horn. Nat Rev Neurosci 2010;11(12):823–836.

29. Ikeda H, et al: Synaptic amplifier of inflammatory pain in the spinal dorsal horn. Science 2006;312(5780):1659–1662.

30. Djouhri L, Lawson SN: Abeta-fiber nociceptive primary afferent neurons: a review of incidence and properties in relation to other afferent A-fiber neurons in mammals. Brain Res Brain Res Rev 2004;46(2):131–145.

31. Zeilhofer HU, Wildner H, Yevenes GE: Fast synaptic inhibition in spinal sensory processing and pain control. Physiol Rev 2012;92(1):193–235.

32. Peirs C, et al: Dorsal horn circuits for persistent mechanical pain. Neuron 2015;87(4):797–812.

33. Schoffnegger D, Ruscheweyh R, Sandkuhler J: Spread of excitation across modality borders in spinal dorsal horn of neuropathic rats. Pain 2008; 135(3):300–310.

34. Laskowski K, et al: A systematic review of intravenous ketamine for postoperative analgesia. Can J Anaesth 2011;58(10):911–923.

35. McNicol ED, Schumann R, Haroutounian, S: A systematic review and meta-analysis of ketamine for the prevention of persistent post-surgical pain. Acta Anaesthesiol Scand 2014;58(10):1199–1213.

36. Bannister K, et al: Diffuse noxious inhibitory controls and nerve injury: restoring an imbalance between descending monoamine inhibitions and facilitations. Pain 2015;156(9):1803–1811.

37. Barbera-Cremades M, et al: P2X7 receptor-stimulation causes fever via PGE2 and IL-1beta release. FASEB J 2012;26(7):2951–2962.

38. Ulmann L, et al: Up-regulation of P2X4 receptors in spinal microglia after peripheral nerve injury mediates BDNF release and neuropathic pain. J Neurosci 2008;28(44):11263–11268.

39. Samad TA, Sapirstein A, Woolf CJ: Prostanoids and pain: unraveling mechanisms and revealing therapeutic targets. Trends Mol Med 2002; 8(8):390–396.

40. Zeilhofer HU, Ralvenius WT, Acuna MA: Restoring the spinal pain gate: GABA(A) receptors as targets for novel analgesics. Adv Pharmacol 2015; 73:71–96.

41. Kahle KT, et al: Therapeutic restoration of spinal inhibition via druggable enhancement of potassium-chloride cotransporter KCC2-mediated chloride extrusion in peripheral neuropathic pain. JAMA Neurol 2014; 71(5):640–645.

42. Abou-Raya A, Abou-Raya S, Khadrawe, T: Methotrexate in the treatment of symptomatic knee osteoarthritis: randomised placebo-controlled trial. Ann Rheum Dis 2014;

43. Landry RP, et al: Propentofylline, a CNS glial modulator does not decrease pain in post-herpetic neuralgia patients: in vitro evidence for differential responses in human and rodent microglia and macrophages. Exp Neurol 2012;234(2):340–350.

44. Melzack R: From the gate to the neuromatrix. Pain 1999(Suppl 6): S121–S126.

45. Tracey I: Can neuroimaging studies identify pain endophenotypes in humans? Nat Rev Neurol 2011;7(3):173–181.

46. Fomberstein K, Qadri S, Ramani, R: Functional MRI and pain. Curr Opin Anaesthesiol 2013;26(5):588–593.

47. Kucyi A, Davis KD: The dynamic pain connectome. Trends Neurosci 2015;38(2):86–95.

48. Helmstetter FJ, et al: Antinociception following opioid stimulation of the basolateral amygdala is expressed through the periaqueductal gray and rostral ventromedial medulla. Brain Res 1998;779(1–2):104–118.

49. Eippert F, et al: Activation of the opioidergic descending pain control system underlies placebo analgesia. Neuron 2009;63(4):533–43.

50. Pertovaara A: Noradrenergic pain modulation. Prog Neurobiol 2006;80(2): 53–83.

51. Villanueva L, Le Bars, D: The activation of bulbo-spinal controls by peripheral nociceptive inputs: diffuse noxious inhibitory controls. Biol Res 1995;28(1):113–125.

52. Kumar K, Wyant GM: Deep brain stimulation for alleviating chronic intractable pain. Can J Surg 1985;28(1):20–22.

53. Roditi D, Robinson, ME: The role of psychological interventions in the management of patients with chronic pain. Psychol Res Behav Manag 2011;4:41–49.

54. Goodin BR, et al: Intranasal oxytocin administration is associated with enhanced endogenous pain inhibition and reduced negative mood states. Clin J Pain 2014;

55. Xu Q, Yaksh, TL: A brief comparison of the pathophysiology of inflammatory versus neuropathic pain. Curr Opin Anaesthesiol 2011; 24(4):400–407.

56. Abbadie C, Brown JL, Mantyh PW, Basbaum AI: Spinal cord substance P receptor immunoreactivity increases in both inflammatory and nerve injury models of persistent pain. Neuroscience 1996;70(1):201–209.

57. Lautenbacher S, Kunz M, et al: Age effects on pain thresholds, temporal summation and spatial summation of heat and pressure pain. Pain. 2005; 115(3):410–418.

58. Prielipp RC and Warner MA: Perioperative nerve injury: a silent scream? Anesthesiology. 2009;111(3):464–466.

59. Mogil JS and Bailey AL: Sex and gender differences in pain and analgesia. Prog Brain Res. 2010;186:141–157.

60. Mogil JS: Pain genetics: past, present and future. Trends Genet. 2012;28(6):258–266.

CHAPTER 74

Pain: Epidemiology, Psychology, and Impact on Function

Trent Emerick and Steven L. Orebaugh

THE IMPACT OF PAIN

Some 30 million surgeries are performed annually in the United States, many resulting in significant acute postoperative pain. There also is an increasing trend toward utilization of oral opioids as the mainstay therapy.[1]

Although most available literature on the prevalence of pain and its effects on patients focuses on chronic, rather than acute, pain, these studies nonetheless provide important insights into the impact of pain on quality of life. The prevalence of chronic pain is estimated to be approximately 4.1% for extremity pain to 10.1% for low back pain, although there is considerable variability among reports.[2,3] The percentage of patients who experience severe pain after surgery is difficult to determine in the literature, although it has been approximated in the 20%-40% range.[4]

Osteoarthritis and rheumatoid arthritis remain two of the most common causes of chronic pain. Chronic pain affects many important aspects of a patient's life. These include sleep, exercise tolerance, activities of daily living, social activities, sexual function, and employment status.[5] In a European study of patients with chronic pain of various types, it was reported that patients with chronic pain lost a mean time of 7.8 days of work over a 6-month period due to their pain.[5] Approximately 60% of patients had visited a physician between two and nine times in the previous 6 months for pain-related issues. In this same study, 21% of respondents stated that they had been diagnosed with depression because of their pain.

Likewise, acute pain has many undesirable effects on patients beyond the unpleasantness of the sensory experience itself (Table 74–1). While the relationship between disturbed sleep and chronic pain remains somewhat difficult to discern, with evidence that either may exacerbate or facilitate the other,[6]

it is reasonably clear that acute, postoperative pain disturbs the sleep cycle,[7] and that this may require time to revert toward normal, especially with regard to restoration of lost rapid-eye-movement sleep.[8] The use of opioids in the perioperative period may further distort normal sleep patterns.[9]

Research suggests that both deep and superficial pain stimuli in muscle increase sympathetic nervous system activity, with concomitant elevations of heart rate and blood pressure.[10] Such adrenergic excitation may predispose older patients with vascular occlusive disease to be at risk for adverse postoperative outcomes, since tachycardia is an independent risk factor for perioperative myocardial infarction.[11] Highly effective analgesic techniques, such as the use of regional anesthesia, have the potential to reduce such complications.[12]

It is difficult to separate the effects of surgical tissue trauma from the pain that invariably accompanies it; as such, the marked elevation of serum markers of stress and inflammation that accompany tissue injury may at least, in part, be related to nociception. Studies suggest that improvements in pain control through regional techniques can attenuate these rises in inflammatory biomolecules,[13] which may also have favorable effects on perioperative outcome.[12]

Poorly controlled acute pain has deleterious effects on activities that patients wish or need to return to after surgery. For instance, on the day of surgery, improved pain control with peripheral nerve blockade results in earlier eating, drinking, ambulation, and discharge from the hospital, among other potential benefit[14,15] (Table 74–2). Although single-shot blocks do not appear to translate into a long-term reduced pain burden once they have resolved,[16] peripheral nerve block (PNB) catheters,[17] various additives, such as dexamethasone,[18] or altered drug formulations, such as liposomal bupivacaine,[19] may extend the duration of single blocks. Preservation

TABLE 74–1. Adverse effects of pain.

Depression
Sleep disturbance
Inactivity
Loss of socialization
Sexual dysfunction
Lost productivity at work
Metabolic stress response
Increased sympathetic activity

of quadriceps muscle strength in association with adequate pain control allows improved function and participation in physical therapy in the acute phase of recovery after total knee arthroplasty.[20] Improved pain control in the early postoperative period may allow patients to return to work earlier as well.[21]

In one large prospective study, younger age, female gender, and preoperative history of chronic pain were all found to be risk factors for more intense postoperative pain independent of the type of surgery.[22] In a large, prospective study in ambulatory surgical patients, Chung et al, reported that younger male patients, American Society of Anesthesiologists (ASA) Physical Status I patients, and patients with a greater body mass index (BMI) had the highest incidence of severe postoperative pain.[23]

Gerbershagen et al,[4] evaluated the level of pain on the first postoperative day among 179 different surgical types, and found that 22 of the top 40 most painful procedures were orthopedic or trauma procedures on the extremities. This underscores the potential of regional anesthesia in decreasing the occurrence of severe postoperative pain. Interestingly, these practitioners also noted that common procedures such as laparoscopic/open appendectomy, open cholecystectomy, and tonsillectomy also ranked in the top 25 most painful procedures. Of note, these procedures ranked worse in pain than open abdominal procedures with the use of neuraxial anesthesia.

Often, anesthesiologists care for acute pain in the recovery room, while surgeons continue to provide analgesia after patients leave the postanesthetic care unit (PACU) to return home or move to the ward, although continuous catheter techniques have resulted in a greater involvement in postoperative care. The current move toward a perioperative surgical home suggests that anesthesiologists will play a larger role in directing perioperative medical therapy and postoperative analgesia.[24]

TABLE 74–2. Benefits of improved perioperative pain control with regional techniques.

Improved patient satisfaction
Bypass of phase I recovery
Earlier discharge from hospital
Improved participation in physical therapy
Earlier return of concentratison
Fewer side effects of opioids
Earlier return of activities, including eating, drinking, ambulation

PAIN PSYCHOLOGY AND BEHAVIORAL EFFECTS OF PAIN

The connection between behavior, personality, and acute postoperative pain is an area of intense interest in pain research. For instance, some studies have shown that the act of catastrophizing (in which a patient treats minor issues as catastrophes) and a lower preoperative mental health score (as measured by a standardized mental health survey) result in worse scores on postoperative function and pain for total knee arthroplasty but not total hip arthroplasty.[25,26] In contrast, the preoperative level of anxiety, personality type, and fear of movement were psychologic symptoms that did not significantly affect the degree of postoperative pain or function.

Pain psychology is a component of a multidisciplinary approach to treatment of chronic pain.[27] Cognitive-behavioral therapy is one of the most commonly utilized approaches to treating a patient with chronic pain through behavioral modification. This therapy analyzes a patient's perception of pain as well as various psychologic variables such as anticipation, avoidance, and mood in an effort to alter how a patient ultimately responds to pain. One important finding of research in this area has been to elucidate that patients can actively process pain information, as opposed to being passive reactors, and that their thoughts can actively alter physiologic responses.[27]

Behavioral assessment is typically conducted through a personal interview with the patient, during which the examiner attempts to develop an understanding of the patient's experience with pain, elicit a detailed psychosocial history, and perform an evaluation of the patient's mood and coping mechanisms. Cognitive behavioral therapy can help patients develop coping skills such as relaxation, breathing exercises, and attention training whereby they concentrate their thinking on a nonpainful stimulus when their pain worsens.

In addition, there are a number of cognitive patterns that have been characterized in the pain psychology literature that are of direct importance to pain perception.[27,28] Examples of these patterns include the polarizing type (in which a patient characterizes a performance or feeling as either perfect or a failure), overgeneralization type (in which a patient assumes a single painful experiences translates into an overall poor outlook), and catastrophizing type.

ASSESSMENT OF PAIN

A myriad of pain-intensity scales have been developed to aid in the assessment and treatment of both acute and chronic pain. It is often noted that no single pain scale has been shown to be more efficacious than another, and these scales are not meant to compare one patient's pain levels to another patient's pain levels. Instead, pain scales should be utilized to compare a single patient's pain intensity at various time points. Many scales incorporate not only an assessment of the patient's pain but also how it impacts their mood and function.

The assessment of pain has become more thorough and complex over the last 20 years. In a speech to the American Pain Society in1995, Dr. James Campbell spoke on the idea of describing pain as the fifth vital sign in an attempt to bring about more effective pain management.[29] This idea was largely adopted by multiple national hospital oversight agencies including the Joint Commission on Accreditation of Healthcare Organizations (JCAHO) and the Veterans Health Administration and is used in hospital quality measures.[30,31] Unfortunately, since the adoption of pain as a fifth vital sign, opioid use has nearly doubled and the incidence of serious side effects due to opioid treatment has substantially increased as well. Morone and Weiner point out that providers will ultimately fall short in the management of a patient's pain if the treatment plan only considers the sensory component; pain is instead an important quality measure because it can impact sensation, mood, function, and cognition.[30] These investigators also note that there is a distinction between acute pain and chronic pain within a context of the vital sign. Chronic pain should not be viewed as a vital sign because it is a simplistic view of a multidimensional problem that often has varying impacts on a patient's life.

The Visual Analog Scale (VAS) is a unidimensional scale that rates a patient's pain on a scale of 0–10. It is very widely used, and its validity has been assessed in numerous patient populations for numerous painful conditions.[32-34] The revised version of the short form of the McGill Pain Questionnaire is a multidimensional validated pain scale that assesses the quality of a patient's neuropathic and nonnociceptive pain through assessment of gnawing, throbbing, or shooting, a pain intensity scale, and labeling pain on a diagram of the body.[35] The Brief Pain Inventory (BPI) also includes a human body pain diagram and questions on mood, function, and psychologic effects of their pain. This scale is widely used for various types of cancer pain and noncancer pain to assess pain and how it impacts a patient's life.[36,37] Furthermore, there are also numerous facial expression scales for evaluating pain in the pediatric population, such as the Wong-Baker FACES Scale.[38] These scales are cited as the preferred method of reporting pain in the pediatric population.[39]

All pain scales, however, have some limitations. First, the patient should have access to their previously reported pain scores to accurately assess their current pain.[40] Interestingly, it has been shown that patients rate their pain differently on using a VAS depending on whether the scale is presented in a vertical or horizontal format.[41] It is also difficult to directly convert a score from one pain scale to a score on a different pain scale.[42] Likewise, the pain score may not directly correlate with patient satisfaction as the data in the emergency medicine literature suggest.[43]

While historically, quantifying pain has taken on increasing importance, scoring alone is not sufficient to direct appropriate therapy and guide future research. Newer scoring systems take into account the alteration in function or activity that a patient experiences, as well as affective responses to the pain, as noted above. The direction of research in postoperative acute pain management is now oriented toward more inclusive assessments, conducted at multiple time periods.[44,45] In 2013, Choi et al evaluated the acute pain literature related to total knee arthroplasty, and found the assessment of postoperative pain and function was seriously deficient, and they called for increased use of more comprehensive scoring systems as well as repeated assessments in the short, intermediate, and long term.[45]

PAIN PHENOTYPING

The future of acute and chronic pain management is evolving toward the ability to tailor a patient's pain regimen in a more individualized fashion. Janda et al recently reported that preoperative fibromyalgia survey scores can predict postoperative opioid consumption in patients having a hysterectomy.[46] The fibromyalgia survey score ranges from 0–31 and incorporates a number of painful body areas (score of 0–19) and associated symptoms such as fatigue and headaches among other factors (score of 0–12). In this study, each 1-point increase in the 31-point fibromyalgia scale equated with an adjusted increase of approximately 7 mg in total morphine dose in the acute inpatient postoperative period. Although only 8.2% of patients in the survey were considered "fibromyalgia positive" based on a total score of 13 or greater of 31, it is important to note that the associations between opioid use and fibromyalgia score could be seen across all scores. For instance, Brummet et al also showed that the fibromyalgia score was predictive of postoperative opioid consumption in the knee and hip arthroplasty population.[47]

Clinical Pearls

- Pain, whether acute or chronic, causes major life disruption for patients, and disturbs many activities of living, leading to significant psychologic consequences.
- Pain may be assessed and quantitated with a number of different scales. However, it is becoming increasingly important to assess not only the degree of discomfort experienced by a patient, but also the severity of functional and psychologic disruption.
- Pain phenotyping seeks to determine which patients may be predisposed to a greater degree of discomfort after a procedure, and this information can be utilized to more effectively plan an analgesic regimen.
- Opioids are useful and effective analgesics, but are limited by adverse effects. Multimodal analgesic techniques allow for a greater diversity of interventions with less reliance on opioids. In acute pain, regional techniques can be particularly effective.

Catastrophizing has been shown to be predictive of increased postoperative opioid requirements. This behavior could potentially be recognized during the preoperative assessment in order to aid in postoperative management.[46] It has been suggested that patients with higher fibromyalgia scores or other preoperative pain phenotyping scores may have intrinsic differences in the functioning of the intrinsic opioid system.[48] These scores could potentially be utilized by the anesthesiologist to customize an intraoperative and postoperative plan that minimizes the likelihood of severe pain.

Individual differences in a patient's endogenous opioid function may dictate a patient's response to exogenous opioids such as morphine. For example, patients with low endogenous opioid function and those with high endogenous opioid function

PART 12

were exposed in one study to two forms of acute evoked painful stimuli. The patients with lower levels of endogenous opioid function at baseline showed a greater response to morphine than those with higher degrees of function at baseline. This may have clinical applications in the future, and methods to test endogenous opioid function may be increasingly more often used.[49] Morphine appears to provide better relief in the treatment of chronic back pain in patients with lower endogenous opioid function as well.[50]

Limitations of Opioid-Based Analgesia

A multimodal treatment plan is of particular benefit to patients' perioperative pain, whether preexisting or not, given the inherent limitations of opioids. The World Health Organization (WHO) has produced an analgesic ladder (originally developed for cancer pain) that helps providers form an algorithm to treat pain in a balanced and multimodal approach—nonopioids for mild to moderate pain, mild opioids for moderate to severe pain, and strong opioids for severe pain.[51]

Common examples of frustrating side effects of opioids include constipation, nausea, pruritus, dysphoria, and urinary retention.[52,53] More serious adverse effects include the development of ileus, with attendant delays in oral intake, as well as oversedation and life-threatening hypoventilation[54] (Table 74–3). Opioids have been associated with numerous deaths during treatment of both acute and chronic pain.[55]

There is a considerable amount of literature that describes not only tolerance to opioids from chronic use but also rapid acute tolerance to perioperatively administered opioids.[56–59] Although there is a decreasing margin of efficacy with opioid medications over time due to opioid tolerance, the connection between chronic pain and addiction/opioid abuse deserves further clarification.[52] Finally, the concern for opioid-induced hyperalgesia both in the acute postoperative pain setting (as well as the chronic pain setting) should not be ignored.[60]

Just as the WHO ladder deemphasized opioids when possible to treat chronic pain, multimodal analgesia should be utilized in the acute setting to minimize perioperative pain. Multimodal analgesia incorporates various pharmacologic

TABLE 74–3. Adverse effects of opioids.

Nausea
Dysphoria
Dizziness
Depression
Confusion
Altered mental status
Pruritus
Ileus
Urinary retention
Hypoventilation
Sedation
Androgen deficiency
Modulation of immune system function

TABLE 74–4. Potential components of multimodal analgesia.

Nonsteroidal anti-inflammatory drugs
Acetaminophen
Cyclooxygenase-2 inhibitors
Tramadol
Tricyclic antidepressants
Topical lidocaine ointment
Serotonin norepinephrine reuptake inhibitors
Systemic opioids
Neuraxial opioids
α_2 agonists (e.g., dexmeditomidine)
Ketamine and dextromethorphan (N-methyl-D-aspartate antagonists)
Magnesium
Local anesthetic parenteral infusion
Gabapentinoids
Beta-blocking agents
Local anesthetic wound injection
Neuraxial local anesthetic infusion
Peripheral nerve blockade

agents such as acetaminophen, nonsteriodal anti-inflammatories, gabapentinoids, and α_2 agonists,[61,62] as well as other analgesic techniques (Table 74–4). For example, both the preoperative use of beta blockers and α_2 agonists have been shown to have anesthesia-sparing and analgesia-sparing effects and reduce postoperative pain and improve cardiovascular stability.[63] In addition, steroids, local anesthetic infusions, and magnesium have all shown some promise in the management of acute pain.[62,64] In addition, there is some evidence that multimodal analgesia may reduce the incidence of chronic postsurgical pain.

Regional anesthesia should be an integral part of a multimodal treatment plan in order to minimize the side-effect burden of opioid medications. Peripheral nerve blockade and/or catheter placement is practical and effective in the perioperative setting for orthopedic and many other painful surgeries.[65,66] Liu et al reported in a meta-analysis that neuraxial and peripheral nerve blockades reduced postoperative pain scores and reduced PACU analgesic administration compared to general anesthesia.[67] Compared with general anesthesia, peripheral nerve blockade has also been shown to increase the ability to bypass PACU, decrease nausea, decrease the number of minutes of stay in PACU, and increased incidence of excellent patient satisfaction.[14,15] Continuous peripheral nerve catheters improve pain control for a longer period, and also favorably affect discharge times for both upper and lower extremity procedures.[68,69]

Considerable debate exists as to whether opioids can alleviate specific types of chronic pain such as neuropathic pain. Furlan et al,[52] as well as other investigators,[70] demonstrated that neuropathic and musculoskeletal pain intensity scores may be decreased by as much as 30% with potent opioids for chronic pain. Many studies evaluating the benefits of long-term opioid use have significant limitations, and further study is required to firmly address this question. Functional improvement is another endpoint which requires ongoing investigation for patients with chronic pain as well, as such benefits have been called into question.[1,70,71]

SUMMARY

Acute, postoperative pain is often inadequately controlled. This is also true for many surgeries that are not routinely thought of as being "painful." Pain, both acute and chronic, has significant effects on a patient's psychology, as well as measurable physiologic effects, including a biomolecular and adrenergic stress response. The impact of pain on patients' daily activities is profound, and serious life disruption is common. Psychologic profiles have given us insight into which patients may have an increased pain burden after surgery, as has pain phenotyping. Both aspects of pain assessment may allow for better and more individualized analgesic regimens in the future. Pain assessment scoring systems have increased in complexity and breadth in order to take into account the impact of pain on the individual, rather than simply allowing quantitative expressions of its severity at a moment in time. Multimodal analgesic techniques with integration of peripheral nerve blockade or other regional anesthesia techniques have the potential for the greatest effect on reducing both pain and its associated adverse outcomes, as well as the many undesirable side effects of high-dose opioids.

REFERENCES

1. Sites BD, Beach ML, Davis MA. Increases in the use of prescription opioids analgesics and the lack of improvement in disability metrics among users Reg Anesth Pain Med 2014;39:6.
2. Hardt J, Jacobsen C, Goldberg J, et al: Prevalence of chronic pain in a representative sample in the united states. Pain Med 2008;9:803.
3. National Center for Health Statistics. United *States Chartbook on Trends in the Health of Americans.* Hyattsville, MD, 2006, p 68.
4. Gerbershagen H, Aduckathil S, van Wijck A, et al: Pain intensity on the first day after surgery: a prospective cohort study comparing 179 surgical procedures. Anesthesiology 2013;118:934.
5. Breivik H, Collett B, Ventafridda V, et al: Survey of chronic pain in Europe: prevalence, impact on daily life, and treatment. Eur. J Pain 2006;10:287.
6. Finan PH, Goodin BR, Smith MT: The association of sleep and pain. J Pain 2013;14:1539.
7. Miller A, Roth T, Roehrs T, et al: Correlation between sleep disruption and postoperative pain. Otol-Head Neck Surg 2015;152:964.
8. Chung F, Liao P, Yegneswaran B, et al: Postoperative changes in sleep-disordered breathing and sleep architecture in patients with obstructive sleep apnea. Anesthesiology 2014;120:287.
9. Cronin AJ, Keifer JC, Davies MF, et al: Postoperative sleep disturbance: influences of opioids and pain in humans. Sleep 2001;24:39.
10. Burton AR, Birznieks I, Bolton PS, et al: Effects of deep and superficial experimentally induced acute pain on muscle sympathetic nerve activity in human subjects. J Physiol 2009;587:183.
11. Devereaux PJ, Xavier D, Pogue J, et al: Characteristics and short-term prognosis of perioperative myocardial infarction in patients undergoing noncardiac surgery: a cohort study. Ann Intern Med 2011;154:523.
12. Memtsoudis SG, Sun X, Chiu YL, et al: Perioperative comparative effectiveness of anesthetic technique in orthopedic patients. Anesthesiology 2013;118:1046.
13. Ezhevskaya AA, Mlyavykh SG, Anderson DG. Effects of continuous epidural anesthesia and postoperative epidural analgesia on pain management and stress response in patients undergoing major spinal surgery. Spine 2013;38:1224.
14. Hadzic A, Arliss J, Kerimoglu B, et al: A comparison of infraclavicular nerve block versus general anesthesia for hand and wrist day-case surgeries. Anesthesiology 2004;101:127.
15. Hadzic A, Williams BA, Caraca PE, et al: For outpatient rotator cuff surgery, nerve block anesthesia provides superior same-day recovery over general anesthesia. Anesthesiology 2005;102:1001.
16. McCarntney CJL, Brull R, Chan VWS, et al: Early but no long-term benefit of regional compared with general anesthesia for ambulatory hand surgery. Anesthesiology 2004;101:461.
17. McGraw III RP, Ilfeld BM: Toward outpatient arthroplasty: accelerating discharge with ambulatory continuous peripheral nerve blocks. Int Anesth Clin 2012;50:111.
18. Choi S, Dodseth R, McCartney CJL: Effects of dexamethasone as a local anaesthetic adjuvant for brachial plexus block: a systematic review and meta-analysis of randomized trials. Br J Anaesth 2014;112:427.
19. Ilfled BM, Jalhotra N, Furnish TJ, et al: Liposomal bupivacaine as a single-injectin peripheral nerve block: a dose response study. Anesth Analg 2013;117:1248.
20. Jaeger P, Zaric D, Fomsgaard JS, et al: Adductor canal block versus femoral nerve block for analgesia after total knee arthroplasty. Reg Anesth Pain Med 2013;38:526.
21. White PF, Kehlet H. Postoperative pain management and patient outcome: time to return to work! Anesth Analg 2007;104:487.
22. Gerbershagen H, Pogatzki-Zahn E, Aduckathil S, et al: Procedure-specific risk factor analysis for the development of severe postoperative pain Anesthesiology 2014;120:1237.
23. Chung F, Ritchie E, Su J: Postoperative Pain in ambulatory surgery. Anesth Analg 1997;85:808.
24. Cyriac J, Cannesson M, Kain Z. Pain management and the perioperative surgical home. Reg Anesth Pain Med 2015;40:1.
25. Vissers M, Bussmann J, Verhaar J, et al: Psychological factors affecting the outcome of total hip and knee arthroplasty: a systematic review. Semin Arthritis Rheum 2012;41:4, 576.
26. Vissers MM, de Groot IB, Reijman M, et al: Functional capacity and actual daily activity do not contribute to patient satisfaction after total knee arthroplasty. BMC Musculoskelet Disord 2010;11:121.
27. Okifuji A, Ackerlind S. Behavioral medicine approaches to pain. Med Clin North Am 2007;91:45.
28. Sullivan MJL, D'Eon JL. Relation between catastrophizing and depression in chronic pain patients. J Abnorm Psychol 1990;99:260.
29. Campbell JN. American Pain Society 1995 presidential address. Pain Forum 1996;5:85.
30. Morone NE, Weiner DK: Pain as the fifth sign: exposing the vital need for patient education. Clin Therap 2013;35:1728.
31. Pain as the 5th Vital Sign Toolkit: 2000 at http://www.va.gov/painmanagement/docs/toolkit.pdf last accessed July 26, 2015.
32. Taddio A, O'Brien L, Ipp M, et al: Reliability and validity of observer ratings of pain using the visual analog scale (VAS) in infants undergoing immunization injections. Pain 2009;147:141.
33. Gallagher EJ, Bijur PE, Latimer C, et al: Reliability and validity of a visual analog scale for acute abdominal pain in the ED. Am J Emerg Med 2002;20:287.
34. Bringuier S, Dadure C, Raux O, et al; The perioperative validity of the visual analog anxiety scale in children: a discriminant and useful instrument in routine clinical practice to optimize postoperative pain management. Anesth Analg 2009;109:737.
35. Dworkin RH, Turk DC, Revicki DA, et al: Development and initial validation of an expanded and revised version of the Short-form McGill Pain Questionnaire (SF-MPQ-2). Pain 2009;144:35.
36. Keller S, Bann CM, Dodd SL, et al: Validity of the brief pain inventory for use in documenting the outcomes of patients with noncancer pain. Clin J Pain 2004;20:309.
37. Cleeland CS, Ryan KM. Pain assessment: global use of the Brief Pain Inventory. Ann Acad Med Singapore 2004;23:129.
38. Chambers CT, Giesbrecht K, Craig KD, et al: A comparison of faces scales for the measurement of pediatric pain: children's and parents' ratings. Pain 1999;83:25.
39. Keck JF, Gerkensmeyer JE, Joyce BA, et al: Validity of the Faces and Word Descriptor scales to measure procedural pain. J Pediatr Nurs. 1996;11:368.
40. Farrar JT, Portenoy RK, Berlin JA, et al. Defining the clinically important difference in pain outcome measures. Pain 2000;88:287.
41. Scott J, Huskisson EC. Vertical or horizontal visual analogue scales. Ann Rheum Dis 1979;38:560.
42. Williamson, A, Hoggart, B. Pain: a review of three commonly used pain rating scales. J Clin Nurs 2005;14:98.
43. Kelly A. Patient satisfaction with pain management does not correlate with initial or discharge VAS pain score, verbal pain rating at discharge, or change in VAS score in the emergency department. J Emerg Med 2000;19:113.

44. Ilfeld BM, Meyer RS, Le LT, et al: Health-related quality of life after tricompartment arthroplasty with and without an extended-duration continuous femoral nerve block: A prospective, 1-year follow up of a randomized, triple-masked, placebo-controlled study. Anesth Analg 2009;108:1320.

45. Choi S, Trang A, McCartney CJL. Reporting functional outcome after knee arthroplasty and regional anesthesia. Reg Anesth Pain Med 2013; 38:340.

46. Janda AM, As-Sanie S, Rajala B, et al: Fibromyalgia survey criteria are associated with increased postoperative opioid consumption in women undergoing hysterectomy. Anesthesiology 2015;122:1103.

47. Brummett CM, Janda AM, Schueller CM, et al: Survey criteria for fibromyalgia independently predict increased postoperative opioid consumption after lower-extremity joint arthroplasty: A prospective, observational cohort study. Anesthesiology 2013;119:1434.

48. Bruehl, S. Personalized pain medicine: pipe dream or reality? Anesthesiology 2015;122:967.

49. Bruehl S, Burns JW, Gupta R, et al: Endogenous opioid function mediates the association between laboratory-evoked pain sensitivity and morphine analgesic responses. Pain 2013;154:1856.

50. Bruehl S, Burns JW, Gupta R, et al: Endogenous opioid inhibition of chronic low-back pain influences degree of back pain relief after morphine administration. Reg Anesth Pain Med 2014;39:120.

51. World Health Organization: *Cancer Pain Relief*, 2nd ed. WHO, Geneva, 1996.

52. Furlan AD, Sandoval JA, Mailis-Gagnon A, et al: Opioids for chronic noncancer pain: a meta-analysis of effectiveness and side effects. Can Med Assoc J 2006;174:1589.

53. White PF. The changing role of non-opioid analgesic techniques in the management of postoperative pain. Anesth Analg 2005;101:S5.

54. Macintyre PE, Loadsman JA, Scott DA. Opioids, ventilation and pain management. Anaesth Int Care 2011;39:545.

55. Centers for Disease Control and Prevention. Vital signs: overdoses of prescription opioid pain relievers, United States, 1999–2008. MMWR 2011;60:1487.

56. Martin WR, Eades CG: Demonstration of tolerance and physical dependence in the dog following a short-term infusion of morphine. J Pharmacol Exp Ther 1961;133:262.

57. Kissin I, Brown PT, Bradley EL: Magnitude of acute tolerance to opioids is not related to their potency. Anesthesiology 1991;75:813.

58. Angst, MS: Intraoperative use of remifentanil for TIVA: postoperative pain, acute tolerance, and opioid-induced hyperalgesia. JCardiothoracic Vasc Anesth 2015;29(Suppl 1):S16.

59. Leah PM, Heath EM, Balleine BW, et al: Chronic morphine reduces surface expression of δ-opioid receptors in subregions of rostral striatum. 2015 June [Epub ahead of print]

60. Prof C., Prof S. Treatment of acute postoperative pain. Lancet 2011; 377:2215.

61. Jin F, Chung F: Multimodal analgesia for postoperative pain control. J Clin Anesth 2001;13:524.

62. Young A, Buvanendran A: Recent advances in multimodal analgesia. Anesth Clin 2012;30:91.

63. White P, Kehlet H, Neal J, et al: The role of the anesthesiologist in fast-track surgery: from multimodal analgesia to perioperative medical care. Anesth Analg 2007;104:1380.

64. De Oliveira Jr. GS, Almeida MD, Benzon HT, et al: Perioperative single does systemic dexamethasoine for postoperative pain. Anesthesiology 2011;115:575.

65. McGraw RP, Ilfeld BM. Toward outpatient arthroplasty: Accelerating discharge with ambulatory continuous nerve blocks. Int Anesth Clin 2012;50:111.

66. Sinatra RS, Torres J, Bustos AM. Pain management after major orthopedic surgery: Current strategies and new concepts. J Am Coll Orthop Surg 2002;10:117.

67. Liu S, Strodbeck W, Richman J, et al: A Comparison of regional versus general anesthesia for ambulatory anesthesia: a meta-analysis of randomized controlled trials. Anesth Analg 2005;101:1634.

68. Ilfeld BM, Morey TE, Enneking FK: Continuous infraclavicular brachial plexus block for postoperative pain control at home: a randomized, double-blinded, placebo-controlled study. Anesthesiology 2002;96:1297, 2002.

69. White PF, Issioui T, Skrivanek GD, et al: The use of a continuous popliteal sciatic nerve block after surgery involving the foot and ankle: does it improve the quality of recovery. Anesth Analg 2003;97:1303, 2003.

70. Kalso E, Edwards J, Moore A, et al: Opioids in chronic non-cancer pain: systematic review of efficacy and safety. Pain 2004;112:372.

71. Caldwell JR, Rapoport RJ, Davis JC, et al: Efficacy and safety of a once-daily morphine formulation in chronic, moderate-to-severe osteoarthritis pain: results from a randomized, placebo-controlled, double-blind trial and an open-label extension trial. J Pain Symp Manag 2002;23:278.

CHAPTER 75

Multimodal Analgesia: Pharmacologic Interventions and Prevention of Persistent Postoperative Pain

Adam C. Young and Asokumar Buvanendran

INTRODUCTION

Multimodal analgesia was popularized in 1993 by Kehlet and Dahl and described as "combined analgesic regimens" in order to achieve "sufficient analgesia due to additive or synergistic effects between different analgesics, with concomitant reduction of side effects."[1] Through the past 20 years, many patients have benefitted from practical implementation of this concept. By modulating multiple receptor-ligand systems involved in the transduction and sensation of pain, we have also appreciated the ability for certain agents to reduce acute postoperative pain and, therefore, reduce the incidence of persistent postsurgical pain. Several individual medications have been identified, although precise dosage, timing, and route of administration have yet to be completely understood. Additionally, there are techniques available, which if used in the perioperative phase, may prevent development of chronic pain after surgery.

MULTIMODAL ANALGESIA

Many analgesic combinations have been shown to demonstrate synergistic analgesia when used in combination, as opposed to the analgesic effects of those agents used individually. Examples include combinations of acetaminophen, nonsteroidal anti-inflammatory drugs (NSAIDs), N-methyl D-aspartate (NMDA)–receptor antagonists, anticonvulsants, and corticosteroids. Other mechanisms of analgesia include the use of regional anesthesia and local wound infiltration.

The sum of these efforts can result in a postoperative course that allows patients undergoing some of the more painful surgical procedures, even total knee arthroplasty, to meet discharge criteria and be discharged the same day as surgery.[2,3]

Surgical stimuli produce a multitude of mediators—leading to inflammation, sensitization, and pain.[4,5] The process begins with tissue damage and the production of prostaglandins (PGs), particularly PGE_2.[4] Other mediators include histamine, bradykinin,[5] substance P, and the excitatory neurotransmitters (glutamate and aspartate).[6] Nociceptors become sensitized as a result of the expression of the c-fos, nitric oxide (NO) synthase, and cyclooxygenase (COX) genes augmenting the sensation of pain and perhaps beginning the process of developing persistent postsurgical pain. By using a multimodal approach to treating acute surgical pain, the various mediators or their targets, optimal pain relief can be achieved both acutely and chronically.

Acetaminophen

Acetaminophen, (paracetamol), produces its analgesic effect by inhibiting central prostaglandin synthesis with minimal inhibition of peripheral prostaglandin synthesis.[7,8] Often labeled as an NSAID, the two substances have some important differences. This includes acetaminophen's weak anti-inflammatory effect[9] and its generally poor ability to inhibit COX in sites of inflammation.[10] Unlike NSAIDs, acetaminophen does not have an adverse effect on platelets[11] or the gastric mucosa.[10]

The use of acetaminophen in the perioperative setting had been limited until intravenous (IV) acetaminophen became available for use. The IV formulation has some benefits over enteral routes of administration; bioavailability is 100% and shorter time peak effect; the onset of 'meaningful' pain relief is less than 30 minutes after administration.[12] In addition, the IV formulation of acetaminophen has been used as the foundation for multimodal analgesia in Europe for years. Since its introduction in the United States, IV acetaminophen has gained praise in the surgical community, and its benefits have been reported in several randomized clinical trials and meta-analyses. The latest shows that IV acetaminophen reduced pain and also the opioid-related side effects.[13]

When used as a combination with NSAIDs, acetaminophen confers superior analgesia compared to either drug alone.[14] This synergism highlights the value of combined central and peripheral COX inhibition. The combination of NSAIDs and acetaminophen has also been proven to decrease pain scores, opioid consumption, sedation, and postoperative nausea and vomiting and improve patient satisfaction in the acute postoperative period.[14,15] Overall, IV acetaminophen has been well received by both patients and physicians and it has become the foundation for multimodal analgesia.

The total daily maximum dose of acetaminophen is 3000 mg to decrease the risk of hepatotoxicity. Prescribers need to take into account combination tablets containing acetaminophen (e.g., Norco, Percocet, or Excedrin) when making this calculation. Liver failure is an absolute contraindication to its administration; relative contraindications include hepatic insufficiency, alcohol abuse, and alcohol dependency.

NSAIDs

Nonselective NSAIDs (e.g., ibuprofen, naproxen, ketorolac) inhibit both the COX-1 and COX-2 isoforms. When cell membranes are damaged, arachadonic acid is liberated; these drugs decrease the conversion of arachadonic acid to prostaglandins and thromboxane. Peripherally, prostaglandin E_1 (PGE_1) and prostaglandin E_2 (PGE_2) sensitize nociceptive sensory nerve endings to histamine and bradykinin.[16,17] The same prostaglandins modulate nociceptors to respond to nonnociceptive stimuli.[18,19] By reducing PGE_1 and PGE_2, NSAIDs decrease inflammation and these processes that lead to sensing pain.

The risks of renal damage, gastrointestinal hemorrhage, and platelet dysfunction[20] have led some physicians to forego using nonspecific NSAIDs in the perioperative period. These effects are due to the inhibition of COX-1, an enzyme that is expressed constitutively. Conversely, the COX-2 isoform is upregulated in damaged tissue,[21] and the desired anti-inflammatory effects of NSAIDs in the periphery can be realized without these posed risks.

Nonspecific COX inhibitors, ibuprofen, and ketorolac have been used intravenously in the acute pain and perioperative setting. Ketorolac has an a COX-1:COX-2 specificity of approximately 330:1,[22] onset of action of 10 minutes, peak analgesic effect at 2–3 hours, and analgesic duration of 6–8 hours.[7] As a single 30-mg preoperative dose, ketorolac has been shown to decrease narcotic consumption and limit nausea. Ketorolac has been incorporated in multimodal pain regimens for total joint arthroplasty and reduced acute postoperative opioid consumption.[18–19] IV ibuprofen may be more attractive for

perioperative pain management given its stronger affinity for the COX-2 isoform (COX-1:COX-2 ratio of 2.5:1).[24] Suggested dosing begins at 400 mg every 6 hours; however, greater analgesia is observed following doses of 800 mg every 6 hours.[23] The current literature includes three small studies that demonstrated IV ibuprofen improves acute pain at rest and with movement, promotes faster times to ambulation, and reduces opioid requirements following surgical procedures.[25,24]

There is only one selective COX-2 inhibitor available to the practitioner in the United States, celecoxib, and it is administered orally. Doses range from 100–200 mg and administration can be taken daily or twice daily. There is a suggestion that initiating a COX-2 inhibitor 2–3 days prior to surgery can lead to accumulation in the cerebrospinal fluid, providing benefit in the perioperative period.[25] Ideally, a COX-2 inhibitor should be continued for at least 2 weeks following surgery, as this coincides with the duration of the acute inflammatory process. Celecoxib has been incorporated in multimodal regimens and consistently demonstrates reduced opioid requirements and correlates with earlier physical activity.[26] In joint arthroplasty, incorporating celecoxib has been correlated with improved outcomes, such as range of motion.[27]

The use of NSAIDs to prevent the development of chronic pain remains controversial. The studies that have investigated NSAIDs have frequently employed ibuprofen or ketorolac in varying doses, and if not administered in a single dose, for short durations postoperatively. The results have favored single-dose ketorolac to reduce pain in the acute postoperative period,[28] although these have failed to demonstrate prevention of chronic pain.[29] With regard to celecoxib, one study did demonstrate a significant difference in pain at rest in patients 12 weeks postoperatively after knee arthroplasty; this difference was not maintained beyond 12 weeks.[29]

Contraindications to NSAIDs include allergy to aspirin as well as to sulfonamides. The dose should be reduced in the elderly or those with reduced renal function. Despite clear evidence, there is concern that NSAIDs in the perioperative period can lead to impaired bone healing.[30] Prior to prescribing an NSAID following a procedure in which bone was manipulated, we suggest consulting with the surgeon.

Anticonvulsants

The gamma-aminobutyric acid analogues, gabapentin and pregabalin, bind to the $\alpha_2\delta$-subunit of the voltage-dependent calcium channel. These drugs inhibit the opening of these channels and reduce the influx of calcium and consequently the release of excitatory neurotransmitters (substance P and calcitonin gene–related peptide). The evidence for incorporating anticonvulsants in multimodal analgesia has increased dramatically. Gabapentin and pregabalin are two of the most commonly used medications in this class; however, there are unique differences to each.

Gabapentin is an orally administered medication that is actively transported across the gastrointestinal mucosa. There are individual differences in the amount of transporters that an individual patient has, and as a consequence patients respond differently to similar doses of gabapentin. As an example, gabapentin 900 mg divided three times per day has an oral bioavailability of nearly 60%. Escalating the dose to 1200, 2400, or 3600 mg results in 47%, 34%, or 33% oral bioavailability, respectively.[31] This point demonstrates the ability of gabapentin to saturate the transporter system assigned to its absorption. Despite the challenges with titrating gabapentin, some studies have shown perioperative gabapentin can lead to improved functional recovery in knee arthroplasty, acutely reducing opioid consumption, and demonstrating fewer opioid-related side effects (nausea, vomiting, and pruritus).

Pregabalin has become popular in the perioperative period on account of its ≥90% oral bioavailability, longer half-life, increased lipid solubility (more readily crossing the blood-brain barrier), and fewer drug interactions.[32] Similar results of opioid-sparing and decreased opioid-related side effects have been seen with pregabalin administered perioperatively.

Voltage-dependent calcium channels may play an important role in developing chronic pain; these receptors are upregulated in the dorsal root ganglia following surgical trauma and are thought to lead to central sensitization.[10] This has been tested in animal models; administering pregabalin has been shown to reduce postoperative hyperalgesia in these studies.[33]

The ability of anticonvulsants to reduce chronic pain has been reviewed with the finding that both gabapentin and pregabalin can reduce the incidence of chronic pain.[34,35] In those reviews, anticonvulsants demonstrated this effect in patients undergoing thyroidectomy, cardiac surgery, abdominal hysterectomy, knee arthroplasty, inguinal hernia repair, or mastectomy. The investigators studying this meta-analysis indicated that pregabalin might have a greater ability to prevent chronic pain compared to gabapentin.

On an outpatient basis, titration of gabapentin is usually accomplished over several weeks to months to achieve satisfactory relief, likely corresponding with adequate serum levels of this drug. This limitation has been expressed in studies investigating single doses of perioperative gabapentin; anywhere from 300–1200 mg have had no impact on chronic postsurgical pain.[31] Even a titration to a median of 2100 mg/day did not have long-term effects in one study.[36] This limitation of gabapentin has been overcome by using pregabalin in the acute postoperative period. Pregabalin given preoperatively and repeated within 24 hours of surgery was effective in reducing chronic pain following discectomy and thyroidectomy.[37–38] Extended courses of pregabalin may prove additional benefit in surgical procedures notorious for inciting chronic postsurgical pain, such as total knee arthroplasty. A single preoperative dose of pregabalin 300 mg followed by a 14-day course of 300 mg divided twice daily reduced the incidence of persistent postsurgical pain to 0% at 6 months following total knee arthroplasty (compared to 5.2% in the placebo group).[39] Of note, the incidence of sedation was significantly higher in the treatment group.

Anticonvulsant use can be limited by side effects. These include dizziness, somnolence, ataxia, blurred vision, weight gain, and fatigue. The best method to minimize these effects is to use the lowest effective dose, titrating to the higher (clinically therapeutic) dosages as tolerated. A reduced dose is indicated in the elderly or patients with impaired renal function, as both gabapentin and pregabalin are excreted renally.

NMDA-Receptor Antagonists

Inhibition of the NMDA receptor is another means of improving pain by prolonging analgesia in the acute setting, potentially attenuating opioid-induced hyperalgesia (OIH), and reducing the incidence of chronic pain. NMDA-receptor antagonism is suspected to interfere with the development of OIH. OIH is a paradoxical effect of the administration of opioids that results in increased sensitivity to noxious stimuli. It has been suggested that OIH develops as a result of changes in both the antinociceptive and pronociceptive systems[40]; NMDA receptors have a role in modulating these processes. It is worth noting that patients with OIH experience postoperative pain that is often difficult to treat. This is of importance as poorly controlled acute pain is an independent risk factor for the development of chronic pain.[41]

Ketamine is a noncompetitive NMDA-receptor antagonist. The discovery of the NMDA receptor and its links to nociceptive pain transmission and central sensitization has renewed interest in ketamine. Ketamine has become the NMDA receptor of choice in the perioperative period. Outside of the operating room, administering ketamine can be difficult as oral preparations are not commonly on formulary and intravenous infusions present a challenge to all personnel involved in patient care.

Ketamine, as part of a multimodal regimen, has been shown to decrease opioid consumption and lower pain scores following spine and hip surgery.[42,43] This is merely part of a growing body of evidence that low-dose ketamine may play an important role when used as an adjunct to opioids, local anesthetics, and other analgesic agents.[44] In combination with IV or epidural opioids, ketamine also prolongs and improves analgesia.

Memantine is available as an oral formulation and could be useful in the acute postoperative period as it is a more potent NMDA-receptor antagonist with a longer half-life. Current studies have not supported perioperative memantine for reducing acute or chronic pain. One study indicated that following traumatic amputation memantine, in combination with regional anesthesia, decreased overall phantom pain intensity for up to 6 months. However, these effects were not maintained beyond 6 months; the treatment group had similar pain scores as the placebo group at 1 year postoperatively.[45]

Ketamine has been shown by prior investigators to reduce the incidence of persistent postsurgical pain in patients undergoing a variety of procedures. A single dose of ketamine 0–0.5 mg/kg followed by an intraoperative and postoperative infusion of 0.7–4.2 mcg/kg/min was able to demonstrate fewer cases of persistent postsurgical pain at 6 months.[44,46,47] A meta-analysis of these data supported not only a preincisional bolus and intraoperative infusion, but an infusion for up to 24 hours.[31] In a separate study, patients undergoing spine surgery received ketamine 0.5 mg/kg followed by an intraoperative ketamine infusion of 10 mcg/kg/min correlated with reduced pain scores compared to placebo at 6 weeks.[45] Although this does not meet the 3-month time mark (which is required to meet the definition of persistent postsurgical pain), this is an impressive finding as these patients were opioid dependent prior to their spine surgery.

Ketamine may have received a "bad rap" with regard to its side effects. It is known that high doses (>2 mg/kg) can cause psychomimetic effects including hallucinations, nightmares, cognitive dysfunction, or excessive sedation. Low-dose ketamine (<1 mg/kg) appears to be associated with less adverse effects and may allow physicians to harness the benefits of perioperative ketamine.

Steroids

Administration of steroids in the perioperative period serves to modulate peripheral inflammatory pathways. By reducing the flood of inflammatory mediators, postoperative pain can be attenuated by adding corticosteroids to a multimodal regimen. Timing of administration to obtain the anti-inflammatory benefits appears to be most effective if steroids are administered preoperatively. The optimal dosage has been debated. Some investigators have obtained a positive effect in reducing acute postoperative pain with dexamethasone 16 mg as part of a multimodal regimen.[48] Half the dose (dexamethasone 8 mg) has provided mixed results; some investigators obtained the same positive result[49] and others have not.[50]

Side effects of corticosteroids have produced some hesitance in investigators using them more widely. These effects include gastrointestinal complications, wound healing complications, hyperglycemia, and potential suppression of the hypothalamic-pituitary-adrenal axis. However, an extensive review concluded that short-term use of corticosteroids for acute postoperative analgesia in relatively healthy individuals is safe.[51]

With regard to the prevention of chronic pain, a recent meta-analysis concluded that high-dose dexamethasone (>0.2 mg/kg) reduces acute pain and demonstrates opioid- sparing effects.[52] Unfortunately, none of the studies included in that meta-analysis reported on pain scores beyond the acute pain phase. Of the few studies that have investigated the effect of perioperative steroids on chronic pain, one study concluded that hydrocortisone 100 mg before open heart surgery followed by a short IV infusion and taper demonstrated significantly reduced pain scores at 6 months.[53]

Opioids With Dual Action

The effects of mu (μ)–receptor agonism in concert with serotonin reuptake inhibition, norepinephrine reuptake inhibition, or NMDA-receptor antagonism have gained interest as these medications when used alone achieve analgesia through multiple mechanisms. The list of dual-action opioids includes tramadol, tapentadol, and methadone.

Tramadol, a weak agonist of the mu-receptor, also inhibits serotonin and norepinephrine reuptake. It has been used successfully to treat chronic neuropathic pain, and it has been suggested that it may be similarly effective in treating acute neuropathic pain. Following oral administration, tramadol must be metabolized to render both serotonin and norepinephrine reuptake inhibition. This is accomplished by the P450 2D6 enzyme; it has been reported that 5%–15% of the population have reduced function of this P450 enzyme, which may explain a variable response between patients. With regard to acute pain, tramadol has been incorporated in multimodal

regimens for total knee arthroplasty[54] and rotator cuff repair[55] with positive results on reducing acute pain. When compared to other analgesics with singular mechanisms of action, tramadol can provide superior analgesia.[56]

Tapentadol has the mechanisms of both mu-receptor agonism and norepinephrine reuptake inhibition. Tapentadol has stronger opioid activity and does not require metabolism of the parent compound to exert its effects. By increasing norepinephrine levels, afferent pain signaling is attenuated leading to improved analgesia. It has been suggested to be as effective as traditional opioids in the acute postoperative setting.[57] Tapentadol holds promise for acute pain stemming from painful procedures, as 100 mg doses are equipotent to oxycodone 15 mg.

Precipitating serotonin syndrome is a potential consequence when starting patients on tramadol or tapentadol if they concomitantly take antidepressants that increase levels of serotonin. Other side effects include nausea, constipation, and sedation (although less sedation than pure mu-receptor agonists).

A substance with mu-receptor agonism and NMDA-receptor antagonism, methadone has historically been used to treat chronic pain. The titration of oral methadone can be complicated as the half-life is variable. However, methadone has been used in the perioperative period as a single dose given IV immediately following induction of anesthesia. Doses have ranged from 0.2[58,59]–0.25 mg/kg.[60] All studies determined single IV doses of methadone were superior to conventional intraoperative opioids. Acute pain scores and opioid consumption were lower in all studies without serious side effects. Potential adverse effects of methadone include those associated with any opioid: nausea, vomiting, constipation, pruritus, somnolence, respiratory depression, and death. A unique concern to chronic methadone use is the prolongation of the QT interval; this can lead to fatal ventricular dysrhythmias.

There are currently no studies investigating dual-action opioids in preventing chronic pain. As mentioned in a previous section, the NMDA receptor appears to be important in the transition from acute to chronic pain. Of the medications mentioned in this section, methadone likely has the largest promise in preventing chronic pain due to its ability to block the NMDA receptor.

Regional Anesthesia

Perioperative regional anesthesia has become popular for a number of reasons. Widespread use of ultrasound has allowed anesthesiologists to perform peripheral nerve blocks that were once impossible with ease. There is emerging evidence that regional anesthesia may be able to reduce not only acute pain, but also the incidence of hyperalgesia, central sensitization, and chronic pain.

A recent meta-analysis on this subject provided some much needed insight into this exciting concept.[61] Epidural anesthesia in 250 (pooled) patients undergoing thoracotomy was shown to have a strong correlation with reduced persistent postsurgical pain; the number needed to treat was 4. Epidural anesthesia also has been studied in abdominal surgery[62]; patients who received epidural anesthesia intraoperatively were pain free at 1 year compared to 28% who received no epidural infusion. Of note, these investigators did include an intraoperative ketamine infusion for patients in all study groups (control and epidural.) Other situations where neuraxial anesthesia has been compared to nonregional methods for pain control include prostatectomy,[63] gynecologic surgery,[64] and lower extremity amputation.[65] One of these studies indicated a positive effect of neuraxial anesthesia; however, the benefits were similar to a group in the study that received systemic opioids and general anesthesia.[68]

Single-shot paravertebral blocks have also been shown to reduce the incidence of persistent postsurgical pain at 4–5 months[66] and 1 year.[67] Both studies were performed on patients undergoing surgery for breast cancer, some including axillary lymph node dissections.

A continuous local wound infiltration at the site of iliac bone graft site for 48 hours after surgery improved pain 4 years postoperatively.[68] The study sample was small at follow-up (19 patients, 9 in the treatment group) but the effects were significant with none of the treatment group experiencing dysesthesias over the harvest site versus 70% of the control group.

Many of the studies investigating regional anesthesia to prevent chronic pain are overall small and provide significant variability in study design.[64] However, there are promising effects of neuraxial blocks, peripheral nerve blocks, and local infiltration to prevent persistent postsurgical pain.

SUMMARY

The concept of multimodal analgesia was described more than 2 decades ago and has gained much support with individual investigators experimenting and developing combinations of analgesics to enhance patient care in the perioperative period. This excitement has led to a variety of combinations tested, albeit with significant variability between studies. The evidence that exists suggests a diverse surgical population can benefit from these interventions.

Chronic pain is costly in terms of both costs to the health care system and to the gross domestic product (GDP) in terms of lost productivity. The 21st century began with a decade of pain research and innovation. Among the many things that came out of this time period was the attention to perioperative pain management. Greater appreciation for the transition from acute pain to chronic pain has led many investigators to investigate the molecular mechanisms responsible for secondary hyperalgesia, central sensitization, and the development of persistent postsurgical pain.

The future of perioperative pain management relies on refining the knowledge accumulated in the past 15 years. Further research is required to determine the maximally effective doses of the medications included in multimodal regimens, as well as the optimal dose to prevent chronic pain. Many of the medications discussed in this chapter have shown a dose-specific effect. Below a certain threshold, the short-term and long-term benefits of a medication could be missed. Large, randomized, prospective trials investigating single agents over appropriate time courses (at least 3 months) at varying doses will help fill this void in our knowledge base. Finally, use of regional anesthesia techniques (peripheral or neuraxial) has gained significant popularity for a number of reasons.

Technology has allowed us to perform continuous blocks with peripheral nerve catheters and elastomeric pumps. What will be interesting is if longer acting local anesthetics will replace this technology and lead to a longer lasting block, and perhaps a longer lasting effect.

Clinical Pearls

- **Acetaminophen**
  - The daily limit of acetaminophen is 3000 mg per day.
- **NSAIDs**
  - Prostaglandins sensitize both nociceptive and nonnociceptive nerve endings, resulting in the two groups of transmitting pain signals regardless of the type of stimulus.
- **Anticonvulsants**
  - Pregabalin's bioavailability and ability to titrate quickly makes it an ideal agent to use in the perioperative phase.
- **NMDA-Receptor Antagonists**
  - Low-dose intraoperative ketamine infusions can have a significant effect on not only acute pain, but also on chronic pain.
- **Steroids**
  - Single doses of corticosteroids given intraoperatively appear to have a dose-effect relationship.
- **Dual-Action Opioids**
  - Norepinephrine reuptake inhibition adds a beneficial effect by reducing ascending nociceptive pathway transmission.
- **Regional Anesthesia**
  - Thoracic epidural anesthesia prevents chronic pain following thoracotomy.
  - Paravertebral blocks reduce chronic pain following breast cancer surgery.

REFERENCES

1. Kehlet H, Dahl JB. The value of "multimodal" or "balanced analgesia" in postoperative pain treatment. Anesth Analg 1993;77:1048–1056.
2. Berger RA, Sanders S, Gerlinger T, et al: Outpatient total knee arthroplasty with a minimally invasive technique. J Arthroplasty 2005;20: 33–38.
3. Buvanendran A, Tuman KJ, McCoy DD, et al: Anesthetic techniques for minimally invasive total knee arthroplasty. J Knee Surg 2006;19:133–136.
4. Samad TA, Sapirstein A, Woolf CJ. Prostanoids and pain: unraveling mechanisms and revealing therapeutic targets. Trends Mol Med 2002;8:390–396.
5. Buvanendran A, Mitchell K, Kroin JS, et al: Cytokine gene expression after total hip arthroplasty: surgical site versus circulating neutrophil response. Anesth Analg 2009;109:959–964.
6. Buvanendran A, Kroin JS, Della Valle CJ, et al: Cerebrospinal fluid neurotransmitter changes during the preoperative period in patients undergoing total knee replacement: a randomized trial. Anesth Analg 2012; 114:434–441.
7. Burke A, Smyth E, Fitzgerald GA. Analgesic-antipyretic and anti-inflammatory agents. In Brunton L, Lazo J, Parker K (eds). *Goodman & Gilman's The Pharmacological Basis of Therapeutics*. 11th ed. New York, NY: McGraw-Hill, 2006, pp 671–716.
8. Graham GG, Scott KF. Mechanism of action of paracetamol. Am J Ther 2005;12:46–55.
9. Keskinbora K, Pekel AF, Aydinli I. Gabapentin and an opioid combination versus opioid alone for the management of neuropathic cancer pain: a randomized open trial. J Pain Symptom Manage 2007;34:183–189.

10. Tiippana EM, Hamunen K, Kontinen VK, et al: Do surgical patients benefit from perioperative gabapentin/pregabalin? A systematic review of efficacy and safety. Anesth Analg 2007;104:1545–1556.

11. Munsterhjelm E, Munsterhjelm NM, Niemi TT, et al: Dose-dependent inhibition of platelet function by acetaminophen in healthy volunteers. Anesthesiology 2005;103:712–717.

12. Sinatra RS, Jahr JS, Reynolds LW, et al: Efficacy and safety of single and repeated administration of 1 gram of intravenous acetaminophen injection (paracetamol) for pain management after major orthopedic surgery. Anesthesiology 2005;102:822–831.

13. Apfel CC, Turan A, Souza K, et al: Intravenous acetaminophen reduces postoperative nausea and vomiting: a systematic review and meta-analysis. Pain 2013;154:677–689.

14. Ong CK, Seymour RA, Lirk P, et al: Combining paracetamol (acetaminophen) with nonsteroidal antiinflammatory drugs: a qualitative systematic review of analgesic efficacy for acute postoperative pain. Anesth Analg 2010;110:1170–1179.

15. Hong JY, Won Han S, Kim WO. Fentanyl sparing effects of combined ketorolac and acetaminophen for outpatient inguinal hernia repair in children. J Urol 2010;183:1551–1555.

16. Issioui T, Klein KW, White PF, et al: The efficacy of premedication with celecoxib and acetaminophen in preventing pain after otolaryngologic surgery. Anesth Analg 2002;94:1188–1193.

17. Rasmussen ML, Mathiesen O, Dierking O, et al: Multimodal analgesia with gabapentin, ketamine and dexamethasone in combination with paracetamol and ketorolac after hip arthroplasty: a preliminary study. Eur J Anaesthesiol 2010;27:324–330.

18. Dorr LD, Raya J, Long WT, et al: Multimodal analgesia without parenteral narcotics for total knee arthroplasty. J Arthroplasty 2008;23: 502–508.

19. Ranawat AS, Ranawat CS. Pain management and accelerated rehabilitation for total hip and total knee arthroplasty. J Arthroplasty 2007;22:12–15.

20. Katz, J. NSAIDs and COX-2-Selective Inhibitors. In Benzon HT, Raja SN, Molloy RE, et al (eds). *Essentials of Pain Medicine and Regional Anesthesia*, 2nd ed. Philadelphia, PA: Elsevier Churchill Livingstone, 2005, pp 141–158.

21. Williams B, Buvanendran A. Non-opioid adjuvants in multimodal therapy for acute perioperative pain. Adv Anesth 2009;27:111–142.

22. Fitzgerald GA, Patrono C. The coxibs, selective inhibitors of cyclooxygenase-2. N Engl J Med 2001;345:433–442.

23. Vane JR, Botting RM. Mechanism of action of nonsteroidal anti-inflammatory drugs. Am J Med 1998;104:2S–8S.

24. Warner TD, Giuliano F, Vojnovic I, et al: Nonsteroid drug selectivities for cyclo-oxygenase-1 rather than cyclo-oxygenase-2 are associated with human gastrointestinal toxicity: a full in vitro analysis. Proc Natl Acad Sci USA 1999;96:7563–7568.

25. Southworth S, Peters J, Rock A, et al: A multicenter, randomized, double-blind, placebo-controlled trial of intravenous ibuprofen 400 and 800 mg every 6 hours in the management of postoperative pain. Clin Ther 2009;31:1922–1935.

26. Kroll PB, Meadows L, Rock A, et al: A multicenter, randomized, double-blind, placebo-controlled trial of intravenous ibuprofen (i.v.-ibuprofen) in the management of postoperative pain following abdominal hysterectomy. Pain Pract 2011;11:23–32.

27. Cortazzo MH, Fishman SM. Major opioids and chronic opioid therapy. In Benzon HT, Rathmell JP, Wu CL, et al (eds). *Raj's Practical Management of Pain*, 4th ed. Philadelphia, PA: Mosby Elsevier, 2008;5:597–611.

28. Sun T, Sacan O, White PF, et al: Perioperative versus postoperative celecoxib on patient outcome after major plastic surgery procedures. Anesth Analg 2008;106:950–958.

29. Schroer WC, Diesfeld PJ, LeMarr AR, Reedy ME: Benefits of prolonged postoperative cyclooxygenase-2 inhibitor administration on total knee arthroplasty recovery: a double-blind, placebo-controlled study. J Arthroplasty 2011;26(6 Suppl):2–7.

30. De Oliveira Jr GS, Agarwal D, Benzon HT. Perioperative single dose ketorolac to prevent postoperative pain: a meta-analysis of randomized trials. Anesth Analg 2012;114:424–433.

31. Chaparro LE, Smith SA, Moore RA, et al: Pharmacotherapy for the prevention of chronic pain after surgery in adults. Cochrane Database Rev 2013;7:1–122.

32. Pountos I, Georgouli T, Calori GM, et al: Do nonsteroidal anti-inflammatory drugs affect bone healing? A critical analysis. Sci World J 2012 ePub ahead of print.

33. Neurontin Package Insert, Pfizer. Accessed April 8, 2014. http://www.pfizer.com/products/product-detail/neurontin

34. Shneker BF, McAuley JW. Pregabalin: a new neuromodulator with broad therapeutic indications. Ann Pharmacother 2005;9:2029–2037.

35. Field MJ, Holloman EF, McCleary S, et al: Evaluation of gabapentin and S-(+)-3-isobutylgaba in a rat model of postoperative pain. J Pharmacol Exp Ther 1997;282:1242–1246.

36. Clarke H, Bonin RP, Orser BA, et al: The prevention of chronic postsurgical pain using gabapentin and pregabalin: a combined systematic review and meta-analysis. Anesth Analg 2012;115:428–442.

37. Buvanendran A. Chronic postsurgical pain: are we closer to understanding the puzzle? Anesth Analg 2012;115:231–232.

38. Nikolajsen L, Finnerup NB, Kramp S, et al: A randomized study of the effects of gabapentin on postamputation pain. Anesthesiology 2006;105:1008–1015.

39. Kim SY, Jeong JJ, Chung WY, et al: Perioperative administration of pregabalin for pain after robot-assisted endoscopic thyroidectomy: a randomized clinical trial: Surg Endosc 2010;24:2776–2781.

40. Burke SM, Shorten GD. Perioperative pregabalin improves pain and functional outcomes 3 months after lumbar discectomy. Anesth Analg 2010;110:1180–1185.

41. Buvanendran A, Kroin JS, Della Valle CJ, et al: Perioperative oral pregabalin reduces chronic pain after total knee arthroplasty: a prospective, randomized, controlled trial. Anesth Analg 2010;110:199–207.

42. Chu LF, Angst MS, Clark D. Opioid-induced hyperalgesia in humans: molecular mechanisms and clinical considerations. Clin J Pain 2008;24:479–496.

43. Kehlet H, Jensen TS, Woolf CJ. Persistent surgical pain: risk factors and prevention. Lancet 2006;367:1618–1625.

44. Remérand F, Le Tendre C, Baud A, et al: The early and delayed analgesic effects of ketamine after total hip arthroplasty: a prospective, randomized, controlled, double-blind study. Anesth Analg 2009;109:1963–1971.

45. Loftus RW, Yeager MP, Clark JA, et al: Intraoperative ketamine reduces perioperative opiate consumption in opiate-dependent patients with chronic back pain undergoing back surgery. Anesthesiology. 2010;113: 639–646.

46. Buvanendran A, Kroin JS. Multimodal analgesia for controlling acute postoperative pain. Curr Opin Anaesthesiol 2009;22:588–593.

47. Schley M, Topfner S, Wiech K, et al: Continuous brachial plexus block in combination with the NMDA receptor antagonist memantine prevents phantom pain in acute traumatic upper limb amputees. Eur J Pain 2007; 11:299–308.

48. De Kock M, Lavand'homme P, Waterloos H. 'Balanced analgesia' in the perioperative period: is there a place for ketamine? Pain 2001;92: 373–380.

49. Katz J, Cohen L. Preventive analgesia is associated with reduced pain disability 3 weeks but not 6 months after major gynecologic surgery by laparotomy. Anesthesiology 2004;101:169–174.

50. Perrin SB, Purcell AN. Intraoperative ketamine may influence persistent pain following knee arthroplasty under combined general and spinal anaesthesia: a pilot study. Anaesth Intensive Care 2009;37:248–253.

51. Kjetil H, Sem TK, Ellen S, et al: The prolonged postoperative analgesic effect when dexamethasone is added to a nonsteroidal anti-inflammatory drug (rofecoxib) before breast surgery. Anesth Analg 2007;105: 481–486.

52. Fukami Y, Terasaki M, Okamoto Y, et al: Efficacy of preoperative dexamethasone in patients with laparoscopic cholecystectomy: a prospective randomized double-blind study. J Hepatobiliary Pancreat Surg 2009;16:367–371.

53. Mathiesen O, Jacobsen LS, Holm HE, et al: Pregabalin and dexamethasone for postoperative pain control: a randomized controlled study in hip arthroplasty. Br J Anaesth 2008;101:535–541.

54. Salerno A, Hermann R. Efficacy and safety of steroid use for postoperative pain relief. Update and review of the medical literature. J Bone Joint Surg Am 2006;88:1361–1372.

55. De Oliveira Jr GS, Almeida MD, Benzon HT, et al: Perioperative single dose systemic dexamethasone for postoperative pain: a meta-analysis of randomized controlled trials. Anesthesiology 2011;115:575–588.

56. Weis F, Kilger E, Roozendaal B, et al: Stress doses of hydrocortisone reduce chronic stress symptoms and improve health-related quality of life in high-risk patients after cardiac surgery: a randomized study. J Thorac Cariovasc Surg 2006;131:277–282.

57. Lamplot JD, Wagner ER, Manning DW. Multimodal pain management in total knee arthroplasty: a prospective randomized controlled trial: J Arthroplasty 2014;29:329–334.

58. Cho CH, Song KS, Min BW, et al: Multimodal approach to postoperative pain control in patients undergoing rotator cuff repair. Knee Surg Sports Traumatol Arthrosc 2011;19:1744–1748.

59. Mitra S, Khandelwal P, Sehgal A. Diclofenac-tramadol vs. diclofenac-acetaminophen combinations for pain relief after caesarean section. Acta Anaesthesiol Scand 2012;56:706–711.

60. Kwong WJ, Ozer-Stillman I, Miller JD, et al: Cost-effectiveness analysis of tapentadol immediate release for the treatment of acute pain. Clin Ther 2010;32:1768–1781.

61. Gottschalk A, Durieux ME, Nemergut E. Intraoperative methadone improves postoperative pain control in patients undergoing complex spine surgery. Anesth Analg 2011;112:218–223.

62. Berde CB, Beyer JE, Bournaki MC, et al: Comparison of morphine and methadone for prevention of postoperative pain in 3- to 7-year-old children. J Pediatr 1991;199:136–141.

63. Chui PT, Gin T. A double-blind randomised trial comparing postoperative analgesia after perioperative loading doses of methadone or morphine. Anaesth Intensive Care 1992;20:46–51.

64. Andreae MH, Andreae DA. Regional anaesthesia to prevent chronic pain after surgery: a Cochrane systematic review and meta-analysis. Br J Anaesth 2013;111:711–720.

65. Lavand'homme P, De Kock M, Waterloos H. Intraoperative epidural analgesia combined with ketamine provides effective preventive analgesia in patients undergoing major digestive surgery. Anesthesiology 2005;103:813–820.

66. Haythornthwaite JA, Raja SN, Fisher B, et al: Pain and quality of life following radical retropubic prostatectomy. J Urol 1998;160:1761–1764.

67. Katz J, Schmid R, Snijdelaar DG, et al: Pre-emptive analgesia using intravenous fentanyl plus low-dose ketamine for radical prostatectomy under general anesthesia does not produce short-term or long-term reductions in pain or analgesic use. Pain 2004;110:707–718.

68. Karanikolas M, Aretha D, Tsolakis I, et al: Optimized perioperative analgesia reduces chronic phantom limb pain intensity, prevalence, and frequency: a prospective, randomized, clinical trial. Anesthesiology 2011;114:1144–1154.

69. Ibarra MM, S-Carralero GC, Vicente GU, et al: Chronic postoperative pain after general anesthesia with or without a single-dose preincisional paravertebral nerve block in radical breast cancer surgery. Rev Esp Anestesiol Reanim 2011;58:290–294.

70. Kairaluoma PM, Bachmann MS, Rosenberg PH, et al: Preincisional paravertebral block reduces the prevalence of chronic pain after breast surgery. Anesth Analg 2006;103:703–708.

71. Singh K, Phillips FM, Kuo E, et al: A prospective, randomized, double-blind study of the efficacy of postoperative continuous local anesthetic infusion at the iliac crest bone graft site after posterior spinal arthrodesis: a minimum of 4-year follow-up. Spine 2007;32:2790–2796.

The Role of Nonopioid Analgesic Infusions in the Management of Postoperative Pain

Gildasio S. De Oliveira, Jr, Honorio T. Benzon, and Paul F. White

INTRODUCTION

Opioids are the most commonly used medications for perioperative pain control. However, opioid-related side effects such as constipation, nausea, vomiting, and respiratory depression often accompany the use opioids. Many studies have evaluated the efficacy of nonopioids such as ketamine, lidocaine, naloxone, and magnesium as perioperative infusions to decrease postoperative pain and minimize the use of opioids after surgery. Infusions of the short-acting beta-blocker esmolol and the α_2 agonist dexmedetomidine have also been investigated as adjuvants to reduce the postoperative opioid requirement. In this chapter, the results of the studies on infusions of ketamine, lidocaine, naloxone, esmolol, α_2 agonists, and magnesium will be summarized, and recommendations on their clinical applicability as part of perioperative pain management will be made.

INTRAVENOUS KETAMINE INFUSION

Ketamine is a noncompetitive N-methyl-D-aspartate glutamate (NMDA) receptor antagonist and a sodium channel blocker.[1] The drug is available as racemic ketamine which contains the S (+) and R (–) stereoisomers. The S (+) ketamine has four times greater affinity for the NMDA receptor than the R (–) ketamine. Ketamine has a half-life of 80–180 minutes. Its metabolite norketamine has a longer half-life life and is one third as potent as the parent compound.[2] Early studies showed ketamine to have analgesic properties at low doses.[3–7]

Ketamine has many qualities as an analgesic. It does not suppress cardiovascular function in the presence of an intact nervous system,[8] does not depress the laryngeal protective reflexes and causes less depression of ventilation compared to opioids,[9] and may even stimulate respiration.[10]

Ketamine has been used in subanesthetic doses as an analgesic.[6] The analgesic effects of ketamine occur at plasma concentrations of 100–150 $ng.mL^{-1}$,[11] The undesirable characteristics of ketamine include postoperative malaise,[12] accumulation of metabolites,[13] development of tolerance,[14] cardiovascular excitation, and the occurrence of psychotomimetic side effects.[15,16] Psychotomimetic effects are the most common feared complication by clinical practitioners but few studies have formally evaluated these side effects.[4-7]

Randomized controlled clinical studies on perioperative IV ketamine showed some beneficial effect. In a study in patients who underwent cervical and lumbar spine surgery, ketamine (1–mg/kg bolus followed by 83 $mcg/kg^{-1}/h^{-1}$) resulted in lower pain scores, less analgesic requirements, and better satisfaction than patients who had saline infusions or those who had lower doses of ketamine infusions (same bolus but with an infusion rate of 42 $mcg/kg^{-1}/h^{-1}$).[17] The same salutary effects were seen in patients who had major abdominal surgery. Perioperative ketamine infusion (0.5–mg/kg bolus followed by 2 $mcg/kg^{-1}/min^{-1}$) for 48 hours after surgery resulted in lower morphine consumption than patients who had saline infusion or those who had the same infusion given intraoperatively.[18] The pain scores were noted to be lower in the ketamine group compared to the control group. To better evaluate the effect of a ketamine bolus on the infusion, Bilgin et al[19] compared ketamine bolus followed by an infusion with ketamine bolus alone given either before the surgical incision or at wound closure. In this study, the patients underwent gynecologic laparotomy. The investigators noted that the patients who had the ketamine bolus and infusion had lower pain scores and lower morphine consumption. Similarly, ketamine infusion reduced postoperative opioid consumption in patients who had spinal anesthesia for cesarean section.[20]

No beneficial effect of ketamine infusion was noted when the general anesthetic consisted of total intravenous anesthesia with remifentanil and propofol infusions.[21] The absence of beneficial effect may be related to the generous use of intraoperative opioids. A systematic review evaluating over 4700 patients demonstrated the efficacy of ketamine in reducing postoperative opioid consumption and pain, especially for thoracic, upper abdominal, and major orthopedic surgical procedures.[22] The investigators demonstrated that despite using less opioid, 25 of 32 treatment groups (78%) experienced less pain than the placebo groups at some point postoperatively when ketamine was efficacious. This finding suggested an improved quality of pain control in addition to decreased opioid consumption.

The effect of perioperative IV ketamine infusion in preventing postamputation pain has been also studied.[23] Ketamine 0.5 mg/kg^{-1} bolus followed by an infusion of 0.5 mg/kg^{-1}/h^{-1} for 72 hours was not effective in reducing morphine consumption or in decreasing the incidence of stump allodynia. At 6-month follow-up, the incidences of phantom pain and stump pain were 47% in the ketamine group compared to 71% and 35% in the control (saline) group. There was no statistical difference in the incidences, so the investigators concluded that IV ketamine did not significantly reduce acute central sensitization or the incidence and severity of postamputation pain.[23]

Ketamine infusion appears to have a beneficial effect on epidural analgesia. The addition of a ketamine infusion to an epidural analgesia in patients who underwent colorectal surgery resulted in less patient-controlled analgesia (PCA) morphine requirements and reduced the area of hyperalgesia.[24] Another group of investigators noted the salutary effect of adding low-dose IV ketamine (0.05 mg/kg^{-1}h^{-1}; approximately 3 mg/h) to epidural analgesia after thoracotomy.[25] In this study, the patients who had the ketamine infusion had less pain and took less analgesics at 3 months after the surgery. Unfortunately, this beneficial effect of ketamine in preventing chronic pain after surgery was not confirmed in other studies.[26,27] In one study, the ketamine infusion (1 mg/kg^{-1} at induction, 1 mg/kg^{-1}/h^{-1} during surgery, then 1 mg/kg^{-1} for 24 hours) in addition to intrapleural ropivacaine improved immediate postoperative pain compared to saline.[26] At 4 months after surgery, however, the analgesic intake and neuropathic pain scores were the same in both groups. In another study, the incidences of moderate and severe postthoracotomy pain syndrome at 3 and 6 months were similar in the ketamine and saline groups.[27]

The addition of ketamine infusion appears to be beneficial in opioid-tolerant patients. An earlier study by Loftus et al showed reduced opioid consumption in the first 48 hours after back surgery in patients who had ketamine bolus ([0.5 mg/kg]) and intraoperative infusion (10 mcg/kg [−1] min [−1]).[28] A more recent study showed that the addition of ketamine infusion (0.2 mg/kg/h) to hydromorphone IV PCA resulted in a statistically significant reduction of "average" pain scores in the opioid-dependent patients.[29] However, "least" and "worst" pain scores and postoperative opioid use did not differ between the ketamine and saline groups.

Most of the studies showed no increased side effects when low-dose ketamine infusions are used. Zakine et al[18] did not observe nightmares, delusions, sleep, or psychiatric disorders in their study. Sleep disturbance and psychomotor were similar between the ketamine infusion group and control group. In a quantitative systematic review, Laskowski and colleagues detected that hallucinations and nightmares were more common with ketamine but sedation was not.[22] They noted that when ketamine was efficacious for pain, postoperative nausea and vomiting were diminished.

Review articles on ketamine infusion noted the small number of patients in the studies, large variations in clinical settings, different ketamine regimens, and different routes of administration.[22,30–34] Most of the randomized controlled studies showed some beneficial effects of a low-dose ketamine infusion. Ketamine infusion appears to improve the efficacy of epidural analgesia. It does not seem to have any effect when the anesthetic technique is total intravenous anesthesia where moderate or substantial amounts of intraoperative opioid are used. IV ketamine may find its use as an adjunct in opioid-tolerant patients, or in patients with a higher incidence of chronic postsurgical pain such as thoracotomy, inguinal herniorraphies, or mastectomies.

> ## Clinical Pearl
>
> - Ketamine intraoperatively is beneficial adjunct in the control of perioperative pain in opioid-dependent patients.

INTRAVENOUS LIDOCAINE INFUSION

Lidocaine has peripheral and central properties that are suitable for pain relief. It decreases albumin extravasation in animal models of chemical peritonitis[35] and inhibits leukocyte migration and metabolic activation.[36] Lidocaine has been shown to modify the neuronal responses in the dorsal horn[37] and selectively suppress synaptic spinal transmission by decreasing C fiber–evoked activity in the spinal cord.[38] Clinically, local anesthetic infusions have been used in the treatment of neuropathic pain[39,40] and pain from burns.[41]

Several studies showed the beneficial effects of intravenous lidocaine in abdominal surgery. In a randomized, double-blind, placebo-controlled study, Cassuto et al[42] showed the analgesic efficacy of a low-dose lidocaine infusion in patients who underwent cholecystectomy. After an intravenous bolus of 100 mg of lidocaine, they infused lidocaine at 2 mg/min, starting at 30 minutes before the surgery, and continued for 24 hours after the surgery. Compared to the group who had saline infusions, the patients who had the lidocaine infusions had significantly lower pain scores during the first day of surgery and required significantly less meperidine during the first 2 postoperative days.[42] Other randomized controlled studies showed the technique to result in lower postoperative pain scores, less opioid consumption, faster return of bowel function, and reduced hospital stay.[43–45] Groudine et al[43] compared lidocaine with saline in patients who had radical retropubic prostatectomy. In the lidocaine group, the patients had 1.5– mg/kg bolus of lidocaine before induction, an intraoperative infusion of either 3 mg/min or 2 mg/min (for patients weighting <70 kg) that was continued until 1 hour postoperatively. Although the analgesic consumption between the patients in the two groups was the same, the patients who had the lidocaine infusion had lower pain scores, a shorter return of bowel movement (62 ± 13 hours vs 74 ± 16 hours) and a shorter hospital stay (4 vs 5 days). In patients who underwent major abdominal surgery, Koppert et al[44] gave a 1.5–mg/kg bolus over 10 minutes, followed by 1.5/mg/kg/h 30 minutes before surgical incision and continued up to 1 hour after the end of surgery. The control group had saline bolus followed by saline infusion. The lidocaine infusion group had lower pain scores, less morphine requirement (130 vs 159 mg) over a 72-hour period, and had bowel movements sooner.[44] The opioid-sparing effect was noted to be most pronounced on the third postoperative day, prompting the investigators to theorize that the lidocaine infusion may have a true preventive analgesic effect. In another study done in patients who had laparoscopic cholecystectomy,[45] the patients were given a lidocaine bolus injection of 1.5 mg/kg at the induction of anesthesia followed by a continuous infusion of 2 mg/kg/h intraoperatively and 1.33 mg/kg/h postoperatively for 24 hours. The control group had saline bolus injections followed by a saline infusion. The times to first flatus (17 vs 28 h), defecation (28 vs 51 h), and hospital discharge (2 vs 3 days) were significantly shorter in the patients who had the lidocaine infusion. In addition, the lidocaine infusion also significantly reduced opioid consumption and postoperative pain and fatigue scores.

Two studies not only looked at pain relief but also the effect of the lidocaine infusion on markers of inflammation and immune response. A randomized study in patients who underwent transabdominal surgery showed less severe postoperative pain in the first 8 hours after surgery, both at rest and during coughing.[46] However, there was no difference in pain scores for the 12–72 hours after surgery between the IV lidocaine and IV saline. The investigators noted less ex vivo production of interleukin-1ra (IL-1ra) and IL-6 and better maintenance of the lymphocyte proliferation response to phytohemagglutinin-M in the intravenous saline group, signifying the ability of lidocaine to reduce surgery-induced immune changes. Another study did not notice improved pain scores but showed other salutary effects when lidocaine infusion is employed in patients undergoing colorectal surgery. Herroeder et al[47] gave an IV bolus of lidocaine 1.5 mg/kg followed by a continuous infusion of 2 mg/min until 4 hours postoperatively. Although the pain ratings were the same compared to a saline control group, the return of bowel function was accelerated and the length of hospital stay was shortened by 1 day. The investigators also noted significant attenuation of the plasma levels of IL-6, IL-8, complement C3a, and IL-1ra as well as expression of CD11b, P-selectin, and platelet-leukocyte aggregates. The findings showed the ability of IV lidocaine to modify the anti-inflammatory activity, which modulates the surgery-induced response.

The salutary effects of IV lidocaine infusion were not duplicated in patients who had a total hip replacement or coronary artery bypass graft surgery. In a randomized, double-blind, placebo-controlled study, 1.5 mg/kg lidocaine bolus was given over 10 minutes at 30 minutes before surgical incision followed

by an infusion of 1.5 mg/kg/h until 1 hour after the end of the surgery.[48] There was no difference between the lidocaine and saline groups in terms of postoperative pain scores and opioid consumption (17 vs 15 mg morphine over 24 hours) and no difference in hip flexion. Low-dose lidocaine infusion was also noted to be ineffective in reducing the supplemental fentanyl, midazolam, or propanolol postoperative requirements in patients who underwent coronary artery bypass.[49] In this study, the lidocaine infusion did not reduce the time to extubation, intensive care unit (ICU) stay, or hospital length of stay. It is not clear if lidocaine infusion has no beneficial effect in coronary artery bypass graft (CABG) or total hip surgery since there is only one study for each surgery. Additional studies are needed to determine if ketamine infusion is really ineffective in these surgical settings.

Initial studies on lidocaine infusion (1.5–mg/kg bolus followed by an infusion of 2 mg/kg^{-1}/h^{-1}) in patients undergoing ambulatory surgery noted that the infusion resulted in less intraoperative opioid use and less pain scores.[50] De Oliveira et al determined that perioperative lidocaine not only reduced postoperative pain and opioid consumption, but also improved overall quality of postsurgical recovery in patients undergoing outpatient laparoscopic gynecologic surgery. Patients who received lidocaine met discharge criteria faster than the group who received saline.[51]

Intravenous lidocaine infusion is not as effective as perioperative epidural analgesia. IV lidocaine was inferior to thoracic epidural analgesia in terms of pain relief and attenuation of cytokine "surge" in patients who underwent colonic surgery. In a nicely done randomized blinded study, Kuo et al[52] showed that thoracic epidural analgesia resulted in better pain relief, lower opioid consumption, earlier return of bowel function, and lesser production of cytokines than IV lidocaine during the 72-hour observation study period. The patients who had the IV lidocaine experienced better pain relief and less cytokine release than the control (saline) group.

A randomized but unblinded study compared IV lidocaine infusion with epidural analgesia in patients who had open colon resection.[53] The IV lidocaine group had infusions of 1–2 mg/min (1 mg/min in <70 kg patients and 2 mg/min in >70 kg patients), while the epidural analgesia group had 10 mL/h of 0.125% bupivacaine and hydromorphone 6 mcg/mL. The infusions were started within 1 hour of the end of surgery and continued until return of bowel function or by the fifth day. There were no statistical differences in the average pain scores (visual analog scale [VAS] of 2.2 in the epidural group vs 3.1 in the IV lidocaine group) and a trend toward greater opioid consumption in the IV lidocaine group. The return of bowel function or the length of hospital stay was not statistically different between the groups.[53] It is interesting to note that two chronic pain patients in the IV lidocaine group were excluded, and an epidural had to be subsequently placed in one of the patients for "further pain treatment."

Two meta-analysis articles showed beneficial effects of perioperative lidocaine infusion. An earlier meta-analysis of eight trials noted improved rehabilitation and shortened hospital stay when a lidocaine infusion is used.[54] The improved recovery was supported by decreased postoperative pain at 24 hours after

TABLE 76-1. Efficacy of perioperative ketamine and lidocaine intravenous infusions.

	Ketamine	Lidocaine
Bolus dose	0.5 –1.0 mg/kg	100 –1.5 mg/kg
Usual infusion dose	40 –100 mgkg^{-1}/h^{-1}	2 –3 mg/min (2 mg/min for patients <70 kg)
Infusion dose with epidural analgesia	0.05 (~3 mg/h)– 0.25 mg/kg^{-1}/h^{-1}	
Efficacy		
Abdominal surgery	Beneficial	Beneficial
Pelvic: gynecologic, urologic	Beneficial	Beneficial
Spine surgery	Beneficial	
Total hip replacement		Not beneficial
Coronary artery bypass surgery		Not beneficial
TIVA	No additional benefit	
Concomitant PCEA	Additional benefit	
Compared to PCEA		Blinded study showed less efficacy[52] while a randomized but unblinded study showed non-statistically significant pain scores and a trend towards greater opioid consumption in the IV lidocaine group.[53]

Source: Reproduced with permission from Benzon HT, Raja SN, Liu SS, et al: *Essentials of Pain Medicine and Regional Anesthesia*, 3rd ed. New York: Elsevier/Churchill Livingstone; 2011.

surgery, lower incidence of nausea and vomiting, and shorter duration of ileus. The ability of IV lidocaine to shorten the duration of ileus was shown clinically; e.g., first passage of gas and feces, and also through radiopaque markers and serial abdominal radiographs.[55] A meta-analysis evaluating over 1700 patients[56] showed that at 6 hours postoperatively, intravenous lidocaine infusion reduced pain at rest (weighted mean difference [WMD] –8.70, 95% confidence intervals [CI] –16.19 to –1.21), during cough (WMD –11.19, 95% CI –17.73 to –4.65), and during movement (WMD –9.56, 95% CI –17.31 to –1.80). Intravenous lidocaine infusion also reduced morphine requirement (WMD –8.44 mg, 95% CI –11.32 to –5.56), time to first flatus (WMD –7.62 hr, 95% CI –10.78 to –4.45), time to first feces (WMD –10.71 hr, 95% CI –16.14 to –5.28), nausea/vomiting (risk ratios = 0.71, 95% CI 0.57– 0.90), and hospital length of stay (WMD –0.17 days, 95% CI –0.41 to –0.07). The investigators concluded that lidocaine infusions used for abdominal surgery was strongly associated with benefits.[56]

The beneficial effects of a perioperative lidocaine infusion in abdominal surgery may be related to its ability to suppress inflammatory processes from the surgery.[46,52] The ability of IV lidocaine to attenuate increased levels of proinflammatory cytokines prevents the development of peripheral and central nervous system sensitization which leads to clinical hyperalgesia.[57]

In terms of prevention of chronic postsurgical pain, systemic perioperative lidocaine has been shown to reduce the development of this postsurgical pain syndrome after mastectomies.[58]

The effect was very large but the study sample size was small (36 subjects). Future larger randomized trials are needed to refute or confirm the role of lidocaine as an effective intervention to reduce chronic postsurgical pain.

The comparable efficacy of perioperative intravenous ketamine and lidocaine infusions is shown in Table 76–1. It can be seen that infusion of either drug is beneficial in abdominal surgery. Ketamine infusion is effective in spine surgery but showed no added benefit when the technique of general anesthesia is total intravenous anesthesia. Lidocaine infusion appears to have no benefit in patients who undergo total hip replacement or coronary artery bypass surgery. A randomized blinded study showed less efficacy of intravenous lidocaine infusion when compared to epidural analgesia.

Clinical Pearl

- Lidocaine infusion can be beneficial in abdominal surgeries but not in total hip surgery. It accelerates the postoperative return of bowel function.

INTRAVENOUS NALOXONE INFUSION

Naloxone is a pure mu-receptor antagonist. Naloxone infusion has been utilized to decrease the incidence of nausea, vomiting, respiratory depression, and urinary retention after epidural[59,60] and intrathecal opioids.[61,62] However, its use comes with the possibility of reversing the analgesia from the opioid.[63] Studies showed that a naloxone infusion at 10 mcg/kg^{-1}/h^{-1} reduced the duration and quality of analgesia from epidural morphine[59] or fentanyl.[60] In patients who had hip surgery under spinal analgesia with bupivacaine and morphine, naloxone infusion at <1 mcg/k^{-1}/h^{-1} was associated with inferior analgesia.[61] Another study showed that the infusion of naloxone at 1 mcgkg^{-1}h^{-1} attenuated the pain relief in the patients who had intrathecal morphine after lumbar laminectomy.[62] In patients who had radical prostatectomy who were given 0.8–1.7 mg intrathecal morphine, the IV infusion of naloxone at 5 mcg/kg/h provided excellent analgesia with infrequent and minor side effects.[64] Unfortunately, the study was retrospective and without a control group.

The efficacy of naloxone infusion in decreasing the incidence of side effects from neuraxial opioids led Gan et al to investigate the effect of naloxone infusion on PCA morphine.[65] In a randomized, double-blind study, 60 patients who underwent hysterectomy were assigned into three groups: (1) PCA morphine, 1 mg/mL, with saline infusion; (2) PCA morphine with low-dose naloxone infusion (0.25 mcg/kg^{-1}/h^{-1}); and (3) PCA morphine with high-dose naloxone infusion (1 mcg/kg^{-1}/h^{-1}).[65] They noted that both naloxone doses were equally effective in reducing the incidence of nausea and vomiting and pruritus compared with placebo. There was no difference in the pain scores between the three groups even though the cumulative morphine usage was significantly lower in the low-dose group (42.3 ± 1 24.1 mg) compared with the placebo (59.1 ± 27.4 mg) or the high-dose group (64.7 ± 33 mg). There was no respiratory depression and no difference in sedation scores, respiratory rate, hemodynamic parameters, or antiemetic use between the three groups.[65] Movafegh et al[66] examined the effect of a 24-hour low-dose naloxone infusion in 90 patients who had hysterectomies. They showed that naloxone significantly reduced morphine consumption over the first 24 postoperative hours compared with the control group (saline). Morphine consumption was also lower, 19.5 (standard deviation [SD] 3.4) mg versus 27.5 (SD 5.9) mg. In addition, the incidence and severity of nausea and vomiting was significantly reduced in the naloxone group, similar to what was observed by Gan et al.[65]

The ability of low doses of naloxone to improve postoperative analgesia is secondary to its dose-dependent effect on pain. Woolf noted that small doses of naloxone produced analgesia in rats while large doses resulted in hyperalgesia.[67] Levine et al also noted that naloxone initially produced analgesia in a dose-dependent manner and then caused hyperalgesia.[68] Other investigators noted this biphasic or dual modulatory effect of naloxone.[69–71] The mechanisms of analgesic effect of naloxone maybe related to the release of endorphins or displacement of endorphins from receptor sites not related to analgesia.[72] Augmentation of the activity of opioid receptors is another possibility, although this upregulation phenomenon has been demonstrated after prolonged naloxone infusion (7 days) and in animals.[73,74] At higher doses, naloxone blocks the action of the released or displaced endorphin at the postsynaptic receptor.

There is no added efficacy when naloxone is administered via IV PCA.[75–77] The different pharmacokinetics of the drug when given intermittently compared to when given as infusion may explain the lack of added benefit. Naloxone has an alpha half-life of 4 minutes and a beta half-life of 55–60 minutes[78,79]; a continuous infusion of the drug, therefore, results in constant plasma levels resulting in a more consistent effect.

The present indication for IV naloxone infusion is to control the side effects of neuraxial opioids. Few studies such as the one by Gan et al[65] and the one from Movafegh et al[66] showed the efficacy of a low-dose naloxone infusion in reducing opioid consumption. Its increased clinical use for postoperative analgesia should await additional controlled studies in different surgical procedures.

Clinical Pearl

- While low-dose naloxone infusion is effective in reducing postoperative opioid consumption, additional studies are needed its role in different surgical settings and whether the analgesic effect of concomitant opioid is diminished.

MAGNESIUM INFUSION

Magnesium is the second most common intracellular ion with a crucial role in maintaining the functions of organisms. Magnesium is an essential component for the function of enzymes, neurotransmission, and cell signaling.[80] Animal studies demonstrated that magnesium is an antagonist of N-methyl-D-aspartate (NMDA) receptors and minimizes the perception and duration of pain.[81] Since dietary intake is the main source of magnesium in humans, long periods of dietary restriction as well as unpredictable operating room schedules are important causes of hypomagnesemia during the perioperative period.[82] In addition, the perioperative administration of intravenous fluids may also contribute to the development of low levels of magnesium.

The effect of systemic magnesium on postoperative analgesia has been examined by different investigators in a large variety of surgical procedures. Two studies looked at the effect of intravenous magnesium to minimize postoperative pain in patients undergoing major abdominal surgery.[83,84] Both studies utilized an initial bolus of magnesium sulfate (50 mg/kg) followed by a postoperative infusion. The study of Jaoua et al examined only 40 patients, and the investigators were not able to detect an opioid-sparing effect of magnesium.[83] In contrast, the study of Amor et al examined 48 patients, and morphine consumption was significantly higher in the control group compared to the magnesium group on the first postoperative day (52 ± −4 mg vs 30 ± −3 mg).[84]

In patients undergoing total abdominal hysterectomy, lower postoperative pain scores and less cumulative postoperative analgesic consumption were noted in patients who received magnesium compared to placebo.[85] Spine surgery is another procedure where perioperative magnesium infusion has been confirmed to improve postoperative analgesia.[86] An area that remains to be investigated is the use of systemic magnesium to minimize postoperative pain in ambulatory surgical patients as there is only one study in this setting. Tramer et al[87] studied 200 patients undergoing ambulatory ilioinguinal hernia repair or varicose vein operation under general anesthesia and randomized them to receive magnesium sulfate 4 g IV or physiologic saline after anesthetic induction. There was no difference in postoperative opioid consumption or pain scores between the study groups. However, it is important to note that patients in the study received a concomitant multimodal analgesic regimen which consisted of diclofenac 100 mg rectally for the patients who underwent varicose vein surgery and a postoperative ilioinguinal-iliohypogastric nerve block for the patients who had hernia repair. Currently, it remains to be determined if perioperative magnesium infusion is a valuable adjunct in minimizing postoperative pain in ambulatory surgical procedures.

Recently, De Oliveira et al performed a meta-analysis to quantitatively assess the effect of perioperative magnesium infusions on postoperative pain outcomes.[88] They evaluated 20 randomized clinical trials, and over 1200 subjects were included in their final analysis. In most of the studies, 30– to 50–mg/kg boluses were initially given followed by an intraoperative infusion of 10–15 mg kg^{-1}/h^{-1}. The overall effect of magnesium on postoperative pain was small for early pain at rest –0.74 (99% CI –1.08 to –0.48) on a 0–10 numerical rating scale. The overall effect of magnesium compared to saline was also small for late pain (24 hours) at rest, –0.36 (99% CI –0.63 to –0.09). In contrast, the effect of magnesium on opioid sparing compared to saline was substantial, –10.52 (99% CI –13.50 to –7.54) mg morphine IV equivalents. After performing a subgroup analysis, the investigators concluded that the intraoperative and postoperative administration of magnesium had greater analgesic effect than a sole intraoperative administration. None of the studies included in the meta-analysis reported signs or symptoms of magnesium toxicity related to high levels of perioperative magnesium.

In summary, magnesium infusion seems to be a promising strategy to minimize postoperative opioid requirement. The lack of reported toxicity also makes it a safe option. However, more studies are still needed to confirm the analgesic effect of systemic magnesium for ambulatory surgical procedures.

Clinical Pearl

- Intraoperative and postoperative administration of magnesium may have an opioid-sparing effect, studies reported no signs of systemic toxicity.

ESMOLOL INFUSION

Esmolol is a cardioselective beta$_1$-receptor blocker commonly used in the anesthesia to treat intraoperative tachyarrhythmias or to blunt the adrenergic response caused by various stimuli during surgery such as in laryngoscopy, intubation, surgical stimulation, and tracheal extubation. The drug has a very rapid onset and short duration of action.[89] Esmolol is rapidly hydrolyzed by plasma esterases at the ester-methyl side chain, which

is the basis for the drug's short duration of action. Esmolol's elimination half-life is about 9 minutes.[90]

The effect of esmolol infusions on postoperative pain outcomes has been examined by several investigators with most studies demonstrating a favorable analgesic effect. Esmolol was first used as an alternative to opioid analgesics in 1991 by White's group in ambulatory arthroscopic procedures.[91] The investigators compared esmolol to alfentanil when used to supplement propofol-N$_2$O-atracurium anesthesia according to a randomized, double-blind protocol, and they concluded that esmolol may be used in place of alfentanil to supplement anesthesia in outpatients undergoing arthroscopic procedures. They noted that avoiding alfentanil did not decrease the incidence of postoperative nausea and vomiting in this outpatient population.[91]

A study examined the influence of perioperative esmolol administration compared to saline on postoperative pain management among patients undergoing hysterectomy.[92] The investigators demonstrated that perioperative esmolol administration during anesthesia reduced the intraoperative use of inhalation anesthetic and fentanyl, decreased hemodynamic responses, and reduced morphine consumption (by 17 mg IV morphine equivalents) for the first 3 postoperative days. Another study compared esmolol with either intermittent fentanyl or continuous remifentanil on postoperative opioid sparing, side effects, and time of discharge in patients undergoing ambulatory cholecystectomy.[93] The investigators concluded that intraoperative IV infusion of esmolol contributes to a significant decrease in postoperative administration of fentanyl and ondansetron and facilitates earlier discharge. More recently, Lee and colleagues confirmed the analgesic properties of esmolol in patients undergoing laparoscopic appendectomy.[94]

The safety of perioperative esmolol infusions has been recently examined by a systematic review of 67 randomized controlled trials.[95] Esmolol infusions titrated to a hemodynamic endpoint was found to be safe and effective in low-risk patients. In contrast, safety data from studies in higher risk patients are needed to establish a perioperative safety and efficacy profile of esmolol.

In summary, esmolol infusions seem to be a valid strategy to ameliorate postoperative pain. The results of randomized studies are particularly encouraging in the ambulatory surgical population.

Clinical Pearl

- Esmolol infusion is a useful an adjuvant in reducing the anesthetic requirement and decreasing acute hemodynamic responses to noxious surgical stimuli. Esmolol can also reduce postoperative opioid requirements and can reduce side effects (e.g., PONV) in ambulatory surgery patients.

α$_2$ AGONISTS

The α$_2$ agonists are often used as anesthetic adjuncts due to its desirable properties including anxiolysis, sedation. and hypnosis.[96] In addition, α$_2$ agonists have also been found to have analgesic properties. Their analgesic effect is attributed to the stimulation of two adrenoreceptors located in the central nervous system and spinal cord. It also has been suggested that systemic α_2 agonists potentiate the analgesic effects of opioids.[97] Systemic clonidine is thought to have opioid-sparing and antiemetic properties, but its routine clinical use as an infusion has been limited by the presence of adverse effects such as hypotension and bradycardia.[98] Another α_2 agonist commonly used in the perioperative setting is dexmedetomidine. Intravenous infusion of dexmedetomidine is commonly initiated with a 1– mcg/kg loading dose, administered over 10 minutes, followed by a maintenance infusion of 0.2–1.0 mcg/kg/h.[99]

The first clinical trial to evaluate the effect of dexmedetomidine infusion on postsurgical pain was performed by Aho and colleagues on patients undergoing laparoscopic tubal ligation.[100] They concluded that intravenously dexmedetomidine relieves pain and reduces the opioid drug requirement but is attended by sedation and a high incidence of bradycardia. Arain et al also detected a beneficial opioid-sparing effect of dexmedetomidine after major inpatient surgery.[101] Another group evaluated dexmedetomidine infusion on pain outcomes in patients undergoing abdominal hysterectomy.[102] In this study, 50 women were randomly assigned to two groups. Group D (n = 25) received a loading dose of dexmedetomidine 1 mcg/kg (–1) IV during induction of anesthesia, followed by a continuous infusion at a rate of 0.5 mcg/kg (–1)/hr (–1) throughout the operation. The investigators demonstrated that continuous IV dexmedetomidine during abdominal surgery provides effective postoperative analgesia, and reduces postoperative morphine requirements without increasing the incidence of side effects.

More recently, Tramer's group performed a meta-analysis of randomized trials on 1792 patients and detected an opioid-sparing effect of dexmedetomidine compared to placebo of –4.1 mg IV morphine equivalents (95% CI –6.0 to –2.2 mg).[103] However, dexmedetomidine increased the risk of postoperative bradycardia (number needed to harm, 3).

In summary, dexmedetomidine appears to be a promising perioperative analgesic, decreasing opioid requirements after surgery. It does not increase side effects, although it can result in bradycardia.

SUMMARY

Several preoperative nonopioid infusions have been adequately studied and can be recommended as part of multimodal approach to post-operative pain management. Ketamine infusions are notable adjuncts in opioid-dependent patients, while lidocaine infusions not only decrease perioperative opioid requirements in abdominal surgeries, but also shorten bowel recovery recovery. Esmolol and dexmedetomidine infusions have well-documented opioid-sparing effects and offer potential advantages in patients with enhanced cardiovascular responses to surgical stimuli. Magnesium may be a viable alternative, but convincing evidence of improved patient outcomes is still lacking. The more widespread use of low-dose naloxone infusions also awaits further studies. The effect of these nonopioid infusions on chronic post-surgical pain awaits further elucidation in clinical trials.

Clinical Pearl

- Infusion of dexmetomidine can reduce both anesthetic and opioid requirements. However, it may result in bradycardia and sedation.

REFERENCES

1. Himmelseher S, Duriex M: Ketamine for perioperative pain management. Anesthesiology 2005;102:211–220.
2. Kohrs R, Durieux M: Ketamine: teaching old drug new tricks. Anesth Analg 1998;1186–1193.
3. White PF: The changing role of non-opioid analgesic techniques in the management of postoperative pain. Anesth Analg 2005;101:S5–S22.
4. Monk TG, Rater JM, White PF: Comparison of alfentanil and ketamine infusions in combination with midazolam for outpatient lithotripsy. Anesthesiology. 1991;74:1023–1028.
5. White PF: Clinical uses of intravenous anesthetic and analgesic infusions. Anesth Analg 1989;68:161–171.
6. White PF, Ham J, Way WL, Trevor AJ: Pharmacology of ketamine isomers in surgical patients Anesthesiology 1980;52:231–239.
7. Javery KB, Ussery TW, Steger HG, Colclough GW: Comparison of morphine and morphine with ketamine for postoperative analgesia. Can J Anaesth 1996;43:212–215.
8. Dowdy EG, Kaya K, Gocho Y: Some pharmacologic similarities of ketamine, lidocaine, and procaine. Anesth Analg 1973;52:839–842.
9. Bourke DL, Mailt LA, Smith TC: Respiratory interactions of ketamine and morphine. Anesthesiology 1987;66:153–156.
10. Reich DL, Silvay G: Ketamine: an update on the first 25 years of clinical experience. Can J Anaesth 1989;36:186–197.
11. Pekoe GM, Smith DJ: The involvement of monoaminergic neuronal systems in the analgesic effects of ketamine. Pain 1982;12:57–73.
12. Bristow A, Orlokowski C: Subcutaneous ketamine analgesia: postoperative analgesia using subcutaneous infusions of ketamine and morphine. Ann R Coll Surg Engl 1989;71:646–666.
13. Leunt LY, Baillie TA: Comparative pharmacology in the rat of ketamine and its two principal metabolites, norketamine and (2)-6-hydroxynorketamine. J Med Chem 1986;29:2396–2399.
14. Slogoff S, Allen GW: The role of baroreceptors in the cardiovascular response to ketamine. Anesth Analg 1974;53:704–707.
15. White PF, Way WL, Trevor AJ: Ketamine—its pharmacology and therapeutic uses. Anesthesiology 1982;56:119–136.
16. Grant IS, Nimmo WS, McNicol LR, Clements JA: Ketamine disposition in children and adults. Br J Anaesth 1995;55:1107–1011.
17. Yamauchi M, Asano M, Watanabe M, et al: Continuous low-dose ketamine improves the analgesic effect of fentanyl patient-controlled analgesia after cervical spine surgery. Anesth Analg 2008;107:1041–1044.
18. Zakine J, Samarcq D, Lorne E, et al: Postoperative ketamine administration decreases morphine consumption in major abdominal surgery: a prospective, randomized, double-blind, controlled study. Anesth Analg 2008;106:1856–1861.
19. Bilgin H, Ozcan B, Bilgin T, et al: The influence of systemic ketamine administration on postoperative morphine consumption. J Clin Anesth 2005;17:592–597.
20. Suppa E, Valente A, Catarci S, et al: A study of low-dose S-ketamine infusion as "preventive" pain treatment for cesarean section with spinal anesthesia: benefits and side effects. Minerva Anestesiol 2012; 78: 774–781.
21. Jaksh W, Lang S, Reichhalter R, et al: Perioperative small-dose S(+)-ketamine has no incremental beneficial effects on postoperative pain when standard-practice opioid infusions are used. Anesth Analg 2002; 94:981–986.
22. Laskowski K, Stirling A, McKay WP, Lim HJ: A systematic review of intravenous ketamine for postoperative analgesia. Can J Anaesth. 2011; 58: 911–923.
23. Hayes C, Armstrong-Brown A, Burstal R: Perioperative ketamine infusion for the prevention of persistent post-amputation pain: a randomized, controlled trial. Anaesth Intensive Care 2004;32:330–338.
24. Lavand'homme P, De Kock M, Waterloos H: Intraoperative epidural analgesia combined with ketamine provides effective preventive analgesia in patients undergoing major digestive surgery. Anesthesiology 2005; 103:813–820.

25. Suzuki M, Haraguti S, Sugimoto K, et al: Low-dose intravenous ketamine potentiates epidural analgesia after thoracotomy. Anesthesiology 2006;105:111–119.

26. Duale C, Sibaud F, Guastella V, et al: Perioperative ketamine does not prevent chronic pain after thoracotomy. Eur J Pain 2009;13:497–505.

27. Mendola C, Cammarota G, Netto R, et al: S+-ketamine for control of perioperative pain and prevention of post thoracotomy pain syndrome: a randomized, double-blind study. Minerva Anestesiol 2012;78: 757–766.

28. Loftus RW, Yeager MP, Clark JA, et al: Intraoperative ketamine reduces perioperative opiate consumption in opiate-dependent patients with chronic back pain undergoing back surgery. Anesthesiology 2010;113:639–646.

29. Barreveld AM, Correll DJ, Liu X, et al: Ketamine decreases postoperative pain scores in patients taking opioids for chronic pain: results of prospective, randomized, double-blind study. Pain Med 2013;14: 925–934.

30. Schmid R, Sandler A, Katz J: Use and efficacy of low-dose ketamine in the management of acute postoperative pain: a review of the current techniques and outcomes. Pain 1999;82:111–125.

31. McCartney C, Sinha A, Katz J: A qualitative review of the role of the NMDA receptor antagonists in preventive analgesia. Anesth Analg 2004;98:1385–1400.

32. Subramanian K, Subramanian B, Steinbrook R: Ketamine as an adjunct analgesic to opioids: a qualitative and quantitative systematic review. Anesth Analg 2004;99:482–295.

33. Elia N, Tramer M: Ketamine and postoperative pain—a quantitative systematic review of randomized trials. Pain 2005;113:61–70.

34. Bell RF, Dahl JB, Moore RA, Kalso E: Perioperative ketamine for acute postoperative pain: a quantitative and qualitative systematic review (Cochrane Review). Acta Anaesthesiol Scand 2005;49:1405–1428.

35. Rimback G, Cassuto J, Wallin G, Westlander G: Inhibition of peritonitis by amide local anesthetics. Anesthesiology 1988;69:881–886.

36. Eriksson AS, Sinclair R, Cassuto J, Thomsen P: Influence of lidocaine on leukocyte function in the surgical wound. Anesthesiology 1992;77: 74–78.

37. Jaffe RA, Rowe MA: Subanesthetic concentrations of lidocaine selectively inhibit a nociceptive response in the isolated rat spinal cord. Pain 1995;60:167–174.

38. Woolf CJ, Wiesenfled-Hallin Z: The systemic administration of local anesthetics produces a selective depression of C-afferent fibre evoked activity in the spinal cord. Pain 1985;23:361–374.

39. Backonja M, Gombar KA: Response of central pain syndromes to intravenous lidocaine. J Pain Symptom Manage 1992;7 :172–178.

40. Ferrante FM, Paggioli J, Cherkuri S, Arthur GR: The analgesic response to intravenous lidocaine in the treatment of neuropathic pain. Anesth Analg 1996;82:91–97.

41. Jonsson A, Cassuto J, Hanson B: Inhibition of burn pain by intravenous lignocaine infusion. Lancet 1991;338:151–152.

42. Cassuto J, Wallin G, Hogstrom S, et al: Inhibition of postoperative pain by continuous low-dose intravenous infusion of lidocaine. Anesth Analg 1985;64:971–974.

43. Groudine SB, Fisher HAG, Kaufman RP, et al: Intravenous lidocaine speeds the return of bowel function, decreases postoperative pain, and shortens hospital stay in patients undergoing radical retropubic prostatectomy. Anesth Analg 1998;86:235–239.

44. Koppert W, Weigard M, Neumann F, et al: Perioperative intravenous lidocaine has preventive effects on postoperative pain and morphine consumption after major abdominal surgery. Anesth Analg 2004;98: 1050–1055.

45. Kaba A, Laurent SR, Detroz BJ, et al: Intravenous lidocaine infusion facilitates acute rehabilitation after laparoscopic colectomy. Anesthesiology 2007;106:11–18.

46. Yardeni IZ, Deilin B, Mayburd E, et al: The effect of perioperative intravenous lidocaine on postoperative pain and immune function. Anesth Analg 2009;109:1464–1469.

47. Herroeder S, Pecher S, Schonherrr E, et al: Systemic lidocaine shortens length of hospital stay after colorectal surgery. Ann Surg 2007;246: 192–200.

48. Martin F, Cheriff K, Gentili ME, et al: Lack of impact of intravenous lidocaine on analgesia, functional recovery, and nociceptive pain threshold after total hip arthroplasty. Anesthesiology 2008;109: 118–123.

49. Insler SR, O'Connor M, Samonte AF, Bazaral MG: Lidocaine and the inhibition of postoperative pain in coronary artery bypass patients. J Cardiothorac Vasc Anaesth 1995;9:541–546.

50. Mckay A, Gottschalk A, Ploppa A, et al: Systemic lidocaine decreased the perioperative opioid analgesic requirements but failed to reduce discharge time after ambulatory surgery. Anesth Analg 2009;109:1805–1808.

51. De Oliveira GS Jr, Fitzgerald P, Streicher LF, et al: Systemic lidocaine to improve postoperative quality of recovery after ambulatory laparoscopic surgery. Anesth Analg 2012;115:262–267.

52. Kuo CP, Jao SW, Chen KM, et al: Comparison of the effects of thoracic epidural analgesia and i.v. infusion with lidocaine on cytokine response, postoperative pain and bowel function in patients undergoing colonic surgery. Br J Anaesth 2006;97:640–646.

53. Swenson BR, Gottaschaljk A, Wells LT, et al: Intravenous lidocaine is as effective as epidural bupivacaine in reducing ileus duration, hospital stay, and pain after colon resection. A randomized clinical trial. Reg Anesth Pain Med 2010;35:370–376.

54. Marret E, Rolin M, Beaussier M, Bonnet F: Meta-analysis of intravenous lidocaine and postoperative recovery after abdominal surgery. Br J Surg 2008;95:1331–1338.

55. Rimback G, Cassuto J, Tollesson PO: Treatment of paralytic ileus by intravenous lidocaine infusion. Anesth Analg 1990;70:414–419.

56. Vigneault L, Turgeon AF, Côté D, et al: Perioperative intravenous lidocaine infusion for postoperative pain control: a meta-analysis of randomized controlled trials. Can J Anaesth 2011;58:22–37.

57. Watkins LR, Maier SF, Goehler LE: Immune activation: the role of pro-inflammatory cytokines in inflammation, illness responses and pathological pain states. Pain 1995;63:289–302.

58. Grigoras A, Lee P, Sattar F, Shorten G: Perioperative intravenous lidocaine decreases the incidence of persistent pain after breast surgery. Clin J Pain 2012; 28:567–72.

59. Rawal N, Schott U, Dahlstrom B, et al: Influence of naloxone infusion on analgesia and respiratory depression following epidural. Anesthesiology 1986;64:194–201.

60. Gueneron JP, Ecoffey C, Carli P, et al: Effect of naloxone infusion on analgesia and respiratory depression after epidural fentanyl. Anesth Analg 1988;67:35–38.

61. Johnson A, Bengtsson M, Lofstrom JB, et al: Influence of postoperative naloxone infusion on respiration and pain relief after intrathecal morphine. Reg Anesth 1988;13:146–151.

62. Wright PM, O'Toole DP, Barron DW: The influence of naloxone infusion on the action of intrathecal diamorphine: low-dose naloxone and neuroendocrine responses. Acta Anaesthesiol Scand 1992;36:230–233.

63. Kendrick WD, Woods AM, Daly MY, et al: Naloxone versus nalbuphine infusion for prophylaxis of epidural morphine-induced pruritus. Anesth Analg 1996;82:641–647.

64. Rebel A, Sloan P, Andrykowski M: Postoperative analgesia after radical prostatectomy with high-dose intrathecal morphine and intravenous naloxone: a retrospective review. J Opioid Manage 2009;5:331–339.

65. Gan TJ, Ginsberg B, Glass PS, et al: Opioid-sparing effects of a low-dose infusion of naloxone in patient-administered morphine sulfate. Anesthesiology 1997;87:1075–1081.

66. Movafegh A, Shocibi G, Ansari M, et al: Naloxone infusion and post-hysterectomy morphine consumption: a double-blind, placebo-controlled study. Acta Anaesthesiol Scand 2012;56:1241–1249.

67. Woolf CJ: Analgesia and hyperalgesia produced in the rat by intrathecal naloxone. Brain Res 1980;189:593–597.

68. Levine JD, Gordon NC, Fields HL: Naloxone dose-dependently produces analgesia and hyperalgesia in postoperative pain. Nature 1979;278:740–741.

69. Ueda H, Fukushima N, Kitao T, et al: Low doses of naloxone produces analgesia in the mouse brain by blocking presynaptic autoinhibition of enkephalin release. Neurosci Lett 1986;65:247–252.

70. Miaskowski C, Taiwo YO, Levine JD: Intracerebroventricular naloxone produces a dose-dependent, monotonic increase in nociceptive threshold in the rat. Brain Res 1990;515:323–325.

71. Crain SM, Shen KF: Ultra-low concentrations of naloxone selectively antagonize excitatory effects of morphine on sensory neurons, thereby increasing its antinociceptive potency and attenuating tolerance/dependence during chronic cotreatment. Proc Natl Acad Sci USA 1995;92:10540–10544.

72. Crain SM, Shen KF: Antagonists of excitatory opioid receptor functions enhance morphine's analgesic potency and attenuate opioid tolerance/dependence liability. Pain 2000;84:121–131.

73. Paronis CA, Holtzmann SG: Increased potency of mu agonists after continuous naloxone infusion in rats. J Pharmacol Exp Ther 1991;259: 582–589.

74. Yoburn BC, Nunes FA, Adler B, et al: Pharmacodynamic supersensitivity and opioid receptor upregulation in the mouse. J Pharmacol Exp Ther 1986;239:132–135.

75. Cepeda MS, Africano JM, Manrique AM, et al: The combination of low dose naloxone and morphine in PCA does not decrease opioid requirements in the postoperative period. Pain 2002;96:73–79.

76. Sartain JB, Barry JJ, Richardson CA, Branagan HC: Effect of combining naloxone and morphine for intravenous patient-controlled analgesia. Anesthesiology 2003;99:148–151.

77. Cepeda MS, Alvarez H, Morales O, Carr DB: Addition of ultralow dose naloxone to postoperative morphine PCA: unchanged analgesia and opioid requirement but decreased incidence of opioid side effects. Pain 2004;107:41–46.

78. Ngai SH, Berkowitz BA, Yang JC, et al: Pharmacokinetics of naloxone in rats and man: basis for its potency and short duration of action. Anesthesiology 1976;44:398–401.

79. Glass PS, Jhaveri RM, Smith LR: Comparison of potency and duration of action of nalmefene and naloxone. Anesth Analg 1994;78:536–541.

80. Fawcett WJ, Haxby EJ, Male DA: Magnesium: physiology and pharmacology. Br J Anaesth 1999;83:302–320.

81. McCarthy RJ, Kroin JS, Tuman KJ, et al: Antinociceptive potentiation and attenuation of tolerance by intrathecal co-infusion of magnesium sulfate and morphine in rats. Anesth Analg 1998; 86:830–836.

82. Rosanoff A, Weaver CM, Rude RK: Suboptimal magnesium status in the United States: are the health consequences underestimated? Nutr Rev 2012; 70:153–164.

83. Jaoua H, Zghidi SM, Wissem L, et al: [Effectiveness of intravenous magnesium on postoperative pain after abdominal surgery versus placebo: double blind randomized controlled trial.] (article in French). Tunis Med 2010;88:317–23.

84. Benhaj Amor M, Barakette M, et al: [Effect of intra and postoperative magnesium sulphate infusion on postoperative pain.] (article in French). Tunis Med 2008;86:550–555.

85. Ryu JH, Kang MH, Park KS, Do SH: Effects of magnesium sulphate on intraoperative anaesthetic requirements and postoperative analgesia in gynaecology patients receiving total intravenous anaesthesia. Br J Anaesth 2008;100:397–403.

86. Levaux Ch, Bonhomme V, Dewandre PY, et al: Effect of intra-operative magnesium sulphate on pain relief and patient comfort after major lumbar orthopaedic surgery. Anaesthesia 2003;58:131–135.

87. Tramèr MR, Glynn CJ: An evaluation of a single dose of magnesium to supplement analgesia after ambulatory surgery: randomized controlled trial. Anesth Analg 2007; 104:1374–1379.

88. De Oliveira GS Jr, Castro-Alves LJ, Khan JH, McCarthy RJ: Perioperative systemic magnesium to minimize postoperative pain: a meta-analysis of randomized controlled trials. Anesthesiology 2013;119:178–190.

89. Deng CY, Lin SG, Zhang WC, et al: Esmolol inhibits Na+ current in rat ventricular myocytes. Methods Find Exp Clin Pharmacol 2006;28: 697–702.

90. Jaillon P, Drici M: Recent antiarrhythmic drugs. Am J Cardiol 1989;64: 65–69.

91. Smith I, Van Hemelrijck J, White PF: Efficacy of esmolol versus alfentanil as a supplement to propofol-nitrous oxide anesthesia. Anesth Analg 1991;73:540–546.

92. Chia YY, Chan MH, Ko NH, Liu K: Role of beta-blockade in anaesthesia and postoperative pain management after hysterectomy. Br J Anaesth. 2004; 93:799–805.

93. Collard V, Mistraletti G, Taqi A: Intraoperative esmolol infusion in the absence of opioids spares postoperative fentanyl in patients undergoing ambulatory laparoscopic cholecystectomy. Anesth Analg 2007;105: 1255–1262.

94. Lee SJ, Lee JN: The effect of perioperative esmolol infusion on the postoperative nausea, vomiting and pain after laparoscopic appendectomy. Korean J Anesthesiol. 2010;59:179–184.

95. Yu SK, Tait G, Karkouti K, et al: The safety of perioperative esmolol: a systematic review and meta-analysis of randomized controlled trials. Anesth Analg 2011;112:267–281.

96. Chan AK, Cheung CW, Chong YK: Alpha-2 agonists in acute pain management. Expert Opin Pharmacother 2010;11:2849–2868.

97. Farrar MW, Lerman J: Novel concepts for analgesia in pediatric surgical patients. Cyclo-oxygenase-2 inhibitors, alpha 2-agonists, and opioids. Anesthesiol Clin North Am 2002;20:59–82.

98. Lui F, Ng KF: Adjuvant analgesics in acute pain. Expert Curr Opin Investig Drugs 2007;8:25–33.

99. Sanders RD, Maze M. Alpha2-adrenoreceptor agonists. Curr Opin Investig Drugs 2007;8:25-33.

100. Aho MS, Erkola OA, Scheinin H: Effect of intravenously administered dexmedetomidine on pain after laparoscopic tubal ligation. Anesth Analg 1991;73:112–118.

101. Arain SR, Ruehlow RM, Uhrich TD, Ebert TJ: The efficacy of dexmedetomidine versus morphine for postoperative analgesia after major inpatient surgery. Anesth Analg 2004;98:153–158.

102. Gurbet A, Basagan-Mogol E, Turker G: Intraoperative infusion of dexmedetomidine reduces perioperative analgesic requirements. Can J Anaesth 2006;53:646–652.

103. Blaudszun G, Lysakowski C, Elia N, Tramèr MR: Effect of perioperative systemic α2 agonists on postoperative morphine consumption and pain intensity: systematic review and meta-analysis of randomized controlled trials. Anesthesiology 2012;116:1312–1322.

CHAPTER 77

Teaching Regional Anesthesia

Ahtsham U. Niazi and Joseph M. Neal

INTRODUCTION

Regional anesthesia enhances patient satisfaction and favorable outcomes, especially in obstetrics and acute pain management. Over the past 20 years, the importance of training anesthesiologists in regional anesthesia has become recognized worldwide, but the actual accomplishment of quality training remains a challenge for residents and fellows, as well as practicing anesthesiologists. Quality training in regional anesthesia is necessary to promote not only clinical competence, but also practitioner confidence in their ability to perform the skill proficiently and safely. Surveys of residency programs demonstrate narrowing variability in training, and recent consensus-based regional anesthesia and acute pain medicine fellowship guidelines may further improve training at all levels. Academic programs have employed conventional and unconventional methods to complement the exposure to regional anesthesia opportunities that residents and fellows receive in the operating room, obstetric suite, and pain clinic. In this chapter, such concepts will be discussed as well as future goals for improving regional anesthesia training for all anesthesiologists.

PAST AND CURRENT TRAINING EXPERIENCE

Evolution of Regional Anesthesia Training

As early as the 1920s, there were dedicated teachers of regional anesthesia. In the United States, both Gaston Labat and John S. Lundy offered 3-month courses to teach the basics to interested practitioners; such teaching influenced many renowned anesthesiologists, including Ralph Waters and Emery Rovenstine.[1] At that time, a few experts promoted regional anesthesia, including the members of the first American Society of Regional Anesthesia, which was founded by Dr. Labat. Yet, prior to the last quarter century, only a few residency programs had officially incorporated regional anesthesia as part of their educational curriculum.

In fact, it was not until 1996 that the Anesthesiology Residency Review Committee (RRC) of the Accreditation Council for Graduate Medical Education (ACGME) formally listed a minimal number of regional anesthetic blocks as a requirement of training in anesthesiology.[2] Prior to that time, there was wide variability in regional anesthesia training in residencies. A survey conducted in 1980 showed that regional anesthesia use ranged from 2.8%–55.7% among responding training programs, with approximately 21% of all cases using regional anesthesia.[3] Indeed, diplomates of well-respected programs could graduate having performed less than a handful of spinal anesthetic procedures. These numbers improved somewhat by 1990, but although regional anesthesia was utilized in more cases (29.8%), primarily reflecting increases in obstetric and pain management applications of regional techniques, the large discrepancy continued with regional techniques contributing 2.8%–58.5% of total caseload experience.[4] By the year 2000, the number of surgical cases with regional anesthetics did not significantly increase (30.2%), nor did the distribution of the types of anesthetics (Figures 77–1 and 77–2), but there was much less disparity in experience between training programs nationwide.[5]

Accreditation Agency Requirements

The current RRC program requirements state that residents must perform 50 epidural, 50 spinal, and 40 peripheral nerve blocks plus an additional 25 nerve blocks for pain management.[2] The most recent survey of residents' experience (2015) shows that over 70% of residents met the minimum for spinal anesthetics. Although all residents performed the minimum number of epidurals, that nearly 80% were from the lumbar approach suggests that most epidural training still occurs in the obstetric suite.[45] These data are encouraging, since studies of clinical competence show it takes between 60 and 90 epidural blocks to reach at least 80% success[6–8] (Figure 77–3).

PART 13

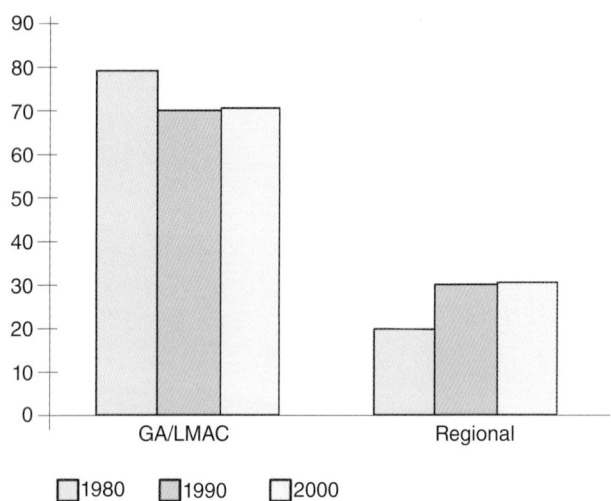

FIGURE 77–1. The use of regional anesthesia in residency training programs compared to general or local anesthesia for cases in 1980 (21.3%), 1990 (29.8%), and 2000 (30.2%).

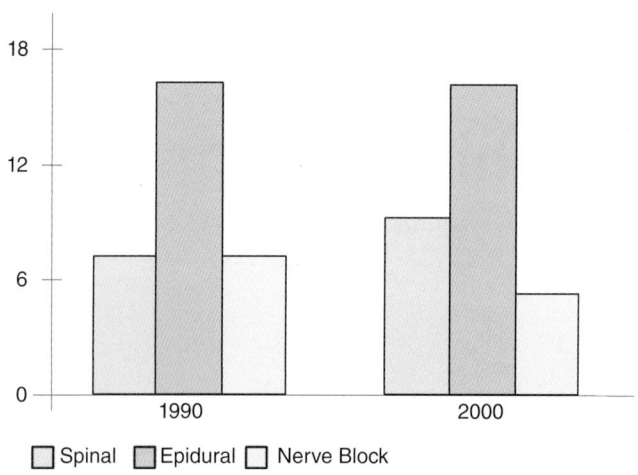

FIGURE 77–2. Distribution of types of regional anesthesia in residency training programs did not change significantly between 1990 and 2000 ($P = .75$).

Achieving a level of competency is reflected in resident confidence, as surveys of graduating residents showed more than 94% were very confident in their lumbar epidural skills.[8–10] Similar evidence exists for spinal blocks, with surveyed residents feeling very confident in their ability to perform spinal anesthesia.[9] Kopacz et al demonstrated that at least 45 spinal anesthetics needed to be performed before at least 90% success rate was attained,[7] a number much closer to the RRC requirement.

The data for peripheral nerve block are encouraging. In the year 2000, approximately 40% of residents reported inadequate experience with peripheral nerve blocks, which had both educational and safety implications.[5] Residents not adequately trained in a particular block are unlikely to use that block in practice[11]; or worse, they may try to use techniques without the proper skills.[9,12] Multiple older surveys have demonstrated that graduating residents did not feel confident in their peripheral

nerve block skills[9] (Figure 77–4). This was especially true of lower extremity nerve blocks[12,13] (Figure 77–5). By the year 2015, nearly 90% of residents reported exceeding the suggested number of continuous and single-injection peripheral nerve blocks by a wide margin, including extensive experience with lower extremity blocks. Not surprisingly, ultrasound-guidance as a nerve localization tool now surpasses by a wide margin peripheral nerve stimulation. [Personal communication: Joseph M. Neal, MD].

Furthermore, the vagueness of "40 peripheral blocks" allows a discrepancy between block types to occur. Because no specific blocks have been named in the core curriculum, it is not possible to ensure that graduates from all resident programs will have comparable expertise in all nerve block procedures. Nearly 34 peripheral nerve block techniques have been suggested as regional anesthesia procedures.[14] If trainees were to perform an equal frequency of each block, they would still not be able to gain competency in any single block in the recommended

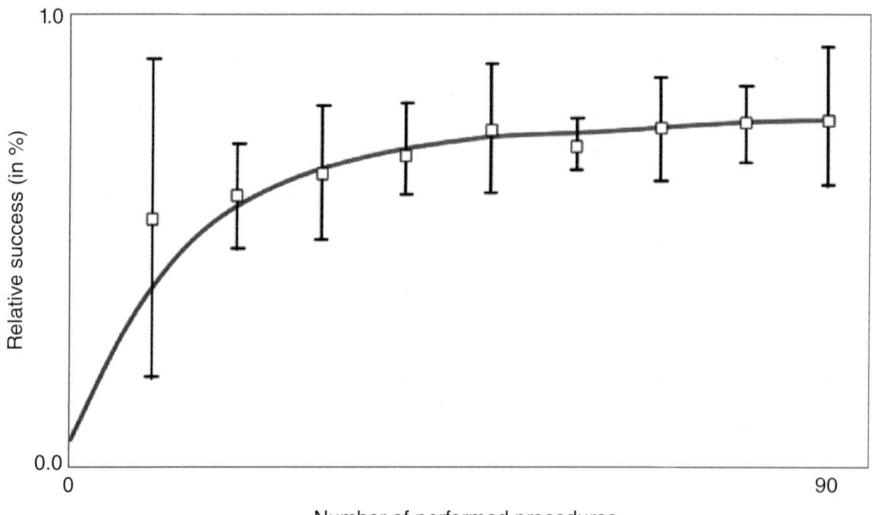

FIGURE 77–3. The learning curve for epidural anesthesia: demonstrating a minimum of 65 blocks to consistently reach 90% success rate.

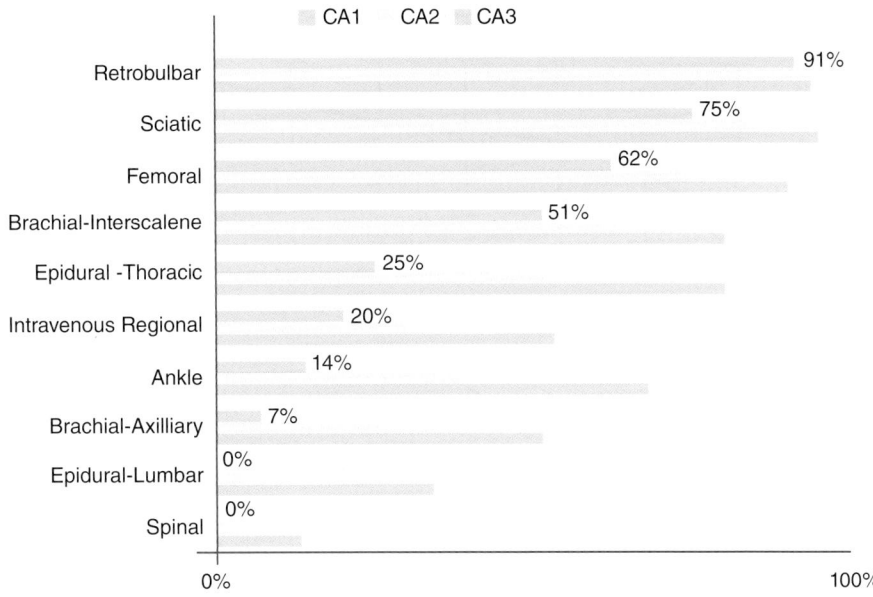

FIGURE 77–4. The percentage of residents, per training year, who categorized themselves as "not confident" in performing a particular block. Exact percentages are listed for the CA-3 resident class. Residents felt least confident with peripheral nerve blocks, and no CA-3 resident admitted to being "not confident" for spinal or lumbar epidural anesthesia.

40 peripheral nerve block performances. In addition, 40 performances of any *one* nerve block may not be suitable to attain competency. Konrad et al demonstrated that 70 axillary blocks are needed before an 85% success rate can be achieved[6] (Figure 77–6). Rosenblatt et al showed that more than 10 interscalene blocks are necessary before the resident attains at least 50% autonomy.[15] Therefore, it is likely that many residents are unable to develop the necessary proficiency because they are not performing enough peripheral nerve blocks. Furthermore, some teaching departments have fewer regional anesthesia teachers than they would prefer. A 2013 survey of department chairs noted that on average they would ideally hire one to three additional regional anesthesia specialists at their faculty.[16]

Clinical Pearl

- Anesthesiology residents trained in the United States are much more likely to fulfill accrediting agency requirements for spinal and epidural anesthesia than for peripheral nerve blocks.

ENRICHING THE EDUCATIONAL EXPERIENCE

Assessing Competency

In addition to a skilled faculty and a culture of using regional anesthesia for surgical cases, learning regional anesthesia

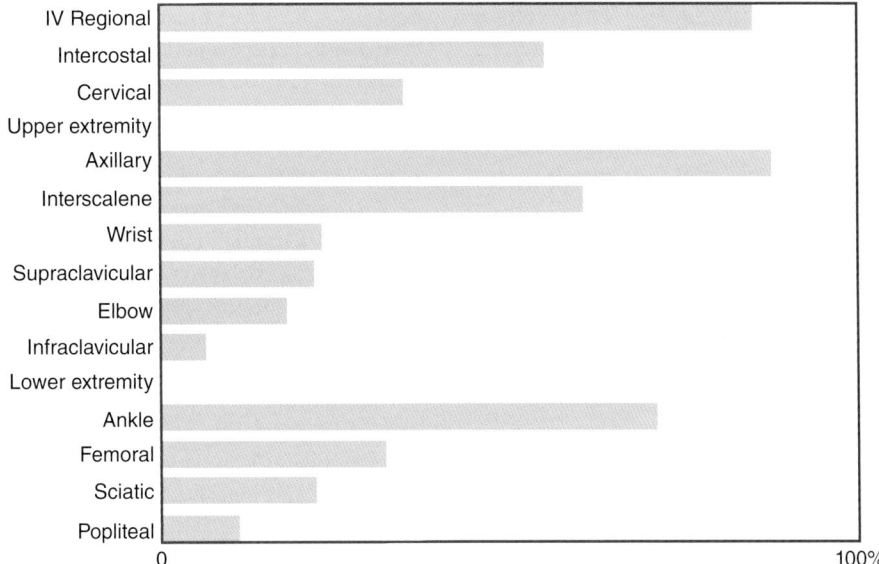

FIGURE 77–5. Percentage of peripheral nerve blocks performed in practice in the United States, as reported by practitioners. (Reproduced with permission from Hadzić A, Vloka JD, Kuroda MM, et al: The practice of peripheral nerve blocks in the United States: a national survey [p2e comments]. *Reg Anesth Pain Med*. 1998 May-Jun;23(3):241–246.)

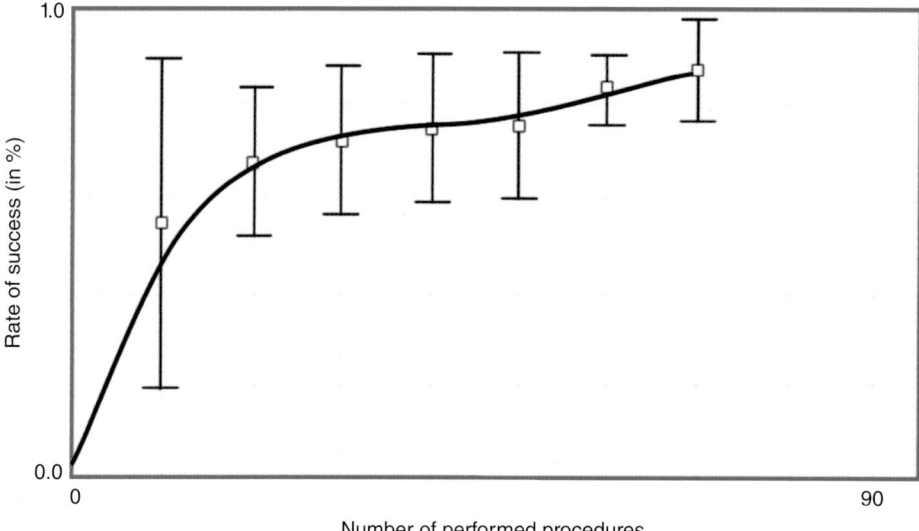

FIGURE 77–6. The learning curve for brachial plexus anesthesia: demonstrating a minimum of 70 blocks to reach 85% success rate.

procedures requires much more than mastering the technical aspects of directing a needle to the intended target. The current RRC focus on the number of blocks performed during training does little to assess actual technical competence, much less nontechnical proficiency. Resident or fellow confidence in the technical aspects of regional anesthesia may not be at all reflective of their overall competence. Indeed, inexperienced trainees may overestimate their technical skills, while at the same time be incompetent in the nontechnical aspects of regional anesthesia. The actual number of blocks performed says little about the trainee's mastery of the physiology and pharmacology of regional anesthesia, intraoperative sedation skills, awareness and management of complications, or overall judgment in selecting which patients should be offered regional techniques.[17] Expertise in regional anesthesia has been defined as not only an ability to have good technical skills but also to have good cognitive skills.[18] These include communicating with the patient, trying to anticipate and minimize their discomfort, and recognizing the limits of safe practice. While competence in cognitive knowledge and problem solving and adaptability can be assessed to some degree by written and oral certifying examinations, respectively, the teaching and assessment of technical and nontechnical aspects of regional anesthesia remain a challenge. Many checklists have been developed for assessment of technical skills for individual peripheral nerve blocks[19,20] and have been validated. However, a need for a single validated checklist for all peripheral nerve blocks remains. Recently, a global checklist has been developed by the Delphi method, which is suitable to assess all ultrasound-guided nerve blocks, and this has been validated in both patients and simulation models. A valid and reliable assessment tool for remote simulation-based ultrasound-guided regional anesthesia.[21] Unfortunately, only limited evidence exists for technical skill assessment in regional anesthesia, and examples have to be obtained from the surgical literature. In surgical training specific and global checklists have been used to grade performance on simulation models,

and they have been proven to be valid, reliable, and cost and time effective.[22]

Alternatives to Bedside Teaching

Anesthesia teaching and learning has traditionally followed the apprenticeship model of "see one, do one, teach one." However, a new paradigm of teaching has emerged which focuses on "see one, practice one, and do one," and this has become an integral part of ultrasound-guided regional anesthesia training programs.[23] This is due to an emphasis on operating room efficiency and patient safety. Specific skills for regional anesthesia can be practiced and assessed on bench model simulators in a "pretraining"[24] period prior to exposure to patients. This provides the student with an unhurried environment that encourages deliberate practice, which is critical process of developing expertise. Deliberate practice calls for repeating a defined task to improve on particular aspects of performance.[25] It allows the teacher to provide immediate feedback and coaching to the trainee and convey their expectations. The use of bench models also allows the task to be broken down to its core components, which can be taught individually.

There is growing evidence that knowledge attained during practice on a simulation model does improve skills in the operating room.[26–28] Barsuk et al have demonstrated that simulation training of central venous catheterization can lead to higher success rates as well as reduce rates of infection in intensive care patients.[29]

Another important area of inquiry concerning simulators is whether high-fidelity simulation training has any advantage over low-fidelity simulation. Friedman et al have shown that low-fidelity and high-fidelity models have an equal impact on teaching of novices.[30] This is interesting as low-fidelity simulation models are cheaper than high-fidelity models and provide similar benefits in the early learning period. However, high-fidelity simulation models do provide some advantage in regional anesthesia. They provide the user with surface anatomy similar to that of real patients. In ultrasound- guided regional anesthesia these models allow the operator to position the transducer and insert the needle in relation to the normal contours of the body. These models also have sophisticated software that allows immediate feedback and also allows the teacher to objectively assess the learner.

Unconventional and inexpensive simulation models can be created with everyday household objects. For example, one model was created with a banana, some slices of bread, and a balloon. As the resident passes the needle through the banana using loss of resistance technique, the fruit mimics the feel of the subcutaneous tissues and ligamentum flavum, and if the resident should advance the needle too far through the bread (epidural space), the balloon (dura) will pop.[31] A foam-block model can be used to teach residents how minimally changing the angle of the needle at the skin greatly affects where the tip of the needle is ultimately placed.[7]

There are also a number of inexpensive simulation models developed from meat,[32] tofu,[33] and gelatin[34] for ultrasound-guided regional anesthesia. Meat models provide realistic tissue feedback, permit injection of local anesthetic and have low background echogenicity, allowing good needle visibility. The gelatin and tofu models provide low background echogenicity but do not reproduce tissue qualities.[35]

Other than simulation bench models, there is a growing trend of using cadavers and virtual reality for teaching skills relevant to regional anesthesia. Unembalmed cadavers are probably the closest phantom media to live human tissue.[35] Embalming of cadavers can change the characteristics of block performance, and it has been seen that Thiel embalmed cadavers provide more realistic simulation than fresh cadavers.[36] This embalming process provides a realistic feeling of passing through fascial planes and also nerve swelling on intraneural injection. Despite their advantages, cadavers are expensive, may provide an infection risk, and teaching has to take place in a remote setting from the operating room. Another disadvantage is that cadaver blood vessels are collapsed and this may impact on their use with ultrasound-guided regional anesthesia. Hocking and his group have described a novel technique to overcome this problem in which gelatin is injected into cadaver blood vessels to prevent them from collapsing.[37]

Virtual reality is another platform of pretraining that can be accessed at one's own time and is an interactive and dynamic form of simulation. A problem with virtual reality for regional anesthesia is that it is expensive and difficult to form an immersion model where the learners feel that they are in a virtual environment. Another problem is feedback from haptic cues. During our clinical practice we rely on touch and pressure feedback that is difficult to incorporate into virtual reality models. Kulcsar et al have developed a virtual reality–based simulator for teaching spinal anesthesia.[38] This model accurately replicates haptic sensations of skin, ligaments, and bone. When used in combination with didactic teaching, this model did not show any benefits to didactic teaching alone when performing spinal anesthesia on a patient. Interestingly, there was, however, a trend toward higher scores on a task-specific checklist and less stress while performing spinal anesthesia in a clinical setting with the group that had trained on the virtual reality simulation model. In ultrasound-guided regional anesthesia virtual reality is still at its preliminary stages. A virtual reality spine model has been developed to teach anatomy and sonoanatomy of the spine.[39] This simulation model allows the user to perform an interactive prepuncture scan on a simulated patient. Anesthesia residents, who had access to the complete module, when compared to those who had access to the anatomy module alone, achieved higher scores on a task-specific checklist while performing a prepuncture scan on live models. The students in the study group were able to identify more key structures such as the vertebral bodies, ligaments, and dura mater, which are important when identifying an ideal intravertebral space to perform neuraxial anesthesia.

Other methods of teaching away from the bedside include interactive graphics on CD-ROMs; a learning tool that is readily at hand (literally, as handheld devices can carry the software) and, therefore, is increasingly popular among residents. Outstanding DVDs are available that allow the student to learn the relevant anatomy and block placement in a three-dimensional mode.[40] Invaluable experience in the placement of continuous perineural catheters can be gained in anesthetized pigs and other animals. Some investigators have described using ultrasound as a visual aid to teach correct needle placement for obstetric lumbar epidural blocks, as such guidance has been shown to improve residents' learning curve.[41]

Residents can also learn from receiving regional anesthesia themselves. Residents participating in compensated volunteer studies learned aspects of regional anesthesia that cannot be taught. After the experience, residents acknowledge that they learned to be more sensitive to patient concerns and to be better communicators with their patients regarding regional anesthesia. Other common observations included the value of sedation, the concept of gentle versus rough touch, and the discomfort caused by local anesthesia infiltration, nerve stimulators, and paresthesias.[42]

Simulation can also be used to teach nontechnical skills. Smith et al have described expertise in regional anesthesia, and have shown that it extends beyond competence in technical skills.[18] To be a true expert one should be able to communicate with the patient, anticipate and minimize their discomfort, and recognize the limits of safe practice. Simulated patients or mannequins can give trainees the ability to practice patient interviews, explanation of regional anesthesia procedures, and crisis management in regional anesthesia. Neal et al have shown that a simulation laboratory scenario can be used to teach residents the use of a specific checklist for local anesthetic toxicity.[43] Hospitals where block rooms are available can perform simulations where team training can take place. This can improve communication and coordination skills between team members and reduce adverse events and improve patient outcome. Figures 77–7 and 77–8 demonstrate several models and simulations commonly used in teaching ultrasound- guided regional anesthesia courses.

Regional Anesthesia Fellowship Training

The ultimate means for a resident to become a highly skilled regional anesthesiologist is to enroll in a fellowship program.

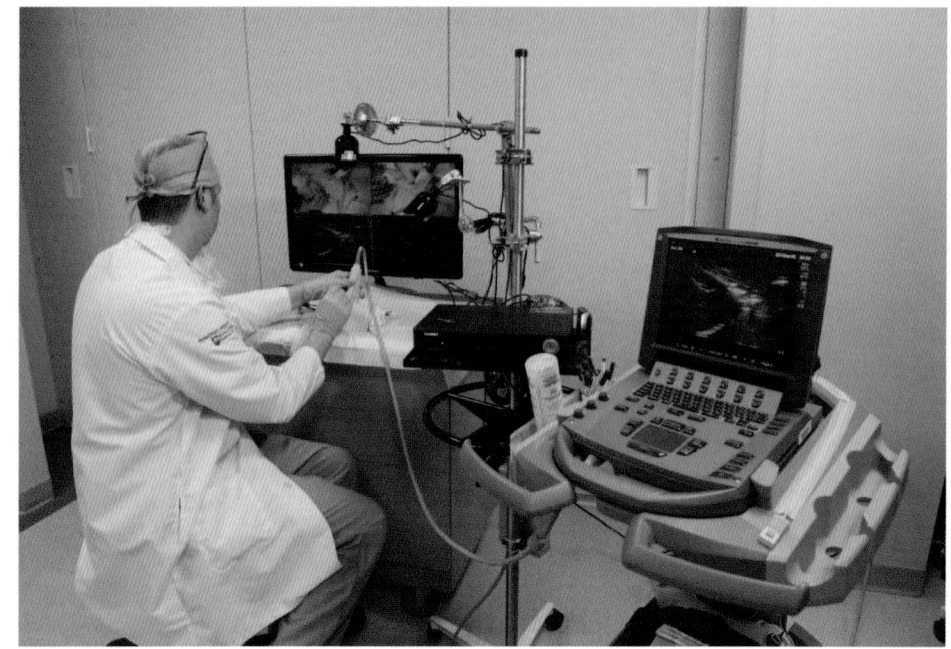

FIGURE 77–7. A simulator for teaching hand–eye coordination during ultrasound-guided regional anesthesia introduced by Adhikary and colleagues.

In 2005, there were approximately 12 active fellowship programs in the United States and Canada.[16] That number has been considerably increased from the two or three training programs that were available prior to the mid- 1990s,[44] and by

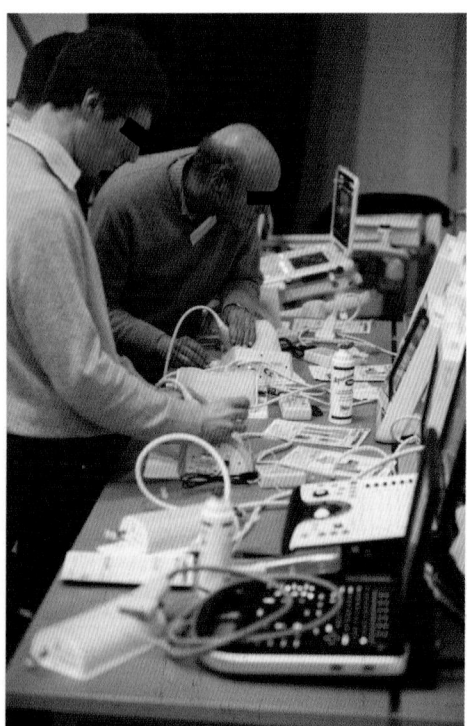

FIGURE 77–8. NYSORA ultrasound-guided nerve blocks and vascular access workshop. A number of nerve block and vascular models as well as tissue models of peripheral nerves are used to simulate the needle guidance under ultrasound and practice core skills in simulated, nonclinical environment.

2013, the number of regional anesthesiology and acute pain medicine programs had grown to 55.[45] Regional anesthesiology and acute pain medicine is likely to be the latest accredited fellowship by the ACGME (full approval expected fall 2016). The training experience and clinical focus of regional anesthesia / acute pain medicine fellows varies considerably from pain medicine fellowship training. Experience and clinical focus varies considerably among programs.[16,44] Until formal accreditation and program requirements are implemented, regional anesthesiology and acute pain medicine fellowship program directors have produced training guidelines periodically to ensure that fellows receive the quality and quantity of regional anesthesia experience they need to become true experts in the field.[44,46] At the time of this book publication, the fellowship in Regional Anesthesia and Acute Pain Medicine is likely to be recognized as ACGME approved and will result in a formal certification.

Continuing Education Opportunities

A final challenge is how best to train postgraduate anesthesiologists in emerging regional techniques. The time-honored method of learning new techniques using patients is less than ideal. To a great extent, continuing medical education programs such as those offered by the American Society of Regional Anesthesia and Pain Medicine and NYSORA serve a valuable role in updating anesthesiologists on the nontechnical aspects of regional anesthesia and pain medicine advances. But technical training is incompletely accomplished in workshop settings. However, the increased availability of cadaver-based anatomy courses and workshops, animal laboratories, and computer-generated imaging technologies are encouraging as future generations of anesthesiologists strive to maintain their skills in an ever-changing subspecialty.

Clinical Pearls

- The numbers of blocks performed or consistently placing a needle near the target nerve are not entirely satisfactory measures of regional anesthesia competency.
- Skills for regional anesthesia should be practiced and assessed on bench model simulators in a "pretraining" period prior to exposure to patients.
- Further development is required to determine means of assessing technical and nontechnical skills required for regional anesthesia.
- Innovative teaching methods are needed not only for resident and fellow training, but also for the continuing education of postgraduate practitioners.

FUTURE DIRECTIONS

Training residents and postgraduates in regional anesthesia has improved remarkably over the past two decades, but many challenges remain. Current research in how regional techniques affect perioperative outcome, as well as the rapid development of continuous perineural catheters, extended-duration local anesthetic and opioid preparations, and ultrasound-assisted nerve localization all point to future anesthesiologists becoming more, not less, involved in regional anesthesia. Certainly, nonpatient training techniques such as bench model simulation, virtual reality, interactive learning programs, and animal laboratories will play an increasing role in the education of future residents and postgraduates alike. The Recommendations for Education and Training in Ultrasound Guided Regional Anesthesia[47] and the *Guidelines for Regional Anesthesia Fellowship Training*[46] should improve the overall quality of regional anesthesia training.

ACKNOWLEDGEMENT

The authors wish to recognize Susan B. McDonald, MD, for her contributions to the original version of this chapter, which appeared in the first edition of this textbook.

REFERENCES

1. Bacon DR, Labat G, Lundy J: Tthe spread of regional anesthesia in America between the World Wars. J Clin Anesth 2002;14:315–320.
2. Accreditation Council for Graduate Medical Education. Program requirements for graduate medical education in anesthesiology. July 2016. Accessed August 29, 2016.
3. Bridenbaugh LD: Are anesthesia resident programs failing regional anesthesia? Reg Anesth 1982;7:26–28.
4. Kopacz DJ, Bridenbaugh LD: Are anesthesia residency programs failing regional anesthesia? The past, present, and future. Reg Anesth 1993;18:84–87.
5. Kopacz DJ, Neal JM: Regional anesthesia and pain medicine: residency training—the year 2000. Reg Anesth Pain Med 2002;27:9–14.
6. Konrad C, Schuepfer G, Wietlisbach M, Gerber H: Learning manual skills in anesthesiology. Is there a recommended number of cases for anesthetic procedures? Anesth Analg 1998;86:635–639.
7. Kopacz DJ, Neal JM, Pollock JE: The regional anesthesia "Learning Curve": What is the minimum number of epidural and spinal blocks to reach consistency? Reg Anesth 1996;21:182–190.
8. Schuepfer G, Konrad C, Schmeck J, et al: Generating a learning curve for pediatric caudal epidural blocks: an empirical evaluation of technical skills in novice and experienced anesthetists. Reg Anesth Pain Med 2000; 25:385–388.
9. Smith MP, Sprung J, Zura A, et al: A survey of exposure to regional anesthesia techniques in American anesthesia residency training programs. Reg Anesth Pain Med 1999;24:11–16.
10. Blumenthal D, Gokhale M, Campbell EG, Weissman JS. Preparedness for clinical practice: reports of graduating residents at academic health centers. JAMA 2001;286:1027–1034.
11. Buffington CW, Ready LB, Horton WG: Training and practice factors influencing the use of regional anesthesia: implications for resident education. Reg Anesth 1986;11:2–6.
12. Hadzic A, Vloka JD, Kuroda MM, et al: The practice of peripheral nerve blocks in the United States: a national survey. Reg Anesth Pain Med 1998;23:241–246.
13. Bouaziz H, Mercier FJ, Narchi P, et al: Survey of regional anesthetic practice among French residents at time of certification. Reg Anesth 1996;22:218–222.
14. Hadzic A, Vloka JD, Koenigsamen J: Training requirements for peripheral nerve blocks. Curr Opin Anaesthesiol 2002;15:669–673.
15. Rosenblatt MA, Fishkind D: Proficiency in interscalene anesthesia—how many blocks are necessary? J Clin Anesth 2003;15:282–288.
16. Neal JM, Kopacz DJ, Liguori GA, et al: The training and careers of regional anesthesia fellows—1983–2002. Reg Anesth Pain Med 2005;30: 226–232.
17. Neal JM: Education in regional anesthesia: caseloads, simulation, journals, and politics: 2011 Carl Koller Lecture. Reg Anesth Pain Med 2012; 37:647–651.
18. Smith AF, Pope C, Goodwin D, Mort M. What defines expertise in regional anaesthesia? An observational analysis of practice. Br J Anaesth 2006;97:401–407.
19. Chin KJ, Tse C, Chan V, et al: Hand motion analysis using the imperial college surgical assessment device: validation of a novel and objective performance measure in ultrasound-guided peripheral nerve blockade. Reg Anesth Pain Med 2011;36:213–219.
20. Naik VN, Perlas A, Chandra DB, et al: An assessment tool for brachial plexus regional anesthesia performance: establishing construct validity and reliability. Reg Anesth Pain Med 2007;32:41–45.
21. Burckett-St Laurent DA, Niazi AU, Cunningham MS, Jaeger M, Abbas S, McVicar J, Chan VW. Reg Anesth Pain Med. 2014 Nov-Dec;39(6): 496–501.
22. Reznick R, Regehr G, MacRae H, et al: Testing technical skill via an innovative "bench station" examination. Am J Surg 1997;173: 226–230.
23. Smith HM, Kopp SL, Jacob AK, et al: Designing and implementing a comprehensive learner-centered regional anesthesia curriculum. Reg Anesth Pain Med 2009;34:88–94.
24. Grantcharov TP, Reznick RK: Teaching procedural skills. BMJ 2008; 336:1129–1131.
25. Ericsson KA: Deliberate practice and acquisition of expert performance: a general overview. Acad Emerg Med Nov 2008;15:988–994.
26. Chandra DB, Savoldelli GL, Joo HS, et al: Fiberoptic oral intubation: the effect of model fidelity on training for transfer to patient care. Anesthesiology 2008;109:1007–1013.
27. Fried GM, Feldman LS, Vassiliou MC, et al: Proving the value of simulation in laparoscopic surgery. Ann Surg 2004;240:518–525; discussion 525–8.
28. Boet S, Bould MD, Schaeffer R, et al: Learning fibreoptic intubation with a virtual computer program transfers to "hands on" improvement. Eur J Anaesthesiol 2010;27:31–35.
29. Barsuk JH, McGaghie WC, Cohen ER, et al: Simulation-based mastery learning reduces complications during central venous catheter insertion in a medical intensive care unit. Crit Care Med 2009;37:2697–2701.
30. Friedman Z, You-Ten KE, Bould MD, Naik V: Teaching lifesaving procedures: the impact of model fidelity on acquisition and transfer of cricothyrotomy skills to performance on cadavers. Anesth Analg 2008; 107:1663–1669.
31. Leighton BL: A greengrocer's model of the epidural space (correspondence). Anesthesiology 1989;70:368–369.
32. Xu D, Abbas S, Chan VW: Ultrasound phantom for hands-on practice. Reg Anesth Pain Med 2005;30:593–594.
33. Pollard BA. New model for learning ultrasound-guided needle to target localization. Reg Anesth Pain Med 2008;33:360–362.
34. Madsen EL, Zagzebski JA, Banjavie RA, Jutila RE: Tissue mimicking materials for ultrasound phantoms. Med Phys 1978;5:391–394.

PART 13

35. Hocking G, Hebard S, Mitchell CH: A review of the benefits and pitfalls of phantoms in ultrasound-guided regional anesthesia. Reg Anesth Pain Med 2011;36:162–170.

36. Benkhadra M, Faust A, Ladoire S, et al: Comparison of fresh and Thiel's embalmed cadavers according to the suitability for ultrasound-guided regional anesthesia of the cervical region. Surg Radiol Anat 2009;31(7):531–535.

37. Hocking G, McIntyre, O: Achieving change in practice by using unembalmed cadavers to teach ultrasound-guided regional anaesthesia. Ultrasound 2011;19:31–35.

38. Kulcsar Z, O'Mahony E, Lovquist E, et al: Preliminary evaluation of a virtual reality-based simulator for learning spinal anesthesia. J Clin Anesth 2013;25:98–105.

39. Niazi AU, Tait G, Carvalho JC, Chan VW: The use of an online three-dimensional model improves performance in ultrasound scanning of the spine: a randomized trial. Can J Anaesth 2013;60:458–464.

40. Peripheral nerve blocks on DVD: Upper and lower limb [computer program]. Philadelphia, PA: Lippincott Williams & Wilkins, 2005.

41. Grau T, Bartusseck E, Conradi R, et al: Ultrasound imaging improves learning curves in obstetric epidural anesthesia: a preliminary study. Can J Anaesth 2003;50:1047–1050.

42. McDonald SB, Thompson GE: "See one, do one, teach one, have one": a novel variation on regional anesthesia training. Reg Anesth Pain Med 2002;27:456–459.

43. Neal JM, Hsiung RL, Mulroy MF, et al: ASRA checklist improves trainee performance during a simulated episode of local anesthetic systemic toxicity. Reg Anesth Pain Med 2012;37:8–15.

44. Hargett MJ, Beckman JD, Liguori GA, Neal JM: Guidelines for regional anesthesia fellowship training. Reg Anesth Pain Med 2005;30:218–225.

45. Neal JM, Liguori GA, Hargett MJ. The training and careers of regional anesthesiology and acute pain medicine fellows, 2013. Reg Anesth Pain Med 2015;40:218–222.

46. Guidelines for fellowship training in regional anesthesiology and acute pain medicine. 3rd ed., 2014. The Regional Anesthesiology and Acute Pain Medicine Fellowship Directors Group. Reg Anesth Pain Med 2015;40:213–217.

47. Sites BD, Chan VW, Neal JM, et al: The American Society of Regional Anesthesia and Pain Medicine and the European Society of Regional Anaesthesia and Pain Therapy Joint Committee recommendations for education and training in ultrasound-guided regional anesthesia. Reg Anesth Pain Med 2009;34:40–46.

Regional Anesthesia and Acute Pain Medicine Fellowship

Jinlei Li and Thomas M. Halaszynski

INTRODUCTION

Regional anesthesia was established early in the history of medicine, but became somewhat obsolete, if not abandoned following the introduction of modern and safer general anesthetics. Acute pain management has regained attention and popularity by anesthesiologists over the past few decades due to several factors, such as significant advances in regional anesthesia technology, patient parameters of a continuing search for improved safety and satisfaction criteria in medicine, and an enhanced accountable evaluation of healthcare system resource utilization. The demand for and acceptance of regional anesthesia practices from both surgeons and patients has also increased over the past few decades. Patients benefit with enhanced approval and outcome and surgeons receive increased patient referrals and decreased perioperative complications with better pain management.[1] Advancement of medical technologies, especially ease and availability of ultrasound developments, have reshaped regional anesthesia into a more accurate, effective, and efficient modality toward enhanced patient care. Trained and experienced anesthesiologists from regional anesthesia fellowship programs are now able to deliver fast, safe, consistent, and reliable regional techniques, especially peripheral nerve blocks, in contrast to the previous conventional (e.g., paresthesia) "hit or miss" methods of regional anesthesia. An enhanced emphasis on effective and adequate pain control, patient autonomy, and patient satisfaction (both surgical and pain management experiences) play a significant role in this continuing transition. Additional benefits of practicing regional anesthesia techniques by fellowship-trained physicians became appreciated by hospital administrators, other healthcare providers besides surgeons, such as earlier ambulation, shorter hospital stay(s), an improved proactive role in rehabilitation, and minimization of adverse side effects often associated with narcotic-based pain medications, to list a few of the clinically relevant advantages. In addition, economic pressure(s) to enhance cost-efficiency of surgical centers, shorten both operating room time and post-anesthesia care unit (PACU) stay, improve Hospital Consumer Assessment of Health Plans Survey (HCAHPS) scores (nationally standardized patient outcome survey), and advance perioperative pain control have all made regional anesthesia/analgesia more appealing as an readily available option toward both patient-specific and procedure-specific anesthesia care. Incorporating regional anesthesia can also provide an alternative for the aging population with complex comorbidities that continue to pose significant risks in healthcare management.

Regional anesthesia continues to play an ever-increasing role and is recognized as a vital component toward more effective patient pain medicine and complementary fulfillment of perioperative medical care. Regional anesthesia/acute pain medicine fellowships are positioned to further emphasize patient and healthcare system value-added when incorporating regional anesthesia/analgesia options into medical management of the surgical patient. The first documented regional anesthesia fellowships were founded at Brigham and Women's Hospital in Boston, Massachusetts (by Benjamin Covino) and at Virginia Mason Medical Center in Seattle, Washington (by Daniel Moore) in the 1980s.[2] The decades that followed were characterized as a continued developmental stage. As of 2007, a total of 11 American Society of Regional Anesthesia/Acute Pain Medicine (ASRA)–recognized regional anesthesia fellowship programs were documented followed by another 10 programs under consideration in the next few subsequent years. Most recently, there has been a continued increase in interest toward regional anesthesia fellowships with 60 programs in 2016 in the United States and 8 in Canada listed on the ASRA website[3] (Table 78–1).

TABLE 78-1. List of regional anesthesia fellowship programs in North America by ASRA.

United States Programs		
State	**Name of Institution**	**No. of Fellows**
Alabama	University of Alabama at Birmington	1
California	UCLA Department of Anesthesia and Perioperative Medicine	1
Colorado	University of Colorado Denver School of Medicine	2
Connecticut	Integrated Anesthesia Associates/Hartford Hospital	2
	St. Francis Hospital and Medical Center	1
Georgia	Emory University Hospital	1
Maryland	University of Maryland	1
Massachusetts	Boston Children's Hospital	2
Michigan	University of Michigan	1
Minnesota	University of Minnesota	1
New York	Westchester Medical Center/ New York Medical College	1
South Carolina	Medical Center of South Carolina	1
Texas	University of Texas Southwestern Medial Center	1
Wisconsin	Medical College of Wisconsin	1
California	Cedars–Sinai Medical Center	2
	University of California at San Diego	3
	University of California, Irvine	3
	University of California, San Francisco	1
	Harbor–University of California, Los Angeles	1
	Stanford University Medical Center	3
	Keck School of Medicine, University of Southern California	2
Connecticut	Yale University School of Medicine	3
District of Columbia	Walter Reed National Military Medical Center	2
Florida	Jackson Memorial Medical Center	2
	The Andrews Institute Surgery Center	1
	Mayo Clinic Mayo School of Graduate Medical Education	2
	University of Florida College of Medicine	4
Illinois	University of Illinois at Chicago	1
	McGaw Medical Center of Northwestern University	2
Iowa	University of Iowa	3
Kansas	Kansas University Medical Center	1
Louisiana	Ochsner Medical Center	1-2
Maryland	Johns Hopkins Medical Center	4
Massachusetts	Massachusetts General Hospital	2
	Brigham and Women's Hospital	2
Minnesota	Mayo Clinic Mayo School of Graduate Medical Education	2

(continued)

TABLE 78–1. List of regional anesthesia fellowship programs in North America by ASRA. (*Continued*)

United States Programs		
State	**Name of Institution**	**No. of Fellows**
Missouri	Washington University	2
New Hampshire	Geisel School of Medicine at Dartmouth	2
New Mexico	University of New Mexico	2
New York	New York–Presbyterian Medical Center Columbia University	2
	Cornell–New York Presbyterian Hospital	3
	Hospital for Special Surgery	9
	Mount Sinai Medical Center	1
	NYU/Hospital for Joint Diseases	1
	NYSORA, The New York School of Regional Anesthesia at St. Luke's-Roosevelt Hospita (1998-2014)	1-2
North Carolina	Duke University Medical Center	3
	University of North Carolina at Chapel Hill	2
	Wake Forest School of Medicine	2
Ohio	Cleveland Clinic	2
	Ohio State University Medical Center	2
Oregon	Oregon Health & Science University	2
Pennsylvania	University of Pittsburgh Medical Center	15
	Drexel University College of Medicine	1
	Thomas Jefferson University	2
	Tennessee Vanderbilt University	2
Texas	University of Texas Health Center at Houston	1
	Utah University of Utah	3
Virginia	University of Virginia	2
Washington	University of Washington	3
	Virginia Mason Medical Center	3
Wisconsin	University of Wisconsin Hospital and Clinics	2
Canada Programs		
Province	**Name of Institution**	**No. of Fellows**
British Columbia	University of British Columbia St Paul's Hospital	1
Nova Scotia	Dalhousie University	1
Qubec	Centre Hospitalier de l'Universite de Montreal	1
Ontario	Toronto Western Hospital	4
	University of Ottawa	2
	University of Toronto Saint Michael's Hospital	4
Alberta	University of Alberta	2

(*continued*)

CHAPTER 78

TABLE 78–1. List of regional anesthesia fellowship programs in North America by ASRA. (*Continued*)

Other Regional Anesthesia Fellowship Programs	
Programs	**State/Province**
Children's Hospital of Philadelphia	Pennsylvania, USA
University of Kentucky	Kentucky, USA
University of Manitoba	Manitoba, Canada

Abbreviation: ASRA: American Society of Regional Anesthesia.

HISTORY AND EVOLUTION OF REGIONAL ANESTHESIA AND REGIONAL ANESTHESIA FELLOWSHIPS

Following innovation of ether and commencement of general anesthesia in 1846, the discovery of local anesthetics marked the introduction of regional anesthesia into medicine and recognition of regional anesthetic techniques separate from general anesthesia.[4] In 1884, cocaine, an extract from coca leaves, made regional techniques possible prior to implementation of modern-day local anesthetics. Subsequent development of various amino ester and then amino amide compounds (with different pharmacodynamics and pharmacokinetics) provided anesthesiologists with additional options to diversify regional techniques.[5] Although spinal and epidural anesthesia has been used since 1899,[6] it was not until 1902 when the term *regional anesthesia* was coined by Harvey Cushing as he started to perform extremity peripheral nerve blockade procedures. A similar analogy (lagging behind in implementation of peripheral nerve blockade) in the history of modern anesthesia is reflective of what is occurring in anesthesiology residency training. Secondary to underutilization and lack of appreciation of peripheral nerve block techniques in clinical practice, regional anesthesia and acute pain medicine training for anesthesia residents largely comes from central neuraxial blockade experience.[1,7] Until relatively recently, most anesthesiology residency programs in the United States and outside of North America were not prepared, equipped, or motivated to provide residents with regional anesthetic technique training beyond constraints of remaining compliant with (ACGME) program requirements. Therefore, it was not until after additional postgraduate training in a regional anesthesia fellowship program that anesthesiology physicians were able to achieve the skill set(s) necessary to safely, effectively, and independently implement regional anesthetic/analgesic techniques.

To fulfill ACGME requirements, anesthesia residents need to perform 50 epidurals, 40 spinals, 40 peripheral nerve blocks (PNBs), and 25 block techniques for chronic pain management. In Germany, a minimum of 100 neuraxial and 50 PNBs are necessary during the training period. There have been many attempts, studies, and program surveys about minimum numbers of procedures for mastery and adeptness at spinal and epidural anesthesia during anesthesiology residency training.

For example, Konrad showed that proficiency with spinal anesthesia requires 70 cases, and 90 cases were necessary to show competency with epidural techniques.[8] However, there is a limited number of studies to investigate and determine minimum numbers of PNBs required to demonstrate proficiency. Among the few available studies on PNBs, Rosenblatt showed that a minimum of 15 interscalene blocks were required to achieve a degree of competency[9] and Schuepfer showed that a minimum of 55 psoas compartment blocks were necessary to achieve a 70% success rate.[10] Clearly, the diversity of PNB procedures requiring different skill set levels makes this matter even more complex to assess and standardize. Nonetheless, it is clear that the ACGME does not yet recognize the need to emphasize proficiency in PNB training, as a total number of 40 PNBs during residency training remains insufficient. Anesthesia house-staff receive more training and emphasis with the more commonly performed neuraxial techniques, and this is not unique for North America. As an example, in a teaching hospital in Australia, first-year anesthesia residents (clinical anesthesia year 1; CA-1) perform on average 6.5 PNB procedures, second-year residents (CA-2) receive training with only 13.5 PNB techniques, CA-3 residents with 14.9 PNBs, CA-4s with an average of 19.1 PNB interventions, and regional fellows achieve higher numbers with an average of 144 PNB techniques.[7] Recently, both the American Society of Anesthesiologists (ASA) and ASRA have jointly launched an ultrasound-guided regional anesthesia (UGRA) education and training initiative for physicians interested in UGRA. In order to receive certification for this UGRA portfolio, a minimum of 10 hours of didactic lectures (knowledge base) is required followed by a written examination of 50 questions, 6 hours of regional anesthesia workshop demonstrating technical skills, and a case log performing 40 PNB techniques. This program is closely reflective of the basic structure and requirements of anesthesia residents in an ACGME-accredited anesthesia-training program.[11]

However, the ASRA membership/administration has not yet petitioned for formalization of recognition, and none of the ASRA regional anesthesia fellowship programs has received either ACGME accreditation or American Board of Medical Specialties (ABMS) certification.[3,12] As a result, regional fellowship programs have candidates performing varying degrees of clinical duties, research endeavors, and patient care responsibilities without receiving formalized certification following completion of their subspecialty training.[3] In addition, some fellowship participants are able to generate a range of revenue potential along with receiving a wide range of compensations during their training periods. This also translates into a variable degree of institutional duties with fellows responsible for minimum or no overnight in-house call to as much as 20%–50% of their training time engaged as junior faculty or clinical instructors. This variability across the regional anesthesia/pain medicine fellowship programs would change once the individual fellowship site would petition for ACGME accreditation. As an example, the duration of fellowship training could range from a mandatory single year to receive a diploma with up to a 2-year optional training period for a research track and the originally offered 3- to 6-month fellowship program would no longer be recognized as fulfillment for a certificate of completion. The proposals for a 2-year fellowship training option (1 research year) would mimic those from the recently developed pediatric anesthesia[13] and critical care medicine[14] anesthesia fellowships.[15]

Despite the variability of structure that exists in the present regional fellowship programs of North American, most of the fellowship candidates rotate through formalized didactics, perform clinical patient care rotations in hospitals and surgical centers, many have research opportunities and occasionally educational rotations to other outside institutions. Several fellowship programs offer clinical patient care incentives and provide support for research. For example, there are programs that offer up to 20% dedicated research time, continuing medical education travel time, and compensation for other academic endeavors. Most regional anesthesia fellowship program directors are collaborative decision data participants who meet several times a year to discuss and exchange current regional fellowship participant activities and concerns applicable to future fellowship candidates in order to maintain a minimum standard of convention and protocol formalization for those programs that wish to participate. This implies that participating programs voluntarily adhere to standards of Regional Anesthesiology and Acute Pain Medicine Fellowship Director Group's "Collaborative Decision Data Agreements" (such as pre and interim training examinations). For those institutions that have such an agreement, it is also stated that no fellowship applicant should be required to accept or decline a fellowship position offer from any participating fellowship program prior to a predetermined date (September) of the previous academic year.[3] The participating programs implemented this initiative in order to improve upon the application process for candidates. Currently (2016), all United States Regional Anesthesia Fellowship Programs collectively generate around 130 formal Regional Anesthesia/Acute Pain Medicine fellowship–trained anesthesiologists annually, and Canada has added another 17 fellowship-trained physicians with an expertise in regional anesthesia. Clearly, regional fellowship training in North American has become more diversified in terms of centers available for trainees and has significantly expanded the opportunities that these centers can provide which has visibly strengthened this subspecialty.[16]

Regional Anesthesia/Acute Pain Medicine Fellowship Curriculum

Following publication of the original version of *Regional Anesthesia Fellowship Training Guidelines* in 2005, regional fellowship program directors across the nation have agreed to grant a regional fellowship diploma to those who have not only finished basic anesthesia training in an ACGME-accredited residency program, but also have been trained for at least a 12-month period in a regional anesthesia fellowship program.[17] Further maturity of the core competencies from anesthesiology residency training remains a vital part of every regional fellow's daily learning and practice and should continue as basic desirable attributes of any regional fellowship program. Regional fellowship training and further perfection of the six core competencies continues beyond that from residency as each fellow is encouraged to apply and practice ALL six of the measures into regional anesthesia daily practices (Table 78–2). In addition, both ASRA and the European Society of Regional Anesthesia (ESRA) committees have developed and incorporated core competencies related to ultrasound-guided regional anesthesia and identified 10 common tasks to be accomplished during UGRA implementation. These 10 tasks summarized the basic procedural and troubleshooting steps in UGRA and emphasized the importance of familiarity with regional anatomy and its variations, direct visualization of needle movement, and local anesthetics distribution patterns as well as adequate patient monitoring.[18,19]

With an emphasis on providing best evidence-based practice, perioperative efficacy, ensuring patient safety, and reducing adverse events/patient complications, regional anesthesiology fellowship training programs have been formally structured with teaching methods in regional anesthesia/acute pain medicine that include, e.g., didactic sessions, cadaver workshops, practice training toward improving ultrasound guidance techniques, and reviewing ultrasound/computed tomography (CT)/magnetic resonance imaging (MRI) video clips.[1] Ultrasound imaging and three-dimentional video clip review has been shown to improve operator performance, and such published guidelines assist in setting the basis for structured fellowship training programs in regional anesthesia.[18,20] In addition, these structured protocols contain the necessary flexibility that permits each individual program to further capitalize and take into account the unique strengths of each academic institution along with considerations for each individual fellow's learning curve and desires in which to tailor pursuit of research endeavors. There are also several regional fellowship programs that incorporate simulation into the curriculum. Simulation in healthcare training has evolved from manual simulation to now include an ability also to focus on nontechnical skills of the trainee.[21] There is evidence supporting the notion that simulation can result in providing better patient care, improving objective measures in technical skill sets of the operator, and an overall enhancement of education for regional fellows.[21,22] Simulator experience has also been shown, e.g., to expedite the learning-skill process, to more effectively familiarize regional fellows with an understanding of applied clinical anatomy, and to allow one to become more efficacious with the necessary physics of ultrasound, sonographic views, and spacial orientation.[23]

TABLE 78–2. Core competencies for training in ultrasound-guided regional anesthesia (UGRA).

Patient care	*Understand the indications and contraindications and use proper judgment in patient selection and exclusion. *Use appropriate monitoring during UGRA: ECG, BP, SPO$_2$. *Provide adequate/appropriate sedation during regional techniques. *Understand and become competent with nerve and nerve plexus localization techniques with and without assistance from other localization techniques. *Develop competent, safe, effective, and efficient peripheral and central neuraxial nerve block techniques.
Ultrasound knowledge	*Become familiar with basic of UGRA techniques. *Become familiar with the physics of ultrasound machines. *Understand key artifacts and pitfall errors associated with UGRA. *Understand benefits and limitations of UGRA techniques and use adjunct techniques as indicated. *Become familiar with in-plane and out-of-plane techniques and apply appropriately into clinical practice. *In depth knowledge of ultrasonographic anatomy of the major neurovascular structures of extremities and trunks.
Interpersonal/ communication skills	*Communicate sensitively and effectively with patients and families regarding risks and benefits and alternatives. *Explain UGRA and PNBs effectively to surgeons and other medical professionals not familiar with PNBs. *Develop leadership skills and executive expertise in establishing and managing a regional anesthesia service.
Professionalism	*Remain current with UGRA techniques and evidence-based literature. *Effective communication skills with patients to explain benefits from PNBs while identifying potential complications. *Develop effective interactions and engagement protocols with surgical teams and other support services.
System-based practice	*Recognize UGRA costs along with UGRA technology limitations. *Collaborate with other members of the healthcare team to ensure quality of perioperative patient care. *Use evidence-based, cost-conscious strategies in caring for patients (e.g., patient-specific and procedure-specific regional techniques).
Practice-based learning and improvement	*Identify, acknowledge, and remedy gaps in personal knowledge and skill-sets in the care of patients presenting for UGRA. *Use reference-based knowledge opportunities such as: textbook, journals, and computer-based resources to broaden the knowledge base of UGRA techniques. *Competence to perform electronic medical literature searches of articles that address medical issues surrounding UGRA. *Understand and critically evaluate outcome studies related to influences of UGRA on perioperative outcome. *Attend, participate, and direct departmental teaching conferences and supervise residents. *Develop time management skills to perform required tasks in a reasonable amount of time with consistent and satisfactory quality.

Abbreviations: BP: blood pressure; ECG: electrocardiogram; PNBs: peripheral nerve blocks; SPO$_2$: functional oxygen saturation pulse oximetry.

Another attribute of advanced regional fellowship training focuses upon the nontechnical skill sets that have been divided into two subgroups: cognitive or mental and social or interpersonal skills. Both technical and nontechnical skills are necessary and equally important for well-trained regional fellows to achieve levels of becoming a competent leader in any regional anesthesia practice.[21] The curriculum that synthesizes regional fellowship training with instruction and practice of nonprocedural aspects of the subspecialty also needs to be emphasized. Regional anesthesia and acute pain medicine fellowship programs will need to continue to focus on the many nontechnical skill training aspects such as research endeavors, career development, and leadership coaching, to name a few. Due to the lack of such training in these various fields during anesthesiology residency, regional anesthesia subspecialty programs are positioned to provide regional fellows with administrative, executive, infrastructural, as well as medicolegal expertise and skills in conflict solving. The above concept will also continue to challenge regional anesthesia program directors to design dynamic program curricula that expand beyond medical knowledge and technical skills with added emphasis on nontechnical domains in order to train regional fellows capable of advancing the subspecialty into the future and moving ahead with trained physicians capable of more than technical expertise.[1,24] Therefore, undertaking a specialized curriculum and providing experiences of advanced regional fellowship training will escalate and solidify a regional fellow's regional anesthesia/analgesia/acute pain-specific knowledge base, achieve a more solid proficiency with technical skills, improve upon the "whole-task" approach to patient care, offer an environment and opportunity toward training of a "balanced" clinician inclusive of nonprocedural skill sets, and provide a foundation recognized as "value-added" to perioperative anesthesia care.

Despite the many efforts made toward standardization in regional anesthesia fellowship training, there has not yet been a well-defined set number of individual PNB procedures or identification of most appropriate types of individual nerve or nerve plexus blockade modalities needed to establish regional fellow proficiency. Suggesting or determining some basic procedural numbers may serve to identify one objective measure of reference for regional fellowship training guidance, but these number specifications alone would not necessarily provide appropriate assessment of regional fellowship candidate qualifications. These predetermined requirements of minimum nerve and nerve plexus blockade techniques would rather simply assist with a degree of objective standardization(s) for regional fellowship training guidelines. Establishing minimum numbers of regional interventions could also serve as one of the many fundamentals that will move forward with regional anesthesia subspecialty recognition and the ACGME accreditation process. In addition, defining minimum numbers could assist as an objective measure assessing a regional fellow candidate's technical skill level. As an example, Chin et al studied regional anesthesia fellow's performance in their first month and then again in the last 3 months of training by measuring time to perform a nerve block procedure, examining ultrasound probe and hand movements, quantifying needle hand movements, and measuring time duration within both ultrasound scan and needling phases.[25] The above study was able to identify that a regional fellow's early performance showed no statistical difference when compared to anesthesia residents. However, these same regional fellow's demonstrated performance during their last 3 months of training revealed no statistically different measurements when compared with regional anesthesiologists with a minimum of 3 years clinical experience when performing an ultrasound-guided supraclavicular nerve blockade.

The current structure of the national ACGME accredited anesthesiology residency programs has traditionally focused on core competencies and evidence-based training of residents with little effort being directed toward research guidance.[26] According to the ACGME, there is no minimum time requirement for anesthesiology residents or fellows to conduct research endeavors, but each resident candidate has to complete an academic assignment. A survey of pediatric fellowship graduates suggested that more responders recommended formal research training during the fellowship period than the number of individuals who actually received such training.[13] As another example, the recently accredited ACGME Obstetric Anesthesia Fellowship requires candidates to take part in at least a 3-month equivalent of time actively engaged in an academic pursuit.[27] The same Obstetric Anesthesia Fellowship Program also requires that more than half of the faculty demonstrate active involvement in research in the format of peer-reviewed journal publication(s), conducting research activities, or developing educational programs.[27] The examples above suggest that regional anesthesiology fellowship programs (those with an aspiration to work toward ACGME accreditation) should focus on objective measures toward developing research initiatives and competencies that can identify quality measures of fellowship programs that have meet ACGME standards.

It may be premature at this stage of regional fellowship training development to make research endeavors mandatory, but those fellowship candidates enthusiastic about research should be carefully supported by the availability of research projects and research mentors. Regional fellowship programs providing such opportunities should be endorsed and encouraged to provide protected research time, along with continuing medical education (CME) time and subspecialty meeting support. There remains several obstacles for fellowship candidates to participate in research such as not enough faculty support and lack of appropriate funding to identify a few of the current hurdles. However, formalized training of regional fellows with both superior clinical skills along with research accomplishments will prove to serve well toward the future of the subspecialty. In addition, if some regional anesthesia fellowship programs could develop and offer an optional 2-year fellowship (with 1 year committed to research) as a way to gain recognition of the subspecialty could further elevate perception and acknowledgement of the specialty. As another example, some cardiac fellowship programs have interdepartmental partnerships (e.g., clinical pharmacology department) that contribute to potential candidate appeal and interest with an additional offer of a master's degree of science specifically designed for young investigators on statistical analysis and clinical trial design.[28]

The regional anesthesia guidelines, originally published in 2005, updated in 2010 and again in 2014, have provided the much needed general guidance for fellowship training[17,20] (Appendix I; pp. 1266-70). In addition, each regional training program recognized on the ASRA web site has identified how it has developed its own unique and comprehensive curriculum that typically incorporates basic and advanced regional techniques along with multi-modal pain management strategies. The individual curriculum and protocols developed by training programs provide guidance for fellows to acquire medical knowledge and cultivate a foundation for clinical and scientific research. With this diversity, some form of standardized examination system will be required to provide uniform direction of this postresidency educational process in order to ensure quality of training (similar to the national board of echocardiography in cardiothoracic anesthesia fellowship training).

CURRENT CHALLENGES AND FUTURE PROSPECTIVE FOR REGIONAL ANESTHESIA FELLOWSHIP TRAINING

Anesthesiology became a recognized medical specialty in the 1930s when anesthesiologists were awarded the first certificates for specialized training. The ABMS formally accepted anesthesiology as a specialty in 1941. The first recognized regional organization, the American Society of Regional Anesthesia, was founded in 1923. However, this early organization of regional anesthesia was practiced predominantly by surgeons and other nonanesthesia-trained physicians. Currently, there are many subspecialties in anesthesiology that offer fellowshiptraining opportunities as listed in Table 78–3. Prior to 2013, the ABMS offered certifications in the first five subspecialties in anesthesiology,[12] and the ACGME accredited four originally, including cardiac, critical care, chronic pain, and pediatric anesthesia. Then in 2013, obstetric anesthesiology became the fifth ACGME-recognized fellowship training program. As of July 2013, there are now nine obstetric anesthesia fellowship programs throughout the United States that have received formal accreditation. Through petition with the ACGME, securing evidence of meeting fellowship-training qualifications,

being awarded endorsement as an approved fellowship program and providing continued evidence of compliance with certification- training mandates; these five anesthesiology subspecialties have the authority and obligation to offer subspecialty training certification by developing and implementing individual specialty specific board examination protocols. Subspecialization in any medical specialty creates an environment for the development of practice parameter expertise and making tremendous strides toward improving healthcare along with advancing patient safety and also providing opportunities for greater further achievements for medical professionals. Other non-ACGME–accredited subspecialty graduates (including regional anesthesia) receive diplomas, but these subspecialties are currently not recognized by the American Board of Anesthesiology (ABA) or the ABMS. Listed in Table 78–3 are the accreditation and certification status of clinical subspecialties in anesthesiology.[3,12,29,30]

At the present, expert training facilities with regional anesthesia pain medicine, as non-ACGME–accredited training programs, cannot compete with those accredited programs that provide ACGME certifications in seeking applicants wishing to receive fellowship opportunities. ACGME recognition, evaluation, approval, and accreditation (recognition from ABA) of regional anesthesia/acute pain medicine fellowship programs will elevate (medical community at large), formalize, and standardize regional subspecialty training. This formal process will also ensure that regional pain medicine fellowship candidates receive superior training that can offer all users (e.g., hospital administration, healthcare paraprofessionals, surgeons, patients) of the service with unique therapy alternatives and clinically relevant

TABLE 78–3. Accreditation and certification status of clinical subspecialties in anesthesiology.

Fellowship	ACGME Accreditation	ABMS Certification	ASA Recognition
Critical care	Yes	Yes	Yes
Pain medicine	Yes	Yes	Yes
Pediatric anesthesia	Yes	Yes	Yes
Hospice and palliative medicine	No	Yes	No
Sleep medicine	No	Yes	No
Cardiothoracic anesthesia	Yes	No	Yes
Obstetric anesthesia	Yes	No	Yes
Ambulatory anesthesia	No	No	Yes
Regional anesthesia	Yes	No	Yes
Neuroanesthesia	No	No	Yes
Liver transplantation	No	No	No
Perioperative echocardiography	No	No	No
Public policy	No	No	Yes
Trauma anesthesia	No	No	Yes

Abbreviations: ABMS: American Board of Medical Specialties; ACGME: Accreditation Council for Graduate Medical Education; ASA: American Society of Anesthesiologists.

treatment options. Therefore, how well regional pain medicine fellows are trained and the ultimate structure of fellowship program along with factors of development toward an ACGME fellowship program will determine what regional anesthesia/pain medicine as a subspecialty will look like in the future. This is exemplified using the example of cardiac anesthesiology fellowship. A survey of faculty from 30 randomly selected cardiac fellowship programs throughout the United States identified faculty from ACGME-accredited programs as producing more scholarly activities in the forms of increased peer-reviewed journal publications, citations, and higher H-indices when compared to those from non-ACGME–recognized programs.[31] However, there are advantages and concerns with ACGME accreditation. The positive aspects are viewed as consistency within the curriculum, potential for graduate medical education (GME) funding, rigorous review process implementation, subspecialty certification, and the potential for more effective fellowship candidate recruitment. Other less favorable aspects may be ACGME accreditation permits less curriculum flexibility, the possibility that Medicare may confer a teaching penalty(s), ACGME hour limitations secondary to program formatting, a faculty practice plan potentially experiencing ineligibility leading to loss of revenue, and lack of opportunities for fellowship candidates to pursue other facets of anesthesiology training. A similar analogy can be portrayed when seeking ABMS certification with advantages including increased clinical expertise, better job satisfaction, and more research opportunities. However, these gains from ABMS certification could result in a cost to collecting medical care dollars, will be associated with an increased duration of training, and risking the potential loss of general anesthesiology skills.[30]

Recent development and implementation of several evidence-based changes have reformed the regional anesthesia community, and has fundamentally reshaped experiences and exposures of candidates during their regional fellowship training. Undoubtedly, foremost of these changes was the embracing of adoption and acceptance of ultrasonography and tailored ultrasound technology implementation into regional anesthesia daily practice and fellowship training. This remains similar to those parameters of cardiothoracic anesthesia fellowship training, where echocardiography experience remains an integral part and plays a major role toward training and proficiency within such programs. Specifically in the situation of regional anesthesia fellowship programs, experiences with real-time ultrasound imaging should be considered an integral part of such fellowship training. Achievement toward goals of expertise and great proficiency with ultrasound utilization during the practice of regional anesthesia/analgesia would be an objective in order to strive toward an evolution of excellence in delivery of healthcare. Incorporation of ultrasound regional techniques into fellowship training will serve to maintain the "state of the art" and high level of development as a device, technique, and scientific field in regional anesthesia/acute pain medicine. In addition, a competent regional fellowship-trained anesthesiologist, with a solid foundation in medical knowledge and ultrasound training, would be prepared to take on, e.g., the challenges of newly developed innovations, nerve block techniques, and cutting-edge modernization, in the field of regional anesthesia.

Similar in scope to other fields of advanced medical education, the intensions of regional fellowship training would be for graduates to continue with a competency of self-education and self-training. In this context, regional trained anesthesia physicians would be better equipped to continue to lead the subspecialty, develop and advance teaching skills, become innovative and/or invent new techniques, tools, research opportunities, and renovate technology related to regional modalities as an added option in the treatment of the surgical patient. In addition, the practice of anesthesiology (especially the subspecialty of regional anesthesia) is currently and will remain into the near future a high-skill set–centered specialty. Both ASRA and ESRA recognize that there are different levels of difficulty for the various procedures and that the mission of and specialty of regional anesthesia fellowship training protocols can vary greatly between the multitude of programs. Therefore, standards and dynamic objective subspecialty regional training characteristics need to be developed and formally implemented that would be capable of addressing some of the numerous hurdles such as (1) deep PNBs (resulting in degradation of ultrasound and block needle tip imaging), (2) strategically addressing those blocks that have the potential to cause serious injury (e.g., pneumothorax, local anesthetic toxicity, unintentional neuraxial injection), (3) nerve blocks that involve smaller distal nerves (often difficult to image), (4) peripheral blocks that involve nerves lacking distinct ultrasonographic interfaces (can often result in difficulties distinguishing nerve structures from surrounding tissues), (5) patient-related factors (e.g., obesity, musculoskeletal disease), and (6) regional catheter-related techniques (e.g., requiring simultaneous transducer stabilization, needle manipulation, catheter threading) along with many other direct and indirect consequences associated with regional anesthesia/acute pain medicine training.

There has been tremendous progress made, e.g., in better understanding of surgical patient trauma, pathophysiologic bases of acute pain, and influence of patient comorbidities related to surgery and anesthesia, but there remains a continued need for clinicians to implement evidence-based procedure-specific multimodal analgesic protocols. Such an approach to patient care modified to meet the needs of individual patients, to enhance the quality of anesthesia services/perioperative pain management, and address clinically relevant patient needs will further complement the accomplishments of our anesthesiology specialty. In addition, there will continue to be a need for collaboration between the various healthcare providers, to integrate improved perioperative medicine with fast-track recovery paradigms; and an innovative approach to improve the quality of the surgical recovery process, reduce length of hospital stay(s) and postoperative morbidity, lead to shorter periods of convalescence, and yield improved patient experiences resulting in higher patient satisfaction.[32,33] Therefore, rather than simply performing systematic reviews and meta-analysis of the literature, an investigational and clinical role of regional anesthesia/acute pain medicine fellowship programs have been well positioned and structured to return to the hard work of performing, e.g., bench research, conducting prospective and randomized clinical trials on a procedure-specific basis, incorporating evidence-based regional anesthesia modalities as anesthetic/analgesic alternatives, and evaluating use of analgesic combinations as part of multimodal analgesic treatment regimens for the perioperative period.[34]

However, there still remains a disparity between the pathophysiologic data on the mechanisms responsible for, e.g., surgical and anesthesia trauma/stress, perioperative pain, and level and degree of medical intervention(s), and the subsequent translation of this evidence into clinically relevant and value-based practices.[35,36] Despite these hurdles, a way forward would be to design, investigate, and show scientific evidence for a necessity to begin to routinely implement procedure-specific, clinically meaningful anesthesia management and pain medicine protocols into the perioperative period by expertly trained physicians.[32,36] This concept provides further evidence as to how such a void could be bridged with regional anesthesia/acute pain medicine, and how well these procedure-specific analgesic care designs could be combined with a fast-track recovery strategy to obtain improvements in surgical and medical patient outcomes. This single important aspect lends further evidence as to how such regional fellowship training programs are positioned for success. In addition, this approach represents a logical next step despite the fact that existing concepts in the literature fail to support unanimous evidence that improvement in pain management automatically leads to enhanced recovery and reduced morbidity.[37] Therefore, it is becoming increasingly more evident that considering all aspects of a perioperative event should prove to yield improved outcomes along with escalated patient satisfaction that can be consistently achieved.[38,39] Once again, this provides additional evidence that subspecialty training with a regional anesthesia fellowship could led toward such an accomplishment and yield clinical results that are meaningful and relevant to the healthcare of surgical patients.

Identified in Table 78–4 are many additional parameters that provide further insight as to the impact that regional

---

TABLE 78–4. List of ongoing and future endeavors of formalized regional anesthesia/acute pain medicine fellowship programs.

1. Increase public awareness of existing deficiencies and possibilities for improving pain management.
2. Educating surgical patients and family members regarding steps they can take to improve quality of perioperative analgesia and facilitate recovery.
3. Provide evidence that immediate along with future solutions to improving the quality of pain management exists at organizational levels.
4. Generate further clinical research to better delineate the essential components of procedure-specific, multimodal, nonopioid analgesic regimens.
5. Conduct the necessary investigation to determine additional potential for evidence of clinical improvement in pain related outcomes by a peripheral approach (targeting pain at the site of origin before centrally mediated changes occur in the spinal cord/cerebral cortex).[40]
6. Study the effects/influences of local application of long-acting local analgesic formulations (e.g., depo-bupivacaine and extended-release bupivacaine,) and topical medications.
7. Design research that may provide evidence and clinical use of novel receptor populations on sensory nerve endings (transient receptor potential binding sites) which may prove to be useful targets for developing new analgesic adjuvants to add to opioid and nonopioid analgesic compounds.
8. Research findings that may led to discovery of other new classes of analgesic drugs and selective analgesic agonists.
9. An important area for future clinical research includes the need to develop a more in-depth understanding of the basis of the large interindividual variability in the pain response to similar noxious surgical stimuli.
10. Continue to show relevance to the concept that improving the quality of clinical outcome may in part require an individualized approach to acute pain management.
11. Is it possible to determine a patient's pain threshold before any surgical intervention?[41]
12. Areas of genetic research that may increase the ability to identify specific genotypes that may influence pharmacodynamics and pharmacokinetics of analgesic choices.[42]
13. Who in the future will be better prepared to investigate pharmacogenetics; an intriguing area for investigations aimed at improving pain management.
14. Study into perioperative pain management related to the influence of metabolic factors, aging, and gender on responses to anesthetic/analgesic interventions.
15. Population of the elderly age category continues to increase at a rapid rate. Therefore, clinical studies are needed to examine the effect of aging on responses to opioid and nonopioid analgesic medications/interventions.
16. Regional fellows are best positioned to continue to study the concept of "preemptive analgesia" and to examine, by randomized trials, any influence on the timing issue of initiating analgesia (medications and/or techniques) before vs after an invasive stimulus.
17. Information is needed regarding optimal duration of postdischarge therapy on a procedure-specific basis and how such treatment should be modified based on individual patient pain response factors.

anesthesia/acute pain medicine fellowship programs will have on the practice of medicine since it is no longer appreciated that implementation of evidenced-based guidelines for pain management protocols alone is sufficient to achieve the desired improvement(s) in patient outcomes. Implications from the several competencies included in Table 78–2, along with many others, and those cultivated from continuing research will advance the expertise and relevance that anesthesia services can provide real clinical value to and for patients receiving perioperative care, surgeons and other members of the healthcare team, hospital administrators, insurance companies, and other governmental regulatory bodies. A structure of this approach would continue to increase public awareness of the existing possibilities to improve anesthesia and surgical care and pain management along with reducing morbidity. It could also serve toward providing evidence to surgical patients and family members of the strides being made to improve the overall quality of anesthesia services and innovative advances to facilitate the recovery process.

SUMMARY

Following anesthesiology residency training, there are a multitude of options for graduating clinicians to consider as they venture forward into their careers as is listed in Table 78–3. A fellowship in regional anesthesia/acute pain medicine is an increasingly popular option that has been selected by anesthesiology fellowship candidates. Interest, enthusiasm, and attraction continues with this anesthesia subspecialty as more and more applicants continue to apply to a limited number a regional fellowship positions and as more academic facilities nationwide and in Canada are creating recognized regional fellowship programs within their institutions. The continued growth of this subspecialty comes partially from evidence-based directives that regional anesthesia/analgesia has become a valuable option for a wide variety of surgical and medical interventions. In addition, the ACGME has made an effort toward having anesthesiology residency programs graduate anesthesiologists with a proficiency in the basics of regional techniques.[43] Although the goals of this certifying organization have not yet been completely fulfilled, initiatives to accomplish ACGME efforts on a nationwide scale continue. Therefore, candidates who have completed an anesthesiology residency and wish to develop an expertise in regional anesthesia/analgesia have an option to pursue additional training in a regional fellowship program. Both professional interests from the medical/surgical community as well as an increasingly larger portion of the educated surgical patient population are making requests and demands for regional anesthesia options when amendable prior to surgical procedures, for postoperative pain management, and during invasive medical interventions. It is this growing enticement with regional anesthesia/analgesia alternatives brought about by public and professional entities that will continue to excite, expand, and inspire continued growth of regional anesthesia and regional anesthesia fellowships.

REFERENCES

1. Broking K, Waurick R: How to teach regional anesthesia. Curr Opin Anaesthesiol 2006;19(5):526–530.
2. Beckman J, Liguori GA: Regional anesthesia fellowships. In Hadzic A (ed): *The New York School of Regional Anesthesia Textbook of Regional Anesthesia and Acute Pain Management.* New York, NY: McGraw-Hill, 2007, pp 1179–1188.
3. ASRA: fellowship programs. http://www.asra.com/residents-fellows.php. Pittsburgh, PA 2013. Last accessed on June 1, 2013.
4. Jacob AK, Kopp SL, Bacon DR, et al: The history of anesthesia. In Barash PG (ed): *Clinical Anesthesia.* Philadelphia, PA: Wolters Kluwer/Lippincott Williams & Wilkinseds, 2009, pp 15–16.
5. Ruetsch YA, Böni T, Borgeat A: From cocaine to ropivacaine: the history of local anesthetic drugs. Curr Top Med Chem 2001;1(3):175–182.
6. Marx GF: The first spinal anesthesia. Who deserves the laurels? Reg Anesth 1994;19(6):429–430.
7. Russell T, Clarke R, Gardner A, et al: Anaesthesia trainees' exposure to regional anaesthesia in an Australian tertiary adult teaching hospital. Anaesth Intensive Care 2011;39(3):472–476.
8. Konrad C, Schüpfer G, Wietlisbach M, et al: Learning manual skills in anesthesiology: Is there a recommended number of cases for anesthetic procedures? Anesth Analg 1998;86(3):635–639.
9. Rosenblatt MA, Fishkind D: Proficiency in interscalene anesthesia—how many blocks are necessary? J Clin Anesth 2003;15(4):285–288.
10. Schuepfer G, Jöhr M: Psoas compartment block (PCB) in children: Part II—generation of an institutional learning curve with a new technique. Paediatr Anaesth 2005;15(6):465–469.
11. ASA: Ultrasound-Guided Regional Anesthesia (UGRA) Education and Clinical Training Portfolio. http://education.asahq.org/usgra. Park Ridge, IL 2013. Last accessed on June 1, 2013.
12. ABMS: Specialties and subspecialties. http://www.abms.org/who_we_help/physicians/specialties.aspx. Chicago, IL, 2013. Last accessed on June 1, 2013.
13. Haberkern CM, Geiduschek JM, Sorensen GK, et al: Multi-institutional survey of graduates of pediatric anesthesia fellowship: assessment of training and current professional activities. Anesth Analg 1997;85(6):1191–1195.
14. Stoltzfus DP, Watson CB, Ries MC: Anesthesiology critical care medicine fellowship training. Anesth Analg 1995;81(3):441–445.
15. Ilfeld BM, Yaksh TL, Neal JM: Mandating two-year regional anesthesia fellowships: fanning the academic flame or extinguishing it? Reg Anesth Pain Med 2007;32(4):275–279.
16. Brown DL: Fellowship training in regional anesthesia. Reg Anesth Pain Med 2005;30(3):215–217.
17. Hargett MJ, Beckman JD, Liguori GA, et al: Guidelines for regional anesthesia fellowship training. Reg Anesth Pain Med 2005;30(3):218–225.
18. Sites BD, Chan VW, Neal JM, et al: The American Society of Regional Anesthesia and Pain Medicine and the European Society of Regional Anaesthesia and Pain Therapy Joint Committee recommendations for education and training in ultrasound-guided regional anesthesia. Reg Anesth Pain Med 201035(2 Suppl):S74–S80.
19. Narouze SN, Provenzano D, Peng P, et al: The American Society of Regional Anesthesia and Pain Medicine, the European Society of Regional Anaesthesia and Pain Therapy, and the Asian Australasian Federation of Pain Societies Joint Committee recommendations for education and training in ultrasound-guided interventional pain procedures. Reg Anesth Pain Med 2012;37(6):657–664.
20. Regional A, Acute Pain Medicine Fellowship Directors G: *Guidelines for Fellowship Training in Regional Anesthesiology and Acute Pain Medicine,* 2nd ed, 2010. Reg Anesth Pain Med 201136(3):282–288.
21. Matveevskii AS, Gravenstein N: Role of simulators, educational programs, and nontechnical skills in anesthesia resident selection, education, and competency assessment. J Crit Care 2008;23(2):167–172.
22. Cheung JJ, Chen EW, Al-Allaq Y, et al: Acquisition of technical skills in ultrasound-guided regional anesthesia using a high-fidelity simulator. Stud Health Technol Inform 2011;163:119–124.
23. Rosenberg AD, Popovic J, Albert DB, et al: Three partial-task simulators for teaching ultrasound-guided regional anesthesia. Reg Anesth Pain Med 2012;37(1):106–110.
24. Edler A, Adamshick M, Fanning R, et al: Leadership lessons from military education for postgraduate medical curricular improvement. Clin Teach 2010;7(1):26–31.
25. Chin KJ, Tse C, Chan V, et al: Hand motion analysis using the imperial college surgical assessment device: validation of a novel and objective

performance measure in ultrasound-guided peripheral nerve blockade. Reg Anesth Pain Med 2011;36(3):213–219.

26. Kluger MT: Trainees' attitudes to research as part of anaesthetic training. Anaesth Intensive Care 1998;26(1):92–95.

27. ACGME: Obstetric Anesthesia. http://www.acgme.org/acgmeweb/Portals/0/PDFs/FAQ/043_obstetric_anesthesiology_FAQs.pdf. Chicago, IL 2013. Last accessed on June 1, 2013.

28. Vanderbilt University: Vanderbilt cardiothoracic anesthesia fellowship program. http://www.mc.vanderbilt.edu/documents/1anesthesiology/files/CT%20Anesth%20Fell%20Brochure%202013-14%20Fillable.pdf. Vanderbuilt, NC 2013. Last accessed on June 1, 2013.

29. ASA: Fellowship opportunities. http://www.asahq.org/For-Students/For-Residents/Fellowship-Opportunities.aspx. Park Ridge, IL 2013. Last accessed on June 18, 2013.

30. Desjardins G, Cahalan MK: Subspecialty accreditation: is being special good? Curr Opin Anaesthesiol 2007;20(6):572–575.

31. Pagel PS, Hudetz JA: Scholarly productivity of united states academic cardiothoracic anesthesiologists: influence of fellowship accreditation and transesophageal echocardiographic credentials on h-index and other citation bibliometrics. J Cardiothorac Vasc Anesth 2011;25(5):761–765.

32. Kehlet H, Wilmore DW: Evidence-based surgical care and the evolution of fast-track surgery. Ann Surg 2008;248(2):189–198.

33. White PF, Kehlet H, Neal JM, et al: The role of the anesthesiologist in fast-track surgery: from multimodal analgesia to perioperative medical care. Anesth Analg 2007;104(6):1380–1396.

34. White PF, Kehlet H: Postoperative pain management and patient outcome: time to return to work! Anesth Analg 2007;104(3):487–489.

35. Apfelbaum JL, Chen C, Mehta SS, et al: Postoperative pain experience: results from a national survey suggest postoperative pain continues to be undermanaged. Anesth Analg 2003.97(2):534–540.

36. White PF, Kehlet H, Liu S: Perioperative analgesia: what do we still know? Anesth Analg 2009;108(5):1364–1367.

37. Liu SS, Wu CL: Effect of postoperative analgesia on major postoperative complications: a systematic update of the evidence. Anesth Analg 2007;104(3):689–702.

38. White PF, Sacan O, Tufanogullari B, et al: Effect of short-term postoperative celecoxib administration on patient outcome after outpatient laparoscopic surgery. Can J Anaesth J 2007;54(5):342–348.

39. Werner MU, Soholm L, Rotboll-Nielsen P, et al: Does an acute pain service improve postoperative outcome? Anesth Analg 2002;95(5):1361–1372.

40. Kehlet H, Liu SS: Continuous local anesthetic wound infusion to improve postoperative outcome: back to the periphery? Anesthesiology 2007;107(3):369–371.

41. Werner MU, Duun P, Kehlet H: Prediction of postoperative pain by preoperative nociceptive responses to heat stimulation. Anesthesiology 2004;100(1):115–119; discussion 115A.

42. Janicki PK, Schuler G, Francis D, et al: A genetic association study of the functional A118G polymorphism of the human mu-opioid receptor gene in patients with acute and chronic pain. Anesth Analg 2006;103(4):1011–1017.

43. Guidelines for Fellowship Training in Regional Anesthesia and Acute Pain Medicine - Third Edition, Regional Anesthesia and Pain Medicine, 2014.

APPENDIX I. GUIDELINES FOR FELLOWSHIP TRAINING IN REGIONAL ANESTHESIOLOGY AND ACUTE PAIN MEDICINE (as adopted from the ASRA website)

Mission Statement

The purpose of this endeavor is to recommend the necessary components of subspecialty fellowship training in regional anesthesiology and acute pain medicine. Although an effort has been made to create a comprehensive set of goals and competency-based objectives, these recommendations may not apply to all programs, nor will they be used for any form of accreditation of fellowship programs. Participating fellowship program directors will ensure the ongoing development of regional anesthesiology and acute pain medicine as a defined subspecialty. Educational curricula, clinical care, and research activities are emphasized.

Programmatic Goals for Fellowship Training in Regional Anesthesiology and Acute Pain Medicine

Outline

I. Organization and Resources
   a. Scope and Duration of Training
   b. Institutional Organization
   c. Program Director and Faculty
   d. Facilities and Resources

II. Education Program
   a. Program Goals
   b. Medical Knowledge
   c. Patient Care
   d. Scholarly Activities/Practice-Based Learning
   e. Interpersonal and Communication Skills
   f. Professionalism
   g. Systems-Based Practice

III. Evaluation Process

I. Organization and Resources
a. Scope and Duration of Training

1. Scope of Training. Regional anesthesiology and acute pain medicine is a subspecialty focused on the perioperative management of patients receiving neuraxial or peripheral neural blockade for anesthesia and/or acute analgesia. Specifically, the setting of this training might include (a) intraoperative application (with or without general anesthesia), (b) postoperative application in inpatients and outpatients, and/or (c) acute pain management of nonsurgical patients. Fellowship training should be concerned with the development of expertise in the practice and theory of regional anesthesiology and acute pain medicine.

2. Duration of Training. The time required for subspecialty training in regional anesthesiology and acute pain medicine shall be 12 months. Program directors are granted flexibility to tailor the program to meet the individual needs of fellows. Specialized clinical rotations of less than 12 months may be made available to interested clinicians, but the minimum amount of training necessary to use "fellowship" in the diploma language shall be 1 year.

b. Institutional Organization

1. Relationship to a Core Program. Institutions with subspecialty training in regional anesthesiology and acute pain medicine must have a direct affiliation with an Accreditation Council for Graduate Medical Education (ACGME) accredited residency in anesthesiology (or similar; e.g., Royal College of Physicians and Surgeons of Canada or Royal College of Anaesthetists). If the institution at which the fellowship is based is other than the primary institution of an accredited residency, a written agreement linking the two is required. An evaluation

protocol consistent with ACGME (or equivalent)–approved standards for residency programs is also a prerequisite.
2. Institutional Policy and Resources. The fellowship should be recognized and approved by the core Department of Anesthesiology and the institution's Department/Division of Medical Education.
3. Institutional Oversight. The core program is encouraged to internally review the fellowship program at least every 5 years to ensure general compliance with these guidelines.

c. Program Director and Faculty

1. Program Director. The director of the fellowship training program must be an American Board of Anesthesiology—certified anesthesiologist (or equivalent) who has completed 1 year of fellowship training in regional anesthesiology and/or acute pain medicine, or is a dedicated and skilled practitioner of these disciplines. The program director must also have an academic and/or clinical affiliation with an ACGME (or equivalent)—accredited institution.
2. Faculty. The majority of the faculty in the training program must be board certified (or equivalent) in anesthesiology. A division of the faculty in the training program must also demonstrate an expertise in regional anesthesiology and/or acute pain medicine. The number of faculty in a program may vary based on the number of fellows in training; however, the program must have a minimum of two regional anesthesiology and/or acute pain medicine faculty.

d. Facilities and Resources

1. Equipment. Suitable equipment for the performance of a wide variety of regional anesthesia/analgesia techniques must be available. Such equipment must include nerve simulators, neuraxial and peripheral block supplies, catheter systems, ultrasound systems, and the basic requirements for conducting general anesthesia according to American Society of Anesthesiologists standards. Dedicated and acceptable on-call facilities must also be maintained, if applicable.
2. Support Services. Appropriate support services may include, but are not limited to, anesthesia technical support and pharmacy support systems.
3. Library. A departmental library, or a portion of the institutional library dedicated to anesthesiology, must be maintained with literature specific to the practice of regional anesthesiology and acute pain medicine.

II. Educational Program
a. Program Goals

Over the course of the 12-month fellowship, the fellow will enhance their cognitive, psychomotor, and affective skills to safely and effectively administer and teach regional anesthesiology and acute pain medicine as a consultant in anesthesiology. The fellow is responsible for decisions related to case and block selection to facilitate the smooth flow of the operating room (OR) cases and to enhance patient recovery. The fellow will be expected to develop and demonstrate the skills needed to establish regional anesthesiology and acute pain medicine as a primary component of their future practice.

b. Medical Knowledge

Upon completion of the program, the fellow should demonstrate knowledge in the following areas sufficient to:

1. Local Anesthetics

a. Describe the pharmacology of local anesthetics with respect to mechanism of action, physicochemical properties, comparative attributes, and appropriate dosing for site of single injection or continuous infusion.
b. Determine the selection and dose of local anesthetics as indicated for specific medical conditions.
c. Compare the dosing, advantages, and disadvantages of local anesthetic adjuncts.
d. Compare toxic risk of local anesthetics and signs, symptoms, and treatment of local anesthetic systemic toxicity or neurotoxicity.

2. Neuraxial and Systemic Opioids, Nonsteroidal Anti-Inflammatory Drugs, and Nonopioid Adjuncts or Analgesia

a. Neuraxial Opioids
  1. Describe indications/contraindications, mechanism of action, physicochemical properties, effective dosing, and duration of action of neuraxial opioids.
  2. Compare extended release epidural morphine with standard preservative-free opioids.
  3. Recognize complications and adverse effects, including related monitoring, prevention, and therapy.
  4. Differentiate intrathecal versus epidural administration relative to dose, effect, and adverse effects.

b. Systemic Opioids
  1. Discuss the pharmacokinetics of opioid analgesics: bioavailability, absorption, distribution, metabolism, and excretion.
  2. Discuss the site and mechanism of action of opioids.
  3. Discuss the differences of chemical structure of the various opioids.
  4. Describe challenges of postprocedure analgesic management in the patient with chronic pain and/or opioid induced hyperalgesia.

c. Nonopioid Analgesics
  1. Describe the concept of multimodal analgesia and its impact on functional restoration after surgery.
  2. Differentiate the pharmacology of nonsteroidal anti-inflammatory drugs (NSAIDs), cyclooxygenase-2 (COX-2) inhibitors, N-methyl-D-aspartic acid antagonists, α_2 agonists, gamma-aminobutyric acid, and pentanoid agents with respect to optimizing postoperative analgesia.

3. Nerve Localization Techniques

a. Explain principles, operation, advantages, and limitations of the peripheral nerve stimulator to localize and anesthetize peripheral nerves.
b. Explain principles, technique, and advantages and disadvantages of paresthesia-seeking, perivascular or transvascular approaches to nerve localization.
c. Explain principles, operation, advantages, and limitations of ultrasound to localize and anesthetize peripheral nerves.

4. Spinal Anesthesia

a. Describe the indications, contraindications, adverse effects, complications, and management of spinal anesthesia.
b. Recognize the cardiovascular and pulmonary physiologic effects of spinal anesthesia.
c. Compare local anesthetics for intrathecal use: agents, dosage, surgical and total duration of action, and adjuvants.
d. Explain the relative importance of factors affecting intensity, extent, and duration of block such as patient position, dose, volume, and baricity of injectate.
e. Define postdural puncture headache, and describe symptoms, etiology, risk factors, and treatment.
f. Differentiate advantages and disadvantages of continuous spinal anesthesia.

5. Epidural Anesthesia (Lumbar, Thoracic, Caudal)

a. Describe the indications, contraindications, adverse effects, complications, and management of epidural anesthesia.
b. Compare the local anesthetics available for epidural use agents, dosage, adjuncts, and duration of action.
c. Differentiate between spinal and epidural anesthesia with regard to reliability, latency, duration, and segmental limitations.
d. Explain the value and techniques of test dosing to minimize certain complications of epidural anesthesia.
e. Interpret the volume-segment relationship and the effect of patient age, pregnancy, position, and site of injection on resultant block.
f. Differentiate combined spinal epidural anesthesia from lumbar epidural anesthesia, including advantages/disadvantages, dose requirements, complications, indications, and contraindications.
g. Categorize outcome benefits of thoracic epidural analgesia for thoracic and abdominal surgery and thoracic trauma.
h. Differentiate caudal epidural and thoracic epidural anesthesia from lumbar epidural anesthesia, including advantages/ disadvantages, dose requirements, complications, indications, and contraindications.
i. Explain the impact of antithrombotic and thrombolytic medications on neuraxial and peripheral anesthesia/analgesia with specific reference to the American Society of Regional Anesthesia and Pain Medicine guidelines: *Regional Anesthesia in the Patient Receiving Antithrombotic or Thrombolytic Therapy.*

6. Upper-Extremity Nerve Block

a. Describe the anatomy and sonoanatomy of the brachial plexus in relation to sensory and motor innervation.
b. Compare local anesthetics for brachial plexus block: agents, dose, duration of action, and adjuvants.
c. Explain the value and techniques of intravascular test dosing to minimize local anesthetic systemic toxicity associated with peripheral nerve block.
d. Differentiate the various brachial plexus (or terminal nerve) block sites, including indications/contraindications, advantages/disadvantages, complications, and management specific to each.
e. Contrast the indications and technique for cervical plexus, suprascapular, or intercostobrachial block as unique blocks, or supplements to brachial plexus block.
f. Summarize the use and advantages/disadvantages specific to continuous brachial plexus anesthesia.

7. Lower-Extremity Nerve Block[9]

a. Describe anatomy and sonoanatomy of the lower extremity: sciatic, femoral, lateral femoral cutaneous, and obturator nerves (and their clinically important branches) in relation to sensory and motor innervation.
b. Compare local anesthetics for lower-extremity block: agents, dose, duration of action, and adjuvants.
c. Explain the value and techniques of intravascular test dosing to minimize local anesthetic systemic toxicity associated with peripheral nerve block.
d. Differentiate the various approaches to lower-extremity blockade, including indications/contraindications, adverse effects, complications, and management specific to each.
e. Summarize the advantages/disadvantages and indications for continuous lower-extremity neural blockade.

8. Truncal Blockade

a. Describe the relevant anatomy for intercostal, paravertebral, ilioinguinal-hypogastric, rectus sheath, and transverses abdominus plane blocks.
b. Compare local anesthetics for truncal blockade: agents, dose, and duration of action.
c. Summarize the indications, contraindications, adverse effects, complications, and management of truncal blockade.

9. Intravenous Regional Anesthesia

a. Review the mechanism of action, indications, contraindications, advantages and disadvantages, adverse effects, complications and management of intravenous regional anesthesia (IVRA).
b. Compare agents for IVRA: local anesthetic choice, dosage, and use of adjuvants.

Hadzic A, Vloka J, Koenigsamen J. Training requirements for peripheral nerve blocks. Curr Opin Anaesthesiol. 2002;15:669Y673.

10. Complications of Regional Anesthesia and Acute Pain Medicine

Discuss those complications specific to regional anesthesia and acute pain medicine practice. A partial list of these complications includes:

a. Hemorrhagic complications in the patient receiving antithrombotic or thrombolytic agents,

b. Infectious complications of neuraxial and peripheral blockade,

c. Neurological complications of regional anesthesia and acute pain medicine,

d. Local anesthetic systemic toxicity, and

e. Opioid-induced respiratory depression.

c. Patient Care

Upon completion of the program, the fellow should be able to:

1. Describe rational selection of regional anesthesia and/or postoperative analgesic techniques for specific clinical situations. Such techniques may involve nontechnical options, such as multimodal analgesia, opioid and nonopioid pharmacologic management, and so on.

2. Debate the advantages/disadvantages of regional versus general anesthesia for various procedures and patients in regard to patient recovery, patient outcome, or efficiency, and cost of care.

3. Recognize and intervene to manage inadequate operative regional anesthetic and postoperative analgesic techniques with supplemental blockade, alternative approaches, and/or pharmacologic intervention.

4. Demonstrate the knowledge and skills necessary to perform and to effectively teach a wide range of advanced practice block techniques, achieving a high success and low complication rate. Examples of blocks in this category, modified from Hadzic et al, include:

   1. Deep cervical plexus block
   2. Suprascapular nerve block
   3. Interscalene block
   4. Supraclavicular block
   5. Infraclavicular block
   6. Continuous interscalene block
   7. Continuous infraclavicular block
   8. Continuous axillary block
   9. Intercostal nerve block
   10. Thoracolumbar paravertebral block: single or continuous
   11. Rectus sheath block
   12. Transversus abdominis plane block
   13. Ilioinguinal-iliohypogastric block
   14. Sciatic nerve block: posterior approaches
   15. Sciatic nerve block: anterior approach
   16. Sciatic popliteal block
   17. Lumbar plexus block
   18. Femoral nerve block
   19. Lateral femoral cutaneous block
   20. Obturator nerve block
   21. Saphenous nerve block
   22. Continuous femoral nerve block
   23. Continuous sciatic nerve block
   24. Continuous popliteal sciatic block

5. Demonstrate an understanding of how the acute pain medicine service addresses (a) surgical regional anesthetic techniques (as placed by the operating room anesthesiologist), (b) the perioperative use of analgesic techniques by the acute pain medicine service, (c) the perioperative management of acute pain medicine interventions, (d) the provision of acute pain medicine services directed toward the chronic pain patient who is now experiencing acute pain, and (e) the provision of acute pain management to select nonsurgical patients, such as those with sickle cell anemia.

6. Demonstrate the ability to direct the acute pain medicine service with attending supervision. Patient management will include multimodal analgesic techniques such as neuraxial and peripheral nerve catheters, local anesthetic and narcotic infusions, and nonnarcotic analgesic adjuvants.

d. Scholarly Activities/Practice-Based Learning
1. Academic Activities

a. Fellows are encouraged to participate in research as a major activity of the year-long fellowship. To accomplish these objectives, the regional anesthesiology and acute pain medicine faculty will mentor the fellow in the production of research, coauthorship of papers as appropriate, and preparation of clinical research proposals with institutional review board approval prior to the start of the fellowship year.

2. Teaching Activities

a. Create and present a lecture during departmental or divisional grand rounds, or a local/regional/national meeting covering a topic or case relevant to regional anesthesia or acute pain medicine.

b. Prepare resident education lectures and journal reviews for regional anesthesiology and/or acute pain medicine subspecialty conference.

c. Participate and direct portions of cadaver anatomy laboratories if available.

d. Develop teaching techniques by instructing residents and/or medical students at the bedside under the supervision of faculty.

e. Review and enhance Web-based teaching resources such as resident teaching materials, curriculum documents, and self-study and testing materials.

3. Practice-Based Learning

a. Evaluate and apply evidence from scientific studies, expert guidelines, and practice pathways to their patients' medical conditions.

b. Apply information technology to obtain and record patient information, access institutional and national policies and guidelines, and participate in self-education.

c. Analyze their own practice with respect to patient outcomes (especially success and complications from regional blockade) and compare with available literature.

e. Interpersonal and Communication Skills

Upon completion of the program, the fellow should be able to:

1. Summarize information to the patient and family with respect to the options, alternatives, risks and benefits of regional anesthesia, and/or acute analgesic techniques in a manner that is clear, understandable, ethical, and appropriate.
2. Develop effective listening skills and answer questions appropriately in the process of obtaining informed consent.
3. Operate effectively in a team environment and communicating and cooperating with surgeons, residents, nurses, pharmacists, physical therapists, and other members of the perioperative team. This requires the fellow to:

    a. Recognize the roles of other members of the team.
    b. Communicate clearly in a collegial manner that facilitates the achievement of care goals.
    c. Help other members of the team to enhance the sharing of important information.
    d. Formulate care plans that utilize the multidisciplinary team skills, such as a plan for facilitated recovery.

f. Professionalism

Upon completion of the program, the fellow should be able to:

1. Continuously conduct the practice of medicine with integrity, honesty, and accountability.
2. Demonstrate a commitment to lifelong learning and excellence in practice.
3. Practice consistent subjugation of self-interest to the good of the patient and the healthcare needs of society.

4. Demonstrate a commitment to ethical principles in providing care, obtaining informed consent, and maintaining patient confidentiality.

g. Systems-Based Practice

Upon completion of the program, the fellow should be able to:

1. Effectively balance the need for operating room efficiency with high-quality patient care. The fellow will effectively choose surgeons, patients, techniques, and approaches to achieve the best balance possible to use regional anesthesia and/or analgesia to improve patient outcomes.
2. Understand the interaction of the acute pain medicine service with other elements of the healthcare system including primary surgical and medical teams and other consultant, nursing, pharmacy, and physical therapy services.
3. Demonstrate awareness of healthcare costs and resource allocation, and the impact of their choices on those costs and resources.
4. Advocate for the patient and their family within the healthcare system and assist them in understanding and negotiating complexities in that system.

III. Evaluation Process

A. Consistent with ACGME residency guidelines, the attending faculty will be evaluated by the fellows at least annually.
B. Written evaluations of fellows by all faculty with whom they have worked shall occur at least every 6 months. The results of these evaluations shall be recorded and reviewed with the fellows by the program director or faculty advisor no less often than every 6 months.
C. A review will be conducted at least twice annually to assess professional development.
D. A 360-degree assessment process will occur at least annually.

STATISTICS AND PRINCIPLES OF RESEARCH DESIGN IN REGIONAL ANESTHESIA AND ACUTE PAIN MEDICINE

CHAPTER 79

Principles of Statistical Methods for Research in Regional Anesthesia

Maxine M. Kuroda

NECESSARY BASICS

Anesthesiologists treat thousands of patients in their busy clinical careers; they also save thousands of lives. However, anesthesiologists also have a place in research where their work is far reaching and can impact the lives of millions of people worldwide. This chapter is dedicated to those anesthesiologists who actively undertake research and who keep abreast of the research literature in order to better serve their patients.

The chapter begins with some very basic principles of statistics that form the foundation for those methods most frequently used in regional anesthesia research. These principles, albeit more theoretic and seemingly abstract, are included in the hopes of offering more than a cookbook approach to the statistical procedures. Several statistical packages are available "to crunch data," yet a minimal number of formulas and calculations are included to illustrate what happens to data when submitted to a statistical program. It is hoped that this chapter will foster more effective dialogue between anesthesiologist and statistician. By the end of the chapter, the reader should have a better understanding of what a statistician needs to know about studies and why this information is crucial to reaching valid research conclusions.

What Is Statistics?

Sir Ronald A. Fisher (1890–1962), the father of modern statistics, considered the science of statistics to be mathematics applied to observational data: "Statistics may be regarded as (i) the study of populations, (ii) as the study of variation, (iii) as the study of methods of the reduction of data."[1] His definition has three important implications for research:

1. Investigators would like to apply their research findings to vast populations, but it is seldom feasible to study an entire population, so they must study samples from it.

2. Each sample studied will be slightly different; i.e., there is variation among samples. Thus, there will be differences among samples even from studies that have used the same design and methods, and even among samples taken from the same population.

3. Investigators summarize and test the data from their study sample in order to reach reasonable conclusions about the parent population that they can communicate to colleagues, to journal editors, and to the public.

Types of Data

The types of data collected in a study determine the types of statistical analyses. Table 79–1 describes the three types of data, what they represent, their typical level of measurement, and their properties.[2]

Quantitative data are on a scale that has equal intervals. For instance, the difference between 35 and 45 years of age is the same as the difference between 60 and 70 years of age. When the scale has a true zero point, it is possible to look at the ratio of measurements; e.g., a patient who weighs 192 lb is twice as heavy as a patient who weighs 96 lb.

Ranked data indicate relative standing. For instance, the American Society of Anesthesiologists (ASA) physical status is assigned to each patient prior to surgery as an indicator of anesthetic risk. Although there is order, we can *not* say that an ASA physical status IV patient is twice as risky as an ASA physical status II patient.

Qualitative data indicate class membership. For instance, women delivering vaginally are in a different category from women delivering by cesarean section. It should be noted that with qualitative data, one category is no better than another. Thus, the vaginal and cesarean section categories merely reflect class membership; they do not reflect amount of risk that may accompany the delivery method.

TABLE 79–1. Properties of three types of data.

Type	Numbers Are	Typical Level of Measurement and Properties
Quantitative	Amount or count	Cardinal (interval-ratio)
		True zero
		Equal intervals
		Order
		Classification
		Frequency distribution
Ranked	Relative standing	Ordinal
		Order
		Classification
		Frequency distribution
Qualitative	Class membership	Nominal
		Classification
		Frequency distribution

Although seemingly elementary, it is often surprisingly difficult to determine what type or types of data variables represent. It is always a wise idea to keep a data dictionary. Table 79–2 illustrates the setup for such a data dictionary with examples of possible variables that might be included. A field for comments (an alphanumeric string variable) is quite useful for recording remarks on individual patients; e.g., "Intraoperative time lengthened because electrocautery device malfunctioned."

Basic Study Designs

Study design plays an important role in ensuring the validity of a study. Table 79–3 describes the four basic study designs.[3] The hallmark of the experimental design is that the investigator manipulates the exposure or treatment (independent variable) to assess its effect on disease or outcome (dependent variable). The cross-sectional, retrospective, case-control, and prospective cohort designs are primarily observational in that the investigator does not manipulate exposures or treatments. For instance, a researcher may want to know whether family infrastructure affects time to return to work following surgery. Since patients cannot be assigned to supportive or nonsupportive families, data must be obtained through interviews or other observational techniques.

There are many other study designs, most of which are variants of these basic ones, and many studies will include a combination of designs. Choice of design depends on the research question or hypothesis as well as feasibility and cost. Each design has its advantages and limitations. Even the

experimental (clinical trial) design, considered to be the "gold standard," is not always ethical, and strictly speaking, results are only generalizable to patients like those who participated in the study. Moreover, no study is immune to bias; i.e., any systematic error that threatens the validity of research findings.[4] For instance, a study's recruitment methods may enroll predominantly employed, upper middle class participants. These subjects tend to be more health conscious, and may have better access to medical care where their health problems can be detected earlier when less severe. Therefore, depending on the particular exposure and outcome being studied, the research findings may be biased by the inclusion of numerous subjects with milder disease. There are endless ways in which a study can contain such systematic errors. Your past experience (or that of your colleagues) may allow you to anticipate certain features of a study that would make it vulnerable to bias. Incorporate this information into your study design because, once a study is biased, its data cannot be "fixed" through statistical wizardry.

Studies in regional anesthesia will often follow the protocols of the experiment or clinical trial. The investigator will typically begin by randomly assigning patients to the "arms" of the experiment. For instance, in order to compare the effectiveness of a new anesthetic with an established standard, an investigator would randomly assign patients to receive one *or* the other of these medications. Similarly, patients might be randomly assigned to receive a novel combination of anesthetics to see whether the new cocktail is more effective or has fewer side effects than standard combinations of the anesthetics.

Random assignment ensures that the overall likelihood of assignment is equivalent for the treatment arms. Because patients are not more likely to be assigned to one arm of the trial than another, the overall effect of random assignment is to reduce confounding by extraneous factors. However, random assignment can occasionally produce atypical groups; say, all male patients are assigned to one group and all female patients to another. If such groups occur following random assignment, subjects should not be reassigned by the investigator; rather, some regression techniques may be useful in adjusting for unbalanced groups. Fortunately, extreme groups are rare, and random assignment typically creates groups that are similar with respect to known (and even unrecognized) confounders.[5]

Random assignment is conducted in several ways. For simple randomization, a popular method is to use sealed envelopes. After consent to participate in the study has been given by the patient, the investigator or an assistant randomly picks an envelope that contains the group assignment for that patient. An equally valid method of random assignment involves the use of a printed table of random numbers (found in many statistics books) or computer-generated random numbers (an option in many statistical packages). A number in the table is pointed to with eyes closed. After this starting point is established by "blind stab," the numbers are consecutively followed in a prespecified direction (top to bottom, left to right, or even diagonally). Numbers are taken in groups of 2s, 3s, or 4s, depending on whether ≤99, 100–999, or 1000+ patients are to be included in the study. If even numbers have been prespecified as the placebo group and odd numbers as the treatment group, any

TABLE 79–2. Data dictionary.

Variable	Label	Definition	Type	Values	Comments
gender	Gender		N	0 = Female 1 = Male	
race	Race		N	1 = White 2 = Black 3 = Hispanic 8 = Other 9 = Unknown	Include "mixed" race in "other" category
dos	Date of surgery		D		Not date of preoperative visit
induct	Induction time (min)	Anesthesia start to anesthesia completed; e.g., spinal anesthetic injected	N		Missing for MAC patients
vas36h	VAS 36 h	VAS 36 hours after PACU discharge	N	1–100	Not available on patients who bypassed PACU
nrs2wk	NRS 2 wk	NRS 2 weeks after hospital discharge	N	1–10	Obtained by phone interview
laconc	LA concentration	Concentration of local anesthetic	N	Values entered as decimal (e.g., 0.0567, not 5.67×10^{-2})	Initial concentration administered
comments	Comments		S		Miscellaneous notes on patients

Abbreviations: D, date; MAC: monitored anesthesia care; N, numeric, PACU: postanesthesia care unit; S, string (alphanumeric); VAS, visual analogue scale; NRS, numeric rating scale.

patient who consents when the number is even is assigned to the placebo group. If the next number is odd, the next patient who consents is assigned to the treatment group; however, if the next number is even, that patient becomes the second individual assigned to the placebo group, and any patient who

consents when the number is odd is assigned to the treatment group. The process continues until all consenting patients are assigned to a group, but may produce unequal numbers in the groups. Modifications to this scheme are incorporated depending on whether three or more groups are being studied. For example, numbers 01–33 could be assigned to the first group, 34–66 to the second group, and 67–99 to the third group.[5]

Other methods, such as blocked, stratified, weighted, or cluster randomization, may be useful[5] and will be mentioned briefly. Blocked randomization is used when the investigator wishes to keep the number of subjects in each group very similar, and is especially useful if a trial could be stopped early. Blocks are developed in which the treatment arms occur the same number of times but in different orders. For instance, because the A, B, and C treatment arms occur twice in the ABCABC and CBABAC blocks, each treatment arm will have the same number of subjects. Stratified randomization is used when there is prior knowledge that it is important to balance a particular characteristic among groups. For example, to study the effects of two different epidurals on laboring women, the researcher may want to assign women by parity status to ensure that similar numbers of

TABLE 79–3. Basic study designs.

1. Experimental (clinical trial)
   Exposure manipulated by the researcher
2. Cross-sectional
   Exposure and disease/outcome obtained at the same time or within a short period of time
3. Retrospective case-control
   Cases and controls selected and past exposures ascertained through interviews, medical records
4. Prospective cohort
   Exposed and unexposed individuals selected and followed to disease/outcome

primiparous and multiparous women are assigned to each of the two epidural groups. Here, the primiparous stratum may be assigned to epidural group 1 or 2 in the 1-2-2-1 order, and the multiparous stratum may be assigned to epidural group in the 2-1-1-2 order.

Weighted randomization is used when there is a reason to have unequal numbers of subjects in the groups (perhaps more subjects are needed in a particular group in order to obtain a precise estimate of a key variable). This is easily accomplished by adapting the methods of simple randomization; e.g., numbers 01–66 could be assigned to the first group and 67–99 to the second group. Finally, cluster randomization can be used to allocate treatment arms to geographic areas rather than to individual subjects. Multicenter clinical trials to evaluate the efficacy of local anesthetics might want to ensure that treatment arms are assigned equivalently among the centers when it is known that approaches to drug delivery and/or monitoring vary in different areas of the country.

Difference Between Descriptive and Inferential Statistics

There are two main subdivisions of statistics. *Descriptive statistics* portray features of the data that are of interest by organizing and summarizing the collection of observations.[6] How this is done depends on the type of data collected. For example, age of patient in years is a quantitative amount and would be presented as a mean and standard deviation of age for each of several peripheral nerve blocks (PNBs); however, gender of patient is a qualitative indicator of class membership and would be presented as a number and percentage for each PNB.

Inferential statistics uses information from study samples to test hypotheses about effects that are thought to be true in the population as a whole.[6] Inferential statistics can be used to answer such questions as whether length of stay in the postanesthesia care unit (PACU) is significantly longer for patients who received femoral or sham block for anterior cruciate ligament repair.

Both areas of statistics are important. The distributional characteristics (i.e., central tendency, spread, and shape) that constitute descriptive statistics are the very foundation of the more "glamorous" inferential statistics. Moreover, because descriptive statistics characterize key features of the data, it is an important tool for data cleaning. Are there missing values? If so, how much information is missing and why? Do the data make sense? Although an equal number of male and female patients may be expected to receive neuraxial anesthesia for lower extremity surgery, it would be an error to find a male receiving an epidural prior to delivering a baby. Are there outliers; if so, are they true outliers or simply typographic errors? Did the patient weigh 702 lb or was weight written sloppily and the patient actually weighed 202 lb? Finally, the assumptions that must be met in order to apply inferential statistics properly are based on the distributional characteristics of descriptive statistics. Thus, statisticians look at these characteristics to decide whether data need to be transformed before inferential statistics can be applied.

Measures of Central Tendency

The three most commonly used measures of central tendency are the mean, median, and mode.[6] The *mean* is the balance point of the distribution and is responsive to the exact position of each score in the distribution. It is an indicator of skewness (i.e., nonbell shapes) when used in conjunction with the median. However, because it is sensitive to each score in the distribution, the mean is more easily influenced by extreme scores than the median or the mode.

The *median* is the point that divides the upper and lower halves of a scale of ordered scores. Since it is not responsive to the exact value of the scores, it is less affected by extreme scores than the mean, and is often a better choice than the mean when describing central tendency for strongly skewed distributions. In fact, it is the only relatively stable measure for open-ended distributions.

The *mode* is simply the most frequently occurring score or the class interval that contains the largest number of subjects. The mode is easily "calculated," and is the only measure suitable for qualitative (class membership) data. Nonetheless, the mode is of little use beyond the descriptive level.

Measures of Spread

The three most commonly used measures of spread are the range, variance, and standard deviation.[6] The *range* is simply the distance spanned by the highest and lowest scores in an ordered distribution. Thus, it does not account for scores that fall between these two extremes. The range is easily "calculated" but is of little use beyond the descriptive level.

As noted by Fisher, *variance* is a key concept in statistics. Simply put, variance is the mean of squared deviations from the mean, $S^2 = [\sum(X - \bar{X})^2] / n$. Each score or observation in a sample is subtracted from the sample mean. These differences (deviations) are squared and summed, and the total is divided by the number of scores. Although vital to statistical inference, variance is of little use for descriptive purposes because people generally find it difficult to think in squared terms.

It is easier to think in terms of the *standard deviation*, which is merely the square root of the variance, $\sqrt{[\sum(X - \bar{X})^2]/n}$. The standard deviation is not only the most important measure to describe spread, but is of great use in inferential statistics. It is responsive to the exact position of each score in the distribution, but is quite resistant to variation among samples. It should also be noted that the standard deviation decreases as sample size increases.

Measures of Shape

Distributions come in many shapes; e.g., J-shaped, U-shaped, rectangular. Shape can be described in terms of skewness and kurtosis.[6] A distribution is positively *skewed* if its values appear to be pulled toward the higher end of the scale; conversely, it is negatively skewed if its values appear to be pulled toward the lower end of the scale (as shown in (E) and (F), respectively, in Figure 79–1). The visual analogue scale (VAS) scores that are used to record patient ratings of pain are often positively skewed immediately after surgery, indicating that

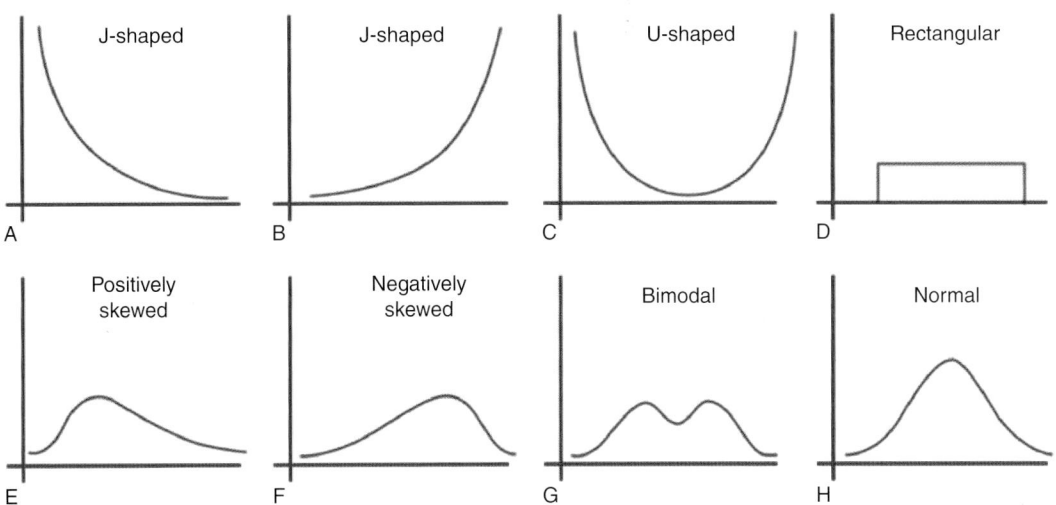

FIGURE 79–1. A few common distributional shapes.

most patients are comfortable right after surgery, and rate their pain at the low end of the distribution. Because the shape of the VAS distribution is not symmetric and bell shaped, it would be appropriate to consider categorizing pain levels into discrete, reasonable ranges; e.g., 0–3 none to mild pain, 4–7 moderate pain, and 8–10 excruciating pain. Nonparametric statistical procedures can be applied to test associations of interest with respect to these categories of pain.

Kurtosis describes peakedness. Leptokurtic distributions have many values in the center and fewer values in the tails of the distribution, giving them a peaked shape with "skinny" tails. In contrast, platykurtic distributions are less peaked, so more values reside in the tails of the distribution, giving them a flatter shape with "fatter" tails. Finally, the mesokurtic distribution is more bell shaped.

The Normal Curve

There is only one standard normal curve. This gaussian curve, named for Carl Friedrich Gauss, a German mathematician (1777–1855), has particular distributional characteristics that are important for inferential statistics. It is symmetric, bell shaped, and has a mean of 0 and a standard deviation of 1. As shown in Figure 79–2, its tails do not touch the horizontal axis because the distribution continues to infinity. Approximately 68% of the scores fall within ± 1 standard deviation of the mean, and roughly 95% of the scores fall within ± 2 standard deviations of the mean; hence, few drawings of the normal curve need to continue beyond ± 3 standard deviations. Figure 79–4 gives areas under the standard normal curve for values of *z*. In particular, note that *z* scores of ± 1.96 correspond to 2.5% in each tail of the curve.

The convenient distributional characteristics of the gaussian curve allow us to calculate standard, or *z* scores; i.e., $z = (X - \bar{X}) / S$. This simple calculation of score minus mean divided by standard deviation gives individual scores their "addresses" on the normal curve. As scores have been standardized to the same curve, we can compare performance on different measures. For example, a score of 95 on an English examination and a score of 75 on a math exam does not necessarily mean that the student performed better on the English exam than on the math exam. If the mean for the English exam was 100 with a standard deviation of 7.5, the student's score of 95 is two thirds of a standard deviation *below* the mean. If the mean for the math exam was 60 with a standard deviation of 10, the student's score of 75 is 1.5 standard deviations *above* the mean. Thus, this student actually performed better on the math exam than on the English exam.

Sampling Distribution of the Mean

Instead of individual scores, the sampling distribution of the mean consists of the *means* of all samples of a specified size taken from the entire population.[2] A particular sample mean's address is located on this distribution.

The hypothetic parent population at the top of Figure 79–3 consists of four scores. The means of every possible sample of size 2 are calculated and distributed into the sampling distribution of the mean at the bottom of the illustration. This allows us to determine the address of any sample mean (here, of size 2) that we might obtain. Thus, a sample mean of 4.5 can be shown to have an address 1.25 standard deviations above the mean on this sampling distribution.

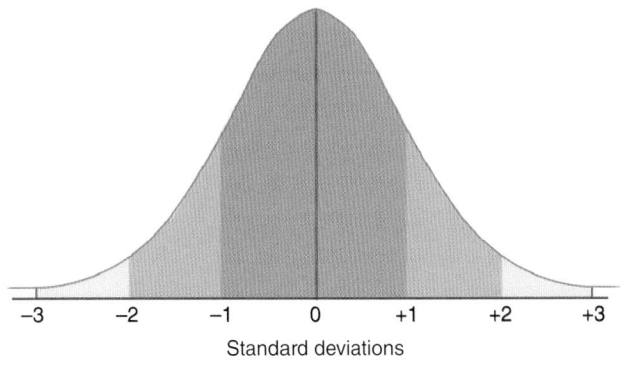

FIGURE 79–2. The gaussian (standard normal) curve.

TABLE 79–4. Type I and Type II errors.

		State of Nature	
		H₀ false	H₀ true
Decision	Retain H₀	Type II (β)[a]	Correct
	Reject H₀	Correct[b]	Type I (α)[c]

[a] "Missing the boat," or failing to convict a guilty person.

[b] "Power" or rejecting H₀ when H₀ is false (1 − β).

[c] "False alarm" or convicting an innocent person.

Central Limit Theorem

In order for the concept of sampling distribution of the mean to be useful, we must also consider the third distributional characteristic, shape. Here, we are fortunate to have an ally known as the central limit theorem. It states that the shape of the sampling distribution of the mean approximates a normal curve if sample size is sufficiently large. So, the question becomes "what is sufficiently large"? This depends on the shape of the parent population. If the parent population is normal, any sample size is sufficiently large. Depending on the extent of

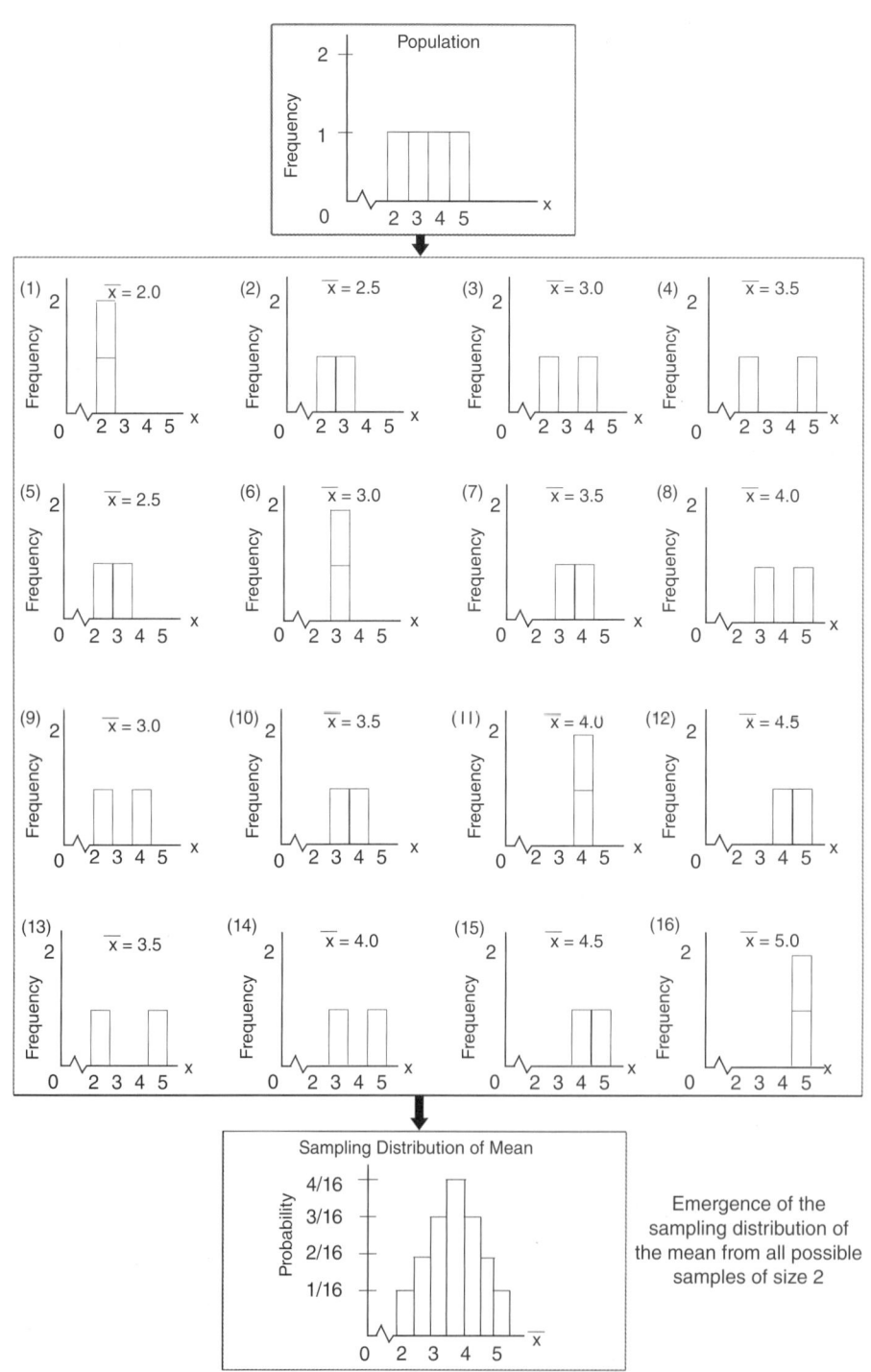

FIGURE 79–3. A sampling distribution of the mean.

abnormality in the parent population, sample sizes between 25 and 100 are typically large enough for the sampling distribution of the mean to have the symmetric bell shape and tapered tails on either side.

Null Hypothesis

The null hypothesis (denoted as H_0) is a statement that there is no effect (e.g., there is no difference in length of PACU stay between patients given regional anesthesia and patients given general anesthesia). H_0 is presumed true until proven false. We must decide whether to reject or retain H_0 based on samples of patients given regional or general anesthesia. Our decision depends on the address of the test statistic on its sampling distribution (Figure 79–4). We are more likely to reject H_0 when our test statistic has an address in the extreme tails of the distribution; conversely, we are more likely to retain H_0 when it has an address in the middle of the distribution. *P*-values indicate how extreme a test statistic is and are used as a guide to rejecting or retaining the null hypothesis.

Alternative Hypotheses

The null hypothesis always makes a claim about one specific value. For example, if we test that there is no difference in time to onset of two anesthetics, we are testing that the difference in onset time between the two anesthetics is literally 0.0000. The alternative, or research, hypothesis (denoted as H_1 or sometimes as H_A) generally complements the null hypothesis and makes a claim about a range of values. Since it is impossible to test infinitesimally every value in a range, we end up testing the specific value of the null hypothesis despite the fact that our real research interest lies in the alternative hypothesis.

The alternative hypothesis comes in three forms: two-sided, one-sided with lower tail critical, one-sided with upper tail critical. If we state that the effect of a new anesthetic on intraoperative blood pressure is different from that of the more established anesthetic, we have not indicated directionality (the new anesthetic may either raise or lower intraoperative blood pressure), so the alternative hypothesis is two-sided. If we state that the effect of a new anesthetic is to lower or to raise intraoperative blood pressure, the alternative hypothesis is one-sided with lower tail critical or with upper tail critical, respectively. Choice of the one-sided alternative hypothesis should be stated when sole concern is about deviations in one direction. However, for most studies, the two-sided alternative hypothesis should be stated, and especially for studies of novel treatments and for early investigations into a new field.

The null hypothesis and *one* of these alternative hypotheses is stated for each research aim of a study. These hypotheses are not questions and should not be written as such. They should not be influenced by preliminary peeks at the data, and ideally should be stated before data are even collected. Once statements about H_0 and H_1 are made, they cannot be changed to accommodate the empirical findings of the study.

Type I and Type II Errors

The type I and type II errors are probabilities:

The type I error is the probability of rejecting H_0 when H_0 is, in fact, true (there actually is no effect). The type II error is the probability of accepting H_0 when H_0 is, in fact, false (there actually is an effect). Neither error can be avoided entirely, so investigators must decide how much error they can tolerate. Is it more important to avoid a type I error (perhaps concluding that a particular anesthetic provides excellent pain relief even at a low dose when it really does not, thus resulting in unnecessary pain for the patient), or is it more important to avoid a type II error (perhaps concluding that a particular anesthetic does not cause bradycardia when it really does, thus endangering the patient during surgery) (Table 79–4)?

After due consideration, the investigator sets the tolerable type I error by specifying α. Typically, this is 0.05, that is, the investigator is willing to take a 5% chance of committing the type I error. Things are a bit more complex with the type II error inasmuch as a number of factors can affect the size of the type II error. The factor over which the investigator has most control is sample size. Studying a larger sample lowers the probability of committing the type II error (Table 79–5).

Principles of Sample Size Estimation

Figure 79–5 shows the underlying sampling distribution of the population means under both the null and alternative hypotheses. For simplicity, only one curve (that for a one-sided lower tail critical test) is shown for the alternative hypothesis. If the researcher has decided to set the type I error at, say, 0.05, the critical value ("address"), denoted in the figure as $\mu_0 - z_0/\sqrt{n}$ is −1.64 for the *z* statistic. Test statistics with addresses to the right of this critical value would result in retention of the null hypothesis, and addresses to the left of the critical value would result in rejection of the null hypothesis.

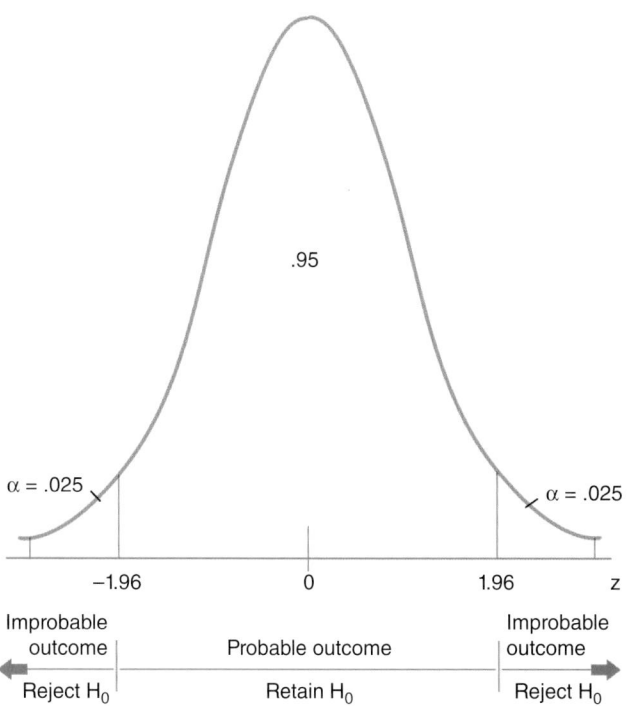

.95

α = .025   α = .025

−1.96   0   1.96   z

| Improbable outcome | Probable outcome | Improbable outcome |
| Reject H_0 | Retain H_0 | Reject H_0 |

FIGURE 79–4. Hypothesized sampling distribution of *z*.

TABLE 79–5. Factors affecting type II error (β).

Sample size: Larger sample size lowers β.

Discrepancy between what is hypothesized and what is true: Larger discrepancy lowers β.

Standard deviation of variable: Smaller σ lowers β.

Relation between samples: Dependent (paired or matched) samples can lower β.

Level of significance: Larger α lowers β.

Choice of H_1: β is smaller for a one-sided test than for a two-sided test.

Source: Data from Minium EW: *Statistical Reasoning in Psychology and Education*, 2nd ed. New York; Wiley & Sons; 1978.

Power (1 − β) is determined by the sampling distribution of the alternative hypothesis. As previously mentioned, increasing sample size decreases variability. Thus, if sample size is increased, both curves pull apart, resulting in less overlap of their tails. The probability of committing a type II error (β) is lessened as the two curves pull apart. However, with too many subjects, the overlap of the curves may be so slight that even a small, clinically unimportant difference can meet or exceed the criterion for statistical significance. Conversely, with too few subjects, the overlap of the curves may be so considerable that it may not be possible to detect any difference, even a sizable one. Therefore, sample size should be reasonable for any study, and grant proposals and manuscripts now require investigators to describe the factors on which the sample size for their study was based. These include criterion for significance (type I error probability, α), desired power (1-type II error probability, β), minimum expected difference with its estimated variability), interest in the one- or two-sided alternative hypothesis, and study design factors (independent *v* paired/matched subjects, number of treatment arms, continuous *v* proportional data collected). Factors that affect sample size are summarized in Table 79–6.

An article by Eng on sample size estimation includes useful suggestions for websites that can be used to estimate sample sizes for some parametric and nonparametric statistics as well as helpful hints on minimizing sample size.[7] However, for descriptive studies (or surveys and polls) in which there is no central hypothesis to test, sample size can be estimated based on an acceptable margin of error (E). This statistic reflects the amount of random sampling error in the results of a survey; hence investigators have more confidence in results with small E (more precision) and less confidence in results with large E (less precision). Several websites contain simple calculators for E; e.g., http://www.raosoft.com/samplesize.html.

Degrees of Freedom

As the name implies, degrees of freedom (df) are the number of values, within a given set of values, that are free to vary. It is a truth in mathematics that differences from a mean must sum to zero; that is, $\sum(X_i - \bar{X}) = 0$. So, given three scores (X_1, X_2, X_3) in the sample, the first deviation $(X_1 - \bar{X})$ might be +4, and the second deviation $(X_2 - \bar{X})$ might be −5. The third deviation $(X_3 - \bar{X})$ must, therefore, be +1. That is, the score X_3 is not free to vary; this sample has only 2 df.

In general, a degree of freedom is used whenever a parameter is estimated, when estimating each regression coefficient in multivariable modeling, and when estimating each treatment and interaction effect in multifactorial analyses of variance. But, importantly, df are also used when estimating error variance ("rubber in the yardstick"). It is little wonder that statisticians worry about having sufficiently large sample sizes to offset the df used during their statistical procedures.

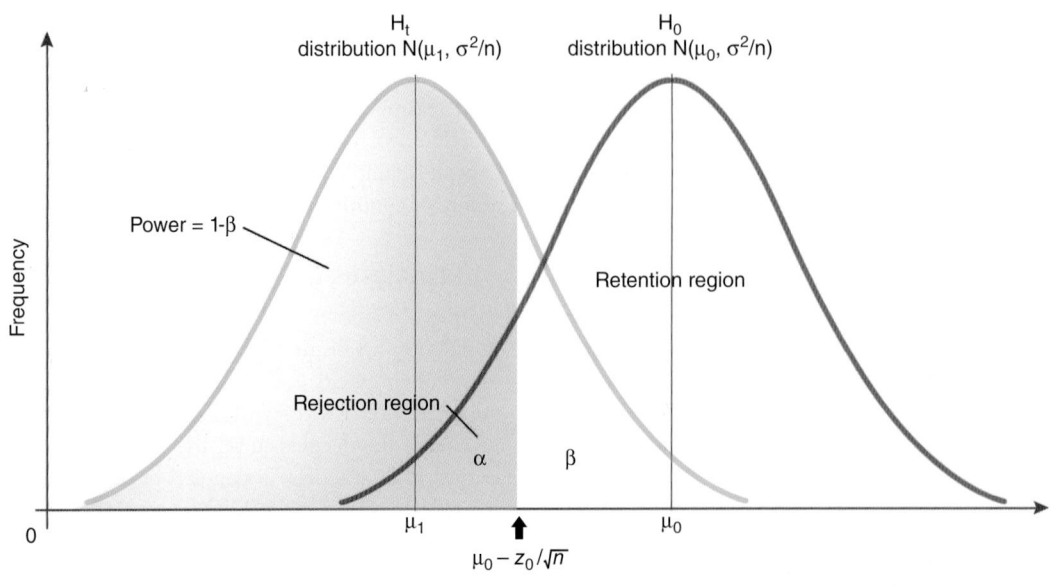

FIGURE 79–5. Sample size estimation.

TABLE 79–6. Factors affecting sample size (n).

n increases as variance (σ^2) increases.

n increases as the significance level is made smaller (i.e., as α decreases).

n increases as the required power is made larger (i.e., as $1 - \beta$ increases).

n decreases with larger absolute value of the distance between the null and alternative means (i.e., as $|\mu_0 - \mu_1|$ increases).

n is larger for two-sided than for one-sided tests.

Source: Data from Minium EW: *Statistical Reasoning in Psychology and Education*, 2nd ed. New York; Wiley & Sons; 1978.

P-Values

Thus far in this chapter, no formal statistical testing has been conducted; however, the concept of critical values has been described: A test statistic is computed and compared to a critical value (the "address" that delineates the retention and rejection regions of H_0). These regions typically contain 2.5% in each tail of the curve for the two-sided test or 5% in one tail for the one-sided test.[8] Although statisticians are not certain how Fisher chose the magical *P*-value of ".05," he may have felt that this is the size of type I error that most researchers could comfortably accept (Table 79–7).

So the *P*-value is the probability of obtaining a test statistic as extreme as or more extreme than the actual test statistic obtained given that H_0 is true. Most statistical software programs automatically provide *P*-values. The computer printout will contain notations attached to test statistics, such as $P = .036$, indicating that the probability of obtaining a test statistic at least as extreme as the one obtained is only 3.6%. And, as this is rather rare, H_0 would be rejected. Note that the *P*-value of .036 should not be interpreted as a 96.4% chance that H_0 is wrong. Put another way, *P*-values are calculated on the assumption that H_0 is true, *but they do not tell us whether that assumption is correct in the first place.*[9]

TABLE 79–7. Guidelines for judging the significance of a *P*-value.

If $01 \leq P < .05$, then the results are *significant*.

If $001 \leq P < .01$, then the results are *highly significant*.

If $P < .001$, then the results are *very highly significant*.

If $P > .05$, then the results are considered *not significant* (sometimes denoted by NS).

However, if $.05 \leq P < .10$, then a trend toward statistical significance is sometimes noted.

Source: Data from Rosner B: *Fundamental of Biostatistics*, 5th ed. Duxbury Press; 2000.

Confidence Intervals

Confidence intervals expand our view beyond *P*-values. Figure 79–6 illustrates that for samples of a given size, intervals can be constructed that may or may not include the population parameter under scrutiny (here, the population mean, μ). Over the collection of all 95% confidence intervals that could be constructed from repeated random samples of a given sample size, 95% of them will contain μ. In reality, you would not be able to construct this figure because you study only a single sample. Consequently, you would not know for certain whether the confidence interval from your particular sample actually does include the population value. You would know, however, that 95% of the intervals from studies such as yours will contain the population parameter. Thus, you will have an estimate of the population parameter with reasonable certainty.

Confidence intervals have several advantages. The *P*-value approach makes a statement about a derived statistic (usually the family of *F*, *r*, or chi-square statistics). This approach merely produces a yes or no answer about whether to reject or retain H_0 and could lead to confusion between statistical significance

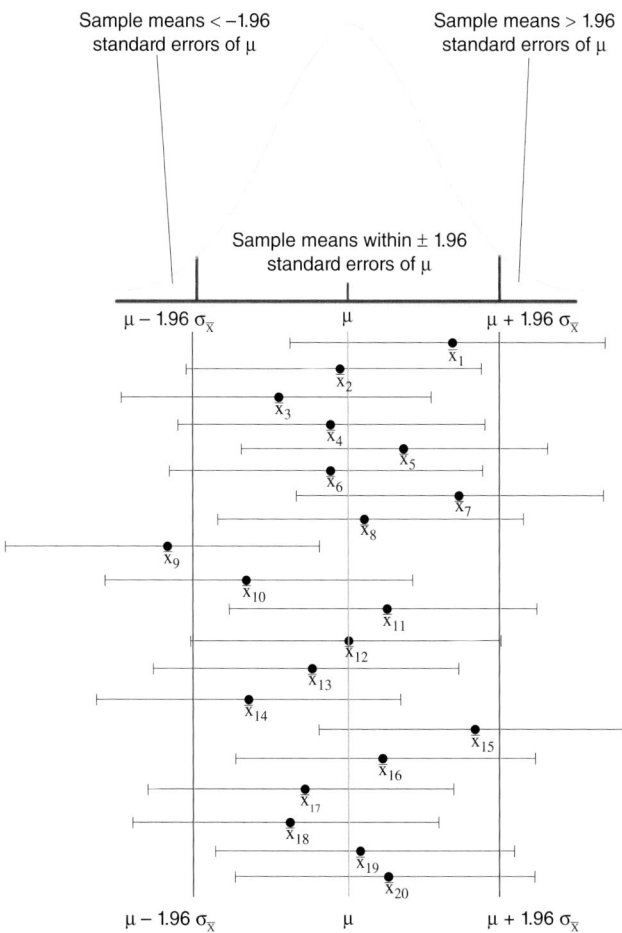

*Although 95% confidence intervals have been constructed for the purpose of illustration, it is possible to construct intervals for any desired certainty (e.g., 90%, 99%).
**Confidence intervals can be constructed for population parameters other than the mean (e.g., for the population correlation coeficient, p (rho)).

FIGURE 79–6. Several 95% confidence intervals arising from the sampling distribution of the mean.

and clinical importance. Confidence intervals, on the other hand, make a statement about the actual parameter of interest. An estimate of the population parameter is produced along with an idea of the precision with which the estimate was made. If the confidence interval is narrow, the estimate was probably based on a sizable number of subjects and precision is good; conversely, if the confidence interval is wide, the estimate was probably based on fewer subjects and precision is not as good.

As noted earlier, the minimum expected difference (MED) that the investigator deems important to detect is a crucial factor in sample size estimation. A simple way of quantifying the MED is to divide it by the standard deviation of the population from which the different treatment groups were taken. This so-called "effect size" (also known as Cohen's d) follows the formula

$$Effect\ size = \frac{(Mean\ of\ experimental\ group) - (Mean\ of\ control\ group)}{Standard\ deviation}$$

where the standard deviation may be estimated either from the control group or pooled from both the experimental and control groups using

$$SD_{pooled} = \sqrt{\frac{(n_e - 1)SD_e^2 + (n_c - 1)SD_c^2}{n_e + n_c - 2}}$$

Effect sizes are standardized (divided by the standard deviation) and, therefore, unitless. An effect size of 0.96 indicates that the average score in the experimental group is nearly a full standard deviation above that of the average score in the control group. (Effect sizes can be negative as, e.g., if the control group provided higher scores than the experimental group in that study.) Cohen has described 0.2 as "small," 0.5 as "medium," and 0.8 as "large" effects.[10] Because they are standardized, effect sizes can be compared (carefully) among different studies such as in meta analyses where they have been most frequently used. Nonetheless, they should be included in most reports as they help us appreciate the "significance" of significance tests. For example, the statement that "the effect of gender on reported pain scores was large, Cohen's d = 2.1, t(12) = 3.2, P < .01" tells us that the impact of gender was sizable despite the small sample size (here, total sample size was 14).

Parametric and Nonparametric Statistical Tests and When to Use Them

A parameter is a characteristic of a population. One of the parameters that we are often interested in is the population mean, μ. Parameters are usually denoted by Greek letters, whereas characteristics of samples are usually denoted by Roman letters (e.g., a sample mean is denoted as $\bar{X}$).

Parametric tests are used with quantitative data and require assumptions about the precise form of the population distribution, e.g., normality and equal variance (also known as homogeneity of variance). Nonparametric tests are used with quantitative, ranked, or qualitative data and require no assumptions about the precise form of the population distribution. These "distribution-free" tests *can be used* with quantitative data that have nonnormal distributions and when variances of the groups are not equal, however, they *must be used* with ranked or qualitative data.

When it is believed that the normality and homogeneity assumptions are met, parametric tests are more powerful than nonparametric tests. However, when sample size is small (say, less than 10), there is a very good possibility that the assumption of normality has been violated. Furthermore, when sample sizes are small *and* unequal, there is a very good possibility that the assumption of equal variance has been violated. Under these circumstances, the nonparametric tests should probably be used. We have already discussed an example of nonnormality with the VAS scores. It was suggested that perhaps the scores should be categorized into levels of pain and submitted to nonparametric tests (as discussed in the section on Nonparametric Tests).

Data Transformations

Raw data may need to be transformed in order to meet the assumptions of the parametric statistical tests. As described throughout this section, data must come from a population with normally distributed values. Thus data that are inconsistent with this assumption should be transformed prior to conducting a parametric statistical test. It is convenient that transforming to normality can reduce the influence of outliers (atypical values) on the analysis, and a nonparametric test may become unnecessary. Another assumption of many parametric tests is that the groups have the same variance; hence, violations to this assumption may require data transformation. A third assumption applies to linear regression (which is covered in the section on Parametric Tests). It states that the model must be a linear combination of variables; hence, transformation must be considered if regression coefficients or raw data suggest a nonlinear (curvilinear) model. It is indeed fortunate that the same transformation often helps to meet the first two assumptions (and sometimes even the third), rather than dealing with one assumption at the expense of the other two.

The only transformation that will be described here is the log transformation as it is by far the most frequently used. Simply, the logarithm of each raw value is computed and used in the inferential statistical analysis. However, results of the analysis are presented in the original scale of measurement. Other transformations require that the square root, reciprocal, square, or even the arcsin of the raw data be obtained prior to analysis.[11] Statistical advice is necessary when using transformations, as certain conditions apply. For instance, a statistician is likely to suggest the log transformation if s/he notes that variance increases as the mean of the groups increases (thereby producing a rather funnel-shaped scatter-plot). However, the statistician will also know that this transformation can only be used with outcome variables that take positive values.

PARAMETRIC TESTS

Our foray into inferential statistics begins with the z test for a single population mean, the most fundamental of the inferential tests. This test is accurate only when the population is normally distributed (or the sample size is large enough to satisfy the central limit theorem), and the population standard deviation, σ, is known. Unfortunately, in regional anesthesia and in other areas of medicine, we rarely know σ, so the z statistic cannot be used. We turn, instead, to the t test for a single sample:

$$z = \frac{\text{(normally distributed variable)} - \text{(constant)}}{\text{(constant)}}$$

$$= \frac{\bar{X} - \mu}{\sigma_{\bar{X}}} \text{ where } \sigma_{\bar{X}} = \frac{\sigma}{\sqrt{n}}$$

$$t = \frac{\text{(normally distributed variable)} - \text{(constant)}}{\text{(variable)}}$$

$$= \frac{\bar{X} - \mu}{s_{\bar{X}}} \text{ where } s_{\bar{X}} = \frac{s}{\sqrt{n}}$$

Not surprisingly, there is a whole family of t curves, one curve for each sample size. As shown in Figure 79–7, although each curve is bell shaped, the area in the tails increases as sample size decreases. Thus, the z score address on a curve with few df must be higher (in the upper tail) and lower (in the lower tail) than the address on a curve with many df. This is to accommodate the thickness of their tails. For the curves shown in the Figure 79–7, the z scores are ± 2.776 and ± 2.228 with 4 and 10 df, respectively, for 2.5% in each tail, as compared to ± 1.96 for the infinite df of the standard normal curve.

The difference between the t and standard normal distributions is greatest for small sample size (usually <30). As sample size increases, the curves converge to that of the standard normal curve because the sample variance (s^2) decreases, and s^2 is better able to approximate the population variance (σ^2).

For our example of the t test for a single sample, we wish to know whether the heart rate of patients undergoing interscalene brachial plexus block differs from the adult norm of 72. Heart rate is recorded on 18 patients (mean 75 beats per minute [bpm] ± 8.8). We calculate $t_{\text{df}=17} = (75 - 72)/(8.8/\sqrt{18}) = 1.45$, which is not significant (P >.05). Thus, heart rate in our sample of patients undergoing interscalene brachial plexus block does not differ from the adult norm of 72 bpm. Note that the test is with 17 df because one degree of freedom was used to estimate s.

Student's *t*

The *Student t* test compares two independent groups with respect to some continuous variable. The test was named for William S. Gosset, a British chemist and statistician

(1876–1937), who worked out the mathematics for the family of t distributions and wrote under the penname of Student. The groups must be independent, so a patient cannot contribute more than one value to a group, nor can a patient contribute values to both groups. The formula to test is basically the same as that for the one sample case, in which the sample mean has been replaced by the sample mean difference, $(\bar{X}_1 - \bar{X}_2)$, the population mean by the population mean difference, $(\mu_1 - \mu_2)$, and the sample standard deviation by the standard error of the mean difference, $S_{\bar{X}_1 - \bar{X}_2}$. It should be noted that $(\mu_1 - \mu_2)$ is regarded as 0 whenever the null hypothesis posits no difference between the groups. It should also be noted that the standard error is essentially a standard deviation; the term *error* is often used to describe variability of computed measures, such as variability in *mean* differences.

For our example, we wish to know whether postoperative heart rate measured in the recovery room differs between patients who receive general anesthesia and those who receive spinal anesthesia. Postoperative heart rate of 10 patients who received general anesthesia (87.7 ± 8.8) is compared with that of 10 patients who received spinal anesthesia (72.7 ± 7.1), $t_{\text{df}=18} = 4.2$, $P = .001$. Thus, postoperative heart rate differs by anesthetic technique (it is higher in patients who receive general anesthesia). Note that df = $(n_1 - 1) + (n_2 - 1) = (10 - 1) + (10 - 1) = 18$, so two df were used estimating s_1 and s_2.

$$t = \frac{(\bar{X}_1 - \bar{X}_2) - (\mu_1 - \mu_2)}{s_{\bar{X}_1 - \bar{X}_2}}$$

$$\text{where } S^2_{\text{Pooled}} = \frac{(n_1 - 1)s_1^2 + (n_2 - 1)s_2^2}{(n_1 - 1)(n_2 - 1)}$$

$$s_{\bar{X}_1 - \bar{X}_2} = \sqrt{\frac{S^2_{\text{Pooled}}}{n_1}} + \sqrt{\frac{S^2_{\text{Pooled}}}{n_2}}, \text{ and}$$

$$\text{df} = (n_1 - 1) + (n_2 - 1)$$

Since,

$$s_p^2 = \frac{(10-1)(8.8^2) + (10-1)(7.1^2)}{(10-1)(10-1)} = 63.925 \text{ and}$$

$$s_{\bar{X}_1 - \bar{X}_2} = \sqrt{\frac{63.925}{10}} + \sqrt{\frac{63.925}{10}} = 3.576,$$

$$\therefore t = \frac{(87.7 - 72.7) - 0}{3.576} = 4.2 (p = .001)$$

Note: The table of z values found in many statistical texts was not included in this chapter; neither were tables of the critical values for the t, F, chi-square (χ^2), and other tests. This is because P-values and confidence intervals for most statistics are included as standard output by the programs used to calculate them, and separate tables are generally not needed.

Dependent (Paired or Matched) *t*

Groups are not independent if subjects are matched on some variable or the same subjects are tested before and after some

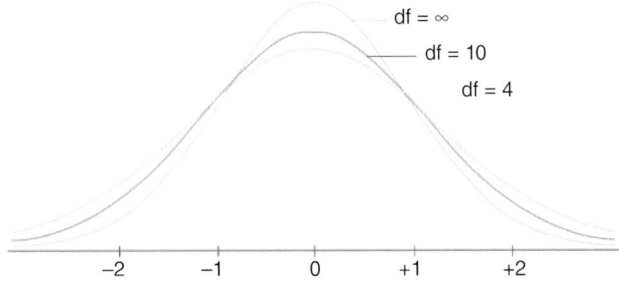

FIGURE 79–7. A couple of t distributions.

intervention, or a cohort of subjects is repeatedly evaluated over an interval of time. For our example, we wish to know whether heart rate differs in 10 patients who received epidural anesthesia at the T1 level before and after a bolus of 15 mL of 2% lidocaine. Heart rate before bolus (78.7 ± 7.4) is compared with heart rate after bolus administration (69.6 ± 6.7) in the same patients, $t_{df = 9} = -10.4$, $P < .001$. Heart rate before bolus differs from heart rate after bolus (it is lower following bolus administration). Note the similarity with the *Student t* formula: The sample mean difference, $(\bar{X}_1 - \bar{X}_2)$ has been replaced by the mean difference between scores, $\bar{D}$, the population mean difference, $(\mu_1 - \mu_2)$, has been replaced by the population difference, μ_D and the standard error of the mean difference, $S_{\bar{X}_1 - \bar{X}_2}$, by $S_{\bar{D}}$. It should also be noted that μ_D is again regarded as 0 because the null hypothesis posits no difference in heart rate before and after boluses of lidocaine.

$$t = \frac{\bar{D} - \mu_D}{S_{\bar{D}}}, \text{ where } s_D = \sqrt{\frac{n(\sum D^2) - (\sum D^2)}{n(n-1)}},$$

$$s_{\bar{D}} = \frac{s_D}{\sqrt{n}}, \text{ and } df = (\text{pairs} - 1).$$

Given $\sum D = -91$, $\sum D^2 = 897$ (calculations not shown),

$$\bar{D} = \frac{-91}{10} = -9.1, s_D = \sqrt{\frac{10(897) - (-91)^2}{10(10-1)}} = 2.7669,$$

$$\text{and } s_{\bar{D}} = \frac{2.7669}{\sqrt{10}} = 0.87496$$

$$\therefore t = \frac{-9.1}{0.87496} = -10.4 \, (p < .001)$$

One-Way Analysis of Variance

One-way analysis of variance (ANOVA) extends the *Student t* test of two population means to three (or more) population means. Whereas the difference in postoperative heart rate between patients randomly assigned to receive one of two different anesthetic techniques might be tested with the *Student t* test, differences in postoperative heart rate among patients randomly assigned to receive one of three (or more) different anesthetic techniques might be tested by one-way ANOVA. The assumptions in ANOVA are the same as those for *Student t*; i.e., all underlying populations are normally distributed with equal variance.

Deviations reflecting random error and the effect of treatment are calculated and compared as a ratio of two variances, known as the *F* ratio in honor of Fisher. When the null hypothesis is true and there is no treatment effect, both the numerator and denominator of the F ratio will reflect sums of squared deviations resulting from random error. As numerator and denominator tend to be similar, the *F* ratio will vary about a value of 1. Conversely, when the null hypothesis is false and there is a treatment effect, the sum of squared deviations that is due to treatment enlarges the numerator and the *F* ratio can become much greater than 1. The F ratio's address is located on

the F distribution (a sampling distribution of variance ratios) in order to determine whether it has become large enough to meet statistical significance. Like the *t* distributions, there is a whole family of F distributions based on the df in the numerator and denominator of the F ratio. Fortunately, levels of significance for the F ratio are automatically provided in statistical output.

For our example, we wish to know whether postoperative heart rate differs among patients who received general or spinal anesthesia or PNB for knee arthroplasty surgery. Postoperative heart rate is studied in patients who are randomly assigned to receive one of the three anesthetic techniques (20 patients per group). We find from the ANOVA that postoperative heart rate differs significantly by anesthetic technique (the critical value for *F* with 2 and 57 df is approximately 5.0 for *P* = .01 and is exceeded by the obtained *F* ratio of 6.5). Subsequent pairwise comparisons reveal that postoperative heart rate is lower in patients given spinal anesthesia (72 bpm) than in those given general anesthesia (88 bpm) but does not differ from that of patients given PNB (78 bpm).

ANOVA Table

Source of Variation	df	Sum of Squares	Mean Square	F	P-Value
Treatment (anesthetic technique)	2	115.6	57.8	6.5	<.01
Error	57	507.4	8.9		
Total	59	623			

Abbreviations: *df*, degrees of freedom; *F*, where $df_{treatment} = (\text{groups} - 1) = (3 - 1) = 2$, $df_{error} = (\text{subjects} - \text{groups} - 1) = (60 - 2 - 1) = 57$, and $df_{total} = (\text{subjects} - 1) = (60 - 1) = 59$.

Factorial ANOVA

Even though we studied three groups in the one-way ANOVA example and could have studied more, we nonetheless looked at a single independent variable (e.g., anesthetic technique). A researcher who wishes to look at more than one independent variable turns to factorial ANOVA. For instance, the researcher interested in the effects of three anesthetic techniques (general or spinal anesthesia or PNB) *and* intake of a beta-blocker (yes/no) on postoperative heart rate would use a 3 × 2 factorial ANOVA. The researcher would be able to look at the effects of anesthetic technique and intake of beta-blocker as well as any interaction between them. These analyses are possible using the same subjects, so factorial designs can be a statistical "best buy."

Factorial ANOVA has the same assumptions as one-way ANOVA. Whereas with one-way ANOVA, there is not much to fear about violating assumptions as long as the group sample sizes are equal and fairly large (>10 per group), factorial ANOVA is not as robust. Even small departures from equal sample sizes could cause extensive computational and interpretation problems. Thus, very complex factorial designs are typically discouraged. For instance, our 3 × 2 factorial could also be assessed by gender and repeated over five time points in a 3 × 2 × 2 × 5 (repeated) design. This and innumerable other complex factorials should be done with a statistician because some may not be as robust as others. Moreover, there will not be much confidence in results from factorials that are difficult to interpret.

Interaction

Interaction occurs when the measure of effect (between exposure and outcome) is modified by the presence of another variable. For our example, the interaction between anesthetic technique and intake of a beta-blocker is statistically significant.

ANOVA Table

Source of Variation	df	Sum of Mean Squares	Mean Square	F	P-Value
Treatment (anesthetic technique)	2	97	48.5	6.1	<.01
Beta-blocker (yes/no)	1	39.6	39.6	5.0	<.05
Interaction (technique × blocker)	2	114	57	7.2	<.01
Error	54	426.6	7.9		
Total	59	677.2			

Abbreviations: df, degree of freedom; F, where $df_{treatment}$ = (groups – 1) = (3-1) = 2, beta-blocker Y/N (2 - 1) = 1, interaction (2 x 1) = 2, and df_{error} = (subjects – groups – 1) = (60-2-1-2-1) = 54, and df_{total} = (subjects – 1) = (60-1) = 59.

Postoperative heart rate is low and fairly stable in patients who received beta-blockers, but is substantially increased in patients given spinal anesthesia or PNB (as illustrated in the left panel of Figure 79–8). Note that when interaction is found, it is the interaction that is of interest and thus described in the report. In our example, the main effects of anesthetic technique and intake of beta-blocker are also statistically significant, but they no longer have "center stage." On the other hand, if there had been *no* interaction (as illustrated by the parallel lines in the right panel of Figure 79–8), the main effects would have been reported separately, as both are statistically significant; e.g., postoperative heart rate differs by anesthetic technique and is decreased in patients who receive beta-blockers prior to surgery regardless of anesthetic technique.

Multiple Comparisons

We return to the one-way ANOVA example of the effects of three different anesthetic techniques on postoperative heart rate. If our F ratio is statistically significant, we know that the three sample means come from different populations; i.e., the anesthetic techniques differ in how they affect postoperative heart rate. However, a significant F ratio does not tell us which group or groups are different. Is postoperative heart rate in patients who receive general anesthesia different from that in patients who receive spinal anesthesia, but not different from that in patients who receive PNB? If specific interest in a comparison (say, between general and spinal anesthetic techniques) had been stated *before looking at the data*, the difference in postoperative heart rate between these two techniques could be followed by the *Student t* test. However, when such a priori comparisons have not been expressed, several comparisons among the groups must be conducted to determine where the significant difference(s) lie. These comparisons are considered post hoc because they involve data that have already been reviewed and analyzed (here, by the one-way ANOVA). But increasing the number of statistical tests increases the risk for committing a type I error (saying there is a difference when there really is none). This is because a null hypothesis rejected at α = 0.05 on a *single* test confers a 5% chance of committing a type I error, but as more and more multiple comparison tests are made, the experiment-wise α rises, and it can rise very fast.

For α set at 0.05, the experiment-wise type I error rate (α_{EW}) rises to nearly 20% by the time four comparisons are made.

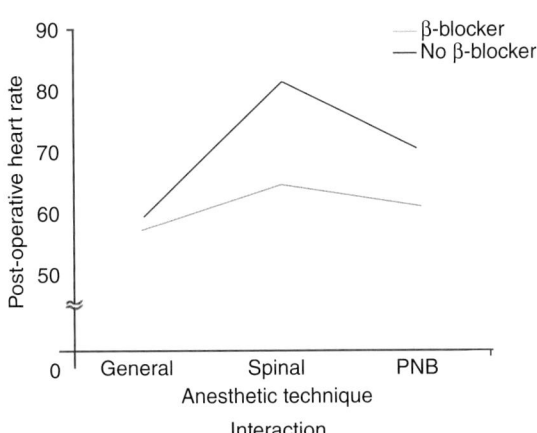

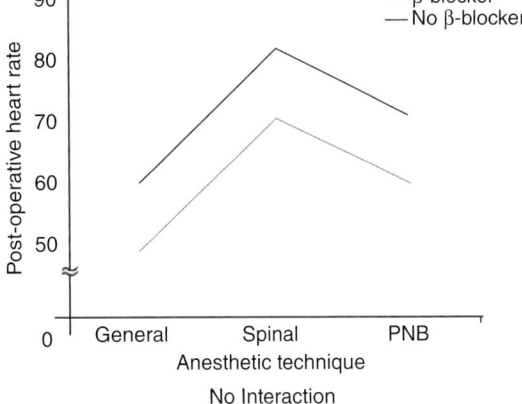

FIGURE 79–8. Interaction vs no interaction.

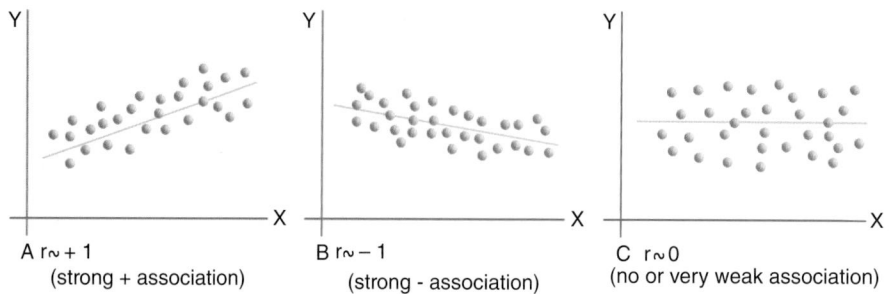

FIGURE 79–9. Pearson product moment correlation coefficient (r).

Most researchers would not be comfortable with a type I error probability this high:

$$\alpha_{EW} = 1 - (1 - 0.05)^1 = 1 - 0.95^1 = 0.05 \text{ for one comparison}$$

$$\alpha_{EW} = 1 - (1 - 0.05)^2 = 1 - 0.95^2 \approx 0.10 \text{ for two comparisons}$$

$$\alpha_{EW} = 1 - (1 - 0.05)^3 = 1 - 0.95^3 \approx 0.14 \text{ for three comparisons}$$

$$\alpha_{EW} = 1 - (1 - 0.05)^4 = 1 - 0.95^4 \approx 0.19 \text{ for four comparisons}$$

Fortunately, a number of tests are designed to help control the experiment-wise error. Three methods are commonly used when the investigator wishes to compare all pairs of means: the Bonferroni approach, the Tukey honestly significant difference test, and the Student-Newman-Keuls comparison test. In the Bonferroni approach, the α level is divided by the number of all possible *pairs* of groups to be compared. For three groups in the experiment (here, simply designated as A, B, and C), α would be divided by 3 (AB, AC, BC); for four groups (A, B, C, D), α would be divided by 6 (AB, AC, AD, BC, BD, CD). Group differences are tested by the *Student t* test using the pooled estimate of the variance (error mean square from the one-way ANOVA). The *t* statistic for each comparison must then exceed the more stringent α in order to be declared statistically significant. The Bonferroni approach tends to be conservative (less powerful) and should be used only when testing a few pairs of means (i.e., not more than five groups). The Tukey and Student-Newman-Keuls tests use range tests to identify homogeneous subsets of means that are not different from one another. They make all possible comparisons between groups and are more powerful when testing a large number of pairs of means. Other popular post hoc comparison methods include the Dunnett test, which is useful when the investigator is not interested in comparing groups among themselves, but instead wishes to compare one control group to each of the other treatment groups. The Scheffé method is useful if the investigator is interested in elaborate comparisons (known as contrasts); e.g., the mean of (A + B + C) vs D; however, it is more conservative than other post hoc tests. Clearly, statistical expertise should be sought when multiple comparison decisions need to be made.

Correlation — Pearson *r*

Numerous statistics can be calculated to assess the extent of association between variables; e.g., Φ coefficient, biserial, point biserial. However, the most well-known and frequently used is

the Pearson product-moment correlation coefficient (simply denoted as r). The Pearson r, named for the British mathematician, Karl Pearson (1857–1936), is a measure of association between two continuous variables (Figure 79–9). Subjects contribute once to each variable; hence subjects are independent in that they do not make multiple contributions to each variable. The coefficient ranges from +1 (perfect positive association) to –1 (perfect negative association). Values around 0 indicate that the two variables are not associated. As r approaches +1, an individual with a high value for one variable is likely to have a high value for the other; an individual with a low value for one variable is likely to have a low value for the other. For instance, time to motor response is positively correlated with distance from nerve at which local anesthetic injection commences. As r approaches –1, an individual with a high value for one variable is likely to have a low value for the other; an individual with a low value for one variable is likely to have a high value for the other. For instance, extent of motor response is negatively correlated with distance from nerve at which the injection commences.

It is important to note, however, that the Pearson r does not measure several things:[11]

- r makes no statement about causality. Even though two variables are strongly associated (either positively or negatively), one did not *cause* the other.
- r is not a measure of the magnitude of the slope of the regression line (Figure 79–10). Both lines indicate perfect association; however, the slope is only impressive for the panel on the left.
- r is not a measure of the appropriateness of the straight-line model (Figure 79–11). Regardless of a high or low r,

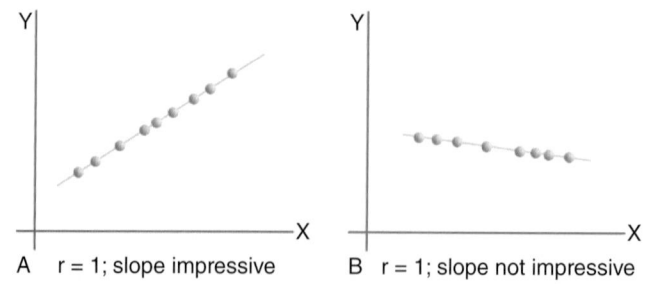

FIGURE 79–10. r Is not a measure of slope.

r close to 0

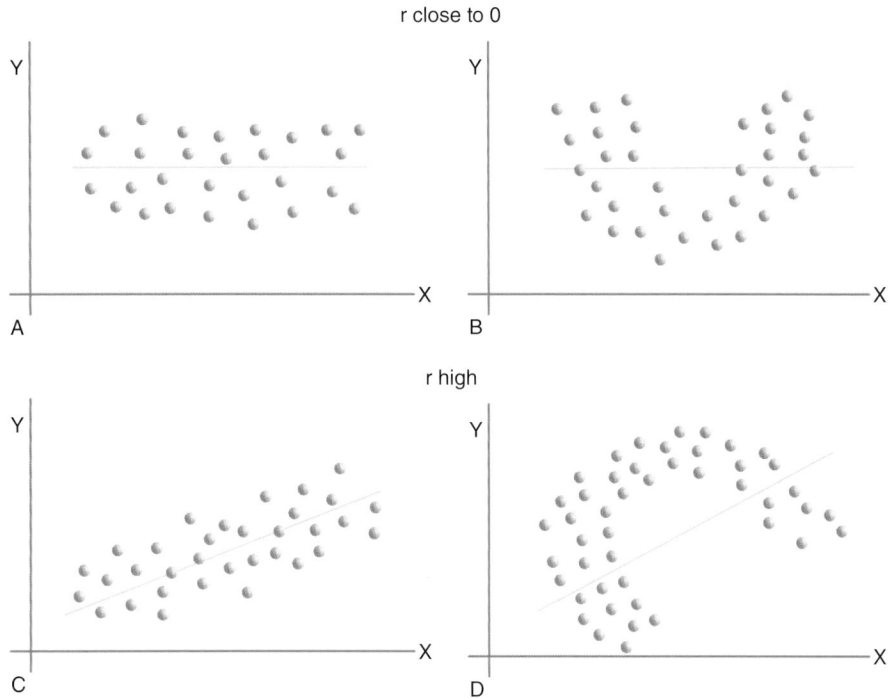

r high

FIGURE 79–11. *r* Is not a measure of appropriateness of straight-line model.

there could be a nonlinear association in the data that is not reflected in the value of *r*. A picture is worth a 1000 words!

Also be aware that:

- r can be sensitive to outliers (i.e., it is easily influenced by them).
- r should not be calculated or should be carefully calculated.
  - Between the time 1 and time 2 measures of the same variable
  - Between two variables at various times (unless time trends have been removed)
  - Between two variables where one variable is included in the other (i.e., if X is part of Y, then r between X and XY should not be calculated)
  - Between a variable and the change in that variable over time (i.e., *r* between X_0 and $X_1 - X_0$ should not be calculated)
- *r* should not be calculated if the research focus is on agreement between two tests or devices as other statistical approaches are more appropriate.[12,13]
- Type I error may increase when many variables are correlated with each other in the same study.

We will not derive the level of significance associated with values of the Pearson *r*. Suffice it to say that *P*-values of Pearson *r* included in the bivariate correlation output derive from testing the null hypothesis that the population correlation (ρ) between the two variables is zero (i.e., H_0: ρ = 0). Researchers who wish to test whether ρ is some value other than zero based on past experience or theory (i.e., H_0: ρ = $ρ_0$ where $ρ_0 \neq 0$) should consult a statistician who will be able to test these

hypotheses and construct the appropriate confidence intervals. Moreover, statistical expertise is advised if your research interest lies in testing the equality of two correlations from independent random samples (i.e., H_0: $ρ_1 = ρ_2$) or two correlations of different variables within the same sample (e.g., H_0: $ρ_{12} = ρ_{13}$).

Least Squares Regression

When the correlation coefficient is 0, we know that *x* is useless in predicting *y*. When the correlation coefficient is +1 or −1, we know that *x* is exactly correct in predicting *y*. However, the value of the correlation coefficient, in and of itself, does not tell us how to go about making the prediction. If the *x* and *y* variables have a linear relationship, a line could be drawn through the scatterplot of points, in which each dot represents the intersection of a subject's *x* and *y* values. The problem is that innumerable lines could be drawn through the scatterplot. Which is the "best fitting" one? Pearson determined this line in such a way that the sum of the squared differences (d_i's) between the line and each scatterplot dot is as small as possible (hence the term, *least squares regression*). That is, the sum of squared discrepancies shown in Figure 79–12 is at a minimum. No other line through that scatterplot has a lower sum of squares.

With bivariate (simple) linear regression, a continuous variable *y* is predicted from a continuous variable *x* based on the equation for a straight line, *y* = α + β*x* + ε. Thus, the components that predict *y* are a constant that indicates the value of *y* when *x* is 0 (known as the intercept of the line, α), a coefficient that indicates the change in *y* for each 1-unit change in *x* (known as the slope, β), and an error term that indicates variability of the observed values from the regression line (ε). For our example, we wish to predict duration of femoral nerve

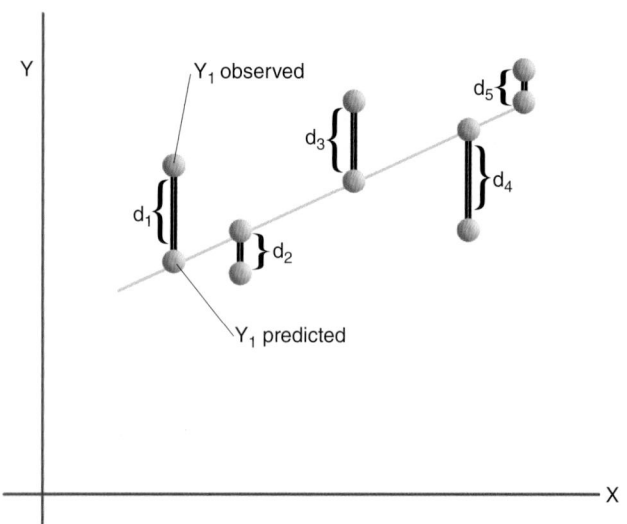

FIGURE 79–12. Least squares regression.

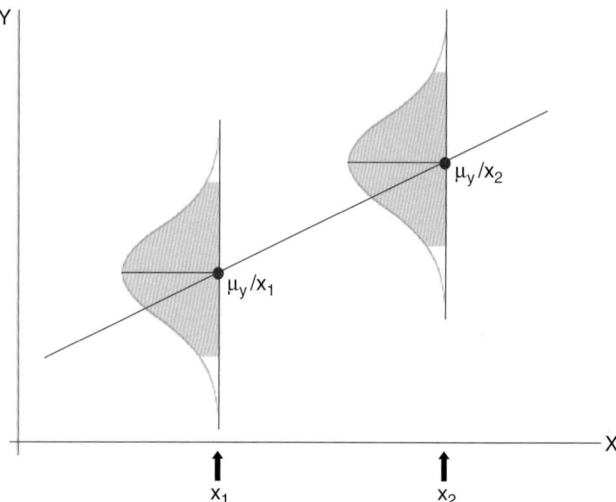

FIGURE 79–13. HEIL Gauss.

blockade from the concentration of 0.5% lidocaine administered. Duration of femoral nerve blockade (in minutes) is measured in 24 patients receiving 0.5%, 1.0%, 1.5%, or 2.0% lidocaine. The model produced is $y = -2.5 + 124 \, x = -2.5 + 124(0.5) = 59.5$ (calculations not shown), indicating an increase of approximately 60 minutes in duration of femoral nerve blockade for every unit increase of 0.5% lidocaine.

With multiple linear regression, a continuous variable y is predicted from a continuous variable x, *while controlling or adjusting for the influence of one or more potentially confounding variables (i.e., other x's in the model)*. When mixed with the exposure and outcome, confounders can strengthen, weaken, or otherwise distort the true association between exposure and outcome.[14] As an example, we found from bivariate linear regression that lidocaine concentration is predictive of duration of femoral blockade. However, concentration of local anesthetic may predict a duration of femoral blockade that is substantially longer or shorter than 60 minutes when a variable reflecting presence or absence of preexisting neuropathy (e.g., diabetic neuropathy) is also included in the model. On the other hand, concentration of local anesthetic may *not* predict duration of femoral blockade when stimulating current at which motor response is observed is included in the model. To determine the relative influence of such potentially confounding covariates and to take a more undisturbed look at the $x - y$ relationship, we construct multiple linear regression models of the form

$$y = \alpha + \beta_1 x_1 + \beta_2 x_2 + \beta_3 x_3 + \ldots + \beta_i x_i + \varepsilon.$$

This would allow us to look at the effect of 0.5% lidocaine concentration on duration of femoral blockade after the effects of preexisting neuropathy and intensity of nerve-stimulating current are controlled.

Covariates can be continuous (e.g., age), ordinal (e.g., level of education), or nominal (e.g., gender). With multiple regression, quadratic terms can be added to model nonlinear relationships (e.g., x_1^2), and product terms can be added to model

interactions (e.g., $x_2 x_3$). If these nonlinear and interaction terms are included in the model, their respective component terms (x_1, x_2, x_3) should also be included in the model; e.g.,

$$y = \alpha + \beta_1 x_1 + \beta_2 x_2 + \beta_3 x_3 + \beta_4 x_1^2 + \beta_5 x_2 x_3 + \varepsilon$$

Assumptions for the Straight-Line Model

Whether we construct a bivariate or multivariable regression model, five assumptions must be met. Students of statistics remember them by the acronym, HEIL Gauss (homoscedasticity, existence, independence, linearity, and normality), even though it seems more logical to describe these assumptions in a different order.[8] So, referring to Figure 79–13, let us begin with "existence." This assumption states that, at any given fixed value of the variable x, there exists a random variable y, and this random variable y has a probability distribution with finite mean and variance. The distribution of y for any fixed value of x has a normal (gaussian) distribution, the variance of y is the same for any of its distributions at x (homoscedasticity is just a fancy term for equal variance), and the mean value of y, i.e., $\mu_{y|x}$, is a straight-line function of x (linearity). Finally, "independence" assumes that patients are not matched on some variable and that the outcome variable is not measured over time on the same patients.

NONPARAMETRIC TESTS

Many of the parametric tests are quite "robust" even though their assumptions are violated, and they are especially robust when the sample size is moderate or large. However, if the violations are sizable and the sample size is small or, if the data are ordinal or qualitative, we turn to the nonparametric tests. The nonparametric tests are more appropriate and can even be more powerful under these circumstances.

Chi-Square

Arguably the most frequently used nonparametric test is the chi-square (χ^2) test. It requires that observations are

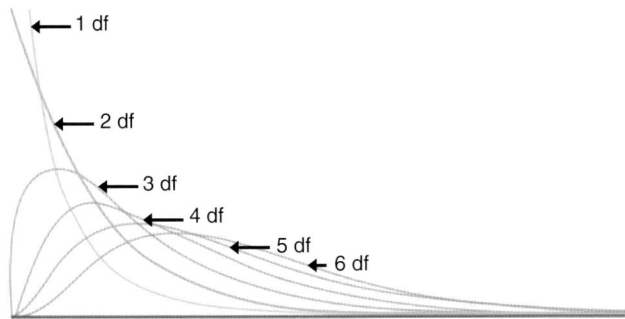

FIGURE 79–14. A family of χ^2 distributions.

independent; i.e., each subject is counted in one, and only one, cell of a contingency table. It also requires that expected frequencies are sufficiently large. So, how are expected frequencies obtained, and what is "sufficiently large"? An expected frequency for a given cell is obtained by multiplying the row and column marginals for that cell and dividing the product by n. Thus, in the 2 × 2 contingency table, the expected frequency for the upper left-hand cell with observed frequency a is $[(a + b)(a + c)]/n$. This process is repeated for each of the remaining three cells. An expected frequency of 5 typically suffices for the test (Figure 79-14A).

Variable A

	Level 1	Level 2	Total
Variable B Level 1	a	b	a+b
Level 2	c	d	c+d
Total	a+c	b+d	N

$$\chi^2 = \sum \frac{(|f_O - f_E| - 0.5)^2}{f_E} \quad \text{where } f_o \text{ is observed frequency and } f_E \text{ is expected frequency}$$

Note: The Yates' correction (0.5) is sometimes subtracted from the observed-expected differences before squaring because the continuous χ^2 distribution is used to test the discrete distribution of sample frequencies. Today, the correction is less frequently used as it may overadjust the χ^2 statistic, making its *P*-value too conservative. Moreover, the Yates' correction only makes a noticeable difference when cell counts are small, and computers can calculate "exact" *P*-values in these instances.

For each cell, the difference between observed and expected frequencies is squared and divided by the expected frequency; the squared quantities are then summed. Since the χ^2 statistic reflects the size of the discrepancies between observed and expected frequencies as a proportion of the expected frequency, large χ^2's indicate differences that are not likely to be due to chance; conversely, small χ^2's indicate differences that could be due to chance. As with the *t* distributions, there is a whole family of χ^2 distributions of different shapes (and, therefore, different areas in their tails) (Figure 79–15). Hence the critical values that delineate statistical significance are based on the χ^2 statistic's df (rows − 1)(columns − 1).

Our example evaluates the association between parity and requests for epidurals during labor; 70% of primiparous women opt for epidurals compared with 55% of multiparous women. Following the calculations just described, the χ^2 statistic has a value of approximately 9. Is this large enough to conclude that the sample did not produce a chance finding? The test statistic exceeds the = 0.05 and the 0.01 levels of significance (3.84 and 6.64, respectively); thus, requests for epidurals is associated with parity (requests are higher from primiparous women than from multiparous women).

$$X^2 = \sum \frac{(|f_O - f_E| - 0.5)^2}{f_E} = \frac{(|140 - 125| - 0.5)^2}{125}$$
$$+ \frac{(|60 - 75| - 0.5)^2}{75} + \frac{(|110 - 125| - 0.5)^2}{125}$$
$$+ \frac{(|90 - 75| - 0.5)^2}{75} = 8.97$$

where f_E = (200)(250)/400 = 125 for cells a and c, and (200)(150)/400 = 75 for cells b and d, and df = (rows − 1) (columns − 1) = (2 − 1)(2 − 1) = 1 (Figure 79-14B).

It should be noted that, although χ^2 is an excellent measure of the statistical *significance* of an association, it does not measure the *extent* of association.[15] Thus, it would be wrong to conclude that primiparous women are about nine times more likely to opt for epidurals than multiparous women. Rather, the odds ratio (a measure of "risk") can be calculated for this 2 × 2 table to estimate risk for epidural request: $[(a)(d)]/[(b)(c)]$ = $[(140)(90)]/[(60)(110)]$ = 1.9, indicating that epidural requests are approximately twofold among primiparous women compared to multiparous women.

Epidural

	Yes	No	Total
Parity Primiparous	140	60	200(50%)
Multiparous	110	90	200(50%)
Total	250(62%)	150(38%)	N

$$\chi^2 = \sum \frac{(|f_O - f_E| - 0.5)^2}{f_E}$$

Chi-square tests can be done on larger tables, such as a 4 × 5 table, following the principles described above. However, if the overall χ^2 statistic is significant, you must conduct several comparisons to determine which cells are different from each other, and you would again be faced with the issue of multiple comparisons. In other instances, you may wish to test a variable that has an intrinsic order. For example, you may wish to examine the association of patient position (supine *vs* sitting) by level of spinal anesthesia, which has an intrinsic quantitative order (e.g., <L1, L1 ≤ T8, >T8). Or, you may wish to examine the association of nerve localization (e.g., nerve stimulator vs "blind") by PNB success, which has an intrinsic qualitative order (e.g., failed, incomplete, complete). A statistician will be able to conduct the χ^2 tests that are appropriate for these situations.

Fisher Exact Test

The "exact" test (more properly, the Fisher-Irwin exact test) applies when the expected value of at least one cell in a 2 × 2 table is <5. Recall that expected frequencies are based on marginal frequencies; but marginals that are small or uneven are less precise and may lead to an inaccurate chi-square test of significance. Thus, the Fisher exact test derives an exact probability (P_{obs}) that is associated with the observed cell frequencies. Exact probabilities are calculated for all other tables that can possibly be constructed using the same marginal frequencies as those in the observed table, and any probabilities that are less than or equal to P_{obs} are summed. This sum is the Fisher exact P-value. As is typical, Fisher exact P-values <.05 are considered to be statistically significant.

The test has been extended to give exact probabilities for tables greater than the 2 × 2. Calculators for such tests, known as the Freeman-Halton extensions of the Fisher exact test, are even available online; e.g., http://vassarstats.net/fisher2x3.html (for the 2 × 3 table) and http://vassarstats.net/fisher2x4.html (for the 2 × 4 table).

McNemar Chi-Square

As noted earlier, χ^2 tests require that subjects are independent; i.e., each is counted in one, and only one, cell. The McNemar χ^2 applies when subjects are matched or their before–after scores are tested. In the example depicted, we wish to know whether block success differs by type of catheter. Interscalene blocks are induced by boluses of local anesthetic through stimulating or nonstimulating catheters. The procedures are performed 2 weeks apart in the same ($n = 20$) volunteers. Intuitively, it can be appreciated that the concordant cells (a and d) do not give us any information about differences in block success by type of catheter. So we look to the discordant cells (b and c) for the test. The value of the McNemar χ^2 test statistic is a mere 0.2. The statistic is referred to the χ^2 critical value of 3.841 with 1 degree of freedom at $\alpha = 0.05$ and is not significant. There is no association between type of catheter and interscalene block success (Figure 79-14C).

	Stimulating catheter	
	Time 1	Time 2
Time 1	a = 3	b = 7
Time 2	c = 5	d = 5

(Non-stimulating catheter)

$$X^2_{McNemar} = \frac{(|b-c|-0.5)^2}{b+c} = \frac{(|7-5|-0.5)^2}{7+5}$$

$$= 0.1875 (NS)$$

Spearman r

The Spearman correlation coefficient (sometimes denoted as r_s) was named for British psychologist Charles E. Spearman (1863–1945) and is the nonparametric counterpart to the Pearson r. It is used to examine the association between two variables when one or both are ordinal or has a very nonnormal shape. Spearman r quantifies the degree of linear association between the ranks of two variables, and varies between +1 and –1.

Since Spearman r is computed on the relative standing of scores within a set of observations (i.e., their ranks), it does not make full use of the quantified scores themselves and may underestimate the degree of association.

For our example, we wish to evaluate the association between pain and function. Patient-reported pain and function scores from 10 subjects are both ranked, and r_s is calculated to be 0.91 (calculations not shown). Its P-value of .02 indicates that the correlation was not likely due to chance and that pain and function are positively correlated.

Kendall Tau (τ)

It is important to note that, unlike the Pearson r, the Spearman r does not estimate a natural population parameter, here, the population correlation, ρ. Hence many statisticians prefer a lesser known correlation coefficient known as the Kendall τ (τ_a is computed when there are no ties in rank; τ_b when there are ties in rank). For our example, two attending physicians rank 12 anesthesia residents at their institution. Concordant and discordant pairs of ranks are computed for a Kendall τ of 0.82 ($P < .001$), indicating high correlation between the ranks of residents assigned by the two attending physicians (calculations not shown).

The Spearman r on the same data is 0.96, which is slightly larger than the Kendall τ. Nonetheless, τ has more accurate P-values and is not overly influenced by a few very discrepant rankings that can influence Spearman r. Importantly, however, Kendall τ does estimate the population variance (the probability of concordance minus the probability of discordance), and, therefore, has an intuitive link from sample to population that Spearman r does not have.

Some Other Nonparametric Tests Commonly Used in Regional Anesthesia Research

Mann-Whitney U (Wilcoxon Rank Sum)

The Student t test has several nonparametric counterparts. The most popular of these is the Mann-Whitney U, a test which is fundamentally equivalent to the Wilcoxon rank sum test. Like Student t, these tests assume that the groups are independent; however, they are immune to violations to normality and equal variance assumptions. The nonparametric tests consider entire population distributions (e.g., ranks throughout the samples) rather than differences among specific population parameters (e.g., difference between two population means). However, if the two population distributions are even moderately similar in shape and variability, the nonparametric tests are excellent tests of central tendency. And, since these tests are based on ranks, they are often interpreted as comparisons of medians.

For the Mann-Whitney U, observations from both groups are combined, and ranks are assigned in ascending order.

(Average rank is assigned whenever scores are tied; however, the number of ties should be small compared with the total number of observations.) The collective ranks for each group would be similar if there is no difference between the underlying populations; i.e., the samples come from the same or similar populations (H_0 is true). Conversely, the collective ranks for each group would be dissimilar if the underlying populations are different; i.e., the samples come from different populations (H_0 is not true). The statistic U is the *smaller of* U1 (the number of times a value in the first group precedes a value in the second group) and U2 (the number of times a value in the second group precedes a value in the first group). Thus, if sample sizes are n_1 and n_2, the quantity U/n_1n_2 is the estimated proportion or probability that a new observation sampled from the first population will be less than a new observation sampled from the second population. When the sample size of either group exceeds 20, U can be used to approximate a z ratio that has the standard normal distribution. Statistical significance is then estimated from the standard normal distribution. Thus, at the 0.05 level of significance, the null hypothesis is rejected if the observed z is more negative than or equal to -1.96 (two-sided test) or -1.645 (one-sided test); otherwise the null hypothesis is retained.

For our example, we wish to know whether the extent of reliable anesthesia for hand surgery differs by method of axillary block (single-injection *vs* multiple-injection) administered to 40 patients randomly assigned to either method (20 patients in each group). The Mann-Whitney U indicates that the mean percent of arm blocked by the single-injection method (85%) differs from that blocked by the multiple-injection method (95%) at $P < .05$ (calculations not shown).

When conducting the nonparametric statistical tests, consult a statistician if many ties occur in your data; complicated corrections should be applied when there are too many ties (say, as many as a third of all scores are tied). Moreover, computer packages should automatically adjust for tied ranks, but not all do. If your sample is small (<10), exact probabilities should be calculated. Beware that computer packages may use the large-sample normal approximation to calculate statistical significance even for small samples.

Sign

The sign test and Wilcoxon signed rank (Wilcoxon T) test are nonparametric counterparts to the dependent *t* test. They apply to studies in which subjects are matched on a potentially confounding variable (and then randomly assigned to treatment groups) or to studies in which the same subjects are assessed at two separate times (e.g., before and after treatment). Half of the subjects are expected to have positive differences and half are expected to have negative differences, so observed and expected frequencies are submitted to a χ^2 test with 1 degree of freedom (χ^2 value 3.841) to determine whether the difference is beyond chance fluctuation. This will be reasonably accurate for 10 or more pairs of scores; smaller numbers of pairs require a small-sample approach (the binomial test). The sign test responds only to the direction of the difference between pairs of scores and is likely to have little utility in regional anesthesia studies.

Wilcoxon Signed Rank (Wilcoxon T)

Unlike the sign test, the Wilcoxon T uses information about the size of the difference as well as directionality. For our example, we wish to know whether the extent of anesthesia for hand surgery differs by method of axillary block (single-injection *vs* multiple-injection) administered to 12 volunteers in randomized order 2 weeks apart. Thus, the same volunteers receive each of the injection methods.

Differences in sensory block by injection method are ranked, and the positive and negative ranks are summed separately. Wilcoxon T is the smaller of these sums, and is 1.5 for the *single*-injection method (calculations not shown). At df = number of pairs with nonzero absolute differences = 10, our Wilcoxon T is significant *at P < .01*; sensory block differs by injection method (sensory block is greater for the *multiple-injection* method).

The Wilcoxon T assumes that there are no ties in rank (even though the test is reasonably robust provided the number of ties is small) and that the *differences* between pairs of scores have a symmetric distribution. This last assumption makes the Wilcoxon T the only nonparametric method whose results can be affected by data transformations. In the case of the Wilcoxon, a transformation should be used only if it makes the distribution of the differences more symmetric. Thus, a statistician should be consulted to determine whether data transformations are appropriate for your data. If the number of nonzero differences is >15, the Wilcoxon can be used to approximate a z ratio that has the standard normal distribution. As described earlier, focus is on the smaller sum, so the value of the observed z will always be negative (or equal to zero). Thus, at the 0.05 level of significance, the null hypothesis is rejected if the observed z is more negative than or equal to -1.96 (two-sided test) or -1.645 (one-sided test); otherwise the null hypothesis is retained. Special small-sample methods are used if the number of nonzero differences is ≤15, and a statistician should again be consulted.

Kruskal-Wallis H

This nonparametric counterpart to one-way ANOVA tests whether three or more independent samples are from the same population. It is an extension of the Mann-Whitney U and assumes independence. Scores from all subgroups are combined and ranked in ascending order. Ties are assigned the mean rank of the scores that are tied. Once ranks have been assigned in the combined group, the subgroups are reconstructed, and the mean rank for each subgroup is compared with the mean rank for the combined group. If the subgroup samples come from identical populations, the subgroup ranks are similar to the overall mean rank. If the samples come from different populations, the subgroup ranks vary more widely from the overall mean rank. Kruskal-Wallis H compares the total magnitude of these discrepancies with what might be expected by chance. Exact probabilities have been worked out for tiny samples. However, in most cases (e.g., with three groups and four or more subjects in each), the χ^2 distribution may be used to evaluate the Kruskal-Wallis H with good approximate results. Like χ^2, Kruskal-Wallis H is nondirectional because it reflects the magnitude of the discrepancies without regard to their direction. So, like χ^2, the region of rejection appropriately lies in the upper tail of the distribution. Finally, it is possible to make multiple comparisons among the groups compared by the Kruskal-Wallis H (with proper cautions regarding inflation of the experiment-wise type I error).

For our example, we wish to know whether opening injection pressure (psi) differs in patients randomly assigned to receive interscalene block for shoulder surgery by three different approaches ($n = 12$ in each group). Variability is uneven among the three groups, so data are analyzed by the Kruskal-Wallis test. The Kruskal-Wallis H is calculated as 4.8 (calculations not shown) and compared to critical values from the chi square distribution with 2 df = (number of groups - 1) = (3 - 1) = 2. The Kruskal-Wallis is not significant ($P > .05$); psi does not differ by the three interscalene approachs studied for shoulder surgery.

A variant of the Kruskal-Wallis H, the Jonckheere trend test (or Jonckheere-Terpstra test) evaluates linear trend in the pattern of observations across three or more ordered groups. The test is more powerful than the Kruskal-Wallis test when there is a priori ordering of the groups. For example, a study may be interested in whether length of stay in the PACU differs by increasing ASA physical status (I–V). A one-tailed alternative hypothesis may state that length of stay *increases* with ASA physical status.

Logistic Regression

As discussed in the section on Parametric Tests above, multivariable linear regression models can contain a number of covariates (independent variables) that help to predict a continuous outcome (dependent variable). It is, however, often the case that the outcome of interest is a dichotomous variable; e.g., the presence or absence of a disease. Logistic regression applies in such instances. Why? If an outcome variable can only take numeric values of 0 or 1, then the mean of these values in a sample of patients is the proportion of patients with the disease (or equivalently, the probability that a patient has the disease of interest). Thus, instead of predicting a continuous outcome, the task of the logistic regression model is to predict the *proportion* of patients with the outcome given the explanatory variables in the model. Unfortunately, this approach can produce impossible probabilities outside the range of 0 to 1, so it is useful to work with a *transformation* of the proportion to be predicted. Logistic regression uses the logit transformation; i.e., the natural logarithm of the odds of the outcome, logit $(p) = \log_e (p/[1 - p])$, where p is the proportion of patients with the outcome and always lies in the range 0 and 1.

Unlike least squares regression, the intercept and coefficients in a logistic regression model are obtained through an iterative process that results in a unique set of maximum likelihood estimates. Among all possible values that could describe the parent population from which the sample emerged, the maximum likelihood estimates are those values that most likely gave rise to the observed data. For our example, logistic regression is used to estimate the risk for severe hypotension (decrease in blood pressure >30% of baseline) *vs* no severe hypotension

following neuraxial blockade. A single binary predictor (dry mucosa *vs* no dry mucosa) is included in the model. The analysis yields a maximum likelihood coefficient, $b_{dry\ mucosa} = 0.6931$, with standard error$_{dry\ mucosa} = 0.1119$. For binary predictors coded 0 or 1, the odds ratio (a widely used measure of risk) can be directly estimated by exponentiating the logistic regression coefficient; i.e., OR = e^b. Thus, if patients without dry mucosae are coded as 0 and patients with dry mucosae as 1, exponentiation of the coefficient, $e^{0.6931} = 2$, indicates a twofold risk for severe hypotension for patients with dry mucosae. Moreover, a confidence interval can be constructed, i.e., $e^{[b \pm (z_{\alpha/2})(s.e._b)]}$, which yields $e^{[0.6931 - (1.96)(0.1119)]} = 1.6$ and $e^{[0.6931 + (1.96)(0.1119)]} = 2.5$ as the lower and upper 95% confidence limits, respectively. Compared with patients without dry mucosae, risk for severe hypotension for patients with dry mucosae is likely to be increased approximately 0.6-fold but no greater than 2.5-fold.

Another expression for the estimated probability of disease, $p = 1/(1 + e^{-\beta\alpha + 1x_1\beta...+)_ix_i})$, can be rearranged in terms of the log odds of disease, i.e., logit$(p) = \alpha + \beta_1 x_1 + ... + \beta_i x_i$, which is reminiscent of the multiple linear regression model, but will always yield values of p that are between 0 and 1. The coefficients (b_i's) denote the amount of increase or decrease in the log odds of the outcome associated with a unit change in the predictor. For instance, a model for the probability of severe hypotension associated with neuraxial blockade might contain the following predictors and their coefficients (Table 79–8).

The log odds for severe hypotension in a 60-year-old hypovolemic patient with preoperative urine output >100 mL/h, preoperative heart rate of 82 bpm, and no dry mucosa is

$$logit(p) = -4.5799 + (0.0296 \times 6) + (-0.6931 \times 0)$$
$$+ (1.6094 \times 1) + (0.6900 \times 1) + (0.5878 \times 0)$$
$$= -2.1029$$

TABLE 79–8. Severe hypotension associated with neuraxial blockade: an example of a patient with specific clinical characteristics.

Predictor	Coefficient	Patient
Intercept	−4.5799	
Age (10-year increments)	0.0296	60 years old
Preoperative urine output (>100 mL/h = 0 vs ≤ 100 mL/h = 1)[a]	−0.6931	>100 mL/h
Hypovolemia (No = 0, Yes = 1)	1.6094	Yes
Preoperative heart rate (10 bpm increments over 72 bpm)	0.6900	82 bpm
Dry mucosa (No = 0, Yes = 1)	0.5878	No

[a] The coefficient for preoperative urine output is negative as the riskier condition (>100 mL/h) is coded as 0.

This patient's probability of severe hypotension is $1/[1 + e^{-(-2.1029)}]$, or about 11%.

It is also possible to compare the risk profiles of two patients using the coefficients in the model. For instance, $\text{logit}(p_1)$ for a patient with dry mucosa can be compared with $\text{logit}(p_2)$ for a patient without dry mucosa (all other predictive characteristics being the same between these patients). That is,

$$\text{logit}(p_1) - \text{logit}(p_2) = \log\left(\frac{p_1}{1 - p_1}\right) - \log\left(\frac{p_2}{1 - p_2}\right)$$

$$= \log\left[\frac{p_1(1 - p_2)}{p_2(1 - p_1)}\right]$$

For our example, the coefficients for the intercept, age, preoperative urine output, hypovolemia, and preoperative heart rate cancel out between these two patients as they are the same for both patients. This results in logit $(p_1) = 0.5878$ for the patient with dry mucosa and logit $(p_2) = 0$ for the patient without dry mucosa. When the difference, logit (p_1) − logit $(p_2) = 0.5878$, is exponentiated, $e^{0.5878} = 1.8$, we obtain the odds ratio (risk) for severe hypotension due to dry mucosa that has been *adjusted for* age, preoperative urine output, hypovolemia, and preoperative heart rate. The adjusted odds ratio of 1.8 is slightly lower than the unadjusted odds ratio of 2 calculated earlier.

Clinical Pearls

1. Know your data. Know the types of variables that you are measuring.
   - Keep a data dictionary.
2. Consult with your statistician at the planning stage of your research study.
   - Strive to use the least complex study design and statistical analyses that will answer your research questions.
3. Remember that bias typically cannot be corrected through statistical methods. So, think carefully and thoroughly about features of your study design that may lead to systematic errors, in particular with respect to (a) ascertainment and selection of your subjects, and (b) measurement of your exposure variables (e.g., vulnerability to recall or interviewer bias).
4. Think carefully about your specific aims and hypotheses. Null and alternative hypotheses are not questions, so write clear, declarative *statements* for your null and alternative hypotheses. Once on paper, they should not be changed to fit the research findings. The two-sided alternative hypothesis is generally more appropriate than the one-sided alternatives, especially so for new areas of research.
5. Have a reasonable idea of the type I and type II error probabilities that you would be willing to tolerate based on your area of research interest and clinical experience.
6. Have some idea of the difference that is clinically meaningful to detect. A literature review may help you estimate this difference and may provide an estimate of variability in the outcome of interest. (If not available, you may need to conduct a preliminary or pilot study to estimate these parameters.) Your statistician will use this information to calculate the sample size required to detect the desired difference at your specified probability of committing a type I error (α) and with sufficient power $(1 - \beta)$.
7. Potential confounding variables must be included during the design phase of the study. Their choice and accuracy of measurement directly affects the extent to which confounding can be controlled by statistical procedures. During your background literature review, consider potential confounders that other investigators have included in their studies. Did they feel that these factors could have influenced their findings? Did they suspect other factors that were not included (or could not be included) in their studies but perhaps should have been?
8. With the help of your statistician, choose between parametric and nonparametric alternatives. You will usually perform one (not both) of these methods to test a given variable. For quantitative data, this will typically be a parametric method unless there are clear indications that the underlying assumptions of normality and equal variance are not met. If violations to these assumptions are noted, your statistician will offer advice with respect to data transformations that may be appropriate for your study prior to running a parametric test. For ranked or qualitative data, descriptive or nonparametric methods must be used.
9. Discuss multiple comparisons with your statistician. If numerous comparisons or contrasts are included in your study, what adjustments are necessary?
10. With the help of your statistician, plan the best ways to present your findings. You may want to feature selected findings in tables and figures.

OBSERVATIONS FROM REVIEWING MANUSCRIPTS SUBMITTED TO ANESTHESIOLOGY JOURNALS

This section describes several common errors found while reviewing manuscripts that have been submitted for publication in anesthesiology journals. Comments pertain to the research (nonclinical) perspective.

Clinical Relevance and Conceptualization

Research questions arise primarily from clinical need, but studies must still be sold to the anesthesiology community. For example, researchers embarking on a study of catheter shearing during removal would have to substantiate the importance of focusing on an occurrence that is exceedingly rare (and perhaps of little clinical interest). Moreover, these researchers must be careful to use catheter shearing forces that could actually be encountered in the clinical setting.

Authors often neglect to explain their choice of study parameters. For instance, if patients must be older than 50 years of age in order to be eligible for a study of cervical plexus block, the authors should provide the reason for this inclusion criterion. Is it because the surgeries for which cervical plexus block is appropriate are rarely performed in individuals younger than 50 years of age? Similarly, choice of drugs is universally explained, but the rationale for choosing specific doses to be studied is sometimes neglected.

Clinical relevance dictates conceptualization of a study in other, often subtle, ways. For instance, when studying ultrasound-guided PNB of the sciatic nerve using different landmarks, it is important to establish the level of experience of the anesthesiologists participating in the study. As their experience may be more extensive with the brachial plexus and femoral nerve blocks than with the sciatic nerve block, it is not sufficient to tell the readers that each anesthesiologist has completed more than 50 ultrasound-guided peripheral nerve blocks. The readers should also be told how much of this experience was specifically with the *sciatic nerve* block, as this is the focus of the study.

Methodology

The two most common problems in methodology are inadequate control for potential confounding variables and inaccuracies in measurement. For instance, a study comparing the length of postoperative analgesia between two local anesthetics administered by popliteal nerve block would have to control for physiologic attributes of the patient (e.g., age, presence of diabetic neuropathy) that could be associated with effectiveness of the drugs and postoperative analgesia. In regional anesthesia studies, this is typically accomplished by randomly assigning patients to receive one or the other of the two local anesthetics, but often the method of randomization and the team members who are blinded to patient assignment are not described. For follow-up, patients are often phoned at home and asked the time that they took their first analgesic medication and NRS scores at specific times following discharge. But even patients discharged with detailed, written directions could misunderstand or fail to record this information. Moreover, accuracy depends heavily on the interviewer's skill with neutral probing as the patient attempts to recall the requested information. Thus, it is necessary to work closely with the patients (providing them with easy-to-follow directions and questionnaires) and with well-trained research assistants in order to collect data as accurately as possible.

Statistics

A statistician may have conducted the statistical analyses, but may have little involvement in writing the manuscript. For instance, a paper may report differences in duration of surgery among three PNBs, but fail to mention the statistical tests used to assess these differences. If a nonparametric statistical procedure was performed instead of a parametric one, it is helpful to explain why the nonparametric counterpart was chosen. For instance, VAS scores may have been categorized and submitted to a χ^2 analysis because of nonnormality of the distribution.

Similarly, less frequently used statistical procedures that may be unfamiliar to the readership should be described with appropriate citation(s) to support their use in the analyses. Statistical packages should be identified with name, version number, and date.

As is frequently done, groups are compared at a series of time points (serial measurements). Because of time dependency in the outcome variable, these studies should consider methods other than t tests or one-way ANOVAs at each time point. A valid alternative approach that is likely to address the study's question(s) calculates a suitable summary response (over time) for each subject. The summary responses are then analyzed as raw data using standard statistical techniques.[16]

Finally, it is important to address data that are missing for any number of reasons, ranging from the subject who withdraws from a study to equipment failure and data entry omissions. Missing data can distort the inferential conclusions drawn in a study. A sample in which data are missing at random may still be representative of the population, whereas a sample in which data are systematically missing is likely to be biased and no longer representative of the population. Ideally, missing data should be avoided in the design phase of the study; e.g., research assistants should check forms for skipped questions before the subject leaves the research setting, and questionnaires can be carefully worded so that specific groups will not be offended and skip any of the items. Datasets containing <5% data missing at random can still be analyzed, but a statistician should be consulted to choose the imputation, interpolation, or deletion technique most appropriate for the analysis.

Presentation of Results

- Investigators should avoid being side-tracked by the *P*-value. Errors of presentation often revolve around the confusion between statistical significance and clinical importance. Writers mistakenly refer to a nonsignificant or insignificant effect as being "clinically unimportant" or as having "little clinical impact."

- Sometimes a test will reach statistical significance that was unanticipated. While it is appropriate to evaluate design, subject, and/or data factors that contributed to the result, the finding may, in fact, be a fluke and not reproducible in future studies. Thus, authors should consider carefully whether the clinical impact of the finding or changes to the direction of the study itself warrant space in the Discussion section of their paper. In any event, hypotheses cannot be changed post hoc to accommodate statistically significant yet surprising findings.

- Conversely, a result that has a *P*-value slightly higher than that required for statistical significance may not receive the attention it deserves. As an example: Investigators might compare quality of recovery between a combined regional anesthesia procedure and general anesthesia. Recovery scores may be higher for the former than for the latter up to postoperative day 6, but may not quite reach the traditional criterion for statistical significance on postoperative day 7 (say, *P* = .08). Given results in the earlier postoperative period and perhaps information in the literature on the combined procedure that prompted the study in the first place, the *P*-value of .08 should not be dismissed so readily. It could be that recovery scores are, in fact, higher for the combined procedure than for general anesthesia *for the entire first postoperative week*.

Tables

- Tables are often "recited" in the text. As readers can read for themselves, short summaries of the table contents are more useful. For instance, if a table includes the information that in the United States, 35% of patients received general anesthesia and 65% received peripheral nerve blocks in 2004, it can be more informative to state, "Nearly twice as many patients received peripheral nerve blocks than general anesthesia in 2004, an increase of 15% from 2000."
- Often the converse is true, i.e., authors include too much verbiage that could be more clearly presented in a table. For instance, stating, "Surgical procedures included open-shoulder stabilization (*n* = 5), hemiarthroplasty (*n* = 10), rotator cuff surgery/decompressions (*n* = 5), other shoulder procedures (*n* = 5)" could be better appreciated as part of the patient demographic and clinical characteristics table. The readers can easily check that the total number of patients (here, *n* = 25) is accounted for.
- Tables often contain unnecessary information; e.g., both standard deviations and ranges when one of these measures of variability usually suffices. A column or row of zeroes to indicate that no block failures occurred may already be in the text and a series of zeroes just looks silly. N(%) for each gender may not be as useful as the male:female ratio. Moreover, if only ASA physical status I or II patients are eligible for a study, it is not entirely necessary to give the *n*(%) of patients in each of these two categories, especially if no comparisons between these categories are relevant to the study. The ASA physical status breakdown in the table becomes superfluous.
- Occasionally, variables that are not continuous measures are presented as though they are. For instance, T11.25 and T9.75 for thoracic positions in the longitudinal plane could be misleading if whole vertebrae were measured and not parts of them.
- Sometimes it is unclear what comparisons a *P*-value refers to in a table. For instance, a table may include measurements on several dorsal locations and several ventral locations. Yet, it is unclear that the *P*-value refers to a comparison of the *mean* measurements of all dorsal locations against the mean measurements of all ventral locations.
- Notations contained in the table may not be explained in the footnotes (and sometimes not even in the text). For instance, asterisks in the table indicate that a footnote applies, yet the footnote or legend may be missing from the table.

Figures

- Journal articles often include an excessive number of figures, many of which are simply unnecessary. The idea is

not to present the same results in different ways. Moreover, a finding can often be described in a single sentence, and each sentence does not need a figure.
- The wrong type of graph may be used to portray the data. For instance, a bar graph (small spaces between bars) is appropriate for nominal categories (e.g., a series of different types of PNBs), whereas a histogram (flush bars) is appropriate for categories of a continuous variable (e.g., age groups, VAS scores that have been categorized).
- Figures are not always consistent with the text. For instance, the text may state that lidocaine kinetics was completed on 15 patients, but the figure may include values for only 10 patients.
- Error bars (typically denoting the 95% confidence interval) should be included with group means for continuous variables. The box and whiskers plots are especially useful when depicting median values. The median value is placed within a "box" where the interquartile range (IQR) (the 75th and 25th percentiles) defines the upper and lower borders of the box. Outliers are identified as values residing above the 75th percentile + (1.5 × IQR) or values residing below the 25th percentile – (1.5 × IQR).

Discussion and Conclusions

Overoptimism appears to be the bane of discussion and concluding statements. Not only do authors have a tendency to *re*state their findings, but they are often tempted to *over*state their findings. For instance, a statement to the effect that 0.5% ropivacaine *is superior to* 1% mepivacaine for a particular block may not be warranted if the study only looked at length of postoperative analgesia. Many other factors go into making one drug "superior" to another (e.g., speed of onset, success rate). The authors should simply state that 0.5% ropivacaine provided longer postoperative analgesia than 1% mepivacaine.

Authors are often tempted to overstep the boundaries of their study. For instance, the conclusion that "Dose of remifentanil for sedation during carotid endarterectomy under cervical plexus block should be reduced in patients older than 70 years of age" may not be warranted if the drug was not tested at lower doses in the study. Satisfactory block may not be achieved in patients older than 70 years of age if the drug is given at lower doses. Similarly, it could not be concluded that "The 12.5-mcg dose of fentanyl is optimal in terms of surgical anesthesia, hemodynamic stability, and reliability of block" if the 12.5-mcg dose was the highest dose tested. Higher doses may be even more "optimal."

Misleading statements are not easy to detect. For instance, stating that the tensile strength of 19- and 20-gauge Brand X epidural catheters differed at *varying* temperatures implies that the catheters were tested on a gradient of temperatures. If only two temperatures were studied, the statement should be revised to reflect that fact (e.g., the tensile strength of 19- and 20-gauge Brand X epidural catheters differed at the two temperatures studied). Similarly, stating that significantly more "technical failures" in nerve stimulation occurred in a specific group may be misleading if the so-called technical failures were only a portion of the total number of block failures that occurred. This is because the total number of block failures may be the primary outcome and may be similar among the groups, but the readers would be left with the impression that one group had more failures (overall) than the others. Finally, it would be misleading to omit some of the parameters tested in a study. For instance, when comparing two approaches to the sciatic nerve block in emergency situations, time to establish landmarks may be significantly shorter by approach A, yet time to perform the block may be shorter by approach B. It would be misleading to conclude that approach A is faster than approach B if time to establish landmarks can be offset by time to perform the block.

REFERENCES

1. Fisher RA: *Statistical Methods for Research Workers*. New York, NY: Hafner, 1948.
2. Witte RS: *Statistics*. Boston, MA: Holt, Rinehart and Winston, Boston, MA; 1980.
3. Lilienfeld AM, Lilienfeld DE: *Foundations of Epidemiology*. Oxford, UK: Oxford University Press, 1980.
4. Mausner JS, Kramer S: *Epidemiology—An Introductory Text*, 2nd ed. Philadelphia, PA: Saunders, 1985.
5. Altman DG: *Practical Statistics for Medical Research*. Chapman & Hall; CRC Texts in Statistical Sciences, Boca Raton, FL, 1991.
6. Minium EW: *Statistical Reasoning in Psychology and Education*, 2nd ed. New York, NY: John Wiley & Sons, 1978.
7. Eng J: Sample size estimation: How many individuals should be studied? Radiology 2003;227(2):309–313.
8. Rosner B: *Fundamentals of Biostatistics*, 5th ed. Pacific Grove, CA: Duxbury Press, 2000.
9. Motulsky H: *Intuitive Biostatistics*. Oxford, UK: Oxford University Press, 1995.
10. Cohen J: *Statistical Power Analysis for the Behavioral Sciences*, 2nd ed. Mahwah, NJ: Lawrence Erlbaum Associates, 1988.
11. Kleinbaum DG, Kupper LL, Muller KE: *Applied Regression Analysis and Other Multivariable Methods*, 2nd ed. Pacific Grove, CA: Duxbury Press, 1988.
12. Bland JM, Altman DG: Statistical methods for assessing agreement between two methods of clinical measurement. Lancet 1986;1(8476): 307–310.
13. Bland JM, Altman DG: Agreement between methods of measurement with multiple observations per individual. J Biopharm Stat 2007;17(4): 571–582.
14. Kelsey JL, Thompson WD, Evans AS: *Methods in Observational Epidemiology. Monographs in Epidemiology and Biostatistics*, vol. 10. Oxford, UK: Oxford University Press, 1986.
15. Fleiss JL: *Statistical Methods for Rates and Proportions*, 2nd ed. New York, NY: John Wiley & Sons, 1981.
16. Matthews JNS, Altman DG, Campbell MJ, Royston P: Analysis of serial measurements in medical research. BMJ 1990;300(6719):230–235.

NERVE STIMULATOR AND SURFACE ANATOMY-BASED NERVE BLOCKS

CHAPTER 80A

Cervical Plexus Block

Jerry D. Vloka, Ann-Sofie Smeets, Tony Tsai, and Cedric Bouts

INTRODUCTION

Cervical plexus anesthesia was developed early in the 20th century with two main approaches being used. In 1912, Kappis described a posterior approach to the cervical and brachial plexus, which attempted to block the nerves at their point of emergence from the vertebral column.[1] The posterior approach was advocated because the vertebral artery and vein lie anterior to the plexus.[2] However, the needle must pass through the extensor muscles of the neck which causes considerable discomfort, and the long path of the needle is more hazardous. Consequently, this technique is not recommended as a routine for cervical or brachial plexus block.

In 1914, Heidenhein described the lateral approach, which has formed the basis for subsequent techniques of anesthetizing the cervical plexus.[6] Victor Pauchet also described a lateral approach to blocking the cervical plexus in 1920 and recommended it over the posterior approach.[7] Winnie revisited the lateral approach to the cervical plexus block in 1975, and described a simplified, single-injection technique.[8] The lateral approach is currently the more commonly used approach and will be described in this chapter.

INDICATIONS AND CONTRAINDICATIONS

Deep and superficial cervical plexus blocks can be used in a variety of surgical procedures, including superficial surgery on the neck and shoulders and thyroid surgery. Its use is most common in carotid endarterectomy, in which an awake patient self-monitors to ensure adequate cerebral blood flow during cross-clamping of the carotid artery (Figure 80A–1).[9,10] Since the description of the first carotid endarterectomy in 1954 by Eastcott, the number of these operations has been growing annually.[11] Regional anesthesia is a viable anesthetic choice for carotid surgery, although debate continues whether it improves patient outcomes.[12–25] The largest randomized trial to date on this topic (GALA trial) showed no difference in 30-day stroke or mortality rates, a conclusion that has been supported by a recent meta-analysis.[26,27]

The superficial cervical plexus block can be used for many superficial surgeries in the neck area, including lymph node dissection, excision of thyroglossal or branchial cleft cysts, carotid endarterectomy, and vascular access surgery.[28]

Comparisons of superficial vs deep cervical plexus blocks for carotid endarterectomy have either shown equivalence or favored the superficial block due to the lower risk of complications.[29–31] Although both the deep and superficial cervical plexus blocks can be performed separately, they have been used by some also in combination for anesthesia and postoperative analgesia for head and neck surgery.[32–34]

Contraindications to performing a cervical plexus block include patient refusal, local infection, and previous surgery or radiation therapy to the neck. Likewise, due to the risk of

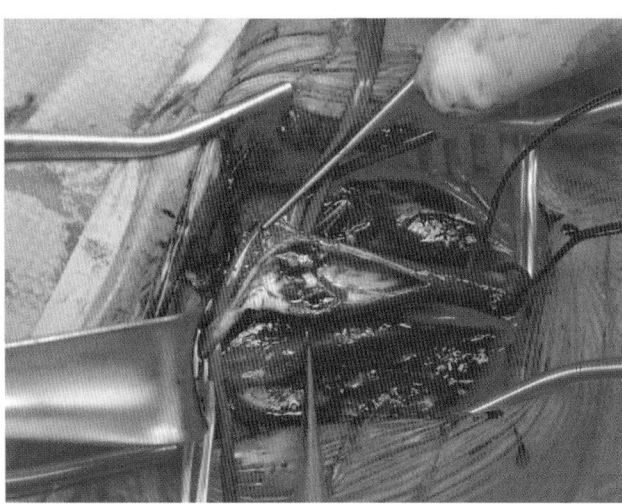

FIGURE 80A–1. Carotid endarterectomy. The image shows open, cross-clamped carotid artery and a plaque inside its wall.

phrenic nerve paresis, the deep cervical plexus block is relatively contraindicated in patients with contralateral phrenic nerve palsy and significant pulmonary compromise.

FUNCTIONAL ANATOMY OF DEEP CERVICAL PLEXUS BLOCKADE

The cervical plexus is formed by the anterior divisions of the four upper cervical nerves (Figure 80A–2). The plexus is situated on the anterior surface of the four upper cervical vertebrae, resting on the levator anguli scapulae and scalenus medius muscles, and is covered by the sternocleidomastoid muscle. The dorsal and ventral roots combine to form spinal nerves as they exit through the intervertebral foramen. The first cervical root is primarily a motor nerve and is of little interest for locoregional anesthesia. The anterior rami of the second through fourth cervical nerves form the cervical plexus. The branches of the superficial cervical plexus innervate the skin and superficial structures of the head, neck, and shoulder (Figure 80A–3). The branches of the deep cervical plexus innervate the deeper structures of the neck, including the muscles of the anterior neck and the diaphragm, which is innervated by the phrenic nerve. The third and fourth cervical nerves send a branch to the spinal accessory nerve, or directly into the deep surface of the trapezius

to supply sensory fibers to this muscle. The fourth cervical nerve may send a branch downward to join the fifth cervical nerve and participate in the formation of the brachial plexus. The cutaneous innervation of both the deep and superficial cervical plexus blocks includes skin of the anterolateral neck and the anteauricular and retroauricular areas (Figure 80A–3).

Anatomic Landmarks

The following three landmarks for a deep cervical plexus block are identified and marked (Figure 80A–4):

1. Mastoid process
2. Chassaignac tubercle (transverse process of the sixth cervical vertebra)
3. Posterior border of the sternocleidomastoid muscle

To estimate the line of needle insertion that overlies the transverse processes, the mastoid process (MP) and the Chassaignac tubercle, which is the transverse process of the sixth cervical vertebra (C6), are identified and marked (Figure 80A–5). The transverse process of C6 is usually easily palpated behind the clavicular head of the sternocleidomastoid muscle at the level just below the cricoid cartilage (Figure 80A–6). Next, a line is drawn connecting the MP to the Chassaignac tubercle. Position the

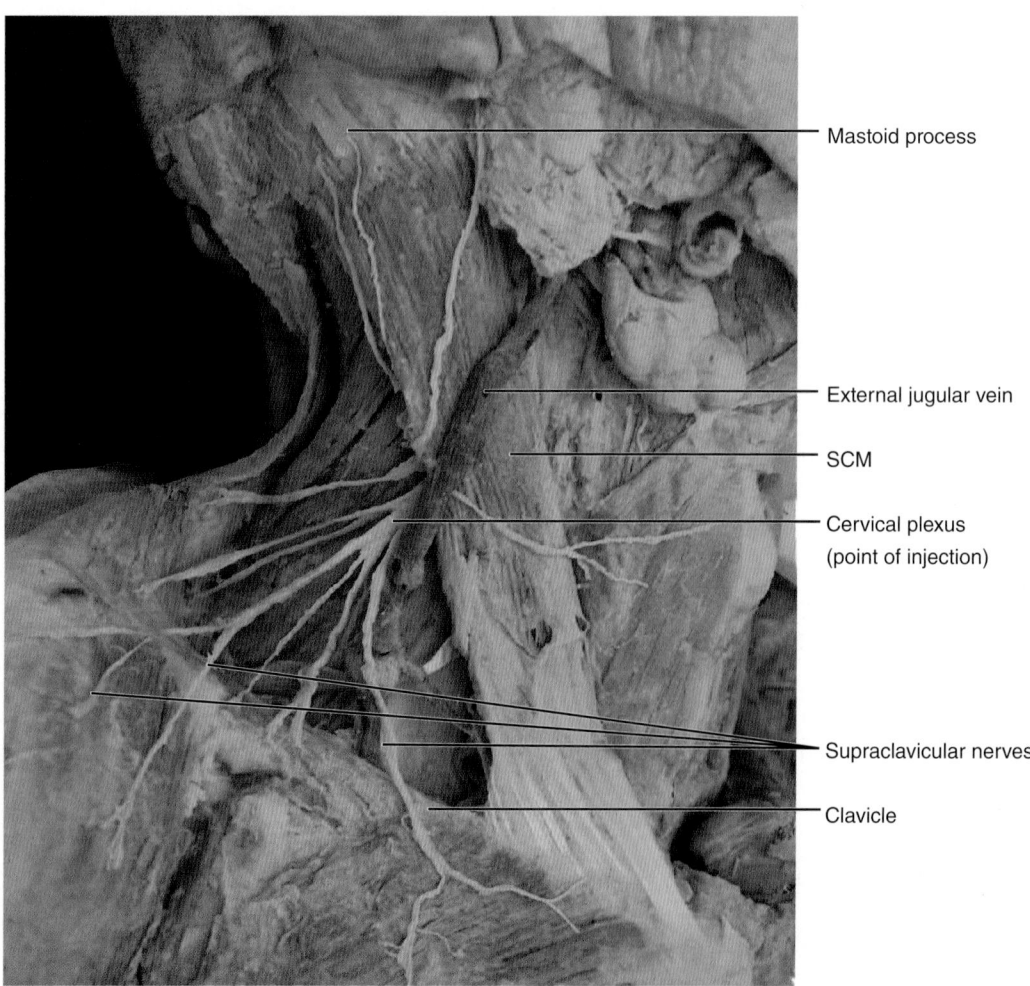

Mastoid process

External jugular vein

SCM

Cervical plexus (point of injection)

Supraclavicular nerves

Clavicle

FIGURE 80A–2. Anatomy of the cervical plexus

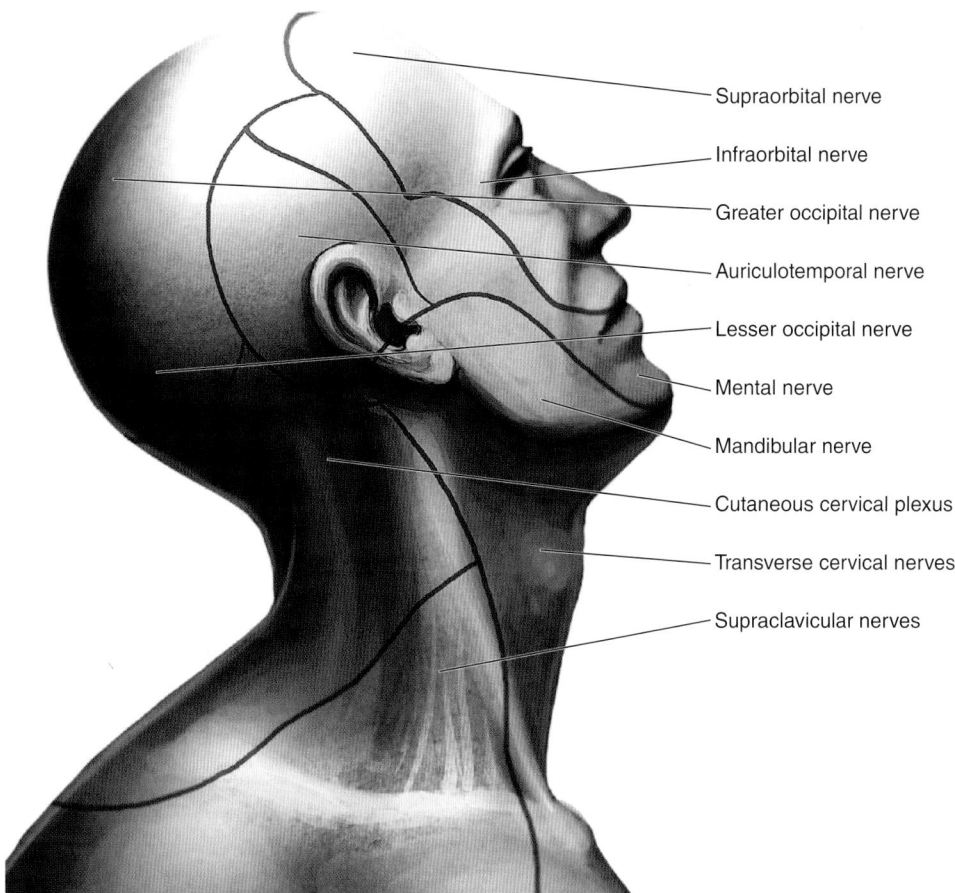

— Supraorbital nerve

— Infraorbital nerve

— Greater occipital nerve

— Auriculotemporal nerve

— Lesser occipital nerve

— Mental nerve

— Mandibular nerve

— Cutaneous cervical plexus

— Transverse cervical nerves

— Supraclavicular nerves

FIGURE 80A–3. Innervation of the head and neck.

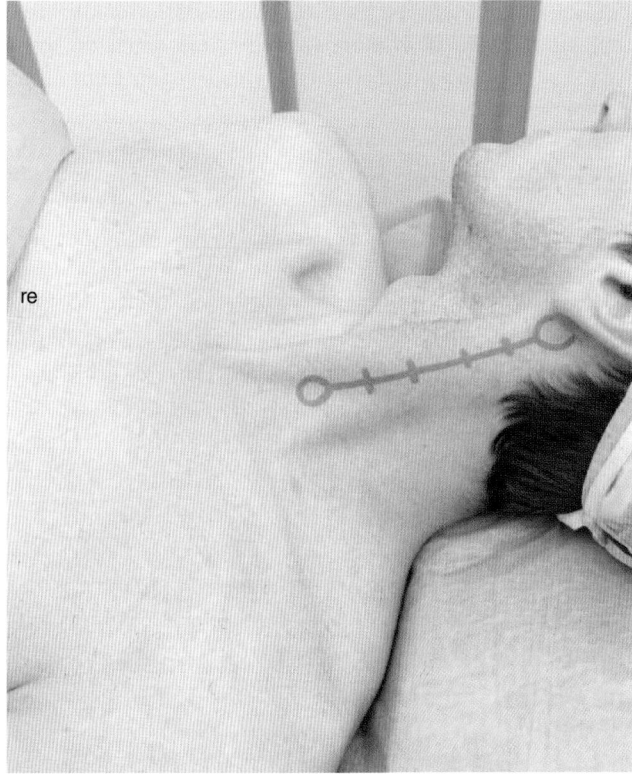

FIGURE 80A–4. Anatomic landmarks for the cervical plexus.
Shown are estimates of the transverse processes C2-C3-C4-C5-C6.

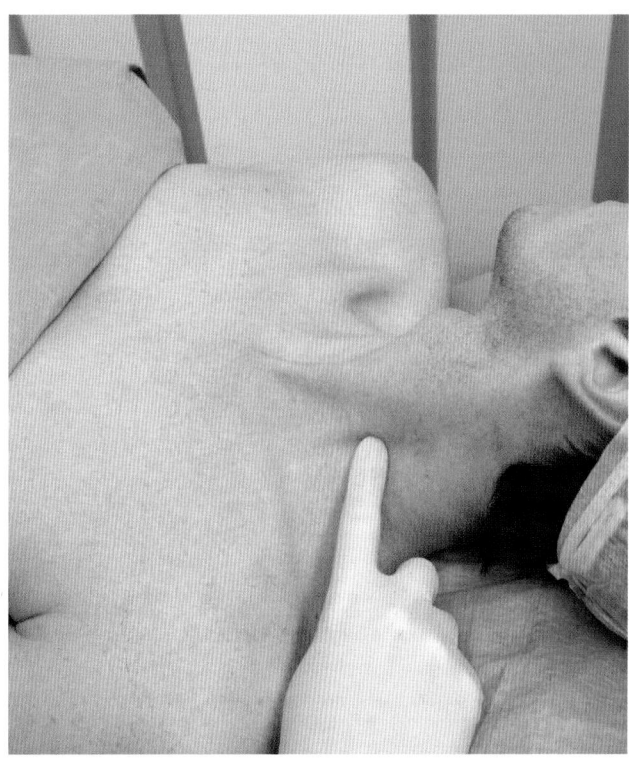

FIGURE 80A–5. Palpation of the transverse process of C6.

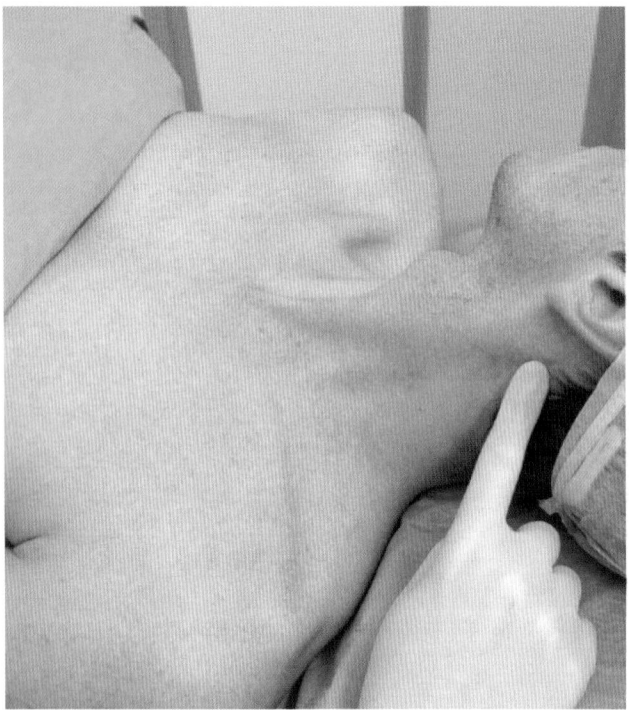

FIGURE 80A–6. Palpation of the mastoid process.

palpating hand just behind the posterior border of the sternoclei-domastoid muscle. Once this line is drawn, label the insertion sites over the C2, C3, and C4, which are respectively located on the MP–C6 line 2 cm, 4 cm, and 6 cm, respectively, caudal to the mastoid process. It is also possible to perform a single injection at the C3 level, which is considered safe and effective.[35]

Clinical Pearls

- The distances specified for spacing along the transverse processes at various levels are estimates at best.
- Once two neighbouring transverse processes are identified, the spacing between the other transverse processes follows a similar pattern.

Choice of Local Anesthetic

A deep cervical plexus block requires 3–5 mL of local anesthetic per level to ensure reliable blockade. Except perhaps with patients with significant respiratory disease who rely on their phrenic nerve to adequately ventilate, most patients benefit from the use of a long-acting local anesthetic. Table 80A–1 shows commonly used local anesthetics with onset and duration of anesthesia and analgesia for deep cervical plexus blocks. Ropivacaine 0.5% provides good quality block of longer duration,[36] and it is one of most common choices for carotid endarterectomy surgery.[37]

Equipment

A standard regional anesthesia tray is prepared with the following equipment:

TABLE 80A–1. Commonly used local anesthetics for deep cervical plexus blocks.

	Onset (min)	Anesthesia (h)	Analgesia (h)
1.5% Mepivacaine (+ HCO_3^- + epinephrine)	10–15	2.0–2.5	3–6
2% Lidocaine (+ HCO_3^- + epinephrine)	10–15	2–3	3–6
0.5% Ropivacaine	10–20	3–4	4–10
0.25% Bupivacaine (+ epinephrine)	10–20	3–4	4–10

- Sterile towels and 4-in. × 4-in. gauze pads
- 20-mL syringe(s) with local anesthetic
- Sterile gloves and marking pen
- One 1.5 -in., 25-gauge needle for skin infiltration
- A 1.5 -in.-long, 22-gauge, short-beveled needle

Technique

After cleaning the skin with an antiseptic solution, local anesthetic is infiltrated subcutaneously along the line estimating the position of the transverse processes. The needle should contact the posterior tubercle of the transverse process where the spinal nerves at the individual levels are located just in front of the transverse process.

The block needle is connected to a syringe with local anesthetic via flexible tubing. The block needle is inserted between the palpating fingers and advanced at an angle perpendicular to the skin. A slight caudal orientation of the needle prevents the inadvertent insertion of the needle toward the cervical spinal cord. The needle should never be oriented cephalad. The needle is advanced slowly until the transverse process is contacted (Figure 80A–7). At this point, the needle is withdrawn 1–2 mm and stabilized for injection of 4 mL of local anesthetic per level after a negative aspiration for blood. The block needle is then removed, and the procedure is repeated at the consecutive levels.

Clinical Pearls

- The transverse process is typically contacted at a depth of 1–2 cm in most patients.
- Never advance the needle beyond 2.5 cm due to the risk of spinal cord injury.
- Paresthesia is often elicited in proximity to the transverse process but should not be relied on as the successful needle placement because of its nonspecific radiating pattern.

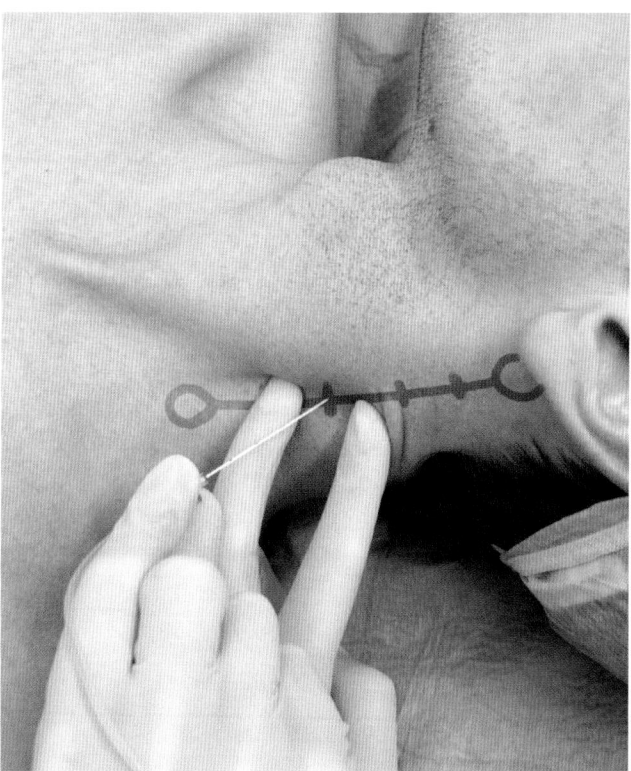

FIGURE 80A–7. Needle insertion to block a single cervical level during deep cervical blockade.

Block Dynamics and Perioperative Management

Although the placement of deep cervical block may be uncomfortable for the patient, excessive sedation should be avoided. During surgery, airway management may be difficult due to the close proximity of the surgical field. Surgeries like carotid endarterectomy require that the patient be cooperative for intraoperative neurologic assessment.[13] Excessive sedation and the consequent lack of patient cooperation can lead to restlessness and patient movement intraoperatively.

The onset time for this block is 10–15 min. The first sign of onset is decreased sensation in the distribution of the respective components of the cervical plexus. It should be noted that due to the complex arrangement of the neuronal coverage of the various layers in the neck area as well as cross coverage from the contralateral side, the anesthesia achieved with cervical plexus block is often incomplete, and its use often requires a knowledgeable surgeon who is skilled in supplementing the block with local anesthetic as necessary.

Clinical Pearl

- Carotid surgery also requires blockade of the glossopharyngeal nerve branches, which is easily accomplished intraoperatively by injecting the local anesthetic inside the carotid artery sheath.

FUNCTIONAL ANATOMY OF SUPERFICIAL CERVICAL PLEXUS BLOCKADE

The superficial cervical plexus innervates the skin of the anterolateral neck (see Figure 80A–3). The terminal branches emerge as four distinct nerves from the posterior border of the sternocleidomastoid muscle. The lesser occipital nerve is usually a direct branch from the main stem of the second cervical nerve. The larger remaining part of this stem then unites with a part of the third cervical nerve to form a trunk that gives rise to the greater auricular and transverse cervical nerves. Another part of the third cervical nerve runs downward to unite with a major part of the fourth cervical nerve to form a supraclavicular trunk, which then divides into the three groups of supraclavicular nerves.

Anatomic Landmarks

A line extending from the mastoid process to C6 is drawn as described above (Figure 80A–8). The site of needle insertion is marked at the midpoint of this line. This is where the branches of the superficial cervical plexus emerge from behind the posterior border of the sternocleidomastoid muscle.

Choice of Local Anesthetic

Superficial cervical plexus block requires 10–15 mL of local anesthetic (3–5 mL per each redirection/injection). Since motor block is not sought with this technique a lower concentration of long-acting local anesthetic is most often used (e.g., 0.2–0.5% ropivacaine or 0.25% bupivacaine). Higher concentration, however, may result in both a greater success rate and a longer duration of blockade.[33]

Table 80A–1 shows choices of local anesthesia, with onset time and duration of anesthesia and analgesia.

Equipment

A standard regional anesthesia tray is prepared with the following equipment:

- Sterile towels and 4-in. × 4-in. gauze pads
- 20-mL syringe with local anesthetic
- Sterile gloves, marking pen
- A 1.5-in., 25-gauge needle for block infiltration

Technique

Anatomic landmarks and the needle insertion point are marked as described above. After cleansing the skin with an antiseptic solution, a skin wheal is raised at the site of needle insertion using a 25-gauge needle. Using a "fan" technique with superior–inferior needle redirections, the local anesthetic is injected alongside the posterior border of the sternocleidomastoid muscle 2–3 cm below and then above the needle insertion site. The goal is to achieve blockade of all four major branches of the superficial cervical plexus.

The goal of the injection is to infiltrate the local anesthetic subcutaneously and behind the sternocleidomastoid muscle. Deep needle insertion should be avoided (e.g., >1–2 cm).

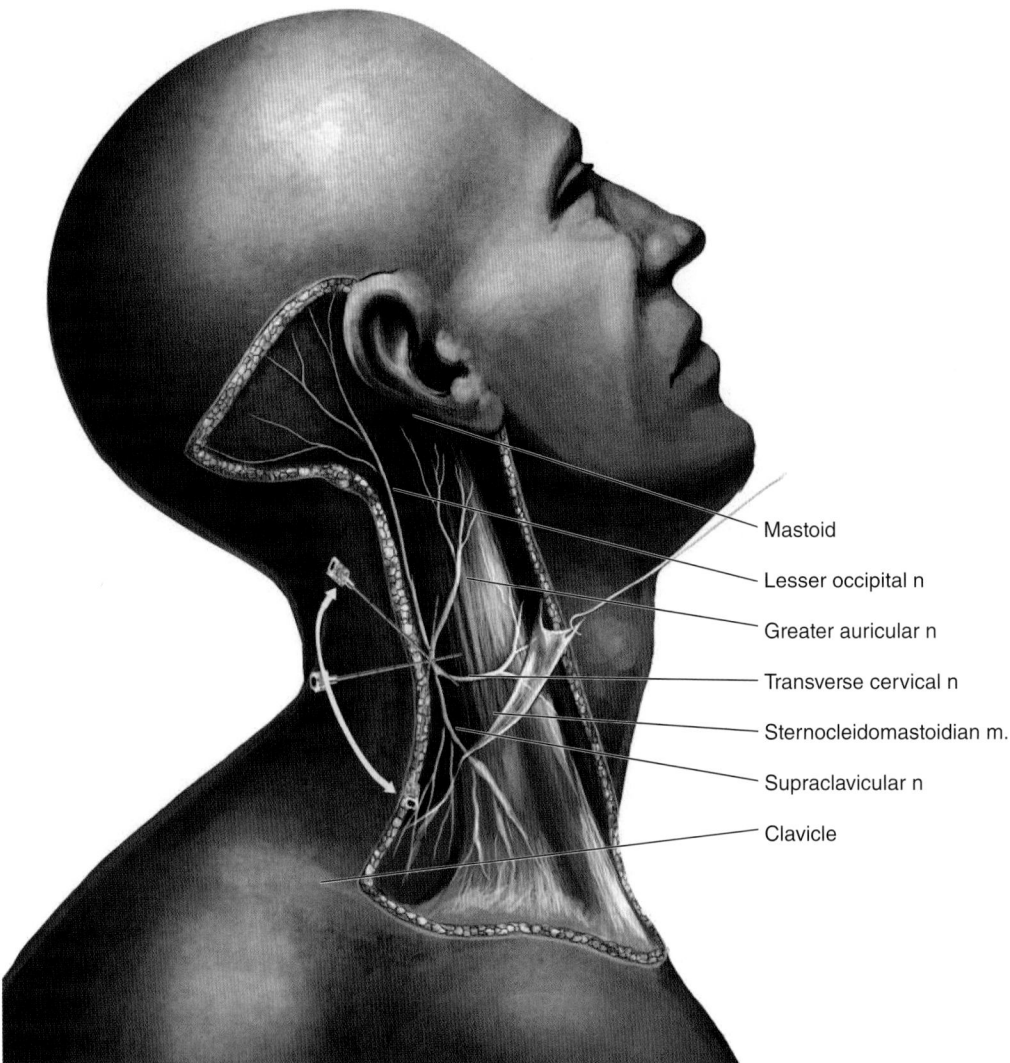

Mastoid

Lesser occipital n

Greater auricular n

Transverse cervical n

Sternocleidomastoidian m.

Supraclavicular n

Clavicle

FIGURE 80A–8. Supraclavicular nerve block. An initial injection of 3 mL local anesthetic is deposited at the midpoint of the sternocleidomastoid muscle, followed by 7 mL injected subcutaneously in a caudad and cephalad direction along the posterior border of the muscle.

▌ Block Dynamics and Perioperative Management

The superficial cervical plexus block is associated with minor patient discomfort, so little or no sedation should be required.

Similar to deep cervical plexus blockade, the sensory coverage of the neck is complex and a degree of cross coverage from the cervical plexus branches from the opposite side of the neck should be expected. The onset time for this block is 10–15 minutes; the first sign of the blockade is decreased sensation in the distribution of the superficial cervical plexus.

Ultrasound guidance can also be used when performing the superficial cervical plexus block, although a studies to date have not demonstrated an advantage over a landmark-based technique.[38,39]

Clinical Pearls

- A subcutaneous midline injection of the local anesthetic extending from the thyroid cartilage distally to the suprasternal notch will also block the branches crossing from the opposite side.
- Superficial cervical plexus can be considered as a "field" block and is very useful for preventing pain from surgical skin retractors on the medial aspect of the neck.

COMPLICATIONS AND HOW TO AVOID THEM

Complications can occur with both deep and superficial cervical plexus blocks (Table 80A–2). Infection, hematoma formation, phrenic nerve block, local anesthetic toxicity, nerve injury, and inadvertent subarachnoid or epidural anesthesia can all occur when performing these blocks.[40-44] In a large prospective study of 1000 blocks for carotid artery surgery, Davies and colleagues reported only 6 blocks (0.6%) showing evidence of intravascular injection.[13] Other possible complications include transient

TABLE 80A–2. Complications of cervical plexus block and means to avoid them.

Infection	• Low risk
	• A strict aseptic technique is used
Hematoma	• Avoid multiple needle insertions, particularly in anticoagulated patients
	• Keep 5 minutes of steady pressure on the site if the carotid artery is inadvertently punctured
Phrenic nerve blockade	• Phrenic nerve blockade (diaphragmatic paresis) invariably occurs with a deep cervical plexus block
	• A deep cervical block should be carefully considered in patients with significant respiratory disease
	• Bilateral deep cervical block in such patients may be contraindicated
	• Blockade of the phrenic nerve does not occur after superficial cervical plexus block
Local anesthetic toxicity	• Central nervous system toxicity is the most serious consequence of the cervical plexus block
	• This complication occurs because of the rich vascularity of the neck, including vertebral and carotid artery vessels and is usually caused by an inadvertent intravascular injection of local anesthetic rather than absorption
	• Careful and frequent aspiration should be performed during the injection
Nerve injury	• Local anesthetic should never be injected against resistance or when the patient complains of severe pain on injection
Spinal anesthesia	• This complication may occur with injection of a larger volume of local anesthetic inside the dural sleeve that accompanies the nerves of the cervical plexus
	• It should be noted that a negative aspiration test for CSF does not rule out the possibility of intrathecal spread of local anesthetic
	• Avoidance of high volume and excessive pressure during injection are the best measures to avoid this complication

Abbreviation: CSF, cerebrospinal fluid.

ischemic attacks either during surgery or in the postoperative period and recurrent laryngeal nerve blockade.[45–47] As with other nerve blocks, the risk of complications can be decreased by meticulous technique and attention to detail.[48–51]

SUMMARY

In summary, cervical plexus blocks have been in clinical use for nearly a century. Although modifications have been made to the approaches first described, the most common approach remains the lateral approach to deep cervical plexus block.

REFERENCES

1. Kappis H: Über Leitunganaesthesie am Bauch, Brust, Arm, und Hals durch injection aus Foramen intervertebrale. Munchen Med Wschr 1912;59:794–796.
2. Boezaart AP, Koorn R, Rosenquist RW: Paravertebral approach to the brachial plexus: An anatomic improvement in technique. Reg Anesth Pain Med 2003;28:241–244.
3. Koorn R, Tenhundfel Fear KM, Miller C, Boezaart A:: The use of cervical paravertebral block as the sole anesthetic for shoulder surgery in a morbid patient: A case report. Reg Anesth Pain Med 2004;29:227–229.
4. Borene SC, Rosenquist RW, Koorn R, et al: An indication for con tinuous cervical paravertebral block (posterior approach to the in-terscalene space). Anesth Analg 2003;97:898–900.
5. Boezaart AP, Koorn R, Borene S, et al: Continuous brachial plexus block using the posterior approach. Reg Anesth Pain Med 2003;28:70–71.
6. Heidenhein L: Operations on the neck. In Braun H (ed): *Local Anesthesia, Its Scientific Basis and Practical Use*. Philadelphia, PA: Lea & Febiger, 1914, pp 268–269.
7. Sherwood-Dunn B: *Regional Anesthesia (Victor Pauchet's Technique)*. Philadelphia, PA: FA Davis, 1920.
8. Winnie AP, Ramamurthy S, Durrani Z, et al: Interscalene cervical plexus block: a single-injection technique. Anesth Analg 1975;54:370–375.
9. Todesco J, Williams RT: Anaesthetic management of a patient with a large neck mass. Can J Anaesth 1994;41:157–160.
10. Kulkarni RS, Braverman LE, Patwardhan NA: Bilateral cervical plexus block for thyroidectomy and parathyroidectomy in healthy and high risk patients. J Endocrinol Invest 1996;19:714–718.
11. Eastcott HH, Pickering GW, Rob CG: Reconstruction of internal carotid artery in a patient with intermittent attacks of hemiplegia. Lancet 1954;267:994–996.
12. Stoneham MD, Knighton JD: Regional anaesthesia for carotid endarterectomy. Br J Anaesth 1999;82:910–919.
13. Davies MJ, Silbert BS, Scott DA, et al: Superficial and deep cervical plexus block for carotid artery surgery: a prospective study of 1000 blocks. Reg Anesth Pain Med 1997;22:442–446.
14. Stoneburner JM, Nishanian GP, Cukingnan RA, et al: Carotid en-darterectomy using regional anesthesia: a benchmark for stenting. Am Surg 2002;68:1120–1123.
15. Harbaugh RE, Pikus HJ: Carotid endarterectomy with regional anes-thesia. Neurosurgery 2001;49:642–645.
16. McCleary AJ, Maritati G, Gough MJ: Carotid endarterectomy; local or general anaesthesia? Eur J Vasc Endovasc Surg 2001;22:1–12.
17. Melliere D, Desgranges P, Becquemin JP, et al: Surgery of the internal carotid: locoregional or general anesthesia? Ann Chir 2000;125:530–538.
18. Stone ME Jr, Kunjummen BJ, Moran JC, et al: Supervised training of general surgery residents in carotid endarterectomy performed on awake patients under regional block is safe and desirable. Am Surg 2000;66:781–786.
19. Knighton JD, Stoneham MD: Carotid endarterectomy. A survey of UK anaesthetic practice. Anaesthesia 2000;55:481–485.
20. Lehot JJ, Durand PG: Anesthesia for carotid endarterectomy. Rev Esp Anestesiol Reanim 2001;48:499–507.
21. Santamaria G, Britti RD, Tescione M, et al: Comparison between local and general anaesthesia for carotid endarterectomy. A retrospective analysis. Minerva Anestesiol 2004;70:771–778.
22. Bowyer MW, Zierold D, Loftus JP, et al: Carotid endarterectomy: a comparison of regional versus general anesthesia in 500 operations. Ann Vasc Surg 2000;14:145–151.

23. Papavasiliou AK, Magnadottir HB, Gonda T, et al: Clinical outcomes after carotid endarterectomy: Comparison of the use of regional and general anesthetics. J Neurosurg 2000;92:291–296.
24. Stoughton J, Nath RL, Abbott WM: Comparison of simultaneous electroencephalographic and mental status monitoring during carotid endarterectomy with regional anesthesia. J Vasc Surg 1998;28:1014–1021.
25. Bonalumi F, Vitiello R, Miglierina L, et al: Carotid endarterectomy under locoregional anesthesia. Ann Ital Chir 1997;68:453–461.
26. GALA Trial Collaborative Group: General anaesthesia versus local anaesthesia for carotid surgery (GALA): a multicentre, randomised controlled trial. Lancet 2008;372:2132–2142.
27. Vaniyapong T, Chongruksut W, Rerkasem K: Local versus general anaesthesia for carotid endarterectomy. Cochrane Database Syst Rev. 2013; 19:12.
28. Brull SJ: Superficial cervical plexus block for pulmonary artery catheter insertion. Crit Care Med 1992;20:1362–1363.
29. Pandit JJ, Bree S, Dillon P, et al: A comparison of superficial versus combined (superficial and deep) cervical plexus block for carotid endarterectomy: a prospective, randomized study. Anesth Analg 2000;91:781–786.
30. Stoneham MD, Doyle AR, Knighton JD, et al: Prospective, randomized comparison of deep or superficial cervical plexus block for carotid endarterectomy surgery. Anesthesiology 1998;89:907–912.
31. JJ Pandit JJ, Satya-Krishna, Gration P: Superficial or deep cervical plexus block for carotid endarterectomy: a systematic review of complications Br J Anaesth, 99 (2007), pp. 159–169.
32. Aunac S, Carlier M, Singelyn F, et al: The analgesic efficacy of bilateral combined superficial and deep cervical plexus block administered before thyroid surgery under general anesthesia. Anesth Analg 2002;95:746–750.
33. Masters RD, Castresana EJ, Castresana MR: Superficial and deep cervical plexus block: Technical considerations. AANA J 1995;63:235–243.
34. Dieudonne N, Gomola A, Bonnichon P, et al: Prevention of post-operative pain after thyroid surgery: a double-blind randomized study of bilateral superficial cervical plexus blocks. Anesth Analg 2001;92:1538–1542.
35. Gratz I, Deal E, Larijani GE, et al: The number of injections does not influence absorption of bupivacaine after cervical plexus block for carotid endarterectomy. J Clin Anesth 2005;17:263–266.
36. Umbrain VJ, van Gorp VL, Schmedding E, et al: Ropivacaine 3.75 mg/ml, 5 mg/ml, or 7.5 mg/ml for cervical plexus block during carotid endarterectomy. Reg Anesth Pain Med 2004;29:312–316.
37. Leoni A, Magrin S, Mascotto G, et al: Cervical plexus anesthesia for carotid endarterectomy: comparison of ropivacaine and mepivacaine. Can J Anaesth 2000;47:185–187.
38. Gürkan Y, Taş Z, Toker K, Solak M: Ultrasound guided bilateral cervical plexus block reduces postoperative opioid consumption following thyroid surgery. J Clin Monit Comput. 2015; 29(5):579–584.
39. Tran DQ, Dugani S, Finlayson RJ: A randomized comparison between ultrasound-guided and landmark-based superficial cervical plexus block. Reg Anesth Pain Med 2010;35(6):539–543.
40. Pandit JJ, McLaren ID, Crider B: Efficacy and safety of the superficial cervical plexus block for carotid endarterectomy. Br J Anaesth 1999;83:970–972.
41. Carling A, Simmonds M: Complications from regional anaesthesia for carotid endarterectomy. Br J Anaesth 2000;84:797–800.
42. Emery G, Handley G, Davies MJ, et al: Incidence of phrenic nerve block and hypercapnia in patients undergoing carotid endarterectomy under cervical plexus block. Anaesth Intensive Care 1998;26:377–381.
43. Stoneham MD, Wakefield TW: Acute respiratory distress after deep cervical plexus block. J Cardiothorac Vasc Anesth 1998;12:197–198.
44. Castresana MR, Masters RD, Castresana EJ, et al: Incidence and clinical significance of hemidiaphragmatic paresis in patients undergoing carotid endarterectomy during cervical plexus block anesthesia. J Neurosurg Anesthesiol 1994;6:21–23.
45. Johnson TR: Transient ischaemic attack during deep cervical plexus block. Br J Anaesth 1999;83:965–967.
46. Lawrence PF, Alves JC, Jicha D, et al: Incidence, timing, and causes of cerebral ischemia during carotid endarterectomy with regional anesthesia. J Vasc Surg 1998;27:329–334.
47. Harris RJ, Benveniste G: Recurrent laryngeal nerve blockade in patients undergoing carotid endarterectomy under cervical plexus block. Anaesth Intensive Care 2000;28: 431–433.
48. Bergeron P, Benichou H, Dupont M, et al: Carotid surgery under cervical block anesthesia. A simple method of heart and brain protection in high risk patients. Int Angiol 1989;8:70–80.
49. Shah DM, Darling RC 3rd, Chang BB, et al: Carotid endarterectomy in awake patients: Its safety, acceptability, and outcome. J Vasc Surg 1994;19:1015–1019.
50. Lee KS, Davis CH Jr, McWhorter JM: Low morbidity and mortality of carotid endarterectomy performed with regional anesthesia. J Neurosurg 1988;69:483–487.
51. Love A, Hollyoak MA: Carotid endarterectomy and local anaesthesia: reducing the disasters. Cardiovasc Surg 2000;8:429–435.

Interscalene Brachial Plexus Block

Alain Borgeat, Matthew Levine, Malikah Latmore, Sam Van Boxstael, and Stephan Blumenthal

INTRODUCTION

The first brachial plexus blocks were performed by William Stewart Halsted, in 1885, at the Roosevelt Hospital in New York City. In 1902, George Washington Crile described an "open approach" to expose the (axillary) plexus facilitating direct application of cocaine. The need for surgical exposure of the brachial plexus led to limited clinical utility of this technique. This changed in the early 1900s when percutaneous access to the brachial plexus was first described. In 1925, July Etienne[1] reported the successful blockade of the brachial plexus by inserting a needle halfway between the lateral border of the sternocleidomastoid muscle and the anterior border of the trapezius muscle at the level of the cricothyroid membrane, making a single injection in the area around the scalene muscles. This approach was most likely the first clinically useful interscalene block technique. In 1970, Alon Winnie[2] described the first consistently effective and technically suitable percutaneous approach to the brachial plexus block. The technique involved palpating the interscalene groove at the level of the cricoid cartilage and injecting local anesthetic between the anterior and middle scalene muscles. Winnie's approach was modified over the years to include slight variations to the technique such as perineural catheter placement.[3] However, the success of this approach and the widespread adoption of the interscalene brachial plexus block as the "unilateral spinal anesthesia for the upper extremity," should be credited solely to Alon Winnie.

More recently, the introduction of ultrasound-guided techniques has allowed for additional refinements and improved block consistency with reduced local anesthetic volumes (see Chapter 32B).[4-6]

Indications

The interscalene block is indicated for procedures on the shoulder and proximal humerus as well as the lateral two thirds of the clavicle. The interscalene block can also be utilized for surgery of the arm or forearm; however, the higher incidence of incomplete blockade of the inferior trunk with this technique may provide inadequate analgesia in the ulnar distribution. The patient's positioning and comfort, the surgeon's preferences, and the duration of surgery may necessitate coadministration of a general anesthetic. An interscalene catheter may be inserted for prolonged postoperative analgesia (Table 80B-1).

Clinical Pearls

- Up to 70% of patients report severe pain on movement after open major shoulder surgery, which is more than after hysterectomy (60%), gastrectomy, or thoracotomy (60%).[7]
- Major shoulder surgery entails massive nociceptive input from the richly innervated joint and periarticular tissues, which produce continuous deep somatic pain and bouts of reflex spasm of muscles.
- Periarticular structures exhibit not only C afferents, but also A alpha and A delta afferents, the latter being poorly blocked by opioids, which explains the relative inefficacy of opioids to control this type of postoperative pain.

Contraindications

Absolute contraindications include patient's refusal, local infection, active bleeding in an anticoagulated patient, and proven allergy to local anesthetic. Relative contraindications include chronic obstructive airway disease, contralateral paresis of the phrenic or recurrent laryngeal nerves, and previous neurologic deficit of the involved arm. The risks and benefits of the chosen anesthetic technique should be discussed with the patient and the surgeon.

TABLE 80B–1. Single-injection vs the choice of technique: interscalene catheter according to surgery.

Type of Surgery	Type of Block	
	Single-Injection	Catheter
Open Surgery		
Arthroplasty	+	+
Rotator cuff repair	+	+
Arthrolysis	+	+
Acromioplasty	+	+
Bankart's repair	+	+
Latarjet	+	+
Proximal humerus osteosynthesis	+	±
Acromioclavicular resection	+	−
Shoulder luxation	+	−
Clavicle osteosynthesis	+ (± superficial cervical block)	−
Arthroscopic Surgery		
Rotator cuff repair	+	+
Arthrolysis	+	+
Bankart's repair	+	±
Acromioplasty	+	±

Skin infiltration of the posterior arthroscopic port site with local anesthetic is often necessary despite a successful interscalene block.

Clinical Pearl

- Skin infiltration of the posterior arthroscopic port site with local anesthetic is often necessary for arthroscopic shoulder surgery in addition to interscalene block.

Anatomy

The plexus is formed by the ventral rami of the fifth to eighth cervical nerves and the greater part of the ventral ramus of the first thoracic nerve (Figure 80B–1). In addition, small contributions may be made by the fourth cervical and the second thoracic nerves. There are multiple complex interconnections between the neural elements of brachial plexus as they course from the interscalene groove to their endpoints in terminal nerves. However, most of what happens to these roots on their way to becoming peripheral nerves is not clinically essential information for the practitioner. However, spatial arrangement of the trunks (superior, middle, and inferior) and interpretation of the motor response with nerve stimulation can be of

importance. (Table 80B–2).The brachial plexus supplies all the motor and most of the sensory functions of the shoulder except the cephalad cutaneous parts of the shoulder. These are innervated by the supraclavicular nerves originating from the lower part of the superficial cervical plexus (C3–4) (Figure 80B–2) which supply sensation to the shoulder above the clavicle, the first two intercostal spaces anteriorly, the posterior cervical triangle and the upper thorax in this area as well as to the tip of the shoulder.[9]

Only three nerves of the brachial plexus innervate the shoulder. The most proximal of these is the upper lateral brachial cutaneous nerve, a branch of the axillary nerve that innervates the lateral side of the shoulder and the skin overlying the deltoid muscle. The upper medial side of the arm is innervated by both the medial brachial cutaneous and the intercostobrachial cutaneous nerves. In the anterior portion of the arm over the biceps muscle, the skin is innervated by the medial antebrachial cutaneous nerve.[9]

Apart from the cutaneous nerve supply to the shoulder, the innervation of the joint deserves special consideration. In general, a nerve crossing a joint gives branches that innervate that joint. Therefore, the nerves supplying the ligaments, capsule, and synovial membrane of the shoulder derive from the axillary, suprascapular, subscapular, and musculocutaneous nerves.[10,11] The relative contributions of these nerves are not constant, and the supply from the musculocutaneus nerve may be very small or completely absent. Anteriorly, the axillary nerve and suprascapular nerve provide most of the nerve supply to the capsule and glenohumeral joint (Figure 80B–3). In some instances, the musculocutaneous nerve may innervate the anterosuperior portion of the joint. In addition, the anterior capsule may be supplied by either the subscapular nerves or the posterior cord of the brachial plexus after piercing the subscapularis muscle. Superiorly, the primary contribution is from two branches of the suprascapular nerve, one branch supplying the acromioclavicular joint and proceeding anteriorly as far as the coracoid process and coracoacromial ligament and the other branch reaching the posterior aspect of the joint. Other nerves contributing to this region of the joint are the axillary nerve and musculocutaneous nerve. Posteriorly, the main nerves are the suprascapular nerve in the upper region and the axillary nerve in the lower region (Figure 80B–4).

Inferiorly, the anterior portion is primarily supplied by the axillary nerve, and the posterior portion is supplied by a combination of the axillary nerve and lower ramifications of the suprascapular nerve.

Clinical Pearls

- **Arthroscopic shoulder surgery:** Nerves of importance to anesthesia: supraclavicular, suprascapular, and axillary (radial) nerves.
- **Open shoulder surgery:** Knowledge of the surgical approach is important because surgery may also involve the territories of the median cutaneous, intercostobrachial, and the median antebrachial cutaneous nerves.

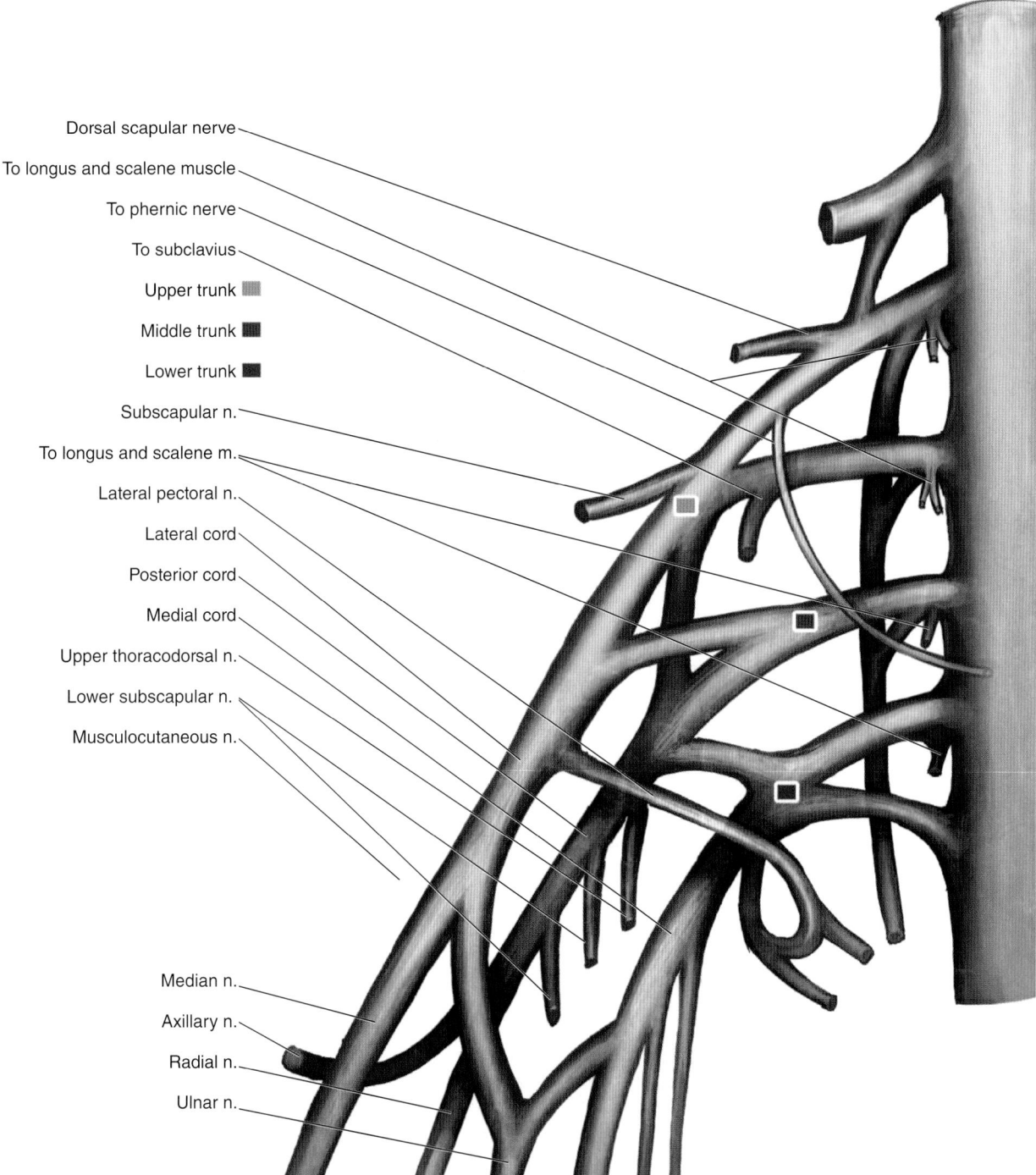

Dorsal scapular nerve
To longus and scalene muscle
To phernic nerve
To subclavius
Upper trunk
Middle trunk
Lower trunk
Subscapular n.
To longus and scalene m.
Lateral pectoral n.
Lateral cord
Posterior cord
Medial cord
Upper thoracodorsal n.
Lower subscapular n.
Musculocutaneous n.
Median n.
Axillary n.
Radial n.
Ulnar n.

FIGURE 80B-1. Organization of the brachial plexus.

Landmarks

The following surface anatomy landmarks are important in identifying the interscalene space:

1. Sternal head of the sternocleidomastoid muscle
2. Clavicular head of the sternocleidomastoid muscle
3. Upper border of the cricoid cartilage
4. Clavicle (Figure 80B–5)

Equipment for Single-Injection Technique

Standard regional anesthesia equipment for a single-shot block consists of the following items (Figure 80B–6):

Marking pen, ruler
Sterile gloves
Peripheral nerve stimulator, surface electrode

TABLE 80B-2. Distribution of the brachial plexus.

Nerve(s)	Spinal Segment(s)	Distribution
Subclavius nerve	C4 through C6	Subclavius muscle
Dorsal scapular nerve	C4–C5	Rhomboid muscles and levator scapulae muscle
Long thoracic nerve	C5 through C7	Serratus anterior muscle
Suprascapular nerve	C4, C5, C6	Supraspinatus and infraspinatus muscles
Pectoralis nerves (medial and lateral)	C5 through T1	Pectoralis muscles
Subscapular nerves	C5, C6	Subscapular and teres major muscles
Thoracodorsal nerve	C6 through C8	Latissimus dorsi muscle
Axillary nerve	C5 and C6	Deltoid and teres minor muscles; skin of shoulder
Radial nerve	C5 through T1	Extensor muscles of the arm and forearm (triceps brachii, extensor carpi radialis, extensor carpi ulnaris) and brachioradialis muscle; digital extension and abductor pollicis muscle; skin over posterolateral surface of the arm
Musculocutaneous nerve	C5 through C7	Flexor muscles of the arm (biceps brachii, brachialis, coracobrachialis); skin over lateral surface of the forearm
Median nerve	C6 through T1	Flexor muscles of the forearm (flexor carpi radialis, palmaris longus); pronator quadratus, and pronator teres muscles; digital flexors (through the palmar interosseous nerve); skin over anterolateral surface of the hand
Ulnar nerve	C8, T1	Flexor carpi ulnaris muscle, adductor pollicis muscle, and small digital muscles, skin over medial surface of the hand

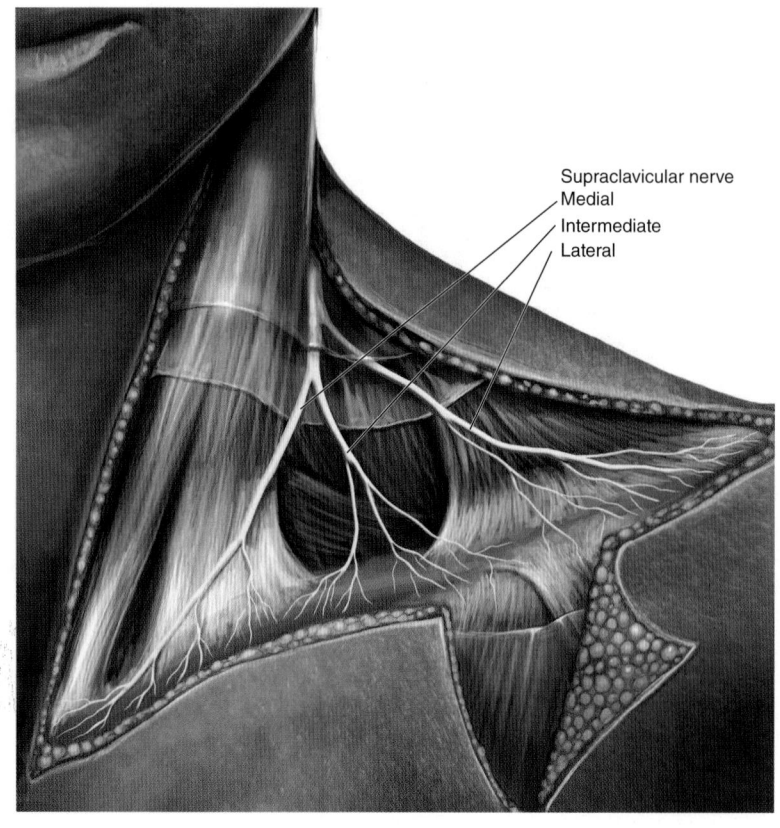

FIGURE 80B-2. The innervation of the skin over the shoulder and clavicle.

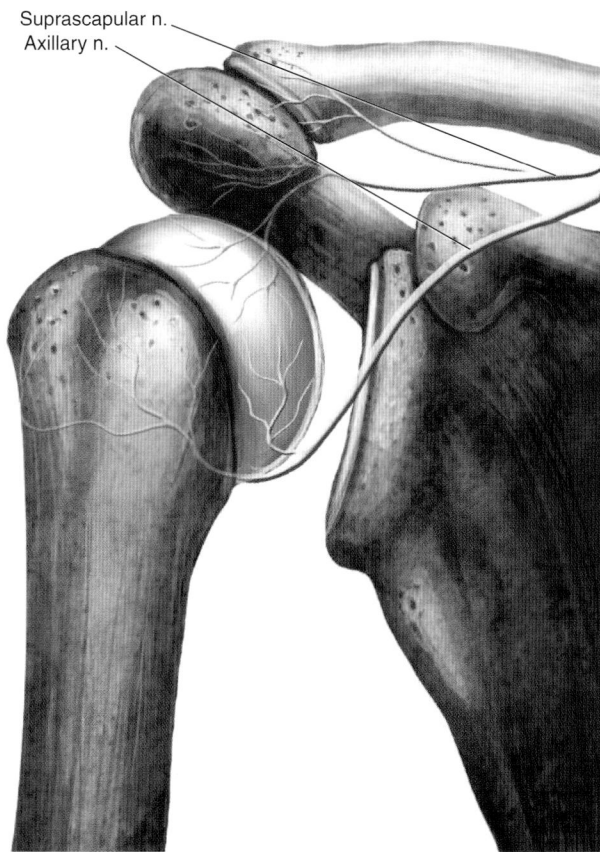

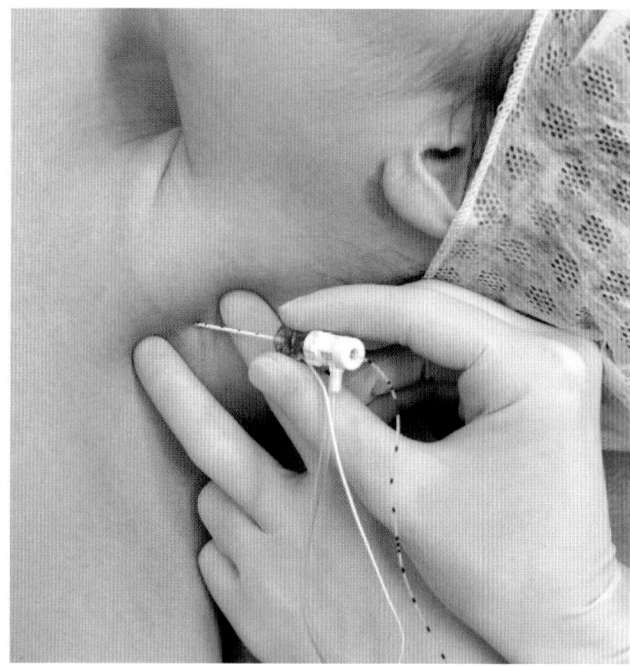

FIGURE 80B–5. Continuous interscalene brachial plexus block. The needle is inserted between anterior and middle scalene muscles in the pictured direction. The needle should not be placed deeper than 2-3 cm in most patients.

FIGURE 80B–3. The innervation of the anterior portion of the shoulder. The axillary and suprascapular nerves form most of the nerve supply to the capsule and the glenohumeral joint.

Disinfection solution and sterile gauze packs
2- to 5-cm, short-bevel, 22-gauge insulated stimulating needle
Syringes with local anesthetic
Injection pressure monitor

Equipment for Continuous Technique

Standard regional anesthesia equipment for a continuous nerve block consists of the following items (Figure 80B–7).

Marking pen, ruler
Peripheral nerve stimulator, surface electrode
Disinfection solution, sterile gauze packs
Sterile transparent drapes
Syringes with local anesthetic for skin infiltration and block injection
25-mm, 25-gauge needle for skin infiltration at puncture point and for tunneling
A set with stimulating needle for continuous nerve block and catheter
Adhesive material for securing the catheter

APPROACHES TO AND TECHNIQUES FOR BRACHIAL PLEXUS BLOCK AT THE LEVEL OF THE NECK

Several approaches to the interscalene brachial plexus block have been described with the use of a nerve stimulator. In this chapter, we describe the, classic (Winnie) technique and common modifications, including the low interscalene approach. The posterior (paravertebral) approach and its modifications

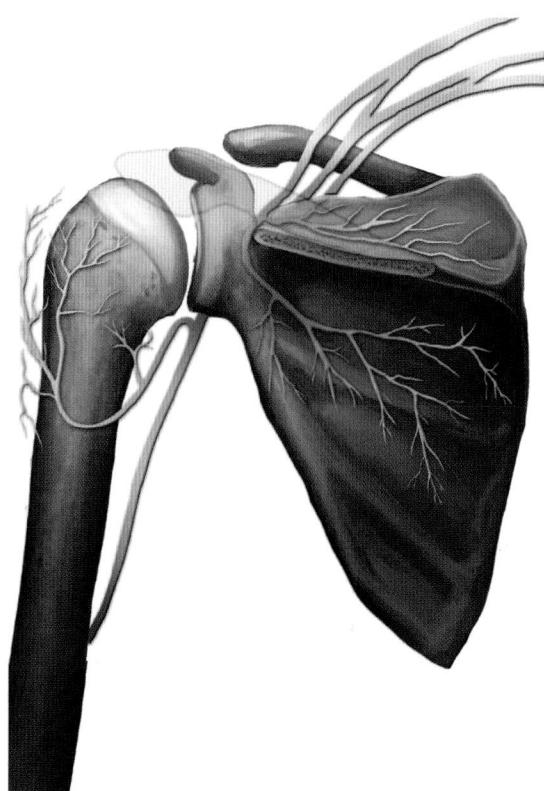

FIGURE 80B–4. The posterior innervation of the shoulder joint. The primary nerves are the suprascapular and the axillary.

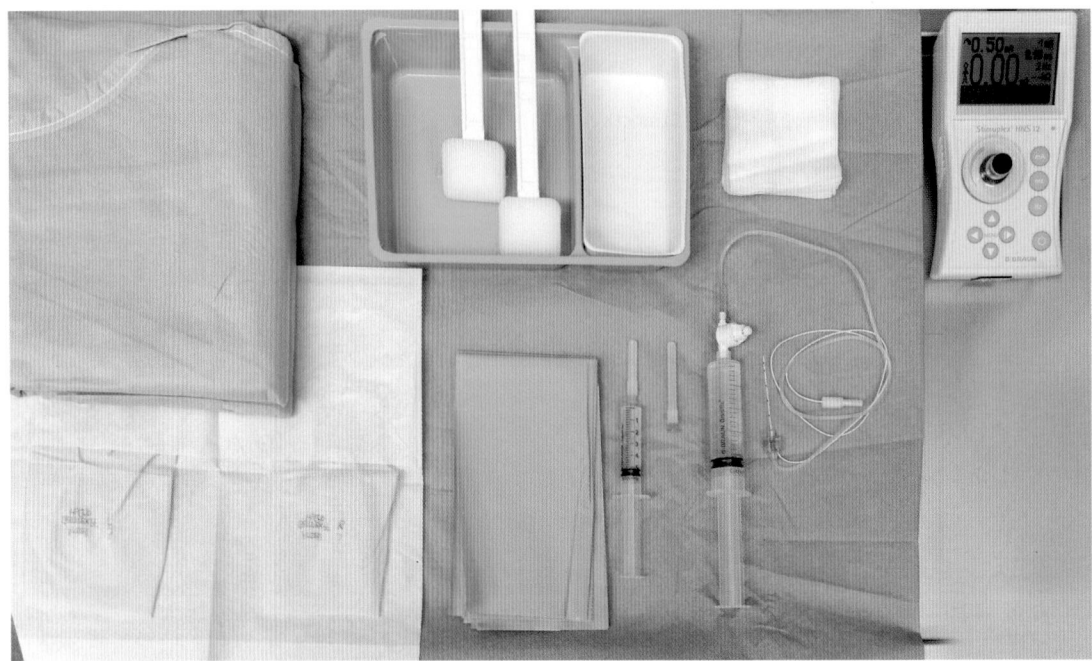

FIGURE 80B-6. Equipment for single-injection interscalene block.

have been largely abandoned for safety reasons and will be omitted from this volume.[16-19]

Classic Technique (Winnie)

The classic approach of Winnie[2] is performed at the level of the sixth cervical vertebra. Winnie originally used a paresthesia technique; however, most practitioners eventually adopted nerve stimulation.

1. The patient is placed in a semisitting or supine position with the head turned away from the side to be blocked.
2. The patient is asked to elevate the head slightly to bring the clavicular head of the sternocleidomastoid muscle into prominence.
3. The index and middle fingers of the nondominant hand are placed immediately behind the lateral edge of the sternocleidomastoid muscle. The patient is instructed to relax so that the palpating fingers can be moved medially

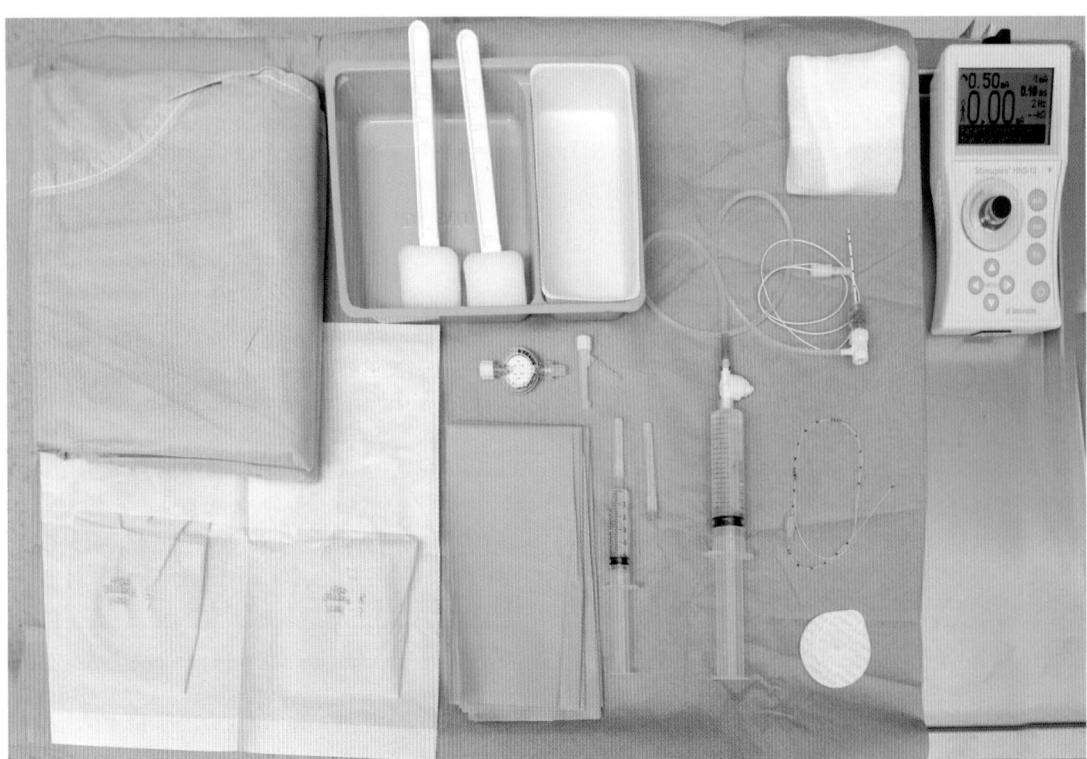

FIGURE 80B-7. Equipment for continuous interscalene block.

behind this muscle and finally lie on the belly of the anterior scalene muscle.

4. The palpating fingers are then rolled laterally across the belly of the anterior scalene muscle until they fall into the interscalene groove (formed by scalene anterior and posterior muscles).

5. With both fingers in the interscalene groove, a 1.5-in., 22- gauge, short-bevel needle is inserted between the fingers at the level of C6 in a direction that is perpendicular to the skin in every plane.

6. After a motor response is obtained, aspiration is carried out to rule out intravascular or intrathecal placement. While the patient is monitored closely for signs of local anaesthetic toxicity or inadvertent subarachnoid injection, 15–20 mL of local anesthetic is slowly injected.

Clinical Pearls

- In Winnie's original description, the needle is advanced slowly until a paresthesia is elicited or until the transverse process is encountered.
- Paresthesia below the level of the shoulder is sought because a paresthesia to the shoulder could result from stimulation of the suprascapular nerve inside or outside the interscalene space.
- If bone is contacted without producing a paresthesia, this is likely the transverse process and the needle should be gently "walked off " anteriorly millimeter by millimeter until a paresthesia or motor response is evoked.

Reported complications with this technique are total spinal anesthesia,[12,13] epidural anesthesia,[14] cervical spinal cord injection with resultant paraplegia, as well as injections into the vertebral artery.[15] These complications are more likely to occur with the classic technique than its modifications because the needle is directed perpendicularly towards the spinal cord. Although an infrequent complication, pneumothorax can also occur. This technique is not well suited for the placement of an interscalene catheter because of the perpendicular approach to the trunks.

Low Interscalene Brachial Plexus Block

The low interscalene technique of brachial plexus block[21] differs in three important aspects from the classic approach and its modifications (Figure 80B-5).[32]

1. Insertion of the needle is significantly lower than with the classic approach, which should reduce the risk of the needle entering the cervical cord or vertebral artery.

2. The brachial plexus is very superficial at this location; the skin to brachial plexus block distance is often less than 1 cm and rarely deeper than 2 cm.

3. The block can be considered a cross between a classic interscalene block (the plexus is approached in the distal interscalene groove) and a supraclavicular block (the needle insertion is slightly above the clavicle).

In contrast to the other approaches, the low interscalene approach provides reliable anesthesia for shoulder, elbow, and forearm surgeries alike.[22]

Landmarks

The landmarks for the low interscalene approach are as follows (Figure 80B–8):

- Clavicle
- Posterior border of the clavicular head of the sternocleidomastoid muscle
- External jugular vein

The landmarks for the low interscalene approach are accentuated by the following maneuvers, which should be routinely performed:

1. Ask the patient to face slightly away from the side to be blocked. This tenses the sternocleidomastoid muscle.
2. Ask the patient to reach the ipsilateral knee on the side to be blocked or pull the patient's wrist toward their knee. This flattens the skin of the neck and helps to identify both the scalene muscles and the external jugular vein.
3. Ask the patient to lift the head off the table while facing away. This tenses the sternocleidomastoid muscle and helps to identify the posterior border of the clavicular head.

Technique

The fingers of the palpating hand should be gently pressed between the anterior and middle scalene muscles to reduce the distance between the skin and brachial plexus (Figure 80B–9). The palpating hand should not be moved during the entire procedure to allow for precise redirections of the needle. A needle connected to a nerve stimulator is inserted between the palpating fingers and advanced at an angle almost perpendicular to the skin and in a slight caudad direction (Figure 80B–10). The nerve stimulator should be initially set to deliver 1 mA (2 Hz, 100 μsec). The needle is advanced slowly. Once any motor response of the brachial plexus is elicited, 15–20 mL of local anesthetic is injected slowly, with intermittent aspiration.

Some common responses to nerve stimulation and the course of action to obtain the proper response are shown in Table 80B–3. The following motor responses can all be accepted as successful localization of the brachial plexus with a similar success rate:

- Pectoralis muscle
- Deltoid muscle
- Triceps muscles
- Any twitch of the hand or forearm
- Biceps muscle

Continuous Interscalene Brachial Plexus Block

The continuous interscalene brachial plexus block is an advanced technique. Paradoxically, although the single-shot interscalene block is one of the easiest intermediate techniques

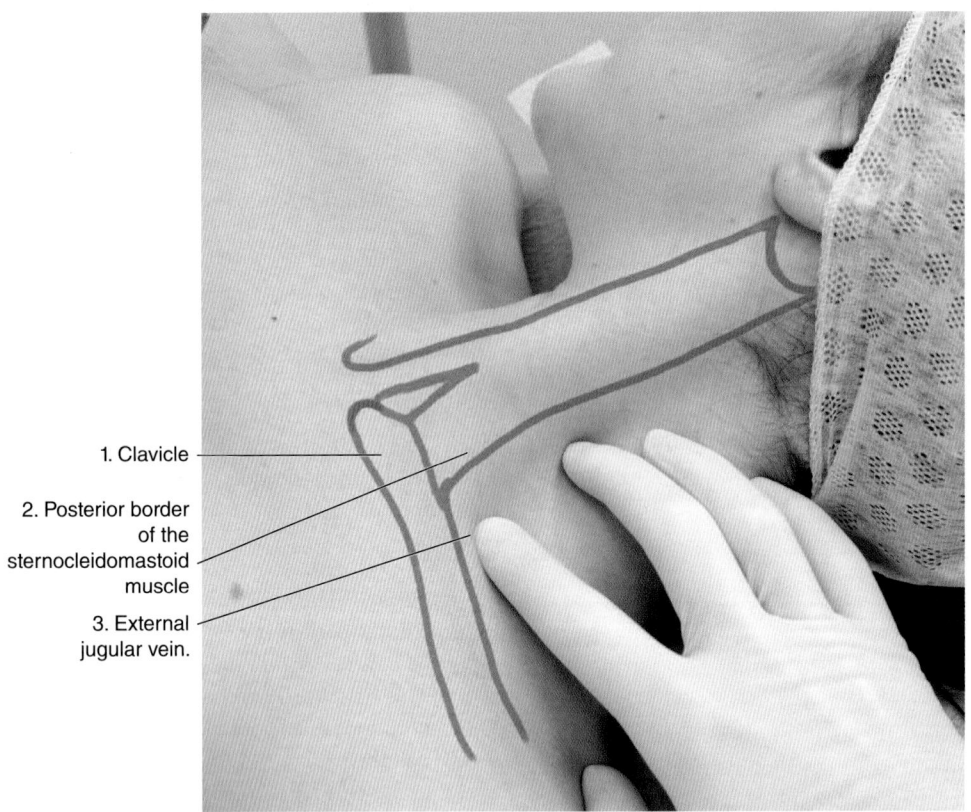

1. Clavicle

2. Posterior border of the sternocleidomastoid muscle

3. External jugular vein.

FIGURE 80B–8. Landmarks for low interscalene approach to brachial plexus block: (1) Clavicle. (2) Posterior border of the sternocleidomastoid muscle. (3) External jugular vein. The palpating fingers are positioned in the scalene "groove" between anterior and middle scalene muscles.

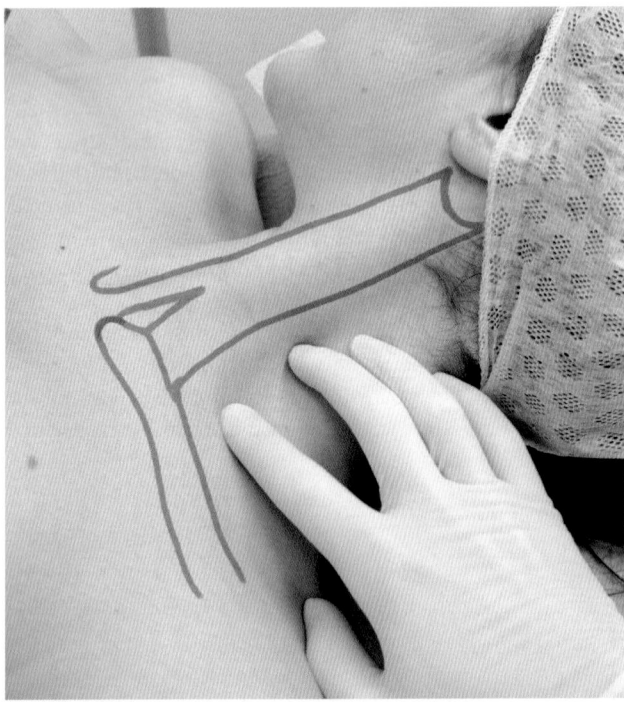

FIGURE 80B–9. Fingers of the palpating hand are positioned in front of the external jugular vein and in the interscalene groove made up of anterior and middle scalene muscles. Interscalene groove is the widest and easiest to palpate in this position.

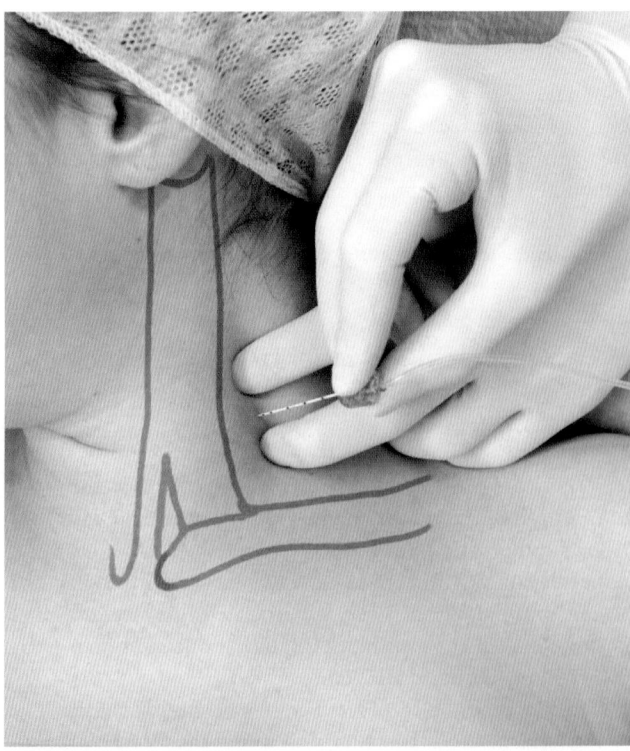

FIGURE 80B–10. Low interscalene block. Proper angle of the needle direction is medial with a slight caudad angulation.

TABLE 80B–3. Guide to troubleshooting interscalene block.

Response Obtained	Interpretation	Problem	Action
Local twitch of the neck muscles	Direct stimulation of the anterior scalene or sternocleoidomastoid muscles	Needle pass is in the wrong plane; usually anterior and medial to the plexus	Withdraw the needle to the skin and reinsert 15 degrees posterior
Needle contacts bone at 1–2 cm depth; no twitches seen	The needle is stopped by the transverse process	The needle is inserted too posterior; the needle contacts anterior tubercles of the transverse process	Withdraw the needle to the skin and reinsert 15 degrees anterior
Twitches of the diaphragm	The result of stimulation of the phrenic nerve	The needle is inserted too anterior and medial	Withdraw the needle and reinsert 15 degrees posterior and lateral
Arterial blood noticed in the tubing	Puncture of the carotid artery (most likely)	The needle insertion and angulation are too anterior	Withdraw the needle and apply pressure for 5 min; reinsert 1–2 cm posterior
Pectoralis muscle twitch	Brachial plexus stimulation (C4–C5)		Accept and inject local anesthetic
Twitch of the scapula	Twitch of the serratus anterior muscle; stimulation of the thoracodorsal nerve	Needle position is posterior/ deep to the brachial plexus	Withdraw the needle to the skin, and reinsert the needle anterior
Trapezius muscle twitches	Accessory nerve stimulation	Needle posterior to the brachial plexus	Withdraw the needle and insert more anteriorly
Twitch of pectorals, deltoid, triceps, biceps, forearm, and hand muscles	Stimulation of the brachial plexus	None	Accept and inject local anesthetic

to perform and master, placement of the catheter in the interscalene groove is much more challenging. This is partially due to the shallow position of the brachial plexus and difficulties in stabilizing the needle during catheter advancement. This technique provides excellent analgesia in patients after shoulder, arm, and elbow surgery.[33]

Technique

The patient is positioned in the same position as in the single-injection technique. After local anesthesia, a 5-cm long needle attached to a nerve stimulator (1.0 mA) is inserted at a slightly caudal angle and advanced until the brachial plexus twitch is elicited at 0.2–0.5 mA (Figure 80B–11). While paying meticulous attention to the position of the needle, the catheter is inserted some 3 cm beyond the tip of the needle and secured to the skin.

The catheter must be carefully checked for intravascular placement before administering large volumes or an infusion of local anesthetics. Before initiating the infusion of local anesthetic, the catheter is first checked for patency, and intravascular placement is ruled out by administering a small volume (2–3 mL of 1% lidocaine with epinephrine 1:300,000). The management of the continuous infusion of local anesthetic is discussed in the section about intraoperative management below.

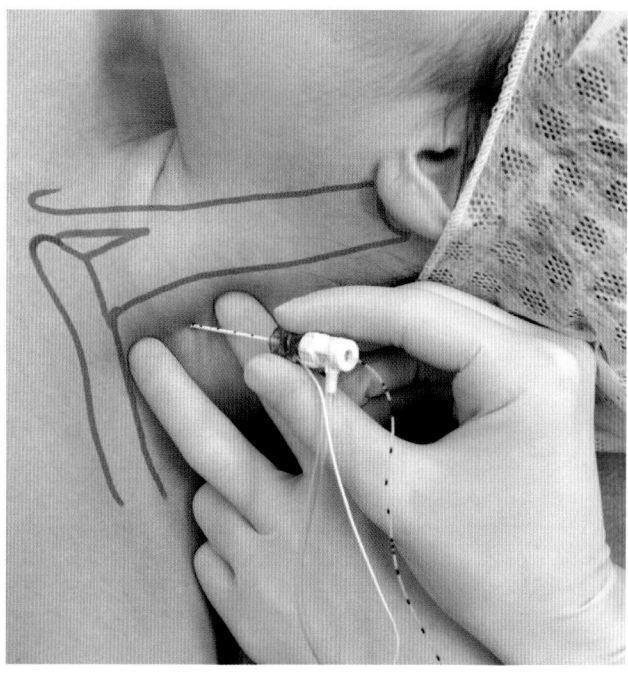

FIGURE 80B-11. Continuous interscalene block. Note the low angle of needle insertion, which is necessary to facilitate insertion of the catheter.

Clinical Pearl

- The following maneuvers help to localize the interscalene groove:
  1. Ask the patient to turn the head away from the side to be blocked and then to lift the head off the table. This maneuver tenses the sternocleidomastoid muscle and helps to identify the lateral border of the clavicular head of the sternocleidomastoid muscle.
  2. In some patients, the clavicular head of the sternocleidomastoid and anterior scalene muscles are packed together. The practitioner can ask the to sniff as the practitioner places the fingers firmly on the muscles. The anterior and middle scalene muscles contract during this maneuver, making their palpation and recognition of the scalene space easier.

INTRAOPERATIVE MANAGEMENT OF AN INTERSCALENE BLOCK DURING SHOULDER SURGERY

Sedation is almost always useful to improve patient comfort and satisfaction. This is in keeping with the preference of most surgeons for their patients to be 'asleep' during surgery, as is also the preference of most patients.

Drugs most commonly used to accomplish this are propofol, midazolam, and an intravenous opioid. A face mask with oxygen (4–6 L/min) should be routinely applied. Patients should be kept warm by using forced air or warm blankets. The onset of shivering can turn a successful regional anesthetic into a significant intraoperative challenge.

Intraoperative use of pneumatic equipment close to the patient's ear can result in noise levels over 100 dB. A significant amount of sedation is needed to mask this noise.[23] The use of earplugs, headphones with or without music, or blankets to protect the patient's ears can make a substantial difference in their comfort, and reduce the amount of sedative drugs required. Hyperhydration should be avoided because the patients are typically not given a urinary catheter, and the sensation of a full bladder can cause considerable discomfort for the patient. It is a good idea to ask patients to empty their bladder before administering any drugs.

Choice of Local Anesthetic

For single-shot techniques, a variety of local anesthetics can be used (Table 80B–4), depending on the desired duration and density of blockade. The typical volume of local anesthetic used for interscalene blocks is 15–20 mL of ropivacaine 0.5% or 0.75%.[25,26,27] Clonidine,[28] but not opioids,[29,30] can prolong the duration of both anesthesia and analgesia with intermediate-acting local anesthetics.[28] The addition of epinephrine also prolongs the duration of action of most local anesthetics.[31]

Continuous infusion of local anesthetics through an interscalene catheter compared with traditional patient-controlled analgesia (PCA) with opioids provides significantly better control of pain, with a lower incidence of side effects and greater

TABLE 80B-4. Local anesthetic mixtures used for single-injection techniques.

	Onset (min)	Anesthesia (h)	Analgesia (h)
3% 2-Chloroprocaine (+ HCO₃ + epinephine)	5–10	1.5	2
1.5% Mepivacaine (+ HCO₃)	10–20	2–3	2–4
1.5% Mepivacaine (+ HCO₃ + epinephrine)	5–15	2.5–4	3–6
2% Lidocaine (+ HCO₃)	10–20	2.5–3	2–5
2% Lidocaine (+ HCO₃ + epinephrine)	5–15	3–6	5–8
0.5% Ropivacaine	15–20	6–8	8–12
0.75% Ropivacaine	5–15	8–10	12–18
0.5% Bupivacaine (+ epinephrine)	20–30	8–10	16–18

patient satisfaction.[34,35] Catheters are typically left in place for 2–3 days. A typical regimen for continuous infusion would be the use of ropivacaine 0.2% at a rate of 5 mL/h with a 5 mL q60min patient controlled bolus.[36-39]

SIDE EFFECTS AND COMPLICATIONS AND HOW TO AVOID THEM

Complications associated with the different techniques of interscalene block are summarized in (Table 80B–5). The most common side effects encountered after interscalene block

TABLE 80B-5. Complications of interscalene block according to approach.

	Winnie	Posterior	Modified Lateral
Spinal injection	++	++	–
Epidural injection	++	++	–
Vertebral artery injection	+	(+)	–
Intravenous injection	+	+	+
Pneumothorax	+	+	+
Discomfort	(+)	++	(+)
Conditions for catheter placement	–	+	++

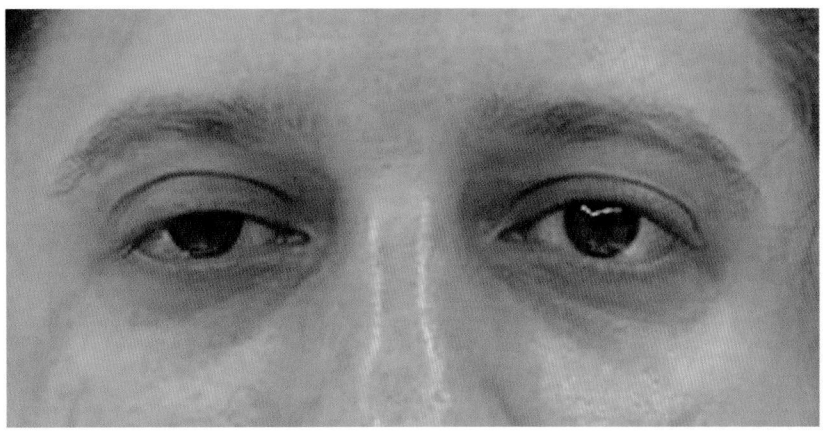

FIGURE 80B-12. Horner syndrome is common after interscalene block and consists of ptosis, myosis, and enophthalmia.

are hoarseness (10%–20%) due to the blockade of the recurrent laryngeal nerve, which occurs more frequently on the right side. Horner syndrome is characterized by ptosis, myosis, and enopthalmia due to the diffusion of the local anesthetic solution on the sympathetic cervical ganglion chain (including the stellatum ganglion) (Figure 80B–12). The reason for this complication is the spread of the local anesthetic around the anterior scalene muscle behind the carotid artery and internal jugular vein toward the longus colli muscle (Figure 80B–13). This results in blockade of the cervical ganglion (Horner syndrome) and phrenic nerve, which are located in this area. In addition, the superior laryngeal nerve (Figure 80B–14) can be affected. It occurs in 40%–60% of patients and resolves with resolution of the block; patient reassurance is all that is needed for management. Ipsilateral hemidiaphragmatic paresis is a common finding and may be present in nearly 100% of patients[40] (Figure 80B–15). However, this rarely presents a problem clinically, and most patients are not aware of it. The paradoxical Bezold-Jarisch reflex (occurrence of bradycardia and hypotension; incidence 15%–30%), can occur when the patient is placed in the sitting position for shoulder surgery and can be prevented by avoiding hypovolemia. It is easily treated by atropine and ephedrine administration.

Early complications (soon after block administration), such as epidural, spinal, or intravascular injection are primarily related to the approach chosen (see Table 80A–5). Late complications include neuropathy, mechanical plexus injury, and infection.

Nerve injuries are a well-recognized complication of anesthesia, although nerve injury directly attributable to interscalene block is extremely rare.[41,42]

Factors related to patient position, such as the use of shoulder braces and the head position, malposition of the arms, and sustained neck extension may increase the risk of injury.[42] Little data are available on the rate of complications related to the use of the continuous interscalene catheters.[43,44] Table 80B–6 lists reported complications of interscalene blocks and suggestions on how to avoid them.

SUMMARY

Interscalene nerve block is one of the most clinically applicable nerve block techniques. With proper training, equipment, and monitoring precautions the technique results in a predictable success rate, excellent anesthesia, and superb postoperative analgesia.

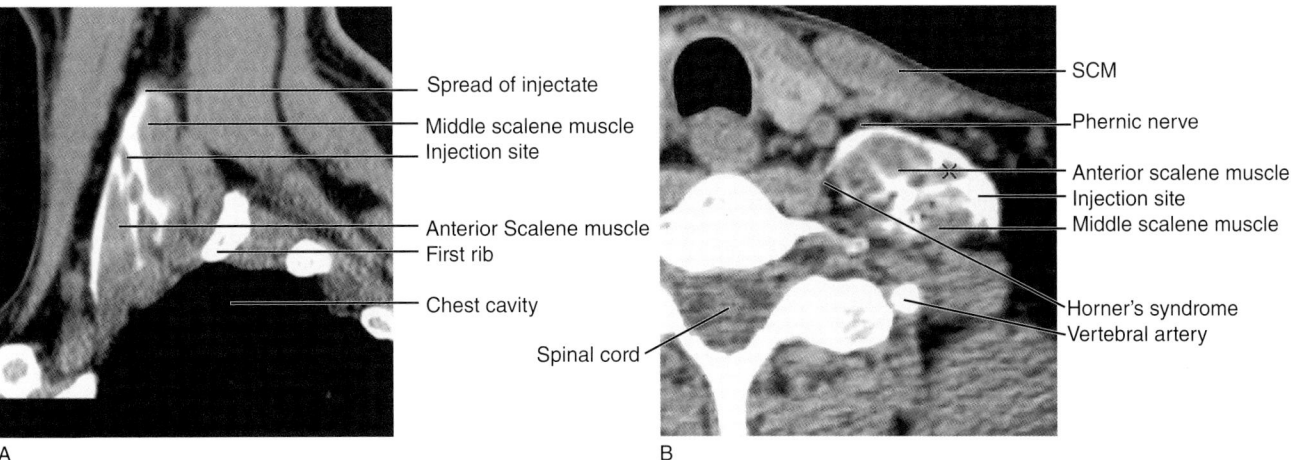

FIGURE 80B–13. Spread of the solution after injection into interscalane space. The contrast is seen in the scalene space around brachial plexus as well as dispersing underneath cervical fascia over anterior and middle scalene muscles. This spread helps explain the common occurrence of phrenic block and Horner's syndrome after ISBPB.

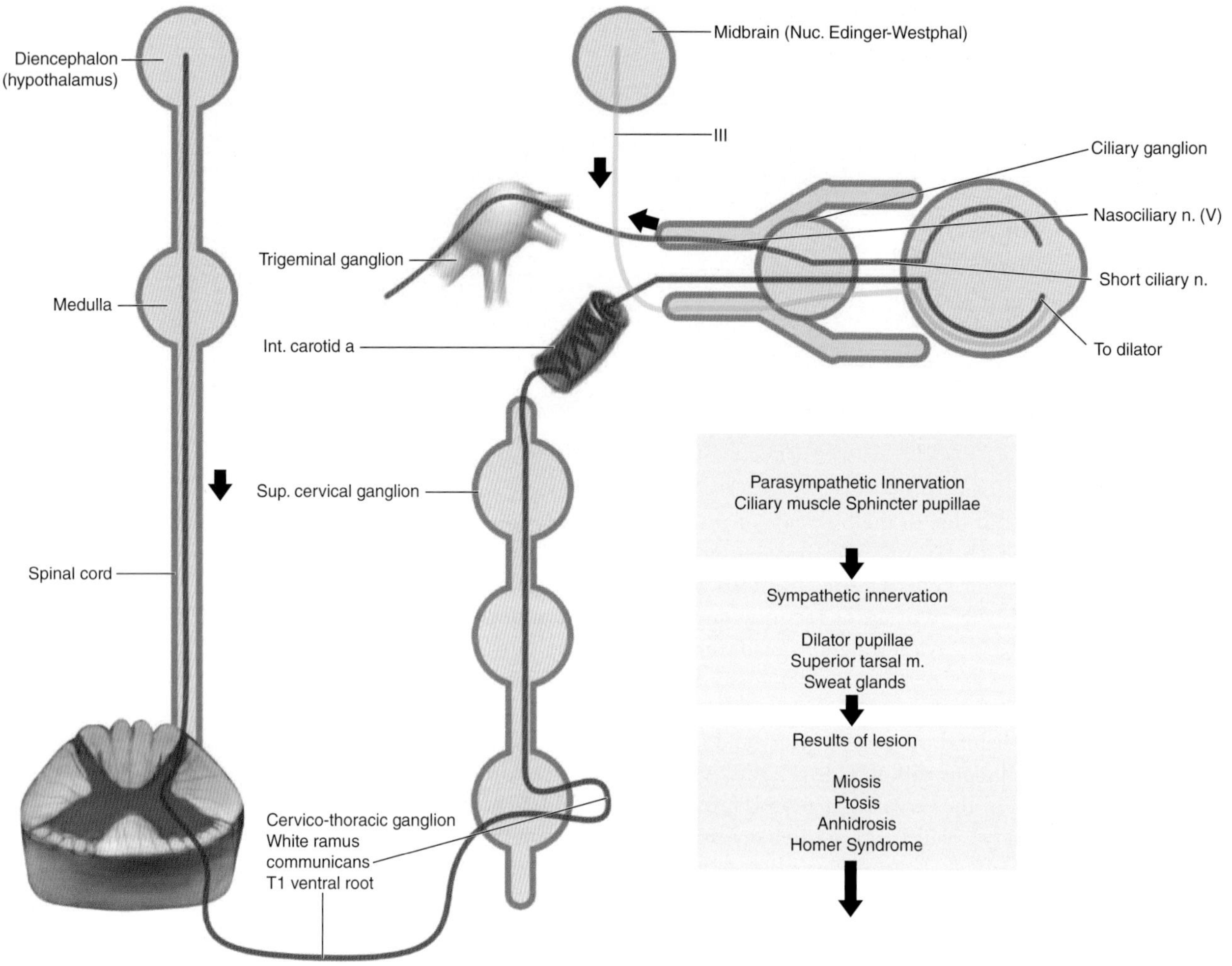

Diencephalon
(hypothalamus)

Midbrain (Nuc. Edinger-Westphal)

III

Ciliary ganglion

Nasociliary n. (V)

Trigeminal ganglion

Short ciliary n.

Medulla

Int. carotid a

To dilator

Sup. cervical ganglion

Spinal cord

Parasympathetic Innervation
Ciliary muscle Sphincter pupillae

Sympathetic innervation

Dilator pupillae
Superior tarsal m.
Sweat glands

Results of lesion

Miosis
Ptosis
Anhidrosis
Homer Syndrome

Cervico-thoracic ganglion
White ramus
communicans
T1 ventral root

FIGURE 80B–14. Horner syndrome results from interruption of the sympathetic pathway anywhere from the hypothalamus (diencephalon) to the eye.

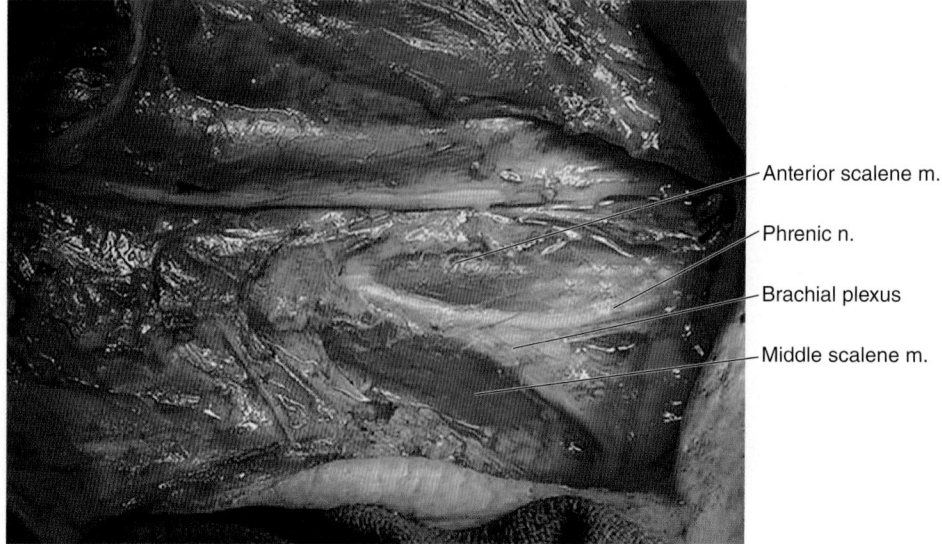

Anterior scalene m.

Phrenic n.

Brachial plexus

Middle scalene m.

FIGURE 80B–15. Neck dissection reveals the relationship of the phrenic nerve, which leaves the brachial plexus anteriorly, and the rest of the brachial plexus, which remains sandwiched between the anterior and middle scalene muscles.

TABLE 80B–6. Complications and how to avoid them.

Infection	• A strict aseptic technique is used
Hematoma	• Avoid multiple needle insertions, particularly in anticoagulated patients • Apply steady pressure for 5 min when carotid artery is inadvertently punctured • Use a smaller gauge needle to localize the brachial plexus in patients with difficult anatomy • In the absence of spontaneous bleeding, the use of anticoagulant therapy should not be regarded as a contraindication for this block
Vascular puncture	• Vascular puncture is not common with this technique • Apply steady pressure for 5 min when the carotid artery is punctured
Local anesthetic toxicity	• Systemic toxicity due to absorption of local anesthetic after interscalene block is rare • Systemic toxicity most commonly occurs during or shortly after injection of local anesthetic; this is most commonly caused by an inadvertent intravascular injection or channeling of forcefully injected local anesthetic into small veins or lymphatic channels cut during needle manipulation • Large volumes of long-acting anesthetic should be reconsidered in older and frail patients. • Careful and frequent aspiration should be performed during the injection • Avoid forceful, fast injection of local anesthetic
Nerve injury	• Never inject local anesthetic when abnormal pressure on injection is encountered (opening pressure >15 psi) • Local anesthetic should never be injected when patient complains of severe pain or exhibits a withdrawal reaction on injection
Total spinal anesthesia	• When stimulation is obtained with current intensity of <0.2 mA, the needle should be pulled back to obtain the same response with current >0.2 mA before injecting local anesthetic to avoid injection into the dural sleeves and the consequent epidural or spinal spread • Never inject local anesthetic when abnormal pressure on injection is encountered
Horner syndrome	• Occurrence of ipsilateral ptosis, hyperemia of the conjunctiva, and nasal congestion is common, and it is dependent on the site of injection (less common with the low interscalene approach) and total volume of local anesthetic injected; patients should be instructed on the occurrence of this syndrome and reassured about its benign nature
Diaphragmatic paralysis	• Commonly present; avoid interscalene blockade or a large volume of local anesthetic in patients

REFERENCES

1. Etienne J: Regional anesthesia: Its application in the surgical treatment of cancer of the breast [French], Faculté de Médecin de Paris, 1925.
2. Winnie AP: Interscalene brachial plexus block. Anesth Analg 1970;49:455–466.
3. Borgeat A, Ekatodramis G: Anaesthesia for shoulder surgery. Best Pract Res Clin Anaesthesiol 2002;16:211–225.
4. Kapral S, Greher M, Huber G, et al: Ultrasonographic guidance improves the success rate of interscalene brachial plexus blockade. Reg Anesth Pain Med 2008;33:253–258.
5. McNaught A, Shastri U, Carmichael N, et al: Ultrasound reduces the minimum effective local anaesthetic volume compared with peripheral nerve stimulation for interscalene block. Br J Anaesth 2011;106:124–130.
6. Gautier P, Vandepitte C, Ramquet C, et al: The minimum effective anaesthetic volume of 0.75% ropivacaine in ultrasound-guided interscalene brachial plexus block. Anesth Analg 2011;113:951–955.
7. Bonica JJ: Anatomic and physiologic basis of nociception and pain. In Bonica JJ (ed). *The Management of Pain*, 2nd ed. Philadelphia, PA: Lea & Febiger, 1990, pp 28–94.
8. Bonica JJ (ed): Postoperative pain. In *The Management of Pain*, 2nd ed. Philadephia, PA: Lea & Febiger, 1990, pp 461–480.
9. Hollinshead WH: Anatomy for Surgeons, 3rd ed. Philadelphia, PA: Harper & Row, 1982

10. DePalma AF: *Surgery of the Shoulder*, 3rd ed. Philadelphia, PA: Lippincott, 1983.
11. Gardner E: The innervation of the shoulder joint. Anat Rec 1948;102:1–18.
12. Dutton RP, Eckhardt WF 3rd, Sunder N: Total spinal anesthesia after interscalene blockade of the brachial plexus. Anesthesiology 1994;80:939–941.
13. Ross S, Scarborough CD: Total spinal anesthesia following brachialplexus block. Anesthesiology 1973;39:458.
14. Scammell SJ: Case report: Inadvertent epidural anaesthesia as a complication of interscalene brachial plexus block. Anaesth Intensive Care 1979;7:56–57.
15. Benumof JL: Permanent loss of cervical cord function associated with interscalene block performed under general anesthesia. Anesthesiology 2000;93:151–154.
16. Pippa P, Cominelli E, Marinelli C, Aito S: Brachial plexus block using the posterior approach. Eur J Anaesthesiol 1990;7:411–420.
17. Dagli G, Guzeldemir ME, Volkan Acar H: The effects and side effects of interscalene brachial plexus block by posterior approach. Reg Anesth Pain Med 1998;23:87–91.
18. Rucci FS, Pippa P, Barbagli R, Doni L: How many interscalenic blocks are there? A comparison between the lateral and posterior approach. Eur J Anaesthesiol 1993;10:303–307.
19. Boezaart AP, De Beer JF, Nell ML: Early experience with continuous cervical paravertebral block using a stimulating catheter. Reg Anesth Pain Med 2003;28:406–413.

20. Meier G, Bauereis C, Heinrich C: [Interscalene brachial plexus catheter for anesthesia and postoperative pain therapy. Experience with a modified technique]. Anaesthesist 1997;46:715–719.

21. Hadzic A, Vloka JD (eds): Interscalene brachial plexus block. In *Peripheral Nerve Blocks: Principles and Practice*. New York, NY: McGraw-Hill, 2003, pp 1009–1029.

22. Low interscalene abstract from ASRA 2005 presentation.

23. Dickerman D, Vloka JD, Koorn R, Hadzic A: Excessive noise levels during orthopedic surgery. Reg Anesth 1997;22:97.

24. Brown AR, Weiss R, Greenberg C, et al: Interscalene block for shoulder arthroscopy: Comparison with general anesthesia. Arthroscopy 1993;9:295–300.

25. Tetzlaff JE, Yoon HJ, O'Hara J, et al: Alkalinization of mepivacaine accelerates onset of interscalene block for shoulder surgery. Reg Anesth Pain Med 1990;15:242–244.

26. Klein SM, Greengrass RA, Steele SM, et al: A comparison of 0.5% bupivacaine, 0.5% ropivacaine, and 0.75% ropivacaine for interscalene brachial plexus block. Anesth Analg 1998;87:1316–1319.

27. Casati A, Borghi B, Fanelli G, et al: Interscalene brachial plexus anesthesia and analgesia for open shoulder surgery: A randomized, double-blinded comparison between levobupivacaine and ropivacaine. Anesth Analg 2003;96:253–259.

28. Singelyn FJ, Gouverneur JM, Robert A: A minimum dose of clonidine added to mepivacaine prolongs the duration of anesthesia and analgesia after axillary brachial plexus block. Anesth Analg 1996;83:1046–1050.

29. Picard PR, Tramer MR, McQuay HJ, Moore RA: Analgesic efficacy of peripheral opioids (all except intra-articular): A qualitative systematic review of randomised controlled trials. Pain 1997;72:309–318.

30. Bouaziz H, Kinirons BP, Macalou D, et al: Sufentanil does not prolong the duration of analgesia in a mepivacaine brachial plexus block: a dose response study. Anesth Analg 2000;90:383–387.

31. Tetzlaff JE, Yoon HJ, Brems J, Javorsky T: Alkalinization of mepivacaine improves the quality of motor block associated with interscalene brachial plexus anesthesia for shoulder surgery. Reg Anesth Pain Med 1995;20:128–132.

32. Hadzic A, Williams BA, Kraca PE, et al: For outpatient rotator cuff surgery, nerve block anesthesia provides superior same-day recovery over general anesthesia. Anesthesiology 2005;102:1001–1007.

33. Klein SM, Grant SA, Greengrass RA, et al: Interscalene brachial plexus block with a continuous catheter insertion system and a disposable infusion pump. Anesth Analg 2000;91:1473–1478.

34. Borgeat A, Schappi B, Biasca N, Gerber C: Patient-controlled analgesia after major shoulder surgery: patient-controlled interscalene analgesia versus patient-controlled analgesia. Anesthesiology 1997;87:1343–1347.

35. Singelyn FJ, Seguy S, Gouverneur JM: Interscalene brachial plexus analgesia after open shoulder surgery: Continuous versus patient-controlled infusion. Anesth Analg 1999;89:1216–1220.

36. Borgeat A, Tewes E, Biasca N, Gerber C: Patient-controlled interscalene analgesia with ropivacaine after major shoulder surgery: PCIA vs PCA. Br J Anaesth 1998;81:603–605.

37. Borgeat A, Kalberer F, Jacob H, et al: Patient-controlled interscalene analgesia with ropivacaine 0.2% versus bupivacaine 0.15% after major open shoulder surgery: The effects on hand motor function. Anesth Analg 2001;92:218–223.

38. Rosenberg PH, Heinonen E: Differential sensitivity of A and C nerve fibres to long-acting amide local anaesthetics. Br J Anaesth 1983;55:163–167.

39. Wildsmith JA, Brown DT, Paul D, Johnson S: Structure-activity relationships in differential nerve block at high and low frequency stimulation. Br J Anaesth 1989;63:444–452.

40. Urmey WF, Talts KH, Shrarock NE: One hundred percent incidence of hemi-diaphragmatic paresis associated with interscalene brachial plexus anesthesia as diagnosed by ultrasonography. Anesth Analg 1991;72:498–503.

41. Todd MM, Brown DL: Regional anesthesia and postoperative pain management: long-term benefits from a short-term intervention. Anesthesiology 1999;91:1–2.

42. Kroll DA, Caplan RA, Posner K, et al: Nerve injury associated with anesthesia. Anesthesiology 1990;73:202–207.

43. Borgeat A, Ekatodramis G, Kalberer F, Benz C: Acute and nonacute complications associated with interscalene block and shoulder surgery: A prospective study. Anesthesiology 2001;95:875–880.

44. Borgeat A, Dullenkopf A, Ekatodramis G, Nagy L: Evaluation of the lateral modified approach for continuous interscalene block after shoulder surgery. Anesthesiology 2003;99:436–442.

CHAPTER 80C

Supraclavicular Brachial Plexus Block

Carlo D. Franco, Bram Byloos, and Ilvana Hasanbegovic

INTRODUCTION

The supraclavicular block is one of several techniques used to anesthetize the brachial plexus. The block is performed at the level of the brachial plexus trunks where almost the entire sensory, motor, and sympathetic innervation of the upper extremity is carried in just three nerve structures confined to a very small surface area. Consequently, this technique typically provides a predictable, dense block with rapid onset.[1-3] In 1911, Georg Hirschel described a surgical approach to the brachial plexus in the axilla. A few months later, Diedrich Kulenkampff, in Germany, performed the first percutaneous supraclavicular approach, reportedly on himself. The technique was published in 1928 by Kulenkampff and Persky.[4] As they described it, the technique was performed with the patient in the sitting position ("a regular chair will suffice") or in the supine position with a pillow between the shoulders. The operator sat on a stool at the side of the patient. The needle was inserted above the midpoint of the clavicle where the pulse of the subclavian artery could be felt and was directed medially toward the spinous process of T2 or T3. Kulenkampff 's familiarity with brachial plexus anatomy allowed him to recognize that "the best way to reach the trunks was in the neighborhood of the subclavian artery over the first rib." His technique was also simple: "all the branches of the plexus could be anesthetized through one injection." These two assertions are still valid today. Unfortunately. his advice on needle direction carried an inherently high risk of pneumothorax. The popularity of the supraclavicular block remained unrivaled during the entire first half of the 20th century until well after World War II. During this time the technique underwent several modifications, most of them intended to reduce the risk of pneumothorax.[1,5-8]

The introduction of axillary techniques by Accardo and Adriani[9] in 1949 and by Burnham[10] in 1958 marked the beginning of the decline in enthusiasm for the supraclavicular block. The axillary block was particularly popularized after a publication in the journal *Anesthesiology* by Rudolph De Jong in 1961[11] The paper was based on cadaver dissections and included the now well-known calculation of 42 mL as the volume needed to fill a cylinder 6 cm long (axillary sheath); according to De Jong, this dose "should be sufficient to completely bathe all branches of the brachial plexus." The article was also critical of the supraclavicular approach. Coincidentally, the same journal published a paper by Brand and Papper,[12] who compared axillary and supraclavicular techniques and warned of the 6.1% rate of pneumothorax frequently quoted for supraclavicular block.

More modern modifications of supraclavicular block include Alon Winnie and Vincent Collins's subclavian perivascular technique[13] and the "plumb-bob" technique of Brown and collaborators.[14] The former is more a concept than a radically different technique, stating that plexus anesthesia is performed around a main vessel (perivascular) and within the confines of a sheath. Otherwise, their technique is similar to Murphey's,[7] who in 1944, described a single-injection technique performed just lateral to the anterior scalene muscle directing the needle caudad. The plumb-bob technique, published in 1993, is based on cadaver dissections and magnetic resonance imaging performed on volunteers. In this technique, the needle is introduced above the clavicle, just lateral to the sternocleidomastoid (SCM) muscle and advanced perpendicularly to the plexus in an anteroposterior direction. If the needle misses the plexus, the pleural dome could be penetrated.

Many investigators appear to perceive the supraclavicular block as being complex and associated with a significant risk of pneumothorax. However, its rapid onset, dense and predictable anesthesia, and high success rate make it a very useful approach, which, according to Brown and collaborators,[14] is "unrivaled" by other techniques. Indeed, in our practice, the supraclavicular approach is the cornerstone of distal upper extremity regional anesthesia, and we use it extensively with a very low rate of complications.[15]

INDICATIONS

The supraclavicular block provides anesthesia and analgesia to the upper extremity below the shoulder. It is an excellent choice for elbow and hand surgery.

CONTRAINDICATIONS

General contraindications to the use of this technique are those that apply to any regional block, such as local infection, significant coagulation abnormalities, and inability to cooperate during block placement or surgery. Like interscalene block, supraclavicular block is not used bilaterally or in patients with respiratory compromise because of the potential risk of pneumothorax or phrenic nerve block.

ANATOMY OF THE BRACHIAL PLEXUS ABOVE THE CLAVICLE

The brachial plexus is formed by five roots originating from the ventral divisions of C5 through T1. The roots lie between the anterior and middle scalene muscles (Figure 80C–1). The anterior scalene muscle originates from the anterior tubercles of the transverse processes of C3 through C6 and inserts on the scalene tubercle of the upper surface of the first rib. The middle scalene muscle originates in the posterior tubercles of the transverse processes of C2 through C7 and

inserts on the upper surface of the first rib behind the subclavian groove. The five roots converge toward one another to form three trunks—upper, middle, and lower—which are stacked one on top of the other as they traverse the triangular interscalene groove, formed between the anterior and middle scalene muscles.

This space becomes wider in the anteroposterior plane as the muscles approach their insertion on the first rib. The subclavian artery accompanies the brachial plexus in the interscalene groove anterior to the lower trunk. Although the roots of the plexus are long, the trunks are almost as short as they are wide, soon giving rise to anterior and posterior divisions as they reach the clavicle. Figure 81C–1 shows the clinical anatomy of the brachial plexus and surrounding structures in the supraclavicular area.

The pleura can potentially be injured in two places during a supraclavicular block; the pleural dome and the first intercostal space. The pleural dome is the apex of the parietal pleura, circumscribed by the first rib. The first rib is a short, broad, and flattened bone shaped like the letter C. It's medial border forms the outer boundary of the pleural dome. The anterior scalene, by inserting in this border of the first rib, comes in contact medially with the pleural dome. There is no pleural dome lateral to the anterior scalene muscle. The first intercostal space on the other hand, is for the most part infraclavicular (see Figure 81C–1) and consequently should not be reached when a supraclavicular block is properly performed.

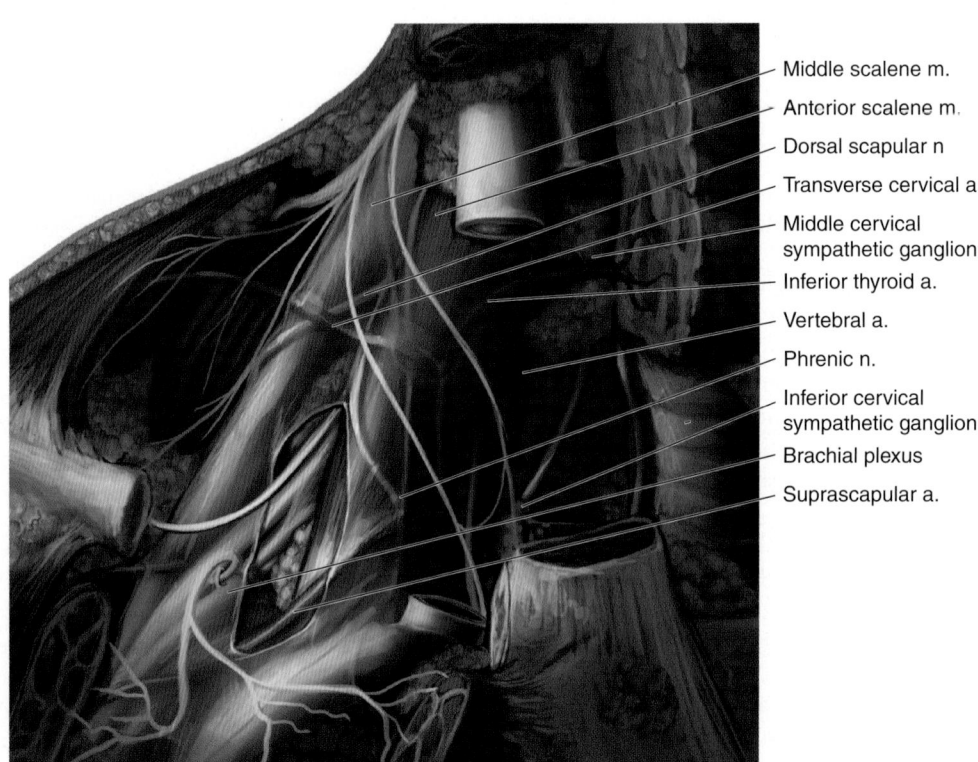

- Middle scalene m.
- Anterior scalene m.
- Dorsal scapular n
- Transverse cervical a.
- Middle cervical sympathetic ganglion
- Inferior thyroid a.
- Vertebral a.
- Phrenic n.
- Inferior cervical sympathetic ganglion
- Brachial plexus
- Suprascapular a.

FIGURE 80C–1. Anatomy of the brachial plexus at the low interscalene space and supraclavicular area.

Clinical Pearls

- With the shoulder pulled down, the three trunks of the brachial plexus are located above the clavicle; therefore, the block needle should never need to reach below the clavicle during a supraclavicular block.
- The first intercostal space is located below the clavicle, thus its penetration is unlikely during a properly performed supraclavicular block.
- The needle should never cross the parasagittal plane medial to the anterior scalene muscle because of the risk of pneumothorax.
- The SCM muscle inserts on the medial third of the clavicle, and the trapezius muscle on the lateral third of it, leaving the middle third for the neurovascular bundle. These proportions are maintained regardless of patient's size.
- Because the brachial plexus moves from medial to lateral as it descends, the higher in the supraclavicular area the more medial (closer to the SCM) the plexus is located.

LANDMARKS

The technique described in this chapter combines the simplicity of the original single-injection Kulenkampff technique with important anatomic principles, which should make the technique safer than the original description. The main landmarks for this block are the lateral insertion of the SCM muscle in the clavicle, the clavicle itself, and the patient's midline. These three landmarks are easily identifiable in the majority of patients.

EQUIPMENT

- Gloves
- Antiseptic solution for skin disinfection

- Marking pen
- Sterile gauze
- Two 20-mL syringes for local anesthetic solution
- One 1-mL syringe with a 25-gauge needle for skin wheal
- One 5-cm, short-beveled, 22-gauge insulated needle
- Surface electrode
- Nerve stimulator
- Injection pressure monitor

TECHNIQUE

Ideally, the block is performed in a room dedicated to regional anesthesia with American Society of Anesthesiologists (ASA) standard monitors, an oxygen source, suctioning, and resuscitation equipment and drugs including lipid emulsion. A contingency plan for emergencies must be in place to deal safely and expeditiously with any emergency that might arise.

If not contraindicated, this block is best performed after premedication (e.g., midazolam 1 mg plus fentanyl 50 mcg IV for the average adult). In young and healthy patients, this dose can be repeated as necessary. The patient is best kept sedated but cooperative and able to relate pain or any undue discomfort.

The block is performed with the patient in a semisitting position with the head rotated to the opposite side as shown in Figure 80C–2A. The semisitting position is more comfortable than the supine position both for the patient and the operator. Because patient positioning is very important in regional anesthesia, the operator should not try to recognize any landmarks until the patient has adopted the desired position. The patient is asked to lower the shoulder and flex the elbow, so the forearm rests on the lap. The wrist is supinated so the palm of the hand faces the patient's face, as shown in Figure 80C–2B. This maneuver allows for detection of any subtle finger movement produced by nerve stimulation. If the patient cannot supinate their wrist, a roll is placed under it so the fingers are free to move.

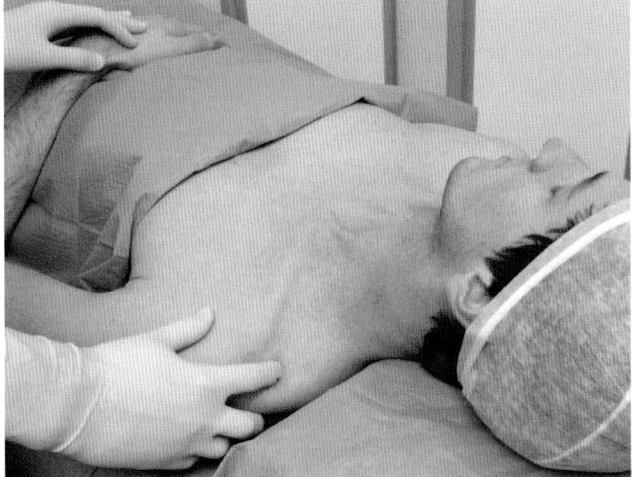

A

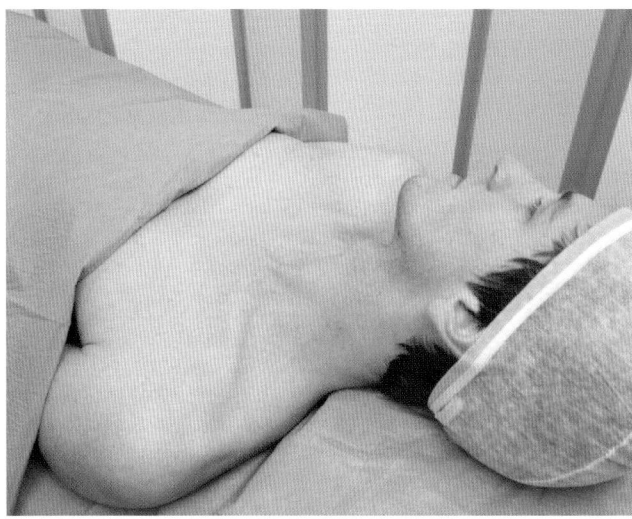

B

FIGURE 80C–2. A: Patient positioning. The patient lies in a semisitting or supine position with the head turned away from the side to be blocked. **B**: The shoulder is down, the elbow is flexed, and the palm of the hand rests on the patient's lap while it is turned toward his face.

The operator usually stands on the side to be blocked, so for a left-side block, the palpation is done with the left hand and the needle is manipulated with the right (see Figure 80C–2B).

For a right-side block, the operator manipulates the needle with the left hand and palpates with the right. However, the operator may choose to manipulate the needle with their preferred hand regardless of the block side.

Point of Needle Entrance

With the patient in the described semisitting position and the shoulder down, the lateral (posterior) border of the SCM muscle is identified and followed distally to the point where it meets the clavicle. This particular point is marked on the skin over the clavicle, as shown in Figure 80C–3. The lateral border of the SCM is usually clearly visible at the level where the external jugular vein crosses it. From this level, the border can be traced caudally to the point where it meets the clavicle. A parasagittal line (parallel to the midline) is drawn at this level to recognize an area medial to it that is at risk for pneumothorax. The point of needle entrance is found lateral to this parasagittal plane, separated by a distance we call "margin of safety." This distance is about 1 in. (2.5 cm) lateral to the insertion of the SCM on the clavicle, as shown in Figure 80C–4. The margin of safety can be alternatively established using a distance equal to the width of the clavicular head of the SCM at its insertion on the clavicle.[16]

The palpating index finger is placed at this site as shown in Figure 80C–5. We customarily draw two arrows at this location pointing to each other. The proximal arrow, above the finger, is used to localize the needle entrance point, the distal one shows the direction of the needle path.

The needle is inserted immediately cephalad to the palpating finger and advanced first perpendicularly to the skin for 2–5 mm (depending on the amount of the patient's subcutaneous tissue) and then turned caudally under the palpating finger to advance it in a direction that is parallel to the midline, as shown in Figure 80C–5.

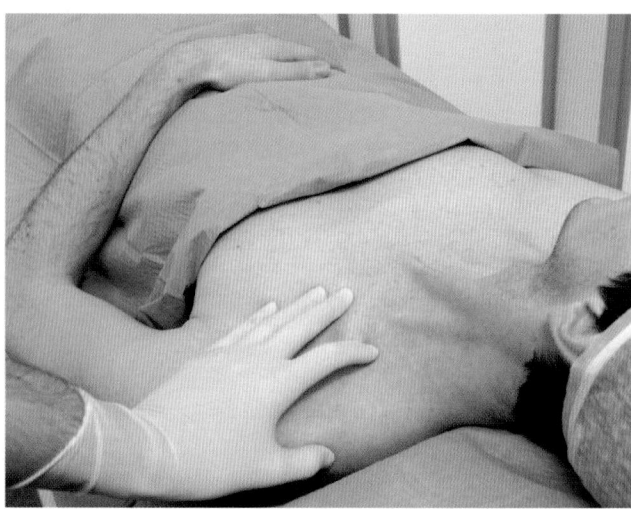

FIGURE 80C–4. Margin of safety. A distance of approximately 1 in. (2.5 cm) is measured laterally from the SCM, to assure the needle placement away from the pleural dome.

The block should take place above the clavicle, under the palpating finger. As a goal we like to elicit an isolated muscle twitch in all fingers either in flexion or extension to confirm needle proximity to the lower trunks of the plexus. Any other response carries a significantly lower success rate.[17]

If repositioning of the needle is necessary, the needle is withdrawn and the angle is adjusted in the anteroposterior plane, but always parallel to the midline and never directed medially.

Nerve Stimulator Settings

The nerve stimulator is initially set to a current intensity of around 0.8 mA and a pulse width of 100 μs. Once the desired response is obtained (i.e., a muscle twitch of the fingers) injection is initiated without reducing the nerve stimulator current.

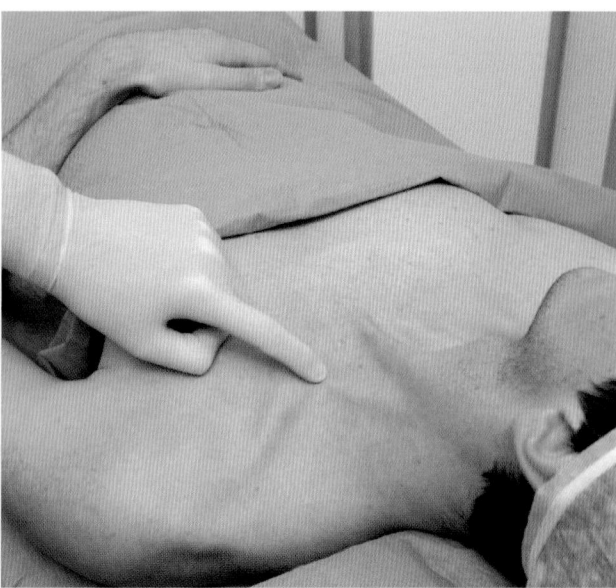

FIGURE 80C–3. Landmarks. The lateral insertion of the SCM to the clavicle is shown underneath the palpating finger.

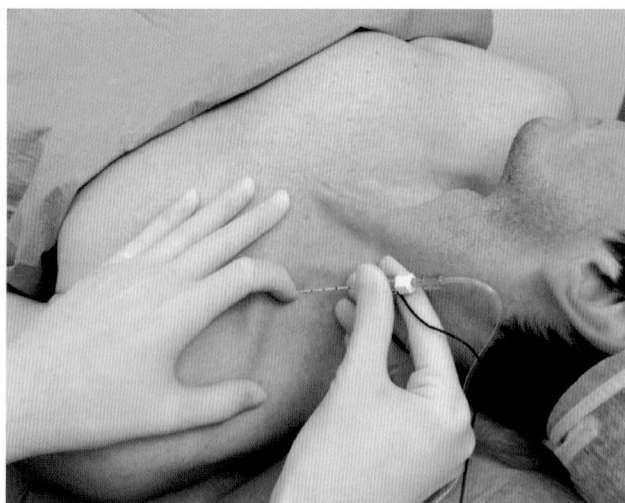

FIGURE 80C–5. Point of needle entrance and direction. The point of needle entrance is located just cephalad to the palpating finger and one fingerbreadth above the clavicle. The needle is first introduced perpendicular to the skin and is then turned and advanced parallel to the midline.

This is a unique characteristic of the supraclavicular block. One study has shown that the onset, duration, and success rate with a supraclavicular block is unaffected by reducing the nerve stimulator to 0.9 mA or less.[18] Supraclavicular and lumbar plexus blocks are the only peripheral nerve blocks in which injecting at a higher current than 0.5 mA is recommended.

Clinical Pearls

- The lateral border of the SCM muscle follows a straight line from the mastoid to the clavicle.
- The needle is inserted in a direction that is parallel to the midline.
- Depending on the patient's weight, the palpating finger needs to exert different amounts of pressure on the deeper tissues. This maneuver helps bring the plexus closer to the skin and makes the trajectory of the needle shorter.
- The needle should never be inserted deeper than 1 in. (2.5 cm) if a twitch from the brachial plexus is not present.
- Because the trunks are contiguous, elicited twitches from one trunk follow the other without interruption. If the twitches instead disappear before reaching the lower trunk, the needle is withdrawn to the point of the previous twitch and advanced with a slight change in the anteroposterior angle of insertion.
- The margin of safety of about 1 in. (2.5 cm) lateral to the insertion of the SCM on the clavicle provides a safe distance lateral to the outer boundary of the pleural dome for the needle to travel. Because of the steep downward direction of the trunks, increasing this distance laterally may prevent the needle from contacting the plexus above the clavicle or miss the short trunks altogether.
- In the supraclavicular block, an initial nerve stimulator current of 0.8 mA is high enough to produce guidance into the plexus, but low enough to assure sufficient proximity for successful blockade.
- The risk of intraneural injection is minimized by using low injection pressures and meticulous technique.
- The injection is performed slowly with frequent aspirations while carefully observing the patient.
- If pain or abnormal pressure is felt at any point during injection, the needle should be withdrawn 1–2 mm, after which a new assessment is made.

CONTINUOUS TECHNIQUE

Traditionally, the supraclavicular technique has not been considered to be an optimal choice for placement of catheters. The great mobility of the neck at this location carries a risk for catheter dislodgement. Tunneling the catheter to the infraclavicular level could help to make the catheter more stable; however, little data are currently available on this topic.

LOCAL ANESTHETIC CHOICES FOR SINGLE-SHOT AND CATHETER TECHNIQUES

Most of upper extremity surgeries performed under regional anesthesia last 1–3 hours. Consequently, we most commonly use 30 mL of 1.5% mepivacaine with 1:200,000 epinephrine, which provides about 3–4 hours of anesthesia. The same anesthetic solution without epinephrine provides about 2–3 hours of anesthesia. To speed block onset, 2 mL of 8.4% sodium bicarbonate may be added to every 20 mL of mepivacaine solution. Solutions of levobupivacaine, ropivacaine, or bupivacaine provide longer acting anesthesia (5–7 hours) when required. Recent studies have suggested that the use of ultrasound guidance may reduce the volume needed for a successful block.[19] For continuous techniques, a bolus dose of about 10–15 mL of local anesthetic solution can be given, followed by an infusion rate of 8–10 mL/h. A solution of 0.2% ropivacaine can be used for this purpose. A patient-controlled bolus of 3–5 Ll every 30–60 minutes can be added, with the basal infusion decreased to around 5 mL/h. Breakthrough pain must be treated with a bolus of local anesthetic because simply increasing the rate of infusion could take several hours to have an effect.

PERIOPERATIVE MANAGEMENT

The patient that receives single-shot blocks can undergo surgery under intravenous sedation titrated to the patient's comfort. The sedation requirements vary from patient to patient and range from small intermittent boluses of midazolam or fentanyl, to a propofol infusion at 25–50 mcg/kg/min, to light general anesthesia.

COMPLICATIONS

Common side effects associated with this technique include phrenic nerve block with diaphragmatic paralysis and sympathetic nerve block with development of Horner syndrome. These are typically self-limiting and do not require intervention. Phrenic nerve block reportedly occurs about 50% of the time, although this may be reduced by the use of ultrasound guidance.[20,21]

Intravascular injection with systemic local anesthetic toxicity and hematoma formation can also occur. To reduce the risk, high level of vigilance is needed due to the risch vascularity of the supraclavicular region.[22] In the case of the supraclavicular block, this can be due to puncture of the subclavian, transverse cervical or dorsal scapular arteries, all of which are located near the plexus at this level.

Pneumothorax occurs as often as 6.1%, which was an incidence reported in 1961 that compared 230 consecutive supraclavicular blocks with 246 consecutive axillary blocks.[12] However, the comparison was neither blinded nor randomized, and the study used several different techniques.[7] In contrast, this complication is rare in the modern literature.[15]

It is frequently mentioned that the pneumothorax complicating a supraclavicular block has a delayed onset.[23,24] Although such cases have been published in the literature, most of the pneumothoraces reported have been diagnosed within a few hours of the procedure and before the patient's discharge.[1,25] Based on the available literature, the pneumothorax associated with supraclavicular block is uncommon, typically small, and it presents within a few hours following the procedure. In some instances its presentation can be delayed up to 12 hours.

SUMMARY

Supraclavicular block is a reliable, rapid-onset approach to brachial plexus anesthesia. The anatomy of the brachial plexus, with its three trunks confined to a much-reduced surface area, affords a high success rate for achieving anesthesia in the upper extremity below the shoulder. A combination of good anatomic knowledge, simple landmarks, and meticulous technique are paramount for consistent success rate and limiting its potential for complications.

REFERENCES

1. Moore D: Supraclavicular approach for block of the brachial plexus. In Moore D (ed): *Regional Block. A Handbook for Use in the Clinical Practice of Medicine and Surgery,* 4th ed. Thomas, Springfield, IL: 1981, pp 221–242.
2. Lanz E, Theiss D, Jankovic D: The extent of blockade following various techniques of brachial plexus block. Anesth Analg 1983;62:55–58.
3. Urmey W: Upper extremity blocks. In Brown D (ed): *Regional Anesthesia and Analgesia.* Philadelphia, PA: Saunders, 1996; pp 254–278.
4. Kulenkampff D, Persky M: Brachial plexus anesthesia. Its indications, technique and dangers. Ann Surg 1928;87:883–891.
5. Labat G: Regional *Anesthesia. Its Technic and Clinical Application.* Philadelphia, PA: Saunders, 1922.
6. Patrick J: The technique of brachial plexus block anesthesia. Br J Surg 1940;27:734–739.
7. Murphey D: Brachial plexus block anesthesia: an improved technic. Ann Surg 1944;119:935–943.
8. Winnie A: *Plexus Anesthesia. Perivascular Techniques of Brachial Plexus Block.* Philadelphia, PA: Saunders, 1993.
9. Accardo N, Adriani J: Brachial plexus block: a simplified technic using the axillary route. South Med J 1949;42:920.
10. Burnham P: Regional anesthesia of the great nerves of the upper arm. Anesthesiology 1958;19:281–284.
11. De Jong R: Axillary block of the brachial plexus. Anesthesiology 1961;22:215–225.
12. Brand L, Papper E: A comparison of supraclavicular and axillary techniques for brachial plexus blocks. Anesthesiology 1961;22:226–229.
13. Winnie A, Collins V: The subclavian perivascular technique of brachial plexus anesthesia. Anesthesiology 1964;25:353–363.
14. Brown DL, Cahill D, Bridenbaugh D: Supraclavicular nerve block: anatomic analysis of a method to prevent pneumothorax. Anesth Analg 1993;76:530–534.
15. Franco C, Vieira Z: 1,001 subclavian perivascular brachial plexus blocks: success with a nerve stimulator. Reg Anesth Pain Med 2000;25:41–46.
16. Franco CD: The subclavian perivascular block. Tech Reg Anesth Pain Manage 1999;3:212–216.
17. Haleem, Shahla; Siddiqui, Ahsan K.; Mowafi, Hany A. Nerve Stimulator Evoked Motor Response Predicting a Successful Supraclavicular Brachial Plexus Block; More Anesthesia & Analgesia. 110(6):1745-1746, June 2010.
18. Franco C, Domashevich V, Voronov G, et al: The supraclavicular block with a nerve stimulator: To decrease or not to decrease, that is the question. Anesth Analg 2004;98:1167–1171.
19. Kant A, Gupta PK, Zohar S, et al: Application of the continual reassessment method to dose-finding studies in regional anesthesia: an estimate of the ED95 dose for 0.5% bupivacaine for ultrasound-guided supraclavicular block. Anesthesiology. 2013;119:29–35.
20. Neal J, Moore J, Kopacz D, et al: Quantitative analysis of respiratory, motor, and sensory function after supraclavicular block. Anesth Analg 1998;86:1239–1244.
21. Renes SH, Spoormans HH, Gielen MJ, et al: Hemidiaphragmatic paresis can be avoided in ultrasound-guided supraclavicular brachial plexus block. Reg Anesth Pain Med. 2009;34:595–599.
22. Murata H, Sakai A, Hadzic A, Sumikawa K.: The presence of transverse cervical and dorsal scapular arteries at three ultrasound probe positions commonly used in supraclavicular brachial plexus blockade. Anesth Analg. 2012;115:470–473.
23. Greengrass R, Steele S, Moretti G, et al: Peripheral nerve blocks. In Raj P (ed): *Textbook of Regional Anesthesia.* New York, NY: Churchill Livingstone, 2002, pp 325–377.
24. Neal J, Hebl J, Gerancher J, et al: Brachial plexus anesthesia: Essentials of our current understanding. Reg Anesth Pain Med 2002;27:402–428.
25. Harley N, Gjessing J: A critical assessment of supraclavicular brachial plexus block. Anesthesia 1969;24:564–570.

Infraclavicular Brachial Plexus Block

Laura Clark

INTRODUCTION

The infraclavicular block provides a block of the arm below the shoulder. Unlike the axillary approach, it can be performed without abduction of the arm, making it useful for patients with limited shoulder mobility. It is amenable to continuous catheter placement by being more accessible and more comfortable for a catheter than the axilla.

Georg Hirschel, in 1911, is considered to have carried out the first percutaneous axillary block because he approached the plexus from the axilla.[1] His goal was to place the local anesthetic on top of the first rib via the axilla. He discovered after his own dissections of the plexus the reason for incompleteness of the axillary block, and was the first to describe that the axillary and musculocutaneous nerves separated from the plexus much higher than in the axilla. However, the needles in the early 1900s were not long enough to reach this area to block those nerves.[2] To remedy this problem in 1911, Diedrich Kulenkampff's supraclavicular description was soon to follow.[2] He felt his technique was safer and more accurate than Hirschel's, but after initial success, the reports of complications of pneumothorax ensued.

In 1914, Bazy[3] described injecting below the clavicle just medial to the coracoid process along a line connecting with the Chassaignac tubercle. The needle trajectory was pointed away from the axilla, close to the clavicle, and was felt to present little chance of pleural damage. Several modifications occurred in the ensuing 8 years. Babitszky said that "to discuss the anatomical relationship and the technique more fully would be superfluous, as it is customary to familiarize oneself with the anatomy of the field in question on the cadaver any time one tends to use an unfamiliar technique."[2] Gaston Labat, in 1922, essentially redescribed Bazy's technique in his textbook, *Regional Anesthesia*,[5] as did Achille Dogliotti[6] in 1939. However, the technique seemed to fade into obscurity. For instance, infraclavicular block was not included in Daniel Moore's *Regional Block*[7] in 1981 or Michael

Cousins and Phillip Bridenbaugh's Neural Blockade in Clinical Anesthesia and Pain Management.[8]

Prithvi Raj[9] is credited with reintroducing the approach in 1973 with modification from the earlier descriptions. He described the initial entry point at the midpoint of the clavicle and directed the needle laterally toward the axilla using a nerve stimulator. His data suggested a virtual absence of risk of pneumothorax with the technique. and a more complete block of musculocutaneous and the ulnar nerves.[9] However, these results were not reproducible in other practitioner's clinical practice.

Kurt Whiffler, in 1981, described what is commonly referred to today as the coracoid block. The injection site was very close to that detailed by Sims,[10] but Whiffler felt that the shoulder should be depressed with the head turned to the opposite side and the arm abducted 45 degrees from the chest wall to make the plexus closer to the coracoid process. To estimate the depth of the plexus one identifies two points. One is the point past the midpoint of the clavicle where the subclavian pulse disappears. The second point is found by determining the highest pulse of the artery in the axilla and placing the thumb of the same hand on the anterior surface of the chest wall that corresponds to that point. Those points are connected, and the needle is then inserted inferior and medial to the coracoid process on that line to the depth that the plexus has been estimated. Whiffler did not use a nerve stimulator because he felt "this simpler approach does not require a nerve stimulator." Incremental injections were used to a total volume of 40 mL, withdrawing the needle 1 cm one to two times.[11]

In 1983, Alon Winnie's book, *Plexus Anesthesia*, describes several infraclavicular approaches including the techniques of Raj (1973), Sims (1977), and Whiffler (1981), although it does not devote a section to infraclavicular block. He states that "none of the infraclavicular techniques appears to offer significant advantages over the more established perivascular techniques …," and documents once again that the sheath can be entered at any level.[12]

The Infraclavicular block gained popularity in the 1990s along with the upsurge of regional anesthesia.

Oivind Klaastad, in 1999, performed a magnetic resonance imaging (MRI) study and determined that if followed exactly as described, the needle was not in close proximity to the cords. In a significant number of cases the cords were caudad and posterior to the target. Furthermore, the needle trajectory's shortest distance to the pleura was only 10 mm, and in one case hit the pleura. Klaastad concluded that a more lateral approach would make it more precise and reduce the risk of complications. This was actually what Raj had found clinically and was suggesting in lectures, but had not published. He had changed the point of needle insertion to be on a line between the pulsation of the subclavian and brachial artery and 2.5 cm from this line, crossing with the inferior border of the clavicle. This is what is commonly referred to as the modified Raj approach.[13]

Four approaches will be described in this chapter: (1) vertical infraclavicular block as described by Kilka and colleagues,[14] (2) the coracoid approach described by Whiffler[11] and modified by Wilson and coworkers,[15] (3) the modified Raj approach,[9] and (4) the lateral and sagittal approach described by Klaastad and associates often used for ultrasound.

INDICATIONS AND CONTRAINDICATIONS

Clinical Pearls

- Distribution of anesthesia consists of the hand, wrist, forearm, elbow, and most of the upper arm.
- Indications are similar to those for axillary block; hand, forearm, elbow, and arteriovenous fistula surgery.
- This approach affords greater applicability due to greater coverage and obviates the need for special arm positioning (abduction).

Indications for infraclavicular block are the same as for axillary blockade but complete anesthesia of the arm is obtained from the lower shoulder to the hand, making it applicable for any surgery up to but not including the shoulder. A tourniquet is well tolerated without supplementation of the intercostobrachial nerve. Bilateral blocks can be carried out without fear of blocking the phrenic nerve. The coracoid process and clavicle landmarks are easily palpable even in obese patients. The technique is also conducive to continuous catheter placement and long-term infusion.

Other than the obligatory contraindications of infection at or near the site or existing coagulopathy, there are no block-specific contraindications to infraclavicular block. Coagulopathy is a relative contraindication and based on the risk-vs-benefit ratio.

FUNCTIONAL ANATOMY

Clinical Pearls

- Block occurs at the level of the cords of the brachial plexus below the clavicle.

- Three cords surround the axillary artery.
- The anatomy of the brachial plexus is complex in this area and variability exists.
- The lateral cord is the most superficial, the posterior cord is encountered next, the medial cord is the deepest and is below the axillary artery.
- The lateral cord and the medial cord each contain half of the median nerve.
- The posterior cord contains all of the radial nerve.
- The musculocutaneous nerve is often outside but very close to the lateral cord.

The pertinent anatomy is illustrated in Figure 80D-1. Divisions exist as the brachial plexus crosses the first rib into the infraclavicular area. They originate from the trunks and divide into anterior and posterior divisions, thus, the origin of the name division. The anterior divisions usually supply flexor muscles (which are most often positioned anterior) and posterior divisions usually supply extensor muscles (which are generally posterior).

The brachial plexus makes most of its major changes in the infraclavicular area in just a few centimeters as it twists and turns from a parallel course in the neck to circumferentially surround the axillary artery in the infraclavicular area and progresses into the axilla as terminal nerves. Mixing of the nerves occurs, and its organization can be quite complex.

Figure 80D–2 shows the course of the brachial plexus from the interscalene to the infraclavicular area. The anatomic terms for the cords are based with the body in anatomic position and relative to its center; this is not how the brachial plexus is encountered clinically. Many textbooks feature two-dimensional rather than three-dimensional diagrams of the plexus in this area, which contributes to the confusion. However, a solid understanding of the three-dimensional organization of the plexus is perhaps the most important factor in its successful blockade.

Divisions, Branches, Cords, and Terminal Nerves

The anterior divisions of the upper (C5 and C6) and middle trunk (C7) unite to form the lateral cord, which lies lateral to the axillary artery and most superficial to the anterior chest. The anterior divisions of the lower trunk (C8 and T1) form the medial cord. It lies medial to the axillary artery and is the deepest from the chest wall. The posterior cord is formed from all of the posterior divisions (C5 through T1) and lies posterior to the artery just under the lateral cord. The cords end in terminal branches that are mixed nerves, which contain both sensory and motor components. They are the musculocutaneous, ulnar, median, axillary, and radial branches.

Other branches also exit the plexus prior to the formation of the terminal nerves. They are not mixed and are unique in that they are either sensory or motor nerves. These nerves are often not addressed but are important because the motor branches can be stimulated during performance of a block and knowing where they originate will help determine where to locate the tip of the needle. Tables 80D–1 and 80D–2 list the branches of the brachial plexus and their innervation.

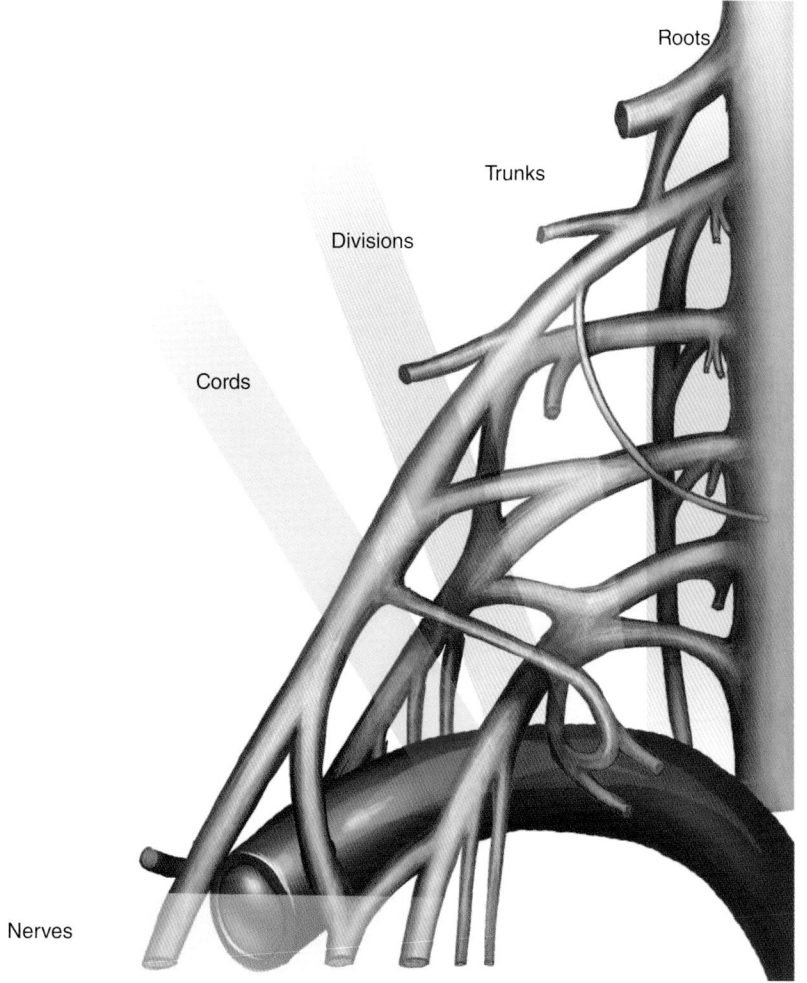

FIGURE 80D-1. Organization of the brachial plexus.

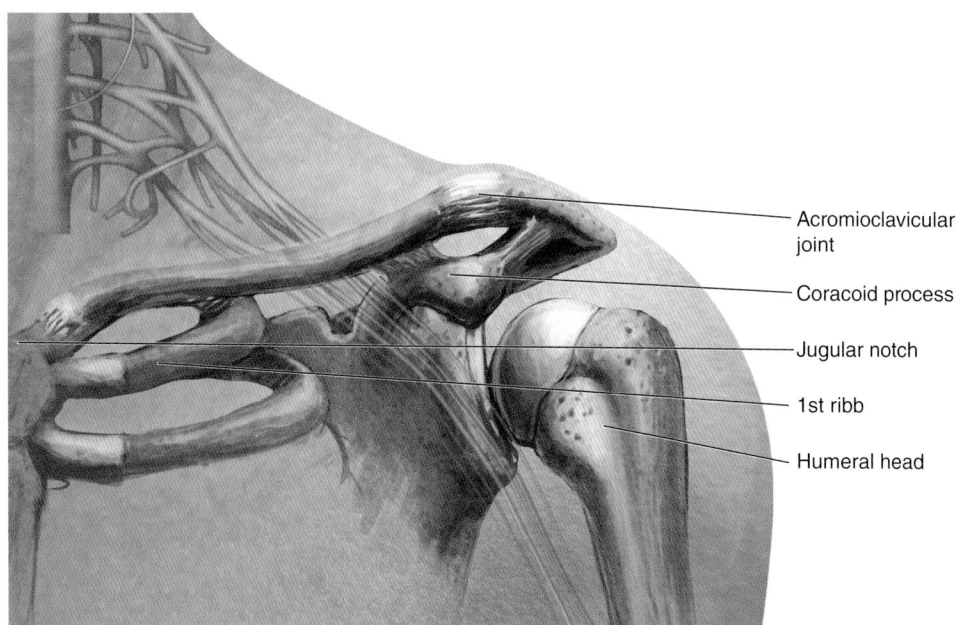

FIGURE 80D-2. Relationship of the brachial plexus, clavicle, and coracoid process.

TABLE 80D–1. Branches of brachial plexus.

	Motor Innervation	Motion Observed	Sensory Innervation
Lateral			
Lateral pectoral nerve	Pectoralis major	Contraction of pectoralis	
Dorsal scapular nerve	Rhomboid major and minor; levator scapulae	Adducts and rotates shoulder, raises scapula	
Posterior			
Upper subscapular	Subscapularis (superomedial part)	Medial rotation or arm	
Thoracodorsal	Latissimus dorsi	Abduction of arm	
Lower subscapular	Subscapularis (lateral part), teres major	Internal rotation, adduction of shoulder	
Axillary	Deltoid, teres minor	Elevation of upper arm	Skin of upper lateral arm
Medial			
Medial pectoral	Pectoralis minor and major	Contraction of pectoralis	
Medial cutaneous nerve of arm			Skin of medial side or arm
Medial cutaneous nerve of forearm			Skin of medial side or forearm

TABLE 80D–2. Terminal nerves of brachial plexus.

	Motor Innervation	Motion Observed	Sensory Innervation
Lateral			
Musculocutaneous	Coracobrachialis, biceps brachii, brachialis	Flexion of elbow	Skin of lateral side of forearm
Median	Flexor digitorum superficialis—all, pronator teres, flexor carpi radialis palmaris longus	Flexion of first fingers, opposition of thumb	Skin of radial half of palm and palmer side of radial three and a half digits
Posterior			
Radial	Brachioradialis, abductor pollicis longus, extensor muscles of the wrist and fingers	Abduction of thumb, extension of wrist and fingers	Skin of posterior arm, forearm and hand
Medial			
Ulnar	Abductor pollicis interossei intrinsic muscles of the hand	Contraction of the 4th and 5th fingers and thumb abduction	Skin of medial side of wrist and hand and ulner one and a half digits
Median	Flexor digitorum superficialis—all, pronator leres, flexor carpi radialis palmaris longus	Flexion of first $3^1/_2$ fingers, opposition of thumb	Skin of radial half of palm and palmer side of radial three and a half digits

Note: *All branches from the medial cord carry C8 and T1 fibers, and that of the higher spinal segments in the brachial plexus (C5 through C6) tend to innnervate muscles more proximal on the upper extremity, whereas the lower segments (C8, T1) tend to innervate more distal muscles, such as those in the hand (T1). Anatomic variation and the comingling of fibers from both lateral and medial cords makes it impossible to tell with certainty which cord is being stimulated with distal median nerve response.*

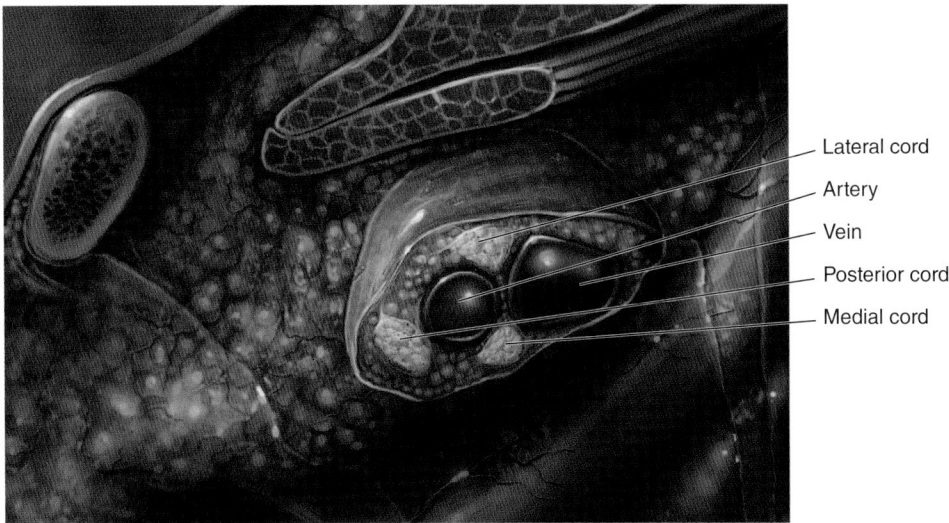

Lateral cord
Artery
Vein
Posterior cord
Medial cord

FIGURE 80D–3. Close-up view of the relationship of the cords of the brachial plexus at the level of infraclavicular blockade to the subclavian/axillary artery.

CLINICAL ANATOMY

A simplified schematic diagram of the plexus is shown in Figure 80D–1. This diagram depicts the plexus as it actually exists and a more clinical representation of how it is encountered when performing infraclavicular block. As shown, the posterior cord is not actually the most posterior cord but instead lies between the lateral and medial cords. The most helpful anatomic picture is in the sagittal plane, as shown in Figure 80D–3. This figure illustrates the brachial plexus at the level of infraclavicular blockade to show this relationship. The relationship shown in Figure 80D–3 is helpful for guiding needle placement while performing this block. The sagittal view shown here illustrates the cords in a close-up view surrounding the artery. Once this relationship is learned, the ability to change the needle directions for correct positioning is based on anatomy, and the need for subsequent passes to achieve successful placement lessens.

The cord that is most often encountered first when performing the infraclavicular block is the lateral cord because it is the most superficial. Just beyond the lateral cord is the posterior cord, which is in close proximity but just a bit deeper than the lateral cord. The medial cord is actually caudal or below the axillary artery, as can be seen in the sagittal view in Figure 80D–3. The schematic diagram of the cord shown in Figure 80D–4 demonstrates the 90-degree angle of needle insertion for the lateral and posterior cord. This figure also illustrates the proximity of the artery and the risk of puncturing the artery when attempting to encounter the medial cord. The anatomy of the plexus varies widely among individuals. The MRI study of Sauter revealed that the cords are found within 2 cm from the center of the artery, approximately within two thirds of a circle Figure 80D–5.

The Lateral Cord

The lateral cord supplies the lateral half of the median nerve and the musculocutaneous and the pectoral nerve branches (see Tables 80D–1 and 80D–2). This lateral portion of the median

nerve is the motor innervation to the flexor muscles in the forearm, flexor carpi radialis, pronator teres (pronation of the forearm), and the thenar muscle of the thumb. It provides sensory innervation for the thumb to the lateral half of the fourth finger including the dorsal tips. The most distal motor response would be flexion of the fingers or flexion and opposition of the thumb.

The thumb has motor innervation from the ulnar nerve as well, which may be confusing if trying to interpret isolated thumb twitch. The ulnar nerve supplies the adductor pollicis, flexor pollicis brevis, and the first dorsal interosseous muscle. These muscles radially adduct the thumb. The flexor pollicis brevis assists in opposition of the thumb. The median nerve's innervation of the flexor pollicis longus, abductor pollicis brevis, and the opponens pollicis are the major flexors for opposition of the thumb.

The musculocutaneous nerve has only muscular branches above the elbow and is purely sensory below the elbow as it becomes the lateral antebrachial cutaneous nerve. The motor response is flexion of the elbow by contraction of the biceps and sensation to the middle to median part of the forearm.

The anatomic relationship of the musculocutaneous nerve to the cords and the coracoid process is pertinent to infraclavicular block. It could be considered a branch because it exits early, but it is more like a terminal nerve because it has sensory and motor innervations. Variations in brachial plexus anatomy are common. Because the musculocutaneous nerve most often exits the lateral cord quite early, the stimulation of this nerve is felt to be an unreliable indicator of stimulation of the lateral cord.[16] It often overlies the lateral cord, which will be stimulated with deeper advancement of the needle as it passes the point of musculocutaneous nerve stimulation. Figure 80D–6 depicts the lateral cord with its stimulated hand motor response.

The Posterior Cord

The posterior cord is just deep or inferior to the lateral cord. The axillary, the thoracodorsal, and upper and lower

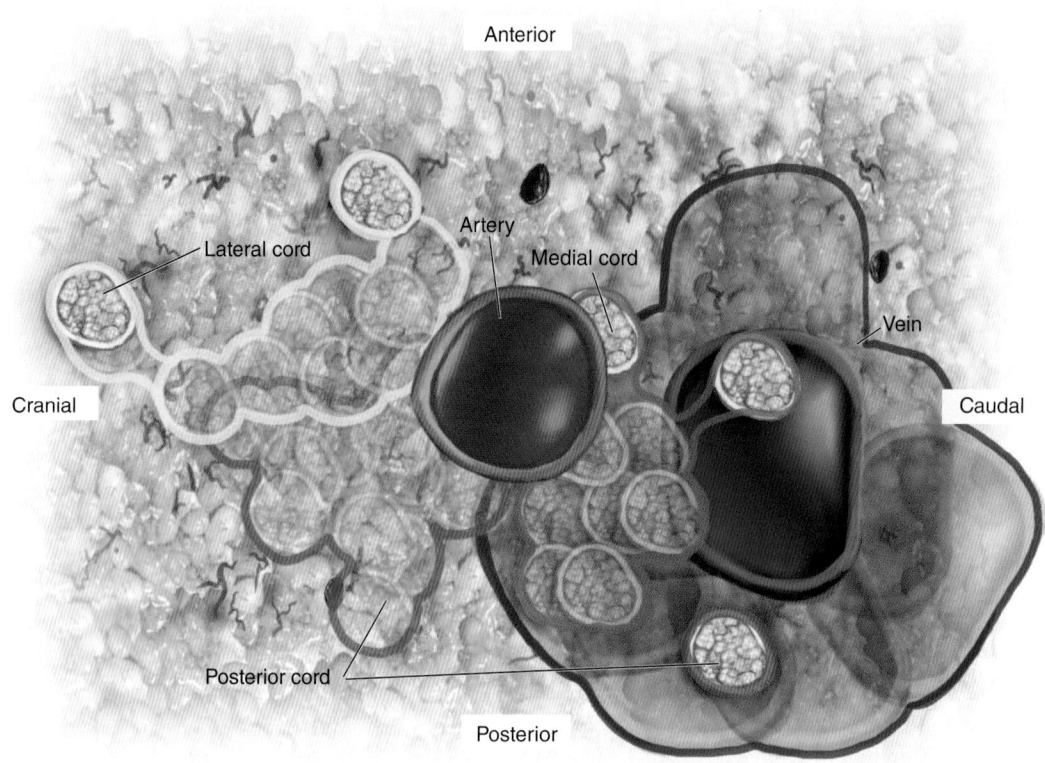

FIGURE 80D–4. Schematic of the relationship of the cords of the brachial plexus to the subclavian/axillary artery.

subscapular nerves are the branches from the posterior cord. They are involved in upper arm movement and shoulder movement and rotation as well as adduction of the shoulder and abduction of the arm. The branch most often encountered is the axillary nerve because it often has separated from the cord prior to the coracoid process. The axillary nerve to the deltoid elevates the upper arm. In addition to its branches, the posterior cord is responsible for the complete radial nerve. The distal responses from stimulation are abduction of the thumb and extension of the wrist and fingers (Figure 80D–7). The

brachioradialis muscle is innervated by the radial nerve and is classified as an extensor. Its stimulation should be characterized because it may be confused as a median nerve response because it actually flexes the elbow joint. Elbow flexion with radial

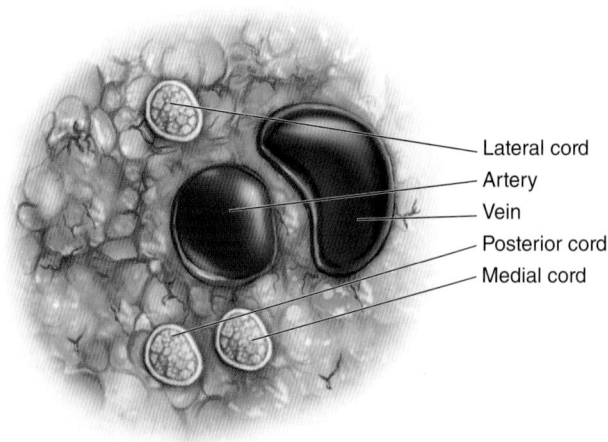

FIGURE 80D–5. Anatomic variations of the infraclavicular brachial plexus among individuals.

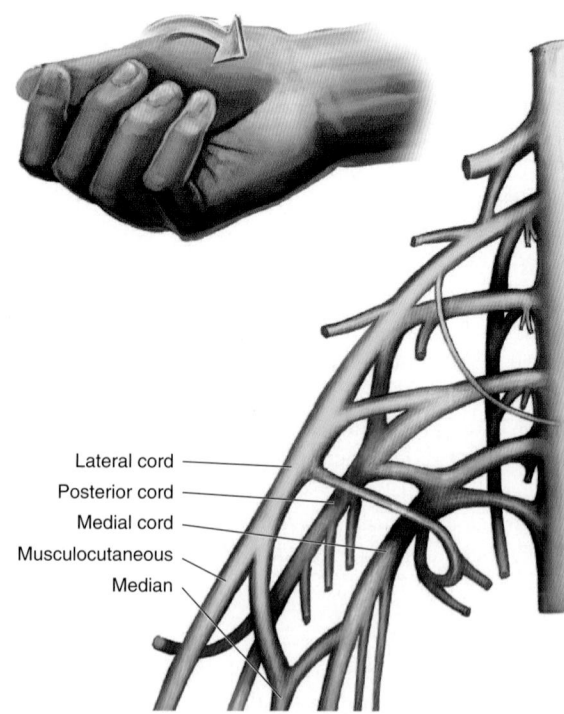

FIGURE 80D–6. Organization and motor response of the lateral cord.

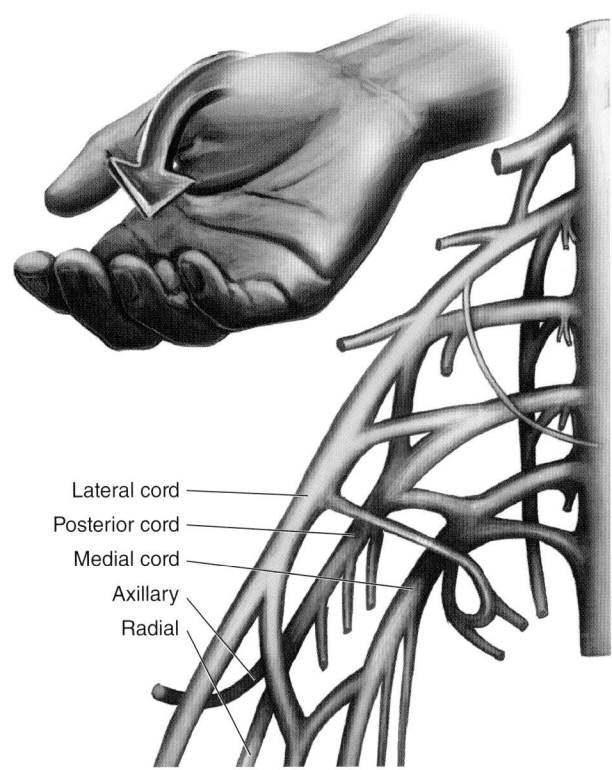

FIGURE 80D–7. Organization and motor response of the posterior cord.

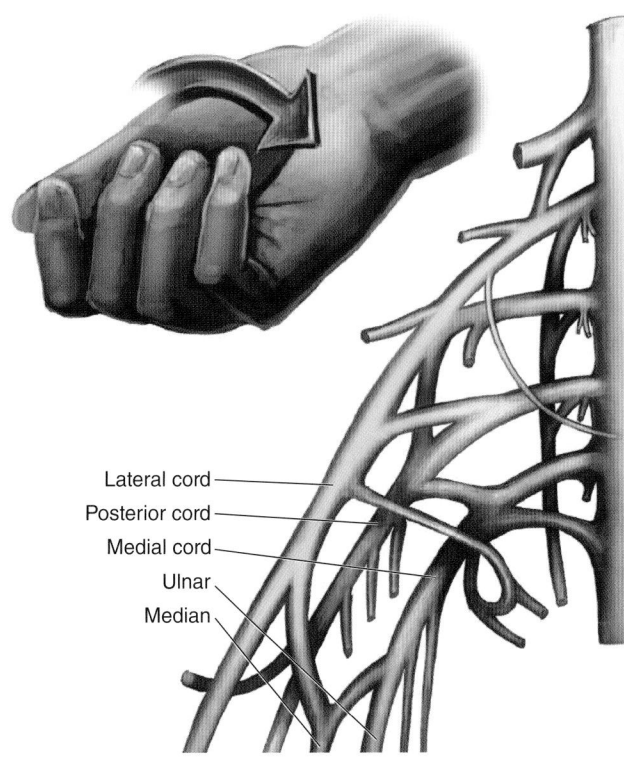

FIGURE 80D–8. Organization and motor response of the medial cord.

deviation of the wrist represents stimulation of the brachioradialis muscle and a posterior cord response. The needle should be readjusted to obtain a more distal response of the radial nerve.

The Medial Cord

The medial cord branches into the ulnar nerve and the medial half of the median nerve. Branches include the medial pectoral, medial brachial cutaneous, and the medial antebrachial cutaneous nerves. These branches innervate the skin of the anterior and medial surfaces of the forearm to the wrist. The ulnar nerve innervates half of the fourth and the fifth fingers, the adductor pollicis, and all interossei, which results in contraction of the fourth and fifth fingers and thumb adduction. Median nerve stimulation results in flexion and sensation of the first three and one half fingers, opposition of the thumb, and sensation of the palm (Figure 80D–8).

Unlike the axillary block, responses to stimulation of the median nerve during infraclavicular block could conceivably arise from either the lateral or medial cord. Classic studies of fiber topography of the median nerve by Sunderland identified pronator teres fibers and flexor carpi radialis in the lateral root, along with nerves to the flexor digitorum profundus, flexor pollicis longus, and intrinsic thenar muscles in the medial root.[17]

Nerve injury studies also suggest that median fibers to the finger flexors are most likely found in the medial cord and medial root of the median nerve.[16] With the most commonly occurring plexus anatomy, finger flexion most likely identifies medial cord (or root) stimulation, but wrist flexion may result from either median or lateral cord (or root) stimulation.[18]

Tables 80D–1 and 80D–2 summarize the cords, branches, terminal nerves, and their motor stimulus response. Because of anatomic variability and the mixing of the median nerve between the medial and lateral cords, the same responses are listed for both nerves. Except in rare variants, the ulnar nerve is carried within the medial cord.

LANDMARKS AND TECHNIQUE

General Guidelines

The bony landmarks used in most approaches are the clavicle, the jugular fossa or notch, the acromioclavicular joint, and the coracoid process, depicted in Figure 80D–9.

MODIFIED RAJ APPROACH

A small amount, approximately 5 mL or less, of local anesthetic is needed for the skin and subcutaneous tissue. Care must be taken to avoid the pleura by never directing the needle in a medial direction. If the plexus is not encountered, the needle should be withdrawn and redirected sequentially by a factor of 10 degrees in either a cephalad or caudad direction. If those maneuvers are not successful, the landmarks should be reassessed before attempting another pass. Initial settings on the nerve stimulator are 1.5 mA, with an acceptable response occurring at less than 0.5 mA. Distal motor responses (below the elbow) are preferable. The infraclavicular block is a large-volume block, and 30 mL of local anesthetic is necessary to block the entire brachial plexus. Some commonly used local anesthetic solutions are listed in Tables 80D–3.

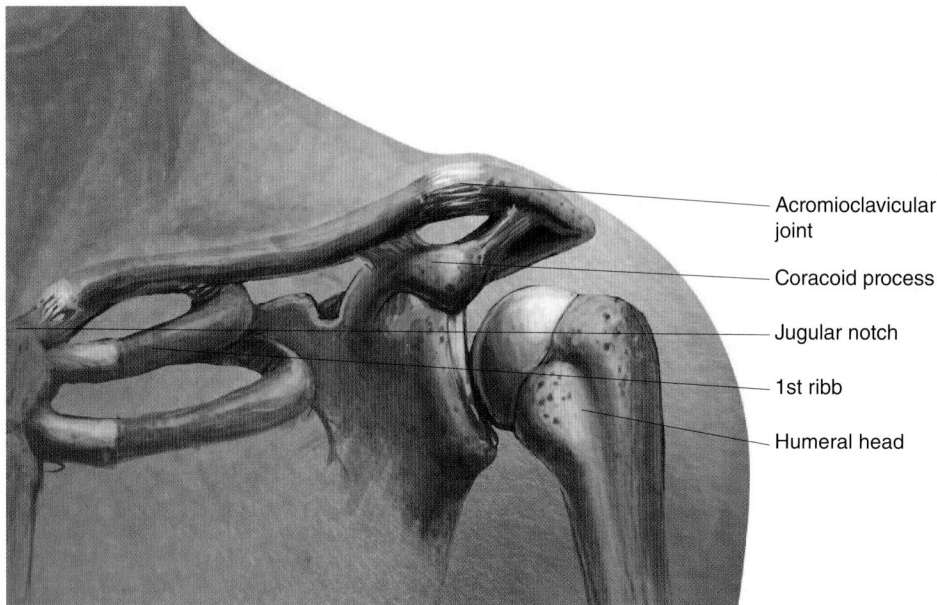

FIGURE 80D–9. Relationship of the jugular (sternal) notch, clavicle and coracoid process.

The patient is in the recumbent position with the head turned away. The subclavian artery is palpated where it crosses the clavicle, or the midpoint of the clavicle is marked. The brachial artery is palpated and marked at the lateral border of the pectoralis muscle. A line joining these two points is made with needle insertion 2.5–3.0 cm below the midpoint of the clavicle at a 45- to 65-degree angle toward the axillary artery (Figure 80D–10).

The operator stands on the opposite side to the site of block placement. The skin is infiltrated with local anesthetic into the skin and pectoralis muscle. The first two fingers of the palpating hand anchor the skin at the point of insertion, and the needle is advanced at a 45- to 65-degree angle toward the point of brachial pulsation or parallel to a line connecting the medial clavicular head with the coracoid process if pulsation cannot be felt (Figure 80D–11).

If the plexus is not encountered, the needle should be withdrawn and redirected 10 degrees cephalad or caudad, depending on the originating angle of insertion. At no time should the needle be pointed medially or posteriorly toward the lung.

VERTICAL INFRACLAVICULAR BLOCK

The vertical infraclavicular block was described by Kilka and coworkers in 1995.[14] The landmarks are the midpoint of a line from the middle of the jugular notch and the ventral process of the acromion (Figure 80D–12). The patient is lying in a supine position with the forearm relaxed on the chest with the head turned slightly to the side.

- Needle insertion is at the midpoint of the line from the jugular fossa to the acromioclavicular joint.
- Insertion is just under the clavicle.
- Needle assumes a 90-degree needle angle.
- A 50-mm needle is used.

TABLE 80D–3. Local anesthetic solutions for infraclavicular block.

Duration	Anesthetic	
Short (1.5–3.0 h)	3% chloroprocaine	
	1.5% lidocaine	
	1.0%–1.5% mepivacaine	
Intermediate (4–5 h)	2% lidocaine + epinephrine	
	1.0%–1.5% mepivacaine	
Long-Lasting (10–14 h)	0.25%–0.50% bupivacaine	(0.0625%–0.1% for infusion)
	0.50% ropivacaine	0.1%–0.2% for infusion)

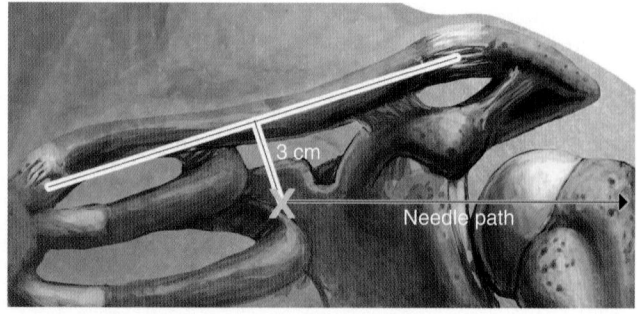

FIGURE 80D–10. Raj approach: Landmarks and needle insertion plane.

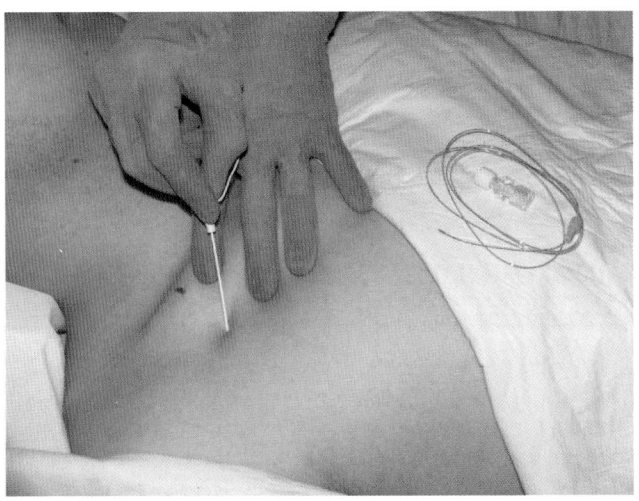

FIGURE 80D-11. Raj approach: Needle insertion and orientation.

A 50-mm needle is inserted close to the clavicle at an angle of 90 degrees (see Figure 80D–12). Local anesthetic is injected after a distal stimulus is obtained at or below 0.5 mA. If on first pass the needle does not encounter the plexus, only the angle is changed while keeping the same plane by 10 degrees caudad or cephalad. The needle is never directed in a medial fashion.

Clinical Pearls

The three most common errors that increase the risk of pneumothorax are[19]:

- Too medial insertion of the needle
- Depth of needle insertion >6 cm
- Medial direction of needle

Adams described an improved success rate by moving the puncture site 1 cm laterally. The rate of unsuccessful block (defined as need for additional analgesic or sedation) was reduced to 8.3%, although this may depend on patient size. Using ultrasonographic assessment, Greher and colleagues

demonstrated topographic anatomy in volunteers and compared the classic approach to a puncture site determined by high-resolution ultrasound location of the plexus. A clear trend was found to a more lateral puncture site, especially in women. They found that when the line from jugular fossa to acromion measured 22.0-22.5 cm the puncture site was exactly at the center of this line. However, for every 1 cm decrease in the length of this line the puncture site moved 2 mm laterally from the center and for every 1 cm increase the puncture site moved 2mm medially.[20]

CORACOID TECHNIQUE (BLOCK)

The coracoid block as described by Whiffler[11] in 1981 used a needle entry site that is most often inferior and medial to the coracoid process. In 1998, Wilson reviewed MRIs and located a point 2 cm medial to the coracoid process and 2 cm caudad. At this skin entry site, direct posterior insertion of the needle makes contact with the cords at a mean range of 4.24 cm ± 1.49 (2.25–7.75 cm) in men and 4.01 ± 1.29 cm (2.25–6.5 cm) in women.[15] As shown in Figure 80D–13, the lateral tip of the coracoid process (not the medial edge) is palpated. Kapral,[19] in 1999, described a lateral approach with the patient in the same position. The point of needle insertion is lateral to the lateral point of the coracoid process. After identifying the coracoid process by touching the bone, the 7-cm needle is withdrawn 2–3 mm and redirected underneath the coracoid process 2–3 cm until the brachial plexus is reached. The usual distance was 5.5–6.5 cm. Rodriguez described his series of coracoid blocks as closer to the coracoid process by making his puncture site 1 cm inferior and 1 cm medial to the coracoid process. He reported a similar success rate.[21,22]

THE LATERAL AND SAGITTAL TECHNIQUE LANDMARKS

In 2004, Klaastad and coworkers described this technique and tested it in an MRI model.[23] The point of needle insertion is the intersection between the clavicle and the coracoid process (see Figure 80D–2). The needle is advanced 15 degrees posteriorly, always strictly in the sagittal plane next to the coracoid process

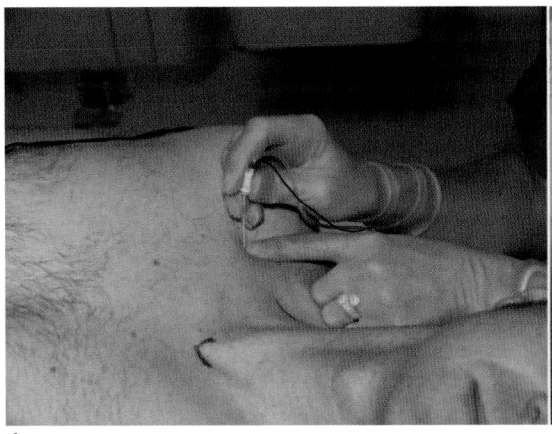
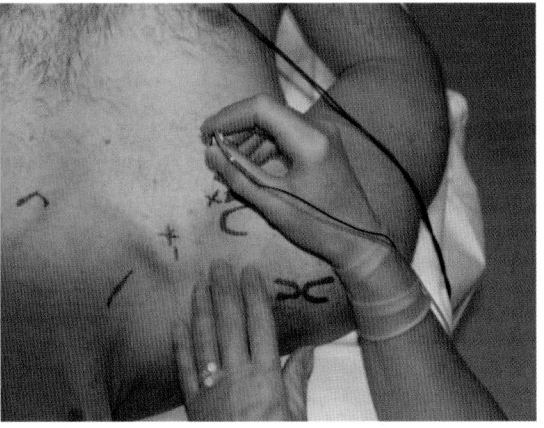

A   B

FIGURE 80D-12. A AND B. Vertical approach: Needle insertion and orientation.

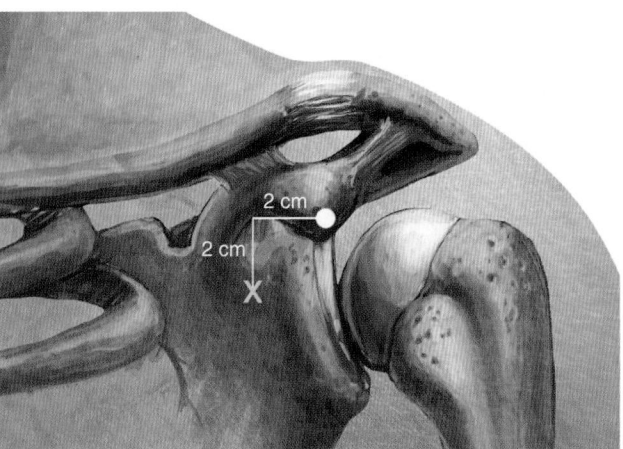

FIGURE 80D–13. Coracoid approach: Landmarks.

while abutting the anteroinferior edge of the clavicle. All needle directions in this method adhere strictly to the sagittal plane through this coracoid prominence. The posterior cord and medial cord were more often reached than the lateral cord. Insertion depth should be no greater than 6.5 cm. Although the cords are usually reached before the axillary artery and vein, puncture of these vessels as well as the cephalic vein is always a possibility.[24] Klaastad and coworkers reported occasionally needing to insert the needle more than 6.5 cm (their estimated maximal safe depth) to obtain satisfactory nerve contact and has not had a case of pneumothorax. The needle can encounter a vessel.[25]

Although initially used with a nerve stimulator, this technique has become the preferred method for use with ultrasound localization of the brachial plexus cords.[14] The cords are superior and posterior to the axillary artery, most commonly at a depth of 4–6 cm. Although it is always possible to puncture the artery, the trajectory of this approach appears to avoid puncture of the axillary vessels because the cords are encountered cephalad to the artery and 2–3 cm cephalad to the pleural cavity. The use of ultrasound may improve block success and decrease morbidity compared with nerve stimulator alone.[26]

SINGLE INJECTION VS MULTIPLE INJECTION AND CONTINUOUS TECHNIQUE

Single stimulation has been reported to have success rates from 82% to 100%.[19,24,27,28] Gaertner and colleagues compared single stimulation to stimulation of all three cords. Multistimulation took slightly longer (9.0 vs 7.5 min); however, 2 of the 40 patients in the multistimulation group were excluded because three cords could not be localized within 15 minutes.[24]

A distal response in the hand or wrist was considered adequate with 10 mL of local anesthetic injected at each site. In the single-stimulation group, 30 mL of local anesthetic was injected after identifying a single response from any cord, (Figure 80D–14). Although their overall success rate was low for both techniques (40.0% for single stimulation and 72.5% for multiple stimulation), Gaertner and colleagues reported that multiple stimulation was significantly more successful than single. The amount of local anesthetic, 30 mL, could have contributed to the overall decreased success rate. However, these researchers attributed the bulk of the difference in overall success to the varying definition of success in the literature. Hand surgery constitutes a large part of the surgeries in these studies. Most hand surgery can be performed with two or three of the nerves to the hand blocked if they are in the correct distribution of the surgery. Gaertner and colleagues felt more stringent criteria should be used. A complete

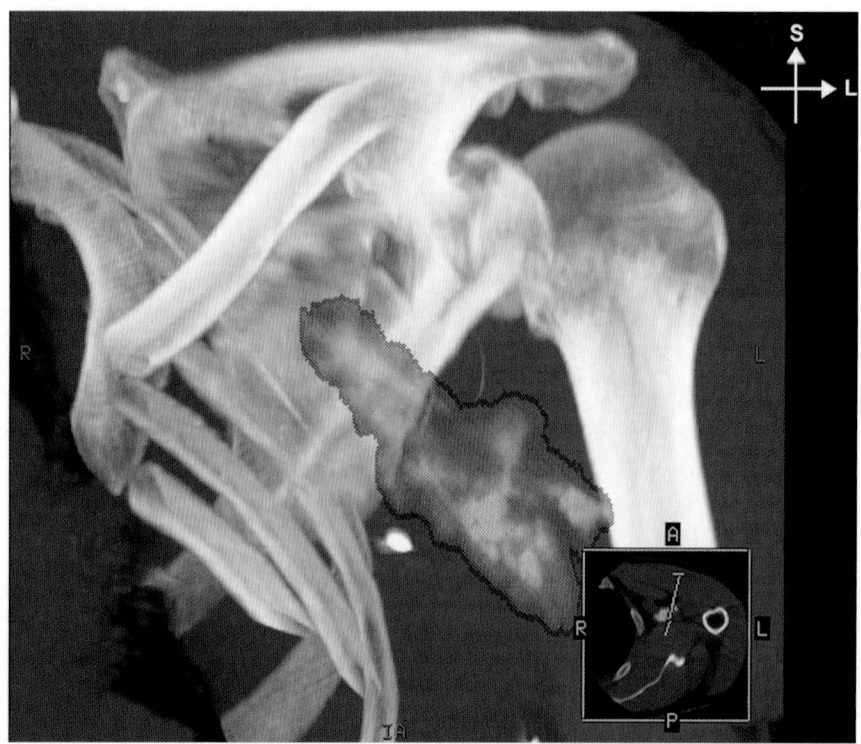

FIGURE 80D–14. Distribution of the local anesthetic after injection through an indwelling catheter.

motor and sensory block of all nerves was necessary for their criteria of success as compared with success defined as completing the procedure without supplementation or the need for general anesthesia.

An example of this criterion is demonstrated by Rodriguez and collaborators[21] in a random controlled trial comparing injection of 42 mL of mepivacaine using a single-, dual-, or triple-injection technique. A significantly less complete motor blockade was found with single injection versus the dual or triple injection. No significant difference was found in the dual- or triple-injection groups. In another study,[22] comparing single and dual stimulation, 22% of the single stimulation group had a musculocutaneous or axillary response. The investigators state that the recommendations for not accepting these responses is based on a published anecdotal report[29] on a noncoracoid approach. Dual injection was suggested as the best balance between efficacy and comfort for patients and resulted in shorter block performance times and decreased vascular puncture rates compared with that for triple-stimulation injection.[30]

Deluze and coworkers found a similar effective rate when comparing single stimulation to triple stimulation by using 40 mL of 0.75% ropivacaine.[31]

Continuous Technique

The infraclavicular block is well suited for continuous nerve block. Patient comfort and catheter securing are easier accomplished with an infraclavicular catheter rather than a dressing in the axillary area. If the distribution of the pain is in the axillary nerve or musculocutaneous areas, the chance of constant sensory blockade of those areas and pain relief are greater.

All approaches have been utilized successfully with a continuous technique, and there is no overwhelming evidence that favors a particular approach.[19,25,32,33]

Clinical Pearl

- The coracoid process can easily be found even in obese patients. The middle finger is placed just below the clavicle and the hand is moved laterally toward the shoulder. The first bony prominence that is felt by the index finger is the coracoid process. The patient's head should be turned to the opposite side.

SUMMARY

The infraclavicular block provides a useful alternative to axillary block for surgery of the arm. The block is reliable for surgery and amenable to ultrasound technique and can be used for continuous as well as single-shot techniques.

REFERENCES

1. Hirschel G: Die Anasthesierung des Plexus brachialis bei Operationen der oberen Extremitat. MMW Munch Med Wochenschr 1911;58:1555–1556.
2. Kulenkampff D: Anasthesie des Plexus brachialis. Zentralbl Chir 1911;8:1337–1350.
3. Bazy L, Pouchet V, Sourdat V, et al: J Anesth Reg 1917;222–225.
4. From Zentralbl Chir 45, 1918. In Winnie AP: *Plexus Anesthesia.* Philadelphia, PA: Saunders, 1983, pp 215–217.
5. *Labat's Regional Anesthesia: Its Technique and Clinical Application,* Philadelphia, PA: Saunders, 1923, p 223.
6. Dogliotti AM: *Anesthesia: Narcosis, Local, Regional, Spinal.* SB Debour: Chicago, 1939.
7. Moore DC: *Regional Block,* 4th ed. Springfield, IL: Thomas, 1981.
8. Cousins MJ, Bridenbaugh PO: *Neural Blockade in Clinical Anesthesia and Pain Management.* Philadelphia, PA: Lippincott, 1980.
9. Raj PP, Montgomery SJ, Nettles D, et al. Infraclaficular brachial plexus block—a new approach. Anesth Analg 1973;52:897–904.
10. Sims JK: A modification of landmarks for infraclavicular approach to brachial plexus block. Anesth Analg 1977;56:554–557.
11. Whiffler K: Coracoid block—a safe and easy technique. Br J Anaesth 1981;53:845.
12. Winnie AP: *Plexus Anesthesia.* Philadelphia, PA: Saunders, 1983.
13. Klaastad O, Lileas FG, Rotnes JS, et al. Magnetic resonance imaging demonstrates lack of precision in needle placement by the infraclavicular brachial plexus block described by Raj et al. Anesth Analg 1999;88:593–598.
14. Kilka HG, Geiger P, Mehrkens HH: Infraclavicular blockade. A new method for anesthesia of the upper extremity: an anatomical and clinical study. Anaesthesist 1995;44:339–344.
15. Wilson JL, Brown DL, Wongy GY: Infraclavicular brachial plexus block: parasagittal anatomy important to the coracoid technique. Anesth Analg 1998;87:870–873.
16. Gelberman RH: *Operative Nerve Repair and Reconstruction.* Philadelphia, PA: Lippincott, 1991, p 1288.
17. Sunderland S: The intraneural topography of the radial, median, and ulnar nerves. Brain 1945;68(pt 4):243–299.
18. Weller RS, Gerancher JC: Brachial plexus block: "best" approach and "best" evoked response—where are we? Reg Anesth Pain Med 2004;29:520–523.
19. Kapral S, Jandrasits O, Schabernig C, et al. Lateral infraclavicular plexus block vs. axillary block for hand and forearm surgery. Acta Anaesthesiol Scand 1999;43:1047–1052.
20. Greher M, Retzl G, Niel P, et al. Ultrasound assessment of topographic anatomy in volunteers suggests a modification of the infraclavicular block. Br J Anaesth 2002;88:621–624.
21. Rodriguez J, Barcena M, Taboada-Muiz M, et al. A comparison of single versus multiple injections on the extent of anesthesia with coracoid infraclavicular brachial plexus block. Anesth Analg 2004;99:1225–1230.
22. Rodriguez J, Barcena M, Lagunilla J, et al. Increased success rate with infraclavicular brachial plexus block using a dual-injection technique. J Clin Anesthesia 2004;16:251–256.
23. Klaastad O, Smith HG, Smedby O, et al. A novel infraclavicular brachial plexus block: the lateral and sagittal technique, developed by magnetic resonance imaging studies. Anesth Analg 2004;98:252–256.
24. Gaertner E, Estebe JP, Zamfir A, et al. Infraclavicular plexus block: multiple injection versus single injection. Reg Anesth Pain Med 2002;27:590–594.
25. Klaastad O, Smith H-J, Smedby O, et al. Response to letter to editor. Anesth Analg 2004;99:950–951.
26. Brull R, McCartney C, Chan V: A novel approach to the infraclavicular brachial plexus block: The ultrasound experience [Letter]. Anesth Analg 2004;99:950.
27. Borgeat A, Ekatodramis G, Dumont C: An evaluation of the infraclavicular block via a modified approach of the Raj technique. Anesth Analg 2001;93:436–441.
28. Jandard C, Gentili ME, Girard F, et al. Infraclavicular block with lateral approach and nerve stimulation: Extent of anesthesia and adverse effects. Reg Anesth Pain Med 2002;27:37–42.
29. Fitzgibbon DR, Deps AD, Erjavec MK: Selective musculocutaneous nerve block and infraclavicular brachial plexus anesthesia. Reg Anesth 1995;20:239–241.
30. Rodriguez J, Taboada-Muiz M, Barcena M, et al. Median versus musculocutaneous nerve response with single-injection infraclavicuar coracoid block. Reg Anesth Pain Med 2004;29:534–538.
31. Deluze A, Gentili ME, et al. A comparison of a single-stimulation lateral infraclavicular plexus block with a triple stimulation axillary block. Reg Anesth Pain Med 2003;28:89–94.
32. Mehrkens HH, Geiger PK: Continuous brachial plexus blockade via the vertical infraclavicular approach. Anaesthesia 1998;53(Suppl 2):19–20.
33. Macaire P, Gaertner E, Capdevila X: Continuous post operative regional analgesia at home. Minerva Anestesiol 2001;67:109–116.

Axillary Brachial Plexus Block

Zbigniew J. Koscielniak-Nielsen and Monika Golebiewski

INTRODUCTION

Brachial plexus block at the level of the axilla is typically chosen for anesthesia of the distal upper limb. Axillary block is one of the most common approaches to brachial plexus blockade. Easy landmarks and simplicity make this block suitable for a wide range of surgical procedures.

HISTORY

The surgical technique of this block was first described by William Hallstead[1] in New York City (Roosevelt Hospital, also the clinical affiliation for NYSORA 1995-2014) in 1884, whereas the percutaneous technique was described by Georg Hirschel[2] in 1911. In 1958, Preston Burnham[3] recognized that filling the neurovascular "sheath" with local anesthetic could simplify the axillary block. He also described the characteristic fascial "click" felt upon needle entry into the axillary sheath. In 1961, while using the formula for a cylinder volume, Rudolph De Jong[4] calculated that in an average adult, 42 mL of local anesthetic (LA) was necessary to fill the fascial compartment to the level of the cords and block all terminal nerves to the arm. A year later, Ejnar Eriksson and Skarby,[5] in an effort to promote the proximal spread of LA, advocated wrapping a rubber tourniquet around the arm, distal to the needle. In 1979, Alon Winnie and coworkers[6] found the tourniquet ineffective and painful and recommended firm distal digital pressure on the neurovascular sheath instead. In addition, they also recommended arm adduction after LA injection, thinking that the head of the abducted humerus com pressed the neurovascular sheath. Both maneuvers were later proved to be clinically ineffective.[7-9] Gale Thompson and Duane Rorie,[10] in 1983, studied brachial plexus using computed tomograms and suggested that the median, ulnar, and radial nerves lie in separate fascial compartments within the neurovascular sheath; this hypothesis provided a rational explanation for incomplete blocks.

However, anatomic studies by Lassale and Ang[11] in 1984 and Vester-Andersen and coworkers[12] in 1986 did not confirm the existence of a true neurovascular sheath. The interfascial space they found contained the median and the ulnar nerves, infrequently the musculocutaneous, and occasionally the radial nerves. Moreover, the space was suggested to communicate proximally only with the medial cord of the plexus. In 1987, Partridge and coworkers[13] found the interneural septa, which were easily broken by injection of dyed latex. In 2002, Oivind Klaastad and coworkers[14] were the first to investigate the spread of the LA through the axillary catheter in studies using magnetic resonance imaging (MRI) scanning. They found that in most patients the spread of LA was uneven and the clinical effect inadequate.

Until the 1960s, the prevalent block techniques were double or multiple axillary injections. After the concept of the neurovascular sheath had been established by De Jong[4] in 1961, the single-injection technique, being the simplest, became standard. However, Vester-Andersen and coworkers[15,16] demonstrated in 1983 and 1984 that despite high volumes of LA, analgesia was often inconsistent ("patchy"). In the early 1990s, the double-injection, transarterial technique was popularized by Urban and Urquhart[17] and Stan and coworkers.[18] More recently, however, development of peripheral nerve stimulators and insulated atraumatic needles has allowed electrolocation and separate blockade (multistimulation technique) of the individual terminal nerves (median, musculocutaneous, ulnar, and radial). This is known as the multiple-nerve stimulation technique. Baranowski and Pither[19] (in 1990), Lavoie and coworkers[20] (in 1992), Koscielniak-Nielsen and coworkers[21,22] (in 1997 and 1998), and Sia and coworkers[23,24] (in 2001 and 2002) independently showed that multiple-nerve stimulation was superior, both to the single- and the double-injection methods by increasing the success rate and shortening the block onset. A recent Cochrane review by Handoll and coworkers[25] validated these findings.

INDICATIONS AND CONTRAINDICATIONS

The most common indications for axillary block include surgery of the forearm, wrist, or hand of moderate to long duration, with or without an arm tourniquet. Relative contraindications to the use of this block are skin infection at the block site, axillary lymphadenopathy, and severe coagulopathy. In addition, this block is best avoided in patients with preexisting neurologic disease of the upper extremity because sensory assessments may be difficult.

PERTINENT ANATOMY

In the apex of the axilla, the three plexus cords (lateral, medial, and posterior) form the main terminal nerves of the upper extremity (axillary, musculocutaneous, median, ulnar, and radial). However, only the last three nerves accompany the blood vessels through the axilla where the blocks are performed (Figure 80E–1), while the axillary and the musculocutaneous nerves leave the plexus approximately at the level of the coracoid process. The axillary nerve departs at a wider angle from the posterior cord, laterally and dorsally, and the musculocutaneous nerve, which originates from the lateral cord, runs obliquely laterally into the coracobrachialis muscle and continues downward. The medial antebrachial cutaneous and brachial cutaneous nerves run subcutaneously parallel to the axillary vessels, although the medial antebrachial cutaneous nerve often follows the median nerve within the neurovascular sheath. In the axilla, the median and musculocutaneous nerves lie superior to the artery, whereas the ulnar and radial nerves lie inferior to it. The depths at which the nerves are found vary. Typically, the median nerve is more superficial than the musculocutaneous, and the ulnar nerve is more superficial than the radial. Occasionally, the radial or the musculocutaneous nerves (or both) are found behind the artery. These two nerves progressively diverge from the neurovascular sheath, continuing down the upper arm, the musculocutaneous above (anterior) and the radial below (posterior) to the humerus, where they can be approached using the mid-humeral approach.[26]

Landmarks

Surface landmarks for the axillary brachial plexus block include (Figure 80E–2):

1. Pulse of the axillary artery
2. Coracobrachialis muscle

3. Pectoralis major muscle
4. Biceps muscle
5. Triceps muscle

EQUIPMENT

- Sterile towels and 4-in. × 4-in. gauze packs
- Sterile gloves, marking pen, and a skin electrode
- 1-in., 25-gauge needle for skin infiltration
- 1- to 1.5-in. atraumatic, insulated stimulating needle
- 20-mL syringes containing LA of choice
- Peripheral nerve stimulator
- Means of assessing opening injection pressure

INJECTION TECHNIQUES

Arm Position for the Block

The arm to be operated on is abducted approximately 90 degrees (see Figure 80E–2). The elbow is flexed and the forearm rests comfortably, supported by a pillow. The arterial pulse is palpated at the level of the major pectoral muscle, and the subcutaneous tissue overlying the artery is infiltrated with 4–5 mL of LA (to block the intercostobrachial and medial cutaneous nerves of the arm). Several techniques and approaches to the brachial plexus block at the level about the axilla have been described; we will describe only some of the well-studied techniques.

A triple-injection axillary block is probably the most efficient technique for axillary brachial plexus blockade.

NERVE STIMULATION TECHNIQUES

Single-Injection (Stimulation) Technique

1. The nerve stimulator is set to deliver 0.5–1.0 mA (2 Hz, 0.1 msec); electrical connections with the needle and the neutral electrode are checked.
2. Depending on the surgical site (palmar and medial or dorsal and lateral aspects of the hand/forearm), the stimulating needle is inserted above the arterial pulse (toward the median nerve) or below the arterial pulse (toward the radial nerve), respectively (Figures 80E–3).
3. As the superficial fascia is penetrated, a characteristic "click" is often felt, and the current amplitude is slowly increased (e.g., at 1-mA increments) until the desired

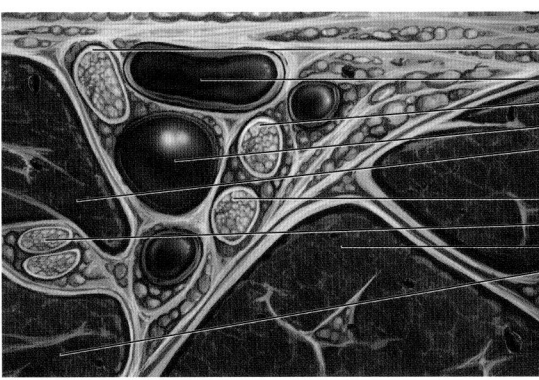

Median nerve
Axillary vein
Ulnar nerve
Axillary artery
Biceps muscle

Radial nerve
Musculocutaneous nerve
Latissimus dorsi muscle
Coracobrachialis muscle

FIGURE 80E–1. Anatomy of the brachial plexus at axilla and at the midhumeral level.

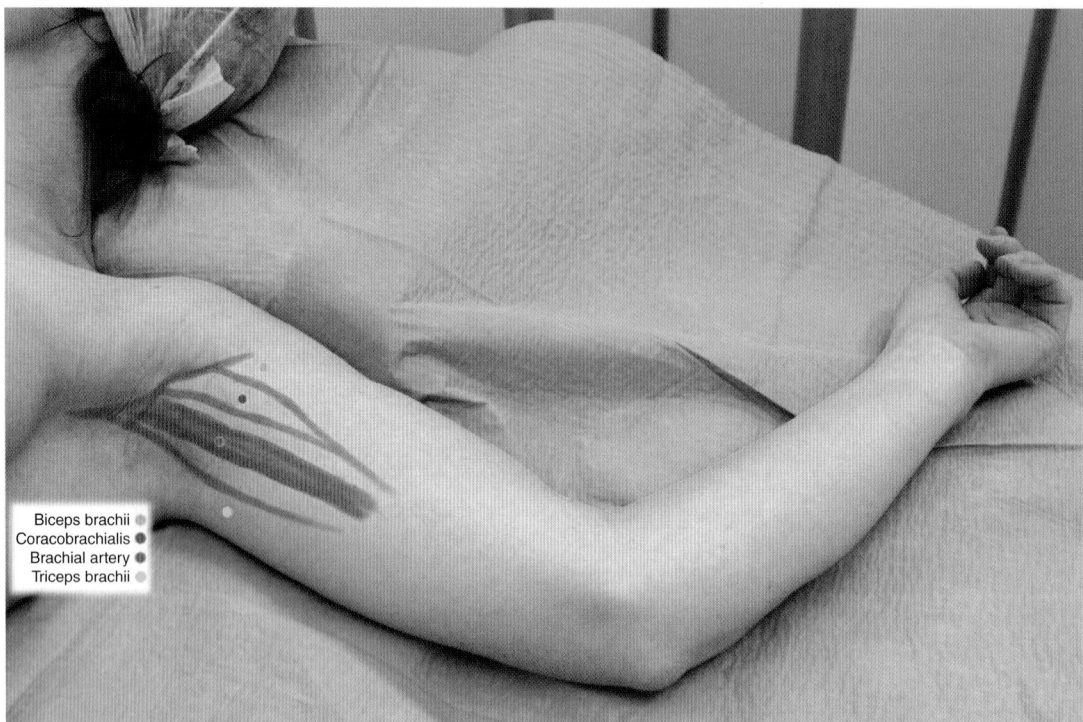

FIGURE 80E-2. Landmarks for the axillary brachial plexus block.

twitch (flexion or extension of the wrist and fingers) is obtained. This helps avoid painful electrical paresthesia when the elastic fascia suddenly "gives in" and the needle enters the neurovascular sheath.[27]

4. After the initial motor response is obtained, the needle is slowly advanced toward the stimulated nerve while reducing the amplitude.

5. Once the stimulation is obtained using a current intensity of 0.3–0.5 mA, the entire volume of LA is injected slowly, while intermittently aspirating to reduce the risk of accidental intravascular injection. This results in substantial spread of the LA within the tissue layers encompassing the brachial plexus (Figure 80E–5).

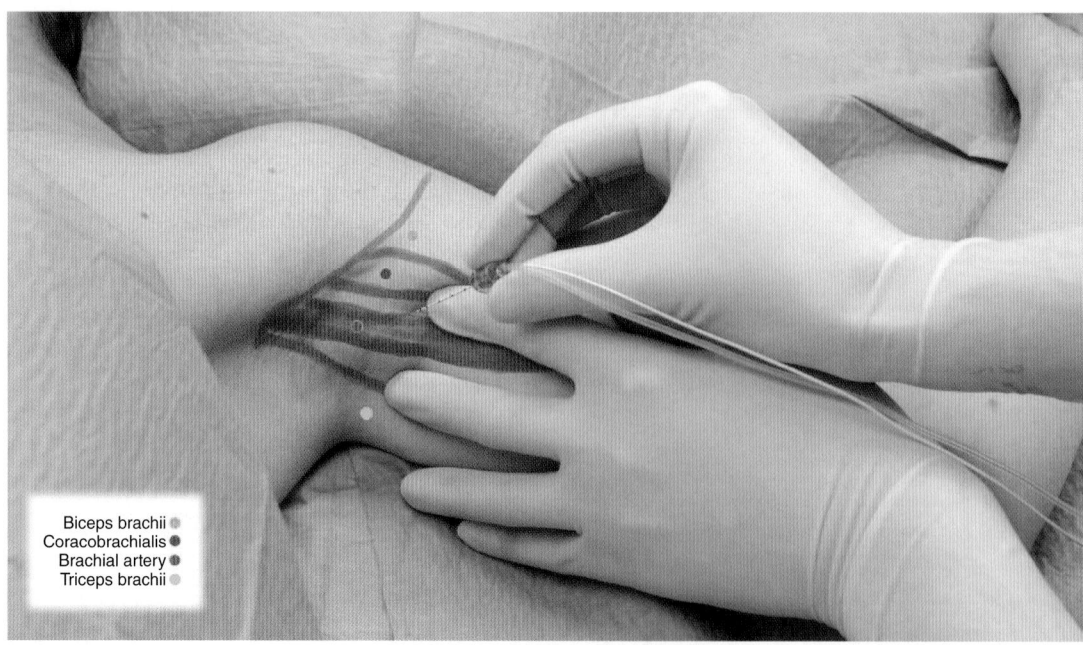

FIGURE 80E-3. Radial nerve block: The needle is inserted above the pulse of the axillary (brachial) artery. CB = coracobrachialis.

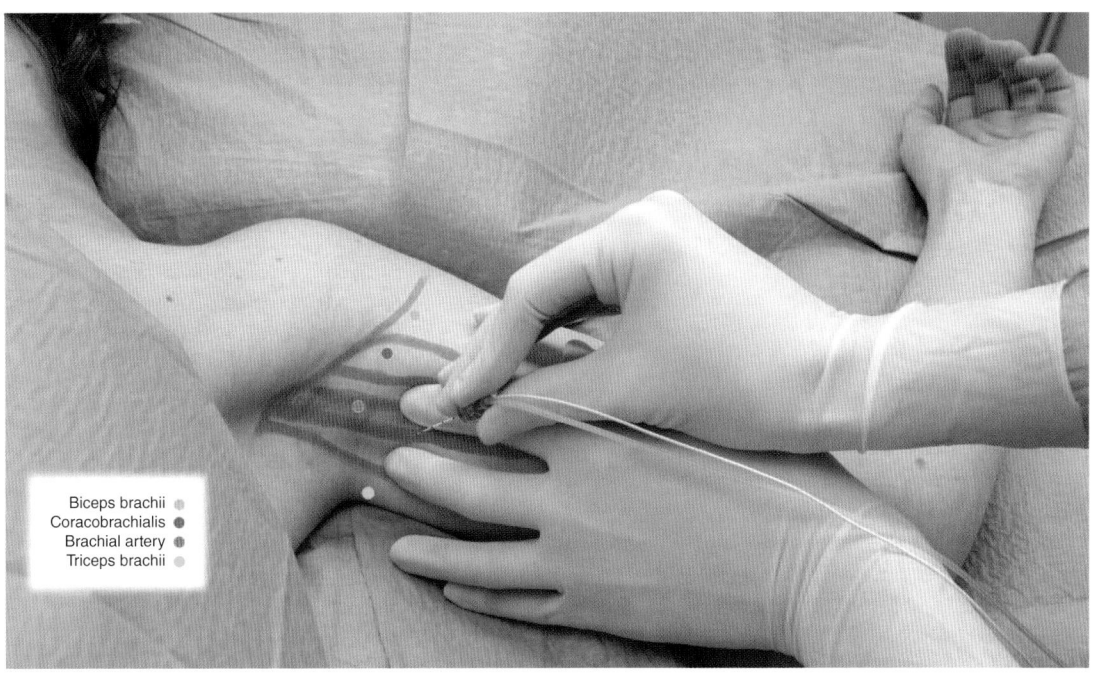

FIGURE 80E–4. Median nerve block: The needle is inserted below the pulse of the axillary (brachial) artery. CB = coracobrachialis.

Biceps brachii ●
Coracobrachialis ●
Brachial artery ●
Triceps brachii ●

Clinical Pearls

- Arterial pulse palpation may prove challenging in some patients. In these patients, the initial motor response can be used to guide needle redirection to achieve the desired response.
- Elbow flexion (stimulation of the coracobrachialis muscle or the musculocutaneous nerve) indicates that the needle is outside the neurovascular sheath; the needle should be redirected downward and more superficially.
- Extension of the wrist and hand (radial nerve) indicates that the needle is below the artery; the median and ulnar nerves are above the artery.

- The more difficult differentiation is between the median and the ulnar nerves, which both result in wrist/finger flexion. In this scenario, the following method can be used to differentiate between the two nerves:
- When flexion is accompanied by forearm pronation, the stimulated nerve is the median (the needle is positioned above the artery).
- Another way to differentiate between these two nerves is by palpation of the flexor tendons at the wrist. Median nerve stimulation produces movements of the palmaris longus and the flexor carpi radialis tendons, which lie in the middle of the wrist, whereas ulnar nerve stimulation produces movement of the flexor carpi ulnaris tendon, which lies medially.
- Decreasing the intensity of the output current of the nerve stimulator helps facilitate differentiation between median and ulnar nerve stimulation.

Double-Injection Technique

1. The stimulating needle is first inserted above the artery, below the coracobrachialis muscle (see Figure 80E–3). After penetrating the fascia, the amplitude is increased until synchronous wrist flexion/pronation and flexion of the first three fingers are obtained (median nerve stimulation). The needle is advanced slowly toward this nerve while reducing the amplitude to 0.3 to 0.5 mA. At this point, half of the planned volume of LA is slowly injected with intermittent aspiration to rule out intravascular injection.
2. The needle is then withdrawn and inserted below the artery and above the triceps muscle (see Figure 80E–4). The fascia is again penetrated and the amplitude slowly increased. The

FIGURE 80E–5. Distribution of local anesthetic injected during axillary brachial plexus blockade. NR = nervus radialis.

S
L

NR

first response is usually either arm extension (muscular branches to the triceps) or thumb adduction and flexion of the last two fingers (ulnar nerve). However, these responses are ignored, and the needle is advanced deeper, often slightly upward, behind the artery (Figure 80E–6) until wrist and finger extension is obtained (radial nerve). After stimulation is obtained using a current intensity lower than 0.5 mA, the remaining volume of LA is slowly injected with intermittent aspiration.

Clinical Pearl

- With ultrasound-guided nerve blocks motor stimulation below 0.5 mA is avoided to decrease the risk of needle–nerve contact or intraneural injection. With nerve stimulator–guided blocks, however, motor response is sought at 0.3—0.5 mA as evoked motor response is the only means of nerve localization, and nerve stimulation does not allow visualization of the tissue spaces or spread of the local anesthetic which is possible with ultrasound guidance.

Multiple-Injection Technique

Needle insertion sites are identical to those for the double-injection technique.

1. After electrolocation of the median nerve, 5–10 mL of the LA volume is injected (see Figure 80E–3).
2. The needle is withdrawn subcutaneously and redirected obliquely, above and into the coracobrachialis muscle. After obtaining stimulation-synchronous biceps flexion, the amplitude is reduced to 0.3–0.5 mA and another 5–10 mL of LA is injected to block the musculocutaneous nerve.
3. The needle is removed and inserted below the artery (see Figure 80E–4). The first stimulated nerve is usually the ulnar nerve, into which 5–10 mL of LA is injected.

4. The needle is advanced deeper until the radial nerve is found (see Double-Injection Technique, p. 1345.).

Clinical Pearls

- Two studies by Sia and colleagues[23,28] suggest that two separate injections below the artery do not improve success rates, and therefore only one such injection is needed. This injection is made close to the radial nerve and should contain half of the planned LA volume.
- Electrolocation of multiple nerves may occasionally take some time. Because the first injection of the LA injection in the vicinity of the median nerve may partially block the ulnar nerve, the search for the nerves should be made expeditiously to minimize the risk of needle–nerve contact or intraneural injection into an anesthetized nerve.
- For these reasons, this technique could be considered an advanced regional anesthesia technique. Careful assessment of resistance to injection by an experienced practitioner or objective monitoring of injection pressure should be used with each injection.

Transarterial Technique

This relatively simple technique does not rely on a nerve stimulator; instead, placement of the needle within the neurovascular sheath is identified by relying on the axillary artery:

- The axillary artery is palpated and stabilized using a two-finger palpation technique.
- As the needle is advanced toward the pulse of the axillary artery, bright red arterial blood is aspirated. A thin, long-beveled needle (typically 1.5-in., 25-gauge) is used to minimize the risk of axillary hematoma.

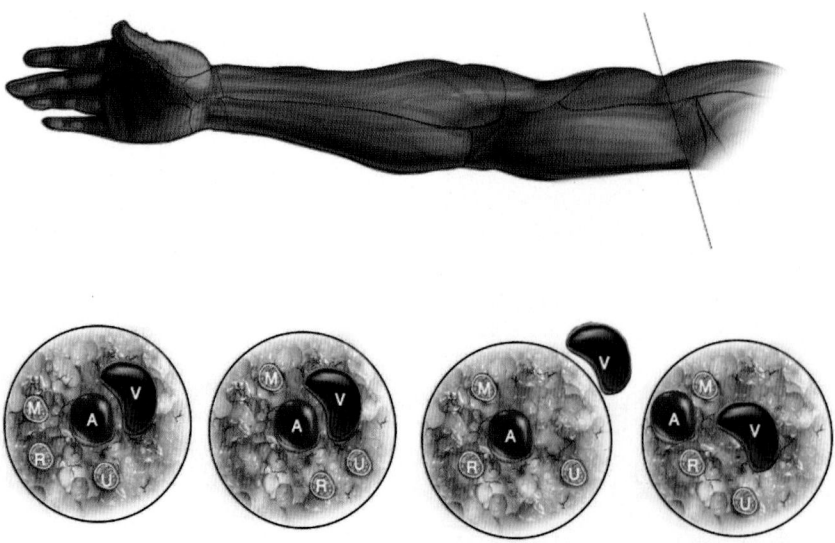

FIGURE 80E–6. Spatial arrangement of the terminal nerves of the brachial plexus in the axilla. M = median nerve, A = artery, V = vein, R = radial nerve, U = ulnar nerve.

- The needle is advanced deeper until blood cannot be aspirated (the tip of the needle has exited the artery) and half of the volume of the LA is injected behind the posterior wall. This should block the radial nerve.
- The needle is slowly withdrawn while aspirating. As the needle enters the axillary artery, bright red blood is again aspirated.
- The withdrawal of the needle is continued until blood cannot be aspirated (the needle exits the artery and its tip is positioned superficial [media] to the artery inside the neurovascular sheath).
- The remaining volume of LA is injected superficial to the anterior wall to block the median and the ulnar nerves.
- A transarterial injection is made as high up in the axilla as possible, and the needle should traverse the artery at an oblique angle. This reduces the risk of making the injection behind the artery intramuscularly and improves the spread of the LA to the plexus cords to block the musculocutaneous nerve.

MIDHUMERAL APPROACH (HUMERAL CANAL BLOCK)

The difference between the multiinjection axillary and the midhumeral (humeral canal) approaches is that in the latter, two terminal nerves, the musculocutaneous and the radial, are blocked separately, above and below the humeral bone, respectively (Figures 80E–1 and 80E–7). With any multistimulation technique, there is always a risk that an intraneural injection may be made into the already anesthetized nerves. Although the four-injection midhumeral block has been found to be more effective than the double-injection axillary technique,[30] either block results in a very high success rate when four injection techniques are used.[24] An advantage of the axillary approach is that incomplete axillary blocks can be supplemented with a midhumeral block.[31] The opposite is not possible, nor is it recommended because electrostimulation may be precluded by blockade distal to the site of nerve localization. An incomplete

midhumeral block, on the other hand, can be supplemented at the elbow or the wrist.

Technique

The injection technique for the midhumeral block is similar to the four-injection axillary technique, except the injections are made more distally. In addition, the musculocutaneous and the radial nerves are sought at a deeper location than in the axillary approach (see Figure 80E–7). Figure 80E–8 demonstrates the spread of the injected local anesthetic in the midhumeral technique.

- The nondominant hand grips the biceps muscle while searching for the musculocutaneous nerve, and the stimulating needle is inserted below the muscle (to avoid direct stimulation).
- When the bone is contacted before eliciting the twitches, the needle is redirected upward, toward the belly of the biceps muscle.
- The triceps muscle is stabilized similarly while attempting stimulation of the radial nerve. It should be kept in mind that the radial nerve winds around the humeral shaft on its way downward, which makes electrolocation of this nerve challenging with distal approaches.

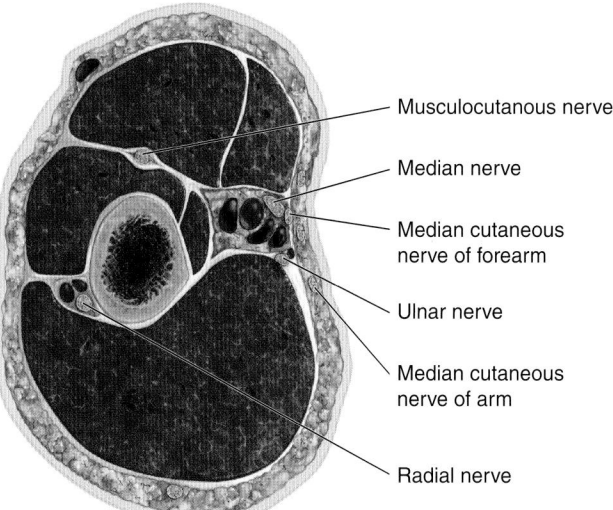

Musculocutanous nerve

Median nerve

Median cutaneous nerve of forearm

Ulnar nerve

Median cutaneous nerve of arm

Radial nerve

FIGURE 80E–7. Spatial arrangement of the terminal nerves of the brachial plexus at the midhumerus.

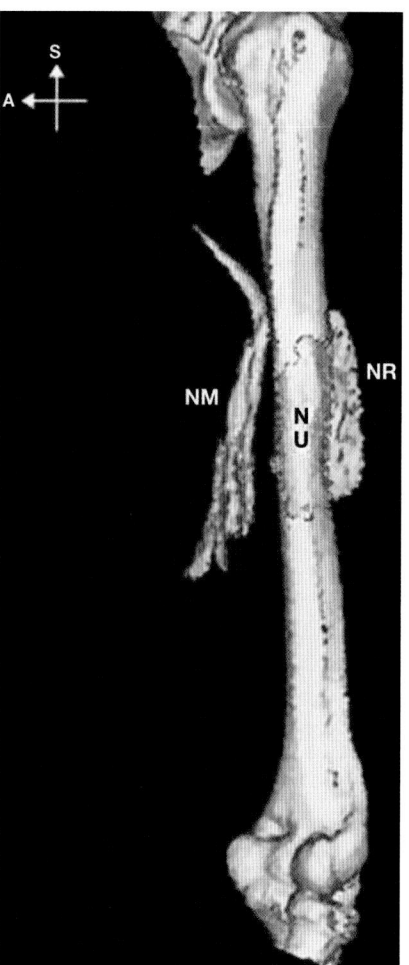

FIGURE 80E–8. Distribution of injectates after midhumeral blockade. NM = nervus medialis, NU = nervus ulnaris, NR = nervus radialis.

CHOICE OF LOCAL ANESTHETIC

The choice of LA depends on the length of surgery and the desired density and duration of blockade. For single-injection blocks, short- and medium-acting LAs (prilocaine, 2-chloro-procaine, lidocaine, or mepivacaine) in concentrations of 1.5%–2% (3% for 2-chloroprocaine), with or without epinephrine or sodium bicarbonate, will provide reliable sensory and motor block of rapid onset (10–20 min) and sufficient duration (3–4 h; 1.5–2 h for 2-chloroprocaine) for most acute and subacute procedures (e.g., wound debridement; closed fracture repositions; ligament-, tendon-, or nerve sutures; finger amputations). For elective procedures of longer duration (e.g., arthrodeses, arthroplasties, osteosyntheses, extensive palmar fasciectomies) ropivacaine 0.5%–0.75% or bupivacaine 0.375%–0.5%, with or without epinephrine, will provide analgesia of slightly slower onset (15–20 min) and longer duration (6–16 h). For specialized hand surgery that may last several hours—for example, multiple joint replacements or reimplantations of severed extremities—a continuous ropivacaine (0.2%–0.375%) infusion via an axillary catheter is probably the best technique. Clonidine (0.5 mcg/kg) may be added to intermediate-acting LAs to prolong analgesia after single-shot blocks.[32]

PERIOPERATIVE MANAGEMENT

The multiple-nerve stimulation technique is uncomfortable for patients[27,33] and should be preceded by adequate premedication (e.g., midazolam + sufentanil).[34] Adequate sedation and analgesia not only improve patients' acceptance of the block but also help relax the arm muscles. This makes precise needle manipulation as well as eliciting and interpreting the motor responses to nerve stimulation significantly easier for the practitioner and more acceptable to patients.

Clinical Pearls

- The first sign of a successful block is weakness of the upper arm muscles, which can be tested immediately after needle withdrawal. This can be done by asking the patient to place the hand on the abdomen or touch the practitioner's finger.
- Loss of coordination signifies that the mantle fascicles of the musculocutaneous and radial nerves, which supply flexors and extensors, are being blocked. Very often patients report an early loss of the position sense in the blocked extremity.

The onset and distribution of analgesia can be tested every 5 or 10 minutes after block administration in the sensory areas of the seven terminal nerves (Figure 80E–9). Thirty minutes after block insertion, the unblocked nerves can be supplemented distal to the initial block site (e.g., elbow blocks).

Clinical Pearls

- Most hand surgery (e.g., palmar fasciectomies and nerve or tendon repair) is performed on the volar aspect and theoretically can be performed with partial blocks (i.e., without the radial or musculocutaneous nerves).
- For elbow surgery, an infraclavicular approach is a better choice then the axillary block.
- Tourniquet analgesia may be more related to the total injected dose of LA rather than to successful block of the medial cutaneous brachial nerves. Most of the injected LA is absorbed into the surrounding muscles, which are the main source of ischemic pain.[35]

CONTINUOUS AXILLARY BLOCK

The indications for continuous axillary block include control of acute postoperative pain, management of chronic pain, and treatment of vascular disease, (e.g., Raynaud syndrome).

Technique

The axillary fossa is shaved and disinfected. After subcutaneous LA infiltration, the specific muscle twitch from the nerve of greatest interest is elicited by a needle or stimulating introducer cannula (see Single-Injection Technique, p. 1343). The intensity of the stimulating current is progressively reduced to 0.5 mA or less, while making fine adjustments to the needle position. A catheter is inserted (under sterile conditions) 5–8 cm cephalad into the neurovascular sheath and either sutured to the skin or tunneled. This helps maintain the catheter in place because the nerves are superficial and the arm sweat makes maintenance of an occlusive dressing difficult.

Clinical Pearl

- Difficulty with catheter insertion usually indicates placement of the needle outside the neurovascular sheath.

Maintenance

Diluted solutions of long-acting LAs (eg, 0.125% bupivacaine or 0.2% ropivacaine) are most often used for continuous infusions. A common infusion regimen includes intermittent bolus of LA (5-10 mL Q 4-6 hrs) of the dilute mixture of LA with or without continuous infusion of 5 mL/h.

Clinical Pearl

- A typical infusion regimen for 0.2% ropivacaine is a basal rate of, for example, 0.1 mL/kg bodyweight per hour (minimum, 5 mL; maximum, 10 mL) and a 5 mL patient-controlled bolus with a lock-out time of 30 minutes.

Complications

Vascular Puncture   Vascular puncture can occur with axillary block but it usually can be detected. However, venous puncture may be undetected if aspiration or palpation pressure collapses the venous lumen.

Intravascular LA Injection   Intravascular LA injection manifests itself as lightheadedness and or tachycardia (ropivacaine- or epinephrine-containing solutions). Note

that intra-arterial injection produces hand paresthesia during injection accompanied by sudden paleness. Slow injection with repeated needle aspirations is mandatory.

Hematoma   Hematoma may occur after arterial puncture. If the artery is punctured, firm, steady pressure should be applied over the puncture site for 5–10 minutes. For the tran-sarterial technique, needles of smaller gauge should be used to minimize the risk of hematoma.

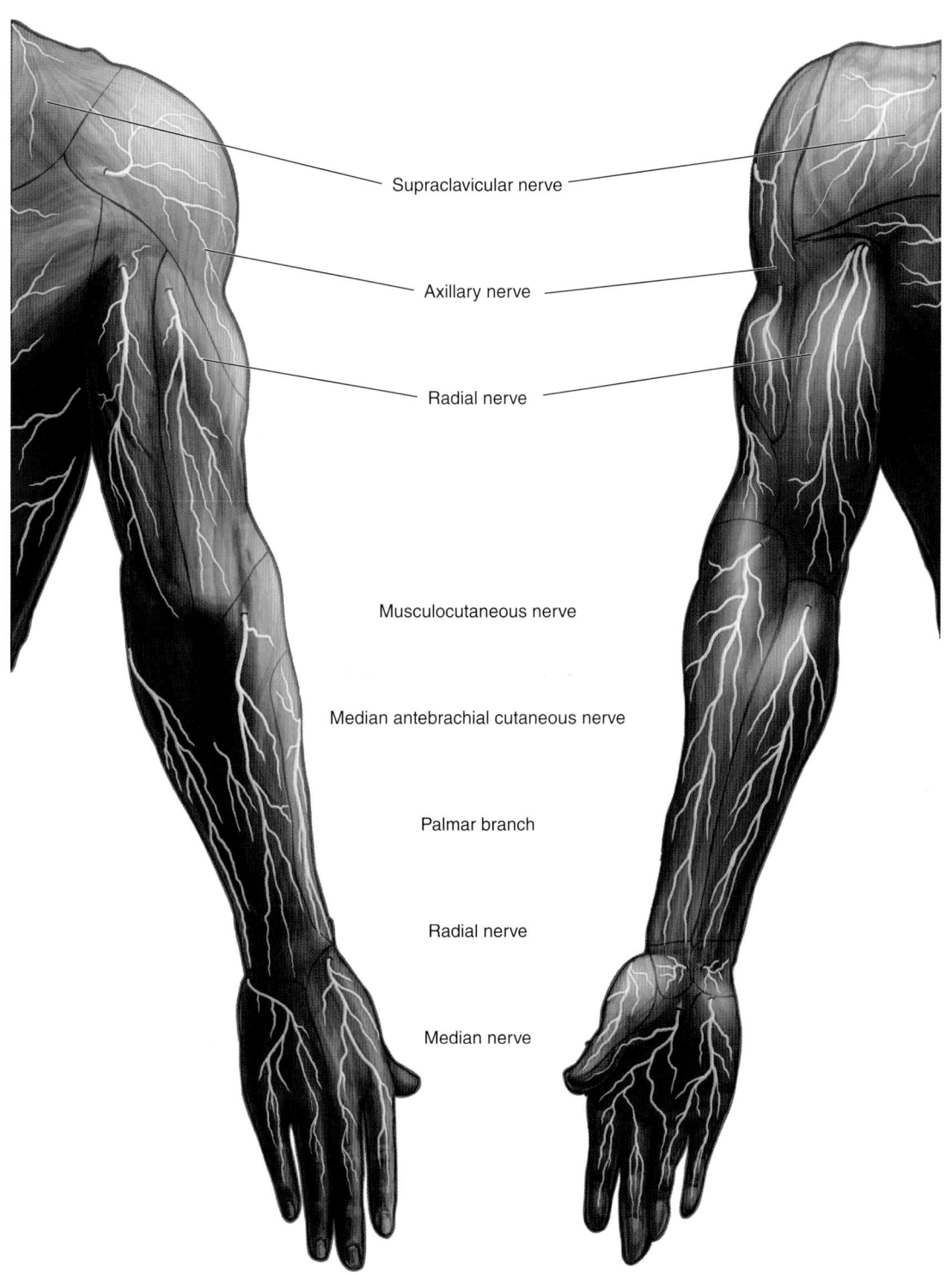

Supraclavicular nerve

Axillary nerve

Radial nerve

Musculocutaneous nerve

Median antebrachial cutaneous nerve

Palmar branch

Radial nerve

Median nerve

FIGURE 80E–9. Sensory innervation of the upper extremity.

Toxicity Due to Absorption of LA Toxicity due to absorption of LA (in contrast to the accidental intravascular injection, which becomes symptomatic during or immediately after the injection) usually becomes symptomatic 5–20 minutes after injection. The symptoms include lightheadedness, dizziness, tunnel vision, circumoral paresthesia, bradycardia or tachycardia, anxiousness (eventually progressing to unconsciousness), and seizures. Oxygen, a sedative/hypnotic in titrated doses, and airway support if necessary should be immediately administered.

Nerve Injury Nerve injury may be caused by the advancing needle, intraneural injection, application of a tourniquet, or a combination of these. Intraneural injections are characterized by pain, extremity withdrawal, and resistance to injection. Needle and injection injuries typically manifest as neurologic deficit in the distribution of the affected nerve. However, ischemic damage caused by prolonged application of the tourniquet more commonly results in a diffuse injury, affects several nerves, and is usually accompanied by soreness of the upper arm. Symptoms of nerve damage (sensory loss and persistent paresthesia) usually appear within a day or two after recovery from the block. Most nerve injuries are neurapraxia (functional damage), which carry a good prognosis and heal within a few weeks.

Clinical Pearls

- When the motor response to nerve stimulation is seen with currents <0.2 mA, the tip of the needle should be slightly withdrawn or repositioned to maintain the twitch with 02–0.5 mA.
- LA should never be injected when abnormal resistance (high opening pressure) to injection is encountered. When this occurs, the needle should be pulled back slightly and the injection reattempted. If the resistance persists, the needle should be completely withdrawn and cleared; it should never be assumed that the cause of the resistance is related only to needle obstruction.

SUMMARY

For axillary brachial plexus block, a triple-injection nerve stimulator technique with electrolocation of median, musculocutaneous, and radial nerves is preferred.[36,37] A double- injection technique is the next best and may be used with or without a nerve stimulator. The midhumeral (a four-injection technique) is probably best suited for supplementing incomplete axillary blocks, although it can be used as a primary technique. For continuous blocks, the catheter should be placed close to the main nerve innervating the surgical site (e.g., the median nerve for surgery of medial and volar surfaces; the radial nerve for surgery of lateral and dorsal surfaces). For more extensive surgery involving the entire circumference of the arm (e.g., major trauma/amputation), an approach higher in the axilla or

infraclavicular block may be better suited. An optimal perineural infusion technique is a basal infusion plus patient-controlled boluses; the suggested LA for this application is ropivacaine 0.2%. An accidental intravascular injection is the most common complication of axillary block. The risk of systemic toxicity of LA can be decreased by avoiding fast, forceful injection and using frequent aspiration to rule out intravascular injection. Pain, paresthesia, extremity withdrawal, or high injection pressure may indicate intraneural needle placement; occurrence of any of these signs and symptoms should prompt immediate cessation of the injection and reevaluation.

REFERENCES

1. Hall RJ: Hydrochlorate of cocaine. NY Med J 1884;40:643.
2. Hirschel G: Die Anästesierung der Plexus Brachialis bei die Operationen an der oberen Extremität. München Med Wochenschr 1911;58: 1555–1556.
3. Burnham PJ: Regional block of the great nerves of the upper arm. Anesthesiology 1958;19:281–284.
4. De Jong RH: Axillary block of the brachial plexus. Anesthesiology 1961;22:215–225.
5. Eriksson E, Skarby HG: A simplified method of axillary brachial plexus block. Nord Med 1962;68:1325.
6. Winnie AP, Radonjic R, Akkineni SR, et al: Factors influencing distribution of local anesthetic injected into the brachial plexus sheath. Anesth Analg 1979;58:225–234.
7. Koscielniak-Nielsen ZJ, Horn A, Rotbøll-Nielsen P: Effect of arm position on the effectiveness of perivascular axillary nerve block. Br J Anaesth 1995;74:387–391.
8. Koscielniak-Nielsen ZJ, Quist Christensen L, Stens-Pedersen HL, et al: Effect of digital pressure on the effectiveness of perivascular axillary block. Br J Anaesth 1995;75:702–706.
9. Yamamoto K, Tsubokawa T, Ohmura S, et al: Effect of arm position on central spread of local anesthetics and on quality of the block with axillary brachial plexus block. Reg Anesth Pain Med 1999;24: 36–42.
10. Thompson GE, Rorie DK: Functional anatomy of the brachial plexus sheaths. Anesthesiology 1983;59:117–122.
11. Lassale B, Ang ET: Particularités de l'organisation du tissus celluleux de la cavité axillaire. Bull Soc Anat Paris 1984;9:57–60.
12. Vester-Andersen T, Broby-Johansen U, Bro-Rasmussen F: Perivascular axillary block VI: The distribution of gelatine solutions injected into the axillary neurovascular sheath of cadavers. Acta Anaesthesiol Scand 1986; 30:18–22.
13. Partrigde B, Katz J, Benirschke K: Functional anatomy of the brachial plexus sheath: Implications for anesthesia. Anesthesiology 1987;66: 743–747.
14. Klaastad O, Smedby O, Thompson GE, et al: Distribution of local anesthetic in axillary brachial plexus block: a clinical and magnetic resonance imaging study. Anesthesiology 2002;96:1315–1324.
15. Vester-Andersen T, Christiansen C, Sørensen M, et al: Perivascular axillary block II: Influence of injected volume of local anaesthetic on neural blockade. Acta Anaesthesiol Scand 1983;27:95–98.
16. Vester-Andersen T, Husum B, Lindeburg T, et al: Perivascular axillary block IV: blockade following 40, 50, or 60 mL mepivacaine 1% with adrenaline. Acta Anaesthesiol Scand 1984;28:99–105.
17. Urban MK, Urquhart B: Evaluation of brachial plexus anesthesia for upper extremity surgery. Reg Anesth Pain Med 1994;19:175–182.
18. Stan TC, Krantz MA, Solomon DL, et al: The incidence of neurovascular complications following axillary brachial plexus block using a transarterial approach. A prospective study of 1000 consecutive patients. Reg Anesth Pain Med 1995;20:486–492.
19. Baranowski AP, Pither CE: A comparison of three methods of axillary brachial plexus anaesthesia. Anaesthesia 1990;45:362–365.
20. Lavoie J, Martin R, Tétrault JP, et al: Axillary plexus block using a peripheral nerve stimulator: single or multiple injections. Can J Anaesth 1992;39:583–586.
21. Koscielniak-Nielsen ZJ, Stens-Pedersen HL, Lippert Knudsen F: Readiness for surgery after axillary block: single or multiple injection techniques. Eur J Anaesthesiol 1997;14:164–171.
22. Koscielniak-Nielsen ZJ, Hesselbjerg L, Fejlberg V: Comparison of transarterial and multiple nerve stimulation techniques for an initial

axillary block by 45 mL of mepivacaine 1% with adrenaline. Acta Anaesthesiol Scand 1998;42:570–575.

23. Sia S, Lepri A, Ponzecchi P: Axillary brachial plexus block using peripheral nerve stimulator: a comparison between double- and triple-injection techniques. Reg Anesth Pain Med 2001;26:499–503.

24. Sia S, Lepri A, Campolo MC, et al: Four-injection brachial plexus block using peripheral nerve stimulator: a comparison between axillary and midhumeral approaches. Anesth Analg 2002;95:1075–1079.

25. Handoll HHG, Koscielniak-Nielsen ZJ. Single, double, or multiple injection techniques for axillary brachial plexus block for hand, wrist, or forearm surgery. Cochrane Database Syst Rev. 2006 Jan 25(1):CD003842. Review.

26. Dupré LJ: Bloc du plexus brachial au canal huméral. Cah Anesth 1994; 42:767–769.

27. Koscielniak-Nielsen ZJ, Rotbøll-Nielsen P, Rasmussen H: Patients' experiences with multiple stimulation axillary block for fast-track ambulatory hand surgery. Acta Anaesthesiol Scand 2002;46:789–793.

28. Sia S, Bartoli M: Selective ulnar nerve localization is not essential for axillary brachial plexus block using a multiple nerve stimulation technique. Reg Anesth Pain Med 2001;26:12–16.

29. Tsui BC, Wagner A, Finucane B: Electrophysiologic effect of injectates on peripheral nerve stimulation. Reg Anesth Pain Med 2004;29:189–193.

30. Bouaziz H, Narchi P, Mercier FJ, et al: The use of selective axillary nerve block for outpatient hand surgery. Anesth Analg 1998;86:746–748.

31. March X, Pardina B, Torres-Bah'ı S, et al: A comparison of triple-injection axillary brachial plexus block with the humeral approach. Reg Anesth Pain Med 2003;28:504–508.

32. Murphy DB, McCartney CJ, Chan VW: Novel analgesic adjuncts for brachial plexus block: a systematic review. Anesth Analg 2000;90:1122–1128.

33. Koscielniak-Nielsen ZJ, Rasmussen H, Nielsen PT: Patients' perception of pain during axillary and humeral blocks using multiple nerve stimulations. Reg Anesth Pain Med 2004;29:328–332.

34. Kinirons BP, Bouaziz H, Paqueron X, et al: Sedation with sufentanil and midazolam decreases pain in patients undergoing upper limb surgery under multiple nerve block. Anesth Analg 2000;90:1118–1121.

35. Koscielniak-Nielsen ZJ, Rotbøll Nielsen P, Sørensen T, et al: Low dose axillary block by targeted injections of the terminal nerves. Can J Anaesth 1999;46:658–664.

36. Sia S, Lepri A, Ponzecchi P: Axillary brachial plexus block using peripheral nerve stimulator: a comparison between double- and triple-injection techniques. Reg Anesth Pain Med 2001;26:499–503.

37. Sia S, Lepri A, Campolo MC, et al: Four-injection brachial plexus block using peripheral nerve stimulator: a comparison between axillary and midhumeral approaches. Anesth Analg 2002;95:1075–1079.

Wrist Block

Paul Hobeika, Tessy Castermans, Joris Duerinckx, and Sam van Boxstael

INTRODUCTION

The wrist block involves anesthesia of the median, ulnar, and radial nerves, including the dorsal sensory branch of the ulnar nerve. The wrist block is simple to perform, essentially devoid of systemic complications, and highly effective for a variety of procedures on the hand and fingers. Wrist blocks can be used in the office or operating room setting. As such, skill in performing a wrist block should be in the armamentarium of every practitioner.[1-9] A study comparing intra-articular and portal infiltration versus wrist block for analgesia after arthroscopy of the wrist has shown that wrist block provides better and more reliable analgesia in patients undergoing arthroscopy of the wrist without exposing patients to the risk of chondrotoxicity.[10]

INDICATIONS & CONTRAINDICATIONS

A wrist block is most commonly used for hand and finger surgery.[11,12] The most common hand surgery in the United States is carpal tunnel release. Sir James Paget described carpal tunnel syndrome in 1853.[1,13] Although Sir James Learmonth reported release of the carpal tunnel at the wrist in 1933, it was not until the 1950s that the surgery became popular through the efforts of George Phalen.[14-16] Because of the ease of performing a wrist block, wrist blocks are used in a variety of settings including the emergency room, outpatient surgery centers, and office-based anesthesia practices. Hand surgeons rely on the wrist block to perform minor procedures in their offices. A wrist block can be used in a patient with a full stomach requiring emergency surgery, thereby obviating the need for general anesthesia and reducing the risk of aspiration.

Although only there are only a few contraindication to wrist blocks, local infection at the site of needle insertion and allergy to local anesthetic are the most cited. Patients are usually able to tolerate a tourniquet on the arm without anesthesia for 20 minutes; a wrist tourniquet can be tolerated for about 120 minutes.

FUNCTIONAL ANATOMY OF WRIST BLOCK

Innervation of the hand is shared by the ulnar, median, and radial nerves (Figure 80F–1). The ulnar nerve innervates more intrinsic muscles than the median nerve, and supplies digital branches to the skin of the medial one and a half digits (Figure 80F–2). A corresponding area of the palm is innervated by palmar branches that arise from the ulnar nerve in the forearm. The deep branch of the ulnar nerve accompanies the deep palmar arch and supplies innervation to the three hypothenar muscles, the medial two lumbrical muscles, all the interossei, and the adductor pollicis. The ulnar nerve also innervates the palmaris brevis muscle.

The median nerve traverses the carpal tunnel and terminates as digital and recurrent branches. The digital branches innervate the skin of the lateral three and a half digits and, usually, the lateral two lumbrical muscles. A corresponding area of the palm is innervated by palmar branches that arise from the median nerve in the forearm. The recurrent branch of the median nerve supplies the three thenar muscles. In the palm, the digital branches of the ulnar and median nerves lie deep in the superficial palmar arch, but in the fingers, they lie anterior to the digital arteries that arise from the superficial arch. Although the innervation of the ring and middle fingers may vary, the skin on the anterior surface of the thumb is always supplied by the median nerve and that of the little finger by the ulnar nerve. The palmar digital branches of the median and ulnar nerves also innervate the nail beds of their respective digits.

The radial nerve passes along the front of the radial side of the forearm. It arises first from the lateral side of the radial

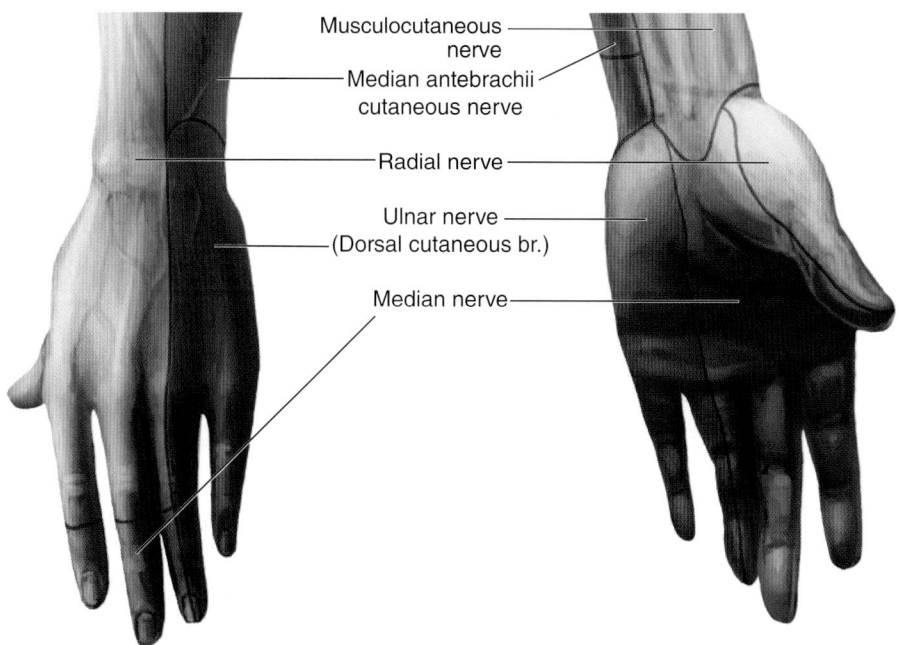

FIGURE 80F-1. Innervation of the hand.

artery and beneath the supinator muscle. About 3 in. above the wrist, it leaves the artery, pierces the deep fascia, and divides into two branches (Figure 80F–3). The superficial branch, the smaller of the two branches, supplies the skin of the radial side and base of the thumb, and joins the anterior branch of the

musculocutaneous nerve. The deep branch of the radial nerve communicates with the posterior branch of the musculocutaneous nerve. On the dorsum of the hand, the deep branch of the radial nerve forms an arch with the dorsal cutaneous branch of the ulnar nerve.

ANATOMIC LANDMARKS

The superficial branch of the radial nerve runs along the medial aspect of the brachioradialis muscle (see Figure 80F–3). It then passes between the tendon of the brachioradialis and radius to pierce the fascia on the dorsal aspect. Just above the styloid process of the radius, it gives off digital branches for the dorsal skin of the thumb, index finger, and lateral half of the middle finger. Several of its branches pass superficially over the anatomic "snuff box."

The median nerve is located between the tendons of the palmaris longus and the flexor carpi radialis (Figures 80F–4; see 80F–2). The palmaris longus tendon is usually the more prominent of the two tendons, and the median nerve passes just lateral to it.

The ulnar nerve passes between the ulnar artery and tendon of the flexor carpi ulnaris (see Figures 80F–2 and 80F–4). The tendon of the flexor carpi ulnaris is superficial to the ulnar nerve.

EQUIPMENT

A standard regional anesthesia tray is prepared with the following equipment:

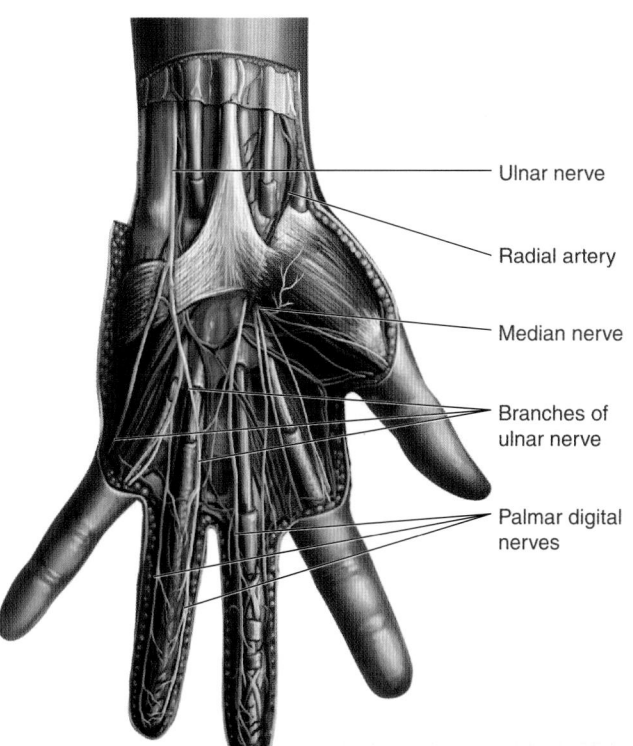

FIGURE 80F-2. Innervation of the hand: The course of the terminal nerves.

- Sterile towels and 4-in. × 4-in. gauze pads
- 10-mL syringes with local anesthetic (LA)
- One 1.5 -in., 25-gauge needle

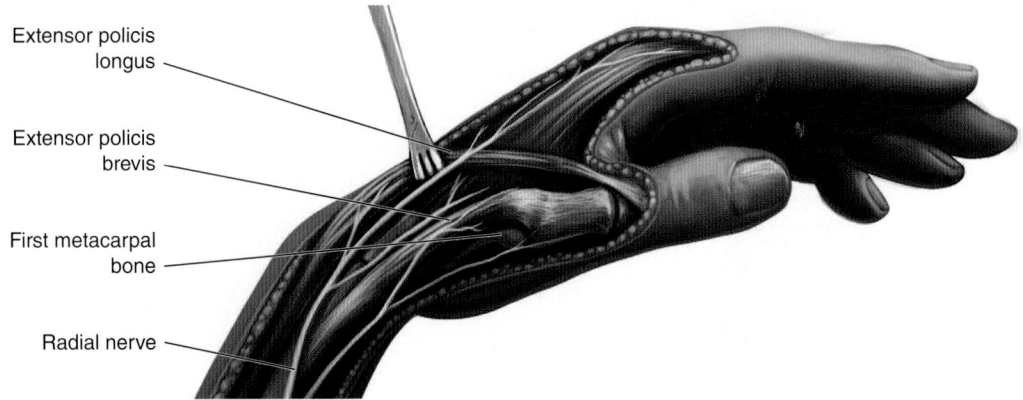

FIGURE 80F–3. Position and course of the radial nerve at the wrist.

TECHNIQUE

The patient is in the supine position with the arm abducted. The wrist should be kept in a slight dorsiflexion.

Block of the Radial Nerve

The radial nerve block is essentially a "field block" and requires a more extensive infiltration because of its less predictable anatomic location and division into multiple, smaller cutaneous branches. Five milliliters of LA is injected subcutaneously just above the radial styloid while advancing the needle medially (Figure 80F–5). The infiltration is then extended laterally, using an additional 5 mL of LA.

Block of the Dorsal Sensory Branch of the Radial Nerve

The dorsal sensory branch of the radial nerve is blocked by inserting the needle 1 cm proximal to the radial styloid, which is radial to the radial artery (Figure 80F–6). This branch of the radial nerve exits from between the brachioradialis and extensor carpi radialis longus 5–8 cm proximal to the radial styloid. The needle is advanced to the Lister tubercle, and if there are no paresthesias, 5 mL of LA is injected subcutaneously throughout this area.

Block of the Ulnar Nerve

The ulnar nerve is anesthetized by inserting the needle under the tendon of the flexor carpi ulnaris muscle close to its

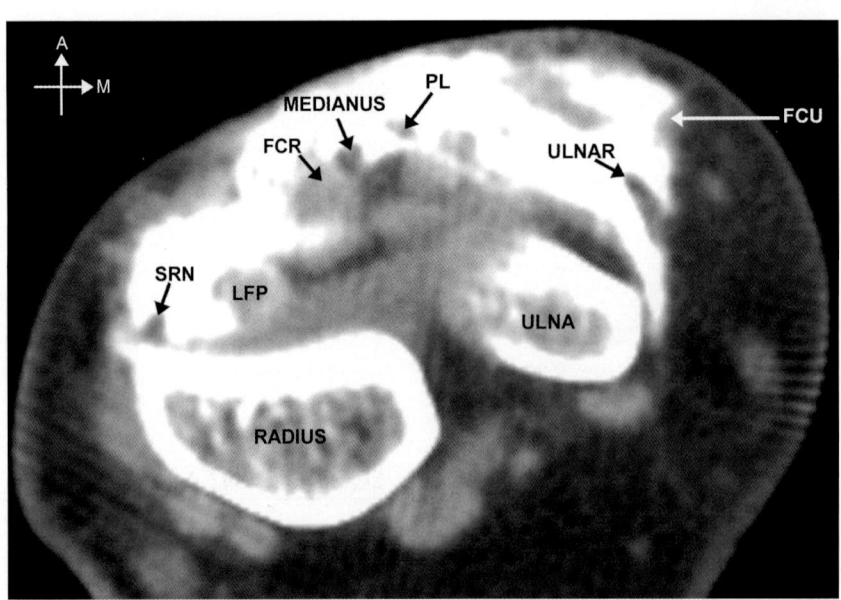

FIGURE 80F–4. Cross-sectional anatomy of the wrist as shown on an MRI scan just above the carpal tunnel. A = anterior, M = medial, SRN = superficial radial nerve, LFP = tendon of the flexor palmaris longus, FCR = flexor carpi radialis, PL = tendon of the palmaris longus, FCU = tendon of the flexor carpi radialis.

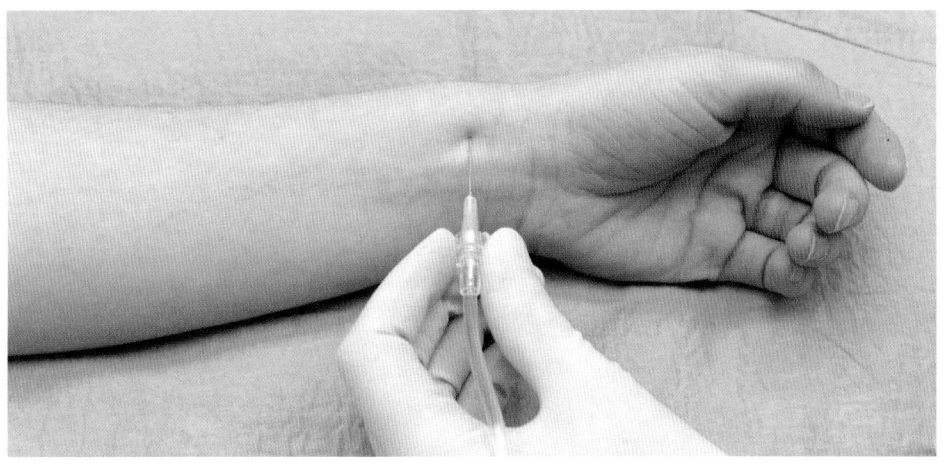

FIGURE 80F–5. Block of the radial nerve above the head of the radius.

distal attachment just above the styloid process of the ulna (Figures 80F–7 and 80F–8; see Figure 80F–4). The needle is advanced 5–10 mm to just past the tendon of the flexor carpi ulnaris. Three to 5 mL of LA solution is injected. A subcutaneous injection of 2–3 mL of local anesthesia just above the tendon of the flexor carpi ulnaris is also advisable in blocking the cutaneous branches of the ulnar nerve, which often extend to the hypothenar area.

Block of the Dorsal Sensory Branch of the Ulnar Nerve

The dorsal sensory branch of the ulnar nerve is blocked by inserting the needle at the level of the ulnar styloid because it travels from palmar to dorsal in the area of the ulnar styloid (Figure 80F–9). Start the injection at the flexor carpi ulnaris and extend subcutaneously dorsally toward the distal radioulnar joint. Five milliliters of LA is injected subcutaneously throughout the area.

Block of the Median Nerve

The median nerve is anesthetized by inserting the needle between the tendons of the palmaris longus and flexor carpi radialis (Figures 80F–10 and 80F–11; see Figure 80F–8). The needle is inserted until it pierces the deep fascia. Three to 5 milliliters of LA is injected. Although the piercing of the deep fascia has been described to result in a fascial "click," it is more reliable to simply insert the needle until it contacts the bone. At that point, the needle is withdrawn 2–3 mm and the LA is injected. Figure 80F–12 demonstrates the spread of the LA after injection of 5 mL using the described technique.

Clinical Pearls

- A "fan" technique is recommended to increase the success rate of the median nerve block.

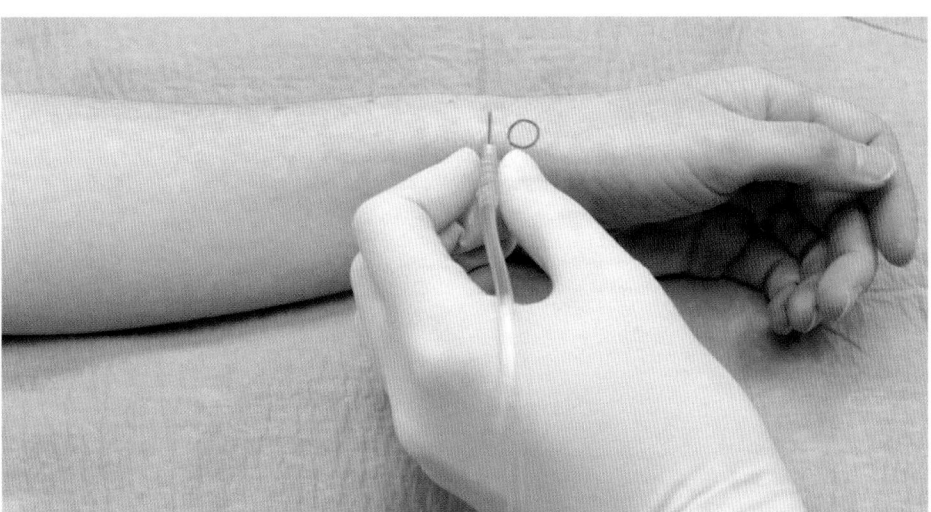

FIGURE 80F–6. Block of the superficial radial nerve

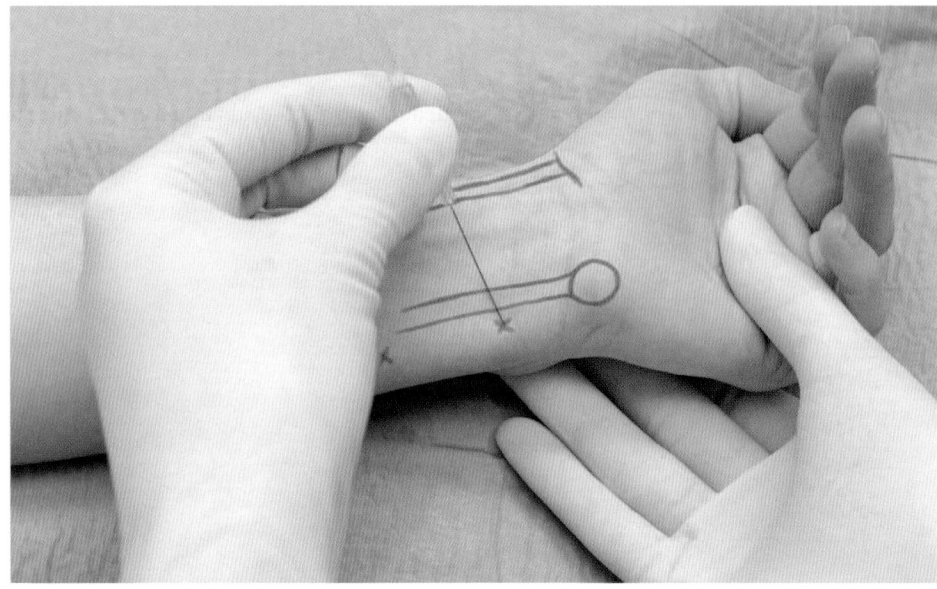

FIGURE 80F–7. Block of the ulnar nerve–the needle is shown inserted just medial to the flexor carpi ulnaris

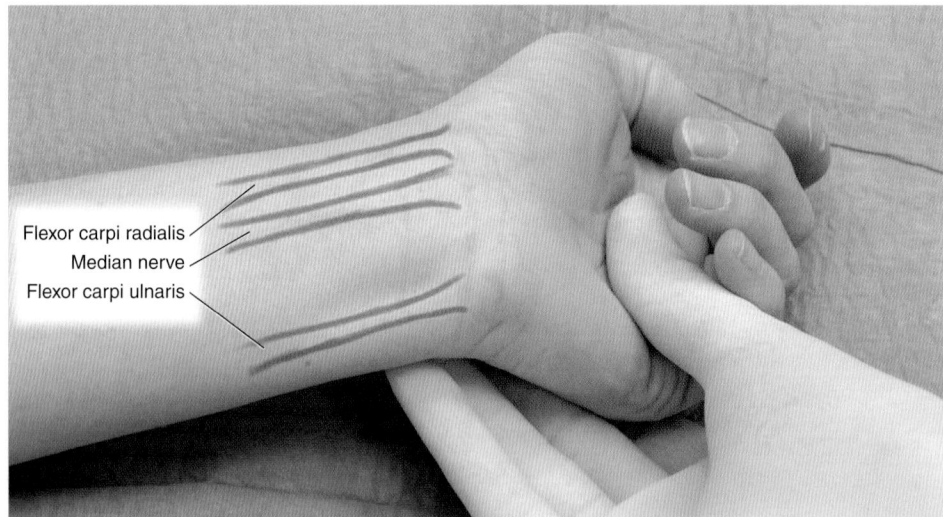

Flexor carpi radialis
Median nerve
Flexor carpi ulnaris

FIGURE 80F–8. Tendons of the wrist flexors and position of the medianus nerve in relationship to the flexor tendons.

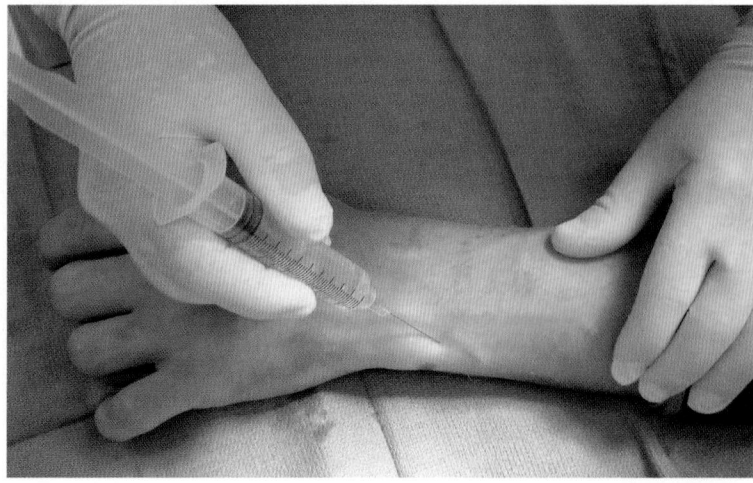

FIGURE 80F–9. Block of the superficial branch of the ulnar nerve.

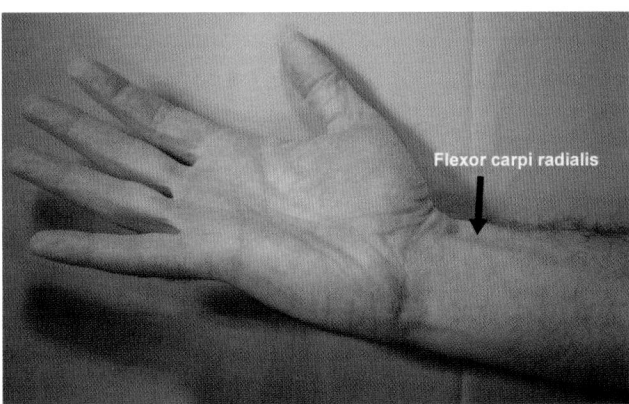

FIGURE 80F–10. A maneuver to accentuate the tendon of the flexor carpi radialis.

- After the initial injection, the needle is withdrawn back to the skin level, redirected 30 degrees laterally, and advanced again to contact the bone.
- After pulling back 1–2 mm off the bone, an additional 2 mL of LA is injected.
- A similar procedure is repeated with a medial redirection of the needle.

Nerve Stimulation Technique

Median and ulnar nerve can also be blocked at the wrist using a nerve stimulator. These blocks may be used for finger flexor tendon repairs, when the surgeon wishes to test their function intraoperatively (function of the forearm muscles is not affected). The median nerve is found in the carpal tunnel between the palmaris longus and the flexor carpi radialis tendons, and the ulnar nerve is found between the flexor carpi ulnaris and the ulnar artery. Twitches are similar to elbow blocks except for the forearm pronation, which is missing. Two to 3 mL of LA is sufficient to block either nerve.

CHOICE OF LOCAL ANESTHETIC

The choice of the type and concentration of LA for wrist blockade is based on the desired duration. Lidocaine is the most used anesthetic for wrist block, but bupivacaine can be used safely, also.[16] Table 80F–1 provides onset times and duration for some commonly used LAs. Clean the entire wrist area with a disinfectant solution. Aspirate prior to injection of LA to avoid intravascular injection.

BLOCK DYNAMICS AND PERIOPERATIVE MANAGEMENT

This technique is associated with moderate patient discomfort because multiple insertions and subcutaneous injections are required. Appropriate sedation and analgesia, midazolam (2–4 mg) and alfentanil (250–500 mcg), are required to ensure the patient's comfort. A typical onset time for a wrist block is 10–15 minutes, depending primarily on the concentration of LA used. Sensory anesthesia of the skin develops faster than the motor block. Placement of an Esmarch latex-free bandage or a tourniquet at the level of the wrist is well tolerated and does not require additional blockade.

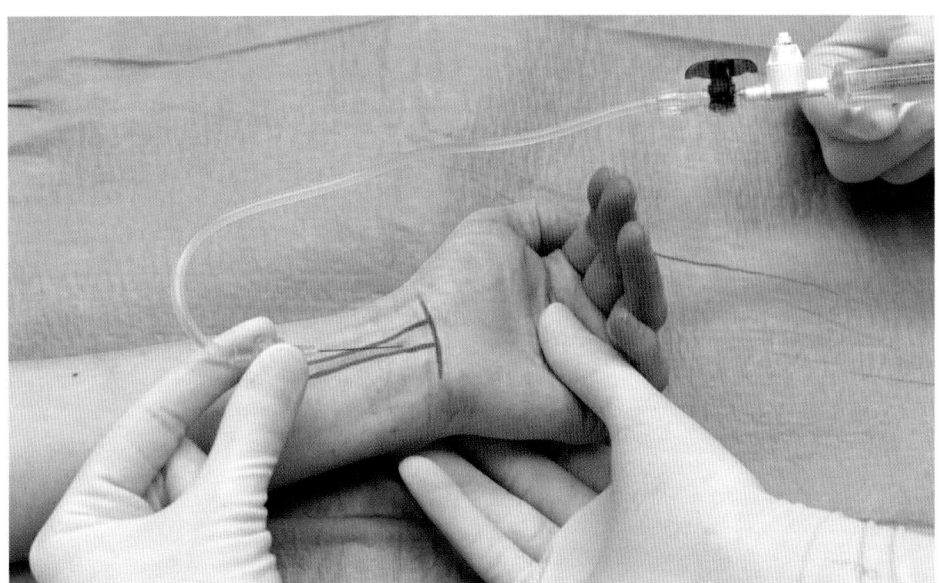

FIGURE 80F–11. Block of the median nerve at the wrist. The needle is shown inserted just medial to the flexor carpi radialis.

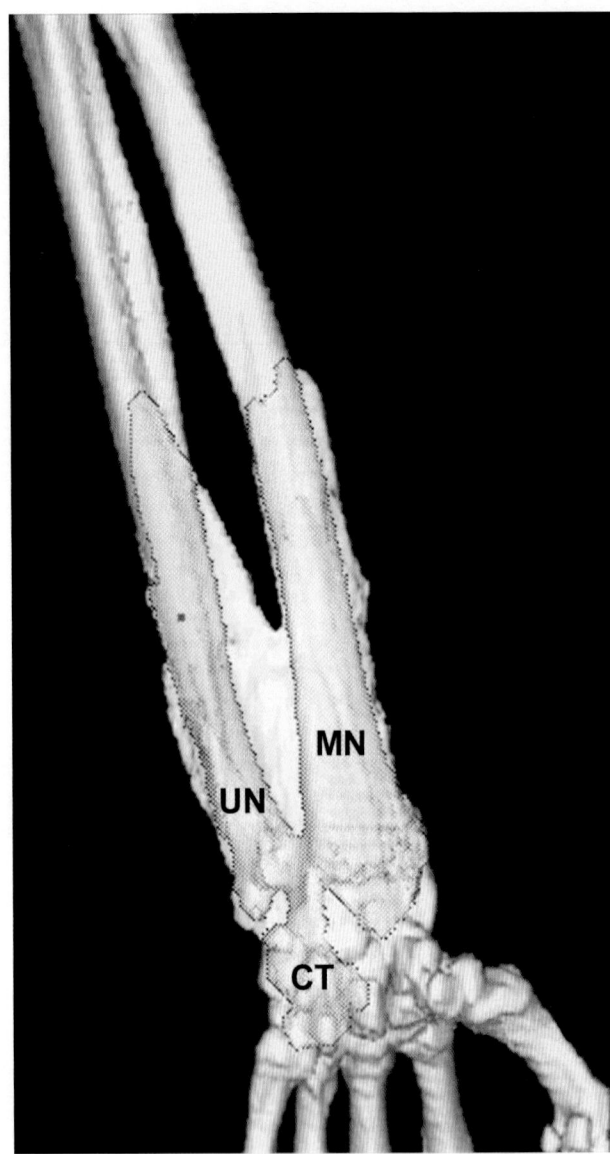

FIGURE 80F–12. Distribution of the dye after wrist block. MN = median nerve, UN = ulnar nerve, CT = carpal tunnel.

TABLE 80F–2. Complications from wrist block.

Infection	This should be very rare with the use of an aseptic technique.
Hematoma	Avoid multiple needle insertions for superficial blocks. Most superficial blocks can be accomplished with one or two needle insertions. Use 25-gauge needle and avoid puncturing superficial veins.
Vascular complications	Do not use epinephrine with wrist and finger blocks.
Nerve injury	Do not inject when the patient complains of pain or high pressure on injection is detected. Do not reinject the median and ulnar nerves.
Other	Instruct the patient on the care of the insensate extremity.

Clinical Pearl

- Both nerves lie quite superficially in tight compartments and cannot move away from the needle. Extra caution should therefore be used when advancing the needle and injecting LA.

COMPLICATIONS AND HOW TO AVOID THEM

Most common complications after wrist block are residual paresthesias due to an inadvertent intraneural injection. Systemic toxicity is rare because of the distal location of the blockade (Table 80F–2).

TABLE 80F–1. Onset times and duration for commonly used local anesthetic mixtures.

	Onset (min)	Anesthesia (h)	Analgesia (h)
1.5% Mepivacaine (+ HCO$_3$)	15–20	2–3	3–5
2% Lidocaine (+ HCO$_3$)	10–20	2–5	3–8
0.5% Ropivacaine	15–30	4–8	5–12
0.75% Ropivacaine	10–15	5–10	6–24
0.5% Bupivacaine (or L-bupivacaine)	15–30	5–15	6–30

REFERENCES

1. Derkash RS, Weaver JK, Berkeley ME, et al: Office carpal tunnel release with wrist block and wrist tourniquet. Orthopedics 1996;19:589–590.
2. Gebhard RE, Al-Samsam T, Greger J, et al: Distal nerve blocks at the wrist for outpatient carpal tunnel surgery offer intraoperative cardiovascular stability and reduce discharge time. Anesth Analg 2002;95:351–355.
3. Martinotti R, Berlanda P, Zanlungo M, et al: Peripheral anesthesia techniques in surgery of the arm. Minerva Chir 1999;54:831–833.
4. Melone CP Jr, Isani A: Anesthesia for hand injuries. Emerg Med Clin North Am 1985;3:235–243.
5. Leversee JH, Bergman JJ: Wrist and digital nerve blocks. J Fam Pract 1981;13:415–421.
6. Dushoff IM: Hand surgery under wrist block and local infiltration anesthesia, using an upper arm tourniquet. Plast Reconstr Surg 1973;51:685–686.
7. Vatashsky E, Aronson HB, Wexler MR, et al: Anesthesia in a hand surgery unit. J Hand Surg [Am] 1980;5:495–497.
8. Klezl Z, Krejca M, Simcik J: Role of sensory innervation variations for wrist block anesthesia. Arch Med Res 2001;32:155–158.

9. Ferrera PC, Chandler R: Anesthesia in the emergency setting: Part I. Hand and foot injuries. Am Fam Physician 1994;50:569–573.

10. Agrawal Y, Russon K, Chakrabarti I, Kocheta A. Intra-articular and portal infiltration versus wrist block for analgesia after arthroscopy of the wrist: a prospective RCT. Bone Joint J. 2015; 97-B(9): 1250–1256.

11. Delaunay L, Chelly JE: Blocks at the wrist provide effective anesthesia for carpal tunnel release. Can J Anaesth 2001;48:656–660.

12. Dupont C, Ciaburro H, Prevost Y, et al: Hand surgery under wrist block and local infiltration anesthesia, using an upper arm tourniquet. Plast Reconstr Surg 1972;50:532–533.

13. Paget J: *Lectures on Surgical Pathology*. Longman, Brown, Green, Longmans/London, 1853.

14. Learmonth JR: The principle of decompression in the treatment of certain diseases of peripheral nerves. Surg Clin North Am 1933;13:905–913.

15. Dellon AL, Amadio PC: James R. Learmonth: The first peripheral nerve surgeon. J Reconstr Microsurg 2000;16:213–217.

16. Phalen GS: Spontaneous compression of the median nerve at the wrist. J Am Med Assoc 1951;145:1128–1133.

17. Nystrom A, Lindstrom G, Reiz S, et al: Bupivacaine: A safe local anesthetic for wrist blocks. J Hand Surg [Am] 1989;14:495–498.

CHAPTER 80G

Digital Block

Sam Van Boxstael, Ann-Sofie Smeets, and Jerry D. Vloka

INTRODUCTION

Strauss[1] provided the first description of the digital block in 1889 for the condition of an ingrown toenail, using 20% cocaine at the base and under the nail. In 1905, Heinrich Braun reported the synergistic advantage of adding epinephrine to local anesthetics.[2,3] However, the use of epinephrine in digital block anesthesia has been avoided due to the theoretical risk of ischemia and possible gangrene. However, Bradon Wilhelmi and colleagues[4] demonstrated the safety and efficacy of epinephrine-containing local anesthetic for digital block. Digital block is one of the most common nerve block techniques. It is frequently used in the emergency department and primary care settings for various procedures such as lacerations of the finger or toe, nail removal, nail bed repair, paronychia drainage, removal of foreign bodies, and any other painful procedures on digits.

In 1990, almost a century after the first publication regarding traditional digital block, David Chiu[5] described a technique of digital block that produced complete finger anesthesia with a single injection into the flexor tendon sheath at the level of the distal palmar crease. In anatomic investigations he showed that after injection of methylene blue into the flexor tendon sheath there was "complete staining of the entire flexor tendon sheath and centrifugal diffusion of the blue dye circumscribing the entire circumference of the proximal phalanx" (see Transthecal Digital Block). The advantages of this technique are (1) rapid onset of action, (2) only a small volume of anesthetic solution is required, (3) only a single injection is required, and (4) absence of risk of direct trauma to the neurovascular bundles.[6–8] Although Chevaleraud and coworkers[9] did not find anesthesia of the dorsum of the finger in all cases, some investigators consider the transthecal method to be as effective as a traditional digital nerve block.[10] Others have found that it results in anesthesia comparable to the newer single-injection subcutaneous digital blocks,[11] both in experimental and clinical situations.[12,13]

Transthecal anesthesia appears to be safe and effective without causing any long-term damage to the tendon sheath.

Several different techniques of digital block and their modifications are available: In this chapter, we describe the two that are most commonly used in our institution.

REGIONAL ANESTHESIA ANATOMY

The common digital nerves are derived from the median and ulnar nerves and divide in the distal palm into the volar aspect, tip, and nail bed area (Figure 80G–1). The main digital nerves, accompanied by digital vessels, run on the ventro-lateral aspect of the finger immediately lateral to the flexor tendon sheath (Figure 80G–2). Small dorsal digital nerves run on the dorso-lateral aspect of the finger and supply innervation to the back of the fingers as far as the proximal joint.

EQUIPMENT

A standard regional anesthesia tray is prepared with the following equipment:

- Sterile towels and 4-in. × 4-in. gauze pads
- A controlled, 10-mL syringe with local anesthetic
- One 1.5 -in., 25-gauge needle

TECHNIQUE

Block of Volar and Dorsal Digital Nerves at the Base of the Finger

A 25-gauge, 1.5 -in. needle is inserted at a point on the dorsolateral aspect of the base of the finger, and a small skin wheal is raised. The needle is then directed anteriorly toward

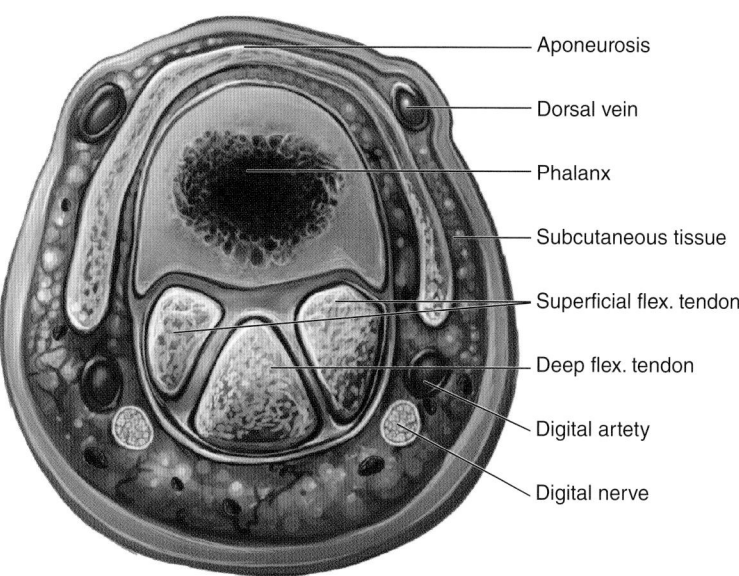

FIGURE 80G–1. The origin and distribution of the digital nerves.

the base of the phalanx (Figures 80G–3 and 80G–4 A and B). The needle is advanced until it contacts the phalanx, while the anesthesiologist observes for any protrusion from the palmar dermis directly opposite the needle path (Figure 80G–5). One milliliter of solution is injected as the needle is withdrawn 1–2 mm from the bone contact. An additional 1 mL is injected continuously as the needle is withdrawn back to the skin. The same procedure is repeated on each side of the base of the finger to achieve anesthesia of the entire finger (Figure 80G–6 A and B).

Transthecal Digital Block

The transthecal digital block is placed by using the flexor tendon sheath for local anesthetic injection. In this technique, the patient's hand is supinated and the flexor tendon is located. Using a 25- to 27-gauge, 1-in. needle, 2 mL of local anesthetic is injected into the flexor tendon sheath at the level of the distal palmar crease (Figures 80G-3 and 80G-7). The needle should puncture the skin at a 45-degree angle. Resistance to the injection suggests that the needle tip is against the flexor tendon. Careful withdrawal of the needle results in the free flow of medication as the potential space between tendon and sheath is entered. Proximal pressure is then applied to the volar surface for the duration of the injection for the diffusion of the medication throughout the synovial sheath.

FIGURE 80G–2. Cross-sectional view of the anatomy of the phalanx.

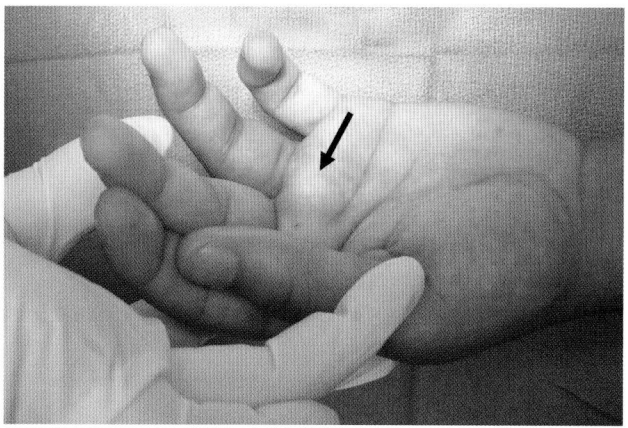

FIGURE 80G–3. Angle of needle insertion for transthecal digital block.

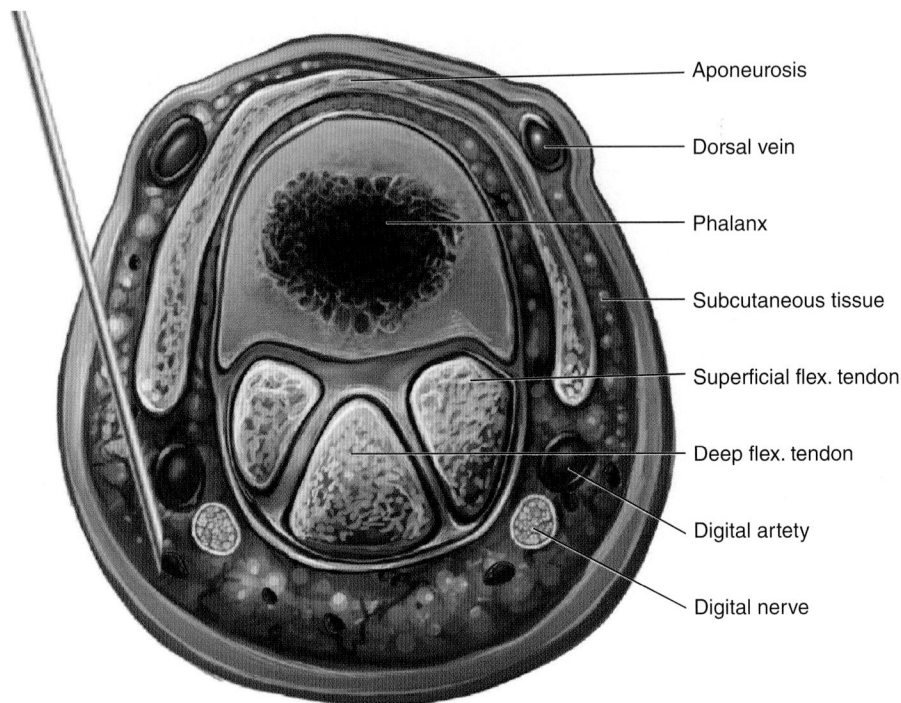

- Aponeurosis
- Dorsal vein
- Phalanx
- Subcutaneous tissue
- Superficial flex. tendon
- Deep flex. tendon
- Digital artety
- Digital nerve

FIGURE 80G–4. The needle is shown inserted at the base of the proximal phalanx to block the medial digital nerve.

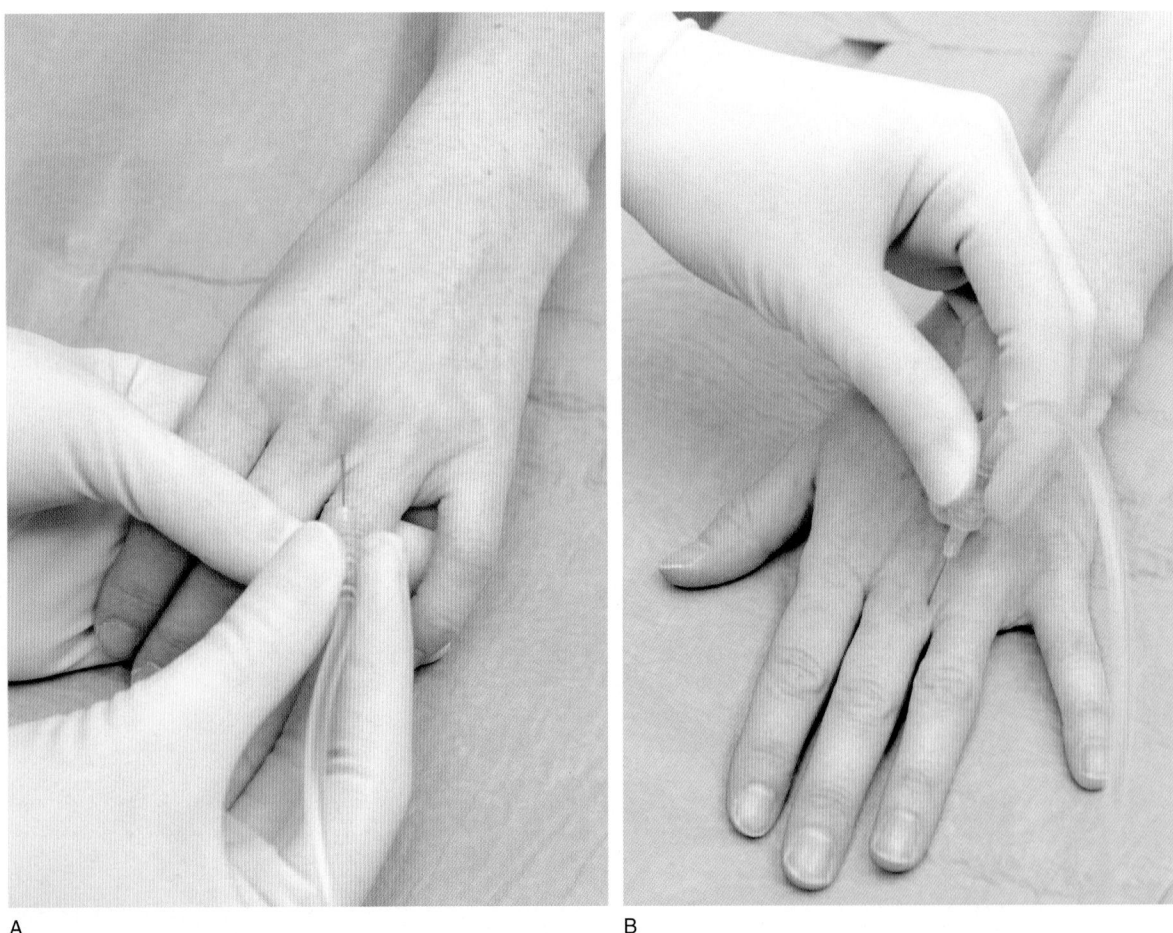

A   B

FIGURE 80G–5. As the needle is inserted and injection is being made, the operator observes the palmar area to stop the advancement of the needle should a protrusion from the palmar dermis opposite the nerve tip be seen.

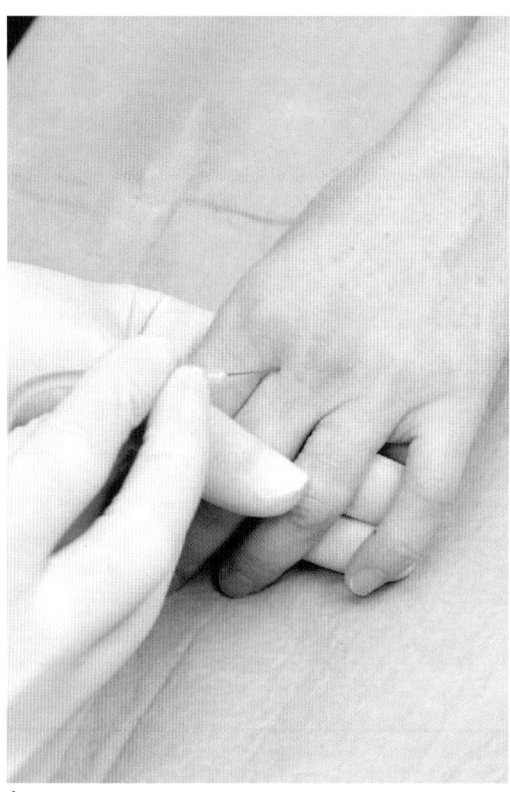 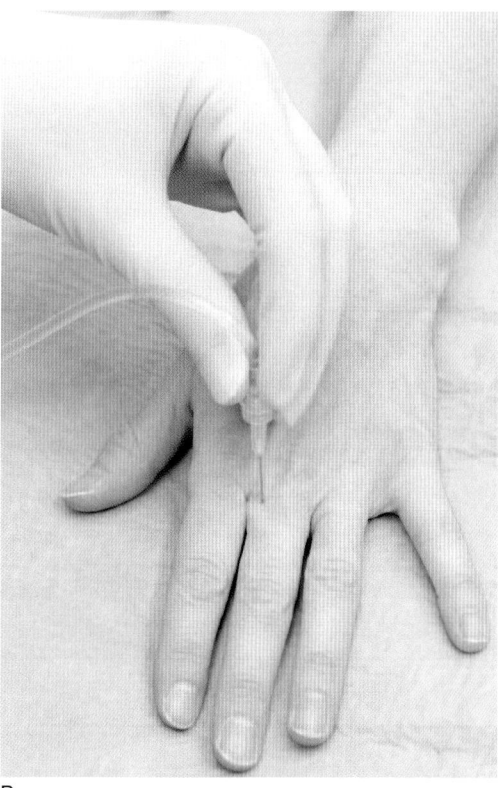

A   B

FIGURE 80G–6. A and B: The identical procedure is repeated on the radial side of the proximal phalanx to block the radial branch of the digital nerve.

Clinical Pearls

- The advantage of this approach is the provision of anesthesia to the entire digit with a single injection and a reportedly higher success rate.
- For more extensive surgery on the finger, it may be advantageous to combine both approaches discussed in this chapter for a greater success rate and more extensive distribution of anesthesia.

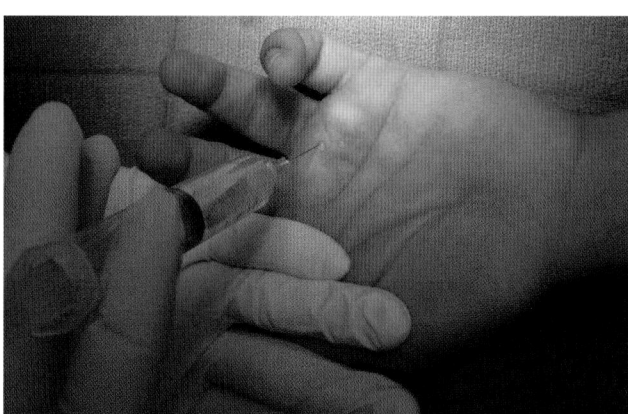

FIGURE 80G–7. Transthecal digital block. The needle is placed into the flexor tendon sheath. To confirm the correct needle placement in the tendon sheath, the needle can be placed without the syringe, in which case the operator flexes and deflexes the finger. This should result in a free and substantial swinging of the needle.

BLOCK DYNAMICS AND PERIOPERATIVE MANAGEMENT

A skin wheal at the point of needle insertion significantly reduces the discomfort during the placement of the block. A digital block requires a small dose of a sedative or a narcotic during placement. Typical onset time for this block is 10–20 min, depending on the concentration and volume of local anesthetic used.

CHOICE OF LOCAL ANESTHETIC

The choice of the type and concentration of local anesthetic for a digital block is based on the desired duration of blockade (Table 80G–1).[14]

TABLE 80G–1. Onset times and duration of anesthesia for some commonly used local anesthetics mixtures.

	Onset (min)	Anesthesia (h)	Analgesia (h)
1.5% Mepivacaine (+ HCO_3^-)	15–20	2–3	3–5
2% Lidocame (+ HCO_3^-)	10–20	2–5	3–8
0.5% Ropivacaine	15–30	4–8	5–12
0.75% Ropivacaine	10–15	5–10	6–24
0.5% Bupivacaine (or L-bupivacaine)	15–30	5–15	6–30

TABLE 80G–2. Complications of digital blocks.

Infection	This should be very rare with use of an aseptic technique.
Hematoma	Avoid multiple needle insertions. Use 25-gauge needle (or smaller) and avoid puncturing superficial veins.
Other	Instruct the patient on the care of the insensate finger.
Gangrene of the digit(s)	The use of epinephrine-containing solutions for this block is avoided by many; the safety of its use is controversial. Limit the injection volume to 3 mL on each side. The mechanical pressure effects of injecting solution into a potentially confined space should always be borne in mind, particularly in blocks at the base of the digit. In patients with small-vessel disease, perhaps an alternative method should be sought in addition to avoidance of digital tourniquet.
Nerve injury	Residual paresthesias are rare and may be due to an inadvertent intraneuronal injection. Systemic toxicity is rare because of the distal location of the blockade and small dose of local anaesthetic used. Do not inject when the patient complains of pain or when high resistance to injection is encountered.

COMPLICATIONS AND HOW TO AVOID THEM

One specific complication of digital blocks is vascular insufficiency and gangrene.[15] This catastrophe is a result of digital artery occlusion together with collateral circulation insufficiency. A series of causative factors is often involved to produce this rare, but serious complication (Table 80G–2).

REFERENCES

1. Strauss L: *Über Gangran nach Lokalanasthesie.* [Inaugural Dissertation]. Berlin, Germany: G. Schade, 1910.
2. Braun H: Zur Anwendung des Adrenalins bei anaethesierenden Gewebsinjektionen. Zentralbl Chir 1903;30:1025.
3. Geddes IC: A review of local anesthetics. Br J Anaesth 1954;26:208.
4. Wilhelmi BJ, Blackwell SJ, Miller JH, et al: Do not use epinephrine in digital blocks: Myth or truth? Plast Reconstr Surg 2001;107:393.
5. Chiu DTW: Transthecal digital block: Flexor tendon sheath used for anesthetic infusion. J Hand Surg 1990;15:471–473.
6. Morrison WG: Transthecal digital block. Arch Emerg Med 1993; 10:35–38.
7. Morros C, Perez D, Raurell A, et al: Digital anaesthesia through the flexor tendon sheath at the palmar level. Int Orthop 1994;17: 273–274.
8. Ramamurathy S Hickey, R: Anestheisa. In Green D (ed): *Operative Hand Surgery*, 3rd ed. Churchill Livingstone. New York, NY: 1993, p 41.
9. Chevaleraud E, Ragot JM, Brunelle E, et al: Anesthesie locale digitale par la gains des flechisseurs. [Local anaesthesia of the finger using the flexor tendon sheath.] Ann Fr Anesth Reanim 1993;12:237–240.
10. Hill RG, Patterson JW, Parker JC, et al: Comparison of transthecal digital block and traditional digital block for anesthesia of the finger. Ann Emerg Med 1995;25:604–607.
11. Whetzel TP, Mabourakh S, Barkhorder R: Modified transthecal digital block. J Hand Surg 1997;22A:361–363.
12. Low CK, Vartany A, Engstrom JW, et al: Comparison of transthecal and subcutaneous single-injection digital block techniques. J Hand Surg 1997a;22A:901–905.
13. Low CK, Wong HP, Low YP: Comparison between single injection transthecal and subcutaneous digital blocks. J Hand Surg 1997b;22B: 582–584.
14. Vinycomb TI, Sahhar LJ. Comparison of local anesthetics for digital nerve blocks: a systematic review. J Hand Surg Am. 2014;39(4):744—751.
15. De Monaco D, De Monaco A, Kammer E, Noever G. Digital nerve block anaesthesia: historical development and two cases of finger-tip necrosis, a rare complication. Handchir Mikrochir Plast Chir. 2002;34(1):59–64. Review."

CHAPTER 80H

Cutaneous Blocks for the Upper Extremity

Joseph M. Neal and Yavuz Gurkan

INTRODUCTION

Although most upper extremity regional anesthesia is accomplished by means of various approaches to the brachial plexus, there are occasions when individual terminal nerves or their branches are blocked selectively. There are generally three instances in which the anesthesiologist desires to perform these selective nerve blocks. First, some surgical sites are partially innervated by sensory nerves that are not part of the brachial plexus or not consistently anesthetized with plexus blocks. This chapter describes how and when to anesthetize the most common of these nerves—the supraclavicular, the suprascapular, and the intercostobrachial. The second indication is when the block of the entire brachial plexus block is not necessary for the planned procedure. In this case, selective upper extremity cutaneous anesthesia or analgesia may involve blocking terminal nerves (radial, median, or ulnar nerves) or their branches (lateral and medial antebrachial cutaneous nerves) distally at the elbow. A final and controversial indication for selective upper extremity nerve blocks is their use as a supplement to an incomplete brachial plexus block.

When considering the application of these various blocks, the reader is reminded that innervation of the upper extremity is often variable and overlapping.[1] Therefore, when faced with the choice of performing a single nerve block versus blocking several adjacent nerves, it is advisable to err on the side of multiple blocks, particularly in those adjacent cutaneous areas that represent potential crossover innervation (Figures 80H–1 and 80H–2). The relevant anatomy will be covered with specific nerve block description.

Local Anesthetic and Adjuvant Selection

Local anesthetics for individual upper extremity nerve blocks are selected for their desired duration of anesthesia and/or analgesia. If intermediate-acting local anesthetics are selected (lidocaine or mepivacaine), duration can be increased with either adjuvant epinephrine (2.5 mcg/mL). Neither adjuvant significantly increases duration if a long-acting local anesthetic such as bupivacaine or ropivacaine is chosen.[1]

SUPRACLAVICULAR NERVE BLOCK INDICATIONS

The supraclavicular nerve provides sensory innervation to the "cape" of the shoulder (Figure 80H–3). Commonly anesthetized as a component of cervical plexus block for carotid surgery, the supraclavicular nerve may also require blockade for surgery involving the shoulder or supraclavicular area. Local anesthetic spread in an interscalene plexus block often blocks the cervical plexus and therefore it is adequate to block the supraclavicular nerve, but the nerve is frequently not anesthetized with a supraclavicular brachial plexus block.

Anatomy

The supraclavicular nerve is derived from the ventral rami of the third and fourth cervical nerve roots (C3–C4); it is thus separate from the brachial plexus. The nerve becomes superficial as it penetrates the midbelly of the sternocleidomastoid muscle, thereafter forming three branches (Figure 80H–3). These branches provide sensory innervation to the cape area, which spans from the midline to the deltoids, and from the second rib anteriorly to the top of the scapula posteriorly.

Technique

Blockade of the supraclavicular nerve is accomplished with 5–10 mL of an intermediate- or long-acting local anesthetic, depending on analgesic requirements. Three milliliters is deposited with a 22- to 25-gauge sharp needle into the midbelly of the sternocleidomastoid. The remaining local anesthetic is then injected subcutaneously in a cephalad and caudad direction along the posterior border of the sternocleidomastoid

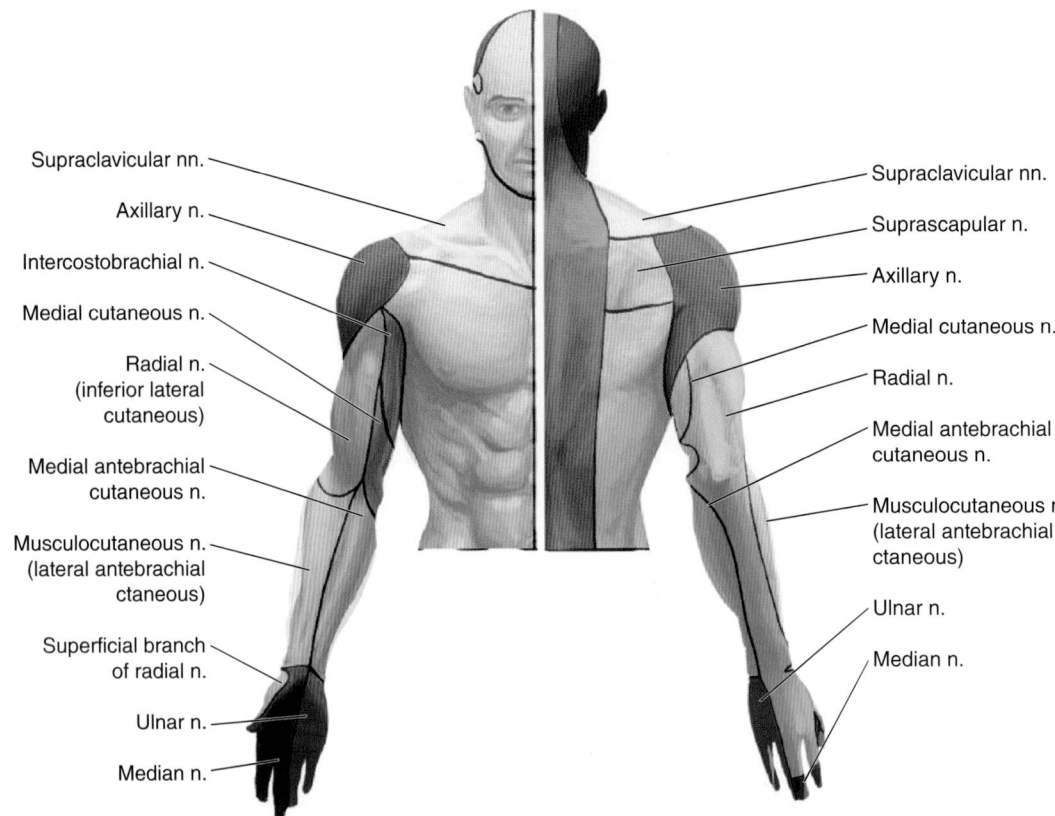

Supraclavicular nn.

Axillary n.

Intercostobrachial n.

Medial cutaneous n.

Radial n.
(inferior lateral
cutaneous)

Medial antebrachial
cutaneous n.

Musculocutaneous n.
(lateral antebrachial
ctaneous)

Superficial branch
of radial n.

Ulnar n.

Median n.

Supraclavicular nn.

Suprascapular n.

Axillary n.

Medial cutaneous n.

Radial n.

Medial antebrachial
cutaneous n.

Musculocutaneous n.
(lateral antebrachial
ctaneous)

Ulnar n.

Median n.

FIGURE 80H–1. Cutaneous innervation of the upper extremity. Actual patients demonstrate large variation in the depicted pattern of innervation and significant crossover between nerves.

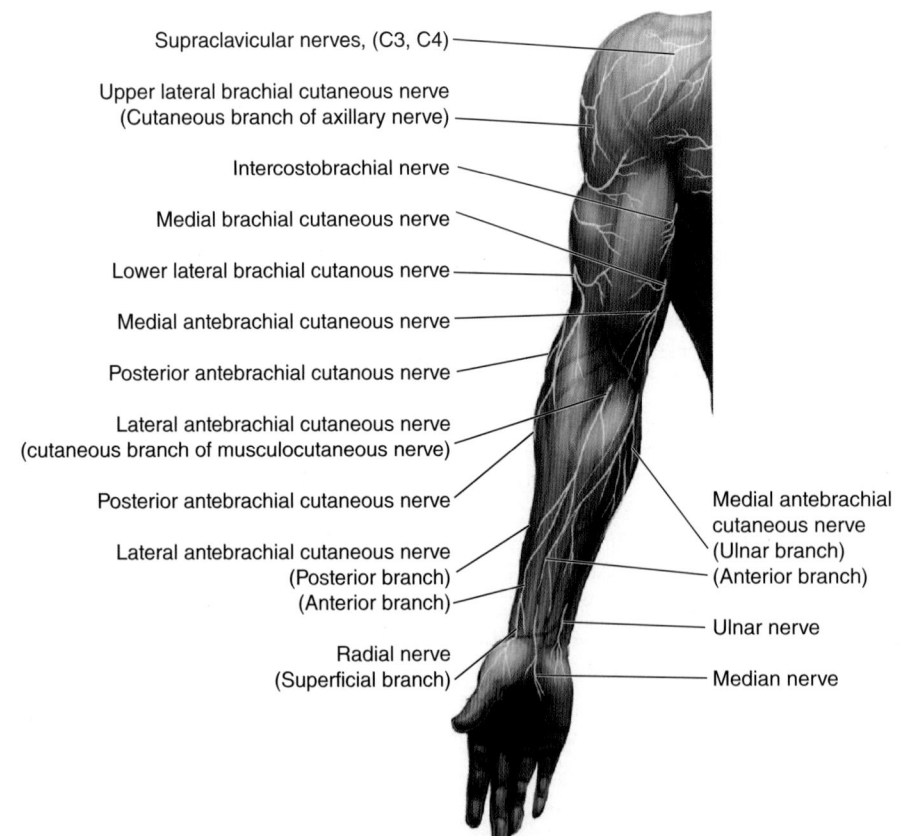

Supraclavicular nerves, (C3, C4)

Upper lateral brachial cutaneous nerve
(Cutaneous branch of axillary nerve)

Intercostobrachial nerve

Medial brachial cutaneous nerve

Lower lateral brachial cutanous nerve

Medial antebrachial cutaneous nerve

Posterior antebrachial cutanous nerve

Lateral antebrachial cutaneous nerve
(cutaneous branch of musculocutaneous nerve)

Posterior antebrachial cutaneous nerve

Lateral antebrachial cutaneous nerve
(Posterior branch)
(Anterior branch)

Radial nerve
(Superficial branch)

Medial antebrachial
cutaneous nerve
(Ulnar branch)
(Anterior branch)

Ulnar nerve

Median nerve

FIGURE 80H–2. Idealized distribution of the cutaneous innervation of the upper arm and forearm.

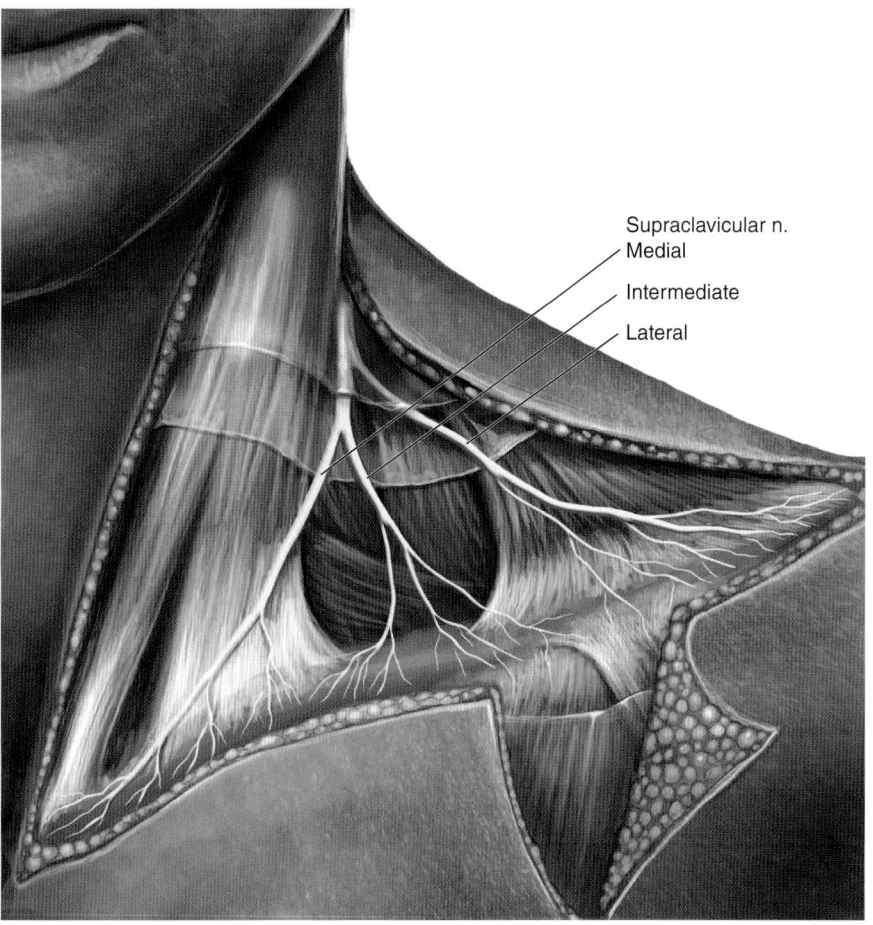

Supraclavicular n.
Medial
Intermediate
Lateral

FIGURE 80H–3. Supraclavicular nerves, derived from C3–C4 nerve roots, is not part of the brachial plexus, and provides sensory innervation of the shoulder "cape."

Complications

Complications of the supraclavicular nerve block are uncommon. The external jugular vein should be avoided to prevent hematoma.

SUPRASCAPULAR NERVE BLOCK

Indications

Suprascapular nerve block (SSNB) can be used as an adjunct to arthroscopic shoulder surgery and total shoulder arthroplasty. When combined with general anesthesia for shoulder arthroscopy, SSNB improves analgesia, reduces opioid-related side effects, and hastens hospital discharge,[2] although SSNB is not superior to interscalene block in this setting.[3]

For anterior open shoulder surgery, supplemental SSNB does not affect outcome when combined with interscalene block.[4]

Anatomy

The suprascapular nerve (C4–C5) branches from the superior trunk of the brachial plexus and, therefore, it is usually anesthetized by an interscalene block. It traverses the suprascapular notch and continues laterally along the superior border of the scapular spine (Figure 80H–5). The supraclavicular nerve

provides sensory innervation to 70% of the posterior-superior shoulder joint, the acromioclavicular joint, and a portion of the anterior axilla in up to 10% of patients.[1]

The suprascapular nerve provides motor innervation to the supraspinatus and infraspinatus muscles, but minimal if any cutaneous innervation over the scapula or posterior shoulder.

Technique

Surface landmarks are identified by drawing one line along the superior border of the scapular spine and then bisecting it with a second line drawn parallel with the vertebral spine. From where these two lines cross, the suprascapular notch underlies a point approximately 2–3 cm toward the middle of the upper/outer quadrant (see Figure 80H–5). A 1.5-in. 22-gauge needle is placed at this entry mark and directed caudad in the sagittal plane until it contacts the scapular spine, followed by injection of 10 mL of a long-acting local anesthetic. If a peripheral nerve stimulator is used, the suprascapular nerve is identified by the motor response of external shoulder rotation.

Complications

Pneumothorax can result from a needle that passes through the suprascapular notch and enters the pleural space. This

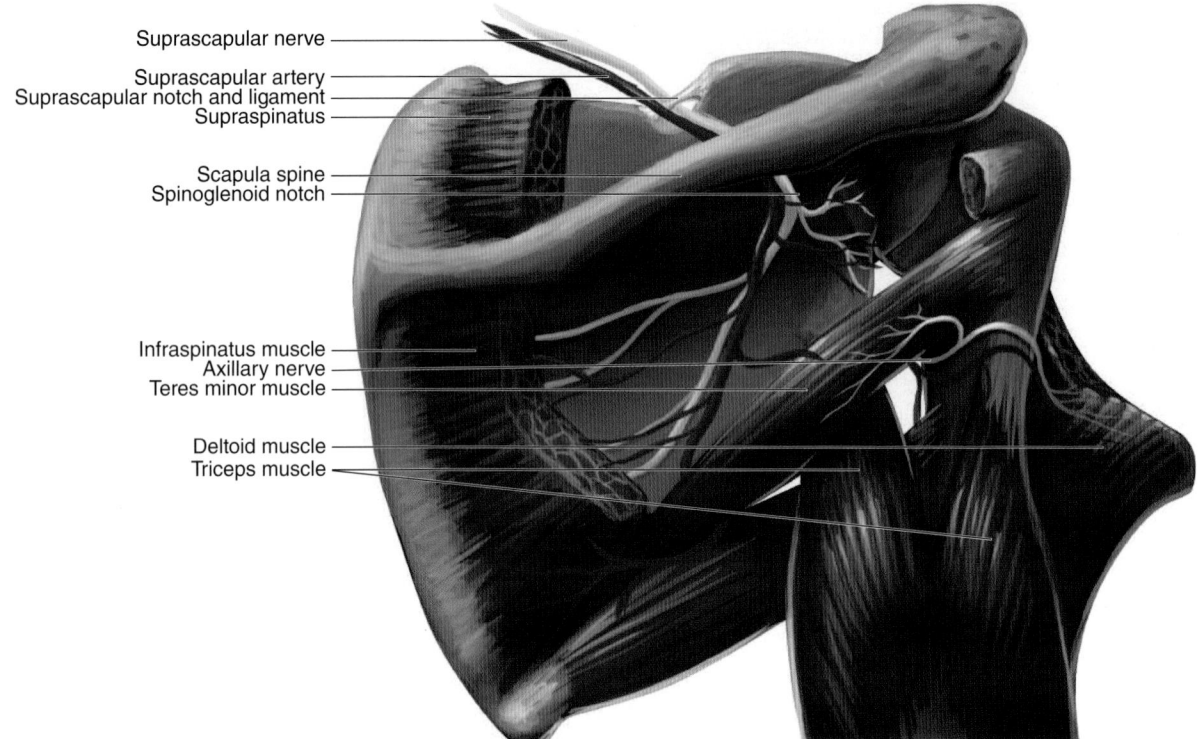

- Suprascapular nerve
- Suprascapular artery
- Suprascapular notch and ligament
- Supraspinatus
- Scapula spine
- Spinoglenoid notch
- Infraspinatus muscle
- Axillary nerve
- Teres minor muscle
- Deltoid muscle
- Triceps muscle

FIGURE 80H–4. Suprascapular nerve block is accomplished by injecting local anesthetic in the suprascapular notch.

complication is largely avoidable by directing the needle in a caudad, rather than anterior, direction.

Clinical Pearls

- Suprascapular nerve block is a valuable analgesic adjunct for shoulder arthroscopy performed with the patient under general anesthesia.
- Suprascapular nerve block does not add value to open shoulder procedures in which an interscalene block is the primary anesthetic.
- Suprascapular nerve block is probably a valuable supplement to interscalene block during total shoulder arthroplasty or in the occasional patient who experiences pain at the anterior arthroscopic port site.

INTERCOSTOBRACHIAL NERVE BLOCK

Indications

The intercostobrachial nerve block is indicated for surgery involving the medial/posterior upper arm and/or for anterior arthroscopic port placement. A secondary indication is to alleviate the sensation resulting from a pneumatic tourniquet applied to the upper arm. Despite commonly held misperception, the intercostobrachial nerve block does not block the ischemic, compressive components that cause tourniquet pain; this is accomplished by brachial plexus block with supplemental intraoperative sedation—additional cutaneous anesthesia is not necessary.

Anatomy

The intercostobrachial nerve arises from the second thoracic (T2 and occasionally T1) nerve root (see Figure 80H–2). As such, it is not a component of the brachial plexus and is, therefore, not anesthetized by any brachial plexus approach. Along with the medial cutaneous nerve of the arm (an intermediary branch of the medial cord), the intercostobrachial nerve provides cutaneous sensation to the upper half of the medial/posterior arm. It also innervates a portion of the anterior axilla (see Figures 80H–1 and 80H–2).

Technique

The intercostobrachial is anesthetized by depositing 5 mL of local anesthetic subcutaneously superiorly and inferiorly along the axillary crease via a 1.5-in. 25-gauge needle (Figure 80H–6).

Complications

Because of its superficial placement, complications of the intercostobrachial nerve block are virtually nonexistent.

Clinical Pearl

- The intercostobrachial nerve block is a useful supplement to any brachial plexus block when surgery involves the upper medial/posterior arm, a pneumatic tourniquet, and/or an anterior arthroscopic port.

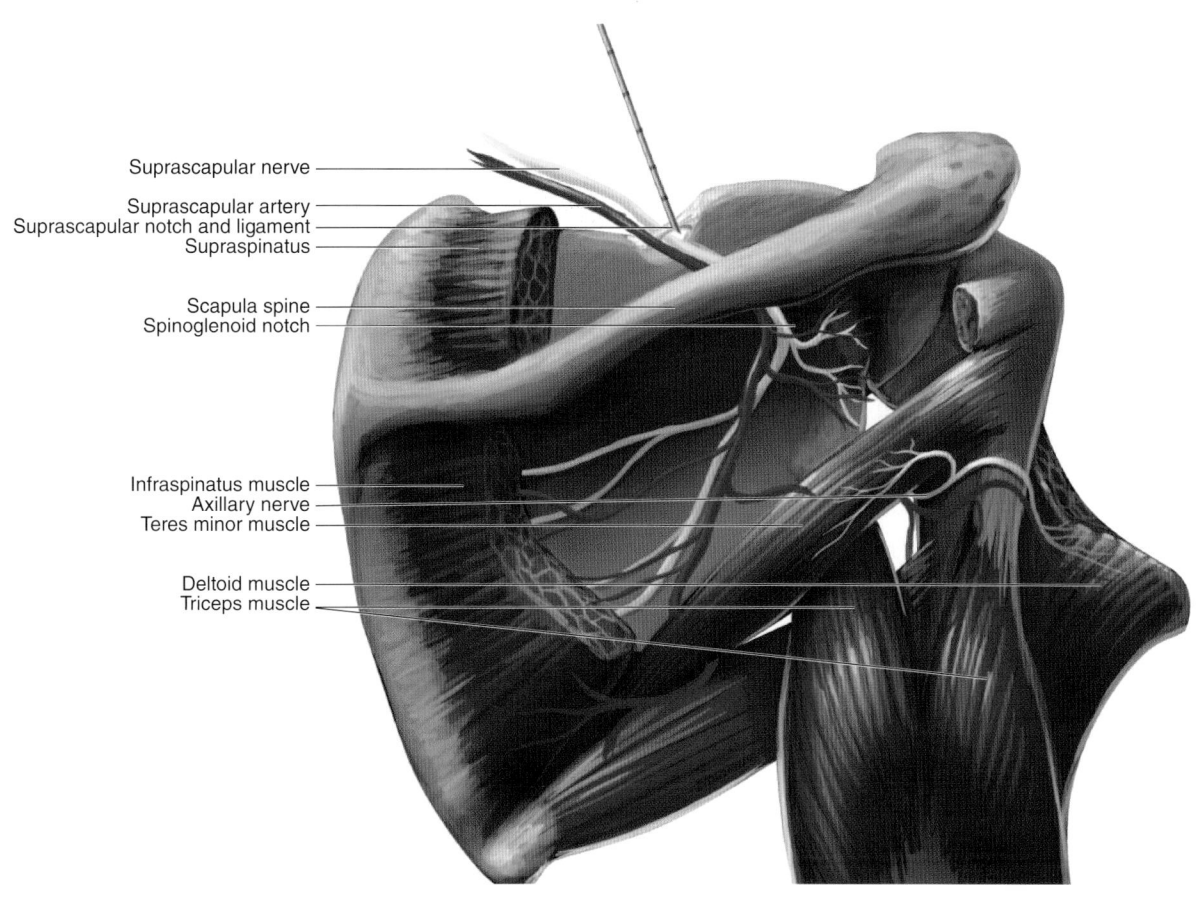

Suprascapular nerve
Suprascapular artery
Suprascapular notch and ligament
Supraspinatus
Scapula spine
Spinoglenoid notch
Infraspinatus muscle
Axillary nerve
Teres minor muscle
Deltoid muscle
Triceps muscle

FIGURE 80H–5. Suprascapular nerve block. The suprascapular nerve is blocked as it emerges from the suprascapular notch. Directing the needle caudally substantially reduces the risk of pneumothorax.

LATERAL AND MEDIAL ANTEBRACHIAL CUTANEOUS NERVE BLOCK

Indications

Local anesthetic blockade of the lateral and medial antebrachial cutaneous nerves is indicated for superficial surgery of the forearm, such as arteriovenous fistula surgery, or as a supplement to incomplete brachial plexus block.

Anatomy

The lateral antebrachial cutaneous nerve of the forearm (LAC) is the primary cutaneous branch of the musculocutaneous nerve. It provides cutaneous innervation to the lateral (radial) half of the volar forearm. The medial antebrachial cutaneous nerve of the forearm (MAC) is an intermediary branch of the medial cord. It provides cutaneous innervation to the medial (ulnar) half of the volar forearm, an area commonly misperceived as innervated by the ulnar nerve (see Figures 80H–1 and 80H–2).

Technique

Considering the unpredictable overlap of forearm cutaneous innervation, it is advisable to perform both LAC and MAC nerve blocks when forearm anesthesia is desired. Blocking the LAC is accomplished with two local anesthetic injections placed along the intercondylar line. The first 5 mL of local anesthetic is

injected just deep to the lateral margin of the biceps tendon; the second 5 mL area injected subcutaneously and lateral from the first injection site, along the elbow crease (Figure 80H–7). The MAC is blocked by injecting a half-ring of 5–7 mL local anesthetic about a quarter of the arm's length above the medial elbow

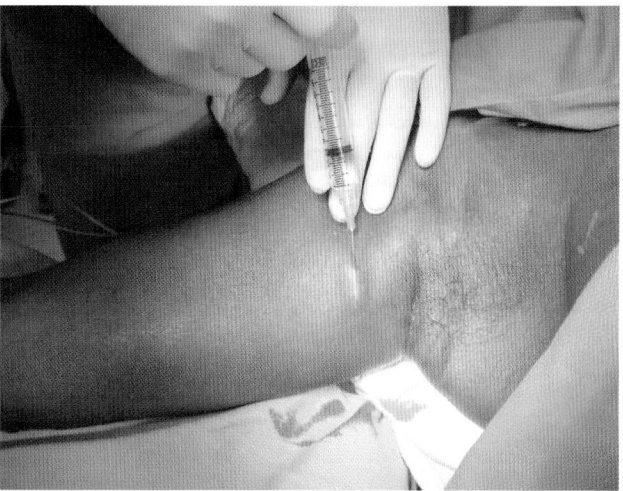

FIGURE 80H–6. Intercostobrachial nerve block. The intercostobrachial nerve is anesthetized by subcutaneous injection of 3–5 mL local anesthetic along the axillary crease.

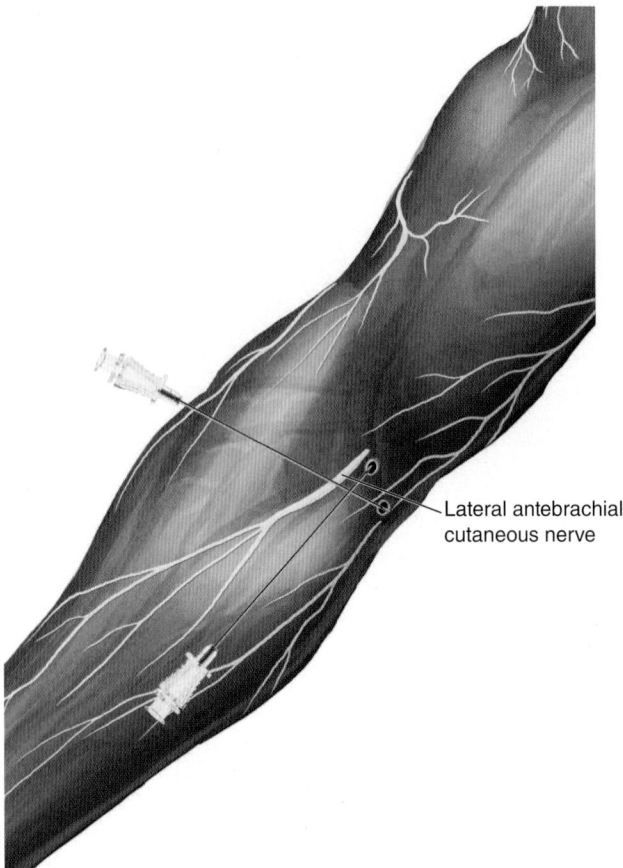

Lateral antebrachial
cutaneous nerve

FIGURE 80H–7. Blocks of the lateral and medial antebrachial cutaneous nerve. Anesthesia for lateral antebrachial cutaneous nerve requires two injections. The first deposits 5 mL local anesthetic just lateral to the border of the biceps tendon. A second 5 mL is then injected subcutaneously and lateral from the first injection site.

(Figure 80H–7). When LAC and/or MAC nerve blocks are supplemental to a previous incomplete brachial plexus block, the additional 15–20 mL of local anesthetic should be well tolerated by patients if injected 20–30 minutes after the primary block.[5]

Complications

Techniques for anesthetizing the LAC and MAC nerves involve only superficial injection of local anesthetic; thus the risk of nerve injury is very low. For this reason, these blocks may be preferable to selective elbow or wrist blocks as a supplement to incomplete brachial plexus anesthesia involving volar forearm cutaneous distribution.

Clinical Pearls

- Medial and lateral antebrachial cutaneous nerve blocks are useful techniques for superficial volar forearm procedures, such as arteriovenous fistula creation.
- The nerve blocks also represent a reasonable alternative for supplementation when proximal brachial plexus block is incomplete.

SELECTIVE NERVE BLOCKS AT THE ELBOW

Indications

Proximal techniques of brachial plexus block are often superior to selective nerve block at the elbow because the latter are more difficult to perform, are more time-consuming and uncomfortable, and potentially carry a greater risk of complications. For instance, the practitioner may rather choose the midhumeral brachial plexus block, where selective application of clonidine[6] or low concentration of long-acting local anesthetics[7] to the median and ulnar nerves prolongs analgesia without concomitant prolongation of motor block. Another reason to avoid selective elbow blocks is the commonly misunderstood cutaneous innervation of the forearm. For example, block of the musculocutaneous nerve must be performed in the axilla to render motor block of the biceps and brachioradialis muscles. But anesthetizing the cutaneous distribution of the musculocutaneous nerve is best accomplished with a LAC nerve block. Anesthetizing the skin of the medial forearm requires blockade of the MAC nerve, not the ulnar nerve at the elbow. A third issue is to avoid elbow blocks to supplement incomplete brachial plexus blocks because this practice theoretically increases the risk of anesthesia-related nerve injury. Indeed, the only indication for elbow approaches is to block forearm flexor and extensor muscles when the surgeon desires immobility of the fingers. Selective nerve blocks can sometimes be used also for pain treatment of minor trauma or surgery. Some authors have even reported selective catheterization to avoid unnecessary motor block or numbness of the uninvolved parts of the upper extremity.[8,9]

Radial Nerve block
Anatomy

The radial nerve supplies sensation to the dorsum of the forearm and hand (see Figures 80H–1 and 80H–2); it also innervates the musculature of the dorsal forearm. The radial nerve descends the posterior arm, traversing from the medial to the lateral side. At the epicondyles, the radial nerve lies relatively deep between the brachialis and brachioradialis muscles (Figure 80H–8).

Technique

The patient is positioned supine for radial nerve block with the arm supinated and abducted. Selective block of the radial nerve is accomplished by placing a needle approximately 1.5 cm lateral to the biceps tendon at the level of the epicondyles (see Figure 80H–8). Three to 5 mL of local anesthetic is injected when a paresthesia to the hand is elicited. If using a peripheral nerve stimulator, one seeks the motor response of wrist extension.

Median Nerve Block
Anatomy

The median nerve provides sensation to the radial palm, the proximal fingers from the thumb to the long finger, and motor control to the forearm flexors (see Figures 80H–1 and 80H–2).

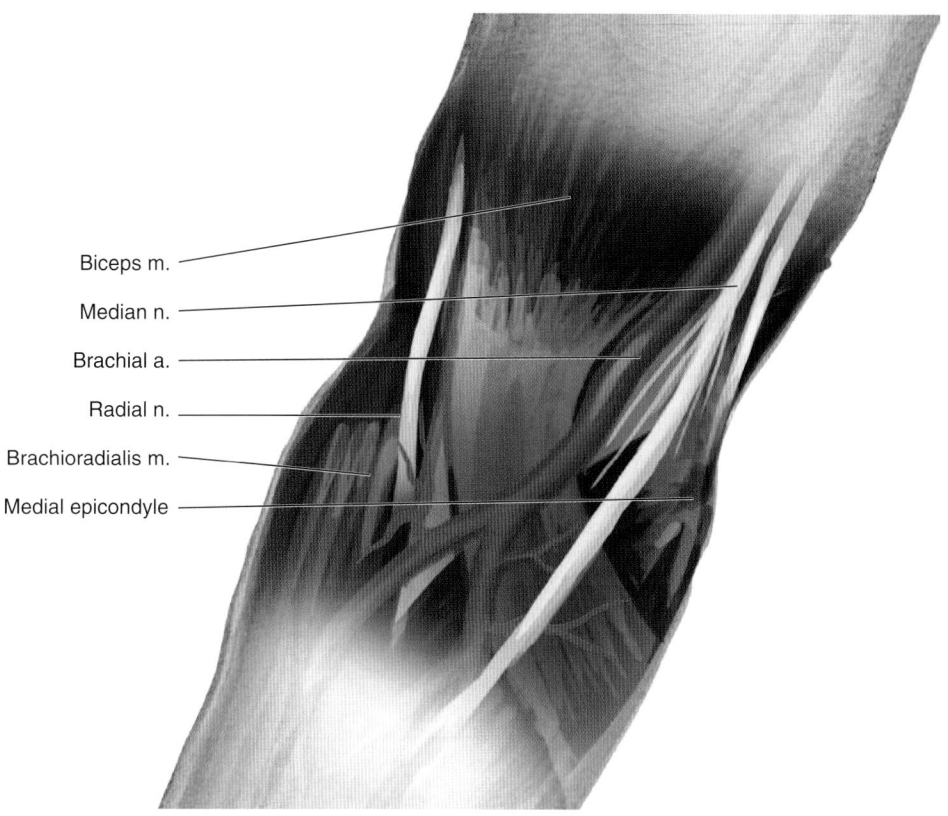

Biceps m.
Median n.
Brachial a.
Radial n.
Brachioradialis m.
Medial epicondyle

FIGURE 80H–8. Radial and median nerves are approached at the level of the epicondyles. The radial nerve is found approximately 1.5 cm lateral to the biceps tendon. The median nerve is more superficial and identified by a needle placed just medial to the brachial artery.

It passes the elbow joint just medial to the brachial artery and in front of the brachialis muscle.

Technique

Median nerve block at the elbow is accomplished with a 1.5-in. needle that is placed just medial to the brachial artery at the level of the epicondyles (see Figure 80H–8). Either a motor response that consists of wrist flexion and/or thumb opposition or a paresthesia to the thumb or index finger is sought before injecting 3–5 mL of local anesthetic.

Ulnar Nerve Block

Anatomy

The ulnar nerve at the elbow is located superficially in the ulnar groove (Figure 80H–9). At this level, blockade of the ulnar nerve results in anesthesia of the little finger and motor block of the intrinsic muscles of the hand.

Technique

The patient is placed supine for ulnar nerve block, and the forearm is flexed at the elbow (see Figure 80H–9). After identification of the ulnar groove, a short needle is placed approximately 1 cm proximal to the epicondyles and directed distally. The desired endpoint is paresthesia to the little finger or a motor response consisting of finger flexion, thumb adduction, and/or ulnar deviation of the wrist. It is suggested that only 2–3 mL of local anesthetic be injected to avoid

excessive pressure within the tight fascial space of the ulnar groove and thereby lessen the possibility of compromising neural blood flow.

Complications

Selective nerve blocks at the elbow may cause hematoma if brachial artery is punctured during procedure.

Clinical Pearls

- Selective nerve blocks at the elbow can be recommended for hand surgery when forearm motor block is desired and motor block of the proximal brachial plexus block is not desired.
- Selective nerve blocks at the elbow to supplement incomplete proximal brachial plexus should be practiced with caution.

PERIOPERATIVE MANAGEMENT

Because cutaneous nerve blocks of the upper extremity require only small amounts of local anesthetic, which are typically injected subcutaneously and not close to major vessels, they can be placed with standard American Society of Anesthesiologists (ASA) monitoring. Patients should be informed to protect their insensate limb from external pressure or temperature extremes.

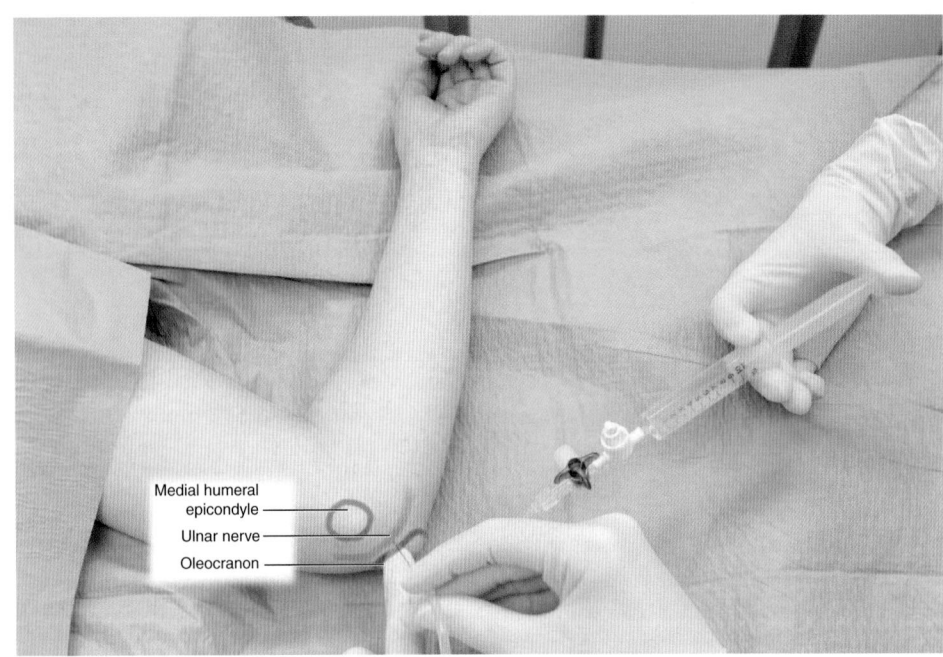

Medial humeral epicondyle
Ulnar nerve
Oleocranon

FIGURE 80H–9. Ulnar nerve block at the elbow. The forearm is flexed, the ulnar groove identified, and a needle is placed 1 cm proximal to the epicondyles and directed distally.

Finally, the advent of ultrasound-guidance has substantially facilitated performance of cutaneous blocks.[10]

SUMMARY

Selective upper extremity nerve blocks can be useful supplements to brachial plexus blocks. Supraclavicular, suprascapular, and intercostobrachial nerve blocks are valuable adjuncts to the anesthesia and/or analgesia primarily provided by a plexus block or general anesthesia. The LAC and MAC nerve blocks can provide either primary anesthesia for superficial forearm operations or supplement an incomplete plexus block. Selective elbow blocks are inferior alternatives to brachial plexus blocks. Their use as a supplement to incomplete plexus blockade should be carefully considered.

REFERENCES

1. Neal JM, Hebl JR, Gerancher JC, Hogan QH: Brachial plexus anesthesia: essentials of our current understanding. Reg Anesth Pain Med 2002; 27:402–428.

2. Ritchie E, Tong D, Chung F, et al: Suprascapular nerve block for post-operative pain relief in arthroscopic shoulder surgery: a new modelity? Anesth Analg 1997;84:1306–1312.

3. Singelyn RJ, Lhotel L, Fabre B: Pain relief after arthroscopic shoulder surgery: acomparison of intraarticular analgesia, suprascapular nerve block, and interscalene brachial plexus block. Anesth Analg 2004;99: 589–592.

4. Neal JM, McDonald SB, Larkin KL, Polissar NL: Suprascapular nerve block prolongs analgesia after nonarthroscopic shoulder surgery, but does not improve outcome. Anesth Analg 2003;96:982–986.

5. Finucane BT, Yilling F: Safety of supplementing axillary plexus blocks. Anesthesiology 1989;70:401–403.

6. Iskandar H, Guillaume E, Dixmerias F, et al: The enhancement of sensory blockade by clonidine selectively added to mepivacaine after midhumeral block. Anesth Analg 2001;93:771–775.

7. Bouaziz H, Narchi P, Mercier FJ, et al: The use of selective axillary nerve block for outpatient hand surgery. Anesth Analg 1998;86:746–748.

8. Frenkel O, Herring AA, Fischer J, Carnell J, Nagdev A. Supracondylar radial nerve block for treatment of distal radius fractures in the emergency department. J Emerg Med. 201;41(4):386–388.

9. Lurf M, Leixnering M. Ultrasound-guided ulnar nerve catheter placement in the forearm for postoperative pain relief and physiotherapy. Acta Anaesthesiol Scand. 2009;53(2):261–263.

10. McCartney CJ, Xu D, Constantinescu C, et al:. Ultrasound examination of peripheral nerves in the forearm. Reg Anesth Pain Med. 2007;32(5): 434–439.

SECTION 2 — Truncal Blocks

CHAPTER 81A

Thoracic & Lumbar Paravertebral Block

Manoj K. Karmakar, Roy A. Greengrass, Malikah Latmore, and Matthew Levin

THORACIC PARAVERTEBRAL BLOCK

Thoracic paravertebral block (TPVB) is the technique of injecting local anesthetic alongside the thoracic vertebra close to where the spinal nerves emerge from the intervertebral foramen.[1,2] This produces unilateral, segmental, somatic, and sympathetic nerve blockade,[3] which is effective for anesthesia and in treating acute and chronic pain of unilateral origin from the chest and abdomen.[1] Hugo Sellheim of Leipzig (1871–1936) is believed to have pioneered TPVB in 1905.[1,2] Kappis, in 1919, developed the technique of paravertebral injection, which is comparable to the one in present day use.

Although paravertebral block (PVB) was fairly popular in the early 1900s, it seemed to have fallen into disfavor during the later part of the century; the reason for which is not known. In 1979, Eason and Wyatt re popularized the technique after describing paravertebral catheter placement.[4] Our understanding of the safety and efficacy of TPVB has improved significantly in the last 25 years, with renewal of interest in this technique. Currently, it is used not only for analgesia but also for surgical anesthesia,[5–7] and its application has been extended to children.[8–10] Introduction of ultrasound to the practice of regional anesthesia led to the renewed efforts to increase safety and consistency of PVBs.

Anatomy

The thoracic paravertebral space (TPVS) is a wedge-shaped space located on either side of the vertebral column (Figure 81A–1). The parietal pleura forms the anterolateral boundary. The base is formed by the vertebral body, intervertebral disc, and the intervertebral foramen with its contents.

The transverse process and the superior costotransverse ligament form the posterior boundary. Lying in between the parietal pleura anteriorly and the superior costotransverse ligament posteriorly is a fibroelastic structure, the endothoracic fascia, which is the deep fascia of the thorax (Figures 81A–1 through 81A–3).[1,11–15] Medially, the endothoracic fascia is attached to the periosteum of the vertebral body. A layer of loose areolar connective tissue, the subserous fascia, lies between the parietal pleura and the endothoracic fascia.

Therefore, there are two potential fascial compartments in the TPVS: the anterior extrapleural paravertebral compartment and the posterior subendothoracic paravertebral compartment (see Figures 81A–1 and 81A–2). The TPVS contains adipose tissue within which lie the intercostal (spinal) nerve, the dorsal ramus, intercostal vessels, and rami communicantes and anteriorly the sympathetic chain. The spinal nerves are segmented into small bundles and lie freely in the adipose tissue of the TPVS, which make them accessible to local anesthetic solutions injected in the TPVS.[16] The TPVS communicates with the epidural space medially[17,18] and with the intercostal space laterally. The TPVSs on either side of the thoracic vertebra also communicate with each other through the epidural and prevertebral space.[1,12,15] The cranial extension of the TPVS is challenging to define and may significantly vary; however, there is direct paravertebral spread of radiopaque contrast medium from the thoracic to the cervical paravertebral space, indicating anatomic continuity. The TPVS also communicates caudally through the medial and lateral arcuate ligaments with the retroperitoneal

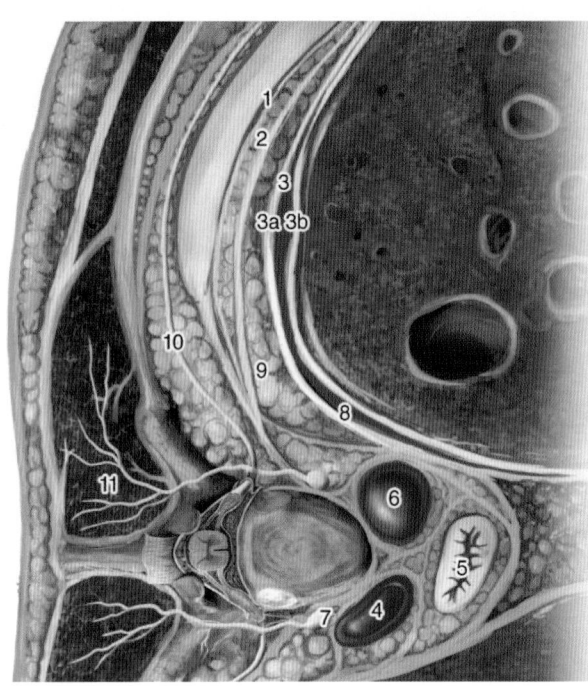

1 Endothoracic fascia
2 Subserous fascia
3 Pleura:
3a - Parietal
3b - Visceral
4 Azygos Vein
5 Esophagus
6 Descending aorta
7 Sympathetic chain
8 Interpleural space
9 Extrapleural compartment
10 Intercostal nerve
11 Posterior primary rami

FIGURE 81A-1. Anatomy of the thoracic paravertebral space, chest cavity and intercostal nerves.

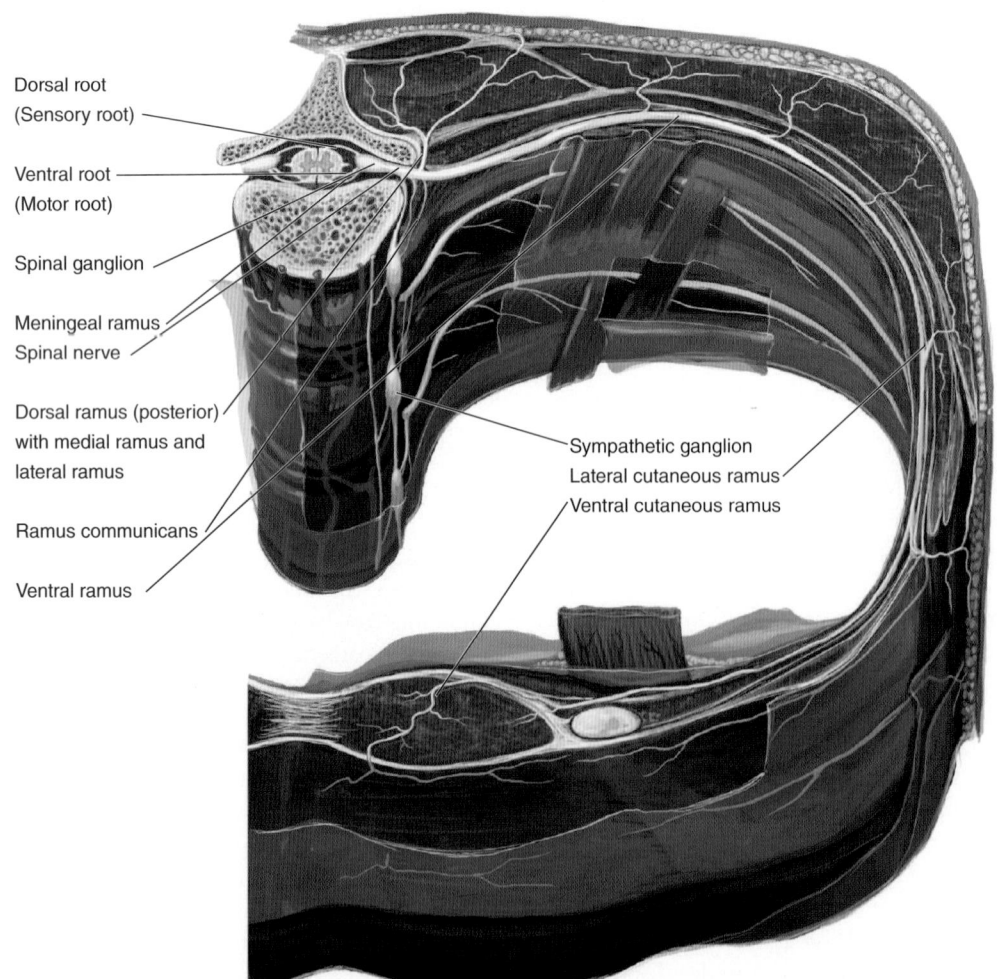

Dorsal root
(Sensory root)

Ventral root
(Motor root)

Spinal ganglion

Meningeal ramus
Spinal nerve

Dorsal ramus (posterior)
with medial ramus and
lateral ramus

Ramus communicans

Ventral ramus

Sympathetic ganglion
Lateral cutaneous ramus
Ventral cutaneous ramus

FIGURE 81A-2. Crossectional anatomy of the vertebra and chest wall demonstrating relationship of paraveretbral space, sympathetic ganglia, spinal and intercostal nerves.

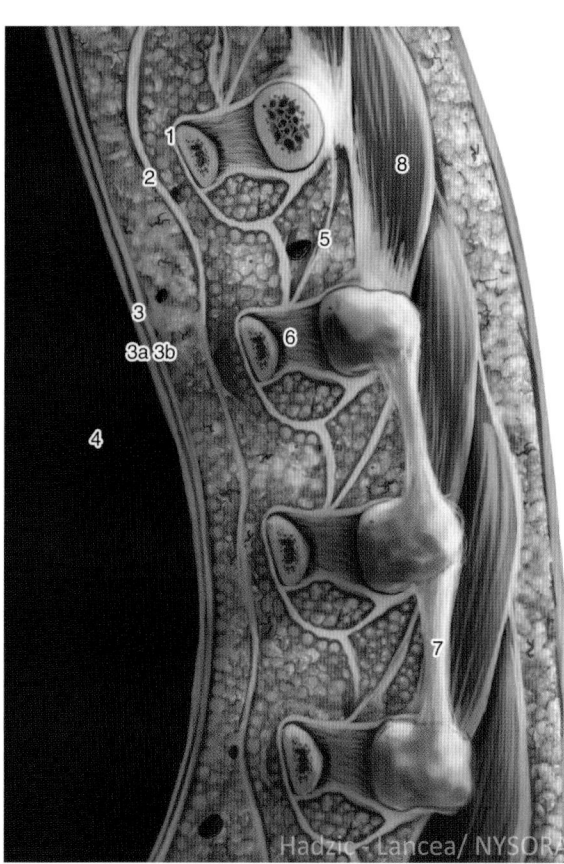

1 Endothoracic fascia

2 Subserous fascia

3 Pleura:

3a - Parietal

3b - Visceral

4 Lung

5 Superior costotransverse
   ligament

6 Lateral costotransverse
   ligament

7 Intertransverse ligament

8 Paraspinal muscle

FIGURE 81A–3. Sagittal section through the thoracic paravertebral space.

space behind the fascia transversalis, where the lumbar spinal nerves are located.[13,19–21]

Mechanism of Block & Distribution of Anesthesia

TPVB produces ipsilateral somatic and sympathetic nerve blockade (Figure 81A–4) due to a direct effect of the local anesthetic on the somatic and sympathetic nerves in the TPVS, extension into the intercostal space laterally, and the epidural space medially. The overall contribution of epidural spread to the dermatomal distribution of anesthesia following a TPVB is not well defined. However, some degree of ipsilateral spread of local anesthetic toward the epidural space probably occurs in the majority of the patients, resulting in a greater distribution of anesthesia than occurs with paravertebral spread alone.[18] The dermatomal distribution of anesthesia following a single injection of a large volume varies and is often unpredictable, but the injected solutions routinely spread both cephalad and caudad to the site of injection to some extent (Figure 81A–5).[1,3,22] Nevertheless, the multiple injection technique, where small volumes (3–4 mL) of local anesthetic are injected at several contiguous thoracic levels, is preferable over single, large-volume injection. This is particularly important when reliable anesthesia over several ipsilateral thoracic dermatomes is desired, such as when TPVB is used for anesthesia during breast surgery. Segmental contralateral anesthesia, adjacent to the site of injection, occurs in approximately 10% of patients after single-injection TPVB and may be due to epidural or prevertebral spread.

Bilateral symmetric anesthesia due to extensive epidural spread or unintentional intrathecal injection into a dural sleeve may occur, particularly when the needle is directed medially or when a larger volume of local anesthetic (>25 mL) is used. For this reason, patients should be monitored using the same vigilance and methods as those employed for injection using the large-volume, single-injection epidural technique. The ipsilateral ilioinguinal and iliohypogastric nerves may also occasionally be involved after lower thoracic paravertebral injections. This is either due to epidural spread or extended subendothoracic fascial spread to the retroperitoneal space where the lumbar spinal nerves are located. The effect of gravity on the dermatomal spread of anesthesia after TPVB is unknown, but there may be a tendency for preferential pooling of injected solution toward the dependent levels.[3,23,24]

Technique

It is preferable to perform TPVB with the patient in the sitting position because the surface anatomy is better visualized and patients are often more comfortable. However, when this is not possible or practical, TPVB can also be performed with the patient in the lateral, or prone position. The number and levels of injections are selected according to the desired spread of local anesthesia. In this example, description of the TPVB for breast surgery is described. Surface landmarks are identified and marked with a skin marker before block placement (Figure 81A–6). Skin markings are also made 2.5 cm lateral to the midline at the thoracic levels that are to be blocked.

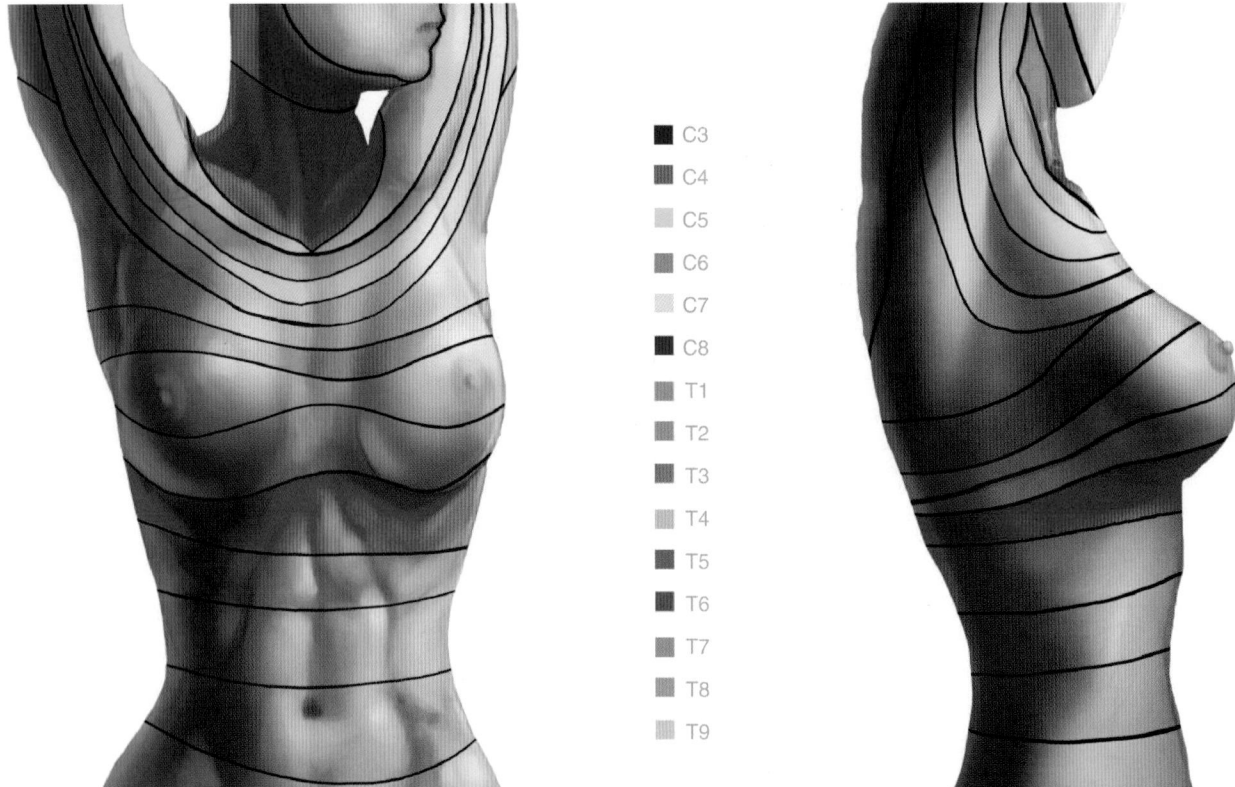

C3
C4
C5
C6
C7
C8
T1
T2
T3
T4
T5
T6
T7
T8
T9

FIGURE 81A-4. Segmental thoracic anesthesia achieved with paravertebral blocks.

These markings indicate the needle insertion sites and should lie over the transverse process of the vertebra (Figure 81A–7). A standard regional anesthesia tray is prepared, and strict asepsis should be maintained during block placement.

A 22-gauge Tuohy needle is recommended for TPVB (Figure 81A–8). Ideally, the needle should have depth markings on its shaft. Alternatively, a depth guard (see Figure 81A–8) is recommended. An epidural set is used if insertion of a catheter

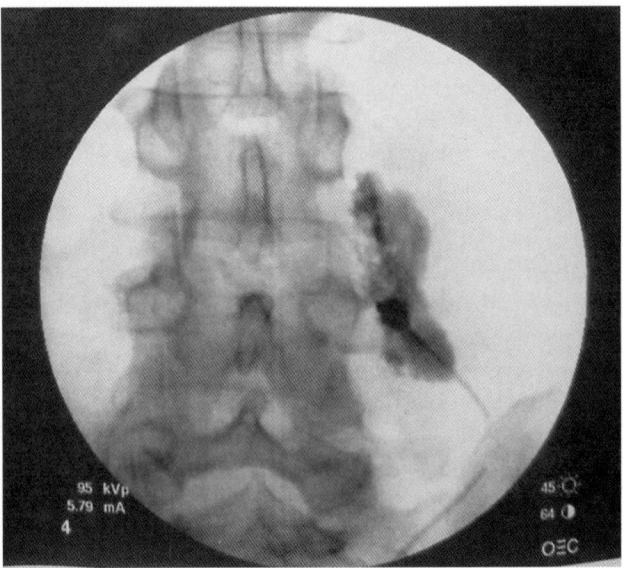

FIGURE 81A-5. Spread of 3 mL of local anesthetic solution in thoracic paravertebral block.

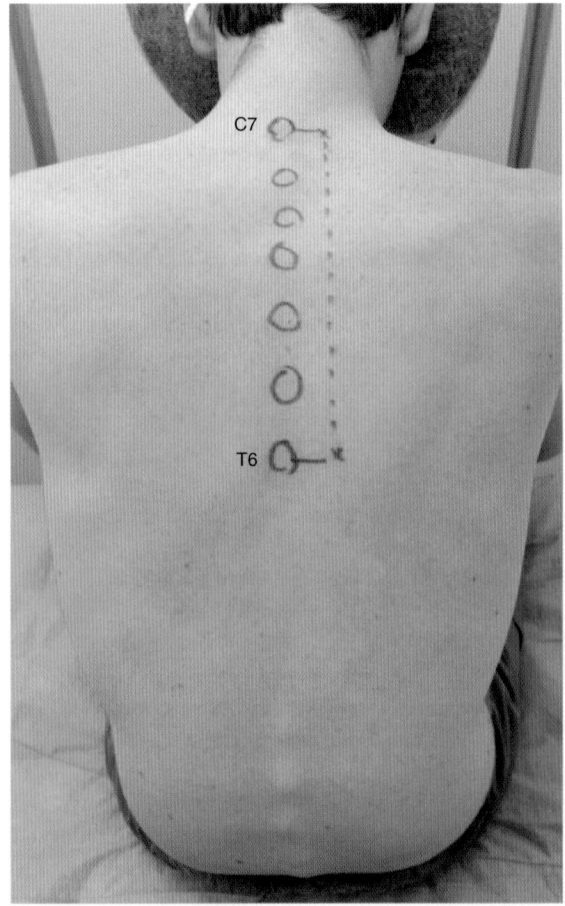

FIGURE 81A-6. Surface landmarks for thoracic paravertebral blocks.

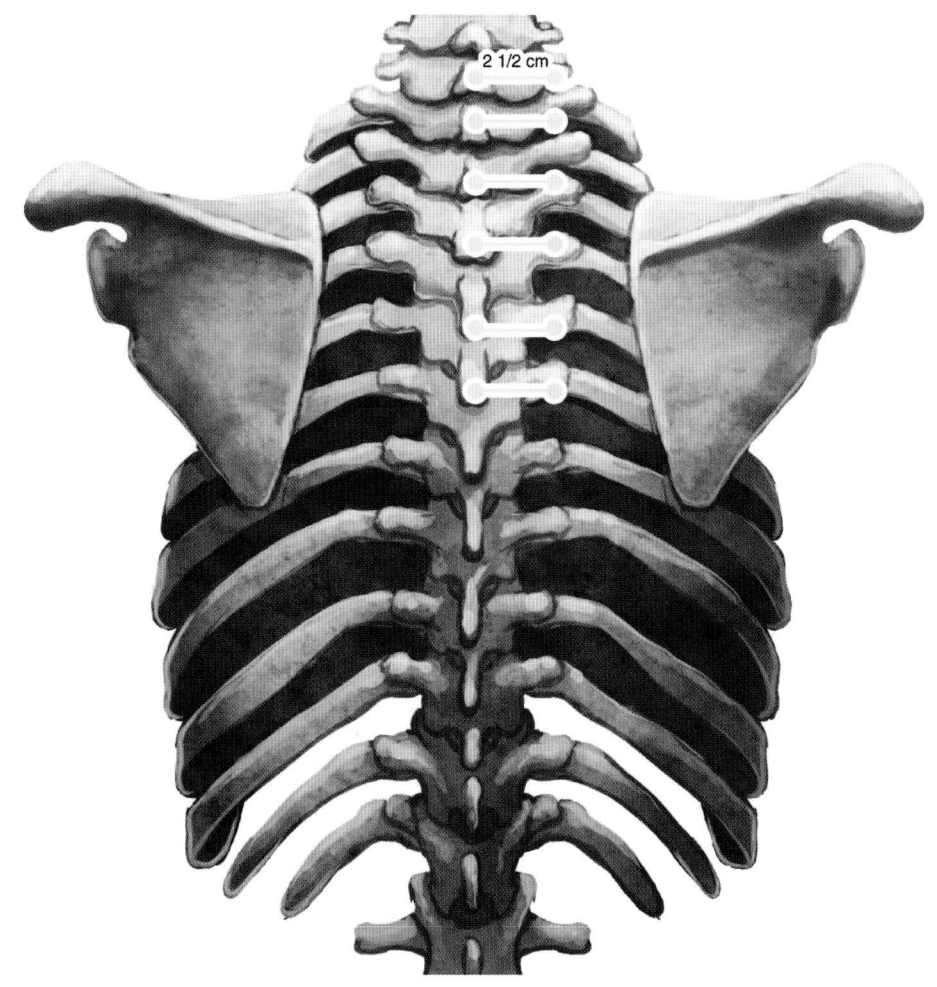

FIGURE 81A–7. Relationship between spinous and transverse processes.

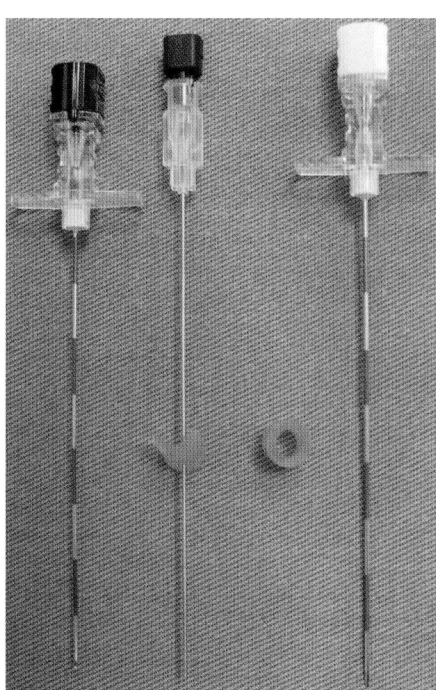

FIGURE 81A–8. Needles commonly used for a single- or multiple-injection thoracic paravertebral block. Note the depth guard that is attached to the needle for assessment of the depth.

into the TPVS is planned. TPVB requires proper premedication to ensure patient acceptance and comfort during block placement.

Loss-of-Resistance Technique

There are several different techniques of TPVB. The classic technique involves eliciting loss of resistance. The skin and underlying tissue is infiltrated with lidocaine 1%, and the block needle is inserted perpendicular to the skin in all planes to contact the transverse process of the vertebra. Note that due to the acute angulation of the thoracic spines in the midthoracic region, the transverse process that is contacted is the one from the lower vertebra (Figures 81A–9 and 81A–10).

The depth at which the transverse process is contacted varies (3–4 cm) and depends on the build of the individual and the level at which the needle is inserted. The depth is deeper at the cervical and lumbar spine level and shallower at the thoracic levels. During needle insertion it is possible to miss the transverse process and inadvertently puncture the pleura. Therefore, it is imperative to search and make contact with the transverse process before advancing the needle too deep and risking pleural puncture. To minimize this complication, the block needle should initially be inserted only to a maximum depth of 4 cm at thoracic and 5 cm at cervical and lumbar levels. If bone is not

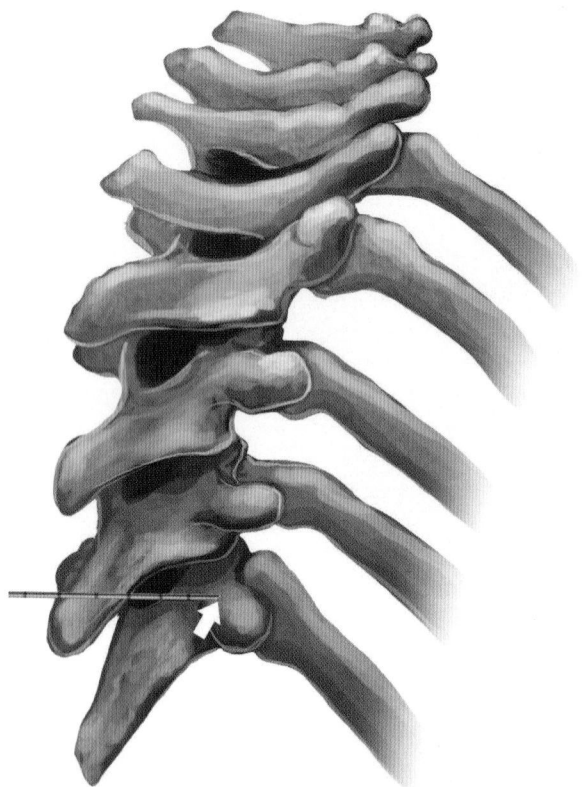

FIGURE 81A–9. Relationship between the spinous and transverse processes at the thoracic level. Due to the steep downward angulation of the spinous processes at the thoracic levels, the needle inserted at the level of the spinous process contacts the transverse process that belongs to the vertebra below it.

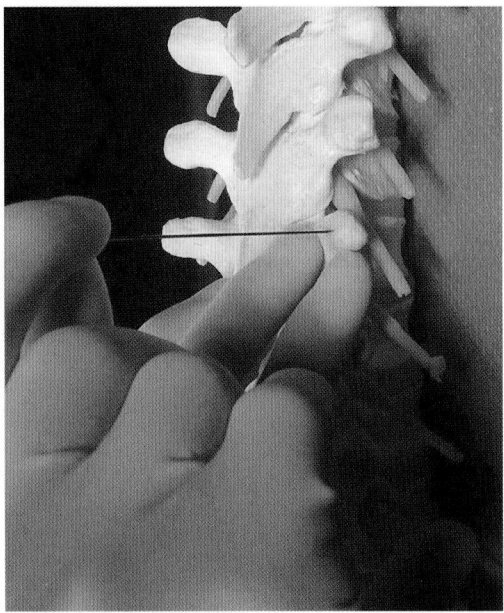

A

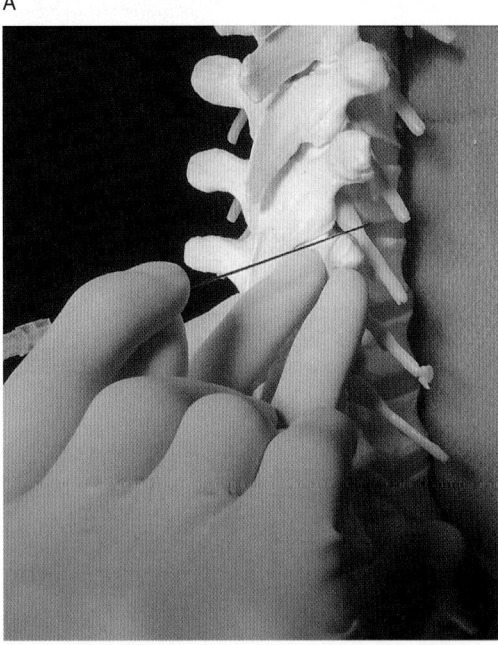

B

FIGURE 81A–10. Technique of "walking off" the transverse process. **A**: The needle is shown contacting the transverse process. **B**: The needle is shown walking off the superior aspect of the transverse process. Walking off the inferiorly may be safer at thoracic level.

contacted, it should be assumed that the needle is in between two adjacent transverse processes. The needle should be withdrawn to the subcutaneous tissue and reinserted with a cephalad or caudad direction to the same depth (4 cm) until bone is contacted. If bone is still not encountered, the needle is advanced a further centimeter and the above procedure repeated until the transverse process is identified. The needle is then walked above or bellow (safer) the transverse process and gradually advanced until a loss of resistance is elicited as the needle traverses the superior costotransverse ligament into the TPVS (Figures 81A–11; see Figure 81A–3).

Clinical Pearls

- "Walking" off the lower aspect of the transverse process is recommended in case the needle has contacted the rib rather than transverse process. When this happens, walking off the rib cephalad may result in pneumothorax.
- This usually occurs within 1.0–1.5 cm from the superior edge of the transverse process (see Figure 81A–3). Although a subtle "pop" or "give" may be appreciated as the needle traverses the superior costotransverse process, this should not be entirely relied on. Instead, the depth of the needle placement should be guided by the initial bone contact (skin-transverse process + 1.0–1.5 cm).

Predetermined Distance Technique

TPVB can also be performed by advancing the needle by a fixed predetermined distance (1 cm) once the needle is walked off the transverse process, without eliciting loss of resistance (Figure 81A–12A and B).[5–7,23] Proponents of this technique have used it very successfully with low risk of pneumothorax. The use of a depth marker is recommended to avoid inadvertent pleural or pulmonary puncture.

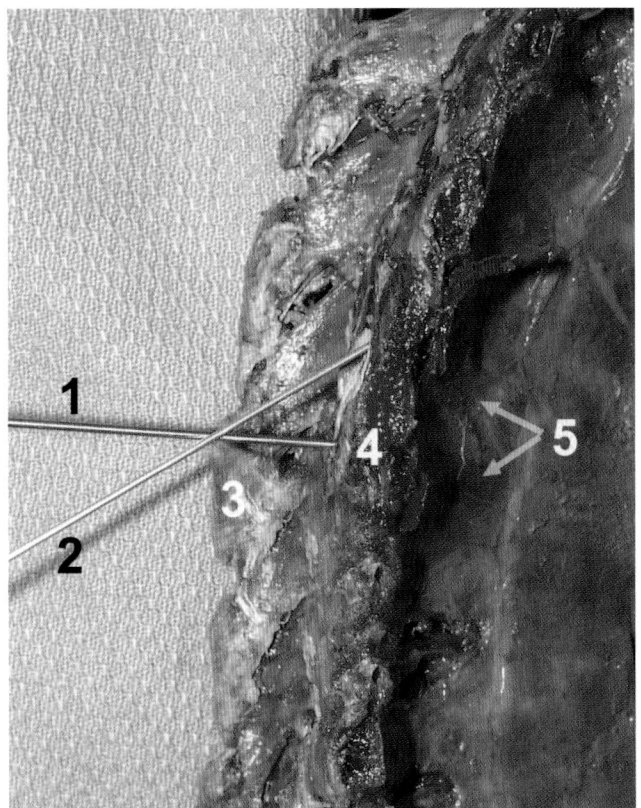

FIGURE 81A–11. Paravertebral block technique. The needle (1) is first advanced to contact the transverse process (4), then redirected cephalad (2) or caudad to walk off the transverse process and enter the paravertebral space. Other structures shown are spinous process (3) and the dispersion of the dye in the paravertebral space and intercostal sulcus.

Clinical Pearls

- Perform TPVB with the patient in the sitting position.
- Surface landmarks should always be identified and marked with a skin marker.
- Use needles with depth markings to facilitate estimation of the depth of insertion.
- It is imperative to search and make contact with the transverse process before advancing the needle any farther.
- The depth at which the transverse process is contacted varies in the same patient at different thoracic levels. It is deepest in the cervical, upper and lower thoracic, and shallowest in the midthoracic region.
- The needle should not be advanced more than 1.5 cm beyond the contact with the transverse process.
- Avoid directing the needle medially to prevent inadvertent epidural or intrathecal needle misadventure.

Placement of Thoracic Paravertebral Catheter

If a continuous TPVB (CTPVB) is planned, a catheter is inserted through a Tuohy needle into the TPVS.[4,22] Unlike epidural catheterization, certain resistance is commonly encountered during insertion of the paravertebral catheter. This can be facilitated by injecting 5–10 mL of saline to create a space before catheter insertion. An unusually seamless passage of catheter should arouse the suspicion of interpleural placement. Perhaps the safest and simplest method of placing a catheter into the TPVS is to place it under direct vision from within the open chest cavity.[8,25] Obviously, this requires an open thorax and is, therefore, done exclusively in patients undergoing a thoracotomy. This technique involves reflecting the parietal pleura from the posterior wound margin onto the vertebral bodies over several thoracic segments, thereby creating an extrapleural paravertebral pocket (Figure 81A–13) into which a percutaneously inserted catheter is placed against the angles of the exposed ribs. The pleura is reapposed to the chest wall, and the thorax is closed. This method can be combined very effectively with a preincisional, single-shot, percutaneous thoracic paravertebral injection to provide perioperative analgesia during thoracic surgery.[26]

Clinical Pearls

- Injecting saline or the bolus dose of the local anesthetic before catheter insertion makes it easier to insert a catheter.
- Very easy passage of catheter (>6 cm) should raise the suspicion of intrapleural placement.
  - Catheter should not be inserted >3 cm to prevent their migration toward epidural space.

Indications

TPVB is indicated for anesthesia and analgesia for unilateral surgical procedures in the chest and abdomen. Commonly reported indications are listed in Table 81A–1. The use of bilateral TPVB has also been reported.

Contraindications

Contraindications for TPVB include infection at the site of injection, allergy to local anesthetic drug, empyema, and a neoplastic mass occupying the paravertebral space. Coagulopathy, bleeding disorders, or patients receiving anticoagulant drugs are relative contraindication for TPVB. One must exercise caution in patients with kyphoscoliosis or deformed spines and those who have had previous thoracic surgery. The chest deformity in the former may predispose to inadvertent thecal or pleural puncture, and the altered paravertebral anatomy due to fibrotic obliteration of the paravertebral space or adhesions of the lung to the chest wall in the latter may predispose to pulmonary puncture.

Choice of Local Anesthetic

Since TPVB does not result in motor weakness of the extremities, long-lasting analgesia is nearly always desirable with TPVB. Consequently, long-acting local anesthetic drugs are typically used. These include bupivacaine or levobupivacaine

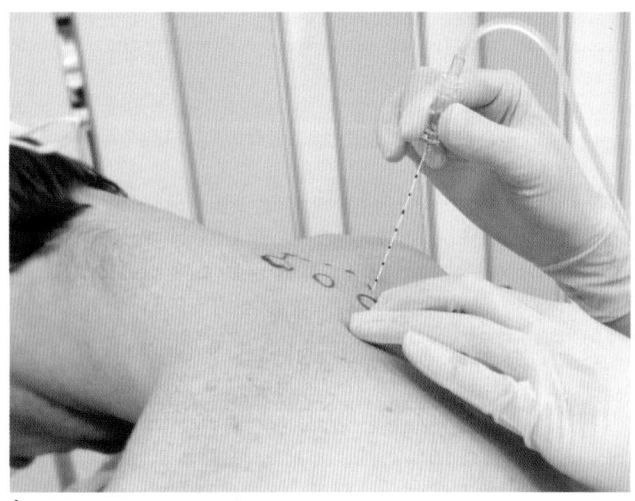
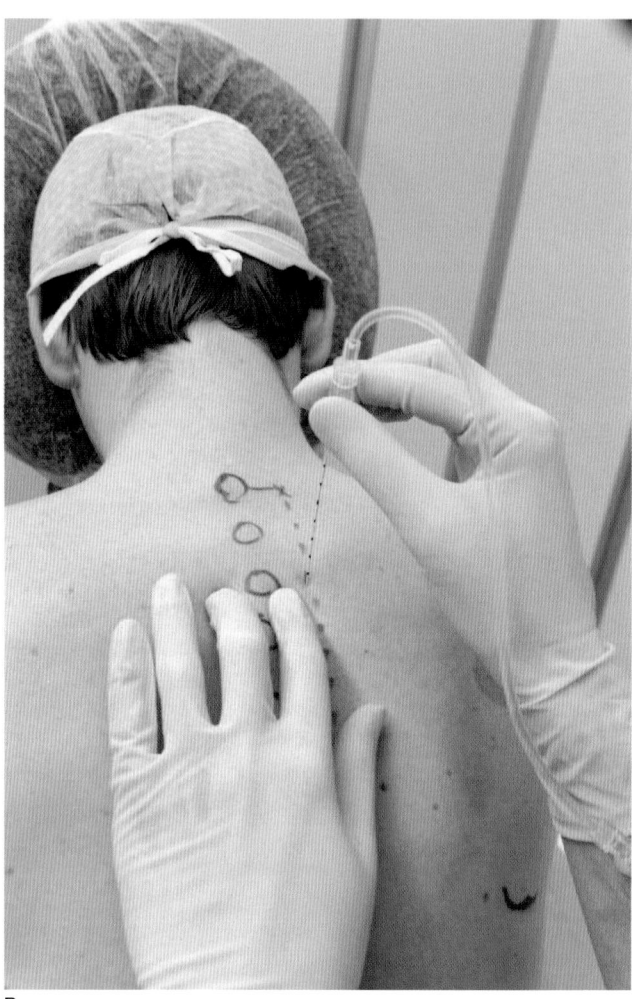

A B

FIGURE 81A–12. Needle angle to contact the transverse process (**A**) and to walk off the transverse process inferiorly (**B**). Once the transverse process is contacted, the needle is walked off and inserted 1.5 cm deeper while paying attention to the depth marks or using a rubber stopper (Figure 81A-8).

0.5% and ropivacaine 0.5%. For single-injection TPVB, 20–25 mL of local anesthetic is injected in aliquots, whereas for multiple-injection TPVB, 4–5 mL of local anesthetic is injected at each level planned.

The maximum dose of local anesthetic must be adjusted in the elderly, poorly nourished, and frail patients. The TPVS is well vascularized, leading to relatively rapid absorption of local anesthetic into the systemic circulation. Consequently, peak plasma concentration of the local anesthetic agent is attained quickly. Epinephrine (2.5–5.0 mcg/mL) containing local anesthetic solutions may be used during the initial injection because it reduces systemic absorption and thereby reduces the potential for toxicity. Epinephrine also helps in increasing the maximum allowable dose of local anesthetic.

The duration of anesthesia after TPVB ranges from 3–4 h, but analgesia often lasts much longer (8–18 h). If a continuous TPVB (CTPVB) is planned, e.g., for postoperative analgesia after thoracotomy or continuous pain relief for multiple fractured ribs, then an infusion of bupivacaine or levobupivacaine 0.25% or ropivacaine 0.2% at 0.1–0.2 mL/kg/h is

started after the initial bolus injection and continued for 3–4 days or as indicated. It is our experience that using a higher concentration of local anesthetic (e.g., bupivacaine 0.5% instead of 0.25%) for the CTPVB does not result in better quality of analgesia, and it may increase the potential for local anesthetic toxicity.

Clinical Pearls

- Consider using lidocaine or chloroprocaine for skin and subcutaneous infiltration to reduce the total dose of the more toxic long- acting local anesthetic.
- Use an epinephrine-containing (e.g., 1:200 000 or 1:400 000) long-acting local anesthetic because it reduces systemic absorption and, therefore, the potential for systemic toxicity.
- Local anesthetic dose should be adjusted in the elderly and those with impairment of hepatic and renal function.

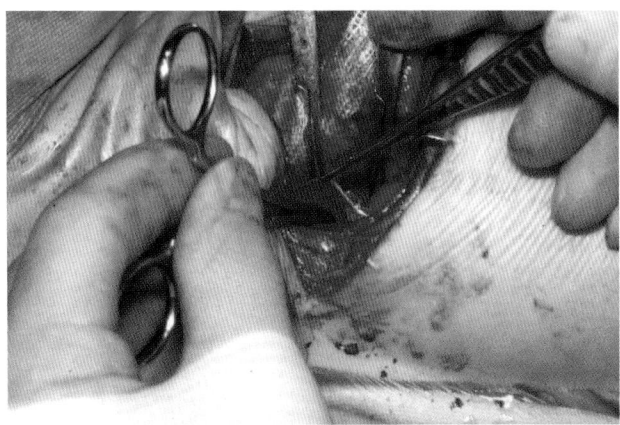

A

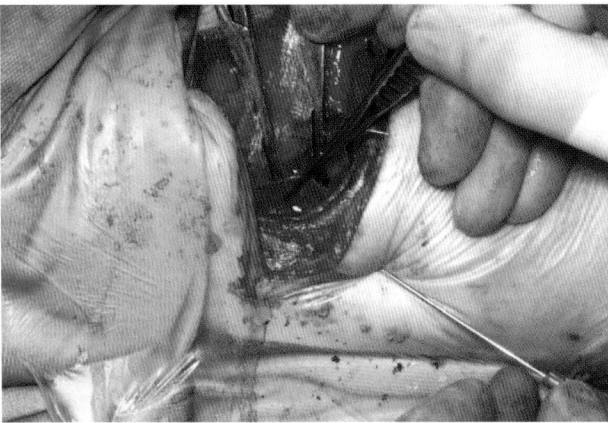

B

FIGURE 81A-13. A: Extrapleural paravertebral catheter placement under direct vision in an infant. Figure shows a curved artery forceps that has been inserted into the extrapleural paravertebral pocket that was created by reflecting the parietal pleura from the posterior wound margin on to the vertebral bodies over several thoracic dermatomes. **B**: Extrapleural paravertebral catheter placement under direct vision in an infant. Figure shows a Tuohy needle that has been inserted from the lower intercostal space into the thoracic paravertebral space; .i.e, the extrapleural paravertebral pocket previously created. A catheter is then inserted through the Tuohy needle and secured in place against the angles of the exposed ribs, after which the pleura is reapposed and the chest is closed.

- Catheter dislodgement is not uncommon and must be excluded whenever a patients complain of breakthrough pain that is not easily controlled.
- Exclude local anesthetic toxicity whenever a patient becomes confused while receiving a continuous thoracic paravertebral infusion.

Practical Management of Thoracic Paravertebral Block

Breast Surgery

Thoracic paravertebral injection of local anesthetic at multiple levels (C7 through T6) in conjunction with intravenous sedation is effective for surgical anesthesia during major breast

TABLE 81A-1. Indications for thoracic paravertebral block.

Anesthesia

- Breast surgery
- Herniorrhaphy (thoracolumbar anesthesia)
- Chest wound exploration

Postoperative Analgesia (as part of a balanced analgesic regimen)

- Thoracotomy
- Thoracoabdominal esophageal surgery
- Video-assisted thoracoscopic surgery
- Cholecystectomy
- Renal surgery
- Breast surgery
- Herniorrhaphy
- Liver resection
- Appendicectomy
- Minimally invasive cardiac surgery
- Conventional cardiac surgery (bilateral TPVB)

Chronic Pain Management

- Benign and malignant neuralgia

Miscellaneous

- Postherpetic neuralgia
- Relief of pleuritic chest pain
- Multiple fractured ribs
- Treatment of hyperhydrosis
- Liver capsule pain after blunt abdominal trauma

Abbreviation: TPVB, thoracic paravertebral block.

surgery (Figure 81A–14).[5,6,27] The C7 spinous process is the most prominent cervical spinous process; the inferior border of the scapula corresponds to T7. Compared with patients who receive only general anesthesia (GA), patients who receive a multiple-injection TPVB for major breast surgery have less postoperative pain, require fewer analgesics, and have less nausea and vomiting after surgery. However, to effectively use the multiple-injection TPVB technique for anesthesia during breast surgery, one must understand the complex innervation of the breast. The anterior and lateral chest wall receives sensory innervation from the anterior and lateral cutaneous branches of the intercostal nerves (T2 through T6), the axilla (T1–T2), the infraclavicular region from the supraclavicular nerves (C4–C5), and the pectoral muscles from the lateral (C5–C6) and medial (C7–C8) pectoral nerves. There also may be overlapping sensory innervation from the contralateral side of the chest. This complex innervation of the breast from the C4–T6 spinal segments explains why TPVB may not provide complete anesthesia for dissection over the pectoral muscle or the infraclavicular region. However, this can be overcome with proper sedation during surgery as well as by injections of local anesthetic by the surgeon intraoperatively into the sensitive areas. Injection of a local anesthetic subcutaneously along the inferior border of the

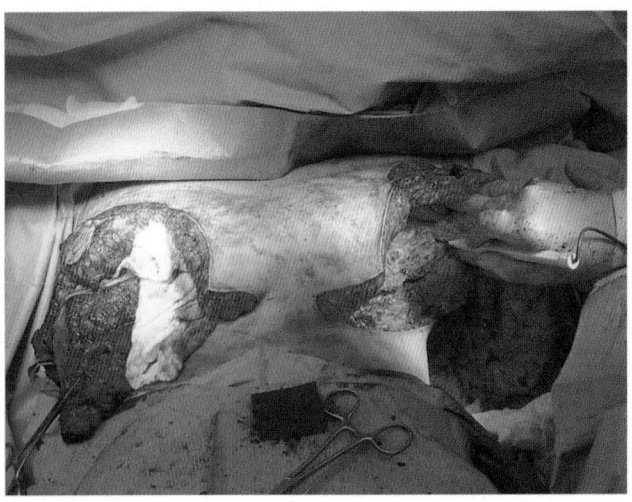
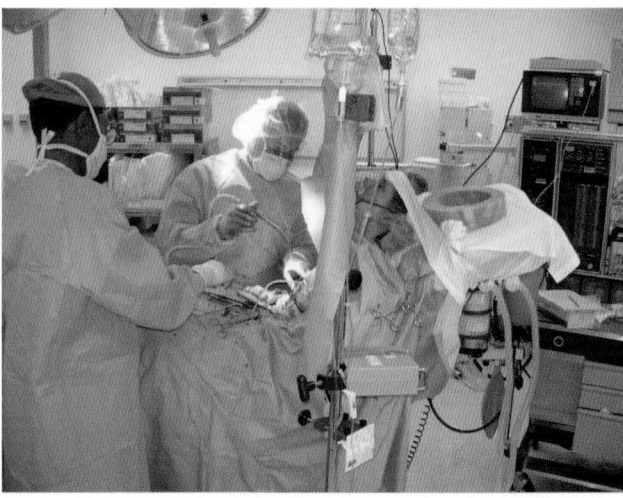

A   B

FIGURE 81A–14. **A**: Extensive breast reconstruction surgery being performed under paravertebral block. **B**: The patient is sedated using propofol infusion. The images demonstrate how potent paravertebral blocks can be both as anesthetic and analgesic techniques.

clavicle or to perform ipsilateral superficial cervical plexus block in order to anaesthetize the supraclavicular nerves (C4–C5) will minimize discomfort and sedative and analgesic requirements during surgery. A combination of midazolam, or propofol infusion, or IV opioid can be used to provide comfort to the patients intraoperatively. Dexmedetomidine, a highly selective α_2-adrenoceptor agonist, with its sedative, analgesic, and minimal or no respiratory depression properties, is a useful alternative for sedation during breast surgery under TPVB.

When combined with general anesthesia, a single injection TPVB with ropivacaine (2 mg/kg diluted to 20 mL with 0.9% saline) with 1:200 000 epinephrine, performed prior to the induction of GA can be used. This provides excellent postoperative analgesia, reduces postoperative analgesic requirement, reduces postoperative vomiting, facilitates the earlier resumption of oral fluid intake, reduces the postoperative decline in respiratory function, and augments the recovery of postoperative respiratory mechanics.

Postthoracotomy Pain Relief

CTPVB is an effective method of providing analgesia after thoracotomy (Figure 81A–15). Ideally, TPVB should be established before the thoracotomy incision, via a catheter that is inserted percutaneously, and continued for 4–5 days after surgery. However, if an extrapleural paravertebral catheter is being placed under direct vision from within the chest during surgery, then a single-injection TPVB can be performed at the level of the thoracotomy incision before the surgical incision, and a continuous infusion of local anesthetic is commenced after the catheter placement.[26] Analgesia achieved by CTPVB is comparable to epidural analgesia but with less hypotension, urinary retention, and the side effects commonly seen with epidural opioid administration.[1,26,28,29] The opioid requirement with such an approach is significantly reduced by the CTPVB, and analgesia is superior to IVPCA alone.[1,30]

Multiple Fractured Ribs

TPVB is an effective method of providing pain relief in patients with unilateral multiple fractured ribs.[1,22,23] A single thoracic paravertebral injection of 25 mL of bupivacaine 0.5% produces pain relief for a mean duration of 10 h and improves respiratory function and arterial blood gases.[1,23] To avoid recurrence of pain and deterioration in respiratory function, a thoracic paravertebral

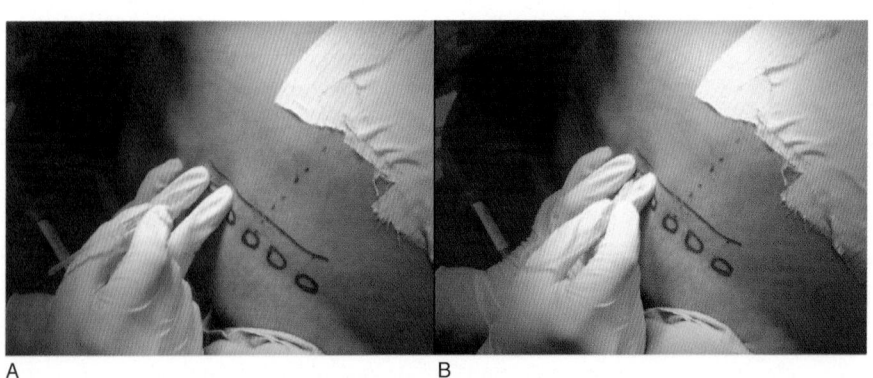

A   B

FIGURE 81A–15. Thoracic paravertebral blocks in patients after thoracotomy. A typical sequence of touching the transverse process (**A**) and walking off 1 cm deeper to the transverse process superiorly or inferiorly (**B**).

catheter can be inserted midway between the highest and the lowest fractured rib, and a CTPVB can be commenced after administration of the initial bolus injection. CTPVB in combination with an NSAID provides continuous pain relief and produces a sustained improvement in respiratory parameters and arterial oxygenation.[22] Since TPVB does not cause urinary retention or affect lower limb motor function, it is useful in patients with multiple fractured ribs who also have concomitant lumbar spinal trauma since it also allows continuous neurologic assessment for signs of spinal cord compression.[31]

Pharmacokinetic Considerations

Relatively large doses of local anesthetics are commonly used during CTPVB. Therefore, there is the potential for local anesthetic toxicity, and patients should be closely monitored during CTPVB and the infusion stopped if signs develop. During a prolonged thoracic paravertebral infusion there is progressive accumulation of local anesthetic in the plasma, and the plasma concentration of the drug may exceed the threshold for central nervous system toxicity (e.g,, 2.0–4.5 mcg/mL for bupivacaine). Despite the systemic accumulation, local anesthetic toxicity is rare. This may be the case because, although the total plasma concentration of the local anesthetic increases postoperatively, the free fraction of the drug remains unchanged[32] and may be due to the postoperative increase in α_1-acid glycoprotein concentration,[32] the protein that binds to local anesthetic drugs. There is also a greater increase in the S-bupivacaine enantiomer,[33,34] which is associated with lower toxicity, than the R-enantiomer. Due to concerns of systemic accumulation and local anesthetic toxicity with prolonged paravertebral infusion, it is preferable to use a local anesthetic with lower potential for toxicity, such as ropivacaine. One must also exercise caution in the elderly and frail patients as well as in patients with impaired hepatic and renal function.

Complications and How to Avoid Them

Based on published data the incidence of complications after TPVB is relatively low and varies from 2.6%–5%.[1,5,35,36] These include vascular puncture (3.8%), hypotension (4.6%), pleural puncture (1.1%), and pneumothorax (0.5%).[35] Unlike with thoracic epidural anesthesia, hypotension is rare in normovolemic patients after TPVB because the sympathetic blockade is unilateral. However, TPVB may unmask hypovolemia and result in hypotension. Therefore, TPVB should be used with caution in patients who are hypovolemic or hemodynamically labile. Nevertheless, hypotension is rare even after bilateral TPVB, probably owing to the segmental nature of the bilateral sympathetic blockade.

Pleural puncture and pneumothorax are two complications that often dissuade anesthesiologists from performing a TPVB. Inadvertent pleural puncture is uncommon after TPVB and may not result in a pneumothorax, which is usually minor and can be managed conservatively. Clues that suggest pleural puncture during a TPVB pronounced loss of resistance as the needle enters chest cavity, cough, onset of sharp chest or shoulder pain, or sudden hyperventilation. Contrary to the common belief, air cannot be aspirated through the needle unless the lung is also inadvertently punctured or air that may have entered the pleural cavity during removal of the stylet is aspirated. Such patients should be closely monitored for the possible development of a pneumothorax. It should be kept in mind that pneumothorax may be delayed in onset and a chest radiograph taken too early to exclude a pneumothorax may not be conclusive. Even a radiologic contrast study using a chest radiograph may be difficult to interpret because the intrapleural contrast disperses rapidly, does not define any specific anatomic plane, and tends to spread to the diaphragmatic angles or horizontal fissure. Systemic local anesthetic toxicity can occur due to inadvertent intravascular injection or from using an excessive dose of local anesthetic. The local anesthetic solution must be injected in aliquots, and the dosage must be adjusted in the elderly and frail patient. An epinephrine-containing local anesthetic solution is suggested to enable the recognition of the intravascular injection and reduce the absorption of the local anesthetic in the systemic circulation. Inadvertent epidural, subdural, or intrathecal injection and spinal anesthesia can also occur. Published data suggest that these complications are more frequent when the needle is directed medially but may also occur with a normally positioned needle due to the close proximity of the needle to the dural cuff and intervertebral foramen. Therefore, the needle must never be directed medially, and care must be taken to exclude intrathecal injection by routinely performing an aspiration test before injection. Transient ipsilateral Horner syndrome can occasionally develop after TPVB. This is due to cephalad spread of the local anesthetic to the stellate ganglion or to the preganglionic fibers of the first few segments of the thoracic spinal cord. Bilateral Horner syndrome has also been reported and may be due to epidural spread or prevertebral spread to the contralateral stellate ganglion. Sensory changes in the arm and lower extremity may also occur after a TPVB. The former is due to spread of local anesthetic to the lower components of the ipsilateral brachial plexus (C8 and T1), and the latter is due to extended subendothoracic fascial spread to the ipsilateral retroperitoneal space where the lumbar spinal nerves are located (discussed earlier), but epidural spread as a cause cannot be excluded. Motor blockade or bilateral symmetric anesthesia involving the lower extremity is rare. It generally suggests significant epidural spread and may be more common if large volumes of local anesthetic (>25–30 mL) are injected at a single level. Therefore, if a wide segmental spread of anesthesia is desired, it is preferable to perform the multiple-injection technique or inject a smaller volume of local anesthetic at several levels a few dermatomes apart.

LUMBAR PARAVERTEBRAL BLOCK

Lumbar paravertebral block (LPVB) is technically similar to a TPVB but due to differences in anatomy between the thoracic and lumbar paravertebral spaces the two paravertebral techniques are described separately. LPVB is used most commonly in combination with a TPVB, as a thoracolumbar paravertebral block, for surgical anesthesia during inguinal herniorrhaphy.

Anatomy

The lumbar paravertebral space (LPVS) is limited anterolaterally by the psoas major muscle; medially by the vertebral bodies, the intervertebral discs, and the intervertebral foramen with its contents; and posteriorly by the transverse process and the ligaments that are interposed between the adjoining transverse processes. Unlike the TPVS, which contains adipose tissue, the LPVS is occupied primarily by the psoas major muscle. The psoas major muscle is made up of a fleshy anterior part that forms the main bulk of the muscle, and a thin accessory posterior part.[37] The main bulk originates from the anterolateral surface of the vertebral bodies and the accessory part originates from the anterior surface of the transverse process.[37] The two parts fuse to form the psoas major muscle except near the vertebral bodies where the two parts are separated by a thin fascia within which lie the lumbar spinal nerve roots and the ascending lumbar veins.[37] The ventral rami of the lumbar spinal nerve roots extend laterally in this intramuscular plane formed by the two parts of the psoas major muscle and form the lumbar plexus within the substance of the psoas major muscle.[37] The psoas muscle is enveloped by a fibrous sheath, "the psoas sheath," which continues laterally as the fascia covering the quadratus lumborum muscle. During a LPVB the local anesthetic is injected anterior to the transverse process into a triangular space between the two parts of the psoas major muscle containing the lumbar spinal nerve root.

The LPVS communicates medially with the epidural space. A series of tendinous arches extends across the constricted parts of the lumbar vertebral bodies, which are traversed by the lumbar arteries and veins and sympathetic fibers. These tendinous arches may provide a pathway for the spread of local anesthetic from the LPVS to the anterolateral surface of the vertebral body, the prevertebral space, and the contralateral side and may be the pathway through which the ipsilateral lumbar sympathetic chain may occasionally be involved.

Mechanism of Block and Distribution of Anesthesia

A lumbar paravertebral injection produces ipsilateral dermatomal anesthesia (Figure 81A–16) by a direct effect of the local anesthetic on the lumbar spinal nerves and by medial extension into the epidural space via the intervertebral foramen. The contribution of epidural spread to the overall distribution of anesthesia after a LPVB is unknown but probably occurs in the

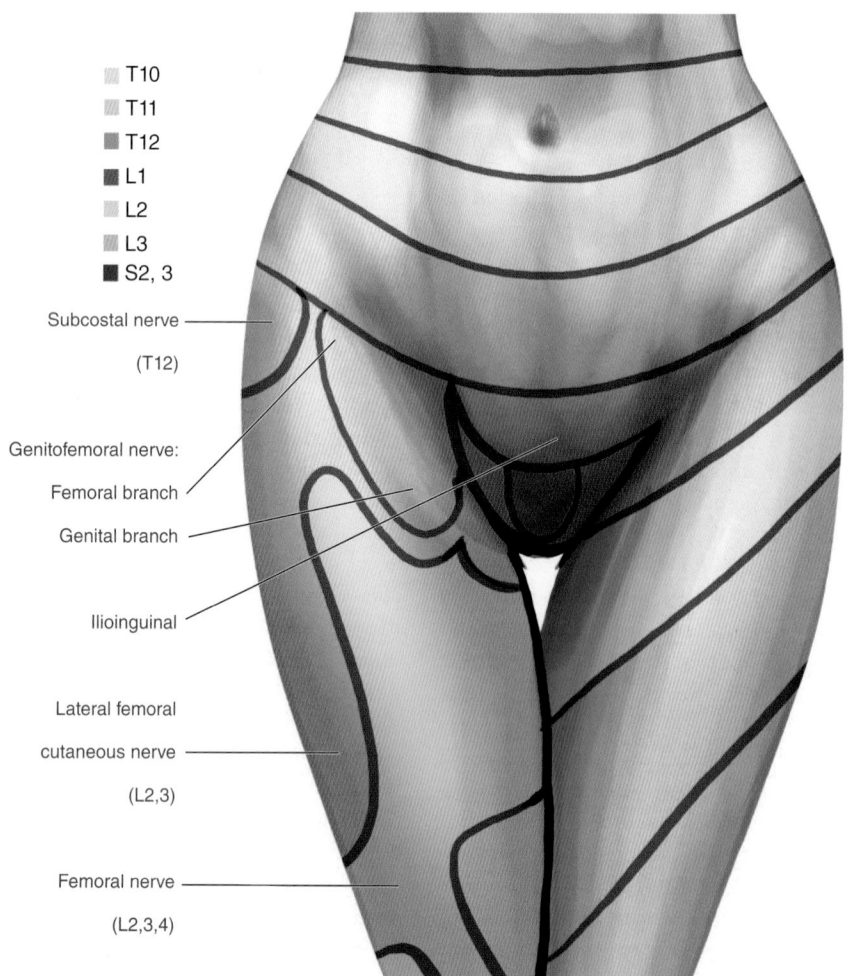

T10
T11
T12
L1
L2
L3
S2, 3

Subcostal nerve

(T12)

Genitofemoral nerve:

Femoral branch

Genital branch

Ilioinguinal

Lateral femoral
cutaneous nerve

(L2,3)

Femoral nerve

(L2,3,4)

FIGURE 81A–16. Segmental distribution of anesthesia with lumbar paravertebral levels.

majority of patients and depends on the volume of local anesthetic injected at a given level. Ipsilateral sympathetic blockade may also occur due to epidural spread or spread of local anesthetic anteriorly via the tendinous arches to the rami communicantes or the lumbar sympathetic chain.

Technique

Lumbar paravertebral block can be performed with the patient in the sitting, lateral, or prone position. Surface landmarks must be identified and marked with a skin marker before block placement. The spinous process of the vertebra at the levels to be blocked represents the midline, the iliac crest corresponds to the L3-L4 interspace, and the tip of scapula corresponds to the T7 spinous process. Skin markings are also made 2.5 cm lateral to the midline at the levels that are to be blocked (Figure 81A–17A) or one can draw a line 2.5 cm lateral to the midline and perform the injections along this line (Figure 81A–17B and C). A standard regional anesthesia tray is prepared; strict asepsis should be maintained during block placement. An 8-cm, 22-gauge, Tuohy tip needle (see Figure 81–1–8) is used for LPVB. Similarly to the recommendations for TPVB, the use of needles with depth markings on the shaft of the needle or a guard indicating the depth (see Figure 81–1–8) is recommended. Advancing the needle by a fixed predetermined distance (1.5–2.0 cm) beyond the transverse process, without eliciting paresthesia, is the method most commonly used to perform LPVB. The block needle is inserted perpendicular to the skin until the transverse process is contacted. The depth at which the transverse process is contacted is variable (4–6 cm) and depends on the build of the patient. Once the transverse process is identified, the marking on the needle is noted or the depth marker is adjusted so that it is 1.5–2.0 cm beyond

the skin–transverse process depth. The needle is then withdrawn to the subcutaneous tissue and reinserted at a 10- to 15-degree superior or inferior angle so that it slides off the superior or inferior edge of the transverse process, similarly to the technique in thoracic paravertebral block (see Figure 81A–11). The needle is advanced by a further 1.5–2.0 cm beyond the contact with the transverse process or until the depth marker is reached. After negative aspiration for blood or cerebrospinal fluid (CSF), the local anesthetic is injected. Since spread of local anesthetic after a single large-volume lumbar paravertebral injection is unpredictable, the multiple-injection technique in which 4–5 mL of local anesthetic is injected at each level is more commonly used.

Choice of Local Anesthetic

As for TPVB, long-acting local anesthetic agents such as bupivacaine 0.5%, ropivacaine 0.5%, or levobupivacaine 0.5% are commonly used for LPVB. During a multiple injection LPVB, 4–5 mL of the local anesthetic is injected at each level. Anesthesia develops in about 15–30 minutes and lasts for 3–6 h. Analgesia is also long-lasting (12–18 h) and generally outlasts the duration of anesthesia. There are no data on the pharmacokinetics of local anesthetic after LPVB. Nevertheless, the addition of epinephrine (2.5–5.0 mcg/mL) to the local anesthetic may reduce systemic absorption and reduce the potential for toxicity.

Indications and Contraindications

LPVB is commonly used in combination with TPVB (T10 through L2) for surgical anesthesia during inguinal herniorrhaphy. It can be also effective for rescue in patients with severe pain after total hip replacement. It can also be used for

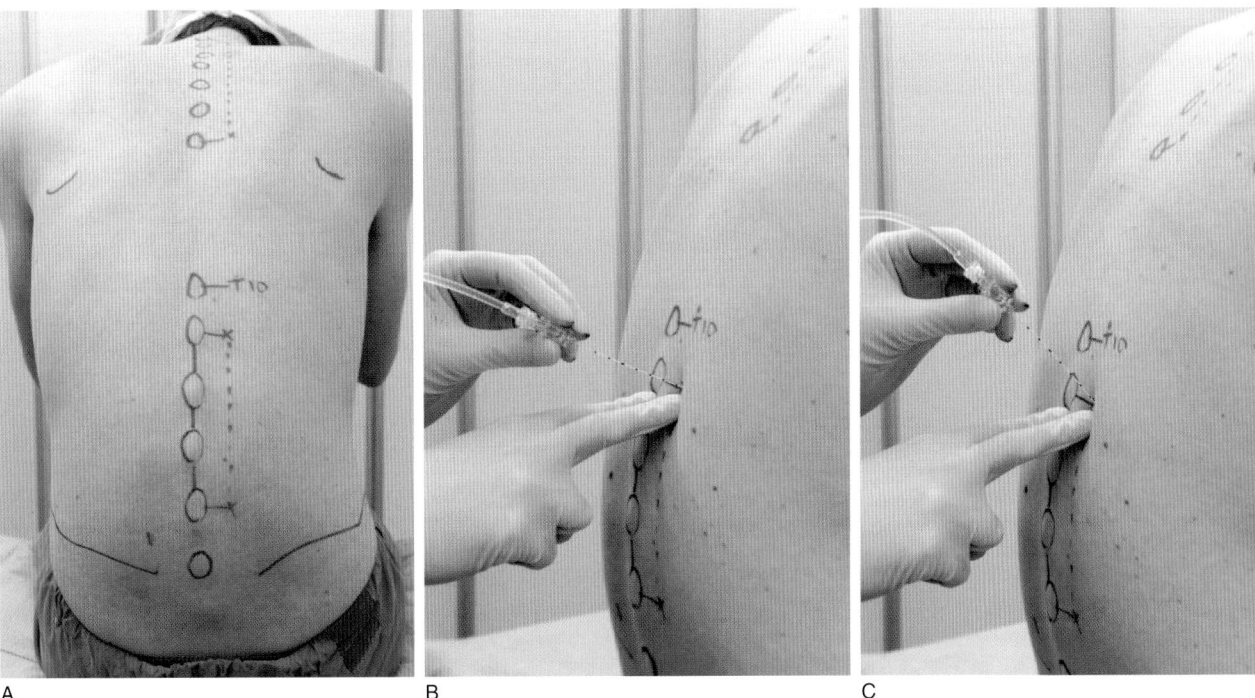

A   B   C

FIGURE 81A–17. A: Surface landmarks and needle insertion sites for lumbar paravertebral block. **B** and **C:** Needle insertion.

diagnostic purpose during evaluation of groin or genital pain, such as that following nerve entrapment syndrome after inguinal herniorrhaphy. Contraindications for LPVB are similar to TPVB, but caution should be exercised in patients who are anticoagulated or are receiving prophylactic anticoagulants since psoas hematoma with lumbar plexopathy has been reported.

Complications and How to Avoid Them

Published data suggest that complication is rare after LPVB.[38,39] Nevertheless, it is possible to inadvertently inject local anesthetic into the intravascular, epidural, or intrathecal spaces during LPVB, and this may be more common if the needle is directed medially. Therefore, the direction of the block needle should be maintained perpendicular to the skin during insertion, and medial angulation should be avoided. Intraperitoneal injection or visceral injury (renal) may also occur, although this can occur only as a result of gross technical error. Motor weakness involving the ipsilateral quadriceps muscle may result if the L2 spinal nerve is blocked (femoral nerve L2–L4).

SUMMARY

Proper training is necessary to acquire stereotactic techniques required to ensure a high success rate. Thoracic paravertebral block produces unilateral somatic and sympathetic nerve blockade that is adequate for surgical anesthesia during breast surgery and for analgesia when pain is of unilateral origin from the chest or abdomen. It has been also described as a rescue analgesic therapy in patients with rib fractures and respiratory compromise.[40] Lumbar paravertebral block is less commonly used in clinical practice. As a thoracolumbar paravertebral block, it is effective for surgical anesthesia during inguinal herniorrhaphy. Hemodynamic stability is usually maintained after a paravertebral block due to the unilateral nature of sympathetic blockade. Bladder and lower limb motor function is also preserved, and no additional nursing vigilance is required during the postoperative period. Successful clinical applications of bilateral paravertebral block have also been reported.

REFERENCES

1. Karmakar MK: Thoracic paravertebral block. Anesthesiology 2001;95:771–780.
2. Richardson J, Lonnqvist PA: Thoracic paravertebral block. Br J Anaesth 1998;81:230–238.
3. Cheema SP, Ilsley D, Richardson J, et al: A thermographic study of paravertebral analgesia. Anesthesia 1995;50:118–121.
4. Eason MJ, Wyatt R: Paravertebral thoracic block—a reappraisal. Anesthesia 1979;34:638–642.
5. Coveney E, Weltz CR, Greengrass R, et al: Use of paravertebral block anesthesia in the surgical management of breast cancer: experience in 156 cases. Ann Surg 1998;227:496–501.
6. Greengrass R, O'Brien F, Lyerly K, et al: Paravertebral block for breast cancer surgery. Can J Anaesth 1996;43:858–861.
7. Klein SM, Bergh A, Steele SM, et al: Thoracic paravertebral block for breast surgery. Anesth Analg 2000;90:1402–1405.
8. Karmakar MK, Booker PD, Franks R, et al: Continuous extrapleural paravertebral infusion of bupivacaine for post-thoracotomy analgesia in young infants. Br J Anaesth 1996;76:811–815.
9. Lonnqvist PA, Hesser U: Radiological and clinical distribution of thoracic paravertebral blockade in infants and children. Paediatr Anaesth 1993;3:83–87.
10. Lonnqvist PA: Continuous paravertebral block in children. Initial experience [see comments]. Anesthesia 1992;47:607–609.
11. Dugan DJ, Samson PC: Surgical significance of the endothoracic fascia. The anatomic basis for empyemectomy and other extrapleural technics. Am J Surg 1975;130:151–158.
12. Karmakar MK, Kwok WH, Kew J: Thoracic paravertebral block: radiological evidence of contralateral spread anterior to the vertebral bodies. Br J Anaesth 2000;84:263–265.
13. Karmakar MK, Chung DC: Variability of a thoracic paravertebral block. Are we ignoring the endothoracic fascia? [letter]. Reg Anesth Pain Med 2000;25:325–327.
14. Moore DC, Bush WH, Scurlock JE: Intercostal nerve block: a roentgenographic anatomic study of technique and absorption in humans. Anesth Analg 1980;59:815–825.
15. Tenicela R, Pollan SB: Paravertebral-peridural block technique: a unilateral thoracic block. Clin J Pain 1990;6:227–234.
16. Nunn JF, Slavin G: Posterior intercostal nerve block for pain relief after cholecystectomy. Anatomical basis and efficacy. Br J Anaesth 1980;52:253–260.
17. Conacher ID: Resin injection of thoracic paravertebral spaces. Br J Anaesth 1988;61:657–661.
18. Purcell-Jones G, Pither CE, Justins DM: Paravertebral somatic nerve block: a clinical, radiographic, and computed tomographic study in chronic pain patients. Anesth Analg 1989;68:32–39.
19. Karmakar MK, Gin T, Ho AM: Ipsilateral thoraco-lumbar anesthesia and paravertebral spread after low thoracic paravertebral injection. Br J Anaesth 2001;87:312–316.
20. Saito T, Gallagher ET, Cutler S, et al: Extended unilateral anesthesia. New technique or paravertebral anesthesia? Reg Anesth 1996;21:304–307.
21. Saito T, Den S, Tanuma K, et al: Anatomical bases for paravertebral anesthetic block: fluid communication between the thoracic and lumbar paravertebral regions. Surg Radiol Anat 1999;21:359–363.
22. Karmakar MK, Critchley LA, Ho AM, et al: Continuous thoracic paravertebral infusion of bupivacaine for pain management in patients with multiple fractured ribs. Chest 2003;123:424–431.
23. Gilbert J, Hultman J: Thoracic paravertebral block: a method of pain control. Acta Anaesthesiol Scand 1989;33:142–145.
24. Richardson J, Jones J, Atkinson R: The effect of thoracic paravertebral blockade on intercostal somatosensory evoked potentials. Anesth Analg 1998;87:373–376.
25. Sabanathan S, Smith PJ, Pradhan GN, et al: Continuous intercostal nerve block for pain relief after thoracotomy. Ann Thorac Surg 1988;46:425–426.
26. Richardson J, Sabanathan S, Jones J, et al: A prospective, randomized comparison of preoperative and continuous balanced epidural or paravertebral bupivacaine on post-thoracotomy pain, pulmonary function and stress responses. Br J Anaesth 1999;83:387–392.
27. Weltz CR, Greengrass RA, Lyerly HK: Ambulatory surgical management of breast carcinoma using paravertebral block. Ann Surg 1995;222:19–26.
28. Sabanathan S, Mearns AJ, Bickford SP, et al: Efficacy of continuous extrapleural intercostal nerve block on post-thoracotomy pain and pulmonary mechanics. Br J Surg 1990;77:221–225.
29. Matthews PJ, Govenden V: Comparison of continuous paravertebral and extradural infusions of bupivacaine for pain relief after thoracotomy. Br J Anaesth 1989;62:204–205.
30. Carabine UA, Gilliland H, Johnston JR, et al: Pain relief for thoracotomy. Comparison of morphine requirements using an extrapleural infusion of bupivacaine. Reg Anesth 1995;20:412–417.
31. Karmakar MK, Chui PT, Joynt GM, et al: Thoracic paravertebral block for management of pain associated with multiple fractured ribs in patients with concomitant lumbar spinal trauma. Reg Anesth Pain Med 2001;26:169–173.
32. Dauphin A, Gupta RN, Young JE, et al: Serum bupivacaine concentrations during continuous extrapleural infusion. Can J Anaesth 1997;44:367–370.
33. Berrisford RG, Sabanathan S, Mearns AJ, et al: Plasma concentrations of bupivacaine and its enantiomers during continuous extrapleural intercostal nerve block. Br J Anaesth 1993;70:201–204.
34. Clark BJ, Hamdi A, Berrisford RG, et al: Reversed-phase and chiral high-performance liquid chromatographic assay of bupivacaine and its enantiomers in clinical samples after continuous extraplural infusion. J Chromatogr 1991;553:383–390.

35. Lonnqvist PA, MacKenzie J, Soni AK, et al: Paravertebral blockade. Failure rate and complications. Anesthesia 1995;50:813–815.

36. Richardson J, Sabanathan S: Thoracic paravertebral analgesia. Acta Anaesthesiol Scand 1995;39:1005–1015.

37. Farny J, Drolet P, Girard M: Anatomy of the posterior approach to the lumbar plexus block. Can J Anaesth 1994;41:480–485.

38. Klein SM, Greengrass RA, Weltz C, et al: Paravertebral somatic nerve block for outpatient inguinal herniorrhaphy: an expanded case report of 22 patients. Reg Anesth Pain Med 1998;23:306–310.

39. Wassef MR, Randazzo T, Ward W: The paravertebral nerve root block for inguinal herniorrhaphy—a comparison with the field block approach. Reg Anesth Pain Med 1998;23:451–456.

40. Murata H, Salviz EA, Chen S, Vandepitte C, Hadzic A. Case report: ultrasound-guided continuous thoracic paravertebral block for outpatient acute pain management of multilevel unilateral rib fractures Anesth Analg. 2013 Jan;116(1):255–257.

CHAPTER 81B

Intercostal Nerve Block

Anthony M.-H. Ho, Robbert Buck, Malikah Latmore, Matthew Levine, and Manoj K. Karmakar

INTRODUCTION

The intercostal nerves (ICNs) innervate the major parts of the skin and musculature of the chest and abdominal wall. The block of these nerves was first described by Braun in 1907 in the textbook *Die Lokalanastesie*.[1] In the 1940s, clinicians noticed that intercostal nerve blocks (ICNBs) can reduce pulmonary complications and in opioid requirements after upper abdominal surgery.[1] In 1981, continuous ICNB was introduced to overcome the problems associated with repeated multiple injections.[1] Today, ICNB is used in a variety of acute and chronic pain conditions affecting the thorax and upper abdomen, including breast and chest wall surgery. Introduction of ultrasound guidance to the practice of regional anesthesia further facilitates its practice. The disadvantages of intercostal block, however, include the requirement for technical expertise, risks of pneumothorax, and local anesthetic toxicity with multiple levels of blockade.

INDICATIONS

ICNB provides excellent analgesia in patients with rib fractures[2,3] and for postsurgical pain after chest and upper abdominal surgery such as thoracotomy, thoracostomy, mastectomy, gastrostomy, and cholecystectomy.[4] Respiratory parameters typically show impressive improvements on relief of pain.[2,3] Blockade of the two dermatomes above and the two below the level of surgical incision is required. ICNB does not block visceral abdominal pain, for which a celiac plexus block is required. Neurolytic ICNB is used to manage chronic pain conditions such as postmastectomy pain (T2) and postthoracotomy pain.

CONTRAINDICATIONS

1. Disorders of coagulation, although this is not an absolute contraindication
2. Local infection, lack of expertise and resuscitating equipment

FUNCTIONAL ANATOMY

As thoracic nerves T1 to T12 emerge from their respective intervertebral foramina, they divide into the following rami (Figure 81B–1):

1. The paired gray and white anterior rami communicantes, which pass anteriorly to the sympathetic ganglion and chain.
2. The posterior cutaneous ramus, supplying skin and muscle in the paravertebral region.
3. The ventral ramus (ICN, the main focus of this chapter).

T1 and T2 send nerve fibers to the upper limbs and the upper thorax, T3 through T6 supply the thorax, T7 through T11 supply the lower thorax and abdomen, and T12 innervates the abdominal wall and the skin of the front part of the gluteal region (Figure 81B–2). Carrying both sensory and motor fibers, the ICN pierces the posterior intercostal membrane about 3 cm (in adults) distal to the intervertebral foramen to enter the subcostal grove where it, for the most part, continues to run parallel to the rib, although branches may often be found anywhere between adjacent ribs. Its course within the thorax is sandwiched between the parietal pleura and innermost intercostal (intercostalis intimus) muscles and the external and internal intercostal muscles (Figures 81B–3 and 81B–4). Just anterior to the midaxillary line, it gives off the lateral cutaneous branch. As the ICN approaches the midline, it turns anteriorly and pierces the overlying muscles and skin to terminate as the anterior cutaneous branch.

However, there are many anatomic variations. The first thoracic nerve (T1) has no anterior cutaneous branch, usually has no lateral cutaneous branch, and most of its fibers leave the intercostal space by crossing the neck of the first rib to join those from C8, while a smaller bundle continues on a genuine intercostal course to supply the muscles of the intercostal space. Some fibers of T2 and T3 give rise to the intercostobrachial

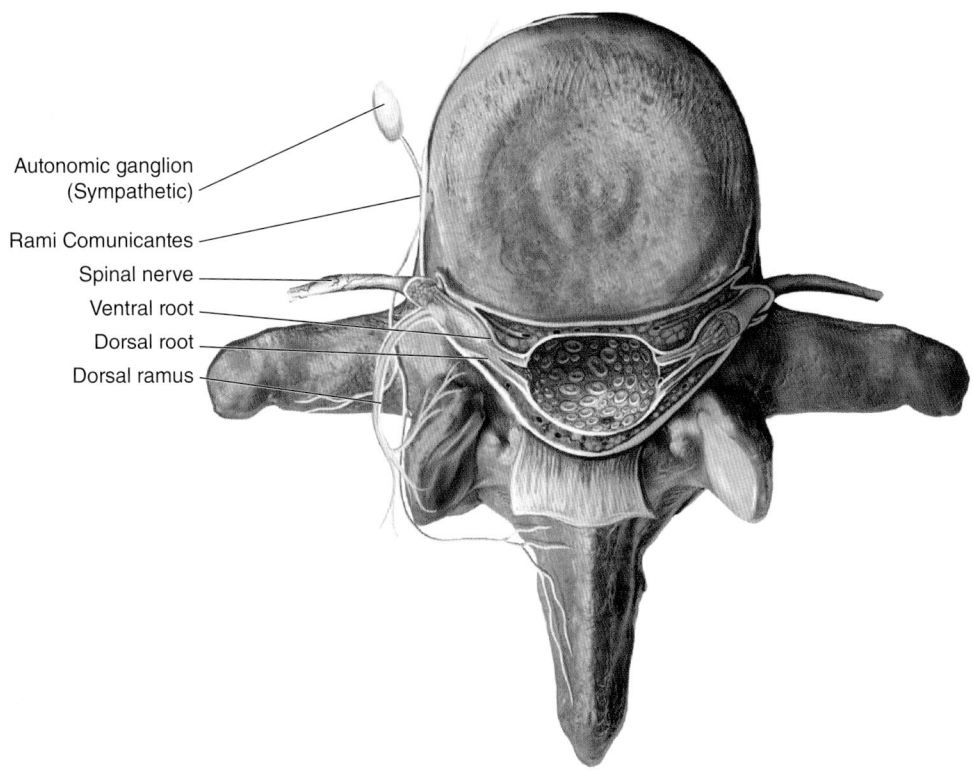

FIGURE 81B-1. Anatomy of the spinal nerve.

nerve, which innervates the axilla and the skin of the medial aspect of the upper arm as far distal as the elbow. In addition, the ventral ramus of T12 is similar to the other ICNs but is called a subcostal nerve because it is not positioned between two ribs.

Lateral Cutaneous Branch

The lateral cutaneous branches of T2 through T11 pierce the internal and external intercostal muscles obliquely before dividing into the anterior and posterior branches (see Figure 81B–4). These branches supply the muscles and skin of the lateral torso. The anterior branches supply of T7–T11 innervate the skin as far forward as the lateral edge of the rectus abdominis. The posterior branches of T7–T11 supply the skin overlying

the latissimus dorsi. The lateral cutaneous branch of T12 does not divide. Most of the ventral ramus of T12 joins that of L1 to form the iliohypogastric, ilioinguinal, and genitofemoral nerves; the rest pierces the transverse abdominal muscle (TAM) to travel between TAM and the internal oblique muscle.

Anterior Cutaneous Branch

The anterior cutaneous branches of T2 through T6 pierce the external intercostals and pectoralis major muscles to enter the superficial fascia near the lateral border of the sternum to supply the skin of the anterior part of the thorax near the midline and slightly beyond (see Figure 81B–4). Smaller branches (T1 through T6) exist to supply the intercostal muscles and parietal

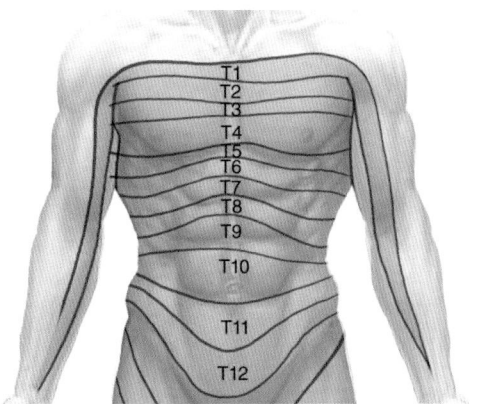

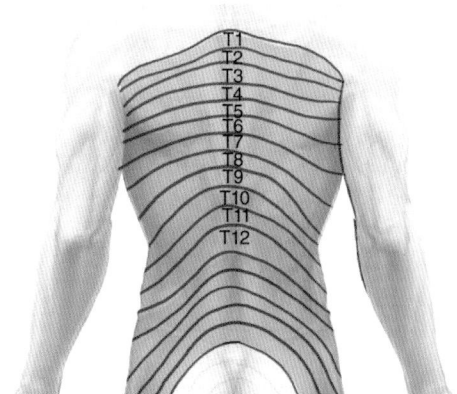

FIGURE 81B-2. Dermatomal distribution of the intercostal nerves.

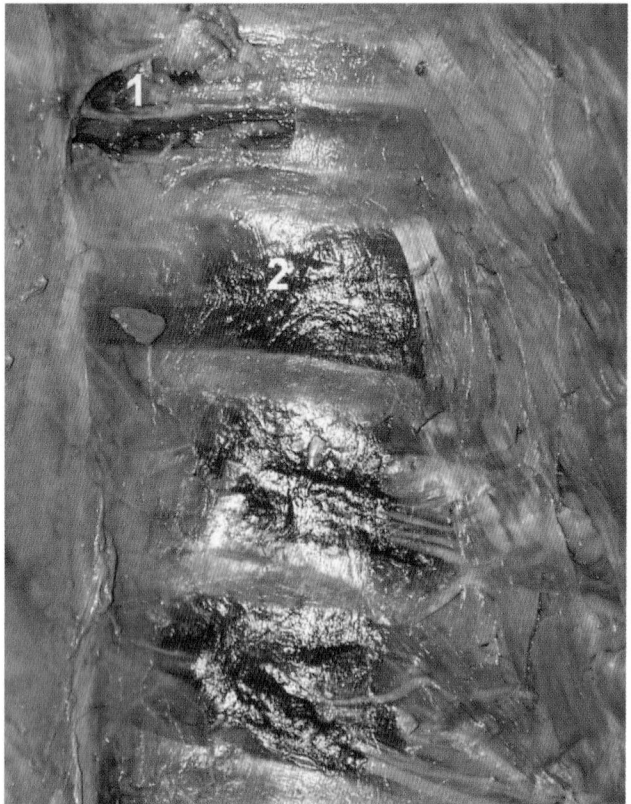

FIGURE 81B-3. Intercostal nerves (accompanied by intercostal artery and vein) shown in the intercostal sulcus as seen from within the open chest cavity in a cadaver. The red dye illustrates spread of solutions injected into the intercostal sulcus during intercostal block. 1. Intercostal nerve. 2. Distribution of the dye after injection into the intracostal sulcus.

pleura, and these branches may cross to adjoining intercostal spaces. The anterior cutaneous branches of T7 through T12 pierce the posterior rectus sheath to supply motor nerves to the rectus muscle and sensory fibers to the skin of the anterior abdominal wall. Some final branches of T7 through T12 continue anteriorly and, together with L1, innervate the parietal peritoneum of the abdominal wall. Their anterior course continues and becomes superficial near the linea alba to provide cutaneous innervation to the midline of the abdomen and a couple of centimeters beyond.

MECHANISM OF BLOCK AND DISTRIBUTION OF ANESTHESIA

ICNB blocks the ipsilateral sensory and motor fibers of the ICNs. Local anesthetic solution injected into the subcostal groove spreads both distally and proximally; some of the injectate may enter paravertebral space as well. (see Figure 81B-3).

TECHNIQUE

An intravenous line should be established, and resuscitation drugs should be readily available. Sedation and analgesia are always used judiciously. ICNB may be performed in an anesthetized patient, although spinal anesthesia has been reported in patients when ICNB was performed under general anesthesia,[4] and there is a concern that the risk of pneumothorax may be increased in a patient under positive pressure ventilation. After the block, the patient should be monitored for potential complications, particularly delayed pneumothorax, local anesthetic toxicity, hematoma, and occurrence of spinal anesthesia (rare).

The ICN can be blocked anywhere proximal to the midaxillary line, where the lateral cutaneous branch takes off. In children, the block is commonly carried out at the posterior axillary line or, alternatively, just lateral to the paraspinal muscles, at the angle of the rib. In adults, the most common site for ICNB is at the angle of the rib (6–8 cm from the spinous processes; Figure 81B-5). At the angle of the rib, the rib is relatively superficial and easy to palpate, and the subcostal groove is the widest. The nerve is inferior to the posterior intercostal artery, which is inferior to the intercostal vein (Figure 81B-6) (mnemonic: VAN [vein/artery/nerve]). VAN are surrounded by adipose tissue and are sandwiched between the internal intercostal and the interior intercostal (intercostalis intimus) muscles. The nerve often runs as three or four separate bundles, without an enclosing endoneural sheath, making it easily accessible to blockade. Blocking intercostal nerves medial to the angle of the rib is not recommended because the nerves lies deep to the posterior intercostal membrane with very little tissue between it and the parietal pleura, and the overlying sacrospinalis muscle makes rib palpation difficult. On the other hand, block distal to the anterior axillary line is more difficult because the nerve has left the subcostal groove and reentered the intercostal space and lies in the substance of the internal intercostal muscle.

ICNB can be performed with the patient in the prone, sitting, or lateral position (block side up). In prone position, a pillow should be placed under the patient's upper abdomen, and the arms are allowed to hang off the sides. The sitting patient should lean slightly forward holding a pillow and be supported. The arms should be forward. The position of the arm in either position is to pull the scapulae laterally and facilitate access to the posterior rib angles above T7 (see Figure 81B-5). Under aseptic conditions, the block sites are identified.

Clinical Pearls

- Ribs can be counted starting from the twelfth rib, or from the seventh rib (inferior tip of the scapula).
- The inferior edges of the ribs to be blocked are marked just lateral to the lateral border of the sacrospinalis (paraspinous) muscle group (usually 6–8 cm from the midline at the lower ribs and 4–7 cm from the midline at the upper ribs), corresponding to the angles of the ribs.

Inferior borders of the ribs to be blocked are palpated and marked (see Figure 81B-5). The needle entry sites are infiltrated with lidocaine 1%–2%. A site of entry is well placed

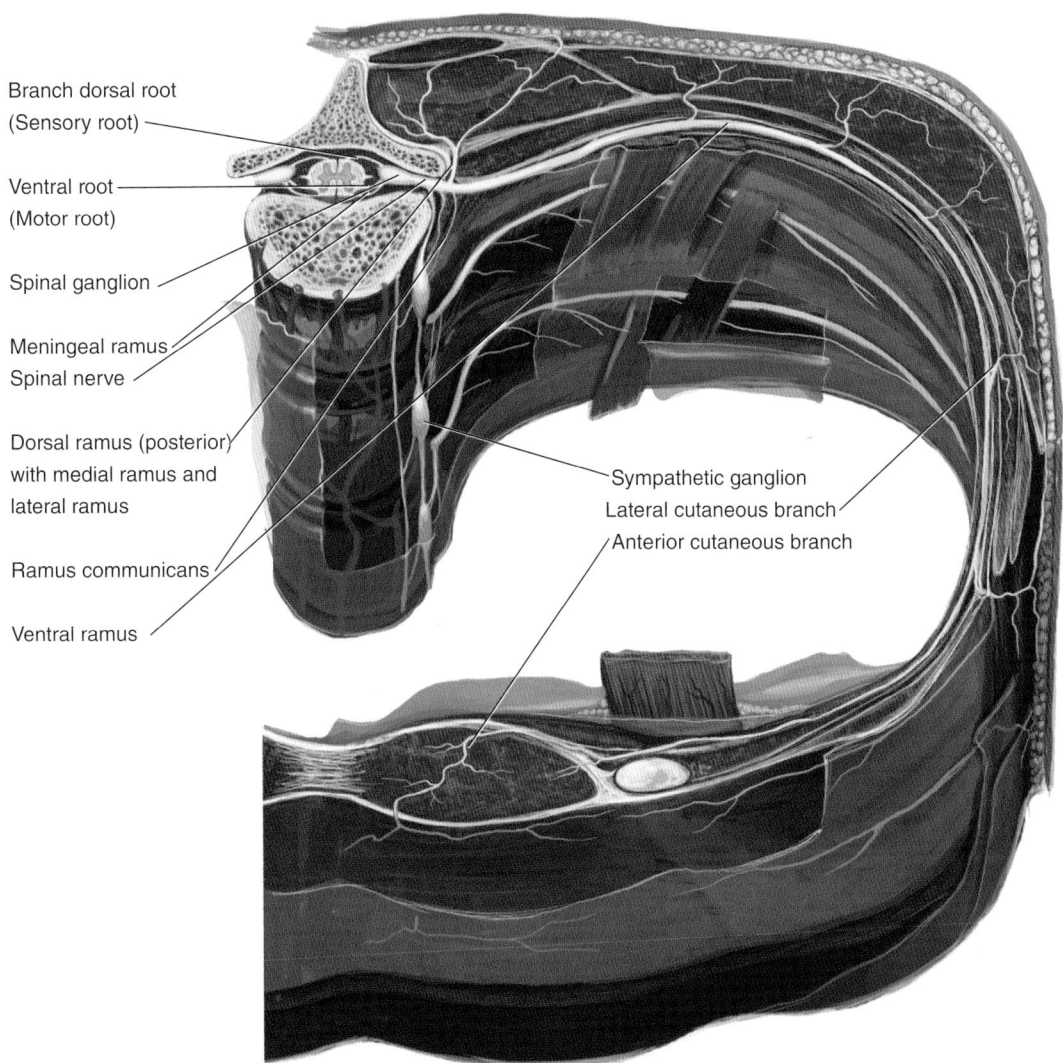

Branch dorsal root
(Sensory root)

Ventral root
(Motor root)

Spinal ganglion

Meningeal ramus
Spinal nerve

Dorsal ramus (posterior)
with medial ramus and
lateral ramus

Ramus communicans

Ventral ramus

Sympathetic ganglion
Lateral cutaneous branch
Anterior cutaneous branch

FIGURE 81B–4. Anatomy of the intercostal nerve.

when a needle introduced through it at 20 degrees cephalad (sagittal plane; see Figure 81B–6) scrapes underneath the inferior border of the rib and reaches the subcostal groove. The skin is first drawn cephalad with the palpating hand by about 1 cm, and a 4- to 5-cm, 22- to 24-gauge (for single-shot injection) needle is introduced through the chosen entry site at a 20-degree cephalad angle with the bevel facing cephalad. The needle is advanced until it contacts the rib at a depth of less than 1 cm in most patients. A small amount of local anesthetic may be injected to anesthetize the periosteum. With the palpating hand holding the needle firmly and resting securely on the patient's back, the injecting hand gently "walks" the needle caudally while the skin is allowed to move back over the rib (Figure 81B–7).

The needle is now advanced farther a few mm, while maintaining the 20-degree tilt angle cephalad (even a slight caudad-pointing angle by the needle greatly reduces the chance of success). A subtle "give" or "pop" of the fascia of the internal intercostal muscle may be felt, especially if a short-beveled

needle is used. As the average distance from the posterior aspect of the rib to the pleura averages 8 mm, advancement of the needle much beyond a few mm increases the risk of pneumothorax.[5] Paresthesia, although not actively sought, occasionally occurs as an additional confirmation of the correct needle placement. Radiologic guidance is advised for neurolytic blocks. At this point, on negative aspiration for blood, 3–5 mL of local anesthetic is injected. For a single ICNB, it is desirable to block at least one ICN cephalad and one caudad because some degree of overlapping innervation from adjacent ICNs is common. To ensure that the tip of the needle remains in the optimal location, unaffected by hand and chest movements, some clinicians prefer to connect extension tubing between the needle and the syringe and have an assistant perform the aspiration and injection.

Blockade of T1 through T7 is technically more challenging because of the scapulae and the rhomboid muscles. For this reason, we prefer to perform a thoracic paravertebral block or an epidural blocks when high thoracic blockade is required.

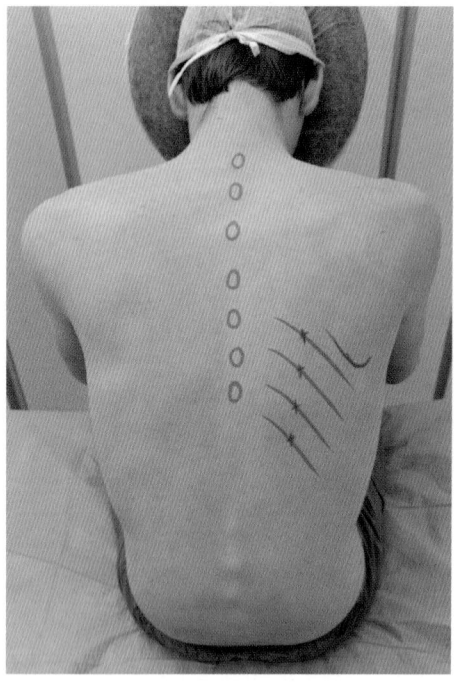

FIGURE 81B-5. The sitting patient should lean slightly forward and be supported. The arms should pull the scapulae laterally to facilitate access to the posterior rib angles above T7. The inferior edges of the ribs to be blocked are marked just lateral to the lateral border of the sacrospinalis (paraspinous) muscle group, corresponding to the angles of the ribs. Points of needle entry are marked at 6–8 cm from the midline in most adults.

EQUIPMENT

Needle: Single shot: 20- to 22-gauge 4- to 5-cm needle (adults)
Catheter placement: 18- to 20-gauge Tuohy needle (adults)
Syringe and needle for local infiltration
Syringe with extension tubing
Sterilizing and resuscitation equipment and drugs, drapes, marking pen, pillow, portable fluoroscope (for neurolytic blocks)

CHOICE OF LOCAL ANESTHETIC

The choice of local anesthetic for single-shot ICNB includes bupivacaine 0.25%–0.5%, lidocaine 1%–2% with epinephrine 1/200,000–1/400,000, and ropivacaine 0.5%. Three to 5 mL of local anesthetic is injected at each level during a multiple-injection ICNB. The duration of action is usually 12 ± 6 h. Addition of epinephrine to bupivacaine or ropivacaine does not significantly prolong the duration of block, but may slow the systemic absorption and increase the maximum allowable dose with a single shot by 30%.[4] Maximum bupivacaine dose is 2 (for plain solution) to 3 (with epinephrine) mg/kg/injection (total at one time)[7] and 7–10 mg/kg/day. Maximum lidocaine dose is up to 5–7 (with epinephrine) mg/kg/injection[7] and 20 mg/kg/day. Volunteers reportedly may tolerate 30% more ropivacaine than bupivacaine before neurologic symptoms

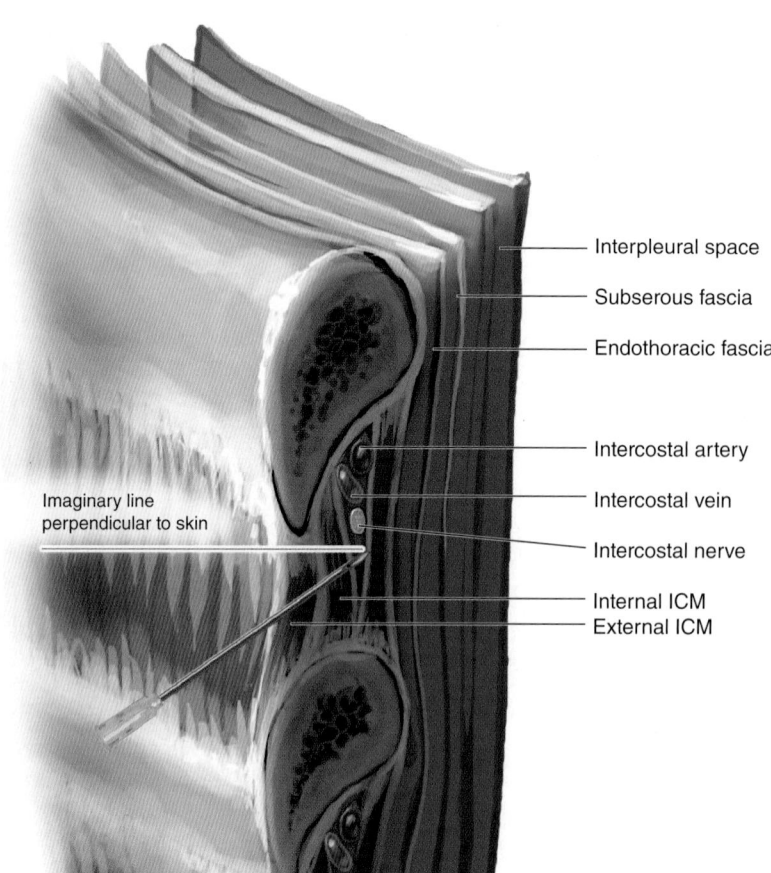

Imaginary line perpendicular to skin

Interpleural space
Subserous fascia
Endothoracic fascia

Intercostal artery
Intercostal vein
Intercostal nerve

Internal ICM
External ICM

FIGURE 81B-6. Needle angle required to enter intercostal sulcus. Note the relationship of the intercostal vessels to the nerve.

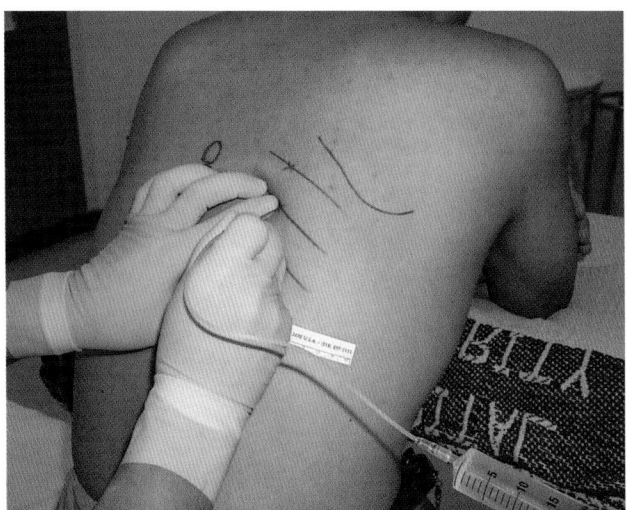

FIGURE 81B–7. With the palpating hand holding the needle firmly and resting securely on the patient's back to control the needle advancement, the injecting hand gently "walks" the needle caudally while the skin is allowed to move back over the rib.

develop.[8] The maximum single injection dose for ropivacaine is 2.5 mg/kg and 4 mg/kg with epinephrine,[7] whereas the maximum daily dose is 9–12 mg/kg/24 h. The maximum single injection of epinephrine as an additive is 4 mcg/kg. Vascular sites favor more rapid local anesthetic absorption, and the blood levels of local anesthetics after ICNB are higher than for most other regional anesthetic procedure. As such, it is advisable to leave a safety margin between the doses given and the maximum recommended dosages, especially in young children; the elderly; debilitated patients; and those with underlying cardiac, hepatic, or renal impairment. For continuous infusion, patients can usually tolerate a gradual build-up of the plasma local anesthetic level better than acute rises. One recommended regimen is a loading dose of 0.3 mL/kg followed by an infusion of 0.1 mL/kg/h of either bupivacaine 0.25% or lidocaine 1%.[5]

Clinical Pearls

- Best needle insertion site for ICNB is the angle of the rib, about 7 cm lateral to midline in adults.
- The ideal angle of entry into the subcostal groove is about 20 degrees cephalad.
- Epidural analgesia may be better suited alternative to bilateral ICNBs because of the risk of bilateral pneumothorax and the potential for local anesthetic toxicity due the large dose of local anesthetic required.
- ICNB above T7 may be difficult because of the scapulae; an alternative technique such as paravertebral or epidural block should be considered.

COMPLICATIONS

The foremost concern is pneumothorax, which may occur in about 1%. Tension pneumothorax and the subsequent need for tube thoracostomy, however, is rare. If an asymptomatic pneumothorax is detected, the best management is observation, reassurance, and, if necessary, supplemental oxygen. The peritoneum and abdominal viscera are at risk of penetration when lower ICNs are blocked. Absorption of local anesthetic from the intercostal space is rapid; arterial plasma concentration peaks in 5-10 minutes, and venous plasma concentration peaks several minutes later.

SUMMARY

ICNB is a useful regional anesthesia technique; which is very effective in the controlling pain involving the thorax and upper abdomen. Although there is the risk of pneumothorax and local anesthetic toxicity, these can be reduced with proper technique and consideration given to the maximum allowable drug dose. The proper use of ICNB includes balancing its advantages and disadvantages against those of alternative techniques such as epidural and paravertebral block. With expertise and proper indications, intercostal nerve block may provide a uniquely suitable anesthetic option in patients in whom general or other regional anesthesia choices may be limited.[9]

REFERENCES

1. Strømskag KE, Kleiven S: Continuous intercostals and interpleural nerve blockades. Tech Reg Anesth Pain Manage 1998;2:79–89.
2. Karmakar MK, Ho AMH: Acute pain management of patients with multiple fractured ribs. J Trauma 2003;54:612–615.
3. Karmakar MK, Critchley LAH, Ho AMH, et al: Continuous thoracic paravertebral infusion of bupivacaine for pain management in patients with multiple fractured ribs. Chest 2003;123:424–431.
4. Kopacz DJ, Thompson GE: Intercostal blocks for thoracic and abdominal surgery. Tech Reg Anesth Pain Manage 1998;2:25–29.
5. Nunn JF, Slavin G: Posterior intercostal nerve block for pain relief after cholecystectomy. Anatomical basis and efficacy. Br J Anaesth 1980;52:253–60.
6. Barron DJ, Tolan MJ, Lea RE: A randomized controlled trial of continuous extra-pleural analgesia post-thoracotomy: efficacy and choice of local anaesthetic. Eur J Anaesthesiol 1999;16:236–245.
7. Lagan G, McLure HA: Review of local anaesthetic agents. Curr Anaesth Crit Care 2004;15:247–254.
8. Scott DB, Lee A, Fagan D, et al: Acute toxicity of ropivacaine compared with that of bupivacaine. Anesth Analg 1989;69:563–569.
9. Vandepitte C, Gautier P, Bellen P, Murata H, Salviz EA, Hadzic A. Use of ultrasound-guided intercostal nerve block as a sole anaesthetic technique in a high-risk patient with Duchenne muscular dystrophy. Acta Anaesthesiol Belg. 2013;64(2):91-94.

CHAPTER 82A

Lumbar Plexus Block

Jerry D. Vloka, Tony Tsai, and Admir Hadzic

INTRODUCTION

Lumbar plexus is an advanced regional anesthesia technique, practiced by relatively few, experienced regional anesthesiologists. This is because these techniques have been challenging to master and resulted in frequent failure.[1–3] Dogliotti[4] pointed out, "the nerve trunks of the lumbar plexus which run into the inferior extremity are at a great distance from each other, so much so that in order to produce anesthesia, multiple procedures are necessary with separate injections, for each nerve trunk." Hence, anesthesiologists preferred the more time-efficient, simpler and reliable techniques of spinal or epidural anesthesia. Several variations of the original technique have been proposed, the main differences in these various approaches being in the level of blockade and the distance from the midline for the needle insertion.[4–6] However, given the deep location of the lumbar plexus, various approaches often represent miniscule technical variations rather than clinically relevant modifications. For instance, Chayen's approach is thought to result in too high incidence of epidural blockade,[7] but another proposed technique also resulted in a 15% incidence of epidural blockade.[8] Although ultrasound guidance may allow visualization of the lumbar plexus, the ultrasound guided technique still requires expertise and is technically challenging; refer Chapter 38.[9–11] Regardless of which technique is followed, certain safety precautions must be used for successful and safe use of this technique.

Indications

Lumbar plexus block has been used for a number of lower extremity procedures. It has been shown to be particularly useful for femoral shaft and neck fractures, knee procedures, and procedures involving the anterior thigh.[1,12–14] However, lumbar plexus block alone cannot provide adequate anesthesia for major surgery of the lower extremity because of the contributing innervation by the sciatic nerve. In one report, even when combined lumbar plexus–sciatic blocks are used for anesthesia in patients undergoing total knee arthroplasty, 22% of patients still required general anesthesia.[15]

Regional Anesthesia Anatomy and Management

The lumbar plexus consists of five nerves on each side, the first of which emerges between the first and second lumbar vertebrae and the last between the last lumbar vertebra and the base of the sacrum. As the L2, L3, and L4 roots of the lumbar plexus split off their spinal nerves and emerge from the intervertebral foramina, they enter the psoas major muscle[16] (Figure 82A–1). Within the muscle, these roots then split into anterior and posterior divisions, which reunite to form the individual branches (nerves) of the plexus.[17] The major branches of the lumbar plexus are the genitofemoral nerve, lateral femoral cutaneous nerve, femoral nerve, and obturator nerve (Figure 82A–2). Within the psoas major muscle, the lateral femoral cutaneous and femoral nerves are separated from the obturator nerve by a muscular fold in more than 50% of patients; anatomic variations are also common.[17,18] The femoral nerve is formed by the posterior divisions of L2–L4 and descends from the plexus lateral to the psoas muscle. The anterior divisions of the same roots unite to form the other major branch of the lumbar plexus, the obturator nerve. The reader is referred to Chapter 39 for more in-depth discussions of anatomy.

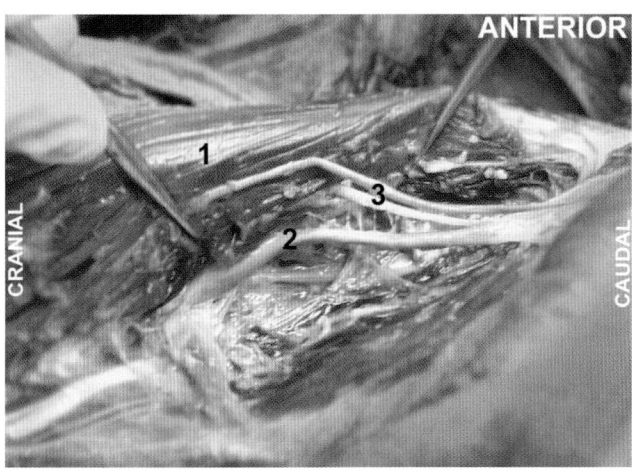

FIGURE 82A-1. Psoas muscle (*1*) is shown exposed from within abdominal cavity with lumbar plexus branches (*2, 3*).

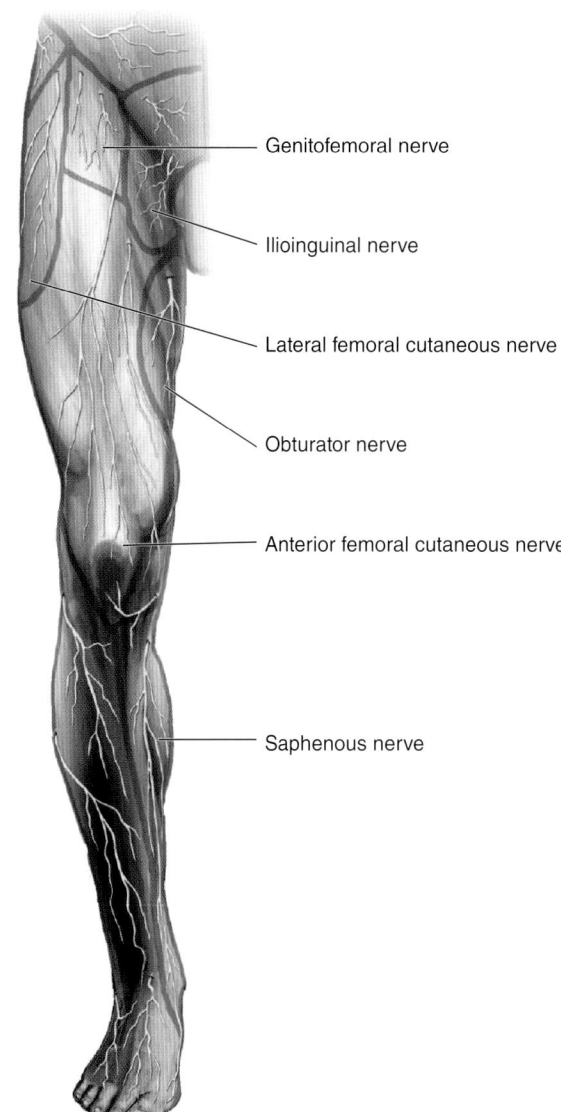

- Genitofemoral nerve
- Ilioinguinal nerve
- Lateral femoral cutaneous nerve
- Obturator nerve
- Anterior femoral cutaneous nerve
- Saphenous nerve

FIGURE 82A-3. Distribution of anesthesia and analgesia after a successful lumbar plexus block.

Distribution of Anesthesia

Injection of local anesthetic during lumbar plexus block most commonly results in spread of the injectate within the body of the psoas muscle around the lumbar branches (L2–L4), with cephalad spread to the lumbar nerve roots.[19]

The femoral nerve supplies motor fibers to the quadriceps muscle (knee extension), the skin of the anteromedial thigh, and the medial aspect of the leg below the knee and foot. The obturator nerve sends motor branches to the adductors of the hip and a highly variable cutaneous area on the medial thigh or knee joint. The lateral femoral cutaneous and genitofemoral nerves are purely cutaneous nerves. Figure 82A–3 illustrates the cutaneous innervation of the lumbar plexus.

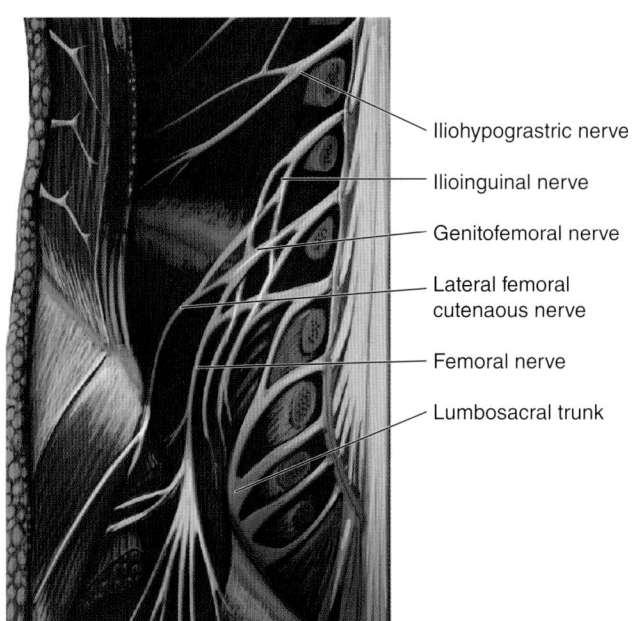

- Iliohypograstric nerve
- Ilioinguinal nerve
- Genitofemoral nerve
- Lateral femoral cutenaous nerve
- Femoral nerve
- Lumbosacral trunk

FIGURE 82A-2. Lumbar plexus branches.

Choice of Local Anesthetic

Lumbar plexus blockade requires a relatively large volume of local anesthetic. The choice of the type and concentration of local anesthetic should be based on whether the block is planned for surgical anesthesia or pain management. Because of the vascular nature of the area and the potential for inadvertent intravascular injection, rapid absorption from the deep muscle beds, and epidural spread, then rapid, forceful injections should be avoided.[20] Epinephrine is almost routinely used as a vascular marker. The most commonly used local anesthetic for this block in our institution for short procedures is alkalinized 2-chloroprocaine 3% with 1:300,000 epinephrine in patients having knee arthroscopy.[21,22] Some common choices of local anesthetics for this block are listed in Table 82A–1.

TABLE 82A-1. Local anesthetic choices for lumbar plexus block.

	Onset (min)	Anesthesia (h)	Analgesia (h)
3% 2-Chloroprocaine (+ HCO₃; + epinephrine)	10–15	1.5	2.0
1.5% Mepivacaine (+ HCO₃)	10–15	2	2–4
1.5% Mepivacaine (+ HCO₃; + epinephrine)	10–15	2.5–3	2–5
2% Lidocaine (+ HCO₃)	10–20	2.5–3	2–5
2% Lidocaine (+ HCO₃ + epinephrine)	10–20	5–6	5–8
0.5% Ropivacaine	15–20	4–6	6–10

Technique

The patient is in the lateral decubitus position with a slight forward tilt (Figure 82A–4). The foot on the side to be blocked should be positioned over the dependent leg so that twitches of the quadriceps muscle and/or patella can be seen easily.

A standard regional anesthesia tray is prepared with the following equipment:

- Sterile towels and 4-in. × 4-in. gauze packs
- 20-mL syringes with local anesthetic
- Sterile gloves, marking pen, and surface electrode
- One 1.5-in., 25-gauge needle for skin infiltration
- A 10-cm long, short-bevel, insulated stimulating needle
- Peripheral nerve stimulator
- Injection pressure monitor

Landmarks for the lumbar plexus block include (Figure 82A–5):

1. Midline (spinous processes)
2. Iliac crest
3. Needle insertion labeled 4-cm lateral to the intersection of landmarks 1 and 2

After cleaning with antiseptic solution, the skin is anesthetized by infiltrating local anesthetic subcutaneously. The fingers of the palpating hand are pressed against the paravertebral muscles to stabilize the landmark and decrease the skin–nerve distance. The needle is inserted at a perpendicular angle to the skin (Figure 82A–6A and B). The nerve stimulator should be initially set to deliver current intensity of 1.5 mA. As the needle is advanced, local twitches of the paravertebral muscles are obtained first at a depth of a few centimeters. The needle is then advanced further until twitches of the quadriceps muscle are obtained (usually at the depth of 6–8 cm). After the twitches are obtained, the current should be lowered to obtain stimulation between 0.5 and 1.0 mA.

At this point, 25–35 mL of local anesthetic is slowly injected with frequent aspiration to rule out inadvertent intravascular placement of the needle. Of note, while ultrasound guidance allowed for reduction of the volume and dose of local anesthetics for most nerve block procedures, this is not the case in the lumbar plexus block.[10]

Clinical Pearls

- Successful lumbar plexus blockade depends on the disposition of the local anesthetic in the fascial plane (psoas muscle) where the roots of the plexus are situated. Nerve stimulation is used to identify this plane by eliciting stimulation of one of the roots.

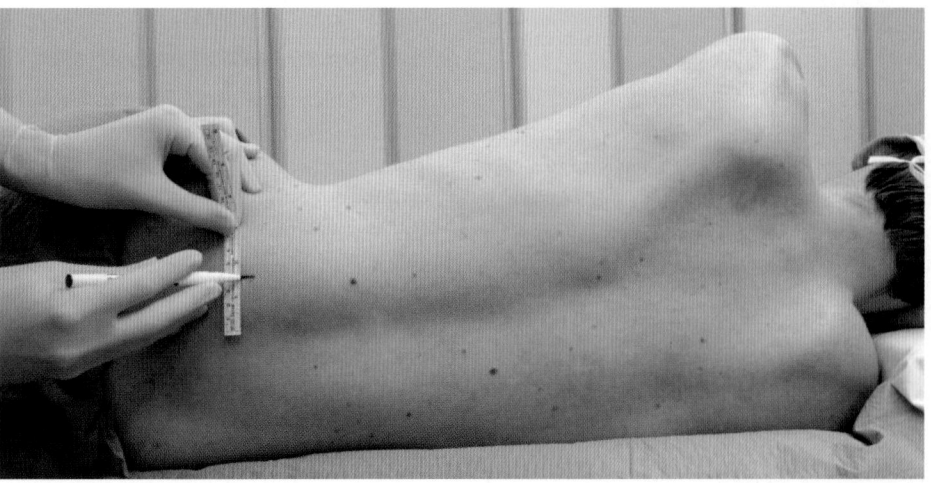

FIGURE 82A-4. Patient position for lumbar plexus block.

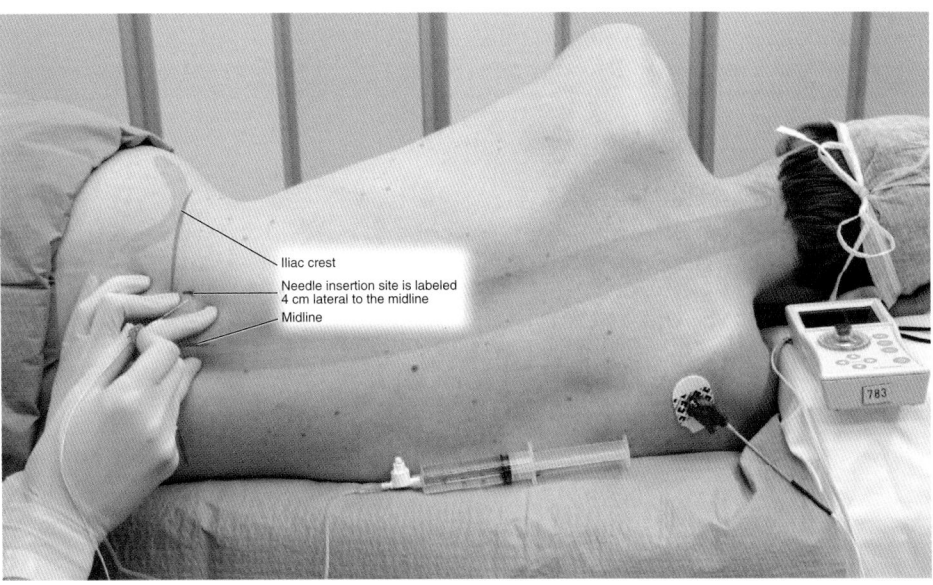

Iliac crest
Needle insertion site is labeled
4 cm lateral to the midline
Midline

FIGURE 82A–5. Landmarks for lumbar plexus block.

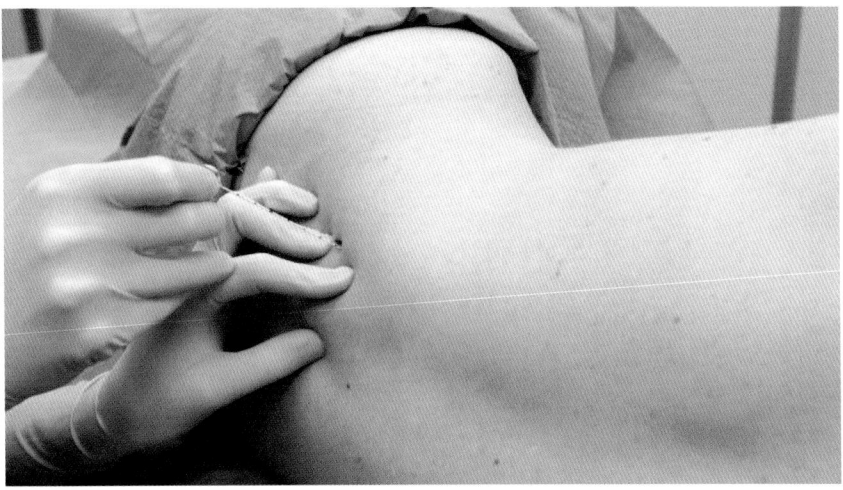

A

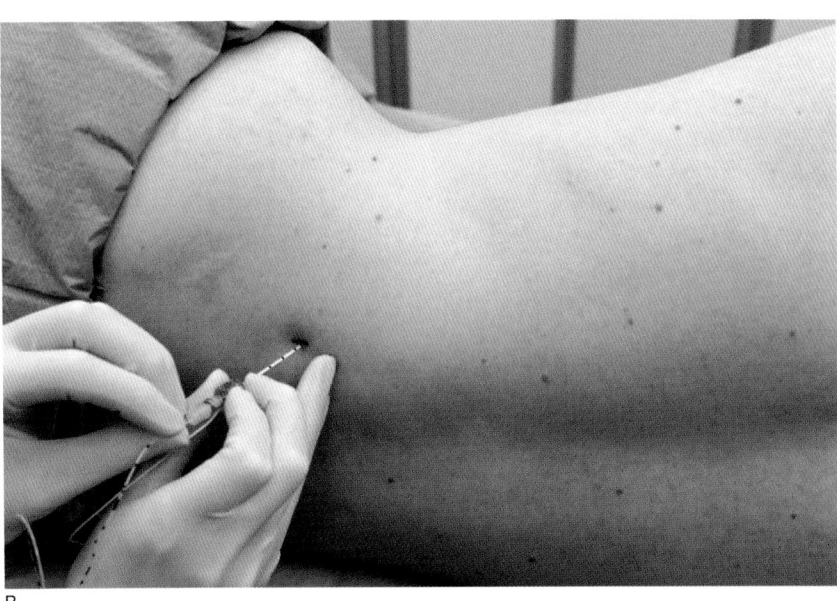

B

FIGURE 82A–6. A and B. Needle insertion for the lumbar plexus block. The needle is inserted perpendicular to the body plane or with a slight medial orientation (shown) (**A**). Catheter placement technique is preceded by similar needle technique (**B**).

TABLE 82A–2. Troubleshooting procedures during lumbar plexus blocks.

Response Obtained	Interpretation	Problem	Action
Local twitch of the paraspinal muscles	Direct stimulation of the paraspinal muscles	Too shallow placement of the needle	Continue advancing the needle
Needle contacts bone at 4–6 cm depth; no twitches are seen	The needle advancement is stopped by the transverse process	Indicates proper needle placement, but requires redirection of the needle	Withdraw the needle to the skin level, and redirect 5 degrees cranially or caudally
Twitches of hamstrings muscles are seen; needle inserted 6–8 cm	Result of stimulation of the roots of the sciatic plexus (sciatic nerve)	Needle inserted too caudally	Withdraw the needle and reinsert 3–5 cm cranially
Flexion of thigh at the depth of > 6–8 cm	This subtle and often missed response is caused by direct stimulation of the psoas muscle	Needle inserted too deep (missed the lumbar plexus roots); further advancement may place the needle intraperitoneally	Stop advancing the needle; withdraw the needle and reinsert using the protocol outlined in the technique description
Needle is placed deep (10 cm), but twitches were not elicited and bone is not contacted	Needle missed the transverse process and roots of the lumbar plexus	Needle placement too lateral	Withdraw the needle and reinsert with a slight medial angulation (5–10 degrees)

• Stimulation at currents less than 0.5 mA should not be sought because stimulation with a low current may indicate placement of the needle inside a dural sleeve. An injection inside this sheath can result in spread of the local anesthetic toward the epidural or subarachnoid space.

When insertion of the needle does not result in quadriceps muscle stimulation, the maneuvers outlined in Table 82A–2 should be followed.

Block Dynamics and Perioperative Management

A lumbar plexus block is uncomfortable for patients owing to the needle passage through multiple muscle planes and adequate premedication is necessary. Typically, we use midazolam 2-4 mg after the patient is positioned and alfentanil 500–750 mcg just before needle insertion. A typical onset time for this block is 15–25 minutes, depending on the type, concentration, and volume of local anesthetic and the level at which the needle is placed.

For example, although an almost immediate onset of anesthesia in the anterior thigh and knee can be achieved with an injection at the L3 level, additional time is required for local anesthetic to block the lateral thigh (L1) or obturator nerve (L5). The first sign of the onset of blockade is usually the loss of sensation in the saphenous nerve territory (medial skin below the knee).

CONTINUOUS LUMBAR PLEXUS BLOCK

Continuous lumbar plexus blockade is an advanced regional anesthesia technique, and adequate experience with the single-shot technique is a prerequisite to ensure its efficacy and safety. Otherwise, the technique is similar to the single-shot injection except that the Tuohy-style tip needle is preferable. The needle opening should be directed cephalad to facilitate threading of the catheter. This technique can be used for postoperative pain management in patients undergoing hip, femur, and knee surgery.[23] However, because a large volume of local anesthetic is required to accomplish analgesia, continuous infusion requires intermittent boluses for success. Consequently, some feel that its advantages over femoral block for postoperative analgesia are questionable at best, and that continuous lumbar plexus block should not be in routine use for postoperative analgesia.[24]

▌ Equipment

A standard regional anesthesia tray is prepared with the following equipment:

• Sterile towels and 4-in. × 4-in. gauze packs
• 20-mL syringe with local anesthetic
• Sterile gloves, marking pen, and surface electrode
• One 1.5-in. 25-gauge needle for skin infiltration
• A 10-cm long, insulated stimulating needle (preferably Tuohy-style tip)
• Catheter
• Peripheral nerve stimulator

Technique

The skin and subcutaneous tissues are anesthetized with local anesthetic. The needle is attached to the nerve stimulator (1.5 mA, 2 Hz, 100 μsec) and to a syringe with local anesthetic. The palpating hand should be firmly pressed and anchored against the paraspinal muscles to facilitate the needle insertion and redirection of the needle when necessary. A 10-cm, Tuohy-style tip, continuous block needle is inserted at a perpendicular angle and advanced until the quadriceps twitch response is obtained at 0.5–1.0 mA current. At this point, the initial volume of local anesthetic is injected (e.g., 15–25 mL), and the catheter is inserted approximately 8–10 cm beyond the needle tip. The needle is then withdrawn back to the skin level, while the catheter is simultaneously advanced. This method prevents inadvertent removal of the catheter and intravascular and intrathecal placement by negative aspiration test.

Clinical Pearl

- The skin in the lumbar area can be mobile; thus insertion of the catheter to a depth of 5–6 cm is necessary to help prevent its removal during patient repositioning.

Continuous Infusion

Continuous infusion is initiated after an initial bolus of dilute local anesthetic through the catheter. For this purpose, we routinely use ropivacaine 0.2% (15–20 mL). The infusion is maintained at 10 mL/h or 5 mL/h when a patient-controlled analgesia (PCA) dose is planned (5 mL/q60min). Figures 82A–7 and 82A–8 show the dispersion of 20 mL of a contrast solution within the psoas sheath.

COMPLICATIONS AND HOW TO AVOID THEM

The lumbar plexus block is an advanced technique with a potential for serious complications. The most common complications reported with lumbar plexus block are epidural spread with a risk of high neuraxial anesthesia,[20,25–28] hypotension, local anesthetic toxicity,[29–31] spinal anesthesia[32] or iliopsoas or renal hematoma.[33–36] Although the plasma concentrations of local anesthetics are not significantly higher after lumbar plexus block compared with other peripheral nerve blocks, there is the potential for rapid absorption and intravascular channeling owing to the large volumes required for this block and intramuscular location of the needle.[37] In addition, this block is best avoided in anticoagulated patients due to the risk of haematoma.[35] Table 82A–3 provides some general and specific instructions on possible complications and methods to avoid.

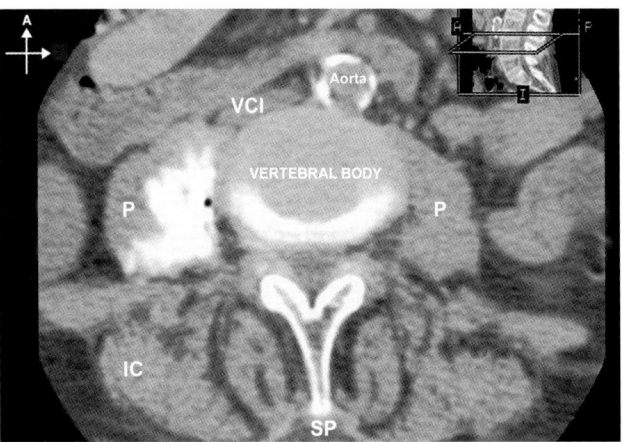

FIGURE 82A–7. Distribution of 20 mL of injectate after lumbar plexus block. A typical fusiform distribution within the psoas muscle is seen.

FIGURE 82A–8. An MRI image demonstrating distribution of local anesthetic after lumbar plexus block. (A, anterior; I, inferior; IC, iliac crest; P, psoas muscle; SP, spinous process; VCI, vena cava inferior.)

TABLE 82A–3. Strategies to decrease the risk of complications.

Complication	Instruction
Infection	• A strict aseptic technique is used
Hematoma	• Avoid multiple needle insertions, particularly in anticoagulated patients • Avoid continuous lumbar plexus blocks in anticoagulated patients • Antiplatelet therapy is not a contraindication for lumbar plexus block in the absence of spontaneous bleeding
Vascular puncture	• Deep needle insertion should be avoided (vena cava, aorta)
Local anesthetic toxicity	• Large volumes of long-acting anesthetic should be reconsidered in older and frail patients • Careful and frequent aspiration should be performed during the injection • Avoid forceful, fast injection of local anesthetic
Nerve injury	• Risk after lumbar plexus block is low • Local anesthetic should never be injected when the patient complains of pain or when abnormally high pressure on injection is noted • When stimulation is obtained with current intensity of <0.5 mA, the needle should be pulled back to obtain the same response with a current of 0.5 mA before injecting local anesthetic to avoid injection into the dural sleeves and the consequent epidural or spinal spread
Hemodynamic consequences	• Lumbar plexus blockade results in unilateral sympathectomy • Spread of the local anesthetic to the epidural space may result in significant hypotension and occurs in up to 15% of patients • Patients receiving a lumbar plexus block should be monitored to the same extent as patients receiving epidural anesthesia

REFERENCES

1. de Takats G: *Local Anesthesia*. Philadelphia, PA: Saunders, 1928.
2. Labat G: *Regional Anesthesia. In Its technic and Clinical Application*, 2nd ed. Philadelphia, PA: Saunders, 1924.
3. Sherwood-Dunn B: *Regional Anesthesia*. Philadelphia, PA: Davis, 1920.
4. Dogliotti A: *Narcosis—Local-Regional-Spinal*. Chicago, IL: Debour, 1939.
5. Mannion S, O'Callaghan S, Walsh M, et al: In with the new, out with the old? Comparison of two approaches for psoas compartment block. Anesth Analg 2005;101:259–264.
6. Awad IT, Duggan EM: Posterior lumbar plexus block: anatomy, approaches, and techniques. Reg Anesth Pain Med 2005;30:143–149.
7. Chayen D, Nathan H, Chayen M: The psoas compartment block. Anesthesiology 1976;45:95–99.
8. Molina Monleon I, Asensio Romero I, Barrio Mataix J, et al: [Epidural anesthesia after posterior lumbar plexus block.] Rev Esp Anestesiol Reanim 2005;52:55–56.
9. Kirchmair L, Entner T, Wissel J, et al: A study of the paravertebral anatomy for ultrasound guided posterior lumbar plexus block. Anesth Analg 2001;93:477–478.
10. Sauter AR, Ullensvang K, Niemi G, et al: The Shamrock lumbar plexus block: A dose finding study. Eur J Anaesthesiol 2015; 32:764–770.
11. Karmakar MK, Li JW, Kwok WH, et al: Sonoanatomy relevant for lumbar plexus block in volunteers correlated with cross-sectional anatomic and magnetic resonance images. Reg Anesth Pain Med 2013;391–397.
12. Capdevilla X, Macaire P, Dadure C, et al: Continuous psoas compartment blocks for postoperative analgesia after total hip arthroplasty: new landmarks, technical guidelines, and clinical evaluation. Anesth Analg 2002;94:1606–1613.
13. Indelli PF, Grant SA, Nielsen K, et al: Regional anesthesia in hip surgery. Clin Orthop Relat Res 2005;441:250–205.
14. Watson MW, Mitra D, McLintock TC, Grant SA: Continuous versus single-injection lumbar plexus blocks: comparison of the effects on morphine use and early recovery after total knee arthroplasty. Reg Anesth Pain Med 2005;30:541–547.
15. Luber MJ, Greengrass R, Vail TP: Patient satisfaction and effectiveness of lumbar plexus and sciatic nerve block for total knee arthroplasty. J Arthroplasty 2001;16:17–21.
16. Di Benedetto P, Pinto G, Arcioni R, De Blasi RA, et al: Anatomy and imaging of lumbar plexus. Minerva Anestesiol 2005;71:549–554.
17. Sim IW, Webb T: Anatomy and anaesthesia of the lumbar somatic plexus. Anaesth Intensive Care 2004;32:178–187.
18. Farny J, Drolet P, Girard M: Anatomy of the posterior approach to the lumbar plexus block. Can J Anaesth 1994;41:480–485.
19. Mannion S, Barrett J, Kelly D, et al: A description of the spread of injectate after psoas compartment block using magnetic resonance imaging. Reg Anesth Pain Med 2005;30:567–571.
20. Gadsden JC, Lindenmuth DM, Hadzic A, et al: Lumbar plexus block using high-pressure injection leads to contralateral and epidural spread. Anesthesiology 2008;683–688.
21. Khy V, Girard M: [The use of 2-chloroprocaine for a combined lumbar plexus and sciatic nerve block.] Can J Anaesth 1994;41:919–924.
22. Hadzic A, Karaca PE, Hobeika P, et al: Peripheral nerve blocks result in superior recovery profile compared with general anesthesia in outpatient knee arthroscopy. Anesth Analg 2005;100:976–981.
23. Chelly JE, Casati A, Al-Samsam T, et al: Continuous lumbar plexus block for acute postoperative pain management after open reduction and internal fixation of acetabular fractures. J Orthop Trauma 2003;17:362–367.
24. Bogoch ER, Henke M, Mackenzie T, et al: Lumbar paravertebral nerve block in the management of pain after total hip and knee arthroplasty: a randomized controlled clinical trial. J Arthroplasty 2002;17:398–401.
25. Litz RJ, Vicent O, Wiessner D, Heller AR: Misplacement of a psoas compartment catheter in the subarachnoid space. Reg Anesth Pain Med 2004;29:60–64.
26. Auroy Y, Benhamou D, Bargues L, et al: Major complications of regional anesthesia in France: The SOS Regional Anesthesia Hotline Service. Anesthesiology 2002;97:1274–1280.
27. Gentili M, Aveline C, Bonnet F: [Total spinal anesthesia after posterior lumbar plexus block.] Ann Fr Anesth Reanim 1998;17:740–742.
28. Farny J, Girard M, Drolet P: Posterior approach to the lumbar plexus combined with a sciatic nerve block using lidocaine. Can J Anaesth 1994;41:486–491.

29. Huet O, Eyrolle LJ, Mazoit JX, Ozier YM: Cardiac arrest after injection of ropivacaine for posterior lumbar plexus blockade. Anesthesiology 2003;99:1451–1453.
30. Mullanu CH, Gaillat F, Scemama F, et al: Acute toxicity of local anesthetic ropivacaine and mepivacaine during a combined lumbar plexus and sciatic block for hip surgery. Acta Anaesthesiol Belg 2002;53: 221–223.
31. Pham-Dang C, Beaumont S, Floch H, et al: [Acute toxic accident following lumbar plexus block with bupivacaine.] Ann Fr Anesth Reanim 2000;19:356–359.
32. Capdevila X, Coimbra C, Choquet O: Approaches to the lumbar plexus: success, risks, and outcome. Reg Anesth Pain Med. 2005; 150–162.

33. Hsu DT: Delayed retroperitoneal haematoma after failed lumbar plexus block. Br J Anaesth 2005;394–395.
34. Aveline C, Bonnet F: Delayed retroperitoneal haematoma after failed lumbar plexus block. Br J Anaesth 2004;93:589–591.
35. Klein SM, D'Ercole F, Greengrass RA, Warner DS: Enoxaparin associated with psoas hematoma and lumbar plexopathy after lumbar plexus block. Anesthesiology 1997;87:1576–1579.
36. Aida S, Takahashi H, Shimoji K: Renal subcapsular hematoma after lumbar plexus block. Anesthesiology 1996;84:452–455.
37. Blumenthal S, Ekatodramis G, Borgeat A: Ropivacaine plasma concentrations are similar during continuous lumbar plexus blockade using two techniques: Pharmacokinetics or pharmacodynamics? Can J Anaesth 2004;51–851.

CHAPTER 82B

Obturator Nerve Block

Herve Bouaziz

INTRODUCTION

Selective obturator nerve block was first described by Gaston Labat in 1922.[1] More interest in obturator nerve block emerged a few years later when Victor Pauchet, Sourdat, and Gaston Labat stated, "obturator nerve block combined with blocks of the sciatic and femoral nerves, anesthetized the entire lower limb." However, a lack of clear anatomic landmarks, the block complexity, and inconsistent results were the reasons why this block had been used infrequently. Historically, Labat's classic technique remained forgotten until 1967, when it was modified by Parks.[2] In 1993, the interadductor approach was described by Wassef,[3] which was further modified by Pinnock in 1996.[4] In 1973, Alon Winnie introduced the concept of the "3-in-1 block," an anterior approach to the lumbar plexus using a simple paravascular inguinal injection to anesthetize the femoral, lateral cutaneous and obturator nerves.[5] Since its description however, many studies have refuted the ability of the 3-in-1 block to reliably block the obturator nerve with this technique. With the introduction of modern nerve stimulators, and particularly ultrasound guidance selective blockade of the obturator nerve has become more reliable.

Indications

Obturator nerve block is used to treat hip joint pain and is also used in the relief of adductor muscle spasm associated with hemiplegia or paraplegia. Muscle spasticity is a relatively common problem among patients suffering from central neurologic problems, such as cerebrovascular pathology, medullar injuries, multiple sclerosis, and cerebral palsy. Spasticity of the adductor muscle induced via the obturator nerve plays a major role in associated pain problems and makes patient hygiene and mobilization very difficult. Tenotomies, cryotherapy, botulinum toxin infiltration, surgical neurolysis, and muscle interpositions

have been suggested to remedy this problem.[6–9] Common clinical practice is to combine a sciatic nerve block with the femoral nerve block for surgical procedures distal to the proximal third of the thigh. When deemed necessary, addition of a selective obturator nerve block may reduce intraoperative discomfort, improve tourniquet tolerance, and improve the quality of postoperative analgesia in these cases.

Obturator nerve block is also occasionally used in urologic surgery to suppress the obturator reflex during transurethral resection of the lateral bladder wall. Direct stimulation of the obturator nerve by the resector as it passes in close proximity to the bladder wall results in a sudden, violent adductor muscle spasm. This is not only distracting to the surgeon, but may increase the risk of complications such as bladder wall perforation, vessel laceration, incomplete tumor resection, and obturator hematomas.[10,11] Prevention strategies include muscle relaxation, reduction in the intensity of the resector, the use of laser resectors, shifting to saline irrigation, periprostate infiltrations, and/or endoscopic transparietal blocks.[12–16] A selective obturator nerve block remains an effective remedy to this problem.[17–22]

Clinical Pearl

- The obturator reflex is not abolished by spinal anesthesia. It can be suppressed only by a selective obturator nerve block.

Neurolytic blocks with alcohol or phenol, performed with the help of a nerve stimulator and/or fluoroscopy, result in a cost-effective and effective reduction of muscle spasms.[3,9,23–26] The main drawback to neurolytic blockade is its temporary duration and the need to repeat the block when the previous block wears off. Selective obturator nerve block has also been used in the diagnosis and treatment of chronic pain states secondary to knee arthrosis or pelvic tumors resistant to conventional analgesic approaches.[27–31]

Contraindications

Patient refusal, inguinal lymphadenopathy, perineal infection, or hematoma at the needle insertion site all are contraindications to obturator nerve blockade. Preexisting obturator neuropathy, clinically manifested by groin pain, pain of the posteromedial aspect at the thigh, and occasionally paresis of the adductor group of muscles, are relative contraindications to this block. Obturator nerve blocks should be avoided in the presence of a coagulopathy.

Anatomy

The obturator nerve is a mixed nerve, which, in most cases, provides motor function to the adductor muscles and cutaneous sensation to a small area behind the knee. It is derived from the anterior primary rami of L2, L3, and L4 (Figure 82B–1). On its initial course, it runs within the psoas major muscle. Taking a vertical course, it emerges from the inner border of the psoas, staying medial and posterior at the pelvis until it crosses at the

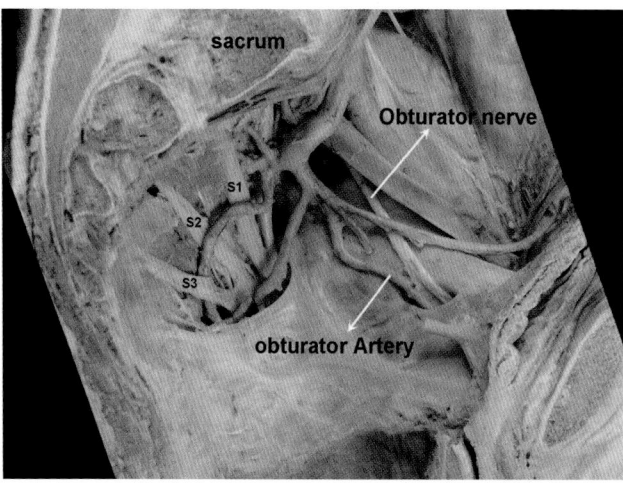

FIGURE 82B–2. Intrapelvic trajectory of the obturator nerve. After crossing under the iliac vessels, the obturator nerve travels toward the obturator foramen via the lateral pelvic wall. During this course, the obturator artery and vein join the nerve, forming the obturator neurovascular bundle.

level of the sacroiliac joint (L5) under the common iliac artery and vein and runs anterior/lateral to the ureter (Figure 82B–2). At this level, it courses close to the wall of the bladder on its inferior/lateral portion and then it takes place anterior to the obturator vessels within the superior part of the obturator foramen, exiting the pelvis below the pubic superior branch. In its intrapelvic course, the obturator nerve is separated from the femoral nerve by the iliopsoas muscle and iliac fascia. It innervates the parietal peritoneum on the lateral pelvic wall and contributes collateral branches to the obturator externus muscle and the hip joint. It leaves the pelvis by passing through the obturator canal before entering the adductor region of the thigh (Figure 82B–3). Here, 2.5–3.5 cm after leaving the obturator foramen, the obturator nerve divides into its two terminal branches, anterior and posterior, providing innervation to the hip adductor compartment (Figure 82B–3).[32]

The anterior branch descends behind the pectineus and adductor longus and in front of the obturator externus and adductor brevis. It gives muscular branches to the adductor longus, adductor brevis, gracilis, and occasionally the pectineus, and it terminates as a small nerve that innervates the femoral artery (Figure 82B–4). In 20% of subjects, it contributes a branch, which anastomoses with branches of the femoral nerve and forms the subsartorial plexus, from which sensory branches emerge to supply sensation to posteromedial aspect of the inferior third of the thigh. The anterior branch contributes articular branches to anteromedial aspect of the hip joint capsule (Figure 82B–5) but does not innervate the knee joint. Under ultrasound guidance, selective block of the anterior or posterior branches can be performed. Block of the anterior branch alone may be adequate for preventing the adductor reflex during bladder surgery."[33–35]

The posterior branch descends between the adductor brevis in front and the adductor magnus behind. It terminates by passing through the adductor hiatus to enter the popliteal fossa, supplying the posterior aspect of the knee joint and the popliteal

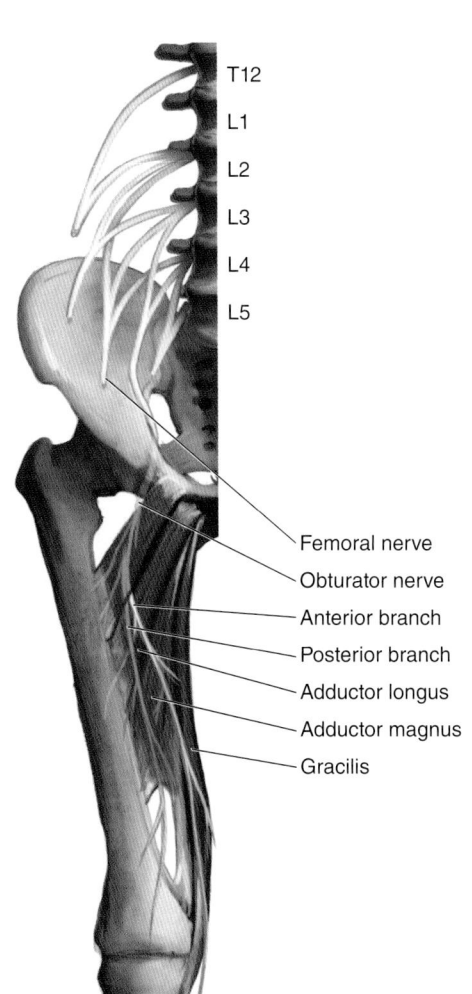

FIGURE 82B–1. Anatomy of the obturator nerve.

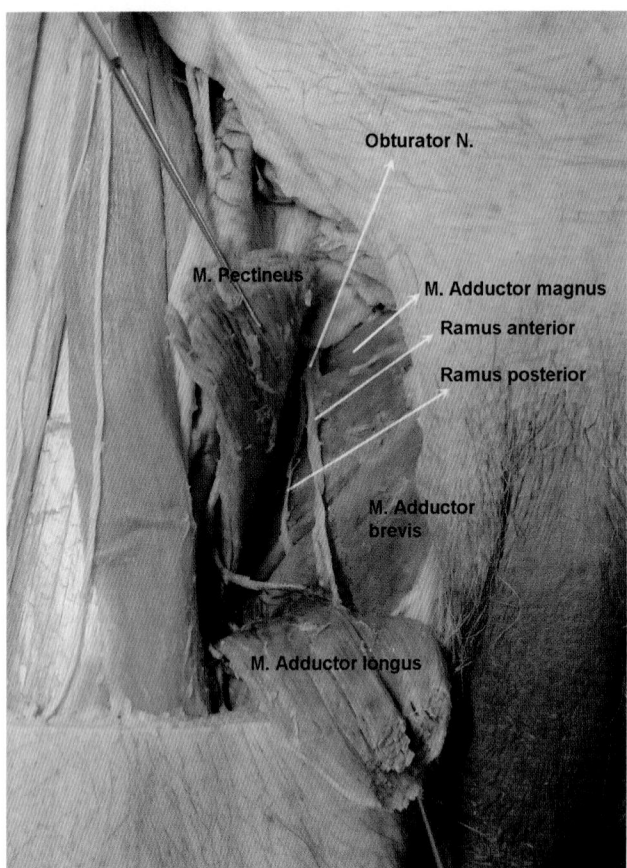

FIGURE 82B–3. Distribution of the anterior and posterior divisions of the obturator nerve after exiting the obturator foramen.

artery. During its course, the posterior branch sends muscular branches to the obturator externus, the adductor magnus, and occasionally the adductor brevis muscles (see Figure 82B–4).

Cutaneous innervation by the obturator nerve varies according to the investigators and is illustrated in Figure 82B–6.

The functions of the muscles innervated by the obturator nerve are adduction of the thigh and assistance with hip flexion. The gracilis muscle assists knee flexion, and the obturator externus aids the lateral rotation of the thigh. To request an active adduction of the thigh, therefore, tests the function of the obturator nerve. The patient should be supine with knees extended. The leg is then adducted against resistance while the examiner supports the contralateral leg. The paralysis (or block) of the nerve is characterized by a severe weakening of the adduction, although it is not completely lost as the adductor magnus (the most powerful adductor muscle) receives fibers from the sciatic nerve and eventually from the femoral nerve.

Anatomic Variants

Numerous variations to the formation, course, and distribution of the obturator nerve can have clinical implications. For instance, in 75% of cases, the obturator nerve divides into its two terminal branches as it passes through the obturator canal. In 10% of cases, this division occurs before the nerve reaches the obturator canal; in the remaining 15% of cases, after entering the thigh.

Occasionally, the anterior and posterior branches descend through the thigh behind the adductor brevis. Note that the sensory cutaneous branch of the obturator nerve is often absent.

Up to 20% of subjects possess an accessory obturator nerve that can be formed from variable combinations of the anterior rami L2–L4 or emanate directly from the trunk of the obturator nerve.[36] It accompanies the obturator nerve as it emerges from the medial border of the psoas, but unlike the obturator, passes in front of the superior pubic ramus to supply a muscular branch, the pectineus. It contributes articular branches to the hip joint and terminates by anastomosing with the obturator nerve itself.

Equipment

To perform a block, the following equipment is required:

- Nerve stimulator
- Insulated stimulating needle (5–8 cm, depending on the approach chosen)
- Local anesthetic: 1% mepivacaine (onset of motor block 15 min, duration 3–4 h) or 0.75% ropivacaine (on-set of motor block 25 min, block duration 8–10 h)
- Sterile fenestrated drape
- Marking pen
- Ruler
- A 10-mL syringe
- Disinfectant
- Sterile gloves

Landmarks

Anatomic landmarks vary depending on the chosen approach. However, it is useful to identify and outline the following landmarks regardless of the approach chosen (Figure 82B–7):

Bony landmarks: Anterior and superior iliac spine and pubic tubercle, inguinal ligament
Vascular landmarks: Femoral artery, femoral crease
Muscular landmarks: Tendon of the adductor longus muscle

Techniques

Several methods can accomplish block of the obturator nerve. These approaches can be grouped into plexus block techniques where the obturator nerve is blocked along with other components of the lumbosacral plexus and specific single-nerve block techniques for the obturator nerve.

3-in-1 Block Technique

Based on the theoretic existence of a suprainguinal compartment, in 1973 Winnie described the lumbar plexus block by an anterior approach or the "3 in 1 block".[5] According to the 3-in-1 concept, a large volume of local anesthetics is injected over the femoral nerve to spread underneath the fascia iliaca. When combined with distal compression, the local anesthetic spreads proximally reaching the lumbar plexus. Unfortunately, studies have repeatedly failed to demonstrate the reliability of

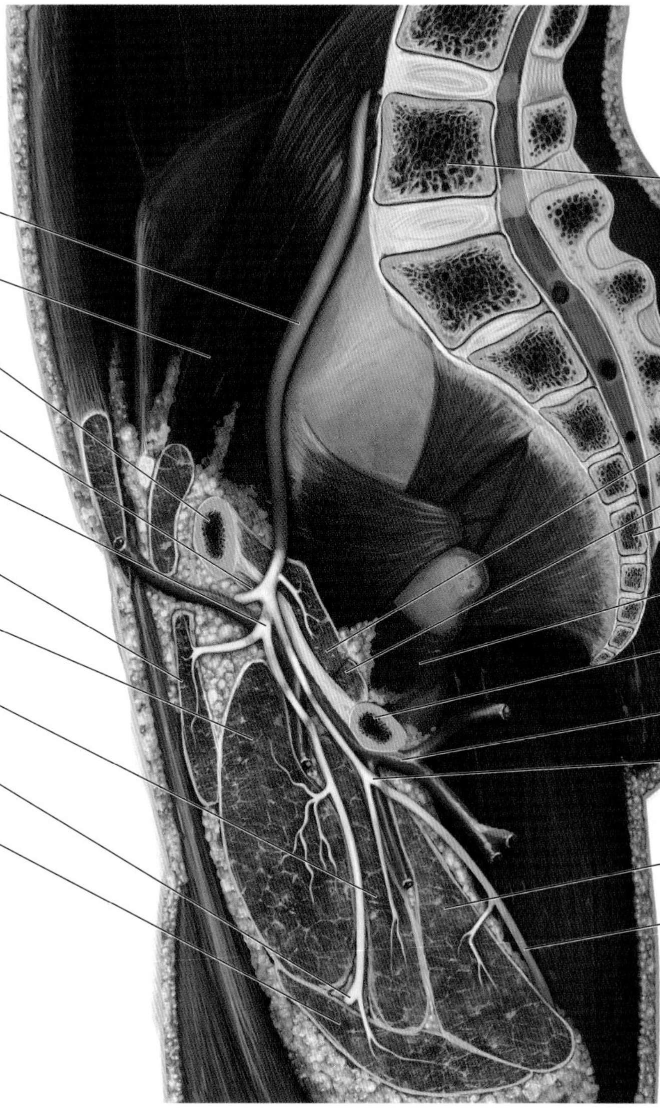

FIGURE 82B–4. Sagittal section demonstrating the relationship of the obturator nerve to the adductor muscles.

Obturator N.
Psoas major
Pubis
Branch to hip joint
Anterior branch
Pectineus
Adductor longus
Adductor brevis
Cutaneus branch
Gracialis

L5
Gluteus maximus
Obturator internus
Obturator externus
Sacrum
Quadratus femoris
Ischium
Medial circumflex artery
Posterior branch
Adductor magnus
Branch to knee joint

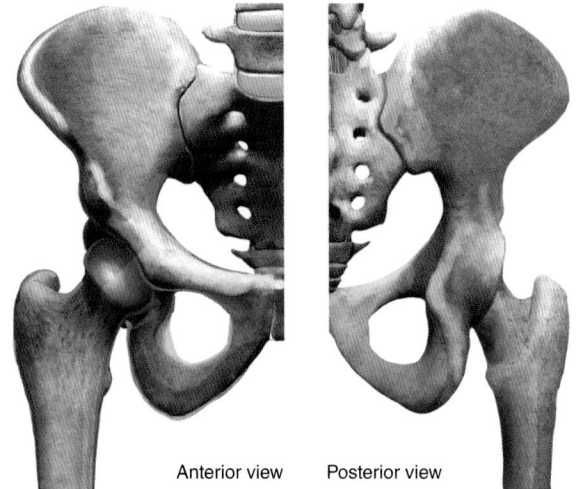

Anterior view   Posterior view

FIGURE 82B–5. The role of the obturator nerve in the sensory innervation of the hip.

this technique to obtain a block of the lumbar plexus or the obturator nerve.[5,37–39] In addition, studies in human cadavers have documented the absence of a fluid-conducting compartment that would allow such an extensive proximal spread of the local anesthetic.[40]

Of note, increasing the volume of injectate does not increase the spread toward the lumbar plexus; no differences were found when local anesthetic injection volumes of 20 or 40 mL were compared.[41]

Theoretically, catheters inserted by an inguinal approach can ascend toward the psoas compartment, however, only a minor percentage (23%) of catheters can be adequately placed in the therapeutic position.[42,43]

Iliofascial Block Technique

Dalens first described this approach in 1989 for use in pediatric patients.[44] Following Winnie's reasoning for the 3-in-1 block,

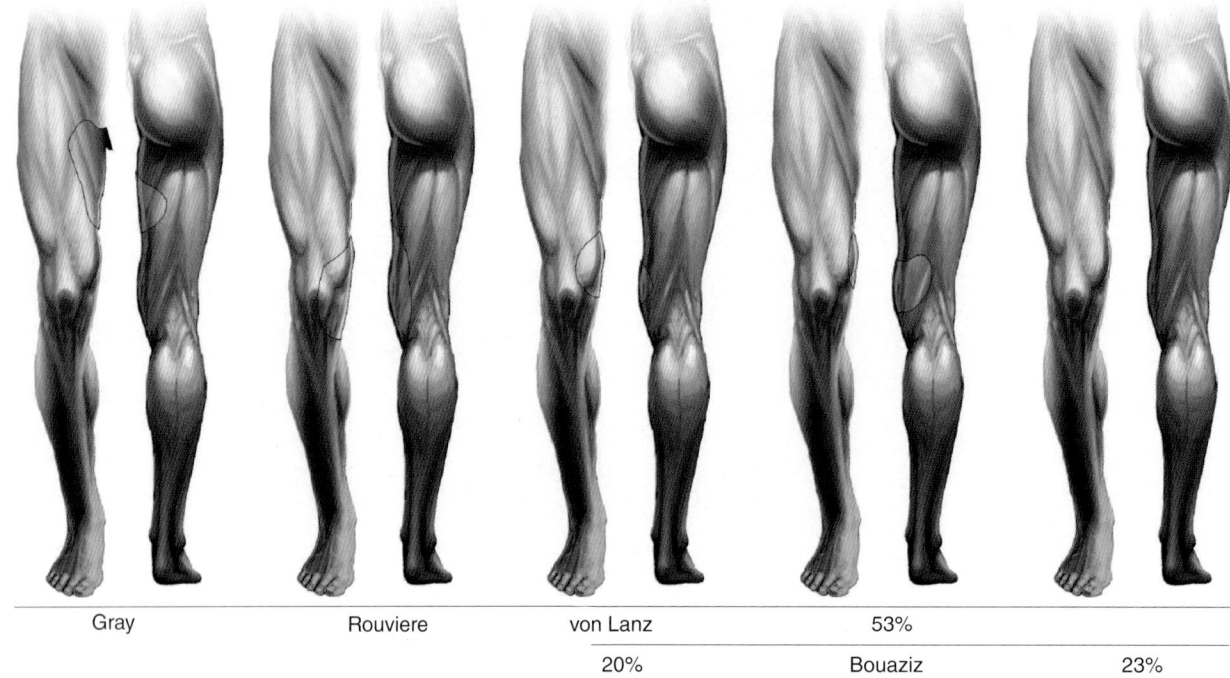

Gray	Rouviere	von Lanz	53%
		20%	Bouaziz	23%

FIGURE 82B–6. Skin innervation by obturator nerve according to different investigators.

he took a more lateral approach and reported a 100% success rate for femoral and femoral cutaneous nerve blockade and 88% success rate for the obturator nerve. However, follow-up studies in adults did not confirm these results.[42,45]

In adults, the iliofascial approach allows more successful blockade of the lateral femoral cutaneous nerve when compared with the 3-in-1 technique. However, the obturator nerve remains spared.[45,46]

Psoas Compartment Block

Since Winnie's description of the posterior approach to the lumbar plexus in 1974 (psoas compartment block), numerous modifications of the technique have been described.[46–50]

The obvious advantage is the ability to obtain a complete lumbar plexus block with a single injection. Indeed, studies have demonstrated femoral nerve block close to 100% plexus

block with this technique, whereas femorocutaneous and obturator nerve blocks are anesthetized 88%–93% of the time.[51,52]

Parasacral Sciatic Block

Mansour initially described this technique in 1993 with the objective of achieving a more complete sciatic nerve block.[53,54] Since this technique is a plexus block, it provides more consistent anesthesia of all branches of the sciatic nerve. It successfully blocks the posterior cutaneous nerve of the thigh, the gluteal superior and inferior nerves, and the pudendal nerve. In addition, the splanchnic nerves, the inferior hypogastric plexus, the proximal portion of sympathetic trunks, and the obturator nerve are located close to the point of injection. Thus, a blockade of all these nervous structures would be theoretically achievable with a single injection. However, recent anatomic and clinical studies suggest that the parietal peritoneum and the pelvic fascia surrounding the sacral plexus are anatomically separated from the obturator nerve that runs along the medial border of the psoas. Consequently, although the parasacral approach to sciatic nerve block should result in a complete block of the sacral plexus, it is not reliable for obturator nerve block.[55]

Selective Block Techniques
Labat's Classic Technique

Labat's classic approach was a common technique before the development of newer approaches that are easier to perform and less uncomfortable to patients. Originally described as a paresthesia method, the advent of nerve stimulation has increased the effectiveness and reduced patient

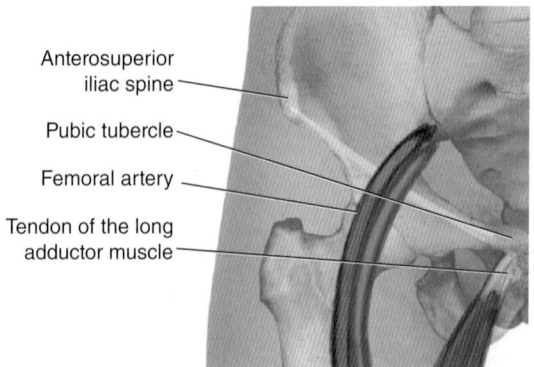

Anterosuperior iliac spine

Pubic tubercle

Femoral artery

Tendon of the long adductor muscle

FIGURE 82B–7. Anatomic landmarks for blockade of the obturator nerve.

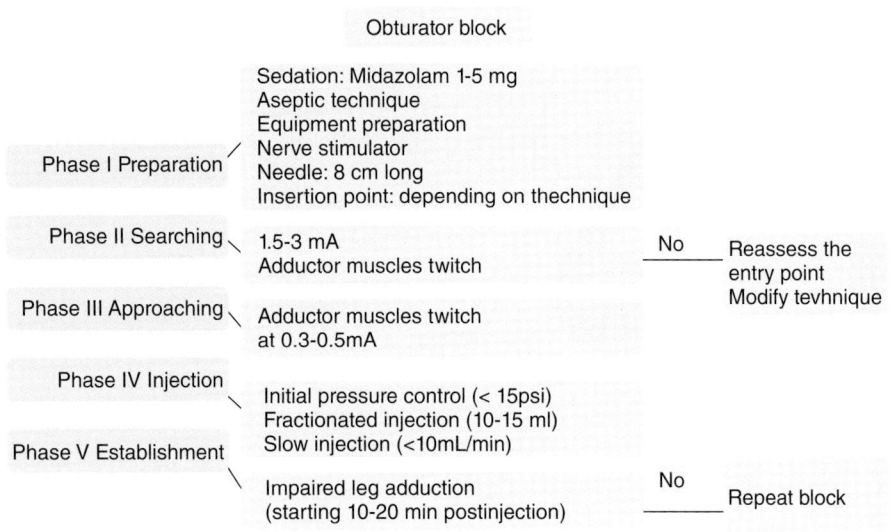

FIGURE 82B-8. A practical algorithm to obturator nerve block.

discomfort, complications, and number of needle insertions. The procedure sequence consists of five phases, depicted in Figure 82B–8.

Nerve stimulation is begun using a current intensity of 2–3 mA (2 Hz, 0.1–0.3 msec) and reduced to 0.3–0.5 mA before injection of local anesthetic. The patient lies supine, with the limb to be blocked at 30 degrees abduction. The pubic tubercle is identified by palpation, and a 1.5-cm long line is drawn laterally and caudally; the injection insertion site is labeled at the tip of the end of the caudal line (Figure 82B–9). The classic approach consists of carrying out three consecutive movements of the needle until the tip of the needle is placed over the top of the obturator foramen, where the nerve runs before splitting into its two terminal branches. With a 22-gauge, 8-cm long needle, the skin is penetrated perpendicularly and the needle is advanced until it makes contact with the inferior border of the superior pubic branch at a depth of 2–4 cm. During the second phase, the needle is

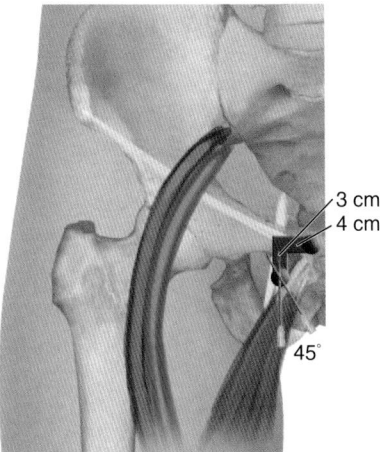

FIGURE 82B-9. Obturator nerve block. Simplified Labat classic technique.

slightly withdrawn and then slipped along the anterior pubic wall (another 2–4 cm). After this, it is redirected anteriorly/posteriorly. Finally, the needle is withdrawn again and slightly redirected (cephalad and laterally) at an angle of 45 degrees for another 2–3 cm until contractions of the thigh adductor muscles are observed.

This technique can be simplified by eliminating the second movement of the needle. Hence, after making contact with the pubic branch, the needle can be redirected 45 degrees laterally to the obturator foramen (see Figure 82B–9).

Paravascular Selective Inguinal Block

This technique consists of a selective block of the two branches of the obturator nerve (anterior and posterior), performed at the inguinal level and slightly more caudad than the previously described techniques.[56] The femoral artery and the tendon of the adductor longus muscle at the pubic tubercle are identified. For tendon identification, extreme leg abduction is required (Figure 82B–10). A line is drawn over the inguinal fold from the pulse of the femoral artery to the tendon of the long adductor muscle. The needle is inserted at the midpoint of this line at an angle of 30 degrees anteriorly/posteriorly and cephalad (Figure 82B–11). By following the needle a few centimeters in depth via the adductor longus muscle, twitches of the adductor longus and gracilis muscles are easily detectable on the posterior and medial aspect of the thigh. Subsequently, the needle is inserted deeper (0.5–1.5 cm) and slightly laterally over the adductor brevis muscle until a response from the adductor magnus muscle is obtained and can be visualized on the posterior-medial aspect of the thigh. After needle insertion, infiltration of 5–7 mL local anesthetic is recommended. Occasionally, a more caudal division of the obturator nerve is found; the two branches are located within the same location at the inguinal fold, and two different motor responses may be observed with a single injection.

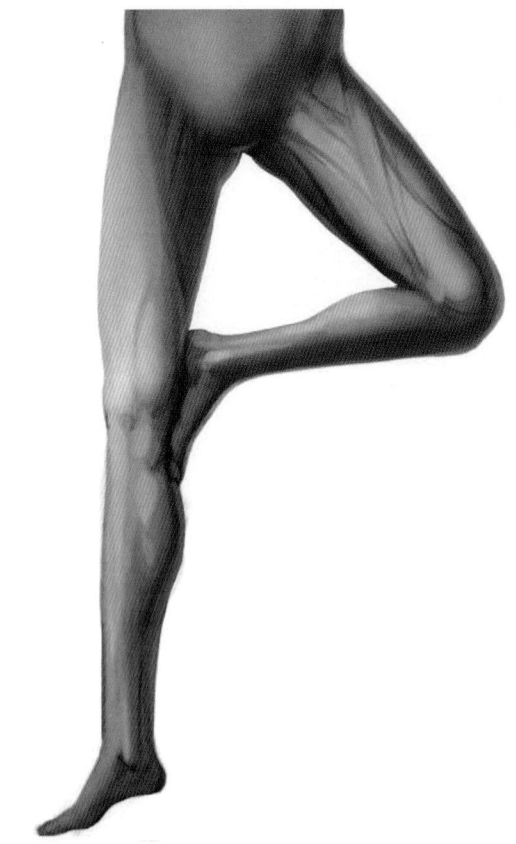

FIGURE 82B–10. Leg abduction.

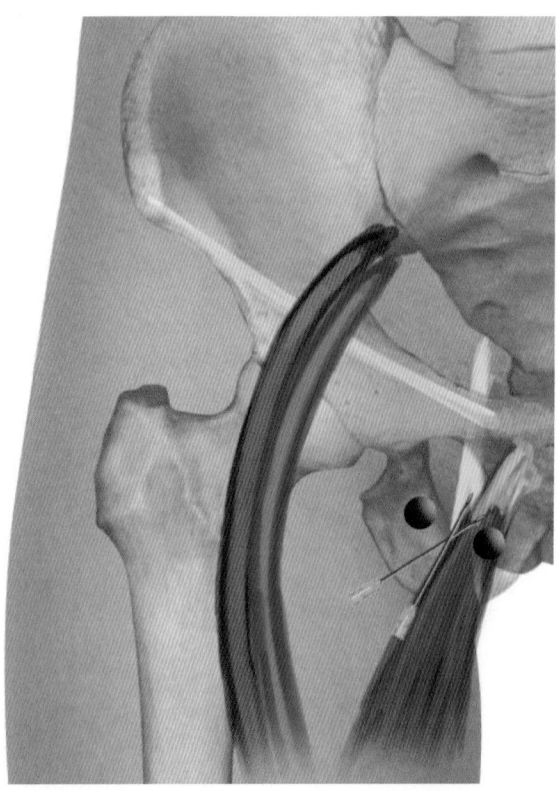

FIGURE 82B–11. Paravascular selective inguinal approach to oobturator nerve. Needle insertion and redirection.

- The inguinal approach to the obturator nerve is easier to perform and more comfortable to the patient.
- The needle insertion site with this approach is away from intrapelvic contents, resulting in a lower risk of complications.
- Articular branches to the hip joint are not blocked with this approach.

Choice of Local Anesthetic

Ten milliliters of local anesthetic is adequate. The type and concentration of the local anesthetic depend on the indication for the block. For diagnostic–therapeutic blockades, highly concentrated neurolytic solutions are used to achieve long-lasting blocks. In the literature, combinations of phenol, ethanol, bupivacaine, levobupivacaine, and/or steroids are well reported.[3,9,23–26]

For lower limb surgeries, the recommended anesthetic technique consists of the administration of medium- to long-lasting local anesthetics that are associated with adequate postoperative analgesia, such as bupivacaine 0.25%–0.5%; ropivacaine 0.25%, and levobupivacaine 0.25%–0.5%. To avoid adductor muscle spasms during transurethral surgery, the use of medium- to long-acting local anesthetics is not required because the surgery does not last more than 2 hours. Therefore, mepivacaine 1%–2% or lidocaine 1%–2% should be adequate for this purpose.[17,57]

BLOCK EVALUATION

The onset of motor blockade is seen approximately 15 minutes after administration of 1% mepivacaine and 25 minutes after injection of 0.5% ropivacaine. Evaluation of an obturator block by sensory testing is unreliable due to the variability in its sensory distribution (see Figure 82B–10). In some cases, the obturator nerve may not contain any sensory branches that can be clinically tested for adequacy of the blockade. In addition, even when a sensory branch is present, there is considerable overlap of cutaneous innervation from the obturator, femoral, and sciatic nerves. It is often erroneously thought that the skin of the medial aspect of the thigh is innervated by the obturator nerve; in fact, sensory branches of the femoral nerve contribute sensory innervation to this region.

- Evaluation of an obturator block by sensory testing can be challenging because of the variability in its sensory distribution.
- The most common sensory innervation of the obturator nerve is the skin in a small region located on the postero-medial aspect of the knee.

- A considerable overlap of cutaneous innervation exists among the obturator, femoral, and sciatic nerves.
- Reduction in adduction strength is the most reliable means of demonstrating successful obturator nerve blockade.

The area of skin most commonly regarded as having exclusive obturator nerve supply is a small region located on the posteromedial aspect of the knee. Also, the strength of the lower limb adductors relies 70% on the obturator nerve. Consequently, reduction in the strength of the adductors of the thigh is the most reliable sign of successful obturator nerve blockade (Figure 82B-10). Adductor muscle strength can be objectively evaluated by comparing the maximal pressure exerted by the patient squeezing a sphygmomanometer that has been preinflated to 40 mm Hg and placed between the legs before and after block performance. Failure to demonstrate a reduction in adductor muscle strength from baseline is synonymous with block failure.

PERIOPERATIVE MANAGEMENT

Patients must be warned that ambulation may be impaired because of the blockade of the thigh adductors.

COMPLICATIONS

There are no reports of complications associated with obturator nerve block. The lack of reported complications, however, is more likely due to the infrequent use of this block rather than to its inherent safety. Needle orientation for the classic pubic approach of Labat is toward the pelvic cavity. Therefore, if advanced too far in a cephalad direction, the needle can pass over the superior pubic ramus and penetrate the pelvic cavity, perforating the bladder, rectum, and spermatic cord. Accidental puncture of the obturator vessels could result in unintentional intravascular injection and hematoma formation. A retropubic anastamosis between the external iliac and obturator arteries (corona Mortis) is present in up to10% of patients: bleeding secondary to puncture of the corona Mortis can be difficult to control. Obturator neuropathy, secondary to needle trauma, intraneural injection, nerve ischemia, or local anesthetic toxicity are also possible, as with other peripheral nerve block techniques.

REFERENCES

1. Labat G: *Regional Anesthesia: Its Technique and Clinical Application.* Philadelphia, PA: Saunders, 1922.
2. Parks CR, Kennedy WF: Obturator nerve block: a simplified approach. Anesthesiology 1967;28:775–778.
3. Wassef M: Interadductor approach to obturator nerve blockade for spastic conditions of adductor thigh muscles. Reg Anesth 1993;18: 13–17.
4. Pinnock CA, Fischer HBJ, Jones RP: *Peripheral Nerve Blockade.* London, UK: Churchill Livingstone, 1996.
5. Winnie AP, Ramamurthy S, Durrani Z: The inguinal paravascular technic of lumbar plexus anaesthesia: the "3-in-1" block. Anesth Analg 1973;52:989–996.
6. Kim PS, Ferrante FM: Cryoanalgesia: A novel treatment for hip adductor spasticity and obturator neuralgia. Anesthesiology 1998;89:534–536.
7. Wheeler ME, Weinstein SL: Adductor tenotomy-obturator neurotomy. J Pediatr Orthop 1984;4:48–51.
8. Benzel EC, Barolat-Romana G, Larson SJ: Femoral obturator and sciatic neurectomy with iliacus and psoas muscle section for spasticity following spinal cord injury. Spine 1988;13:905–908.
9. Pelissier J: Chemical neurolysis using alcohol in the treatment of spasticity in the hemiplegic. Cah Anesthesiol 1993;41;139–143.
10. Akat T, Murakami J, Yoshinaga A: Life-threatening haemorrhage following obturator artery injury during transurethral bladder surgery: sequel of an unsuccessful obturator nerve block. Acta Anaesthesiol Scand 1999; 43:784–788.
11. Shulm MS: Simultaneous bilateral obturator nerve stimulation during transurethral electrovaporizacion of the prostate. J Clin Anesth 1998; 10:518–521.
12. Prentiss RJ: Massive adductor muscle contraction in transurethral surgery: cause and prevention; development of new electrical circuit. Trans Am Assoc Genitourin Surg 1964;56:64–72.
13. Shiozawa H: A new transurethral resection system: operating in saline environment precludes obturator nerve reflex. J Urol 2002;168: 2665–2657.
14. Biserte J: Treatment of superficial bladder tumors using the argon laser. Acta Urol Belg 1989;57:697–701.
15. Brunken C, Qiu H, Tauber R: Transurethral resection of bladder tumours in physiological saline. Urologe 2004;43:1101–1105.
16. Hobika JH, Clarke BG: Use of neuromuscular blocking drugs to counteract thigh-adductor spasm induced by electrical shocks of obturator nerve during transurethral resection of bladder tumors. J Urol 1961; 85:295–296.
17. Atanassoff PG, Weiss BM, Brull SJ: Lidocaine plasma levels following two techniques of obturator nerve block. J Clin Anesth 1996;8:535–539.
18. Kakinohana M: Interadductor approach to obturator nerve block for transurethral resection procedure: comparison with traditional approach. J Anesth 2002;16:123–126.
19. Deliveliotis C, Alexopoulou K, Picramenos D, et al: The contribution of the obturator nerve block in the transurethral resection of bladder tumor. Acta Urol Belg 1995;63:51–54.
20. Schwilick R, Wingartner K, Kissler GV, et al: Elimination of the obturator reflex as a specific indication for dilute solution of etidocaine. A study of the suitability of a local anesthetic for reflex elimination in the 3-in-1 block technic. Reg Anesth 1990;13–610.
21. Rubial M, Molins N, Rubio P, et al: Obturator nerve block in transurethral surgery. Actas Urol Esp 1989;13:79–81.
22. Gasparich JP, Mason JT, Berger RE: Use of nerve stimulator for simple and accurate obturator nerve block before transurethral resection. J Urol 1984;132:291–293.
23. Viel E, Pelissier J, Pellas F, et al: Alcohol neurolytic blocks for pain and muscle spasticity. Neurochirurgie 2003;49:256–262.
24. Viel E.J, Peennou D, Ripart J, et al: Neurolytic blockade of the obturator nerve for intractable spasticity of adductor thigh muscle. Eur J Pain 2002; 6:97–104.498
25. Kirazli Y, On AY, Kismali B, et al: Comparison of phenol block and botulinus toxin type A in the treatment of spastic foot aster stroke. A randomized double-blind trial. Am J Phys Med Rehabil 1998;77: 510–515.
26. Loubser PG: Neurolytic interventions for upper extremity spasticity associated with head injury. Reg Anesth 1997;22:386–387.
27. Heywang-Kobrunner SH, Amaya B, Okoniewski M, et al: CT-guided obturator nerve block for diagnosis and treatment of painful conditions of the hip. Eur Radiol 2001;11:1047–1053.
28. Hong Y, O'Grady T, Lopresti D, et al: Diagnostic obturator nerve block for inguinal and back pain: a recovered opinion. Pain 1996;67:507–509.
29. Edmonds-Seal J, Turner A, Khodadadeh S, et al: Regional hip blockade in osteoarthrosis. Effects on pain perception. Anaesthesia 1982;37: 147–151.
30. James CDT, Little TF: Regional hip blockade. A simplified technique for the relief of intractable osteoarthritic pain. Anaesthesia 1976;31: 1060–1070.
31. Sunderland S: Obturator nerve. In Sunderland S (ed): *Nerves and Nerve Injuries.* Edinburgh, Scotland: Livingstone, 1968, pp 1096–1109.
32. Whiteside JL, Walters MD: Anatomy of the obturator region: Relations to a trans-obturatorsling. Int Urogynecol J Pelvic Floor Dys- funct 2004;15:223–226.
33. Sinha SK, Abrams JH, Houle TT, Weller RS: Ultrasound-guided obturator nerve block: an interfascial injection approach without nerve stimulation. Reg Anesth Pain Med 2009;34:261–264.

34. Taha AM: Brief reports: ultrasound-guided obturator nerve block: a proximal interfascial technique.. Anesth Analg 2012;114:236–239.

35. Manassero A, Bossolasco M, Ugues S: Ultrasound-guided obturator nerve block: interfascial injection versus a neurostimulation-assisted technique. Reg Anesth Pain Med. 2012;37:67–71.

36. Falsenthal G: Nerve blocks in the lower extremities: anatomic considerations. Arch Phys Med Rehabil 1974;55:504–507.

37. Parkinson SK, Mueller JB, Little WL, et al: Extend of blockade with various approaches to the lumbar plexus. Anesth Analg 1989;68:243–248.

38. Brindenbaugh PO, Wedel DJ. The lower extremity. Somatic blockade. In Cousins MJ, Brindenbaugh PO (eds): *Neural Blockage in Clinical Anesthesia and Management of Pain*. Philadelphia, PA: Lippincott-Raven, 1998, pp 373–394.

39. Atanassoff PG, Weiss BM, Brull SJ, et al: Electromyographic comparison of obturator nerve block to three-in-one block. Anesth Analg 1995;81:529–533.

40. Ritter JW: Femoral nerve "sheath" form inguinal paravascular plexus block is not found in human cadavers. J Clin Anesth 1995;7:470–473.

41. Seeberger MD, Urwyler A: Paravascular lumbar plexus extension after femoral nerve stimulation and injection of 20 vs 40 ml mepivacaine 10 mg/kg. Acta Anesthesia Scand 1995;39:769–813.

42. Singelyn FJ, Gouverneur JM, Gribomont BF: A high position of the catheter increases the success rate of continuous 3-in-1 block. Anesthesiology 1996;85:A723.

43. Capdevila X, Biboulet P, Morau D, et al: Continuous 3-in-1 block for postoperative pain after lower limb orthopedic surgery: where did the catheter go? Anesth Analg 2002;94:1001–1006.

44. Dalens B, Vanneuville G, Tanguy A: Comparison of the fascia iliac block with the 3-in-1 block in children. Anesth Analg 1989;69:705–713.

45. Morau D, Lopez S, Biboulet P, et al: Comparison of continuous 3-in-1 and fascia iliaca compartment blocks for postoperative analgesia: feasibility, catheter migration, distribution of sensory block, and analgesic efficacy. Reg Anesth Pain Med 2003;28:309–314.

46. Capdevila X, Biboulet P, Bouregba M, et al: Compartment of the 3-in-1 and fascia iliaca compartment block in adults: clinical and radiographic analysis. Anesth Analg 1998;86:1039–1044.

47. Winnie AP, Ramamurthy S, Durrani Z, et al: Plexus blocks for lower extremity surgery. Anesthesiol Rev 1974;1:1–6.

48. Chayen D, Nathan H, Chayen M: The posterior compartment block. Anesthesiology 1976;45:95–99.

49. Hanna MH, Peat SJ, D'Costa F: Lumbar pexus block: an anatomical study. Anaesthesia 1993;48:675–678.

50. Schupfer G, Jöhr M: Psoas compartment block in children: Part I—Description of the technique. Pediatric Anesth 2005;15:461–464.

51. Pandin PC, Vandesteen A, d'Hollander AA: Lumbar plexus posterior approach: a catheter placement description using electrical nerve stimulation. Anesth Analg 2002;95:1428–1431.

52. Awad IT, Duggan EM: Posterior lumbar plexus block: anatomy, approaches, and techniques. Reg Anesth Pain Med 2005;30:143–149.

53. Mansour NY: Reevaluating the sciatic nerve block: Another landmark for consideration. Reg Anesth 1993;18:322–323.

54. Morris GF, Lang SA, Dust WN, et al: The parasacral sciatic nerve block. Reg Anesth 1997;22:223–228.

55. Jochum D, Iohom G, Choquet, et al: Adding a selective obturator nerve block to the parasacral sciatic nerve block: an evaluation. Anesth Analg 2004;99:1544–1549.

56. Choquet O, Nazarian S, Manelli H: Bloc obturateur au pli in- guinal: étude anatomique. Ann Fr Anesth Réanim 2001;20:131s.

57. Fujita Y, Kimura K, Furukawa Y, et al: Plasma concentrations of lignocaine alter obturator nerve block combined with spinal anaesthesia in patient undergoing transurethral resection procedures. Br J Anaesth 1992;68:596–598.

Femoral Nerve Block

Jerry D. Vloka, Admir Hadzic, and Philippe Gautier

INTRODUCTION

The femoral nerve block is one of the most clinically applicable nerve block techniques that it is relatively simple to perform, carries a low risk of complications, and results in a high success rate.

Indications
Single-Injection Technique

Femoral nerve block is well suited for surgery on the anterior aspect of the thigh and for superficial surgery on the medial aspect of the leg below the knee. Some examples include repair of the quadriceps tendon or quadriceps muscle biopsy, long saphenous vein stripping, and postoperative pain management after femur and knee surgery. A perineural catheter can be placed to provide prolonged analgesia for patients with fractures on the femoral neck or shaft. Femoral nerve block provides effective analgesia following total knee arthroplasty. Femoral nerve block can also be used to supplement a sciatic or popliteal block to provide complete anesthesia of the lower leg and ankle.[1–4]

Continuous Technique

The primary indication of continuous femoral nerve block is pain management after major femur or knee surgery.[5–21]

In addition, when compared with a single-dose technique or placebo, continuous femoral nerve block significantly reduces postoperative morphine consumption in patients having total hip replacement.[22,23]

Continuous femoral nerve block provides excellent analgesia in patients with femoral shaft or femoral neck fractures.[13,14,20,24] Its relative simplicity makes it uniquely suitable for use to provide analgesia in the emergency room and facilitate physical and radiologic examinations as well as manipulations of the fractured femur or hip.

After major knee surgery, continuous femoral nerve block provides better pain relief than parenteral administration of opioids (IV PCA, intramuscular)[6,11,15,16,19] or intra-articular analgesia.[17,25] For knee surgery, continuous femoral block is as effective as continuous lumbar plexus block[26] or continuous epidural analgesia,[11,19] but causes fewer complications.[27]

Contraindications

Relative contraindications for femoral nerve block include previous ilioinguinal surgery (femoral vascular graft, kidney transplantation), large inguinal lymph nodes or tumor, local infection, peritoneal infection, and preexisting femoral neuropathy.

Anatomy

The femoral nerve is the largest branch of the lumbar plexus. It is formed by the dorsal divisions of the anterior rami of the L2, L3, and L4 spinal nerves. It emerges from the lateral border of the psoas muscle, approximately at the junction of the middle and lower thirds of that muscle. Along its course to the thigh, it remains deep to the fascia iliaca. It enters the thigh posterior to the inguinal ligament, where it is positioned immediately lateral and slightly posterior to the femoral artery (Figure 82C–1). At this level, it is situated deep to both fascia lata and fascia iliaca (Figure 82C–2). As the nerve passes into the thigh, it divides into anterior and posterior branches (Figure 82C–3). Located above the fascia iliaca, the anterior branches innervate the sartorius and pectineus muscles (Figure 82C–4) and the skin of the anterior and medial aspects of the thigh.

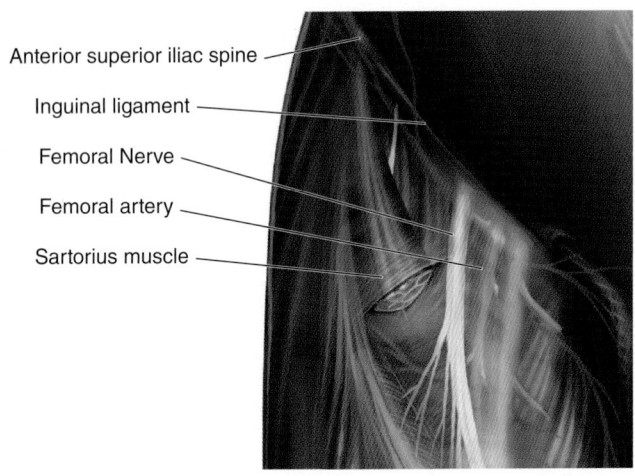

FIGURE 82C–1. Anatomic relationship in the femoral triangle.

Labels: Anterior superior iliac spine, Inguinal ligament, Femoral Nerve, Femoral artery, Sartorius muscle

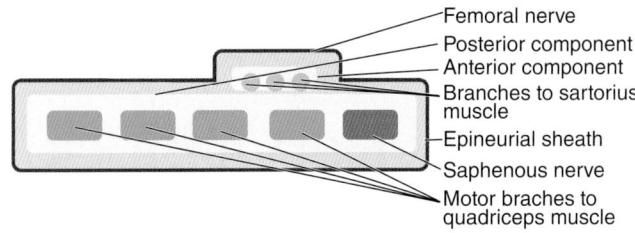

FIGURE 82C–3. Composition of the femoral nerve at the level of blockade.

Labels: Femoral nerve, Posterior component, Anterior component, Branches to sartorius muscle, Epineurial sheath, Saphenous nerve, Motor branches to quadriceps muscle

Clinical Pearl

- In obese patients, the identification of the inguinal crease can be facilitated by asking an assistant to retract the lower abdomen laterally (see Figure 82C–7).

Equipment

A standard regional anesthesia tray is prepared with the following equipment:

- Sterile towels and gauze packs
- 20-mL syringe with local anesthetic
- Sterile gloves, marking pen
- One 25-gauge, 1.5-in. needle for skin infiltration
- A 5-cm long, short-bevel, insulated stimulating needle
- A peripheral nerve stimulator and a surface electrode
- Injection pressure monitor

BLOCK TECHNIQUE

Patient position. The patient lies in the supine position. The ipsilateral extremity is abducted 10–20 degrees and slightly externally rotated with the lateral side of the foot resting on the table.

Site of needle insertion. The site of needle insertion (Figure 82C–6) is located at the femoral crease but below the inguinal crease and immediately lateral (1 cm) to the pulse of the femoral artery.

Located under the fascia iliaca, the posterior branches innervate the quadriceps muscle and the knee joint and give off the saphenous nerve. The saphenous nerve supplies the skin of the medial aspect of the leg below the knee (Figure 82C–5).

Landmarks

The following landmarks are used to determine the site of needle insertion: inguinal ligament, inguinal crease, femoral artery (see Figure 82C–6).

Clinical Pearls

- It is useful to think of the mnemonic VAN (vein, artery, nerve) going from medial to lateral when recalling the relationship of the femoral nerve to vessels at the inguinal crease.

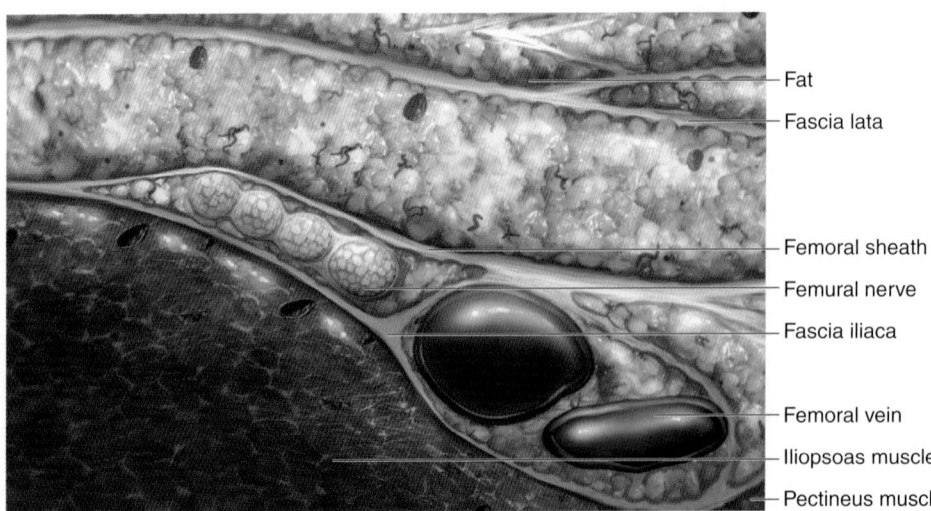

FIGURE 82C–2. Tissue sheaths and femoral nerve, artery and vein relationships.

Labels: Fat, Fascia lata, Femoral sheath, Femoral nerve, Fascia iliaca, Femoral vein, Iliopsoas muscle, Pectineus muscle

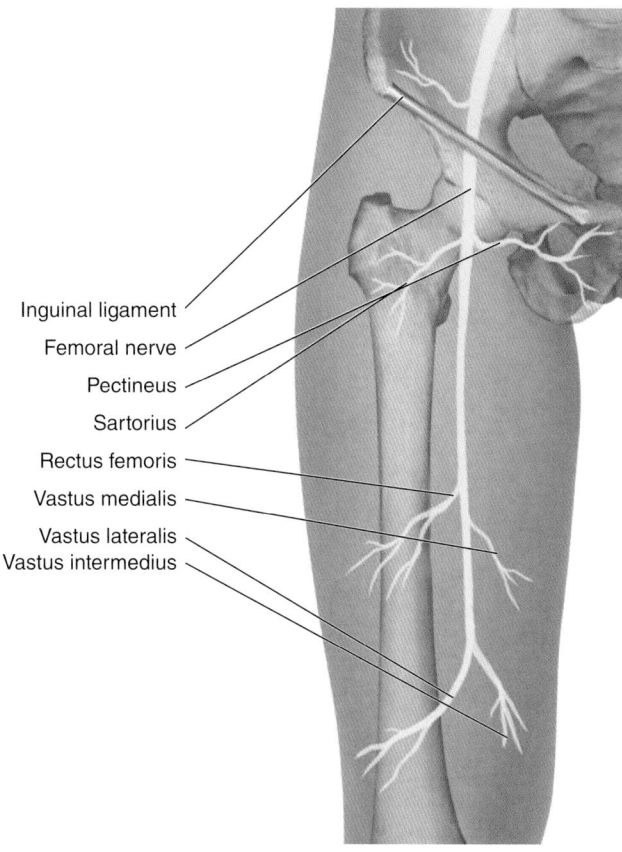

FIGURE 82C–4. Motor branches of the femoral nerve.

Inguinal ligament
Femoral nerve
Pectineus
Sartorius
Rectus femoris
Vastus medialis
Vastus lateralis
Vastus intermedius

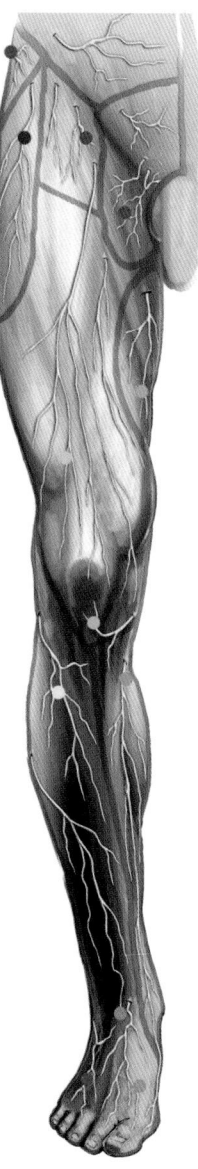

Blocked with femoral nerve block
- Anterior femoral cutaneous nerves
- Infrapattelar branch of the saphenous
- Saphenous nerve

Not blocked with femoral nerve block
- Subcostal nerve
- Femoral branch of genitofemoral
- Genital branch of genitofemoral
- Lateral femoral cutaneous nerve
- Cutaneous branches of the obturator
- Lateral sural cutaneous nerves
- Superficial peroneal nerve
- Deep peroneal nerve
- Lateral dorsal cutaneous nerve

FIGURE 82C–5. Sensory innervation of the femoral nerve and distribution of anesthesia with femoral nerve block.

- The femoral nerve is approached at the femoral crease, rather than at the inguinal ligament.

Single-Injection Technique

In obese patients, the lower abdomen is retracted laterally to allow access to the inguinal area (Figure 82C–7). The needle is connected to a nerve stimulator set at a current intensity of 1 mA (0.1 msec/2 Hz) and introduced at a 30- to 45-degree angle to the skin in a cephalad direction (Figure 82C–8). The needle is advanced through the fascia lata and iliaca, often associated with a certain feeling of a "pop" as the needle pierces the fasciae.

As the quadriceps muscle contractions (i.e., patellar twitch) are obtained, the current is gradually decreased while the needle is advanced. The position of the needle is adequate when patellar twitches are elicited with current output between 0.3 and 0.5 mA. After negative aspiration; 15–20 mL of local anesthetic is injected. Some common responses to nerve stimulation and appropriate action to troubleshoot are featured in Table 82C–1.

Multiple injection techniques have also been described, where vastus lateralis, intermedius, and medialis twitches are individually identified and separate injections of local anesthetic made at each nerve branch.[30,31] When compared with a single injection, the total volume of local anesthetic required and the block onset time were significantly reduced. However, 14% of patients reported paresthesia, and 28%

reported discomfort during block performance.[32] Consequently, this technique has been largely abandoned as being unnecessary.

Clinical Pearls

- The needle tip must be positioned below fascia iliaca to obtain a complete femoral nerve block.
- Larger volume than 15-20 mL is not necessary because it is not associated with a better success rate.[33]

Continuous Femoral Nerve Block

The continuous technique is similar to the single-injection technique. After passage through both fascia lata and iliaca, the needle is advanced to elicit a patellar twitch using a current output between 0.3 and 0.5 mA (0.1 msec) (Figure 82C–9).

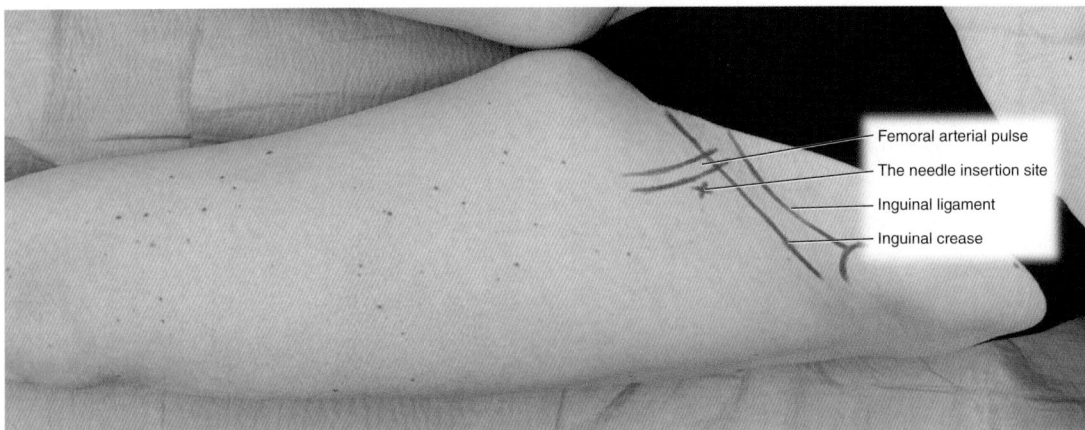

FIGURE 82C–6. Anatomic landmarks for femoral nerve block. The needle insertion site (X) is located just below the inguinal crease, 1–2 cm lateral to the pulse of the femoral artery.

The catheter is then inserted 5 cm beyond the tip of the needle and secured in place. After a negative aspiration test for blood, a bolus dose of 10 mL of local anesthetic is injected and followed by a continuous infusion of dilute local anesthetic and/or intermittent boluses of 5 ml hourly. (Figure 82C–10).

- Catheter insertion under the fascia iliaca should be without resistance. When this is not the case, the needle is probably not under the fascia iliaca. The needle should be withdrawn to the skin and reinserted.

Block Assessment

Sensory blockade is assessed by cold or pin prick test on the anterior and medial aspect of the thigh (femoral nerve) and on the medial aspect of the lower leg (saphenous nerve). Motor blockade is evaluated by asking the patient to extend the knee (e.g., to elevate the foot from the table).

CHOICE OF LOCAL ANESTHETIC

Single-Injection Technique

For surgical anesthesia, mepivacaine or lidocaine 1.5–2.0% or ropivacaine 0.5%–0.75% are frequently used, depending on the expected duration of surgery. For postoperative analgesia alone, a more dilute concentration of long acting local anesthetic (eg ropivacaine or bupivacaine 0.2%–0.25%) is appropriate. Onset times and mean duration of both anesthesia and analgesia with different types and concentrations of local anesthetic solution are presented in Table 82C–2.

Continuous Technique

The initial bolus of 10–15 mL is followed by an infusion of dilute concentration (e.g., ropivacaine 0.2%). A typical infusion regimen is 5 mL/h basal infusion with a 5 mL/q60min patient-controlled bolus.

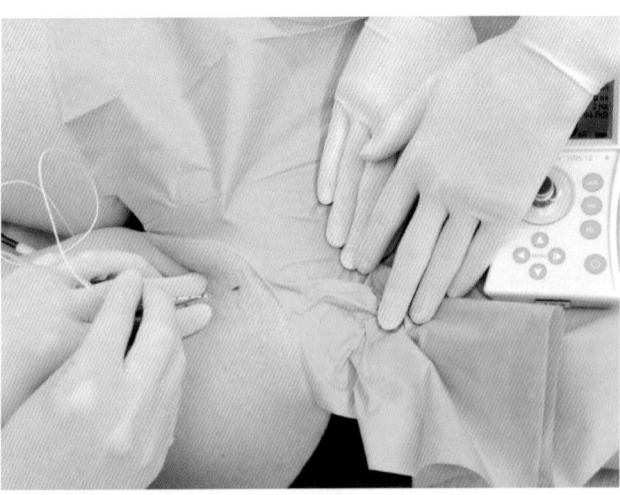

FIGURE 82C–7. The abdomen is retracted laterally to facilitate exposure of the anatomy during femoral nerve blockade.

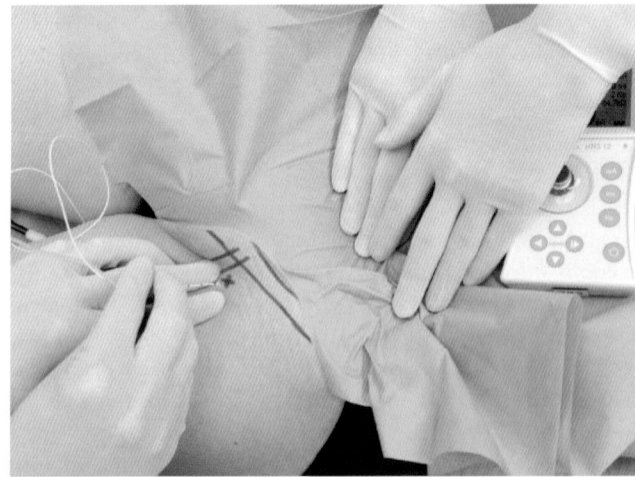

FIGURE 82C–8. The needle is connected to a nerve stimulator set at 1 mA current intensity and introduced at a 30- to 45-degree angle to the skin in a cephalad direction.

TABLE 82C–1. Common responses to nerve stimulation and action to obtain femoral nerve twitch.

Response Obtained	Interpretation	Problem	Action
No response	The needle is inserted either too medially or to laterally	Femoral artery not properly localized	Follow the systematic lateral angulation and reinsertion of the needle as described in the technique
Bone contact	The needle contacts hip or superior ramus of the pubic bone	The needle is inserted too deep	Withdraw to the level of the skin and reinsert in another direction
Local twitch	Direct stimulation of the illiopsoas or pectineus muscle	Too deep insertion	Withdraw to the level of the skin and re-insert in another direction
Twitch of the sartorius muscle	Sartorius muscle twitch	The needle tip is slightly anterior and medial to the main trunk of the femoral nerve	Redirect the needle laterally and advance deeper 1–3 mm
Vascular puncture	Needle placement into the femoral or femoral circumflex artery, less commonly - femoral vein	Too medial needle placement	Withdraw and reinsert laterally 1 cm
Patella twitch	Stimulation of the main trunk of the femoral nerve	None	Accept and inject local anesthetic

PERIOPERATIVE MANAGEMENT OF FEMORAL NERVE BLOCKS

The performance of femoral nerve block is associated with minor patient discomfort because the needle passes only through the skin and adipose of the inguinal region. Femoral nerve block is associated with weakness of the quadriceps muscle, leading to the decrease in its use in some practices, particularly where ultrasound is available for adductor canal blocks. This is because knee extension and weight bearing on the blocked side are impaired with femoral nerve block, which must be clearly explained to the patient to reduce the risk of falls. The use of a knee immobilizer for ambulation following femoral nerve block has been shown to reduce the risk of falls, particularly following total knee arthroplasty.[34,35]

Complications and How to Avoid Them

Complications of femoral nerve block include[13] vascular puncture,[33] femoral nerve compression by a hematoma,[36] diffusion of

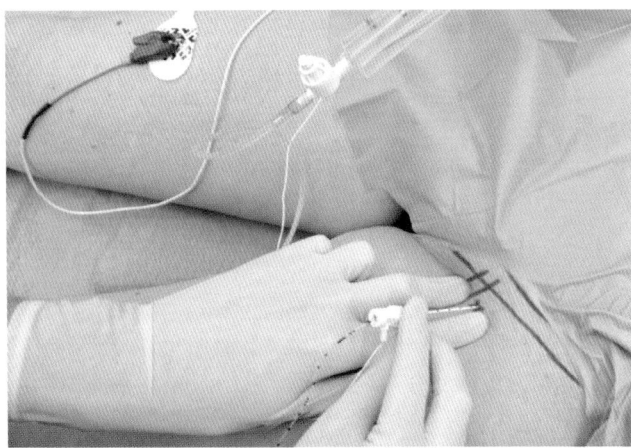

FIGURE 82C–9. Continuous femoral nerve block: Needle insertion.

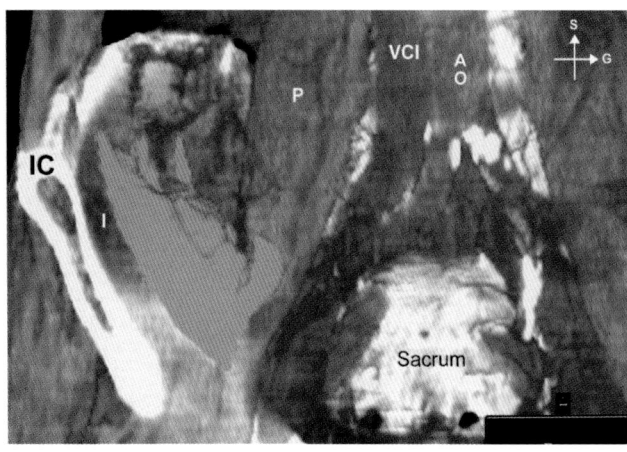

FIGURE 82C–10. Spread of the injectate underneath the fascia iliaca after injection through the femoral catheter. (Used with permission from Dr. Philippe Gauiter, Bruxelles, BE.)

TABLE 82C-2. Onset and duration of 20 ml of local anesthetic in femoral block.

	Onset (min)	Anesthesia (h)	Analgesia (h)
3% 2-Chloroprocaine	10–15	1	2
3% 2-Chloroprocaine (+ HCO₃ + epi)	10–15	1.5–2	2–3
1.5% Mepivacaine	15–20	2–3	3–5
1.5% Mepivacaine (+ HCO₃ + epi)	15–20	2–5	3–8
2% Lidocaine	10–20	2–5	3–8
0.5% Ropivacaine	15–30	4–8	5–12
0.75% Ropivacaine	10–15	5–10	6–24
0.5 Bupivacaine	15–30	5–15	8–30

TABLE 82C-3. Femoral nerve block: complications.

Hematoma	• When the femoral artery or vein is punctured, the procedure should be stopped and pressure applied over the puncture site for 2–3 min.
Vascular puncture	• Maintain a palpating finger on the femoral pulse and insert the needle just lateral and parallel to the pulse. • The needle should never be directed medially.
Nerve injury	• Use a nerve stimulator avoid injection when motor response is present at <0.3 mA (0.1 msec). • Do not seek paresthesia as method of localization of FN because paresthesia is rarely elicited with femoral nerve block and should not be sought or relied on to indicate an intraneural injection. However, should severe pain on injection be reported, abort the injection. • Do not inject when high pressures on injection are encountered. • Use the minimal efficient volume and concentration of local anesthetic (15-20 mL).
Catheter infection	• Use strict aseptic technique during catheter insertion. • Sterile drapes should be used with continuous techniques. • Remove the catheter after 48–72 h (risk of infection increases with time).
Prevention of Falls	• Instruct patient on the inability to bear weight on the blocked extremity.

the local anesthetic solution into the epidural space with resultant epidural block,[37] catheter shearing,[38] and femoral nerve injury (incidence of 0.25%).[12,39,40] With regard to continuous catheters, bacterial contamination of the catheters commonly occurs after 48 hours.[32,39,40] However, local or systemic infection remains rare, with the estimated risk of 0.13%[41], Table 82C-3.

SUMMARY

Femoral nerve block is easy to perform and associated with a low risk of complications. It is suitable for catheter insertion. When used alone, it is effective for surgery on the anterior thigh and for postoperative pain management after femur and knee surgery. When combined with sciatic and/or obturator nerve blocks, anesthesia of almost the entire lower limb from the midthigh level can be achieved.

REFERENCES

1. Kwofie MK, Shastri UD, Gadsden JC, et al: The effects of ultrasound-guided adductor canal block versus femoral nerve block on quadriceps strength and fall risk: a blinded, randomized trial of volunteers. Reg Anesth Pain Med 2013;38:321–325..
2. Jæger P, Zaric D, Fomsgaard JS, et al: Adductor canal block versus femoral nerve block for analgesia after total knee arthroplasty: a randomized, double-blind study. Reg Anesth Pain Med 2013;38:526-532.
3. Shah NA, Jain NP: Is continuous adductor canal block better than continuous femoral nerve block after total knee arthroplasty? effect on ambulation ability, early functional recovery and pain control: a randomized controlled trial. J Arthroplasty 2014 Jun 19. pii: S0883-540 [Epub ahead of print]
4. Perlas A, Kirkham KR, Billing R, et al: The impact of analgesic modality on early ambulation following total knee arthroplasty. Reg Anesth Pain Med 2013;38:334–339..
5. Anker-Møller E, Spangsberg N, Dahl J, et al: Continuous blockade of the lumbar plexus after knee surgery: a comparison of the plasma concentrations and analgesic effect of bupivacaine 0.250% and 0.125%. Acta Anaesthesiol Scand 1990;34:468–472.
6. Ganapathy S, Wasserman R, Watson J, et al: Modified continuous femoral three-in-one block for postoperative pain after total knee arthroplasty. Anesth Analg 1999;89:1197–1202.
7. Singelyn F, Gouverneur JM: Extended "3-in-1" block after total knee arthroplasty: continuous versus patient-controlled techniques. Anesth Analg 2000;91:176–180.
8. Eledjam JJ, Cuvillon P, Capdevila X, et al: Postoperative analgesia by femoral nerve block with ropivacaine 0.2% after major knee surgery: continuous versus patient-controlled techniques. Reg Anesth Pain Med 2002;27:604–611.
9. Singelyn F, Vanderelst P, Gouverneur JM: Extended femoral nerve sheath block after total hip arthroplasty: continuous vs patient-controlled techniques. Anesth Analg 2001;92:455–459.
10. Tetzlaff J, Andrish J, O'Hara J, et al: Effectiveness of bupivacaine administered via femoral nerve catheter for pain control after anterior cruciate ligament repair. J Clin Anesth 1997;9:542–545.
11. Capdevila X, Barthelet Y, Biboulet P, et al: Effects of perioperative analgesic technique on the surgical outcome and duration of rehabilitation after major knee surgery. Anesthesiology 1999;91:8–15.
12. Singelyn F, Gouverneur JM: Postoperative analgesia after total hip arthroplasty: IV PCA with morphine, patient-controlled epidural analgesia, or continuous "3-in-1" block? A prospective evaluation by our acute pain service in more than 1300 patients. J Clin Anesth 1999;11:550–554.
13. Ben-David B, Croituru M: Psoas block for surgical repair of hip fracture: a case report and description of a catheter technique. Anesth Analg 1990;71:298–301.
14. Capdevila X, Biboulet P, Bouregba M, et al: Bilateral continuous 3-in-1 nerve blockade for postoperative pain relief after bilateral femoral shaft surgery. J Clin Anesth 1998;10:606–609.
15. Serpell M, Millar F, Thomson M: Comparison of lumbar plexus block versus conventional opioid analgesia after total knee replacement. Anaesthesia 1991;46:275–277.

16. Dahl J, Christiansen C, Daugaard J, et al: Continuous blockade of the lumbar plexus after knee surgery—postoperative analgesia and bupivacaine plasma concentrations. Anaesthesia 1988;43:1015–1018.

17. De Andrés J, Bellver J, Barrera L, et al: A comparative study of analgesia after knee surgery with intraarticular bupivacaine, intraarticular morphine, and lumbar plexus block. Anesth Analg 1993;77:727–730.

18. Schultz P, Christensen E, Anker-Møller E, et al: Postoperative pain treatment after open knee surgery: continuous lumbar plexus block with bupivacaine versus epidural morphine. Reg Anesth Pain Med 1991;16:34–37.

19. Singelyn F, Deyaert M, Joris D, et al: Effects of intravenous patient-controlled analgesia with morphine, continuous epidural analgesia, and continuous "3-in-1" block on postoperative pain and knee rehabilitation after unilateral total knee arthroplasty. Anesth Analg 1998;87:88–92.

20. Johnson C: Continuous femoral nerve blockade for analgesia in children with femoral fractures. Anaesth Intensive Care 1994;22:281–283.

21. Capdevila X, Biboulet P, Bouregba M, et al: Comparison of the three-in-one and fascia iliaca compartment blocks in adults: clinical and radiographic analysis. Anesth Analg 1998;86:1039–1044.

22. Singelyn FJ, Ebongo F, Symens B, et al: Influence of the analgesic technique on postoperative rehabilitation after total hip replacement. Reg Anesth Pain Med 2001;26–39.

23. Boujlel S, Delbos A, Singelyn F: Continuous but not single-dose femoral nerve sheath block provides efficient pain relief after total hip replacement (THR). Reg Anesth Pain Med 2001;26–135.

24. Chudinov A, Berkenstadt H, Salai M, et al: Continuous psoas compartment block for anesthesia and perioperative analgesia in patients with hip fractures. Reg Anesth Pain Med 1999;24:563–568.

25. Dauri M, Polzoni M, Fabbi E, et al: Comparison of epidural, continu- ous femoral block and intraarticular analgesia after anterior cruciate ligament reconstruction. Acta Anaesthesiol Scand 2003;47:20–25.

26. Kaloul I, Guay J, Côtré C, et al: The posterior lumbar plexus (psoas compartment) block and the three-in-one femoral nerve block provide similar postoperative analgesia after total knee replacement. Can J Anaesth 2004;51:45–51.

27. Chelly J, Greger J, Gebhard R, et al: Continuous femoral blocks improve recovery and outcome of patients undergoing total knee arthroplasty. J Arthroplasty 2001;16:436–445.

28. Winnie AP, Ramamurthy S, Durrani Z: The inguinal paravascular technic of lumbar plexus anesthesia. The "3-in-1 block." Anesth Analg 1973;52:989–996.

29. Vloka JD, Hadzic A, Drobnik L, et al Anatomical landmarks for femoral nerve block: a comparison of four needle insertion sites. Anesth Analg 1999;89:1467–1470.

30. Casati A, Fanelli G, Beccaria P, et al: The effects of single or multiple injections on the volume of 0.5% ropivacaine required for femoral nerve blockade. Anesth Analg 2001;93:183–186.

31. Casati A, Fanelli G, Beccaria P, et al: The effects of the single or multiple injection technique on the onset time of femoral nerve block with 0.75 % ropivacaine. Anesth Analg 2000;91:181–184.

32. Fanelli G, Casati A, Garancini P, et al: Nerve stimulator and multi- ple injection technique for upper and lower limb blockade: Failure rate, patient acceptance and neurologic complications. Anesth Analg 1999;88:847–852.

33. Seeberger M, Urwyler A: Paravascular lumbar plexus block: Block extension after femoral nerve stimulation and injection of 20 vs. 40 mL mepivacaine 10 mg/mL. Acta Anaesthesiol Scand 1995;39: 769–773.

34. Beebe MJ, Allen R, Anderson MB, et al: Continuous femoral nerve block using 0.125% bupivacaine does not prevent early ambulation after total knee arthroplasty. Clin Orthop Relat Res. 2014;472:1394–1399..

35. Cui Q, Schapiro LH, Kinney MC, et al: Reducing costly falls of total knee replacement patients. Am J Med Qual. 2013;28:335–338. Epub 2013 Jan 15.

36. Jôhr M: A complication of continuous femoral nerve block. Reg Anaesth 1987;10:37–38.

37. Singelyn F, Contreras V, Gouverneur JM: Epidural anesthesia complicating continuous 3-in-1 lumbar plexus blockade. Anesthesiolgy 1995;83: 217–220.

38. Lee B, Goucke C: Shearing of a peripheral nerve catheter. Anesth Analg 2002;95:760–761.

39. Cuvillon P, Ripart J, Lalourcey L, et al: The continuous femoral nerve block catheter for postoperative analgesia: bacterial colonization, infectious rate and adverse effects. Anesth Analg 2001;93:1045–1049.

40. Pirat P, Branchereau S, Bernard N, et al: Suivi prospectif descriptif des effets adverses non infectieux liés aux blocs nerveux périphériques continus: á propos de 1416 patients. Ann Fr Anesth Réanim 2002; 21:R010.

41. Bernard N, Pirat P, Branchereau S, et al: Suivi multicentrique prospectif des effets adverses d'ordre infectieux sur 1416 blocs nerveux périphériques continus. Ann Fr Anesth Réanim 2002;21:R076.

Sciatic Nerve Block

Elizabeth Gartner, Elisabeth Fouché, Olivier Choquet,
Admir Hadzic, and Jerry D. Vloka

INTRODUCTION

Victor Pauchet, a French surgeon, first described the sciatic nerve block in *L'Anesthesie Regionale* in 1920: "the site of needle insertion for blocking the sciatic nerve at the level of hip: 3 cm along the perpendicular that bisects a line drawn between the greater trochanter and the posterior superior iliac spine."[1] This technique has since been referred to as "The classic approach of Labat," possibly because it was first described in the English language literature in 1923 by Gaston Labat, a student of Pauchet, in his book *Regional Anesthesia: Its Technic and Clinical Application*.[2] Labat's book went through several reprints of the first edition of one of the first English-language textbooks of regional anesthesia. Curiously, this book was very similar to *L'Anesthesie Regionale*.[3] In the same year, Labat founded the American Society of Regional Anesthesia (ASRA). Anecdotally, Labat intended to name the new group "The Labat Society" in his own honor, but the name ASRA remains today as we know it.

Alon Winnie eventually modified the Labat approach in 1975.[4] Alternatives, such as the anterior approach described by George Beck in 1963 and the lithotomy approach described by Prithvi Raj in 1975, were devised to allow the sciatic nerve to be blocked in the supine patient.[5,6] A number of other approaches have been proposed, most of which include minor modifications. The most useful of these newer techniques are likely the subgluteal and parasacral approach introduced by Pia di Benedetto and Philippe Cuvillon, respectively.[7,8] In this chapter, we focus on the classic approach to sciatic nerve block, parasacral and subgluteal modifications, and the anterior approach.

Indications and Contraindications

Indications for sciatic nerve block include lower-limb surgery, combined with a femoral or psoas compartment block.[9] For distal surgery of the lower extremity, however, more distal approaches such as ankle block or popliteal sciatic nerve block are preferable whenever feasible. Note that the sciatic nerve block often needs to be combined with additional blocks, such as lumbar plexus (femoral or saphenous nerve) when anesthesia of the entire lower extremity is desired.

Contraindications to sciatic nerve block may include include local infection and bed sores at the site of insertion, coagulopathy, preexisting central or peripheral nervous systems disorders, and allergy to local anesthesia.

Functional Anatomy

The union of the lumbosacral trunk with the first three sacral nerves forms the sacral plexus (Figure 82D–1). The lumbosacral trunk originates from the anastomosis of the last two lumbar nerves with the anterior branch of the first sacral nerve. This structure receives the anterior branches of the second and third sacral nerves, forming the sacral plexus. The sacral plexus is shaped like a triangle pointing toward the sciatic notch, with its base spanning across the anterior sacral foramina. It rests on the anterior aspect of the piriformis muscle and is covered by the pelvic fascia, which separates it from the hypogastric vessels and pelvic organs. Seven nerves stem from the sacral plexus: six collateral branches and one terminal branch—the sciatic nerve, the largest nerve of the plexus (Figure 82D–2).

The sciatic nerve is the largest peripheral nerve in the body and measures more than 1 cm in width at its origin. It exits the pelvis through the greater sciatic notch below the piriformis muscle, then descends between the greater trochanter of the femur and the ischial tuberosity. The nerve then runs along the posterior thigh to the lower third of the femur, where it diverges into two large branches, the tibial and common peroneal nerves. This division may occur at any level proximal to the lower third of the femur.[10,11] The common peroneal and tibial nerves are separated from their onset at the sacral plexus (15%); in this case, the common peroneal nerve typically pierces the piriformis muscle. The course of the sciatic nerve can be

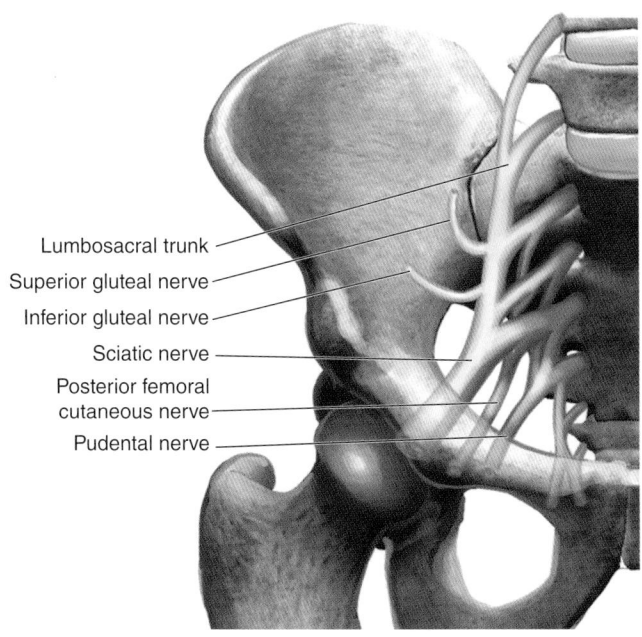

FIGURE 82D-1. Formation of the sacral plexus.

Lumbosacral trunk
Superior gluteal nerve
Inferior gluteal nerve
Sciatic nerve
Posterior femoral cutaneous nerve
Pudental nerve

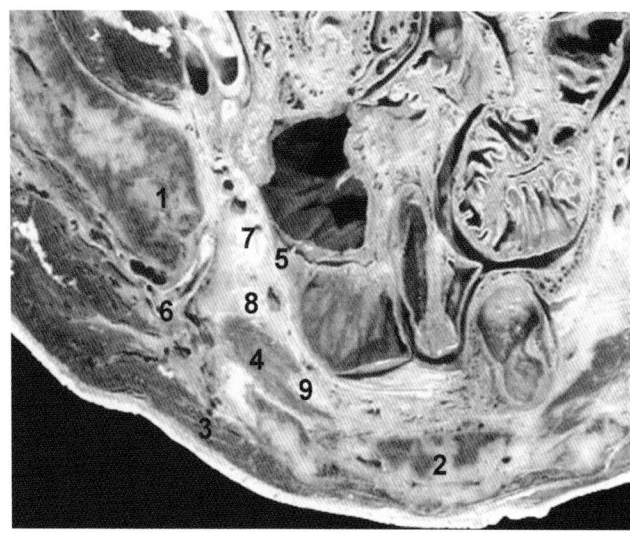

FIGURE 82D-3. Parasacral area. Transversal section at the S3 level. *1*, Iliac bone; *2*, sacrum; *3*, gluteal muscle; *4*, piriformis muscle; *5*, pelvic aponeurosis; *6*, inferior gluteal plexus; *7*, lumbosacral trunk; *8*, first sacral root; *9*, second sacral root.

estimated by drawing a line on the back of the thigh beginning from the apex of the popliteal fossa to the midpoint of the line joining the ischial tuberosity to the apex of the greater trochanter. From its onset, the sciatic nerve also gives off numerous articular (hip, knee) and muscular branches.

In the upper part of its course, the sciatic nerve lies deep in the gluteus maximus muscle and rests on the posterior surface of the ischium (Figures 82D–3 and 82D–4). The sciatic

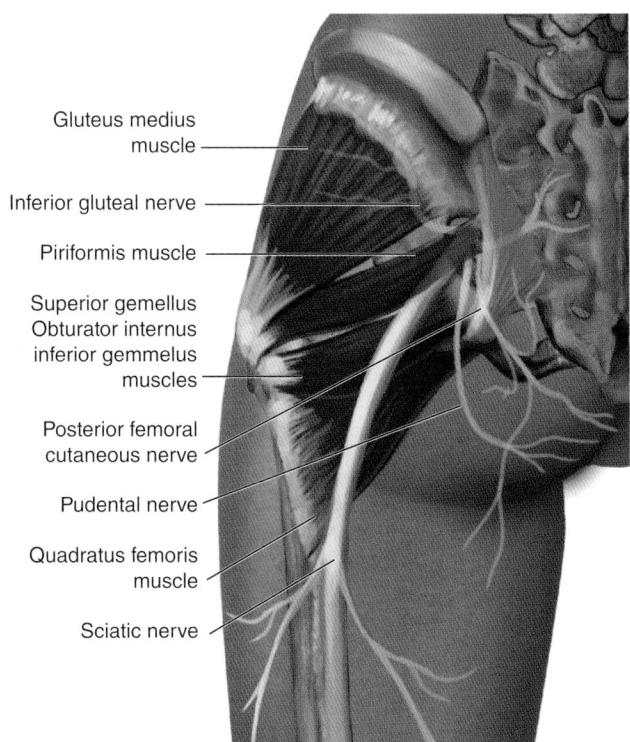

Gluteus medius muscle
Inferior gluteal nerve
Piriformis muscle
Superior gemellus
Obturator internus
inferior gemmelus muscles
Posterior femoral cutaneous nerve
Pudental nerve
Quadratus femoris muscle
Sciatic nerve

FIGURE 82D-2. Course of the sciatic nerve at the exit from the pelvis.

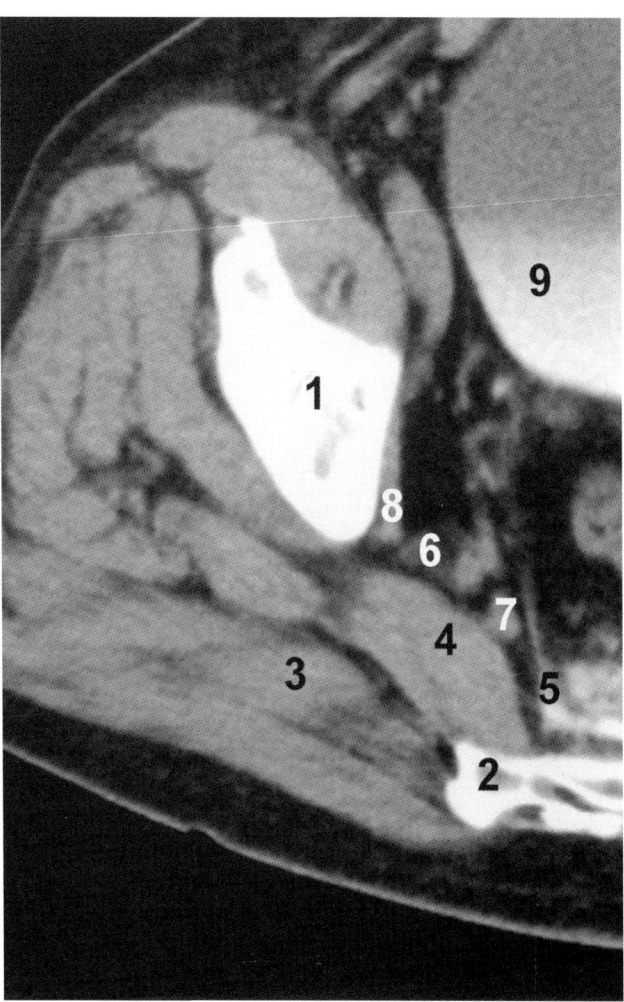

FIGURE 82D-4. Computed tomographic (CT) scan of the parasacral area, at the S3 level. *1*, Iliac bone; *2*, sacrum; *3*, gluteal muscle; *4*, piriformis muscle; *5*, pelvic aponeurosis; *6*, inferior gluteal plexus; *7*, lumbosacral trunk; *8*, first sacral root; *9*, bladder.

nerve crosses the external rotators, obturator internus, and gemelli muscles, then passes on to the quadratus femoris. The quadratus femoris separates the sciatic nerve from the obturator externus and the hip joint. Medially, the posterior cutaneous nerve of the thigh and the inferior gluteal plexus accompany the sciatic nerve, whereas more distally the sciatic nerve lies on the adductor magnus. The long head of the biceps femoris crosses the sciatic nerve obliquely. The articular branches of the sciatic nerve arise from the upper part of the nerve and supply the hip joint by perforating the posterior part of its capsule. However, the articular branches are sometimes derived directly from the sacral plexus. The muscular branches of the sciatic nerve innervate the gluteus, the biceps femoris, the ischial head of the adductor magnus, the semitendinosus, and the semimembranosus muscles (Figure 82D–5; Table 82D–1). The branches for the ischial head of the adductor magnus and semimembranosus muscles arise from a common trunk. The nerve to the short head of the biceps femoris comes from the common peroneal division, whereas the other muscular branches arise from the tibial division of the sciatic nerve.

The parasacral area is delineated by the ventral aponeurosis of the piriformis muscle dorsally, by the pelvic aponeurosis medially, and by the aponeurosis of the obturator internis

TABLE 82D–1. Branches, source, and motor innervation of the sacral plexus.

Nerve	Source	Muscular Innervation
Nerve to obturator internus muscle	Lumbosacral trunk and S1	Obturator internus
Superior gluteal nerve	Lumbosacral trunk and S1	Gluteus medius
		Gluteus minimus
		Tensor fasciae lata
Nerve to piriformis muscle	S2	Piriformis
Nerve to biceps femoris superior	Anterior portion of plexus	Biceps femoris superior
Nerve to biceps femoris inferior and quadratus femoris	Anterior portion of plexus	Biceps femoris inferior
		Quadratus femoris
		Branch to coxofemoral articulation
Posterior femoral cutaneous nerve (lesser sciatic nerve)	Lumbosacral trunk, S1, S2	Inferior gluteal n. to gluteus maximus muscle
		Sensory branch to buttock, thigh, popliteal fossa, and lateral aspect of knee

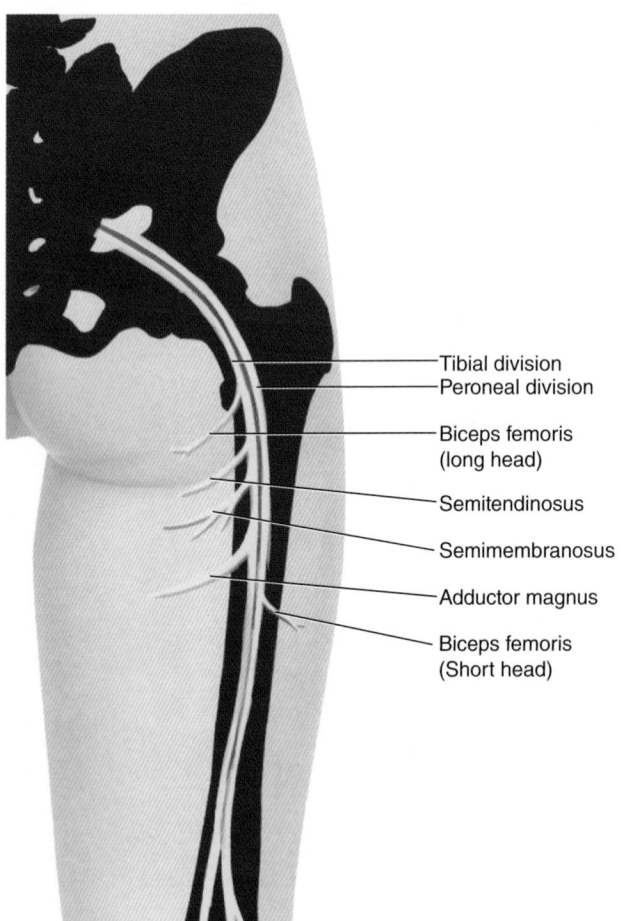

FIGURE 82D–5. Sciatic nerve. Downward course and motor branches to the hamstrings muscles.

Tibial division
Peroneal division
Biceps femoris (long head)
Semitendinosus
Semimembranosus
Adductor magnus
Biceps femoris (Short head)

muscle laterally.[8] The common peroneal component passes through the piriformis muscle or above it, and only the tibial component passes below the muscle.

The tibial and common peroneal elements of the sciatic nerve each have their own outer layer of epineurium. Both components are further enclosed by a dense layer of connective tissue, which runs from the origin of the sciatic nerve to its bifurcation. This layer has been given several names over the years, but lately it is commonly referred to as the "paraneural sheath" of the sciatic nerve. Injection of local anesthetic deep to this sheath (but outside the epineurium of the tibial or common peroneal nerves) has been shown to spread a considerable distance proximally and distally, and result in a rapid onset, dense block. This is not considered an "intraneural" injection as the injection occurs outside of the epineurium.[12–14]

TABLE 82D–2. Local anesthetic choices for sciatic nerve block: duration of anesthesia and analgesia.

	Onset (min)	Anesthesia (h)	Analgesia (h)
3% 2-Chloroprocaine	10–15	2	2.5
1.5% Mepivacaine	10–15	4–5	5–8
2% Lidocaine	10–20	5–6	5–8
0.5% Ropivacaine	15–20	6–12	6–24
0.75% Ropivacaine	10–15	8–12	8–24
0.5% Bupivacaine	15–30	8–16	10–48

Choice of Local Anesthetic

Despite its large size, sciatic block requires a relatively low volume of local anesthetic to achieve anesthesia of the entire trunk of the nerve.[15] Generally, 20–25 mL of local anesthetic is sufficient. The choice of the type and concentration of local anesthetic should be based on whether the block is planned for surgical anesthesia or pain management[16] (Table 82D–2). When seeking prolonged pain relief, longer-acting local anesthetic may be more appropriate.[17,18] Addition of epinephrine may be justified in patients undergoing above the knee amputation, in whom prolonged analgesia is desired.

Equipment

As with all regional anesthesia techniques, the heart rate, blood pressure, and pulse oximetry are routinely monitored before performing the block. Resuscitation equipment and emergency medications must be immediately available and ready to use. Supplemental oxygen via face mask is routinely used before giving sedation. A standard regional anesthesia tray is prepared with the following equipment:

- Sterile towels and 4-in. × 4-in. gauze packs
- 20-mL syringe with local anesthetic
- Sterile gloves, marking pen, and surface electrode
- One 1.5 -in., 25-gauge needle for skin infiltration
- A 10-cm long, short-bevel, insulated stimulating needle (15 cm for anterior approach)
- Peripheral nerve stimulator
- Injection pressure monitor

Interpreting Responses to Nerve Stimulation

Twitches of the hamstrings, calf, foot, or toes at 0.3–0.5 mA current all can be used as signs of successful localization of the sciatic plexus (nerve). Table 82D–3 presents common responses to nerve stimulation and the course of action to take to obtain the proper response.[19]

BLOCK DYNAMICS AND PERIOPERATIVE MANAGEMENT

Sciatic nerve block may cause patient discomfort because the needle passes through the gluteus muscles. Adequate sedation and analgesia are important to ensure patient comfort. Midazolam 2–4 mg can be given for patient positioning, and

TABLE 82D–3. Common responses to nerve stimulation and action to take.

Response Obtained	Interpretation	Problem	Action
Local twitch of the gluteus muscle	Direct stimulation of the gluteus muscle	Too shallow (superficial) placement of the needle	Continue advancing the needle
Needle contacts bone but local twitch of the gluteus muscle not elicited	Needle inserted close to the caudal aspect of the iliac bone or the lateral aspect of the sacrum	Too superior or too medial needle insertion	Slightly laterally and caudally redirect the needle
Needle encounters bone and sciatic twitches elicited	Needle missed the plane of the sciatic nerve and is stopped by the hip joint or ischial bone	Needle inserted too laterally (hip joint) or medially (ischial bone)	Withdraw the needle and redirect slightly medially or laterally (5–10 degrees)
Hamstring twitch	Stimulation of the main trunk of the sciatic nerve	None. These branches are within the sciatic nerve sheath at this level	Accept and inject local anesthetic
The needle placed deep (10 cm) but no twitches elicited and no bone contact	Needle has passed through the sciatic notch	Too inferior needle placement	Withdraw and redirect the needle slightly laterally, or cephalad
Paresthesia of the genital organs	Needle is stimulating the inferior roots of the sacral plexus (pudendal nerve)	Too inferior and too medial needle placement	Withdraw and redirect the needle slightly cephalad and laterally

alfentanil 500–750 mcg is given just before needle insertion. A typical onset time for this block is 10–25 minutes, depending on the type, concentration, and volume of local anesthetic used. The first signs of block onset are usually reported by the patient as a feeling that the foot is "different" or that they cannot wiggle their toes.

Clinical Pearl

- Inadequate skin anesthesia despite an apparent timely onset of the blockade can occur. Local infiltration at the site of the incision by the surgeon is often all that is needed to allow the surgery to proceed.

POSTERIOR APPROACHES TO SCIATIC NERVE BLOCK

General Considerations

The posterior approach to sciatic block has wide clinical applicability for surgery and pain management of the lower extremity. The block require expertise with more basic nerve blocks for successful and safe practice.[20,21] It is particularly well suited for surgery on the knee, calf, Achilles tendon, ankle, and foot. It provides complete anesthesia of the leg below the knee with the exception of the medial strip of skin, which is innervated by the saphenous nerve (Figure 82D–6). When combined with a femoral nerve or lumbar plexus block, anesthesia of almost the entire leg can be achieved.

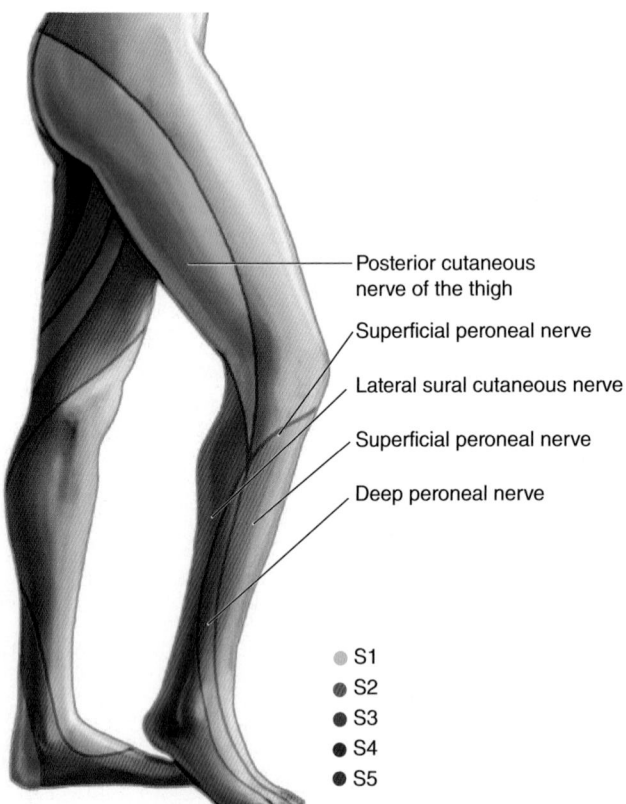

Posterior cutaneous nerve of the thigh

Superficial peroneal nerve

Lateral sural cutaneous nerve

Superficial peroneal nerve

Deep peroneal nerve

- S1
- S2
- S3
- S4
- S5

FIGURE 82D–6. Sciatic nerve. Cutaneous innervation.

Distribution of Anesthesia

Sciatic nerve block results in anesthesia of the skin of the posterior aspect of the thigh, hamstrings, and biceps muscles, part of the hip and knee joints, and the entire leg below the knee, with the exception of the skin of the medial aspect of the lower leg (see Figure 82D–6). Depending on the level of surgery, the addition of a saphenous or femoral nerve block may be required.

Classic Posterior Approach
Anatomic Landmarks

Landmarks for the posterior approach to sciatic blockade are easily identified in most patients (Figure 82D–7A, B). Proper palpation technique is of utmost importance because the adipose tissue over the gluteal area may obscure these bony prominences. The landmarks are outlined by a marking pen:

1. Greater trochanter
2. Posterior superior iliac spine
3. Needle insertion site 4 cm distal to the midpoint between the two landmarks

Technique

The patient is in the lateral decubitus position with a slight forward tilt–this prevents the "sag" of the soft tissues in the gluteal area and significantly facilitates block placement. The foot on the side to be blocked should be positioned over the dependent leg so that twitches of the foot or toes can be easily noted. After cleaning with an antiseptic solution, local anesthetic is infiltrated subcutaneously at the determined needle insertion site.

Clinical Pearl

- Raise the height of the bed enough and assume an ergonomic position to allow a comfortable and stable position for the patient during block placement and for observation of the motor responses to nerve stimulation.

The fingers of the palpating hand should be firmly pressed on the gluteus muscle to decrease the skin–nerve distance (Figure 82D–8). The palpating hand should not be moved during block placement; even small movements of the palpating hand can substantially change the position of the needle insertion site because the skin and soft tissues in the gluteal region are highly mobile. The needle is introduced at an angle perpendicular to the spherical skin plane (Figure 82D–8A and B). The nerve stimulator should be initially set to deliver 1.0–1.5 mA current (2 Hz, 100 μsec) to allow detection of twitches of the gluteal muscles and stimulation of the sciatic nerve.

As the needle is advanced, the first twitches observed are from the gluteal muscles. These twitches merely indicate that the needle position is still too shallow. The goal is to achieve

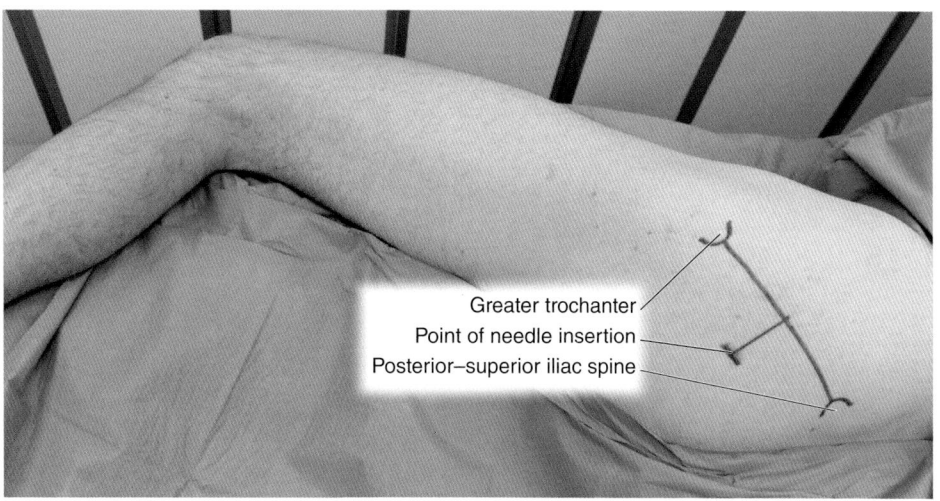

FIGURE 82D–7. Sciatic nerve block, posterior approach.

visible or palpable twitches of the hamstrings, calf muscles, foot, or toes at 0.3–0.5 mA current. Twitches of the hamstrings are equally acceptable because this approach blocks the nerve proximal to the separation of the neuronal branches to the hamstrings muscle. Once the gluteal twitches disappear, brisk response of the sciatic nerve to stimulation is observed (hamstrings, calf, foot, or toe twitches). After the initial stimulation of the sciatic nerve is obtained, the stimulating current is gradually decreased until twitches are still seen or felt at 0.3–0.5 mA current. This typically occurs at a depth of 5–8 cm.

After negative aspiration for blood, 15–25 mL of local anesthetic is injected (Figure 82D–9). Any resistance to the injection of local anesthetic should prompt needle withdrawal by 1 mm. The injection is then reattempted. Persistent resistance to injections should prompt complete needle withdrawal and ensuring needle patency before reintroduction.

Clinical Pearls

- Since the level of the blockade with this approach is above the departure of the branches for hamstring muscles, twitch of any of the hamstring muscles can be accepted as a reliable sign of localization of the sciatic nerve without deliberately seeking foot response.
- When the first needle pass does not result in nerve localization, do not regard it as a failure. Instead, use a systematic approach to troubleshooting:
- Ascertain the nerve stimulator is functional, properly connected, and set to deliver the desired current.
- Mentally visualize the plane of the initial needle insertion, and redirect the needle in a slightly caudal direction (5–10 degrees) to the initial insertion plane.
- If the above maneuver fails, withdraw the needle to the skin and redirect it slightly cephalad (5–10 degrees) to the initial insertion plane.
- Failure to obtain hamstrings or foot response to nerve stimulation should prompt a reassessment of the landmarks and patient position.

Continuous Block

The continuous sciatic nerve block is an advanced regional anesthesia technique, and experience with the single-shot technique is recommended to ensure its efficacy and safety. Continuous sciatic nerve block was described by Gross in 1956.[22] The current technique used is similar to the single-shot injection; however, slight angulation of the needle in the caudal direction is necessary to facilitate threading of the catheter. Securing and maintenance of the catheter are easy and convenient. This technique can be used for surgery and postoperative pain management in patients undergoing a wide variety of lower leg, foot, and ankle surgeries. Perhaps the single most important indication for use of this block is for amputation of the lower extremity.

Technique

Patient positioning, marking of landmarks, skin preparation and local anesthetic infiltration are performed as described above. An 8–10 cm long, insulated stimulating needle (preferably Tuohy-style tip) is inserted in the same manner as for the single-injection technique. The opening of the needle should face distally (pointing toward the patient's foot) to facilitate catheter insertion.

Clinical Pearls

- When insertion of the catheter proves difficult, lowering the angle of the needle can be helpful.
- It is useful to inject some local anesthetic intramuscularly to prevent pain on advancement of larger gauge and blunt-tipped needles typically used for this block.

After obtaining the motor response at a current of 0.3–0.5 mA, a 20-mL bolus of local anesthetic is injected. This is followed by insertion of the catheter 5 cm beyond the needle tip (Figure 82D–10). The catheter is then aspirated to check for inadvertent intravascular placement.

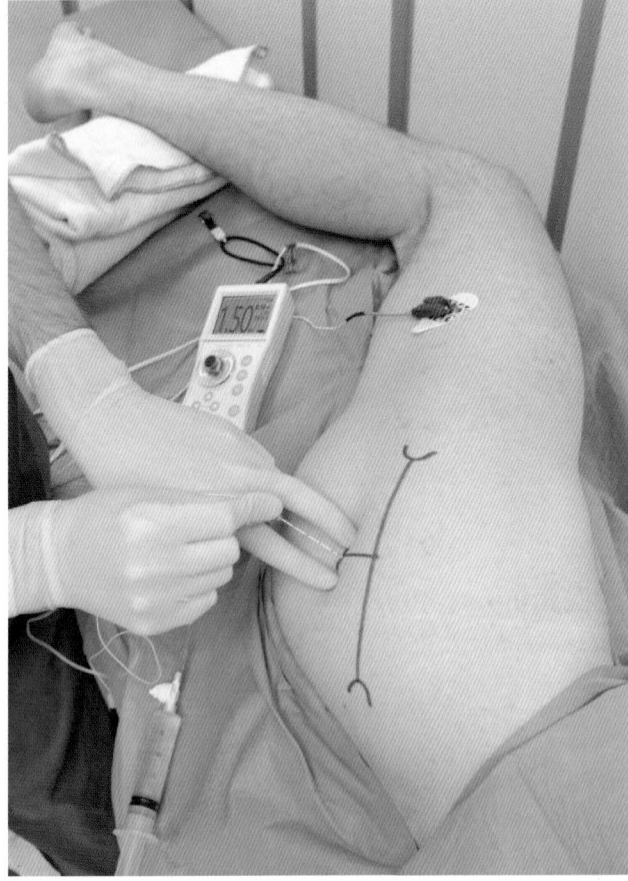

A

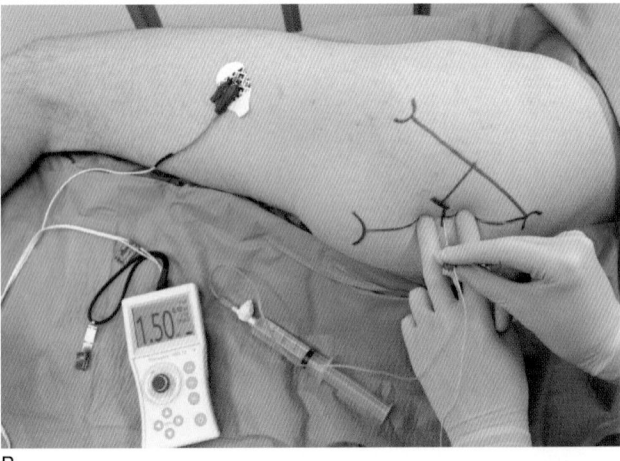

B

FIGURE 82D-8. A and B. Sciatic nerve block, posterior approach. Needle insertion is in the perpendicular plane; the palpating hand is firmly pressed to decrease the skin–nerve distance and stabilize the anatomy.

A number of techniques to secure the catheter to the skin have been proposed. A benzoin skin preparation followed by application of a clear dressing and a cloth tape is one such simple and efficacious method. The infusion port should be clearly marked as "continuous sciatic block."

Continuous Infusion

Continuous infusion is always initiated after an initial bolus of dilute local anesthetic through the catheter. Ropivacaine 0.2%

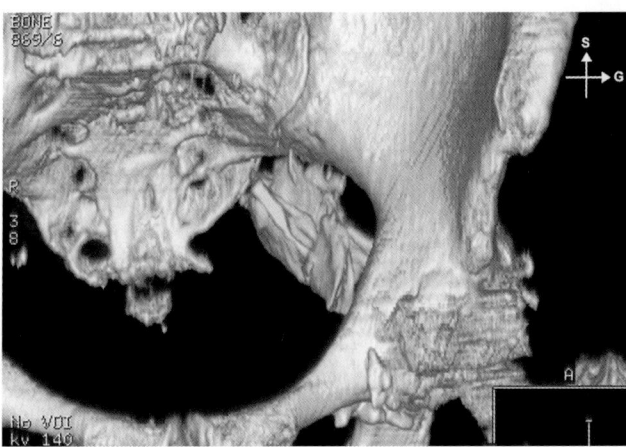

FIGURE 82D-9. Sciatic nerve block, posterior approach. Dispersion of the local anesthetic after injection.

is commonly used for this purpose (15–20 mL). Diluted solutions of bupivacaine or L-bupivacaine are also suitable, but can result in undesirably greater motor blockade. The infusion is initiated at 10 mL/h or 5 mL/h when a patient-controlled analgesia (PCA) dose is planned (5 mL).[23,24]

Parasacral Approach

Described by Mansour in 1993, the parasacral sciatic nerve block is well suited for continuous infusion of local anesthetic.[9,25–30] In addition, this block has characteristics of a

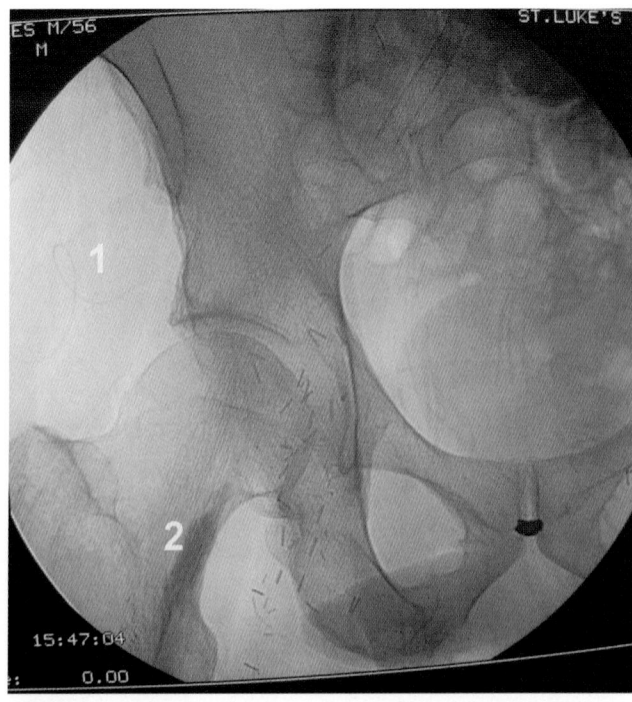

FIGURE 82D-10. Continuous sciatic nerve block, posterior approach. Shown is the course of the catheter (*1*) and the fusiform-shaped contrast area indicating the spread of the local anesthetic in the sheath of the sciatic nerve (*2*). In this example, a mere 2 mL of the local anesthetic is injected.

plexus block and yields anesthesia of the entire sacral plexus, and obturator nerve.[26,2731] Ripart[25] reported a 94% success rate in his series of 400 parasacral sciatic nerve block cases.

The parasacral approach to sciatic blockade has a wide clinical applicability for surgery and pain management of the lower extremity, particularly when combined with a femoral or psoas compartment block.[26,31] This technique is associated with a high success rate and is particularly well suited for surgery on the popliteal fossa and the knee.[32]

Distribution of Anesthesia

Parasacral sciatic nerve blockade results in anesthesia of the skin of the posterior thigh, hamstrings, and biceps femoris muscles; part of the hip and knee joint; and the entire leg below the knee except the medial cutaneous skin of the lower leg (see Figure 82D–6). Morris[26] demonstrated extension of anesthesia to the obturator nerve after sciatic nerve block, as tested by the presence of adductor muscle weakness on a numeric scale. Jochum however,[32] suggested that the obturator nerve is sporadically affected by the parasacral sciatic nerve block.

Anatomic Landmarks

Landmarks for the parasacral approach to sciatic blockade are easily identified in most patients (Figure 82D–11). Careful palpation technique is important because the adipose tissue over the gluteal area may obscure these bony prominences (Figures 82D–12 and 82D–13). The following landmarks are outlined by a marking pen:

- Posterior–superior iliac spine (PSIS)
- Ischial tuberosity (IT)
- A line between the PSIS and the IT is drawn. The needle insertion point lies 6 cm caudad to the PSIS on this line. The insulated needle is inserted at this point and advanced in a sagittal plane.

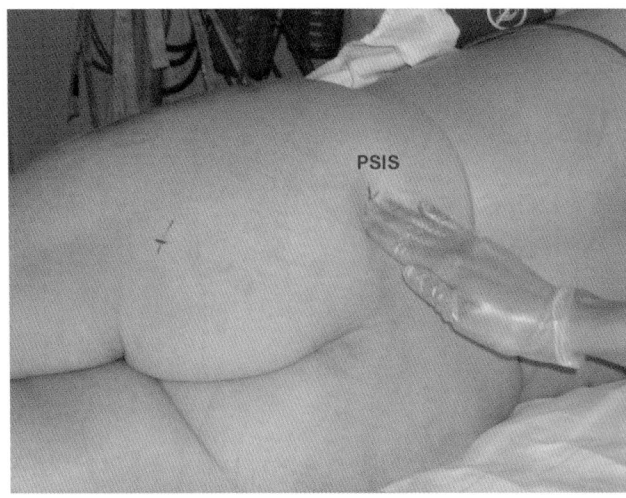

FIGURE 82D–12. Parasacral sciatic nerve block. Palpation technique to identify posterior superior iliac spine (PSIS).

Technique

The patient is positioned in a lateral decubitus position, similar to the position required for the classic posterior approach to sciatic block (Figure 82D–13). The dependent limb is kept straight while the limb to be blocked is flexed at both the hip and knee. Appropriate sedation and analgesia are mandatory to ensure the patient's comfort throughout the procedure. After cleaning with an antiseptic solution, local anesthetic is infiltrated subcutaneously at the determined needle insertion site.

- Contact with the bone usually indicates the needle contact with the wings of the sacrum or the iliac bone, superior to and near the greater sciatic notch.
- In this case, the needle is withdrawn and redirected slightly caudally and laterally.
- Contact with the bone can be used as a depth test. The needle depth is noted; the needle should not be advanced

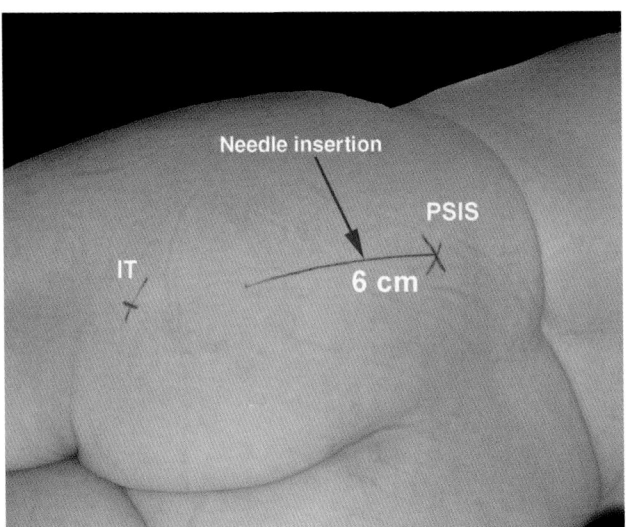

FIGURE 82D–11. Parasacral approach to sciatic nerve block. Shown are the posterior superior iliac spine (PSIS) and the ischial tuberosity (IT). The needle insertion site is marked as 6 cm caudad to the PSIS on the line connecting PSIS with IT.

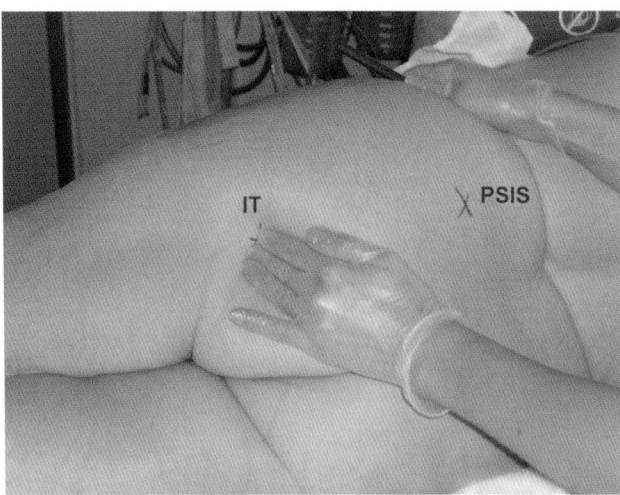

FIGURE 82D–13. Parasacral sciatic nerve block. Proper palpation technique to identify the ischial tuberosity. (IT, ischial tuberosity; PSIS, posterior superior iliac spine.)

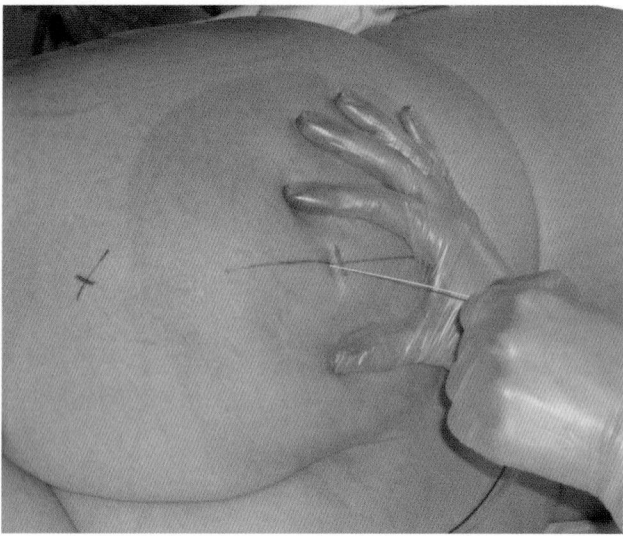

FIGURE 82D–14. Parasacral sciatic nerve block. Needle insertion is perpendicular to the horizontal plane.

more than 2 cm beyond this depth. At this site, the sciatic nerve is approached at the top of the greater sciatic foramen while leaving the pelvis. Advancing the needle deeper may expose pelvic viscera and vessels to risk of injury.

The needle is inserted perpendicular to the skin and advanced slowly (Figure 82D–14). The motor response of the sciatic plexus is usually obtained at a depth between 6 and 8 cm. The goal is to achieve visible or palpable twitches of the hamstrings, calf muscles, foot, or toes at the current intensity of 0.3–0.5 mA. The distal motor response may be either a tibial or a peroneal response—it is not necessary to stimulate both components (Figure 82D–15).[33,34] Twitches of the hamstrings are equally acceptable because this approach blocks the sciatic

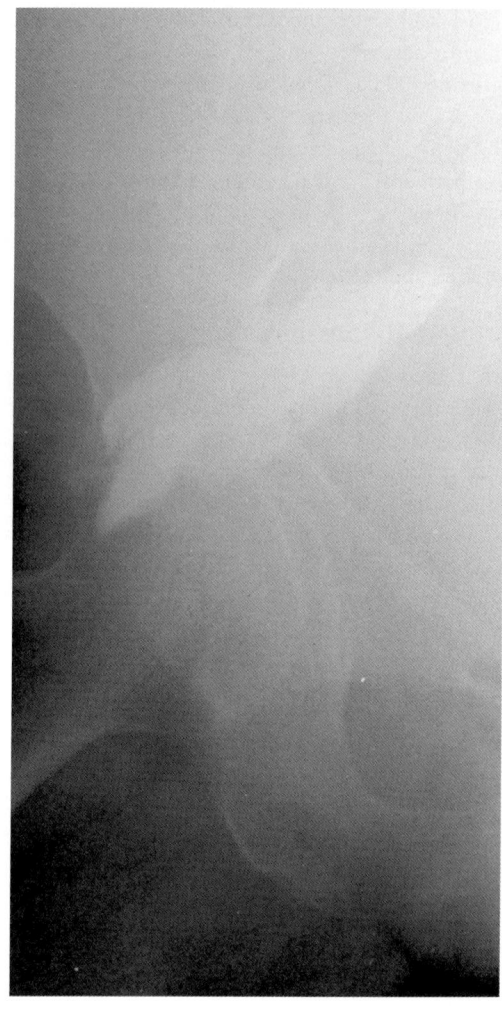

FIGURE 82D–16. Parasacral nerve block: dispersion of the contrast after injection, the "negative" contrast sign, and a typical fusiform distribution of the injectate.

nerve proximal to the separation of the neuronal branches to the hamstring muscles.

Once an appropriate response is obtained, 20-25 mL of local anesthetic is injected slowly with intermittent aspiration (Figure 82D–16).

Cuvillon et al.[8] compared the parasacral sciatic nerve block with Winnie's approach with one or two stimulations. Winnie's approach using the double-injection technique required more time to perform the block compared with Winnie's single-injection technique and the parasacral method. Although the onset of sensory and motor blocks were significantly faster with the double-injection method, the additional time needed to perform the double-injection block eliminated the advantage of the faster onset.

Continuous Parasacral Sciatic Nerve Block

The continuous parasacral sciatic nerve block is similar to the single-shot injection; however, slight caudal angulation of the needle is necessary to facilitate threading of the catheter. Securing and maintenance of the catheter are easy and convenient.[36] This technique can be used for surgery and postoperative pain

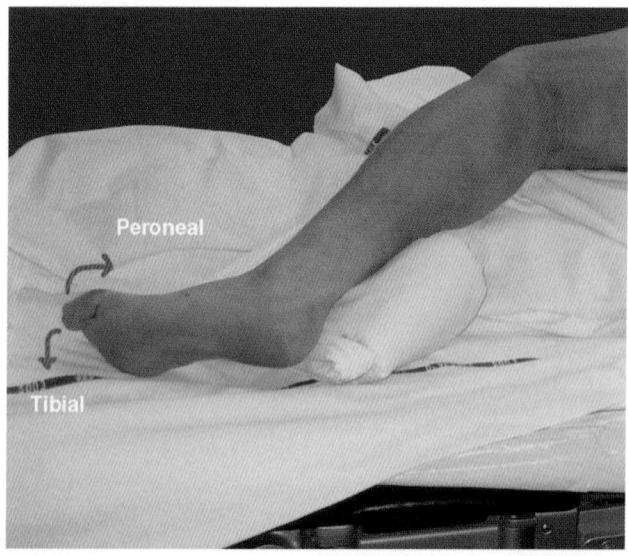

FIGURE 82D–15. Sciatic nerve stimulation: motor response of the common peroneal and tibial nerves indicate proper localization of the sciatic nerve.

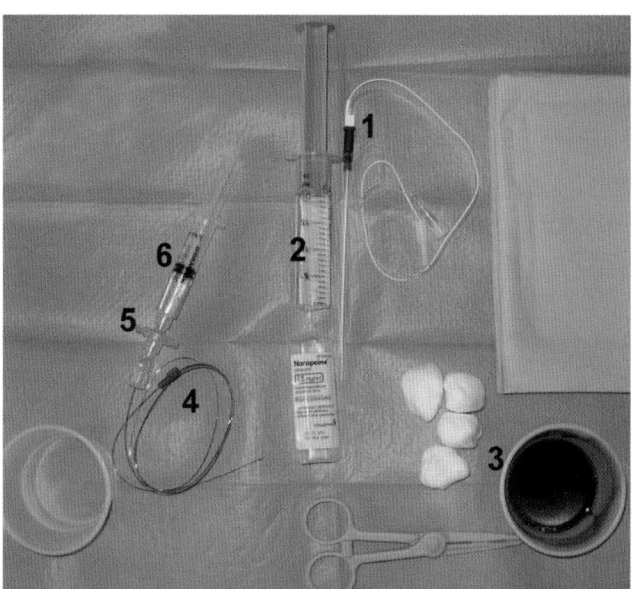

FIGURE 82D–17. Equipment for continuous sciatic block.

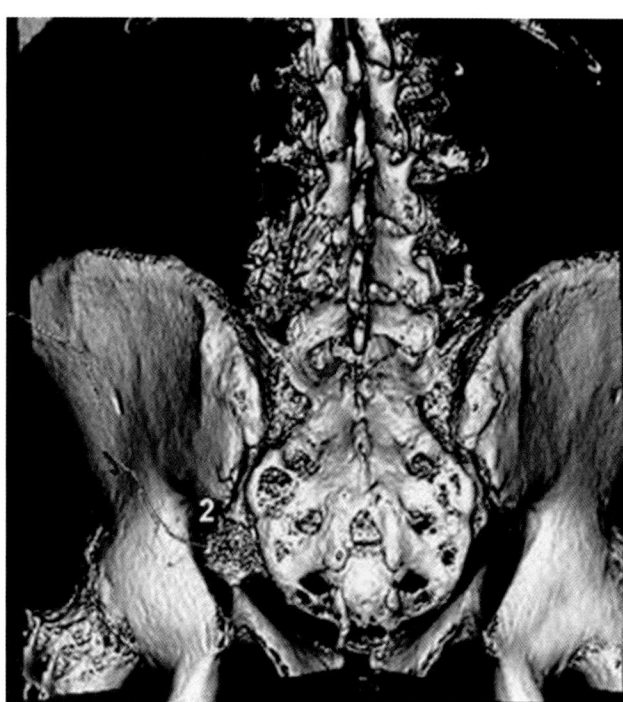

FIGURE 82D–18. Parasacral sciatic block: shown is the course of the catheter and visualization of the injectate around the sciatic nerve.

management in patients undergoing a wide variety of knee, lower leg, foot, and ankle surgeries.

The technique is identical to the single injection technique, except a continuous-block needle is used (Figure 82D–17). The opening of the needle should face distally to facilitate catheter insertion.[37] The initial intensity of the stimulating current should be 1.0–1.5 mA.

Clinical Pearl

- It is useful to inject some local anesthetic intramuscularly to decrease pain during placement of the continuous nerve block needle.

After obtaining the motor response at 0.3–0.5 mA, a 20 mL bolus of local anesthetic is injected and the catheter inserted 3-5 cm beyond the needle tip. If confirmation of catheter placement is desired, contrast media can be injected through the catheter and radiographic images can be studied.[31] The presence of a spindle 2–3 cm in length with an oblique orientation crossing the sciatic notch on the anteroposterior radiograph and/or shadowing of the sacral roots are considered to indicate injection into the correct plane and adequate placement of the catheter (see Figure 82D–18). After securing the catheter, an infusion (e.g., ropivacaine 0.2% at 5 mL/hr with 5 mL/q60min patient-controlled bolus) is initiated.

ALTERNATIVE POSTERIOR APPROACHES

Di Benedetto[38] described a subgluteal approach to the sciatic nerve block in 2002. This technique is a good alternative to the more proximal approaches to the sciatic nerve, with the potential for reducing the discomfort experienced by the patient during block placement. The landmarks with the subgluteal approach are the greater trochanter of the femur, the ischial tuberosity, and a line between the two with the midpoint marked. From the midpoint, another line is drawn perpendicularly and extended 4 cm in the caudal direction to identify the needle insertion point. A 20-gauge, 10-cm needle and nerve stimulator are used for this approach, and 20 mL of local anesthetic is injected when twitches of the sciatic nerve are obtained at ≤0.5 mA current.

Of note, ultrasound-guided subgluteal approach to sciatic block has become one of the most common sciatic nerve block techniques in modern regional anesthesia. Traditional approaches to the sciatic nerve at the pelvic level require identification of pelvic bone structures. Although the size of the buttocks is variable among different individuals and in the same individual over time, the relation of the sciatic nerve to the pelvis is constant throughout life. Using this premise, Franco has suggested a more simplified approach to the sciatic nerve block that does not require palpation of deep bony structures. The landmarks with this approach are the midline of the intergluteal sulcus, and a point 10 cm lateral to the midline of the intergluteal sulcus where the block needle will be inserted. The curvature of the buttocks is disregarded when locating the needle insertion point. Care must be taken not to stretch the soft tissues when marking the needle insertion site as subsequent recoil of the tissues will occur, causing the distance to the nerve to be underestimated. The patient is either in the prone or lateral position and the needle is inserted parallel to the midline.[39]

Complications in Posterior Approaches and How to Avoid Them

Table 82D–4 lists instructions on possible complications of sciatic nerve blockade and methods to decrease the risk.

TABLE 82D–4. Complications and how to avoid them.

Infection	Use strict aseptic technique
Hematoma	Avoid multiple needle insertions, particularly in anticoagulated patients
Vascular puncture	Avoid deep needle insertion (pelvic vessels)
Local anesthetic toxicity	Avoid using large volumes and doses of local anesthetic owing to the proximity of the large vessels and the potential for rapid absorption
	Injection of local anesthetic should be carried out slowly and with frequent aspiration to rule out intravascular injection
Nerve injury	Sciatic nerve has a unique predisposition for mechanical and pressure injury
	Use nerve stimulation and slow needle advancement
	Never inject local anesthesia when the patient complains of pain or when abnormally high pressure on injection is noted
	Never assume that the needle is obstructed with tissue debris when resistance to injection is met
	When stimulation is obtained with a current intensity of <0.2 mA, withdraw the needle slightly to obtain the same response with a current intensity of >0.2 mA before injecting local anesthetic
Nerve injury	Advance the needle slowly when twitches of the gluteus muscle cease to avoid impaling the sciatic nerve on a rapidly advancing needle
Other	Instruct the patient and nursing staff on the care of the insensate extremity
	Explain the need for frequent body repositioning to avoid stretching and prolonged ischemia (sitting) on the anesthetized sciatic nerve
	Advise heel padding during prolonged bed rest or sleep to prevent pressure sores from developing
Perforation of pelvic organs	Directing the needle medially should be exercised with this complication in mind
Anesthesia of the pudendal nerve	The pudendal nerve, a branch of the sacral plexus, may be anesthetized by the parasacral nerve block owing to diffusion of the injected local anesthesia
	Inform patients that this problem is transient
Tourniquet	Injection of the local anesthetic within the sciatic nerve sheath, epinephrine, and a tourniquet over the site of injection all can combine to cause ischemia of the sciatic nerve

ANTERIOR APPROACH

General Considerations

The anterior approach to a sciatic block is an advanced nerve block technique. The block is suited for surgery on the leg below the knee, particularly on the ankle and foot. It provides complete anesthesia of the leg below the knee with the exception of the medial strip of skin innervated by the saphenous nerve (Figure 82D–19). When combined with a femoral nerve block, anesthesia of the entire knee and lower leg is achieved.[40] The anterior approach is much less clinically applicable than posterior approaches because the distribution of anesthesia is more limited and a higher level of skill is required. In addition, this technique is not suitable for catheter insertion because of the deep location and perpendicular angle of needle insertion required to reach the sciatic nerve. Consequently, this block is best reserved for patients who cannot easily be moved to the lateral position needed for the posterior approach; e.g., patients with spinal injuries or under general anesthesia.[41,42]

Since the original description by Beck[5] several clinicians have attempted to devise more reliable landmarks and technique for this block. However, all described approaches derive the needle insertion site at nearly identical points regardless of whether they use bony prominences, soft tissue, or femoral artery as landmarks.[40,43–47] In addition, even if these different approaches varied slightly in the site of needle insertion, the long path by the needle required to reach the sciatic nerve (8–12 cm) and the tendency of long, blunt-tipped needles to bend on insertion through the tissues make any such differences meaningless when it comes to increasing the precision of the technique.

Equipment

A standard regional anesthesia tray is prepared with the following equipment:

- Sterile towels and 4-in.× 4-in. gauze packs
- 20-mL syringes with local anesthetic

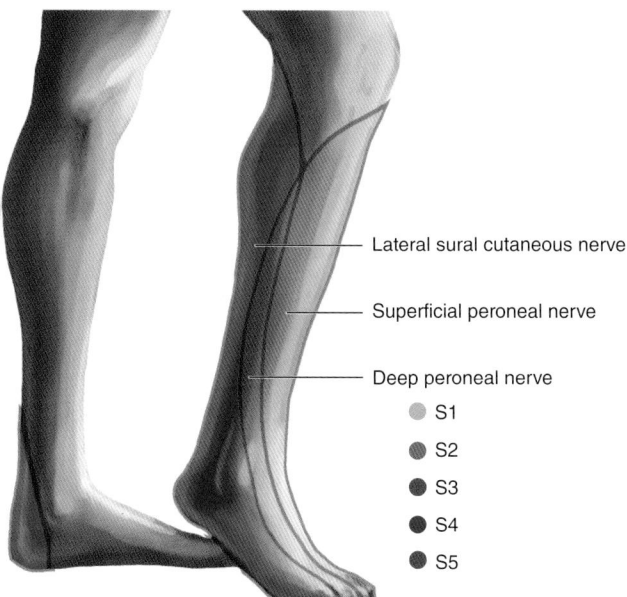

FIGURE 82D–19. Distribution of anesthesia with anterior approach to sciatic nerve block.

- Sterile gloves, marking pen, and surface electrode
- One 1.5-in., 25-gauge needle for skin infiltration
- A 15-cm long, short-bevel, insulated stimulating needle
- Peripheral nerve stimulator

Anatomic Landmarks

The following landmarks should routinely be outlined using a marking pen (Figure 82D–20):

1. Femoral crease
2. Femoral artery pulse
3. Needle insertion point marked 4–5 cm distally on the line passing through the pulse of the femoral artery and perpendicular to the femoral crease

Technique

The leg is fully extended on the table with the patient in the supine position. After cleaning the area with an antiseptic solution, local anesthetic is infiltrated subcutaneously at the needle insertion site. The fingers of the palpating hand should be firmly pressed against the quadriceps muscle to decrease the skin–nerve distance. The block needle (connected to a nerve stimulator set to deliver a current of 1.5 mA) is introduced at a perpendicular angle to the skin plane (Figure 82D–21). Motor response of the sciatic nerve is typically obtained at a depth of 8–12 cm. Acceptable responses are visible or palpable twitches of the calf muscles, foot, or toes at a current of 0.3–0.5 mA. After negative aspiration for blood, 20 mL of local anesthetic is slowly injected. If high injection pressure is detected, the needle should be withdrawn by 1 mm and injection attempted again. If high injection pressure persists, the needle should be withdrawn and flushed prior to further attempts.

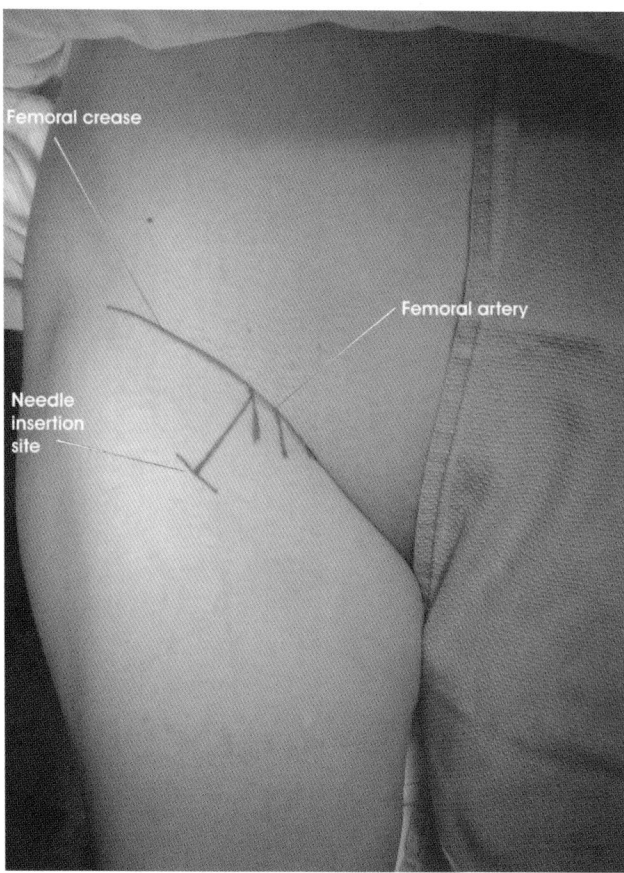

FIGURE 82D–20. Sciatic nerve block through the anterior approach.

Clinical Pearls

- Local twitches of the quadriceps muscle are often elicited during needle advancement. The needle should be advanced past these twitches.
- Although there is a concern of femoral nerve injury with further needle advancement, at this level, the femoral nerve is divided into smaller terminal branches that are movable and unlikely to be penetrated by a slowly advancing, blunt-tipped needle.
- Resting the patient's heel on the bed surface may prevent the foot from twitching even when the sciatic nerve is stimulated. This can be prevented by placing the ankle on a footrest or by having an assistant continuously palpate the calf or Achilles tendon.
- Because branches to the hamstring muscle may depart the main trunk of the sciatic nerve at the level of needle insertion, twitches of the hamstrings should not be accepted as a reliable sign of sciatic nerve localization.

Bone contact is frequently encountered during needle advancement. This indicates that the needle has contacted the femur (usually lesser trochanter). In this case, the foot is first rotated laterally, which should swing the lesser trochanter out of the path of the needle and allow deeper advancement of the

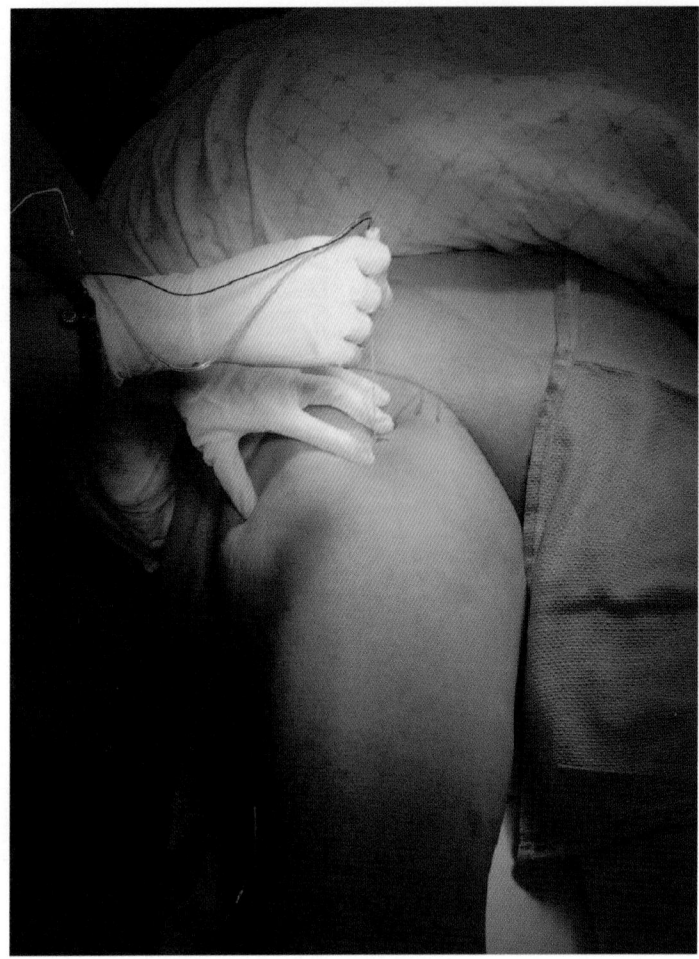

FIGURE 82D–21. Sciatic nerve block through the anterior approach. Needle insertion.

TABLE 82D–5. Interpreting responses to nerve stimulation.

Response Obtained	Interpretation	Problem	Action
Twitch of the quadriceps muscle (patella twitch)	Common; stimulation of the branches of the femoral nerve	Too shallow (superficial) placement of needle	Continue advancing the needle
Local twitch at the femoral crease area	Direct stimulation of the iliopsoas or pectineus muscles	Too superior insertion of needle	Stop the procedure and reassess the landmarks
Hamstring twitch	Needle may be stimulating branch(es) of the sciatic nerve to the hamstring muscle; direct stimulation of the hamstrings with higher current is also possible	Unreliable-difficult to determine whether the needle is in the proximity of the sciatic nerve	Withdraw the needle and redirect slightly medially or laterally (5–10 degrees)
The needle is placed deep (12–15 cm) but twitches were not elicited and bone is not contacted	The needle is likely too medial		Withdraw and redirect slightly laterally
Twitches of the calf, foot, or toes	Stimulation of the sciatic nerve	None	Accept and inject local anesthetic

needle and nerve localization. If this maneuver fails, the needle is redirected slightly medially or reinserted more medially. Table 82D–5 lists some common responses to nerve stimulation and the course of action to take to obtain the proper response.

SUMMARY

Although the sciatic nerve block was described in 1920, many practitioners avoided this block because of its perceived complexity. Sciatic nerve block is an important technique for the regional anesthesiologist to master because the combination of this block and a femoral nerve block or lumbar plexus block can anesthetize almost the entire leg. Although the posterior sciatic nerve block has an intermediate level of difficulty, with practice and knowledge of anatomy, high success rates can be achieved. Many approaches have been proposed; the most relevant have been presented in this chapter. Finally, nearly all described approaches are similar in clinical efficacy; therefore, learning one single approach well is recommended as this would suffice for most clinical indications.

REFERENCES

1. Sherwood-Dunn B: *Regional Anesthesia: (Victor Pauchet's Technique)*. Philadelphia, PA: Davis, 1921.
2. Labat G: *Regional Anesthesia: Its Technic and Clinical Application*. Philadelphia, PA: Saunders, 1924.
3. Côté AV, Vachon CA, Horlocker TT: From Victor Pauchet to Gaston Labat: The Transformation of Regional Anesthesia from a Surgeon's Practice to the Physician Anesthesiologist. Anesth Analg 2003;96(4):1193-1200.
4. Winnie AP: Regional anesthesia. Surg Clin North Am 1975;55:861–892.
5. Beck GP: Anterior approach to sciatic nerve block. Anesthesiology 1963;24:222–224.
6. Raj PP, Parks RI, Watson TD, Jenkins MT: A new single-position supine approach to sciatic-femoral nerve block. Anesth Analg 1975;54:489–493.
7. di Benedetto P, Bertini L, Casati A, et al: A new posterior approach to the sciatic nerve block: a prospective, randomized comparison with the classic posterior approach. Anesth Analg 2001;93:1040–1044.
8. Cuvillon P, Ripart J, Jeannes P, et al: Comparison of the parasacral approach and the posterior approach, with single- and double-injection techniques, to block the sciatic nerve. Anesthesiology 2003;98:1436–1441.
9. Mansour NY, Bennetts FE: An observational study of combined continuous lumbar plexus and single-shot sciatic nerve blocks for post-knee surgery analgesia. Reg Anesth 1996;21:287–291.
10. Babinski MA, Machado FA, Costa WS: A rare variation in the high division of the sciatic nerve surrounding the superior gemellus muscle. Eur J Morphol 2003;41:41–42.
11. Vloka JD, Hadzic A, April EW, et al: Division of the sciatic nerve in the popliteal fossa and its possible implications in the popliteal nerve blockade. Anesth Analg 2001;92:215–217.
12. Andersen HL, Andersen SL, Tranum-Jensen J: Injection inside the paraneural sheath of the sciatic nerve: direct comparison among ultrasound imaging, macroscopic anatomy, and histologic analysis. Reg Anesth Pain Med. 2012;37:410–413.
13. Vloka JD, Hadzić A, Lesser JB: A common epineural sheath for the nerves in the popliteal fossa and its possible implications for sciatic nerve block. Anesth Analg. 1997;84:387–390.
14. Franco CD: Connective tissues associated with peripheral nerves. Reg Anesth Pain Med. 2012;37:363–365.
15. Smith BE, Siggins D: Low volume, high concentration block of the sciatic nerve. Anaesthesia 1988;43:8–11.
16. Sinnott CJ, Strichartz GR: Levobupivacaine versus ropivacaine for sciatic nerve block in the rat. Reg Anesth Pain Med 2003;28:294–303.
17. Eledjam JJ, Ripart J, Viel E: Clinical application of ropivacaine for the lower extremity. Curr Top Med Chem 2001;1:227–231.
18. Casati A, Fanelli G, Borghi B, Torri G: Ropivacaine or 2% mepivacaine for lower limb peripheral nerve blocks. Study Group on Orthopedic Anesthesia of the Italian Society of Anesthesia, Analgesia, and Intensive Care. Anesthesiology 1999;90:1047–1152.
19. Hadzic A, Vloka J: *Peripheral Nerve Blocks: Principles and Practice*. New York, NY: McGraw-Hill, 2004.
20. Bruelle P, Muller L, Bassoul B, Eledjam JJ: Block of the sciatic nerve. Cah Anesthesiol 1994;42:785–791.
21. Dalens B, Tanguy A, Vanneuville G: Sciatic nerve blocks in children: comparison of the posterior, anterior, and lateral approaches in 180 pediatric patients. Anesth Analg 1990;70:131–137.
22. Gross G: Continuous sciatic nerve block. Br J Anaesth 1956;28:373–376.
23. Ilfeld BM, Thannikary LJ, Morey TE, et al: Popliteal sciatic perineural local anesthetic infusion: a comparison of three dosing regimens for postoperative analgesia. Anesthesiology 2004;101:970–977.
24. di Benedetto P, Casati A, Bertini L: Continuous subgluteus sciatic nerve block after orthopedic foot and ankle surgery: comparison of two infusion techniques. Reg Anesth Pain Med 2002;27:168–172.
25. Mansour NY: Reevaluating the sciatic nerve blocK: another landmark for consideration. Reg Anesth 1993;18:322–323.
26. Morris GF, Lang SA: Continuous parasacral sciatic nerve block: two case reports. Reg Anesth 1997;22:469–472.
27. Morris GF, Lang SA, Dust WN, Van der Wal M: The parasacral sciatic nerve block. Reg Anesth 1997;22:223–228.
28. Ripart J, Cuvillon P, Nouvellon E, et al: Parasacral approach to block the sciatic nerve: a 400-case survey. Reg Anesth Pain Med 2005;30:193–197.
29. Bertini L, Borghi B, Grossi P, et al: Continuous peripheral block in foot surgery. Minerva Anestesiol 2001;67:103–108.
30. di Benedetto P, Borghi B, Ricci A, van Oven H: Loco-regional anaesthesia of the lower limbs. Minerva Anestesiol 2001;67:56–64.
31. Ho AM, Karmakar MK: Combined paravertebral lumbar plexus and parasacral sciatic nerve block for reduction of hip fracture in a patient with severe aortic stenosis. Can J Anaesth 2002;49:946–950.
32. Jochum D, Iohom G, Choquet O, et al: Adding a selective obturator nerve block to the parasacral sciatic nerve block: an evaluation. Anesth Analg 2004;99:1544–1549.
33. Bailey SL, Parkinson SK, Little WL, Simmerman SR: Sciatic nerve block. A comparison of single versus double injection technique. Reg Anesth 1994;19:9–13.
34. Gaertner E, Lascurain P, Venet C, et al: Continuous parasacral sciatic block : a radiographic study. Anesth Analg 2004;98:831–834.
35. Bendtsen TF, Lönnqvist PA, Jepsen KV: Preliminary results of a new ultrasound-guided approach to block the sacral plexus: the parasacral parallel shift. Br J Anaesth. 2011;107:278–280.
36. Souron V, Eyrolle L, Rosencher N: The Mansour's sacral plexus block: an effective technique for continuous block. Reg Anesth Pain Med 2000;25:208–209.
37. Chelly J, Fanelli G, Casati A (eds): *Continuous Peripheral Nerve Blocks : an Illustrated Guide*. St. Louis, MO: Mosby, 2001.
38. di Benedetto P, Casati A, Bertini L, Fanelli G: Posterior subgluteal approach to block the sciatic nerve: description of the technique and initial clinical experiences. Eur J Anaesthesiol 2002;19:682–686.
39. Franco CD: Posterior approach to the sciatic nerve in adults: is euclidean geometry still necessary? Anesthesiology 2003;98:723–728.
40. Magora F, Pessachovitch B, Shoham I: Sciatic nerve block by the anterior approach for operations on the lower extremity. Br J Anaesth 1974;46:121–123.
41. McNicol LR: Anterior approach to sciatic nerve block in children: loss of resistance or nerve stimulator for identifying the neurovascular compartment. Anesth Analg 1987;66:1199–1200.
42. McNicol LR: Sciatic nerve block for children. Sciatic nerve block by the anterior approach for postoperative pain relief. Anaesthesia 1985;40:410–414.
43. Mansour NY: Anterior approach revisited and another new sciatic nerve block in the supine position. Reg Anesth 1993;18:265–266.
44. Chelly JE, Delaunay L: A new anterior approach to the sciatic nerve block. Anesthesiology 1999;91:1655–1660.
45. Vloka JD, Hadzic A, April E, Thys DM: Anterior approach to the sciatic nerve block: the effects of leg rotation. Anesth Analg 2001;92:460–462.
46. Van Elstraete AC, Poey C, Lebrun T, Pastureau F: New landmarks for the anterior approach to the sciatic nerve block: Imaging and clinical study. Anesth Analg 2002;95:214–218.
47. Hadzic A, Vloka JD: Anterior approach to sciatic nerve block. In: Hadzic A, Vloka J (eds): *Peripheral Nerve Blocks*. New York, NY: McGraw-Hill, 2004.

CHAPTER 82E

Block of the Sciatic Nerve in the Popliteal Fossa

Jerry D. Vloka and Admir Hadzic

INTRODUCTION

Distal sciatic nerve block (popliteal fossa block) is a very clinically valuable technique that results in anesthesia of the calf, tibia, fibula, ankle, and foot.[1-3] The sciatic nerve can be approached from either the posterior approach, described by Duane Keith Rorie,[3] or the lateral approach, described by Jerry Vloka.[1] Both approaches provide equivalent anesthesia and are suitable for catheter placement. Overall, however, the posterior approach is easier for trainees to learn.[1,2]

Popliteal fossa block performed with long-acting local anesthetics such as ropivacaine can provide 12–24 hours of analgesia after foot surgery.[3,4]

When used as a sole technique popliteal fossa block provides excellent anesthesia and postoperative analgesia, allows use of a calf tourniquet, and avoids the disadvantages of neuraxial blockade.[5]

Analgesia with popliteal fossa blocks lasts significantly longer than with ankle blocks. For instance, David H. McLeod found that lateral popliteal fossa block with 0.5% bupivacaine lasted 18 hours when compared with ankle block, which lasted only 6.2 hours.[6] Popliteal fossa block has also been used as an effective analgesic technique in children.[7] In a study of the efficacy of the popliteal sciatic nerve blockade (0.75 mL/kg of ropivacaine 0.2%) after foot and ankle surgery, 19 of 20 children required no analgesic agents during the first 8–12 hours postoperatively.

Indications and Contraindications

The popliteal block is one of the most commonly used techniques in regional anesthesia practice. Some common indications include corrective foot surgery, foot debridement, short saphenous vein stripping, repair of the Achilles tendon, and others.[8] As opposed to the more proximal block of the sciatic nerve,

popliteal fossa block anesthetizes the leg distal to the hamstring muscles, allowing patients to retain knee flexion.[9,10]

Functional Anatomy

The sciatic nerve consists of two separate nerve trunks: the tibial and common peroneal nerves. A common paraneural sheath envelops these two nerves from their origin in the pelvis, which is distinctly separate from the epineurium of each nerve.[11] Studies utilizing ultrasound imaging have shown that injecting local anesthetic within this sheath consistently gives a rapid onset, safe, and effective block.[12] This is not considered to be an intraneural injection as long as the epineurium of the individual nerves is not breached.[13,14] As the sciatic nerve descends toward the knee, the two components eventually diverge just proximal to the popliteal fossa, giving rise to the tibial and common peroneal nerves (Figure 82E–1). This division of the sciatic nerve usually occurs between 50 and 120 mm proximal to the popliteal fossa crease.[15,16] Following its divergence from the sciatic nerve, the common peroneal nerve continues its path laterally and descends along the head and neck of the fibula. Its major branches in this region are branches to the knee joint and cutaneous branches that form the sural nerve. Its terminal branches are the superficial and deep peroneal nerves. The tibial nerve is the larger of the two divisions of the sciatic nerve and continues its path vertically through the popliteal fossa. Its terminal branches are the medial and lateral plantar nerves. Its collateral branches give rise to the cutaneous sural nerves, muscular branches to the muscles to the calf, and articular branches to the ankle joint. The tibial nerve is enveloped by a well-defined paraneural sheath; consequently, a single injection of a large volume of local anesthetic into the sheath of the tibial nerve may carry a higher success rate than an injection into the sheath of the common peroneal nerve.[11] Note that in contrast to the

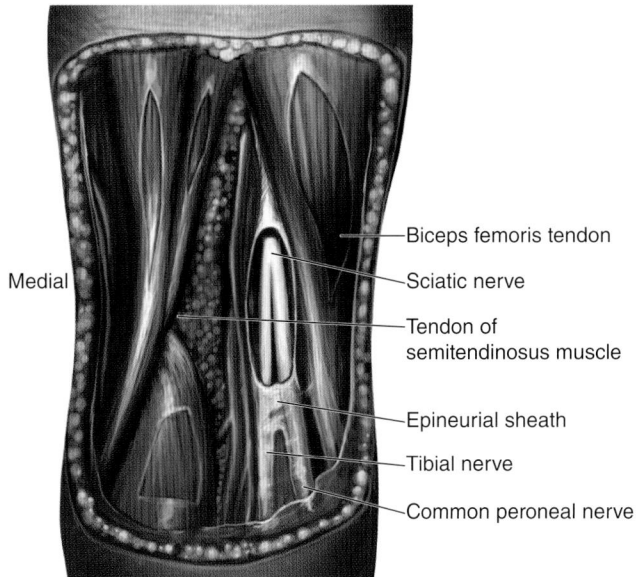

FIGURE 82E–1. Anatomy of the distal sciatic nerve. The sciatic nerve descends between the hamstring muscles and diverges as tibial and common peroneal nerves approximately at or below 7–8 cm above the popliteal fossa crease. A common epineural sheath that serves as a conduit for injected local anesthetic is shown dissected.

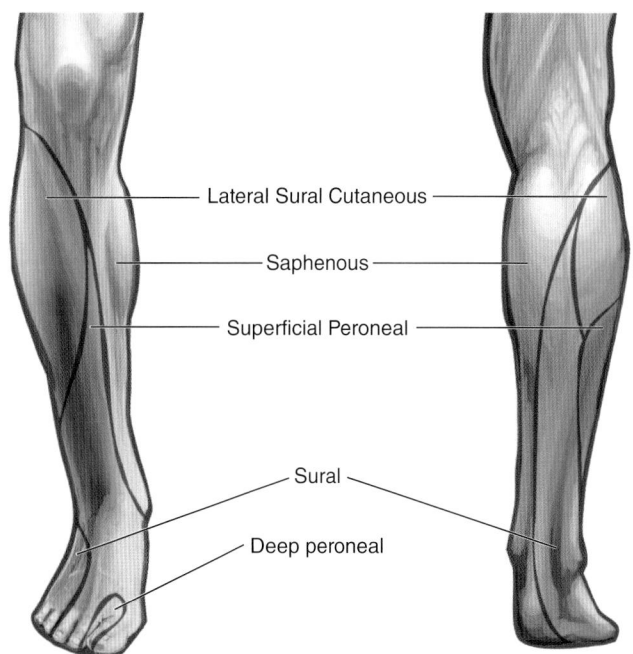

FIGURE 82E–2. Sensory distribution of anesthesia after popliteal blockade. Popliteal block results in anesthesia of all shaded areas except that of the saphenous nerve (femoral).

common assumption, the sciatic nerve is not enveloped by the same tissue sheath as are the popliteal vessels; consequently, the concept of the neurovascular sheath is not applicable to this block.[11] Instead, in the popliteal fossa, the sciatic nerve components are lateral and superficial to the popliteal artery and vein. This anatomic characteristic is important in understanding why vascular punctures and systemic toxicity are so rare after popliteal blockade.

Distribution of Anesthesia

Popliteal block results in anesthesia of the entire distal two thirds of the lower extremity, with the exception of the medial aspect of the leg[17] (Figure 82E–2). Cutaneous innervation of the medial leg below the knee is provided by the saphenous nerve, a superficial terminal extension of the femoral nerve. Depending on the location of surgery, the addition of a saphenous nerve block may be required. Saphenous nerve block is not generally required for patients to tolerate tourniquet pain below the knee because this pain is the result of pressure and ischemia of the deep muscle beds.

Choice of Local Anesthetic

Popliteal blockade requires a larger volume of local anesthetic (20 mL) to achieve anesthesia of both divisions of the nerve.[5] The choice of type, volume, and concentration of local anesthetic should be based on the patient's size and general condition and whether the block is planned for surgical anesthesia or pain management. The type and concentration of local anesthetics and the choice of additives to local anesthetic influence the onset and, particularly, the duration of the blockade (Table 82E–1).

TECHNIQUES

Intertendinous (Posterior) Approach

The patient is in the prone position.[18] The foot on the side to be blocked should be positioned so that even the slightest movement of the foot or toes can be easily observed. This is best achieved by allowing the foot to protrude off the edge of the bed.

Equipment

A standard regional anesthesia tray is prepared with the following equipment:

TABLE 82E–1. Local anesthetics choice for popliteal block.

	Onset (min)	Anesthesia (h)	Analgesia (h)
3% 2-Chloroprocaine	10–15	1	2
1.5% Mepivacaine	15–20	2–3	3–5
1.5% Mepivacaine epinephrine	15–20	2–5	3–8
2% Lidocaine epinephrine	10–20	2–5	3–8
0.5% Ropivacaine	15–30	4–8	5–12
0.75% Ropivacaine	10–15	5–10	6–24
0.5 (L) Bupivacaine	15–30	5–15	6–30

- Sterile towels and 4-in. × 4-in. gauze packs
- One 20-mL syringes with local anesthetic
- Sterile gloves, marking pen, and surface electrode
- One 1.5-in., 25-gauge needle for skin infiltration
- A 5-cm long, short-bevel, insulated stimulating needle
- Peripheral nerve stimulator
- Injection pressure monitor

Anatomic Landmarks

Landmarks for this approach are easily identified, even in obese patients (Figure 82E–3). The landmarks should be routinely outlined by a marking pen: (1) popliteal fossa crease, (2) tendon of biceps femoris (laterally), and (3) tendons of semitendinosus and semimembranosus (medially).

The needle insertion point is marked at 7 cm above the popliteal fossa crease at the midpoint between the tendons. This point is just above the sciatic nerve in the popliteal fossa in nearly two thirds of patients (Figure 82E–4).

Clinical Pearls

- Relying on tendons (rather than on subjective interpretation of the "popliteal fossa triangle" as described elsewhere) gives a much more precise and consistent localization of the popliteal nerve.

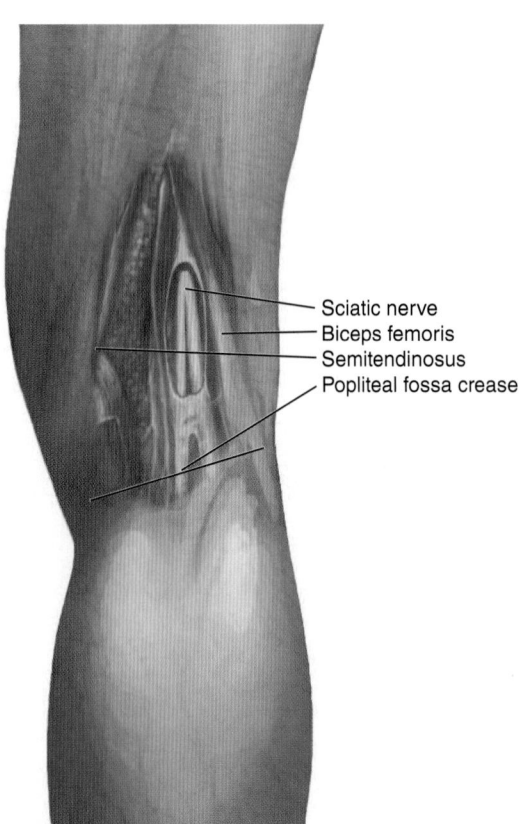

Sciatic nerve
Biceps femoris
Semitendinosus
Popliteal fossa crease

FIGURE 82E–3. Popliteal block. Landmarks for the intertendinous approach.

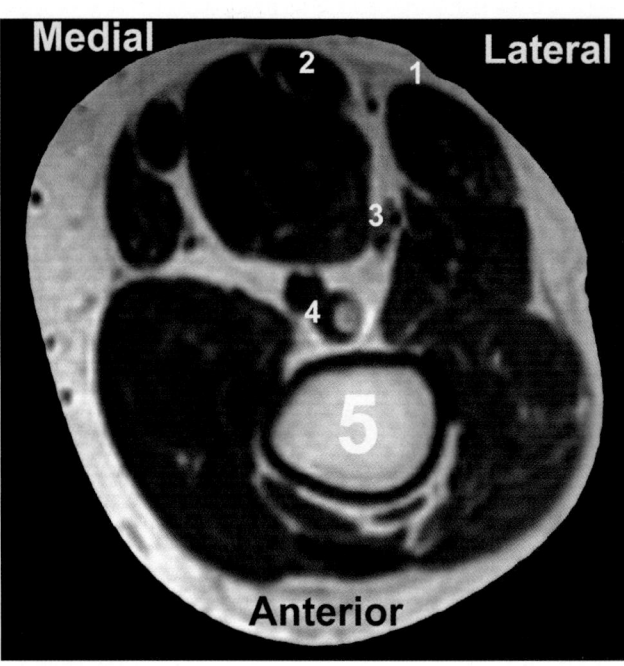

FIGURE 82E–4. Magnetic resonance image (MRI) of the popliteal fossa 7 cm above the popliteal fossa crease. *1*, Tendon of the biceps femoris muscle; *2*, tendon of the semitendinosus muscle; *3*, sciatic nerve in the popliteal fossa (shown are both components: the tibial nerve is positioned more anteriorly and medially, whereas the common peroneal nerve is more posterior and lateral); *4*, popliteal artery and vein; *5*, femur.

- The landmarks can be accentuated by asking the patient to flex the knee joint (Figure 82E–5). This maneuver tightens the hamstring muscles and facilitates more accurate palpation of the tendons.

Technique

The practitioner is best positioned on the side of the patient with the palpating hand on the biceps femoris muscle while observing the motor response of the foot and toes

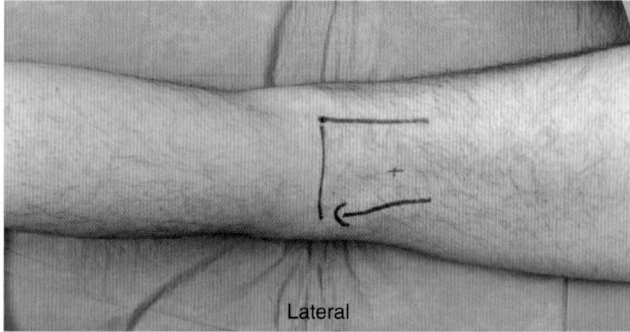

FIGURE 82E–5. Landmarks for the popliteal block, intertendinous approach. The landmarks can be accentuated by asking the patient to flex the leg. The arrow indicates attachment of the biceps femoris tendon; + sign indicates site of needle placement.

(Figure 82E–6A–C). The needle is introduced at the midpoint between the tendons. The nerve stimulator should be initially set to deliver 1.5 mA current (2 Hz, 100 μsec). When the needle is inserted in the correct plane, advancement of the needle should not result in any local muscular twitches; the first response to nerve stimulation is typically that of the sciatic nerve (foot twitch). The stimulating current is gradually decreased and the needle repositioned until twitches are still seen or felt at 0.2–0.5 mA. This typically occurs at a depth of 3–5 cm from the skin. After negative aspiration for blood, 20 mL of local anesthetic is slowly injected.

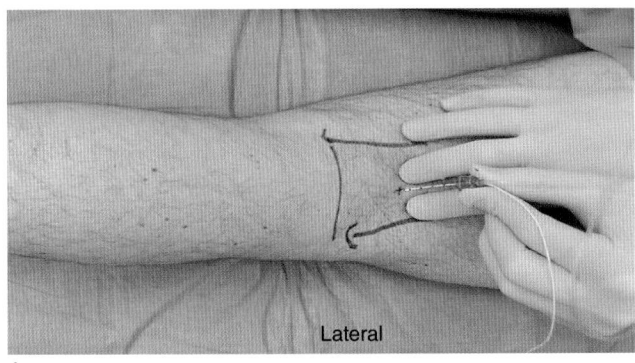

A

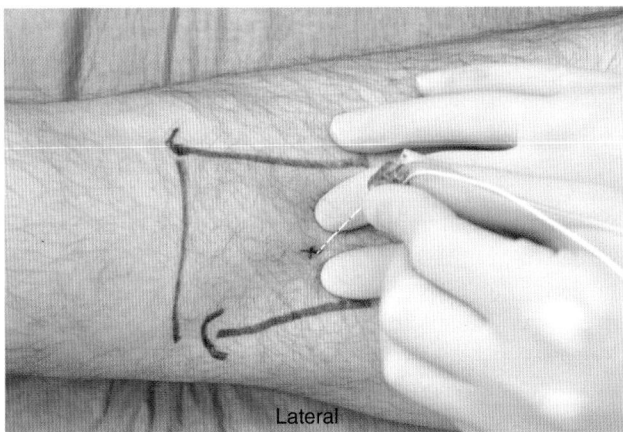

B

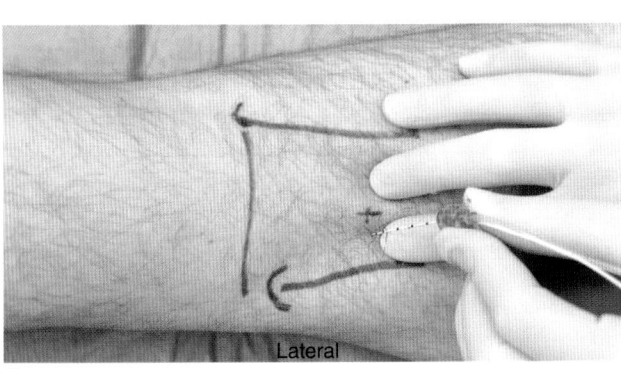

C

FIGURE 82E–6. A. Popliteal block, intertendinous approach. The needle is inserted perpendicularly between tendons of the biceps femoris and semitendinosus muscles. **B.** In case no foot or toe twitch can be elicited, withdraw and redirect 15 degrees laterally. **C.** In case no foot or toe twitch can be elicited after redirection, withdraw needle completely, reinsert 1 cm laterally, and repeat the procedure starting with perpendicular needle insertion.

Clinical Pearls

- In patients with long-standing diabetes mellitus, peripheral neuropathy, sepsis, or severe peripheral vascular disease. Stimulating currents up to 1 mA can be accepted.
- When a rather small change in the needle position (e.g.,1 mm) results in a change of the motor response from that of the popliteal nerve (plantar flexion of the foot) to that of the common peroneal nerve (dorsiflexion of the foot), the needle tip is above the divergence of the sciatic into tibial and common peroneal nerves.

  - Entrance of the needle into the sciatic sheath is almost always associated with a "fascial click." The skilled practitioner should use this sign as a valuable clue in conjunction with the nerve stimulation information to ascertain proper needle position.
  - Absence of high opening injection pressure is essential to assure extrafascicular needle placement as motor response may be absent after injection.

There are two types of motor responses that can be elicited with sciatic nerve stimulation at the level of the popliteal fossa. Common peroneal nerve stimulation results in dorsiflexion and eversion of the foot, whereas stimulation of the tibial nerve results in plantar flexion and inversion (Figure 82E–7). As the

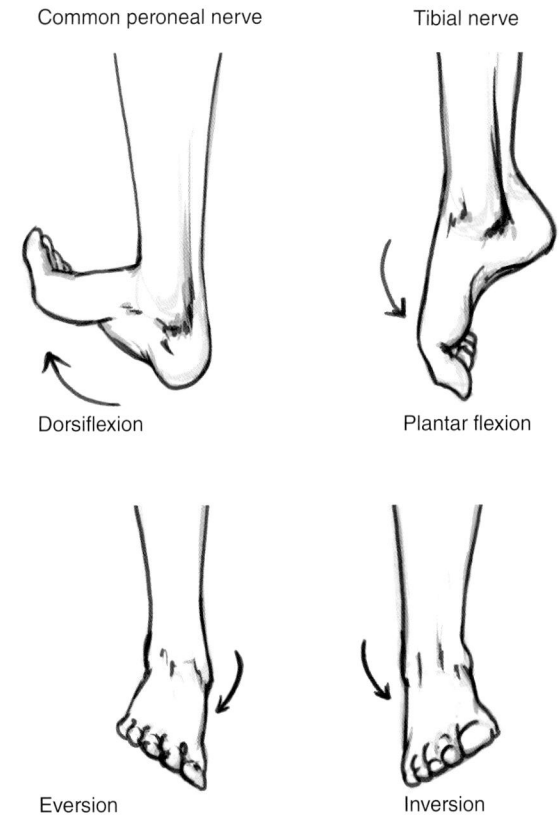

FIGURE 82E–7. Motor responses obtained on stimulation of the sciatic nerve in the popliteal fossa.

TABLE 82E–2. Intertendinous popliteal block: troubleshooting.

Response Obtained	Interpretation	Problem	Corrective Action
Local twitch of the biceps muscle	Direct stimulation of the biceps femoris muscle	Too lateral placement of the needle	Withdraw the needle and redirect slightly medially (5–10 degrees)
Local twitch of the semitendinosus/membranosus muscles	Direct stimulation of the semitendinosus/membranosus muscles	Too medial placement of the needle	Withdraw the needle and redirect slightly laterally (5–10 degrees)
Twitch of the calf muscles without foot or toe movement	Stimulation of the muscular branches of the sciatic nerve	These small branches are often outside the sciatic sheath	Disregard and continue advancing the needle until the foot/toes twitches are obtained
Vascular puncture	Blood in the syringe most commonly indicates placement into the popliteal artery or vein	Too medial or too deep needle placement	Withdraw and redirect laterally
Bone contact	The needle encounters the femur	Too deep needle insertion—either the nerve was missed or motor response was not appreciated	Withdraw the needle slowly and look for the foot twitch; if twitches are not seen, reinsert in another direction

stimulating current is being decreased, the twitch of the great toe often remains the only motor response seen with currents of <0.5 mA. Either response is adequate when the response is still present with current intensity of 0.2–0.4 mA (0.1 msec) as long as a large volume of local anesthetic is used. Some common responses to nerve stimulation and the course of action to obtain the proper response are shown in Table 82E–2.[19]

Block Dynamics and Perioperative Management

The intertendinous approach to the popliteal block is associated with relatively minor patient discomfort because the needle passes only through the adipose tissue of the popliteal fossa. Regardless, adequate sedation and analgesia are always important to ensure a still and tranquil patient. Midazolam 1–2 mg after the patient is positioned and alfentanil 250–500 mcg or 5 mg ketamine just before block placement suffices for most patients. A typical onset time for this block is 10–25 minutes, depending on the type, concentration, and volume of local anesthetic used. The first signs of block onset are usually that the patient reports that the foot "feels different" or that they are unable to wiggle the toes. Sensory anesthesia of the skin with this block is often the last to develop. Inadequate skin anesthesia despite the apparent timely onset of the blockade is common because it may take up to 30 minutes for full blockade to develop. However, local infiltration at the site of the incision is often all that is needed to allow the surgery to proceed.

Continuous Popliteal Block

Continuous popliteal block is an advanced regional anesthesia technique, and adequate experience with the single-shot technique is necessary to ensure its efficacy. The technique is similar

to the single-shot injection; however, slight angulation of the needle cephalad is necessary to facilitate insertion of the catheter. This technique can be used for surgery and postoperative pain management in patients undergoing a wide variety of lower leg, foot, and ankle surgeries.

Ilfeld[9] reported excellent postoperative analgesia using a continuous catheter in the popliteal fossa and a portable infusion pump for outpatients having moderately painful, lower extremity orthopedic surgery. The patients who received ropivacaine experienced a significant decrease in sleep disturbances, oral opioid use, and opioid-related adverse effects, and had a high rate of satisfaction with the technique.[20]

Klein et al.[21] examined the efficacy and complications of long-acting popliteal nerve block after discharge home. This prospective study included 1791 patients who had received an upper- or lower-extremity nerve block with 0.5% ropivacaine and were discharged on the day of surgery. The results showed that long-acting popliteal nerve block may be used in the ambulatory setting with a high degree of efficacy, safety, and satisfaction.

Chelly et al.[22] documented the benefits of a continuous lateral popliteal sciatic nerve block infusion technique for postoperative analgesia in patients who had undergone open reduction and internal fixation of the ankle. Continuous infusion of ropivacaine 0.2% was associated with a significant reduction of morphine consumption by 29% and 62% during postoperative days 1 and 2, respectively.

Technique

After insertion, the block needle is advanced slowly with a slight cranial direction while seeking a motor response. After

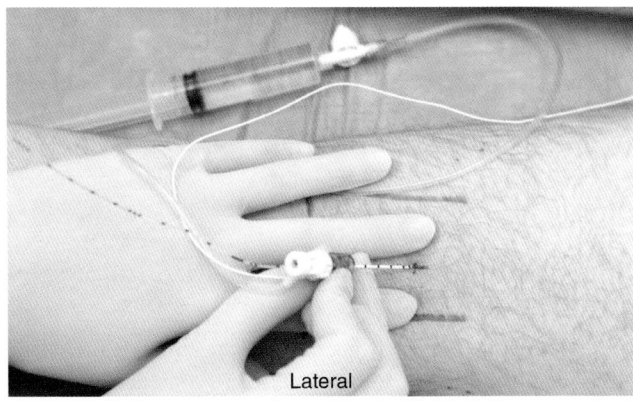

FIGURE 82E–8. Image depicts a non-sterile catheter field. Popliteal block, intertendinous approach. Catheter insertion.

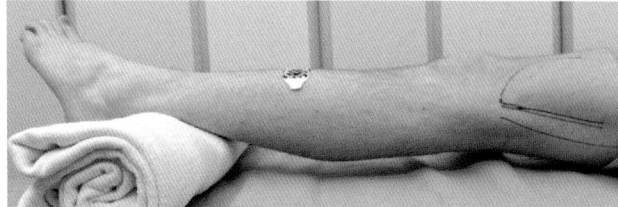

FIGURE 82E–9. Popliteal block, lateral approach. Landmarks for this technique include vastus lateralis (VL), biceps femoris (BF), and popliteal fossa crease. The needle insertion site is marked 8 cm above the popliteal fossa crease (*thick vertical line*).

obtaining an appropriate motor response at a current of 0.5 mA, a bolus of local anesthetic is injected (10-15 ml) and the catheter advanced 5 cm beyond the needle tip (Figure 82E–8). The catheter is aspirated to check for inadvertent intravascular placement, then an infusion can be started. A typical infusion regimen is ropivacaine 0.2% at 5 mL/h with a 5 mL/q60min patient-controlled bolus.

Clinical Pearls

- Breakthrough pain in patients on continuous infusion is always managed by administering a bolus of local anesthetic. Increasing only the rate of infusion is never adequate.
- Patients receiving continuous nerve block infusion should also be prescribed an alternative oral or intravenous (e.g., intravenous patient-controlled analgesia [IV PCA]) pain management protocol because incomplete analgesia and catheter dislodgement can occur leaving the patient without a back-up option.

Popliteal (Lateral) Approach

The main advantage of the lateral approach, described by Jerry Vloka is that the patient does not need to be positioned in the prone position.[6,1923]

Regional Anesthesia Anatomy

The sciatic nerve is located between the biceps and semitendinosus muscles (see Figure 82E–4). During block performance, stimulation of the common peroneal nerve is usually obtained first (65%) because this nerve is positioned more lateral and superficial than the tibial nerve.

Patient Positioning

The patient is in the supine position. The foot on the side to be blocked should be positioned so that even the slightest movement of the foot or toes can be easily observed. This is best achieved by placing the foot on a footrest.

Equipment

The equipment is identical to that for the posterior intertendinous approach except that a 10-cm stimulating needle is used.

Anatomic Landmarks

Landmarks for the lateral approach to popliteal block include the popliteal fossa crease, vastus lateralis muscle, and biceps femoris muscle (Figure 82E–9). The needle insertion site is marked in the groove between the vastus lateralis and biceps femoris muscles, 8 cm proximal to the popliteal crease (Figure 82E–10).

Technique

The operator should be seated, facing the side to be blocked. The height of the patient's bed is adjusted to allow for an ergonomic position and greater precision during block placement. This position also allows the operator to simultaneously monitor both the patient and the responses to nerve stimulation. The site of needle insertion is cleaned with an antiseptic solution and infiltrated with local anesthetic.

A 10-cm, 22-gauge needle is connected to a nerve stimulator inserted in a horizontal plane between the vastus lateralis and biceps femoris muscles, and advanced to contact the femur (see Figure 82E–10). The contact with the femur is important because it provides information on the depth of the nerve (typically 1–2 cm beyond the skin–femur distance) as well as on the angle at which the needle will need to be redirected

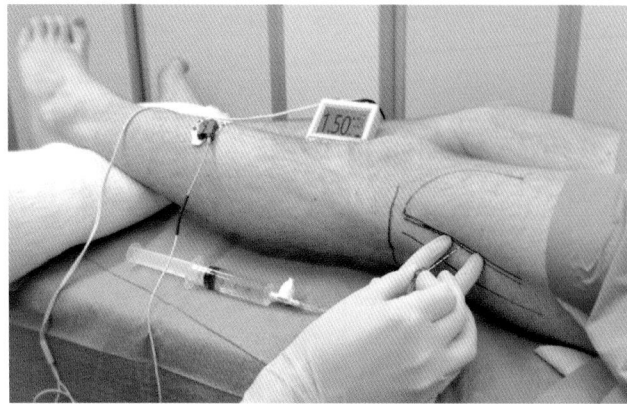

FIGURE 82E–10. Popliteal block, lateral approach. The needle is inserted between vastus lateralis (VL) and biceps femoris in the horizontal plane to contact the femur.

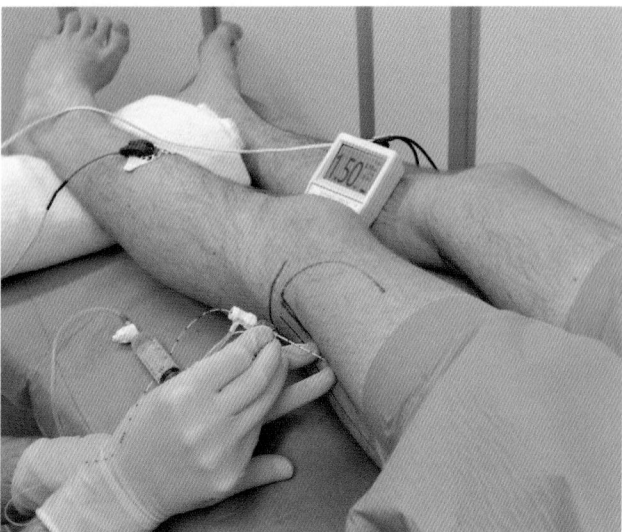

FIGURE 82E–11. After the femur is contacted, the needle is redirected 30 degrees posterior to the plane in which the femur was contacted. VL, vastus.

posterior to stimulate the nerve. The current intensity is initially set at 1.5 mA. Keeping the fingers of the palpating hands firmly pressed and immobile in the groove, the needle is then withdrawn to the skin, redirected 30 degrees posterior to the angle at which the femur was contacted, and advanced toward the nerve (Figure 82E–11).

When the sciatic nerve is not localized on the first needle pass, the needle is withdrawn to the skin level and the following procedure is followed:

Clinical Pearls

- Assure that the nerve stimulator is functional and properly connected to the patient and to the needle and that it is set to deliver current of desired intensity.
- Assure that the leg is not externally rotated at the hip joint and that the foot forms a 90-degree angle to the horizontal plane of the table. Any deviation from this angle changes the relationship of the sciatic nerve to the femur and biceps femoris muscle.
- Mentally visualize the plane of the initial needle insertion and redirect the needle in a slightly posterior direction (5–10 degrees posterior angulation).
- If the above maneuver fails, withdraw the needle and reinsert with an additional 5–10 degrees posterior redirection.
- If the above maneuvers fail, withdraw the needle to the skin and reinsert 1 cm inferior to the initial insertion site; then repeat the above steps.
- Failure to obtain foot response to nerve stimulation should prompt reassessment of the landmarks and leg position. In addition, the stimulating current should be increased to 2 mA.

After the initial stimulation of the sciatic nerve is obtained, the stimulating current is gradually decreased until motor response of

the foot or toes is still seen or felt at 0.5 mA. This typically occurs at a depth of 5–7 cm. Entrance of the needle into the sheath with a Touhy-style tip needle is often accompanied by a perceptible "click." At this point, the needle should be stabilized, and after negative aspiration for blood, 20 mL of local anesthetic is slowly injected. The hands should be kept as immobile as possible to prevent injection outside the sheath of the sciatic nerve.

Continuous Popliteal Block Through the Lateral Approach

The continuous popliteal block technique through the lateral approach is similar to the single-injection technique, except that a 10-cm Touhy-style tip needle is used. When the needle is directed towards the sciatic nerve, a slight cranial angulation should be taken to facilitate catheter insertion (Figure 82E–12).

After obtaining appropriate twitches at 0.2–0.5 mA, a bolus of local anesthetic is injected and the catheter advanced 5–7 cm beyond the tip of the needle. The management of the catheter is similar to that of the intertendinous technique.

Clinical Pearls

- In some patients, the biceps muscle may be atrophic and the iliotibial aponeurosis may be more prominent. In such cases, the needle insertion site is labeled in the groove between the vastus lateralis and the iliotibial tract.
- Flexing the patient's leg in the knee helps with identification of the popliteal fossa crease and the biceps and vastus lateralis muscles (Figure 82E–13).

Some common responses during block placement using a nerve stimulator and the course of proper action to obtain twitches of the foot (Table 82E–3).

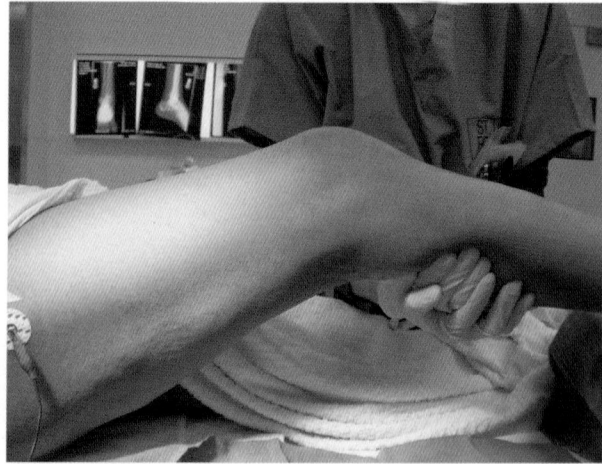

FIGURE 82E–12. Popliteal block, lateral approach. Continuous technique is similar to the single-injection method except that a larger needle is used. The needle opening should be directed cephalad, and a slight cephalad needle angulation is used after localization of the sciatic nerve; these maneuvers facilitate insertion of the catheter.

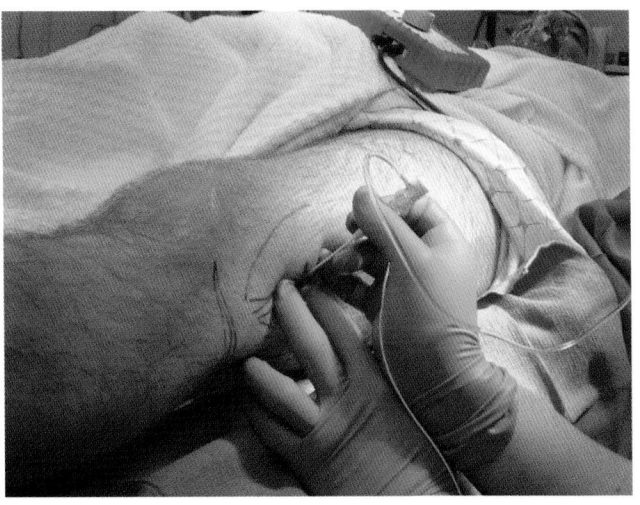

FIGURE 82E–13. Popliteal block, lateral approach. Asking the patient to flex the leg in the knee joint facilitates identification of the landmarks (popliteal fossa crease, vastus lateralis, and biceps femoris).

TABLE 82E–3. Lateral popliteal block: troubleshooting.

Response Obtained	Interpretation	Problem	Corrective Action
Local twitch of the biceps muscle	Direct stimulation of the biceps femoris muscle	Too shallow placement of the needle	Advance the needle deeper
Local twitch of the vastus lateralis muscle	Direct stimulation of the vastus lateralis muscles	Too anterior placement of the needle	Withdraw the needle and reinsert posterior
Twitch of the calf muscles without foot or toe movement	Stimulation of the muscular branches of the sciatic nerve	These small branches are often outside the sciatic sheath	Disregard and continue advancing the needle until the foot/toes twitches are obtained
Vascular puncture	Blood in the syringe most commonly indicates placement into the popliteal artery or vein	Too deep and anterior placement of the needle placement	Withdraw and redirect laterally
Twitches of the foot or toes	Stimulation of the sciatic nerve	None	Accept and inject local anesthetic

TABLE 82–4. Complications of popliteal block and measures to prevent them.

Infection	• Use strict aseptic technique
Hematoma	• Avoid multiple needle passes with a continuous block needle; the larger needle diameter and/or Tuohy design may result in a hematoma of the biceps femoris or vastus lateralis muscles
Vascular puncture	• Avoid too deep insertion of needle because the vascular sheath is positioned medially and deeper to the sciatic nerve
	• When the nerve is not localized within 2 cm after the local twitches of the biceps muscle cease, the needle should be withdrawn and reinserted at a different angle, rather than advanced deeper
Nerve injury	• Use nerve stimulation and slow needle advancement; do not inject when patient complains of pain or high pressures on injection are met; do not inject when stimulation is obtained at <0.2 mA current (100 μsec)
Pressure necrosis of the heel	• Instruct patient on the care of the insensate extremity
	• Use heel padding and frequent repositioning

COMPLICATIONS AND HOW TO AVOID THEM

A retrospective review of 400 continuous popliteal catheters revealed one case of infection (abscess formation requiring surgical drainage) and two cases of nerve injury resulting in paresthesias.[24]. Table 82E–4 provides specific instructions on possible complications and how to avoid them. Special attention should be paid when common peroneal response is elicited as most neurologic injuries occur to this nerve, probably because of its composition where there is often one or two large fascicles that present a greater risk for an intrafascicular needle placement.

SUMMARY

Popliteal sciatic block is useful technique to accomplish anesthesia and analgesia for ankle and foot surgery. Posterior and lateral approaches are both highly effective and applicable in numerous clinical scenarios.

REFERENCES

1. Hadzic A, Vloka JD: A comparison of the posterior versus lateral approaches to the block of the sciatic nerve in the popliteal fossa. Anesthesiology 1998;88:1480–1486.
2. Rongstad K, Mann RA, Prieskorn D, et al: Popliteal sciatic nerve block for postoperative analgesia. Foot Ankle Int 1996;17:378–382.
3. Rorie DK, Byer DK, Nelson DO, et al: Assessment of block of the sciatic nerve in the popliteal fossa. Anesth Analg 1980;59:371–376.
4. Singelyn FJ, Gouverneur JM, Gribomont BF: Politeal sciatic nerve block aided by a nerve stimulator: a reliable technique for foot and ankle surgery. Reg Anesth 1991;16:278–281.
5. Hansen E, Eshelman MR, Cracchiolo A: Popliteal fossa neural blockade as the sole anesthetic technique for outpatient foot and ankle surgery. Foot Ankle Int 2000;21:38–44.
6. McLeod DH, Wong DH, Claridge RJ, Merrick PM: Lateral popliteal sciatic nerve block compared with subcutaneous infiltration for analgesia following foot surgery. Can J Anaesth 1994;41:673–676.
7. Tobias JD, Mencio GA: Popliteal fossa block for postoperative analgesia after foot surgery in infants and children. J Pediatr Orthop 1999;19:511–514.
8. Vloka JD, Hadzic A, Mulcare R, et al: Combined blocks of the sciatic nerve at the popliteal fossa and posterior cutaneous nerve of the thigh for short saphenous vein stripping in outpatients: an alternative to spinal anesthesia. J Clin Anesth 1997;9:618–622.
9. Ilfeld BM, Morey TE, Wang DR, Enneking F K: Continuous popliteal sciatic nerve block for postoperative pain control at home: a randomized, double-blinded, placebo-controlled study. Anesthesiology 2002;97:959–965.
10. Mulroy MF, McDonald SB: Regional anesthesia for outpatient surgery. Anesthesiol Clin North Am 2003;21:289–303.
11. Vloka JD, Hadzic A, Lesser JB, et al: A common epineural sheath for the nerves in the popliteal fossa and its possible implications for sciatic nerve block. Anesth Analg 1997;84:387–390.
12. Perlas A, Wong P, Abdallah F: Ultrasound-guided popliteal block through a common paraneural sheath versus conventional injection: a prospective, randomized, double-blind study. Reg Anesth Pain Med. 2013;38:218–225.
13. Andersen HL, Andersen SL, Tranum-Jensen J: Injection inside the paraneural sheath of the sciatic nerve: direct comparison among ultrasound imaging, macroscopic anatomy, and histologic analysis. Reg Anesth Pain Med. 2012;37:410–414.
14. Franco D: Connective tissues associated with peripheral nerves. Reg Anesth Pain Med. 201;37:363–365.
15. Sunderland S: The sciatic nerve and its tibial and common peroneal divisions. anatomical features. In: Sunderland S (ed): *Nerves and Nerve Injurie*. Edenburgh, Scotland: Livingstone, 1968, 543:1012–1095.
16. Vloka JD, Hadzic A, April EW, et al: Division of the sciatic nerve in the popliteal fossa and its possible implications in the popliteal nerve blockade. Anesth Analg 2001;92:215–217.
17. Benzon HT, Kim C, Benzon HP, et al: Correlation between evoked motor response of the sciatic nerve and sensory blockade. Anesthesiology 1997;87:548–552.
18. Vloka JD, Hadzic A, Koorn R, Thys D: Supine approach to the sciatic nerve in the popliteal fossa. Can J Anaesth 1996;43:964–967.
19. Hadzic A, Vloka JD: Popliteal block. In: Hadzic A, Vloka J (eds): *Peripheral Nerve Blocks: Principles and Practice*. New York, NY: McGraw-Hill, 2004.
20. Saporito A, Sturini E, Borgeat A, Aguirre J: The effect of continuous popliteal sciatic nerve block on unplanned postoperative visits and readmissions after foot surgery –a randomised, controlled study comparing day-care and inpatient management. Anaesthesia. 2014;69:1197–1205.
21. Klein SM, Nielsen KC, Greengrass RA: Ambulatory discharge after long-acting peripheral nerve blockade: 2382 blocks with ropivacaine. Anesth Analg 2002;94:65–70.
22. Chelly JE, Greger J, Casati A: Continuous lateral sciatic blocks for acute postoperative pain management after major ankle and foot surgery. Foot Ankle Int 2002;23:749–752.
23. Zetlaoui PJ, Bouaziz H: Lateral approach to the sciatic nerve in the popliteal fossa. Anesth Analg 1998;87:79–82.
24. Compére V, Rey N, Baert O, et al: Major complications after 400 continuous popliteal sciatic nerve blocks for post-operative analgesia. Acta Anaesthesiol Scand. 2009;53:339–345.

Ankle Block

Joseph Kay, Rick Delmonte, and Paul M. Greenberg

INTRODUCTION

Anesthesia of the foot can be accomplished by blocking the five peripheral nerves that innervate the area at the level of the ankle.[1-5] This technique relies on anatomic landmarks that are easily identified. It does not require special equipment, paresthesia elicitation, nerve stimulation, special positioning, or patient cooperation.[1-5] The ankle block can be used for all types of foot surgery and is safe and reliable, and has a high success rate.[2,3,5-9]

Ankle block impairs ambulation on the affected leg, but to a lesser degree than sciatic or popliteal block, and patients can be discharged home before the block wears off.[4] Long-acting local anesthetics with ankle block can provide excellent postoperative analgesia.[6,9]

Indications and Contraindications

All types of foot surgeries can be carried out with ankle block, including bunionectomy, forefoot reconstruction, arthroplasty, osteotomy, and amputation.[1-10] Ankle block can also provide analgesia for fracture and soft tissue injuries[11] and or gout arthritis.[12] Moreover, it can be used for diagnostic and therapeutic purposes with spastic equinovarus[13] and sympathetically mediated pain.[14] Because motor block of the proximal leg and calf is avoided, ankle block may be preferable to sciatic/femoral (saphenous) nerve block for outpatient forefoot surgery.[15]

Ankle block should be avoided in patients with local infection, infection, edema, burn, soft tissue trauma, or distorted anatomy with scarring in the area of block placement.

Clinical Pearls

- Ankle block is well suited for ambulatory foot surgery.
- Ankle block can be life saving by avoiding the risks of general anesthesia in very ill patients having foot surgery (e.g. toes amputation, debridment).

Clinical Anatomy

The foot is innervated by five nerves (Figures 82F–1 and 82F–2). The medial aspect is innervated by the saphenous nerve, a terminal branch of the femoral nerve (Figure 82F–3). The rest of the foot is innervated by branches of the sciatic nerve:

- The lateral aspect is innervated by the sural nerve arising from the tibial and communicating superficial peroneal branches (Figure 82F–4).
- The deep ventral structures, muscles, and sole of the foot are innervated by the posterior tibial nerve, arising from the tibial branch (Figure 82F–5).
- The dorsum of the foot is innervated by the superficial peroneal nerve, arising from the common peroneal branch (Figure 82F–6).
- The deep dorsal structures and web space between the first and second toes are innervated by the deep peroneal nerve (see Figure 82F–2).[16,17]

At the level of the malleoli, the saphenous, superficial peroneal, and sural nerves are relatively superficial and subcutaneous. The posterior tibial and deep peroneal nerves are deep to the flexor and extensor retinaculi, respectively, and are more difficult to locate.

The posterior tibial nerve passes with the artery posterior to the medial malleolus deep to the flexor retinaculum, giving off a medial calcaneal branch to supply the lower and posterior surface of the heel.[18] The nerve and artery then become superficial and more accessible as they curve behind and underneath the sustentaculum tali, a bony ridge on the calcaneus about 2–3 cm below the medial malleolus. The nerve then divides into medial and lateral plantar nerves.[2]

The deep peroneal nerve passes lateral to the anterior tibial artery, extensor hallucis longus, and tibialis anterior tendons, and medial to the extensor digitorum longus tendon, deep to the extensor retinaculum. It becomes more superficial to travel

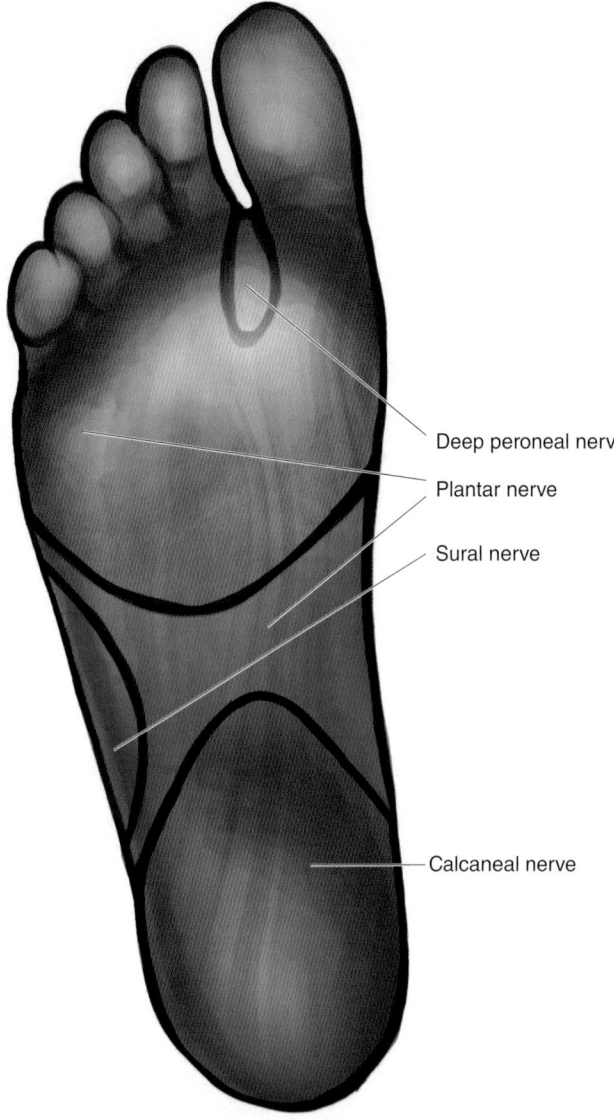

FIGURE 82F–1. Sensory innervation of the sole of the foot.

with the dorsalis pedis artery on the dorsum of the foot, where it is easily accessible.

Sensory innervation of the foot is highly variable. For example, in a study of 100 patients, 40% had the sural nerve

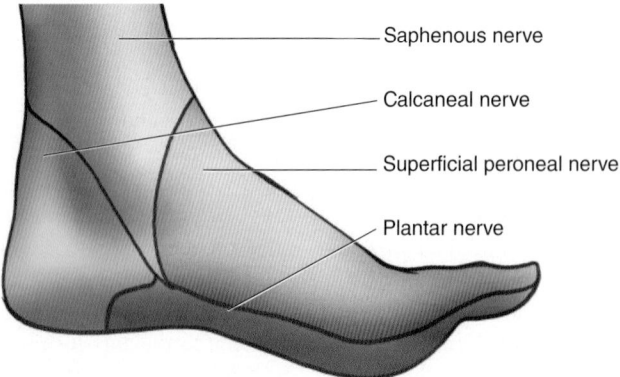

FIGURE 82F–2. Sensory innervation of the medial aspect of the foot.

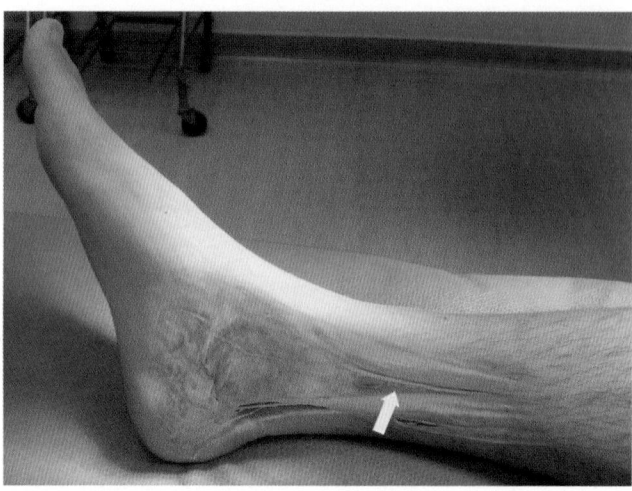

FIGURE 82F–3. Saphenous nerve at the level of the ankle (*white arrow*).

extend medially to involve the fourth toe, and 10% had the saphenous nerve extend distally to involve the first metatarsophalangeal joint and occasionally the great toe.[18]

Because the deep structures of the foot are supplied by the deep peroneal and posterior tibial nerves and because cutaneous innervation is variable, it has been suggested that all five nerves should be blocked for any foot surgery, especially if a tourniquet is used.[19] The one exception would be purely cutaneous surgery without tourniquet in the distribution of the sural, saphenous, or superficial peroneal nerves.[20] Selective versus complete ankle block for forefoot surgery under ankle tourniquet demonstrated that 43% versus 89% of patients were pain free during surgery, suggesting that complete ankle block is preferable under these conditions.[12] In contrast, another study has demonstrated that saphenous nerve block is not necessary for bunion surgery in 97% of patients).[21]

Landmarks

The landmarks for ankle block are the medial and lateral malleoli, the Achilles tendon, extensor hallucis longus tendon (identified by having the patient extend the great toe) (Figure 82F–7), the posterior tibial and dorsalis pedis arteries, and the

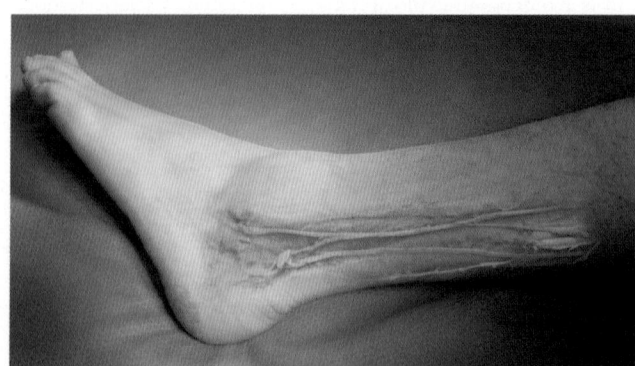

FIGURE 82F–4. Sural nerve at the level of the ankle.

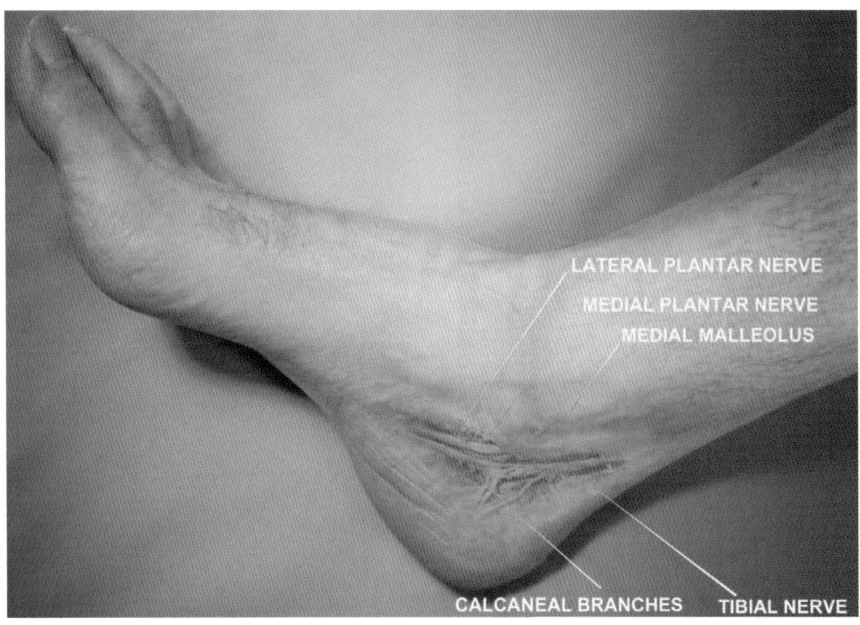

FIGURE 82F-5. Posterior tibial nerve at the level of the medial malleolus.

sustenaculum tali (a bony medial calcaneal ridge 2–3 cm below the malleolus).

For blockade at the level of the malleoli, the saphenous, sural, and superficial peroneal nerves are blocked with a circumferential subcutaneous injection of 10–15 mL of local anesthetic along a line just proximal to the malleoli and anterior from the Achilles tendon medially to laterally (Figures 82F–8 through 82F–10). The deep peroneal nerve is blocked by injection of 5 mL of local anesthetic just lateral to the extensor hallucis longus tendon deep to the retinaculum along the same circumferential line (Figure 82F–11). The posterior tibial nerve is blocked by injection of the same volume of local anesthetic just posterior to the posterior tibial artery if palpable, or midway between the Achilles tendon and medial malleolus deep to the retinaculum (Figure 82F–12).

For block at the midtarsal level, the saphenous, sural, and superficial peroneal nerves are blocked with a circumferential

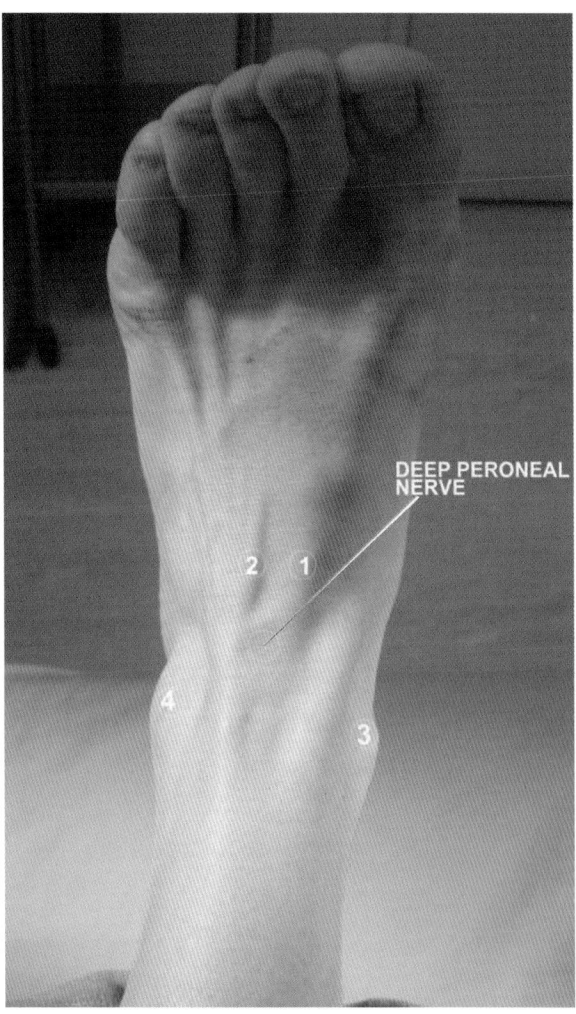

FIGURE 82F-7. Maneuver to accentuate the landmarks for the deep peroneal nerve block. *1,* Extensor hallucis longus; *2,* extensor digitorum longus; *3,* medial malleolus; *4,* lateral malleolus.

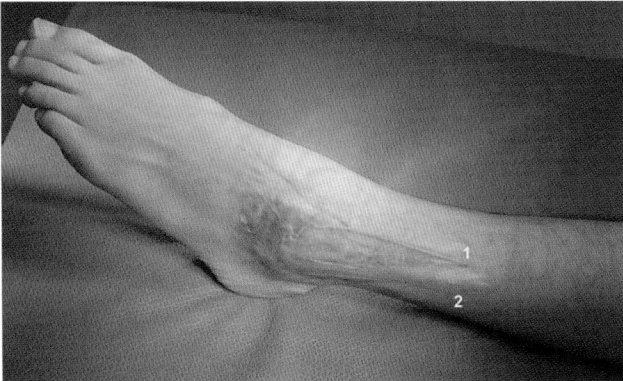

FIGURE 82F-6. Superficial peroneal nerve. Shown is the emergence of the superficial nerve and its distribution on the dorsum of the foot. *1,* Superficial peroneal nerve; *2,* sural nerve.

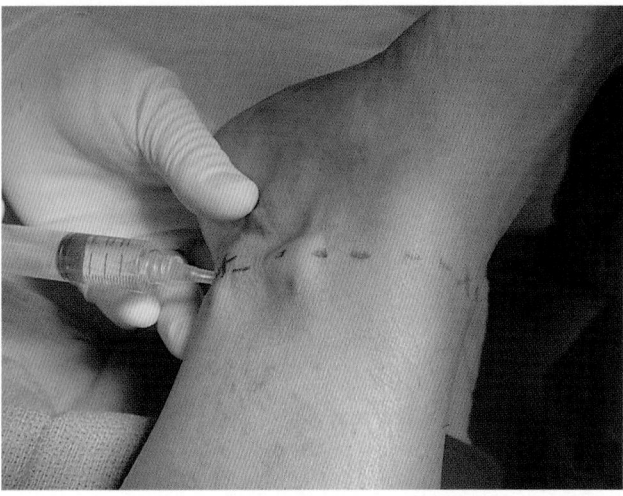

FIGURE 82F–8. Saphenous nerve block is accomplished by injection of 5 mL of local anesthetic subcutaneously at the level of the medial melleolus.

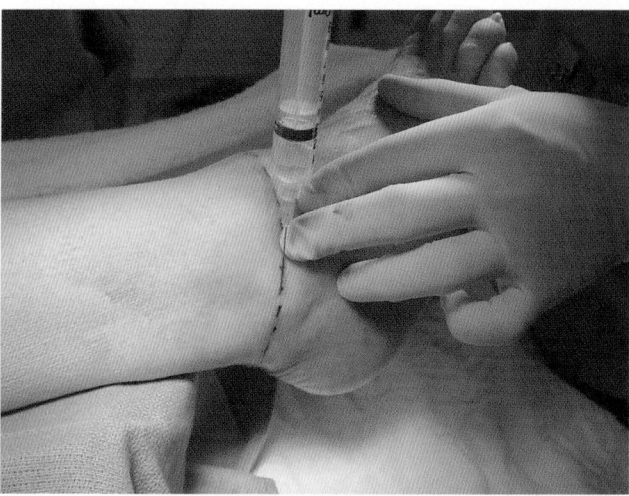

FIGURE 82F–10. Block of the sural nerve.

subcutaneous injection of 10–15 mL of local anesthetic along a line distal to the malleoli from the Achilles tendon medially to laterally. The deep peroneal nerve is blocked just lateral to the extensor hallucis longus tendon and medial to the dorsalis pedis artery. The posterior tibial nerve is blocked on either side of the posterior tibial artery (if palpable).

Equipment

No special equipment other than disinfectant, gauze, and 10-mL syringes with 1.5-in., 25-gauge needles is required for ankle block. Although nerve stimulation is not necessary for distal approaches, it has been described for the proximal approach to the posterior tibial nerve.[22]

If a tourniquet is required for surgery, a pneumatic ankle tourniquet should be used rather than an Esmarch bandage, because pressures with the latter are variable, are unknown, and may be extremely high, up to 380 mm Hg.[23,24]

Tourniquet pressures just above the malleoli between 200 and 250 mm Hg should ensure a bloodless field and maximize safety.[25,26] Ankle tourniquets are tolerated better than those placed at the midcalf or thigh, with less pain and no increase in neurologic complications.[27–30] An audit of 1000 cases of ankle block revealed that with proper tourniquet application and the option of sedation, only 3.1% of patients complained of tourniquet pain. Risk factors for tourniquet pain were age over 70 and tourniquet times greater than 30 minutes.[30]

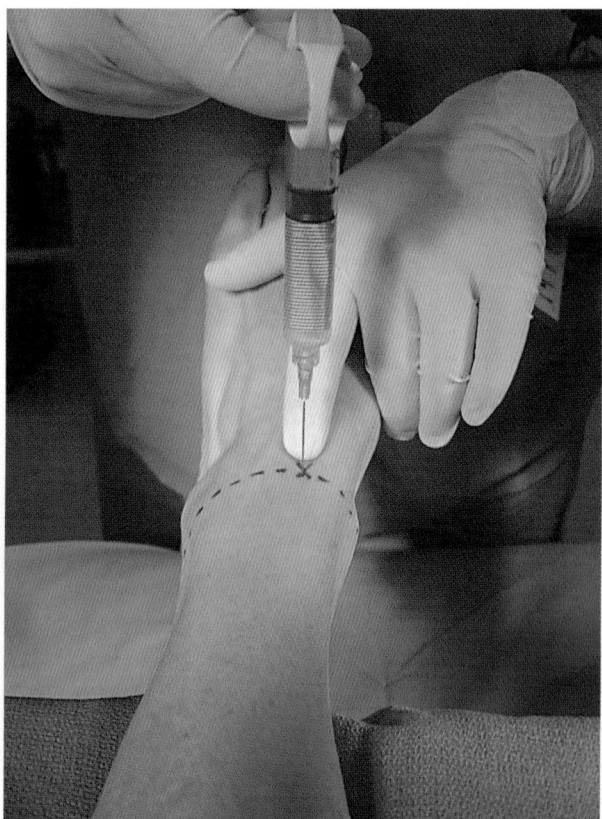

FIGURE 82F–11. Block of the deep peroneal nerve.

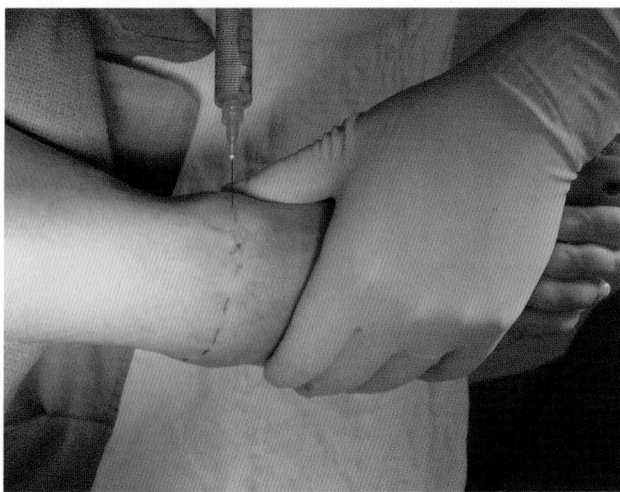

FIGURE 82F–9. Superficial peroneal block.

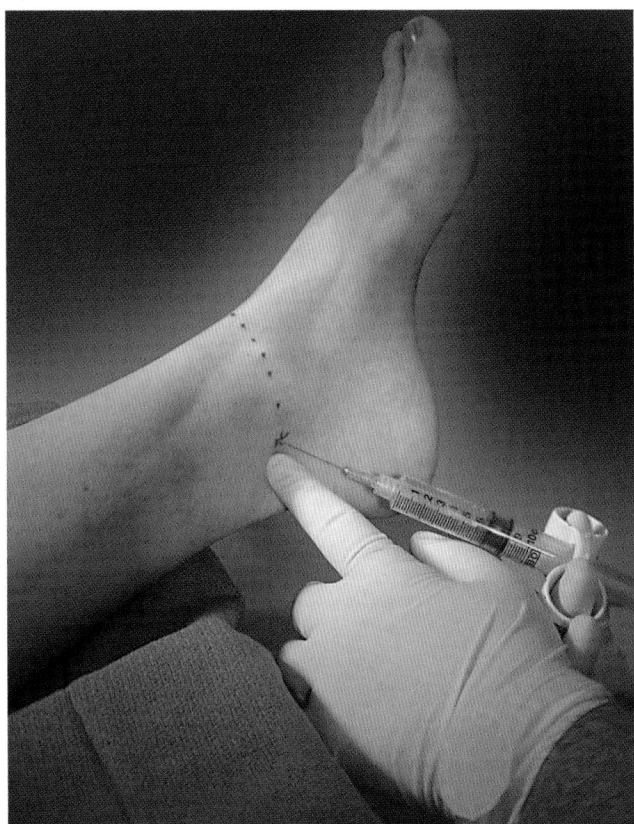

FIGURE 82F–12. Block of the posterior tibial nerve.

Clinical Pearl

- Always ensure that when a tourniquet is required, a padded ankle tourniquet is used to maximize patient comfort, minimize sedation, and prevent general anesthesia.

Technique

There are several techniques for performing ankle block; they can be classified as *perimalleolar* or *midtarsal* (inframalleolar) blocks. The location of the block determines the procedures that can be done; forefoot surgery is easily accomplished under a midtarsal block, but midfoot and more proximal foot surgery require a perimalleolar block. Success rates are higher with the midtarsal technique because the deep peroneal and posterior tibial nerves are more superficial, so this technique is preferable for forefoot surgery.[2,3]

For all approaches, the patient can be supine, with a pillow under the calf to facilitate access.

Saphenous, Superficial Peroneal, and Sural Nerve Blocks

The saphenous, superficial peroneal, and sural nerves are already subcutaneous just proximal to the malleoli, and all can be blocked by a subcutaneous ring of local anesthetic at this location from just anterior to the Achilles tendon medially to laterally (see Figures 82F–8 through 82F–10). The advantage

of blocking these nerves here is that the area under an ankle tourniquet will be anesthetized and tourniquet pain is less likely. By injecting slowly and continuously advancing a 1.5-in., 25-gauge needle into the previously injected area, the number of injections and discomfort from them can be minimized. This subcutaneous ring of local anesthetic can also be performed distal to the malleoli for a midtarsal block.

Deep Peroneal Nerve Block

For the perimalleolar approach, the patient is asked to extend the great toe, which will tense and identify the extensor hallucis tendon (see Figure 82F–7). A 1.5-in., 25-gauge needle is inserted immediately lateral to the tendon, perpendicular to the tibia, and is advanced until it contacts bone (see Figure 82F–11). The needle is then withdrawn a few millimeters, and after negative aspiration, 5 mL of local anesthetic is injected.

For the midtarsal approach, the extensor hallucis tendon is identified as mentioned above, but more distally, and the pulse of the dorsalis pedis artery is identified on the top of the foot as well. A 1.5-in., 25-gauge needle is inserted immediately lateral to the tendon and medial to the artery, and after negative aspiration, 5 mL of local anesthetic is injected.

Posterior Tibial Nerve Block

For the perimalleolar approach, a 1.5-in., 25-gauge needle is inserted just posterior to the pulse of the posterior tibial artery behind the medial malleolus, or if it cannot be palpated, midway between the Achilles tendon and the posterior aspect of the medial malleolus (see Figure 82F–12). The needle is directed toward the tibia at a 45-degree angle to contact bone. The needle is then withdrawn a few millimeters, and after negative aspiration, 5 mL of local anesthetic is injected.

For the midtarsal approach, there are two approaches. Either the posterior tibial artery is identified below and distal to the medial malleolus on the calcaneus, or the sustentaculum tali is identified. The needle is directed toward the calcaneus, slightly under the bony shelf of the sustentaculum tali, or on either side of the tibial artery. After contact with bone, the needle is withdrawn 2 mm, and 5 mL of local anesthetic is injected.

Clinical Pearl

- Because the posterior tibial artery is not palpable in all individuals, the sustentaculum tali is a more consistent, easily palpable landmark for posterior tibial nerve block.

MAYO BLOCK

Clinical Anatomy

The Mayo block is a combination of the nerve block and a field block that involves the infiltration of local anesthesia through the tissues proximal to a surgical site in a ring shape around the first metatarsal (most commonly) or a lesser metatarsal base.[30] When the Mayo block is used around the first metatarsal base, the nerves that are anesthetized include the medial dorsal cutaneous nerve and the deep peroneal nerve on the dorsal aspect. The first and second branches of the common plantar digital nerves, which are superficial branches of the medial plantar nerve, provide sensation to the plantar aspect of the first metatarsal.

Indications

The Mayo block is commonly used in podiatric office surgery to anesthetize the area before performing bunion or hallux surgery. The injection can be used with or without epinephrine.

Technique

The Mayo block consists of three or four separate injections. The block is performed by raising a wheal of local anesthetic proximally and dorsally in the first intermetatarsal space and advancing the needle in the plantar direction while injecting 3–5 mL of local anesthetic (Figure 82F–13). The needle is then withdrawn partially and redirected medially, raising a subcutaneous wheal along its course (3–5 mL) (Figure 82F–14). The needle is then removed and reentered and directed laterally to raise a subcutaneous wheal along the course (3–5 mL) (Figure 82F–15). Finally, the needle is removed and directed plantar-medially to the metatarsal and injected from medial to lateral underneath the metatarsal bone (3–5 mL) (Figure 82F–16). The block encircles the entire metatarsal bone.

Choice of Local Anesthetic

The decision regarding which local anesthetic solution to use depends on the anticipated duration of surgery and the degree of postoperative pain. Commonly used solutions include lidocaine 2% for shorter, less painful procedures and ropivacaine 0.5% for longer or more painful procedures.

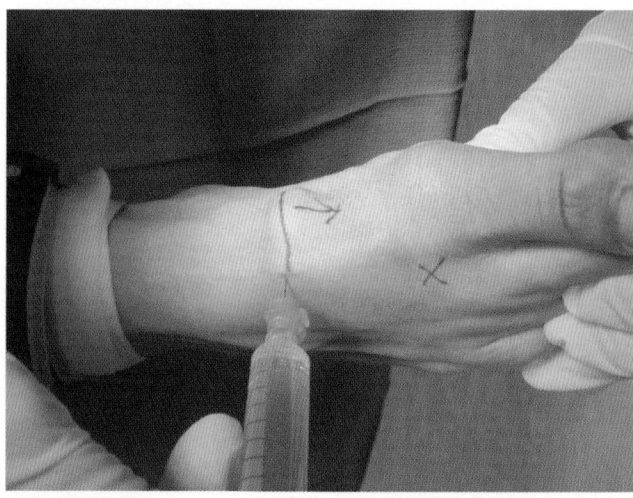

FIGURE 82F–14. Mayo block, step 1. The needle is entered subcutaneously dorsomedially raising a wheal along the course. (Arrow, First metatarsal bone; X, first metarsal space.)

Blood levels of plain local anesthetic are well below toxic levels, even when large amounts are used. Bilateral midtarsal blocks performed with up to 30 mL of plain 0.75% bupivacaine resulted in peak venous blood levels of 0.5 mcg/mL[-1], whereas 13 mL of 2% lidocaine for unilateral block resulted in 1.1 mcg/mL.[-19] No adverse local anesthetic effects were reported in a series of 66 patients receiving bilateral ankle blocks with mixtures of plain lidocaine and ropivacaine 0.75%, ropivacaine 0.75% or ropivacaine 0.75% with clonidine 1 mcg/kg.[-16] The addition of epinephrine with ankle block remains controversial. The preponderance of the literature suggests that epinephrine should not be used in distal extremity local anesthesia.[31,33] However, low concentrations of epinephrine in local anesthetic solutions have been used with remarkable safety.[33] The overall incidence of severe vascular complications after injection of epinephrine-containing local anesthetics has been estimated to be 1 per 132,000 injections.

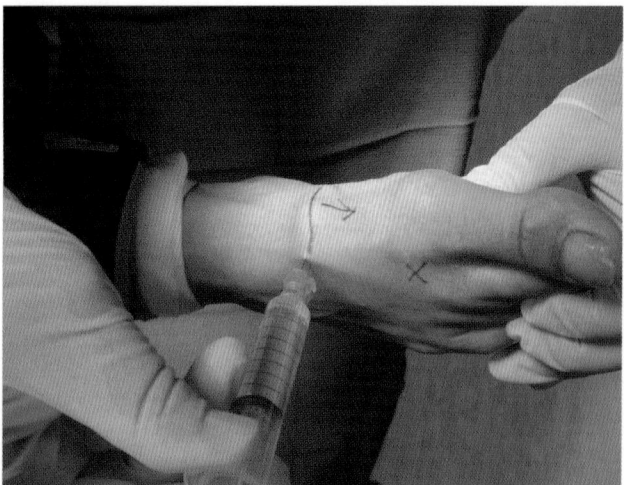

FIGURE 82F–13. Mayo block, step 2. After a wheal of local anesthesia is raised at the level of the first intermetatarsal space, the needle is advanced in the plantar direction and 3–5 mL of local anesthetic is injected. (Arrow, First metatarsal bone; X, first metatarsal space.)

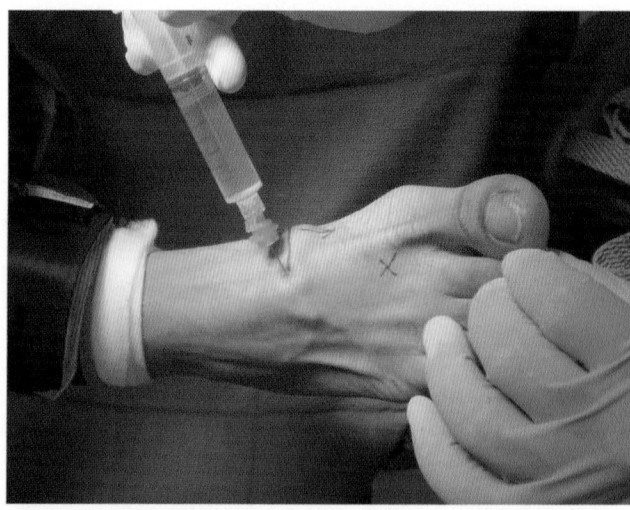

FIGURE 82F–15. Mayo block, step 3. The needle is directed medial to lateral subcutaneously and 3–5 mL is injected. (Arrow, First metatarsal bone; X, first metarsal space.)

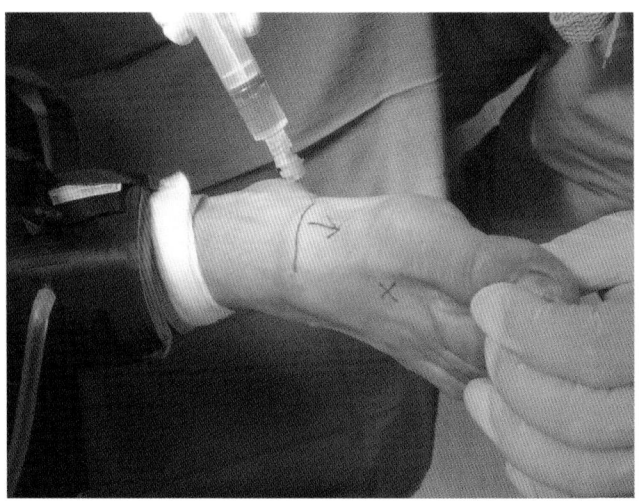

FIGURE 82F–16. Mayo block, step 4. The needle is directed medial to lateral and plantar underneath the metatarsal bone while injecting 3–5 mL of local anesthetic. (Arrow, First metatarsal bone; X, first metarsal space.)

Note that the use of 1:100,000 solutions of epinephrine has a 2.5 greater risk of complications compared with 1:200,000, suggesting that when epinephrine is indicated, it should be used only as dilute concentrations (i.e., 1:300,000 or less). Regardless, epinephrine is probably best avoided altogether in patients with peripheral vascular disease or compromised circulation.

The high-efficacy, prolonged postoperative analgesia and safety of plain bupivacaine and ropivacaine suggest that these drugs should be the choice for surgery in which postoperative pain is expected. However, blocks should be performed 30 minutes before surgery (minimum of 20 minutes) when using bupivacaine or ropivacaine to maximize success rate. In a prospective analysis of 1000 patients, the failure rate was significantly lower after waiting 20 minutes after the injection, with the lowest failure rates occurring after 50 minutes.[7]

Clinical Pearl

- When using ropivacaine or bupivacaine, perform the block at least 30 minutes before surgery to allow adequate time for block onset.

PERIOPERATIVE MANAGEMENT

Because performing an ankle block requires more than one injection and requires subcutaneous infiltration, it can cause more discomfort than single-injection blocks. In addition to gentle, slow injection, patients usually benefit from anxiolysis and analgesia with midazolam 1–4 mg and fentanyl 25–100 mcg. Before starting surgery, the block should be checked in all five nerve distributions, and supplemental local anesthetic can be injected if necessary.

Tourniquets should have a soft lining or padding and should be placed just above the malleoli. Ankle tourniquets are

tolerated better than those placed at the midcalf or thigh, with less pain and no increase in neurologic complications.[27–30] An audit of 1000 cases of ankle block revealed that with proper tourniquet application and the option of sedation, only 3.1% of patients complained of tourniquet pain.[30]

Supplementation by the surgeon intraoperatively may rescue an incomplete block.

Postoperatively, acetaminophen and a nonsteroidal anti-inflammatory drug (NSAID) can be continued routinely. Depending on the extent and type of surgery, small doses of a long-acting opioid such as controlled-release oxycodone may provide a smooth transition from block to postoperative analgesia and may facilitate rehabilitation.[34] Ambulation with crutches is possible right after surgery. Elevation of the leg, when not ambulating, may further decrease postoperative pain.

COMPLICATIONS AND HOW TO AVOID THEM

Because most surgery is done under tourniquet, it is difficult to differentiate the cause of neurologic complications. In a retrospective study of 3027 patients with pneumatic ankle tourniquet at relatively high pressures of 325 mm Hg, there were three cases (0.1%) of posttourniquet syndrome.[29] Ankle tourniquets have been used routinely with as little as 200 mm Hg pressure,[5] although a bloodless surgical field may require 218.6 ± 34.6 mm Hg, with younger normotensive patients requiring only 203.9 ± 22.3 mm Hg.[26] Thus, no more than 250 mm Hg pressure is necessary, and more pressure may be harmful.

The incidence of complications after ankle block is low and is usually in the form of transient paresthesias, which almost always resolve. The incidence is usually less than 1%, although it ranges from 0%–10%, depending on the source of the data. Complications may occur from injection or from application of the tourniquet. In a prospective survey of 284 patients with posterior tibial, sural, and saphenous blocks at the ankle and common peroneal block at the knee, no patient developed postanesthetic neuralgia or other complications. In three other studies with a total of 120 patients who received ankle blocks, no patients developed complications.[2,5,10] After midtarsal ankle block in 71 of 100 patients available for follow-up, 1 patient developed transient posterior tibial paresthesias, which resolved in 4 weeks.[3] In another study of 40 patients, 1 developed paresthesias lasting 6 weeks, which resolved.[1] In a retrospective study of 1373 patients who received ankle block followed by a posterior tibial nerve catheter for postoperative analgesia, 5 patients had transient paresthesias, with 1 patient developing neurolysis (probably related to the catheter insertion) but with complete recovery.[22] In a prospective randomized trial of 32 patients (40 total feet) undergoing forefoot surgery under ankle tourniquet (inflation pressure 100 mm Hg over systolic) under complete or selective ankle block of which 26 patients (33 total feet) were available for follow-up to injection or tourniquet, 1 had ankle pain, and 1 had cold toes.[8]

Local anesthetic systemic toxicity would be expected to be rare, given the low blood levels after injection. In the retrospective series of 1373 patients previously mentioned, 1 patient had a convulsion, thought to be secondary to an intravascular injection.[22] In another series of 1295 patients who received standard and modified ankle blocks as well as digital nerve blocks, 3 patients had vasovagal reactions and 1 had an episode of hypotension and supraventricular tachycardia, thought by the investigators to be from lidocaine toxicity. No other complications were seen in this series.[4]

There are single case reports of injection-related complications such as an Achilles tendon avulsion from tibial nerve block in a patient with spastic talipes equinovarus,[13] and acute compartment syndrome from ankle block in a patient with previous scarring from forefoot arthroplasty.[32]

Both of these patients had an altered anatomy, which may have predisposed them to the complication.

Clinical Pearls

- Ensure that the patient's anatomy is normal before injection and avoid injecting in scarred or swollen areas.
- Avoid injection of large volumes; most ankle blocks can be performed with less than 30 mL of local anesthetic.
- There should be no resistance to injection at any time. If there is, stop the injection and reposition the needle.

REFERENCES

1. Schurman DJ: Ankle block anesthesia for foot surgery. Anesthesiology 1976;44:348–352.
2. Wassef MR: Posterior tibial nerve block. A new approach using the bony landmark of the sustentaculum tali. Anaesthesia 1991;46:841–844.
3. Sharrock NE, Waller JF, Fierro LE: Midtarsal block for surgery of the forefoot. Br J Anaesthesia 1986;58:37–40.
4. Myerson MS, Ruland CM, Allon SM: Regional anesthesia for foot and ankle surgery. Foot Ankle 1992;13:282–288.
5. Sarrafian SK, Ibrahim IN, Breihan JH: Ankle-foot peripheral nerve block for mid and forefoot surgery. Foot Ankle 1993;4:86–90.
6. Rudkin GE, Rudkin AK, Dracopoulos GC: Bilateral ankle blocks: a prospective audit. ANZ Surg 2005;75:39–42.
7. Rudkin GE, Rudkin AK, Dracopoulos GC: Ankle block success rate: a prospective analysis of 1,000 patients. Can J Anesth 2005;52:209–210.
8. Delgado-Martinez AD, Marchal JM, Molina M, et al: Forefoot surgery with ankle tourniquet: complete or selective ankle block? Reg Anesth Pain Med 2001;26:184–186.
9. Mineo R, Sharrock NE: Venous levels of lidocaine and bupivacaine after mid-tarsal ankle block. Reg Anesth Pain Med 1992;17:47–49.
10. Needoff M, Radford P, Costigan P: Local anesthesia for postoperative pain relief after foot surgery: A prospective clinical trial. Foot Ankle Int 1995;16:11–13.
11. Winiecke DG, Louis JM: Local anesthetic nerve blocks in the treatment of foot fractures. J Am Podiatr Med Assoc 1977;67:87–90.
12. Haber GR, Johnson DR, Nashel DJ, et al: Lidocaine regional block in the treatment of gouty arthritis of the foot. J Am Podiatr Med Assoc 1985;75:492–493.
13. Deltombe T, Nisolle JF, De Cloedt P, et al: Tibial nerve block with anesthetics resulting in Achilles tendon avulsion. Am J Phys Rehabil 2004;83:331–334.
14. Harvey CK: Dilute lidocaine ankle blocks in the diagnosis of sympathetically mediated pain. J Am Podiatr Med Assoc 1997;87:473–477.
15. McLeod DH, Wong DHW, Vaghadia H, et al: Lateral popliteal sciatic nerve block compared with ankle block for analgesia following foot surgery. Can J Anaesth 1995;42:765–769.
16. Agur AMR, Lee MJ: *Grant's Atlas of Anatomy*, 9th ed. Philadelphia, PA: Williams & Wilkins, 1991, pp 255–352.
17. Clemente CD: *Anatomy: A Regional Atlas of the Human Body*, 4th ed. Philadelphia, PA: Williams & Wilkins, 1997, pp 309–402.
18. McCutcheon R: Regional anaesthesia for the foot. Can Anesth Soc J 1965;12:465–474.
19. Hoerster, W: Blocks in the area of the ankle. In: Zenz M, Panhans C, Niesel HC et al, (eds.) Regional Anesthesia. Year Book Medical Publishers, Inc, Chicago, IL; 1988:88.
20. Cohen SJ, Roenigk RK: Nerve blocks for cutaneous surgery on the foot. J Dermatol Surg Oncol 1991;17:527–534.
21. López AM, Sala-Blanch X, Magaldi M, et al: Ultrasound-guided ankle block for forefoot surgery: the contribution of the saphenous nerve. Reg Anesth Pain Med. 2012;37:554–557.
22. Frederic A, Bouchon Y: Analgesia in surgery of the foot. Can Anesthesiol 1996;44:115–118.
23. Biehl WC, Morgan JM, Wagner FW, et al: The safety of the Esmarch tourniquet. Foot Ankle 1993;14:278–283.
24. Finsen V, Kasseth AM: Tourniquets in forefoot surgery. Less pain when placed at the ankle. J Bone Jt Surg Br 1997;79B:99–101.
25. Pauers RS, Carocci MA: Low pressure pneumatic tourniquets: Effectiveness at minimum recommended inflation pressures. J Foot Ankle Surg 1994;33:605–609.
26. Diamond EL, Sherman M, Lenet M: A quantitative method of determining the pneumatic ankle tourniquet setting. J Foot Surg 1985;24:330–334.
27. Lichtenfeld NS: The pneumatic ankle tourniquet with ankle block anesthesia for foot surgery. Foot Ankle 1992;13:344–349.
28. Chu J, Fox I, Jassen M: Pneumatic ankle tourniquet: clinical and electrophysiologic study. Arch Phys Med Rehabil 1981;62(11):570-575.
29. Derner R, Buckholz J: Surgical hemostasis by pneumatic ankle tourniquet during 3027 podiatric operations. J Foot Ankle Surg 1995;34:236–246.
30. McGlamry DE, Banks AS, Downey M: Ankle block. In: McGlamry DE, Banks AS, Downey M (eds): *Comprehensive Textbook of Foot Surgery*, 2nd ed. Philadelphia, PA: Williams & Wilkins, 1992, pp 243–244.
31. Wylie WD: *A Practice of Anesthesia*. Yearbook, 1972, pp 1166–1172.
32. Hardy JD: *Rhoads Textbook of Surgery Principles and Practice*, 5th ed. Philadelphia, PA: Lippincott, 1973, pp 2310–2315.
33. Roth RD: Utilization of epinephrine-containing anesthetic solutions in the toes. J Am Podiatr Med Assoc 1981;71:189–199.
34. Reinhart DJ, Wang W, Stagg KS, et al: Postoperative analgesia after peripheral nerve block for podiatric surgery: clinical efficacy and chemical stability of lidocaine alone versus lidocaine plus clonidine. Anesth Analg 1996;83:760–765.

Cutaneous Nerve Blocks of the Lower Extremity

Jerry D. Vloka and Luc Van Keer

INTRODUCTION

Blocks of the lateral femoral cutaneous, posterior femoral cutaneous, saphenous, sural, and superficial peroneal nerves are useful anesthetic techniques for a variety of superficial surgical procedures and carry a low risk of complications.[1,2]

Indications and Contraindications

The lateral femoral cutaneous nerve block has been used to provide anesthesia for pediatric patients undergoing muscle biopsy[3] and to provide analgesia after femoral neck surgery in older patients.[4,5] The posterior femoral cutaneous nerve block is used for any surgical procedure performed on the posterior aspect of the thigh.[6] The saphenous, sural, and superficial peroneal nerve blocks can be used as part of an ankle block to provide complete anesthesia to the foot and ankle, or they can be used separately to provide anesthesia to specific portions of the foot and ankle.

The contraindications to performing cutaneous nerve blocks of the lower extremity are few, but include local infection at the sites of needle insertion, and allergy to local anesthetic.

Functional Anatomy

The cutaneous nerves of the extremities are blocked by injection of local anesthetic in the subcutaneous layers above the muscle fascia. The subcutaneous tissue contains a variable amount of fat, superficial nerves, and vessels. Deep to this area lies a tough membranous layer, deep fascia of the lower extremity enclosing muscles of the leg. This deep fascia is penetrated by numerous superficial nerves and vessels.

The cutaneous innervation of the lower extremity is accomplished by nerves that are part of the lumbar and sciatic plexuses (Figures 82G–1 and 82G–2). A more detailed review of the relevant anatomy is provided with a description of the individual block procedures in Chapter 3.

Choice of Local Anesthetic

Any local anesthetic can be used for cutaneous blocks of the lower extremity; the choice is based primarily on the desired duration of blockade. Because these blocks do not result in motor block, longer-cting local anesthetics are most commonly chosen (e.g., 0.2%–0.5% ropivacaine or 0.25%-0.5% bupivacaine). When performing blocks in the ankle area, it is always prudent to avoid using epinephrine owing to the risk of decreasing blood flow to the toes. Onset time for the block depends on the local anesthetic used[7] (Table 82G–1).

LATERAL FEMORAL CUTANEOUS NERVE BLOCK

General Considerations

This block can be used to provide complete anesthesia in patients undergoing skin graft on the lateral aspect of the thigh, or it can be combined with femoral block[8–10] or sciatic block. Its use has also been reported as a diagnostic tool for meralgia paresthetica, neuralgia of the lateral femoral cutaneous nerve of the thigh.

Distribution of Anesthesia

The lateral femoral cutaneous nerve provides sensation to the anterolateral aspect of the thigh (see Figure 82G–1). In some patients however, the nerve can provide surprisingly large innervation territory of the anterior thigh as well.

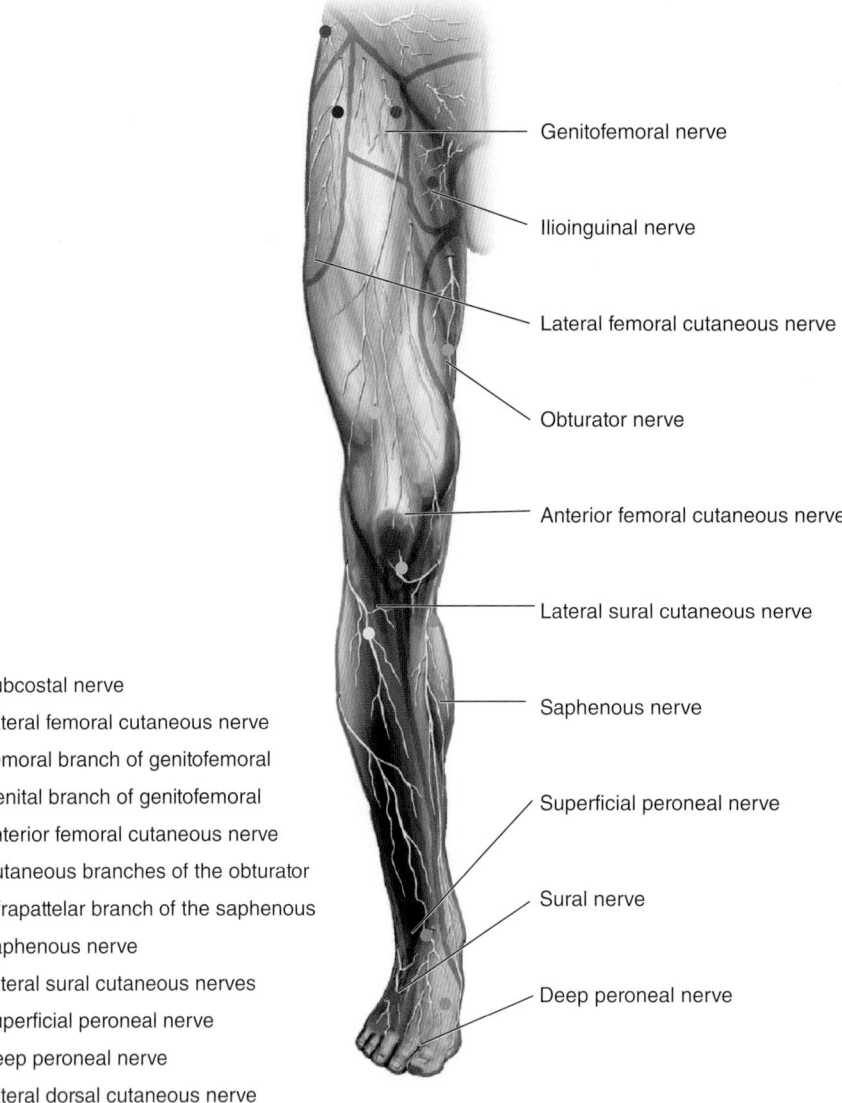

- Subcostal nerve
- Lateral femoral cutaneous nerve
- Femoral branch of genitofemoral
- Genital branch of genitofemoral
- Anterior femoral cutaneous nerve
- Cutaneous branches of the obturator
- Infrapattelar branch of the saphenous
- Saphenous nerve
- Lateral sural cutaneous nerves
- Superficial peroneal nerve
- Deep peroneal nerve
- Lateral dorsal cutaneous nerve

Genitofemoral nerve

Ilioinguinal nerve

Lateral femoral cutaneous nerve

Obturator nerve

Anterior femoral cutaneous nerve

Lateral sural cutaneous nerve

Saphenous nerve

Superficial peroneal nerve

Sural nerve

Deep peroneal nerve

FIGURE 82G–1. Cutaneous innervation of the lower extremity, anterior view.

Patient Positioning

The patient is in a supine position and the anterior superior iliac spine is palpated and marked.

Anatomic Landmarks

The main landmark for lateral femoral cutaneous nerve blockade is the anterior superior iliac spine. The lateral femoral cutaneous nerve emerges from the lateral border of the psoas major muscle and crosses the iliacus muscle obliquely toward the anterior superior iliac spine, where it supplies the parietal peritoneum of the iliac fossa. The nerve then passes into the thigh behind or through the inguinal ligament, variably medial to the anterior iliac spine (typically about 1 cm) or through the tendinous origin of the sartorius muscle, dividing into anterior and posterior branches.

The anterior branch becomes superficial about 10 cm distal to the anterior superior iliac spine supplying innervation to the skin of the anterior and lateral thigh as far as the knee. It connects terminally with the cutaneous branches of the anterior division of the femoral nerve and the infrapatellar branch of the saphenous nerve, forming the patellar plexus. The posterior branch pierces the fascia lata higher than the anterior, dividing to supply the skin on the lateral surface from the greater trochanter to about the middle of the thigh and occasionally also supplying the gluteal skin.

Technique

A 22-25 gauge needle is inserted 2 cm medial and 2 cm distal to the anterior superior iliac spine (Figure 82G–3). The needle is advanced until a loss of resistance or a "pop" is felt as the needle passes through the fascia lata. Because this fascia "give" is not consistent and its perception may vary among practioners, local anesthetic is injected in a fanwise fashion both above and below the fascia lata from medial to lateral. A volume of 10 mL of local anesthetic is injected for this block. Although the lateral femoral cutaneous nerve is a sensory nerve, relatively higher

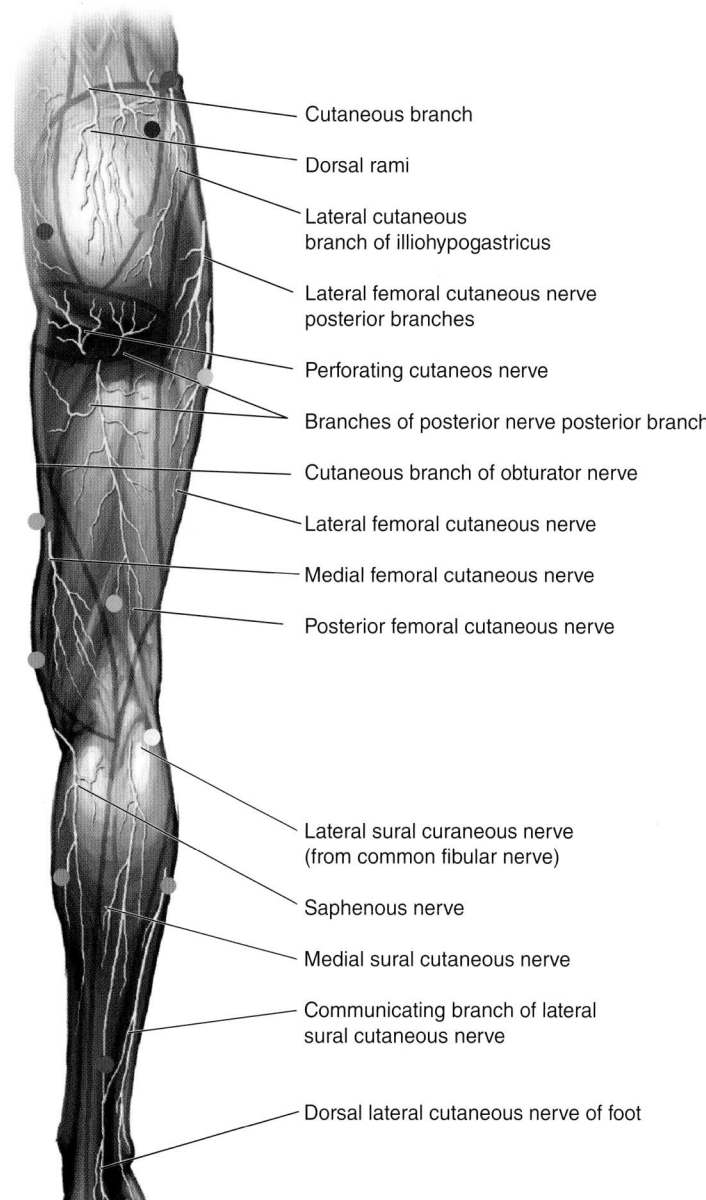

- ● 1st Thoracic
- ● Illiohypogastric
- ● Posterior division of S1, 2, 3
- ● Posterior division of L1, 2, 3
- ● Lateral Femoral Cutaneous
- ● Anterior Femoral cutaneous
- ● Posterior femoral cutaneous nerve (of the thigh)
- ● Obturator
- Lateral sural cutaneous
- ● Saphenous
- ● Superficial peroneal
- ● Sural
- ▒ Medial plantar
- ● Medial sural cutaneous

Cutaneous branch

Dorsal rami

Lateral cutaneous branch of illiohypogastricus

Lateral femoral cutaneous nerve posterior branches

Perforating cutaneos nerve

Branches of posterior nerve posterior branches

Cutaneous branch of obturator nerve

Lateral femoral cutaneous nerve

Medial femoral cutaneous nerve

Posterior femoral cutaneous nerve

Lateral sural curaneous nerve (from common fibular nerve)

Saphenous nerve

Medial sural cutaneous nerve

Communicating branch of lateral sural cutaneous nerve

Dorsal lateral cutaneous nerve of foot

FIGURE 82G–2. Cutaneous innervation of the lower extremity, posterior view.

TABLE 80G–1. Choice of anesthetic for cutaneous nerve block of the lower extremity.

	Onset (min)	Anesthesia (h)	Analgesia (h)
1.5% Mepivacaine	15–20	2–3	3–5
2% Lidocaine	10–20	2–5	3–8
0.5% Ropivacaine	15–30	4–8	5–12
0.75% Ropivacaine	10–15	5–10	6–24
0.5% (L) Bupivacaine	15–30	5–15	6–30

concentrations of long-acting local anesthetic are useful to increase the success rate (0.5% ropivacaine or bupivacaine) because this is essentially a "blind" technique. Alternatively, nerve stimulator (2 mA, 1msec) can be used to elicit paresthesia sensation in the typical distribution of the nerve to assure its location.

When used to provide anesthesia for a skin graft harvest site on the lateral thigh, the peripheral innervation of the lateral femoral cutaneous nerve in specific patients is outlined before beginning skin harvesting.

Because no larger vascular structures or other organs are nearby, blockade of the lateral femoral cutaneous nerve carries a minimal risk of complications.

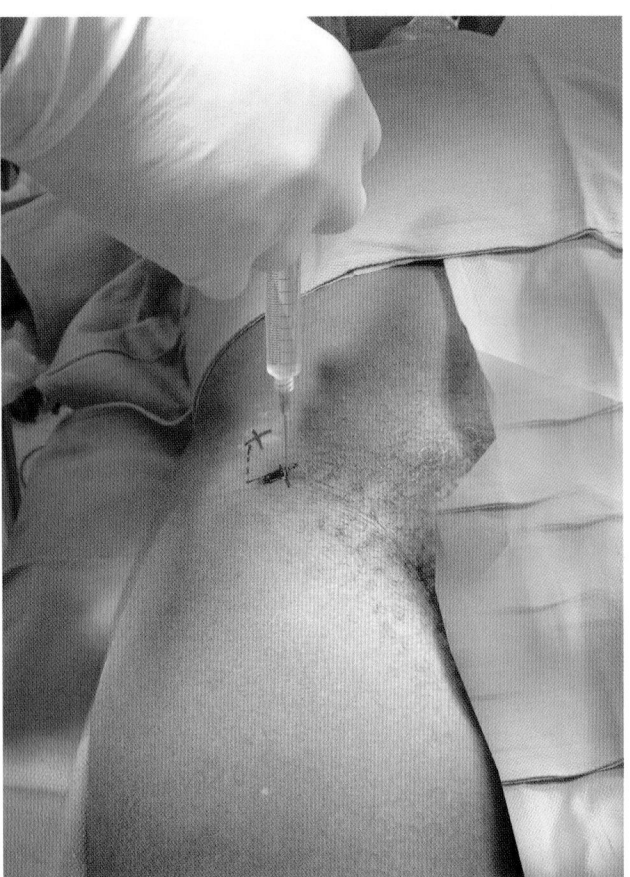

FIGURE 82G–3. Lateral femoral cutaneous nerve block. The landmark for this block is the anterior superior iliac spine.

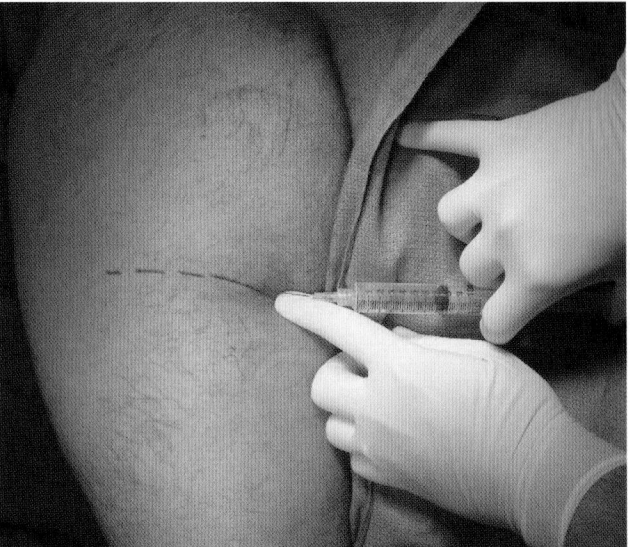

FIGURE 82G–4. Posterior cutaneous nerve of the thigh block, subgluteal approach.

It runs through the greater sciatic foramen below the piriformis and descends under the gluteus maximus muscle with the inferior gluteal vessels, posterior or medial to the sciatic nerve. The nerve then descends in the back of the thigh deep to the

POSTERIOR CUTANEOUS NERVE OF THE THIGH BLOCK

General Considerations

This block has been used in burn patients with donor skin for grafting taken from the posterior thigh or as part of a popliteal/posterior femoral cutaneous nerve block in short saphenous vein stripping.[11]

Distribution of Anesthesia

The posterior cutaneous nerve of the thigh innervates the skin over the posterior thigh between the lateral femoral cutaneous and anterior femoral cutaneous nerves (see Figure 82G–2).

Patient Positioning

The patient can be positioned prone, in the lateral decubitus position (shown in Figures 82G–4 and 82G–5), or supine with the leg elevated 90 degrees.

Anatomic Landmarks

The posterior femoral cutaneous nerve originates from the dorsal branches of the first and second sacral rami and from the ventral branches of the second and third sacral rami.

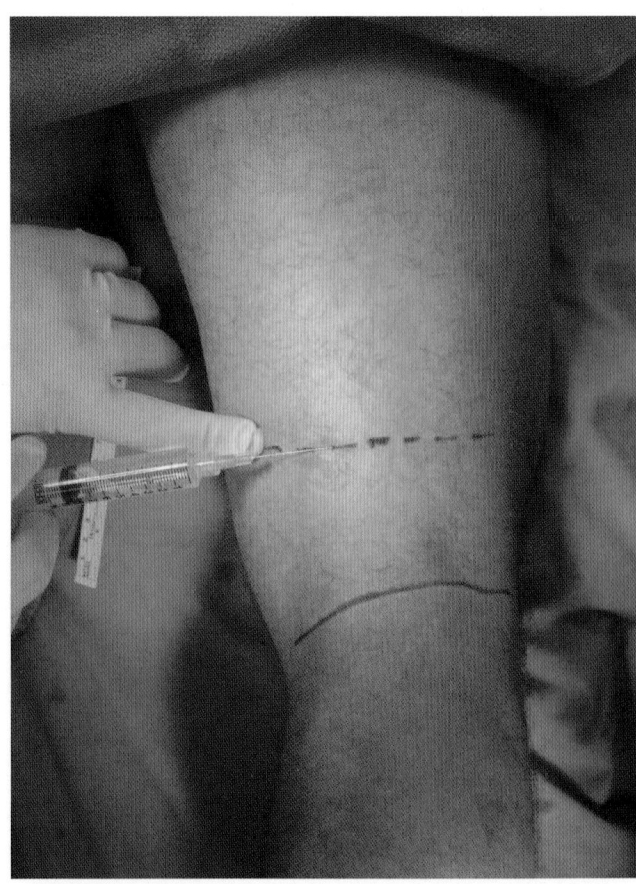

FIGURE 82G–5. Posterior cutaneous nerve of the thigh block, midthigh approach.

fascia lata. Its branches are all cutaneous and are distributed to the gluteal region, the perineum, and the flexor aspect of the thigh and leg.

Technique

The gluteal fold is identified and 10 mL of local anesthetic is injected subcutaneously to raise a skin wheal (see Figure 82G–4). In addition, at the midpoint of the gluteal crease, 5 mL of local anesthetic is injected at a deeper level, using a fan technique to reach the nerve that has not emerged through the deep fascia.

To block the posterior cutaneous nerve of the thigh above the knee level, as for short saphenous vein stripping (as a complement to popliteal block),[11] 10 mL of local anesthetic is injected subcutaneously along a line 5 cm above and parallel with the popliteal crease (see Figure 82G–5).

SAPHENOUS NERVE BLOCK

General Considerations

The saphenous nerve block is most commonly used in combination with a sciatic nerve block or popliteal block to complement anesthesia of the lower leg for various vascular, orthopedic, and podiatric procedures. The saphenous nerve is a terminal cutaneous branch of the femoral nerve. Its course is in the subcutaneous tissue of the skin on the medial aspect of the ankle and foot. All cutaneous nerves of the foot should be thought of as a neuronal network rather than well defined innervation territories of specific nerves.

Distribution of Anesthesia

The saphenous nerve innervates the skin over the medial, anteromedial, and posteromedial aspects of the lower leg from above the knee (part of the patellar plexus) to as low as the first metatarsophalangeal joint in some instances (Figures 80G–1 and 80G–7).

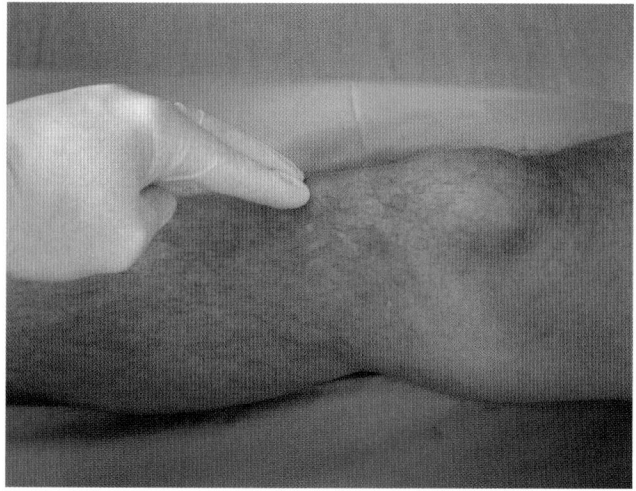

FIGURE 82G–6. Tibial tuberosity. Palpation of the landmark for the saphenous nerve block.

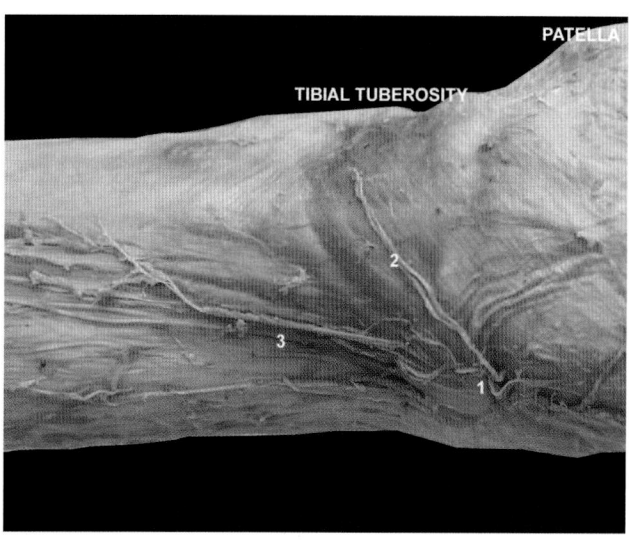

FIGURE 82G–7. Saphenous nerve anatomy. Saphenous nerve pierces through the sartorius muscle (1), subpatellar branch (2), saphenous nerve in its descent on the medial aspect of the thigh (3).

Patient Positioning

The patient is placed supine with the leg to be blocked supported by a footrest.

Anatomic Landmarks

The main landmark for this block is the tibial tuberosity, an easily recognizable and palpable bony prominence on the anterior aspect of the tibia, a few centimeters distal from the patella (Figure 82G–6). The saphenous nerve is the largest cutaneous branch of the femoral nerve. It descends lateral to the femoral artery into the adductor canal, where it crosses anteriorly to become medial to the artery. It proceeds vertically along the medial side of the knee behind the sartorius, pierces the fascia lata between the tendons of the sartorius and gracilis, and then becomes subcutaneous. From here, it descends on the medial side of the leg with the long saphenous vein. Note that the saphenous nerve divides into numerous small branches as it enters the subcutaneous space, and, as such, it is often difficult to achieve block of the entire extensive saphenous nerve network.

Techniques

The below-knee field block is performed with the patient in thesupine position. Five to 10 mL of local anesthetic is injected as a ring deeply subcutaneously, starting at the medial surface of the tibial condyle and ending at the dorsomedial aspect of the upper calf (Figure 82G–8).

A perivenous technique has also been described, which is based on the close relation of the saphenous vein and nerve, to achieve a higher success rate. First, the saphenous vein is identified using a tourniquet around the leg in dependent position. The technique involves injection of 5 mL of local anesthetic in a fanlike fashion around the vein on the medial side of the leg just distal from the patella.[12] This technique, however, carries a small risk of creating a hematoma if the saphenous vein is punctured.

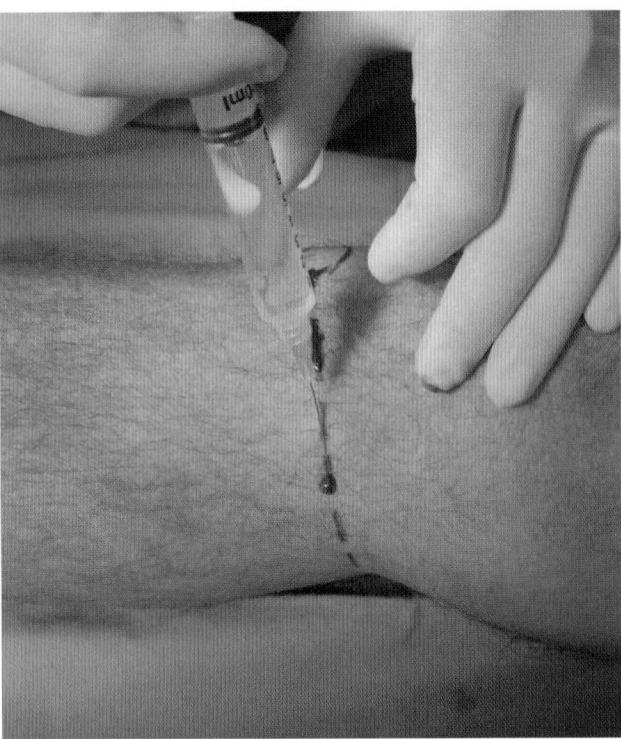

FIGURE 82G–8. Saphenous nerve block. Shown is a subcutaneous injection of 10 mL of local anesthetic in a circumferential fashion on the medial aspect of the leg at the level of the tibial tuberosity.

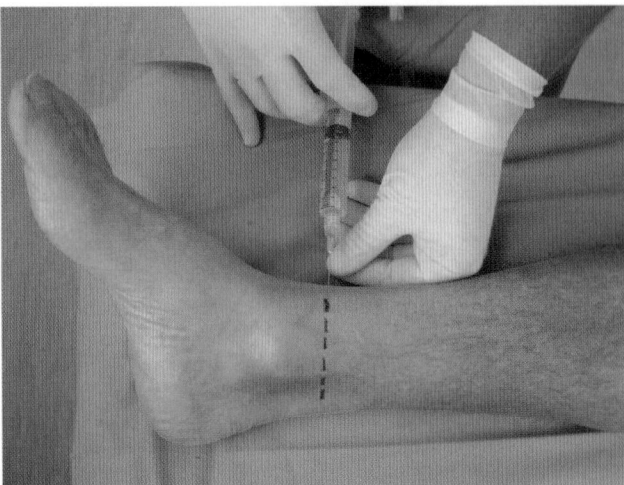

FIGURE 82G–9. Saphenous nerve block, distal approach above the medial malleolus.

Clinical Pearls

- The most effective method of blocking the saphenous nerve is a low-volume femoral nerve block.
- Injection of 10 mL of local anesthetic upon obtaining twitches of the patella or vastus medialis muscle results in a high success rate.

In the transsartorial approach, with the patient in the supine position, a skin wheal is raised over the sartorius muscle belly. The sartorius muscle can be palpated just above the knee with the leg extended and actively elevated. The needle is inserted at 1 finger-width above the patella slightly posterior to the coronal plane and slightly caudad through the muscle belly of the sartorius until a loss of resistance identifies the subsartorial adipose tissue. The depth of insertion is typically between 1.5 and 3.0 cm. After negative aspiration for blood, 10 mL of local anesthetic is injected.

For surgery on the foot, the saphenous nerve is best blocked just above the medial malleolus, similar to the technique in ankle block (Figure 82G–9). Using a 1.5-in. needle, 6–8 mL of local anesthetic is injected subcutaneously immediately above the medial malleolus in a ring-like fashion. The most commonly reported complication of this block is a hematoma of the saphenous vein at the injection site.

The saphenous nerve can also be blocked by using a nerve stimulator technique and performing a low-volume femoral nerve block (see Chapter 82C). Injection of 10 mL of local anesthetic after obtaining either a medial muscle response, signified by contraction of the vastus medialis muscle, or an anterior muscle response, signified by contraction of the rectus femoris muscle and elevation of the patella, results in a high rate of block success.[13,14] Neurostimulation of the medial compartment of the femoral nerve requires even less volume of local anesthetic, compared with that of a standard femoral block.[15]

In a comparison of the different approaches to saphenous nerve block, the transsartorial approach resulted in 100% sensory blockade of the medial aspect of the leg, whereas the perifemoral and the below-knee field block were successful only in 70%. The medial femoral condyle block resulted in 40% of the patients having sensory blockade of the medial aspect of the leg with only 25% having complete anesthesia at the medial malleolus.[16] This supported the findings of a previous study in which 94% of patients had complete anesthesia of the medial malleolus after a transsartorial saphenous nerve block.[17] However, saphenous nerve often does not reach the level of the medial malleolus.[18] The introduction of ultrasound-guided techniques and several studies supporting its use as an alternative to femoral block for total knee arthroplasty have greatly increased the interest in the transsartorial (or "adductor canal") approach to the saphenous nerve.[19,20]

SURAL NERVE BLOCK

General Considerations

The sural nerve block is used for superficial surgery on the lateral aspect of the ankle and foot and in conjunction with ankle block for foot and toe surgery.

Distribution of Anesthesia

The sural nerve innervates the posterior and lateral skin of the distal third of the leg along the lateral side of the foot and little toe (see Figure 82G–1).

Patient Positioning

For the block procedure, the patient can be positioned prone or supine with the ankle supported by a footrest.

Anatomic Landmarks

The sural nerve, a branch of the tibial nerve, pierces the deep fascia proximally in the leg and is joined by a branch of the common peroneal nerve. It descends near the lesser saphenous vein and between the lateral malleolus and the calcaneus.

Technique

Using a 1.5-in., 25-gauge needle, a skin wheal is raised lateral to the Achilles tendon and just above the lateral malleolus (Figure 82G–10). The needle is then inserted through the wheal and advanced toward the fibula while injecting 6–8 mL of local anesthetic.

SUPERFICIAL PERONEAL BLOCK

General Considerations

A superficial peroneal block is used alone or in combination with other blocks for foot surgery or ascending venography.[21,22]

Distribution of Anesthesia

The superficial peroneal branches supply innervation to the dorsal skin of all the toes except that of the lateral side of the fifth and

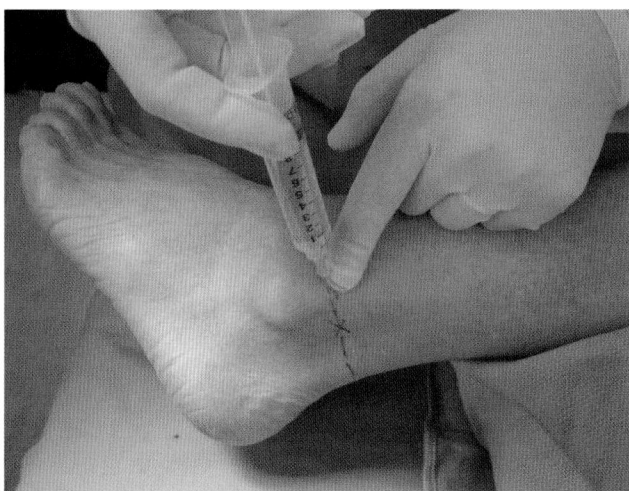

FIGURE 82G–10. Sural nerve block.

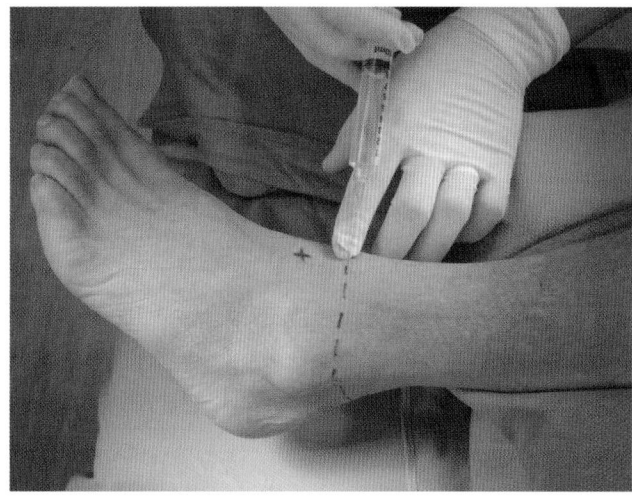

FIGURE 82G–11. Superficial peroneal block.

adjoining sides of the first and second toes (see Figures 82G–1 and 82G–2).

Anatomic Landmarks

The superficial peroneal nerve begins at the common peroneal bifurcation. It pierces the deep fascia in the distal third of the leg. It descends the leg adjacent to the extensor digitorum longus muscle, where it divides into terminal branches above the ankle.

Patient Positioning

For the block procedure, the patient can be positioned supine with the ankle supported by a footrest.

Technique

The superficial peroneal nerve is blocked immediately above and medial to the lateral malleolus. 5–10 mL of local anesthetic is injected to form a subcutaneous wheal from the extensor hallucis longus tendon to the anterior surface of the lateral malleolus (Figure 82G–11).

COMPLICATIONS

Few complications result from performing cutaneous nerve blocks of the lower extremity. Possible complications and suggestions for how to avoid them are outlined in Table 82G–2.

SUMMARY

There are many uses for cutaneous nerve blocks of the lower extremity in everyday clinical practice. These blocks are easy to perform and are nearly devoid of complications.

TABLE 80G-2. Possible complications from cutaneous nerve blocks of the lower extremity.

Systemic toxicity of local anesthetic	• Risk is small and may be of concern only when higher volumes are used in conjunction with other high-volume major conduction blocks
Hematoma	• Avoid multiple needle insertions and insertion of the needle through superficial veins
Nerve injury	• Usually manifested as transient paresthesias or dysesthesias
	• Avoid injecting when high pressures on injection are felt or when the patient reports pain in the distribution of the nerve

REFERENCES

1. Hopkins P, Ellis F, Halsall P: Evaluation of local anaesthetic blockade of the lateral femoral cutaneous nerve. Anaesthesia 1991;46:95–96.
2. Coad N: Postoperative analgesia following femoral-neck surgery: A comparison between 3 in 1 femoral nerve block and lateral cutaneous nerve block. Eur J Anaesthesiol 1991;8:287–290.
3. Maccani R, Wedel D, Melton A, Gronert G: Femoral and lateral femoral cutaneous nerve block for muscle biopsies in children. Paediatr Anaesth 1995;5:223–227.
4. Jones S, White A: Analgesia following femoral neck surgery. Lateral cutaneous nerve block as an alternative to narcotics in the elderly. Anaesthesia 1985;40:682–685.
5. Hood G, Edbrooke D, Gerrish S: Postoperative analgesia after triple nerve block for fractured neck of femur. Anaesthesia 1991;46:
6. Hughes P, Brown T: An approach to posterior femoral cutaneous nerve block. Anaesth Intensive Care 1986;14:350–351.
7. Elmas C, Elmas Y, Gautschi P, Uehlinger P: Combined sciatic 3-in-1 block. Application in lower limb orthopedic surgery. Anaesthetist 1992;41:639–643.
8. McNicol L: Lower limb blocks for children. Lateral cutaneous and femoral nerve blocks for postoperative pain relief in paediatric practice. Anaesthesia 1986;41:27–31.
9. Wardrop P, Nishikawa H: Lateral cutaneous nerve of the thigh blockade as primary anaesthesia for harvesting skin grafts. Br J Plast Surg 1995;48:597–600.
10. Brown T, Dickens D: A new approach to lateral cutaneous nerve of thigh block. Anaesth Intensive Care 1986;14:126–127.
11. Vloka J, Hadzic A, Mulcare R, et al: Combined popliteal and posterior cutaneous nerve of the thigh blocks for short saphenous vein stripping in outpatients: an alternative to spinal anesthesia. J Clin Anesth 1997;9:618–622.
12. De Mey J, Deruyck L, Cammu G, et al: A paravenous approach for the saphenous nerve block. Reg Anesth Pain Med 2001;26:504–506.
13. Comfort V, Lang S, Yip R: Saphenous nerve anaesthesia: a nerve stimulator technique. Can J Anaesth 1996;43:852–857.
14. Mansour N: Subsartorial saphenous nerve block with the aid of nerve stimulator. Reg Anesth Pain Med 1993;18:266–268.
15. Chassery C, Gilbert M, Minville V, et al: Neurostimulation does not increase the success rate of saphenous nerve blocks. Can J Anaesth 2005;52:269–275.
16. Benzon H, Sharma S, Calimaran A: Comparison of the different approaches to saphenous nerve block. Anesthesiology 2005;102:633–638.
17. van der Wal M, Lang S, Yip R: Transsartorial approach for saphenous nerve block. Can J Anaesth 1993;40:542–546.
18. López AM1, Sala-Blanch X, Magaldi M, Poggio D, Asuncion J, Franco CD: Ultrasound-guided ankle block for forefoot surgery: the contribution of the saphenous nerve. Reg Anesth Pain Med. 2012 37(5):554-7.
19. Jœger P, Zaric D, Fomsgaard JS, et al: Adductor canal block versus femoral nerve block for analgesia after total knee arthroplasty: a randomized, double-blind study. Reg Anesth Pain Med. 2013;38:526–532.
20. Shah NA, Jain NP: Is Continuous Adductor Canal Block Better Than Continuous Femoral Nerve Block After Total Knee Arthroplasty? Effect on Ambulation Ability, Early Functional Recovery and Pain Control: A Randomized Controlled Trial. J Arthroplasty. 2014 Jun 19 [Epub ahead of print].
21. Mussurakis S: Combined superficial peroneal and saphenous nerve block for ascending venography. Eur J Radiol 1992;14:56–59.
22. Lieberman R, Kaplan P: Superficial peroneal nerve block for leg venography. Radiology 1987;165:578–579.

APPENDICES

APPENDIX 1

European Recommendations for Use of Regional Anesthesia in the Setting of Anticoagulation

Luc Van Keer, Dimitri Dylst, and Ine Leunen

Abbreviations Table 1A and B:

ACT: Activated clotting time

ACS: Acute coronary syndrome

Afib: Atrial fibrillation

Anesth.: Anesthesia

aPTT : Activated partial thromboplastin time

ASA: Acetylsalicylic acid

ATE: Arterial thromboembolism

BMS: Bare metal stent

COX: cyclooxygenase

CrCl : Creatinine clearance

CV: CHA_2DS_2-VASc

CVA: Cerebral vascular accident

CYP3A4: Cytochrome P450 3A4

DES: Drug eluting stent

DVT: Deep venous thrombosis

GP IIb-IIIa: glycoprotein IIb-IIIa

HB: HAS-BLED score

ICD: implantable cardioverter defibrillator

INR: International normalized ratio

IV: Intravenous

LMWH: Low molecular weight heparin

NOACs: New oral anticoagulants

OBR: Intra operative bleeding risk

Prim.: primary

PCI: Percutaneous coronary intervention

PE: Pulmonary embolism

P-gp: P-glycoprotein

PT: Prothrombin time

Prev.: prevention

PO: Per Os

RA: Regional anaesthesia

SC: Subcutaneous

Sec.: secondary

TER: Thrombo embolic risk

TIA: Transient ischemic attack

UFH: Unfractionated heparin

VKA: Vitamin K antagonist

VTE: Venous thromboembolism

⊗ time interval between drug stop and procedure

⊚ time interval to restart the drug after procedure

TABLE 1–1A. Overview of antiplatelet agents and anticoagulants with clinically useful information about dosage and perioperative management of patients using this type of drug. The overview was composed from a perspective of medical practice in western europe (Belgium).

Product (T½ in Hours)	Brand Name	Normal Dose	⊗	⊙	Bridging	Comments Concerning RA
COX inhibitors (ASA) PO						
Aspirin (3)	Asaflow®	Prim. prevention: 80 mg 1x/d	5 d	24 h	Don't bridge with LMWH	**Spinal anesthesia: OK**
		Sec. prevention: 80 mg 1x/d	do not stop	24 h		**Epidural anesthesia: OK**
						Aggrenox® = ASA + Dipyridamole ≈ ASA
P2Y12 inhibitors PO		Prim. prevention: No indication				
Clopidogrel (7)	Plavix®	Sec. prevention: 75 mg po 1x/d	7 d	24 h	Asaflow® 80 mg po 1x/d	**Neuraxial anaesthesia: NO**
Ticlopidine (12)	Ticlid®	250 mg po 2x/d	10 d	24 h	Asaflow® 80 mg po 1x/d	**Combi-therapie: ASA x P2Y12**
Prasugrel (7)	Efient®	10 mg po 1x/d	10 d	24 h	Asaflow® 80 mg po 1x/d	(see Table 1-1B)
Ticagrelor (7)	Brilique®	90 mg po 2x/d	7 d	24 h	Asaflow® 80 mg po 1x/d	
GP IIb-IIIa inhibitors						
Abciximab (20)	Reopro®	iv	48 h	4 h	Don't bridge with LMWH	**Neuraxial anaesthesia: NO**
Eptifibatid (2,5)	Integrilin®	iv	12 h	4 h		Platelet count ≥ 70x10⁹/L
Tirofiban (2)	Aggrastat®	iv	12 h	4 h		
VKA PO					LMWH according to TER	
Acenocoumarol (8)	Sintrom®	1-8 mg po 1x/d	4 d	72 h	Low: Clexane® profylactic	**Neuraxial anesthesia if INR ≤ 1.4 / PT ≥ 60%**
Warfarine (40)	Marevan®	1,5-5 mg po 1x/d	7 d	72 h	Intermediate: Clexane® Intermediate	LMWH according to TER (see Table 1-1B)
Fenprocoumol (120)	Marcoumar®	1,5-6 mg po 1x/d	10 d	72 h	High: Clexane® therapeutic	Start bridging when INR ≤ 2
						see section on LMWH below
UFH IV						
Heparin (1,5)	Heparine®	ACT, aPTT	4 h	60 min		**Heparin IV ≥ 60 min after neuraxial anesthesia**
						Platelet count ≥ 70x10⁹/L
LMWH SC						
Enoxaparine (4)	Clexane®					**Prophylactic dose as long as catheter in situ**
Profylactic		50 IU anti-Xa/kg = 0.5 mg/kg 1x/d	12 h	8 h		Half the dosage if CrCl ≤ 30 mL/m
Intermediate		100 IU anti-Xa/kg = 1.0 mg/kg 1x/d	24 h	24 h		Platelet count ≥ 70x10⁹/L
Therapeutic		100 IU anti-Xa/kg = 1.0 mg/kg 2x/d	24 h	72 h		
Thrombolytics IV						
Urokinase (15')	Actosolv®	iv	14 d	10 d		**Neuraxial aneshesia: NO**
Tenecteplase (25')	Metalyse®	iv	14 d	10 d		Platelet count ≥ 70x10⁹/L
Alteplase (35')	Actilyse®	iv	14 d	10 d		

Anti IIa PO

Dabigatran (17) — Pradaxa®

Indication / Dose	Time
Prim. prev. VTE 220 mg po 1×/d	(see Table 1-1B)
Dose reduction* 150 mg po 1×/d	72 h
Prev. ATE in AFib 150 mg po 2×/d	72 h
Dose reduction* 110 mg po 1×/d	72 h
	72 h

PREOPERATIVELY: Don't Bridge
OBR = low: Don't stop NOAC
= intermediate: OK, accurate timing
= high: OK, accurate timing
POSTOPERATIVELY: LMWH according to TER see section on VKA

Neuraxial anesthesia: (see Table 1-1B)
Start LMWH postoperatively: Profylactic 8 h
Intermediate 24 h
Therapeutic 72 h

Dose adjustment: P-gp inductors/inhibitors
*Dose reduction: ≥ 75 y, CrCl 30-49 mL/min, verapamil
Not indicated: CrCl ≤ 30 mL/min

Anti-Xa SC

Fundaparinux (17) — Arixtra®

Indication / Dose	Time	
Prim. prev. VTE 2.5 mg sc 1×/d	36 h	7 h

Spinal anesthesia: OK; Epidural anesthesia: NO

Anti-Xa PO

Apixaban (12) — Eliquis®
Edoxaban (11) — Lixiana®
Rivaroxaban (12) — Xarelto®

Indication / Dose	Time
Prim. prev. VTE 2.5 mg po 2×/d	(see Table 1-1B)
Prev. AVT in AFib 5.0 mg po 2×/d	72 h
Prev. AVT in AFib 60 mg po 1×/d	72 h
Dose reduction* 30 mg po 1×/d	72 h
Prim. prev. VTE 10 mg po 1×/d	72 h
Prev. AVT in AFib 20 mg po 1×/d	72 h
Treatment VTE 15 mg po 2×/d	72 h
Sec. prev. VTE 20 mg po 1×/d	72 h

PREOPERATIVELY: Don't bridge
OBR = low: Don't stop NOAC
= intermediate: OK, accurate timing
= high: OK, accurate timing
POSTOPERATIVELY: LMWH according to TER see section on VKA

Neuraxial anesthesia: (see Table 1-1B)
Start LMWH postoperatively: Prophylactic 8 h
Intermediate 24 h
Therapeutic 72 h

Dose adjustment: P-gp and CYP3A4
*Dose reduction: HB ≥ 3, CrCl 30-49 mL/min
Not indicated: CrCl ≤ 15 mL/min

APPENDICES

TABLE 1–1B. Risk stratification and guide to management of patients undergoing surgical or diagnostic procedures in the presence of antiplatelet agents or new oral anticoagulants. The overview was composed from a perspective of medical practice in western europe (Belgium).

Intraoperative Bleeding Risk (OBR)

Low
- Minor dental procedures
- Superficial dermatologic procedures
- Cataract and glaucoma under topical anesth
- Diagnostic gastroscopy
- Diagnostic bronchoscopy without biopsies
- Coronarography or PCI by radial artery
- Replacement pacemaker or ICD

Standard
- Endoscopy with biopsies
- Bladder biopsy
- Phlebologic procedures
- Angiography
- Implantation pacemaker or ICD
- Coronarography or PCI by femoral artery
- Electrophysiologic examination ± ablation

High
- Neuraxial anesthesia, lumbar puncture
- Cardiac surgery
- Intracranial and spinal surgery (1)
- Thoracic and major abdominal surgery
- Peripheral and other major vascular surgery
- Hip and knee arthroplasty, cruciate ligament reconstruction
- Reconstructive and plastic surgery
- Major oncologic surgery
- Prostate and bladder surgery (2)
- Endoscopic resection of colon polyps
- Prostate, kidney, and liver biopsy
- Endoscopic sphincterotomy

Thrombo Embolic Risk (TER)

	Heart Valve Prosthesis	Atrial Fibrillation	Venous Thrombo Embolism
High ATE > 10%/y VTE > 10%/y	Mitral valve prosthesis, old aortic valve prosthesis (monoleaflet or ball prosthesis)	CV > 5; CVA/TIA (< 6 m) Rheumatic valve disease	DVT/PE < 3 mths Severe thrombophilia
Moderate ATE 5-10%/y VTE < 10%/y	Bileaflet aortic valve prosthesis	CV = 4 - 5 CVA/TIA > 6 m	DVT/PE 3 - 12 mths Recurrent DVT/PE Active Oncology Mild thrombophilia
Low ATE 2-5%/Y VTE < 2%/Y		CV ≤ 3 **and** no CVA/TIA	DVT/PE once > 12 mths **and** no thrombophilia

$CHA2DS_2$-VASc (CV)

	Points	Total Score	Stroke % / y
C: Congestive heart failure	1	0	0
H: Hypertension	1	1	1.3
A_2: Age > 75	2	2	2.2
D: Diabetes	1	3	3.2
S_2: CVA/TIA/VTE	2	4	4.0
V: Vascular disease	1	5	6.7
A: Age 65 - 74	1	6	9.8
Sc: Sex category Female	1	7	9.6
		8	6.7
		9	15.2

HAS-BLED (HB)

	Points	Total score	Bleeding % / y
H: Hypertension	1	0	1.13
A: Abnormal renal function / Abnormal liver function	1	1	1.02
S: Stroke	1	2	1.88
B: Bleeding	1	3	3.74
L: Labile INR	1	4	8.70
E: Elderly	1		
D: Drugs / Alcohol	1		

NOACs interruption of therapy for elective surgery

If OBR = low: do not interrupt NOACs. Perform procedure 12 – 16 h after last intake. Normal dosage will be taken in the evening after surgery. NOACs should always be taken in the evening.

CrCl	Dabigatran Pradaxa® Standard	High	Abigatran Eliquis® Standard	High	Edoxaban Lixiana® Standard	High	Rivaroxaban Xarelto® Standard	High
>80 mL/min	24 h	48 h	24 h	48 h	24 h	48 h	24 h	48 h
50 - 80 mL/min	36 h	72 h	24 h	48 h	24 h	48 h	24 h	48 h
30 - 50 mL/min	48 h	96 h	24 h	48 h	24 h	48 h	24 h	48 h
15 - 30 mL/min	-	-	36 h	48 h	36 h	48 h	36 h	48 h
< 15 mL/min	-	-	-	-	-	-	-	-

Combination Therapy of Platelet Antiaggregation ASA x P2Y12

	OBR	ASA	P2Y12
Recent coronary stenting BMS < 1 mths DES < 6 mths ACS ≤ 6 wks	High	Only lifesaving surgery after advice	Continue
	Standard	Only urgent surgery	Continue
	Low	Elective surgery can proceed	Continue
No recent stenting	High	Only to be stopped in case of (see OBR (1) and (2))	Stop
	Standard	Continue	Stop
	Low	Continue	Stop

Thrombophilia

Severe	Antithrombine deficiency; ≥ 2 mild thrombophilia factors, homozygous factor V Leiden or protrombine gene variant G20210A, antifosfolipid syndrome
Mild	Protein C or S deficiency, high factor VIII, heterozygous factor V Leiden or protrombine gene variant G20210A

Disposition of Injectate with Common Regional Anesthesia Techniques

Philippe Gautier

The outcome of regional anesthesia technique is ultimately dependent on the distribution of the local anesthetic in the relevant tissue space that contains the nerve(s) of interest. Prior to the introduction of ultrasound in regional anesthesia, our understanding of the disposition of the local anesthetic had been limited due to the lack of technology that could allow such monitoring. This addendum features studies of computed tomographic (CT) images that we painstakingly acquired by the author over a period of nearly 2 decades in attempt to elucidate the disposition of local anesthetic injections with nerve block injections and their relationship to the outcome of regional anesthesia. The maldistribution of local anesthetic associated with block failures and/or complications due to the spillage of local anesthetic to the undesired places, such as, for example, the phrenic nerv and neuraxial space are also demonstrated. A uniquely educational aspect of these images is the relationship of the volume of the injectate and its physical spread in the tissue spaces.

The all original material presented in this appendix is organized in clusters of images of distribution of local anesthetic containing radiopaque solution. In addition to images of the expected, desired distribution, the images of the maldistribution of local anesthetic are also included as well. Wherever available, images of desired distribution and maldistribution are presented in several imaging planes, as well as in three-dimensional (3D) reconstruction. Importantly, the distribution patterns presented in the images cannot be fully or reliably studied by ultrasonography; hence their relevance in the era of ultrasound-guided regional anesthesia.

CERVICAL PLEXUS BLOCK

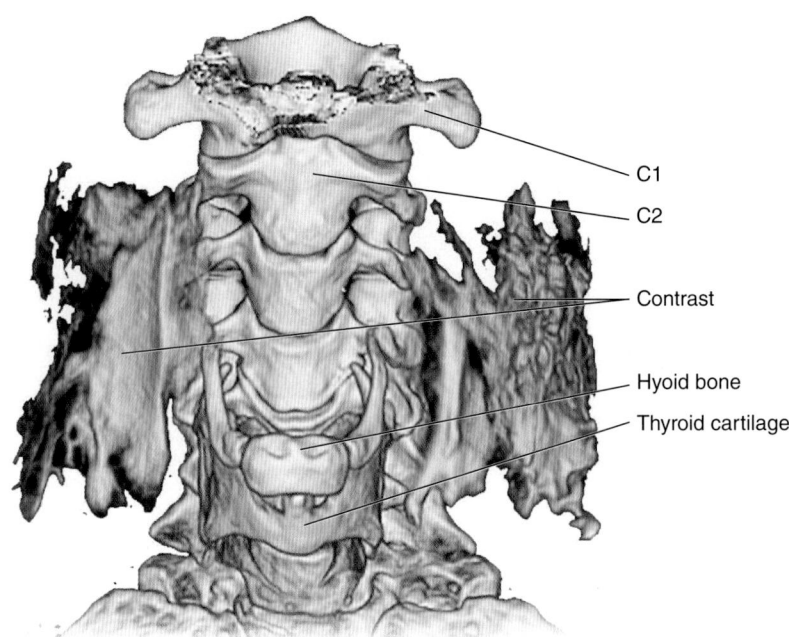

FIGURE 2–1. Five milliliters of local anesthetic solution containing radiopaque contrast was injected after insertion of the needle at the level of C4, behind the posterior aspect of the sternocleidomastoid muscle. An additional 10 mL was injected behind the sternocleidomastoid muscle. The 3D CT imaging shows bilateral distribution of the injectate from C2–C5 levels.

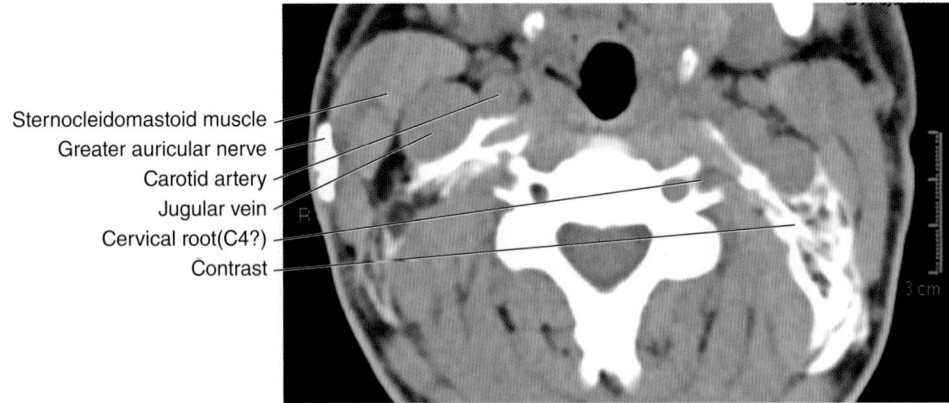

FIGURE 2–2. Injection of 15 mL of local anesthetic solution containing radi-opaque contrast behind the sternocleidomastoid muscle demonstrates substantial distribution of injectate in deeper tissue planes, resulting is contrast contacting cervical roots.

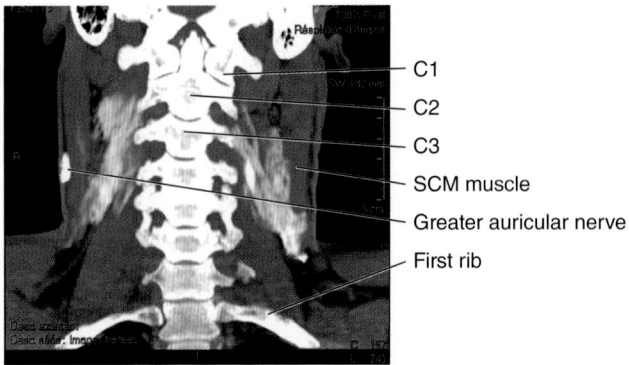

FIGURE 2–3. The same injection—frontal view. Injection of 15 mL of local anesthetic solution containing radiopaque contrast behind the sternocleidomastoid muscle demonstrates substantial distribution of injectate in deeper tissue planes, resulting is contrast contacting cervical roots.

INTERSCALENE BRACHIAL PLEXUS BLOCK

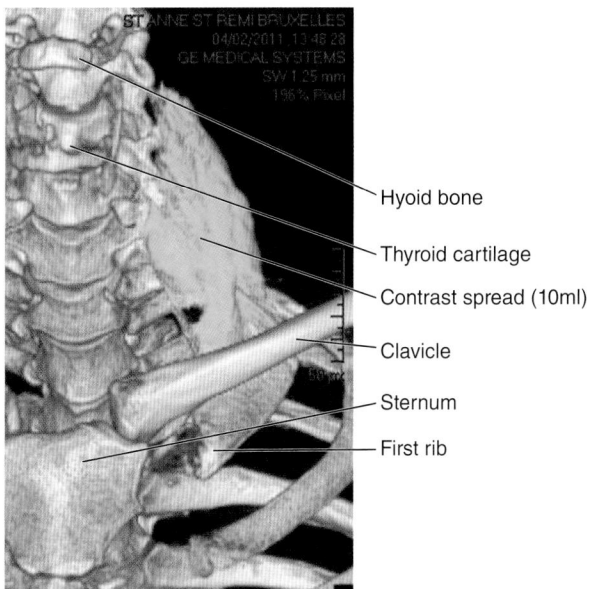

Hyoid bone

Thyroid cartilage

Contrast spread (10ml)

Clavicle

Sternum

First rib

FIGURE 2–4. The image demonstrates typical contrast spread after injection of 10 mL of the solution in interscalene space for brachial plexus block. The contrast is seen spreading from C5 to the clavicle.

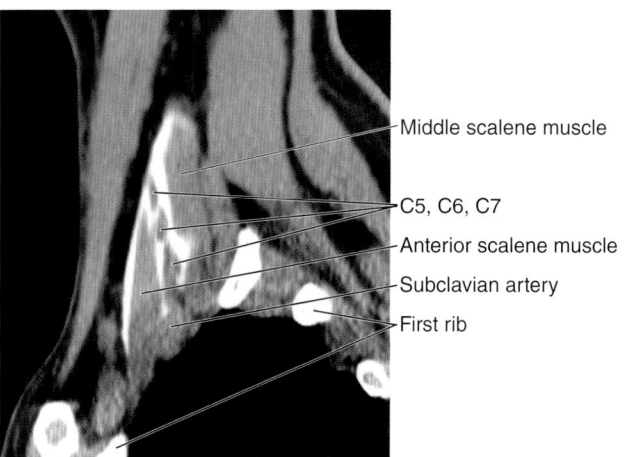

Middle scalene muscle

C5, C6, C7

Anterior scalene muscle

Subclavian artery

First rib

FIGURE 2–6. CT image—sagittal view of expected contrast spread after injection of 10 mL of the solution in interscalene space for brachial plexus block. The contrast is in the scalene space in contact with three roots of the brachial plexus (C5–C6). Also, the contrast is seen underneath fascia of the middle and anterior scalene muscles encountering phrenic nerve.

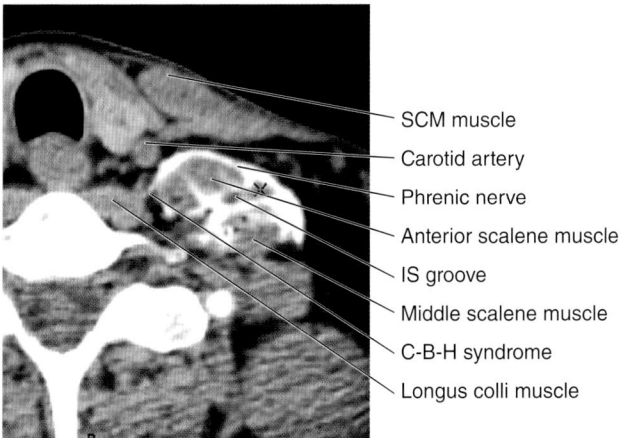

SCM muscle

Carotid artery

Phrenic nerve

Anterior scalene muscle

IS groove

Middle scalene muscle

C-B-H syndrome

Longus colli muscle

FIGURE 2–5. An axial CT image of expected contrast spread after injection of 10 mL of the solution in interscalene space for brachial plexus block. The contrast is in the scalene space in contact with three roots of the brachial plexus. Also, the contrast is seen underneath fascia of the middle and anterior scalene muscles encountering phrenic nerve. Claude-Bernard-Horner syndrome results from the block of the sympathetic fibers (C-B-H).

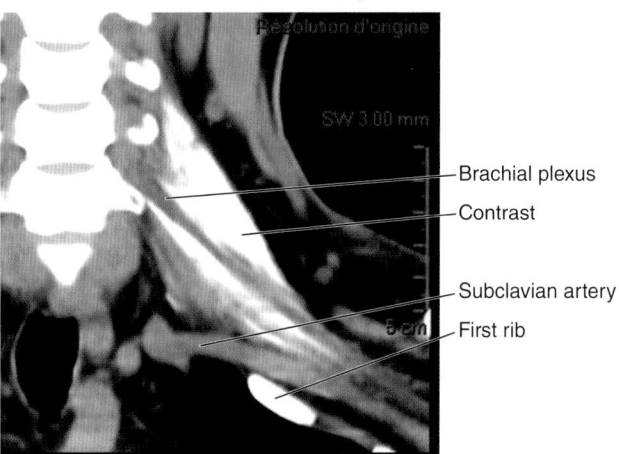

Brachial plexus

Contrast

Subclavian artery

First rib

FIGURE 2–7. CT—frontal view of adequate spread of the contrast after injection of 10 mL of the solution in interscalene space for brachial plexus block. The contrast is in the scalene space in contact with all relevant roots of the brachial plexus. The roots are (brachial plexus) seen as negative contrast image. Distal spread toward the supraclavicular and infraclavicular spaces is seen as well, (see spread over the first rib) demonstrating the anatomical continuity of the brachial plexus sheath.

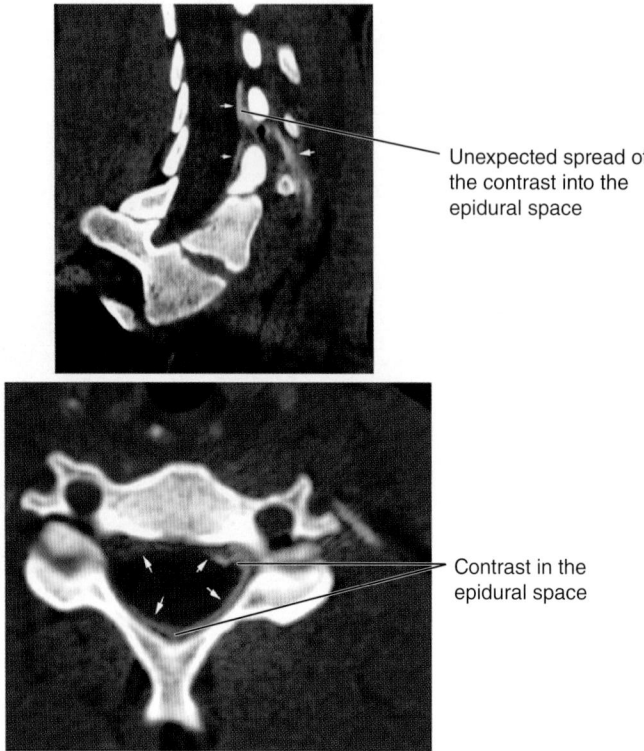

Unexpected spread of
the contrast into the
epidural space

Contrast in the
epidural space

FIGURE 2-8. Epidural spread of the contrast after high-pressure (>25 psi) injection into the scalene brachial plexus. These images may explain the mechanism of the high neuraxial block that occasionally occurs after an interscalene brachial plexus injection.

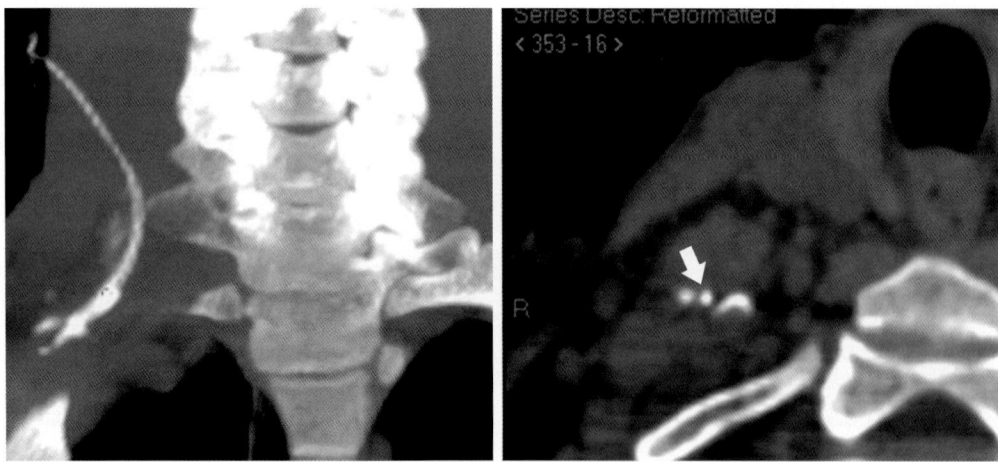

FIGURE 2-9. Course of the interscalene brachial plexus catheter . The catheter is seen curving and properly positioned in the scalene space 2–3 cm (*arrow*). The tip of the catheter is properly located between anterior and middle scalene muscles. Shown is opacification after injection of 0.15 mL of the contrast.

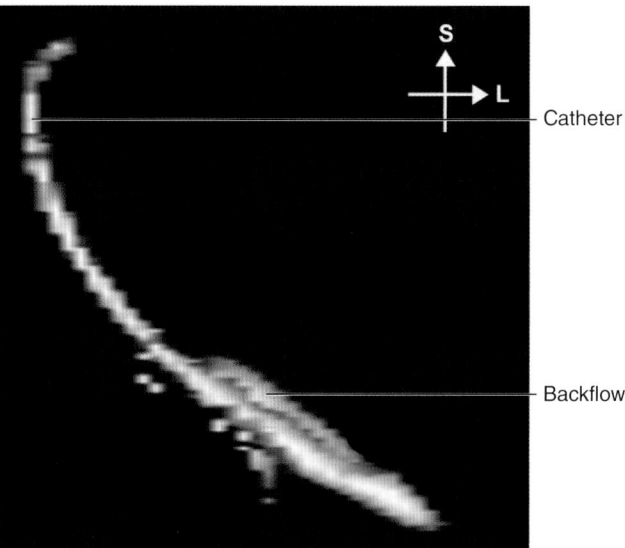

FIGURE 2–10. Course of the catheter inserted in an out of plane approach. After an injection of 0.2 mL of the contrast, the solution is seen inside the catheter, as well as backtracking alongside the catheter insertion track. This helps explain the mechanism of local anesthetic leakage around the catheter insertion site.

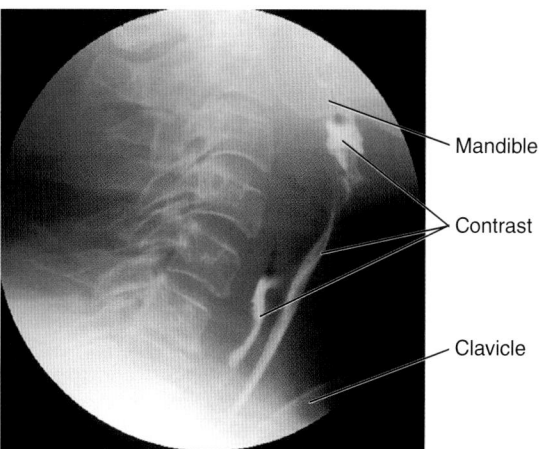

FIGURE 2–13. Catheter misadventure: The wire- reinforced catheter was intended to be placed into the interscalene space. However, the catheter was advanced too far, resulting in a distribution of the contrast in the paraesophageal space.

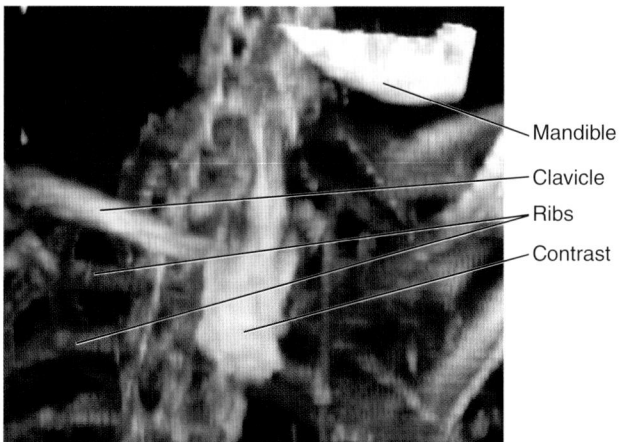

FIGURE 2–11. Maldistribution of the contrast injected through the catheter (20 mL) after the wire-reinforced catheter was advanced too far into the scalene space. The patient developed horse voice. The CT images shows contrast disposition paratracheally.

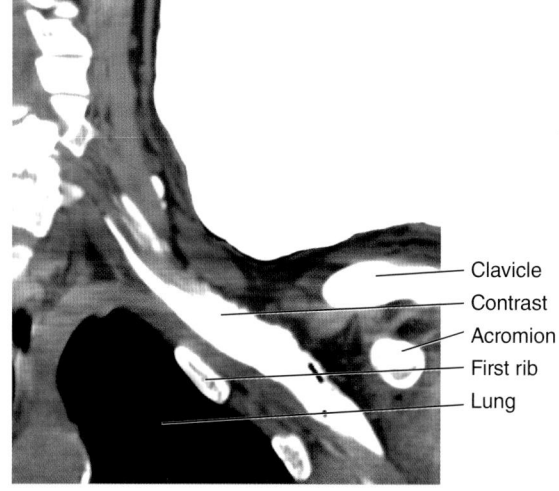

FIGURE 2–14. Too distal spread of the injectate into the infraclavicular and axillary brachial plexus sheath. The catheter was placed into the interscalene space, advancement of the catheter resulted in absence of the spread in the scalene space. These images demonstrate that the position of the tip of the catheter or distribution of the injectate should be checked by ultrasound to assure catheter functionality.

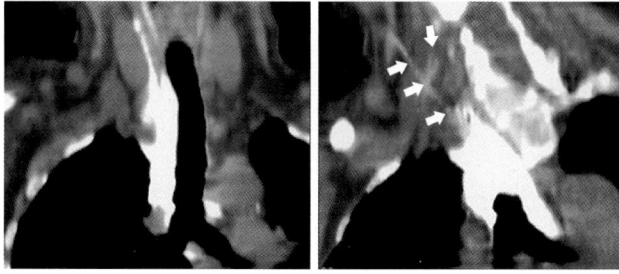

FIGURE 2–12. Maldistribution of the contrast in the same patient as in Figure 2–11, in oblique-frontal view. The catheter is seen passing through the scalene space into the paratracheal space. The dark areas represent lungs, trachea, and carina.

SUPRACLAVICULAR BLOCK

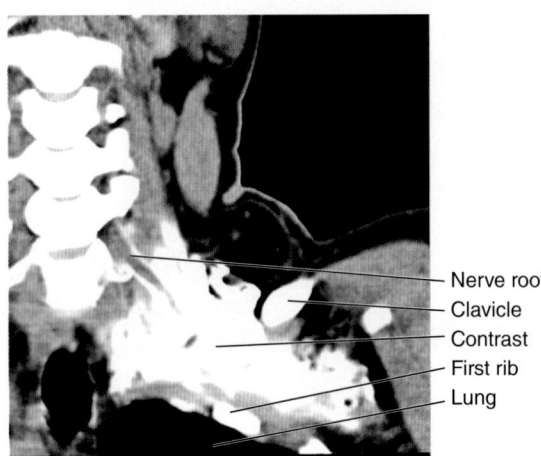

- Nerve root
- Clavicle
- Contrast
- First rib
- Lung

FIGURE 2–15. Twenty milliliters of injectate containing radiopaque contrast was injected into the supraclavicular brachial plexus sheath. The contrast is seen throughout the sheath, along with the negative contrast of one C7 root.

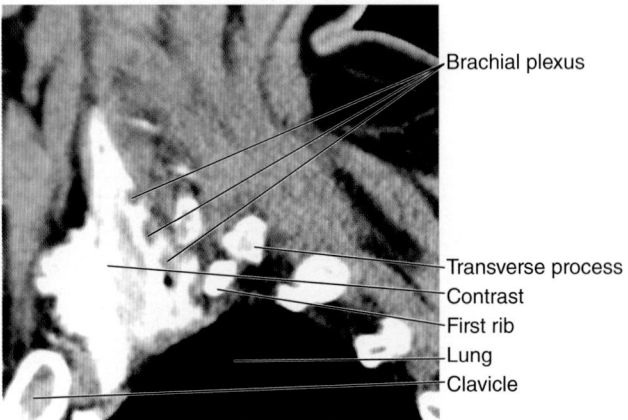

- Brachial plexus
- Transverse process
- Contrast
- First rib
- Lung
- Clavicle

FIGURE 2–16. CT image in a parasagittal view of an injection of 20 mL of the contrast for the supraclavicular brachial plexus resulted in the expected spread within the supraclavicular brachial plexus sheath. In addition, the injection also resulted in a significant spread proximally alongside the brachial plexus sheath, into the lower interscalene space and bathing the C5-C7 nerve roots. This finding demonstrates that (a) brachial plexus sheath is continuous and (b) supraclavicular and low interscalene brachial plexus blocks share common clinical features as the injection of larger volume into either may result in both blocks simultaneously.

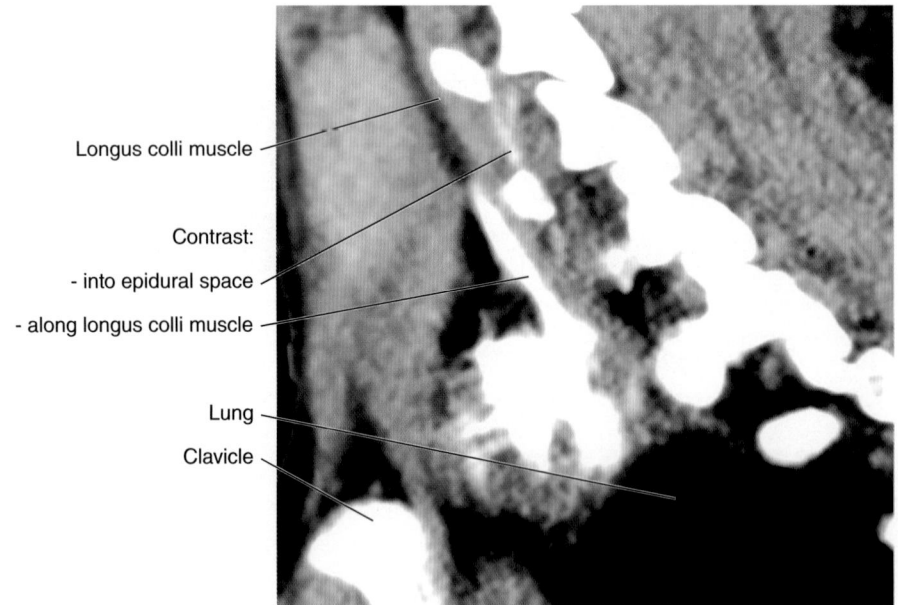

- Longus colli muscle
- Contrast:
- - into epidural space
- - along longus colli muscle
- Lung
- Clavicle

FIGURE 2–17. Supraclavicular block injection with a spread of the local anesthetic (sagittal view) alongside the longus coli muscle and even into the epidural space. This unexpected finding is rather common as large volumes of local anesthetic tend to continue to travel alongside tissue planes. Disposition of the injectate alongside the longus coli muscle contributes to the sympathectomy often obtained with supraclavicular blockade.

INFRACLAVICULAR BLOCK

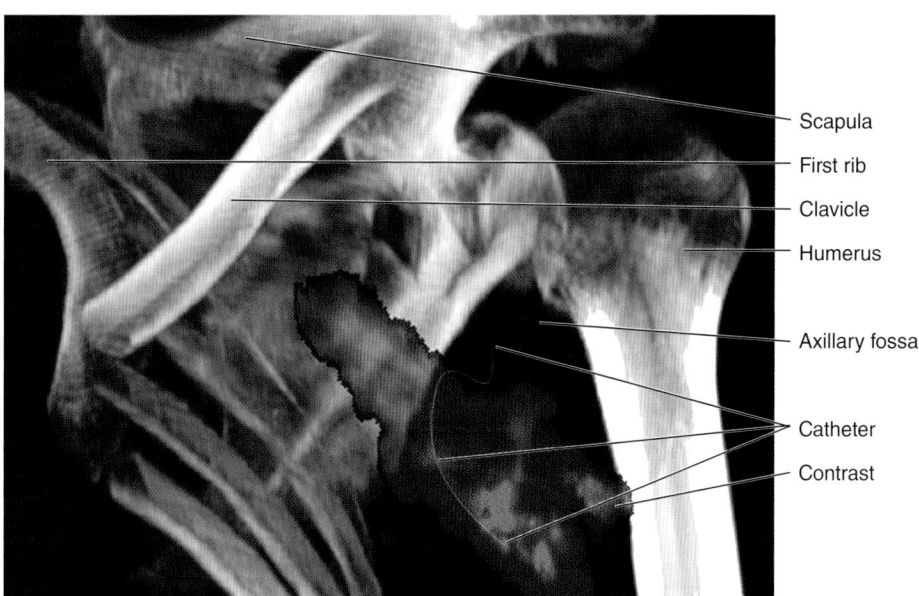

Scapula
First rib
Clavicle
Humerus

Axillary fossa

Catheter
Contrast

FIGURE 2–18. Spread of 20 mL of contrast around the subclavian artery, underneath the pectoralis minor muscle and within the infraclavicular brachial plexus space.

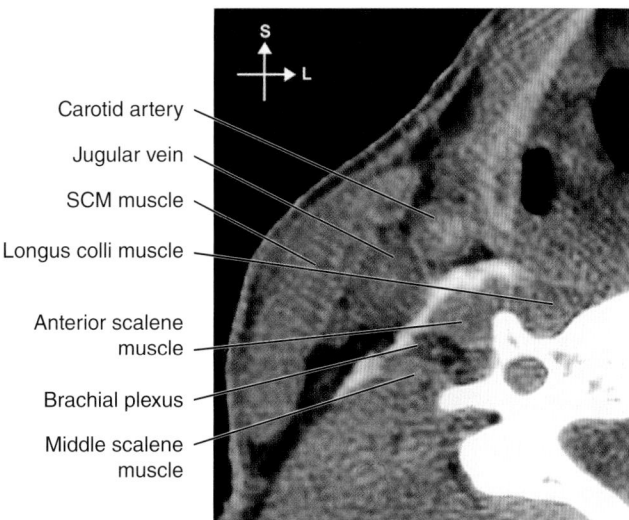

Carotid artery
Jugular vein
SCM muscle
Longus colli muscle

Anterior scalene muscle

Brachial plexus

Middle scalene muscle

FIGURE 2–19. The spread of 20 mL of contrast around the subclavian artery, underneath the pectoralis minor muscle and within the infraclavicular brachial plexus space.

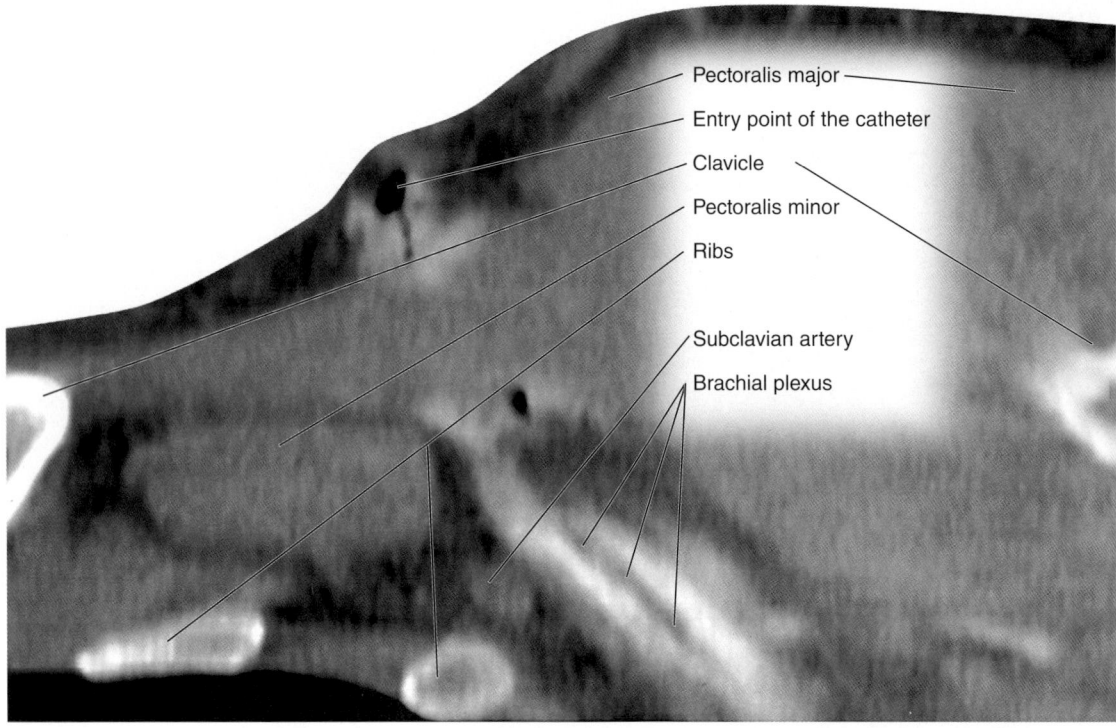

Pectoralis major
Entry point of the catheter
Clavicle
Pectoralis minor
Ribs
Subclavian artery
Brachial plexus

FIGURE 2–20. Anatomic distribution of 20 mL of contrast through the catheter placed in the infraclavicular space. Catheter insertion site is also seen in the image.

AXILLARY BLOCK MIDHUMERAL APPROACH

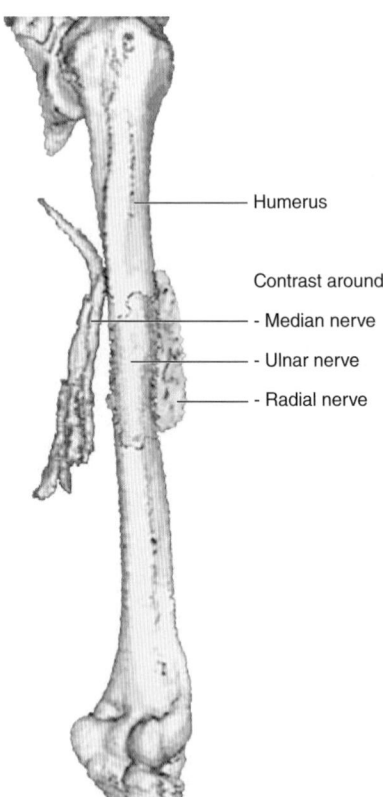

Humerus

Contrast around
- Median nerve
- Ulnar nerve
- Radial nerve

FIGURE 2–21. Distribution of the contrast alongside the medial, ulnar and radial nerves is demonstrated in this 3D CT image.

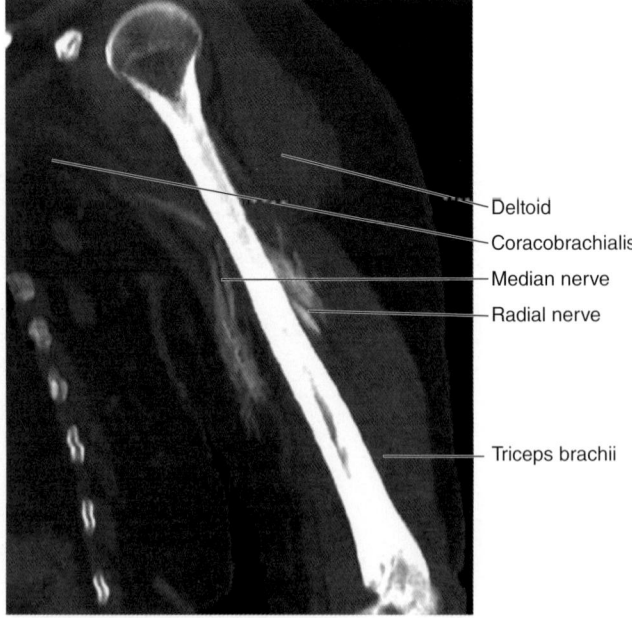

Deltoid
Coracobrachialis
Median nerve
Radial nerve

Triceps brachii

FIGURE 2–22. Negative radiocontrast image in the same patient demonstrating the distribution of 5 mL of radiocontrast after injections for radial and median nerves. Negative cotrast imprint is seen highlighting both nerves.

ELBOW BLOCK

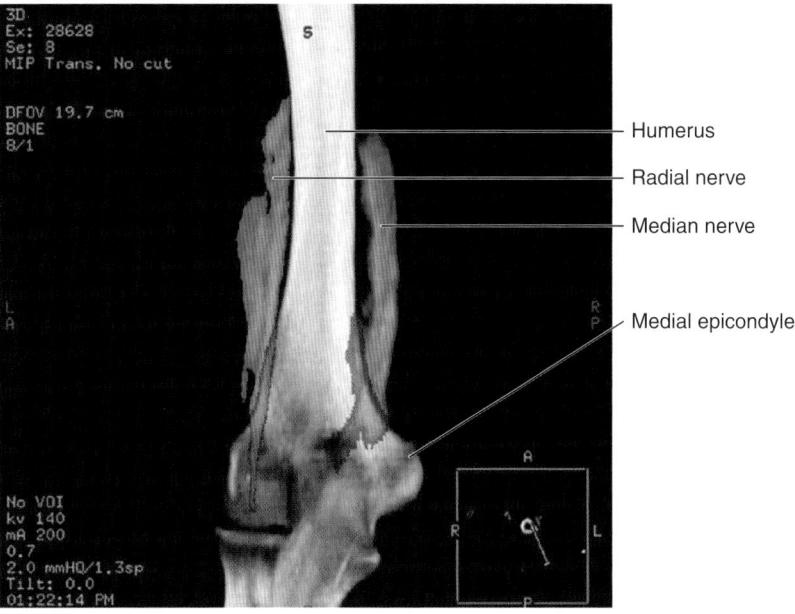

FIGURE 2–23. 3D CT image demonstrating spread of the injectate after radial and median nerve blocks (10 mL each) at the level of the elbow.

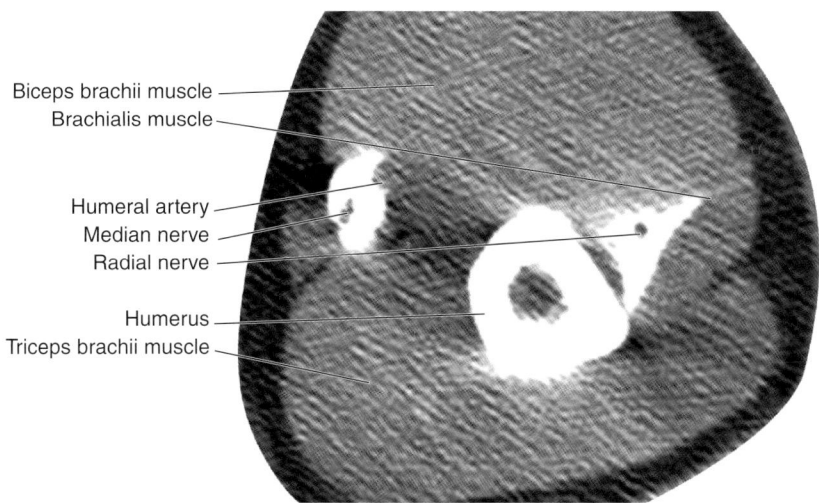

FIGURE 2–24. Axial view of the same patient as in Figure 2–23. The image demonstrates spread of the injectate after radial and median nerve blocks (10 mL each) at the level of the elbow.

PARAVERTEBRAL BLOCK

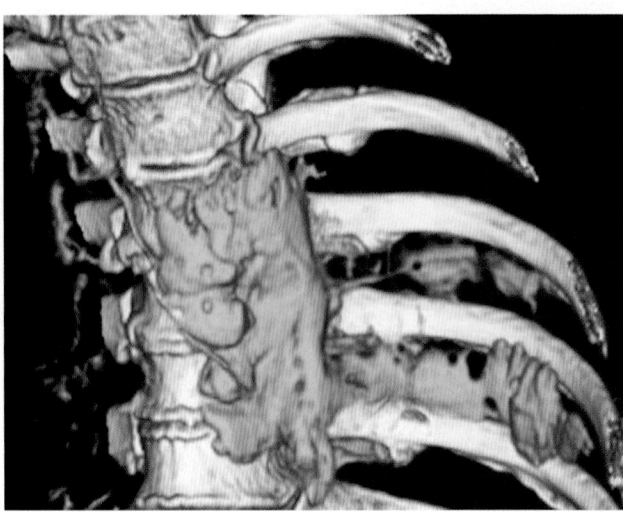

FIGURE 2–25. 3D CT image of 10 mL of the contrast demonstrating four levels of the blockade of the sympathetic chain and spread of the injectate out of the paravertebral space into two intercostal spaces.

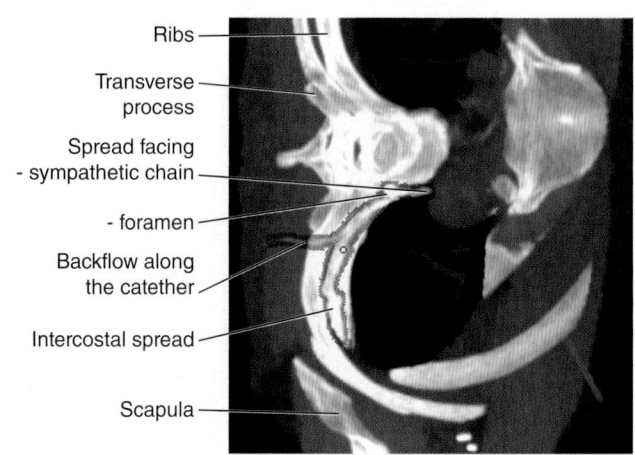

Ribs
Transverse process
Spread facing
- sympathetic chain
- foramen
Backflow along the catheter
Intercostal spread
Scapula

FIGURE 2–27. An axial CT images demonstrating the catheter tip position and the distribution of the injectate toward the sympathetic chain and paravertebral and intercostal spaces, explaining the mechanism of action of the paravertebral block. The backflow alongside the catheter insertion path is also seen.

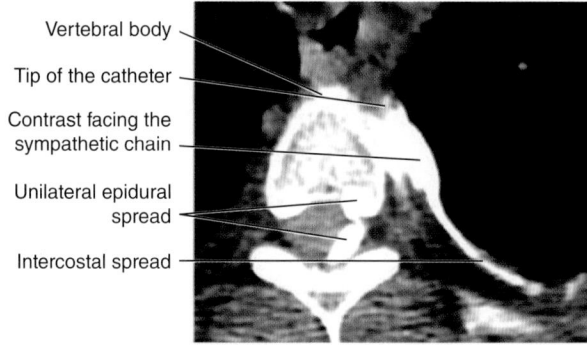

Vertebral body
Tip of the catheter
Contrast facing the sympathetic chain
Unilateral epidural spread
Intercostal spread

FIGURE 2–28. An axial image demonstrating the disposition of the injectate at the thoracic (T4) paravertebral space. Of note, spread to the epidural space, as seen in this image, is a common occurrence.

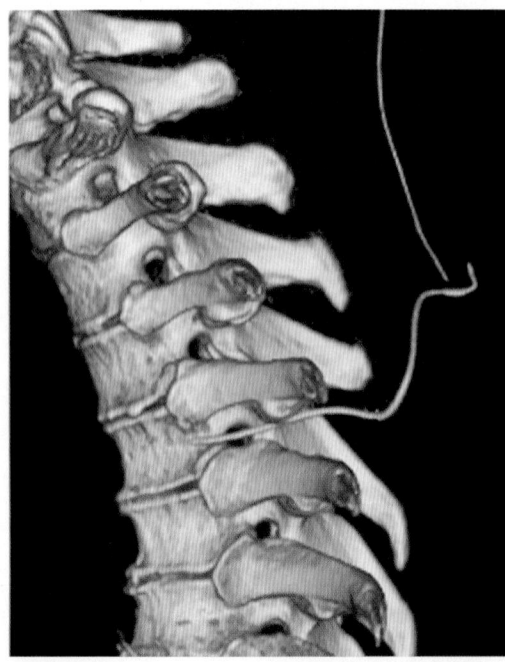

FIGURE 2–26. Catheter placed in the paravertebral space. The entry point is at 4 cm from the midline, the Tuohy needle is advanced toward the articular process, walked off the process, and advanced an additional 1 cm. The catheter is then inserted 3–4 cm. In this case, the catheter tip is seen in the vicinity of the anterior aspect of the foramen.

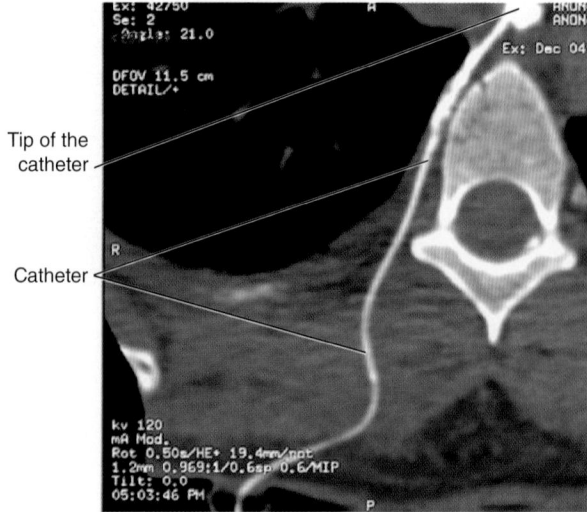

Tip of the catheter
Catheter

FIGURE 2–29. Malposition of the thoracic paravertebral catheter. The catheter is shown in the mediastinum. This image suggests the importance of avoiding insertion of the catheter too deeply too deeply (>4 cm).

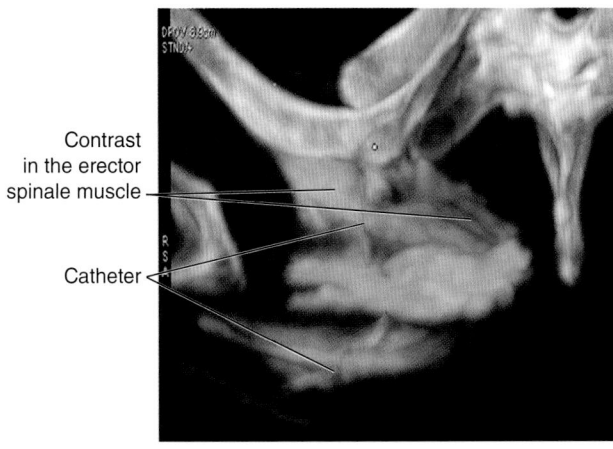

Contrast
in the erector
spinale muscle

Catheter

FIGURE 2–30. Malposition of the thoracic paravertebral catheter. In this case, the catheter was advanced only 2 cm beyond the tip of the needle, resulting in catheter migration out of the paravertebral space into the erector spinae muscle. Paravertebral skin and muscles are highly mobile, and sufficient depth of the catheter placement is necessary to prevent dislodgement outside of the paravertebral space.

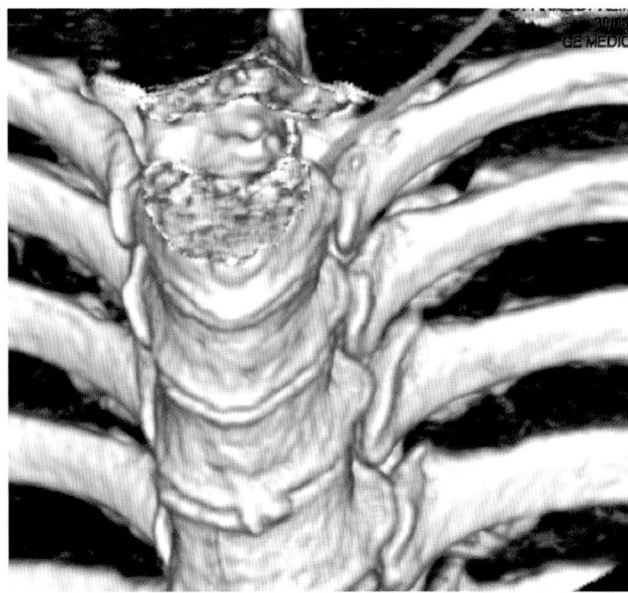

FIGURE 2–32. Reconstruction of the needle path in the Shibata-Renes approach. This 3D CT reconstruction illustrates the importance of avoiding needle advancement beyond the transverse process as this path may lead to the needle entry toward central neuraxis.

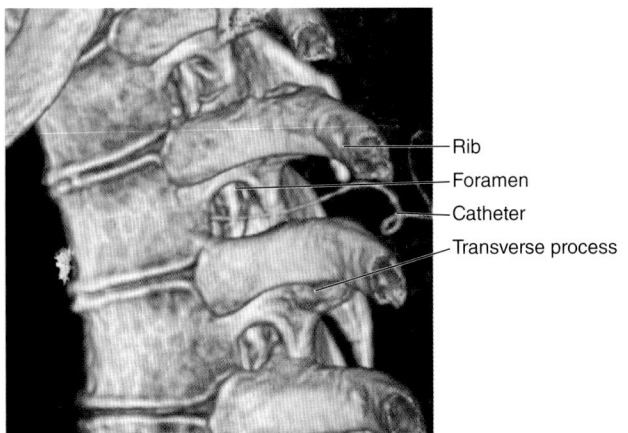

Rib
Foramen
Catheter
Transverse process

FIGURE 2–31. Malposition of the thoracic paravertebral catheter in the epidural space through the intervertebral foramen.

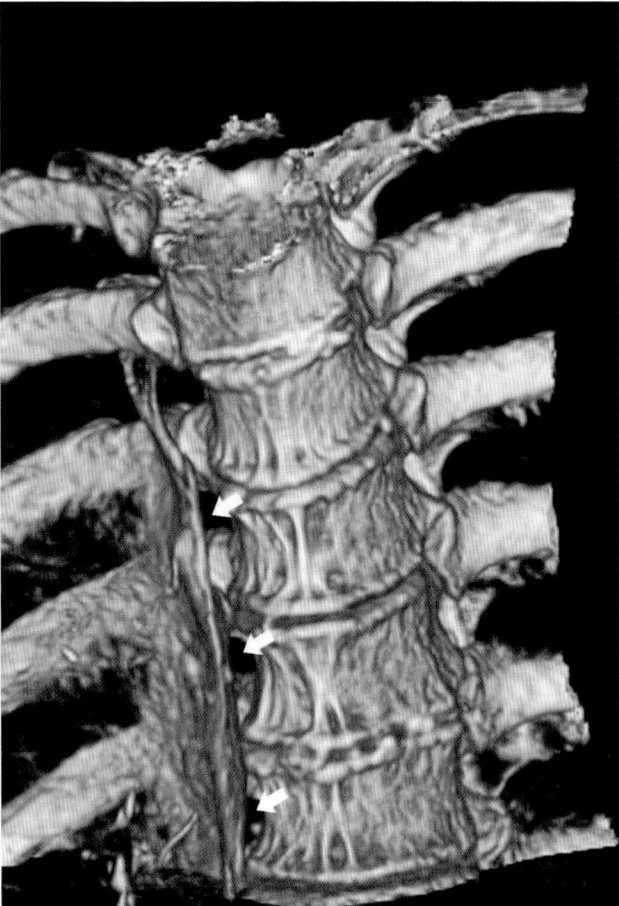

FIGURE 2–33. Malposition of the thoracic paravertebral catheter. The image demonstrate an intrapleural catheter placement (*arrows*), probably caused by too lateral needle insertion.

LUMBAR PLEXUS BLOCK

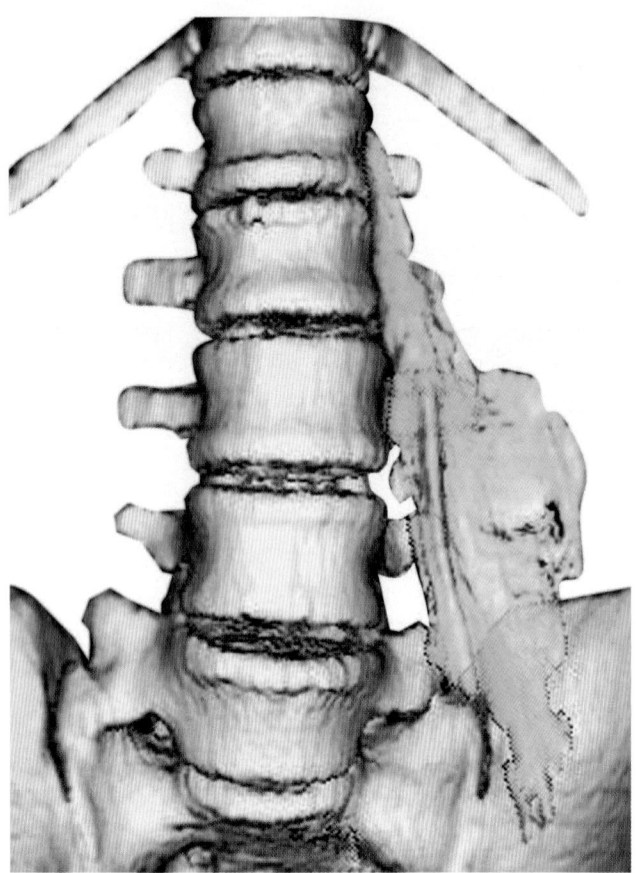

FIGURE 2–34. A typical fusiform injectate distribution from L1 to sacroiliac joint within lumbar plexus sheath.

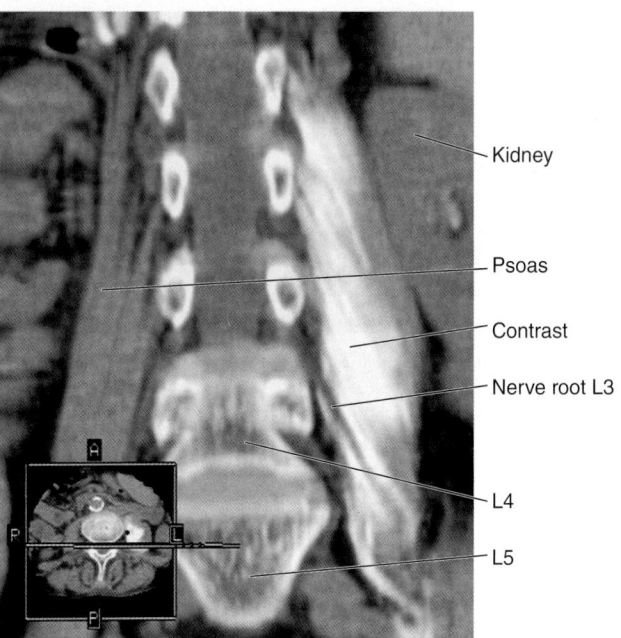

FIGURE 2–35. A desirable disposition of the injectate within the psoas sheath. Negative imprint of the L3 root is seen as well as a substantial spread of the injectate in the fusiform fashion, necessary for successful blockade of the lumbar plexus.

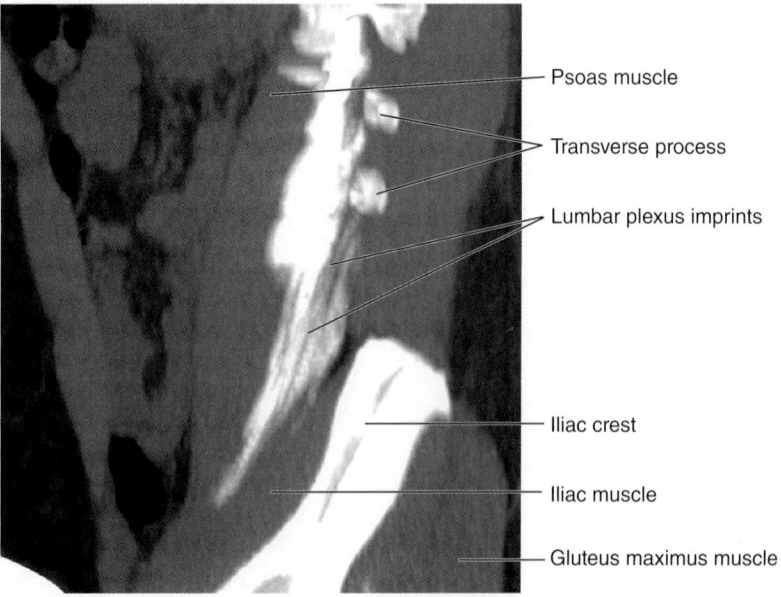

FIGURE 2–36. Proper disposition of the injectate within the psoas sheath,—sagittal view. Negative imprint of the lumbar roots is seen, as well as spread of the injectate in the fusiform fashion within the posterior aspects of the psoas sheath.

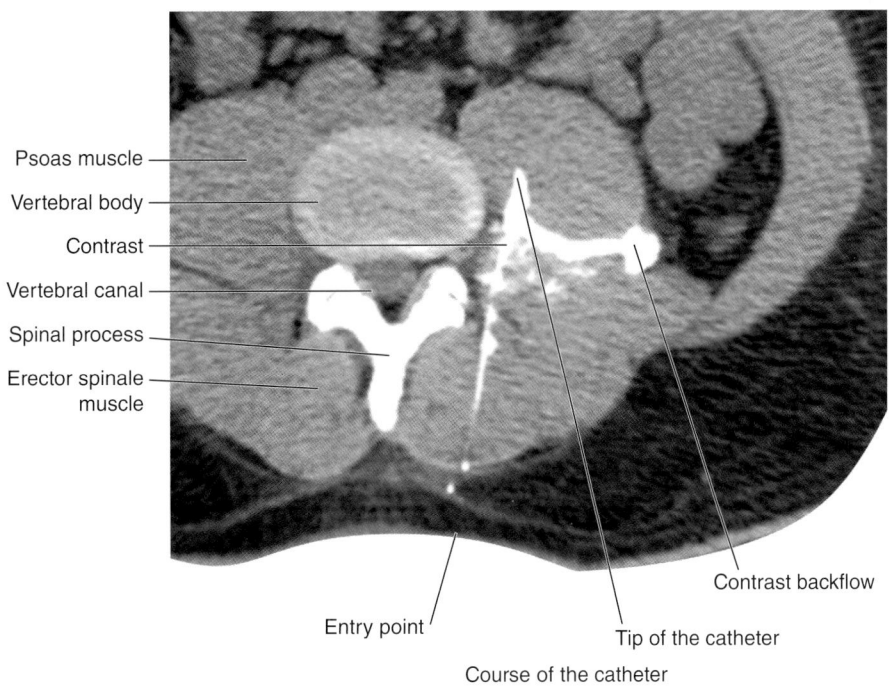

Psoas muscle
Vertebral body
Contrast
Vertebral canal
Spinal process
Erector spinale muscle

Contrast backflow

Entry point
Tip of the catheter

Course of the catheter

FIGURE 2–37. A proper position of the catheter for lumbar plexus block. The needle was inserted to the level of the nerve. The consequent insertion of the catheter brought the catheter tip in the posteromedial aspect of the psoas muscle. The spread of the contrast is seen in the vicinity of the neural foramen and outlining the outer surface of the psoas muscle underneath its posterolateral fascia.

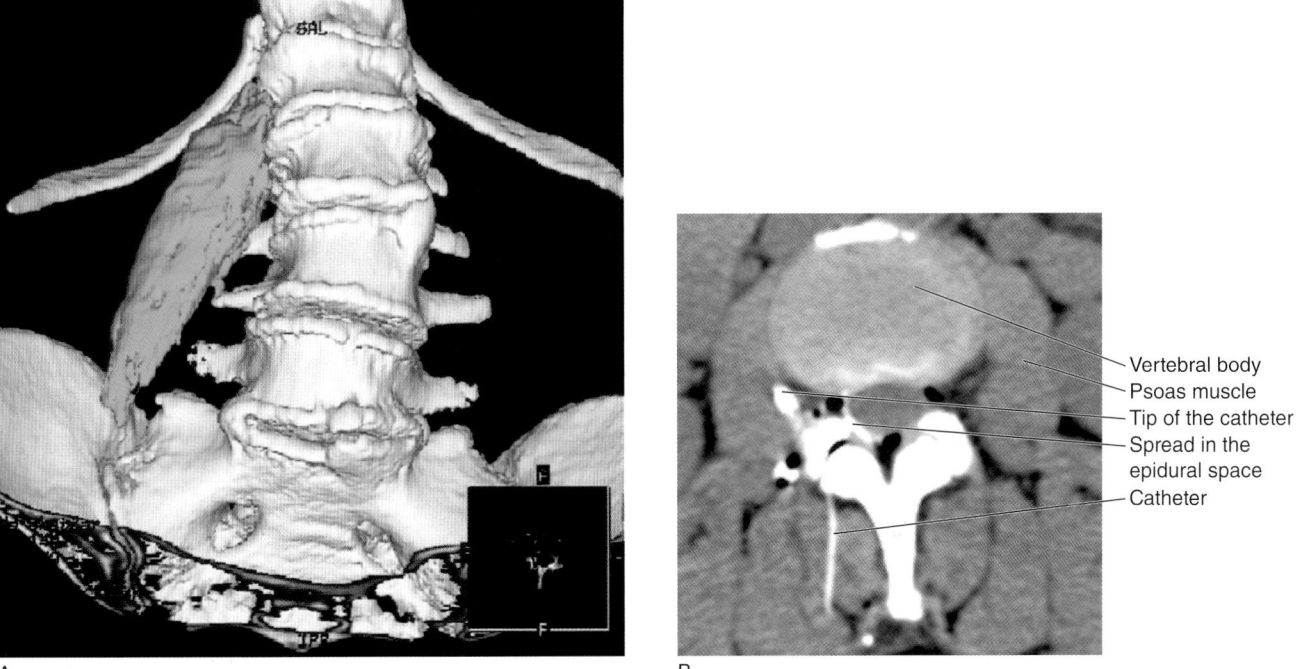

A

B

Vertebral body
Psoas muscle
Tip of the catheter
Spread in the epidural space
Catheter

FIGURE 2–38A AND B. Maldistribution of the lumbar plexus block injection. The injectate is seen in the anterolateral aspect of the muscle underneath fascia, leading to block failure.

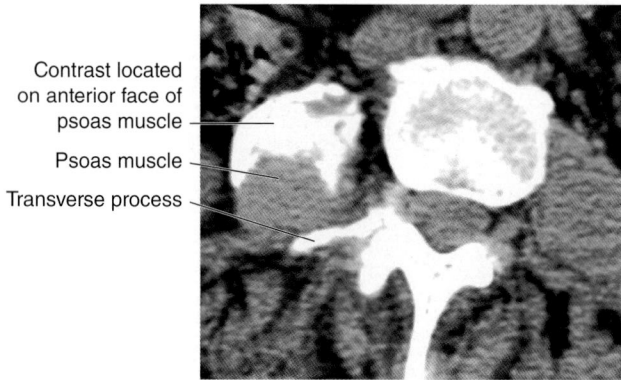

Contrast located
on anterior face of
psoas muscle

Psoas muscle

Transverse process

FIGURE 2–39. Same patient as in Figure 2–39 but with an axial image demonstrating maldistribution of the injectate in the anterolateral aspect of the muscle underneath fascia, resulting in block failure.

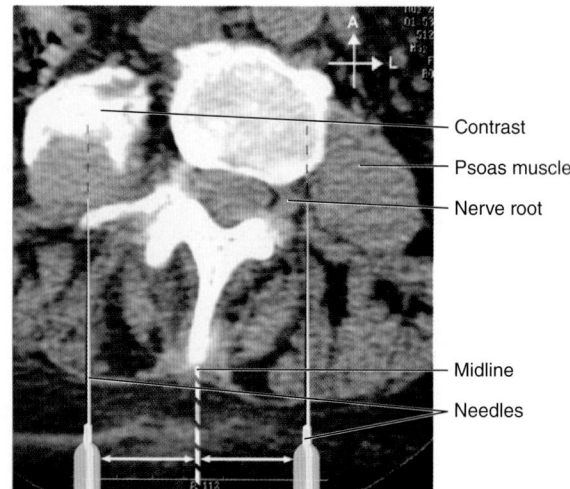

Contrast

Psoas muscle

Nerve root

Midline

Needles

FIGURE 2–41. Simulation of the lumbar plexus block in a patient with scoliosis. Shown is estimated needle reach using customary landmark in a patient with scoliosis. Left: the contrast is seen in the anterolateral aspect of the muscle (failure), whereas on the right the needle is nearly entering the foramen. Since patients with a relatively minor scoliosis are common in daily practice, this possibility should be kept in mind when practicing lumbar plexus block.

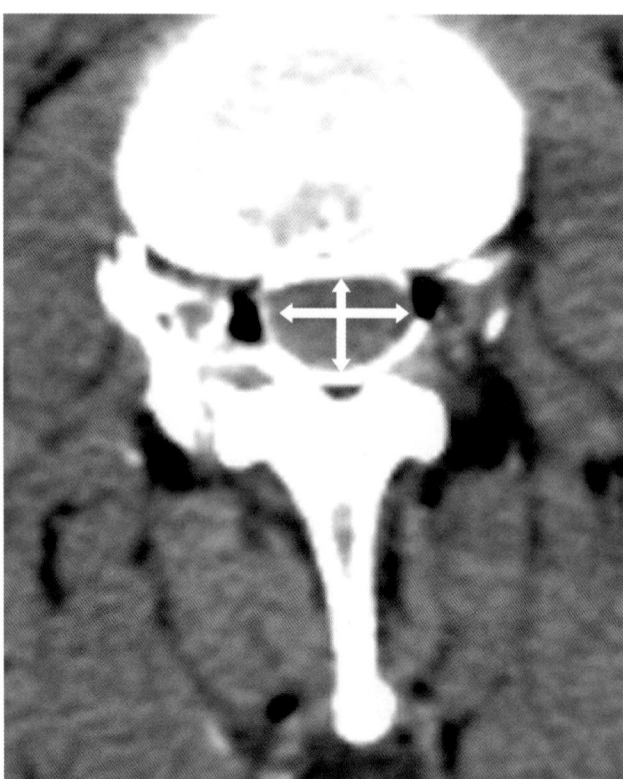

FIGURE 2–40. In this example, the spread of the local anesthetic injection through the catheter is seen in the epidural space. This observation is probably common and, in fact, may be contributory to the mechanism of action of lumbar plexus. High epidural spread may occur with high injection pressure injections.

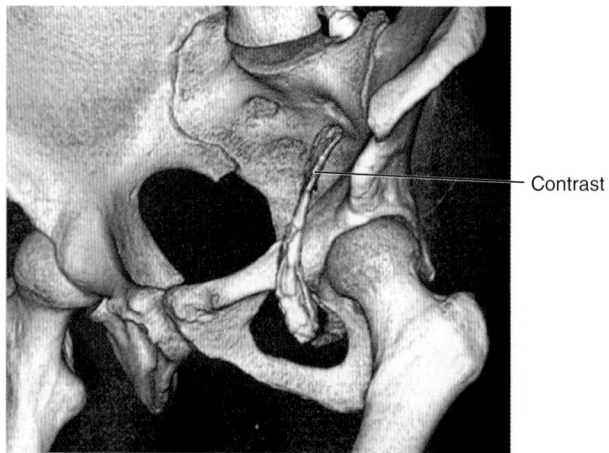

Contrast

FIGURE 2–42. Spread of the injectate after femoral nerve block. The contrast is seen tracking proximally along the femoral nerve.

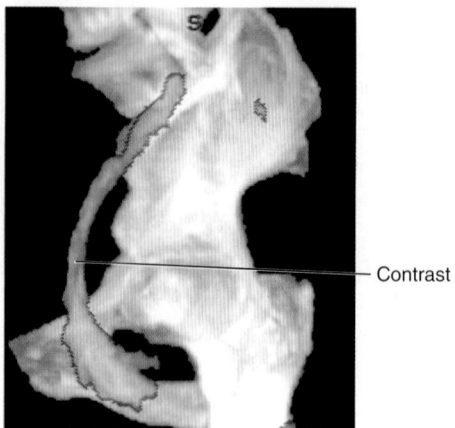

Contrast

FIGURE 2–43. Femoral nerve block. The contrast (10 mL) is seen underneath iliacus fascia following femoral nerve nearly to L5 vertebra.

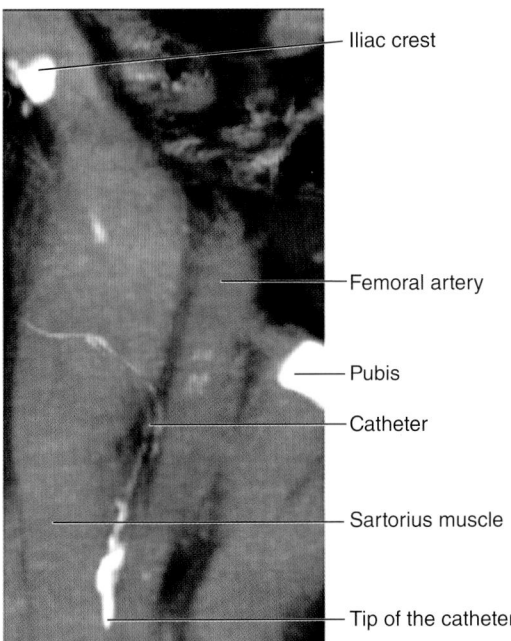

Iliac crest

Femoral artery

Pubis

Catheter

Sartorius muscle

Tip of the catheter

FIGURE 2–44. Femoral nerve catheter. The catheter is seen coursing alongside the femoral nerve. The iliopectineal ligament prevents the course of the catheter too medially; therefore, insertion of the femoral catheter 3–5 cm to prevent catheter withdrawal is desirable in this location.

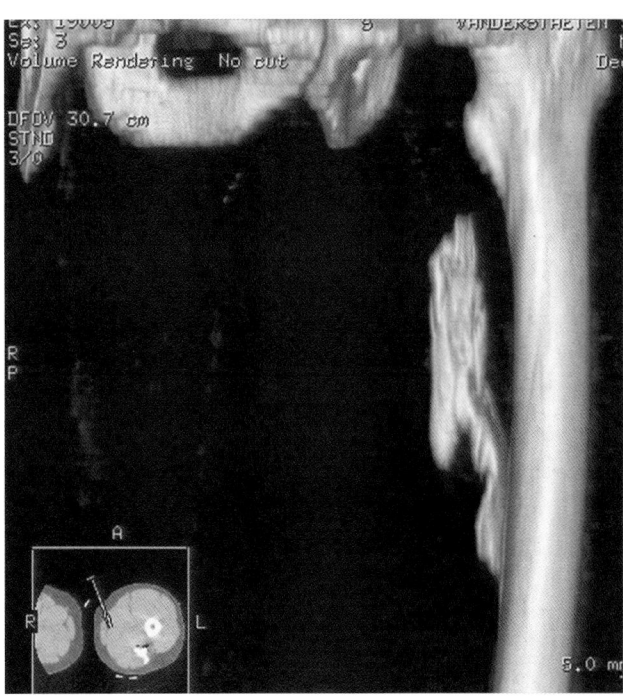

FIGURE 2–46. Subgluteal block —the contrast is seen in the frontal view with a typical distribution in the intermuscular canal, forming the sciatic nerve sheath. Twenty milliliters of the contrast-containing local anesthetic was injected

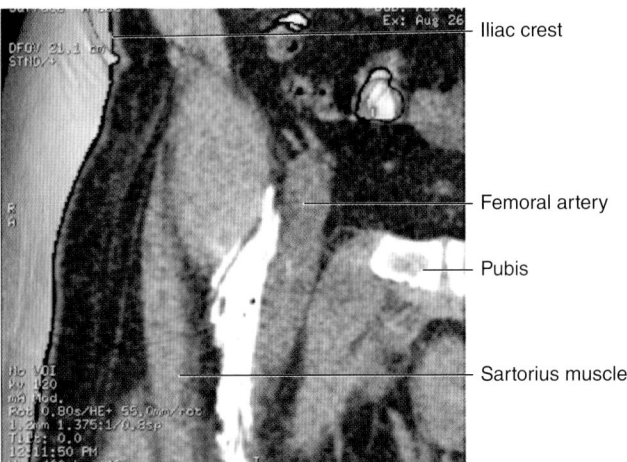

Iliac crest

Femoral artery

Pubis

Sartorius muscle

FIGURE 2–45. The same patient and catheter as in Figure 2–45, in frontal view. The distribution of the contrast (20 mL) is in the space between sartorius muscle and femoral artery.

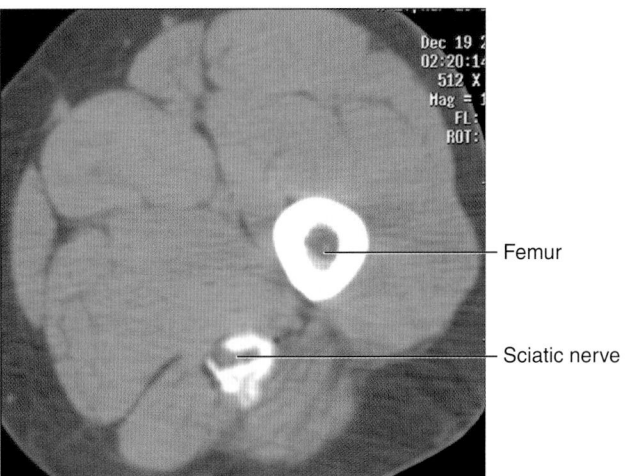

Femur

Sciatic nerve

FIGURE 2–47. The same patient as in Figure 2–11 in a cross-sectional view. The contrast is seen surrounding the sciatic nerve in its intermuscular sheath.

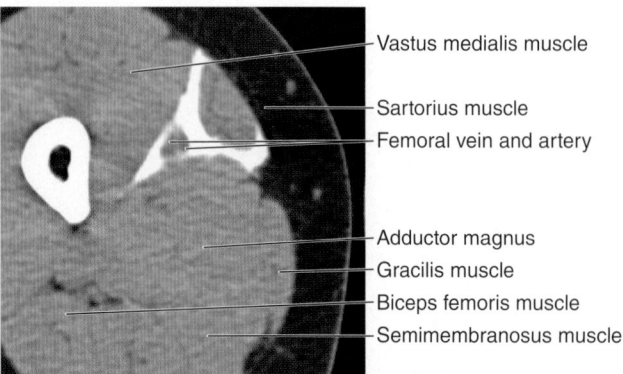

Vastus medialis muscle

Sartorius muscle
Femoral vein and artery

Adductor magnus
Gracilis muscle
Biceps femoris muscle
Semimembranosus muscle

FIGURE 2–48. Adductor canal block. An injection of 20 mL of contrast injected the lower hiatus spreads extensively in the canal underneath the sartorius muscle and around the femoral artery in the canal.

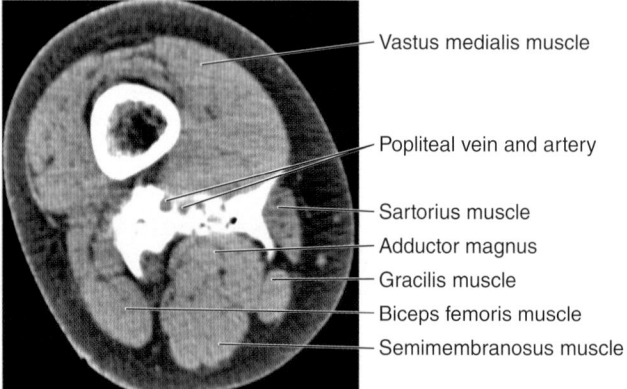

Vastus medialis muscle

Popliteal vein and artery

Sartorius muscle
Adductor magnus
Gracilis muscle
Biceps femoris muscle
Semimembranosus muscle

FIGURE 2–49. Adductor canal block. After injection of 20 mL of the contrast, the spread of the injectate is seen also reaching the popliteal fossa. This extensive spread alongside the tissue sheaths and into the fossa may help explain additional analgesic benefits of the adductor canal block, beyond the block of the saphenous nerve as the contrast reached the sciatic nerve.

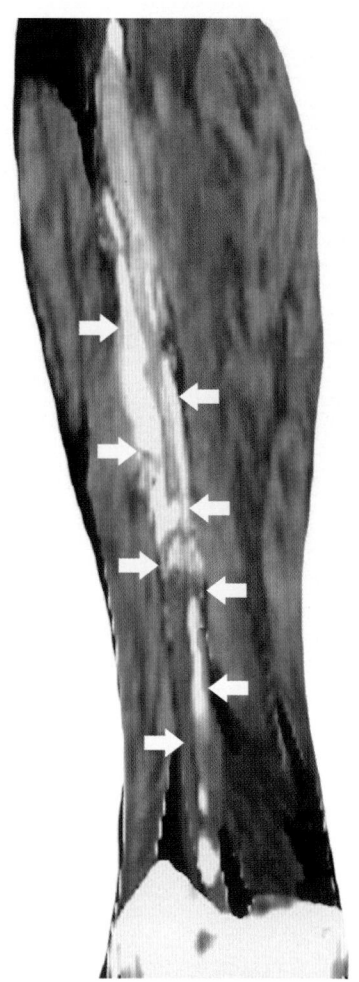

FIGURE 2–50. Popliteal block. Extensive spread of 20 mL of contrast injected into the sheath of the sciatic nerve resulted in a spiral spread around the sciatic nerve.

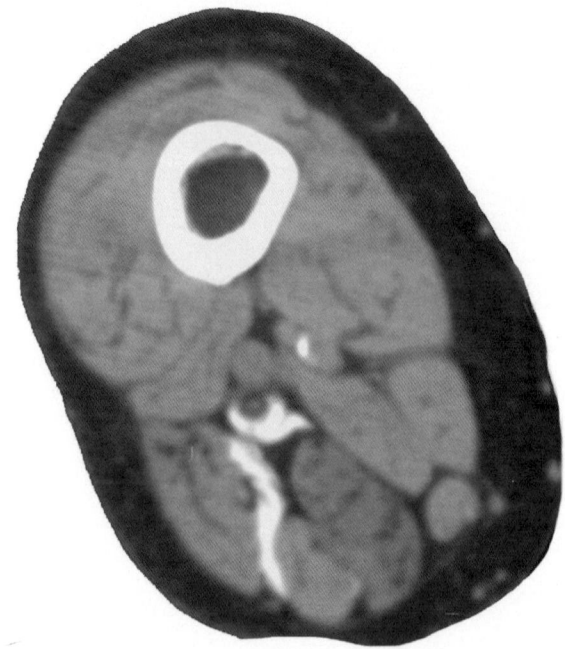

FIGURE 2–51. The same patient as in Figure 2–47 in axial view. Shown is the catheter path alongside with a backflow of the contrast. The circumferential spread of the contrast is seen within the sciatic nerve sheath.

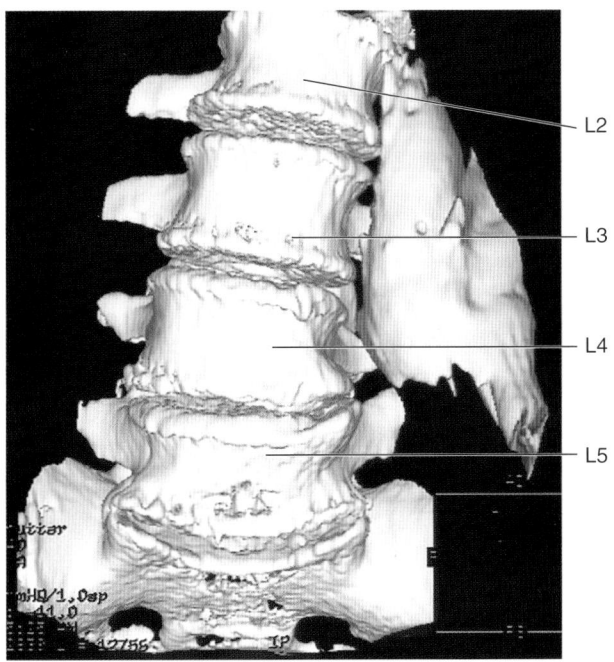

FIGURE 2-52. Tibial nerve: Injection of 10 mL of the contrast for tibial nerve block. The contrast is seen within the sheath of the tibial nerve, formed by the intermuscular canal.

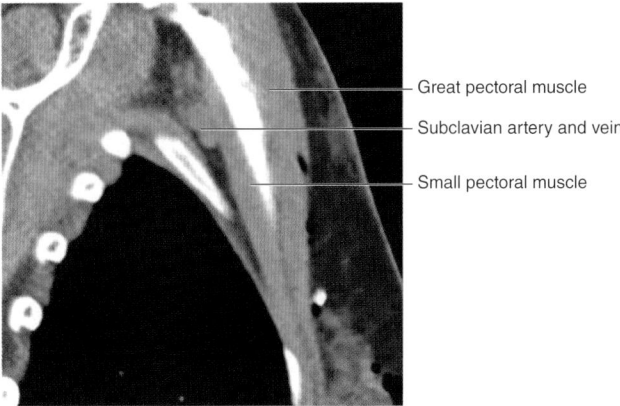

FIGURE 2-54. The same patient as in Figure 2-54, in a sagittal view. The contrast is seen spreading between pectoralis major and minor muscles.

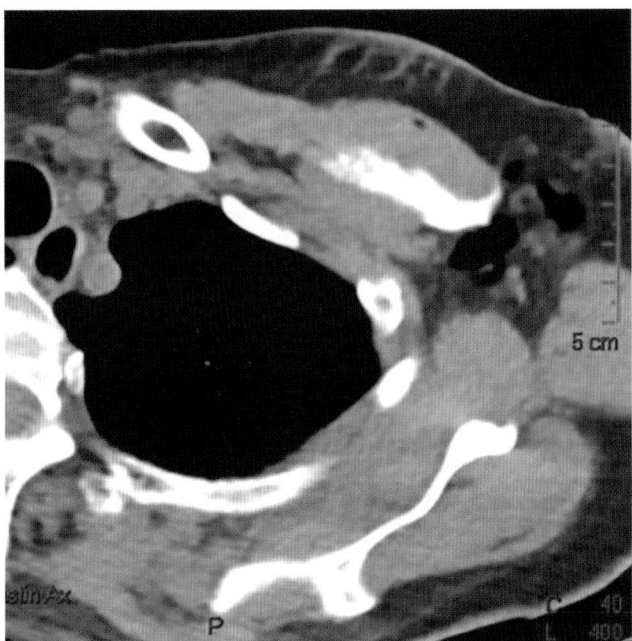

FIGURE 2-53. Pectoralis block (PEC I)—10 mL of the contrast was injected between pectoralis major and pectoralis minor muscles. Of note, the contrast did not spread toward the axillary fossa, possibly because of the barrier formed by the ligament of Gerdy (suspensory ligament of the axilla).

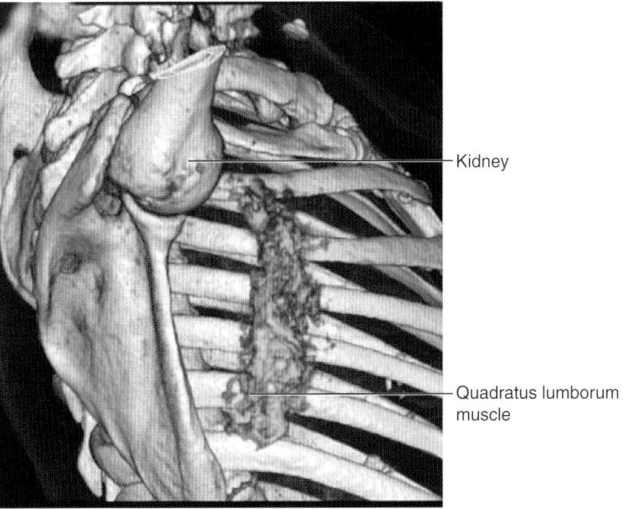

FIGURE 2-55. 3D image of pectoralis muscle block (PEC II). Injection occurred below the pectoralis minor muscle at the level of the 3rd rib in the anterior axillary line. Thirty milliliters of the contrast-containing local anesthetic was injected and resulted in the spread between third to seventh ribs.

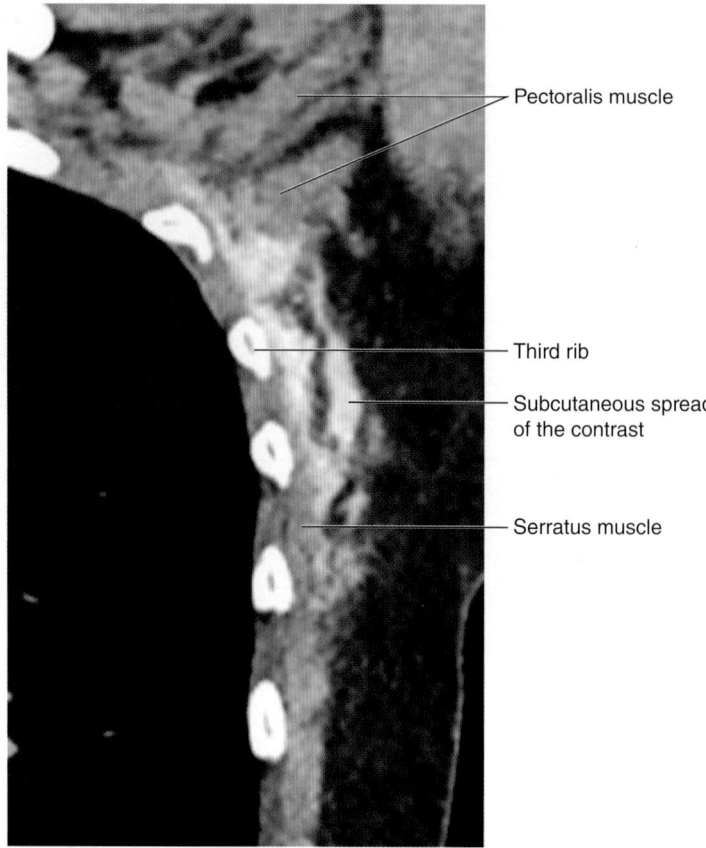

FIGGURE 2–56. The same patient as in Figure 2–56 but in a frontal view. Insertion of the pectoralis minor is seen as well as the spread of the contrast subcutaneously, superficial to the serratus muscles.

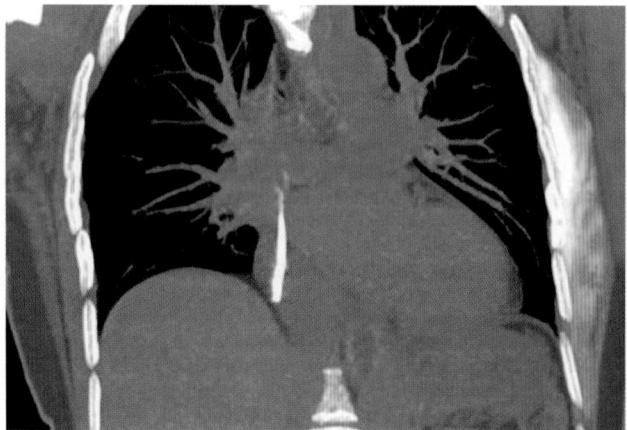

FIGGURE 2–57. Serratus block. Thirty milliliters of the contrast-containing local anesthetic was injected at the level of the forth and fifth ribs, between the ribs and the serratus muscle. The contrast is seen spreading distally to the seventh rib in the plane between the ribs and serratus muscle.

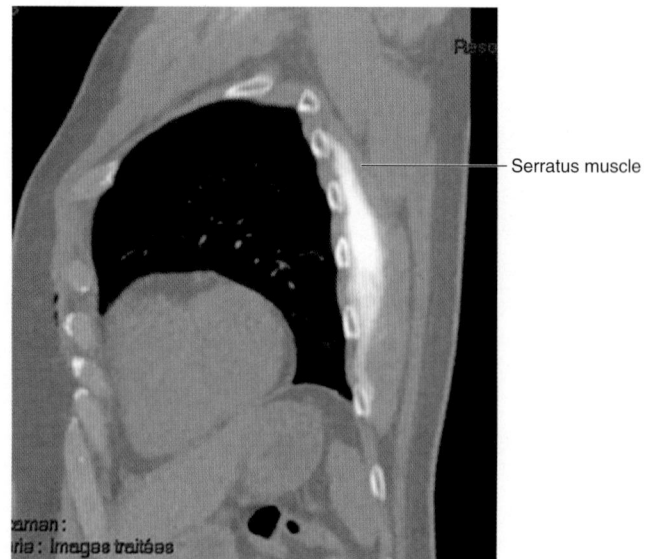

FIGURE 2–58. Serratus block, same patient as in Figure 2–58, but a sagittal view. The spread of 30 mL of contrast is shown deep to the serratus muscles and in the plane between the serratus muscles and the ribs.

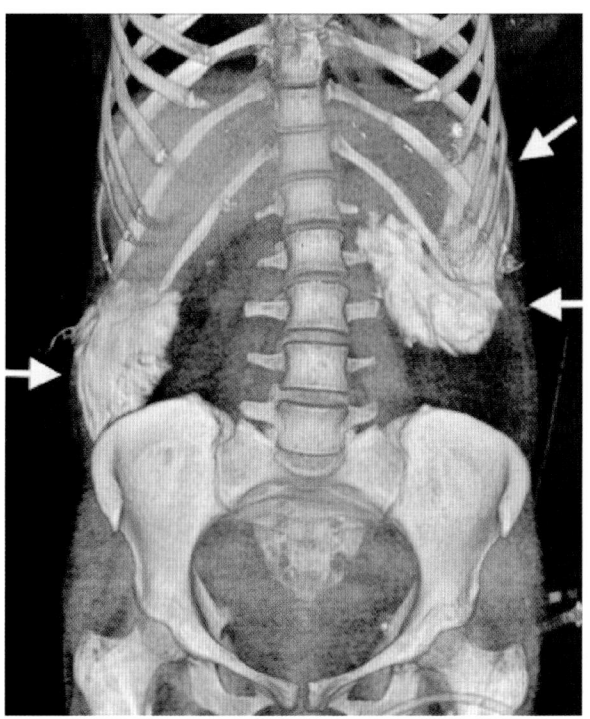

FIGURE 2-59. Quadratus lumborum space (QL1) injection.

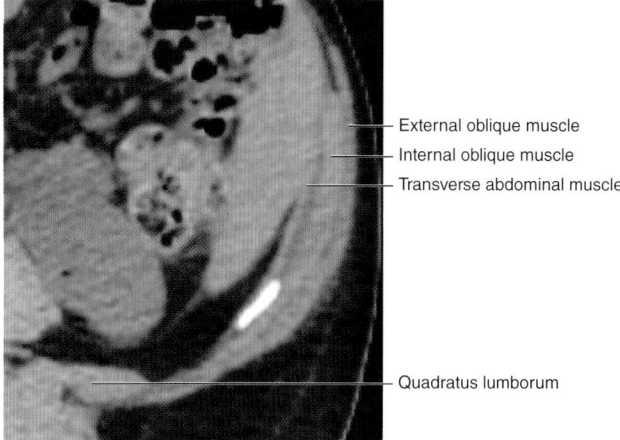

External oblique muscle
Internal oblique muscle
Transverse abdominal muscle

Quadratus lumborum

FIGURE 2-61. Transversus abdominis plane (TAP) block, axial view. An injection of 1 mL of radiocontrast is seen spreading in the plane between transversus abdominis and internal oblique muscles.

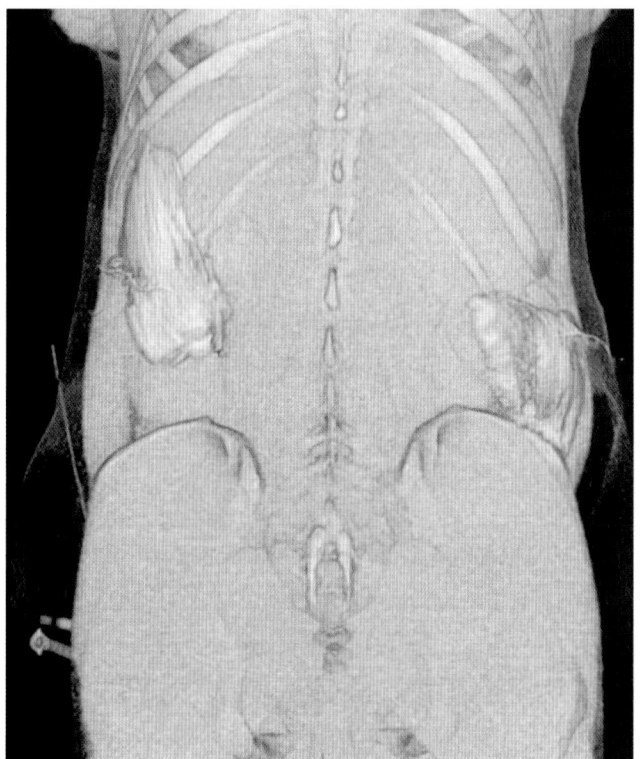

FIGURE 2-60. Transversus abdominis plane (TAP) block. The spread of the 20 mL of radiocontrast is injected bilaterally. The spread of the contrast on the patient's right side is after injection in the traditional TAP plane. The contrast spread on the patient's left side is after quadratus lumborum injection.

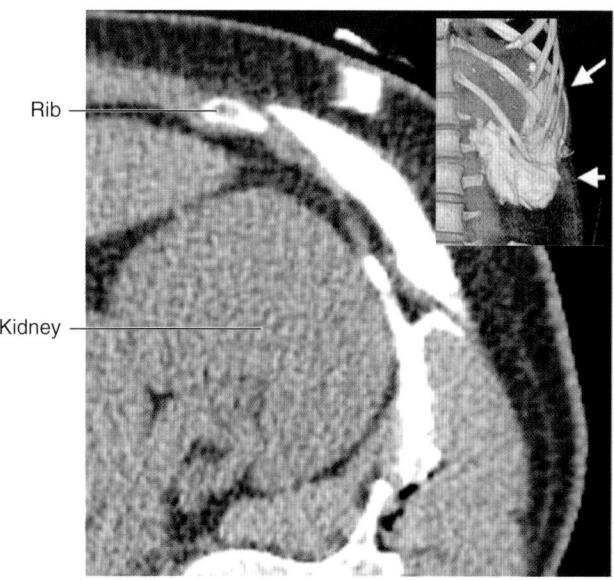

Rib

Kidney

FIGURE 2-62. Quadratus lumborum block QL1. The contrast solution was injected at the lateral edge of the QL muscle at the L2 level, spreading to the posterior aspect of the QL muscle and medially toward the transverse process (see the 3D CT insert in the right upper corner). The dye solution spreads medially from the quadratus-lumborum space, cranially into the the thoraco-lumbar fascia up to the the 12th and 11th ribs.

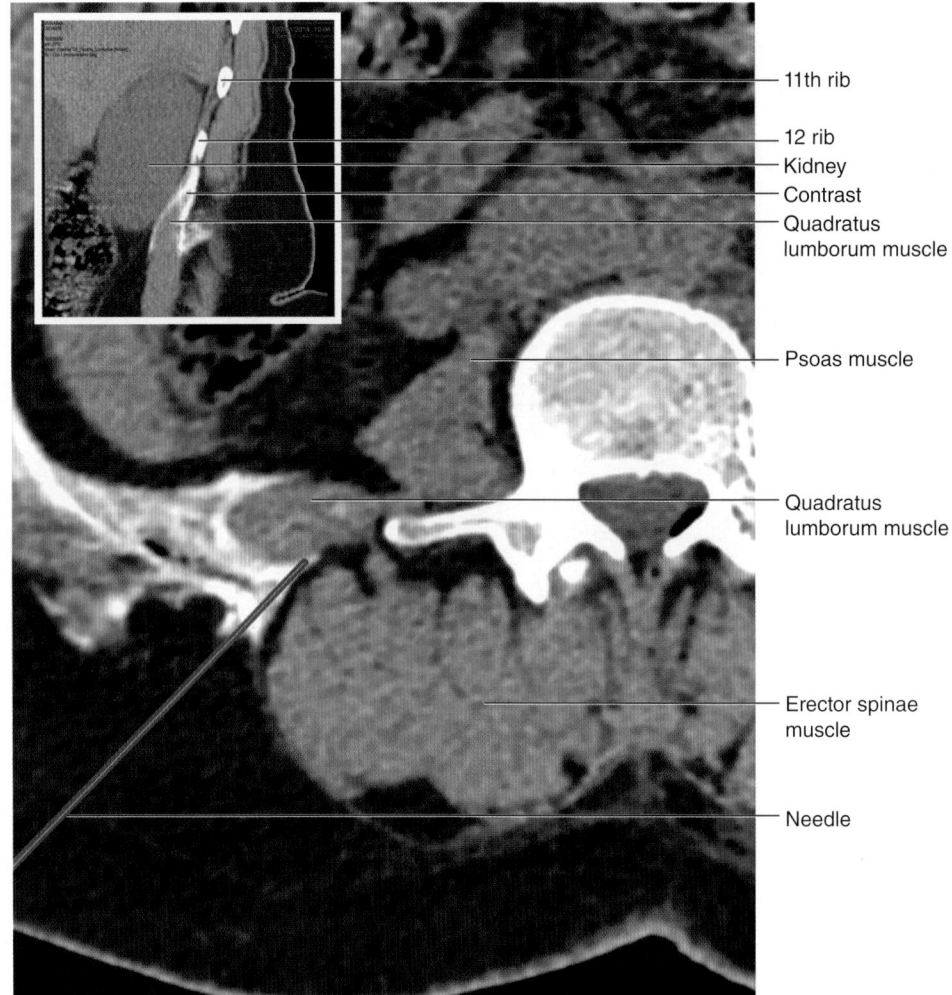

FIGURE 2–63. Quadratus Lumborum block QL2. Axial view of the distribution of 20 mL contrast after QL2 block. The injection was performed at the posterior aspect of the QL muscle. The contrast is seen on the anterolateral aspect of the quadratus muscle and laterally into the transversus abdominis plane. The insert (3D CT) in the left upper corner of the image shows the proximal extent of the injectate around QL muscle in the same patient.

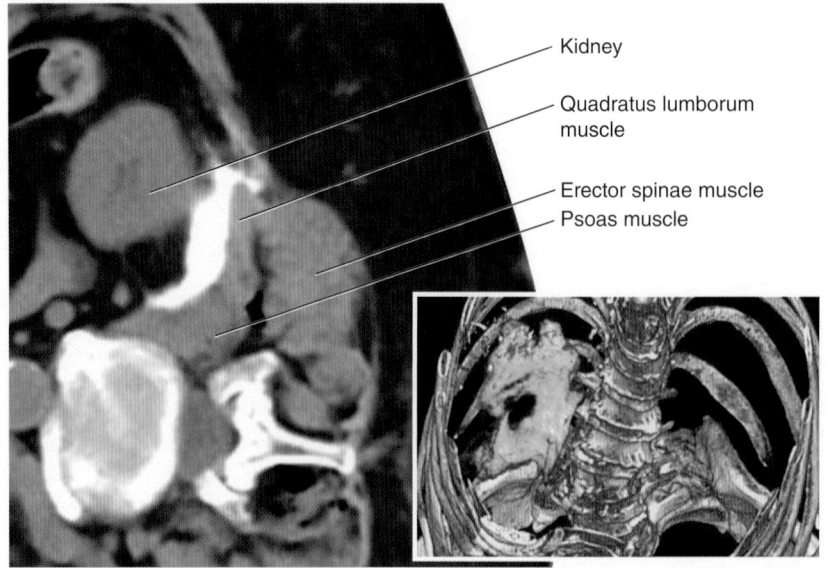

FIGURE 2–64. Quadratus lumborum block QL3. Twenty milliliters of contrast was injected between QL and psoas major muscles ("Shamrock" techniques). The injectate is seen between the QL and psoas major muscles and alongside the anterior aspect of the QL muscle without spread toward the paravertebral space is seen. The insert in the right lower corner of the image shows the proximal extent of the injectate in the same patient on a 3D CT.

INDEX

Note: Page numbers followed by *f*, *t*, or *b* refer to the page location of figures, tables, or boxes, respectively.